THIRD EDITION

▼▼▼▼▼▼▼▼▼The Molecular Basis of Blood Diseases

George Stamatoyannopoulos, MD, DrSci

Professor of Medicine
Department of Medicine
Division of Medical Genetics
University of Washington School of Medicine
Seattle, Washington

Philip W. Majerus, MD

Professor of Medicine and Biological Chemistry
Division of Hematology-Oncology
Washington University School of Medicine
St. Louis, Missouri

Roger M. Perlmutter, MD, PhD

Executive Vice Pesident of Basic Research
Merck Research Laboratories
Rahway, New Jersey

Harold Varmus, MD

President and Chief Executive Officer
Memorial Sloan-Kettering Cancer Center
Professor of Cell Biology and Genetics
Cornell Medical School
New York, New York

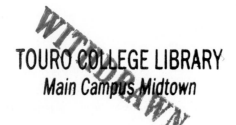
W.B. SAUNDERS COMPANY
A Harcourt Health Sciences Company
Philadelphia London New York St. Louis Sydney Toronto

MT

W.B. SAUNDERS COMPANY
A Harcourt Health Sciences Company

The Curtis Center
Independence Square West
Philadelphia, Pennsylvania 19106

Library of Congress Cataloging-in-Publication Data

The molecular basis of blood diseases / [edited by] George Stamatoyannopoulos
. . . [et al.].—3rd ed.

p.   cm.

Includes bibliographical references and index.

ISBN 0–7216–7671–5

1. Blood—Diseases—Molecular aspects.   I. Stamatoyannopoulos, George.
  [DNLM: 1. Hematologic Diseases—genetics. WH 120 M718 2001]

RC636.M57 2001   616.1′507—dc21

DNLM/DLC   00-029714

Acquisitions Editor: Marc Strauss
Manuscript Editors: Thomas Stringer, Jennifer Ehlers
Senior Production Manager: Peter Faber
Illustration Specialist: Lisa Lambert

THE MOLECULAR BASIS OF BLOOD DISEASES   ISBN 0–7216–7671–5

Last digit is the print number: 9   8   7   6   5   4   3   2   1

▼▼▼▼ CONTRIBUTORS

▼ **John P. Atkinson, MD**
Samuel B. Grant Professor of Medicine, Professor of Molecular Microbiology, Washington University School of Medicine; Physician, Barnes-Jewish Hospital, St. Louis, Missouri
Paroxysmal Nocturnal Hemoglobinuria

▼ **Edward J. Benz, Jr, MD**
Sir William Osler Professor of Medicine, Director, Department of Medicine, Professor of Molecular Biology and Genetics, Johns Hopkins University School of Medicine; Physician-In-Chief, Johns Hopkins Hospital, Baltimore, Maryland
The Erythrocyte Membrane and Cytoskeleton: Structure, Function, and Disorders

▼ **Monica Bessler, MD, PhD**
Assistant Professor, Internal Medicine, Hematology; Assistant Professor, Pharmacology and Molecular Biology, Washington University School of Medicine, St. Louis, Missouri
Paroxysmal Nocturnal Hemoglobinuria

▼ **George J. Broze, Jr, MD**
Professor, Departments of Medicine and Cell Biology and Physiology, Washington University; Attending Physician, Barnes-Jewish Hospital, St. Louis, Missouri
Regulation of Blood Coagulation by Protease Inhibitors

▼ **Eric Bruening, PhD**
Postdoctoral Researcher, Parke Davis Pharmaceuticals, Ann Arbor, Michigan
Viral Pathogenesis of Hematological Disorders (Herpesviruses)

▼ **H. Franklin Bunn, MD**
Professor of Medicine, Harvard Medical School; Physician, Director of Hematology Research, Brigham and Women's Hospital, Boston, Massachusetts
Human Hemoglobins: Sickle Hemoglobin and Other Mutants

▼ **D. Collen, MD, PhD**
Professor of Medicine, Faculty of Medicine, University of Leuven, Leuven, Belgium
Fibrinolysis and the Control of Hemostasis

▼ **John T. Curnutte, MD, PhD**
Clinical Professor of Pediatrics, Department of Pediatrics, Stanford University School of Medicine, Stanford, California; Senior Director, Department of Immunology, Genentech, Inc., South San Francisco, California
Genetic Disorders of Phagocyte Killing

▼ **Björn Dahlbäck, MD, PhD**
Professor of Blood Coagulation Research, Lund University, Department of Clinical Chemistry, University Hospital, Malmö, Malmö, Sweden
Vitamin K–Dependent Proteins in Blood Coagulation; The Protein C Anticoagulant System

▼ **Earl W. Davie, PhD**
Professor of Biochemistry, University of Washington, Seattle, Washington
Hemophilia A, Hemophilia B, and von Willebrand Disease

▼ **Mary C. Dinauer, MD, PhD**
Nora Letzter Professor of Pediatrics, and Medical and Molecular Genetics; Herman B. Wells Center for Pediatric Research; James Whitcomb Riley Hospital for Children, Indiana University School of Medicine, Indianapolis, Indiana
Genetic Disorders of Phagocyte Killing

▼ **Russell F. Doolittle, PhD**
Research Professor, Center of Molecular Genetics, University of California, San Diego, La Jolla, California
The Molecular Basis of Fibrin

▼ **Eric O. Freed, PhD**
Investigator, National Institute of Allergy and Infectious Diseases, National Institutes of Health, Bethesda, Maryland
The Molecular and Biological Properties of the Human Immunodeficiency Virus

▼ **Patrick G. Gallagher, MD**
Assistant Professor, Department of Pediatrics, Yale University School of Medicine; Attending Physician, Yale–New Haven Hospital, New Haven, Connecticut
The Erythrocyte Membrane and Cytoskeleton: Structure, Function, and Disorders

▼ **Craig Gerard, MD**
Associate Professor, Department of Pediatrics, Harvard Medical School; Director, Ina Sue Perlmutter Laboratory, Children's Hospital, Boston, Massachusetts
Chemokines and Their Receptors

▼ **Mark H. Ginsberg, MD**
Professor, The Scripps Research Institute; Adjunct Professor, University of California, San Diego, La Jolla, California
Integrins in Hematology

▼ **Frank Grosveld, PhD**
Professor in Molecular Cell Biology, Erasmus University, Department of Cell Biology, Rotterdam, The Netherlands
Hemoglobin Switching

▼ **James Ihle, MD, PhD**
Chairman, Department of Biochemistry; Investigator,
Howard Hughes Medical Institute/St. Jude Children's
Research Hospital, Memphis, Tennessee
Signal Transduction in the Regulation of Hematopoiesis

▼ **David I. Jarmin, MD**
Postdoctoral Fellow, Ina Sue Perlmutter Laboratory,
Children's Hospital, Boston, Massachusetts
Chemokines and Their Receptors

▼ **Kenneth Kaushansky, MD**
Professor of Medicine, Adjunct Professor of Biochemistry,
University of Washington; Attending Physician, University
Hospital, Seattle, Washington
Hematopoietic Growth Factors and Receptors

▼ **Ilan R. Kirsch, MD**
Chair, Genetics Department, Medicine Branch, Division of
Clinical Sciences, National Cancer Institute, Bethesda,
Maryland
Gene Rearrangements in Lymphoid Cells

▼ **Richard D. Klausner, MD**
Director, National Cancer Institute, National Institutes of
Health, Bethesda, Maryland
Molecular Basis of Iron Metabolism

▼ **W. Michael Kuehl, MD**
Section Chief, Genetics Department, Medicine Branch,
Division of Clinical Sciences, National Cancer Institute,
Bethesda, Maryland
Gene Rearrangements in Lymphoid Cells

▼ **Ihor Lemischka, PhD**
Associate Professor, Department of Molecular Biology,
Princeton University, Princeton, New Jersey
Stem Cell Biology

▼ **H. R. Lijnen, PhD**
Professor, Faculty of Medicine, University of Leuven,
Leuven, Belgium
Fibrinolysis and the Control of Hemostasis

▼ **John B. Lowe, MD**
Professor of Pathology, Warner-Lambert/Parke-Davis
Professor in Medicine, University of Michigan Medical
School; Investigator, Howard Hughes Medical Institute,
Ann Arbor, Michigan
Red Cell Membrane Antigens

▼ **Douglas R. Lowy, MD**
Deputy Director, National Cancer Institute, Division of
Basic Sciences, National Institutes of Health, Bethesda,
Maryland
Molecular Aspects of Oncogenesis

▼ **Philip W. Majerus, MD**
Professor of Medicine, Professor of Biochemistry and
Molecular Biophysics, Co-Director, Division of
Hematology, Washington University School of Medicine,
St. Louis, Missouri
Platelets

▼ **Malcolm A. Martin, MD**
Chief, Laboratory of Molecular Microbiology, National
Institute of Allergy and Infectious Diseases, National
Institutes of Health, Bethesda, Maryland
*The Molecular and Biological Properties of the Human
Immunodeficiency Virus*

▼ **Arthur W. Nienhuis, MD**
Director, St. Jude Children's Research Hospital, Memphis,
Tennessee
Gene Therapy for Hematopoietic Diseases

▼ **Stuart H. Orkin, MD**
Leland Fikes Professor of Pediatric Medicine, Harvard
Medical School; Investigator, Howard Hughes Medical
Institute, Boston, Massachusetts
Transcription Factors That Regulate Lineage Decisions

▼ **Thalia Papayannopoulou, MD, DrSci**
Professor of Medicine, Division of Hematology,
Department of Medicine, University of Washington, Seattle,
Washington
Stem Cell Biology

▼ **Roger M. Perlmutter, MD, PhD**
Executive Vice President, Worldwide Basic Research and
Preclinical Development, Merck Research Laboratories,
Rahway, New Jersey
Antigen Processing and T-Cell Effector Mechanisms

▼ **David M. Rose, DVM, PhD**
Research Associate, Department of Vascular Biology, The
Scripps Research Institute, La Jolla, California
Integrins in Hematology

▼ **Tracey A. Rouault, MD**
Chief, Section on Human Iron Metabolism, Cell Biology
and Metabolism Branch, National Institute of Child Health
and Human Development, Bethesda, Maryland
Molecular Basis of Iron Metabolism

▼ **J. Evan Sadler, MD, PhD**
Professor, Department of Medicine, Department of
Biochemistry & Molecular Biophysics, Washington
University School of Medicine; Investigator, Howard
Hughes Medical Institute, Washington University School of
Medicine, St. Louis, Missouri
Hemophilia A, Hemophilia B, and von Willebrand Disease

▼ **Charles L. Sawyers, MD**
Professor, Division of Hematology/Oncology, UCLA
School of Medicine, Los Angeles, California
Mechanisms of Leukemogenesis

▼ **Gerald Siu, PhD, MD**
Assistant Professor of Microbiology, Columbia University,
College of Physicians and Surgeons, New York, New York
Lymphocyte Development

▼ **Brian P. Sorrentino, MD**
Associate Member, St. Jude Children's Research Hospital,
Memphis, Tennessee
Gene Therapy for Hematopoietic Diseases

▼ **George Stamatoyannopoulos, MD, DrSci**
Professor of Medicine, Department of Medicine, Division of Medical Genetics, University of Washington School of Medicine, Seattle, Washington
Hemoglobin Switching

▼ **Johan Stenflo, MD, PhD**
Professor, Lund University, Department of Clinical Chemistry, University Hospital, Malmö, Malmö, Sweden
Vitamin K–Dependent Proteins in Blood Coagulation; The Protein C Anticoagulant System

▼ **Bill Sugden, PhD**
Professor of Oncology, McArdle Laboratory for Cancer Research, University of Wisconsin–Madison, Madison, Wisconsin
Viral Pathogenesis of Hematological Disorders (Herpesviruses)

▼ **Douglas M. Tollefsen, MD, PhD**
Professor, Departments of Medicine and Biochemistry and Molecular Biophysics, Washington University Medical School; Attending Physician, Barnes-Jewish Hospital, St. Louis, Missouri
Regulation of Blood Coagulation by Protease Inhibitors

▼ **D. J. Weatherall, MD**
Regius Professor of Medicine and Honorary Director of the Institute of Molecular Medicine, University of Oxford, Oxford, United Kingdom
The Thalassemias

▼ **Owen N. Witte, MD**
Professor, Microbiology, Immunology and Molecular Genetics, President's Chair in Developmental Immunology, University of California, Los Angeles; Investigator, Howard Hughes Medical Institute, University of California–Los Angeles, Los Angeles, California
Mechanisms of Leukemogenesis

▼ **Linda Wolff, PhD**
Chief, Leukemogenesis Section, Laboratory of Cellular Oncology, National Cancer Institute, National Institutes of Health, Bethesda, Maryland
Molecular Aspects of Oncogenesis

▼ **Mitsuaki Yoshida, PhD**
Professor, Institute of Medical Science, University of Tokyo, Tokyo, Japan
Viral Pathogenesis of Hematological Disorders (Retroviruses [HTLVs])

▼ **Neal Young, MD**
Chief, Hematology Branch, National Heart, Lung, and Blood Institute, Bethesda, Maryland
Viral Pathogenesis of Hematological Disorders (B19 Parvoviruses)

▼ **Roy Zent, MD, PhD**
Clinical Scholar, Division of Nephrology, University of California, San Diego; Research Associate, Department of Vascular Biology, The Scripps Research Institute, La Jolla, California
Integrins in Hematology

▾▾▾▾ **PREFACE**

Since the second edition of this book was published in 1994, knowledge of the molecular basis of blood diseases has grown exponentially. This is reflected in the contents of the third edition of the book. Seven new chapters, on Stem Cell Biology, on Hematopoietic Growth Factors and Receptors, on Hematopoietic Transcriptional Factors, on Signal Transduction in the Regulation of Hematopoiesis, on Integrins in Hematology, on Paroxysmal Nocturnal Hemoglobinuria, and on Gene Therapy of Blood Diseases, have been added. All other chapters have been rewritten or extensively updated to reflect the explosion of knowledge. The first two editions established *The Molecular Basis of Blood Diseases* as a very useful resource for all individuals with an interest in hematology. We hope that the expanded and extensively updated third edition will be useful to a diverse audience, including established scientists, individuals engaged in teaching and the practice of hematology, postdoctoral fellows, and residents as well as medical and graduate students.

THE EDITORS

▼▼▼▼ PREFACE to the Second Edition

Molecular biology has revolutionized hematology research. The first edition of this book, published in 1987, was among the first texts to examine the impact of molecular biology on disease mechanisms. In the intervening six years, the body of knowledge about proteins, cells and organisms gained by manipulation and characterization of DNA and RNA has grown exponentially. The challenge now is not only to understand disease mechanisms but also to apply this new knowledge to find more effective therapies.

Virtually all facets of hematology have now been subjected to study by molecular genetic techniques. Most inherited and many acquired diseases are now at least partially understood at the molecular level. Fundamental cellular mechanisms such as transcriptional regulation, signal transduction, antigen processing, and cell motility are coming to be understood. Our purpose with this second edition remains the same, namely to assemble this body of knowledge about gene structure, function, and organization and about disease mechanisms that form the basis for a molecular approach to hematology. The growth in information and our desire to provide a comprehensive exposition of principles has resulted in substantial increase in size of this second edition. Again we have relied on experts with broad perspective to write chapters related to their own areas of expertise.

The knowledge acquired by molecular techniques has broadened the scope of this edition of "The Molecular Basis of Blood Diseases." However, it, like the first edition, is not a textbook of hematology. No effort has been made to describe diseases for which molecular biological and sophisticated cell biological approaches have not yet yielded relevant information about disease mechanisms.

The book begins with a section, "Basic Concepts," that contains three chapters of broad relevance. An understanding of methods remains essential to comprehend the body of knowledge acquired by molecular techniques. Accordingly, Chapter 1 provides a general description of the methodology of molecular biology and serves as an introduction to gene structure and function. The mechanisms by which regulatory proteins interact with one another and with nucleic acids to regulate gene expression in determining patterns of cellular differentiation is addressed in Chapter 2. Blood-forming tissues are a dispersed hematopoietic organ that respond to microenvironmental influences including cytokines, negative regulators, and cytoadhesive molecules to achieve controlled production of red cells, lymphocytes, phagocytic cells including neutrophils, and platelets. Thereby the number of these elements remain fairly constant in circulating blood. Chapter 3 provides a comprehensive introduction to hematopoietic mechanisms.

Several chapters are included in the section on red cells. Effective treatment of sickle cell anemia and severe β

thalassemia could be achieved if the fetal to adult switch during the perinatal period that initiates disease manifestations in affected individuals were reversed. Progress toward this goal achieved by application of molecular and cellular techniques provides a paradigm for understanding regulation of gene expression during development. Knowledge of the thalassemias, disorders reflecting deficient globin synthesis, illustrates the level of understanding about disease manifestations that can be achieved by consistent application of molecular methods. Sickle cell anemia, the first molecular disease for which the amino acid and nucleotide substitutions were known, remains challenging with respect to the pathophysiology of disease causing vaso-occlusive episodes. Since the first edition, there has been substantial progress in defining the structure of membrane proteins and surface antigens and mutations that lead to membrane dysfunction. Red cell enzyme defects, defined by classic biochemical techniques, have now come to be defined at the molecular level. New chapters on each of these topics have been included. Much progress has also been achieved in understanding how cells control iron uptake and storage to ensure availability for critical functions as described in the final chapter in this section.

Consideration of immunoglobulin and T-cell receptor gene rearrangements, lymphopoiesis, and the effector arm of the immune response has been expanded in Section III. These chapters are meant to provide a comprehensive account of important principles that have emerged as molecular knowledge about the immune system has grown. The function of phagocytic cells including endocytosis, the oxidative burst, and cell motility required much expanded consideration in the two chapters of Section IV.

Much progress has also been achieved in the study of hemostasis and its pathological counterpart, thrombosis, by application of molecular methods. The genes for the proteins involved in hemostasis and thrombosis have been characterized and mutations identified in individuals with deficiencies providing insights into protein structure and function. There is now a better understanding of the fibrinolytic mechanism and new therapies have been applied. Many new platelet functions have been characterized and these cellular fragments continue to provide novel insights into signaling mechanisms and cellular activation. The several chapters in Section V are designed to capture these new developments.

Neoplasms have come to be understood as acquired diseases with gene defects. Chromosome rearrangements create novel oncoproteins, and point mutations, gene amplification, or gene deletion either activate, increase or decrease critical cellular proteins. Each neoplastic cell has several mutations that interact in causing uncontrolled growth. Our approach, in Section VI, has been to emphasize important principles with representative examples providing the framework to allow the interested reader to learn details through further reading.

Viruses manage to evade the immune system in establishing and maintaining infection, thereby creating disease by unique mechanisms. Section VII has been expanded to provide a comprehensive chapter on AIDS and a second chapter that covers other viruses that may invade and cause disease in both normal and immunocompromised individuals.

The size and weight of this book is one testimony to the impact of molecular biology on our understanding of the fundamental properties of the blood, bone marrow, and lymphoid organs and the elucidation of hematological diseases. What about therapy? Coagulation factor replacement, use of cytokines to stimulate hematopoiesis, and various fibrinolytic agents are current products of the molecular biological revolution. In the future, one hopes that pharmaceutical agents that target specific defective gene products or cellular functions will be discovered based on an appreciation of the molecular basis of blood diseases. The use of genes as investigative or therapeutic agents is already a clinical reality. Our decision not to cover this emerging area of research reflects the current status in which most research has focused on developing methodology and testing vectors in animal models. Undoubtedly future editions of this book will contain many examples of the successful use of gene therapy and other therapeutic approaches derived from molecular knowledge.

We hope that individuals of diverse backgrounds will find this book useful. For the serious student of hematology, whether medical student, resident or fellow, it will serve as a supplement to standard textbooks. Individuals engaged in the practice of teaching of hematology should find the book useful in learning and applying the principles of molecular biology in their discipline. The text should also be valuable to the graduate student, postdoctoral fellow, or established scientist with a working knowledge of molecular biology who desires to learn about the molecular basis of various blood diseases.

GEORGE STAMATOYANNOPOULOS
ARTHUR W. NIENHUIS
PHILIP W. MAJERUS
HAROLD VARMUS

▼▼▼▼ CONTENTS

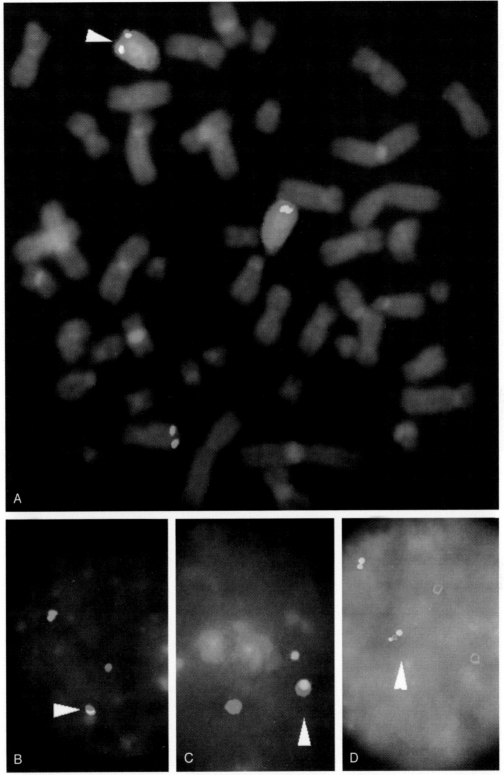

Plate 11–1. More sensitive identification of Ig translocations by metaphase or interphase fluorescent in situ hybridization (FISH) analyses. FISH of two myeloma cell lines was performed with a chromosome 14 painting probe (purple in A); a CH BAC probe (green in all panels) that includes Igα and Eα sequences from the centromeric end of the IgH locus (see Fig. 11–11); a c-myc plasmid probe (orange in A and B); a VH cosmid from the telomeric end of the VH locus (orange in C); and a pair of BAC probes that flank cyclin DI and are separated by about 100 kb (orange in D). The first myeloma line (panels A–C) has a t(8;14) translocation. A, The arrow indicates juxtaposition of c-myc and CH on metaphase chromosome 14, plus a normal chromosome 14 with CH and a normal 8 with c-myc. B, The arrow indicates the t(8;14) translocation as manifested by close juxtaposition (red/yellow/green signal) of c-myc and CH in interphase nuclei. C, The split VH and CH signals demonstrate the presence of a translocation, with the arrow indicating the normal juxtaposition of CH and VH probes as an overlapping yellow/green signal. D, A second myeloma line shows CH sequences inserted between two sequences that flank the cyclin DI oncogene, as indicated by the arrow. Molecular cloning showed that the CH sequences in D include Eα1 and other intervening sequences released during intrachromosomal switching from μ to ε in this tumor (see text and Fig. 11–11).[206, 212] The pictures were kindly provided by A. Gabrea and Y. Shou.

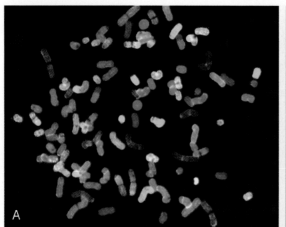
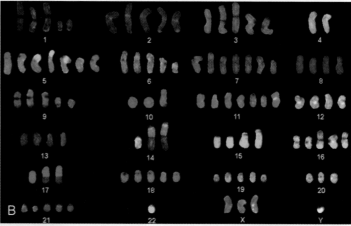
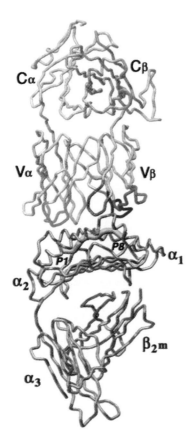

Plate 11-2. Spectral karyotyping (SKY) of a metaphase from a multiple myeloma cell line. *A*, Visualization of a metaphase spread with simultaneous identification of each distinct chromosome in different colors after hybridization with 24 combinatorially labeled chromosome painting probes. Chromosome painting probes were prepared in a two-step degenerate oligonucleotide primed (DOP) PCR of a human chromosome library, using combinations of different fluorochromes for labeling.[240] Spectral image acquisition and analysis were performed on a Leica DMRXA microscope equipped with the SD200 SpectraCube system and related software (Applied Spectral Imaging).

B, Ordered arrangement of the metaphase in *A*.

C, Karyotype of *B* shown in "classification" colors. A spectrum-based classification algorithm allows unambiguous identification of all pixels in the image that have the same or similar spectra. All pixels with the same spectrum are assigned the same classification color. The origin of all rearranged chromosomes was identified in this experiment. The numbers next to the aberrant chromosomes indicate the origin of translocated material. (These pictures and analysis were kindly provided by A. Roschke.)

Plate 13-1. Structure of the T-cell receptor visualized by X-ray crystallography. Shown is a backbone rendering of the mouse 2C T-cell receptor binding to its cognate ligand, an ovalbumin-derived peptide presented by the H-2K^b class I gene. The T-cell receptor constant regions are at the top of the figure, viewed from a perspective perpendicular to the plane of the cell membrane, with the class I-peptide complex immediately juxtaposed. The hypervariable loops of the Vα and Vβ regions interact with both the peptide and the α1 and α2 regions of the class I molecule. Reproduced from [146] with permission of the publisher.

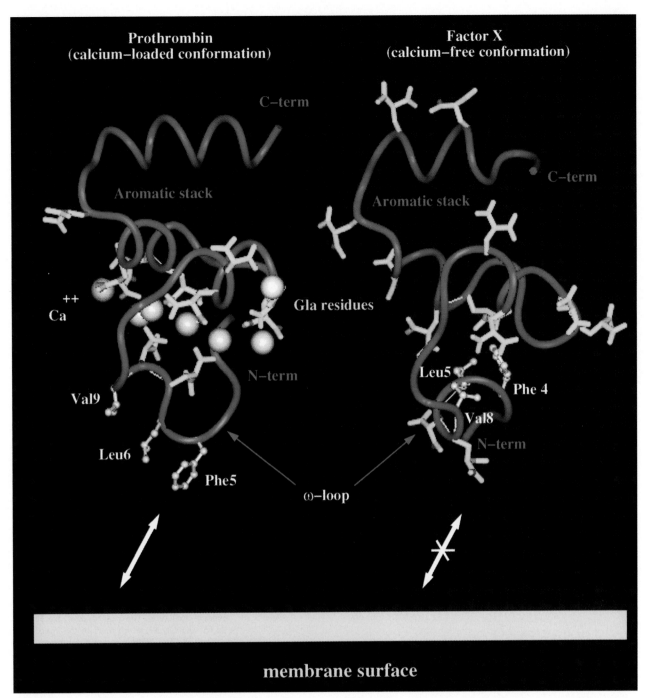

**Prothrombin
(calcium–loaded conformation)**

**Factor X
(calcium–free conformation)**

C–term

Aromatic stack

Aromatic stack

C–term

Ca $^{++}$

Gla residues

Leu5

Phe 4

Val9

Val8

N–term

Leu6

N–term

Phe5

ω–loop

membrane surface

Plate 18–1. The NMR structure of the calcium-free form of the Gla module of factor X (bovine) is represented on the right. With the same orientation, the X-ray structure of the calcium-loaded form of the Gla module of prothrombin is displayed on the left side. Few side chains are shown to simplify the figure. The calcium ions are presented as spheres. Upon calcium binding, an important conformational change occurs mainly at the level of the N-terminal ω loop and results in the internalization of some negatively charged Gla residues (in yellow) and the exposure of three hydrophobic side chains (in light gray). The residues are Phe4, Leu5, and Val8 in factor X and in prothrombin the corresponding residues are 5, 6, and 9.

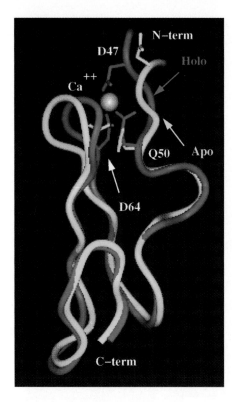

Plate 18–2. Schematic diagram showing the overall structure of the first EGF module of human factor IX. The X-ray structure of the holo form (red) of human factor IX[262] was superimposed onto the minimized average NMR structure of the same module in its apo form (yellow).[245] The key residues whose side chains are involved in calcium binding induce conformational changes within the N-terminal region of the module.

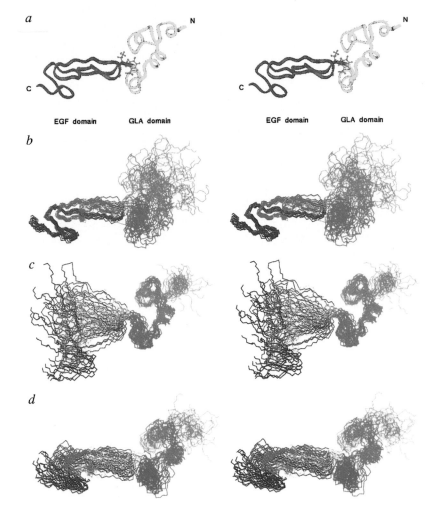

Plate 18–3. The GlaEGF module pair. *A,* Stereo ribbon drawing or the energy-minimized average structure. The red residues are Phe 40, Ile 65, and Gly 66, which mediate the interdomain contact. *B,* The NMR structures (obtained in the absence of calcium) were superimposed by minimizing the r.m.s.d. for the backbone atoms of residues 45-86 in the EGF module to the average structure. *C,* A family of NMR structures superimposed on the Gla module (residues 4-44). *D,* The family of NMR structures superimposed on the entire module pair (residues 4-86). Residues 1-19 are colored orange, 20-31 red, 32-44 magenta, 45-55 pink, 56-65 green, 66-75 blue, and 76-86 dark blue. Although the individual modules in the pair are well defined, their relative orientation is very poorly defined, indicating that they are joined by a flexible hinge region. The hinge is locked by binding of a single Ca^{2+} to the site in the EGF module.

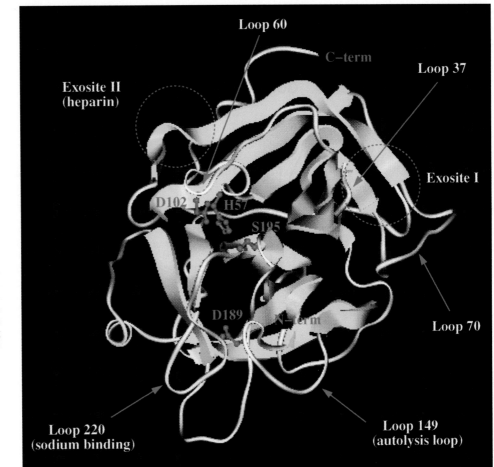

Plate 18–4. Thrombin structure. Richardson diagram of the B-chain of human thrombin with a view down the active side cleft.[37] Residues of the catalytic triad together with the residue at the bottom of the specificity pocket are shown in ball-and-stick representation (magenta). Important loop regions of the protein are noted. The anion-binding exosite I, important for the interaction with TM, fibrinogen, hirudin, and the thrombin receptors, is labeled. The anion-binding exosite II, known to interact with heparin, is also shown. The loop centered around residue 70 is homologous to the calcium-binding loop of trypsin, factors VII, IX, and X, and protein C.

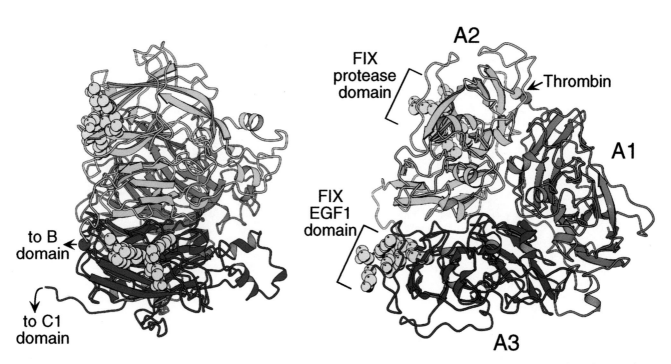

Plate 21–1. Molecular model of the factor VIII A domains. Two views are shown that differ by rotation of 90 degrees about the vertical axis. The right-hand view is looking down the pseudo threefold axis of symmetry. Domain A1 (red), A2 (yellow), and A3 (blue) are labeled. Helices are represented as coils, and the strands of β-sheets are represented as arrows. Side chains of residues proposed to interact with the factor IX protease domain and the first EGF-like domain are shown in space-filling (CPK) spheres. The termini of chains cleaved by thrombin also are indicated by spheres. In the left-hand view, termini that connect to domains not represented in the model are indicated. The carboxyl terminus of domain A1 continues into the B domain, and the carboxyl terminus of domain A3 continues into domain C1. The model was drawn with the program MOLSCRIPT[528] using the coordinates of Pemberton et al.[32]

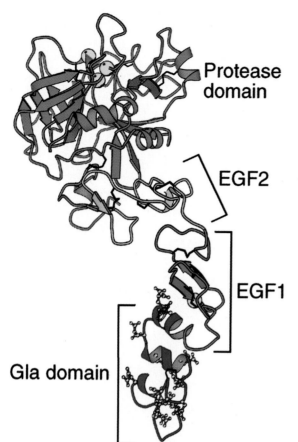

Plate 21–2. Three dimensional structure of porcine factor IXa. Domains of factor IXa are labeled: Gla domain (blue), the first EGF-like domain (EGF1, red), the second EGF-like domain (EFG2, yellow), and the serine protease domain (red). Gla residues are shown as ball and stick. The position of a β-hydroxyaspartic acid residue in EGF1 is shown as a gray sphere. Disulfide bonds are shown as black lines. The positions of α-carbons for the active site residues of the serine protease domain are shown as spheres. The domains shown in red (EGF1, Protease domain) appear to interact with specific sites in factor VIIIa. The model was drawn with the program MOLSCRIPT[528] using the coordinates of Brandstetter et al.[529]

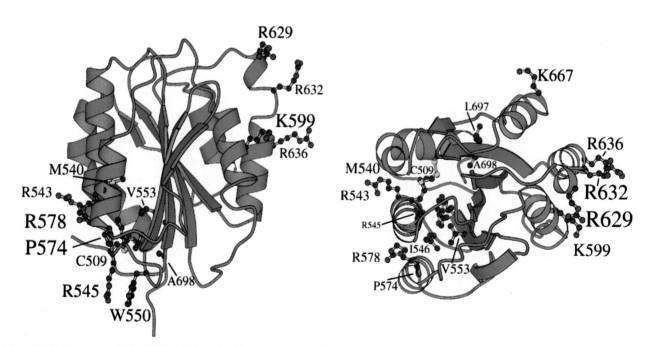

Plate 21–3. Structure of the VWF A1 domain. The two views differ by rotation of 90 degrees about the horizontal axis, so that the view on the right looks down on the top of the view at the left. Selected amino acids are shown by their side chains (ball and stick) and residue numbers (numbering from the amino terminus of the mature subunit). Mutagenesis studies suggest that Lys599 at the upper right interacts with platelet GPIbα, and that R636 and K667 interact with botrocetin; R629 and R632 may interact with either of these ligands. The residues clustered at the lower left (left panel) are mutated in VWD type 2B and may mark the location of a regulatory site that inhibits binding to GPIbα until VWF first interacts with connective tissue or certain soluble modulators. This figure was prepared with the program MOLSCRIPT[528] using the coordinates of Celikel et al.[411]

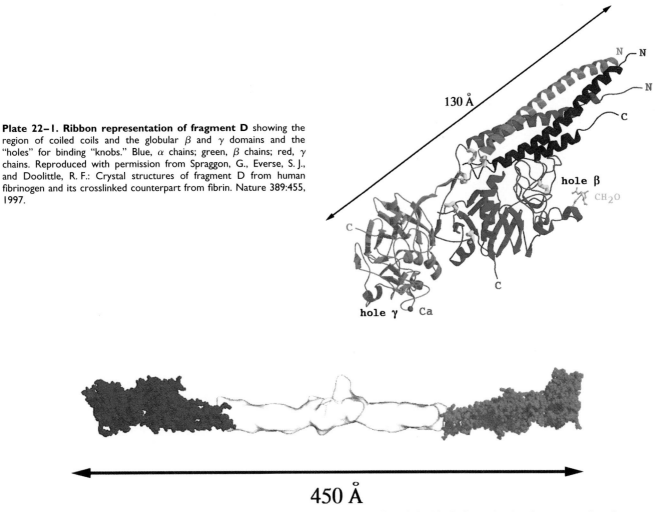

Plate 22–1. Ribbon representation of fragment D showing the region of coiled coils and the globular β and γ domains and the "holes" for binding "knobs." Blue, α chains; green, β chains; red, γ chains. Reproduced with permission from Spraggon, G., Everse, S. J., and Doolittle, R. F.: Crystal structures of fragment D from human fibrinogen and its crosslinked counterpart from fibrin. Nature 389:455, 1997.

Plate 22–2. Reconstruction of fragment X based on structures of fragments D and double-D. Reproduced with permission from Spraggon, G., Everse, S. J., and Doolittle, R. F.: Crystal structures of fragment D from human fibrinogen and its crosslinked counterpart from fibrin. Nature 389: 455, 1997.

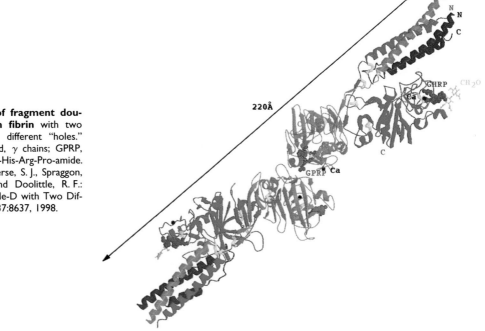

Plate 22–3. Ribbon structure of fragment double-D from cross-linked human fibrin with two different peptide ligands bound in different "holes." Blue, α chains; green, β chains; red, γ chains; GPRP, Gly-Pro-Arg-Pro-amide; GHRP, Gly-His-Arg-Pro-amide. Reprinted with permission from Everse, S. J., Spraggon, G., Veerapandian, L., Riley, M., and Doolittle, R. F.: Crystal Structure of Fragment Double-D with Two Different Bound Ligands. Biochemistry 37:8637, 1998.

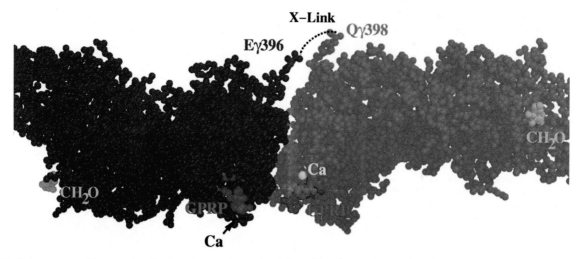

Plate 22–4. Structure of interacting D domains as determined from X-ray crystallography of fragment double-D. Reproduced with permission from Spraggon, G., Everse, S. J., and Doolittle, R. F.: Crystal structures of fragment D from human fibrinogen and its crosslinked counterpart from fibrin. Nature 389:455, 1997.

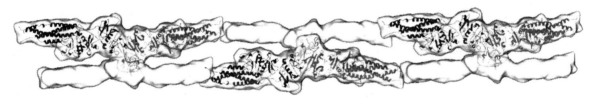

Plate 22–5. Reconstruction of a protofibril as modeled from structures of fragment double-D with bound peptide ligands. Reproduced with permission from Spraggon, G., Everse, S. J., and Doolittle, R. F.: Crystal structures of fragment D from human fibrinogen and its crosslinked counterpart from fibrin. Nature 389:455, 1997.

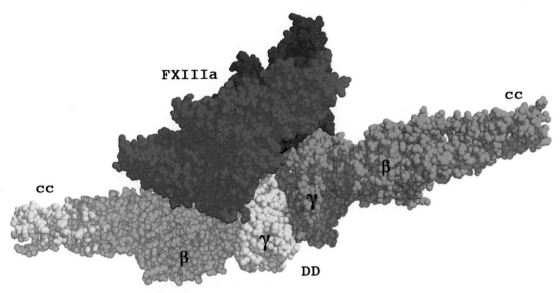

Plate 22–6. Model of factor XIII docked with a model of fragment double-D in a position appropriate for incorporating a γ-γ crosslink. Reprinted with permission from Doolittle, R. F., Spraggon, G. S., and Everse, S. J.: Three-dimensional structure studies on fragments from fibrinogen and fibrin. Current Opinion in Structural Biology. 8:792, 1998.

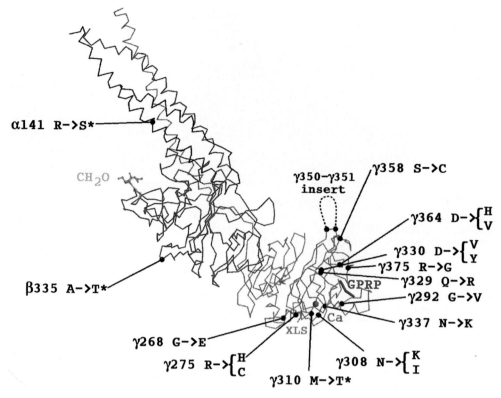

α141 R->S*

CH₂O

β335 A->T*

γ350-γ351
insert

γ358 S->C

γ364 D->{ H
          V

γ330 D->{ V
          Y

γ375 R->G

γ329 Q->R

GPRP

γ292 G->V

γ337 N->K

Ca

XLS

γ268 G->E

γ275 R->{ H
          C

γ310 M->T*

γ308 N->{ K
          I

Plate 22–7. Backbone trace of fragment D showing the positions of some known genetic variants. Asterisks (*) indicate asparagines that become glycosylated because of serine or threonine replacements two residues away. Blue, α chain; green, β chain; red, γ chain; XLS, crosslinking site. Reprinted with permission from Everse, S. J., Spraggon, G., and Doolittle, R. F.: A three-dimensional consideration of variant human fibrinogens. Thromb. Haemostasis 80:1, 1998.

Part I
HEMATOPOIESIS

1 Stem Cell Biology

Thalia Papayannopoulou and
Ihor Lemischka

Vertebrate hematopoiesis is a multitiered developmental system whose overall spatial and temporal organization ensures the normal production of all mature blood cell elements. Because the mature hematopoietic cell types have variable, though finite, life spans, they are continually replenished by new cells produced within the bone marrow from a small number of stem or progenitor cells. Immature cells remain confined within the extravascular spaces of the bone marrow, whereas mature cells and a small number of stem cells (i.e., the two ends of the spectrum of hematopoietic development) leave the bone marrow and circulate in a finely tuned "cruise control" state. Not only is there continuous renewal of all cell components throughout adult life, similar to some other developmental systems (e.g., skin, intestinal epithelium, or the male germ line); there is also a developmental regulation of hematopoiesis and intriguing migration patterns during ontogeny with successively recruited anatomical sites for their growth and development. Because of these attributes, hematopoiesis has been a very attractive and unique biological system for study.

The collective cellular composition of the bone marrow and the peripheral blood is exceedingly diverse. The key to understanding the global production of these diverse cell populations seems to lie in the multilayered organization of the entire hematopoietic system. Many years of effort have been devoted to describing this organization both in terms of distinct cellular compartments and in terms of the regulatory mechanisms that control the sizes of these compartments and the transitions between them.

The flow of cells from the stem cell to the irreversibly committed progenitor compartment, their proliferation and differentiation to mature cells, and their rapid expansion on demand are collectively controlled by glycoprotein regulators, a responsive intrinsic cell program, and cues derived from their microenvironment. Because many of the hemato-

poietic growth factors have now been isolated in pure recombinant form and several transcriptional regulators have been identified for hematopoietic cells, our understanding of the regulatory aspects of hematopoiesis has been considerably expanded.

Organization of Hematopoiesis

▼ CELL COMPARTMENTS: GENERAL FEATURES

Through a series of amplification divisions beginning from a multipotential stem cell, several heterogeneous populations of cells representing the entire differentiation sequence along each of the hematopoietic lineages are present at any given time. For operational reasons, these populations have been categorized into distinct hematopoietic cellular compartments. Three main compartments are generally accepted for hematopoiesis: the stem cell compartment, the committed progenitor cell compartment, and the precursor cell compartment. Each compartment includes a spectrum of cells, but it has distinctive features that set it apart from the next hierarchical compartment.

The *stem cell* compartment is composed of very rare cells endowed with certain fundamental properties (discussed in detail later), but mainly their ability to both self-renew and provide multilineage hematopoiesis for the life of the animal. Several physical characteristics have been ascribed to the stem cells, and these have aided both their purification and the assays used to define them in different transplantation systems.[1] For example, human stem cells are believed to express a set of antigens, and these include the expression of Thy-1,[2] the expression of Flk-1/KDR receptor,[3] and a fluctuating expression of CD34.[4] Lineage markers are absent from these cells, and they normally are found in a quiescent state or are turning over very slowly. Stem cells are also equipped with a regimen of critical transcriptional factors (e.g., SCL, GATA-2, PU-1, Myb, CBF) that are important in the execution of their fundamental cellular functions of cell renewal and multilineage differentiation (see Chapter 3).

The *progenitor cell* compartment contains cells that are found at a higher frequency than the stem cells and, like stem cells, are not morphologically distinguishable. Their existence is revealed by their ability to give rise to differentiated progeny in vitro in well-defined functional assays.[5] The progenitor cell compartment is derived from stem cells through a process of commitment to different lineage pathways. The precise molecular events that dictate stem cells to commit irreversibly to multilineage or unilineage pathways are not understood. A large body of experimental data suggests that transition of stem cells to cells of the committed compartment is achieved not by acquisition of new characteristics or new proteins but by enhancement of certain molecular pathways, already primed in these cells, and abrogation of others.[6] Instrumental in the commitment process are the functional status of key transcriptional regulators and the influence of hematopoietic cytokines in securing the survival of committed cells and the execution of selected pathways down the line (see Chapter 2). Within each lineage, a spectrum of progenitor cells exists, and these are hierarchically categorized on the basis of their proliferative potential, maturation time, response to a set of cytokines, and type of differentiated progeny, as revealed through in vitro clonogenic cultures. For example, multilineage progenitors giving rise to multiple lineages in vitro (e.g., colony-forming unit–granulocytic, erythroid, eosinophil, macrophage, megakaryocyte [CFU-GEEMM]) are presumed to be more primitive than unilineage progenitors committed only to a single lineage. As such, they are able to give rise to large colonies in vitro, because of their higher proliferative potential, and with a delayed maturation profile. By contrast, more mature progenitors give rise to smaller colonies and in a shorter time in culture. Because a high proportion of later, more mature progenitors is already cycling, a shortened maturation time is required in vitro, compared with more primitive progenitors, among which only a small fraction is actively cycling. In the erythroid lineage, for example, the burst-forming unit–erythroid (BFU-E) is the most primitive class of unilineage progenitor cells, characterized by multiclustered, large colonies and a delayed hemoglobinization profile with a peak at 2 to 3 weeks in culture.[7] The most mature set of erythroid progenitors, the colony-forming unit–erythroid (CFU-E), gives rise to small colonies and in a shorter time in culture. Although the two classes of progenitor cells, BFU-E and CFU-E, are distinct, in reality, erythroid progenitors constitute a continuum with graded changes in their properties. Primitive progenitors of other lineages (granulocytic, megakaryocytic, lymphoid) have similar properties, such as increased proliferative potential, low rate of cycling, and response to a combination of cytokines instead of a single cytokine for the very late progenitors.

The surface antigens and the molecular characteristics of progenitor cells have been defined through the use of monoclonal antibodies, their adhesion and migration properties in vitro, and molecular analyses. It is the combination of these properties that characterizes primitive versus more mature progenitors, rather than a single antigen or a single characteristic. Primitive progenitors of different lineages display many shared properties regarding the expression of surface antigens, growth factor receptors, transcriptional factors, or signaling molecules. These features explain the synergistic and overlapping properties of growth factors in these cells. The central role of transcriptional regulators and proto-oncogenes present in these progenitors has been increasingly appreciated as chromosomal translocations have been characterized in leukemic cells and studied further by genetic analyses in mice.[8, 9]

As progenitor cells differentiate, they acquire more distinctive features characteristic of each lineage and move away from shared primitive progenitor characteristics. For example, unipotent erythroid progenitors (BFU-E) are mainly CD45RA −/CD33 −/CD71 high, whereas unipotent myeloid progenitors are CD45RA +/CD33 +. Likewise, B lymphoid progenitors are CD34 +/CD20 +. Most mature progenitors (CFU-E) express Rh antigens and ABH antigens and an increased abundance of erythropoietin receptors; that is, they show the enhancement of lineage-specific characteristics, with a diminished or absent expression of multilineage properties (e.g., expression of growth factor receptors other than Epo-R). Progenitor cells of each lineage are internally programmed to ensure their own survival, but external cues are frequently impinged on these internal programs that control differentiation, maturation, and survival.

The *precursor cell* compartment, in contrast to stem and progenitor cell compartments, is defined by morphological criteria and contains cells at different maturational stages; the cells may be capable of undergoing a few rounds of cell division, or they may be end-stage, non-mitotic cells with a finite life span. The morphological characteristics of these cells reflect the accumulation of lineage-specific proteins and organelles and the decline of nuclear activity, which gives them a unique appearance. Furthermore, precursor cells for each lineage follow a unique maturation sequence; for example, in erythroid cells, the end product is an enucleated red cell, as the nuclei are expelled before terminal maturation. By contrast, terminally mature white cells remain nucleated. Also, cells of megakaryocytic lineage undergo unique endoreduplication cycles, forming large cells with multilobulated nuclei. The maturation sequence for each lineage requires a specific time frame, but there is enough plasticity to allow for faster than normal production of end-stage effector cells. Such deviations from the normal sequence are dictated by stress, which demands quick delivery of specialized (mainly white) cells into the periphery. Cytokines must also be finely tuned to accommodate the urgent demands for increased production of white cells.

A large pool of maturing progenitors for each lineage is stored within the marrow, and this allows for rapid recruitment and export at times of stress. Although this is largely true for white cells (with the exception of monocytes), it is not true for the erythroid cells or megakaryocytic cells. Every day, 8.7×10^8 polymorphonuclear neutrophil leukocytes (PMNs) per kilogram are produced, plus 5.7×10^6 monocytes, this production rate, together with an increased storage pool within the bone marrow, can quickly accommodate urgent needs. Crucial among precursor cells for each lineage is the expression of functional receptors specific for that lineage, such as Epo receptors for erythroid cells and G or GM receptors for myeloid cells[10] (see Chapter 2). In addition, certain transcriptional factors or proto-oncogenes influence their differentiation to specific lineages, as their downstream targets are many lineage-affiliated proteins. For example, GATA-1, FOG, and EKLF are important in erythroid differentiation.[8] In general, each lineage has a complex regulation and maturation process, and the increased understanding of the regulation of lineage differentiation has had an immediate impact in clinical medicine, with effective strategies being implemented for therapeutic management. How the constant number of maturing cells for each lineage is maintained, both in the periphery and within the bone marrow, is poorly understood. It has been speculated that feedback signals from the maturing population limit their production, but the detailed mechanisms have not been delineated. Recently, at least for the erythroid lineage, a paradigm has been presented that may have applicability to other lineages.[11] A Fas ligand produced by mature erythroid cells can have an impact on Fas receptor expressed on erythroid progenitors, with a negative influence on their survival, by targeting pivotal transcriptional factors, such as GATA-1. Similar mechanisms could be envisioned for other lineages, but no specific information has been presented.

In addition to intrinsic cellular pathways, great influence (positive or negative) on hematopoietic cell development is exercised by cues derived from the microenvironment, both during ontogeny and in the adult, within the bone marrow. Such effects are largely mediated through cytoadhesive interaction and signaling between hematopoietic cells bearing cognate receptors for diverse ligands that are presented, secreted, or sequestered by microenvironmental cells and their extracellular matrix.[12–16]

Hematopoietic regulation by growth factors and their receptors, as well as the emerging molecular requirements in hematopoiesis, are discussed in detail in separate chapters. This chapter deals mainly with hematopoiesis as an organ, its origin during ontogeny, and the distinctive features of intrauterine versus adult hematopoiesis; it engages current concepts and controversies regarding stem cell issues. The availability of new culture techniques, cell micromanipulations, and sensitive molecular analyses and the discovery of new regulators with in vivo testing using mouse genetics have provided significant new information germane to issues discussed in this chapter.

Emergence of Hematopoiesis and Relationship to Vascular Cells

Since its inception, hematopoiesis has been intimately associated with blood vessels. The anatomical links and the "budding" of blood cells within the vascular channels have been emphasized in all species examined. The ontogenic development of hematopoietic and vascular cells has been coordinately regulated, so that differentiated blood cells begin to circulate as soon as vascular channels are established. These anatomical and temporal associations during ontogeny led to the concept that both endothelial cells and hematopoietic cells arise from a common precursor. Thus a theory of "simultaneous formation of endothelium and blood cells from the same common source" had already been formulated at the turn of the twentieth century,[17–19] and the term *heman-*

gioblast had been coined to denote this common progenitor cell. This theory has been revived several times over the last 10 to 20 years, as new experimental approaches became available. Early experiments in birds and amphibians provided the first supportive evidence.[20–25] Using heterospecies grafts or quail chick chimeras, it was shown that mesoderm in the splachnopleural (SP) region is capable of giving rise to both endothelial cells and hematopoietic cells.[25, 26] Furthermore, single cell labeling with chick cells was found to generate both vascular endothelial cells and hematopoietic cells in vitro,[27] and both lineages could be induced in vitro when cells from dissociated quail blastodiscs were used.[26, 28] Quail monoclonal antibodies (QH1 and MB1) recognize surface epitopes present in endothelial and blood cells, and both cell types express the Flk-homologue in quail (Quek1).[20, 21] In zebrafish, a single ventral marginal zone cell of the blastula can give rise to both endothelial and hematopoietic cells.[29, 30] Evidence in the mouse and higher vertebrates was less apparent early on. The situation has changed in the last few years, however, as mice with targeted mutations of either vascular or hematopoietic genes were studied or other technical advances in in vitro approaches were used. Mice deficient in Flk-1 (vascular endothelial growth factor [VEGF]-R2), the receptor for VEGF, die between 8.5 and 9.5 days post conception (dpc) owing to a lack of endothelial cells as well as hematopoietic cells in the yolk sac.[31] Thus the presence of Flk-1 receptor in a presumed common progenitor cell was deemed absolutely necessary for the development of both lineages. Similar data were obtained when its ligand, VEGF, was ablated.[32] In zebrafish, the gene *cloche* affects both endothelial and hematopoietic cells acting upstream of Flk-1.[33] Because of their interrelationships, however, one may think that a defect in one lineage (endothelial) may have secondary effects in the other lineage (hematopoietic). A series of subsequent examples, however, suggest that this is only partially true. As discussed later, severe impairments in blood vessel development do not necessarily lead to hematopoietic defects, and vice versa.

A regulatory hierarchy in the molecular requirements for vasculogenesis (differentiation of mesodermal precursors into endothelial cells and their subsequent assembly into a capillary plexus) or angiogenesis (the remodeling of primary vessels into a larger, complex network) has recently been uncovered by gene targeting experiments. Thus, although Flk-1 was found to be necessary for vasculogenesis and hematopoiesis,[34, 35] the ablation of several other genes downstream of Flk-1 did not affect the origin of vasculogenesis, but it did lead to a variety of defects in vascular development with no significant influence on hematopoiesis. In general, these type of genes fall into several different categories. Some are receptor-ligand pairs important for the interaction of endothelial cells with their surrounding mesenchymal cells, such as Tie-2,[36] its ligand angiopoietin-1,[37] the tissue factor (TF, ligand for factor VII/VIIa),[38] or the Flt-1 (VEGF-R1) receptor.[39] Other genes represent transcription factors or signaling molecules important in angiogenesis. In this category, lung Kruppel-like factor,[40] stem cell leukemia/T-cell acute leukemia-1,[41] aromatic hydrocarbon receptor nuclear translocator,[42] and the G protein Gα-13[43] are examples. Two gene products, Tie-2 and SCL, seem to affect angiogenesis similarly by a cell autonomous defect and generate similar yolk sac phenotypes. However, one of these, Tie-2, leads to no apparent hematopoietic defects,[44] whereas SCL affects the development of hematopoietic cells and of vitelline vessels as well.[41, 45] As such, SCL, in contrast to all other genes downstream of Flk-1 that affect angiogenesis only, is placed at the interphase between vasculogenesis and angiogenesis; at the same time, it appears to be highly critical for hematopoietic development. Although SCL is expressed in endothelial cells and was originally considered dispensable for blood vessel formation, following selective hematopoietic lineage rescue in SCL−/− mice, it was shown that SCL is also important for remodeling of the yolk sac vascular network.[41, 45] This experience is highly instructive of in vivo effects potentially missed when early embryonic lethality is encountered and raises the possibility that even for the other genes affecting angiogenesis, subtle hematopoietic effects may be present but not yet uncovered. Another example is the Tie-2 targeted ablation, which was reported not to affect hematopoiesis.[44] More recent evidence suggests that it may impair definitive hematopoiesis.[46] Angiopoietin-1 enhanced the adhesion of Tie-2+ hematopoietic cells that were sorted from 9.5 dpc embryos, implying that Tie-2 and angiopoietin-1 signals may play a critical role in the development of definitive hematopoiesis as well as angiogenesis.[46] Nevertheless, analysis of hematopoietic progenitors present in the yolk sac, the aorta-gonad-mesonephros area, or the fetal liver in angiopoietin-1 and angiopoietin-2 knockout mice showed no quantitative hematopoietic defects.[47] In the same vein, the block in hematopoiesis in Flk-1−/− mice is not absolute, as hemoglobinized cells do develop from embryoid body differentiation of Flk-1−/− embryonic stem cells.[34] Because Flk-1 is required for both the differentiation of endothelial cells and the migration of primitive precursors of endothelial cells from the posterior primitive streak to the yolk sac, one may claim that the lack of hematopoietic cell development is due to the failure of these cells to migrate into a microenvironment that is permissive for hematopoiesis.[35]

Despite the associations listed above, rigorous experimental support for the isolation and identification of a single bipotent progenitor cell has remained elusive. Recently, however, experimental data have been presented that seem to satisfy several critics who doubted its existence. First, it was shown that disrupted embryoid bodies, 3 to 3.5 days after culture of ES cells, generate blast-type colonies with both definitive and primitive hematopoietic potential.[48] In addition, these blast cell colonies, derived in the presence of VEGF and kit ligand, can give rise to both endothelial and hematopoietic cells. (ES cells were differentiated for 3 to 3.5 days, and the embryoid bodies were dispersed and replated in the presence of VEGF, kit ligand, and conditioned medium from a supportive endothelial line D4T.) Adherent cells derived from these colonies were composed mainly of endothelial cells, although some macrophages were also present.[49] Their endothelial cell identity was confirmed by the expression of Flk-1, Tie-1, and Tie-2. Although these experiments demonstrated that endothelial and hematopoietic cells arose from colonies of a presumed single cell origin, they did not convincingly show that a single cell can generate both types of colonies. This claim has been presented by another group of scientists who used mesodermic yolk sac cells for culture.[50] Single cells with the phenotypic properties of endothelial cells (i.e., VE-cadherin+/CD45−) and with coexpression of Flk-1, CD31, and CD34 were isolated from 9.5 dpc embryos, and these can give rise to hematopoietic cells. Such endothelial cells were present in both the yolk sac and the embryo proper—that is, at sites associated with the first hematopoietic cell development. These data, together with the earlier observations with the use of ES cells, provide the first in vitro demonstration that such a common progenitor cell exists early in development. One may argue that endothelial cells in the above in vitro experiments have the phenotypic characteristics of endothelial cells but not the functional requirements for blood vessel formation (did not form lumen in culture). Therefore, it is unclear whether they behave the same way in vivo. It is of interest that only endothelial cells in the specific mesodermic areas where hematopoiesis arises have this property. The same phenotype in other sites does not give rise to hematopoietic cells—probably only to endothelial cells.[26, 50] The issue of whether VE-cadherin–positive cells represent "hemangioblasts" or just "hemogenic endothelial cells"[51] is moot at this point. It is conceivable, as proposed in another study, that blocking of the Flk-1 receptor by VEGF in a common precursor precludes activation of the other pathway, and vice versa.[24] For example, experiments with Flk-1+ cells in vitro gave rise to either hematopoietic or endothelial colonies, but not both. The authors have suggested that both endothelial and hematopoietic precursors display the Flk-1 receptor, but two factors—VEGF or an unknown factor that competes for the same receptor—are crucial for the fate of these precursor cells. Nevertheless, the experiments with ES cells[49] and the murine mesodermic yolk sac cells[50] mentioned earlier do not support this argument.

Histological observations suggest that the putative hemangioblasts differentiate in two directions; the peripheral ones form angioblasts, and the more central ones form the hematopoietic blast cells.[25, 26] There is a brief window during which the two lines are interdependent, and then each can proceed independently of the other. Mesodermal induction by several factors is considered critical for hemangioblast differentiation. Several molecules have been identified as inducers, such as basic fibroblast growth factor, activin, bone morphogenetic protein–4, or transforming growth factor–1β.[52] Mesodermic induction has been studied most extensively in *Xenopus*. All hematopoietic cells in *Xenopus* are derived from ventral mesoderm and populate two sites of the embryo: the ventral blood islands (VBIs) and the dorsal lateral plate (DLP), analogous to the yolk sac and the AGM, respectively, in higher vertebrates. BMP-4 was shown to induce patterning in ventral mesoderm, but cooperative effects with other inducers gave optimal results.[52] Studies of genetic mutants in zebrafish also provided insight into the early mesodermal induction of hematopoiesis. Homozygous *cloche* embryos lack endothelial cells (head and trunk endothelial cells) and blood but retain some tail endothelial cells.[52] Flk-1 expression is delayed in these embryos, suggesting that *cloche* is developmentally the earliest upstream gene important for vascular and hematopoietic cell mesodermal induction. Mice generated by targeted disruption of the BMP-4 gene die between about 7.5 and 10.5 dpc and show abnormalities in the extraembryonic mesoderm of the yolk sac,[53] thus implicating BMP-4 in the induction of hematopoiesis from mesoderm. TGF-β null mice also have defective yolk sac hematopoiesis,[54] but data with activin *null* mice do not show hematopoietic abnormalities.[55] Contribution of maternally derived activin may play a role. Although more attention has been given to signals for mesodermal induction, recent evidence suggests that prior signaling through primitive endoderm is necessary for embryonic hematopoiesis. Classical transplantation experiments in chick embryos have implicated primitive endoderm in the formation of blood and vascular tissue by extraembryonic mesoderm,[56] but in mammalian embryos its involvement has been unclear. More recent observations in the mouse suggest that molecular determinants for these lineages are present in primitive endoderm 6.5 dpc, at least 18 hours before blood cells are detectable, and they target hemangioblasts. Furthermore, within a narrow window of time, signals from the endoderm can reprogram anterior ectoderm to develop into hemangioblastic lineages.[57]

The close interrelationships between vascular and hematopoietic cells in mesodermal sites during ontogeny do not terminate when hematopoiesis is established in subsequent anatomical sites, such as fetal liver or bone marrow. In the fetal liver, hematopoietic cells develop in the extravascular space, similar to bone marrow hematopoiesis. However, all hematopoietic sites share one cell in common: the endothelial cell. Endothelial cell lines from yolk sac, AGM, or fetal liver[58–61] support hematopoiesis in vitro and maintain long-term repopulating cells. This support requires direct contact, thus reproducing the in vivo physical contact between endothelial and hematopoietic cells. Moreover, a significant body of data also demonstrates the supportive role of adult bone marrow endothelium in hematopoiesis in adults.[62] Endothelial cells constitutively express high levels of growth factors such as stem cell factor (kit ligand), granulocyte colony-stimulating factor, granulocyte-macrophage colony-stimulating factor, and interleukin-6, and endothelial stromal cell layers from bone marrow have been shown to support proliferation and differentiation of hematopoietic cells in vitro.[63] Expression and display of endothelial cell adhesion molecules in addition to growth factors may also be important for hematopoietic cell function and for the trafficking and homing of progenitor cells. In this context, it is of interest that endothelial cells in bone marrow display exclusive properties not shared by endothelial cells in other tissue. For example, they constitutively express VCAM-1, E-selectin, and higher levels of stromal cell derived factor-1, in contrast to endothelial cells from other tissues.[64, 65] Furthermore, endothelial cells express receptors for several growth factors (IL-3, SCF, erythropoietin, and thrombopoietin) and show functional responses to IL-3 and erythropoietin, implying a reciprocal role in trophic signals between endothelial and hematopoietic cells.[66]

Primitive and Definitive Hematopoiesis

▼ PRIMITIVE/EMBRYONIC

The first site of appearance of differentiated hematopoietic cells during ontogeny is the blood islands of the yolk sac. Beginning at 7.5 to 8 dpc in the mouse (approximately at day 15 in humans), clusters of hematopoietic cells arise from the inner lining of blood vessels in the yolk sac. The intravascular origin of red cells was first described in 1892 by van der Stricht,[67] and this view was adopted and expanded upon by Dantschakoff and Maximov between 1907 and 1910.[68–71] The development and differentiation of erythroid cells within the yolk sac blood islands are virtually synonymous with the term *embryonic* or *primitive hematopoiesis*.

It lasts only a few days in the mouse or a few weeks in humans, then develops exclusively intravascularly, and distributes throughout the embryo following the newly developed circulatory channels.

Embryonic or primitive hematopoiesis has a unique constellation of morphological, biochemical, and molecular features that will never reappear together during the subsequent period of organism development. Terminally differentiated human embryonic red cells, in contrast to those appearing later in life, do not enucleate and thus resemble those in lower vertebrates. They are very large cells (mean corpuscular volume >140) with a high hemoglobin content, a distinct membrane, and a brilliant red color under the microscope. These nucleated red cells contain a combination of embryonic hemoglobins (hemoglobin Gower I [$\epsilon_2\zeta_2$] and Gower II [$\alpha_2\epsilon_2$] and hemoglobin Portland [$\zeta_2\gamma_2$]) exclusively. Although small quantities of embryonic globin chains (ϵ or ζ) or embryonic hemoglobins can be synthesized in erythroid cells later in life, no terminally differentiated cells with the same morphology and exclusive embryonic hemoglobin content have ever been seen in adult life either normally or in leukemic states. Differentiation of erythroid cells within the yolk sac blood islands appears synchronous, so that cells with blast appearance are first evident, followed by a population of basophilic erythroblasts, which in turn mature to polychromatophilic and orthochromatic nucleated red cells that are exclusively found in circulation later on.

In addition to differentiated erythroid cells in the yolk sac, multipotent progenitors giving rise to erythroid and several non-erythroid lineages appear in the yolk sac at approximately the same time that similar progenitor cells are detected within the embryo proper, in the AGM area.[52, 72, 73] These progenitors in the yolk sac have the appearance of blast cells and in clonogenic semisolid media in vitro give rise to differentiated descendents of granulocytic, monocytic/macrophage, erythroid, and lymphoid lineages. Multipotent and oligopotent progenitors giving rise to colonies of more than one lineage are very dominant in the yolk sac, especially the bipotent erythroid/megakaryocytic progenitors.[74] It is important to stress that when these progenitors give rise to erythroid descendents in vitro, they do not form colonies of embryonic erythroblasts, but the erythroid colonies or the bursts formed are of the definitive lineage similar to ones from AGM or fetal liver. As such, they produce adult-type hemoglobin in the mouse, or mostly fetal and some adult hemoglobin in humans. Thus, in the yolk sac, one simultaneously finds differentiated cells representing embryonic hematopoiesis and progenitor cells that belong to the definitive lineage. Cells of the embryonic lineage can form only small CFU-E–like colonies with brilliant red color within the first 3 to 5 days in culture and are phenotypically[62, 75] distinct from CFU-Es arising from definitive-type progenitors. Thus, the distinction between primitive and definitive lineage cells rests not so much on the basis of the specific time or specific site of their appearance during ontogeny (Fig. 1–1), but mainly on their ability to complete terminal differentiation in vivo and on the several discriminatory features between these two lineages.

The coexistence in the yolk sac of undifferentiated progenitors of definitive lineage together with terminally differentiated erythroid cells of primitive lineage could imply a common progenitor for both cell lineages with a distinct microenvironmental induction of only embryonic erythropoi-

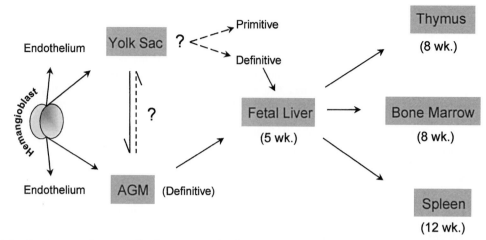

Figure 1–1. Models of ontogeny of mammalian hematopoiesis. Currently available evidence in mice and man suggests the early appearance of hematopoietic cells (from hemogenic endothelium) both in the extraembryonic yolk sac and within the embryo proper, in the aorta-gonad-mesonephros (AGM) area. Whether they appear first in yolk sac and then migrate to AGM after circulation is established is disputed at present.[72, 72a] In yolk sac, differentiated erythroid cells and macrophages, as well as their progenitor cells, appear first, and soon after, definitive progenitors of several lineages (differentiating only in vitro) are detected both in yolk sac and AGM. The wave of primitive erythroid cells is transient and synchronous. Primitive cells may or may not share a common progenitor with cells of definitive lineage.[48, 76, 77] Definitive progenitor cells present in circulation colonize the liver at ~5–6 weeks, and full development of liver hematopoiesis is established by 8–9 weeks and maintained until about 12 weeks, when bone marrow and spleen are colonized. Bone marrow is the exclusive site of hematopoiesis in the adult animal.

esis in the yolk sac, or it could be due to the autonomous development of the two lineages by distinct mesodermal precursor cells. Whether one or the other view is correct remains debatable, and experimental data in support of both views have been presented.[48, 76, 77] One of the strongest arguments in support of an autonomous and distinct origin of embryonic cells in the yolk sac is their molecular requirements, which sharply distinguish them from the definitive progenitors present on the same site. Such requirements have been uncovered in the last few years, mainly through the use of targeted ablation of several molecules in mice or through the in vitro differentiation of the ES/embryoid body system.[78] There is a growing list of proteins (transcriptional factors, signaling molecules, oncogenes, growth factors, and so forth) that influence the development of cells of definitive lineage but are dispensable for the embryonic lineage (for example, AML-1/CBF-β, Myb, Rb, PU-1, JAK-2, SOCS3, Caspase 8, kit, BclX).[79–91] Either no or sparse definitive progenitors are present in the yolk sac, in AGM, or in fetal liver in the absence of these proteins. However, embryonic erythropoiesis develops normally. The fact that within the same anatomical site (the yolk sac blood islands) embryonic erythroid cells develop normally but definitive progenitors are absent argues against a common progenitor for definitive and embryonic cells with an environmental influence only on embryonic cells. However, the nature of the effect by many of the factors, for example, the CCAAT-binding factor complex, has not yet been addressed, and it is not clear whether definitive cells are not generated or are generated but are unresponsive to growth factors needed for their detection in vitro. Although the core binding factors (CAFα2/CBFβ) are important for all types of definitive progenitors and appear to be among the most upstream required for their development, a number of other factors show a preferential requirement for certain lineages among definitive cells. Ablation of these factors leaves embryonic hematopoiesis in the yolk sac unaffected. The c-myb and the PU-1 transcription factors are

included in this category (for details, see Chapter 3). In the absence of c-myb, normal megakaryocytopoiesis is maintained, but all other lineages are affected,[83] and if PU-1 is absent, normal fetal liver erythroid and megakaryocytes are seen, but myeloid development is severely impaired.[85, 86] Targeted ablation of other transcription factors, such as GATA-2, causes global quantitative defects, especially for the definitive progenitors and less so for the embryonic ones.[92] Conversely, signaling molecules such as jak-2[87] or gp130,[93] the common β chain of IL-6, GM-CSF, and IL-11, impair maturational aspects of definitive progenitors and less so of embryonic ones. It is of interest that certain factors, such as SOCS3[88] or Caspase 8,[91] influence fetal liver erythropoiesis in a negative fashion, with overproduction of erythroid cells in their absence. Finally, other factors, such as jumonji[94] and Nrf-1,[95] may cause not a cell-autonomous effect but an environmentally induced effect with a quantitative impact only on definitive hematopoiesis.

The in vitro requirements of primitive versus definitive progenitors also are distinct. Whereas progenitors have an absolute requirement in vitro for certain growth factors, the small CFU-E–like colonies arising from embryonic progenitors do not appear to have the same requirements, and only factors promoting their in vitro survival and terminal differentiation could be important. In this context, it is of interest that thrombopoietin has been found in high concentration in yolk sac blood islands[96] and, when present in culture as a single factor, seems to influence the proliferation and differentiation of erythroid colonies from the yolk sac but not those from fetal liver or adult bone marrow.[96] Nevertheless, these colonies are of definitive lineage and are not embryonic cell derived. Also, both kit and kit ligand are detectable in the yolk sac at days 8 to 9 dpc; however, this pathway appears to be more important for cells of definitive lineage.[89] Other factors such as VEGF or macrophage colony-stimulating factor are produced by cells in close contact with the embryonic erythroid cells (macrophages, endothelial cells), but the influence of these factors on embryonic erythropoiesis is unclear. Erythropoietin is not detectable in the yolk sac, but definitive colonies developing in vitro are dependent on Epo for their subsequent differentiation. In this context, it is of extreme interest that overexpression of Epo in the yolk sac leads to in vivo differentiation of definitive erythroid progenitors at that site.[97] These results give credence to the view that the environment in the yolk sac in vivo does not promote the downstream differentiation of definitive cells.

▼ DEFINITIVE

Fetal liver is the main site of complete development of definitive hematopoiesis in intrauterine life. As indicated previously, fetal liver is colonized by progenitor cells already developed earlier in the AGM or yolk sac.[52, 72, 73] Initiation of hematopoiesis in the liver is heralded by the appearance of undifferentiated blast cells in the hepatic cords. This population of blasts expands exponentially (between day 11 and 12 in the mouse) within the extravascular spaces of the developing liver. In contrast to yolk sac blood islands, fetal liver contains the full hierarchy of both hematopoietic progenitors and precursor cells, but at distinct proportions from those found later in adult bone marrow. Progenitor cells present in fetal liver, like those present in the AGM or yolk sac, are detectable by functional endpoints in semisolid assays and include erythroid, megakaryocytic, granulocytic, and multilineage colony-forming cells. In addition to these progenitor cells, cells able to engraft allogeneic or xenogeneic recipients with multilineage long-term reconstitution potential are present in fetal liver from day 11 onward.[52, 72, 73] At the same day, long-term repopulating cells (LTRCs) are also detectable in the other hematopoietic sites—the AGM and the yolk sac. Before day 11, such stem cells can be detected in the AGM or yolk sac when only neonatal recipients are used.[98, 99]

In vivo, fetal liver is characterized by a predominance of erythroid cells at different stages of maturation. Although erythropoiesis predominates in fetal liver, it lacks the synchronicity observed in the yolk sac, and the final product, the fetal red cell, is a smaller, enucleated cell containing predominantly fetal hemoglobin. The fact that differentiation in fetal liver is predominantly erythropoietic reflects either an increased intrinsic probability to commit to the erythroid pathway or an increased propensity of already committed erythroid progenitors for differentiation and expansion within the fetal liver microenvironment in vivo. Certainly the proportion of erythroid bursts, especially of mature ones and of CFU-E, is found increased in culture.[100] Furthermore, fetal liver cells are characterized by a dramatic expansion per progenitor cell occurring at earlier times in vitro (colonies become large within a short time) and with a fuller maturation profile. This indicates not only an increased output per progenitor cell but also that the fetal cells, as they complete their maturation, are less susceptible to conditions in vitro that cause apoptosis in adult cells. In addition to quantitative predominance of erythroid progenitor and precursor cells in fetal liver, there is an increased proportion of multipotential progenitors detected in vitro and an increased frequency of bipotent erythroid/megakaryocytic progenitors.

These findings are qualitatively similar to progenitors present in the yolk sac or AGM.[101]

Hematopoiesis in the liver is fully developed between days 12 and 15 in the mouse (8 to 9 weeks in humans). Following that time, hematopoietic cells migrating through the circulation settle in the spleen and, after day 17 or so, in the developing bone marrow of mice. Hematopoiesis in the murine spleen is found until the end of gestation and a few weeks thereafter. In humans, fetal liver remains the main hematopoietic organ for about 12 weeks (12 to 23 weeks). The spleen becomes hematopoietically active after 19 weeks but ceases to be hematopoietic after birth. The final destination of hematopoietic cells in the fetus is the bone marrow. The development of the bone marrow is subsequent to invasion of avascular cartilage by vascular mesenchyme. The invading mesenchyme is necessary for the rudimentary bone development and calcification of cartilage. Hematopoiesis in the bone marrow is heralded by the appearance of undifferentiated basophilic cells in dilated marrow sinuses. This occurs at day 17 to 18 in the mouse and begins at about week 20 of gestation in humans. In the mouse, hematopoiesis in the bone marrow is predominantly granulocytopoietic in utero, but after birth, bone marrow gains in erythroid function, so that the E to G ratio is 1:5. In humans, however, bone marrow hematopoiesis in utero displays erythropoietic activity from the beginning.

Comparisons of progenitor cells in fetal liver to those in adult bone marrow have revealed differences in their surface phenotype,[102, 103] in their responsiveness to growth factors,[104–108] in their turnover rate, and in their rate of regeneration post-transplant.[109, 110] Several of these aspects have been studied in detail in mice, and similar differences seem to exist between human fetal and adult hematopoietic cells.[101, 111, 111a] Phenotypic analysis of cells from the AGM region and the fetal liver at day 11 shows that all the long-term repopulating activity in the mouse is found within the kit-positive population.[112] The kit-negative population never provided reconstitution in irradiated recipients. However, human fetal CD34+CD38− stem cells are highly heterogeneous in their expression of c-kit.[109] In the mouse, the long-term repopulating activity peaks in the AGM at day 11, whereas in the liver it peaks at day 12, possibly reflecting migration of massive numbers of progenitor cells at that time.[113] Kit-positive cells contain some Sca-1+ cells (less than 1 per cent in the AGM and liver); CD44 and Mac-1 are detected in significant proportions in the kit-positive population (94 per cent of the kit-positive cells in the fetal liver, but about 20 per cent of the kit-positive cells in the AGM area). Less frequent are other antigens such as CD34 and the AA4.1 among kit-positive cells.

The phenotypic characteristics of LTRCs residing in fetal liver versus adult bone marrow show rather minor differences. There was high expression of CD44 in the fetal liver,[113] and long-term repopulating activity can be found both in Mac-1+ and Mac-1− cells in fetal liver and AGM, in contrast to bone marrow cells.[113] (Seventy-six per cent of kit+/34+ are MAC-1+ at day 11 in the fetal liver, but only 54 per cent in the AGM.) It is noteworthy that LTRCs in the yolk sac are kit positive and AA4.1 positive, but they are Sca-1 negative and CD44 negative.[98, 102, 112–114] As such, they differ from both fetal liver and bone marrow cells. The putative role of Mac-1 as an important adhesion molecule within these fetal sites is unclear. Alternatively, an association between its expression and the cycling activity of these progenitors cannot be excluded. Furthermore, it is not clear whether a real difference exists between fetal and adult cells in CD34 expression. Long-term repopulating activity was noted in CD34− donor cells in adult mice,[115] but very little such activity was found in fetal liver cells.[112] Also, the longevity of CD34− human cells transplanted in fetal sheep was found to be superior to that of CD34+ cells.[116] Kit continues to be expressed on virtually all hematopoietic progenitors from the embryonic period and throughout adult life. Anti-kit antibody treatment in vivo decreases colony-forming cell (CFC) numbers in the developing fetal liver[117] and both CFC and colony-forming unit–spleen (CFU-S) numbers in the adult mouse.[118, 119] Mutant mice with mutations of kit are compromised in their ability to regenerate hematopoiesis in transplanted myeloablated +/+ recipients.[110] For example, transplantation of W42/W42 cells with a complete abrogation of the tyrosine kinase activity of the kit receptor showed only transient hematopoietic activity in primary recipients; thus, later on, stem cells appear to be increasingly dependent on kit ligand.[110] Also, Steel mice (Sl/Sl^d) with an absence of membrane-bound kit ligand[120] show impaired hematopoiesis that is exaggerated when these mice are used as irradiated recipients of normal donor cells.[121] Therefore, membrane-bound kit ligand may be particularly important for sustaining cell renewal in vivo in adults. All these experiments have provided ample evidence of an important role for the kit/kit ligand pathway in the activation and maintenance of most primitive hematopoietic cells. However, embryonic hematopoiesis and, to a large extent, early progenitor compartments in fetal liver hematopoiesis are not significantly compromised in the absence of kit/kit ligand signals.[89, 122] This apparent discrepancy can be explained by differences between fetal and adult stem cells in the sensitivity to kit ligand either alone or in combination with other cytokines.[62] However, even at these early periods of hematopoiesis, all the transplantable hematopoietic activity was present only among c-kit–positive cells.[112] It is of interest that stem cell factor or kit ligand is present in the ductular cells around the portal vein during the late stages of fetal liver development. In the adult liver, both bile ducts and bile ductules are positive for kit ligand and kit.[123] Thus, it appears that the kit/kit ligand signaling transduction system is involved in the development of bile ducts and in the biology of liver stem cells, in addition to their role in hematopoiesis. This system, therefore, may exercise a unique environmental effect on fetal liver hematopoiesis. As both hepatic differentiation and hematopoiesis occur simultaneously, the impact of the kit/kit ligand system on hematopoiesis during liver development is complicated. Likewise, in the AGM area, some kit-positive cells are likely primordial germ cells.[124] It is of interest that these cells can generate in vitro hematopoietic colonies like the ones from the AGM or fetal liver.[72]

The adhesive phenotype and adhesive behavior of bone marrow progenitor cells (colony-forming unit–culture [CFU-C]) versus those from fetal liver have also been studied, and differences between these two cell sources have been noted. Bone marrow CFU-Cs adhere better to bone marrow stroma in vitro than do fetal liver cells.[103] By contrast, fetal liver CFU-Cs adhere to collagen IV (through $\alpha_2 \beta_1$ integrin), to which bone marrow cells do not adhere.[103] Also, more primitive progenitors, long-term culture initiating cells (LTC-IC), and CFU-C from both sources adhere to vascular cell adhesion molecule (VCAM-1) and to fibronectin present within the bone marrow stroma through $\alpha_4 \beta_1$ and $\alpha_5 \beta_1$ integrins.[125] Additional adhesive interactions in vitro and likely in vivo are mediated through β_2 integrins, selectins, CD44, and proteoglycans expressed by hematopoietic progenitors. Overall, bone marrow cells express less L-selectin and CD44 compared with fetal liver cells, although the significance of this is unclear. The lack of α_4 in α_4 "null" mice was originally reported to affect only lymphoid development,[126] however, recent data suggest a major role for α_4 in the maintenance and expansion of fetal and especially adult hematopoiesis.[126a] These data are consistent with functional abrogation of α_4 in pregnant mice treated with anti-α_4 antibodies, leading to severely diminished fetal liver erythropoiesis.[117] Furthermore, it was recently noted that expression of α_4 was abrogated in fetal liver in c-myb-deficient mice[127] which display defective definitive hematopoiesis within fetal liver, but the contribution of a lack of α_4 in this defect is unclear.

Hematopoietic Stem Cells

▼ GENERAL PRINCIPLES

The underlying dogma of the hematopoietic system is the existence of a population of stem cells, which are collectively responsible for sustained, lifelong production of all mature blood cell types.[1, 128, 129] An understanding of the functional properties and physical characteristics of stem cells is key to unraveling the cellular and molecular mechanisms that globally regulate normal hematopoiesis and that go awry in pathological conditions such as myelodysplasias and leukemias. An understanding of basic stem cell biology also has an impact on the development of more effective clinical transplantation strategies and the eventual application of gene therapy for inherited as well as acquired hematological disorders.

The hallmark functional properties traditionally ascribed to the stem cell compartment are the following. First, at least operationally, the stem cell compartment is self-renewing. This follows from the staggering and continuous rate of new mature blood cell production necessitated by the finite half-lives of these cells in the periphery and the obvious requirement for these cells throughout adult life. In the human, for example, approximately 250 billion red cells are produced per day. Correlated with self-renewal ability is a very high proliferative potential. Second, at least at the population level, the stem cell compartment must be multipotential, given the existence of at least eight distinct lineages of mature blood cells. Third, the functional abilities of the stem cell population must be tightly controlled to ensure the proper balance of self-renewal versus commitment to differentiation. The production of the various mature cell populations in their physiologically correct proportions must also be guaranteed by stringent control mechanisms. At the same time, these control mechanisms must be flexible in order to respond appropriately to situations of hematological stress, which may be global or lineage specific in nature.

At its most fundamental level, the biology of hematopoietic stem cells is a function of cell-fate choice mechanisms with many similarities to other developmental systems.[1, 8, 128–136] As in all these systems, cell-fate choice regulatory mechanisms have cell-autonomous and non-cell-autonomous components.[132, 138–145] In addition, the regulatory mechanisms may be stochastic, deterministic, instructive, or a combination of these.[2, 129, 132, 139, 146] It has been suggested that the hematopoietic stem cell system may, at least in part, be regulated by mechanisms that are similar to those first described in invertebrates.[132, 147–149]

▼ HIERARCHICAL ORGANIZATION OF THE STEM CELL COMPARTMENT

Two additional features of the stem cell compartment that deserve mention at this point are the extremely rare nature of primitive stem cells and the functionally hierarchical organization of the entire stem cell population.[150–152] The former feature has the practical consequence that stem cells have traditionally been difficult to study directly. The latter feature provides a convenient intellectual framework within which to interrelate self-renewal, commitment to differentiation, and proliferation. This interrelation has been used to functionally define more and less primitive subsets of the stem cell hierarchy; the more primitive a stem cell, the higher its self-renewal potential and its ability to produce very large populations of mature cells encompassing all distinct lineages.[2, 129, 132, 133, 153] In short, all primitive stem cells are highly self-renewing and multipotent. Additionally, the more primitive the stem cell, the greater its tendency to be quiescent or slowly cycling during steady-state adult hematopoiesis.[154–159] It follows from this that the most primitive stem cells are also the rarest. A tendency to be relatively quiescent is not a necessary characteristic of all hematopoietic stem cells, because the stem cell compartment from fetal liver tends to be in an active cell cycle.[159] It has been shown that these cells are at least as primitive as adult bone marrow stem cells.[160–162] It is important to stress at this point that the hierarchical organization of the stem cell compartment can be extended to the entire hematopoietic system, including the penultimate progenitors of all individual mature blood cell lineages.

How the stem cell and the entire hematopoietic hierarchy is correctly established and globally regulated is a question of major basic and clinical importance. Before considering these issues, it is critical to address the experimental bases on which the existence, the functional properties, and the organizational features of the stem cell hierarchy have been established. Implicit in this is the exact definition of the experimental criteria that provide measures of self-renewal ability, multipotentiality, and proliferative potential and the fact that the relevant experimental criteria must also be quantitative.

▼ STEM CELL ASSAY SYSTEMS

General Principles

In the following sections, the various techniques for measuring the in vivo properties of stem cells are discussed. All these assay systems share certain features but differ in others. In general, their similarities have permitted a rigorous con-

sensus on stem cell functional properties to be established. In contrast, their differences, in particular the distinct, assay-specific demands imposed on stem cells, may reveal differences in the functional abilities of distinct stem cell subsets, but also raise other important questions. Collectively, the availability of different stem cell assay systems permits the analysis of the same population of cells in very different contexts. This has led to a broader range of insights and therefore represents a strength in diversity. All these issues are discussed in considerable detail below.

It is not possible to exhaustively cover more than four decades of hematopoietic stem cell research. Rather, an effort is made to describe how the hallmark properties of stem cells have been defined and are manifest from each assay system. In addition, each distinct stem cell assay system is described in the context of its unique contribution to the field of stem cell biology. In the following sections, the focus is exclusively on in vivo stem cell analysis in the mouse.

What are the exact experimental assays that have been used to define stem cells? The modus operandi of all murine stem cell assays is the transplantation of normal hematopoietic tissue into irradiated or genetically stem cell–ablated recipient hosts. More recently, it has been shown that minimally or completely non-ablated hosts can be used, although it is not yet clear how this system differs from the others in revealing stem cell properties.[163, 164] In essence, all stem cell assay systems rely on the ability to transfer a fully functional hematopoietic system from a donor to a recipient host animal. This necessitates the ability to distinguish donor-derived hematopoietic cells from their residual host counterparts. Thus, a hallmark feature of all stem cell assay systems is the presence of suitable markers. The nature of these markers, as will become evident later, is the defining factor that determines the ultimate resolution of each individual assay system.

In general, a source of donor hematopoietic stem cells is introduced into the recipient, and their resultant, fully mature donor-derived progeny are measured. Therefore, most hematopoietic stem cell assays deal only with the two extreme poles of the hematopoietic hierarchy. As discussed in a subsequent section, this has important implications. Very little information can be directly obtained concerning the myriad complex processes or steps required to establish the hematopoietic hierarchy in vivo from the most primitive transplanted stem cells. Nevertheless, clever and elegant exploitation of the known properties of the fully mature hematopoietic cell populations (in particular, their half-lives in the periphery and their population numbers), together with the analysis of donor cells over time, has led to a number of fundamental insights into the developmental properties of the most primitive stem cell compartment. In addition, a few of the assays permit conclusions regarding the early events that occur during the establishment of the hematopoietic hierarchy.[155, 165]

There are basically three categories of in vivo stem cell assays: radioprotection, engraftment into genetically compromised recipients, and competitive repopulation.[150, 166–168] Each of these can be subdivided according to the type of marker systems employed: donor versus host markers or clonotypic markers.[168, 169] The latter has the crucial property that the progeny of single stem cells can be identified, and it may be geographically distinct and isolatable, as in CFU-S assays (see below).

All the stem cell assays also have differences. The roles and importance of these differences are highlighted where appropriate—in particular, situations in which the unique features of a particular assay system have led to important biological insights.

How do the functional properties of these cells translate into measurable experimental information? Before delving into these questions, four points deserve mention. First, stem cells and the assays in which they are measured are codependent, in the sense that in many cases the nature of the assay system—in particular, its demands and constraints—may influence the observed biological properties. This means that the measurable functional characteristics of stem cells are a function of the intrinsic properties of these cells *and* the exact experimental context in which they are analyzed. In the extreme case, a given cell population may be defined as stem cells in one assay system but not show any such functional capacity in another. Examples of this are discussed later.

Second, all stem cell assay systems are retroactive and indirect; that is, the existence and functional properties of a stem cell are defined exclusively as a function of the more mature cells produced by the stem cell in a given assay system. Simply stated, a stem cell is defined as any cell capable of producing a population of mature cells that is large enough to be shown as clonally related. Therefore, the definition of a stem cell is intimately dependent on the resolution and sensitivity of the particular assay system used to determine clonal relatedness among members of a cell population. An obvious consequence of this is the impossibility of measuring the direct cellular or physical properties of an individual candidate stem cell and simultaneously verifying its hallmark stem cell functional abilities.

Third, as described below, all stem cell assay systems are highly manipulated and far removed from the normal setting. Therefore, there is no guarantee that stem cell function is similar in an unperturbed hematopoietic system. It is possible, for example, that the property of multipotentiality is manifested only upon transplantation and that in a normal context individual stem cells contribute only to selected subsets of mature hematopoietic cell lineages.

Finally, as discussed in more detail below, stem cells can be accurately defined only by their in vivo function. Therefore, the existence and virtually all functional properties of stem cells have been best defined in the mouse system. Remarkably, in spite of their differences and unique characteristics, the hallmarks of multipotentiality, self-renewal, and proliferative properties of stem cells have been consistently revealed by all the assay systems. Therefore, it is safe to say that these are true stem cell characteristics that are intrinsic to these cells and/or to the interplay of stem cells with their microenvironments. Although it is highly likely that murine and human hematopoietic stem cells share fundamental properties, there may be important species-specific differences. It is important to keep this in mind when extrapolating experimental results from the mouse system to the clinically relevant human system.

The following discussion is focused on describing various murine stem cell assay systems, how stem cell functional properties are revealed in these systems, and how the individual systems differ with respect to revealing these properties. Emphasis is also placed on how the different assay systems can be used to reveal distinct functional compartments of the stem cell hierarchy and thus define its existence and overall organization. The discussion is centered on assays that measure the properties of stem cells after they have been specified during embryonic development—that is, those that are relevant for their lifelong hematopoietic activity.

Transplantation Assays

The most primitive stem cells have traditionally been studied by transplantation into radiologically or genetically ablated hosts. In these systems, the engrafting donor stem cells are required to rescue the host animal from radiation-induced bone marrow aplasia or to compete effectively with their genetically compromised resident counterparts. Remarkably, using early and crude versions of this basic assay system, it was possible to define all the basic properties of stem cells, including self-renewal potential, multipotential differentiation ability, proliferative capacity, tissue sources, and approximate numbers. Additionally, important insights into the stochastic and/or deterministic nature of stem cell–fate choice regulation, as well as evidence for the existence of other, less primitive intermediate compartments of the hierarchy, were obtained. In all these experiments, the donor source of stem cells was whole, unfractionated bone marrow or, in some cases, fetal liver tissue. The donor and host must vary in some diagnostic, genetically determined karyotypic or other marker, such as an isozyme or hemoglobin variant. After transplantation, the presence of the donor marker in a large proportion of mature blood cells defines the existence of stem cells in the cell population used in the transplant. The presence of the marker in different myeloid and lymphoid cell lineages defines multipotentiality, at least at the level of the entire transplanted stem cell population. The definition of a stem cell in the context of this assay is any cell that is capable of giving rise to substantial, easily detectable numbers of mature progeny. Similarly, the persistence of the marker in mature cells with short half-lives over long post-transplant time intervals strongly suggests a self-renewal process occurring in some compartment of the transplanted donor cell population. Self-renewal is therefore experimentally and operationally defined as the ability to give rise to mature cells at a later point in time.

Measuring Multipotentiality and Self-Renewal at the Clonal Level

Extensions of this basic strategy that used random chromosomal aberrations introduced into the donor cell population by limited doses of radiation allowed the functional in vivo analysis of single stem cells.[169] The mature donor-derived cells that contain a given chromosomal aberration must have their origin in a single, initially marked stem cell. These studies demonstrated two important stem cell properties. First, because the same marker could be detected in both myeloid and lymphoid cell populations, the initially marked stem cells are multipotent. Second, the overall proportion of mature cells with a given marker is a direct and quantitative measure of the ability of a single stem cell to give rise to large populations of functional, terminally differentiated blood cells. It was also possible to directly demonstrate self-renewal at the level of the multipotent stem cell by retransplantation of the bone marrow of a primary transplanted animal into a cohort of secondary mice. The detection of the same marker in mature cells of the primary animal and in several secondary recipients strongly argues that the initially engrafted stem cell formed a clone of undifferentiated stem cells in the bone marrow of the primary recipient.

At this point, it is worth considering what exactly is required of the transplanted stem cell in order for its properties to be defined in this type of experimental context. The purpose of this exercise is to highlight the dramatic potential of the assay system to influence the experimental observations and, therefore, our definitions of stem cell properties. Donor hematopoietic cells are introduced into the recipients via the circulation; therefore, the stem cells must find their way to the appropriate bone marrow microenvironments or niches. Although little is known about the cellular nature of these niches, there is reason to think that they may be quite specific. This implies that only a donor stem cell that has avoided non-specific entrapment in organs such as the liver and homed to bone marrow can interact with specific and possibly limited microenvironments. Thus, only those stem cells that have successfully completed this process can possibly be measured in the assay. The homing and localization process is thought to occur rapidly, with a time frame of several hours. The overall efficiency of bone marrow homing is difficult to measure with accuracy, although a number of studies have suggested an estimate of 5 to 10 per cent.[170, 171] It is easy to see how this ambiguity complicates any efforts to precisely enumerate stem cells. This complication becomes particularly significant in the stem cell purification studies, which are discussed in a later section.

Although the random chromosome marker studies discussed above established many of the hallmark properties of stem cells, they suffer from several drawbacks that impose considerable limitations. The efficiency of the marking procedure is low and consequently does not permit the simultaneous analysis of numerous, uniquely marked stem cells in individual recipient mice. Several issues, including how individual members of a population of stem cells are organized over time in their hematopoietic function, cannot be easily addressed. In addition, the low marking efficiency does not permit the detection of other, possibly more mature and transiently functional stem cell populations. Because of these concerns and possible damage incurred during the marking procedures, the use of genetically anemic (W) host recipient animals was introduced.[169] However, in these mice, the endogenous stem cell compartment is only partially compromised; therefore, it is not possible to quantitatively measure the absolute extent to which a single stem cell can reconstitute an entire, fully functional hematopoietic system.

Defining the Properties of Stem Cells Using Retroviral Markers

The introduction of retroviral marker technology expanded on the concept of random clonal marking by providing a much higher level of resolution.[172–174] Though powerful, the

application of this technology to the analysis of in vivo stem cell behavior served primarily to confirm previous observations and to extend them in a temporal and more quantitative direction. As such, these studies provided an accurate dynamic picture of a transplanted reconstituted hematopoietic system and an accurate quantitative estimate of what a stem cell can do.[129, 173]

The strategy and features of retroviral marking in stem cell biology have been reviewed in detail elsewhere.[129] Only several particularly relevant issues are highlighted here. There are three major advantages to retroviral marking that are relevant to stem cell analyses. The first advantage of this approach is its relatively benign nature; the retroviruses can be engineered to be transcriptionally silent and to contain no gene products capable of harmful effects, such as those resulting from viral spread. Therefore, marking occurs only once—in vitro prior to transplantation. The marker provirus is incapable of being mobilized even in the presence of the endogenous retroviruses often found in the murine germline. The transcriptional silence of the provirus does not permit the potential activation of adjacent chromosomal genes. Moreover, although the in vitro culture period necessary to introduce the retrovirus has some disadvantages, in general, it does not severely debilitate the in vivo capabilities of stem cells. The second advantage is the largely random nature or at least the very large number of potential retroviral integration sites in the genomic DNA. This ensures that each transduced or marked cell is uniquely "tagged" with a diagnostic provirus. This tag is usually revealed by Southern blots designed to show the size of the provirus plus its flanking chromosomal sequences and performed on DNA isolated from the clonal progeny of single cells. Additionally, the marker provirus is rarely, if ever, deleted from the chromosomal DNA. Formally, therefore, retroviral marking of stem cells is equivalent to inducing random chromosomal aberrations by radiation, although it is much more benign. The third advantage is the efficiency of the marking procedure. Although retroviral transduction of primitive stem or progenitor cells has been problematic in the human system, in the mouse, it is feasible to mark virtually all stem cells. A fourth advantage is the ability to detect the provirus in all progeny of a marked cell, not only those in mitosis from which metaphase spreads can be karyotypically analyzed. This also implies that the analytical method is quantitative; that is, the intensity of a diagnostic individual proviral integrant on a Southern blot provides an accurate measure for the absolute proportion of a given cell population that shares a clonal relationship.

As a somewhat formal exercise, it is instructive to consider how the existence and various hallmark properties of stem cells are defined within the context of the retroviral marking assay. Generally, the marked stem cells are transplanted into a lethally irradiated recipient, usually not in limiting-dilution quantities. After a suitable time interval, an aliquot of peripheral blood is obtained and fractionated into representative myeloid and lymphoid lineages, and the samples are processed and analyzed by Southern blots for the presence and the molarity of individual proviral integrants. The existence of a stem cell in the donor cell population is defined by the presence of a detectable proviral integrant. Such a proviral-containing DNA fragment visible in the mature peripheral blood cells must, by definition, have initially been present in a single cell before engraftment. Therefore, the mature cells that contain this provirus represent the clonal progeny of this cell. A stem cell is thus defined retroactively as any cell capable of giving rise in vivo to a clone of progeny large enough to yield an amount of DNA permissive for the detection of a haploid content of a specific proviral insertion. Inherent in this is a lower limit to the proliferative or clonogenic potential that must be met by the given cell to qualify it for stem cell status. Because of the limited sensitivity of the Southern blot, this means that the cell must give rise to at least 5 to 10 per cent of the total nucleated cells present in the peripheral blood at the time of analysis. This fairly large proportion constitutes a rather stringent criterion for a cell's clonogenic capacity in order for it to be defined as a stem cell. Recently, it has been possible to substantially improve the sensitivity of specific integration site detection by using inverse polymerase chain reaction (PCR).[175] It is not clear, however, whether this dramatically increased sensitivity is useful, because the ability to contribute to a large proportion of mature cells seems a priori to be a necessary defining criterion for a stem cell. It should be pointed out that this also sets an upper limit of 10 to 20 for the number of stem cells whose activities can, in principle, be monitored in a single host by standard Southern blot techniques.

The property of multipotentiality is defined by detection of the same integration position in myeloid as well as lymphoid cell populations. By similar logic, an integrant in only some lineages but not others may be diagnostic of a lineage-restricted stem cell. As discussed in more detail later, such an interpretation is not straightforward. Because the exact proportion of each lineage harboring a discrete integrant can be easily determined, it is possible to estimate the equal or unequal contribution of a single multipotent stem cell to distinct lineage compartments. This, in turn, may reflect on the choice of particular commitment decisions. As in the case of a restricted lineage distribution of a proviral integrant based on its detection in a subset of lineages, such interpretations are complicated.

A major contribution of retroviral marking studies was an unprecedented level of resolution and quantitation in defining the property of stem cell self-renewal at the level of single stem cell clones. As mentioned previously, self-renewal can be operationally defined as the ability of a stem cell to contribute to mature cell populations over time. This is particularly true for mature cells with short half-lives, such as those in the myeloid lineages. It is possible to measure the persistence of discrete proviral integrants in neutrophils, monocyte macrophages, and T and B lymphocytes all obtained from a a single small aliquot of peripheral blood. Therefore, a cohort of animals can be analyzed at 6- to 8-week intervals for overall periods of at least a year. The persistence of the same proviral integrant in myeloid cells throughout this entire period constitutes strong evidence for a self-renewal process. Frequently, the same spectrum of proviral integrants was detected at the same levels in all lineages throughout the entire time course. Each of these integrants is therefore proof of the continuous function of a single multipotent stem cell clone for near lifelong intervals. The remarkable qualitative as well as quantitative stability and lack of fluctuation of the proviral integrant patterns are also strong indications that the marked stem cell clone has

given rise to a hematopoietic hierarchy where self-renewal and commitment are exquisitely balanced.

Measuring the Number of Stem Cells

A critical question in hematopoietic biology concerns the exact numbers of stem cells in a given hematopoietic tissue as well as in the intact organism. A simple arithmetical calculation involving stem cell numbers, the daily birthrate of mature cells of all blood cell lineages, and the average life span of an organism provides such an estimate. This value represents a lower limit, because its calculation does not take into account turnover rates in the numerous intermediate compartments of the hematopoietic hierarchy, and it assumes that all stem cells function simultaneously and equally throughout life. Nevertheless, all compartments of the hierarchy have their origin in a single type of cell, and single stem cells are necessary and sufficient for a normally and permanently functional hematopoietic system, as shown in the retroviral marking experiments. Therefore, such calculations reflect on the proliferative potential that is ultimately inherent in the stem cell. Knowing the number of cells in the most primitive stem cell population provides a quantitative baseline with which to begin estimating the degree of cell proliferation that occurs with the establishment of successively more mature compartments of the hematopoietic hierarchy from single stem cells. Another reason why estimates of stem cell numbers are important is more practical. As discussed in a subsequent section, knowing this value has a great impact on various strategies aimed at physically purifying the most primitive stem cell compartment, as well as separating and subdividing other members of the hierarchy.

How are stem cell numbers measured experimentally? Because stem cells can be assayed only by in vivo transplantation, this is a difficult question, for the reasons discussed above. A number of studies nevertheless provided reasonable estimates. All these are grounded in limiting-dilution or more sophisticated statistical calculations. It should be kept in mind that these estimates are lower limits, given the complexities of in vivo transplantation.

Radioprotection ability—that is, how many total donor versus host-distinguishable bone marrow cells are required to save the lives of irradiated mice and to persistently contribute to peripheral blood populations—is one way to measure stem cell frequency. For obvious reasons, this is a demanding assay and therefore is not easily amenable to statistical calculations. A more permissive, genetically anemic W/W^v host system circumvents these limitations. These mice, although anemic and compromised at the stem cell level, are nonetheless viable. Engrafted wild-type stem cells eventually outcompete their mutant, host-derived counterparts. The traditional readout in this assay is the permanent cure of the anemia, which is taken as evidence for engraftment with the most primitive stem cell. Limiting-dilution transplantation into W/W^v animals provided an estimate of stem cell frequency of about one in 10,000 to one in 100,000 total bone marrow cells.[150] More recently, it has been possible to essentially confirm and extend these estimates using the similarly anemic and viable W^{41}/W^{41} recipient host, together with congenic protein difference markers as direct evidence of long-term engraftment.[176] Largely based on these types of studies, there is now general agreement on the above range of frequency estimates. Therefore, if there are on average 100 million total marrow cells in a mouse, then there are approximately 1000 to 10,000 total stem cells. An interesting question is, why so many? As clearly demonstrated by retroviral marking and limiting-dilution studies, a single cell is both necessary and sufficient.

Measuring the Properties of Stem Cells by Competitive Repopulation

Similar values were obtained in a different transplantation assay called competitive repopulation. This assay is generally based on a lethally irradiated mouse; however, unlike the radioprotection system, it does not require life-sparing function from the cell population whose stem cell content is to be measured. In this case, this population, designated as the tester, is evaluated for net stem cell activity relative to a competitor population that is present in greater than radio-protecting quantities. Both these donor populations are generally non-compromised and are transplanted as a mixture into the same hosts. Obviously, a key ingredient here is the ability to distinguish the mature tester-derived hematopoietic donor cell progeny from the competitor in the same host. This is accomplished by congenic markers distributed among the tester, competitor, and host mouse strains. Two such systems are hemoglobin and glucose phosphate isomerase electrophoretic variants and Ly5.1/Ly5.2 cell surface marker variants, which can be revealed by specific antibodies.[168, 177] The latter system has the advantage that Ly5 is expressed on all nucleated peripheral blood cell populations and can therefore be measured by flow cytometry, usually in multicolor combinations with lineage-specific markers to reveal not only total contribution by the tester cells but also their multilineage repopulating activity.[178] In general, the competitor cell population carries the same congenic marker as the recipient host; however, this is not a serious complication. It should be noted that there are variations on the competitive repopulation assay that use compromised competitor cells. In general, these are one-time transplanted bone marrow cell populations that provide short-term post-transplant support but lack substantial long-term stem cell abilities. Because of this feature, this variation may be more sensitive in revealing tester stem cell activity, although this has not been demonstrated conclusively. The most important advantage of all competitive repopulation assay systems is their ability to effectively uncouple radioprotection from long-term functional activity as defining criteria for stem cells in a completely hematopoietically ablated host. As discussed in a subsequent section, this has proved to be instrumental in the definition and separation of short- and long-term functional and other primitive compartments of the hematopoietic hierarchy.

How are the content of stem cells and their biological properties actually measured by competitive repopulation? Conceptually, the assay is simple. When a mixture of Ly5.1 (tester) and Ly5.2 (competitor) cells is transplanted into an irradiated Ly5.2 host and equal numbers of Ly5.1 and Ly5.2 cells are observed in the periphery after a suitable time, the stem cell content in the tester population is equivalent to that in the competitor (plus any, usually minimal, radioresistant host-derived contribution). In short, the stem cell content in the tester is measured relative to a fixed standard. In general, this value is quantitatively represented as competitive repopulating units (CRUs) per 100,000 total tester cells.[167, 168] An important advantage of this system is the ability to measure stem cell content in different sources of stem cells, such as fetal liver and bone marrow, relative to the same standard. This permits an evaluation of the relative in vivo functional abilities of different stem cell populations. An example is the use of this assay system to demonstrate the long-term in vivo superiority of fetal versus adult stem cells.[160–162] The statistical treatment of data from competitive repopulation experiments is rigorous and well developed and has been extensively reviewed.[167, 168]

There are a number of issues that must be kept in mind when thinking about the competitive repopulation system. First and most important, the assay system rests on the assumption that all transplanted stem cells present in the tester and competitor function simultaneously, continuously, and to an approximately equal extent in repopulating the mature cell populations in peripheral blood. Moreover, it is assumed that on a per cell basis, these cells contribute equally to the different myeloid and lymphoid subpopulations. Although dose-response and statistical correlation arguments have been made to support these assumptions,[167, 168] it is also true that, as described above in the discussion of retroviral marking experiments, a major theme is clonal dominance.[179] In almost all these studies, the long-term reconstituted hematopoietic system is oligoclonal, often originating almost entirely from a few—sometimes single—marked stem cell clones. It is also evident from the retroviral studies that single stem cell clones in a transplant recipient can contribute equally to all lineages, but to varying overall proportions of these populations. This suggests that in a transplanted stem cell population, not all individual members are functional to the same extent. Currently, the reasons for such discrepancies are not clear, but it is likely that they reflect in part the potentially subtle differences between the donor versus host and clonotypic marking and stem cell transplantation strategies.

Other considerations in competitive repopulation revolve around the quantitative degree to which a stem cell contributes, as evidenced by the presence of tester-derived cells in the periphery. Does the persistent presence of minimal—say, 1 per cent—tester Ly5–type marked mature cells represent the function of a stem cell? What is the appropriate quantitative cutoff to define a stem cell? Are minimally contributing stem cells equivalent on a per cell basis to those that are robust in their repopulating activities? Would a minimally contributing stem cell exhibit different repopulating abilities in a different host or assay system? Such questions have not been adequately resolved and impose a degree of qualitative subjectivity and arbitrariness onto this otherwise quantitatively rigorous stem cell assay system. As will become evident, these questions become even more problematic when competitive repopulation is used to assess the degree of stem cell enrichment in a variety of purification schemes. In a nutshell, the sensitivity and permissive nature of this assay system are both its main advantages and its drawbacks.

CFU-S Assay

Interestingly, the first attempts to quantify stem cells were made considerably earlier than the efforts described above.

It was noticed that irradiated mice transplanted with limiting doses of bone marrow contained splenic nodules at short postengraftment times. An elegant series of chromosomal marker and dose-response linearity experiments proved that these nodules were in fact clonal and were therefore the progeny of a class of stem cells designated as colony-forming unit–spleen, or CFU-S.[180-184] The nodules contained large numbers of mature cells composed of erythroid and often myeloid cell types. The CFU-S assay was the first to establish the long tradition of quantitative clonal analysis, which is a hallmark of hematopoietic research. Although, for reasons discussed later, the use of this assay has fallen out of fashion, the historical importance of the CFU-S assay is difficult to overstate. In short, because the nodules are geographically discrete, it provided a way to physically analyze the clonal progeny of a single cell with at least some of the properties characteristic of the most primitive stem cell. As will become evident, it is highly likely that the CFU-S is not equivalent to the most primitive stem cell. But remarkably, most of the canonical general properties of stem cells were first defined and quantitated in the context of this assay. Among the significant insights obtained using the CFU-S assay, several deserve specific mention. First, it was shown that in addition to the various terminally maturing cell types, the CFU-S–derived colonies contain progenitor cells that are measurable in vitro and have a much more limited clonogenic potential. These progenitors were therefore the progeny of the CFU-S and thus represent and define later stages of the developing hierarchy and directly establish a precursor-product relationship. Second, the CFU-S assay provided the first direct demonstration of a self-renewal process. Retransplantation of a single spleen colony into secondary animals yielded additional CFU-S–derived colonies—a formal definition of self-renewal within the constraints of this assay. Plotting the frequency of such secondary CFU-S present in a large series of primary spleen colonies led to a numerical distribution that could be approximated by a probabilistic function.[185] This constituted the first indication that self-renewal versus commitment cell-fate choices are governed at least in part by stochastic mechanisms. It was also possible to calculate the average probability of self-renewal as a function of the cell proliferation occurring during the formation of the spleen colony. Third, clever experiments using recipient mice in which segments of bone were implanted into the spleens showed that the microenvironment can play an instructive role in the differentiation outcome of a CFU-S.[144] Fourth, retransplantation experiments also provided a first seeding-factor estimate for the efficiency of a transplantation process.[186] Although it was later shown that the CFU-S is not likely equivalent to the long-term engrafting stem cell, most of the general stem cell concepts were and still can be measured using this assay system.

What is the evidence that CFU-S represents a more mature stem cell compartment of the hematopoietic hierarchy? This issue has been addressed in several ways. First, there are no conclusive data that the lineage repertoire of a CFU-S includes lymphoid cells. Although this may be a consequence of the assay system's inability to reveal such potential, it seems more likely that the CFU-S is already intrinsically restricted to the myeloid and erythroid pathways. Second and more compelling, although the CFU-S has the capacity to self-renew into other CFU-S entities, it has not been possible to demonstrate the complete and long-term reconstitution of a hematopoietic system with individual spleen colonies retransplanted into secondary irradiated hosts. As always, it is important to evaluate these results in the context of the exact assay system—in this case, radioprotection. It is possible that a more permissive and less demanding transplantation assay would reveal some degree of long-term and multilineage functional ability.

Implicit in this discussion is the notion that the most primitive stem cells, CFU-S, and other members of the hematopoietic hierarchy exist as discrete compartments. From a functional point of view, these compartments are revealed by the different assay systems. From a cellular point of view, these discrete compartments have remained largely undefined. This issue is discussed further in a subsequent section. One indication that CFU-S represents a discrete population of cells is obtained from its numbers; that is, on a per cell basis, spleen colony-forming ability is about 10-fold higher in bone marrow than is long-term repopulating capacity.[187] This is in line with one of the hallmark features of the overall hematopoietic hierarchy—that is, that progressively more mature cell compartments are more numerous. In addition, the existence of large populations of even more mature progenitor cells in the collective progeny of a CFU-S is consistent with this property of the hierarchy.

The indistinct boundary and the somewhat elusive nature of the differences between the most primitive stem cells and CFU-S are illustrated in studies that analyzed the appearance of spleen colonies over time.[188] These studies adopted a kinetic approach and were able to show that the post-transplant time window in which CFU-S–derived spleen colonies appear can be directly linked to the primitiveness of the colony–founding clonogenic cell. Spleen colonies that are observed at early points in time are generally composed of a single mature cell lineage and are smaller than those that appear at later times and contain multiple myeloid and erythroid cell types. In addition, the early colonies are transient, which may be indicative of limited self-renewal ability. Moreover, one of these studies provided further evidence that the CFU-S population is at least largely distinct from the most primitive stem cells.[155] Specifically, it was shown that the cycle-active drug 5-fluorouracil introduced in vivo spares the late-appearing spleen colonies to a much larger extent than the early-appearing ones. This is consistent with the origin of the former class from more quiescent precursors.

In the same study, an elegant set of experiments in which radioactive strontium was incorporated into the bone environment of the recipient mice before whole-body irradiation and transplantation showed that the late-appearing spleen colonies were eliminated. Because the early spleen colonies were largely unaffected, this argued that the stem cell ultimately responsible for late spleen colony formation first had to migrate to and reside in the bone marrow. Subsequently, it—or, more likely, its immediate progeny—finds its way to the spleen and initiates colony formation. One interpretation of these experiments is that they reveal very early events in the establishment of the hematopoietic hierarchy.

▼ ASSAYS FOR HUMAN HEMATOPOIETIC STEM CELLS

The mouse and human hematopoietic systems are very similar in most of their overall properties. Clearly, it is not possible to perform the kinds of transplantation assays that have been described for mouse stem cells in the human system. How are human stem cells defined, and how are their biological properties analyzed? There have been a number of in vitro systems suggested as suitable surrogate assays for human stem cells.[137, 189–198] Although these have been very useful, in the human system, as in the mouse, the only rigorous measure of stem cell activity is by in vivo transplantation. As a consequence, several xenogeneic transplantation systems have been developed.[199–202] Three of these use immunodeficient mouse strains as recipients for human stem cell material. The humanized severe combined immunodeficient (hu-scid) murine model relies on engrafted fragments of human bone and thymus to provide a natural environment for subsequently introduced human hematopoietic stem cells.[137] The other two murine models are the beige-nude xid (bnx) mouse and the non-obese diabetic severe combined immunodeficient (nod/scid) mouse.[199–201] Engraftment and proliferation of adult human hematopoietic cells in the bnx and the nod/scid systems are commonly facilitated by the addition of recombinant human cytokines. The use of these murine models in limiting-dilution engraftment studies, together with the appropriate antigenic markers to reveal the presence of human hematopoietic cells, has defined a scid repopulating cell (SRC) activity in a number of human tissue sources, including bone marrow, umbilical cord blood, mobilized peripheral blood, and fetal liver. In addition to enumerating the frequency of this activity, many studies have demonstrated long-term engraftment and the generation of numerous hematopoietic lineages of human origin. In one very elegant study, it was possible to demonstrate a common clonal origin of human myeloid and T-lymphoid cell types in the engrafted mice.[175] The murine immunodeficient models have also been widely used to assess the cell surface phenotype of the SRC activity.[3]

Although the murine xenogeneic transplant systems have been very useful, it is still somewhat premature to conclude that they are measuring the "true" human stem cell. It must be kept in mind that these systems are highly artificial, and as such, they compound the assay-dependent complications discussed earlier. In addition, the small size of the mouse recipient does not permit a measure of the proliferative potential of the engrafting human cells. As mentioned earlier, the ability of single murine stem cells to reconstitute an entire hematopoietic system has been a useful assessment of the developmental potential of these cells. In spite of these limitations, the murine systems are of value primarily because they can be readily used in many individual laboratories.

A second xenogeneic system involves in utero transplantation of human stem cells into sheep fetuses.[202, 203] The recipient fetus is immunologically permissive, and in some cases, high levels of chimerism have been detected both postnatally and in adult life. It has also been possible to subsequently retransplant human hematopoietic cells into secondary recipient fetuses.[116, 204] Because it is a large animal model, it would seem that, in principle, the sheep would be a better assay system than the mouse for human stem cell activity. However, it must be pointed out that a rigorous side-by-side comparison of these xenogeneic model systems has not been performed. In addition, the sheep system cannot be readily implemented in most hematopoietic stem cell laboratories.

Although it is not the purpose of this chapter to provide a thorough discussion of in vitro surrogate assays for human stem cell activity, several points deserve mention. First, necessity has been the mother of invention; therefore, these assays have been developed to a very high level of sophistication. In addition, they have been widely used and have provided much valuable information. Second, with the advent of the xenogeneic assays described above, it has been possible to compare the activities that read out in vivo and in vitro. In general, and in agreement with the data from the mouse system, the activities that can be measured in vitro are more abundant than those that engraft in vivo in any given tissue or cell source. These observations have permitted the overall description of a hematopoietic hierarchy in the human system. Finally, in more recent studies, very long-term in vitro systems have been described that appear to measure a cell population that at least overlaps with the in vivo engrafting cell population.[191] In addition, culture systems have been developed that permit the generation of both myeloid and lymphoid lineages from single human candidate stem cells.[195]

▼ PHYSICAL PURIFICATION OF STEM CELL ACTIVITY

Converting a Biological Activity Into a Cellular Entity

In all the above studies, the existence and the properties of stem cells were measured indirectly—that is, solely by analysis of their more mature progeny in the transplant recipient. Even in situations employing clonal markers, the properties of individual stem cells could only be inferred retroactively. This limitation prevented direct experiments to address the biology of the stem cell population in terms of cellular and physical properties as well as regulatory mechanisms. A major leap forward was achieved by the development of strategies designed to physically purify the stem cell biological activity.[115, 154, 156, 160, 161, 173, 178, 205–215] The establishment of all these techniques began with the demonstration that the transplantable activity could be segregated to a cell fraction that possessed some physically distinguishable property, such as a distinct cell density or a differential expression of immunochemically identifiable cell surface markers. A general feature of all stem cell purification techniques is the judicious combination of a variety of physical properties, each of which individually serves as a positive or negative marker for in vivo biological activity. To date, no unique marker for the stem cell population has been described; however, enrichments of 1000- to 2000-fold are routinely feasible in numerous laboratories.

Individual studies that use stem cell enrichment are too numerous to review in this chapter. Rather, a summary of the significant advances facilitated by the enrichments and a discussion of several general issues are presented. Clearly, the most significant benefit of stem cell purification is that a biological activity has been ascribed a precise cellular phenotype; in other words, the stem cell became an actual cell amenable to the experimental tools of cellular and molecular biology. In practice, this has permitted several specific and fruitful avenues of investigation. First, it has been possible to perform engraftments with very few physically purified cells, either alone or in competition with unfractionated competitor material.[115, 178, 214] In fact, the 1000- to 2000-fold purification value commonly encountered in the literature is most easily obtained in a competitive repopulation context.

It is relevant at this point to ask whether the degree of enrichment by any individual protocol approaches homogeneity. Quite clearly, most purified stem cell populations are heterogeneous in terms of stem cell content and also contain somewhat more mature, though still primitive, members of the hematopoietic hierarchy, such as CFU-S.[154, 216–218] Several studies have segregated the most primitive stem cell activity from less primitive progenitor activities.[115, 187, 211, 212] In one case, it was possible to establish a precursor-product relationship between these various physically separable activities.[2, 132] In spite of such progress, the issue of stem cell homogeneity is difficult to address experimentally, given that the in vivo assay system is the only true measure of stem cell activity.

Several studies have attempted to engraft mice with very few, sometimes single, purified stem cells.[115, 178, 214] As discussed in a previous section, retroviral marking approaches have demonstrated that single stem cells are both necessary and sufficient to yield a normal hematopoietic system in a transplanted mouse. Consistent with this, in one study using single purified stem cells, it was possible to demonstrate high-level engraftment in about 20 per cent of the animals.[115] Although clearly this particular purified stem cell population is highly enriched in biological activity, it is not possible to say whether the absolute purity is one in five or whether factors such as seeding efficiency and other phenomena are responsible for the observed engraftment frequency.

Similar considerations can be extended to the exact choice of transplantation assay. A good example of this can be found in a comparison of bone marrow stem cell frequencies revealed by transplantation into irradiated or into genetically anemic recipient mice.[176] In the latter case, the apparent frequencies were considerably higher.

In summary, stem cell purification strategies are effective; however, it is important to keep in mind the role of the exact assay systems when evaluating experimental results, particularly when comparing data from different individual efforts. An additional complication in evaluating the homogeneity of purified stem cell populations arises from conceptual models that describe the organization of the hematopoietic stem cell population in a stochastic manner.[129, 139, 146] In these models, primitive stem cells exist in probability states that may be distributed along a continuum. Thus, individual members of a "homogeneous" stem cell population may not read out in the same way when measured at the single cell level. In fact, evidence for the stochastic in vivo behavior of both CFU-S and the most primitive stem cell compartment has been obtained.[129, 146] In practice, if stem cell properties are regulated in a stochastic manner, it may not be possible to "cleanly" segregate discrete biological activities into de-monstrably homogeneous physically purified compartments. Recently it has been shown that certain cell surface molecules can be expressed in a fluctuating manner on stem cells, suggesting that there may not be a uniform physical phenotype for the entire stem cell population.[4, 219]

In Vitro Studies With Purified Hematopoietic Stem Cells

An area of research that has greatly benefited from stem cell purification strategies is the intensive effort to define the regulatory mechanisms that act at the level of the primitive stem cell. In general, these studies have focused on defining ex vivo culture systems in which transplantable stem cell activity can be maintained or expanded during prolonged periods. The driving forces behind these efforts are both purely scientific and clinically oriented. In the former case, the development of such systems is a necessary prerequisite to defining the exact cellular and molecular regulatory mechanisms; in the latter case, the ability to maintain or expand stem cell activity ex vivo would have profound implications for therapeutic transplantation. Over the past decade, numerous studies have explored the activities of a large variety of cytokines, either alone or in combination, in supporting in vitro cultures initiated with purified stem cells. The vast majority of these studies have yielded disappointing results. A general theme that emerges from these efforts is that stem cell exposure to cytokine combinations almost invariably results in the loss of their ability to function in vivo.[220–224] It has been suggested that this is a manifestation of in vitro differentiation. Such an interpretation is supported by the concomitant expansion of more committed cells still capable of generating large numbers of mature hematopoietic progeny. In some cases, it has been clearly demonstrated that the addition of certain cytokines to cultures of multipotent stem cells results in lineage-specific differentiation defects.[224] Other studies that use cell-cycle synchronization have suggested that stem cells stimulated into the active cell cycle lose their engraftment abilities as a function of their exact position in the cell cycle.[225] Possible reasons for this impairment are alterations in homing properties.[226] In these cases, the engraftment defect is reversible and fluctuates as a function of position in the cell cycle.[164, 227] These examples highlight the role played by the exact parameters and requirements of a given assay system in defining the stem cell nature of a cell population.

Is it reasonable to expect that any well-defined ex vivo culture system will be capable of stem cell maintenance and/or expansion? Several recent reports suggest a reason for optimism. In these studies, combinations of c-kit ligand, Flt3/Flk2 ligand, interleukin-11, and interleukin-6 are sufficient to maintain approximately input levels of transplantable activity in short-term cultures initiated with highly purified stem cell populations.[228] Because the input cells were highly enriched, it is likely that these cytokines are acting directly on the stem cell. As shown by naturally occurring and engineered genetic lesions, the ckit/ckit ligand and the Flt3/Flk2/Flt3/Flk2 ligand signaling pathways are likely to play a role in stem cell regulation in normal in vivo hematopoietic systems.[229, 230] More recently, it has been shown that thrombopoietin alone is sufficient for a similar degree of ex vivo stem cell maintenance.[231] Significantly, because engineered mice containing mutations in either thrombopoietin or its receptor cMpl have defects in primitive stem cell or progenitor cell compartments,[232] it is likely that this signaling pathway also plays a role in normal in vivo stem cell regulation. In all these studies, it appears that the maintenance of stem cell activity is not accompanied by extensive cell proliferation.

The above studies are encouraging, but they do not provide evidence for extensive self-renewal in a defined ex vivo context. One report demonstrated that highly purified stem cells can initiate colony formation in vitro without a dramatic loss of engrafting ability.[176] Although these data fall short of demonstrating self-renewal, they do suggest that at least limited stem cell division in a defined culture system is not necessarily incompatible with the maintenance of in vivo functional ability. Clearly, during normal development and during a post-transplantation time interval, extensive expansion of the stem pool must occur in vivo.[233] It is therefore reasonable to assume that a better definition of the in vivo signals that govern such expansion should provide novel, more effective, and more physiologically relevant ex vivo culture systems for stem cell expansion. Efforts to define such in vivo signals began with the development of the Dexter culture system supported by a stromal cell layer that can be viewed as representative of the normal hematopoietic microenvironment.[189, 234] In this culture system, hematopoiesis, as measured by the production of mature myeloid cells, is maintained for many months. This suggests that self-renewal and commitment to differentiation can both occur ex vivo. A direct and strong indication for the self-renewal of transplantable stem cells in a Dexter culture system was provided by studies that used retroviral markers.[235, 236] In these experiments, several mice transplanted with retrovirally marked cells from a single culture contained the same proviral integrant in their mature peripheral blood cells. The only interpretation for these observations is that an initially marked stem cell must have undergone at least one self-renewal division during the culture period. In spite of these encouraging results, it has not been possible to demonstrate a net increase in transplantable stem cell activity during the course of the culture period. Other, more quantitative competitive repopulation studies have shown that the overall stem cell activity decreases over time in the Dexter culture system.[237, 238] A likely interpretation of the collective data is that self-renewal and commitment to differentiation are balanced in this culture system.

The cellular composition of the supporting stromal monolayer in the traditional Dexter culture system is exceedingly heterogeneous, and most studies using this culture system do not begin with highly purified input stem cell populations. Because of these complications, it has not been possible to precisely identify the cellular and molecular mechanisms responsible for the supportive properties of the culture system. Numerous studies have sought to dissect the supportive stromal monolayer into clonal cell lines. The underlying hypothesis for this approach is that distinct cell types within the complex monolayer promote or facilitate different aspects of stem cell behavior. Many stromal cell lines have been described, and they are indeed widely heterogeneous in terms of their abilities to support in vitro hematopoiesis and to maintain in vivo transplantable stem cells.[239–242] Stromal cell lines that effectively maintain trans-

plantable stem cells are infrequent, whereas those that support the production of mature hematopoietic cells at the expense of stem cell activity are much more abundant. Interestingly, in one study there was no dramatic difference observed in the mRNA expression levels for a panel of 15 cytokines between cell lines with widely different supportive abilities.[240] In some cases, the stromal cell lines have been used in conjunction with highly purified stem cell populations.[241, 242] Somewhat of a "holy grail" for this type of culture system would be to define a clonal cell line that, when seeded with highly purified stem cells, would support the self-renewal expansion of transplantable activity without commitment or differentiation. Has such a system been described, and if not, is it reasonable to expect that one will?

One fetal liver–derived stromal cell line is particularly effective in the qualitative and quantitative maintenance of the input transplantable stem cell activity present in a highly purified cell population obtained from either fetal liver or adult bone marrow.[242] Moreover, this activity can be maintained for prolonged periods of at least 6 weeks. The cultured cells are identical to freshly isolated cells in their in vivo multilineage engraftment abilities, as measured by competitive repopulation. By all established criteria, including secondary engraftment capability, the stem cell properties of the long-term cultured cells are undiminished. As described above, there are no obvious differences in the mRNA levels for a variety of cytokines present in this cell line, in comparison with the levels detected in a non-supporting cell line obtained from the same source. Interestingly, the maintenance of input in vivo stem cell activity in these cultures is accompanied by the dramatic expansion of primitive committed progenitors for myeloid as well as lymphoid lineages. Taken together, the results from these studies support a model in which the entire primitive portion of the hematopoietic hierachy can be established from the most primitive stem cell in a culture system supported by a single stromal cell type. It is interesting that the numerical content of more and less primitive cells typical of the in vivo hematopoietic hierarchy is also recapitulated in vitro, at least to a first approximation. A number of studies have shown that this murine cell line is also very effective in supporting long-term in vitro human hematopoiesis initiated by purified human stem cells from several different sources.[192, 195, 243]

The above model predicts that the input stem cell population is actively dividing and that this cell division is accompanied by a balance of self-renewal and commitment to differentiation. If these notions are correct, then the idea that there will be a defined system in which net stem cell expansion can be easily achieved needs to be reconsidered.

▼ THE FLEXIBILITY OF STEM CELLS

The hematopoietic system is not unique in its ability to generate large numbers of mature cells continuously throughout life. The intestinal epithelium, the skin epithelium, and the male germline all share this property.[132, 136] Other tissue systems such as the liver, the muscles, the vasculature, and the nervous system have the ability to regenerate mature cells in response to injury or stress. Although they are less well developed than the hematopoietic system, studies focused on some of these tissues have defined candidate stem cell populations. Noteworthy examples include muscle satellite cells, central nervous system stem cells, peripheral nervous system stem cells, and mesenchymal stem cells.[244-256]

A common dogma for all these tissue systems is that the relevant stem cell populations, though endowed with self-renewal, proliferative, and differentiation abilities, would nonetheless be "dedicated" to the tissue in question. Thus, a hematopoietic stem cell would be limited to the production of blood cells, whereas other stem cells would be limited to the production of muscle, skin epithelium, intestinal epithelium, and so on. This dogma is based on embryological considerations, on the availability of appropriate assay systems, and on intellectual preconceptions. Recently, several reports suggested that the lineage differentiation abilities of stem cell populations may be considerably broader. In one study, it was shown that highly purified murine bone marrow stem cell populations could contribute to muscle tissue as well as to hematopoietic cell populations in the appropriate host recipient system—the irradiated mdx mouse, a model for the human disorder Duschenne muscular dystrophy.[257] Similarly, these studies showed that a cell population isolated from muscle contained hematopoietic repopulating activity. Remarkably, a recent report demonstrated that short-term cultured muscle tissue contains approximately 10 times more hematopoietic activity than fresh bone marrow.[258] This was shown by the stringent competitive repopulation assay discussed in a previous section. An even more remarkable study suggested that clonally derived cultured central nervous system stem cells are capable of hematopoietic function in transplanted irradiated mouse recipients.[259]

Do these surprising observations warrant a rethinking of the current stem cell dogma? At this point, the answer is no—or at least, not yet.[260] In order to understand the rationale for this conclusion, it is necessary to highlight again the role that clonal analysis has played in defining the hematopoietic stem cell. Simply stated, the experiments showing that a single cell population can yield hematopoietic as well as muscle tissue were not performed at the level of single cells. One possibility is that the bone marrow contains some amount of stem cells dedicated to muscle and that, conversely, the muscle contains hematopoietic stem cells. Although it is difficult to explain why this should be the case, this possibility needs to be rigorously excluded before a significant revision of existing stem cell concepts is called for.

REFERENCES

1. Morrison, S.J., Uchida, N., and Weissman, I.L.: The biology of hematopoietic stem cells. Annu. Rev. Cell. Dev. Biol. 11:35, 1995.
2. Morrison, S.J., and Weissman, I.L.: The long-term repopulating subset of hematopoietic stem cells is deterministic and isolatable by phenotype. Immunity 1:661, 1994.
3. Ziegler, B., Valtieri, M., Porada, G., De Maria, R., Mueller, R., Masella, B., Gabbianelli, M., Casella, I., Pelosi, E., Bock, T., Zanjani, E., and Peschle, C.: KDR receptor: a key marker defining hematopoietic stem cells. Science 285:1553, 1999.
4. Sato, T., Laver, J.H., and Ogawa, M.: Reversible expression of CD34 by murine hematopoietic stem cells. Blood 94:2548, 1999.
5. Terstappen, L., Huang, S., Safford, M., Lansdorp, P., and Loken, M.: Sequential generations of hematopoietic colonies derived from single nonlineage-committed CD34 + CD38 − progenitor cells. Blood 77:1218, 1991.
6. Hu, M., Krause, D., Greaves, M., Sharkis, S., Dexter, M., Heyworth, C., and Enver, T.: Multilineage gene expression precedes commitment in the hemopoietic system. Genes Dev. 11:774, 1997.
7. Gregory, C., and Eaves, A.: Human marrow cells capable of erythropoietic differentiation in vitro: definition of three erythroid colony responses. Blood 49:855, 1977.
8. Shivdasani, R.A., and Orkin, S.H.: The transcriptional control of hematopoiesis. Blood 87:4025, 1996.
9. Engel, I., and Murre, C.: Transcription factors in hematopoiesis. Curr. Opin. Genet. Dev. 9:575, 1999.
10. Bagby, G.C., Jr., and Heinrich, M.C.: Growth factors, cytokines, and the control of hematopoiesis. In Hoffman, R., Benz, E., Shattil, S., Furie, B., Cohen, H., Silberstein, L., and McGlave, P. (Eds.): Hematology—Basic Principles and Practice. 3rd ed. Philadelphia, Churchill Livingstone, 2000, p. 154.
11. De Maria, R., Zeuner, A., Eramo, A., Domenichelli, C., Bonci, D., Grignani, F., Srinivasula, S., Alnemri, E., Testa, U., and Peschle, C.: Negative regulation of erythropoiesis by caspase-mediated cleavage of GATA-1. Nature 401:489, 1999.
12. Long, M.W.: Blood cell cytoadhesion molecules. Exp. Hematol. 20:288, 1992.
13. Yoder, M.C., and Williams, D.A.: Matrix molecule interactions with hematopoietic stem cells. Exp. Hematol. 23:961, 1995.
14. Klein, G.: The extracellular matrix of the hematopoietic microenvironment. Experientia 51:914, 1995.
15. Papayannopoulou, T., and Craddock, C.: Homing and trafficking of hematopoietic progenitor cells. Acta Haematol. 97:97, 1997.
16. Verfaillie, C.: Anatomy and physiology of hematopoiesis. In Hoffman, R., Benz, E., Shattil, S., Furie, B., Cohen, H., Silberstein, L., and McGlave, P. (Eds.): Hematology—Basic Principles and Practice. 3rd ed. Philadelphia, Churchill Livingstone, 2000, p. 139–154.
17. Sabin, F.R.: Studies on the origin of blood vessels and of red corpuscles as seen in the living blastoderm of the chick during the second day of incubation. Contrib. Embryol. 9:213, 1920.
18. Maximov, A.A.: Relation of blood cells to connective tissues and endothelium. Physiol. Rev. 4:533, 1924.
19. Murray, P.D.F.: The development in vitro of the blood of the early chick embryo. Proc. R. Soc. Lond. 11:497, 1932.
20. Péault, B., Coltey, M., and Le Douarin, N.: Ontogenic emergence of a quail leukocyte/endothelium cell surface antigen. Cell Differ. 23:165, 1988.
21. Péault, B., Thiery, J.P., and Le Douarin, N.M.: A surface marker for the hemopoietic and endothelial cell lineages in the quail species defined by a monoclonal antibody. Proc. Natl. Acad. Sci. USA 80:2976, 1983.
22. Flamme, I., and Risau, W.: Induction of vasculogenesis and hematopoiesis in vitro. Development 116:435, 1992.
23. Paranaud, L., and Dieterlen-Lièvre, F.: Emergence of endothelial and hemopoietic cells in the avian embryo. Anat. Embryol. 187:107, 1993.
24. Eichmann, A., Corbel, C., Nataf, V., Vaigot, P., Breant, C., and Le Douarin, N.M.: Ligand-dependent development of the endothelial and hemopoietic lineages from embryonic mesodermal cells expressing VEGF-receptor 2. Proc. Natl. Acad. Sci. USA 94:5141, 1997.
25. Pardanaud, L., Yassine, F., and Dieterlen-Lièvre, F.: Relationship between vasculogenesis, angiogenesis and haemopoiesis during avian ontogeny. Development 105:473, 1989.
26. Pardanaud, L., Luton, D., Prigent, M., Bourcheix, L.M., Catala, M., and Dieterlen-Lièvre, F.: Two distinct endothelial lineages in ontogeny, one of them related to hemopoiesis. Development 122:1363, 1996.
27. Stern, C.D., Fraser, S.E., Keynes, R.J., and Primmett, D.R.N.: A cell analysis of segmentation in the chick embryo. Development 104:231, 1988.
28. Dieterlen-Lièvre, F., Godin, I., and Pardanaud, L.: Where do hemopoietic stem cells come from? Int. Arch. Allergy Immunol. 112:3, 1997.
29. Lee, R.K., Stainier, D.Y., Weinstein, B.M., and Fishman, M.C.: Cardiovascular development in the zebrafish. II. Endocardial progenitors are sequestered within the heart field. Development 120:3361, 1994.
30. Stainier, D.Y., Lee, R.K., and Fishman, M.C.: Cardiovascular development in the zebrafish. I. Myocardial fate map and heart tube formation. Development 119:31, 1993.
31. Shalaby, F., Rossant, J., Yamaguchi, T.P., Gertsenstein, M., Wu, X.F., Breitman, M.L., and Schuh, A.C.: Failure of blood island formation and vasculogenesis in Flk-1 deficient mice. Nature 376:62, 1995.
32. Carmeliet, P., Ferreira, V., Breier, G., Pollefeyt, S., Kieckens, L., Gertsenstein, M., Fahrig, M., Vandenhoeck, A., Hapal, K., Eberhardt,

C., Declercq, C., Pawling, J., Moons, L., Collen, D., Risau, W., and Nagy, A.: Abnormal blood vessel development and lethality in embryos lacking a single VEGF allele. Nature 380:435, 1996.

33. Liao, W., Bisgrove, B.W., Sawyer, H., Hug, B., Bell, B., Peters, K., Grunwald, D.J., and Stainier, D.Y.: The zebrafish gene cloche acts upstream of a Flk-1 homologue to regulate endothelial cell differentiation. Development 124:381, 1997.

34. Shalaby, F., Ho, J., Stanford, W.L., Fischer, K.D., Schuh, A.C., Schwartz, L., Bernstein, A., and Rossant, J.: A requirement for Flk1 in primitive and definitive hematopoiesis and vasculogenesis. Cell 89:981,1997.

35. Hidaka, M., Stanford, W., and Bernstein, A.: Conditional requirement for the Flk-1 receptor in the in vitro generation of early hematopoietic cells. Proc. Natl. Acad. Sci. USA 96:7370, 1999.

36. Dumont, D.J., Gradwohl, G., Fong, G.-H., Puri, M.C., Gerstenstein, M., Auerbach, A., and Breitman, M.L.: Dominant-negative and targeted null mutations in the endothelial receptor tyrosine kinase, tek, reveal a critical role in vasculogenesis of the embryo. Genes Dev. 8:1897, 1994.

37. Suri, C., Jones, P.F., Patan, S., Bartunkova, S., Maisonpierre, P.C., Davis, S., Sato, T.N., and Yancopoulos, G.D.: Requisite role of angiopoietin-1, a ligand for the TIE2 receptor, during embryonic angiogenesis. Cell 87:1171, 1996.

38. Carmeliet, P., Mackman, N., Moons, L., Luther, T., Gressens, P., Van Vlaenderen, I., Demunck, H., Kasper, M., Breier, G., Evrard, P., Muller, M., Risau, W., Edgington, T., and Collen, D.: Role of tissue factor in embryonic blood vessel development. Nature 383:73, 1996.

39. Fong, G.H., Rossant, J., Gerstenstein, M., and Breitman, M.L.: Role of the Flt-1 receptor tyrosine kinase in regulating assembly of vascular endothelium. Nature 376:66, 1995.

40. Kuo, C.T., Veselits, M.L., Barton, K.P., Lu, M.M., Clendenin, C., and Leiden, J.M.: The LKLF transcription factor is required for normal tunica media formation and blood vessel stabilization during murine embryogenesis. Genes Dev. 11:2996, 1997.

41. Visvader, J.E., Fujiwara, Y., and Orkin, S.H.: Unsuspected role for the T-cell leukemia protein SCL/tal-1 in vascular development. Genes Dev. 12:473, 1998.

42. Kozak, K.R., Abbott, B., and Hankinson, O.: ARNT-deficient mice and placental differentiation. Dev. Biol. 191:297, 1997.

43. Offermanns, S., Mancino, V., Revel, J.-P., and Simon, M.I.: Vascular system defects and impaired cell chemokinesis as a result of $G\alpha_{13}$ deficiency. Science 275:533, 1997.

44. Sato, T.N., Tozawa, Y., Deutsch, U., Wolburg-Buchholz, K., Fujiwara, Y., Gendron-Maguire, M., Gridley, T., Wolburg, H., Risau, W., and Qin, Y.: Distinct roles of the receptor tyrosine kinases Tie-1 and Tie-2 in blood vessel formation. Nature 376:70, 1995.

45. Porcher, C., Swat, W., Rockwell, K., Fujiwara, Y., Alt, F.W., and Orkin, S.H.: The T cell leukemia oncoprotein SCL/tal-1 is essential for development of all hematopoietic lineages. Cell 86:47, 1996.

46. Sato, A., Iwama, A., Takakura, N., Nishio, H., Yancopoulos, G.D., and Suda, T.: Characterization of TEK receptor tyrosine kinase and its ligands, angiopoietins, in human hematopoietic progenitor cells. Int. Immunol. 10:1217, 1998.

47. Papayannopoulou, T., and Yancopoulos, G.D.: Unpublished data, 1997.

48. Kennedy, M., Firpo, M., Choi, K., Wall, C., Robertson, S., Kabrun, N., and Keller, G.: A common precursor for primitive erythropoiesis. Nature 386:488, 1997.

49. Choi, K., Kennedy, M., Kazarov, A., Papadimitriou, J.C., and Keller, G.: A common precursor for hematopoietic and endothlial cells. Development 125:725, 1998.

50. Nishikawa, S.-I., Nishikawa, S., Hirashima, M., Matsuyoshi, N., and Kodama, H.: Progressive lineage analysis by cell sorting and culture identifies FLK1⁺VE-cadherin + cells at a diverging point of endothelial and hemopoietic lineages. Development 125:1747, 1998.

51. Dieterlen-Lièvre, F.: Intraembryonic hematopoietic stem cells. Hematol. Oncol. Clin. North Am. 11:1149, 1997.

52. Zon, L.I.: Developmental biology of hematopoiesis. Blood 86:2876, 1995.

53. Winnier, G., Blessing, M., Labosky, P.A., and Hogan, B.L.: Bone morphogenetic protein-4 is required for mesoderm formation and patterning in the mouse. Genes Dev. 9:2105, 1995.

54. Dickson, M.C., Martin, J.S., Cousins, F.M., Kulkarni, A.B., Karlsson, S., and Akhurst, R.J.: Defective haematopoiesis and vasculogenesis in transforming growth factor-β1 knock out mice. Development 121:1845, 1995.

55. Matzuk, M.M., Kumar, T.R., Shou, W., Coerver, K.A., Lau, A.L., Behringer, R.R., and Finegold, M.J.: Transgenic models to study the roles of inhibins and activins in reproduction, oncogenesis, and development. Recent Prog. Horm. Res. 51:123, 1996.

56. Miura, Y., and Wilt, F.H.: Tissue interaction and the formation of the first erythroblasts of the chick embryo. Dev. Biol. 19:201, 1969.

57. Belaoussoff, M., Farrington, S.M., and Baron, M.H.: Hematopoietic induction and respecification of A-P identity by visceral endoderm signaling in the mouse embryo. Development 125:5009, 1998.

58. Fennie, C., Cheng, J., Dowbenko, D., Young, P., and Lasky, L.A.: CD34 + endothelial cell lines derived from murine yolk sac induce the proliferation and differentiation of yolk sac CD34 + hematopoietic progenitors. Blood 86:4454, 1995.

59. Xu, M.J., Tsuji, K., Ueda, T., Mukouyama, Y.S., Hara, T., Yang, F.C., Ebihara, Y., Matsuoka, S., Manabe, A., Kikuchi, A., Ito, M., Miyajima, A., and Nakahata, T.: Stimulation of mouse and human primitive hematopoiesis by murine embryonic aorta-gonad-mesonephros–derived stromal cell lines. Blood 92:2032, 1998.

60. Ohneda, O., Fennie, C., Zheng, Z., Donahue, C., La, H., Villacorta, R., Cairns, B., and Lasky, L.A.: Hematopoietic stem cell maintenance and differentiation are supported by embryonic aorta-gonad-mesonephros region–derived endothelium. Blood 92:908, 1998.

61. Sato, Y., Hong, H.N., Yanai, N., and Obinata, M.: Involvement of stromal membrane–associated protein (SMAP-1) in erythropoietic microenvironment. J. Biochem. (Tokyo) 124:209, 1998.

62. Migliaccio, A.R., and Papayannopoulou, T.: Erythropoiesis. In Bunn, H.F., and Forget, B.G. (Eds.): Hemoglobin: Molecular, Genetic and Clinical Aspects. Philadelphia, W.B. Saunders (in press).

63. Rafii, S., Shapiro, F., Pettengell, R., Ferris, B., Nachman, R.L., Moore, M.A., and Asch, A.S.: Human bone marrow microvascular endothelial cells support long-term proliferation and differentiation of myeloid and megakaryocytic progenitors. Blood 86:3353, 1995.

64. Schweitzer, K.M., Drager, A.M., van der Valk, P., Thijsen, S.F.T., Zevenbergen, A., Theijsmeijer, A.R., van der Schoot, C.E., and Langenbuijen, M.M.A.C.: Constitutive expression of E-selectin and vascular cell adhesion molecule-1 on endothelial cells of hematopoietic tissues. Am. J. Pathol. 148:165, 1996.

65. Peled, A., Grabovsky, V., Habler, L., Sandbank, J., Arenzana-Seisdedos, F., Petit, I., Ben-Hur, H., Lapidot, T., and Alon, R.: The chemokine SDF-1 stimulates integrin-mediated arrest of CD-34⁺ cells on vascular endothelium under shear flow. J. Clin. Invest. 104:1199, 1999.

66. Karsan, A., and Harlan, J.M.: The blood vessel wall. In Hoffman, R., Benze, E.J., Jr., Shattil, S.J., Furie, B., Cohen, H.J., Silberstein, L.E., and McGlave, P. (Eds.): Hematology—Basic Principles and Practice. 3rd ed. New York, Churchill Livingstone, 2000, pp. 1770–1782.

67. Van der Stricht, O.: Nouvelles recherches sur la genese des globules rouges et des globules blancs due sang. Arch. Biol. (Liege) 12:199, 1892.

68. Dantschakoff, W.: Über das erste Auftreten der Blutelemente im Hühnerembryo. Folia Haematol. 4(Suppl.):159, 1907.

69. Dantschakoff, W.: Untersuchungen über die Entwickelung des Blutes und Bindegewebes bei den Vogeln. Anat. Hefte 1(Abt. 37):471, 1908.

70. Maximov, A.: Untersuchungen über Blut und Bindegewebe. 1. Die frühesten Entwickelungstadien der Blut- und Bindegewebszellen beim Saugetierembryo bis zum Angang der Blutbildung in der Leber. Arch. Mikr. Anat. 73:444, 1909.

71. Maximov, A.: Untersuchungen über die Blut und Bindegewebe. III. Die embryonale Histogenese des Knockenmarks der Saugetiere. Arch. Mikr. Anat. 76:1, 1910.

72. Müller, A.M., Medvinsky, A., Strouboulis, J., Grosveld, F., and Dzierzak, E.: Development of hematopoietic stem cell activity in the mouse embryo. Immunity 1:291, 1994.

72a. Palis, J., Robertson, S., Kennedy, M., Wall, C., Keller, G.: Development of erythroid and myeloid progenitors in the yolk sac and embryo proper of the mouse. Development 126:5073, 1999.

73. Godin, I., Dieterlen-Lièvre, F., and Cuman, A.: Emergence of multipotent hemopoietic cells in the yolk sac and paraaortic splanchnopleura in mouse embryos, beginning at 8.5 days postcoitus. Proc. Natl. Acad. Sci. USA 92:773, 1995.

74. Papayannopoulou, T: Unpublished observations, 1997.

75. Keller, G., Kennedy, M., Papayannopoulou, T., and Wiles, M.V.: Hematopoietic commitment during embryonic stem cell differentiation in culture. Mol. Cell. Biol. 13:473, 1993.

76. Nakano, T., Kodama, H., and Honjo, T.: In vitro development of primitive and definitive erythrocytes from different precursors. Science 272:722, 1996.

77. Turpen, J.B., Kelly, C.M., Mead, P.E., and Zon, L.I.: Bipotential primitive-definitive hematopoietic progenitors in the vertebrate embryo. Immunity 7:325, 1997.

78. Orkin, S.H.: Embryonic stem cells and transgenic mice in the study of hematopoiesis. Int. J. Dev. Biol. 42:927, 1998.

79. Okuda, T., van Deursen, J., Hiebert, S.W., Grosveld, G., and Downing, J.R.: AML1, the target of multiple chromosomal translocations in human leukemia, is essential for normal fetal liver hematopoiesis. Cell 84:321, 1996.

80. Wang, Q., Stancy, T., Binder, M., Marín-Padilla, M., Sharpe, A.H., and Speck, N.A.: Disruption of the CbFa2 gene causes necrosis and hemorrhaging in the central nervous system and blocks definitive hematopoiesis. Proc. Natl. Acad. Sci. USA 93:3444, 1996.

81. Sasaki, K., Yagi, H., Bronson, R.T., Tominaga, K., Matsunashi, T., Deguchi, K., Tani, Y., Kishimoto, T., and Komori, T.: Absence of fetal liver hematopoiesis in mice deficient in transcriptional coactivator core binding factor β. Proc. Natl. Acad. Sci. USA 93:12359, 1996.

82. Wang, Q., Stacy, T., Miller, J.D., Lewis, A.F., Gu, T.L., Huang, X., Bushweller, J.H., Bories, J.C., Alt, F.W., Ryan, G., Liu, P.P., Wynshaw-Boris, A., Binder, M., Marín-Padilla, M., Sharpe, A.H., and Speck, N.A.: The CBFβ subunit is essential for CBFα2 (AML1) function in vivo. Cell 87:697, 1996.

83. Allen, R.D., III, Bender, T.P., and Siu, G.: c-Myb is essential for early T cell development. Genes Dev. 13:1073, 1999.

84. Lee, E.Y., Chang, C.Y., Hu, N., Wang, Y.C., Lai, C.C., Herrup, K., Lee, W.H., and Bradley, A.: Mice deficient for Rb are nonviable and show defects in neurogenesis and haematopoiesis. Nature 359:288, 1992.

85. McKercher, S.R., Torbett, B.E., Anderson, K.L., Henkel, G.W., Vestal, D.J., Baribault, H., Klemsz, M., Feeney, A.J., Wu, G.E., Paige, C.J., and Maki, R.A.: Targeted disruption of the PU.1 gene results in multiple hematopoietic abnormalities. EMBO J. 15:5647, 1996.

86. Scott, E.W., Simon, M.C., Anastasi, J., and Singh, H.: Requirements of transcription factor PU.1 in the development of multiple hematopoietic lineages. Science 265:1573, 1994.

87. Parganas, E., Wang, D., Stravopodis, D., Topham, D.J., Marine, J.-C., Tegulund, S., Vanin, E.F., Bodner, S., Colamonici, O.R., van Deursen, J.M., Grosveld, G., and Ihle, J.N.: Jak2 is essential for signaling through a variety of cytokine receptors. Cell 93:385, 1998.

88. Marine, J.C., McKay, C., Wang, D., Topham, D.J., Parganas, E., Nakajima, H., Pendeville, H., Yasukawa, H., Sasaki, A., Yoshimura, A., and Ihle, J.N.: SOCS3 is essential in the regulation of fetal liver erythropoiesis. Cell 98:617, 1999.

89. Galli, S.J., Zsebo, K.M., and Geissler, E.N.: The kit ligand, stem cell factor. Adv. Immunol. 55:1, 1994.

90. Motoyama, N., Wang, F., Roth, K.A., Sawa, H., Nakayama, K., Nakayama, K., Negishi, I., Senju, S., Zhang, Q., Fujii, S., and Loh, D.Y.: Massive cell death of immature hematopoietic cells and neurons in Bcl-x-deficient mice. Science 267:1506, 1995.

91. Varfolomeev, E.E., Schuchmann, M., Luria, V., Chiannilkulchai, N., Beckmann, J.S., Mett, I.L., Rebrikov, D., Brodianski, V.M., Kemper, O.C., Kollet, O., Lapidot, T., Soffer, D., Sobe, T., Avraham, K.B., Goncharov, T., Holtmann, H., Lonai, P., and Wallach, D.: Targeted disruption of the mouse caspase 8 gene ablates cell death induction by the TNF receptors, Fas/Apol, and DR3 and is lethal prenatally. Immunity 9:267, 1998.

92. Tsai, F.Y., and Orkin, S.H.: Transcription factor GATA-2 is required for proliferation/survival of early hematopoietic cells and mast cell formation, but not for erythroid and myeloid terminal differentiation. Blood 89:3636, 1997.

93. Yoshida, K., Taga, T., Saito, M., Suematsu, S., Kumanogoh, A., Tanaka, T., Fujiwara, H., Hirata, M., Yamagami, T., Nakahata, T., Hirabayashi, T., Yoneda, Y., Tanaka, K., Wang, W.Z., Mori, C., Shiota, K., Yoshida, N., and Kishimoto, T.: Targeted disruption of gp130, a common signal transducer for the interleukin 6 family of cytokines, leads to myocardial and hematological disorders. Proc. Natl. Acad. Sci. USA 93:407, 1996.

94. Kitajima, K., Kojima, M., Nakajima, K., Kondo, S., Hara, T., Miyajima, A., and Takeuchi, T.: Definitive but not primitive hematopoiesis is impaired in jumonji mutant mice. Blood 93:87, 1999.

95. Chan, J.Y., Kwong, M., Lu, R., Chang, J., Wang, B., Yen, T.S., and Kan, Y.W.: Targeted disruption of the ubiquitous CNC-bZIP transcription factor, Nrf-1, results in anemia and embryonic lethality in mice. EMBO J. 17:1779, 1998.

96. Kieran, M.W., Perkins, A.C., Orkin, S.H., and Zon, L.I.: Thrombopoietin rescues in vitro erythroid colony formation from mouse embryos lacking the erythropoietin receptor. Proc. Natl. Acad. Sci. USA 93:9126, 1996.

97. Lee, R., Kertesz, N., Joseph, S.B., Jegalian, A., and Wu, H.: Early activation of erythropoietin receptor initiates the premature switch from primitive to definitive erythropoiesis in vivo. Blood 94:652a, 1999.

98. Yoder, M.C., Hiatt, K., Dutt, P., Mukherjee, P., Bodine, D.M., and Orlic, D.: Characterization of definitive lymphohematopoietic stem cells in the day 9 murine yolk sac. Immunity 7:335, 1997.

99. Yoder, M.C., and Hiatt, K.: Engraftment of embryonic hematopoietic cells in conditioned newborn recipients. Blood 89:2176, 1997.

100. Migliaccio, G., Migliaccio, A.R., Petti, S., Mavilio, F., Russo, G., Lazzaro, D., Testa, U., Marinucci, M., and Peschle, C.: Human embryonic hemopoiesis. Kinetics of progenitors and precursors underlying the yolk sac–liver transition. J. Clin. Invest. 78:51, 1986.

101. Charbord, P., Tavian, M., Humeau, L., and Peault, B.: Early ontogeny of the human marrow from long bones: an immunohistochemical study of hematopoiesis and its microenvironment. Blood 87:4109, 1996.

102. Marcos, M.A.R., Morales-Alcelay, S., Godin, I.E., Dieterlen-Lièvre, F., Copin, S.G., and Gaspar, M.L.: Antigenic phenotype and gene expression pattern of lymphohemopoietic progenitors during early mouse ontogeny. J. Immunol. 158:2627, 1997.

103. Roy, V., and Verfaillie, C.M.: Expression and function of cell adhesion molecules on fetal liver, cord blood and bone marrow hematopoietic progenitors: implications for anatomical localization and developmental stage specific regulation of hematopoiesis. Exp. Hematol. 27:302, 1999.

104. Valtieri, M., Gabbianelli, M., Pelosi, E., Bassano, E., Petti, S., Russo, G., Testa, U., and Peschle, C.: Erythopoietin alone induces erythroid burst formation by human embryonic but not adult BFU-E in unicellular serum-free culture. Blood 74:460, 1989.

105. Migliaccio, G., Baiocchi, M., Hamel, N., Eddleman, K., and Migliaccio, A.R.: Circulating progenitor cells in human ontogenesis response to growth factors and replating potential. J. Hematother. 5:161, 1996.

106. Migliaccio, A.R., and Migliaccio, G.: Human embryonic hemopoiesis control mechanisms underlying progenitor differentiation in vitro. Dev. Biol. 125:127, 1988.

107. Zandstra, P.W., Conneally, E., Piret, J.M., and Eaves, C.J.: Ontogeny-associated changes in the cytokine responses of primitive human haemopoietic cells. Br. J. Haematol. 101:770, 1998.

108. Kurata, H., Mancini, G.C., Alespeti, G., Migliaccio, A.R., and Migliaccio, G.: Stem cell factor induces proliferation and differentiation of fetal progenitor cells in the mouse. Br. J. Haematol. 101:676, 1998.

109. Lansdorp, P.M., Dragowska, W., and Mayani, H.: Ontogeny-related changes in proliferative potential of human hematopoietic cells. J. Exp. Med. 178:787, 1993.

110. Miller, C.L., Rebel, V.I., Helgason, C.D., Lansdorp, P.M., and Eaves, C.J.: Impaired steel factor responsiveness differentially affects the detection and long-term maintenance of fetal liver hematopoietic stem cells in vivo. Blood 89:1214, 1997.

111. Tavian, M., Coulombel, L., Luton, D., Clemente, H.S., Dieterlen-Lièvre, F., and Peault, B.: Aorta-associated CD34+ hematopoietic cells in the early human embryo. Blood 87:67, 1996.

111a. Huyhn, A., Dommergues, M., Izac, B., Croisille, L., Katz, A., Vainchenker, W., and Coulombel, L.: Characterization of hematopoietic progenitors from human yolk sacs and embryos. Blood 86:4474, 1995.

112. Medvinsky, A., and Dzierzak, E.: Definitive hematopoiesis is autonomously initiated by the AGM region. Cell 86:897, 1996.

113. Sanchez, M.J., Holmes, A., Miles, C., and Dzierzak, E.: Characterization of the first definitive hematopoietic stem cells in the AGM and liver of the mouse embryo. Immunity 5:513, 1996.

114. Petrenko, O., Beavis, A., Klaine, M., Kittappa, R., Godin, I., and Lemischka, I.R.: The molecular characterization of the fetal stem cell marker AA4. Immunity 10:691, 1999.

115. Osawa, M., Hanada, K., Hamada, H., and Nakauchi, H.: Long-term lymphohematopoietic reconstitution by a single CD34-low/negative hematopoietic stem cell. Science 273:242, 1996.

116. Zanjani, E.D., Almeida-Porada, G., Livingston, A.G., Flake, A.W., and Ogawa, M.: Human bone marrow CD34− cells engraft in vivo and undergo multilineage expression that includes giving rise to CD34+ cells. Exp. Hematol. 26:353, 1998.

117. Hamamura, K., Matsuda, H., Takeuchi, Y., Habu, S., Yagita, H., and Okumura, K.: A critical role of VLA-4 in erythropoiesis in vivo. Blood 87:2513, 1996.

118. Ogawa, M., Nishikawa, S., Yoshinaga, K., Hayashi, S.-I., Kunisada, T., Nakao, J., Kina, T., Sudo, T., Kodama, H., and Nishikawa, S.-I.: Development and function of c-kit in fetal hemopoietic progenitor cells: transition from the early c-kit-independent to the late c-kit-dependent wave of hemopoiesis in the murine embryo. Development 117:1089, 1993.

119. Ogawa, M., Matsuzaki, Y., Nishikawa, S., Hayashi, S.I., Kunisada, T., Sudo, T., Kina, T., Nakuchi, H., and Nishikawa, S.I.: Expression and function of c-kit in hemopoietic progenitor cells. J. Exp. Med. 174:63, 1991.

120. Brannon, C.I., Lyman, S.D., Williams, D.E., Eisenman, J., Anderson, D.M., Cosman, D., Bedell, M.A., Jenkins, N.A., and Copeland, N.G.: Steel-Dickie mutation encodes a c-kit ligand lacking transmembrane and cytoplasmic domains. Proc. Natl. Acad. Sci. USA 88:4671, 1991.

121. McCulloch, E.A., Siminovitch, L., Till, J.E., Russell, E.S., and Bernstein, S.E.: The cellular basis of the genetically determined hemopoietic defect in anemic mice of genotype $S1^d/S1^d$. Blood 26:399, 1965.

122. Russell, E.S.: Hereditary anemias of the mouse: a review for geneticists. Adv. Genet. 20:357, 1979.

123. Omori, M., Omori, N., Evarts, R.P., Teramoto, T., and Thorgeirsson, S.S.: Coexpression of flt-3 ligand/flt3 and SCF/c-kit signal transduction system in bile-duct-ligated Sl and W mice. Am. J. Pathol. 150:1179, 1997.

124. Rich, I.N.: Primordial germ cells are capable of producing cells of the hematopoietic system in vitro. Blood 86:463, 1995.

125. Oostendorp, R.A.J., and Dörmer, P.: VLA-4-mediated interactions between normal human hematopoietic progenitors and stromal cells. Leuk. Lymphoma 24:423, 1997.

126. Arroyo, A.G., Yang, J.T., Rayburn, H., and Hynes, R.O.: Differential requirements for α4 integrins in hematopoiesis. Cell 85:997, 1996.

126a. Arroyo, A.G., Yang, J.T., Rayburn, H., and Hynes, R.O.: α4 Integrins regulate the proliferation/differentiation balance of multilineage hematopoietic progenitors in vivo. Immunity 11:555, 1999

127. Sheppard, A.M., Onken, M.D., Rosen, G.D., Noakes, P.G., and Dean, D.C.: Expanding roles for α4 integrin and its ligands in development. Cell Adhes. Commun. 2:27, 1994.

128. Dexter, T.M., and Spooncer, E.: Growth and differentiation in the hemopoietic system. Annu. Rev. Cell. Biol. 3:423, 1987.

129. Lemischka, I.R.: The haematopoietic stem cell and its clonal progeny: mechanisms regulating the hierarchy of primitive haematopoietic cells. Cancer Surv. 15:3, 1992.

130. Domen, J., and Weissman, I.: Self-renewal, differentiation or death: regulation and manipulation of hematopoietic stem cell fate. Mol. Med. Today 5:201, 1999.

131. Metcalf, D.: The Molecular Control of Blood Cells. Cambridge, Harvard University Press, 1988.

132. Morrison, S.J., Shah, N.M., and Anderson, D.J.: Regulatory mechanisms in stem cell biology. Cell 88:287, 1997.

133. Morrison, S.J., Wright, D.E., Cheshier, S.H., and Weissman, I.L.: Hematopoietic stem cells: challenges to expectations. Curr. Opin. Immunol. 9:216, 1997.

134. Ogawa, M.: Hematopoiesis. J. Allergy Clin. Immunol. 94:645, 1994.

135. Orkin, S.H.: Development of the hematopoietic system. Curr. Opin. Genet. Dev. 6:597, 1996.

136. Potten, C.S., and Loeffler, M.: Stem cells: attributes, cycles, spirals, pitfalls and uncertainties. Lessons for and from the crypt. Development 110:1001, 1990.

137. Chen, B.P., Galy, A., Kyoizumi, S., Namikawa, R., Scarborough, J., Webb, S., Ford, B., Cen, D.Z., and Chen, S.C.: Engraftment of human hemopoietic precursor cells with secondary transfer potential in SCID-hu mice. Blood 84:2497, 1994.

138. Muller-Sieburg, C.E., and Riblet, R.: Genetic control of the frequency of hematopoietic stem cells in mice: mapping of a candidate locus to chromosome 1. J. Exp. Med. 83:1141, 1996.

139. Ogawa, M.: Differentiation and proliferation of hematopoietic stem cells. Blood 81:2844, 1993.

140. Phillips, R.L., Reinhart, A.J., and Van Zant, G.: Genetic control of murine hematopoietic stem cell pool sizes and cycling kinetics. Proc. Natl. Acad. Sci. USA 89:11607, 1992.

141. Phillips, R.L., Couzens, M.S., and Van Zant, G.: Genetic factors influencing murine hematopoietic productivity in culture. J. Cell. Physiol. 164:99, 1995.

142. de Haan, G., and Van Zant, G.: Intrinsic and extrinsic control of hemopoietic stem cell numbers: mapping of a stem cell gene. J. Exp. Med. 186:529, 1997.

143. de Haan, G., Nijhof, W., and Van Zant, G.: Mouse strain-dependent changes in frequency and proliferation of hematopoietic stem cells during aging: correlation between lifespan and cycling activity. Blood 89:1543, 1997.

144. Trentin, J.J.: Influence of hematopoietic organ stroma (hematopoietic inductive microenvironments) on stem cell differentiation. In Gordon, A. (ed.): Regulation of Hematopoiesis. New York, Appleton-Century-Crofts, 1970, pp 161–186.

145. Lemischka, I.R.: Microenvironmental regulation of hematopoietic stem cells. Stem Cells 15 (Suppl. 1):63, 1997.

146. Abkowitz, J.L., Catlin, S.N., and Guttorp, P.: Evidence that hematopoiesis may be a stochastic process in vivo. Nat. Med. 2:190, 1996.

147. Artavanis-Tsakonas, S., Rand, M.D., and Lake, R.J.: Notch signaling: cell fate control and signal integration in development. Science 284:770, 1999.

148. Milner, L.A., Kopan, R., Martin, D.I., and Bernstein, I.D.: A human homologue of the Drosophila developmental gene, Notch, is expressed in CD34+ hematopoietic precursors. Blood 83:2057, 1994.

149. Milner, L.A., and Bigas, A.: Notch as a mediator of cell fate determination in hematopoiesis: evidence and speculation. Blood 93:2431, 1999.

150. Boggs, D.R., Boggs, S.S., Saxe, D.F., Gress, L.A., and Canfield, D.R.: Hematopoietic stem cells with high proliferative potential. Assay of their concentration in marrow by the frequency and duration of cure of W/Wv mice. J. Clin. Invest. 70:242, 1982.

151. Hodgson, G.S., and Bradley, T.R.: Properties of haematopoietic stem cells surviving 5-fluorouracil treatment: evidence for a pre-CFU-S cell? Nature 281:381, 1979.

152. Rosendaal, M., Hodgson, G.S., and Bradley, T.R.: Organization of haemopoietic stem cells: the generation-age hypothesis. Cell Tissue Kinet. 12:17, 1979.

153. Morrison, S.J., Wandycz, A.M., Hemmati, H.D., Wright, D.E., and Weissman, I.L.: Identification of a lineage of multipotent hematopoietic progenitors. Development 124:1929, 1997.

154. Spangrude, G.J., and Johnson, G.R.: Resting and activated subsets of mouse multipotent hematopoietic stem cells. Proc. Natl. Acad. Sci. USA 87:7433, 1990.

155. Van Zant, G.: Studies of hematopoietic stem cells spared by 5-fluorouracil. J. Exp. Med. 159:679, 1984.

156. Wolf, N.S., Kone, A., Priestley, G.V., and Bartelmez, S.H.: In vivo and in vitro characterization of long-term repopulating primitive hematopoietic cells isolated by sequential Hoechst 33342-rhodamine 123 FACS selection. Exp. Hematol. 21:614, 1993.

157. Bradford, G.B., Williams, B., Rossi, R., and Bertoncello, I.: Quiescence, cycling, and turnover in the primitive hematopoietic stem cell compartment. Exp. Hematol. 24:445, 1997.

158. Cashman, J.D., Lapidot, T., Wang, J.C., Doedens, M., Shultz, L.D., Lansdorp, P., Dick, J.E., and Eaves, C.J.: Kinetic evidence of the regeneration of multilineage hematopoiesis from primitive cells in normal human bone marrow transplanted into immunodeficient mice. Blood 89:4307, 1997.

159. Fleming, W.H., Alpern, E.J., Uchida, N., Ikuta, K., Spangrude, G.J., and Weissman, I.L.: Functional heterogeneity is associated with the cell cycle status of murine hematopoietic stem cells. J. Cell. Biol. 122:897, 1993.

160. Jordan, C.T., Astle, C.M., Zawadzki, J., Mackarehtschian, K., Lemischka, I.R., and Harrison, D.E.: Long-term repopulating abilities of enriched fetal liver stem cells measured by competitive repopulation. Exp. Hematol. 23:1011, 1995.

161. Harrison, D.E., Zhong, R.K., Jordan, C.T., Lemischka, I.R., and Astle, C.M.: Relative to adult marrow, fetal liver repopulates nearly five times more effectively long-term than short-term. Exp. Hematol. 25:293, 1997.

162. Pawliuk, R., Eaves, C., and Humphries, R.K.: Evidence of both ontogeny and transplant dose-regulated expansion of hematopoietic stem cells in vivo. Blood 88:2852, 1996.

163. Stewart, F.M., Zhong, S., Wuu, J., Hsieh, C., Nilsson, S.K., and Quesenberry, P.J.: Lymphohematopoietic engraftment in minimally myeloablated hosts. Blood 91:3681, 1998.

164. Quesenberry, P., Becker, P., Nilsson, S., Stewart, M., Zhong, S., Grimaldi, C., Reilly, J., Hababian, H., Dooner, M., Peters, S., and Ramshaw, H.: Stem cell engraftment and cell cycle phenotype. Leukemia 13(Suppl. 1):S92, 1999.

165. Spangrude, G.J.: The pre-spleen colony-forming unit assay: measurement of spleen colony-forming unit regeneration. Curr. Top. Microbiol. Immunol. 177:31, 1992.

166. Harrison, D.E.: Competitive repopulation: a new assay for long-term stem cell functional capacity. Blood 55:77, 1980.

167. Harrison, D.E.: Evaluating functional abilities of primitive hematopoietic stem cell populations. *In* Muller-Sieburg, C., Torok-Storb, B., Visser, J., and Storb, R. (Eds.): Hematopoietic Stem Cells, Animal Models and Human Transplantation: Current Topics in Microbiology and Immunology. Berlin, Springer-Verlag, 1992, pp. 13–30.

168. Harrison, D.E., Jordan, C.T., Zhong, R.K., and Astle, C.M.: Primitive hemopoietic stem cells: direct assay of most productive populations by competitive repopulation with simple binomial, correlation and covariance calculations. Exp. Hematol. 21:206, 1993.

169. Abramson, S., Miller, R.G., and Phillips, R.A.: The identification in adult bone marrow of pluripotent and restricted stem cells of the myeloid and lymphoid systems. J. Exp. Med. 145:1567, 1977.

170. Lanzkron, S.M., Collector, M.I., and Sharkis, S.J.: Hematopoietic stem-cell tracking in vivo: a comparison of short-term and long-term repopulating cells. Blood 93:1916, 1999.

171. Szilvassy, S.J., Bass, M.J., Van Zant, G., and Grimes, B.: Organ-selective homing defines engraftment kinetics of murine hematopoietic stem cells and is compromised by ex vivo expansion. Blood 93:1557, 1999.

172. Lemischka, I.R., Raulet, D.H., and Mulligan, R.C.: Developmental potential and dynamic behavior of hematopoietic stem cells. Cell 45:917, 1986.

173. Jordan, C.T., McKearn, J.P., and Lemischka, I.R.: Cellular and developmental properties of fetal hematopoietic stem cells. Cell 61:953, 1990.

174. Jordan, C.T., and Lemischka, I.R.: Clonal and systemic analysis of long-term hematopoiesis in the mouse. Genes Dev. 4:220, 1990.

175. Nolta, J.A., Dao, M.A., Wells, S., Smogorzewska, E.M., and Kohn, D.B.: Transduction of pluripotent human hematopoietic stem cells demonstrated by clonal analysis after engraftment in immune-deficient mice. Proc. Natl. Acad. Sci. USA 93:2414, 1996.

176. Trevisan, M., Yan, X.Q., and Iscove, N.N.: Cycle initiation and colony formation in culture by murine marrow cells with long-term reconstituting potential in vivo. Blood 88:4149, 1996.

177. Schied, M.P., and Triglia, D.: Further description of the Ly5 system. Immunogenetics 9:423, 1979.

178. Spangrude, G.J., Brooks, D.M., and Tumas, D.B.: Long-term repopulation of irradiated mice with limiting numbers of purified hematopoietic stem cells: in vivo expansion of stem cell phenotype but not function. Blood 85:1006, 1995.

179. Lemischka, I.R.: What we have learned from retroviral marking of hematopoietic stem cells. Curr. Top. Microbiol. Immunol. 177:59, 1992.

180. Till, J.E., and McCulloch, E.A.: A direct measurement of the radiation sensitivity of normal mouse bone marrow cells. Radiat. Res. 14:213, 1961.

181. Becker, A., McCulloch, E., and Till, J.: Cytological demonstration of the clonal nature of spleen colonies derived from transplanted mouse marrow cells. Nature 197:452, 1963.

182. Wu, A.M., Till, J.E., Siminovitch, L., and McCulloch, E.A.: A cytological study of the capacity for differentiation of normal hemopoietic colony-forming cells. J. Cell. Physiol. 69:177, 1967.

183. Wu, A.M., Siminovitch, L., Till, J.E., and McCulloch, E.A.: Evidence for a relationship between mouse hemopoietic stem cells and cells forming colonies in culture. Proc. Natl. Acad. Sci. USA 59:1209, 1968.

184. Wu, A.M., Till, J.E., Siminovitch, L., and McCulloch, E.A.: Cytological evidence for a relationship between normal hematopoietic colony-forming cells and cells of the lymphoid system. J. Exp. Med. 127:455, 1968.

185. Siminovitch, L., McCulloch, E.A., and Till, J.E.: The distribution of colony-forming cells among spleen colonies, J. Cell. Physiol. 62:327, 1963.

186. Till, J.E., and McCulloch, E.A.: The "f-factor" of the spleen-colony assay for hemopoietic stem cells. Ser. Haematol. 5:15, 1972.

187. Ploemacher, R.E., and Brons, R.H.: Separation of CFU-S from primitive cells responsible for reconstitution of the bone marrow hemopoietic stem cell compartment following irradiation: evidence for a pre-CFU-S cell. Exp. Hematol. 17:263, 1989.

188. Magli, M.C., Iscove, N.N., and Odartchenko, N.: Transient nature of early haematopoietic spleen colonies. Nature 295:527, 1982.

189. Dexter, T.M., Spooncer, E., Simons, P., and Allen, T.D.: Long-term marrow culture: an overview of techniques and experience. *In* Wright, D.G., and Greenberger, J.S. (Eds.): Long Term Bone Marrow Culture. New York, Alan R. Liss, 1984, pp. 57–96.

190. Hao, Q.L., Shah, A.J., Thiemann, F.T., Smogorzewska, E.M., and Crooks, G.M.: A functional comparison of CD34 + CD38 − cells in cord blood and bone marrow. Blood 86:3745, 1995.

191. Hao, Q.L., Thiemann, F.T., Petersen, D., Smogorzewska, E.M., and Crooks, G.M.: Extended long-term culture reveals a highly quiescent and primitive human hematopoietic progenitor population. Blood 88:3306, 1996.

192. Miller, J.S., McCullar, V., Punzel, M., Lemischka, I.R., and Moore, K.A.: Single adult human CD34 + /Lin − /CD38 − progenitors give rise to natural killer cells, B-lineage cells, dendritic cells, and myeloid cells. Blood 93:96, 1999.

193. Nordon, R.E., Ginsberg, S.S., and Eaves, C.J.: High-resolution cell division tracking demonstrates the FLt3-ligand-dependence of human marrow CD34 + CD38 − cell production in vitro. Br. J. Haematol. 98:528, 1997.

194. Petzer, A.L., Hogge, D.E., Landsdorp, P.M., Reid, D.S., and Eaves, C.J.: Self-renewal of primitive human hematopoietic cells (long-term-culture-initiating cells) in vitro and their expansion in defined medium. Proc. Natl. Acad. Sci. USA 93:1470, 1996.

195. Punzel, M., Wissink, S.D., Miller, J.S., Moore, K.A., Lemischka, I.R., and Verfaillie, C.M.: The myeloid-lymphoid initiating cell (ML-IC) assay assesses the fate of multipotent human progenitors in vitro. Blood 93:3750, 1999.

196. Shah, A.J., Smogorzewska, E.M., Hannum, C., and Crooks, G.M.: Flt3 ligand induces proliferation of quiescent human bone marrow CD34 + CD38 − cells and maintains progenitor cells in vitro. Blood 87:3563, 1996.

197. Sutherland, H.J., Eaves, C.J., Eaves, A.C., Dragowska, W., and Lansdorp, P.M.: Characterization and partial purification of human marrow cells capable of initiating long-term hematopoiesis in vitro. Blood 74:1563, 1989.

198. Young, J.C., Varma, A., DiGiusto, D., and Backer, M.P.: Retention of quiescent hematopoietic cells with high proliferative potential during ex vivo stem cell culture. Blood 87:545, 1996.

199. Bhatia, M., Wang, J.C.Y., Kapp, U., Bonnet, D., and Dick, J.E.: Purification of primitive human hematopoietic cells capable of repopulating immune-deficient mice. Proc. Natl. Acad. Sci. USA 94:5320, 1997.

200. Larochelle, A., Vormoor, J., Hanenberg, H., Wang, J.C., Bhatia, M., Lapidot, T., Moritz, T., Murdoch, B., Xiao, X.L., Kato, I., Williams, D.A., and Dick, J.E.: Identification of primitive human hematopoietic cells capable of repopulating NOD/SCID mouse bone marrow: implications for gene therapy. Nat. Med. 2:1329, 1996.

201. Turner, C.W., Yeager, A.M., Waller, E.K., Wingard, J.R., and Fleming, W.H.: Engraftment potential of different sources of human hematopoietic progenitor cells in BNX mice. Blood 87:3237, 1996.

202. Zanjani, E.D., Almeida-Porada, G., and Flake, A.W.: The human/sheep xenograft model: a large animal model of human hematopoiesis. Int J. Hematol. 63:179–192, 1996.

203. Zanjani, E.D., Almeida-Porada, G., Ascensao, J.L., MacKintosh, F.R., and Flake, A.W.: Transplantation of hematopoietic stem cells in utero. Stem Cells 15:79, 1997.

204. Zanjani, E.D., Almeida-Porada, G., Livingston, A.G., Porada, C.D., and Ogawa, M.: Engraftment and multilineage expression of human bone marrow CD34 − cells in vivo. Ann. N.Y. Acad. Sci. 872:220, 1999.

205. Visser, J.W., Bauman, J.G., Mulder, A.H., Eliason, J.F., and deLeeuw, A.M.: Isolation of murine pluripotent hemopoietic stem cells. J. Exp. Med. 59:1576, 1984.

206. Bauman, J.G., de Vries, P., Pronk, B., and Visser, J.W.: Purification of murine hemopoietic stem cells and committed progenitors by fluorescence activated cell sorting using wheat germ agglutinin and monoclonal antibodies. Acta Histochem. Suppl. 36:241, 1988.

207. Spangrude, G.J., Heimfeld, S., and Weissman, I.L.: Purification and characterization of mouse hematopoietic stem cells. Science 241:58, 1988.

208. Uchida, N., and Weissman, I.L.: Searching for stem cells: evidence that Thy-1.1 loLin-Sca + cells are the only stem cells in C57BL/Ka-Thy-1.1 bone marrow. J. Exp. Med. 175:175, 1992.

209. Lemischka, I.R.: Purification and properties of fetal hematopoietic stem cells. Dev. Biol. 4:379, 1993.

210. Morrison, S.J., Hemmati, H.D., Wandycz, A.M., and Weissman, I.L.: The purification and characterization of fetal liver hematopoietic stem cells. Proc. Natl. Acad. Sci. USA 92:10302, 1995.

211. Jones, R.J., Wagner, J.E., Celano, P., Zicha, M.S., and Sharkis, S.J.: Separation of pluripotent haematopoietic stem cells from spleen colony-forming cells. Nature 347:188, 1990.

212. Jones, R.J., Collector, M.I., Barber, J.P., Vala, M.S., Fackler, M.J., May, W.S., Griffin, C.A., Hawkins, A.L., Zehnbauer, B.A., Hilton, J., Colvin, O.M., and Sharkis, S.J.: Characterization of mouse lympho-hematopoietic stem cells lacking spleen colony-forming activity. Blood 88:487, 1996.

213. Trevisan, M., and Iscove, N.N.: Phenotypic analysis of murine long-term hemopoietic reconstituting cells quantitated competitively in vivo and comparison with more advanced colony-forming progeny. J. Exp. Med. 181:93, 1995.

214. Smith, L.G., Weissman, I.L., and Heimfeld, S.: Clonal analysis of hematopoietic stem-cell differentiation in vivo. Proc. Natl. Acad. Sci. USA 88:2788, 1991.

215. Goodell, M.A., Brose, K., Paradis, G., Conner, A.S., and Mulligan, R.C.: Isolation and functional properties of murine hematopoietic stem cells that are replicating in vivo. J. Exp. Med. 183:1797, 1996.

216. Uchida, N., Fleming, W.H., Alpern, E.J., and Weissman, I.L.: Heterogeneity of hematopoietic stem cells. Curr. Opin. Immunol. 5:177, 1993.

217. Morrison, S.J., and Weissman, I.L.: Heterogeneity of hematopoietic stem cells: implications for clinical applications. Proc. Assoc. Am. Physicians 107:187, 1995.

218. Li, C.L., and Johnson, G.R.: Rhodamine[123] reveals heterogeneity within murine Lin-, Sca-1 + hemopoietic stem cells. J. Exp. Med. 175:1443, 1992.

219. Goodell, M.A.: Introduction: focus on hematology. CD34(+) or CD34(−): does it really matter? Blood 94:2545, 1999.

220. Knobel, K.M., McNally, M.A., Berson, A.E., Rood, D., Chen, K., Kilinski, L., Tran, K., Okarma, T.B., and Lebkowski, J.S.: Long-term reconstitution of mice after ex vivo expansion of bone marrow cells: differential activity of cultured bone marrow and enriched stem cell populations. Exp. Hematol. 22:1227, 1994.

221. Peters, S.O., Kittler, E.L., Ramshaw, H.S., and Quesenberry, P.J.: Murine marrow cells expanded in culture with IL-3, IL-6, IL-11, and SCF acquire an engraftment defect in normal hosts. Exp. Hematol. 23:461, 1995.

222. Traycoff, C.M., Cornetta, K., Yoder, M.C., Davidson, A., and Srour, E.F.: Ex vivo expansion of murine hematopoietic progenitor cells generates classes of expanded cells possessing different levels of bone marrow repopulating potential. Exp. Hematol. 24:299, 1996.

223. Williams, D.A.: Ex vivo expansion of hematopoietic stem and progenitor cells—robbing Peter to pay Paul? Blood 81:3169, 1993.

224. Yonemura, Y., Ku, H., Hirayama, F., Souza, L.M., and Ogawa, M.: Interleukin 3 or interleukin 1 abrogates the reconstituting ability of hematopoietic stem cells. Proc. Natl. Acad. Sci. USA 93:4040, 1996.

225. Reddy, G.P., Tiarks, C.Y., Pang, L., Wuu, J., Hsieh, C.C., and Quesenberry, P.J.: Cell cycle analysis and synchronization of pluripotent hematopoietic progenitor stem cells. Blood 90:2293, 1997.

226. Becker, P.S., Nilsson, S.K., Li, Z., Berrios, V.M., Dooner, M.S., Cooper, C.L., Hsieh, C.C., and Quesenberry, P.J.: Adhesion receptor expression by hematopoietic cell lines and murine progenitors: modulation by cytokines and cell cycle status. Exp. Hematol. 27:533, 1999.

227. Habibian, H.K., Peters, S.O., Hsieh, C.C., Wuu, J., Vergilis, K., Grimaldi, C.I., Reilly, J., Carlson, J.E., Frimberger, A.E., Stewart, F.M., and Quesenberry, P.J.: The fluctuating phenotype of the lympho-hematopoietic stem cell with cell cycle transit. J. Exp. Med. 188:393, 1998.

228. Ku, H., Yonemura, Y., Kaushansky, K., and Ogawa, M.: Thrombopoietin, the ligand for the Mpl receptor, synergizes with steel factor and other early acting cytokines in supporting proliferation of primitive hematopoietic progenitors of mice. Blood 87:4544, 1996.

229. Lyman, S.D., and Jabobsen, S.E.: c-kit Ligand and Flt3 ligand: stem/progenitor cell factors with overlapping yet distinct activities. Blood 91:1101, 1998.

230. Mackarehtschian, K., Hardin, J.D., Moore, K.A., Boast, S., Goff, S.P., and Lemischka, I.R.: Targeted disruption of the flk2/flt3 gene leads to deficiencies in primitive hematopoietic progenitors. Immunity 3:147, 1995.

231. Matsunaga, T., Kato, T., Miyazaki, H., and Ogawa, M.: Thrombopoie-tin promotes the survival of murine hematopoietic long-term reconstituting cells: comparison with the effects of Flt3/Flk-2 ligand and interleukin-6. Blood 92:452, 1998.

232. Kaushansky, K.: Thrombopoietin and the hematopoietic stem cell. Blood 92:1, 1998.

233. Iscove, N.N., and Nawa, K.: Hematopoietic stem cells expand during serial transplantation in vivo without apparent exhaustion. Curr. Biol. 7:805, 1997.

234. Dexter, T.M., Allen, T.D., and Lajtha, L.G.: Conditions controlling the proliferation of haemopoietic stem cells in vitro. J. Cell. Physiol. 91:335, 1977.

235. Fraser, C.C., Eaves, C.J., Szilvassy, S.J., and Humphries, R.K.: Expansion in vitro of retrovirally marked totipotent hematopoietic stem cells. Blood 76:1071, 1990.

236. Fraser, C.C., Szilvassy, S.J., Eaves, C.J., and Humphries, R.K.: Proliferation of totipotent hematopoietic stem cells in vitro with retention of long-term competitive in vivo reconstituting ability. Proc. Natl. Acad. Sci. USA 89:1968, 1992.

237. van der Sluijs, J.P., van den Bos, C., Baert, M.R., van Beurden, C.A., and Ploemacher, R.E.: Loss of long-term repopulating ability in long-term bone marrow culture. Leukemia 7:725, 1993.

238. Harrison, D.E., Lerner, C.P., and Spooncer, E.: Erythropoietic repopulating ability of stem cells from long-term marrow culture. Blood 69:1021, 1987.

239. Wineman, J.P., Nishikawa, S.I., and Muller-Sieburg, C.E.: Maintenance of high levels of pluripotent hematopoietic stem cells in vitro: effect of stromal cells and c-kit. Blood 81:365, 1993.

240. Wineman, J., Moore, K., Lemischka, I., and Muller-Sieburg, C.: Functional heterogeneity of the hematopoietic microenvironment: rare stromal elements maintain long-term repopulating stem cells. Blood 87:4082, 1996.

241. Szilvassy, S.J., Weller, K.P., Lin, W., Sharma, A.K., Ho, A.S., Tsukamoto, A., Hoffman, R., Leiby, K.R., and Gearing, D.P.: Leukemia inhibitory factor upregulates cytokine expression by a murine stromal cell line enabling the maintenance of highly enriched competitive repopulating stem cells. Blood 87:4618, 1996.

242. Moore, K.A., Ema, H., and Lemischka, I.R.: In vitro maintenance of highly purified, transplantable hematopoietic stem cells. Blood 89:4337–4347, 1997.

243. Thiemann, F.T., Moore, K.A., Smogorzewska, E.M., Lemischka, I.R., and Crooks, G.M.: The murine stromal cell line AFT024 acts specifically on human CD34 + CD38 − progenitors to maintain primitive function and immunophenotype in vitro. Exp. Hematol. 26:612, 1998.

244. Overturf, K., al-Dhalimy, M., Ou, C.N., Finegold, M., and Grompe, M.: Serial transplantation reveals the stem-cell-like regenerative potential of adult mouse hepatocytes. Am. J. Pathol. 151:1273, 1997.

245. Shi, Q., Rafii, S., Wu, M.H., Wijelath, E.S., Yu, C., Ishida, A., Fujita, Y., Kothari, S., Mohle, R., Sauvage, L.R., Moore, M.A., Storb, R.F., and Hammond, W.P.: Evidence for circulating bone marrow–derived endothelial cells. Blood 92:362, 1998.

246. Temple, S., and Alvarez-Buylla, A.: Stem cells in the adult mammalian nervous system. Curr. Opin. Neurobiol. 9:135, 1999.

247. Brill, S., Zvibel, I., and Reid, L.M.: Expansion conditions for early hepatic progenitor cells from embryonal and neonatal rat livers. Dig. Dis. Sci. 44:364, 1999.

248. Cameron, H.A., and McKay, R.: Stem cells and neurogenesis in the adult brain. Curr. Opin. Neurobiol. 8:677, 1998.

249. Doetsch, F., Caille, I., Lim, D.A., Garcia-Verdugo, J.M., and Alvarez-Buylla, A.: Subventricular zone astrocytes are neural stem cells in the adult mammalian brain. Cell 97:703, 1999.

250. Gage, F.H.: Stem cells of the central nervous system. Curr. Opin. Neurobiol. 8:671, 1998.

251. Johansson, C.B., Momma, S., Clarke, D.L., Risling, M., Lendahl, U., and Frisen, J.: Identification of a neural stem cell in the adult mammalian central nervous system. Cell 96:25, 1999.

252. Morrison, S.J., White, P.M., Zock, C., and Anderson, D.J.: Prospective identification, isolation by flow cytometry, and in vivo self-renewal of multipotent mammalian neural crest stem cells. Cell 96:737, 1999.

253. Petersen, B.E., Bowen, W.C., Patrene, K.D., Mars, W.M., Sullivan, A.K., Murase, N., Boggs, S.S., Greenberger, J.S., and Goff, J.P.: Bone marrow as a potential source of hepatic oval cells. Science 284:1168, 1999.

254. Asahara, T., Murohara, T., Sullivan, A., Silver, M., van der Zee, R., Li, T., Witzenbichler, B., Schatteman, G., and Isner, J.M.: Isolation of

putative progenitor endothelial cells for angiogenesis. Science 275:964, 1997.

255. Baroffio, A., Hamann, M., Bernheim, L., Bochaton-Piallat, M.L., Gabbiani, G., and Bader, C.R.: Identification of self-renewing myoblasts in the progeny of single human muscle satellite cells. Differentiation 60:47, 1996.

256. Pittenger, M.F., Mackay, A.M., Beck, S.C., Jaiswal, R.K., Douglas, R., Mosca, J.D., Moorman, M.A., Simonetti, D.W., Craig, S., and Marshak, D.R.: Multilineage potential of adult human mesenchymal stem cells. Science 284:143, 1999.

257. Gussoni, E., Soneoka, Y., Strickland, C.D., Buzney, E.A., Khan, M.K., Flint, A.F., Kunkel, L.M., and Mulligan, R.C.: Dystrophin expression in the mdx mouse restored by stem cell transplantation. Nature 401:390, 1999.

258. Jackson, K.A., Mi, T., and Goodell, M.A.: Hematopoietic potential of stem cells isolated from murine skeletal muscle. Proc. Natl. Acad. Sci. USA 96:14482, 1999.

259. Bjornson, C.R., Rietze, R.L., Reynolds, B.A., Magli, M.C., and Vescovi, A.L.: Turning brain into blood: a hematopoietic fate adopted by adult neural stem cells in vivo. Science 283:534, 1999.

260. Lemischka, I.R.: The power of stem cells reconsidered? Proc. Natl. Acad. Sci. USA 96:14193, 1999.

2 Hematopoietic Growth Factors and Receptors

▼▼▼▼ Kenneth Kaushansky

▼ ▼

Hematopoiesis, the production of blood cells from their marrow progenitors, is a complex process requiring the productive interaction of marrow stem and progenitor cells, hematopoietic growth factors, and the cells and proteins of the marrow microenvironment. This chapter examines the growth factors and their receptors and how disordered production or function of these molecules can lead to hematopoietic failure, excess, or transformation. The discussion is organized into several distinct segments. Paradigms in the Hematopoietic Growth Factors and Receptors draws together the similarities of form and function of these molecules gleaned from several decades of research. Once the general rules by which these molecules operate are presented, details of each of the specific molecules important for normal hematopoiesis are discussed. Finally, the last two sections of the chapter are devoted to the role of disordered growth factor or growth factor receptor structure or function in blood diseases.

Paradigms in the Hematopoietic Growth Factors and Receptors

A great many signals have an impact on hematopoietic stem and progenitor cells, inducing a variety of responses including survival, proliferation, differentiation, activation, apoptosis, and quiescence. This segment considers the prop-erties shared by those proteins responsible for supporting the survival and proliferation of hematopoietic cells and those that influence their terminal maturation. Depending on the activity assay used for their discovery or the physiological source of production, these proteins have been termed interleukins (ILs), colony-stimulating factors (CSFs), or endocrine hormones. However, given our increasing understanding of the physiology of these proteins, a classification scheme based on whether the protein acts on progenitors with a capacity to develop into multiple hematopoietic cell types or on cells committed to a single lineage should be considered. Another useful classification might be based on the biochemistry of the proteins. However, despite there being two major and seemingly distinct classes of hematopoietic receptors (the non–kinase-containing hematopoietic cytokine receptor family and the receptor tyrosine kinases), there appears to be but a single structural scaffold on which minor diversity generates a myriad of distinct receptor/ligand interactions. Finally, it is also clear that hematopoietic growth factors are presented to cells in several ways: as soluble blood-borne or paracrine hormones, as cell surface molecules requiring direct cell-cell contact, and adsorbed onto glycosaminoglycans as part of the microenvironment. The biological impact of each of these signaling routes differs and must be carefully considered to fully appreciate the subtlety of hematopoietic control.

▼ HEMATOPOIETIC GROWTH FACTOR PRODUCTION: MULTIPLE SOURCES AND LEVELS OF REGULATION

The proteins essential for hematopoietic stem and progenitor cell development are derived from both distant organs and adjacent marrow stromal cells. There are three major patterns of cytokine production that work to ensure an adequate supply of blood cells. Under steady-state conditions, basal levels of several hematopoietic growth factors can be detected, including stem cell factor (SCF; also termed steel factor, mast cell growth factor, and Kit ligand), Flt3 ligand (FL), erythropoietin (EPO), granulocyte (G)–CSF, macrophage (M)–CSF, and thrombopoietin (TPO). In response to an isolated cytopenia induced by loss or destruction of a single cell type, blood levels of the corresponding hormone (EPO for red cells, G-CSF for neutrophils, and TPO for platelets) increase. Under inflammatory conditions, levels of several additional cytokines increase, including IL-3, granulocyte-monocyte (GM)–CSF, IL-5, IL-6, and IL-11, cytokines that work in synergy with the lineage-dominant hormones to augment multiple types of blood cells. Virtually every known mechanism of gene regulation is employed by cells responsible for hematopoietic growth factor production.

Hematopoietic growth factors issue from three major sites: the liver and kidney; the immune system; and the marrow microenvironment, a complex of macrophages, fibroblasts, and endothelial cells[1] that can secrete nearly every (except EPO) hematopoietic growth factor.[2–8] The marrow stroma contributes to hematopoietic development by providing adhesion molecules, complex glycoproteins, and both soluble and cell-bound growth factors. The importance of the stroma in hematopoiesis can be demonstrated in several ways. For example, marrow stromal cell lines have been identified that support hematopoietic stem cells for weeks without the addition of soluble growth factors.[9] Because such cells are rare within the stroma,[10] this example also serves to point out the heterogeneity of marrow stromal cells. In addition, the marrow microenvironment provides unique signals: Although stromal cells produce both soluble and membrane-bound SCF, a comparison of *Sl/Sl^d* (soluble SCF only, viable but severely anemic) and normal mice indicates that the stromal, cell-bound form of some growth factors may be more important than their soluble counterparts. The glycosaminoglycans secreted into the matrix of the marrow may also play an important role in stem and progenitor cell biology. Growth factors such as GM-CSF and M-CSF can localize to the matrix,[11, 12] and one of the "stimulatory" hematopoietic effects of the marrow stroma may rest in the ability of its glycosaminoglycans to neutralize transforming growth factor-β (TGF-β).[13]

▼ HEMATOPOIETIC GROWTH FACTOR STRUCTURE: THE HEMATOPOIETIC CYTOKINE MOTIF

A primary sequence alignment of the hematopoietic cytokines reveals little homology. With the exception of a high degree of homology between EPO and TPO, the majority of hematopoietic cytokines bear little primary structural similarity to one another. However, with the availability of their tertiary structures, it is now clear that all of the hematopoietic cytokines bear a remarkable resemblance to one another.

The first hematopoietic cytokine for which a tertiary structure became available was porcine growth hormone,[14] a protein only retrospectively assigned to the hematopoietic family of cytokines. The structure of porcine and human growth hormone consists of a "left-handed" four α helix barrel. The first and second α helices and the third and fourth run parallel to each other, the second and third antiparallel. This arrangement requires the structure to make two long loops, between the first and second and between the third and fourth helices, with a short intervening loop between the second and third. At the time of its initial description, this structure was unique. A short time later, the structure of the first hematopoietic cytokine was solved, that for IL-2. However, although it contained four α helices, the initial structure indicated that all four were antiparallel,[15] a structural fold distinct from all other proteins, including growth hormone. Subsequently, in a remarkable theoretical analysis, Bazan[16] argued that the IL-2 structure must resemble that of growth hormone, a proposal confirmed by a reassessment of the experimental data.[17] Since that time, every hematopoietic cytokine structure solved (including GM-CSF,[18] IL-4,[19] M-CSF,[20] G-CSF,[21] IL-5,[22] leukemia inhibitory factor[23] [LIF], IL-3,[24] IL-6,[25] ciliary neurotrophic factor,[26] and oncostatin M[27]) has conformed to the same basic structural pattern (Fig. 2–1), although two subfamilies based on relative helical lengths have been described.[28, 29] In addition, the sites for functionally critical residues are shared by all of these proteins. Surface residues on the first and fourth helices and the AB loop compose a receptor-interactive face that can bind to receptor with low affinity, and amino acids located on the surface of the first and third helices form another interactive surface capable of recruiting a second receptor subunit. However, despite their common structural scaffold, and by extrapolation their common evolutionary origin, each cytokine displays a unique set of surface residues enabling it to interact with one and only one cytokine receptor. Several reviews have been published on this topic.[28, 30, 31]

▼ HEMATOPOIETIC GROWTH FACTOR RECEPTOR STRUCTURE: THE HEMATOPOIETIC CYTOKINE RECEPTOR AND RECEPTOR PROTEIN TYROSINE KINASE FAMILIES

On the basis of the recurring presence of predicted β-pleated sheet structures, Bazan[32] predicted the general form of the hematopoietic cytokine receptors many years before their tertiary structures were established by physical means. The binding domain of these receptors contains two barrel-like structures, each composed of seven β-pleated sheets, and includes the EPO, G-CSF, TPO, IL-3, GM-CSF, IL-5, IL-6, IL-11, and LIF receptors. The family also includes receptors for cytokines not usually associated with hematopoiesis, such as those for growth hormone and leptin.[32, 33] In fact, our greatest understanding of this family of proteins derives from Wells and colleagues' work with growth hormone receptor (reviewed in Wells[34]). As gleaned from the co-crystal structure of growth hormone and its receptor, two molecules of receptor each make six distinct contacts with

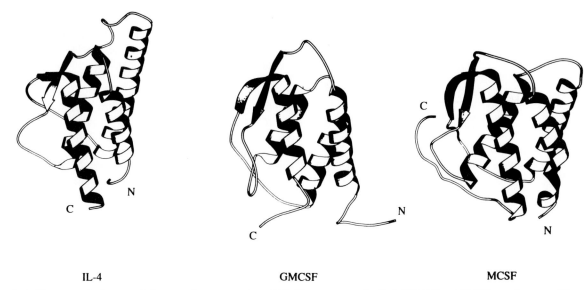

IL-4   GMCSF   MCSF

Figure 2–1. Hematopoietic growth factors share a tertiary fold. The structures for IL-4, GM-CSF, and M-CSF are shown as ribbon diagrams representing the α carbon backbones. All are left-handed four α-helical bundles, are members of the "short helix" subclass of hematopoietic cytokines, and can be overlaid with as little as 1.5 Å mean deviation for the helical bundle. This degree of structural homology is remarkable, especially given that the receptors for the three molecules differ considerably (see text). (From Kaushansky, K., and Karplus, A.: The hematopoietic growth factors: understanding functional diversity in structural terms. Blood 82:8229, 1993; with permission.)

two different faces of a single hormone molecule,[35] sites on the receptor for the most part localized to the short protruding loops between sheets. This work has been extended to determination of the receptor residues that interact with other hematopoietic cytokines.[36–39] All have been put into the context of the seven β sheet model of Bazan and have identified critical ligand binding residues on the AB loop, EF loop, G β sheet, B′C′ loop, C′ β sheet, E′F′ loop and adjacent β sheets, and F′G′ loop. In addition, it appears that ligand binding induces a conformational change in the receptor.[40] Many efforts at modeling the receptor/ligand complex have been published,[41–45] all based on the initial description of the growth hormone/growth hormone receptor cocrystal structure.[35]

Several studies have begun to provide insights into how cytokine binding begins the process of receptor signal transduction. It is clear that receptor activation begins with dimerization of two signaling receptor subunits. However, several pieces of evidence suggest that ligand binding plays a dynamic role, more complex than simply inducing receptor dimerization. For example, β_C receptor dimers exist before signaling in the GM-CSF receptor[46]; these data argue that ligand binding must induce a critical receptor conformational change necessary for signal transduction. Moreover, because truncation of the extracellular domain of several growth factor receptors can contribute to constitutive activation,[47–49] it has been proposed that one or more regions of the extracytoplasmic domain inhibit association of the receptor components necessary for signaling[50]; ligand binding acts to relieve this critical barrier to receptor activation.

Hematopoietic cytokine receptors display tremendous variability in the length of the cytoplasmic domain (from 54 to 569 residues) and share little primary sequence homology. The family can be divided into two function-based subgroups (Fig. 2–2). The first subfamily consists of receptors that bind ligand with low affinity but by themselves are insufficient to transmit a proliferative, antiapoptotic, or dif-

ferentiative signal. Examples of this subfamily include the GM-CSF, IL-3, IL-5, IL-6, and IL-11 receptors; each is termed an α subunit. Some of these receptors require their intracytoplasmic domain for full function (e.g., GM-CSFRα, IL-3Rα, IL-5Rα), but others do not (IL-6Rα, IL-11Rα). The second subfamily, β subunits, are directly responsible for recruitment and docking of the intermediary molecules necessary for signal transduction. The sites at which these events occur include the box1 and box2 motifs, critical for cytoplasmic tyrosine kinase binding; a box3 motif, thought to be required for binding of differentiation mediators; and SH2, SH3, and PTB domains. (See Chapter 4.) Some of these signaling receptor subunits bind ligand with high affinity (e.g., EPO-R, TPO-R, G-CSF-R), but others do so only with low affinity or not at all (e.g., LIF-R, gp130, and β_C). Many excellent reviews on hematopoietic cytokine receptors have been published.[51–54]

The extracellular domains of members of the receptor tyrosine kinase family are composed of a variable number of immunoglobulin-like domains (five each for the M-CSF, SCF, and FL receptors). Interdomain swapping experiments have revealed the fourth and fifth immunoglobulin domains to be critical for receptor specificity (see below). The cytoplasmic segment of these receptors also contains a tyrosine kinase domain, which differs from many other receptor tyrosine kinases (e.g., receptors for insulin or epidermal growth factor) in being split by an "insert region." The significance of this structure is unknown. However, in the absence of phosphorylation, the kinase is inactive. Each ligand that uses members of the hematopoietic RTK family is dimeric, allowing it to cross-link two monomeric receptors. By bringing two inactive kinase domains into close juxtaposition, the ligand induces receptor *trans*-phosphorylation, activating the kinase activity of each, triggering signal transduction. In addition to the intrinsic receptor kinase activity, other cytoplasmic kinases participate in M-CSF, SCF, and FL signaling, including some of the same kinases responsible for signaling in the hematopoietic cytokine receptor family.

Extracellular Domains

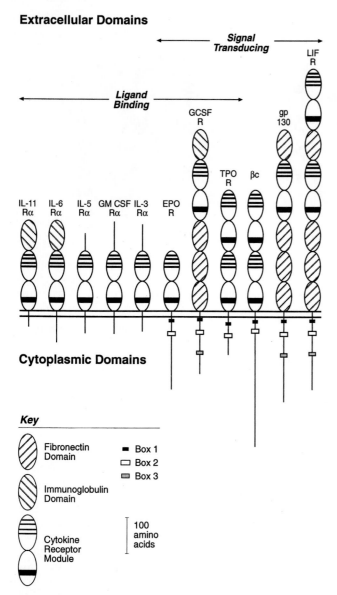

Figure 2–2. The modular structure of hematopoietic receptors. Three types of modules compose the extracellular domains of hematopoietic cytokine receptors: fibronectin, immunoglobulin, and the cytokine receptor motif. The last is a 200 amino acid domain composed of two seven–β sheet structures. The intracytoplasmic domains are composed of 54 to 424 residues and include only three small regions of homology, the box1, box2, and box3 motifs. The models are drawn to scale.

Most members of both families of hematopoietic growth factor receptors have been shown to be capable of giving rise to soluble forms that circulate. Theoretically, soluble receptors could serve as cytokine antagonists, carriers of ligand, or even enhancers of ligand action. Levels of soluble receptors have ranged from non-detectable to enough to theoretically bind all of the corresponding cytokine in the plasma.[55] When they are expressed as recombinant proteins, most of these soluble receptors act to neutralize their cognate ligand.[56–59] However, notable exceptions are the low-affinity receptors that employ gp130 as a signal transduction subunit (e.g., IL-6 and IL-11). Because the cytoplasmic domain of these low-affinity α subunits is not required for receptor function, and the α subunit/ligand complex can bind to

gp130 through its extracellular domain alone, such complexes are actually stimulatory to *every* cell that bears the gp130 receptor.[53, 60] However, the precise function of the soluble receptors remains unclear.[61]

▼ HEMATOPOIETIC GROWTH FACTORS: FUNCTION

It is commonly stated that hematopoietic growth factors support the survival, proliferation, and differentiation of hematopoietic progenitor cells. Whereas this is true in toto, a useful paradigm for their function has been revealed by careful study of all of the requirements for erythropoiesis in vivo and in vitro. It has long been assumed that EPO is the primary regulator of erythropoiesis. Studies of the inverse relationship between red cell mass and EPO levels, administration of the hormone to animals and people, and analysis of mice engineered to eliminate expression of the hormone or its receptor have confirmed this prediction. However, erythroid progenitors can develop in vivo in the absence of the EPO receptor,[62] and animals in which other hematopoietic growth factor genes are eliminated also display an anemic phenotype. The most notable of these are the W and Sl mice, deficient in the c-Kit receptor and its ligand, SCF.

The use of isolated erythroid progenitors of high purity has allowed investigators to examine the role of each of the erythropoietic cytokines in the survival, proliferation, or differentiation of these cells. This approach has shed important light on the highly cooperative actions of hematopoietic growth factors. It has been suggested that programmed cell death (apoptosis) is a default program in normal cells that must be actively blocked. Under serum-free culture conditions, purified erythroid progenitors are highly dependent on EPO for survival, the hormone acting to prevent their apoptotic death.[63] In fact, using graded doses of the hormone, the same investigators established that within a population of erythroid progenitors, there exists heterogeneity with respect to EPO sensitivity. Some cells survive and can develop in the presence of low levels of EPO; at the other end of the spectrum are cells that require extremely high concentrations of the hormone to avoid apoptosis. This finding suggests a model of hematopoietic regulation. If hematopoietic progenitors are differentially sensitive to the apoptosis-sparing effects of their corresponding growth factor, it follows that in times of erythroid cell excess and EPO deficiency, few progenitors survive and net red cell production falls. Conversely, under anemic conditions, EPO levels are high, resulting in the survival of most erythroid progenitors and hence increased red cell production. Increased EPO levels "stimulate" increased erythropoiesis by allowing a higher proportion of erythroid progenitor cells to survive than at times of reduced hormone concentrations. This model is so compelling that it has been adapted to virtually all hematopoietic lineages. Interestingly, the suppression of apoptosis appears to be the primary function of EPO. When added alone to cultures of purified erythroid progenitors, EPO supports little erythroid cell proliferation.[64] In contrast, the addition of SCF, itself a poor mediator of cell survival, is required for optimal progenitor cell cycling, and insulin-like growth factor (IGF)–1 is required for optimal erythroid differentiation (as measured by globin synthesis and enucleation). Thus, EPO deficiency leads to erythroid failure, but EPO alone does not appear to support the proliferation and differentiation of the lineage.

A second important paradigm in hematopoietic growth factor function is that the cytokines that stimulate the progenitor cells of any given lineage often prime the resultant mature cells to become functionally active. For example, GM-CSF reduces the threshold for neutrophil and monocyte oxidative metabolism and killing when these cells are confronted with immune complexes or opsonized microorganisms.[65-67] This function of many of the hematopoietic cytokines helps to explain their production at sites other than the marrow microenvironment (i.e., they participate in local reactions) and in some cases may represent their primary role. Indeed, genetic elimination of GM-CSF has no apparent effect on neutrophil or monocyte production. Rather, the function of a highly specialized monocyte, the pulmonary alveolar macrophage, is critically affected by GM-CSF,[68] and GM-CSF deficiency leads to pulmonary alveolar proteinosis because of deficiency of the cell.[69]

A third important paradigm for hematopoiesis is that although many of the hormones and cytokines appear to influence overlapping populations of cells to develop similar functional capacities, hematopoietic growth factor functions are not strictly redundant. On the surface, GM-CSF appears redundant. The cytokine supports the production of neutrophils and monocytes and the early development of erythroid and megakaryocytic lineages. However, neutrophil production is primarily supported by G-CSF, monocyte production is supported by M-CSF, and the erythroid and megakaryocytic activities of GM-CSF are supported by other early-acting and late-acting cytokines and hormones. Moreover, GM-CSF knockout mice display normal numbers of all of these cells,[69] under both steady-state and stressed conditions, arguing that even if GM-CSF plays a role in blood cell production, it can be readily compensated for by other cytokines. However, the pulmonary alveolar macrophage defect of the GM-CSF nullizygous mouse attests to the importance of the cytokine for at least this aspect of normal homeostasis. Each of the hematopoietic cytokine knockout mice have displayed one or more specific hematological phenotypes (Table 2–1).

Finally, a fourth important paradigm in hematopoiesis is that the proximate outcome of ligand binding to hematopoietic growth factor receptor is signaling subunit dimerization and activation, and the ultimate consequence of this event is growth and development of the hematopoietic cell in which the receptor is expressed. Whether the signal that originates from each receptor is distinct (i.e., unique pathways are activated) or the signals activated by one receptor are interchangeable with those of another remains one of the contentious questions of current hematopoietic research. Evidence on both sides of the argument can be persuasive. For example, the pluripotent hematopoietic cell line FDCP-Mix can develop into neutrophils in the presence of G-CSF, monocytes if treated with M-CSF, or erythrocytes if given EPO. However, if first engineered to express the antiapoptotic *bcl-2* gene, it spontaneously develops into all three hematopoietic lineages,[70] arguing that all three cytokines provide an identical (survival) signal. However, other data suggest that growth factors exert a unique signal. For example, the addition of IL-3 but not other cytokines to a culture of primitive

Table 2–1. Hematopoietic Phenotypes of the Hematopoietic Growth Factor Nullizygous Mice

Growth Factor or Receptor	Primary Hematological Deficiency State
EPO	Erythroid failure[62]
G-CSF	Neutropenia[127, 128]
M-CSF	Osteopetrosis[866]
GM-CSF	Pulmonary alveolar proteinosis[69]
IL-3	Diminished delayed hypersensitivity[867]
IL-5	Eosinophil deficiency[225]
TPO	Thrombocytopenia[164, 868]
SCF	Severe macrocytic anemia[294-299]
FL	Dendritic cell deficiency[356]
IL-6	Modest reduction in neutrophil production[129]
IL-11	None yet reported[428]
LIF	None yet reported[433]

hematopoietic cells clearly skews the progeny away from a lymphoid phenotype.[71] This ongoing controversy has recently been summarized.[72]

The Physiology of Specific Hematopoietic Growth Factors and Their Receptors

This section considers the biochemistry and physiology of each of the cytokines and hormones that has an impact on hematopoietic stem and progenitor cells. Emphasis is placed on the physiological properties observed in studies that use purified cytokines and enriched or purified populations of target cells in vitro, because many if not most of the hematopoietic cytokines can mediate both direct and indirect physiological effects. As a result, the net effect of any individual hematopoietic growth factor in vivo can be extremely complex.

▼ ERYTHROPOIETIN AND THE ERYTHROPOIETIN RECEPTOR

The primary regulator of erythrocyte production was postulated to exist in 1906,[73] but reports of its cloning did not appear until 1985.[74, 75] The cDNA predicts a polypeptide of 193 amino acids that includes a 27 amino acid leader sequence, resulting in a 166 residue secreted polypeptide. As the carboxyl-terminal arginine residue is cleaved, the mature circulating hormone is composed of 165 amino acids of predicted M_r 18.2 kDa. However, when it is produced in mammalian cells, the actual M_r approximates 34 kDa, the result of carbohydrate modification at a single serine and three asparagine residues. Key biochemical features of the protein are summarized in Table 2–2.

EPO is produced in the kidney and to a lesser extent in the liver, although the precise cellular localization in these organs is still debated. Using in situ hybridization, two groups have demonstrated production by the peritubular cells of the renal cortex, thought to be either interstitial[76] or endothelial[77] in origin. However, using the EPO promoter linked to a reporter gene, another group has challenged this view, suggesting production by renal proximal tubular cells.[78] Other studies using a similar strategy and greater amounts

Table 2–2. Biochemical Properties of Primary Regulators of Hematopoiesis

Hormone/Cytokine	No. Amino Acids		Polypeptide M_r (kDa)	Actual M_r (kDa)	Disulfide Location	Carbohydrate (No. and Type)	Chromosome Location	Critical Receptor Binding Residues
	PREDICTED	MATURE PROTEIN						
EPO[74, 75, 869–871]	193	165	18.2	34	C_7–C_{161} C_{29}–C_{33}	3 N 1 O	7q11	R_{14}, Y_{15}, R_{45}, S_{100}, R_{103}, N_{147}, G_{151}
G-CSF[106–108, 872, 873]	204	174	19.2	19	C_{36}–C_{42} C_{64}–C_{74}	1 O	17q11	L_{15}, E_{19}, K_{40}, V_{48}, L_{49}, D_{112}, F_{144}
TPO[57, 141, 874, 875]	356	332	36	70	C_7–C_{151} C_{29}–C_{85}	6 N $\geq$5 O	3q21	D_8, K_{14}, K_{52}, K_{59}, K_{136}, K_{138}, R_{140}

of the EPO 5′ flanking region have confirmed peritubular localization of EPO production (14 kb of 5′ flanking sequence was required to recapitulate the endogenous renal EPO production pattern[79]).

Blood levels of EPO vary inversely with the oxygen-carrying capacity of the blood, climbing at an exponential rate as the degree of anemia progresses.[80] It is clear that the primary stimulus for its production is tissue hypoxia; responsiveness is mediated by a heme protein or flavoprotein,[81, 82] and increased production is driven primarily by an increase in transcription of the EPO gene.[83] The human and murine EPO genes are highly conserved, especially in the coding sequence, first intron, and 3′ flanking regions, suggesting important regulatory functions for these last two regions. The 3′ flanking region of the EPO gene contains a hypoxia-inducible element,[84] a 50 nucleotide motif also present in the vascular endothelial growth factor and the glucose transporter-1 genes.[85] This region corresponds to a DNAse hypersensitive site specific to hepatic cells, indicating its accessibility to the transcriptional machinery.[86] The hypoxia-inducible element of the EPO gene provides a scaffold on which a trimolecular complex forms, composed of the hypoxia-inducible factor-1 (HIF-1) (regulated by hypoxia-mediated protein stabilization), the constitutively expressed hepatic nuclear factor-4 (HNF-4), and the general transcriptional activator p300.[85, 87]

The 5′ flanking region of the EPO gene also contains transcriptionally important sequences. A minimal 117 nucleotide promoter has been identified, which is modestly inducible by hypoxia in hepatic cells.[88] This region includes sites for the HNF-4 protein, potentially providing a bridge between the 3′ enhancer and the promoter regions of the gene. Unfortunately, because a suitable EPO-producing renal cell line has not been established, detailed studies of the type performed in hepatic cells are not available. However, use of primary renal cell protein extracts in an in vitro transcription assay has also indicated the presence of a hypoxia-inducible transcriptional activator that operates on the promoter region of the EPO gene.[89]

Regulation of mRNA stability may also play a role in the regulation of EPO production. A hypoxia-induced protein has been identified that binds to the 3′ untranslated region (UTR) of EPO mRNA, which acts to prolong message stability.[90] However, further work will be required, including cloning of cDNA for this protein, before the precise role of post-transcriptional modulation of EPO mRNA levels can be fully assessed.

EPO acts to increase erythrocyte levels in three ways. Immediately, infusion of EPO stimulates the early release of maturing normoblasts from their marrow sites of development. Second, EPO increases the amount of hemoglobin synthesized per erythrocyte. Most important, however, EPO stimulates the expansion of late erythroid burst-forming units (BFU-E) and all erythroid colony-forming units (CFU-E) into mature red cells. At least one of the primary mechanisms by which this is accomplished, and perhaps the most important, is its suppression of programmed erythroid cell death. The role played by EPO in the suppression of programmed cell death and its implications for erythroid growth regulation are discussed above.

The physiological importance of EPO was established when genetic elimination of the gene for the hormone or its receptor was shown to result in embryonic lethality. Homozygote embryos die by day 13 owing to severe anemia.[91, 92] However, EPO does not appear to be absolutely essential for the development of erythroid progenitor cells; erythroid colony-forming cells can be demonstrated among fetal liver cells just before intrauterine death by culturing EPO knockout mouse cells in EPO or EPO-R knockout cells in SCF and TPO.[62] These findings are consistent with the model of erythropoiesis noted above[64]; EPO alone prevents apoptosis but does little to expand progenitor numbers or lead to their expression of differentiation programs (globin synthesis or enucleation).

Using a novel functional expression cloning system, D'Andrea and colleagues[93] obtained cDNA for the EPO-R in 1989, not only opening a window on the molecular mechanisms of hematopoietic cytokine action but also providing a useful strategy for obtaining cDNA representing additional, equally elusive receptors.[94] The gene for the human EPO-R resides on chromosome 19p[95] and encodes a cell surface protein of approximately 55 kDa (see Fig. 2–2). Multiple forms of the receptor (M_r = 64, 66, 70, and 78 kDa) can be identified in EPO-R–bearing cells, which differ by the degree of glycosylation present.[96] Compelling evidence has been presented that only the highest M_r forms of the receptor bind hormone and signal.[96] The weight of available evidence also suggests that a homodimeric EPO-R is necessary and sufficient for responsiveness to EPO,[97, 98] the most persuasive of which is the tertiary structure of the EPO-R complexed to an EPO-mimetic peptide.[99] However, in addition to the homodimeric signaling complex, evidence is accumulating that the EPO-R functionally and physically interacts with the c-Kit receptor[100] and the β chain of the IL-3 receptor.[101]

Within the erythroid lineage, constitutive expression of the EPO-R is first noted at the level of the late BFU-E (~300 receptors/cell); receptor numbers rise in CFU-E and erythroblasts (~1100 receptors/cell) and are almost absent on reticulocytes.[102] This low level of receptor expression is characteristic of the family. However, careful calculations indicate that receptor occupancy levels of just 5 to 10 per cent are sufficient to trigger signal transduction. Receptor levels within these cells are also subject to modulation; EPO withdrawal increases receptor expression threefold.[103] As with other erythroid-specific proteins, expression of the EPO-R is dependent on the transcription factor GATA-1. Modification of receptor expression correlates with modulation of GATA-1 levels. There are also Sp1 and CACCC binding sites within the 256 bp promoter region that are important for expression.[104, 105] Regulation of expression may also be directed by additional *cis*-acting elements located within DNAse hypersensitivity sites 0.5 and 2.4 kb upstream of the transcription initiation site.

▼ G-CSF AND ITS RECEPTOR

G-CSF was purified from several cell lines and cloned more than 10 years ago.[106–108] The human gene localizes to chromosome 17q11[109] and encodes a polypeptide of 204 amino acids. After cleavage of the 30 residue secretory leader sequence, the resultant 19 kDa polypeptide is distinct from most of the other hematopoietic proteins; only a single Thr residue carries an O-glycan side chain.[110] The biochemical features of G-CSF are summarized in Table 2–2. Soon after cloning of the initial cDNA, a second form of G-CSF was described, containing a Val-Ser-Glu tripeptide insertion after Leu 35. The longer form of the hormone is approximately 50-fold less active than the shorter form in vitro because of reduced receptor binding.[111] Moreover, the longer splicoform is not generated by murine cells,[110] which makes its significance uncertain.

The sources of G-CSF production are ubiquitous. Multiple cell types, including fibroblasts and endothelial cells of the marrow stroma, express specific transcripts for the cytokine. However, few studies have demonstrated constitutive expression of the gene. Rather, the cytokine is easily inducible by mediators of the inflammatory response (including lipopolysaccharide [LPS], IL-1, and tumor necrosis factor-α [TNF-α][112–115]). Moreover, local production of the cytokine in response to regional inflammatory conditions[116] may also contribute hormone that activates neutrophils.

Transcriptional, post-transcriptional, and receptor-mediated mechanisms regulate expression of G-CSF production. A complex region 200 to 165 nucleotides upstream of the G-CSF cap site is necessary for induction of cytokine production in fibroblasts, a sequence that contains both κB and NF-IL-6 sites. This region cooperatively binds the Rel-related protein p65 (but not p50) and C/EBPβ, both of which are induced by IL-1 and TNF in fibroblasts.[117, 118] In addition to transcriptional regulation, stabilization of G-CSF message is also influenced by a number of inflammatory mediators, further enhancing the steady-state levels of specific mRNA.[119] Being the physiological regulator of neutrophil production, G-CSF levels are inversely related to neutrophil counts and are elevated in the presence of infection.[120–124] The level of G-CSF in physiological fluids, like that of all cytokines and hormones, is the net result of production and destruction. Neutrophils metabolize G-CSF by receptor uptake and internalization,[125] making these cells effective regulators of cytokine concentrations.

Although the term G-CSF implies that the protein induces the production of colonies of all types of granulocytes, G-CSF supports the proliferation and maturation only of hematopoietic progenitors exclusively committed to the neutrophilic lineage. Eosinophils require GM-CSF or IL-5, and basophilic colonies are dependent on the presence of SCF or IL-3 (see below). This selectivity is demonstrated in vivo; administration of G-CSF to animals and humans results exclusively in a neutrophilic leukocytosis,[126] and genetic elimination of G-CSF or its receptor reduces only neutrophil levels.[127, 128] However, G-CSF is not absolutely essential for neutrophil formation. Although genetic elimination of G-CSF or its receptor reduces neutrophil counts to about 15 per cent of normal, the remaining cells are fully developed. The number of committed granulocyte-macrophage progenitor cells is only modestly (50 per cent) reduced in the mice, arguing that the cytokine is also not essential for lineage commitment. Rather, G-CSF appears to serve as an amplifier of a developmental pathway that can be qualitatively maintained by other cytokines. As discussed below, one of the candidates to fill this role was IL-6, but results argue that although this cytokine aids neutrophil generation under conditions of G-CSF deficiency, it is not essential for the process.[129]

In addition to supporting the expansion and maturation of neutrophilic progenitor cells, G-CSF also acts in synergy with other cytokines to prime neutrophils for enhanced functional activity and to expand primitive hematopoietic progenitor cells. Neutrophils respond to a number of biological mediators by enhancing phagocytic capacity, intracellular killing, and antibody-dependent cellular cytotoxicity. G-CSF acts to prime leukocytes to respond to these direct activators,[67, 130, 131] which include the chemokines IL-8 and macrophage inflammatory protein-1α (MIP-1α) and bacterial products such as the peptide f-Met–Leu—Phe. Local production of G-CSF (and GM-CSF, which shares this neutrophil priming capacity) is thought to play an important role in the host response to inflammatory stimuli through this priming effect. Somewhat unexpectedly, G-CSF was also found to act in synergy with IL-3 or SCF to enhance the proliferation of primitive hematopoietic progenitor cells.[132, 133] The physiological implications of this finding are uncertain. It has been speculated that it represents a mechanism by which the need for neutrophils "signals" the more primitive progenitor compartment to expand.

One basis for myeloid lineage–specific development appears to lie in the differential presence of the transcription factors necessary for myeloid growth factor receptor expression. The G-CSF receptor (G-CSF-R) gene is located on human chromosome 1p32[134] and encodes an 812 residue polypeptide composed of a 601 amino acid extracellular domain (including an immunoglobulin domain, a hematopoietic cytokine receptor motif, and three fibronectin domains), a 25 residue transmembrane sequence, and a 186 amino acid intracellular domain[135] (see Fig. 2–2). The G-CSF-R binds G-CSF with high affinity, and its cytoplasmic domain includes box1 and box2 homologies, allowing it to signal without partner molecules.[136] G-CSF-R expression is developmentally regulated by the transcription factors C/EBP and PU.1, as are the GM-CSF and M-CSF receptors.[137, 138] Models of lineage commitment have been put forward suggesting that the alternative expression of C/EBP and PU.1 versus GATA-1 and NF-E2 might determine cellular fate by driving expression of either myeloid (M-CSF-R, G-CSF-R, GM-CSF-R) or erythroid and megakaryocytic (EPO-R, TPO-R) growth factor receptors, respectively.[139] These classes of transcription factors, GATA-1 for erythroid and megakaryocytic cells, and PU.1 for myeloid cells, appear also to induce specific unresponsiveness to alternative lineage choices. For example, PU.1 expression in erythroid lines blocks erythroid differentiation, and overexpression of GATA-1 in myeloid cells interrupts myeloid development. However, the molecular mechanisms that allow separate development of the four myeloid cell classes—monocytic, neutrophilic, eosinophilic, and basophilic—are poorly understood. This topic is more thoroughly discussed in Chapter 3.

▼ THROMBOPOIETIN AND ITS RECEPTOR, c-Mpl

The cloned human TPO cDNA encodes 353 amino acids, which includes a 21 amino acid secretory leader sequence. The TPO gene localizes to human chromosome 3q21, a region shown to be abnormal in a patient with thrombocytosis and blastic transformation of chronic myeloid leukemia.[140] The polypeptide can be conveniently divided into two domains; the amino-terminal 154 residues of the mature polypeptide bear striking sequence homology with EPO and bind to the Mpl receptor. The carboxyl-terminal domain bears no resemblance to any known proteins but contains multiple sites of both N- and O-linked carbohydrate. This feature accounts for the large discrepancy between the predicted and actual M_r of the protein; nearly 50 per cent of the 70 kDa TPO molecule is carbohydrate. Functions for the carbohydrate-containing carboxyl-terminal domain include increasing the circulatory survival and improving secretory efficiency of TPO. These and other features of TPO are summarized in Table 2–2.

The preponderance of available data indicates that TPO blood levels vary inversely with the combined megakaryocyte and platelet mass. The explanation for the inverse relationship is relatively straightforward; TPO-specific transcripts can be found in many organs[57, 141, 142] as a result of its production by hepatocytes, endothelial cells, and fibroblasts. In most organs, including the liver, the richest source of the protein, production is constitutive.[143, 144] This gives rise to a relatively fixed total body TPO production rate. Platelets and megakaryocytes contain high-affinity TPO-Rs,[145, 146] which can consume and destroy the hormone.[147, 148] Hence, in states of thrombocytosis, the large platelet mass metabolizes the majority of TPO before its impact on marrow megakaryocytes, limiting new platelet production. In contrast, during thrombocytopenic states, elimination of TPO by the reduced platelet mass is greatly diminished, leaving increased blood levels to support increased marrow megakaryocyte and platelet production. The contribution of megakaryocytes to TPO metabolism appears to become important during consumptive thrombocytopenias. The compensatory megakaryocytic hyperplasia seen in states of platelet destruction is thought to be responsible for the relatively low TPO blood levels detected in immune thrombocytopenia.[149] However, it is also possible that the reduced level of TPO in some of these states is responsible for the thrombocytopenia per se. For instance, about one quarter of patients with what is otherwise typical idiopathic thrombocytopenic purpura do not display increased platelet turnover or megakaryocytic hyperplasia.[150] TPO levels have not been checked in this subset of patients, but reduced TPO levels (by either immune targeting or other mechanisms) could account for their thrombocytopenia. In addition, other

mechanisms for the regulation of TPO exist. These findings are summarized in Figure 2–3.

TPO is the major regulator of megakaryocyte maturation,[151] supporting the formation of platelet-specific granules, demarcation membranes, and platelet fields[152]; the expression of platelet-specific membrane proteins, such as the fibrinogen receptor glycoprotein IIb/IIIa[153] and the von Willebrand receptor glycoprotein Ib/V/IX[154]; the enhancement of megakaryocyte adhesion through activation of glycoprotein IIb/IIIa and very late antigens 4 (VLA-4) and 5 (VLA-5)[155, 156]; and the promotion of endomitosis and its resultant polyploid state.[152] Other cytokines fail to induce similar levels of megakaryocyte maturation if endogenous TPO effects are blocked. The hormone is also a potent inducer of proliferation of megakaryocytic progenitor cells. At optimal levels, the hormone by itself can induce the proliferation of up to 75 per cent of all marrow progenitor cells fully or in part committed to the megakaryocyte lineage.[154, 157, 158] At lower levels, the hormone acts synergistically to enhance megakaryocyte colony formation in combination with IL-3, SCF, IL-11, and EPO.[159] At least one of the mechanisms by which TPO acts, like that for EPO, is by suppression of progenitor cell apoptosis.[160]

Somewhat surprisingly, TPO can support the survival of a candidate hematopoietic stem cell population and acts in synergy with IL-3 and SCF to induce these cells into the cell cycle and increase their output of both primitive and committed hematopoietic progenitor cells of all lineages.[161–163a] These in vitro effects are reflective of in vivo events; genetic elimination of TPO or its receptor is associated with reduction of the numbers of marrow hematopoietic stem and progenitor cells of all lineages to approximately 25 per cent of normal values.[164–166]

The TPO-R was initially cloned as the homologue of the murine transforming oncogene v-mpl.[49] Recognized as a hematopoietic growth factor receptor by virtue of its characteristically spaced Cys residues and "WSXWS box," several features of c-mpl suggested an important role in megakaryocyte formation,[49, 167, 168] a conclusion confirmed with the cloning of TPO. Equilibrium binding experiments with radiolabeled TPO revealed a single class of receptors with a binding affinity of approximately 100 pmol; platelets display approximately 25 receptors per cell.[145, 146] Megakaryocytes

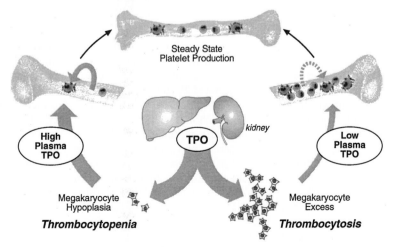

Figure 2–3. A model of thrombopoietin regulation. The liver and kidney produce TPO constitutively[57, 141, 143, 144] and release it into the circulation. Platelets destroy the hormone by receptor-mediated uptake from the circulation.[146] In states of thrombocytopenia, as depicted on the left, little of the released TPO is metabolized, leaving high plasma levels to affect hematopoiesis. In addition, marrow stroma produces TPO during thrombocytopenia.[144, 349, 893] High TPO levels help to restore megakaryocyte and platelet production. In contrast, during thrombocytosis, depicted on the right, high platelet levels remove most of the TPO in the circulation and marrow stromal cell production ceases, leaving little of the hormone to act on marrow megakaryopoiesis. The model has been adapted from one proposed by Kuter and Rosenberg[147] and is similar to ones proposed to account for the regulation of M-CSF by monocytes[267] and G-CSF by neutrophils.[125]

display far greater numbers of receptors, although precise quantitation has been technically challenging.

In addition to the most abundant signaling form of Mpl illustrated in Figure 2–2, a soluble form arises by splicing out of the exon encoding the WSXWS and transmembrane regions,[169] and another form of the receptor (the K form) is derived from an alternative reading frame that eliminates the box1/box2 and all other signaling motifs of the intracytoplasmic domain of the receptor.[49] It is unlikely that any of the alternative forms of Mpl bind TPO (e.g., mutation of the WSXWS region of the growth hormone and EPO receptors unfolds the proteins[170, 171]) or signal, potentially making their presence splicing artifacts. It is formally possible, however, that the K form of Mpl acts as a decoy receptor.

▼ INTERLEUKIN-3, GM-CSF, INTERLEUKIN-5, AND THE β_c FAMILY OF RECEPTORS

IL-3 is a monomeric 25 to 30 kDa polypeptide produced almost exclusively by T lymphocytes, natural killer (NK) cells, and mast cells. The human IL-3 gene is present on the long arm of human chromosome 5 adjacent to that of GM-CSF[172] and encodes a 152 amino acid polypeptide that is processed to a mature 133 residue cytokine.[173] As in many of the other hematopoietic cytokines, significant amounts of N-linked carbohydrate modification account for approximately 40 per cent of its apparent M_r. The biochemical features of IL-3 and the related molecules GM-CSF and IL-5 are summarized in Table 2–3.

IL-3 is produced almost exclusively by T lymphocytes of all subsets,[174, 175] although the stimuli adequate for secretion may differ subtly.[176–178] Most studies indicate that T-cell production of IL-3 must be induced by antigen receptor stimulation. However, two studies demonstrated that long-term marrow cultures produce IL-3 at low levels without the addition of standard T-cell stimuli.[5, 179] Much is known of the *cis*-acting and *trans*-acting elements that act on IL-3 gene expression, which include both positive and negative control regions located both proximal and distal to the transcription initiation site.[180–186]

By use of in vitro assays, IL-3 has been shown to possess a number of hematopoietic activities. Cultures of marrow cells containing IL-3 develop colonies composed of basophils, eosinophils, neutrophils, monocytes, and megakaryocytes, alone and in combination, and if EPO is added, both large erythroid bursts and small erythroid colonies also develop.[187–191] Colony formation is also significantly enhanced when IL-3 is used in combination with other cytokines and hormones. Like many other hematopoietic cytokines, IL-3 acts to prime the mature cells it helps produce to become functionally activated[192]; and like all hematopoietic growth factors, IL-3 is thought to act, at least in part, by inhibiting programmed cell death in its target cells. Initial insights into this process have been reported. One effect of IL-3 receptor activation is serine phosphorylation of the antiapoptotic molecule Bcl-2 at position 70.[193] Alanine to Ser 70 mutants of Bcl-2 fail to suppress apoptosis, which suggests its phosphorylation by IL-3 to be a critical functional event. In addition, IL-3 also indirectly induces the phosphorylation of BAD,[194] a dimerization partner of Bcl-2 that blocks its antiapoptotic properties. Serine and threonine

phosphorylation of BAD prevents its inhibition of Bcl-2 and is mediated by an IL-3–initiated pathway involving sequential activation of phosphatidylinositol 3′ (PI3) kinase and Akt, the serine-threonine kinase that phosphorylates BAD.

GM-CSF, an 18 to 30 kDa monomeric protein, is produced by T lymphocytes, endothelial cells, monocytes, and fibroblasts. Like IL-3, GM-CSF is highly modified with both N-linked and O-linked carbohydrate.[195] The human GM-CSF gene is localized on chromosome 5q, just 9 kb downstream of the IL-3 gene,[172] and predicts a polypeptide of 144 amino acids, including a 17 residue secretory leader.[196] The regulation of GM-CSF expression is both similar to and distinct from that of its closest evolutionary homologue, IL-3. Although both genes are transcriptionally upregulated in T lymphocytes in response to similar stimuli (which is at least partly explained by the presence of an NFAT-containing enhancer located 3 and 14 kb upstream of the two genes, respectively), GM-CSF is also produced by fibroblasts, endothelial cells, and monocytes, including those present in the marrow stroma.[197–204] Both transcriptional and post-transcriptional mechanisms are responsible for enhanced expression of GM-CSF[199, 203, 205]; the post-transcriptional mechanisms take the form of alterations in mRNA half-life.[205–207] Although several putative RNA-binding proteins have been identified by a number of techniques,[208–211] including one that correlates with GM-CSF mRNA stability,[212] a complete understanding of how GM-CSF transcript stability is regulated is far from realized.

As its name implies, GM-CSF can support the growth of colonies containing all types of granulocytes and monocytes, alone and in combination. However, the polypeptide can also act in synergy with EPO to support the development of erythroid bursts and with TPO to stimulate the production of megakaryocyte-containing colonies.[213, 214] Many but not all of the effects of GM-CSF are shared with IL-3. GM-CSF has also been shown to prime neutrophils, eosinophils, and monocytes for functional activity.[65, 215] This role appears to be its most important, or at least its only unique physiological function. Data for this contention come from two quarters. Although genetic elimination of the GM-CSF gene in mice fails to affect granulocyte or monocyte production, it is associated with pulmonary alveolar proteinosis,[69] thought to be related to inadequate pulmonary alveolar macrophage function. In addition, about half of humans with the disease harbor a mutation in the β_c chain (see below) of the GM-CSF receptor.[216] Further support for a critical role in macrophage function is the finding that mice deficient in GM-CSF display increased tolerance to LPS-induced sepsis syndromes[217]; peritoneal macrophages were shown to produce less IL-1 and nitric oxide in response to LPS than the phagocytes from control animals.

The gene for human IL-5 localizes to human chromosome 5, close to those of the related cytokines IL-3 and GM-CSF.[172] IL-5 is produced by T lymphocytes, in response to antigenic stimulation. Studies with T-cell clones suggest that a specific subset of T cells, Th2, produce the cytokine[218] and that upregulation is accomplished by transcriptional enhancement.[219] The mature protein is composed of two identical disulfide-linked 115 residue polypeptides, each derived from a 134 amino acid precursor.[220, 221] The M_r of the mature protein is 40 to 45 kDa, half of which is carbohydrate, a modification not essential for cytokine function.[222, 223] The

Table 2–3. Biochemical Properties of the β_c-Related Cytokines

Hormone/Cytokine	No. Amino Acids		Polypeptide M_r (kDa)	Actual M_r (kDa)	Disulfide Location	Carbohydrate (No. and Type)	Chromosome Location	Critical Receptor Binding Residues
	PREDICTED	MATURE PROTEIN						
IL-3[24, 173, 876, 877]	152	133	15.1	25–30	C_{16}–C_{84}	4 N ≥2 O	5q23	D_{21}, E_{22}, E_{43}, D_{44}, I_{47}, E_{50}, R_{54}, R_{94}, E_{119}, N_{120}
GM-CSF[18, 41, 172, 195, 196, 878, 879]	144	127	14.5	18–25	C_{54}–C_{96} C_{88}–C_{121}	2 N ≥3 O	5q23	E_{21}, E_{108}, D_{112}
IL-5[22, 172, 220–223, 880, 881]	134	116	13.2	40	C_{45}–C_{45}* C_{87}–C_{87}*	2 N 1 O	5q23	T_{14}, A_{18}, M_{65}, R_{90}, E_{90}

*Interchain disulfide bonds.

IL-5 homodimer is structurally unique among the hematopoietic cytokines; each monomer contains a four α helix bundle resembling that found in GM-CSF and other hematopoietic cytokines, but the first three helices of each monomer are derived from one subunit and the fourth helix is derived from the partner subunit.[22]

The term initially applied to IL-5 was eosinophil differentiation factor, which aptly describes its function. The administration of neutralizing antibody to the cytokine eliminates parasite-induced eosinophilia,[224] as does its genetic elimination.[225] In vitro, IL-5 supports the development of eosinophilic colony-forming cells, blocks apoptosis of mature eosinophils, and is chemotactic for and activates eosinophils to produce superoxide anion.[226–228] Blood levels of IL-5 are elevated in a proportion of individuals with eosinophilia.[229] Two other cytokines, IL-3 and GM-CSF, have been reported to have potent in vitro and in vivo effects on eosinophil production (see above). Studies in semisolid and suspension cultures have suggested slightly different roles for GM-CSF and IL-3 than for IL-5; GM-CSF and IL-3 act to expand the number of eosinophilic progenitor cells to a greater extent than does IL-5, but because eosinophil output in suspension culture is far greater in the presence of IL-5 than with either of the other two cytokines, IL-5 is thought to have a greater effect on the expansion of developmentally more mature eosinophilic precursors.[189] Although GM-CSF and IL-3 can stimulate eosinophil colony formation in vitro, and administration of either cytokine increases eosinophil levels in mouse and man, they are not essential for eosinophilopoiesis, because genetic elimination of either GM-CSF or IL-3 in mice has no effect on eosinophil production.[230] In contrast, genetic elimination of the IL-5 gene abolishes eosinophil production.[225]

In addition to its effects on eosinophil production, IL-5 activates mature eosinophils.[231] IL-5 also affects B-lymphocyte production and function. B lymphocytes bear IL-5 receptors[232, 233] and respond to IL-5 by proliferation and maturation into immunoglobulin-secreting cells.[234] Part of the effect of IL-5 on lymphocytes may be mediated by IL-5R/IL-2R cross-talk. Introduction of a functional IL-2 receptor into IL-5–dependent cells allows IL-5 to induce phosphorylation of the IL-2R.[235] Of considerable interest, chronic overproduction of IL-5 in a transgenic mouse induces elevated serum levels of immunoglobulins M, E, and A; elevates the numbers of Ly1+/B220+ splenic lymphocytes; and leads to a massive eosinophilia.[236, 237] However, the cells appear normal, and there are no apparent untoward effects of the massive tissue eosinophilic infiltration.[238] Thus, eosinophilia, per se, does not appear to be pathological.

The receptors for IL-3, GM-CSF, and IL-5 are heterodimeric; each consists of a unique polypeptide (GM-CSF-Rα,[94] IL-3-Rα,[239] IL-5-Rα[240]), which binds ligand with low affinity, and one shared by the three receptors, which converts binding to high affinity and transduces signals.[241–244] Because the high-affinity IL-3, GM-CSF, and IL-5 receptors share a common component, their ligands display mutual cross-competition for receptor binding.[245, 246] The low-affinity binding subunits are now termed α chains; the shared, affinity-converting, signaling subunit is specified β$_C$. Many excellent reviews on this topic have been published.[51, 52]

The cloned human IL-3-Rα, GM-CSF-Rα, and IL-5-Rα subunits consist of 378, 400, and 420 amino acids, respectively, and share homology with members of the hematopoietic cytokine receptor family[32] (see Fig. 2–2). Mutagenesis studies have indicated that the cytoplasmic domains of IL-3-Rα, GM-CSF-Rα, and IL-5-Rα are required for full receptor function.[244, 247–250] β$_C$ is 897 amino acids in length and contains an extracellular tandem repeat of the cytokine receptor motif and 438 cytoplasmic residues.[242] The structural basis for β$_C$ action has been reviewed[251] and is discussed at greater length in Chapter 4. However, it must be pointed out here that dimerization of two β$_C$ chains and ligand-induced disulfide bonding between an α and a β subunit[252] are essential for receptor signaling. On the basis of several structural considerations and analogy to the IL-6/IL-6 receptor stoichiometry, it has been proposed that the signaling GM-CSF, IL-3, or IL-5 receptor complexes are composed of two receptor α chains, two β$_C$ polypeptides, and two molecules of ligand.[251, 252]

As for most of the hematopoietic cytokine receptors, soluble forms of GM-CSF-Rα and IL-5-Rα have been described.[240, 243, 253] It is clear that the soluble receptors inhibit the activity of their corresponding ligand[58] by sequestering ligand, blocking its access to the cell surface receptor. The role of these forms in normal physiology was, until recently, poorly understood.[61] However, possible insights into soluble IL-5-Rα function have now been reported. Normally, the soluble form of IL-5-Rα is the more abundant transcript present in activated T cells.[240, 243] However, in asthmatic patients, the level of expression of the transmembrane receptor is directly correlated with the severity of asthma, and the soluble form is inversely related to disease.[254] These findings suggest that the differential expression of the two forms of IL-5-Rα can influence eosinophil-mediated disease and that the two forms might be differentially regulated. A more formal test of this hypothesis is necessary, but if confirmed, the results may point to physiological and pathological roles for soluble forms of hematopoietic receptors.

Finally, in addition to the well-characterized association of the various components of the IL-3, GM-CSF, and IL-5 receptors, studies have begun to suggest that β$_C$ may associate with other hematopoietic receptors, including the EPO and TPO receptors. Evidence for both functional and physical interaction has been presented.[101, 255]

▼ M-CSF AND ITS RECEPTOR, c-Fms

Purification of a soluble form of M-CSF (also termed CSF-1) was accomplished in 1981,[256] but cDNA for the protein was not cloned until several years later.[196, 257] The gene for human M-CSF resides on the short arm of chromosome 1.[258] The secreted mature growth factor is a homodimer composed of two disulfide-linked 165 amino acid polypeptides. As noted above, the M-CSF receptor belongs to the receptor tyrosine kinase family, distinct from the protein family that binds most of the hematopoietic cytokines. Thus, it was surprising to find the tertiary structure of M-CSF to be virtually superimposable on the structures of most of the hematopoietic cytokines.[20] For example, the structural cores of an M-CSF monomer and GM-CSF can be aligned with a mean deviation of only 1.8 Å.[31] The biochemistry of M-CSF and the related cytokines SCF and FL is summarized in Table 2–4.

Table 2–4. Biochemical Properties* of the RTK-Related Hematopoietic Cytokines

Hormone/Cytokine	No. Amino Acids		Polypeptide M_r‡ (kDa)	Actual M_r‡ (kDa)	Disulfide Location	Carbohydrate (No. and Type)	Chromosome Location	Critical Receptor Binding Residues
	PREDICTED	MATURE PROTEIN						
M-CSF[20, 258, 882–884]	554	191–218‡	24.5	45–70	C_7—C_{90} C_{48}—C_{139} C_{102}—C_{146} C_{31}—C_{31}§	2 N ≥2 O	1p13	H_9, H_{15}, V_{78}
SCF[329]	248	165	18.5	45–70	C_4—C_{89} C_{43}—C_{138}	2 N ≥2 O	12q	
FL[344, 346, 885]	235	133–156‡	18	65	C_4—C_{85} C_{44}—C_{132}	2 N ≥2 O	19q13	

* Properties of the soluble isoforms.
† Dimeric M_r given, whether covalent or non-covalent.
‡ Limits of size, precise cleavage site not yet known.
§ Interchain disulfide bond.

M-CSF production is complex. The cytokine is produced by many cell types, including fibroblasts, endothelial cells, and monocytes. Both constitutive and inflammatory mediator-induced expression patterns have been described,[119, 259, 260] using both transcriptional and post-transcriptional mechanisms of regulation.[261–263] M-CSF circulates in the plasma at 3 to 8 ng/ml, levels that increase in a number of myeloproliferative disorders.[264–266] Regulation of circulating levels of the hormone is also mediated by macrophage uptake and destruction of M-CSF.[267]

In addition to circulating M-CSF, transmembrane-bound forms of the cytokine also exist. Multiple mRNA species for M-CSF that encode polypeptides of different fates have been described on the basis of alternative splicing of the primary transcription product (Fig. 2–4). The longest form of the spliced M-CSF transcript encodes a 554 amino acid polypeptide, which is inserted into the cell membrane as a homodimer after removal of the secretory leader sequence. The inclusion of part of intron V with exon 6 during the generation of this splicoform presumably encodes a recognition

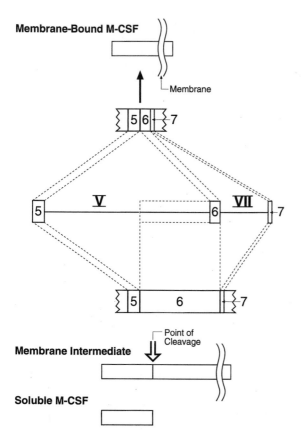

Figure 2–4. Alternative splicing of the primary M-CSF transcript. The germline configuration of the M-CSF locus from exons 5 through 7 is shown, along with two alternative transcription products. Inclusion of part of intron V with the usual exon 6 results in translation of a 554 residue transmembrane polypeptide,[894] a protein released from the cell membrane by cleavage at a site located 191 to 218 residues from its amino terminus.[882] Elimination of the intron V–derived sequence gives rise to a 256 amino acid polypeptide, removing the protease recognition signal or site. This membrane-bound form of the cytokine is only slowly released from the cell surface.[268, 269] Nearly identical mechanisms are likely to account for the generation of soluble and membrane-bound forms of SCF and FL. Exons are drawn to scale, introns are half-size. The proteolytic cleavage site is indicated by a broad arrow.

sequence that allows the rapid release of M-CSF from the cell surface,[268, 269] probably by the same or a similar protease that cleaves membrane-bound SCF a fixed distance from the cell surface.[270] The relationship of this ectodomain shedding protease to the KUZ and TACE proteases involved in Notch and TNF-α processing, respectively, is presently unclear.[271] Elimination of the intron V–derived cleavage signal results in a polypeptide only poorly released from the cell surface.

Two additional levels of M-CSF complexity exist. Alternative splicing of exons 9 and 10 of the M-CSF transcription product has also been described, resulting in differing 3′ UTR of the mRNA molecules. Inclusion of exon 10 adds an AU-rich sequence, possibly affecting protein production by virtue of a reduced mRNA half-life.[206] Finally, post-translational modification of M-CSF also occurs; a proteoglycan version to which chondroitin sulfate has been added can be extracted from marrow stroma.[12] Although the relative biological activities of the various forms of M-CSF have not been studied extensively, it is clear from investigations of the highly homologous SCF polypeptide (see below) that the membrane-bound form of M-CSF is likely to exert a much more prolonged and critical biological effect than the soluble form of the cytokine.

M-CSF was the first colony-stimulating factor purified and was shown to support the growth of monocyte-containing colonies. In addition, like many of the other colony-stimulating factors, M-CSF also functionally activates the mature cells it helps form,[272–275] although not under all circumstances.[276, 277] Mice deficient in M-CSF have reduced numbers of monocytes,[278] but they are not absolutely monocytopenic, nor are double M-CSF/GM-CSF knockout animals. Thus, other pathways to monocyte production remain to be discovered. However, studies of the mutant *op/op* (osteopetrotic) mouse point to the unique physiological contribution of the cytokine. In this naturally occurring mutation of the M-CSF locus, osteopetrosis is due to inadequate function of the osteoclast, a cell derived from marrow monocytes.[278, 279] Thus, like the pulmonary macrophage defect of GM-CSF deficiency, M-CSF appears particularly critical for activating a highly specific developmental program in a mature progeny cell.

The M-CSF receptor was initially identified as the cellular counterpart of the viral oncogene v-*fms*, the transforming gene of the HZ5 feline sarcoma virus.[280, 281] Sequence analysis revealed it to contain five immunoglobulin motifs in its extracellular domain, a single membrane-spanning region, and an interrupted tyrosine kinase motif in its intracytoplasmic domain. The gene is located on the long arm of chromosome 5, close to the platelet-derived growth factor (PDGF) β receptor.[282] Two promoters for the M-CSF receptor have been identified, each responsible for distinct tissue-specific expression.[283, 284] Like many other monocytic genes, activation of the M-CSF receptor promoter is mediated by PU.1 and the C/EBP-AML1 complex[84, 285, 286] and by an enhancer localized to the second intron of the gene.[287]

▼ STEM CELL FACTOR AND THE c-Kit RECEPTOR

Alterations at either the *W* or the *Sl* locus of mice produce variable degrees of anemia, sterility, and changes in coat pigment. Analysis of transplantation studies between normal and the mutant mice[288–291] indicated that *W* probably encoded a hematopoietic receptor and *Sl* its ligand. This hypothesis was confirmed with the cloning and analysis of the c-Kit receptor (*W* locus[292, 293]) and SCF (*Sl* locus[294–299]) genes. An excellent review of the properties of SCF and its receptor has been published.[300]

The cloning of SCF was first reported under a variety of names (SCF, mast cell growth factor, Kit ligand, and steel factor), reflecting the diverse nature of the assays used to identify the protein. The importance of the protein to hematopoiesis is easily demonstrated; although nullizygous mice (*Sl/Sl*) are embryonic lethal owing to a number of developmental defects, the presence of a partially functional allele (*Sl^d*) allows compound heterozygotes (*Sl/Sl^d*) to survive gestation. However, the resultant mice are severely anemic[288] because of diminished numbers of primitive and lineage-committed hematopoietic progenitors in the marrow and spleen.[301–303] In addition to its critical role in hematopoietic ontogeny, treatment of adult mice with a neutralizing monoclonal antibody to the SCF receptor also results in severe pancytopenia,[304] indicating an important hematopoietic role for the receptor/ligand pair throughout life.

The gene for human SCF is located on chromosome 12q and encodes a primary transcript that by alternative splicing can yield at least two polypeptides (SCF[248] and SCF[220]) differing in a 28 amino acid segment midway through the coding region. The ratio of the two forms of SCF transcripts varies widely between tissues,[305, 306] with SCF[248] predominating in marrow stromal cells.[307] Like M-CSF, both splicoforms of SCF first localize to the cell membrane; the longer form is then cleaved by a group of metalloproteases to release a soluble growth factor.[308] Both membrane-bound and soluble SCF exist in equilibrium between monomeric and homodimeric forms, although the monomer predominates at physiological concentrations.[309] However, only the dimeric form is active; mutation to lessen dimer formation reduced SCF activity, forced dimerization enhanced it.

By itself, SCF is only a weak stimulator of hematopoiesis, both in vitro and in vivo, primarily inducing the development of mast cells. However, in the presence of IL-3 or other cytokines (including IL-6, IL-11, G-CSF, and TPO), SCF exerts profound effects on the generation of hematopoietic progenitor cells of all lineages,[310–315] pointing to primitive hematopoietic cells as critical targets. SCF also displays prominent effects on the growth of colony-forming cells. SCF increases both the number of cells per colony and the number of colonies that develop in the presence of EPO, IL-3, GM-CSF, IL-6, IL-11, and TPO.[159, 310, 316–319] The molecular mechanisms of such synergy are beginning to emerge. A physical association of the SCF-R and EPO-R has been detected after SCF stimulation of cells bearing both receptors, an event that is essential for their functional synergy.[100] Moreover, stimulation of cells bearing both receptors with EPO results in SCF-R dimerization.[320] However, despite much progress in understanding the basis for the effects of SCF on hematopoietic progenitor cells, the physiological role of SCF on hematopoietic stem cell survival and expansion has been more difficult to document. For example, although SCF can expand splenic colony-forming units (CFU-S) manyfold[321] and support the survival of highly enriched populations of stem cells,[322] other factors produced

by marrow stromal cells can support hematopoietic stem cell survival when SCF function is eliminated.[323] Moreover, although the biological effects of the membrane-bound form of SCF are greater than those of the soluble growth factor[6, 324] because of prolonged signaling,[325] fibroblasts derived from mice deficient in membrane-bound SCF (*Sl/Sl^d*; see below) can support the survival of primitive hematopoietic cells as well as normal stromal cells.[326]

A number of cell types produce SCF, including endothelial cells, fibroblasts, and purified marrow stromal cells.[307, 327] Inflammatory mediators, such as IL-1β or TNF-α, only minimally affect gene expression, although TGF-β reduces its expression from endothelial cells.[328] These in vitro results are mirrored in vivo; levels of the cytokine (normally 3 ng/ml[329]) do not change with any physiological or pathological state.[330, 331] It is not known whether the proportion of soluble and membrane-bound forms of the growth factor is altered under any stimulus.

The c-Kit receptor, a 145 kDa member of the type III receptor tyrosine kinase family, is expressed in virtually all hematopoietic progenitor cells[292, 332–334] and in many other cells and tissues.[335, 336] Expression levels are low in hematopoietic stem cells, increase and peak at the lineage-committed progenitor cell stage, and then decline in maturing blood cells.[333] Other than its down-modulation secondary to SCF binding or exposure of cells to TGF-β or TNF-α,[337, 338] Kit expression does not appear to be a major target for hematopoietic regulation. Like the other hematopoietic members of this family of proteins, Kit contains five extracellular immunoglobulin domains, the first three of which are important for SCF binding.[339–341] The fourth immunoglobulin domain of Kit has been proposed to facilitate receptor dimerization,[341] but this role is currently disputed.[342] It is clear, however, that the extracellular domain of Kit is necessary and sufficient for ligand-induced dimerization,[343] and the stoichiometry of the interaction is 2:2.[342]

Like so many other hematopoietic cytokine receptors, a soluble form of the Kit receptor exists, is derived from proteolytic cleavage of the membrane-bound form, and circulates at levels 30-fold in excess of its corresponding ligand.[55] Kinetic studies have shown that soluble Kit binds SCF as avidly as the cell surface receptor[59] and can compete with membrane-bound receptor for SCF. However, like many other soluble hematopoietic receptors, the physiological role of soluble Kit is unknown.

▼ Flt3 LIGAND AND THE Flt3/Flk2 RECEPTOR

Flt3 ligand was cloned[344] as the binding partner for a recently identified novel orphan receptor, a protein most closely related to the receptor for SCF (hence Flt, *f*ms-*l*ike *t*yrosine kinase). The protein shares 13 per cent sequence identity with SCF and 10 per cent identity with M-CSF. The gene for FL resides on human chromosome 19q13 and contains 10 exons.[345, 346] The primary FL transcript can undergo at least five forms of alternative splicing, three of which result in variation in the 3′ UTR. However, two distinct forms, which either include or exclude the fifth intron, result in mRNA species that encode 231 or 220 amino acid polypeptides, respectively.[345–347] The first identified form of FL removes the fifth intron, yielding a protein that is transiently expressed on the cell membrane but is then cleaved to yield a soluble homodimeric protein of 60 kDa. Each monomer contains 12 kDa of carbohydrate, which is required for the long plasma half-life of the protein, and two critical disulfide bonds. Inclusion of the fifth intron yields a distinct carboxyl terminus of the polypeptide, which is hydrophobic and inserts into the cell membrane, from which it cannot be removed. Thus, like SCF and M-CSF, both soluble and membrane-bound forms of FL exist, but it remains to be determined whether the biological properties of the two forms differ as for SCF.

FL was initially derived from T cells[344, 348]; subsequent studies indicate that the cytokine is also produced by marrow stromal cells.[8, 349] Blood levels of FL are approximately 15 pg/ml in normal animals and humans; levels can rise to 2500 pg/ml in response to pancytopenia.[345] Interestingly, only pancytopenia, and not individual lineage deficiencies, causes an increase in blood FL concentrations.

Like SCF, FL appears to act on hematopoietic cells only in synergy with other hematopoietic cytokines or hormones.[350, 351] Administration of the recombinant protein to animals and man results in a modest rise in lymphocyte levels, a moderate increase in neutrophils, and a marked increase in monocytes (especially NK and dendritic cells[352, 353]). In particular, these antigen-presenting cells seem particularly dependent on FL, because the combination of FL and TGF-β can generate dendritic cells from CD34-selected marrow cells in serum-free culture.[354] FL also counteracts the inhibitory effects of TGF-β on primitive hematopoietic cells.[355] As expected from the in vitro and in vivo administration experiments, targeted disruption of the FL gene substantially reduces the number of splenic NK and dendritic cells.[352, 356, 357] Like many other hematopoietic cytokines, FL exerts a profound effect on mobilization of hematopoietic stem and progenitor cells.[358, 359] After a 10 day course of FL administration, CD34+ cell levels climb 30-fold above baseline values, and committed colony-forming cells approximately 200- to 300-fold.

The human Flt3 receptor is a 993 amino acid transmembrane polypeptide that belongs to the class III receptor tyrosine kinase family.[360, 361] The gene is located on human chromosome 13q12 and shares 18 per cent and 19 per cent identity with the SCF and M-CSF receptors in their extracellular domains, respectively, including 63 to 64 per cent in the tyrosine kinase domains. Flt3 receptor expression is, for the most part, confined to the hematopoietic system. It is weakly expressed in mature granulocytes and monocytes, is absent from mature T and B cells, but is abundant on primitive hematopoietic cell populations and cell lines representing primitive cell types.[362–364]

▼ INTERLEUKIN-6, INTERLEUKIN-11, LEUKEMIA INHIBITORY FACTOR, AND THE gp130 FAMILY OF RECEPTORS

IL-6, cloned by several groups of investigators with use of several different assays (antiviral activity, myeloma cell growth, hepatocyte growth, immunoglobulin secretion), was later found to affect megakaryocytic and primitive hematopoietic cells.[365] The IL-6 gene is present on the short arm of human chromosome 7 and encodes a 26 kDa polypeptide

produced in almost all tissues from T cells, fibroblasts, macrophages, and stromal cells.[365] The mature protein is composed of 184 amino acids, contains two disulfide bonds, and displays both N-linked and O-linked carbohydrate modification. These and other biochemical features of IL-6 and the related cytokines IL-11 and LIF are presented in Table 2–5.

IL-6 is produced in response to inflammatory (mediated by IL-1 and TNF) and mitogenic stimuli, primarily by transcriptional upregulation. Regulatory elements responsible for IL-6 promoter activation include nuclear factor-κB (NF-κB), activator protein-1 (AP-1)[366, 367] and two forms of CAATT binding proteins, C/EBPβ (formerly known as NF-IL6)[117, 368] and C/EBPδ (formerly known as NF-IL6β).[369, 370] Similar regulatory sites are also present in many other hematopoietic and inflammatory response genes (e.g., TNF, IL-8, and G-CSF[117]). Of interest, many of these transcriptional activators can also be induced by IL-6, thus contributing to a positive feedback loop designed to maintain or amplify the inflammatory response.

Alone, IL-6 fails to exert any significant hematopoietic effects in vitro. However, it acts in synergy with SCF or IL-3 to induce primitive hematopoietic cells into the cell cycle,[315, 371] to augment myelopoiesis,[372, 373] and to modestly enhance megakaryocyte development.[190, 374, 375] The role of IL-6 in steady-state hematopoiesis is uncertain. The predominant phenotype of IL-6–deficient mice is liver failure and defective hepatic regeneration,[376] but the animals also display a modest reduction in the number of T lymphocytes. In contrast, myeloid cell numbers are normal.[377] However, the combined genetic elimination of G-CSF and IL-6 was shown to produce a more severe neutropenia than that found in the G-CSF receptor knockout mouse.[129] It is also clear that IL-6 plays a critical role in neutrophil activation, because genetic IL-6 deficiency obviates the neutrophilic response to *Listeria* or *Candida* infections.[377–379]

IL-11 was cloned as a gibbon marrow stromal cell–derived activity that induced the differentiation of an IL-6–responsive myeloma cell line.[4] However, it was also shown to act in synergy with IL-3 to stimulate megakaryocyte colony formation,[4, 380, 381] enlisting it in the ranks of hematopoietic cytokines. The human IL-11 gene is located on the long arm of chromosome 19[382] and encodes a mature protein containing 199 amino acids. Unlike the other hematopoietic growth factors, IL-11 is devoid of cysteine residues and does not contain sites of N-linked carbohydrate modification.[383] As such, the M_r of IL-11 is close to that predicted by its amino acid sequence, 23 kDa.

IL-11 is constitutively produced from cells of the marrow stroma, especially fibroblasts, and production increases when these cells are stimulated with IL-1, TGF-β, or calcium ionophore.[384, 385] This appears to occur in vivo, because high levels of the cytokine were found in rheumatoid synovial fluid.[386] Blood levels of IL-11 are thought to react to other stimuli; some[387, 388] but not all investigators[389] have found increased IL-11 blood levels in thrombocytopenic patients. The molecular basis for its regulation is only just becoming better understood. The promoter region of the IL-11 gene contains a TATA sequence and an AP-1 site, which promote basal level transcription,[390] and two NF-κB sites, essential for IL-11 induction in response to viral infection in lung epithelial cells.[391] In addition, post-transcriptional mecha-

Table 2–5. Biochemical Properties of the gp130-Related Hematopoietic Cytokines

Hormone/Cytokine	No. Amino Acids		Polypeptide M_r (kDa)	Actual M_r (kDa)	Disulfide Location	Carbohydrate (No. and Type)	Chromosome Location	Critical Receptor Binding Residues
	PREDICTED	MATURE PROTEIN						
IL-6[29, 886–888]	266	185	20.9	26	C_{45}–C_{51} C_{74}–C_{84}	2 N 1 O	7p21	R_{24}, K_{27}, Q_{28}, Y_{31}, G_{35}, E_{52}, S_{53}, S_{54}, K_{55}, E_{56}, L_{57}, E_{59}, K_{66}, A_{68}, E_{69}, K_{70}, Q_{75}, S_{76}, S_{118}, V_{121}, F_{125}, W_{157}, T_{162}, R_{180}, Q_{183}
IL-11[4, 382, 383, 392, 889]	220	199	19.6	23	0	≥2 O	19q13	P_{13}, E_{16}, L_{17}, L_{22}, R_{25}, L_{28}, T_{31}, R_{32}, L_{34}, R_{39}, K_{41}, K_{98}, R_{150}, H_{153}, D_{164}, W_{165}, R_{168}
LIF[408, 890–892]	196	179	19.6	38–67	C_{13}–C_{135} C_{19}–C_{132} C_{61}–C_{64}	7 N ? O	22q12	Q_{25}, S_{28}, Q_{32}, D_{120}, I_{121}, G_{124}, S_{127}, F_{156}, K_{159}, V_{175}

nisms of regulation have also been identified[392]; like that for GM-CSF and other inflammatory response hematopoietic cytokines, marrow stromal cell–derived IL-11 mRNA is stabilized by treatment with IL-1 and by stimulation of protein kinase C.[390]

IL-11 is a pleiotropic cytokine that exerts a multitude of growth stimulatory effects on diverse organs[383, 393–396]; however, the most well studied effects are hematopoietic. Like IL-6, IL-11 acts in synergy with IL-3, SCF, or FL to induce primitive hematopoietic cells into the cell cycle,[133, 397, 398] resulting in expansion in the subsequent numbers of committed progenitor cells.[315, 399, 400] IL-11 acts together with IL-3 or SCF to enhance erythropoiesis[401]; with SCF and G-CSF to augment myelopoiesis[392, 402]; and with IL-3, SCF, or TPO to promote megakaryocyte development.[4, 159, 380, 381, 403] The hematopoietic effects of IL-3 and IL-11 are similar to those reported for IL-3 and IL-6[397] and can be readily explained on the basis of the common receptor signaling components of the complete IL-6 and IL-11 receptors (see below). However, one exception to this general rule may be the differential effects of IL-6 and IL-11 on platelet function. When administered to animals, IL-6 activates platelets, shifting their dose response to platelet agonists.[404, 405] However, such effects have not been reported for IL-11. The explanation for this apparent discrepancy may be the differential expression of the IL-6-Rα and IL-11-Rα subunits.[406]

LIF was initially cloned as an activity that induced leukemic M1 cells to differentiate, thereby to cease proliferation, and independently as a *h*uman *inter*leukin that induced *DA*-1 cells to proliferate (hence the alternative name HILDA).[407] The LIF gene is located on the long arm of human chromosome 22.[408] It encodes a protein composed of 180 amino acids; contains three disulfide bonds; and has seven sites of N-linked carbohydrate modification,[409] a feature that is responsible for its highly heterogeneous molecular mass of 38 to 67 kDa. LIF is produced by monocytes and other marrow stromal cells in response to stimulation with IL-1, TNF-α, or TGF-β.[410, 411] Its effects on hematopoietic cells are similar to those of IL-6 and IL-11[403, 412–414] and so are not discussed further.

With only a few exceptions, the hematopoietic effects of IL-6, IL-11, and LIF are identical. This finding led investigators to propose that the receptors for these cytokines might be related. Subsequent studies revealed this to be the case; the receptors for IL-6, IL-11, and LIF are heterodimers, each composed of a distinct ligand-binding subunit (IL-6-Rα, IL-11-Rα, and LIF-R) and the affinity-converting and signal-transducing subunit gp130.[415–417] The stoichiometry of the final signaling complex appears to be 2:2:2, because IL-6 binding induces gp130 homodimerization, a step required for receptor transphosphorylation and signaling.[418, 419]

The ligand-binding IL-6-Rα polypeptide contains 468 amino acids,[420] including a short cytoplasmic tail that lacks any recognizable homologies (see Fig. 2–2). The transmembrane and cytoplasmic domains are not necessary for function, as demonstrated by the stimulatory effect of soluble forms of the receptor (see below). The M_r of the mature cell surface receptor is 80 kDa, but nearly 40 per cent of its mass is accounted for by carbohydrate modification.[421] Several of the IL-6 binding sites of the IL-6-Rα polypeptide have been mapped by mutagenesis studies[36, 422–424] and align with those

identified in the related receptors for growth hormone, EPO and β_c.

There are two isoforms of the ligand-binding IL-11-R polypeptide (termed α and $\alpha2$) that are 99 per cent identical but somewhat unexpectedly arise from two distinct loci (α[425]; $\alpha2$[426]) on the short arm of human chromosome 9.[427] Interestingly, the two IL-11-R genes are expressed at different sites; IL-11-Rα is expressed widely, and it is the only form in hematopoietic cells; IL-11-R$\alpha2$ transcripts have been identified only in the testis, thymus, and lymph nodes and possibly in the kidney. The relative importance of the two receptors has not been fully evaluated. In addition, a cDNA that encodes a severely truncated version of the receptor has been reported, one that retains its transmembrane but not its intracytoplasmic domain.[427] Whether this protein is actually synthesized and its biological role have not been determined.

Expression of the IL-11-Rα polypeptide (the hematopoietic version) has been eliminated in mice by standard gene targeting strategies.[428] The expected number of $-/-$ pups were born, and no effect on life span was noted. However, $-/-$ females were reported to be infertile. Hematological analysis was unremarkable. Specifically, the $-/-$ mice had normal distributions of B and T cells of all subtypes; there were normal red cell, granulocyte, and platelet levels in peripheral blood; and the marrow cellularity was normal, as was that of the spleen. By use of in vitro colony-forming assays and in vivo assessment of splenic colonies, hematopoietic progenitor cell levels were normal, both under steady-state and stress (after 5-FU and after hydrazine hemolysis recovery experiments) conditions. Thus, unique functions for IL-11 are presently being sought.

Although IL-6, IL-11, and LIF can bind to their respective receptors, the interaction is of low affinity and fails to produce any biological effect. The added presence of gp130 converts each of the receptors to a high-affinity binding complex, one capable of transmitting both proliferative and differentiative signals (see Taga and Kishimoto[54] for an excellent review). The gp130 polypeptide is constitutively present on many if not most hematopoietic cells and is composed of 918 amino acids including several recognizable structural motifs[415] (see Fig. 2–2). The box1 and box2 motifs so critical for signal initiation (see Chapter 4) were first recognized in gp130,[429] as was the box3 domain,[430] a region that serves to dock signaling molecules necessary for the cellular differentiation events that follow binding of ligand to this family of receptors.

The gp130 family of cytokines appears to be essential for hematopoietic development; although targeted disruption of the gp130 locus in mice leads to embryonic lethality because of failure of cardiac development (one member of the gp130 family of receptors is cardiotropin-1), significant reductions in the number of pluripotent hematopoietic progenitors (CFU-S$_{11}$) and variable levels of anemia[431] are also present. Moreover, the importance of the hematopoietic effects of gp130-related cytokines is reinforced by the finding that transgenic expression of both IL-6 and IL-6-Rα in mice expands the numbers of primitive hematopoietic progenitor cells.[432] Unfortunately, which of the gp130-related cytokines is responsible for this aspect of hematopoiesis remains uncertain. Because of the substantial overlap in hematopoietic functions displayed by IL-6, IL-11, and LIF and their ubiquitous patterns of expression, individual cytokine receptor knockout experiments may fail to produce any hematopoietic defects (e.g., targeted disruption of neither IL-11-Rα nor LIF results in any hematopoietic phenotype).[428, 433] However, an important caveat to note before accepting the importance of gp130 in hematopoiesis is that these cytokines may play an important role only during development and not during adult hematopoiesis. Support for this notion comes from the much greater effect of oncostatin M, a gp130-related cytokine, on fetal hematopoietic progenitor development than on adult cells.[434]

▼ INTERLEUKIN-1 AND ITS RECEPTORS

Interleukin-1 is the quintessential multifunctional cytokine. It has effects on virtually every organ, acting in concert with other tissue-specific and pleiotropic agents to enhance the inflammatory response. Because much of blood cell production is devoted to host defense, IL-1 exerts considerable influence on hematopoiesis. The effects of the cytokine have been extensively reviewed.[435]

There are three IL-1–related polypeptides (Fig. 2–5), IL-1α, IL-1β, and IL-1 receptor antagonist (IL-1-Ra). All three are evolutionarily related as evidenced by their clustering within 430 kb on human chromosome 2q.[436] IL-1α and IL-1β are synthesized as 31 kDa precursor polypeptides rich in β-pleated sheet structure. Unlike most of the hematopoietic cytokines, the IL-1 polypeptides do not contain secretory leader sequences. Rather, the IL-1α and IL-1β precursor forms are cleaved intracellularly, by calpain or interleukin-1β–converting enzyme (ICE), respectively, to form the 17 kDa proteins found in the circulation. In contrast, IL-1-Ra has evolved to contain a leader peptide and is secreted from the cell soon after its synthesis. Being the only secreted protein among the three, only IL-1-Ra contains carbohydrate modification, increasing its M_r to 22 kDa.

IL-1α, IL-1β, and IL-1-Ra share at most 26 per cent amino acid sequence identity, although the tertiary structures of all three are similar,[437–439] and all bind to the IL-1 receptor with similar high affinity.[440, 441] IL-1α is produced by monocytes in response to cellular activation, with a broad range of proximate stimuli including phagocytosis, adhesion, hypoxia, thermal injury, radiation, inflammatory complement components, fibrin degradation products, other cytokines (TNF-α, IL-2, or GM-CSF), and surface membrane integrin engagement. IL-1 plasma levels rise in response to pathological inflammatory states, including sepsis, thermal burns, autoimmune disease, and graft rejection, and IL-1 appears to be a critical component of the host response. For example, the administration of IL-1Ra to LPS-injected patients leads to a 50 per cent reduction in the induced neutrophilia.[442] There are several points in the IL-1α and IL-1β biosynthetic pathways subject to regulatory control, including their rate of transcription, mRNA stability, translation efficiency, subcellular localization, and proteolytic processing.[211, 443–449]

Once synthesized, IL-1α is fully active[450] but must be released from its cell of origin to gain access to conventional target cells. One mechanism is its release from dying cells. In addition, a fraction of IL-1α is localized to the cell membrane by myristoylation,[451] allowing its release on calpain-mediated proteolysis.[452] However, the major circulating form of IL-1 is IL-1β, forcing investigators to consider other roles for IL-1α. Evidence is accumulating for its role as an intracellular autocrine stimulator of multiple cellular processes.[453–455] Moreover, an intriguing mechanism is in place to provide an intracellular autocrine loop; on cleavage by calpain, the IL-1α propiece (which contains a nuclear localization signal and a DNA-binding segment) or possibly the mature IL-1α bound to intracellular IL-1-RI is retained in the cell and translocated to the nucleus.[455, 456] Unfortunately, the nature of the signals generated by this mechanism is not yet understood.

Unlike IL-1α, the majority of IL-1β precursor is inactive until processed to the mature form by ICE,[457, 458] although alternative processing events mediated by other proteases have also been described.[459–461] The regulation of ICE activity is not well understood; LPS increases its activity,[462] increased intracellular potassium may do the same,[463] and maturation of monocytes into macrophages reduces their capacity to process proIL-1β.[464] Once processed, mature IL-1β is released by the cell, although this event is also poorly understood, because the polypeptide lacks any obvious secretory signal.[465]

Of the two cytokines, IL-1β appears to be more important than IL-1α. For example, IL-1α knockout mice continue to mount an acute phase and febrile response to inflammatory stimuli; IL-1β–deficient animals do not, nor do they develop collagen-induced arthritis. IL-1β appears to function as a hormone, designed to evoke a systemic inflammatory response, including the hematopoietic system.[466, 467] Its success in doing so is moderated by three proteins: soluble IL-1-R, which sequesters the cytokine, preventing its access to the cell surface receptor; IL-1-Ra, which competes directly with IL-1β for binding to IL-1-R; and IL-1-RII, which binds IL-1β but does not lead to a productive signal (see Fig. 2–5).

The physiological response to IL-1, once it is bound to the complex of IL-1-RI and its accessory binding protein (IL-1R-AcP), is dictated by the cellular target. IL-1-RI is

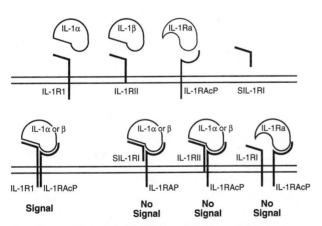

Figure 2–5. The IL-1 system of ligands and receptors. Three IL-1 ligands and four receptor-like proteins compose the system. There are two IL-1 receptors, type I and II, each derived from a distinct gene.[895] A soluble (s) form of these receptors also exists. IL-1-R-AcP, which does not bind IL-1 itself but increases IL-1-RI binding affinity for the cytokine,[896] is required to trigger a productive signal. Only engagement of IL-1-RI and IL-1-R-AcP together by IL-1α or IL-1β induces a productive signal. Although IL-1-RII can bind IL-1α or IL-1β with an affinity equal to that of IL-1-RI, it fails to signal because of an inadequate intracytoplasmic domain. Engagement of IL-1-R-AcP by IL-1-Ra fails to recruit IL-1-RI, again acting to block signaling.

expressed on endothelial cells, smooth muscle cells, fibroblasts, monocytes, and T lymphocytes. IL-1 and TGF-β down-modulate and prostaglandin E_2, IL-2, IL-4, and dexamethasone increase IL-1-RI expression.[468–470] However, this discussion is restricted to the hematopoietic system and its supporting microenvironment. IL-1 exerts its effects through increasing gene expression, either by increasing transcription or by decreasing mRNA degradation. Target genes important for hematopoiesis include cytokines (GM-CSF,[2, 114, 199, 200] G-CSF,[2, 114, 199] M-CSF,[199, 471] IL-6,[472–477] LIF,[475] interferon-γ [IFN-γ],[476, 477] and IL-8 and other chemokines[478–480]); cytokine receptors (IL-2-Rα,[481] c-Kit,[482, 483] $β_C$[484]); proto-oncogenes involved in hematopoietic cell proliferation and differentiation (c-*jun*,[485, 486] c-*abl*,[487] c-*myc*,[488] c-*fos*[489, 490]); and adhesion molecules present on leukocytes, hematopoietic progenitors, and marrow stromal cells (intercellular adhesion molecule-1,[479] endothelial leukocyte adhesion molecule-1,[491] vascular cell adhesion molecule-1,[492] and L-selectin[493]). In addition to its indirect effects on hematopoiesis, IL-1 acts directly on primitive hematopoietic cells to enhance the response to other cytokines. When added to marrow cell cultures containing M-CSF or GM-CSF, IL-1β profoundly augments the proliferative potential of cells capable of forming leukocyte-containing colonies.[494, 495] The net hematopoietic result is myelopoietic stimulation (e.g., enhanced expression of G-CSF, GM-CSF, M-CSF), leukocyte activation (through chemokines, integrins, and selectins), and erythropoietic inhibition (indirectly through IFN-γ).

▼ TUMOR NECROSIS FACTORS AND THEIR RECEPTORS

TNF-α is one of a family of proteins related by virtue of common receptor structures. Other members of the family play important roles in the immune response and include CD40 and its ligand, mutation of which results in the immunodeficiency/hyperimmunoglobulin M syndrome, and Fas and its ligand, deficiency of which results in autoimmunity due to insufficient apoptotic elimination of autoreactive lymphocyte clones. Although few of the ligands for these receptors display structural homology, TNF-α is related to lymphotoxin (also termed TNF-β), with which it shares an adjacent (1 kb away) chromosomal locus and 30 per cent sequence homology; because of an identical receptor structure, it has been presumed that the only differences in the biology of the two are the cells in which they are produced and the kinetics of their release. However, deficiency of TNF-β leads to a developmental deficiency of peripheral lymph nodes, a function that apparently cannot be fully compensated by an intact TNF-α gene.[496] Excellent reviews discussing the biology of the TNFs and their receptors have appeared.[497–499]

The genes for TNF-α and TNF-β localize to the human major histocompatibility locus on chromosome 6.[499] The structures of both proteins have been determined by X-ray crystallography.[500, 501] The active form of each is trimeric; each monomer is composed primarily of two sheets, each consisting of eight β strands. The overall organization is termed the β-jellyroll fold. The structure of TNF-β bound to its p55 receptor subunit has also been solved[502] and reveals receptor trimerization induced by ligand binding. It is presumed that the ligand-induced clustering of the three receptor monomers is responsible for signal transduction.

Activated macrophages and lymphocytes are the most important sources of TNF-α and TNF-β, respectively. Events and agents known to activate macrophages to produce TNF-α include LPS,[503] phagocytosis of opsonized (antibody-coated) and non-opsonized particles,[504] cross-linking of the Fc receptor,[505] and exposure of cells to cytokines.[201, 506] IFN-γ augments macrophage TNF-α production in the presence of any of these other stimulatory agents.[507] Multiple mechanisms account for enhanced expression of the TNF genes and include transcriptional, post-transcriptional, translational, and post-translational processes.[435, 508–514]

Like IL-1, TNF qualifies as a quintessential pleiotropic cytokine. Virtually every type of cell seems capable of responding to TNFs, because all bear receptors. The cytokine plays an important role in numerous physiological and pathological reactions including sepsis, graft-versus-host disease, granulomatous disorders, and autoimmunity. Important target cells are macrophages and neutrophils, of which TNF is a potent inflammatory activator of the superoxide and nitric oxide pathways,[515, 516] and endothelial cells and fibroblasts, which are induced to display integrins, become procoagulant, and produce hematopoietic growth factors.[497, 517–519] TNF-α is also an important direct inhibitor of hematopoietic progenitor cells.

TNF-α and TNF-β are inducers of GM-CSF, G-CSF, and M-CSF production by endothelial cells and fibroblasts,[199, 506] IL-1 and IL-6 production by smooth muscle and endothelial cells,[497, 520, 521] IFN-γ from lymphocytes (in conjunction with IL-2[522]), and chemokines including IL-8 from dermal fibroblasts and keratinocytes.[523, 524] However, not all of its effects are stimulatory. In general, the *direct* effects of TNF-α are to inhibit hematopoietic stem and progenitor cells; the net effect of TNF on any given hematopoietic cell type is the result of opposing actions. For example, although TNF-α directly inhibits stem cells, it also acts to eliminate TGF-β expression, and because TGF-β is an important inhibitor of stem cell cycling, at low levels TNF-α actually stimulates stem cell expansion.[525] In a similar way, the direct inhibitory effects of TNF-α on granulocyte-macrophage progenitor cell growth is overcome by its stimulatory effects on GM-CSF and G-CSF production, the net result being increased leukocyte production. In contrast, because TNF-α directly inhibits erythroid progenitor cell growth[526] and reduces EPO production,[527–529] the net effect on erythropoiesis is inhibitory.

There are two distinct TNF receptors, of M_r 55 and 75 kDa, each containing three or four (respectively) of the 40 amino acid motifs that characterize this receptor family. The two receptors bind TNF-α and TNF-β with comparable affinities, despite sharing only 27 per cent amino acid identity. Like most other hematopoietic growth factor receptors, the TNF receptors do not contain recognizable tyrosine kinase motifs. However, the most remarkable feature of the cytoplasmic region of most of the receptors in this family is the "death domain," a sequence present in p55 but not p75, capable of triggering programmed cell death. The absence of this domain in p75 suggests differential effects of the two receptors, although this aspect of TNF biology is presently incompletely understood. However, it is clear that p55 plays a distinct physiological role; genetic elimination of the gene leads to resistance to the toxic effects of TNF during sepsis and to a specific defect in the ability of macrophages to kill intracellular pathogens such as *Listeria*.[530, 531] At least for these two effects of TNF, p75 cannot substitute.

▼ INTERFERONS AND THE INTERFERON RECEPTOR FAMILY

The interferons are proteins first defined by their ability to induce an antiviral state in mammalian cells. Biochemical fractionation has revealed three classes of interferons: IFN-α, a family of 17 distinct but highly homologous molecules; IFN-β, a single molecule more distantly related to the various isoforms of IFN-α; and IFN-γ, a unique molecule that shares functional properties but not structure with the others. Because IFN-γ exerts the most profound hematological effects of the three classes of proteins, it is the focus of this discussion. Several excellent and comprehensive reviews on IFN-γ have been published.[532-534]

The human IFN-γ gene localizes to chromosome 12[535] and encodes a 166 amino acid polypeptide that includes a 23 residue secretory leader sequence.[536] The mature polypeptide forms a non–covalently linked homodimer consisting of two 17 kDa subunits, each modified with three N-linked carbohydrate side chains yielding a 50 kDa protein.[536] The crystal structure of IFN-γ has been solved[537, 538] and reveals an antiparallel dimer of two highly α-helical subunits. The carbohydrate modification appears to aid in the proper alignment of the dimer, but once the dimer is formed, carbohydrate does not affect the biological activity of the protein.[539] The dimeric structure allows a single IFN-γ to simultaneously bind two IFN-γ Rα subunits.[540]

IFN-γ is produced by activated T lymphocytes and NK cells in response to T-cell antigen cross-linking and in response to stimulation by TNF-α, IL-12, or IL-15.[541-544] The cytokine displays pleiotropic effects, because more than 200 genes are known to be regulated by IFN-γ.[534] Prominent hematological effects include activation of macrophages to assume an inflammatory phenotype (e.g., secretion of TNF-α and enhanced tumor cell killing); upregulation of major histocompatibility complex class I and class II molecules, enhancing antigen recognition responses; and inhibition of proliferative responses in a wide variety of cell types. All of the effects of the cytokine can be viewed as part of a coordinated immune response to infectious disease. This statement is supported by analysis of animals in which IFN-γ, its receptor, or STAT1 (the primary intracellular signal-transducing molecule employed by the IFN-γ receptor) is genetically eliminated; all have subtle defects of immune function that are made obvious by infectious challenge.[545-548]

Of particular importance for blood cell production, IFN-γ inhibits hematopoietic colony growth[549, 550] by several mechanisms. First, the cytokine can directly induce programmed cell death in hematopoietic progenitor cells[551] by inducing a Fas-based suicide loop.[552] Second, the cytokine can induce apoptosis through induction of other death-associated proteins (DAP1 to DAP5[553-556]), although their relevance for hematopoiesis is not yet certain. Third, IFN-γ inhibits primitive hematopoietic cells by inducing nitric oxide and interferon regulatory factor-1 in CD34+ cells.[557] Finally, IFN-γ indirectly affects hematopoietic progenitors

by inducing the expression of inhibitory chemokines, such as IP-10.[558]

The gene for the primary IFN-γ receptor (termed IFN-γ-Rα) resides on human chromosome 6,[559] and the encoded polypeptide binds its ligand with high affinity. However, genetic evidence suggested that a distinct molecule encoded by a gene on human chromosome 21 is also required for cellular responses to IFN-γ. The cloning of IFN-γ-Rβ confirmed this hypothesis.[560] Nearly all cells express the IFN-γ-Rα polypeptide. Cell surface expression of the polypeptide does not appear be modulated, a finding reinforced by analysis of the promoter, which resembles that of many housekeeping genes.[533] In contrast to that for IFN-γ-Rα, the promoter region of IFN-γ-Rβ includes the binding sites for many inflammatory response mediators, indicating that a cell's capacity to respond to IFN-γ is a controlled event, regulated at the level of IFN-γ-Rβ expression.[533] A third subunit, also located on human chromosome 21, is required for transmission of some (e.g., initiating an antiviral state) but not all signals emanating from the IFN-γ receptor complex.[560]

IFN-γ-Rα binds its ligand with high affinity, further increased about fourfold in the presence of IFN-γ-Rβ.[533] Moreover, the cytoplasmic domain of IFN-γ-Rβ probably provides a critical component of the signaling complex, because analysis of the structure of an IFN-γ/IFN-γ-Rα co-crystal provides much room for α/β interactions.[533] Once bound, IFN-γ is quickly internalized and destroyed, allowing the receptor to recycle to the cell surface. However, this event is not essential for signaling; mutations in the IFN-γ-Rα subunit that fail to internalize are still competent to signal.[561]

▼ TRANSFORMING GROWTH FACTOR-β AND ITS RECEPTORS

Five isoforms of TGF-β have been described, β1 to β5, which share 60 to 80 per cent homology. Most tissues produce one or more forms of TGF-β; hematopoietic tissues produce primarily TGF-β1.[562] Each of the TGF-β isoforms is a disulfide-linked homodimer, each subunit containing 112 residues. The disulfide linkage pattern (one interchain and four intrachain bonds) is identical in each isoform of the protein, which serves to maintain a highly elongated tertiary structure.[563]

The biochemistry of active TGF-β production is complex. TGF-β subunits are synthesized as inactive 390 amino acid precursors, which dimerize and are proteolyzed to an inactive complex containing a dimeric TGF and its two amino-terminal dimeric remnants.[564] In many tissues, an additional inhibitory 125 kDa polypeptide, termed latent TGF-binding protein (LTBP), binds to the TGF-β complex. Both of these forms of TGF-β are inactive. Removal of the inhibitory remnant dimer (because of its function, the remnant is termed a latency-associated peptide [LAP]) and LTBP requires strong physical or chemical treatment; as such, the cellular processes that normally lead to the release and activation of circulating TGF-β are poorly understood. Evidence for additional proteolysis has been presented.

Once liberated of its corresponding LAPs and LTBP, each isoform of TGF-β can bind to a variety of cell surface

TGF-β receptors. There are presently at least five receptor classes described (cDNA from three of the classes has been cloned[565, 566]), which demonstrate a limited degree of tissue specificity (e.g., type III receptors are not expressed in hematopoietic cells, and type IV are displayed only in the pituitary). Only modest structural homology is shown across the different classes of TGF-β receptors (primarily the clusters of cysteine residues), although the type I receptors are closely related to one another. Most of the receptors are serine-threonine kinases (type III being the exception), and most cells display both type I and type II receptors. A number of experimental approaches have shown that TGF-β acts to bring together type I and II receptors, although recent evidence suggests that a tetramer of two type I dimers and two type II dimers may constitute the active receptor complex.[567] Once engaged, the TGF-β receptor complex induces phosphorylation of a number of substrates. The best understood TGF pathways involve Rb and p27. By indirectly reducing phosphorylation of Rb,[568] TGF-β maintains the transcription factors necessary for entry into S phase in an inactive, sequestered state.[569] And by enhancing expression of p27, an inhibitor of the cyclin E/Cdk2 kinase complex, TGF-β blocks the step critical for progression from G_1 to S.[570] The net result is a late G_1 cell cycle arrest. The importance of its antiproliferative effect on inflammatory cells becomes most apparent by examination of the TGF-β1 knockout mouse; the animals die within 4 weeks of birth of an overexuberant inflammatory reaction.[571]

The hematopoietic effects of TGF-β are primarily inhibitory, at least for progenitor cells derived from adult bone marrow.[525, 572–574] Because hematopoietic cells secrete TGF-β and bear receptors for it, the potential for an inhibitory autocrine loop exists. Support for this concept comes from many investigators. The addition of a neutralizing antibody to TGF-β enhances total cell output 5- to 20-fold from long-term marrow cultures,[575] erythroid colony growth 3- to 25-fold from purified erythroid progenitors,[576] and multilineage hematopoietic colony formation from highly purified (CD34 + +/CD38 −) adult marrow cells.[525] However, the developmental stage of the hematopoietic cells must be taken into account in considering the effects of any cytokine. A similar population of highly purified (CD34 + +/CD38 −) hematopoietic cells derived from fetal liver was hardly affected by neutralizing the cytokine.[525] In contrast to its effects on primitive hematopoietic colony-forming cells, TGF-β fails in some but not all studies to affect cells committed to a single hematopoietic lineage.[562]

In addition to the direct effects of TGF-β on cell cycle regulators of primitive hematopoietic progenitor cells, the cytokine can exert indirect effects on hematopoiesis. For example, TGF-β is a potent inhibitor of the production of SCF[328] and can down-modulate the expression of receptors for many hematopoietic growth factors.[328, 577] This effect can be balanced by other cytokines (e.g., TNF-α) that act to stimulate growth factor release from the marrow stroma. Somewhat paradoxically, TGF-β also stimulates the production of other hematopoietic growth factors from marrow stromal cells.[578] Obviously, the net effect of TGF-β on hematopoiesis is complex and is dependent on the developmental stage of the cell under study and the precise growth factor and cytokine environment in which it is placed.

▼ CHEMOKINES AND THEIR RECEPTORS

Although chemokines were initially thought to primarily affect leukocyte trafficking, our appreciation of the scope of chemokine action has broadened considerably in recent years. Genetic evidence suggests that as many as 50 chemokines may eventually be characterized. An excellent review of the chemokines has been published.[579]

At present, four subfamilies of chemokines can be recognized on the basis of biochemical and genetic criteria. For the most part, chemokines are small polypeptides containing four cysteine residues, of M_r ranging from 8 to 12 kDa. The CXC chemokines, so named because of their characteristic spacing of amino-terminal cysteine residues (Cys-anything-Cys), cluster on the long arm of chromosome 14, with the exception of stromal cell–derived factor-1 (SDF-1). In addition to the CXC homology, members of this subfamily also contain three β sheets and two other spatially conserved cysteine residues. The CC subfamily shares most structural features with the CXC family, except that it has adjacent rather than spaced cysteine residues in the amino terminus. The CC subfamily of chemokines maps to the long arm of human chromosome 17. Each of the remaining two subfamilies consists of a single member at present. Lymphotactin,[580] a potent attractant for T lymphocytes but not for monocytes, is the only member of the C subfamily, containing only two of the four characteristic cysteine residues, only one of which is in the amino terminus. The gene maps to chromosome 1q23. Neurotactin,[581] the only member of what is now termed the CX_3C subfamily, retains the four cysteine residues and three β sheets characteristic of chemokines but is part of a large mucinous transmembrane protein, containing a "chemokine domain" at its amino terminus. The neurotaxin gene maps to chromosome 16.

The chemokines share significant amino acid sequence homology and highly similar tertiary folds. The multimer state of the active molecule is presently controversial. Although chemokines are homodimeric in crystalline form,[579] some investigators argue that monomeric chemokines bind more avidly to chemokine receptors than to their partner molecule.[582] Moreover, mutant forms of IL-8 that can no longer dimerize remain fully active.[583] However, mutant forms of monocyte chemoattractant protein-1 (MCP-1) that no longer bind to chemokine receptors inhibit the activity of the native molecule. This finding suggests that such mutants act in a dominant negative fashion, necessitating dimeric biology.[584]

The prototypical CXC chemokine is IL-8, a polypeptide with potent neutrophil-specific chemotactic activity,[585] a property shared with other CXC chemokines bearing an amino-terminal Glu-Leu-Arg (ELR) tripeptide.[586] Both the ELR sequence and its close proximity to the amino terminus of the protein are necessary for neutrophil chemotactic activity.[579] IL-8 is a 72 amino acid peptide synthesized by monocytes, lymphocytes, neutrophils, and endothelial cells, although endothelial cells produce a 77 residue peptide containing an amino terminal extension. The long form of IL-8 is thought to play a role in leukocyte diapedesis through the endothelium.[587] A second CXC chemokine is GRO-α,[588] a molecule with potent neutrophil chemotactic activity. GRO-α was initially identified in a number of assays (as the PDGF-inducible gene *KC,* as melanocyte growth stimulatory activity, and as a differentially expressed gene in tumor cells[588-590]), reflecting its multiple activities. Other amino-terminal ELR chemokines include neutrophil-activating peptide-2 (NAP-2), GRO-β, GRO-γ, epithelial cell–derived neutrophil attractant-78 (ENA-78), and granulocyte chemotactic protein-2 (GCP-2). Overproduction of IL-8 in a transgenic mouse blocks neutrophil mobilization in response to a local challenge by overwhelming the local concentration gradients of the chemokine on which chemotaxis is based. This and other experiments administering IL-8 to mice[591] attest to the importance of this chemokine in neutrophil recruitment.[592]

Additional CXC chemokines display a myriad of actions. Human platelet basic protein (PBP) contains 94 amino acids, including an ELR tripeptide 26 residues from the amino terminus. Hence, PBP is not a neutrophil chemoattractant. However, proteolysis of nine amino-terminal residues of PBP yields connective tissue–activating peptide III (CTAP-III), a weak fibroblast mitogen and potent inducer of matrix glycoprotein production. Removal of four additional residues from CTAP-III yields β-thromboglobulin, a chemoattractant for fibroblasts, and removal of a total of 24 amino acids from PBP yields NAP-2. Once cleaved to NAP-2, the ELR sequence becomes residues 2 to 4 of the peptide, which converts it to a potent chemoattractant for neutrophils. In purified platelets, CTAP-III predominates, with only 10 to 30 per cent of the protein full-length PBP.[593] Platelet factor-4 (PF-4), found in platelet α granules, is a weak fibroblast chemoattractant[594] but potently inhibits endothelial cell proliferation after further proteolytic processing.[595] IP-10 is produced by many IFN-γ–stimulated cells, including monocytes, lymphocytes, and endothelial cells, and acts to inhibit angiogenesis[596, 597] and to attract certain classes of lymphocytes.[598] Finally, SDF-1α and SDF-1β were cloned from a bone marrow stromal cell line.[599] SDF-1α has gained much notoriety as the ligand that binds to lymphocyte CXCR4, a co-receptor for the human immunodeficiency virus.[600, 601] SDF-1α stimulates the growth of pre-B lymphocytes (hence, its alternative name PBSF) and displays potent chemoattractant effects on CD34+ hematopoietic progenitor cells,[602] possibly explaining mechanisms of stem cell localization to the marrow. The phenotype of SDF-1α nullizygous mice is consistent with these activities; the mice display greatly reduced numbers of B lymphocytes and myeloid progenitor cells.[603] More recently, SDF-1α has been shown to augment TPO-induced megakaryocyte formation[604] and to promote proplatelet formation and transmigration of mature megakaryocytes through bone marrow endothelial cells.[605] Neither TPO nor SCF displays these activities.

MCP-1 is a CC chemokine first purified from smooth muscle cells.[606] As its name (monocyte chemoattractant protein) implies, MCP-1 induces expression of the monocyte integrins necessary for chemotaxis.[607, 608] The protein also attracts T but not B cells toward endothelial cells and helps generate and induce granule release from NK cells.[609] MCP-1 is also a potent stimulus of basophil histamine release.[471] Like the results with transgenic overexpression of IL-8, overexpression of MCP-1 in vivo makes monocytes resistant to the local concentration gradients of the chemokine, rendering the mice more susceptible to organisms normally disposed by monocyte-based killing.[610] MCP-2 and MCP-3 display activities similar to those of MCP-1, although the chemotaxis and cellular activation profile of MCP-2 and

MCP-3 is slightly greater (activating eosinophils and dendritic cells as well as monocytes[611]). MCP-4 and MCP-5 have been cloned more recently[612, 613] and display varying chemoattractant potencies for monocytes, T lymphocytes, and eosinophils. Despite these seemingly distinct profiles of activities, the structure-function relationships of the MCPs are subtle. For example, full-length MCP-1 induces the release of basophil but not eosinophil granules; removal of only the amino-terminal residue nearly eliminates basophil activity but converts the chemokine to a potent activator of eosinophils.[614] This finding suggests that regulated proteolysis of chemokines may be capable of tailoring the leukocyte response to specific insults.

MIP-1α and MIP-1β were first identified in LPS-stimulated monocytes (hence the designation macrophage inflammatory proteins[615, 616]) and attract and activate monocytes and neutrophils. Both also attract lymphocytes; MIP-1α affects CD8+ cells, and MIP-1β primarily affects CD4+ cells.[617] Other human CC chemokines that exert overlapping activities on monocytes, granulocytes, and lymphocytes include RANTES,[618] eotaxin,[619] TARC,[620] and I309.[621]

In addition to their effects on the migration of mature hematopoietic cells, both CXC and CC chemokines play an important role in hematopoietic cell development.[622] Many of the chemokines are produced in marrow stromal cells, and expression can be upregulated in response to inflammatory cytokines by multiple mechanisms.[578, 623, 624] MCP-1, MIP-1α, GRO-β, IP-10, PF-4, ENA-78, IL-8, and lymphotaxin have been reported to inhibit colony formation from CFU-GEMM (granulocytes, erythroid cells, macrophages, and megakaryocytes), CFU-GM, and BFU-E[558, 625-627] and hematopoiesis in vivo.[628] Interestingly, in most cases, the chemokines inhibit colony formation in response to combinations of stimulatory cytokines (e.g., SCF plus GM-CSF) but not to single cytokines, findings that imply the chemokines primarily inhibit immature progenitor cells. Chemokines that bear an amino-terminal ELR sequence (IL-8, NAP-2, MIP-1α, MIP-1β) are particularly effective at inhibiting megakaryocyte colony formation.[629] Although active alone, chemokines display profound inhibitory synergy, with up to 2500-fold enhanced potency when present in combination in vitro and in vivo.[628] Hematopoietic stem cells also appear to be inhibited by the chemokines,[630] effects that can be observed in vivo; the administration of chemokines to animals protects hematopoietic stem and progenitor cells from S phase–specific chemotherapeutic agents.[631]

One of the most complex features of chemokine physiology is their receptor promiscuity. At present, four CXC and seven CC receptors have been identified. All are members of the seven transmembrane domain, G protein–coupled receptor family. Like many other similar receptors, ligand engagement induces a fall in cyclic adenosine monophosphate levels, but other second message pathways, including PI3 kinase and mitogen-activated protein (MAP) kinase, are also involved in chemokine signaling.[632] Multiple chemokines bind to individual receptors, and a single chemokine can bind to multiple receptors. For example, of the four CXC receptors, IL-8 uses CXCR1 and CXCR2; GRO, NAP-2, and ENA bind CXCR2; CXCR3 is engaged by IP-10 and monokine induced by IFN-γ (MIG); and SDF-1α uses CXCR4.[579] The seven CC receptors also display substantial cross-reactivity. However, some specificity exists; CCR3 was cloned from eosinophils, and only the eosinophilic chemoattractants (eotaxin, RANTES, MCP-2, MCP-3, and MCP-4) bind with high affinity. Nonetheless, given this level of ligand promiscuity, studies with targeted gene disruption are required to determine the unique and redundant aspects of each chemokine/chemokine receptor interaction. Such studies have begun to provide insights. Elimination of CCR1 prevents response to MIP-1α, resulting in abnormal leukocyte trafficking and impaired response to fungal and parasitic infection.[633] In contrast, other chemokine receptors are inhibitory; genetic elimination of CXCR2 leads to a large expansion of hematopoietic progenitors in vivo.[634]

▼ Jagged AND ITS RECEPTOR, Notch

Notch was first identified in *Drosophila melanogaster* and *Caenorhabditis elegans* as a gene critical for decisions of cell fate. In general, *Notch* and its paralogues are concerned not with directing precursor cells along specific lineages but rather with modulating their ability to respond to specific lineage-inducing signals. The field of signaling from Notch proteins has been reviewed.[635]

A mammalian homologue of *Notch* was first recognized as *Tan-1*, a gene present at the t(7;9) breakpoint of several T-cell leukemias.[636–638] The oncoprotein encoded by the rearranged gene is a truncated version of a human *Notch* homologue, its normally large extracellular domain eliminated. When introduced into marrow cells, the rearranged gene induces a nearly identical T-cell leukemia.[639] Normal Notch protein homologues have now been identified in many tissues of mammals. Constitutively active mutant forms of Notch have been shown to profoundly affect hematopoietic lineage decisions.[640, 641] However, although such gain of function experiments suggest that the normal genes may play a role in hematopoiesis, they do not establish it. Therefore, although the following discussion of the role of Notch in hematopoiesis is likely to be correct in concept, it is subject to changes in detail. Notch and its ligands clearly represent a hematological work in progress.

Human paralogues of *Notch* genes encode large (~300 kDa) transmembrane receptors composed of several (~36) epidermal growth factor motifs in their extracellular domains and an intracellular domain that interacts with transcriptional regulators.[642] Six distinct mammalian ligands for Notch receptors have been identified, including homologues of the *Drosophila delta* and *serrate* genes.[643–645] The mechanism by which Notch signals is hotly debated. By use of constitutively active forms of the natural receptor, initial studies suggested that nuclear translocation of all or part of the receptor was necessary for Notch function.[646] Proposed models to explain this requirement include ligand-induced release of cell membrane–sequestered transcription factors and cleavage of the extracellular domain by the KUZ protease (in mammalian systems also termed MDC/ADAM10), allowing the intracellular domain to travel to the nucleus to directly interact with the transcriptional apparatus.[647, 648] Major targets of Notch appear to be members of the helix-loop-helix family of transcription factors, such as MyoD.[646] However, it is unlikely that Notch interacts directly with either DNA or MyoD; rather, evidence has been presented that an intermediary protein, suppressor of hairless, plays this role.[649]

Recent findings suggest that Notch and its ligands play a role in hematopoiesis. Both Notch-1 and Notch-2 have been identified on CD34-selected hematopoietic progenitor cells,[650] and Jagged-1 has been localized to marrow stromal cells.[651–653] Moreover, Jagged-2 localizes with Notch-1 in the developing thymus, suggesting involvement in T-cell development.[645] The interaction of these receptor/ligand systems with other hematopoietic growth factors is also under active investigation.

Co-culture of primitive hematopoietic progenitor cells (Lin⁻/Sca⁺/Kit⁺) in SCF, FL, IL-6, and IL-11 with stromal cells engineered to express Jagged enhanced the output of both HPP-Mix and CFU-GM fourfold above a similar co-culture with stromal cells that did not express Jagged.[651] Expression of an autoactivated (extracellular truncation mutant) form of Notch in 32D cells inhibits G-CSF–induced granulocytic differentiation[641] while expanding the uncommitted cells in the culture. Similar results with use of the normal form of the receptor and both membrane-bound and soluble Jagged-1 were reported.[641] These effects are similar to those of *Drosophila Notch* genes on neurogenesis and myogenesis. Clearly, many exciting experiments lie ahead for these new receptor/ligand systems, but the initial impression is that these systems serve to skew the decision away from differentiation toward expansion.

▼ THE HEMATOPOIETIC STROMA

The preceding sections of this chapter have dealt with the hematopoietic growth factors produced by or presented on the surface of cells of the marrow microenvironment. In addition, these cells elaborate a number of complex carbohydrate–containing matrix proteins[654] that affect hematopoiesis either indirectly, by binding growth factors[11, 655] or their inhibitors,[13] or directly by promoting hematopoietic cell growth. For example, both heparin and chondroitin sulfate B expand the number of cord blood–derived CD34+ cells when present as an underlayer in cultures containing IL-3 and SCF. Genetic elimination of tenascin C, another matrix glycoprotein, reduces the self-renewal capacity of hematopoietic stem cells in long-term marrow culture.[656] The marrow microenvironment has also been shown to exert a negative effect on progenitor cell proliferation. Studies have suggested that this is due to the binding of fibronectin to $\alpha_4\beta_1$ and $\alpha_5\beta_1$ integrins present on CD34+ cells, an effect that requires immobilization of the integrins. Unfortunately, little is known about the mechanism that serves to control the influence of stromal glycoproteins (if one exists) in times of increased hematopoietic need.

Hematopoietic Growth Factors in Pathological Conditions

▼ HEMATOPOIETIC GROWTH FACTOR DEFICIENCY STATES

The Anemia of Renal Failure

As discussed earlier, EPO is produced in response to tissue hypoxia from cells of the juxtaglomerular region of the kidney. Hence, renal failure is almost always associated with varying degrees of anemia (the only exception being polycystic kidney disease, which can be associated with polycythemia because of excess EPO production from hypoxic renal tissue distal to an obstructing renal cyst). The anemia of patients with renal insufficiency can range from mild to requiring transfusional support but only roughly parallels the degree of renal insufficiency.

Other Hypoproliferative Anemias

Although reduced output of EPO best characterizes the anemia of renal failure, there are many patients with other hypoproliferative anemias in whom the level of plasma EPO is low relative to that found in patients with normal renal function and otherwise similar degrees of anemia. Many of these patients have acquired immunodeficiency syndrome, chronic diseases, or cancer. This state of relative EPO deficiency is poorly understood but may be related to the capacity of IL-1 (and possibly other inflammatory cytokines) to suppress EPO production.[528, 529] As such, treatment with EPO (often requiring high doses) can sometimes improve the anemia in such patients.

Thrombocytopenia in Hepatic Failure

Although previous explanations for the thrombocytopenia associated with hepatic failure focused on reduced platelet survival, due to splenic sequestration, and increased consumption due to low-grade chronic disseminated intravascular coagulopathy, more recent studies indicate that hepatic production of TPO is impaired in patients with liver failure. The most compelling data are derived from patients undergoing orthotopic liver transplantation. TPO levels are nearly always undetectable in such patients.[657, 658] Although orthotopic liver transplantation is associated with increased platelet consumption in the perioperative period,[659] it leads to an immediate increase in blood TPO levels and prompt recovery from thrombocytopenia,[657–659] the kinetics of which are consistent with simple TPO replacement therapy. Confirmation of this pathophysiological explanation will come with clinical trials of the recombinant hormone in patients with liver failure not undergoing transplantation, results that should become available soon.

The 5q− Syndrome

The 5q− syndrome is a myelodysplastic state characterized by a specific cytogenetic abnormality, anemia, leukopenia, thrombocytosis, female predominance, and a relatively prolonged survival but a low incidence of transformation to acute leukemia.[660] A large number of hematopoietic cytokine, cytokine receptor, and cytokine responsive genes (including GM-CSF, IL-3, IL-4, IL-5, IL-9, the M-CSF receptor, the tyrosine kinase Fer, and CD14) reside on the long arm of human chromosome 5. In addition, a potential protooncogene, interferon regulatory factor-2, has also been identified in this region, leading many to postulate that loss of one or more of these genes may lead to the marrow failure and myelodysplastic syndrome seen in a number of patients in association with the partial loss of 5q.[661, 662] However, careful mapping of the sites of chromosome loss in many such patients has indicated that none of these genes is consistently lost in all of the patients. Thus, although the idea was initially tempting, it is not presently clear whether the loss of any of these genes plays any role in this syndrome.

▼ STATES OF HEMATOPOIETIC GROWTH FACTOR EXCESS

Polycythemia

A number of polycythemic conditions are secondary to increased EPO production due to either tissue hypoxia (e.g., congestive heart failure, right to left cardiac shunts, abnormal hemoglobins with increased oxygen affinity, cigarette smoking, chronic carbon monoxide poisoning) or autonomous production of the hormone (hepatoma, cerebellar hemangioblastoma, renal cysts, renal carcinomas). In contrast, there is no evidence that polycythemia vera is caused by excess production of EPO or any other known hematopoietic cytokine.

Post-transplantation polycythemia is the term given to patients who develop erythrocytosis after successful renal transplantation. The disorder occurs in approximately 10 per cent of renal transplant recipients and can be treated with angiotensin-converting enzyme inhibitors or theophylline.[663–665] Some studies implicate overproduction of EPO from the renal graft,[666] but others call these data into question.[663, 667] In addition to overproduction of EPO, three alternative hypotheses have been advanced. Elevated IGF-1 levels have been detected in patients with post-transplantation polycythemia,[668] a finding congruent with the important effects of that cytokine on erythropoiesis.[64] Heightened sensitivity of erythroid progenitor cells, perhaps due to the chronic low EPO levels that characterize renal failure, has also been blamed. Treatment of patients with EPO during their pretransplantation period appears to reduce the likelihood of development of post-transplantation polycythemia, supporting a role for heightened EPO sensitivity. Third, angiotensin II has been demonstrated to enhance the formation of early erythroid colonies (BFU-E) from CD34+ cells, implicating an abnormal renin-angiotensin system in patients after renal transplantation and potentially helping to explain the favorable effect of angiotensin inhibitors on the disorder.[669]

Eosinophilia

Significant blood levels of IL-5 are seen in some patients with hypereosinophilic syndrome (HES),[670] Hodgkin disease,[671, 672] T-cell lymphoma,[673] episodic angioedema and eosinophilia,[674] angiolymphoid hyperplasia (Kimura disease[675]) or after the use of L-tryptophan[676, 677] or IL-2.[678] Eosinophils are known to produce IL-5 in certain pathological states,[679] including patients with HES, so it is unclear whether the overproduction of IL-5 in some of these disorders drives the eosinophilia, or vice versa. However, at least for HES, the pathophysiological process is more complex than simple overproduction of IL-5, because transgenic expression of the cytokine fails to recapitulate the tissue infiltration and destruction characteristic of HES.[236, 238] It is possible that one or more of the eosinophil-active chemokines could provide a second signal in this disorder. For example, eotaxin is constitutively produced in heart and lung and can be further induced by allergic stimulation,[680, 681] leading to tissue eosinophilic infiltration in states of IL-5 excess.[682]

Overproduction of IL-3 appears to be the mechanism of eosinophilia in patients with acute lymphoblastic leukemia who harbor the t(5;14) translocation.[683] The rearrangement brings the immunoglobulin heavy chain promoter region of chromosome 14, active in the leukemic lymphoblasts, into juxtaposition with the IL-3 gene located on chromosome 5. The result is constitutive activation of IL-3 gene expression and eosinophilia.

Familial Essential Thrombocythemia

Essential thrombocythemia is a clonal marrow disorder in which uncontrolled platelet production is the major hematological abnormality. Morbidity and mortality are secondary to thrombosis or pathological bleeding or, rarely, conversion to acute myeloid leukemia. The diagnosis of the disease is one of exclusion; reactive thrombocytosis due to iron deficiency, inflammation, or tumor or signs of other myeloproliferative diseases (polycythemia vera, chronic myelogenous leukemia [CML], or agnogenic myeloid metaplasia) must be absent.

Because it is the rarest of the myeloproliferative disorders, and usually the most benign, few molecular insights have been generated into the pathogenesis of essential thrombocythemia. Occasional patients report a familial history, and it is this subgroup in which progress in understanding the molecular mechanisms of disease has been made. Two groups have described patients with inherited thrombocytosis who display much higher than expected levels of plasma TPO.[684, 685] Different mutations have been uncovered in the two pedigrees. In one, a one nucleotide deletion in the 5′ UTR of the TPO gene results in its enhanced expression; in the other, a mutation in the splice acceptor site of the third intron of the TPO gene leads to elimination of the third exon, causing initiation from an upstream ATG and enhanced production of the hormone. These studies represent the first opportunity we have to understand this enigmatic disease. However, it is not yet clear whether these patients have the clonal myeloproliferative disease termed essential thrombocythemia or simply hereditary thrombocytosis. The distinction is not just semantic; if the patients overproduce TPO, benign thrombocytosis would be the expected outcome. However, if overproduction of TPO results in a clonal neoplastic disease, the pathogenic and therapeutic implications are far greater. Findings from transgenic mice that overproduce TPO may eventually shed some light on this question. When marrow cells were engineered to express high levels of TPO, then transplanted into lethally irradiated recipient mice, the result was a myeloproliferative disorder that resembled agnogenic myeloid metaplasia with myelofibrosis.[686] Unfortunately, the investigators have not yet reported whether the murine disease is clonal or whether platelet function is abnormal, as it often is in the human disease.

Secondary Thrombocytosis

A number of conditions are associated with thrombocytosis, including iron deficiency, inflammation, active bleeding, and a number of tumors. With the availability of enzyme-linked immunosorbent assays for cytokines known to affect platelet production (IL-1, IL-6, IL-11, TPO), the role of these cytokines in the thrombocytosis can be assessed. At present, there is little evidence that elevated levels of any of these cytokines can account for the thrombocytosis of iron deficiency or active bleeding. However, elevated levels of IL-1 and IL-6 are seen in a large number of inflammatory states, perhaps helping to explain the modestly elevated platelet counts in these conditions.[687–689] Many patients with underlying malignant neoplasms are thrombocytotic. Elevated IL-1 and IL-6 levels have been found in some of these patients.[690–695] More recently, because the liver is the predominant site of TPO production, the role of the hormone in thrombocytosis associated with hepatoma has been investigated. In seven patients with hepatocellular carcinoma and thrombocytosis, serum TPO concentrations were elevated; the level tended to correlate with the degree of thrombocytosis.[696]

The Anemia of Chronic Disease

The chronic administration of IL-1 to mice results in anemia.[697] Moreover, the degree of anemia in patients with chronic inflammatory disorders is roughly proportional to circulating IL-1β and TNF-α levels.[698] Inflammatory cytokine levels are higher in patients with rheumatoid arthritis and anemia than in rheumatoid arthritis patients with normal blood cell production.[699] There are many potential ways in which IL-1 could affect erythropoiesis (Fig. 2–6). IL-1 suppresses EPO production, blocks its effects on late erythroid progenitor cells, and works together with IFN to inhibit the proliferation of CFU-E.[528, 529, 700, 701] IL-1 also induces chemokine production (MCP-1 and IP-10) from marrow stromal cells,[702] proteins known to inhibit primitive erythroid colony formation.[625, 627] Perhaps more important, IL-1 also induces production of TNF-α and IFN-γ,[476, 477, 703, 704]

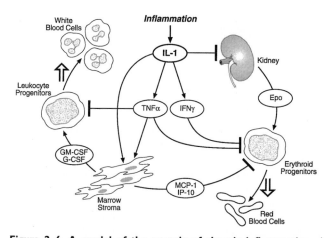

Figure 2–6. A model of the anemia of chronic inflammation. A wide range of inflammatory conditions elevate plasma IL-1β and TNF-α levels. Although both cytokines directly inhibit myeloid progenitor cell proliferation, they also both lead to enhanced production of hematopoietic growth factors such as GM-CSF and G-CSF from the marrow stroma. The net effect is stimulation of myelopoiesis. In contrast, both TNF-α and IL-1β inhibit erythroid progenitor cell expansion by multiple mechanisms and suppress renal EPO production; both effects lead to reduced erythropoiesis and anemia.

cytokines that display even more potent antagonistic effects on erythropoietic progenitor cell growth[526, 552, 705–708] by both direct and indirect mechanisms.[700, 709] In addition, TNF-α can reduce red cell survival.[710] IFN-γ acts to downregulate SCF and EPO receptors on erythroid progenitor cells,[711] thereby limiting the means to overcome cytokine inhibition of erythroid progenitor cell survival and expansion.

Fanconi Anemia

Fanconi anemia (FA) is a rare, autosomal recessive, phenotypically and genotypically heterogeneous disorder in which patients manifest a diverse assortment of congenital abnormalities, bone marrow failure, and a predisposition to cancer, especially acute myeloid leukemia. The mean survival is 16 years; patients usually succumb to complications of marrow failure. An excellent review of some of the newer aspects of the clinical course, diagnosis, and pathophysiology of FA has been published.[712]

The standard diagnostic test of FA is heightened susceptibility of somatic cells to DNA cross-linking agents. Such damaged cells rapidly undergo programmed cell death. By use of DNA cross-linking assays and cell fusion experiments, five complementation groups have been identified (A through E), suggesting that a number of distinct genes have an impact on the final common pathway leading to this disorder.[712] Significant progress has been made with the cloning of two of the genes (A and C) whose deficiency gives rise to FA.[713, 714] The FA-A and FA-C genes do not resemble any known proteins and are predicted to localize to the nucleus and cytoplasm of the cell, respectively.

FA-C encodes a 558 amino acid polypeptide of M_r 63 kDa and maps to 80 kb of the long arm of human chromosome 9.[713, 715] At present, only seven different mutations in this gene have been identified in patients.[712] FA-C localizes to the cytoplasm of most cells and interacts with several, mostly unidentified proteins.[716] However, two interacting proteins are known, the G_2/M cell cycle kinase Cdc2[717] and the molecular chaperone GRP94,[718] suggesting roles in the G_2/M transition and protein transport. FA-A cDNA was obtained in 1996,[714, 719] predicts a polypeptide of 1455 amino acids including two nuclear localization signals, and maps to the long arm of human chromosome 16.[720] Studies using specific antisera have revealed that FA-C and FA-A associate in the cytoplasm and are then translocated to the nucleus,[721] possibly providing a structural explanation for their involvement in the same functional pathway.

Much early attention focused on the sensitivity of cells from patients with FA to DNA cross-linking agents. It was postulated that the defective genes were important in DNA repair; the marrow failure so characteristic of the disease was thus due to accumulated DNA damage in hematopoietic stem and progenitor cells. Studies in which both FA-A and FA-C translocate to the nucleus are consistent with a role in DNA repair. Moreover, cells from patients with FA groups A, B, and D are deficient in a 230 kDa polypeptide that composes part of an endonuclease complex that binds to and excises cross-linked DNA.[722] However, the cloned genes do not resemble known DNA repair enzymes, and one localizes to the cytoplasm, forcing a re-evaluation of the pathogenesis of marrow failure in FA. More recently, much attention has been focused on the effects of hematopoietic cytokines on the marrow cells of these patients.

Mouse models of FA complementation group C have been developed by gene targeting.[723, 724] The nullizygous mice display the same sensitivity to DNA cross-linking agents and display a delayed (compared with humans) age-related decrease in hematopoietic progenitor cell numbers.[724] The mechanism of marrow failure in FA is under active investigation. Hematopoietic progenitors derived from FA-C nullizygous mice are hypersensitive to the apoptotic effects of IFN-γ.[724] This is also true of children with FA-C; progenitor cell proliferation can be inhibited by 20- to 100-fold less IFN-γ than that required to inhibit progenitor cells from normal individuals[725] and is due to IFN-γ–induced apoptosis.[653] Fas plays a key role in this effect, because an anti-Fas antibody eliminated IFN-γ–induced progenitor cell inhibition. In normal cells, signaling intermediates are inactivated by dephosphorylation soon after their activation. In FA-C–derived cells, STAT1 dephosphorylation (the primary mediator of IFN-γ signal transduction) after IFN-γ stimulation is significantly delayed, suggesting that the IFN-γ signal is unusually prolonged in these cells and potentially provides a mechanism for the aplastic anemia characteristic of FA.[725] Critical tests of this hypothesis are required before it can be accepted, but at present, it represents an attractive explanation for this enigmatic disorder.

Severe Aplastic Anemia

A complete discussion of the etiology, diagnosis, and management of severe aplastic anemia (SAA) is beyond the scope of this chapter. The reader is referred to an excellent review on the subject.[726] However, an important pathophysiological aspect of the disease, the role played by hematopoietic cytokines, is discussed here.

For many decades, an immunological basis for SAA was suspected, and many lines of evidence support this conclusion. First, many if not most patients with SAA respond to immunosuppressive therapy.[727, 728] Consistent with this finding, marrow transplantation for SAA from identical sibling donors fails in about half of cases unless immunosuppression is given to the recipient.[729] Second, although hematopoietic progenitor cells derived from the marrow of patients with SAA develop poorly, removal of T lymphocytes restores colony formation in most samples.[730, 731] Although these reports have been criticized for concentrating on previously transfused patients, in whom transfusion-induced sensitization may have been responsible for the T-cell suppression of growth, subsequent studies have revealed much evidence incriminating the T cells of patients with SAA. These include inverted T-helper/T-suppressor lymphocyte ratios in peripheral blood of SAA patients[732, 733] and increased suppressor and NK cell activities in the marrow of such patients.[734] Third, T-suppressor cell and monocyte-derived IFN-γ has been widely implicated in the pathogenesis of the disease.

Some of the earliest studies of immune-mediated hematopoietic failure identified soluble lymphokines as mediating hematopoietic suppression[735]; the active component was identified as IFN-γ.[736] As detailed in an earlier section of this chapter, numerous studies have convincingly demonstrated that IFN-γ suppresses hematopoietic progenitor cell development.[549-551, 737, 738] Monocytes derived from patients with SAA overproduce IFN-γ, both spontaneously and in response to minimal stimulation, and levels of IFN-γ are elevated in patients with SAA.[739] The origin of the IFN-γ appears to be, at least in part, the bone marrow. Using reverse transcription–polymerase chain reaction (RT-PCR), Young's laboratory found elevated marrow signals for IFN-γ mRNA in 14 of 18 patients with SAA, in 4 of 7 with moderate severity AA, but in none of the bone marrow samples from normal or heavily transfused individuals tested.[740] The marrow origin of the IFN-γ appears to be particularly important; expression from marrow stromal cells, even at low levels, profoundly affects hematopoietic development, much greater than that exerted by far higher blood levels of the cytokine.[741] Taken together, these data indicate that an overabundance of IFN-γ, derived from activated lymphocytes or marrow stroma, mediates much of the immune suppression of hematopoiesis in SAA.

▼ HEMATOPOIETIC GROWTH FACTORS AS AUTOCRINE FACTORS IN MYELOPROLIFERATIVE DISORDERS

Twenty years ago, Todaro and colleagues[742, 743] proposed that cells might become autonomous, independent of the need for an exogenous supply of support, by expressing their own requisite growth factors. This step might be all or part of the process necessary for a cell to transform to malignancy. A corollary of this "autocrine hypothesis" of tumorigenicity implies that autoactivation of the receptor for that requisite growth factor has the same effects. Although not truly autocrine, such a mechanism would employ the same pathways used in autocrine growth. The hypothesis received support from the finding of TGF-α production in K-*ras* oncogene–transformed rodent cells[744, 745] and the finding that the sarcoma-inducing gene v-*sis* is an altered form of PDGF,[746, 747] an oncogene that transforms only PDGF receptor–bearing cells.[748]

Proof of the principle of autocrine growth in the hematopoietic system was derived from studies of a number of factor-dependent hematopoietic cell lines. Although such factor-dependent cells (e.g., FDC-P1, BaF3, 32D) can proliferate in vitro in the presence of one or another of the hematopoietic growth factors, the cells are not transformed in the classical sense; their injection into nude mice does not lead to leukemia. However, if the requisite growth factor is autonomously expressed,[749, 750] or if a mutated, constitutively activated cytokine receptor is introduced (see below), the cells become factor independent in vitro and tumorigenic in vivo. It is now well established that human hematopoietic neoplasms can arise from cells that produce their own growth factors and can stimulate neighboring cells to do so (a paracrine mechanism) or from the expression of altered forms of hematopoietic cytokine receptors that deliver ligand-independent, constitutive proliferative signals. However, whether such autocrine signals must transit the cell membrane is uncertain; evidence both for[750, 751] and against[752] internal signaling has been presented. The mechanism of autocrine production of growth factors in leukemic cells is also unclear; in the majority of cases, the cytokine locus under study does not appear rearranged.[753] Instead, increased

cytokine production may relate to increased transcript stability.[754] The frequency with which such mechanisms contribute to human disease is also poorly understood. Nevertheless, autocrine and paracrine mechanisms of disease provide new strategies (anticytokine or anti–cytokine receptor reagents such as neutralizing antibodies, cytokine antagonists, soluble receptors, and antisense DNA) for the treatment of hematological neoplasms.

Acute Myelogenous Leukemia

In humans, acute myelogenous leukemia (AML) represents a spectrum of heterogeneous disorders of immature hematopoietic cells, with varying immune phenotype, histology, and clinical characteristics. This diversity probably represents the effects of a variety of etiological factors and pathogenetic mechanisms. Although significant progress has been made in the treatment of these disorders, particularly for patients with "favorable" prognostic indicators, the majority of patients with AML ultimately succumb to their disease. Many excellent reviews on the diagnostic classification, prognosis, and treatment of AML have been published.[755-757]

As in normal hematopoiesis, most leukemic cells are derived from a relatively small pool of progenitor cells with high proliferative capacity, cells that are, in turn, derived from the putative "leukemic stem cell." Examination of this cell is clearly critical if one is to understand and intervene in the leukemogenic process. Unfortunately, it is presently unclear whether the capacity of leukemic cells to form colonies in semisolid medium (the AML-CFU assay) measures the properties of the theoretical leukemic stem cell.

Despite uncontrolled cellular proliferation in vivo, the proliferation of most but not all AML-CFU remains dependent on hematopoietic growth factors in vitro. The clonogenic cells from samples of different patients display a great deal of heterogeneity, differentially responding to single or multiple cytokines including GM-CSF, IL-3, G-CSF, M-CSF, SCF, TPO, and IL-1.[758-763] Moreover, although neither IL-6 nor EPO supports the growth of leukemic cells when it is used alone, they can act in synergy with the other colony-stimulating factors.[764, 765] However, marrow cells from about one third of patients with AML can form clusters of leukemic cells in semisolid culture in the absence of exogenous growth factors.[766-769] The proliferation or survival of these cells is potentially driven by autocrine mechanisms, and such cases have received much investigative attention. Three questions remain paramount: Can autocrine production of a requisite growth factor lead to tumorigenicity in humans? What are the mechanisms responsible? If autocrine growth has a pathogenic role in human acute leukemia, does it influence the clinical course of the disease?

More than 10 years ago, Griffin and colleagues[767] began to report that fresh AML cells produced and responded to GM-CSF, and their autonomous growth could be inhibited by a neutralizing monoclonal antibody to the cytokine. Several additional reports confirmed these findings,[753, 770, 771] and others extended the hypothesis to include autocrine production of IL-11,[772] IL-6,[773] TPO,[762] and G-CSF.[774] However, other work revealed many cases of AML that secreted multiple cytokines,[775] making the significance of each difficult to discern. Soon after GM-CSF production in AML cells was described, IL-1 production by leukemic samples was also noted.[776] Of considerable interest, IL-1 cannot be detected by RT-PCR in the peripheral blood mononuclear cells of normal individuals[777] but is detectable by use of far less sensitive techniques in 35 to 80 per cent of blast cells from patients with AML.[778, 779] Because IL-1 is known to stimulate marrow stromal cells to produce GM-CSF and G-CSF,[2, 202, 780, 781] it was postulated that leukemic cell–derived IL-1 stimulates adjacent marrow stromal cells to produce the GM-CSF or other cytokines on which the leukemic cells are dependent.[776] Alternatively, the IL-1 could stimulate the leukemic cells themselves to produce their own GM-CSF,[782, 783] the importance of which was demonstrated by inhibition of autonomous leukemic cell growth by neutralizing GM-CSF antibodies. Both of these mechanisms have now been confirmed; the addition of IL-1-Ra, soluble IL-1-R, or neutralizing IL-1β antibodies to spontaneously growing cultures of fresh leukemic blast cells inhibited growth and, in some, inhibited the production of both GM-CSF and IL-1.[778, 784] Moreover, inhibition of the protease responsible for IL-1β activation, ICE, also inhibited spontaneous AML colony growth.[785] The autocrine production of M-CSF has also been established in a radiation-induced model of leukemia in the SJL/J mouse.[786] Evidence for autocrine production of M-CSF by leukemic cells, expression of its receptor on the same cell, elevated circulating levels of the cytokine in vivo before the development of frank leukemia, and inhibition of leukemogenesis by the administration of neutralizing M-CSF antibodies both in vitro and in vivo provide a compelling case for the role of autocrine loops in murine leukemia. Although some authors contend that the process of cell preparation can induce cytokine production from cells that were not producing it in vivo,[770] the weight of available evidence strongly suggests that the autocrine and paracrine production of hematopoietic growth factors can play a role in the pathogenesis of myeloid leukemia.

In addition to the foregoing evidence of autocrine production of hematopoietic growth factors in leukemia, the mechanism by which these autocrine loops act has begun to be explored. Analysis of a human myeloid leukemic cell line revealed autocrine production of GM-CSF and evidence that the GM-CSF receptor signaled in the cells.[787] In a study of several cases of AML that display factor-independent growth and a GM-CSF autocrine loop, higher levels of bcl-2 expression were found, potentially providing a mechanistic link between autonomous growth factor stimulation and increased leukemic cell survival.[788]

It is also important to consider whether autocrine growth is necessarily sufficient for malignant transformation. In most cases in which non-malignant factor-dependent hematopoietic cell lines have been engineered to express their requisite growth factor, leukemic transformation has ensued on introduction into syngeneic or nude mice.[789–791] However, this is not invariant. Introduction of an M-CSF expression plasmid into an M-CSF–dependent macrophage line led to growth factor–independent proliferation, but the resultant cells failed to induce leukemia in nude mice.[792] A second genetic event also seemed to be necessary in an experiment involving an IL-3–dependent cell line and GM-CSF.[793] Transgenic expression of hematopoietic growth factors such as GM-CSF, IL-3, and TPO in hematopoietic cells leads to myeloproliferative syndromes[686, 790, 794–796] but not to frank leukemia. Thus, in addition to acquiring the capacity for

hematopoietic cytokine-induced autocrine growth, there appear to be additional genetic steps in the leukemogenic progression.[793, 797] This phenomenon is presently poorly understood but appears to involve uncoupling of proliferation and differentiation.[769, 798] Nevertheless, the conservative conclusion from all of these data is that autocrine pathways to hematopoietic cell proliferation may remove one of the normal mechanisms of cellular growth regulation, rendering the cell one step closer to a fully malignant phenotype.

Of the mechanism of autocrine growth factor production, precious little is understood. One established mechanism is viral insertional mutagenesis; the murine myelomonocytic leukemia cell line WEHI-3B produces IL-3 by virtue of a retroviral insertion just upstream of the IL-3 locus.[799] A chromosomal event, t(5;14), is also responsible for autoactivation of the IL-3 gene in a human case of acute lymphoid leukemia with eosinophilia.[683] However, little else exploring the mechanisms behind leukemic cell production of hematopoietic growth factors has been reported.

Finally, the consequence of autocrine mechanisms on the clinical course of acute leukemia has begun to be studied. In an analysis of 114 cases of AML, those cases that demonstrated spontaneous growth in culture displayed a worse prognosis than those that did not.[769] Similar results were reported in two additional studies of patients with AML.[638, 800]

Chronic Myelogenous Leukemia

It is clear that the pathophysiological process of CML is heavily or entirely invested in the bcr-abl chromosomal rearrangement. Because the novel oncogene is a dysregulated tyrosine kinase that interacts with several of the intermediates involved in growth factor receptor signaling, much of what is known of the pathogenesis of the disease is discussed in Chapter 26. However, one intriguing observation pertains to the potential for the aberrant gene product to introduce autocrine growth in hematopoietic cells. Introduction of a bcr-abl gene into factor-dependent hematopoietic cell lines relieves their dependence on exogenous growth factors.[801] Of considerable interest, at least in M07E cells, the mechanism appears to be the autocrine production of GM-CSF and IL-3.[802] Whether this finding extends to samples from patients is not certain at present. Similar considerations may apply to the accelerated phase of CML[410, 803]; like the results in the study of samples from AML patients, IL-1-Ra, soluble IL-1-R, and neutralizing IL-1β antibodies blocked spontaneous proliferation of CML blast cells.[804, 805]

Juvenile Chronic Myelogenous Leukemia and Chronic Myelomonocytic Leukemia

Juvenile chronic myelogenous leukemia (JCML), is a rare disease of young children, presenting with weight loss, fever, night sweats, and infectious complications. The peripheral blood contains excess numbers of immature myeloid cells and prominent numbers of monocytes. The bone marrow is hypercellular without signs of dysplasia. Chronic myelomonocytic leukemia (CMML), a myelodysplastic syndrome seen primarily in older adults, presents with weight loss or complaints related to anemia. Splenomegaly is usually prominent, and hypogranular or bilobed neutrophils (Pelger-Huët anomaly) and monocytosis predominate in the peripheral blood smear. The bone marrow is hypercellular, with prominent dysplastic erythroid, myeloid, and megakaryocytic precursors. In some respects, these two disorders resemble one another. Both are chronic diseases of the hematopoietic stem cell but neither is associated with the Ph[1] chromosome, both display a far higher incidence of spontaneous growth in culture than does AML (spontaneous colony growth is considered a hallmark of JCML),[806] and both display prominent monocytosis. The two disorders also appear to meet at the IL-1/GM-CSF pathway. Spontaneous colony formation in JCML appears to be dependent on paracrine mechanisms; elimination of accessory cells from marrow cells of patients with JCML eliminates spontaneous colony formation.[491] Because the leukemic monocytes of JCML samples produce IL-1, an IL-1–induced stromal cell cytokine is thought to be responsible for leukemic cell growth. Recent evidence argues persuasively that this cytokine is GM-CSF, because a GM-CSF antagonist induces apoptosis of JCML cells.[807] Similar mechanisms can be uncovered in samples from patients with CMML.[808]

Of considerable interest, autonomous production of GM-CSF from CMML cells can be regulated. In normal marrow mononuclear cells, IL-10 inhibits the release of cytokines such as GM-CSF. In one study, the spontaneous production of GM-CSF in 10 of 11 cases of CMML was inhibited by the addition of IL-10 to culture, resulting in substantially reduced autonomous leukemic cell growth, an effect mimicked by a neutralizing GM-CSF antibody and that could be overcome by the addition of exogenous GM-CSF.[809] This result strongly supports the role of GM-CSF in the pathogenesis of CMML and provides a potentially novel therapeutic approach to the disease.

TNF also appears to play a pathogenic role in JCML. In six newly diagnosed patients with the disorder, tissue culture supernatant from marrow cells was found to contain TNF-α, which acted to inhibit the proliferation of BFU-E, CFU-GM, CFU-MK, and CFU-GEMM from normal marrow but did not adversely affect the growth of progenitors from the leukemic marrow cells.[810] In fact, the supernatant also contained GM-CSF, derived from the leukemic cells, which stimulated growth of leukemic progenitors. Thus, JCML cell elaboration of and resistance to TNF-α might help to explain the spontaneous growth of marrow cells in this disorder and the suppression of normal hematopoiesis so characteristic of the myeloproliferative disorders.

Hematopoietic Growth Factor Receptors in Hematological Disease

As discussed above, hematopoietic growth factor receptors play an important role in the survival and proliferation of hematopoietic cells. Thus, it is not surprising that mutagenic autoactivation of such receptors might play a pathogenic role in the uncontrolled expansion of hematopoietic cells characteristic of many of the myeloproliferative syndromes.

Hematopoietic growth factor action begins with the activation of either intrinsic or receptor-associated tyrosine kinases, all of which require multimerization for initial activation. Three lines of evidence support a potentially important role for altered cytokine receptors in the pathogenesis of human hematological diseases (for review, see Gonda and

D'Andrea[50]). First, a number of cytokine receptors are expressed in hematopoietic stem or primitive progenitor cells, placing them in the cells in which the transforming events of acute leukemia take place. Second, many naturally occurring hematopoietic receptor mutations in mice have been identified by analysis of viral oncogenes, including transforming versions of the M-CSF (v-*fms*), SCF (v-*kit*), and TPO (v-*mpl*) receptors. Third, the introduction of site-directed mutants of most if not all of the hematopoietic growth factor receptors can lead to growth factor independence of factor-dependent myeloid cell lines and lead to their tumorigenicity on injection into animals. Examples of this mechanism extend to the EPO, TPO, and β_C of the GM-CSF, IL-3, and IL-5 receptors. Proof of this principle has come from the identification of several naturally occurring mutations of hematopoietic growth factor receptors in pathological states in man (see below). It is likely that additional examples of this process will be identified in the near future.

▼ NATURALLY OCCURRING AND INDUCED RECEPTOR MUTATIONS CAUSING TRANSFORMING EVENTS IN VITRO

Several autonomously functioning versions of the EPO-R have been described. The first was obtained as part of a selection strategy to identify receptors that could function independently of ligand. The remainder were derived from generating similar mutations in the receptor at sites adjacent to the initial mutation. Substitution of Arg 129 by an unpaired Cys allows receptor dimerization and constitutive activity.[811] This residue can be aligned with the dimer interface region of the growth hormone receptor. A similar substitution of the closely adjacent positions 132 and 133 results in a similar receptor phenotype.[97]

Infection with the murine myeloproliferative leukemia virus rapidly leads to massive proliferation of all hematopoietic lineages, eventually resulting in hematopoietic failure due to acute leukemia.[812] The responsible viral gene, v-*mpl*, is a fusion of the retroviral envelope gene and a short region of the extracytoplasmic domain and the entire transmembrane and cytoplasmic domains of the murine c-*mpl* locus, a gene that displays critical sequence homology with members of the hematopoietic cytokine receptor family.[49] The mechanism of *env-mpl* fusion gene function is similar to that of the constitutively active EPO-R. The presence of an unpaired Cys residue derived from the *env* gene leads to v-*mpl* protein dimerization and constitutive activity.[813] Removal of the Cys residue by mutagenesis neutralizes the constitutive activity of the fusion receptor and its transforming capacity.[50] Engineering of an unpaired Cys residue in the predicted dimer interface region of the normal cellular receptor gene, c-*mpl*, also results in autonomously functioning receptors. Using a screening strategy similar to that which identified the initial Arg 129 to Cys EPO-R mutation, Onishi and colleagues[814] identified an autonomously functioning Mpl receptor mutant, in this case, a Ser 498 to Asn 498 substitution mutation in the transmembrane domain that leads to spontaneous receptor dimerization.

Several mutations of β_C are associated with ligand-independent receptor function. Introduction of a β_C receptor containing a duplication of 37 residues of the membrane proximal cytokine receptor motif[815] led to autonomous growth of FDC-P1 cells. The duplicated sequence does not include the predicted dimer interface region; rather, it involves residues downstream of this region, arguing that an alternative mechanism forms the basis of ligand-independent function of this mutant receptor. A number of other activating single–amino acid substitution mutants of this same domain of β_C have also been described. Disruption of a complex interaction of the third and fourth cytokine receptor barrel structures appears to underlie the effects of these autonomous receptors.[50]

Alterations in the receptor tyrosine kinase family of hematopoietic receptors can also lead to cellular transformation. Point mutations in the cytoplasmic domain of the c-Kit receptor have resulted in autonomous growth and tumorigenicity in both human and murine cell lines,[816, 817] mutant receptors that when introduced into normal hematopoietic cells cause their transformation.[818] One but not the only difference between v-*fms* and c-*fms* is a loss of 40 c-*fms*–specific cytoplasmic domain residues and their replacement by 11 unrelated amino acids. As a result, the transforming gene no longer encodes Tyr 969 of the M-CSF receptor.[281] Subsequent study of c-*fms* revealed this to be a site of ligand-induced phosphorylation, elimination of which leads to increased M-CSF signaling.[819] However, this mutation alone does not completely explain the oncogenicity of v-*fms*; cells bearing receptors containing only this mutation are not tumorigenic. Another site that appears to be involved in the activation of the M-CSF receptor is Leu 301.[820] Mutation to serine converts the receptor to an oncogenic version when it is introduced into 3T3 fibroblasts, although its role in myeloid transformation has not been established. Nevertheless, these elegant studies established that hematopoietic growth factor receptors could participate in the pathogenesis of malignant transformation.

▼ CYTOKINE RECEPTOR MUTATIONS IN HUMAN DISEASE

Congenital Erythrocytosis

"Erythropoietin Receptor Mutations and Olympic Glory" read the title of the editorial.[821] Congenital erythrocytosis is distinguished from polycythemia vera by its genetics but more importantly by the absence of other signs of panmyeloid expansion (basophilia, eosinophilia, splenomegaly) and the absence of pathological bleeding or thrombosis.

Several pedigrees of individuals with congenital polycythemia have now been identified that display a mutant EPO-R. One such family included a Gold medal winner from the 1948 Winter Olympics. As described in Chapter 4, the carboxyl terminus of the EPO-R appears to limit the action of hormone binding by serving as a docking site for a receptor-deactivating phosphatase. Although multiple mutations have been described, all of the reported pedigrees display variable deletions in this region of the EPO-R.[822–824] The disorder caused by these genetic events is an isolated erythrocytosis, very much resembling congenital and acquired cases of secondary polycythemia. In particular, such individuals do not display the expansion of other myeloid lineages, the progenitor cell hypersensitivity to hematopoietic growth factors, the hypercoagulability, or the propensity

for development of acute leukemia shown by patients with authentic polycythemia vera.

Polycythemia Vera

A number of lines of evidence suggest that hematopoietic growth factor receptors may play a role in the pathogenesis of polycythemia vera. The disease is characterized by a panmyeloid disturbance; abnormalities of all hematopoietic lineages can be detected in patients with the disease. Hematopoiesis is clonal; all lineages derive from a single cell, most easily proven by analysis of X-linked genes such as glucose-6-phosphate dehydrogenase[825] or other highly allelic genetic markers.[826] Hematopoietic progenitor cells are no longer dependent on the cytokines and hormones normally required to induce colony growth in semisolid medium. Such "endogenous erythroid colony" formation, which provides a useful diagnostic test for myeloproliferative disorders such as polycythemia vera,[827, 828] is not truly factor independence but rather factor hypersensitivity.[829, 830]

Initial studies focused on the sensitivity of erythroid progenitor cells to EPO; most studies[831, 832] but not all (reviewed in Heimpel[833]) demonstrated that erythroid progenitors were hypersensitive to the proliferative effects of the hormone. The logical outgrowth of these studies was to analyze the EPO-R in polycythemia vera; such studies have failed to detect either receptor-binding or molecular-signaling defects.[832, 834–836] Additional study revealed that erythroid and other progenitor cell types derived from patients with polycythemia vera display a heightened sensitivity to other growth factors, including IL-3,[837, 838] GM-CSF,[839] SCF,[840] and IGF-1.[841] Analysis of several of these receptors in patients with polycythemia vera has also been unrevealing,[840] and given the sensitivity of erythroid and other hematopoietic precursors to many growth factors, it is logical to propose that polycythemia vera represents a disorder of a signaling pathway common to all of these receptors. Current research has focused on the phosphatases activated after growth factor receptor stimulation, because some of the receptors considered in this segment display heightened baseline phosphorylation and enhanced phosphorylation in response to minimal concentrations of their respective growth factors.[842] Evidence that a counterregulatory phosphatase may be abnormal in polycythemia vera progenitor cells has been presented,[843, 844] but the nature or relevance of this pathway has not been discerned. Equally intriguing is the finding of reduced levels of a naturally occurring truncated form of the EPO-R in the blood cells of patients with polycythemia vera.[845] Because a truncated receptor would be expected to act as a dominant negative form, loss of such a normally limiting mechanism would be expected to enhance sensitivity to EPO. The ultimate role of such alternative forms of receptors or phosphatases in myeloproliferative disorders is under active investigation.

Acute Myelogenous Leukemia After Congenital Neutropenia

Severe congenital neutropenia (SCN or Kostmann syndrome) is characterized by severe neutropenic infections from birth (often the first manifestation is an umbilical stump infection) but without any other hematopoietic defect.

Patients with idiopathic (acquired) neutropenia and cyclic neutropenia are not included in this diagnostic category. The etiology is unknown, but germline defects in G-CSF and G-CSF-R have been excluded. It is suspected but not proven that a G-CSF-R signaling defect is responsible. Until 10 years ago, children with SCN usually succumbed to infectious complications unless a bone marrow transplant could be performed. Despite normal production of G-CSF and a normal G-CSF-R, the administration of pharmacological doses of G-CSF has dramatically improved the prognosis of these patients; 90 to 95 per cent experience a profoundly improved quality of life. However, during the past 6 years, numerous cases of AML have been reported in these patients, prompting re-examination of the role of G-CSF in this condition.

The risk for development of AML or myelodysplasia in a patient with Kostmann syndrome receiving G-CSF therapy is approximately 9 per cent during a mean follow-up period of 4.5 years.[846] In contrast, none of more than 250 patients treated with G-CSF for cyclic neutropenia or idiopathic acquired neutropenia has had this unfortunate outcome. Before the use of G-CSF, an occasional patient with Kostmann syndrome developed AML, attesting to a natural tendency for this event, but most patients did not because their life expectancy was short. Starting in 1994, patients with Kostmann syndrome and AML were noted to harbor nonsense mutations in the gene encoding their G-CSF receptor.[847] The mutations resulted in truncation of the cytoplasmic domain of the receptor, eliminating the box3 domain associated with G-CSF–induced maturation. (See Chapter 4.) In contrast, this mutation is rare in patients with spontaneously occurring AML.[848] An update of two groups has brought the number of cases of a mutated G-CSF-R in Kostmann syndrome to 16 (of 59 patients tested) and the number with an associated AML or myelodysplastic syndrome to 8.[849] In one patient, the mutation was noted before the development of AML.[850] However, in other reports, patients with the mutation have remained healthy, and some individuals with AML do not bear the truncated receptor. Because of this finding, the role of the mutation in the pathogenesis of the AML that follows Kostmann syndrome remains controversial.

Because the region of the G-CSF-R deleted in these patients mediates cellular maturation and ligand internalization and destruction,[851, 852] its elimination should result in a mutant receptor that supports a hyperproliferative growth response and exerts a dominant negative effect on differentiation.[847] Studies with G-CSF–responsive leukemic cell lines have confirmed this prediction.[850] However, more recently, homologous recombination of a truncated receptor into one or both of the G-CSF-R alleles of normal mice has been accomplished.[853] Analysis of these mice has failed to confirm a defect in neutrophil differentiation; only the enhanced G-CSF–induced in vitro and in vivo proliferation of granulocytic precursor cells could be identified. It is not yet known whether these mice will develop AML, but their ongoing study should help settle the controversy surrounding this field.

Kit Mutations in Mastocytosis

Loss of function or reduced function c-*kit* mutations are well known, producing the W phenotype in mice[854] and pie-baldism in humans.[855] The v-*kit* oncogene encodes an autonomously active tyrosine kinase. Compared with the feline c-*kit* gene, from which it was derived, the v-Kit protein contains deletions in the extracellular, transmembrane, and distal cytoplasmic domains and two potentially important deletions within the cytoplasmic domain, at a site where Src kinases bind in homologous receptors.[856] Autophosphorylating mutations of the c-Kit receptor gene have also been described in transformed cell lines, the HMC-1 human mast cell leukemia and the P-815 murine mastocytoma.[816, 817] Both mutations mapped to Asp 816 (Asp 814 in mouse), a residue in the intracytoplasmic kinase domain of the receptor.

Several somatic gain of function mutations in the c-Kit receptor have now been reported in patients with mastocytosis. In two reports,[857, 858] five patients with myelodysplastic syndrome and mastocytosis or skin mastocytosis alone were found to have an Asp 816 → Val mutation in the c-Kit receptor. A different group again identified Asp 816 → Val as the activating c-Kit receptor mutation in a patient with urticaria pigmentosa and aggressive mast cell infiltration of the marrow.[859] A nearby mutation, Asp 820 → Gly, again in the phosphotransferase domain of c-Kit, was identified in a patient with aggressive mastocytosis and bone marrow infiltration.[860]

Flt3 Mutations in Acute Myeloid Leukemia

Several reports have now appeared linking internal tandem duplications of the Flt3 receptor to acute leukemia.[861, 862] In one paper, internal duplications were found in 20 per cent of patients with acute myeloid leukemia and in patients with myelodysplastic syndromes evolving to acute leukemia. In all of these series, the internal duplications involved a juxtamembrane region and, although not completely consistent in location, always involved either Tyr 591 or Tyr 599. This region is predicted (by homology to the PDGF receptor) to be phosphorylated and serve as an SH2 docking site. As such, it could increase signal intensity on FL binding, or the duplication could disrupt a negative regulatory domain. Unfortunately, much work remains to decipher the role of this receptor mutation in the pathogenesis of leukemia. It is of interest, however, that the presence of the duplication is associated with higher leukocyte counts, higher lactate dehydrogenase levels, lower fibrinogen levels, and a poor prognosis.[862]

Fms Mutations in Myelodysplastic Diseases

Two sites in the M-CSF receptor have been shown to cooperate in generating autonomous receptor activity, Leu 301 and Tyr 969.[820] Two surveys of more than 150 patients with myelodysplastic and myeloproliferative syndromes[863, 864] revealed only two examples of a Leu 301 mutation of c-*fms*, and those mutations (Leu to Phe or Val) do not introduce transforming activity into the receptor.[820] Rather, the two studies did reveal that 20 of the patients displayed mutations of Tyr 969, all of which would be expected to abolish the "braking" activity on receptor activation that phosphorylation at this site normally generates. However, because a Tyr 969 mutation alone is not sufficient to convert c-*fms* into a transforming gene,[820] and the presence of a similar mutation in a seemingly normal individual[863] argues that the c-*fms* mutation in these patients may be only part of the transforming event.

▼ LOST RECEPTORS IN HUMAN DISEASE

Amegakaryocytic Thrombocytopenia

Children with amegakaryocytic thrombocytopenia are usually variably pancytopenic and often progress to myelodysplasia or frank leukemia within a few years of presentation. It is highly likely that such patients have a myelodysplastic stem cell disorder. However, a single patient has now been described with amegakaryocytic thrombocytopenia that lacks the Mpl receptor.[865] The child is mildly anemic and severely thrombocytopenic (platelet count of 14,000/mm³). RT-PCR analysis of peripheral blood mononuclear cells failed to reveal a band specific for the Mpl receptor. Of additional interest, the concentration of hematopoietic progenitors of all cell lineages was greatly reduced in this patient, consistent with the panhematopoietic activities of this receptor/ligand system.

REFERENCES

1. Penn, P.E., Jiang, D.Z., Fei, R.G., Sitnicka, E., and Wolf, N.S.: Dissecting the hematopoietic microenvironment. IX. Further characterization of murine bone marrow stromal cells. Blood 81:1205, 1993.
2. Fibbe, W.E., van Damme, J., Billiau, A., Goselink, H.M., Voogt, P.J., van Eeden, G., Ralph, P., Altrock, B.W., and Falkenbur, J.H.F.: Interleukin 1 induces human marrow stromal cells in long-term culture to produce granulocyte colony-stimulating factor and macrophage colony-stimulating factor. Blood 71:430, 1988.
3. Kohama, T., Handa, H., and Harigaya, K.: A burst-promoting activity derived from the human bone marrow stromal cell line KM 102 is identical to the human granulocyte-macrophage colony-stimulating factor. Exp. Hematol. 16:603, 1988.
4. Paul, S.R., Bennett, F., Calvetti, J.A., Kelleher, K., Wood, C.R., O'Hara, R.M., Jr., Leary, A.C., Sibley, B., Clark, S.C., Williams, D.A., and Yang, Y.C.: Molecular cloning of a cDNA encoding interleukin 11, a stromal cell–derived lymphopoietic and hematopoietic cytokine. Proc. Natl. Acad. Sci. USA 87:7512, 1990.
5. Kittler, E.L., McGrath, H., Temeles, D., Crittenden, R.B., Kister, V.K., and Quesenbery, P.J.: Biological significance of constitutive and subliminal growth factor production by bone marrow stroma. Blood 79:3168, 1992.
6. Toksoz, D., Zsebo, K.M., Smith, K.A., Hu, S., Brankow, D., Suggs, S.V., Martin, F.H., and Williams, D.A.: Support of human hematopoiesis in long-term bone marrow cultures by murine stromal cells selectively expressing the membrane-bound and secreted forms of the human homolog of the steel gene product, stem cell factor. Proc. Natl. Acad. Sci. USA. 89:7350, 1992.
7. Nagahisa, H., Nagata, Y., Ohnuki, T., Osada, M., Nagasawa, T., Abe, T., and Todokoro, K.: Bone marrow stromal cells produce thrombopoietin and stimulate megakaryocyte growth and maturation but suppress proplatelet formation. Blood 87:1309, 1996.
8. Lemieux, M.E., Chappel, S.M., Miller, C.L., and Eaves, C.J.: Differential ability of flt3-ligand, interleukin-11, and Steel factor to support the generation of B cell progenitors and myeloid cells from primitive murine fetal liver cells. Exp. Hematol. 25:951, 1997.
9. Moore, K.A., and Lemischka, I.R.: The molecular profile of a stem cell supporting microenvironment. Exp. Hematol. 25:736, 1997.
10. Wineman, J., Moore, K., Lemischka, I., and Muller-Sieberg, C.: Functional heterogeneity of the hematopoietic microenvironment: rare stromal elements maintain long-term repopulating stem cells. Blood 87:4082, 1996.
11. Gordon, M.Y., Riley, G.P., Watt, S.M., and Greaves, M.F.: Compart-mentalization of a hematopoietic growth factor (GM-CSF) by glycosaminoglycans in the bone marrow microenvironment. Nature 326:403, 1987.
12. Ohtsuki, T., Suzu, S., Hatake, K., Nagata, N., Miura, Y., and Motoyoshi, K.: A proteoglycan form of macrophage colony-stimulating factor that binds to bone-derived collagens and can be extracted from bone matrix. Biochem. Biophys. Res. Commun. 190:215, 1993.
13. Han, Z.C., Bellucci, S., Shen, Z.X., Maffrand, J.P., Pascal, M., Petitou, M., Lormeau, J., and Caen, J.P.: Glycosaminoglycans enhance megakaryocytopoiesis by modifying the activities of hematopoietic growth regulators. J. Cell. Physiol. 168:97, 1996.
14. Abdel-Meguid, S.S., Shieh, H.S., Smith, W.W., Dayringer, H.E., Violand, B.N., and Bentle, L.A.: Three dimensional structure of a genetically engineered variant of porcine growth hormone. Proc. Natl. Acad. Sci. USA. 84:6434, 1987.
15. Brandhuber, B.J., Boone, T., Kenney, W.C., and McKay, D.B.: Three dimensional structure of interleukin 2. Science 238:1707, 1987.
16. Bazan, J.F.: Unraveling the structure of IL-2. Science 257:410, 1992.
17. McKay, D.B.: Unraveling the structure of IL-2. Response. Science 257:412, 1992.
18. Diederichs, K., Boone, T., and Karplus, P.A.: Novel fold and putative receptor binding site of granulocyte-macrophage colony-stimulating factor. Science 254:1779, 1991.
19. Powers, R., Garret, D.S., March, C.J., Frieden, E.A., Gronenborn, A., and Clore, G.M.: Three-dimensional solution structure of human interleukin-4 by multidimensional heteronuclear magnetic resonance spectroscopy. Science 256:1673, 1992.
20. Pandit, J., Bohm, A., Jancarik, J., Halenbeck, R., Koths, K., and Kim, S.H.: Three-dimensional structure of dimeric human recombinant macrophage colony-stimulating factor. Science 258:1358, 1992.
21. Hill, C.P., Osslund, T.D., and Eisenberg, D.: The structure of granulocyte colony-stimulating factor and its relationship to other growth factors. Proc. Natl. Acad. Sci. USA 90:5167, 1993.
22. Milburn, M.V., Hassell, A.M., Lambert, M.H., Jordan, S.P., Proudfoot, A.E.I., Graber, P., and Wells, T.N.: A novel dimer configuration revealed by the crystal structure at 2.4ÅA resolution of human interleukin-5. Nature 363:172, 1993.
23. Robinson, R.C., Grey, L.M., Staunton, D., Vankelecom, H., Vernallis, A.B., Moreau, J.F., Stuart, D.I., Heath, J.K., and Jones, E.Y.: The crystal structure and biological function of leukemia inhibitory factor: implications for receptor binding. Cell 77:1101, 1994.
24. Feng, Y., Klein, B.K., Vu, L., Aykent, S., and McWherter, C.A.: ¹H, ¹³C, and ¹⁵N NMR resonance assignments, secondary structure, and backbone topology of a variant of human interleukin-3. Biochemistry 34:6540, 1995.
25. Somers, W., Stahl, M., and Seehra, J.S.: A crystal structure of interleukin 6: implications for a novel mode of receptor dimerization and signaling. EMBO J. 16:989, 1997.
26. McDonald, N.Q., Panayotatas, N., and Hendrickson, W.A.: Crystal structure of dimeric human ciliary neurotrophic factor determined by MAD phasing. EMBO J. 14:2689, 1995.
27. Hoffman, R.C., Moy, F.J., Price, V., Richardson, J., Kaubisch, D., Frieden, E.A., Krakover, J.D., Castner, B.J., King, J., March, C.J., and Powers, R.: Resonance assignments for Oncostatin M, a 24-kDa alphahelical protein. J. Biomol. NMR 7:273, 1996.
28. Rozwarski, D.A., Gronenborn, A.M., Clore, G.M., Bazan, J.F., Bohm, A., Wlodawer, A., Hatada, M., and Karplus, P.A.: Structural comparisons among the short-chain helical cytokines. Structure 2:159, 1994.
29. Simpson, R.J., Hammacher, A., Smith, D.K., Matthews, J.M., and Ward, L.D.: Interleukin-6: structure-function relationships. Protein Sci. 6:929, 1997.
30. Bazan, J.F.: Genetic and structural homology of stem cell factor and macrophage colony-stimulating factor. Cell 65:9, 1991.
31. Kaushansky, K., and Karplus, A.: The hematopoietic growth factors: understanding functional diversity in structural terms. Blood 82:8229, 1993.
32. Bazan, J.F.: Structural design and molecular evolution of a cytokine receptor family. Proc. Natl. Acad. Sci. USA 87:6934, 1990.
33. Tartaglia, L.A., Dembski, M., Weng, X., Deng, N., Culpepper, J., Devos, R., Richards, G.J., Campfield, L.A., Clark, F.T., Deeds, J., Muir, C., Sander, S., Moriarty, A., Moore, K.J., Smutko, J.S., Mays, G.G., Woolf, E.A., Monroe, C.A., and Tepper, R.I.: Identification and expression cloning of a leptin receptor, OB-R. Cell 83:1263, 1995.
34. Wells, J.A.: Binding in the growth hormone receptor complex. Proc. Natl. Acad. Sci. USA 93:1, 1996.

35. de Vos, A.M., Ultsch, M., and Kossiakoff, A.A.: Human growth hormone and extracellular domain of its receptor: crystal structure of the complex. Science 255:306, 1992.
36. Yawata, H., Yasukawa, K., Natsuka, S., Murakami, M., Yamasaki, K., Hibi, M., Taga, T., and Kishimoto, T.: Structure-function analysis of human IL-6 receptor: dissociation of amino acid residues required for IL-6 binding for IL-6 signal transduction through gp130. EMBO J. 12:1705, 1993.
37. Woodcock, J.M., Zacharakis, B., Plaetinck, G., Bagley, C.J., Qiyu, S., Hercus, T.R., Tavernier, J., and Lopez, A.F.: Three residues in the common β chain of the human GM-CSF, IL-3 and IL-5 receptors are essential for GM-CSF and IL-5 but not IL-3 with high affinity binding and interact with Glu21 of GM-CSF. EMBO J. 13:5176, 1994.
38. Cornelis, S., Plaetinck, G., Devos, R., Van der Heyden, J., Tavernier, J., Sanderson, C.J., Guisez, Y., and Fiers, W.: Detailed analysis of the IL-5–IL-5Rα interaction: characterization of crucial residues on the ligand and the receptor. EMBO J. 14:3395, 1995.
39. Middleton, S.A., Johnson, D.L., Jin, R., McMahon, F.J., Collins, A., Tullai, J., Gruninger, R.H., Jolliffe, L.K., and Mulcahy, L.S.: Identification of a critical ligand binding determinant of the human erythropoietin receptor. J. Biol. Chem. 271:14045, 1996.
40. Mellado, M., Rodriguez-Frade, J.M., Kremer, L., von Kobbe, C., de Ana, A.M., Mérida, I., and Martinez, A.C.: Conformational changes required in the human growth hormone receptor for growth hormone signaling. J. Biol. Chem. 272:9189, 1997.
41. Goodall, G.J., Bagley, C.J., Vadas, M.A., and Lopez, A.F.: A model for the interaction of the GM-CSF, IL-3, and IL-5 receptors with their ligands. Growth Factors 8:87, 1993.
42. Gustchina, A., Zdanov, Z., Schalk-Hik, C., and Wlodawer, A.: A model of the complex between interleukin-4 and its receptors. Proteins 21:140, 1995.
43. Lyne, P.D., Bamborough, P., Duncan, D., and Richards, W.G.: Molecular modeling of the GM-CSF and IL-3 receptor complexes. Protein Sci. 4:2223, 1995.
44. Caravella, J.A., Lyne, P.D., and Richards, W.G.: A partial model of the erythropoietin receptor complex. Proteins 24:394, 1996.
45. Klein, B.K., Feng, Y., McWherter, C.A., Hood, W.F., Paik, K., and McKearn, J.P.: The receptor binding site of human interleukin-3 defined by mutagenesis and molecular modeling. J. Biol. Chem. 272:22630, 1997.
46. Muto, A., Watanabe, S., Miyajima, A., Yokota, T., and Arai, K.: The β subunit of human granulocyte-macrophage colony-stimulating factor receptor forms a homodimer and is activated via association with the subunit. J. Exp. Med. 183:1911, 1996.
47. Roussel, M.F., Downing, J.R., Ashmun, R.A., Rettenmier, C.W., and Sherr, C.J.: Colony-stimulating factor 1–mediated regulation of a chimeric c-fms/v-fms receptor containing the c-fms encoded tyrosine kinase domain. Proc. Natl. Acad. Sci. USA 85:5903, 1988.
48. Qiu, F.H., Ray, P., Brown, K., Barker, P.E., Jhanwar, S., Ruddle, F.H., and Besmer, P.: Primary structure of c-kit: relationship with the CSF-1/PDGF receptor kinase family—oncogenic activation of v-kit involves deletion of extracellular domain and C terminus. EMBO J. 7:1003, 1988.
49. Vigon, I., Mornon, J.-P., Cocault, L., Mitjavila, M.-T., Tambourin, P., Gisselbrecht, S., and Souyri, M.: Molecular cloning and characterization of MPL, the human homolog of the v mpl oncogene: identification of a member of the hematopoietic growth factor receptor superfamily. Proc. Natl. Acad. Sci. USA 89:5640, 1992.
50. Gonda, T.J., and D'Andrea, R.J.: Activating mutations in cytokine receptors: implications for receptor function and role in disease. Blood 89:355, 1997.
51. Miyajima, A., Mui, A.L.F., Ogorochi, T., and Sakamaki, K.: Receptors for granulocyte-macrophage colony-stimulating factor, interleukin-3 and interleukin-5. Blood 82:1960, 1993.
52. Cosman, D.: The hematopoietin receptor superfamily. Cytokine 5:95, 1993.
53. Kishimoto, T., Akira, S., Narazaki, M., and Taga, T.: Interleukin-6 family of cytokines and gp130. Blood 86:1243, 1995.
54. Taga, T., and Kishimoto, T.: gp130 and the interleukin-6 family of cytokines. Annu. Rev. Immunol. 15:797, 1997.
55. Wypych, J., Bennett, L.G., Schwartz, M.G., Clogston, C.L., Lu, H.S., Broudy, V.C., Bartley, T.D., Parker, V.P., and Langley, K.E.: Soluble Kit receptor in human serum. Blood 85:66, 1995.
56. Tsuruoka, N., Yamashiro, K., and Tsujimoto, M.: Purification of soluble murine interleukin 5 receptor alpha expressed in Chinese hamster ovary cells and its action as an IL-5 antagonist. Arch. Biochem. Biophys. 307:133, 1993.
57. Lok, S., Kaushansky, K., Holly, R.D., Kuijper, J.L., Lofton-Day, C.E., Oort, P.J., Grant, F.J., Heipel, M.D., Burkhead, S.K., Kramer, J.M., Bell, L.A., Sprecher, C.A., Blumberg, H., Johnson, R., Prunkard, D., Ching, A.F.T., Mathewes, S.L., Bailey, M.C., Forstrom, J.W., Buddle, M.M., Osborn, S.G., Evans, S.J., Sheppard, P.O., Presnell, S.R., O'Hara, P.J., Hagen, F.S., Roth, G.J., and Foster, D.C.: Cloning and expression of murine thrombopoietin cDNA and stimulation of platelet production in vivo. Nature 369:565, 1994.
58. Brown, C.B., Beaudry, P., Dickinson-Laing, T., Shoemaker, S., and Kaushansky, K.: In vitro characterization of the human recombinant soluble GM-CSF receptor. Blood 85:1488, 1995.
59. Turner, A.M., Bennett, L.G., Lin, N.L., Wypych, J., Bartley, T.D., Hunt, R.W., Atkins, H.L., Langley, K.E., Parker, V., Martin, F., and Broudy, V.C.: Identification and characterization of a soluble c-kit receptor produced by human hematopoietic cell lines. Blood 85:2052, 1995.
60. Baumann, H., Wang, Y., Morella, K.K., Lai, C.F., Dams, H., Hilton, D.J., Hawley, R.G., and Mackiewicz, A.: Complex of the soluble IL-11 receptor and Il-11 acts as IL-6-type cytokine in hepatic and nonhepatic cells. J. Immunol. 157:284, 1996.
61. Heaney, M.L., and Golde, D.W.: Soluble cytokine receptors. Blood 87:847, 1996.
62. Kieran, M.W., Perkins, A.C., Orkin, S.H., and Zon, L.I.: Thrombopoietin rescues in vitro erythroid colony formation from mouse embryos lacking erythropoietin receptor. Proc. Natl. Acad. Sci. USA 93:9126, 1996.
63. Koury, M.J., and Bondurant, M.C.: Erythropoietin retards DNA breakdown and prevents programmed death in erythroid progenitor cells. Science 248:378, 1990.
64. Muta, K., Krantz, S.B., Bondurant, M.C., and Wickrema, A.: Distinct roles of erythropoietin, insulin-like growth factor I, and stem cell factor in the development of erythroid progenitor cells. J. Clin. Invest. 94:34, 1994.
65. Weisbart, R.H., Kwan, L., Golde, D.W., and Gasson, J.C.: Human GM-CSF primes neutrophils for enhanced oxidative metabolism in response to the major physiological chemoattractants. Blood 69:18, 1987.
66. Fabian, I., Kletter, Y., Mor, S., Geller-Bernstein, C., Ben-Yaakov, M., Volovitz, B., and Golde, D.W.: Activation of human eosinophil and neutrophil functions by haematopoietic growth factors: comparisons of IL-1, IL-3, IL-5 and GM-CSF. Br. J. Haematol. 80:137, 1992.
67. Wiltschke, C., Krainer, M., Wagner, A., Linkesch, W., and Zielinski, C.C.: Influence of in vivo administration of GM-CSF and G-CSF on monocyte cytotoxicity. Exp. Hematol. 23:402, 1995.
68. Chen, B.D.M., Mueller, M., and Chou, T.H.: Role of granulocyte/macrophage of colony-stimulating factor in the regulation of murine alveolar macrophage proliferation and differentiation. J. Immunol. 141:139, 1988.
69. Dranoff, G., Crawford, A.D., Sadelain, M., Ream, B., Rashid, A., Bronson, R.T., Dickersin, G.R., Bachurski, C.J., Mark, E.L., Whitsett, J.A., and Mulligan, R.C.: Involvement of granulocyte-macrophage colony-stimulating factor in pulmonary homeostasis. Science 264:713, 1994.
70. Fairbairn, L.J., Cowling, G.J., Reipert, B.M., and Dexter, T.M.: Suppression of apoptosis allows differentiation and development of a multipotent hematopoietic cell line in the absence of added growth factors. Cell 74:823, 1993.
71. Hirayama, F., Lyman, S.D., Clark, S.C., and Ogawa, M.: The flt3 ligand supports proliferation of lymphohematopoietic progenitors and early B-lymphoid progenitors. Blood 85:1762, 1995.
72. Metcalf, D., Enver, T., Heyworth, C.M., and Dexter, T.M.: Growth factors and hematopoietic cell fate. Blood 92:345, 1998.
73. Carnot, P., and Deflandre, C.: Sur l'activite hematopoietique des serum au cours de la regeneration du sang. Acad. Sci. M. 3:384, 1906.
74. Jacobs, K., Shoemaker, C., Rudersdorf, R., Neill, S.D., Kaufman, R.J., Mufson, A., Seehra, J., Jones, S.S., Hewick, R., Fritsch, E.F., Kawakita, M., Shimizu, T., and Miyake, T.: Isolation and characterization of genomic and cDNA clones of human erythropoietin. Nature 313:806, 1985.
75. Lin, F.K., Suggs, S., Lin, C.H., Browne, J.K., Smalling, R., Egrie, J.C., Chen, K.K., Fox, G.M., Martin, F., Stabinsky, Z., Badrawi, S.M., Lai, P.H., and Goldwasser, E.: Cloning and expression of the human erythropoietin gene. Proc. Natl. Acad. Sci. USA. 82:7580, 1985.

76. Koury, S.T., Bondurant, M.C., and Koury, M.J.: Localization of erythropoietin synthesizing cells in murine kidneys using in situ hybridization. Blood 71:524, 1988.

77. Lacombe, C., Da Silva, J., Bruneval, P., Fournier, J., Wendling, F., Casadevall, N., Camilleri, J.P., Bariety, J., Varet, B., and Tambourin, P.: Peritubular cells are the site of erythropoietin synthesis in murine hypoxic kidneys. J. Clin. Invest. 81:620, 1988.

78. Loya, F., Yang, Y., Lin, H., Goldwasser, E., and Albitar, M.: Transgenic mice carrying the erythropoietin gene promoter linked to *lacZ* express the reporter in proximal convoluted tubule cells after hypoxia. Blood 84:1831, 1994.

79. Semenza, G.L.: Erythropoietin gene expression in transgenic mice and human hepatoma cells. Ann. N. Y. Acad. Sci. 718:41, 1994.

80. Erslev, A.J.: Erythropoietin titers in health and disease. Semin. Hematol. 28:2, 1991.

81. Goldberg, M.A., Dunning, S.P., and Bunn, H.F.: Regulation of the erythropoietin gene: evidence that the oxygen sensor is a heme protein. Science 242:1412, 1988.

82. Gleadle, J.M., Ebert, B.L., and Ratcliffe, P.J.: Diphenylene iodonium inhibits the induction of erythropoietin and other mammalian genes by hypoxia. Implications for the mechanism of oxygen sensing. Eur. J. Biochem. 234:99, 1995.

83. Schuster, S.J., Badiavas, E.V., Costa-Giomi, P., Weinmann, R., Erslev, A.J., and Caro, J.: Stimulation of erythropoietin gene transcription during hypoxia and cobalt exposure. Blood 73:13, 1989.

84. Bunn, H.F., Gu, J., Huang, L.E., Park, J.W., and Zhu, H.: Erythropoietin: a model system for studying oxygen-dependent gene regulation. J. Exp. Biol. 201:1197, 1998.

85. Huang, L.E., Ho, V., Arany, Z., Krainc, D., Galson, D., Tendler, D., Livingston, D.M., and Bunn, H.F.: Erythropoietin gene regulation depends on heme-dependent oxygen sensing and assembly of interacting transcription factors. Kidney Int. 5:548, 1997.

86. Semenza, G.L., Nejfelt, M.K., Chi, S.M., and Antonarakis, S.E.: Hypoxia-inducible factors bind to an enhnancer element located 3′ to the human erythropoietin gene. Proc. Natl. Acad. Sci. USA 88:5680, 1991.

87. Huang, L.E., Gu, J., Schau, M., and Bunn, H.F.: Erythropoietin gene is regulated by modulating HIF-1α stability through an oxygen-dependent destabilization domain. Blood 90(suppl. 1):303a, 1997.

88. Blanchard, K.L., Acquaviva, A.M., Galson, D.L., and Bunn, H.F.: Hypoxic induction of the human erythropoietin gene: cooperation between the promoter and enhancer, each of which contains steroid receptor response elements. Mol. Cell. Biol. 12:5373, 1992.

89. Tsuchiya, T., Ochiai, H., Imajoh-Ohmi, S., Ueda, M., Suda, T., Nakamura, M., and Kanegasaki, S.: In vitro reconstitution of an erythropoietin gene transcription system using its 5′ flanking sequence and a nuclear extract from anemic kidney. Biochem. Biophys. Res. Commun. 182:137, 1992.

90. McGary, E.C., Rondon, I.J., and Beckman, B.S.: Post-transcriptional regulation of erythropoietin mRNA stability by erythropoietin mRNA-binding protein. J. Biol. Chem. 272:8628, 1997.

91. Wu, H., Liu, X., Jaenisch, R., and Lodish, H.F.: Generation of committed erythroid BFU-E and CFU-E progenitors does not require erythropoietin or the erythropoietin receptor. Cell 83:59, 1995.

92. Lin, C.S., Lim, S.K., D'Agati, V., and Constantini, F.: Differential effects of an erythropoietin receptor gene disruption on primitive and definitive erythropoiesis. Genes Dev. 10:154, 1996.

93. D'Andrea, A.D., Lodish, H.F., and Wong, G.G.: Expression cloning of the murine erythropoietin receptor. Cell 57:277, 1989.

94. Gearing, D.P., King, J.A., Gough, N.M., and Nicola, N.A.: Expression cloning of a receptor for human granulocyte-macrophage colony-stimulating factor. EMBO J. 8:3667, 1989.

95. Winkelmann, J.C., Penny, L.A., Deaven, L.L., Forget, B.G., and Jenkens, R.B.: The gene for the human erythropoietin receptor: analysis of the coding sequence and assignment to chromosome 19p. Blood 76:24, 1990.

96. Sawyer, S.T., and Hankis, W.D.: The functional form of the erythropoietin receptor is 78-kDa protein: correlation with cell surface expression, endocytosis, and phosphorylation. Proc. Natl. Acad. Sci. USA 90:6849, 1993.

97. Watowich, S.S., Yoshimura, A., Longmore, G.D., Hilton, D.J., Yoshimura, Y., and Lodish, H.F.: Homodimerization and constitutive activation of the erythropoietin receptor. Proc. Natl. Acad. Sci. USA 89:2140, 1992.

98. Schneider, H., Chaovapong, W., Matthews, D.J., Karkaria, C., Cass, R.T., Zhan, H., Boyle, M., Lorenzini, T., Elliott, S.G., and Giebel, L.B.: Homodimerization of erythropoietin receptor by a bivalent monoclonal antibody triggers cell proliferation and differentiation of erythroid precursors. Blood 89:473, 1997.

99. Livnah, O., Stura, E.A., Johnson, D.L., Middleton, S.A., Mulcahy, L.S., Wrighton, N.C., Dower, W.J., Jolliffe, L.K., and Wilson, I.A.: Functional mimicry of a protein hormone by a peptide agonist: the EPO receptor complex at 2.8 Å. Science 273:464, 1996.

100. Wu, H., Klingmüller, U., Acurio, A., Hsiao, J.G., and Lodish, H.F.: Functional interaction of erythropoietin and stem cell factor receptor is essential for erythroid colony formation. Proc. Natl. Acad. Sci. USA. 94:1806, 1997.

101. Jubinsky, P.T., Krijanovski, O.I., Nathan, D.G., Tavernier, J., and Sieff, C.A.: The β chain of the interleukin-3 receptor functionally associates with the erythropoietin receptor. Blood 90:1867, 1997.

102. Broudy, V.C., Lin, N., Brice, M., Nakamoto, B., and Papayannopoulou, T.: Erythropoietin receptor characteristics on primary human erythroid cells. Blood 12:2583, 1991.

103. Migliaccio, A.R., Jiang, Y., Migliaccio, G., Nicolis, S., Crotta, S., Ronchi, A., Ottolenghi, S., and Adamson, J.W.: Transcriptional and posttranscriptional regulation of the expression of the erythropoietin receptor gene in human erythropoietin-responsive cell lines. Blood 82:3760, 1993.

104. Youssoufian, H.: Further characterization of *cis*-acting regulatory sequences in the genomic locus of the murine erythropoietin receptor: evidence for stage-specific regulation. Blood 83:1428, 1994.

105. Chin, K., Oda, N., Shen, K., and Noguchi, C.T.: Regulation of transcription of the human erythropoietin receptor gene by proteins binding to GATA-1 and Sp1 motifs. Nucleic Acids Res. 23:3041, 1995.

106. Welte, K., Platzer, E., Lu, L., Gabrilove, J.L., Levi, E., Mertelsmann, R., and Moore, M.A.S.: Purification and biochemical characterization of human pluripotent hematopoietic colony-stimulating factor. Proc. Natl. Acad. Sci. USA 82:1526, 1985.

107. Souza, L.M., Boone, T.C., Gabrilove, J., Lai, P.H., Zsebo, K.M., Murdock, D.C., Chazin, V.R., Bruszewski, J., Lu, H., and Chen, K.K.: Recombinant human granulocyte colony-stimulating factor: effects on normal and leukemic myeloid cells. Science 232:61, 1986.

108. Nagata, S., Tsuchiya, M., Asano, S., Kaziro, Y., Yamakazi, T., Yamamoto, O., Hirata, Y., Kubota, N., Oheda, M., and Nomura, H.: Molecular cloning and expression of cDNA for human granulocyte colony-stimulating factor. Nature 319:415, 1986.

109. Simmers, R.N., Smith, J., Shannon, M.F., Wong, G., Lopez, A.F., Baker, E., Sutherland, G.R., and Vadas, M.A.: Localization of the human G-CSF gene to the region of the breakpoint in the translocation typical of acute promyelocytic leukemia. Hum. Genet. 78:134, 1988.

110. Nagata, S.: Gene structure and function of granulocyte colony-stimulating factor. Bioessays 10:113, 1989.

111. Arakawa, T., Horan, T.P., Leong, K., Prestrelski, S.J., Narhi, L.O., and Hu, S.: Structure and activity of granulocyte colony-stimulating factor derived from CHO cells containing cDNA coding for alternatively spliced sequences. Arch. Biochem. Biophys. 316:285, 1995.

112. Rennick, D., Yang, G., Gemmell, L., and Lee, F.: Control of hemopoiesis by a bone marrow stromal cell clone: lipopolysaccharide- and interleukin-1–inducible production of colony-stimulating factors. Blood 69:682, 1987.

113. Koeffler, H.P., Gasson, J., Ranyard, J., Souza, L., Shepard, M., and Munker, R.: Recombinant human TNF alpha stimulates production of granulocyte colony-stimulating factor. Blood 70:55, 1987.

114. Kaushansky, K., Lin, N., and Adamson, J.W.: IL-1 stimulates fibroblasts to synthesize granulocyte/macrophage (GM) and granulocyte (G) colony-stimulating factors: a mechanism for the hematopoietic response to inflammation. J. Clin. Invest. 81:92, 1988.

115. Yang, Y.C., Tsai, S., Wong, G.G., and Clark, S.C.: Interleukin-1 regulation of hematopoietic growth factor production by human stromal fibroblasts. J. Cell. Physiol. 134:292, 1988.

116. Rugo, H.S., O'Hanley, P., Bishop, A.G., Pearce, M.K., Abrams, J.S., Howard, M., and O'Garra, A.: Local cytokine production in a murine model of *Escherichia coli* pyelonephritis. J. Clin. Invest. 89:1032, 1992.

117. Akira, S., Isshiki, H., Sugita, T., Tanabe, O.K.S., Nishio, Y., Nakajima, T., Hirano, T., and Kishimoto, T.: A nuclear factor for IL-6 expression (NF-IL6) is a member of a C/EBP family. EMBO J. 9:1897, 1990.

118. Shannon, M.F., Coles, L.S., Fielke, R.K., Goodall, G.J., Lagnado, C.A., and Vadas, M.A.: Three essential promoter elements mediate

tumor necrosis factor and interleukin-1 activation of the granulocyte colony-stimulating factor gene. Growth Factors 7:181, 1992.

119. Ernst, T.J., Ritchie, A.R., Demetri, G.D., and Griffin, J.D.: Regulation of granulocyte and monocyte colony-stimulating factor mRNA levels in human blood monocytes is mediated primarily at a post-transcriptional level. J. Biol. Chem. 264:5700, 1989.

120. Kawakami, M., Tsutsumi, H., Kumakawa, T., Abe, H., Hirai, M., Kurosawa, S., Mori, M., and Fukushima, M.: Levels of serum granulocyte colony-stimulating factor in patients with infections. Blood 76:1962, 1990.

121. Mempel, K., Pietsch, T., Menzel, T., Zeidler, C., and Welte, K.: Increased serum levels of granulocyte colony-stimulating factor in patients with severe congenital neutropenia. Blood 77:1919, 1991.

122. Cairo, M.S., Suen, Y., Sender, L., Gillan, E.R., Ho, W., Plunkett, J.M., and Van de Ven, C.: Circulating granulocyte colony-stimulating factor (G-CSF) levels after allogeneic and autologous bone marrow transplantation: endogenous G-CSF production correlates with myeloid engraftment. Blood 79:1869, 1992.

123. Miksits, K., Beyer, J., and Siegert, W.: Serum concentrations of G-CSF during high-dose chemotherapy with autologous stem cell rescue. Bone Marrow Transplant. 11:375, 1993.

124. Kojima, S., Matsuyama, T., Kodera, Y., Nishihara, H., Ueda, K., Shimbo, T., and Nakahata, T.: Measurement of endogenous granulocyte colony-stimulating factor in patients with acquired aplastic anemia by a sensitive chemiluminescent immunoassay. Blood 87:1303, 1996.

125. Sallerfors, B.: Endogenous production and peripheral blood levels of granulocyte-macrophage (GM-) and granulocyte (G-) colony stimulating factors. Leuk. Lymphoma 13:235, 1994.

126. Morstyn, G., Campbell, L., Souza, L.M., Alton, N.K., Keech, J., Green, M., Sheridan, W., Metcalf, D., and Fox, R.: Effect of granulocyte colony stimulating factor on neutropenia induced by cytotoxic chemotherapy. Lancet 1:667, 1988.

127. Lieschke, G.J., Grail, D., Hodgson, D., Metcalf, D., Stanley, E., Cheers, C., Fowler, K.J., Basu, S., Zhan, Y.F., and Dunn, A.R.: Mice lacking granulocyte colony-stimulating factor have chronic neutropenia, granulocyte and macrophage progenitor cell deficiency, and impaired neutrophil mobilization. Blood 84:1737, 1994.

128. Liu, F., Wu, H.Y., Wesselschmidt, R., Kornaga, T., and Link, D.: Impaired production and increased apoptosis of neutrophils in granulocyte colony-stimulating factor receptor deficient mice. Immunity 5:491, 1996.

129. Liu, F., Poursine-Laurent, J., Wu, H.Y., and Link, D.C.: Interleukin-6 and the granulocyte colony-stimulating factor receptor are major independent regulators of granulopoiesis in vivo but are not required for lineage commitment or terminal differentiation. Blood 90:2583, 1997.

130. Balazovich, K.J., Almeida, H.I., and Boxer, L.A.: Recombinant human G-CSF and GM-CSF prime human neutrophils for superoxide production through different signal transduction methods. J. Lab. Clin. Med. 118:576, 1991.

131. Ohsaka, A., Kitagawa, S., Yuo, A., Motoyoshi, K., Furasawa, S., Miura, Y., Takaku, F., and Saito, M.: Effects of granulocyte colony stimulating factor on respiratory burst activity of neutrophils in patients with myelodysplastic syndromes. Clin. Exp. Immunol. 91:308, 1993.

132. Ikebuchi, K., Clark, S.C., Ihle, J.N., Souza, L.M., and Ogawa, M.: Granulocyte colony-stimulating factor enhances interleukin 3–dependent proliferation of multipotential hemopoietic progenitors. Proc. Natl. Acad. Sci. USA 85:3445, 1988.

133. Leary, A.G., Zeng, H.Q., Clark, S.C., and Ogawa, M.: Growth factor requirements for survival in G0 and entry into the cell cycle of primitive human hematopoietic progenitors. Proc. Natl. Acad. Sci. USA 89:4013, 1992.

134. Tweardy, D.J., Anderson, K., Cannizzaro, L.A., Steinman, R.A., Croce, C.M., and Huebner, K.: Molecular cloning of cDNAs for the human granulocyte colony-stimulating factor receptor from HL-60 and mapping of the gene to chromosome 1p32–34. Blood 79:1148, 1992.

135. Fukunaga, R., Seto, Y., Mizushima, S., and Nagata, S.: Three different mRNAs encoding human granulocyte colony-stimulating factor receptor. Proc. Natl. Acad. Sci. USA 87:8702, 1990.

136. Fukunaga, R., Ishizaka-Ikeda, E., Pan, C.X., Seto, Y., and Nagata, S.: Functional domains of the granulocyte colony stimulating factor receptor. EMBO J. 10:2855, 1991.

137. Zhang, D.E., Hohaus, S., Vovo, M.T., Chen, H.M., Smith, L.T., Heth-

138. erington, C.J., and Tenen, D.G.: Function of PU.1 (Spi-1), C/EBP, and AML1 in early myelopoiesis: regulation of multiple myeloid CSF receptor promoters. Curr. Top. Microbiol. Immunol. 211:137, 1996.

138. Smith, L.T., Hohaus, S., Gonzalez, D.A., Dziennes, S.E., and Tenen, D.G.: PU.1 (Spi-1) and C/EBP alpha regulate the granulocyte colony stimulating factor promoter in myeloid cells. Blood 88:1234, 1996.

139. Tenen, D.G., Hromas, R., Licht, J.D., and Zhang, D.E.: Transcription factors, normal myeloid development and leukemia. Blood 90:489, 1997.

140. Bernstein, R., Bagg, A., Pinto, M., Lewis, D., and Mendelow, B.: Chromosome 3q21 abnormalities associated with hyperactive thrombopoiesis in acute blastic transformation of chronic myeloid leukemia. Blood 68:652, 1986.

141. de Sauvage, F.J., Hass, P.E., Spencer, S.D., Malloy, B.E., Gurney, A.L., Spencer, S.A., Darbonne, W.C., Henzel, W.J., Wong, S.C., Kuang, W.J., Oles, K.J., Hultgren, B., Solberg, L.A., Jr., Goeddel, D.V., and Eaton, D.L.: Stimulation of megakaryocytopoiesis and thrombopoiesis by the c-Mpl ligand. Nature 369:533, 1994.

142. Bartley, T.D., Bogenberger, J., Hunt, P., Li, Y.-S., Lu, H.S., Martin, F., Chang, M.-S., Samal, B., Nichol, J.L., Swift, S., Johnson, M.J., Hsu, R.-Y., Parker, V.P., Suggs, S., Skrine, J.D., Merewether, L.A., Clogston, C., Hsu, E., Hokom, M.M., Hornkohl, A., Choi, E., Pangelinan, M., Sun, Y., Mar, V., McNinch, J., Simonet, L., Jacobsen, F., Xie, C., Shutter, J., Chute, H., Basu, R., Selander, L., Trollinger, D., Sieu, L., Padilla, D., Trail, G., Elliott, G., Izumi, R., Covey, T., Crouse, J., Garcia, A., Xu, W., del Castillo, J., Biron, J., Cole, S., Hu, M.C.-T., Pacifici, R., Ponting, I., Saris, C., Wen, D., Yung, Y.P., Lin, H., and Bosselman, R.A.: Identification and cloning of a megakaryocyte growth and development factor that is a ligand for the cytokine receptor Mpl. Cell 77:1117, 1994.

143. Ulich, T.R., del Castillo, J., Yin, S., Swift, S., Padilla, D., Senaldi, G., Bennett, L., Shutter, J., Bogenberger, J., Sun, D., Samal, B., Shimamoto, G., Lee, R., Steinbrink, R., Boone, T., Sheridan, W.T., and Hunt, P.: Megakaryocyte growth and development factor ameliorates carboplatin-induced thrombocytopenia in mice. Blood 86:971, 1995.

144. McCarty, J.M., Sprugel, K.H., Fox, N.E., Sabath, D.E., and Kaushansky, K.: Murine thrombopoietin mRNA levels are modulated by platelet count. Blood 86:3668, 1995.

145. Broudy, V.C., Lin, N.L., Sabath, D.F., Papayannopoulou, T.H., and Kaushansky, K.: Human platelets display high affinity receptors for thrombopoietin. Blood 89:1896, 1997.

146. Fielder, P.J., Hass, P., Nagel, M., Stefanich, E., Widmer, R., Bennett, G.L., Keller, G.A., de Sauvage, F.J., and Eaton, D.: Human platelets as a model for the binding and degradation of thrombopoietin. Blood 89:2782, 1997.

147. Kuter, D.J., and Rosenberg, R.D.: The reciprocal relationship of thrombopoietin (c-Mpl ligand) to changes in the platelet mass during busulfan-induced thrombocytopenia in the rabbit. Blood 85:2720, 1995.

148. Fielder, P.J., Gurney, A.L., Stefanich, E., Marian, M., Moore, M.W., Carver-Moore, K., and de Sauvage, F.J.: Regulation of thrombopoietin levels by c-mpl–mediated binding to platelets. Blood 71:430, 1996.

149. Emmons, R.V.B., Reid, D.M., Cohen, R.L., Meng, G., Young, N.S., Dunbar, C.E., and Shulman, N.R.: Human thrombopoietin levels are high when thrombocytopenia is due to megakaryocyte deficiency and low when due to increased platelet destruction. Blood 87:4068, 1996.

150. Gernsheimer, T., Stratton, J., Ballem, P.J., and Slichter, S.J.: Mechanisms of response to treatment in autoimmune thrombocytopenic purpura. N. Engl. J. Med. 320:974, 1989.

151. Kaushansky, K.: Thrombopoietin. Drug Therapy Series. N. Engl. J. Med. 339:746, 1998.

152. Kaushansky, K., Broudy, V.C., Lin, N., Jorgensen, M.J., McCarty, J., Fox, N., Zucker-Franklin, D., and Lofton-Day, C.: Thrombopoietin, the Mpl-ligand, is essential for full megakaryocyte development. Proc. Natl. Acad. Sci. USA 92:3234, 1995.

153. Komatsu, N., Kirito, K., Shimizu, R., Kunitama, M., Yamada, M., Uchida, M., Takatoku, M., Eguchi, M., and Miura, Y.: In vitro development of erythroid and megakaryocytic cells from a UT-7 subline, UT-7/GM. Blood 89:4021, 1997.

154. Kaushansky, K., Lok, S., Holly, R.D., Broudy, V.C., Lin, N., Bailey, M.C., Forstrom, J.W., Buddle, M., Oort, P.J., Hagen, F.S., Roth, G.J., Papayannopoulou, Th., and Foster, D.C.: Promotion of megakaryocyte progenitor expansion and differentiation by the c-Mpl ligand thrombopoietin. Nature 369:568, 1994.

155. Zauli, G., Bassini, A., Vitale, M., Gibellini, D., Celeghini, C., Cara-

melli, E., Pierpaoli, S., Guidotti, L., and Capitani, S.: Thrombopoietin enhances the $\alpha_{IIb} \beta_3$-dependent adhesion of megakaryocytic cells to fibrinogen or fibronectin through PI 3 kinase. Blood 89:883, 1997.

156. Cui, L., Ramsfjell, V., Borge, O.J., Veiby, O.P., Lok, S., and Jacobsen, S.E.W.: Thrombopoietin promotes adhesion of primitive human hemopoietic cells to fibronectin and vascular cell adhesion molecule-1. J. Immunol. 159:1961, 1997.

157. Nichol, J., Hokom, M., Hornkohl, A., Sheridan, W.P., Ohashi, H., Kato, T., Li, Y.S., Bartley, T.D., Choi, E., Bogenberger, J., Skrine, J.D., Knudten, A., Chen, J., Trail, G., Sleeman, L., Cole, S., Grampp, G., and Hunt, P.: Megakaryocyte growth and development factor: analysis of in vitro effects on human megakaryopoiesis and endogenous serum levels during chemotherapy induced thrombocytopenia. J. Clin. Invest. 95:2973, 1995.

158. Angchaisuksiri, P., Carlson, P.L., and Dessypris, E.N.: Effects of recombinant thrombopoietin on megakaryocyte colony formation and megakaryocyte ploidy by human CD34 + cells in a serum free system. Br. J. Haematol. 93:13, 1996.

159. Broudy, V.C., Lin, N.L., and Kaushansky, K.: Thrombopoietin (c-*mpl* ligand) acts synergistically with erythropoietin, stem cell factor, and Il-11 to enhance murine megakaryocyte colony growth and increases megakaryocyte ploidy in vitro. Blood 85:1719, 1995.

160. Nagasawa, T., Osada, M., Komeno, T., Kojima, H., Ninomiya, H., Todokoro, K., and Abe, T.: In vitro and in vivo deprivation of thrombopoietin induces megakaryocytic apoptosis and regulates platelet production. Exp. Hematol. 25:897, 1997.

161. Ku, H., Yonemura, Y., Kaushansky, K., and Ogawa, M.: Thrombopoietin, the ligand for the Mpl receptor, synergy with steel factor and other early-acting cytokines in supporting proliferation of primitive hematopoietic progenitors of mice. Blood 87:4544, 1996.

162. Sitnicka, E., Lin, N., Priestley, G.V., Fox, N., Broudy, V.C., Wolf, N.S., and Kaushansky, K.: The effect of thrombopoietin on the proliferation and differentiation of murine hematopoietic stem cells. Blood 87:4998, 1996.

163. Kobayashi, M., Laver, J.H., Kato, T., Miyazaki, H., and Ogawa, M.: Thrombopoietin supports proliferation of human primitive hematopoietic cells in synergy with steel factor and/or interleukin-3. Blood 88:429, 1996.

163a. Yagi, M., Ritchie, K.A., Sitnicka, E., Storey, C., Roth, G.J., and Bartelmez, S.: Sustained ex vivo expansion of hematopoietic stem cells mediated by thrombopoietin. Proc. Natl. Acad. Sci. USA 96:8126, 1999.

164. Alexander, W.S., Roberts, A.W., and Nicola, N.A.: Deficiencies in progenitor cells of multiple hematopoietic lineages and defective megakaryocytopoiesis in mice lacking the thrombopoietin receptor c-Mpl. Blood 87:2162, 1996.

165. Carver-Moore, K., Broxmeyer, H.E., Luoh, S.M., Cooper, S., Peng, J., Burstein, S.A., Moore, M.W., and de Sauvage, F.J.: Low levels of erythroid and myeloid progenitors in thrombopoietin and mpl-deficient mice. Blood 88:803, 1996.

166. de Sauvage, F.J.: Multiple roles of Tpo revealed by gene targeting. Acta Hematol. 98(suppl. 1):36, 1997.

167. Methia, N., Louache, F., Vainchenker, W., and Wendling, F.: Oligodeoxynucleotides antisense to the proto-oncogene c-*mpl* specifically inhibit in vitro. Blood 82:1395, 1993.

168. Vigon, I., Florindo, C., Fichelson, S., Guenet, J.-L., Mattei, M.-G., Souyri, M., Cosman, D., and Gisselbrecht, S.: Characterization of the murine *Mpl* proto-oncogene, a member of the hematopoietic cytokine receptor family: molecular cloning, chromosomal location and evidence for a function in cell growth. Oncogene 8:2607, 1993.

169. Skoda, R.C., Seldin, D.C., Chiang, M.K., Peichel, C.L., Vogt, T.F., and Leder, P.: Murine c-*mpl*: a member of the hematopoietic growth factor receptor superfamily that transduces a proliferative signal. EMBO J. 12:2645, 1993.

170. Baumgartner, J.W., Wells, C.A., Chen, C.M., and Waters, M.J.: The role of the SWXWS equivalent motif in growth hormone receptor function. J. Biol. Chem. 269:29094, 1994.

171. Hilton, D.J., Watowich, S.S., Katz, L., and Lodish, H.F.: Saturation mutagenesis of the WSXWS motif of the erythropoietin receptor. J. Biol. Chem. 271:4699, 1996.

172. Van Leeuwen, B.H., Martinson, M.E., Webb, G.C., and Young, I.G.: Molecular organization of the cytokine gene cluster, involving the human IL-3, IL-4, IL-5 and GM-CSF genes, on human chromosome 5. Blood 73:1142, 1989.

173. Yang, Y.C., Ciarletta, A.B., Temple, P.A., Chung, M.P., Kovacic, S., Witek-Giannotti, J.S., Leary, A.C., Kriz, R., Donahue, R.E., Wong, G.G., and Clark, S.C.: Human IL-3 (multi-CSF): Identification by expression cloning of a novel hematopoietic growth factor related to murine IL-3. Cell 47:3, 1986.

174. Kelso, A., and Gough, N.M.: Coexpression of granulocyte-macrophage colony-stimulating factor, δinterferon, and interleukins 3 and 4 is random in murine alloreactive T-lymphocyte clones. Proc. Natl. Acad. Sci. USA 85:9189, 1988.

175. Niemeyer, C.M., Sieff, C.A., Mathey-Prevot, B., Wimperis, J.Z., Bierer, B.E., Clark, S.C., and Nathan, D.G.: Expression of human interleukin-3 (multi-CSF) is restricted to human lymphocytes and T-cell tumor lines. Blood 73:945, 1989.

176. Kelso, A., Metcalf, D., and Gough, N.M.: Independent regulation of granulocyte-macrophage colony-stimulating factor and multi-lineage colony-stimulating factor production in T lymphocyte clones. J. Immunol. 136:1718, 1986.

177. Kelso, A., and Owens, T.: Production of two hemopoietic growth factors is differentially regulated in single T lymphocytes activated with an anti–T cell receptor antibody. J. Immunol. 140:1159, 1988.

178. Guba, S.C., Stella, G., Turka, L.A., June, C.H., Thompson, C.B., and Emerson, S.G.: Regulation of interleukin 3 gene induction in normal human T cells. J. Clin. Invest. 84:1701, 1989.

179. Gibson, F.M., Scopes, J., Daly, S., Rizzo, S., Ball, S.E., and Gordon-Smith, E.C.: IL-3 is produced by normal stroma in long-term bone marrow cultures. Br. J. Haematol. 90:518, 1995.

180. Mathey-Prevot, B., Andrews, N.C., Murphy, H.S., Kreissman, S.G., and Nathan, D.G.: Positive and negative elements regulate human interleukin 3 expression. Proc. Natl. Acad. Sci. USA 87:5046, 1990.

181. Shoemaker, S.G., Hromas, R., and Kaushansky, K.: IL-3 gene expression is dependent upon AP-1 and a novel transcriptional regulator, NF-IL3-A, in human T-lymphocytes. Proc. Natl. Acad. Sci. USA 87:9650, 1990.

182. Cockerill, P.N., Shannon, M.F., Bert, A.G., Ryan, G.R., and Vadas, M.A.: The granulocyte-macrophage colony-stimulating factor/interleukin 3 locus is regulated by an inducible cyclosporin A–sensitive enhancer. Proc. Natl. Acad. Sci. USA 90:2466, 1993.

183. Engeland, K., Andrews, N.C., and Mathey-Prevot, B.: Multiple proteins interact with the nuclear inhibitor protein repressor element in the human interleukin-3 promoter. J. Biol. Chem. 270:24572, 1995.

184. Gerondakis, S., Strasser, A., Metcalf, D., Grigoriadis, G., Scheerlinck, J.P.Y., and Grumont, R.J.: Rel-deficient T cells exhibit defects in production of interleukin 3 and granulocyte-macrophage colony-stimulating factor. Proc. Natl. Acad. Sci. USA 93:3405, 1996.

185. Duncliffe, K.N., Bert, A.G., and Vadas, M.A.: A T cell–specific enhancer in the interleukin-3 locus is activated cooperatively by Oct and NFAT elements within a DNase I–hypersensitive site. Immunity 6:175, 1997.

186. Uchida, H., Zhang, J., and Nimer, S.D.: AML1A and AML1B can transactivate the human IL-3 promoter. J. Immunol. 158:2251, 1997.

187. Kindler, V., Thorens, B., de Kossodo, S., Allet, B., Eliason, J.F., Thatcher, D., Farber, N., and Vassalli, P.: Stimulation of hematopoiesis in vivo by recombinant bacterial murine interleukin 3. Proc. Natl. Acad. Sci. USA 83:1001, 1986.

188. Broxmeyer, H.E., Williams, D.E., Hangoc, G., Cooper, S., Gillis, S., Shadduck, R.K., and Bicknell, D.C.: Synergistic myelopoietic actions in vivo after administration to mice of combinations of purified natural murine colony-stimulating factor 1, recombinant murine interleukin 3 and recombinant murine granulocyte/macrophage colony-stimulating factor. Proc. Natl. Acad. Sci. USA 84:3871, 1987.

189. Clutterbuck, E.J., Hirst, E.M.A., and Sanderson, C.J.: Human interleukin-5 (IL-5) regulates the production of eosinophils in human bone marrow cultures: comparison and interaction with IL-1, IL-3, IL-6, and GMCSF. Blood 73:1504, 1989.

190. Carrington, P.A., Hill, R.J., Stenberg, P.E., Levin, J., Corash, L., Scheurs, J., Baker, G., and Levin, F.C.: Multiple in vivo effects of interleukin 3 and interleukin 6 on mouse megakaryocytopoiesis. Blood 77:34, 1991.

191. Yonemura, Y., Kawakita, M., Masuda, T., Fujimoto, T., Kato, K., and Takatsuki, K.: Synergistic effects of interleukin 3 and interleukin 11 on murine megakaryopoiesis in serum-free culture. Exp. Hematol. 20:1011, 1992.

192. Valent, P., Besemer, J., Muhm, M., Majdic, O., Lechner, K., and Bettelheim, P.: Interleukin 3 activates human blood basophils via high-affinity binding sites. Proc. Natl. Acad. Sci. USA 86:5542, 1989.

193. Deng, X., Ito, T., Carr, B., and May, W.S.: Dynamic phosphorylation

of Bcl2 associated with survival phenotype. Exp. Hematol. 25:897, 1997.

194. del Peso, L., González-Garcia, M., Page, C., Herrera, R., and Nuñez, G.: Interleukin-3–induced phosphorylation of BAD through the protein kinase Akt. Science 278:687, 1997.

195. Kaushansky, K., O'Hara, P.J., Hart, C.E., Forstrom, J.W., and Hagen, F.S.: Role of carbohydrate in the function of human granulocyte-macrophage colony-stimulating factor. Biochemistry 26:4861, 1987.

196. Wong, G.G., Witek, J.S., Temple, P.A., Wilkens, K.M., Leary, A.C., Luxenberg, P.D., Jones, S.S., Brown, E.L., Kay, R.M., Orr, E.C., Shoemaker, C., Golde, D.W., Kaufman, R.J., Hewick, R.M., Wang, E.A., and Clark, S.C.: Human GM-CSF: molecular cloning of the complementary DNA and purification of the natural and recombinant proteins. Science 228:810, 1985.

197. Munker, R., Gasson, J., Ogawa, M., and Koeffler, H.P.: Recombinant human TNF induces production of granulocyte-monocyte colony-stimulating factor. Nature 323:79, 1986.

198. Broudy, V.C., Kaushansky, K., Segal, G.M., Harlan, J.M., and Adamson, J.W.: Tumor necrosis factor type alpha stimulates human endothelial cells to produce granulocyte/macrophage colony-stimulating factor. Proc. Natl. Acad. Sci. USA 83:7467, 1986.

199. Seelantag, W.K., Mermod, J.J., Montesano, R., and Vassalli, P.: Additive effects of interleukin 1 and tumour necrosis factor-α on the accumulation of the three granulocyte and macrophage colony-stimulating factor mRNAs in human endothelial cells. EMBO J. 6:2261, 1987.

200. Sieff, C.A., Tsai, S., and Faller, D.V.: Interleukin 1 induces cultured human endothelial cell production of granulocyte-macrophage colony-stimulating factor. J. Clin. Invest. 79:48, 1987.

201. Cannistra, S.A., Rambaldi, A., Spriggs, D.R., Hermann, F., Kufe, D., and Griffin, J.D.: Human granulocyte-macrophage colony-stimulating factor induces expression of the tumor necrosis factor gene by the U937 cell line and by normal human monocytes. J. Clin. Invest. 79:1720, 1987.

202. Zsebo, K.M., Yuschenkoff, V.N., Schiffer, S., Chang, D., McCall, E., Dinarello, C.A., Brown, M.A., Altrock, B., and Bagby, G.C., Jr.: Vascular endothelial cells and granulopoiesis: interleukin-1 stimulates release of G-CSF and GM-CSF. Blood 71:99, 1988.

203. Kaushansky, K.: Control of granulocyte-macrophage colony stimulating factor production in normal endothelial cells by positive and negative elements. J. Immunol. 143:2525, 1989.

204. de Wynter, E., Allen, T., Coutinho, L., Flavell, D., Flavell, S.U., and Dexter, T.M.: Localisation of granulocyte macrophage colony-stimulating factor in human long-term bone marrow cultures. J. Cell Sci. 106:761, 1993.

205. Koeffler, H.P., Gasson, J., and Tobler, A.: Transcriptional and post-transcriptional modulation of myeloid colony-stimulating factor expression by tumor necrosis factor and other agents. Mol. Cell. Biol. 8:3432, 1988.

206. Shaw, G., and Kamen, R.: A conserved AU sequence from the 3' untranslated region of GM-CSF mRNA mediates selective mRNA degradation. Cell 46:659, 1986.

207. Thorens, B., Mermod, J.J., and Vassalli, P.: Phagocytosis and inflammatory stimuli induce GMCSF mRNA in macrophages through post-transcriptional regulation. Cell 48:671, 1987.

208. Zhang, W., Wagner, B.J., Ehrenman, K., Schaefer, A.W., DeMaria, C.T., Crater, D., DeHaven, K., Long, L., and Brewer, G.: Purification, characterization, and cDNA cloning of an AU-rich element RNA-binding protein, AUF1. Mol. Cell. Biol. 13:7652, 1993.

209. Rajagopalan, L.E., and Malter, J.S.: Modulation of granulocyte-macrophage colony-stimulating factor mRNA stability in vitro by the adenosine-uridine binding factor. J. Biol. Chem. 269:23882, 1994.

210. Bichsel, V.E., Walz, A., and Bickel, M.: Identification of proteins binding specifically to the 3'-untranslated region of granulocyte/macrophage-colony stimulating factor mRNA. Nucleic Acids Res. 25:2417, 1997.

211. Sirenko, O.I., Lofquist, A.K., DeMaria, C.T., Morris, J.S., Brewer, G., and Haskill, J.S.: Adhesion-dependent regulation of an A + U–rich element-binding activity associated with AUF1. Mol. Cell. Biol. 17:3898, 1997.

212. Buzby, J.S., Lee, S.M., DeMaria, C.T., Brewer, G., and Cairo, M.S.: Increased GM-CSF mRNA instability in cord vs adult mononuclear cells is translation dependent and associated wtih increased levels of A + U–rich element binding factor (AUF1). Blood 88:2889, 1996.

213. Kaushansky, K., O'Hara, P.J., Berkner, K., Segal, G.M., Hagen, F.S.,

and Adamson, J.W.: Genomic cloning, characterization, and multilineage expression of human granulocyte-macrophage colony-stimulating factor. Proc. Natl. Acad. Sci. USA 83:3101, 1986.

214. Emerson, S.G., Yang, Y.C., Clark, S.C., and Long, M.W.: Human recombinant granulocyte-macrophage colony stimulating factor and interleukin-3 have overlapping but distinct hematopoietic activity. J. Clin. Invest. 82:1282, 1988.

215. DiPersio, J.F., Billing, P., Williams, R., and Gasson, J.C.: Human granulocyte-macrophage colony-stimulating factor and other cytokines prime human neutrophils for enhanced arachidonic acid release and leukotriene B₄ synthesis. J. Immunol. 140:4315, 1988.

216. Dirksen, U., Nishinakamura, R., Groneck, P., Hattenhorst, U., Nogee, L., Murray, R., and Burdach, S.: Human pulmonary alveolar proteinosis associated wtih a defect in GM-CSF/IL-3/IL-5 receptor common chain expression. J. Clin. Invest. 100:2211, 1997.

217. Basu, S., Dunn, A.R., Marino, M.W., Savoia, H., Hodgson, G., Lieschke, G.J., and Cebon, J.: Increased tolerance to endotoxin by granulocyte-macrophage colony-stimulating factor–deficient mice. J. Immunol. 159:1412, 1997.

218. Coffman, R.L., Seymour, B.W.P., Lebman, D.A., Hiraki, D.D., Christiansen, J.A., Shrader, B., Cherwinski, H.M., Savelkoul, H.F.J., Finkelman, F.D., Bond, M.W., and Mosmann, T.R.: The role of helper T cell products in mouse B cell differentiation and isotype regulation. Immunol. Rev. 102:5, 1988.

219. Karlen, S., Mordvinov, V.A., and Sanderson, C.J.: How is expression of the IL-5 gene regulated? Immunol. Cell Biol. 74:218, 1996.

220. Tanabe, T., Konishi, M., Mizuta, T., Noma, T., and Honjo, T.: Molecular cloning and structure of the human interleukin-5 gene. J. Biol. Chem. 262:16580, 1987.

221. Campbell, H.D., Tucker, W.Q.J., Hort, Y., Martinson, M.E., Mayo, G., Clutterbuck, E.J., Sanderson, C.J., and Young, I.G.: Molecular cloning, nucleotide sequence, and expression of the gene encoding human eosinophil differentiation factor (interleukin 5). Proc. Natl. Acad. Sci. USA 84:6629, 1987.

222. Tominaga, A., Takahashi, T., Kikuchi, Y., Mita, S., Naomi, S., Harada, N., Yamaguchi, N., and Takatsu, K.: Role of carbohydrate moiety of IL-5. J. Immunol. 144:1345, 1990.

223. Sanderson, C.J.: Interleukin-5, eosinophils, and disease. Blood 79: 3101, 1992.

224. Coffman, R.L., Seymour, B.W.P., Hudak, S., Jackson, J., and Rennick, D.: Antibody to interleukin-5 inhibits helminth-induced eosinophilia in mice. Science 245:308, 1989.

225. Kopf, M., Brombacher, F., Hodgkin, P.D., Ramsey, A.J., Milbourne, E.A., Dai, W.J., Ovington, K.S., Behm, C.A., Kohler, G., Young, I.G., and Matthaei, K.I.: IL-5 deficient mice have a developmental defect in CD5+ B-1 cells and lack eosinophilia but have normal antibody and cytotoxic T cell responses. Immunity 4:15, 1996.

226. Yamaguchi, Y., Suda, T., Suda, J., Eguchi, M., Miura, Y., Harada, N., Tominaga, A., and Takatsu, K.: Purified interleukin 5 supports the terminal differentiation and proliferation of murine eosinophilic precursors. J. Exp. Med. 167:43, 1988.

227. Yamaguchi, Y., Hayashi, Y., Sugama, Y., Miura, Y., Kasahara, T., Torisu, M., Mita, S., Tominaga, A., Takatsu, K., and Suda, T.: Highly purified murine interleukin (IL-5) stimulates eosinophil function and prolongs in vitro survival: IL-5 as an eosinophil chemotactic factor. J. Exp. Med. 167:1737, 1988.

228. Yamaguchi, Y., Suda, T., Ohta, S., Tominaga, K., Miura, Y., and Kasahara, T.: Analysis of the survival of mature human eosinophils: interleukin-5 prevents apoptosis in mature human eosinophils. Blood 78:2542, 1991.

229. Koike, T., Enokihara, H., Arimura, H., Ninomiya, H., Yamashiro, K., Tsuruoka, N., Tsujimoto, M., Aoyagi, M., Watanabe, K., Nakamura, Y., Saitou, K., Furusawa, S., and Shishido, H.: Serum concentrations of IL-5, GM-CSF and IL-3 and the production of lymphocytes in various eosinophilia. Am. J. Hematol. 50:98, 1995.

230. Nishinakamura, R., Miyajima, A., Mee, P.J., Tybulewicz, V.L.J., and Murray, R.: Hematopoiesis in mice lacking the entire granulocyte-macrophage colony-stimulating factor/interleukin 3/interleukin 5 functions. Blood 88:2458, 1996.

231. Walsh, G.M., Hartnell, A., Wardlaw, A.J., Kurihara, K., Sanderson, C.J., and Kay, A.B.: IL-5 enhances the in vitro adhesion of eosinophils, but not neutrophils, in a leukocyte integrin (CD11/CD18) dependent manner. Immunology 71:258, 1990.

232. Hitoshi, Y., Yamaguchi, N., Mita, S., Sonoda, E., Takaki, S., Tominaga, A., and Takatsu, K.: Distribution of IL-5 receptor positive B

cells: expression of IL-5 receptor on Ly-1(CD5+) B cells. J. Immunol. 144:4218, 1990.

233. Huston, M.M., Moore, J.P., Mettes, H.J., Tavana, G., and Huston, D.P.: Human B cells express IL-5 receptor messenger ribonucleic acid and respond to IL-5 with enhanced IgM production after mitogenic stimulation with *Moraxella catarrhalis*. J. Immunol. 156:1392, 1996.

234. Randall, T.D., Lund, F.E., Brewer, J.W., Aldridge, C., Wall, R., and Corley, R.B.: Interleukin 5 (IL-5) and IL-6 define two molecularly distinct pathways of B cell differentiation. Mol. Cell. Biol. 13:3929, 1993.

235. Ohbo, K., Asao, H., Kouro, T., Nakamura, M., Takakai, S., Kikuchi, Y., Hirokawa, K., Tominaga, A., Takatsu, K., and Sugamura, K.: Demonstration of a cross-talk between IL-2 and IL-5 in phosphorylation of IL-2 and IL-5 receptor beta chains. Int. Immunol. 8:951, 1996.

236. Dent, L.A., Strath, M., Mellor, A.L., and Sanderson, C.J.: Eosinophilia in transgenic mice expressing interleukin 5. J. Exp. Med. 172:1425, 1990.

237. Lee, N.A., McGarry, M.P., Larson, K.A., Horton, M.A., Kirstensen, A.B., and Lee, J.J.: Expression of IL-5 in thymocytes/T cells leads to the development of a massive eosinophilia, extramedullary eosinophilopoiesis, and unique histopathologies. J. Immunol. 158:1332, 1997.

238. Tominaga, A., Takaki, S., Koyama, N., Katoh, S., Matsumoto, R., Migita, M., Hitoshi, Y., Hosoya, Y., Yamaguchi, S., Kanai, Y., Miyazaki, J.-I., Usuku, G., Yamamura, K.-I., and Takatsu, K.: Transgenic mice expressing a B cell growth and differentiation factor (interleukin 5) develop eosinophilia and autoantibody formation. J. Exp. Med. 173:429, 1991.

239. Itoh, N., Yonehara, S., Scheurs, J., Gorman, D.M., Maruyama, K., Ishii, A., Yahara, I., Arai, K., and Miyajima, A.: Cloning of an interleukin 3 receptor gene: a member of a distinct receptor gene family. Science 247:324, 1990.

240. Murata, Y., Takaki, S., Migita, M., Kikuchi, Y., Mita, S., Sonoda, E., Yamaguchi, N., and Takatsu, K.: Molecular cloning and expression of the murine interleukin-5 receptor. J. Exp. Med. 175:341, 1992.

241. Gorman, D.M., Itoh, M., Kitamura, T., Schreurs, J., Yonehara, S., Yahara, I., Arai, K., and Miyajima, A.: Cloning and expression of a gene encoding an interleukin 3 receptor–like protein: identification of another member of the cytokine receptor family. Proc. Natl. Acad. Sci. USA 87:5459, 1990.

242. Hayashida, K., Kitamura, T., Gorman, D.M., Arai, K., Yokota, T., and Miyajima, A.: Molecular cloning of a second subunit of the receptor for human granulocyte-macrophage colony-stimulating factor (GM-CSF): reconstitution of a high affinity GM-CSF receptor. Proc. Natl. Acad. Sci. USA 87:9655, 1990.

243. Tavernier, J., Devos, R., Cornelis, S., Tuypens, T., Van der Heyden, J., Fiers, W., and Plaetinck, G.: A human high affinity interleukin-5 receptor (IL5R) is composed of an IL5-specific α-chain and a β-chain shared with the receptor for GM-CSF. Cell 66:1175, 1991.

244. Takaki, S., Murata, Y., Kitamura, T., Miyajima, A., Tominaga, A., and Takatsu, K.: Reconstitution of the functional receptors for murine and human interleukin 5. J. Exp. Med. 177:1523, 1993.

245. Park, L.S., Waldron, P.E., Friend, D., Sassenfeld, H.M., Price, V., Anderson, D., Cosman, D., Andrews, R.G., Bernstein, I.D., and Urdal, D.L.: Interleukin-3, GM-CSF, and G-CSF receptor expression on cell lines and primary leukemia cells: receptor heterogeneity and relationship to growth factor responsiveness. Blood 74:56, 1989.

246. Lopez, A.F., Eglinton, J.M., Gillis, D., Park, L.S., Clark, S., and Vadas, M.A.: Reciprocal inhibition of binding between interleukin 3 and granulocyte-macrophage colony-stimulating factor to human eosinophils. Proc. Natl. Acad. Sci. USA 86:7022, 1989.

247. Weiss, M., Yokohama, C., Shikama, Y., Naugle, C., Druker, B., and Sieff, C.A.: Human granulocyte-macrophage colony-stimulating factor receptor signal transduction requires the proximal cytoplasmic domains of the α and β subunits. Blood 82:3298, 1993.

248. Mire-Sluis, A., Page, L.A., Wadhwa, M., and Thorpe, R.: Evidence for a signaling role for the α chains of granulocyte-macrophage colony-stimulating factor (GM-CSF), interleukin-3 (IL-3), and IL-5 receptors: divergent signaling pathways between GM-CSF/IL-3 and IL-5. Blood 86:2679, 1995.

249. Matsuguchi, T., Zhao, Y., Lilly, M.B., and Kraft, A.S.: The cytoplasmic domain of granulocyte-macrophage colony-stimulating factor (GM-CSF) receptor subunit is essential for both GM-CSF–mediated growth and differentiation. J. Biol. Chem. 272:17450, 1997.

250. Pless, M., Palmer, D., Callus, B., Rebel, V., and Mathey-Prevot, B.:

The cytoplasmic α-chain of the interleukin-5 receptor determines selectivity in the signaling receptor. Blood 90(suppl. 1):433a, 1997.

251. Bagley, C.J., Woodcock, J.M., Stomski, F.C., and Lopez, A.F.: The structural and functional basis of cytokine receptor activation: lessons from the common β subunit of the granulocyte-macrophage colony-stimulating factor, interleukin-3 (IL-3), and IL-5 receptors. Blood 89:1471, 1997.

252. Stomski, F., Woodcock, J., Bagley, C., and Lopez, A.: The mechanism of activation of the human GM-CSF receptor. Blood 90 (suppl. 1):57a, 1997.

253. Raines, M.A., Liu, L., Quan, S.G., Joe, V., DiPersio, J.F., and Golde, D.W.: Identification and molecular cloning of a soluble human granulocyte-macrophage colony-stimulating factor receptor. Proc. Natl. Acad. Sci. USA 88:8203, 1991.

254. Yasruel, Z., Humbert, M., Kotsimbos, T.C., Ploysongsang, Y., Minshall, E., Durham, S.R., Pfister, R., Menz, G., Tavernier, J., and Kay, A.B.: Membrane-bound and soluble alpha IL-5 receptor mRNA in the bronchial mucosa of atopic and nonatopic asthmatics. Am. J. Respir. Crit. Care Med. 155:1413, 1997.

255. Ooi, J., Tojo, A., Asano, S., Sato, Y., and Oka, Y.: Thrombopoietin induces tyrosine phosphorylation of a common beta subunit of GM-CSF receptor and its association with Stat5 in TF-1/TPO cells. Biochem. Biophys. Res. Commun. 246:132, 1998.

256. Stanley, E.R., and Guilbert, L.J.: Methods for the purification, assay, characterization and target cell binding of a colony-stimulating factor (CSF-1). J. Immunol. Methods 42:253, 1981.

257. Kawasaki, E.S., Ladner, M.B., Wang, A.M., Van Arsdell, J., Warren, M.K., Coyne, M.Y., Schweickart, V.L., Lee, M.T., Wilson, K.J., Boosman, A., Stanley, E.R., Ralph, P., and Mark, D.F.: Molecular cloning of a complementary DNA encoding human macrophage colony-stimulating factor. CSF-1. Science 230:291, 1985.

258. Morris, S.W., Valentine, M.B., Shapiro, D.N., Sublett, J.E., Deaven, L.L., Foust, J.T., Roberts, W.M., Cerretti, D.P., and Look, A.T.: Reassignment of the human CSF-1 gene to the chromosome 1p13–p21. Blood 78:2013, 1991.

259. Sieff, C.A., Niemeyer, C.M., Mentzer, S.J., and Faller, D.V.: Interleukin-1, tumor necrosis factor, and the production of colony stimulating factors by cultured mesenchymal cells. Blood 72:1316, 1988.

260. Gruber, M.F., and Gerrard, T.L.: Production of macrophage colony-stimulating factor (M-CSF) by human monocytes is differentially regulated by GM-CSF, TNFα and IFN-γ. Cell. Immunol. 142:361, 1992.

261. Sherman, M.L., Weber, B.L., Datta, R., and Kufe, D.W.: Transcriptional and post transcriptional regulation of macrophage-specific colony-stimulating factor gene expression by tumor necrosis factor. Involvement of arachidonic acid metabolites. J. Clin. Invest. 58:442, 1990.

262. Yamada, H., Iwase, S., Mohri, M., and Kufe, D.: Involvement of a nuclear NF-κB–like protein in induction of the macrophage colony-stimulating factor gene by tumor necrosis factor. Blood 78:1988, 1991.

263. Chambers, S.K., Gilmore-Hebert, M., Wang, Y., Rodov, S., Benz, E.J., Jr., and Kacinski, B.M.: Posttranscriptional regulation of colony-stimulating factor 1 (CSF-1) and CSF-1 receptor gene expression during inhibition of phorbol-ester–induced monocytic differentiation by dexamethasone and cyclosporin A: potential involvement of a destabilizing protein. Exp. Hematol. 21:1328, 1993.

264. Hanamura, T., Motoyoshi, K., Yoshida, K., Saito, M., Miura, Y., Kawashima, T., Nishida, M., and Takaku, F.: Quantitation and identification of human monocytic colony-stimulating factor in human serum by enzyme-linked immunosorbent assay. Blood 72:886, 1988.

265. Gilbert, H.S., Praloran, V., and Stanley, E.R.: Increased circulating CSF-1 (M-CSF) in myeloproliferative disease: association with myeloid metaplasia and peripheral bone marrow extension. Blood 74:1231, 1989.

266. Janowska-Wieczorek, A., Belch, A.R., Jacobs, A., Bowen, D., Padua, R.A., Paietta, E., and Stanley, E.R.: Increased circulating colony-stimulating factor-1 in patients with preleukemia, leukemia, and lymphoid malignancies. Blood 77:1796, 1991.

267. Bartocci, A., Mastrogiannis, D.S., Migliorati, G., Stockert, R.J., Wolkoff, A.W., and Stanley, E.R.: Macrophages specifically regulate the concentration of their own growth factor in the circulation. Proc. Natl. Acad. Sci. USA 84:6179, 1987.

268. Rettenmier, C.W., and Roussel, M.F.: Differential processing of colony stimulating factor 1 precursors encoded by two human cDNAs. Mol. Cell. Biol. 8:5026, 1988.

269. Manos, M.M.: Expression and processing of a recombinant human macrophage colony-stimulating factor in mouse cells. Mol. Cell. Biol. 8:5035, 1988.

270. Cheng, H.J., and Flanagan, J.G.: Transmembrane kit ligand cleavage does not require a signal in the cytoplasmic domain and occurs at a site dependent on spacing from the membrane. Mol. Biol. Cell 5:943, 1994.

271. Blobel, C.P.: Metalloprotease-disintegrins: links to cell adhesion and cleavage of TNF and Notch. Cell 90:589, 1997.

272. Cheers, C., Hill, M., Haigh, A.M., and Stanley, E.R.: Stimulation of macrophage phagocytic but not bacteriocidal activity of colony stimulating factor 1. Infect. Immun. 57:1512, 1989.

273. Curley, S.A., Roh, M.S., Kleinerman, E., and Klostergaard, J.: Human recombinant macrophage colony-stimulating factor activates murine Kupffer cells to a cytotoxic state. Lymphokine Res. 9:355, 1990.

274. James, S.L., Cook, K.W., and Lazdins, J.K.: Activation of human monocyte-derived macrophages to kill schistosomules of *Schistosoma mansoni* in vitro. J. Immunol. 145:2686, 1990.

275. Nishimura, Y., Higashi, N., Tsuji, T., Higuchi, M., and Osawa, T.: Activation of human monocytes by interleukin-2 and various cytokines. J. Immunother. 12:90, 1992.

276. Belosevic, M., Davis, C.E., Meltzer, M.S., and Nacy, C.Y.: Regulation of activated macrophage antimicrobial activities: identification of lymphokines that cooperate with IFN-gamma for induction of resistance to infection. J. Immunol. 141:890, 1988.

277. Denis, M.: Killing of *Mycobacterium tuberculosis* within human monocytes: activation by cytokines and calcitriol. Clin. Exp. Immunol. 84:200, 1991.

278. Stanley, E.R., Berg, K.J., Einstein, D.B., Lee, P.S., and Yeung, Y.G.: The biology and action of colony-stimulating factor-1. Stem Cells 12(suppl. 1):15, 1994.

279. Takahashi, N., Udagawa, N., Akatsu, T., Tanaka, H., Isogai, Y., and Suda, T.: Deficiency of osteoclasts in osteopetrotic mice is due to a defect in the local microenvironment provided by osteoblastic cells. Endocrinology 128:1792, 1991.

280. Sherr, C.J., Rettenmier, C.W., Sacca, R., Roussel, M.F., Look, A.T., and Stanley, E.R.: The c-*fms* proto-oncogene product is related to the receptor for the mononuclear phagocyte growth factor, CSF-1. Cell 41:665, 1985.

281. Coussens, L., Van Beveren, C., Smith, D., Chen, E., Mitchell, R.L., and Isacke, C.M.: Structural alteration of viral homologue of receptor proto-oncogene *fms* at carboxyl terminus. Nature 320:277, 1986.

282. Roberts, W.M., Look, A.T., Roussel, M.F., and Sherr, C.J.: Tandem linkage of human CSF-1 receptor (c-*fms*) and PDGF receptor genes. Cell 55:655, 1988.

283. Visvader, J., and Verma, J.M.: Differential transcription of exon 1 of the human c-*fms* gene in placental trophoblasts and monocytes. Mol. Cell. Biol. 9:1336, 1989.

284. Roberts, W.M., Shapiro, L.H., Ashmun, R.A., and Look, A.T.: Transcription of the human colony-stimulating factor-1 receptor gene is regulated by separate tissue-specific promoters. Blood 79:586, 1992.

285. Reddy, M.A., Yang, B.S., Yue, X., Barnett, C.J., Ross, I.L., Sweet, M.J., Hume, D.A., and Ostrowski, M.C.: Opposing actions of c-ets/ PU.1 and c-myb proto-oncogene products in regulating the macrophage-specific promoters of the human and mouse colony-stimulating factor-1 receptor (c-*fms*) genes. J. Exp. Med. 180:2309, 1994.

286. Celada, A., Borras, F.E., Soler, C., Lloberas, J., Klemsz, M., Van Beveren, C., McKercher, S., and Maki, R.A.: The transcription factor PU.1 is involved in macrophage proliferation. J. Exp. Med. 184:61, 1996.

287. Yue, X., Favot, P., Dunn, T.L., Cassady, A.I., and Hume, D.A.: Expression of mRNA encoding the macrophage colony-stimulating factor receptor (c-*fms*) is controlled by a constitutive promoter and tissue-specific transcription elongation. Mol. Cell. Biol. 13:3191, 1993.

288. Russell, E.S.: Hereditary anemias of the mouse: a review for geneticists. Adv. Genet. 20:357, 1979.

289. Bernstein, S.E.: Tissue transplantation as an analytic and therapeutic tool in hereditary anemias. Am. J. Surg. 119:448, 1970.

290. Dexter, T.M., and Moore, M.A.S.: In vitro duplication and "cure" of haemopoietic defects in genetically anaemic mice. Nature 269:412, 1977.

291. Wolf, N.S.: Dissecting the hematopoietic microenvironment III. Evidence for a short range stimulus for cellular proliferation. Cell Tissue Kinet. 11:335, 1978.

292. Nocka, K., Majumder, S., Chabot, B., Ray, P., Cervone, M., Bernstein, A., and Besmer, P.: Expression of c-*kit* gene products in known cellular targets of W mutations in normal and W mutant mice—evidence for an impaired c-*kit* kinase in mutant mice. Genes Dev. 3:816, 1989.

293. Sherr, C.: Colony-stimulating factor-1 receptor. Blood 75:1, 1990.

294. Anderson, D.M., Lyman, S.D., Baird, A., Wignall, J.M., Eisenman, J., Rauch, C., March, C.J., Boswell, H.S., Gimpel, S.D., Cosman, D., and Williams, D.E.: Molecular cloning of mast cell growth factor, a hemopoietin that is active in both membrane bound and soluble forms. Cell 63:235, 1990.

295. Copeland, N.G., Gilbert, D.J., Cho, B.C., Donovan, P.J., Jenkins, N.A., Cosman, D., Anderson, D., Lyman, S.D., and Williams, D.E.: Mast cell growth factor maps near the steel locus on mouse chromosome 10 and is deleted in a number of steel alleles. Cell 63:175, 1990.

296. Flanagan, J.G., and Leder, P.: The kit ligand: a cell surface molecule altered in steel mutant fibroblasts. Cell 63:185, 1990.

297. Huang, E., Nocka, K., Beier, D.R., Chu, T.Y., Buck, J., Lahm, H.W., Wellner, D., Leder, P., and Besmer, P.: The hematopoietic growth factor KL is encoded by the *Sl* locus and is the ligand of the c-*kit* receptor, the gene product of the *W* locus. Cell 63:225, 1990.

298. Martin, F.H., Suggs, S.V., Langley, K.E., Lu, H.S., Ting, J., Okino, K.H., Morris, C.F., McNiece, I.K., Jacobsen, F.W., Mendiaz, E.A., Birkett, N.C., Smith, K.A., Johnson, M.J., Parker, V.P., Flores, J.C., Patel, A.C., Fisher, E.F., Erjavec, H.O., Pope, J.A., Leslie, I., Wen, D., Lin, C.H., Cupplies, R.L., and Zsebo, K.M.: Primary structure and functional expression of rat and human stem cell factor. Cell 63:203, 1990.

299. Zsebo, K.M., Williams, D.A., Geissler, E.N., Broudy, V.C., Martin, F.H., Atkins, H.L., Hsu, R.-Y., Birkett, N.C., Okino, K.H., Murdock, D.C., Jacobsen, F.W., Langley, K.E., Smith, K.A., Takeishi, T., Cattanach, B.M., Galli, S.J., and Suggs, S.V.: Stem cell factor is encoded at the *Sl* locus of the mouse and is the ligand for the c-*kit* tyrosine kinase receptor. Cell 63:213, 1990.

300. Broudy, V.C.: Stem cell factor and hematopoiesis. Blood 90:1345, 1997.

301. McCulloch, E.A., Siminovitch, L., and Till, J.E.: Spleen-colony formation in anemic mice of genotype WWV. Science 144:844, 1964.

302. Lewis, J.P., O'Grady, L.F., Bernstein, S.E., Russell, E.S., and Trobaugh, F.E., Jr.: Growth and differentiation of transplanted W/Wv marrow. Blood 30:601, 1967.

303. Barker, J.E.: *Sl/Sl^d* hematopoietic progenitors are deficient in situ. Exp. Hematol. 22:174, 1994.

304. Ogawa, M., Matsuzawa, Y., Nishikawa, S., Hayashi, S.I., Kunisada, T., Sudo, T., Kina, T., Nakauchi, H., and Nishikawa, S.I.: Expression and function of c-*kit* in hemopoietic progenitor cells. J. Exp. Med. 174:63, 1991.

305. Huang, E.J., Nocka, K.H., Buck, J., and Besmer, P.: Differential expression and processing of two cell associated forms of the kit-ligand: KL-1 and KL-2. Mol. Biol. Cell 3:349, 1992.

306. Huang, E.J., Manova, K., Packer, A.I., Sanchez, S., Bachvarova, R.F., and Besmer, P.: The murine steel panda mutation affects kit ligand expression and growth of early ovarian follicles. Dev. Biol. 157:100, 1993.

307. Linenberger, M.L., Jacobsen, F.W., Broudy, V.C., Martin, F.H., and Abkowitz, J.L.: Stem cell factor production by human marrow stromal fibroblasts. Exp. Hematol. 23:1104, 1995.

308. Arribas, J., Coodly, L., Vollmer, P., Kishimoto, T.K., Rose-John, S., and Massagué, J.: Diverse cell surface protein ectodomains are shed by a system sensitive to metalloprotease inhibitors. J. Biol. Chem. 271:11376, 1996.

309. Hsu, Y.R., Wu, G.M., Mendiaz, E.A., Syed, R., Wypych, J., Toso, R., Mann, M.B., Boone, T.C., Narhi, L.O., Lu, H.S., and Langley, K.E.: The majority of stem cell factor exists as monomer under physiological conditions. J. Biol. Chem. 272:6406, 1997.

310. Bernstein, I.D., Andrews, R.G., and Zsebo, K.M.: Recombinant human stem cell factor enhances the formation of colonies by CD34+ and CD34+lin− cells, and the generation of colony-forming cell progeny from CD34+lin− cells cultured with interleukin-3, granulocyte colony-stimulating factor, or granulocyte-macrophage colony-stimulating factor. Blood 77:2316, 1991.

311. Migliaccio, G., Migliaccio, A.R., Druzin, M.L., Giardina, P.J.V., Zsebo, K.M., and Adamson, J.W.: Long-term generation of colony-forming cells in liquid culture of CD34+ cord blood cells in the presence of recombinant human stem cell factor. Blood 79:2620, 1992.

312. Haylock, D.N., To, L.B., Dowse, T.L., and Juttner, C.A.: Ex vivo expansion and maturation of peripheral blood CD34+ cells into the myeloid lineage. Blood 80:1405, 1992.

313. Brandt, J., Briddell, R.A., Srour, E.F., Leemhuis, T.B., and Hoffman, R.: Role of c-*kit* ligand in the expansion of human hematopoietic progenitor cells. Blood 79:634, 1992.

314. Brugger, W., Möcklin, W., Heimfeld, S., Berenson, R.J., Mertelsmann, R., and Kanz, L.: Ex vivo expansion of enriched peripheral blood CD34+ progenitor cells by stem cell factor, interleukin-1β (IL-1β), IL-6, IL-3, interferon-γ, and erythropoietin. Blood 81:2579, 1993.

315. Ariyama, Y., Misawa, S., and Sonoda, Y.: Synergistic effects of stem cell factor and interleukin 6 or interleukin 11 on the expansion of murine hematopoietic progenitors in liquid suspension culture. Stem Cells 13:404, 1995.

316. Broxmeyer, H.E., Hangoc, G., Cooper, S., Anderson, D., Cosman, D., Lyman, S.D., and Williams, D.E.: Influence of murine mast cell growth factor (c-*kit* ligand) on colony formation by mouse marrow hematopoietic progenitor cells. Exp. Hematol. 19:143, 1991.

317. Briddell, R.A., Bruno, E., Cooper, R.J., Brandt, J.E., and Hoffman, R.: Effect of c-*kit* ligand on in vitro human megakaryocytopoiesis. Blood 78:2854, 1991.

318. Metcalf, D., and Nicola, N.A.: Direct proliferative actions of stem cell factor on murine bone marrow cells in vitro: effects of combination with colony-stimulating factors. Proc. Natl. Acad. Sci. USA 88:6239, 1991.

319. Debili, N., Massé, J.M., Katz, A., Guichard, J., Breton-Gorius, J., and Vainchenker, W.: Effects of the recombinant hematopoietic growth factors interleukin-3, interleukin-6, stem cell factor, and leukemia inhibitory factor on the megakaryocytic differentiation of CD34+ cells. Blood 82:84, 1993.

320. Broudy, V.C., Lin, N., Buhring, H.J., Komatsu, N., and Kavanaugh, T.J.: Analysis of c-kit receptor dimerization by fluorescence resonance energy transfer. Blood 91:898, 1998.

321. de Vries, P., Brasel, K.A., Eisenman, J.R., Alpert, A.R., and Williams, D.E.: The effect of recombinant mast cell growth factor on purified murine hematopoietic stem cells. J. Exp. Med. 173:1205, 1991.

322. Li, C.L., and Johnson, G.R.: Stem cell factor enhances the survival but not the self-renewal of murine hematopoietic long-term repopulating cells. Blood 84:408, 1994.

323. Wineman, J.P., Nishikawa, S.-I., and Müeller-Sieberg, C.E.: Maintenance of high levels of pluripotent hematopoietic stem cells in vitro: effect of stromal cells and c-*kit*. Blood 81:365, 1993.

324. Kapur, R., Xiao, X., McAndrews-Hill, M., and Williams, D.A.: Sustained activation of erythropoietin receptor by membrane presentation of stem cell factor: a unique in vivo role for membrane-associated SCF in erythropoiesis. Exp. Hematol. 25:882, 1997.

325. Miyazawa, K., Williams, D.A., Gotoh, A., Nishimaki, J., Broxmeyer, H.E., and Toyama, K.: Membrane bound steel factor induces more persistent tyrosine kinase activation and longer life span of c-kit gene encoded protein than its soluble form. Blood 85:641, 1995.

326. Sutherland, H.J., Hogge, D.E., Cook, D., and Eaves, C.J.: Alternative mechanisms with and without steel factor support primitive human hematopoiesis. Blood 81:1465, 1993.

327. Heinrich, M.C., Dooley, D.C., Freed, A.C., Band, L., Hoatlin, M.E., Keeble, W.W., Peters, S.T., Silvey, K.V., Ey, F.S., Kabat, D., Maziarz, R.T., and Bagby, G.C., Jr.: Constitutive expression of steel factor gene by human stromal cells. Blood 82:771, 1993.

328. Heinrich, M.C., Dooley, D.C., and Keeble, W.W.: Transforming growth factor β1 inhibits expression of the gene products for steel factor and its receptor (c-*kit*). Blood 85:1769, 1995.

329. Langley, K.E., Bennett, L.G., Wypych, J., Yancik, S.A., Liu, X.D., Westcott, K.R., Chang, D.G., Smith, K.A., and Zsebo, K.M.: Soluble stem cell factor in human serum. Blood 81:656, 1993.

330. Wodnar-Filipowicz, A., Yancik, S., Moser, Y., dalle Carbonare, V., Gratwohl, A., Tichelli, A., Speck, B., and Nissen, C.: Levels of soluble stem cell factor in serum of patients with aplastic anemia. Blood 81:3259, 1993.

331. Bowen, D., Yancik, S., Bennett, L., Culligan, D., and Resser, K.: Serum stem cell factor concentration in patients with myelodysplastic syndromes. Br. J. Haematol. 85:63, 1993.

332. Ashman, L.K., Cambareri, A.C., To, L.B., Levinsky, R.J., and Juttner, C.A.: Expression of the YB5.B8 antigen (c-*kit* proto-oncogene product) in normal human bone marrow. Blood 78:30, 1991.

333. Broudy, V.C., Lin, N., Zsebo, K.M., Birkett, N.C., and Smith, K.A.: Isolation and characterization of a monoclonal antibody that recognizes the human c-*kit* receptor. Blood 79:338, 1992.

334. Palacios, R., and Nishikawa, S.I.: Developmentally regulated cell surface expression and function of c-*kit* receptor during lymphocyte ontogeny in the embryo and adult mice. Development 115:1133, 1992.

335. Manova, K., Bachvarova, R.F., Huang, E.J., Sanchez, S., Pronovost, S.M., Velazquez, E., McGuire, B., and Besmer, P.: c-*kit* receptor and ligand expression in postnatal development of the mouse cerebellum suggests a function for c-*kit* in inhibitory interneurons. J. Neurosci. 12:4663, 1992.

336. Broudy, V.C., Kovach, N.L., Bennett, L.G., Lin, N., Jacobsen, F.W., and Kidd, P.G.: Human umbilical vein endothelial cells display high-affinity c-*kit* receptors and produce a soluble form of the c-*kit* receptor. Blood 83:2145, 1994.

337. Dubois, C.M., Ruscetti, F.W., Stankova, J., and Keller, J.R.: Transforming growth factor-β regulates c-*kit* message stability and cell-surface protein expression in hematopoietic progenitors. Blood 83:3138, 1994.

338. Rusten, L.S., Smeland, E.B., Jacobsen, F.W., Lien, E., Lesslauer, W., Loetscher, H., Dubois, C.M., and Jacobsen, S.E.W.: Tumor necrosis factor-α inhibits stem cell factor–induced proliferation of human bone marrow progenitor cells in vitro. J. Clin. Invest. 94:165, 1994.

339. Blechman, J.M., Lev, S., Brizzi, M.F., Leitner, O., Pegoraro, L., Givol, D., and Yarden, Y.: Soluble c-kit proteins and antireceptor monoclonal antibodies confine the binding site of the stem cell factor. J. Biol. Chem. 268:4399, 1993.

340. Lev, S., Blechman, J., Nishikawa, S.I., Givol, D., and Yarden, Y.: Interspecies molecular chimeras of kit help define the binding site of the stem cell factor. Mol. Cell. Biol. 13:2224, 1993.

341. Blechman, J.M., Lev, S., Eisenstein, M., Vaks, B., Vogel, Z., Givol, D., and Yarden, Y.: The fourth immunoglobin domain of the stem cell factor receptor couples ligand binding to signal transduction. Cell 80:103, 1995.

342. Lemmon, M.A., Pinchasi, D., Zhou, M., Lax, I., and Schlessinger, J.: Kit receptor dimerization is driven by bivalent binding of stem cell factor. J. Biol. Chem. 272:6311, 1997.

343. Lev, S., Yarden, Y., and Givol, D.: Dimerization and activation of the kit receptor by monovalent and bivalent binding of the stem cell factor. J. Biol. Chem. 267:15970, 1992.

344. Lyman, S.D., James, L., Vanden Bos, T., de Vries, P., Brasel, K., Gliniak, B., Hollingsworth, L.T., Picha, K.S., McKenna, H.J., Splett, R.R., Fletcher, F.A., Marakovsky, E., Farrah, T., Foxworthe, D., Williams, D.E., Beckmann, M.P.: Molecular cloning of a ligand for the flt3/flk2 tyrosine kinase receptor: a proliferative factor for primitive hematopoietic cells. Cell 75:1157, 1993.

345. Lyman, S.D., Seaberg, M., Hanna, R., Zappone, J., Brasel, K., Abkowitz, J.L., Prchal, J.T., Schultz, J.C., and Shahidi, N.T.: Plasma/serum levels of flt3 ligand are low in normal individuals and highly elevated in patients with Fanconi anemia and acquired aplastic anemia. Blood 86:4091, 1995.

346. McClanahan, T., Culpepper, J., Campbell, D., Wagner, J., Franz-Bacon, K., Mattson, J., Tsai, S., Luh, J., Guimaraes, M.J., Mattei, M.G., Rosnet, O., Birnbaum, D., and Hannum, C.H.: Biochemical and genetic characterization of multiple splice variants of the Flt3 ligand. Blood 88:3371, 1996.

347. Hannum, C., Culpepper, J., Campbell, D., McClanahan, T., Zurawski, S., Bazan, J.F., Kastelein, R., Hudak, S., Wagner, J., Mattson, J., Luh, J., Duda, G., Martina, N., Peterson, D., Menon, S., Shanafelt, A., Muench, M., Kelner, G., Namikawa, R., Rennick, D., Roncarolo, M.-G., Zlotnik, A., Rosnet, O., Dubreuil, P., Birnbaum, D., and Lee, F.: Ligand for FLT3/FLK2 receptor tyrosine kinase regulates growth of haematopoietic stem cells and is encoded by variant RNAs. Nature 368:643, 1994.

348. Lyman, S.D., James, L., Johnson, L., Brasel, K., de Vries, P., Escobar, S.S., Downey, H., Splett, R.R., Beckmann, M.P., and McKenna, H.J.: Cloning of the human homologue of the murine flt3 ligand: a growth factor for early hematopoietic progenitor cells. Blood 83:2795, 1994.

349. Guerriero, A., Worford, L., Holland, H.K., Guo, G.-R., Sheehan, K., and Waller, E.K.: Thrombopoietin is synthesized by bone marrow stromal cells. Blood 90:3444, 1997.

350. Muench, M.O., Roncarolo, M.G., Menon, S., Xu, Y., Kastelein, R., Zurawski, S., Hannum, C.H., Culpepper, J., Lee, F., and Namikawa, R.: FLK-2/FLT-3 ligand regulates the growth of early myeloid progenitors isolated from human fetal liver. Blood 85:963, 1995.

351. Rasko, J.E., Metcalf, D., Rossner, M.T., Begley, C.G., and Nicola, N.A.: The flt3/flk-2 ligand: receptor distribution and action on murine haemopoietic cell survival and proliferation. Leukemia 9:2058, 1995.

352. Maraskovsky, E., Brasel, K., Teepe, M., Roux, E.R., Lyman, S.D., Shortman, K., and McKenna, H.J.: Dramatic increases in the number of functionally mature dendritic cells in Flt3 ligand treated mice: multiple dendritic cell populations identified. J. Exp. Med. 184:1953, 1996.

353. Maraskovsky, E., Roux, E., Teepe, M., Braddy, S., Hoek, J., Lebsack, M., and McKenna, H.J.: Flt3 ligand increases peripheral blood dendritic cells in healthy volunteers. Blood 90(suppl. 1):581a, 1997.

354. Strobl, H., Bello-Fernandez, C., Riedl, E., Pickl, W.F., Majdic, O., Lyman, S.D., and Knapp, W.: flt3 ligand in cooperation with transforming growth factor-1 potentiates in vitro development of Langerhans-type dendritic cells and allows single-cell dendritic cell cluster formation under serum-free conditions. Blood 90:1425, 1997.

355. Xiao, M., Oppenlander, B.K., and Dooley, D.C.: Flt3 ligand (FL) counteracts the inhibitory activity of transforming growth factor-β1 (TGF-1) on primitive human hematopoietic CD34$^+$CD38^{dim} cells. Blood 90(suppl. 1):476a, 1997.

356. McKenna, H.J., Miller, R.E., Brasel, K.E., Maraskovsky, E., Maliszewski, C., Pulendran, B., Lynch, D., Teepe, M., Roux, E.R., Smith, J., Williams, D.E., Lyman, S.D., Peschon, J.J., and Stocking, K.: Targeted disruption of the flt3 ligand gene in mice affects multiple hematopoietic lineages, including natural killer cells, B lymphocytes, and dendritic cells. Blood 88(suppl. 1):474a, 1996.

357. Lyman, S.D., Brasel, K., Maraskovsky, E., Miller, R.E., Schuh, J., Maliszewski, C., Pulendran, B., Stocking, K., Peachon, J., Lynch, D., and McKenna, H.: Biological activities of flt3 ligand. Exp. Hematol. 25:729, 1997.

358. Molineux, G., McCrea, C., Yan, X.Q., Kerzic, P., and McNiece, I.: Flt-3 ligand synergizes with granulocyte colony-stimulating factor to increase neutrophil numbers and to mobilize peripheral blood stem cells with long-term repopulating potential. Blood 89:3998, 1997.

359. Papayannopoulou, T., Nakamoto, B., Andrews, R.G., Lyman, S.D., and Lee, M.Y.: In vivo effects of flt/flk2 ligand on mobilization of hematopoietic progenitors in primates and potent synergistic enhancement with granulocyte colony-stimulating factor. Blood 90:620, 1997.

360. Matthews, W., Jordan, C.T., Gavin, M., Jenkins, N.A., Copeland, N.G., and Lemischka, I.R.: A receptor tyrosine kinase cDNA isolated from a population of enriched primitive hematopoietic cells and exhibiting close genetic linkage to c-kit. Proc. Natl. Acad. Sci. USA 88:9026, 1991.

361. Rosnet, O., Schiff, C., Marchetto, S., Tonnelle, C., Toiron, Y., Birg, F., and Birnbaum, D.: Human FLT3/FLK2 gene: cDNA cloning and expression in hematopoietic cells. Blood 82:1110, 1993.

362. Matthews, W., Jordan, C.T., Wiegand, G.W., Pardoll, D., and Lemischka, I.R.: A receptor tyrosine kinase specific to hematopoietic stem and progenitor cell-enriched populations. Cell 65:1143, 1991.

363. Small, D., Levenstein, M., Kim, E., Carow, C., Amin, S., Rockwell, P., Witte, L., Burrow, C., Ratajczak, M.Z., Gewirtz, A.M., and Civin, C.I.: STK-1, the human homolog of Flk-2/Flt-3 is selectively expressed in CD34+ human bone marrow cells and is involved in the proliferation of early progenitor/stem cells. Proc. Natl. Acad. Sci. USA 91:459, 1994.

364. Turner, A.M., Lin, N.L., Issarachai, S., Lyman, S.D., and Broudy, V.C.: FLT3 receptor expression on the surface of normal and malignant human hematopoietic cells. Blood 88:3383, 1996.

365. Kishimoto, T.: The biology of interleukin-6. Blood 74:1, 1989.

366. Libermann, T.A., Baltimore, D.: Activation of interleukin-6 gene expression through the NF-κB transcription factor. Mol. Cell. Biol. 10:2327, 1990.

367. Nakayama, K., Shimizu, H., Mitomo, K., Watanabe, T., Okamoto, S., and Yamamoto, K.I.: A lymphoid cell-specific nuclear factor containing c-Rel–like proteins preferentially interacts with interleukin-6 κB-related motifs whose activities are repressed in lymphoid cells. Mol. Cell. Biol. 12:1736, 1992.

368. Poli, V., and Mancini, F.P.: IL-6 DBP, a nuclear protein involved in interleukin-6 signal transduction, defines a new family of leucine zipper proteins related to C/EBP. Cell 63:643, 1990.

369. Kinoshita, S., Akira, S., and Kishimoto, T.: A member of the C/EBP family, NF-IL6, forms a heterodimer and transcriptionally synergizes with NF-IL6. Proc. Natl. Acad. Sci. USA 89:1473, 1992.

370. Ramji, D.P., Vitelli, A., Tronche, F., Cortese, R., and Ciliberto, G.: The two C/EBP isoforms, IL-6DBP/NF-IL6 and C/EBPδ/NF-IL6β, are induced by IL-6 to promote acute phase gene transcription via different mechanisms. Nucleic Acids Res. 21:289, 1993.

371. Ikebuchi, K., Wong, G.G., Clark, C.S., Ihle, J.N., Hirai, Y., and Ogawa, M.: Interleukin-6 enhancement of interleukin-3–dependent proliferation of multipotential hemopoietic progenitors. Proc. Natl. Acad. Sci. USA 84:9035, 1987.

372. Ulich, T.R., del Castillo, J., and Guo, K.Z.: In vivo hematologic effects of recombinant interleukin 6 on hematopoiesis and circulating numbers of RBCs and WBCs. Blood 73:108, 1989.

373. Hudak, S., Thompson-Snipes, L., Rocco, C., Jackson, J., Pearce, M., and Rennick, D.: Anti–IL-6 antibodies suppress myeloid cell production and the generation of CFU-c in long term bone marrow cultures. Exp. Hematol. 20:412, 1992.

374. Ishibashi, T., Kimura, H., Uchida, T., Kariyone, S., Friese, P., and Burstein, S.A.: Human interleukin 6 is a direct promoter of maturation of megakaryocytes in vitro. Proc. Natl. Acad. Sci. USA 86:5953, 1989.

375. Hill, R.J., Warren, M.K., and Levin, J.: Stimulation of thrombopoiesis in mice by human recombinant interleukin 6. J. Clin. Invest. 85:1242, 1990.

376. Cressman, D.E., Greenbaum, L.E., DeAngelis, A., Ciliberto, G., Furth, E.E., and Poli, V.: Liver failure and defective hepatocyte regeneration in interleukin-6–deficient mice. Science 274:1379, 1996.

377. Bluethmann, H., Rothe, J., Schultze, N., Tkachuk, M., and Koebel, P.: Establishment of the role of IL-6 and TNF receptor 1 using gene knockout mice. J. Leukoc. Biol. 56:565, 1994.

378. Dalrymple, S.A., Lucian, L.A., Slattery, R., McNeil, T., Aud, D.M., Fuehino, S., Lee, F., and Murray, R.: Interleukin-6–deficient mice are highly susceptible to Listeria monocytogenes infection: correlation with ineffecient neutrophilia. Infect. Immun. 63:2262, 1995.

379. Romani, L., Mencacci, A., Cenci, E., Spaccapelo, R., Toniatti, C., Puccetti, P., Bistoni, F., and Poli, V.: Impaired neutrophil response and CD4+ T helper cell 1 development in interleukin 6–deficient mice infected with Candida albicans. J. Exp. Med. 183:1345, 1996.

380. Bruno, E., Briddell, R.A., Cooper, R.J., and Hoffman, R.: Effects of recombinant interleukin 11 on human megakaryocyte progenitor cells. Exp. Hematol. 19:378, 1991.

381. Teramura, M., Kobayashi, S., Hoshino, S., Oshimi, K., and Mizoguchi, H.: Interleukin 11 enhances human megakaryocytopoiesis in vitro. Blood 79:327, 1992.

382. McKinley, D., Wu, Q., Yang-Feng, T., and Yang, Y.C.: Genomic sequence and chromosomal location of human interleukin-11 gene (IL11). Genomics 13:814, 1992.

383. Du, X.X., and Williams, D.A.: Interleukin 11: A multifunctional growth factor derived from the hematopoietic microenvironment. Blood 83:2023, 1994.

384. Elias, J.A., Zheng, T., Whiting, N.L., Trow, T.K., Merrill, W.W., Zitnik, R., Ray, P., and Alderman, E.M.: IL-1 and transforming growth factor beta regulation of fibroblast derived IL-11. J. Immunol. 152:2421, 1994.

385. Murphy, G.M., Jr., Bitting, L., Majewska, A., Schmidt, K., Song, Y., and Wood, C.R.: Expression of interleukin 11 and its encoding mRNA by glioblastoma cells. Neurosci. Lett. 196:153, 1995.

386. Okamoto, H., Yamamura, M., Morita, Y., Harada, S., Makino, H., and Ota, Z.: The synovial expression and serum levels of interleukin-6, interleukin-11, leukemia inhibitory factor, and oncostatin M in rheumatoid arthritis. Arthritis Rheum. 40:1096, 1997.

387. Chang, M., Suen, Y., Meng, G., Buzby, J.S., Bussel, J., Shen, V., Van de Ven, C., and Cairo, M.S.: Differential mechanisms in the regulation of endogenous levels of thrombopoietin and interleukin 11 during thrombocytopenia: insight into the regulation of platelet production. Blood 88:3354, 1996.

388. Endo, S., Inada, K., Arakawa, N., Yamada, Y., Nakae, H., Takakuwa, T., Namiki, M., Inoue, Y., Shimamura, T., Suzuki, T., Taniguchi, S., and Yoshida, M.: Interleukin 11 levels in patients wth disseminated intravascular coagulation. Res. Commun. Mol. Pathol. Pharmacol. 91:253, 1996.

389. Heits, F., Katschinski, D.M., Wilmsen, U., Wiedemann, G.J., and Jelkmann, W.: Serum thrombopoietin and interleukin 6 concentrations in tumour patients and response to chemotherapy-induced thrombocytopenia. Eur. J. Haematol. 59:53, 1997.

390. Yang, L., and Yang, Y.-C.: Regulation of interleukin (IL)–11 gene expression in IL-1 induced primate bone marrow stromal cells. J. Biol. Chem. 269:32732, 1994.

391. Bitko, V., Velazquez, A., Yang, L., Yang, Y.C., and Barik, S.: Transcriptional induction of multiple cytokines by human respiratory syncytial virus requires activation of NF-κB and is inhibited by sodium salicylate and aspirin. Virology 232:369, 1997.

392. Du, X.X., and Williams, D.A.: Interleukin-11: review of molecular, cell biology and clinical use. Blood 89:3897, 1997.

393. Baumann, H., and Schendel, P.: Interleukin-11 regulates the hepatic expression of the same plasma protein genes as interleukin-6. J. Biol. Chem. 226:20424, 1991.

394. Mehler, M.F., Rozental, R., Dougherty, M., Spray, D.C., and Kessler, J.A.: Cytokine regulation of neuronal differentiation of hippocampal progenitor cells. Nature 362:62, 1993.

395. Keller, D.C., Du, X.X., Srour, E.F., Hoffman, R., and Williams, D.A.: Interleukin-11 inhibits adipogenesis and stimulates myelopoiesis in human long-term marrow cultures. Blood 82:1428, 1993.

396. Hughes, F.J., and Howells, G.L.: Interleukin-11 inhibits bone formation in vitro. Calcif. Tissue Int. 53:362, 1993.

397. Musashi, M., Yang, Y.C., Paul, S.R., Clark, S.C., Sudo, T., and Ogawa, M.: Direct and synergistic effects of interleukin 11 on murine hemopoiesis in culture. Proc. Natl. Acad. Sci. USA 88:765, 1991.

398. Jacobsen, S.E., Okkenhaug, C., Myklebust, J., Veiby, O.P., and Lyman, S.D.: The FLT3 ligand potently and directly stimulates the growth and expansion of primitive murine bone marrow progenitor cells in vitro: synergistic interactions with interleukin (IL) 11, IL-12, and other hematopoietic growth factors. J. Exp. Med. 181:1357, 1995.

399. Neben, S., Donaldson, D., Sieff, C., Mauch, P., Bodine, D., Ferrara, J., Yetz-Aldape, J., and Turner, K.: Synergistic effects of interleukin-11 with other growth factors on the expansion of murine hematopoietic progenitors and maintenance of stem cells in liquid culture. Exp. Hematol. 22:353, 1994.

400. Du, X.X., Scott, D., Yang, Z.X., Cooper, R., Xiao, X.L., and Williams, D.A.: Interleukin-11 stimulates multilineage progenitors, but not stem cells, in murine and human long-term marrow cultures. Blood 86:128, 1995.

401. Quesniaux, V.F.J., Clark, S.C., Turner, K., and Fagg, B.: Interleukin-11 stimulates multiple phases of erythropoiesis in vitro. Blood 80:1218, 1992.

402. Cairo, M.S., Plunkett, J.M., Schendel, P., and Van de Ven, C.: The combined effects of interleukin-11, stem cell factor, and granulocyte colony-stimulating factor on newborn rat hematopoiesis. Significant enhancement of the absolute neutrophil count. Exp. Hematol. 22:1118, 1994.

403. Burstein, S.A., Mei, R.L., Henthorn, J., Friese, P., and Turner, K.: Leukemia inhibitory factor and interleukin-11 promote maturation of murine and human megakaryocytes in vitro. J. Cell. Physiol. 153:305, 1992.

404. Peng, J., Friese, P., George, J.N., Dale, G.L., and Burstein, S.A.: Alteration of platelet function in dogs mediated by interleukin 6. Blood 83:398, 1994.

405. Peng, J., Friese, P., Wolf, R.F., Harrison, P., Downs, T., Lok, S., Dale, G.L., and Burstein, S.A.: Relative reactivity of platelets from thrombopoietin and interleukin-6 treated dogs. Blood 87:4158, 1996.

406. Weich, N.S., Wang, A., Fitzgerald, M., Neben, T.Y., Donaldson, D., Giannotti, J.A., Yetz-Aldape, J., Leven, R.M., and Turner, K.J.: Recombinant human interleukin 11 directly promotes megakaryocytopoiesis in vitro. Blood 90:3893, 1997.

407. Moreau, J.F., Donaldson, D.D., Bennett, F., Witek-Giannotti, J., Clark, S.C., and Wong, G.G.: Leukaemia inhibitory factor is identical to the myeloid growth factor human interleukin for DA cells. Nature 336:690, 1988.

408. Sutherland, G.R., Baker, E., Hyland, V.J., Callen, D.F., Stahl, J., and Gough, N.M.: The gene for human leukemia inhibitory factor (LIF) maps to 22q12. Leukemia 3:9, 1989.

409. Gough, N.M.: Molecular genetics of leukemia inhibitory factor (LIF) and its receptor. Growth Factors 7:175, 1992.

410. Wetzler, M., Kurrzock, R., Low, D.G., Kantarjian, H., Gutterman, J.U., and Talpaz, M.: Alteration in bone marrow adherent layer growth factor expression: a novel mechanism of chronic myelogenous leukemia progression. Blood 78:2400, 1991.

411. Grolleau, D., Soulillou, J.P., and Anegon, I.: Control of HILDA/LIF gene expression in activated human monocytes. Ann. N. Y. Acad. Sci. 628:19, 1991.

412. Metcalf, D., Waring, P., and Nicola, N.A.: Actions of leukaemia inhibitory factor on megakaryocyte and platelet formation. Ciba Found. Symp. 167:174, 1992.

413. Keller, J.R., Gooya, J.M., and Ruscetti, F.W.: Direct synergistic effects of leukemia inhibitory factor on hematopoietic progenitor cell growth: comparison with other hematopoietins that use the gp130 receptor subunit. Blood 88:863, 1996.

414. Akiyama, Y., Kajimura, N., Matsuzaki, J., Kikuchi, Y., Imai, N., Tanigawa, M., and Yamaguchi, K.: In vivo effect of recombinant human leukemia inhibitory factor in primates. Jpn. J. Cancer Res. 88:578, 1997.

415. Hibi, M., Murakami, M., Saito, M., Hirano, T., Taga, T., and Kishimoto, T.: Molecular cloning and expression of an IL-6 signal transducer, gp130. Cell 63:1149, 1990.

416. Saito, M., Yoshida, K., Hibi, M., Taga, T., and Kishimoto, T.: Molecular cloning of a murine IL-6 receptor–associated signal transducer, gp130, and its regulated expression in vivo. J. Immunol. 148:4066, 1992.

417. Nandurkar, H.H., Hilton, D.J., Nathan, P., Willson, T., Nicola, N., and Begley, C.G.: The human IL-11 receptor requires gp130 for signaling: demonstration by molecular cloning of the receptor. Oncogene 12:585, 1996.

418. Murakami, M., Hibi, M., Nakagawa, T., Yasukawa, K., Yamanishi, K., Taga, T., and Kishimoto, T.: IL-6–induced homodimerization of gp130 and associated activation of a tyrosine kinase. Science 260:1808, 1993.

419. Paonessa, G., Graziani, R., De Serio, A., Savino, R., Ciapponi, L., Lahm, A., Salvati, A.L., Toniatti, C., and Ciliberto, G.: Two distinct and independent sites on IL-6 trigger gp130 dimer formation and signaling. EMBO J. 14:1942, 1995.

420. Yamasaki, K., Taga, T., Hirata, Y., Yawata, W., Kawanishi, Y., Seed, B., Taniguchi, T., Hirano, T., and Kishimoto, T.: Cloning and expression of the human interleukin 6 (BSF-2/IFN beta 2) receptor. Science 241:825, 1988.

421. Hirata, Y., Taga, T., Hibi, M., Nakano, N., Hirano, T., and Kishimoto, T.: Characterization of IL-6 receptor expression by monoclonal and polyclonal antibodies. J. Immunol. 143:2900, 1989.

422. Kalai, M., Montero-Julian, F.A., Grotzinger, J., Wollmer, A., Morelle, D., Brochier, J., Rose-John, S., Heinrich, P.C., Brailly, H., and Content, J.: Participation of two Ser-Ser-Phe-Tyr repeats in interleukin-6 (IL-6)–binding sites of the human IL-6 receptor. Eur. J. Biochem. 238:714, 1996.

423. Ehlers, M., Grotzinger, J., Fischer, M., Boss, H.K., Brakenhoff, J.P., and Rose-John, S.: Identification of single amino acid residues of human IL-6 involved in receptor binding and signal initiation. J. Interferon Cytokine Res. 16:569, 1996.

424. Kalai, M., Montero-Julian, F.A., Grotzinger, J., Fontaine, V., Vandenbussche, P., Deschutyeneer, R., Wollmer, A., Brailly, H., and Content, J.: Analysis of the human interleukin-6/human interleukin-6 receptor binding interface at the amino acid level: proposed mechanism of interaction. Blood 89:1319, 1997.

425. Hilton, D.J., Hilton, A.A., Raicevic, A., Raker, S., Harrison-Smith, M., Gough, N.M., Begley, C.G., Nicola, N.A., and Wilson, T.A.: Cloning of a murine IL-11 receptor alpha chain; requirement for gp130 for high affinity binding and signal transduction. EMBO J. 13:4765, 1994.

426. Bilinski, P., Hall, M.A., Neuhaus, H., Gissel, C., Heath, J.K., and Gossler, A.: Two differentially expressed interleukin-11 receptor genes in the mouse genome. Biochem. J. 320:359, 1996.

427. Chérel, M., Sorel, M., Apiou, F., Lebeau, B., Dubois, S., Jacques, Y., and Minvielle, S.: The human interleukin-11 receptor alpha gene (IL11RA): genomic organization and chromosome mapping. Genomics 32:49, 1996.

428. Nandurkar, H.H., Robb, L., Tarlinton, D., Barnett, L., Köntgen, F., and Begley, C.G.: Adult mice with targeted mutation of the interleukin-11 receptor (IL11R) display normal hematopoiesis. Blood 90:2148, 1997.

429. Murakami, M., Narazaki, M., Hibi, M., Yawata, H., Yasukawa, K., Hamaguchi, M., Taga, T., and Kishimoto, T.: Critical cytoplasmic region of the interleukin 6 signal transducer gp130 is conserved in the cytokine receptor family. Proc. Natl. Acad. Sci. USA 88:11349, 1991.

430. Baumann, H., Gearing, D., and Ziegler, S.F.: Signaling by the cytoplasmic domain of hematopoietin receptors involves two distinguishable mechanisms in hepatic cells. J. Biol. Chem. 269:16297, 1994.

431. Akira, S., Yoshida, K., Tanaka, T., Taga, T., and Kishimoto, T.: Targeted disruption of the IL-6 related genes: gp130 and NF–IL-6. J. Exp. Med. 148:221, 1995.

432. Peters, M., Schirmacher, P., Goldschmitt, J., Odenthal, M., Peschel, C., Fattori, E., Ciliberto, G., Dienes, H.P., Meyer-zum-Buschenfelde, K.H., and Rose-John, S.: Extramedullary expansion of hematopoietic progenitor cells in interleukin (IL)–6 sIL-6R double transgenic mice. J. Exp. Med. 185:755, 1997.

433. Owczarek, C.M., Layton, M.J., Robb, L.G., Nicola, N.A., and Begley, C.G.: Molecular basis of the soluble and membrane bound forms of the murine leukemia inhibitory factor alpha chain. Expression in

normal, gestating and leukemia inhibitory factor nullizygous mice. J. Biol. Chem. 271:5495, 1996.

434. Mukouyama, Y., Hara, T., Xu, M., Tamura, K., Donovan, P.J., Kim, H., Kogo, H., Tsuji, K., Nakahata, T., and Miyajima, A.: In vitro expansion of murine multipotential hematopoietic progenitors from the embryonic aorta-gonad-mesonephros region. Immunity 8:105, 1998.

435. Dinarello, C.A.: Biologic basis for interleukin-1 in disease. Blood 87:2095, 1996.

436. Modi, W.S., Masuda, A., Yamada, M., Oppenheim, J.J., Matsushima, K., and O'Brien, S.J.: Chromosomal localization of the human interleukin 1 alpha (IL-1 alpha) gene. Genomics 2:310, 1988.

437. Priestle, J.P., Schar, H.P., and Grutter, M.G.: Crystallographic refinement of interleukin 1 beta at 2.0 Å resolution. Proc. Natl. Acad. Sci. USA 86:9667, 1989.

438. Graves, G.J., Hatada, H.H., Hendrickson, W.A., Miller, J.K., Madison, V.S., and Satow, Y.: Structure of interleukin-1 at 2.7Å resolution. Biochemistry 29:2679, 1990.

439. Vigers, G.P., Caffes, P., Evans, R.J., Thompson, R.C., Eisenberg, S.P., and Brandhuber, B.J.: X-ray structure of interleukin-1 receptor antagonist at 2.0-Å resolution. J. Biol. Chem. 269:12874, 1994.

440. Hannum, C.H., Wilcox, C.J., Arend, W.P., Joslin, F.G., Dripps, D.J., Heimdal, P.L., Armes, L.G., Sommer, A., Eisenberg, S.P., and Thompson, R.C.: Interleukin-1 receptor antagonist activity of a human interleukin-1 inhibitor. Nature 343:336, 1990.

441. Eisenberg, S.P., Evans, R.J., Arend, W.P., Verderber, E., Brewer, M.T., Hannum, C.H., and Thompson, R.C.: Primary structure and functional expression from complementary DNA of a human interleukin-1 receptor antagonist. Nature 343:341, 1990.

442. Granowitz, E.V., Porat, R., Mier, J.W., Orencole, S.F., Callahan, M.V., Cannon, J.G., Lynch, E.A., Ye, K., Poutsiaka, D.D., Vannier, E., Shapiro, L., Pribble, J.P., Stiles, D.M., Catalano, M.A., Wolf, S.M., and Dinarello, C.A.: Hematological and immunomodulatory effects of an interleukin-1 receptor antagonist coinfusion during low-dose endotoxemia in healthy humans. Blood 82:2985, 1993.

443. Fenton, M.J., Vermeulen, M.W., Clark, B.D., Webb, A.C., and Auron, P.E.: Human pro-IL-1 beta gene expression in monocytic cells is regulated by two distinct pathways. J. Immunol. 140:2267, 1988.

444. Mora, M., Carinci, V., Bensi, G., Raugei, G., Buonamassa, D.T., and Melli, M.: Differential expression of the human IL-1 alpha and beta genes. Prog. Clin. Biol. Res. 349:205, 1990.

445. Schindler, R., Ghezzi, P., and Dinarello, C.A.: IL-1 induces IL-1. IV. IFN-γ suppresses IL-1 but not lipopolysaccharide-induced transcription of IL-1. J. Immunol. 144:2216, 1990.

446. Ghezzi, P., Dinarello, C.A., Bianchi, M., Rosandich, M.E., Repine, J.E., and White, C.W.: Hypoxia increases production of interleukin-1 and tumor necrosis factor by human mononuclear cells. Cytokine 3:189, 1991.

447. Serkkola, E., and Hurme, M.: Synergism between protein-kinase C and cAMP-dependent pathways in the expression of the interleukin 1β gene is mediated via the activator-protein-1 (AP-1) enhancer activity. Eur. J. Biochem. 213:243, 1993.

448. Auron, P.E., and Webb, A.C.: Interleukin-1: a gene expression system regulated at multiple levels. Eur. Cytokine Netw. 5:573, 1994.

449. Kominato, Y., Galson, D.L., Waterman, W.R., Webb, A.C., and Auron, P.E.: Monocyte expression of the prointerleukin 1 beta gene dependent on promoter sequences which bind the hematopoietic transcription factor Spi-1/PU.1. Mol. Cell. Biol. 15:59, 1995.

450. Mosley, B., Urdal, D.I., Prickett, K.S., Larsen, A., Cosman, D., Conlon, P.J., Gillis, S., and Dower, S.K.: The interleukin-1 receptor binds the human interleukin-1α precursor but not the interleukin-1β precursor. J. Biol. Chem. 262:2941, 1987.

451. Stevenson, F.T., Bursten, S.I., Fanton, C., Locksley, R.M., and Lovett, D.M.: The 31-kDa precursor of interleukin-1 is myristoylated on specific lysines within the 16-kDa N-terminal propiece. Proc. Natl. Acad. Sci. USA 90:7245, 1993.

452. Kobayashi, Y., Yamamoto, K., Saido, T., Kawasaki, H., Oppenheim, J.J., and Matsushima, K.: Identification of calcium-activated neutral protease as a processing enzyme of human interleukin 1 alpha. Proc. Natl. Acad. Sci. USA 87:5548, 1990.

453. Maier, J.A.M., Voulalas, P., Roeder, D., Maciag, T.: Extension of the life span of human endothelial cells by an interleukin-1α antisense oligomer. Science 249:1570, 1990.

454. Zubiaga, A.M., Munoz, E., and Huber, B.T.: Production of IL-1 by activated Th type 2 cells. Its role as an autocrine growth factor. J. Immunol. 146:3849, 1991.

455. Maier, J.A.M., Statuto, M., and Ragnotti, G.: Endogenous interleukin-1 alpha must be transported to the nucleus to exert its activity in human endothelial cells. Mol. Cell. Biol. 14:1845, 1994.

456. Stevenson, F.T., Torrano, F., Locksley, R.M., and Lovett, D.H.: The patterns of translation and intracellular distribution support alternative secretory mechanisms. J. Cell. Physiol. 152:223, 1992.

457. Cerretti, D.P., Kozlosky, C.J., Mosley, B., Nelson, N., Van Ness, K., Greenstreet, T.A., March, C.J., Kronheim, S.R., Druck, T., Cannizzaro, L.A., Huebner, K., and Black, R.A.: Molecular cloning of the IL-1β processing enzyme. Science 256:97, 1992.

458. Kuida, K., Lippke, J.A., Ku, G., Harding, M.W., Livingston, D.J., Su, M.S.S., and Flavell, R.A.: Altered cytokine export and apoptosis in mice deficient in interleukin-1 converting enzyme. Science 267:2000, 1995.

459. Dinarello, C.A., Cannon, J.G., Mier, J.W., Bernheim, H.A., LoPreste, G., Lynn, D.L., Love, R.N., Webb, A.C., Auron, P.E., Reuben, R.C., Rich, A., Wolf, S.M., and Putney, S.D.: Multiple biological activities of human recombinant interleukin-1. J. Clin. Invest. 77:1734, 1986.

460. Hazuda, D.J., Strickler, J., Kueppers, F., Simon, P.L., and Young, P.R.: Processing of precursor interleukin-1 beta and inflammatory disease. J. Biol. Chem. 265:6318, 1990.

461. Irmler, M., Hertig, S., MacDonald, H.R., Sadoul, R., Becherer, J.D., Proudfoot, A., Solari, R., and Tschopp, J.: Granzyme A is an interleukin-1β–converting enzyme. J. Exp. Med. 181:1917, 1995.

462. Higgins, G.C., Foster, J.L., and Postlethwaite, A.E.: Interleukin-1 beta propeptide is detected intracellularly and extracellularly when human monocytes are stimulated with LPS in vitro. J. Exp. Med. 180:607, 1994.

463. Perregaux, D., Barberia, J., Lanzetti, A.J., Geoghegan, K.F., Carty, T.J., and Gabel, C.A.: IL-1β maturation: evidence that mature cytokine formation can be induced specifically by nigercin. J. Immunol. 149:1294, 1992.

464. Aznar, C., Fitting, C., and Cavaillon, J.M.: Lipopolysaccharide-induced production of cytokines by bone-marrow-derived macrophages: dissociation between intracellular interleukin-1 production and interleukin-1 release. Cytokine 2:259, 1990.

465. Singer, I.I., Bayne, E.K., Chin, J., Limjuco, G., Weidner, J., Miller, D.K., Chapman, K., and Kostura, M.J.: The interleukin-1 beta–converting enzyme (ICE) is localized on the external cell surface membranes and in the cytoplasmic ground substance of human monocytes by immuno-electron microscopy. J. Exp. Med. 182:1447, 1995.

466. Neta, R., Vogel, S.N., Plocinski, J.M., Parenes, S., Benjamin, W., Caizzonite, R., and Pilcher, M.: In vivo modulation with anti IL-1 receptor (p80) antibody 35E5 of the response to IL-1. Blood 76:57, 1990.

467. Henricson, B.E., Neta, R., and Vogel, S.N.: An interleukin-1 receptor antagonist blocks lipopolysaccharide-induced colony stimulating factor production and early endotoxin tolerance. Infect. Immun. 59:1188, 1991.

468. Dubois, C.M., Ruscetti, F.W., Palaszynski, E.W., Falk, L.A., Oppenheim, J.J., and Keller, J.R.: Transforming growth factor β is a potent inhibitor of interleukin-1 (IL-1) receptor expression: proposed mechanism of inhibition of IL-1 action. J. Exp. Med. 172:737, 1990.

469. Koch, K.C., Ye, K., Clark, B.D., and Dinarello, C.A.: Interleukin (IL) 4 up-regulates gene and surface IL-1 receptor type 1 in murine T helper type 2 cells. Eur. J. Immunol. 22:153, 1992.

470. Takii, T., Hayashi, H., Marunouchi, T., and Onozaki, K.: Interleukin-1 downregulates type 1 interleukin-1 receptor mRNA expression in a human fibroblast cell line TIG-1 in the absence of prostaglandin E_2 synthesis. Lymphokine Cytokine Res. 13:213, 1994.

471. Kuna, P., Reddigari, S.R., Rucinski, D., Oppenheim, J.J., and Kaplan, A.P.: Monocyte chemotactic and activating factor is a potent histamine-releasing factor for human basophils. J. Exp. Med. 175:489, 1992.

472. Neta, R., Vogel, S.N., Sipe, J.D., Wong, G.G., and Nordan, R.P.: Comparison of in vivo effects of human recombinant IL1 and human recombinant IL6 in mice. Lymphokine Res. 7:403, 1988.

473. Sironi, M., Breviario, F., Proserpio, P., Biondi, A., Vecchi, A., van Damme, J., Dejana, E., and Mantovani, A.: IL-1 stimulates IL-6 production in endothelial cells. J. Immunol. 142:549, 1989.

474. Helle, M., Boeije, L., and Aarden, L.A.: Il-6 is an intermediate in IL-1 induced thymocyte proliferation. J. Immunol. 142:4335, 1989.

475. Hamilton, J.A., Waring, P.M., and Filonzi, E.L.: Induction of leukemia inhibitory factor in human synovial fibroblasts by IL-1 and tumor necrosis factor-alpha. J. Immunol. 150:1496, 1993.

476. Le, J., Lin, J.X., Henriksen-DeStefano, D., and Vilcek, J.: Bacterial lipopolysaccharide-induced interferon-gamma production: roles of interleukin 1 and interleukin 2. J. Immunol. 136:4525, 1986.

477. Altmeyer, A., and Dumont, F.J.: Rapamycin inhibits IL-1 mediated interferon-gamma production in the YAC-1 T cell lymphoma. Cytokine 5:133, 1993.

478. Lukacs, N.W., Kunkel, S.L., Burdick, M.D., Lincoln, P.M., and Streiter, R.M.: Interleukin-1 receptor antagonist blocks chemokine production in the mixed lymphocyte reaction. Blood 82:3668, 1993.

479. Sciacca, F.L., Sturzl, M., Bussolino, F., Sironi, M., Brandstetter, H., Zietz, C., Zhou, D., Matteucci, C., Peri, G., Sozzani, S., Bennelli, R., Arese, M., Albini, A., Colotta, F., and Montovani, A.: Expression of adhesion molecules, platelet-activating factor, and chemokines by Kaposi's sarcoma cells. J. Immunol. 153:4816, 1994.

480. Seitz, M., Loetscher, P., Dewald, B., Towbin, H., Ceska, M., and Baggiolini, M.: Production of interleukin-1 receptor antagonist, inflammatory chemotactic proteins, and prostaglandin E by rheumatoid and osteoarthritis synoviocytes—regulation by IFN-gamma and IL-4. J. Immunol. 152:2060, 1994.

481. Shirakawa, F., Tanaka, Y., Eto, S., Suzuki, H., Yodoi, J., and Yamashita, U.: Effect of interleukin 1 on the expression of interleukin 2 receptor (Tac antigen) on human natural killer cells and natural killer–like cell line (YT cells). J. Immunol. 137:551, 1986.

482. Buzby, J.S., Knoppel, E.M., and Cairo, M.S.: Coordinate regulation of Steel factor, its receptor (Kit), and cytoadhesion molecule (ICAM-1 and ELAM-1) mRNA expression in human vascular endothelial cells of differing origins. Exp. Hematol. 22:122, 1994.

483. Konig, A., Corbacioglu, S., Ballmaier, M., and Welte, K.: Downregulation of c-kit expression in human endothelial cells by inflammatory stimuli. Blood 90:148, 1997.

484. Watanabe, Y., Kitamura, T., Hayashida, K., and Miyajima, A.: Monoclonal antibody against the common beta subunit (beta c) of the human interleukin-3 (IL-3), IL-5, and granulocyte-macrophage colony-stimulating factor receptors shows upregulation of beta c by IL-1 and tumor necrosis factor-alpha. Blood 80:2215, 1992.

485. Conca, W., Kaplan, P.B., and Krane, S.M.: Increases in levels of procollagenase messenger RNA in cultured fibroblasts induced by human recombinant interleukin 1 beta or serum follow c-jun expression and are dependent on new protein synthesis. J. Clin. Invest. 83:1753, 1989.

486. Ku, J.C., Liu, M.Y., and Wu, M.C.: Stimulation of macrophage colony-stimulating factor synthesis by interleukin-1. Arch. Biochem. Biophys. 295:42, 1992.

487. Guy, G.R., Cao, X., Chua, S.P., and Tan, Y.H.: Okadaic acid mimics multiple changes in early protein phosphorylation and gene expression induced by tumor necrosis factor or interleukin-1. J. Biol. Chem. 267:1846, 1992.

488. Escriou, N., Jankovic, D.L., and Theze, J.: Interleukin-1 and interleukin-6 synergize in preparing resting murine B cells to respond to antimu: correlation wth c-myc expression. Cell. Immunol. 141:243, 1992.

489. Lafyatis, R., Kim, S.J., Angel, P., Roberts, A.B., Sporn, M.B., Karin, M., and Wilder, R.L.: Interleukin-1 stimulates and all-trans-retinoic acid inhibits collagenase gene expression through its 5 activator protein-1-binding site. Mol. Endocrinol. 4:973, 1990.

490. Munoz, E., Zubiago, A.M., and Huber, B.T.: Interleukin-1 induces c-fos and c-jun gene expression in T helper type II cells through different signal transmission pathways. Eur. J. Immunol. 22:2101, 1992.

491. Bagby, G.C., Jr.: Interleukin-1 and hematopoiesis. Blood Rev. 3:152, 1989.

492. Osborn, L., Hession, C., Tizard, R., Vassallo, C., Luhowskyj, S., Chi-Rosso, G., and Lobb, R.: Direct expression cloning of vascular cell adhesion molecule 1, a cytokine-induced endothelial protein that binds to lymphocytes. Cell 59:1203, 1989.

493. Spertini, O., Luscinskas, F.W., Kansas, G.S., Munro, J.M., Griffin, J.D., Gimbrone, M.A., Jr., and Tedder, T.F.: Leukocyte adhesion molecule-1 (LAM-1, L-selectin) interacts with an inducible endothelial cell ligand to support leukocyte adhesion. J. Immunol. 147:2565, 1991.

494. Jubinsky, P.T., and Stanley, E.R.: Purification of hemopoietin 1: a multilineage hemopoietic growth factor. Proc. Natl. Acad. Sci. USA 82:2764, 1985.

495. Mochizuki, D.Y., Eisenman, J.R., Conlon, P.J., Larsen, A.D., and Tushinski, R.J.: Interleukin 1 regulates hematopoietic activity, a role previously ascribed to hemopoietin 1. Proc. Natl. Acad. Sci. USA 84:5267, 1987.

496. De Togni, P., Goellner, J., Ruddle, N.H., Streeter, P.R., Fick, A., Mariathasan, S., Smith, S.C., Carlson, R., Shornick, L.P., Strauss-Schoenberger, J., Russell, J.H., Karr, R., and Chaplin, D.D.: Abnormal development of peripheral lymphoid organs in mice deficient in lymphotoxin. Science 264:703, 1994.

497. Beutler, B., and Cerami, A.: The biology of cachectin/TNFα primary mediator of the host response. Annu. Rev. Immunol. 7:625, 1989.

498. Vassalli, P.: The pathophysiology of tumor necrosis factors. Annu. Rev. Immunol. 10:411, 1992.

499. Cosman, D.: A family of ligands for the TNF receptor superfamily. Stem Cells 12:440, 1994.

500. Eck, M.J., and Sprang, S.R.: The structure of tumor necrosis factor-α at 2.6Å resolution. Implications for receptor binding. J. Biol. Chem. 267:2119, 1989.

501. Eck, M.J., Ultsch, M., Rinderknecht, E., de Vos, A.M., and Sprang, S.R.: The structure of human lymphotoxin (tumor necrosis factor-β) at 1.9-Å resolution. J. Biol. Chem. 267:2119, 1992.

502. Banner, D.W., D'Arcy, A., Janes, W., Gentz, R., Schoenfeld, H.J., Broger, C., Loetscher, H., and Lesslauer, W.: Crystal structure of the soluble human 55kD TNF receptor–human TNFβ complex: implications for TNF receptor activation. Cell 73:431, 1993.

503. Old, L.J.: Tumor necrosis factor (TNF). Science 230:630, 1985.

504. Chensue, S., Otterness, I., Higashi, G., Forsch, C., and Kunkel, S.: Monokine production by hypersensitivity (Schistosoma mansoni egg) and foreign body (Sephadex bead)–type granuloma macrophages. Evidence for sequential production of IL-1 and tumor necrosis factor. J. Immunol. 142:1281, 1989.

505. Stein, M., and Gordon, S.: Regulation of tumor necrosis factor (TNF) release by murine peritoneal macrophages: role of cell stimulation and specific phagocytic plasma membrane receptors. Eur. J. Immunol. 21:431, 1991.

506. Warren, M.K., and Ralph, P.: Macrophage growth factor CSF-1 stimulates human monocyte production of interferon, tumor necrosis factor, and colony stimulating activity. J. Immunol. 137:2281, 1986.

507. Philip, R., and Epstein, L.B.: Tumor necrosis factor as immunomodulator and mediator of monocyte cytotoxicity induced by itself, gamma-interferon and interleukin-1. Nature 323:86, 1986.

508. Sung, S., Bjorndahl, J., Wang, C., Kao, H., and Fu, S.: Production of tumor necrosis factor/cachectin by human T cell lines and peripheral blood T lymphocytes stimulated by phobol myristate acetate and anti-CD3 antibody. J. Exp. Med. 167:937, 1988.

509. Collart, M.A., Baeuerle, P., and Vassalli, P.: Regulation of tumor necrosis factor alpha transcription in macrophages: involvement of four κB-like motifs and of constitutive and inducible forms of NF-κB. Mol. Cell. Biol. 10:1498, 1990.

510. Ulich, T.R., Guo, K.Z., Irwin, B., Remick, D.G., and Davatelis, G.N.: Endotoxin-induced cytokine gene expression in vivo. II. Regulation of tumor necrosis factor and interleukin-1 alpha/beta expression and suppression. Am. J. Pathol. 137:1173, 1990.

511. Bogdan, C., Paik, J., Vodovotz, Y., and Nathan, C.: Contrasting mechanisms for suppression of macrophage cytokine release by transforming growth factor-beta and interleukin-10. J. Biol. Chem. 267:23301, 1992.

512. Newell, C.L., Deisseroth, A.B., and Lopez-Berestein, G.: Interaction of nuclear proteins with an AP-1/CRE-like promoter sequence in the human TNF-alpha gene. J. Leukoc. Biol. 56:27, 1994.

513. Hayes, M.P., Freeman, S.L., and Donnelly, R.P.: IFN-gamma priming of monocytes enhances LPS-induced TNF production by augmenting both transcription and mRNA stability. Cytokine 7:427, 1995.

514. Moss, M.L., Jin, S.L., Milla, M.E., Bickett, D.M., Burkhart, W., Carter, H.L., Chen, W.J., Clay, W.C., Didsbury, J.R., Hassler, D., Hoffman, C.R., Kost, T.A., Lambert, M.H., Leesnitzer, M.A., McCauley, P., McGeehan, G., Mitchell, J., Moyer, M., Pahel, G., Rocque, W., Overton, L.K., Schoenen, F., Seaton, T., Su, J.L., and Becherer, J.D.: Cloning of a disintegrin metalloproteinase that processes precursor tumour-necrosis factor-alpha. Nature 385:733, 1997.

515. Drapier, J.C., Wietzerbin, J., and Hibbs, J.: Interferon-γ and tumour necrosis factor induce the L-arginine–dependent cytotoxic effector mechanism in murine macrophages. Eur. J. Immunol. 18:1587, 1988.

516. Ding, A.H., Nathan, C.F., and Stuehr, D.J.: Release of reactive nitrogen intermediates and reactive oxygen intermediates from mouse peritoneal macrophages. Comparison of activating cytokines and evidence for independent production. J. Immunol. 141:2407, 1988.

517. Doukas, J., and Pober, J.S.: IFN-γ enhances endothelial activation induced by tumor necrosis factor but not IL-1. J. Immunol. 145:1727, 1990.

518. Osborn, L.: Leukocyte adhesion to endothelium in inflammation. Cell 62:3, 1990.

519. Van der Poll, T., Büller, H.R., ten Cate, H., Wortel, C.H., Bauer, K.A., van Deventer, S.J.H., Hack, C.E., Sauerwein, H.P., Rosenberg, R.D., and ten Cate, J.W.: Activation of coagulation after administration of tumor necrosis factor to normal subjects. N. Engl. J. Med. 322:1622, 1990.

520. Warner, S.J.C., and Libby, P.: Human vascular smooth muscle cells. Target for and source of tumor necrosis factor. J. Immunol. 142:100, 1989.

521. Jirik, F.R., Podor, T.J., Hirano, T., Kishimoto, T., Loskutoff, D.J., Carson, D.A., and Lotz, M.: Bacterial lipopolysaccharide and inflammatory mediators augment IL-6 secretion by human endothelial cells. J. Immunol. 142:144, 1989.

522. Scheurich, P., Thoma, B., Ucer, U., and Pfizenmaier, K.: Immunoregulatory activity of recombinant human tumor necrosis factor (TNF)-α: induction of TNF receptors on human T cells and TNF-α–mediated enhancement of T cell responses. J. Immunol. 138:1786, 1987.

523. Pillai, S., Bikkle, D., Eessalu, T., Aggarwal, B., and Elias, P.: Binding and biological effects of tumor necrosis factor alpha on cultured human neonatal foreskin keratinocytes. J. Clin. Invest. 83:816, 1989.

524. Schröder, J.M., Sticherling, M., Heineicke, H.H., Preissner, W.C., and Christophers, E.: IL-1 or tumor necrosis factor-α stimulate releases of three NAP-1/IL-8–related neutrophil chemotactic proteins in human dermal fibroblasts. J. Immunol. 144:2223, 1990.

525. Weekx, S., Plum, J., Van Bockstaele, D.R., Nijs, G., Lenjou, M., Vandenabeele, P., Berneman, Z.N., and Snoeck, H.W.: Differences in autocrine TGF-β effects and in TNF-α modulation correlate with myelopoietic growth properties of human fetal and adult hematopoietic stem cells. Blood 90(suppl. 1):476a, 1997.

526. Roodman, G.D., Bird, A., Hutzler, D., and Montgomery, W.: Tumor necrosis factor-alpha and hematopoietic progenitors: effects of tumor necrosis factor on the growth of erythroid progenitors CFU-E and BFU-E and the hematopoietic cell lines K562, HL60, and HEL cells. Exp. Hematol. 15:928, 1987.

527. Fandrey, J., and Jelkmann, W.E.: Interleukin-1 and tumor necrosis factor-alpha inhibit erythropoietin production in vitro. Ann. N. Y. Acad. Sci. 628:250, 1991.

528. Faquin, W.C., Schneider, T.J., and Goldberg, M.A.: Effect of inflammatory cytokines on hypoxia-induced erythropoietin production. Blood 79:1987, 1992.

529. Jelkmann, W., Wolff, M., and Fandrey, J.: Inhibition of erythropoietin production by cytokines and chemotherapy may contribute to the anemia in malignant disease. Adv. Exp. Med. Biol. 345:525, 1994.

530. Pfeffer, A., Matsuyama, T., Kundig, T.M., Wakeham, A., Kishihara, K., Shahinian, A., Wiegmann, K., Ohashi, P.S., Kronke, M., and Mak, T.W.: Mice deficient for the 55 kD tumor necrosis factor receptor are resistant to endotoxic shock, yet succumb to *L. monocytogenes* infection. Cell 73:457, 1993.

531. Rothe, J., Lesslauer, W., Lotscher, H., Lang, Y., Koebel, P., Kontgen, F., Althage, A., Zinkernagel, R., Steinmetz, M., and Bluethmann, H.: Mice lacking the tumour necrosis factor receptor 1 are resistant to TNF-mediated toxicity but highly susceptible to infection by *Listeria monocytogenes*. Nature 364:798, 1993.

532. Billiau, A.: Interferon-γ: biology and role in pathogenesis. Adv. Immunol. 62:61, 1996.

533. Bach, E.A., Aguet, M., and Schreiber, R.D.: The IFNγ receptor: a paradigm for cytokine receptor signaling. Annu. Rev. Immunol. 15:563, 1997.

534. Boehm, U., Klamp, T., Groot, M., Howard, J.C.: Cellular responses to interferon-γ. Annu. Rev. Immunol. 15:749, 1997.

535. Naylor, S.L., Gray, P.W., and Lalley, P.A.: Mouse immune interferon (IFN-gamma) gene is on chromosome 10. Somat. Cell Mol. Genet. 10:531, 1984.

536. Rinderknecht, E., O'Connor, B.H., and Rodriguez, H.: Natural human interferon-γ. Complete amino acid sequence and determination of sites of glycosylation. J. Biol. Chem. 259:6790, 1984.

537. Samudzi, C.T., Burton, L.E., and Rubin, J.R.: Crystal structure of recombinant rabbit interferon-gamma at 2.7-Å resolution. J. Biol. Chem. 266:21791, 1991.

538. Ealick, S.E., Cook, W.J., Vijay-Kumar, S., Carson, M., Nagabhushan, T.L., Trotta, P.P., and Bugg, C.E.: Three-dimensional structure of recombinant human interferon-γ. Science 252:268, 1991.

539. Sareneva, T., Pirhonen, J., Cantell, K., Kalkkinen, N., and Julkunen, I.: Role of *N*-glycosylation in the synthesis, dimerization and secretion of human interferon-gamma. Biochem. J. 303:831, 1994.

540. Walter, M.R., Windsor, W.T., Nagabhushan, T.L., Lundell, D.J., Lunn, C.A., Zauodny, P.J., and Narula, S.K.: Crystal structure of a complex between interferon-gamma and its soluble high-affinity receptor. Nature 376:230, 1995.

541. Mosmann, T.R., and Coffman, R.L.: TH1 and TH2 cells: different patterns of lymphokine secretion lead to different functional properties. Annu. Rev. Immunol. 7:145, 1989.

542. Sad, S., Marcotte, R., and Mosmann, T.R.: Cytokine-induced differentiation of precursor mouse CD8+ T cells into cytotoxic CD8+ T cells secreting Th1 or T2 cytokines. Immunity 2:271, 1995.

543. Trinchieri, G.: Interleukin-12: a proinflammatory cytokine with immunoregulatory functions that bridge innate resistance and antigen-specific adaptive immunity. Annu. Rev. Immunol. 13:251, 1995.

544. Carson, W.E., Ross, M.E., Baiocchi, R.A., Marica, M.J., Bolani, N., Grabstein, K., and Caligiuri, M.A.: Endogenous production of interleukin 15 by activated human monocytes is critical for optimal production of interferon-gamma by natural killer cells in vitro. J. Clin. Invest. 96:2578, 1995.

545. Dalton, D.K., Pitts-Meek, S., Keshav, S., Figari, I.S., Bradley, A., and Stewart, T.A.: Multiple defects of immune cell function in mice with disrupted interferon-γ genes. Science 259:1739, 1993.

546. Huang, S., Hendriks, W., Althage, A., Hemmi, S., Bluethmann, H., Kamijo, R., Vilcek, J., Zinkernagel, R.M., and Aguet, M.: Immune response in mice that lack the interferon-γ receptor. Science 259:1742, 1993.

547. Meraz, M.A., White, J.M., Sheehan, K.C.F., Bach, E.A., Rodig, S.J., Dighe, A.S., Kaplan, D.H., Riley, J.K., Greenlund, A.C., Campbell, D., Carver-Moore, K., DuBois, R.N., Clark, R., Aguet, M., and Schreiber, R.D.: Targeted disruption of the *Stat1* gene in mice reveals unexpected physiological specificity in the JAK-STAT signaling pathway. Cell 84:431, 1996.

548. Durbin, J.E., Hackenmiller, R., Simon, M.C., and Levy, D.E.: Targeted disruption of the mouse *Stat1* gene results in compromised innate immunity to viral disease. Cell 84:443, 1996.

549. Broxmeyer, H.E., Cooper, S., Rubin, B.Y., and Taylor, M.W.: The synergistic influence of human interferon-gamma and interferon-alpha on suppression of hematopoietic progenitor cells is additive with the enhanced sensitivity of these cells to inhibition by interferons at low oxygen tension in vitro. J. Immunol. 135:2502, 1985.

550. Ganser, A., Carlo-Stella, C., Greher, J., Volkers, B., and Hoelzer, D.: Effect of recombinant interferons alpha and gamma on human bone marrow–derived megakaryocytic progenitor cells. Blood 70:1173, 1987.

551. Taniguchi, S., Dai, C.H., and Krantz, S.B.: Specific binding of interferon-gamma to high affinity receptors on human erythroid colony-forming cells. Exp. Hematol. 25:193, 1997.

552. Dai, C.H., Price, J.O., Abdel-Meguid, S.S., Brunner, T., and Krantz, S.B.: Fas ligand is present in human erythroid colony-forming cells and interacts wtih Fas induced by interferon to produce erythroid cell apoptosis. Blood 91:1235, 1998.

553. Deiss, L.P., Feinstein, E., Berissi, H., Cohen, O., and Kimchi, A.: Identification of a novel serine/threonine kinase and a novel 15-kD protein as potential mediators of the γ-interferon–induced cell death. Genes Dev. 9:15, 1995.

554. Feinstein, E., Wallach, D., Boldin, M., Varfolomeev, E., and Kimchi, A.: The death domain: a module shared by proteins with diverse cellular functions. Trends Biochem. Sci. 20:342, 1995.

555. Kissil, J.L., Deiss, L.P., Bayewitch, M., Raveh, T., Khaspekov, G., and Kimchi, A.: Isolation of DAP-3, a novel mediator of interferon-γ–induced cell death. J. Biol. Chem. 270:27932, 1995.

556. Levy-Strumpf, N., Deiss, L.P., Berissi, H., and Kimchi, A.: DAP-5, a novel homolog of eukaryotic translation initiation factor 4G isolated as a putative modulator of gamma interferon induced programmed cell death. Mol. Cell. Biol. 17:1615, 1997.

557. Sato, T., Selleri, C., Young, N.S., and Maciejewski, J.P.: Hematopoietic inhibition by interferon-γ is partially mediated through interferon responsive factor-1. Blood 86:3373, 1995.

558. Sarris, A.H., Broxmeyer, H.E., Wirthmueller, U., Karasavvas, N., Cooper, S., Lu, L., Krueger, J., and Ravetch, J.V.: Human interferon-inducible protein 10: expression and purification of recombinant protein demonstrate inhibition of early human hematopoietic progenitors. J. Exp. Med. 178:1127, 1993.

559. Le Coniat, M., Alcaide-Loridan, C., Fellous, M., and Berger, R.: Human interferon gamma receptor 1 (IFNGR1) gene maps to chromosome region 6q23–6q24. Hum. Genet. 84:92, 1989.

560. Soh, J., Donnelly, R.O., Kotenko, S., Mariano, T.M., Cook, J.R., Wang, N., Emanuel, S., Schwartz, B., Miki, T., and Pestka, S.: Identification and sequence of an accessory factor required for activation of the human interferon γ receptor. Cell 76:793, 1994.

561. Farrar, M.A., Fernandez-Luna, J., and Schreiber, R.D.: Identification of two regions within the cytoplasmic domain of the human interferon-gamma receptor required for function. J. Biol. Chem. 266:19626, 1991.

562. Keller, J.R., Jacobsen, S.E.W., Dubois, C.M., Hestdal, K., and Ruscetti, F.W.: Transforming growth factor-β: a bidirectional regulator of hematopoietic cell growth. Int. J. Cell Cloning 10:2, 1992.

563. Daopin, S., Piez, K.A., Ogawa, Y., and Davies, D.R.: Crystal structure of transforming growth factor-β2: an unusual fold for the superfamily. Science 257:369, 1992.

564. Derynck, R., Jarrett, J.A., Chen, E.Y., Eaton, D.H., Bell, J.R., Assoian, R.K., Roberts, A.B., Sporn, M.B., and Goeddel, D.V.: Human transforming growth factor-β complementary DNA sequence and expression in normal and transformed cells. Nature 316:701, 1985.

565. Franz'en, P., ten Dijke, P., Ichijo, H., Yamashita, H., Schulz, P., Heldin, C.H., and Miyazono, K.: Cloning of a TGF beta type I receptor that forms a heteromeric complex with the TGF beta type II receptor. Cell 75:681, 1993.

566. López-Casillas, F., Cheifetz, S., Doody, J., Andres, J.L., Lane, W.S., and Massagué, J.: Structure and expression of the membrane proteoglycan betaglycan, a component of the TGF-β receptor system. Cell 67:785, 1991.

567. Yamashita, H., ten Dijke, P., Franz'en, P., Miyazono, K., and Heldin, C.H.: Formation of hetero-oligomeric complexes of type I and type II receptors for transforming growth factor beta. J. Biol. Chem. 269:20172, 1994.

568. Laiho, M., DeCaprio, J.A., Ludlow, J.W., Livingston, D.M., and Massagué, J.: Growth inhibition by TGF-β linked to suppression of retinoblastoma protein phosphorylation. Cell 62:175, 1990.

569. Weinberg, R.A.: The retinoblastoma protein and cell cycle control. Cell 81:323, 1995.

570. Polyak, K., Kato, J.Y., Solomon, M.J., Sherr, C.J., Massagué, J., Roberts, J.M., and Koff, A.: p27Kip1, a cyclin-Cdk inhibitor, links transforming growth factor-beta and contact inhibition to cell cycle arrest. Genes Dev. 8:9, 1994.

571. Shull, M.M., Ormsby, I., Kier, A.B., Pawlowski, S., Diebold, R.J., Yin, M., Allen, R., Sidman, C., Proetzel, G., Calvin, D., Annunziata, N., and Doetschman, T.: Targeted disruption of the mouse transforming growth factor-beta 1 gene results in multifocal inflammatory disease. Nature 359:693, 1992.

572. Ohta, M., Greenberger, J.S., Anklesaria, P., Bassols, A., and Massagué, J.: Two forms of transforming growth factor distinguished by multipotential haematopoietic progenitor cells. Nature 329:539, 1987.

573. Keller, J.R., Mantel, C., Sing, G.K., Ellingsworth, L.R., Ruscetti, S.K., and Ruscetti, F.W.: Transforming growth factor β1 selectively regulates early murine hematopoietic progenitors and inhibits the growth of IL-3–dependent myeloid leukemia cell lines. J. Exp. Med. 168:737, 1988.

574. Jackson, H., Williams, N., Westcott, K.R., and Green, R.: Differential effects of transforming growth factor-beta 1 on distinct developmental stages of murine megakaryocytopoiesis. J. Cell. Physiol. 161:312, 1994.

575. Waegell, W.O., Higley, H.R., Kincade, P.W., and Dasch, J.R.: Growth acceleration and stem cell expansion in Dexter-type cultures by neutralization of TGF-β. Exp. Hematol. 22:1051, 1994.

576. Dybedal, I., and Jacobsen, S.E.W.: Transforming growth factor β (TFG-β), a potent inhibitor of erythropoiesis: neutralizing TGF-β antibodies show erythropoietin as a potent stimulator of murine burst-forming unit erythroid colony formation in the absence of a burst-promoting activity. Blood 86:949, 1995.

577. Jacobsen, S.E.W., Ruscetti, F.W., Dubois, C.M., Lee, J., Boone, T.C., and Keller, J.R.: Transforming growth factor-β trans-modulates the expression of colony stimulating factor receptors on murine hematopoietic progenitor cell lines. Blood 77:1706, 1991.

578. Pindolia, K.R., Noth, C.J., Xu, Y.X., Janakiraman, N., Chapman, R.A., and Gautam, S.C.: IL-4 upregulates IL-1–induced chemokine gene expression in bone marrow stromal cells by enhancing NF-κB activation. Hematopathol. Mol. Hematol. 10:171, 1996.

579. Rollins, B.J.: Chemokines. Blood 90:909, 1997.

580. Kelner, G.S., Kennedy, J., Bacon, K.B., Kleyensteuber, S., Largaespada, D.A., Jenkins, N.A., Copeland, N.G., Bazan, J.F., Moore, K.W., Schall, T.J., and Zlotnik, A.: Lymphotactin: a cytokine that represents a new class of chemokine. Science 266:1395, 1994.

581. Pan, Y., Lloyd, C., Zhou, H., Dolich, S., Deeds, J., Gonzalo, J.A., Vath, J., Gosselin, M., Ma, J., Dussault, B., Woolf, E., Alperin, G., Culpepper, J., Gutierrez-Ramos, J.C., and Gearing, D.: Neurotactin, a membrane-anchored chemokine upregulated in brain inflammation. Nature 387:611, 1997.

582. Burrows, S.D., Doyle, M.L., Murphy, K.P., Franklin, S.G., White, J.R., Brooks, I., McNulty, D.E., Scott, M.O., Knutson, J.R., Porter, D., Young, P.R., and Hensley, P.: Determination of the monomer-dimer equilibrium of interleukin-8 reveals it is a monomer at physiological concentrations. Biochemistry 33:12741, 1994.

583. Rajarathnam, K., Sykes, B.D., Kay, C.M., Dewald, B., Geiser, T., Baggiolini, M., and Clark-Lewis, I.: Neutrophil activation by monomeric interleukin-8. Science 264:90, 1994.

584. Zhang, Y., and Rollins, B.J.: A dominant negative inhibitor indicates that monocyte chemoattractant protein 1 functions as a dimer. Mol. Cell. Biol. 15:4851, 1995.

585. Yoshimura, T., Matsushima, K., Tanaka, S., Robinson, E.A., Appella, E., Oppenheim, J.J., and Leonard, E.J.: Purification of a human monocyte-derived neutrophil chemotactic factor that has peptide sequence similarity to other host defense cytokines. Proc. Natl. Acad. Sci. USA 84:9233, 1987.

586. Hebert, C.A., Viytangcol, R.V., and Baker, J.B.: Scanning mutagenesis of interleukin-8 identifies a cluster of residues required for receptor binding. J. Biol. Chem. 266:18989, 1991.

587. Huber, A.R., Kunkel, S.L., Todd, R.F., Weiss, S.J.: Regulation of transendothelial neutrophil migration by endogenous interleukin-8. Science 254:99, 1991.

588. Anisowicz, A., Bardwell, L., and Sager, R.: Constitutive overexpression of a growth-regulated gene in transformed Chinese hamster and human cells. Proc. Natl. Acad. Sci. USA 84:7188, 1987.

589. Richmond, A., Belentien, E., Thomas, H.G., Flaggs, G., Barton, D.E., Spiess, J., Bordoni, R., Francke, U., and Derynck, R.: Molecular characterization and chromosomal mapping of melanoma growth stimulatory activity, a growth factor structurally related to β-thromboglobulin. EMBO J. 7:2025, 1988.

590. Oquendo, P., Alberta, J., Wen, D., Graycar, J.L., Derynck, R., and Stiles, C.D.: The platelet-derived growth factor–inducible KC gene encodes a secretory protein related to platelet α-granule proteins. J. Biol. Chem. 264:4133, 1989.

591. Hechtman, D.J., Cybulsky, M.I., Fuchs, H.J., Baker, J.B., and Gimbrone, M.A.: Intravascular IL-8: inhibitor of polymorphonuclear leukocyte accumulation at sites of acute inflammation. J. Immunol. 147:883, 1991.

592. Simonet, W.S., Hughes, T.M., Nguyen, H.Q., Trebasky, L.D., Danilenko, D.M., and Medlock, E.S.: Long-term impaired neutrophil migration in mice overexpressing human interleukin-8. J. Clin. Invest. 94:1310, 1994.

593. Holt, J.C., Harris, M.E., Holt, A.M., Lange, E., Henschen, A., and Niewiarowski, S.: Characterization of human platelet basic protein, a precursor form of low-affinity platelet factor 4 and β-thromboglobulin. Biochemistry 25:1988, 1986.

594. Deuel, T.F., Senior, R.M., Chang, D., Griffin, G.L., Henrikson, R.L., and Kaiser, E.T.: Platelet factor 4 is chemotactic for neutrophils and monocytes. Proc. Natl. Acad. Sci. USA 78:4584, 1981.

595. Gupta, S.K., Hassel, T., and Singh, J.P.: A potent inhibitor of endothelial cell proliferation is generated by proteolytic cleavage of the chemokine platelet factor 4. Proc. Natl. Acad. Sci. USA 92:7799, 1995.

596. Luster, A.D., Unkeless, J.C., and Ravetch, J.V.: γ-Interferon transcriptionally regulates an early-response gene containing homology to platelet proteins. Nature 315:672, 1985.

597. Narumi, S., Wyner, L., Stoler, M.H., Tannenbaum, C.S., and Hamilton, T.A.: Tissue-specific expression of murine IP-10 mRNA following systemic treatment with interferon γ. J. Leukoc. Biol. 52:27, 1992.

598. Taub, D.D., Longo, D.L., and Murphy, W.J.: Human interferon-inducible protein-10 induces mononuclear cell infiltration in mice and promotes the migration of human T lymphocytes into the peripheral tissues and human peripheral blood lymphocytes—SCID mice. Blood 87:1423, 1996.

599. Tashiro, K., Tada, H., Heilker, R., Shirozu, M., Nakano, T., and Honjo, T.: Signal sequence trap: a cloning strategy for secreted proteins and type I membrane proteins. Science 261:600, 1993.

600. Bleul, C.C., Farzan, M., Choe, H., Parolin, C., Clark-Lewis, I., So-

droski, J., and Sprinter, T.A.: The lymphocyte chemoattractant SDF-1 is a ligand for LESTR/fusin and blocks HIV-1 entry. Nature 382:829, 1996.

601. Oberlin, E., Amara, A., Bachelerie, F., Bessia, C., Virelizier, J.L., Arenzana-Seisdedos, F., Schwartz, O., Heard, J.M., Clark-Lewis, I., Legler, D.F., Loetscher, M., Baggiolini, M., and Moser, B.: The CXC chemokine SDF-1 is the ligand for LESTR/fusin and prevents infection by T-cell-line-adapted HIV-1. Nature 382:833, 1996.

602. Aiuti, A., Webb, I.J., Bleul, C., Springer, T., and Gutierrez-Ramos, J.C.: The chemokine SDF-1 is a chemoattractant for human CD34+ hematopoietic progenitor cells and provides a new mechanism to explain the mobilization of CD34+ progenitors to peripheral blood. J. Exp. Med. 185:111, 1997.

603. Nagasawa, T., Hirota, S., Tachibana, K., Takakura, N., Nishikawa, S., Kitamura, Y., Yoshida, N., Kikutani, H., and Kishimoto, T.: Defects of B-cell lymphopoiesis and bone-marrow myelopoiesis in mice lacking the CXC chemokine PBSF/SDF-1. Nature 382:635, 1996.

604. Wang, J.F., Liu, Z.Y., and Groopman, J.E.: The α-chemokine receptor CXCR4 is expressed on the megakaryocytic lineage from progenitors to platelets and modulates migration and adhesion. Blood 92:756, 1998.

605. Hamada, T., Möhle, R., Hesselgesser, J., Hoxie, J., Nachman, R.L., Moore, M.A.S., and Rafii, S.: Stromal derived factor-1 (SDF-1) induces chemotaxis, proplatelet formation and transmigration of mature polyploid megakaryocytes through bone marrow endothelial cells. J. Exp. Med. 188:539, 1998.

606. Valente, A.J., Graves, D.T., Vialle-Valentin, C.E., Delgado, R., and Schwartz, C.J.: Purification of a monocyte chemotactic factor secreted by nonhuman primate vascular cells in culture. Biochemistry 27:4162, 1988.

607. Jiang, Y., Beller, D.I., Frendl, G., and Graves, D.T.: Monocyte chemoattractant protein-1 regulates adhesion molecule expression and cytokine production in human monocytes. J. Immunol. 148:2423, 1992.

608. Vaddi, K., and Newton, R.C.: Regulation of monocyte integrin expression by β-family chemokines. J. Immunol. 153:4721, 1994.

609. Carr, M.W., Roth, S.J., Luther, E., Rose, S.S., and Springer, T.A.: Monocyte chemoattractant protein 1 acts as a T-lymphocyte chemoattractant. Proc. Natl. Acad. Sci. USA 91:3652, 1994.

610. Rutledge, B.J., Rayburn, H., Rosenberg, R., North, R.J., Gladue, R.P., Corless, C.L., and Rollins, B.J.: High level monocyte chemoattractant protein-1 expression in transgenic mice increases their susceptibility to intracellular pathogens. J. Immunol. 155:4838, 1995.

611. Dahinden, C.A., Geiser, T., Brunner, T., von Tscharner, V., Caput, D., Ferrara, P., Minty, A., and Baggiolini, M.: Monocyte chemotactic protein 3 is a most effective basophil- and eosinophil-activating chemokine. J. Exp. Med. 179:751, 1994.

612. Uguccioni, M., Loetscher, P., Forssmann, U., Dewald, B., Li, H., Lima, S.H., Li, Y., Kreider, B., Garrota, G., Thelen, M., and Baggiolini, M.: Monocyte chemotactic protein 4 (MCP-4), a novel structural and functional analogue of MCP-3 and eotaxin. J. Exp. Med. 183:2379, 1996.

613. Sarafi, M.N., Garcia-Zepeda, E.A., MacLean, J.A., Charo, I.F., and Luster, A.D.: Murine monocyte chemoattractant protein (MCP)-5: a novel CC chemokine that is a structural and functional homologue of human MCP-1. J. Exp. Med. 185:99, 1997.

614. Weber, M., Uguccioni, M., Baggiolini, M., Clark-Lewis, I., and Dahinden, C.A.: Deletion of the NH₂-terminal residue converts monocyte chemotactic protein 1 from an activator of basophil mediator release to an eosinophil chemoattractant. J. Exp. Med. 183:681, 1996.

615. Wolpe, S.D., Davatelis, G., Sherry, B., Beutler, B., Hesse, D.G., Nguyen, H.T., Moldawer, L.L., Nathan, C.F., Lowry, S.F., and Cerami, A.: Macrophages secrete a novel heparin-binding protein with inflammatory and neutrophil chemotactic properties. J. Exp. Med. 167:570, 1988.

616. Sherry, B., Tekamp-Olson, P., Gallegos, C., Bauer, D., Davatelis, G., Wolpe, S.D., Masiarz, F., Coit, D., and Cerami, A.: Resolution of the two components of macrophage inflammatory protein 1β, and cloning and characterization of one of those components, macrophage inflammatory protein 1β. J. Exp. Med. 168:2251, 1988.

617. Taub, D.D., Conlon, K., Lloyd, A.R., Oppenheim, J.J., and Kelvin, D.J.: Preferential migration of activated CD4+ and CD8+ T cells in response to MIP-1α and MIP-1β. Science 260:355, 1993.

618. Schall, T.J., Jongstra, J., Dyer, B.J., Jorgensen, J., Clayberger, C., Davis, M.M., and Krensky, A.M.: A human T cell–specific molecule is a member of a new gene family. J. Immunol. 141:1018, 1988.

619. Jose, P.J., Griffiths-Johnson, D.S., Collins, P.D., Walsh, D.T., Moqbel, R., Totty, N.F., Truong, O., Hsuan, J.J., and Williams, T.J.: Eotaxin: a potent eosinophil chemoattractant cytokine detected in a guinea pig model of allergic airways inflammation. J. Exp. Med. 179:881, 1994.

620. Imai, T., Yoshida, T., Baba, M., Nishimura, M., Kakizaki, M., and Yoshie, O.: Molecular cloning of a novel T-cell–directed CC chemokine expressed in thymus by signal sequence trap using Epstein-Barr virus vector. J. Biol. Chem. 271:21514, 1996.

621. Miller, M.D., and Krangel, M.S.: The human cytokine I-309 is a monocyte chemoattractant. Proc. Natl. Acad. Sci. USA 89:2950, 1992.

622. Graham, G.J., Wright, E.G., Hewick, R., Wolpe, S.D., Wilkie, N.M., Donaldson, D., Lorimore, S., and Pragnell, I.B.: Identification and characterization of an inhibitor of haemopoietic stem cell proliferation. Nature 344:442, 1990.

623. Ohmori, Y., Fukumoto, S., and Hamilton, T.A.: Two structurally distinct kappa B sequence motifs cooperatively control LPS-induced KC gene transcription in mouse macrophages. J. Immunol. 155:3593, 1995.

624. Shi, M.M., Godleski, J.J., and Paulauskis, J.D.: Molecular cloning and posttranscriptional regulation of macrophage inflammatory protein-1 alpha in alveolar macrophages. Biochem. Biophys. Res. Commun. 211:289, 1995.

625. Broxmeyer, H.E., Sherry, B., Cooper, S., Lu, L., Maze, R., Beckmann, M.P., Cerami, A., and Ralph, P.: Comparative analysis of the human macrophage inflammatory protein family of cytokines (chemokines) on proliferation of human myeloid progenitor cells. Interacting effects involving suppression, synergistic suppression, and blocking of suppression. J. Immunol. 150:3448, 1993.

626. Lu, L., Xiao, M., Grigsby, S., Wang, W.X., Wu, B., Shen, R.N., and Broxmeyer, H.E.: Comparative effects of suppressive cytokines on isolated single CD34(3+) stem/progenitor cells from human bone marrow and umbilical cord blood plated with and without serum. Exp. Hematol. 21:1442, 1993.

627. Su, S., Mukaida, N., Wang, J., Zhang, Y., Takami, A., Nakao, S., and Matsushima, K.: Inhibition of immature erythroid progenitor cell proliferation by macrophage inflammatory protein-1 alpha by interacting mainly with a C-C chemokine receptor, CCR1. Blood 90:605, 1997.

628. Broxmeyer, H.E.: Preclinical and clinical studies on the biology and mechanisms of action of chemokines as suppressors of hematopoiesis—review and update. Exp. Hematol. 25:777, 1997.

629. Gewirtz, A.M., Zhang, J., Ratajczak, J., Ratajczak, M., Park, K.S., Li, C., Yan, Z., and Poncz, M.: Chemokine regulation of human megakaryocytopoiesis. Blood 86:2559, 1995.

630. Verfaille, C.M., Catanzarro, P.M., and Li, W.N.: Macrophage inflammatory protein 1 alpha, interleukin 3 and diffusible marrow stromal factors maintain human hematopoietic stem cells for at least eight weeks in vitro. J. Exp. Med. 179:643, 1994.

631. Han, Z.C., Li, J.M., Lecomte, L., Alemany, M., Bovan, B., and Caen, J.P.: CXC-chemokines and derived peptides support the survival of hematopoietic progenitor cells and reduce their chemosensitivity to cytotoxic agents. Exp. Hematol. 25:836, 1997.

632. Yen, H., Penfold, S., Zhang, Y., and Rollins, B.J.: MCP-1–mediated chemotaxis requires activation of non-overlapping signal transduction pathways. J. Leukoc. Biol. 61:529, 1997.

633. Gao, J.L., Wynn, T.A., Chang, Y., Lee, E.J., Broxmeyer, H.E., Cooper, S., Tiffany, H.L., Westphal, H., Kwon-Chung, J., and Murphy, P.M.: Impaired host defense, hematopoiesis, granulomatous inflammation and type 1–type 2 cytokine balance in mice lacking CC chemokine receptor. J. Exp. Med. 185:1959, 1997.

634. Broxmeyer, H.E., Cooper, S., Cacalano, G., Hague, N.L., Bailish, E., and Moore, M.W.: Involvement of interleukin (IL) 8 receptor in negative regulation of myeloid progenitor cells in vivo: evidence from mice lacking the murine IL-8 receptor homologue. J. Exp. Med. 184:1825, 1996.

635. Artavanis-Tsakonas, S., Matsuno, K., and Fortini, M.E.: Notch signaling. Science 268:225, 1995.

636. Ellisen, L.W., Bird, J., West, D.C., Soreng, A.L., Reynolds, T.C., Smith, S.D., and Sklar, J.: TAN-1, the human homolog of the Drosophilia notch gene, is broken by chromosomal translocations in T lymphoblastic neoplasms. Cell 66:649, 1991.

637. Larsson, C., Lardelli, M., White, I., and Lendahl, U.: The human Notch 1, 2 and 3 genes are located at chromosome positions 9q34, 1p13-p11, and 19p13.2-p13.1 in regions of neoplasia associated translocations. Genomics 24:253, 1994.

638. Aster, J., Peat, W., Hasserjian, R., Erba, H., Davi, F., Luo, B., Scott, M., Baltimore, D., and Sklar, J.: Functional analysis of the TAN-1 gene, a human homolog of *Drosophila* notch. Cold Spring Harb. Symp. Quant. Biol. 59:125, 1994.

639. Pear, W.S., Aster, J.C., Scott, M.L., Hasserjian, R.P., Soffer, B., Sklar, J., and Baltimore, D.: Exclusive development of T cell neoplasms in mice transplanted with bone marrow expressing activated *Notch* alleles. J. Exp. Med. 183:2283, 1996.

640. Robey, E., Chang, D., Itano, A., Cado, D., Alexander, H., Lans, D., Weinmaster, G., and Salmon, P.: An activated form of Notch influences the choice between CD4 and CD8 T cell lineages. Cell 87:483, 1996.

641. Milner, L.A., Li, L., Hood, L., and Torok-Storb, B.: Activation of *Notch1* by its ligand, Jagged1, inhibits granulocytic differentiation and permits expansion of immature myeloid progenitors. Blood 90(suppl. 1):571a, 1997.

642. Robey, E.: Notch in vertebrates. Curr. Opin. Genet. Dev. 7:551, 1997.

643. Lindsell, C.E., Shawber, C.J., Boulter, J., and Weinmaster, G.: Jagged: a mammalian ligand that activates Notch1. Cell 80:909, 1995.

644. Nye, J.S., and Kopan, R.: Vertebrate ligands for Notch. Curr. Biol. 5:966, 1995.

645. Shawber, C., Boulter, J., Lindsell, C.E., and Weinmaster, G.: *Jagged*2: a serrate-like gene expressed during rat embryogenesis. Dev. Biol. 180:370, 1996.

646. Kopan, R., Nye, J.S., and Weinbraub, H.: The intracellular domain of mouse Notch: a constitutively activated repressor of myogenesis directed at the basic helix-loop-helix region of MyoD. Development 120:2385, 1994.

647. Pan, D., and Rubin, G.M.: Kuzbanian controls proteolytic processing of notch and mediates lateral inhibition during *Drosophilia* and vertebrate neurogenesis. Cell 90:271, 1997.

648. Blaumueller, C.M., Qi, H., Zagouras, P., and Artavanis-Tsakonas, S.: Intracellular cleavage of notch leads to a heterodimeric receptor on the plasma membrane. Cell 90:281, 1997.

649. Fortini, M.E., and Artavanis-Tsakonas, S.: The suppressor of Hairless participates in Notch receptor signaling. Cell 79:273, 1994.

650. Flowers, D., Wilson, D., Zagouras, P., Myerson, D., Varnum-Finney, B., Artavanis-Tsakonas, A., and Bernstein, I: The expression pattern of Notch 1 and 2 on hematopoietic cells suggests their involvement in coordinating the development of individual lineages. Unpublished work, 1999.

651. Varnum-Finney, B., Purton, L., Gray, G., Mann, R., Artavanis-Tsakonas, S., and Bernstein, I.: The notch ligand, jagged-1, promotes the formation of increased numbers of a primitive hematopoietic precursor cell. Blood 90(suppl. 1):162a, 1997.

652. Li, L., Iwata, M., Deng, Y., Graf, L., Milner, L., Hood, L., and Torok-Storb, B.: Human Jagged1 expressed by marrow stroma is a ligand for Notch1. Blood 90(suppl. 1):480a, 1997.

653. Rathbun, R.K., Faulkner, G.R., Ostroski, M.H., Christianson, T.A., Hughes, G., Jones, G., Cahn, R., Maziarz, R., Royle, G., Keeble, W., Heinrich, M.C., Grompe, M., Tower, P.A., and Bagby, G.C.: Inactivation of the Fanconi anemia group C gene augments interferon-gamma–induced apoptotic responses in hematopoietic cells. Blood 90:974, 1997.

654. Klein, G.: The extracellular matrix of the hematopoietic microenvironment. Experientia 51:914, 1995.

655. Bruno, E., Luikart, S.D., Long, M.W., and Hoffman, R.: Marrow derived heparan sulfate proteoglycan mediates the adhesion of hematopoietic progenitor cells to cytokines. Exp. Hematol. 23:1212, 1995.

656. Ohta, M., Sakai, T., Saga, Y., Aizawa, S., and Saito, M.: Tenascin-C gene-knockout mice, apparently born normally and developed as well, show significant suppression of hematopoietic activity in long term bone marrow cultures. Blood 91:4074, 1998.

657. Peck-Radosavljevic, M., Zacherl, J., Meng, Y.G., Pidlich, J., Lipinski, E., Langle, F., Steininger, R., Muhlbacher, F., and Gangl, A.: Is inadequate thrombopoietin a major cause of thrombocytopenia in cirrhosis of the liver? J. Hepatol. 72:127, 1997.

658. Martin, T.G., III, Somberg, K.A., Meng, Y.G., Cohen, R.L., Heid, C.A., de Sauvage, F.J., and Shuman, M.A.: Thrombopoietin levels in patients with cirrhosis before and after orthotopic liver transplantation. Ann. Intern. Med. 128:285, 1997.

659. Richards, E.M., Alexander, G.J.M., Calne, R.Y., and Baglin, T.P.: Thrombocytopenia following liver transplantation is associated with platelet consumption and thrombin generation. Br. J. Haematol. 98:315, 1997.

660. Van den Berge, H., and Michaux, L.: 5q−, 25 years later: a synopsis. Cancer Genet. Cytogenet. 94:1, 1997.

661. Le Beau, M.M., Westbrook, C.A., Diaz, M.O., Larson, R.A., Rowley, J.D., Gasson, J.C., Golde, D.W., and Sherr, C.J.: Evidence for the involvement of GM-CSF and FMS in the deletion (5q) in myeloid disorders. Science 231:984, 1986.

662. Sutherland, G.R., Baker, E., Callen, D.F., Campbell, H.D., Young, I.G., Sanderson, C.J., Garson, O.M., and Lopez, A.F.: Interleukin-5 is at 5q31 and is deleted in the 5q− syndrome. Blood 71:1150, 1988.

663. Beckingham, I.J., Woodrow, G., Hinwood, M., Rigg, K.M., Morgan, A.G., Burden, R.P., and Broughton-Pipkin, F.: A randomized placebo controlled study of enalapril in the treatment of erythrocytosis after renal transplantation. Nephrol. Dial. Transplant. 10:2316, 1995.

664. Perazella, M., McPhedran, P., Klinger, A., Lorber, M., Levy, E., and Bia, M.J.: Enalapril treatment of post-transplant erythrocytosis: efficacy independent of circulating erythropoietin levels. Am. J. Kidney Dis. 26:495, 1995.

665. Mulhern, J.G., Lipkowitz, G.S., Braden, G.L., Madden, R.L., O'Shea, M.H., Harvilchuck, H., Guarnera, J.M., and Germain, M.J.: Association of post-transplant erythrocytosis and microalbuminuria: response to angiotensin converting enzyme inhibition. Am. J. Nephrol. 15:318, 1995.

666. Oymak, O., Demiroglu, H., Akpolat, T., Erdem, Y., Yasavul, Y., Turgan, C., Caglar, S., Dundar, S., and Kirazli, S.: Increased erythropoietin response to venesection in erythrocytosic renal transplant patients. Int. Urol. Nephrol. 27:223, 1995.

667. Kessler, M.: Erythropoietin and erythropoiesis in renal transplantation. Nephrol. Dial. Transplant. 10(suppl. 6):114, 1995.

668. Marrone, L.F., Di Paolo, S., Logoluso, F., Schena, A., Stallone, G., Giogino, F., and Schena, F.P.: Interference of angiotensin converting enzyme inhibitors on erythropoiesis in kidney transplant patients: role of growth factors and cytokines. Transplantation 64:913, 1997.

669. Mrug, M., Stopka, T., Julian, B.A., Prchal, J.F., and Prchal, J.T.: Angiotensin II stimulates proliferation of normal early erythroid progenitors. J. Clin. Invest. 100:2310, 1997.

670. Owen, W.F., Rothenberg, M.E., Petersen, J., Weller, P.F., Silberstein, D., Sheffer, A.L., Stevens, R.L., Soberman, R.J., and Austen, K.F.: Interleukin 5 and phenotypically altered eosinophils in the blood of patients with the idiopathic hypereosinophilic syndrome. J. Exp. Med. 170:343, 1989.

671. Samoszuk, M., and Nansen, L.: Detection of interleukin 5 messenger RNA in Reed Sternberg cells of Hodgkin's disease with eosinophilia. Blood 75:13, 1990.

672. Di Biagio, E., Sanchez-Borges, M., Desenne, J.J., Suarez-Chacon, R., Somoza, R., and Acquatella, G.: Eosinophilia in Hodgkin's disease: a role for interleukin 5. Int. Arch. Allergy Immunol. 110:244, 1996.

673. Samoszuk, M., Ramzi, E., and Cooper, D.L.: Interleukin 5 mRNA in three T cell lymphomas with eosinophilia. Am. J. Hematol. 42:402, 1993.

674. Butterfield, J.H., Leiferman, K.M., Abrams, J., Silver, J.E., Bower, J., Gonchoroff, N., and Gleich, G.J.: Elevated serum levels of interleukin-5 in patients with the syndrome of episodic angioedema and eosinophilia. Blood 79:688, 1992.

675. Terada, N., Konno, A., Shirotori, K., Fujisawa, T., Atsuta, J., Ichimi, R., Kikuchi, Y., Takaki, S., Takatsu, K., and Togawa, K.: Mechanism of eosinophil infiltration in the patient with subcutaneous angioblastic lymphoid hyperplasia with eosinophilia (Kimura's disease): mechanisms of eosinophil chemotaxis mediated by candida antigen and IL-5. Int. Arch. Allergy Immunol. 104(suppl. 1):18, 1994.

676. Owen, W.F., Jr., Petersen, J., Sheff, D.M., Folkerth, R.D., Anderson, R.J., Corson, J.M., Sheffer, A.L., and Austen, K.F.: Hypodense eosinophils and interleukin 5 activity in the blood of patients with the eosinophilia-myalgia syndrome. Proc. Natl. Acad. Sci. USA 87:8647, 1990.

677. Yamaoka, K.A., Miyasaka, N., Inuo, G., Saito, I., Kolb, J.P., Fujita, K., and Kaashiwazaki, S.: 1,1′-Ethylidenebis (tryptophan) (Peak E) induces functional activation of human eosinophils and interleukin 5 production from T lymphocytes: association of eosinophilia-myalgia syndrome with an L-tryptophan contaminant. J. Clin. Immunol. 14:50, 1994.

678. Yamaguchi, Y., Suda, T., Shiozaki, H., Miura, Y., Hitoshi, Y., Tominaga, A., Takatsu, K., and Kasahara, T.: Role of IL-5 in IL-2–induced eosinophilia in vivo and in vitro expression of IL-5 mRNA by IL-2. J. Immunol. 145:873, 1990.

679. Desreumaux, P., Janin, A., Dubucquoi, S., Copin, M.C., Torpier, G.,

Capron, A., Capron, M., and Prin, L.: Synthesis of interleukin-5 by activated eosinophils in patients with eosinophilic heart diseases. Blood 82:1553, 1993.

680. Rothenberg, M.E., Luster, A.D., Lilly, C.M., Drazen, J.M., and Leder, P.: Constitutive and allergen-induced expression of eotaxin mRNA in the guinea pig lung. J. Exp. Med. 181:1211, 1995.

681. Gonzalo, J.A., Jia, G.Q., Aguirre, V., Friend, D., Coyle, A.J., Jenkins, N.A., Lin, G.S., Katz, H., Lichtman, A., Copeland, N., Kopf, M., and Gutierrez-Ramos, J.C.: Mouse eotaxin expression parallels eosinophil accumulation during lung allergic inflammation but it is not restricted to a Th2-type response. Immunity 4:1, 1996.

682. Rothenberg, M.E., Ownbey, R., Mehlhop, P.D., Loiselle, P.M., van de Rijn, M., Bonventre, J.V., Oettgen, H.C., Leder, P., and Luster, A.D.: Eotaxin triggers eosinophil selective chemotaxis and calcium flux via a distinct receptor and induces pulmonary eosinophilia in the presence of interleukin 5 in mice. Mol. Med. 2:334, 1996.

683. Meeker, T.C., Hardy, D., William, C., Hogan, T., and Abrams, J.: Activation of the interleukin-3 gene by chromosome translocation in acute lymphocytic leukemia with eosinophilia. Blood 76:285, 1990.

684. Wiestner, A., Schlemper, R.J., van der Maas, A.P.C., and Skoda, R.C.: An activating splice donor mutation in the thrombopoietin gene causes hereditary thrombocythemia. Nat. Genet. 18:49, 1998.

685. Kondo, T., Okabe, M., Sanada, M., Suzuki, S., Kurosawa, M., Kobayashi, M., Hosokawa, M., and Asaka, M.: Familial essential thrombocythemia associated with a one bone deletion in the 5' untranslated region of the thrombopoietin gene. Blood 92:1091, 1998.

686. Yan, X.-Q., Lacey, D., Hill, D., Chen, Y., Fletcher, F., Hawley, R.G., and McNiece, I.K.: A model of myelofibrosis and osteosclerosis in mice induced by overexpressing thrombopoietin (mpl ligand): reversal of disease by bone marrow transplant. Blood 88:402, 1996.

687. Straneva, J.E., van Besien, K.W., Derigs, G., and Hoffman, R.: Is interleukin 6 the physiological regulator of thrombopoiesis? Exp. Hematol. 20:47, 1992.

688. Yasumoto, S., Imayama, S., and Hori, Y.: Increased serum level of interleukin-6 in patients with psoriatic arthritis and thrombocytosis. J. Dermatol. 22:718, 1995.

689. Ertenli, I., Haznedaroglu, I.C., Kiraz, S., Celik, I., Calguneri, M., and Kirazhi, S.: Cytokines affecting megakaryocytopoiesis in rheumatoid arthritis with thrombocytosis. Rheumatol. Int. 16:5, 1996.

690. Gastl, G., Plante, M., Finstad, C.L., Wong, G.Y., Frederici, M.H., Bander, N.H., and Rubin, S.C.: High IL-6 levels in ascitic fluid correlate with reactive thrombocytosis in patients with epithelial ovarian cancer. Br. J. Haematol. 83:433, 1993.

691. Blay, J.Y., Favrot, M., Rossi, J.F., and Wijidenes, J.: Role of interleukin-6 in paraneoplastic thrombocytosis. Blood 82:2261, 1993.

692. Tefferi, A., Ho, T.C., Ahmann, G.J., Katzmann, J.A., and Greipp, P.R.: Plasma interleukin-6 and C-reactive protein levels in reactive versus clonal thrombocytosis. Am. J. Med. 97:374, 1994.

693. Tange, T., Hasegawa, Y., Oka, T., Sunaga, S., Higashihara, M., Matsuo, K., Miyazaki, H., Shimosaka, A., and Okano, A.: Establishment and characterization of a new human mesothelioma cell line (T-85) from malignant peritoneal mesothelioma with remarkable thrombocytosis. Pathol. Int. 45:791, 1995.

694. Blay, J.Y., Rossi, J.F., Wijdenes, J., Menetrier-Caux, C., Schemann, S., N'egrier, S., Philip, T., and Favrot, M.: Role of interleukin-6 in the paraneoplastic inflammatory syndrome associated wtih renal-cell carcinoma. Int. J. Cancer 72:424, 1997.

695. Takagi, M., Egawa, T., Motomura, T., Sakuma-Mochizuki, J., Nishimoto, N., Kasayama, S., Hayashi, S., Koga, M., Yoshizaki, K., Yoshioka, T., Okuyama, A., and Kishimoto, T.: Interleukin-6 secreting phaeochromocytoma associated with clinical markers of inflammation. Clin. Endocrinol. 46:507, 1996.

696. Komura-Naito, E., Matsumura, T., Sawada, T., Kato, T., and Tahara, T.: Thrombopoietin in patients with hepatoblastoma. Blood 90:2849, 1997.

697. Furmanski, P., and Johnson, C.S.: Macrophage control of normal and leukemic erythropoiesis. Identification of the macrophage derived erythroid suppressing activity as interleukin-1 and the mediator of its effect as tumor necrosis factor. Blood 75:2328, 1990.

698. Eastgate, J.A., Symons, J.A., Wood, N.C., Grinlinton, F.M., di Giovine, F.S., and Duff, G.W.: Correlation of plasma interleukin 1 levels with disease activity in rheumatoid arthritis. Lancet 2:706, 1988.

699. Jongen-Lavrencic, M., Peeters, H.R., Wognum, A., Vreugdenhil, G., Breedveld, F.C., and Swaak, A.J.: Elevated levels of inflammatory cytokines in bone marrow of patients with rheumatoid arthritis and anemia of chronic disease. J. Rheumatol. 24:1504, 1997.

700. Means, R.T., Jr., and Krantz, S.B.: Inhibition of human erythroid colony-forming units by tumor necrosis factor requires beta interferon. J. Clin. Invest. 91:416, 1993.

701. Means, R.T.: Pathogenesis of the anemia of chronic disease: a cytokine mediated anemia. Stem Cells 13:32, 1995.

702. Gautam, S.C., Pindolia, K.R., Noth, C.J., Janakiraman, N., Xu, Y.X., and Chapman, R.A.: Chemokine gene expression in bone marrow stromal cells: downregulation with sodium salicylate. Blood 86:2541, 1995.

703. Ikejima, T., Ikusawa, S., Ghezzi, P., van der Meer, J.W.M., and Dinarello, C.A.: IL-1 induces TNF in human PBMC in vitro and a circulating TNF-like activity in rabbits. J. Infect. Dis. 162:215, 1990.

704. Delwel, R., van Buitenen, C., Salem, M., Oosterom, R., Touw, I., and Löwenberg, B.: Hemopoietin-1 activity of interleukin-1 (IL-1) on acute myeloid leukemia colony-forming cells (AML-CFU) in vitro: IL-1 induces production of tumor necrosis factor-alpha which synergizes with IL-3 or granulocyte-macrophage colony-stimulating factor. Leukemia 4:557, 1990.

705. Broxmeyer, H.E., Williams, D.E., Lu, L., Cooper, S., Anderson, S.L., Beyer, G.S., Hoffman, R., and Rubin, B.Y.: The suppressive influences of human tumor necrosis factors on bone marrow hematopoietic progenitor cells from normal donors and patients with leukemia: synergism of tumor necrosis factor and interferon-gamma. J. Immunol. 136:4487, 1986.

706. Means, R.T., Dessypris, E.N., and Krantz, S.B.: Inhibition of human erythroid colony-stimulating units by interleukin-1 is mediated by interferon-γ. J. Cell. Physiol. 150:159, 1992.

707. Katevas, P., Andonopoulos, A.P., Kourakli-Symeonidis, A., Lafi, T., Makri, M., and Zoumbos, N.C.: Peripheral blood mononuclear cells from patients with rheumatoid arthritis suppress erythropoiesis in vitro via the production of tumor necrosis factor alpha. Eur. J. Haematol. 53:26, 1994.

708. Jongen-Lavrencic, M., Peeters, H.R., Backx, B., Touw, I.P., Vreugdenhil, G., and Swaak, A.J.: Rh erythropoietin counteracts the inhibition of in vitro erythropoiesis by tumour necrosis factor alpha in patients with rheumatoid arthritis. Rheumatol. Int. 14:109, 1994.

709. Rusten, L.S., and Jacobsen, S.E.: Tumor necrosis factor (TNF)–alpha directly inhibits human erythropoiesis in vitro: role of p55 and p75 TNF receptors. Blood 85:989, 1995.

710. Moldawer, L.L., Marano, M.A., Wei, H., Fong, Y., Silen, M.L., Kuo, G., Manogue, K.R., Vlassara, H., Cohen, H., Cerami, A., and Lowry, S.F.: Cachectin/tumor necrosis factor-alpha alters red blood cell kinetics and induces anemia in vivo. FASEB J. 3:1637, 1989.

711. Taniguchi, S., Dai, C., Price, J.O., and Krantz, S.B.: Interferon γ downregulates stem cell factor and erythropoietin receptors but not insulin-like growth factor-I receptors in human erythroid colony-forming cells. Blood 90:2244, 1997.

712. D'Andrea, A.D., and Grompe, M.: Molecular biology of Fanconi anemia: implications for diagnosis and therapy. Blood 90:1725, 1997.

713. Strathdee, C.A., Gavish, H., Shannon, W.R., and Buchwald, M.: Cloning of cDNAs for Fanconi's anaemia by functional complementation. Nature 356:763, 1992.

714. Lo Ten Foe, J.R., Rooimans, M.A., Bosnoyan-Collins, L., Alon, N., Wijker, M., Parker, L., Lightfoot, J., Carreau, M., Callen, D.F., Savoia, A., Cheng, N.C., van Berkel, C.G., Strunk, M.H., Gille, J.J., Pals, G., Kruyt, F.A., Pronk, J.C., Arwert, F., Buchwald, M., and Joenje, H.: Expression cloning of a cDNA for the major Fanconi anaemia gene, FAA. Nat. Genet. 14:320, 1996.

715. Gibson, R.A., Buchwald, M., Roberts, R.G., and Mathew, C.G.: Characterisation of the exon structure of the Fanconi anaemia group C gene by vectorette PCR. Hum. Mol. Genet. 2:35, 1993.

716. Youssoufian, H., Auerbach, A.D., Verlander, P.C., Steimle, V., and Mach, B.: Identification of cytosolic proteins that bind to the Fanconi anemia complementation group C polypeptide in vitro. J. Biol. Chem. 270:9876, 1995.

717. Kupfer, G.M., Yamashita, T., Asano, S., Suliman, A., and D'Andrea, A.D.: The Fanconi anemia protein, FAC, binds to the cyclin-dependent kinase, cdc2. Blood 90:1047, 1997.

718. Hoshino, T., Youssoufian, H., Wang, J., Devetten, M.P., Iwata, N., Kajigaya, S., Wise, R.J., and Liu, J.M.: The molecular chaperone GRP94 binds to the Fanconi anemia group C protein and regulates its intracellular expression. Blood 91:4379, 1998.

719. Apostolou, S., Whitmore, S.A., Crawford, J., Alon, N., Wijker, M., Parker, L., Lightfoot, J., Carreau, M., Callen, D.F., Savoia, A., Cheng, N.C., van Berkel, C.G.M., Strunk, M.H.P., Gille, J.J.P., Pals, G.,

Kruyt, F.A.E., Pronk, J.C., Arwert, F., Buchwald, M., and Joenje, H.: Positional cloning of the Fanconi anaemia group A gene. Nat. Genet. 14:324, 1996.

720. Pronk, J.C., Gibson, R.A., Savoia, A., Wijker, M., Morgan, N.S., Melchionda, S., Ford, D., Temtamy, S., Ortega, J.J., Jansen, S., Harenga, C., Cohn, R.J., de Ravel, T.J., Roberts, I., Westerveld, A., Easton, D.J., Joenje, H., Mathew, C.G., and Arwert, F.: Localization of the Fanconi anemia complementation group A gene to chromosome 16q24.3. Nat. Genet. 11:338, 1995.

721. Kupfer, G.M., Näf, D., Suliman, A., Pulsipher, M., and D'Andrea, A.D.: The Fanconi anaemia proteins, FAA and FAC, interact to form a nuclear complex. Nat. Genet. 17:487, 1997.

722. Hang, B., Yeung, A.T., and Lambert, M.W.: A damage-recognition protein which binds to DNA containing interstrand cross-links is absent or defective in Fanconi anemia, complementation group A, cells. Nucleic Acids Res. 21:4187, 1993.

723. Chen, M., Tomkins, D.J., Auerbach, W., McKerlie, C., Youssoufian, H., Liu, L., Gan, O., Carreau, M., Auerbach, A., Groves, T., Guidos, C.J., Freeman, M.H., Cross, J., Percy, D.H., Dick, J.E., Joyner, A.L., and Buchwald, M.: Inactivation of FAC in mice produces inducible chromosomal instability and reduced fertility reminiscent of Fanconi anaemia. Nat. Genet. 12:448, 1996.

724. Whitney, M.A., Royle, G., Low, M.J., Kelly, M.A., Axthelm, M.K., Reifsteck, C., Olson, S., Braun, R.E., Heinrich, M.C., Rathbun, R.K., Bagby, G.C., and Grompe, M.: Germ cell defects and hematopoietic hypersensitivity to gamma interferon in mice with a targeted disruption of the Fanconi anemia C gene. Blood 88:49, 1996.

725. Rathbun, K., Christianson, T.A., Faulkner, G.R., Ostroski, M.H., Hughes, G., Heinrich, M.C., Grompe, M., Tower, P.A., and Bagby, G.C.: Molecular pathogenesis of bone marrow failure in Fanconi anemia of the C-type. Exp. Hematol. 25:883, 1997.

726. Young, N.S., and Maciejewski, J.: The pathophysiology of acquired aplastic anemia. N. Engl. J. Med. 336:1365, 1997.

727. Frickhofen, N., Kaltwasser, J.P., Schrezenmeier, H., Raghavachar, A., Vogt, H.G., Herrmann, F., Freund, M., Meusers, P., Salama, A., and Heimpel, H.: Treatment of aplastic anemia with antilymphocyte globulin and methylprednisolone with or without cyclosporine. N. Engl. J. Med. 324:1297, 1991.

728. Colby, C., Stoukides, C.A., and Spitzer, T.R.: Antithymocyte immunoglobulin in severe aplastic anemia and bone marrow transplantation. Ann. Pharmacother. 30:1164, 1996.

729. Champlin, R.E., Feig, S.A., Sparkes, R.S., and Gale, R.P.: Bone marrow transplantation from identical twins in the treatment of aplastic anaemia: implication for the pathogenesis of the disease. Br. J. Haematol. 56:455, 1984.

730. Kagan, W.A., Ascensao, J.A., Pahwa, R.N., Hansen, J.A., Goldstein, G., Valera, E.B., Incefy, G.S., Moore, M.A., and Good, R.A.: Aplastic anemia: presence in human bone marrow of cells that suppress myelopoiesis. Proc. Natl. Acad. Sci. USA 73:2890, 1976.

731. Hoffman, R.A., Zanjani, E.D., Lutton, J.D., Zalusky, R., and Wasserman, L.R.: Suppression of erythroid-colony formation by lymphocytes from patients with aplastic anemia. N. Engl. J. Med. 296:10, 1977.

732. Zoumbos, N.C., Ferris, W.O., Hsu, S.-M., Goodman, S., Griffith, P., Sharrow, S.O., Humphries, R.K., Nienhuis, A.W., and Young, N.: Analysis of lymphocyte subsets in patients with aplastic anaemia. Br. J. Haematol. 58:95, 1984.

733. Ruiz-Arguelles, G.J., Katzmann, J.A., Greipp, P.R., Marin-Lopez, A., Gonzalez-Llaven, J., and Cano-Castellanos, R.: Lymphocyte subsets in patients with aplastic anemia. Am. J. Hematol. 16:267, 1984.

734. Maciejewski, J.P., Hibbs, J.R., Anderson, S., Katevas, P., and Young, N.S.: Bone marrow and peripheral blood lymphocyte phenotype in patients with bone marrow failure. Exp. Hematol. 22:1102, 1994.

735. Bacigalupo, A., Podesta, M., Frassoni, F., Piaggio, G., Van-Lint, M.T., Raffo, M.R., Repetto, M., and Marmont, A.: Generation of CFU-C suppressed T cells in vitro. Br. J. Haematol. 52:421, 1982.

736. Zoumbos, N.C., Djeu, J.Y., and Young, N.S.: Interferon is the suppressor of hematopoiesis generated by stimulated lymphocytes in vitro. J. Immunol. 133:769, 1984.

737. Rigby, W.F., Ball, E.D., Guyre, P.M., and Fanger, M.W.: The effects of recombinant-DNA–derived interferons on the growth of myeloid progenitor cells. Blood 65:858, 1985.

738. Maciejewski, J.P., Selleri, C., Sato, T., Cho, H.J., Keefer, L.K., Nathan, C.F., and Young, N.S.: Nitric oxide suppression of human hematopoiesis in vitro: contribution to inhibitory action of interferon-γ and tumor necrosis factor-α. J. Clin. Invest. 96:1085, 1996.

739. Zoumbos, N., Gascon, P., Djeu, J., and Young, N.S.: Interferon is a mediator of hematopoietic suppression in aplastic anemia in vitro and possibly in vivo. Proc. Natl. Acad. Sci. USA 82:188, 1985.

740. Nisticò, A., and Young, N.S.: Gamma-interferon gene expression in the bone marrow of patients with aplastic anemia. Ann. Intern. Med. 120:463, 1994.

741. Selleri, C., Maciejewski, J.P., Sato, T., and Young, N.S.: Interferon-gamma constitutively expressed in the stromal microenvironment of human marrow cultures mediates potent hematopoietic inhibition. Blood 87:4149, 1996.

742. Sporn, M.B., and Todaro, G.J.: Autocrine secretion and malignant transformation of cells. N. Engl. J. Med. 303:878, 1980.

743. Sporn, M.B., and Roberts, A.B.: Autocrine growth factors and cancer. Nature 313:745, 1985.

744. De Larco, J.E., and Todaro, G.J.: Growth factors from murine sarcoma virus–transformed cells. Proc. Natl. Acad. Sci. USA 75:4001, 1978.

745. Ozanne, B., Fulton, R.J., and Kaplan, P.L.: Kirsten murine sarcoma virus transformed cell lines and a spontaneously transformed rat cell-line produce transforming factors. J. Cell. Physiol. 105:163, 1980.

746. Doolittle, R.F., Hunkapiller, M.W., Hood, L.E., Devare, S.G., Robbins, K.C., Aaronson, S.A., and Antoniades, H.N.: Simian sarcoma virus onc gene, v-sis, is derived from the gene (or genes) encoding a platelet-derived growth factor. Science 221:275, 1983.

747. Waterfield, M.D., Scrace, G.T., Whittle, N., Stroobant, P., Johnsson, A., Wasteson, A., Westermark, B., Heldin, C.H., Huang, J.S., and Deuel, T.F.: Platelet-derived growth factor is structurally related to the putative transforming protein p28^{cis} of simian sarcoma virus. Nature 304:35, 1983.

748. Garrett, J.S., Coughlin, S.R., Niman, H.L., Tremble, P.M., Giles, G.M., and Willimas, L.T.: Blockade of autocrine stimulation in simian sarcoma virus–transformed cells reverses down-regulation of platelet-derived growth factor receptors. Proc. Natl. Acad. Sci. USA 81:7466, 1984.

749. Hapel, A.J., Van de Woude, G., Campbell, H.D., Young, I.G., and Robins, T.: Generation of an autocrine leukemia using a retroviral expression vector carrying the interleukin-3 gene. Lymphokine Res. 5:249, 1986.

750. Dunbar, C.E., Browder, T.M., Abrams, J.S., and Nienhuis, A.W.: COOH-terminal–modified interleukin-3 is retained intracellularly and stimulates autocrine growth. Science 245:1493, 1989.

751. Rogers, S.Y., Bradbury, D., Kozlowski, R., and Russell, N.H.: Evidence for internal autocrine regulation of growth in acute myeloblastic leukemia cells. Exp. Hematol. 22:593, 1994.

752. Villeval, J.L., Mitjavila, M.-T., Dusanter-Fourte, I., Wendling, F., Mayeux, P., and Vainchenker, W.: Autocrine stimulation by erythropoietin (Epo) requires Epo secretion. Blood 84:2649, 1994.

753. Falcinelli, F., Onorato, M., Falzetti, F., Ciurnelli, R., Gabert, J., Mannoni, P., Martelli, M.F., and Tabilio, A.: Activation of the granulocyte-monocyte colony stimulating factor gene in acute myeloid leukemia cells is not related to gene rearrangement. Leuk. Res. 15:957, 1991.

754. Ernst, T.J., Ritchie, A.R., O'Rourke, R., and Griffin, J.D.: Colony-stimulating factor gene expression in human acute myeloblastic leukemia cells is post-transcriptionally regulated. Leukemia 3:620, 1989.

755. Smith, F.O., Raskind, W.H., Fialkow, P.J., and Bernstein, I.D.: Cellular biology of acute myelogenous leukemia. J. Pediatr. Hematol. Oncol. 17:113, 1995.

756. Wolin, M.J., and Gale, R.P.: Therapy of acute myelogenous leukemia: understanding the question, understanding the answer. Leuk. Res. 21:3, 1997.

757. Preisler, H.D., Bi, S., Venugopal, P., and Raza, A.: Cytokines, molecular biological abnormalities, and acute myelogenous leukemia. Leuk. Res. 21:299, 1997.

758. Hoang, T., Haman, A., Goncalves, O., Letendre, F., Mathieu, M., Wong, G.G., and Clark, S.C.: Interleukin 1 enhances growth factor-dependent proliferation of the clonogenic cells in acute myeloblastic leukemia and normal human primitive hemopoietic precursors. J. Exp. Med. 168:463, 1988.

759. Delwel, R., Salem, M., Dorssers, I., Wagemaker, G., Clark, S., and Löwenberg, B.: Growth regulation of human acute myeloid leukemia: effects of five recombinant hematopoietic factors in a serum-free culture system. Blood 72:1944, 1988.

760. Pebusque, M.J., Lopez, M., Torres, H., Carotti, A., Guilbert, I., and Mannom, P.: Growth response of human myeloid leukemia cells to colony stimulating factors. Exp. Hematol. 16:360, 1988.

761. Ikeda, H., Kanakura, Y., Tamaki, T., Kuriu, A., Kitayama, H., Ishi-

kawa, J., Kanayama, Y., Yonezawa, T., Tarui, S., and Griffin, J.D.: Expression and functional role of the proto-oncogene c-kit in acute myeloblastic leukemia cells. Blood 78:2962, 1991.

762. Matsumura, I., Kanakura, Y., Ideda, H., Ishikawa, J., Yoshida, H., Nishiura, T., Tahara, T., Kato, T., Miyazaki, H., and Matsuzawa, Y.: Coexpression of thrombopoietin and c-mpl genes in human acute myeloblastic leukemia cells. Leukemia 10:91, 1996.

763. Li, Y., Hetet, G., Kiladjian, J.J., Gardin, C., Grandchamp, B., and Briere, J.: Proto-oncogene cmpl is involved in spontaneous mega-karyocytopoiesis in myeloproliferative disorders. Br. J. Haematol. 92:60, 1996.

764. Asano, Y., Harada, M., Okamura, S., Shibuya, T., and Niho, Y.: Growth of clonogenic myeloblastic leukemic cells in the presence of human recombinant erythropoietin in addition to various human recombinant hemopoietic growth factors. Blood 72:1682, 1988.

765. Hoang, T., Haman, A., Goncalves, O., Wong, G.G., and Clark, S.C.: Interleukin-6 enhances growth factor–dependent proliferation of the blast cells of acute myeloblastic leukemia. Blood 72:823, 1988.

766. Griffin, J.D., and Lowenberg, B.: Clonogenic cells in acute myeloblastic leukemia. Blood 68:1185, 1986.

767. Young, D.C., Wagner, K., and Griffin, J.D.: Constitutive expression of the granulocyte-macrophage colony-stimulating factor gene in acute myeloblastic leukemia. J. Clin. Invest. 79:100, 1987.

768. Demetri, G.D., and Griffin, J.D.: Hemopoietins and leukemia. Hematol. Oncol. Clin. North Am. 3:535, 1989.

769. Löwenberg, B., and Touw, I.P.: Hematopoietic growth factors and their receptors in acute leukemia. Blood 81:281, 1993.

770. Kaufman, D., Baer, M., Gao, X.Z., Wang, Z., and Preisler, H.D.: Enhanced expression of granulocyte-macrophage colony stimulating factor gene in acute myeloblastic leukemia cells following in vitro blast cell enrichment. Blood 72:1329, 1988.

771. Cheng, G.Y.M., Kelleher, C.A., Miyauchi, J., Wang, C., Wong, G., Clark, S.C., McCulloch, E.A., and Minden, M.D.: Structure and expression genes of GM-CSF and G-CSF in blast cells from patients with acute myeloblastic leukemia. Blood 71:35, 1988.

772. Kobayashi, S., Teramura, M., Sugawara, I., Oshimi, K., and Mizoguchi, H.: Interleukin-11 acts as an autocrine growth factor for human megakaryoblastic cell lines. Blood 81:889, 1993.

773. Sugiyama, H., Inoue, K., Ogawa, H., Yamagami, T., Soma, T., Miyake, S., Hirata, M., and Kishimoto, T.: The expression of IL-6 and its related genes in acute leukemia. Leuk. Lymphoma 21:49, 1996.

774. Asano, Y., Yokoyama, T., Shibata, S., Kobayashi, S., Shimoda, K., Nakashima, H., Okamura, S., and Niho, Y.: Effect of the chimeric soluble granulocyte colony-stimulating factor receptor on the proliferation of leukemic blast cells from patients with acute myeloblastic leukemia. Cancer Res. 57:3395, 1997.

775. Oster, W., Cicco, N.A., Klein, H., Hirano, T., Kishimoto, T., Lindemann, A., Mertelsmann, R.H., and Herrmann, F.: Participation of cytokines interleukin-6, tumour necrosis factor-alpha and interleukin-1-beta secreted by acute myelogenous leukemia blasts in autocrine and paracrine leukemia growth control. J. Clin. Invest. 84:451, 1989.

776. Griffin, J.D., Rambaldi, A., Vellenga, E., Young, D.C., Ostapovicz, D., and Cannistra, S.A.: Secretion of interleukin-1 by acute myeloblastic leukemia cells in vitro induces endothelial cells to secrete colony stimulating factors. Blood 70:1218, 1987.

777. Mileno, M.D., Magolis, N.H., Clark, B.D., Dinarello, C.A., Burke, J.F., and Gelfand, J.A.: Coagulation of whole blood stimulates interleukin-1 gene expression: absence of gene transcripts in anticoagulated blood. J. Infect. Dis. 172:308, 1995.

778. Rambaldi, A., Torcia, M., Bettoni, S., Vannier, E., Barbui, T., Shaw, A.R., Dinarello, C.A., and Cozzolino, F.: Modulation of cell proliferation and cytokine production in acute myeloblastic leukemia by interleukin-1 receptor antagonist and lack of its expression by leukemic cells. Blood 78:3248, 1991.

779. Kurzrock, R., Kantarjian, H., Wetzler, M., Estrov, Z., Estey, E., Troutman-Worden, K., Gutterman, J.U., and Talpaz, M.: Ubiquitous expression of cytokines in diverse leukemias of lymphoid and myeloid lineage. Exp. Hematol. 21:80, 1993.

780. Bagby, G.C., Jr., McCall, E., Bergstrom, K.A., and Burger, D.: A monokine regulates colony-stimulating activity production by vascular endothelial cells. Blood 62:663, 1983.

781. Broudy, V.C., Kaushansky, K., Harlan, J.M., and Adamson, J.W.: Interleukin 1 stimulates human endothelial cells to produce granulocyte-macrophage colony-stimulating factor and granulocyte colony-stimulating factor. J. Immunol. 139:464, 1987.

782. Delwel, R., van Buitenen, C., Salem, S., Bot, F., Gillis, S., Kaushansky, K., Altrock, B., and Löwenberg, B.: Interleukin-1 stimulates proliferation of acute myeloblastic leukemia cells by induction of granulocyte-macrophage colony-stimulating factor release. Blood 74:586, 1989.

783. Bradbury, D., Rogers, S., Kozlowski, R., Bowen, G., Reilly, I.A.G., and Russell, N.H.: Interleukin-1 is one factor which regulates the autocrine production of GM-CSF by blast cells of acute myeloblastic leukaemia. Br. J. Haematol. 76:488, 1990.

784. Estrov, Z., Kurzrock, R., Estey, E., Wetzler, M., Ferrajoli, A., Harris, D., Blake, M., Gutterman, J.U., and Talpaz, M.: Inhibition of acute myelogenous leukemia blast proliferation by interleukin-1 (IL-1) receptor antagonist and soluble IL-1 receptors. Blood 79:1938, 1992.

785. Estrov, Z., and Talpaz, M.: Role of interleukin-1 beta converting enzyme (ICE) in acute myelogenous leukemia cell proliferation and programmed cell death. Leuk. Lymphoma 24:379, 1997.

786. Haran-Ghera, N., Krautghamer, R., Lapidot, T., Peland, A., Dominguez, M.G., and Stanley, E.R.: Increased circulating colony-stimulating factor-1 (CSF-1) in SJL/J mice with radiation-induced acute myeloid leukemia (AML) is associated with autocrine regulation of AML cells by CSF-1. Blood 89:2537, 1997.

787. Paul, C.C., Mahrer, S., McMannama, K., and Baumann, M.A.: Autocrine activation of the IL3/GM-CSF/IL-5 signaling pathway in leukemic cells. Am. J. Hematol. 56:79, 1997.

788. Bradbury, D.A., Zhu, Y.M., and Russell, N.H.: Bcl-2 expression in acute myeloblastic leukemia: relationship with autonomous growth and CD34 antigen expression. Leuk. Lymphoma 24:221, 1997.

789. Schrader, J.W., and Crapper, R.M.: Autogenous production of a hemopoietic growth factor, persisting-cell-stimulating factor, as a mechanism for transformation of bone marrow–derived cells. Proc. Natl. Acad. Sci. USA 80:6892, 1983.

790. Lang, R.A., Metcalf, D., Gough, N.M., Dunn, A.R., and Gonda, T.J.: Expression of a hemopoietic growth factor cDNA in a factor-dependent cell line results in autonomous growth and tumorigenicity. Cell 43:531, 1985.

791. Jirik, F.R., Burstein, S.A., Treger, L., and Sorge, J.A.: Transfection of a factor-dependent cell line with the murine interleukin-3 (IL-3) cDNA results in autonomous growth and tumorigenesis. Leuk. Res. 11:1127, 1987.

792. Roussel, M.F., Rettenmier, C.W., and Sherr, C.J.: Introduction of a human colony stimulating factor-1 gene into a mouse macrophage cell line induces CSF-1 independence but not tumorigenicity. Blood 71:1218, 1988.

793. Laker, C., Stocking, C., Bergholz, U., Hess, N., DeLamarter, J.F., and Ostertag, W.: Autocrine stimulation after transfer of the granulocyte/macrophage colony-stimulating factor gene and autonomous growth are distinct but interdependent steps in the oncogenic pathway. Proc. Natl. Acad. Sci. USA 84:8458, 1987.

794. Johnson, G.R., Gonda, T.J., Metcalf, D., Hiriharan, I.K., and Cory, S.: A lethal myeloproliferative syndrome in mice transplanted with bone marrow cells infected with a retrovirus expressing GM-CSF. EMBO J. 8:441, 1988.

795. Chang, J.M., Metcalf, D., Lang, R.A., Gonda, R.J., and Johnson, G.R.: Nonneoplastic hematopoietic myeloproliferative syndrome induced by dysregulated multi-CSF (IL-3 expression). Blood 73:1487, 1989.

796. Wong, P.M.C., Chung, S., Dunbar, C.E., Bodine, D.M., Ruscetti, S.R., and Nienhuis, A.W.: Retrovirus mediated transfer and expression of the IL-3 gene in mouse hematopoietic cells results in a myeloproliferative disorder. Mol. Cell. Biol. 9:797, 1989.

797. Moreau-Gachelin, F., Wendling, F., Molina, T., Denis, N., Titeux, M., Grimber, G., Briand, P., Vainchenker, W., and Tavitian, A.: Spi-1/PU.1 transgenic mice develop multistep erythroleukemias. Mol. Cell. Biol. 16:2453, 1996.

798. Metcalf, D.: The Charlotte Friend Memorial Lecture. The role of hematopoietic growth factors in the development and suppression of myeloid leukemias. Leukemia 11:1599, 1997.

799. Leslie, K.B., Lee, F., and Schrader, J.W.: Intracisternal A-type particle-mediated activations of cytokine genes in a murine myelomonocytic leukemia: generation of functional cytokine mRNAs by retroviral splicing events. Mol. Cell. Biol. 11:5562, 1991.

800. Hunter, A.E., Rogers, S.Y., Roberts, I.A., Barrett, A.J., and Russell, N.: Autonomous growth of blast cells is associated with reduced survival in acute myeloblastic leukemia. Blood 82:899, 1993.

801. Hallek, M., Danhauser-Riedl, S., Herbst, R., Warmuth, M., Winkler, A., Kolb, H.J., Druker, B., Griffin, J.D., Emmerich, B., and Ullrich,

A.: Interaction of the receptor tyrosine kinase p145c-kit with the p210bcr/abl kinase in myeloid cells. Br. J. Haematol. 94:5, 1996.

802. Sirard, C., Laneuville, P., and Dick, J.E.: Expression of bcr-abl abrogates factor-dependent growth of human hematopoietic M07E cells by an autocrine mechanism. Blood 83:1575, 1994.

803. Specchia, G., Liso, V., Capalbo, S., Fazioli, F., Bettoni, S., Bassan, R., Vicero, P., Barbui, T., and Rambaldi, A.: Constitutive expression of IL1 beta, M-CSF and c-fms during myeloid blastic phase of chronic myelogenous leukemia. Br. J. Haematol. 80:310, 1992.

804. Bagby, G.C., Jr., Dinarello, C.A., Neerhout, R.C., Ridgway, D., and McCall, E.: Interleukin-1 dependent paracrine granulopoiesis in chronic granulocytic leukemia of the juvenile type. J. Clin. Invest. 82:1430, 1988.

805. Estrov, Z., Kurzrock, R., Wetzler, M., Kantarjian, H., Blake, M., Harris, D., Gutterman, J.U., and Talpaz, M.: Suppression of chronic myelogenous leukemia colony growth by IL-1 receptor antagonist and soluble IL-1 receptors. A novel application for inhibitors of IL-1 activity. Blood 78:1476, 1991.

806. Estrov, Z., Grunberger, T., Chan, H.S.L., and Freeman, M.H.: Juvenile chronic myelogenous leukemia: characterization of the disease using cell cultures. Blood 67:1382, 1986.

807. Iversen, P.O., Rodwell, R.L., Pitcher, L., Taylor, K.M., and Lopez, A.F.: Inhibition of proliferation and induction of apoptosis in juvenile myelomonocytic leukemic cells by the granulocyte-macrophage colony-stimulating factor analogue E21R. Blood 88:2634, 1996.

808. Everson, M.P., Brown, C.B., and Lilly, M.B.: Interleukin-6 and granulocyte-macrophage colony-stimulating factor are candidate growth factors for chronic myelomonocytic leukemia cells. Blood 74:1472, 1989.

809. Geissler, K., Ohler, L., Fodinger, M., Virgolini, I., Leimer, M., Kabrna, E., Kollars, M., Skoupy, S., Bohle, B., Rogy, M., and Lechner, K.: Interleukin 10 inhibits growth and granulocyte/macrophage colony-stimulating factor production in chronic myelomonocytic leukemia cells. J. Exp. Med. 184:1377, 1996.

810. Freedman, M.H., Cohen, A., Grunberger, T., Bunin, N., Luddy, R.E., Saunders, E.F., Shahidi, N., Lau, A., and Estrov, Z.: Central role of tumour necrosis factor, GM-CSF, and interleukin 1 in the pathogenesis of juvenile chronic myelogenous leukaemia. J. Haematol. 80:40, 1992.

811. Yoshimura, A., Longmore, G., and Lodish, H.F.: Point mutation in the exoplasmic domain of the erythropoietin receptor resulting in hormone-independent activation and tumorigenicity. Nature 348:647, 1990.

812. Wendling, F., Varlet, P., Charon, M., and Tambourin, P.: A retrovirus complex inducing an acute myeloproliferative leukemia disorder in mice. Virology 149:242, 1986.

813. Souyri, M., Vigon, I., Penciolelli, J.F., Tambourin, P., and Wendling, F.: A putative truncated cytokine receptor gene transduced by the myeloproliferative leukemia virus immortalizes hematopoietic progenitors. Cell 63:1137, 1990.

814. Onishi, M., Mui, A.L.F., Morikawa, Y., Cho, L., Kinoshita, S., Nolan, G.P., Gorman, D.M., Miyajima, A., and Kitamura, T.: Identification of an oncogenic form of the thrombopoietin receptor using retrovirus-mediated gene transfer. Blood 88:1399, 1996.

815. D'Andrea, A.D., Rayner, J., Moretti, P., Lopez, A., Goodall, G.J., Gonda, T.J., and Vadas, M.A.: A mutation of the common receptor subunit for interleukin 3 (IL-3), granulocyte-macrophage colony-stimulating factor, and IL-5 that leads to ligand independence and tumorigenicity. Blood 83:2802, 1994.

816. Furitsu, T., Tsujimura, T., Tono, T., Ideda, H., Kitayama, H., Koshimizu, U., Sugahara, H., Butterfield, J.H., Ashman, L.K., Kanayama, Y., Matsuzawa, Y., Kitamura, Y., Kanakura, Y.: Identification of mutations in the coding sequence of the proto-oncogene c-kit in human mast cell leukemia cell line causing ligand-independent activation of c-kit product. J. Clin. Invest. 92:1736, 1993.

817. Tsujimura, T., Furitsu, T., Morimoto, M., Isozaki, K., Nomura, S., Matsuzawa, Y., Kitamura, Y., and Kanakura, Y.: Ligand-independent activation of c-kit receptor tyrosine kinase in a murine mastocytoma cell line P-815 generated by a point mutation. Blood 83:2619, 1994.

818. Kitayama, H., Tsujimura, T., Matsumura, I., Oritani, K., Ikeda, H., Ishikawa, J., Okabe, M., Suzuki, M., Yamamura, K.I., Matsuzawa, Y., Kitamura, Y., and Kanakura, Y.: Neoplastic transformation of normal hematopoietic cells by constitutively activating mutations of c-kit receptor tyrosine kinase. Blood 88:995, 1996.

819. Roussel, M.F., Dull, T.J., Rettenmier, C.W., Ralph, P., Ullrich, A., and Sherr, C.J.: Transforming potential of the c-fms proto-oncogene (CSF-1 receptor). Nature 325:549, 1987.

820. Roussel, M.F., Downing, J.R., and Sherr, C.J.: Transforming activities of human CSF-1 receptors with different point mutations at codon 301 in their extracellular domains. Oncogene 5:25, 1990.

821. Longmore, G.: Erythropoietin receptor mutations and Olympic glory. Nat. Genet. 4:108, 1993.

822. de la Chapelle, A., Traskelin, A.L., and Juvonen, E.: Truncated erythropoietin receptor causes dominantly inherited benign human erythrocytosis. Proc. Natl. Acad. Sci. USA 90:4495, 1993.

823. Sokol, L., Luhovy, M., Guan, Y., Prchal, J.F., Semenza, G.L., Prchal, J.T.: Primary familial polycythemia: a frameshift mutation in the erythropoietin receptor gene and increased sensitivity of erythroid progenitors to erythropoietin. Blood 86:15, 1995.

824. Kralovics, R., Indrak, K., Stopka, T., Berman, B.W., Prchal, J.F., and Prchal, J.T.: Two new EPO receptor mutations: truncated EPO receptor mutations are most commonly associated with primary familial and congenital polycythemias. Blood 90:2057, 1997.

825. Adamson, J.W., Fialkow, P.J., Murphy, S., Prchal, J.F., and Steinmann, L.: Polycythemia vera. Stem-cell and probably clonal origin of disease. N. Engl. J. Med. 295:913, 1976.

826. Hodges, E., Howell, W.M., Boyd, Y., and Smith, J.L.: Variable X-chromosome DNA methylation patterns detected with probe M27 beta in a series of lymphoid and myeloid malignancies. Br. J. Haematol. 77:315, 1991.

827. Prchal, J.F., and Axelrad, A.A.: Bone marrow responses in polycythemia vera. N. Engl. J. Med. 290:1382, 1974.

828. Lemoine, F., Najman, A., Baillou, C., Stachowiak, J., Boffa, G., Aegerter, P., Douay, L., Laporte, J.P., Gorin, N.C., and Duhamel, G.: A prospective study of the value of bone marrow erythroid progenitor cultures in polycythemia. Blood 68:995, 1986.

829. Zanjani, E.D., Lutton, J.D., Hoffman, R., and Wasserman, L.R.: Erythroid colony formation by polycythemia vera bone marrow in vitro: dependence on erythropoietin. J. Clin. Invest. 59:841, 1977.

830. Casadevall, N., Vainchenker, W., Lacombe, C., Vinci, G., Chapman, J., Breton-Gorius, J., and Varet, B.: Erythroid progenitors in polycythemia vera: demonstration of their hypersensitivity to erythropoietin using serum free cultures. Blood 59:447, 1982.

831. Lamperi, S., Carozzi, S., and Icardi, A.: Polycythaemia is erythropoietin-independent after renal transplantation. Proc. Eur. Dial. Transplant. Assoc. Eur. Ren. Assoc. 21:928, 1985.

832. Means, R.T., Jr., Krantz, S.B., Sawyer, S.T., and Gilbert, H.S.: Erythropoietin receptors in polycythemia vera. J. Clin. Invest. 84:1340, 1989.

833. Heimpel, H.: The present state of pathophysiology and therapeutic trials in polycythemia vera. Int. J. Hematol. 64:153, 1996.

834. Emanuel, P.D., Eaves, C.J., Broudy, V.C., Papayannopoulou, T., Moore, M.R., D'Andrea, A.D., Prchal, J.F., Eaves, A.C., and Prchal, J.T.: Familial and congenital polycythemia in three unrelated families. Blood 79:3019, 1992.

835. Hess, G., Rose, P., Gamm, H., Papadileris, S., Huber, C., and Seliger, B.: Molecular analysis of the erythropoietin receptor system in patients with polycythaemia vera. Br. J. Haematol. 88:794, 1994.

836. Mittelman, M., Gardyn, J., Carmel, M., Malovani, H., Barak, Y., and Nir, U.: Analysis of the erythropoietin receptor gene in patients with myeloproliferative and myelodysplastic syndromes. Leuk. Res. 20:459, 1996.

837. Dai, C.H., Krantz, S.B., and Zsebo, K.M.: Human burst forming units–erythroid need direct interaction with stem cell factor for further development. Blood 78:2493, 1991.

838. Kobayashi, S., Teramura, M., Hoshino, S., Motoji, T., Oshimi, K., and Mizoguchi, H.: Circulating megakaryocyte progenitors in myeloproliferative disorders are hypersensitive to interleukin-3. Br. J. Haematol. 83:539, 1993.

839. Dai, C.H., Krantz, S.B., Dessypris, E.N., Means, R.T., Jr., Horn, S.T., and Gilbert, H.S.: Hypersensitivity of bone marrow erythroid, granulocyte-macrophage, and megakaryocyte progenitor cells to interleukin-3 and granulocyte-macrophage colony-stimulating factor. Blood 80:891, 1992.

840. Dai, C.H., Krantz, S.B., Koury, S.T., and Kollar, K.: Polycythaemia vera. Specific binding of stem cell factor to normal and polycythaemia vera highly purified erythroid progenitor cells. Br. J. Haematol. 88:497, 1994.

841. Correa, P.N., Eskinazi, D., Axelrad, A.A.: Circulating erythroid progenitors in polycythemia vera are hypersensitive to insulin-like growth factor-1 in vitro: studies in an improved serum-free medium. Blood 83:99, 1994.

842. Mirza, A.M., Correa, P.N., and Axelrad, A.A.: Increased basal and induced tyrosine phosphorylation of the insulin-like growth factor I receptor subunit in circulating mononuclear cells of patients with polycythemia vera. Blood 86:877, 1995.

843. Dai, C., Krantz, S.B., and Sawyer, S.T.: Enhanced proliferation and phosphorylation due to vanadate are diminished in polycythemia vera erythroid progenitor cells: a possible defect of phosphatase activity in polycythemia vera. Blood 89:3574, 1997.

844. Sui, X., Krantz, S.B., and Zhao, Z.: Identification of increased protein tyrosine phosphatase activity in polycythemia vera erythroid progenitor cells. Blood 90:651, 1997.

845. Chiba, S., Takahashi, T., Takeshita, K., Minowada, J., Yazaki, Y., Ruddle, F.H., and Hirai, H.: Selective expression of mRNA coding for the truncated form of erythropoietin receptor in hematopoietic cells and its decrease in patients with polycythemia vera. Blood 90:97, 1997.

846. Freedman, M.H.: Safety of long term administration of granulocyte colony stimulating factor for severe congenital neutropenia. Curr. Opin. Hematol. 4:217, 1997.

847. Dong, F., Hoefsloot, L.H., Schelen, A.M., Broeders, C.A., Meijer, Y., Veerman, A.J., Touw, I.P., and Löwenberg, B.: Identification of a nonsense mutation in the granulocyte colony stimulating factor receptor in severe congenital neutropenia. Proc. Natl. Acad. Sci. USA 91:4480, 1994.

848. Carapeti, M., Soede-Bobok, A., Hockhaus, A., Sill, H., Touw, I.P., and Goldman, J.M.: Rarity of dominant negative mutations of the G-CSF receptor in patients with blast crisis of CML or de novo acute leukemia. Leukemia 11:1005, 1997.

849. Tidow, N., and Welte, K.: Advances in understanding postreceptor signaling in response to granulocyte colony-stimulating factor. Curr. Opin. Hematol. 4:171, 1997.

850. Dong, F., Brynes, R.K., Tidow, N., Welte, K., Löwenberg, B., and Touw, I.P.: Mutations in the gene for the G-CSF receptor in patients with acute myeloid leukemia preceded by severe congenital neutropenia. N. Engl. J. Med. 333:487, 1995.

851. Avalos, B.R.: Molecular analysis of the granulocyte colony-stimulating factor receptor. Blood 88:761, 1996.

852. Hunter, M., and Avalos, B.: A dileucine motif in the G-CSFR may mediate the dominant negative phenotype in SCN/AML. Blood 90(suppl. 1):443a, 1997.

853. McLemore, M.L., Poursine-Laurent, J., and Link, D.C.: Increased granulocyte colony-stimulating factor responsiveness but normal resting granulopoiesis in mice carrying a targeted granulocyte colony-stimulating factor receptor mutation derived from a patient with severe congenital neutropenia. J. Clin. Invest. 102:483, 1998.

854. Bernstein, A., Chabot, B., Dubreuil, P., Reith, A., Nocka, K., Majumder, S., Ray, P., and Besmer, P.: The mouse W/kit locus. Ciba Found. Symp. 148:158, 1990.

855. Spritz, R.A., Holmes, S.A., Ramesar, R., Greenberg, J., Curtis, D., and Beighton, P.: Mutations of the kit (mast/stem cell growth factor receptor) proto-oncogene account for a continuous range of phenotypes in human piebaldism. Am. J. Hum. Genet. 51:1058, 1992.

856. Herbst, R., Munemitsu, S., and Ullrich, A.: Oncogenic activation of v-kit involves deletion of a putative tyrosine-substrate interaction site. Oncogene 10:369, 1995.

857. Nagata, H., Worobec, A.S., Oh, C.K., Chowdhury, B.A., Tannenbaum, S., Suzuki, Y., and Metcalfe, D.D.: Identification of a point mutation in the catalytic domain of the protooncogene c-kit in peripheral blood mononuclear cells of patients who have mastocytosis with an associated hematologic disorder. Proc. Natl. Acad. Sci. USA 92:10560, 1995.

858. Nagata, H., Okata, T., Worobec, A.S., Semere, T., and Metcalfe, D.D.: c-kit mutation in a population of patients with mastocytosis. Int. Arch. Allergy Immunol. 113:184, 1997.

859. Longley, B.J., Tyrrell, L., Lu, S.Z., Ma, Y.S., Langley, K., Ding, T.G., Duffy, T., Jacobs, P., Tang, L.H., and Modlin, I.: Somatic c-KIT activating mutation in urticaria pigmentosa and aggressive mastocytosis: establishment of clonality in a human mast cell neoplasm. Nat. Genet. 12:312, 1996.

860. Pignon, J.M., Giraudier, S., Duquesnoy, P., Jouault, H., Imbert, M., Vainchenker, W., Vernant, J.P., and Tulliez, M.: A new c-kit mutation in a case of aggressive mast cell disease. Br. J. Haematol. 96:374, 1997.

861. Nakao, M., Yokota, S., Iwai, T., Kaneko, H., Horiike, S., Kashima, K., Sonoda, Y., Fujimoto, T., and Misawa, S.: Internal tandem duplica-tion of the flt3 gene found in acute myeloid leukemia. Leukemia 10:1911, 1996.

862. Horiike, S., Yokoto, S., Nakao, M., Iwai, T., Sasai, Y., Kaneko, H., Taniwaki, M., Kashima, K., Fujii, H., Abe, T., and Misawa, S.: Tandem duplications of the FLT3 receptor gene are associated with leukemic transformation of myelodysplasia. Leukemia 11:1442, 1997.

863. Ridge, S.A., Worwood, M., Oscier, D., Jacobs, A., and Padua, R.A.: FMS mutations in myelodysplastic leukemic and normal subjects. Proc. Natl. Acad. Sci. USA 87:1377, 1990.

864. Tobal, K., Pagliuca, A., Bhatt, B., Baily, N., Layton, D.M., and Mufti, G.J.: Mutation of the human fms gene (M-CSF receptor) in myelodysplastic syndromes and acute myeloid leukemia. Leukemia 4:486, 1990.

865. Muraoka, K., Ishii, E., Tsuji, K., Yamamoto, S., Yamaguchi, H., Hara, T., Koga, H., Nakahata, T., and Miyazaki, S.: Defective response to thrombopoietin and impaired expression of cmpl mRNA of bone marrow cells in congenital amegakaryocytic thrombocytopenia. Br. J. Haematol. 96:287, 1997.

866. Yoshida, H., Hayashi, S.I., Kunisada, T., Ogawa, M., Nishikawa, S., Okamura, H., Sudo, T., and Shultz, L.D.: The murine mutation osteopetrosis is in the coding region of the macrophage colony-stimulating factor gene. Nature 345:442, 1990.

867. Mach, N., Lantz, C.S., Galli, S.J., Reznikoff, G., Mihm, M., Small, C., Granstein, R., Beissert, S., Sadelain, M., Mulligan, R.C., and Dranoff, G.: Involvement of interleukin-3 in delayed-type hypersensitivity. Blood 91:778, 1998.

868. Gurney, A.L., Carver-Moore, K., de Sauvage, F.J., and Moore, M.W.: Thrombocytopenia in c-mpl–deficient mice. Science 265:1445, 1994.

869. Powell, J.S., Berkener, K.L., Lebo, R.V., and Adamson, J.W.: Human erythropoietin gene: high level expression in stably transfected mammalian cells and chromosome localization. Proc. Natl. Acad. Sci. USA 83:6465, 1986.

870. Elliott, S., Lorenzini, T., Chang, D., Barzilay, J., Delorme, E., Giffin, J., and Hesterberg, L.: Fine-structure epitope mapping of antierythropoietin monoclonal antibodies reveals a model of recombinant human erythropoietin structure. Blood 87:2702, 1996.

871. Elliott, S., Lorenzini, T., Chang, D., Barzilay, J., and Delorme, E.: Mapping of the active site of recombinant human erythropoietin. Blood 89:493, 1997.

872. Lu, H.S., Boone, T.C., Souza, L.M., and Lai, P.H.: Disulfide and secondary structures of recombinant human granulocyte colony stimulating factor. Arch. Biochem. Biophys. 268:81, 1989.

873. Reidhaar-Olson, J.F., De Souza-Hart, J.A., and Selick, H.E.: Identification of residues critical to the activity of human granulocyte colony-stimulating factor. Biochemistry 35:9034, 1996.

874. Hoffman, R.C., Andersen, H., Walker, K., Krakover, J.D., Patel, S., Stamm, M.R., and Osborn, S.G.: Peptide, disulfide and glycosylation mapping of recombinant human thrombopoietin from Ser1 to Arg246. Biochemistry 35:14849, 1996.

875. Pearce, K.H., Potts, B.J., Presta, L.G., Bald, L.N., Fendly, B.M., and Wells, J.A.: Mutational analysis of thrombopoietin for identification of receptor and neutralizing antibody sites. J. Biol. Chem. 272:20595, 1997.

876. Clark-Lewis, I., Hood, L.E., and Kent, S.B.: Role of disulfide bridges in determining the biological activity of interleukin-3. Proc. Natl. Acad. Sci. USA 85:7897, 1988.

877. Olins, P.O., Bauer, C., Braford-Goldberg, S., Sterbenz, K., Polazzi, J.O., Caparon, M.H., Klein, B.K., Easton, A.M., Paik, K., Klover, J.A., Thiele, B.R., and McKearn, J.P.: Saturation mutagenesis of human interleukin-3. J. Biol. Chem. 270:23754, 1995.

878. Hercus, T.R., Bagley, C.J., Cambareri, B., Dottore, M., Woodcock, J.M., Vadas, M.A., Shannon, M.F., and Lopez, A.F.: Specific human granulocyte-macrophage colony-stimulating factor antagonists. Proc. Natl. Acad. Sci. USA 91:5838, 1994.

879. Rajotte, D., Cadieux, C., Haman, A., Woodcock, J.A., Lopez, A., and Hoang, T.: Crucial role of the residue R280 at the F′-G′ loop of the human granulocyte-macrophage colony stimulating factor receptor alpha chain for ligand recognition. J. Exp. Med. 185:1939, 1997.

880. Morton, T., Li, J., Cook, R., and Chaiken, I.: Mutagenesis in the C-terminal region of human interleukin 5 reveals a central patch for receptor α chain recognition. Proc. Natl. Acad. Sci. USA 92:10879, 1995.

881. Dickason, R.R., Huston, M.M., and Huston, D.P.: Delineation of domains predicted to engage the IL-5 receptor complex. J. Immunol. 156:1030, 1996.

882. Wong, G.G., Temple, P.A., Leary, A.C., Witek-Giannotti, J., Yang, Y.C., Ciarletta, A.B., Chung, M., Murtha, P., Kriz, R., Kaufman, R.J., Ferenz, C.R., Sibley, B.S., Turner, K.J., Hewick, R.M., Clark, S.C., Yanai, N., Yokota, H., Yamada, M., Saito, M., Motoyoshi, K., and Takaku, F.: Human CSF-1: molecular cloning and expression of 4-kb cDNA encoding the urinary protein. Science 235:1504, 1987.

883. Glocker, M.O., Arbogast, B., Schreurs, J., and Deinzer, M.L.: Assignment of the inter- and intramolecular disulfide linkages in recombinant macrophage colony stimulating factor using fast atom bombardment mass spectrometry. Biochemistry 32:482, 1993.

884. Koths, K.: Structure-function studies on human macrophage colony-stimulating factor (M-CSF). Mol. Reprod. Dev. 46:31, 1997.

885. Lyman, S.D., James, L., Escobar, S., Downey, H., de Vries, P., Brasel, K., Stocking, K., Beckmann, M.P., Copeland, N.G., Cleveland, L.S., Jenkins, N.A., Belmont, J.W., and Davison, B.L.: Identification of soluble and membrane-bound isoforms of the murine flt3 ligand generated by alternative splicing of mRNAs. Oncogene 10:149, 1995.

886. Bowcock, A.M., Kidd, J.R., Lathrop, G.M., Daneshvar, L., May, L.T., Ray, A., Sehgal, P.B., Kidd, K.K., and Cavalli-Sforza, L.L.: The human interferon beta 2/hepatocyte stimulating factor/interleukin 6 gene: DNA polymorphism studies and localization to chromosome 7p21. Genomics 3:8, 1988.

887. Orita, T., Oh-eta, M., Hasegawa, M., Kuboniwa, H., Esaki, K., and Ochi, N.: Polypeptide and carbohydrate structure of recombinant human interleukin 6 produced in Chinese hamster ovary cells. J. Biochem. (Tokyo) 115:345, 1994.

888. Sporeno, E., Savino, R., Ciapponi, L., Paonessa, G., Cabibbo, A., Lahm, A., Pulkki, K., Sun, R.-X., Toniatti, C., Klein, B., and Ciliberto, G.: Human interleukin-6 receptor super-antagonists with high potency and wide spectrum on multiple myeloma cells. Blood 87:4510, 1996.

889. Czupryn, M.J., McCoy, J.M., and Scoble, H.A.: Structure-function relationships in human interleukin-11. J. Biol. Chem. 270:978, 1995.

890. Nicola, N.A., Cross, B., Simpson, R.J.: The disulfide bond arrangement of leukemia inhibitory factor: homology to oncostatin M and structural implications. Biochem. Biophys. Res. Commun. 190:20, 1993.

891. Giovannini, M., Selleri, L., Hermanson, G.G., and Evans, G.A.: Localization of the human oncostatin M gene (SM) to chromosome 22q12, distal to the Ewing's sarcoma breakpoint. Cytogenet. Cell Genet. 62:32, 1993.

892. Hudson, K.R., Vernallis, A.B., and Heath, J.K.: Characterization of the receptor binding sites of human leukemia inhibitory factor and creation of antagonists. J. Biol. Chem. 271:11971, 1996.

893. Sungaran, R., Markovic, B., and Chong, B.H.: Localization and regulation of thrombopoietin mRNA expression in human kidney, liver, bone marrow and spleen using in situ hybridization. Blood 89:101, 1997.

894. Ladner, M.B., Martin, G.A., Noble, J.A., Nikoloff, D.M., Tal, R., Kawasaki, E.S., and White, T.J.: Human CSF-1: gene structure and alternative splicing of mRNA precursors. EMBO J. 6:2693, 1987.

895. Sims, J.E., Painter, S.L., and Gow, I.R.: Genomic organization of the type I and type II IL-1 receptors. Cytokine 7:483, 1995.

896. Greenfeder, S.A., Nunes, P., Kwee, L., Labow, M., Chizzonite, R.A., and Ju, G.: Molecular cloning and characterization of a second subunit of the interleukin-1 receptor complex. J. Biol. Chem. 270:13757, 1995.

3
Transcription Factors That Regulate Lineage Decisions

Stuart H. Orkin

EARLY HEMATOPOIETIC DEVELOPMENT AND LINEAGE COMMITMENT: A DISTINCTION

IDENTIFICATION OF RELEVANT GENES AND THEIR FUNCTIONAL ANALYSIS

FACTORS REQUIRED FOR FORMATION OR MAINTENANCE OF THE EARLIEST PROGENITORS OF THE HEMATOPOIETIC STEM CELL
- ▼ SCL/Tal-1
- ▼ Rbtn2/Lmo2
- ▼ Core Binding Factor

FACTORS INFLUENCING EXPANSION OF IMMATURE PROGENITORS
- ▼ GATA-2
- ▼ Homeobox Proteins
- ▼ c-Myb

TRANSCRIPTION FACTORS REQUIRED IN ONE OR MULTIPLE MYELOERYTHROID LINEAGES FOR LINEAGE SELECTION OR CELLULAR MATURATION
- ▼ GATA-1: A Factor Required for Both Erythroid and Megakaryocytic Development
- ▼ FOG: A GATA-1 Cofactor Required for Both Erythroid and Megakaryocytic Development
- ▼ EKLF: A Factor Required for β Globin Expression and Definitive Red Cell Maturation

- ▼ NF-E2: A Factor Essential for Megakaryocyte Development and Platelet Biogenesis but Largely Dispensable for Erythropoiesis
- ▼ Mi: A Factor Required for Production of Normal Mast Cells
- ▼ PU.1: An Ets-Related Factor Required for Both Myeloid and Lymphoid Development
- ▼ CCAAT/Enhancer Binding Proteins: Factors Required for Granulopoiesis

FACTORS REQUIRED FOR THE DEVELOPMENT OF LYMPHOID LINEAGES
- ▼ Factors Involved Broadly in Lymphoid Development
  PU.1
  Ikaros and Related Proteins
- ▼ Factors Required for B-cell Development
  Pax-5/BSAP
  E2A
  Oct-2 and Its Coactivator
  Early B-Cell Factor
- ▼ Factors Essential for T-Lymphocyte Development
  LEF-1 and TCF-1
  GATA-3

POSSIBLE MECHANISMS OF LINEAGE SELECTION

▼ ▼

Among the greatest and most fascinating challenges in the field of hematopoiesis is understanding how enormous diversity at the cellular level is programmed from a single progenitor, the hematopoietic stem cell (HSC).[1, 2] Red cell precursors devoted to synthesizing hemoglobin would seem to share little with immunoglobulin-producing B-lymphoid cells. Yet both lineages are descendants of the HSC. Highly evolved cellular programs are presumed to exist that specify differentiation along one path, as opposed to the many other options ultimately available. Whether lineage decisions in the hematopoietic system are "instructed" by cytokines or dependent on "intrinsic" regulatory networks remains an issue of considerable interest and debate (see references 3 and 4). The current weight of evidence favors a "permissive" role of cytokines in fostering cell survival and proliferation. From this perspective, attention shifts to the nucleus and in particular to the role of transcriptional regulatory proteins in lineage choice and cellular differentiation. Because the entire repertoire of relevant proteins remains to be defined, an understanding of how hematopoietic development is programmed is admittedly incomplete, although greatly enriched by recent findings. In this chapter, specific transcription factors and their functions in hematopoiesis are reviewed with the goal of providing a framework in which to consider models of normal and aberrant hematopoiesis. The intrinsic role in normal blood cell development of several proteins first discovered in the context of chromosome translocations in human leukemias suggests immediate clinical relevance of the topics discussed below.

Early Hematopoietic Development and Lineage Commitment: A Distinction

The establishment of the hematopoietic system reflects a series of developmental events followed by expansion of immature progenitors or HSCs and the subsequent commitment of later progenitors to differentiation along selected pathways. For clarity, it is best to consider separately the steps leading to the formation of the HSC and the processes involved in lineage selection and cellular maturation. Although some aspects may be shared, as evidenced by the possible involvement of some transcription factors in both, there are compelling reasons for making an explicit distinction. The formation of the first blood cells and HSCs within the developing embryo very likely represents the culmination of inductive events involving local growth factors that specify mesoderm to a hematopoietic fate (Fig. 3–1). Specific transcription factors are induced or activated and serve to execute their downstream programs by regulating expression of their target genes. Once HSCs are formed, however, lineage choice and differentiation may result from the action of these, or other, transcription factors operating largely within intrinsic regulatory networks and apparently less subject to direct growth factor influences (Fig. 3–2).

As described elsewhere (Chapter 1), the site of hematopoiesis shifts during development from the yolk sac blood islands to the fetal liver, then to the bone marrow in the perinatal period. Primitive hematopoiesis, that associated with the production of nucleated embryonic red blood cells, occurs in the blood islands. Definitive hematopoiesis, charac-

Induction/Specification

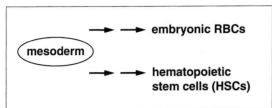

Figure 3–1. Induction or specification of the hematopoietic system. Hematopoietic cells are derived from mesoderm. Within the yolk sac, embryonic red blood cells (RBCs) are produced, possibly without generation of a long-term repopulating hematopoietic stem cell (HSC). In the embyo proper, HSCs are generated within selected regions (AGM, vitelline artery, umbilical artery). The arrows represent successive, as yet incompletely defined, steps in the pathways.

terized by enucleated erythrocytes, first takes place in the fetal liver. HSCs, as defined by reconstitution of adult recipients, can be identified within the mouse embryo in the aortic/gonad/mesonephros (AGM) region on embryonic day (E) 12 but not in the yolk sac.[5–7] By transplantation into fetal recipients, long-term repopulating cells may be found in the yolk sac as early as E9 to E10.[8] The precise relationship between these two compartments of presumptive HSCs remains to be defined. Culture evidence suggests, however, that primitive and definitive progenitors have a common origin.[9]

Blood islands are derived from aggregates of mesodermal cells that colonize the developing yolk sac on approximately E7. The close temporal and physical emergence of the first hematopoietic and vascular cells shortly thereafter is consistent with the hypothesis that they arise from a common precursor, the hemangioblast.[10] Data in favor of a common precursor from mouse embryonic stem (ES) cells[11] and possibly also from the AGM region have been reported.[12] For the purposes of this review, I consider a common origin of hematopoietic and vascular cells to be established. This stance is consistent with the requirement for the vascular endothelial growth factor receptor, Flk1, in both vasculogenesis and hematopoiesis[13] as well as the involvement of some transcription factors in both lineages (see below). Culture data from ES cells differentiated in vitro and from endothelial cells purified from early embryos support the existence of the hemangioblast and derivation of hematopoietic cells from endothelial-like cells.[11, 12]

Whereas the presumptive hemangioblast may have two options available, HSCs have at least eight (erythroid, megakaryocytic, mast, neutrophil, monocyte/macrophage, eosinophil, B-lymphoid, and T-lymphoid). One remarkable feature of hematopoietic progenitors, as exemplified by colony assays, is their myriad commitment patterns and plasticity. In principle, lineage selection might be achieved from two different "ground" states. Individual lineages might need to be "specified" by activation or expression of a particular transcription factor on an otherwise naive background. Alternatively, HSCs or early progenitors might activate multiple programs simultaneously, sequentially, or at random, only to select out a single one for subsequent consolidation. These models are considered later in the context of specific recent findings.

Identification of Relevant Genes and Their Functional Analysis

Those genes shown to be important to transcriptional regulation in hematopoietic development have been identified principally in one of two ways. First, study of lineage markers expressed in a cell-restricted manner (e.g., globins or immunoglobulins) has led to characterization of *cis*-regulatory elements and ultimately the transcription factors binding to them.[14] This directed strategy has as an explicit aim the identification of transcription factors controlling end-stage markers of a lineage. It has proved useful in dissecting development because many of such factors are employed in multiple ways, such that earlier regulatory events are also under their aegis. These complex relationships often thwart efforts to construct a simple regulatory hierarchy and also must be taken into account in interpreting genetic ablation of individual components in mice. A second approach relies on the isolation of genes involved in chromosome translocations in leukemia.[15] Whereas a priori there is no reason that the products of such genes would need to be involved intrinsically in normal hematopoiesis, experience has shown that this is more often than not the case. A direct implication of these observations is that leukemias arise through perturbation of normal regulatory networks operative in hematopoietic progenitors or HSCs. With the widespread sequencing of cDNA clones from various sources, including immature hematopoietic cells, gene discovery through genomics may soon provide additional genes that will be found to be required for critical aspects of hematopoiesis.

Among the methods for assaying gene function, targeted mutation in ES cells and mice (knockout technology) has been particularly informative in establishing in vivo roles for specific genes.[16] In addition to conventional interbreeding of heterozygous mice to generate homozygous mutants, ES cells rendered null for expression of a given gene can be subjected to in vitro differentiation or to chimera analysis.[17, 18] By the former approach, hematopoietic colonies are generated from ES cells within a 10 to 14 day period, thereby allowing analysis of the consequences of gene mutation apart from the viability of the intact mutant animal or embryo. Structure-function analyses can be performed either by rescue of mutant ES cells with transgenes or by use of immortalized cell lines derived from mutant ES cells.[19, 20] Chimera analysis, in which null ES cells are injected into wild-type host blastocysts, is particularly useful for assessing the developmental potential of cells within the context of a developing, intact mouse.[21] In such experiments, the ability

Lineage Selection/Differentiation

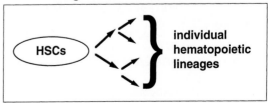

Figure 3–2. Lineage selection and differentiation of hematopoietic progenitors. HSCs, which are typically quiescent, enter the progenitor pool (indicated by the multiple arrows), eventually giving rise to precursors committed to individual hematopoietic lineages.

of ES cells to contribute to specific cell lineages provides a measure of their capacity to differentiate within the normal milieu and discriminates cell autonomous from non–cell autonomous effects of gene mutation. A compilation of the requirement for specific transcription factors in hematopoiesis is provided in Table 3–1.

Besides knockout experiments, gain of function or forced expression assays also provide clues to the possible function of particular transcription factors. This approach, which relies on the notion that expression of one component may divert or alter cellular differentiation, is analogous to experiments in which myogenic transcription factors serve to convert fibroblasts or many other cell types into myoblasts.[22]

Although differentiation even in the muscle system is now considered to be more complex than originally appreciated, forced expression experiments may often provide useful insights, particularly if favorable recipient cells are available. As described more fully below, experiments in which the transcription factors GATA-1, PU.1, SCL/Tal-1, and C/EBP have been expressed in various hematopoietic progenitors, cell lines, or embryos have defined dominantly acting functions of these factors in differentiation.[23–31] The findings, which are elaborated on below, are summarized in Figure 3–3. In addition to expression of exogenous genes in cell lines, gain of function experiments may be performed in transgenic mice. These have been most informative tradition-

Table 3–1. Summary of Transcription Factors and Their Requirements in Hematopoiesis*

Factor	Class	Associated Proteins (or Interacting)	Expression Pattern	Where Required
SCL/Tal-1	bHLH	E2A (E12, E47) Rbtn2/Lmo2	Progenitors, E, Mast, Meg Vascular and CNS	All hematopoiesis Angiogenesis
Rbtn2/Lmo2	LIM only	SCL/Tal-1 Ldb-1 GATA-1	Hematopoietic enriched (not fully defined)	All hematopoiesis
Cbfa2/AML1	Runt	Cbfb	Sites of definitive hematopoiesis Vascular (not fully defined)	Definitive hematopoiesis ? Vascular integrity
GATA-2	GATA family	Other GATAs CBP/p300	Widespread HSCs, progenitors, Meg, Mast	Hematopoietic progenitors
c-Myb	Myb	CBP/p300 p100	Progenitors	Definitive hematopoiesis (? except Megs)
GATA-1	GATA family	FOG Other GATAs, CBP/p300 Sp1, EKLF	E, Mast, Meg, Eos, progenitors Sertoli cells	E and Meg maturation
FOG	FOG/u-shaped	GATA-1	E, Meg, progenitors	E maturation Meg formation
EKLF	Kruppel family	GATA-1	E	β globin expression and definitive E maturation
p45 NF-E2	bZIP	p18 NF-E2 TAFIII-130 WW-proteins	E, Meg, Mast, progenitors	Platelet formation Meg maturation (slight E hypochromia)
Mi	bHLH-zipper	bHLH-zipper factors	Mast, melanocytes	Mast cell production Melanocyte survival
PU.1	Ets family	NF-EM5/Pip Other interactors	Mono/mac, B-lymphoid (low-level: G, E, meg)	Mac, B lymphopoiesis (G, T lymphopoiesis)
Ikaros-related proteins	Ikaros/zinc family	Ikaros members	Progenitors, lymphoid cells	Lymphopoiesis
Pax-5/BSAP	Pax family		B cells, CNS	B lymphopoiesis CNS
E2A	bHLH	SCL/Tal-1, other bHLHs	Ubiquitous	B lymphopoiesis T-cell homeostasis
Oct-2	POU homeodomain	OCA-B/OBF-1/Bob-1	B cells, other sites	Selected B-cell properties
OCA-B/OBF-1/Bob-1		Oct-2/Oct-1	B cells	Selected B-cell properties
EBF	Novel		B cells	B lymphopoiesis
LEF-1 and TCF-1	HMG family	ALY, β-catenin	T cells Other sites (LEF-1)	T lymphopoiesis Skin
GATA-3	GATA family		T cells, other sites	T lymphopoiesis CNS

CNS, central nervous system; E, erythroid cells; Eos, eosinophils; G, granulocytes; HSCs, hematopoietic stem cells; Mast, mast cells; Meg, megakaryocytes; Mono/mac, monocytes/macrophages.
* See text corresponding to each factor for details.

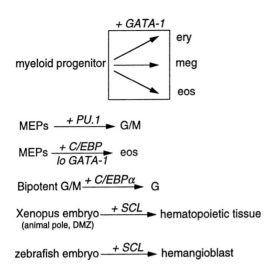

Figure 3–3. Dominant lineage programming (or reprogramming) by hematopoietic transcription factors. Forced expression of various transcription factors alters cellular phenotypes. Details of these experiments are discussed in the text. ery, erythroid cells; meg, megakaryocytes; eos, eosinophils; MEPs, multipotential chicken progenitors; G/M, myeloid cells; G, granulocytes; DMZ, dorsal marginal zone.

ally in mimicking leukemias[32] but hold promise for revealing mechanisms of progenitor regulation and lineage selection.[33]

Factors Required for Formation or Maintenance of the Earliest Progenitors of the Hematopoietic Stem Cell

Lying at the top of a regulatory hierarchy would appear to be those genes that are required for the formation of all hematopoietic lineages. Such genes might act at the pre-HSC level, for example, within mesoderm or the hemangioblast, to specify a hematopoietic "fate" or within the HSC to foster survival or proliferation. Genes in this general class encode the transcription factors known as SCL/Tal-1, Rbtn2/Lmo2, and core binding factor (CBF). Remarkably, these are all targeted by translocations seen in human leukemias, perhaps predictive of their critical roles in normal hematopoiesis.

▼ SCL/Tal-1

This gene was first identified in humans at the site of chromosome translocations associated with T-cell acute lymphoblastic leukemia (T-ALL; hence its name, stem cell leukemia).[34, 35] The locus is frequently activated at the transcriptional level in T-ALL by translocation or upstream interstitial deletions involving another locus, designated *sil*.[36, 37] The encoded SCL/Tal-1 polypeptide is a member of the basic helix-loop-helix (bHLH) class of transcription factors, which includes cell-specific regulators of muscle or neuron differentiation, such as MyoD and Mash-1, respectively, and ubiquitous proteins, such as E2A, with established roles in development.[35, 38–40] Expression of SCL/Tal-1 is cell restricted, limited to hematopoietic and endothelial cells[41, 42] as well as selected sites in the central nervous system. Within

the hematopoietic system, SCL/Tal-1 is expressed in a distribution remarkably similar to that of GATA-1 (see below), that is, within erythroid, mast, and megakaryocytic lineages. SCL/Tal-1 interacts with DNA in a sequence-specific manner as a heterodimer with products of the E2A gene (E12 and E47) and presumably other related polypeptides.[43] The consensus site recognized by the SCL/Tal-1 heterodimer conforms to an E box motif, CANNTG, although gene targets in large part remain to be identified (see below). Consistent with its implied involvement in T-ALL, expression of SCL/Tal-1 directed to early lymphoid cells by the Lck promoter in transgenic mice leads to lymphoma after a long latency.[44, 45] Oncogenic transformation by SCL/Tal-1 is potentiated by casein kinase II[44] or by coexpression of one of its interacting proteins, Rbtn2/Lmo2.[46]

The pattern of expression of SCL/Tal-1 in *Xenopus* and zebra fish embryos is consistent with an important role in blood cell development. In *Xenopus*, SCL/Tal-1 mRNA is expressed in a domain within which the ventral blood island (an analogue of the mammalian yolk sac) is destined to develop.[25] In zebra fish embryos, mRNA is found in a region, the intermediate cell mass, that is thought to give rise to immature progenitors or HSCs.[47] Gain of function experiments also point to possible functions for SCL/Tal-1. When its expression is forced in cultured mouse Friend virus–transformed erythroleukemia cells, erythroid maturation is enhanced.[48] Moreover, expression after microinjection in *Xenopus* animal cap assays has been interpreted to suggest that SCL/Tal-1 is able to specify mesoderm to a hematopoietic fate.[25]

Loss of function or knockout experiments in mice have been particularly revealing with regard to SCL/Tal-1's in vivo roles. Remarkably, embryos and yolk sacs lacking SCL/Tal-1 are entirely bloodless and consequently die by E10.[49, 50] In vitro differentiation and chimera analyses with SCL/Tal-1 null ES cells established a requirement for formation of all adult lineages as well.[51, 52] SCL/tal$^{-/-}$ cells are unable to generate erythroid, myeloid, or lymphoid cells at any developmental stage. Thus, the protein is required at the earliest definable step in hematopoiesis. Because endothelial cells are present in SCL/Tal-1$^{-/-}$ yolk sac, signifying specification of vascular development, it was initially inferred that SCL/Tal-1 acts primarily or solely within the hematopoietic pathway, even if it were expressed within the hemangioblast. Subsequent analysis using mouse chimeras, however, revealed a failure in reorganization of the primary yolk sac capillary network in the absence of SCL/Tal-1, an unsuspected angiogenic defect.[53] A role in both hematopoiesis and vascular development was supported by experiments in zebra fish embryos in which it was shown that exogenous SCL/Tal-1 expressed from an injected plasmid can partially rescue both blood and vessel defects of the cloche (*clo*) mutant.[27] Accordingly, SCL/Tal-1 is hypothesized to act downstream of the unknown *clo* gene in both hematopoietic and vascular lineages. Moreover, injection of SCL/Tal-1 RNA appears to promote conversion of mesoderm to hematopoietic and vascular lineages, a finding compatible with a role for the protein in the induction of hemangioblast development.[26] A summary of the genetic experiments aimed at defining the in vivo roles of SCL/Tal-1 is presented in Figure 3–4.

The simplest interpretation of the genetic tests of function is that SCL/Tal-1 serves as a "master" regulator of

Deduced Roles for SCL/tal-1 in Development

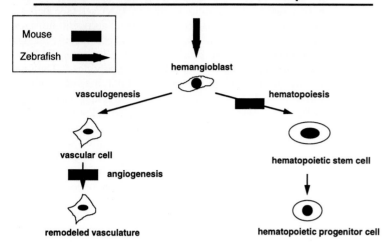

Figure 3–4. Deduced roles for SCL/Tal-1 in development. See text for specific details. The boxes indicate the stage of vascular development or hematopoiesis at which a block is evident in the mouse in the absence of SCL/Tal-1. The arrow in the box indicates that SCL/Tal-1 appears to promote hemangioblast formation from mesoderm in the zebra fish.

blood cell development and is required for specification of hematopoietic development from the hemangioblast. Although this remains a strong possibility, others are not excluded. Alternatively, SCL/Tal-1 might be required for maintenance of HSCs once formed, their response to growth factor stimulation, or survival. Current limitations in the understanding of SCL/Tal-1's roles in development include the paucity of defined target genes and convenient assays of protein function. How its normal role in blood cell development relates to leukemogenesis is uncertain. Two different models have now been distinguished. SCL/Tal-1 may incite leukemia directly by activating an "early" hematopoietic program on its deregulated expression or indirectly by sequestering E2A-related proteins and, secondarily, influencing cellular growth properties.

It has been difficult until recently to identify target genes regulated directly by SCL/Tal-1. By chromatin immunoselection methods, one putative target gene, *otogelin,* was identified.[54] Within an intron of this mucin-related gene, a binding site for a potential pentameric protein complex containing SCL/Tal-1 (see below) was found. The relevance of *otogelin* to hematopoietic functions of SCL/Tal-1 is as yet unclear. Recently, however, the gene encoding c-Kit, the receptor for stem cell factor (Kit ligand), has also been proposed as a possible target for SCL/Tal-1 on the basis of forced experiments in hematopoietic cell lines.[55] If the gene encoding c-Kit can be validated as a target, a direct connection will have been established between this transcription factor and growth factor regulation of immature hematopoietic progenitors.

▼ Rbtn2/Lmo2

This member of the zinc finger LIM family of proteins has important connections to SCL/Tal-1. First, the gene was discovered in association with chromosome translocation in acute T-ALL.[56, 57] Second, its expression is deregulated by the rearrangement. Whereas expression of Rbtn2/Lmo2 is not normally restricted to the hematopoietic system, it is highest in extraembryonic mesoderm, yolk sac, and fetal liver erythroid cells and absent in T lymphocytes. Like SCL/

Tal-1, Rbtn2/Lmo2 transcripts are localized within presumptive early hematopoietic progenitors in zebrafish.[47] Third, despite its inability to bind DNA on its own, Rbtn2/Lmo2 protein strongly interacts with SCL/Tal-1 in erythroid cell nuclei.[58] Indeed, binding site selection assays performed in vitro reveal that Rbtn2/Lmo2 and SCL/Tal-1 assemble together with at least three other proteins (GATA-1, E47, and the LIM-interacting protein Lbd1/NL1) on a bipartite DNA motif composed of an E box (CAGGTG) followed 7 to 9 bp downstream by a GATA site[59] (Fig. 3–5). These findings have been interpreted to suggest that Rbtn2/Lmo2 serves as a "bridging" protein within larger transcriptional complexes. T cell–directed expression of Rbtn2/Lmo2 leads to lymphoma and cooperates with SCL/Tal-1 in oncogenesis.[46]

A functional connection between Rbtn2/Lmo2 and SCL/Tal-1 is supported by the consequences of a loss of function mutation in mice. Embryos lacking Rbtn2/Lmo2 are also bloodless. Furthermore, like SCL/Tal-1$^{-/-}$ cells, Rbtn2/Lmo2$^{-/-}$ cells fail to give rise to adult blood lineages.[60] Thus, the hematological consequences of loss of Rbtn2/Lmo2 and SCL/Tal-1 appear indistinguishable. Whether Rbtn2/Lmo2 also functions in vascular development is presently unknown. SCL/Tal-1 and Rbtn2/Lmo2 appear to function together within an essential protein complex and regulatory program to control target genes required within the earliest hematopoietic compartment during embryogenesis.

A Pentameric Hematopoietic Protein Complex?

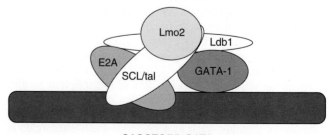

CAGGTG(N)₉GATA

Figure 3–5. Proposed multiprotein complex assembled on an E box–GATA composite DNA-binding site. See text for details.

The block to blood cell formation in the absence of either protein is envisioned to impair a precursor common to both primitive erythropoiesis and definitive hematopoiesis.

▼ CORE BINDING FACTOR

CBF, also known as PEBP2, provides yet another example of a leukemia-associated gene that plays a critical role in development of the most immature hematopoietic progenitors.[61–64] CBF is a heterodimeric factor consisting of a DNA-binding subunit (Cbfa2, also known as AML1) that is homologous to the product of the *Drosophila runt* gene and an unrelated partner protein (Cbfb) that enhances DNA-binding affinity. The *runt* domain mediates interaction with both DNA and Cbfb. The Cbf2a and Cbfb loci are involved in translocations in acute myeloid leukemia.[65] In these instances, rather than merely activating expression, chromosome rearrangements generate novel chimeric (or fusion) proteins (see Chapter 26) that appear to act largely as *trans*-dominant inhibitors of normal CBF function.[66–68] Remarkably, loss of function mutations of either Cbf2a or Cbfb lead to identical phenotypes in mice: a complete failure of *definitive* hematopoiesis.[69–71] Yolk sac hematopoiesis is unaffected because of either the presence of other *runt*-like proteins that substitute in the absence of CBF or CBF-independent transcriptional programs in embryonic red cell progenitors. It is likely that CBF function is essential to the emergence, maintenance, or survival of the earliest adult hematopoietic progenitors of HSCs. The differential in vivo effects of CBF loss point to potentially important differences in primitive and adult hematopoietic regulatory programs.

The role of Cbf2a or AML1 in hematopoietic development appears to be conserved in that the *Xenopus* homologue is expressed in the developing ventral blood island and a truncated mutant interferes with primitive hematopoiesis.[72] Although the critical target genes regulated by CBF in definitive hematopoietic cells are largely undefined, growth factor receptor genes, such as that encoding macrophage colony-stimulating factor (M-CSF), are likely candidates on the basis of promoter analysis. Study of the M-CSF promoter suggests that CBF interacts with and works in concert with other myeloid transcription factors, such as PU.1 and C/EBPα, and with more general coactivators, such as p300/CREB-binding protein (CBP), to activate transcription.[73–75]

The point at which CBF is required for definitive hematopoiesis has been defined more precisely by an elegant gene knockin experiment in which the bacterial β-galactosidase gene *(lacZ)* has been introduced into the gene encoding Cbf2a.[76] In this instance, *lacZ* serves two functions: knockout of the CBF function and also a marker for cells expressing the Cbf2a locus. In heterozygous animals, *lacZ* staining is seen in the area of the dorsal aorta (the vicinity of the AGM) in endothelial cells from which presumptive hematopoietic cells bud off as grape-like clusters. In homozygous animals, *lacZ* staining is seen in the endothelial cells, but budding of hematopoietic cells is not. These findings strongly suggest that CBF is required for the emergence of the first definitive hematopoietic cells from "hemogenic" endothelium, the functional equivalent of a hemangioblast.

Factors Influencing Expansion of Immature Progenitors

A critical feature of the establishment of the hematopoietic system is expansion of progenitors, in effect to provide an adequate pool from which precursor cells are chosen for subsequent differentiation. Expansion of progenitors is necessary during growth and development of the embryo and also for sustaining blood cell production in the adult individual. Several transcription factors, representing different protein classes, seem to function at this level.

▼ GATA-2

GATA-2, a member of the zinc finger GATA family of factors,[77] appears to be required for the proliferation and survival of multipotential progenitors of both primitive and definitive origins.[78] GATA-2 transcripts are expressed widely in different cell types but are particularly abundant in immature progenitors and very likely in HSCs. In addition, they are found in early (but not late) erythroid precursors, mast cells, and megakaryocytes. During embryonic development in mice, *Xenopus,* and zebra fish, GATA-2 expression marks cells presumed to represent early progenitors of HSCs.[47] Expression of GATA-2 in progenitors is downregulated as they switch from a proliferative state and commit to erythroid maturation. Consistent with a proposed role in controlling cellular proliferation or participating in a choice between self-renewal and differentiation, forced expression of GATA-2 in chicken progenitor cells blocks erythroid development.[79]

Loss of GATA-2 function in mice leads to embryonic lethality associated with reduced hematopoiesis and a marked decrease in the number of multipotential progenitors.[78] The phenotype of such embryos is similar to but much more severe and earlier in onset than that seen in classical *W* or *steel* mutant mice. In chimera experiments, the contribution of GATA-2$^{-/-}$ cells to adult hematopoietic lineages is nearly undetectable. In addition to a quantitative loss of multipotential progenitors, GATA-2 loss ablates mast cell commitment or development.[80] GATA-2 is required for the intrinsic differentiation of other lineages. On the basis of in vitro ES cell differentiation experiments, it has been concluded that GATA-2 is necessary in the earliest progenitors (so-called blast-like colonies)[80] where it is believed to control responses of these cells to stimulation by cytokines or pathways of cell survival (or self-renewal).

▼ HOMEOBOX PROTEINS

Given the prominence of homeodomain-containing transcription factors in embryonic development, it is not surprising that they have also garnered attention with respect to potential roles in hematopoiesis. The multiplicity of homeobox proteins, particularly those within the conventional *HOX* clusters, has confounded assigning specific and non-redundant functions in blood cells. Surveys of gene expression patterns have described restricted expression of some *HOX* genes in hematopoietic cell lines.[81] These studies implicate *HOXB (B2, B4, B6–B9), HOXC (C6, C8),* and *HOXA (A5)* in erythropoiesis; *HOXA–C* in lymphopoiesis; and *A9, A10, B3, B7,* and *B8* in myelomonocytic differentiation.

Several lines of evidence, however, have provided more substantive connections between homeobox factors and hematopoiesis. In a gain of function experiment, *HOXB4* overexpression in transduced murine bone marrow cells led to a more than 50-fold increase in HSC number without perturbation of specific lineages or the development of leukemia.[82] Thus, homeobox factors might regulate aspects of progenitor cell self-renewal. Overexpression of another *HOX* gene, *HOXA10,* in murine bone marrow disturbs myeloid and B-cell development and leads to acute myeloid leukemia with a prolonged latency.[83] Loss of function of *HOXA9* perturbs early T-cell development,[84] whereas forced expression transforms primary bone marrow cells.[85] The variety and complex patterns of homeobox factor expression in progenitors and specific lineages provide ample room for intricate regulatory interactions and overlapping functions in vivo.

Homeobox genes are also rearranged in leukemias, as in the fusion of *HOXA9* with nucleoporin NUP98 in myeloid leukemia.[86, 87] In a variation of this theme, a putative regulator of *HOX* genes, a homologue of the *Drosophila* trithorax gene *Mll* (also known as *HRX* and *ALL-1*), is involved in translocations associated with mixed-lineage leukemia. Apparent Mll haploinsufficiency leads to perturbed hematopoiesis, characterized by decreased numbers of red blood cells, platelets, and B lymphocytes.[88] Hematopoietic colonies derived from Mll$^{-/-}$ murine yolk sacs and fetal liver are reduced in number, small, and delayed in their formation.[89, 90] Whether these effects of Mll on hematopoiesis are mediated through control of *HOX* gene expression is unproven.

Other classes of homeobox factors may also be involved in hematopoiesis, but in less direct ways. Studies in *Xenopus* embryos have shown that a bone morphogenetic protein-4 growth factor–induced paired-class homeobox protein known as Mix.1 can induce ventral mesoderm and potentiate blood formation.[91] This homeobox protein may lie far upstream in a hierarchy that converges on hematopoietic development. A member of the LIM homeobox family, Lhx2, has been shown to be required for normal fetal liver erythropoiesis.[92] However, the consequences of loss of function in this instance are non–cell autonomous, suggesting that Lhx2 functions within the fetal liver microenvironment.

▼ c-Myb

Immature hematopoietic progenitor cells express high levels of the cellular homologue of the v-Myb nuclear oncoprotein, c-Myb. Expression of several myeloid-expressed genes have been shown to be dependent on the action of c-Myb in concert with C/EBP, CBF, or Ets family proteins.[93–95] In chicken cells, c-Myb cooperates with NF-M, the mammalian homologue of C/EBPβ, to activate transcription of the Mim-1 promoter.[96] Like many other factors, c-Myb appears to require the transcriptional coactivator CBP.[94, 97] Moreover, c-Myb interacts with a ubiquitous coactivator, designated p100, that influences its transcriptional activity.[98] In turn, Pim-1, an oncogenic serine-threonine kinase, phosphorylates p100, leading to the formation of a stable complex with c-Myb and enhancing c-Myb's transcriptional activity.[99] Expression of c-Myb can profoundly affect hematopoi-

etic differentiation. Overexpression of c-Myb blocks erythroid differentiation in cell culture,[100] whereas antisense oligonucleotide inhibition leads to growth arrest and reduced colony formation. A retrovirus carrying both v-Myb and Ets transforms chicken progenitor cells.[101] Taken together, these observations predict a function for c-Myb in hematopoiesis, which was confirmed by a mouse knockout. In mice lacking c-Myb, definitive hematopoiesis except for megakaryopoiesis in the fetal liver is defective.[102] Primitive hematopoiesis is unaffected. Whereas these findings have been interpreted as supporting a role for c-Myb in controlling the proliferation of immature progenitors, they are also consistent with independent requirements for c-Myb in multiple lineages.

Transcription Factors Required in One or Multiple Myeloerythroid Lineages for Lineage Selection or Cellular Maturation

Several transcription factors characterized to date exhibit restricted patterns of expression among the maturing precursor cells and are specifically required for development of one or more hematopoietic lineages. Because the expression of some of these factors overlaps other family members, the consequences of loss of function mutations may be somewhat narrower than the hematopoietic domain in which they actually participate in transcriptional control. The sharing of transcriptional responsibilities by family members and dynamic regulation of individual members most likely serve to fine-tune differentiation within highly plastic progenitors. The following survey of factors is meant to be illustrative rather than comprehensive.

▼ GATA-1: A FACTOR REQUIRED FOR BOTH ERYTHROID AND MEGAKARYOCYTIC DEVELOPMENT

GATA-1, the founding member of the GATA family of transcription factors,[14, 103, 104] is related to GATA-2 by virtue of a highly homologous two–zinc finger DNA-binding domain. Except for Sertoli cells of the testis, in which its function is uncertain,[105] GATA-1's expression is tightly restricted to the hematopoietic system. GATA-1 is abundant in erythroid precursors, megakaryocytes, eosinophils, and mast cells. Multipotential progenitors express lower levels. GATA-1 is probably absent in HSCs. During embryonic development, GATA-1 is expressed in extraembryonic mesoderm of the developing yolk sac blood islands and in embryonic erythroblasts.[106] The onset of expression may be slightly later than that of SCL/Tal-1, GATA-2, or Rbtn2/Lmo2, although this conclusion should be considered tentative because differences in sensitivity of RNA transcript detection cannot be excluded. Within the zebra fish embryo, GATA-1 transcripts mark the earliest circulating hematopoietic cells, although they appear to be absent in the presumptive stem cell population that is positive for SCL/Tal-1 and GATA-2.[47] When the primary sequences of GATA-1 proteins of different species are compared, marked divergence is noted except within the zinc finger region (Fig. 3–6). This unexpected "evolutionary" finding is consistent with experimental evi-

GATA-1: Sequence Comparison

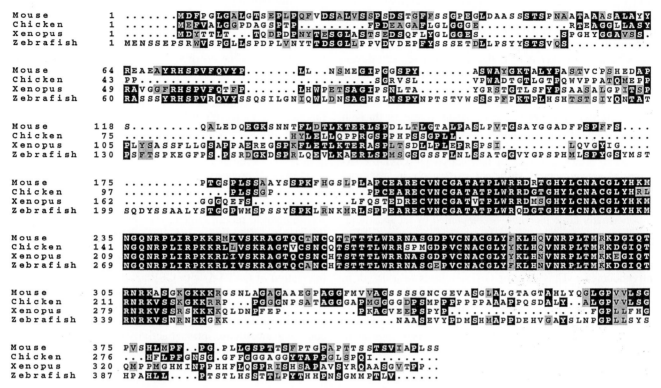

Figure 3–6. Comparison of primary amino acid sequences of GATA-1 of different species. Blackened amino acids demonstrate identities, whereas gray shading depicts similar residues.

dence suggesting that the principal functions of GATA-1 are concentrated within this domain.

GATA-1 was first discovered as a nuclear factor that binds a consensus sequence, {(T/A)GATA(A/G)}, found in the promoters or enhancers of globin genes of all species.[14, 103, 107] Subsequent work has revealed that GATA motifs are found in critical *cis*-regulatory elements of virtually all genes expressed specifically in erythroid cells. Shortly after cloning of its cDNA, its expression was detected in megakaryocytes and mast cells.[108, 109] Indeed, more recent findings indicate that the majority of megakaryocyte-specific genes, as well as several mast and eosinophil-specific genes, are regulated in part through GATA-1. Thus, although GATA-1 has been considered an "erythroid" transcription factor, it functions in multiple lineages that are related to one another through bipotential or tripotential progenitors (such as the erythroid/megakaryocyte or erythroid/megakaryocyte/mast cell progenitors).

Evidence also suggests that GATA-1 can exert dominant effects on lineage selection. Among the hematopoietic transcription factors examined, GATA-1 is particularly potent in altering the phenotype of progenitor cells in which it is expressed. For example, introduction of expressible GATA-1 into a murine myeloid cell line 416B induces megakaryocytic differentiation.[24] Moreover, forced expression reprograms *myb-ets* transformed chicken progenitors along erythroid, eosinophilic, and thromboblastic (megakaryocytic) pathways.[23] In both situations, lineage switching is accompanied by downregulation of myeloid markers. In the chicken

system, lineage reprogramming seems to depend on the concentration at which GATA-1 is ultimately expressed. Also, stable expression of GATA-1 and the erythropoietin receptor in a myeloid derivative of mouse FDC cells (a multipotential cell line) is associated with activation of endogenous GATA-1, erythroid Kruppel-like factor (EKLF, see below), and β globin genes.[110] The effects of GATA-1 expression on cellular phenotype implicate GATA-1 in regulating a cascade of downstream pathways in cellular differentiation. The identification of critical GATA-binding sites in promoters of the SCL/Tal-1[48] and EKLF[111] (see below) transcription factors and the erythropoietin receptor genes is compatible with this concept.

Gene targeting experiments involving the GATA-1 locus have been particularly insightful with regard to GATA-1's in vivo functions. Embryos lacking GATA-1 die by E10 to E11 owing to extreme anemia.[21, 112] Rather than entirely ablating erythroid cell commitment as one might anticipate, loss of GATA-1 is accompanied by the production of primitive (or definitive) erythroid precursors that are arrested at a proerythroblast-like stage.[112, 113] These cells undergo apoptosis, thereby providing a link between GATA-1 action and cell survival. In the absence of GATA-1, arrested erythroid precursors contain high levels of GATA-2, approximately more than 50-fold beyond that seen in wild-type proerythroblasts. It is reasonable to presume, although unproven, that erythroid commitment in the absence of GATA-1 occurs under the aegis of GATA-2. The elevation of GATA-2 levels in precursors lacking GATA-1 demonstrates cross-talk between these GATA factors.[113] GATA-1 serves to repress (either directly or indirectly) the expression of GATA-2. The downregulation of GATA-2 correlates normally with the transition from proliferation to differentiation. In the absence of GATA-1, the program of terminal erythroid maturation cannot be completed.

Whereas GATA-1 is essential for proper red cell development, its role in other lineages has been more difficult to assess conclusively because of the embryonic lethality of GATA-1 knockout mice. A requirement for GATA-1 in megakaryocyte development was established, however, through study of a unique mouse mutant generated by deletion of an upstream region of the GATA-1 locus.[114] This targeted mutation led to a selective loss of megakaryocyte GATA-1 expression, yet preserved sufficient expression in erythroid precursors to complete red cell development. Mice lacking megakaryocyte GATA-1 expression have reduced numbers of abnormally large platelets, accompanied by an accumulation of megakaryocytes in spleen and bone marrow. GATA-1$^-$ megakaryocytes are markedly retarded in their cellular maturation and exhibit enhanced proliferation in culture with thrombopoietin. Thus, loss of GATA-1 leads to a defect in megakaryocyte development, which superficially resembles that seen in GATA-1$^-$ erythroid cells, whereas precursors display unrestrained growth rather than apoptosis. Apoptosis and proliferation may be viewed as alternative responses to impaired cellular differentiation in the absence of GATA-1. Loss of function mutations for GATA-1 have not as yet revealed effects on lineage commitment, as might be predicted from the gain of function experiments summarized above. This may reflect unique features of the progenitor cell lines used to demonstrate dominant lineage effects of GATA-1 expression or the existence of compensatory mechanisms operating in vivo in the absence of GATA-1. Analysis of the development and function of mast cells and eosinophils lacking GATA-1 has not proceeded far enough for firm conclusions to be drawn regarding the requirement for the factor in these lineages.

How GATA-1 functions in transcriptional control is of particular interest. Whereas GATA binding sites are often found in promoters, they are also present within distant regulatory elements such as the core regions of globin locus control regions (LCRs).[115] These are sites of DNase I superhypersensitivity, a correlation that implicates GATA-1 in organizing the proper assembly of chromatin-associated complexes. In conventional reporter assays in heterologous cells, GATA-1 behaves like a conventional transcriptional activator.[116] Nonetheless, structure-function experiments in which various forms of GATA-1 were tested for rescue of differentiation in GATA-1$^-$ erythroid precursor cells dissociate transcriptional activation from the capacity to drive erythroid maturation. These observations have led to a model in which GATA-1 requires a transcriptional cofactor (or set of cofactors) to function in erythroid and very likely also megakaryocytic cells.[20]

Consistent with the notion that GATA-1 acts in part through interaction with other proteins, the zinc finger domain has been demonstrated to associate with several other nuclear proteins. These include Kruppel family zinc finger proteins, the ubiquitous factor Sp1 and erythroid-restricted factor EKLF[117] (see below), as well as the general transcriptional coactivators (or integrators) known as p300/CBP.[118]

Although firm evidence that GATA-1 interactions with Sp1 or EKLF are required for erythroid development is lacking, cell culture findings support a role for p300/CBP in erythroid differentiation.[118] Protein interactive screening of erythroid cDNAs yielded the postulated GATA-1 cofactor, a novel gene product dubbed FOG (Friend of GATA-1)[119] (see below). The appreciation of the multiple protein interactions operating through the DNA-binding domain of GATA-1 suggests an alternative view of how GATA-1 participates in transcriptional control. It seems likely that one of its primary functions is to recruit proteins into larger hematopoietic-specific complexes at specific chromosome sites. Thus, GATA-1 is poised to control the expression of diverse genes at different developmental stages in multiple lineages.

GATA-1 orchestrates multiple programs of erythroid development, including control of cell cycle and apoptosis, as well as differentiation. At the biochemical level, GATA-1 is thought to recruit critical proteins to target sites. Within the globin LCR elements, GATA sites figure prominently, consistent with the notion that GATA-1 bound to these regions might alter chromatin structure or function. The interaction of GATA-1 with CBP/p300 suggests at least one mechanism by which histone acetylases might be brought to specific sites.[118] By modifying chromatin-bound histones or perhaps by modification of GATA-1 itself,[120] acetylases could enhance transcriptional activity of globin loci. In this context, GATA-1 might be viewed more as an "architectural" factor rather than a traditional transcriptional activator.

▼ FOG: A GATA-1 COFACTOR REQUIRED FOR BOTH ERYTHROID AND MEGAKARYOCYTIC DEVELOPMENT

FOG is a complex zinc finger protein that interacts physically with the amino (N)–zinc finger of GATA-1.[119] The zinc fingers of FOG differ from the GATA-type zinc finger in their primary sequences and are composed of both C_2H_2 and C_2HC fingers. During embryogenesis, FOG is coexpressed at high level with GATA-1 in the embryonic erythroblasts in the yolk sac blood islands and in erythroid precursors in the fetal liver. Among hematopoietic lineages, its pattern of expression overlaps that of GATA-1. FOG is expressed in erythroid and megakaryocytic lineages, as well as in multipotential progenitors, but is not detected in mast cells. Cell culture experiments demonstrate that FOG is able to synergize with GATA-1 in GATA-1–dependent erythroid or megakaryocytic maturation of GATA-1$^-$ erythroid precursors or murine 416B cells, respectively. These findings are consistent with a possible role for FOG in GATA-1–dependent differentiation but fail to address the extent to which development relies on the presence of FOG.

If FOG were dedicated solely to mediating the transcriptional effects of GATA-1, the consequences of FOG or GATA-1 loss would be indistinguishable. In practice, FOG knockout embryos and cells closely resemble GATA-1$^-$ mutants with some notable exceptions. FOG$^{-/-}$ mice are embryonic lethal because of severe anemia.[121] However, in contrast to GATA-1$^-$ embryos, some hemoglobinization of erythroid precursors is appreciated on visual inspection. Erythroid precursor cells are largely arrested at the proerythroblast stage, but some differentiation beyond the block is also seen. Thus, FOG$^{-/-}$ erythroid precursors appear similar to those lacking GATA-1, but the developmental block is not as stringent. These findings are consistent with the postulated function of FOG as the principal cofactor for GATA-1 in erythroid cells. The somewhat attenuated severity of the mutation could be accounted for either by some FOG-independent functions of GATA-1 or by the limited action of other potential cofactors within the cell.

The effects of FOG loss on megakaryocyte development are more severe and unique among transcription factors critical for hematopoiesis.[121] Rather than producing hyperproliferative, developmentally arrested megakaryocytes, FOG deficiency ablates megakaryocyte colony formation. No megakaryocytes can be obtained either from FOG$^{-/-}$ embryos or from in vitro differentiation of mutant ES cells. RNA transcripts for the megakaryocyte-specific product glycoprotein IIb are absent, and those for platelet factor-4 are vastly reduced. These observations signify a GATA-1–independent function for FOG in megakaryocyte development, imposed earlier than the block to maturation seen in the absence of GATA-1. Whereas these data demonstrate a requirement for FOG at the earliest steps in megakaryocyte development, they do not preclude FOG's functioning as a GATA-1 cofactor during mid-megakaryocyte development. It is likely, therefore, that FOG is critical to megakaryocyte gene transcription at multiple points in the development and maturation of the lineage.

The intricacies of the physical interaction of GATA-1 and FOG have been examined in depth by extensive mutagenesis of the N-finger of GATA-1.[122, 123] Several important amino acid residues have been identified within the N-finger that mediate interaction with finger-6 (or finger-1) of FOG. These lie on a contiguous surface projecting opposite to the face of the GATA-1 N-finger involved in DNA recognition. Altered specificity mutants of GATA-1 have been selected in yeast that disrupt interaction with FOG but preserve other properties of GATA-1, most notably normal DNA binding.[123] Forced expression of these novel GATA-1 mutants, together with suppressor or second-site FOG mutants that are restored for interaction, demonstrates that physical association of GATA-1 and FOG is, indeed, essential for proper terminal erythroid differentiation. In the absence of the GATA-1/FOG interaction, numerous GATA-1 target genes are not regulated appropriately. Nonetheless, a subset of targets, including EKLF (see below) and FOG itself, are largely FOG independent in their expression in erythroid cells. The use of altered specificity mutational analysis offers a stringent means of testing the biological relevance of pairwise protein associations in vivo.

The physical association of GATA-1 and FOG is a paradigm for the interaction of GATA factors with a novel class of complex zinc finger proteins. In *Drosophila,* the function of the GATA factor Pannier is controlled by a FOG-like polypeptide known as u-shaped (Ush).[124, 125] Like FOG, Ush interacts with the N-finger of Pannier. However, unlike FOG's effect on GATA-1 in erythroid cells, Ush appears to inhibit Pannier's function in neuronal development. Given the multiplicity of GATA factors in vertebrates, it seems likely that their transcriptional activities will be modulated either positively or negatively by an array of FOG/Ush-like proteins. These interactions provide a combinatorial basis for the function of GATA factors in different developmental contexts.

▼ EKLF: A FACTOR REQUIRED FOR β GLOBIN EXPRESSION AND DEFINITIVE RED CELL MATURATION

Gene promoters often contain CACC motifs within critical regions. These are bound by a variety of nuclear proteins, including the ubiquitous factor Sp1 and other Kruppel-related proteins. cDNA subtraction between erythroid and lymphoid transcripts culminated in the identification of a novel predicted protein, designated erythroid Kruppel-like factor (EKLF),[126] whose expression is highly restricted to erythroid cells of both primitive and definitive origin.[127] The EKLF gene promoter contains critical GATA motifs, consistent with the hypothesis that EKLF lies downstream of GATA-1 in a transcriptional hierarchy.[111] Moreover, an upstream enhancer of the gene contains a critical composite GATA–E box–GATA element that is required for maximal activity in vivo.[128]

EKLF binds avidly to an extended CACC motif present in the promoter of the adult β globin gene and serves as a transcriptional activator of reporter constructs bearing this element.[129] The CACC motifs to which EKLF binds are also sites of naturally occurring mutations in patients with β thalassemia.[130] Such variant CACC boxes are poorly bound by EKLF, consistent with a model in which EKLF serves as a specific activator of β globin gene expression. The β globin CACC box appears to be context dependent; that is, its introduction into the β globin promoter does not confer high-level sensitivity to expressed EKLF.[131, 132] Thus, interactions with other proteins binding the β globin promoter are likely to influence EKLF-dependent transcription.

Targeted mutation of the mouse EKLF leads to an embryonic lethal phenotype characterized by severe anemia at the fetal liver stage due to a failure in production of normal red blood cells and marked deficiency of β globin synthesis.[133, 134] This thalassemia-like phenotype supports the hypothesis that EKLF is required as a direct activator of β globin transcription. Although EKLF transcripts and protein are present in embryonic erythroblasts,[133] primitive erythropoiesis is not ostensibly impaired, reflecting either the lack of critical EKLF target genes in these cells or inactivity of EKLF itself. Experiments in which an LCR–β globin gene transgene was bred into an EKLF$^{-/-}$ background demonstrate, however, that EKLF is active and functional in embryonic cells.[135] Whether critical target genes for EKLF other than β globin exist in definitive erythroid cells is not established, although it is likely. Thus, EKLF is required for normal erythroid development.

Recent findings also suggest that EKLF is indirectly involved in regulating the switch from γ to β globin expression during the fetal-adult transition.[136, 137] Study of the pattern of expression of human globin transgenes in an EKLF$^{-/-}$ environment demonstrates that downregulation of γ globin expression in fetal liver erythroblasts is retarded in the absence of EKLF. Although it is clear that EKLF is not required to initiate the globin switch, its presence influences the shutoff of fetal globin expression, most likely by reducing competition for the globin LCR in its absence. It is envisioned that an association between the β globin promoter and the LCR takes place on gene activation, perhaps in part mediated by EKLF protein in a larger protein complex. In effect, this reduces the availability of the LCR for the γ globin gene regulatory elements and fosters extinction of fetal globin expression.

Some evidence suggests that EKLF function may be influenced by protein modifications, including phosphorylation within a postulated N-terminal interaction domain[138] and acetylation through association with histone acetyltransferases such as CBP/p300.[139] The extent to which these modifications contribute to EKLF's effects in vivo is uncertain. The concept that histone acetyltransferases are involved, however, fits well with data suggesting that transcriptional activation by EKLF in vitro requires association with a chromatin remodeling complex (E-RC1).[140] The interplay between EKLF and chromatin is further emphasized by altered DNA-binding specificity mutant analysis that implicates EKLF as an activator functioning through a site within hypersensitive site 3 (HS3) of the human β locus control region.[141]

▼ NF-E2: A FACTOR ESSENTIAL FOR MEGAKARYOCYTE DEVELOPMENT AND PLATELET BIOGENESIS BUT LARGELY DISPENSABLE FOR ERYTHROPOIESIS

The second erythroid transcription factor to be identified,[142] nuclear factor erythroid-2 (NF-E2) provides an interesting example of a factor considered likely to be critical in one lineage but subsequently found, instead, to be essential in another. NF-E2 was initially discovered as an erythroid-restricted activity that bound to AP-1–like sites in the promoter of the human porphobilinogen deaminase gene. Interest was stimulated by the demonstration that dimeric AP-1–like sites are present in HS2 of the human β-LCR and mediate enhancer action in transfected cells.[143] Further evidence from transgenic mouse studies indicated that HS2 could direct high-level globin gene expression in vivo, an activity also dependent on presumptive NF-E2 binding sites.[144]

Protein purification led to characterization of NF-E2 as an obligate heterodimer of a hematopoietic-restricted component (p45 NF-E2) and a more widely expressed polypeptide (p18 NF-E2, also known as MafK[145]).[146, 147] Both subunits are members of the basic leucine zipper (bZIP) family of factors. p45 NF-E2 is related in its primary sequence to a *Drosophila* protein, cap 'n' collar (CNC), and with it defines a subfamily of bZIP factors. p18 NF-E2 is related to a chicken viral oncoprotein v-*maf* and the retinal protein Nrl, and it defines the small Maf polypeptide family. The NF-E2 heterodimer recognizes an asymmetric, extended AP-1–like site. The p18 NF-E2 subunit, which lacks a transcriptional activation domain, confers specificity for the larger portion of the site. p45 NF-E2 provides an activation domain to the heterodimer.

Experiments in cultured mouse erythroleukemia (MEL) cells support an important role for NF-E2 in globin gene expression. Notably, MEL cells harboring integrated Friend virus sequences in the p45 NF-E2 locus do not express p45 NF-E2 and are not able to synthesize α or β globins at high level.[148] Reintroduction of p45 NF-E2 cDNA restores globin expression. Moreover, dominant negative forms of p18 NF-E2 impair globin expression when expressed in wild-type MEL cells.[149] Multiple regions of the amino terminus of p45 NF-E2 are required for rescue of globin expression,[150] suggesting that specific and multiple interactions are necessary for NF-E2–mediated transcription in vivo. One candidate for a mediator of NF-E2's transcriptional effects is the TAF component known as TAFIII-130.[151] Other interacting proteins include WW domain–containing proteins.[152] Additional in vitro studies also suggest that the NF-E2 complex is able to modulate chromatin structure in an adenosine triphosphate–dependent fashion, thereby possibly facilitating binding of other transcription factors, such as GATA-1, to critical elements (e.g., globin LCR HS2).[150, 153] The in vivo contribution of these interactions and phenomena to NF-E2 function remains to be established.

Despite the persuasive evidence linking NF-E2 to globin and erythroid gene expression, knockout of p45 NF-E2 in mice has only subtle effects on erythroid development; slight hypochromia, indicative of mildly reduced globin expression, is seen.[154] In this instance, it was demonstrated that loss of the p45 NF-E2 subunit alone abolished detectable NF-E2 DNA-binding activity in erythroid cells. Mice deficient in p18 NF-E2 are entirely normal, presumably owing to the presence of other small Maf polypeptides that substitute in heterodimer assembly with p45 NF-E2.[155] Remarkably, however, mice lacking p45 NF-E2 fail to produce circulating platelets and frequently succumb to severe bleeding in the immediate perinatal period.[156] This defect reflects delayed megakaryocyte maturation, accompanied by failure to form platelet territories and bud platelets. Thus, p45 NF-E2, like GATA-1 and FOG, is required for proper megakaryopoiesis. The block, however, appears somewhat later and does not affect megakaryocyte proliferation or the expression of early markers of the lineage. These roles for NF-E2 are compatible with the observed induction of p45 NF-E2 during megakaryocyte differentiation.

In normal megakaryocytes, p18 NF-E2/MafK constitutes only a minor fraction of the small Maf proteins in complex with p45 NF-E2.[157, 158] This is consistent with perturbed megakaryopoiesis seen in the absence of MafG.

Why NF-E2 appears not to be rate limiting for erythropoiesis in vivo is not yet fully explained. Although p45 NF-E2–like polypeptides, designated Nrf1 (LCRF1) and Nrf2, have been characterized, they do not substitute in its absence, as shown by the phenotypes and interbreeding of knockout mice and attempts to rescue globin expression in MEL cells lacking NF-E2.[159–164] Whether additional p45 NF-E2–related proteins known as Bach1 and Bach2 might substitute functionally in erythroid cells in its absence remains to be determined.[165] Further studies are needed to resolve the enigma of NF-E2's role in erythropoiesis.

▼ Mi: A FACTOR REQUIRED FOR PRODUCTION OF NORMAL MAST CELLS

Mast cells, as well as melanocytes, are deficient in the classical mouse mutants, *W* and *steel*, corresponding to defects in the c-Kit and c-Kit ligand (stem cell factor) loci. These cell types are also deficient in a mouse mutant *mi*-

crophthalmia (Mi), which also has reduced eye size, osteopetrosis, and early-onset deafness.[166] The similarities between these melanocyte and mast cell phenotypes suggested that the Mi locus might encode a protein required for transducing signals mediated by the c-Kit receptor.[167] Transgenic insertional mutagenesis led to identification of the Mi gene as a novel bHLH-zipper protein, which is expressed in anatomical sites affected in Mi mice.[166, 168] Mutations in the human counterpart of the Mi gene are seen in Waardenburg syndrome II, a form of human deafness.

The Mi protein appears to function as a major regulator of melanocyte development; it controls target genes encoding pigmentation enzymes[169] and also confers melanocyte characteristics to transfected fibroblasts.[170] Besides a deficiency of mast cells in Mi mice, specific mast cell proteases are reduced in their expression.[171, 172] For example, the E box bind motif for Mi is found in the protease 5 and 6 promoters. Of particular interest is the connection between the Mi protein and the c-Kit signaling pathway. Although current findings have been obtained in melanocytes, the general principles are likely to apply to Mi's function in mast cell transcription. Treatment of cells with c-Kit ligand leads to activation of mitogen-activated protein kinase and phosphorylation of Mi at a consensus target serine residue, which in turn upregulates Mi-dependent transactivation of a promoter reporter construct.[173] In part, this upregulation of Mi transactivation potential may be mediated through a phosphorylation-dependent interaction with CBP/p300.[174, 175] The modification of Mi protein by phosphorylation provides a mechanism by which signals received at the c-Kit receptor are transmitted to the transcriptional machinery. Presumably, failure of such signaling impairs mast cell proliferation in response to growth factors and leads to mast cell deficiency seen in Mi mutant mice.

▼ PU.1: AN Ets-RELATED FACTOR REQUIRED FOR BOTH MYELOID AND LYMPHOID DEVELOPMENT

PU.1 is a tissue-specific Ets family member,[176] which is encoded by the *spi-1* locus, whose deregulated expression caused by insertion of spleen focus-forming provirus leads to erythroleukemia in mice.[177] PU.1 is expressed principally in monocytes/macrophages and B lymphocytes. Lower level expression is also seen in granulocytes, early erythroid precursors, and megakaryocytes.[178] PU.1 recognizes a purine-rich sequence, GAGGAA (the PU box).[176] Numerous potential target genes for PU.1 have been identified on the basis of promoter analyses,[74] including immunoglobulin λ light chain; the integrin CD11b; and receptors for granulocyte-monocyte (GM)–CSF, granulocyte (G)–CSF, and M-CSF. At a selected set of sites, PU.1 recruits another factor, NF-EM5/Pip, dependent on phosphorylation of its PEST domain.[179, 180] PU.1 has been demonstrated to interact with a variety of other proteins, including the TATA-binding protein, retinoblastoma (Rb), NF-IL6, and high-mobility group (HMG) domain proteins, although the in vivo relevance of these associations remains to be tested.

Genetic experiments have provided conclusive evidence in support of PU.1's roles in both myeloid and lymphoid development, although the features of two different reported knockouts are not in complete agreement.[181, 182] Mutation of the locus in both instances leads to the failure to produce both B cells and macrophages. One of the mutant mouse strains is embryonic lethal late in gestation, although the basis for this is not clear. These mice have no T-cell development, and neutrophils are not detectable. In the other mutant strain, some T cells and neutrophils appear on treatment of newborn mice with antibiotics. Whether the phenotypic differences between the two PU.1 mutants can be accounted for by low-level residual expression in that with the milder phenotype is uncertain.[181] Nonetheless, taken together, these findings point to defects in multiple lineages, including both myeloid and lymphoid cells, in the absence (or near absence) of PU.1. Subsequent chimera experiments with homozygous mutant ES cells demonstrated that the hematopoietic defect is at the multipotential progenitor cell level, a finding that lends support to the existence of a common lymphoid and myeloid progenitor in the fetal liver.[183] Moreover, PU.1 appears to be required for development of osteoclasts, because its deficiency leads to osteopetrosis.[184]

The precise mechanisms through which PU.1 is essential for various lineages are under investigation. Experiments in chicken progenitors are interpreted to suggest that PU.1 can induce myeloid commitment by a coordinated series of events leading to activation of numerous myeloid genes and downregulation of non-myeloid regulators, most notably GATA-1.[28] In this system, these effects are dependent on the presence of an intact transactivation domain in PU.1. In vitro differentiation of homozygous mutant ES cells, however, suggests that myeloid (neutrophil/macrophage) progenitors arise in the absence of PU.1 but that these progenitors are not responsive to the myeloid-specific cytokines GM-CSF, G-CSF, and M-CSF.[185] Taken together, current data indicate that PU.1 controls both proliferation and differentiation pathways during myelopoiesis.[186]

▼ CCAAT/ENHANCER BINDING PROTEINS: FACTORS REQUIRED FOR GRANULOPOIESIS

The family of CCAAT/enhancer binding proteins[187] (C/EBPs) is composed of six bZIP-type transcription factors, which act either positively or negatively to control their target genes. Although they are expressed in diverse tissues,[188] specific C/EBPs, notably α and ε, are expressed in the myeloid lineage.[189, 190] Whereas C/EBPα is found in several different tissues, C/EBPε appears to be highly restricted to the hematopoietic system, and particularly within granulocytes and eosinophils.[191] C/EBP polypeptides bind DNA as heterodimers and homodimers, providing a high degree of complexity to regulation through this family. C/EBPα interacts and synergizes with other myeloid transcription factors, such as PU.1 and CBF, in the transcription of myeloid gene promoters.[74, 75] In addition, the DNA-binding domains of C/EBPα and Ets-1 interact and function in concert with GATA-1 to regulate eosinophil-specific promoters, such as that for the chicken EOS47 gene.[30]

Forced expression studies in several cell systems also provide evidence that C/EBP members activate expression of critical myeloid genes and may direct lineage selection.[31, 189] For example, expression of C/EBPε in a multipotential mouse cell line (EML-C1) stimulated expression of the receptor for M-CSF. Also, expression of C/EBPα in bipotential (granulocytic/monocytic) myeloid cells triggers granulocytic differentiation, upregulates the G-CSF receptor and secondary granule proteins, and blocks the monocytic program.

Genetic experiments reveal non-redundant roles for C/EBPα and C/EBPε in terminal myeloid development. Although animals lacking C/EBPα suffer from multiple abnormalities and succumb to impaired glycogenesis by the liver, this isoform is specifically required for neutrophil and eosinophil maturation.[192] Blast-like precursors are produced in the absence of this factor. The developmental block observed may in part relate to impaired expression of the G-CSF receptor. Likewise, neutrophil and eosinophil differentiation is also perturbed in the absence of C/EBPε.[193] In this instance, however, growth factor receptor expression may be increased, rather than reduced. Although C/EBPα and C/EBPε overlap in their expression, these genetic experiments reveal unique individual requirements and also place C/EBPε downstream of C/EBPα in the pathway to neutrophils and eosinophils.

Factors Required for the Development of Lymphoid Lineages

As with the myeloerythroid lineages, several transcription factors have been identified as essential regulators of lymphoid development. Given the more precise definition of subpopulations of lymphoid cells with numerous markers for which monoclonal antibodies have been obtained, the stages at which development is perturbed in gene knockout experiments have been more clearly elucidated. As with the myeloerythroid lineages, a multiplicity of factors of different protein classes have been identified. The discussion provided below is meant to be an introduction to the transcriptional regulation of lymphoid development.

▼ FACTORS INVOLVED BROADLY IN LYMPHOID DEVELOPMENT

PU.1

As noted above, loss of PU.1 function results in abnormalities of lymphoid development, principally absence of B lymphocytes. This defect appears to be manifest at the level of multipotential lymphoid-myeloid progenitors.[183] The role in T-lymphoid development is less certain, given the difference in phenotype of the two reported knockout strains.[181, 182] In one, T cells are absent; in the other, normal-appearing T cells are generated if mice are maintained with antibiotics.

Ikaros and Related Proteins

Zinc finger polypeptides of the Ikaros family are particularly interesting in relation to lymphopoiesis.[194] These proteins are characterized by two sets of Kruppel-like fingers, one that mediates dimer formation and another required for sequence-specific DNA binding.[195–197] The family includes three polypeptides (plus additional isoforms generated by alternative splicing): Ikaros, Aiolos, and Helios.[198–200] Ikaros was first identified through cDNA cloning of a T cell–enriched nuclear factor that interacts with the CD3 enhancer and isolated independently as a factor (LyF-1) binding to the terminal

deoxynucleotidyl transferase (TdT) promoter in B and T cells.[194, 196] The precise expression patterns of the various Ikaros family members are still being defined. Ikaros appears to be expressed from pluripotential progenitors (or HSCs) through mature lymphocytes, whereas Aiolos is first detected in committed progenitors with lymphoid potential. Thus, it has been suggested that Ikaros and Aiolos, as homomeric and heteromeric complexes, regulate target genes in lymphoid cells. Helios appears to be expressed also within immature progenitors and T but not B cells. Helios is stoichiometrically associated with Ikaros in T cells.

Whereas Ikaros proteins have potential binding sites in the promoters of numerous lymphoid-expressed genes and have been reported to activate transcription in reporter assays, the mechanisms by which they participate in gene regulation are uncertain. It was recently shown that rather than being associated with euchromatin, as would be anticipated for a positively acting transcription factor, Ikaros and Helios are specifically found in centromeric heterochromatin.[198, 201, 202] These observations support a model of nuclear organization in which genes that are repressed are selectively recruited into centromeric domains, in part through Ikaros proteins. The variation in isoform composition during lymphoid development and within lymphoid subpopulations predicts a complex role for Ikaros family polypeptides in lymphopoiesis.

An understanding of the in vivo roles of Ikaros through knockout studies has evolved with increasing appreciation of the complexity of Ikaros isoforms and biology. A mutation in the Ikaros DNA-binding domain was initially generated through gene targeting.[203] Homozygous mice lacked mature lymphoid cells and their progenitors, a finding interpreted as defining an essential role for Ikaros is all lymphoid lineages. Subsequent studies revealed that this initial modification of the locus generated a dominant negative mutation, such that homodimeric and heterodimeric complexes unable to bind DNA were formed. In mice heterozygous for this mutation, lymphopoiesis was deranged, leading to rapid accumulation of T lymphoblasts and eventual neoplastic transformation.[204] A null mutation at the Ikaros locus, on the other hand, displays defects in fetal T lymphocytes and fetal and adult B lymphocytes.[205] Natural killer cells are also absent. Thus, Ikaros function is differentially required in fetal and postnatal T-cell development. The differences between the original dominant negative and null phenotypes point to overlapping roles for Ikaros-related factors in the lymphoid system. Loss of Aiolos function in the mouse perturbs B-cell activation and maturation.[206] In the periphery, B cells show an activated cell surface phenotype. In contrast to conventional B cells, those of the peritoneum, the marginal zone, and the recirculating bone marrow population are reduced in number. Further studies of mice lacking Helios, and various combinations of these Ikaros-related factors, should elucidate precise requirements and the extent of "redundancy" in immature multipotential progenitors as well as in lymphoid lineages.

▼ FACTORS REQUIRED FOR B-CELL DEVELOPMENT

Pax-5/BSAP

A novel B cell–specific transcription factor, originally known as BSAP, was first identified as a mammalian homologue of a sea urchin protein that bound histone promoters.[207] On purification and cDNA cloning, BSAP was shown to encode Pax-5, a member of the paired domain family of DNA-binding protein.[208] Apart from its B-cell specificity, Pax-5/BSAP is expressed in the developing central nervous system, specifically within the mesencephalon and the spinal cord. Numerous potential target genes for Pax-5/BSAP in B cells have been identified by conventional reporter assays, including CD19.

Knockout of Pax-5/BSAP leads to a complete block of early B-lymphoid cell differentiation and to altered patterning of the posterior midbrain.[209] This role of Pax-5 overlaps that of Pax-2, as shown by interbreeding of Pax-2 and Pax-5 knockout strains.[210] Within the B-lymphoid compartment, Pax-5 function appears to differ during fetal and adult stages. In the bone marrow, B-cell development is arrested at the early pro-B cell stage and is characterized by absence of the markers CD19, CD25, and BP-1 but retention of expression of c-Kit, CD43, and $\lambda 5$.[211] Despite the inability to detect B-lymphoid progenitors in Pax-5$^{-/-}$ fetal livers, deficient fetal liver cells give rise to pre-B cells on bone marrow transplantation. In bone marrow cells, Pax-5$^{-/-}$ cells undergo D(H) to J(H) rearrangements, but V(H) to D(H)J(H) rearrangements are markedly reduced. Thus, Pax-5 is necessary in the pathway controlling V to DJ recombination.

The mechanisms of gene regulation by Pax-5 are multiple and complex. With rescue of differentiation of Pax-5$^{-/-}$ cells by introduction of conditional Pax-5 proteins, target genes have been identified.[212] The genes encoding the B-cell receptor component mb-1 (immunoglobulin subunit α) and transcription factors N-Myc and LEF-1 (see below) are positively regulated by the protein, whereas that for the cell surface protein PD-1 is repressed. Restoration of CD19 synthesis was highly dependent on the concentration of Pax-5. N-Myc expression was rescued only in the presence of full-length protein, whereas the DNA-binding portion of Pax-5 was sufficient to restore expression of mb-1 and LEF-1. Presumably, the DNA-binding domain recruits other proteins to an active transcriptional complex. Thus, Pax-5 acts both positively and negatively to regulate genes critical to B-lymphoid development.

E2A

Proteins expressed from the E2A locus, designated E12 and E47, are bHLH factors that form homodimers or heterodimers capable of binding E box sequences (CANNTG).[213, 214] The E box–binding family of proteins include ubiquitously expressed factors such as E12 and E47 and tissue-restricted factors such as MyoD and SCL/Tal-1. Functional studies have shown that the tissue-restricted factors (e.g., MyoD) require heterodimerization with E12 and E47 for biological activity.[215] In the case of SCL/Tal-1, it has been presumed that E12 and E47 represent the in vivo partners, although proteins related to E12 and E47 (e.g., HEB, E2-2) might also function. This must be the case, because the phenotypes of the E2A and SCL/Tal-1 knockouts in mice are not equivalent (see below). In some cases of human pre-B cell ALL harboring a t(1;19) translocation, E2A coding sequences outside its DNA-binding/dimerization regions are fused to the Prl homeoprotein.[216, 217]

Despite the widespread expression of E2A in tissues,

knockout of the gene in mice leads to a failure of B-lymphoid cell development.[218, 219] The block occurs at a relatively early stage of B-cell development, before D(H) to J(H) rearrangement and expression of B220. Heterozygous mice contain a reduced number of B cells, consistent with a gene-dosage effect. Knockout of other related and widely expressed factors (HEB and E2-2) alone, however, does not impair B-cell lymphopoiesis.[220] Replacement of the E2A gene with HEB sequences restores B-cell development, suggesting that the functional divergence of these proteins in different cell types is partially defined by the context of gene expression. Studies have revealed additional consequences of E2A loss in vivo, which point to an additional role in T-cell development. E2A$^{-/-}$ mice display a partial block in early T cells, which ultimately leads to the development of T-cell lymphomas.[221, 222] Thus, E2A function appears critical for maintaining the homeostasis of T lymphocytes. Inactivation of E2A function may be a common feature of T-cell malignant neoplasms, perhaps including those involving the heterodimeric partners SCL/Tal-1 and Lyl-1.

Oct-2 and Its Coactivator

Early experiments in cell-specific transcription demonstrated that a consensus octamer sequence plays a critical role in immunoglobulin gene expression in B lymphocytes. This led to the discovery of a cell-restricted homeodomain protein, Oct-2, one of the founding members of the subgroup containing a POU domain.[223–225] The POU homeodomain represents a bipartite DNA-binding motif. Determination of the precise transcriptional roles of Oct-2 is complicated by the existence of a ubiquitous factor, Oct-1.[226, 227]

Despite the initial suspicion that Oct-2 might fulfill broad functions in B cells, loss of function experiments suggested a more limited requirement. In null mice (which were neonatal lethal for unknown reasons), normal numbers of B cells are produced but a modest deficiency of immunoglobulin M$^+$ B cells is seen.[228] These B cells are significantly impaired in their capacity to secrete immunoglobulin on mitogenic stimulation. Although one might presume that the failure to observe a more striking effect on immunoglobulin gene expression in the knockout is due to redundancy by Oct-1 (which can activate transcription from immunoglobulin promoters in test assays), the situation may not be so simple. Targeted mutation of the Oct-2 locus in a murine B-cell line showed that reporters containing multiple octamer motifs were poorly expressed.[229] Thus, both Oct-2–dependent and Oct-2–independent pathways of octamer-mediated gene activation exist. Subsequent studies of Oct-2$^{-/-}$ mice have also shown that Oct-2 is required for the maintenance of peritoneal B-1 lymphocytes and for normal antigen-driven maturation of conventional B cells.[230] CD36 appears to be an authentic direct target of Oct-2 action in B cells.[231]

How specificity for B-cell transcription is conferred in the presence of two octamer-binding factors, Oct-1 and Oct-2, has been the subject of attention. In vitro transcription studies demonstrated the presence of a B-cell nuclear extract–enriched coactivator for these factors.[232] Subsequently, this novel protein, variously called OCA-B, OBF-1, or Bob-1, was identified both through protein purification and by protein interaction screening using Oct-2.[233, 234] As anticipated, this coactivator is B-cell restricted in its expression and acts along with Oct-1 or Oct-2 to drive octamer-dependent transcription. OCA-B/OBF-1/Bob-1 forms a ternary complex with Oct-1 or Oct-2 to recognize a subset of octamer sequences, thereby implicating the coactivator in a distinct set of B cell–expressed genes.[235, 236] B lymphocytes lacking OCA-B/OBF-1/Bob-1 are impaired in several respects.[237–239] Antigen-dependent B-cell maturation is affected, largely because of reduced levels of transcription from normally switched immunoglobulin heavy chain genes. In association with defective isotype production, germinal center formation is absent.

Early B-Cell Factor

Analysis of the promoter elements controlling expression of the mb-1 gene, which encodes a protein associated with membrane-bound antibody, led to the discovery of early B-cell factor (EBF).[240, 241] The binding site recognized by this factor is also present in the promoters of major histocompatibility complex and class II A α-D promoters. The protein is specifically expressed in pre-B and B cells but also within olfactory neuronal cells. In the latter setting, the identical protein was identified as Olf-1. DNA binding by EBF is mediated by a novel cysteine-rich zinc coordination motif, which also allows homodimerization.[242] Coexpression of EBF and the bHLH factor E47 in immature hematopoietic BaF3 cells induces expression of the endogenous immunoglobulin surrogate light chain genes λ5 and VpreB, whereas other pre-B cell–specific genes remain silent.[243] These findings suggest that the two proteins act in concert to control a subset of genes expressed during an early stage of B-cell development. Knockout of the EBF gene in mice has established its importance in vivo. EBF[−/−] mice lack B cells with rearranged immunoglobulin D and JH gene segments.[244] Nonetheless, they contain B220[+]/CD433[+] progenitor cells. Thus, EBF is essential at a stage before immunoglobulin gene rearrangement but subsequent to the commitment of progenitors to the B-cell lineage.

▼ FACTORS ESSENTIAL FOR T-LYMPHOCYTE DEVELOPMENT

LEF-1 and TCF-1

These proteins are closely related members of the HMG family, a set of regulators of cell specialization including the mammalian testis-determining factor SRY.[245] Binding sites for these factors are present in the T-cell antigen receptor α (TCRα) enhancer among others. Expression is seen in pre-B and T lymphocytes but not in more mature B cells. Most non-lymphoid tissues do not express these factors. Lymphoid enhancer factor-1 (LEF-1), however, is expressed in neural crest, mesencephalon, tooth germs, whisker follicles, and several other sites during embryogenesis. One of the most striking features of these proteins is their ability to bend DNA and, thereby, facilitate the assembly of protein complexes.[246] LEF-1, for example, is unable to activate transcription by itself on binding to DNA, suggesting that it serves an architectural role in organizing higher order nucleoprotein structures. Of particular interest, it has been demonstrated that LEF-1 interacts with β-catenin, a homologue of the *Drosophila* protein Armadillo, the most downstream compo-

nent defined in the wingless (Wnt) signaling pathway.[247, 248] Expressed LEF-1 and β-catenin form a complex within the nucleus. Whereas this interaction is likely to be important in many aspects of LEF-1 function, the interaction of LEF-1 and β-catenin does not appear important in the regulation of the TCRα enhancer. Rather, another cofactor, ALY, seems to associate with LEF-1 in this context.[249] Present data suggest, therefore, that LEF-1 (and presumably the closely related T-cell factor-1 [TCF-1]) subserve diverse regulatory functions by association with different protein cofactors.

Knockout of LEF-1 alone does not lead to defects of lymphoid development in mice. Instead, mutant mice lack teeth, mammary glands, whiskers, hair, and the mesencephalic nucleus of the trigeminal nerve.[250] Loss of TCF-1, on the other hand, leads to a partial block in thymocyte development at the transition from CD8[+], immature single-positive T cells to CD4[+]/CD8[+] cells.[251] Hence, the number of immunocompetent T cells in peripheral lymphoid organs is significantly reduced. The similarity of LEF-1 and TCF-1 in their structure and pattern of expression in lymphoid cells suggested potential redundancy. Loss of either protein alone does not affect TCRα gene expression. Combined deficiency of LEF-1 and TCF-1, however, leads to complete arrest at the immature CD8[+] stage.[252] Moreover, TCRα gene transcription is markedly reduced. Thus, LEF-1 and TCR-1 are overlapping in their function in T-cell development.

GATA-3

The enhancer for the TCRα gene is also bound by GATA-3, one of the three GATA family proteins expressed in hematopoietic lineages.[253] Whereas GATA-3 expression has been detected in multipotential progenitors, particularly in chicken, it is best characterized in T cells, where it is expressed exceedingly early in the lineage and apparently coexpressed with TCF-1. Like other enhancer binding proteins, GATA-3 appears to act in concert with other factors as part of a larger nucleoprotein complex.

Germline knockout of GATA-3 is embryonic lethal in the mouse because of complex developmental abnormalities at midgestation.[254] More specific analysis of the effects of GATA-3 loss on lymphoid development with use of chimeric mice demonstrates that GATA-3[−/−] cells cannot give rise to detectable T-cell progenitors.[255] Differentiation is blocked before the earliest double-negative CD4[−]/CD8[−] stage, whereas development of other hematopoietic lineages is ostensibly normal. Thus, GATA-3 is an essential regulator of very early thymocyte development. More recent studies demonstrate that GATA-3 is selectively expressed in the CD4[+] T-helper 2 (Th2) population, which produces various cytokines including interleukins 4 and 5. GATA-3 expression is extinguished in the Th1 subset.[256] Antisense inhibition of GATA-3 inhibits cytokine expression, whereas elevated expression of GATA-3 in the CD4 cells of transgenic mice induces Th2 cytokine expression in Th1 cells. Therefore, GATA-3 functions later within lymphoid development to drive Th2 cytokine gene expression. GATA-3 provides a clear example of a regulatory factor used selectively at different stages of development of a lineage.

Possible Mechanisms of Lineage Selection

Through the studies reviewed above, the in vivo requirements for numerous transcription factors in hematopoietic development have been established, as summarized schematically on the traditional developmental hierarchy in Figure 3–7. Blocks in development provide compelling evidence of the involvement of these factors but fail to convey the inherent complexity and regulatory interactions operative during the progression of stem cells to single lineage–committed precursors. Blocks early in the hierarchy obscure later roles for many factors, whereas late blocks underestimate early functions that may be partially compensated by the action of related factors or other pathways. Nonetheless, the establishment of in vivo requirements lays the foundation for considering how hematopoietic development is achieved at a dynamic level.

How are specific hematopoietic lineage programs established? In considering this central question, it is useful to review some of the principles that are emerging from studies of regulatory factors in hematopoietic cells. Four sets of observations underlie current model building.

First, hematopoietic progenitors and cell lines are highly plastic in their developmental potentials.[257] Thus, although conventional hierarchy diagrams of hematopoiesis are widely presented, there appears to be no unique and simple set of roadmaps from multipotential progenitor to unilineage-committed precursor.

Second, whereas single transcription factors do not fulfill all criteria of "master" regulators in converting any cell type to a unique blood lineage, single factors, or pairs of factors, are potent in altering the phenotype of hematopoietic cells under defined circumstances. As noted previously, the transcription factors GATA-1, PU.1, SCL/Tal-1, and C/EBP act as dominant regulators of phenotype in various test systems.[23–31] Often, such lineage effects are potentiated by the coexpression of another protein, such as in the augmentation of GATA-1 function on addition of FOG,[119] or blunted, as in the inhibition of Ets-1 transactivation by MafB.[258] Thus, combinatorial control is exercised at the level of pairs (or greater numbers) of cell-specific regulators.

Third, multiple lines of evidence now indicate that protein/protein interactions and the formation of multiprotein hematopoietic-specific protein complexes are important determinants of transcription in hematopoietic cells. At their simplest, these may include protein pairs, such as GATA-1 and FOG, or Ets-1 and MafB. The assembly of a larger complex containing GATA-1, SCL/Tal-1, E12, Rbtn2/Lmo2, and Ldb1 on a composite GATA–E box DNA element[59] and the ability of GATA-1, and several other transcription factors, to recruit additional proteins, such as CBP/p300,[118] predict the existence of numerous, and heterogeneous, hematopoietic-specific complexes. Although direct data are lacking, it is most likely that the critical hematopoietic transcription factors are present in multiple complexes of different composition, rather than in a single complex. Moreover, given the dynamic expression of many factors throughout hematopoietic development, the composition of these complexes probably changes during progression from HSCs to committed precursors. In many instances, members of a transcription factor family may be exchanged within a multiprotein complex. For example, GATA-1 may replace GATA-2 during the shift from HSCs to later progenitors, or different C/EBP polypeptides may predominate at different stages of myeloid development. The assembly and disassembly of multiprotein complexes provides a dynamic means by which transcriptional control may be modulated by changing transcription factor levels or interaction affinities rather than by the mere presence or absence of single regulators.[1, 2, 259]

Finally, multilineage gene expression programs are activated in progenitors before unilineage commitment. For example, single-cell transcript analysis demonstrates the simultaneous expression of erythroid- and myeloid-specific markers[260] and the simultaneous accessibility of globin and immunoglobulin loci[261] in multipotential progenitors. At subsequent stages of lineage commitment, unilineage patterns of chromatin accessibility and gene expression are evident. This "promiscuity" in multipotential progenitors is in agreement with the observed expression of many lineage-restricted transcription factors (e.g., GATA-1, FOG, PU.1, Ikaros, NF-E2) in progenitors that have not yet committed to a single pathway. Whether multilineage gene activation

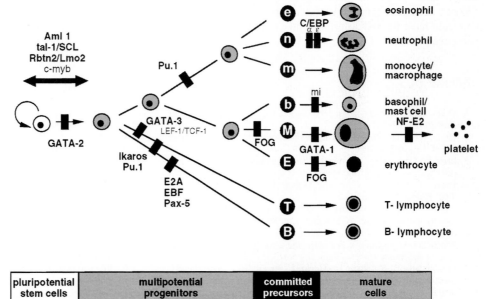

Figure 3–7. Transcription factor requirements in hematopoiesis. Schematic representation of in vivo roles of transcription factors. See text and Table 3–1 for details. Black boxes depict arrests in development in the absence of each factor.

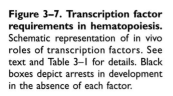

reflects priming of specific loci for later expression or is incidental to the action of multiprotein transcriptional complexes is uncertain. One view is that multipotential progenitors are rehearsing for the "final" performance.

Taking these features together, we are led to a model of hematopoietic development in which combinatorial control is exercised not only at the level of expression of lineage-enriched transcriptional regulators but also through multiple, yet selective, protein/protein interactions. The pivotal involvement of multiprotein complexes, although seemingly unnecessarily convoluted, provides many potential advantages. By preassembly of some complexes, or portions of complexes, multipotential progenitors are poised for lineage commitment by the addition, or replacement, of one component without the need to initiate their formation from "scratch." Furthermore, as long as one protein within a complex is competent to bind DNA in a sequence-specific manner, the recruitment of transcription factors to complexes through protein/protein interaction provides a versatility to otherwise conventional nuclear factors. That is, DNA binding by all factors may not be required at some *cis*-regulatory elements. The compartmentalization of the nucleus, as exemplified by the findings with Ikaros proteins,[198, 202] suggests that the action of protein complexes may vary, depending on their context. If, as seems probable, multiprotein complexes are fundamental to the transcriptional determination of lineage and cellular maturation, their changing compositions are predicted to drive development from pluripotent stem cells to committed precursors through hematopoiesis. An obvious implication of such models is that mere definition of expression profiles of RNAs in progenitor subpopulations is unlikely to elucidate the mechanisms by which cells commit to particular developmental pathways.

Current models of hematopoietic development are readily reconciled with the consistent involvement of transcription factors in leukemogenesis. Ectopic expression of critical factors or expression of chimeric proteins in leukemias would be expected to upset the finely tuned balance of regulators and, in effect, "freeze" cells and render them unable to complete their developmental programs.[262] This convergence of normal and leukemic differentiation may account for why genes discovered first in the context of leukemia have figured so prominently in normal hematopoietic development.

REFERENCES

1. Orkin, S.H.: Hematopoiesis: how does it happen? Curr. Opin. Cell Biol. 7:870, 1995.
2. Orkin, S.H.: Development of the hematopoietic system. Curr. Opin. Genet. Dev. 6:597, 1996.
3. Metcalf, D.: Lineage commitment and maturation in hematopoietic cells: the case for extrinsic regulation. Blood 92:345, 1998.
4. Enver, T., Heyworth, C.M., and Dexter, T.M.: Do stem cells play dice? Blood 92:348, 1998.
5. Medvinsky, A., and Dzierzak, E.: Definitive hematopoiesis is autonomously initiated by the AGM region. Cell 86:897, 1996.
6. Sanchez, M.-J., Holmes, A., Miles, C., and Dzierzak, E.: Characterization of the first definitive hematopoietic stem cells in the AGM and liver of the mouse embryo. Immunity 5:513, 1996.
7. Mukouyama, Y.-S., Hara, T., Xu, M.-J., Tamura, K., Donovan, P.J., Nakahata, T., and Miyajima, A.: In vitro expansion of murine multipotential hematopoietic progenitors from the embryonic aorta-gonad-mesonephros region. Immunity 8:105, 1998.
8. Yoder, M.C., Hiatt, K., Dutt, P., Mukherjee, P., Bodine, D.M., and Orlic, D.: Characterization of definitive lymphohematopoietic stem cells in the day 9 murine yolk sac. Immunity 7:335, 1997.
9. Kennedy, M., Firpo, M., Choi, K., Wall, C., Robertson, S., Kabrun, N., and Keller, G.: A common precursor for primitive erythropoiesis and definitive hematopoiesis. Nature 386:488, 1997.
10. Pardanaud, L., Yassine, F., and Dieterlen-Lievre, F.: Relationship between vasculogenesis, angiogenesis, and haemopoiesis during avian ontogeny. Development 105:473, 1989.
11. Choi, K., Kennedy, M., Kazarov, A., Papadimitriou, J.C., and Keller, G.: A common precursor for hematopoietic and endothelial cells. Development 125:725, 1998.
12. Nishikawa, S.-I., Nishikawa, S., Kawamoto, H., Yoshida, H., Kizumoto, M., Kataoka, H., and Katsura, Y.: In vitro generation of lymphohematopoietic cells from endothelial cells purified from murine embryos. Immunity 8:761, 1998.
13. Shalaby, F., Rossant, J., Yamaguchi, T.P., Breitman, M.L., and Schuh, A.C.: Failure of blood island formation and vasculogenesis in flk-1 deficient mice. Nature 376:62, 1995.
14. Tsai, S.F., Martin, D.I., Zon, L.I., D'Andrea, A.D., Wong, G.G., and Orkin, S.H.: Cloning of cDNA for the major DNA-binding protein of the erythroid lineage through expression in mammalian cells. Nature 339:446, 1989.
15. Rabbitts, T.H.: Chromosomal translocations in human cancer. Nature 372:143, 1994.
16. Capecchi, M.R.: Altering the genome by homologous recombination. Science 244:1288, 1989.
17. Keller, G., Kennedy, M., Papayannopoulou, T., and Wiles, M.V.: Hematopoietic differentiation during embryonic stem cell differentiation in culture. Mol. Cell. Biol. 13:472, 1993.
18. Weiss, M.J., and Orkin, S.H.: In vitro differentiation of murine embryonic stem cells. New approaches to old problems. J. Clin. Invest. 97:591, 1996.
19. Keller, G., Wall, C., Fong, A.Z.C., Hawley, T.S., and Hawley, R.G.: Overexpression of HOX11 leads to the immortalization of embryonic precursors with both primitive and definitive hematopoietic potential. Blood 92:877, 1998.
20. Weiss, M.J., Yu, C., and Orkin, S.H.: Erythroid-cell-specific properties of transcription factor GATA-1 revealed by phenotypic rescue of a gene-targeted cell line. Mol. Cell. Biol. 17:1642, 1997.
21. Pevny, L., Simon, M.C., Robertson, E., Klein, W.H., Tsai, S.-F., D'Agati, V., Orkin, S.H., and Costantini, F.: Erythroid differentiation in chimeric mice blocked by a targeted mutation in the gene for transcription factor GATA-1. Nature 349:257, 1991.
22. Weintraub, H., Davis, R., Tapscott, S., Thayer, M., Krause, M., Benezra, R., Blackwell, T.K., Turner, D., Rupp, R., and Hollenberg, S.: The myoD gene family: nodal point during specification of the muscle cell lineage. Science 251:761, 1991.
23. Kulessa, H., Frampton, J., and Graf, T.: GATA-1 reprograms avian myelomonocytic cells into eosinophils, thromboblasts and erythroblasts. Genes Dev. 9:1250, 1995.
24. Visvader, J.E., Elefanty, A.G., Strasser, A., and Adams, J.M.: GATA-1 but not SCL induces megakaryocytic differentiation in an early myeloid line. EMBO J. 11:4557, 1992.
25. Mead, P.E., Kelley, C.M., Hahn, P.S., Piedad, O., and Zon, L.I.: SCL specifies hematopoietic mesoderm in *Xenopus* embryos. Development 125:2611, 1998.
26. Gering, M., Rodaway, A.R.F., Gottgens, B., Patient, R.K., and Green, A.R.: The SCL gene specifies haemangioblast development from early mesoderm. EMBO J. 17:4029, 1998.
27. Liao, E.C., Paw, B.H., Oates, A.C., Pratt, S.J., Postlethwait, J.H., and Zon, L.I.: SCL/Tal-1 transcription factor acts downstream of *cloche* to specify hematopoietic and vascular progenitors in zebrafish. Genes Dev. 12:621, 1998.
28. Nerlov, C., and Graf, T.: PU.1 induces myeloid lineage commitment in multipotent hematopoietic progenitors. Genes Dev. 12:2403, 1998.
29. Muller, C., Kowenz-Leutz, E., Grieser-Ade, S., Graf, T., and Leutz, A.: NF-M (chicken C/EBP) induces eosinophilic differentiation and apoptosis in a hematopoietic progenitor cell line. EMBO J. 14:6127, 1995.
30. McNagny, K.M., Sieweke, M.H., Doderlein, G., Graf, T., and Nerlov, C.: Regulation of eosinophil-specific gene expression by a C/EBP-Ets complex and GATA-1. EMBO J. 17:3669, 1998.
31. Radomska, H.S., Huettner, C.S., Zhang, P., Cheng, T., Scadden, D.T., and Tenen, D.G.: CCAAT/enhancer binding protein is a regulatory

switch sufficient for induction of granulocytic development from bipotential myeloid progenitors. Mol. Cell. Biol. 18:4301, 1998.

32. Look, A.T.: Oncogenic transcription factors in the human acute leukemias. Science 278:1059, 1997.

33. Helgason, C.D., Sauvageau, G., Lawrence, H.J., Largman, C., and Humphries, R.K.: Overexpression of HOXB4 enhances the hematopoietic potential of embryonic stem cells differentiated in vitro. Blood 87:2740, 1996.

34. Chen, Q., Cheng, J.-T., Tsai, L.-H., Schneider, N., Buchanan, G., Carroll, A., Crist, W., Ozanne, B., Siciliano, M.J., and Baer, R.: The tal gene undergoes chromosome translocation in T cell leukemia and potentially encodes a helix-loop-helix protein. EMBO J. 9:415, 1990.

35. Begley, C.G., Aplan, P.D., Denning, S.M., Haynes, B.F., Waldmann, T.A., and Kirsch, I.R.: The gene SCL is expressed during early hematopoiesis and encodes a differentiation-related DNA-binding motif. Proc. Natl. Acad. Sci. USA 86:10128, 1989.

36. Brown, L., Cheng, J.-T., Chen, Q., Siciliano, M.J., Crist, W., Buchanan, G., and Baer, R.: Site-specific recombination of the tal-1 gene is a common occurrence in human T cell leukemia. EMBO J. 9:3343, 1990.

37. Aplan, P.D., Lombardi, D.P., and Kirsch, I.R.: Structural characterization of SIL, a gene frequently disrupted in T-cell acute lymphoblastic leukemia. Mol. Cell. Biol. 11:5462, 1991.

38. Visvader, J., Begley, C.G., and Adams, J.M.: Differential expression of the Lyl, SCL, and E2a helix-loop-helix genes within the hemopoietic system. Oncogene 6:187, 1991.

39. Green, A.R., Salvaris, E., and Begley, C.G.: Erythroid expression of the helix-loop-helix gene, SCL. Oncogene 6:475, 1991.

40. Green, A.R., Lints, T., Visvader, J., Harvey, R., and Begley, C.G.: *SCL* is coexpressed with GATA-1 in hemopoietic cells but is also expressed in developing brain. Oncogene 6:475, 1992.

41. Kallianpur, A.R., Jordan, J.E., and Brandt, S.J.: The SCL/TAL-1 gene is expressed in progenitors of both the hematopoietic and vascular systems during embryogenesis. Blood 83:1200, 1994.

42. Drake, C.J., Brandt, S.J., Trusk, T.C., and Little, C.D.: TAL1/SCL is expressed in endothelial progenitor cells/angioblasts and defines a dorsal-to-ventral gradient of vasculogenesis. Dev. Biol. 192:17, 1997.

43. Hsu, H.-L., Cheng, J.-T., Chen, Q., and Baer, R.: Enhancer-binding activity of the tal-1 oncoprotein in association with the E47/E12 helix-loop-helix proteins. Mol. Cell. Biol. 11:3037, 1991.

44. Kelliher, M.A., Seldin, D.C., and Leder, P.: Tal-1 induces T cell acute lymphoblastic leukemia accelerated by casein kinase II. EMBO J. 115:5160, 1996.

45. Condorelli, G.L., Facchiano, F., Valtieri, M., Proietti, E., Vitelli, L., Lulli, V., Huebner, K., Peschle, C., and Croce, C.M.: T-cell-directed TAL-1 expression induces T-cell malignancies in transgenic mice. Cancer Res. 56:5113, 1996.

46. Larson, R.C., Lavenir, I., Larson, T.A., Baer, R., Warren, A.J., Wadman, I., Nottage, K., and Rabbitts, T.H.: Protein dimerization between Lmo2 (Rbtn2) and Tal1 alters thymocyte development and potentiates T cell tumorigenesis in transgenic mice. EMBO J. 15:1021, 1996.

47. Detrich, H.W., Kieran, M.W., Chan, F.W., Barone, L.M., Yee, K., Rundstadler, J.A., Pratt, S., Ransom, D., and Zon, L.I.: Intra-embryonic hematopoietic cell migration during vertebrate development. Proc. Natl. Acad. Sci. USA 92:10713, 1995.

48. Aplan, P.D., Nakahara, K., Orkin, S.H., and Kirsch, I.R.: The SCL gene product: a positive regulator of erythroid differentiation. EMBO J. 11:4073, 1992.

49. Shivdasani, R., Mayer, E., and Orkin, S.H.: Absence of blood formation in mice lacking the T-cell leukemia oncoprotein tal-1/SCL. Nature 373:432, 1995.

50. Robb, L., Lyons, I., Li, R., Hartley, L., Kontgen, F., Harvey, R.P., Metcalf, D., and Begley, C.G.: Absence of yolk sac hematopoiesis from mice with a targeted disruption of the scl gene. Proc. Natl. Acad. Sci. USA 92:7075, 1995.

51. Robb, L., Elwood, N.J., Elefanty, A.G., Kontgen, F., Li, R., Barnett, L.D., and Begley, C.G.: The scl gene product is required for the generation of all hematopoietic lineages in the adult mouse. EMBO J. 15:4123, 1996.

52. Porcher, C., Swat, W., Rockwell, K., Fujiwara, Y., Alt, F.W., and Orkin, S.H.: The T-cell leukemia oncoprotein SCL/tal-1 is essential for development of all hematopoietic lineages. Cell 86:47, 1996.

53. Visvader, J.E., Fujiwara, Y., and Orkin, S.H.: Unsuspected role for the T-cell leukemia protein SCL/tal-1 in vascular development. Genes Dev. 12:473, 1998.

54. Cohen-Kaminsky, S., Maouche-Chretien, L., Vitelli, L., Vinit, M.A., Blanchard, I., Yamamoto, M., Peschle, C., and Romeo, P.H.: Chromatin immunoselection defines a TAL-1 target gene. EMBO J. 17:5151, 1998.

55. Krosl, G., He, G., Lefrancois, M., Charron, F., Romeo, P.H., Jolicoeur, P., Kirsch, I.R., Nemer, M., and Hoang, T.: Transcription factor SCL is required for c-kit expression and c-Kit function in hemopoietic cells. J. Exp. Med. 188:439, 1998.

56. Boehm, T., Foroni, L., Kaneko, Y., Perutz, M.P., and Rabbitts, T.H.: The rhombotin family of cysteine-rich LIM-domain oncogenes: distinct members are involved in T-cell translocations to human chromosomes 11p15 and 11p13. Proc. Natl. Acad. Sci. USA 88:4367, 1991.

57. Royer-Pokora, B., Loos, U., and Ludwig, W.-D.: TTG-2, a new gene encoding a cysteine-rich protein with the LIM motif, is overexpressed in acute T-cell leukaemia with the t(11;14)(p13;q11). Oncogene 6:1887, 1991.

58. Valge-Archer, V.E., Osada, H., Warren, A.J., Forster, A., Li, J., Baer, R., and Rabbitts, T.H.: The LIM protein RBTN2 and the basic helix-loop-helix protein TAL1 are present in a complex in erythroid cells. Proc. Natl. Acad. Sci. USA 91:8617, 1994.

59. Wadman, I.S., Osada, H., Grutz, G.G., Agulnick, A.D., Westphal, H., Forster, A., and Rabbitts, T.H.: The LIM-only protein Lmo2 is a bridging molecule assembling an erythroid, DNA-binding complex which includes TAL1, E47, GATA-1, and Ldb1/NL1 proteins. EMBO J. 16:3145, 1997.

60. Yamada, Y., Warren, A.J., Dobson, C., Forster, A., Pannell, R., and Rabbitts, T.H.: The T cell leukemia LIM protein Lmo2 is necessary for adult mouse hematopoiesis. Proc. Natl. Acad. Sci. USA 95:3890, 1998.

61. Wang, S.W., and Speck, N.A.: Purification of core-binding factor, a protein that binds the conserved core site in murine leukemia virus enhancers. Mol. Cell. Biol. 12:89, 1992.

62. Ogawa, E., Inuzuka, M., Maruyama, M., Satake, M., Naito-Fujimoto, M., Ito, Y., and Shigesada, K.: Molecular cloning and characterization of PEBP2β, the heterodimeric partner of a novel *Drosophila* runt-related DNA binding protein PEBP2α. Virology 194:314, 1993.

63. Ogawa, E., Maruyama, M., Kagoshima, H., Inuzuka, M., Lu, J., Satake, M., Shigesada, K., and Ito, Y.: PEBP2/PEA2 represents a new family of transcription factor homologous to the products of the *Drosophila* runt and the human AML1 gene. Proc. Natl. Acad. Sci. USA 90:6859, 1993.

64. Wang, S., Wang, Q., Crute, B.E., Melnikova, I.N., Keller, S.R., and Speck, N.A.: Cloning and characterization of subunits of the T-cell receptor and murine leukemia virus enhancer core-binding factor. Mol. Cell. Biol. 13:3324, 1993.

65. Liu, P., Tarle, S.A., Hajra, A., Claxton, D.F., Marlton, P., Freedman, M., Siciliano, M.J., and Collins, F.S.: Fusion between transcription factor CBFb/PEBP2b and a myosin heavy chain in acute myeloid leukemia. Science 261:1041, 1993.

66. Yergeau, D.A., Hetherington, C.J., Wang, Q., Zhang, P., Sharpe, A.H., Binder, M., Marin-Padilla, M., Tenen, D.G., Speck, N.A., and Zhang, D.-E.: Embryonic lethality and impairment of haematopoiesis in mice heterozygous for an AML1-ETO fusion gene. Nat. Genet. 15:303, 1997.

67. Castilla, L., Wijmenga, C., Wang, Q., Stacy, T., Speck, N.A., Eckhaus, M., Marin-Padilla, M., Collins, F.S., Wynshaw-Boris, A., and Liu, P.P.: Failure of embryonic hematopoiesis and lethal hemorrhages in mouse embryos heterozyous for a knocked-in leukemia gene CBFB-MYH11. Cell 87:687, 1996.

68. Okuda, T., Cai, Z., Yang, S., Lenny, N., Lyu, C.J., van Deursen, J.M., Harada, H., and Downing, J.R.: Expression of a knocked-in AML1-ETO leukemia gene inhibits the establishment of normal definitive hematopoiesis and directly generates dysplastic hematopoietic progenitors. Blood 91:3134, 1998.

69. Okuda, T., Deursen, J.V., Hiebert, S.W., Grosveld, G., and Downing, J.R.: AML1, the target of multiple chromosomal translocations in human leukemia, is essential for normal fetal liver hematopoiesis. Cell 84:321, 1996.

70. Wang, Q., Stacy, T., Miller, J.D., Lewis, A.F., Gu, T.L., Huang, X., Bushweller, J.H., Bories, J.C., Alt, F.W., Ryan, G., Liu, P.P., Wynshaw-Boris, A., Binder, M., Marin-Padilla, M., Sharpe, A.H., and Speck, N.A.: The CBFβ subunit is essential for CBFα2(AML1) function in vivo. Cell 87:697, 1996.

71. Wang, Q., Stacy, T., Binder, M., Marin-Padilla, M., Sharpe, A.H., and Speck, N.A.: Disruption of the *Cbfa2* gene causes necrosis and

hemorrhaging in the central nervous system and blocks definitive hematopoiesis. Proc. Natl. Acad. Sci. USA 93:3444, 1996.

72. Tracey, W.D.J., Pepling, M.E., Horb, M.E., Thomsen, G.H., and Gergen, J.P.: A *Xenopus* homologue of aml-1 reveals unexpected patterning mechanisms leading to the formation of embryonic blood. Development 125:1371, 1998.

73. Kitabayashi, I., Yokoyama, A., Shimizu, K., and Ohki, M.: Interaction and functional cooperation of the leukemia-associated factors AML1 and p300 in myeloid cell differentiation. EMBO J. 17:2994, 1998.

74. Petrovick, M.S., Hiebert, S.W., Friedman, A.D., Hetherington, C.J., Tenen, D.G., and Zhang, D.E.: Multiple functional domains of AML1: PU.1 and C/EBPalpha synergize with different regions of AML1. Mol. Cell. Biol. 18:3915, 1998.

75. Zhang, D.E., Hetherington, C.J., Meyers, S., Rhoades, K.L., Larson, C.J., Chen, H.M., Hiebert, S.W., and Tenen, D.G.: CCAAT enhancer-binding protein (C/EBP) and AML1 (CBFalpha2) synergistically activate the macrophage colony-stimulating factor receptor promoter. Mol. Cell. Biol. 16:1231, 1996.

76. North, T.E., Gu, T.-L., Stacy, T., Wang, Q., Howard, L., Binder, M., Marin-Padilla, M., and Speck, N.A.: Cbfa2 is required for the formation of intra-aortic hematopoietic clusters. Development 126:2563, 1999.

77. Dorfman, D.M., Wilson, D.B., Bruns, G.A., and Orkin, S.H.: Human transcription factor GATA-2. Evidence for regulation of preproendothelin-1 gene expression in endothelial cells. J. Biol. Chem. 267:1279, 1992.

78. Tsai, F.-Y., Keller, G., Kuo, F.C., Weiss, M.J., Chen, J.-Z., Rosenblatt, M., Alt, F., and Orkin, S.H.: An early haematopoietic defect in mice lacking the transcription factor GATA-2. Nature 371:221, 1994.

79. Briegel, K., Lim, K.-C., Plank, C., Beug, H., Engel, J., and Zenke, M.: Ectopic expression of a conditional GATA-2/estrogen receptor chimera arrests erythroid differentiation in a hormone-dependent manner. Genes Dev. 7:1097, 1993.

80. Tsai, F.-Y., and Orkin, S.H.: Transcription factor GATA-2 is required for proliferation/survival of early hematopoietic cells and mast cell formation, but not for erythroid and myeloid terminal differentiation. Blood 89:3636, 1997.

81. Shen, W.-F., Largman, C., Lowney, P., Corral, J.C., Detmer, K., Hauser, C.A., Simonitchk, T.A., Hack, F.M., and Lawrence, H.J.: Lineage-restricted expression of homeobox-containing genes in human hematopoietic cell lines. Proc. Natl. Acad. Sci. USA 86:8536, 1989.

82. Sauvageau, G., Thorsteinsdottir, U., Eaves, C.J., Lawrence, H.J., Largman, C., Landsorp, P.M., and Humphries, R.K.: Overexpression of HOXB4 in hematopoietic cells causes the selective expansion of more primitive populations in vitro and in vivo. Genes Dev. 9:1753, 1995.

83. Thorsteinsdottir, U., Sauvageau, G., Hough, M.R., Dragowska, W., Lansdorp, P.M., Lawrence, H.J., Largman, C., and Humphries, R.K.: Overexpression of HOXA10 in murine hematopoietic cells perturbs both myeloid and lymphoid differentiation and leads to acute myeloid leukemia. Mol. Cell. Biol. 17:495, 1997.

84. Izon, D.J., Rozenfeld, S., Fong, S.T., Komuves, L., Largman, C., and Lawrence, H.J.: Loss of function of the homeobox gene Hoxa-9 perturbs early T-cell development and induces apoptosis in primitive thymocytes. Blood 92:383, 1998.

85. Kroon, E., Krosl, J., Thorsteinsdottir, U., Baban, S., Buchberg, A., and Sauvageau, G.: Hoxa9 transforms primary bone marrow cells through specific collaboration with Meis1a but not Pbx1b. EMBO J. 17:3714, 1998.

86. Nakamura, T., Largaespada, D.A., Lee, M.P., Johnson, L.A., Ohyashiki, K., Toyama, K., Chen, S.J., Willman, C.L., Chen, I.M., Feinberg, A.P., Jenkins, N.A., Copeland, N.G., and Shaughnessy, J.D. Jr.: Fusion of the nucleoporin gene NUP98 to HOXA9 by the chromosome translocation t(7;11)(p15;p15) in human myeloid leukemia. Nat. Genet. 12:154, 1996.

87. Borrow, J., Shearman, A.M., Stanton, V.P. Jr., Becher, R., Collins, T., Williams, A.J., Dube, I., Katz, F., Kwong, Y.L., Morris, C., Ohyashiki, K., Toyama, K., Rowley, J., and Housman, D.E.: The t(7;11)(p15;p15) translocation in acute myeloid leukemia fuses the genes for nucleoporin NUP98 and class I homeoprotein HOXA9. Nat. Genet. 12:159, 1996.

88. Yu, B.D., Hess, J.L., Horning, S.E., Brown, G.A.J., and Korsmeyer, S.J.: Altered Hox expression and segmental identity in Mll-mutant mice. Nature 378:505, 1995.

89. Hess, J.L., Yu, B.D., Li, B., Hanson, R., and Korsmeyer, S.J.: Defects in yolk sac hematopoiesis in Mll-null embryos. Blood 90:1799, 1997.

90. Yagi, H., Deguchi, K., Aono, A., Tani, Y., Kishimoto, T., and Komori, T.: Growth disturbance in fetal liver hematopoiesis of Mll-mutant mice. Blood 92:108, 1998.

91. Mead, P.E., Brinvanlou, I.H., Kelley, C.M., and Zon, L.I.: BMP-4 responsive regulation of dorsoventral patterning by the homeobox protein Mix.1. Nature 382:357, 1996.

92. Porter, F.D., Drago, J., Xu, Y., Cheema, S.S., Wassif, C., Huang, S.P., Lee, E., Grinberg, A., Massalas, J.S., Bodine, D., Alt, F., and Westphal, H.: Lhx2, a LIM homeobox gene, is required for eye, forebrain, and definitive erythrocyte development. Development 124:2935, 1997.

93. Shapiro, L.H.: Myb and Ets proteins cooperate to transactivate an early myeloid gene. J. Biol. Chem. 270:8763, 1995.

94. Oelgeschlager, M., Janknecht, R., Krieg, J., Schreek, S., and Luscher, B.: Interaction of the co-activator CBP with Myb proteins: effects on Myb-specific transactivation and on the cooperativity with NF-M. EMBO J. 15:2771, 1996.

95. Britos-Bray, M., and Friedman, A.D.: Core binding factor cannot synergistically activate the myeloperoxidase proximal enhancer in immature myeloid cells without c-Myb. Mol. Cell. Biol. 17:5127, 1997.

96. Ness, S.A., Kowenz, L.E., Casini, T., Graf, T., and Leutz, A.: Myb and NF-M: combinatorial activators of myeloid genes in heterologous cell types. Genes Dev. 7:749, 1993.

97. Dai, P., Akimaru, H., Tanaka, Y., Hou, D.X., Yasukawa, T., Kanei-Ishii, C., Takahashi, T., and Ishii, S.: CBP as a transcriptional coactivator of c-Myb. Genes Dev. 10:528, 1996.

98. Dash, A.B., Orrico, F.C., and Ness, S.A.: The EVES motif mediates both intermolecular and intramolecular regulation of c-Myb. Genes Dev 10:1858, 1996.

99. Leverson, J.D., Koskinen, P.J., Orrico, F.C., Rainio, E.M., Jalkanen, K.J., Dash, A.B., Eisenman, R.N., and Ness, S.A.: Pim-1 kinase and p100 cooperate to enhance c-Myb activity. Mol. Cell 2:417, 1998.

100. Clarke, M.F., Kukowska-Latallo, J.F., Westin, E., Smith, M., and Prochownik, E.V.: Constitutive expression of a c-myb cDNA blocks Friend murine erythroleukemia cell differentiation. Mol. Cell. Biol. 8:884, 1988.

101. Graf, T., McNagny, K.M., Brady, G., and Frampton, J.: Chicken "erythroid" cells transformed by the gag-myb-ets–encoding E26 leukemia virus are multipotent. Cell 70:201, 1992.

102. Mucenski, M.L., McLain, K., Kier, A.B., Swerdlow, S.H., Schreiner, C.M., Miller, T.A., Pietryga, D.W., Scott, J., W.J., and Potter, S.S.: A functional c-myb gene is required for normal fetal hepatic hematopoiesis. Cell 65:677, 1991.

103. Evans, T., and Felsenfeld, G.: The erythroid-specific transcription factor eryf1: a new finger protein. Cell 58:877, 1989.

104. Orkin, S.H.: Globin gene regulation and switching: circa 1990. Cell 63:665, 1990.

105. Ito, E., Toki, T., Ishihara, H., Ohtani, H., Gu, L., Yokoyama, M., Engel, J.D., and Yamamoto, M.: Erythroid transcription factor GATA-1 is abundantly transcribed in mouse testis. Nature 362:466, 1993.

106. Silver, L., and Palis, J.: Initiation of murine embryonic erythropoiesis: a spatial analysis. Blood 89:1154, 1997.

107. Evans, T., Reitman, M., and Felsenfeld, G.: An erythrocyte-specific DNA-binding factor recognizes a regulatory sequence common to all chicken globin genes. Proc. Natl. Acad. Sci. USA 85:5976, 1988.

108. Martin, D.I.K., Zon, L.I., Mutter, G., and Orkin, S.H.: Expression of an erythroid transcription factor in megakaryocytic and mast cell lineages. Nature 344:444, 1990.

109. Romeo, P.-H., Prandini, M.-H., Joulin, V., Mignotte, V., Prenant, M., Vainchenker, W., Marguerie, G., and Uzan, G.: Megakaryocytic and erythrocytic lineages share specific transcription factors. Nature 344:447, 1990.

110. Seshasayee, D., Gaines, P., and Wojchowski, D.M.: GATA-1 dominantly activates a program of erythroid gene expression in factor-dependent myeloid FDCW2 cells. Mol. Cell. Biol. 18:32780, 1998.

111. Crossley, M., Tsang, A.P., Bieker, J.J., and Orkin, S.H.: Regulation of the erythroid Kruppel-like factor (EKLF) gene promoter by the erythroid transcription factor GATA-1. J. Biol. Chem. 269:15440, 1994.

112. Fujiwara, Y., Browne, C.P., Cunniff, K., Goff, S.C., and Orkin, S.H.: Arrested development of embryonic red cell precursors in mouse embryos lacking transcription factor GATA-1. Proc. Natl. Acad. Sci. USA 93:12355, 1996.

113. Weiss, M.J., Keller, G., and Orkin, S.H.: Novel insights into erythroid development revealed through in vitro differentiation of GATA-1 embryonic stem cells. Genes Dev. 8:1184, 1994.

114. Shivdasani, R.A., Fujiwara, Y., McDevitt, M.A., and Orkin, S.H.: A lineage-selective knockout establishes the critical role of transcription factor GATA-1 in megakaryocyte growth and platelet development. EMBO J. 16:3965, 1997.

115. Philipsen, S., Talbot, D., Fraser, P., and Grosveld, F.: The β-globin dominant control region: hypersensitive site 2. EMBO J. 9:2159, 1990.

116. Martin, D.I.K., and Orkin, S.H.: Transcriptional activation and DNA-binding by the erythroid factor GF-1/NF-E1/Eryf 1. Genes Dev. 4:1886, 1990.

117. Merika, M., and Orkin, S.H.: Functional synergy and physical interactions of the erythroid transcription factor GATA-1 and Kruppel family proteins, Sp1 and EKLF. Mol. Cell. Biol. 15:2437, 1995.

118. Blobel, G.A., Nakajima, T., Eckner, R., Montminy, M., and Orkin, S.H.: CREB-binding protein cooperates with transcription factor GATA-1 and is required for erythroid differentiation. Proc. Natl. Acad. Sci. USA 95:2061, 1998.

119. Tsang, A.C., Visvader, J.E., Turner, C.A., Fujiwara, Y., Yu, C., Weiss, M.J., Crossley, M., and Orkin, S.H.: FOG, a multitype zinc finger protein, acts as a cofactor for transcription factor GATA-1 in erythroid and megakaryocytic differentiation. Cell 90:109, 1997.

120. Boyes, J., Byfield, P., Nakatani, Y., and Ogryzko, V.: Regulation of activity of the transcription factor GATA-1 by acetylation. Nature 396:594, 1998.

121. Tsang, A.P., Fujiwara, Y., Hom, D.B., and Orkin, S.H.: Failure of megakaryopoiesis and arrested erythropoiesis in mice lacking the GATA-1 transcriptional cofactor FOG. Genes Dev. 12:1176, 1998.

122. Fox, A.H., Kowalski, K., King, G.F., Mackay, J.P., and Crossley, M.: Key residues characteristic of GATA N-fingers are recognized by FOG. J. Biol. Chem. 273:33595, 1998.

123. Crispino, J.D., Lodish, M.B., MacKay, J.P., and Orkin, S.H.: Use of altered specificity mutants to probe a specific protein-protein interaction in differentiation: the GATA-1:FOG complex. Mol. Cell 3:219, 1999.

124. Cubadda, Y., Heitzler, P., Ray, R.P., Bourouis, M., Ramain, P., Gelbart, W., Simpson, P., and Haenlin, M.: u-shaped encodes a zinc finger protein that regulates the proneural genes achaete and scute during the formation of bristles in *Drosophila*. Genes Dev. 11:3083, 1997.

125. Haenlin, M., Cubadda, Y., Blondeau, F., Heitzler, P., Lutz, Y., Simpson, P., and Ramain, P.: Transcriptional activity of Pannier is regulated negatively by heterodimerization of the GATA DNA-binding domain with a cofactor encoded by the u-shaped gene of *Drosophila*. Genes Dev. 11:3096, 1997.

126. Miller, I.J., and Bieker, J.J.: A novel, erythroid cell–specific murine transcription factor that binds to the CACCC element and is related to the Kruppel family of nuclear proteins. Mol. Cell. Biol. 13:2776, 1993.

127. Southwood, C.M., Downs, K.M., and Bieker, J.J.: Erythroid Kruppel-like factor exhibits an early and sequentially localized pattern of expression during mammalian erythroid ontogeny. Dev. Dyn. 206:248, 1996.

128. Anderson, K.P., Crable, S.C., and Lingrel, J.B.: Multiple proteins binding to a GATA-E box-GATA motif regulate the erythroid Kruppel-like factor (EKLF) gene. J. Biol. Chem. 273:14347, 1998.

129. Feng, W.C., Southwood, C.M., and Bieker, J.J.: Analyses of β-thalassemia mutant DNA interactions with erythroid Kruppel-like factor (EKLF), an erythroid cell–specific transcription factor. J. Biol. Chem. 269:1493, 1994.

130. Orkin, S.H., and Kazazian, H.H., Jr.: The mutation and polymorphism of the human beta-globin gene and its surrounding DNA. Annu. Rev. Genet. 18:131, 1984.

131. Bieker, J.J., and Southwood, C.M.: The erythroid Kruppel-like factor transactivation domain is a critical component for cell-specific inducibility of a β-globin promoter. Mol. Cell. Biol. 15:852, 1995.

132. Asano, H., and Stamatoyannopoulos, G.: Activation of beta-globin promoter by erythroid Kruppel-like factor. Mol. Cell. Biol. 18:102, 1998.

133. Perkins, A.C., Sharpe, A.H., and Orkin, S.H.: Lethal β-thalassemia in mice lacking the erythroid CACCC-transcription factor EKLF. Nature 375:318, 1995.

134. Nuez, B., Michalovich, D., Bygrave, A., Ploemacher, R., and Grosveld, F.: Defective haematopoiesis in fetal liver resulting from inactivation of the EKLF gene. Nature 375:316, 1995.

135. Guy, L.-G., Mei, Q., Perkins, A.C., Orkin, S.H., and Wall, L.: Erythroid Kruppel-like factor is essential for β-globin gene expression even in absence of gene competition, but is not sufficient to induce the switch from γ-globin to β-globin gene expression. Blood 91:2259, 1998.

136. Wijgerde, M., Gribnau, J., Trimborn, T., Nuez, B., Philipsen, S., Grosveld, F., and Fraser, P.: The role of EKLF in human β-globin gene competition. Genes Dev. 10:2894, 1996.

137. Perkins, A.C., Gaensler, K.M.L., and Orkin, S.H.: Silencing of human fetal globin expression is impaired in the absence of the adult β-globin gene activator protein EKLF. Proc. Natl. Acad. Sci. USA 93:12267, 1996.

138. Ouyang, L., Chen, X., and Bieker, J.J.: Regulation of erythroid Kruppel-like factor (EKLF) transcriptional activity by phosphorylation of a protein kinase casein kinase II site within its interaction domain. J. Biol. Chem. 273:23019, 1998.

139. Zhang, W., and Bieker, J.J.: Acetylation and modulation of erythroid Kruppel-like factor (EKLF) activity by interaction with histone acetyltransferases. Proc. Natl. Acad. Sci. USA 95:9855, 1998.

140. Armstrong, J.A., Bieker, J.J., and Emerson, B.M.: A SWI/SNF-related chromatin remodeling complex, E-RC1, is required for tissue-specific transcriptional regulation by EKLF in vitro. Cell 95:93, 1998.

141. Gillemans, N., Tewari, R., Lindeboom, F., Rottier, R., de Wit, T., Wijgerde, M., Grosveld, F., and Philipsen, S.: Altered DNA-binding specificity mutants of EKLF and Sp1 show that EKLF is an activator of the beta-globin locus control region in vivo. Genes Dev. 12:2863, 1998.

142. Mignotte, V., Wall, L., deBoer, E., Grosveld, F., and Romeo, P.-H.: Two tissue-specific factors bind the erythroid promoter of the human porphobilinogen deaminase gene. Nucleic Acids Res. 17:37, 1989.

143. Ney, P.A., Sorrentino, B.P., McDonagh, K.T., and Nienhuis, A.W.: Tandem AP-1–binding sites within the human β-globin dominant control region function as an inducible enhancer in erythroid cells. Genes Dev. 4:993, 1990.

144. Caterina, J.J., Donze, D., Sun, C.-W., Ciavatta, D.J., and Townes, T.M.: Cloning and functional characterization of LCR-F1: a bZIP transcription factor that activates erythroid-specific, human globin gene expression. Nucleic Acids Res. 22:2383, 1994.

145. Igarashi, K., Kataoka, K., Itoh, K., Hayashi, N., Nishizawa, M., and Yamamoto, M.: Regulation of transcription by dimerization of erythroid factor NF-E2 p45 with small Maf proteins. Nature 367:568, 1994.

146. Andrews, N.C., Erdjument-Bromage, H., Davidson, M.B., Tempst, P., and Orkin, S.H.: Erythroid transcription factor (NF-E2) is a haematopoietic-specific basic-leucine zipper protein. Nature 362:722, 1993.

147. Andrews, N.C., Kotkow, K.J., Ney, P.A., Erdjument-Bromage, H., Tempst, P., and Orkin, S.H.: The ubiquitous subunit of erythroid transcription factor NF-E2 is a small basic-leucine zipper protein related to the *v-maf* oncogene. Proc. Natl. Acad. Sci. USA 90:11488, 1993.

148. Lu, S.-J., Rowan, S., Bani, M.R., and Ben-David, Y.: Retroviral integration within the *Fli-2* locus results in inactivation of the erythroid transcription factor NF-E2 in Friend erythroleukemias: evidence that NF-E2 is essential for globin expression. Proc. Natl. Acad. Sci. USA 91:8398, 1994.

149. Kotkow, K.J., and Orkin, S.H.: Dependence of globin gene expression in mouse erythroleukemia cells on the NF-E2 heterodimer. Mol. Cell. Biol. 15:4640, 1995.

150. Bean, T.L., and Ney, P.A.: Multiple regions of p45NF-E2 are required for β-globin gene expression in erythroid cells. Nucleic Acids Res. 25:2509, 1997.

151. Amrolia, R.J., Ramamurthy, L., Saluja, D., Tanese, N., Jane, S.M., and Cunningham, J.M.: The activation domain of the enhancer binding protein p45NF-E2 interacts with TAFIII130 and mediates long-range activation of the alpha- and beta-globin gene loci in an erythroid cell line. Proc. Natl. Acad. Sci. USA 94:10051, 1997.

152. Gavva, N.R., Gavva, R., Ermekova, K., Sudol, M., and Shen, C.-K., J.: Interaction of WW domains with hematopoietic transcription factor p45/NF-E2 and RNA polymerase II. J. Biol. Chem. 272:24105, 1997.

153. Gong, Q.H., McDowell, J.C., and Dean, A.: Essential role of NF-E2 in remodeling of chromatin structure and transcriptional activation of the epsilon-globin gene in vivo by 5′ hypersensitive site 2 of the beta-globin locus control region. Mol. Cell. Biol. 16:6055, 1996.

154. Shivdasani, R., and Orkin, S.H.: Erythropoiesis and globin gene expression in mice lacking the transcription factor NF-E2. Proc. Natl. Acad. Sci. USA 92:8690, 1995.

155. Kotkow, K.J., and Orkin, S.H.: Complexity of the erythroid transcription factor NF-E2 as revealed by gene targeting of the mouse p18 NF-E2 locus. Proc. Natl. Acad. Sci. USA 93:3514, 1996.

156. Shivdasani, R.A., Rosenblatt, M.F., Zucker-Franklin, D., Jackson,

C.W., Hunt, P., Saris, C.J.M., and Orkin, S.H.: Transcription factor NF-E2 is required for platelet formation independent of the actions of thrombopoietin/MGDF in megakaryocyte development. Cell 81:695, 1995.

157. Lecine, P., Blank, V., and Shivdasani, R.: Characterization of the hematopoietic transcription factor NF-E2 in primary murine megakaryocytes. J. Biol. Chem. 273:7572, 1998.

158. Shavit, J.A., Motohashi, H., Onodera, K., Akasaka, J., Yamamoto, M., and Engel, J.D.: Impaired megakaryopoiesis and behavioral defects in mafG-null mutant mice. Genes Dev. 12:2164, 1998.

159. Chan, J.Y., Han, X.-L., and Kan, Y.W.: Cloning of Nrf1, an NF-E2–related transcription factor, by genetic selection in yeast. Proc. Natl. Acad. Sci. USA 90:11371, 1993.

160. Moi, P., Chan, K., Asunis, I., Cao, A., and Kan, Y.W.: Isolation of NF-E2–related factor 2 (Nrf2), a NF-E2–like basic leucine zipper transcriptional activator that binds to the tandem NF-E2/AP1 repeat of the β-globin locus control region. Proc. Natl. Acad. Sci. USA 91:9926, 1994.

161. Chui, D.H.K., Tang, W., and Orkin, S.H.: cDNA cloning of murine Nrf2 gene, coding for a p45 NF-E2 related transcription factor. Biochem. Biophys. Res. Commun. 209:40, 1995.

162. Chan, K., Lu, R., Chang, J.C., and Kan, Y.W.: NRF2, a member of the NFE2 family of transcription factors, is not essential for murine erythropoiesis, growth, and development. Proc. Natl. Acad. Sci. USA 93:13943, 1996.

163. Farmer, S.C., Sun, C.-W., Winnier, G.E., Hogan, B.L.M., and Townes, T.M.: The bZIP transcription factor LCR-F1 is essential for mesoderm formation in mouse development. Genes Dev. 11:786, 1997.

164. Chan, J.Y., Kwong, M., Lu, R., Chang, J., Wang, B., Yen, T.S.B., and Kan, Y.W.: Targeted disruption of the ubiquitous CNC-bZIP transcription factor, Nrf-1, results in anemia and embryonic lethality in mice. EMBO J. 17:1779, 1998.

165. Igarashi, K., Hoshino, H., Muto, A., Suwabe, N.N., S., Kakauchi, H., and Yamamoto, M.: Multivalent DNA binding complex generated by small Maf and Bach1 as a possible biochemical basis for beta-globin locus control region complex. J. Biol. Chem. 273:11783, 1998.

166. Hodgkinson, C.A., Moore, K.J., Nakayama, A., Steingrimsson, E., Copeland, N.G., Jenkins, N.A., and Arnheiter, H.: Mutations at the mouse microphthalmia locus are associated with defects in a gene encoding a novel basic-helix-loop-helix-zipper protein. Cell 74:395, 1993.

167. Dubreuil, P., Forrester, L., Rottapel, R., Reedijk, M., Fujita, J., and Bernstein, A.: The c-fms gene complements the mitogenic defect in mast cells derived from mutant W mice but not mi (microphthalmia) mice. Proc. Natl. Acad. Sci. USA 88:2341, 1991.

168. Hughes, M.J., Lingrel, J.B., Krakowsky, J.M., and Anderson, K.P.: A helix-loop-helix transcription factor–like gene is located at the mi locus. J. Biol. Chem. 268:20687, 1993.

169. Hemesath, T.J., Steingrimsson, E., McGill, G., Hansen, M.J., Vaught, J., Hodgkinson, C.A., Arnheiter, H., Copeland, N.G., Jenkins, N.A., and Fisher, D.E.: Microphthalmia, a critical factor in melanocyte development, defines a discrete transcription factor family. Genes Dev 8:2770, 1994.

170. Tachibana, M., Takeda, K., Nobukuni, Y., Urabe, K., Long, J.E., Meyers, K.A., Aaronson, S.A., and Miki, T.: Ectopic expression of MITF, a gene for Waardenburg syndrome type 2, converts fibroblasts to cells with melanocyte characteristics. Nat. Genet. 14:50, 1996.

171. Morii, E., Tsujimura, T., Jippo, T., Hashimoto, K., Takebayashi, K., Tsujino, K., Nomura, S., Yamamoto, M., and Kitamura, Y.: Regulation of mouse mast cell protease 6 gene expression by transcription factor encoded by the mi locus. Blood 88:2488, 1996.

172. Morii, E., Jippo, T., Tsujimura, T., Hashimoto, K., Kim, D.K., Lee, Y.M., Ogihara, H., Tsujino, K., Kim, H.M., and Kitamura, Y.: Abnormal expression of mouse mast cell protease 5 gene in cultured mast cells derived from mutant mi/mi mice. Blood 90:3057, 1997.

173. Hemesath, T.J., Price, E.R., Takemoto, C., Badalian, T., and Fisher, D.E.: MAP kinase links the transcription factor Microphthalmia to c-Kit signalling in melanocytes. Nature 391:298, 1998.

174. Price, E.R., Ding, H.F., Badalian, T., Bhattacharya, S., Takemoto, C., Yao, T.P., Hemesath, T.J., and Fisher, D.E.: Lineage-specific signaling in melanocytes. C-kit stimulation recruits p300/cbp to microphthalmia. J. Biol. Chem. 273:17983, 1998.

175. Sato, S., Roberts, K., Gambino, G., Cook, A., Kouzarides, T., and Goding, C.R.: CBP/p300 as a co-factor for the Microphthalmia transcription factor. Oncogene 14:3083, 1997.

176. Klemsz, M.J., McKercher, S.R., Celada, A., Van Beveren, C., and Maki, R.A.: The macrophage and B cell–specific transcription factor PU.1 is related to the ets oncogene. Cell 61:113, 1990.

177. Moreau-Gachelin, F., Ray, D., Tambourin, P., Tavitian, A., Klemsz, M.J., McKercher, S.R., Celada, A., Van Beveren, C., and Maki, R.A.: The Pu.1 transcription factor is the product of the putative oncogene Spi-1. Cell 61:1166, 1990.

178. Hromas, R., Orazi, A., Neiman, R.S., Maki, R., Van Beveran, C., Moore, J., and Klemsz, M.: Hematopoietic lineage- and stage-restricted expression of the ETS oncogene family member PU.1. Blood 82:2998, 1993.

179. Pongaba, J.M., Nagulapalli, S., Klemsz, M.J., McKercher, S.R., Maki, R.A., and Atchison, M.L.: PU.1 recruits a second nuclear factor to a site important for immunoglobulin κ3′ enhancer activity. Mol. Cell. Biol. 12:368, 1992.

180. Eisenbeis, C.F., Singh, H., and Storb, U.: Pip, a novel IRF family member, is a lymphoid-specific, PU.1-dependent transcriptional activator. Genes Dev. 9:1377, 1995.

181. McKercher, S.R., Torbett, B.E., Anderson, K.L., Henkel, G.W., Vestal, D.J., Baribault, H., Klemsz, M., Feeney, A.J., Wu, G.E., Paige, C.J., and Maki, R.A.: Targeted disruption of the PU.1 gene results in multiple hematopoietic abnormalities. EMBO J. 15:5647, 1996.

182. Scott, E.W., Simon, M.C., Anastasi, J., and Singh, H.: Requirement of transcription factor PU.1 in the development of multiple hematopoietic lineages. Science 265:1573, 1994.

183. Scott, E.W., Fisher, R.C., Olson, M.C., Kehrli, E.W., Simon, M.C., and Singh, H.: PU.1 functions in a cell-autonomous manner to control the differentiation of multipotential lymphoid-myeloid progenitors. Immunity 6:437, 1997.

184. Tondravi, M.M., McKercher, S.R., Anderson, K., Erdmann, J.M., Quiroz, M., Maki, R., and Teitelbaum, S.L.: Osteopetrosis in mice lacking haematopoietic transcription factor PU.1. Nature 386:81, 1997.

185. DeKoter, R.P., Walsh, J.C., and Singh, H.: PU.1 regulates both cytokine dependent proliferation and differentiation of granulocyte/macrophage progenitors. EMBO J. 17:4456, 1998.

186. Anderson, K.L., Smith, K.A., McKercher, S.R., Maki, R.A., and Torbett, B.E.: Myeloid development is selectively disrupted in PU.1 null mice. Blood 91:3702, 1998.

187. Landschultz, W.H., Johnson, P.F., Adashi, E.Y., Graves, B.J., and McKnight, S.L.: Isolation of a recombinant copy of the gene encoding C/EBP. Genes Dev. 2:786, 1988.

188. Friedman, A.D., Landschultz, W.H., and McKnight, S.L.: C/EBP activates the promoter of the serum albumin gene in cultured hepatoma cells. Genes Dev. 3:1314, 1989.

189. Williams, S.C., Du, Y., Schwartz, R.C., Weiler, S.R., Ortiz, M., Keller, J.R., and Johnson, P.F.: C/EBPepsilon is a myeloid-specific activator of cytokine, chemokine, and macrophage-colony-stimulating factor receptor genes. J. Biol. Chem. 273:13493, 1998.

190. Katz, S., Kowenz, L.E., Muller, C., Meese, K., Ness, S.A., and Leutz, A.: The NF-M transcription factor is related to C/EBPβ and plays a role in signal transduction, differentiation and leukemogenesis of avian myelomonocytic cells. EMBO J. 12:1321, 1993.

191. Yamanaka, R., Kim, G.D., Radomska, H.S., Lekstrom-Himes, J., Smith, L.T., Antonson, P., Tenen, D.G., and Xanthopoulos, K.G.: CCAAT/enhancer binding protein epsilon is preferentially up-regulated during granulocytic differentiation and its functional versatility is determined by alternative use of promoters and differential splicing. Proc. Natl. Acad. Sci. USA 94:6462, 1997.

192. Zhang, D.Z., Zhang, P., Wang, N.D., Hetherinton, C.J., Darlington, G., and Tenen, D.: Absence of granulocyte colony-stimulating signaling and neutrophil development in CCAAT enhancer binding protein-α deficient mice. Proc. Natl. Acad. Sci. USA 94:569, 1997.

193. Yamanaka, R., Barlow, C., Lekstrom-Himes, J., Castilla, L.H., Liu, P.P., Eckhaus, M., Decker, T., Wynshaw-Boris, A., and Xanthopoulos, K.G.: Impaired granulopoiesis, myelodysplasia, and early lethality in CCAAT/enhancer binding protein ε–deficient mice. Proc. Natl. Acad. Sci. USA 94:13187, 1997.

194. Georgopoulos, K., Moore, D.D., and Defler, B.: Ikaros, an early lymphoid-specific transcription factor and a putative mediator for T cell commitment. Science 258:808, 1992.

195. Molnar, A., and Georgopoulos, K.: The Ikaros gene encodes a family of functionally diverse zinc finger DNA-binding proteins. Mol. Cell. Biol. 14:8292, 1994.

196. Hahm, K., Ernst, P., Lo, K., Kim, G.S., Turck, C., and Smale, S.T.: The lymphoid transcription factor LyF-1 is encoded by specific, alter-

natively spliced mRNAs derived from the Ikaros gene. Mol. Cell. Biol. 14:7111, 1994.

197. Sun, L., Liu, A., and Georgopoulos, K.: Zinc finger–mediated protein interactions modulate Ikaros activity, a molecular control of lymphocyte development. EMBO J. 15:5358, 1996.

198. Hahm, K., Cobb, B.S., McCarty, A.S., Brown, K.E., Klug, C.A., Lee, R., Akashi, K., Weissman, I.L., Fisher, A.G., and Smale, S.T.: Helios, a T cell–restricted Ikaros family member that quantitatively associates with Ikaros at centromeric heterochromatin. Genes Dev. 12:782, 1998.

199. Kelley, C.M., Ikeda, T., Koipally, J., Avitahl, N., Wu, L., Georgopoulos, K., and Morgan, B.A.: Helios, a novel dimerization partner of Ikaros expressed in the earliest hematopoietic progenitors. Curr. Biol. 8:508, 1998.

200. Morgan, B., Sun, L., Avitahl, N., Andrikopoulos, K., Ikeda, T., Gonzales, E., Wu, P., Neben, S., and Georgopoulos, K.: Aiolos, a lymphoid restricted transcription factor that interacts with Ikaros to regulate lymphocyte differentiation. EMBO J. 16:2004, 1997.

201. Brown, K.E., Guest, S.S., Smale, S.T., Hahm, K., Merkenschlager, M., and Fisher, A.G.: Association of transcriptionally silent genes with Ikaros complexes at centromeric heterochromatin. Cell 91:845, 1997.

202. Klug, C.A., Morrison, S.J., Masek, M., Hahm, K., Smale, S.T., and Weissman, I.L.: Hematopoietic stem cells and lymphoid progenitors express different Ikaros isoforms, and Ikaros is localized to heterochromatin in immature lymphocytes. Proc. Natl. Acad. Sci. USA 95:657, 1998.

203. Georgopoulos, K., Bigby, M., Wang, J.-H., Molnar, A., Wu, P., Winandy, S., and Sharpe, A.: The Ikaros gene is required for the development of all lymphoid lineages. Cell 79:143, 1994.

204. Winandy, S., Wu, P., and Georgopoulos, K.: A dominant mutation in the Ikaros gene leads to rapid development of leukemia and lymphoma. Cell 83:289, 1995.

205. Wang, J.H., Nichogiannopoulou, A., Wu, L., Sun, L., Sharpe, A.H., Bigby, M., and Georgopoulos, K.: Selective defects in the development of the fetal and adult lymphoid system in mice with an Ikaros null mutation. Immunity 5:537, 1996.

206. Wang, J.H., Avitahl, N., Cariappa, A., Friedrich, C., Ikeda, T., Renold, A., Andrikopoulos, K., Liang, L., Pillai, S., Morgan, B., and Georgopoulos, K.: Aiolos regulates B cell activation and maturation to effector state. Immunity 9:543, 1998.

207. Barberis, A., Widenhorn, K., Vitelli, L., and Busslinger, M.: A novel B-cell lineage–specific transcription factor present at early but not late stages of differentiation. Genes Dev. 4:849, 1990.

208. Adams, B., Dorfler, P., Aguzzi, A., Kozmik, Z., Urbanek, P., Maurer-Fogy, I., and Busslinger, M.: Pax-5 encodes the transcription factor BSAP and is expressed in B lymphocytes, the developing CNS, and adult testis. Genes Dev. 6:1589, 1992.

209. Urbanek, P., Wang, Z.-Q., Fetka, I., Wagner, E.R., and Busslinger, M.: Complete block of early B cell differentiation and altered patterning of the posterior midbrain in mice lacking Pax5/BSAP. Cell 79:901, 1994.

210. Schwartz, M., Alvarez-Bolado, G., Urbanek, P., Busslinger, M., and Gruss, P.: Conserved biological function between Pax-2 and Pax-5 in midbrain and cerebellum development: evidence from targeted mutations. Proc. Natl. Acad. Sci. USA 94:14518, 1997.

211. Nutt, S.L., Urbanek, P., Rolink, A., and Busslinger, M.: Essential functions of Pax5 (BSAP) in pro-B cell development: difference between fetal and adult B lymphopoiesis and reduced V-to-DJ recombination at the IgH locus. Genes Dev. 11:476, 1997.

212. Nutt, S.L., Morrison, A.M., Dorfler, P., Rolink, A., and Busslinger, M.: Identification of BSAP (Pax-5) target genes in early B-cell development by loss- and gain-of-function experiments. EMBO J. 17:2319, 1998.

213. Murre, C., McCaw, P.S., and Baltimore, D.: A new DNA binding and dimerization motif in immunoglobin enhancer binding, daughterless, MyoD, and myc proteins. Cell 56:777, 1989.

214. Murre, C., McCaw, P.S., Vaessin, H., Caudy, M., Jan, L.Y., Jan, Y.N., Cabrera, C.V., Buskin, J.N., Hauschka, S.D., Lassar, A.B., et al.: Interactions between heterologous helix-loop-helix proteins generate complexes that bind specifically to a common DNA sequence. Cell 58:537, 1989.

215. Lassar, A.B., Davis, R.L., Wright, W.E., Kadesch, T., Murre, C., Voronova, A., Baltimore, D., and Weintraub, H.: Functional activity of myogenic HLH proteins requires hetero-oligomerization with E12/E47-like proteins in vivo. Cell 66:305, 1991.

216. Mellentin, J.D., Murre, C., Donlon, T.A., McCaw, P.S., Smith, S.D., Carroll, A.J., McDonald, M.E., Baltimore, D., and Cleary, M.L.: The gene for enhancer binding proteins E12/E47 lies at the t(1;19) breakpoint in acute leukemias. Science 246:379, 1989.

217. Kamps, M.P., Murre, C., Sun, X.H., and Baltimore, D.: A new homeobox gene contributes the DNA binding domain of the t(1;19) translocation protein in pre-B ALL. Cell 60:547, 1990.

218. Bain, G., Maandag, E.C., Izon, D.J., Amsen, D., Kruisbeek, A.M., Weintraub, B.C., Krop, I., Schlissel, M.S., Feeney, A.J., and van Roon, M.: E2A proteins are required for proper B cell development and initiation of immunoglobulin gene rearrangements. Cell 79:885, 1994.

219. Zhuang, Y., Soriano, P., and Weintraub, H.: The helix-loop-helix gene E2A is required for B cell formation. Cell 79:875, 1994.

220. Zhuang, Y., Barndt, R.J., Pan, L., Kelley, R., and Dai, M.: Functional replacement of the mouse E2A gene with a human HEB cDNA. Mol. Cell. Biol. 18:3340, 1998.

221. Yan, W., Young, A.Z., Soares, V.C., Kelley, R., Benezra, R., and Zhuang, Y.: High incidence of T-cell tumors in E2A-null mice and E2A/Id1 double-knockout mice. Mol. Cell. Biol. 17:7317, 1997.

222. Bain, G., Engel, I., Robanus, M.E.C., te Riele, H.P., Voland, J.R., Sharp, L.L., Chun, J., Huey, B., Pinkel, D., and Murre, C.: E2A deficiency leads to abnormalities in alpha/beta T-cell development and to rapid development of T-cell lymphomas. Mol. Cell. Biol. 17:4782, 1997.

223. Staudt, L.M., Clerc, R.G., Singh, H., LeBowitz, J.H., Sharp, P.A., and Baltimore, D.: Cloning of a lymphoid-specific cDNA encoding a protein binding the regulatory octamer DNA motif. Science 241:577, 1988.

224. Scheidereit, C., Cromlish, J.A., Gerster, T., Kawakami, K., Balmaceda, C.-G., Currie, R.A., and Roeder, R.G.: A human lymphoid-specific transcription factor that activates immunoglobulin genes is a homeobox protein. Nature 336:551, 1988.

225. Scheidereit, C., Heguy, A., and Roeder, R.G.: Identification and purification of a human lymphoid-specific octamer-binding protein (OTF-2) that activates transcription of an immunoglobulin promoter in vitro. Cell 51:783, 1987.

226. Sturm, R.A., Das, G., and Herr, W.: The ubiquitous octamer-binding protein Oct-1 contains a POU domain with a homeo subdomain. Genes Dev. 2:1582, 1988.

227. Clerc, R.G., Corcoran, L.M., LeBowitz, J.H., Baltimore, D., and Sharp, P.A.: The B-cell specific Oct-2 protein contains POU-box and homeo-box-type domains. Genes Dev. 2:1570, 1988.

228. Corcoran, L.M., Karvelas, M., Nossal, G.J., Ye, Z.S., Jacks, T., and Baltimore, D.: Oct-2, although not required for early B-cell development, is critical for later B-cell maturation and for postnatal survival. Genes Dev. 7:570, 1993.

229. Feldhaus, A.L., Klug, C.A., Arvin, K.L., and Singh, H.: Targeted disruption of the Oct-2 locus in a B cell provides genetic evidence for two distinct cell type–specific pathways of octamer element–mediated gene activation. EMBO J. 12:2763, 1993.

230. Humbert, P.O., and Corcoran, L.M.: Oct-2 gene disruption eliminates the peritoneal B-1 lymphocyte lineage and attenuates B-3 cell maturation and function. J. Immunol. 159:5273, 1997.

231. Konig, H., Pfisterer, P., Corcoran, L.M., and Wirth, T.: Identification of CD36 as the first gene dependent on the B-cell differentiation factor Oct-2. Genes Dev. 9:1598, 1995.

232. Luo, Y., Fujii, H., Gerster, T., and Roeder, R.G.: A novel B cell–derived coactivator potentiates the activation of immunoglobulin promoters by octamer-binding transcription factors. Cell 71:231, 1992.

233. Gstaiger, M., Knoepfel, L., Georgiev, O., Schaffner, W., and Hovens, C.M.: A B-cell coactivator of octamer-binding transcription factors. Nature 373:360, 1995.

234. Luo, Y., and Roeder, R.G.: Cloning, functional characterization, and mechanism of action of the B-cell–specific transcriptional coactivator OCA-B. Mol. Cell. Biol. 15:4115, 1995.

235. Cepek, K.L., Chasman, D.I., and Sharp, P.A.: Sequence-specific DNA binding of the B-cell–specific coactivator OCA-B. Genes Dev. 10:2079, 1996.

236. Gstaiger, M., Georgiev, O., van Leeuwen, H., van der Vliet, P., and Schaffner, W.: The B cell coactivator Bob1 shows DNA sequence-dependent complex formation with Oct-1/Oct-2 factors, leading to differential promoter activation. EMBO J. 15:2781, 1996.

237. Kim, U., Qin, X.F., Gong, S., Stevens, S., Luo, Y., Nussenzweig, M., and Roeder, R.G.: The B-cell–specific transcription coactivator OCA-B/OBF-1/Bob-1 is essential for normal production of immunoglobulin isotypes. Nature 383:542, 1996.

238. Schubart, D.B., Rolink, A., Kosco-Vilbois, M.H., Botteri, F., and

Matthias, P.: B-cell–specific coactivator OBF-1/OCA-B/Bob1 required for immune response and germinal centre formation. Nature 383:534, 1996.

239. Nielsen, P.J., Georgiev, O., Lorenz, B., and Schaffner, W.: B lymphocytes are impaired in mice lacking the transcriptional co-activator Bob1/OCA-B/OBF1. Eur. J. Immunol. 26:3214, 1996.

240. Hagman, J., Travis, A., and Grosschedl, R.: A novel lineage-specific nuclear factor regulates mb-1 gene transcription at the early stages of B cell differentiation. EMBO J. 10:3409, 1991.

241. Hagman, J., Belanger, C., Travis, A., Turck, C.W., and Grosschedl, R.: Cloning and functional characterization of early B-cell factor, a regulator of lymphocyte-specific gene expression. Genes Dev 7:760, 1993.

242. Hagman, J., Gutch, M.J., Lin, H., and Grosschedl, R.: EBF contains a novel zinc coordination motif and multiple dimerization and transcriptional activation domains. EMBO J. 14:2907, 1995.

243. Sigvardsson, M., O'Riordan, M., and Grosschedl, R.: EBF and E47 collaborate to induce expression of the endogenous immunoglobulin surrogate light chain genes. Immunity 7:25, 1997.

244. Lin, H., and Grosschedl, R.: Failure of B-cell differentiation in mice lacking the transcription factor EBF. Nature 376:263, 1995.

245. Travis, A., Amsterdam, A., Belanger, C., and Grosschedl.: LEF-1, a gene encoding a lymphoid-specific protein with an HMG domain, regulates T-cell receptor α enhancer function. Genes Dev. 5:880, 1991.

246. Giese, K., Cox, J., and Grosschedl, R.: The HMG domain of lymphoid enhancer factor 1 bends DNA and facilitates assembly of functional nucleoprotein structures. Cell 69:185, 1992.

247. Brunner, E., Peter, O., Schweizer, L., and Basler, K.: Pangolin encodes a Lef-1 homologue that acts downstream of Armadillo to transduce the Wingless signal in *Drosophila*. Nature 385:829, 1997.

248. Behrens, J., von Kries, J.P., Kuhl, M., Bruhn, L., Wedlich, D., Grosschedl, R., and Birchmeier, W.: Functional interaction of beta-catenin with the transcription factor LEF-1. Nature 382:638, 1996.

249. Hsu, S.C., Galceran, J., and Grosschedl, R.: Modulation of transcriptional regulation by LEF-1 in response to wnt-1 signaling and association with beta-catenin. Mol. Cell. Biol. 18:4807, 1998.

250. van Genderen, C., Okamura, R.M., Farinas, I., Quo, R.-G., Parslow, T.G., Bruhn, L., and Grosschedl, R.: Development of several organs that require inductive epithelial-mesenchymal interactions is impaired in LEF-1–deficient mice. Genes Dev. 8:2691, 1994.

251. Verbeek, S., Izon, D., Hofhuis, F., Robanus-Maandag, E., te Riele, H., van de Wetering, M., Oosterwegel, M., Wilson, A., MacDonald, H.R., and Clevers, H.: An HMG-box–containing T-cell factor required for thymocyte differentiation. Nature 374:70, 1995.

252. Okamura, R.M., Sigvardsson, M., Galceran, J., Verbeek, S., Clevers, H., and Grosschedl, R.: Redundant regulation of T cell differentiation and TCRalpha gene expression by the transcription factors LEF-1 and TCF-1. Immunity 8:11, 1998.

253. Ho, I.-C., Vorhees, P., Marin, N., Oakley, B.K., Tsai, S.-F., Orkin, S.H., and Leiden, J.M.: Human GATA-3: a lineage-restricted transcription factor that regulates the expression of the T cell receptor a gene. EMBO J. 10:1187, 1991.

254. Pandolfi, P.P., Roth, M.E., Karis, A., Leonard, M.W., Dzierzak, E., Grosveld, F.G., Engel, J.D., and Lindenbaum, M.H.: Targeted disruption of the GATA3 gene causes severe abnormalities in the nervous system and in fetal liver haematopoiesis. Nat. Genet. 11:40, 1995.

255. Ting, C.-N., Olson, M.C., Barton, K.P., and Leiden, J.M.: Transcription factor GATA-3 is required for development of the T-cell lineage. Nature 384:474, 1996.

256. Zheng, W., and Flavell, R.A.: The transcription factor GATA-3 is necessary and sufficient for Th2 cytokine gene expression in CD4 T cells. Cell 89:587, 1997.

257. Suda, J., Suda, T., and Ogawa, M.: Analysis of differentiation of mouse hemopoietic stem cells in culture by sequential replating of paired progenitors. Blood 64:393, 1984.

258. Sieweke, M.H., Tekotte, H., Frampton, J., and Graf, T.: MafB is an interaction partner and repressor of Ets-1 that inhibits erythroid differentiation. Cell 84:49, 1996.

259. Sieweke, M.H., and Graf, T.: Dynamic changes of transcription factor interactions in blood cell differentiation: a cocktail party scenario. Curr. Opin. Genet. Dev. 8:545, 1998.

260. Hu, M., Kruase, D., Greaves, M., Sharkis, S., Dexter, M., Heyworth, C., and Enver, T.: Multilineage gene expression precedes commitment in the hemopoietic system. Genes Dev. 11:774, 1997.

261. Jimenez, G., Griffiths, S.D., Ford, A.M., Greaves, M.F., and Enver, T.: Activation of the β-globin locus control region precedes commitment to the erythroid lineage. Proc. Natl. Acad. Sci. USA 89:10618, 1992.

262. Enver, T., and Greaves, M.: Loops, lineage, and leukemia. Cell 94:9, 1998.

4 Signal Transduction in the Regulation of Hematopoiesis

James N. Ihle

Introduction

Hematopoiesis is stringently regulated through the availability and function of a wide variety of growth factors, cytokines or chemokines. Their functions can be generically described as being required for the expansion of differentiating progenitors through the regulation of cell cycle progression; the regulation of the susceptibility of cells to apoptosis; or the regulation of the function of differentiated cells. Progressively, the challenges have been to identify the factors involved, a process that has resulted in the identification and characterization of literally hundreds of factors. The second challenge was to identify the cellular receptors that mediate the effects through their ability to bind ligand and initiate cellular responses. This challenge has similarly resulted in the cloning and characterization of a large number of receptors and the demonstration that they consist of a limited number of structurally and functionally defined families. The most recent challenge has been to understand the cellular consequences of binding of ligand to receptors, an area of research referred to as signal transduction. Only in the last few years have major advances been made in this area of research. Even with these advances however, only infrequently do we understand an entire signal transduction pathway to the extent that we understand the biochemical events in the pathway and the consequences of its activation in cellular responses.

Receptors can be grouped on both structural and functional similarities (Table 4–1). As detailed below, there are signal transduction pathways that are dedicated to the function of specific families of receptors as well as many that are shared. The receptor tyrosine kinases and the cytokine receptor superfamily members mediate their effects through the induction of tyrosine phosphorylation. In contrast, the TGFβ family of receptors relies on serine and threonine phosphorylation. Chemokines and the wnt factors utilize the serpentine receptors that function through their ability to activate G-protein coupled signaling events. Members of the TNF receptor and Fas family typically activate caspase based pathways and NF-κB transcription factors through signaling pathways that are just beginning to be understood. The IL-1 receptor family may utilize signaling intermediates that are common to the TNF/FAS systems. The notch family of receptors regulates gene expression through a novel mechanism that appears to involve the liberation of a transcription factor complex component from the cytoplasmic domain of the receptor.

The biochemical consequences of receptor engagement have been studied intensely over the past several years. These studies have resulted in the identification of a large number of proteins that are modified following receptor activation or that associate with the receptor complex. In many cases, it has not been apparent what role individual proteins play in specific aspects of the cellular responses. However, the ability to derive mice lacking a specific gene has provided an essential means to assess function. As noted below this has helped to define not only responses that require a specific protein but also has identified situations where activation of a particular pathway may have no essential function.

Receptor Tyrosine Kinases

The protein tyrosine kinase receptors constitute one of the largest families of cellular ligand receptors.[1] The family is characterized by receptors that have a single transmembrane spanning domain and a cytoplasmic domain that contains a protein tyrosine kinase catalytic domain. The protein tyrosine kinase receptors are further subdivided into subfamilies based on the structure of the extracellular domains. The defining domains include fibronectin-like repeats, EGF-like domains, immunoglobulin-like domains, cysteine rich domains, leucine-rich domains, or acidic box domains.

Table 4-1. Receptor Families

Receptor tyrosine kinases
Cytokine receptor superfamily members
TGFβ receptor family
Frizzled receptor family
Serpentine, G-protein coupled receptors
TNF/FAS receptor family
IL-1 receptor family
Notch family receptors

A number of tyrosine kinase receptors are implicated in the regulation of hematopoiesis including the receptor for colony stimulating factor-1 (CSF-1), a major regulator of macrophage function, and the receptor for stem cell factor (SCF), a factor that contributes to the expansion of early hematopoietic progenitor cells. Flt-1 is related in structure to the CSF-1 and SCF receptors and is the receptor for vascular endothelial factor. Recent studies have demonstrated that flt-1 plays an essential role in early hematopoiesis.[2] In contrast, c-kit disruption results in severe anemia and perinatal or late embryonic death, but some level of hematopoiesis is maintained. In addition, tyrosine kinase receptors have been identfed in early hematopoietic stem cells such as fetal liver kinase-2 (flk-2), which is also known as flt-3. Interestingly, mice deficient in the CSF-1 or flt-3 are viable and have only quantative reductions in hematopoietic functions indicating a contribution but not an essential, nonredundant function in hematopoiesis.[3, 4]

The activation of signaling by the tyrosine kinase receptors involves four steps: 1) ligand induced oligomerization of the receptor, 2) transphosphorylation of the activation loop, 3) phosphorylation of additional sites and recruitment of proteins to the receptor complex, and 4) most frequently, phosphorylation of substrates (Fig. 4–1). The primary function of the ligand is to induce the dimerization or oligomerization of the receptor. This results in the juxtaposition of the cytoplasmic catalytic domains in such a manner as to allow transphosphorylation and activation of kinase activity.[5–9] The mechanisms by which ligand induces oligomeriza-

tion can be one of several. The ligand may exist normally as a dimer and therefore binds two receptor chains in a symmetrical manner, as is the case for CSF-1 or SCF. Alternatively, a ligand may have two binding sites for the receptor. Lastly, many ligands are cell associated and thereby can induce receptor oligomerization. Irrespective of the mechanism utilized, the key function of the ligand is to drive receptor oligomerization.

The mechanism of activation of receptor tyrosine kinases almost invariably involves the transphosphorylation of a critical tyrosine in the kinase domain in a region referred to as the activation loop. The recent determination of the molecular structures of receptor tyrosine kinase catalytic domains has provided insights into the basis for activation. In the case of the insulin receptor,[10] the critical regulatory tyrosine resides in a loop that is very near the substrate binding site and thereby can interfere with the ability of the ATP binding loop to have access to the catalytic site. The phosphorylation of the tyrosine is speculated to result in a change of conformation that results in the swinging out of this inhibitory loop from the catalytic site, thereby allowing substrates to bind and to be phosphorylated. More recently, the structure for the fibroblast growth factor receptor has been solved.[10, 11] Although the orientation of the tyrosine relative to the substrate binding site and the ATP binding loop is somewhat different, the unphosphorylated form can be hypothesized to primarily interfere with access of the ATP binding loop to the catalytic site. The structure of the kinase domain and the critical role that tyrosine phosphorylation plays in receptor activation provide important target sites for small molecule inhibitors. As noted below this same theme appears to apply to the kinases that associate with receptors of the cytokine receptor superfamily.

The activation of kinase activity is followed by phosphorylation of a variety of sites within the cytoplasmic domain of the receptor. These sites are critical for receptor function by serving as "docking" sites for a variety of proteins that are either substrates for the kinases or are activated through their recruitment into the receptor complex.[12] The majority of the proteins recruited to the receptor

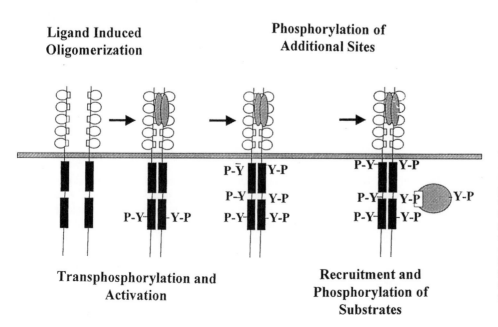

Ligand Induced Oligomerization

Phosphorylation of Additional Sites

Transphosphorylation and Activation

Recruitment and Phosphorylation of Substrates

Figure 4–1. Sequence of reactions in activation of tyrosine kinase receptors. The activation of tyrosine kinase receptors is initiated by the binding of the ligand to the extracellular domain resulting in the aggregation of the receptors. When aggregated the kinase domains are brought into proximity, allowing the transphosphorylation of sites with the activation loop domain, resulting in the activation of kinase activity. The activated kinases phosphorylate additional sites within the intracellular domain creating potential "docking" sites for the recruitment of phosphotyrosine-binding proteins into the activated receptor complex. The recruited substrates are, in turn, phosphorylated on tyrosines that either activates their function or allows them to associate with proteins whose function is affected by binding.

complex are recruited through the interaction of src homology 2 (SH2) domains with specific sites of tyrosine phosphorylation. SH2 domains consist of 100 amino acid domains that contain a binding pocket that recognizes phosphotyrosine and generally three to six carboxyl-located amino acid residues that provide the specificity of interaction. The structures of several SH2 domains have been solved and provide important insights into the interactions involved in phosphotyrosine binding and specificity.[13, 14] More recently, a second domain, termed the phosphotyrosine binding domain or PTB domain, has been identified.[15, 16] The binding properties of PTB domains are quite different from SH2 domains and are much less frequently encountered than SH2 domains.

The concept of receptor recruitment of substrates has two important consequences. First, the requirement to recruit substrates to a site of active tyrosine phosphorylation provides an essential mechanism of providing specificity for signaling. Only those pathways will be activated for which the components can be recruited to the receptor complex. Secondly, the requirement for receptor tyrosine phosphorylation ensures that phosphorylation of signaling components will only occur within the context of ligand driven receptor activation. Thus the critical requirements for both ligand-dependent and ligand/receptor-specific activation are obtained. The importance of this is readily evident when comparing the properties of the wild type receptors with altered receptors that are mutated or fused with aggregation inducing partners as occurs in a variety of transformed cells. In these cases not only is activation of kinase activity independent of ligand but frequently also results in the phosphorylation and activation of substrates that are not seen in the responses to the normal ligand.

Essential to a regulated response is the ability to deactivate ligand activated receptor complexes. One mechanism of inactivation is internalization of the ligand-receptor complex. This often involves internalization through clathrin-coated pits and internalization to the endosomes. In the endosomes, receptor-ligand complexes dissociate and are either degraded or the receptor can be recycled back to the membrane.[17] In some cases ligand-induced receptor activation results in ubiquitination of the receptor that targets it for degradation by the proteosomes. Lastly, dephosphorylation of the receptor may be responsible for its down-regulation, particularly dephosphorylation of the critical tyrosines in the activation loop. Of particular interest in this regard are the tyrosine phosphatases that contain SH2 domains and therefore can be specifically recruited to the receptor complex. Although some evidence supports such a mechanism for the tyrosine protein receptor kinases,[18] a critical role for such phosphatases is evident in the function of the cytokine receptor superfamily as noted below.

The proposed roles of receptor tyrosine kinases in hematopoiesis would be anticipated to have an associated role in transformation. Consistent with this, at least two translocations involve activation of tyrosine kinase receptors. In a subgroup of chronic myelomonocytic leukemia, characterized by a t(5;12)(q33;p13) balanced translocation, the kinase domain of the PDGF receptor on chromosome 5 is fused to the helix loop helix domain of the ets transcription family member termed Tel on chromosome 12.[19] Similarly, in anaplastic large-cell lymphomas that contain a t(2;5)(p23;q35) translocation,

there is a fusion of nucleophosmin (NPM) on chromosome 5 with an orphan tyrosine kinase receptor termed anaplastic lymphoma kinase (ALK) on chromosome 2.[20] In both cases, the fusion results in the constitutive activation of the kinase domain through the ability of the partner (Tel or NPM) to promote dimerization, resulting in transphorylation within the activation loop sequences. Interestingly, Tel has also been shown to fuse with the abelson cytoplasmic tyrosine kinase in a case of acute undifferentiated myeloid leukemia with a t(9;12;14)(q34;p13;q22). The fusion product causes oligomerization of the Abl kinase domain and results in its constitutive activation.[21] The biological consequence may be similar to the much more common Bcr/Abl fusion associated with chronic myelogenous leukemia in cases with t(9;22) translocations. The Tel gene is also involved in the activation of the Jak2 cytoplasmic tyrosine kinase as described below. These forms of activation of tyrosine kinases are distinct from the altered expression, without structural modification, of the src family member kinase lck, by translocations that place the Lck locus under the transcriptional control of retroviral promoters.[22]

Cytokine Receptors and Janus Protein Tyrosine Kinases

One of the larger receptor families involved in hematopoiesis is the cytokine receptor superfamily. Members of this receptor family mediate the cellular responses of essential cytokines such as erythropoietin (Epo), thrombopoietin (Tpo), granulocyte-specific colony-stimulating factor (G-CSF), and IL-7, among a wide variety of other cytokines. Initially it had not been expected that this group of cytokines would utilize structurally and functionally related receptors. Indeed, it was only with the initial purification and cloning of several of the receptors that it was realized that they mediated their effects through a very distinct family of receptors. The receptors were initially recognized as a family through conserved motifs that were found in the extracellular domains[23, 24] (Fig. 4–2). These included four positionally conserved cysteine residues and the characteristic tryptophan, serine, any amino acid, tryptophan serine (WSXWS) motif, located normally near the transmembrane domain. Indeed, these motifs are now used to predict that a newly identified protein will be a receptor of this family of receptors.

The crystal structures for several cytokine receptors, complexed with ligands, have been determined. The first structure established was that of the growth hormone receptor.[25] The structure was somewhat surprising in revealing that growth hormone ligates the receptor through interaction with two different sites. The extracellular domains of the receptors consist of a tandem repeat of fibronectin type III-like modules, each containing the characteristic cysteines. From the structure the role of the WSXWS motif cannot be deduced. The structure of growth hormone complexed to the prolactin receptor has also been determined.[26] The structure illustrates a remarkable similarity in structure to the growth hormone receptor although the two receptors contain only 28% identical amino acids in the extracellular domain. More recently the structure of the Epo receptor has been determined, ligated with a peptide that is capable of activing receptor function.[27] Again the structure emphasized the re-

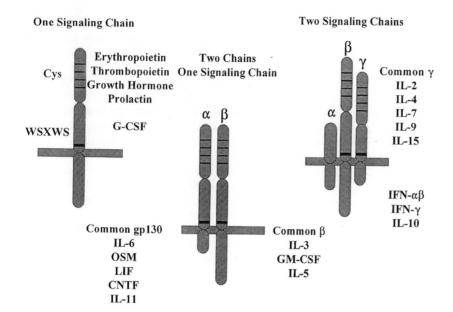

One Signaling Chain

Two Signaling Chains

Figure 4–2. Structures of cytokine receptor superfamily members. The organization of a variety of receptors of the cytokine receptor superfamily is illustrated. The receptors for erythropoietin, thrombopoietin, growth hormone, prolactin, and granulocyte-specific colony stimulating factor (G-CSF) consist of single chains that contain the characteristic, positionally conserved cysteine residues and the WSXWS motif. The receptors for many cytokines consist of two chains, one of which is cytokine specific and one of which is a shared component (gp130 or LIFR for the IL-6 family of cytokines or the common β chain for IL-3, GM-CSF, and IL-5). The family of cytokines that affect lymphoid functions consists of a common γ chain and a ligand-specific component referred to as an α or β chain. In addition, the receptor for IL-2 contains another chain, the α chain, which does not contain the characteristic motifs associated with the other receptor chains. Lastly, the receptors for IFN-αβ, IFN-γ, and IL-10 contain two ligand-specific chains, both of which are essential for signal transduction.

markable similarity of the overall structure of the extracellular domain to the other cytokine receptors. The structure further demonstrated that relatively few contacts were involved in the binding of the peptide miminic leading to the suggestion that activation of cytokine receptors may be accomplished by relatively small molecules, hormone miminics. This concept has been recently established by the identification of a small molecule that is a G-CSF miminic both in vitro and in vivo and functions by binding to a relatively small extracellular domain of the receptor just distal from the transmembrane domain.[28]

Independent of the work on the cytokine receptors, similar efforts were being made to characterize the receptors for the interferons (IFNs). With the purification and cloning of the receptors it became obvious that they were structurally most related to the newly growing family of cytokine receptors with some modification of the extracellular characteristic motifs. For this reason the cytokine receptor superfamily is now generally divided into the cytokine receptor classes I and II, the latter containing the highly related receptors for IFNα, IFNβ, IFNγ, and IL-10.

In spite of the similarity of the extracellular domains, the cytokine receptors have cytoplasmic domains that vary considerably in both structure and size. Indeed, the most disappointing observation was that none of the receptors contained any obvious catalytic domains in the cytoplasmic domain, thus not making it apparent how these receptors might function. The only structural similarity was limited to the membrane proximal domain and consisted of what is often referred to as the box 1 and box 2 motifs.[29] These motifs are very loosely defined and the box 1 "conserved" motif is limited to a pro, any amino acid, pro (P × P) motif. Irrespective of the limited conservation of the sequence, mutational analysis of this region of all the receptors examined indicated that this region was essential for all receptor functions.

Cytokine receptors can consist of one or more chains (see Fig. 4–2). For example, the receptors for Epo, growth hormone, prolactin, and Tpo consist of single chains that are highly related in tertiary structure and therefore have been

suggested to have been derived from a common progenitor. This is particularly likely in the case of the growth hormone and prolactin receptors that genetically colocalize and thus can be envisioned to have arisen from a recent gene duplication event.

The receptors for a number of cytokines consist of multiple chains and often involve the utilization of a ligand-specific chain and a chain that is shared among a number of receptors. For example, the IL-3, GM-CSF and IL-5 receptors all utilize a common β chain that associates with a ligand specific α chain.[30] In addition, in mice, there is an IL-3 specific β chain. Similarily, a large number of cytokines are structurally related to the IL-6 receptor. The IL-6 receptor itself consists of an α chain that functions either as a membrane bound receptor or as a soluble, extracellular ligand binding protein.[31] Either membrane associated or ligated with IL-6 in a soluble complex, the IL-6/α chain complex is required to induce the oligomerization of gp130. In a very similar manner, the receptors for OSM and CNTF consist of a ligand specific component that associates with the common gp130 signaling chain or a highly related signaling chain referred to as the LIFRβ chain.

The cytokines that affect lymphoid cells utilize receptors that have unique receptor components. The structure of the IL-2 receptor was the first to be determined and, as indicated in Figure 4–2, consists of three chains.[32] The first chain identified, termed the α chain or CD25, interestingly does not contain any of the structural motifs of the other receptor chains and, indeed, is not essential for IL-2 signal transduction. It is required to increase the affinity of the β/γ subunits by a factor of one log. The β chain is only found in the receptors of IL-2 and the highly related cytokine IL-15 and provides the ligand specificity of the receptor complex. Signal transduction by the IL-2 receptor complex is absolutely dependent upon the presence of the γ chain that is also required for the function of the majority of the cytokines that affect lymphoid function. Indeed mutation of the γ chain is the most frequent cause of severe combined immunodeficiency (SCID). The receptors for IL-7, IL-7, and IL-9 consist of a ligand specific α chain and the common γ chain initially identified in the IL-2 receptor. Lastly, the IFN receptors each contain two distinct chains that are both required for signal transduction.[33] However, irrespective of the number of chains involved, the common function of the ligand is to drive the aggregation of the receptor chains.

Studies with a variety of the cytokine receptors indicated that receptor function is dependent upon the ability of the receptor to mediate ligand induced activation of tyrosine phosphorylation. Moreover, the induction of tyrosine phosphorylation was dependent upon the conserved membrane proximal region of the cytoplasmic domains of the receptors. These observations prompted the search for cytoplasmic protein tyrosine kinases that might associate with the receptors and mediate the critical first steps in signal transduction. The identification of the critical kinases came from two independent approaches. The first came from studies directed at defining the pathways involved in interferon mediated gene regulation. Initially a number of cell lines were established through an insightful approach to obtain mutant cell lines defective in signaling.[34] These were further defined as constituting a number of independent complementation groups. To identify the genes involved, a complementation screen was done by genomic DNA transfections. Using this approach it was demonstrated that Tyk2, a member of a newly evolving family of protein tyrosine kinases, was able to complement one mutant.[35] This led to the concept that the IFNα/β receptor associated with Tyk2 and mediated its acivation following IFN binding.

Independently, groups were using biochemical approaches to identify the cytoplasmic protein kinases that associated with cytokine receptors and were activated following ligand binding. Although several kinases were implicated by these approaches, many were not significantly activated nor could they be shown to associate with the receptors or activation failed to correlate among receptor mutants. It was only with the development of reagents for the *Janus* kinases that all the criteria were fulfilled. Initially this was demonstrated for Jak2 activation in the response to Epo[36] as well as growth hormone.[37] Subsequent to these studies it has been shown that one or another of the Jak family of kinases associates with all the receptors of the cytokine receptor superfamily.

The Jak family of kinases consists of four members. The family members have a large amino-terminal domain that contains regions of sequence identity. These blocks of homology are found among family members but not with other proteins (Fig. 4–3). This domain has been shown to associate with the cytoplasmic domains of the cytokine receptors and is critical for function within the context of the receptor. The carboxyl-terminal region contains a characteristic protein tyrosine kinase catalytic domain. Amino-terminal to the kinase domain is a pseudokinase domain that contains significant homology to the catalytic domain but which does not have kinase activity. The role of the pseudokinase domain is not known although some studies indicate that it may negatively affect the kinase domain. Three of the family members, Jak1, Jak2, and Tyk2, are ubiquitously expressed while Jak3 is primarily expressed in hematopoietic cells.

The model that has emerged envisions the constitutive association of one or more of the Jaks with specific cytokine receptor chains through the conserved membrane proximal

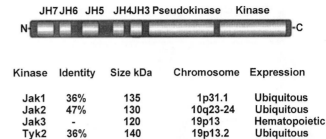

Kinase	Identity	Size kDa	Chromosome	Expression
Jak1	36%	135	1p31.1	Ubiquitous
Jak2	47%	130	10q23-24	Ubiquitous
Jak3	-	120	19p13	Hematopoietic
Tyk2	36%	140	19p13.2	Ubiquitous

Figure 4–3. Structure and properties of the *Janus* family of protein tyrosine kinases. The structural organization of members of the *Janus* family of protein tyrosine kinases is illustrated at the top. The family members have a functional kinase catalytic domain at the carboxyl-tail of the protein. Immediately amino-terminal to the kinase domain is a domain that has the characteristic subdomains found in tyrosine kinase catalytic domains. However, the pseudokinase domain has amino acid changes that would suggest the lack of functional activity, consistent with the inability to demonstrate kinase activity by the pseudokinase domain. The large amino-terminal domain consists of blocks of similarities among the family members. These are referred to as Jak homology domains and are not found in other proteins. The amino-terminal domain is involved in association with the cytoplasmic domain of cytokine receptors. The bottom section indicates the pattern of expression, the chromosomal location of the human genes, the apparent protein size, and the percent identity of various family members to Jak3.

region (Fig. 4–4). For example, the Epo, Tpo, GH, and prolactin receptors associate with Jak2 through the membrane proximal domain. The ligand is envisioned to drive aggregation of the receptor complex, bringing into close proximity the associated Jak2. Transphosphorylation can then occur and result in the activation of kinase activity. A variety of studies with receptor and Jak mutants support this model of ligand induced activation.

One of the unique receptor systems is that associated with the IL-6 subfamily of cytokines. In this case, the receptors consist of ligand specific components and a shared receptor chain referred to as gp130 or the highly related chain LIFRβ. These receptor chains can bind multiple Jaks and mediate their ligand dependent activation. In this context it is important to note that the single chain receptor for G-CSF is much more related to that of the gp130 receptor chain than to the receptors for Epo, Tpo, prolactin, or growth hormone and, like gp130, binds multiple Jaks.

Lastly, several of the receptors that utilize multiple chains also utilize multiple Jaks. For example, the IL-2 subfamily of cytokines activates both Jak1 and Jak3. This is through the ability of Jak3 to bind to the common γ chain and by the binding of Jak1 to the ligand specific α chains, such as in the case of IL-7 or IL-4, or to the β chain in the case of the receptors for IL-2 and IL-15. The activation however is still envisioned to involve ligand induced receptor aggregation resulting in placing the Jaks in sufficient proximity to allow their activation.

The activation of the Jaks, in each case, involves the transphosphorylation of a critical tyrosine within the activation loop of the kinase domain. Although the molecular structures of the Jaks have not been determined, the sequence of the kinase domain is highly related to that of the receptor tyrosine kinases, particularly in the activation loop region of the kinase domain. Consistent with a role for tyrosine phosphorylation of sites within the activation loop, mutation

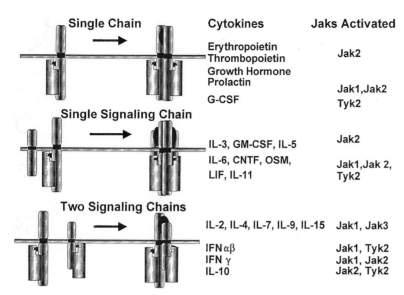

Figure 4–4. Mechanisms of activation of cytokine receptor superfamily members. The activation of cytokine receptor superfamily members involves the ligand induced aggregation of receptor chains and the transphosphorylation and activation of the associated Jak family kinases. Receptors consist of signal chains that associate specifically with Jak2 or the G-CSF receptor that can associate with three of the family members. Receptors consisting of a ligand-specific binding chain and the signal transducing chain are illustrated in the middle. The common β chain of the IL-3 related cytokine receptors uniquely associates with Jak2 while gp130, or the related signaling chain LIFRβ, can associate with multiple Jaks. Lastly, the IL-2 family of lymphoid cytokine receptors has a ligand-specific chain that associates with Jak1 while the common γ chain associates with Jak3. The IFN related receptors consist of two essential signaling chains, each of which associates with a specific Jak family member as indicated.

of the presumed critical sites results in the virtual elimination of catalytic activity.[38–40]

A confirmation for the critical role of the Jaks in cytokine signaling has come from studies of humans and mice that lack specific Jaks. In particular, Jak3 is unique among the Jaks in that it has only been shown to bind to the γ_c chain and thus would only be hypothesized to function within the context of the cytokines that use this receptor chain. This group of cytokines, which includes IL-2, IL-4, IL-7, IL-9, and IL-15, predominantly functions within the context of the immune system. In particular, IL-7 is known to be essential for the amplification of early progenitors. Loss of IL-7, or its receptor chains, results in a phenotype of SCID.[41] The observation that mice deficient in Jak3 also have a phenotype of SCID supports a critical role for Jak3 in IL-7 signaling.[42, 43] Moreover, the phenotype of mice lacking Jak3 indicates that this kinase is not required for any other functions including normal development in general or myeloid lineage development in particular.

SCID is also a genetically acquired disease in humans. Although the most frequent form of human SCID is associated with mutations in the IL-2 receptor γ_c chain, it has recently been shown that some SCID patients have inherited mutations that disrupt the Jak3 gene.[44–46] Based on the essential role for Jak3 in the amplification of the earliest lymphoid progenitors, it might be anticipated that a deficiency in Jak3 would be correctable through gene therapy. Indeed, recent studies with a murine model have shown that retroviral mediated transfer of the Jak3 gene to early hematopoietic stem cells and reconstitution into deficient mice can rapidly correct the immunodeficiency.[47] It will be of considerable interest to determine whether the same degree of efficacy is observed in human SCID, Jak3-deficient patients.

More recent studies have focused on the role of the Jak1 and Jak2 through the derivation of mice that are deficient in these family members. Mice that are deficient in Jak1 are born viable and die shortly thereafter.[48] Although the actual cause of lethality is not known, a number of receptor systems have been examined. For example, receptor signaling through the IL-2 subfamily of cytokines is defective, consistent with an essential role for both Jak1, as well as Jak3, in

the receptors for these cytokines. Similarly, all the IFN receptors have been shown to activate Jak1 and to have a receptor chain that associates with Jak1. In the knockout mice these functions are also lost. Perhaps more relevant to the early lethality, however, is the observation that signaling through the IL-6 family of receptors is severely affected by the absence of Jak1. This is particularly interesting since all these receptors also associate with and activate Jak2 or Tyk2. Thus, for reasons yet to be defined, the IL-6 family of receptors uniquely requires Jak1 activation.

The absence of Jak2 is more profound and results in an embryonic lethality at 10–12 days of development.[49, 50] In this case lethality is due to the lack of production of definitive erythrocytes and, indeed, the phenotype is similar but perhaps more profound, than the phenotype seen in mice lacking either the Epo receptor or Epo.[51] The ability of fetal liver cells to respond to cytokines that had been shown to activate Jak2 was also lost including the responses to Tpo, IL-3, IL-5, and GM-CSF. Importantly, other aspects of embryonic development were normal. Also the ability of members of the IL-6 family of receptors, the IL-2 family of receptors, G-CSF, and IFNα/β were not affected. However, the ability to respond to IFNγ was lost, as predicted by the unique activation of Jak2 by this IFN. Together the results establish the critical role of Jak2 in a very defined group of cytokines that utilizes receptors that associate with Jak2.

Following receptor aggregation and activation of the Jaks through phosphorylation within the activation loop, phosphorylation of the receptor is observed as well as phosphorylation of a variety of cellular substrates. The emerging models for receptor complex activation and signaling specificity are virtually identical to those proposed for the protein tyrosine kinase receptors. Namely, tyrosine phosphorylation sites on the receptor chains are "docking" sites that allow the recruitment of potential substrates and signal transducers to the receptor complex in a receptor specific manner. In addition, however, the Jaks are themselves tyrosine phosphorylated at multiple sites and, although yet to be clearly demonstrated, it can be hypothesized that one or more of these sites will also be important in recruiting signaling proteins to the receptor complex.

Like the tyrosine kinase receptors, it is important to consider the mechanisms by which the cytokine receptor complexes are downregulated. In this case considerable evidence exists to indicate that one of the tyrosine specific phosphatases plays a key role. In particular, the SH2 domain containing phosphatase SHP-1 is recruited to many of the receptor complexes through its ability to interact with sites of tyrosine phosphorylation on the receptor through its SH2 domains. Recruitment of the phosphatase to the Epo receptor complex has been shown to be associated with receptor down-regulation and specifically with the de-phosphorylation of the associated Jak2.[52] However, the most dramatic evidence comes from the phenotype of mice in which the SHP-1 gene is mutated.[53, 54] These mice die within a few weeks after birth and have a variety of defects of the hematopoietic system that collectively are associated with overproliferation. The results are consistent with a broad role for SHP-1 in the regulation of cytokine signaling.

Recent studies[55, 56] have indicated that the Jaks may also be involved in leukemias. In particular, fusions of the ets transcription factor family member Tel with the kinase domain of Jak2 have been shown to occur in lymphoid leukemias containing a t(9;12) translocation and in a t(9;15;12) translocation in a patient with myeloid disease. As in the cases with the fusions to the PDGF receptor or abl, the consequence of the fusion is the constitutive activation of the Jak2 kinase catalytic domain. The fusion protein is able to abrogate the growth factor dependence of myeloid or lymphoid factor dependent cell lines. It might be anticipated that translocations will be identified that involve other Jak family members.

Potential Regulators of Cytokine Receptor Signaling: JABs, SOCS, CIS

Recent studies have raised the provocative hypothesis that a family of structurally related, immediate early genes are involved in the negative regulation of cytokine receptor signal transduction. Initially, an immediate early gene was identified in the response to erythropoietin, the expresssion of which was regulated by the activation of the transcription factors Stat5a or Stat5b (see below). The gene product CIS (cytokine-inducible SH2-containing protein) consists of a relatively small protein containing an SH2 domain[57] that binds to phosphorylation sites on the Epo receptor. Based on these observations it was proposed that Epo, by activating the Stat5 transcription factors, induces the expression of CIS which, in turn, binds to the receptor complex and down-regulates its activity. Presumably, CIS would mediate a comparable affect in the response to other cytokines that induce its expression including Tpo, growth hormone, prolactin, IL-3, and GM-CSF, among others.

Subsequent to the identification of CIS, a structurally related protein was identified independently by three groups, which, unfortunately, resulted in three names for the same gene product, JAB1, SOCS1, and SSI1. In one case the gene was identified by its ability to bind to phosphorylated Jak2 (Jak binding protein 1, JAB-1).[58] In another laboratory it was isolated as a gene product that could suppress IL-6–induced myeloid cell line differentiation (SOCS-1, suppressor of cytokine signaling).[59] Lastly, the gene was identi-

fied in attempts to isolate novel Stat proteins using an antibody against the SH2 domain of Stat3, SSI1 (Stat-induced Stat inhibitor-1).[60] JAB1 has homology to CIS in being a relatively small, SH2 containing protein. In addition there is a region of homology at the carboxyl-region that is now referred to as the SOCS homology domain. Searching of data bases resulted in the identification of at least 20 proteins that contain the SOCS homology domain, eight of which contain an SH2 domain. Other proteins that contain SOCS domains contain various additional motifs that allow them to be divided into four distinct families.

The biological roles of the members of the CIS/JAB family of genes are based on both the means by which they were identified as well as results derived from overexpression of the genes in various biological assays. In general, the results have suggested that the members of this family bind in activated receptor complexes with either the Jaks, the receptor, or presumably substrates of tyrosine phosphorylation within the complex. As noted above, these interactions are speculated to suppress cytokine signaling. Targeted gene disruptions have only recently begun to provide another vantage point from which to assess function. In the case of CIS, mice lacking the gene have no detectable phenotype (S. Teglund, C. Marine, J.N. Ihle, unpublished data). More recently, mice deficient in SOCS-1 (JAB1, SSI1) have been derived.[61, 62] The phenotype is quite complex and the mice exhibit stunted growth and die before weaning with fatty degeneration of the liver and monocytic infiltration of several organs. In addition, there is a marked loss of both B cells and T cells.

Substrates of Tyrosine Kinases

The activation of receptor tyrosine kinases results in the recruitment and phosphorylation of a variety of substrates that have been identified over the last several years (Table 4–2). Importantly, many of these proteins are also substrates in response to ligands that activate receptors of the cytokine receptor superfamily as well as substrates for tyrosine phosphorylation by the kinases associated with T and B cell receptors and with the Fc receptors. Although identified as

Table 4–2. Tyr-Kinase Substrates

Phospholipase C γ1 and γ2
p85α and p85β; regulatory subunits of PI-3 kinase
SH2-containing tyrosine phosphatase (SHP-2)
Vav
SHC adapter protein
Stam
SHIP
Cbl
Insulin response substrates (IRS)
Signal transducers and activators of transcription (Stats)
Crk, Crkl
p130Cas, p105Casl
Hepatocyte growth factor regulated kinase substrate (Hrs)
Linker for activation of T cells (LAK)
Lnk
SH2 domain-containing leukocyte protein of 76 kDa (SLP-76)
IL-4 receptor interacting protein (FRIP)
p62^{dok}

substrates, the roles of many of these substrates of phosphorylation are only now becoming obvious. In many cases, tyrosine phosphorylation of a substrate allows it to associate with other proteins and thus the concept has evolved of adapter or linker proteins. When phosphorylated these proteins allow the formation of complexes that are involved in signal transduction. Alternatively, tyrosine phosphorylation may alter the enzyme activity of a protein or, in the case of the Stat proteins, allow dimerization, nuclear translocation, and DNA binding activity.

Regulatory Subunits of PI-3K

The phosphoinositides are components of membrane lipids and serve as critical signaling molecules in a variety of settings. Two principle modifications are induced in response to ligands, including the phosphorylation/dephosphorylation and the hydrolysis of the inositol moiety (Fig. 4–5). The phosphorylations are mediated by kinases that are specific for the 3, 4, or 5 positions of inositol. Among these, many receptor systems affect the function of the enzymes that phosphorylate the 3 position. More recently, a phosphatase that is specific for the 5 position has been identified as a substrate of tyrosine phosphorylation. The cleavage of the inositol moiety is mediated by phospholipases. The lipid products of PI-3 kinases have been implicated in a variety of signaling pathways[63]; several critical ones are indicated below.

One of the common receptor mediated events is the activation of phosphoinositide 3-kinase activity. Such activity is seen with protein tyrosine kinase receptors and the cytokine receptor superfamily, as well as with several of the G-protein coupled receptors. The interest in phosphatidylinositol phosphorylation originated with the observation that phosphatidylinositol (PtdIns) kinase activity was associated with the polyoma middle T complexes with c-src.[64] It was speculated that such activity might contribute to the mechanism by which middle T transforms cells. Subsequently, it was demonstrated that an avian transforming virus had transduced the PI 3-kinase catalytic subunit and that increased activity was required for transforming activity.[65] Therefore the biological data suggest that the ability to regulate the production of 3-phosphoinositols can influence cell proliferation. The focus therefore has been to determine how receptor complexes regulate the activity and utilize phospholipids in cellular signaling.[66]

In mammals there are several different enzymes that can mediate the PtdIns 3-kinase reaction.[67, 68] Two enzymes mediate a specific PtdIns 3-kinase reaction and are not known to be regulated by any signaling system. However, a p120 PI 3-kinase is known to be activated by both the α and βγ heterotrimeric G protein complexes. In addition, three catalytic subunits, p110α, p110β, and p110*, have PI 3-kinase activity that is regulated through the association with regulatory subunits. The p110* isoform is of interest since, unlike the other isoforms, it is primarily expressed in the lymphoid lineages.[69] Importantly the regulatory subunit isoforms (p85α, p85β, and p55[PIK]) contain two SH2 domains as well as an SH3 domain in the case of p85α and p85β, and two proline rich domains. The model currently envisions that the regulatory subunit is recruited to an activated receptor complex through interaction of the SH2 domains with sites of tyrosine phosphorylation on the receptor. This interaction recruits the catalytic p110 subunit to the membrane associated receptor complex and in contact with its potential substrates. This ultimately results in the generation of PtdIns (3) P, PtdIns (3,4) P, and PtdIns (3,4,5) P. These signaling molecules are then available to propagate a signal or as indicated below, cause the recruitment of other proteins to the membrane.

Studies of the role of the PI 3-kinases in cellular responses have been greatly aided by the identification of inhibitors that are relatively specific. Wortmannin is a steroid-like toxin isolated from a soil bacterium, while LY294002 is a bioflavonoid derived from quercitin. As with any inhibitors, however, caution in interpretation of results must be used since the affects may reflect activity against unknown additional targets.

Precisely how the 3-phosphorylated lipids function as second messengers is not known. Studies have identified at least two potential links in signal transduction. First, it has been shown that Ras interacts with the catalytic subunit of PI 3-kinase in a GTP-dependent manner and may influence the catalytic activity of PI 3-kinase.[70] The ras dependent activation of PI 3-kinase is speculated to be essential for the membrane ruffling seen in ras transformed cells. The second potential signaling linked pathway is with apoptosis. Specifically, 3-phosphorylated lipids bind to and activate the Akt (also termed protein kinase B, PKB) serine/threonine kinase. Activated Akt has been found to phosphorylate a protein termed Bad.[71, 72] Bad, in the nonphosphorylated form, binds to Bcl-2 and inactivates its ability to suppress apoptosis.[73] The functions of Bcl-2 in preventing apoptosis are discussed in greater detail below. Thus ligand-mediated activation of Akt, through the activation of PI 3-kinase, is hypothesized to be able to suppress cell death.

Alternatively, the essential function of PI 3-kinase may be to generate 3-phosphorylated lipids themselves. These lipids bind proteins with plecstrin homology domains and SH2 domains. Such binding would result in the translocation of various proteins to the inner membrane surface where

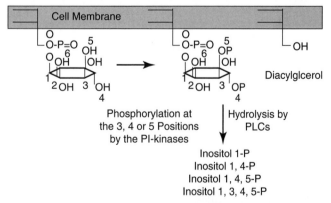

Phosphorylation at the 3, 4 or 5 Positions by the PI-kinases

Hydrolysis by PLCs

Inositol 1-P
Inositol 1, 4-P
Inositol 1, 4, 5-P
Inositol 1, 3, 4, 5-P

Figure 4–5. Phosphoinositide metabolism in signal transduction. Phosphoinositides are components of membrane lipids and their modification is a common feature of activation of cytokine receptors. The modifications can involve the phosphorylation of the inositol moiety at one or several positions. Receptor engagement is also often associated with the hydrolysis of the inositol moiety by C-type phospholipases, resulting in the liberation of diacylglcerol that is capable of activating protein kinase C.

activation may occur and result in the membrane reorganization or other membrane-associated changes. There have been a number of proteins shown to bind phospholipids through their plecstrin homology domains including Btk (Bruton's tyrosine kinase), a cytoplasmic kinase that is essential for B-cell development. In the absence of Btk, or in the presence of mutations within the plecstrin homology domain, B-cell development is impaired resulting in agammaglobulinemia.[74, 75] As noted above, the role of PI 3-kinase activity in fundamental aspects of cell function is indicated by the observations that a transforming avian retrovirus transduced an activated form of the catalytic subunit. More recently a p55-activated, transforming form of the p85α regulatory subunit has been identified in a thymoma.[76]

The role of phosphorylation of lipids in general cellular regulation has also been supported by studies of the tumor suppressor gene termed PTEN. The gene was initially identified as a gene mapping to a tumor suppressor locus on 10q23.3 and mutations of the PTEN gene were identified in a wide variety of tumor types.[77, 78] Although initially characterized as a potential dual-specific phosphatase,[79] it was subsequently shown that PTEN was phospholipid phosphatase capable of dephosphorylating the 3 position of the phosphatidylinositol 3,4,5-trisphosphate.[80] The deletion of PTEN results in an embryonic lethality at embryonic day 9.5 that is characterized by an overgrowth of the cephalic and caudal areas of the developing brain.[81] The defect is associated with enhanced proliferation and decreased apoptosis. Fibroblasts from deficient embryos are remarkably resistant to a number of inducers of apoptosis. The key to the relationship came from the observation that in deficient fibroblasts, Akt is hyperphosphorylated and constitutively active. Thus the model has emerged that PTEN is required to dephosphorylate IP_3, thereby reducing activation of Akt and consequently increasing the susceptibility of the cells to apoptosis.

More recently, the role of one of the regulatory subunits of PI 3-kinase activity has been assessed by the derivation of mice lacking one or all isoforms.[82, 83] Specifically, the p8α gene encodes three proteins, derived by alternative splicing of p85, p55, or p50. Disruption of the gene in such a manner as to only remove the p85 form results in the derivation of viable mice that have impaired B-cell development that is nearly identical to mice in which the Btk gene is disrupted. Disruption of the gene in a manner that removes all isoforms results in a perinatal lethality of undefined origin. Reconstitution of the lymphoid lineages with cells lacking all isoforms had a similar phenotype to that observed in mice lacking only the p85 isoform, demonstrating that among the various splice variants, p85 uniquely plays an essential role in B-cell development through its regulation of Btk activity or localization.

Phospholipases

A wide variety of tyrosine kinase receptors, as well as activated Jak kinases, phosphorylate phospholipase C γ1 or γ2 on tyrosines. The enzymes are recruited to the receptor complex through SH2 domains that recognize specific sites of tyrosine phosphorylation in the receptor complex. The subsequent phosphorylation has been shown to increase the catalytic activity of PLC-γ1,[84] and it is presumed that PLC-γ2 is comparably regulated. However, it should be noted that the in vitro phosphorylation of PLC-γ1 by the EGF receptor, although occurring on the same sites as in vivo, did not affect catalytic activity,[85] suggesting an indirect, unknown, mechanism of activation in vivo.

The PLC enzymes mediate the liberation of phosphatidylinositol 1,4,5-trisphosphate (IP_3) from membrane phospholipids and the production of diacylglycerol (DAG) (see Fig. 4–5).[86] Following the release of IP_3 into the cytosol, IP_3 binds receptors on the endoplasmic reticulum resulting in an efflux of Ca^{++}. The increased Ca^{++} levels then affect a variety of enzymes that are regulated by Ca^{++} including calmodulin, which regulates the activity of CaM kinases. The kinases, in turn, regulate the activity of downstream targets. For example, CaM kinase II phosphorylates the transcription factor, cyclic AMP response element binding protein (CREB). The DAG that is produced activates serine/threonine kinases of the protein kinase C family. Protein kinase C is also the physiological substrate of the tumor promoting phorbol esters. The activation of PKC has been associated with the phosphorylation of several substrates and, indirectly, with the activation of NF-κB.

The role of PLC-γ1 in signaling has been explored through the derivation of mice lacking the gene. Unfortunately, the disruption of the gene results in an embryonic lethality at approximately 9 days of development.[87] The basis for lethality has not been determined although fibroblasts derived from mutant embryos respond normally to fibroblast growth factor and epidermal growth factor, both of which induce the tyrosine phosphorylation and activation of PLC-γ1 activity.[88] Comparable studies have not been published for PLC-γ2 that, unlike PLC-γ1, is predominantly expressed in hematopoietic cells. Recent studies[89] have implicated this isoform in signal transduction from the CSF-1 receptor and may contribute to signaling that is required for differentiation.

▼ SHIP

SHIP (SH2 containing inositol 5-phosphatase) had been initially identified as a substrate of tyrosine phosphorylation that associated with SHC in the response to various cytokines[90, 91] and was recently cloned. It contains an amino-terminal SH2 domain, a central 5′-phosphoinositol phosphatase domain, two PTB domains, and a proline rich carboxyl tail. A wide variety of growth factors (i.e. SCF, CSF-1) and cytokines (i.e. Epo, IL-3, Tpo) as well as the T cell and B cell receptors induce SHIP phosphorylation. SHIP selectively hydrolyzes the 5′-phosphate from inositol 1,3,4,5-tetraphosphate and the 3,4,5-trisphosphate. Phosphorylations do not appear to affect enzyme activity but may be important in recruiting components into the complex.

Mice have recently been obtained that are deficient for SHIP by homologous recombination in ES cells.[92] Viable mice can be obtained, thus indicating that SHIP is not non-redundantly essential for normal development. However, the mice fail to survive for normal times and die with massive myeloid cell infiltration of the lungs. Studies of the hematopoietic progenitors are consistent with the hypothesis that SHIP normally negatively affects cytokine responses. More studies will be required to precisely define the role of SHIP in signal transduction.

▼ SHP-1 AND SHP-2

Two tyrosine specific phosphatases have been consistently implicated in signal transduction by receptors that activate tyrosine phosphorylation. The two structurally similar proteins, SHP-1 and SHP-2, contain a carboxyl-localized tyrosine phosphatase catalytic domain.[93–95] In addition both proteins contain two amino-terminal localized SH2 domains. In spite of the structural similarity the proposed roles in signal transduction are speculated to be quite different. SHP-1 is recruited to a variety of receptor complexes through the interaction of the SH2 domains with sites of tyrosine phosphorylation. With binding, the catalytic activity is increased and is responsible for the dephosphorylation of the receptor and, in the case of cytokine receptors, the kinase responsible for activation of signal transduction. The model therefore is that the recruitment of SHP-1 to the receptor complexes is essential for down-regulating receptor function.

The model for SHP-1 has been largely confirmed by the characterization of a naturally occurring mutant of mice, termed *motheaten*, in which a mutation inactivates SHP-1.[53, 54] The phenotype is complex and involves multiple lineages but is consistent with the excessive proliferation of a variety of hematopoietic lineages. As a consequence the mice survive for only a few weeks.

In contrast to SHP-1, SHP-2 is hypothesized to contribute positively to cellular responses although precisely how is not known. SHP-2 is tyrosine phosphorylated when recruited to receptor complexes and has been proposed to act as an adapter protein and does not require catalytic activity. Unfortunately, the derivation of mice deficient in SHP-2 has not provided much insight into its function. Although the mutation results in an embryonic lethal, it has not been possible to precisely define the receptor systems that are affected.[96]

The regulation of SHP-2 activity by binding to phosphotyrosine motifs has been determined by obtaining the crystal structure of SHP-2.[97] The structure has revealed that the amino-terminal SH2 domain binds intramolecularly to the catalytic domain and blocks the active site. Binding of a phosphopeptide to the amino terminal SH2 domain releases this inhibition and stimulates catalytic activity 10 fold. Binding of phosphopeptides to both SH2 domains further increases catalytic activity to 100 fold that of the non-engaged phosphatase. Thus the model hypothesizes that binding to the receptor complex activates the tyrosine phosphatase activity toward substrates.

▼ Vav

The gene *Vav* was initially identified by its contribution to a fusion protein that was associated with transforming activity.[98] Subsequently it was shown that *Vav* is rapidly tyrosine phosphorylated in the response to cytokines or growth factors that utilize either cytokine receptor superfamily members or receptor tyrosine kinases. The ability of a particular receptor complex to mediate *Vav* phosphorylation again is dependent upon the existence of receptor-phosphorylated tyrosines that can recruit the protein through the *Vav* SH2 domain.

The biochemical functions of *Vav*, phosphorylated or unphosphorylated, are not fully defined. Evidence has been presented that *Vav* is a guanine nucleotide exchange factor (GEF) for ras and thus could potentially link *Vav* to the ras signaling pathway.[99] However, subsequent studies have failed to establish this link although *Vav* may function as a GEF for another ras family member. In addition, it has been suggested that *Vav* is associated with phosphatidylinositol 3-kinase activity and thus may link receptor activation to phosphatidylinositol signaling.[100] These types of observations indicate the considerable difficulty that is often seen when trying to determine how a particular protein fits in cellular signaling.

Although a variety of studies, using various approaches, had suggested a broadly significant role for *Vav* in cytokine and growth factor signaling, the phenotype of mice that lack the *Vav* gene indicates a more proscribed function.[101–103] Mice lacking *Vav* die during early embryogenesis[104]; however, the role in hematopoiesis has been examined by reconstitution experiments. In particular, the only defect that was identified was a loss of function of T and B cells in signaling through the antigen specific receptors. Conversely, no defects were detectable in hematopoiesis although a variety of cytokines, such as Epo, induce the tyrosine phosphorylation of *Vav*.

▼ INSULIN RESPONSE SUBSTRATES

The insulin response substrates (IRS-1 and IRS-2) were initially identified in studies of the substrates of insulin-induced tyrosine phosphorylation.[105, 106] This initially led to the cloning of IRS-1 and the subsequent identification of a highly related protein termed IRS-2. More recently, a smaller protein of 60 kDa has been identified that structurally is related to the IRS proteins and is speculated to be a member of the family, referred to as IRS-3. Both the IRS-1 and IRS-2 proteins are common substrates of ligand induced tyrosine phosphorylation in the response to a variety of growth hormones as well as cytokines. The phosphorylation of IRS proteins has been shown to be critical for IL-4 induced proliferation of myeloid lineage cells.[107] Both IRS-1 and IRS-2 contain a pleckstrin homology domain at the amino-terminal and multiple sites of tyrosine phosphorylation throughout the remainder of the protein. The IRS proteins are generally regarded as adapter proteins that can recruit a variety of signaling proteins to the receptor complex through the interaction of phosphotyrosine binding domains with sites of IRS phosphorylation, thus providing surrogate "docking" sites.

The roles of phosphorylation of the IRS proteins in many of the situations in which their phosphorylation is seen are not known. However, mice that are deficient in IRS-1 are severely growth retarded due to insulin-like growth factor 1 resistance as well as insulin resistance.[108, 109] More recently, mice have been derived that are deficient in IRS-2.[110] The deletion results in impaired peripheral insulin signaling and pancreatic β-cell function that results in progressive diabetes similar in pathology to human type 2 diabetes. It is anticipated that mice that lack both IRS-1 and IRS-2 may have a more severe phenotype. Interesting mice that are heterozygous for the loss of IRS-1 and the insulin receptor develop a noninsulin-dependent diabetes mellitus with age.[111] Irrespective the data suggest that IRS-1 functions primarily within the context of the insulin and insulin-like growth factor receptors. The significance of ligand induced IRS phosphorylation in the context of other receptors such as Epo or IL-4 is much less clear.

▼ SIGNAL TRANSDUCERS AND ACTIVATORS OF TRANSCRIPTION

The signal transducers and activators of transcription (Stats) were discovered in studies to identify the IFN-regulated transcription factors that mediated the gene inductions associated with the establishment of an antiviral response.[34] Subsequent studies both identified additional members of the family and implicated these proteins in regulation of gene transcription by a variety of cytokines that utilize cytokine receptors as well as growth factors and cytokines that utilize tyrosine kinase receptors. Although most commonly associated with cytokine responses that utilize receptors of the cytokine receptor superfamily, a variety of reports have appeared that demonstrate that these proteins can also be activated by members of the tyrosine kinase receptor family. As detailed below, the significance of these latter observations, if any, is not apparent at this time.

The structure of the Stat proteins is shown in Figure 4–6. The Stats consist of a centrally located, conserved DNA binding domain that binds a palindromic sequence with the consensus sequence of TTT NC N NN NAA, which is referred to as the IFN activated sequence (GAS). This DNA binding domain, although highly conserved among the Stats, is not found in any other DNA binding proteins. In addition, the Stats contain a phosphotyrosine binding, SH2 domain that is highly conserved among the various family members. As noted below, this domain is critical for a number of Stat functions. Immediately after the SH2 domain is a positionally conserved tyrosine that is critical for function. The carboxyl-domains are highly diverse but in all cases are required for transcriptional activation. The amino-terminal

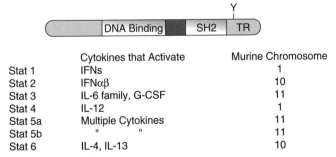

	Cytokines that Activate	Murine Chromosome
Stat 1	IFNs	1
Stat 2	IFNαβ	10
Stat 3	IL-6 family, G-CSF	11
Stat 4	IL-12	1
Stat 5a	Multiple Cytokines	11
Stat 5b	" "	11
Stat 6	IL-4, IL-13	10

Figure 4–6. Structure and members of the family of signal transducers and activators of transcription. The domain organization of members of the Stat family is illustrated at the top. The Stat specific DNA binding domain resides in the middle of the protein. The critical SH2 domain resides carboxyl to the DNA binding domain and near a critical tyrosine that, in its phosphorylated state, is essential for dimer formation, nuclear translocation, and gene activation. The carboxyl-tail region contains a transcriptional activation domain that is essential for function.

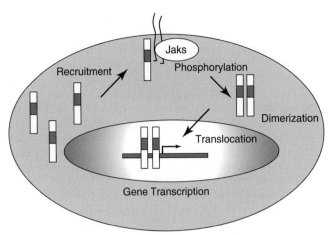

Figure 4–7. Activation of Stats by receptor complexes. The sequence of events in the activation of Stat proteins is illustrated. The Stat proteins exist as cytoplasmic latent proteins that are recruited to an activated receptor complex through the interaction of their SH2 domains with specific sites of tyrosine phosphorylation on the receptor chains. Following recruitment the Stats are phosphorylated on a critical carboxyl-terminal tyrosine, either by cytokine receptor associated Jaks or by receptor tyrosine kinases. Following phosphorylation, the Stats homo- or heterodimerize through the interaction of the carboxyl phosphotyrosine with the SH2 domain of the partner molecule. The dimer then translocates to the nucleus through unknown mechanisms, binds specifics sites on DNA, and either induces or suppresses gene transcription depending upon the transcription complex.

domain contains conserved elements and is likely to be involved in stabilization of dimers and translocation of the dimer to the nucleus.

The molecular structures of two Stat family members have been recently determined.[112, 113] The structure is quite remarkable in several aspects. Dimer formation is essential for DNA binding and as indicated below, this requires tyrosine phosphorylation of a critical carboxyl tyrosine. The structural data show that this tyrosine is on a flexible loop that bends in such a manner as to allow its binding by the SH2 domain of the partner molecule and thereby "fixes" the dimer conformation. The DNA binding domains straddle the DNA with the dimerization region positioned above the minor groove of the DNA. In overall structure the Stat DNA binding complex is very similar to that observed with the NF-κB transcription family members.

The model for the Jak-Stat signaling pathway is remarkably elegant in its simplicity (Fig. 4–7).[114–116] The Stat proteins exist as latent cytoplasmic proteins that are widely expressed. Ligand binding and receptor complex activation result in the creation of phosphotyrosine docking sites that are recognized by the SH2 domains of the Stats. Each Stat recognizes different phosphotyrosine sites, based on the flanking sequences, and thus only certain Stats are recruited to a particular receptor complex. This specificity is elegantly illustrated by the ability to move such sites to different receptors and thereby change the pattern of Stat recruitment.[117] Once the Stat is recruited to the complex, it is phosphorylated on the critical tyrosine that is carboxyl to the SH2 domain. This phosphorylation is mediated by the Jaks and requires the Stat SH2 domain for recognition by the Jak. Importantly, there is no apparent specificity of a particular Jak for a particular Stat, thus emphasizing that all the specificity for activation is dependent upon the receptor structure.

Following the tyrosine phosphorylation of the Stat, they form homo- or heterodimers through the interaction of the SH2 domains with the carboxyl phosphotyrosine site. This interaction is of particularly high affinity and drives the reaction toward the accumulation of the dimers. As dimers, the Stats are able to bind DNA, whereas the monomers have no detectable DNA binding activity, consistent with the symmetrical DNA binding motif. Also as dimers the Stats translocate to the nucleus where they contribute to the activation of gene expression. The mechanisms involved in the ultimate turnover of the proteins in the nucleus are not known but have been speculated to involve either a proteosome dependent pathway or dephosphorylation and recycling of the protein to the cytoplasm.

Certain Stats have been found to heterodimerize with other Stats. For example, a commonly observed heterodimer is one consisting of Stat1 and Stat3. However, there are limitations and thus, for example, the only heterodimers of Stat5 proteins that have been observed are those that occur between the two very highly related Stat5 genes referred to as Stat5a and Stat5b. Therefore, although heterodimerization has the potential to significantly expand the spectrum of transcriptional complexes that can be generated, the extent to which this occurs is not clear.

The significance of Stat activation has largely come from the analysis of mice that lack individual Stat family members. As indicated in Figure 4–6, there have been seven mammalian Stat genes identified and to date mutant mice have been generated for each of the Stats with the exception of Stat2. The first mutant mice generated were deficient in Stat1.[118] Stat1 is activated in the responses to both IFNα/β as well as IFNγ and was identified as the transcription factor that was activated in the responses of IFNs and mediated the transcriptional activation of genes involved in the establishment of an antiviral response. A variety of reports, however, demonstrated that Stat1 could be activated in other responses, both in the context of cytokine receptor superfamily members as well as members of the receptor tyrosine kinases.

The phenotype of mice that are deficient in Stat1 was quite striking in that the mice, under pathogen-free living conditions, developed completely normally.[118, 119] Therefore Stat1 is either not required, or is redundant to another factor, for any aspect of normal developmental physiology. However, the mice were found to be extremely sensitive to infection by a variety of viruses and bacteria. The sensitivity to some viruses was increased a dramatic 10,000 fold. The results have emphasized, in a striking manner, the critical role that the IFN system, through its ability to activate Stat1, plays in our daily effort to survive infectious agents.

Stat3 is primarily activated within the context of members of the IL-6 subfamily of cytokines including cytokines such as leptin and leukemia inhibitory factor (LIF). Within the context of IL-6, Stat3 is required for the expression of a wide variety of genes collectively referred to as the acute phase response genes. Mutant mice lacking Stat3 die early during embryogenesis, probably prior to gastrulation, indicating an essential role for some aspect of early embryogenesis.[120] Although relatively little information is available, it has been suggested that in these mice mesoderm fails to

develop. In this context it is important to note that one of the cytokines that strongly activates Stat4 is LIF and derivation of mice lacking LIF has demonstrated its essential maternal role in supporting implantation.[121] Thus, it could be envisioned that maternally derived LIF is signaling embryonic tissues through the activation of Stat3 for critical events in implantation. It will be of some interest to develop conditional mutant mice such that the function of Stat3 in adult physiology can be examined. For example, recently mice were derived in which Stat3 was deleted in the T-cell lineage, resulting in a very minor phenotype.[122]

Stat4 was initially cloned by homology with Stat1 and for a considerable time it was an orphan Stat for which a ligand was not identified that would induce its tyrosine phosphorylation and activation.[123, 124] However, it was ultimately shown that, among the approximately 50 cytokines that utilize receptors of the cytokine receptor superfamily, IL-12 induced the activation of Stat4.[125, 126] In addition to its activation by IL-12, however, Stat4 had a number of interesting properties including the loss of expression in differentiating hematopoietic cells and high levels of expression during the terminal stages of spermatogenesis. Irrespective, the Stat4 deficient mice were not deficient in either hematopoiesis or in spermatogenesis. Indeed the primary defects in these mice were specifically related to the biological functions of IL-12.[127, 128] The defects included a loss of upregulation of NK cytolytic activity of spleen cells in response to IL-12. In addition, IL-12–induced Th$_1$ differentiation was disrupted. Indeed, the phenotype of the mice was virtually identical to that of mice that lacked IL-12.[129]

Stat6 was initially cloned as an IL-4 induced Stat like activity[130] and by searching databases of expressed sequences.[131] The induction of tyrosine phosphorylation of Stat4 is primarily seen in the response of lymphocytes to IL-4 or to IL-13. The specificity of Stat4 activation by IL-4 is related to the presence of a docking site for the IL-4 SH2 domain within the IL-4 receptor α chain. To assess the biological function of Stat6, mice lacking Stat4 were generated.[132–134] The Stat4 deficient mice are viable and lack any gross abnormalities. However, virtually all the biological functions associated with IL-4 or IL-13 are deficient in these mice. For example, splenic T cells are unable to respond to IL-4 by generating Th$_2$ cells. More strikingly, a variety of stimuli are unable to induce IgE production in these mice. This observation supports a previous hypothesis that Stat6 regulated the transcription of the nonrearranged IgE isotype region of the heavy chain locus and that such transcription was required for efficient rearrangement during the process of class switching. In addition, a number of cell surface antigens that are normally upregulated during immune responses as a consequence of IL-4 production are not upregulated in the deficient mice. Again, somewhat remarkably, the phenotype was very similar to the phenotype of mice in which the IL-4 gene had been deleted.

In contrast to the above Stat genes, the two highly related Stat5 gene products are activated in the response to a wide variety of cytokines, including cytokines such as Epo, Tpo, IL-7, growth hormone, prolactin, and IL-2, among a few. Therefore it was anticipated that Stat5 would have a more general, broadly significant spectrum of activity. The analysis of Stat5 function was somewhat complicated, however, by the existence of the two genes that are approximately 95% identical in amino acid sequence and that genetically co-localize. Indeed it can be reasonably speculated that the two genes arose through a relatively recent genomic duplication event. Irrespective, the analysis required the generation of mutant mice for each of the genes by targeting each gene in embryonal stem cells and then using double targeting in embryonic stem cells to obtain mice deficient in both genes.

The analysis of the various mutant mice revealed some striking and unexpected phenotypes. Mice deficient in Stat5a[135] are defective in mammary gland development, particularly during lactation. This phenotype is consistent with a critical role for Stat5a in prolactin regulation of mammary gland development. Mice deficient in Stat5b[136] have two phenotypes that include a decreased size of the males, comparable with the size differences associated with growth hormone defects. The second phenotype is an altered pattern of liver enzyme expression, a phenotype that is also consistent with a role in growth hormone signal transduction.

The phenotype of mutant mice in which both genes were disrupted further supported a key role in both prolactin and growth hormone function as well as revealing an essential role in T cell activation.[137] The mutation of both Stat5 genes resulted in a reduced size of both male and female mice, now fully consistent with the phenotype seen in growth hormone deficient mice. In addition, the females were sterile and failed to develop corpus lutea, consistent with another known function of prolactin. Thus in these mice virtually all the physiological functions associated with growth hormone and prolactin are deficient. In addition, however, mature T cells from the mice fail to mitogenically respond to IL-2 in synergy with stimulation of the T cell receptor.[138] As a consequence the immune system is defective and with time the mice develop manifestations of an altered immune response. Taken together the results indicate that the Stat signaling pathways mediate very precise functions, each associated with a relatively few cytokines. This contrasts quite distinctly from pathways such as the ras pathway that is speculated to provide a common mechanism by which cytokines regulate cell growth and differentiation.

▼ Cas AND Crk FAMILIES OF PROTEINS

The c-crk protein was identified as the proto-oncogene of v-crk, a transforming gene of the CT10 virus.[139] Subsequently a second family member was identified termed crk-like (Crkl).[140] Both proteins consist of one SH2 domain and two SH3 domains. P130 Cas (crk associated protein) was identified as a heavily tyrosine phosphorylated protein that associates with Crk.[141] Again, related proteins termed Cas-like (CasL), HEF1,[142] and Efs/Sin[143, 144] have been identified. The crk proteins bind to a variety of receptors through interaction with sites of receptor tyrosine phosphorylation. In addition, they interact, through the SH2 and SH3 domains, with a variety of signaling proteins, including Cbl, paxillin, and SOS, as well as another guanine nucleotide exchange factor termed C3G that activates the ras related small G protein termed Rap1.[145] As with many substrates of tyrosine phosphorylation, the precise roles that these proteins play in signal transduction are not known. However, accumulating evidence suggests that these families of proteins are involved in the regulation of cell shape and motility by transmitting information between receptor complexes and focal adhesions.

▼ Cbl

The c-cbl protein is a substrate of tyrosine phosphorylation in the response to a wide variety of growth factors and cytokines, and through stimulation of the B-cell and T-cell receptors. C-cbl was initially identified as the cellular homolog of the v-cbl oncogene identified as a retrovirally transduced transforming gene.[146, 147] The 120 kDa c-cbl protein contains a nuclear localization signal although it is primarily cytoplasmic, a zinc-finger like motif, and a carboxyl-terminal leucine zipper. In addition there is a large proline rich domain that mediates its interaction with a number of SH3 containing proteins including Grb2 and members of the src family of cytoplasmic kinases.

The significance of the participation of c-cbl in complexes that are affected by signal transduction are largely unknown. C-cbl has been proposed to be an essential component that is downstream from c-src signaling in bone resorption.[148] Alternatively, c-cbl has been proposed to be a negative regulator of the syk tyrosine kinase in signaling in T and B cells.[149] As with many of the signaling proteins, it took the recent derivation of mice deficient in c-cbl to begin to understand the situations in which its tyrosine phosphorylation may play an important role.[150] C-cbl deficient mice are viable, fertile, and outwardly normal. Specifically, bone development and remodelling were normal and therefore inconsistent with a previously proposed role in osteoclast function. The mice did exhibit lymphoid hyperplasia and splenic extramedullary hemopoiesis as well as increased ductal density and branching in the mammary glands. The hyperplastic consequences of deletion of c-cbl have suggested the possibility that c-cbl negatively influences signal transduction rather than the previously presumed positive role in signal transduction.

▼ OTHER SUBSTRATES OF TYROSINE PHOSPHORYLATION

A number of additional substrates of tyrosine phosphorylation have been identified but for which little functional information is available. Examples include hepatocyte growth factor-regulated tyrosine kinase substrate (Hrs), a 115 kDa protein with a putative zinc finger domain.[151] Stam (signal transducing adapter molecule) is a 70 kDa phosphotyrosine protein that contains an SH3 domain and immunoreceptor tyrosine based activation motif (ITAM).[152] Linker for activation of T cells (LAT) is a 36–38 kDa substrate of tyrosine phosphorylation.[153] Following phosphorylation LAT associates with Grb2, PLC-γ1 and the p85 subunit of PI-3 kinase. Similar functions have been suggested for the small phosphoprotein termed Lnk (Linker protein).[154] The protein p97/Gab2, a scaffolding protein, is tyrosine phosphorylated in many cytokine respones and associates with a variety of SH2 containing proteins including SHP2.[155] It can be anticipated that the derivation of mice that lack these genes will be required to provide additional insights into their role in the various signal transduction systems in which they are inducibly tyrosine phosphorylated. A tyrosine-phosphorylated protein, p62[dok], has been identified that is characteristically seen in chronic myelogenous leukemia cells and associates with GAP.[156] The significance to bcr-abl mediated transformation is yet to be established. More recently, the gene for a substrate of IL-4 induced tyrosine phosphorylation has been cloned, termed IL-four receptor interacting protein (*frip*).[157] The protein has significant identities to p62[dok] in the pleckstrin homology domain and in the phosphotyrosine binding domain.

The SLP-76 (SH2 domain-containing leukocyte protein of 76 kDa) protein is a substrate of the kinases associated with the T cell receptor complex. SLP-76 forms a complex with *Vav* and is constitutively associated with Grb2.[158] The gene is primarily expressed in T cells, macrophages and natural killer cells. The importance of SLP-76 in T-cell development has been revealed by deriving mice that lack the gene product. SLP-76[−/−] mice lack peripheral T cells as a result of a block in early thymocyte development. Interestingly, macrophage and natural killer cell populations and function are normal. The critical biochemical roles for SLP-76 are not known, although, as noted above, the deletion of *Vav* in lymphocytes results in a defect in both T- and B-cell functioning.

TGFβ Signal Transduction

A considerable amount of information has been obtained during the last 2 years regarding the mechanisms by which the TGFβ family of cytokines functions. This family includes ligands that mediate a wide variety of physiological functions and includes the TGFβs, the activins and inhibins, and the bone morphogenetic proteins (BMPs). The TGFβ related factors bind to receptors that consist of two distinct serine/threonine kinase chains. The type I receptors have a region that is rich in glycine and serine in the juxtamembrane domain (GS-domain) that is not found in the type II receptors. The ligand initially binds to the type II receptor chain (Fig. 4–8). Subsequently, the type I receptor is recruited into the complex where it is phosphorylated in the GS-domain and activated by the type I kinase. Unique type I and II receptors exist that mediate the affects of the bone morphogenetic proteins, the activins as well as TGFβ.[159]

Following the activation of the receptor complex, the critical substrates of TGFβ signaling are recruited to the complex and activated by phosphorylation. Remarkably, the primary functions of the TGFβ receptors are to phosphorylate members of a single family of transcription factors, termed the SMAD family of transcription factors. The term SMAD is a fusion of the names for the related transcription factors identified in either *Drosophila*, Mad (mothers against decapentaplegic), or *C. elegans*, Sma. The SMAD family consists of eight known mammalian proteins of 40 to 60 kDa that share a carboxyl-terminal homology domain that is referred to as an MH2 domain. The molecular structure of the MH2 domain of SMAD4 has been determined.[160] In addition, several SMADs contain a related amino-terminal domain that has DNA binding activity and is referred to as the MH1 domain. The MH1 and MH2 domains are connected by a region termed the linker. The SMADs can be

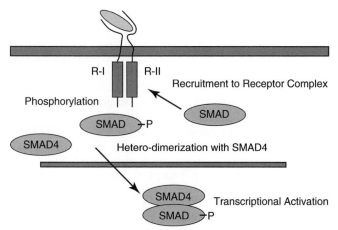

Figure 4–8. Signaling through the TGFβ receptor family. The receptors for the TGFβ family of cytokines consist of two serine/threonine kinase proteins. The ligand initally binds the type II receptor chain and, as a consequence, the type I receptor chain is recruited into the complex. The constitutively active type II receptor then phosphorylates the type I receptor in the juxtamembrane region, activating its kinase activity. The receptor activated SMADs are then recruited to the complex through recognition of the phosphorylated type I receptor and are phosphorylated. The receptor activated SMAD then associates with the common SMAD (SMAD4) and the heterodimeric complex translocates to the nucleus where the complex binds specific DNA sequences and activates, or suppresses, gene expression.

divided into three functional groups. The R-SMADs are receptor-regulated through phosphorylation, confer the receptor specificity, and all contain the MH1 domain. The C-SMAD is a common SMAD, which is required for the function of the R-SMADs as described below. Lastly, inhibitory SMADs function to suppress receptor signaling and are characterized by the absence of the MH1 domain. The MH1 domain has been shown to bind DNA while the MH2 domain is required for transcriptional activation. The linker region contains sites of phosphorylation by MAP kinases that are hypothesized to inhibit translocation to the nucleus and thus suppress TGFβ signaling.

Although many details of activation need to be further elucidated, a remarkably simply picture is emerging in which the R-SMADs are initially recruited to the receptor complex through the interaction of a small domain in the carboxyl-domain of the SMADs with the receptor complex. The receptor recognition is defined by as few as two amino acid differences in the domain.[161] Once recruited to the receptor complex the SMADs are directly phosphorylated by the type II receptor kinase, translocate to the nucleus and activate, or in some cases, suppress gene transcription.[162] Phosphorylation of the R-SMADs occurs in the carboxyl-terminal at a characteristic Ser-Ser-X-Ser motif. The translocation and transcriptional activation require the association of the common SMAD, SMAD4, with the activated SMADs. SMAD4, unlike the other SMADs, does not contain the SSXS motif and has not been shown to be recruited into the receptor complex. Thus the model that is emerging is that pathway receptor–regulated SMADs (1, 2, 3, 5, 9) are recruited, through their ability to recognize specific receptor complexes, to the receptor complex, are phosphorylated, and then associate with the common mediator, SMAD4, to translocate and regulate gene expression.

In addition to activators, inhibitory SMADs have also been identified and are characterized by the absence of the MH2 domain. These SMADs are often induced by TGFβ signaling and are hypothesized to therefore control the extent and duration of signaling. The mechanism of repression by SMAD6 and SMAD7 appears to involve binding to type I receptors, thereby interfering with the phosphorylation of other receptor specific SMADs.[163, 164] Their inability to dissociate from the receptor complex is speculated to be due to the absence of the canonical phosphorylation site in the carboxyl-terminus.

The SMADs represent another example of a receptor specific system of transcription factors and, in many aspects, are very much like the Stat proteins in cytokine receptor superfamily signaling. It should be noted that recent studies have indicated that SMAD1 may also be phosphorylated by the mitogen activated kinases (MAPKs) following activation of the MAPK by signaling through other receptor systems.[165] These phosphorylations inhibit nuclear accumulation and therefore can negatively affect SMAD signaling. In addition, recent studies have identified a potentially important co-activator for the SMAD proteins termed FAST-1.[166–168]

The biological roles of the TGF family of cytokines have been documented through the derivation of mice lacking individual cytokines, receptors, and, more recently, the SMADs. In particular, mice deficient in TGFβ1, TGFβ2, TGFβ3, BMP-4, BMP-2, activin/inhibin βA, activin/inhibin βB, and inhibin α have been reported.[169–175] The majority of the phenotypes provide dramatic illustrations of the essential roles for these cytokines in normal development. The one exception is TGFβ1, which, when deleted, results in a wasting syndrome accompanied by multifocal, mixed inflammatory cell responses and extensive tissue necrosis leading to organ failure. In addition, the critical role of the activin type II and type I receptors in activin signaling has been demonstrated by the derivation of mice that lack the receptor.[176, 177]

More recently the essential functions of the SMADs have also begun to be examined by the derivation of mice that lack specific genes. The available mutants strongly reinforce the essential role for the SMADs in TGFβ cytokine signaling. For example, the absence of SMAD4 is associated with an embryonic lethal phenotype associated with a defect in gastrulation.[178] Similarly the derivation of mice lacking SMAD2 has demonstrated its essential role in mesoderm formation in the embryo by specifying the anterior-posterior polarity of the embryo.[179, 180]

TGFβ signaling has also been implicated in cancer. For example, the human SMAD4 gene was initially identified as a tumor suppressor gene (DPC4) on chromosome 18q21.1 that is associated with pancreatic and possibly other human cancers.[181] More strikingly, mice deficient in SMAD3, although otherwise normal and without a phenotype, develop colorectal adenocarcinomas at between 4 to 6 months.[182] It is hypothesized that inactivation of TGFβ signaling relieves some epithelial cells from differentiation signals and thereby allows the maintenance of a proliferative state, conducive to tumor formation.

Chemokine Receptor Signal Transduction

The chemokine receptors mediate the function of a large number of chemokines, which now includes at least 40 proteins.[183–186] Many of the cytokines are involved in aspects of hematopoiesis, such as IL-8, the monocyte chemotactic proteins (MCPs), and the macrophage inhibitory proteins (MIPs), to name a few subfamilies. Importantly, these receptors have also been recently shown to serve as receptors for the human immunodeficiency viruses.[187–192] In addition, receptors of this family mediate the cellular responses of a variety of peptide hormones such as glucagon, thrombin, and angiotensin and small molecules such as platelet activating factor, the cannabinoids, and serotonin.

All the receptors are structurally related in consisting of cell surface proteins containing seven membrane spanning domains, the so-called serpentine receptors. There are approximately 15 receptors that are named based on the class of chemokines for which they function. The receptors CXCR1-5 bind the CXC subgroup of chemokines, the CCR1-8 receptors bind the CC subgroup, and the XCR1 receptor binds the C subgroup chemokine, while the CX_3CR1 receptor binds CX_3C chemokine. Depending upon the ligand, one or more of the extracellular domains may be involved in ligand binding, although the large amino-terminal extracellular fragment is consistently involved in ligand binding. The effect of ligand binding is speculated to cause a sequential change in the conformation of the receptor that initiates its function as a signal transducing protein.

All the chemokine receptors function by mediating G protein–coupled events.[194] As a general model, ligand binding induces a conformational change in the receptor, resulting in the dissociation of GDP from the α subunit of the associated heterotrimeric G protein.[195] The subsequent binding of GTP to the α subunit induces a conformational change that results in the dissociation of the α subunit from the receptor as well as the βγ subunits. The GTP bound α subunit and the βγ subunit complex are then capable of interacting with various effector proteins. The cycle is completed with the hydrolysis of the α subunit–bound GTP, which can be accelerated by various effector proteins interacting with the GTP bound α subunit, and the reassociation with the βγ complex.

The diversity of signaling associated with the chemokine receptors is due to the complexity of the G proteins available for receptor association. For example, 20 mammalian G-protein α subunits have been identified; some of these are highly restricted in their pattern of expression while others are widely expressed. Similarly, five β subunits and ten γ subunits have been identified in mammals that similarly show both restricted and wide patterns of expression. With some exceptions, various β subunits associate with various γ subunits and the βγ complexes can associate with various α subunits to generate a wide variety of heterotrimeric combinations. Inhibition studies suggest that defined αβγ combinations are associated with specific functions. This is important since specific receptors can associate with different heterotrimeric complexes and thereby activate a variety of cellular responses.

Downstream of the receptor, the dissociation of the GTP-α subunit and the βγ subunit are responsible for the activation of the various effector functions. The classical targets of the Gα proteins are the adenylyl cyclases that are regulated both positively and negatively through direct interaction. The activated adenylyl cyclases then generate cAMP that allosterically activates protein kinase A (PKA).

Many chemokine receptors also lead to the stimulation of phospholipase C activity and the hydrolysis of phosphatidyl-4,5-bisphosphate to generate inositol-1,4,5-trisphosphate and diacylglyerol. This occurs through the regulation of members of the PLC-β family of phospholipase C enzymes through their interaction, in a family member dependent pattern of interaction, with G proteins. As noted above, another subfamily of phospholipase C enzymes, the PLC-γ subfamily, is regulated through phosphorylation by other receptor families.

In addition to the classic G-protein associated responses, it has been shown that the chemokine receptors can activate other signaling pathways in a pertussis toxin, G-protein independent manner. For example, RANTES and MIP-1α have been shown to activate Stat1 and Stat3 in T cells.[196] Also in T cells, RANTES has been shown to induce the tyrosine kinase activities of the cell adhesion associated kinase p125[FAK] and the T cell receptor associated kinase ZAP-70.[197] Similarly the angiotensin II receptor has been shown to activate members of the Jak family of protein tyrosine kinases.[198] As discussed in detail below, one of the most consistently activated pathways in the responses to a wide variety of cytokines is the MAP kinase cascade. This pathway has been strongly linked to growth and is frequently a target for transforming events. Recently a variety of G protein coupled receptors have been shown to lead to the activation of members of the MAP kinase family. Although still being examined, recent studies have indicated that this may involve rc tyrosine kinase and Pyk2.[199] The functional significances of any of these biochemical responses to biological readouts are not known.

Signal Transduction by the Frizzled Family of Receptors

Although generally not considered within the context of hematopoietic signal transduction, it is important to briefly summarize the current status of this growing class of receptors (frizzled) that transduce signals from a number of proteins related to the ligand termed wingless (wng) that was initially identified in *Drosophila*. To some extent, the initial interest in this *Drosophila* factor originated from the observation that the retrovirally transduced mammary gland transforming gene termed *int-1* was the mammalian homologue of wng.[200, 201] The frizzled receptors share in common an amino-terminal signal sequence followed by a domain of approximately 120 amino acids with an invariant pattern of ten cysteine residues. This is followed by a seven membrane-spanning domain and a conserved carboxyl-terminal domain.

The players in signal transduction through the frizzled receptors have been identified both genetically and by biochemical studies.[202–204] The critical components include proteins related to the *Drosophila* gene *armadillo* that includes β-catenin and plakogloblin in vertebrates, proteins related to the *Drosophila* gene product *disheveled*, glycogen synthase kinase 3β, the tumor suppressor gene *adenomatous polyposis coli* (*APC*), and members of the T cell factor (TCF) transcription factors or the related lymphoid enhancer-binding factors (LEFs). The TCF/LEFs alone poorly bind DNA and only weakly, if at all, activate gene transcription. However, binding of β-catenin dramatically affects both functions,

indicating that the active transcription factor is a heterodimer of TCF/LEFs and β-catenin.[205, 206] The formation of this transcriptionally active complex is dependent upon the availability of β-catenin. Normally β-catenin exists in a complex with *APC* and GSK-3β that targets β-catenin for degradation. The role of GSK-3β is both to phosphorylate *APC* and increase its affinity for β-catenin as well as to phosphorylate β-catenin and thereby promote its destruction. The engagement of the receptor is envisioned to modify the function of the disheveled proteins, possibly through phosphorylation, to allow the inhibition of GSK-3β function to allow the accumulation of β-catenin and, in turn, the increase in transcriptionally active complexes containing β-catenin.

The frizzled receptors may also function very similarly to the G-coupled receptors. Recent studies have shown that some members of the receptor superfamily can stimulate phosphatidylinositol signaling through a conventional heterotrimeric G-protein complex.[207] The ability to activate Gβγ and Gα subunits would suggest that these receptors could couple wnt binding to the activation of a number of additional pathways, including the activation of protein kinase C.

The potential relevance of this pathway to hematopoiesis is indicated by the phenotype of mice that lack TCF-1.[208] Postnatal expression of TCF-1 is restricted to the T cell lineage. Consistent with a role in T cell development, mice lacking the gene have defective thymocyte differentiation. The block appears to occur at the transition from immature single positive cells to the major double positive population. It is not known what ligands or receptors regulate TCF-1 function in these cells.

Signal Transduction by the Death Domain–Containing and Related Receptors

This subfamily of receptors was first identified as the receptors for the tumor necrosis factors (TNFs) and the receptor for the FAS ligand were characterized. The identifying conserved motif resides in the extracellular domain and consists of a six cysteine-containing domain. This family includes receptors for CD40, CD30, CD27, and OX-40 as well as the TNFs and FAS ligand. Among the receptors, the TNFR1, FAS, and NGFR p75 also contain a conserved cytoplasmic domain referred to as the death domain, since this region is critical for the ability of the receptors to couple ligand binding to the induction of apoptosis. More recently, the receptors for TRAMP (DR3), TRAIL (DR4), and a related receptor DR5 have also been shown to contain cytoplasmic death domains. The death domains can be moved among various receptors and retain their ability to induce an apoptotic response. The emerging model is one in which ligand drives aggregation of the receptors, altering the confirmation of the receptors in such a way as to now recruit various proteins to the receptor complex. The major consequences of receptor activation are the induction of NF-κB transcription factor activity and, in the case of the death domain containing receptors, the activation of caspases, which in turn proteolytically cleave and activate a cascade of additional caspases that mediate cell death. The exact biochemical mechanisms involved are not known but over the past 2 years potentially key components have been identified.

▼ NF-κB ACTIVATION

The activation of NK-κB activity is brought about by the degradation of IκB proteins that bind NF-κB and retain it in the cytoplasm. Following dissociation, NF-κB translocates to the nucleus and activates gene expression. The destruction of IκB is dependent upon phosphorylation at two sites in the amino-terminal region of the protein. Following phosphorylation at these sites, polyubiquitination occurs and targets the proteins for rapid degradation by the 2κS proteosome. Recent studies[209, 210] have identified two related serine kinases, termed IκB kinases (IKKα and IKKβ), that can phosphorylate IκB at the critical sites (reviewed in ref. 211). Upstream of the IKKs is another kinase that is thought to regulate the activity of the IKKs. This kinase, termed NF-κB inducing kinase (NIK), was identified as a kinase that is able to bind to one of the TNF receptor associated proteins described below (TRAF2).[212] Thus the current model envisions the activation of NIK by receptor aggregation, its activation of the IKKs, the subsequent phosphorylation of IκBs, and the translocation of NF-κB to the nucleus, resulting in the activation of gene expression.

The significance of the activation of NF-κB has been, in part, revealed through the derivation of mice that lack NF-κB components. The NF-κB family of proteins include the two components of the classically defined NF-κB complex, p50 (NF-κB1) and pκ5 (RelA) as well as c-Rel, RelB, and p52 (NF-κB2). Mice lacking RelB are viable and development is normal. However, with age, they develop multi-organ inflammation and myeloid hyperplasia, all of which are dependent upon an altered T cell response.[213, 214] Mice that lack the p50 subunit of NF-κB similarly are born viable and development is largely normal. However, the mice exhibit a number of defects in B cell development[215] and nonspecific responses to infections. The absence of RelA results in embryonic lethality that is associated with a defect in liver development.[216] Lastly, mice that lack c-rel have mature B and T cells, but the cells are unresponsive to most mitogenic stimuli and the induction of cytokines in T cells is deficient.[217, 218] The derivation of mice that lack IκB, the regulatory subunit of the NF-κB family members, has also been accomplished[219] and support the critical role that members of this family of transcription factors play in lymphoid regulation.

▼ RECEPTOR ASSOCIATED PROTEINS

The use of yeast two-hybrid screening for proteins that can bind to the death domains of various receptors has resulted in the identification of a number of proteins that may be important in signaling uniquely through this group of receptors (Fig. 4–9). The independent isolation of several of the proteins by different groups has led to the use of different names for the same protein. In general the proteins can be classified into structurally and often functionally related families. The most important are the caspases as detailed below. FADD and Casper share some structural similarities with the caspases. The TRAFs constitute another family of receptor associated proteins. Two structurally related kinases, RIP and RIP2, have been found to associate with the receptor

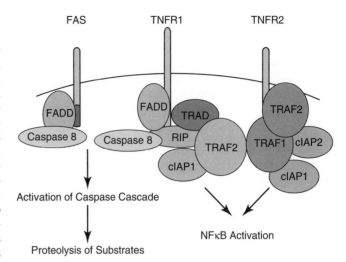

Figure 4–9. Components in TNF signaling complexes. The binding of Fas ligand or TNF to their respective receptors induces the recruitment of a variety of proteins that have been identified as receptor associating proteins. The functional consequences of receptor engagement consist of the activation of caspase cascades, normally resulting in the induction of apoptosis. In addition, TNF induces the activation of NK-κB, which contributes to a variety of biological responses, including responses that can protect cells from apoptosis.

complex. Lastly, additional "adapter" proteins have been identified, including TRADD.

The current model envisions that receptor activation results in receptor death domains binding the adapter protein termed FADD (Fas-associated death domain containing protein), which contains an amino terminal death effector domain (DED) that associates with DEDs in other proteins that are associated with apoptosis. Importantly, this group of proteins includes caspase-8 that is hypothesized to be essential for apoptosis. Twelve members of the caspase family of proteases have been identified, termed caspases 1–12, and many when overexpressed can mediate cell death. They share in common a conserved catalytic site motif that includes a critical cysteine residue that contributes to the active site. The caspases are synthesized as proenzymes that require proteolytic cleavage for activation. Activation and amplification of the caspases result in the degradation of a number of target proteins that together mediate the characteristic pattern of apoptotic cell death. A number of excellent reviews of the biochemistry of the caspases have been published.[220–222]

The role of the caspase family of proteases in mediating cell death has emerged over the past 2 years. The first member identified was the interleukin 1β converting enzyme (ICE).[223] Subsequent to the cloning of ICE, a gene (ced3) involved in apoptosis during differentiation in nematodes was cloned and found to be related structurally to ICE.[224] Subsequently FLICE, now known as caspase 8, was identified through its binding of FADD (FADD-like ICE).[225] The unique role of ICE in regulating IL-1 release is nicely illustrated by the phenotype of mutant mice lacking ICE.[226] The mice develop normally but have a major defect in the production of IL-1β, and to a lesser extent the production of IL-1α, in response to stimulation. This inability is speculated to be the basis for the resistance of the mice to LPS induced endotoxic shock. The phenotype also illustrates the lack of a nonredundant role for this member of the family in other cellular systems.

The role of FADD in signaling through the TNF family members has been examined through the derivation of mice that lack the gene.[227] Rather remarkably, deficiency of FADD is associated with embryonic lethality at about 10–11 days of development. This was surprising since the deletion of neither the TNF receptor nor FAS results in embryonic lethality, suggesting that FADD may be involved in yet unknown functions. The basis for the lethality is not well defined although there are major defects in cardiac development. In addition, there is a profound erythrocytosis suggesting that embryonic erythropoiesis is, in part, regulated by the elimination of a significant fraction of proliferating erythroblasts. Using fibroblasts from deficient mice, it was found that the ability of Fas, TNFR1 and DR3, but not DR4, to mediate apoptosis was dramatically reduced, consistent with a role in signaling apoptosis. However, the ability of a variety of other agents to induce apoptosis was unaffected.

In the case of FAS, the emerging model is relatively simple in that aggregation of Fas by Fas ligand causes the recruitment and/or aggregation of FADD and the associated caspase 8 resulting in, potentially, the autocatalytic activation of caspase 8. Activated caspase 8 can then activate other caspases and/or substrates of the caspases. One intriguing substrate is the inhibitor of the caspase activated DNase.[228, 229] Cleavage of the inhibitor liberates the active DNase that then cleaves DNA, resulting in the characteristic nucleosomal degradation that has long characterized cells undergoing induced apoptosis.

The critical role that caspase 8 plays in apoptosis is illustrated by the phenotype of mice that are deficient in caspase 8.[230] The mutation results in an embryonic lethality at midgestation. The embryos display a dramatic erythrocytosis that is virtually identical to that seen in the FADD deficient embryos. Again, since neither Fas nor TNF have been implicated in regulating embryonic erythropoiesis, it must be presumed that another related receptor/ligand system exists that also utilizes FADD and caspase 8. Also, similar to the results with the FADD deficient embryos, fibroblasts from caspase 8 deficient embryos were resistant to Fas, TNF, and DR3 receptor activation induced cell death. However the ability of these receptor systems to activate Jun kinases, or to trigger IκB phosphorylation and degradation, were unaffected.

Other proteins that associate with death domain containing receptors include the TRADD (TNFR1-associated death domain protein), which was isolated by its ability to bind to TNFR1. TRADD does not contain a death effector domain, but TRADD binds to FADD and is hypothesized to be critical for the recruitment of FADD to the TNFR1. Casper was identified by sequence similarity to FADD although when full clones were obtained it was found to also be related to caspase 8, and thus was termed caspase 8 related protein.[231] Somewhat remarkably Casper interacts with FADD, caspase-8, caspase-3, TRAF1, and TRAF2, all through different domains.

RIP was initially identified as a protein that interacted with Fas.[232] RIP consists of an amino-terminal kinase domain, an α-helical center domain, and a carboxyl death domain. Again, the derivation of mice lacking RIP has provided a somewhat different view for this kinase than

was initially derived from the biochemical studies.[233] RIP deficient mice are normal at birth but fail to thrive and die at 1–3 days. Unexpectedly there was extensive apoptosis in both lymphoid and adipose tissues. Indeed, the cells are highly sensitive to TNFα induced cell death. Importantly, however, TNFα is not capable of inducing NF-κB activation in the cell from the mutant mice. Thus RIP is presumably in the receptor complex and is essential for the signaling pathway that results in NF-κB activation. More recently a highly related kinase (RIP2) has been identified and shown to be capable of activating NF-κB.[234]

The TRAF (TNF receptor-associated factors) proteins is another group of proteins that associates with the TNF receptor family. The TRAF family is characterized by a conserved carboxyl-terminal domain, termed the TRAF-C domain, and an α-helical domain termed the TRAF-N domain. In addition, all but TRAF1 contain an amino-terminal RING finger domain, a domain that is found in a wide variety of proteins but the function of which is yet to be defined. The TRAF family currently consists of six members.[235] A recently identified family member has been shown to be involved in IL-1 signaling.[235] Overexpression of many of the members of the family can induce NF-κB activation and therefore may be important as adapter proteins in the formation of complexes that activate NIK or the IKKs.

The precise role of the TRAF family members is currently being examined by the derivation of mutant mice. Mice that lack TRAF3 die shortly after birth.[236] The mice are runted and the peripheral white cell counts decrease dramatically within a few days after birth. Fetal liver cells can completely reconstitute the hematopoietic system but the T cells are defective in such mice. The phenotype of the T cells is consistent with the hypothesis that TRAF3 is critical for a T cell proliferative response of T cells. The phenotype of the T cell defects has suggested that CD30 may be the receptor with which TRAF3 interacts.

In addition to ligand/receptor mediated induction of apoptosis, a variety of agents can induce apoptosis through lesser understood pathways. In some cases, one of the major functions of cytokine receptor signaling is to suppress this form of apoptosis. As above, only recently have potential components of these systems been identified and experiments done to provide possible models. For example, one emerging model has as its critical components caspase 9 and a protein termed Apaf1. The relationship between these components was, in part, derived from studies that sought to identify the proteins that were required for an in vitro model of apoptosis. Among the required components were cytochrome c, caspase 9, and Apaf1. Importantly, the *C. elegans* homologue of Apaf1 had been previously identified as a necessary component of the *C. elegans* death pathway.[237] The model that emerged from these studies envisioned the release of cytochrome c from mitochondria under "stress" conditions that evoked apoptosis. Cytochrome c would then associate with a complex consisting of Apaf1 and caspase 9, resulting in the activation of caspase 9.[238] Caspase 9, in turn, would activate caspase 3 and initiate the apoptotic response.

The correctness of the above model is supported by the phenotypes of mutant mice that lack caspase 9[239, 240] or Apaf1.[241, 242] Both mutations result in an embryonic lethality that is associated with abnormal brain development due to excessive accumulation of cells in the brain. Embryonic fibroblasts from embryos of either mutant strain are resistant to a variety of stimuli that normally induce apoptosis including UV and γ irradiation. Interestingly, however, thymocytes are not resistant to UV induced apoptosis but are resistant to dexamethasone and γ irradiation. The model that emerges in this case is that Apaf1 and caspase 9 play a major role in inducing apoptosis with the developing brain in a similar manner to the role of caspase 8 in embryonic erythropoiesis.

From the above descriptions, it should be apparent that a number of proteins have been identified that interact with receptors of the TNF receptor family, and it should be equally obvious that much of the details and significance of these interactions are yet to be obtained. The essential questions involve which of these receptor-associated proteins are required for the specific functions associated with the activation of the receptors of this family. The two major functions are the activation of the caspase proteolytic cascade and the induction of apoptosis or the activation of the NF-κB factors. Moreover, considerable evidence exists to indicate that one of the consequences of NF-κB activation is the expression of genes that can inhibit the activation of the apoptosis pathway. Irrespective of the specifics involved, it is clear from the phenotype of the mice in which the various components have been deleted that these genes play critical roles in maintaining the critical balances between promoting differentiation and eliminating autoreactive clones that exist within lymphoid lineages.

Bcl Family Members and Cytokine Signaling

One of the functions of cytokine signaling is the suppression of apoptosis, and a considerable amount of work has been directed at linking the biochemical events associated with apoptosis and the biochemical events associated with receptor activation. At present, the most consistent link is that of cytokine induced expression of the genes encoding Bcl family members and their interaction with the basic machinery of apoptosis. Extensive reviews have been written regarding the Bcl family of proteins[243, 244]; consequently, only the emerging models will be considered.

The prevailing model implicates members of the Bcl family of proteins in mitochondrial function and maintenance. A review concerning this aspect of the Bcl family function has been published.[245, 246] Although the details are lacking, it is suggested that Bcl-2 and Bcl-X are important for the maintenance of mitochondrial function and, in their absence, cytochrome C is released. As noted above, the released cytochrome C is then envisioned to associate with Apaf1 and caspase 9 resulting in the activation of caspase 9 that, in turn, activates caspase 3, initiating apoptosis. Precisely what the functions of the Bcl proteins are in this pathway, however, are not known. In C. elegans, the Bcl-X homologue suppresses the function of Apaf1 and the associated caspases and this may be the result of direct interaction of Bcl proteins with the complex to inhibit the ability of cytochrome c to activate the complex.[247] Consistent with this, a ternary complex of caspase-9, Bcl-X, and Apaf1 has been shown to exist.[248] Alternatively, the Bcl proteins have been proposed to be ion channel regulating proteins in the mitochondrial membrane. The absence of sufficient Bcl proteins, or their inactivation, would result in altered mitochrondrial permeability, loss of cytochrome C, and activation of apoptosis. As noted below, the phenotype of the Bcl-X deficient mice is not similar to that of the Apaf1 or caspase 9 deficient mice and thus, at this level, the results are inconsistent with the ternary complex model.

A potential link between Fas and mitochondrial damage has been proposed in the way of the BID protein.[249–251] BID was identified as a caspase 8 substrate and, independently, as a Bcl-2 binding protein. It contains a region that has sequence similarity to a region (BH3) of the Bcl family of proteins. Following Fas receptor engagement, BID is cleaved and translocates to the mitochondrial membranes. The model envisioned is one in which BID is cleaved, translocates to the mitochondria, interacts with Bcl family members, and thereby blocks their ability to suppress cytochrome C activation of the Apaf1/caspase 9 complex.

As noted above, one consequence of cytokine receptor engagement is often the increased transcription of the genes of Bcl family members. Enforced expression of Bcl family members suppresses the apoptosis seen with the removal of cytokines, demonstrating a clear functional role for their induction. Unfortunately, virtually nothing is known concerning the signaling pathways that are involved in this transcription regulation. Another model envisions cytokine-induced phosphorylation of the Bcl family member Bad.[244] Following phosphorylation, Bad is sequestered in the cytosol by the 14-3-3 proteins; this precludes its interaction with Bcl-X, thus allowing Bcl-X to protect against apoptosis. More recently it has been proposed that Akt is the kinase responsible for the ligand induced phosphorylation of Bad.[244] Thus, the pathway would involve receptor recruitment and phosphorylation of p85, the regulatory subunit of PI-3 kinase, the production of IP4 and activation of Akt, the phosphorylation of Bad, the release of Bcl-X and the suppression of the release of cytochrome C, and activation of the caspase 9/Apaf1 complex. Clearly much work remains to confirm the existence of this pathway as detailed here.

The specificity with which each of the Bcl family members participates in cellular functions has been most dramatically illustrated by the derivation of mice lacking each of the family members. For example, although Bcl-2 expression is widespread in both development and in adult animals, Bcl-2 deficient mice develop normally, and it is only with age that they develop a marked lymphoid apoptosis as well as melanocytic, neuronal, and intestinal lesions.[252] The phenotype is consistent with the hypothesis that Bcl-2 is critical for the maintenance of peripheral T cell populations. In contrast, deficiency of Bcl-X results in an embryonic lethality.[253] The lethality is, in part, due to failure of erythropoiesis associated with extensive apoptosis of fetal liver hematopoietic progenitors. Interestingly, this is the opposite phenotype from that seen with deficiencies in FADD or caspase 8. Moreover, Bcl-X expression is normally very high in fetal liver hematopoietic progenitors and this expression is dependent upon Epo signaling. Thus the data are consistent with the concept that embryonic erythropoiesis is regulated through a delicate balance of inducing apoptosis or providing factors that can suppress this apoptosis. Lastly, deficiency in Bcl-w results in male infertility due to extensive apoptosis in germ cells and supporting Sertoli cells without any other detectable deficiency.[254] Deficiency of the pro-apoptotic gene, Bax, results in an increase in some cell types, including granulosa cells, certain neurons, lymphocytes, and immature germ cells.[255] Crosses of Bax and Bcl-2 deficient mice support the concept that Bax is responsible for much of the lymphoid loss, while crosses of Bax and Bcl-X deficient mice suggest that Bax is responsible for only a portion of the apoptosis seen in the Bcl-X deficient mice.[256]

IL-1 Receptor Mediated Signal Transduction

IL-1 was one of the first cytokines identified and is a prototype for the proinflammatory cytokines. The initial IL-1 family consisted of three separate genes encoding IL-1α and IL-1β as well as a receptor antagonist termed IL-1ra. The biological consequences of IL-1 production are diverse and excellent reviews have appeared that have detailed the responses.[257, 258] More recently IL-18 was identified as an interferon-γ–inducing factor that was found to have structural similarity to IL-1; both structurally and functionally it is of the IL-1 family. Both IL-1 and IL-18 are synthesized as inactive precursors that require cleavage by the IL-1β converting enzyme (ICE) for maturation and release. The phenotype of mice lacking IL-18 has recently been reported and consists of defects in NK function and Th1 type helper T cell responses.[259]

IL-1 binding activity is associated with two related proteins termed the IL-1 type I receptor and the type II receptor. Importantly, the cytoplasmic domain of the type II receptor is only 29 amino acids compared with the type I receptor with a cytoplasmic domain of 210 amino acids. All the functions of IL-1 are associated with binding to the type I receptor. Then cytoplasmic domain of the type I IL-1 receptor was initially noted to have a rather striking sequence similarity to the cytoplasmic domain of a *Drosophila* gene termed *toll*.[260] *Toll* encodes a receptor that utilizes the kinase gene *pelle* and a gene termed *tube*, which encodes a receptor adapter protein to activate the function of the gene product of *dorsal*. Importantly, *dorsal* is the fly homologue of NK-κB. Consistent with a functional similarity of the IL-1 signaling pathway and the fly *toll* pathway, IL-1 is a potent inducer of NF-κB transcriptional activity. In addition to activating NK-κB, IL-1 also induces the acivity of the mitogen activated kinases. Functionally these pathways contribute to the IL-1 induced expression of genes such as the acute phase proteins, cytokines, and adhesion molecules.

In addition to the type I and II IL-1 receptors a number of related receptors have been identified. These include an IL-1 receptor–related protein (IL-1Rrp) that is the receptor for IL-18, IL-Rrp2, T1/ST2, and the five *toll*-related receptors (TLR1-5).[261–265] Importantly, although the ligand is unknown, a constitutively activated human homologue of the *Drosophila toll* gene was found to induce the activation of NF-κb, again emphasizing the functional relationship among this family of receptors.

As mentioned above, in *Drosophila*, the receptor (*toll*) associates following ligand binding with an adapter protein (*tube*) that recruits a serine/threonine kinase (*pelle*) to ultimately activate the NK-κB homologue (*dorsal*). The first mammalian homologue of *pelle* to be identifed was the IL-1

receptor associated kinase (IRAK).[266] Subsequently a second related kinase was identified, IRAK-2, that was found to associate with the receptor complex in combination with an adapter protein termed *MyD88*.[267] Importantly, *MyD88* is structurally related to the *Drosophila tube* protein. The importance of *MyD88* is evident from the phenotype of mice lacking the gene, which consists of a complete loss of IL-1 and IL-18 mediated functions.[268] In addition to *MyD88*, a member of the TRAF family of proteins has been identifed, TRAF6, which may be involved in IL-1 signaling through its interaction with IRAK.[266]

Notch Receptor Signaling

The *notch* receptor gene family was initially identified in studies dealing with cell fate decisions during differentiation in *Drosophila*, and its role in both flies and nematodes has been extensively studied biologically.[269] Interest in the mammalian notch family members arose with the demonstration that the chromosomal translocation t(7;9)(q34;q34.3) in T-cell lymphoblastic leukemia involves the fusion of the T-cell receptor β locus with the cytoplasmic domain of the a mammalian notch homologue, now referred to as the mammalian *notch1* gene.[270] Subsequently, three additional mammalian family members have been identified, including *notch2, notch3* and *notch4*. Importantly, *notch1* is also activated in thymic lymphomas by retroviral insertions,[271] *notch2* has been implicated in a feline leukemia virus induced lymphoma, and *notch4* was identified as the gene associated with a common mammary tumor virus integration site in tumors (int3). Lastly, *notch3* has been implicated in an hereditary, adult-onset condition causing stroke and dementia.[272]

Relatively little is known regarding the normal functions of the mammalian *notch* family members. However, *notch1* is expressed on hematopoietic stem cells and, based on its role in cell fate determination in other species, has been speculated to control hematopoietic stem cell decisions. *Notch1* has also been implicated in T cell development based on its high level of expression in the thymus, the involvement in T cell leukemias, and the observation that overexpression of an activated form of *notch1* affects CD4/CD8[273] and αβ/γδ[274] fate specification. Moreover, an activated form of *notch* can induce T cell neoplasmia in mice.[275] The targeted mutation of *notch1* in mice results in an embryonic lethality at day 9 due to defects in somite segmentation, and analysis of the embryos further supports a critical role in neurogenesis.[276, 277]

The *notch* family of receptors are large transmembrane proteins of approximately 300 kDa that contain 36 tandem EGF-like repeats and three repeats of a motif termed the lin-12 repeat in the extracellular domain. The cytoplasmic domain characteristically consists of a number of ankyrin-like repeats, a glutamine rich domain, and a region that is rich in glutamine, serine, and threonine referred to as PEST domain. Transformation of various cell types by *notch* family members is associated with the overexpression of the cytoplasmic domain.

Relatively less is known regarding the mammalian ligands for the *notch* receptors. Two ligands, Jagged1[278] and Jagged2,[279] have been cloned based on homology with the ligands for the *Drosophila notch* receptor, delta and serrate. The ligands contain several unique motifs and properties. The amino terminal contains a signal peptide that is followed by a novel motif shared with the *Drosophila* serrate (DSL) and 16 EGF-like repeats comparable with those found in the receptors. In addition the extracellular portion contains a cysteine rich domain followed by the transmembrane domain. The cytoplasmic domain consists of approximately 130 amino acids without distinguishing motifs. Both Jagged1 and Jagged2 are expressed in a variety of tissues. The cell membrane association of the ligands and the existence of a relatively large cytoplasmic domain suggests the interesting possibility that the ligand may also initiate intracellular signaling events. In flies, a secreted protein termed *fringe* regulates signaling by delta and serrate. A murine homologue has been identified and shown to be critical for somite formation by gene disruption studies.[280, 281]

The *notch* receptors are speculated to signal by a quite unique mechanism. Ligand binding is speculated to induce an intracellular cleavage, releasing the cytoplasmic domain to translocate the nucleus and to regulate gene transcription through its interaction with a DNA binding protein variably termed RBP-Jκ (recombination signal sequence binding protein for Jκ genes), CBF1 (C-promoter binding factor 1), or KBF2 (kappa binding factor 2). RBP-Jκ binds the promoters of several viral and cellular genes and suppresses their transcription. Importantly, RBP-Jκ is the mammalian homologue of a DNA binding protein suppressor of hairless (Su(H)) that has been implicated in the signaling by the *Drosophila notch* receptor. The current model[282] envisions that the intracellular cleavage product of *notch*, through the membrane proximal region, interacts with a repression domain of RBP-Jκ. Association with RBP-Jκ both suppresses its activity as a repressor of transcription and may provide transcriptional activator activity. The ability to associate with and activate the transcriptional activity of RBP-Jκ is also a property of the EBV protein EBNA2.[283] It should be noted that studies of the *Drosophila notch* signaling suggest that the cytoplasmic domain of the unligated *notch* retains Su(H) and, following ligand binding, Su(H) is released and translocates to the nucleus. Gene disruption studies have demonstrated that RBP-Jκ is critical for early embryonic development.[284]

The MAP Kinase Cascade

Perhaps one of the most studied signaling pathways is one often referred to as the mitogen activated protein kinase (MAPK) cascade. Unfortunately, this area of signal transduction is also plagued by incredibly difficult and duplicative terminology that significantly hinders a nonspecialist from easily following the literature. The cascade actually consists of several related and overlapping pathways of kinase activations that are highly conserved in evolution and that are activated in the context of a wide variety of cytokines and growth factors as well as conditions of cellular stress. This can be derived from a wide variety of growth factor receptor signaling, as detailed below, cellular stress, or receptors that mediate pro-inflammatory responses. Irrespective of the nature of the initial input, the primary function is the activation of a kinase that has the ability to subsequently activate another kinase of the family of related kinases, the MKKs,

which in turn activate the structurally and functionally related Erk, Jnk, and p38 kinases. The latter, when activated, can translocate to the nucleus and phosphorylate transcription factors, thereby regulating gene expression.

The kinase cascades function to induce the tyrosine and threonine phosphorylation of a group of structurally and functionally related kinases that includes the extracellular signal–regulated kinases, Erk (Erk1, Erk2, Erk5), the c-jun kinases, Jnk (Jnk1, Jnk2, Jnk3), and the p38 group of kinases (p38α, p38β, p38γ, p38*). This group of kinases is frequently referred to as the mitogen activated protein (MAP) kinases. The kinases are structurally related and are relatively small, ranging from 38 kDa to approximately 45 kDa with specificity for phosphorylation on threonine or serine. All also share the property that their activity is dramatically affected by phosphorylation of threonine and tyrosine within the kinase catalytic domain. In Erks, the essential sequence is a TEY, in Jnks the sequence is TPY, and in p38 kinases the sequence is TGY. Phosphorylation of these sites can increase catalytic activity 1000 fold and the mechanism is hypothesized to be very similar to the phosphorylation within the activation loop of the kinase domain of tyrosine kinases, as discussed above. In particular, in Erk2, binding of its activating kinase, Mek, alters the conformation of the subdomain VIII loop and exposes Y^{185} for phosphorylation. Its phosphorylation would then release the block for substrate binding with the subsequent T^{183} phosphorylation further activating the enzyme by facilitating the correct alignment of the catalytic residues. Once the MAP kinases are phosphorylated they translocate to the nucleus through a mechanism that involves dimer formation,[285] and phosphorylate a number of substrates including a variety of transcription factors.

Numerous substrates have been identified for the activated Erks, Jnks, and p38 kinases, many being transcriptional factors. Some of the substrates are unique for a particular family member, while other substrates can be phosphorylated by more than one family member. A few examples will illustrate the function of the pathway as well as illustrating the importance of the pathways. Perhaps the classic example is the regulation of the immediate early gene, *c-fos*, a gene that is highly and transiently induced in the response to a wide variety of cellular stimulants. The serum-induced expression of *c-fos* is dependent upon a serum response element (SRE), which binds a serum response factor (SRF). The induction of *c-fos* expression requires the recruitment to SRF of a factor to form a ternary complex. The recruited factor is an ets family member termed SAP-1 or the highly related family member Elk-1.[286] The ability of Elk-1 or SAP-1 to be recruited into the complex is dependent upon phosphorylation of a cluster of serine and threonine in the carboxyl-terminal region. These phosphorylations can be mediated by both the Erk family members[287, 288] and Jnk members.[289] Thus within the context of serum stimulation, growth factor or cytokine *c-fos* activation is mediated by the Erks while the induction of *c-fos* by UV light, stress, TNFα, IL-1, or osmotic shock is mediated by the Jnks. Another transcription factor that is activated following serine phosphorylation at two sites in the amino-terminal is c-jun. Importantly, the Jnks were initially identified from the cloning of novel Erk-related kinases that could mediate this phosphorylation.[290, 291] Other transcription factors that are regulated by phosphorylation include ATF2 by the Jnks,[292] CHOP by p38,[293] and MEF2C by p38[294] as well as by Erk5.[295] Lastly, two intracellular receptors, the estrogen receptor[296] and the PPARγ receptor,[297] are functionally modified by phosphorylation by the MAP kinases.

The importance of this family of kinases is also illustrated by the series of events leading to the cloning of p38. This began with the identification of a compound that was found to inhibit the production of IL-1 and TNFα by human monocytes in response to LPS. The compound was used in affinity labeling to identify a 45 kDa protein that was the major, if not sole, protein labeled by the compound. The gene was subsequently cloned based on peptide sequence from the affinity-purified protein.

The activities of the MAP kinases are regulated through their phosphorylation as well as through their dephosphorylation. The dephosphorylation is mediated by a group of dual-specificity phosphatases capable of dephosphorylating both tyrosine and threonine at the activation domain of the MAP kinases. The first MAP kinase phosphatases (MKP) were identified as immediate early genes in response to growth factors or serum.[298-300] Thus it is curious that serum induces the activation of the MAP kinases and subsequently this pathway, or others, induces the transcription of genes that encode the phosphatases that will inactivate the pathway. Many of the phosphatases show remarkable specificity for particular MAP kinases and this appears to be due to the requirement for interaction of a noncatalytic domain of the phosphatase with the MAP kinase. This interaction is required for the activation of phosphatase activity.[301] There are currently up to nine mammalian dual-specificity phosphatases including MKP-1, MKP-2, MKP-3, MKP-4, and PAC-1, all of which are specific for MAP kinases.

The activation of the MAP kinases is mediated by a family of dual-specificity kinases that is capable of phosphorylating the critical threonine and tyrosine residues in the activation domain. The kinases of this family are generally referred to as MAP kinase kinases (MKKs), although a variety of nonmenclatures exist, including MEK and MAPKK. The MKKs exhibit varying specificities for the various MAP kinases. MKK1 and MKK2 specifically phosphorylate the Erk MAP kinases. MKK3 and MKK6 phosphorylate the p38 MAP kinases. MKK4 and MKK7 phosphorylate the Jnk MAP kinases. Recently, mice deficient in MKK4 (also termed SEK1, JNKK) have been generated. The absence of MKK4 results in an embryonic lethality, relatively late in development at day 14.[302] Importantly, the ability of heat shock or the protein synthesis inhibitor anisomycin to induce JNK activation is lost, demonstrating the essential, nonredundant role for MKK4 in these signaling pathways. However, the ability to activate JNK in the response to a number of additional inducers was not affected. The role of MKK4 in lymphoid cells was examined in chimeric rag$^{-/-}$ mice.[303, 304] Relatively minor phenotypes were observed that suggest that MKK4 might be involved in aspects of CD28-mediated IL-2 production and/or provide some slight degree of protection from fas and CD3 mediated apoptosis.

The MKKs are, in turn, activated by a wide variety of kinases, minimally 14, that are activated in the responses to growth factors and stress. At this level, the terminology becomes even more complex and a consistent nomenclature has not emerged. A number of examples will be given to illustrate the classic pathways and the newly emerging kinases that are capable of activating one or more of the MAP kinase pathways. The classic pathway is the growth factor associated ras/raf activation of the Erks. The activation of the pathway begins with the recruitment of an "adapter" protein to an activated receptor complex. In the case of the tyrosine kinase receptors, the adapter protein is most frequently one termed Grb2, while in the case of most cytokine receptors the adapter protein SHC is recruited to the receptor complex. In either case, recruitment involves the recognition of specific sites of tyrosine phosphorylation on the receptor by the SH2 domains of the adapter protein. In the case of the recruitment of SHC, the adapter is phosphorylated and Grb2 is recruited to the complex through its interaction with the tyrosine phosphorylated SHC. Grb2 subsequently recruits the GTP exchange factor SOS to the complex, resulting in the exchange of GDP for GTP on ras. Recent studies of the structural of a Ras/Sos complex have begun to provide insights into the mechanisms by which SOS promotes nucleotide exchange.[305]

In an unspecified manner, GTP-ras recruits Raf-1 to the membrane and mediates its activation.[306, 307] It should be noted that simply targeting Raf-1 to the membrane will result in its activation and subsequent activation of the pathway.[308] Activated Raf-1 is directly capable of activating MKK1 or MKK2[309] that, as discussed above, activates the Erks. It is presumed that the activation of the two additional Raf family members, Raf-A and Raf-B, occur in a similar manner.

A series of protein kinases, termed MEKK1, MEKK2, MEKK3, and MEKK4, have been identified based on homology with yeast kinases involved in MAP kinase signaling pathways. MEKK1 is able to specifically activate the Erk MAP kinase pathway through the phosphorylation of MKK1[310] and the Jnk MAP kinase pathway through MKK4.[311, 312] The activation of MEKK1 binds Ras in a GTP-dependent manner as well as Cdc42 and Rac. Evidence exists to indicate that the activation of MEKK1 by EGF requires ras. In quite distinct contrast from this mechanism, MEKK1 has also been shown to be activated by cleavage by caspases.[313] In this case, the activation of MEKK1 is associated with the induction of apoptosis. Lastly, a kinase (Nck interacting kinase, NIK) has been identified that binds to an adapter protein termed Nck and is capable of activating MEKK1.[314] It can be anticipated that the derivation of mice deficient in MEKKs will help to resolve the biological roles of these kinases as well as provide insights into their role in activation of the various MAP kinase pathways.

Another group of kinases that is involved in the activation of MAP kinase pathways, possibly through the phosphorylation of MKKs, is the PAK kinases (p21-activated kinases) (PAK1, PAK2, PAK3). The PAKs regulate morphological and cytoskeletal changes in a variety of cell types. Their activities are regulated by Rac and Cdc42. PAK2 has also been shown to be activated by caspase cleavage.[315] Activated forms of the PAKs have been shown to activate the Jnk and p38, but not the Erk, MAP kinase pathways,[314] and this may be independent of Rac and Cdc42 activation.[316]

Other kinases that have been implicated in activation of the MAP kinase pathways include apoptosis signal-regulating kinase (Ask1),[317] the proto-oncogene Tpl-2,[318] hematopoietic progenitor kinase 1 (Hpk1),[319] members of the mixed lineage kinases (MLK),[320] and germinal center kinase

(GCK).[321] In addition, Tab1 and Tak1 are implicated in TGFβ induced activation of MAP kinase pathways.

Summary and Conclusions

The last several years have seen a dramatic increase in our understanding of the mechanisms by which extracellular signals are interpreted by cells. The concept that nature has chosen to use a relatively few specific mechanisms for signal transduction is consoling, although the bewildering array of permutations on these few themes makes it a challenge to follow the specifics. One of the somewhat surprising emerging concepts is that everything that happens as a consequence of receptor engagement may not always play a nonredundant essential role. One extreme example of this concept is the observation that a wide variety of growth factors and cytokines can induce the expression of the immediate early gene *Egr-1*. However, mice that lack *Egr-1* have a single striking phenotype consisting of the inability to produce luteinizing hormone,[322] suggesting that the *Egr-1* has evolved to regulate the expression of one gene in a nonredundant manner. The same concept applies to the induction of the tyrosine phosphorylation of specific substrates. For example, although Epo, Tpo, and many other cytokines induce the tyrosine phosphorylation and activation of the Stat5 proteins, gene disruption studies demonstrate that it is only in the responses to growth hormone and prolactin that they play a nonredundant essential role. Conversely, although IL-7 activates a wide variety of signaling pathways, the ability to rescue T cell development in an IL-7 receptor knockout mouse by a Bcl-2 transgene would suggest that among all the pathways activated, the essential one is that associated with the upregulation of Bcl-2.[323-325] Clearly the possibility exists in many cases that pathways redundantly regulate critical events. Appropriate crosses of mutant mice should allow the identification of such situations.

A number of technological advances have significantly impacted the studies of signal transduction. Advances in the areas of protein isolation, sequence analysis, and structural determination have had a dramatic impact on the ease with which investigators can identify proteins involved in signaling. Equally important has been the development of a large number of extensive libraries of expressed sequences. This has allowed the rapid identification of members of families of proteins that share particular motifs. Extensive studies of the functions of protein family members have supported the concept that structural similarity almost always predicts a functional similarity. Indeed, family members often differ only in the lineages in which a common function is mediated. For example, the receptors for Epo, Tpo, growth hormone, and prolactin are both structurally and functionally highly related and, when examined, each can mediate the function of the other when expressed in the appropriate lineages. Relative to signal transduction, it is important to note, however, that the ability of the prolactin receptor to activate Stat5 is its essential function when expressed on mammary epithelial cells, while this function is not relevant to its ability to support erythropoiesis.

The last several years have focused on developing the means to rapidly assess the function of a particular signaling component in cellular responses. As noted throughout the chapter, the approaches include the use of "specific" inhibitors, the use of a variety of antisense types of approaches, and the use of various dominant negative types of approaches. It is becoming increasing obvious that these approaches may have significant limitations and should not be used as the only means to assess the function of proteins. Thus inhibitors are clearly only "specific" with regard to what can be measured, and unfortunately all potential targets cannot be assessed either for practical reasons or because a number of potential targets are yet to be identified. The same concerns exist with regard to all the antisense types of approaches. The dominant negative approaches have potentially a better chance for specificity but overexpression of mutants has the potential to interfere with other functions.

The potential concerns with the above approaches have been brought to light because the ability to target mutations in germline genes has provided the unique and essential means by which the specific functions of genes can be assessed. Advances in the ability to target mutations to specific lineages or stage of development will greatly expand the utility of this approach in assessing gene function. There are potential limitations, however, including the redundancy of functions and selection for compensating mutations that, for example, might select for inappropriate or higher levels of expression of family members. Irrespective, the advances in assessing gene function will continue to extend not only the rate with which cellular signaling can be accomplished but also the precision.

Knowledge of the specifics of signal transduction has provided additional avenues for the development of drugs for the treatment of a variety of conditions. For example, the concept that the function of a ligand is often to drive the aggregation of receptors has led to the search for small molecules that can also accomplish this function. These searches are beginning to identify such compounds that could conceivably become orally active drugs that mimic the function of such physiologically important regulators as erythropoietin, thrombopoietin, growth hormone, and insulin. Knowledge of the specifics in signaling pathways allows an increasing number of potential points for intervention in cellular responses. For example, the critical role that specific caspases play in both normal development and innate and acquired immunity strongly supports efforts to identy specific inhibitors. Newly discovered potential drug targets include the SMADs, Stats, and IκB kinases, just to name a few. In this area, the ability to create mutant strains of mice lacking specific genes is also playing a critical role in defining potential targets. In particular, a mutant strain or conditional deletion of a particular gene in time or lineage theoretically defines the in vivo consequences of administering a truly specific gene product targeted drug. For example, a drug that specifically inhibited the function of Stat6 should have the affect of eliminating IL-4/IL-13 associated physiological functions based on the phenotype of mice lacking Stat6. Any additional affects must be ascribed to secondary targets.

REFERENCES

1. Heldin, C.H.: Protein tyrosine kinase receptors. Cancer Surv. 27:7–24:7, 1996.

2. Shalaby, F., Ho, J., Stanford, W.L., Fischer, K.-D., Schuh, A.C., Schwartz, L., Bernstein, A., and Rossant, J.: A requirement for Flk1 in primitive and definitive hematopoiesis and vasculogenesis. Cell 89:981, 1997.

3. Yoshida, H., Hayashi, S., Kunisada, T., Ogawa, M., Nishikawa, S., Okamura, H., Sudo, T., and Shultz, L.D.: The murine mutation osteopetrosis is in the coding region of the macrophage colony stimulating factor gene. Nature 345:442, 1990.

4. Mackarehtschian, K., Hardin, J.D., Moore, K.A., Boast, S., Goff, S.P., and Lemischka, I.R.: Targeted disruption of the *flk2/flt3* gene leads to deficiencies in primitive hematopoietic progenitors. Immunity 3:147, 1995.

5. Heldin, C.H., and Ostman, A.: Ligand-induced dimerization of growth factor receptors: Variations on the theme. Cytokine Growth Factor Rev. 7:3, 1996.

6. Weiss, F.U., Daub, H., and Ullrich, A.: Novel mechanisms of RTK signal generation. Curr. Opin. Genet. Dev. 7:80, 1997.

7. Lemmon, M.A., and Schlessinger, J.: Regulation of signal transduction and signal diversity by receptor oligomerization. Trends Biochem. Sci. 19:459, 1994.

8. Ullrich, A., and Schlessinger, J.: Signal transduction by receptors with tyrosine kinase activity. Cell 61:203, 1990.

9. Heldin, C.H.: Dimerization of cell surface receptors in signal transduction. Cell 80:213, 1995.

10. Hubbard, S.R., Wei, L., Ellis, L., and Hendrickson, W.A.: Crystal structure of the tyrosine kinase domain of the human insulin receptor. Nature 372:746, 1994.

11. Mohammadi, M., Schlessinger, J., and Hubbard, S.R.: Structure of the FGF receptor tyrosine kinase domain reveals a novel autoinhibitory mechanism. Cell 86:577, 1996.

12. Pawson, T.: Protein modules and signalling networks. Nature 373:573, 1995.

13. Booker, G.W., Breeze, A.L., Downing, A.K., Panayotou, G., Gout, I., Waterfield, M.D., and Campbell, I.D.: Structure of an SH2 domain of the p85 alpha subunit of phosphatidylinositol-3-OH kinase. Nature 358:684, 1992.

14. Waksman, G., Kominos, D., Robertson, D.R., Pant, N., Baltimore, D., Birge, R.B., Cowburn, D., Hanafusa, H., Mayer, B.J., Overduin, M., Resh, M.D., Rios, C.B., Silverman, L., and Kuriyan, J.: Crystal structure of the phosphotyrosine recognition domain SH2 of v-src complexed with tyrosine-phosphorylated peptides. Nature 358:646, 1992.

15. Kavanaugh, W.M., and Williams, L.T.: An alternative to SH2 domains for binding tyrosine-phosphorylated proteins. Science 266:1862, 1995.

16. van der Geer, P., and Pawson, T.: The PTB domain: A new protein module implicated in signal transduction. Tibs 20:277, 1995.

17. Sherr, C.J.: Colony-stimulating factor-1 receptor. Blood 75:1, 1990.

18. Kozlowski, M., Larose, L., Lee, F., Le, D.M., Rottapel, R., and Siminovitch, K.A.: SHP-1 binds and negatively modulates the c-Kit receptor by interaction with tyrosine 569 in the c-Kit juxtamembrane domain. Mol. Cell. Biol. 18:2089, 1998.

19. Golub, T.R., Barker, G.F., Lovett, M., and Gilliland, D.G.: Fusion of PDGF receptor beta to a novel ets-like gene, tel, in chronic myelomonocytic leukemia with t(5;12) chromosomal translocation. Cell 77:307, 1994.

20. Morris, S.W., Kirstein, M.N., Valentine, M.B., Dittmer, K.G., Shapiro, D.N., Saltman, D.L., and Look, A.T.: Fusion of a kinase gene, ALK, to a nucleolar protein gene, NPM, in non-Hodgkin's lymphoma [published erratum appears in Science 1995 Jan 20;267(5196):316–7]. Science 263:1281, 1994.

21. Golub, T.R., Goga, A., Barker, G.F., Afar, D.E., McLaughlin, J., Bohlander, S.K., Rowley, J.D., Witte, O.N., and Gilliland, D.G.: Oligomerization of the ABL tyrosine kinase by the Ets protein TEL in human leukemia. Mol. Cell. Biol. 16:4107, 1996.

22. Garvin, A.M., Pawar, S., Marth, J.D., and Perlmutter, R.M.: Structure of the murine lck gene and its rearrangement in a murine lymphoma cell line. Mol. Cell. Biol. 8:3058, 1988.

23. Bazan, J.F.: A novel family of growth factor receptors: A common binding domain in the growth hormone, prolactin, erythropoietin and IL-6 receptors, and the p75 IL-2 receptor beta-chain. Biochem. Biophys. Res. Commun. 164:788, 1989.

24. Bazan, J.F.: Emerging families of cytokines and receptors. Curr. Biol. 3:603, 1997.

25. De Vos, A.M., Ultsch, M., and Kossiakoff, A.A.: Human growth hormone and extracellular domain of its receptor: Crystal structure of the complex. Science 255:306, 1992.

26. Somers, W., Ultsch, M., De Vos, A.M., and Kossiakoff, A.A.: The X-ray structure of a growth hormone-prolactin receptor complex. Nature 372:478, 1994.

27. Livnah, O., Stura, E.A., Johnson, D.L., Middleton, S.A., Mulcahy, L.S., Wrighton, N.C., Dower, W.J., Jolliffe, L.K., and Wilson, I.A.: Functional mimicry of a protein hormone by a peptide agonist: The EPO receptor complex at 2.8 A [see comments]. Science 273:464, 1996.

28. Tian, S.S., Lamb, P., King, A.G., Miller, S.G., Kessler, L., Luengo, J.I., Averill, L., Johnson, R.K., Gleason, J.G., Pelus, L.M., Dillon, S.B., and Rosen, J.: A small, nonpeptidyl mimic of granulocyte-colony-stimulating factor [see comments]. Science 281:257, 1998.

29. Murakami, M., Narazaki, M., Hibi, M., Yawata, H., Yasukawa, K., Hamaguchi, M., Taga, T., and Kishimoto, T.: Critical cytoplasmic region of the interleukin 6 signal transducer gp130 is conserved in the cytokine receptor family. Proc. Natl. Acad. Sci. U.S.A. 88:11349, 1991.

30. Miyajima, A., Mui, A.L.F., Ogorochi, T., and Sakamaki, K.: Receptors for granulocyte-macrophage colony-stimulating factor, interleukin-3, and interleukin-5. Blood 82:1960, 1993.

31. Kishimoto, T., Akira, S., Narazaki, M., and Taga, T.: Interleukin-6 family of cytokines and gp130. Blood 86:1243, 1995.

32. Leonard, W.J., Shores, E.W., and Love, P.E.: Role of the common cytokine receptor gamma chain in cytokine signaling and lymphoid development. Immunol. Rev. 148:97, 1995.

33. Bach, E.A., Aguet, M., and Schreiber, R.D.: The IFN gamma receptor: A paradigm for cytokine receptor signaling. Annu. Rev. Immunol. 15:563–91:563, 1997.

34. Darnell, J.E., Jr., Kerr, I.M., and Stark, G.R.: Jak-STAT pathways and transcriptional activation in response to IFNs and other extracellular signaling proteins. Science 264:1415, 1994.

35. Pellegrini, S., John, J., Shearer, M., Kerr, I.M., and Stark, G.R.: Use of a selectable marker regulated by alpha interferon to obtain mutations in the signaling pathway. Mol. Cell. Biol. 9:4605, 1989.

36. Witthuhn, B., Quelle, F.W., Silvennoinen, O., Yi, T., Tang, B., Miura, O., and Ihle, J.N.: JAK2 associates with the erythropoietin receptor and is tyrosine phosphorylated and activated following EPO stimulation. Cell 74:227, 1993.

37. Artgetsinger, L.S., Campbell, G.S., Yang, X., Witthuhn, B.A., Silvennoinen, O., Ihle, J.N., and Carter-Su, C.: Identification of JAK2 as a growth hormone receptor-associated tyrosine kinase. Cell 74:237, 1993.

38. Feng, J., Witthuhn, B.A., Matsuda, T., Kohlhuber, F., Kerr, I.M., and Ihle, J.N.: Activation of Jak2 catalytic activity requires phosphorylation of Y^{1007} in the kinase activation loop. Mol. Cell. Biol. 17:2497, 1997.

39. Gauzzi, M.C., Velazquez, L., McKendry, R., Mogensen, K.E., Fellous, M., and Pellegrini, S.: Interferon-α-dependent activation of Tyk2 requires phosphorylation of positive regulatory tyrosines by another kinase. J. Biol. Chem. 271:20494, 1996.

40. Zhou, Y.J., Hanson, E.P., Chen, Y.Q., Magnuson, K., Chen, M., Swann, P.G., Wange, R.L., Changelian, P.S., and O'Shea, J.J.: Distinct tyrosine phosphorylation sites in JAK3 kinase domain positively and negatively regulate its enzymatic activity. Proc. Natl. Acad. Sci. U.S.A. 94:13850, 1997.

41. von Freeden-Jeffry, U., Vieria, P., Lucian, L.A., McNeil, T., Burdach, S.E.G., and Murray, R.: Lymphopenia in interleukin (IL)-7 gene-deleted mice identifies IL-7 as a nonredundant cytokine. J. Exp. Med. 181:1519, 1995.

42. Nosaka, T., van Deursen, J.M.A., Tripp, R.A., Thierfelder, W.E., Witthuhn, B.A., McMickle, A.P., Doherty, P.C., Grosveld, G.C., and Ihle, J.N.: Defective lymphoid development in mice lacking Jak3. Science 270:800, 1995.

43. Thomis, D.C., Gurniak, C.B., Tivol, E., Sharpe, A.H., and Berg, L.J.: Mice lacking Jak3 have defects in B lymphocyte maturation and T lymphocyte activation. Science 270:794, 1995.

44. Asao, H., Tanaka, N., Ishii, N., Higuchi, M., Takeshita, T., Nakamura, M., Shirasawa, T., and Sugamura, K.: Interleukin 2-induced activation of JAK3: possible involvement in signal transduction for c-myc induction and cell proliferation. FEBS Lett. 351:201, 1994.

45. Macchi, P., Villa, A., Giliani, S., Sacco, M.G., Frattini, A., Porta, F., Ugazio, A.G., Johnston, J.A., Candotti, F., O'Shea, J.J., Vezzoni, P., and Notarangelo, L.D.: Mutations of Jak-3 gene in patients with autosomal severe combined immune deficiency (SCID). Nature 377:65, 1995.

46. Russell, S.M., Tayebi, N., Nakajima, H., Riedy, M.C., Roberts, J.L., Aman, M.J., Migone, T.-S., Noguchi, M., Markert, M.L., Buckley, R.H., O'Shea, J.J., and Leonard, W.J.: Mutation of Jak3 in a patient with SCID: Essential role of Jak3 in lymphoid development. Science 270:797, 1995.

47. Bunting, K.D., Sangster, M.Y., Ihle, J.N., and Sorrentino, B.P.: Restoration of lymphocyte function in Janus kinase 3-deficient mice by retroviral-mediated gene transfer [see comments]. Nat. Med. 4:58, 1998.

48. Rodig, S.J., Meraz, M.A., White, J.M., Lampe, P.A., Riley, J.K., Arthur, C., King, K.L., Sheehan, K.C.F., Yin, L., Pennica, D., Johnson, E.M. Jr., and Schreiber, R.D.: Targeted disruption of the Jak1 gene demonstrates obligatory and nonredundant roles of Janus kinases in mediating cytokine induced biologic responses. Cell 93:373, 1998.

49. Neubauer, H., Cumano, A., Muller, M., Wu, H., Huffstadt, U., and Pfeffer, K.: Jak2 deficiency defines an essential developmental checkpoint in definitive hematopoiesis. Cell 93:397, 1998.

50. Parganas, E., Wang, D., Stravopodis, D., Topham, D.J., Marine, J.-C., Teglund, S., Vanin, E.F., Bodner, S., Colamonici, O.R., van Deursen, J.M., Grosveld, G., and Ihle, J.N.: Jak2 is essential for signaling through a variety of cytokine receptors. Cell 93:385, 1998.

51. Wu, H., Liu, X., Jaenisch, R., and Lodish, H.F.: Generation of committed erythroid BFU-E and CFU-E progenitors does not require erythropoietin or the erythropoietin receptor. Cell 83:59, 1995.

52. Klingmuller, U., Lorenz, U., Cantley, L.C., Neel, B.G., and Lodish, H.F.: Specific recruitment of the hematopoietic protein tyrosine phosphatase SH-PTP1 to the erythropoietin receptor causes inactivation of JAK2 and termination of proliferative signals. Cell 80:729, 1995.

53. Shultz, L.D., Schweitzer, P.A., Rajan, T.V., Yi, T., Ihle, J.N., Matthews, R.J., Thomas, M.L., and Beier, D.R.: Mutations at the murine motheaten locus are within the hematopoietic cell protein tyrosine phosphatase (Hcph) gene. Cell 73:1445, 1993.

54. Tsui, H.W., Siminovitch, K.A., de Souza, L., and Tsui, F.W.L.: Motheaten and viable motheaten mice have mutations in the haematopoietic cell phosphatase gene. Nat. Gen. 4:124, 1993.

55. Lacronique, V., Boureux, A., Valle, V.D., Poirel, H., Quang, C.T., Mauchauffe, M., Berthou, C., Lessard, M., Berger, R., Ghysdael, J., and Bernard, O.A.: A TEL-JAK2 fusion protein with constitutive kinase activity in human leukemia. Science 278:1309, 1997.

56. Peeters, P., Raynaud, S.D., Cools, J., Wlodarska, I., Grosgeorge, J., Philip, P., Monpoux, F., Rompaey, L., Baens, M., Berghe, H., and Marynen, P.: Fusion of TEL, the ETS-variant gene 6 (ETV6), to the receptor-associated kinase JAK2 as a result of t(9;12) in a lymphoid and t(9;15;12) in a myeloid leukemia. Blood 90:2535, 1997.

57. Yoshimura, A., Ohkubo, T., Kiguchi, T., Jenkins, N.A., Gilbert, D.J., Copeland, N.G., Hara, T., and Miyajima, A.: A novel cytokine-inducible gene CIS encodes an SH2-containing protein that binds to tyrosine-phosphorylated interleukin-3 and erythropoietin receptors. EMBO J. 14:2816, 1995.

58. Endo, T.A., Masuhara, M., Yokouchi, M., Suzuki, R., Sakamoto, H., Mitsui, K., Matsumoto, A., Tanimura, S., Ohtsubo, M., Misawa, H., Miyazaki, T., Leonor, N., Taniguchi, T., Fujita, T., Kanakura, Y., Komiya, S., and Yoshimura, A.: A new protein containing an SH2 domain that inhibits JAK kinases. Nature 387:921, 1997.

59. Starr, R., Willson, T.A., Viney, E.M., Murray, L.J., Rayner, J.R., Jenkins, B.J., Gonda, T.J., Alexander, W.S., Metcalf, D., Nicola, N.A., and Hilton, D.J.: A family of cytokine-inducible inhibitors of signalling. Nature 387:917, 1997.

60. Naka, T., Narazaki, M., Hirata, M., Matsumoto, T., Minamoto, S., Aono, A., Nishimoto, N., Kajita, T., Taga, T., Yoshizaki, K., Akira, S., and Kishimoto, T.: Structure and function of a new STAT-induced STAT inhibitor. Nature 387:924, 1997.

61. Starr, R., Metcalf, D., Elefanty, A.G., Brysha, M., Willson, T.A., Nicola, N.A., Hilton, D.J., and Alexander, W.S.: Liver degeneration and lymphoid deficiencies in mice lacking suppressor of cytokine signaling-1. Proc. Natl. Acad. Sci. U.S.A. 95:14395, 1998.

62. Naka, T., Matsumoto, T., Narazaki, M., Fujimoto, M., Morita, Y., Ohsawa, Y., Saito, H., Nagasawa, T., Uchiyama, Y., and Kishimoto, T.: Accelerated apoptosis of lymphocytes by augmented induction of Bax in SSI-1 (STAT-induced STAT inhibitor-1) deficient mice. Proc. Natl. Acad. Sci. U.S.A. 95:15577, 1998.

63. Toker, A., and Cantley, L.C.: Signalling through the lipid products of phosphoinositide-3-OH kinase. Nature 387:673, 1997.

64. Whitman, M., Kaplan, D., Roberts, T., and Cantley, L.: Evidence for two distinct phosphatidylinositol kinases in fibroblasts. Implications for cellular regulation. Biochem. J. 247:165, 1987.

65. Chang, H.W., Aoki, M., Fruman, D., Auger, K.R., Bellacosa, A., Tsichlis, P.N., Cantley, L.C., Roberts, T.M., and Vogt, P.K.: Transformation of chicken cells by the gene encoding the catalytic subunit of PI 3-kinase. Science 276:1848, 1997.

66. Divecha, N., and Irvine, R.F.: Phospholipid signaling. Cell 80:269, 1997.

67. Vanhaesebroeck, B., Leevers, S.J., Panayotou, G., and Waterfield, M.D.: Phosphoinositide 3-kinases: A conserved family of signal transducers. Trends. Biochem. Sci. 22:267, 1997.

68. Vanhaesebroeck, B., Stein, R.C., and Waterfield, M.D.: The study of phosphoinositide 3-kinase function. Cancer Surv. 27:249–70:249, 1996.

69. Chantry, D., Vojtek, A., Kashishian, A., Holtzman, D.A., Wood, C., Gray, P.W., Cooper, J.A., and Hoekstra, M.F.: p110delta, a novel phosphatidylinositol 3-kinase catalytic subunit that associates with p85 and is expressed predominantly in leukocytes. J. Biol. Chem. 272:19236, 1997.

70. Rodriguez-Viciana, P., Warne, P.H., Vanhaesebroeck, B., Waterfield, M.D., and Downward, J.: Activation of phosphoinositide 3-kinase by interaction with Ras and by point mutation. EMBO J. 15:2442, 1996.

71. Datta, S.R., Dudek, H., Tao, X., Masters, S., Fu, H., Gotoh, Y., and Greenberg, M.E.: Akt phosphorylation of BAD couples survival signals to the cell-intrinsic death machinery. Cell 91:231, 1997.

72. Peso, L., Gonzalez-Garcia, M., Page, C., Herrera, R., and Nunez, G.: Interleukin-3-induced phosphorylation of BAD through the protein kinase Akt. Science 278:687, 1997.

73. Zha, J., Harada, H., Yang, E., Jockel, J., and Korsmeyer, S.J.: Serine phosphorylation of death agonist BAD in response to survival factor results in binding to 14-3-3 not BCL-X$_L$. Cell 87:619, 1996.

74. Thomas, J.D., Sideras, P., Smith, C.I., Vorechovsky, I., Chapman, V., and Paul, W.E.: Colocalization of X-linked agammaglobulinemia and X-linked immunodeficiency genes. Science 261:355, 1993.

75. Tsukada, S., Saffran, D.C., Rawlings, D.J., Parolini, O., Allen, R.C., Klisak, I., Kubagawa, H., Mohandas, T., Quan, S., Belmont, J.W., Cooper, M.D., Conley, M.E., and Witte, O.N.: Deficient expression of a B-cell cytoplasmic tyrosine kinase in human X-linked agammaglobulinemia. Cell 72:279, 1993.

76. Jimenez, C., Jones, D.R., Rodriguez-Viciana, P., Gonzalez-Garcia, A., Leonardo, E., Wennstrom, S., Kobbe, C., Toran, J.L., Borlado, L., Calvo, V., Copin, S.G., Albar, J.P., Gaspar, M.L., Diez, E., Marcos, M.A., Downward, J., Martinez, A., Merida, I., and Carrera, A.C.: Identification and characterization of a new oncogene derived from the regulatory subunit of phosphoinositide 3-kinase. EMBO J. 17:743, 1998.

77. Li, J., Yen, C., Liaw, D., Podsypanina, K., Bose, S., Wang, S.I., Puc, J., Miliaresis, C., Rodgers, L., McCombie, R., Bigner, S.H., Giovanella, B.C., Ittmann, M., Tycko, B., Hibshoosh, H., Wigler, M.H., and Parsons, R.: PTEN, a putative protein tyrosine phosphatase gene mutated in human brain, breast, and prostate cancer. Science 275:1943, 1997.

78. Steck, P.A., Pershouse, M.A., Jasser, S.A., Yung, W.K., Lin, H., Ligon, A.H., Langford, L.A., Baumgard, M.L., Hattier, T., Davis, T., Frye, C., Hu, R., Swedlund, B., Teng, D.H., and Tavtigian, S.V.: Identification of a candidate tumour suppressor gene, MMAC1, at chromosome 10q23.3 that is mutated in multiple advanced cancers. Nat. Genet. 15:356, 1997.

79. Myers, M.P., Stolarov, J.P., Eng, C., Li, J., Wang, S.I., Wigler, M.H., Parsons, R., and Tonks, N.K.: P-TEN, the tumor suppressor from human chromosome 10q23, is a dual-specificity phosphatase. Proc. Natl. Acad. Sci. U.S.A. 94:9052, 1997.

80. Maehama, T., and Dixon, J.E.: The tumor suppressor, PTEN/MMAC1, dephosphorylates the lipid second messenger, phosphatidylinositol 3,4,5-trisphosphate. J. Biol. Chem. 273:13375, 1998.

81. Stambolic, V., Suzuki, A., de la Pompa, J.L., Brothers, G.M., Mirtsos, C., Sasaki, T., Ruland, J., Penninger, J.M., Siderovski, D.P., and Mak, T.W.: Negative regulation of PKB/Akt-dependent cell survival by the tumor suppressor PTEN. Cell 95:29, 1998.

82. Fruman, D.A., Snapper, S.B., Yballe, C.M., Davidson, L., Yu, J.Y., Alt, F.W., and Cantley, L.C.: Impaired B cell development and proliferation in absence of phosphoinositide 3-kinase p85alpha. Science 283:393, 1999.

83. Suzuki, H., Terauchi, Y., Fujiwara, M., Aizawa, S., Yazaki, Y., Kadowaki, T., and Koyasu, S.: Xid-like immunodeficiency in mice with disruption of the p85alpha subunit of phosphoinositide 3-kinase. Science 283:390, 1999.

84. Nishibe, S., Wahlm, M.I., Hernandez-Soromayor, S.M.T., Tonks, N.K., Rhee, S.G., and Carpenter, G.: Increase of the catalytic activity of phospholipase C-gamma1 by tyrosine phosphorylation. Science 250:1253, 1990.

85. Kim, J.W., Sim, S.S., Kim, U.H., Nishibe, S., Wahl, M.I., Carpenter, G., and Rhee, S.G.: Tyrosine residues in bovine phospholipase C-gamma phosphorylated by the epidermal growth factor receptor in vitro. J. Biol. Chem. 265:3940, 1990.

86. Joseph, S.K.: The inositol triphosphate receptor family. Cell Signal 8:1, 1996.

87. Ji, Q.-S., Winnier, G.E., Niswender, K.D., Horstman, D., Wisdom, R., Magnuson, M.A., and Carpenter, G.: Essential role of the tyrosine kinase substrate phospholipase C-delta1 in mammalian growth and development. Proc. Natl. Acad. Sci. U.S.A. 94:2999, 1997.

88. Ji, Q.-S., Ermini, S., Baulida, J., Sun, F., and Carpenter, G.: Epidermal growth factor signaling and mitogenesis in Plcg1 null mouse embryonic fibroblasts. Mol. Biol. Cell 9:749, 1997.

89. Bourette, R.P., Myles, G.M., Choi, J.L., and Rohrschneider, L.R.: Sequential activation of phosphatidylinositol 3-kinase and phospholipase C-gamma2 by the M-CSF receptor is necessary for differentiation signaling. EMBO J. 16:5880, 1997.

90. Damen, J.E., Liu, L., Rosten, P., Humphries, R.K., Jefferson, A.B., Majerus, P.W., and Krystal, G.: The 145-kDa protein induced to associate with Shc by multiple cytokines is an inositol tetraphosphate and phosphatidylinositol 3,4,5-triphosphate 5-phosphatase. Proc. Natl. Acad. Sci. U.S.A. 93:1689, 1996.

91. Lioubin, M.N., Algate, P.A., Tsai, S., Carlberg, K., Aebersold, A., and Rohrschneider, L.R.: p150Ship, a signal transduction molecule with inositol polyphosphate-5-phosphatase activity. Genes Dev. 10:1084, 1996.

92. Helgalson, C.D., Damen, J.E., Rosten, P., Grewal, R., Sorensen, P., Chappel, S.M., Borowski, A., Jirik, F., Krystal, G., and Humphries, R.K.: Targeted disruption of SHIP leads to hemopoietic perturbations, lung pathology and a shortened lifespan. Genes Dev. 12:1610, 1998.

93. Shen, S.H., Bastien, L., Posner, B.I., and Chrëtien, P.: A protein-tyrosine phosphatase with sequence similarity to the SH2 domain of the protein-tyrosine kinases. Nature 352:736, 1991.

94. Yi, T., Cleveland, J.L., and Ihle, J.N.: Identification of novel protein tyrosine phosphatases of hematopoietic cells by PCR amplification. Blood 78:2222, 1991.

95. Feng, G.-S., Hui, C.-C., and Pawson, T.: SH2-containing phosphotyrosine phosphatase as a target of protein-tyrosine kinases. Science 259:1607, 1993.

96. Saxton, T.M., Henkemeyer, M., Gasca, S., Shen, R., Rossi, D.J., Shalaby, F., Feng, G.S., and Pawson, T.: Abnormal mesoderm patterning in mouse embryos mutant for the SH2 tyrosine phosphatase Shp-2. EMBO J. 16:2352, 1997.

97. Hof, P., Pluskey, S., Dhe-Paganon, S., Eck, M.J., and Shoelson, S.E.: Crystal structure of the tyrosine phosphatase SHP-2. Cell 92:441, 1998.

98. Katzav, S., Martin-Zanca, D., and Barbacid, M.: Vav, a novel human oncogene derived from a locus ubiquitously expressed in hematopoietic cells. EMBO J. 8:2283, 1989.

99. Gulbins, E., Coggeshall, K., Baier, G., Katzav, S., Burn, P., and Altman, A.: Tyrosine kinase-stimulated guanine nucleotide exchange activity of vav in T cell activation. Science 260:822, 1993.

100. Shigematsu, H., Iwasaki, H., Otsuka, T., Ohno, Y., Arima, F., and Niho, Y.: Role of the *vav* proto-oncogene product (Vav) in erythropoietin-mediated cell proliferation and phosphatidylinositol 3-kinase activity. J. Biol. Chem. 272:14334, 1997.

101. Fischer, K.-D., Zmuidzinas, A., Gardner, S., Barbacid, M., Bernstein, A., Guidos, C.: Defective T-cell receptor signalling and positive selection of Vav-deficient CD4+CD8+ thymoctyes. Nature 374:474, 1995.

102. Tarakhovsky, A., Turner, M., Schall, S., Mee, P.J., Duddy, L.P., Rajewsky, K., and Tybulewicz, L.J.: Defective antigen receptor-mediated proliferation of B and T cells in the absence of Vav. Nature 374:467, 1995.

103. Zhang, R., Alt, F.W., Davidson, L., Orkin, S.H., and Swat, W.: Defective signalling through the T- and B-cell antigen receptors in lymphoid cells lacking the vav proto-oncogene. Nature 374:470, 1995.

104. Zmuidzinas, A., Fischer, K.-D., Lira, S.A., Forrester, L., Bryant, S., Bernstein, A., and Barbacid, M.: The *vav* proto-oncogene is required early in embryogenesis but not for hematopoietic development *in vitro*. EMBO J. 14:1, 1995.

105. Myers, M.G., Jr., Xiao, J.S., and White, M.F.: The IRS-1 signaling system. Trends Biochem. Sci. 19:289, 1994.

106. Yenush, L., and White, M.F.: The IRS-signalling system during insulin and cytokine action. Bioessays 19:491, 1997.

107. Keegan, A.D., Nelms, K., White, M., Wang, L.-M., Pierce, J.H., and Paul, W.E.: An IL-4 receptor region containing an insulin receptor motif is important for IL-4-mediated IRS-1 phosphorylation and cell growth. Cell 76:811, 1994.

108. Araki, E., Lipes, M.A., Patti, M.E., Bruning, J.C., Haag, B., Johnson, R.S., and Kahn, C.R.: Alternative pathway of insulin signalling in mice with targeted disruption of the IRS-1 gene [see comments]. Nature 372:186, 1994.

109. Tamemoto, H., Kadowaki, T., Tobe, K., Yagi, T., Sakura, H., Hayakawa, T., Terauchi, Y., Ueki, K., Kaburagi, Y., and Satoh, S.: Insulin resistance and growth retardation in mice lacking insulin receptor substrate-1 [see comments]. Nature 372:182, 1994.

110. Withers, D.J., Gutierrez, J.S., Towery, H., Burks, D.J., Ren, J.M., Previs, S., Zhang, Y., Bernal, D., Pons, S., Shulman, G.I., Bonner-Weir, S., and White, M.F.: Disruption of IRS-2 causes type 2 diabetes in mice. Nature 391:900, 1998.

111. Bruning, J.C., Winnay, J., Bonner-Weir, S., Taylor, S.I., Accili, D., and Kahn, C.R.: Development of a novel polygenic model of NIDDM in mice heterozygous for IR and IRS-1 null alleles. Cell 88:561, 1997.

112. Becker, S., Groner, B., and Müller, C.W.: Three-dimensional structure of the Stat3β homodimer bound to DNA. Nature 394:145, 1998.

113. Chen, X., Vinkemeier, U., Zhao, Y., Jeruzalmi, D., Darnell, J.E.J., and Kuriyan, J.: Crystal structure of a tyrosine phosphorylated STAT-1 dimer bound to DNA. Cell 93:827, 1998.

114. Allen, J.B., Walberg, M.W., Edwards, M.C., and Elledge, S.J.: Finding prospective partners in the library: The two-hybrid system and phage display find a match. Trends Biochem. Sci. 20:511, 1995.

115. Darnell, J.E.J.: STATs and gene regulation. Science 277:1630, 1997.

116. Ihle, J.N.: STATs: Signal transducers and activators of transcription. Cell 84:331, 1996.

117. Stahl, N., Farruggella, T.J., Boulton, T.G., Zhong, Z., Darnell, J.E., Jr., and Yancopoulos, G.D.: Modular tyrosine-based motifs in cytokine receptors specify choice of stats and other substrates. Science 267:1349, 1995.

118. Durbin, J.E., Hackenmiller, R., Simon, M.C., and Levy, D.E.: Targeted disruption of the mouse Stat1 gene results in compromised innate immunity to viral disease. Cell 84:443, 1996.

119. Meraz, M.A., White, J.M., Sheehan, K.C.F., Bach, E.A., Rodig, S.J., Dighe, A.S., Kaplan, D.H., Riley, J.K., Greenlund, A.C., Campbell, D., Carver-Moore, K., Dubois, R.N., Clark, R., Aguet, M., and Schreiber, R.D.: Targeted disruption of the Stat1 gene in mice reveals unexpected physiologic specificity in the JAK-STAT signaling pathway. Cell 84:431, 1996.

120. Takeda, K., Noguchi, K., Shi, W., Tanaka, T., Matsumoto, M., Yoshida, N., Kishimoto, T., and Akira, S.: Targeted disruption of the mouse stat3 gene leads to early embryonic lethality. Proc. Natl. Acad. Sci. U.S.A. 94:3801, 1997.

121. Stewart, C.L., Kaspar, P., Brunet, L.J., Bhatt, H., Gadi, I., Kontgen, F., and Abbondanzo, S.J.: Blastocyst implantation depends on maternal expression of leukaemia inhibitory factor [see comments]. Nature 359:76, 1992.

122. Takeda, K., Kaisho, T., Yoshida, N., Takeda, J., Kishimoto, T., and Akira, S.: Stat3 activation is responsible for IL-6-dependent T cell proliferation through preventing apoptosis: Generation and characterization of T cell-specific Stat3-deficient mice. J. Immunol. 161:4652, 1998.

123. Zhong, Z., Wen, Z., and Darnell, J.E. Jr.: Stat3 and Stat4: Members of the family of signal transducers and activators of transcription. Proc. Natl. Acad. Sci. USA 91:4806, 1994.

124. Yamamoto, K., Quelle, F.W., Thierfelder, W.E., Kreider, B.L., Gilbert, D.J., Jenkins, N.A., Copeland, N.G., Silvennoinen, O., and Ihle, J.N.: Stat4: A novel GAS binding protein expressed in early myeloid differentiation. Mol. Cell. Biol. 14:4342, 1994.

125. Jacobson, N.G., Szabo, S., Weber-Nordt, R.M., Zhong, Z., Schreiber, R.D., Darnell, J.E., Jr., and Murphy, K.M.: Interleukin 12 activates Stat3 and Stat4 by tyrosine phosphorylation in T cells. J. Exp. Med. 181:1755, 1995.

126. Bacon, C.M., McVicar, D.W., Ortaldo, J.R., Rees, R.C., O'Shea, J.J., and Johnston, J.A.: Interleukin-12 induces tyrosine phosphorylation of JAK2 and TYK2: Differential use of Janus tyrosine kinases by interleukin-2 and interleukin-12. J. Exp. Med. 181:399, 1995.

127. Kaplan, M.H., Sun, Y.-L., Hoey, T., and Grusby, M.J.: Impaired IL-12 responses and enhanced development of Th2 cells in Stat4-deficient mice. Nature 382:174, 1996.

128. Thierfelder, W.E., van Deursen, J., Yamamoto, K., Tripp, R.A., Sarawar, S.R., Carson, R.T., Sangster, M.Y., Vignali, D.A.A., Doherty, P.C., Grosveld, G., and Ihle, J.N.: Stat4 is required for IL-12 mediated responses of NK and T-cells. Nature 382:171, 1996.

129. Wolf, S.F., Sieburth, D., and Sypek, J.: Interleukin-12: A key modulator of immune function. Stem Cells 12:154, 1994.

130. Hou, J., Schindler, U., Henzel, W.J., Wong, S.C., and McKnight, S.L.: Identification and purification of human Stat proteins activated in response to interleukin-2. Immunity 2:321, 1995.

131. Quelle, F.W., Shimoda, K., Thierfelder, W., Fischer, C., Kim, A., Ruben, S.M., Cleveland, J.L., Pierce, J.H., Keegan, A.D., Nelms, K., Paul, W.E., and Ihle, J.N.: Cloning of murine Stat6 and human Stat6, stat proteins that are tyrosine phosphorylated in responses to IL-4 and IL-3 but are not required for mitogenesis. Mol. Cell. Biol. 15:3336, 1995.

132. Shimoda, K., van Deursen, J., Sangster, M.Y., Sarawar, S.R., Carson, R.T., Tripp, R.A., Chu, C., Quelle, F.W., Nosaka, T., Vignali, D.A.A., Doherty, P.C., Grosveld, G., Paul, W.E., and Ihle, J.N.: Lack of IL-4-induced Th2 response and IgE class switching in mice with disrupted Stat6 gene. Nature 380:630, 1996.

133. Kaplan, M.H., Schindler, U., Smiley, S.T., and Grusby, M.J.: Stat6 is required for mediating responses to IL-4 and for the development of Th2 cells. Immunity 4:313, 1996.

134. Kopf, M., Le Gros, G., Bachmann, M., Lamers, M.C., Bluethmann, H., and Kohler, G.: Disruption of the murine IL-4 gene blocks Th2 cytokine responses. Nature 362:245, 1993.

135. Liu, X., Robinson, G.W., Wagner, K.U., Garrett, L., Wynshaw-Boris, A., and Hennighausen, L.: Stat5a is mandatory for adult mammary gland development and lactogenesis. Genes Dev. 11:179, 1997.

136. Udy, G.B., Snell, R.G., Wilkins, R.J., Park, S.-H., Ram, P.A., Waxman, D.J., and Davey, H.W.: Requirement of STAT5b for sexual dimorphism of body growth rates and liver gene expression. Proc. Natl. Acad. Sci. U.S.A. 94:7239, 1997.

137. Teglund, S., McKay, C., Schuetz, E., van Deursen, J., Stravopodis, D., Wang, D., Brown, M., Bodner, S., Grosveld, G., and Ihle, J.N.: Stat5a and Stat5b proteins have essential and non-essential, or redundant, roles in cytokine responses. Cell 93:841, 1998.

138. Moriggl, R., Topham, D.J., Teglund, S., Sexl, V., McKay, C., Wang, D., Hoffmeyer, A., van Deursen, J., Sangster, M.Y., Bunting, K.D., Grosveld, G.C., and Ihle, J.N.: Stat5 is required for IL-2 induced cell cycle progression of peripheral T cells. Immunity In press:1999.

139. Mayer, B.J., Hamaguchi, M., and Hanafusa, H.: A novel viral oncogene with structural similarity to phospholipase C. Nature 332:272, 1988.

140. Hoeve, J., Morris, C., Heisterkamp, N., and Groffen, J.: Isolation and chromosomal localization of CRKL, a human crk-like gene. Oncogene 8:2469, 1993.

141. Sakai, R., Iwamatsu, A., Hirano, N., Ogawa, S., Tanaka, T., Mano, H., Yazaki, Y., and Hirai, H.: A novel signaling molecule, p130, forms stable complexes in vivo with v-Crk and v-Src in a tyrosine phosphorylation-dependent manner. EMBO J. 13:3748, 1994.

142. Law, S.F., Estojak, J., Wang, B., Mysliwiec, T., Kruh, G., and Golemis, E.A.: Human enhancer of filamentation 1, a novel p130cas-like docking protein, associates with focal adhesion kinase and induces pseudohyphal growth in Saccharomyces cerevisiae. Mol. Cell. Biol. 16:3327, 1996.

143. Ishino, M., Ohba, T., Sasaki, H., and Sasaki, T.: Molecular cloning of a cDNA encoding a phosphoprotein, Efs, which contains a Src homology 3 domain and associates with Fyn. Oncogene 11:2331, 1995.

144. Alexandropoulos, K., and Baltimore, D.: Coordinate activation of c-Src by SH3- and SH2-binding sites on a novel p130Cas-related protein, Sin. Genes Dev. 10:1341, 1996.

145. Tanaka, S., Morishita, T., Hashimoto, Y., Hattori, S., Nakamura, S., Shibuya, M., Matuoka, K., Takenawa, T., Kurata, T., and Nagashima, K.: C3G, a guanine nucleotide-releasing protein expressed ubiquitously, binds to the Src homology 3 domains of CRK and GRB2/ASH proteins. Proc. Natl. Acad. Sci. U.S.A. 91:3443, 1994.

146. Blake, T.J., Shapiro, M., Morse, H.C., and Langdon, W.Y.: The sequences of the human and mouse c-cbl proto-oncogenes show v-cbl was generated by a large truncation encompassing a proline-rich domain and a leucine zipper-like motif. Oncogene 6:653, 1991.

147. Langdon, W.Y., Hartley, J.W., Klinken, S.P., Ruscetti, S.K., and Morse, III, H.C.: v-cbl, an oncogene from a dual-recombinant murine retrovirus that induces early B-lineage lymphomas. Proc. Natl. Acad. Sci. U.S.A. 86:1168, 1989.

148. Tanaka, S., Amling, M., Neff, L., Peyman, A., Uhlmann, E., Levy, J.B., and Baron, R.: c-Cbl is downstream of c-Src in a signalling pathway necessary for bone resorption. Nature 383:528, 1996.

149. Ota, Y., and Samelson, L.E.: The product of the proto-oncogene c-cbl: A negative regulator of the Syk tyrosine kinase. Science 276:418, 1997.

150. Murphy, M.A., Schnall, R.G., Venter, D.J., Barnett, L., Bertoncello, I., Thien, C.B., Langdon, W.Y., and Bowtell, D.D.: Tissue hyperplasia and enhanced T-cell signalling via ZAP-70 in c-Cbl-deficient mice. Mol. Cell. Biol. 18:4872, 1998.

151. Komada, M., and Kitamura, N.: Growth factor-induced tyrosine phosphorylation of Hrs, a novel 115-kilodalton protein with a structurally conserved putative zinc finger domain. Mol. Cell. Biol. 15:6213, 1995.

152. Takeshita, T., Arita, T., Higuchi, M., Asao, H., Endo, K., Kuroda, H., Tanaka, N., Murata, K., Ishii, N., and Sugamura, K.: STAM, signal transducing adaptor molecule, is associated with janus kinases and involved in signaling for cell growth and c-myc induction. Immunity 6:449, 1997.

153. Zhang, W., Sloan-Lancaster, J., Kitchen, J., Trible, R.P., and Samelson, L.E.: LAT: The ZAP-70 tyrosine kinase substrate that links T cell receptor to cellular activation. Cell 92:83, 1998.

154. Huang, X., Li, Y., Tanaka, K., Moore, K.G., and Hayashi, J.I.: Cloning and characterization of Lnk, a signal transduction protein that links T-cell receptor activation signal to phospholipase C gamma 1, Grb2, and phosphatidylinositol 3-kinase. Proc. Natl. Acad. Sci. U.S.A. 92:11618, 1995.

155. Gu, H., Pratt, J.C., Burakoff, S.J., and Neel, B.G.: Cloning of p97/Gab2, the major SHP2-binding protein in hematopoietic cells, reveals a novel pathway for cytokine-induced gene activation. Mol. Cell 2:729, 1998.

156. Carpino, N., Wisniewski, D., Strife, A., Marshak, D., Kobayashi, R., Stillman, B., and Clarkson, B.: p62(dok): A constitutively tyrosine-phosphorylated, GAP-associated protein in chronic myelogenous leukemia progenitor cells. Cell 88:197, 1997.

157. Nelms, K., Snow, A.L., Hu-Li, J., and Paul, W.E.: FRIP, a hematopoietic cell-specific rasGAP-interacting protein phosphorylated in response to cytokine stimulation. Immunity 9:13, 1998.

158. Clements, J.L., Yang, B., Ross-Barta, S.E., Eliason, S.L., Hrstka, R.F., Williamson, R.A., and Koretzky, G.A.: Requirement for the leukocyte-specific adapter protein SLP-76 for normal T cell development. Science 281:416, 1998.

159. Massague, J.: TGFbeta signaling: Receptors, transducers, and Mad proteins. Cell 85:947, 1996.

160. Shi, Y., Hata, A., Lo, R.S., Massague, J., and Pavletich, N.P.: A structural basis for mutational inactivation of the tumour suppressor Smad4 [see comments]. Nature 388:87, 1997.

161. Lo, R.S., Chen, Y.G., Shi, Y., Pavletich, N.P., and Massague, J.: The L3 loop: A structural motif determining specific interactions between SMAD proteins and TGF-beta receptors. EMBO J. 17:996, 1998.

162. Heldin, C.H., Miyazono, K., Dijke, P.: TGF-beta signalling from cell membrane to nucleus through SMAD proteins. Nature 390:465, 1997.

163. Nakao, A., Afrakhte, M., Moren, A., Nakayama, T., Christian, J.L., Heuchel, R., Itoh, S., Kawabata, M., Heldin, N.E., Heldin, C.H., and Dijke, P.: Identification of Smad7, a TGFbeta-inducible antagonist of TGF-beta signalling [see comments]. Nature 389:631, 1997.

164. Imamura, T., Takase, M., Nishihara, A., Oeda, E., Hanai, J., Kawabata, M., and Miyazono, K.: Smad6 inhibits signalling by the TGF-beta superfamily [see comments]. Nature 389:622, 1997.

165. Kretzschmar, M., Doody, J., and Massague, J.: Opposing BMP and EGF signalling pathways converge on the TGF-beta family mediator Smad1. Nature 389:618, 1997.

166. Ali, S., Chen, Z., Lebrun, J.J., Vogel, W., Kharitonenkov, A., Kelly, P.A., and Ullrich, A.: PTP1D is a positive regulator of the prolactin signal leading to beta-casein promoter activation. EMBO J. 15:135, 1996.

167. Chen, X., Rubock, M.J., and Whitman, M.: A transcriptional partner for MAD proteins in TGF-beta signalling [published erratum appears in Nature 1996 Dec 19–26;384(6610):648]. Nature 383:691, 1996.

168. Chen, X., Weisberg, E., Fridmacher, V., Watanabe, M., Naco, G., and Whitman, M.: Smad4 and FAST-1 in the assembly of activin-responsive factor. Nature 389:85, 1997.

169. Shull, M.M., Ormsby, I., Kier, A.B., Pawlowski, S., Diebold, R.J., Yin, M., Allen, R., Sidman, C., Proetzel, G., and Calvin, D.: Targeted disruption of the mouse transforming growth factor-beta 1 gene results in multifocal inflammatory disease. Nature 359:693, 1992.

170. Sanford, L.P., Ormsby, I., Gittenberger-de Groot, A.C., Sariola, H., Friedman, R., Boivin, G.P., Cardell, E.L., and Doetschman, T.: TGFbeta2 knockout mice have multiple developmental defects that are non-overlapping with other TGFbeta knockout phenotypes. Development 124:2659, 1997.

171. Winnier, G., Blessing, M., Labosky, P.A., and Hogan, B.L.: Bone morphogenetic protein-4 is required for mesoderm formation and patterning in the mouse. Genes Dev. 9:2105, 1995.

172. Zhang, H., and Bradley, A.: Mice deficient for BMP2 are nonviable and have defects in amnion/chorion and cardiac development. Development 122:2977, 1996.

173. Matzuk, M.M., Kumar, T.R., Vassalli, A., Bickenbach, J.R., Roop, D.R., Jaenisch, R., and Bradley, A.: Functional analysis of activins during mammalian development [see comments]. Nature 374:354, 1995.

174. Vassalli, A., Matzuk, M.M., Gardner, H.A., Lee, K.F., and Jaenisch, R.: Activin/inhibin beta B subunit gene disruption leads to defects in eyelid development and female reproduction. Genes Dev. 8:414, 1994.

175. Matzuk, M.M., Finegold, M.J., Su, J.G., Hsueh, A.J., and Bradley, A.: Alpha-inhibin is a tumour-suppressor gene with gonadal specificity in mice. Nature 360:313, 1992.

176. Matzuk, M.M., Kumar, T.R., and Bradley, A.: Different phenotypes for mice deficient in either activins or activin receptor type II [see comments]. Nature 374:356, 1995.

177. Gu, Z., Nomura, M., Simpson, B.B., Lei, H., Feijen, A., Eijnden-van Raaij, J., Donahoe, P.K., and Li, E.: The type I activin receptor ActRIB is required for egg cylinder organization and gastrulation in the mouse. Genes Dev. 12:844, 1998.

178. Sirard, C., Pompa, J.L., Elia, A., Itie, A., Mirtsos, C., Cheung, A., Hahn, S., Wakeham, A., Schwartz, L., Kern, S.E., Rossant, J., and Mak, T.W.: The tumor suppressor gene Smad4/Dpc4 is required for gastrulation and later for anterior development of the mouse embryo. Genes Dev. 12:107, 1998.

179. Nomura, M., and Li, E.: Smad2 role in mesoderm formation, left-right patterning and craniofacial development [see comments]. Nature 393:786, 1998.

180. Waldrip, W.R., Bikoff, E.K., Hoodless, P.A., Wrana, J.L., and Robertson, E.J.: Smad2 signaling in extraembryonic tissues determines anterior-posterior polarity of the early mouse embryo. Cell 92:797, 1998.

181. Hahn, S.A., Schutte, M., Hoque, A.T., Moskaluk, C.A., Costa, L.T., Rozenblum, E., Weinstein, C.L., Fischer, A., Yeo, C.J., Hruban, R.H., and Kern, S.E.: DPC4, a candidate tumor suppressor gene at human chromosome 18q21.1 [see comments]. Science 271:350, 1996.

182. Zhu, Y., Richardson, J.A., Parada, L.F., and Graff, J.M.: Smad3 mutant mice develop metastatic colorectal cancer. Cell 94:703, 1998.

183. Baggiolini, M., Dewald, B., and Moser, B.: Human chemokines: An update. Annu. Rev. Immunol. 15:675, 1997.

184. Howard, O.M., Ben-Baruch, A., and Oppenheim, J.J.: Chemokines: Progress toward identifying molecular targets for therapeutic agents. Trends Biotechnol. 14:46, 1996.

185. Strosberg, A.D.: G protein coupled R7G receptors. Cancer Surv. 27:65, 1997.

186. Taub, D.D., and Oppenheim, J.J.: Chemokines, inflammation and the immune system. Ther. Immunol. 1:229, 1994.

187. Balter, M.: A second coreceptor for HIV in early stages of infection [news]. Science 272:1740, 1996.

188. Deng, H., Liu, R., Ellmeier, W., Choe, S., Unutmaz, D., Burkhart, M., Di Marzio, P., Marmon, S., Sutton, R.E., Hill, C.M., Davis, C.B., Peiper, S.C., Schall, T.J., Littman, D.R., and Landau, N.R.: Identification of a major co-receptor for primary isolates of HIV-1 [see comments]. Nature 381:661, 1996.

189. Doranz, B.J., Rucker, J., Yi, Y., Smyth, R.J., Samson, M., Peiper, S.C., Parmentier, M., Collman, R.G., and Doms, R.W.: A dual-tropic primary HIV-1 isolate that uses fusin and the beta-chemokine receptors CKR-5, CKR-3, and CKR-2b as fusion cofactors. Cell 85:1149, 1996.

190. Dragic, T., Litwin, V., Allaway, G.P., Martin, S.R., Huang, Y., Nagashima, K.A., Cayanan, C., Maddon, P.J., Koup, R.A., Moore, J.P., and Paxton, W.A.: HIV-1 entry into CD4+ cells is mediated by the chemokine receptor CC-CKR-5 [see comments]. Nature 381:667, 1996.

191. Liu, R., Paxton, W.A., Choe, S., Ceradini, D., Martin, S.R., Horuk, R., MacDonald, M.E., Stuhlmann, H., Koup, R.A., and Landau, N.R.: Homozygous defect in HIV-1 coreceptor accounts for resistance of some multiply-exposed individuals to HIV-1 infection. Cell 86:367, 1996.

192. Samson, M., Libert, F., Doranz, B.J., Rucker, J., Liesnard, C., Farber, C.M., Saragosti, S., Lapoumeroulie, C., Cognaux, J., Forceille, C., Muyldermans, G., Verhofstede, C., Burtonboy, G., Georges, M., Imai, T., Rana, S., Yi, Y., Smyth, R.J., Collman, R.G., Doms, R.W., Vassart, G., and Parmentier, M.: Resistance to HIV-1 infection in caucasian individuals bearing mutant alleles of the CCR-5 chemokine receptor gene [see comments]. Nature 382:722, 1996.

193. Ward, S.G., Bacon, K., and Westwick, J.: Chemokines and T lymphocytes: More than an attraction. Immunity 9:1, 1998.

194. Offermanns, S., and Simon, M.I.: Organization of transmembrane signalling by heterotrimeric G proteins. Cancer Surv. 27:177, 1996.

195. Liri, T., Farfel, Z., and Bourne, H.R.: G-protein diseases furnish a model for the turn-on switch. Nature 394:35, 1998.

196. Wong, M., and Fish, E.N.: RANTES and MIP-1α activate STATS in T cells. J. Biol. Chem. 273:309, 1998.

197. Bacon, K.B., Szabo, M.C., Yssel, H., Bolen, J., and Schall, T.J.: RANTES induces tyrosine kinase activity of stably complexed p125FAK and ZAP-70 in human T cells. J. Exp. Med. 184:873, 1996.

198. Paxton, W.G., Marrero, M.B., Klein, J.D., Delafontaine, P., Berk, B.C., and Bernstein, K.E.: The angiotensin II AT1 receptor is tyrosine and serine phosphorylated and can serve as a substrate for the src family of tyrosine kinases. Biochem. Biophys. Res. Commun. 200:260, 1994.

199. Dikic, I., Tokiwa, G., Lev, S., Courtneidge, S.A., and Schlessinger, J.: A role for Pyk2 and Src in linking g-protein-coupled receptors with MAP kinase activation. Nature 383:547, 1996.

200. Nusse, R., van Ooyen, A., Cox, D., Fung, Y.K., and Varmus, H.: Mode of proviral activation of a putative mammary oncogene (int-1) on mouse chromosome 15. Nature 307:131, 1984.

201. Rijsewijk, F., Schuermann, M., Wagenaar, E., Parren, P., Weigel, D., and Nusse, R.: The Drosophila homolog of the mouse mammary oncogene int-1 is identical to the segment polarity gene wingless. Cell 50:649, 1987.

202. Nusse, R.: A versatile transcriptional effector of Wingless signaling. Cell 89:321, 1997.

203. Siegfried, E., Wilder, E.L., and Perrimon, N.: Components of wingless signalling in Drosophila. Nature 367:76, 1994.

204. Cadigan, K.M., and Nusse, R.: Wingless signaling in the Drosophila eye and embryonic epidermis. Development 122:2801, 1996.

205. Huber, O., Korn, R., McLaughlin, J., Ohsugi, M., Herrmann, B.G., and Kemler, R.: Nuclear localization of beta-catenin by interaction with transcription factor LEF-1. Mech. Dev. 59:3, 1996.

206. Behrens, J., von Kries, J.P., Kuhl, M., Bruhn, L., Wedlich, D., Grosschedl, R., and Birchmeier, W.: Functional interaction of beta-catenin with the transcription factor LEF-1. Nature 382:638, 1996.

207. Slusarski, D.C., Corces, V.G., and Moon, R.T.: Interaction of Wnt and a Frizzled homologue triggers G-protein-linked phosphatidylinositol signalling. Nature 390:410, 1997.

208. Verbeek, S., Izon, D., Hofhuis, F., Robanus-Maandag, E., te Riele, H., van de Wetering, M., Oosterwegel, M., Wilson, A., MacDonald, H.R., and Clevers, H.: An HMG-box-containing T-cell factor required for thymocyte differentiation. Nature 374:70, 1995.

209. DiDonato, J.A., Hayakawa, M., Rothwarf, D.M., Zandi, E., and Karin, M.: A cytokine-responsive IkappaB kinase that activates the transcription factor NF-kappaB [see comments]. Nature 388:548, 1997.

210. Regnier, C.H., Song, H.Y., Gao, X., Goeddel, D.V., Cao, Z., and Rothe, M.: Identification and characterization of an IkappaB kinase. Cell 90:373, 1997.

211. Stancovski, I., and Baltimore, D.: NF-kB Activation: The IkB kinase revealed? Cell 91:299, 1997.

212. Malinin, N.L., Boldin, M.P., Kovalenko, A.V., and Wallach, D.: MAP3K-related kinase involved in NF-kappaB induction by TNF, CD95 and IL-1. Nature 385:540, 1997.

213. Weih, F., Carrasco, D., Durham, S.K., Barton, D.S., Rizzo, C.A., Ryseck, R.P., Lira, S.A., and Bravo, R.: Multiorgan inflammation and hematopoietic abnormalities in mice with a targeted disruption of RelB, a member of the NF-kappaB/Rel family. Cell 80:331, 1995.

214. Weih, F., Durham, S.K., Barton, D.S., Sha, W.C., Baltimore, D., and Bravo, R.: Both multiorgan inflammation and myeloid hyperplasia in RelB-deficient mice are T cell dependent. J. Immunol. 157:3974, 1996.

215. Sha, W.C., Liou, H.-C., Tuomanen, E.I., and Baltimore, D.: Targeted disruption of the p50 subunit of NF-kappaB leads to multifocal defects in immune responses. Cell 80:321, 1995.

216. Beg, A.A., Sha, W.C., Bronson, R.T., Ghosh, S., and Baltimore, D.: Embryonic lethality and liver degeneration in mice lacking the RelA component of NF-kappa B. Nature 376:167, 1995.

217. Gerondakis, S., Strasser, A., Metcalf, D., Grigoriadis, G., Scheerlinck, J.Y., and Grumont, R.J.: Rel-deficient T cells exhibit defects in production of interleukin 3 and granulocyte-macrophage colony-stimulating factor. Proc. Natl. Acad. Sci. U.S.A. 93:3405, 1996.

218. Kontgen, F., Grumont, R.J., Strasser, A., Metcalf, D., Li, R., Tarlinton, D., and Gerondakis, S.: Mice lacking the c-rel proto-oncogene exhibit defects in lymphocyte proliferation, humoral immunity, and interleukin-2 expression. Genes Dev. 9:1965, 1995.

219. Beg, A.A., Sha, W.C., Bronson, R.T., and Baltimore, D.: Constitutive NF-kappa B activation, enhanced granulopoiesis, and neonatal lethality in I kappa B alpha-deficient mice. Genes Dev. 9:2736, 1995.

220. Salvesen, G.S., and Dixit, V.M.: Caspases: Intracellular signaling by proteolysis. Cell 91:443, 1997.

221. Ashkenazi, A., and Dixit, V.M.: Death receptors: Signaling and modulation. Science 281:1305, 1998.

222. Thornberry, N.A., and Lazebnik, Y.: Caspases: Enemies within. Science 281:1312, 1998.

223. Cerretti, D.P., Kozlosky, C.J., Mosley, B., Nelson, N., Ness, K., Greenstreet, T.A., March, C.J., Kronheim, S.R., Druck, T., and Cannizzaro, L.A.: Molecular cloning of the interleukin-1 beta converting enzyme. Science 256:97, 1992.

224. Yuan, J., Shaham, S., Ledoux, S., Ellis, H.M., and Horvitz, H.R.: The C. elegans cell death gene ced-3 encodes a protein similar to mammalian interleukin-1β-converting enzyme. Cell 75:641, 1993.

225. Muzio, M., Chinnaiyan, A.M., Kischkel, F.C., O'Rourke, K., Shevchenko, A., Ni, J., Scaffidi, C., Bretz, J.D., Zhang, M., Gentz, R., Mann, M., Krammer, P.H., Peter, M.E., and Dixit, V.M.: FLICE, a novel FADD-homologous ICE/CED-3-like protease, is recruited to the CD95 (Fas/APO-1) death-inducing signaling complex. Cell 85:817, 1996.

226. Li, P., Allen, H., Banerjee, S., Franklin, S., Herzog, L., Johnston, C., McDowell, J., Paskind, M., Rodman, L., Salfeld, J., Towne, E., Tracey, D., and Wardwell, S.: Mice deficient in IL-1β-converting enzyme are defective in production of mature IL-1β and resistant to endotoxic shock. Cell 80:401, 1995.

227. Yeh, W.-C., de la Pompa, J.L., McCurrach, M.E., Shu, H., Elia, A.J., Shahinian, A., Ng, M., Wakeham, A., Khoo, W., Mitchell, K., El-Deiry, W.S., Lowe, S.W., Goeddel, D.V., and Mak, T.W.: FADD: Essential for embryo development and signaling from some, but not all, inducers of apoptosis. Science 279:1954, 1998.

228. Sakahira, H., Enari, M., and Nagata, S.: Cleavage of CAD inhibitor in CAD activation and DNA degradation during apoptosis [see comments]. Nature 391:96, 1998.

229. Enari, M., Sakahira, H., Yokoyama, H., Okawa, K., Iwamatsu, A., and Nagata, S.: A caspase-activated DNase that degrades DNA during apoptosis, and its inhibitor ICAD [see comments]. Nature 391:43, 1998.

230. Varfolomeev, E.E., Schuchmann, M., Luria, V., Chiannilkulchai, N., Beckmann, J.S., Mett, I.L., Rebrikov, D., Brodianski, V.M., Kemper, O.C., Kollet, O., Lapidot, T., Soffer, D., Sobe, T., Avraham, K.B., Goncharov, T., Holtmann, H., Lonai, P., and Wallach, D.: Targeted disruption of the mouse caspase 8 gene ablates cell death induction by the TNF receptors, Fas/Apo1, and DR3 and is lethal prenatally. Immunity 9:267, 1998.

231. Shu, H., Halpin, D.R., and Goeddel, D.V.: Casper is a FADD- and caspase-related inducer of apoptosis. Immunity 6:751, 1997.

232. Stanger, B.Z., Leder, P., Lee, T.-H., and Seed, B.: RIP: A novel "death domain"-containing protein kinase that interacts with Fas/APO-1 (CD95) and causes cell death. Cell 81:513, 1995.

233. Kelliher, M.A., Grimm, S., Ishida, Y., Kuo, F., Stanger, B.Z., and Leder, P.: The death domain kinase RIP mediates the TNF-induced NF-κB signal. Immunity 8:297, 1998.

234. McCarthy, J.V., Ni, J., and Dixit, V.M.: RIP2 is a novel NF-kappaB-activating and cell death-inducing kinase. J. Biol. Chem. 273:16968, 1998.

235. Cao, Z., Xiong, J., Takeuchi, M., Kurama, T., and Goeddel, D.V.: TRAF6 is a signal transducer for interleukin-1. Nature 383:443, 1996.

236. Xu, Y., Cheng, G., and Baltimore, D.: Targeted disruption of TRAF3 leads to postnatal lethality and defective T-dependent immune responses. Immunity 5:407, 1996.

237. Zou, H., Henzel, W.J., Liu, X., Lutschg, A., and Wang, X.: Apaf-1, a human protein homologous to C. elegans CED-4, participates in cytochrome c-dependent activation of caspase-3 [see comments]. Cell 90:405, 1997.

238. Li, P., Nijhawan, D., Budihardjo, I., Srinivasula, S.M., Ahmad, M., Alnemri, E.S., and Wang, X.: Cytochrome c and dATP-dependent formation of Apaf-1/caspase-9 complex initiates an apoptotic protease cascade. Cell 91:479, 1997.

239. Hakem, R., Hakem, A., Duncan, G.S., Henderson, J.T., Woo, M., Soengas, M.S., Elia, A., Pompa, J.L., Kagi, D., Khoo, W., Potter, J., Yoshida, R., Kaufman, S.A., Lowe, S.W., Penninger, J.M., and Mak, T.W.: Differential requirement for caspase 9 in apoptotic pathways in vivo. Cell 94:339, 1998.

240. Kuida, K., Haydar, T.F., Kuan, C.Y., Gu, Y., Taya, C., Karasuyama, H., Su, M.S., Rakic, P., and Flavell, R.A.: Reduced apoptosis and cytochrome c-mediated caspase activation in mice lacking caspase 9. Cell 94:325, 1998.

241. Yoshida, H., Kong, Y.Y., Yoshida, R., Elia, A.J., Hakem, A., Hakem, R., Penninger, J.M., and Mak, T.W.: Apaf1 is required for mitochondrial pathways of apoptosis and brain development. Cell 94:739, 1998.

242. Cecconi, F., Alvarez-Bolado, G., Meyer, B.I., Roth, K.A., and Gruss, P.: Apaf1 (CED-4 homolog) regulates programmed cell death in mammalian development. Cell 94:727, 1998.

243. Adams, J.M., and Cory, S.: The Bcl-2 protein family: Arbiters of cell survival. Science 281:1322, 1998.

244. Chao, D.T., and Korsmeyer, S.J.: BCL-2 family: Regulators of cell death. Annu. Rev. Immunol. 16:395, 1998.

245. Green, D.R., and Reed, J.C.: Mitochondria and apoptosis. Science 281:1309, 1998.

246. Green, D.R.: Apoptotic pathways: The roads to ruin. Cell 94:695, 1998.

247. Chinnaiyan, A.M., O'Rourke, K., Lane, B.R., and Dixit, V.M.: Interaction of CED-4 with CED-3 and CED-9: A molecular framework for cell death [see comments]. Science 275:1122, 1997.

248. Pan, G., O'Rourke, K., and Dixit, V.M.: Caspase-9, Bcl-XL, and Apaf-1 form a ternary complex. J. Biol. Chem. 273:5841, 1998.

249. Wang, K., Yin, X.M., Chao, D.T., Milliman, C.L., and Korsmeyer, S.J.: BID: A novel BH3 domain-only death agonist. Genes Dev. 10:2859, 1996.

250. Luo, X., Budihardjo, I., Zou, H., Slaughter, C., and Wang, X.: Bid, a Bcl2 interacting protein, mediates cytochrome c release from mitochondria in response to activation of cell surface death receptors. Cell 94:481, 1998.

251. Li, H., Zhu, H., Xu, C.J., and Yuan, J.: Cleavage of BID by caspase 8 mediates the mitochondrial damage in the Fas pathway of apoptosis. Cell 94:491, 1998.

252. Veis, D.J., Sorenson, C.M., Shutter, J.R., and Korsmeyer, S.J.: Bcl-2-deficient mice demonstrate fulminant lymphoid apoptosis, polycystic kidneys, and hypopigmented hair. Cell 75:229, 1993.

253. Motoyama, N., Wang, F., Roth, K.A., Sawa, H., Nakayama, K., Nakayama, K., Negishi, I., Senju, S., Zhang, Q., Fujii, S., and Loh, D.Y.: Massive cell death of immature hematopoietic cells and neurons in Bcl-x-deficient mice. Science 267:1506, 1995.

254. Ross, A.J., Waymire, K.G., Moss, J.E., Parlow, A.F., Skinner, M.K., Russell, L.D., and MacGregor, G.R.: Testicular degeneration in Bclw-deficient mice [see comments]. Nat. Genet. 18:251, 1998.

255. Knudson, C.M., Tung, K.S.K., Tourtellotte, W.G., Brown, G.A.J., and Korsmeyer, S.J.: Bax-deficient mice with lymphoid hyperplasia and male germ cell death. Science 270:96, 1995.

256. Knudson, C.M., and Korsmeyer, S.J.: Bcl-2 and Bax function independently to regulate cell death. Nat. Genet. 16:358, 1997.

257. Dinarello, C.A.: Biologic basis for interleukin-1 in disease. Blood 87:2095, 1996.

258. Dinarello, C.A.: Interleukin-1 and interleukin-1 antagonism. Blood 77:1627, 1991.

259. Takeda, K., Tsutsui, H., Yoshimoto, T., Adachi, O., Yoshida, N., Kishimoto, T., Okamura, H., Nakanishi, K., and Akira, S.: Defective NK cell activity and Th1 response in IL-18-deficient mice. Immunity 8:383, 1998.

260. Gay, N.J., and Keith, F.J.: Drosophila Toll and IL-1 receptor [letter]. Nature 351:355, 1991.

261. Lovenberg, T.W., Crowe, P.D., Liu, C., Chalmers, D.T., Liu, X.J., Liaw, C., Clevenger, W., Oltersdorf, T., Souza, E.B., and Maki, R.A.: Cloning of a cDNA encoding a novel interleukin-1 receptor related protein (IL 1R-rp2). J. Neuroimmunol. 70:113, 1996.

262. Medzhitov, R., Preston-Hurlburt, P., and Janeway, C.A.J.: A human homologue of the Drosophila Toll protein signals activation of adaptive immunity [see comments]. Nature 388:394, 1997.

263. Mitcham, J.L., Parnet, P., Bonnert, T.P., Garka, K.E., Gerhart, M.J., Slack, J.L., Gayle, M.A., Dower, S.K., and Sims, J.E.: T1/ST2 signal-

ing establishes it as a member of an expanding interleukin-1 receptor family. J. Biol. Chem. 271:5777, 1996.

264. Parnet, P., Garka, K.E., Bonnert, T.P., Dower, S.K., and Sims, J.E.: IL-1Rrp is a novel receptor-like molecule similar to the type I interleukin-1 receptor and its homologues T1/ST2 and IL-1R AcP. J. Biol. Chem. 271:3967, 1996.

265. Rock, F.L., Hardiman, G., Timans, J.C., Kastelein, R.A., and Bazan, J.F.: A family of human receptors structurally related to Drosophila Toll. Proc. Natl. Acad. Sci. U.S.A. 95:588, 1998.

266. Cao, Z., Henzel, W.J., and Gao, X.: IRAK: A kinase associated with the interleukin-1 receptor. Science 271:1128, 1996.

267. Muzio, M., Ni, J., Feng, P., and Dixit, V.M.: IRAK (Pelle) family member IRAK-2 and MyD88 as proximal mediators of IL-1 signaling. Science 278:1612, 1997.

268. Adachi, O., Kawai, T., Takeda, K., Matsumoto, M., Tsutsui, H., Sakagami, M., Nakanishi, K., and Akira, S.: Targeted disruption of the *MyD88* gene results in loss of IL-1- and IL-18-mediated function. Immunity 9:143, 1998.

269. Artavanis-Tsakonas, S., Matsuno, K., and Fortini, M.E.: Notch signaling. Science 268:225, 1995.

270. Ellisen, L.W., Bird, J., West, D.C., Soreng, A.L., Reynolds, T.C., Smith, S.D., and Sklar, J.: TAN-1, the human homolog of the Drosophila notch gene, is broken by chromosomal translocations in T lymphoblastic neoplasms. Cell 66:649, 1991.

271. Girard, L., Hanna, Z., Beaulieu, N., Hoemann, C.D., Simard, C., Kozak, C.A., and Jolicoeur, P.: Frequent provirus insertional mutagenesis of Notch1 in thymomas of MMTVD/myc transgenic mice suggests a collaboration of c-myc and Notch1 for oncogenesis. Genes Dev. 10:1930, 1996.

272. Joutel, A., Corpechot, C., Ducros, A., Vahedi, K., Chabriat, H., Mouton, P., Alamowitch, S., Domenga, V., Cecillion, M., Marechal, E., Maciazek, J., Vayssiere, C., Cruaud, C., Cabanis, E.A., Ruchoux, M.M., Weissenbach, J., Bach, J.F., Bousser, M.G., and Tournier-Lasserve, E.: Notch3 mutations in CADASIL, a hereditary adult-onset condition causing stroke and dementia [see comments]. Nature 383:707, 1996.

273. Robey, E., Chang, D., Itano, A., Cado, D., Alexander, H., Lans, D., Weinmaster, G., and Salmon, P.: An activated form of Notch influences the choice between CD4 and CD8 T cell lineages. Cell 87:483, 1996.

274. Washburn, T., Schweighoffer, E., Gridley, T., Chang, D., Fowlkes, B.J., Cado, D., and Robey, E.: Notch activity influences the αβ versus gamma delta T cell lineage decision. Cell 88:833, 1997.

275. Pear, W.S., Aster, J.C., Scott, M.L., Hasserjian, R.P., Soffer, B., Sklar, J., and Baltimore, D.: Exclusive development of T cell neoplasms in mice transplanted with bone marrow expressing activated Notch alleles. J. Exp. Med. 183:2283, 1996.

276. Conlon, R.A., Reaume, A.G., and Rossant, J.: Notch1 is required for the coordinate segmentation of somites. Development 121:1533, 1995.

277. Pompa, J.L., Wakeham, A., Correia, K.M., Samper, E., Brown, S., Aguilera, R.J., Nakano, T., Honjo, T., Mak, T.W., Rossant, J., and Conlon, R.A.: Conservation of the Notch signalling pathway in mammalian neurogenesis. Development 124:1139, 1997.

278. Lindsell, C.E., Shawber, C.J., Boulter, J., and Weinmaster, G.: Jagged: A mammalian ligand that activates Notch1. Cell 80:909, 1995.

279. Shawber, C., Boulter, J., Lindsell, C.E., and Weinmaster, G.: Jagged2: A serrate-like gene expressed during rat embryogenesis. Dev. Biol. 180:370, 1996.

280. Evrard, Y.A., Lun, Y., Aulehla, A., Gan, L., and Johnson, R.L.: *Lunatic fringe* is an essential mediator of somite segmentation and patterning. Nature 394:377, 1998.

281. Zhang, N., and Gridley, T.: Defects in somite formation in *lunatic fringe*-deficient mice. Nature 394:374, 1998.

282. Jarriault, S., Brou, C., Logeat, F., Schroeter, E.H., Kopan, R., and Israel, A.: Signalling downstream of activated mammalian Notch [see comments]. Nature 377:355, 1995.

283. Hsieh, J.J., Henkel, T., Salmon, P., Robey, E., Peterson, M.G., and Hayward, S.D.: Truncated mammalian Notch1 activates CBF1/RBPJk-repressed genes by a mechanism resembling that of Epstein-Barr virus EBNA2. Mol. Cell. Biol. 16:952, 1996.

284. Oka, C., Nakano, T., Wakeham, A., de la Pompa, J.L., Mori, C., Sakai, T., Okazaki, S., Kawaichi, M., Shiota, K., Mak, T.W., and Honjo, T.: Disruption of the mouse RBP-J kappa gene results in early embryonic death. Development 121:3291, 1995.

285. Khokhlatchev, A.V., Canagarajah, B., Wilsbacher, J., Robinson, M.,

Atkinson, M., Goldsmith, E., and Cobb, M.H.: Phosphorylation of the MAP kinase ERK2 promotes its homodimerization and nuclear translocation. Cell 93:605, 1998.

286. Hill, C.S., and Treisman, R.: Transcriptional regulation by extracellular signals: Mechanisms and specificity. Cell 80:199, 1995.

287. Gille, H., Sharrocks, A.D., and Shaw, P.E.: Phosphorylation of transcription factor p62^{TCF} by MAP kinase stimulates ternary complex formation at c-fos promoter. Nature 358:414, 1992.

288. Gille, H., Kortenjann, M., Thomae, O., Moomaw, C., Slaughter, C., Cobb, M.H., and Shaw, P.E.: ERK phosphorylation potentiates Elk-1-mediated ternary complex formation and transactivation. EMBO J. 14:951, 1995.

289. Cavigelli, M., Dolfi, F., Claret, F.X., and Karin, M.: Induction of c-fos expression through JNK-mediated TCF/Elk-1 phosphorylation. EMBO J. 14:5957, 1995.

290. Derijard, B., Hibi, M., Wu, I.H., Barrett, T., Su, B., Deng, T., Karin, M., and Davis, R.J.: JNK1: A protein kinase stimulated by UV light and Ha-Ras that binds and phosphorylates the c-Jun activation domain. Cell 76:1025, 1994.

291. Hibi, M., Lin, A., Smeal, T., Minden, A., and Karin, M.: Identification of an oncoprotein- and UV-responsive protein kinase that binds and potentiates the c-Jun activation domain. Genes Dev. 7:2135, 1993.

292. Gupta, S., Campbell, D., Derijard, B., and Davis, R.J.: Transcription factor ATF2 regulation by the JNK signal transduction pathway. Science 267:389, 1995.

293. Wang, X.Z., and Ron, D.: Stress-induced phosphorylation and activation of the transcription factor CHOP (GADD153) by p38 MAP kinase. Science 272:1347, 1996.

294. Han, J., Jiang, Y., Li, Z., Kravchenko, V.V., and Ulevitch, R.J.: Activation of the transcription factor MEF2C by the MAP kinase p38 in inflammation. Nature 386:296, 1997.

295. Kato, Y., Kravchenko, V.V., Tapping, R.I., Han, J., Ulevitch, R.J., and Lee, J.D.: BMK1/ERK5 regulates serum-induced early gene expression through transcription factor MEF2C. EMBO J. 16:7054, 1997.

296. Kato, S., Endoh, H., Masuhiro, Y., Kitamoto, T., Uchiyama, S., Sasaki, H., Masushige, S., Gotoh, Y., Nishida, E., and Kawashima, H.: Activation of the estrogen receptor through phosphorylation by mitogen-activated protein kinase. Science 270:1491, 1995.

297. Hu, M.C., Qiu, W.R., Wang, X., Meyer, C.F., and Tan, T.H.: Human HPK1, a novel human hematopoietic progenitor kinase that activates the JNK/SAPK kinase cascade. Genes Dev. 10:2251, 1996.

298. Charles, C.H., Sun, H., Lau, L.F., and Tonks, N.K.: The growth factor-inducible immediate-early gene 3CH134 encodes a protein-tyrosine-phosphatase. Proc. Natl. Acad. Sci. U.S.A. 90:5292, 1993.

299. Sun, H., Charles, C.H., Lau, L.F., and Tonks, N.K.: MKP-1 (3CH134), an immediate early gene product, is a dual specificity phosphatase that dephosphorylates MAP kinase in vivo. Cell 75:487, 1993..

300. Yoon, J.K., and Lau, L.F.: Involvement of JunD in transcriptional activation of the orphan receptor gene *nur77* by nerve growth factor and membrane depolarization in PC12 cells. Mol. Cell. Biol. 14:7731, 1994.

301. Camps, M., Nichols, A., Gillieron, C., Antonsson, B., Muda, M., Chabert, C., Boschert, U., and Arkinstall, S.: Catalytic activation of the phosphatase MKP-3 by ERK2 mitogen-activated protein kinase [see comments]. Science 280:1262, 1998.

302. Yang, D., Tournier, C., Wysk, M., Lu, H.T., Xu, J., Davis, R.J., and Flavell, R.A.: Targeted disruption of the MKK4 gene causes embryonic death, inhibition of c-Jun NH2-terminal kinase activation, and defects in AP-1 transcriptional activity. Proc. Natl. Acad. Sci. U.S.A. 94:3004, 1997.

303. Nishina, H., Bachmann, M., Oliveira, d.S.A., Kozieradzki, I., Fischer, K.D., Odermatt, B., Wakeham, A., Shahinian, A., Takimoto, H., Bernstein, A., Mak, T.W., Woodgett, J.R., Ohashi, P.S., and Penninger, J.M.: Impaired CD28-mediated interleukin 2 production and proliferation in stress kinase SAPK/ERK1 kinase (SEK1)/mitogen-activated protein kinase kinase 4 (MKK4)-deficient T lymphocytes. J. Exp. Med. 186:941, 1997.

304. Nishina, H., Fischer, K.D., Radvanyi, L., Shahinian, A., Hakem, R., Rubie, E.A., Bernstein, A., Mak, T.W., Woodgett, J.R., and Penninger, J.M.: Stress-signalling kinase Sek1 protects thymocytes from apoptosis mediated by CD95 and CD3. Nature 385:350, 1997.

305. Boriack, P.A., Margarit, S.M., Bar-Sagi, D., and Kuriyan, J.: The structural basis of the activation of ras by sos. Nature 394:337, 1998.

306. Vojtek, A.B., Hollenberg, S.M., and Cooper, J.A.: Mammalian ras interacts directly with the serine/threonine kinase raf. Cell 74:205, 1993.

307. Zhang, X.F., Settleman, J., Kyriakis, J.M., Takeuchi-Suzuki, E., Elledge, S.J., Marshall, M.S., Bruder, J.T., Rapp, U.R, and Avruch, J.: Normal and oncogenic p21ras proteins bind to the amino-terminal regulatory domain of c-Raf-1. Nature 364:308, 1993.

308. Stokoe, D., Macdonald, S.G., Cadwallader, K., Symons, M., and Hancock, J.F.: Activation of raf as a result of recruitment to the plasma membrane. Science 264:1463, 1994.

309. Kyriakis, J.M., App, H., Zhang, X.F., Banerjee, P., Brautigan, D.L., Rapp, U.R., and Avruch, J.: Raf-1 activates MAP kinase-kinase. Nature 358:417, 1992.

310. Lange-Carter, C.A., Pleiman, C.M., Gardner, A.M., Blumer, K.J., and Johnson, G.L.: A divergence in the MAP kinase regulatory network defined by MEK kinase and Raf. Science 260:315, 1993.

311. Yan, M., Dai, T., Deak, J.C., Kyriakis, J.M., Zon, L.I., Woodgett, J.R., and Templeton, D.J.: Activation of stress-activated protein kinase by MEKK1 phosphorylation of its activator SEK1. Nature 372:798, 1994.

312. Minden, A., Lin, A., Claret, F.X., Abo, A., Karin, M.: Selective activation of the JNK signaling cascade and c-Jun transcriptional activity by the small GTPases Rac and Cdc42Hs. Cell 81:1147, 1995.

313. Pharr, P.N., and Hofbauer, A.: Loss of flk-2/flt3 expression during commitment of multipotent mouse hematopoietic progenitor cells to the mast cell lineage. Exp. Hematol. 25:620, 1997.

314. Su, Y.C., Han, J., Xu, S., Cobb, M., and Skolnik, E.Y.: NIK is a new Ste20-related kinase that binds NCK and MEKK1 and activates the SAPK/JNK cascade via a conserved regulatory domain. EMBO J. 16:1279, 1997.

315. Rudel, T., and Bokoch, G.M.: Membrane and morphological changes in apoptotic cells regulated by caspase-mediated activation of pak2. Science 276:1571, 1997.

316. Lamarche, N., Tapon, N., Stowers, L., Burbelo, P.D., Aspenstrom, P., Bridges, T., Chant, J., and Hall, A.: Rac and Cdc42 induce actin polymerization and G1 cell cycle progression independently of p65PAK and the JNK/SAPK MAP kinase cascade. Cell 87:519, 1996.

317. Ichijo, H., Nishida, E., Irie, K., Dijke, P., Saitoh, M., Moriguchi, T., Takagi, M., Matsumoto, K., Miyazono, K., and Gotoh, Y.: Induction of apoptosis by ASK1, a mammalian MAPKKK that activates SAPK/JNK and p38 signaling pathways. Science 275:90, 1997.

318. Salmeron, A., Ahmad, T.B., Carlile, G.W., Pappin, D., Narsimhan, R.P., and Ley, S.C.: Activation of MEK-1 and SEK-1 by Tpl-2 proto-oncoprotein, a novel MAP kinase kinase kinase. EMBO J. 15:817, 1996.

319. Kiefer, F., Tibbles, L.A., Anafi, M., Janssen, A., Zanke, B.W., Lassam, N., Pawson, T., Woodgett, J.R., and Iscove, N.N.: HPK1, a hematopoietic protein kinase activating the SAPK/JNK pathway. EMBO J. 15:7013, 1996.

320. Rana, A., Gallo, K., Godowski, P., Hirai, S., Ohno, S., Zon, L., Kyriakis, J.M., and Avruch, J.: The mixed lineage kinase SPRK phosphorylates and activates the stress-activated protein kinase activator, SEK-1. J. Biol. Chem. 271:19025, 1996.

321. Pombo, C.M., Kehrl, J.H., Sanchez, I., Katz, P., Avruch, J., Zon, L.I., Woodgett, J.R., Force, T., and Kyriakis, J.M.: Activation of the SAPK pathway by the human STE20 homologue germinal centre kinase. Nature 377:750, 1995.

322. Lee, S.L., Sadovsky, Y., Swirnoff, A.H., Polish, J.A., Goda, P., Gavrilina, G., and Milbrandt, J.: Luteinizing hormone deficiency and female infertility in mice lacking the transcription factor NGFI-A (Egr-1). Science 273:1219, 1996.

323. Akashi, K., Kondo, M., von Freeden-Jeffry, U., Murray, R., and Weissman, I.L.: Bcl-2 rescues T lymphopoiesis in interleukin-7 receptor-deficient mice. Cell 89:1033, 1997.

324. Kondo, M., Akashi, K., Domen, J., Sugamura, K., and Weissman, I.L.: Bcl-2 rescues T lymphopoiesis, but not B or NK cell development, in common gamma chain-deficient mice. Immunity 7:155, 1997.

325. Maraskovsky, E., O'Reilly, L.A., Teepe, M., Corcoran, L., Peschon, J.J., and Strasser, A.: Bcl-2 can rescue T lymphocyte development in interleukin-7 receptor-deficient mice but not in mutant rag-1-/- mice. Cell 89:1011, 1997.

Part II

RED CELLS

5 Hemoglobin Switching
▼▼▼▼
G e o r g e   S t a m a t o y a n n o p o u l o s   a n d
F r a n k   G r o s v e l d

▼ ▼

All animals that use hemoglobin for oxygen transport have different hemoglobin species during the early and later stages of development.[1] In humans, two gene clusters direct the synthesis of hemoglobins during development: the α locus, which contains the embryonic ζ gene plus the two adult α genes, and the β cluster, which consist of the ϵ, $^{G}\gamma$, $^{A}\gamma$, δ, and β genes (Fig. 5–1). Both loci are controlled by major regulatory elements placed upstream of the structural genes: the β locus control region (LCR) placed 6 to 20 kb upstream of the ϵ globin gene and the HS-40 regulatory element placed 40 kb upstream of the ζ gene. The structure and function of these regulatory elements is described in a later section of this chapter.

Two globin gene switches occur during development: the embryonic to fetal globin switch, coinciding with the transition from embryonic (yolk sac) to definitive (fetal liver) hematopoiesis, and the fetal to adult switch, occurring near the perinatal period. The switches from ϵ to γ and γ to β globin gene expression are controlled exclusively at the transcriptional level. The ζ to α switch is controlled predominantly at the transcriptional level, although post-transcriptional mechanisms also play a role.[2] Unlike humans, most species have only one switch from embryonic to definitive globin expression occurring early in development. Expres-

sion of the γ gene during the fetal period is a rather recent evolutionary event, occurring 35 to 55 million years ago, during primate evolution.[3]

The globin genes are arranged from 5' to 3' according to the order of their expression during ontogeny. Two genes of the β locus, the $^{G}\gamma$ and $^{A}\gamma$ genes, and two genes of the α locus, the α_1 and α_2 genes, are structurally identical products of gene duplication and gene conversion. The two types of γ chains can be distinguished only at amino acid position 136, where the $^{G}\gamma$ gene encodes for glycine but the $^{A}\gamma$ gene encodes for alanine.[4] The relative synthesis of $^{G}\gamma$ and $^{A}\gamma$ chains changes during the perinatal switch from fetal to adult hemoglobin; the $^{G}\gamma$ to $^{A}\gamma$ ratio of 3:1 found in fetal red cells becomes 2:3 in the small amounts of fetal hemoglobin in adult red cells.[5–7] Unequal expression is also characteristic of the two genes of the α locus, with the α_2 showing higher expression than α_1 throughout development.[8] The higher expression of the 5' placed members of the duplicated γ and α genes perhaps is a result of their preferential interaction with the LCR because of their proximity to this regulatory element.[9]

Red cells containing hemoglobin F (Hb F) exhibit a higher oxygen affinity than cells containing hemoglobin A (Hb A), mainly because Hb F does not bind 2,3-diphospho-

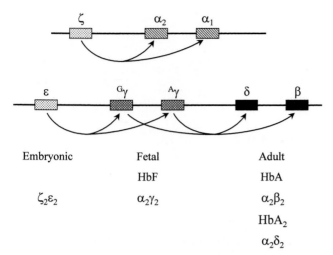

Figure 5–1. Human globin genes and hemoglobins produced during human development.

glycerate (2,3-DPG).[10] (See Chapter 7.) The higher oxygen affinity of fetal blood compared with maternal blood may facilitate oxygen transport across the placenta. This differential oxygen affinity is not obligatory, however, because normal infants have been born of mothers who have a high-affinity hemoglobin variant.[11]

Hemoglobin Production During Development

Erythropoiesis in the human begins in the yolk sac, but at about 5 weeks of gestation, the site of hematopoiesis changes from the yolk sac islands to the liver. The liver remains the predominant site of erythropoiesis in the fetus until about the twentieth week of gestation (Fig. 5–2). Hematopoiesis subsequently occurs in the spleen and the bone marrow, and by the time of birth, the bone marrow is the main hematopoietic organ.[12–14]

Shifts in the site of erythropoiesis are characteristic during development of all species.[1] In amphibians, the first red cells arise from the ventral blood islands of the embryo. Subsequently, the kidneys become erythropoietically active,

and the liver ultimately becomes the main erythropoietic organ in amphibian larvae.[15–19] In the juvenile frog, the liver is the primary erythropoietic site, whereas in the adult frog, erythropoiesis resides in the bone marrow.[17, 19, 20, 21] In chickens, precursors to the erythroid series are found in the primary mesenchyme, whereas descendants of these precursors become part of the yolk sac; late in embryonic life and after hatching, the bone marrow becomes the predominant site of erythropoiesis.[22, 23]

In all species, the shifting sites of erythropoiesis coincide with changes in the hemoglobin composition of red cells and also with changes in other morphological and biochemical characteristics. In the human, embryonic erythrocytes are very large nucleated cells (average volume about 200 μl^3). The volume of human fetal red cells is approximately 125 μl^3, whereas adult red cells are significantly smaller, with an average volume of 80 μl^3. The membrane carbohydrate profile also changes strikingly. (See Chapter 9.) For example, the unbranched carbohydrate of the i antigenic determinant is found on fetal red cells, whereas adult red cells have the branched structure reflecting the acquisition of a branching enzyme, present in adult red cells but absent from the red cells of the fetus. The i antigenic determinant may be detected on adult red cells,[24] but these red cells differ from fetal red cells in that they also fully express the I antigenic determinant. The activity of several glycolytic enzymes is lower in fetal red cells than in those of adult individuals, and characteristic changes in isozyme profiles, such as those exhibited by carbonic anhydrase, may also be observed.[25, 26]

In humans, the switch from ϵ to γ globin production begins very early in gestation,[27, 28] and it is completed well before 10 weeks of gestation.[27, 29] Staining of embryonic and fetal erythroblasts from 38- to 60- day human fetuses shows that ϵ globin expression is restricted in yolk sac cells, whereas the γ and β globins are restricted to erythroblasts of liver origin.[30, 31] β globin expression starts early in human development, and small amounts of Hb A can be detected by biosynthetic or immunochemical methods even in the smallest human fetuses studied.[30–33] Expression of the γ gene in the fetus is approximately 50 times higher than β gene expression. Double immunofluorescent staining of erythroblasts and fetal red cells shows that γ and β globins are

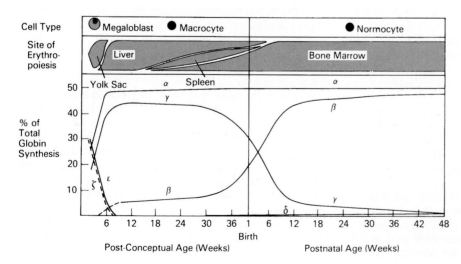

Figure 5–2. Changes in globin chain production, sites of hematopoiesis, red cell morphology, and size of erythrocytes during the course of development. (From Wood, D. G.: Haemoglobin synthesis during human fetal development. Br. Med. Bull. 32:282, 1976; with permission.)

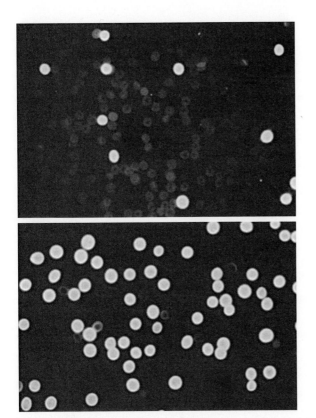

Figure 5–3. Detection of F cells in the blood from an adult by staining with fluorescent anti-γ globin chain monoclonal antibodies. *Upper,* Normal adult. *Lower,* Juvenile chronic myeloid leukemia (CML).

coexpressed in the same cell.[31] Synthesis of the β chain increases progressively during intrauterine development to approximately 10 per cent of γ chain synthesis by 30 to 35 weeks. Then β chain synthesis increases sharply, and γ chain production falls steadily. At birth, Hb F comprises 60 to 80 per cent of the total hemoglobin. In the 16 to 20 week old infant, Hb F constitutes about 3 per cent of all hemoglobin synthesized.[34] It takes about 2 years to reach the level of Hb F that is characteristic of adult red cells.

Only 0.5 to 1 per cent of the total hemoglobin in human adult red cells is Hb F; it is restricted to a few erythrocytes called *F cells*[35, 36] (Fig. 5–3). Approximately 3 to 7 per cent of erythrocytes are F cells,[36] and each contains about 4 to 8 picograms (pg) of Hb F, along with 22 to 26 pg of Hb A.[35] The number of F cells and the amount of Hb F in each F cell may be increased in various acquired and genetic conditions characterized by elevated Hb F levels.

The developmental switch in the genes of the α locus more or less parallels the ε to γ switch in the β locus, but there are differences. First, ζ and α genes appear to be coexpressed in embryonic red cells, although α gene expression is much lower compared with ζ. Second, ζ gene transcription continues in the definitive erythropoiesis of the fetal liver, as shown by the detection of ζ mRNA.[37] Third, synthesis of ζ chains can be detected in normal newborns[38] and even in adult carriers of α thalassemia.[39] The absolute restriction of the ε gene expression in the yolk sac erythropoiesis that is characteristic of the β locus does not apply to the embryonic gene of the α locus.

The mouse has been used extensively to study the regu-

lation of globin gene expression by creation of transgenic animals. In this species, the embryonic to adult switch takes place at 10.5 days of gestation.[40, 41] The yolk sac erythrocytes of the embryo contain ζ and α globin chains, the two embryonic globins (βh1 and εy), but no adult β globin chains. The murine εy gene is orthologous to the human ε, and the βh1 gene is orthologous to the human γ gene. The expression of the γ-like gene of the mouse (i.e., βh1) is restricted to the cells of the embryonic erythropoiesis. The definitive fetal liver erythroblasts of the murine fetus produce α globin, the two adult-type β globins (β major and β minor), but no embryonic globin chains.

Mutations Affecting Switching

Many insights into the regulation of hemoglobin switching have been acquired by the study of mutations that increase fetal hemoglobin production during adult life. These mutations are clinically relevant, because increased synthesis of Hb F in individuals with sickle cell anemia or β thalassemia reduces disease severity. More than 60 such mutations have been discovered. The hematological characteristics of heterozygotes for these mutations are given in Table 5–1.

Several parameters may be used in classifying these mutations. Many mutations reflect deletion of a portion of the β globin gene cluster, whereas others reflect point mutations within the cluster. These are called *deletion* (Table 5–2) and *non-deletion* (Table 5–3) mutations, respectively. Among the deletion and the non-deletion classes are mutations that result in a more or less uniform distribution of Hb F in peripheral blood cells (pancellular) and those that result in a non-uniform increase in Hb F (heterocellular). Mutations that cause a heterocellular increase in Hb F may lead to an increase in the percentage of F cells and/or an increase in the average amount of Hb F per F cell. Some mutations result in an increase in $^G\gamma$ globin only, others in an increase in $^A\gamma$ globin only, and still others in a more or less equal increase in both globins. Mutations that increase Hb F production may be categorized by whether they are characterized by hypochromic and microcytic red cells or by morphologically normal red cells in heterozygous individuals (see Table 5–1). The first are the thalassemia mutations, and the second are called the hereditary persistence of fetal hemoglobin (HPFH) type of mutations.

Much of the older literature on mutations that increase Hb F synthesis is highly descriptive, with classifications relying on phenotypic features rather than molecular characterization. For example, when the HPFH-type mutations were recognized, an African form[42] and a Greek form[43] were

Table 5–1. Phenotypes of HPFH and δβ Thalassemia Heterozygotes

	HPFH	**δβ Thalassemia**
Red cell morphology	Normal	Abnormal
Mean corpuscular hemoglobin (MCH)	Near normal	Decreased
Hematocrit	Normal	Decreased
Distribution of Hb F in red cells	Pancellular	Heterocellular

HPFH, hereditary persistence of fetal hemoglobin.

Table 5–2. Deletion Mutations of the β Globin Gene Cluster

Type	Ethnic Group	Hb F Level in Heterozygotes (%)	References
A. Hereditary persistence of fetal hemoglobin (HPFH)			
HPFH-1	American black	20–30	48–52
HPFH-2	Ghanian	20–30	48, 50–56
HPFH-3	Indian	22–23	56–58
HPFH-4	Italian	14–30	59
HPFH-5	Sicilian	16–20	60
HPFH-6	Vietnamese	18–27	61
Hb Kenya		5–15	62–65
B. (δβ)⁰ thalassemia			
1	Japanese	5–7	69–70
2	Spanish	5–15	71–73
3	Indian	5–15	74–75
4	Turkish	15	76
5	Macedonian/Turkish	7–14	77–79
6	Black	25	80, 81
7	Eastern European	13–18	82
8	Laotian	11	83
9	Thai	10	84
10	Mediterranean/Sicilian	2–15	49, 55, 85, 86
11	Hb Lepore	1–5	87
C. (ᴬγδβ)⁰ thalassemia			
1	Cantonese	19–20	88
2	Malaysian (1)	Unknown	89
3	Malaysian (2)	Unknown	90
4	Chinese	9–20	89, 91, 92
5	Yunnanese	9–17	93, 94
6	Thai	17–23	95, 96
7	German	10–13	97
8	Belgian	14–15	98
9	Italian		99
10	Turkish	10–14	50, 55, 100
11	American black	6–21	55, 101
12	Indian	10–18	89, 102
D. (εγδβ)⁰ thalassemia			
1	Mexican		103
2	Scotch-Irish		104
3	Yugoslavian		105
4	Canadian		105
5	Irish		106
6	Dutch		107
E. β⁰ thalassemia*			
0.3 kb	Turkish/Bulgarian	2.7–3.3	108
0.5 kb	African American	0.2	109
1.6 kb	Croatian	5.8–8.5	110
1.4 kb	African American	1.8–7.1	111
3.5 kb	Thai	4.5	112
4.2 kb	Czech	3.3–5.7	113
7.6 kb	Turkish	1.0–1.9	114
10.3 kb	Asian Indian	3.2–4.7	115
12 kb	Australian	2.5–7.2	116
12.6 kb	Dutch	4.1–10.9	117
27 kb	Southeast Asian	14.1–23.8	118
45 kb	Filippino	3.8–9.1	119
67 kb	Italian	9.0	120
F. Deletions removing sequences of the locus control region (LCR)†			
HS1 to 5	Dutch		121, 122
HS1 to 5	Anglosaxon		122, 123
HS1 to 5	English		124
HS2 to 5	Hispanic		125
HS1 only			126

*β Gene deletions that also remove the β gene promoter. The β gene deletion length is given in kilobases.

†Deleted DNase I hypersensitive sites (HS). Deletions that include HS2 to HS5 have the phenotype of (εγδβ)⁰ thalassemia. Deletion of HS1 only does not produce an abnormal hematological phenotype.

Table 5–3. Non-deletion Mutants of Hereditary Persistence of Fetal Hemoglobin

Type and Ethnic Group	Mutation	Hb F in Heterozygotes (%)	References
Gγ HPFH			
Japanese	Gγ-114 C to T	11–14	135
Australian	Gγ-114 C to G	8.6	136
Black/Sardinian	Gγ-175 T to C	17–30	137, 138
Tunisian	Gγ-200 + C	18–49	139
Black	Gγ-202 C to G	15–25	140
Aγ HPFH			
Georgian	Aγ-114 C to T	3–6.5	141
Black	Aγ-114 to −102 Deleted	30–32	142
Greek	Aγ-117 G to A	10–20	43, 143, 144
Cretan	Aγ-158 C to T	2.9–5.1	145
Black	Aγ-175 T to C	36–41	146
Brazilian	Aγ-195 C to G	4.5–7	147
Chinese/Italian	Aγ-196 C to T	14–21	148–150
British	Aγ-198 To to C	3.5–10	151
Georgian	Aγ-202 C to T	1.6–3.9	152

defined. The African variety was subsequently subdivided into a common variant in which the $^{G}\gamma$ and $^{A}\gamma$ chains were present ($^{G}\gamma^{A}\gamma$ HPFH) and a rare variant exhibiting only $^{G}\gamma$ chains ($^{G}\gamma$ HPFH).[44] The Hb F in Greek HPFH contains predominantly $^{A}\gamma$ chains[45]—hence this variant was named $^{A}\gamma$HPFH. The African $^{G}\gamma^{A}\gamma$ and $^{G}\gamma$ variants and the Greek $^{A}\gamma$ variant display a pancellular distribution of Hb F, whereas other forms of HPFH display heterocellular distributions.[46] The term $\delta\beta$ thalassemia was reserved for the form of thalassemia in which heterozygotes have relatively high levels of Hb F and normal levels of Hb A$_2$. (See Chapter 6.) Because of its high F phenotype, this condition was initially called *F thalassemia*.[47] Subsequent molecular characterization has revealed an extraordinary complexity to these mutations.

▼ DELETION MUTATIONS

Deletion Hereditary Persistence of Fetal Hemoglobin

$^{G}\gamma^{A}\gamma$ HPFH is found among individuals of African, Asiatic, and European descent (see Table 5–2 and Fig. 5–4).[48–60] These mutations are characterized by total absence of δ and β globin synthesis *cis* to the HPFH determinant. The $^{G}\gamma$ and $^{A}\gamma$ globins are produced in almost equal proportion. Heterozygotes produce 14 to 30 per cent Hb F and are clinically and hematologically normal. Although homozygotes were found to produce 100 per cent Hb F,[66, 67] their red cells failed to show other properties of fetal erythrocytes. Such individuals are healthy, although their hemoglobin levels and red cell counts are higher than normal, reflecting the increased oxygen affinity of blood in which the red cells contain only Hb F. The only additional hematological manifestations in homozygotes are microcytosis, hypochromia (mean corpuscular hemoglobin of 23 to 27 pg), and a slightly increased α to γ biosynthetic ratio.[68] Structural studies have identified six deletions producing $^{G}\gamma^{A}\gamma$ HPFH phenotypes (see Table 5–2 and Fig. 5–4).

Kenya HPFH results from an unequal crossing over between the $^{A}\gamma$ gene and the β gene that deletes the $^{A}\gamma$ to β region and leads to the production of a new fusion globin. The ($^{A}\gamma\beta$) chain of Hb Kenya is a fusion protein containing amino acids 1 to 80 of the $^{A}\gamma$ chain and 81 to 146 of the β chain.[62–65] Heterozygotes produce 7 to 25 per cent Hb Kenya and 5 to 15 per cent Hb F. Fetal hemoglobin contains α and only $^{G}\gamma$ chains, and it is pancellularly distributed in the red cells.[64] Red cell morphology and hematological indices are normal.

Deletion Thalassemias

In the most common variant, found in Mediterranean populations, heterozygotes produce 2 to 15 per cent Hb F, which is heterogeneously distributed among the red cells (see Table 5–2 and Fig. 5–4). Heterozygotes also have very mild anemia and abnormalities of red cell morphology. Because δ and β globin chain production *cis* to the thalassemia determinant is absent, homozygotes produce only Hb F. Hemoglobin levels of homozygotes usually range from 8 to 11 g/dl, and the α to γ biosynthetic ratio averages 2.4:1. The "thalassemic" hematological findings in heterozygotes and clinical manifestations in the homozygotes indicate that production of γ chains is inefficient and cannot fully compensate for the lack of β globin.

Several mutations that cause $(\delta\beta)°$ thalassemia have been analyzed structurally, and an extensive variability in the 5′ and 3′ breakpoints and in the size of deletions has been discovered (see Fig. 5–4). The deletions in the Spanish and Japanese $(\delta\beta)°$ thalassemia mutants are even larger than those of HPFH-1 and -2, whereas other mutants delete the δ and β genes and limited flanking upstream and downstream sequences. There is considerable variation among mutants in the level of Hb F production in heterozygotes and in the severity of hematological manifestations in homozygotes, indicating that individual mutations may variably affect the efficiency of γ gene expression in the adult.

The $(^{A}\gamma\delta\beta)°$ thalassemias are found in several ethnic groups. Heterozygotes produce 6 to 23 per cent Hb F. Homozygotes produce Hb F that contains only $^{G}\gamma$ chains. The 12

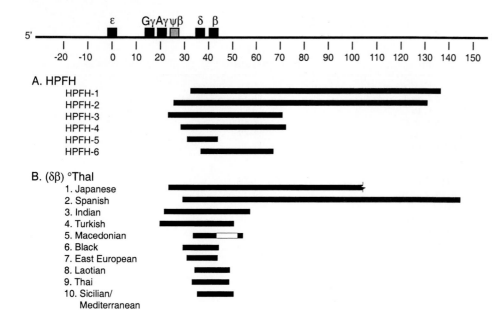

A. HPFH

B. (δβ) °Thal

Figure 5–4. Location and size of deletion mutants of *(A)* hereditary persistence of fetal hemoglobin (HPFH) and *(B)* δβ thalassemia.

mutants that have been characterized (see Table 5–2) display considerable variation in the 5′ and 3′ breakpoints (Fig. 5–5). There are also differences in the efficiency of γ globin production among mutants. The Chinese and Yunnanese mutants delete about 100 kilobases of the β locus. The homozygote for the Chinese mutant presented with severe anemia requiring frequent transfusions and a splenectomy, whereas the homozygote for the Yunnanese mutant had moderate anemia (hemoglobin value of 10 g/dl), no other clinical manifestations, and no need for transfusions.[93]

The (εγδβ)° thalassemias result from deletions that remove all the genes of the β locus and therefore are characterized by complete absence of ε, γ, δ, and β chain production. Heterozygotes present during the perinatal period with transient hemolytic anemia.[103] Subsequently, their red cells display the characteristics of β thalassemia trait. Presumably, homozygotes for these mutations die in utero.

Several mutations remove all or a portion of the β globin gene and produce the phenotype of β° thalassemia. Shown in Table 5–2 are β° thalassemia mutants in which the deletion includes the β promoter. Notice that the elevated fetal hemoglobin level in heterozygotes is characteristic of all but one mutation. As expected from the competition

mechanism of globin gene switching (discussed later), in the absence of β gene promoter, the γ gene competes more favorably for interaction with the LCR, resulting in increased expression in the adult heterozygotes.

An informative category of mutations delete sequences of the LCR (see Table 5–2). The contribution of these mutations to the understanding of the function of the LCR is described in a later section of this chapter.

▼ MOLECULAR BASIS OF ELEVATED HEMOGLOBIN F IN DELETION HEREDITARY PERSISTENCE OF FETAL HEMOGLOBIN AND DELETION (δβ)° THALASSEMIA

Several hypotheses have been proposed to explain why in HPFH the deletion of δ and β genes is associated with high levels of Hb F distributed homogeneously in the red cell (pancellular HPFH) while in (δβ)° thalassemia the levels of Hb F are lower, they vary considerably between mutants, and they are distributed heterogeneously in the red cells. An early hypothesis proposed that a regulatory sequence located between ^Aγ and δ genes is responsible for γ gene silenc-

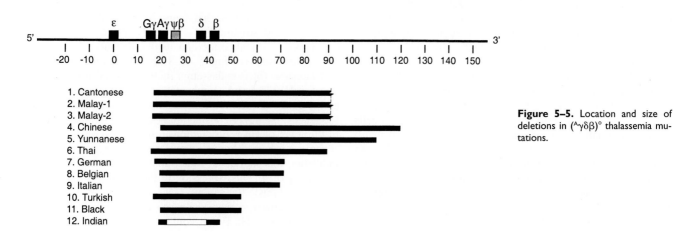

Figure 5–5. Location and size of deletions in (^Aγδβ)° thalassemia mutations.

ing.[127] Presumably, this sequence is deleted in deletional HPFH (hence the high levels of Hb F in the heterozygotes) but it is not removed in deletional δβ thalassemia (hence Hb F is low, resulting in an inadequate compensation for the absence of β gene expression). Evidence against this hypothesis has been obtained from observations of mutants that delete the putative regulatory region and are not associated with significant elevations of Hb F.[128] This hypothesis has been disproved by the results of studies in transgenic mice carrying human β loci from which the hypothetical regulatory sequence is deleted; these mice do not display elevated γ gene expression.[129–131]

An alternative hypothesis proposes that the high levels of Hb F in HPFH result from powerful fetal enhancer elements that are located downstream to the globin locus and, because of the deletion of the intervening large segments of DNA, are juxtaposed to the $^A\gamma$ gene.[48] Sequences having the properties of enhancers have been localized near the 3′ breakpoint of deletional HPFHs.[132, 133] Direct evidence in support of this hypothesis was obtained from studies in transgenic mice using constructs in which the enhancer element located downstream to the 3′ breakpoint of HPFH-1 was juxtaposed to the $^A\gamma$ gene.[134] Adult mice carrying this construct displayed high levels of γ mRNA, but γ gene expression was barely detectable in control animals carrying γ genes without the downstream enhancer.[134]

▼ NON-DELETION HEREDITARY PERSISTENCE OF FETAL HEMOGLOBIN MUTATIONS

Non-deletion HPFHs are caused by mutations affecting the promoter of $^G\gamma$ or $^A\gamma$ genes (see Table 5–3). Individuals with these mutations have normal red cell morphology and red cell counts and no clinical abnormalities. The δ and β globin genes are expressed *cis* to the $^G\gamma$ and the $^A\gamma$ HPFH determinants. The $^G\gamma$ HPFHs have mutations affecting the $^G\gamma$ promoter, whereas the $^A\gamma$ HPFHs affect the $^A\gamma$ promoter. Heterogeneity in γ gene expression is characteristic.

Experimental evidence proving that the γ gene promoter mutations associated with HPFH are the cause of the activation of γ gene expression in the adult has been obtained in studies of transgenic mice. Mice carrying human β locus yeast artificial chromosomes (βYACs) typically transcribe the human β gene, but they fail to express the γ genes in the adult stage.[153, 154] However, mice carrying a β locus YAC containing the −117 G→A base-pair substitution in the $^A\gamma$ gene promoter continue to express the $^A\gamma$ gene in the adult stage; they have the phenotype of $^A\gamma$ HPFH.[129]

▼ HEREDITARY PERSISTENCE OF FETAL HEMOGLOBIN MUTATIONS LOCATED OUTSIDE THE GLOBIN GENE CLUSTER

Certain HPFH variants are characterized by production of low levels of Hb F, distributed in a heterocellular pattern without an identified mutation in the β globin gene cluster.[155–163] Little is known about the molecular biology of these variants. Initial family studies suggested linkage with the β globin cluster.[157–159, 164] Analyses of other families have

suggested free recombination between the HPFH determinant and the globin structural genes.[160–163, 165–171]

This form of HPFH probably is genetically heterogeneous and composed of several variants, some of which may be linked to the β cluster and others found at more distant chromosomal positions. Population genetic studies have raised the possibility that a locus that increases the number of F cells in the adult is located on the X chromosome[172–174] at Xp22.2.[173] Studies of a large Asian Indian family have revealed a major gene for heterocellular HPFH,[175] which is located in chromosome 6, at 6q22.3-q24.[170]

▼ CLINICAL SIGNIFICANCE

Mutations that increase Hb F levels modulate the effects of the β thalassemia and Hb S genes. (See Chapters 6 and 7.) Compound heterozygotes have a much milder clinical syndrome than do homozygous individuals with thalassemia or sickle cell anemia. For example, individuals with $^G\gamma^A\gamma$ HPFH and a β thalassemia or an Hb S allele are asymptomatic, and they are detected by chance during population screening. The combination of Greek HPFH with β thalassemia produces a hemolytic anemia of mild to moderate severity.[43] Even heterocellular HPFHs that modestly increase Hb F levels have ameliorating effects in individuals homozygous for the β thalassemia or the Hb S genes.[156, 165, 176–179]

Regulation of the Globin Genes

The globin genes are relatively small genes comprising three coding exons and two introns. The exons code for 141 and 146 amino acids in the α- and β-like globin chains, respectively. The exons correspond to functional domains in the proteins; for example, exon 2 codes for the part of the globin chains involved in heme binding and tetramer formation, and exon 3 codes for many of the amino acids required for cooperative binding of heme and interactions between tetramer subunits.[180, 181] The introns vary from 117 to 1264 bp. In addition to the normal splicing function, at least in the case of the β globin gene, intron 2 appears to be important for polyadenylation and release of the transcript from the template to allow transport from the nucleus to the cytoplasm.[182, 183]

The tissue- and developmental-specific expression pattern of the individual globin genes is achieved through the action of transcription factors on regulatory sequences that are immediately flanking the individual genes and on more distant sequences that are important for the regulation of all the genes of the locus. Analogous to what has been observed in other tissues, the factors that regulate globin genes are either tissue restricted or ubiquitous with respect to their expression pattern. Only a few factors have been studied in detail for their role in the transcription of the globin genes. Several factors effect globin gene transcription through their importance in hematopoietic or erythroid differentiation in general. (See Chapter 3.) Several factors are important for globin gene transcription, but they are ubiquitous and influence the expression of many genes, most of which are not erythroid specific. The latter two categories of factors are not discussed in this chapter.

▼ ERYTHROID TRANSCRIPTION FACTORS AND GLOBIN GENE REGULATION

GATA-1

GATA-1, a transcriptional factor, was the first of a family of DNA-binding proteins with a central consensus binding motif of GATA.[184] Binding sites with this motif are present at many positions in the α and β globin loci, and they have also been found in many other genes. (See Chapter 3.) The GATA motif is present in one or more copies in almost all the regulatory elements of the globin genes that have been identified. At first, GATA-1 was thought to be an erythroid-specific protein, but it subsequently was shown to be present in other hematopoietic lineages[185-189] (e.g., mast cells, megakaryocytes) and the testis.[190] A GATA motif is often accompanied by a G-rich motif[191] in erythroid specific regulatory sequences, suggesting that GATA-1 specifies an erythroid specific combination in concert with members of the Krüppel-like family of zinc finger proteins, which includes Sp1 and erythroid Krüppel–like factor (EKLF).[192] In megakaryocytes, GATA-1 is accompanied by binding sites for the ETS family of protein binding sites.[193]

The family of GATA proteins is characterized by two zinc fingers that interact with specific nucleotides in the major groove of the DNA helix.[194] The carboxy-terminal finger is required for the binding to the GATA motif, and this binding is stabilized by the N-terminal finger of the protein.[195-198] The N-terminal finger also has DNA-binding properties (to a different sequence[199]), but its main function appears to be a specific interaction with another zinc finger that is present in the protein FOG-1.[200, 201] A second protein complex of GATA-1 with E47, Tal1, Lmo2, and Ldb1 has been described, and this combination specifically binds a GATA consensus in combination with an E-box motif.[202] This motif has yet to be found in a naturally occurring gene, and the function of this complex in globin transcription or erythroid differentiation is unknown. GATA-1 can also interact with itself,[203] E-box proteins,[204] and cofactors such as CBP, a histone acetyltransferase.[205]

GATA-1 was identified as a transcription factor by virtue of its ability to transactivate a minimal promoter in non-erythroid cells, provided it contained the N-terminal and C-terminal zinc fingers.[206-208] It appears that the C-terminal DNA-binding activity provides a platform on the DNA for interacting proteins such as FOG-1 to bind and exert their action on the transcriptional machinery. GATA-1 is phosphorylated[209] throughout the nucleus, but in addition, a high concentration of the protein is present in a few nuclear foci of unknown function.[210] The DNA-binding activity of GATA-1 changes during the cell cycle: it is low in G_1, peaks in S phase, and decreases during G_2/M.[211]

Five other GATA genes (GATA-2 to -6) have been isolated by virtue of their homology in the zinc fingers, and of these, only GATA-2 and -3 are also expressed in the hematopoietic system in addition to many other tissues.[212-216] Within a single species, the GATA proteins are completely diverged outside the DNA-binding domain, although with the exception of GATA-1, these areas are conserved between the individual GATA factors between species.[217] All GATA factors have been shown to be transcriptional activators when cotransfected with a plasmid having a minimal promoter containing a minimal GATA motif.[184]

GATA-1 is essential for fetal (definitive) erythroid differentiation. Inactivation of the GATA-1 gene by homologous recombination in embryonic stem cells leads to a fatal defect. Chimeras made with GATA-1–deficient cells show a complete absence of any contribution to the erythroid lineage.[218] The GATA-1–deficient cells fail to mature beyond the proerythroblast stage in primitive and definitive cells and go into apoptosis.[219-222] Differentiation of the wild-type cells is also disturbed by the presence of GATA-1–deficient cells in the chimera.[219] Macrophage, neutrophil, mast cell, and megakaryocyte differentiation appears to be unaffected, although there is a higher abundance of megakaryocytes.[223, 224] Overexpression of GATA-1 at that stage leads to the opposite effect in erythroid cells; it stimulates the proliferation of proerythroblast cells and inhibits differentiation,[225, 226] an effect that is also seen in non-erythroid cells.[227] This effect appears to be exerted through cyclin A_2, leading to a hyperphosphorylation of *Rb* and early entry into the S phase. Transgenic mice overexpressing GATA-1 in late erythroid cells show a similar phenotype in mice lacking the retinoblastoma gene, *Rb*[228-230] and they die of anemia around day 13 of gestation. The presence of overexpressing cells does not change the proliferation and differentiation of the wild-type cells. These results suggest that GATA-1 has a crucial function in determining the balance between erythroid cell proliferation and cell differentiation and that this balance is regulated by a feedback signal from the differentiating cells.[226]

Inactivation of GATA-2 results in an embryonic lethal phenotype in vivo, and differentiation experiments in vitro indicate that the protein is essential for the proliferation and survival[212] of early multipotential hematopoietic progenitor cells, although not for the terminal differentiation of erythroid cells. This result implies that GATA-2 is not directly involved in the expression of globin genes. Inactivation of GATA-3 also leads to early hematopoietic defects,[216] but there is no evidence that it is involved in the regulation of globin genes. GATA-3 is important for the maturation of T-cells.[231-233]

FOG Protein

The gene coding for the protein FOG was identified after a search for proteins that interact with GATA-1.[200] The FOG gene was found on the basis of the function of the N-terminal finger of GATA-1 in a yeast two hybrid screen. It contains nine zinc fingers of two types, of which zinc finger 6 specifically interacts to form a complex with the N-terminal finger af GATA-1 in vivo and in vitro. FOG is coexpressed with GATA-1 during development, and it is present in erythroid and megakaryocytic cells. In cell culture, it cooperates with GATA-1 to promote erythroid and megakaryocytic differentiation. Inactivation of FOG in the mouse leads to a fatal anemia in the fetal stage of hematopoiesis. Similar to GATA-deficient erythroid cells, FOG-deficient red cells show a partial block of maturation. Megakaryocytes also fail to develop in the absence of FOG, indicating that FOG is probably not a cofactor of GATA-1 in the megakaryocytic lineage, but it is required earlier in megakaryocytic differentiation.[201]

Nuclear Factor–Erythroid 2

Nuclear factor–erythroid 2 (NF-E2) was the second protein that was identified through DNA-binding studies in vitro after GATA-1 (initially called NF-E1) and was thought to be erythroid specific.[186, 234–236] It was discovered through its binding to an AP-1 motif[234, 235] in the promoter of the porphobilinogen deaminase gene and was somewhat ignored until it was shown that this factor could bind to the hypersensitive site 2 (HS2) region of the LCR of the β globin locus.[236, 237] The AP-1 consensus sequence at this position is largely responsible for the activity of HS2, and it was shown that NF-E2 binding requires a G residue two nucleotides upstream of the AP-1 consensus sequence with an ideal consensus of (T/C)GCTGA(C/G)TCA(T/C).[238]

The gene coding for NF-E2 was cloned after microsequencing of the purified protein,[238] and it is expressed in several hematopoietic lineages, including erythroid, mast, and megakaryocytic cells. It also is expressed in the intestine of anemic mice and may be involved in iron metabolism.[238, 239] It is a 45 kDa protein with a basic DNA-binding domain, an adjacent leucine zipper domain, an N-terminal proline-rich domain, and a CNC domain necessary for transcriptional activation.[240, 241]

NF-E2 heterodimerizes with members of the family of small, ubiquitously expressed 18 kDa proteins, the Maf proteins, which themselves have no transcriptional activation domain but which are essential for binding site recognition.[242–245] The leucine zipper of the 45 kDa protein is also capable of interacting with the DNA-binding domain of the thyroid (T3) and retinoic acid (RAR) receptors stimulating transactivation by T3 or RAR. This interaction is prevented by Maf but stimulated by the cognate hormone. The latter requires the NF-E2 transactivation domain and a strong interaction with a domain in the coactivator CBP that is responsible for mediating inhibition of transcription by AP-1 factors.[246]

NF-E2 is capable of binding in vitro reconstituted chromatin by disrupting the nucleosome structure in an ATP-dependent process and forming a DNase I hypersensitive site, similar to those observed in vivo.[247] Disruption of the gene coding for the 45 kDa subunit of NF-E2 leads to an absence of circulating platelets and to hemorrhage.[248] The mice only show a small change in hemoglobin content per cell and have a normal balanced globin gene synthesis and normal globin gene switching.[248] Disruption of one of the genes coding for one of the Maf subunits shows no phenotype, most likely because of compensation by one of the other Maf proteins.[249]

NRF-1, LCRF-1, NRF-2, ECH, BACH-1, and BACH-2

Several other proteins containing a CNC- and leucine zipper domain were identified as binding to the NF-E2/AP1 motif and were named NRF-1,[250–253] NRF-2,[250, 254] ECH,[255] LCRF-1,[256] and BCH-1 and -2.[257] Some are restricted to a small number of tissues, but none is erythroid specific. Like NF-E2, these proteins heterodimerize with an 18 kDa Maf subunit.[255] Inactivation of the *NRF1* gene leads to an early embryonic lethal phenotype: the embryos fail to form a primitive streak and have no detectable mesoderm. However, NRF-1–deficient embryonic stem cells contribute to meso-

dermally derived tissues including erythroid cells. These cells have normal levels of hemoglobin, suggesting that NRF-1 is not essential for globin gene expression.[258, 259] Inactivation of the *NRF2* gene does not result in any clear phenotype, suggesting that NRF-2 is not essential for globin gene expression.[260] It is unknown whether the BACH proteins play any role in globin gene expression, although they are capable of activating (BACH-1) and repressing (BACH-2), a reporter gene carrying an NF-E2 binding site in the promoter.[257]

EKLF

EKLF is a member of the Sp1 family of zinc finger proteins. These proteins typically contain three fingers, each of which recognizes a 3 bp sequence on the DNA,[261] giving a binding site of nine consecutive base-pair binding sequences.[262] EKLF binds to the sequence CCACACCCT, which is found in the promoter of the β globin gene and related sequences.[263] However, the specificity of activation of the β promoter by EKLF is determined by the overall context of the β promoter rather than solely by the sequence of the β gene CACCC box.[264] Like other members of this family of proteins, EKLF acts as a transcriptional activator in reporter assays through a proline-rich domain that can be subdivided in stimulatory and inhibitory subdomains.

EKLF is the most restricted factor with respect to its expression pattern and is only found in the erythroid pathway. It is already functional in primitive erythroid cells,[265–266] although the β globin gene is its only known target gene. Absence of EKLF by inactivation of the gene results in a lethal phenotype at the fetal stage because of the absence of β globin gene expression.[267, 268] Overexpression of EKLF in erythroid cells in transgenic mice results in a reduction of the number of circulating platelets, suggesting that EKLF may have a role in determining the balance between megakaryocytic and erythroid lineages, perhaps by prematurely activating erythroid lineage-specific genes.[266] Data indicate that EKLF may also have a role in the activation of the LCR[269] by interacting with the G-rich sequence in HS3 (see below). This hypersensitive site is capable of remodeling chromatin,[270] which would fit with another set of data indicating that EKLF interacts with members of the SWI/SNF family of chromatin-modifying proteins.[271]

Other DNA-Binding Proteins

Several other binding activities have been identified during study of various regulatory elements. These include a number of ill-defined "suppressor" factors and well-known factors involved in the silencing of the embryonic and fetal genes. For example, the embryonic ε globin gene contains an upstream silencer element that binds the ubiquitously expressed YY1 (and GATA-1).[272–275] High-affinity YY1 motifs have also been identified in several regions of the β locus.[276] A factor designated NF-E3[277–278] has been identified as a possible repressor complex of the γ globin gene. Other factors that are important for globin gene expression are mentioned later in the discussion of individual regulatory sequences.

In addition to the factors that bind directly to the DNA, there exist several cofactors, some of which may provide erythroid specificity to their cognate DNA-binding factor. Most are factors expressed in many tissues, and perhaps the best characterized of these as important for erythroid expression is the factor XH-2, which was found through the analysis of patients with the ATR-X syndrome.[279] This is an X-linked disorder comprising a number of abnormalities, including α thalassemia, and it is caused by mutations in the gene coding for the helicase XH-2. (See Chapter 6.) The phenotype of ATR-X patients indicates that the XH-2 gene is a general transcriptional cofactor that when mutated becomes rate limiting in the expression of a number of genes in different cell types, including the α globin genes in erythroid cells.[279, 280] The protein contains a PHD interaction domain[280] and is a member of the SNF2 family of helicases.

▼ REGULATORY ELEMENTS OF THE INDIVIDUAL GLOBIN GENES

Each globin gene has a number of regulatory elements—a promoter, enhancers, or silencers—that are important for its precise developmental regulation. These elements are thought to interact with the more distant β globin LCR or the HS-40 in the α locus to achieve high levels of gene expression. Each regulatory element is composed of binding motifs for multiple erythroid-restricted and ubiquitously expressed transcriptional activators or suppressors. These factors interact and synergize with each other and other cofactors such as CBP or XH-2 to result in multimeric complexes that change chromatin structure to allow complex interactions resulting in the action of the basic transcription machinery and the formation of an initiation complex. The initiation complex is assembled at the TATA box, which is located approximately 30 bp upstream from the initiation site of each of the globin genes. The frequency of initiation of individual genes is determined by the interaction of this complex with other factors bound to the promoter and the other more distant regulatory sequences.

ε Globin Gene

Like the promoters of other globin genes, the promoter of the ε globin gene contains a number of binding sites for erythroid restricted and ubiquitously expressed transcription factors responsible for tissue-specific expression (Fig. 5–6). Expression of the gene depends on the presence of the LCR, which provides an additional layer of tissue specificity. The TATA box is situated 30 bp upstream of the initiation site, followed by a canonical CAAT and CACCC boxes at approximately 70 and 110 bp from the initiation site, respectively. A number of experiments with transfection systems indicated that these elements, in conjunction with the GATA sites of the ε gene promoter, are required for expression.[281–283] However, it is unknown which factors interact with these

sequences in vivo. For example the CACCC box, which is required for expression,[284, 285] binds the ubiquitous factor Sp1,[284] but inactivation of Sp1 in vivo[286] does not result in defective ε gene expression. Either a different factor is responsible for normal expression or a multitude of factors can normally bind this sequence and compensate for the loss of Sp1. Two factors belonging to the EKLF/Sp1 family, named FKLF[287] and FKLF-2,[288] interact with the CACCC box of the γ and ε genes. FKLF activates ε gene expression in transient assays and in stable transfections. Whether FKLF participates in regulation of ε gene expression in vivo remains to be determined.

The ε promoter contains a number of GATA sites. These sites appear to have different functions. Mutations of the GATA sites at position −163 and −269 decrease ε gene expression in embryonic cells of transgenic mice, but mutations of the site at −208 inhibit ε gene silencing.[272] Presumably, when GATA-1 binds at −208, it acts as a repressor, and when it binds at −163 or −269, it can act as an activator. The function of the −163 and −269 GATA sites appears to be more complex, because inactivation of GATA-1 does not lead to a loss of ε gene expression.[218]

The CAAT box of the ε gene binds CP1; destruction of the CCAAT motif leads to substantial reduction in ε expression in the embryonic erythroid cells of transgenic mice, suggesting that CP1 activates ε gene expression.[289] In the region of the CCAAT box of the embryonic and fetal, but not of adult, globin gene promoters, there exist one or two direct repeats of a short motif that is analogous to DR-1 binding sites for non-steroid nuclear hormone receptors.[289] NF-E3[290] is immunologically related to COUP-TF orphan nuclear receptors[289] and binds to the DR-1 element of the ε gene promoter.[289] Destruction of the DR-1 element of the ε promoter yields a striking increase in ε expression in adult transgenic mice, indicating that the NF-E3 complex acts as a developmental repressor of the ε gene.[289]

A number of other proteins play roles in the regulation of the ε promoter, including factors such as PREIIBF, which has DNA-bending properties and binds in the upstream part of the promoter.[291, 292, 293]

The ε gene requires the LCR for expression.[294, 295] The contribution of LCR sequences on ε gene activation has been shown in studies of βYAC transgenic mice. Deletion of the core element of HS3 in the context of a β locus YAC results in total absence of ε expression in day 9 embryonic cells,[296] suggesting that sequences of the core element of HS3 are necessary for interaction with the ε gene and activation of ε gene transcription.

ε gene expression is totally restricted in the embryonic yolk sac cells. The developmental control of the ε globin gene is autonomous; all the sequences required for the silencing of ε gene expression in the cells of definitive erythropoiesis are contained in the sequences flanking the gene.[294, 295, 297, 298] Regulatory sequences mediating this autonomous

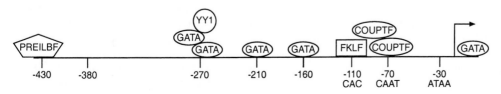

Figure 5–6. The ε gene promoter, showing the locations of conserved "boxes" and binding motifs for various proteins.

Figure 5–7. The γ globin gene promoter, showing the positions of conserved "boxes" and binding motifs for various proteins.

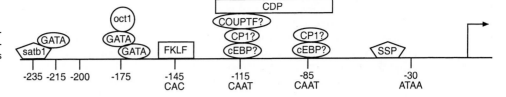

silicing of ε gene expression in definitive erythroid cells have been mapped to four regions: about −3000 relative to the cap site,[299] between −2000 and −460,[300] between −460 and −180,[272, 274, 299, 300] and in the proximal promoter.[300] Deletions[300] or point mutations[272] of these negative elements yield detectable ε globin transcription in adult cells of transgenic mice.

The first silencing element to be studied in transgenic mice[301] was initially identified as a negative regulatory element in transfection assays in cultured cells.[302] This silencer is located between −182 and −467 bp from the initiation site, and it contains three binding motifs important for suppression: a GATA site at −208, a YY1 site at −269, and a CACCC motif at −379.[272, 275] Disruption of a GATA-1 or a YY1 binding site is sufficient for derepression of ε gene expression in adult transgenic mice.[272] Overexpression of GATA-1 in transgenic mice results in a specific decrease of a human ε globin expression.[273] YY1 acts as a repressor in several systems,[303, 304] but the finding that GATA-1 may have a suppressive role in this context was surprising. Thus, several proteins appear to play a role in the silencing of the ε gene presumably by disrupting the interaction between the ε promoter and the LCR.

When the suppressor region (−304 to −179) was deleted from a YAC containing the entire β globin locus, ε transgene expression was essentially abolished, raising the possibility that this region contains elements that are important for the activation of the ε globin gene.[305] Another study, however, found that deletions from a βYAC of a −182 to −467 bp region of the ε promoter did not decrease ε gene expression in embryonic cells.[306] The reasons for such contradictory results are not apparent.

γ Globin Genes

The regulation of the γ globin genes is of special interest because of the ameliorating effects of the synthesis of fetal hemoglobin in patients with β thalassemia syndromes and in those with sickle cell disease (Fig. 5–7). Therefore, the study of the γ promoters has been intense. A large number of proteins has been identified as capable of binding the first 300 bp of the promoter, and many point mutations that produce hereditary persistence of fetal hemoglobin have been identified. Most of these HPFH mutations occur in transcription factor binding sites, and they create new factor binding motifs, or they destroy existing ones. The two γ globin gene promoters are identical in sequence. Each contains a canonical TATA box, a duplicated CAAT box within a 27 bp segment, and a single CACCC box.

The proximal promoter region contains a G-rich sequence between the CAAT box and the TATA box, which has been shown to bind Sp1, and a binding activity called stage selector protein (SSP).[307, 308] Sp1 is not functionally

important in vivo, or it can be replaced by another protein, because the γ globin gene is still expressed in transgenic mice that contain the human β locus but lack Sp1.[286] In contrast, the SSP complex appears to be important. It was originally defined by homology to an element called stage selector element (SSE) found in the chicken γ globin gene promoter.[309] In chickens, a binding activity, NF-E4, interacts with the SSE and, in the adult stage, confers a competitive advantage to the β globin gene promoter over the ε globin gene promoter for interaction with the β/ε enhancer.[309] A sequence between −53 and −34 of the γ gene promoter is conserved in species that express the γ gene in fetal stage, but it diverges in species in which the γ gene homologue is expressed in embryonic cells.[310] This sequence is considered to be analogous to the chicken SSE; SSP binds to this sequence. On the basis of cell transfection experiments, it has been proposed that the γ gene SSE has a similar role to the chicken β gene SSE and that, when SSP binds to SSE, it provides to the γ globin gene a competitive advantage over the β globin gene.[307] Experiments using transgenic mice show that mutations in the SSE that prevent the binding of SSP result in downregulation of the γ globin gene only when it is in competition with β globin gene expression during the switch (Ristaldi and Grosveld, unpublished data).

SSP has been partially purified and appears to be a heterodimeric protein composed of the ubiquitously expressed factor CP2 and a protein from an not yet cloned erythroid-specific gene.[311] The binding of Sp1 and SSP on SSE appears to be mutually exclusive,[308] and the balance of this competition may be regulated during development by the methylation of the two CpG dinucleotides that occur between −55 and −50 in this region. These dinucleotides are frequently methylated in human embryonic and adult cells, although not in human fetal erythroid cells.[312, 313] Methylation of the CpG sequences causes a 10-fold enhancement of Sp1 binding, suggesting, in agreement with the SSE mutation data, that SSP could be an activator at the fetal stage, possibly to be replaced by Sp1 as a repressor at the adult stage. This, however, would only be a secondary effect, because the available data suggest that the γ globin genes are turned off before methylation takes place.[314]

The CAAT box region of the γ globin genes has been subjected to intense studies because point mutations in this region result in HPFH (see Table 5–3). The CAAT box region interacts with a number of proteins.[135, 278, 315–318] CP1, a ubiquitously expressed protein heterodimer, binds to both CAAT boxes and is thought to act as a positive transcriptional activator, although no in vivo functional data on its role are available. CAAT displacement protein (CDP) binds over a broad region, including both CAAT boxes, competitively displacing CP1. CDP acts in vitro as a transcriptional repressor.[319] On the basis of studies using K562 cells, it was claimed that the derepression of the γ globin genes by sodium butyrate (discussed later) was associated with a decrease in the level of CDP,[317] but data in transgenic mice indicate that this reactivation is associated with the upstream part of the γ gene promoter.[320] This contradictory situation may be resolved by the inactivation of the gene coding for CDP and measurement of the effect of the inactivation on derepression of the γ globin genes in transgenic mice.

NF-E3 and GATA-1 have also been associated with γ globin gene suppression, because their binding is decreased by the −117 G to A mutation at the distal CAAT box.[315, 316, 290, 318] However, the introduction of novel mutations that decrease GATA-1 or NF-E3 binding in the CAAT box did not lead to any (GATA-1) or a very small (NF-E3) persistence of expression of the γ globin gene at the adult stage in transgenic mice.[321] A factor designated NF-E6[318] is a member of the cEBP family of proteins[322, 323] and may act as a positive regulator of the γ globin genes.

Destruction or deletion of the γ CACCC box produces only minor decrease in γ gene expression in the embryonic erythroid cells of transgenic mice, but it strikingly decreases γ gene expression in the cells of definitive erythropoiesis of fetal liver and adult marrow.[324, 325] Such data indicate that this motif plays a role in γ gene expression at the fetal stage of definitive hematopoiesis, when the major synthesis of fetal hemoglobin takes place in humans. In vitro studies have shown that several proteins bind to the CACCC box. Sp1 and Sp3 bind to this motif, but they do not appear to play a role in vivo.[286] BKLF/TEF2,[326] which is homologous to EKLF, is expressed in several cell types including erythroid cells; there is no evidence that BKLF effects γ gene expression. FKLF[287] and FKLF-2[288] bind to the γ CACCC box, but their role in the control of γ gene expression in vivo has not been determined.

The upstream part of the γ globin gene promoter contains a number of additional sites for binding of transcription factors, and some of these sites have been uncovered through mutations that result in the phenotype of HPFH. A T to C substitution at −175 of the γ gene promoter is associated with a large increase in γ globin gene expression in the adult.[137, 146] The −175 mutation alters the interaction of this region with GATA-1 and removes a binding site for octamer proteins in vitro,[327, 328] but a direct correlation between GATA-1 binding activity and promoter activity has been difficult, suggesting that another factor may be involved.

The −200 region has several mutations that increase the level of expression of the γ globin genes. Some of these, such as the −198 T to C or −202 C to G substitutions, create improved or new binding sites for Sp1 and SSP, respectively.[308, 329] The improved Sp1 binding site is associated with an increase in promoter activity in a heterologous assay,[330] and the novel SSP site can functionally replace the −50 region in transfection assays in mouse erythroleukemia (MEL) cells.[308] One possible explanation of these results is that these novel binding sites may in part overcome suppression of the γ gene promoter in the adult stage. A second explanation is that mutations of this region operate by altering the DNA conformation. This region of the promoter is capable of forming a triple-stranded structure, leaving the −206 γ to −217 γ region of the promoter single stranded.[331] This structure is thought to be the binding site for a repressor complex that is displaced by the transcription factors that bind to the novel sequences created by the HPFH muta-

tions.[331, 332] In support of the triple-stranded repressor complex are mutations such as an insertion of an additional C at −200, which does not change the profile of factor binding in vitro but which would destabilize triple-strand formation.[139] The two effects, disturbance of triple-strand formation and the creation of new binding sites, could synergize to increase the level of γ globin gene expression.

The further upstream part of the γ promoter contains a large number of potential binding sites for proteins.[310, 326, 333] Experiments with transgenic mice have largely confirmed the role of the different regions of the γ globin gene promoter and revealed a possible upstream region required for proper silencing of the gene.[324] The promoter region also contains a number of polymorphisms that correlate with the level of residual γ globin gene expression in the adult.[334–341]

Transfection experiments have identified an "enhancer" element 750 bp downstream from the $^A\gamma$ gene.[342] This element is sensitive to nuclease digestion in erythroid cells[343] and contains binding sites for GATA-1 and SATB-1, a nuclear matrix–associated protein.[344, 345] Experiments in transgenic mice carrying β locus YAC constructs from which this element was deleted indicate that it has no role in enhancing γ gene expression.[346] This element may be involved in γ gene silencing, because in transgenic mice carrying a γ globin construct containing this 3′ element, the γ gene is silenced autonomously,[347] but in transgenic mice carrying a γ globin gene lacking the 3′ element, γ gene expression continues in the adult stage.[348] However, these experiments are not directly comparable because of differences in the DNA constructs. It is likely that this 3′ element has a functional role, because its presence in μLCR γ gene constructs protects the γ gene from position effects[349, 350] perhaps by stabilizing the interaction between the LCR and the γ gene.[350]

δ Globin Gene

The δ globin gene is normally expressed at very low levels in adults because of a very weak promoter. The major reason for its low level of expression is the absence of a functional CACCC box that would be capable of binding EKLF.[351, 352] Insertion of the β globin gene CACCC box at the normal position of the δ globin gene increases its expression approximately 10-fold.[351]

β Globin Gene

The proximal part of the β globin gene promoter contains an initiator sequence, a TATA box at −30, a G-rich sequence at −50, a CAAT box at −75, and two CACCC boxes at −90 to −110 (Fig. 5–8). The initiator element was discovered through in vitro analysis of promoter mutations and a β thalassemia due to a point mutation at the +1 site of the gene.[353, 354] A G-rich sequence called the "β DRE repeats" is in a position homologous to the SSE binding site in the γ globin gene promoter, and it has been highly conserved during evolution.[355] Mutations of the repeats affect promoter function in transfection assays in erythroid cells, and a DNA-binding activity has been associated with the element.[356]

The CAAT box region is important for promoter function in erythroid cells[357] and has been shown to bind several

Figure 5–8. The β globin gene promoter, showing the position of conserved "boxes" and the binding motifs for functionally important transcriptional activators.

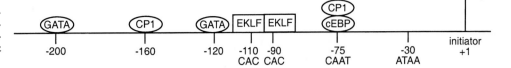

different factors: CP1, GATA-1, and a factor called NF-E6 or DSF.[357–359, 318, 322] CP1 is thought to be a positive regulator of the CAAT box, but as in the case of the γ globin genes, this has not been confirmed in vivo. Similar to what was observed in the case of the γ globin genes, GATA-1 binds fairly weakly at the CAAT box and probably is not functionally important at this position.[290] NF-E6/DSF is cEBP γ[322, 323] and appears to play a role in vivo. Overexpression of a dominant negative mutant of cEBP in transgenic mice leads to a defect in erythropoiesis in general and to a shift in the ratio of γ to β gene expression.[323]

Of the two CACCC boxes, the proximal appears to be more important for function. The CACCC box binds several factors in vitro,[360] but the functional protein in vivo is the transcription factor EKLF.[262, 263] The β globin CACCC box has a higher binding affinity for EKLF than the ε or γ globin CACCC boxes, and mutations that substantially lower the binding affinity of the CACCC box for EKLF produce a thalassemic phenotype.[361] Inactivation of the gene coding for EKLF in mice leads to a fatal anemia because of a failure to express the adult mouse β globin genes.[267, 268] When crossed to mice carrying the human β globin locus, the absence of EKLF affects the expression of the β but not the ε or γ globin genes,[362, 363] even though EKLF is present and active during the embryonic stages of development.[266] Mice that are heterozygous for EKLF express the β gene at a reduced level, although only when in competition with the γ globin gene. Absence or reduction of EKLF does not affect the timing of γ globin gene silencing.[362, 363]

The upstream part of the promoter contains additional binding sites for GATA-1 (at −120 and −200) and CP1 (−160), and these appear to be important for inducible β promoter activity in erythroleukemia cells.[357, 359] In contrast, the gene remains inducible when the LCR is coupled directly to the minimal (−100) promoter.[357] The role of these sequences in the context of the entire locus has yet to be established.

The β globin gene has been reported to contain two enhancer elements, one located near the junction of the second intron and the third exon and another a few hundred bases downstream from the poly-A site of the gene.[358, 359, 364] The activity of the first enhancer has been established by transfection experiments in erythroleukemia cells[358] and in transgenic mice.[364] However, its role has not been confirmed in the context of the LCR or the entire locus, and it is difficult to study because the 3′ half of the intron also contains sequences that are required for polyadenylation and release of the transcript from the template.[183] The role of this enhancer remains obscure. The second enhancer contains four GATA-1 binding sites and stimulates the activity of a linked promoter in transfection experiments.[358] It also functions as an adult-stage–specific activator in transgenic mouse experiments when the transgene is not linked to the LCR.[364–369] When the 3′ enhancer is deleted from a β globin YAC containing the entire locus, expression of the β globin gene

is severely affected in transgenic mice.[305] This element appears to play an important role in the expression of the β globin gene.

ζ Globin Gene

The proximal part of the ζ globin gene promoter contains a TATA box (−28), a CAAT box (−66), and a CACCC box (−95) analogous to those found in the other globin genes. The CAAT box binds CP2,[370] and the CACCC box region binds Sp1-like proteins.[371, 372] Like the ε promoter, the ζ promoter contains DR-1 repeats.[289] The Sp1 binding site overlaps with a strong binding site for GATA-1, and the two proteins bind in a competitive manner. Another GATA-1 binding site is found in the upstream part of the promoter (−230). Transient transfection experiments showed that the two GATA-1 sites are required for the interaction with the HS-40.[373] A positive regulatory element has been identified between −207 and −417.[374] It contains a GATA site at −230, which is flanked at the 3′ side by a CACCC box that binds Sp1 and an unknown factor different from EKLF or BKLF.[375] Another unknown factor, designated URE-BF, that may interact with GATA-1[375] binds just 5′ of the GATA site.

The developmental control of the ζ globin gene is autonomous; all the sequences required for silencing are contained in the gene or the sequences flanking the gene.[376–378] When linked to the HS2 of the β globin LCR, the ζ gene is expressed in primitive erythroid cells but not definitive cells in transgenic mice. This pattern is maintained even when only 128 bp of the promoter are present, suggesting that at least some of the sequences important for suppression of the gene in definitive cells are located close to the gene.[376] Subsequent analysis of this promoter region failed to identify the elements involved in gene silencing. It appears that transcriptional and post-transcriptional mechanisms participate in the silencing of the ζ gene.[2] Synthesis of ζ mRNA continues in the cells of definitive erythropoiesis,[37] but the mRNA is unstable, and it is cleared quickly. Responsible for the accelerated clearance is the decreased affinity of a messenger ribonucleoprotein (mRNP) stability-determining complex to determinants located in the transcribed region and in the 3′ flanking region of the ζ gene.[379–381] In contrast, high-affinity *cis* elements within the α globin mRNA UTR assemble the mRNP complexes efficiently, resulting in stabilization of the α globin mRNA.

α Globin Gene

The α globin gene promoter shows some notable exceptions in structure compared with other globin genes. It lacks a CACCC box, but it has a CG-rich promoter area as part of a methylation free island that extends into the gene.[382, 383] This may explain why, in contrast to the β genes, the α gene is expressed after transfection into non-erythroid cells without the addition of an enhancer.[384, 385] However, the α

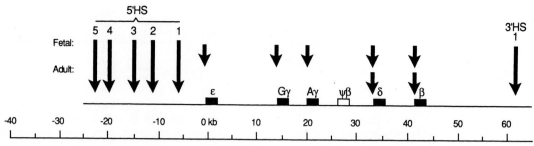

Figure 5–9. Locations of nuclease-hypersensitive sites within the β globin gene cluster. These sites mark the position of nucleosome-free DNase sequences. Developmentally stable hypersensitive sites flank the cluster; 5' hypersensitive sites 1 to 4 are erythroid specific and contain the locus control region (LCR) activity. Each promoter has a hypersensitive site in fetal stage erythroid cells, but only the δ and β genes are nuclease sensitive in adult-stage erythroid cells.

gene requires the presence of the HS-40 or the β globin LCR to be expressed in transgenic mice.[386–390] The α globin promoter binds a number of proteins also bound by the β-like promoters, such as GATA-1 (-185) or CP1 (-90), and a few proteins that are different, such as the inverted repeat protein and CP2.[370, 391–393]

The Locus Control Region

Attention to the region 5 to 25 kb upstream from the ε globin gene was drawn by the discovery of an erythroid-specific, developmentally stable DNase I HS in the chromatin of this region[343, 394] (Fig. 5–9). These sites are numbered 5'HS1 to 5'HS5 from 3' to 5'. HS1 to HS4 are erythroid lineage specific.[343, 394] HS5 was initially considered to be constitutive,[394] but subsequent studies showed that it is expressed mostly in hemopoietic cells.[395, 396] Two new sites, HS6 and HS7, located 6 and 12 kb upstream of the human 5'HS5 have been described,[397] but it is unclear whether they constitute components of the β globin LCR.

The first clue to the existence of important regulatory sequences upstream from the individual globin genes was provided by characterization of deletion mutants that removed sequences to the 5' of the locus but left the globin genes intact[121–126] (Fig. 5–10). The Dutch (εγδβ)° thalassemia has a deletion of about 100 kb of DNA, including the complete LCR and the ε, γ, and δ genes, but it leaves the β globin gene, 2.5kb of the 5' flanking region, and the entire 3' side of the β locus intact. The β gene functions normally in vitro,[398] but in vivo, it is silent, and it is embedded in an inactive chromatin structure.[399] Other deletions of this type have been found (see Table 5–3). In the Hispanic (εγδβ)° thalassemia,[125] a deletion that begins 8 kb 5' to the ε globin gene, leaving the entire gene cluster and the first erythroid-specific HS intact, was shown to silence the entire β cluster.[400]

The seminal observation that conclusively identified the LCR was the demonstration that, when coupled to a β globin gene and introduced into transgenic mice, this region resulted in copy number–dependent, full expression of the gene, independent of the position of integration of the transgene in the host genome.[401] A large body of data obtained by gene transfer into cultured cells and by creation of transgenic animals showed that the activities of the LCR are mostly localized to the core elements of the HSs, which are approximately 300 bp long.

The β globin LCR was the first to be discovered. Subsequently, an erythroid-specific HS localized 40 kb upstream from the ζ globin gene that is required for α-like globin gene expression was detected.[386] This LCR-like element appears to lack the characteristic property of the β globin cluster LCR: the ability to confer integration position-independent, copy number–dependent expression on a linked gene.[402] The LCR is not unique to the globin loci, because a number of LCRs have been described for other genes that are expressed in a variety of tissues.[403–415] Many genes are likely to have regulatory elements that have one or more functions of the LCR.

▼ PROPERTIES OF THE β GLOBIN LOCUS CONTROL REGION

The unique property of the LCR that distinguishes it from a classical enhancer is its capacity to confer integration position-independent expression on a linked gene.[401, 401a] In earlier studies, globin genes without the LCR were expressed in only about one half of transgenic mouse lines and then only at the level ranging from 0.1 to 3 per cent that of a

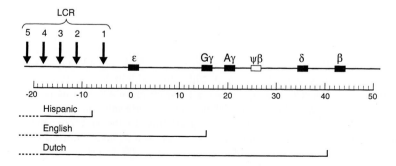

Figure 5–10. The (εγδβ)° thalassemias are caused by a deletion that removes the 5' of the β globin locus, including DNase I hypersensitive sites of the locus control region.

normal mouse globin gene.[366–369, 416] The lack of expression or the variable expression was thought to reflect the influence of chromatin structure or the influence of nearby regulatory elements at the site where the globin transgene had integrated in the host genome.

When integrated in an accessible chromatin structure, such a transgene was expressed, albeit at low levels, but it was silenced when in a non-accessible or heterochromatin environment. Such effects, known as *position effects*,[417] appear to be overcome by the LCR in a dominant manner by always establishing an active chromatin structure and activating the nearby genes.[18, 401a, 419] In this context, the LCR differs from boundary elements, such as described in *Drosophila*,[420, 421] which appear to function by insulating the gene from other regulatory sequences present in the host genome. This does not mean that such sequences are not present in the LCR, because there are good indications that HS4 in the chicken β globin locus does have insulating properties (see below). In addition, experiments with the chicken lysozyme locus in transgenic mice indicate that the locus contains insulating-type sequences in addition to sequences possessing LCR-type activating properties.[422] The insulating sequences of the lysozyme gene appear to prevent position effects in the tissues in which the lysozyme gene is not normally expressed.[422] Thus, the first property of the LCR is an activating function allowing expression of a linked gene in erythroid tissues. The activating function of the LCR leads to structural changes in the chromatin before any transcription is apparent.[423]

Recently, the concept that the LCR is required to open the chromatin structure of the locus has been challenged.[424–426] In contrast to the thalassemia mutants due to LCR deletions,[121–125, 400] which show that the LCR is required for the "opening" of a closed chromatin structure during development and that a failure to do so results in the absence of transcription in vivo, deletions of the LCR from the endogenous murine locus by homologous recombination have shown that the globin genes are still expressed, albeit at a very low level and that DNase sensitivity of the locus is maintained.[425, 426] The results from the knockout experiments were interpreted to suggest that the LCR is not required for the opening of chromosomal domain, and still unidentified elements may be responsible for activation. The reasons for such discrepant results remain unclear.[427, 428]

Another property of the LCR is its ability to confer tissue-specific expression on linked, heterologous promoters.[388] For example, the herpes simplex thymidine kinase gene promoter exhibits erythroid-specific expression in transgenic mice when linked to the LCR, and, furthermore, the promoter becomes inducible during erythroid maturation. The human γ and β globin genes by themselves exhibit erythroid-specific and developmentally restricted expression,[366–369, 416] but the LCR is clearly able to complement this inherent specificity in achieving high-level expression.

The LCR may also have a role in establishing the pattern of early DNA replication that characterizes the locus in erythroid but not in non-erythroid cells.[429–431] The entire β locus, with the exception of sites between the two γ globin genes, and sites 20 kb 5′ to the ε globin gene and 20 kb 3′ to the β globin gene, replicates very early in S phase. In the Hispanic (εγδβ)° thalassemia, this whole region of DNA is replicated late in S phase.[400]

▼ DNASE I HYPERSENSITIVE SITES OF THE LOCUS CONTROL REGION

Mapping of individual HS has shown that 250 to 500 bp of DNA is exposed to nuclease action at each site.[191, 433–436] Formation of these sites is thought to represent displacement of one or two nucleosomes, the number usually associated with this length of DNA. Each HS contains one or more binding motifs for the two erythroid-restricted transcriptional activators, GATA-1 and NF-E2, and for other ubiquitous DNA-binding proteins, most notably those associated with the CACC/GTGG class of binding motifs (Fig. 5–11).

Only one of the HSs, HS2, appears to act as a strong, classical enhancer element[236, 437] in transient transfection reporter experiments in erythroid cells. This property is mediated by a tandem NF-E2/AP-1 binding site[236, 434] that is not found (as a tandem) in any of the other HS. The other elements have very low or no classical enhancer properties, but all of the elements have activating properties when integrated in the genome, after transfection and selection for integration, or in transgenic mice (for review, see reference 438).

HS3 appears to be the most powerful element in conferring an active chromatin structure. With the exception of HS3, individual elements have to be present in multiple copies to activate gene expression.[270, 439]

HSs can exist without being linked to a gene; these sites appear to be independent of transcription.[440] However, it was not excluded in any of these experiments that the HS did not induce the transcription of a host gene at the site of integration or the transcription of flanking sequences or the LCR element itself, particularly since it is known that intergenic transcription takes place in the locus.[441] It is therefore not clear whether the individual HSs of the LCR are capable of establishing hypersensitivity independent of transcription.

The activity of the individual HSs is additive when linked together[438] and increases to levels equal to that observed with the complete genomic 20 kb LCR when all four individual sites are present.

▼ STRUCTURES OF THE INDIVIDUAL HYPERSENSITIVE SITES

The HSs have been extensively characterized with respect to their factor-binding properties in vitro and in vivo.[432–436, 442–447] The proteins bound by the different HSs (see Fig. 5–11) include tissue-restricted and ubiquitously expressed proteins.

One or more GATA-1–binding motifs are found within each HS. The inverted GATA-1 sites in HS4 are required for HS formation.[435, 436] Two of the GATA-1 motifs in HS3, those placed around position 100 on the diagram in Figure 5–11 and flanking the GT motif, are required for LCR activity of a minimal HS3 fragment in transgenic mice.[448] Mutagenesis of the GATA-1 sites at position 230 to 250 of

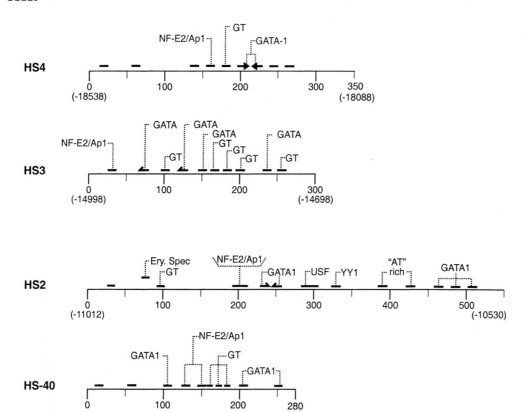

Figure 5–11. Position of binding motifs for various proteins within individual hypersensitive sites.

HS2 reduces the activity of a minimal fragment of HS2 when linked to a β globin gene transferred into mouse erythroleukemia cells.[439] The same mutation has no effect on β gene expression in transgenic mice or on expression of a linked γ globin gene in human erythroleukemia cells. This apparent contradiction may reflect limitations of the assays. Overall, the data suggest critical roles for GATA proteins in LCR function pertaining both to chromatin structure and to gene activity. Although these roles are generally ascribed to GATA-1, note should be made that GATA-2 is also expressed in primitive hematopoietic cells.

The combination of GATA-1 binding sites and a GGTGG motif occurs a number of times and appears to be associated with erythroid specificity. Each characterized HS has binding motifs of this type. GT motifs in each HS are protein bound in intact cells, as shown by in vivo footprinting.[449, 450] Experiments with HS3 in transgenic mice show that EKLF is the active factor at the GT site in vivo and that the binding of EKLF induces a change in chromatin structure detected by DNase I sensitivity.[269] This correlates well with the fact that EKLF binds to members of the SWI/SNF family of proteins, which modify chromatin structure.[271] The transcription factor Sp1 does not have such a role in the minimal HS3 and appears not to have a function in globin gene expression,[286] even though the concentration of Sp1 strongly affects globin gene expression in transgenic mice that carry a mutated LCR and that are subject to position effects[419] (Millot and colleagues, unpublished data). It is unknown whether EKLF is the only "GT" protein active at these sites. A number of other activities have been detected

to bind these sequences, but it is unknown whether any of these are functional in vivo.

Another important binding motif is AP1/NF-E2. The binding motif for NF-E2 is also found in each of the characterized HSs.[436] In the β globin LCR HS2, tandem motifs are phased at a 10 bp interval, establishing binding sites on successive turns of the DNA double helix.[236, 237, 433, 451, 452] These binding motifs for NF-E2 are required for inducible enhancer activity of HS2, as demonstrated in transient assays and after gene integration in human erythroleukemia cells. Furthermore, NF-E2 binding to these sites is also necessary for full LCR activity of HS2 in transgenic mice.[451, 453] Mutations that eliminate NF-E2 but preserve AP-1 binding markedly reduce HS2 activity in each of these assays. Two closely spaced NF-E2 binding sites in α HS-40[373, 454–456] (see Fig. 5–11) play a similar role in the ability of this HS to enhance gene expression.[373] The role, if any, of the NF-E2/Ap-1 motifs in 5′ HS3, HS4, and HS5 has not been defined. Other widely expressed proteins, such as USF and YY1, have been shown to interact with the LCR, but the functional relevance of such interactions has not been defined.

In summary, the LCR is a collection of structurally and functionally different HSs, each containing clustered motifs for several DNA-binding proteins. Three transcriptional activators, GATA-1, EKLF, and NF-E2, with limited cellular distribution of expression that includes red cells, have been directly implicated in the regulation of erythroid cell development and hemoglobin synthesis. Other proteins that interact with the LCR are likely to be ubiquitously expressed. Some protein-DNA interactions defined primarily by in vitro methods may not be functionally relevant or may not even occur in vivo. Only HS2 has strong classical enhancer properties, and HS3 appears to have the strongest chromatin opening capabilities.

▼ GLOBIN LOCUS CONTROL REGIONS OF OTHER SPECIES

The LCRs of several species have been molecularly cloned and sequenced, permitting comparison with the human LCR.[457–463] The general organization and spatial array of the individual sites have been conserved, although the goat genome appears to lack the 5′ HS4. The goat and human LCR share 6.5 kb that are approximately 68 per cent conserved. The homology is between 80 and 90 per cent within and adjacent to the individual HS and specific binding motifs; for example, the NF-E2 sites in HS2 are nearly identical.

The mouse and human LCRs have an identical organization, although insertion of repetitive sequences within this region during evolution has altered the exact distances between sites.[459–461] There are extended regions of significant homology, with the highest conservation within and adjacent to the individual HSs. Overall, the evolutionary comparison suggests that the functionally important sequences extend beyond the core elements of the HSs required for LCR activity in cultured cells and transgenic mice.[463]

The LCR of the chicken β globin gene cluster has also been well characterized.[464–466] It contains four upstream HSs designated 5′ HS1 to 5′ HS4. The chicken LCR confers integration position–independent and copy number–dependent expression on a linked human β globin gene in transgenic mice.[466, 467] A significant difference from the human LCR concerns the function of HS4. This HS marks the 5′ border of the chicken β locus domain (i.e., the transition from DNase I sensitive to DNase I resistant chromatin) and has clear cut properties of a chromatin insulator.[468–472] A 250 bp core fragment accounts for a significant portion of the insulator activity, and a 42 bp fragment within this core is necessary and sufficient for the enhancer blocking activity of the insulator.[469] This sequence is the binding site of CTFCC (i.e., CCCTC-binding factor), a highly conserved ubiquitous DNA-binding protein.[470] Chicken HS4 acts also as an insulator in retroviral vectors.[473]

▼ TRANSGENIC MICE CARRYING β LOCUS YEAST ARTIFICIAL CHROMOSOMES

Regulation of the β locus can be best investigated in transgenic mice using constructs in which the LCR and the globin genes are contained in their normal spatial organization. This was achieved by constructing cosmids containing the entire 70 kb β locus[474] or by using yeast artificial chromosomes.[153, 154, 475–478] Initially, a 248 kb YAC containing the entire β locus, 35 kb of upstream and about 100 kb of downstream sequences, was used.[153] The globin genes of this β YAC exhibit normal developmental regulation. The γ genes are expressed predominantly in the embryonic cells and in the fetal liver cells of definitive erythropoiesis, and they are switched off after birth, while the β gene is expressed only in the cells of the definitive erythropoiesis.[153,]

[479, 476, 478] Globin gene expression is independent of the position of integration of the transgene, and the level of expression per gene copy approximates that of the endogenous murine genes.[478] A smaller YAC, 150 kb long, has also been used for production of transgenic mice with similar results.[154, 478]

YACs provide several advantages for studies of developmental control because of the facility of producing mutations in the locus using the efficient recombination system of the yeast.[153, 478] Single base-pair substitutions[129] or deletions of various sizes (see below) have been introduced in β locus YACs. However, YACs have a tendency to rearrange during the DNA purification or during the process of microinjection of the DNA into the nucleus of the murine oocytes.[478] Integrated YAC transgenes need to be carefully analyzed to verify the structural integrity of the locus. Recently, 150 kb β locus YACs have been produced that contain a rare restriction site in their arms, greatly facilitating structural analysis of the integrated transgenes using pulse field gel electrophoresis.[478] After their introduction for the analysis of the β globin locus, YACs were extensively applied in the analysis of function of several other loci in transgenic mice (for citation see reference 478).

▼ DELETIONS OF INDIVIDUAL HYPERSENSITIVE SITES FROM THE COMPLETE β LOCUS

Deletions of Individual Hypersensitive Sites

Deletion of HSs from the 70 kb locus showed that an intact LCR is required to protect the transgenes from position effects, especially when the transgene is integrated in a strong heterochromatic region, such as the centromere.[419] Deletion of about 2 kb of DNA including the HS3 from a β locus YAC decreased ε gene expression in embryonic cells and β gene expression in the erythrocytes of adult transgenic mice, whereas deletion of about 2 kb of DNA including the HS2 produced a small reduction in expression of all human genes.[479] Another approach was to delete an HS from the murine LCR through homologous recombination. Targeted deletions of HS2 or HS3 from the murine LCR resulted in only moderate reduction of β gene expression.[480, 481] These results suggested that the LCR contains functionally redundant elements and that formation of an LCR complex does not require the presence of all HSs.[479]

Deletions of the Core Elements of the Hypersensitive Sites

In contrast to the deletion of large DNA regions containing an HS, significant phenotypical effects appear when the core elements of individual HSs are deleted in the context of a β locus YAC. Initially, it was reported that deletion of the 200 to 300 bp core element of HS3 and HS4 had catastrophic effects on globin gene expression in all stages of development.[482] A similar catastrophic effect was reported for the deletion of the core element of HS2.[483] These results led to the suggestion that the cores of HSs interact with each other for the formation of the LCR holocomplex and that, when one core is mutated, the whole LCR complex malfunctions.[482] Recent studies including detailed structural analyses of the integrated mutant YACs provide a different picture. Thus, deletion of the 250 bp core element of HS4 shows no effect on ε and γ gene expression in the embryonic cells and position-dependent β and γ gene expression in the adult cells,[484] raising the possibility that the previously reported catastrophic effect of HS4 deletion may have been caused by rearrangements of the YAC DNA.

Deletion of the core element of HS3 produces a specific phenotype characterized by absence of ε gene expression but normal γ gene expression in the cells of the embryonic erythropoiesis and total absence of γ gene expression in the cells of fetal liver erythropoiesis.[296] β gene expression in these mice is position dependent.[296] It appears that the core of HS3 is necessary for ε gene transcription in embryonic cells and for γ gene transcription in definitive cells.[296] These results and those of previous studies[485] provide evidence for developmental stage specificity of the interaction of the HSs with the globin genes.

▼ LOCUS CONTROL REGIONS AND LINEAGE COMMITMENT

Hemopoietic lineage commitment usually is thought to be associated with the expression of new properties not existing in pluripotential stem cells. Alternatively, multipotentiality may be associated with the activation of all chromatin domains required for gene expression in the different lineages, and lineage commitment represents the shut down of the domains not used in a particular lineage upon differentiation.[486] In vitro and in vivo observations on the LCR appear to support the latter model, first proposed by Till.[487] Studies using established lines[488] and CD34+ cells[489] suggest that the HSs are already formed in multipotential hematopoietic progenitor cells; induction of differentiation down a non-erythroid pathway causes a progressive loss of hypersensitivity of the LCR.[488] This concept is supported by in vivo studies in transgenic mice showing that the LCR is active in multipotent (CUFGEMM), bipotent (erythroid-megakaryocytic), and monopotent erythroid progenitors but not in myeloid progenitors.[490] Analysis of the LCR function after transfer of β locus YACs in erythroid or non-erythroid cell lines is also compatible with the possibility that normal activation of the LCR requires interactions with the transcriptional environment of uncommitted progenitor cells.[491]

▼ THE REGULATORY ELEMENT OF THE α GLOBIN GENE CLUSTER

Like the individual genes of the β cluster, the α globin genes exhibit tissue-specific and developmentally modulated gene expression. However, despite similar tissue restriction and developmental modulation, regulatory mechanisms operative in controlling the α globin gene cluster differ in many significant respects from those that control β gene expression.[492, 493]

The α gene cluster lies a short distance (170 to 340 kb) from the telomere of the short arm of chromosome 16.[494] Unlike the β cluster, this region has very high GC content (54%), has a high density of Alu repeats (26% of the entire sequence), and has several CpG islands.[382, 495, 496] A contiguous 300 kb segment containing the α cluster has been sequenced[382]; four constitutively expressed genes lie between the α cluster and the telomere, and five other genes are located in the centromeric site of the α cluster (Fig. 5–12).[382] A large portion of the 300 kb region exists as open chromatin.[495, 497] Several erythroid-specific HSs are found upstream from the α globin gene cluster, within a constitutively active chromatin domain. HS-40, the one HS that has been shown to be functionally relevant to α globin regulation, lies within an intron of a constitutively transcribed gene (see Fig. 5–12).[386, 402, 495]

Several lines of evidence have established that HS-40 is the major regulatory element of the α globin gene locus. Several deletion mutants that remove upstream sequences have been described (see Chapter 6); these mutants leave the cluster intact but nonetheless silence the linked globin genes.[492, 493, 496, 498, 499] When the ζ gene or α globin gene is integrated into MEL cells, α globin gene expression is undetectable or barely detectable after induction, but consistently high levels of α mRNA are measured when the α genes are linked to HS-40.[386] Deletion, by homologous recombination, of a 1 kb sequence containing the HS-40 of a human chromosome contained in a mouse erythroleukemia cell line results in severe downregulation of the α genes.[500] In transgenic mice, the α genes are not expressed in the absence of HS-40, but they are always expressed in an erythroid lineage–specific manner when linked to HS-40.[386, 289, 502] The HS-40 acts as a powerful erythroid-specific enhancer of linked gene expression.[386, 402, 501, 503] However, in contrast to mice containing α genes driven by the β globin LCR,[389, 502] in mice carrying HS-40α gene constructs, the level of α gene expression is suboptimal; it declines with

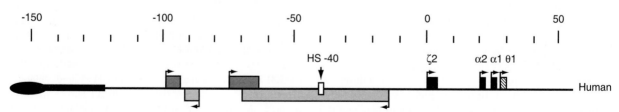

Figure 5–12. Structure of the human α globin gene cluster in 16p13.3. The telomere is shown as an oval and the subtelomeric region as a thick black horizontal bar. The globin genes are shown as black boxes, the θ1 gene as a hatched box, and four widely expressed genes as stippled boxes. The direction of transcription of each gene is indicated by an arrow. The α globin regulatory element (HS-40) is shown as an open box and lies within an intron of the −14 gene. (Adapted from Higgs, D.R., Sharpe, J.A., Gourdon, G., Craddock, C.F., Vyas, P., Picketts, D.J., Barbour, V., Ayyub, H., and Wood, W.G.: Expression of the human α-globin cluster in transgenic mice. In Stamatoyannopoulos, G. [ed]: Hemoglobin Switching. Andover, Intercept, 1995, pp. 165–178; with permission.)

development and is not copy number dependent, particularly at high gene copy numbers. In contrast to the deletions of the β locus LCR, deletions of HS-40 have no effect on DNA methylation or the DNase I sensitivity of the locus; even the DNase I hypersensitive sites of the α gene promoters are formed.[497, 500]

The HS-40 appears to function very much like 5′ HS2 of the β gene cluster rather than the β locus LCR. Similar to the HSs of the β LCR, in vitro data and in vivo footprinting[454–456, 505] have shown that the functional domain of HS-40 is contained in a 300 bp stretch of DNA sequence that includes a number of factor-binding motifs for GATA-1–, NFE-2/Ap1–, and GT-binding proteins.

It is unknown what other sequences in the α globin region are required for continued high expression of the genes. Extensive studies of the locus in transgenic mice using 70 kb cosmids[504] or 150 kb PACS[492] have failed to identify such sequences. One possibility is that sequences downstream of the cluster are required to prevent loss of activity during development through activating properties similar to those of HS-40 or by acting as insulators.

Molecular Control of Switching

Analysis of the developmental expression of the human globin genes in transgenic mice has provided many insights into the mechanism of switching. The mouse is in principle not the ideal system, because there is only a single switch in gene expression from embryonic, primitive cells to fetal or adult definitive cells. The embryonic εy and βh1 genes are expressed in the primitive cells derived from the yolk sack, followed by a single switch to the adult β globin genes starting at day 10.5 in the fetal liver. The human γ and β globin genes without the LCR are expressed at very low levels when introduced in transgenic mice, but they show tissue- and developmental stage–specific expression.[364–368, 416, 506] The expression of the γ and β genes is restricted to erythroid cells, and the flanking regions of the genes appear to contain the elements responsible for stage specificity.

With the discovery of the LCR,[401] the question arose about how the genes are developmentally regulated under the control of this powerful regulatory element. The subsequent studies by a number of laboratories have led to the proposal of a dual mechanism of control of hemoglobin switching: gene silencing and gene competition.

▼ GLOBIN GENE SILENCING

Transgenic mice containing only the ε globin gene with 2 kb 5′ and 150 bp 3′ flanking sequences fail to express the ε gene at any stage of development. When linked to the LCR, the ε gene is expressed specifically in yolk sac–derived primitive erythrocytes, albeit at lower levels than the mouse εy gene.[294, 295] This result indicates that the gene is silenced autonomously, and when the sequences containing a putative silencing element[302] were deleted from the ε gene,[301] expression continued into definitive erythroid cells, albeit at a low level.[301] Autonomous silencing has also been demonstrated for the ζ globin gene,[376–378] but a deletion analysis up to −128 bp in the promoter[376] failed to show the presence of a silencer element similar to that observed in the ε gene. The α gene requires elements from the β LCR or the HS-40 from the α locus to be expressed in transgenic mice. When co-injected with a condensed version of the β LCR, the α gene is not expressed at day 9 of development but is expressed on day 11.[377] When directly linked to the complete or condensed form of the β LCR and a β globin gene, it is already expressed at day 9 of development,[502] although its expression is increased at day 11. Although the results do not quite agree, they nevertheless suggest that the α globin gene has some autonomous stage-specific control.

The γ globin gene is silenced or only expressed at very low levels in adult transgenic mice when linked to the LCR,[347, 348, 507, 508] indicating that the control of the γ globin gene is largely autonomous. The promoter of the γ globin gene is involved in this process, because mutations that cause a non-deletion HPFH in humans also result in high levels of persistent γ globin gene expression in adult mice.[318, 321, 129] The normal silencing in transgenic mice is also overridden when an enhancer region placed downstream to the 3′ breakpoint of HPFH-1[132, 133] is juxtaposed to the ᴬγ globin gene.[134] As discussed earlier, attempts to characterize the sequences and proteins involved in the silencing process have been only partially successful.

The β globin gene is not silent at the embryonic stage of development but is immediately activated when coupled to the LCR[507, 508] and does not appear to be under autonomous control. Instead, it needs the other genes to remain silent at the embryonic stage.

▼ GENE COMPETITION

The finding that silencing the β globin gene requires the presence of the γ globin gene in its normal configuration led to the proposal that the β globin gene is regulated through competition with the γ globin genes.[507–510] It was proposed that the probability of LCR interaction with the γ promoter or the β promoter is primarily determined by the *trans*-acting environment. The gene that successfully competes for the LCR is expressed; the unsuccessful gene is switched off. In the embryonic stage, the LCR interacts with the ε globin gene. In the fetus, ε is silenced, and the LCR interacts with the ᴳγ and ᴬγ genes. In the adult, the γ genes are silenced, and the LCR recognizes β, the last available gene (Fig. 5–13). The concept of gene competition was developed earlier on the basis of transfection experiments with reporter plasmids[511, 512] and the chicken globin genes.[309]

The competitive switching mechanism allows the output of the α and β globin loci to be kept in balance throughout development. Competition ensures that the amount of product lost from the early genes through silencing is automatically replaced by the same amount of product from the next gene. Good evidence for such a competitive mechanism has been obtained from studies of non-deletion HPFHs, showing that the increased production of γ globin chains is balanced by a loss of β globin chains from the β globin gene in *cis* but not in *trans*.[148]

Experiments using changes in gene distances[9, 510] led to the proposal that proximity to the LCR is an important factor in the gene's ability to compete. Introduction of a second β globin gene in the human locus showed that competition

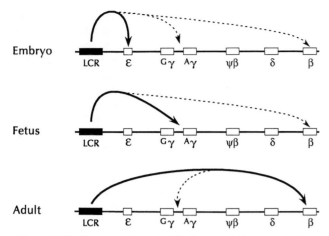

Figure 5–13. The competition model of human globin gene switching.

operated over the entire locus and that the β globin gene is already expressed in the embryo when is present in a position close to the LCR.[513, 514] Similar results were obtained when a heterologous gene was integrated in the human or murine β globin locus:[515, 516] the globin genes are downregulated, and the more proximally to the LCR integrated heterologous genes have the strongest effect on downstream gene downregulation.

Thus, a dual mechanism appears to be operative in the locus to achieve stage specific expression; the major mechanism is autonomous silencing, particularly of the early genes, and the secondary mechanism is gene competition.

▼ MODELS OF REGULATION

The fact that a dual mechanism controls globin gene switching has propelled attempts to decipher how the LCR regulates the genes at a distance. Competition is difficult to explain by some of the mechanisms that have been proposed for the action of distant regulatory sequences. Three different models have been put forward to explain the available data: a binary activation model, a tracking model, and a looping model.[516a]

The binary model implies that when the locus is activated each gene is capable of binding transcription factors

in a stochastic fashion; the genes behave independently of each other and competition does not take place. An additional parameter was proposed to explain why proximal genes have an advantage over more distal genes; transcription of the upstream gene leads to undefined downstream changes that interfere with the transcription of downstream genes. Developmental silencing of the upstream genes permits transcription of the downstream genes. The LCR therefore strictly functions in generating and maintaining an active chromatin domain.[517, 518]

The tracking model proposes that the LCR functions as an entry site for some components of the transcriptional machinery that track along the DNA until it reaches a gene to activate transcription. This pattern provides the proximal genes with an advantage over more distal genes.[519, 520] As in all the other models, the LCR plays an important role in generating an active chromatin structure.

The looping model (Fig. 5–14) proposes that initiation of transcription is achieved by an interaction between the LCR and the genes, looping out the intervening DNA. It is unclear whether the different elements of the LCR form a holocomplex[270, 516a, 521] that interacts as one unit with the gene or a different part of the LCR interacts with different regulatory sequences in or surrounding the gene. Transcription initiation only takes place while the interaction is maintained, and the level of transcription of the globin genes is the product of the frequency of interaction of the LCR with a given gene and the stability of the interaction.

The data obtained by manipulating the human globin locus have shown that there is a clear-cut distance dependence of the gene and LCR that affects the frequency of transcription.[513, 514] They have also shown that the genes on the same allele are interdependent and not transcribed in a stochastic fashion, with only one gene being transcribed at any time.[521, 522] These properties are best explained by a looping model in which the stability of the interactions is most important for the developmental regulation, with an important role for suppression factors that destabilize the interactions.

Cell Biology of Switching

The switches in hemoglobin phenotypes during development were known to physiologists working on oxygen transport

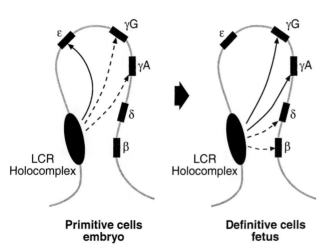
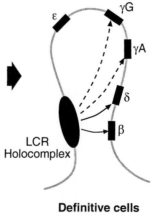

Primitive cells embryo   **Definitive cells fetus**   **Definitive cells adult**

Figure 5–14. The looping model of function of the locus control region.

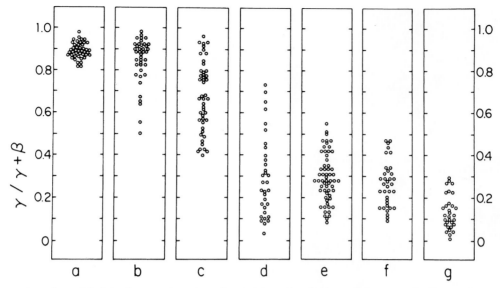

Figure 5–15. Proportions of γ and β chains (expressed as γ/γ + β ratios) in erythroid colonies from various developmental stages. Each open circle represents a measurement in a single colony. a, fetus; g, adult; b–f, newborns.

in amphibians since the 1930s.[523, 524] When simple electrophoretic techniques became available in the 1950s, many new observations were made about the pattern of hemoglobins during the development of various species. Questions such as whether switching is controlled by an intrinsic mechanism or by an inductive extracellular environment or whether it relates to changes in hematopoietic cell lineages were addressed. These questions were again asked in the 1970s and 1980s, when more sophisticated cell biological techniques were introduced. This section of the chapter reviews the major insights obtained from the studies of the cell biology of switching during the past 20 years.

▼ GLOBIN GENE SWITCHING AS AN INTRINSIC PROPERTY OF HEMATOPOIETIC CELLS

When clonal hematopoietic cell cultures were introduced for the study of erythropoiesis, progenitors from various developmental stages were analyzed to gain insights into the cellular control of hemoglobin switching. The levels of Hb F and Hb A observed in colonies derived from fetal, neonatal, or adult burst-forming units–erythroid (BFUe) were generally the expected ones for the ontogenic stage from which the clones were derived.[525] In cultures of adult BFUe, moderate levels of Hb F are produced, but these are distinctly lower than those observed in cultures of fetal or neonatal progenitors (Fig. 5–15). In adult BFUe colonies, Hb F is restricted to a subset of the total cells within the burst that are distributed in a segmental pattern (Fig. 5–16). In contrast, BFUe from human fetal liver give rise to erythroid colonies that make 90 to 95 per cent Hb F. Intermediate Hb F levels are produced in BFUe colonies of neonates (see Fig. 5–15). Apparently, erythroid progenitors encode developmental programs of globin gene expression that are characteristic for each developmental stage, suggesting that switching is an intrinsic property of hematopoietic cells.

▼ SWITCHING OCCURS IN CELLS OF A SINGLE HEMATOPOIETIC CELL LINEAGE

Early models of the control of embryonic to adult globin switching in chickens and in amphibians assumed the existence of two hematopoietic cell lineages: primitive and definitive.[526] The primitive lineage was thought to be irreversibly committed to expression of the embryonic globin program, whereas the definitive lineage was thought to be committed to expression of the adult globin program. Hemoglobin switching was attributed to the replacement of the primitive by the definitive hematopoietic cell lineage. The transitions in major erythropoietic sites during ontogeny seem to support this hypothesis.

Several observations argue against the clonal evolution model of switching. The model predicts a restriction of embryonic globins to primitive cells and of adult globins to definitive cells, but no such restriction occurs. During switching in chickens, erythrocytes of the definitive erythropoiesis coexpress embryonic and definitive globin chains.[527] In the mouse, the primitive erythrocytes of the yolk sac origin, which continue to circulate in the fetal blood after the onset of definitive erythropoiesis, coexpress embryonic and adult globins.[528] In quail chick chimeras,[529] the yolk sac and intraembryonic stem cells generate erythroblasts containing embryonic and definitive hemoglobins.[530] In humans, embryonic ζ chains are observed even in erythroid cells of neonates[38] (i.e., cells of the definitive hematopoietic lineage).

Evidence against the clonal evolution model has also been obtained from studies of clonal erythroid cell cultures. Each colony originates from a single committed progenitor. If there are separate stem cell lineages, embryonic, fetal, and adult globins should be produced in separate erythroid colonies. However, colonies formed by plating progenitors from early human fetuses coexpress ε and γ globins,[531, 532] indicating that during the ε to γ switch the progenitor cells have a program allowing coexpression of γ and ε genes.

Clonal evolution models based on the existence of sepa-

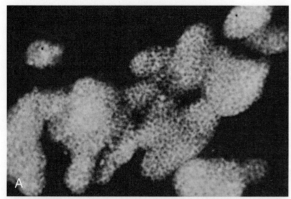

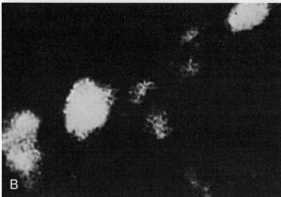

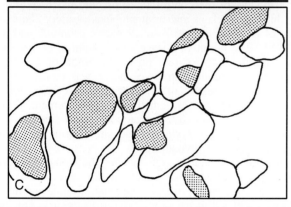

Figure 5–16. An adult erythroid colony (an erythroid burst from a plasma clot culture) composed of many subcolonies has been stained with anti-β (A) and anti-γ globin (B) fluorescent antibodies. All the subcolonies are homogeneously stained in A, whereas only sectors are stained in B. C, The sectors expressing fetal hemoglobin are shown. Such data show that F cells and non-F cells are progeny of a single burst-forming unit-erythroid (BFUe).

rate fetal and adult stem cell lineages were also proposed to explain the γ to β switch.[533–536] Evidence against these models has been obtained from analyses of globins in single neonatal erythroid colonies. If the γ to β switch resulted from replacement of a fetal stem cell lineage by an adult stem cell lineage, there should be a discontinuous change in the pattern of Hb F synthesis in BFUe-derived colonies during the neonatal period. In contrast, if the erythroid progenitors of the fetal, neonatal, and adult stages derived from a single stem cell lineage, a continuous distribution of Hb F values in erythroid colonies is expected during the switching period. Most experimental data support the latter interpretation. The amounts of Hb F in erythroid burst colonies derived from umbilical cord blood BFUe have a continuous

distribution intermediate between the Hb F contents of fetal and adult progenitor-derived colonies[525, 537] (see Fig. 5–15). Although other studies[536, 538] have yielded data interpreted to support the clonal evolution hypothesis, the weight of evidence indicates that globin gene switching occurs in a single stem cell population. Direct experimental evidence against the clonal evolution model comes from analyses of human globin expression in hybrids produced by fusing human fetal erythroid cells with MEL cells.

Heterospecific Hybrids

Somatic cell hybrids produced by fusion of MEL cells with human cells inherit the unlimited proliferative potential of MEL cells and the capacity of this cell line to undergo erythroid maturation after exposure to a variety of inducers. There is rapid segregation of human chromosomes after fusion, and after several generations of growth, only a few human chromosomes are retained by the hybrids. A specific human chromosome can be retained if culture conditions that select for hybrids containing that chromosome are used.

There is no culture condition that can select hybrids containing human chromosome 11. An alternative system based on immunochemical detection of a chromosome 11–linked cell surface determinant allows maintenance of chromosome 11–containing hybrids using immune adherence or cell sorting.[539] When the human chromosome 11 transferred into MEL cells is derived from adult erythroid or non-erythroid cells (fibroblasts or lymphoblasts), only the β globin gene is activated[540–544]; the human fetal globin genes are not expressed in these hybrids. There is, however, human γ globin gene expression when the human chromosome 11 is derived from HEL cells, i.e., a human erythroleukemia cell line producing γ globin.[545] Human γ globin is also produced when the transferred human β locus contains an HPFH mutation.[546] Hybrids that contain a deletion ᴬγᴳγ HPFH chromosome produce ᴳγ and ᴬγ human globins, whereas those containing a −117 ᴬγ HPFH chromosome produce ᴬγ and β globin, as expected from the molecular lesions underlying these mutations.[546]

The most interesting observations have been made when MEL cells were fused with human fetal erythroblasts.[539] Such hybrids produce only fetal or predominantly fetal human globin (Fig. 5–17). Apparently, the human fetal erythroid cell transmits to the hybrids a program that determines that there will be high γ and low β gene transcription. Whether the hybrids express this program because they inherit from the fetal cells a locus producing a *trans*-acting factor that induces γ gene expression remains to be determined. When these hybrids are propagated in culture, a "switch" from γ to β expression is observed (Fig. 5–18). One interpretation of this switch is that the chromosome containing the locus for the *trans*-acting factor required for γ gene expression is initially present in the hybrids but is subsequently lost by chromosomal segregation. However, cytogenetic and restriction fragment length polymorphism (RFLP) studies[547] have failed to support this suggestion. Other possibilities are that a γ gene transactivating locus is present on chromosome 11 and turns off as culture time advances or that the molecular mechanism that controls switching acts primarily in *cis*.[539]

Each hybrid originates from a single cell. The fact that

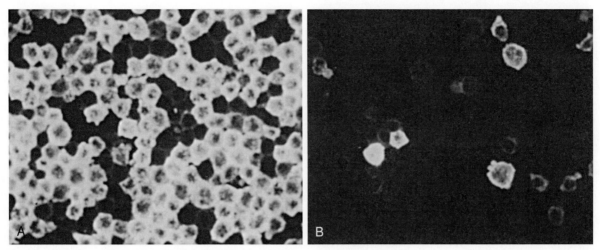

Figure 5–17. Staining of a human fetal erythroid × mouse erythroleukemia (MEL) hybrid with anti-human γ *(left)* and anti-human β *(right)* fluorescent antibodies. Notice the abundance of γ-positive cells on the left and the rarity of β-positive cells on the right. (From Papayannopoulou, Th., Brice, M., and Stamatoyannopoulos, G.: Analysis of human globin switching in MEL × human fetal erythroid cell hybrids. Cell 46:469, 1986; with permission.)

the γ to β switch occurs during the propagation of single-cell clones (see Fig. 5–18) provides direct evidence that the γ to β gene switching occurs in cells of a single lineage.

▼ THE TIME OF SWITCHING IS DETERMINED BY THE DEVELOPMENTAL MATURITY OF THE FETUS

Many observations of human fetuses have been made to detect factors that influence switching. It is possible that switching is related to the rate of hematopoietic cell regeneration, which is very high in the fetus and slows after birth. However, acceleration of erythropoiesis in the fetus has no significant effect on the rate of switching. Thus, infants with hemolytic disease due to blood group incompatibility or newborns with severe hypoxemia from congenital heart disease exhibit a normal switching pattern.[548, 549] A delay in switching is often observed in cases of placental insuffi-

ciency or maternal hypoxia.[550, 551] One cannot conclude that there is a direct relationship between these conditions and switching, because infants affected by these conditions exhibit generalized developmental retardation.

The proportion of Hb F in newborns is related to their age from conception rather than to birth itself.[552–554] Premature newborns have very high levels of Hb F; such newborns switch to Hb A at a time corresponding to the end of their normal gestational period.[555] This observation suggests that the switch is developmentally determined independent of the intrauterine or extrauterine status of the individual; rather, the degree of developmental maturity of the fetus determines the rate and the timing of γ to β switch.

▼ SWITCHING MAY BE CONTROLLED BY A DEVELOPMENTAL CLOCK

The model of developmental clock assumes that hemoglobin switching represents a developmental progression intrinsic to cells that form the erythroid lineage.[525] The clock is set as embryogenesis begins and proceeds inevitably, regardless of external influences. Two sets of observations support this concept.

As described earlier, hybrids produced by fusion of MEL cells with fetal erythroblasts initially produce high levels of fetal globin but several weeks later switch to adult globin synthesis. The rate of the switch of these hybrids correlates to the age of the fetus from which the erythroblasts were derived.[539] Thus, hybrids produced using cells of younger fetuses switch slower than do hybrids produced using cells of older fetuses (Fig. 5–19). It is as if the human fetal erythroid cells "know" whether they belong to an early or to a late developmental time, and they transmit this information into the hybrid cells. The analyses of chromosomal composition of somatic cell hybrids[547] suggest that the developmental clock of switching is located on chromosome 11. The second line of evidence comes from the results of hematopoietic cell transplantation experiments.

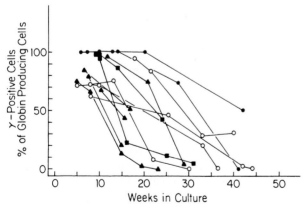

Figure 5–18. Time-related switching of human fetal erythroid × MEL hybrids in culture. Proportion of γ globin–positive cells is shown as the percentage of total cells expressing human globin. Identical symbols represent different hybrids from the same fusion. These results prove that switching occurs in the cells of a single lineage, perhaps by a developmental clock type of mechanism. (From Papayannopoulou, Th., Brice, M., and Stamatoyannopoulos, G.: Analysis of human globin switching in MEL × human fetal erythroid cell hybrids. Cell 46:469, 1986; with permission.)

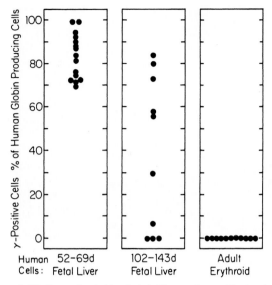

Figure 5–19. Rate of switching in hybrids correlates with the developmental age of the human erythroblasts used for hybrid production. (From Papayannopoulou, Th., Brice, M., and Stamatoyannopoulos, G.: Analysis of human globin switching in MEL × human fetal erythroid cell hybrids. Cell 46:469, 1986; with permission.)

The Transplantation Model

These experiments were designed to distinguish between the mechanisms of "developmental clock" and "inductive environment." The model of the inductive environment assumes that hemoglobin switching reflects physiological changes occurring within the fetus. The hematopoietic environment acts on erythroid progenitors and determines the pattern of hemoglobin synthesis in their progeny erythroblasts.[525] Switching reflects changes in the environment to which the erythroid lineage responds.

Adult bone marrow cells injected into fetal sheep in utero resulted in the formation of erythroid cells containing adult-type hemoglobin.[556] This was interpreted as indicating that the fetal environment failed to influence the program of adult cells.

Another experimental approach has been the injection of hemopoietic cells from sheep fetuses into lethally irradiated adult sheep.[557–559] Analogous observations have been made in humans transplanted with fetal liver cells.[560, 561] In transplanted sheep, Hb F is initially produced. Subsequently, there is a switch to adult hemoglobin production by the transplanted cells. However, the rate of the switch depends on the gestational age of the donor fetus.

The fetal to adult sheep transplantation experiments led to two conclusions. First, the perinatal switch from fetal to adult hemoglobin synthesis is not dependent directly on changes occurring in the organism at that time. Second, the transplanted fetal stem cells appear to know their developmental age and switch slower or faster, depending on the age of the fetus from which they derive.

▼ THE RATE OF SWITCHING CAN BE MODULATED BY THE ENVIRONMENT

Several observations suggest that the developmental clock of switching can be modulated by the environment. Among

the more dramatic changes that occur in the fetus are those of the endocrine system. Fetal thyroidectomy, nephrectomy, adrenalectomy, and hypophysectomy have all been performed in sheep in an effort to influence the rate of switch.[562, 563] With hypophysectomy, there is general developmental retardation; such abnormal sheep fetuses exhibit a delay in the γ to β switch. Removal of the adrenal inhibits the normal increase in plasma cortisol that precedes birth.[563] The γ to β switch in such adrenalectomized animals is delayed, although the animals are grossly normal with respect to developmental progression.[563] Administration of cortisol to establish levels approximating those found in fetuses with normal adrenals allows the switch to progress with normal kinetics.

Attempts have also been made to modulate the rate of switch in MEL × fetal erythroid hybrids. Conditions that accelerate or retard the rate of cell divisions on these hybrids were employed, but there were no differences in switching. External factors, however, could influence the rate of switch. Serum deprivation or addition of dexamethasone in the culture media strikingly accelerated the γ to β switch. Addition of sodium butyrate inhibited switching.[564]

One of the most spectacular manipulations of γ to β switching was done in fetal sheep.[565] In this species, the γ to β switch starts around gestational day 120, and it is completed quickly, so by day 145 when the animal is born, predominantly β chain is synthesized. Preswitch fetuses were cannulated and sodium butyrate was infused. In these fetuses, the γ to β switch was essentially arrested, and lambs with high levels of Hb F were born.[565] As expected, the inhibition of switching was transient, and the switch occurred after birth. These experiments provided proof of the principle that the perinatal γ to β switch can be arrested with pharmacological treatments of the fetus.

Fetal Hemoglobin in the Adult

The γ to β switch is "leaky" in that low levels of γ globin continue to be produced in the adult stage of development. This γ globin is restricted to a minority of cells, called *F cells* (see Fig. 5–3). Activation of γ globin expression occurs in several inherited and acquired conditions and in clonal cultures of adult erythroid progenitors.

▼ HEMOGLOBIN F PRODUCTION IS ACTIVATED BY ACUTE ERYTHROPOIETIC STRESS

Observations in several pathological conditions and physiological states suggest that rapid regeneration of the erythroid marrow induces F-cell production.[566–575] Transient erythroblastopenia of childhood is a condition characterized by an arrest in erythropoiesis. The bone marrow of such children is severely erythroblastopenic but suddenly and spontaneously recovers, and vigorous erythropoiesis appears. This recovery is typically associated with increased F-cell production.[567, 568] Increased F-cell production is also characteristic of bone marrow regeneration after bone marrow transplantation.[569, 576–578] Induction of Hb F also follows the chemotherapeutic ablation of bone marrow.[570] Enhanced F-cell production may also be observed during expansion of erythropoiesis. For example, in severe, untreated iron deficiency anemia, the levels of F cells are within normal limits; after treatment with iron, there is a sharp reticulocyte response, and during this stage of erythroid expansion, F cells are preferentially produced.[566] Acute hemolysis also results in elevated F-cell production,[568] although acquired or congenital chronic hemolytic anemias are only rarely associated with increased Hb F. A kinetic model based on our knowledge of the regulation of F-cell production during erythroid progenitor differentiation has been developed to account for these observations and is discussed in a later section.

An increase in F-cell production early during the second trimester of pregnancy is characteristic.[579, 580] The idea that humoral factors of fetal origin may affect the maternal bone marrow with respect to F-cell production has found no experimental support. Rather, the increase in F cells occurs during a period when the blood volume (and therefore red cell production) in the pregnant woman increases sharply. Hence, the enhanced F-cell production during pregnancy may be analogous to that observed in other situations in which there is acute expansion of erythropoiesis.

The relation between rapid erythroid regeneration and activation of γ globin expression has been documented experimentally. Acute bleeding in baboons or in humans activates γ globin production.[568, 571–575] The induction of fetal hemoglobin by acute erythropoietic stress has also been reproduced in vivo by administration of high doses of recombinant erythropoietin.[581, 582]

▼ HEMOGLOBIN F IN CHRONIC ANEMIA

The consistent activation of Hb F in acute erythropoietic expansion should be contrasted to the findings in chronic anemias. With the exception of hemoglobinopathies and congenital hypoplastic anemias, there is no elevation of Hb F in most patients with chronic anemias.[583] Administration of low doses of erythropoietin to baboons increases the hematocrit but fails to induce Hb F.[581] After bleeding, there is a surge of F-reticulocyte production, but when chronic anemia is instituted, the number of F reticulocytes falls.[573, 575] The difference in the rates of F-cell formation between acute and chronic erythropoietic stress suggests that the *kinetics* of erythroid regeneration influence whether a cell will become an F cell or an A cell.

Among the chronic anemias, fetal hemoglobin is typically increased in individuals with thalassemia or sickle cell syndromes. The major factor in the activated production of Hb F is the intense erythropoietic stress of these syndromes. The levels of Hb F in the peripheral blood reflect the increased rate of F-cell production but mainly the preferential survival of erythrocytes containing fetal hemoglobin.

Sickle Cell Syndromes

Several factors account for the striking variation in the amount of Hb F found in the blood of patients with sickling disorders. One significant influence is the heterogeneous distribution of Hb F in the red cells of patients with these disorders. F cells have a lower concentration of Hb S, and Hb F inhibits polymerization, directly accounting for the lower propensity of F cells to form intracellular polymer and undergo sickling. (See Chapter 7.) Hence, there is selective survival of sickle red cells containing Hb F, leading to amplification of the F-cell population.

There is also marked variability in the intrinsic capacity for Hb F synthesis among individuals with the various Hb S syndromes.[176–179] Co-inheritance of a non-deletion HPFH is likely in many patients who have high levels of Hb F production. Particular chromosomal haplotypes, as defined by restriction enzyme polymorphisms, have been associated with relatively high levels of Hb F and a correspondingly mild clinical syndrome in sickle cell anemia patients of diverse ethnic origins.[584–586] A unique chromosomal haplotype is observed in individuals with sickle cell anemia from Saudi Arabia and the subcontinent of India.[586] The Saudi patients have high levels of Hb F and are more or less free of symptoms resulting from vaso-occlusive episodes.[177, 586, 588] Although the increase in the amount of Hb F in Saudis with homozygous Hb S disease has a genetic basis, it is exhibited only in the presence of accelerated erythropoiesis.

Thalassemia Syndromes

Individuals who are homozygous for β thalassemia have a striking increase in Hb F that is of diagnostic significance. The proportion of Hb F in the blood may range from 10 to 98 per cent, depending on whether the patient has inherited thalassemia mutations of the β or β° variety. The amount of Hb F in peripheral blood grossly misrepresents the actual production of γ chains in the patient's bone marrow.[589] Characteristic of the thalassemic marrow is the heterogeneous synthesis of Hb F by erythroid cells. Those erythroblasts lacking capacity for γ chain synthesis are eliminated in the bone marrow because of the toxic effects of excess α chains. The minority of cells capable of producing γ chains in significant quantity (F erythroblasts) survive preferentially in the bone marrow and in peripheral blood. There may be as much as a 40-fold amplification of Hb F levels compared with the intrinsic capacity for γ chain synthesis.

Patients with homozygous β thalassemia may also inherit a determinant that increases Hb F.[157, 165] The same chromosomal haplotypes observed in individuals with a sickle cell syndrome with high Hb F have also been associated with an increased capacity for Hb F production in thalassemic individuals. Interaction of the β thalassemia genes with mutations that increase Hb F in compound heterozygotes may give rise to thalassemia syndromes of moderate severity. Hb F and F-cell numbers are also above normal in several β thalassemia heterozygotes, although the mechanism for this increase is unknown.

Congenital Hypoplastic or Aplastic Anemias

Congenital hypoplastic anemia (i.e., Diamond-Blackfan syndrome) affects only the erythroid series and occurs as autosomal recessive, autosomal dominant, and sporadic forms.[590] Untransfused individuals with this disorder have elevated Hb F that is heterogeneously distributed among red cells. These patients often improve with corticosteroid treatment and exhibit further increases in Hb F levels. Hematologically normal parents of patients with the autosomal recessive form of Diamond-Blackfan syndrome have no increase in Hb F levels. The mechanism of increased γ chain synthesis in these patients may reflect disordered erythroid progenitor maturation.

Pancytopenia is characteristic of Fanconi's anemia, an autosomal recessive condition that affects all three hematopoietic lineages.[590] Distortions of cell kinetics early in erythropoiesis may form the basis for increased Hb F synthesis.

▼ HEMATOPOIETIC MALIGNANCY CAN INDUCE A FETAL GLOBIN PROGRAM

Juvenile chronic myelogenous leukemia is characterized by striking increases in Hb F production[534, 591, 592]; Hb F may represent 70 to 90 per cent of the total hemoglobin. The red cells of these patients exhibit other "fetal" characteristics, such as low glycolytic enzyme activity, the carbonic anhydrase isozyme characteristic of fetal red cell, and the absence of I antigen. Initially, these features suggested a reversion to true fetal erythropoiesis.[534, 591] However, careful study of red cell populations has shown that the various "fetal" characteristics are not expressed in a coordinated fashion. Some cells having predominantly Hb F may express the I antigen, whereas other cells lacking Hb F express the i antigen. Apparently, there is a gross distortion in the coordinate regulation of gene expression in this syndrome rather than a simple reversion to fetal erythropoiesis.[593, 594] Some patients with a myeloproliferative disorder or a preleukemia syndrome exhibit a striking increase in Hb F production.[595, 596] Their red cells may resemble those found in patients with juvenile chronic myelogenous leukemia with respect to enzyme activity and antigen expression.

Rarely, Hb F synthesis may be increased in patients with solid tumors. Choriocarcinomas of the testes or placenta, adenocarcinomas of the lung, and hepatomas are among the tumors in which this phenomenon has been observed.[597–601] An increased capacity for Hb F production, observed in individuals without anemia who are not being treated with chemotherapeutic agents, suggests the production by the tumor of a humoral substance that influences F-cell production. There is no experimental evidence to support this hypothesis, however.

The increase of F cells in hematopoietic malignancy has been attributed to transformation of "fetal stem cells" that happen to still reside in the bone marrow of the patients.[533, 570, 596] In view of the evidence against the existence of separate fetal and adult stem cell lineages summarized earlier in this chapter, other explanations should be considered. It is possible that malignancy in some way activates the fetal globin program. Alternatively, these fetal phenotypes may reveal the primitive programs of globin expression that are encoded by the transformed progenitors or the stem cells from which the malignant cell population is derived. This hypothesis has also been proposed to explain why a fetal or embryonic globin program is typical of all the human erythroleukemia lines characterized to date.

Human Erythroleukemia Lines

Several human erythroleukemia lines have been established (Table 5–4) by culturing cells of adult patients with hematopoietic malignancies. Typical of all these lines is the expression of a primitive globin program characterized by synthesis

Table 5–4. Human Erythroleukemia Lines

Line	Globin Phenotype	References
K562	ϵ, γ, δ, ζ, α	602–604
HEL	ϵ, γ, ζ, α	604–606
KMOE	γ, β	604, 607
OCIM1	γ, α	604, 608
OCIM2	γ, δ (β), ζ, α	604, 608
RM10	ϵ, γ, δ, ζ†	609
KU-812	γ, β, α	610
CMK	γ^+	611
UT-7	γ (β)#	612, 613
JK-1	ϵ, γ, β, ζ, α	614
MB-02	ϵ, γ, β, α	615
F-36	γ, β, ζ	616
LAMA-84*	γ†	617
MEG-01*	γ†	618, 619
TF-1*	γ†	620

*Phenotype from published reports only. For the rest of the lines, the data are derived from testing in our laboratory.[621]

†These lines have not been analyzed for the presence of the remaining globin species.

( ), Barely detectable; #, presumed positive but not yet tested in our laboratory.

of predominantly fetal and some embryonic globin chains. The K562 cells produce $^G\gamma$, $^A\gamma$, and ϵ chains but no β chains. Human erythroleukemia (HEL) cells produce $^G\gamma$ and $^A\gamma$ chains but no ϵ chains. A variant of the HEL line, HEL-R, shows considerable ϵ gene expression. KMOE cells express mainly γ globin. Predominant γ globin expression is characteristic of OCI-M1 and OCI-M2 cells. These lines also have multiple myeloid-erythroid-megakaryocytic potentialities. HEL cells have monocytic/macrophagic properties.

▼ HEMOGLOBIN F PRODUCTION IN ADULT PROGENITOR CELL-DERIVED COLONIES

Application of the clonal hematopoietic culture methodology to the analysis of hemoglobin synthesis in human progenitor-derived colonies immediately identified higher levels of Hb F production in culture than in vivo.[622] Hb F is not uniformly distributed. Some subclones of the erythroid colonies produce Hb F in all cells, and others have no detectable Hb F, whereas most clones are composed of erythroblasts that contain Hb F (F erythroblasts) and those that contain only Hb A (A erythroblasts) (see Fig. 5–16). Statistical analyses are compatible with the assumption that expression of Hb F in erythroid progenitors depends on random or stochastic events occurring during the first few cell divisions of the progenitor that forms the colony.[623] If the stochastic event occurs with the first cell division, a colony may be formed that is composed of erythroblasts, all or none of which contain Hb F. If stochastic events occur during several subsequent cell cycles, sectorial distribution of Hb F within the erythroid burst-derived colony would be predicted, as is observed.

It has been proposed that one factor influencing the stochastic process by which F-cell production is determined is the stage at which a progenitor cell enters the erythroblast compartment.[623] A "short circuit" of the normal continuum from BFUe to colony-forming unit–erythroid (CFUe) to proerythroblasts may enhance the probability for F-cell formation (Fig. 5–20).

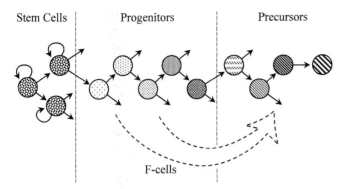

Stem Cells   Progenitors   Precursors

F-cells

Figure 5–20. Model of Hb F synthesis during erythroid maturation and progenitor cell differentiation. The diagram illustrates the hypothesis that F cells are formed by a premature commitment of earlier progenitor cells.

Stochastic events, although apparently random, depend on many parameters. The amount of Hb F in adult human progenitor-derived erythroid colonies may be influenced by conditions within the culture medium. Many of these are poorly defined and undoubtedly account for the different results obtained by various laboratories interested in the switching problem. Other factors that control the amount of Hb F produced in clonal culture without affecting colony development have emerged from well-designed experiments.[624] Sera from sheep fetuses strikingly decrease (or even abolish) fetal hemoglobin in adult or neonatal BFUe-derived colonies.[625] Conversely, fetal calf serum contains inducers of Hb F expression.[626–629] Growth factors such as granulocyte-macrophage colony-stimulating factor (GM-CSF) or stem cell factor have been implicated in γ globin activation in BFUe-derived colonies,[630, 631] although the experimental results have not been consistent.[628]

▼ THERE IS A γ TO β SWITCH DURING ERYTHROID CELL MATURATION

Whenever fetal and adult hemoglobins are coexpressed in human cells, they are produced asynchronously during maturation of erythroblasts.[632–636] Synthesis of γ globin occurs in proerythroblasts and basophilic erythroblasts predominantly, whereas β globin synthesis begins slightly later. There is a hemoglobin switch within the compartment of erythroblasts, but both globins are produced in the peripheral blood reticulocytes.

▼ MODELS OF CELLULAR CONTROL

The heterocellular distribution of Hb F in normal adults and those with many hematological disorders fostered the notion that F cells and cells lacking Hb F might be derived from different stem cell or progenitor cell populations.[533, 535, 536] The finding of F erythroblasts and A erythroblasts in colonies derived from a single progenitor (see Fig. 5–16) disproves this hypothesis.[637] Further evidence against this hypothesis was derived from the study of clonal hematopoietic stem cell disorders such as chronic myelogenous leukemia, polycythemia vera, or paroxysmal nocturnal hemoglobinuria.[638–641] These hematopoietic diseases are of single stem cell origin. Nonetheless, individuals with these disorders exhibit a heterocellular distribution of Hb F, providing further evidence that determination with respect to this phenotypic characteristic occurs after commitment of progenitors to the erythroid lineage.[638–641]

Another hypothesis about the control of Hb F in the adult assumes that early progenitors encode a program allowing expression of fetal globin genes, but this program is changed to one allowing only adult globin expression during the downstream differentiation and maturation of erythroid progenitor cells[637, 642] (Fig. 5–21). Presumably, the earlier progenitor cells contain *trans*-acting factors that favor γ globin expression, whereas the late progenitors have *trans*-acting factors that favor β globin expression. F cells are produced when earlier progenitors become committed prematurely.[642] This hypothesis predicts that, in acute erythropoietic stress, accelerated erythropoiesis increases the chance of premature commitment of early progenitors, resulting in an increment in production of F cells. In contrast, in chronic anemia, the kinetics of differentiation are less distorted, recruitment of early progenitors is diminished, and there is a lower rate of F-cell formation compared with the acute erythropoietic stress.

In support of this hypothesis is the induction of F-cell formation in acute marrow regeneration[566–575] and after administration of high doses of recombinant erythropoietin.[581, 582] Experimental evidence has also been obtained by sequential daily measurements of erythroid progenitor pools in baboons treated with high doses of recombinant erythropoietin.[582] These studies showed that the major effect of erythropoietin is an acute expansion of the late erythroid progenitors and a mobilization of BFUe. An increase in F-programmed CFUe (F-CFUe) accounts for almost all the expansion of CFUe. The increase in F-CFUe is followed by a striking increase in F-positive erythroid clusters, which precedes the appearance of F reticulocytes in the circulation.[582]

Experiments in culture were interpreted to suggest an inverse relationship between fetal hemoglobin expression and the degree of differentiation of the progenitors that form the colonies[637, 642]; alternative hypotheses and variations of this hypothesis have also been proposed.[643–646] Experimental support for this relationship has been obtained in baboon bone marrow cultures in which BFUe-derived colonies produce the highest levels of fetal globin, whereas the most mature progenitors produce the lowest levels.[647] The overall evidence thoroughly supports the hypothesis that the less differentiated erythroid cells have a transcriptional program that permits γ globin gene transcription.

▼ GENETIC CONTROL OF F CELLS

That the F cells of the normal adult are genetically controlled is indicated by the existence of mutants not linked to the β locus that are manifested by increased F-cell numbers. Two loci, one on the X chromosome[173] and one on chromosome 6,[170] have been identified. The ability of individuals to respond with high or low levels of F cells when erythropoiesis is stressed may also be under genetic control. Genetic control of the degree of F-cell response to stress has been shown in baboons; these animals segregate to high F-cell responders

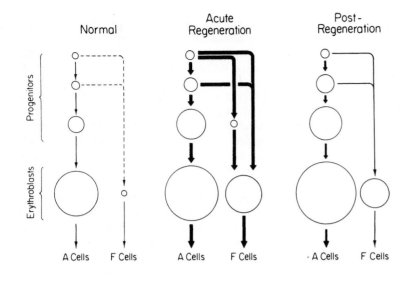

Normal   Acute Regeneration   Post-Regeneration

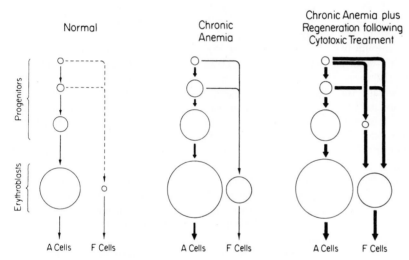

Normal   Chronic Anemia   Chronic Anemia plus Regeneration following Cytotoxic Treatment

Figure 5–21. Model of formation of F cells in the normal adult, in acute erythroid regeneration, in the postregeneration period (or in chronic anemia), and after cytotoxic drug treatment. Normally, only a rare cell becomes an F cell. Acute regeneration forces cells to commit prematurely (to meet the peripheral demand); as a result, F cell production is induced. Expansion of erythropoiesis in the postregeneration stage satisfies the peripheral demand with less distortion of differentiation kinetics; compared with the acute regeneration stage, fewer F cells are formed.

or to low F-cell responders after an acute erythropoietic stress, and this phenotype is transmitted as a simple mendelian trait.[574] Genetic control of the response to acute stress is also indicated by the differences in F-cell response among species. Baboons usually exhibit striking F-cell increases when their erythropoiesis is stressed,[571–574] whereas monkeys (unpublished data) and humans[568] show modest F-cell induction.

Certain β globin locus haplotypes are associated with a higher level of Hb F production in patients with sickle cell anemia or β thalassemia (reviewed by Nagel and colleagues[586]). A reasonable explanation for this association is that haplotypes are linked to variants of *cis*-acting elements that modulate γ gene expression. Such elements may be located in the regulatory regions of the β locus. The activation of γ genes by these variants may depend on *trans*-acting factors present in higher concentration during stressed erythropoiesis. This is a necessary assumption because normal persons who carry these haplotypes have normal numbers of F cells. Observations derived from studies of erythroid progenitors of these individuals in clonogenic erythroid cultures[587] support this interpretation.

Pharmacological Manipulation of Hemoglobin F Synthesis

Considerable progress has been achieved in the last two decades in the pharmacologic induction of fetal hemoglobin synthesis in animal models and in patients with β chain hemoglobinopathies.[648] In contrast to other fields in which therapeutic advances are frequently serendipitous, all the discoveries of Hb F inducers have been hypothesis driven. It was the hypothesis that DNA demethylation can reactivate a dormant gene that led to the use of 5-azazytidine for induction of Hb F in primates[649] and in humans.[650] It was the hypothesis[637, 642] and the subsequent experimental evidence that rapid erythroid regeneration induces Hb F production that led to the use of cytotoxic compounds such as arabinosylcytosine (ara-C)[651] and hydroxyurea[651, 652] for induction of Hb F in primates.

▼ 5-AZACYTIDINE

5-Azacytidine causes DNA demethylation by substituting for cytosine residues in DNA. The incorporated 5-azazytidine inhibits the activity of the methyltransferase that methylates cytosine in newly synthesized DNA.[653, 654] There is a general correlation between cytosine methylation and gene expression; active genes are usually hypomethylated, whereas inactive genes are more frequently methylated, but several exceptions to this rule exist. Globin gene expression correlates with DNA methylation,[312, 313] but DNA methylation does not appear to be a primary mechanism controlling globin gene switching.[314]

The first attempt at pharmacological induction of Hb F synthesis was done by DeSimone and associates,[649] who treated anemic juvenile baboons with escalating doses of 5-azacytidine; a striking augmentation of Hb F production occurred.[649, 655] This effect of 5-azacytidine was observed only in anemic animals, suggesting that optimal drug action required the presence of an expanded erythropoiesis. Subsequently, Ley and colleagues[650] treated a patient with severe homozygous β thalassemia with a 7 day course of 5-azacytidine; a sevenfold increase in γ globin mRNA synthesis, a decrease in α chain excess, and a transient increase in hemoglobin concentration were observed. Induction of fetal hemoglobin was subsequently demonstrated in patients with homozygous Hb S or S/β thalassemia or homozygous β thalassemia.[650, 656–659] Because of concerns about risks of carcinogenicity,[660] this compound has been used only for compassionate treatment of patients with end-stage homozygous β thalassemia. In a patient with severe congestive heart failure due to cardiomyopathy from iron overload, periodic infusion of 5-azacytidine over 2 years reduced ineffective erythropoiesis and increased hemoglobin levels from 6.0 g/dl to 10 to 12 g/dl, allowing the institution of an iron mobilization regimen consisting of chelation and periodic phlebotomies.[661] Another patient who had developed multiple autoantibodies and alloantibodies and severe anemia was treated with 5-azacytidine for 21 months, with substantial hematological improvement.[661]

The mechanism of action of 5-azacytidine has been debated. This cytotoxic compound is expected to kill the most actively cycling erythroid cells. The resulting decrease in late erythroid progenitor cells could trigger rapid erythroid regeneration and induce F-cell formation.[662] Measurements of erythroid progenitor cell pools in baboons treated with 5-azacytidine are compatible with this hypothesis.[662] A direct effect on erythroid progenitors or early erythroblasts is also suggested by studies in culture.[663–665] It is likely that a combined effect on erythropoiesis and on the methylation status of regulatory elements of the β locus is the cause for the superior in vivo induction of Hb F by 5-azacytidine.

▼ HYDROXYUREA

The discovery of Hb F induction by hydroxyurea was a consequence of the debate on the mechanism of action of 5-azacytidine. It was argued that, if cytoreduction and secondary regeneration were the cause of Hb F induction by 5-azacytidine, other cytotoxic compounds producing similar perturbations of erythropoiesis but not DNA demethylation would also induce F-cell formation.[651] Baboons treated with cytotoxic doses of ara-C responded with striking elevations of F reticulocytes with kinetics indistinguishable from those elicited by 5-azacytidine.[651] Induction of γ globin also oc-

curred in monkeys or baboons treated with hydroxyurea.[651, 652] Vinblastine, an M-stage–specific agent that arrests cells in mitosis, also produces perturbations of erythropoiesis and stimulates Hb F synthesis in baboons.[666] Administration of cytotoxic doses of hydroxyurea or ara-C to Hb S homozygotes stimulated γ globin production.[667, 668] Stimulation of Hb F synthesis by cell cycle–specific drugs was transient and associated initially with a reduction and subsequently an expansion of the late erythroid progenitor pools.[664, 667] Following these studies, hydroxyurea, a readily available drug that can be taken orally, that probably is not carcinogenic, and that has been extensively used in the treatment of myeloproliferative disorders, was used for induction of Hb F in patients with sickle cell disease and β thalassemia.

Treatment of Patients With Sickle Cell Disease

Various regimens have been used to define schedules and doses that can produce maximal F-cell stimulation in sickle cell disease.[669–674] The most effective regimen requires a daily administration of hydroxyurea.[674] Highest levels of Hb F are achieved when myelotoxic doses of the compound are used[673, 674]; myelotoxicity mainly manifests with moderate granulocytopenia and is reversible.[673, 674] There is considerable variation in the maximal tolerated dose of hydroxyurea; in general, the levels of Hb F achieved correlate with the dose of hydroxyurea tolerated. Several patients fail to respond to hydroxyurea with a significant increase in F cells.[673, 674] A 4 to 12 week lag period between the initiation of treatment and maximal increase in fetal hemoglobin has been observed.[673, 674]

Several objective measurements suggest that hydroxyurea treatment is beneficial in treating sickle cell disease. A decrease in hemolysis, improvement of red cell survival, decrease in the calculated amount of Hb S polymer in F cells, and virtual disappearance of dense cells from the circulation and of irreversibly sickled erythrocytes from the blood smear have been reported.[673–676] Considerable data were collected from a multicenter, randomized, placebo-controlled trial of the efficacy of hydroxyurea in decreasing painful crises in severely affected adults with sickle cell anemia.[677–681] The trial was stopped a few months ahead of time because of the statistically significant reduction of painful crises in the group of hydroxyurea-treated patients compared with controls. However, not all patients benefited from the treatment. The mean increase of Hb F in all patients was about twofold over the baseline pretreatment level. Few patients achieved levels of Hb F above 20%.[680] More striking elevations of Hb F have been observed after administration of hydroxyurea to pediatric groups of patients with sickle cell disease.[682–687] In addition to the induction of fetal hemoglobin synthesis, other factors such as the alteration of adhesive receptors present on red blood cells and vascular endothelium[688] and the reduction of the white blood cell counts due to the myeloblastic effects of the drug may contribute to the beneficial effects of this compound in sickle cell disease.[681, 689]

The induction of F-cell formation by hydroxyurea was expected under the hypothesis linking F-cell induction to erythroid regeneration.[637, 642] The finding that optimal F-cell responses are achieved with myelosuppressive doses of this drug[679–681] is compatible with this mechanism.

Treatment of Patients With Thalassemia

There are only limited studies on the effect of hydroxyurea on thalassemia major, but it appears that this compound increases the total hemoglobin and fetal hemoglobin in patients with intermediate thalassemia.[690–694] Most impressive results have been reported for patients with HbS/β thalassemia.[695, 696] Increased fetal hemoglobin production and improved erythropoiesis have also been reported for β thalassemia/Hb E patients treated with hydroxyurea.[697]

▼ ERYTHROPOIETIN

Erythropoietin was used to stimulate F-cell production according to the hypothesis that this compound induces rapid erythroid regeneration accompanied by an increase in fetal hemoglobin production.[581] Relatively low doses of erythropoietin failed to induce F cells in baboons. To produce acute regeneration kinetics, high doses of erythropoietin (1500 IU/kg and higher) were used and caused sharp elevations of F reticulocytes.[581] F-reticulocyte induction correlated with the degree of reticulocytosis and the dose of erythropoietin.[581, 698] In contrast to the findings in baboons, erythropoietin produced only minor induction of F cells in patients with sickle cell disease.[699, 700] Patients treated with 800 to 1500 IU/kg/day responded with twofold to threefold elevations of F reticulocytes.[700] Induction of fetal hemoglobin requires iron supplementation.[700]

Treatment of baboons with erythropoietin and hydroxyurea increases fetal hemoglobin in an additive fashion,[701, 702] suggesting that this combination treatment could increase Hb F levels in patients on lower doses of hydroxyurea or increase F-cell production in patients who responded poorly to hydroxyurea alone. It was initially reported that patients treated with maximally tolerated doses of hydroxyurea and erythropoietin failed to show F-cell induction above the level achieved by hydroxyurea alone.[676] Two other studies,[703, 704] however, showed that this combination treatment increases Hb F and F cells above the levels achieved by hydroxyurea. The difference between the two studies may be attributed to differences in the degree of marrow perturbation induced by hydroxyurea. When this compound produces a maximal F-cell stimulation, erythropoietin may fail to increase F-cell production. When F-cell stimulation by hydroxyurea is suboptimal, erythropoietin may further stimulate erythropoiesis to reach its maximal capacity of F-cell formation.

Erythropoietin has been proposed as a method of treatment of thalassemia intermedia.[705, 706] There has been a moderate increase in total hemoglobin in several patients and variable effects on fetal hemoglobin synthesis. The most likely reason for the increase in total hemoglobin is the rescue of thalassemic erythroblasts destined to die in situ; any simulation of γ chain production results in consumption of α chains that, if left unbound, will produce membrane damage and cell death. Such erythroblasts will survive, contributing to the increase in total hemoblast levels. Paradoxically, if such "rescued" erythroblasts also produce β chains, there may not be an increase in fetal hemoglobin, despite the fact that it was the γ gene induction that allowed the erythroblast to survive.

It is questionable whether a treatment that would further expand the already highly expanded erythroid marrow of patients with intermediate thalassemia is desirable. Most beneficial is expected to be the combination of erythropoietin with a cytotoxic drug such as hydroxyurea, and this form of treatment appears to be beneficial in patients with the combination of HbS with β thalassemia.[695]

▼ OTHER HEMATOPOIETINS

Administration of other hematopoietins, such as GM-CSF, interleukin-3 (IL-3), or stem cell factor, has failed to induce Hb F in baboons when these compounds were administered alone. A combination treatment of IL-3 and erythropoietin was tried according to the hypothesis that IL-3 can expand the early progenitor cell pools on which erythropoietin acts. An increase in the absolute numbers of F reticulocytes was observed, but there was no increase in the percentage of F reticulocytes.[707] Another study showed that a combination of hydroxyurea, IL-3, and GM-CSF induced F cells above the level induced by hydroxyurea alone.[702]

▼ BUTYRATE AND OTHER SHORT-CHAIN FATTY ACIDS

Butyrate affects gene expression in many mammalian cell types and induces erythroid differentiation in murine and human erythroleukemia cells[708–710] and embryonic chain production in anemic chickens.[711] Bard and Prosmanne[712] and Perrine and associates[713] observed that the γ to β switch is strikingly delayed in infants of diabetic mothers. With experiments in sheep fetuses, Perrine showed that α-aminobutyric acid, which is elevated in maternal diabetes, is responsible for the delayed γ to β switch.[565] Subsequent studies showed that butyrate stimulated γ globin production in adult baboons.[714, 715] Butyrate also induced γ globin in neonatal erythroid colonies or in colonies formed by erythroid progenitors from adult animals or patients with sickle cell anemia.[714–716] Coadministration of butyrate and erythropoietin in baboons increased fetal hemoglobin in an additive fashion, whereas treatment with 5-azacytidine and butyrate increased fetal hemoglobin in a synergistic fashion.[714, 715, 717]

Subsequent studies showed that several other short-chain fatty acids increase fetal hemoglobin in adult BFUe cultures and in baboons.[718, 719] Derivatives of short-chain fatty acid such as phenylbutyrate[720, 721] and valproic acid[719, 722] induce Hb F in vivo. In vivo accumulation of propionate in patients with propionic acidemia is associated with elevated Hb F in the absence of anemia.[723] Elevation of Hb F has been also observed in patients with conditions associated with increased levels of β-hydroxybutyrate.[724] Other compounds with short carbon chains, such as phenylacetic and phenylalkyl acids,[725] induce Hb F in cultures and in primates.

How short-chain fatty acids induce γ gene expression remains unclear. The prevailing hypothesis is that they exert their effect through inhibition of histone deacetylase.[726] Butyrate is a well-known inhibitor of histone deacetylase in vitro,[727] and it is this function that has been linked to γ globin gene induction. Cloning of histone acetyltransferases and histone deacetylases has provided insights on how acetylation allows activation of gene transcription and, conversely, how histone deacetylate affects gene silencing. Histone acetyltransferases (HATs) catalyze the transfer of acetyl groups to the epsilon amino residues of lysine side chains of the core histones.[728–730] It is believed that histone acetylation leads to gene activation by weakening the binding of histone tail regions to nucleosomal DNA, which makes the DNA accessible to transcription factors.[731] Unlike HAT-mediated gene activation, histone deacetylases are believed to largely mediate gene repression, because deacetylation of histones would allow the histone tails to bind more tightly to the nucleosomal DNA and displace transcription factors. Specificity of repression may be obtained by recruitment of a deacetylase to promoter regions targeted by sequence-specific DNA-binding factors.[732] Targeting HAT or histone deacetylase activities to specific regions of the globin locus would likely alter the acetylation status of histones packaging globin genes and thereby modulate transcriptional factor binding. Hb F induction observed with compounds having histone deacetylase inhibition activity may occur through mechanisms involving increased histone acetylation levels. Fetal globin is induced by histone deacetylase inhibitors in K562 cells, human primary cells,[733, 734] and heterospecific hybrids.[734a] However, it remains to be demonstrated whether alteration of acetylation levels of histones packaging the globin locus specifically affects globin gene expression.

Several clinical studies have been done with sickle cell disease or β thalassemia patients treated with butyrate or butyrate derivatives. Phenylbutyrate[720, 721] or isobutyramide[735] produce only minor induction of Hb F in these patients. A homozygous Hb Lepore patient treated with intravenous administration of arginine butyrate (arginine is added to adjust the pH of the sodium butyrate solution) for more than 50 days increased the hemoglobin concentration from 4.7 to 10.2 g/dl.[736] Apparently, γ globin induction had a profound effect on red cell survival and on the ineffective erythropoiesis in that patient. Another clinical study[737] failed to observe beneficial effects of prolonged intravenous administration of butyrate in patients with severe thalassemia. Other patients, however, responded to butyrate treatment with Hb F induction and significant hematological improvement.[738] The differences between studies perhaps reflect variation in the response to butyrate between patients or differences in the mode of administration of this compound.

Studies in baboons treated with short-chain fatty acids have shown that a decline in F cell production follows the initial induction of Hb F despite continued administration of the inducer to the animal.[718, 719] If treatment stops and is reinstituted a few days later, F-cell production is again induced.[718, 719] It is therefore unlikely that sustained induction of Hb F can be achieved in patients treated for prolonged periods with continuous intravenous administration of butyrate. Most recently it has been shown that intermittent administration of butyrate to patients with sickle cell disease results in sustained induction of fetal hemoglobin synthesis in the majority of treated patients.[743]

Future Prospects

Hydroxyurea and butyrate are first-generation inducers of fetal hemoglobin, and they have undesirable properties. Hydroxyurea is ineffective in several patients with sickle cell disease, and it is of minor benefit in β thalassemia; in addition, life-long treatment of patients with a cytotoxic drug is clearly undesirable. Butyrate is ineffective in several patients, and its requirement for intravenous administration makes it undesirable as a treatment modality for patients with chronic disorders.

New and potent Hb F inducers that have no toxicity or have low toxicity and can be administered orally are required. It is likely that such compounds will be discovered with studies of derivatives or analogues of short-chain fatty acids. It is also expected that the delineation of the *cis* elements and *trans* factors that are involved in γ gene silencing will lead to discovery of new approaches for pharmacologic inhibition of γ gene silencing. Similarly, the cloning and characterization of transcriptional activators and coactivators of γ gene expression is expected to lead to the discovery of a new generation of Hb F inducers of γ gene transcription.

Sickle cell anemia and β thalassemia are unique among human genetic disorders in that nature has shown the way to treat them through the production of fetal hemoglobin synthesis. The challenge to the field of cell and molecular biology of hemoglobin switching is to develop a cure for these diseases by improving on the method discovered in nature.

REFERENCES

1. Stamatoyannopoulos, G., and Nienhuis, A.W. (eds.): Hemoglobins in Development and Differentiation. New York, Alan R. Liss, 1981.
2. Liebhaber, S.A., Wang, Z., Cash, F.E., Monks, B., and Russell, J.E.: Developmental silencing of the embryonic ζ-globin gene: concerted action of the promoter and the 3′-flanking region combined with stage-specific silencing by the transcribed segment. Mol. Cell. Biol. 16:2637, 1996.
3. TomHon, C., Zhu, W., Millinoff, D., Hayasaka, K., Slighton, J.L., Goodman, M., and Gumucio, D.L.: Evolution of a fetal expression pattern via *cis* changes near the γ globin gene. J. Biol. Chem. 272:14062, 1997.
4. Schroeder, W.A., Huisman, T.H.J., Shelton, J.R., Shelton, J.B., Kleihauer, E.F., Dozy, A.M., and Robberson, B.: Evidence for multiple structural genes for the γ chain of human fetal hemoglobin. Proc. Natl. Acad. Sci. USA 60:537, 1968.
5. Huisman, T.H.J., Harris, H., and Gravely, M.: The chemical heterogeneity of the fetal hemoglobin in normal newborn infants and in adults. Mol. Cell. Biochem. 17:45, 1977.
6. Schroeder, W.A.: The synthesis and chemical heterogeneity of human fetal hemoglobin. Hemoglobin 4:431, 1980.
7. Nute, P.E., Pataryas, H.A., and Stamatoyannopoulos, G.: The Gγ and Aγ hemoglobin chains during human fetal development. Am. J. Hum. Genet. 25:271, 1973.
8. Orkin, S.H., and Goff, S.C.: The duplicated human α globin genes: their relative expression as measured by RNA analysis. Cell 24:345, 1981.
9. Peterson, K.R., and Stamatoyannopoulos, G.: Role of gene order in developmental control of human γ and β-globin gene expression. Mol. Cell. Biol. 13:4836, 1993.
10. Adachi, K., Konitzer, P., Pang., J., Reddy, K.S., and Surrey, S.: Amino acids responsible for decreased 2,3-biphosphoglycerate binding to fetal hemoglobin. Blood 90:2916, 1997.
11. Parer, J.T.: Reversed relationship of oxygen affinity in maternal and fetal blood. Am. J. Obstet. Gynecol. 108:323, 1970.
12. Bloom, W., and Bartelmez, G.W.: Hematopoiesis in young human embryos. Am. J. Anat. 67:21, 1940.
13. Knoll, W., and Pingel, E.: Der Gang der Erythropoese beim Menschlichenembryo. Acta Haematol. 2:369, 1949.
14. Wintrobe, M.M., and Shumacker, H.B., Jr.: Comparison of hematopoi-

esis in the fetus and during recovery from pernicious anemia. J. Clin. Invest. 14:837, 1935.

15. Hollyfield, J.G.: The origin of erythroblasts in *Rana pipiens* tadpoles. Dev. Biol. 14:461, 1966.

16. Turpen, J.B., Turpen, C.J., and Flajnik, M.: Experimental analysis of hematopoietic cell development of the liver of larval *Rana pipiens*. Dev. Biol. 69:466, 1979.

17. Maniatis, G.M., and Ingram, V.M.: Erythropoiesis during amphibian metamorphosis. I. Site of maturation of erythrocytes in *Rana catesbeiana*. J. Cell. Biol. 49:372, 1971.

18. Broyles, R.H., Johnson, G.M., Maples, P.B., and Kindell, G.R.: Two erythropoietic microenvironments and two larval red cell lines in bullfrog tadpoles. Dev. Biol. 81:299, 1981.

19. Broyles, R.H.: Changes in the blood during amphibian metamorphosis. *In* Gilbert, L.I., and Friden, E. (eds.): Metamorphosis: A Problem in Developmental Biology. New York, Plenum Press, 1981, pp. 461–490.

20. Maniatis, G.M., and Ingram, V.M.: Erythropoiesis during amphibian metamorphosis. III. Immunochemical detection of the tadpole and frog hemoglobins *(Rana catesbeiana)* in single erythrocytes. J. Cell. Biol. 49:390, 1971.

21. Broyles, R.H., Dorn, A.R., Maples, P.B., Johnson, G.M., Kindell, G.R., and Parkinson, A.M.: Choice of hemoglobin type in erythroid cells of *Rana catesbeiana. In* Stamatoyannopoulos, G., and Nienhuis, A.W. (eds.): Hemoglobins in Development and Differentiation. New York, Alan R. Liss, 1981, pp. 179–191.

22. Ingram, V.M.: Hemoglobin switching in amphibians and birds. *In* Stamatoyannopoulos, G., and Nienhuis, A.W. (eds.): Hemoglobins in Development and Differentiation. New York, Alan R. Liss, 1981, pp. 147–160.

23. Bruns, G.A.P., and Ingram, V.M.: The erythroid cells and hemoglobins of the chick embryo. Philos. Trans. R. Soc. Lond. (Biol.) 266:225, 1973.

24. Papayannopoulou, Th., Chen, P., Maniatis, A., and Stamatoyannopoulos, G.: Simultaneous assessment of i-antigenic expression and fetal hemoglobin in single red cells by immunofluorescence. Blood 55:221, 1980.

25. Chen, S.-H., Anderson, J.E., Giblett, E.R., and Stamatoyannopoulos, G.: Isozyme patterns in erythrocytes from human fetuses. Am. J. Hematol. 2:23, 1977.

26. Tashian, R.E.: Biochemical genetics of carbonic anhydrase. Hum. Genet. 7:1, 1976.

27. Huehns, E.R., Dance, N., Beaven, G.H., Keil, J.V., Hecht, F., and Motulsky, A.G.: Human embryonic haemoglobins. Nature 201:1095, 1964.

28. Hecht, F., Motulsky, A.G., Lemire, R.J., and Shepard, T.E.: Predominance of hemoglobin Gower 1 in early human embryonic development. Science 152:91, 1966.

29. Gale, R.E., Clegg, J.B., and Huehns, E.R.: Human embryonic haemoglobins Gower 1 and Gower 2. Nature 280:162, 1979.

30. Papayannopoulou, Th., Shepard, T.H., and Stamatoyannopoulos, G.: Studies of hemoglobin expression in erythroid cells of early human fetuses using anti-γ and anti-γ-globin chain fluorescent antibodies. *In* Stamatoyannopoulos, G., and Nienhuis, A.W. (eds.): Globin Gene Expression and Hemopoietic Differentiation. New York, Alan R. Liss, 1983, pp. 421–430.

31. Papayannopoulou, Th., and Stamatoyannopoulos, G.: Unpublished data.

32. Kazazian, H.H., Jr., and Woodhead, A.P.: Hemoglobin A synthesis in the developing fetus. N. Engl. J. Med. 289:58, 1973.

33. Cividalli, G., Nathan, D.G., Kan, Y.W., Santamarina, B., and Frigoletto, F.: Relation of β to γ synthesis during the first trimester: an approach to prenatal diagnosis of thalassemia. Pediatr. Res. 8:553, 1974.

34. Bard, H.: The postnatal decline of hemoglobin F synthesis in normal full-term infants. J. Clin. Invest. 55:395, 1975.

35. Boyer, S.H., Belding, T.K., Margolet, L., and Noyes, A.N.: Fetal hemoglobin restriction to a few erythrocytes (F cells) in normal human adults. Science 188:361, 1975.

36. Wood, W.G., Stamatoyannopoulos, G., Lim, G., and Nute, P.E.: F-cells in the adult: normal values and levels in individuals with hereditary and acquired elevations of Hb F. Blood 46:671, 1975.

37. Yagi, M., Gelinas, R., Elder, J.T., Peretz, M., Papayannopoulou, Th., Stamatoyannopoulos, G., and Groudine, M.: Chromatin structure and developmental expression of the human α-globin cluster. Mol. Cell. Biol. 6:1108, 1986.

38. Chui, D.H., Mentzer, W.C., Patterson, M., Iarocci, T.A., Embury, S.H., Perrine, S.P., Mibasan, R.S., and Higgs, D.R.: Human embryonic ζ-globin chains in fetal and newborn blood. Blood 74:1409, 1989.

39. Chung, S.W., Wong, S.C., Clarke, B.J., Patterson, M., Walker, W.H., and Chui, D.H.: Human embryonic ζ-globin chains in adult patients with α-thalassemias. Proc. Natl. Acad. Sci. USA 19:6188, 1984.

40. Farace, M.G., Brown, B.A., Raschella, G., Alexander, J., Gambari, R., Fantoni, A., Hardies, S.C., Hutchison III, C.A., and Edgell, M.H.: The mouse βh1 gene codes for the z chain of embryonic hemoglobin. J. Biol. Chem. 259:7123, 1984.

41. Chada, K., Magram, J., and Costantini, F.: An embryonic pattern of expression of a human fetal globin gene in transgenic mice. Nature 319:685, 1986.

42. Conley, C.L., Weatherall, D.J., Richardson, S.N., Shepard, M.K., and Charache, S.: Hereditary persistence of fetal hemoglobin: a study of 79 affected persons in 15 Negro families in Baltimore. Blood 21:261, 1963.

43. Fessas, P., and Stamatoyannopoulos, G.: Hereditary persistence of fetal hemoglobin in Greece: a study and a comparison. Blood 24:223, 1964.

44. Huisman, T.H.J., Schroeder, W.A., Dozy, A.M., Shelton, J.R., Shelton, J.B., Boyd, E.M., and Apell, G.: Evidence for multiple structural genes for the γ-chain of human fetal hemoglobin in hereditary persistence of fetal hemoglobin. Ann. N.Y. Acad. Sci. 165:320, 1969.

45. Huisman, T.H.J., Schroeder, W.A., Stamatoyannopoulos, G., Bouver, N., Shelton, J.R., Shelton, J.B., and Apell, G.: Nature of fetal hemoglobin in the Greek type of hereditary persistence of fetal hemoglobin with and without concurrent β thalassemia. J. Clin. Invest. 49:1035, 1970.

46. Boyer, S.H., Margolet, L., Boyer, M.L., Huisman, T.H.J., Schroeder, W.A., Wood, W.G., Weatherall, D.J., Clegg, J.B., and Cartner, R.: Inheritance of F cell frequency in heterocellular hereditary persistence of fetal hemoglobin: an example of allelic exclusion. Am. J. Hum. Genet. 29:256, 1977.

47. Stamatoyannopoulos, G., Fessas, Ph., and Papayannopoulou, Th.: F-thalassemia: a study of thirty-one families with simple heterozygotes and combinations of F-thalassemia with A₂-thalassemia. Am. J. Med. 47:194, 1969.

48. Feingold, E.A., and Forget, B.G.: The breakpoint of a large deletion causing hereditary persistence of fetal hemoglobin occurs within an erythroid DNA domain remote from the β-globin gene cluster. Blood 74:2178, 1989.

49. Tuan, D., Feingold, E., Newman, M., Weissman, S.M., and Forget, B.G.: Different 3′ end points of deletions causing δβ-thalassemia and hereditary persistence of fetal hemoglobin: implications for the control of γ-globin gene expression in man. Proc. Natl. Acad. Sci. USA 80:6937, 1983.

50. Fritsch, E.F., Lawn, R.M., and Maniatis, T.: Characterization of deletions which affect the expression of fetal globin genes in man. Nature 279:598, 1979.

51. Bernards, R., and Flavell, R.A.: Physical mapping of the globin gene deletion in hereditary persistence of foetal hemoglobin (HPFH). Nucleic Acids Res. 8:1521, 1980.

52. Jagadeeswaran, P., Tuan, D., Forget, B.G., and Weissman, S.M.: A gene deletion ending at the midpoint of a repetitive DNA sequence in one form of hereditary persistence of fetal hemoglobin. Nature 296:469, 1982.

53. Tuan, D., Murnane, M.J., deRiel, J.L., and Forget, B.G.: Heterogeneity in the molecular basis of hereditary persistence of fetal hemoglobin. Nature 285:335, 1980.

54. Collins, F.S., Cole, J.L., Lockwood, W.K., and Iannuzzi, M.C.: The deletion in both common types of hereditary persistence of fetal hemoglobin is approximately 105 kilobases. Blood 70:1797, 1987.

55. Henthorn, P.S., Smithies, O., and Mager, D.L.: Molecular analysis of deletions in the human β-globin gene cluster: deletion junctions and locations of breakpoints. Genomics 6:226, 1990.

56. Kutlar, A., Gardiner, M.B., Headlee, M.G., Reese, A.L., Cleek, M.P., Nagle, S., Sukumaran, P.K., and Huisman, T.H.J.: Heterogeneity in the molecular basis of three types of hereditary persistence of fetal hemoglobin and the relative synthesis of the Gγ and Aγ types of chains. Biochem. Genet. 22:21, 1984.

57. Wainscoat, J.S., Old, J.M., Wood, W.G., Trent, R.J., and Weatherall, D.J.: Characterization of an Indian (δβ)° thalassemia. Br. J. Haematol. 58:353, 1984.

58. Henthorn, P.S., Mager, D., Huisman, T.H.J., and Smithies, O.: A gene deletion ending within a complex array of repeated sequences 3′

to the human β-globin gene cluster. Proc. Natl. Acad. Sci. USA 83:5194, 1986.

59. Saglio, G., Camaschella, C., Serra, A., Bertero, T., Rege Cambrin, G., Guerrasio, A., Mazza, U., Izzo, P., Terragni, F., Giglioni, B., Comi, P., and Ottolenghi, S.: Italian type of deletional hereditary persistence of fetal hemoglobin. Blood 68:646, 1986.

60. Camaschella, C., Serra, A., Gottardi, E., Alfarano, A., Revello, D., Mazza, U., and Saglio, G.: A new hereditary persistence of fetal hemoglobin deletion has the breakpoint within the 3′ β-globin gene enhancer. Blood 75:1000, 1990.

61. Motum, P.I., Hamilton, T.J., Lindeman, R., Le, H., and Trent, R.J.: Molecular characterization of Vietnamese HPFH. Hum. Mutat. 2:179, 1993.

62. Huisman, T.H.J., Wrightstone, R.N., Wilson, J.B., Schroeder, W.A., and Kendall, A.G.: Hemoglobin Kenya: the product of fusion of γ- and β-polypeptide chains. Arch. Biochem. Biophys. 152:850, 1972.

63. Kendall, A.G., Ojwang, P.J., Schroeder, W.A., and Huisman, T.H.J.: Hemoglobin Kenya, the product of a γδ fusion gene: studies of the family. Am. J. Hum. Genet. 25:548, 1973.

64. Nute, P.E., Wood, W.G., Stamatoyannopoulos, G., Olweny, C., and Fialkow, P.J.: The Kenya form of hereditary persistence of fetal hemoglobin: structural studies and evidence for homogeneous distribution of haemoglobin F using fluorescent anti-haemoglobin F antibodies. Br. J. Haematol. 32:55, 1976.

65. Ojwang, P.J., Nakatsuji, T., Gardiner, M.B., Reese, A.L., Gilman, J.G., and Huisman, T.H.J.: Gene deletion as the molecular basis for the Kenya-γ-HPFH condition. Hemoglobin 7:115, 1983.

66. Baglioni, C.: A child homozygous for persistence of foetal haemoglobin. Nature 298:1177, 1963.

67. Huisman, T.H.J., Schroeder, W.A., Charache, S., Bethlen-Falvay, N.C., Bouver, N., Shelton, J.R., Shelton, J.B., and Apell, G.: Hereditary persistence of fetal hemoglobin: heterogeneity of fetal hemoglobin in homozygotes and in conjunction with β-thalassemia. N. Engl. J. Med. 285:711, 1971.

68. Charache, S., Clegg, J.B., and Weatherall, D.J.: The Negro variety of hereditary persistence of fetal hemoglobin is a mild form of thalassemia. Br. J. Haematol. 34:527, 1976.

69. Matsunaga, E., Kimura, A., Yamada, H., Fukumaki, Y., and Takagi, Y.: A novel deletion in δβ-thalassemia found in Japan. Biochem. Biophys. Res. Commun. 126:185, 1985.

70. Shiokawa, S., Yamada, H., Takihara, Y., Matsunaga, E., Ohba, Y., Yamamoto, K., and Fukumaki, Y.: Molecular analysis of Japanese δβ-thalassemia. Blood 72:1771, 1988.

71. Ottolenghi, S., and Giglioni, B.: The deletion in a type of δβ thalassemia begins in an inverted Alu I repeat. Nature 300:770, 1982.

72. Ottolenghi, S., Giglioni, B., Taramelli, R., Comi, P., Mazza, U., Saglio, G., Camaschella, C., Izzo, P., Cao, A., Galanello, R., Gimferrer, E., Baiget, M., and Gianni, A.M.: Molecular comparison of δβ thalassemia and hereditary persistence of fetal hemoglobin DNAs: evidence of a regulatory area? Proc. Natl. Acad. Sci. USA 79:2347, 1982.

73. Camaschella, C., Serra, A., Saglio, G., Baiget, M., Malgaretti, N., Mantoveni, R., and Ottolenghi, S.: The 3′ ends of the deletions of Spanish δβ°-thalassemia and Black HPFH 1 and 2 lie within 17 kilobases. Blood 70:593, 1987.

74. Mishima, N., Landman, H., Huisman, T.H., and Gilman, J.G.: The DNA deletion in an Indian delta beta-thalassaemia begins one kilobase from the A gamma globin gene and ends in an L1 repetitive sequence. Br. J. Haematol. 73:375, 1989.

75. Gilman, J.G., Brinson, E.C., and Mishima, N.: The 32.6 kb Indian delta beta-thalassaemia deletion ends in a 3.4 kb L1 element downstream of the beta-globin gene. Br. J. Haematol. 82:417, 1992.

76. Oner, R., Oner, C., Erdem, G., Balkan, H., Ozdag, H., Erkan, M., Gumruk, F., Gurgey, A., and Altay, C.: A novel (δβ)°-thalassemia due to a approximately 30-kb deletion observed in a Turkish family. Acta Haematol. 96:232, 1996.

77. Kulozik, A.E., Bellan-Koch, A., Kohne, E., and Kleihauer, E.: A deletion/inversion rearrangement of the β-globin gene cluster in a Turkish family with δβ-thalassemia intermedia. Blood 79:2455, 1992.

78. Efremov, G.D., Nikolov, N., Hattori, Y., Bakioglu, I., and Huisman, T.H.J.: The 18- to 23-kb deletion of the Macedonian δβ-thalassemia includes the entire δ and β globin genes. Blood 68:971, 1986.

79. Craig, J.E., Efremov, G.D., Fisher, C., and Thein, S.L.: Macedonian (δβ)° thalassemia has the same molecular basis as Turkish inversion-deletion (δβ)° thalassemia. Blood 85:1146, 1995.

80. Anagnou, N.P., Papayannopoulou, Th., Stamatoyannopoulos, G., and Nienhuis, A.W.: Structurally diverse molecular deletions in the β-globin gene cluster exhibit an identical phenotype on interaction with the β^s gene. Blood 65:1245, 1985.

81. Waye, J.S., Eng, B., Coleman, M.B., Steinberg, M.H., and Alter, B.P.: δβ-Thalassemia in an African-American: identification of the deletion endpoints and PCR-based diagnosis. Hemoglobin 18:389, 1994.

82. Palena, A., Blau, A., Stamatoyannopoulos, G., and Anagnou, N.P.: Eastern European (δβ)°-thalassemia: molecular characterization of a novel 9.1-kb deletion resulting in high levels of fetal hemoglobin in the adult. Blood 85:1146, 1995.

83. Zhang, J.-W., Stamatoyannopoulos, G., and Anagnou, N.P.: Laotian (δβ)°-thalassemia: molecular characterization of a novel deletion associated with increased production of fetal hemoglobin. Blood 72:983, 1988.

84. Trent, R.J., Svirklys, L., and Jones, P.: Thai (δβ)°-thalassemia and its interaction with γ-thalassemia. Hemoglobin 12:101, 1988.

85. Ottolenghi, S., and Giglioni, B.: γβ Thalassemia is due to a gene deletion. Cell 9:71, 1976.

86. Bernards, R., Kooter, J.M., and Flavell, R.A.: Physical mapping of the globin gene deletion in δβ thalassemia. Gene 6:265, 1979.

87. Baglioni, C.: The fusion of two peptide chains in hemoglobin Lepore and its interpretation as a genetic deletion. Proc. Natl. Acad. Sci. USA 48:1880, 1962.

88. Zeng, Y.T., Huang, S.Z., Chen, B., Liang, Y.C., Chang, Z.M., Harano, T., and Huisman, T.H.J.: Hereditary persistence of fetal hemoglobin or (δβ)°-thalassemia: three types observed in South-Chinese families. Blood 66:1430, 1985.

89. Trent, R.J., Jones, R.W., Clegg, J.B., Weatherall, D.J., Davidson, R., and Wood, W.G.: (^Aγδβ) Thalassaemia: similarity of phenotype in four different molecular defects, including one newly described. Br. J. Haematol. 57:279, 1984.

90. George, E., Faridah, K., Trent, R.J., Padanilam, B.J., Huang, H.J., and Huisman, T.H.J.: Homozygosity for a new type of ^Gγ (^Aγδβ)°-thalassemia in a Malaysian male. Hemoglobin 10:353, 1986.

91. Jones, R.W., Old, J.M., Trent, R.J., Clegg, J.B., and Weatherall, D.J.: Restriction mapping of a new deletion responsible for ^Gγ (δβ)° thalassemia. Nucleic Acids Res. 9:6813, 1981.

92. Mager, D.L., Henthorn, P.S., and Smithies, O.: A Chinese ^Gγ (^Aγδβ)° thalassemia deletion: comparison to other deletions in the human β-globin gene cluster and sequence analysis of the breakpoints. Nucleic Acids Res. 13:6559, 1985.

93. Zhang, J.-W., Song, W.-F., Zhao, Y.-J., Wu, G.-Y., Qiu, Z.-M., Wang, F.-N., Chen, S.-S., and Stamatoyannopoulos, G.: Molecular characterization of a novel form of (^Aγδβ)° thalassemia deletion in a Chinese family. Blood 81:1624, 1993.

94. Zhang, X.-Q., and Zhang, J.W.: The 3′ breakpoint of the Yunnanese (^Aγδβ)°-thalassemia deletion lies in an L1 family sequence: implications for the mechanism of deletion and the reactivation of the ^Gγ-globin gene. Hum. Genet. 103:90, 1998.

95. Fucharoen, S., Winichagoon, P., Chaicharoen, S., and Wasi, P.: Different molecular defects of ^Gγ(^Aγδβ)°-thalassemia in Thailand. Eur. J. Haematol. 39:154, 1987.

96. Winichagoon, P., Fucharoen, S., Thonglairoam, V., and Wasi, P.: Thai ^Gγ(^Aγδβ)°-thalassemia and its interaction with a single γ-globin gene on a chromosome carrying β°-thalassemia. Hemoglobin 14:185, 1990.

97. Anagnou, N.P., Papayannopoulou Th., Nienhuis, A.W., and Stamatoyannopoulos, G.: Molecular characterization of a novel form of (^Aγδβ)°-thalassemia deletion with a 3′ breakpoint close to those of HPFH-3 and HPFH-4: insights for a common regulatory mechanism. Nucleic Acids Res. 16:6057, 1988.

98. Losekoot, M., Fodde, R., Gerritsen, E.J.A., van de Kuit, I., Schreuder, A., Giordina, P.C., Vossen, J.M., and Bernini, L.F.: Interaction of two different disorders in the β-globin gene cluster associated with an increased Hb F production: a novel deletion type of ^Gγ+(^Aγδβ)°-thalassemia and a δ° hereditary persistence of fetal hemoglobin determinant. Blood 77:861, 1991.

99. De Angioletti, M., Lacerra, G., and Carestia, C.: Breakpoint characterization of the Italian (^Aγδβ)° thalassemia showing 3′ breakpoint clustering with those of Indian HPFH and Belgian (^Aγδβ)° thalassemia. Abstracts of the Sixth International Conference on Thalassemia. Malta, 1997, p. 146.

100. Orkin, S.H., Alter, B.P., and Altay, C.: Deletion of the ^Aγ gene in ^Gγδβ thalassemia. J. Clin. Invest. 64:866, 1979.

101. Henthorn, P.S., Smithies, O., Nakatsuji, T., Felice, A.E., Gardiner, M.B., Reese, A.L., and Huisman, T.H.J.: (^Aγδβ)°-Thalassemia in

blacks is due to a deletion of 34 kbp of DNA. Br. J. Haematol. 59:343, 1985.

102. Jennings, M.W., Jones, R.W., Wood, W.G., and Weatherall, D.J.: Analysis of an inversion with the human β globin gene cluster. Nucleic Acids Res. 13:2897, 1985.

103. Pirastu, M., Kan, Y.W., Lin, C.C., Baine, R.M., and Holbrook, C.T.: Hemolytic disease of the newborn caused by a new deletion of the entire β-globin cluster. J. Clin. Invest. 72:602, 1983.

104. Fearon, E.R., Kazazian, H.H., Jr., Waber, P.G., Lee, J.I., Antonarakis, S.E., Orkin, S.H., Vanin, E.F., Henthorn, P.S., Grosveld, F.G., Scott, A.F., and Buchanan, G.R.: The entire β-globin gene cluster is deleted in a form of γδβ-thalassemia. Blood 61:1269, 1983.

105. Diaz-Chico, J.C., Huang, H.J., Juri, D., Efremov, G.D., Wadsworth, L.D., and Huisman, T.H.J.: Two new large deletions resulting in εγδβ-thalassemia. Acta Haematol. 80:79, 1988.

106. Fortina, P., Delgrosso, K., Werner, E., Haines, K., Rappaport, E., Schwarts, E., and Surrey, S.: A greater than 200 kb deletion removing the entire beta-like globin gene cluster in a family of Irish descent. Hemoglobin 15:23, 1991.

107. Abels, J., Michiels, J.J., Giordano, P.C., Bernini, L.F., Baysal, E., Smetanina, N.S., Kazanetz, E.G., Leonova, J.Y., and Huisman, T.H.: A de novo deletion causing εγδβ-thalassemia in a Dutch patient. Acta Haematol. 96:108, 1996.

108. Aulehla-Scholz, C., Spiegelberg, R., and Horst, J.: A β-thalassemia mutant caused by a 300-bp deletion in the human beta globin gene. Hum. Genet. 81:298, 1989.

109. Waye, J.S., Cai, S.P., Eng, B., Clark, C., Adams, J.G., III, Chui, D.H., and Steinberg, M.H.: High hemoglobin A₂β°-thalassemia due to a 532-basepair deletion of the 5′ β globin gene region. Blood 77:1100, 1991.

110. Dimovski, A.J., Efremov, D.G., Jankovich, L., Plaseka, D., Juricic, D., and Efremov, G.D.: A β°-thalassemia due to a 1605 bp deletion of the 5′ β-globin gene region. Br. J. Haematol. 85:143, 1993.

111. Waye, J.S., Chui, D.H., Eng, B., Cai, S.P., Coleman, M.B., Adams, J.G., III, and Steinberg, M.H.: Hb S/β°-thalassemia due to the approximately 1.4-kb deletion is associated with a relatively mild phenotype. Am. J. Hematol. 38:108, 1991.

112. Lynch, J.R., Brown, J.M., Best, S., Jennings, M.W., and Weatherall, D.J.: Characterization of the breakpoint of a 3.5-kb deletion of the β-globin gene. Genomics 10:509, 1991.

113. Popovich, B.W., Rosenblatt, D.S., Kendall, A.G., and Nishioka, Y.: Molecular characterization of an atypical β-thalassemia caused by a large deletion in the 5′ β-globin gene region. Am. J. Hum. Genet. 39:797, 1986.

114. Oner, C., Oner, R., Gurgey, A., and Altay, C.: A new Turkish type of β-thalassemia major with homozygosity for two non-consecutive 7.6 kb deletions of the psi beta and beta genes and an intact delta gene. Br. J. Haematol. 89:306, 1995.

115. Craig, J.E., Kelly, S.J., Barnetson, R., and Thein, S.L.: Molecular characterization of a novel 10.3 kb deletion causing β-thalassemia with unusually high Hb A₂. Br. J. Haematol. 82:735, 1992.

116. Motum, P.I., Lindeman, R., Hamilton, T.J., and Trent, R.J.: Australian β°-thalassaemia: a high haemoglobin A₂ β°-thalassaemia due to a 12 kb deletion commencing 5′ to the β-globin gene. Br. J. Haematol. 82:107, 1992.

117. Gilman, J.G.: The 12.6 kilobase DNA deletion in Dutch β°-thalassemia. Br. J. Haematol. 67:369, 1987.

118. Dimovski, A.J., Divoky, V., Adekile, A.D., Baysal, E., Wilson, J.B., Prior, J.F., Raven, J.L., and Huisman, T.H.: A novel deletion of approximately 27 kb including the β-globin gene and the locus control region 3′ HS-1 regulatory sequence: β°-thalassemia or hereditary persistence of fetal hemoglobin? Blood 83:822, 1994.

119. Motum, P.I., Kearney, A., Hamilton, T.J., and Trent, R.J.: Filipino β° thalassemia: a high Hb A₂ β° thalassaemia resulting from a large deletion of the 5′ beta globin gene region. J. Med. Genet. 30:240, 1993.

120. Lacerra, G., De Angioletti, M., Sabato, V., Schettini, F., and Caraestia, C.: Abstracts of the Sixth International Conference on Thalassaemia and the Haemoglobinopathies. Malta, 1997.

121. Van der Ploeg, L.H., Konings, A., Oort, M., Roos, D., Bernini, L., and Flavell, R.A.: γ-β-thalassemia studies showing that deletion of the γ- and δ-genes influence β-globin gene expression in man. Nature 283:637, 1980.

122. Vanin, E.F., Henthorn, P.S., Kioussis, D., Grosveld, F., and Smithies, O.: Unexpected relationships between four large deletions in the human β-globin gene cluster. Cell 35:701, 1983.

123. Orkin, S.H., Goff, S.C., and Nathan, D.G.: Heterogeneity of the DNA deletion in γδβ-thalassemia. J. Clin. Invest. 67:878, 1981.

124. Curtin, P., Pirastu, M., Kan, Y.W., Gobert-Jones, J.A., Stephens, A.D., and Lehmann, H.: A distant gene deletion affects β-globin gene function in an atypical γδβ-thalassemia. J. Clin. Invest. 76:1554, 1985.

125. Driscoll, M.C., Dobkin, C.S., and Alter, B.P.: γδβ-Thalassemia due to a de novo mutation deleting the 5′ β-globin gene activation-region hypersensitive sites. Proc. Natl. Acad. Sci. USA 86:7470, 1989.

126. Kulozik, A.E., Bail, S., Bellan-Koch, A., Bartram, C.R., Kohne, E., and Kleihauer, E.: The proximal element of the β-globin locus control region is not functionally required in vivo. J. Clin. Invest. 87:2142, 1991.

127. Huisman, T.H.J., Schroeder, W.A., and Efremov, G.D.: The present status of the heterogeneity of fetal hemoglobin in β-thalassaemia: an attempt to unify some observations on thalassemia and related conditions. Ann. N.Y. Acad. Sci. 232:107, 1974.

128. Galanello, R., Melis, M.A., Podda, A., Monne, M., Perseu, L., Loudianos, G., Cao, A., Pirastu, M., and Piga, A.: Deletion delta-thalassemia: the 7.2 kb deletion of Corfu delta-beta-thalassemia in a non-beta-thalassemia chromosome. Blood 75:1747, 1990.

129. Peterson, K.R., Li, Q., Clegg, C.H., Furukawa, T., Navas, P.A., Norton, E.J., Kimbrough, T.G., and Stamatoyannopoulos, G.: Use of YACs in studies of development: production of β-globin locus YAC mice carrying human globin developmental mutants. Proc. Natl. Acad. Sci. USA. 92:5655, 1995.

130. Zhang, Z., Ling, C., Wang, S., and Gaensler, K.M.L.: Globin gene switching in β-globin YAC transgenic with a 12.5 kb deletion of the region between the ᴬγ and δ genes. Blood 90:129a, 1997.

131. Calzolari, R., McMorrow, T., Yannoutsos, N., Langeveld, A., and Grosveld, F.: Deletion of a region that is a candidate for the difference between the deletion forms of hereditary persistence of fetal hemoglobin and δβ-thalassemia affects β- but not γ-globin gene expression. EMBO J. 15:949, 1999.

132. Anagnou, N.P., Perez-Stable, C., Gelinas, R., Costantini, F., Liapaki, K., Constantopoulou, M., Kosteas, T., Moschonas, N.K., and Stamatoyannopoulos, G.: Sequences located 3′ to the breakpoint of the hereditary persistence of fetal hemoglobin-3 deletion exhibit enhancer activity and can modify the developmental expression of the human ᴬγ globin gene in transgenic mice. J. Biol. Chem. 270:10256, 1995.

133. Kosteas, T., Palena, A., and Anagnou, N.P.: Molecular cloning of the breakpoints of the hereditary persistence of fetal hemoglobin type-6 (HPFH-6) deletion and sequence analysis of the novel juxtaposed region from the 3′ end of the β-globin gene cluster. Hum. Genet. 100:441, 1997.

134. Arcasoy, M.O., Romana, M., Fabry, M.E., Skarpidi, E., Nagel, R.L., and Forget, B.G.: High levels of human γ-globin gene expression in adult mice carrying a transgene of deletion-type hereditary persistence of fetal hemoglobin. Mol. Cell. Biol. 17:2076, 1997.

135. Fucharoen, S., Shimizu, K., and Fukumaki, Y.: A novel C-T transition within the distal CCAAT motif of the ᴳγ-globin gene in the Japanese HPFH: implication of factor binding in elevated fetal globin expression. Nucleic Acids Res. 18:5245, 1990.

136. Motum, P.I., Deng, Z.M., Huong, L., Trent, R.J.: The Australian type of nondeletional ᴳγ-HPFH has a C→G substitution at nucleotide −114 of the ᴳγ gene. Br. J. Haematol. 86:219, 1994.

137. Surrey, S., Delgrosso, K., Malladi, P., and Schwartz, E.: A single base change at position −175 in the 5′-flanking region of the ᴳγ-globin gene from a black with ᴳγβ⁺-HPFH. Blood 71:807, 1988.

138. Ottolenghi, S., Nicolis, S., Taramelli, R., Malgaretti, N., Mantovani, R., Comi, P., Giglioni, B., Longinotti, M., Dore, F., Oggiano, L., Pistidda, P., Serra, C., Camaschella, C., and Saglio, G.: Sardinian ᴳγ-HPFH: A T→C substitution in a conserved "octamer" sequence in the ᴳγ-globin promoter. Blood 71:815, 1988.

139. Pissard, S., M'rad, A., Beuzard, Y., and Romeo, P.H.: A new type of hereditary persistence of fetal haemoglobin (HPFH): HPFH Tunisia β+ (+C-200) ᴳγ. Br. J. Haematol. 95:67, 1996.

140. Collins, F.S., Stoeckert, C.J., Jr., Serjeant, G.R., Forget, B.G., and Weissman, S.M.: ᴳγβ⁺ Hereditary persistence of fetal hemoglobin: cosmid cloning and identification of a specific mutation 5′ to the ᴳγ gene. Proc. Natl. Acad. Sci. USA 81:4894, 1984.

141. Oner, R., Kutlar, F., Gu, L.-H., and Huisman, T.H.J.: The Georgia type of nondeletional hereditary persistence of fetal hemoglobin has a C→T mutation at nucleotide −114 of the ᴬγ-globin gene. Blood 77:1124, 1991.

142. Gilman, J.G., Mishima, N., Wen, X.J., Stoming, T.A., Lobel, J., and

Huisman, T.H.J.: Distal CCAAT box deletion in the ^Aγ globin gene of two black adolescents with elevated fetal ^Aγ globin. Nucleic Acids Res. 16:10635, 1988.

143. Gelinas, R., Endlich, B., Pfeiffer, C., Yagi, M., and Stamatoyanno-poulos, G.: G to A substitution in the distal CCAAT box of the ^Aγ-globin gene in Greek hereditary persistence of fetal haemoglobin. Nature 313:323, 1985.

144. Collins, F.S., Metherall, J.E., Yamakawa, M., Pan, J., Weissman, S.M., and Forget, B.G.: A point mutation in the ^Aγ-globin gene promoter in Greek hereditary persistence of fetal haemoglobin. Nature 313:325, 1985.

145. Patrinos, G.P., Kollia, P., Loutradi-Anagnostou, A., Loukopoulos, D., and Papadakis, M.N.: The Cretan type of non-deletional hereditary persistence of fetal hemoglobin (Aγ-158C→T) results from two inde-pendent gene conversion events. Hum. Genet. 102:629, 1998.

146. Stoming, T.A., Stoming, G.S., Lanclos, K.D., Fei, Y.I., Altay, C., Kutlar, F., and Huisman, T.H.J.: An ^Aγ type of nondeletional hereditary persistence of fetal hemoglobin with a T→C mutation at position −175 to the cap site of the ^Aγ globin gene. Blood 73:329, 1989.

147. Costa, F.F., Zago, M.A., Cheng, G., Nechtman, J.F., Stoming, T.A., and Huisman, T.H.J.: The Brazilian type of nondeletional ^Aγ-fetal hemoglobin has a C-G substitution at nucleotide −195 of the ^Aγ-globin gene. Blood 76:1896, 1990.

148. Giglioni, B., Casini, C., Mantovani, R., Merli, S., Comi, P., Ottolenghi, S., Saglio, G., Camaschella, C., and Mazza, U.: A molecular study of a family with Greek hereditary persistence of fetal hemoglobin and β-thalassemia. EMBO J 3:2641, 1984.

149. Farquhar, M., Gelinas, R., Tatsis, B., Murray, J., Yagi, M., Mueller, R., and Stamatoyannopoulos, G.: Restriction endonuclease mapping of γδβ globin region in ^Gγβ+ HPFH and a Chinese ^Aγ HPFH variant. Am. J. Hum. Genet. 35:611, 1983.

150. Gelinas, R., Bender, M., Lotshaw, C., Waber, P., Kazazian, H., Jr., and Stamatoyannopoulos, G.: Chinese ^Aγ HPFH: C to T substitution at position −196 of the ^Aγ gene promoter. Blood 67:1777, 1986.

151. Tate, V.E., Wood, W.G., and Weatherall, D.J.: The British form of hereditary persistence of fetal hemoglobin results from a single base pair mutation adjacent to an S1 hypersensitive site 5′ to the ^Aγ globin gene. Blood 68:1389, 1986.

152. Gilman, J.G., Mishima, N., Wen, X.J., Kutlar, F., and Huisman, T.H.J.: Upstream promoter mutation associated with modest elevation of fetal hemoglobin expression in human adults. Blood 72:78, 1988.

153. Peterson, K.R., Clegg, C.H., Huxley, C., Josephson, B.M., Haugen, H.S., Furukawa, T., Stamatoyannopoulos, G.: Transgenic mice con-taining a 248 kb human β locus yeast artificial chromosome display proper developmental control of human globin genes. Proc. Natl. Acad. Sci. USA 90:7593, 1993.

154. Gaensler, K.M., Kitamura, M., and Kan, Y.W.: Germ-line transmission and developmental regulation of a 150-kb yeast artificial chromosome containing the human β-globin locus in transgenic mice. Proc. Natl. Acad. Sci. USA 23:11381, 1993.

155. Marti, H.R.: Normale und anormale menschliche Hämoglobine. Ber-lin, Springer-Verlag, 1987, pp. 81–89.

156. Stamatoyannopoulos, G., Wood, W.G., Papayannopoulou, Th., and Nute, P.E.: A new form of hereditary persistence of fetal hemoglobin in blacks and its association with sickle cell trait. Blood 46:683, 1975.

157. Wood, W.G., Weatherall, D.J., and Clegg, J.B.: Interaction of hetero-cellular hereditary persistence of foetal haemoglobin with β thalas-semia and sickle cell anaemia. Nature 264:247, 1976.

158. Zago, M.A., Wood, W.G., Clegg, J.B., Weatherall, D.J., O'Sullivan, M., and Gunson, H.: Genetic control of F cells in human adults. Blood 53:977, 1979.

159. Milner, P.F., Leibfarth, J.D., Ford, J., Barton, B.P., Grenett, H.E., and Garver, F.A.: Increased Hb in sickle cell anemia is determined by a factor linked to the β^s gene from one parent. Blood 63:64, 1984.

160. Gianni, A.M., Bregni, M., Cappellini, M.D., Fiorelli, G., Taramelli, R., Giglioni, B., Comi, P., and Ottolenghi, S.: A gene controlling fetal hemoglobin expression in adults is not linked to the non-α globin cluster. EMBO J. 2:921, 1983.

161. Giampaolo, A., Mavilio, F., Sposi, N.M., Care, A., Massa, A., Cianetti, L., Petrini, M., Russo, R., Cappellini, M.D., and Marinucci, M.: Heterocellular hereditary persistence of fetal hemoglobin (HPFH): molecular mechanisms of abnormal γ-gene expression in association with β thalassemia and linkage relationship with the β-globin gene cluster. Hum. Genet. 66:151, 1984.

162. Cappellini, M.D., Fiorelli, G., and Bernini, L.F.: Interaction between

163. homozygous β° thalassemia and the Swiss type of hereditary persis-tence of fetal haemoglobin. Br. J. Haematol. 48:561, 1981.

163. Martinez, G., Novelletto, A., DiRienzo, A., Felicetti, L., and Colombo, B.: A case of hereditary persistence of fetal hemoglobin caused by a gene not linked to the β-globin cluster. Hum. Genet. 82:335, 1989.

164. Dover, G.J., Boyer, S.H., and Pembrey, M.E.: F-cell production in sickle cell anemia: regulation by genes linked to β-hemoglobin locus. Science 211:1441, 1981.

165. Prchal, J., and Stamatoyannopoulos, G.: Two siblings with unusually mild homozygous β-thalassemia: a didactic example of the effect of a nonallelic modifier gene on the expressivity of a monogenic disorder. Am. J. Med. Genet. 10:291, 1981.

166. Boyer, S.H., Dover, G.J., Sergeant, G.R., Smith, K.D., Antonarakis, S.E., Embury, S.H., Margolet, L., Noyes, A.N., Boyer, M.L., and Bias, W.B.: Production of F cells in sickle cell anemia: regulation by a genetic locus or loci separate from the β-globin gene cluster. Blood 64:1053, 1984.

167. Thein, S.L., and Weatherall, D.J.: A non-deletion hereditary persis-tence of fetal hemoglobin (HPFH) determinant not linked to the β-globin gene complex. Prog. Clin. Biol. Res. 316B:97, 1989.

168. Oppenheim, A., Yaari, A., Rund, D., Rachmilewitz, E.A., Nathan, D., Wong, C., Kazazian, H.H., Jr., and Miller, B.: Intrinsic potential for high fetal hemoglobin production in a Druz family with β-thalassemia is due to an unlinked genetic determinant. Hum. Genet. 86:175, 1990.

169. Seltzer, W.K., Abshire, T.C., Lane, P.A., Roloff, J.S., and Githens, J.H.: Molecular genetic studies in black families with sickle cell anemia and unusually high levels of fetal hemoglobin. Hemoglobin 16:363, 1992.

170. Craig, J.E., Rochette, J., Fisher, C.A., Weatherall, D.J., Marc S., Lathrop, G.M., Demenais, F., and Thein, S.: Dissecting the loci con-trolling fetal haemoglobin production on chromosomes 11p and 6q by the regressive approach. Nat. Genet. 12:58, 1996.

171. Craig, J.E., Rochette, J., Sampietro, M., Wilkie, A.O., Barnetson, R., Hatton, C.S., Demenais, F., and Thein, S.L.: Genetic heterogeneity in heterocellular hereditary persistence of fetal hemoglobin. Blood 90:428, 1997.

172. Miyoshi, K., Kaneto, Y., Kawai, H., Ohchi, H., Niki, S., Hasegawa, K., Shirakami, A., and Yamano, T.: X-linked dominant control of F-cells in normal adult life: characterization of the Swiss type as heredi-tary persistence of fetal hemoglobin regulated dominantly by gene(s) on X chromosome. Blood 72:1854, 1988.

173. Dover, G.J., Smith, K.D., Chang, Y.C., Purvis, S., Mays, A., Meyers, D.A., Sheils, C., and Serjeant, G.: Fetal hemoglobin levels in sickle cell disease and normal individuals are partially controlled by an X-linked gene located at Xp22.2. Blood 80:816, 1992.

174. Chang, Y.C., Smith, K.D., Moore, R.D., Serjeant, G.R., and Dover, G.J.: An analysis of fetal hemoglobin variation in sickle cell disease: the relative contributions of the X-linked factor, β-globin haplotypes, α-globin gene number, gender, and age. Blood 85:1111, 1995.

175. Thein, S.L., Sampietro, M., Rohde, K., Rochette, J., Weatherall, D.J., Lathrop, G.M., and Demenais, F.: Detection of a major gene for heterocellular hereditary persistence of fetal hemoglobin after account-ing for genetic modifiers. Am. J. Hum. Genet. 54:214, 1994.

176. Serjeant, G.R., Serjeant, B.E., and Mason, K.: Heterocellular heredi-tary persistence of fetal haemoglobin and homozygous sickle-cell disease. Lancet 1:795, 1977.

177. Perrine, R.P., Brown, M.J., Clegg, J.B., Weatherall, D.J., and May, A.: Benign sickle-cell anaemia. Lancet 2:1163, 1972.

178. Wood, W.G., Pembrey, M.E., Serjeant, G.R., Perrine, R.P., and Weath-erall, D.J.: Hb F synthesis in sickle cell anaemia: a comparison of Saudi Arabian cases with those of African origin. Br. J. Haematol. 45:431, 1980.

179. Ali, S.A.: Milder variant of sickle-cell disease in Arabs in Kuwait associated with unusually high level of foetal haemoglobin. Br. J. Haematol. 19:613, 1970.

180. Eaton, W.A.: The relationship between coding sequences and function in hemoglobin. Nature 284:183, 1980.

181. Go, M.: Correlation of DNA exonic regions with protein structural units in hemoglobin. Nature 291:90, 1981.

182. Collis, P., Antoniou, M., and Grosveld, F.: Definition of the minimal requirements within the human beta-globin gene and the dominant control region for high level expression. EMBO J. 9:233, 1990.

183. Antoniou, M., Geraghtry, F., Hurst, J., and Grosveld, F.: Efficient 3′-end formation of human beta-globin mRNA in vivo requires sequences within the last intron but occurs independently of the splicing reaction. Nucleic Acids Res. 26:721, 1998.

184. Orkin, S.H.: GATA-binding transcription factors in hematopoietic cells. Blood 80:575, 1992.

185. Martin, D.I.K., Zon, L.I., Mutter, G., and Orkin, S.H.: Expression of an erythroid transcription factor in megakaryocytic and mast cell lineages. Nature 344:444, 1990.

186. Romeo, P.-H., Prandini, M.-H., Joulin, V., Mignotte, V., Prenant, M., Vainchenker, W., Marguerie, G., and Uzan, G.: Megakaryocytic and erythrocytic lineages share specific transcription factors. Nature 344:447, 1990.

187. Mouthon, M.-A., Bernard, O., Mitjavila, M.-T., Romeo, P.-H., Vainchenker, W., and Mathieu-Mahul, D.: Expression of tal-1 and GATA-binding proteins during human hematopoiesis. Blood 81:647, 1993.

188. Sposi, N.M., Zon, L.I., Care, A., Valtieri, M., Testa, U., Gabbianelli, M., Mariani, G., Bottero, L., Mather, C., Orkin, S.H., and Peschle, C.: Cell cycle–dependent initiation and lineage-dependent abrogation of GATA-1 expression in pure differentiating hematopoietic progenitors. Proc. Natl. Acad. Sci. USA 89:6353, 1992.

189. Crotta, S., Nicolis, S., Ronchi, A., Ottolenghi, S., Ruzzi, L., Shimada, Y., Migliaccio, A.R., and Migliaccio, G.: Progressive inactivation of the expression of an erythroid transcriptional factor in GM- and G-CSF–dependent myeloid cell lines. Nucleic Acids Res. 18:6863, 1990.

190. Ito, E., Toki, T., Ishihara, H., Ohtani, H., Gu, L., Yokoyama, M., Engel, J.D., and Yamamoto, M.: Erythroid transcription factor GATA-1 is abundantly transcribed in mouse testis. Nature 362:466, 1993.

191. Philipsen, S., Talbot, D., Fraser, P., and Grosveld, F.: The beta-globin dominant control region: hypersensitive site 2. EMBO J. 9:2159, 1990.

192. Merika, M., and Orkin, S.H.: Functional synergy and physical interactions of the erythroid transcription factor GATA-1 with the Kruppel family proteins Sp1 and EKLF. Mol. Cell. Biol. 15:2437, 1995.

193. Lemarchandel, V., Ghysdael, J., Mignotte, V., Rahuel, C., and Romeo, P.H.: GATA and Ets cis-acting sequences mediate megakaryocyte-specific expression. Mol. Cell. Biol. 13:668, 1993.

194. Omichinski, J.G., Clore, G.M., Schaad, O., Felsenfeld, G., Trainor, C., Appella, E., Stahl, S.J., and Gronenborn, A.M.: NMR structure of a specific DNA complex of Zn-containing DNA binding domain of GATA-1. Science 261:438, 1993.

195. Tsai, S.-F., Martin, D.I.K., Zon, L.I., D'Andrea, A.D., Wong, G.G., and Orkin, S.H.: Cloning of cDNA for the major DNA-binding protein of the erythroid lineage through expression in mammalian cells. Nature 339:446, 1989.

196. Zon, L.I., Tsai, S.-F., Burgess, S., Matsudaira, P., Bruns, G.A.P., and Orkin, S.H.: The major human erythroid DNA-binding protein (GF-1): primary sequence and localization of the gene to the X chromosome. Proc. Natl. Acad. Sci. USA 87:668, 1990.

197. Evans, T., and Felsenfeld, G.: The erythroid-specific transcription factor ERYF1: a new finger protein. Cell 58:877, 1989.

198. Trainor, C.D., Evans, T., Felsenfeld, G., and Boguski, M.S.: Structure and evolution of a human erythroid transcription factor. Nature 343:92, 1990.

199. Whyatt, D.J., deBoer, E., and Grosveld, F.: The two zinc finger-like domains of GATA-1 have different DNA binding specificities. EMBO J. 12:4993, 1993.

200. Tsang, A.P., Visvader, J.E., Turner, C.A., Fujiwara, Y., Yu, C., Weiss, M.J., Crossley, M., and Orkin, S.H.: FOG, a multitype zinc finger protein, acts as a cofactor for transcription factor GATA-1 in erythroid and megakaryocytic differentiation. Cell 90:109, 1997.

201. Tsang, A.P., Fujiwara, Y., Hom, D.B., and Orkin, S.H.: Failure of megakaryopoiesis and arrested erythropoiesis in mice lacking the GATA-1 transcriptional cofactor FOG. Genes Dev. 12:1176 1998.

202. Wadman, I.A., Osada, H., Grutz, G.G., Agulnick, A.D., Westphal, H., Forster, A., and Rabbitts, T.H.: The LIM-only protein Lmo2 is a bridging molecule assembling an erythroid, DNA-binding complex which includes the TAL1, E47, GATA-1 and Ldb1/NLI proteins. EMBO J. 16:3145, 1997.

203. Crossley, M., Merika, M., and Orkin, S.H.: Self-association of the erythroid transcription factor GATA-1 mediated by its zinc finger domains. Mol. Cell. Biol. 15:2448, 1995.

204. Anderson, K.P., Crable, S.C., and Lingrel, J.B.: Multiple proteins binding to a GATA-E box-GATA motif regulate the erythroid Kruppel-like factor (EKLF) gene. J. Biol. Chem. 273:14347, 1998.

205. Blobel, G.A., Nakajima, T., Eckner, R., Montminy, M., and Orkin, S.H.: CREB-binding protein cooperates with transcription factor GATA-1 and is required for erythroid differentiation. Proc. Natl. Acad. Sci. USA 3:2061, 1998.

206. Evans, T., and Felsenfeld, G.: Trans-activation of a globin promoter in nonerythroid cells. Mol. Cell. Biol. 11:843, 1991.

207. Martin, D.I.K., and Orkin, S.H.: Transcriptional activation and DNA binding by the erythroid factor GF-1/NF-E1/ERYF 1. Genes Dev. 4:1886, 1990.

208. Yang, H.Y., and Evans, T.: Distinct roles for the two cGATA-1 finger domains. Mol. Cell. Biol. 12:4562, 1992.

209. Crossley, M., and Orkin, S.H.: Phosphorylation of the erythroid transcription factor GATA-1. J. Biol. Chem. 269:16589, 1994.

210. Elefanty, A.G., Antoniou, M., Custodio, N., Carmo-Fonseca, M., and Grosveld, F.: GATA transcription factors associate with a novel class of nuclear bodies in erythroblasts and megakaryocytes. EMBO J. 15:319, 1996.

211. Cullen, M.E., and Patient, R.K.: GATA-1 DNA binding activity is down-regulated in late S phase in erythroid cells. J. Biol. Chem. 272:2464, 1997.

212. Tsai, F.Y., Keller, G., Kuo, F.C., Weiss, M., Chen, J., Rosenblatt, M., Alt, F.W., and Orkin, S.H.: An early haematopoietic defect in mice lacking the transcription factor GATA-2. Nature 371:221, 1994.

213. Ma, G.T., Roth, M.E., Groskopf, J.C., Tsai, F.Y., Orkin, S.H., Grosveld, F., Engel, J.D., and Linzer, D.I.: GATA-2 and GATA-3 regulate trophoblast-specific gene expression in vivo. Development 124:907, 1997.

214. Oosterwegel, M., Timmerman, J., Leiden, J., and Clevers, H.: Expression of GATA-3 during lymphocyte differentiation and mouse embryogenesis. Dev. Immunol. 3:1, 1992.

215. George, K.M., Leonard, M.W., Roth, M.E., Lieuw, K.H., Kioussis, D., Grosveld, F., and Engel, J.D.: Embryonic expression and cloning of the murine GATA-3 gene. Development 120:2673, 1994.

216. Pandolfi, P.P., Roth, M.E., Karis, A., Leonard, M.W., Dzierzak, E., Grosveld, F., Engel, J.D., and Lindenbaum, M.H.: Targeted disruption of the GATA-3 gene causes severe abnormalities in the nervous system and in fetal liver haematopoiesis. Nat. Genet. 11:40, 1995.

217. Yamamoto, M., Ko, L.J., Leonard, M.W., Beug, H., Orkin, S.H., and Engel, J.D.: Activity and tissue-specific expression of the transcription factor NF-E1 multigene family. Genes Dev. 4:1650, 1990.

218. Pevny, L., Simon, M.C., Robertson, E., Klein, W.H., Tsai, S.F., d'Agati, V., Orkin, S.H., and Costantini, F.: Erythroid differentiation in chimaeric mice blocked by a targeted mutation in the gene for transcription factor GATA-1. Nature 349:257, 1991.

219. Pevny, L., Lin, C.S., d'Agati, V., Simon, M.C., Orkin, S.H., and Costantini, F.: Development of hematopoietic cells lacking transcription factor GATA-1. Development 121:163, 1995.

220. Fujiwara, Y., Browne, C.P., Cunniff, K., Goff, S.C., and Orkin, S.H.: Arrested development of embryonic red cell precursors in mouse embryos lacking transcription factor GATA-1. Proc. Natl. Acad. Sci. USA 93:12355, 1996.

221. Blobel, G.A., and Orkin, S.H.: Estrogen-induced apoptosis by inhibition of the erythroid transcription factor GATA-1. Mol. Cell. Biol. 4:1687, 1996.

222. Weiss, M.J., and Orkin, S.H.: Transcription factor GATA-1 permits survival and maturation of erythroid precursors by preventing apoptosis. Proc. Natl. Acad. Sci. USA 92:9623, 1995.

223. Visvader, J.E., Crossley, M., Hill, J., Orkin, S.H., and Adams, J.M.: The C-terminal zinc finger of GATA-1 or GATA-2 is sufficient to induce megakaryocytic differentiation of an early myeloid cell line. Mol. Cell. Biol. 15:634, 1995.

224. Takahashi, S., Komeno, T., Suwabe, N., Yoh, K., Nakajima, O., Nishimura, S., Kuroha, T., Nagasawa, T., and Yamamoto, M.: Role of GATA-1 in proliferation and differentiation of definitive erythroid and megakaryocytic cells in vivo. Blood 92:434, 1998.

225. Whyatt, D.J., Karis, A., Harkes, I.C., Verkerk, A., Elephanty, A., Ploemacher, R., Philipsen, S., and Grosveld, F.: The level of the tissue-specific factor GATA-1 affects the cell cycle machinery. Genes Funct. 1:11, 1997.

226. Whyatt, D.J., and Grosveld, F.: Unpublished data.

227. Dubart, A., Romeo, P.H., Vainchenker, W., and Dumenil, D.: Constitutive expression of GATA-1 interferes with the cell-cycle regulation. Blood, 87:3711, 1996.

228. Clarke, A.R., Maandag, E.R., van Roon, M., van der Lugt, N.W., van der Valk, M., Hooper, M.L., Berns, A., and te Riele, H.: Requirement for a functional Rb-1 gene in murine development. Nature 359:328, 1992.

229. Jacks, T., Fazeli, A., Schmitt, E.M., Bronson, R.T., Goodell, M.A., and Weinberg, R.A.: Effects of an Rb mutation in the mouse. Nature 359:295, 1992.

230. Williams, B.O., Schmitt, E.M., Remington, L., Bronson, R.T., Albert,

D.M., Weinberg, R.A., and Jacks, T.: Extensive contribution of Rb-deficient cells to adult chimeric mice with limited histopathological consequences. EMBO J. 13:4251, 1994.

231. Hattori, N., Kawamoto, H., and Katsura, Y.: Isolation of the most immature population of murine fetal thymocytes that includes progenitors capable of generating T, B, and myeloid cells. J. Exp. Med. 184:1901, 1996.

232. Ting, C.N., Olson, M.C., Barton, K.P., and Leiden, J.M.: Transcription factor GATA3 is required for development of the T-cell lineage. Nature 384:474, 1996.

233. Zhang, D.H., Cohn, L., Ray, P., Bottomly, K., and Ray, A.: Transcription factor GATA-3 is differentially expressed in murine Th1 and Th2 cells and controls Th2-specific expression of the interleukin-5 gene. J. Biol. Chem. 272:21597, 1997.

234. Mignotte, V., Eleouet, J.F., Raich, N., and Romeo, P.H.: *Cis*- and *trans*-acting elements involved in the regulation of the erythroid promoter of the human porphobilinogen deaminase gene. Proc. Natl. Acad. Sci. USA 86:6548, 1989.

235. Mignotte, V., Wall, L., de Boer, E., Grosveld, F., and Romeo, P.H.: Two tissue-specific factors bind the erythroid promoter of the human porphobilinogen deaminase gene. Nucleic Acids Res. 17:37, 1989.

236. Ney, P.A., Sorrentino, B.P., McDonagh, K.T., and Nienhuis, A.W.: Tandem AP-1-binding sites within the human β-globin dominant control region function as an inducible enhancer in erythroid cells. Genes Dev. 4:993, 1990.

237. Ney, P.A., Sorrentino, B.P., Lowrey, C.H., and Nienhuis, A.W.: Inducibility of the HS II enhancer depends on binding of an erythroid specific nuclear protein. Nucleic Acids Res. 18:6011, 1990.

238. Andrews, N.C., Erdjument-Bromage, H., Davidson, M.B., Tempst, P., and Orkin, S.H.: Globin locus control region enhancer binding factor (NF-E2): an hematopoietic-specific basic-leucine zipper protein. Nature 362:722, 1993.

239. Ney, P.A., Andrews, N.C., Jane, S.M., Safer, B., Purucker, M.E., Weremowicz, S., Morton, C.C., Goff, S.C., Orkin, S.H., Nienhuis, A.W.: Purification of the human NF-E2 complex: cDNA cloning of the hematopoietic cell-specific subunit and evidence for an associated partner. Mol. Cell. Biol. 13:5604, 1993.

240. Amrolia, P.J., Ramamurthy, L., Saluja, D., Tanese, N., Jane, S.M., and Cunningham, J.M.: The activation domain of the enhancer binding protein p45NF-E2 interacts with TAFII130 and mediates long-range activation of the alpha- and beta-globin loci in an erythroid cell line. Proc. Natl. Acad. Sci. USA 94:10051, 1997.

241. Bean, T.L., and Ney, P.A.: Multiple regions of p45 NF-E2 are required for beta-globin gene expression in erythroid cells. Nucleic Acids Res. 25:2509, 1997.

242. Motohashi, H., Shavit, J.A., Igarashi, K., Yamamoto, M., and Engel, J.D.: The world according to Maf. Nucleic Acids Res. 25:2953, 1997.

243. Johnsen, O., Murphy, P., Prydz, H., and Kolsto, A.B.: Interaction of the CNC-bZIP factor TCF11/LCR-F1/Nrf1 with MafG: binding-site selection and regulation of transcription. Nucleic Acids Res. 26:512, 1998.

244. Igarashi, K., Itoh, K., Motohashi, H., Hayashi, N., Matuzaki, Y., Nakauchi, H., Nishizawa, M., and Yamamoto, M.: Activity and expression of murine small Maf family protein MafK. J. Biol. Chem. 270:7615, 1995.

245. Blank, V., Kim, M.J., and Andrews, N.C.: Human MafG is a functional partner for p45 NF-E2 in activating globin gene expression. Blood 89:3925, 1997.

246. Cheng, X., Reginato, M.J., Andrews, N.C., and Lazar, M.A.: The transcriptional integrator CREB-binding protein mediates positive cross talk between nuclear hormone receptors and the hematopoietic bZip protein p45/NF-E2. Mol. Cell. Biol. 17:1407, 1997.

247. Armstrong, J.A., and Emerson, B.M.: NF-E2 disrupts chromatin structure at human beta-globin locus control region hypersensitive site 2 in vitro. Mol. Cell. Biol. 16:5634, 1996.

248. Shivdasani, R.A., and Orkin, S.H.: Erythropoiesis and globin gene expression in mice lacking the transcription factor NF-E2. Proc. Natl. Acad. Sci. USA 92:8690, 1992.

249. Kotkow, K.J., and Orkin, S.H.: Complexity of the erythroid transcription factor NF-E2 as revealed by gene targeting of the mouse p18 NF-E2 locus. Proc. Natl. Acad. Sci. USA 93:3514, 1996.

250. Chan, J., Han, X., and Kan, Y.: Cloning NRF1 an NF-E2 related transcription factor by genetic selection in yeast. Proc. Natl. Acad. Sci. USA 90:11371, 1990.

251. Chan, J.Y., Han, X.L., and Kan, Y.W.: Isolation of cDNA encoding the human NF-E2 protein. Proc. Natl. Acad. Sci. USA 90:11366, 1993.

252. Luna, L., Johnsen, O., Skartlien, A.H., Pedeutour, F., Turc-Carel, C., Prydz, H., and Kolsto, A.B.: Molecular cloning of a putative novel human bZIP transcription factor on chromosome 17q22. Genomics 22:553, 1994.

253. McKie, J., Johnstone, K., Mattei, M.G., and Scambler, P.: Cloning and mapping of murine Nfe2l1. Genomics 25:716, 1995.

254. Moi, P., Chan, K., Asunis, I., Cao, A., and Kan, Y.W.: Isolation of NF-E2-related factor 2 (Nrf2), a NF-E2-like basic leucine zipper transcriptional activator that binds to the tandem NF-E2/AP1 repeat of the beta-globin locus control region. Proc. Natl. Acad. Sci. USA 91:9926, 1994.

255. Itoh, K., Igarashi, K., Hayashi, N., Nishizawa, M., Yamamoto, M.: Cloning and characterization of a novel erythroid cell-derived CNC family transcription factor heterodimerizing with the small Maf family proteins. Mol. Cell Biol. 15:4184, 1995.

256. Caterina, J.J., Donze, D., Sun, C.W., Ciavatta, D.J., and Townes, T.M.: Cloning and functional characterization of LCR-F1: a bZIP transcription factor that activates erythroid-specific, human globin gene expression. Nucleic Acids Res. 22:2383, 1994.

257. Oyake, T., Itoh, K., Motohashi, H., Hayashi, N., Hoshino, H., Nishizawa, M., Yamamoto, M., and Igarashi, K.: Bach proteins belong to a novel family of BTB-basic leucine zipper transcription factors that interact with MafK and regulate transcription through the NF-E2 site. Mol. Cell. Biol. 16:6083, 1996.

258. Farmer, S.C., Sun, C.W., Winnier, G.E., Hogan, B.L., and Townes, T.M.: The bZIP transcription factor LCR-F1 is essential for mesoderm formation in mouse development. Genes Dev. 11:786, 1997.

259. Chan, J.Y., Kwong, M., Lu, R., Chang, J., Wang, B., Yen, T.S., and Kan, Y.W.: Targeted disruption of the ubiquitous CNC-bZIP transcription factor, Nrf-2, results in anemia and embryonic lethality in mice. EMBO J. 17:1779, 1998.

260. Chan, K., Lu, R., Chang, J.C., and Kan, Y.W.: NRF2, a member of the NFE2 family of transcription factors, is not essential for murine erythropoiesis, growth and development. Proc. Natl. Acad. Sci. USA 93:13943, 1996.

261. Pavletich, N.P., and Pabo, C.O.: Zinc finger-DNA recognition: crystal structure of a Zif268-DNA complex at 2.1 A. Science 252:809, 1991.

262. Miller, I.J., and Bieker, J.J.: A novel, erythroid cell-specific murine transcription factor that binds to the CACCC element and is related to the Kruppel family of nuclear proteins. Mol. Cell. Biol. 13:2776, 1993.

263. Feng, W.C., Southwood, C.M., and Bieker, J.J.: Analyses of beta-thalassemia mutant DNA interactions with erythroid Krüppel-like factor (EKLF), an erythroid cell-specific transcription factor. J. Biol. Chem. 269:1493, 1994.

264. Asano, H., and Stamatoyannopoulos, G.: Activation of β-globin promoter by erythroid Krüppel-like factor. Mol. Cell. Biol. 18:102, 1998.

265. Southwood, C.M., Downs, K.M., and Bieker, J.J.: Erythroid Krüppel-like factor exhibits an early and sequentially localized pattern of expression during mammalian erythroid ontogeny. Dev. Dyn. 206:248, 1996.

266. Tewari, R., Gillemans, N., Wijgerde, M., Nuez, B., von Lindern, M., Grosveld, F., and Philipsen, S.: Erythroid Krüppel-like Factor (EKLF) is active in primitive and definitive erythroid cells and is required for the function of 5′ HS3 of the β-globin locus control region. EMBO J. 17:2334, 1998.

267. Nuez, B., Michalovich, D., Bygrave, A., Ploemacher, R., and Grosveld, F.: Defective haematopoiesis in fetal liver resulting from inactivation of the EKLF gene. Nature 375:316, 1995.

268. Perkins, A.C., Sharpe, A.H., and Orkin, S.H.: Lethal beta-thalassemia in mice lacking the erythroid CACCC-transcription factor EKLF. Nature 375:318, 1995.

269. Gillemans, N., Tewari, R., Lindeboom, F., Rottier, R., de Wit, T., Wijgerde, M., Grosveld, F., and Philipsen, S.: Altered DNA-binding specificity mutants of EKLF and Sp1 show that EKLF is an activator of the beta-globin locus control region in vivo. Genes Dev. 12:2863, 1998.

270. Ellis, J., Tan-Un, K.C., Harper, A., Michalovich, D., Yannoutsos, N., Philipsen, S., Grosveld, F.: A dominant chromatin-opening activity in 5′ hypersensitive site 3 of the human beta-globin locus control region. EMBO J. 15:562, 1996.

271. Emerson, B., personal communication.

272. Raich, N., Clegg, C.H., Grofti, J., Romeo, P.H., and Stamatoyannopoulos, G.: GATA1 and YY1 are developmental repressors of the human epsilon-globin gene. EMBO J. 14:801, 1995.

273. Li, Q., Clegg, C., Peterson, K., Shaw, S., Raich, N., and Stamatoyan-

nopoulos, G.: Binary transgenic mouse model for studying the trans control of globin gene switching: evidence that GATA-1 is an in vivo repressor of human epsilon gene expression. Proc. Natl. Acad. Sci. USA 94:2444, 1997.

274. Wada-Kiyama, Y., Peters, B., and Noguchi, C.T.: The ε-globin gene silencer. J. Biol. Chem. 267:11532, 1992.

275. Peters, B., Merezhinskaya, N., Diffley, J.F.X., and Noguchi, C.T.: Protein-DNA interactions in the ε-globin gene silencer. J. Biol. Chem. 268:3430, 1993.

276. Yant, S.R., Zhu, W., Millinoff, D., Slightom, J.L., Goodman, M., and Gumucio, D.L.: High affinity YY1 binding motifs: identification of two core types (ACAT and CCAT) and distribution of potential binding sites within the human beta globin cluster. Nucleic Acids Res. 11:4353, 1995.

277. Mantovani, R., Malgaretti, N., Nicolis, S., Giglioni, B., Comi, P., Cappellini, N., Bertero, M.T., Caligaris-Cappio, F., and Ottolenghi, S.: An erythroid specific nuclear factor binding to the proximal CACCC box of the β-globin gene promoter. Nucleic Acids Res. 16:4299, 1988.

278. Mantovani, R., Superti-Furga, G., Gilman, J., and Ottolenghi, S.: The deletion of the distal CCAAT box region of the ^Aγ-globin gene in black HPFH abolishes the binding of the erythroid specific protein NFE3 and of the CCAAT displacement protein. Nucleic Acids Res. 17:6681, 1989.

279. Gibbons, R.J., Picketts, D.J., Villard, L., and Higgs, D.R.: Mutations in a putative global transcriptional regulator cause X-linked mental retardation with alpha-thalassemia (ATR-X syndrome). Cell 80:837, 1995.

280. Gibbons, R.J., Bachoo, S., Picketts, D.J., Aftimos, S., Asenbauer, B., Bergoffen, J., Berry, S.A., Dahl, N., Fryer, A., Keppler, K., Kurosawa, K., Levin, M.L., Masuno, M., Neri, G., Pierpont, M.E., Slaney, S.F., and Higgs, D.R.: Mutations in transcriptional regulator ATRX establish the functional significance of a PHD-like domain. Nat. Genet. 17:146, 1997.

281. Gong, Q., and Dean, A.: Enhancer-dependent transcription of the ε-globin promoter requires promoter-bound GATA-1 and enhancer-bound AP-1/NF-E2. Mol. Cell. Biol. 13:911, 1993.

282. Gong, Q.-H., Stern, J., and Dean, A.: Transcriptional role of a conserved GATA-1 site in the human ε-globin gene promoter. Mol. Cell. Biol. 11:2558, 1991.

283. Walters, M., and Martin, D.I.K.: Functional erythroid promoters created by interaction of the transcription factor GATA-1 with CACCC and AP-1/NFE-2 elements. Proc. Natl. Acad. Sci. USA 89:10444, 1992.

284. Yu, C.-Y., Motamed, K., Chen, J., Bailey, A.D., and Shen, C.-K.J.: The CACC box upstream of human embryonic ε globin gene binds Sp1 and is a functional promoter element in vitro and in vivo. J. Biol. Chem. 266:8907, 1991.

285. Motamed, K., Bastiani, C., Zhang, Q., Bailey, A., and Chen, C.K.: CACC box and enhancer response of the human embryonic epsilon globin promoter. Gene 123:235, 1993.

286. Marin, M., Karis, A., Visser, P., Grosveld, F., and Philipsen, S.: Transcription factor Sp1 is essential for early embryonic development but dispensable for cell growth and differentiation. Cell 89:619, 1997.

287. Asano, H., Li, X.S., and Stamatoyannopoulos, G.: FKLF, a novel Krüppel-like factor that activates human embryonic and fetal β-like globin genes. Mol. Cell. Biol. 19:3571, 1999.

288. Asano, H., Li, X.S., Stamatoyannopoulos, G.: FKLFf-2: a novel Krüppel-like factor that activates globin and other erythroid lineage genes. Blood (in press).

289. Filipe, A., Li, Q., Deveaux, S., Godin, I., Romeo, P-H., Stamatoyannopoulos, G., and Mignotte, V.: Regulation of embryonic/fetal globin genes by nuclear hormone receptors: a novel perspective on hemoglobin switching. EMBO J. 18:687, 1999.

290. Ronchi, A.E., Bottardi, S., Mazzucchelli, C., Ottolenghi, S., and Santoro, C.: Differential binding of the NFE3 and CP1/NFY transcription factors to the human gamma- and epsilon-globin CCAAT boxes. J. Biol. Chem. 270:21934, 1995.

291. Trepicchio, W.L., Dyer, M.A., and Baron, M.H.: Developmental regulation of the human embryonic beta-like globin gene is mediated by synergistic interactions among multiple tissue- and stage-specific elements. Mol. Cell. Biol. 13:7457, 1993.

292. Dyer, M.A., Naidoo, R., Hayes, R.J., Larson, C.J., Verdine, G.L., and Baron, M.H.: A DNA-binding protein interacts with an essential upstream regulatory element of the human embryonic beta-like globin gene. Mol. Cell. Biol. 16:829, 1996.

293. Dyer, M.A., Hayes, P.J., and Baron, M.H.: The HMG domain protein SSRP1/PREIIBF is involved in activation of the human embryonic β-like globin gene. Mol. Cell. Biol. 18:2617, 1998.

294. Raich, N., Enver, T., Nakamoto, B., Josephson, B., Papayannopoulou, Th., and Stamatoyannopoulos, G.: Autonomous developmental control of human embryonic globin gene switching in transgenic mice. Science 250:1147, 1990.

295. Shih, D.M., Wall, R.J., and Shapiro, S.G.: Developmentally regulated and erythroid-specific expression of the human embryonic β-globin gene in transgenic mice. Nucleic Acids Res. 18:5465, 1990.

296. Navas, P.A., Peterson, K.R., Li, Q., Skarpidi, E., Rohde, A., Shaw, S.E., Clegg, C.H., Asano, H., and Stamatoyannopoulos, G.: Developmental specificity of the interaction between the locus control region and embryonic or fetal globin genes in transgenic mice with an HS3 core deletion. Mol. Cell. Biol. 18:4188, 1998.

297. Lindenbaum, M.H., and Grosveld, F.: An in vitro globin gene switching model based on differentiated embryonic stem cells. Genes Dev. 4:2075, 1990.

298. Shih, D.M., Wall, R.J., and Shapiro, S.G.: A 5' control region of the human ε-globin gene is sufficient for embryonic specificity in transgenic mice. J. Biol. Chem. 268:3066, 1993.

299. Li, J., Noguchi, C.T., Miller, W., Hardison, R., and Schechter, A.N.: Multiple regulatory elements in the 5' flanking sequence of the human epsilon-globin gene. J. Biol. Chem. 273:10202, 1998.

300. Li, Q., Blau, C.A., Clegg, C.H., Rohde, A., and Stamatoyannopoulos, G.: Multiple ε-promoter elements participate in the developmental control of ε-globin genes in transgenic mice. J. Biol. Chem. 273:17361, 1998.

301. Raich, N., Papayannopoulou, T., Stamatoyannopoulos, G., and Enver, T.: Demonstration of a human ε-globin gene silencer with studies in transgenic mice. Blood 79:861, 1992.

302. Cao, S.X., Gutman, P.D., Davie, H.P., and Schechter, A.N.: Identification of a transcriptional silencer in the 5'-flanking region of the human ε-globin gene. Proc. Natl. Acad. Sci. USA 86:5306, 1989.

303. Park, K., and Atchison, M.L.: Isolation of a candidate repressor/activator, NF-E1 (YY-1δ), that binds to the immunoglobulin k3' enhancer and the immunoglobulin heavy-chain μE1 site. Proc. Natl. Acad. Sci. USA 88:9804, 1991.

304. Shi, Y., Seto, E., Chang, L.-S., and Shenk, T.: Transcriptional repression by YY1, a human GLI-Krüppel–related protein, and relief of repression by adenovirus E1A protein. Cell 67:377, 1991.

305. Liu, Q., Bungert, J., and Engel, J.D.: Mutation of gene-proximal regulatory elements disrupts human epsilon-, gamma- and beta-globin expression in yeast artificial chromosome transgenic mice. Proc. Natl. Acad. Sci. USA 94:169, 1997.

306. Navas, P.A., and Stamatoyannopoulos, G.: unpublished data.

307. Jane, S.M., Ney, P.A., Vanin, E.F., Gumucio, D.L., and Nienhuis, A.W.: Identification of a stage selector element in the human γ-globin gene promoter that fosters preferential interaction with the 5' HS2 enhancer when in competition with the β-promoter. EMBO J. 11:2961, 1992.

308. Jane, S.M., Gumucio, D.L., Ney, P.A., Cunningham, J.M., and Nienhuis, A.W.: Methylation enhanced binding of Sp1 to the stage selector element of the human γ-globin gene promoter may regulate developmental specificity of expression. Mol. Cell. Biol. 13:3272, 1993.

309. Choi, O.R., and Engel, J.D.: Developmental regulation of β-globin gene switching. Cell 55:17, 1988.

310. Gumucio, D.L., Heilstedt-Williamson, H., Gray, T.A., Tarlé, S.A., Shelton, D.A., Table, D.A., Slightom, J.L., Goodman, M., and Collins, F.S.: Phylogenetic footprinting reveals a nuclear protein which binds to silencer sequences in the human γ and ε globin genes. Mol. Cell. Biol. 12:4919, 1992.

311. Jane, S.M., Nienhuis, A.W., and Cunningham, J.M.: Hemoglobin switching in man and chicken is mediated by a heteromeric complex between the ubiquitous transcription factor CP2 and a developmentally specific protein. EMBO J. 14:97, 1995.

312. van der Ploeg, L.H., and Flavell, R.A.: DNA methylation in the human γδβ-globin locus in erythroid and nonerythroid tissues. Cell 19:947, 1980.

313. Mavilio, F., Giampaolo, A., Car, E.A., Migliaccio, G., Calandrini, M., Russo, G., Pagliardi, G.L., Mastroberardino, G., Marinucci, M., and Peschle, C.: Molecular mechanisms of human hemoglobin switching: selective undermethylation and expression of globin genes in embryonic, fetal, and adult erythroblasts. Proc. Natl. Acad. Sci. USA 80:6907, 1983.

314. Enver, T., Zhang, J.-W., Papayannopoulou, Th., and Stamatoyannopoulos, G.: DNA methylation: a secondary event in globin gene switching? Genes Dev. 2:698, 1988.

315. Gumucio, D.L., Rood, K.L., Gray, T.A., Riordan, M.F., Sartor, C.I., and Collins, F.S.: Nuclear proteins that bind the human γ-globin gene promoter: alterations in binding produced by point mutations associated with hereditary persistence of fetal hemoglobin. Mol. Cell. Biol. 8:5310, 1988.

316. Mantovani, R., Malgaretti, N., Nicolis, S., Ronchi, A., Giglioni, B., and Ottolenghi, S.: The effects of HPFH mutations in the human γ-globin promoter on binding of ubiquitous and erythroid specific nuclear factors. Nucleic Acids Res. 16:7783, 1988.

317. McDonagh, K.T., and Nienhuis, A.W.: Induction of the human γ-globin gene promoter in K562 cells by sodium butyrate: Reversal of repression by CCAAT displacement protein. Blood 78:255a, 1991.

318. Berry, M., Grosveld, F., and Dillon, N.A.: A single point mutation is the cause of the Greek form of hereditary persistence of foetal haemoglobin. Nature 358:499, 1992.

319. Skalnik, D.G., Strauss, E.C., and Orkin, S.H.: CCAAT displacement protein as a repressor of the myelomonocytic-specific gp91-phox gene promoter. J. Biol. Chem. 266:16736, 1991.

320. Pace, B.S., Li, Q., and Stamatoyannopoulos, G.: In vivo search for butyrate responsiveness sequences using transgenic mice carrying Aγ gene promoter mutants. Blood 88:1079, 1996.

321. Ronchi, A., Berry, M., Raguz, S., Imam, A., Yannoutsos, N., Ottolenghi, S., Grosveld, F., and Dillon, N.: Role of the duplicated CCAAT box region in γ-globin gene regulation and hereditary persistence of fetal haemoglobin. EMBO J. 15:143, 1996.

322. Wall, L., Destroismaisons, N., Delvoye, N., and Guy, L.G.: CAAT/enhancer-binding proteins are involved in beta-globin gene expression and are differently expressed in murine erythroleukemia and K562 cells. J. Biol. Chem. 271:16477, 1996.

323. Zafarana, G., and Grosveld, F.: Unpublished data.

324. Stamatoyannopoulos, G., Josephson, B., Zhang, J-W., and Li, Q.: Developmental regulation of human γ-globin genes in transgenic mice. Mol. Cell. Biol. 13:7636, 1993.

325. Duan, Z-J., Stamatoyannopoulos, G., and Li, Q.: Role of the CACCC box in developmental regulation of human γ-globin gene expression (Submitted).

326. Crossley, M., Whitelaw, E., Perkins, A., Williams, G., Fujiwara, Y., and Orkin, S.H.: Isolation and characterization of the cDNA encoding BKLF/TEF-2, a major CACCC-box-binding protein in erythroid cells and selected other cells. Mol. Cell. Biol. 16:1695, 1996.

327. McDonagh, K.T., Lin, H.J., Lowrey, C.H., Bodine, D.M., and Nienhuis, A.W.: The upstream region of the human γ-globin gene promoter: identification and functional analysis of nuclear protein binding sites. J. Biol. Chem. 266:11965, 1991.

328. Magis, W., and Martin, D.I.: HMG-I binds to GATA motifs: implications for an HPFH syndrome. Biochem. Biophys. Res. Commun. 214:927, 1995.

329. Ronchi, A., Nicholis, S., Santoro, C., and Ottolenghi, S.: Increased Sp1 binding mediates erythroid-specific overexpression of a mutated (HPFH) γ-globin promoter. Nucleic Acids Res. 17:10231, 1989.

330. Gumucio, D.L., Rook, K.L., Blanchard-McQuate, K.L., Gray, T.A., Saulino, A., and Collins, F.S.: Interaction of Sp1 with the human γ globin promoter: binding and transactivation of normal and mutant promoters. Blood 78:1853, 1991.

331. Ulrich, M.J., Gray, W.J., and Ley, T.J.: An intramolecular DNA triplex is disrupted by point mutations associated with hereditary persistence of fetal hemoglobin. J. Biol. Chem. 267:18649, 1992.

332. Bacolla, A., Ulrich, M.J., Larson, J.E., Ley, T.J., Wells, R.D.: An intramolecular triplex in the human gamma-globin 5'-flanking region is altered by point mutations associated with hereditary persistence of fetal hemoglobin. J. Biol. Chem. 270:24556, 1995.

333. Ponce, E., Lloyd, J.A., Pierani, A., Roeder, R.G., and Lingrel, J.B.: Transcription factor OTF-1 interacts with two distinct DNA elements in the A γ-globin gene promoter. Biochemistry 30:2961, 1991.

334. Gilman, J.G., and Huisman, T.H.: DNA sequence variation associated with elevated fetal Gγ globin production. Blood 66:783, 1985.

335. Lanclos, K.D., Oner, C., Dimovski, A.J., Gu, Y.C., and Huisman, T.H.: Sequence variations in the 5' flanking and IVS-II regions of the Gγ- and Aγ-globin genes of βs chromosomes with five different haplotypes. Blood 77:2488, 1991.

336. Sampietro, M., Thein, S.L., Contreras, M., and Pazmany, L.: Variation of Hb F and F-cell number with the Gγ Xmn I (C→T) polymorphism in normal individuals. Blood 79:832, 1992.

337. Harvey, M.P., Motum, P., Lindeman, R., and Trent, R.J.: An Aγ globin promoter (four base-pair deletion) mutant shows linked polymorphic changes throughout the Aγ gene. Exp. Hematol. 20:320, 1992.

338. Pissard, S., and Beuzard, Y.: A potential regulatory region for the expression of fetal hemoglobin in sickle cell disease. Blood 84:331, 1994.

339. Ballas, S.K., Talacki, C.A., Adachi, K., Schwartz, E., Surrey, S., and Rappaport, E.: The Xmn I site (−158, C→T) 5' to the Gγ gene: correlation with the Senegalese haplotype and Gγ globin expression. Hemoglobin 15:393, 1991.

340. Lu, Z.H., and Steinberg, M.H.: Fetal hemoglobin in sickle cell anemia: relation to regulatory sequences cis to the β-globin gene: multicenter study of hydroxyurea. Blood 87:1604, 1996.

341. Peri, K.G., Ganon, J., Gagnon, C., and Bard, H.: Association of −158 (C→T) (XmnI) DNA polymorphism in G gamma-globin promoter with delayed switchover from fetal to adult hemoglobin synthesis. Pediatr. Res. 41:214, 1997.

342. Bodine, D.M., and Ley, T.J.: An enhancer element lies 3' to the human ^Aγ globin gene. EMBO J. 6:2997, 1987.

343. Forrester, W.C., Thompson, C., Elder, J.T., and Groudine, M.: A developmentally stable chromatin structure in the human β-globin gene cluster. Proc. Natl. Acad. Sci. USA 83:1359, 1986.

344. Dickinson, L.A., Joh, T., Kohwi, Y., and Kohwi-Shigematsu, T.: A tissue-specific MAR/SAR DNA-binding protein with unusual binding site recognition. Cell 70:631, 1992.

345. Purucker, M., Bodine, D., Lin, H., McDonagh, K., and Nienhuis, A.W.: Structure and function of the enhancer 3' to the human Aγ globin gene. Nucleic Acids Res. 18:7407, 1990.

346. Liu, Q., Tanimoto, K., Bunger, J., and Engel, J.D.: The Aγ-globin 3' element provides no unique function(s) for human β-globin locus gene regulation. Proc. Natl. Acad. Sci. USA 95:9944, 1998.

347. Dillon, N., and Grosveld, F.: Human γ-globin genes silenced independently of other genes in the β-globin locus. Nature 350:252, 1991.

348. Enver, T., Ebens, A.J., Forrester, W.C., Stamatoyannopoulos, G.: The human β-globin locus activating region alters the developmental fate of a human fetal globin gene in transgenic mice. Proc. Natl. Acad. Sci. USA 86:7033, 1989.

349. Li, Q., and Stamatoyannopoulos, J.A.: Position independence and proper developmental control of γ-globin gene expression require both a 5' locus control region and a downstream sequence element. Mol. Cell. Biol. 14:6087, 1994.

350. Stamatoyannopoulos, J., Clegg, C.H., and Li, Q.: Sheltering of γ-globin expression from position effects requires both an upstream locus control region and a regulatory element 3' to the ^Aγ-globin gene. Mol. Cell. Biol. 17:240, 1997.

351. Donze, D., Jeancake, P.H., and Townes, T.M.: Activation of δ-globin gene expression by erythroid Krüpple-like factor: a potential approach for gene therapy of sickle cell disease. Blood 88:4051, 1996.

352. Tang, D.C., Ebb, D., Hardison, R.C., and Rodgers, G.P.: Restoration of the CCAAT box or insertion of the CACCC motif activates [corrected] δ-globin gene expression. Blood 90:421, 1997.

353. Antoniou, M., De Boer, E., Spanopoulou, E., and Grosveld, F.: TBP binding and the rate of transcription initiation from the human β-globin gene. Nucleic Acids Res. 23:3473, 1995.

354. Lewis, B.A., and Orkin, S.H.: A functional initiator element in the human β-globin promoter. J. Biol. Chem. 270:28139, 1995.

355. Stuve, L.L., and Myers, R.M.: A directly repeated sequence in the β-globin promoter regulates transcription in murine erythroleukemia cells. Mol. Cell. Biol. 10:972, 1990.

356. Myers, R.M., Cowie, A., Stuve, L., Hartzog, G., and Gaensler, K.: Genetic and biochemical analysis of the mouse β-major globin promoter. Prog. Clin. Biol. Res. 316A:117, 1989.

357. Antoniou, M., and Grosveld, F.: β-Globin dominant control region interacts differently with distal and proximal promoter elements. Genes Dev. 4:1007, 1990.

358. Antoniou, M., deBoer, E., Habets, G., and Grosveld, F.: The human β-globin gene contains multiple regulatory regions: identification of one promoter and two downstream enhancers. EMBO J. 7:377, 1988.

359. deBoer, E., Antoniou, M., Mignotte, V., Wall, L., and Grosveld, F.: The human β-globin promoter; nuclear protein factors and erythroid specific induction of transcription. EMBO J. 7:4203, 1988.

360. Hartzog, G.A., and Myers, R.M.: Discrimination among potential activators of the β-globin CACCC element by correlation of binding and transcriptional properties. Mol. Cell. Biol. 13:44, 1993.

361. Donze, D., Townes, T.M., and Bieker, J.J.: Role of erythroid Krüppel-

like factor in human γ- to β-globin gene switching. J. Biol. Chem. 270:1955, 1995.

362. Wijgerde, M., Gribnau, J., Trimborn, T., Nuez, B., Philipsen, S., Grosveld, F., and Fraser, P.: The role of EKLF in human β-globin gene competition. Genes Dev. 10:2894, 1996.

363. Perkins, A.C., Gaensler, K.M., and Orkin, S.H.: Silencing of human fetal globin expression is impaired in the absence of the adult β-globin gene activator protein EKLF. Proc. Natl. Acad. Sci. USA 93:12267, 1996.

364. Behringer, R.R., Hammer, R.E., Brinster, R.L., Palmiter, R.D., and Townes, T.M.: Two 3′ sequences direct adult erythroid-specific expression of human β-globin genes in transgenic mice. Proc. Natl. Acad. Sci. USA 84:7056, 1987.

365. Kollias, G., Hurst, J., deBoer, E., Grosveld, F.: The human beta-globin gene contains a downstream developmental specific enhancer. Nucleic Acids Res. 15:5739, 1987.

366. Kollias, G., Wrighton, N., Hurst, J., and Grosveld, F.: Regulated expression of human A γ-, β-, and hybrid γ β-globin genes in transgenic mice: manipulation of the developmental expression patterns. Cell 46:89, 1986.

367. Trudel, M., and Costantini, F.: A 3′ enhancer contributes to the stage-specific expression of the human β-globin gene. Genes Dev. 1:954, 1987.

368. Trudel, M., Magram, J., Bruckner, L., and Costantini, F.: Upstream G γ-globin and downstream β-globin sequences required for stage-specific expression in transgenic mice. Mol. Cell. Biol. 7:4024, 1987.

369. Magram, J., Niederreither, K., and Costantini, F.: β-Globin enhancers target expression of a heterologous gene to erythroid tissues of transgenic mice. Mol. Cell. Biol. 9:4581, 1989.

370. Lim, L.C., Swendeman, S.L., and Sheffery, M.: Molecular cloning of the α-globin transcription factor CP2. Mol. Cell. Biol. 12:828, 1992.

371. Watt, P., Lamb, P., Squire, L., and Proudfoot, N.: A factor binding GATAAG confers tissue specificity on the promoter of the human ζ-globin gene. Nucleic Acids Res. 18:1339, 1990.

372. Yu, C.Y., Chen, J., Lin, L.I., Tam, M., and Shen, C.K.: Cell type–specific protein-DNA interactions in the human ζ-globin upstream promoter region: displacement of Sp1 by the erythroid cell-specific factor NF-E1. Mol. Cell. Biol. 10:282, 1990.

373. Zhang, Q., Reddy, P.M., Yu, C.Y., Bastiani, C., Higgs, D., Stamatoyannopoulos, G., Papayannopoulou, T., and Shen, C.K.: Transcriptional activation of human zeta 2 globin promoter by the alpha globin regulatory elements (HS-40): functional role of specific nuclear factor-DNA complexes. Mol. Cell. Biol. 13:2298, 1993.

374. Sabath, D.E., Koehler, K.M., Yang, W.Q., Patton, K., and Stamatoyannopoulos, G.: Identification of a major positive regulatory element located 5′ to the human ζ-globin gene. Blood 85:2587, 1995.

375. Sabath, D.E., Koehler, K.M., and Yang, W.Q.: Structure and function of the ζ-globin upstream regulatory element. Nucleic Acids Res. 24:4978, 1996.

376. Sabath, D.E., Spangler, E.A., Rubin, E.M., and Stamatoyannopoulos, G.: Analysis of the human zeta-globin gene promoter in transgenic mice. Blood 82:2899. 1993.

377. Albitar, M., Katsumata, M., and Liebhaber, S.A.: Human alpha-globin genes demonstrate autonomous developmental regulation in transgenic mice. Mol. Cell. Biol. 11:3786, 1991.

378. Pondel, M.D., Proudfoot, N.J., Whitelaw, C., and Whitelaw, E.: The developmental regulation of the human zeta-globin gene in transgenic mice employing beta-galactosidase as a reporter gene. Nucleic Acids Res. 20:5655, 1992.

379. Russell, J.E., Morales, J., Makeyev, A.V., and Liebhaber, S.A.: Sequence divergence in the 3′ untranslated regions of human ζ- and α-globin mRNAs mediates a difference in their stabilities and contributes to efficient a-to-z gene developmental switching. Mol. Cell. Biol. 18:2173, 1998.

380. Wang, Z., and Liebhaber, S.A.: A 3′-flanking NF-κB site mediates developmental silencing of the human ζ-globin gene. EMBO J. 18:2218, 1999.

381. Chkheidze, A.N., Lyakhov, D.L., Makeyev, A.V., Morales, J., Kong, J., and Liebhaber, S.A.: Assembly of the alpha-globin mRNA stability complex reflects binary interaction between the pyrimidine-rich 3′ untranslated region determinant and poly(C) binding protein alphaCP. Mol. Cell. Biol. 19:4572, 1999.

382. Flint, J., Thomas, K., Micklem, G., Raynham, H., Clark, K., Doggett, N.A., King, A., and Higgs, D.R.: The relationship between chromosome structure and function at a human telomeric region. Nat. Genet. 15:252, 1997.

383. Shewchuk, B.M., and Hardison, R.C.: CpG islands from the alpha-globin gene cluster increase gene expression in an integration-dependent manner. Mol. Cell. Biol. 17:5856, 1997.

384. Humphries, R.K., Ley, T., Turner, P., Moulton, A.D., and Nienhuis, A.W.: Differences in human α-, β-, and δ-globin gene expression in monkey kidney cells. Cell 30:173, 1982.

385. Brickner, H.E., Zhu, X.X., and Atweh, G.F.: A novel regulatory element of the human α-globin gene responsible for its constitutive expression. J. Biol. Chem. 266:15363, 1991.

386. Higgs, D.R., Wood, W.G., Jarman, A.P., Sharpe, J., Lida, J., Pretorius, I.-M., and Ayyub, H.: A major positive regulatory region located far upstream of the human α-globin gene locus. Genes Dev. 4:1588, 1990.

387. Sharpe, J.A., Wells, D.J., Whitelaw, E., Vyas, P., Higgs, D.R., and Wood, W.G.: Analysis of the human α-globin gene cluster in transgenic mice. Proc. Natl. Acad. Sci. USA 90:11262, 1993.

388. Blom van Assendelft, G., Hanscombe, O., Grosveld, F., and Greaves, D.R.: The β-globin dominant control region activates homologous and heterologous promoters in a tissue-specific manner. Cell 56:969, 1989.

389. Ryan, T.M., Behringer, R.R., Townes, T.M., Palmiter, R.D., and Brinster, R.L.: High-level erythroid expression of human alpha-globin genes in transgenic mice. Proc. Natl. Acad. Sci. USA 86:37, 1989.

390. Talbot, D., Collis, P., Antoniou, M., Vidal, M., Grosveld, F., and Greaves, D.R.: A dominant control region from the human beta-globin locus conferring integration site-independent gene expression. Nature 338:6213, 1989.

391. Kim, C.G., Swendeman, S.L., Barnhart, K.M., and Sheffery, M.: Promoter elements and erythroid cell nuclear factors that regulate α-globin gene transcription in vitro. Mol. Cell. Biol. 10:5958, 1990.

392. Lim, L.C., Fang, L., Swendeman, S.L., Sheffery, M.: Characterization of the molecularly cloned murine α-globin transcription factor CP2. J. Biol. Chem. 268:18008, 1993.

393. Swendeman, S.L., Spielholz, C., Jenkins, N.A., Gilbert, D.J., Copeland, N.G., and Sheffery, M.: Characterization of the genomic structure, chromosomal location, promoter, and development expression of the alpha-globin transcription factor CP2. J. Biol. Chem. 269:11663, 1994.

394. Tuan, D., Solomon, W., Li, Q., and London, I.M.: The "β-like-globin" gene domain in human erythroid cells. Proc. Natl. Acad. Sci. USA 82:6384, 1985.

395. Li, Q., Zhang, M., Stamatoyannopoulos, G.: Structural analysis and mapping of DNase I hypersensitivity of the HS5 of the β-globin locus control region. Genomics 61:183, 1999.

396. Zafarana, G., Raguz, S., Pruzina, S., Grosveld, F., and Meijer, D.: The regulation of human β-globin gene expression: the analysis of hypersensitive site 5 (HS5) in the LCR. In: Developmental Control of Globin Genes. Andover, U.K., Intercept, 1995, p. 39.

397. Bulger, M., von Doorninck, J.H., Saitoh, N., Telling, A., Farrell, C., Bender, M.A., Felsenfeld, G., Axel, R., and Groudine, M.: Conservation of sequence and structure flanking the mouse and human β-globin loci: the β-globin genes are embedded within an array of odorant receptor genes. Proc. Natl. Acad. Sci. USA 96:5129, 1999.

398. Wright, S., deBoer, E., Rosenthal, A., Flavell, R.A., and Grosveld, F.G.: DNA sequences required for regulated expression of the β-globin genes in murine erythroleukaemia cells. Phil. Trans. Royal Soc. Lond. B307:271, 1984.

399. Kioussis, D., Vanin, E., deLange, T., Flavell, R.A., and Grosveld, F.G.: β-Globin gene inactivation by DNA translocation in γδβ-thalassemia. Nature 306:662, 1983.

400. Forrester, W.C., Epner, E., Driscoll, M.C., Enver, T., Brice, M., Papayannopoulou, Th., and Groudine, M.: A deletion of the human β-globin locus activation region causes a major alteration in chromatin structure and replication across the entire β-globin locus. Genes Dev. 4:1637, 1990.

401a. Fraser, P., Grosveld, F.: Locus control regions, chromatin activation and transcription. Curr. Opin. Cell Biol. 10:361, 1998.

401. Grosveld, F., van Assendelft, G.B., Greaves, D.R., and Kollias, G.: Position-independent, high-level expression of the human β-globin gene in transgenic mice. Cell 51:975, 1987.

402. Sharpe, J.A., Chan-Thomas, P.S., Lida, J., Ayyub, H., Wood, W.G., and Higgs, D.R.: Analysis of the human α globin upstream regulatory element (HS-40) in transgenic mice. EMBO J. 11:4565, 1992.

403. Greaves, D.R., Wilson, F.D., Lang, G., and Kioussis, D.: Human CD2 3′-flanking sequences confer high-level, T cell-specific, position-independent gene expression in transgenic mice. Cell 56:979, 1989.

404. Lang, G., Mamalaki, C., Greenberg, D., Yannoutsos, N., and Kioussis,

D.: Deletion analysis of the human CD2 gene locus control region in transgenic mice. Nucleic Acids Res. 19:5851, 1991.

405. Aronow, B.J., Silbiger, R.N., Dusing, M.R., Stock, J.L., Yager, K.L., Potter, S.S., Hutton, J.J., and Wiginton, D.A.: Functional analysis of the human adenosine deaminase gene thymic regulatory region and its ability to generate position independent transgene expression. Mol. Cell. Biol. 12:4170, 1992.

406. Wang, Y., Macke, J.P., Merbs, S.L., Zack, D.J., Klaunberg, B., Bennett, J., Gearhart, J., and Nathans, J.: A locus control region adjacent to the human red and green visual pigment genes. Neuron 9:429, 1992.

407. Madisen, L., and Groudine, M.: Identification of a locus control region in the immunoglobulin heavy-chain locus that deregulates c-*myc* expression in plasmacytoma and Burkitt's lymphoma cells. Genes Dev. 8:2212, 1994.

408. Dang, Q., Walker, D., Taylor, S., Allan, C., Chin, P., Fan, J., and Taylor, J.: Structure of the hepatic control region of the human apolipoprotein E/C-I gene locus. J. Biol. Chem. 270:22577, 1995.

409. Jones, B.K., Monks, B.R., Liebhaber, S.A., and Cooke, N.E.: The human growth hormone gene is regulated by a multicomponent locus control region. Mol. Cell. Biol. 15:7010, 1995.

410. Montoliu, L., Umland, T., and Schutz, G.: A locus control region at −12 kb of the tyrosinase gene. EMBO J. 15:6026, 1996.

411. Kushida, M.M., Dey, A., Zhang, X.L., Campbell, J., Heeney, M., Carlyle, J., Ganguly, S., Ozato, K., Vasavada, H., and Chamberlain, J.W.: A 150-base pair 5′ region of the MHC class I HLA-B7 gene is sufficient to direct tissue-specific expression and locus control region activity: the alpha site determines efficient expression and in vivo occupancy at multiple cis-active sites throughout this region. J. Immunol. 159:4913, 1997.

412. Raguz, S., Hobbs, C., Yague, E., Ioannou, P.A., Walsh, F.S., and Antonious, M.: Muscle-specific locus control region activity associated with the human desmin gene. Dev. Biol. 201:26, 1998.

413. Madisen, L., Krumm, A., Hebbes, T.R., and Groudine, M.: The immunoglobulin heavy chain locus control region increases histone acetylation along like c-*myc* genes. Mol. Cell. Biol. 18:6281, 1998.

414. Radomska, H.S., Satterthwaite, A.B., Burn, T.C., Oliff, I.A., and Tenen, D.G.: Multiple control elements are required for expression of the human CD34 gene. Gene 222:305, 1998.

415. Kioussis, D., and Festenstein, R.: Locus control regions: overcoming heterochromatin-induced gene inactivation in mammals. Curr. Opin. Genet. Dev. 7:614, 1997.

416. Townes, T.M., Lingrel, J.B., Chen, H.Y., Brinster, R.L., and Palmiter, R.D.: Erythroid-specific expression of human β-globin genes in transgenic mice. EMBO J. 4:1715, 1985.

417. Milot, E., Fraser, P., and Grosveld, F.: Position effects and genetic disease. Trends Genet. 12:123, 1996.

418. Festenstein, R., Tolaini, M., Corbella, P., Mamalaki, C., Parrington, J., Fox, M., Miliou, A., Jones, M., and Kioussis, D.: Locus control region function and heterochromatin-induced position effect variegation. Science 271:1123, 1996.

419. Milot, E., Strouboulis, J., Trimborn, T., Wijgerde, M., de Boer, E., Langeveld, A., Tan-Un, K., Vergeer, W., Yannoutsos, N., Grosveld, F., and Fraser, P.: Heterochromatin effects on the frequency and duration of LCR-mediated gene transcription. Cell 87:105, 1996.

420. Kellum, R., and Schedl, P.: A position-effect assay for boundaries of higher order chromosomal domains. Cell 64:941, 1991.

421. Geyer, P.K., and Corces, V.G.: DNA position-specific repression of transcription by a *Drosophila* zinc finger protein. Genes Dev. 6:1865, 1992.

422. Bonifer, C., Yannoutsos, N., Kruger, G., Grosveld, F., and Sippel, A.E.: Dissection of the locus control function located on the chicken lysozyme gene domain in transgenic mice. Nucleic Acids Res. 22:4202, 1994.

423. Forrester, W.C., Takegawa, S., Papayannopoulou, Th., Stamatoyannopoulos, G., and Groudine, M.: Evidence for a locus activation region: the formation of developmentally stable hypersensitive sites in globin-expressing hybrids. Nucleic Acids Res. 24:10159, 1987.

424. Reik, A., Telling, A., Zitnik, G., Cimbora, D., Epner, E., and Groudine, M.: The locus control region is necessary for gene expression in the human beta-globin locus but not the maintenance of an open chromatin structure in erythroid cells. Mol. Cell. Biol. 18:5992, 1998.

425. Epner, E., Reik, A., Cimbora, D., Telling, A., Bender, M.A., Fiering, S, Enver, T., Martin, D.I., Kennedy, M., Keller, G., Groudine, M.: The β-globin LCR is not necessary for an open chromatin structure or developmentally regulated transcription of the native mouse beta-globin locus. Mol. Cell. 2:447, 1998.

426. Bender, M.A., Bulger, M., Halow, J., Telling, A., Close, J., Groudine, M.: Globin gene switching and DNase I sensitivity of the endogenous β-globin locus in mice does not require the locus control region. Mol. Cell, in press.

427. Higgs, D.R.: Do LCRs open chromatin domains? Cell 95:299, 1998.

428. Grosveld, F.: Activation by locus control regions? Curr. Opin. Genet. Dev. 9:152, 1999.

429. Epner, E., Forrester, W.C., and Groudine, M.: Asynchronous DNA replication within the human β-globin gene locus. Proc. Natl. Acad. Sci. USA 85:8081, 1988.

430. Dhar, V., Mager, D., Iqbal, A., and Schildkraut, C.L.: The coordinate replication of the human β-globin gene domain reflects its transcriptional activity and nuclease hypersensitivity. Mol. Cell. Biol. 8:4958, 1988.

431. Aladjem, M.I., Groudine, M., Brody, L.L., Dieken, E.S., Fournier, R.E.K., Wahl, G.M., and Epner, E.M.: Participation of the human β-globin locus control region in initiation of DNA replication. Science 270:815, 1995.

432. Talbot, D., Philipsen, S., Fraser, P., and Grosveld, F.: Detailed analysis of the site 3 region of the human β-globin dominant control region. EMBO J. 9:2169, 1990.

433. Talbot, D., Grosveld, F.: The 5′HS2 of the globin locus control region enhances transcription through the interaction of a multimeric complex binding at two functionally distinct NF-E2 binding sites. EMBO J. 10:1391, 1991.

434. Pruzina, S., Hanscombe, O., Whyatt, D., Grosveld, F., and Philipsen, S.: Hypersensitive site 4 of the human β globin locus control region. Nucleic Acids Res. 19:1413, 1991.

435. Lowrey, C.H., Bodine, D.M., and Nienhuis, A.W.: Mechanism of DNase I hypersensitive site formation within the human globin locus control region. Proc. Natl. Acad. Sci. USA 89:1143, 1992.

436. Stamatoyannopoulos, J.A., Goodwin, A.J., Joyce, T.M., and Lowrey, C.H.: Characterization of a DNAse I hypersensitive-site forming element from the human β-globin locus control region. *In* Stamatoyannopoulos, G. (ed.): Molecular Biology of Hemoglobin Switching. Andover, U.K., Intercept, 1995, pp. 71–86.

437. Tuan, D., Solomon, W.B., London, I.M., and Lee, D.P.: An erythroid-specific, developmental-stage–independent enhancer far upstream of the human "β-like globin" genes. Proc. Natl. Acad. Sci. USA 86:2554, 1989.

438. Grosveld, F., Dillon, N., and Higgs, D.: The regulation of human globin gene expression. Baillieres Clin. Haematol. 6:31, 1993.

439. Ellis, J., Talbot, D., Dillon, N., and Grosveld, F.: Synthetic human beta-globin 5′ HS2 constructs function as locus control regions only in multicopy transgene concatamers. EMBO J. 12:127, 1993.

440. Pawlik, K.M., and Townes, T.M: Autonomous, erythroid-specific DNase I hypersensitive site formed by human beta-globin locus control region (LCR) 5′ HS 2 in transgenic mice. Dev. Biol. 169:728, 1996.

441. Ashe, H.L., Monks, J., Wijgerde, M., Fraser, P., and Proudfoot, N.J: Intergenic transcription and transinduction of the human beta-globin locus. Genes Dev. 11:2494, 1997.

442. Walters, M., Kim, C., and Gelinas, R.: Characterization of a DNA binding activity in DNase I hypersensitive site 4 of the human globin locus control region. Nucleic Acids Res. 19:5385, 1991.

443. Strauss, E.C., and Orkin, S.H.: In vivo protein-DNA interactions at hypersensitive site 3 of the human β-globin locus control region. Proc. Natl. Acad. Sci. USA 89:5809, 1992.

444. Ikuta, T., and Kan, Y.W.: In vivo protein-DNA interactions at the β-globin gene locus. Proc. Natl. Acad. Sci. USA 88:10188, 1991.

445. Reddy, P.M., and Shen, C.K.: Protein-DNA interactions in vivo of an erythroid-specific, human β-globin locus enhancer. Proc. Natl. Acad. Sci. USA 88:8676, 1991.

446. Stamatoyannopoulos, J.A., Goodwin, A., Joyce, T., and Lowrey, C.H.: NF-E2 and GATA binding motifs are required for the formation of DNase I hypersensitive site 4 of the human beta-globin locus control region. EMBO J. 14:106, 1995.

447. Pomerantz, O., Goodwin, A.J., Joyce, T., and Lowrey, C.H.: Conserved elements containing NF-E2 and tandem GATA binding sites are required for erythroid-specific chromatin structure reorganization within the human beta-globin locus control region. Nucleic Acids Res. 26:5684, 1998.

448. Philipsen, S., Pruzina, S., and Grosveld, F.: The minimal requirements for activity in transgenic mice of hypersensitive site 3 of the β globin locus control region. EMBO J. 12:1077, 1993.

449. Reddy, P.M.S., Stamatoyannopoulos, G., Papayannopoulou, Th., and Shen, C.-K.J.: Genomic footprinting and sequencing of human β-globin locus: tissue specificity and cell line artifact. J. Biol. Chem. 269:8287, 1994.

450. Ikuta, T., Papayannopoulou, Th., Stamatoyannopoulos, G., and Kan, Y.W.: Globin gene switching. In vivo protein-DNA interactions of the human β-globin locus in erythroid cells expressing the fetal or the adult globin gene program. J. Biol. Chem. 271:14082, 1996.

451. Caterina, J.J., Ryan, T.M., Pawlik, K.M., Palmiter, R.D., Brinster, R.L., Behringer, R.R., and Townes, T.M.: Human β-globin locus control region: analysis of the 5′ DNase I hypersensitive site HS2 in transgenic mice. Proc. Natl. Acad. Sci. USA 88:1626, 1991.

452. Moi, P., and Kan, Y.W.: Synergistic enhancement of globin gene expression by activator protein-1–like proteins. Proc. Natl. Acad. Sci. USA 87:9000, 1990.

453. Liu, D., Chang, J.C., Moi, P., Liu, W., Kan, Y.W., and Curtin, P.T.: Dissection of the enhancer activity of β-globin 5′ DNase I-hypersensitive site 2 in transgenic mice. Proc. Natl. Acad. Sci. USA 89:3899, 1992.

454. Jarman, A.P., Wood, W.G., Sharpe, J.A., Gourdon, G., Ayyub, H., and Higgs, D.R.: Characterization of the major regulatory element upstream of the human α-globin gene cluster. Mol. Cell. Biol. 11:4679, 1991.

455. Strauss, E.C., Andrews, N.C., Higgs, D.R., and Orkin, S.H.: In vivo footprinting of the human α-globin locus upstream regulatory element by guanine and adenine ligation-mediated polymerase chain reaction. Mol. Cell. Biol. 12:2135, 1992.

456. Rombel, I., Yu, K-H., Zhang, Q., Papayannopoulou, Th., Stamatoyannopoulos, G., Shen, C-K.J.: Transcriptional activation of human adult α-globin genes by hypersensitive site-40 enhancer: function of nuclear factor-binding motifs occupied in erythroid cells. Proc. Natl. Acad. Sci. USA 92:6454, 1995.

457. Li, Q., Zhou, B., Powers, P., Enver, T., and Stamatoyannopoulos, G.: Primary structure of the goat β-globin locus control region. Genomics 9:488, 1991.

458. Li, Q.L., Zhou, B., Powers, P., Enver, T., and Stamatoyannopoulos, G.: β-Globin locus activation regions: conservation of organization, structure, and function. Proc. Natl. Acad. Sci. USA 87:8207, 1990.

459. Moon, A.M., and Ley, T.J.: Conservation of the primary structure, organization, and function of the human and mouse β-globin locus-activating regions. Proc. Natl. Acad. Sci. USA 87:7693, 1990.

460. Hug, B.A., Moon, A.M., and Ley, T.J.: Structure and function of the murine β-globin locus control region 5′ HS-3. Nucleic Acids Res. 20:5771, 1992.

461. Jimenez, G., Gale, K.B., and Enver, T.: The mouse β-globin locus control region: hypersensitive sites 3 and 4. Nucleic Acids Res. 20:5797, 1992.

462. Slightom, J.L., Bock, J.H., Tagle, D.A., Gumucio, D.L., Goodman, M., Stojanovic, N., Jackson, J., Miller, W., and Hardison, R.: The complete sequences of the galago and rabbit beta-globin locus control regions: extended sequence and functional conservation outside the cores of DNase hypersensitive sites. Genomics 39:90, 1997.

463. Hardison, R., Slightom, J.L., Gumucio, D.L., Goodman, M., Stojanovic, N., Miller, W.: Locus control regions of mammalian beta-globin gene clusters: combining phylogenetic analyses and experimental results to gain functional insights. Gene 205:73, 1997.

464. Evans, T., Felsenfeld, G., and Reitman, M.: Control of globin gene transcription. Annu. Rev. Cell Biol. 6:95, 1990.

465. Mason, M.M., Abruzzo, L.V., and Reitman, M.: Regulation of the chicken β- globin gene cluster. In Stamatoyannopoulos, G. (ed.): Molecular Biology of Hemoglobin Switching. Andover, U.K., Intercept, 1995, pp. 13–22.

466. Mason, M.M., Lee. E., Westphal, H., and Reitman, M.: Expression of the chicken beta-globin gene cluster in mice: correct developmental expression and distributed control. Mol. Cell. Biol. 15:407, 1995.

467. Reitman, M., Lee, E., Westphal, H., and Felsenfeld, G.: Site independent expression of the chicken β A-globin gene in transgenic mice. Nature 348:749, 1990.

468. Chung, J.H., Whiteley, M., and Felsenfeld, G.: A 5′ element of the chicken beta-globin domain serves as an insulator in human erythroid cells and protects against position effect in Drosophila. Cell 74:505, 1993.

469. Chung, J.H., Bell, A.C., and Felsenfeld, G.: Characterization of the chicken beta-globin insulator. Proc. Natl. Acad. Sci. USA 94:575, 1997.

470. Bell, A.C., West, A.G., and Felsenfeld, G.: The protein CTCF is required for the enhancer blocking activity of vertebrate insulators. Cell 98:387, 1999.

471. Prioleau, M.N., Nony, P., Simpson, M., and Felsenfeld, G.: An insulator element and condensed chromatin region separate the chicken beta-globin locus from an independently regulated erythroid-specific folate receptor gene. EMBO J. 18:4035, 1999.

472. Bell, A.C., and Felsenfeld, G.: Stopped at the border: boundaries and insulators. Curr. Opin. Genet. Dev. 9:191, 1999.

473. Emery, D.W., Yannaki, E., Tubb, J., and Stamatoyannopoulos, G.: A chromatin insulator protects retrovirus vectors from position effects. Submitted.

474. Strouboulis, J., Dillon, N., and Grosveld, F.: Developmental regulation of a complete 70-kb human beta-globin locus in transgenic mice. Genes Dev. 6:1857, 1992.

475. Peterson, K.R., Clegg, C.H., Li, Q., and Stamatoyannopoulos, G.: Production of transgenic mice with yeast artificial chromosomes. Trends Genet. 13:61, 1997.

476. Peterson, K.R., Zitnik, G., Huxley, C., Gnirke, A., Leppig, K.A., Papayannopoulou, Th., and Stamatoyannopoulos, G.: Use of yeast artificial chromosomes (YACs) for studying control of gene expression: correct regulation of the genes of a human β-globin locus YAC following transfer to mouse erythroleukemia lines. Proc. Natl. Acad. Sci. USA 90:11207, 1993.

477. Porcu, S., Kitamura, M., Witkowska, E., Zhang, Z., Utero, A., Lin, C., Chang, J., and Gaensler, K.M: The human beta globin locus introduced by YAC transfer exhibits a specific and reproducible pattern of developmental regulation in transgenic mice. Blood 90:4602, 1997.

478. Peterson, K.R., Navas, P.A., Li, Q., and Stamatoyannopoulos, G.: LCR-dependent gene expression in β-globin YAC transgenics: detailed structural studies validate functional analysis even in the presence of fragmented YACs. Hum. Mol. Genet. 7:2079, 1998.

479. Peterson, K.R., Clegg, C.H., Navas, P.A., Norton, E.J., Kimborough, T.G., and Stamatoyannopoulos, G.: Effect of deletion of 5′HS3 or 5′HS2 of the human β-globin locus yeast artificial chromosome transgenic mice. Proc. Natl. Acad. Sci. USA 93:6605, 1996.

480. Fiering, S., Epner, E., Robinson, K., Zhuang, Y., Telling, A., Hu, M., Martin, D.I., Enver, T., Ley, T.J., and Groudine, M.: Targeted deletion of 5′HS2 of the murine beta-globin LCR reveals that it is not essential for proper regulation of the beta-globin locus. Genes Dev. 9:2203, 1995.

481. Hug, B.A., Wesselschmidt, R.L., Fiering, S., Bender, M.A., Epner, E., Groudine, M., and Ley, T.J.: Analysis of mice containing a targeted deletion of beta-globin locus control region 5′ hypersensitive site 3. Mol. Cell. Biol. 16:2906, 1996.

482. Bungert, J., Davé, U., Lim, K.-C., Lieuw, K.H., Shavit, J.A., Liu, Q., and Engel, J.D.: Synergistic regulation of human beta-globin gene switching by locus control region elements HS3 and HS4. Genes Dev. 9:3083, 1995.

483. Bungert, J., Tanimoto, K., Patel, S., Liu, Q., Fear, M., and Engel, J.D.: Hypersensitive site 2 specifies a unique function within the human beta-globin locus control region to stimulate globin gene transcription. Mol. Cell. Biol. 19:3062, 1999.

484. Navas, P., and Stamatoyannopoulos, G.: Unpublished data.

485. Fraser, P., Pruzina, S., Antoniou, M., Grosveld, F.: Each hypersensitive site of the human β-globin locus control region confers a different developmental pattern of expression on the globin genes. Genes Dev. 7:106, 1993.

486. Cross, M.A., and Enver, T.: The lineage commitment of haemopoietic progenitor cells. Curr. Opin. Genet. Dev. 7:609, 1997.

487. Till, J.E.: Regulation of hemopoietic stem cells. In Cairnie, A.B., Lala, P.K., and Osmond, D.G. (eds.): Stem Cells of Renewing Cell Populations. New York, Academic Press, 1976, pp. 143–155.

488. Jimenez, G., Griffiths, S.D., Ford, A.M., Greaves, M.F., and Enver, T.: Activation of the β-globin locus control region precedes commitment to the erythroid lineage. Proc. Natl. Acad. Sci. USA 89:10618, 1992.

489. Hu, M., Krause, D., Greaves, M., Sharkis, S., Dexter, M., Heyworth, C., and Enver, T.: Multilineage gene expression precedes commitment in the hemopoietic system. Genes Dev. 11:774, 1997.

490. Papayannopoulou, Th., Nakamoto, B., Peterson, K., and Priestley, G.: Functional in vivo evidence that an erythroid specific enhancer can be activated in all types of hemopoietic progenitors in vivo with extinction later in white cells but consolidation of expression in erythroid and megakaryocytic cells. Blood 90:428a, 1997.

491. Vassilopoulos, G., Navas, P.A., Skarpidi, E., Peterson, K.R., Lowrey, C.H., and Stamatoyannopoulos, G.: Correct function of the locus control region may require passage through a non-erythroid cellular environment. Blood 93:703, 1999.
492. Higgs, D.R., Sharpe, J.A., Gourdon, G., Craddock, C.F., Vyas, P., Picketts, D.J., Barbour, V., Ayyub, H., and Wood, W.G.: Expression of the human α-globin cluster in transgenic mice. In Stamatoyannopoulos, G. (ed.): Hemoglobin Switching. Andover, U.K., Intercept, 1995, pp. 165–178.
493. Higgs, D.R., Sharpe, J.A., and Wood, W.G.: Understanding α globin gene expression: a step towards effective gene therapy. Semin. Hematol. 35:93, 1998.
494. Wilkie, A.O., Higgs, D.R., Rack, K.A., Buckle, V.J., Spun, N.K., Fischel-Ghodsian, N., Ceccherini, I., Brown, W.R., and Harris, P.C.: Stable length polymorphism of up to 260 kb at the tip of the short arm of human chromosome 16. Cell 65:595, 1991.
495. Vyas, P., Vickers, M.A., Simmons, D.L., Ayyub, H., Craddock, C.F., and Higgs, D.R.: Cis-acting sequences regulating expression of the human α-globin cluster lie within constitutively open chromatin. Cell 69:781, 1992.
496. Higgs, D.R., Vickers, M.A., Wilkie, A.O., Pretorius, I.M., Jarman, A.P., and Weatherall, D.J.: A review of the molecular genetics of the human α-globin gene cluster. Blood 73:1081, 1989.
497. Craddock, C.F., Vyas, P., Sharpe, J.A., Ayyub, H., Wood, W.G., and Higgs, D.R.: Contrasting effects of alpha and beta globin regulatory elements on chromatin structure may be related to their different chromosomal environments. EMBO J. 154:1718, 1995.
498. Romeo, L., Osorio-Almeida, L., Higgs, D.R., Lavinha, J., and Liebhaber, S.A.: α-Thalassemia resulting from deletion of regulatory sequences far upstream of the α-globin structural genes. Blood 78:1589, 1991.
499. Hatton, C.S., Wilkie, A.O., Drysdale, H.C., Wood, W.G., Vickers, M.A., Sharpe, J., Ayyub, H., Pretorius, I.M., Buckle, V.J., and Higgs, D.R.: α-Thalassemia caused by a large (62 kb) deletion upstream of the human α globin gene cluster. Blood 76:221, 1990.
500. Bernet, A., Sabatier, S., Picketts, D.J., Ouazana, R., Morlé, F., Higgs, D.R., and Godet, J.: Targeted inactivation of the major positive regulatory element (HS-40) of the human alpha-globin gene locus. Blood 86:1202, 1995.
501. Ren, S., Lou, X.-N., and Atweh, G.F.: The major regulatory element upstream of the alpha-globin gene has classical and inducible enhancer activity. Blood 81:1058, 1993.
502. Hanscombe, O., Vidal, M., Kaeda, J., Luzzatto, L., Greaves, D.R., and Grosveld, F.: High-level, erythroid-specific expression of the human hemoglobin in murine erythrocytes. Genes Dev. 3:1572, 1989.
503. Pondel, M.D., George, M., and Proudfoot, N.J.: The LCR-like alpha-globin positive regulatory element functions as an enhancer in transiently transfected cells during erythroid differentiation. Nucleic Acids Res. 20:237, 1992.
504. Gourdon, G., Sharpe, J.A., Wells, D., Wood, W.G., and Higgs, D.R.: Analysis of a 70 kb segment of DNA containing the human zeta and alpha-globin genes linked to their regulatory element (HS-40) in transgenic mice. Nucleic Acids Res. 22:4139, 1994.
505. Zhang, Q., Rombel, I., Reddy, G.N., Gang, J.B., and Shen, C.K.: Functional roles of in vivo footprinted DNA motifs within an alpha-globin enhancer: erythroid lineage and developmental stage specificities. J. Biol. Chem. 270:8501, 1995.
506. Costantini, F., Radice, G., Magram, J., Stamatoyannopoulos, G., Papayannopoulou, Th., and Chada, K.: Developmental regulation of human globin genes in transgenic mice. Cold Spring Harb. Symp. Quant. Biol. 50:361, 1985.
507. Enver, T., Raich, N., Ebens, A.J., Papayannopoulou, Th., Costantini, F., and Stamatoyannopoulos, G.: Developmental regulation of human fetal-to-adult globin gene switching in transgenic mice. Nature 344:309, 1990.
508. Behringer, R.R., Ryan, T.M., Palmiter, R.D., Brinster, R.L., and Townes, T.M.: Human γ- to β-globin gene switching in transgenic mice. Genes Dev. 4:380, 1990.
509. Stamatoyannopoulos, G.: Human hemoglobin switching. Science 252:383, 1991.
510. Hanscombe, O., Whyatt, D., Fraser, P., Yannoutsos, N., Greaves, D., Dillon, N., and Grosveld, F.: Importance of globin gene order for correct developmental expression. Genes Dev. 5:1387, 1991.
511. Wasylyk, B., Wasylyk, C., Augereau, P., and Chambon, P.: The SV40 72 bp repeat preferentially potentiates transcription starting from proximal natural or substitute promoter elements. Cell 32:503, 1983.
512. de Villiers, J., Olson, L., Banerji, J., and Schaffner, W.: Analysis of the transcriptional enhancer effect. Cold Spring Harb. Symp. Quant. Biol. 47(Pt 2):911, 1983.
513. Dillon, N., Trimborn, T., Strouboulis, J., Fraser, P., and Grosveld, F.: The effect of distance on long-range chromatin interactions. Mol. Cell. 1:131, 1997.
514. Peterson, K.R., Navas, P.A., and Stamatoyannopoulos, G.: Cis-control of globin gene switching resides in gene-specific sequences, as well as in gene order. Blood 94:614a, 1999.
515. Kim, C.G., Epner, E.M., Forrester, W.C., and Groudine, M.: Inactivation of the human beta-globin gene by targeted insertion into the beta-globin locus control region. Genes Dev. 6:928, 1992.
516. Shehee, W.R., Oliver, P., and Smithies, O.: Lethal thalassemia after insertional disruption of the mouse major adult beta-globin gene. Proc. Natl. Acad. Sci. USA 90:3177, 1993.
516a. Fraser, P., Gribnau, J., Trimborn, T.: Mechanisms of developmental regulation of globin loci. Curr. Opin. Hematol. 5:139, 1998.
517. Groudine, M., and Weintraub, H.: Propagation of globin DNase I-hypersensitive sites in absence of factors required for induction: a possible mechanism for determination. Cell 30:131, 1982.
518. Martin, D.I., Fiering, S., and Groudine, M.: Regulation of beta-globin gene expression: straightening out the locus. Curr. Opin. Genet. Dev. 6:488, 1996.
519. Herendeen, D.R., Kassavetis, G.A., and Geiduschek, E.P.: A transcriptional enhancer whose function imposes a requirement that proteins track along DNA. Science 256:1298, 1992.
520. Tuan, D., Kong, S., and Hu, K.: Transcription of the hypersensitive site HS2 enhancer in erythroid cells. Proc. Natl. Acad. Sci. USA 89:11219, 1992.
521. Wijgerde, M., Grosvedl, F., and Fraser, P.: Transcription complex stability and chromatin dynamics in vivo. Nature 377:209, 1995.
522. Gribnau, J., de Boer, E., Trimborn, T., Wijgerde, M., Milot, E., Grosveld, F., and Fraser, P.: Chromatin interaction mechanism of transcriptional control in vivo. EMBO J. 17:6020, 1998.
523. Svedberg, T., and Hedenius, A.: The sedimentation constants of the respiratory proteins. Biol. Bull. 66:191, 1934.
524. McCutcheon, F.H.: Hemoglobin function during the life history of the bullfrog. J. Cell. Comp. Physiol. 8:63, 1936.
525. Stamatoyannopoulos, G., Papayannopoulou, Th., Brice, M., Kurachi, S., Nakamoto, B., Lim, G., and Farquhar, M.: Cell biology of hemoglobin switching. I. The switch from fetal to adult hemoglobin formation during ontogeny. In Stamatoyannopoulos, G., and Nienhuis, A.W. (eds.): Hemoglobins in Development and Differentiation. New York, Alan R. Liss, 1981, pp. 287–305.
526. Ingram, V.M.: Embryonic red cell formation. Nature 235:338, 1972.
527. Chapman, B.S., and Tobin, A.J.: Distribution of developmentally regulated hemoglobins in embryonic erythroid populations. Dev. Biol. 69:375, 1979.
528. Brotherton, T.W., Chui, D.H.K., Gauldie, J., and Patterson, M.: Hemoglobin ontogeny during normal mouse fetal development. Proc. Natl. Acad. Sci. USA 76:2853, 1979.
529. Le Douarin, N.: Ontogeny of hematopoietic organs studied in avian embryo interspecific chimeras. In Clarkson, B., Marks, P.A., and Till, J. (eds.): Differentiation in Normal and Neoplastic Hemopoietic Cells. New York, Cold Spring Harbor, 1978, pp. 5–31.
530. Beaupain, D., Martin, C., and Dieterlen-Lievre, F.: Origin and evolution of hemopoietic stem cells in the avian embryo. In Stamatoyannopoulos, G., and Nienhuis, A.W. (eds.): Hemoglobins in Development and Differentiation. New York, Alan R. Liss, 1981, pp. 161–169.
531. Peschle, C., Migliaccio, A.R., Migliaccio, G., Petrini, M., Calandrini, M., Russo, G., Mastroberardino, G., Presta, M., Gianni, A.M., Comi, P., Giglioni, B., and Ottolenghi, S.: Embryonic to fetal Hb switch in humans: studies on erythroid bursts generated by embryonic progenitors from yolk sac and liver. Proc. Natl. Acad. Sci. USA 81:2416, 1984.
532. Stamatoyannopoulos, G., Constantoulakis, P., Brice, M., Kurachi, S., and Papayannopoulou, Th.: Coexpression of embryonic, fetal, and adult globins in erythroid cells of human embryos: relevance to cell-lineage models of globin switching. Dev. Biol. 123:191, 1987.
533. Weatherall, D.J., Clegg, J.B., and Wood, W.G.: A model for the persistence or reactivation of fetal haemoglobin production. Lancet 2:660, 1976.
534. Weatherall, D.J., Edwards, J.A., and Donohoe, W.T.A.: Haemoglobin and red cell enzyme changes in juvenile myeloid leukaemia. Br. Med. J. 1:679, 1968.

535. Alter, B.P., Jackson, B.T., Lipton, J.M., Piasecki, G.J., Jackson, P.L., Kudisch, M., and Nathan, D.G.: Control of simian fetal hemoglobin switch at the progenitor cell level. J. Clin. Invest. 67:458, 1981.

536. Alter, B.P., Jackson, B.T., Lipton, J.M., Piasecki, G.J., Jackson, P.L., Kudisch, M., and Nathan, D.G.: Three classes of erythroid progenitors that regulate hemoglobin synthesis during ontogeny in the primate. *In* Stamatoyannopoulos, G., and Nienhuis, A.W. (eds.): Hemoglobins in Development and Differentiation. New York, Alan R. Liss, 1981, pp. 331–340.

537. Kidoguchi, K., Ogawa, M., Karam, J.D., McNeil, J.S., and Fitch, M.S.: Hemoglobin biosynthesis in individual bursts in culture: studies of human umbilical cord blood. Blood 53:519, 1979.

538. Weinberg, R.S., Goldberg, J.D., Schofield, M.J., Lenes, A.L., Styczynski, R., and Alter, B.P.: Switch from fetal to adult hemoglobin is associated with a change in progenitor cell population. J. Clin. Invest. 71:785, 1983.

539. Papayannopoulou, Th., Brice, M., and Stamatoyannopoulos, G.: Analysis of human globin switching in MEL × human fetal erythroid cell hybrids. Cell 46:469, 1986.

540. Willing, M.C., Nienhuis, A.W., and Anderson, W.F.: Selective activation of human β- but not γ-globin gene in human fibroblast × mouse erythroleukaemia cell hybrids. Nature 277:534, 1979.

541. Pyati, J., Kucherlapati, R.S., and Skoultchi, A.I.: Activation of human β-globin genes from nonerythroid cells by fusion with murine erythroleukemia cells. Proc. Natl. Acad. Sci. USA 77:3435, 1980.

542. Ley, T.J., Chiang, Y.L., Haidaris, D., Anagnou, N.P., Wilson, V.L., and Anderson, W.F.: DNA methylation and regulation of the human β-globin–like genes in mouse erythroleukemia cells containing human chromosome. Proc. Natl. Acad. Sci. USA 81:6618, 1984.

543. Chiang, Y.L., Ley, T.J., Sanders-Haigh, L., and Anderson, W.F.: Human globin gene expression in hybrid 2S MEL × human fibroblast cells. Somatic Cell. Mol. Genet. 10:399, 1984.

544. Takegawa, S., Brice, M., Stamatoyannopoulos, G., and Papayannopoulou, Th.: Only adult hemoglobin is produced in fetal non-erythroid × MEL cell hybrids. Blood 68:1384, 1986.

545. Papayannopoulou, Th., Lindsley, D., Kurachi, S., Lewison, K., Hemenway, T., Melis, M., Anagnou, N.P., and Najfeld, V.: Adult and fetal human globin genes are expressed following chromosomal transfer into MEL cells. Proc. Natl. Acad. Sci. USA 82:780, 1985.

546. Papayannopoulou, Th., Enver, T., Takegawa, S., Anagnou, N.P., and Stamatoyannopoulos, G.: Activation of developmentally mutated human globin genes by cell fusion. Science 242:1056, 1988.

547. Melis, M., Demopulos, G., Najfeld, V., Zhang, J., Brice, M., Papayannopoulou, Th., and Stamatoyannopoulos, G.: A chromosome 11-linked determinant controls fetal globin expression and the fetal to adult globin switch. Proc. Natl. Acad. Sci. USA 84:8105, 1987.

548. Oppe, T.E., and Fraser, I.D.: Foetal haemoglobin in haemolytic disease of the newborn. Arch. Dis. Child. 36:507, 1961.

549. Bard, H.: Postnatal synthesis of adult and fetal hemoglobin in infants with congenital cyanotic heart disease. Biol. Neonate 28:219, 1976.

550. Bard, H.: The effect of placental insufficiency on fetal and adult hemoglobin synthesis. Am. J. Obstet. Gynecol. 120:67, 1974.

551. Bromberg, Y.M., Abrahamov, A., and Salzberger, M.: The effect of maternal anoxaemia on the foetal haemoglobin of the newborn. J. Obstet. Gynecol. 63:875, 1956.

552. Bischoff, H.: Untersuchungen über die Resistenz des Hämoglobins des Menschenblutes mit besonderer Berücksichtigung des Sauglingsalters. Z. Gesamte Exp. Med. 48:472, 1925.

553. della Torre, L., and Meroni, P.: Studi sul sangue fetole nota I: Livelli di emoglobina fetale e adulta nella gravidanza fisio-logica; relazione con la maturita fetal. Ann. Ostet. Ginecol. 91:148, 1969.

554. Bard, H., Makowski, E.L., Meschia, G., and Battaglia, F.C.: The relative rates of synthesis of hemoglobins A and F in immature red cells of newborn infants. Pediatrics 45:766, 1970.

555. Bard, H.: Postnatal fetal and adult hemoglobin synthesis in early preterm newborn infants. J. Clin. Invest. 52:1789, 1973.

556. Zanjani, E.D., Lim, G., McGlave, P.B., Clapp, J.F., Mann, L.I., Norwood, T.H., and Stamatoyannopoulos, G.: Adult haematopoietic cells transplanted to sheep fetuses continue to produce adult globins. Nature 295:244, 1982.

557. Zanjani, E.D., McGlave, P.B., Bhakthavathsalan, A., and Stamatoyannopoulos, G.: Sheep fetal haematopoietic cells produce adult haemoglobin when transplanted in the adult animal. Nature 280:495, 1979.

558. Bunch, C., Wood, W.G., Weatherall, D.J., Robinson, J.S., and Corp, M.J.: Haemoglobin synthesis by fetal erythroid cells in an adult environment. Br. J. Haematol. 49:325, 1981.

559. Wood, W.G., Bunch, C., Kelly, S., Gunn, Y., and Breckon, G.: Control of haemoglobin switching by a developmental clock? Nature 313:320, 1985.

560. Papayannopoulou, Th., Nakamoto, B., Agostinelli, F., Manna, M., Lucarelli, G., and Stamatoyannopoulos, G.: Fetal to adult hemopoietic cell transplantation in man: insights into hemoglobin switching. Blood 67:99, 1986.

561. Delfini, C., Saglio, G., Mazza, U., Muretto, P., Filippetti, A., and Lucarelli, G.: Fetal haemoglobin synthesis following fetal liver transplantation in man. Br. J. Haematol. 55:609, 1983.

562. Wood, W.G., Nash, J., Weatherall, D.J., Robinson, J.S., and Harrison, F.A.: The sheep as an animal model for the switch from fetal to adult hemoglobins. *In* Stamatoyannopoulos, G., and Nienhuis, A.W. (eds.): Cellular and Molecular Regulation of Hemoglobin Switching. New York, Grune & Stratton, 1979, pp. 153–167.

563. Wintour, E.M., Smith, M.B., Bell, R.J., McDougall, J.G., and Cauchi, M.N.: The role of fetal adrenal hormones in the switch from fetal to adult globin synthesis in the sheep. J. Endocrinol. 104:165, 1985.

564. Zitnik, G., Peterson, K., Stamatoyannopoulos, G., and Papayannopoulou, Th.: Effects of butyrate and glucocorticoids on gamma- to beta-globin gene switching in somatic cell hybrids. Mol. Cell. Biol. 15:790, 1995.

565. Perrine, S.P., Rudolph, A., Faller, D.V., Roman, C., Cohen, R.A., Chen, S.J., and Kan, Y.W.: Butyrate infusions in the ovine fetus delay the biological clock for globin gene switching. Proc. Natl. Acad. Sci. USA 85:8540, 1988.

566. Dover, G.J., Boyer, S.H., and Zinkham, W.H.: Production of erythrocytes that contain fetal hemoglobin in anemia. J. Clin. Invest. 63:173, 1979.

567. Alter, B.P.: Fetal erythropoiesis in stress hematopoiesis. Exp. Hematol. 7:200, 1979.

568. Papayannopoulou, Th., Vichinsky, E., and Stamatoyannopoulos, G.: Fetal Hb production during acute erythroid expansion. I. Observations in patients with transient erythroblastopenia and post-phlebotomy. Br. J. Haematol. 44:535, 1980.

569. Alter, B.P., Rappeport, J.M., Huisman, T.H.J., Schroeder, W.A., and Nathan, D.G.: Fetal erythropoiesis following bone marrow transplantation. Blood 48:843, 1976.

570. Sheridan, B.L., Weatherall, D.J., Clegg, J.B., Pritchard, J., Wood, W.G., Callender, S.T., Durrant, I.J., McWhirter, W.R., Ali, M., Partridge, J.W., and Thompson, E.N.: The patterns of fetal haemoglobin production in leukaemia. Br. J. Haematol. 32:487, 1976.

571. DeSimone, J., Biel, S.I., and Heller, P.: Stimulation of fetal hemoglobin synthesis in baboons by hemolysis and hypoxia. Proc. Natl. Acad. Sci. USA 75:2937, 1978.

572. DeSimone, J., Biel, M., and Heller, P.: Maintenance of fetal hemoglobin (HbF) elevations in the baboon by prolonged erythropoietic stress. Blood 60:519, 1982.

573. Nute, P.E., Papayannopoulou, Th., Chen, P., and Stamatoyannopoulos, G.: Acceleration of F-cell production in response to experimentally induced anemia in adult baboons (*Papio cynocephalus*). Am. J. Hematol. 8:157, 1980.

574. DeSimone, J., Heller, P., Biel, M., and Zwiers, D.: Genetic relationship between fetal Hb levels in normal and erythropoietically stressed baboons. Br. J. Haematol. 49:175, 1981.

575. Stamatoyannopoulos, G., Veith, R., Galanello, R., and Papayannopoulou, Th.: Hb F production in stressed erythropoiesis: observations and kinetic models. Ann. N.Y. Acad. Sci. 445:188, 1985.

576. Galanello, R., Barella, S., Maccioni, L., Paglietti, E., Melis, M.A., Rosatelli, M.C., Argiolu, F., and Cao, A.: Erythropoiesis following bone marrow transplantation from donors heterozygous for beta-thalassaemia. Br. J. Haematol. 72:561, 1989.

577. Ferster, A., Corazza, F., Vertongen, F., Bujan, W., Devalck, C., Fondu, P., Cochaux, P., Lambermont, M., Khaladji, Z., and Sariban, E.: Transplanted sickle-cell disease patients with autologous bone marrow recovery after graft failure develop increased levels of fetal haemoglobin which corrects disease severity. Br. J. Haematol. 90:804, 1995.

578. Meletis, J., Papavasiliou, S., Yataganas, X., Vavourakis, S., Konstantopoulos, K., Poziopoulos, C., Samarkos, M., Michali, E., Dalekou, M., Eliopoulos, G.: "Fetal" erythropoiesis following bone marrow transplantation as estimated by the number of F cells in the peripheral blood. Bone Marrow Transplant. 14:737, 1994.

579. Pembrey, M.E., Weatherall, D.J., and Clegg, J.B.: Maternal synthesis of haemoglobin F in pregnancy. Lancet 1:1350, 1973.

580. Popat, N., Wood, W.G., Weatherall, D.J., and Turnbull, A.C.: Pattern of maternal F-cell production during pregnancy. Lancet 2:377, 1977.

581. Al-Khatti, A., Veith, R.W., Papayannopoulou, Th., Fritsch, E.F., Gold-wasser, E., and Stamatoyannopoulos, G.: Stimulation of fetal hemoglobin synthesis by erythropoietin in baboons. N. Engl. J. Med. 317:415, 1987.

582. Umemura, T., Al-Khatti, A., Papayannopoulou, Th., and Stamatoyannopoulos, G.: Fetal hemoglobin synthesis in vivo: direct evidence for control at the level of erythroid progenitors. Proc. Natl. Acad. Sci. USA 85:9278, 1988.

583. Ellis, M.J., and White, J.C.: Studies on human foetal haemoglobin. II. Foetal haemoglobin levels in healthy children and adults and in certain haematological disorders. J. Haematol. 6:201, 1960.

584. Labie, D., Pagnier, J., Lapoumeroulie, C., Rouabhi, F., Dunda-Belkhodja, O., Chardin, P., Beldjord, C., Wajcman, H., Fabry, M.E., and Nagel, R.L.: Common haplotype dependency of high G γ-globin gene expression and high Hb F levels in β-thalassemia and sickle cell anemia patients. Proc. Natl. Acad. Sci. USA 82:2111, 1985.

585. Nagel, R.L., Fabry, M.E., Pagnier, J., Zohoun, I., Wajcman, H., Baudin, V., and Labie, D.: Hematologically and genetically distinct forms of sickle cell anemia in Africa. N. Engl. J. Med. 312:880, 1985.

586. Nagel, R.L., and Ranney, H.M.: Genetic epidemiology of structural mutations of the β-globin gene. Semin. Hematol. 37:342, 1990.

587. Miller, B.A., Salameh, M., Ahmed, M., Wainscoat, J., Antognetti, G., Orkin, S., Weatherall, D., and Nathan, D.: High fetal hemoglobin production in sickle cell anemia in the eastern province of Saudi Arabia is genetically determined. Blood 67:1404, 1986.

588. Pembrey, M.E., Wood, W.G., Weatherall, D.J., and Perrine, R.P.: Fetal haemoglobin production and the sickle gene in the oases of eastern Saudi Arabia. Br. J. Haematol. 40:415, 1978.

589. Fessas, P.: Thalassemia: clinical and patho-physiological considerations. Trans. R. Soc. Trop. Med. Hyg. 61:164, 1967.

590. Alter, B.P., Rappeport, J.M., and Parkman, R.: The bone marrow failure syndromes. In Nathan, D.G., and Oski, F.A. (eds.): Hematology of Infancy and Childhood. 5th ed. Philadelphia, W.B. Saunders, 1998, pp. 237–335.

591. Maurer, H.S., Vida, L.N., and Honig, G.R.: Similarities of the erythrocytes in juvenile chronic myelogenous leukemia to fetal erythrocytes. Blood 39:778, 1972.

592. Dover, G.J., Boyer, S.H., Zinkham, W.H., Kazazian, H.H., Jr., Pinney, D.J., and Sigler, A.: Changing erythrocyte populations in juvenile chronic myelocytic leukemia: evidence for disordered regulation. Blood 49:355, 1977.

593. Papayannopoulou, Th., Halfpap, L., Chen, S.H., Fukuda, M., Hoffman, R., Dow, L., and Hill, S.: Fetal red cell markers and their relationships in patients with hematologic malignancies. In Stamatoyannopoulos, G., and Nienhuis, A.W. (eds.): Hemoglobins in Development and Differentiation. New York, Alan R. Liss, 1981, pp. 443–456.

594. Papayannopoulou, T., Nakamoto, B., Anagnou, N.P., Chui, D., Dow, L., and Sanders, J.: Expression of embryonic globins by erythroid cells in juvenile chronic myelocytic leukemia. Blood 77:2569, 1991.

595. Bagby, G.C., Jr., Richert-Boe, K., and Koler, R.D.: 32P and acute leukemia: development of leukemia in a patient with hemoglobin Yakima. Blood 52:350, 1978.

596. Pagnier, J., Lopez, M., Mathiot, C., Habibi, B., Zamet, P., Varet, B., and Labie, D.: An unusual case of leukemia with high fetal hemoglobin: demonstration of abnormal hemoglobin synthesis localized in a red cell clone. Blood 50:249, 1977.

597. Krauss, J.S., Rodriguez, A.R., and Milner, P.F.: Erythroleukemia with high fetal hemoglobin after therapy for ovarian carcinoma. Am. J. Clin. Pathol. 76:721, 1981.

598. Chudwin, D.S., Rucknagel, D.L., Scholnik, A.P., Waldmann, T.A., and McIntire, K.R.: Fetal hemoglobin and α-fetoprotein in various malignancies. Acta Haematol. 58:288, 1977.

599. Dainiak, N., and Hoffman, R.: Hemoglobin-F production in testicular malignancy. Cancer 45:2177, 1980.

600. Nyman, M., Skolling, R., and Steiner, H.: Acquired macrocytic anemia and hemoglobinopathy—a paraneoplastic manifestation? Am. J. Med. 41:815, 1966.

601. Stewart, T.C.: The occurrence of foetal haemoglobin in a patient with hepatoma. Med. J. Aust. 2:664, 1971.

602. Lozzio, C., and Lozzio, B.: Human chronic myelogenous leukemia cell line with a positive Philadelphia chromosome. Blood 45:321, 1975.

603. Rutherford, T., Clegg, J.B., Higgs, D.R., Jones, R.W., Thompson, J., and Weatherall, D.J.: Embryonic erythroid differentiation in the human cell line K562. Proc. Natl. Acad. Sci. USA 78:348, 1981.

604. Enver, T., Zhang, J., Anagnou, N.P., Stamatoyannopoulos, G., and Papayannopoulou, Th.: Developmental programs of human erythroleukemia cells: globin gene expression and methylation. Mol. Cell. Biol. 8:4917, 1988.

605. Martin, P., and Papayannopoulou, Th.: HEL cells: a new human erythroleukemia cell line with spontaneous and induced globin expression. Science 216:1233, 1982.

606. Papayannopoulou, Th., Nakamoto, B., Kurachi, S., and Nelson, R.: Analysis of the erythroid phenotype of HEL cells: clonal variation and the effect of inducers. Blood 6:1764, 1987.

607. Okano, H., Okamura, J., Yagawa, K., Tasaka, H., and Motomura, S.: Human erythroid cell lines derived from a patient with acute erythremia. Cancer Res. Clin. Oncol. 102:49, 1981.

608. Papayannopoulou, Th., Nakamoto, B., Kurachi, S., Tweeddale, M., and Messner, H.: Surface antigenic profile and globin phenotype of two new human erythroleukemia lines: characterization and interpretations. Blood 72:1029, 1988.

609. Hirata, J., Sato, H., Takahira, H., Shiokawa, S., Endo, T., Nishimura, J., Katsuno, M., Masuda, S., Sasaki, R., Fukumaki, Y., Nawata, H., and Okano, H.: A novel CD10-positive erythroid cell line, RM10, established from a patient with chronic myelogenous leukemia. Leukemia 4:365, 1990.

610. Fukuda, T., Kishi, K., Ohnishi, Y., and Shibata, A.: Bipotential cell differentiation of KU-812: evidence of a hybrid line that differentiates into basophils and macrophage-like cells. Blood 70:612, 1987.

611. Sato, T., Fuse, A., Eguchi, M., Hayashi, Y., Ryo, R., Adachi, M., Kishimoto, Y., Teramura, M., Mozoguchi, H., Shima, Y., Komori, I., Sunami, S., Okimoto, Y., and Nakajima, H.: Establishment of a human leukaemic cell line (CMK) with megakaryocytic characteristics from a Down's syndrome patient with acute megakaryoblastic leukaemia. Br. J. Hematol. 72:184, 1989.

612. Komatsu, N., Nakauchi, H., Miwa, A., Ishihara, T., Eguchi, M., Moroi, M., Okada, M., Sato, Y., Wada, H., Yawata, Y., Suda, T., and Miura, Y.: Establishment and characterization of a human leukemic cell line with megakaryocytic features: dependency on granulocyte-macrophage colony-stimulating factor, interleukin 3, or erythropoietin for growth and survival. Cancer Res. 51:341, 1991.

613. Miura, Y., Komatsu, N., and Suda, T.: Growth and differentiation of two human megakaryoblastic cell lines: CMK and UT-7. Prog. Clin. Biol. Res. 356:259, 1990.

614. Hitomi, K., Fujita, K., Sasaki, R., Chiba, H., Okuno, Y., Ichiba, S., Takahashi, T., and Imura, H.: Erythropoietin receptor of a human leukemic cell line with erythroid characteristics. Biochem. Biophys. Res. Commun. 154:902, 1988.

615. Morgan, D., Gumucio, D.L., and Brodsky, I.: Granulocyte-macrophage colony-stimulating factor–dependent growth and erythropoietin-induced differentiation of a human cell line MB-02. Blood 78:2860, 1991.

616. Chiba, S., Takaku, F., Tange, T., Shibuya, K., Misawa, C., Sasaki, K., Miyagawa, K., Yazaki, Y., and Hirai, H.: Establishment and erythroid differentiation of a cytokine-dependent human leukemic cell line F-36: a parental line requiring granulocyte-macrophage colony-stimulating factor or interleukin-3, and a subline requiring erythropoietin. Blood 78:2261, 1991.

617. Seigneurin, D., Champelovier, P., Mouchiroud, G., Berthier, R., Leroux, D., Prenant, M., McGregor, J., Starck, J., Morle, F., Micoiun, C., Pietrantuono, A., and Kolodie, L.: Human chronic myeloid leukemia cell line with positive Philadelphia chromosome exhibits megakaryocytic and erythroid characteristics. Exp. Hematol. 15:822, 1987.

618. Ogura, M., Morishima, Y., Ohno, R., Kato, Y., Hirabayashi, N., Nagura, H., and Saito, H.: Establishment of a novel human megakaryoblastic leukemia cell line, MEG-01, with positive Philadelphia chromosome. Blood 66:1384, 1985.

619. Morle, R., Laverriere, A.C., and Godet, J.: Globin genes are actively transcribed in the human megakaryoblastic leukemia cell line MEG-01. Blood 70:3094, 1992.

620. Kitamura, T., Tange, T., Terasawa, T., Chiba, T., Kuwaki, T., Miyagawa, K., Piao, Y-F., Miyazono, K., Urabe, A., and Takaku, F.: Establishment and characterization of a unique human cell line that proliferates dependently on GM-CSF, IL-3, or erythropoietin. J. Cell. Physiol. 140:323, 1989.

621. Papayannopoulou, Th.: Unpublished data.

622. Papayannopoulou, Th., Brice, M., and Stamatoyannopoulos, G.: Stimulation of fetal hemoglobin synthesis in bone marrow cultures from adult individuals. Proc. Natl. Acad. Sci. USA 73:2033, 1976.

623. Stamatoyannopoulos, G., Kurnit, D.M., and Papayannopoulou, Th.:

Stochastic expression of fetal hemoglobin in adult erythroid cells. Proc. Natl. Acad. Sci. USA 78:7005, 1981.

624. Constantoulakis, P., Walmsley, M., Patient, R., Papayannopoulou, Th., Enver, T., and Stamatoyannopoulos, G.: Cell lines produce factors that induce fetal hemoglobin in human BFUe-derived colonies. Blood 80:2650, 1992.

625. Papayannopoulou, Th., Kurachi, S., Nakamoto, B., Zanjani, E.D., and Stamatoyannopoulos, G.: Hemoglobin switching in culture: evidence for a humoral factor that induces switching in adult and neonatal but not fetal erythroid cells. Proc. Natl. Acad. Sci. USA 79:6579, 1982.

626. Rosenblum, B.B., Strahler, J.R., Hanash, S.M., Whitten, C.F., Butkunas-Puskorius, R., and Roberts, A.: Peripheral blood erythroid progenitors from patients with sickle cell anemia: HPLC separation of hemoglobins and the effect of a Hb F switching factor. *In* Stamatoyannopoulos, G., and Nienhuis, A.W. (eds.): Experimental Approaches for the Study of Hemoglobin Switching. New York, Alan R. Liss, 1981, pp. 397–410.

627. Constantoulakis, P., Nakamoto, B., Papayannopoulou, Th., and Stamatoyannopoulos, G.: Fetal calf serum contains activities which induce fetal hemoglobin in adult erythroid cell cultures. Blood 75:1862, 1990.

628. Migliaccio, A-R., Migliaccio, G., Brice, M., Constantoulakis, P., Stamatoyannopoulos, G., and Papayannopoulou, Th.: Influence of recombinant hemopoietins and of fetal calf serum on the globin synthetic pattern of human BFUe. Blood 76:1150, 1990.

629. Fujimori, Y., Ogawa, M., Clark, S.C., and Dover, G.J.: Serum-free culture of enriched hematopoietic progenitors reflects physiologic levels of fetal hemoglobin biosynthesis. Blood 745:1718, 1990.

630. Gabbianelli, M., Pelosi, E., Labbaye, C., Valtieri, M., Testa, U., and Peschle, C.: Reactivation of Hb F synthesis in normal adult erythroid bursts by IL-3. Br. J. Haematol. 74:114, 1986.

631. Miller, B.A., Perrine, S.P., Bernstein, A., Lyman, S.D., Williams, D.E., Bell, L.L., and Olivieri, N.F.: Influence of Steel factor on hemoglobin synthesis in sickle cell disease. Blood 79:1861, 1992.

632. Papayannopoulou, Th., Kalamantis, T., and Stamatoyannopoulos, G.: Cellular regulation of hemoglobin switching: evidence for inverse relationship between fetal hemoglobin synthesis and degree of maturity of human erythroid cells. Proc. Natl. Acad. Sci. USA 76:6420, 1979.

633. Chui, D.H.K., Wong, S.C., Enkin, M.W., Patterson, M., and Ives, R.A.: Proportion of fetal hemoglobin synthesis decreases during erythroid cell maturation. Proc. Natl. Acad. Sci. USA 77:2757, 1980.

634. Dover, G.J., and Boyer, S.H.: Quantitation of hemoglobins within individual red cells: asynchronous biosynthesis of fetal and adult hemoglobin during erythroid maturation in normal subjects. Blood 56:1082, 1980.

635. Wood, W.G., and Jones, R.W.: Erythropoiesis and hemoglobin production: a unifying model involving sequential gene activation. *In* Stamatoyannopoulos, G., and Nienhuis, A.W. (eds.): Hemoglobins in Development and Differentiation. New York, Alan R. Liss, 1981, pp. 243–261.

636. Farquhar, M.N., Turner, P.A., Papayannopoulou, Th., Brice, M., Nienhuis, A.W., and Stamatoyannopoulos, G.: The asynchrony of γ- and β-chain synthesis during human erythroid cell maturation. Dev. Biol. 85:403, 1981.

637. Papayannopoulou, Th., Brice, M., and Stamatoyannopoulos, G.: Hemoglobin F synthesis in vitro: evidence for control at the level of primitive erythroid stem cells. Proc. Natl. Acad. Sci. USA 74:2923, 1977.

638. Papayannopoulou, Th., Bunn, H.F., and Stamatoyannopoulos, G.: Cellular distribution of hemoglobin F in a clonal hemopoietic stem-cell disorder. N. Engl. J. Med. 298:72, 1978.

639. Papayannopoulou, Th., Rosse, W., Stamatoyannopoulos, G., Chen, P., and Adams, J.: Fetal hemoglobin in paroxysmal nocturnal hemoglobinuria (PNH): evidence for derivation of Hb F-containing erythrocytes (F cells) from the PNH clone as well as from normal hemopoietic stem cell lines. Blood 52:740, 1978.

640. Bunch, C., Wood, W.G., Weatherall, D.J., and Adamson, J.W.: Cellular origins of the fetal-haemoglobin–containing cells of normal adults. Lancet 1:1163, 1979.

641. Hoffman, R., Papayannopoulou, Th., Landaw, S., Wasserman, L.R., DeMarsh, Q.B., Chen, P., and Stamatoyannopoulos, G.: Fetal hemoglobin in polycythemia vera: cellular distribution in 50 unselected patients. Blood 53:1148, 1979.

642. Stamatoyannopoulos, G., and Papayannopoulou, Th.: Fetal hemoglobin and the erythroid stem cell differentiation process. *In* Stamatoyan-

nopoulos, G., and Nienhuis, A.W. (eds.): Cellular and Molecular Regulation of Hemoglobin Switching. New York, Grune & Stratton, 1979, pp. 323–349.

643. Macklis, R.M., Javid, J., Lipton, J.M., Kudisch, M., Pettis, P., and Nathan, D.G.: Synthesis of hemoglobin F in adult simian erythroid progenitor–derived colonies. J. Clin. Invest. 70:752, 1982.

644. Dover, G.J., and Ogawa, M.: Cellular mechanisms for increased fetal hemoglobin production in culture. J. Clin. Invest. 66:1175, 1980.

645. Kidoguchi, K., Ogawa, M., and Karam, J.D.: Hemoglobin biosynthesis in individual erythropoietic bursts in culture. J. Clin. Invest. 63:804, 1979.

646. Peschle, C., Migliaccio, G., Covelli, A., Lettieri, F., Migliaccio, A.R., Condorelli, M., Comi, P., Pozzoli, M.L., Giglioni, B., Ottolenghi, S., Cappellini, M.D., Polli, E., and Gianni, A.M.: Hemoglobin synthesis in individual bursts from normal adult blood: all bursts and subcolonies synthesize ᴳγ- and ᴬγ-globin chains. Blood 56:218, 1980.

647. Torrealba de Ron, A., Papayannopoulou, Th., and Stamatoyannopoulos, G.: Studies of Hb F in adult nonanemic baboons: Hb F expression in erythroid colonies decreases as the level of maturation of erythroid progenitors advances. Exp. Hematol. 13:919, 1985.

648. Stamatoyannopoulos, J.A., and Nienhuis, A.W.: Therapeutic approaches to hemoglobin switching in treatment of hemoglobinopathies. Annu. Rev. Med. 43:497, 1992.

649. DeSimone, J., Heller, P., Hall, L., and Zwiers, D.: 5-Azacytidine stimulates fetal hemoglobin synthesis in anemic baboons. Proc. Natl. Acad. Sci. USA 79:4428, 1982.

650. Ley, T.J., DeSimone, J., Anagnou, N.P., Keller, G.H., Humphries, R.K., Turner, P.H., Young, N.S., Heller, P., and Nienhuis, A.W.: 5-Azacytidine selectively increases γ globin synthesis in a patient with β⁺ thalassemia. N. Engl. J. Med. 307:1469, 1982.

651. Papayannopoulou, Th., Torrealba de Ron, A., Veith, R., Knitter, G., and Stamatoyannopoulos, G.: Arabinosylcytosine induces fetal hemoglobin in baboons by perturbing erythroid cell differentiation kinetics. Science 224:617, 1984.

652. Letvin, N.L., Linch, D.C., Beardsley, G.P., McIntyre, K.W., and Nathan, D.G.: Augmentation of fetal-hemoglobin production in anemic monkeys by hydroxyurea. N. Engl. J. Med. 310:869, 1984.

653. Vesel, Y.J.: Mode of action and effects of 5-azacytidine and of its derivatives in eukaryotic cells. Pharmacol. Ther. 28:227, 1985.

654. Jones, P.A.: Effects of 5-azacytidine and its 2'-deoxyderivative on cell differentiation and DNA methylation. Pharmacol. Ther. 28:17, 1985.

655. DeSimone, J., Heller, P., Schimenti, J.C., and Duncan, C.H.: Fetal hemoglobin production in adult baboons by 5-azacytidine or by phenylhydrazine-induced hemolysis is associated with hypomethylation of globin gene DNA. *In* Stamatoyannopoulos, G., and Nienhuis, A.W. (eds.): Globin Gene Expression and Hematopoietic Differentiation. New York, Alan R. Liss, 1983, pp. 489–500.

656. Nienhuis, A.W., Ley, T.J., Humphries, R.K., Young, N.S., and Dover, G.: Pharmacological manipulation of fetal hemoglobin synthesis in patients with severe β-thalassemia. Ann. N.Y. Acad. Sci. 445:198, 1985.

657. Charache, S., Dover, G., Smith, K., Talbot, Jr., C.C., Moyer, M., and Boyer, S.: Treatment of sickle cell anemia with 5-azacytidine results in increased fetal hemoglobin production and is associated with nonrandom hypomethylation of DNA around the γ-δ-β-globin gene complex. Proc. Natl. Acad. Sci. USA 80:4842, 1983.

658. Dover, G.J., Charache, S., Boyer, S.H., Vogelsang, G., and Moyer, M.: 5-Azacytidine increases Hb F production and reduces anemia in sickle cell disease: dose-response analysis of subcutaneous and oral dosage regimens. Blood 66:527, 1985.

659. Ley, T.J., and Nienhuis, A.W.: Induction of hemoglobin F synthesis in patients with β-thalassemia. Annu. Rev. Med. 36:485, 1985.

660. Editorial: 5-azacytidine for beta-thalassemia? Lancet 1:36, 1983.

661. Lowrey, C.H., and Nienhuis, A.W.: Brief report: treatment with azacitidine of patients with end-stage beta-thalassemia. N. Engl. J. Med. 329:845, 1993.

662. Torrealba de Ron, A., Papayannopoulou, Th., Knapp, M.S., Fu, M., Knitter, G., and Stamatoyannopoulos, G.: Perturbations in the erythroid marrow progenitor cell pools may play a role in the augmentation of Hb F by 5-azacytidine. Blood 63:201, 1984.

663. Humphries, R.K., Dover, G., Young, N.S., Moore, J.G., Charache, S., Ley, T., and Nienhuis, A.W.: 5-Azacytidine acts directly on both erythroid precursors and progenitors to increase production of fetal hemoglobin. J. Clin. Invest. 75:547, 1985.

664. Galanello, R., Stamatoyannopoulos, G., and Papayannopoulou, Th.:

Mechanism of Hb F stimulation by S-stage compounds: in vitro studies with bone marrow cells exposed to 5-azacytidine, ara-C or hydroxyurea. J. Clin. Invest. 81:1209, 1988.

665. Miller, B.A., Platt, O., Hope, S., Dover, G., and Nathan, D.G.: Influence of hydroxyurea on fetal hemoglobin production in vitro. Blood 70:1824, 1987.

666. Veith, R., Papayannopoulou, Th., Kurachi, S., and Stamatoyannopoulos, G.: Treatment of baboon with vinblastine: insights into the mechanisms of pharmacologic stimulation of Hb F in the adult. Blood 66:456, 1985.

667. Veith, R., Galanello, R., Papayannopoulou, Th., and Stamatoyannopoulos, G.: Stimulation of F-cell production in Hb S patients treated with Ara-C or hydroxyurea. N. Engl. J. Med. 313:1571, 1985.

668. Platt, O.S., Orkin, S.H., Dover, G., Beardsley, G.P., Miller, B., and Nathan, D.G.: Hydroxyurea enhances fetal hemoglobin production in sickle cell anemia. J. Clin. Invest. 74:652, 1984.

669. Kaufman, R.E.: Hydroxyurea: specific therapy for sickle cell anemia? Blood 79:2503, 1992.

670. Charache, S., Dover, G.J., Moyer, M.A., and Moore, J.W.: Hydroxyurea-induced augmentation of fetal hemoglobin production in patients with sickle cell anemia. Blood 69:109, 1987.

671. Dover, G.J., Humphries, R.K., Moore, J.G., Ley, T.J., Young, N.S., Charache, S., and Nienhuis, A.W.: Hydroxyurea induction of hemoglobin F production in sickle cell disease: relationship between cytotoxicity and F cell production. Blood 67:735, 1986.

672. Rodgers, G.P.: Recent approaches to the treatment of sickle cell anemia. JAMA 265:2097, 1991.

673. Rodgers, G.P., Dover, G.J., Noguchi, C.T., Schechter, A.N., and Nienhuis, A.W.: Hematologic responses of patients with sickle cell disease to treatment with hydroxyurea. N. Engl. J. Med. 322:1037, 1990.

674. Charache, S., Dover, G.J., Moore, R.D., Eckert, S., Ballas, S.K., Koshy, M., Milner, P.F.A., Orringer, E.P., Phillips G., Jr., Platt, O.S., and Thomas, G.H.: Hydroxyurea: effects on hemoglobin F production in patients with sickle cell anemia. Blood 79:2555, 1992.

675. Ballas, S.K., Dover, G.J., and Charache, S.: The effect of hydroxyurea on the rheological properties of sickle erythrocytes in vivo. Am. J. Hematol. 32:104, 1989.

676. Goldberg, M.A., Brugnara, C., Dover, G.J., Schapira, L., Carache, S., and Bunn, H.F.: Treatment of sickle cell anemia with hydroxyurea and erythropoietin. N. Engl. J. Med. 323:366, 1990.

677. Charache, S., Terrin, M.L., Moore, R.D., Dover, G.J., McMahon, R.P., Barton, F.B., Waclawiw, M., and Eckert, S.V.: Design of the multicenter study of hydroxyurea in sickle cell anemia. Control. Clin. Trials 16:432, 1995.

678. Charache, S., Terrin, M.L., Moore, R.D., Dover, G.J., Barton, F.B., Eckert, S.V., McMahon, R.P., and Bonds, D.R.: Effect of hydroxyurea on the frequency of painful crises in sickle cell anemia. N. Engl. J. Med. 332:1317, 1995.

679. Charache, S., Barton, F.B., Moore, R.D., Terrin, M.L., Steinberg, M.H., Dover, G.J., Ballas, S.K., McMahon, R.P., Castro, O., and Orringer, E.P.: Hydroxyurea and sickle cell anemia: clinical utility of a myelosuppressive "switching" agent. The multicenter study of hydroxyurea in sickle cell anemia. Medicine (Baltimore) 75:300, 1996.

680. Steinberg, M.H., Ju, Z.H., Barton, F.B., Terrin, M.L., Charache, S., and Dover, G.J.: Fetal hemoglobin in sickle cell anemia: determinants of response to hydroxyurea. Multicenter study of hydroxyurea. Blood 89:1078, 1997.

681. Charache, S.: Mechanism of action of hydroxyurea in the management of sickle cell anemia in adults. Semin. Hematol. 34:15, 1997.

682. Rogers, Z.R.: Hydroxyurea therapy for diverse pediatric populations with sickle cell disease. Semin. Hematol. 34:42, 1997.

683. Vichinsky, E.P.: Hydroxyurea in children: present and future. Semin. Hematol. 34:22, 1997.

684. Maier-Redelsperger, M., de Montalembert, M., Flahault, A., Neonato, M.G., Ducrocq, R., Masson, M.P., Girot, R., and Elion, J.: Fetal hemoglobin and F-cell responses to long-term hydroxyurea treatment in young sickle cell patients. The French study group on sickle cell disease. Blood 91:4472, 1998.

685. Maier-Redelsperger, M., Labie, D., and Elion, J.: Long-term hydroxyurea treatment in young sickle cell patients. Curr. Opin. Hematol. 6:115, 1999.

686. Koren, A., Segal-Kupershmit, D., Zalman, L., Levin, C., Abu Hana, M., Palmor, H., Luder, A., and Attias, D.: Effect of hydroxyurea in sickle cell anemia: a clinical trial in children and teenagers with severe sickle cell anemia and sickle cell beta-thalassemia. Pediatr. Hematol. Oncol. 16:221, 1999.

687. Scott, J.P., Hillery, C.A., Brown, E.R., Misiewicz, V., and Labotka, R.J.: Hydroxyurea therapy in children severely affected with sickle cell disease. J. Pediatr. 128:820, 1996.

688. Styles, L.A., Lubin, B., Vichinsky, E., Lawrence, S., Hua, M., Test, S., and Kuypers, F.: Decrease of very late activation antigen-4 and CD36 on reticulocytes in sickle cell patients treated with hydroxyurea. Blood 89:2554, 1997.

689. Abboud, M., Laver, J., and Blau, C.A.: Granulocytosis causing sickle-cell crisis. Lancet 351:959, 1998.

690. Arruda, V.R., Lima, C.S., Saad, S.T., and Costa, F.F.: Successful use of hydroxyurea in beta-thalassemia major. N. Engl. J. Med. 336:964, 1997.

691. Rigano, P., Manfre, L., La Galla, R., Renda, D., Renda, M.C., Calabrese, A., Calzolari, R., and Maggio, A.: Clinical and hematological response to hydroxyurea in a patient with Hb Lepore/beta-thalassemia. Hemoglobin 21:219, 1997.

692. Saxon, B.R., Rees, D., and Olivieri, N.F.: Regression of extramedullary haemopoiesis and augmentation of fetal haemoglobin concentration during hydroxyurea therapy in beta thalassemia. Br. J. Haematol. 101:416, 1998.

693. Saxon, B.R., Waye, J.S., and Olivieri, N.F.: Increase in hemoglobin concentration during therapy with hydroxyurea in Cooley's anemia. Ann. N.Y. Acad. Sci. 850:459, 1998.

694. Styles, L., Lewis, B., Foote, D., Cuda, L., and Vichinsky, E.P.: Preliminary report: hydroxyurea produces significant clinical response in thalassemia intermedia. Ann. N.Y. Acad. Sci. 850:461, 1998.

695. Loukopoulos, D., Voskaridou, E., Stamoulakatou, A., Papassotiriou, Y., Kalotychou, V., Loutradi, A., Cozma, G., Tsiarta, H., and Pavlides, N.: Hydroxyurea therapy in thalassemia. Ann. N.Y. Acad. Sci. 850:120, 1998.

696. Voskaridou, E., Kalotychou, V., and Loukopoulos, D.: Clinical and laboratory effects of long-term administration of hydroxyurea to patients with sickle-cell beta-thalassaemia. Br. J. Haematol. 89:479, 1995.

697. Fucharoen, S., Siritanaratkul, N., Winichagoon, P., Chowthaworn, J., Siriboon, W., Muangsup, W., Chaicharoen, S., Poolsup, N., Chindavijak, B., Pootrakul, P., Piankijagum, A., Schechter, A.N., and Rodgers, G.P.: Hydroxyurea increases hemoglobin F levels and improves the effectiveness of erythropoiesis in beta-thalassemia/hemoglobin E disease. Blood 87:887, 1996.

698. Blau, C.A., Constantoulakis, P., Al-Khatti, A., Spadaccino, E., Goldwasser, E., Papayannopoulou, Th., and Stamatoyannopoulos, G.: Fetal hemoglobin in acute and chronic states of erythroid expansion. Blood 81:227, 1993.

699. Al-Khatti, A., Umemura, T., Clow, J., Abels, R.I., Vance, J., Papayannopoulou, Th., and Stamatoyannopoulos, G.: Erythropoietin stimulates F-reticulocyte formation in sickle cell anemia. Trans. Assoc. Am. Physicians 101:54, 1988.

700. Nagel, R.L., Vichinsky, E., Shah, M., Johnson, R., Spadaccino, E., Fabry, M.E., Mangahas, L., Abel, R., and Stamatoyannopoulos, G.: F reticulocyte response in sickle cell anemia treated with recombinant human erythropoietin: a double blind study. Blood 81:9, 1993.

701. Al-Khatti, A., Papayannopoulou, Th., Knitter, G., Fritsch, E.F., and Stamatoyannopoulos, G.: Cooperative enhancement of F-cell formation in baboons treated with erythropoietin and hydroxyurea. Blood 72:817, 1988.

702. McDonagh, K.T., Dover, G.J., Donahue, R.E., Nathan, D.G., Agricola, B., Byrne, E., and Nienhuis, A.W.: Hydroxyurea-induced Hb F production in anemic primates: augmentation by erythropoietin, hematopoietic growth factors, and sodium butyrate. Exp. Hematol. 20:1156, 1992.

703. Rodgers, G.P., Dover, G.J., Uyesaka, N., Noguchi, C.T., Schechter, A.N., and Nienhuis, A.W.: Augmentation by erythropoietin of the fetal-hemoglobin response to hydroxyurea in sickle cell disease. N. Engl. J. Med. 328:73, 1993.

704. el-Hazmi, M.A., al-Momen, A., Warsy, A.S., Kandaswamy, S., Huraib, S., Harakati, M., and al-Mohareb, F.: The pharmacological manipulation of fetal haemoglobin: trials using hydroxyurea and recombinant human erythropoietin. Acta Haematol. 93:57, 1995.

705. Bourantas, K., Economou, G., and Georgiou, J.: Administration of high doses of recombinant human erythropoietin to patients with beta-thalassemia intermedia: a preliminary trial. Eur. J. Haematol. 58:22, 1997.

706. Rachmilewitz, E.A., and Aker, M.: The role of recombinant human erythropoietin in the treatment of thalassemia. Ann. N.Y. Acad. Sci. 850:129, 1998.

707. Umemura, T., Al-Khatti, A., Donahue, R.E., Papayannopoulou, Th., and Stamatoyannopoulos, G.: Effects of interleukin-3 and erythropoietin on in vivo erythropoiesis and F-cell formation in primates. Blood 74:1571, 1989.

708. Kruh, J.: Effects of sodium butyrate, a new pharmacologic agent, on cells in culture. Mol. Cell. Biochem. 42:65, 1982.

709. Leder, A., and Leder, P.: Butyric acid, a potent inducer of erythroid differentiation in cultured erythroleukemic cells. Cell 5:319, 1975.

710. Papayannopoulou, Th., Nakamoto, B., Kurachi, S., and Nelson, R.: Analysis of the erythroid phenotype of HEL cells: clonal variation and the effect of inducers. Blood 70:1764, 1987.

711. Ginder, G.D., Whitters, M.J., and Pohlman, J.K.: Activation of a chicken embryonic globin gene in adult erythroid cells by 5-azacytidine and sodium butyrate. Proc. Natl. Acad. Sci. USA 81:3954, 1984.

712. Bard, H., and Prosmanne, J.: Relative rates of fetal hemoglobin and adult hemoglobin synthesis in cord blood of infants of insulin dependent diabetic mothers. Pediatrics 75:1143, 1985.

713. Perrine, S.P., Greene, M.F., and Faller, D.V.: Delay in the fetal globin switch in infants of diabetic mothers. N. Engl. J. Med. 312:334, 1985.

714. Constantoulakis, P., Papayannopoulou, Th., and Stamatoyannopoulos, G.: α-Amino-N-butyric acid stimulates fetal hemoglobin in the adult. Blood 72:1961, 1988.

715. Constantoulakis, P., Knitter, G., and Stamatoyannopoulos, G.: On the induction of fetal hemoglobin by butyrates: in vivo and in vitro studies with sodium butyrate and comparison of combination treatments with 5-AzaC and AraC. Blood 74:1963, 1989.

716. Perrine, S.P., Miller, B.A., Faller, D.V., Cohen, R.A., Vichinsky, E.P., Hurst, D., Lubin, B.H., and Papayannopoulou, Th.: Sodium butyrate enhances fetal globin gene expression in erythroid progenitors of patients with Hb SS and β thalassemia. Blood 74:454, 1989.

717. Blau, C.A., Constantoulakis, P., Shaw, C.M., and Stamatoyannopoulos, G.: Fetal hemoglobin induction with butyric acid: efficacy and toxicity. Blood 81:529, 1993.

718. Stamatoyannopoulos, G., Blau, C.A., Nakamoto, B., Josephson, B., Li, Q., Liakopoulou, E., Pace, B., Papayannopoulou, T., Brusilow, S.W., and Dover, G.: Fetal hemoglobin induction by acetate, a product of butyrate catabolism. Blood 84:3198, 1994.

719. Liakopoulou, E., Blau, C.A., Li, Q., Josephson, B., Wolf, J.A., Fournarakis, B., Raisys, V., Dover, G., Papayannopoulou, T., and Stamatoyannopoulos, G.: Stimulation of fetal hemoglobin production by short chain fatty acids. Blood 86:3227, 1995.

720. Dover, G.J., Brusilow, S., and Charache, S.: Induction of fetal hemoglobin production in subjects with sickle cell anemia by oral sodium phenylbutyrate. Blood 84:339, 1994.

721. Collins, A.F., Pearson, H.A., Giardina, P., McDonagh, K.T., Brusilow, S.W., and Dover, G.J.: Oral sodium phenylbutyrate therapy in homozygous beta thalassemia: a clinical trial. Blood 85:43, 1995.

722. Collins, A.F., Dover, G.J., and Luban, N.L.: Increased fetal hemoglobin production in patients receiving valproic acid for epilepsy. Blood 84:1690, 1994.

723. Little, J.A., Dempsey, N.J., Tuchman, M., and Ginder, G.D.: Metabolic persistence of fetal hemoglobin. Blood 85:1712, 1995.

724. Peters, A., Rohloff, D., Kohlmann, T., Renner, F., Jantschek, G., Kerner, W., and Fehm, H.L.: Fetal hemoglobin in starvation ketosis of young women. Blood 91:691, 1998.

725. Torkelson, S., White, B., Faller, D.V., Phipps, K., Pantazis, C., and Perrine, S.P.: Erythroid progenitor proliferation is stimulated by phenoxyacetic and phenylalkyl acids. Blood Cells Mol. Dis. 22:150, 1996.

726. Swank, R.A., and Stamatoyannopoulos, G.: Fetal gene reactivation. Curr. Opin. Genet. Dev. 8:366, 1998.

727. Sealy, L., and Chalkley, R.: The effect of sodium butyrate on histone modification. Cell 14:115, 1978.

728. Kuo, M.H., Brownell, J.E., Sobel, R.E., Ranalli, T.A., Cook, R.G., Edmondson, D.G., Roth, S.Y., and Allis, C.D.: Transcription-linked acetylation by Gen5p of histones H3 and H4 at specific lysines. Nature 383:269, 1996.

729. Mizzen, C.A., Yang, X.J., Kokubo, T., Brownell, J.E., Bannister, A.J., Owen-Hughes, T., Workman, J., Wang, L., Berger, S.L., Kouzarides, T., Nakatani, Y., and Allis, C.D.: The TAF(II)250 subunit of TFIID has histone acetyltransferase activity. Cell 87:1261, 1996.

730. Ogryzko, V.V., Schiltz, R.L., Russanova, V., Howard, B.H., and Nakatani, Y.: The transcriptional coactivators p300 and CBP are histone acetyltransferases. Cell 87:953, 1996.

731. Vettese-Dadey, M., Grant, P.A., Hebbes, T.R., Crane-Robinson, C., Attis, C.D., and Workman, J.L.: Acetylation of histone H4 plays a primary role in enhancing transcription factor binding to nucleosomal DNA in vitro. EMBO J. 15:2508, 1996.

732. Pazin, M.J., and Kadonaga, J.T.: What's up and down with histone deacetylation and transcription? Cell 89:325, 1997.

733. McCaffrey, P.G., Newsome, D.A., Fibach, E., Yoshida, M., and Su, M.S.: Induction of gamma-globin by histone deacetylase inhibitors. Blood 90:2075, 1997.

734. Swank, R.A., Skarpidi, E., and Stamatoyannopoulos, G.: Inhibition of histone deacetylase increases γ globin synthesis in human BFUE cultures. (Submitted.)

734a. Swank, R.A., Skarpidi, E., O'Neill, L., Turner, B., Papayannopoulou, Th., and Stamatoyannopoulos, G.: β globin locus acetylation: locus-wide rather than gene specific changes are associated with γ globin gene reactivation. (Submitted.)

735. Cappellini, M.D., Graziadei, G., Ciceri, L., Comino, A., Bianchi, P., Pomati, M., and Fiorelli, G.: Butyrate trials. Ann. N.Y. Acad. Sci. 850:110, 1998.

736. Perrine, S.P., Ginder, G.D., Faller, D.V., Dover, G.H., Ikuta, T., Witkowska, H.E., Cai, S.-P., Vichinsky, E.P., and Oliveri, N.F.: A short-term trial of butyrate to stimulate fetal-globin-gene expression in the β-globin disorders. N. Engl. J. Med. 328:81, 1993.

737. Sher, G.D., Ginder, G.D., Little, J., Yang, S., Dover, G.J., and Olivieri, N.F.: Extended therapy with intravenous arginine butyrate in patients with beta-hemoglobinopathies. N. Engl. J. Med. 332:1606, 1995.

738. Faller, D.V., and Perrine, S.P.: Butyrate in the treatment of sickle cell disease and beta-thalassemia. Curr. Opin. Hematol. 2:109, 1995.

739. Atweh, G.F., Sutton, M., Nassif, I., Boosalis, V., Dover, G.J., Wallenstein, S., Wright, E., McMahon, L., Stamatoyannopoulos, G., Faller, D.V., and Perrine, S.P.: Sustained induction of fetal hemoglobin by pulse butyrate therapy in sickle cell disease. Blood 93:1790, 1999.

6 The Thalassemias

▼▼▼▼ D. J. Weatherall

▼ ▼

The thalassemias are the most common single-gene disorders in the world population. They were among the first diseases to be studied by the methods of molecular biology and remain the prime model for understanding the relationship between molecular pathology and phenotypic diversity. Because of their particularly high frequency in many parts of the developing world, the control of the thalassemias presents a major opportunity and challenge for the application of the methods of molecular genetics to clinical practice.

Historical Perspective[1]

A form of severe anemia occurring early in life and associated with splenomegaly and characteristic bone changes was first described by Thomas Cooley and Pearl Lee in 1925.[2] A similar but milder condition was identified independently by several Italian physicians at about the same time.[1] The disorder described by Cooley was later named thalassemia, from θαλασσα, "the sea," by George Whipple because the first cases on which he carried out autopsies were all of Mediterranean background.[3] In the English literature on the field, the milder variety became known as thalassemia intermedia. It was only after 1940 that the true genetic nature of thalassemia was fully appreciated. It became clear that the disease described by Cooley and Lee is the homozygous state for a recessive autosomal gene. It was subsequently found that thalassemia is not restricted to the Mediterranean but occurs widely throughout the Mediterranean region, the Middle East, the Indian subcontinent, and Southeast Asia.[1]

In the early 1950s, after the discovery of the molecular basis of sickle cell anemia by Linus Pauling and colleagues,[4] the hemoglobin of patients with different clinical forms of thalassemia was studied in many parts of the world. It was soon realized that thalassemia is not a single disease but that it is extremely heterogeneous. Analyses of the hemoglobin patterns of patients with different types of thalassemia who had also inherited structural hemoglobin variants led to the suggestion by Vernon Ingram and Anthony Stretton that there might be two main types, α and β thalassemia.[5] The development of methods for studying hemoglobin synthesis in vitro led to the experimental validation of this hypothesis and to the further analysis of thalassemia,[6] so that it was apparent by the early 1970s that there are many different forms, all associated with defective synthesis of one or more of the globin chains of hemoglobin.

By the early 1970s, a great deal was known about the genetic control of human hemoglobin, many structural variants had been characterized, and the biosynthetic defects and remarkable heterogeneity of the thalassemias had been established.[7] The human hemoglobin field was, therefore, an ideal testing ground for the application of the new techniques of recombinant DNA. First, by soluble hybridization, it was possible to demonstrate reduced amounts of globin messenger RNA (mRNA) and, later, deletions of the globin genes in some forms of thalassemia. Later, the advent of Southern blotting and cloning technology led to the definition of the molecular pathology of many forms of thalassemia, so paving the way for an understanding of the molecular basis for many human single-gene disorders.

Definition and Classification

The thalassemias are defined as a heterogeneous group of inherited disorders of hemoglobin synthesis, all characterized by the absence or reduced output of one or more of the globin chains of hemoglobin. They can be classified at several levels. First, there is a clinical classification, which simply describes the degree of severity. Second, the thalassemias can be defined by the particular globin chain that is synthesized at a reduced rate. Finally, it is now often possible to subclassify them according to the particular mutation that is responsible for defective globin chain synthesis.[7, 8]

▼ CLINICAL CLASSIFICATION

The descriptive classification of thalassemia, although it has no strict genetic basis, is still useful in clinical practice. The thalassemias are divided into the major forms of the illness, which are severe and transfusion dependent, and the symptomless minor forms, which usually represent the carrier state, or trait. Thalassemia major results either from the homozygous inheritance of a particular mutation or from the compound heterozygous state for two different mutations.

Thalassemia intermedia describes conditions that are associated with a more severe degree of anemia than the trait, although they are not as severe as the major forms. In practice, this term encompasses a wide clinical spectrum ranging from disorders that are almost as serious as the major forms to asymptomatic conditions that are only slightly more severe than the trait.

Finally, there are some forms of thalassemia trait that are clinically and hematologically completely silent; they are designated "silent" carrier states.

▼ GENETIC CLASSIFICATION

The thalassemias are classified according to their genetic basis by describing the globin chain that is synthesized at a reduced rate. A classification of the thalassemia syndromes is shown in Table 6–1.

Table 6–1. The Thalassemias and Related Disorders

α Thalassemia
$\quad \alpha^0$
$\quad \alpha^+$
$\qquad$ Deletion ($-\alpha$)
$\qquad$ Non-deletion (α^T)
β Thalassemia
$\quad \beta^0$
$\quad \beta^+$
$\quad$ Normal Hb A_2
$\quad$ "Silent"
$\delta\beta$ Thalassemia
$\quad (\delta\beta)^+$
$\quad (\delta\beta)^0$
$\quad (^A\gamma\delta\beta)^0$
γ Thalassemia
δ Thalassemia
$\quad \delta^0$
$\quad \delta^+$
$\epsilon\gamma\delta\beta$ Thalassemia
Hereditary persistence of fetal hemoglobin
$\quad$ Deletion
$\qquad (\delta\beta)^0$
$\qquad$ G$\gamma(\gamma\beta)^+$ (Hb Kenya)
$\quad$ Non-deletion
$\qquad$ Linked to β globin genes
$\qquad \quad {}^G\gamma\beta^+$
$\qquad \quad {}^A\gamma\beta^+$
$\qquad$ Unlinked to β globin genes

The structure and genetic control of human hemoglobin is summarized in Figure 6–1. Human adult hemoglobin is a mixture of proteins consisting of a major component, hemoglobin A (Hb A), and a minor component, Hb A_2, which constitutes about 2.5 per cent of the total. During early development, there are several embryonic hemoglobins, after which the main hemoglobin during intrauterine life is Hb F.

The structure of these hemoglobins is similar. Each consists of two separate pairs of identical globin chains. Except for some of the embryonic hemoglobins, all the normal human hemoglobins have one pair of α chains: in Hb A, they are combined with β chains ($\alpha_2\beta_2$); in Hb A_2, with δ chains ($\alpha_2\delta_2$); and in Hb F, with γ chains ($\alpha_2\gamma_2$). Human hemoglobin shows further heterogeneity, particularly in fetal life, an observation that has important implications for understanding the thalassemias. Hb F is a mixture of two molecular forms with the formulas $\alpha_2\gamma_2^{136Gly}$ and $\alpha_2\gamma_2^{136Ala}$. The γ chains containing glycine at position 136 are designated $^G\gamma$ chains, and those containing alanine at this position are called $^A\gamma$ chains.

Before the eighth week of intrauterine life, there are three embryonic hemoglobins, Hb Gower 1 ($\zeta_2\epsilon_2$), Hb Gower 2 ($\alpha_2\epsilon_2$), and Hb Portland ($\zeta_2\gamma_2$). The ζ and ϵ chains are the embryonic counterparts of the adult α and β, γ, and δ chains, respectively. Although thalassemia involving the embryonic globin genes has not been described, they are of importance in the thalassemia field because in some forms of α thalassemia, there is persistence of ζ chain synthesis.

The classification of the thalassemias according to which chain is produced at a reduced rate reflects the structure of the globin gene clusters that are involved in their synthesis (see Fig. 6–1). The β-like globin chains are controlled by a gene cluster on chromosome 11 in which the different genes are arranged in the order 5'-ϵ-$^G\gamma$-$^A\gamma$-$\psi\beta$-δ-β-3'. The α-like gene cluster is on chromosome 16, p13.3, and the genes are arranged in the order $5'-\zeta-\psi\zeta-\varphi\alpha-\alpha2-\alpha1-\theta-3'$.

As shown in Table 6–1, the thalassemias are classified into α, β, γ, $\delta\beta$, δ, and $\epsilon\gamma\delta\beta$ varieties, depending on which chain or chains are synthesized at a reduced rate.

α Thalassemia. Because there are two α globin genes per haploid genome, four in all, the α thalassemias are classified according to the relative output of both α genes. When both α globin genes on a chromosome are inactivated, the condition is called α^0 thalassemia. The heterozygous genotype can be written $--/\alpha\alpha$. When one of the linked α globin genes is inactivated, the condition is called α^+ thalassemia, and the genotype can be written $-\alpha/\alpha\alpha$ in cases in which one of the α globin genes in deleted, or $\alpha^T\alpha/\alpha\alpha$ if one of the linked α genes is inactivated by a mutation. In other words, α^0 and α^+ thalassemia describe an α globin haplotype, that is, the state of the *two* linked α globin genes on a particular chromosome: in α^0 thalassemia, there is no output of α globin from the particular chromosome; in α^+ thalassemia, there is some output, but usually only the product of a single α globin locus. In some descriptions of α thalassemia, the less logical terms α thalassemia 1 and 2 are used to describe α^0 and α^+ thalassemia, respectively.

β Thalassemia. There are two main varieties of β thalassemia, β^0 thalassemia, in which no β globin chains are produced, and β^+ thalassemia, in which some β chains are produced but at a reduced rate. Some forms of β thalassemia are designated β^{++} to indicate that the defect in β chain production is particularly mild.

The diagnostic feature of β thalassemia is an elevated level of Hb A_2 in heterozygotes, which is found in most forms of β^0 and β^+ thalassemia. There are, however, less common forms of β thalassemia in which the Hb A_2 level is normal in heterozygotes. These so-called normal Hb A_2 β thalassemias are also heterogeneous. They are classified into two varieties: type 1, in which there are no associated hematological changes; and type 2, in which the hematological findings are typical of β thalassemia trait with a raised Hb A_2 level. Type 1 normal Hb A_2 β thalassemia is also called silent β thalassemia. Both these forms of β thalassemia with normal Hb A_2 levels are heterogeneous at the molecular level.

δβ Thalassemia. The $\delta\beta$ thalassemias are also heterogeneous. In some cases, no δ or β chains are synthesized. In the past, it was customary to classify these conditions according to the structure of the γ chains of the Hb F that are produced, $^G\gamma^A\gamma(\delta\beta)^0$ and $^G\gamma(\delta\beta)^0$ thalassemia, for example. This was illogical and out of line with the classification of thalassemia according to the chain that is ineffectively synthesized. Thus, these conditions are best described as $(\delta\beta)^0$ and $(^A\gamma\delta\beta)^0$ thalassemias.

There are also $(\delta\beta)^+$ forms of $\delta\beta$ thalassemia. In many of these conditions, an abnormal hemoglobin is produced that has normal α chains combined with non-α chains that are constituted by the N-terminal residues of the δ chain fused to the C-terminal residues of the β chain. These $\delta\beta$ fusion variants, collectively called the Lepore hemoglobins, are synthesized inefficiently and produce the clinical phenotype of $\delta\beta$ thalassemia.

δ Thalassemia. Several different mutations give rise to a reduced output of δ chains and hence a reduced level of Hb A_2. These conditions are clinically silent and are of importance only insomuch that when they are inherited together with β thalassemia, they may prevent an elevation of the level of Hb A_2.

εγδβ Thalassemia. This rare form of thalassemia results from loss of either the whole or part of the β-like globin gene cluster. Homozygotes have not been encountered, presumably because the condition would not be compatible with life; heterozygotes have the clinical phenotype of β thalassemia with a normal Hb A_2 level.

γ Thalassemia. There have been a few reports of deletions involving one or the other γ globin genes.[8] They have been identified by determining the level of $^G\gamma$ and $^A\gamma$ chains in Hb F and do not appear to be of clinical significance. They are not considered further in this chapter.

Hereditary Persistence of Fetal Hemoglobin (HPFH) as a Form of β or δβ Thalassemia. This is another heterogeneous group of disorders of hemoglobin synthesis that are characterized by persistent fetal hemoglobin synthesis in adult life in the absence of major hematological abnormalities. They are described in detail in Chapter 5. By virtue of their interaction with the β thalassemias, and from other evidence, it is apparent that many of these conditions are extremely well compensated forms of β or $\delta\beta$ thalassemia. In addition, HPFH is important in the thalassemia field because of the way in which it can modify the clinical phenotype of the β thalassemias.

As shown in Table 6–1, HPFH is classified along lines similar to the thalassemias. First, there are those forms in which no δ or β globin chains are produced but in which there is almost complete compensation by a high output of γ

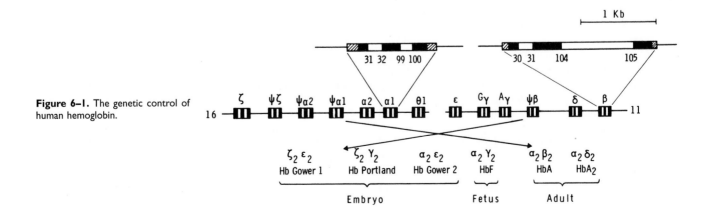

Figure 6–1. The genetic control of human hemoglobin.

chains; these conditions are designated $(\delta\beta)^0$ HPFH. Second, there is a family of HPFH variants in which there is β and probably δ chain synthesis in *cis* to the HPFH determinant. These conditions are designated $^G\gamma\beta^+$ or $^A\gamma\beta^+$ HPFH, depending on the structure of the Hb F. Finally, there is a group of conditions, also heterogeneous, in which much lower levels of Hb F are found in otherwise normal individuals. There is increasing evidence that the genetic determinant for at least some types of this form of HPFH may not be linked to the β globin gene cluster.

The first two types of HPFH are characterized by relatively high levels of Hb F production in heterozygotes, usually 15 to 25 per cent of the total hemoglobin, which is relatively homogeneously distributed among the red cells. In the last group, there are much lower levels of persistent Hb F production, in the 2 to 10 per cent range, usually heterogeneously distributed among the red cells. Thus, HPFH is also classified as either pancellular or heterocellular, although this subdivision is becoming less useful as knowledge of its molecular pathology increases.

▼ MOLECULAR CLASSIFICATION

As their molecular pathology has been worked out, it has been feasible to develop a more accurate approach to the designation of the different types of α and β thalassemia. For example, in many cases, it is now possible to describe the genotype of a patient with the clinical picture of β thalassemia major according to the particular mutations at the homologous pairs of β globin chain loci. Homozygotes for a common Mediterranean nonsense mutation would have the genotype $\alpha\alpha/\beta^{39C \rightarrow T}\beta^{39C \rightarrow T}$. On the other hand, compound heterozygotes for this mutation and another common Mediterranean RNA processing mutation would have the genotype $\alpha\alpha/\beta^{39C \rightarrow T}\beta^{IVS-1,1G \rightarrow A}$.

The molecular classification of different forms of thalassemia is considered in more detail as their molecular pathology is described in later sections.

The Complexity of the Thalassemias: The Thalassemia Syndromes

It is clear from the classification of the thalassemias outlined in the previous section that all the common forms of thalassemia, particularly the α, β, and $\delta\beta$ thalassemias, are extremely heterogeneous. However, the complexity of these disorders does not end there. In many populations in which thalassemia is common, there is also a high frequency of structural hemoglobin variants, particularly Hb S, Hb C, or Hb E. Thus, it is common for an individual to inherit thalassemia from one parent and a structural hemoglobin variant from another. Similarly, both α and β thalassemia occur at a high frequency, and therefore individuals may inherit one or more different α thalassemia alleles and β thalassemia as well.

In countries like Thailand, where there is a high frequency of all forms of thalassemia and a particular structural hemoglobin variant, in this case Hb E, the many different interactions of these different mutations produce a bewilderingly complex series of clinical phenotypes ranging from

disorders that are lethal to those that are symptomless and are recognized only by mild anemia or morphological changes of the red cells.[7, 8]

In the sections that follow, I describe each of the different types of thalassemia separately and then attempt to define the clinical phenotypes produced by their interactions. As will become apparent, although we have a sophisticated understanding of the molecular pathology of many of these disorders, our knowledge about the clinical consequences of their interaction is, in many cases, still fragmentary.

α Thalassemia

▼ BACKGROUND AND CLASSIFICATION

The evolution of our understanding of the α thalassemias[1, 7–10] has taken longer than for β thalassemia, largely because for many years it was not appreciated that normal individuals have four α globin genes, two per haploid genome. The first intimation of the existence of α thalassemia came from the discovery of patients with thalassemia-like blood pictures and varying amounts of a hemoglobin variant that was later shown to be a homotetramer composed of four β chains (β_4). This abnormal hemoglobin was discovered in the mid-1950s, when new electrophoretic hemoglobin variants were designated by letters of the alphabet, and was called Hb H. A few years later, another variant of this type, in this case a homotetramer of γ chains, γ_4, was discovered in an anemic baby at St. Bartholomew's Hospital, London. By then, there were no letters of the alphabet left for new hemoglobins, which had to be named by their place of discovery; the γ_4 variant was called Hb Bart's, the abbreviated form of St. Bartholomew's Hospital! Thus, it appeared that Hb Bart's and Hb H might reflect defective α chain production, α thalassemia, in fetal and adult life, respectively.

Subsequently it became apparent that there are two main clinical forms of α thalassemia. First, there is the Hb Bart's hydrops fetalis syndrome, a disorder characterized by a severe deficiency of α chains and death late in uterine life. The second important variety, Hb H disease, is characterized by a moderately severe anemia associated with variable amounts of Hb H in the blood. Analysis of the parents of patients with the Hb Bart's hydrops fetalis syndrome or Hb H disease led to the idea that there are two types of α thalassemia trait, a severe form, which was called α thalassemia 1, and a much milder condition, α thalassemia 2, which may be hematologically silent.

When it was realized that there are two α globin genes on each of the homologous pairs of chromosomes 16, and when methods for their direct analysis became available, it was possible to clarify the genetics of α thalassemia. It became clear that there are two types: α^0 thalassemia, in which no normal α globin is produced from the α globin gene complex; and α^+ thalassemia, in which the output is reduced. Further work showed that α^+ thalassemia usually results from the deletion or inactivation by a mutation of one of the linked pairs of α globin gene. Thus, the terms α thalassemia 1 and α thalassemia 2 should be replaced by α^0 thalassemia and α^+ thalassemia, respectively.

A general model of the interaction of the α^0 and α^+ thalassemias is shown in Figure 6–2. The Hb Bart's hydrops

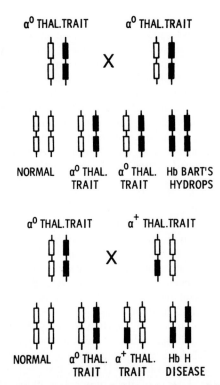

Figure 6–2. The genetics of α thalassemia. The α globin genes are represented as boxes. The black α genes represent gene deletions or otherwise inactivated α genes. The open boxes represent normal α genes. The terms α⁰ thalassemia and α⁺ thalassemia are defined in the text.

syndrome results from the homozygous state for α⁰ thalassemia, whereas Hb H disease usually reflects the compound heterozygous state for α⁰ and α⁺ thalassemia.

Now that the molecular pathology of the α globin genes is worked out, it is possible to further classify the α thalassemias.[9] The normal α globin haplotype may be written αα, representing the α2 and α1 genes, respectively. Therefore, a normal individual has the genotype αα/αα. A deletion involving one (– α) or both (– –) α genes may be further

classified on the basis of its size, written as a superscript; thus – α³·⁷ indicates a deletion of 3.7 kb of DNA including one α gene. When the size of a deletion has not yet been established, a superscript describing the geographical or individual origin of the deletion is used; thus, – –ᴹᴱᴰ describes a deletion of both α genes first identified in individuals of Mediterranean origin. Finally, in those α thalassemic haplotypes in which both linked α globin genes are intact, the nomenclature αᵀα or ααᵀ is used, indicating a thalassemia mutation at one or the other of the linked α genes. When the precise molecular defect is known, as in the α globin chain termination mutant Hb Constant Spring, for example, αᵀα can be replaced by the more precise αᶜˢα.

This nomenclature has provided a useful shorthand way of describing the complex interactions of the different forms of α thalassemia. For example, the genotype – –ˢᴱᴬ/αᶜˢα denotes the interaction of a chromosome containing the Hb Constant Spring mutation with a chromosome containing the common Southeast Asian form of α⁰ thalassemia, a common finding in patients with Hb H disease.

▼ THE STRUCTURE OF THE α GLOBIN GENE COMPLEX

The α globin gene cluster lies near the tip of chromosome 16 and has been assigned to 16p13.3. The distance from the telomere varies from 170 to 430 kb, reflecting common length polymorphisms in this region.[11, 12] The cluster includes the duplicated α genes, α2 and α1; an embryonic α-like gene (ζ2); and three pseudogenes, ψζ1, ψα1, and ψα2, arranged in the order 5'-ζ2-ψζ1-ψα2-ψα1-α2-α1-θ-3' (Fig. 6–3; see also Fig. 6–1). Analysis of the normal map of this region and that of a patient with a deletion of the terminal part of chromosome 16 has shown that the α complex is arranged with the ζ2 gene at the telomeric end of the array and the α1 gene at the centromeric end.

The 26 kb segment of DNA that contains the α globin genes and an extended cloned segment flanking the cluster are part of a long G + C rich isochore.[9] The α globin

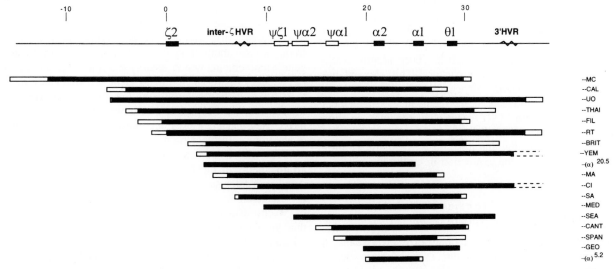

Figure 6–3. The deletions of the α globin genes that result in α⁰ thalassemia. References to the original descriptions are given in references 12 and 38. (Prepared by Dr. D. R. Higgs.)

cluster and its boundaries have many of the characteristics of such regions; it is G + C rich, early replicating, within a Giemsa-negative band, and it contains many *Alu* family repeats. Such regions of the genome are usually thought to contain a high proportion of housekeeping genes; at least four widely expressed genes have been identified between the α gene cluster and the telomere.[10, 12]

Structure and Expression of the α-Like Globin Genes

The α globin gene family has evolved through a series of gene duplications and sequence divergences so that now the functional α and ζ genes show only 58 per cent homology in their 141 amino acids.[9, 10, 12, 13] In contrast, the α1 and α2 genes are highly homologous, encode identical proteins, and differ in sequence only within intervening sequence 2 (IVS-2) and in their 3′ non-coding regions. Like all globin genes, the α genes are divided into three exons by two non-coding intervening sequences. All the α-like globin genes and their flanking regions have been sequenced, and the entire region from the telomere of 16p to beyond the α globin gene complex has been cloned and partially mapped. A region stretching nearly 300,000 bp from the telomere has been sequenced, providing a detailed picture of the structural and functional organization of a telomeric region.[14]

Both α and ζ genes are expressed in the primitive erythroblasts of the yolk sac up to 6 or 7 weeks of gestation, although ζ globin synthesis predominates during this period; definitive-line erythroblasts synthesize α globin almost exclusively. The expression of the α2 gene predominates over the α1 gene by approximately 3:1 throughout all stages of development and in adult life. By use of sensitive assays, low levels of ζ globin expression can be detected throughout fetal life and in up to 80 per cent of cord blood samples. Although the function of the θ gene is unknown, θ mRNA can be detected at all stages of development.[9]

Each of the α genes contain typical promoter box structures at their 5-terminal flanking regions. Studies of α globin synthesis in mouse erythroleukemia cells and in transgenic mice, combined with an analysis of the position of DNase I hypersensitive sites and naturally occurring deletions upstream from the α globin gene complex, have defined an element 40 kb upstream from the α globin gene cluster (HS40) that has some of the properties of a locus control region (LCR) similar to that which has been identified upstream from the β globin gene cluster.[15] This element has been sequenced and shown to contain binding sites for NF-E2/AP-1, GATA-1, and CAC box proteins in an arrangement similar to the β globin LCR. As we shall see later, deletion of the α LCR sequences completely inactivates the α globin gene complex, suggesting that it is a major regulatory region involved in α globin gene expression in erythroid tissues.

Polymorphisms and Normal Variability at the α Globin Gene Complex

In interpreting the molecular pathology of α thalassemia, it is important to appreciate structural variability in the α globin gene cluster that is not associated with any hematological abnormalities. Its structure is highly polymor-phic.[9–14, 16] There are numerous point mutations, rearrangements, and gene conversions that have no apparent effect on the expression of the α globin genes. Analysis of the patterns of these polymorphisms in chromosomes derived from individuals representing 25 different populations has led to the definition of a number of specific α globin haplotypes that are extremely valuable for anthropological and population studies and, in particular, for tracing the origins and distribution of the α thalassemia mutations.[7, 9, 10]

Length Variation at the Telomere of Chromosome 16p. As mentioned earlier, there are common length variation alleles involving the end of chromosome 16. These lie at 170 kb, 245 kb, 350 kb, and 430 kb from the 16p telomeric repeats.[11, 12]

Chromosome Rearrangements Involving 16p13.3. Translocations involving 16p.13.3 may move the α globin locus to the tip of another chromosome. If these are balanced, there are no associated clinical features, and in no case has there been any evidence of α thalassemia. This topic is expanded in a later section that deals with the α thalassemia mental retardation syndromes.

Variable Numbers of Tandem Repeats (VNTRs). The α globin gene cluster contains several tandemly repeated segments of DNA, or minisatellites. They were first identified as highly variable regions (HVRs), later called VNTRs, located at the 3′ end of the complex (α globin 3-HVR), between the ζ2 and ψζ1 genes (interζ HVR), and within the introns of the ζ-like genes (ζ intron HVRs).[16] More recently, similar regions have been located in the 5′ flanking region of the cluster; a particularly informative polymorphic locus lies 70 kb upstream of the ζ2 gene, a region that has been designated the 5′ HVR.[17] At least 10 VNTRs have been identified in the terminal 300 kb of chromosome 16. Together with other polymorphisms, these regions have been of great value in the genetic analysis of the α globin cluster.

Variation in the Number of α-Like Globin Genes.[9, 10, 12] As a result of unequal genetic exchange, phenotypically normal individuals may have four, five, or six α genes and three, four, five, or six ζ-like genes. The ααα chromosome arrangement occurs at a relatively high frequency, 0.01 to 0.08 in most populations. Even in the homozygous state for the triplicated α gene arrangement, there are no hematological abnormalities.

Chromosomes carrying a single ζ gene instead of the usual ζ2-ψζ1 arrangement are also common, with a gene frequency of about 0.05 in West Africa. The triplicated ζ gene arrangement, which usually has the structure ζ2-φζ1-φζ, occurs in parts of Southeast Asia at a frequency of 0.09 to 0.20; it is particularly common throughout Melanesia, Micronesia, and Polynesia, where phenotypically normal homozygotes (ζζζ/ζζζ) have been described. This arrangement is uncommon in other parts of the world.

The molecular basis for the generation of these novel arrangements of the ζ and α globin genes is considered in detail in a later section that describes the deletion forms of α+ thalassemia.

Gene Conversions.[9, 10, 12] Sequence analyses suggest that gene conversion events have taken place between the α1 and α2 and the ζ2 and ψζ1 genes during evolution.

Studies of the downstream ζ-like gene in several populations have shown that it exists in two distinct forms, one typically that of a pseudogene (ψζ1), the other in which the ψζ1 gene has undergone a gene conversion by the ζ2 gene such that it becomes similar to the functional ζ gene. The frequency of the ζ2-ζ1 chromosome varies between populations, and normal individuals homozygous for either the ζ2-ψζ1 or ζ2-ζ1 chromosomes have been observed. There are also several examples of conversions between the α2 and α1 genes.

Deletions and Insertions in the α Globin Complex.[10, 12] Several phenotypically silent deletions and insertions have been identified in the α globin complex. There are no hematological abnormalities. It is important to recognize that these changes can be found in normal individuals if they are not to be misinterpreted as the cause of unusual types of α thalassemia.

▼ MOLECULAR PATHOLOGY

In defining the molecular pathology of the α thalassemias, it is necessary to describe the molecular events that cause the loss of both α globin genes and hence produce the phenotype of α^0 thalassemia, and those that lead to the inactivation of one of the linked pairs of α genes and underlie the phenotype of α^+ thalassemia (Table 6–2). It turns out that the α^0 thalassemias are due to a heterogeneous series of deletions involving either the α globin gene complex itself or the α globin LCR. On the other hand, the α^+ thalassemias may result either from deletions of one or the other of the linked pairs of α globin genes or from mutations that cause their partial or complete inactivation although they leave the genes intact.

α^0 Thalassemia

Deletions That Remove All or Part of the α Globin Gene Cluster

To date, 18 different lesions have been described that remove both α globin genes[9, 10, 12] (see Fig. 6–3). The majority of these lesions remove both α genes, although in two cases they remove one gene and part of the other; in some cases, the ζ globin genes are lost. It is clear, therefore, that chromosomes containing these deletions can produce no α globin chains, and hence molecular lesions of this type are all associated with the phenotype of α^0 thalassemia. As mentioned earlier, the terminal 300 kb of chromosome 16 has now been sequenced,[14] and the full extent of some of these deletions, which extend from 100 to 250 kb, has been defined. In some cases, they remove other genes that flank the cluster, including those for a DNA repair enzyme, an inhibitor of GPD dissociation from Rho, and a protein disulfide isomerase.[12, 14]

In contrast to the α^+ thalassemia deletions, which are described later, the α^0 thalassemia deletions are limited in their geographical distribution. For example, the − −[BRIT] mutation has been observed in 36 different families, all of which come from a small region in the north of England.[18] Analysis of polymorphic markers upstream of the common α^0 thalassemias of Southeast Asia and the Mediterranean region, − −[SEA] and − −[MED], suggests that each of these mutations has arisen only once during evolution and reached their current high frequency by selection.[9, 12]

Detailed analyses of the sequences across the breakpoints of these deletions have provided some evidence about the molecular events that have produced them.[9, 10, 19] A number of mechanisms have been demonstrated, including illegitimate recombination, reciprocal translocation, and truncation of chromosome 16. Hence, the study of these lesions has provided valuable information about the ways in which deletions of human chromosomes may occur.

It turns out that several of the 3′ breakpoints of the α^0 thalassemia deletions fall within a 6 to 8 kb region at the 3′ end of the α globin complex, suggesting that this may represent a breakpoint cluster region *(bcr)*, similar to those observed in the chromosomal translocations associated with certain forms of leukemia. In some of the deletions, − −[MED], − −[SEA], − −[20.5], − −[SA], and − −[BRIT], the 5′ breakpoints also appear to cluster (see Fig. 6–3). It appears, therefore, that the 5′ breakpoints are located approximately the same distance apart and in the same order along the chromosome as their respective 3′ breakpoints.[19] These observations are consistent with similar findings in a group of deletions of the β globin gene cluster. It has been suggested that such staggered deletions may result from illegitimate recombination events, which lead to the deletion of an integral number of chromatin loops as they pass through their nuclear attachment points during replication.[20]

One of these deletions, − −[MED], also involves a more complex rearrangement in which a new piece of DNA bridges the two breakpoints in the α globin gene cluster.[19] The inserted sequence originates upstream from the α globin gene cluster, where it normally exists in an inverted orientation to that found between the breakpoints of the deletion. Thus, it appears to have been incorporated into the junction in a way that reflects its close proximity to the deletion breakpoint regions during replication.

Table 6–2. Classes of Mutations That Cause α^+ Thalassemia*

α^0 Thalassemia
    Deletions involving α globin gene cluster
    Truncations of telomeric region of 16p
    Deletions of HS40 region
α^+ Thalassemia
    Deletions involving α2 or α1 genes
    Point mutations involving α2 or α1 genes
      mRNA processing
        IVS-1 donor
        IVS-1 acceptor
        Poly(A) signal
      mRNA translation
        Initiation codon
        Exon 1 or 2
        Termination codon
      Post-translational
        Unstable α globin
α Thalassemia mental retardation
    ATR-16
      Deletions/telomeric truncations of 16p
      Translocations
    ATR-X
      Mutations of *XH2*
      Deletions
      Missense
      Nonsense
      Splice site

* Complete lists of individual mutations are found in references 10, 12, and 38.

Further sequence analyses have shown that members of the dispersed family of *Alu* repeats are found frequently at or near the breakpoints of these deletions. One deletion, $\alpha\alpha^{RA}$, seems to have resulted from simple homologous recombination between two *Alu* repeats that are usually 62 kb apart.[19] *Alu* family repeats have been involved in similar recombinational events elsewhere in the genome.

Another mechanism for the generation of α^0 thalassemia has been identified.[21] In this case, there is a terminal truncation of the short arm of chromosome 16 to a site 50 kb distal to the α globin genes. Interestingly, the telomeric consensus sequence $(TTAGGG)_n$ had been added directly to the site of the break. Because this mutation was shown to be stably inherited, it appears that telomeric DNA alone is sufficient to stabilize the broken chromosome end. This observation raises the possibility that other genetic diseases may result from chromosome truncations.

Deletions Involving the α Globin LCR

Several deletions have been identified that appear to down-regulate the α globin genes by removal of the α globin LCR[22–24] (Fig. 6–4). In each case, the α globin genes are left intact, although in RA, the 3' breakpoint is found between the $\zeta2$ and $\psi\zeta1$ genes, thus removing the $\zeta2$ gene.[23] It appears that these deletions completely inactivate the α globin gene complex. They have not been observed in the homozygous state, presumably because it would be lethal.

Deletions Downstream of the α Globin Gene Cluster

One deletion, 18 kb, has been found to involve the $\alpha1$ and θ genes and a region downstream from the α gene cluster.[25] It appears to inactivate the remaining $\alpha2$ gene; the mechanism has not yet been determined. It is possible that a downstream regulatory region has been removed by the deletion.

α+ Thalassemia

So far, all the α^+ thalassemias have been found to result either from deletions of one or the other of the duplicated α globin genes or from mutations that inactivate them.

α+ Thalassemia Due to Deletions

The most common types of α^+ thalassemia involve the deletion of one or the other of the duplicated α globin genes, $-\alpha^{3.7}$ and $-\alpha^{4.2}$ (Fig. 6–5). These conditions are among the most common human genetic disorders and are found in every population in which α thalassemia is common.

The mechanism that has led to the generation of the α^+ thalassemia deletions reflects the underlying structure of the α globin gene complex.[13, 26] Each α gene lies within a boundary of homology approximately 4 kb long, interrupted by two small non-homologous regions. The homologous regions were probably generated by an ancient duplication and then, subsequently, were subdivided, presumably by insertions and deletions, to give three homologous subsegments that are designated X, Y, and Z (Fig. 6–6). The duplicated Z boxes are 3.7 kb apart, and the X boxes are 4.2 kb apart. As shown in Figure 6–6, misalignment and reciprocal cross-over between these segments at meiosis produce a chromosome with either single ($-\alpha$) or triplicated ($\alpha\alpha\alpha$) α globin genes. If the cross-over occurs between homologous Z boxes, 3.7 kb of DNA are lost, an event that is described as a rightward deletion, $-\alpha^{3.7}$. A similar process occurring between the two X boxes deletes 4.2 kb, the leftward deletion, $-\alpha^{4.2}$. The corresponding triplicated α gene arrangements are called $\alpha\alpha\alpha^{anti-3.7}$ and $\alpha\alpha\alpha^{anti-4.2}$.[27–30] Chromosomes with four α genes, $\alpha\alpha\alpha\alpha^{anti-3.7}$ or $\alpha\alpha\alpha\alpha^{anti-4.2}$, presumably arose from similar types of cross-overs involving the $\alpha\alpha\alpha^{anti-3.7}$ and $\alpha\alpha\alpha^{anti-4.2}$ chromosomes, respectively.[31]

Rearrangements involving the Z box are more frequent than those involving the X or Y regions. The Z box rearrangements can be subdivided into three types, $-\alpha^{3.7I}$, $-\alpha^{3.7II}$, and $-\alpha^{3.7III}$, depending on the site of the cross-over with respect to three restriction enzyme sites that differ between the $\alpha2$ and $\alpha1$ Z boxes.[32] From population data, it appears that the frequency of each of these subtypes is related to the length of homology within each subsegment.

In addition to the three $-\alpha^{3.7}$ and the $-\alpha^{4.2}$ deletions, three additional rare deletions that produce α^+ thalassemia have been described. One that removes the entire $\alpha1$ gene and its flanking DNA ($-\alpha^{3.5}$) has been found in two Asian Indians.[33] The breakpoints of this deletion have not yet been defined in detail. A second deletion, referred to as $\alpha(\alpha^{5.3})$,

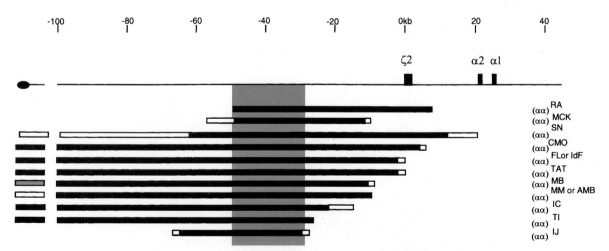

Figure 6–4. Deletions upstream from the α globin genes that inactivate the α globin gene complex by removing HS40. Original descriptions in reference 12. (Prepared by Dr. D. R. Higgs.)

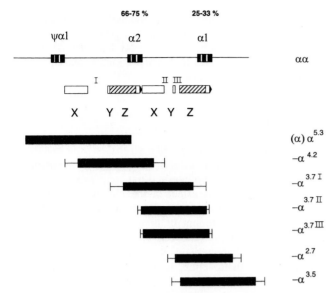

Figure 6–5. The deletions that underlie the α^+ thalassemias.

all lead to a reduced output of α chains from the affected chromosome (see Fig. 6–5). Because the output of the $\alpha2$ gene is two to three times greater than that of the $\alpha1$ gene, it would be expected that there would be phenotypic differences between these conditions. Interestingly, the phenotypes of homozygotes for the $-\alpha^{4.2}$ and $-\alpha^{3.7III}$ determinants are similar, suggesting that removal of the $\alpha2$ gene results in a partial compensatory increase in the expression of the remaining $\alpha1$ gene on the $-\alpha^{4.2}$ chromosome.[36] In fact, a compensatory increase in expression of the $\alpha1$ gene when the $\alpha2$ gene is deleted has been demonstrated at the RNA level.[37] Thus, the phenotypic effects of these deletions follow the pattern of all lesions of this type involving the globin gene clusters in that they exert an effect on the expression of nearby genes.

It appears, therefore, that homologous genetic recombination occurs relatively frequently within the human α globin gene cluster. It is not known whether such rearrangements occur between misaligned chromosomes or between chromatids during meiosis. The finding of a triplicated α globin gene arrangement, $\alpha\alpha\alpha$, in most populations at a low frequency suggests that the single α globin gene arrangement that forms the basis for the deletion form of α^+ thalassemia has come under strong selection in those parts of the world where α^+ thalassemia is common. We shall return to this theme later in the chapter when the population genetics of the α thalassemias is considered.

removes the 5′ end of the $\alpha2$ globin gene; the 5′ breakpoint lies 22 bp upstream from the mRNA cap site of the $\alpha1$ gene, whereas the 3′ breakpoint is located in IVS-1 of the $\alpha2$ gene.[34] This deletion appears to have arisen by an illegitimate recombination event. A third rare α^+ thalassemia deletion involves 2.7 kb that removes the $\alpha1$ gene; the breakpoints have not been sequenced.[35]

The seven deletions involving single α globin genes, $(\alpha)\alpha^{5.3}, -\alpha^{3.7I}, -\alpha^{3.7II}, -\alpha^{3.7III}, -\alpha^{4.2}, -\alpha^{3.5}$, and $-\alpha^{2.7}$,

Non-Deletion Types of α^+ Thalassemia

Non-deletion α^+ thalassemias are conditions in which the output of α globin from one of the linked α globin genes is defective yet the affected gene is grossly intact. These disorders result from single or oligonucleotide mutations of the particular α globin gene. The majority involve the $\alpha2$ gene, but because the output from this locus is two to three times greater than that from the $\alpha1$ gene, this may reflect ascertainment bias due to a greater effect on the phenotype and, possibly, a greater selective advantage. Unlike the effects of deletions of the $\alpha2$ gene that underlie the $-\alpha^{4.2}$ form of α^+ thalassemia, there appears to be no compensatory increase in expression of the $\alpha1$ gene when the $\alpha2$ gene is inactivated by a point mutation. It follows, therefore, that the non-deletion α^+ thalassemias have a greater phenotypic effect than the deletion forms do.

Complete catalogues of these mutations have been compiled,[12, 38] and only those of particular functional interest are described here.

The varieties of mutations that cause non-deletion α^+ thalassemia are summarized in Table 6–2. They are much less common than the deletion forms of α^+ thalassemia, and their geographical distribution is limited. Depending on their site, they may exert their effect at the translational level or by interfering with processing of α globin mRNA.

Several types of mutations involving the $\alpha2$ gene interfere with the translation of its mRNA. First, there are those that involve initiation. In two cases, for example, the initiation codon is completely inactivated, ATG $\rightarrow$ ACG or GTG.[39, 40] In another, the efficiency of initiation is reduced by a dinucleotide deletion in the consensus sequence around the start signal (CCCACCATG $\rightarrow$ CCCCATG).[41] Another family of mutations involves substitutions in the $\alpha2$ globin

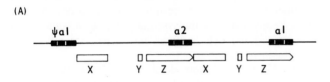

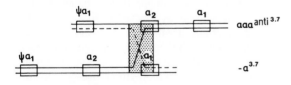

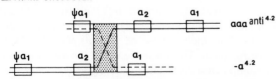

Figure 6–6. The mechanisms of unequal cross-over that give rise to the $-\alpha^{3.7}$ and $-\alpha^{4.2}$ deletions. A, The fine structure of the duplicated α globin genes with the positions of the homology boxes X, Y, and Z. B, The rightward cross-over occurs when genetic exchange takes place between misaligned homologous Z boxes, giving rise to a chromosome with either one ($-\alpha^{3.7}$) or three ($\alpha\alpha\alpha^{anti-3.7}$) α globin genes. C, The leftward cross-over occurs when genetic exchange takes place between the misaligned homologous X boxes, giving rise to a chromosome with either one ($\alpha^{4.2}$) or three ($\alpha\alpha\alpha^{anti-4.2}$) α globin genes.

termination codon, TAA.[42] Each replacement specifically changes this codon so that an amino acid is inserted instead of the chain's terminating. This is followed by readthrough of α globin mRNA that is not normally translated until another in-phase stop codon is reached. The result is an elongated α globin chain with 31 additional residues at the C-terminal end. Five variants of this kind have been identified, hemoglobins Constant Spring, Icaria, Koya Dora, Seal Rock, and Paksé.[43–47] They are identical except for the residue at position 142, which reflects different substitutions in the chain termination codon (Fig. 6–7). Although it is not absolutely clear why the readthrough of normally untranslated mRNA leads to a reduced output from the α2 gene, there is considerable evidence that in some way it destabilizes the mRNA. Whatever the mechanism, the output from the α2 gene is markedly reduced; in homozygotes for Hb Constant Spring, the level of the variant hemoglobin, representing the output of both α2 genes, is only about 5 per cent of the total hemoglobin.[42] Finally, there are several internal mutations that lead to premature chain termination or otherwise inactivate the α globin mRNA. For example, a mutation identified in a black patient from Mississippi causes premature termination of translation by changing codon 116 in exon 3 to an in-phase termination codon (GAG → UAG),[48] and a two-nucleotide deletion, also found in a black patient, leads to a shift in the α globin mRNA reading frame.[49]

Other mutations that produce non-deletion forms of α[+] thalassemia involve the processing of the α globin mRNA transcript. One results from a pentanucleotide deletion including the 5′ splice site of IVS-1 of the α2 gene. This deletion involves the invariant GT donor splicing sequence (G*GT*GAGGCT → GGCT) and abolishes the removal of IVS-1 during processing.[50, 51] Another splice mutation involves the acceptor site of IVS-1 of the α2 gene, with retention of IVS-1 and the generation of a new stop signal at codon 31.[52]

Another group of mutations involve substitutions in the poly(A) addition signal (AATAA*A* → AATAA*G*) and downregulate the α2 gene by interfering with the 3′ end processing of its mRNA and possibly with termination of transcription.[53, 54] Like other non-deletion forms of α thalassemia involving the α2 gene, this mutation seems to downregulate both α2 and α1 globin genes.

Finally, the phenotype of non-deletion α[+] thalassemia can be caused by mutations in the α2 gene that give rise to highly unstable α globin variants. At least 19 variants of this kind have been identified. Their structure and properties are the subject of several reviews.[14, 38, 55]

▼ PATHOPHYSIOLOGY

The α thalassemia mutations, like all thalassemia mutations, lead to their phenotypic effects, in particular the anemia of varying severity, in two ways. First, and most important, there is the deleterious effect of the globin chains that are produced in excess on red cell production and survival. Second, a reduced amount of hemoglobin production contributes to the anemia and causes the hypochromic blood picture that is characteristic of all the thalassemias. As in the case of β thalassemia, however, the critical factor in determining the severity of the phenotype in α thalassemia is the degree of imbalanced globin chain synthesis.

The pathophysiological process of α thalassemia differs fundamentally from that of β thalassemia because of the properties of the globin chains that are produced in excess. Excess γ chains in fetal life or β chains in adults form homotetramers, Hb Bart's and Hb H. Although, particularly in the case of Hb H, they are unstable, unlike the excess α chains produced in β thalassemia, they do not precipitate to any important degree in the red cell precursors in the bone marrow. Thus, unlike in the β thalassemias, ineffective erythropoiesis due to destruction of developing red cells is not a major feature of α thalassemia. Rather, Hb H tends to precipitate and form inclusion bodies in mature red cells as they age in the circulation. Cells containing inclusions of this type are trapped in the spleen and other parts of the reticuloendothelial system, resulting in a hemolytic anemia. Thus, the anemia of α thalassemia is due to a combination of shortened red cell survival and a reduced amount of hemoglobin production.

As discussed in more detail in a later section dealing with the pathophysiology of β thalassemia, it is now clear that globin chain precipitation has profound effects on red cell membrane function, in addition to the mechanical consequences of inclusion body formation. Evidence is accumulating that these effects are different in α and β thalassaemia.[56] For example, although the red cell membranes are extremely rigid in both disorders, they are mechanically unstable in β thalassemia yet hyperstable in Hb H disease. This difference is interpreted as reflecting the state of protein 4.1, a major component of the membrane skeleton that controls its crosslinking; it is partially oxidized in β thalassemia but not in α thalassemia. Furthermore, whereas β thalassemic erythrocytes are dehydrated, those of patients with Hb H disease are overhydrated. Thus, it is clear that the accumulation of α or β globin genes has widely different effects on erythrocyte channels that control cellular hydration, particularly the K:Cl cotransporter. These effects appear to be even more marked in the red cells of individuals with Hb Constant Spring, an observation that has been related to the presence of oxidized α[CS] chains attached to the membrane and its skeleton.

The other major pathophysiological mechanism that may have a profound phenotypic effect in α thalassemia is the functional properties of Hb Bart's and Hb H.[7] Because

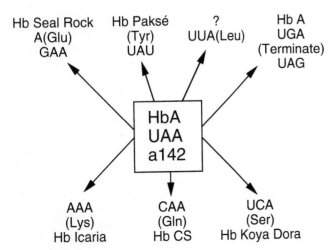

Figure 6–7. The α globin chain termination mutations.

they are homotetramers, they show no heme/heme interaction and they have an extremely high oxygen affinity, which makes them physiologically useless as oxygen transporters. Thus, the clinical picture of α thalassemia reflects a complex combination of hypochromic anemia, hemolysis, and defective oxygen transport due to the properties of varying amounts of physiologically ineffective hemoglobin in the red cells. The resulting degree of tissue hypoxia may, therefore, be much greater than might be expected for the degree of anemia, a phenomenon that is well exemplified by the findings in the homozygous states for α⁰ thalassemia, the Hb Bart's hydrops syndrome.

Another factor that adds to the complexity of the pathophysiology of the α thalassemias is that a critical level of reduction of α globin output is required for the production of homotetramers of γ or β chains. Furthermore, regardless of the type of α thalassemia mutation, the degree of globin chain imbalance seems to vary at different stages of development. For example, in many but not all infants who are heterozygous for deletion forms of α⁺ thalassemia (– α/αα), it is possible to demonstrate small amounts of Hb Bart's in the cord blood, and homozygotes for this condition have approximately 5 to 10 per cent Hb Bart's at birth. Yet in both cases, the Hb Bart's disappears during the first few months of life and is not replaced by a similar amount of Hb H.[7–9] These observations suggest that during this phase of development, any defect in α globin chain production may be exaggerated, possibly because there is some imbalance of α and non-α chain synthesis in many normal infants during the transition from γ to β chain production.

It is also clear that a critical level of reduction of α chain production is required before Hb H appears in a soluble form in the red cells. The most sensitive way of identifying trace amounts of Hb H is by finding inclusion bodies in the red cells after incubation with redox agents like the dye brilliant cresyl blue. Although inclusions of this type can be found in heterozygotes for α⁰ thalassemia, they are rarely present in α⁺ thalassemia heterozygotes or homozygotes.[57] The presence of sufficient Hb H to be demonstrated by electrophoresis usually requires the deletion of three of the four α globin genes (– α/– –) or the homozygous state for non-deletion mutations that seem to downregulate both α2 and α1 genes ($\alpha^T\alpha/\alpha^T\alpha$). Thus, the production of soluble homotetramers depends both on the stage of development and on subtle factors involving the precise level of excess β chain production in adults.

Another curious feature about the pathophysiology of Hb H disease is that many patients with this condition appear to produce Hb Bart's in adult life. This suggests that there may be a modest increase in γ chain production after the neonatal period.[7] As is the case with Hb F production in β thalassemia (see later section), γ chain production appears to be heterogeneously distributed among the red cells. It is possible that the presence of Hb Bart's in Hb H disease may reflect a low level of γ chain production, and also, because the γ_4 tetramer is more stable than the β_4 tetramer, there may be some selective survival of cells containing Hb Bart's.

It is against this complex background that the relationships between the molecular pathology and the phenotypic findings in the different clinical forms of α thalassemia have to be interpreted.

▼ INTERACTION OF THE α THALASSEMIA HAPLOTYPES AND THE CLINICAL PHENOTYPES OF α THALASSEMIA

As mentioned earlier, it is convenient to describe α thalassemia mutations as haplotypes, that is, the overall effect of a particular mutation on the output of both linked α globin genes. Although this is self-evident in the case of the deletions that remove both of them, it is equally valid for describing the effect of point mutations in one gene, particularly because many of them have an effect on the output of their normal partner in *cis*.

Currently, more than 30 different α thalassemia haplotypes have been described, and because these can interact with any other haplotype on the homologous chromosome 16, there is the potential for between 400 and 500 different phenotypes.[7–10, 12] In practice, these interactions produce a remarkable degree of clinical variability, ranging from complete normality to death during intrauterine life. Despite this complexity, for clinical purposes, the α thalassemias can be divided into the Hb Bart's hydrops fetalis syndrome, Hb H disease, the homozygous state for Hb Constant Spring, α thalassemia minor, and the silent carrier states. These different clinical forms of α thalassemia together with their underlying α globin haplotypes are summarized in Table 6–3.

The Hb Bart's Hydrops Fetalis Syndrome

This condition occurs commonly in Southeast Asia and in the Mediterranean region.[7, 10, 58] It usually results from the homozygous inheritance of the two forms of α⁰ thalassemia that are common in these regions, – –ˢᴱᴬ/– –ˢᴱᴬ or – –ᴹᴱᴰ/– –ᴹᴱᴰ. Hence, fetuses with this disorder produce no α globin chains, and their hemoglobin consists of about 80 per cent Hb Bart's and about 20 per cent Hb Portland, the synthesis of which persists up to birth in this condition.[7] A few exceptions to this rule have been described, however. There have been reports of hydropic infants from Greece and Southeast Asia who have low levels of α chain synthesis. Preliminary gene mapping analyses suggest that these infants have a common α⁰ thalassemia determinant on one chromosome and a non-deletion mutation on the other; the nature of the latter has yet to be determined.[59] As mentioned earlier, mutations of this kind reduce the output of both linked α globin genes.

Babies with this syndrome die either in utero between

Table 6–3. Interactions of α Thalassemia Haplotypes

		α⁰	α⁺				
			αα	ααᵀ	– α	αᵀα	– αᵀ
α⁰		Hy	T	H	H	H, Hy	—
α⁺	– αᵀ		T	–	H	T	H
	αᵀα		T	–	T	H	–
	– α		T	–	T		
	ααᵀ		T	–			
	αα		N				

Hy, Hb Bart's hydrops; H, Hb H disease; T, α thalassemia trait.

30 and 40 weeks' gestation or soon after birth. Several cases have been reported in which they were delivered early, transfused, and nursed intensively; they have been maintained with regular blood transfusions and have survived to develop normally.[60, 61]

The clinical picture is characterized by a pale, edematous infant with signs of cardiac failure and severe intrauterine hypoxia.[7, 10, 62] There is massive hypertrophy of the placenta. Hepatosplenomegaly is always found, and there is a significant increase in other congenital abnormalities. The hemoglobin level at birth ranges from 3 to 10 g/dl, and the blood film is characterized by variation in the shape and size of the red cells, which are grossly hypochromic; there are large numbers of nucleated red cells in the peripheral blood.

The other important feature of this syndrome is the high frequency of maternal complications including hypertension, antepartum hemorrhage, malpresentation, difficult vaginal delivery often necessitating cesarean section, retained placenta, and postpartum hemorrhage.[62]

It is clear, therefore, that the pathological changes in the Hb Bart's hydrops fetalis syndrome are the result of gross intrauterine hypoxia. These changes are not always seen in infants who are born with similar hemoglobin levels for other reasons and reflect the hemoglobin constitution of these babies. As mentioned earlier, Hb Bart's is physiologically useless, and hence the only way that oxygen can be transported is by Hb Portland, which usually makes up only about 20 per cent of the hemoglobin. Functionally, therefore, these babies are profoundly anemic, and it is surprising that so many of them survive to term.

Hb H Disease

Hb H disease usually results from the interaction of α^+ and α^0 thalassemia and is therefore found predominantly in Southeast Asia ($--^{SEA}/-\alpha^{3.7}$) and the Mediterranean region ($--^{MED}/-\alpha^{3.7}$).[7–10] In Southeast Asia, it also results from the inheritance of α^0 thalassemia and Hb Constant Spring ($--/\alpha^{CS}\alpha$).[42] It may also result from the homozygous inheritance of non-deletion mutations that affect the predominant $\alpha2$ gene, $\alpha^T\alpha/\alpha^T\alpha$.[39, 54, 63] In Algeria, homozygotes for chromosomes carrying the $-\alpha^{3.7II}$ deletion together with a non-deletion α thalassemia mutation on the remaining α gene ($-\alpha^T/-\alpha^T$) seem to have typical Hb H disease.[64]

As evidenced from the deletion forms of Hb H disease, $--^{SEA}/-\alpha$, for example, the loss of three of four α genes leads to a sufficient excess of β chains to generate viable β_4 tetramers. The same overall deficit of α chains must occur in the homozygous state for the non-deletion forms of α^+ thalassemia. On the other hand, homozygotes for the deletion forms of α^+ thalassemia, $-\alpha/-\alpha$, do not have Hb H disease. When the $\alpha2$ gene is inactivated by a mutation, the $\alpha1$ gene does not increase its output in the way that it does when the $\alpha2$ gene is deleted (Fig. 6–8). This may reflect the fact that there is competition between the α genes for activating factors that bind to their promoters, both of which are retained in the non-deletion α^+ thalassemias, or a more subtle effect reflecting the position of the $\alpha1$ gene relative to HS40 on the deletion chromosomes. Whatever the mechanism, the overall deficit of α chains in non-deletion α^+ thalassemia homozygotes is sufficient to lead to the phenotype of Hb H disease (see Fig. 6–8).

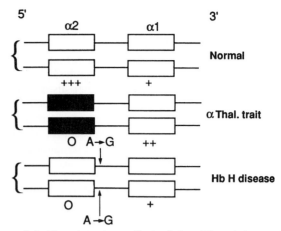

Figure 6–8. The phenotype effect of the different types of α^+ thalassemia. Normally, the output from the $\alpha2$ gene exceeds that from the $\alpha1$ gene by 3:1. In the homozygous state for α^+ thalassemia due to a deletion of the $\alpha2$ gene, the output from the remaining $\alpha1$ genes is increased, and hence there is a mild phenotype similar to thalassemia trait. However, when both $\alpha2$ genes have a point mutation—in this case, in the poly (A) addition site—the output of the linked $\alpha1$ gene is not increased, and hence the phenotype is much more severe.

Hemoglobin H disease is characterized by anemia and splenomegaly together with typical thalassemic changes of the red cells, which contain variable amounts of Hb H. This clinical picture is extremely variable, however. Some patients with Hb H disease are asymptomatic, whereas others have severe anemia and require blood transfusions. Considering how much is known about the molecular pathology of this condition, it is disappointing to reflect on our lack of understanding about the reasons for this clinical heterogeneity. It appears that overall, Hb H disease due to compound heterozygosity for α^0 and α^+ thalassemia is milder than if the disorder results from the interaction of α^0 thalassemia with a haplotype that carries a non-deletion form of α^+ thalassemia.[9, 10, 65] For example, in Southeast Asia, there is evidence that individuals with the former type of Hb H disease are less anemic and have, on average, lower levels of Hb H than those who have the genotype $--^{SEA}/\alpha^{CS}\alpha$.[9, 66, 67] This difference may reflect the milder defect in α chain production from the $-\alpha$ chromosome compared with the $\alpha^{CS}\alpha$ haplotype or the properties of Hb Constant Spring. Otherwise, there is little information about the reason for the clinical variability of Hb H disease, even between individuals who have the same molecular lesions.

The hematological findings in Hb H disease are characterized by a variable degree of anemia, hypochromic microcytic red cells, and levels of Hb H ranging from 2 to 40 per cent; when the cells are incubated with redox dyes, this is reflected in the number of them that contain typical Hb H inclusions. Overall, fetal hemoglobin levels appear to be normal in this condition, although in many patients, in addition to Hb H, small amounts of Hb Bart's have been observed, suggesting that there may be slightly increased γ chain production after birth. For reasons that are not absolutely clear, there have been occasional reports of individuals with the phenotype of Hb H disease in which the level of Bart's is higher than that of the level of Hb H.[7] The level of Hb A_2 is either normal or subnormal.

The most common complication of Hb H disease is the

development of increasing splenomegaly and hypersplenism. Others include infection, leg ulcers, gallstones, and folic acid deficiency. Progressive iron loading, which is so common in β thalassemia, is not a major feature, although older patients may have significantly raised serum ferritin levels. Because of the sensitivity of Hb H to redox agents, there may be exacerbation of the hemolysis after the administration of drugs with redox potential.

The Homozygous State for Hb Constant Spring

We have already seen how the homozygous states for some non-deletion forms of α^+ thalassemia are associated with the clinical picture of Hb H disease. This is presumably because they involve the dominant α2 gene and also because they seem to downregulate the linked α1 gene, or at least prevent the compensatory increase in its output that occurs when the α2 gene is lost by a deletion. The homozygous state for the non-deletion form of α^+ thalassemia due to the Hb Constant Spring mutation on the α2 gene has a different phenotype, however. Because this α globin chain termination variant occurs at a high frequency in many parts of Southeast Asia, the homozygous state has been encountered often enough for its clinical phenotype to have been well established.[7, 68, 69]

The clinical picture is characterized by a moderate degree of anemia, mild icterus, and splenomegaly. The red cells are hypochromic and show variation in shape and size with marked basophilic stippling. The reticulocyte count is elevated, usually in the region of 10 per cent. The red cell survival is considerably reduced, but ferrokinetic studies indicate only a mild degree of ineffective erythropoiesis.[69]

The hemoglobin consists of 5 to 8 per cent Hb Constant Spring, normal levels of Hb A_2 and Hb F, and the persistence of Hb Bart's into adult life at about 1 to 2 per cent of the total.

Hemoglobin biosynthetic studies demonstrate an overall defect in α globin chain synthesis that becomes more marked during erythroid maturation, suggesting that α globin mRNA from the α^{CS} locus is unstable.[69] Hb Constant Spring is not unstable, and therefore the anemia seems to result mainly from defective α chain production consequent on the instability of α^{CS} mRNA. This, in turn, presumably results from the translation of a 3' α globin mRNA sequence that is not normally used. Biosynthetic studies clearly demonstrate a pool of free β chains in the cells of these patients, but it is not usually possible to demonstrate Hb H in the peripheral blood. Why they produce small amounts of Hb Bart's and not Hb H has not been satisfactorily explained. We shall encounter this problem again when the interactions of α thalassemia with some of the β globin variants, such as Hb E, are considered. It appears that under certain conditions, excess β chains do not form stable β_4 tetramers, but why this occurs is not clear.

As mentioned earlier, work on the pathophysiology of the red cell membranes in α thalassemia[56] suggests that the red cells of patients with Hb Constant Spring are overhydrated and hyperstable; it has been suggested that these changes reflect the interaction of Hb Constant Spring with the red cell membrane. Although these findings are of great interest, it is difficult to equate them with the large body of

biosynthetic evidence suggesting that Hb Constant Spring is not unstable. It is possible the α^{CS} chains combine relatively inefficiently with β chains and that some are bound to the red cell membranes in red cell precursors; once a tetramer is formed, however, it appears to be stable.

Homozygous or Compound Heterozygous States for α^+ Thalassemia[7–10]

The clinical phenotype of the homozygous states for α^+ thalassemia varies, depending on the particular type of α thalassemia variant. Homozygotes for the deletion forms of α^+ thalassemia, $-\alpha^{3.7}/-\alpha^{3.7}$, for example, have a phenotype typical of thalassemia trait. Their red cells are hypochromic and microcytic and they may be mildly anemic, but otherwise their adult hemoglobin pattern is normal. At birth, there is 5 to 10 per cent Hb Bart's, which disappears during the first few months of life, not to be replaced by Hb H.

As already mentioned, homozygotes for at least some non-deletion forms of α^+ thalassemia have a more severe deficit of α chains and may show the clinical phenotype of Hb H disease. It is clear, therefore, that if the α2 globin genes are inactivated by mutations but are otherwise intact, the overall deficit of α chains is much greater than if the same genes are deleted.

The compound heterozygous states for deletion and non-deletion forms of α^+ thalassemia have been well characterized in the Saudi Arabian population.[54] The genotype $-\alpha/\alpha^{Saudi}\alpha$, in which α^{Saudi} represents a polyA addition site mutation in the α2 gene, is characterized by findings typical of a thalassemia trait.

α^0 Thalassemia Trait

This condition is characterized by a mild anemia and a reduction in the mean cell hemoglobin (MCH) and mean cell volume (MCV). In adult life, there are no changes in the hemoglobin pattern, but at birth, there is 5 to 10 per cent Hb Bart's. This is not replaced by electrophoretically demonstrable amounts of Hb H in adult life, although a few cells containing Hb H inclusion bodies can usually be found on incubation of the red cells with redox dyes. In cases in which the embryonic ζ genes are spared, trace amounts of ζ chains can be demonstrated in the red cells.[9]

α^+ Thalassemia Trait

The α^+ thalassemia traits are all associated with extremely mild hematological changes, and the hemoglobin level and red cell indices are usually normal. Studies of newborn infants with this condition have shown that some of them have a slight elevation of Hb Bart's, in the 1 to 2 per cent range, but this is not always the case and it is not possible to identify this condition with certainty in the neonatal period, or at any other time, other than by DNA analysis. The only exception to this rule is the heterozygous state for Hb Constant Spring or related chain termination variants in which it is possible to observe 0.1 to 1.5 per cent of the variant hemoglobin by sensitive methods of hemoglobin electrophoresis.

▼ INTERACTION OF α THALASSEMIA WITH STRUCTURAL HEMOGLOBIN VARIANTS

Because the inherited disorders of hemoglobin occur commonly in many parts of the world, it is common for individuals to inherit more than one condition of this type. The results of the inheritance of both α and β thalassemia are considered later in this chapter. Here, I review briefly the various phenotypes that result from the inheritance of α thalassemia with either α or β globin structural variants. It is beyond the scope of this chapter to describe all these interactions in detail. Readers who wish to learn more about this subject are referred to several reviews and monographs.[7-10] However, now that the molecular pathology of α thalassemia has been worked out by direct analysis of the structure of the α globin genes, it is possible to derive some general principles from the study of these interesting experiments of nature.

α Thalassemia With α Chain Variants[7-10]

Some of the α globin chain variants that have been found in association with α thalassemia are summarized in Table 6–4. Unless the variants are unstable, the associated clinical phenotype is simply that of the particular form of α thalassemia. Because normal individuals have four α globin genes, if one of them carries a mutation for a structural hemoglobin variant, in heterozygotes the abnormal hemoglobin should make up approximately 25 per cent of the total. Although there is some variability, depending on whether the mutation involves the α2 or α1 gene, this expectation has been borne out in most of these interactions. If the variant occurs on a chromosome in which the linked α globin gene is deleted, that is, on one with a deletion form of α^+ thalassemia, the relative level of the variant in heterozygotes will be higher, approximately 30 per cent of the total hemoglobin. Homozygotes for α globin variants, Hb J Tongariki, for example, on chromosomes of this type have no Hb A because their genotype is $-\alpha^J/-\alpha^J$. Similarly, their inheritance together with a chromosome carrying an α^0 thalassemia deletion results in the clinical phenotype of Hb H disease in which the hemoglobin consists only of the variant form, and again there is no Hb A ($--/-\alpha^X$).

Table 6–4. α Globin Variants Associated With Deletional Forms of α Thalassemia*

Variant		Genotype	Population
Hb Evanston	α^{14} Trp→Arg	$-\alpha^{3.7}$	Black
Hb Hasharon	α^{47} Asp→His	$-\alpha^{3.7}$ and αα	Mediterranean, Ashkenazy Jews
Hb G Philadelphia	α^{68} Asn→Lys	$-\alpha^{3.7}$ and αα	Algerian, Mediterranean, black, Melanesian
Hb Q (Mahidol)	α^{74} Asp→His	$-\alpha^{4.2}$	Southeast Asian
Hb Duan	α^{75} Asp→Ala	$-\alpha^{4.2}$	Chinese
Hb Nigeria	α^{81} Ser→Lys	Not determined	Black
Hb J Capetown	α^{92} Arg→Gln	$-\alpha^{3.7I}$	South African
Hb J Tongariki	α^{115} Ala→Asp	$-\alpha^{3.7III}$	Melanesian

* Original descriptions in references 10 and 12.

As shown in Table 6–4, many of the α globin chain variants have been found on chromosomes with α thalassemia. Some occur on several different types of chromosomes, indicating that they represent independent mutations. For example, Hb G Philadelphia ($\alpha^{68\text{Asn} \rightarrow \text{Lys}}$) has been found in at least four different racial groups and on both normal and α^+ thalassemia chromosomes.

α Thalassemia With β Chain Variants[8]

Because α thalassemia occurs so frequently in Africa and Southeast Asia, it is often encountered in individuals who also have the β chain hemoglobin variants that occur commonly in these populations. The clinical phenotypes resulting from the inheritance of α thalassemia with the sickle cell trait or sickle cell anemia have been well characterized in individuals of African background. Similarly, the consequences of inheriting different types of α thalassemia with Hb E have been well documented in Thailand. The only phenotypic effects of these complex interactions on the sickle cell or Hb E trait are the hematological characteristics of the particular form of α thalassemia and a lower level of the β globin variant than is usually found in heterozygotes. The reason for the latter finding lies in the differential affinity of α chains for normal and variant β chains. It appears that α chains have a higher affinity for normal β chains than for β^S or β^E chains. Thus, if there is an overall deficit of α chains, those that are synthesized bind preferentially to β^A chains, and therefore there is a relatively lower level of the abnormal hemoglobin than is usually found in heterozygotes.

This differential affinity of α chains for normal or variant β chains also explains the findings in individuals who have the genotype of Hb H disease but who also have the Hb S or Hb E traits. The hematological picture is similar to Hb H disease, and the hemoglobin consists of Hb A with a low level, in the 10 per cent range, of Hb S or Hb E. Hb H is never seen in the red cells in these interactions, although it is usual to find small amounts of Hb Bart's. Presumably, with a severe degree of α chain deficiency, such α chains as are synthesized combine preferentially with normal β chains to produce Hb A. The resulting excess β^S or β^E chains are unable to form stable tetramers and hence do not appear in the peripheral blood. Similarly, because α chains have a higher affinity for β than for γ chains, if γ chain synthesis persists, excess γ chains produce Hb Bart's (γ_4).

Because of the high frequency of Hb E together with α^0 and α^+ thalassemia in Thailand and other parts of Southeast Asia, a variety of different clinical phenotypes have been defined that result from the co-inheritance of the Hb E gene with different combinations of α thalassemia.[7] Because the mutation that causes Hb E also produces a mild form of thalassemia, some of these conditions have severe clinical phenotypes. As mentioned before, the inheritance of the Hb E trait with the genotype of Hb H disease gives rise to a well-defined disorder that is clinically similar to Hb H disease but in which the hemoglobin pattern consists of Hb A + Hb E + Hb Bart's. The homozygous state for Hb E together with the genotype of Hb H disease is associated with a severe form of thalassemia intermedia in which the hemoglobin pattern consists of Hb E + Hb Bart's with an elevated level of Hb F.

The clinical effects of the inheritance of α thalassemia on sickle cell anemia have been characterized in several populations.[70] Comparisons of patients with sickle cell anemia who are homozygous for α^+ thalassemia with those who do not have α thalassemia have shown that the α thalassemic group has a higher hemoglobin level, typical thalassemic red cell indices, a greater likelihood of splenomegaly after early childhood, and, possibly, fewer episodes of the acute chest syndrome and chronic leg ulceration. They also have lower levels of Hb F. In vitro studies have shown that the deformability of sickle cells is enhanced if α thalassemia is also present, thus providing a cellular basis for these observations.[71]

▼ WORLD DISTRIBUTION AND POPULATION GENETICS

Because of the difficulties of identifying the genotypes of α thalassemia from their hematological phenotypes, it is only after the advent of DNA analysis that it has been possible to start to determine the distribution and frequency of α thalassemia in different parts of the world.[7, 72] The approximate frequency of α^+ and α^0 thalassemia among the world populations is illustrated in Figure 6–9. It is clear that α^+ thalassemia occurs commonly across tropical Africa, the Middle East, and certain regions of India and throughout Southeast Asia. The disorder reaches its highest frequency in some of the Pacific Islands populations. Although detailed population analyses of the varieties of α^+ thalassemia have been limited, it appears that the $-\alpha^{3.7}$ types predominate in Africa whereas both $-\alpha^{3.7}$ and $-\alpha^{4.2}$ mutations occur frequently throughout Southeast Asia and the Pacific Islands. The variant of the $-\alpha^{3.7}$ deletion, $-\alpha^{3.7III}$, is found commonly in Melanesia.

α^0 Thalassemia, on the other hand, is limited in its distribution to the Mediterranean region and parts of Southeast Asia, particularly southern China, Thailand, and Vietnam. This accounts for the uneven distribution of the Hb Bart's hydrops fetalis syndrome and Hb H disease in the world population. These conditions are found frequently only in regions where α^0 thalassemia occurs, that is, in Southeast Asia and in the Mediterranean populations. In Saudi Arabia, Hb H disease occurs commonly, but this reflects a high frequency of the non-deletion form of α^+ thalassemia due to a mutation in the poly(A) addition site of the α2 gene that, in the homozygous state, produces typical Hb H disease.[53, 63] Where there is a relatively high frequency of both deletion and non-deletion forms of α thalassemia, a number of complex genotypes are observed, including the heterozygous and homozygous states for the deletion forms of α^+ thalassemia, $-\alpha/\alpha\alpha$ and $-\alpha/-\alpha$; the compound heterozygous state for the deletion and non-deletion forms, $-\alpha/\alpha^T\alpha$; and the homozygous state for the non-deletion form of α^+ thalassemia, $\alpha^T\alpha/\alpha^T\alpha$.[63] Sporadic cases of Hb H due to the homozygous state for other non-deletion forms of α^+ thalassemia have been found in several racial groups.[7]

The occurrence of the different triplicated α globin gene arrangements ($\alpha\alpha\alpha^{anti-3.7}$, $\alpha\alpha\alpha^{anti-4.2}$) in most populations suggests that the cross-over events leading to the deletion forms of α^+ thalassemia occur frequently.[7] Analysis of the α globin restriction fragment length polymorphism (RFLP) haplotypes associated with these disorders also indicates that they have had multiple origins within both the same and different populations. The finding of extremely high frequencies of the deletion chromosomes in some populations suggests that they may have come under selection. In recent years, the application of DNA analysis to this problem has provided strong circumstantial evidence that a major factor responsible for the high frequency of α thalassemia is protection against *Plasmodium falciparum* malaria. Most of this evidence comes from work in the Pacific Islands populations.

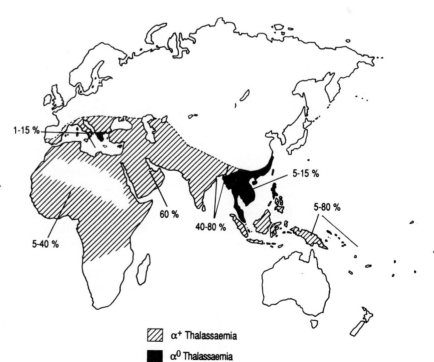

Figure 6–9. The world distribution of α thalassemia.

1-15 %

5-15 %

60 %

5-80 %

40-80 %

5-40 %

▨ α^+ Thalassaemia

■ α^0 Thalassaemia

It has been firmly established that there is a strong positive correlation throughout Melanesia between malarial endemicity and the frequency of α thalassemia.[73] In Papua New Guinea, where α thalassemia affects more than 80 per cent of the population in some regions, the relationship is altitude dependent. Throughout Melanesia, there is a north to south, east to west decrease in malarial endemicity that is closely paralleled by a decrease in the gene frequency of α thalassemia. A number of other loci, not linked to the α globin gene cluster, have been analyzed to see whether any other polymorphisms have this particular distribution pattern, but none has been found. Furthermore, investigation of the molecular structure of α+ thalassemia in this region shows that a few types, – α$^{4.2}$, two haplotypes with – α$^{3.7I}$, and the – α$^{3.7III}$ variant, predominate.[73] Furthermore, all these mutations are found on α globin gene haplotypes, that is, particular combinations of RFLPs, that are common to Melanesia and extremely rare elsewhere. These findings suggest that the α+ thalassemia determinants found throughout this malaria cline originated in Melanesia and were amplified to a high frequency by a locally operating selective mechanism rather than being imported by population migrations from outside the region, from Southeast Asia, for example.

In a series of parallel studies, α thalassemia gene frequencies have been analyzed in areas where malaria has never been recorded.[74, 75] These include Iceland and Japan and many of the island archipelagoes of Micronesia and Polynesia as Oceanic controls. There is virtually no α thalassemia in either Iceland or Japan, but, surprisingly, gene frequencies as high as 12 per cent are seen in parts of Polynesia. However, population studies suggest that the variant has been carried into the eastern Pacific during the migrations of proto-Polynesian colonizers.[75]

It appears, therefore, that there is a strong correlation between the frequency of α thalassemia and present or past *P. falciparum* malaria. Recently, further progress has been made toward defining this relationship. In a case-control study in northern Papua New Guinea, it was found that homozygous α+ thalassemic children are significantly protected against severe *P. falciparum* malaria. Interestingly, in the same study, it was observed that this genotype also offered some protection against other infective illnesses, particularly those involving the respiratory tract.[76] In a large cohort study carried out at the same time in one of the Vanuatuan islands, in which babies with different α globin genotypes were observed for the first 5 years of life together with detailed health records, it was found, surprisingly, that babies homozygous for α^0 thalassemia were *more* prone to malaria due to both *P. falciparum* and *P. vivax* in the first 2 years of life, whereas later they appeared to be protected, at least against *P. falciparum*.[77]

These studies suggest that during the first 2 years of life, infants homozygous for α thalassemia, although they are protected from the severe effects of malaria in other ways, may be more prone to contract both *P. vivax* and *P. falciparum* malaria. It is possible, therefore, that this provides early immunization against subsequent infection.[77] Interestingly, in the Vanuatuan population, as elsewhere, babies tend to contract *P. vivax* malaria earlier than that due to *P. falciparum,* and there may be some cross-immunity between the two species.[78] These observations also suggest that it is homozygotes for α+ thalassemia who come under most

intense selection, although in all the studies there has been a trend for some degree of heterozygote protection. This may reflect a transient polymorphism, rather than the more usual type of balanced polymorphism that occurs in these conditions; given time, and if malaria persists, it will go to fixation within the population. However, this interpretation assumes that homozygotes for α+ thalassemia show no reduction in fitness; this is still not absolutely certain.[78]

▼ α THALASSEMIA AND MENTAL RETARDATION

In 1980, three patients were described who had varying degrees of mental retardation associated with the phenotype of Hb H disease.[79] Subsequently, there were several reports of a similar syndrome.[80, 81] There were some unusual features about this particular form of α thalassemia. First, the patients were all of Caucasian origin, which as we have seen is unusual for α thalassemia. Second, although one parent showed evidence of a mild form of α thalassemia, the other was completely normal. Thus, it appeared that this condition was unlike the forms of Hb H disease described in other populations, in both its genetic transmission and the associated mental retardation, which is not seen in the inherited types of Hb H disease. It was suggested that these patients might have a de novo mutation, which had occurred in the germ cells of one of their parents, that was responsible for both α thalassemia and mental retardation. Because the condition had been identified only because of the chance inheritance of α thalassemia from the one parent, leading to the phenotype of Hb H disease, it was predicted that individuals would be found with mental retardation and the phenotype of α^0 thalassemia trait. Later, this prediction was borne out, and more patients and families with this syndrome were identified.

It is now clear that there are two different varieties of the α thalassemia mental retardation (ATR) syndrome[82, 83] (see Table 6–2). First, there is a group of patients who have relatively mild mental handicap and a variable constellation of facial and skeletal dysmorphisms. These individuals have long deletions involving the α globin gene cluster, removing at least 1 Mb. It appears that this condition can arise in several ways, including unbalanced translocation involving chromosome 16, truncation of the tip of chromosome 16, and loss of the α globin gene cluster and parts of its flanking regions by other mechanisms. These findings localize a region of about 1.7 Mb in band 16p13.3 proximal to the α globin genes as being involved in mental handicap. This condition is now called ATR-16.

The second group is characterized by defective α globin synthesis associated with severe mental retardation and a strikingly homogeneous pattern of dysmorphology including similar facial appearances and genital abnormalities.[83] These patients have a relatively mild form of Hb H disease, and so far all have had a male karyotype. Extensive structural studies have shown no abnormalities of the α globin genes, the activity of which appears to be reduced both in *cis* and *trans*. Family studies indicate that the transmission is X linked.[84] There seems to be extreme inactivation of the affected X chromosome in the female carriers. Further linkage analyses localized the disease locus to the region Xq13.1–q21.1 and ultimately led to the identification of the gene responsible for the ATR-X syndrome as *XH2*, a member of the DNA helicase family.[85–87] Sequencing studies indicate that this is a member of the SNF2 subgroup of a superfamily of proteins with similar adenosine triphosphatase and helicase motifs.[87] Among the many mutations that have been documented as the cause of this condition, there are missense, nonsense, splicing, and frameshift mutations and one small (2.0 kb) deletion. These are unevenly distributed throughout the gene; a considerable number of them are concentrated in the 5′-terminal zinc finger (PHD) domain and in the ATPase/helicase domains.[88]

It seems likely that the *XH2* gene product plays a role in α globin gene transcription. Furthermore, it is widely expressed during early fetal development, particularly in the brain and urogenital system, and therefore it must play a key role in embryogenesis because its mutations give rise to such a diverse series of developmental abnormalities in these regions.

▼ α THALASSEMIA AND LEUKEMIA

The association of the phenotype of Hb H disease with myeloproliferative disorders is well established.[89, 90] There is a strong predominance of males, and the condition occurs in older populations. It is usually seen in the setting of the myelodysplastic syndrome, although some patients have developed a more florid form of acute leukemia.

It appears that this is a clonal disorder involving the neoplastic cell line. The peripheral blood picture is dimorphic, with both normal and hypochromic populations. In some patients, the hypochromic population expands such that there is an almost complete absence of α chain synthesis in the red cell progenitors and reticulocytes.[89] Thus, it appears that the deficiency of α chains is mediated in both *cis* and *trans*. Cell fusion experiments have suggested that it can be corrected when the affected human chromosomes 16 are transferred into mouse erythroleukemia cells,[90] although these results must be interpreted with caution because of difficulties in defining the origin of the human cells. In all cases that have been studied in detail, the α globin genes have been intact, and extensive mapping studies have shown no abnormalities. Thus, the findings are not unlike those observed in ATR-X; further work is required to determine the location of the factor responsible for defective α chain synthesis.

β Thalassemia

The β thalassemias are among the most intensively studied monogenic disorders in man. Over 180 different mutations that give rise to the clinical phenotype of β thalassemia have been identified. Although the elucidation of the molecular pathology of the first few cases of β thalassemia that were studied involved sequencing random β thalassemia genes, the identification of new mutations was greatly facilitated by the observation that within any population, each β thalassemia mutation is in strong linkage disequilibrium with specific arrangements of RFLPs in the β globin complex, called haplotypes.[91] Furthermore, as different populations were studied, it was found that the bulk of β thalassemias result

from a small number of common mutations together with varying numbers of rare ones in every case and that each ethnic group has its particular β thalassemia alleles. It has been inferred from these observations that the β thalassemias originated independently in these populations and were then subjected to positive selection, presumably because heterozygotes were protected against *P. falciparum* malaria. It turns out that about 20 different alleles account for more than 80 per cent of β thalassemia genes in the world population.

Because there are several different common β thalassemia mutations in all the populations in which there is a high frequency of the disorder, it follows that many patients with β thalassemia major, rather than being homozygous for a particular mutation, are compound heterozygotes for two different β thalassemia alleles. The only exception to this rule is in populations in which there is a high frequency of consanguineous marriages. Because the mutations that underlie β+ thalassemia vary widely in their effect on β chain production, it follows that there is considerable possibility for phenotypic diversity based on different interactions of β thalassemia alleles in compound heterozygotes.

▼ THE β GLOBIN GENE CLUSTER

The β globin gene cluster on chromosome 11 contains the non-α globin genes arranged in the following order: ε-Gγ-Aγ-ψβ-δ-β (see Fig. 6–1). Much of this region of DNA has been sequenced, and many of the major regulatory regions have been defined.[92] It contains many RFLPs, although unlike in the α globin gene cluster, no minisatellite (hypervariable) sequences have been identified. The arrangement of RFLPs is not random between different populations. Rather, each population has a limited number of common arrangements of RFLPs, or β globin haplotypes, a finding that has been of considerable value in evolutionary studies of human populations and of the β globin genes.[91]

The first indication of the existence of major regulatory sequences in this gene cluster came from studies that identified DNase I hypersensitive sites, five located far upstream and one far downstream from the cluster itself. These sites are erythroid specific but developmentally stable, that is, they represent regions of chromatin that are open at all stages of development. As described earlier for the α globin gene cluster, the region identified by DNase sensitivity 5′ to the cluster has been characterized in detail and designated the LCR.[92, 93] It seems to be of major importance in regulating the expression of the entire β globin gene cluster in erythroid tissue and, in addition, appears to have classical enhancer-like function that is relatively specific for cells of erythroid origin. A number of other sequences with enhancer-like properties have been defined within the β globin gene cluster.

▼ MOLECULAR PATHOLOGY

The deficiency or absence of β globin chains that characterizes β thalassemia reflects the action of mutations that affect every level of β globin gene function, that is, transcription, mRNA processing, translation, and post-translational stability of the β globin chain product. Some of these mutations

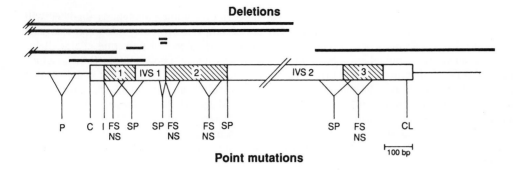

Figure 6–10. The major classes of mutations of the β globin gene that cause β thalassemia. P = Promoter boxes; C = CAP site; I = initiation codon; FS = frameshift; NS = non-sense; SP = splice junction, consensus sequence, or cryptic splice site; CL = RNA cleavage (poly [A]) site.

are illustrated in Figure 6–10 and classified in Table 6–5, grouped according to the mechanism by which they affect β globin gene expression. They have been the subject of several reviews,[38, 94, 95] and only those of particular phenotypic importance are described here.

Nearly all the different β thalassemia mutations that have been identified so far behave like alleles of the β globin gene and involve it directly. As we shall see in a later section, mutations many kilobases upstream from the β globin locus may cause its defective function, as occurs in some of the α thalassemias, but these lesions also involve γ and δ chain production and therefore do not give rise to the clinical phenotype of β thalassemia.

Gene Deletions

Unlike in the α thalassemias, gene deletion is an uncommon cause of β thalassemia. Only a handful of different deletions affecting only the β globin gene have been described (Fig. 6–11). Of these, only a 619 bp deletion involving the 3′ end of the β globin gene is common, and even this is restricted to the Sind populations of India and Pakistan, where it constitutes about 30 per cent of the β thalassemia alleles.[96] The other deletions that result in β thalassemia are extremely rare.[38, 95, 97–102] In each case, the 5′ end of the β globin gene is lost while the δ gene remains intact. As we shall see later, these deletions are of particular phenotypic interest because they are all associated with an unusually high level of Hb A$_2$ production in heterozygotes.

Mutations in Promoter Regions of the β Globin Gene

Several mutations have been observed in or around the highly conserved sequences 5′ to the β globin gene that constitute the various promoter boxes.[38, 95, 103–105] They involve single nucleotide substitutions in the TATA box, at around −30 nucleotides (nt) from the transcription start site, or in the proximal or distal promoter elements, CACACCC

at −90 nt and −105 nt. These mutations result in decreased β globin mRNA production in transient expression systems, ranging from 10 to 25 per cent of the output from a normal β globin gene, indicating that they are responsible for the associated β thalassemia phenotype. Interestingly, no mutations have yet been observed in the CCAAT box at −70 nt.

One mutation, C → T at position −101 nt to the β globin gene, appears to cause an extremely mild deficit of β globin mRNA.[106] As we shall see later, this allele is so mild that it is completely silent in carriers, but it can be identified by its interaction with more severe β thalassemia alleles in compound heterozygotes.

Cap Site Mutations

The single reported incidence of a mutation at the β globin gene mRNA cap site, cap + 1 nt (A → C), has an extremely mild effect on β globin gene transcription. A homozygote has hematological values similar to the β thalassemia trait.[107] The +1 nucleotide is the start site for transcription as well as the site at which capping of the β globin mRNA precursor occurs. It is possible that this mutation functions at either the transcriptional or processing level or at both levels.

Mutation of the 5′ Untranslated Region of the β Globin Gene

Several mutations involving the 5′ untranslated region of the β globin gene have been described.[38, 108, 109] They are associated with variable phenotypes. In some cases, they are completely silent in heterozygotes; in others, the heterozygous phenotype is more similar to that of other forms of β thalassemia, although the red cell indices are less abnormal and the Hb A$_2$ levels are only marginally elevated. In the +33 (C → G) mutation, the findings in the heterozygote are almost completely normal except for a slightly reduced MCH level; the Hb A$_2$ levels are in the normal range, and there is no globin chain imbalance. However, it is clear that when this class of mutations interacts with other forms of

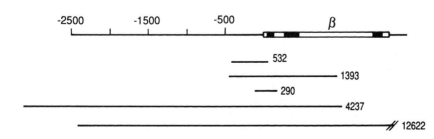

Figure 6–11. Illustrative deletions of the β globin gene that cause β^0 thalassemia.

Table 6–5. Molecular Pathology of the β Thalassemias*

    β⁰ or β⁺ Thalassemia
      Gene deletions
      Promoter regions
      Cap site
      5′ Untranslated region
      Intron/exon boundaries
      Splice site consensus sequences
      Cryptic sites in exons
      Cryptic sites in introns
      Poly(A) signal
      Translation of β globin mRNA
        Initiation
        Nonsense
        Frameshift
      Unstable β globin chains
    Normal Hb A₂ β thalassemia
      β Thalassemia + δ thalassemia, *cis or trans*
      "Silent" β thalassemia
        Some promoter mutations
        Cap + 1
        Cap + 33
        5′ Untranslated regions
        Splice mutation IVS-2 844 C→G
        Termination codon + 6
    Dominant β thalassemia
      Single base substitutions—highly unstable products
      Codon deletions
      Premature termination, exon 3
      Frameshifts—elongated, unstable products

* Full list of mutations given in reference 38.

thalassemia, a more severe phenotype occurs. Thus, they must be regarded as either silent or extremely mild β thalassemias. The mechanism for defective β globin production is not clear but appears to involve a decreased rate of β mRNA transcription.

Splice Site Mutations Involving Intron/Exon Boundaries

The boundaries between exons and introns are characterized by the invariant dinucleotides G–T at the donor (5′) site and A–G at the acceptor (3′) site. Mutations that affect either of these sites completely abolish normal splicing and give rise to the phenotype of β⁰ thalassemia.[38, 103, 110] The transcription of genes carrying these mutations appears to be normal, but there is a complete inactivation of splicing at the altered junction. In every case, other donor-like sequences located elsewhere in the mRNA precursor are employed in splicing. Because these sites are not normally involved, they are referred to as cryptic splice sites. For this reason, abnormally processed products accumulate at low levels, in both erythroid precursors in vivo and in vitro expression systems, as a result of splicing to the cryptic sites in the surrounding exons or introns.

Mutations Involving Splice Site Consensus Sequences

Although only the G–T dinucleotide is invariant at the donor splice site, there is conservation of adjacent nucleotides, and a consensus sequence of these regions can be identified. Mutations within this sequence can reduce the efficiency of splicing to varying degrees and lead to alternative splicing at the surrounding cryptic sites.[38, 91, 111–114] For example, mutations at position 5 of IVS-1, G to C or T, result in a moderately severe reduction of β chain production and in the phenotype of severe β⁺ thalassemia.[91] On the other hand, the substitution of C for T at position 6 in IVS-1 leads to a mild reduction in the output of β chains.[91] This mutation, which is called the Portuguese form of β thalassemia, is particularly common in the Mediterranean population.[115] Interestingly, far more mutations have been found in the consensus donor sequence of IVS-1 than IVS-2.

Mutations at Cryptic Sites in Exons

One of the cryptic splice sites involved in alternative splicing in mutations affecting the IVS-1 donor site spans codons 24 to 27 of exon 1 of the β globin gene. This site contains a G–T dinucleotide, and adjacent substitutions that alter it so that it more closely resembles the consensus donor splice site result in its activation, even though the normal splice site is intact. For example, a mutation at codon 24, GGT to GGA, although it does not alter the amino acid that is normally found at this position in the β globin chain (glycine), allows some splicing to occur at this site instead of the exon/intron boundary. This results in the production of both normal and abnormally spliced β globin mRNA and in the clinical phenotype of severe β⁺ thalassemia.[116]

Mutations at codons 19 (A → G), 26 (G → A), and 27 (G → T) result in a reduced production of mRNA due to abnormal splicing and an amino acid substitution when the mRNA that is spliced normally is translated into protein (Fig. 6–12). The abnormal hemoglobins produced are Hb Malay, Hb E, and Hb Knossos, respectively.[117–119] All these variants are associated with a mild β thalassemia–like phenotype.

Mutations that involve the cryptic donor splice site in exon 1 illustrate how sequence changes in coding rather than intervening sequences may influence RNA processing. Furthermore, they underline the importance of competition between potential splice site sequences in generating both normal and abnormal varieties of β globin mRNA.

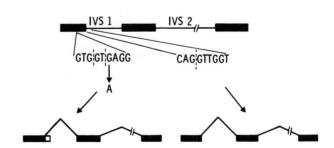

Figure 6–12. Activation of a cryptic splice site in exon 1 of the β globin gene as the basis for the thalassemic phenotype associated with Hb E. Splicing occurs at both the normal splice junction and the cryptic splice site with the production of both normal and abnormal types of mRNA.

Mutations at Cryptic Sites in Introns

Cryptic splice sites in introns may also carry mutations that activate them even though the normal site remains intact. The first mutation of this type to be characterized involved a base substitution at position 110 in IVS-1.[120, 121] This region contains a sequence similar to a 3' acceptor splice site although it lacks the invariant A–G dinucleotide (Fig. 6–13). The change of the G to A at position 110 creates this dinucleotide. The result is that about 90 per cent of the RNA transcript splices to this particular site and only 10 per cent to the normal site, producing the phenotype of severe β^+ thalassemia. The product of the abnormal splicing is a nonfunctional β globin mRNA that contains an extra 19 nucleotides derived from IVS-1. It can be detected in low amounts in reticulocyte or marrow RNA.

Several β thalassemia mutations have been described that generate new donor sites within IVS-2 of the β globin gene.[91, 111] Their effects are complex. In each case, a cryptic acceptor site within IVS-2 following nucleotide 580 is used for processing abnormal transcripts. No normal β globin mRNA appears to be processed from a gene with an A → G substitution at IVS-2 position 654, and hence the clinical phenotype is β^0 thalassemia.[111] This is a curious observation because the IVS-2 donor and acceptor sites are entirely normal. It appears that all stable transcripts are spliced from the normal IVS-2 donor to the cryptic acceptor site and from the abnormal new donor site to the normal IVS-2 acceptor. The processed β globin mRNA contains an insertion derived from IVS-2. It is not clear why splicing from the normal donor to acceptor sites does not occur.

Polyadenylation Signal Mutations

The sequence AAUAAA in the 3' untranslated region of β globin mRNA is the signal for cleavage and polyadenylation of the β gene transcript. Several different mutations of this region have been described.[38, 122–125] For example, a T → C substitution in the β globin gene in this sequence leads to only one tenth of the normal amount of β globin mRNA transcript and hence to a phenotype of moderately severe β^+ thalassemia.[122] A small amount of an extended β globin mRNA molecule can be found in reticulocytes, presumably polyadenylated at a downstream site.

Mutations That Result in Abnormal Translation of β Globin mRNA

There are three main classes of mutations of this kind. Base substitutions that change an amino acid codon to a chain termination codon prevent translation of β globin mRNA and result in the phenotype of β^0 thalassemia.[38, 126, 127] Several mutations of this kind have been described, the most common being a codon 17 mutation, which occurs widely throughout Southeast Asia,[127] and a codon 39 mutation, which is common in the Mediterranean populations.[126] Curiously, low levels of nuclear and cytoplasmic β globin mRNA have been found in red cell precursors in association with these mutations.[128, 129] It is not clear how the generation of a premature chain termination codon could reduce the overall amount of β globin mRNA that is synthesized.

The second group of mutations of this class involve the insertion or deletion of one, two, or four nucleotides in the coding region of the β globin gene.[37, 91, 125] These disrupt the normal reading frame, cause a frameshift, and therefore interfere with the translation of β globin mRNA. The end result is the insertion of anomalous amino acids after the frameshift until a termination codon is reached in the new reading frame. This type of mutation always leads to the phenotype of β^0 thalassemia.

Finally, there are two mutations that involve the β globin initiation codon, ATG → AGG or ACG, and presumably reduce the efficacy of translation.[91, 123]

Unstable β Globin Chain Variants

Just as is the case of the unstable α globin variants, it might be expected that the synthesis of a highly unstable β globin variant that is incapable of forming a stable tetramer, and which is rapidly degraded, might produce the phenotype of β^0 thalassemia.[130–133] In many of these conditions, no abnormal globin chain product can be demonstrated by protein analysis or globin synthesis studies, and the molecular pathology has to be interpreted simply on the basis of a derived sequence of the variant β chain obtained from DNA analysis. In some cases, small quantities of abnormal globin chains have been identified by hemoglobin synthesis studies.

Studies have started to shed some light on the complex clinical phenotypes that may result from the synthesis of unstable β globin products. It turns out that there is a spectrum of disorders ranging from a family of exon 3 mutations that give rise to a moderately severe form of thalassemia in heterozygotes, through conditions that are characterized as mild hypochromic anemia, to those in which the major feature is hemolysis due to precipitation of unstable β chain hemoglobin variants in the peripheral circulation. We shall return to this theme later in this chapter.

▼ PATHOPHYSIOLOGY

The pathophysiological process of β thalassemia has been the subject of several extensive reviews.[7, 56, 134–138] Only those aspects of the topic essential for an understanding of the relationship between the molecular pathology and the clinical phenotypes are summarized here.

The main cause of the anemia of β thalassemia is

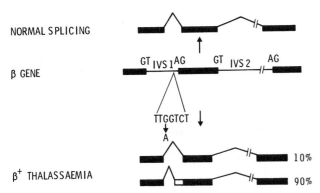

Figure 6–13. The activation of a splice site in IVS-I of the β globin gene due to a G→A change at position 110. Since the abnormal splice site is utilized to a greater extent than the normal site, and hence a large amount of abnormal β globin mRNA is generated, this mutation results in a severe β^+ thalassemia phenotype.

imbalanced globin chain synthesis and the deleterious effects of the excess of α chains on erythroid maturation and survival. It follows, therefore, that the major factor in determining the clinical phenotype is the magnitude of α chain excess in the red cell precursors. Although this reflects the degree of defective β chain production, there are other factors involved, particularly the level of γ chain synthesis and, much less important, δ chain production. The degree of globin chain imbalance may also be modified by the level of α chain synthesis, in particular the coexistence of α thalassemia. Although it has been suggested that other factors such as differences in the rate of proteolysis of excess α chains may also modify the phenotype of β thalassemia, it has been much more difficult to obtain solid evidence to this effect.

The Consequences of Imbalanced Globin Chain Synthesis

Measurements of in vitro globin chain synthesis in the blood or bone marrow of patients with different types of β thalassemia have shown either an absence or a reduction of β chains together with the synthesis of a variable excess of α chains.[7] Unpaired α chains are unable to form a viable hemoglobin tetramer and hence precipitate in red cell precursors.[139] The resulting inclusion bodies can be demonstrated by both light and electron microscopy.[140] In the bone marrow, α chain precipitation occurs in the earliest hemoglobinized precursors and throughout the erythroid maturation pathway.[141] These inclusions are responsible for the intramedullary destruction of red cell precursors and hence the ineffective erythropoiesis that characterizes all the β thalassemias. It has been calculated that a large proportion of the developing erythroblasts are destroyed in the bone marrow in severe forms of β thalassemia.[142] α Chain precipitation can also be demonstrated in the red cell progenitors of β thalassemia heterozygotes, although they are scanty. The bulk of excess α chains is presumably degraded by proteolytic enzymes; notwithstanding, there is a mild degree of ineffective erythropoiesis.[143]

There is also a hemolytic component to the anemia of β thalassemia. Such red cells as enter the circulation contain inclusions that result in their damage as they pass through the microcirculation, particularly the spleen. In addition to this physical mechanism for hemolysis, many abnormalities of metabolism of red cells and their precursors have been demonstrated, in both severe and mild forms of β thalassemia.[56, 134–138, 144] In short, it appears that damage to the red cell and its membrane follows from two major processes. First, the heme and hemichromes of the membrane-bound denatured α globin result in oxidation and clustering of protein band 3, thus providing a site for immunoglobulin G and C3 binding, with immune removal of erythrocytes. Second, through the degradation of hemoglobin with the production of heme and iron, a variety of reactive oxygen species are generated that result in lipid peroxidation with subsequent damage to a variety of components of the red cell and its membranes. Isolated membranes are mechanically unstable, probably reflecting damage to the membrane proteins, notably protein 4.1, a major component of the cytoskeleton that is oxidized in β thalassemia. The β thalassemic red cell also loses potassium and accumulates calcium

and, as mentioned earlier, unlike the red cell in α thalassemia, is dehydrated.

It appears, therefore, that the shortened red cell survival in β thalassemia is the consequence of both physical damage due to the presence of inclusion bodies and a complex series of secondary metabolic changes resulting from the effects of hemoglobin precipitation and damage to the red cell membranes. As we shall see, all these changes vary in severity between the heterogeneous cell populations that are found in the peripheral blood in severe forms of β thalassemia.

Persistent Fetal Hemoglobin Production and Cellular Heterogeneity

One of the earliest observations on the hemoglobin patterns of children with severe β thalassemia was that there is a variable amount of Hb F production that persists into childhood and later life.[7] Indeed, in the β⁰ thalassemias, except for small amounts of Hb A₂, Hb F is the only hemoglobin produced. Examination of the peripheral blood by use of staining methods specific for Hb F shows that it is heterogeneously distributed among the red cells. There are still many unanswered questions about the mechanism of persistent γ chain synthesis in the β thalassemias. From such evidence as is available, it is clear that both cell selection and genetic factors that modify γ chain production are involved.

Cell Selection

Normal adults produce small quantities of Hb F that is also heterogeneously distributed among the red cells; cells with demonstrable Hb F are called F cells. It is clear that one important mechanism for the apparent persistence of Hb F production in β thalassemia is cell selection. As mentioned earlier, the major cause of ineffective erythropoiesis and shortened red cell survival is the deleterious effect of excess α chains on erythroid maturation and survival of red cells in the blood. It follows, therefore, that any red cell precursors that produce significant numbers of γ chains will be at an advantage in an environment in which there are excess α chains; the α chains will combine with γ chains to produce Hb F, and therefore the magnitude of α chain precipitation will be less. Differential centrifugation experiments and in vivo labeling studies have shown that populations of red cells with relatively large amounts of Hb F are more efficiently produced and survive longer in the blood than those with low levels or no Hb F.[7, 145, 146] This is one of the main reasons for the heterogeneity of cell populations in the peripheral blood of patients with severe β thalassemia. They show remarkable differences with respect to their survival; there are those that contain predominantly Hb A or virtually no hemoglobin that are rapidly destroyed in the spleen and elsewhere, cells with a longer survival that contain relatively more Hb F, and cells of intermediate survival and hemoglobin constitution. These changes in hemoglobin content and constitution are mirrored by variability in the associated metabolic abnormalities.[147]

Whether cell selection of this type is the only mechanism for the presence of relatively large amounts of Hb F in the blood of transfusion-dependent patients with β thalassemia is not clear. Because of the gross destruction of red cell progenitors, the marked expansion of the erythron, and the cellular heterogeneity of distribution of Hb F, it is difficult to calculate absolute amounts of Hb F production in this disease. Although it has been suggested that the marked increase in the turnover of red cell progenitors and the increased rate of red cell maturation may create an environment that favors γ chain production, it has not been possible to obtain any definite evidence that this is the case. Other dyserythropoietic and hemolytic anemias are not associated with high levels of Hb F production, although of course in these disorders there is no reason for selection of progenitors that are synthesizing γ chains. It remains a possibility, however, that there may be an absolute increase in Hb F production; this is certainly so in some milder forms of homozygous β thalassemia, but as we shall see, there may be other genetic factors that are responsible for the relatively high level of γ chain synthesis in these conditions.

Genetic Factors That Modify γ Chain Synthesis

Despite that it has been evident for a long time that genetic factors play a major role in determining the level of Hb F production in β thalassemia, knowledge about their nature remains incomplete. However, from such information as is available, it is clear that they fall into three major groups. First, there is growing evidence that the mutations involving the β globin genes or their flanking regions that give rise to β thalassemia may themselves have some effect on the output of Hb F. Second, it appears that polymorphisms involving the εγδβ globin gene cluster may modify the amount of Hb F produced in the face of defective β chain production. Finally, there are genetic determinants unlinked to the cluster that seem to modify the level of Hb F production in adult life, in both normal and β thalassemic individuals. These different mechanisms for modifying Hb F production in β thalassemia are summarized in Figure 6–14.

One approach to determining the effect of individual β thalassemia mutations on γ chain synthesis is to analyze Hb F levels in homozygotes or compound heterozygotes for those mutations that produce a mild deficit of β chains. Because imbalanced globin chain synthesis and cell selection play an important role in determining the level of Hb F in β thalassemia, it might be expected that it would be relatively low in such individuals. This is borne out by careful phenotypic analysis of homozygotes for the common IVS-1 position 6 (T → C) β^+ thalassemia mutation, the Portuguese

mutation, which occurs widely in the Mediterranean. Such persons have a mild phenotype with levels of Hb F in the 10 to 20 per cent range.[115] On the other hand, it has been realized for many years that β thalassemia is particularly mild in black populations.[7] Many homozygotes have been described with hemoglobin levels of 9 to 12 g/dl. Yet nearly all these persons have Hb F levels between 40 and 60 per cent of the total hemoglobin.[7, 112] It is now clear that most of them are either homozygotes or compound heterozygotes for two common promoter mutations, − 29 (A → G) and − 88 (C → T).[85, 91] Homozygotes or compound heterozygotes for these mutations, whether they occur in blacks[112] or other populations,[148] usually have inappropriately high levels of Hb F for the degree of imbalanced globin chain synthesis. It is possible, therefore, that in conditions of relative hematopoietic stress, in which γ chain synthesis is more likely to occur, the level of γ chain production may be modified by competition for transcriptional regulatory proteins between the γ and β chain loci; mutations in or near these transcriptional boxes that cause β thalassemia may favor γ chain production. This hypothesis is strengthened by the observation that heterozygotes for the deletion forms of β thalassemia that remove the 5′ flanking regions of the β globin genes, in addition to unusually high levels of δ chain production, have, on average, higher levels of Hb F than is usual in β thalassemia heterozygotes.[95, 149]

Analyses of this kind are complicated, however, by increasing evidence that polymorphisms or mutations of the γ globin genes *cis* to the β globin genes that contain β thalassemia mutations may have a considerable effect in modifying γ chain production. An extreme example of this kind is the finding of the common nonsense mutation at codon 39 in the β globin gene associated with a point mutation at position − 196 upstream of the $^A\gamma$ gene on the same chromosome in Sardinian patients with a form of β^0 thalassemia associated with a mild phenotype and high levels of γ chain production. We will consider the way in which this type of chromosome has been generated in a later section, which deals with the pathogenesis of δβ thalassemia.

One approach to asking whether *cis*-acting sequences may modify γ chain production is to determine whether there are any particular β globin RFLP haplotypes associated with β thalassemia and unusually high levels of Hb F.[150] This is based on the notion that if this is the case, it is likely that the genetic determinant responsible for the increased level of Hb F production is within or close to the εγδβ

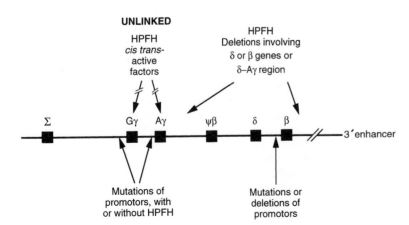

Figure 6–14. A summary of some of the genetic mechanisms that modify the level of Hb F production in β thalassemia.

globin gene cluster. There has been particular interest in the relationship between Hb F production and a C → T polymorphism at position 158 in the $^G\gamma$ globin gene. This substitution can be identified with the restriction enzyme *Xmn*I, which makes it possible to analyze large populations for its presence or absence.[151] Studies in Asian, Mediterranean, and Middle Eastern populations have shown that this polymorphism is associated predominantly with one common β globin RFLP haplotype and is not found on chromosomes carrying the other common haplotypes in these regions.[152] Extensive analysis of β thalassemics of Afro-Asian, Mediterranean, and Turkish backgrounds has shown a strong but not absolute correlation between increased γ chain production and the presence of the *Xmn*I polymorphism.[152–154]

Similar although less consistent observations have been made on Hb F production in sickle cell anemia in relationship to this polymorphism.[155–157] The lack of an absolute association between haplotype and Hb F production, and the clear demonstration in Indian[158, 159] and Saudi Arabian[160] populations that other genetic factors are involved in setting the fetal hemoglobin level in β thalassemia and sickle cell anemia, suggest that Hb F response to the β chain disorders reflects the complex interactions of a number of different genetic determinants. Whereas some of these may be encoded in the β globin gene cluster and reflect complex duplications or other rearrangements of the γ globin genes,[38] it is becoming increasingly clear that others are not linked to this cluster. One condition of particular importance in this respect is heterocellular HPFH.

There is strong evidence that there is a small group of otherwise normal individuals in all populations who have slightly elevated levels of Hb F and that this phenomenon is inherited.[161] Extensive family data indicate that the co-inheritance of this type of HPFH with β thalassemia causes β thalassemia heterozygotes to have an unusually high level of Hb F; homozygotes have a mild phenotype, presumably owing to the large amounts of Hb F that they produce.[162, 163] It appears that this form of HPFH is also heterogeneous; there is some but not unequivocal evidence that at least one form is encoded by the X chromosome[164]; there is equally clear evidence that other forms are not.[165]

Some progress has been made in dissecting the genetics of heterocellular HPFH. The position regarding X chromosome determinants remains uncertain. There is some evidence that the level of F cells, that is, cells that contain Hb F, and the level of Hb F in normal adults are controlled by a locus on the X chromosome,[166] although the relationship of this locus to the putative locus for heterocellular HPFH[164] is not clear. However, there is good evidence for a locus on chromosome 6 that is involved in the generation of at least one form of HPFH that can interact with β thalassemia.[167, 168] Furthermore, at least one extensive pedigree has been reported in which there is no evidence of linkage of the heterocellular HPFH determinant to the X chromosome, the β globin gene cluster on chromosome 11, or chromosome 6.[169]

It is clear, therefore, that the genetic factors modifying Hb F production in β thalassemia are extremely complex and are still not fully worked out. For example, as mentioned earlier, there are extensive data to suggest that, by and large, the β globin promoter mutations that cause mild forms of thalassemia are associated with relatively high levels of

γ chain production. Interpretation of these observations is complicated by the finding that at least some of the common promoter mutations that occur in black populations occur on a chromosome that carries the *Xmn* polymorphism. On the other hand, it seems unlikely that this is the only reason for the high level of Hb F production in these individuals because homozygotes for the promoter mutations in other populations also produce unusually high levels of Hb F. Perhaps both mechanisms are involved. It is also possible that the C → T change at position 158 acts as a more efficient promoter for γ chain production in conditions of increased red cell production and turnover.

In summary, the Hb F response to β thalassemia probably reflects a complex series of genetic variables including the nature of the individual β thalassemic mutation, polymorphisms of the γ globin genes *cis* to the affected β globin gene, and the interaction of other genes unlinked to the β globin gene cluster, set against a background of cell selection and an increased likelihood of producing γ chains because of the accelerated level of erythropoiesis consequent to the destruction of a red cell precursor due to the underlying β thalassemic mutation.

Variability in α Chain Production

It is clear that the major pathophysiological mechanism that leads to the anemia of β thalassemia is the deleterious effects of the excess α chains on red cell maturation. It follows, therefore, that a relative deficit of α chain production should ameliorate the clinical phenotype of β thalassemia. As we shall see later in this chapter, many experiments of nature have been encountered that provide clear-cut evidence that it is the excess of α chains that is the major factor in the pathogenesis of β thalassemia. Individuals who inherit one or more α thalassemia determinants together with β thalassemia have a milder clinical phenotype than do patients with β thalassemia who have four intact α genes.[170] Similarly, β thalassemia carriers who inherit chromosomes with three α genes (ααα) have an unusually severe phenotype.[170] I describe the phenotypic consequences of these interactions in a later section.

Acquired Factors[7]

In trying to assess the genotype/phenotype relationships in β thalassemia, it is important to remember that many acquired and environmental factors may modify the clinical phenotype. Indeed, unless these are carefully controlled, it is almost impossible to compare patients with the same molecular defects in an attempt to relate molecular lesions to clinical phenotypes.

The constant bombardment of the spleen with abnormal red cells in β thalassemics gives rise to the phenomenon of "work hypertrophy." Progressive splenomegaly may exacerbate the anemia. Enlarged spleens act as a sump for red cells and may sequestrate a considerable proportion of the peripheral red cell mass. Furthermore, splenomegaly may cause plasma volume expansion, a complication that may be exacerbated by massive hypertrophy of the erythroid bone marrow; this may also lead to folate deficiency. All these factors may combine to cause considerable worsening of the anemia in β thalassemia.

In β thalassemia homozygotes who are severely anemic, there is an increase in intestinal iron absorption related to the degree of expansion of the red cell precursor population.[7] Iron may also accumulate after regular blood transfusion. Iron accumulation occurs in the parenchymal cells of the liver, in endocrine glands, in the pancreas, and, most important, in the myocardium. The consequences of iron loading include diabetes, hyperparathyroidism, hypogonadism, and cardiac failure.[7, 8, 138]

Thus, in attempting to relate the genotype to the phenotype of β thalassemia, it is essential to take into consideration the widespread secondary complications of the disease that may modify the phenotype.

▼ GENOTYPE/PHENOTYPE RELATIONSHIPS FOR THE β THALASSEMIAS

Given the considerable molecular heterogeneity of β thalassemia and the many other genetic and acquired factors that have the potential to modify its phenotype, it is not surprising that the clinical spectrum produced by different β thalassemia mutations is so broad. Homozygotes or compound heterozygotes for different β thalassemia mutations may show a clinical picture ranging from a disease that is lethal in the first few months of life to a completely asymptomatic disorder that may be ascertained only by routine hematological analysis. Similarly, although the heterozygous states are usually asymptomatic, it is now apparent that a small subset of carriers have a moderately severe disease that is clearly inherited in a dominant fashion.

Severe Transfusion-Dependent Forms of β Thalassemia

Because most racial groups with a high frequency of β thalassemia have only a few common mutations, the severe phenotypes usually result from the homozygous or compound heterozygous states for those that produce a severe deficit of β chain production. In the Mediterranean population, for example, severe disease is seen frequently in homozygotes for codon 39 (C → T) or position 110 of IVS-1 (G → A) mutations or in compound heterozygotes who have received one of these mutations from each parent. In Melanesia, where there is only one common mutation, in this case G → C at position 5 of IVS-1, all severely affected individuals are homozygous for this particular allele.

In populations such as those of the Mediterranean in which there is a relatively high frequency of a mild β thalassemia allele, in this case IVS-1 position 6 (T → C), many compound heterozygotes are encountered who have received this mutation from one parent and a more severe β thalassemia allele from the other. As experience of these interactions is growing, it is becoming possible to define the resulting clinical phenotypes. For example, although the co-inheritance of the codon 39 (C → T) mutation with the IVS-1 position 6 (T → C) mutation produces a slightly milder phenotype, it is usually transfusion dependent. On the other hand, many patients who are compound heterozygotes for IVS-1 position 6 (T → C) mutation and the IVS-1 position 110 (G → A) mutation have the phenotype of non–transfusion-dependent thalassemia intermedia (see below).

Intermediate Forms of β Thalassemia

These conditions are extremely heterogeneous,[7, 170] with respect to both their underlying genotype and the spectrum of their clinical phenotypes, which range from a relatively severe degree of anemia requiring intermittent blood transfusion to an asymptomatic condition that is identified by chance hematological study. Some of the different genotypes associated with the phenotype of thalassemia intermedia are summarized in Table 6–6, and the mechanisms that modify the severity of β thalassemia are summarized in Figure 6–15.

Mild β Thalassemia Mutations

The homozygous state for particularly mild mutations such as IVS-1 position 6 (T → C) and those involving the promoter regions −88 (C → T) and −29 (A → G) are usually characterized by mild clinical phenotypes.[112, 115] This probably reflects the moderate reduction in the output of β globin chains, although in the case of the promoter box mutations, it may also depend to some degree on relatively high levels of γ chain production. When these particular forms of thalassemia are present with more severe β thalassemia mutations in compound heterozygotes, there is a greater degree of anemia and a more severe form of β thalassemia intermedia. As mentioned earlier, the results of these interactions depend on whether the more severe β thalassemia mutation is of the β+ or β0 variety. For example, there are many compound heterozygotes for the IVS-1 position 6 (T → C) mutation and the IVS-1 position 110 (G → A) β+ thalassemia mutation who, although anemic, survive with only intermittent transfusions.

However, as more experience of these interactions is gained, it is becoming clear that there is remarkable heterogeneity even within patients with well-defined mutations. For example, in an extensive series of patients homozygous for the IVS-1 position 6 (T → C) mutation in Israel, the clinical phenotype has ranged from a transfusion-dependent thalassemia to a mild form of thalassemia intermedia; no

Table 6–6. β Thalassemia Intermedia

Mild (including "silent") forms of β thalassemia
    Homozygosity for mild β+ thalassemia alleles
    Compound heterozygosity for two mild β+ thalassemia alleles
    Compound heterozygosity for a mild and more severe β thalassemia
        allele
Inheritance of α and β thalassemia
    Homozygous or compound heterozygous β+ thalassemia with α0
        thalassemia (− −/αα) or α+ thalassemia (−α/αα or −α/−α)
    Homozygous or compound heterozygous β+ thalassemia with genotype
        of Hb H disease (− −/−α)
β Thalassemia with elevated γ chain synthesis
    Homozygous or compound heterozygous β thalassemia with
        heterocellular HPFH
    Homozygous or compound heterozygous β thalassemia with γ gene
        promoter mutations
    Compound heterozygosity for β thalassemia and deletion forms of
        HPFH
Compound heterozygosity for β thalassemia and β chain variants
    Hb E/β thalassemia
    Other interactions with rare β chain variants
Heterozygous β thalassemia with triplicated α chain genes (ααα)
Dominant forms of β thalassemia
Interactions of β, (δβ)+, (δβ)0, and (γδβ)0 thalassemia

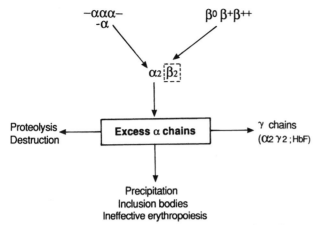

Figure 6–15. Major factors that modify the phenotype of β thalassemia.

factors have been identified to explain this remarkable phenotypic diversity.[171]

Coexistent α Thalassemia

Extensive data collected from the populations of the Mediterranean and Southeast Asia indicate that the coexistence of α thalassemia may modify the phenotype of homozygotes or compound heterozygotes for different β thalassemia mutations.[172–177] Again, the phenotypes are complex and depend on the number of α globin genes that are inactivated together with whether the β thalassemia is of the β^0 or β^+ variety. For example, it is clear that the coexistence of the heterozygous state for α^+ thalassemia and the homozygous state for β^0 thalassemia has little effect on the phenotype. On the other hand, individuals who are either α^+ thalassemia homozygotes or α^0 thalassemia heterozygotes, and who also are homozygous for β^+ thalassemia, may have a mild form of β thalassemia intermedia that is not transfusion dependent. The same applies even to patients who have the genotype of Hb H disease together with homozygous β^+ or compound heterozygous β^+/β^0 thalassemia. These remarkable experiments of nature are the best evidence we have that the most important factor in determining the phenotype of β thalassemia is the degree of imbalanced globin chain synthesis.

β Thalassemia With Unusually High Levels of Hb F Production

As mentioned earlier, many genetic factors may modify the level of Hb F production in β thalassemia (see Fig. 6–14). Perhaps the most extreme example is β^0 thalassemia in patients of Afro-Asian or Middle Eastern origin who are asymptomatic with hemoglobin values of 9 to 11 g/dl and whose hemoglobin consists almost entirely of Hb F with a small amount of Hb A_2.[153–155] Family studies have shown no evidence of HPFH. Many but not all of these individuals seem to be homozygous or heterozygous for the β globin RFLP haplotype that carries the *Xmn*I polymorphism. It is likely, but by no means certain, that these mild phenotypes result from the fact that the β thalassemia mutation is on a chromosome carrying the C → T change at position 158 in the $^G\gamma$ globin gene. Studies of the Hb F have shown a predominance of $^G\gamma$ chains, in keeping with this hypothesis.

In addition to mild forms of β thalassemia of this type, there are many examples of the co-inheritance of definable forms of non-deletion types of HPFH together with β thalassemia that give rise to a phenotype of β thalassemia intermedia.[162, 163] In these cases, β thalassemia homozygotes or compound heterozygotes seem to have an increased production of Hb F both *cis* and *trans* because of the action of the HPFH determinant.

Compound Heterozygous States for β Thalassemia and "Silent" β Thalassemia

In a few patients with the phenotype of mild β thalassemia intermedia, genetic studies suggest that affected individuals have received a severe β thalassemia allele from one parent and a completely silent allele from the other. Sequence analyses of the silent allele have, in some cases, revealed no abnormality, although genetic studies indicate that β chain synthesis is defective. In some families, the silent allele represents the C → T mutation at position −101 in the β globin gene promoter,[106, 178] whereas others result from mutations in the 5′ untranslated region[38, 107–109] or at IVS-2 position 844 (C → G)[178] (see Table 6–5). Although there have been reports that a genetic determinant for the silent allele segregates independently of the β globin gene cluster,[179] these remain to be confirmed. The nature of the silent β thalassemia alleles, at least in some families, is unknown.

Triplicated α Globin Genes Together With β Thalassemia

Triplicated α globin gene arrangements, ααα, occur in most populations at a low frequency. When they are inherited together with β thalassemia trait, they may produce the picture of thalassemia intermedia.[180–184] The clinical phenotypes vary, depending on the nature of the β thalassemia allele. If it is a β^+ thalassemia, the condition is mild; the most severe interaction is with exon 3 mutations that produce dominantly inherited forms of β thalassemia,[185] as described in the following section.

Dominant Forms of β Thalassemia

In some families, particularly of northern European and Japanese origin, a form of β thalassemia intermedia is inherited as a mendelian dominant.[186, 187] A disorder characterized by moderately severe anemia with jaundice and splenomegaly can be traced vertically and horizontally through different generations, indicating that the phenotype is due to the inheritance of a single gene and not the co-inheritance of two different alleles.[186, 187] This condition is also characterized by the presence of inclusion bodies in the red cell precursors and has therefore also been called inclusion body β thalassemia.[187] However, because all severe forms of β thalassemia have inclusions in the red cell precursors, dominantly inherited β thalassemia is the preferred term.

Some insights into the molecular pathology of these conditions have been obtained. With use of β globin RFLP linkage analysis, it has been found that they segregate with the β globin gene, indicating that they are due to mutations at or near this locus.[185] Sequence analysis has shown that they are heterogeneous at the molecular level but that the majority of them involve mutations of exon 3 of the β globin gene (see Table 6–5). These include frameshifts, premature chain termination (nonsense) mutations, and complex rearrangements that lead to the synthesis of truncated or elongated and highly unstable β globin gene products.[38, 95, 130–133, 185, 188–197] The most common mutation of this type is a GAA → TAA change at codon 121 that leads to the synthesis of a truncated β globin chain.[191] Although it is unusual to demonstrate an abnormal β chain product from loci affected by mutations of this type, many of these conditions have been designated hemoglobin variants.

A comparison of the lengths of abnormal gene products due to nonsense or frameshift mutations in the β globin gene (Fig. 6–16A) has suggested a mechanism to explain why most heterozygous forms of β thalassemia are mild whereas those due to mutations that involve exon 3 are more severe.[185] Nonsense or frameshift mutations that produce truncated β chains up to about 72 residues in length are usually associated with a mild phenotype in heterozygotes. These short β chain fragments are presumably degraded, and the resulting small excess of α chains is removed in the same way. However, many exon 3 mutations produce longer products; it is likely that the associated phenotypes reflect their heme binding properties and stability. Those with only 72 residues or less cannot bind heme, whereas those truncated to residue 120 or longer should bind heme because only helix H is missing. Such heme-containing products should have secondary structure and hence be less susceptible to proteolytic degradation. Furthermore, the lack of helix H, which would expose one of the hydrophobic patches of helix G and those of helices E and F, would also lead to aggregation. It was suggested, therefore, that the large inclusions in the red cell progenitors of these patients consist of aggre-

gates of precipitated β chain products together with excess α chains (Fig. 6–16B),[185] a prediction that was confirmed recently.[198] This explains the marked degree of dyserythropoiesis observed in this interesting condition. Their relative rarity and their occurrence mainly in northern Europeans suggest that they have had no selective value. Indeed, some of them represent de novo mutations.

Some unstable β globin variants, as exemplified by Hb Showa-Yakushiji, $\beta^{110Leu\rightarrow Pro}$, produce a phenotype much more like that of β thalassemia trait.[131] There is a mild anemia with hypochromic red cells and no evidence of ineffective erythropoiesis. This variant introduces a proline residue into the middle of the G helix that would disrupt all four α_1-β_1 contact points in the helix and hence may lead to rapid post-translational catabolism.

The pattern emerging from these studies is that there is a spectrum of disorders of β globin synthesis ranging, in the heterozygous state, from typical β thalassemia trait with hypochromic red cells, through the pattern of dominantly inherited β thalassemia with severe ineffective erythropoiesis, to a pure hemolytic anemia with effective erythropoiesis and destruction of the red cells in the peripheral blood due to instability of β globin chain variants. The main factors that determine the phenotype appear to be the length of the primary globin gene product, its ability to bind heme and to form an αβ dimer and tetramer, and the stability of the tetramer in the developing red cell precursor and peripheral circulation.

Interaction of β Thalassemia With δβ Thalassemia[7]

The δβ thalassemias are described in a later section. The co-inheritance of β and δβ thalassemia is associated with a variable phenotype, depending on the particular type of δβ

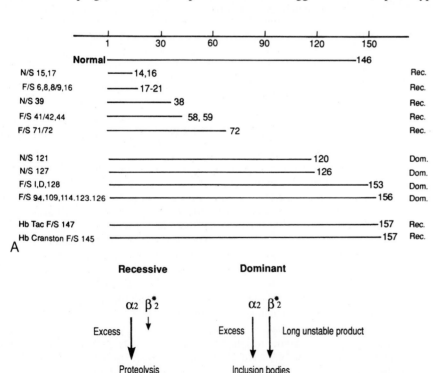

Figure 6–16. The molecular mechanisms for the dominant forms of β thalassemia. *A,* Mutations that result in truncated β globin gene products up to 70 residues are associated with the phenotype of β^0 thalassemia trait. The family of mutations that involve exon 3, many of which lead to elongated and highly unstable gene products, are associated with the genotype of dominant β thalassemia. *B,* The cellular basis for dominant β thalassemia.

thalassemia mutation. For example, the co-inheritance of β thalassemia with (δβ)$^+$ thalassemia of the Lepore variety, in which the output of γ chains from the Hb Lepore–containing chromosome is low, is often associated with a severe transfusion-dependent form of β thalassemia. On the other hand, the co-inheritance of β thalassemia with a deletion form of (δβ)^0 thalassemia leads to a milder phenotype because of the high output of γ chains generated by the chromosome containing the (δβ)^0 thalassemia mutation.

β Thalassemia in Association With Structural Variants of β Globin[7]

The consequences of the compound inheritance of β thalassemia with β globin chain variants depend on the nature of the particular structural variant. For example, because the action of the β thalassemia gene is to reduce the output of Hb A, the phenotypes of sickle cell β thalassemia and Hb C β thalassemia depend mainly on the properties of Hb S and Hb C. In interactions between β^0 thalassemia and these variants, the hemoglobin consists almost entirely of S and C. On the other hand, in the interactions of β$^+$ thalassemia, the level of hemoglobin A depends on the severity of the β thalassemia mutation.[199] The sickling disorders are described in Chapter 7.

The most important interaction of this type is Hb E β thalassemia, which, globally, may become the most common serious form of thalassemia in the future.[200] This condition is widely distributed throughout the eastern part of the Indian subcontinent and Southeast Asia. As mentioned earlier, Hb E results from a mutation in exon 1 that activates a cryptic splice site. Hence, it is associated with the phenotype of a mild form of β thalassemia. When this variant interacts with β^0 thalassemia or the severe forms of β$^+$ thalassemia, a marked deficit of β globin chains follows, resulting in the phenotype of a more severe form of β thalassemia. However, because the homozygous state for hemoglobin E is associated with the hematological findings of β thalassemia trait, it is not clear why this interaction is so severe. In the steady state, it does not appear to result from the innate instability of Hb E, although its remarkable heat instability may play a role in the worsening of the anemia that is associated with intercurrent infection.[201]

Although much remains to be learned about the natural history of Hb E β thalassemia, both early descriptions[202] and more recent series[203–206] indicate that it is a remarkably heterogeneous condition. At one end of the spectrum, the clinical picture is indistinguishable from severe transfusion-dependent thalassemia major; at the other extreme, patients grow and survive normally and are ascertained only by chance or family studies.[206] Although the co-inheritance of α thalassemia may play some part in this heterogeneity in Southeast Asia,[203] this is not the case in the eastern populations of the Indian subcontinent, in which at least some of the variability of severity seems to be related to the steady-state level of Hb F production.[206] The protean clinical manifestations and complications of this disease have been reviewed.[7]

β Globin Chain Variant Genes That Also Contain β Thalassemia Mutations

Several examples have been found in which a β globin gene containing a sickle mutation has also been found to carry a

β$^+$ thalassemia mutation.[207] Affected individuals have the phenotype of β thalassemia trait with an elevated level of Hb A$_2$ and an unusually low level of Hb S, in the 10 per cent range. In one example of this type, the β$^+$ thalassemia mutation was found to be the -88 C → T, which is a common form of β$^+$ thalassemia in black populations. The same β$^+$ thalassemia mutation has also been found in a β globin gene carrying the mutation β$^{75 Leu → 0}$ that is responsible for the unstable variant Hb Vicksburg.[208] The phenotype in this case is more severe and resembles thalassemia intermedia.

β Thalassemia Trait

The β thalassemia traits, whether β$^+$ or β^0, are usually characterized by mild anemia and small, poorly hemoglobinized red cells. There is an elevation of Hb A$_2$ to about twice the normal level. This is the result of both a relative deficiency of β chains and an absolute increase in the output of δ chains, both *cis* and *trans* to the β thalassemia mutation.[7] There is a slight elevation of Hb F in about 50 per cent of cases.

There are rarer variant forms of β thalassemia trait, many of which have now been analyzed at the molecular level.

β Thalassemia Trait With Unusually High Levels of Hb A$_2$

This condition almost invariably results from deletions that remove part or all of the β globin gene, including its 5′ promoter sequences, but leave the δ globin gene intact. It appears, therefore, that in the absence of the β globin gene promoter, there is an absolute increase in δ chain synthesis above that seen in the usual forms of β thalassemia trait. This may reflect the availability of regulatory elements that normally compete for the promoters of the β and δ globin genes.

Normal A$_2$ β Thalassemia

In populations in which β thalassemia is common, individuals are encountered occasionally who have the features of β thalassemia trait but with a normal Hb A$_2$ level. The molecular mechanisms for this form of β thalassemia are, again, heterogeneous.[95] The bulk of cases seem to result from the co-inheritance of both β and δ thalassemia; the mutations that give rise to δ thalassemia are considered in a later section.

Another relatively common cause of normal Hb A$_2$ β thalassemia in Middle Eastern and Mediterranean populations is the mutation at codon 26, GCC → TCC, that generates Hb Knossos, a variant not detectable by electrophoresis under standard conditions. As is the case for Hb E, this mutation results in both the insertion of a different amino acid and a reduced production of β globin mRNA.[119] However, although it is associated with a β thalassemia–like disorder, the Hb A$_2$ level is not elevated. It turns out that the chromosome that carries the Hb Knossos mutation also has a mutation of the δ globin gene, the loss of an A in codon 59, which completely inactivates it.[209] Because most patients with Hb Knossos seem to share the same β globin RFLP haplotype, it appears that the δ^0/β^{Knossos} allele has been disseminated throughout the Mediterranean region.

Finally, under "normal A_2 β thalassemia" should be included the silent β thalassemias, which are described earlier, and the carrier state for εγδβ thalassemia, a condition described later in this chapter.

As mentioned earlier, it has been customary to define the normal Hb A_2 β thalassemias into type 1, or silent β thalassemia, and type 2, in which the hematological picture is typical of β thalassemia trait. As will have become apparent from this discussion, this classification, although still useful clinically, has little genetic meaning.

▼ CLINICAL AND HEMATOLOGICAL FEATURES OF THE β THALASSEMIAS

It is beyond the scope of this chapter to consider the clinical features of the β thalassemias in detail. They are the subject of several monographs,[7, 134, 210] and readers who wish to obtain a detailed account of this aspect of the thalassemia field are referred to these sources. Here, I simply outline the major clinical features of the three main clinical groups of β thalassemias, the molecular basis and pathophysiology of which have been considered in the previous sections.

The Major Forms of β Thalassemia

These conditions often present during the first year as the level of Hb F declines. They usually declare themselves by failure to thrive, pallor, or anemia that is discovered during an intercurrent illness such as an infection. Left untreated, affected infants are incapable of maintaining a hemoglobin level above 5 g/dl. Their subsequent clinical course and physical findings depend on whether they are prescribed an adequate transfusion regimen at this stage or whether they are given insufficient blood to develop normally.

The standard textbook picture of the major form of thalassemia, Cooley's anemia, describes the disease as it is seen in children who have been inadequately transfused. They show early growth retardation, pallor, icterus, and, as they grow older, brown pigmentation of the skin. Progressive expansion of the bone marrow in response to anemia leads to characteristic skeletal changes, including bossing of the skull, overgrowth of the zygomata, and protrusion of the jaws. These changes may ultimately lead to the classical thalassemic facies. They are associated with characteristic radiological abnormalities including a "hair on end" appearance of the skull and thinning and trabeculation of the bones of the hands and the long bones. The bone changes may become so marked as to lead to repeated pathological fractures. There is progressive hepatosplenomegaly, and this may lead to a secondary dilutional anemia, with leukopenia and thrombocytopenia. These poorly developed children are particularly prone to infection, which during the early years of life is the most common cause of morbidity and mortality.[171]

In children who have been transfused regularly to maintain hemoglobin levels above 9 to 10 g/dl, growth and development are usually normal until early puberty. The splenomegaly that is common in inadequately transfused children is not so prominent, and hypersplenism rarely develops. However, by the age of 10 to 15 years, patients treated in this way, unless they have received regular chelation therapy to remove excess iron derived from transfusions,

start to show signs of progressive hepatic, cardiac, and endocrine dysfunction associated with a reduced pubertal growth spurt and failure of sexual maturation. On the other hand, children who have been adequately chelated may have normal sexual maturation. Even they often have some growth retardation, however.

The hematological findings are also dependent on the type of transfusion regimen. In inadequately transfused children, the peripheral blood shows typical thalassemic red cell morphology with anisocytosis and poikilocytosis, target cells, and red cell fragments, all set against a background of marked hypochromia. Nucleated red cells are usually present and after splenectomy may become frequent. The white cell and platelet count varies, depending on the degree of hypersplenism. In adequately transfused children, the peripheral blood count is often remarkably normal, simply reflecting the suppression of the patient's bone marrow.

The bone marrow shows intense erythroid hyperplasia. The red cell precursors have nuclear and cytoplasmic abnormalities and contain inclusions formed from precipitated α chains. Ferrokinetic and erythrokinetic studies demonstrate an extreme degree of ineffective erythropoiesis with a reduced survival of red cells in the peripheral blood.

In untransfused or inadequately transfused patients, the hemoglobin consists of a variable amount of Hb F; in patients with no β chain production, there is no Hb A and the hemoglobin consists entirely of Hb F with a small proportion of Hb A_2. The level of Hb A_2 in homozygotes or compound heterozygotes for severe forms of β thalassemia is of no diagnostic value. It tends to be low in red cells that contain predominantly Hb F and relatively higher in those that contain Hb A; the level of Hb A_2 in the blood represents an average of its different distribution in these heterogeneous cell populations.[7]

β Thalassemia Intermedia

As might be expected from the heterogeneity of its molecular basis,[170] this is an ill-defined clinical entity with a broad spectrum ranging from a condition little different from thalassemia major to a symptomless disorder that is discovered only by chance examination of the blood. One of the most useful indications that β thalassemia is likely to follow a milder course is its time of presentation; babies with β thalassemia intermedia tend to present late in the first year and often well into the second year of life.[210] Otherwise, the clinical features are characterized by a varying degree of anemia and splenomegaly and, in the more severe forms, bone changes similar to the major form of the illness.

At the severe end of the spectrum, the hemoglobin level settles down to 5 to 7 g/dl, and by the age of 2 and 3 years, it is clear that development is not normal; there are already signs of the skeletal changes, particularly deformity of the skull and face, characteristic of untreated thalassemia major. If these children are transfused, which may not need to be as frequent as for those with thalassemia major, these changes can be arrested and future skeletal development is normal. However, at the other end of the spectrum, patients may not become symptomatic until they reach adult life and may remain transfusion free, with hemoglobin levels at 8 to 12 g/dl. However, they may develop complications as they get older, including increasing splenomegaly and hypersplenism, iron loading due to increased absorption, painful arthritis, gallstones, leg ulcers, and an increased proneness to infection.[7]

The hematological picture is similar to thalassemia major. The hemoglobin composition is extremely variable. Those who are homozygous for β^0 thalassemia have only Hb F and Hb A_2, whereas others who have inherited mild β^+ thalassemia mutations may have Hb F levels as low as 5 to 10 per cent. The relationship of the level of Hb F to particular mutations is considered earlier in this chapter.

Dominantly Inherited β Thalassemia

This condition has a different phenotype from other forms of β thalassemia intermedia in several respects.[186, 187] There is a variable degree of anemia, splenomegaly, and morphological changes of the red cells. The bone marrow shows marked erythroid hyperplasia with well-formed inclusion bodies in the red cell precursors. However, hemoglobin analysis is characterized by a raised level of Hb A_2 but normal or only slightly elevated levels of Hb F. These findings, together with the pattern of dominant inheritance, are diagnostic.

β Thalassemia Trait

The heterozygous states for β^0 and β^+ thalassemia are invariably asymptomatic and, despite their molecular heterogeneity, show a remarkably uniform hematological picture. There is microcytosis and hypochromia with low MCV and MCH values together with an increased level of Hb A_2. There is a slightly increased level of Hb F in about 50 per cent of cases. The only exceptions are β thalassemia heterozygotes who also have α thalassemia trait in whom, for reasons that are not clear, the MCH and MCV are much closer to normal. The Hb A_2 level is elevated, however.

The hematological findings in the subtypes of β thalassemia, such as those with unusually high levels of Hb A_2 or normal levels of Hb A_2, are similar. These conditions are defined by the Hb A_2 levels.

▼ WORLD DISTRIBUTION AND POPULATION GENETICS

The world distribution of the β thalassemias and the mutations that occur in different populations are shown in Figure 6–17 and have been summarized in reviews[38, 72] and a monograph.[7]

Gene frequency data for β thalassemia in different parts of the world are often based on small samples, and there are only sporadic reports of individual cases for many populations. It is clear, however, that with a few exceptions, such as Liberia, the condition occurs at a low frequency throughout tropical Africa, although higher frequencies have been observed in North Africa. It is particularly common throughout the Mediterranean region, parts of the Middle East, and India and Burma.[7] It is also common throughout Southeast Asia in a line starting in southern China, stretching through Thailand, Cambodia, and Laos, and down the Malay peninsula into Indonesia. It is distributed sporadically in Melanesia.

In each of the high-frequency areas, there are a few common mutations together with a varying number of rare ones (see Fig. 6–17). Furthermore, in each of these populations, the pattern of mutations is different.[103, 110, 112, 154, 211–215] Even where the same mutation occurs in different populations, it is usually found together with a different β globin gene RFLP haplotype. It is likely, therefore, that the β thalassemia mutations have arisen independently in different populations and achieved their high frequency by selection. Although there may have been some movement of the β thalassemia genes between populations, by drift and so on,

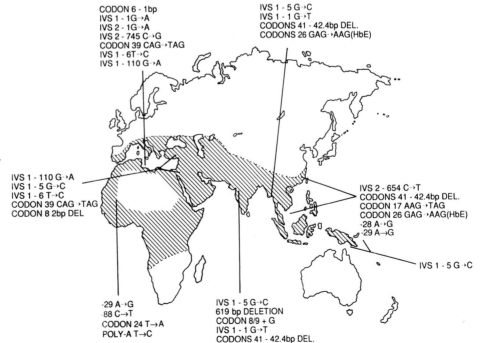

Figure 6–17. The world distribution of the different β thalassemia mutations. Nomenclature is described in the text.

there is little doubt that independent mutation and selection have been the major factors responsible for the world distribution of the β thalassemias.

Population studies suggest that a major factor that has maintained the β thalassemia polymorphism is protection of heterozygotes against *P. falciparum* malaria.[72] Studies in Melanesia have shown that there is a frequency-dependent altitude correlation with malaria just as has been shown for α thalassemia,[113] an observation noted earlier in other populations.[72] However, the data that would relate β thalassemia and Hb E to heterozygote protection against *P. falciparum* malaria are not nearly as strong as those described earlier in this chapter for α thalassemia. It will be necessary to carry out the same types of investigations that have demonstrated the protective effect of α thalassemia in populations in which β thalassemia and Hb E are common.

The δβ Thalassemias

Globally, the δβ thalassemias are much less common than the β thalassemias.[7] Like the β thalassemias, they are extremely heterogeneous in their molecular pathology and clinical phenotype.

▼ CLASSIFICATION

It is useful to divide the δβ thalassemias into the (δβ)$^+$ and (δβ)^0 thalassemias to indicate whether there is any output of δ and β chains from the affected chromosome (see Table 6–1).

The (δβ)$^+$ thalassemias fall into two main classes. First, there are those that result from abnormal crossing over and the production of δβ fusion hemoglobin variants, of which Hb Lepore is the prototype. Second, there are complex disorders that result from the presence of two different mutations in the ϵγδβ globin gene cluster; one leads to either the δ or β globin genes being partially or completely inactivated, and the other involves the promoter region of the γ globin genes or another site and results in increased γ gene expression. As knowledge of the molecular pathology of these rare conditions has increased, it has become apparent that many of them are not true δβ thalassemias, but because they appear in the thalassemia literature under this heading, they are considered in this section.

The (δβ)^0 thalassemias usually result from long deletions involving the ϵγδβ globin gene cluster that remove the β and δ genes but leave either one or both of the γ globin genes intact. If only the β and δ genes are deleted, they are referred to as $^Gγ^Aγ(δβ)^0$ thalassemias, or more simply as (δβ)^0 thalassemias. If the $^Aγ$ gene is lost as well, they are called ($^Aγδβ)^0$ thalassemia. They produce a phenotype similar to the deletion forms of HPFH, which are described in detail in Chapter 5, that is, there is a high output of γ chains from the γ locus or loci *cis* to the mutation. Indeed, HPFH can be looked on as a form of (δβ)^0 thalassemia in which there is almost, but not complete, compensation for defective β chain synthesis by persistent γ chain production.

▼ MOLECULAR PATHOLOGY

The molecular pathology of the δβ thalassemias, although of interest for its own sake, has been studied in particular

detail because it was hoped that it might help to define the regions of the ϵγδβ globin gene cluster involved in the regulation of the transition from γ to β globin chain synthesis during development. This is of particular interest with respect to the lengths and sites of the deletions that underlie the deletion forms of δβ thalassemia as compared with HPFH.

(δβ)$^+$ Thalassemia

Fusion Chain Variants

There is a family of hemoglobin variants that have arisen by non-homologous crossing over within the ϵγδβ globin gene complex (Fig. 6–18). The first to be discovered, Hb Lepore, named after the family in which it was found, contains normal α chains and non-α chains that consist of the first 50 to 80 amino acid residues of the δ chain and the last 60 to 90 residues of the normal C-terminal sequence of the β chains.[216] Thus, the Hb Lepore non-α chain is a δβ fusion chain. Three different variants of Hb Lepore have been described in which the transition from δ to β sequences occurs at different points.[7, 217] Hemoglobin Kenya is analogous except that in this case, the abnormal hybrid chain contains γ and β sequences, that is, it is a γβ fusion chain.[7]

These fusion globin chains have arisen by non-homologous crossing over between part of the δ locus on one chromosome and part of the β locus on the complementary chromosome (see Fig. 6–18). This event results from misalignment of chromosome pairs during meiosis so that a δ chain gene pairs with a β chain gene instead of its homologous partner. As shown in Figure 6–18, this mechanism should give rise to two abnormal chromosomes. The Lepore chromosome has no normal δ or β loci and carries a δβ fusion gene. On the opposite of the homologous pairs of chromosomes, there is an anti-Lepore (βδ) fusion gene together with normal δ and β loci. Similarly, in the generation of the γβ fusion variant, Hb Kenya, an anti-Kenya chromosome with intact $^Aγ$, δ, and β loci is produced. A variety of anti-Lepore–like hemoglobins have been discovered, including hemoglobins Miwada, P-Congo, Lincoln Park, and P-Nilotic.[217]

Another variant with δβ chains, Hb Parchman, is more complex in that the non-α chain has δ sequences at the N-*and* C-terminal ends and β sequences in the middle. It is likely that this arose by a double cross-over event.[217]

The different cross-over regions that generate the Lepore and anti-Lepore hemoglobins have been defined at the molecular level.[218] The δ fusion chains are synthesized ineffectively and hence give rise to the clinical phenotype of δβ thalassemia. It seems likely that this reflects that the composite δβ fusion gene contains the 5′ flanking region regulatory elements of the δ gene. In particular, there is a potentially important change in the CAAT box, which in the case of the δ globin gene promoter has the sequence CCAAC.[219] It is believed that this change may be the cause of the low-level expression of the δ globin gene, although it has been observed that there is no erythroid Kruppel-like factor binding site related to the δ globin as compared with the β globin genes.[220] These sequence differences, and other possible differences, notably in δ IVS-2,[221] may explain the marked reduction of the δβ fusion product. Unlike in the (δβ)^0 thalassemias, there is little compensation by the γ globin genes on the same chromosome, and hence the homozygous

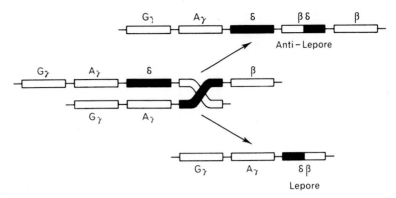

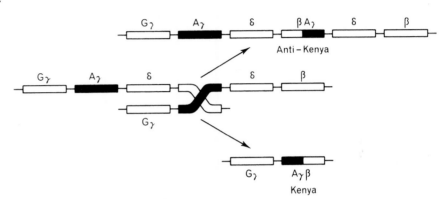

Figure 6–18. The abnormal crossing over mechanisms involved in the generation of the Lepore and anti-Lepore hemoglobins and Hb Kenya.

state for Hb Lepore is often associated with a severe clinical disorder. On the other hand, the chromosome carrying the $^A\gamma\beta$ fusion product, Hb Kenya, is not associated with an abnormal phenotype because there is a high output of γ chains and hence the clinical picture of HPFH.

$(\delta\beta)^+$ Thalassemia–Like Disorders Due to Two Mutations in the β Globin Gene Cluster

A heterogeneous family of non-deletion $\delta\beta$ thalassemias has been described that result from two mutations in the $\epsilon\gamma\delta\beta$ globin gene cluster. Strictly speaking, not all are $\delta\beta$ thalassemias, but because their phenotypes resemble the deletion forms of $(\delta\beta)^0$ thalassemia that are described in the next section, they appear in the literature under this title.

In the Sardinian form of $\delta\beta$ thalassemia,[222] the β globin gene has the common Mediterranean codon 39 nonsense mutation that leads to an absence of β globin synthesis. However, there is a relatively high expression of the $^A\gamma$ gene in *cis,* which gives this condition the phenotype of $\delta^+\beta^0$ thalassemia; this is because there is a point mutation at position -196 upstream from the $^A\gamma$ gene. Heterozygotes for this condition have thalassemic red cell changes, 15 to 20 per cent Hb F, and normal levels of Hb A_2. Thus, this disorder is a phenocopy of $\delta\beta$ thalassemia.

Another condition that has the phenotype of $\delta\beta$ thalassemia, with more than 20 per cent Hb F in heterozygotes, has been described in a Chinese patient in whom defective β globin gene synthesis appears to be due to an A → G change in the ATA sequence in the promoter region of the β globin gene.[223] The increased γ chain synthesis, which appears to involve both $^G\gamma$ and $^A\gamma$ genes *cis* to this mutation, remains unexplained.

Another condition that was originally called $\delta\beta$ thalas-

semia has been described in the Corfu population.[224] Again, this results from two mutations in the β globin gene cluster.[225] First, there is a 7201 bp deletion that starts in the δ globin gene, IVS-2 position 818 to 822, and extends upstream to a 5' breakpoint located 1719 to 1722 bp 3' to the $\psi\beta$ gene termination codon. In addition, there is G → A mutation at position 5 in the donor site consensus region of IVS-1 of the β globin gene. The output from this novel chromosome consists of relatively high levels of γ chains with low levels of β chains. The $^A\gamma$ and $^G\gamma$ globin genes have been sequenced, including the upstream promoter regions from position -360 to the cap sites, but no other mutations have been found. It is presumed, therefore, that the high level of γ chain production from this chromosome in adult life is related to the deletion.

Homozygotes for the Corfu form of thalassemia have almost 100 per cent Hb F with traces of Hb A but no Hb A_2. Curiously, heterozygotes have only slightly elevated levels of Hb F; the phenotype is similar to normal Hb A_2 β thalassemia. Thus, strictly speaking, this condition is a $\delta^0\beta^+$ thalassemia with unusually high levels of Hb F in homozygotes.

$(\delta\beta)^0$ and $(^A\gamma\delta\beta)^0$ Thalassemia

These conditions result from deletions of various lengths that remove the δ and β globin genes. They are classified into the $(\delta\beta)^0$ and $(^A\gamma\delta\beta)^0$ thalassemias depending on the length of the deletion, that is, whether the $^A\gamma$ genes are involved or not (see Table 6–1). The extent of these deletions is illustrated in Figure 6–19. The molecular basis and original descriptions of these diseases have been catalogued,[38] and details of their associated clinical and hematological findings and various interactions have also been reviewed.[7]

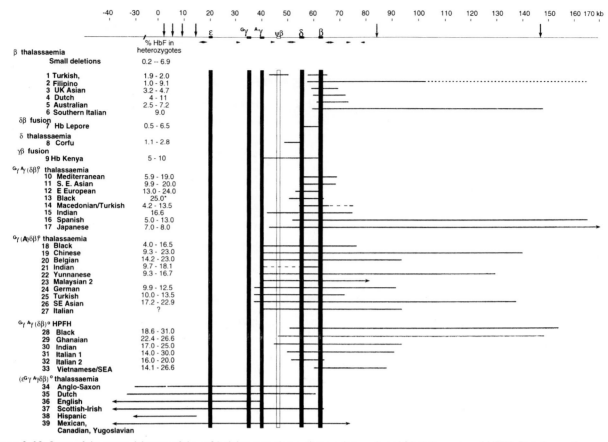

Figure 6–19. Some of the major deletions of the εγδβ globin gene cluster that result in γ, β, and δβ thalassemia and HPFH. Data from references given in text and reference 38. (Prepared by Dr. W. G. Wood.)

(δβ)⁰ Thalassemia

These conditions result from deletions involving the δ and β globin genes, which are categorized by the racial origin of the individual in whom they were first described: Indian,[226] Japanese,[227] Spanish,[228] black,[229] east European,[230] Laotian,[231] Thai,[232] Sicilian,[233] Macedonian,[234] and Turkish.[235] The majority of the deletions that underlie these conditions are relatively small and are contained within the β globin gene cluster. The one exception is the Spanish variety, in which the deletion extends much farther to the 3′ side, and beyond the 3′ end of the (δβ)⁰ hereditary persistence of fetal hemoglobin lesions.[228]

The homozygous states for these conditions are characterized by a mild form of β thalassemia intermedia; no Hb A or A₂ is produced. The heterozygous phenotypes are remarkably consistent, showing the hematological changes of β thalassemia trait with Hb F values in the 5 to 20 per cent range and normal Hb A₂ levels.

(^Aγδβ)⁰ Thalassemia

These conditions, which also result from long deletions or more complex rearrangements involving the β globin gene cluster, are designated by the country of origin of the first individual in whom they were reported: Indian,[236] German,[237] Cantonese,[238] Malay-1,[239] Turkish,[240] Malay-2,[241] Belgian,[242] black,[243] Chinese,[244] Yunnanese,[245] Thai,[246] and Italian.[247] The deletions that underlie these conditions extend into or beyond the ^Aγ gene on the 5′ side, as well as removing the δ

and β genes. Where it has been determined, the 3′ extent of the deletions usually terminates within 20 kb of the β gene, although the Chinese variety extends much farther. The Indian form is not a simple deletion but results from a complex rearrangement with two deletions, one affecting the ^Aγ gene and the other the δ and β genes; the intervening region remains but is inverted. Incidentally, this was the first example of a major gene inversion underlying a genetic disease in man.

The homozygous state is similar to that for (δβ)⁰ thalassemia, with the clinical picture of thalassemia intermedia and hemoglobin values in the few reported cases ranging between 8 and 11 g/dl. Heterozygotes have thalassemic red cell changes, and their Hb F values cluster tightly in the 11 to 14 per cent range.

Overall, although these two forms of δβ thalassemia have similar clinical phenotypes, it appears that (^Aγδβ)⁰ thalassemia runs a slightly more severe course, a conclusion that is strengthened by a detailed comparison of their interactions with β thalassemia.[7]

▼ GENOTYPE/PHENOTYPE RELATIONS IN δβ THALASSEMIA

The major phenotypic difference between the β and most of the δβ thalassemias reflects the relatively high output of γ globin chain production that occurs in δβ thalassemia and leads to a milder disorder. The exception is the Hb Lepore disorders, in which there is a low output of γ chains and a severe deficit of non-α chain production leading to a clinical phenotype similar to β thalassemia. In all the other δβ thalassemias, there is a relatively high output of either $^{G}\gamma$ and $^{A}\gamma$ or $^{G}\gamma$ chains. With the exception of the Sardinian and Chinese phenocopies, in which upstream mutations involving the γ globin gene similar to those observed in the non-deletion forms of HPFH (see Chapter 5) have been demonstrated, there is no obvious reason for the high output of γ chains and it is assumed, therefore, that this must be due to the effect of the extensive deletions of the β-like globin gene cluster.

As described in Chapter 5, there is a family of deletion forms of HPFH that produce a clinical picture similar to (δβ)⁰ thalassemia but in which the output of γ chains is higher, and therefore the phenotype is even milder. The two African forms of (δβ)⁰ HPFH are both due to extensive deletions, of similar length but with staggered ends, differing phenotypically only in the proportions of γ chains produced. A third form of HPFH of this type, found in Indians, is associated with a more severe phenotype, particularly when it is co-inherited with β thalassemia (see Fig. 6–19). The difference between the output of γ chains in HPFH and δβ thalassemia is only a matter of degree; homozygotes for the deletion forms of HPFH have small red cells and imbalanced globin chain synthesis.[248]

Because of the problems of cell selection due to imbalanced globin chain synthesis found in δβ thalassemia homozygotes, and even to some degree in HPFH homozygotes, the most valid comparisons of the phenotypic expression of these conditions are made in heterozygotes. Heterozygotes for (δβ)⁰ thalassemia have levels of Hb F that greatly exceed those of β thalassemia heterozygotes, usually in the range of 5 to 15 per cent. On the other hand, heterozygotes for deletion forms of HPFH have Hb F values in the range 15 to 25 per cent. Clearly, therefore, γ chain output is more effective in HPFH. However, detailed analyses of the underlying deletions have not provided a unifying hypothesis to explain these differences. In general, deletions that start within the β globin gene complex and extend 3′ to it appear to leave the surviving γ genes active in adult life. Whereas this could reflect the effects of newly opposed 3′ promoter sequences on γ chain synthesis, the large number of different deletions of this type makes it difficult to imagine that each one mediates its effect in the same way. Furthermore, two of the deletions, those associated with Hb Kenya and the Indian form of ($^{A}\gamma\delta\beta$)⁰ thalassemia, leave the 3′ end of the β gene and beyond intact (see Fig. 6–19). Comparison of (δβ)⁰ thalassemia and (δβ)⁰ HPFH does not identify any single region between the $^{A}\gamma$ and δ genes that remains intact in one condition but that is lost in the other, and it has not been possible to identify a sequence in the gene cluster that might be involved in modifying γ chain output in these different conditions. Similarly, models that implicate the altered spatial relationships between the LCR and the genes of the β cluster consequent on these deletions do not fully account for the phenotypic differences between (δβ)⁰ thalassemia and (δβ)⁰ HPFH.

δ Thalassemia

Thalassemia involving the δ globin locus is of no clinical significance except insofar as when it is inherited together with β thalassemia, it may prevent the usual elevation of Hb A₂ that occurs in β thalassemia heterozygotes. As mentioned earlier, the co-inheritance of β and δ thalassemia is one of the most common causes of normal Hb A₂ β thalassemia.

▼ MOLECULAR PATHOLOGY

Like other forms of thalassemia, δ thalassemia can be classified into δ⁰ and δ⁺ thalassemia, depending on the particular molecular lesion. Some of the mutations that cause δ thalassemia are summarized in Figure 6–20, and the references to their original descriptions are given in 38, 209, and 249.

One type of δ⁰ thalassemia that occurs in the Mediterranean population is due to a partial deletion of the δ globin gene. This particular lesion is described in the previous section as part of the molecular pathology of the Corfu form of δβ thalassemia.[225] The deletion involves the loss of 7201 bp with a 5′ breakpoint at a site 3′ to the ψβ globin gene and a 3′ breakpoint in the middle of IVS-2 of the δ globin gene. This deletion has been observed on chromosomes with a normal β globin gene in patients in the Mediterranean population.[249] Presumably, the Corfu form of δβ thalassemia arose as a recombinational event with a chromosome containing a β gene with the IVS-1 position 5 G → A mutation. Several other molecular forms of δ⁰ thalassemia have been described as shown in Figure 6–20. Similarly, there are several mutations that should give rise to the phenotype of δ⁺ thalassemia because they are similar to those in the β globin gene that cause its partial inactivation.

Interestingly, at least three of the mutations that have been found in δ thalassemia have their equivalents in the same position in the β globin chain in β thalassemia. These are δ⁺27, δ⁰ IVS-1 position 1, and G → C at codon 30.[249] It is presumed that identical nucleotide substitutions in the β and δ genes have arisen, either as independent mutations or as the result of gene conversion events. Most of the δ thalassemias have been observed in *trans* to β thalassemia. However, the δ⁺27 mutation has been observed in both *cis* and *trans*. As mentioned in an earlier section, the form of δ thalassemia that results from a loss of an A in codon 59 occurs on the same chromosome as the Hb Knossos muta-

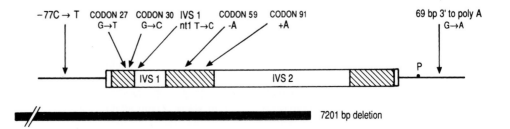

Figure 6–20. The mutations that cause δ thalassemia. (Data from Olds, R. J., et al.: A novel δ⁰ mutation in *cis* with Hb Knossos: A study of different genetic interactions in three Egyptian families. Br. J. Haematol. 78:430, 1991; and Piratsu, M., et al.: Molecular analysis of atypical β-thalassemia heterozygotes. Ann. N. Y. Acad. Sci. 612:90, 1990.)

tion, thus explaining the normal level of Hb A_2 associated with this mild form of β thalassemia.[209]

▼ CLINICAL AND HEMATOLOGICAL IMPLICATIONS

The δ thalassemias are not associated with any hematological changes. Because they prevent an elevation of Hb A_2 when they are inherited together with β thalassemia, they are of diagnostic importance for genetic counseling and screening. Although there have been no population surveys, it seems likely that they occur at a low frequency because there is no reason for them to have come under any form of selection.

εγδβ Thalassemia

This is a rare form of thalassemia that results from six different long deletions starting approximately 50 to 100 kb upstream from the globin gene cluster and extending 3′ where they remove all or part of the cluster. Because even if they spare the β globin gene it is inactivated, they are all (εγδβ)⁰ thalassemias.

The approximate extent of these deletions is illustrated in Figure 6–19. In cases in which the deletion spares the β globin gene, the Dutch[250] and English[251] forms, for example, no β chain production occurs, even though the gene is expressed in heterologous systems. Similarly, the Hispanic deletion, which extends upstream 5′ from the ε gene, is also associated with defective β chain production.[252]

The reason for the inactivation of the β globin gene *cis* to these deletions was clarified by the discovery of the LCR about 50 kb upstream from the εγδβ globin gene cluster.[75] Just as occurs when the α globin LCR is inactivated by a deletion, as described earlier, the removal of this critical regulatory region seems to completely inactivate the downstream globin gene complex. The Hispanic form[252] results from a deletion that includes most of the LCR including four of the five DNase I hypersensitive sites. These lesions appear to close down the chromatin domain that is usually open in erythroid tissues. They also delay the replication of the β genes in the cell cycle. Thus, although these are rare mutations, they have been of considerable importance; it was the analysis of the Dutch deletion that first pointed to the possibility of there being a major control region upstream from the β-like globin gene cluster and ultimately led to the discovery of the β globin LCR.

The clinical and hematological phenotypes associated with (εγδβ)⁰ thalassemia vary, depending on the stage of development.[253] The homozygous states presumably would not be compatible with fetal survival. At birth, heterozygotes are sometimes anemic with hypochromic red cells and a variable degree of hemolysis. In some cases, this has necessitated blood transfusion in the neonatal period. Three of nine infants with the Dutch variety of the disorder died. Five of the six living children with this condition required blood transfusions after delivery, whereas the remaining one survived with no treatment.

In adult life, the condition is characterized by the hematological picture of β thalassemia trait with a normal Hb A_2 level. The reason that this condition is so severe in some but not all heterozygotes in the neonatal period remains unexplained.

Thalassemias for Which the Cause Has Not Been Determined

Despite intensive work in many laboratories during the last 15 years, a significant number of thalassemia-like disorders remain for which the cause has not yet been determined. Most laboratories that study the disorder have encountered on the order of 5 per cent of cases in which the hematological findings and globin synthesis data suggest a thalassemic defect, yet complete sequence analysis of the appropriate globin gene and its flanking regions has revealed no abnormality.

It seems likely that some of these disorders will be due to mutations involving HS40 or the LCR for the α or β globin genes, respectively. The strategy of studying these areas in unusual cases of α thalassemia has already disclosed several different deletions involving this region. It seems likely that similar lesions will be found in the β globin LCR. Unlike the extensive deletions involving this region that have been found to date, there may be more subtle deletions or even point mutations. It is also possible, of course, that there are regulatory regions controlling expression of the globin genes that are not close to the globin gene clusters or are even on other chromosomes. The discovery that one form of α thalassemia associated with mental retardation is due to a lesion on the X chromosome suggests that such regulatory loci exist and that they may be involved in the genesis of some thalassemic disorders.

The Control and Treatment of the Thalassemias

The hemoglobin disorders are probably the most common single-gene diseases in the world population. Because they occur with a particularly high frequency in the developing world where the rate of population increase is the greatest, it is likely that their prevalence will tend to increase, even if the major selective force that has maintained these polymorphisms in the past is removed. With the resurgence of malaria in many parts of the world, it may be a long time before this occurs. Indeed, the World Health Organization has estimated that by the year 2000, approximately 7 per cent of the world's population will be carriers for important globin disorders.

It is beyond the scope of this chapter to deal with the population control and clinical management of the thalassemias in detail. Here, I concentrate on those aspects based on an understanding of its molecular basis.

▼ SCREENING AND PRENATAL DIAGNOSIS

In many ways, the thalassemias are ideal recessive disorders for developing population screening programs and prenatal diagnosis.[254, 255] The carrier states for the important α and β thalassemias can be identified hematologically and by hemoglobin analysis in the majority of cases. Occasionally, difficulty may be encountered in distinguishing these traits from iron deficiency, and complex interactions, particularly the co-inheritance of α and β thalassemia, may cause problems for screening, but overall the carrier states can be identified by any hematology laboratory with appropriately trained personnel.

Because the treatment of the important forms of α and β thalassemia is still unsatisfactory, the most important approach to their control is screening followed by prenatal diagnosis. Originally, this was done by obtaining fetal blood from the placenta or umbilical cord followed by globin chain synthesis analysis.[254] In this way, it was possible to identify the important varieties of α thalassemia and the β⁰ and β⁺ thalassemias. Despite the technical difficulties involved, this technique was applied widely and successfully in many populations.[254–258] Its main disadvantage is that fetal blood sampling cannot be carried out until well into the second trimester of pregnancy. Hence, if the fetus is affected with a form of severe thalassemia, the pregnancy has to be terminated toward the end of the second trimester, which may be extremely distressing for the mother.

With the advent of DNA technology, prenatal diagnosis was carried out on fetal DNA, first obtained from amniotic fluid[259] and later by chorionic villus sampling (CVS) between 9 and 12 weeks of pregnancy.[260, 261] Although studies have suggested that the fetal loss rate is slightly higher after CVS than after amniocentesis, many women are still willing to accept this rather than endure the trauma of a second trimester diagnosis. For this reason, many centers now use CVS as their first line and retain amniocentesis or fetal blood sampling for those pregnancies in which the mother presents too late for CVS.

The diagnostic techniques used for fetal DNA analysis have evolved during the last 10 years.[255] The earliest prenatal diagnoses were carried out by Southern blotting of fetal DNA using either RFLP linkage analysis[259–261] or, in those cases in which a mutation could be identified directly, a specific oligonucleotide probe.[261, 262] The use of RFLP analysis for prenatal detection of genetic disease entails three steps. First, an appropriate RFLP marker is chosen that is either within or closely linked to the disease locus and for which an individual at risk of transmitting the disease is heterozygous. Second, it is necessary to determine which of the marker alleles is on the chromosome carrying the disease allele; this involves the study of family members, ideally a previously affected or normal child. Finally, with use of the markers, fetal DNA is examined to see whether the fetus has inherited the chromosome carrying the gene for the particular form of thalassemia or its normal allele. The disadvantage of this method is that it is necessary to establish, by a family study, that appropriate markers are available. Although it has been largely superseded by more direct approaches of identifying thalassemia mutations in fetal DNA, it is still a valuable fallback in families at risk for having children with rare forms of thalassemia. α⁰ Thalassemia and the few forms of β⁰ thalassemia that result from gene deletions can be identified directly by Southern blotting.[254, 255] In addition, there are approximately 20 different β thalassemia mutations that alter a particular restriction enzyme site and can therefore be identified in the same way.[255]

Later, after the development of the polymerase chain reaction (PCR), the identification of thalassemia mutations in fetal DNA was greatly facilitated.[263–265] For example, it can be used for the rapid detection of mutations that alter restriction enzyme cutting sites. The appropriate fragment of the β globin gene is amplified approximately 30 times, after which the DNA fragments are digested with an appropriate enzyme and separated by electrophoresis. Because PCR produces so much DNA, these fragments can be detected by either ethidium bromide or silver staining of DNA bands on gels; no radioactive probes are required.

Now that the mutations have been determined in so many different forms of α and β thalassemia, most centers running prenatal diagnosis programs are using the direct detection of these mutations as their first-line approach. Because most racial groups have only a few common β thalassemia mutations, in many cases it is possible to determine the mutations in the parents and then to analyze fetal DNA for their presence. The development of PCR combined with the use of oligonucleotide probes to detect individual mutations has offered a variety of new approaches for facilitating the speed and accuracy of carrier detection and prenatal diagnosis. For example, diagnoses can be made by hybridization of specific ³²P end–labeled oligonucleotides to an amplified region of the β globin gene dotted onto a nylon membrane.[255] Because the β globin gene sequence of interest is amplified more than 10⁶-fold, hybridization time can be limited to 1 hour and the entire procedure can be carried out in 2 hours.

A number of variations on this theme have been developed. For example, another approach for the identification of mutations with use of PCR, called the amplification refractory mutation system, also allows the diagnosis to be made in 1 to 2 hours.[266] This is based on the observation that, in many cases, oligonucleotides for the 3′ mismatched residue will, under appropriate conditions, not function as primers in the PCR. This method makes use of two primers. The normal one is refractory to PCR on mutant template DNA; the mutant sequence is refractory to PCR on normal DNA. The difference between normal DNA and that carrying a particular mutation is identified by size differences of the amplified fragments (Fig. 6–21). Other modifications of the PCR involve the use of non–radioactively labeled probes.[267, 268] For example, it is feasible to use horseradish peroxidase labeling of the 5′ end of oligonucleotides designed to detect mutations. A further simplification of this approach, reverse oligonucleotide hybridization,[269] uses membrane-bound, allele-specific oligonucleotide probes that hybridize to the complementary sequence of a PCR product prepared against the patient's DNA as the starting template.

In establishing a prenatal diagnosis program, it is first necessary to determine the common α or β thalassemia mutations in the population. It is then possible to identify the majority of them by dot blotting with use of PCR and radioactively labeled probes. There will be a few rare β thalassemias in each population that can be analyzed by rapid sequencing methods or, if they are not available, by RFLP linkage analysis or by fetal blood sampling and globin chain synthesis.

The error rate with use of these different approaches varies, depending on a number of factors, particularly the experience of the laboratory. Fetal blood sampling with globin synthesis analysis is usually associated with an error rate

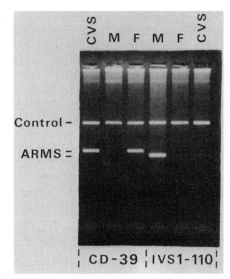

Figure 6–21. The rapid prenatal diagnosis of β thalassemia by the ARMS (*a*mplification *r*efractory *m*utation *s*ystem), a development for the rapid identification of mutations based on the polymerase chain reaction. One parent has the common Mediterranean codon 39 C→T (CD) mutation, the other the IVS-I-110-G→A mutation. The fetus is heterozygous for the codon 39 mutation. M = mother; F = father; CVS = fetal DNA from chorionic villus sampling.

of 2 to 3 per cent, although this may be reduced to less than 1 per cent in experienced hands. Low error rates, less than 1 per cent, have been reported from most laboratories using fetal DNA analysis.[255] Potential sources of error include maternal contamination of fetal DNA, non-paternity, and genetic recombination in cases in which RFLP linkage analysis is used.

Despite the apparent "high technology" of some of these approaches, they have been established successfully in many countries, and the overall reduction in the birth of babies with β thalassemia is a remarkable testament to their effectiveness (Fig. 6–22). The majority of centers that are carrying out this work have switched successfully from fetal blood sampling to DNA diagnostic techniques. Provided that one center can develop simple dot blot technology, it is possible to establish a prenatal diagnosis program that will cover 80 or 90 per cent of cases. Centers in Greece, Cyprus, and Italy have succeeded in lowering the birth rate of β thalassemic babies to 10 per cent or less of the prescreening levels (see Fig. 6–22).

Major prevention programs have started in Israel, China, and Thailand. However, in many countries, particularly those with large Islamic populations, this approach to the control of genetic disease is incompatible with religious beliefs. This problem is highlighted in the United Kingdom where there are large Cypriot and Afro-Asian populations; new cases of thalassemia have become rare in the Cypriot population, but there has been virtually no reduction in the birth of β thalassemics in Afro-Asians.

▼ TREATMENT

Because the α thalassemias cause either intrauterine death or a relatively mild disorder in adult life, they do not pose a major health burden in countries in which they are common. The major public health problem for countries in which the thalassemias are common is the management of the severe forms of β thalassemia.

Symptomatic

For many years, the standard approach to managing severe β thalassemia has been regular blood transfusion, chelation therapy to remove excess iron, and the judicious use of splenectomy.[7, 270] Children who are treated in this way survive into adult life, have a normal puberty, and may have children.[270] However, all this is at a great price to both the patients and their families. The only proven form of chelation therapy is deferoxamine given as an overnight infusion.[271] Many children cannot cope with this regimen, and particularly as they grow older, there is a high level of noncompliance.[272] For children who are not able to manage regular chelation therapy, the prognosis is poor, and few of them survive after the age of 20 years; death usually results from iron loading of the myocardium and either acute or chronic cardiac failure, often precipitated by infection. The recent development of new families of oral chelating agents may improve the situation,[271] although the safety and efficiency of these drugs for long-term administration have yet to be determined. For these reasons, the symptomatic treatment of β thalassemia is still far from satisfactory.

Marrow Transplantation

In recent years, there has been increasing interest in the use of bone marrow transplantation for β thalassemia. Good results have been obtained, particularly if the procedure is carried out early in life.[273–275] Unfortunately, however, successful engraftment requires the availability of a sibling or relative with a complete HLA match, and therefore this form of treatment is available only to a proportion of children with thalassemia.

Experimental Approaches

A number of experimental approaches to the management of thalassemia are under evaluation. Because it is clear that the production of high levels of fetal hemoglobin can protect β thalassemics, there has been much interest in finding ways to stimulate Hb F production. The methods being explored are based on earlier observations that there is a transient reversal to fetal hemoglobin synthesis during recovery from marrow suppression after the use of cytotoxic drugs for the treatment of leukemia[276] or after bone marrow transplantation.[277] These studies, and a number of related animal experiments, suggested that in a rapidly regenerating or expanding bone marrow, the pattern of erythropoiesis is perturbed in such a way that it favors the expression of the γ globin genes.[278] Another approach has been based on a completely different series of observations. It was found that there is a delay in the switch from fetal to adult hemoglobin production in infants of diabetic mothers, and it was suggested that this might reflect the higher levels of butyrate to which these infants were exposed.[279] This possibility was strengthened by the observation that butyrate infusions in the bovine fetus delay gene switching.[280] Hence, it was reasoned that it might

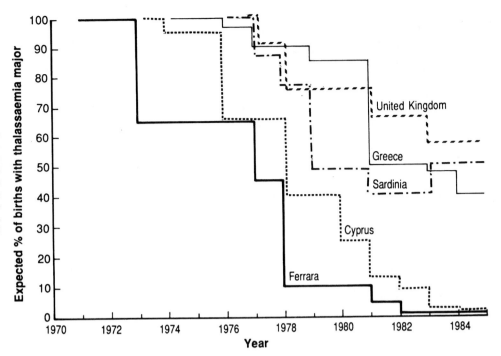

Figure 6–22. The effects of the development of prenatal diagnosis programs in different countries on the births of homozygous β thalassemic persons. (Reproduced by permission from Modell B., and Bulyzhenkov, V.: Distribution and control of some genetic disorders. World Health Stat. Q. 41:209–218, 1988, Fig. 4, p. 217.)

be possible to modify or reactivate fetal hemoglobin production by the administration of butyrate analogues.

In recent years, extensive studies have been directed toward attempts to increase the level of fetal hemoglobin in both sickle cell anemia and β thalassemia.[275, 278, 281] The first large-scale trials were carried out in adult patients with sickle cell anemia and demonstrated a reduced frequency of painful crises associated with long-term administration of hydroxyurea. Although this was associated with a modest increase in fetal hemoglobin, it still is not clear whether this is the only reason for the clinical improvement in these patients.[282] A number of observational studies have been carried out to determine the effect of agents such as 5-azacytidine, hydroxyurea, erythropoietin, and butyrate analogues in patients with various forms of β thalassemia.[281] With one exception, the results have not been impressive, although in some cases there has been a modest rise in the level of fetal hemoglobin, but not such that would lead to any significant clinical benefit.

The one exceptional response to these agents was a severely affected Hb Lepore homozygote who had a dramatic rise in fetal hemoglobin after the administration of intravenous arginine butyrate.[283] Although it was not possible to continue this therapy, she showed a further response to oral butyrate and hydroxyurea and has now lived independently of blood transfusion with an almost normal hemoglobin level for more than 4 years.[284] Subsequently, this patient's brother, with the same form of thalassemia, was treated with oral butyrate and hydroxyurea, which was followed by a rise in the level of Hb F of almost 5 g/dl; he, too, has remained transfusion independent for nearly 2 years.[284] There were no other obvious reasons for an unusual response of this type in this family, and therefore these observations raise the possibility that the deletion of the β globin gene cluster that underlies the generation of the δβ fusion chain of Hb Lepore may be in some way responsible for this remarkable pharmacological effect; there is evidence

that this condition is associated with a slightly more effective γ globin chain response than are many other forms of β thalassemia.[7] There have also been preliminary reports of improved responses to butyrate and hydroxyurea by intermittent dosage[285] or suggesting that certain phenoxyacetic acids, cinnamic acids, and dimethyl fatty acids may have the ability to stimulate γ globin chain synthesis without the side effects of suppression of erythropoiesis.[286]

Although it is early days, these studies are encouraging and suggest that at least if the right combination of drugs can be found, it may be possible to produce a useful elevation of Hb F production, at least in some forms of β thalassemia.

The other major area of investigation for the management of the thalassemias and other single-gene disorders is somatic gene therapy. Here the idea is to try to replace or correct defective globin genes in the patient's hematopoietic stem cells. For gene replacement therapy, one or more copies of a normal globin gene would be inserted into the hematopoietic stem cell to produce sufficient amounts of the missing gene product to correct the disorder, or at least to convert it into a heterozygous phenotype. On the other hand, correction therapy involves lining up a normal globin gene with the defective gene under conditions that would favor a recombination event between the two genes and hence correct the thalassemic defect.

The present status of somatic gene therapy, particularly as it relates to hematopoietic stem cells, has been the subject of several reviews.[287, 288] There has been a considerable amount of progress in the isolation and in vitro culture of human hematopoietic progenitors with at least some of the repopulating characteristics required of a stem cell. Although most of the work in this field has used vectors based on the Moloney murine leukemia virus, there is much current interest in the development of vectors that can infect non-dividing cells. It has been established for some time that the genes for viral proteins, which compose nearly 80 per cent of the retroviral genome, can be deleted and replaced by DNA sequences encoding the gene to be transferred. Of course, cells containing such a recombinant retrovirus are not able to produce infectious particles unless the structural viral proteins are supplied from elsewhere. This problem has been overcome by the development of specific packaging lines. Bone marrow progenitors from mice, primates, and humans have been transfected with a variety of retroviral vectors containing different human genes. Whereas the results of these experiments have been encouraging, the selection of retroviral producer clones on the basis of expression in murine fibroblast cell lines has not always correlated with what happens in primary hematopoietic cells. Indeed, although excellent expression can be obtained in fibroblasts or hematopoietic cell lines, it has been found that there is often a low level of expression in primary murine hematopoietic cells.

Although the discovery of the β globin LCR has been a major advance toward gene therapy, it is still uncertain whether all the regulatory regions that are required for gene transfer have been identified. Even when the LCR is included, globin gene transfer may be unpredictable, with multiple gene rearrangements. Although attempts have been made to identify *cis*-acting sequences that may be responsible, and systematically to eliminate them by deletion by site-directed mutagenesis, these problems have still not been overcome. However, steady progress is being made toward a better understanding of the regulation of the globin gene clusters and of the sequences required for their long-term, high-level expression.

Efforts to insert globin gene sequences into the human β globin locus by site-directed homologous recombination have also met with some success,[289] although, currently, the major problem with this approach is its extremely low efficiency. Similarly, considerable progress has been made toward the development of mammalian artificial chromosomes, but although many of the problems of telomere physiology have been solved, the construction of sequences with the properties of the centromere remains problematic.[287]

Thus, although this work must continue, the thalassemias will present a major public health problem for many of the poorer tropical countries in the next millennium. The approaches to gene therapy, if they come to fruition, are likely to be extremely expensive. In the interim, resources should be concentrated on screening and prenatal diagnosis where this is acceptable, together with major efforts toward finding agents what will stimulate fetal hemoglobin production, particularly in the intermediate forms of thalassemia such as Hb E thalassemia, which will present such a major challenge in the future.

REFERENCES

1. Weatherall, D.J.: Historical introduction: the thalassaemia syndromes. *In* Weatherall, D.J., and Clegg, J.B. (eds): The Thalassaemia Syndromes. 4th ed. Oxford, Blackwell Science (in press).
2. Cooley, T.B., and Lee, P.: A series of cases of splenomegaly in children with anemia and peculiar bone changes. Trans. Am. Pediatr. Soc. 37:29, 1925.
3. Whipple, G.H., and Bradford, W.L.: Mediterranean disease–thalassemia (erythroblastic anemia of Cooley); associated pigment abnormalities simulating hemochromatosis. J. Pediatr. 9:279, 1933.
4. Pauling, L., Itano, H.A., Singer, S.J., and Wells, I.C.: Sickle-cell anemia, a molecular disease. Science 10:543, 1949.
5. Ingram, V.M., and Stretton, A.O.W.: Genetic basis of the thalassaemia diseases. Nature 184:1903, 1959.
6. Weatherall, D.J, Clegg, J.B, and Naughton M.A.: Globin synthesis in thalassaemia: an in vitro study. Nature 208:1061, 1965.
7. Weatherall, D.J., and Clegg, J.B. (eds): The Thalassaemia Syndromes. 4th ed. Oxford, Blackwell Science (in press).
8. Weatherall, D.J., Clegg, J.B., Higgs, D.R., and Wood, W.G.: The hemoglobinopathies. *In* Scriver, C.R., Beaudet, A.L., Sly, W.S., Valle, D. (eds): The Metabolic Basis of Inherited Disease, 7th ed. New York, McGraw-Hill Book Co., 1995, pp. 3417–3484.
9. Higgs, D.R., Vickers, M.A., Wilkie, A.O.M., Pretorius, I.-M., Jarman, A.P., and Weatherall, D.J.: A review of the molecular genetics of the human α globin gene cluster. Blood 73:1081, 1989.
10. Higgs, D.R.: α-Thalassaemia. *In* Higgs, D.R., and Weatherall, D.J. (eds): Baillière's Clinical Haematology. International Practice and Research: The Haemoglobinopathies. London, Baillière Tindall, 1993, pp. 117–150.
11. Wilkie, A.O.M., Higgs, D.R., Rack, K.A., Buckle, V.J., Spurr, N., Fischel-Ghodsian, N., Ceccherini, I., Brown, W.R.A., and Harris, P.C.: Stable length polymorphism of up to 260 kb at the tip of the short arm of chromosome 16. Cell 64:595, 1991.
12. Higgs, D.R.: α-Thalassaemia. *In* Weatherall, D.J., and Clegg, J.B. (eds): The Thalassaemia Syndromes. 4th ed. Oxford, Blackwell Science (in press).
13. Lauer, J., Shen, C-K.J., and Maniatis, T.: The chromosomal arrangement of human α-like globin genes: sequence homology and α-globin gene deletions. Cell 20:119, 1980.
14. Flint, J., Thomas, K., Micklem, G., Raynham, H., Clark, K., Doggett, N.A., King, A., and Higgs, D.R.: The relationship between chromosome structure and function at a human telomeric region. Nat. Genet. 15:252, 1997.
15. Higgs, D.R., Wood, W.G., Jarman, A.P., Sharpe, J., Lida, J., Pretorius, I.-M., and Ayyub, H.: A major positive regulatory region located far upstream of the human α-globin gene locus. Genes Dev. 4:1588, 1990.
16. Higgs, D.R., Wainscoat, J.S., Flint, J., Hill, A.V.S., Thein, S.L., Nicholls, R.D., Teal, H., Ayyub, H., Peto, T.E.A., Jarman, A., Clegg, J.B., and Weatherall, D.J.: Analysis of the human α globin gene cluster reveals a highly informative genetic locus. Proc. Natl. Acad. Sci. USA 83:5165, 1986.
17. Jarman, A.P., and Higgs D.R.: A new hypervariable marker for the human α-globin gene cluster. Am. J. Hum. Genet. 42:249, 1988.
18. Higgs, D.R., Ayyub, H., Clegg, J.B., Hill, A.V.S., Nicholls, R.D., Teal, H., Wainscoat, J.S., and Weatherall, D.J.: α-Thalassaemia in British people. Br. Med. J. 290:1303, 1985.
19. Nicholls, R.D., Fischel-Ghodsian, N., and Higgs, D.R.: Recombination at the human α-globin gene cluster: sequence features and topological constraints. Cell 49:369, 1987.
20. Vanin, E.F., Henthorn, P.S., Kioussis, G., Grosveld, F., and Smithies, O.: Unexpected relationships between four large deletions in the human β-globin gene cluster. Cell 35:701, 1983.
21. Wilkie, A.O.M., Lamb, J., Harris, P.C., Finney, R.D., and Higgs, D.R.: A truncated human chromosome 16 associated with α thalassaemia is stabilized by addition of telomeric repeat (TTAGGG)$_n$. Nature 346:868, 1990.
22. Hatton, C.S.R., Wilkie, A.O.M., Drysdale, H.C., Wood, W.G., Vickers, M.A., Sharpe, J., Ayyub, H., Pretorius, I.-M., Buckle, V.J., and Higgs, D.R.: α-Thalassaemia caused by a large (62 kb) deletion upstream of the human α globin gene cluster. Blood 76:221, 1990.
23. Liebhaber, S.A., Griese, E-U., Weiss, I., Cash, F.E., Ayyub, H., Higgs, D.R., and Horst J.: Inactivation of human α-globin gene expression by a de novo deletion located upstream of the α-globin gene cluster. Proc. Natl. Acad. Sci. USA 87:9431, 1990.
24. Romao, L., Osorio-Almeida, L., Higgs, D.R., Lavinha, J., and Liebhaber, S.A.: α-Thalassaemia resulting from deletion of regulatory sequences far upstream of the α-globin structural gene. Blood 78:1589, 1991.
25. Indrak, K., Gu, Y.-C., Novotny, J., Huisman, T.H.J.: A new α-thalassaemia-2 deletion resulting in microcytosis and hypochromia and in vitro chain imbalance in the heterozygote. Am. J. Hematol. 43:144, 1993.
26. Embury, S.H., Miller, J.A., Dozy, A.M., Kan, Y.W., Chan, V., and Todd, D.: Two different molecular organizations account for the single α-globin gene of the α-thalassaemia-2 genotype. J. Clin. Invest. 66:1319, 1980.
27. Higgs, D.R., Old, J.M., Pressley, L., Clegg, J.B., and Weatherall D.J.: A novel α-globin gene arrangement in man. Nature 284:632, 1980.

28. Goossens, M., Dozy, A.M., Embury, S.H., Zachariades, Z., Hadjiminas, M.G., Stamatoyannopoulos, G., and Kan, Y.W.: Triplicated α-globin loci in humans. Proc. Natl. Acad. Sci. USA 77:518, 1980.

29. Trent, R.J., Higgs, D.R., Clegg, J.B., and Weatherall D.J.: A new triplicated α-globin gene arrangement in man. Br. J. Haematol. 49:149, 1981.

30. Lie-Injo, L.E., Herrera, A.R., and Kan, Y.W.: Two types of triplicated α globin loci in humans. Nucleic Acids Res. 9:3707, 1981.

31. Gu, Y.C., Landman, H., and Huisman, T.H.J.: Two different quadruplicated α globin gene arrangements. Br. J. Haematol. 66:245, 1987.

32. Higgs, D.R., Hill, A.V.S., Bowden, D.K., Weatherall, D.J., and Clegg, J.B.: Independent recombination events between duplicated human α globin genes: implications for their concerted evolution. Nucleic Acids Res. 12:6965, 1984.

33. Kulozik, A., Kar, B.C., Serjeant, B.E., Serjeant, G.R., and Weatherall, D.J.: The molecular basis of α-thalassemia in India: its interaction with sickle cell disease. Blood 71:467, 1988.

34. Lacerra, G., Fioretti, G., De Angioletti, M., Pagano, L., Guarino, E., De Bonis, C., Viola, A., Magione, G., Scarollo, A., De Rose, L., and Carestia, C.: A novel α$^+$-thalassaemia deletion with the breakpoints in the α2-globin gene and in close proximity to an Alu family repeat between the φα2- and φα1-globin genes. Blood 78:2740, 1991.

35. Zhao, J.B., Zhao, L., Fei, Y.J., Liu, J.C., and Huisman, T.H.: A novel α-thalassemia-2 (-2.7 kb) observed in a Chinese patient with Hb H disease. Am. J. Hematol. 38:248, 1991.

36. Bowden, D.K., Hill, A.V.S., Higgs, D.R., Oppenheimer, S.J., Weatherall, D.J., and Clegg J.B.: Different hematologic phenotypes are associated with leftward (-α$^{4.2}$) and rightward (-α$^{3.7}$) α$^+$-thalassemia deletions. J. Clin. Invest. 79:39, 1987.

37. Liebhaber, S.A., Cash, F.E., and Main D.M.: Compensatory increase in α1-globin gene expression in individuals heterozygous for the α-thalassemia-2 deletion. J. Clin. Invest. 76:1057, 1985.

38. Huisman, T.H.J., Carver, M.F.H., and Baysal, E.: A Syllabus of Thalassemia Mutations. Augusta, GA, The Sickle Cell Anemia Foundation, 1997.

39. Pirastu, M., Saglio, G., Chang, J.C., Cao, A., and Kan, Y.W.: Initiation codon mutation as a cause of α thalassemia. J. Biol. Chem. 259:12315, 1984.

40. Moi, P., Cash, F.E., Liebhaber, S.A., Cao, A., and Pirastu, M.: An initiation codon mutation (AUG→GUG) of the human α1-globin gene: structural characterisation and evidence for a mild thalassemic phenotype. J. Clin. Invest. 80:1416, 1987.

41. Morle, F., Lopez, B., Henni, T., and Godet, J.: α-Thalassemia associated with the deletion of two nucleotides at position -2 and -3 preceding the AUG codon. EMBO J. 4:1245, 1985.

42. Weatherall, D.J., and Clegg, J.B.: The α-chain termination mutants and their relationship to the α-thalassaemias. Philos. Trans. R. Soc. Lond. B. Biol. Sci. 271:411, 1975.

43. Milner, P.F., Clegg, J.B., and Weatherall, D.J.: Haemoglobin H disease due to a unique haemoglobin variant with an elongated α chain. Lancet 1:729, 1971.

44. Clegg, J.B., Weatherall, D.J., Contopoulos-Griva, I., Caroutsos, K., Poungouras, P., and Tsevrenis, H.: Haemoglobin Icaria, a new chain termination mutant which causes α-thalassaemia. Nature 251:245, 1974.

45. De Jong, W.W., Khan, P.M., and Bernini, L.F.: Hemoglobin Koya Dora; high frequency of a chain termination mutant. Am. J. Hum. Genet. 27:81, 1975.

46. Bradley, T.B., Wohl, R.C., and Smith, G.J.: Elongation of the α-globin chain in a black family: interaction with Hb G Philadelphia. Clin. Res. 23:131, 1975.

47. Waye, J.S., Eng, B., Patterson, M., Chui, D.H.K., and Olivieri, N.F.: Identification of a novel termination codon mutation (TAA→TAT, Term→Tyr) in the α2 globin gene of a Laotian girl with hemoglobin H disease. Blood 83:3418, 1994.

48. Liebhaber, S.A., Coleman, M.B., Adams, J.G., III, Cash, F.E., and Steinberg, M.H.: Molecular basis for non-deletion α-thalassemia in American blacks α2$^{116GAG->UAG}$ J. Clin. Invest. 80:154, 1987.

49. Safaya, S., and Rieder, R.F.: Dysfunctional α-globin gene in hemoglobin H disease in blacks. J. Biol. Chem. 263:4328, 1988.

50. Orkin, S.H., Goff, S.C., and Hechtman, R.L.: Mutation in an intevening sequence splice junction in man. Proc. Natl. Acad. Sci. USA 78:5041, 1981.

51. Felber, B.K., Orkin, S.H., and Hamer, D.H.: Abnormal RNA splicing causes one form of α thalassemia. Cell 29:895, 1982.

52. Harteveld, C.L., Heister, J.G., Giordano, P.C., Batelaan, D., von-Delft, P., Haak, H.L., Wijermans, P.W., Losekoot, M., and Bernini, L.F.: An IVS1-116 (A→G) acceptor splice site mutation in the α2 globin gene causing α$^+$ thalassaemia in two Dutch families. Br. J. Haematol. 95:461, 1996.

53. Higgs, D.R., Goodbourn, S.E.Y., Lamb, J, Clegg, J.B., Weatherall, D.J., and Proudfoot, N.J.: α-Thalassaemia caused by a polyadenylation signal mutation. Nature 306:398, 1983.

54. Thein, S.L., Wallace, R.B., Pressley, L., Clegg, J.B., Weatherall, D.J., and Higgs D.R.: The polyadenylation site mutation in the α-globin gene cluster. Blood 71:313, 1988.

55. Adams, J.G., III, and Coleman, M.B.: Structural hemoglobin variants that produce the phenotype of thalassemia. Semin. Hematol. 27:229, 1990.

56. Schrier, S.L.: Thalassemia: pathophysiology of red cell changes. Annu. Rev. Med. 45:211, 1994.

57. Galanello, R., Paglietti, E., Melis, M.A., Giagu, L., and Cao, A.: Hemoglobin inclusions in heterozigous α-thalassemia according to their α-globin genotype. Acta Haematol. 72:34, 1984.

58. Pootrakul, S., Wasi, P., and Na-Nakorn, S.: Haemoglobin Bart's hydrops foetalis in Thailand. Ann. Hum. Genet. 30:283, 1967.

59. Sharma, R.S., Yu, V., and Walters, W.A.W.: Haemoglobin Bart's hydrops fetalis syndrome in an infant of Greek origin and prenatal diagnosis of alpha-thalassaemia. Med. J. Aust. 2:404, 433, 1979.

60. Beaudry, M.A., Ferguson, D.J., Pearse, K., Yanofsky, R.A., Rubin, E.M., and Kan, Y.W.: Survival of a hydropic infant with homozygous α-thalassemia-1. J. Pediatr. 108:713, 1986.

61. Bianchi, D.W., Beyer, E.C., Start, A.R., Saffan, D., Sachs, B.P., and Wolfe, L.: Normal long-term survival with α-thalassemia. J. Pediatr. 108:716, 1986.

62. Liang, S.T., Wong, V.C.W., So, W.W.K., Ma, H.K., Chan, V., and Todd, D.: Homozygous α-thalassaemia: clinical presentation, diagnosis and management. A review of 46 cases. Br. J. Obstet. Gynaecol. 92:680, 1985.

63. Pressley, L., Higgs, D.R., Clegg, J.B., Perrine, R.P., Pembrey, M.E., and Weatherall, D.J.: A new genetic basis for hemoglobin-H disease. N. Engl. J. Med. 303:1383, 1980.

64. Henni, T., Morle, F., Lopez, B., Colonna, P., and Godet, J.: α-Thalassemia haplotypes in the Algerian population. Hum. Genet. 75:272, 1987.

65. Galanello, R., Pirastu, M., Melis, M.A., Paglietti, E., Moi, P., and Cao, A.: Phenotype-genotype correlation in haemoglobin H disease in childhood. J. Med. Genet. 20:425, 1983.

66. Winichagoon, P., Adirojnanon, P., and Wasi, P.: Levels of haemoglobin H and proportions of red cells with inclusion bodies in the two types of haemoglobin H disease. Br. J. Haematol. 46:507, 1980.

67. Styles, L., Foote, D.H., Kleman, K.M., Klumpp, C.J., Heer, N.B., and Vichinsky, E.P.: Hemoglobin H–Constant Spring Disease: an under recognized, severe form of α thalassemia. Int. J. Pediatr. Hematol. Oncol. 4:69, 1997.

68. Pootrakul, P., Winichagoon, P., Fucharoen, S., Pravatmuang, P., Piankijagum, A., and Wasi, P.: Homozygous haemoglobin Constant Spring: a need for revision of concept. Hum. Genet. 59:250, 1981.

69. Derry, S., Wood, W.G., Pippard, M., Clegg, J.B., Weatherall, D.J., Wickramasinghe, S., Darley, J., Winichagoon, P., and Wasi, P.: Hematologic and biosynthetic studies in homozygous hemoglobin Constant Spring. J. Clin. Invest. 73:1673, 1984.

70. Higgs, D.R., Aldridge, B.E., Lamb, J., Clegg, J.B., Weatherall, D.J., Hayes, R.J., Grandison, Y., Lowrie, Y., Mason, K.P., Serjeant, B.E., and Serjeant, G.R.: The interaction of alpha-thalassemia and homozygous sickle-cell disease. N. Engl. J. Med. 306:1441, 1982.

71. Noguchi, C.T., Dover, G.J., Rodgers, G.P., Serjeant, G.R., Antonarakis, S.E., Anagnou, N.P., Higgs, D.R., Weatherall, D.J., and Schechter, A.N.: α Thalassemia changes erythrocyte heterogeneity in sickle cell disease. J. Clin. Invest. 75:1632, 1985.

72. Flint, J., Harding, R.M., Boyce, A.J., and Clegg, J.B.: The population genetics of the haemoglobinopathies. In Higgs, D.R., and Weatherall, D.J. (eds): Ballière's Clinical Haemotology. The Haemoglobinopathies. London, Ballière Tindall, 1993, pp. 215–262.

73. Flint, J., Hill, A.V.S., Bowden, D.K., Oppenheimer, S.J., Sill, P.R., Serjeantson, S.W., Bana-Koiri, J., Bhatia, K., Alpers, M.P., Boyce, A.J., Weatherall, D.J., and Clegg, J.B.: High frequencies of α thalassemia are the result of natural selection by malaria. Nature 321:744, 1986.

74. Flint, J., Hill, A.V.S., Weatherall, D.J., Clegg, J.B., and Higgs, D.R.:

Alpha globin genotypes in two North European populations. Br. J. Haematol. 63:796, 1986.

75. O'Shaughnessy, D.F., Hill, A.V.S., Bowden, D.K., Weatherall, D.J., and Clegg, J.B.: Globin genes in Micronesia: origin and affinities of Pacific Island peoples. Am. J. Hum. Genet. 46:44, 1990.

76. Allen, S.J., O'Donell, A., Alexander, N.D.E., Alpers, M.P., Peto, T.E.A., Clegg, J.B., and Weatherall, D.J.: α⁺-Thalassaemia protects children against disease due to malaria and other infections. Proc. Natl. Acad. Sci. USA 94:14736, 1997.

77. Williams, T.N., Maitland, K., Bennett, S., Ganczakowski, M., Peto, T.E.A., Newbold, C.I., Bowden, D.K., Weatherall, D.J., and Clegg, J.B.: High incidence of malaria in α-thalassaemic children. Nature 383:522, 1996.

78. Weatherall, D.J., Clegg, J.B., and Kwiatkowski D.: The role of genomics in studying genetic susceptibility to infectious disease. Genome Res. 7:967, 1997.

79. Weatherall, D.J., Higgs, D.R., Bunch, C., Old, J.B., Hunt, D.M., Pressley, L., Clegg, J.B., Bethlenfalvay, N.C., Sjolin, S., Koler, R.D., Magenic, E., Francis, J.L., and Bebbington, D.: Hemoglobin H disease and mental retardation. A new syndrome or a remarkable coincidence? N. Engl. J. Med. 305:607, 1981.

80. Hutz, M.H., Marmitt, C.R., Schuler, L., and Salzano, F.M.: Hereditary anemias in Brazil—new case of Hb H disease with mental retardation [abstract]. Seventh International Congress of Human Genetics; Berlin, Germany; September 22–26, 1986, p. 458.

81. Bowcock, A.M., Tonder, S.V., and Jenkins T.: The hemoglobin H disease mental retardation syndrome: molecular studies on the South African case. Br. J. Haematol. 56:69, 1984.

82. Wilkie, A.O.M., Buckle, V.J., Harris, P.C., Lamb, J., Bartin, N.J., Reeders, S.T., Lindenbaum, R.H., Nicholls, R.D., Barrow, M., Bethlenfalvay, N.C., Hutz, M.H., Tolmie, J.L., Weatherall, D.J., and Higgs D.R.: Clinical features and molecular analysis of the α thalassemia/mental retardation syndromes. I. Cases due to deletions involving chromosome band 16p13.3. Am. J. Hum. Genet. 46:1112, 1990.

83. Wilkie, A.O.M., Zeitlin, H.C., Lindenbaum, R.H., Buckle, V.J., Fischel-Ghodsian, N., Chui, D.H.K., Gardner-Medwin, D., MacGillivray, M.H., Weatherall, D.J., and Higgs, D.R.: Clinical features and molecular analysis of the α thalassemia/mental retardation syndromes. II. Cases without detectable abnormality of the α globin complex. Am. J. Hum. Genet. 46:1127, 1990.

84. Gibbons, R.J., Wilkie, A.O.M., Weatherall, D.J., and Higgs, D.R.: A new defined X-linked mental retardation syndrome associated with α thalassaemia. J. Med. Genet. 28:729, 1991.

85. Gibbons, R.J., Suthers, G.K., Wilkie, A.O.M., Buckle, V.J., and Higgs, D.R.: X-linked α thalassemia/mental retardation (ATR-X) syndrome: localization to Xq12–21.31 by X-inactivation and linkage analysis. Am. J. Hum. Genet. 51:1136, 1992.

86. Gibbons, R.J., Picketts, D.J., Villard, L., and Higgs, D.R.: Mutations in a putative global transcriptional regulator cause X-linked mental retardation with α-thalassemia (ATR-X syndrome). Cell 80:837, 1995.

87. Picketts, D.J., Higgs, D.R., Bachoo, S., Blake, D.J., Quarrell, O.W.J., and Gibbons, R.J.: ATRX encodes a novel member of the SNF2 family of proteins: mutations point to a common mechanism underlying the ATR-X syndrome. Hum. Mol. Genet. 5:1899, 1996.

88. Gibbons, R.J., Bachoo, S., Picketts, D.J., Aftimos, S., Asenbauer, B., Bergoffen, J., Berry, S.A., Dahl, N., Fryer, A., Keppler, K., Kurosawa, K., Levin, M.L., Masuno, M., Neri, G., Pierpont, M.E., Slaney, S.F., and Higgs, D.R.: Mutations in transcriptional regulator *ATRX* establish the functional significance of a PHD-like domain. Nat. Genet. 17:146, 1997.

89. Higgs, D.R., Wood, W.G., Barton, C., and Weatherall, D.J.: Clinical features and molecular analysis of acquired Hb H disease. Am. J. Med. 75:181, 1983.

90. Anagnou, N.P., Ley, T.J., Chesbro, B., Wright, G., Kitchens, C., Liebhaber, S., Nienhuis, A.W., and Deisseroth, A.B.: Acquired α-thalassemia in preleukemia is due to decreased expression of all four α-globin genes. Proc. Natl. Acad. Sci. USA 80:6051, 1983.

91. Orkin, S.H., Kazazian, H.H., Jr., Antonarakis, S.E., Goff, S.C., Boehm, C.D., Sexton, J.P., Waber, P.G., and Giardina, P.J.V.: Linkage of β-thalassemic mutations and β-globin gene polymorphisms with DNA polymorphisms in the human β-globin gene cluster. Nature 296:727, 1982.

92. Grosveld, F., Dillon, N., and Higgs, D.: The regulation of human globin gene expression. Clin. Haematol. 6:31, 1993.

93. Grosveld, F., van Assendelft, G.B., Greaves, D.R., and Kollias G.: Position-independent, high-level expression of the human β-globin gene in transgenic mice. Cell 51:975, 1987.

94. Kazazian, H.H.: The thalassemia syndromes: molecular basis and prenatal diagnosis in 1990. Semin. Hematol. 27:209, 1990.

95. Thein, S.L.: β-Thalassaemia. Clin. Haematol. 6:151, 1993.

96. Thein, S.L., Old, J.M., Wainscoat, J.S., and Weatherall, D.J.: Population and genetic studies suggest a single origin for the Indian deletion β⁰ thalassaemia. Br. J. Haematol. 57:271, 1984.

97. Anand, R., Boehm, C.D., Kazazian, H.H., Jr., and Vanin, E.F.: Molecular characterization of a β⁰-thalassemia resulting from a 1.4 kb deletion. Blood 72:636, 1988.

98. Aulehla-Scholtz, C., Spielberg, R., and Horst, J.: A β-thalassemia mutant caused by a 300 bp deletion in the human β-globin gene. Hum. Genet. 81:298, 1989.

99. Diaz-Chico, J.C., Yang, K.G., Kutlar, A., Reese, A.L., Aksoy, M., and Huisman, T.H.J.: A 300 bp deletion involving part of the 5′ β-globin gene region is observed in members of a Turkish family with β-thalassaemia. Blood 70:583, 1987.

100. Gilman, J.G.: The 12.6 kilobase deletion in Dutch β⁰-thalassemia. Br. J. Haematol. 67:369, 1987.

101. Padanilam, B.J., Felice, A.E., and Huisman, T.H.J.: Partial deletion of the 5′ β-globin gene region causes β⁰-thalassemia in members of an American black family. Blood 64:941, 1984.

102. Popovich, B.W., Rosenblatt, D.S., Kendall, A.G., and Nishioka, Y.: Molecular characterization of an atypical β-thalassemia caused by a large deletion in the 5′ β-globin gene region. Am. J. Hum. Genet. 39:797, 1986.

103. Antonarakis, S.E., Orkin, S.H., Cheng, T-C., Scott, A.F., Sexton, J.P., Trusco, S.P., Charache, S., and Kazazian, H.H.: β-Thalassemia in American blacks: novel mutations in the TATA box and IVS-2 acceptor splice site. Proc. Natl. Acad. Sci. USA 81:1154, 1984.

104. Orkin, S.H., Antonarakis, S.E., and Kazazian, H.H., Jr.: Base substitution at position −88 in a β-thalassemic globin gene: further evidence for the role of distal promoter element ACACCC. J. Biol. Chem. 259:8679, 1984.

105. Orkin, S.H., Sexton, J.P., Cheng, T-C., Goff, S., Giardina, P.J.V., Lee, J.I., and Kazazian, H.H.: ATA box transcription mutation in β-thalassemia. Nucleic Acids Res. 11:4727, 1983.

106. Gonzalez-Redondo, J.H., Stoming, T.A., Kutlar, F., Lanclos, K.D., Howard, E.F., Fei, Y.J., Aksoy, M., Altay, C., Gurgey, A., Basak, A.N., Efremov, G.D., Petkov, G., and Huisman, T.H.J.: A C→T substitution at nt −101 in a conserved DNA sequence of the promoter region of the β-globin gene is associated with "silent" β-thalassemia. Blood 73:1705, 1989.

107. Wong, C., Dowling, C.E., Saiki, R.K., Higuchi, R.G., Erlich, H.A., and Kasasian, H.H.: Characterization of beta-thalassemia mutations using direct genomic sequencing of amplified single copy DNA. Nature 330:384, 1987.

108. Cai, S.-P., Eng, B., Francombe, W.H., Olivieri, N.F., Kendall, A.G., Waye, J.S., and Chui, D.H.K.: Two novel β-thalassemia mutations in the 5′ and 3′ noncoding regions of the β-globin gene. Blood 79:1342, 1992.

109. Ho, P.J., Rochette, J., Fisher, C.A., Wonke, B., Jarvis, M.K., Yardumian, A., and Thein, S.L.: Moderate reduction of β-globin gene transcript by a novel mutation in the 5′ untranslated region: a study of its interaction with other genotypes in two families. Blood 87:1170, 1996.

110. Kazazian, H.H., Jr., Orkin, S.H., Antonarakis, S.E., Sexton, J.P., Boehm, C.D., Goff, S.C., and Waber, P.G.: Molecular characterization of seven β-thalassemia mutations in Asian Indians. EMBO J. 3:593, 1984.

111. Cheng, T., Orkin, S.H., Antonarakis, S.E., Potter, M.J., Sexton, J.P., Markham, A.F., Giardina, P.J.V., Lia, A., and Kazazian, H.H.: β-Thalassemia in Chinese: use of in vivo RNA analysis and oligonucleotide hybridization in systematic characterization of molecular defects. Proc. Natl. Acad. Sci. USA 81:2821, 1984.

112. Gonzalez-Redondo, J.H., Stoming, T.A., Lanclos, K.D., Gu, Y.C., Kutlar, A., Kutlar, F., Nakasuji, T., Deng, B., Han, I.S., McKie, V.C., and Huisman, T.H.J.: Clinical and genetic heterogeneity in Black patients with homozygous β-thalassemia from the Southeastern United States. Blood 72:1007, 1988.

113. Hill, A.V.S., Bowden, D.K., O'Shaughnessy, D.F., Weatherall, D.J., and Clegg, J.B.: β-Thalassemia in Melanesia: association with malaria and characterization of a common variant. Blood 72:9, 1988.

114. Lapoumeroulie, C., Pagnier, J., Bank, A., Labie, D., and Krishnamoor-

thy, R.: β-Thalassemia due to a novel mutation in IVS-1 sequence donor site consensus sequence creating a restriction site. Biochem. Biophys. Res. Commun. 139:709, 1986.

115. Tamagnini, G.P., Lopes, M.C., Castanheira, M.E., Wainscoat, J.S., and Wood, W.G.: β+ Thalassaemia—Portuguese type: clinical, haematological and molecular studies of a newly defined form of β thalassaemia. Br. J. Haematol. 54:189, 1983.

116. Goldsmith, M.E., Humphries, R.K., Ley, T., Cline, A., Kantor, J.A., and Nienhuis, A.W.: Silent substitution in β+-thalassemia gene activating a cryptic splice site in β-globin RNA coding sequence. Proc. Natl. Acad. Sci. USA 80:2318, 1983.

117. Yang, K.G., Kutlar, F., George, E., Wilson, J.B., Kutlar, A., Stoming, T.A., Gonzalez-Redondo, J.M., and Huisman, T.H.J.: Molecular characterization of β-globin gene mutations in Malay patients with Hb E-β-thalassaemia and thalassaemia major. Br. J. Haematol. 72:73, 1989.

118. Orkin, S.H., Kazazian, H.H., Jr., Antonarakis, S.E., Oster, H., Goff, S.C., and Sexton, J.P.: Abnormal RNA processing due to the exon mutation of the βE-globin gene. Nature 300:768, 1982.

119. Orkin, S.H., Antonarakis, S.E., and Loukopoulos, D.: Abnormal processing of βKnossos RNA. Blood 64:311, 1984.

120. Spritz, R.A., Jagadeeswaran, P., Choudary, P.V., Biro, P.A., Elder, J.D., de Riel, J.K., Manley, J.L., Gefter, M.L., Forget, B.G., and Weissman, S.M.: Base substitution in an intervening sequence of a β+-thalassemic human globin gene. Proc. Natl. Acad. Sci. USA 78:2455, 1981.

121. Westaway, D., and Williamson, R.: An intron nucleotide sequence variant in a cloned β+-thalassemia globin gene. Nucleic Acids Res. 9:1777, 1981.

122. Orkin, S.H., Cheng, T.-C., Antonarakis, S.E., and Kazazian, H.H.: Thalassemia due to a mutation in the cleavage-polyadenylation signal of the human β-globin gene. EMBO J. 4:453, 1985.

123. Jankovic, L., Efremov, G.D., Petkov, G., Kattamis, C., George, E., Yang, K.-G., Stoming, T.A., and Huisman, T.H.J.: Three novel mutations leading to β-thalassemia. Blood 24:226A, 1989.

124. Rund, D., Filon, D., Rachmilewitz, E.A., Cohan, T., Dowling, C., Kazazian, H.H., and Oppenheim, A.: Molecular analysis of β-thalassemia in Kurdish Jews: novel mutations and expression studies. Blood 74:821A, 1989.

125. Wong, C., Antonarakis, S.E., Goff, S.C., Orkin, S.H., Boehm, C.D., and Kazazian, H.H.: On the origin and spread of β-thalassemia: recurrent observation of four mutations in different ethnic groups. Proc. Natl. Acad. Sci. USA 83:6529, 1986.

126. Trecartin, R.F., Liebhaber, S.A., Chang, J.C., Lee, K.Y., Kan, Y.W., Furbetta, A., Angius, A., and Cao, A.: β0-Thalassemia in Sardinia is caused by a nonsense mutation. J. Clin. Invest. 68:1012, 1981.

127. Chang, J.C., and Kan, Y.W.: β0-Thalassemia, a nonsense mutation in man. Proc. Natl. Acad Sci. USA 76:2886, 1979.

128. Takeshita, K., Forget, B.G., Scarpa, A., and Benz, E.J.: Intranuclear defect in β globin mRNA accumulation to a premature termination codon. Blood 64:13, 1984.

129. Humphries, R.K., Ley, T.J., Anagnou, N.P., Baur, A.W., and Nienhuis A.W.: β0 − 39-Thalassemia gene: a premature termination codon causes β mRNA deficiency without changing cytoplasmic β mRNA stability. Blood 64:23, 1984.

130. Adams, J.G., Steinberg, M.H., Boxer, L.A., Baehner, R.L., Forget, B.G., and Tsistrakis, G.A.: The structure of hemoglobin Indianapolis [β112 (G14) arginine]. An unstable variant detectable only by isotopic labeling. J. Biol. Chem. 254:3479, 1979.

131. Kobayashi, Y., Fukumaki, Y., Komatsu, N., Ohba, Y., Miyaji, T., and Miura, Y.: A novel globin structural mutant, Showa-Yakushiji (β110 Leu-Pro) causing a β-thalassemia phenotype. Blood 70:1688, 1987.

132. Hall, G.W., Franklin, I.M., Sura, T., and Thein, S.L.: A novel mutation (Nonsense β127) in exon 3 of the β globin gene produces a variable thalassaemia phenotype. Br. J. Haematol 79:342, 1991

133. Park, S.S., Barnetson, R., Kim, S.W., Weatherall, D.J., and Thein, S.L.: A spontaneous deletion of β33/34 val in exon 2 of the β globin gene (Hb Korea) produces the phenotype of dominant β thalassaemia. Br. J. Haematol. 78:581, 1991.

134. Bunn, H., and Forget, B.G.: Hemoglobin: Molecular, Genetic and Clinical Aspects. Philadelphia, W.B. Saunders, 1986.

135. Shinar, E., Rachmilewitz, E.A., and Lux, S.E.: Different erythrocyte membrane skeletal protein defects in alpha and beta thalassemia. J. Clin. Invest. 83:1190, 1989.

136. Shinar, E., and Rachmilewitz, E.A.: Oxidative denaturation of red blood cells in thalassemia. Semin. Hematol. 27:70, 1990.

137. Shinar, E., and Rachmilewitz, E.A.: Haemoglobinopathies and red cell membrane function. Clin. Haematol. 6:357, 1993.

138. Weatherall, D.J.: Pathophysiology of β thalassaemia. Clin. Haematol. (in press).

139. Fessas, P.: Inclusions of hemoglobin in erythroblasts and erythrocytes of thalassemia. Blood 21:21, 1963.

140. Wickramasinghe, S.N., and Hughes, M.: Some features of bone marrow macrophages in patients with homozygous β-thalassemia. Br. J. Haematol. 38:23, 1978.

141. Yataganas, X., and Fessas, P.: The pattern of hemoglobin precipitation in thalassemia and its significance. Ann. N. Y. Acad. Sci. 165:270, 1969.

142. Finch, C.A., Deubelbeiss, K., Cook, J.D., Eschbach, J.W., Harker, L.A., Funk, D.D., Marsaglia, G., Hillman, R.S., Slichter, S., Adamson, J.W., Ganzoni, A., and Giblett, E.R.: Ferrokinetics in man. Medicine (Baltimore) 49:17, 1970.

143. Chalevelakis, G., Clegg, J.B., and Weatherall, D.J.: Imbalanced globin chain synthesis in β-thalassemic bone marrow. Proc. Natl. Acad. Sci. USA 72:3853, 1975.

144. Nathan, D.G., Stossel, T.B., Gunn, R.B., Zarkowsky, H.S., and Laforet, M.T.: Influence of hemoglobin precipitation in alpa and beta thalassemica J. Clin. Invest. 48:33, 1969.

145. Gabuzda, T.G., Nathan, D.G., and Gardner, F.H.: The turnover of hemoglobins A, F and A2 in the peripheral blood of three patients with thalassemia. J. Clin. Invest. 42:1678, 1963.

146. Loukopoulos, D., and Fessas, P.: The distribution of hemoglobin types in thalassemic erythrocyte. J. Clin. Invest. 44:231, 1965.

147. Nathan, D.G., and Gunn, R.B.: Thalassemia: the consequences of unbalanced hemoglobin synthesis. Am. J. Med. 41:815, 1966.

148. Camaschella, C., Alfarano, A., Gottardi, E., Serra, A., Revello, D., and Saglio, G.: The homozygous state for the −87 C→G β+ thalassemia. Br. J. Haematol. 75:132, 1990.

149. Thein, S.L., Hesketh, C., Brown, J.M., Anstey, A.V., and Weatherall, D.J.: Molecular characterisation of a high A2 β thalassemia by direct sequencing of single strand enriched amplified genomic DNA. Blood 73:924, 1989.

150. Wainscoat, J.S., Thein, S.L., Higgs, D.R., Bell, J.I., Weatherall, D.J., Al-Awamy, B., and Serjeant, G.: A genetic marker for elevated levels of haemoglobin F in homozygous sickle cell disease. Br. J. Haematol. 60:261, 1985.

151. Gilman, J.G., and Huisman, T.H.J.: DNA sequence variation associated with elevated fetal Gγ globin production. Blood 66:783, 1985.

152. Thein, S.L., Sampietro, M., Old, J.M., Cappellini, M.D., Fiorelli, G., Modell, B., and Weatherall, D.J.: Association of thalassaemia intermedia with a beta-globin gene halptype. Br. J. Haematol. 65:367, 1987.

153. Thein, S.L., Hesketh, C., Wallace, R.B., and Weatherall, D.J.: The molecular basis of thalassaemia major and thalassaemia intermedia in Asian Indians: application to prenatal diagnosis. Br. J. Haematol. 70:225, 1988.

154. Diaz-Chico, J.C., Yang, K.G., Stoming, T.A., Efremov, D.G., Kutlar, A., Kutlar, F., Aksoy, N., Altay, C., Gurgey, A., Kining, Y., and Huisman, T.H.J.: Mild and severe β-thalassemia among homozygotes from Turkey: identification of the types by hybridization of amplified DNA with synthetic probes. Blood 71:248, 1988.

155. Kulozik, A.E., Wainscoat, J.S., Serjeant, G.R., Al-Awamy, B., Essan, F., Falusi, Y., Haque, S.K., Hilali, A.M., Kate, S., Sanasinghe, W.A.E.P., and Weatherall, D.J.: Geographical survey of βS-globin gene haplotypes: evidence for an independent Asian origin of the sickle-cell mutation. Am. J. Hum. Genet. 39:239, 1986.

156. Nagel, R.L., Fabry, M.E., Pagnier, J., Zohoun, I., Wajcman, H., Baudin, V., and Labie, D.: Hematologically and genetically distinct forms of sickle cell anemia in Africa. N. Engl. J. Med. 312:880, 1985.

157. Labie, D., Dunda-Belkhodja, O., Rouabhi, F., Pagnier, J., Ragusa, A., and Nagel, R.L.: The −158 site 5′ to the Gγ gene and Gγ expression. Blood 66:1463, 1985.

158. Kulozik, A.E., Kar, B.C., Satapathy, R.K., Serjeant, B.E., Serjeant, G.R., and Weatherall, D.J.: Fetal hemoglobin levels and βS globin haplotypes in an Indian population with sickle cell disease. Blood 69:1742, 1987.

159. Kulozik, A.E., Thein, S.L., Kar, B.C., Wainscoat, J.S., Serjeant, G.R., and Weatherall, D.J.: Raised Hb F levels in sickle cell disease are caused by a determinant linked to the β globin gene cluster. In Stamatoyannopoulos G (ed): Hemoglobin Switching. 5th ed. New York, Alan R. Liss, 1987, pp. 427–439.

160. Miller, B.A., Salameh, M., Ahmen, M., Wainscoat, J.S., Antognetti,

G., Orkin, S., Weatherall, D.J., and Nathan, D.G.: High fetal hemoglobin production in sickle cell anemia in the eastern province of Saudi Arabia is genetically determined. Blood 67:1404, 1986.

161. Zago, M.A., Wood, W.G., Clegg, J.B., Weatherall, D.J., O'Sullivan, M., and Gunson, H.H.: Genetic control of F-cells in human adults. Blood 53:977, 1979.

162. Wood, W.G., Weatherall, D.J., and Clegg, J.B.: Interaction of heterocellular hereditary persistence of foetal haemoglobin with β thalassaemia and sickle cell anaemia. Nature 264:247, 1976.

163. Cappellini, M.D., Fiorelli, G., and Bernini, L.F.: Interaction between homozygous β° thalassaemia and the Swiss type of hereditary persistence of fetal haemoglobin. Br. J. Haematol. 48:561, 1981.

164. Miyoshi, K., Kaneto, Y., Kawai, H., Ohchi, H., Niki, S., Haseqawa, K., Shirakami, A., and Yamano, T.: X-linked dominant control of F cells in normal adult life: characterization of the Swiss type as hereditary persistence of fetal hemoglobin regulated dominantly by gene(s) on X-chromosome. Blood 72:1854, 1988.

165. Jeffreys, A.J., Wilson, V., Thein, S.L., Weatherall, D.J., and Ponder, B.A.J.: DNA "fingerprints" and segregation analysis of multiple markers in human pedigrees. Am. J. Hum. Genet. 39:11, 1986.

166. Dover, G.J., Smith, K.D., Chang, Y.C., Purvis, S., Mays, A., Meyers, D.A., Sheils, C., and Serjeant, G: Fetal hemoglobin levels in sickle cell disease and normal individuals are partially controlled by an X-linked gene located at Xp22.2. Blood 80:816, 1992.

167. Thein, S.L., Sampietro, M., Rohde, K., Weatherall, D.J., Lathrop, G.M., and Demenais, F.: Detection of a major gene for heterocellular HPFH after accounting for genetic modifiers. Am. J. Hum. Genet. 54:14, 1994.

168. Craig, J.E., Rochette, J., Fisher, C.A., Weatherall, D.J., Marc, S., Lathrop, G.M., Demenais, F., and Thein, S.L.: Haemoglobin switch: dissecting the loci controlling fetal haemoglobin production on chromosomes 11p and 6q by the regressive approach. Nat. Genet. 12:58, 1996.

169. Craig, J.E., Rochette, J., Sampietro, M., Wilkie, A.O.M., Barnetson, R., Hatton, C.S.R., Demenais, F., and Thein S.L.: Genetic heterogeneity in heterocellular hereditary persistence of fetal hemoglobin. Blood 90:428, 1997.

170. Weatherall, D.J.: Overview: mechanisms for the heterogeneity of the thalassemias. Int. J. Pediatr. Hematol. Oncol. 4:3, 1997.

171. Rund, D., Oron-Karni, V., Filon, D., Goldfarb, A., Rachmilewitz, E., and Oppenheim, A.: Genetic analysis of β-thalassemia intermedia in Israel: diversity of mechanisms and unpredictability of phenotype. Am. J. Hematol. 54:16, 1997.

172. Weatherall, D.J., Pressley, L., Wood, W.G., Higgs, D.R., and Clegg, J.B.: The molecular basis for mild forms of homozygous β thalassaemia. Lancet 1:527, 1981.

173. Wainscoat, J.S., Old, J.M., Weatherall, D.J., and Orkin, S.H.: The molecular basis for the clinical diversity of β thalassaemia in Cypriots. Lancet 1:1235, 1983.

174. Kanavakis, E., Wainscoat, J.S., Wood, W.G., Weatherall, D.J., Cao, A., Furbeta, M., Galanello, R., Georgiou, D., and Sophocleous, T.: The interaction of α thalassaemia with heterozygous β thalassaemia. Br. J. Haematol. 52:465, 1982.

175. Rosatelli, C., Falchi, A.M., Scalas, M.T., Tuveri, T., Furbetta, M., and Cao, A.: Hematological phenotype of double heterozygous state for alpha and beta thalassemia. Hemoglobin 8:25, 1984.

176. Wainscoat, J.S., Bell, J.I., Old, J.M., Weatherall, D.J., Furbetta, M., Galanello, R., and Cao, A.: Globin gene mapping studies in Sardinian patients homozygous for β° thalassaemia. Mol. Biol. Med. 1:1, 1983.

177. Wainscoat, J.S., Kanavakis, E., Wood, W.G., Letsky, E.A., Huehns, E.R., Marsh, G.W., Higgs, D.R., Clegg, J.B., and Weatherall, D.J.: Thalassaemia intermedia in Cyprus—the interaction of α- and β-thalassaemia. Br. J. Haematol. 53:411, 1983.

178. Bianco, I., Cappabianca, M.P., Foglietta, E., Lerone, M., Deidda, G., Morlupi, L., Grisanti, P., Ponzoni, D., Rinaldi, S., and Graziani, B.: Silent thalassemias: genotypes and phenotypes. Haematologica 82:269, 1997.

179. Semenza, G.L., Delgrosso, K., Poncz, M., Malladi, P., Schwartz, E., and Surrey, S.: The silent carrier allele: β-thalassemia without a mutation in the β-globin gene or its immediate flanking regions. Cell 39:123, 1984.

180. Kanavakis, E., Metaxatou-Mavromati, A., Kattamis, C., Wainscoat, J.S., and Wood, W.G.: The triplicated α gene locus and β thalassaemia. Br. J. Haematol. 54:201, 1983.

181. Sampietro, M., Cazzola, M., Cappellini, M.D., and Fiorelli G.: The triplicated alpha-gene locus and heterozygous beta thalassaemia: a case of thalassaemia intermedia. Br. J. Haematol. 55:709, 1983.

182. Kulozik, A.E., Thein, S.L., Wainscoat, J.S., Gale, R., Kay, L., Weatherall, D.J., Wood, J.K., and Huehns, E.R.: Thalassaemia intermedia: interaction of the triple α-globin gene arrangement and heterozygous β-thalassaemia. Br. J. Haematol. 66:109, 1987.

183. Camaschella, C., Bertero, M.T., Serra, A., Dall'Acqua, M., Gasparini, P., Trento, M., Vettore, L., Perona, G., Saglio, G., and Mazza, U.: A benign form of thalassemia intermedia may be determined by the interaction of triplicated α locus and heterozygous β thalassemia. Br. J. Haematol. 66:103, 1987.

184. Galanello, R., Ruggeri, R., Paglietti, E., Addis, M., Melis, A., and Cao, A.: A family with segregating triplicated alpha globin loci and beta thalassemia. Blood 62:1035, 1983.

185. Thein, S.L., Hesketh, C., Taylor, P., Temperley, P., Hutchison, R.M., Old, J.M., Wood, W.G., Clegg, J.B., and Weatherall, D.J.: Molecular basis for dominantly inherited inclusion body β thalassaemia. Proc. Natl. Acad. Sci. USA 87:3924, 1990.

186. Weatherall, D.J., Clegg, J.B., Knox-Macaulay, H.H.M., Bunch, C., Hopkins, C.R., and Temperley, I.J.: A genetically determined disorder with features both of thalassaemia and congenital diserythropoietic anaemia. Br. J. Haematol. 24:679, 1973.

187. Stamatoyannopoulos, G., Woodson, R., Papayannopoulou, T., Heywood, D., and Kurachi, M.S.: Inclusion-body β-thalassaemia trait. A form of β thalassaemia producing clinical manifestations in simple heterozygotes. N. Engl. J. Med. 290:939, 1974.

188. Beris, R.P., Miescher, P.A., Diaz-Chico, J.C., Han, I.-S., Kutlar, A., Hu, H., Wilson, J.B., and Huisman, T.H.J.: Inclusion body β-thalassemia trait in a Swiss family is caused by an abnormal hemoglobin (Geneva) with an altered and extended β chain carboxy-terminus due to a modification in codon β114. Blood 72:801, 1988.

189. Kazazian, H.H., Jr., Dowling, C.E., Hurwitz, R.L., Coleman, M., and Adams, J.G., III: Thalassemia mutations in exon 3 of the β-globin gene often cause a dominant form of thalassemia and show no predilection for malarial-endemic regions of the world. Am. J. Hum. Genet. 45:A242, 1989.

190. Fei, Y.J., Stoming, T.A., Kutlar, A., Huisman, T.H.J., and Stamatoyannopoulos, G.: One form of inclusion body β-thalassemia is due to a GAA→TAA mutation at codon 121 of the β chain. Blood 73:1075, 1989.

191. Murru, S., Loudianos, G., Deiana, M., Camaschella, C., Sciarratta, G.V., Agosti, S., Parodi, M.I., Cerruti, P., Cao, A., and Pirastu, M.: Molecular characterization of β-thalassemia intermedia in patients of Italian descent and identification of three novel β-thalassemia mutations. Blood 77:1342, 1991.

192. Ristaldi, M.S., Pirastu, M., Murru, S., Casula, L., Loudianos, G., Cao, A., Sciarratta, G.V., Agosti, S., Parodi, M.I., Leone, D., and Melesendi, C.: A spontaneous mutation produced a novel elongated β° globin chain structural variant (Hb Agnana) with a thalassemia-like phenotype. Blood 75:1378, 1990.

193. Fucharoen, S., Kobayashi, Y., Fucharoen, G., Ohba, Y., Miyazono, K., Fukumaki, Y., and Takaku, F.: A single nucleotide deletion in codon 123 of the β-globin gene causes an inclusion body β-thalassemia trait: a novel elongated globin chain β^Makabe. Br. J. Haematol. 75:393, 1990.

194. Fucharoen, G., Fucharoen, S., Jetsrisuparb, A., and Fukumaki, Y.: Eight-base deletion of the β-globin gene produced a novel variant (β Khon Kaen) with an inclusion body β-thalassemia trait. Blood 78:537, 1991.

195. Thein, S.L., Best, S., Sharpe, J., Paul, B., Clark, D.J., and Brown, M.J.: Hemoglobin Chesterfield (β28 Leu→Arg) produces the phenotype of inclusion body β thalassemia. Blood 77:2791, 1991.

196. Podda, A., Galanello, R., Maccioni, L., Melis, M.A., Rosatelli, C., Perseu, L., and Cao, A.: Hemoglobin Cagliari (β69 [E4] VAL→GLU): a novel unstable thalassemic hemoglobinopathy. Blood 77:371, 1991.

197. Fucharoen, S., Fucharoen, G., Fukumaki, Y., Nakamaya, Y., Hattori, Y., Yamamoto, K., and Ohba Y.: Three-base deletion in exon 3 of the β-globin gene produced a novel variant (βGunma) with a thalassemia-like phenotype. Blood 76:1894, 1990.

198. Wickramasinghe, S.N., Lee, M.J., Furukawa, T., Eguchi, M., and Reid, C.D.L.: Composition of the intra-erythroblastic precipitates in thalassaemia and congenital dyserythropoietic anaemia (CDA): identification of a new type of CDA with intra-erythroblastic precipitates not reacting with monoclonal antibodies to α- and β-globin chains. Br. J. Haematol. 93:576, 1996.

199. Gonzalez-Redondo, J.M., Kutlar, A., Stoming, T.A., de Pablos, J.M., Kilinc, Y., Huisman, T.H.J.: Hb S(C)-β⁺-thalassaemia: different mutations are associated with different levels of normal Hb A. Br. J. Haematol. 70:85, 1988.

200. Weatherall, D.J., and Clegg, J.B.: Thalassemia—a global public health problem. Nat. Med. 2:847, 1996.

201. Rees, D.C., Clegg, J.B., and Weatherall, D.J.: Is hemoglobin instability important in the interaction between hemoglobin E and β thalassemia? Blood 92:2141, 1998.

202. Wasi, P., Na-Nakorn, S., Pootrakul, S., Sookanek, M., Disthasongcham, P., Pornpatkul, M., and Manich, V.: Alpha- and beta-thalassemia in Thailand. Ann. N. Y. Acad. Sci. 165:60, 1969.

203. Fucharoen, S., Winichagoon, P., Pootrakul, P., Piankijagum, A., and Wasi, P.: Variable severity of Southeast Asian β⁰-thalassemia/Hb E disease. Birth Defects 23:241, 1988.

204. Khanh, N.C., Thu, L.T., Truc, D.B., Hoa, D.P., Hoa, T.T., and Ha, T.H.: Beta-thalassemia/haemoglobin E disease in Vietnam. J. Trop. Pediatr. 36:43, 1990.

205. Agarwal, S., Gulati, R., and Singh, K.: Hemoglobin E-beta thalassemia in Utta Pradesh. Indian Pediatar. 34:287, 1997.

206. Baklouti, F., Ouazana, R., Gonnet, C., Lapillonne, A., Delaunay, J., and Godet, J.: The hemoglobin E syndromes. Ann. N. Y. Acad. Sci. 850:334, 1998.

207. Baklouti, F., Ouazana, R., Gonnet, C., Lapillonne, A., Delaunay, J., and Godet, J.: β⁺-thalassemia in cis of a sickle cell gene: occurrence of a promoter mutation on a βˢ chromosome. Blood 74:1817, 1989.

208. Adams, J.G., III, Steinberg, M.H., Newman, M.V., Morrison, W.T., Benz, E.J., and Iyer, R.: β-Thalassemia present in cis to a new β-chain structural variant: Hb Vicksburg [β75 (E19) leu→0]. Proc. Natl. Acad. Sci. USA 78:469, 1981.

209. Olds, R.J., Sura, T., Jackson, B., Wonke, B., Hoffbrand, A.V., and Thein, S.L.: A novel δ⁰ mutation in cis with Hb Knossos: a study of different genetic interactions in three Egyptian families. Br. J. Haematol. 78:430, 1991.

210. Modell, C.B., and Berdoukas, V.A.: The Clinical Approach to Thalassemia. New York, Grune & Stratton, 1981.

211. Chehab, F.F., Der Kaloustian, V., Khouri, F.P., Deeb, S.S., and Kan, Y.W.: The molecular basis of β-thalassemia in Lebanon: application to prenatal diagnosis. Blood 69:1141, 1987.

212. Kazazian, H.H., Jr., Orkin, S.H., Markham, A.F., Chapman, C.R., Youssoufian, H., and Waber, P.G.: Quantification of the close association between DNA haplotypes and specific β-thalassemia mutations in Mediterraneans. Nature 310:152, 1984.

213. Thein, S.L., Hesketh, C., and Weatherall, D.J.: The molecular basis of β-thalassemia in UK Asian Indians: applications to prenatal diagnosis. Br. J. Haematol. 70:225, 1988.

214. Thein, S.L., Winichagoon, P., Hesketh, C., Fucharoen, S., Wasi, P., and Weatherall, D.J.: The molecular baais of β thalassemia in Thailand: application to prenatal diagnosis. Am. J. Hum. Genet. 47:369, 1990.

215. Clegg, J.B.: The world distribution and population genetics of thalassaemia. In Weatherall, D.J., and Clegg, J.B. (eds): The Thalassaemia Syndromes. 4th ed. Oxford, Blackwell Science (in press).

216. Baglioni, C.: The fusion of two peptide chains in hemoglobin Lepore and its interpretation as a genetic deletion. Proc. Natl. Acad. Sci. USA 48:1880, 1962.

217. Efremov, G.D.: Hemoglobins Lepore and anti-Lepore. Hemoglobin 2:197, 1978.

218. Huisman, T.H.J.: Compound heterozygosity for Hb S and the hybrid Hbs Lepore, P-Nilotic, and Kenya; comparison of hematological and hemoglobin composition data. Hemoglobin 21:249, 1997.

219. Spritz, R.A., DeRiel, J.K., Forget, B.G., and Weissman, S.M.: Complete nucleotide sequence of the human δ-globin gene. Cell 21:639, 1980.

220. Tang, D.C., Ebb, D., Hardison, R.C., and Rodgers, G.P.F.: Restoration of the CCAAT box or insertion of the CACCC motif activates δ-globin gene expression. Blood 90:421, 1997.

221. LaFlamme, S., Acuto, S., Markowitz, D., Vick, L., Landschultz, W., and Bank, A.: Expression of chimeric human beta and delta-globin genes during erythroid differentiation. J. Biol. Chem. 262:4819, 1987.

222. Ottolenghi, S., Giglioni, B., Pulazzini, A., Comi, P., Camaschella, C., Serra, A., Guerrasio, A., and Saglio, G.: Sardinian δβ⁰-thalassemia: a further example of a C to T substitution at position −196 of the ᴬγ globin gene promoter. Blood 69:1058, 1987.

223. Atweh, G.F., Zhu, X-X., Brickner, H.W., Dowling, C.H., Kazazian, H.H., Jr., and Forget, B.G.: The β-globin gene on the Chinese δβ-thalassemia chromosome carries a promoter mutation. Blood 70:1470, 1987.

224. Wainscoat, J.S., Thein, S.L., Wood, W.G., Weatherall, D.J., Tzotos, S., Kanavakis, E., Metaxatou-Mavromati, A., and Kattamis, C.: A novel deletion in the β globin gene complex. Ann. N. Y. Acad. Sci. 445:20, 1985.

225. Kulozik, A., Yarwood, N., and Jones, R.W.: The Corfu δβ⁰ thalassemia: a small deletion acts at a distance to selectively abolish β globin gene expression. Blood 71:457, 1988.

226. Mishima, N., Landman, H., Huisman, T.H.J., and Gilman, J.G.: The DNA deletion in an Indian delta beta-thalassemia begins one kilobase from the A gamma globin gene and ends in an L1 repetitive sequence. Br. J. Haematol. 73:375, 1989.

227. Matsunaga, E., Kimura, A., Yamada, H., Fukumaki, Y., and Takagi, Y.: A novel deletion in δβ-thalassemia found in Japan. Biochem. Biophys. Res. Commun. 126:185, 1985.

228. Ottolenghi, S., Giglioni, B., Taramelli, R., Comi, P., Massa, U., Saglio, G., Camaschella, C., Izzo, P., Cao, A., Galanello, R., Gimferrer, E., Baiget, M., and Gianni, A.M.: Molecular comparison of δβ-thalassemia and hereditary persistence of fetal hemoglobin DNAs: evidence of a regulatory area? Proc. Natl. Acad. Sci. USA 79:2347, 1982.

229. Anagnou, N.P., Papayannopolou, T., Stamatoyannopoulos, G., and Nienhuis, A.W.: Structurally diverse molecular deletions in the β-globin gene cluster exhibit an identical phenotype on interaction with the βˢ-gene. Blood 65:1254, 1985.

230. Palena, A., Blau, A., Stamatoyannopoulos, G., and Anagnou, N.P.: Easetrn European (δβ)⁰ thalassemia: molecular characterization of a novel 9.1 kb deletion resulting in high levels of fetal hemoglobin in the adult. Blood 83:3738, 1994.

231. Zhang, J.-W., Stamatoyannopoulos, G., and Anagnou, N.P.: Laotian (δβ)⁰ thalassemia: molecular characterization of a novel deletion associated with increased production of fetal hemoglobin. Blood 72:983, 1988.

232. Trent, R.J., Svirklys, L., and Jones, P.: Thai (δβ)⁰ thalassemia and its interaction with γ-thalassemia. Hemoglobin 12:101, 1988.

233. Ottolenghi, S., Giglioni, B., Comi, P., Gianni, A.M., Polli, E., Acquaye, C.T.A., Oldham, J.H., and Masera, G.: Globin gene deletion in HPFH, δ⁰β⁰ thalassemia and Hb Lepore disease. Nature 278:654, 1979.

234. Efremov, G.D., Nikolov, N., Bakioglu, I., and Huisman, T.H.J.: The 18- to 23-kb deletion of the Macedonian δβ-thalassemia includes the entire δ and β globin genes. Blood 68:971, 1986.

235. Öner, R., Öner, C., Erdem, G., Balkan, H., Özdag, H., Erkan, M., Gümrük, F., Gürgey, A., and Altay C.: A novel (δβ)⁰-thalassemia due to an approximately 30-kb deletion observed in a Turkish family. Acta Haematol. 96:232, 1996.

236. Jones, R.W., Old, J.M., Trent, R.J., Clegg, J.B., and Weatherall, D.J.: Major rearrangement in the human β-globin gene cluster. Nature 291:39, 1981.

237. Anagnou, N.P., Papayannopoulou, T., Nienhuis, A.W., and Stamatoyannopoulos G.: Molecular characterization of a novel form of (ᴬγδβ)⁰-thalassemia deletion with a 3′ breakpoint close to those of HPFH-3 and HPFA-4: insights for a common regulatory mechanism. Nucleic Acids Res. 16:6057, 1988.

238. Zeng, Y.-T., Huang, S.-Z., Chen, B., Kiang, Y.-C., Chang, Z.-M., Harano, T., and Huisman, T.H.J.: Heriditary persistence of fetal hemoglobin or (δβ)⁰-thalassemia: three types observed in South-Chinese families. Blood 66:1430, 1985.

239. Trent, R.J., Jones, R.W., Clegg, J.B., Weatherall, D.J., Davidson, R., and Wood, W.G.: (ᴬγδβ) Thalassaemia: similarity of phenotype in four different molecular defects, including one newly described. Br. J. Haematol. 57:279, 1984.

240. Orkin, S.H., Alter, B.P., Altay, C., Mahoney, M.J., Lazarus, H., Hobbins, J.C., and Nathan, D.G.: Application of endonuclease mapping to the analysis and prenatal diagnosis of thalassemias caused by globin-gene deletion. N. Engl. J. Med. 299:166, 1978.

241. George, E., Faridah, K., Trent, R.J., Padanilam, B.J., Huang, H.J., and Huisman, T.H.J.: Homozygosity for a new type of ᴳγ(ᴬγδβ)⁰-thalassemia in a Malaysian male. Hemoglobin 10:353, 1986.

242. Losekoot, M., Fodde, R., Gerritsen, E.J.A., van de Juit, I., Schreuder, A., Giordina, P.C., Vossen, J.M., and Bernini, L.F.: Interaction of two different disorders in the β-globin gene cluster associated with an increased hemoglobin F production: a novel deletion type of ᴳγ + (ᴬγδβ)⁰-thalassemia and δ⁰-hereditary persistence of fetal hemoglobin determinant. Blood 77:861, 1991.

243. Henthorn, P.S., Smithies, O., and Mager, D.L.: Molecular analysis of deletions in the human β-globin gene cluster: deletion junctions and locations of breakpoints. Genomics 6:226, 1990.

244. Jones, R.W., Old, J.M., Trent, R.J., Clegg, J.B., and Weatherall, D.J.: Restriction mapping of a new deletion responsible for $^{G}\gamma(\delta\beta)^{0}$ thalassemia. Nucleic Acids Res. 9:6813, 1981.

245. Zhang, J.-W., Song, W.-F., Zhao, Y.-J., We, G.-Y., Qiu, Z.-M., Wang, F.-N., Chen, S.-S., and Stamatoyannopoulos, G.: Molecular characterization of a novel form of $(^{A}\gamma\delta\beta)^{0}$ thalassemia deletion in a Chinese family. Blood 81:1624, 1993.

246. Fucharoen, S., Winichagoon, P., Chaicharoen, S., and Wasi, P.: Different molecular defects of $^{G}\gamma(^{A}\gamma\delta\beta)^{0}$-thalassemia in Thailand. Eur. J. Haematol. 39:154, 1987.

247. De Angioletti, M., Lacerra, G., and Carestia, C.: Abstract 148. Sixth International Conference on Thalassaemia and Haemoglobinopathies; Malta; personal communication, 1997.

248. Charache, S., Clegg, J.B., and Weatherall, D.J.: The Negro variety of hereditary persistence of fetal haemoglobin is a mild form of thalassaemia. Br. J. Haematol. 34:527, 1976.

249. Pirastu, M., Ristaldi, M.S., Loudianos, G., Murru, S., Sciarratta, G.V., Parodi, M.I., Leone, D., Agosti, S., and Cao, A.: Molecular analysis of atypical β-thalassemia heterozygotes. Ann. N. Y. Acad. Sci. 612:90, 1990.

250. Van Der Ploeg, L.H.T., Konings, A., Cort, M., Roos, D., Bernini, L., and Flavel, R.A.:γ-β-Thalassaemia studies showing that deletion of the γ- and δ-genes influence β-globin gene expression in man. Nature 283:637, 1980.

251. Curtin, P., Pirastu, M., Kan, Y.W., Gobert-Jones, J.A., Stephens, A.D., and Lehmann, H.: A distant gene deletion affects β-globin gene function in an atypical γδβ-thalassaemia. J. Clin. Invest. 76:1554, 1985.

252. Driscoll, M.C., Dobkin, C.S., and Alter, B.P.: γδβ-thalassaemia due to a de novo mutation deleting the 5′ β-globin gene activation-region hypersensitive sites. Proc. Natl. Acad. Sci. USA 86:7470, 1989.

253. Trent, R.J., Williams, B.G., Kearney, A., Wilkinson, T., and Harris, P.: Molecular and hematological characterisation of Scottish-Irish type (εγδβ)⁰ thalassemia. Blood 76:2132, 1990.

254. Weatherall, D.J.: Prenatal diagnosis of haematological disease. *In* Hann, I.M., Gibson, B.E.S., and Letsky, E.A. (eds): Fetal and Neonatal Haematology. London, Baillière Tindall, 1991, pp. 285–314.

255. Cao, A., and Rosatelli, M.C.: Screening and prenatal diagnosis of the haemoglobinopathies. Clin. Haematol. 6:263, 1993.

256. Cao, A, Rosatelli, M.C., Battista, G, Tuveri, T., Scalas, M.T., Monni, G., Olla, G., and Galanello, R.: Antenatal diagnosis of β-thalassemia in Sardinia. Ann. N. Y. Acad. Sci. 612:215, 1990.

257. Loukopoulos, D., Hadji, A., Papadakis, M., Karababa, P., Sinopoulou, K., Boussiou, M., Kollia, P., Xenakis, M., Antsaklis, A., Mesoghitis, S., Loutradi, A., and Fessas, P.: Prenatal diagnosis of thalassemia and of the sickle cell syndromes in Greece. Ann. N. Y. Acad. Sci. 612:226, 1990.

258. Alter, B.P.: Antenatal diagnosis: summary of results. Ann. N. Y. Acad. Sci. 612:237, 1990.

259. Kazazian, H.H., Jr., Phillips, J.A., III, Boehm, C.D., Vik, T., Mahoney, M.J., and Ritchey, A.K.: Prenatal diagnosis of β-thalassemia by amniocentesis: linkage analysis of multiple polymorphic restriction endonuclease sites. Blood 56:926, 1980.

260. Old, J.M., Ward, R.H.T., Petrou, M., Karagozlu, F., Modell, B., and Weatherall, D.J.: First trimester diagnosis for haemoglobinopathies: a report of 3 cases. Lancet 2:1413, 1982.

261. Old, J.M., Fitches, A., Heath, C., Thein, S.L., Weatherall, D.J., Warren, R., McKenzie, C., Rodeck, C.H., Modell, B., Petrou, M., and Ward, R.H.T.: First trimester fetal diagnosis for haemoglobinopathies: report on 200 cases. Lancet 2:763, 1986.

262. Pirastu, M., Kan, Y.W., Cao, A., Conner, B.J., Teplitz, R.L., and Wallace, R.B.: Prenatal diagnosis of β-thalassemia: detection of a single nucleotide mutation in DNA. N. Engl. J. Med. 309:284, 1983.

263. Kogan, S.C., Doherty, M., and Gitschier, J.: An improved method for prenatal diagnosis of genetic diseases by analysis of amplified DNA sequences: application to hemophilia A. N. Engl. J. Med. 317:985, 1987.

264. Chehab, F., Doherty, M., Cai, S., Cooper, S., and Rubin, E.: Detection of sickle cell anemia and thalassaemia. Nature 329:293, 1987.

265. Saiki, R.K., Chang, C.-A., Levenson, C.H., Warren, T.C., Boehm, C.D., Kazazian, H.H., Jr., and Erlich, H.A.: Diagnosis of sickle cell anemia and β-thalassemia with enzymatically amplified DNA and non-radioactive allele-specific oligonucleotide probes. N. Engl. J. Med. 319:537, 1988.

266. Old, J.M., Varawalla, N.Y., and Weatherall, D.J.: The rapid detection and prenatal diagnosis of β-thalassaemia in the Asian Indian and Cypriot populations in the UK. Lancet 336:834, 1990.

267. Cai, S.P., Chang, C.A., Zhang, J.Z., Saiki, R.K., Erlich, H.A., and Kan, Y.W.: Rapid prenatal diagnosis of β-thalassemia using DNA amplification and nonradioactive probes. Blood 73:372, 1989.

268. Saiki, R.K., Walsh, P.S., Levenson, C.H., and Erlich, H.A.: Genetic analysis of amplified DNA with immobilized sequence-specific oligonucleotide probes. Proc. Natl. Acad. Sci. USA 86:6230, 1989.

269. Saiki, R.K., Walsh, P.S., Levenson, C.H., and Erlich H.A.: Genetic analysis of amplified DNA with immobilized sequence-specific oligonucleotide probes. Proc. Natl. Acad. Sci. USA 86:6230, 1989.

270. Piornelli, S.: Management of Cooley's anaemia. Clin. Haematol. 6:287, 1993.

271. Oliveiri, N.F., Brittenham, G.M.: Iron-chelating therapy and the treatment of thalassemia. Blood 89:739, 1997.

272. Vullo, C., and Di Palma, A.: Compliance with therapy in Cooley's anemia. *In* Buckner, C.D., Gale, R.P., and Lucarelli, G. (eds): Progress in Clinical and Biological Research. Vol. 309. Advances and Controversies in Thalassemia Therapy. New York, Alan R. Liss, 1989, pp. 43–49.

273. Thomas, E.D., Buckner, C.D., Sanders, J.E., Papayannopoulou, T., Borgna-Pignatti, C., de Stafano, P., Sullivan, K.M., Clift, R.A., and Storb, R.: Marrow transplantation for thalassaemia. Lancet 2:227, 1982.

274. Lucarelli, G., Galimberti, M., Polchi, P., Angelucci, E., Baronciani, D., Giardini, C., Politi, P., Durazzi, S.M.T., Muretto, P., and Albertini, F.: Bone marrow transplantation in patients with thalassemia. N. Engl. J. Med. 322:417, 1990.

275. Giardini, C.: Treatment of β-thalassemia. Curr. Opin. Hematol. 4:79, 1997.

276. Sheridan, B.L., Weatherall, D.J., Clegg, J.B., Pritchard, J., Wood, W.G., Callender, S.T., Durrant, I.J., McWhirter, W.R., Ali, M., Partridge, J.W., and Thompson, E.N.: The patterns of fetal haemoglobin production in leukaemia. Br. J. Haematol. 32:487, 1976.

277. Alter, B.P., Rappeport, J.M., Huisman, T.H.J., Schroeder, W.A., and Nathan, D.G.: Fetal erythropoiesis following bone marrow transplantation. Blood 48:843, 1976.

278. Ley, T.J.: The pharmacology of hemoglobin switching: of mice and men. Blood 77:1146, 1991.

279. Perrine, S.P., Greene, M.F., and Faller, D.V.: Delay in the fetal globin switch in infants of diabetic mothers. N. Engl. J. Med. 312:334, 1985.

280. Perrine, S.P., Rudolph, A., Faller, D.V., Roman, C., Cohen, R.A., Shen, S.-J., and Kan, Y.W.: Butyrate infusions in the ovine fetus delay the biologic clock for globin gene switching. Proc. Natl. Acad. Sci. USA 85:8540, 1988.

281. Olivieri, N.F.: Reactivation of fetal hemoglobin in patients with β thalassemia. Semin. Hematol. 33:24, 1996.

282. Charache, S., Terrin, M.L., Moore, R.D., Dover, G.J., Barton, F.B., Eckert, S.V., McMahon, R.P., and Bonds, D.R.: Effect of hydroxyurea on the frequency of painful crises in sickle cell anemia. N. Engl. J. Med. 332:1317, 1995.

283. Perrine, S.P., Ginder, G.D., Faller, D.V., Dover, G.H., Ikuta, T., Witkowska, E., Cai, S.-P., Vichinsky, E.P., and Olivieri, N.F.: A short-term trial of butyrate to stimulate fetal-globin-gene expression in the β-globin disorders. N. Engl. J. Med. 328:81, 1993.

284. Olivieri, N.F., Rees, D.C., Ginder, G.D., Thein, S.L., Brittenham, G.M., Waye, J.S., and Weatherall, D.J.: Treatment of thalassaemia major with phenylbutyrate and hydroxyurea. Lancet 350:491, 1997.

285. Atweh, G.F., Dover, G.J., Faller, G., Stamatoyannopoulos, G., Fournarakis, B., and Perrine, S.P.: Sustained hematologic response to pulse butyrate therapy in beta globin disorders. Blood 88(suppl.):652a, 1996.

286. Pace, B.S., DaFonseca, S., White, G.L., Dover, G.J., and Perrine, S.P.: Induction of γ globin and erythropoiesis in transgenic mice and anemic baboons with oral hemokines. Blood 90(suppl.):131a, 1997.

287. Lever, A.M.L., and Goodfellow, P.: Gene therapy. Br. Med. Bull. 51:1, 1995.

288. Karlsson, G.: Gene therapy of haemotopoietic cells. J. Intern. Med. Suppl. 740:95, 1997.

289. Smithies, P., Gregg, R.G., Boggs, S.S., Koralewski, M.A., and Kucherlapati, R.S.: Insertion of DNA sequences into the human chromosomal β-globin locus by homologous recombination. Nature 317:230, 1985.

7 Human Hemoglobins: Sickle Hemoglobin and Other Mutants

H. Franklin Bunn

▼ ▼

The study of hemoglobins, both normal and mutant, has provided fundamental and continued insights into structure-function relationships of proteins in general and the molecular basis of oxygen transport in particular. The discovery by Pauling and Itano[1] that sickle hemoglobin has an abnormal electrophoretic mobility ushered us into the era of molecular medicine. With the advent of recombinant DNA technology, research on hemoglobin provided early and important information about the organization and regulation of genes as well as insights as to how ontogeny affects gene expression. The switch from fetal to adult hemoglobin production, a topic of vital importance in developmental biology, is discussed in Chapter 5; Chapter 6 covers the thalassemias, inherited defects in globin biosynthesis.

This chapter begins with a description of normal human hemoglobin, its structure and physiological function. The minor hemoglobin components are also discussed because measurement of these species can offer valuable clues to the diagnosis of both congenital and acquired disorders. Human hemoglobin mutants are considered first in terms of the underlying mutations in globin gene structure and then in terms of their phenotypic expression. A major portion of the chapter is devoted to sickle hemoglobin and sickle cell disease because contemporary molecular biology has had a major and growing impact on our understanding of the pathogenesis of this important disease and the development of rational approaches to therapy.

Normal Human Hemoglobin

▼ STRUCTURE

Hemoglobin is a 64.4 kDa tetramer composed of two pairs of unlike globin polypeptide chains designated by Greek letters (e.g., $\alpha_2\beta_2$). A heme group, ferroprotoporphyrin IX, is linked covalently at a specific site to each chain. In the reduced (ferrous) state, it can bind reversibly with gaseous ligands, such as oxygen or carbon monoxide. Approximately 75 per cent of hemoglobin in its native state is in the form of α helix (Fig. 7–1). Individual residues can be assigned to one of eight helices or to adjacent non-helical stretches. This has greatly facilitated establishment of homology between globin subunits. Thus, in all hemoglobins whose primary structure is known, the heme iron is linked covalently to a histidine at the eighth residue of the F helix. In human hemoglobins, His F8 is residue 87 of the α chain and 92 of the β chain (see Fig. 7–1). Residues that have charged side groups, such as lysine, arginine, and glutamic acid, lie on the surface of the molecule in contact with the surrounding water solvent. Uncharged residues are generally oriented toward the hydrophobic interior of the molecule. Unlike most proteins, hemoglobin contains no disulfide bonds.

From X-ray analyses of crystals of hemoglobins, Max Perutz at the Medical Research Council Laboratory in Cambridge, England, determined the three-dimensional structure of human hemoglobin.[2] This remarkable achievement, which earned Perutz the Nobel prize, has enabled a thorough understanding of the relationship between structure and function. The hemoglobin tetramer is a globular molecule ($5.0 \times 5.4 \times 6.4$ nm) with a single (dyad) axis of symmetry. The polypeptide chains are themselves folded in such a way that the four heme groups lie in clefts on the surface of the molecule equidistant from one another. Subsequent, more refined X-ray analyses are of sufficiently high resolution that the coordinates of all atoms in the molecule are known to within 0.2 nm.[3, 4] As shown in Figure 7–2, the molecule undergoes a marked change in conformation on deoxygenation. The β chains rotate apart by about 0.7 nm. In contrast, liganded forms, including oxyhemoglobin, carboxyhemoglo-

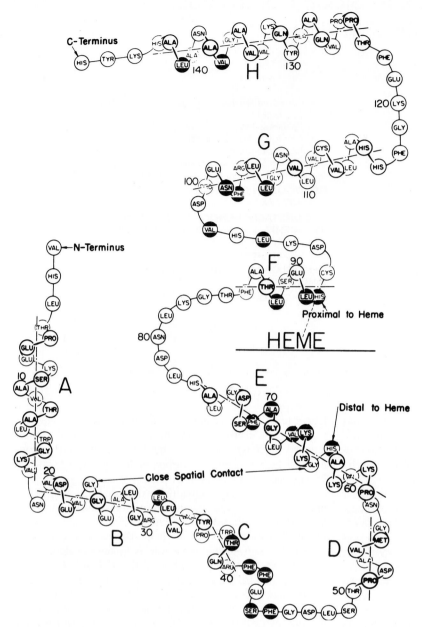

Figure 7–1. Primary and secondary structure of the β chain of human hemoglobin. The eight helices are shown, designated A through H. The iron atom of the heme group is covalently attached to the "proximal histidine," residue 92, with the helical location F8. (From Huisman, T.H.J., and Schroeder, W.A.: New Aspects of the Structure, Function and Synthesis of Hemoglobins. Boca Raton, FL, CRC Press, 1971; with permission. Copyright CRC Press, Inc., Boca Raton, FL.)

bin, and cyanmethemoglobin, appear to be isomorphous. The conformational change that occurs on removal and addition of ligand accounts for the many known differences in physical and chemical properties of oxyhemoglobin and deoxyhemoglobin. Perutz[2] has shown that deoxyhemoglobin is stabilized in a constrained or taut (T) configuration by the presence of intersubunit and intrasubunit salt bonds (Fig. 7–3). These include residues responsible for the Bohr effect (Fig. 7–3B) and for the binding of 2,3-bisphosphoglycerate (2,3-BPG) (discussed below). On the addition of ligand, such as oxygen, these salt bonds are sequentially broken. The fully liganded hemoglobin is in the so-called relaxed (R) configuration. In this state, there is considerably less bonding energy between subunits, and the liganded molecule is able to dissociate reversibly according to the reaction $\alpha_2\beta_2 \leftrightarrow 2\alpha\beta$. The formation of αβ dimers is required for hemoglobin to bind to haptoglobin and to traverse renal glomeruli.[5] As shown in Figure 7–2, each subunit in the tetramer is oriented toward the two unlike subunits in different ways (i.e., $\alpha_1\beta_1$ and $\alpha_1\beta_2$). The dissociation of the liganded tetramer into dimers occurs at the $\alpha_1\beta_2$ interface. Thus, there is stronger binding between α_1 and β_1 subunits than between α_1 and β_2 subunits. Furthermore, during oxygenation and deoxygenation (T = R), there is considerable movement along the $\alpha_1\beta_2$ interface. As will be discussed, hemoglobin mutants having an amino acid substitution in this interface are likely to have markedly abnormal functional properties.

▼ FUNCTIONAL PROPERTIES

The oxygenation of hemoglobin, as depicted by the classical sigmoid oxyhemoglobin dissociation curve shown in Figure 7–4, can be characterized by two important properties: oxygen affinity and cooperativity.

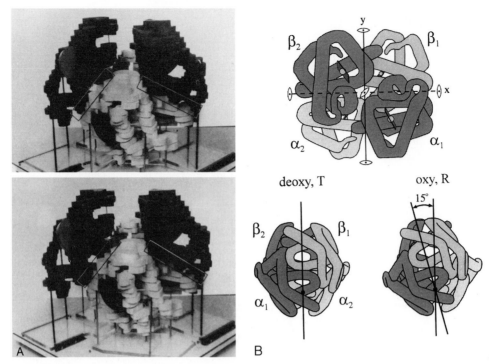

Figure 7–2. *A,* A three-dimensional model of hemoglobin, based on early x-ray crystallographic analysis. The a chains are shown in white, the b chains in black; the boxed areas are the ab contact areas. The heme groups are depicted as disks inserted into each subunit. There is an axis of symmetry that is parallel to the plane of the paper. Note the difference in conformation between oxyhemoglobin and deoxyhemoglobin. (From Muirhead, H., Cox, J.M., Mazzarella, L.: Structure and function of haemoglobin. 3. A three-dimensional fourier synthesis of human deoxyhaemoglobin at 5.5 Angstrom resolution. J. Mol. Biol. 28:117, 1967; with permission.) *B,* Schematic structures of hemoglobin, adapted from R.E. Dickerson and I. Geis, *Hemoglobin: Structure, Function, Evolution and Pathology* (Benjamin Cummings, Menlo Park, CA, 1983). These diagrams are oriented the same way as the solid model shown in *A.* The two panels at the bottom depict the change in quaternary structure upon oxygenation which involves a rotation of the symmetrically related $\alpha\beta$ dimers by about 15° relative to each other and a translation by about 0.1 nm along the rotation axis. (From W.A. Eaton, E.R. Henry, J. Hofrichter, A. Mozarelli, Nature Structural Biology, in press.)

A convenient index of oxygen affinity is P_{50} or partial pressure of oxygen at which hemoglobin is half saturated. If the oxyhemoglobin dissociation curve is shifted to the right, P_{50} is increased and oxygen affinity is decreased. Thus, P_{50} varies inversely with oxygen affinity. As discussed in detail in this section, P_{50} depends on temperature, pH, organic phosphates, and P_{CO_2}. Under physiological conditions (37°C, pH 7.40, 2,3-BPG = 5 mmol, P_{CO_2} = 40 mm Hg), the P_{50} of normal adult blood is 26 mm Hg.

The sigmoid shape of the oxyhemoglobin binding curve indicates that hemoglobin binds oxygen in a cooperative fashion. Cooperativity means that when hemoglobin is partially saturated with oxygen, the affinity of the remaining hemes on the tetramer for oxygen increases markedly. This phenomenon can be considered in terms of two hemoglobin conformations: deoxy (or T) and oxy (or R). The T form has a lower affinity for ligands such as oxygen and carbon monoxide than the R form has. At some point during the sequential addition of oxygen to the four hemes of the molecule, a transition from the T to the R conformation occurs. At this point, the oxygen affinity of the partially liganded molecule increases markedly. In this way, hemoglobin can be considered a prototype of a more general class of allosteric enzymes, in which the binding of a ligand to a protein alters the affinity for the ligand at a different site on the same macromolecule.[6]

During the last 25 years, a generation of biochemists and biophysicists have focused intently on the question of whether the oxygenation of hemoglobin faithfully adheres to the two-state model of Monod, Wyman, and Changeux (MWC).[6] Owing to the concerted transition implicit in a highly cooperative molecule, only the unligated (deoxy) and the fully ligated hemoglobins are present in sufficient amounts for structural and functional analyses. Because the partially oxygenated intermediates are present in such low abundance, investigators have gone to great lengths to prepare and study hybrid molecules in which heme groups have been modified in ways that stably impose on the subunit either the deoxy or liganded tertiary structure. In general, the properties of these hybrid hemoglobins are in reasonable agreement with the MWC two-state model, although some minor deviations have been noted.*

When two or three molecules of oxygen are bound, the $\alpha_1\beta_2$ interface is sufficiently destabilized to flip the quaternary structure from T to R, thereby increasing the affinity of the remaining hemes for oxygen. How can the seemingly small structural perturbation resulting from the oxygenation

---

*Ackers and colleagues[7] have coupled the preparation of hybrid hemoglobins with meticulous measurements of dimer-tetramer equilibria, which, through thermodynamic linkage considerations, provide a valid measurement of the free energy of subunit cooperativity. They find that certain partially ligated species depart significantly from the pure T (deoxy) and R (oxy) quaternary states. They present evidence for a third allosteric state (and quaternary structure) consisting of either singly ligated species or the tetramer in which an $\alpha\beta$ dimer is fully oxygenated and the other is unligated.

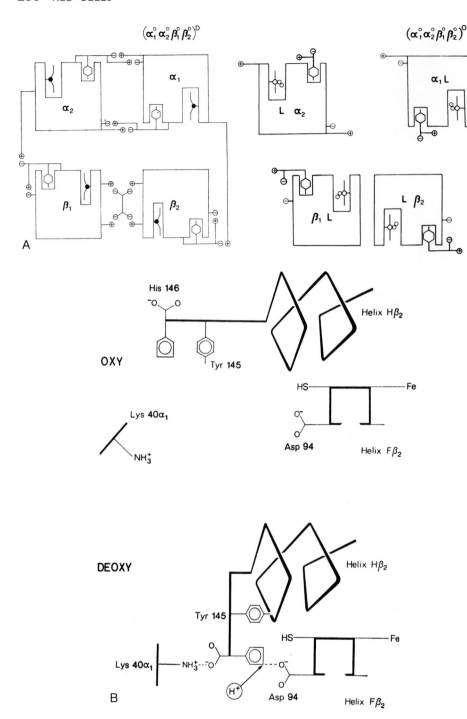

$(\alpha_1^D \alpha_2^D \beta_1^D \beta_2^D)^D$

$(\alpha_1^o \alpha_2^o \beta_1^o \beta_2^o)^O$

Figure 7–3. *A,* Diagrammatic representation of the quaternary configurations of deoxyhemoglobin *(left)* and oxyhemoglobin *(right).* A molecule of 2,3-BPG is depicted between the β subunits. Its negatively charged groups interact with positively charged residues on the β subunits. Intrasubunit and intersubunit salt bonds are broken on oxygenation. *B,* Effect of oxygenation on the contacts of C-terminal residues of the β chain. The salt bridges of β[146His] break when the quaternary structure changes from T to R or when the β chain hemes take up oxygen, whichever comes first. The proton shown in this figure, as explained in the text, is a major contributor to the Bohr effect. (*A* modified and *B* reprinted by permission from *Nature,* Vol. 228, p. 734; copyright © 1970 Macmillan Magazines Limited.)

of two or three heme groups cause sufficient alteration in the protein conformation to have an impact on subunit interactions? This question persistently occupied Perutz's attention during the 25 years that elapsed since he solved the structures of oxyhemoglobin and deoxyhemoglobin. In deoxyhemoglobin, the iron atoms lie outside the plane of the porphyrin ring by about 0.038 nm.[8] The trigger that effects this allosteric transition appears to be the decrease in the atomic radius of heme iron on the addition of ligand. The smaller iron atom is now able to snap into the plane of the porphyrin ring. The resulting alteration in heme configuration is amplified by an intramolecular path that transduces this chemical signal to the $\alpha_1\beta_2$ interface, resulting in in-

creased ligand affinity. Under physiological conditions (i.e., in the presence of organic phosphates), when deoxyhemoglobin binds oxygen, the α chain hemes are favored.

During the past several years, a considerable amount has been learned about the environment within the heme pocket, thanks to a combination of (1) high-resolution structural analyses of hemoglobin and model ("picket fence") heme compounds; (2) studies on site-directed mutants of hemoglobin, which can be produced in high quantities in *Escherichia coli*[9–11]; and (3) ultrafast measurements of the kinetics of ligand binding and conformational transitions.[12, 13] This collective body of information has provided fresh and penetrating insights about physiologically important proper-

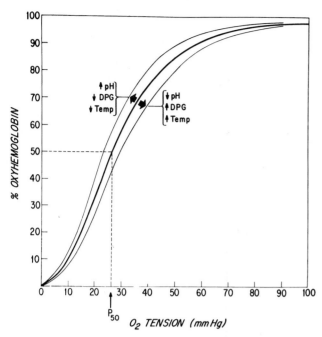

Figure 7–4. The principal factors that influence the position of the oxyhemoglobin dissociation curve in red cells: temperature, pH, and the intracellular concentration of 2,3-BPG.

ties of hemoglobin, such as the relative affinity of hemoglobin for oxygen versus carbon monoxide and the rate of auto-oxidation of hemoglobin. In free heme, the affinity for oxygen is several thousand–fold lower than that for carbon monoxide. Such a molecule could not serve as a physiological oxygen transporter because it would remain saturated by the carbon monoxide that is continually produced by heme catabolism. Accordingly, one of the challenges in the evolutionary engineering of hemoglobin was to increase oxygen affinity relative to carbon monoxide.* In the α chains of hemoglobin, a nitrogen atom on the imidazole of the distal (E7) histidine forms a hydrogen bond with the bound oxygen, thereby significantly increasing oxygen affinity. When an E7 His is replaced with a glycine residue by means of site-directed mutagenesis, the affinity for carbon monoxide increases fourfold.[9] Mutagenesis at E7 His has also provided insights into hemoglobin's remarkable ability to resist spontaneous oxidation of its heme iron atoms, resulting in the conversion to non-functional methemoglobin. Auto-oxidation is considerably facilitated by protons. Perutz[14] has suggested that the distal histidine acts as proton trap and shuttle, protecting the ferrous heme iron from auto-oxidation. No other amino acid side chain could function in this way. "Evolution is a brilliant chemist."[14]

Cooperativity (or heme/heme interaction) depends on interaction between unlike globin subunits. This phenomenon has considerable physiological importance. The familiar sigmoid shape of the oxyhemoglobin dissociation curve (see Fig. 7–4) allows a considerable amount of oxygen to be released over a relatively small drop in oxygen tension. In contrast, heme proteins, such as myoglobin and hemoglobins

H (β_4) and Bart's (γ_4), which lack cooperativity, have a hyperbolic curve, which allows much less oxygen unloading.

▼ EFFECTORS OF HEMOGLOBIN FUNCTION

Inside the red cell, oxygen affinity of hemoglobin is modulated by protons, carbon dioxide, and 2,3-BPG. As will be explained, these allosteric effectors bind preferentially to deoxyhemoglobin and alter the equilibrium between T and R quaternary structures.

Protons. In 1904, Bohr and colleagues[15] discovered that the oxygen affinity of hemoglobin decreased with increasing carbon dioxide tension. It was later shown that this phenomenon depends primarily on pH. Thus, over a pH range of 6 to 8.5, oxygen affinity varies directly with pH. A thermodynamic corollary of this statement is that deoxyhemoglobin binds protons more strongly than does oxyhemoglobin. Under physiological conditions, a molecule of hemoglobin releases about 2.8 protons on oxygenation:

$$Hb \cdot H + 4\ O_2 \leftrightarrow Hb(O_2)_4 + 2.8\ H^+$$

High-resolution X-ray data in conjunction with experiments on chemically modified hemoglobins[16] have permitted the identification of specific acid groups on hemoglobin that yield Bohr protons. After nearly a decade of controversy, high-resolution proton nuclear magnetic resonance (NMR) analyses[17] have confirmed one of Perutz's earliest and boldest predictions: A substantial portion of the Bohr effect is due to an intrasubunit salt bond between the positively charged imidazole of β146 histidine and the negatively charged carboxyl of β94 aspartate. This salt bridge is one of the important bonds that stabilize the deoxy conformation (see Fig. 7–3B). When hemoglobin is oxygenated, these bonds are broken and protons are released.

The Bohr effect offers a physiological advantage in facilitating oxygen unloading. At the tissue level, the drop in pH due to carbon dioxide influx lowers oxygen affinity, thereby enhancing oxygen release. In contrast, at the pulmonary level, the increase in pH due to the efflux of carbon dioxide increases oxygen affinity and uptake.

Carbamino Adducts. Carbon dioxide can bind free amino groups on hemoglobin to form carbamino complexes according to the following reaction:

$$RNH_2 + CO_2 \leftrightarrow RNHCOO^- + H^+$$

Only nonprotonated amino groups can react with carbon dioxide. The only amino groups in globin whose pK values are low enough to be partially nonprotonated at physiological pH are at the N termini of the α and β chains. Deoxyhemoglobin forms carbamino complexes more readily than does oxyhemoglobin. From this, it follows that at a given pH, carbon dioxide lowers oxygen affinity. Under physiological conditions, only about 10 per cent of the carbon dioxide produced by tissue metabolism is transported to the lungs in the form of carbamino hemoglobin.[5] In crocodiles, bicarbonate, rather than carbon dioxide, plays a physiologically important role in binding to a specific site on hemoglobin, lowering its oxygen affinity, thus enabling the animal to unload extra oxygen during periods when it is submerged and unable to breathe.[18]

2,3-Bisphosphoglycerate. The red cell contains an un-

---

*The Haldane coefficient (K_{CO}/K_{O_2}) for the hemoglobins of man and other mammals is about 210, at least 10-fold lower than that of free heme.

usually high concentration of 2,3-BPG (about 5 mmol/l). This compound is a potent modifier of hemoglobin function.[19] The addition of increasing amounts of 2,3-BPG to a solution of purified Hb A results in a progressive lowering of oxygen affinity. This helps explain the long-known fact that the whole blood has a lower oxygen affinity than a solution of dialyzed hemoglobin, studied under comparable conditions. The mechanism by which 2,3-BPG lowers oxygen affinity can be explained by the fact that it binds to human deoxyhemoglobin avidly ($K_d = 2 \times 10^{-5}$ M) in a 1:1 molar ratio but only weakly to oxyhemoglobin. Model fitting and X-ray diffraction measurements[20] have established the sites on hemoglobin involved in 2,3-BPG binding. 2,3-BPG is situated in the central cavity between the two β chains. Its negative charges are neutralized by the positively charged groups: β NH$_2$ terminus, β2 histidine, β82 lysine, and β143 histidine. This information on the binding of 2,3-BPG to hemoglobin suggests the following simple reaction:

$$Hb \cdot BPG + 4\ O_2 \leftrightarrow Hb(O_2)_4 + BPG$$

(Note the similarity of this equation and that for the Bohr effect previously shown.) This equilibrium expresses both the preferential binding of 2,3-BPG for deoxyhemoglobin and the 1:1 stoichiometry. Furthermore, changing concentrations of 2,3-BPG shift the oxygen-binding equilibrium in accord with the experimental results cited.

The position of the oxyhemoglobin dissociation curve is influenced by a number of factors. As depicted in Figure 7–4, the three most important are temperature, pH, and red cell 2,3-BPG concentration. Oxygen affinity varies inversely with temperature. This phenomenon is physiologically appropriate because during a period of relative hyperthermia, oxygen requirement is likely to be increased. The decrease in oxygen affinity at elevated body temperature would facilitate unloading of oxygen to tissues. The effects of pH and 2,3-BPG on hemoglobin function have already been discussed. Conventionally, whole blood oxygen saturation curves are corrected to pH 7.4, 37°C. Thus, the main variable leading to fluctuation in the position of the standardized oxygen dissociation curve is red cell 2,3-BPG concentration.

How does the oxygen affinity of the blood affect the delivery of oxygen to tissues? This subject has been reviewed in detail.[5, 21] At a given blood flow and hemoglobin concentration, the amount of oxygen that is unloaded depends on the position of the oxyhemoglobin dissociation curve. As shown in Figure 7–4, red cells that are right-shifted have enhanced oxygen release when going from a normal arterial Po$_2$ (95 mm Hg) to a normal mixed venous Po$_2$ (40 mm Hg). This is due to the fact that with this decrease in Po$_2$, a steeper portion of the oxygen dissociation curve is encompassed. In contrast, if the oxyhemoglobin dissociation curve is shifted to the left, less oxygen is unloaded. This phenomenon bears on several clinical states, including hemoglobin mutants associated with polycythemia, discussed at the end of this chapter.

SNO Adduct. As discussed in the preceding section, molecular evolution has endowed the hemoglobin molecule with properties that optimize oxygen transport, such as cooperative oxygen binding, the Bohr effect, and interaction with 2,3-BPG. Remarkably, hemoglobin may subserve yet another important function: the regulation of vasomotor tone.

During the past decade, there has been an explosive

amount of new information on the biological properties of nitric oxide (NO), which includes, *primus inter pares*, its role as a potent vasodilator. The oxidized nitrosyl derivative of NO (NO$^+$) can form adducts with proteins including sulfhydryl groups on cysteine residues. Hemoglobins of virtually all mammals and many other vertebrates contain a highly conserved cysteine on the β subunit, close to the heme pocket (β[93Cys]). When hemoglobin is oxygenated (R quaternary structure), this SH group has free access to chemical modification, whereas it is sterically blocked when the molecule is deoxygenated (T structure). These facts led Stamler and colleagues[22–24a] to propose that the allosterically linked SNO adduct enables release of NO into the microcirculation, where it dilates blood vessels. As depicted in Figure 7–5, NO, produced in pulmonary arteries and arterioles, binds to the β[93Cys] SH group, forming the SNO derivative. As the blood traverses the peripheral arterioles and precapillaries, the unloading of oxygen to tissues results in the formation of deoxy or T state hemoglobin, which precludes NO binding to β[93Cys]. This NO is thus ejected from hemoglobin and diffuses out of the red cell into the lumen of arteriolar and precapillary resistance vessels, where it serves as a local vasodilating agent. As deoxyhemoglobin recirculates back to the lungs, it is reoxygenated and its β[93Cys] SH group is again available for forming an SNO adduct. This dynamic cycle would thus enable efficient transport of NO to the small blood vessels, enhancing flow and oxygen delivery to respiring tissues.

Experimental model systems support the claim that SNO

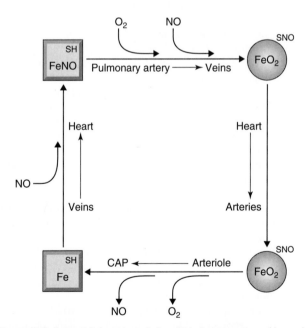

Figure 7–5. Proposed dynamic cycle by which deoxygenation of hemoglobin is linked to release of vasoactive NO to precapillary resistance vessels. Hemoglobin molecules that are deoxygenated and in the T quaternary structure are shown as purple squares; hemoglobin molecules that are oxygenated and in the R quaternary structure are shown as red circles. The β[93Cys] sulfhydryl group is shown either buried and unreactive in T hemoglobin or accessible and reactive in the R structure. NO is taken up in the pulmonary arteries and arterioles, and oxygen is taken up in the lungs. NO is released in the precapillaries, enabling vasodilatation to occur and enhanced blood flow. Oxygen is released in both precapillaries and capillaries.

hemoglobin can provide a source of vasoactive NO.[22–24] Direct measurements indicate that arterial blood contains about 0.0005 mol of the SNO adduct per mole of hemoglobin tetramer, whereas mixed venous blood contains considerably less. Moreover hemoglobin is capable of transferring its SNO adduct to reduced glutathione, which is abundant in the red cell, thereby facilitating diffusion and egress of NO from the red cell. The spectroscopic studies[24] suggesting that NO can be transferred from heme to the β^{93Cys} SH group are difficult to interpret and need further in-depth investigation.

Notwithstanding the great appeal of this novel regulatory mechanism, many more rigorous biochemical and physiological measurements are required to verify its role in vivo. Experimental verification is inherently difficult because of the extremely small mole fraction of endogenous SNO adduct on hemoglobin and because of the oxidative reactions of NO that greatly complicate interpretation of spectroscopic data. Moreover, meticulous attention must be paid to the kinetics of NO reactions with heme versus those with thiol groups on hemoglobin and glutathione. It will be a formidable challenge to critically assess whether there is oxygen-linked net release of NO from red cells during the rapid transit time (<0.5 second) from the arteries through the precapillary circulation.

▼ OTHER HEMOGLOBIN COMPONENTS

In red cells of adults and children older than 6 months, Hb A ($\alpha_2\beta_2$) accounts for more than 90 per cent of the total hemoglobin. However, other globin genes are preferentially expressed during embryonic and fetal development. The ontogeny and regulation of globin gene expression are discussed in Chapter 5. Several of these hemoglobins provide information useful in the diagnosis of a variety of congenital and acquired hematological disorders. Furthermore, posttranslational modifications of hemoglobin have been exploited in the monitoring of certain non-hematological disorders.

Hemoglobin F. After the eighth week of gestation, Hb F ($\alpha_2\gamma_2$) becomes the predominant hemoglobin. Other primates and ruminants also have structurally different γ chains. In humans, the γ chain differs from the β chain in 39 of 146 residues. Unlike the other human globin subunits, the γ chain has structural heterogeneity.[25] In newborns, about two thirds of the γ chains have glycine at position 136, whereas the remaining γ chains have alanine. This ratio falls during the switch from γ to β chain production. The two F hemoglobins ($\alpha_2{}^G\gamma_2$ and $\alpha_2{}^A\gamma_2$) have similar properties.[26] The $^G\gamma$ and $^A\gamma$ chains are products of adjacent genes located between the ϵ and δ genes. In addition, there is structural heterogeneity at position 75; in certain populations, the γ chain contains threonine instead of isoleucine.[27] The incidence of this substitution in different populations ranges from 0 to 40 per cent. Only the $^A\gamma$ chain carries this polymorphism. The determination of these differences in primary sequences has provided insights into the thalassemias and hereditary persistence of fetal hemoglobin (see Chapters 5 and 6).

About 20 per cent of Hb F in the developing fetus has a post-translational modification: the N terminus of the γ chain is acetylated (Hb F).[28] In contrast, no other human globin subunits are acetylated, except for mutants that have substitutions of the N-terminal residue.[5]

Fetal red cells have a considerably higher oxygen affinity than do adult red cells. This phenomenon, which has been observed in a number of mammalian species,[5] may facilitate the transport of oxygen across the placenta. In the human, this discrepancy in relative oxygen affinities is due to the diminished interaction of Hb F with red cell organic phosphates[29–31] (discussed earlier). Hemoglobin F has the special property of being remarkably resistant to denaturation at extremes of pH. The measurement of alkali-resistant hemoglobin has proved a useful although indirect way of estimating the content of Hb F within a hemolysate.

The red cells of the newborn contain about 80 per cent Hb F, 20 per cent Hb A (Fig. 7–6A). By the time individuals are older than 6 months, Hb F constitutes less than 1 per cent of the total hemoglobin and is distributed unevenly among red cells.[32, 33] Normally, only 0.1 to 7 per cent of red cells contain detectable amounts of fetal hemoglobin. These

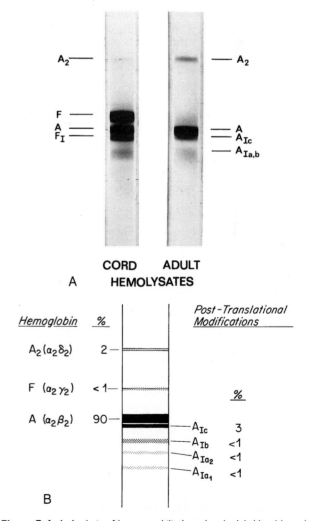

Figure 7–6. A, Analysis of human umbilical cord and adult blood hemolysates by gel electrofocusing. The gels have been overloaded to demonstrate Hb A₂. B, Separation of hemoglobin components in a normal hemolysate by means of gel electrofocusing. Glycated hemoglobins are shown on the right, along with the percentage of components in normal individuals. (A from Bunn, H.F., and Forget, B.G.: Hemoglobin: Molecular, Genetic, and Clinical Aspects. Philadelphia, W.B. Saunders Co., 1986, p. 62.)

"F cells" contain about 5 pg of Hb F, approximately 20 per cent of the total hemoglobin in the cell. As explained in more detail in Chapter 5, F cell production is genetically controlled.

Hemoglobin F is increased to a variable extent in several hereditary disorders, including β thalassemia, hereditary persistence of fetal hemoglobin (Chapter 6), and sickle cell anemia (discussed below).

Hemoglobin A$_2$. About 2.5 per cent of the hemoglobin in normal red cells is Hb A$_2$ ($\alpha_2\delta_2$). It can be readily separated from Hb A by electrophoresis or ion-exchange chromatography (Fig. 7–6). This minor component is evenly distributed among red cells, and its functional behavior is similar to that of Hb A.[5] The δ and β chains have identical sequence in all but 10 of 146 residues. The level of Hb A$_2$ is altered in a variety of congenital and acquired diseases.[34] The increased percentage of A$_2$ in β thalassemia is a useful diagnostic aid (see Chapter 6). In addition, Hb A$_2$ is slightly increased in megaloblastic anemia. By contrast, Hb A$_2$ is decreased in α thalassemia as well as in iron deficiency and sideroblastic anemias. The relative rate of synthesis of this minor component is markedly curtailed in the final stages of erythroid development.[35, 36] The level of Hb A$_2$ appears to depend on the rate of assembly of hemoglobin subunits, as discussed later.

Glycated Hemoglobins. When the hemoglobin from normal adult red cells is carefully analyzed by column chromatography,[37, 38] several minor components can be detected that have lower isoelectric points than the main Hb A (Fig. 7–6B). These are designated A$_{Ia1}$, A$_{Ia2}$, A$_{Ib}$, and A$_{Ic}$. Hemoglobin A$_{Ic}$ accounts for approximately 3 per cent of the hemoglobin in normal adult red cells.[39] This minor component differs from Hb A only at the N-terminal amino group of each β chain where glucose is attached non-enzymatically by a ketoamine linkage.[40, 41] In addition, approximately 5 per cent of hemoglobin molecules have glucose linked to certain lysine residues. These adducts cannot be separated from unmodified hemoglobins by ordinary chromatography or electrophoresis, but they can be isolated by means of an affinity resin containing phenylboronate that binds to sugar hydroxyl groups.

In like manner, sugar phosphates and other red cell metabolites combine with hemoglobin at the β N terminus to form less abundant adducts. Hb A$_{Ib}$ is an adduct of pyruvate with the β N terminus.[42] These hemoglobins are formed slowly and continuously throughout the 120-day life span of the red cell. Consequently, individuals who have increased red cell turnover (hemolysis) have decreased levels of these minor hemoglobin components.[43]

Patients with diabetes mellitus have levels of Hb A$_{Ic}$ that are two to three times higher than normal. The measurement of Hb A$_{Ic}$ has proved a useful independent assessment of the degree of diabetic control, because it is not subject to fluctuations of the blood glucose level.[44] Furthermore, Hb A$_{Ic}$ is a prototype of glycosylation of other proteins, which could contribute to the long-term complications of the disease.

During a period of weeks to months, glycated hemoglobin can undergo further rearrangement reactions to form fluorescent advanced glycation end products.[45] Such products in other tissues may contribute importantly to the long-term complications of diabetes.

Other Post-Translational Modifications. Although glucose adducts are by far the most common and abundant type of chemical modification of hemoglobin, other small molecules are also capable of forming covalent linkages and thereby may reflect significant metabolic perturbations. Examples include cyanate adducts in uremic patients,[46] acetaldehyde adducts in alcoholic patients,[47, 48] and porphyrin-substituted hemoglobin in patients with lead poisoning.[49, 50]

Human Hemoglobin Mutants

More than 500 structurally different human hemoglobin mutants have been discovered to date.[51] They are classified in Table 7–1 according to type of mutation and affected subunit.

In heterozygotes, the β globin mutant hemoglobin generally composes about half of the total hemoglobin in the red cell, in keeping with the presence of two β globin genes. In contrast, normal individuals have four α globin genes. Accordingly, α globin mutants usually compose about 25 per cent of the hemolysate. This fraction increases with concurrent α thalassemia. The two tandem α globin genes differ significantly in transcriptional efficiency: α2 > α1. Therefore, stable mutants expressed by the α2 gene tend to be relatively more abundant than those expressed by the α1 gene.[52]

There are nearly twice as many known β chain mutants as α chain mutants. This may seem surprising because of the greater number of α globin genes. However, α globin mutants, because of their relatively low abundance, often escape clinical detection. On occasion, δ chain and γ chain mutants have been encountered and characterized, but again, the frequency of detection is limited by their low abundance.

Table 7–1. Molecular Mechanisms Underlying Globin Mutations*

Mechanism	α	β	γ	δ
Single base substitution → amino acid replacements (e.g., S, C, E)	208	344	70	29
Two replacements in same subunit (e.g., C-Harlem)	1	18		
Fusion hemoglobins δβ—3 (Lepore variants) βδ—5 (e.g., Miyada, P-Congo) δβδ—1 (Parchman) γβ—1 (Kenya)				
Deletion or insertions (e.g., Gun Hill)	4	13		
Insertion (Grady, Koriyama, Catonsville)	4	2		
Deletion/insertion (Montreal, Galacia, Birmingham)		3		
Extended subunit Termination codon mutation (e.g., Constant Spring)	5			
Frameshift (Wayne, Tak, Cranston, Saverne)	1	3		
N-terminal mutation → retention of initiator methionine (e.g., Long Island–Marseille)	1	3		

*As of August 1997. International Hemoglobin Information Center; Variant List. Hemoglobin 21:505, 1997.

The majority of these hemoglobin mutants are not associated with any clinical manifestations. Many were discovered during the course of large population surveys. The simplest and most practical diagnostic tool for the detection of new hemoglobin mutants is zone electrophoresis, which separates proteins that differ in charge. However, in recent years, a number of more sophisticated techniques have been applied to the detection of mutant hemoglobins, including high-performance liquid chromatography,[53, 54] mass spectrometry,[54] and sequencing of DNA fragments generated by the polymerase chain reaction.[55–57]

Assembly of Mutant Hemoglobins. The proportion of normal and mutant hemoglobins in red cells of heterozygotes provides insight into the assembly of human hemoglobins.[58, 59] The great majority of β chain mutants are synthesized at the same rate as β^A[60] and have normal stability. Therefore, heterozygotes would be expected to have equal amounts of normal and mutant hemoglobin. However, measurements of the proportion of normal and abnormal hemoglobins in heterozygotes have revealed unexpected variability. Figure 7–7A shows a comparison of stable β chain mutants. The positively charged mutants, such as hemoglobins S, C, D–Los Angeles, and E, constitute significantly less than half of the total hemoglobin in heterozygotes and are reduced further in the presence of α thalassemia (Fig. 7–7B).[58, 59, 61] In contrast, many of the negatively charged mutants are present in amounts exceeding that of Hb A. In two heterozygotes who had a negatively charged mutant (Hb J-Baltimore or Hb J-Iran) in conjunction with α thalassemia, the proportion of the mutant hemoglobin was found to be further increased. This analysis of the proportion

of β chain mutant in heterozygotes suggests that alterations in surface charge contribute to different rates of assembly of the hemoglobin tetramer. This hypothesis is supported by in vitro mixing experiments on normal and mutant β subunits showing that when α chains are present in limiting amounts (mimicking α thalassemia), negatively charged mutants are formed much more readily than are positively charged mutants.[62, 63]

This electrostatic model of hemoglobin assembly has clinical implications. Differences in rates of assembly explain not only the low proportion of Hb S in sickle trait (AS) but also the higher proportion of Hb S in sickle C (SC) disease. The prominent clinical manifestations of SC disease and their absence in sickle trait can be attributed in part to differences in the intracellular content of Hb S.[58] This model also provides an explanation for differences in the levels of Hb A_2[58] and Hb F[64, 65] that accompany certain hematological disorders.

Clinical Phenotypes. Individuals with hemoglobin mutants come to the attention of physicians because the mutation affects hemoglobin solubility, oxygenation, or synthesis (Table 7–2). In this clinical classification of the hemoglobinopathies, by far the most important are the sickle syndromes, either homozygous (SS) disease or the compound heterozygous states SC and S/β thalassemia. Hb S causes morbidity by its propensity, when deoxygenated, to aggregate into rigid polymers, thereby occluding flow in the microcirculation. Hb C is also less soluble than Hb A, forming crystals rather than long polymers (reference 66 and references therein). More important, Hb C, either in the homozygous state (CC) or in heterozygous states (SC, AC),

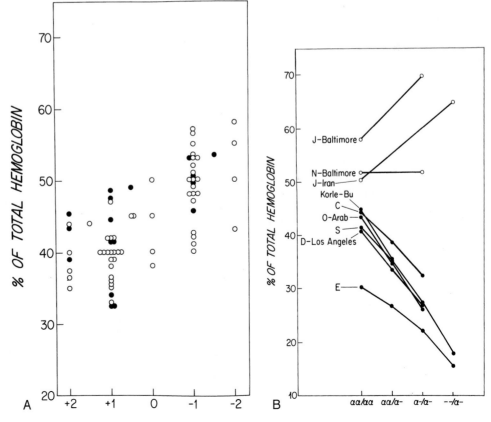

Figure 7–7. *A,* Effect of charge on the proportion of abnormal hemoglobin in individuals heterozygous for 72 stable β globin variants. Each data point represents a mean value for a given variant. The solid circles denote measurements of Huisman (Am. J. Hematol. 14:393, 1983), using high-resolution chromatography. Substitutions involving a histidine residue were scored as a change of one half charge. The −1 group differs significantly from the +1 group ($p < .001$) and from the 0 group ($p \leq .05$). (From Bunn, H.F., and Forget, B.G.: Hemoglobin: Molecular, Genetic, and Clinical Aspects. Philadelphia, W.B. Saunders Co., 1986, p. 420.) *B,* Effect of α thalassemia on the proportion of six positively charged β chain variants *(solid circles)* and of three negatively charged variants *(open circles).* (Modified and updated by permission from *Nature,* Vol. 306, p. 498; copyright © 1983 Macmillan Magazines Limited.)

Table 7–2. Clinically Important Hemoglobin Mutants

The sickle syndromes
  Sickle cell trait
  Sickle cell disease
    SS
    SC
    S/β thalassemia
Structural mutants that result in a thalassemic phenotype (approximately
  15 mutants)
The unstable hemoglobins (congenital Heinz body anemia) (approximately
  80 mutants)
Mutants with abnormal oxygen affinity
  High affinity (familial erythrocytosis) (approximately 3.5 mutants)
  Low affinity (Hb Kansas, Hb Beth Israel → familial cyanosis)
  The M hemoglobins → familial cyanosis (7 mutants)

induces red cell dehydration.[67–69] The sickle syndromes and Hb C are discussed in detail below. The unstable mutants are also relatively insoluble. Rather than forming ordered polymers or crystals, these mutant molecules aggregate into amorphous precipitates (Heinz bodies) that cause hemolysis because they impair red cell pliability and damage the erythrocyte membrane. Hemoglobin mutants with abnormally high oxygen affinity are associated with secondary erythrocytosis owing to impaired oxygen delivery to tissues, whereas the much less common low-affinity mutants are sometimes so unsaturated with oxygen that they may cause cyanosis. Cyanosis may also be due to mutants (the M hemoglobins) in which the heme iron is locked in the ferric or methemoglobin form. Finally, if a mutant hemoglobin has impaired synthesis, it may be associated with a thalassemic phenotype. These clinical phenotyes are discussed in the remainder of this chapter.

Sickle Hemoglobin and Sickle Cell Disease

▼ MOLECULAR PATHOGENESIS

The packaging of a high concentration (32 to 34 g/dl) of hemoglobin into red cells requires that the protein be extraordinarily soluble. The substitution of valine for glutamic acid at β6 results in a marked decrease in the solubility of Hb S when it is deoxygenated. The polymerization of deoxy Hb S is the primary event in the molecular pathogenesis of sickle cell disease. Under physiological conditions of pH, ionic strength, and temperature extant in the circulating red blood cell, the polymer assumes the form of an elongated rope-like fiber that usually aligns with other fibers, resulting in distortion into the classical crescent or sickle shape and a marked decrease in cell deformability. These rigid cells are responsible for the vaso-occlusive phenomena that are the hallmark of sickle cell disease.

Structure of the Sickle Fiber

After deoxygenation, Hb S–containing cells assume a variety of interesting shapes readily appreciated by light microscopy and even more clearly by scanning electron microscopy, as shown in Figure 7–8. To understand the molecular events responsible for these morphological changes, much higher resolution is necessary. Transmission electron microscopy provides structural information at roughly 3 nm resolution.

Analyses of deoxygenated sickle cells reveal the presence of parallel bundles of long fibers that are oriented along the axis of sickling.[70–73] In cells that assume a holly leaf shape, bundles of Hb S fibers point in the direction of each projection. Higher resolution electron micrographs with negative staining showed that the sickle fiber is a solid structure.[74] The high quality of these electron micrographs enabled Edelstein and colleagues[75] to use optical diffraction and image reconstruction to obtain a three-dimensional structure of the fiber. This analysis showed that individual fibers have an elliptical cross-section with a maximal diameter of about 23 nm and a minimal diameter of about 18 nm. Because hemoglobin tetramers are globular molecules with a diameter of about 5.5 nm, one can calculate that up to about 15 molecules could be packed into a cross-sectional area. Longitudinal views, as shown in Figure 7–9A, reveal a subtle but regular undulating pattern, in keeping with the elliptical cross-section and suggestive of a helical structure.[75] The helix has a high pitch with a periodicity of about 300 nm. The twisted rope-like structure, shown in Figure 7–9B, is composed of 14 strands, an inner core of 4 surrounded by a sheath of 10. Each strand is a string of deoxy Hb S beads aligned in head-to-tail (or axial) array. Even higher resolution views revealed additional structural features: a hexagonal cross-section composed of seven pairs of molecules[76, 77] (Fig. 7–10A). Verification of the double strand as the primary structural unit in the sickle fiber was provided by the finding of occasional fibers that lack one pair of strands (or even two) but no fibers that lack only a single strand.[74] These elegant electron micrographs provided sufficient detail to establish the directionality or polarity of the double strands as shown in Figure 7–10B.[76, 77] Such information on polarity is essential in determining intermolecular contacts in the fiber, compared with those in the crystal, described below.

Although these electron microscopy and optical diffraction studies have provided critical information on the packing of the sickle fiber, they lack sufficient resolution to address two important issues: the orientation of the hemoglobin tetramer in the polymer and the contacts with neighboring tetramers. Earlier optical measurements[78, 79] indicated that the long molecular X-axis (6.5 nm dimension) was within 20° of the fiber axis.*

To address these questions in detail, it was necessary to employ X-ray diffraction. X-ray analyses of sickle fibers in gels of deoxy Hb S[80] provided independent evidence for the presence of double strands but lacked sufficient resolution to convey information on molecular orientation or contacts. Love and associates[81] prepared crystals of deoxy Hb S in 10 to 15 per cent polyethylene glycol and performed X-ray diffraction analysis, initially at 0.5 nm resolution. Subsequently, the structure was solved at 0.3 nm resolution and then extensively refined,[82, 83] recently at 0.2 nm resolution.[84] The primary structural unit in the crystal is a double strand in which hemoglobin molecules are half-staggered. Adjacent molecules in the unit cell are related to one another by a 180° (twofold) screw symmetry. This finding motivated the search for and identification of comparable double strands in the fiber. The crystal contains alternate layers of double strands of opposite polarity. The structure of individual tetra-

---

*Accordingly, the dyad axis of symmetry would be nearly perpendicular to the fiber axis.

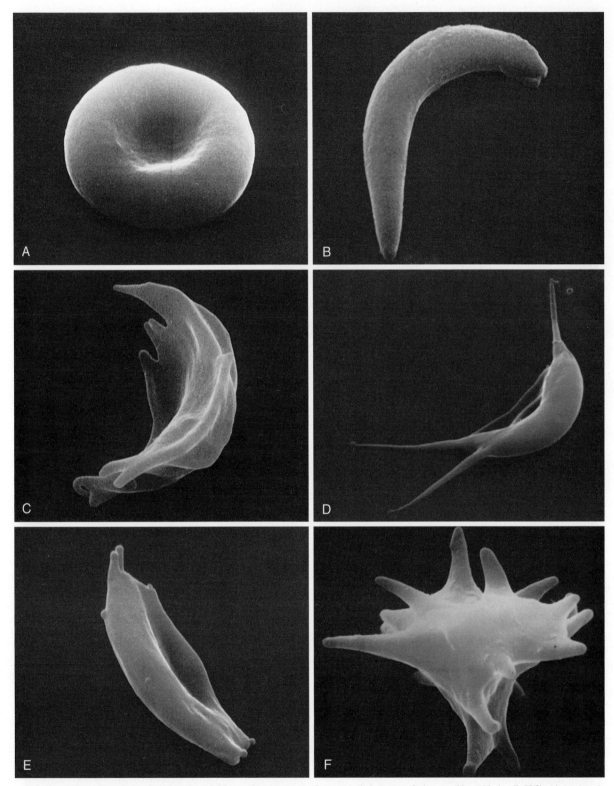

Figure 7–8. Scanning electron micrographs of SS erythrocytes. *A*, Oxygenated discocyte. *B*, Irreversibly sickled cell (ISC). Note the elongated shape and smooth contour. *C–F*, Deoxygenated discocytes (reversibly sickled cells). Cell D has a few elongated spiculated projections, giving rise to an elongated sickle shape, whereas cell F has multiple projections, giving rise to a holly leaf shape. (Prepared by Dr. James White. For further information, see Arch. Intern. Med. 133:545, 1974.)

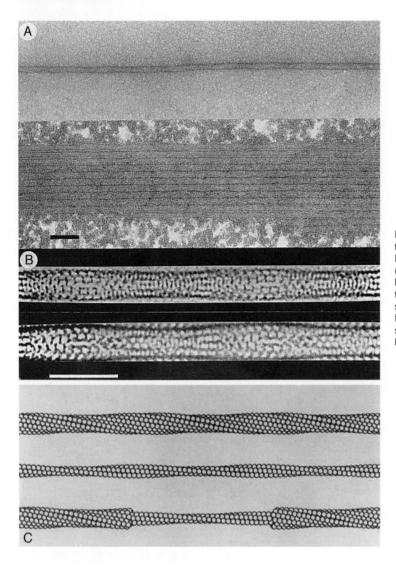

Figure 7–9. *A,* Electron micrographs of negatively stained sickle fibers. A single fiber and multiple aligned fibers are shown. *B,* Fiber images showing the twist of the strands within each fiber. (*A* and *B* from Rodgers, D.W., Crepeau, R.H., and Edelstein, S.J.: Pairings and polarities of the 14 strands in sickle cell hemoglobin fibers. Proc. Natl. Acad. Sci. USA 84:6157, 1987; with permission.) *C,* Three-dimensional image reconstruction of the fiber. Each sphere represents a Hb S tetramer. The inner core of 4 strands and the outer sheath of 10 strands are shown. (Prepared by Dr. S. Edelstein.)

mers of deoxy Hb S is indistinguishable from that of deoxy Hb A except for a shift in the A helix of one of the β subunits that enables contact with the β E and F helices of the neighboring molecule in the other strand (Fig. 7–11). The hemoglobin tetramer $\alpha_1\beta_1\alpha_2\beta_2$ is oriented in such a way that the 6(A3) Val of one of the two β subunits (β_2) forms a hydrophobic contact with a complementary or acceptor site at 70(E14) Ala, 85(F1) Phe, and 88(F4) Leu on the β_1 subunit of a tetramer in the partner strand.*

Importantly, the 6 Val of the β_1 subunit makes no contacts in the crystal structure or in the fiber structure. As discussed below, this observation bears directly on the participation of non-S hemoglobins in the polymerization process. Moreover, the contact between β^{6Val} and an acceptor site on the partner strand is possible only when Hb S is in the T or deoxy conformation. R or oxygenated molecules cannot fit into the polymeric structure.

There is convincing evidence that the structure of the double strand in the crystal, including intermolecular contacts, is nearly identical to that in the fiber. Accordingly, the high-resolution information available from the crystal

structure can be applied directly to the fiber, which as stated before is the physiologically relevant structure. The double strands that are stacked in an antiparallel linear array in the crystal are slightly twisted in the fiber (Fig. 7–12). Stretching of the outer strands in the fiber limits its size to seven pairs.

Before these direct structural analyses, a considerable body of important information on the contacts between molecules in the polymer was generated by Bookchin and Nagel,[85–87] who studied the gelation of mixtures of Hb S with Hb A, HbA₂, HbF, and a large number of β globin mutants. Subsequently, Benesch and Benesch[88, 89] performed similar experiments with α globin mutants. When Hb S ($\alpha_2\beta^S_2$) and a β globin mutant ($\alpha_2\beta^X_2$) are mixed, the tetramers readily dissociate into αβ dimers that can then reassociate to form hybrid tetramers ($\alpha_2\beta^S\beta^X$)[90] as well as the parent tetramers. Because only one β^{6Val} is required for polymerization at position β_2, the participation of the hybrid tetramer in the gel provides unambiguous information about contacts in the β_1 *(trans)* subunit. Taken together, the results of these gelation experiments are in remarkably good agreement with the X-ray analyses. The mutants that are indistinguishable from Hb A when mixed with Hb S generally have amino acid substitutions at sites not involved in contacts. The β globin mutants that do affect gelation tend to be on the β_1 or *trans*

---
*Similar but not identical contacts are made with 6 Val of β_2 in the other strand: 70(E14) Ala, 73(E17) Asp, and 88(F4) Leu.

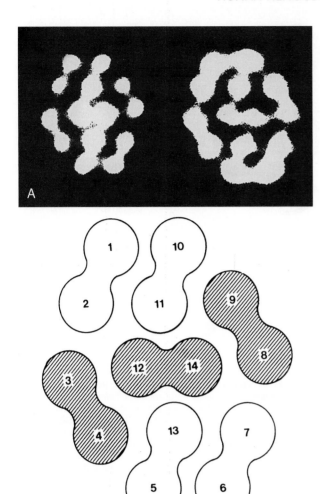

Figure 7–10. *A,* Cross-sectional views calculated from correlated images of fibers. *B,* Relationship between the cross-sectional views and strand pairing and the polarity of the pairs. (*B* from Rodgers, D.W., Crepeau, R.H., and Edelstein, S.J.: Pairings and polarities of the 14 strands in sickle cell hemoglobin fibers. Proc. Natl. Acad. Sci. USA 84:6157, 1987; with permission.)

even more readily than Hb S.[95] In contrast, replacement of β^{6Glu} by tryptophan results in inhibition of polymerization.[95a] Other site-directed mutants have been developed to test other contacts within the sickle fiber[96, 97] and the sites on γ and δ chains responsible for inhibition of polymerization.[98, 99]

Sickle Hemoglobin Polymerization

The polymerization of sickle hemoglobin involves the self-association of identical molecules. The detailed information on the structure of the polymer summarized in the preceding section indicates that no accessory molecules are involved. Accordingly, the assembly process should and does obey simple chemical rules. During the last 15 years, a rigorous body of thermodynamic and kinetic measurements, primarily from the laboratory of Eaton and Hofrichter,* provided a thorough understanding of the mechanistic pathway for Hb S polymerization in pure solution as well as in intact red cell. This information is critical to an understanding of the pathogenesis of the vaso-occlusive events in sickle cell disease.

Equilibrium Measurements

When a gelled solution of deoxygenated Hb S is carefully examined by various physical-chemical probes, large polymers (fibers) and free tetramers can be readily demonstrated, but species of intermediate size cannot be detected. This indicates that the polymerization of Hb S is a highly concerted process and therefore can be regarded as a simple phase change. Accordingly, the equilibrium between sol and gel can be studied by a measurement of the concentration of free hemoglobin in solution after segregating the polymer, such as by high-speed centrifugation[93, 102, 103] (Fig. 7–13). As in any bona fide solubility measurement, the result is independent of the total hemoglobin concentration.† For pure deoxy Hb S at pH 7, 20°C, the solubility is 20 g/dl, considerably lower than the concentration of hemoglobin inside the red cell. Such solubility measurements have provided highly reliable information on the effect of a number of physiologically relevant parameters, such as fractional oxygenation, pH, temperature, ionic strength, organic phosphates, and the presence of non-S hemoglobins.

Fractional Oxygenation. Because the crystal structure of Hb S is nearly identical with that of Hb A, it is not surprising that in dilute solution, the two hemoglobins have identical oxygen-binding curves under a variety of solvent conditions.[104] However, at concentrations above the solubility of deoxy Hb S, the oxygen-binding curve is progressively right shifted.[105–107] Because Hb S polymerizes only when it is in the T quaternary conformation, it is not surprising that the polymer binds oxygen non-cooperatively and with low affinity.[108] The principles of thermodynamic linkage dictate that oxygen affinity is lowered in direct proportion to the amount of polymer formed. Moreover, because of the reciprocal relationship between oxygen binding and polymeriza-

subunit and involve either lateral contacts between partners of the double strand or axial contacts between members of a single strand. In contrast, α chain contacts tend to be either axial or between double strands.[91, 92*]

The preparation and testing of genetically engineered site-directed globin mutants are providing further information about the contacts in the polymer. For example, the double mutant β^{6Val}, β^{121Gln} polymerizes much more readily than does Hb S.[94] This experimental result explains why individuals heterozygous for this double mutant (HbS-Oman) have a clinical phenotype nearly as severe as that of SS homozygote.[94a] These findings are fully consistent with the earlier finding of enhanced polymerization in a mixture of Hb S and Hb O-Arab (β^{121Gln}), confirming this site as a contact in the fiber. Another mutagenesis experiment has shown that β^{6Val} is not required for polymerization. Replacement of β^{6Glu} (in Hb A) by another hydrophobic residue, isoleucine, results in a hemoglobin ($\alpha_2\beta^{6Ile}_2$) that polymerizes

*For a complete compilation of the experimental data on mixtures of Hb S with naturally occurring hemoglobin mutants, see references 92 and 93.

---

*For a definitive review of this topic, see reference 93; and for reviews that are less detailed and comprehensive, see references 100 and 101.
†As explained below, this statement does not hold for partially oxygenated solutions or mixtures of S and non-S hemoglobins, owing to considerations of non-ideality and differences in the composition of the polymer and solution phases.

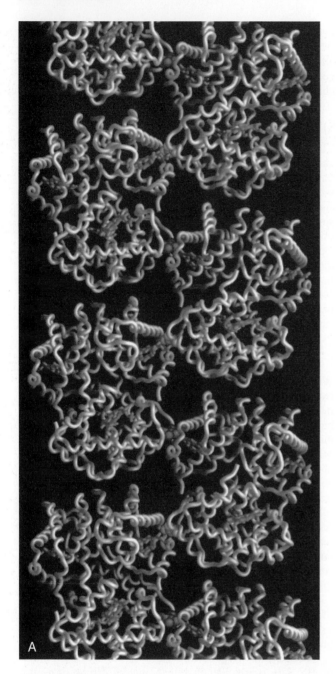

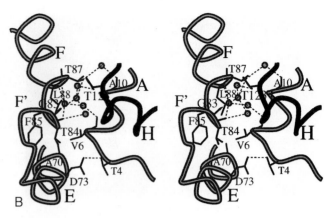

Figure 7–11. *A,* Intermolecular contacts in the sickle double strand. The protein backbones are shown as white coils. The heme groups are colored red, the β^{6Val} is colored blue. One β^{6Val} in each hemoglobin tetramer interacts with a complementary site on a β subunit on an adjacent strand, forming a lateral contact. Axial contacts are located within a single strand in a vertical direction. *B,* Stereo diagram of the β^{6Val} involvement in a lateral contact. The β^{6Val} (V6) on helix A interacts with β^{845Phe} (F84) and β^{88Leu} (L88) on helix F of a β subunit on an adjacent strand. (Prepared by Drs. William Royer and Daniel Harrington. From Harrington, D.J., Adachi, K., and Royer, W.E., Jr.: The high resolution crystal structure of deoxyhemoglobin S. J. Mol. Biol. 272:398, 1997; with permission.)

tion, it follows that the solubility of Hb S increases directly with oxygen saturation. Fully oxygenated molecules of Hb S or partially oxygenated molecules that assume the R conformation cannot be incorporated into the polymer but indirectly lower the solubility because their large excluded volume greatly increases the chemical activity of the coexisting T-state molecules,[109] thereby favoring their aggregation. This non-ideality consideration[109, 110] applies equally well to the solubility of mixtures of S and non-S hemoglobins and is a particularly important determinant of polymer formation at high hemoglobin concentrations, such as in red blood cells.

pH. The solubility of deoxy Hb S is lowest between pH 6.0 and 7.2 and rises sharply at higher and lower pH values.[111, 112] Accordingly, in the pH range 6.5 to 7.5, the alkaline Bohr effect is enhanced in concentrated solutions of Hb S as well as in SS red cells.[113]

Temperature. The polymerization of Hb S is an endothermic process,[110, 114, 115] consistent with the importance of hydrophobic interactions. Therefore, polymer formation is entropically driven, resulting from the release of ordered water molecules from the surface of free hemoglobin. Sickle polymers are melted by cooling. Accordingly, a temperature jump is a simple and effective way of initiating polymerization, thereby enabling kinetic measurements.

Ionic Strength. The solubility of deoxy Hb S depends on salt and buffer conditions. At salt concentrations spanning the physiological range, solubility increases with ionic strength,[116] but it decreases markedly at high ionic

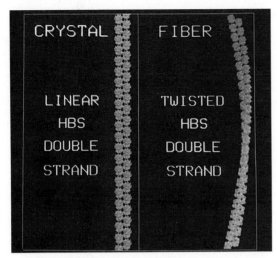

Figure 7–12. Comparison between the linear double strand in the deoxy Hb S crystal and the twisted double strand in the deoxy Hb S fiber. (Prepared by Drs. S. Watowich, L. Grass, and Robert Josephs.)

strength.[116, 117] This salting out effect allows experiments to be performed with relatively small amounts of hemoglobin. In general, the solubility data obtained in high phosphate buffers agree well but not perfectly[118] with measurements made under physiological conditions.

Organic Phosphates. As mentioned in the beginning of this chapter, the primary modulator of oxygen affinity in the red cell is 2,3-BPG. An increase in red cell 2,3-BPG favors Hb S polymerization in three ways: lowered oxygen affinity and a reduction in intracellular pH (both of which increase deoxy Hb S) and a direct effect on the conformation of deoxy Hb S.[119, 120]

Non-S Hemoglobins. A considerable amount has been learned about intermolecular contacts from measurements of the gelation or solubility of mixtures of S and non-S hemoglobins. Of particular and practical importance is the effect of hemoglobins F, A, and C that commonly coexist in high concentration in the red cells of patients with various sickle genotypes. Information on the co-polymerization of Hb S with these hemoglobins has provided important insights into the pathogenesis and clinical severity of the various sickle syndromes, including SS with increased levels of Hb F, S/β^0 thalassemia, S/β^+ thalassemia, SC disease, ·and AS (sickle trait). Moreover, as mentioned previously,

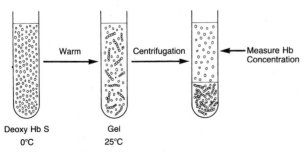

Figure 7–13. Measurement of the solubility of deoxy Hb S. A concentrated hemoglobin solution is warmed from 0°C to 25°C, allowing gelation to occur. After high-speed centrifugation, Hb S polymer forms a pellet at the bottom of the tube. The concentration of hemoglobin in the supernatant provides an accurate measurement of the solubility.

these studies have provided early and reliable information on the intermolecular contacts in the sickle fiber. The solubility of a mixture of equal amounts of Hb S and Hb A (and that of Hb S + Hb C) is only about 40 per cent higher than that of Hb S alone. In this mixture, half of the hemoglobin is composed of asymmetrical hybrid tetramers ($\alpha_2\beta^S\beta^A$). Because only one of the two $\beta6$ valines is engaged in an intermolecular contact, there is a 50 per cent chance that the hybrid tetramer will enter the polymer in such a way that all the proper contacts are made. Indeed, incorporation of Hb A into the sickle polymer has been experimentally documented.[111] In contrast, the Hb A tetramers ($\alpha_2\beta_2$), which compose 25 per cent of the mixture, fail to be incorporated into the polymer. Nevertheless, by virtue of their excluded volume,[109] the solubility is further lowered.

In contrast to Hb A and Hb C, Hb F and Hb A_2 inhibit polymerization. Accordingly, the hybrid tetramers $\alpha_2\beta\gamma$ and $\alpha_2\beta\delta$ fail to be incorporated into the sickle polymer. Because Hb F ($\alpha_2\gamma_2$) affects polymerization by means of the asymmetrical hybrid $\alpha_2\beta^S\gamma$,[111, 121] the inhibition is *trans* to the β^{6Val} contact. Nagel and colleagues[86] have presented evidence that γ^{87} is one of the important inhibitory sites. This residue constitutes one of the lateral contacts in the double strand of the sickle fiber.

Kinetics of Polymerization

The information presented thus far on the structure of the sickle fiber as well as on the thermodynamics of gelation may lead to the false impression of a static process. In fact, the polymerization of sickle hemoglobin is a remarkably dynamic event. Rigorous measurements, primarily by Eaton and Hofrichter and colleagues,[122, 123] of the kinetics of polymer formation, both in pure Hb S solutions and in sickle erythrocytes, have provided critical insights into the pathogenesis of vaso-occlusive crises, which play such a dominant role in sickle cell disease. Their studies led directly to information on the nucleation mechanism responsible for fiber formation. Their experiments on intact red cells have provided an explanation at the molecular level of the morphological changes that are observed after the deoxygenation of cells, both in vitro and in vivo. Finally, understanding the kinetics of polymerization has enabled them to propose a novel and workable approach to the assessment of new antisickling therapy.

Solution Studies. The time course for polymerization of a concentrated solution of Hb S can be monitored after rapid removal of ligand, such as by photolysis, or (as mentioned above) by rapidly increasing the temperature of deoxy Hb S, taking advantage of the markedly endothermic nature of the process. The formation of sickle fibers can be documented by a variety of physical-chemical techniques including turbidity, light scattering, calorimetry, and NMR spectroscopy. The subsequent alignment of fibers is best monitored by measurement of birefringence. After ligand removal or temperature jump, there is a clearly measurable lag time before a signal reflecting the presence of detectable polymer. Simultaneous calorimetry and birefringence measurements document formation of fibers and their subsequent alignment. The progress of polymer formation is exponential. During the delay time, there is insufficient amount of polymer to provide a signal, owing to limitations of

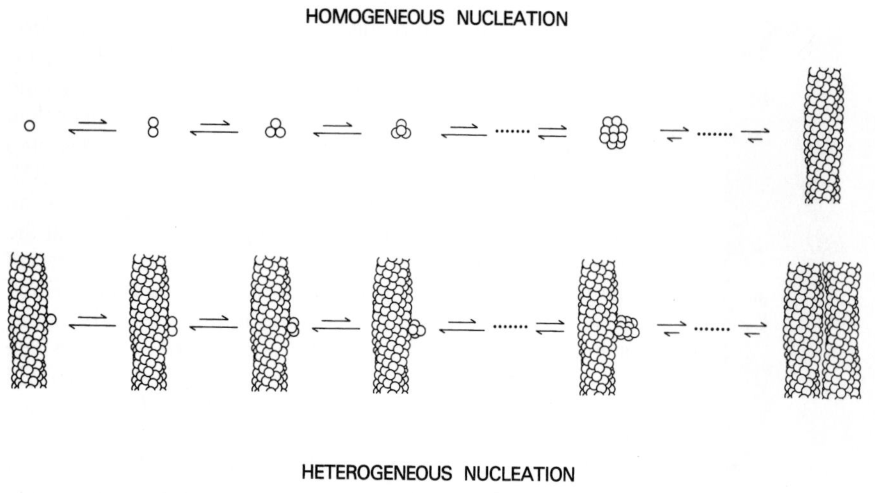

HOMOGENEOUS NUCLEATION

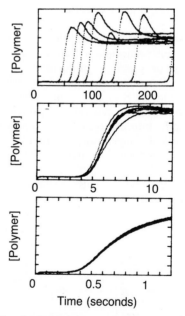

Figure 7–14. Schematic representation of homogeneous and heterogeneous nucleation. In the homogeneous pathway, nuclei form in solution, whereas in the heterogeneous pathway, nuclei form on the surface of existing fibers. Initially, the formation of small aggregates is thermodynamically unfavorable. As the aggregate increases in size, each participating hemoglobin molecule has relatively more contacts, providing enhanced stability, which overcomes the unfavorable entropic forces. Once this critical nucleus is formed, propagation of the polymer is rapid. (Prepared by Dr. William A. Eaton. From Bunn, H.F., and Forget, B.G.: Hemoglobin: Molecular, Genetic, and Clinical Aspects. Philadelphia, W.B. Saunders Co., 1986, p. 472.)

HETEROGENEOUS NUCLEATION

sensitivity of the methods for monitoring. Fiber formation begins with a nucleation process, shown in Figure 7–14, in which a relatively small number of hemoglobin molecules assemble to form a lattice on which fiber growth can take place. The number of molecules in the nucleus is proportional to the slope of the concentration dependence of the delay time (Fig. 7–15). At high concentration of hemoglobin, the estimated slope is about 15, whereas at lower concentrations, this number increases to about 30. As shown in Figure 7–14, aggregates smaller than the critical nucleus are thermodynamically unfavored. In contrast, once the nucleus is formed, subsequent addition of molecules is highly favored and fiber growth becomes rapid (approximately 250 hemoglobin tetramers per second).[124] Ferrone and colleagues[125]

observed that delay times on relatively concentrated solutions, although short, were highly reproducible; whereas, to their surprise, when measurements were made on small volumes of more dilute solutions, the longer delay times varied markedly. This stochastic behavior, shown in Figure 7–16, suggested to them that each signal had been amplified from a single nucleation event. Statistical thermodynamic modeling of their results[125, 126] led these investigators to propose two pathways for the nucleation of sickle hemoglobin fibers. In one, nucleation of individual fibers occurs in the bulk solution phase and is called homogeneous nucle-

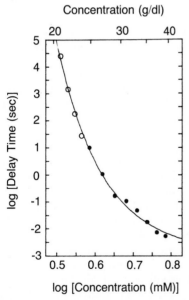

Figure 7–15. Concentration dependence of the delay time of polymerization of deoxy Hb S from laser photolysis of concentrated solutions *(solid circles)* and temperature jump measurements of less concentrated solutions *(open circles)*. The slope of this curve provides an approximation of the "order" of the polymerization reaction and therefore of the size of the critical nucleus. (From Eaton, W.A., and Hofrichter, J.: Hemoglobin S gelation and sickle cell disease. Blood 70:1245, 1987; with permission.)

Figure 7–16. Kinetic plots of the progress curves for the polymerization of deoxy Hb S. In a concentrated solution *(bottom panel)*, where the delay time is short (approximately 0.4 second), replicate experiments are highly reproducible. In contrast, in a more dilute solution *(top panel)*, replicate experiments are highly variable, with delay times ranging from 40 to 175 seconds. This stochastic behavior reflects the formation and propagation of a single polymer domain. (From Eaton, W.A., and Hofrichter, J.: Hemoglobin S gelation and sickle cell disease. Blood 70:1245, 1987; with permission.)

ation. In the second, nucleation occurs on the surface of existing polymers, which leads to autocatalytic formation of fibers and hence the delay period. This second pathway is called heterogeneous nucleation. As shown in Figure 7–14, in highly concentrated solutions of deoxy Hb S, homogeneous nucleation is favored. Polarizing microscopy reveals multiple domains of polymers giving rise to birefringent spherulites. These are probably the tactoids that Harris[127] first observed in solutions of deoxy Hb S. In less concentrated solutions of deoxy Hb S, heterogeneous nucleation predominates, leading to fewer domains of aligned sickle fibers. The kinetics of formation of individual fibers has been observed directly by means of video-enhanced differential interference contrast microscopy.[124] The growth of new fibers from branch points provides direct support for a heterogeneous nucleation mechanism.

Cellular Studies. The extension of the equilibrium and kinetic studies of polymerization to erythrocytes is greatly complicated by marked heterogeneity of SS cells, owing to a wide range of oxygen affinity, an even wider distribution of intracellular hemoglobin concentration (20 to 50 g/dl), and the heterogeneous distribution of Hb F. However, when these variables are taken into account, the delay times of SS red cells and the amount of polymer per cell at equilibrium are remarkably close to what is encountered in hemoglobin solutions.[128] This conclusion is consistent with the finding that the cytosolic surface of the red cell membrane has no effect on the delay time.[129]

The kinetics of polymerization plays a critical role in the rheology and morphology of circulating red cells.[130] Equilibrium measurements of polymer content of red cells, whether by oxygen-binding curves,[131] by NMR spectroscopy,[132, 133] or by differential polarization microscopy,[134] grossly overestimate the amount of intracellular polymer that is formed in vivo as SS red cells are deoxygenated in the arterioles and capillaries. Because the range of transit times in the microcirculation is short, relative to the range of delay times of SS red cells, the great majority (perhaps 95 per cent) of cells fail to form polymer during their flow through arterioles and capillaries.[130] In contrast, if these cells were equilibrated at the oxygen tensions in the microcirculation, virtually all of them would contain polymer and as a result would have markedly decreased deformability.

As shown in Figure 7–17, kinetics is the critical determinant of cell shape and morphology. A number of early experiments clearly demonstrated that when SS red cells are deoxygenated slowly, they form classical elongated (sickle) shapes. This observation is a vivid demonstration of homogeneous nucleation, wherein one domain propagates by fiber growth and alignment to distort the cell into a classical sickle shape. With somewhat more rapid deoxygenation, a few independent domains will induce a more irregular shape.[135] In contrast, when deoxygenation is rapid, multiple spherulitic domains result in a granular or cobblestone texture with no gross distortion of cell shape. Because the shape of the sickled cell is so dependent on the number of independent polymer domains, it is possible to convert a holly leaf cell into an elongated sickle shape by partial reoxygenation![136] As discussed in detail below, the distortion of cell shape by projections of aligned Hb S fibers plays a critical role in the pathogenesis of the membrane lesion.

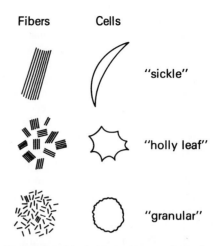

Figure 7–17. Relationship between the number of polymer domains and the shape of the sickled cell. *Top,* When cells sickle slowly, there is likely to be a single polymer domain, which propagates into long fibers with further alignment of fibers along a single long axis, giving rise to the classical banana or sickle shape. *Middle,* With intermediate rates of polymerization, there will be several polymer domains composed of shortened aligned fibers, resulting in multiple spiculated projections and a holly leaf shape (see Fig. 7–8). When polymerization is rapid, there will be multiple domains with randomly oriented fibers, resulting in a granular appearance with no projections from the cell surface. (From Eaton, W.A., and Hofrichter, J.: Hemoglobin S gelation and sickle cell disease. Blood 70:1245, 1987; with permission.)

▼ THE ERYTHROCYTE MEMBRANE IN SICKLE CELL DISEASE

Although information on the kinetics and thermodynamics of Hb S polymerization has provided remarkably penetrating insights into the pathogenesis of sickle cell disease, a fuller understanding depends on reckoning with the complexities of the flow of sickle erythrocytes in the microcirculation. The red cell membrane is the fulcrum that links primary intracellular events (polymer formation, growth, and orientation) with secondary changes that have an impact on red cell deformability as well as interactions with the vascular endothelium. Several hundred papers have been written on this subject during the past decade. For more detailed coverage than is possible in this chapter, see reviews by Hebbel.[137, 138]

Membrane Proteins

Lipid Bilayer–Skeleton Uncoupling. The red cell skeleton is composed of a two-dimensional hexagonal lattice of interacting spectrin tetramers, stabilized by actin and protein 4.1. This flexible yet sturdy "geodesic dome" is covered snugly by a lipid bilayer in which is embedded a variety of proteins, such as erythroid-specific glycophorins and transport proteins including the anion channel (protein 3), Na^+,K^+-ATPase, and other cation channels. Ankyrin provides a bridge between spectrin and protein 3; protein 4.1 is linked to glycophorins A and C and to aminophospholipids on the cytoplasmic side of the lipid bilayer. The spicules that are observed after slow deoxygenation of SS erythrocytes contain protein 3 but not spectrin.[139] These spicules represent the penetration of bundles of aligned sickle fibers through the skeleton, thereby dissociating it from the lipid bilayer.[139]* When the red cell is reoxygenated, the sickle polymers melt, and the bilayer lipids at the tip of the spicule are occasionally released from the cells in the form of hemoglobin-rich lipid vesicles. A large proportion of the additional perturbations in the structure and function of red cell membrane proteins and lipids discussed in this section are a direct consequence of the draconian distortions imposed by projections of sickle polymer.

Irreversibly Sickled Cells. The earliest evidence of impaired structure and function of SS erythrocyte membranes came with the recognition of irreversibly sickled cells (ISC) that remain locked in an elongated shape despite full oxygenation and absence of polymer. Unlike reversibly sickled cells, which usually contain multiple sharp projections (see Fig. 7–8), ISCs have a relatively smooth contour. The persistence of the elongated (sickled) shape, even after removal of the membrane lipid by a detergent, provided convincing evidence that the architecture of the skeleton was irreversibly perturbed.[141] This shape change is a consequence of plastic deformation of membrane skeletal proteins induced by rearrangement of spectrin heterodimers.[142]

Anywhere between 1 and 50 per cent of the red cells in blood films from patients with SS disease have an elongated shape. However, about half of these cells are reversibly sickled, having such low oxygen affinity that polymerized Hb S persists during the preparation of the specimen.[143] Truly *irreversibly* sickled cells are those that retain an elongated shape after all of the intracellular polymer has been melted by equilibrating the blood specimen with carbon monoxide before preparing the microscope slide.[143]

ISCs are generally dense cells with mean corpuscular hemoglobin concentration (MCHC) as high as 50 g/dl. In a given patient, ISCs have lower levels of Hb F than less dense cells.[144] Moreover, among a large group of SS patients, in the absence of concurrent α thalassemia, the percentage of ISCs correlates inversely with percentage of Hb F.[145, 146] SS red cells lacking Hb F have a much higher potential for forming polymer than do SS F cells, for reasons discussed above. Therefore, it is likely that the ISC is the pickled consequence of repeated cycles of in vivo sickling. In vitro experiments provide support for this claim. ISCs can be formed in vitro by repetitive cycles of deoxygenation (references 147 and 148 and references therein) and, importantly, by a single deoxygenation step if the oxygen removal is slow enough to allow the SS cell to assume an elongated "sickle" shape.[135] Under these conditions, K^+ leak exceeds Na^+ gain and the cell becomes dehydrated, contributing further to deoxy Hb S polymerization. Earlier reports notwithstanding, ATP depletion is not necessary for in vitro ISC formation, whereas external Ca^{2+} is required.[135] This finding suggests that the Gardos channel may contribute to the K^+ loss that accompanies ISC formation (see Disordered Volume Control).

ISCs tend to be young red cells.[149] Moreover, because of their high MCHC and stiff membrane, they are inordinately rigid cells that understandably have a markedly shortened life span. Thus, these cells are morphological reminders

of the autocatalytic processes that are such a fundamental feature of sickle cell disease.

Disordered Membrane Protein Interactions. The structure and function of a number of membrane proteins are perturbed in SS red cells. The demonstration that inside-out vesicles from SS red cells show decreased binding to normal spectrin implies an abnormality in ankyrin.[150] Likewise, protein 4.1 from SS red cells has decreased capability for binding to normal inside-out vesicles that have been depleted of endogenous protein 4.1. Moreover, SS vesicles have a decreased content of protein 4.1.[151] It is not clear whether these findings reflect impaired binding of protein 4.1 to amino phospholipids or to glycophorin. The altered function of protein 4.1 from SS red cells may be due to oxidative damage (see below).[151] The interaction of Hb S with the cytosolic surface may also contribute to disordered membrane function. Hb S binds more readily than Hb A to normal inside-out vesicles (references 152 and 153 and references therein). Nevertheless, this interaction does not appear to alter the kinetics of intracellular polymerization of Hb S.[129] A small amount of globin appears to be covalently linked to spectrin in SS red cells as well as in other types of dehydrated cells.[154] The adherence of Hb S to the red cell membrane contributes significantly to the static rigidity of SS red cells.[155]

These abnormalities in the organization of proteins on the cytoplasmic surface of SS membranes are accompanied by equally striking alterations on the cell surface. In particular, glycophorin[156, 157] and protein 3[157] are abnormally clustered. The aggregates of protein 3 may lead to the enhanced binding of immunoglobulin that has been observed on the surface of circulating SS red cells. It has been suggested but not yet proved that clustering of glycophorin and protein 3 may be provoked by the formation of Heinz bodies (aggregates of denatured Hb S).[137] The abnormal distribution of these highly charged surface proteins in SS red cells may contribute significantly to the pathogenesis of vaso-occlusion because of adhesion to endothelial cells or, less likely, as a source of procoagulant. The enhanced binding of immunoglobulin to SS red cells may trigger accelerated clearance by the mononuclear phagocyte system.

Oxidation of SS Membrane Proteins. Considerable effort has been expended seeking and documenting oxidant damage to membranes of SS red cells.[137] There is a significant although modest reduction in free sulfhydryl groups of SS membrane proteins.[158, 159] However, the formation of interprotein disulfide bonds cannot be extensive because protein sizing gels reveal many fewer high molecular weight aggregates compared with the number observed with oxidant-type hemolytic anemia. Oxidant damage can impose other structural alterations on specific proteins in SS membranes. For example, in protein 4.1, decreased free sulfhydryl content is accompanied by large protein aggregates, half of which appeared to be disulfide cross-links, and also by oxidized amino acids.[151] Treatment of SS red cells with the reducing agent *N*-acetylcysteine results in conversion of ISCs to biconcave discs.[160] This result suggests that the dysregulation of red cell volume in ISCs is due to sulfhydryl oxidation of membrane channel proteins.

Why should SS red cells be unduly susceptible to oxidant damage? In an attempt to answer this question, Hebbel[137] and colleagues have amassed experimental data indi-

---

*In like manner, the vesicles that are shed after repeated cycles of in vitro sickling are free of spectrin.[140]

cating that oxidized Hb S is the culprit. They found that purified Hb S auto-oxidized 1.7 times faster than Hb A purified from the same AS donor[161] and that Hb S had a faster rate of dissociation of heme comparable to the rate of methemoglobin formation. These investigators propose that these abnormalities are responsible for the twofold increased deposition of heme and heme proteins, such as hemichromes, that has been documented on the membranes of SS red cells.[162, 163] Because these heme moieties can serve as a biological Fenton reagent, they may be responsible for the enhanced rate of hydroxyl radical generated from superoxide and peroxide in SS red cells.[164, 165] Sickle red cell membranes have increased iron, not only free molecular iron bound to phosphatidylserine on the inner lipid bilayer but also free heme as well as hemichrome that aggregates with clusters of band 3.[166] Sickle cell membranes promote auto-oxidation of Hb S and accumulation of heme unless they are stripped of iron.[167]

Two issues remain controversial: (1) the mechanisms responsible for the formation of hemichrome and activated oxygen compounds in SS red cells and (2) the contribution of these phenomena to the damage of SS membranes. It is not at all clear that the modest increase in the rate of auto-oxidation of Hb S[161] is the cause of the twofold increase in the generation of superoxide and hydroxyl radical. Current understanding of the three-dimensional structure of hemoglobin and the molecular events responsible for auto-oxidation and hemichrome formation does not predict that the $\beta^{6Glu \rightarrow Val}$ replacement would have any impact. Moreover, there are stable mutants, such as Hb Kansas, that have markedly higher rates of hemoglobin auto-oxidation than that reported for Hb S and yet are not associated with any apparent red cell membrane damage or hemolysis. Moreover, like SS individuals, Hb Kansas heterozygotes have no detectable methemoglobinemia. Rather than auto-oxidation, another more striking abnormality of Hb S may be responsible for hemichrome formation: On mechanical shaking in room air, Hb S denatures more readily than Hb A and other common mutants[168, 169] with a twofold increase in the release of hemin.[170] This enhanced denaturation at the liquid/gas interface may have a parallel at the cytosol/membrane interface within the red cell.

There is general agreement that hemichromes (irreversibly oxidized hemoglobin) are modestly increased (twofold to threefold) in SS red cells. How much do these products contribute to the multiplicity of structural and functional perturbations in SS membranes? Much higher levels of hemichromes are encountered in red cells of individuals having unstable hemoglobin mutants, and yet the clinical and laboratory phenotype in this disorder bears only superficial similarity to sickle cell disease. In vitro loading of hemin onto normal red cell cytoskeletons does induce membrane defects similar to what has been reported in SS red cells.[171, 172] However, differences in the dose of hemin and its presentation in the membrane raise concern about the relevance of these in vitro experiments to the pathophysiology of sickle cell disease. A similar concern may be raised about the pathophysiological significance of the comparably modest (twofold) increase in the production of superoxide and hydroxyl radical by SS red cells. However, it may be that in SS red cells, the enhanced production of activated oxygen compounds synergizes with the increased levels of

heme and non-heme iron in the membrane, resulting in significant oxidant damage.[137] If so, therapeutic removal of iron bound to SS red cell membranes would be expected to result in amelioration of the membrane lesion. The iron is bound to the inner leaflet of the membrane with high affinity.[173] However, deferiprone (L1), a chelator that unlike deferoxamine can enter cells, is effective in vitro in removal of iron deposits from SS red cell membranes.[174] It will be of considerable interest to ascertain whether the administration of deferiprone to SS patients results in hematological and clinical improvement.

Membrane Lipids

Instability of the Lipid Bilayer. In a variety of biological membranes, the distribution of phospholipids is asymmetrical. In the lipid bilayer of the human red cell, more than 75 per cent of the choline-containing phospholipids (phosphatidylcholine [PC] and sphingomyelin) are on the outer leaflet, whereas more than 80 per cent of phosphatidylethanolamine (PE) and all of phosphatidylserine (PS) are on the inner leaflet. This asymmetry is maintained by two independent mechanisms: (1) an adenosine triphosphate (ATP)–dependent aminophospholipid translocase that catalyzes the transfer of PE and PS from the plasma across the outer leaflet to the inner leaflet[175]; and (2) the binding of the aminophospholipids (PE and PS) to proteins of the skeleton (spectrin and protein 4.1). The importance of the second mechanism is controversial (reference 176 and references therein).

In a variety of hemolytic disorders including SS disease, reduction of membrane stability has been documented by a decrease in phospholipid asymmetry and by increased rates of transit of choline phospholipids across the bilayer. In SS red cells, aminophospholipids have been noted in the outer leaflet of ISCs as well as in discoid SS cells that have been induced to sickle.[177] The precise extent of the flip-flop is unclear because the methods used to monitor phospholipid asymmetry are likely to perturb the equilibrium between phospholipids in the inner and outer leaflets. In ISCs and in deoxygenated discoid SS cells, reduction of phospholipid asymmetry is accompanied by an increase in PC translocation.[178-180] These phenomena appear to be a direct result of the marked upheaval in the organization of the skeleton, as discussed in detail above. Polymerization-induced deformation of red cell shape is necessary to induce both enhanced PC translocation and loss of phospholipid asymmetry. When discoid SS cells are deoxygenated under conditions that produce multiple domains of polymer but no spicules or gross membrane distortion, the stability of the lipid bilayer is maintained.[179, 180] Moreover, when SS cells have been stressed by multiple cycles of deoxygenation and reoxygenation, the vesicles that are formed from the shed spicules have markedly decreased phospholipid asymmetry, whereas the remnant despiculated cell appears to have normal membrane stability.[178] These findings again underscore the primacy of polymerization-induced distortion of cell shape in the pathogenesis of the membrane lesion in sickle cell disease.

The loss of phospholipid asymmetry in SS red cells may contribute to the vaso-occlusive manifestations of the disease. ISCs, sickled discocytes, and the vesicles shed from sickled cells, like PE-enriched liposomes, are potent proco-agulants.[175, 181, 182] There is a large and confusing literature on abnormalities in hemostasis in sickle cell disease. The aggregate of clinical and labortory data suggests that thrombosis may play a significant albeit secondary role (see review by Ballas and Narla[183]).

Lipid Peroxidation. Oxidant stress affects the structure not only of proteins but also of lipids. Membranes of SS red cell have about twofold higher levels of lipid peroxidation than normal red cells.[184, 185] Moreover, ISCs have a novel phospholipid composed of PE and PS cross-linked by malondialdehyde,[186] a product of lipid peroxidation. It is likely that increased amounts of denatured hemoglobin[187] as well as of non-heme iron[188] in SS membranes generate activated oxygen compounds responsible for increased lipid peroxidation.

The pathophysiological significance of a twofold increase in lipid peroxidation is not clear. Considering the fact that such a tiny mole fraction of membrane lipid is modified, it seems plausible that this phenomenon is overshadowed by the impact of oxidant stress on the structure and function of SS membrane proteins. However, lipid peroxidation may induce enhanced recognition of SS red cells by macrophages, thereby contributing to the shortened in vivo survival of SS red cells.[189]

Disordered Volume Control*

The rate and extent of polymer formation in a circulating SS red cell depend on three primary variables: the cell's hemoglobin composition,† its degree of deoxygenation, and its intracellular hemoglobin concentration (MCHC). During their 120-day survival, circulating normal AA red cells lose a small amount of solute and water with a concomitant small increase in MCHC. Therefore, normal red cells have a narrow distribution of MCHC and density that depend in part on in vivo aging. Although the MCHC and mean cell density of the overall population of SS red cells are close to what is found in normal red cells, the density distribution of SS red cells is unusually broad. The increase in the least dense SS cells is due primarily to a high number of reticulocytes that have a relatively low MCHC. The marked increase in dense cells is a result of enhanced dehydration of a substantial proportion of circulating cells. The ISC is the final stage of this process. Because the polymerization of deoxy Hb S is so markedly dependent on hemoglobin concentration, dense SS cells are much more prone to sickle and thus contribute disproportionately to the vaso-occlusive and hemolytic aspects of the disease. Arguably, this accelerated in vivo dehydration is the most relevant pathophysiological consequence of perturbations in the structure of the membrane in SS red cells.

There is convincing evidence that four independent phenomena contribute to dehydration of SS red cells: K:Cl cotransport, calcium-activated K+ efflux, passive K+ and Na+ leak, and decrease in osmotic pressure. All but the first of these are triggered by intracellular polymerization of Hb S.‡

---

*For more detailed coverage of this topic, see the review by Bookchin and coworkers.[190]

†In particular, whether Hb F is present in the SS red cell, and if so, its concentration.

‡All of the multiple leak pathways that have been identified in sickle red cells, as described in this section, can also be activated in normal red cells by the membrane stretch that accompanies hypotonic swelling.[191]

K:Cl Cotransport. Sheep erythrocytes that are genetically low in K+ have a ouabain- and bumetanide-resistant transport system that is a major pathway for the flux of K+ and Cl−.[192, 193] K:Cl cotransport was first demonstrated in human red cells by Brugnara and colleagues.[69, 194] In normal AA red cells, this channel is active only in reticulocytes[195, 196] and may contribute to the decrease in MCHC that accompanies normal in vivo red cell aging. Much higher levels of K:Cl cotransport are observed in CC[69, 197] and SS[194, 197] red cells. This finding cannot be due merely to hemolysis with an increase in young red cells because K:Cl cotransport is also elevated in AC and AS red cells,[198] which have normal life spans. Thus, it is likely that the function of this transporter is affected by these mutants, which are known to have enhanced binding to the cytosolic surface of the red cell membrane.[152] K:Cl cotransport is induced by hypo-osmolarity and also by a modest decrease in pH (to 7.0). As discussed in more detail below, this stimulus probably pertains in vivo, particularly at sites of stagnant circulation. Conversely, the pathway is inhibited by divalent cations[202, 203] as well as by DIOA.[199]* The latter agent is not fully specific because it also inhibits the anion channel.

K:Cl cotransport probably plays a major role in the marked dehydration that is a hallmark of CC[69] and SC[200] red cells. In SS cells, this pathway is particularly active in those cells lacking Hb F and thus could contribute to progressive dehydration of these cells.[201] Nevertheless, Hb F does not directly inhibit this pathway.[149] K:Cl cotransport is significantly inhibited by deoxygenation, probably because of the accompanying rise in free cytosolic Mg2+.[202, 203] The overall contribution of K:Cl cotransport to the dehydration of SS red cells must be weighed against sickling-induced mechanisms discussed below.

Calcium-Dependent K+ Channel. SS red cells have increased amounts of Ca2+,[204, 205] which is compartmentalized within intracellular vesicles.[206, 207] The steady-state level of free ionized Ca2+ in the cytosol is normal.[190] However, when cells undergo sickling, there is an increase in the permeability of a number of cations including not only Ca2+[190] but also K+, Na+,[208] and Mg2+.[209] This leak appears to be limited to cations because sickling fails to affect the permeability for sulfate anion, erythritol, mannitol, or arabinose.[210] Similar to other perturbations in SS membrane structure and function, discussed above, this non-specific leak in cations requires not only the formation of sickle polymer but also the distortion of the membrane by elongated spicules. ATP is maintained at normal levels in SS red cells, and therefore the Ca2+-ATPase that efficiently pumps Ca2+ out of the cell or into vesicles remains fully active. However, when the cell membrane is stretched by sickling, the transient increase in free cytosolic Ca2+ is sufficient to trigger the Ca2+-dependent (Gardos) K+ channel, thereby providing a pathway for sickling-induced loss of K+ and water, leading to cell dehydration. This process could be accentuated by inhibition of Ca2+-ATPase. Although Ca2+-ATPase levels are probably normal in SS red cells (reviewed in reference 190), enzyme activity could be low in vulnerable SS cells because the enzyme is susceptible to both reversible and permanent damage by oxidants known to be produced by SS cells.[211]

---

*[(DihydroIndenyl)Oxy]Alkanoic acid.

Passive K⁺ and Na⁺ Leak. Forty-five years ago, Tosteson[212] showed that when SS cells were deoxygenated, they became leaky to Na⁺ and K⁺. These ion movements are unaffected by furosemide or by anion replacement and do not involve a Na⁺-K⁺ exchange mechanism. The Na⁺ and K⁺ leak can be inhibited by stilbene disulfonates such as DIDS* but in a manner independent of inhibition of the anion channel (protein 3).[213] As mentioned, this increase in cation permeability requires true sickling with gross deformation and stretching of the cell membrane.[208] Subsequent measurements confirmed that sickling-induced passive influx of K⁺ and efflux of Na⁺ are almost precisely balanced.[214] However, because the red cell sodium pump (Na⁺,K⁺-ATPase) has a stoichiometry of 3 K⁺ out for 2 Na⁺ in, repeated cycles of sickling should result in a net loss of total cation and water. Modeling studies[190, 215] suggest that the dehydration caused by sickling-induced K⁺ and Na⁺ leak is likely to be slow and modest and probably does not account for the rapid transition from young reticulocyte to dense ISC that has been noted in vivo[149] (see below). Simulation experiments suggest that oxidant damage to SS membrane may act synergistically with mechanical distortion to magnify cation leaks.[216, 217]

Decrease in Osmotic Pressure. A fourth mechanism for sickling-induced cell dehydration evolves directly from thermodynamic principles. As sickle hemoglobin polymerizes inside the red cell, there may be a significant change in osmolarity with an accompanying shift in water across the cell membrane. The solute concentration in the water that is trapped within sickle polymers does not appear to differ significantly from that in the free cytosol.[218] Accordingly, intracellular polymerization of Hb S should be associated with a fall in osmolarity and therefore with prompt cell shrinkage. Previous measurements of this phenomenon have given conflicting results owing to pH changes and difficulties in accurately measuring red cell volumes. However, carefully obtained measurements verify that deoxygenation of SS red cells is associated with a small but significant degree of cell shrinkage. Because the kinetics of deoxy Hb S polymerization is so exquisitely dependent on hemoglobin concentration, this phenomenon could be an amplification factor, increasing the rate and extent of polymerization during flow in the microcirculation. Note that this process depends on polymer formation but unlike Ca²⁺-induced K⁺ efflux or passive Na⁺ and K⁺ leaks does not depend on sickling-

*4,4′Diisothiocyano-2,2′disulfostilbene.

induced distortion of the cell membrane. Moreover, unlike the other three means for dehydration of SS cells, the polymerization-induced change in osmolarity is instantaneous and fully reversible.

Model of Dehydration. Bookchin and Lew[149, 215, 219] have presented an integrated model that places in perspective the four independent mechanisms, discussed above, that can induce rapid dehydration of young SS red cells. In contrast to mature red cells, reticulocytes do not return to their original steady state after transient perturbations. Brief spurts of either acidosis or sickling-induced Ca²⁺ influx can trigger K⁺ and water efflux. As shown in Figure 7–18, there is positive cooperativity between these two processes, leading to "fast-track" dehydration of young SS red cells.[219] K⁺ efflux is accompanied by an equivalent Cl⁻ efflux that is compensated by co-influx of Cl⁻ and protons through the Jacobs-Stewart mechanism. This secondary acidosis would trigger further K⁺ and water loss through K:Cl cotransport. In essence, red cells in general and reticulocytes in particular do not have an effective way of dealing with K⁺ loss. A transient period of sickling can set in motion K⁺ and water loss through cooperation of the Gardos and K:Cl cotransport channels, resulting in hysteresis and drift, setting the young SS cell on a downhill trajectory leading eventually to the ISC. This fast-track dehydration of young SS red cells pertains mainly to those lacking Hb F,[220] a finding consistent with the critical role of polymerization in triggering the Gardos pathway.

The rapid conversion of SS reticulocytes to ISCs has been documented in vivo by clinical observation that oxygen therapy during pain crisis acutely suppressed erythropoiesis.[221] Cessation of oxygen administration was associated with a sequential increase in plasma erythropoietin levels, reticulocytes, and ISCs.

▼ IN VIVO SICKLING

The two salient clinical manifestations of sickle cell disease are severe hemolysis and vaso-occlusive episodes. Just as an understanding of the molecular basis of sickle hemoglobin polymerization helps to explain many of the complex perturbations of SS membranes, these membrane abnormalities provide insights into how sickle red cells might interact with other cells in ways that contribute to the pathophysiology of the disease. Specifically, enhanced binding of SS erythrocytes to monocytes/macrophages may contribute importantly

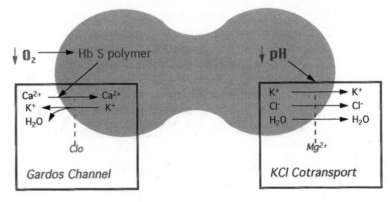

Figure 7–18. Scheme of the major pathways leading to dehydration of sickle red cells. K⁺ and Cl⁻ efflux is triggered either by sickling-induced Ca²⁺ influx, which activates the Gardos channel *(left-hand box)*, or by transient acidosis, which triggers the K:Cl cotransport pathway *(right-hand box)*. The latter is particularly active in reticulocytes. The Gardos pathway is inhibited by clotrimazole (Clo), and K:Cl cotransport is inhibited by magnesium ion (Mg²⁺).

to hemolysis; more important, the adherence of SS red cells to vascular endothelial cells appears to play a critical role in vaso-occlusive crises. The most mysterious and challenging aspect of the disease is the episodic and unpredictable nature of these events, both temporally and spatially. Although the unique kinetic features of Hb S polymerization are likely to be the primary determinant of the stochastic nature of these vaso-occlusive events, complex secondary phenomena such as membrane changes, cell/cell interactions, and vicissitudes in the microcirculation are probably important additional contributors.

Adherence of SS Erythrocytes to Macrophages

Red cell destruction in sickle cell disease is primarily extravascular, in keeping with only modest elevation of plasma hemoglobin. The enhanced rigidity of ISCs and sickled discocytes leads to extravascular destruction, akin to that of rigid cells encountered in a host of other hemolytic disorders such as hereditary spherocytosis and congenital Heinz body hemolytic anemia (see below). In addition, hemolysis in SS disease may be amplified by immune recognition and clearance. SS red cells have enhanced adherence to monocytes and macrophages[185, 222] and more readily undergo erythrophagocytosis.[185, 223] Two mechanisms have been proffered to explain these phenomena.

The external surface of a subpopulation of SS red cells has increased deposits of γ globulin (IgG)[185, 224, 225] that appear to be abnormally clumped[226] and thereby more susceptible to recognition by Fc receptors on macrophages. Adherence and phagocytosis can be inhibited either by Fc blockade[185] or by elution of IgG.[225] Alternatively, monocytes and macrophages may recognize the abnormal display of PE and PS in the outer membrane leaflet of sickled cells[222] (see Membrane Lipids). This may explain why the adherence of monocytes to deoxygenated SS cells is reversed on oxygenation. In general, there is a strong correlation between monocyte adherence and maneuvers that increase the display of surface PS on SS cells as well as on normal red cells. Moreover, this process can be partially blocked by preincubation of monocytes with PS liposomes.

Adherence of SS Erythrocytes to Endothelial Cells

The potential for a sickled cell to initiate a vaso-occlusive event depends primarily on whether the delay time for sickling is within the range of the capillary transit time.[100] Therefore, any secondary phenomenon that retards the transit of SS red cells in the microcirculation would promote polymerization and consequent vaso-occlusion. Accordingly, there has been considerable interest in studies demonstrating enhanced adherence of SS red cells to endothelial cells.[156, 227, 228] Moreover, independent of sickling, such adherence would narrow the lumen of arterioles and capillaries and therefore contribute to vaso-occlusion. Most of the experiments described below have used human umbilical vein endothelial cells [HUVEC][156, 228–231] or endothelium from bovine aorta.[227, 232]*

Initially, Hebbel and colleagues measured adherence by incubating radiolabeled sickle and normal red cells with a HUVEC monolayer, followed by successive washings. Subsequently, the development of flow chambers has provided a more physiological way to study the adherence of red cells to endothelial cells.[229–231] Mohandas and Evans[232, 234, 235] devised a micropipette technique that enabled them to make direct measurements on individual red cells, including the quantitation of strength of adherence at shear forces that would be anticipated in the microcirculation. Irregularly shaped discocytes are more adherent than regularly shaped discocytes. These micropipette experiments confirmed that ISCs are the least adherent,[156, 234] probably because their rigidity precludes their forming extensive surface contact with the endothelial cell. This consideration may explain why deoxygenated sickled discocytes also have relatively weak adherence.[156]

In a flow chamber, shear stresses can be applied that simulate in vivo flow in the microcirculation. At low shear rates, simulating flow in capillaries and venules, high-density SS red cells adhered to HUVEC less readily than did low-density cells,[230] probably owing in part to the poor binding of ISCs. This finding could be an explanation for why pain crises appear to be more frequent in SS patients with a greater percentage of more deformable low-density cells.[236, 237] All populations of SS red cells were markedly more adherent than AA or AS cells. However, high-reticulocyte AA red cells behaved similarly to SS red cells. Thus, there appear to be surface determinants on young red cells, independent of hemoglobin composition, that facilitate adherence to endothelium. The fact that patients with other types of hemolytic anemia do not have sickle-type crises argues that adherence of SS cells to vascular endothelium is not sufficient for the development of vaso-occlusive events.

In addition to red cell age, other intrinsic properties more specific to SS erythrocytes have been implicated as contributors to endothelial cell adherence. These include glycophorin clustering, oxidation of membrane proteins or lipids, aminophospholipid externalization, red cell dehydration,[137] and density of adhesive molecules on SS reticulocytes.[238, 239]

Plasma appears to be required for optimal adherence,[234, 240] even though in an albumin-buffer medium, SS red cells are more adherent than normal cells. SS plasma, particularly samples obtained during crises, supports adherence more than normal plasma does.[229, 240] These results implicate the participation of acute phase reactants in the plasma. Fibrinogen has been suggested to be an important plasma contributor because adherence is strengthened by addition and weakened by depletion of this abundant plasma protein.[240] Experiments showing that adherence is inhibited by EDTA and restored by excess calcium[234] suggest that adhesive molecules such as the integrins are involved in this phenomenon. The demonstration that adherence can be partially blocked by removal of collagen-binding proteins[234] or by the addition of RGDS peptide* lends further support to this conclusion.[231, 235, 241] There is circumstantial evidence that high molecular weight multimers of von Willebrand protein (vWF) play a critical role. Specific depletion of this protein markedly inhibits adhesion,[229, 231] as does the addition

---

*As discussed below, SS erythrocytes have also been shown to have increased adherence in vivo to vascular endothelium of rat mesentery.[233]

*Arg-Gly-Asp-Ser.

of antibodies to glycoprotein Ib or IIb/IIIa,[242] platelet plasma membrane molecules that bind to vWF. Ex vivo adherence of SS red cells to the endothelium of rat mesentery is enhanced by pretreating the animal with desamino-8-D-arginine vasopressin (DDAVP),[243] an agent that enhances the secretion of vWF multimers from endothelial cells. Von Willebrand multimer is a particularly appealing mediator of adherence because its huge size would permit bridging between red cell and endothelial cell over a distance sufficient to minimize repulsion due to the negative charge on the surfaces of the two cells. However, as indicated below, VWF assays, under certain circumstances, inhibit adhesion of SS red blood cells to the endothelium.

Studies have begun to delineate the molecular interactions responsible for adhesion of SS red cells to endothelium, the best documented of which are shown in Figure 7–19. Reticulocytes, especially those from SS patients, have on their surface the integrin complex $\alpha_4\beta_1$ (VLA-4) that binds to both fibronectin[244] and vascular cell adhesion molecule-1 (VCAM-1),[245, 246] molecules expressed on the surface of endothelial cells, particularly after activation by inflammatory cytokines such as tumor necrosis factor-α. In addition, both microvascular endothelial cells and a subpopulation of sickle reticulocytes display CD36,[238] which binds to thrombospondin secreted by activated platelets.[247, 248] It is likely that sickle cell patients have enhanced release of thrombospondin from activated platelets, especially during pain crises when plasma levels of thrombospondin rise and platelet levels fall.[249] Thrombospondin also binds to sulfated glycans on SS red cells.[250, 251] This interaction can be inhibited by soluble anionic polysaccharides.[251a] Von Willebrand protein can bind to thrombospondin, thereby inhibiting red cell adhesion.[252] Thus, the relative concentrations of vWF and thrombospondin at specific sites in the microcirculation may be a determinant of red cell adhesion to the endothelium.

It is likely that activation of endothelial cells plays an important role in sickle cell adherence and in the pathogenesis of acute vaso-occlusive events. Circulating endothelial cells are both elevated and activated in sickle cell patients, especially during pain crisis.[253] Moreover, these cells have

increased expression of tissue factor, at both the mRNA and protein levels,[254] a finding consistent with elevated tissue factor procoagulant activity in the blood of SS patients.[255] Thus, the activated endothelial cell is likely to be the proximal cause of the induction of the coagulation cascade in sickle cell patients, particularly during crisis (see review of Ballas and Narla[183]).

In addition to their interaction with endothelial cells, SS erythrocytes also have enhanced binding to the subendothelial matrix, in particular laminin[251] and immobilized thrombospondin.[255a] These molecules may be exposed within gaps formed by tissue injury or by retraction of activated endothelial cells.[255b] Sickle red cells have enhanced surface expression of lutheran antigen,[255c] which binds specifically to the alpha5 chain of laminin.[255d]

Roughly 20 per cent of acute vaso-occlusive events are triggered by infection. During inflammatory stress, adhesion of SS red cells to endothelial cells is likely to be increased owing to increases in the plasma proteins as well as upregulation of VCAM-1 expression and other relevant adhesive molecules on activated endothelial cells. Moreover, infectious agents may directly condition endothelial cells. Double-stranded RNA viruses induce VCAM-1 on endothelial cells and consequently increase their adherence to SS red cells.[256] Furthermore, HUVEC cells infected with herpes simplex virus type 1 have enhanced adherence to SS red cells, mediated through an increase in the expression of receptors for the Fc portion of IgG.[257]

As mentioned in the section on sickle cell membrane, intracellular polymerization induces marked perturbations in the topology and structure of transmembrane proteins, potentially creating targets for cell/cell adhesion. Band 3, which is known to be aggregated in SS membranes, appears to be a culprit because adherence to endothelial cells can be blocked by peptide loops of band 3 that are displayed on the external surface of the red cell.[258]

Neutrophils from SS patients also appear to be sticky, probably owing to the action of inflammatory cytokines during vaso-occlusive events. Enhanced adhesion of SS neutrophils to vascular endothelium during pain crises appears

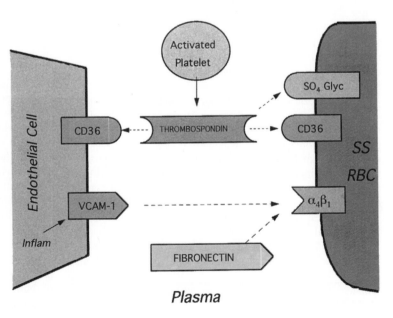

Figure 7–19. Principal interactions responsible for the adhesion of a sickle red cell to the microvascular endothelium. Activation of platelets releases thrombospondin, which can act as a bridging molecule, binding to CD36 on the endothelial cell and to CD36 or to sulfated glycans on the sickle reticulocyte. Inflammatory cytokines induce the expression of VCAM-1 on endothelial cells. This adhesive molecule can bind directly to the $\alpha_4\beta_1$ integrin on the sickle reticulocyte.

to be due in part to increased expression of CD64, the high-affinity immunoglobulin Fc receptor.[259] Moreover, SS neutrophils have increased binding to fibronectin.[260] These interactions may contribute to vaso-occlusive episodes.

The pathophysiological importance of the adherence of SS red cells to endothelium is underscored by the finding that unlike a host of other laboratory parameters that have been examined, the degree of adherence correlates strongly with clinical severity in a large number of patients with SS disease and other sickle genotypes.[228]

Sickling in the Microcirculation

The neural and humoral control of blood flow in the microcirculation, coupled with temporal and spatial variability in oxygen consumption, adds greatly to the complexity of in vivo sickling.* Significant advances have been made in the development of in vivo or ex vivo models of sickle vaso-occlusion. Kaul and colleagues[233, 243, 262, 263] have studied the behavior of SS and AA red cells infused into the vascular bed of rat mesocecum. This preparation permits both direct microscopic visualization of the transit of individual red cells in the microcirculation and measurements of pressure, flow, and vascular resistance. More recently, these investigators have studied the microcirculation of the cremaster muscle in a transgenic sickle mouse model.[264] Taken together, these experiments have shown convincingly that the enhanced adherence of SS red cells, described before, pertains to in vivo blood flow. The extent of adherence of oxygenated cells varied inversely with blood flow. Consistent with in vitro results in a flow chamber,[230] adherence varied inversely with red cell density, with reticulocytes and young discocytes being the most adherent, particularly in immediate postcapillary venules and at vessel bendings and near vessel junctions. Shear rates would be expected to be significantly lower here than in the arterioles or capillaries, thereby reducing the chance for red cell detachment. Adherence was associated with an increase in peripheral resistance, particularly when the infusate included the most dense cells, which are the least adherent. Thus, it is likely that the adherence of low-density discocytes results in secondary trapping of rigid dense SS cells including the ISCs (Fig. 7–20). Preferential trapping of dense SS cells has been observed during perfusion of the femoral artery in the rat.[262] [31]P magnetic resonance measurements showed that the vaso-occlusion was associated with acidosis and edema, both indicators of tissue ischemia.

Nitric oxide is likely to be an important determinant of blood flow in sickle cell disease. An ex vivo study of the rat cerebral microcirculation has demonstrated that SS red cells were more adherent than normal AA red cells,[265] and that patency of flow was dependent on endogenous production of NO since infusion of *N*-nitro-L-arginine methyl ester (L-NAME), an inhibitor of NO synthase, resulted in marked decrease in blood flow and cerebral infarcts. These experiments suggest that the NO pathway for vasoregulation may be a critical determinant of stroke in sickle cell disease. Studies in vivo with transgenic sickle mice suggest that NO may protect the liver from ischemic damage[266] and also

---

*For more detailed information, see reviews by Eaton and Hofrichter[100] and by Francis and Johnson.[261]

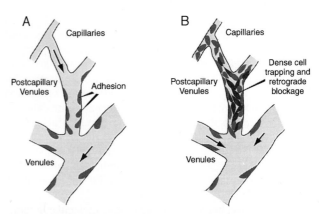

Figure 7–20. A sequential model of vaso-occlusion in sickle cell disease. *A* shows preferential adhesion of light and normal density SS red cells, especially reticulocytes, to postcapillary venules, followed by trapping of dense and irreversibly sickled cells (shown in *B*) with retrograde obstruction. (Modified by Drs. R.E. Kaul, M.E. Fabry, and R.L. Nagel from their review: The pathophysiology of vascular obstruction in the sickle syndromes. Blood Rev. 10:29, 1996.)

contribute to increased glomerular filtration in the kidney.[267] In addition to its direct effect as a local vasodilator, NO may also enhance blood flow by inhibiting the upregulation of the endothelial cell adhesion molecule VCAM-1. During acute chest syndrome, SS patients have a concomitant increase in soluble VCAM-1 and a decrease in NO metabolites.[267a] Thus inhalational NO therapy may not only enhance vessel patency in the pulmonary microcirculation, but also inhibit adhesion of sickle red cells to the endothelium.

Rodgers and colleagues[268–270] have applied a number of non-invasive methods to compare in vivo blood flow in SS patients with that in other sickle syndromes as well as in normal individuals. Cutaneous microvascular flow can be monitored by laser-Doppler velocimetry.[268, 269, 271] About 50 per cent of SS patients, 12 per cent of SC patients,[271] and an occasional AA individual[272] have oscillations in blood flow termed periodic microcirculatory flow. This phenomenon is thought to represent a compensatory response to impaired blood flow caused by sickle vaso-occlusion. When SS patients are subjected to progressive periods of partial occlusion of forearm blood flow, the post-occlusive hyperemia was associated with proportional increases in blood flow and in the magnitude of the flow oscillations and with a significant delay in the peak level of blood flow.[269] It is of interest that a similar pattern was observed in two patients with homozygous Hb C disease,[269, 271] in whom red cells are dehydrated but not subject to sickling. In one SS patient, the abnormal flow pattern was reversed by exchange transfusion.[269]

Studies of in vivo blood flow can be complemented by non-invasive assessment of tissue function and metabolism. For example, positron emission tomography has demonstrated focal abnormalities in cerebral metabolic rate in sites not identified by conventional computed tomographic scans.[273]

The application of these accurate non-invasive techniques to studies of vaso-occlusion in sickle cell disease provides a special opportunity to make objective assessments of both conventional and new therapeutic modalities. For example, the administration of an arteriolar vasodilator, nifedipine, was shown to result in significant improvement in microvascular flow in the retina and conjunctiva.[270] The development of transgenic animal models for sickle cell disease (discussed below) will also be useful in assessing whether therapeutic maneuvers result in improvement of blood flow in the microcirculation and in prevention of vaso-occlusive events.

Pathogenesis of Sickle Crises. Among the protean manifestations of sickle cell disease, the feature that is most enigmatic to clinicians is the acute pain crisis. In a given patient, none of the many readily available laboratory or diagnostic parameters currently in use correlates with the frequency of crises or serves as a predictor for their onset. Analyses of large numbers of SS patients indicate that the frequency of crises varies directly with hemoglobin level[237, 274, 275] and inversely with the level of Hb F.[275] Surprisingly, the potential of a patient's red cells to form sickle polymer is sometimes *not* a good predictor of pain crises.[276] For example, the frequency of acute crises in S/β^0 thalassemia appears to be greater than in SS disease,[275, 276] even though the degree of polymer formation would be less, owing to the lower intracellular hemoglobin concentration. For this reason, it is doubtful whether sophisticated (yet greatly oversimplified) numerical calculations of intracellular polymer fraction[277–279a] offer additional insight into the pathophysiology of the vaso-occlusive complications of sickle cell disease. It is likely that acute pain crises reflect perturbations in the macrocirculation and microcirculation sufficiently complex and multifactorial to elude current understanding. From decades of careful clinical observations, Sergeant[276] has proposed that pain crises are sometimes triggered by circulatory reflexes. The acute onset of pain in an extremity after cold exposure may result in the diversion of blood flow away from the skin and bone marrow to shunts in the muscle with subsequent vaso-occlusion in the marrow. This mechanism would explain the remarkable symmetry of the distribution of pain, swelling, and osteonecrosis in the hand-foot syndrome as well as a significant proportion of pain crises in older patients. This interesting hypothesis begs for rigorous investigation in the whole organism.

There is confusion in the literature about the relationship between acute pain crises and the properties of SS red cells. There appears to be no consistent change in the percentage of circulating ISCs with the development of pain crises, although some of the ISCs have been noted to acquire a spiculated (echinocytic) shape during crisis.[280] The filterability of partially and fully oxygenated SS red cells is significantly decreased for several days after the onset of crises.[281–283] Because MCHC is the main determinant of red cell deformability, these observations are consistent with the report of a 54 per cent increase in the fraction of dense cells 3 to 4 days after crisis.[284] These density distribution measurements are difficult to reconcile with reports from another institution of a 51 per cent *decrease* in the fraction of dense cells 3 to 4 days after the onset of acute pain crisis (reference 285 and references therein).

Recent studies have addressed the relationship between acute pain crisis and the levels of inflammatory mediators in the plasma.[285a, 285b] Endothelin-1, a mediator of vasoconstriction, prostaglandin E_2,[285a] and the neuropeptide substance P[285c] are all elevated during crises. The challenge is to learn whether any of these molecules play a causal role in vaso-occlusive crises rather than reflecting a secondary response.

Transgenic Mouse Model. The large chasm between our thorough knowledge of the molecular basis of polymerization of Hb S and our rudimentary understanding of the temporal, regional, humoral, and neural factors that affect in vivo sickling is unlikely to be bridged by "traditional" investigations either at the laboratory bench or at the bedside. There is a critical need for an animal model that faithfully duplicates the hematological and vaso-occlusive manifestations of the disease. The development of transgenic mice bearing the β^S gene is a major advance toward achieving this end. It appears increasingly likely that this model will provide not only a deeper understanding of the pathogenesis of sickle cell disease but also an efficient and rigorous way of testing new and innovative therapies, before clinical trials in patients.[285d]

In the application of this technology to the study of globin gene regulation, considerable effort has been devoted toward the identification and characterization of the important tissue- and development-specific *cis*-acting elements of the human α and β genes that are responsible for their high-level expression in erythroid cells.*

A number of independent research groups have made transgenic mice that express the β^S gene. In an initial report,[286] only a small amount of β^S was expressed in the homozygote because the transgene lacked the control elements. The red cells failed to sickle in part because β^S/total β was only 10 per cent and in part because the hybrid tetramer $\alpha^M_2\beta^S_2$ lacks the appropriate α subunit contacts[287] owing to differences in primary sequence between mouse and man. These early experiments showed that it is necessary for the mouse red cells to contain high levels of human Hb S. Increased expression of Hb S has been achieved by injecting both α and β^S transgenes that each contain the appropriate globin gene control elements.[288, 289] These animals have 30 per cent to as much as 80 per cent Hb S in their red cells. Although they are not anemic or hemolytic, their red cells form polymer and assume classical sickle shapes when they are deoxygenated. The relative amount of Hb S in these transgenic animals can be further improved by breeding them into a background of mouse β thalassemia[286, 289, 290] and α thalassemia. Indeed, the β thalassemic mice that express the β^S transgene enjoy a partial correction of their anemia and red cell abnormalities owing to an improvement in chain imbalance.[291]

Additional strategies are available to further increase sickling to make the transgenic animal mimic the SS patient. One approach is to breed the Hb S–bearing transgene into mice that have left-shifted oxygen-binding curves owing to naturally occurring mutant mouse hemoglobins.[292] This would enhance the proportion of oxygen released from the Hb S and therefore promote sickling. Another option is to add mutations other than β^{6Val} that would further promote polymerization (see Structure of the Sickle Fiber). The naturally occurring mutant $\beta^{S \, Antilles}$ sickles more readily than β^S because the β^{6Val} substitution is combined with β^{23Ile}, which further stabilizes the sickle polymer.[293] Transgenic mice having 50 per cent $\beta^{S \, Antilles}$ (in a β thalassemic background) had readily demonstrable in vitro sickling and a widening of

---

*For further information on this topic, see Chapter 5.

their red cell volume profile when they were exposed to 10 days of hypoxia.[294] Mice have been prepared with a transgene containing β^{6Val}, β^{23Ile}, and a third mutation, β^{121Gln} (D–Los Angeles), which also promotes polymerization.[295] When bred into a homozygous β thalassemia background and a heterozygous α thalassemia background, the resulting SAD[0] transgenic mice have a severe hemolytic disease having several features in common with SS disease including hemolytic anemia and splenomegaly.[295–297] When the SAD transgene was bred into mice that have a high oxygen affinity hemoglobin mutant, the phenotype was even closer to that in human SS patients.[292]

The complicated genetic manipulations described in the preceding paragraph would be unnecessary if a transgenic mouse produced only human hemoglobin. Indeed, two laboratories have succeeded in preparing mice in which the endogenous α and β globin genes have been knocked out and in which the human transgene expresses both γ and β^S globin with the physiological fetal to adult switch.[298, 299] As a result, these animals have a "clinical" phenotype close to that of human SS disease and indeed have abnormalities in blood flow[299a] that approximate those observed in patients with SS disease. This impressive technological advance should greatly enhance the relevance and utility of the transgenic mouse model of sickle cell disease.

▼ EPIDEMIOLOGY OF SICKLE CELL DISEASE

Origin of the β^S Gene

In 1978, Kan and Dozy[300] discovered that in African-Americans with SS disease, the β^S gene is linked to a polymorphic restriction site *(HpaI)* in the 5′ flanking region. This finding led to the use of additional restriction enzymes that identified other β globin polymorphisms in populations with common hemoglobin disorders, particularly the thalassemias* and sickle cell disease. Populations in which large-scale migrations have been absent or limited have only a small number of specific polymorphism patterns, called haplotypes. These can be regarded as ancestral sequences of DNA. Description of haplotypes of the β globin gene complex has provided valuable information on important and diverse issues, such as the antenatal diagnosis of β thalassemia, the origin of the β^S and other β globin mutations, the migration of affected populations, and the phenotypic contribution of other genes or regulatory elements in *cis* to the β globin gene.

Labie, Nagel, and colleagues[301–303] have conducted extensive field trips in Africa to explore the genetic background of β^S genes and its impact on phenotype.† They have identified regions in central Africa, shown in Figure 7–21A, designated (from west to east) Senegal, Benin, and Central African Republic (CAR), also called Bantu, in which the β^S gene is nearly exclusively associated with a single and specific haplotype (Fig. 7–21B).‡

In each region, individuals with β^A genes have not only

this haplotype but also a few others. Therefore, it can be assumed that in each of these regions, the β^S gene arose as a spontaneous mutation in a chromosome bearing this haplotype. Because the gene confers fitness to malaria (see below), it became fixed in this region with a high frequency. Haplotypes identified by restriction site polymorphisms have been verified and refined by the association of specific variable tandem repeat polymorphisms.[303] These collective data strongly suggest that the β^S gene arose independently in at least three different times and locations in central Africa.

Further detailed analyses of these haplotypes have revealed subtle variations within each of these three population groups. In the Senegal and CAR areas, less than 10 per cent of the β^S chromosomes have atypical polymorphism patterns. About 80 per cent of the β^S CAR chromosomes have undergone a conversion event between the $^G\gamma$ and $^A\gamma$ genes.[305] Of these, about half have a 6 bp deletion 5′ to the $^G\gamma$ gene.[306] Heterogeneity at the 5′ end of the CAR haplotype can be explained by recombination in a hot spot in the $\psi\beta$ pseudogene 5′ to the β gene.[307]

Population Migrations. The study of β^S haplotypes has provided valuable insights into the history and route of movement of populations. For example, the geographical distribution of the CAR haplotype supports earlier linguistic evidence for the eastward and southward spread of the Negroes originally located in West Africa.[304] In contrast, populations sharing the Benin β^S haplotype migrated northward to Morocco, Algeria, and Egypt as well as across the Mediterranean to Sicily,[308] Greece,[309] and Turkey.* The fact that 100 per cent of the β^S chromosomes have the Benin haplotype in Sicily, whereas none of the β^A chromosomes does, provides compelling evidence for this northward migration.[308] β^S chromosomes in the western Arabian peninsula also have the Benin haplotype, indicating that the migration also extended northeastward across the Red Sea (Fig. 7–21A).

In contrast, in the eastern Arabian peninsula, individuals who have the β^S gene share a common and unique haplotype with those in the subcontinent of India. The frequency of the β^S gene is high among the scheduled tribes that are distributed throughout central and southern India. These tribal peoples live apart, outside of the mainstream of the Indian caste system.[304] The finding that these widely dispersed tribes share a common β^S haplotype provides evidence not only for a unicentric origin of the β^S gene in India but also for a common ancestry among the tribes.[310] The fact that all β^S chromosomes in eastern Arabia also share this haplotype begs the question of the actual origin of this mutation and the direction of the subsequent migration.

Investigation of β^S haplotypes also provides independent information about the slave trade to the New World. Analyses of β^S haplotypes in Jamaica, Cuba, and the United States are in remarkably good agreement with historical records from the 17th to 19th century of the place of origin of the slaves.[304]

Malaria and the Sickle Gene. Both the high frequency of the β^S gene in central Africa and its origination in at least three different locations can be explained by the fact that in

---

*For discussion of globin polymorphisms in the thalassemias, see Chapter 6.

†See review by Nagel and Ranney[304] for more detailed coverage of this topic.

‡A fourth African haplotype, differing from the other three in both 5′ and 3′ regions, has been found in a specific and restricted ethnic group designated Eton, originating in Cameroon.[304]

---

*In Portugal, all three haplotypes are found in association with the β^S gene, in keeping with the impact of frequent and extensive maritime voyages on the gene pool.[304]

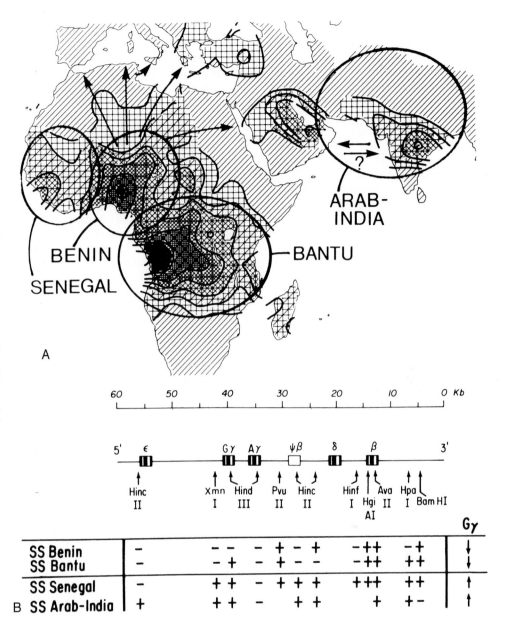

Figure 7–21. *A,* Map of Africa and Asia Minor and the Indian subcontinent. Regions of high frequency of the β^s gene are depicted by the dark-hatched textures. The four major β^s haplotypes are labeled according to their respective locales. The arrows depict flow of the β^s gene to North Africa, the Mediterranean, and the Arabian Peninsula. *B,* The β globin gene cluster and the major restriction fragment length polymorphisms (RFLPs) that determine the four major β^s-linked haplotypes. (*A* and *B* from Nagel, R.L., and Ranney, H.M.: Genetic epidemiology of structural mutations of the β-globin gene. Semin. Hematol. 27:342, 1990; with permission.)

	Hinc II	Xmn I	Hind III	Pvu II	Hinc II	Hinf I	Hgi AI	Ava II	Hpa I Bam HI	Gγ
SS Benin	–	–	–	–	+	–	+	–++	– +	↓
SS Bantu	–	–	+	–	+	–	–	–++	++	↓
SS Senegal	–	+	+	–	+	+	+	+++	++	↑
SS Arab-India	+	+	+	–		+	+	+	+–	↑

heterozygotes, the gene confers increased fitness, almost certainly by enhancing resistance against malaria.[311, 312] In evolutionary terms, the high morbidity and mortality of the SS homozygote is a small price to pay for improved survival of the much more common heterozygote. This phenomenon is probably the best studied and understood example in human biology of "balanced polymorphism." AS heterozygotes become infected with *Plasmodium falciparum* at about the same rate as AA individuals do, but fewer die of the infection.[313] Experiments have demonstrated that transgenic mice expressing sickle hemoglobin are protected from lethal malaria.[314]

The molecular basis for this enhanced resistance is still not fully understood. In 1970, Luzzato and colleagues[315] reported that parasitization of AS red cells greatly accelerated their rate of sickling. The enhanced clearance of these rigid cells thus facilitated the host's destruction of the parasite. The sickling of parasitized AS red cells may be further enhanced by the adherence of trophozoite-induced knobs to the venular endothelium.[316] The decreased rate of growth of *P. falciparum* in AS red cells compared with AA red cells has been attributed to a lower level of intracellular K^+ induced by sickling. However, it is likely that intracellular polymerization rather than cation content is the primary deterrent to parasite growth.[311] Sickle polymers are a poor substrate for malarial proteases.

Genetic Modulators of Sickle Cell Disease

Relation of β^s Haplotype to Phenotype. The demonstration of multiple origins of the β^s gene raises questions about whether, among these genes, there are differences in *cis* that have a significant impact on disease phenotype. To answer this question, Nagel and colleagues as well as others have collected a considerable amount of genetic and clinical data both in the United States and all over the world. There is solid agreement that the β^s haplotype has a significant bearing on the ratio of $^G\gamma$ to $^A\gamma$ production, which is normally about 60:40 at birth but after about 4 months of life changes to about 40:60 (see Chapter 5). The Senegal and the Arab-Indian haplotypes are associated with maintenance of the newborn ratio into adult life, whereas the Benin and CAR haplotypes are associated with a normal switch after birth.[146, 317]

SS individuals homozygous for the Senegal β^S haplotype also appear to have higher levels of Hb F compared with Benin and CAR homozygotes, although there is considerable spread in the data.[146, 304, 318] This relationship may be stronger for African patients[146, 317] than for SS patients in the United States, where conflicting results have been obtained.[319-321] An even more complex issue is whether the β^S haplotype affects the degree of anemia and clinical course of SS homozygotes. Again, conflicting results have been reported.[319-321] In interpreting these reports, two separate issues are relevant. There may be additional genetic modulators, not linked to the β^S gene, that are fixed in African populations and independently affect the severity of SS disease among the Senegals, Benins, and CARs. Second, despite the large number of American and Jamaican patients studied (60 in reference 319, 113 in reference 320), the results are confounded by genetic admixture. The Benin haplotype is strongly favored. Therefore, there is ample access to Benin homozygotes, whereas there is a relative paucity of Americans and Jamaicans homozygous for the Senegal and CAR haplotypes. Results on the remaining heterozygotes are difficult to interpret.

SS homozygotes from eastern Arabia and India, who share a common and distinct β globin haplotype, have unusually mild disease, owing primarily to high levels of Hb F and perhaps also to a high gene frequency for α thalassemia (see below). The high Hb F appears to be linked to the β^S gene.[322] Thus, the Arab-Indian haplotype can be considered a marker for increased expression of Hb F.* Hemolytic stress is apparently required for this effect because it is seen only in SS homozygotes. AS heterozygotes bearing this haplotype have normal levels of Hb F. In addition, there may be other genetic modulators that have an impact on γ gene expression in these populations.

X-Linked Determinant of Hb F Production. A survey of a large number of people in Japan revealed that the distribution of Hb F and F cells was affected by gender.[323] Relatively high levels (>0.7 per cent Hb F and >4.4 per cent F cells) were encountered in about 10 per cent of men and 20 per cent of women. Family studies on these high F individuals strongly suggested an X-linked determinant of Hb F production. Dover and colleagues[324] have confirmed these findings in African-Americans. From analysis of polymorphic restriction sites on sib pairs of SS homozygotes, they have shown that this Hb F production gene is controlled by a locus on Xp22.2. This gene accounts for 40 per cent of the variation in Hb F among sickle cell homozygotes.[325]

Concurrent α Thalassemia. As explained in detail in Chapter 6, deletion of one of the two tandem α globin genes

is commonly encountered among all populations in which the β^S gene is fixed at high frequency. About 30 per cent of Afro-Americans are heterozygotes ($-\alpha/\alpha\alpha$) and about 3 per cent are homozygotes ($-\alpha/-\alpha$).[326, 327] The frequency of α thalassemia is even higher among Arabs and Asian Indians who have the β^S gene. Among Africans, the majority have the "rightward deletion" $-\alpha$ haplotype[328] (also see Chapter 6), although the "leftward deletion" has been reported.[329] Deletion of both α globin genes ($--$) occurs rarely in Africans.[330] Accordingly, α thalassemia is of little clinical significance among Africans. However, the coexistence of the $-\alpha/\alpha\alpha$ or the $-\alpha/-\alpha$ in Africans with the β^S gene affects the phenotype of both sickle trait (AS) and homozygous (SS) disease.

There is a trimodal distribution of Hb S and Hb A in red cells of AS heterozygotes that correlates strongly with the number of α globin genes. Non-thalassemic AS individuals have about 40 per cent Hb S, whereas those with $-\alpha/\alpha\alpha$ have about 35 per cent and those with $-\alpha/-\alpha$ have about 28 per cent (see Fig. 7–7B). The most reliable and uniform manifestation of in vivo sickling in AS individuals is a defect in the ability of the renal medulla to produce concentrated urine. This defect varies directly with the percentage of Hb S in the AS red cells and therefore with the number of α globin genes.[331]

The impact of α thalassemia on SS disease is more complex.* As expected, the mean corpuscular volume (MCV) decreases in proportion to the number of α globin genes deleted. Of note is a parallel reduction in the severity of anemia. SS patients with the $-\alpha/-\alpha$ genotype have a mean hemoglobin of 9.0 g/dl, compared with 7.9 g/dl in those without α thalassemia.[334-336] α Thalassemia ameliorates the degree of hemolysis[337] primarily by a reduction in dense cells, in ISCs, and in intracellular hemoglobin concentration, phenomena that greatly inhibit intracellular polymerization. The combination of fewer reticulocytes (light cells) and fewer dense cells results in a more narrow red cell density distribution profile.[338] Cation leak in deoxygenated SS cells is significantly reduced in the presence of α thalassemia,[318] in keeping with decreased potential for intracellular polymerization. In like manner, the deformability of SS red cells is increased in proportion to the number of α globin genes deleted.[339] However, at a given density fraction, deformability is unaffected by α thalassemia.[339] Thus, α thalassemia affects the properties of SS red cell primarily through its impact on cell density and intracellular hemoglobin concentration. The coexistence of α thalassemia is associated with a slight decrease in the percentage of Hb F and F cells, in keeping with a comparatively slight reduction in the preferential survival of F cells.[338, 340] Because of their lower MCHC, the non-F cells do not undergo such a rapid transition to dense cells[338] and therefore have improved survival.

Despite the significant impact of α thalassemia on hematological values in SS disease and on the properties of SS red cells, it has little impact on the clinical manifestations of the disease. Specifically, three studies[321, 335, 336] agree that the incidence of acute pain crises is not affected by the α globin gene number. Concurrent α thalassemia may be associated with a lower incidence of leg ulcers[321, 335] and

---

*This contention is supported by the observation that although the Arab-Indian haplotype is encountered only rarely in Jamaican SS patients, it is invariably associated with high levels of Hb F.[322] Non-linked genes for enhanced γ globin expression in the Arab-Indian populations would be diluted out in these Jamaican patients.

---

*For more information on this topic, see reviews by Steinberg and Embury[332] and by Embury.[333]

protection against sickle cell glomerulopathy,[340a] but with an increased risk for development of avascular bone necrosis[341, 342] and perhaps retinopathy.[343] It is of interest that these last two complications also occur often in SC disease and S/β thalassemia. The development of bone necrosis and retinopathy may be enhanced by a relatively high hemoglobin level, a feature shared by all three of these forms of sickle cell disease. Because α thalassemia has such little impact on the clinical manifestation of SS disease, it is surprising that it has been associated with improved survival.[344] This report needs to be verified by the study of a larger, well-characterized population.

It may be overly simplistic to assume that the effects of α thalassemia on SS disease all stem from reduction in cell density and intracellular hemoglobin concentration. The low MCV or the more redundant red cell membrane in SS patients with α thalassemia might independently affect the hematological or clinical SS phenotype.[333]

Glucose-6-Phosphate Dehydrogenase Deficiency. The most common genetic abnormality among populations with a high frequency of the β^S gene is deficiency of erythrocyte glucose-6-phosphate dehydrogenase (G6PD). About 10 per cent of African-American males are deficient in this enzyme, which is encoded by a gene on the X chromosome. About the same proportion of American males with SS disease are G6PD deficient. Past reports (cited in reference 345) have been conflicting, claiming that the deficiency state has beneficial, harmful, or no influence on the hematological or clinical manifestations of SS disease. The Cooperative Study of Sickle Cell Disease has settled this issue by a definitive analysis of a large number (801) of male patients with SS disease.[345] G6PD deficiency had no effect on the hematological values, morbidity (pain crises, episodes of sepsis, anemic crises), or mortality of these SS patients.

▼ COMPOUND HETEROZYGOUS STATES: SC AND S/βTHAL

SC Disease

Hemoglobin C. To understand the molecular pathogenesis of SC disease, it is necessary to first discuss the properties and phenotypic features of Hb C ($\beta^{6Glu \rightarrow Lys}$), the third most commonly encountered mutant worldwide, next to Hb S and Hb E. The frequency of the β^C gene in areas of West Africa, particularly Ghana and Upper Volta, approaches 0.15.[5] Among American blacks, the gene frequency is 0.010 to 0.012. AC heterozygotes have no clinical manifestations and normal hematological values except for slightly dehydrated and dense red cells, which appear as target cells on stained blood films. CC homozygotes have a mild hemolytic anemia and moderate splenic enlargement.[346] CC red cells are markedly dehydrated with increased MCHC. The primary morphological feature is the presence of plump target cells.

The clinical and hematological phenotype of AC and CC individuals can be explained by two relevant properties of Hb C. The replacement of β6 glutamic acid by lysine results in a significant decrease in solubility of both oxygenated and deoxy forms, resulting in the formation of crystals. In CC patients who have undergone splenectomy, occasional red cells will contain elongated rectangular crystals of oxy-

hemoglobin.[66] Larger and more frequent crystals can be induced by incubating CC red cells in a hypertonic medium. The crystallization of oxy Hb C is inhibited by the presence of Hb F, primarily at γ^{87Gln}.[347] Accordingly, no Hb F is incorporated into the crystal. In contrast, the presence of Hb S increases the rate at which Hb C forms crystals.[348] Moreover, such crystals contain Hb S in addition to Hb C. The other relevant property of Hb C is its ability to stimulate K:Cl cotransport to an even greater extent than Hb S[69] (see earlier section, Disordered Volume Control). As a result of K^+ efflux and accompanying water loss, CC red cells rapidly become dehydrated, dense, and targeted. It is not known why CC and even AC red cells have enhanced K:Cl cotransport. It is noteworthy that Hb C binds more avidly than does Hb A to protein 3 on the inner surface of the red cell membrane.[349]

Clinical Features of SC Disease. Among American blacks, the β^S gene occurs about three times as frequently as the β^C gene. However, the prevalence of SC disease is nearly that of SS disease, owing to the higher mortality of the homozygous state. SC patients have a mild hemolytic anemia. The peripheral blood smear reveals plump target cells. Some are pointed at opposite ends, resembling broad-beamed canoes. Classical ISCs are not seen. Occasional cells contain crystals, and others may have round hemoglobin aggregates (billiard ball cells).[200, 350] Patients with SC disease may develop any of the vaso-occlusive complications seen in SS homozygotes, although such events are generally less frequent and severe. However, a few exceptions are noteworthy. Proliferative retinopathy is more common in SC patients than in SS homozygotes. Aseptic necrosis of the femoral head and hematuria from renal medullary infarction occur almost as frequently in SC disease as in SS disease.

Pathogenesis of SC Disease. Why do SC individuals have significantly more morbidity than AS individuals? When incubated at decreased oxygen tensions, SC cells sickle much more readily than AS cells. The increased tendency to form polymer cannot be explained by enhanced co-polymerization of Hb S with Hb C.[68, 351] Rather, the enhanced sickling of SC cells can be attributed to two independent phenomena.[68] First, SC cells contain about 25 per cent more Hb S than do AS cells owing to a slower rate of assembly of Hb C compared with Hb A.[59] Second, SC red cells have a higher MCHC and a significantly higher proportion of dense cells, compared with AS cells,[67, 68] owing to the contribution of Hb C to increased K:Cl cotransport, which, as explained before (see Disordered Volume Control), leads to K^+ and water loss.[69, 350] In view of the importance of intracellular hemoglobin concentration on the kinetics of polymerization of Hb S, it is not surprising that a patient with both SC disease and concurrent hereditary spherocytosis* had unusually severe clinical manifestations and laboratory evidence of enhanced sickling.[352]

S/β Thalassemia

Individuals who inherit the β^S gene from one parent and a β thalassemia gene from the other have a disorder that is highly variable in severity and laboratory manifestations. If

---

*This congenital disorder of the red cell skeleton is associated with increased intracellular hemoglobin concentration.

the β thalassemia allele is incapable of producing any normal subunit, the patient will have S/β⁰ thalassemia and red cells containing Hb S (80 to 95 per cent), Hb F (2 to 20 per cent), and Hb A_2 (2 to 4 per cent). In contrast, if the β thalassemia allele is capable of some synthesis of βᴬ, the patient will have S/β⁺ thalassemia and red cells containing Hb S (55 to 75 per cent), Hb A (10 to 30 per cent), Hb F (1 to 13 per cent), and Hb A_2 (3 to 6 per cent). Large-scale clinical studies both in the United States and in Jamaica have demonstrated that the clinical and hematological severity of S/β⁰ thalassemia is on a par with that of SS disease, although milder in certain features and perhaps more severe in others. As mentioned above, patients with S/β⁰ thalassemia apparently have more frequent pain crises than have those with SS disease.[275, 276] In contrast, patients with S/β⁺ thalassemia have relatively mild clinical manifestations. As in SC disease, S/β⁺ thalassemia patients have a high incidence of proliferative retinopathy.

The marked clinical severity of S/β⁰ thalassemia is puzzling. Measurements of red cell indices consistently show a reduction in MCHC. Accordingly, the rate and extent of polymer formation should be correspondingly reduced. There is a need for careful measurements of cell density distributions in S/β⁰ thalassemia blood specimens. The fact that ISCs are commonly encountered must mean that accelerated cell dehydration is taking place. It may be that the α subunits, present in excess because of the imbalance in hemoglobin synthesis, triggers K:Cl cotransport, leading to increased K⁺ and water loss.

▼ ADVANCES IN MANAGEMENT OF SICKLE CELL DISEASE

Antenatal Diagnosis*

A family who is at risk for having a baby with SS disease might decide to interrupt the pregnancy if the diagnosis were established safely, accurately, and early in gestation. Clearly, this is a highly sensitive issue that requires skilled and empathetic counseling coupled with access to up-to-date diagnostic facilities.

Considerable advances have been made in the technology for the antenatal diagnosis of the hemoglobinopathies. Initially, it was necessary to assess globin chain synthesis in a sample of fetal blood to establish diagnoses in utero of sickle cell disease or one of the clinically significant thalassemias. This approach has been supplanted by analysis of globin DNA.[354] Adaptation of the polymerase chain reaction[355, 356] has enabled accurate diagnoses of the SS, AS, and AA genotypes to be made simply and rapidly on small amounts of DNA. The development of chorionic villus biopsy[357] permits samples to be obtained safely during weeks 6 to 10 of gestation, whereas amniocentesis cannot be performed before the 15th week.

In a worldwide survey of all antenatal diagnoses done for hemoglobinopathies from 1974 through 1989, 2800 or 14 per cent were on fetuses at risk for sickle cell disease.[358] Nearly all of these cases were from the United States and Canada. In recent years, more than 90 per cent of sickle cell cases used analyses of DNA rather than fetal blood. Even though the accuracy of diagnosis has increased to more than

99.5 per cent and the incidence of fetal loss has fallen, the procedure has thus far had little impact on the prevention of SS disease. Only a small fraction of the families in the United States at risk for having a baby with SS disease have taken advantage of antenatal diagnosis. Moreover, even when the diagnosis of SS disease is established in a fetus, approximately one third of families surveyed[358] have elected to continue the pregnancy. This percentage depends in part on the effectiveness of the diagnostic and counseling services that are provided to the families at risk. In contrast, a recent study from Africa reveals that 96 per cent of women carrying a fetus with SS disease elect to terminate the pregnancy.[358a]

Newborn Screening and Prophylaxis

During the last decade, considerable advances have been made in reducing the morbidity and mortality of SS disease, particularly during the first 10 years of life. Because the Hb F to Hb S switch does not occur until about 6 months after birth, SS newborns are clinically and phenotypically normal. Nevertheless, the diagnosis of SS disease and of the clinically significant compound heterozygous states can be readily made on a small sample of cord blood either by routine electrophoretic methods or by analysis of DNA.[359] There is ample evidence that early diagnosis as a result of screening newborns has greatly improved the care of children with sickle cell disease.[360, 361] Parents benefit from an orderly and comprehensive education about the disease, including relevant preventive measures (see below) and advice on when and how to seek medical help. The child has a greater chance of enrolling into a health care system that is experienced and knowledgeable about sickle cell disease. Newborn screening and follow-up appear to be cost-effective in regions that have a relatively high incidence of the βˢ gene[361] but probably not in regions where sickle cell disease is infrequently encountered.[362]

During infancy and early childhood, infections, especially due to *Streptococcus pneumoniae*, are the major cause of morbidity and mortality. The incidence and severity of pneumococcal sepsis are retarded but not eliminated by polyvalent vaccination. Large-scale clinical trials[363, 364] have provided conclusive evidence for the efficacy of prophylactic penicillin. In comparison to a placebo group, those receiving oral penicillin G had an 84 per cent reduction in the incidence of pneumococcal sepsis.[364]

Rational Approaches to Antisickling Therapy

The preceding portion of this chapter presents a synopsis of biochemical, genetic, and clinical studies that have greatly advanced our understanding of the molecular and cellular pathogenesis of sickle cell disease. From the current body of information, three independent rational approaches to therapy have been developed: chemical inhibition of Hb S polymerization, reduction of intracellular hemoglobin concentration (MCHC), and pharmacological induction of fetal hemoglobin (Hb F). This topic has recently been reviewed by Bunn[364a] and by Steinberg.[364b]

Inhibitors of Hb S Polymerization

Detailed information on the three-dimensional structure of the Hb S polymer (see Figs. 7–9 to 7–11) has facilitated the

---

*For more information on this topic, see review by Old and colleagues.[353]

design and development of compounds that inhibit polymerization.[365–368] Although a review of the large literature on this topic is beyond the scope of this chapter, a few underlying principles merit discussion. Inhibitors of sickling can be classified as covalent versus non-covalent and also by their mechanism of action. Compounds that bind covalently to hemoglobin are more likely to have therapeutic potential. The non-covalent inhibitors described to date would not be effective drugs because they bind relatively weakly to Hb S, and therefore a high plasma concentration would be required for a significant fraction of the hemoglobin to be modified. However, it is possible that a non-covalent inhibitor could be designed that binds to Hb S with such high affinity that the plasma concentration would be relatively low and non-toxic.

Inhibitors of sickling could work either by increasing oxygen affinity, thereby decreasing the relative amount of deoxy Hb S in the red cell, or by binding to contact sites on the Hb S fiber, thereby inhibiting polymer assembly or growth. The in vivo administration of gaseous NO was reported to increase the whole blood oxygen affinity of sickle cell patients but with no effect on normal AA blood.[369] However, this finding could not be confirmed in a subsequent study.[369a] The decreased P_{50} of SS red cells after NO treatment is puzzling. The strategy of treating sickle cell disease by increasing red cell oxygen affinity may be a problem because any compound that significantly increases oxygen affinity is likely to induce an increase in red cell production. As discussed elsewhere in this chapter, there is good clinical evidence that an increase in red cell mass has a significant negative impact on the clinical course of sickle cell disease.

The design of a safe and effective inhibitor of Hb S polymer assembly is a formidable challenge. The ideal agent should be readily absorbed through the gastrointestinal tract, circulate in the plasma without strong binding to plasma proteins, readily penetrate the erythrocyte membrane, bind strongly and specifically to Hb S in a way that will inhibit polymerization but not affect physiological oxygen transport, and bind minimally to other biologically important molecules. Unfortunately, an Ehrlichian "magic bullet" for sickle cell disease still eludes us. No antisickling agents tested thus far can be regarded as safe and effective therapy.

Reduction of MCHC

Because the rate of polymerization of sickle hemoglobin is so exquisitely dependent on Hb S concentration (see Fig. 7–15), any treatment that lowers MCHC has a sound rationale. The simplest approach is induction of hyponatremia, thereby causing osmotic swelling of red cells.[370] Although with careful monitoring this treatment appears to be effective, it is too cumbersome and risky to be adapted to chronic outpatient care.[371]

Considerable progress has been made in the development of drugs that inhibit K^+ and water loss from SS red cells, thereby resulting in a reduction in intracellular hemoglobin concentration. The Gardos channel is specifically inhibited by the widely used antifungal drug clotrimazole. The efficacy of this drug has been demonstrated by in vitro incubation experiments,[372] studies in transgenic mice with sickle cell disease,[373] and observations on SS patients.[374] At lower doses than those used for antifungal therapy, clotri-

mazole treatment of five SS patients resulted in a prompt and striking reduction in dense and irreversibly sickled cells and an increase in intracellular K^+, accompanied by a modest increase in hemoglobin concentration and a significant decrease in serum unconjugated bilirubin concentration, indicating amelioration of hemolysis.

There is no known pharmacological inhibitor of K:Cl cotransport, the other major pathway for K^+ efflux and dehydration. However, intracellular divalent cations, particularly Mg^{2+}, effectively retard K^+ and water loss from SS red cells in vitro.[202] In vivo administration of magnesium supplements to transgenic mice with sickle cell disease[375] and to 11 patients with SS disease resulted in approximately 50 per cent inhibition of K:Cl cotransport, accompanied by a significant decrease in dense erythrocytes and an increase in hemoglobin concentration.[376]

The efficacy of clotrimazole and magnesium therapies in lowering the fraction of dense SS red cells provides strong evidence of the importance of the Gardos and K:Cl cotransport pathways in the pathogenesis of cell dehydration.

Induction of Hb F

In 1948, Watson reported that the red corpuscles of newborns with sickle cell anemia did not sickle as readily as those of older children with the disease.[377] She attributed this to the high percentage of fetal hemoglobin (Hb F) that is still present at the time of birth. Subsequent studies (see Sickle Hemoglobin Polymerization, Non-S Hemoglobins) confirmed that Hb F is indeed a potent inhibitor of polymerization of deoxyhemoglobin S. In certain populations, such as Bedouin Arabs and Veddoid Indians, SS homozygotes produce relatively high amounts of Hb F (see Genetic Modulators of Sickle Cell Disease). In view of the marked effect of Hb F in impeding Hb S polymerization, it is not surprising that these patients have relatively mild clinical manifestations. The inhibitory effect of Hb F extends to all homozygotes. A study of the natural history of SS patients in the United States showed that the frequency of pain crises correlated inversely with the level of Hb F.[275]

Because of the compelling biochemical and clinical evidence that Hb F inhibits sickling, therapeutic agents that increase Hb F production would be expected to benefit patients with sickle cell disease. Indeed, recent studies with biotin-labeled SS red cells show that the F cells have an in vivo survival of 6 to 8 weeks whereas those lacking HbF have a life span of about 2 weeks.[377a] The first drug to be tested was 5-azacytidine, an antineoplastic drug known to inhibit maintenance methylation of DNA. DeSimone and colleagues[378] knew that actively expressed genes are generally hypomethylated and that in erythroid cells, with the developmental switch from γ globin to β globin production, the inactive γ gene becomes methylated. Therefore, they reasoned that the administration of 5-azacytidine might turn on dormant γ globin production. They showed that anemic baboons developed a marked increase in Hb F a few weeks after receiving the drug. These results prompted limited clinical trials demonstrating significant, albeit somewhat less dramatic, induction of Hb F production in patients with homozygous β thalassemia and sickle cell disease.[379–381]

Hydroxyurea. Subsequently, other antitumor agents including cytosine arabinoside[382, 383] and hydroxyurea[384, 385] have also been shown to induce increased production of fetal hemoglobin in primates[382, 384] as well as in man.[383, 385–393] Because these agents are not known to be a direct cause of hypomethylation, the molecular mechanism through which they induce Hb F production remains enigmatic.

Despite the considerable interest in alternative means of inducing Hb F in sickle cell patients, hydroxyurea is currently the only agent shown to provide safe and effective therapy. It is relatively non-toxic, its myelosuppressive effects are readily reversible, and it is not known to induce secondary malignant neoplasms. During the last 20 years, the major use of hydroxyurea has been in myeloproliferative diseases, in which it has been noted to induce modest increases in Hb F levels.[394] Much more impressive increases in Hb F have been noted in sickle cell disease.[385–393] Among 32 SS patients treated with hydroxyurea, the mean Hb F level was 14.9 per cent compared with a mean value of 3.7 per cent before treatment.[393] The great majority of SS patients who are given sufficient doses to cause mild myelosuppression develop a marked increase in F cells and percentage of Hb F[386–392] as well as an increase in Hb F per F cell.[389, 391] This effect is accompanied by an increase in hemoglobin coupled with a decreased reticulocyte count indicative of a decrease in hemolytic rate. Prolonged survival of ^{51}Cr-labeled autologous red cells and reduction in serum non-conjugated bilirubin and lactate dehydrogenase document the decrease in hemolysis.[390, 391]

These improvements in hematological parameters during hydroxyurea therapy are accompanied by objective evidence of inhibition of intracellular polymerization of Hb S. There is a significant decrease in irreversibly sickled cells[391, 392] and dense cells[390–392] as well as in vitro measurements of sickling.[391] There are conflicting reports on whether hydroxyurea therapy affects the cation content of SS red cells.[390–392] Preliminary data on a small number of SS patients indicated that treatment results in amelioration of pain crises.[388, 391]

A national multicenter 2-year clinical trial of hydroxyurea in 299 adult patients with sickle cell disease revealed it to be relatively non-toxic and effective not only in increasing Hb F levels[395–397] but also in reducing the frequency and severity of pain crises, along with decreasing the incidence of acute chest syndrome and the need for transfusions.[395, 396] A cross-over study of 22 children with sickle cell disease also demonstrated a substantial reduction in clinical events requiring hospitalization.[398] Subsequently, larger clinical studies have verified the efficacy[398a] and safety[398b] of hydroxyurea administered to children over an approximately 2-year period.

It is generally assumed that the beneficial effects of hydroxyurea treatment of patients with sickle cell disease are due to the induction of Hb F. However, a detailed multivariable analysis of data from the multicenter study showed that the percentage of F cells correlated inversely with rate of pain crises only during the initial 3 months of therapy. In contrast, there was a strong correlation between neutrophil count and crisis rate throughout the 2-year study.[396] Thus, the modest neutropenia that accompanies hydroxyurea treatment may contribute to the drug's efficacy. This finding may be linked to the experimental observation (discussed above) that SS neutrophils have enhanced binding to fibronectin.[260] In addition, the benefit of hydroxyurea therapy may be due in part to a reduction in reticulocytes

and young, low-density SS red cells, because these cells are particularly likely to adhere to vascular endothelium. Indeed, after initiation of treatment with hydroxyurea, the adhesion of patients' red cells to cultured endothelial cells decreased markedly within 2 weeks, long before there is a significant induction of Hb F.[399] This result may be due to suppression by hydroxyurea of expression of $\alpha_4\beta_1$ and CD36 on the surface of reticulocytes.[239] Because hydroxyurea treatment also partially suppresses erythropoiesis, this reduction of young adherent cells is accompanied by only a modest increase in red cell mass. A full compensatory response to the reduction in hemolysis might have adverse rheological consequences.

As experience with long-term treatment of patients with sickle cell disease with hydroxyurea increases, there is appropriate concern about the possible induction of tumors. The risk appears to be small in patients with myeloproliferative disorders who have taken the drug for up to 10 years. Despite 2 years of hydroxyurea treatment in 32 patients with sickle cell disease, no increase in chromosome abnormalities in bone marrow cells was seen.[393]

Erythropoietin. Even though hydroxyurea is relatively non-toxic, there are legitimate concerns about long-term administration of any antitumor drug to patients with a congenital non-malignant disorder. Accordingly, there is considerable interest in identifying safe alternatives for inducing Hb F production. Recombinant human erythropoietin (rhEPO) has proved to be both extremely effective and remarkably non-toxic therapy for the anemia of chronic renal disease.[400, 401] Preliminary studies indicated that rhEPO stimulated Hb F production not only in primates[402] but also in patients with sickle cell anemia.[388] When six SS patients were treated with weekly high-dose rhEPO, there was no increase of F reticulocytes, F cells, or percentage of Hb F.[391] Subsequently, the same dosage schedule of rhEPO was given to nine SS patients.[403] Five had no significant response. In four patients who also received supplemental iron therapy, rhEPO treatment was associated with a significant increase in F reticulocytes but no significant increase in F cells.

SS patients might derive benefit from a combination of hydroxyurea and rhEPO. Three patients who had achieved maximal induction of Hb F from daily treatment with hydroxyurea had no significant increment from the addition of weekly high-dose rhEPO.[391] However, high-dose rhEPO, in combination with iron supplementation, induces further Hb F production in patients receiving pulse hydroxyurea therapy (four consecutive days per week).[404] It is likely that this dose of hydroxyurea was suboptimal, because of intermittent administration as well as the possibility that iron therapy partially offset the drug's inhibition of ribonucleotide reductase.[405] Further treatment trials with different dose schedules are needed to assess whether the addition of rhEPO will provide an effective and sustained increment in Hb F production, thereby permitting the use of lower and less toxic doses of hydroxyurea.

Butyrates. There has been considerable interest in the physiological and pharmacological roles of butyric acid and analogues thereof in the regulation of Hb F production. Ginder and colleagues[406, 407] found that when adult anemic chickens were treated with a combination of 5-azacytidine and sodium butyrate, there was selective hypomethylation and reactivation of embryonic globin gene expression. Perrine and coworkers[408] showed that the switch from Hb F to Hb A is delayed in infants of diabetic mothers in association with increased levels of a amino-N-butyric acid. They found that the addition of this metabolite enhanced γ globin and suppressed β globin expression in cultured neonatal human cells.[409] Moreover, this metabolite as well as sodium butyrate enhanced γ globin gene expression in erythroid progenitors of patients with SS disease and β thalassemia.[410] These in vitro results led to in vivo infusions of butyrate into fetuses of sheep[411] and normal baboons.[412] In both animal models, there were substantial increases of Hb F production. These promising animal studies prompted further investigation of butyrate compounds in patients with hemoglobin disorders. There are conflicting reports regarding efficacy of arginine butyrate in patients with β thalassemia and sickle cell disease.[413, 414] both the efficacy and safety of arginine butyrate appear to be enhanced by intermittent or pulse therapy.[414a] Analogues of butyrate as well as of acetate[415] and other short chain fatty acid derivatives[416, 417] also appear to induce Hb F. Clearly, more studies are needed to assess the efficacy and safety of these potentially non-teratogenic and non-mutagenic means of inducing Hb F production.

Hemoglobin Mutants With a Thalassemia Phenotype

Thus far, about 30 human hemoglobin mutants have been found to be associated with a thalassemia-like red cell morphology including microcytosis, hypochromia, and often stippling.[418, 419]* These include 14 α globin mutants, 13 β globin mutants, and 3 $\delta\beta$ fusion mutants (the Lepore hemoglobins). Clinical severity in heterozygotes varies considerably from normal hemoglobin levels and reticulocyte counts to marked hemolysis or ineffective erythropoiesis.

Some of these thalassemia-like mutants have arisen because of interesting molecular mechanisms. These include elongated subunits, such as Hb Constant Spring, because of the mutations in the termination codon; the $\delta\beta$ fusion products because of non-homologous cross-over; and mutations such as Hb E that cause abnormal splicing.

Hb E is the most commonly encountered hemoglobin mutant worldwide. The frequency of the Hb E gene approaches 0.5 in regions of Laos and Thailand.[304] As discussed in detail in Chapter 6, the production of Hb E, both at the mRNA level and at the protein level, is impaired because the base substitution giving rise to $\beta^{26Glu \rightarrow Lys}$ also created a surrogate splice junction leading to a reduction in the level of correctly spliced mRNA. Hb EE homozygotes have microcytic red cells but no significant anemia, hemolysis, or clinical problems. Hb E poses a problem only when it coexists in the compound heterozygous state with β thalassemia.

Several of the α globin mutants have a thalassemia phenotype because they are invariably linked to a tandem α globin gene deletion. The most common of these are Hb G Philadelphia and Hb Hasharon.

Some mutants consist of single amino acid replacements that confer such instability that the mutant subunit can be detected only by special techniques, such as by radioactive labeling of newly synthesized transient subunits. Both the mutant β chain and its normal α chain partner precipitate in erythroblasts, shortly after their synthesis.[420] The first and best known example of this is Hb Terra Haute ($\beta^{112Leu \rightarrow Arg}$), originally called Hb Indianapolis.* Most of these mutants involve exon 3 of the β-globin gene.[419]

As information accumulates on well-characterized mutant hemoglobins, it is becoming apparent that there is a continuum that blurs the boundaries between those inducing a thalassemia phenotype and those that give rise to congenital Heinz body hemolysis. The former mutants (described above) have such extreme instability that they are readily degraded in bone marrow precursor cells, resulting in a thalassemia phenotype with ineffective erythropoiesis. The latter mutants, described in the next section, have intermediate stability and form Heinz bodies in circulating red blood cells, resulting in hemolysis.

The Unstable Hemoglobin Mutants (Congenital Heinz Body Hemolytic Anemia)

In 1952, Cathie[422] described a patient with congenital nonspherocytic hemolytic anemia associated with jaundice, splenomegaly, and pigmenturia. Subsequently, other patients with similar clinical findings were suspected of having a structurally abnormal hemoglobin because their hemolysates formed a precipitate readily on heating. In most cases, structural analyses have demonstrated mutant hemoglobins. So-called congenital Heinz body hemolytic anemia (CHBA) constitutes an important type of congenital hemolytic disease. Although the term is widely used, CHBA is a misnomer. Because of its variable severity, clinical manifestations may not appear until later in childhood or in adulthood, and Heinz bodies are not always present.

Unstable hemoglobinopathy has an autosomal dominant pattern of inheritance. Thus, affected individuals are heterozygotes. The unstable hemoglobin constitutes only a minority (10 to 30 per cent) of the total. As expected in the heterozygous state, the remaining hemoglobin is predominantly normal Hb A. A sizable minority of cases of unstable hemoglobinopathy appear to have arisen because of a spontaneous mutation, with both parents being unaffected.[423] Viewed another way, of the instances of apparent spontaneous mutations among hemoglobin mutants reported to date, approximately two thirds involve patients with unstable hemoglobins. This is not surprising because many cases are sufficiently severe that medical attention and evaluation are sought. In contrast, the chances are remote of finding an asymptomatic individual with a hemoglobin mutant due to a spontaneous mutation. Furthermore, the potential of patients

---

*These mutants are discussed in more detail in Chapter 6. In addition, see reviews by Adams and Coleman[418] and by Kazazian and associates.[419]

*By means of elegant high-resolution analyses of radiolabeled peptides, Adams and colleagues concluded that this mutant was $\beta^{112Cys \rightarrow Arg}$. However, a second report of a mutant with this replacement but without a thalassemic phenotype prompted Adams and colleagues[421] to re-examine their case. The patient was deceased and the only available specimen was some old bone marrow slides. Analysis of minute amounts of DNA from cells scraped off these slides by means of the polymerase chain reaction showed conclusively that the correct replacement was $\beta^{106Leu \rightarrow Arg}$.

with severe unstable hemoglobinopathy to have healthy offspring may be slightly decreased.

▼ PATHOGENESIS

Thus far, more than 100 structurally different unstable hemoglobin mutants have been documented. Many of these show only mild instability in vitro and are not associated with any significant clinical manifestations. About three fourths of these are β chain mutants. Many of them are amino acid replacements in the vicinity of the heme pocket (Fig. 7–22). The majority are neutral replacements, such as Hb Köln (β$^{98Val \rightarrow Met}$). Such an alteration in primary structure may cause considerable perturbations in the hydrophobic interior of the molecule. Considering the nature of such amino acid replacements, one is not surprised that many of these mutants have electrophoretic mobility identical to that of Hb A. Others may appear as single or multiple bands having isoelectric points higher than that of Hb A. If these bands are no longer visible after the addition of hemin to the hemolysate, it is likely that the abnormal electrophoretic mobility was due to heme loss (or heme displacement) rather than to an alteration in the charge of a globin subunit. About one fifth of the unstable mutants involve a replacement by proline. Proline residues can prevent the formation or extension of an α helix. Thus, instability may result from disruption of the secondary structure of the subunit. Some unstable mutants contain deletions of one to five amino acids in sequence (see Table 7–1) and probably arose because of frameshift mutagenesis in the region of reiterated nucleotide sequence.[5] This mechanism is supported by the finding of "mirror-image" mutants: Hb Gun Hill, which has a five-residue deletion at position 93–97, and Hb Koriyama, which has a tandem insertion of the same five residues.[56] A few unstable mutants have insertions within deletions (see Table 7–1).

The mechanism by which red cells hemolyze is not fully understood. Much of the red cell destruction occurs in the bone marrow.[424] There is convincing evidence that normally placed hemes confer considerable stability to their respective globin subunits. In many of the unstable hemoglobin mutants, the amino acid substitution prevents a normal heme/globin linkage. Once the heme becomes detached from its normal position in the cleft on the surface of the involved subunit, it probably binds nonspecifically to another site on the globin. Both spectrophotometric and electron spin resonance measurements indicate that the formation of hemichrome may be an intermediate step in the denaturation of unstable hemoglobins.[425] After heme displacement, the globin subunits aggregate to form a coccoid precipitate having the morphological characteristics of a Heinz body. The Heinz bodies and the heat-induced precipitate contain equal amounts of α and β chains and probably a normal complement of heme.[426] Red cells containing Heinz bodies have reduced deformability[427] and are likely to be entrapped in the microcirculation. There is convincing morphological evidence that these Heinz bodies become selectively removed, or "pitted," during circulation through the sinusoids of the spleen.[428] Therefore, it is not surprising that patients who have undergone splenectomy have an increased number of Heinz bodies and, in most cases, an increase in the amount of the hemoglobin mutant relative to normal Hb A.

The intracellular release of heme from these unstable mutants may contribute to decreased deformability of CHBA red cells and therefore to the rate of hemolysis. The release of reactive oxidants, such as hydrogen peroxide, superoxide, and hydroxyl radical, may damage the red cell membrane by both lipid peroxidation and cross-linking of membrane proteins.[429, 430]

Because the degree of instability of these hemoglobin mutants spans a wide range, the extent of hemolysis varies considerably. In some, such as Hb Zürich, an additional oxidant stress, such as the ingestion of certain drugs, is required for significant hemolysis. Fever may also increase the hemolytic rate.[431] Many patients, however, have continuous and marked red cell breakdown. The degree of anemia is influenced not only by the severity of the hemolysis but also by the ability of the blood to unload oxygen.[5] Thus, patients having unstable mutants of high oxygen affinity,

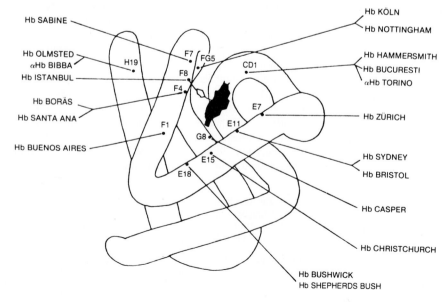

Figure 7–22. Three-dimensional representation of β chain showing sites of amino acid substitutions at the heme pocket that make the mutant hemoglobins unstable. (From Milner, P.F., and Wrightstone, R.N.: *In* Wallach, D. [ed.]: The Function of Red Blood Cells. New York, Alan R. Liss, 1981. Copyright © 1981 by John Wiley & Sons, Inc. Reprinted by permission of John Wiley & Sons, Inc.)

such as Hb Köln, may have a nearly normal hemoglobin level (i.e., compensated hemolysis). In contrast, the hemoglobin level is apt to be much lower in patients having mutants with decreased oxygen affinity, such as Hb Hammersmith.

The structural alteration in Hb Zürich leads to particularly interesting functional and clinical consequences.[432, 433] The replacement of the distal histidine by arginine at βE7 causes a larger space in the heme pocket where gas ligands bind. Accordingly, carbon monoxide is able to bind in a nonconstrained fashion and with much higher affinity. Carbon monoxide protects this mutant from oxidative denaturation. Individuals with Hb Zürich who smoke tend to accumulate high levels of carboxyhemoglobin and have less hemolysis than affected family members who do not smoke.

A few hemoglobin mutants are so unstable that virtually no mutant gene product can be detected in the hemolysate. Examples include Hb Terra Haute,[421] Hb Showa-Yakushiji,[434] and Hb Geneva.[435] As mentioned earlier, heterozygotes have a phenotype of thalassemia intermedia with moderate anemia, splenomegaly, microcytic red cells, Heinz bodies, and elevated Hb A_2.

▼ CLINICAL FEATURES

These pathophysiological considerations explain a number of the clinical features of this disorder. Patients usually present in early childhood with a hemolytic anemia accompanied by jaundice and splenomegaly. In some cases, hemolysis is markedly aggravated by fever or the ingestion of an oxidant-type drug. The red cell morphology is somewhat variable. Often, patients with a functioning spleen have normal-looking red cells. Slight hypochromia and prominent basophilic stippling are common features. Indeed, the intensity of the basophilic stippling may equal or even exceed that noted in pyrimidine 5′-nucleotidase deficiency. In both conditions, the stippling may be due to excessive clumping of ribosomes. The blood may have to be incubated to demonstrate Heinz bodies. In some cases, it appears as if a bite had been taken from a margin of the red cells, and it is tempting to speculate that a Heinz body had been pitted at this site. After splenectomy, red cells appear much more abnormal. Heinz bodies are larger and more numerous. The extent of symptoms varies considerably in keeping with the degree of anemia. As mentioned earlier, one of the two parents is affected in about two thirds of the cases. Some patients give a history of passing dark urine. Although this pigment has not been completely characterized, it appears to be a dipyrrole (mesobilifuscin) and may be the consequence of aberrant (perhaps non-enzymatic) heme catabolism. Dipyrroles have also been detected by fluorescence microscopy of CHBA red cells.[436]

Hemoglobin Mutants With Abnormal Oxygen Binding

In 1966, Charache and coworkers[437] described a family with erythrocytosis due to the presence of a hemoglobin mutant, Hb Chesapeake ($\alpha^{92\text{Arg} \rightarrow \text{Leu}}$). Oxygen equilibria done on both whole blood and the isolated abnormal hemoglobin

revealed a marked increase in oxygen affinity and a reduction in subunit cooperativity. Because of the "shift to the left" and consequent reduction in oxygen unloading, individuals with a high-affinity hemoglobin mutant have compensatory erythrocytosis through increased production of erythropoietin.[438] To date, more than 50 other mutants with high oxygen affinity have been discovered. In each case, affected family members have erythrocytosis. Unlike the unstable hemoglobins, which also may have abnormal oxygen affinity, these mutants are not associated with any hemolysis or abnormal red cell morphology. This group of mutants has provided a wealth of information on structure-function relationships of hemoglobin and physiological oxygen transport in man.

The location and nature of the amino acid substitutions in the high oxygen affinity mutants have been useful in establishing specific sites on the hemoglobin molecule that are critical to its function. A number of these mutants, including Hb Kempsey, have substitutions at the $\alpha_1\beta_2$ interface. As Figure 7–23 shows, in normal Hb A, the interaction of $\beta^{99\text{Asp}}$ with $\alpha^{42\text{Tyr}}$ at this subunit interface contributes to the stability of the T structure. In Hb Kempsey, the substitution $\beta^{99\text{Asp} \rightarrow \text{Asn}}$ prevents this interaction. There is good experimental evidence that the high oxygen affinity of Hb Kempsey is due to destabilization of the T (deoxy) conformation. In contrast, the oxy or R conformation of Hb A is stabilized by an interaction at the $\alpha_1\beta_2$ interface between $\beta^{102\text{Asn}}$ and $\alpha^{94\text{Asp}}$ (Fig. 7–23). The *low* oxygen affinity of Hb Kansas can be attributed to decreased stability of the R form, owing to the replacement of β102 asparagine by threonine.[5] A second group of high oxygen mutants have substitutions at the C terminus of the abnormal subunit. As explained at the beginning of this chapter and depicted in Figure 7–3B, electrostatic interactions at the C terminus of the β subunit are important contributors to the stability of the T quaternary conformation and to the Bohr effect. Hb Hiroshima ($\beta^{146\text{His} \rightarrow \text{Asp}}$) is one of several mutants in which replacement of the C-terminal histidine gives rise to increased oxygen affinity and diminished Bohr effect (Fig. 7–24). A third group of high oxygen affinity mutants has substitutions at the 2,3-BPG binding site, which results in impaired binding to 2,3-BPG and increased intracellular oxygen affinity.[5]

Other than erythrocytosis, affected individuals have minimal clinical manifestations. In most cases, the increase in red cell mass is probably appropriate to ensure tissue oxygenation. Hemodynamic studies of these individuals have produced somewhat variable results. Some patients have had increased cardiac output or low mixed venous Po_2, or both, when subjected to graded exercise or bled down to a normal red cell mass.[5] Packed cell volumes seldom reach high enough levels so that increased blood viscosity necessitates therapeutic phlebotomy. There are many reports of affected mothers carrying unaffected offspring to term. In these cases, the oxygen affinity of the maternal blood was probably greater than that of the fetus. The lack of any untoward complications[439] argues against the physiological importance of increased oxygen affinity of fetal blood.

The possibility of a functionally abnormal hemoglobin should be considered in any case of unexplained erythrocytosis. A positive family history and an abnormal hemoglobin electrophoresis are helpful. However, I have seen one child in whom neither of these findings was present. She

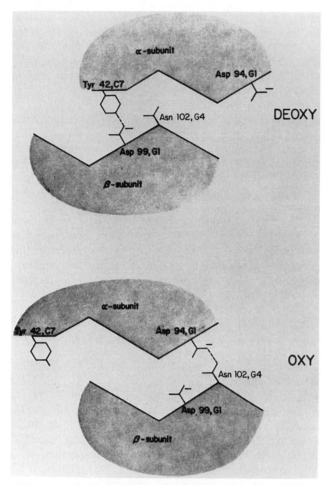

Figure 7–23. Mechanism by which substitutions at the $\alpha_1\beta_2$ interface affect oxygen affinity. On oxygenation, the area of contact between subunits shifts in a dovetail fashion. Deoxyhemoglobin is normally stabilized by a hydrogen bond between α^{42Tyr} and β^{99Asp}. This bond cannot form in a set of high oxygen mutants, including Hb Kempsey ($\beta^{99Asp \rightarrow Asn}$). Conversely, oxyhemoglobin is stabilized by a bond between α^{94Asp} and β^{102Asn}. This bond cannot form in Hb Kansas ($\beta^{102Asn \rightarrow Thr}$), Hb Beth Israel ($\beta^{102Asn \rightarrow Thr}$), and Hb Titusville ($\alpha^{94Asp \rightarrow Asn}$). (From Perutz, M.F.: New Scient. Sci. J., June 1971; with permission.)

was found to have Hb Bethesda, which apparently arose as a spontaneous mutation. In such cases, a measurement of oxygen affinity is required to establish the diagnosis. Not all familial erythrocytosis is due to a functionally abnormal hemoglobin mutant; in some families, enhanced production of erythropoietin has been documented.[440, 441] In other families, the polycythemia is due to mutations of the erythropoietin receptor leading to enhanced sensitivity to erythropoietin.[442]

M Hemoglobins

The appearance of blue or dusky skin and mucous membranes is a common and informative finding on physical examination. In the majority of cases, cyanosis is due to an excess of deoxyhemoglobin in the blood, owing to cardiac or pulmonary dysfunction and rarely to a stable mutant hemoglobin (such as Hb Kansas) that has unusually low oxygen affinity.

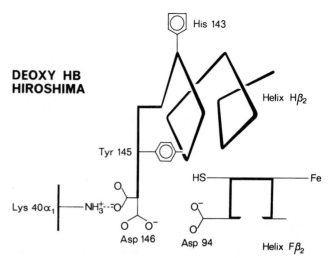

DEOXY HB HIROSHIMA

Figure 7–24. Diagram of the contacts of $\beta^{Hiroshima}$ in which the C-terminal 146 histidine is replaced by aspartic acid. Compare with Figure 7–3B. The substitution prevents the salt bond with β^{Asp94} and explains why Hb Hiroshima has high oxygen affinity and half-normal Bohr effect. (From Perutz, M.F.: Molecular anatomy, physiology, and pathology of hemoglobin. *In* Stamatoyannopoulos, G., Nienhuis, A.W., Leder, P., and Majerus, P.W.: The Molecular Basis of Blood Diseases. Philadelphia, W.B. Saunders Co., 1981, p. 127.)

Much less often, cyanosis is due to oxidized hemoglobin (methemoglobin or sulfhemoglobin) in circulating red cells. Congenital methemoglobinemia is usually caused by a deficiency of the enzyme cytochrome b_5 reductase (also called diaphorase I or NADH-dependent methemoglobin reductase), which enables red cell hemoglobin to be maintained in the reduced form. A more uncommon cause of congenital methemoglobinemia is the presence of one of the M hemoglobins. Like the other two classes of functionally abnormal hemoglobins discussed in detail in this chapter, the M hemoglobins are inherited according to an autosomal dominant pattern. Affected individuals present with cyanosis but are otherwise asymptomatic. In general, there is no evidence of anemia. The blood has a peculiar mahogany color "like that of Japanese soy sauce."[443] Spectral examination of the hemoglobin shows an abnormal pattern that is similar to, but not identical with, that of methemoglobin. Hemoglobin electrophoresis reveals an abnormal band with a slightly anodal mobility. The normal A and abnormal M hemoglobins may be separated more readily if the entire hemolysate is converted to methemoglobin before the electrophoresis.

Seven M hemoglobins have been described (Table 7–3). The α and β chain mutants have been detected in unrelated

Table 7–3. Properties of the M Hemoglobins

Hemoglobin	Structure	Helical Residue	Oxygen Affinity at P_{50}	Bohr Effect
M-Boston	$\alpha58$ His $\rightarrow$ Tyr	E7	Decreased	Decreased
M-Iwate	$\alpha87$ His $\rightarrow$ Tyr	F8	Decreased	Decreased
M-Saskatoon	$\beta63$ His $\rightarrow$ Tyr	E7	Normal	Present
M-Hyde Park	$\beta92$ His $\rightarrow$ Tyr	F8	Normal	Present
M-Milwaukee-I	$\beta67$ Val $\rightarrow$ Glu	E11	Decreased	Present
FM-Osaka	$\gamma63$ His $\rightarrow$ Tyr	E7		
FM-Fort Ripley	$\gamma92$ His $\rightarrow$ Tyr	F8		

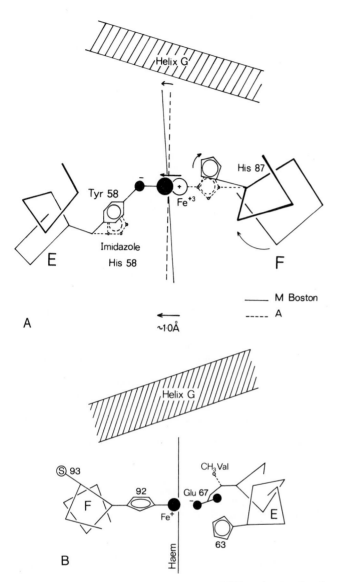

Figure 7–25. *A*, Diagram of the heme pocket of $\beta^{M\text{-}Boston}$ showing that the oxidized (Fe^{3+}) iron atom forms a bond with the substituted tyrosine at $\alpha 58$ (E7) on the distal side of the heme rather than with the proximal F8 histidine. (From Pulsinelli, P.D., Perutz, M.F., and Nagel, R.L.: Structure of hemoglobin M Boston, a variant with a five-coordinated ferric heme. Proc. Natl. Acad. Sci. USA 70:3870, 1973; with permission.) *B*, Comparable diagram of $\beta^{M\text{-}Milwaukee\text{-}I}$ showing the binding of the carboxyl group of the substituted $\beta 67$ glutamic acid with the oxidized heme iron. (Reprinted by permission from *Nature* [New Biol], Vol. 237, p. 259; copyright © 1972 Macmillan Magazines Limited.)

should not be confused with some of the unstable mutants, such as Hb Freiburg and Hb St. Louis, in which a high proportion of the abnormal subunit oxidizes to methemoglobin. Hb FM-Osaka ($\gamma^{63His \rightarrow Tyr}$)[444] and Hb FM–Fort Ripley ($\gamma^{92His \rightarrow Tyr}$)[445] were discovered in cyanotic newborns. The cyanosis disappeared during the first few months of life as β chains replaced γ chains.

In this disorder, treatment is neither indicated nor possible. The M hemoglobins are perhaps of more interest and concern to molecular biologists than to the individuals affected.

ACKNOWLEDGMENTS

I thank Rosemary LaFratta for skilled secretarial and editorial assistance. The preparation of this chapter was greatly facilitated by the cooperation of a number of colleagues who generously supplied reprints and preprints. Drs. Stuart Edelstein, Robert Josephs, Daniel Harrington, William Royer, Dhananjaya Kaul, and James White kindly prepared figures for this chapter. Drs. Carlo Brugnara, Robert Hebbel, and John Olson provided critical comments on portions of the chapter.

REFERENCES

1. Pauling, L., Itano, H., Singer, S.J., and Wells, I.C.: Sickle cell anemia: a molecular disease. Science 110:543, 1949.
2. Perutz, M.F.: Molecular anatomy, physiology, and pathology of hemoglobin. *In* Stamatoyannopoulos, G., and Nienhuis, A.W. (eds): The Molecular Basis of Blood Diseases. Philadelphia, W.B. Saunders Co., 1987, p. 127.
3. Shaanan, B.: The structure of human oxyhaemoglobin at 2.1 Å resolution. J. Mol. Biol. 171:31, 1983.
4. Fermi, G., Perutz, M.F., and Shaanan, B.: The crystal structure of human deoxyhemoglobin at 1.74 Å resolution. J. Mol. Biol. 175:159, 1984.
5. Bunn, H.F., and Forget, B.G.: Hemoglobin: Molecular, Genetic and Clinical Aspects. Philadelphia, W.B. Saunders Co., 1986.
6. Monod, J., Wyman, J., and Changeux, J.P.: On the nature of allosteric transitions: a plausible model. J. Mol. Biol. 12:88, 1965.
7. Ackers, G.K., Doyle, M.L., Myers, D., and Daugherty, M.A.: Molecular code for cooperativity in hemoglobin. Science 255:54, 1992.
8. Fermi, G., Perutz, M.F., and Shulman, R.G.: Iron distances in hemoglobin: comparison of x-ray crystallographic and extended x-ray absorption fine structure studies. Proc. Natl. Acad. Sci. USA 84:6167, 1987.
9. Nagai, K., Perutz, M.F., and Poyart, C.: Studies of haemoglobin functions by site-directed mutagenesis. Philos. Trans. R. Soc. Lond. A 317:443, 1986.
10. Nagai, K., Luisi, B., Shih, D., Miyazaki, G., Imai, K., Poyart, C., De, Y.A., Kwiatkowsky, L., Noble, R.W., Lin, S.H., et al.: Distal residues in the oxygen binding site of haemoglobin studied by protein engineering. Nature 329:858, 1987.
11. Hoffman, S.J., Looker, D.L., Roehrich, J.M., Cozart, P.E., Durfee, S.L., Tedesco, J.L., and Stetler, G.L.: Expression of fully functional tetrameric human hemoglobin in *Escherichia coli*. Proc. Natl. Acad. Sci. USA 87:8521, 1990.
12. Murray, L.P., Hofrichter, J., Henry, E.R., Ikeda, S.M., Kitagishi, K., Yonetani, T., and Eaton, W.A.: The effect of quaternary structure on the kinetics of conformational changes and nanosecond geminate rebinding of carbon monoxide to hemoglobin. Proc. Natl. Acad. Sci. USA 85:2151, 1988.
13. Murray, L.P., Hofrichter, J., Henry, E.R., and Eaton, W.A.: Time-resolved optical spectroscopy and structural dynamics following photodissociation of carbonmonoxyhemoglobin. Biophys. Chem. 29:63, 1988.
14. Perutz, M.F.: Mechanisms regulating the reactions of human hemoglo-

families all over the world. Six of the seven M hemoglobins represent substitution of either the proximal (F8) or distal (E7) histidine by tyrosine. It is likely that the side group of the substituted tyrosine can serve as an internal ligand, stabilizing the heme iron in the ferric form (Fig. 7–25). As anticipated, the M hemoglobins are functionally abnormal. Both α chain mutants have decreased oxygen affinity and decreased Bohr effect.[5] The whole blood oxygen affinity of individuals with Hb M may be markedly decreased, owing in part to the intrinsic functional abnormality of the hemoglobin mutant and in part to increased 2,3-BPG in the red cell.[5] Furthermore, individuals who have one of the M hemoglobins may have mild hemolysis. However, the M hemoglobins bin with oxygen and carbon monoxide. Annu. Rev. Physiol. 52:1, 1990.

15. Bohr, C., Hasselbalch, K., and Krogh, A.: Über einen in biologischer Beziehung wichtigen Einfluss. Den die Kohlen-sauerespannung des Blutes auf dessen Sauerstoffbinding ubt. Skand. Arch. Physiol. 16:402, 1904.

16. Riggs, A.F.: The Bohr effect. Annu. Rev. Physiol. 50:181, 1988.

17. Busch, M.R., Mace, J.E., Ho, N.T., and Ho, C.: Roles of the beta 146 histidyl residue in the molecular basis of the Bohr effect of hemoglobin: a proton nuclear magnetic resonance study. Biochemistry 30:1865, 1991.

18. Komiyama, N.H., Miyazaki, G., Tame, J., and Nagai, K.: Transplanting a unique allosteric effect from crocodile into human haemoglobin. Nature 373:244, 1995.

19. Benesch, R., and Benesch, R.E.: Intracellular organic phosphates as regulators of oxygen release by haemoglobin. Nature 221:618, 1969.

20. Arnone, A.: X-ray diffraction study of binding of 2,3-diphosphoglycerate to human deoxyhaemoglobin. Nature 237:146, 1972.

21. Adamson, J.W., and Finch, C.A.: Hemoglobin function, oxygen affinity, and erythropoietin. Annu. Rev. Physiol. 38:351, 1975.

22. Jia, L., Bonaventura, C., Bonaventura, J., and Stamler, J.S.: S-Nitrosohaemoglobin: a dynamic activity of blood involved in vascular control. Nature 380:221, 1996.

23. Stamler, J.S., Jia, L., Eu, J.P., McMahon, T.J., Demchenko, I.T., Bonaventura, J., Gernert, K., and Piantadosi, C.A.: Blood flow regulation by S-nitrosohemoglobin in the physiological oxygen gradient. Science 276:2034, 1997.

24. Gow, A.J., and Stamler, J.S.: Reactions between nitric oxide and haemoglobin under physiological conditions. Nature 391:169, 1998.

24a. Gow, A.J., Luchsinger, B.P., Pawloski, J.R., Singel, D.J., and Stamler, J.S.: The oxyhemoglobin reaction of nitric oxide. Proc. Natl. Acad. Sci. USA 96:9027, 1999.

25. Huisman, T.H., Schroeder, W.A., Bannister, W.H., and Grech, J.L.: Evidence for four nonallelic structural genes for the chain of human fetal hemoglobin Biochem. Genet. 7:131, 1972.

26. Adachi, K., Kim, J., Asakura, T., and Schwartz, E.: Characterization of two types of fetal hemoglobin: alpha 2G gamma 2 and alpha 2A gamma 2. Blood 75:2070, 1990.

27. Ricco, G., Mazza, U., Turi, R.M., Pich, P.G., Camaschella, C., Saglio, G., and Bernini, L.F.: Significance of a new type of human fetal hemoglobin carrying a replacement isoleucine replaced by threonine at position 75 (E 19) of the gamma chain. Hum. Genet. 32:305, 1976.

28. Schroeder, W.A., Cua, J.T., Matsuda, G., and Fenninger, W.D.: Hemoglobin F₁, an acetyl-containing hemoglobin. Biochem. Biophys. Acta 63:532, 1962.

29. Bauer, C., Ludwig, I., and Ludwig, M.: Different effects of 2,3-diphosphoglycerate and adenosine triphosphate on the oxygen affinity of adult and fetal human hemoglobin. Life Sci. 7:1339, 1968.

30. Tyuma, I., and Shimizu, K.: Different response to organic phosphates of human fetal and adult hemoglobins. Arch. Biochem. Biophys. 129:404, 1969.

31. Adachi, K., Konitzer, P., Pang, J., Reddy, K.S., and Surrey, S.: Amino acids responsible for decreased 2,3-biphosphoglycerate binding to fetal hemoglobin. Blood 90:2916, 1997.

32. Boyer, S.H., Belding, T.K., Margolet, L., and Noyes, A.N.: Fetal hemoglobin restriction to a few erythrocytes (F cells) in normal human adults. Science 188:361, 1975.

33. Wood, W.G., Stamatoyannopoulos, G., Lim, G., and Nute, P.E.: F-cells in the adult: normal values and levels in individuals with hereditary and acquired elevations of Hb F. Blood 46:671, 1975.

34. Steinberg, M.H., and Adams, J.D.: Hemoglobin A₂: origin, evolution, and aftermath. Blood 78:2165, 1991.

35. Rieder, R.F., and Weatherall, D.J.: Studies on hemoglobin biosynthesis: asynchronous synthesis of hemoglobin A and hemoglobin A₂ by erythrocyte precursors. J. Clin. Invest. 44:42, 1965.

36. Roberts, A.V., Weatherall, D.J., and Clegg, J.B.: The synthesis of human haemoglobin A₂ during erythroid maturation. Biochem. Biophys. Res. Commun. 47:81, 1972.

37. Allen, D.W., Schroeder, W.A., and Balog, J.: Observations on the chromatographic heterogeneity of normal adult and fetal human hemoglobins. J. Am. Chem. Soc. 80:1628, 1958.

38. McDonald, M.J., Shapiro, R., Bleichman, M., Solway, J., and Bunn, H.F.: Glycosylated minor components of human adult hemoglobin. Purification, identification, and partial structural analysis. J. Biol. Chem. 253:2327, 1978.

39. Garlick, R.L., Mazer, J.S., Higgins, P.J., and Bunn, H.F.: Characterization of glycosylated hemoglobins. Relevance to monitoring of diabetic control and analysis of other proteins. J. Clin. Invest. 71:1062, 1983.

40. Bookchin, R.M., and Gallop, P.M.: Structure of hemoglobin A₁c: nature of the N-terminal beta chain blocking group. Biochem. Biophys. Res. Commun. 32:86, 1968.

41. Bunn, H.F., Haney, D.N., Gabbay, K.H., and Gallop, P.M.: Further identification of the nature and linkage of the carbohydrate in hemoglobin A₁c. Biochem. Biophys. Res. Commun. 67:103, 1975.

42. Prome, D., Blouquit, Y., Ponthus, C., Prome, J.C., and Rosa, J.: Structure of the human adult hemoglobin minor fraction A₁b by electrospray and secondary ion mass spectrometry. Pyruvic acid as amino-terminal blocking group. J. Biol. Chem. 266:13050, 1991.

43. Bunn, H.F., Haney, D.N., Kamin, S., Gabbay, K.H., and Gallop, P.M.: The biosynthesis of human hemoglobin A₁c. Slow glycosylation of hemoglobin in vivo. J. Clin. Invest. 57:1652, 1976.

44. Bunn, H.F., Gabbay, K.H., and Gallop, P.M.: The glycosylation of hemoglobin: relevance to diabetes mellitus. Science 200:21, 1978.

45. Makita, Z., Vlassara, H., Rayfield, E., Cartwright, K., Friedman, E., Rodby, R., Cerami, A., and Bucala, R.: Hemoglobin-AGE: a circulating marker of advanced glycosylation. Science 258:651, 1992.

46. Fluckiger, R., Harmon, W., Meier, W., Loo, S., and Gabbay, K.H.: Hemoglobin carbamylation in uremia. N. Engl. J. Med. 304:823, 1981.

47. Stevens, V.J., Fantl, W.J., Newman, C.B., Sims, R.V., Cerami, A., and Peterson, C.M.: Acetaldehyde adducts with hemoglobin. J. Clin. Invest. 67:361, 1981.

48. Hoberman, H.D.: Post-translational modification of hemoglobin in alcoholism. Biochem. Biophys. Res. Commun. 113:1004, 1983.

49. Charache, S., and Weatherall, D.J.: Fast hemoglobin in lead poisoning. Blood 28:377, 1966.

50. Lamola, A.A., Piomelli, S., Poh, F.M., Yamane, T., and Harber, L.C.: Erythropoietic protoporphyria and lead intoxication: the molecular basis for difference in cutaneous photosensitivity. II. Different binding of erythrocyte protoporphyrin to hemoglobin. J. Clin. Invest. 56:1528, 1975.

51. Hemoglobin: International Hemoglobin Information Center: List of hemoglobin variants. Hemoglobin 15:139, 1991.

52. Cash, F.E., Monplaisir, N., Goossens, M., and Liebhaber, S.A.: Locus assignment of two alpha-globin structural mutants from the Caribbean basin: alpha Fort de France (alpha 45 Arg) and alpha Spanish Town (alpha 27 Val). Blood 74:833, 1989.

53. Wilson, J.B., Chen, S.S., Webber, B.B., Kutlar, A., Kutlar, F., Villegas, A., and Huisman, T.H.: The identification of five rare beta-chain abnormal hemoglobins by high performance liquid chromatographic procedures. Hemoglobin 10:49, 1986.

54. Lubin, B.H., Witkowska, E., and Kleman, K.: Laboratory diagnosis of hemoglobinopathies. Clin. Biochem. 24:363, 1991.

55. Schnee, J., Aulehla, S.C., Eigel, A., and Horst, J.: Hb D Los Angeles (D-Punjab) and Hb Presbyterian: analysis of the defect at the DNA level. Hum. Genet. 84:365, 1990.

56. Codrington, J.F., Kutlar, F., Harris, H.F., Wilson, J.B., Stoming, T.A., and Huisman, T.H.: Hb A₂-Wrens or alpha 2 delta 2 98(FG5) Val—Met, an unstable delta chain variant identified by sequence analysis of amplified DNA. Biochim. Biophys. Acta 1009:87, 1989.

57. Camaschella, C., and Saglio, G.: Recent advances in diagnosis of hemoglobinopathies. Crit. Rev. Oncol. Hematol. 14:89, 1993.

58. Bunn, H.F., and McDonald, M.J.: Electrostatic interactions in the assembly of haemoglobin. Nature 306:498, 1983.

59. Bunn, H.F.: Subunit assembly of hemoglobin: an important determinant of hematologic phenotype. Blood 69:1, 1987.

60. Liebhaber, S.A., Cash, F.E., and Cornfield, D.B.: Evidence for post-translational control of Hb C synthesis in an individual with Hb C trait and alpha-thalassemia. Blood 71:502, 1988.

61. Huisman, T.H.: Percentages of abnormal hemoglobins in adults with a heterozygosity for an alpha-chain and/or a beta-chain variant. Am J Hematol 14:393, 1983.

62. Mrabet, N.T., McDonald, M.J., Turci, S., Sarkar, R., Szabo, A., and Bunn, H.F.: Electrostatic attraction governs the dimer assembly of human hemoglobin. J. Biol. Chem. 261:5222, 1986.

63. Adachi, K., Yamaguchi, T., Pang, J., and Surrey, S.: Effects of increased anionic charge in the β-globin chain on the assembly of human hemoglobin in vitro. Blood 91:1438, 1998.

64. Adams, J.D., Coleman, M.B., Hayes, J., Morrison, W.T., and Steinberg, M.H.: Modulation of fetal hemoglobin synthesis by iron deficiency. N. Engl. J. Med. 313:1402, 1985.

65. Chui, D.H., Patterson, M., Dowling, C.E., Kazazian, H.J., and Kendall, A.G.: Hemoglobin Bart's disease in an Italian boy. Interaction between alpha-thalassemia and hereditary persistence of fetal hemoglobin. N. Engl. J. Med. 323:179, 1990.

66. Hirsch, R.E., Raventos, S.C., Olson, J.A., and Nagel, R.L.: Ligand state of intraerythrocytic circulating HbC crystals in homozygote CC patients. Blood 66:775, 1985.

67. Fabry, M.E., Kaul, D.K., Raventos, S.C., Chang, H., and Nagel, R.L.: SC erythrocytes have an abnormally high intracellular hemoglobin concentration. Pathophysiological consequences. J. Clin. Invest. 70:1315, 1982.

68. Bunn, H.F., Noguchi, C.T., Hofrichter, J., Schechter, G.P., Schechter, A.N., and Eaton, W.A.: Molecular and cellular pathogenesis of hemoglobin SC disease. Proc. Natl. Acad. Sci. USA 79:7527, 1982.

69. Brugnara, C., Kopin, A.S., Bunn, H.F., and Tosteson, D.C.: Regulation of cation content and cell volume in hemoglobin erythrocytes from patients with homozygous hemoglobin C disease. J. Clin. Invest. 75:1608, 1985.

70. White, J.G.: The fine structure of sickled hemoglobin in situ. Blood 31:561, 1968.

71. Bertles, J.F., and Dobler, J.: Reversible and irreversible sickling: a distinction by electron microscopy. Blood 33:884, 1969.

72. Edelstein, S.J., Telford, J.N., and Crepeau, R.H.: Structure of fibers of sickle cell hemoglobin. Proc. Natl. Acad. Sci. USA 70:1104, 1973.

73. Dykes, G., Crepeau, R.H., and Edelstein, S.J.: Three-dimensional reconstruction of the fibres of sickle cell haemoglobin. Nature 272:506, 1978.

74. Garrell, R.L., Crepeau, R.H., and Edelstein, S.J.: Cross-sectional views of hemoglobin S fibers by electron microscopy and computer modeling. Proc. Natl. Acad. Sci. USA 76:1140, 1979.

75. Dykes, G.W., Crepeau, R.H., and Edelstein, S.J.: Three-dimensional reconstruction of the 14-filament fibers of hemoglobin S. J. Mol. Biol. 130:451, 1979.

76. Rodgers, D.W., Crepeau, R.H., and Edelstein, S.J.: Pairings and polarities of the 14 strands in sickle cell hemoglobin fibers. Proc. Natl. Acad. Sci. USA 84:6157, 1987.

77. Carragher, B., Bluemke, D.A., Gabriel, B., Potel, M.J., and Josephs, R.: Structural analysis of polymers of sickle cell hemoglobin. I. Sickle hemoglobin fibers. J. Mol. Biol. 199:315, 1988.

78. Perutz, M.F., and Mitchison, J.M.: State of haemoglobin in sickle-cell anemia. Nature 166:677, 1950.

79. Hofrichter, J., Hendricker, D.G., and Eaton, W.A.: Structure of hemoglobin S fibers: optical determination of the molecular orientation in sickled erythrocytes. Proc. Natl. Acad. Sci. USA 70:3604, 1973.

80. Magdoff, F.B., and Chiu, C.C.: X-ray diffraction studies of fibers and crystals of deoxygenated sickle cell hemoglobin. Proc. Natl. Acad. Sci. USA 76:223, 1979.

81. Wishner, B.C., Ward, K.B., Lattman, E.E., and Love, W.E.: Crystal structure of sickle-cell deoxyhemoglobin at 5 Å resolution. J. Mol. Biol. 98:179, 1975.

82. Padlan, E.A., and Love, W.E.: Refined crystal structure of deoxyhemoglobin S. II. Molecular interactions in the crystal. J. Biol. Chem. 260:8280, 1985.

83. Padlan, E.A., and Love, W.E.: Refined crystal structure of deoxyhemoglobin S. I. Restrained least-squares refinement at 3.0-Å resolution. J. Biol. Chem. 260:8272, 1985.

84. Harrington, D.J., Adachi, K., and Royer, W.E., Jr.: The high resolution crystal structure of deoxyhemoglobin S. J. Mol. Biol. 272:398, 1997.

85. Bookchin, R.M., Nagel, R.L., and Ranney, H.M.: Structure and properties of hemoglobin C-Harlem, a human hemoglobin variant with amino acid substitutions in 2 residues of the beta-polypeptide chain. J. Biol. Chem. 242:248, 1967.

86. Nagel, R.L., Bookchin, R.M., Johnson, J., Labie, D., Wajcman, H., Isaac, S.W., Honig, G.R., Schiliro, G., Crookston, J.H., and Matsutomo, K.: Structural bases of the inhibitory effects of hemoglobin F and hemoglobin A$_2$ on the polymerization of hemoglobin S. Proc. Natl. Acad. Sci. USA 76:670, 1979.

87. Nagel, R.L., Johnson, J., Bookchin, R.M., Garel, M.C., Rosa, J., Schiliro, G., Wajcman, H., Labie, D., Moo, P.W., and Castro, O.: Beta-chain contact sites in the haemoglobin S polymer. Nature 283:832, 1980.

88. Benesch, R.E., Yung, S., Benesch, R., Mack, J., and Schneider, R.G.: alpha-Chain contacts in the polymerisation of sickle haemoglobin. Nature 260:219, 1976.

89. Benesch, R.E., Kwong, S., and Benesch, R.: The effects of alpha chain mutations cis and trans to the beta6 mutation on the polymerization of sickle cell haemoglobin. Nature 299:231, 1982.

90. Bunn, H.F., and McDonough, M.: Asymmetrical hemoglobin hybrids. An approach to the study of subunit interactions. Biochemistry 13:988, 1974.

91. Edelstein, S.J.: Molecular topology in crystals and fibers of hemoglobin S. J. Mol. Biol. 150:557, 1981.

92. Watowich, S.J., Gross, L.J., and Josephs, R.: Intermolecular contacts within sickle hemoglobin fibers. J. Mol. Biol. 209:821, 1989.

93. Eaton, W.A., and Hofrichter, J.: Sickle cell hemoglobin polymerization. Adv. Protein Chem. 40:63, 1990.

94. Adachi, K., Kim, J., Ballas, S., Surrey, S., and Asakura, T.: Facilitation of Hb S polymerization by the substitution of Glu for Gln at beta 121. J. Biol. Chem. 263:5607, 1988.

94a. Nagel, R.L., Daar, S., Romero, J.R., Suzuka, S.M., Gravell, D., Bouhassira, E., Schwartz, R.S., Fabry, M.E., and Krishnamoorthy, R.: HbS-Oman heterozygote: a new dominant sickle syndrome. Blood 92:4375, 1998.

95. Baudin, C.V., Pagnier, J., Marden, M., Bohn, B., Lacaze, N., Kister, J., Schaad, O., Edelstein, S.J., and Poyart, C.: Enhanced polymerization of recombinant human deoxyhemoglobin beta 6 Glu→Ile. Proc. Natl. Acad. Sci. USA 87:1845, 1990.

95a. Harrington, D.J., Adachi, K., and Royer, W.E.: Crystal structure of deoxy-human hemoglobin beta6 Glu→Trp. Implications for the structure and formation of the sickle cell fiber. J. Biol. Chem. 273:32690, 1998.

96. Himanen, J.-P., Popowicz, A.M., and Manning, J.M.: Recombinant sickle hemoglobin containing a lysine substitution at Asp-85(α): expression in yeast, functional properties, and participation in gel formation. Blood 89:4196, 1997.

97. Li, X., Mirza, U.A., Chait, B.T., and Manning, J.M.: Systematic enhancement of polymerization of recombinant sickle hemoglobin mutants: implications for transgenic mouse model for sickle cell anemia. Blood 90:4620, 1997.

98. Adachi, K., Pang, J., Konitzer, P., and Surrey, S.: Polymerization of recombinant hemoglobin F γE6V and hemoglobin F γE6V, γQ87T alone, and in mixtures with hemoglobin S. Blood 87:1617, 1996.

99. Adachi, K., Pang, J., Reddy, L.R., Bradley, L.E., Chen, Q., Trifillis, P., Schwartz, E., and Surrey, S.: Polymerization of three hemoglobin A$_2$ variants containing Val^{86} and inhibition of hemoglobin S polymerization by hemoglobin A$_2$. J. Biol. Chem. 271:24557, 1996.

100. Eaton, W.A., and Hofrichter, J.: Hemoglobin S gelation and sickle cell disease. Blood 70:1245, 1987.

101. Briehl, R.W.: Sickle-cell hemoglobin. In Encyclopedia of Human Biology. Vol. 7. San Diego, Academic Press, 1991, p. 1.

102. Bertles, J.F., Rabinowitz, R., and Dobler, J.: Hemoglobin interaction: modification of solid phase composition in the sickling phenomenon. Science 169:375, 1970.

103. Briehl, R.W., and Ewert, S.: Effects of pH, 2,3-diphosphoglycerate and salts on gelation of sickle cell deoxyhemoglobin. J. Mol. Biol. 80:445, 1973.

104. Bunn, H.F.: The interaction of sickle hemoglobin with DPG, CO$_2$ and other hemoglobins: formation of asymmetrical hybrids. Adv. Exp. Med. Biol. 28:41, 1975.

105. Gill, S.J., Skold, R., Fall, L., Shaeffer, T., Spokane, P., and Wyman, J.: Aggregation effects on oxygen binding of sickle cell hemoglobin. Science 201:362, 1978.

106. Benesch, R.E., Edalji, R., Kwong, S., and Benesch, R.: Oxygen affinity as an index of hemoglobin S polymerization: a new micromethod. Anal. Biochem. 89:162, 1978.

107. Gill, S.J., Benedict, R.C., Fall, L., Spokane, R., and Wyman, J.: Oxygen binding to sickle cell hemoglobin. J. Mol. Biol. 130:175, 1979.

108. Sunshine, H.R., Hofrichter, J., Ferrone, F.A., and Eaton, W.A.: Oxygen binding by sickle cell hemoglobin polymers. J. Mol. Biol. 158:251, 1982.

109. Minton, A.P.: Non-ideality and the thermodynamics of sickle-cell hemoglobin gelation. J. Mol. Biol. 110:89, 1977.

110. Ross, P.D., Hofrichter, J., and Eaton, W.A.: Thermodynamics of gelation of sickle cell deoxyhemoglobin. J. Mol. Biol. 115:111, 1977.

111. Goldberg, M.A., Husson, M.A., and Bunn, H.F.: Participation of hemoglobins A and F in polymerization of sickle hemoglobin. J. Biol. Chem. 252:3414, 1977.

112. Briehl, R.W.: Gelation of sickle cell hemoglobin. IV. Phase transitions in hemoglobin S gels: separate measures of aggregation and solution-gel equilibrium. J. Mol. Biol. 123:521, 1978.

113. Ueda, Y., and Bookchin, R.M.: Effects of carbon dioxide and pH variations in vitro on blood respiratory function, red cell volume, transmembrane pH gradients and sickling in sickle cell anemia. J. Lab. Clin. Med. 104:146, 1984.

114. Ross, P.D., Hofrichter, J., and Eaton, W.A.: Calorimetric and optical characterization of sickle cell hemoglobin gelation. J. Mol. Biol. 96:239, 1975.

115. Magdoff, F.B., Poillon, W.N., Li, T., and Bertles, J.F.: Thermodynamic studies of polymerization of deoxygenated sickle cell hemoglobin. Proc. Natl. Acad. Sci. USA 73:990, 1976.

116. Poillon, W.N., and Bertles, J.F.: Deoxygenated sickle hemoglobin. Effects of lyotropic salts on its solubility. J. Biol. Chem. 254:3462, 1979.

117. Adachi, K., Ozguc, M., and Asakura, T.: Nucleation-controlled aggregation of deoxyhemoglobin S. Participation of hemoglobin A in the aggregation of deoxyhemoglobin S in concentrated phosphate buffer. J. Biol. Chem. 255:3092, 1980.

118. Roth, E.F.J., Bookchin, R.M., and Nagel, R.L.: Deoxyhemoglobin S gelation and insolubility at high ionic strength are distinct phenomena. J. Lab. Clin. Med. 93:867, 1979.

119. Swerdlow, P.H., Bryan, R.A., Bertles, J.F., Poillon, W.N., Magdoff-Fairchild, B., and Milner, P.F.: Effect of 2,3-diphosphoglycerate on the solubility of deoxy sickle hemoglobin. Hemoglobin 1:527, 1977.

120. Poillon, W.N., and Kim, B.C.: 2,3-Diphosphoglycerate and intracellular pH as interdependent determinants of the physiologic solubility of deoxyhemoglobin S. Blood 76:1028, 1990.

121. Bookchin, R.M., Nagel, R.L., and Balazs, T.: Role of hybrid tetramer formation in gelation of haemoglobin S. Nature 256:667, 1975.

122. Hofrichter, J., Ross, P.D., and Eaton, W.A.: Kinetics and mechanism of deoxyhemoglobin S gelation: a new approach to understanding sickle cell disease. Proc. Natl. Acad. Sci. USA 71:4864, 1974.

123. Hofrichter, J., Ross, P.D., and Eaton, W.A.: Supersaturation in sickle cell hemoglobin solutions. Proc. Natl. Acad. Sci. USA 73:3035, 1976.

124. Samuel, R.E., Salmon, E.D., and Briehl, R.W.: Nucleation and growth of fibres and gel formation in sickle cell haemoglobin. Nature 345:833, 1990.

125. Ferrone, F.A., Hofrichter, J., Sunshine, H.R., and Eaton, W.A.: Kinetic studies on photolysis-induced gelation of sickle cell hemoglobin suggest a new mechanism. Biophys. J. 32:361, 1980.

126. Hofrichter, J.: Kinetics of sickle hemoglobin polymerization. III. Nucleation rates determined from stochastic fluctuations in polymerization progress curves. J. Mol. Biol. 189:553, 1986.

127. Harris, J.W.: Studies on the destruction of red blood cells. VII. Molecular orientation in sickle cell hemoglobin solutions. Proc. Soc. Exp. Biol. Med. 75:197, 1950.

128. Coletta, M., Hofrichter, J., Ferrone, F.A., and Eaton, W.A.: Kinetics of sickle haemoglobin polymerization in single red cells. Nature 300:194, 1982.

129. Goldberg, M.A., Lalos, A.T., and Bunn, H.F.: The effect of erythrocyte membrane preparations on the polymerization of sickle hemoglobin. J. Biol. Chem. 256:193, 1981.

130. Mozzarelli, A., Hofrichter, J., and Eaton, W.A.: Delay time of hemoglobin S polymerization prevents most cells from sickling in vivo. Science 237:500, 1987.

131. Winslow, R.M.: Hemoglobin interactions and whole blood oxygen equilibrium curves in sickling disorders. In Caughey, W.S. (ed.): Clinical and Biochemical Aspects of Hemoglobin Abnormalities. New York, Academic Press, 1978, p. 369.

132. Noguchi, C.T., Torchia, D.A., and Schechter, A.N.: Determination of deoxyhemoglobin S polymer in sickle erythrocytes upon deoxygenation. Proc. Natl. Acad. Sci. USA 77:5487, 1980.

133. Noguchi, C.T., Torchia, D.A., and Schechter, A.N.: Intracellular polymerization of sickle hemoglobin. Effects of cell heterogeneity. J. Clin. Invest. 72:846, 1983.

134. Mickols, W.E., Corbett, J.D., Maestre, M.F., Tinoco, I.J., Kropp, J., and Embury, S.H.: The effect of speed of deoxygenation on the percentage of aligned hemoglobin in sickle cells. Application of differential polarization microscopy. J. Biol. Chem. 263:4338, 1988.

135. Horiuchi, K., Ballas, S.K., and Asakura, T.: The effect of deoxygenation rate on the formation of irreversibly sickled cells. Blood 71:46, 1988.

136. Horiuchi, K., and Asakura, T.: Oxygen promotes sickling of SS cells. Ann. N. Y. Acad. Sci. 565:395, 1989.

137. Hebbel, R.P.: Beyond hemoglobin polymerization: the red blood cell membrane and sickle disease pathophysiology. Blood 77:214, 1991.

138. Hebbel, R.P., and Vercellotti, G.M.: The endothelial biology of sickle cell disease J. Lab. Clin. Med. 129:288, 1997.

139. Liu, S.C., Derick, L.H., Zhai, S., and Palek, J.: Uncoupling of the spectrin-based skeleton from the lipid bilayer in sickled red cells. Science 252:574, 1991.

140. Allan, D., Limbrick, A.R., Thomas, P., and Westerman, M.P.: Release of spectrin-free spicules on reoxygenation of sickled erythrocytes. Nature 295:612, 1982.

141. Lux, S.E., John, K.M., and Karnovsky, M.J.: Irreversible deformation of the spectrin-actin lattice in irreversibly sickled cells. J. Clin. Invest. 58:955, 1976.

142. Liu, S.C., Derick, L.H., Zhai, S., and Palek, J.: Ultrastructural anatomy of the red cell membrane lesion in sickle cells: penetration of the hemoglobin S polymers through the membrane skeleton and the reorganization of the skeletal lattice. Blood 74(suppl. 1):44a, 1989.

143. Rodgers, G.P., Noguchi, C.T., and Schechter, A.M.: Irreversibly sickled erythrocytes in sickle cell anemia: a quantitative reappraisal. Am. J. Hematol. 207:17, 1985.

144. Bertles, J.F., and Milner, P.F.: Irreversibly sickled erythrocytes: a consequence of the heterogeneous distribution of hemoglobin types in sickle-cell anemia. J. Clin. Invest. 47:1731, 1968.

145. Fabry, M.E., Mears, J.G., Patel, P., Schaefer, R.K., Carmichael, L.D., Martinez, G., and Nagel, R.L.: Dense cells in sickle cell anemia: the effects of gene interaction. Blood 64:1042, 1984.

146. Nagel, R.L., Fabry, M.E., Pagnier, J., Zohoun, I., Wajcman, H., Baudin, V., and Labie, D.: Hematologically and genetically distinct forms of sickle cell anemia in Africa. The Senegal type and the Benin type. N. Engl. J. Med. 312:880, 1985.

147. Horiuchi, K., and Asakura, T.: Formation of light irreversibly sickled cells during deoxygenation-oxygenation cycles. J. Lab. Clin. Med. 110:653, 1987.

148. Horiuchi, K., Ohata, J., Hirano, Y., and Asakura, T.: Morphologic studies of sickle erythrocytes by image analysis. J. Lab. Clin. Med. 115:613, 1990.

149. Bookchin, R.M., Ortiz, O.E., and Lew, V.L.: Evidence for a direct reticulocyte origin of dense red cells in sickle cell anemia. J. Clin. Invest. 87:113, 1991.

150. Platt, O.S., Falcone, J.F., and Lux, S.E.: Molecular defect in the sickle erythrocyte skeleton. Abnormal spectrin binding to sickle inside-out vesicles. J. Clin. Invest. 75:266, 1985.

151. Schwartz, R.S., Rybicki, A.C., Heath, R.H., and Lubin, B.H.: Protein 4.1 in sickle erythrocytes. Evidence for oxidative damage. J. Biol. Chem. 262:15666, 1987.

152. Klipstein, F.A., and Ranney, H.M.: Electrophoretic components of the hemoglobin of red cell membranes. J. Clin. Invest. 39:1894, 1960.

153. Fung, L.W.-M., Litvin, S.D., and Reid, T.M.: Spin-label detection of sickle hemoglobin-membrane interaction at physiological pH. Biochemistry 22:864, 1983.

154. Fortier, N., Snyder, L.M., Garver, F., Kiefer, C., McKenney, J., and Mohandas, N.: The relationship between in vivo generated hemoglobin skeletal protein complex and increased red cell membrane rigidity. Blood 71:1427, 1988.

155. Evans, E.A., and Mohandas, N.: Membrane-associated sickle hemoglobin: a major determinant of sickle erythrocyte rigidity. Blood 70:1443, 1987.

156. Hebbel, R.P., Yamada, O., Moldow, C.F., Jacob, H.S., White, J.G., and Eaton, J.W.: Abnormal adherence of sickle erythrocytes to cultured vascular endothelium: possible mechanism for microvascular occlusion in sickle cell disease. J. Clin. Invest. 65:154, 1980.

157. Waugh, S.M., Willardson, B.M., Kannan, R., Labotka, R.J., and Low, P.S.: Heinz bodies induce clustering of band 3, glycophorin, and ankyrin in sickle cell erythrocytes. J. Clin. Invest. 78:1155, 1986.

158. Rank, B.H., Carlsson, J., and Hebbel, R.P.: Abnormal redox status of membrane-protein thiols in sickle erythrocytes. J. Clin. Invest. 75:1531, 1985.

159. Rice, E.C., Omorphos, S.C., and Baysal, E.: Sickle cell membranes and oxidative damage. Biochem. J. 237:265, 1986.

160. Gibson, X.A., Shartava, A., McIntyre, J., Monteiro, C.A., Zhang, Y., Shah, A., Campbell, N.F., and Goodman, S.R.: The efficacy of reducing agents or antioxidants in blocking the formation of dense cells and irreversibly sickled cells in vitro. Blood 91:4373, 1998.

161. Hebbel, R.P., Morgan, W.T., Eaton, J.W., and Hedlund, B.E.: Accelerated autoxidation and heme loss due to instability of sickle hemoglobin. Proc. Natl. Acad. Sci. USA 85:237, 1988.

162. Asakura, T., Minakata, K., Adachi, K., Russell, M.O., and Schwartz,

E.: Denatured hemoglobin in sickle erythrocytes. J. Clin. Invest. 59:633, 1977.

163. Kuross, S.A., Rank, B.H., and Hebbel, R.P.: Excess heme in sickle erythrocyte inside-out membranes: possible role in thiol oxidation. Blood 71:876, 1988.

164. Hebbel, R.P., Eaton, J.W., Balasingam, M., and Steinberg, M.H.: Spontaneous oxygen radical generation by sickle erythrocytes. J. Clin. Invest. 70:1253, 1982.

165. Repka, T., and Hebbel, R.P.: Hydroxyl radical formation by sickle erythrocyte membranes: role of pathologic iron deposits and cytoplasmic reducing agents. Blood 78:2753, 1991.

166. Browne, P., Shalev, O., and Hebbel, R.P.: The molecular pathobiology of cell membrane iron: the sickle red cell as a model. Free Radic. Biol. Med. 24:1040, 1998.

167. Shalev, O., and Hebbel, R.P.: Catalysis of soluble hemoglobin oxidation by free iron on sickle red cell membranes. Blood 87:3948, 1996.

168. Asakura, T., Agarwal, P.L., Relman, D.A., McCray, J.A., Chance, B., Schwartz, E., Friedman, S., and Lubin, B.: Mechanical instability of the oxy-form of sickle haemoglobin. Nature 244:437, 1973.

169. Asakura, T., Onishi, T., Friedman, S., and Schwartz, E.: Abnormal precipitation of oxyhemoglobin S by mechanical shaking. Proc. Natl. Acad. Sci. USA 71:1594, 1974.

170. Liu, S.C., Zhai, S., and Palek, J.: Detection of hemin release during hemoglobin S denaturation. Blood 71:1755, 1988.

171. Liu, S.C., Zhai, S., Lawler, J., and Palek, J.: Hemin-mediated dissociation of erythrocyte membrane skeletal proteins. J. Biol. Chem. 260:12234, 1985.

172. Jarolim, P., Lahav, M., Liu, S.C., and Palek, J.: Effect of hemoglobin oxidation products on the stability of red cell membrane skeletons and the associations of skeletal proteins: correlation with a release of hemin. Blood 76:2125, 1990.

173. Shalev, O., and Hebbel, R.P.: Extremely high avidity association of Fe(III) with the sickle red cell membrane. Blood 88:349, 1996.

174. Shalev, O., Repka, T., Goldfarb, A., Grinberg, L., Abrahamov, A., Olivieri, N.F., Rachmilewitz, E.A., and Hebbel, R.P.: Deferiprone (L1) chelates pathologic iron deposits from membranes of intact thalassemic and sickle red blood cells both in vitro and in vivo. Blood 86:2008, 1995.

175. Middelkoop, E., Lubin, B.H., Bevers, E.M., Op den Kamp, J.A., Comfurius, P., Chiu, D.T., Zwaal, R.F., van Deenen, L.L., and Roelofsen, B.: Studies on sickled erythrocytes provide evidence that the asymmetric distribution of phosphatidylserine in the red cell membrane is maintained by both ATP-dependent translocation and interaction with membrane skeletal proteins. Biochim. Biophys. Acta 937:281, 1988.

176. Devaux, P.F.: Static and dynamic lipid asymmetry in cell membranes. Biochemistry 30:1163, 1991.

177. Lubin, B., Chiu, D., Bastacky, J., Roelofsen, B., and van Deenen, L.L.: Abnormalities in membrane phospholipid organization in sickled erythrocytes. J. Clin. Invest. 67:1643, 1981.

178. Franck, P.F., Bevers, E.M., Lubin, B.H., Comfurius, P., Chiu, D.T., Op den Kamp, J.A., Zwaal, R.F., Van, D.L., and Roelofsen, B.: Uncoupling of the membrane skeleton from the lipid bilayer. The cause of accelerated phospholipid flip-flop leading to an enhanced procoagulant activity of sickled cells. J. Clin. Invest. 75:183, 1985.

179. Mohandas, N., Rossi, M., Bernstein, S., Ballas, S., Ravindranath, Y., Wyatt, J., and Mentzer, W.: The structural organization of skeletal proteins influences lipid translocation across erythrocyte membrane. J. Biol. Chem. 260:14264, 1985.

180. Blumenfeld, N., Zachowski, A., Galacteros, F., Beuzard, Y., and Devaux, P.F.: Transmembrane mobility of phospholipids in sickle erythrocytes: effect of deoxygenation on diffusion and asymmetry. Blood 77:849, 1991.

181. Chiu, D., Lubin, B., Roelofsen, B., and Van, D.L.: Sickled erythrocytes accelerate clotting in vitro: an effect of abnormal membrane lipid asymmetry. Blood 58:398, 1981.

182. Westerman, M.P., Cole, E.R., and Wu, K.: The effect of spicules obtained from sickle red cells on clotting activity. Br. J. Haematol. 56:557, 1984.

183. Ballas, S.K., and Mohandas, N.: Pathophysiology of vaso-occlusion. Hematol. Oncol. Clin. North Am. 10:1221, 1996.

184. Das, S.K., and Nair, R.C.: Superoxide dismutase, glutathione peroxidase, catalase and lipid peroxidation of normal and sickled erythrocytes. Br. J. Haematol. 44:87, 1980.

185. Hebbel, R.P., and Miller, W.J.: Phagocytosis of sickle erythrocytes: immunologic and oxidative determinants of hemolytic anemia. Blood 64:733, 1984.

186. Jain, S.K., and Shohet, S.B.: A novel phospholipid in irreversibly sickled cells: evidence for in vivo peroxidative membrane damage in sickle cell disease. Blood 63:362, 1984.

187. Van den Berg, J.J.M., Kuypers, F.A., Qju, J.H., Chiu, D., Lubin, B., Roelofsen, B., and Op den Kamp, J.A.: The use of cis-parinaric acid to determine lipid peroxidation in human erythrocyte membranes. Comparison of normal and sickle erythrocyte membranes. Biochim. Biophys. Acta 944:29, 1988.

188. Kuross, S.A., and Hebbel, R.P.: Nonheme iron in sickle erythrocyte membranes: association with phospholipids and potential role in lipid peroxidation. Blood 72:1278, 1988.

189. Hebbel, R.P., and Miller, W.J.: Unique promotion of erythrophagocytosis by malondialdehyde. Am. J. Hematol. 29:222, 1988.

190. Bookchin, R.M., Ortiz, O.E., and Lew, V.L.: Mechanisms of red cell dehydration in sickle cell anemia. Application of an integrated red cell model. In Raess, B.U., and Tunnicliff, G. (eds.): The Red Cell Membrane: A Model for Solute Transport. Clifton, NJ, Humana Press, 1989.

191. Sugihara, T., Yawata, Y., and Hebbel, R.P.: Deformation of swollen erythrocytes provides a model of sickling-induced leak pathways, including a novel bromide-sensitive component. Blood 83:2684, 1994.

192. Lauf, P.K., and Theg, B.E.: A chloride dependent K+ flux induced by N-ethylmaleimide in genetically low K+ sheep and goat erythrocytes. Biochem. Biophys. Res. Commun. 92:1422, 1980.

193. Dunham, P.B., and Ellory, J.C.: Passive potassium transport in low potassium sheep red cells: dependence upon cell volume and chloride. J. Physiol. 318:511, 1981.

194. Brugnara, C., Bunn, H.F., and Tosteson, D.C.: Regulation of erythrocyte cation and water content in sickle cell anemia. Science 232:388, 1986.

195. Hall, A.C., and Ellory, J.C.: Evidence for the presence of volume-sensitive KCl transport in 'young' human red cells. Biochim. Biophys. Acta 858:317, 1986.

196. Brugnara, C., and Tosteson, D.C.: Cell volume, K+ transport and cell density. Am. J. Physiol. 21:C269, 1987.

197. Canessa, M., Spalvins, A., and Nagel, R.L.: Volume-dependent and NEM-stimulated K+,Cl- transport is elevated in oxygenated SS, SC and CC human red cells. FEBS Lett 200:197, 1986.

198. Olivieri, O., Vitoux, D., Galacteros, F., Bachir, D., Blouquit, Y., Beuzard, Y., and Brugnara, C.: Hemoglobin variants and activity of the (K+Cl-) cotransport system in human erythrocytes. Blood 79:793, 1992.

199. Vitoux, D., Olivieri, O., Garay, R.P., Cragoe, E.J., Galacteros, F., and Beuzard, Y.: Inhibition of K+ efflux and dehydration of sickle cells by [(dihydroindenyl)oxy]alkanoic acid: an inhibitor of the K+Cl- cotransport system. Proc. Natl. Acad. Sci. USA 86:4273, 1989.

200. Lawrence, C., Fabry, M.E., and Nagel, R.L.: The unique red cell heterogeneity of SC disease: crystal formation, dense reticulocytes, and unusual morphology. Blood 78:2104, 1991.

201. Fabry, M.E., Romero, J.R., Buchanan, I.D., Suzuka, S.M., Stamatoyannopoulos, G., Nagel, R.L., and Canessa, M.: Rapid increase in red blood cell density driven by K:Cl cotransport in a subset of sickle cell anemia reticulocytes and discocytes. Blood 78:217, 1991.

202. Brugnara, C., and Tosteson, D.C.: Inhibition of K transport by divalent cations in sickle erythrocytes. Blood 70:1810, 1987.

203. Canessa, M., Fabry, M.E., and Nagel, R.L.: Deoxygenation inhibits the volume-stimulated, Cl--dependent K+ efflux in SS and young AA cells: a cytosolic Mg2+ modulation. Blood 70:1861, 1987.

204. Eaton, J.W., Skelton, T.D., Swofford, H.S., Kolpin, C.E., and Jacob, H.S.: Elevated erythrocyte calcium in sickle cell disease. Nature 246:105, 1973.

205. Palek, J., Thomae, M., and Ozog, D.: Red cell calcium content and transmembrane calcium movements in sickle cell anemia. J. Lab. Clin. Med. 89:1365, 1977.

206. Lew, V.L., Hockaday, A., Sepulveda, M.I., Somlyo, A.P., Somlyo, A.V., Ortiz, O.E., and Bookchin, R.M.: Compartmentalization of sickle-cell calcium in endocytic inside-out vesicles. Nature 315:586, 1985.

207. Williamson, P., Puchulu, E., Westerman, M., and Schlegel, R.A.: Erythrocyte membrane abnormalities in sickle cell disease. Biotechnol. Appl. Biochem. 12:523, 1990.

208. Mohandas, N., Rossi, M.E., and Clark, M.R.: Association between morphologic distortion of sickle cells and deoxygenation-induced cation permeability increase. Blood 68:450, 1986.

209. Ortiz, O.E., Lew, V.L., and Bookchin, R.M.: Deoxygenation permeabilizes sickle cell anaemia red cells to magnesium and reverses its gradient in the dense cells. J. Physiol. 427:211, 1990.
210. Clark, M.R., and Rossi, M.E.: Permeability characteristics of deoxygenated sickle cells. Blood 76:2139, 1990.
211. Hebbel, R.P., Shalev, O., Foker, W., and Rank, B.H.: Inhibition of erythrocyte Ca^{2+} − ATPase by activated oxygen through thiol- and lipid-dependent mechanisms. Biochim. Biophys. Acta 862:8, 1986.
212. Tosteson, D.C., Shea, E., and Darling, R.C.: Potassium and sodium of red blood cells in sickle cell anemia. J. Clin. Invest. 31:406, 1952.
213. Joiner, C.H.: Deoxygenation-induced cation fluxes in sickle cells: II. Inhibition by stilbene disulfonates. Blood 76:212, 1990.
214. Joiner, C.H., Platt, O.S., and Lux, S.T.: Cation depletion by the sodium pump in red cells with pathologic cation leaks. Sickle cells and xerocytes. J. Clin. Invest. 78:1487, 1986.
215. Lew, V.L., Freeman, C.J., Ortiz, O.E., and Bookchin, R.M.: A mathematical model of the volume, pH, and ion content regulation in reticulocytes. Application to the pathophysiology of sickle cell dehydration. J. Clin. Invest. 87:100, 1991.
216. Ney, P.A., Christopher, M.M., and Hebbel, R.P.: Synergistic effects of oxidation and deformation on erythrocyte monovalent cation leak. Blood 75:1192, 1990.
217. Sugicara, T., Rawicz, W., Evans, E.A., and Hebbel, R.P.: Lipid hydroperoxides permit deformation-dependent leak of monovalent cation from erythrocytes. Blood 77:2757, 1991.
218. Lew, V.L., and Bookchin, R.M.: Osmotic effects of protein polymerization: analysis of volume changes in sickle cell anemia red cells following deoxy-hemoglobin S polymerization. J. Membr. Biol. 122:55, 1991.
219. Bookchin, R.M., and Lew, V.L.: Pathophysiology of sickle cell anemia. Hematol. Oncol. Clin. North Am. 10:1241, 1996.
220. Franco, R.S., Thompson, H., Palascak, M., and Joiner, C.H.: The formation of transferrin receptor-positive sickle reticulocytes with intermediate density is not determined by fetal hemoglobin content. Blood 90:3195, 1997.
221. Embury, S.H., Garcia, J.F., Mohandas, N., Pennathur-Das, R., and Clark, M.R.: Oxygen inhalation by subjects with sickle cell anemia. Effects of endogenous erythropoietin kinetics, erythropoiesis, and pathophysiologic properties of sickle blood. N. Engl. J. Med. 311:291, 1984.
222. Schwartz, R.S., Tanaka, Y., Fidler, I.J., Chiu, D.T., Lubin, B., and Schroit, A.J.: Increased adherence of sickled and phosphatidylserine-enriched human erythrocytes to cultured human peripheral blood monocytes. J. Clin. Invest. 75:1965, 1985.
223. Solanki, D.L.: Erythrophagocytosis in vivo sickle cell anemia. Am. J. Hematol. 20:353, 1985.
224. Petz, L.D., Yam, P., Wilkinson, L., Garratty, G., Lubin, B., and Mentzer, W.: Increased IgG molecules bound to the surface of red blood cells of patients with sickle cell anemia. Blood 64:301, 1984.
225. Galili, U., Clark, M.R., and Shohet, S.B.: Excessive binding of natural anti-alpha-galactosyl immunoglobin G to sickle erythrocytes may contribute to extravascular cell destruction. J. Clin. Invest. 77:27, 1986.
226. Schluter, K., and Drenckhahn, D.: Co-clustering of denatured hemoglobin with band 3: its role in binding of autoantibodies against band 3 to abnormal and aged erythrocytes. Proc. Natl. Acad. Sci. USA 83:6137, 1986.
227. Hoover, R., Rubin, R., Wise, G., and Warren, R.: Adhesion of normal and sickle erythrocytes to endothelial monolayer cultures. Blood 54:872, 1979.
228. Hebbel, R.P., Boogaerts, M.A.B., Eaton, J.W., and Steinberg, M.H.: Erythrocyte adherence to endothelium in sickle cell anemia: possible determinant of disease severity. N. Engl. J. Med. 302:992, 1980.
229. Smith, B.D., and La, C.P.: Erythrocyte-endothelial cell adherence in sickle cell disorders. Blood 68:1050, 1986.
230. Barabino, G.A., McIntire, L.V., Eskin, S.G., Sears, D.A., and Udden, M.: Endothelial cell interactions with sickle cell, sickle trait, mechanically injured, and normal erythrocytes under controlled flow. Blood 70:152, 1987.
231. Wick, T.M., Moake, J.L., Udden, M.M., Eskin, S.G., Sears, D.A., and McIntire, L.V.: Unusually large von Willebrand factor multimers increase adhesion of sickle erythrocytes to human endothelial cells under controlled flow. J. Clin. Invest. 80:905, 1987.
232. Mohandas, N., and Evans, E.: Adherence of sickle erythrocytes to vascular endothelial cells: requirement for both cell membrane changes and plasma factors. Blood 64:282, 1984.
233. Kaul, D.K., Fabry, M.E., and Nagel, R.L.: Microvascular sites and characteristics of sickle cell adhesion to vascular endothelium in shear flow conditions: pathophysiological implications. Proc. Natl. Acad. Sci. USA 86:3356, 1989.
234. Mohandas, N., and Evans, E.: Sickle erythrocyte adherence to vascular endothelium. Morphologic correlates and the requirement for divalent cations and collagen-binding plasma proteins. J. Clin. Invest. 76:1605, 1985.
235. Mohandas, N., and Evans, E.: Rheological and adherence properties of sickle cells. Potential contribution to hematologic manifestations of the disease. Ann. N. Y. Acad. Sci. 565:327, 1989.
236. Ballas, S.K., Larner, J., and Smith, E.D.: Rheologic predictors of the severity of the painful sickle cell crisis. Blood 72:1216, 1988.
237. Lande, W.M., Andrews, D.L., Clark, M.R., Braham, N.V., Black, D.M., Embury, S.H., and Mentzer, W.C.: The incidence of painful crisis in homozygous sickle cell disease: correlation with red cell deformability. Blood 72:2056, 1988.
238. Browne, P.V., and Hebbel, R.P.: CD36-positive stress reticulocytosis in sickle cell anemia. J. Lab. Clin. Med. 127:340, 1996.
239. Styles, L.A., Lubin, B., Vichinsky, E., Lawrence, S., Hua, M., Test, S., and Kuypers, F.: Decrease of very late activation antigen-4 and CD36 on reticulocytes in sickle cell patients treated with hydroxyurea. Blood 89:2554, 1997.
240. Wick, T.M., Moake, J.L., Udden, M.M., and McIntire, L.V.: Unusually large vWF multimers preferentially promote young sickle and non-sickle erythrocyte adhesion to endothelial cells. Am. J. Hematol. 284, 1993.
241. Kumar, A., Eckman, J.R., and Wick, T.M.: Inhibition of plasma-mediated adherence of sickle erythrocytes to microvascular endothelium by conformationally constrained RGD-containing peptides. Am. J. Hematol. 53:92, 1996.
242. Hebbel, R.P., Moldow, C.F., and Steinberg, M.H.: Modulation of erythrocyte-endothelial interactions and the vasocclusive severity of sickling disorders. Blood 58:947, 1981.
243. Kaul, D.K., Nagel, R.L., Chen, D., and Tsai, H.M.: Sickle erythrocyte-endothelial interactions in microcirculation: the role of von Willebrand factor and implications for vasoocclusion. Blood 81:2429, 1993.
244. Kumar, A., Eckmann, J.R., Swerlick, R.A., and Wick, T.M.: Phorbol ester stimulation increases sickle erythrocyte adherence to endothelium: a novel pathway involving $\alpha_4\beta_1$ integrin receptors on sickle reticulocytes and fibronectin. Blood 88:4348, 1996.
245. Swerlick, R.A., Eckman, J.R., Kumar, A., Jeitler, M., and Wick, T.M.: $\alpha_4\beta_1$-Integrin expression on sickle reticulocytes: vascular cell adhesion molecule-1−dependent binding to endothelium. Blood 82:1891, 1993.
246. Gee, B.E., and Platt, O.S.: Sickle reticulocytes adhere to VCAM-1. Blood 85:268, 1995.
247. Sugihara, K., Sugihara, T., Mohandas, N., and Hebbel, R.P.: Thrombospondin mediates adherence of CD36 + sickle reticulocytes to endothelial cells. Blood 80:2634, 1992.
248. Brittain, H.A., Eckman, J.R., Swerlick, R.A., Howard, R.J., and Wick, T.M.: Thrombospondin from activated platelets promotes sickle erythrocyte adherence to human microvascular endothelium under physiologic flow: a potential role for platelet activation in sickle cell vasoocclusion. Blood 81:2137, 1993.
249. Browne, P.V., Mosher, D.F., Steinberg, M.H., and Hebbel, R.P.: Disturbance of plasma and platelet thrombospondin levels in sickle cell disease. Am. J. Hematol. 51:296, 1996.
250. Joneckis, C.C., Shock, D.D., Cunningham, M.L., Orringer, E.P., and Parise, L.V.: Glycoprotein IV–independent adhesion of sickle red blood cells to immobilized thrombospondin under flow conditions. Blood 87:4862, 1996.
251. Hillery, C.A., Du, M.C., Montgomery, R.R., and Scott, J.P.: Increased adhesion of erythrocytes to components of the extracellular matrix: isolation and characterization of a red blood cell lipid that binds thrombospondin and laminin. Blood 87:4879, 1996.
251a. Barabino, G.A., Liu, X.D., Ewenstein, B.M., and Kaul, D.K.: Anionic polysaccharides inhibit adhesion of sickle erythrocytes to the vascular endothelium and result in improved hemodynamic behavior. Blood 93:1422, 1999.
252. Barabino, G.A., Wise, R.J., Woodbury, V.A., Zhang, B., Bridges, K.A., Hebbel, R.P., Lawler, J., and Ewenstein, B.M.: Inhibition of sickle erythrocyte adhesion to immobilized thrombospondin by von Willebrand factor under dynamic flow conditions. Blood 89:2560, 1997.
253. Solovey, A., Lin, Y., Browne, P., Choong, S., Wayner, E., and Hebbel,

R.P.: Circulating activated endothelial cells in sickle cell anemia. N. Engl. J. Med. 337:1584, 1997.

254. Solovey, A., Gui, L., Key, N.S., and Hebbel, R.P.: Tissue factor expression by endothelial cells in sickle cell anemia J. Clin. Invest. 101:1899, 1998.

255. Key, N.S., Slungaard, A., Dandelet, L., Nelson, S.C., Moertel, C., Styles, L.A., Kuypers, F.A., and Bach, R.R.: Whole blood tissue factor procoagulant activity is elevated in patients with sickle cell disease. Blood 91:4216, 1998.

255a. Hillery, C.A., Scott, J.P., and Du, M.D.: The carboxy-terminal cell-binding domain of thrombospondin is essential for sickle red blood cell adhesion. Blood 94:302, 1999.

255b. Manodori, A.B., Matsui, N.M., Chen, J.Y., and Embury, S.H.: Enhanced adherence of sickle erythrocytes to thrombin-treated endothelial cells involves interendothelial cell gap formation. Blood 92:3445, 1998.

255c. Udani, M., Zen, Q., Cottman, M., Leonard, N., Jefferson, S., Daymont, C., Truskey, G., and Telen, M.J.: Basal cell adhesion moleculae/lutheran protein. The receptor critical for sickle cell adhesion to laminin. J. Clin. Invest. 101:2550, 1998.

255d. Lee, S.P., Cunningham, M.L., Hines, P.C., Joneckis, C.C., Orringer, E.P., and Parise, L.V.: Sickle cell adhesion to laminin: potential role for the alpha5 chain. Blood 92:2951, 1998.

256. Smolinski, P.A., Offermann, M.K., Eckman, J.R., and Wick, T.M.: Double-stranded RNA induces sickle erythrocyte adherence to endothelium: a potential role for viral infection in vaso-occlusive pain episodes in sickle cell anemia. Blood 85:2945, 1995.

257. Hebbel, R.P., Visser, M.R., Goodman, J.L., Jacob, H.S., and Vercellotti, G.M.: Potentiated adherence of sickle erythrocytes to endothelium infected by virus. J. Clin. Invest. 80:1503, 1987.

258. Thevenin, B.J.-M., Crandall, I., Ballas, S., Sherman, I.W., and Shohet, S.B.: Band 3 peptides block the adherence of sickle cells to endothelial cells in vitro. Blood 90:4172, 1997.

259. Fadlon, E., Vordermeier, S., Pearson, T.C., Mire-Sluis, A.R., Dumonde, D.C., Phillips, J., Fishlock, K., and Brown, K.A.: Blood polymorphonuclear leukocytes from the majority of sickle cell patients in the crisis phase of the disease show enhanced adhesion to vascular endothelium and increased expression of CD64. Blood 91:266, 1998.

260. Kasschau, M.R., Barabino, G.A., Bridges, K.R., and Golan, D.E.: Adhesion of sickle neutrophils and erythrocytes to fibronectin. Blood 87:771, 1996.

261. Francis, R.J., and Johnson, C.S.: Vascular occlusion in sickle cell disease: current concepts and unanswered questions. Blood 77:1405, 1991.

262. Fabry, M.E., Rajanayagam, V., Fine, E., Holland, S., Gore, J.C., Nagel, R.L., and Kaul, D.K.: Modeling sickle cell vasoocclusion in the rat leg: quantification of trapped sickle cells and correlation with 31P metabolic and 1H magnetic resonance imaging changes. Proc. Natl. Acad. Sci. USA 86:3808, 1989.

263. Kaul, D.K., Chen, D., and Zhan, J.: Adhesion of sickle cells to vascular endothelium is critically dependent on changes in density and shape of the cells. Blood 83:3006, 1994.

264. Kaul, D.K., Fabry, M.E., Costantini, F., Rubin, E.M., and Nagel, R.L.: In vivo demonstration of red cell–endothelial interaction, sickling and altered microvascular response to oxygen in the sickle transgenic mouse. J. Clin. Invest. 96:2845, 1995.

265. French, J.A.I., Kenny, D., Scott, J.P., Hoffman, R.G., Wood, J.D., Hudetz, A.G., and Hillery, C.A.: Mechanisms of stroke in sickle cell disease: sickle erythrocytes decrease cerebral blood flow in rats after nitric oxide synthase inhibition. Blood 89:4591, 1997.

266. Osei, S.Y., Ahima, R.S., Fabry, M.E., Nagel, R.L., and Bank, N.: Immunohistochemical localization of hepatic nitric oxide synthase in normal and transgenic sickle cell mice: the effect of hypoxia. Blood 88:3583, 1996.

267. Bank, N., Aynedjian, H.S., Qiu, J.-H., Osei, S.Y., Ahima, R.S., Fabry, M.E., and Nagel, R.L.: Renal nitric oxide synthases in transgenic sickle cell mice. Kidney Int. 50:184, 1996.

267a. Stuart, M.J., and Setty, B.N.: Sickle cell acute chest syndrome: pathogenesis and rationale for treatment. Blood 94:1555, 1999.

268. Rodgers, G.P., Schechter, A.N., Noguchi, C.T., Klein, H.G., Nienhuis, A.W., and Bonner, R.F.: Periodic microcirculatory flow in patients with sickle cell disease. N. Engl. J. Med. 311:1534, 1984.

269. Rodgers, G.P., Schechter, A.N., Noguchi, C.T., Klein, H.G., Nienhuis, A.W., and Bonner, R.F.: Microcirculatory adaptations in sickle cell anemia: reactive hyperemia response. Am. J. Physiol. 258:H113, 1990.

270. Rodgers, G.P., Roy, M.S., Noguchi, C.T., and Schechter, A.N.: Is there a role for selective vasodilation in the management of sickle cell disease? Blood 71:597, 1988.

271. Kennedy, A.P., Williams, B., Meydrech, E.F., and Steinberg, M.H.: Regional and temporal variation in oscillatory blood flow in sickle cell disease. Am. J. Hematol. 28:92, 1988.

272. Brody, A.S., Embury, S.H., Mentzer, W.C., Winkler, M.L., and Gooding, C.A.: Preservation of sickle cell blood-flow patterns during MR imaging: an in vivo study. Am. J. Radiol. 151:139, 1988.

273. Rodgers, G.P., Clark, C.M., Larson, S.M., Rapoport, S.I., Nienhuis, A.W., and Schechter, A.N.: Brain glucose metabolism in neurologically normal patients with sickle cell disease. Arch. Neurol. 45:78, 1988.

274. Baum, K.F., Dunn, D.T., Maude, G.H., and Serjeant, G.R.: The painful crisis of homozygous sickle cell disease. A study of the risk factors. Arch. Intern. Med. 147:1231, 1987.

275. Platt, O.S., Thorington, B.D., Brambilla, D.J., Milner, P.F., Rosse, W.F., Vichinsky, E., and Kinney, T.R.: Pain in sickle cell disease: rates and risk factors. N. Engl. J. Med. 325:11, 1991.

276. Sergeant, G.R., and Chalmers, R.M.: Current concerns in hematology 1. Is the painful crisis of sickle cell disease a "steal" syndrome? Clin. Pathol. 43:789, 1990.

277. Brittenham, G.M., Schechter, A.N., and Noguchi, C.T.: Hemoglobin S polymerization: primary determinant of the hemolytic and clinical severity of the sickling syndromes. Blood 65:183, 1985.

278. Noguchi, C.T., Rodgers, G.P., Sergeant, G., and Schechter, A.N.: Levels of fetal hemoglobin necessary for treatment of sickle cell disease. N. Engl. J. Med. 318:96, 1988.

279. Keidan, A.J., Sowter, M.C., Johnson, C.S., Noguchi, C.T., Girling, A.J., Stevens, S.M., and Stuart, J.: Effect of polymerization tendency on haematological, rheological and clinical parameters in sickle cell anaemia. Br. J. Haematol. 71:551, 1989.

279a. Poillon, W.N., Kim, B.C., and Castro, O.: Intracellular hemoglobin S polymerization and the clinical severity of sickle cell anemia. Blood 91:1777, 1998.

280. Warth, J.A., and Rucknagel, D.L.: Density ultracentrifugation of sickle cells during and after pain crisis: increased dense echinocytes in crisis. Blood 64:507, 1984.

281. Rieber, E.E., Veliz, G., and Pollack, S.: Red cells in sickle cell crisis: observations on the pathophysiology of crisis. Blood 49:967, 1977.

282. Kenney, M.W., Meaken, M., Worthington, D.J., and Stuart, J.: Erythrocyte deformability in sickle crisis. Br. J. Haematol. 49:103, 1981.

283. Lucas, G.S., Caldwell, N.M., and Stuart, J.: Fluctuating deformability of oxygenated sickle erythrocytes in the asymptomatic state and in painful crisis. Br. J. Haematol. 59:363, 1985.

284. Ballas, S.K., and Smith, E.D.: Red blood cell changes during the evolution of the sickle cell painful crisis. Blood 79:2154, 1992.

285. Billett, H.H., Nagel, R.L., and Fabry, M.E.: Evolution of laboratory parameters during sickle cell painful crisis: evidence compatible with dense red cells sequestration without thrombosis. Am. J. Med. Sci. 296:293, 1988.

285a. Graido-Gonzalez, E., Doherty, J.C., Bergreen, E.W., Organ, G., Telfer, M., and McMillen, M.A.: Plasma endothelin-1, cytokine and prostaglandin E_2 levels in sickle cell disease and acute vaso-occlusive sickle crisis. Blood 92:2551, 1998.

285b. Rybicki, A.C., and Benjamin, L.J.: Increased levels of endothelin-1 in plasma of sickle cell anemia patients. Blood 92:2594, 1998.

285c. Michaels, L.A., Ohene-Frempong, K., Zhao, H., and Douglas, S.D.: Serum levels of substance P are elevated in patients with sickle cell disease and increase further during vaso-occlusive crisis. Blood 92:3148, 1998.

285d. Nagel, R.L.: A knockout of a transgenic mouse—animal models of sickle cell anemia. N. Engl. J. Med. 339:194, 1998.

286. Rubin, E.M., Lu, R.H., Cooper, S., Mohandas, N., and Kan, Y.W.: Introduction and expression of the human β^s-globin gene in transgenic mice. Am. J. Hum. Genet. 42:585, 1988.

287. Rhoda, M.D., Domenget, C., Vidaud, M., Bardakdjian-Michau, J., Rouyer-Fessard, P., Rosa, J., and Beuzard, Y.: Mouse α chains inhibit polymerization of hemoglobin induced by human β^s or $\beta^{s\ Antilles}$ chains. Biochim. Biophys. Acta 952:208, 1988.

288. Greaves, D.R., Fraser, P., Vidal, M.A., Hedges, M.J., Ropers, D., Luzzatto, L., and Grosveld, F.: A transgenic mouse model of sickle cell disorder [see comments]. Nature 343:183, 1990.

289. Ryan, T.M., Townes, T.M., Reilly, M.P., Asakura, T., Palmiter, R.D., Brinster, R.L., and Behringer, R.R.: Human sickle hemoglobin in transgenic mice. Science 247:566, 1990.

290. Fabry, M.E., Nagel, R.L., Pachnis, A., Suzuka, S.M., and Costantini, F.: High expression of human beta S- and alpha-globins in transgenic mice: hemoglobin composition and hematological consequences. Proc. Natl. Acad. Sci. USA 89:12150, 1992.

291. Rubin, E.M., Kan, Y.W., and Mohandas, N.: Effect of human beta s-globin chains on cellular properties of red cells from beta-thalassemic mice. J. Clin. Invest. 82:1129, 1988.

292. Popp, R.A., Popp, D.M., Shinpock, S.G., Yang, M.Y., Mural, J.G., Aguinaga, M.D.P., Kopsombut, P., Roa, P.D., Turner, E.A., and Rubin, E.M.: A transgenic mouse model of hemoglobin S Antilles disease. Blood 89:4204, 1997.

293. Monplaisir, N., Merault, G., Poyart, C., Rhoda, M.D., Craescu, C., Vidaud, M., Galacteros, F., Blouquit, Y., and Rosa, J.: Hemoglobin S Antilles: a variant with lower solubility than hemoglobin S and producing sickle cell disease in heterozygotes. Proc. Natl. Acad. Sci. USA 83:9363, 1986.

294. Rubin, E.M., Witkowska, H.E., Spangler, E., Curtin, P., Lubin, B.H., Mohandas, N., and Clift, S.M.: Hypoxia-induced in vivo sickling of transgenic mouse red cells. J. Clin. Invest. 87:639, 1991.

295. Trudel, M., Saadane, N., Garel, M.C., Bardakdjian, M.J., Blouquit, Y., Guerquin, K.J., Rouyer, F.P., Vidaud, D., Pachnis, A., Romeo, P.H.: Towards a transgenic mouse model of sickle cell disease: hemoglobin SAD. EMBO. J. 10:3157, 1991.

296. Saadane, N., Trudel, M., Garel, M.-C., Bardakdjian-Michau, J., Blouquit, Y., Guerquin-Kern, J.-L., Rouyer-Fessard, P., Vichaud, D., Pachnis, A., Romeo, P.-H., Constantini, F., and Beuzard, Y.: Sickle cell anemia in transgenic SAD mice. Blood 78:369a, 1991.

297. Trudel, M., Paepe, M.E.D., Chretien, N., Saadane, N., Jacmain, J., Sorette, M., Hoang, T., and Beuzard, Y.: Sickle cell disease of transgenic SAD mice. Blood 84:3189, 1994.

298. Ryan, T.M., Ciavatta, D.J., and Townes, T.M.: Knockout-transgenic mouse model of sickle cell disease. Science 278:873, 1997.

299. Paszty, C., Brion, C.M., Manci, E., Witkowska, H.E., Stevens, M.E., Mohandas, N., and Rubin, E.M.: Transgenic knockout mice with exclusively human sickle hemoglobin and sickle cell disease. Science 278:876, 1997.

299a. Embury, S.H., Mohandas, N., Paszty, C., Cooper, P., and Cheung, A.T.: In vivo blood flow abnormalities in the transgenic knockout sickle cell mouse. J. Clin. Invest. 103:915, 1999.

300. Kan, Y.W., and Dozy, A.M.: Polymorphism of DNA sequence adjacent to human beta-globin structural gene: relationship to sickle mutation. Proc. Natl. Acad. Sci. USA 75:5631, 1978.

301. Pagnier, J., Mears, J.G., Dunda, B.O., Schaefer, R.K., Beldjord, C., Nagel, R.L., and Labie, D.: Evidence for the multicentric origin of the sickle cell hemoglobin gene in Africa. Proc. Natl. Acad. Sci. USA 81:1771, 1984.

302. Labie, D., Pagnier, J., Lapoumeroulie, C., Rouabhi, F., Dunda, B.O., Chardin, P., Beldjord, C., Wajcman, H., Fabry, M.E., and Nagel, R.L.: Common haplotype dependency of high G gamma-globin gene expression and high Hb F levels in beta-thalassemia and sickle cell anemia patients. Proc. Natl. Acad. Sci. USA 82:2111, 1985.

303. Chebloune, Y., Pagnier, J., Trabuchet, G., Faure, C., Verdier, G., Labie, D., and Nigon, V.: Structural analysis of the 5′ flanking region of the beta-globin gene in African sickle cell anemia patients: further evidence for three origins of the sickle cell mutation in Africa. Proc. Natl. Acad. Sci. USA 85:4431, 1988.

304. Nagel, R.L., and Ranney, H.M.: Genetic epidemiology of structural mutations of the beta-globin gene. Semin. Hematol. 27:342, 1990.

305. Bouhassira, E.E., Lachman, H., Krishnamoorthy, R., Labie, D., and Nagel, R.L.: A gene conversion located 5′ to the A gamma gene in linkage disequilibrium with the Bantu haplotype in sickle cell anemia. J. Clin. Invest. 83:2070, 1989.

306. Bouhassira, E.E., and Nagel, R.L.: A 6-bp deletion 5′ to the G gamma globin gene in beta S chromosomes bearing the Bantu haplotype. Am. J. Hum. Genet. 47:161, 1990.

307. Srinivas, R., Dunda, O., Krishnamoorthy, R., Fabry, M.E., Georges, A., Labie, D., and Nagel, R.L.: Atypical haplotypes linked to the beta S gene in Africa are likely to be the product of recombination. Am. J. Hematol. 29:60, 1988.

308. Ragusa, A., Lombardo, M., Sortino, G., Lombardo, T., Nagel, R.L., and Labie, D.: Beta S gene in Sicily is in linkage disequilibrium with the Benin haplotype: implications for gene flow. Am. J. Hematol. 27:139, 1988.

309. Boussiou, M., Loukopoulos, D., Christakis, J., and Fessas, P.: The origin of the sickle mutation in Greece; evidence from beta S globin gene cluster polymorphisms. Hemoglobin 15:459, 1991.

310. Labie, D., Srinivas, R., Dunda, O., Dode, C., Lapoumeroulie, C., Devi, V., Devi, S., Ramasami, K., Elion, J., Ducrocq, R., et al.: Haplotypes in tribal Indians bearing the sickle gene: evidence for the unicentric origin of the beta S mutation and the unicentric origin of the tribal populations of India. Hum. Biol. 61:479, 1989.

311. Nagel, R.L., and Roth, E.J.: Malaria and red cell genetic defects. Blood 74:1213, 1989.

312. Nagel, R.L.: Innate resistance to malaria: the intraerythrocytic cycle. Blood Cells 16:321, 1990.

313. Allison, A.C.: Protection afforded by sickle-cell trait against subtertian malarial infection. Br. Med. J. 1:190, 1954.

314. Hood, A.T., Fabry, M.E., Costantini, F., Nagel, R.L., and Shear, H.L.: Protection from lethal malaria in transgenic mice expressing sickle hemoglobin. Blood 87:1600, 1996.

315. Luzzatto, L., Nwachuku, J.E., and Reddy, S.: Increased sickling of parasitised erythrocytes as mechanism of resistance against malaria in the sickle-cell trait. Lancet 1:319, 1970.

316. Raventos, S.C., Kaul, D.K., Macaluso, F., and Nagel, R.L.: Membrane knobs are required for the microcirculatory obstruction induced by *Plasmodium falciparum*–infected erythrocytes. Proc. Natl. Acad. Sci. USA 82:3829, 1985.

317. Nagel, R.L., Rao, S.K., Dunda, B.O., Connolly, M.M., Fabry, M.E., Georges, A., Krishnamoorthy, R., and Labie, D.: The hematologic characteristics of sickle cell anemia bearing the Bantu haplotype: the relationship between G gamma and HbF level. Blood 69:1026, 1987.

318. Embury, S.H., Backer, K., and Glader, B.E.: Monovalent cation changes in sickle erythrocytes: a direct reflection of alpha-globin gene number. J. Lab. Clin. Med. 106:75, 1985.

319. Nagel, R.L., Erlingsson, S., Fabry, M.E., Croizat, H., Susuka, S.M., Lachman, H., Sutton, M., Driscoll, C., Bouhassira, E., and Billett, H.H.: The Senegal DNA haplotype is associated with the amelioration of anemia in African-American sickle cell anemia patients. Blood 77:1371, 1991.

320. Rieder, R.F., Safaya, S., Gillette, P., Fryd, S., Hsu, H., Adams, J.D., and Steinberg, M.H.: Effect of beta-globin gene cluster haplotype on the hematological and clinical features of sickle cell anemia [see comments]. Am. J. Hematol. 36:184, 1991.

321. Powars, D., Chan, L.S., and Schroeder, W.A.: The variable expression of sickle cell disease is genetically determined. Semin. Hematol. 27:360, 1990.

322. Wainscoat, J.S., Thein, S.L., Higgs, D.R., Bell, J.I., Weatherall, D.J., Al-Awamy, B., and Serjeant, G.R.: A genetic marker for elevated levels of haemoglobin F in homozygous sickle cell disease? Br. J. Haematol. 60:261, 1985.

323. Miyoshi, K., Kaneto, Y., Kawai, H., Ohchi, H., Niki, S., Hasegawa, K., Shirakami, A., and Yamano, T.: X-linked dominant control of F-cells in normal adult life: characterization of the Swiss type as hereditary persistence of fetal hemoglobin regulated dominantly by gene(s) on X chromosome. Blood 72:1854, 1988.

324. Dover, G.J., Smith, K.D., Chang, Y.C., Purvis, S., Mays, A., Meyers, D.A., Sheils, C., and Serjeant, G.: Fetal hemoglobin levels in sickle cell disease and normal individuals are partially controlled by an X-linked gene located at Xp22.2. Blood 80:816, 1992.

325. Chang, Y.C., Smith, K.D., Moore, R.D., Serjeant, G.R., and Dover, G.J.: An analysis of fetal hemoglobin variation in sickle cell disease: the relative contributions of the X-linked factor, beta-globin haplotypes, alpha-globin gene number, gender, and age. Blood 85:1111, 1995.

326. Davis, J.R., Dozy, A.M., Lubin, B., Koenig, H.M., Pierce, H.I., Stamatoyannopoulos, G., and Kan, Y.W.: Alpha thalassemia in blacks is due to gene deletion. Am. J. Hum. Genet. 31:569, 1979.

327. Dozy, A.M., Kan, Y.W., Embury, S.H., Mentzer, W.C., Wang, W.C., Lubin, B., Davis, J.J., and Koenig, H.M.: alpha-Globin gene organisation in blacks precludes the severe form of alpha-thalassaemia. Nature 280:605, 1979.

328. Embury, S.H., Miller, J.A., Dozy, A.M., Kan, Y.W., Chan, V., and Todd, D.: Two different molecular organizations account for the single alpha-globin gene of the alpha-thalassemia-2 genotype. J. Clin. Invest. 66:1319, 1980.

329. Embury, S.H., Gholson, M.A., Gillette, P., and Rieder, R.F.: The leftward deletion alpha-thal-2 haplotype in a black subject with hemoglobin SS. Blood 65:769, 1985.

330. Steinberg, M.H., Coleman, M.B., Adams, J.D., Hartmann, R.C., Saba, H., and Anagnou, N.P.: A new gene deletion in the alpha-like globin gene cluster as the molecular basis for the rare alpha-thalassemia-

1($--$/alpha alpha) in blacks: HbH disease in sickle cell trait. Blood 67:469, 1986.

331. Gupta, A.K., Kirchner, K.A., Nicholson, R., Adams, J.D., Schechter, A.N., Noguchi, C.T., and Steinberg, M.H.: Effects of alpha-thalassemia and sickle polymerization tendency on the urine-concentrating defect of individuals with sickle cell trait. J. Clin. Invest. 88:1963, 1991.

332. Steinberg, M.H., and Embury, S.H.: Alpha-thalassemia in blacks: genetic and clinical aspects and interactions with the sickle hemoglobin gene. Blood 68:985, 1986.

333. Embury, S.H.: Alpha thalassemia, a modifier of sickle cell disease. Ann. N. Y. Acad. Sci. 565:213, 1989.

334. Embury, S.H., Dozy, A.M., Miller, J., Davis, J.J., Kleman, K.M., Preisler, H., Vichinsky, E., Lande, W.N., Lubin, B.H., Kan, Y.W., and Mentzer, W.C.: Concurrent sickle-cell anemia and alpha-thalassemia: effect on severity of anemia. N. Engl. J. Med. 306:270, 1982.

335. Higgs, D.R., Aldridge, B.E., Lamb, J., Clegg, J.B., Weatherall, D.J., Hayes, R.J., Grandison, Y., Lowrie, Y., Mason, K.P., Serjeant, B.E., and Serjeant, G.R.: The interaction of alpha-thalassemia and homozygous sickle-cell disease. N. Engl. J. Med. 306:1441, 1982.

336. Steinberg, M.H., Rosenstock, W., Coleman, M.B., Adams, J.G., Platica, O., Cedeno, M., Rieder, R.F., Wilson, J.T., Milner, P., and West, S.: Effects of thalassemia and microcytosis on the hematologic and vasoocclusive severity of sickle cell anemia. Blood 63:1353, 1984.

337. DeCeulear, K., Higgs, D.R., Weatherall, D.J., Hayes, R.J., Serjeant, B.E., and Serjeant, G.R.: α-Thalassemia reduces the hemolytic rate in homozygous sickle cell disease. N. Engl. J. Med. 309:189, 1984.

338. Noguchi, C.T., Dover, G.J., Rodgers, G.P., Serjeant, G.R., Antonarakis, S.E., Anagnou, N.P., Higgs, D.R., Weatherall, D.J., and Schechter, A.N.: Alpha thalassemia changes erythrocyte heterogeneity in sickle cell disease. J. Clin. Invest. 75:1632, 1985.

339. Embury, S.H., Clark, M.R., Monroy, G., and Mohandas, N.: Concurrent sickle cell anemia and alpha-thalassemia. Effect on pathological properties of sickle erythrocytes. J. Clin. Invest. 73:116, 1984.

340. Dover, G.J., Chang, V.T., Boyer, S.H., Serjeant, G.R., Antonarakis, S., and Higgs, D.R.: The cellular basis for different fetal hemoglobin levels among sickle cell individuals with two, three, and four alpha-globin genes. Blood 69:341, 1987.

340a. Guasch, A., Zayas, C.F., Eckman, J.R., Muralidharan, K., Zhang, W., and Elsas, L.J.: Evidence that microdeletions in the alpha globin gene protect against the development of sickle cell glomerulopathy in humans. J. Am. Soc. Nephrol. 10:1014, 1999.

341. Hawker, H., Neilson, H., Hayes, R.J., and Serjeant, G.R.: Haematological factors associated with avascular necrosis of the femoral head in homozygous sickle cell disease. Br. J. Haematol. 50:29, 1982.

342. Milner, P.F., Kraus, A.P., Sebes, J.I., Sleeper, L.A., Dukes, K.A., Embury, S.H., Bellevue, R., Koshy, M., Moohr, J.W., and Smith, J.: Sickle cell disease as a cause of osteonecrosis of the femoral head. N. Engl. J. Med. 325:1476, 1991.

343. Hayes, R.J., Condon, P.I., and Serjeant, G.R.: Haematological factors associated with proliferative retinopathy in homozygous sickle cell disease. Br. J. Ophthalmol. 65:29, 1981.

344. Mears, J.G., Lachman, H.M., Labie, D., and Nagel, R.L.: Alpha-thalassemia is related to prolonged survival in sickle cell anemia. Blood 62:286, 1983.

345. Steinberg, M.H., West, M.S., Gallagher, D., and Mentzer, W.: Effects of glucose-6-phosphate dehydrogenase deficiency upon sickle cell anemia. Blood 71:748, 1988.

346. Olson, J.F., Ware, R.E., Schultz, W.H., and Kinney, T.R.: Hemoglobin C disease in infancy and childhood. J. Pediatr. 125:745, 1994.

347. Hirsch, R.E., Lin, M.J., and Nagel, R.L.: The inhibition of hemoglobin C crystallization by hemoglobin. F. J. Biol. Chem. 263:5936, 1988.

348. Liń, M.J., Nagel, R.L., and Hirsch, R.E.: Acceleration of hemoglobin C crystallization by hemoglobin S. Blood 74:1823, 1989.

349. Reiss, G.H., Ranney, H.M., and Shaklai, N.: Association of hemoglobin C with erythrocyte ghosts. J. Clin. Invest. 70:946, 1982.

350. Diggs, L.W., and Bell, A.: Intraerythrocytic hemoglobin crystals in sickle cell hemoglobin C disease. Blood 25:218, 1965.

351. Bookchin, R.M., and Balazs, T.: Ionic strength dependence of the polymer solubilities of deoxyhemoglobin S + C and S + A mixtures. Blood 67:887, 1986.

352. Warkentin, T.E., Barr, R.D., Ali, M.A., and Mohandas, N.: Recurrent acute splenic sequestration crisis due to interacting genetic defects: hemoglobin SC disease and hereditary spherocytosis. Blood 75:266, 1990.

353. Old, J.M., Thein, S.L., Weatherall, D.J., Cao, A., and Loukopoulos, D.: Prenatal diagnosis of the major haemoglobin disorders. Mol. Biol. Med. 6:55, 1989.

354. Chang, J.C., and Kan, Y.W.: A sensitive new prenatal test for sickle-cell anemia. N. Engl. J. Med. 307:30, 1982.

355. Embury, S.H., Scharf, S.J., Saiki, R.K., Gholson, M.A., Golbus, M., Arnheim, N., and Erlich, H.A.: Rapid prenatal diagnosis of sickle cell anemia by a new method of DNA analysis. N. Engl. J. Med. 316:656, 1987.

356. Chehab, F.F., Doherty, M., Cai, S.P., Kan, Y.W., Cooper, S., and Rubin, E.M.: Detection of sickle cell anaemia and thalassaemias [letter] [published erratum appears in Nature 329:678, 1987]. Nature 329:293, 1987.

357. Rhoads, G.G., Jackson, J.G., Schlesselman, S.E., de la Cruz, F.F., Desnick, R.J., Golbus, M.S., Ledbetter, D.H., Lubs, H.A., Mahoney, M.J., Pergament, E., Simpson, J.L., Carpenter, R.J., Elias, S., Ginsberg, N.A., Goldberg, J.D., Hobbins, J.C., Lynch, L., Shiono, P.H., Wapner, R.J., and Zachary, J.M.: The safety and efficacy of chorionic villus sampling for early prenatal diagnosis of cytogenic abnormalities. N. Engl. J. Med. 320:609, 1989.

358. Alter, B.P.: Antenatal diagnosis. Summary of results. Ann. N. Y. Acad. Sci. 612:237, 1990.

358a. Akinyanju, O.O., Disu, R.F., Akinde, J.A., Adewole, T.A., Otaigbe, A.I., and Emuveyan, E.E.: Initiation of prenatal diagnosis of sickle-cell disorders in Africa. Prenat. Diagn. 19:299, 1999.

359. Rubin, E.M., Andrews, K.A., and Kan, Y.W.: Newborn screening by DNA analysis of dried blood spots. Hum. Genet. 82:134, 1989.

360. Pearson, H.: A neonatal program for sickle cell anemia. Adv. Pediatr. 33:381, 1986.

361. Vichinsky, E., Hurst, D., Earles, A., Kleman, K., and Lubin, B.: Newborn screening for sickle cell disease: effect on mortality. Pediatrics 81:749, 1988.

362. Tsevat, J., Wong, J.B., Pauker, S.G., and Steinberg, M.H.: Neonatal screening for sickle cell disease: a cost-effective analysis. J. Pediatr. 118:546, 1991.

363. John, A.B., Ramlal, A., Jackson, H., Maude, G.H., WaightSharma, A., and Serjeant, G.R.: Prevention of pneumococcal infection in children with homozygous sickle cell disease. Br. Med. J. 288:1567, 1984.

364. Gaston, M.H., Verter, J.I., Woods, G., Peglow, C., Kelleher, J., Presbury, G., Zarkowsky, H., Vichinsky, E., Iyer, R., Lobel, J.S., Diamond, S., Gill, S., and Falletta, J.M.: Prophylaxis with oral penicillin in children with sickle cell anemia: a randomized trial. N. Engl. J. Med. 314:1593, 1986.

364a. Bunn, H.F.: Pathogenesis and treatment of sickle cell disease. N. Engl. J. Med. 337:762, 1997.

364b. Steinberg, M.H.: Management of sickle cell disease. N. Engl. J. Med. 340:1021, 1999.

365. Cerami, A., and Manning, J.M.: Potassium cyanate as an inhibitor of the sickling of erythrocytes in vitro. Proc. Natl. Acad. Sci. USA 68:1180, 1971.

366. Walder, J.A., Zaugg, R.H., Walder, R.Y., Steele, J.M., and Klotz, I.M.: Diaspirins that cross-link beta chains of hemoglobin: bis(3,5-dibromosalicyl) succinate and bis(3,5-dibromosalicyl) fumarate. Biochemistry 18:4265, 1979.

367. Abraham, D.J., Perutz, M.F., and Phillips, S.E.: Physiological and x-ray studies of potential antisickling agents. Proc. Natl. Acad. Sci. USA 80:324, 1983.

368. Manning, J.M.: Covalent inhibitors of the gelatin of sickle cell hemoglobin and their effects on function. Adv. Enzymol. Rel. Areas Mol. Biol. 64:55, 1991.

369. Head, C.A., Brugnara, C., Martinez-Ruiz, R., Kacmarek, R.M., Bridges, K.R., Kuter, D., Bloch, K.D., and Zapol, W.M.: Low concentrations of nitric oxide increase oxygen affinity of sickle erythrocytes in vitro and in vivo. J. Clin. Invest. 100:955, 1997.

369a. Gladwin, M.T., Schechter, A.N., Shelhamer, J.H., Pannell, D.A., Conway, B.W., Hrinczenko, J.S., Pease-Fye, M.D., Noguchi, C.T., Rodgers, G.P., and Ognibene, F.P.: Inhaled nitric oxide augments nitric oxide transport on sickle cell hemoglobin without affecting oxygen affinity. J. Clin. Invest. 104:937, 1999.

370. Rosa, R.M., Bierer, B.E., Thomas, R., Stoff, J.S., Kruskall, M., Robinson, S., Bunn, H.F., and Epstein, F.H.: A study of induced hyponatremia in the prevention and treatment of sickle cell crises. N. Engl. J. Med. 303:1138, 1980.

371. Charache, S., and Walker, W.G.: Failure of desmopressin to lower serum sodium or prevent crisis in patients with sickle cell anemia. Blood 58:892, 1981.

372. Brugnara, C., de Franceschi, F.L., and Alper, S.L.: Inhibition of Ca^{2+}-dependent K^+ transport and cell dehydration in sickle erythrocytes by clotrimazole and other imidazole derivatives. J. Clin. Invest. 92:520, 1993.

373. De Franceschi, L., Saadane, N., Trudel, M., Alper, S.L., Brugnara, C., and Beuzard, Y.: Treatment with oral clotrimazole blocks Ca^{2+}-activated K^+ transport and reverses erythrocyte dehydration in transgenic SAD mice. A model for therapy of sickle cell disease. J. Clin. Invest. 93:1670, 1994.

374. Brugnara, C., Gee, B., Armsby, C.C., Kurth, S., Sakamoto, M., Rifai, N., Alper, S., and Platt, O.S.: Therapy with oral clotrimazole induces inhibition of the Gardos channel and reduction of erythrocyte dehydration in patients with sickle cell disease. J. Clin. Invest. 97:1227, 1996.

375. De Franceschi, L., Beuzard, Y., Jouault, H., and Brugnara, C.: Modulation of erythrocyte potassium chloride cotransport, potassium content, and density by dietary magnesium intake in transgenic SAD mouse. Blood 88:2738, 1996.

376. De Franceschi, L., Bachir, D., Galacteros, F., Tchernia, G., Cynober, T., Alper, S., Platt, O., Beuzard, Y., and Brugnara, C.: Oral magnesium supplements reduce erythrocyte dehydration in patients with sickle cell disease. J. Clin. Invest. 100:1847, 1997.

377. Watson, J., Stahman, A.W., and Bilello, F.P.: The significance of the paucity of sickle cells in newborn Negro infants. Am. J. Med. Sci. 215:419, 1948.

377a. Franco, R.S., Lohmann, J., Silberstein, E.B., Mayfield-Pratt, G., Palascak, M., Nemeth, T.A., Joiner, C.H., Weiner, M., and Rucknagel, D.L.: Time-dependent changes in the density and hemoglobin F content of biotin-labeled sickle cells. J. Clin. Invest. 101:2730, 1998.

378. DeSimone, J., Heller, P., Hall, L., and Zwiers, D.: 5-Azacytidine stimulates fetal hemoglobin synthesis in anemic baboons. Proc. Natl. Acad. Sci. USA 79:4428, 1982.

379. Ley, T.J., DeSimone, J., Anagnou, N.P., Keller, G.H., Humphries, R.K., Turner, P.H., Young, N.S., Keller, P., and Nienhuis, A.W.: 5-Azacytidine selectively increases gamma-globin synthesis in a patient with beta$^+$ thalassemia. N. Engl. J. Med. 307:1469, 1982.

380. Ley, T.J., DeSimone, J., Noguchi, C.T., Turner, P.H., Schechter, A.N., Heller, P., and Nienhuis, A.W.: 5-Azacytidine increases gamma-globin synthesis and reduces the proportion of dense cells in patients with sickle cell anemia. Blood 62:370, 1983.

381. Dover, G.J., Charache, S., Boyer, S.H., Vogelsang, G., and Moyer, M.: 5-Azacytidine increases HbF production and reduces anemia in sickle cell disease: dose-response analysis of subcutaneous and oral dosage regimens. Blood 66:527, 1985.

382. Papayannopoulou, T., Torrealba de Ron, A., Veith, R., Knitter, G., and Stamatoyannopoulos, G.: Arabinosylcytosine induces fetal hemoglobin in baboons by perturbing erythroid cell differentiation kinetics. Science 224:617, 1984.

383. Veith, R., Galanello, R., Papayannopoulou, T., and Stamatoyannopoulos, G.: Stimulation of F-cell production in patients with sickle cell anemia treated with cytarabine or hydroxyurea. N. Engl. J. Med. 313:1571, 1985.

384. Letvin, N.L., Linch, D.C., Beardsley, G.P., McIntyre, K.W., and Nathan, D.G.: Augmentation of fetal-hemoglobin production in anemic monkeys by hydroxyurea. N. Engl. J. Med. 310:869, 1984.

385. Platt, O.S., Orkin, S.H., Dover, G., Beardsley, G.P., Miller, B., and Nathan, D.G.: Hydroxyurea enhances fetal hemoglobin production in sickle cell anemia. J. Clin. Invest. 74:652, 1984.

386. Sumoza, A., and Bisotti, R.S.: Treatment of sickle cell anemia with hydroxyurea: results in 26 patients. Blood 68:67a, 1986.

387. Dover, G.J., Humphries, R.K., Moore, J.G., Ley, T.J., Young, N.S., Charache, S., and Nienhuis, A.W.: Hydroxyurea induction of hemoglobin F production in sickle cell disease: relationship between cytotoxicity and F cell production. Blood 67:735, 1986.

388. Charache, S., Dover, G.J., Moyer, M.A., and Moore, J.W.: Hydroxyurea-induced augmentation of fetal hemoglobin production in patients with sickle cell anemia. Blood 69:109, 1987.

389. Rodgers, G.P., Dover, G.J., Noguchi, C.T., Schechter, A.N., and Nienhuis, A.W.: Hematological responses of sickle cell patients treated with hydroxyurea. N. Engl. J. Med. 322:1037, 1990.

390. Ballas, S.K., Dover, G.J., and Charache, S.: Effect of hydroxyurea on the rheological properties of sickle erythrocytes in vivo. Am. J. Hematol. 32:104, 1989.

391. Goldberg, M.A., Brugnara, C., Dover, G.J., Schapira, L., Charache, S., and Bunn, H.F.: Treatment of sickle cell anemia with hydroxyurea and erythropoietin. N. Engl. J. Med. 323:366, 1990.

392. Orringer, E.P., Blythe, D.S., Johnson, A.E., Phillips, G.J., Dover, G.J., and Parker, J.C.: Effects of hydroxyurea on hemoglobin F and water content in the red blood cells of dogs and of patients with sickle cell anemia. Blood 78:212, 1991.

393. Charache, S., Dover, G.J., Moore, R.D., Eckert, S., Ballas, S.K., Koshy, M., Milner, P.F., Orringer, E.P., Phillips, G.J., Platt, O.S., et al.: Hydroxyurea: effects on hemoglobin F production in patients with sickle cell anemia. Blood 79:2555, 1992.

394. Alter, B.P., and Gilbert, H.S.: The effect of hydroxyurea on hemoglobin F in patients with myeloproliferative syndromes. Blood 66:373, 1985.

395. Charache, S., Terrin, M.L., Moore, R.D., Dover, G.J., Barton, F.B., Eckert, S.V., McMahon, R.P., and Bonds, D.R.: Effect of hydroxyurea on the frequency of painful crisis in sickle cell anemia. N. Engl. J. Med. 332:1317, 1995.

396. Charache, S., Barton, F.B., Moore, R.D., Terrin, M.L., Steinberg, M.H., Dover, G.J., Ballas, S.K., McMahon, R.P., Castro, O., and Orringer, E.P.: Hydroxyurea and sickle cell anemia: clinical utility of a myelosuppressive "switching agent." Medicine (Baltimore) 75:320, 1996.

397. Steinberg, M.H., Lu, Z.-H., Barton, F.B., Terrin, M.L., Charache, S., and Dover, G.J.: Fetal hemoglobin in sickle cell anemia: determinants of response to hydroxyurea. Blood 89:1078, 1997.

398. Ferster, A., Vermylen, C., Cornu, G., Buyse, M., Corazza, F., Devalck, C., Fondu, P., Toppet, M., and Sariban, E.: Hydroxyurea for treatment of severe sickle cell anemia: a pediatric clinical trial. Blood 88:1960, 1996.

398a. Maier-Redelsperger, M., deMontalambert, M., Flahault, A., Neonato, M.G., Ducrocq, R., Masson, M.-P., Girot, R., and Elion, J.: Fetal hemoglobin and F-cell responses to long-term hydroxyurea treatment in young sickle cell patients. The French Study Group on Sickle Cell Disease. Blood 91:4472, 1998.

398b. Kinney, T.R., Helms, R.W., O'Branski, E.E., Ohene-Frempong, K., Wang, W., Daeschner, C., Vichinsky, E., Redding-Lallinger, R., Gee, B., Platt, O.S., and Ware, R.E.: Safety of hydroxyurea in children with sickle cell anemia: results of the HUG-KIDS study, a phase I/II trial. Blood 94:1550, 1999.

399. Bridges, K.R., Barabino, G.D., Brugnara, C., Cho, M.R., Christoph, G.W., Dover, G., Ewenstein, B.M., Golan, D.E., Guttmann, C.R.G., Hofrichter, J., Mulkern, R.V., Zhang, B., and Eaton, W.A.: A multiparameter analysis of sickle erythrocytes in patients undergoing hydroxyurea therapy. Blood 88:4701, 1996.

400. Eshbach, J.W., Egrie, J.C., Downing, M.R., Browne, J.K., and Adamson, J.W.: Correction of the anemia of end-stage renal disease with recombinant human erythropoietin. N. Engl. J. Med. 316:73, 1987.

401. Winearls, C.G., Pippard, M.J., Downing, M.R., Oliver, D.O., Reid, C., and Cotes, P.M.: Effect of human erythropoietin derived from recombinant DNA on the anaemia of patients maintained by chronic haemodialysis. Lancet 2:1175, 1986.

402. Al-Khatti, A., Veith, R.W., Papayannopoulou, T., Fritsch, E.F., Goldwasser, E., and Stamatoyannopoulos, G.: Stimulation of fetal hemoglobin synthesis by erythropoietin in baboons. N. Engl. J. Med. 317:415, 1987.

403. Vichinsky, E., Nagel, R.L., Shah, M., Johnson, R., Spadacino, E., Fabry, M.F., Mangahas, L., and Stamtoyannopoulos, G.: The stimulation of fetal hemoglobin by rhErythropoietin in sickle cell anemia: a double blind study. In Stamatoyannopoulos, G., and Nienhuis, A. (eds.): The Regulation of Hemoglobin Switching. Proceedings of the Seventh Conference on Hemoglobin Switching. Baltimore, Johns Hopkins University Press, 1991, p. 394.

404. Rodgers, G.P., Dover, G.J., Uyesaka, N., Noguchi, C.T., Schechter, A.N., and Nienhuis, A.W.: Augmentation by erythropoietin of fetal hemoglobin response to hydroxyurea in sickle cell patients. N. Engl. J. Med. 328:73, 1993.

405. Oblender, M., and Carpentieri, U.: Effects of iron, copper and zinc on the activity of ribonucleotide reductase in normal and leukemic human lymphocytes. Anticancer Res. 10:123, 1990.

406. Ginder, G.D., Whitters, M.J., and Pohlman, J.K.: Activation of a chicken embryonic globin gene in adult erythroid cells by 5-azacytidine and sodium butyrate. Proc. Natl. Acad. Sci. USA 81:3954, 1984.

407. Burns, L.J., Glauber, J.G., and Ginder, G.D.: Butyrate induces selective transcriptional activation of a hypomethylated embryonic globin gene in adult erythroid cells. Blood 72:1536, 1988.

408. Perrine, S.P., Greene, M.F., and Faller, D.V.: Delay in the fetal globin switch in infants of diabetic mothers. N. Engl. J. Med. 312:334, 1985.

409. Perrine, S.P., Miller, B.A., Greene, M.F., Cohen, R.A., Cook, N., Shackleton, C., and Faller, D.V.: Butyric acid analogues augment gamma globin gene expression in neonatal erythroid progenitors. Biochem. Biophys. Res. Commun. 148:694, 1987.

410. Perrine, S.P., Miller, B.A., Faller, D.V., Cohen, R.A., Vichinsky, E.P., Hurst, D., Lubin, B.H., and Papayannopoulou, T.: Sodium butyrate enhances fetal globin gene expression in erythroid progenitors of patients with Hb SS and beta thalassemia. Blood 74:454, 1989.

411. Perrine, S.P., Rudolph, A., Faller, D.V., Roman, C., Cohen, R.A., Chen, S.J., and Kan, Y.W.: Butyrate infusions in the ovine fetus delay the biologic clock for globin gene switching. Proc. Natl. Acad. Sci. USA 85:8540, 1988.

412. Constantoulakis, P., Knitter, G., and Stamatoyannopoulos, G.: On the induction of fetal hemoglobin by butyrates: in vivo and in vitro studies with sodium butyrate and comparison of combination treatments with 5-AzaC and AraC. Blood 74:1963, 1989.

413. Perrine, S.P., Ginder, G.D., Faller, D.V., Dover, G., Ikuta, T., Witkowska, H.E., Cai, S., Vichinshy, E., and Olivieri, N.: A short-term trial of butyrate to stimulate fetal-globin-gene expression in the β-globin disorders. N. Engl. J. Med. 328:81, 1993.

414. Sher, G.D., Ginder, G.D., Little, J., Yang, S., Dover, G.J., and Olivieri, N.F.: Extended therapy with intravenous arginine butyrate in patients with beta-hemoglobinopathies. N. Engl. J. Med. 332:1606, 1995.

414a. Atweh, G.F., Sutton, M., Nassif, I., Boosalis, V., Dover, G.J., Wallenstein, S., Wright, E., McMahon, L., Stamatoyannopoulos, G., Faller, D.V., and Perrine, S.P.: Sustained induction of fetal hemoglobin by pulse butyrate therapy in sickle cell disease. Blood 93:1790, 1999.

415. Stamatoyannopoulos, G., Blau, C.A., Nakamoto, B., Josephson, B., Li, Q., Liakopoulou, E., Pace, B., Papayannopoulou, T., Brusilow, S.W., and Dover, G.: Fetal hemoglobin induction by acetate, a product of butyrate catabolism. Blood 84:3198, 1994.

416. Little, J.A., Dempsey, N.J., Tuchman, M., and Ginder, G.D.: Metabolic persistence of fetal hemoglobin. Blood 85:1712, 1995.

417. Liakopoulou, E., Blau, C.A., Li, Q., Josephson, B., Wolf, J.A., Fournarakis, B., Raisys, V., Dover, G., Papayannopoulou, T., and Stamatoyannopoulos, G.: Stimulation of fetal hemoglobin production by short chain fatty acids. Blood 86:3227, 1995.

418. Adams, J.G., and Coleman, M.B.: Structural hemoglobin variants that produce the phenotype of thalassemia. Semin. Hematol. 27:229, 1990.

419. Kazazian, H.H., Jr., Dowling, C.E., Hurwitz, R.L., Coleman, M., Stopeck, A., and Adams, J.G., III: Dominant thalassemia-like phenotypes associated with mutations in exon 3 of the β-globin gene. Blood 79:3014, 1992.

420. Ho, P.J., Wickramasinghe, S.N., Rees, D.C., Lee, M.J., Eden, A., and Thein, S.L.: Erythroblastic inclusions in dominantly inherited β-thalassemias. Blood 89:322, 1997.

421. Coleman, M.B., Steinberg, M.H., and Adams, J.D.: Hemoglobin Terre Haute arginine beta 106. A posthumous correction to the original structure of hemoglobin Indianapolis. J. Biol. Chem. 266:5798, 1991.

422. Cathie, I.A.B.: Apparent idiopathic Heinz body anemia. Great Ormond St. J. 3:43, 1952.

423. Stamatoyannopoulos, G., Nute, P.E., and Miller, M.: De novo mutations producing unstable hemoglobins or hemoglobins M. I. Establishment of a depository and use of data to test for an association of de novo mutation with advanced parental age. Hum. Genet. 58:396, 1981.

424. Vissers, M.C., Winterbourn, C.C., and Carrell, R.W.: Rapid proteolysis of unstable globins in human bone marrow. Br. J. Haematol. 53:417, 1983.

425. Rachmilewitz, E.A.: Denaturation of the normal and abnormal hemoglobin molecule. Semin. Hematol. 11:441, 1974.

426. Winterbourn, C.C., and Carrell, R.W.: Characterization of Heinz bodies in unstable hemoglobin. Nature 240:150, 1972.

427. Jandl, J.H., Simmons, R.L., and Castle, W.B.: Red cell filtration and the pathogenesis of certain hemolytic anemias. Blood 18:133, 1961.

428. Rivkind, R.A.: Heinz body anemia: an ultrastructural study. II. Red cell sequestration and destruction. Blood 26:433, 1965.

429. Flynn, T.P., Allen, D.W., Johnson, G.J., and White, J.G.: Oxidant damage of the lipids and proteins of the erythrocyte membranes in unstable hemoglobin disease. Evidence for the role of lipid peroxidation. J. Clin. Invest. 71:1215, 1983.

430. Allen, D.W., Burgoyne, C.F., Groat, J.D., Smith, C.D., and White, J.G.: Comparison of hemoglobin Köln erythrocyte membranes with malondialdehyde-reacted normal erythrocyte membranes. Blood 64:1263, 1984.

431. Winterbourn, C.C., Williamson, D., Vissers, M.C., and Carrell, R.W.: Unstable haemoglobin haemolytic crises: contributions of pyrexia and neutrophil oxidants. Br. J. Haematol. 49:111, 1981.

432. Tucker, P.W., Phillips, S.E., Perutz, M.F., Houtchens, R., and Caughey, W.S.: Structure of hemoglobins Zurich [His E7(63)beta replaced by Arg] and Sydney [Val E11(67)beta replaced by Ala] and role of the distal residues in ligand binding. Proc. Natl. Acad. Sci. USA 75:1076, 1978.

433. Zinkham, W.H., Houtchens, R.A., and Caughey, W.S.: Carboxyhemoglobin levels in an unstable hemoglobin disorder (Hb Zurich): effect on phenotypic expression. Science 209:406, 1980.

434. Kobayashi, Y., Fukumaki, Y., Komatsu, N., Ohba, Y., Miyaji, T., and Miura, Y.: A novel globin structural mutant, Showa-Yakushiji (beta 110 Leu-Pro) causing a beta-thalassemia phenotype. Blood 70:1688, 1987.

435. Beris, P., Miescher, P.A., Diaz, C.J., Han, I.S., Kutlar, A., Hu, H., Wilson, J.B., and Huisman, T.H.: Inclusion body beta-thalassemia trait in a Swiss family is caused by an abnormal hemoglobin (Geneva) with an altered and extended beta chain carboxy-terminus due to a modification in codon beta 114. Blood 72:801, 1988.

436. Eisinger, J., Flores, J., Tyson, J.A., and Shohet, S.B.: Fluorescent cytoplasm and Heinz bodies of hemoglobin Köln erythrocytes: evidence for intracellular heme catabolism. Blood 65:886, 1985.

437. Charache, S., Weatherall, D.J., and Clegg, J.B.: Polycythemia associated with a hemoglobinopathy. J. Clin. Invest. 45:813, 1966.

438. Adamson, J.W., Parer, J.T., and Stamatoyannopoulos, G.: Erythrocytosis associated with hemoglobin Rainier: oxygen equilibria and marrow regulation. J. Clin. Invest. 48:1376, 1969.

439. Charache, S., Catalano, P., Burns, S., Jones, R.T., Koler, R.D., Rutstein, R., and Williams, R.R.: Pregnancy in carriers of high-affinity hemoglobins. Blood 65:713, 1985.

440. Adamson, J.W.: Familial polycythemia. Semin. Hematol. 12:383, 1975.

441. Sergeyeva, A., Gordeuk, V.R., Tokarev, Y.N., Sokol, L., Prchal, J.F., and Prchal, J.T.: Congenital polycythemia in Chuvashia. Blood 89:2148, 1997.

442. de la Chapelle, A., Traskelin, A.-L., and Juvonen, E.: Truncated erythropoietin receptor causes dominantly inherited benign human erythrocytosis. Proc. Natl. Acad. Sci. USA 90:4495, 1993.

443. Shibata, S., Miyaji, T., Iuchi, I., Ohba, Y., and Yamamoto, K.: Hemoglobins M of the Japanese. Bull. Yamaguchi Med. School 14:141, 1967.

444. Priest, J.R., Watterson, J., Jones, R.T., Faassen, A.E., and Hedlund, B.E.: Mutant fetal hemoglobin causing cyanosis in a newborn. Pediatrics 83:734, 1989.

445. Hayashi, A., Fujita, T., Fujimura, M., and Titani, K.: A new abnormal fetal hemoglobin, Hb FM Osaka ($\alpha_2\gamma_2^{63His-Tyr}$). Hemoglobin 4:447, 1980.

8 ▼▼▼▼ The Erythrocyte Membrane and Cytoskeleton: Structure, Function, and Disorders

Patrick G. Gallagher
and Edward J. Benz, Jr.

▼ ▼

Introduction

The plasma membrane (plasma lemma) is the integument of the cell. It demarcates the boundary between the cell's interior milieu and the external environment in which it must survive and function. Membranes are fluid, semipermeable, lipid-protein mosaics whose biochemical properties allow them to act both as a barrier to diffusion and as the surface through which regulated entry and egress of nutrients, macromolecules, hormones, ions, and information can occur. These features place the plasma membrane at the center of many life sustaining processes. Selective permeability provides for retention of essential intracellular components, exclusion of unwanted toxins, uptake of nutrients, and excretion of metabolic by-products. Channels and pumps embedded in membranes modulate intracellular ion content, which in turn determines each cell's osmotic pressure and electrical potential. The plasma membrane also functions as the primary site for interaction and communication with the external environment. For example, the ability of hematopoietic cells of a given lineage to respond to hormones or growth factors depends in part on the presence and density of appropriate receptor proteins embedded in the lipid bilayer. Cell-cell and cell-matrix interactions essential for stem cell homing phenomena, hematopoiesis, or contact-dependent cellular activation depend on the topological array of membrane bound cell adhesion molecules and their receptors.

Immune recognition by antibodies or effector cells requires presentation of antigens and cofactor proteins on the exterior face of the membrane. An intact and functioning plasma lemma is, therefore, indispensable for cellular life.

The concept of membranes as static, passive, semipermeable structures surrounding cells and organelles is incomplete. The plasma membrane is a dynamic entity utilized as a major locus for organizing, localizing, and regulating metabolic processes. Membranes have the capacity to compartmentalize and sequester key molecules involved in metabolic regulation. In some cases, enzymes or cofactors attach to membranes to form topological arrays that modulate the efficiency of a particular metabolic process, for example, electron transport along the inner leaflet mitochondrial cristae. Conversely, reversible attachment to membranes can sequester proteins until their activity is appropriate to cellular function.

Membranes are highly ordered yet fluid structures that spontaneously form thin hydrophobic sheets or layers when suspended in aqueous fluids. (To conserve space, references for some aspects of the material in these introductory sections that summarize well-established principles are limited to reviews of the relevant topics.[1-7]) They are non-covalent, self-assembling, and self-sealing mosaics composed of several types of lipids and many types of proteins. Lipid-protein complexes do not themselves possess sufficient tensile strength or rigidity to confer stability of shape, physical

275

tolerance to shear stress, or topological order on the membrane. These properties are attained by attachment to underlying protein complexes that form a firm, elastic network called the cytoskeleton (Fig. 8–1). The cortical cytoskeleton is that portion that forms the interior lining of the plasma membrane. Analogous skeletal networks also penetrate further into the interior of cells and form the structural underpinnings of organelles such as the Golgi apparatus, the endoplasmic reticulum, mitochondria and nuclei. The protein-lipid bilayer complex thus provides a hydrophobic barrier and membrane fluidity, whereas the cytoskeleton plays the major role in defining the size and shape and compartmentalization of the encased space. Tensile strength, elasticity, and exterior topology of the entire cell are determined by the interaction between the bilayer and cytoskeleton.

Any attempt to understand the physiology of hematopoietic cells or the pathophysiology of their diseases must include a thorough examination of the biology of hematopoietic cell membranes. This chapter summarizes current knowledge about the structure and function of a particular membrane, the erythrocyte membrane, its cytoskeleton, and disorders attributable to their derangement. At the present time, erythrocytes are the cells about which the most detailed information is available concerning the normal structure and function of their cytoskeleton and about the molecular pathology of disorders due primarily to abnormal membrane

or cytoskeletal structure. The erythrocyte membrane remains the paradigm for ongoing studies of other cell types.

We first consider the basic elements of membranes and cytoskeletal structures. We then discuss unique features that adapt the red cell to withstand the prolonged physical and metabolic stresses associated with extended life in the circulation. Finally, we survey current understanding of the pathophysiology and molecular basis of representative disorders of the red cell membrane and cytoskeleton.

Structure and Function of Cell Membranes

To a first approximation, membrane lipids sustain barrier function, whereas protein components provide the receptors, channels, and pumps by which the barrier can be breached for purposes of solute transport and exterior-to-interior communication. The hydrophobicity of the lipid bilayer is the essential property that provides for the diffusion barrier.[4] Most cells live in an aqueous external environment; intracellular metabolic reactions also occur largely in the aqueous phase. Most substances that are soluble in water cannot traverse the highly hydrophobic environment of the lipid bilayer. The bilayer thus prevents dispersion of vital intracellular components and precludes their random admixture with molecules on the outside.

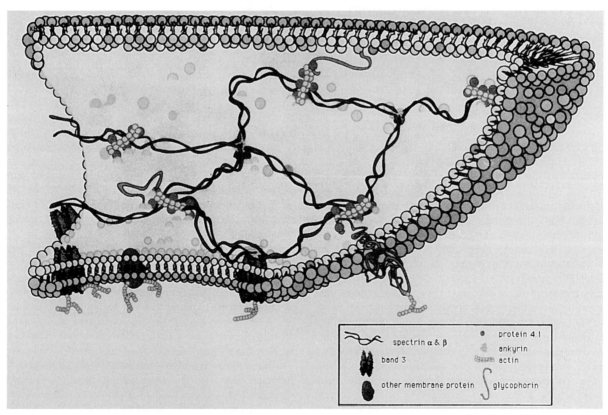

spectrin α & β

band 3

other membrane protein

protein 4.1

ankyrin

actin

glycophorin

Figure 8–1. A three-dimensional view of the cell membrane from the interior and exterior of the cell. The lipid bilayer is shown as hydrophilic head groups (shaded circles) attached to hydrophobic tails, forming the lipid bilayer. The underlying cytoskeletal meshwork, consisting of spectrin fibers arranged in a hexagonal, anastomosing lattice, is attached to the bilayer by means of band 3, actin, protein 4.1, and ankyrin. The principal transmembrane proteins at which the cytoskeleton is attached, band 3 and glycophorin, are shown spanning the lipid bilayer. The lipid components of the membrane are presented in more detail in Figure 8–2, and the arrangements of proteins, in Figures 8–3 and 8–4. (From Morrow, J.: Plasma membrane dynamics and organization. *In* Hoffman, R., Benz, E.J., Jr., Shattil, S., Furie, B., and Cohen, H. [eds.]: Hematology: Basic Principles and Practice. New York, Churchill Livingstone, 1991, pp. 36–50; with permission.)

Proteins embedded in, or attached to, the bilayer provide the means by which both substances and information can traverse the bilayer.[1-3] Substances enter via transmembrane pumps or channels, or by internalization of materials that contact the outer membrane (e.g., receptor-ligand complexes). Membrane-spanning proteins also convey information to the interior of the cell by undergoing allosteric conformational changes of their cytoplasmic domains upon binding to substances on the exterior face. These changes signify the occurrence of external events to signal transduction elements on the inside, without the need for the provoking molecule to enter the cell.

▼ MEMBRANE LIPIDS

Membrane lipids consist of cholesterol and two types of amphipathic lipids: phospholipids and glycolipids.[1, 3, 4] The term amphipathic refers to the possession of both hydrophobic and hydrophilic tendencies. Most amphipathic lipids contain aliphatic carbon chains or tails at one end of the molecule attached to polar head groups, consisting of more highly charged moieties, such as acidic, phosphate, or sugar residues. The hydrophobic tails of these molecules tend to associate with one another to exclude water and form a nonaqueous interior, whereas the polar head groups remain in contact with the aqueous solution. This arrangement leads to the formation of micelles (Fig. 8–2).

Free fatty acids, the simplest amphipathic lipids, are not usually found in cell membranes because they form spherical globules lacking the flexibility and linearity essential for a viable membrane. Membrane lipids generally have highly polar head groups and bulky hydrophobic tails; they can satisfy their need to exist in a hydrophobic environment only by aligning in linear micelles[1] (see Fig. 8–2A).

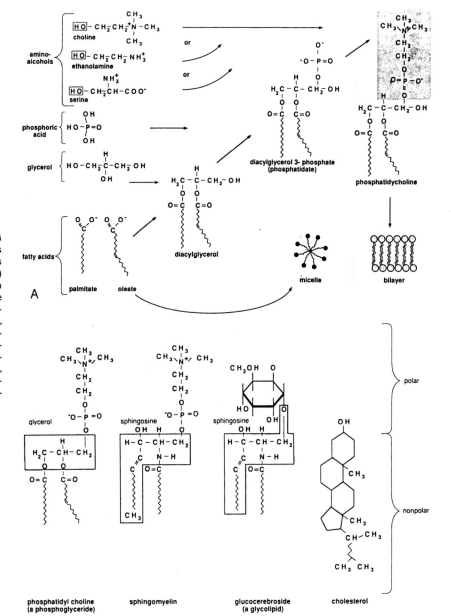

Figure 8–2. Lipid components of membranes. *A* shows the basic chemical structures of lipids found in membranes. The bulky polar head groups of lipids actually found in membranes (cf. text) favor exclusion of water in such a way as to form a lipid bilayer, rather than the spherical micelle formed by simple fatty acids. *B* shows the structures of the major phospholipid, sphingomyelin, glycolipid, and cholesterol moieties found in naturally occurring membranes. (Adapted from Morrow, J.: Plasma membrane dynamics and organization. *In* Hoffman, R., Benz, E.J., Jr., Shattil, S., Furie, B., and Cohen, H. [eds.]: Hematology: Basic Principles and Practice. New York, Churchill Livingstone, 1991, pp. 36–50; with permission.)

Two types of phospholipids account for most of the amphipathic lipid membranes: phosphoglycerides, derived from glycerol, and sphingomyelin (SM), derived from ceramide, a derivative of sphingosine[1, 3] (see Fig. 8–2B). The most abundant phospholipid is phosphatidylcholine (PC). Other major components include phosphatidylethanolamine (PE), phosphatidylserine (PS), and phosphatidylinositol (PIP). The long hydrocarbon tails of these lipids are modified to varying degrees by the formation of double bonds between carbon moieties, creating unsaturated phospholipids. As the degree of desaturation increases, the packing of hydrophobic tails in the core of the bilayer is increasingly disrupted, thereby enhancing the fluidity of the membrane.

The glycolipids present in eukaryotic membranes are largely based on sphingosine and therefore are called glycosphingolipids.[2, 4] Glucocerebroside and galactocerebroside are the simplest examples; more complex arrangements of sugar residues or the lipid core result in the formation of substances called gangliosides. Glycolipids tend to be located almost exclusively on the extracellular face of the plasma membrane, with the result that the sugar residues protrude into the extracellular space. The precise biological importance of this asymmetry is unknown. Asymmetry of and in itself may permit biochemical discrimination between the interior and exterior faces of the membrane.

Cholesterol, the third lipid component, is unique among membrane lipids because it is almost entirely hydrophobic. Its primary role appears to be to control membrane fluidity. Interspersion of cholesterol among the phospholipids and glycolipids interferes with packing of their hydrophobic tails into highly ordered arrays. Cholesterol contributes to maintenance of membrane fluidity, even under conditions, such as low temperature, that might lead to phospholipid crystallization and rigidification of the bilayer.

Lipids account for 50–60 per cent of membrane mass. The remainder is protein. Although lipids are clearly critical for the membrane organization, disease states due primarily to derangements in membrane lipids are uncommon. A few illustrative examples are discussed later. The remainder of this chapter focused primarily on proteins associated with the membrane. Proteins play the predominant role in conferring tensile strength and specialized functional properties on membranes of individual cell types. Most "membrane diseases" that have been well characterized are due to abnormal membrane proteins.

▼ MEMBRANE PROTEINS

Membrane proteins are classified according to the ease with which they can be removed from membranes.[1, 5, 6] Peripheral proteins are more loosely associated; they are extractable by high- or low-salt or high-pH extraction (Fig. 8–3A). Integral proteins are firmly embedded into or through the lipid bilayer by hydrophobic domains within their amino acid sequences. They can be extracted only by harsh reagents such as chaotropic solvents or detergents.[5, 6] Peripheral proteins are typically associated with only one face of the membrane (i.e., exterior or extracellular versus interior or cytoplasmic), whereas many integral proteins often protrude into both spaces.

The intimacy with which proteins associate with the

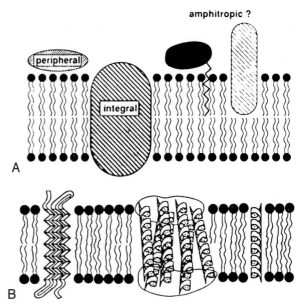

Figure 8–3. Types of membrane proteins and their interactions with membranes. The schematic A illustrates the different types of membrane proteins, based on the intimacy of their relationship to the lipid bilayer. Peripheral proteins, shown at the far left, are reversibly attached by non-covalent weak forces or by non-covalent binding to more firmly embedded proteins. At the other extreme, integral proteins are firmly embedded in the membrane by virtue of their extensive regions of hydrophobic α helices of β-pleated sheets. Amphitropic proteins, shown at the right, are partially or more reversibly embedded in the membrane by virtue of less extensive hydrophobic domains (illustrated on the far right) or reversible attachments to fatty acid moieties (proteins shown second from the right). These interactions are discussed in more detail in the text. B illustrates the helical and β-pleated sheet motifs characteristic of firmly embedded proteins. On the far left is shown a protein with a single bilayer spanning the α helix (e.g., glycophorin); in the center is shown a globular protein with multiple membrane-spanning helices (e.g. band 3); and on the right is shown a β-pleated sheet (e.g., porin). (See text for details.) (Adapted from Morrow, J.: Plasma membrane dynamics and organization. In Hoffman, R., Benz, E.J., Jr., Shattil, S., Furie, B., and Cohen, H. [eds.]: Hematology: Basic Principles and Practice. New York, Churchill Livingstone, 1991, pp. 36–50; with permission.)

membrane is not a static property. Rather, proteins can become more or less tightly bound according to their state of phosphorylation, methylation, glycosylation, or lipid modification (myristylation, palmitylation, or farnesylation).[1] The term amphitropic (see Fig. 8–3) is used to describe the changeable affinity of these proteins for the hydrophobic environment of the lipid bilayer.[6]

Integral proteins may be embedded in the membrane or anchored to it.[1, 5–7] *Embedded* proteins are intimately, and usually permanently, associated with the lipid bilayer by virtue of extensive amphipathic α helical or β-pleated sheet structures within their amino acid sequences (see Fig. 8–3B). Examples include transmembrane proteins such as growth factor receptors, transport ATPases, and bacterial rhodopsin. *Anchored* proteins associate by means of covalent reversible attachments to the bilayer. Examples include the phosphoinositide (GPI) linkages that attach complement modulating proteins (CD59, etc.), leukocyte alkaline phosphatase, or the CD4 antigen to the exterior surface of the membrane, or certain metabolic enzymes that become reversibly anchored in the lipid bilayer by farnesylation or myristylation.[2, 8] Loss of GPI proteins (due to mutations of the *pig-A* gene that encodes a key intermediate in the anchoring process) is a hallmark of the classic hematologic disease, paroxysmal nocturnal hemoglobinuria (PNH).[9] Peripheral proteins are attached indirectly to the lipid bilayer by means of covalent or non-covalent binding to the (usually) cytoplasmic domains of embedded or anchored proteins.

Embedded proteins generally contain large domains of hydrophobic residues. Some, like the prototype glycophorin A, form α helices approximately 20 amino acids long, spanning a distance just sufficient to traverse the lipid bilayer.[9, 10] Others, such as the bacterial membrane protein porin, utilize β-pleated sheet structures for the same purpose.[11] One or both ends of the protein are typically hydrophilic. The generic structure of an embedded protein is thus one in which hydrophobic domains are insinuated in the lipid bilayer, whereas the more hydrophilic extremities of the molecule protrude either into the extracellular or the cytoplasmic space or into both.

Anchored proteins, on the other hand, tend to possess short consensus sequences at their NH_2- or COOH-termini that serve as recognition sites for myristylation, farnesylation, or attachment of phosphoinositides. They fall into two general classes: those attached by direct covalent bonding between the lipid bilayer and amino acid residues on the protein, and those insinuated into the bilayer by covalent linkage to a lipid moiety. The former are exemplified by proteins, such as CD4 that bind to phosphoinositide.[2] The latter possess conserved structural motifs at the amino- or carboxyl-terminus that promote covalent modification by lipid moieties such as palmitate or myristate.[8] These moieties confer hydrophobic tendencies that favor partial insertion into the lipid bilayer. This association can be reversed by cleavage of the bond between the protein and its lipid modifier. Myristylation and farnesylation are being increasingly recognized as mechanisms whereby proteins can be anchored or sequestered in order to enhance, compartmentalize, or diminish their availability for metabolic impact on cells.

Anchored proteins bind reversibly to the membrane by covalent or non-covalent linkage to the cytoplasmic domains of embedded or anchored proteins.[1, 12] Attached proteins are often multivalent, permitting reversible assembly of complex multi-molecular aggregates. Assembly is a dynamic process because binding affinities can be readily modulated by modifications such as methylation, phosphorylation, attachment of phosphoinositide groups, and/or conformational changes induced by interaction of the attached proteins with other proteins, cofactors, metabolites, or ions.

▼ MAINTENANCE OF ASYMMETRY AND TOPOLOGICAL ORGANIZATION OF THE MEMBRANE

Lipids and embedded membrane proteins are freely diffusible in *lateral* directions along the plane of the lipid bilayer. Phospholipids or proteins embedded in the bilayer could, based on a typical diffusion constant, circumnavigate the red cell membrane in a matter of seconds.[13] In contrast, *transverse* mobility is highly constrained because of the bulkiness of polar head groups, amino acid side chains, or end modifications, such as sugar residues.[14] The free energy expenditure required to drag these bulky hydrophilic groups *through* the hydrophobic membrane prohibits spontaneous "flip flopping" across the bilayer. These chemical constraints maintain asymmetry of the interior and exterior faces of the membrane; this is critical for communication and regulatory functions.

In red cells, the aminophospholipids, PS and PE are almost exclusively found in the inner monolayer, while SM and PC are predominantly in the outer monolayer.[7, 15] Maintenance of this asymmetry appears to be important, at least for normal regulation of hemostasis, because appearance of PS on the outer leaflet causes the red cell surface to become prothrombotic, by providing exposed PS for prothrombinase binding; indeed, phospholipid "flipping" could conceivably contribute to the thrombotic diatheses in conditions like sickle cell disease. Appearance of PS on the outer surface is one of the earliest changes occurring in apoptosis; it has also been correlated with complement activation and red cell clearance by macrophages. Lipid asymmetry is now thought to be a widespread property of eukaryotic membranes, one potentially critical to normal interaction of the cell with its outer environment.

Enzymes called "flippases" actively translocate PS and PE to the inner leaflet; "floppases" catalyze translocation to the outer leaflet. Asymmetry seems to depend on the fact that "flipping" occurs at a higher rate than "flopping." Flippase activity is mediated by a 130 kDa integral membrane protein that is a member of the Mg^{++}-dependent, P-glycoprotein ATPases.[16] Floppase activity in red cell membranes appears to be mediated by the multidrug resistance protein 1 (MRP1).[17, 18] Experiments with erythrocytes from mice with targeted disruption of the multidrug resistance P-glycoproteins Mdr1a/1b, Mdr2, and Mrp1, revealed that Mrp1 is responsible for the flop of labeled lipid analogues in the membrane. A "scramblase" activated by elevated intracellular calcium that promotes randomization and loss of asymmetry has been isolated and cloned.[19, 20] This scramblase mediates redistribution of membrane phospholipids in activated, injured or apoptotic cells and is activated by calcium via an EF motif.[21–23] Derangements within the red cell often raise intracellular calcium by direct or indirect damage to ion channels and pumps. Scott's syndrome is a congenital bleeding disorder in which red cells and platelets expose subnormal amounts of PS on the outer surface in response to calcium, but it does not appear to be due to scramblase deficiency.[24, 25]

Even though many integral membrane proteins should be freely diffusible in the lateral plane, their actual mobilities are usually far more restricted (e.g., by binding to the cytoskeleton) than their potential.[26] Restricted mobility begets non-random aggregation and clustering of proteins in specific parts of the membrane, thus allowing development of localized functions, cell polarity, formation of pseudopods for cell motility, pinocytosis, and other organized behaviors.[3]

Membrane organization arises from interactions between integral membrane proteins and other molecules contacting the hydrophilic faces of the membrane, and by protein-protein or protein-lipid interactions within the bilayer itself. The best studied examples of *exterior* interactions are those that occur when multivalent extracellular ligands or antibodies bind to their receptors or epitopes, forming clusters or patches of receptor multimers, or antigen-antibody complexes.[27] Antigen capping and the formation of receptor dimers or oligomers that activate signal transduction events are widely known examples.[28, 29]

Integral membrane proteins can interact with one another or with lipids *within* the lipid bilayer. Stable associations between the subunits of multi-component channels and pumps are often maintained by interaction of the transmembrane segments with one another, whereas other proteins maintain association with one another by interacting with lipids such as phosphatidylinositol 4,5-bisphosphate (PIP$_2$). An important membrane cytoskeletal protein, protein 4.1, regulates one of its affinities for membranes via this type of lipid interaction.

Interactions on the *cytoplasmic* face of the protein are usually mediated by the cortical cytoskeleton. This structure consists of a submembranous scaffold of spectrin-actin fibers connected to the membrane at multiple points by the multivalent linking proteins ankyrin and protein 4.1. Ankyrin and protein 4.1 attach by binding to spectrin or complexes of spectrin and actin, on the one hand, and to the cytoplasmic domains of integral membrane proteins, such as band 3, glycophorin, and Na$^+$K$^+$ATPase, on the other. Proteins like p55, protein 4.2, dematin, and adducin seem to augment or stabilize these interactions, or to facilitate reversible attachment to additional components. The avidity of the attachments is modulated by posttranslational modifications of the participating proteins, such as phosphorylation.[1, 12, 30]

By utilizing the cytoplasmic domains of embedded proteins as attachment points, the cytoskeleton not only affixes itself to the lipid bilayer but also provides a means to order the topological arrangement of the transmembrane proteins; the act of attachment constrains motion along the transverse plane. For example, the localization of the Na$^+$K$^+$ATPase to the basolateral, but not the apical, surface of renal epithelial cells is achieved in part by fixing the enzyme to recognition domains on ankyrin and thereby to the spectrin-actin cytoskeleton.[31]

The Erythrocyte Membrane and Its Cytoskeleton

Red cells circulate for 120 days, devoid of a nucleus, mitochondria, polyribosomes, or nucleic acids.[32, 33] They have no capacity to synthesize new proteins to replace those lost or damaged by life in the blood stream. During this odyssey, they traverse the circulation more than 100,000 times, facing enormous mechanical and metabolic challenges during each passage. For example, many capillary beds have interior diameters smaller than the 7.5 µm diameter of the red cell. The red cell must deform to squeeze through these capillaries and then resume its normal shape upon emergence into more capacious venules at the distal end of the capillaries. The enormous burden of intracellular protein (hemoglobin) creates a large oncotic pressure gradient. Erythrocytes thus tend to swell in isotonic solutions and to shrivel in hypertonic solutions. In the distal tubules and collecting system of the kidney, red cells pass through zones having molarities ranging from isotonic to nearly six times isotonic and back again in a matter of milliseconds. Iron and hemichromes released from damaged hemoglobin molecules add further redox stresses, intensified by marked changes in the pH and Po$_2$, that must be endured in the kidney, spleen, and muscle.[34, 35]

These challenges demand that red cells possess several properties to remain structurally sound. The membrane must be highly pliable yet sufficiently resilient to resist fragmentation in the face of substantial shear stresses. It must be distensible enough to accommodate rapid changes in osmotic pressure. In addition, the bilayer and its underpinnings (the cortical cytoskeleton) must be resistant to damage resulting from oxidation, proteolysis, or other noxious stimuli in the circulation, since no replacement of damaged proteins is possible. The erythrocyte membrane is highly adapted to meet these demands.

▼ PHYSICAL AND MECHANICAL PROPERTIES OF ERYTHROCYTES

From a physiological and clinical perspective, the single most important property of red cells required for normal survival is cellular deformability.[36] This term refers to the ability of the erythrocyte to undergo distortions and deformations and then to resume its normal shape without fragmentation or loss of integrity. Red cells normally have a biconcave discoid shape. Under the hydrostatic pressure of the circulation, the erythrocyte is distorted to an ellipsoidal shape when it must pass through narrow vascular conduits in the capillary beds; upon entering more capacious vessels on the venous side of the circulation, normal red cells resume their discoid shape. Normal red cells must also be able to swell and shrink in response to changes in osmolality without bursting or imploding. The *cellular* deformability of erythrocytes is now known to depend predominantly on three variables: geometry (biconcave disc shape), cytoplasmic viscosity, and *membrane* deformability."

The *biconcave disc shape* of red cells is critical for their survival. Objects with this surface geometry have a high ratio of surface area to enclosed volume. In the red cell, for example, the normal volume is ~90 µm^3; the minimum surface area that could encase this volume would be a sphere of ~98 µm^3.[33] The surface area of a biconcave disc enclosing this volume is ~140 µm^3. Thus, shape alone provides the red cell with a considerable amount of redundant membrane and cytoskeleton. This feature provides for the extra membrane area needed when red cells swell. More importantly, the geometrical arrangement allows red cells to be stretched as they undergo deformation and distortion in response to mechanical stress. Loss of membrane, by partial phagocytosis in immune hemolytic anemias or by fragmentation of bits of membrane from the cell in patients with cytoskeletal defects, leads to elliptocytic or spherocytic shapes having greatly reduced surface area and, therefore, much less deformability.[33, 37, 38] The consequent reduction in tolerance of these cells to osmotic stress explains why anemias due to membrane defects are often accompanied by osmotic fragility, the basis for a useful clinical laboratory test. Conversely, if erythrocytes are engorged with water, they become macrospherocytic and less deformable.

Red cell viscosity is largely determined by hemoglobin content.[33, 37] At normal intracellular concentrations (27 to 35 g/dl), viscosity contributes very little to cellular deformability. When erythrocytes become dehydrated, the effective intracellular hemoglobin concentration rises, and viscosity increases exponentially. Membrane pumps and channels normally maintain intracellular volumes that hold hemoglobin concentrations below the level at which cytoplasmic viscosity has an impact on deformability. Inherited anomalies of pumps or channels (e.g., hereditary xerocytosis[7]) or derangements of them by polymerized or crystallized hemoglobin (e.g., sickle cell anemia or HbC disease)[37, 38] lead to cellular dehydration and greatly increased red cell viscosity.

Red cells experience mechanical stress when forced through the narrow conduits of small capillaries and venules under hydrostatic pressure. This force, which can be mimicked by laboratory devices such as the ektacytometer,[7] deforms the discoid erythrocyte to an elliptocytic shape, which reverts to the normal disc when the force is removed.[39, 40] Excessive or prolonged application of force exceeds deformability, resulting in permanent deformation; application of even higher levels of force begins to produce red cell fragmentation.

Membrane deformability[39–41] is the material property of the membrane-cytoskeletal unit that determines the extent to which the membrane is distorted by application of a defined level of force. The *stability* of the membrane, in contrast, is defined as the maximum extent of deformation that is reversible.[7, 39] In other words, membrane stability reflects the maximum force that can be tolerated before the membrane becomes irreversibly deformed by application of force. Decreased deformability results in rigid red cells, whereas decreased membrane stability results in increased susceptibility to fragmentation under normal circulating stresses.[40] Defects of integral membrane and cytoskeletal proteins have been shown to cause temporary deformation, permanent (plastic) deformation, and/or fragmentation at lower than normal forces.[37, 39]

▼ THE RED CELL CYTOSKELETON: THE MOLECULAR BASIS FOR RED CELL DEFORMABILITY AND STABILITY

The deformability and stability of red cells depend on the topology of the cytoskeleton and the means by which it is attached to the fragile lipid bilayer. The basic structure of the cytoskeleton is a hexagonal latticework[42] composed of spectrin and actin filaments onto which are attached additional proteins that fasten the lattice to the lipid bilayer[1, 32, 39] (Figs. 8–1 and 8–4). Additional proteins intersect at the attachment points to stabilize or weaken the attachment. Attachment occurs at regular intervals by means of multivalent proteins (ankyrin, protein 4.1, protein 4.2, p55) that bind to the lattice, to the cytoplasmic domains for the integral proteins glycophorin and band 3, and, sometimes, to the lipid bilayer.[5, 32, 43]

The spectrin and actin filaments can be regarded as firm but spring-like rods. In the resting state, the folded helical segments of spectrin (described later) are in a relatively highly coiled state.[33, 37] Deformation is accompanied by a rearrangement of the network. Some spectrin molecules become uncoiled and extended, whereas others become more compressed and folded, resulting in no net change in surface area. Thus, shape changes but surface area does not. The extent to which this stretching and compression are possible determines the extent of deformability. Further distortion of shape requires an increase in membrane surface area, which

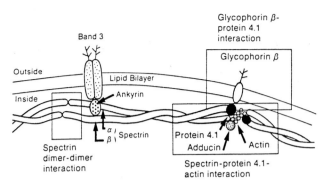

Figure 8–4. Arrangement of the major membrane and cytoskeletal proteins within and attached to the erythrocyte membrane. This diagram is best appreciated by comparison to Figure 8–1. The transmembrane proteins band 3 and glycophorin are shown traversing the lipid bilayer. The spectrin latticework illustrated in Figure 8–1 is represented here by the shaded intertwined α and β subunits, shown with the spectrin-spectrin association between the NH_2-terminus of the α subunit and the COOH-terminus of the β subunit. Attachment of the latticework to the membrane is mediated by the formation of spectrin/actin/protein 4.1 junctional complexes that in turn attach to the cytoplasmic domain of glycophorin, and the binding of ankyrin to both spectrin and the cytoplasmic domain of band 3, an interaction thought to be facilitated by protein 4.2.

can occur only if the attachments to the cytoskeleton are broken at the protein 4.1/glycophorin/spectrin/actin junction points (described later).[39, 43] At this point, the membrane fails, becoming permanently deformed or fragmented.

Clearly, deformability will be increased or decreased by increasing or decreasing the chemical associations of the spectrin-actin hexagonal network with molecules influencing their ability to coil or uncoil. Membrane stability will be decreased by any state or event that weakens the junctional complexes. Mutations or acquired alterations of membrane and cytoskeletal proteins could exert either or both effects. Thus a single mutation might simultaneously exert adverse effects on deformability and stability.

▼ COMPONENTS OF THE ERYTHROCYTE MEMBRANE AND UNDERLYING CYTOSKELETON

Lipid Components

The red cell membrane consists of 52% protein, 40% lipid, and 8% carbohydrate, proportions typical of most mammalian membranes.[44, 45] The lipid component consists of roughly equimolar quantities of phospholipids and unesterified cholesterol and minimal amounts of free fatty acids and glycolipids (see Fig. 8–2). The four major phospholipids are phosphatidlycholine (PC, 30%), sphingomyelin (SM, 25%), phosophatidylethanolamine (PE, 28%), and phosphatidylserine (PS, 14%). Other phospholipids, such as phophatidylinositol 4,5-bisphosphate (PIP_2), constitute only small amounts, 2–3%. These lipids are highly asymmetrical with respect to the interior and exterior faces of the membrane. As already mentioned, the relatively uncharged phospholipids, PC and SM, exist largely in the outer monolayer (leaflet); 80% of the highly charged (amino) phospholipids, PE and PS, are localized to the inner leaflet. Cholesterol freely diffuses into and through the bilayer.

Red cells have no capacity to synthesize new lipids, but lipids in the circulation exchange relatively freely with the membrane, resulting in considerable turnover, usually without significant changes in overall lipid composition. This mechanism provides for rejuvenation and renewal of the lipid components. In certain pathological situations, such as advanced cirrhosis and abetalipoproteinemia, abnormal circulating lipid profiles and/or abnormal mechanisms of exchange can generate morphological abnormalities (e.g., acanthocytosis) or actual hemolytic anemia.[33]

Protein Components

Mild detergent extraction of red cell membranes removes lipids, leaving behind the hexagonal protein latticework of the cortical cytoskeleton.[1] The individual proteins composing this structure were first named according to their mobility in a sodium dodecyl sulfate (SDS)-acrylamide gel system described by Fairbanks.[5, 6] The slowest migrating band was band 1 (or protein 1), the next slowest band, band 2 (or protein 2), and so on (Fig. 8–5). Subbands were designated with decimals. Thus, for example, the terms protein 4.1 and 4.2 designated two subbands constituting a zone at the position of the fourth most slowly migrating band (see Fig. 8–5). Some of these proteins were later renamed when they were better characterized. For example, proteins 1 and 2 are the α and β chains of spectrin, protein 3 is the anion transport channel, and protein 5 is actin. Other proteins critical to red cell function, such as proteins 4.1 and 4.2, have never been renamed.

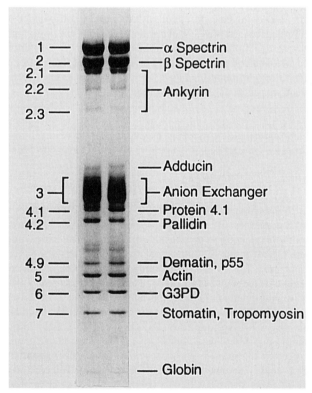

Figure 8–5. Protein composition of the red blood cell membrane skeleton. The major components of the erythrocyte membrane are separated by sodium dodecyl sulfate-polyacrylamide gel electrophoresis (SDS-PAGE) and revealed by Coomassie blue staining. (Adapted from Gallagher, P.G., Tse, W.T., and Forget, B.G.: Clinical and molecular aspects of disorders of the erythrocyte membrane skeleton. Semin. Perinatol. 1990;14:352.)

The original Fairbanks gels resolved about a dozen major cytoskeletal proteins.[5, 6] Many more proteins have subsequently been found, but only a few merit detailed consideration because of their quantity, function, or role in hereditary anemias. Currently, the most notable of these are the two spectrin subunits (α, and β), ankyrin, protein 4.1, actin, the glycophorins, band 3, protein 4.2, the adducins, p55, protein 4.9, and aquaporin. Other potentially important proteins, such as the Rh D antigen core protein, Na^+K^+ ATPase, or the Gardos channel, are either insufficiently understood or insufficiently abundant to warrant detailed discussion at this time.

The major embedded red cell proteins of relevance to this chapter are band 3 and the glycophorins. The other cytoskeletal proteins are attached to and arrayed along the inner (cytoplasmic) leaflet of the lipid bilayer (see Figs. 8–1 and 8–4). They associate to form a cytoskeletal lattice that is composed largely of tetrameric spectrin filaments, connected to one another at nodes that also contain F-actin filaments and protein 4. 1. The nodes attach to the overlying lipid bilayer by the binding of protein 4.1 to glycophorin and of the multivalent linking protein ankyrin to both spectrin and the cytoplasmic tail of band 3. The attachments are dynamic, subject to modification by phosphorylation or direct interaction with lipids such as PIP_2. The adducins, p55, protein 4.2, and protein 4.9 appear to stabilize the interaction of spectrin and actin with these complexes or with the lipid bilayer, or to modulate the bundling of actin.

▼ MAJOR INTEGRAL MEMBRANE PROTEINS

Band 3

Band 3 (also called protein 3 or Anion Exchanger-1, AE1), a transmembrane glycoprotein with a molecular mass of 100 kDa,[29, 47, 48] is the major anion transport protein in erythrocytes (Fig. 8–6).[1] It is also being increasingly appreciated as a critical regulator of red cell deformability, membrane assembly, intermediary metabolism, and red cell senescence.[46–49] It is highly abundant (10^6 copies per erythrocyte).[46] The NH_2-terminal end of the protein encodes a 43 kDa cytoplasmic domain[50, 51] and the remainder of the protein folds into helices and β sheets to form 12 to 14 membrane-spanning segments containing the anion transport channels. The boundary between the cytoplasmic tail and the first membrane-spanning segment (amino acids 400 to 404) is highly conserved in erythrocytes of diverse species.[46, 52] In particular, the proline at position 403 is thought to be critical for creating either a β bend or a random coil at the membrane junction, thereby giving the tail freedom of movement (inter-domain hinge).[49, 53] This feature is essential for red cell flexibility; mutations in this region produce rigid erythrocytes (Fig. 8–7). The physiologically functional form in which interactions with cytoplasmic molecules occur most efficiently appears to be a tetramer.[54]

There is considerable evidence to suggest that band 3 is of central importance to red cell homeostasis.[48, 49] It is the major anion (chloride-bicarbonate) exchanger. It may regulate metabolic pathways by sequestering key pathway enzymes, such as the glycolytic enzymes glyceraldehyde-3-phosphate dehydrogenase, phosphoglycerate kinase, and aldolase, as well as carbonic anhydrase II.[7, 55] There is evi-

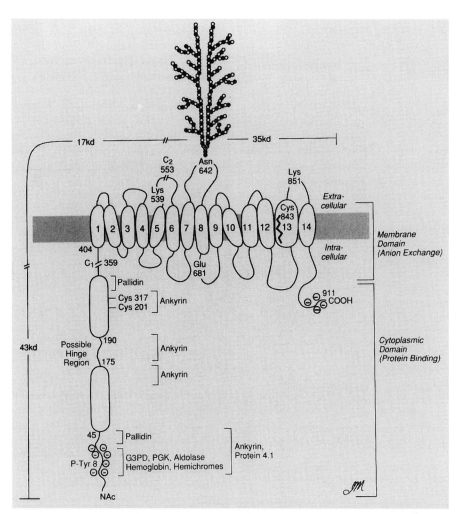

Figure 8–6. Organizational model of band 3, or AEl, the human erythrocyte anion exchange protein. The protein is divided into two structurally and functionally distinct domains: an approximately 43-kDa cytoplasmic domain which contains binding sites for several cellular proteins and an approximately 52-kDa transmembrane domain which forms the anion exchange channel. The two regions can be separated by chymotrypsin cleavage at the inner membrane (C_1). A second chymotryptic site (C_2) is accessible at the external surface. *Cytoplasmic Domain.* The highly acidic NH_2 terminal region (amino acids 1 to 45) binds hemoglobin, hemichromes, protein 4.1, and several glycolytic enzymes. Enzyme attachment is blocked by phosphorylation of tyrosine 8. Ankyrin and probably protein 4.2 binding involves several noncontiguous regions scattered throughout the cytoplasmic domain, which suggests that these binding sites are formed by protein folding. A functional hinge exists in the middle of the domain. *Transmembrane Domain.* Band 3 contains 12–14 transmembrane segments. Their orientation with respect to the inside and outside of the membrane has been extensively studied, but almost nothing is known about how they are positioned, relative to each other, to form the anion channel. Lys^{539} and Lys^{851} are probably the sites where H_2-DIDS, a covalent inhibitor of anion transport, attaches to band 3. Glu^{681} is probably one of the specific sites involved in anion exchange. A fatty acid, indicated by the zig-zag symbol, is esterified to Cys^{843}, and a complex carbohydrate structure is attached to Asn^{642}. Within the carbohydrate structure, solid circles represent N-acetylglucosamine; hatched circles, mannose; and open circles, galactose. (From Lux, S.E., and Palek, J.: Disorders of the red cell membrane. *In* Handin, R.J., Lux, S.E., and Stossel, T.P. [eds.]: Blood: Principles and Practice of Hematology. Philadelphia, W.B. Saunders Co., 1995, pp 1701–1818.)

dence that band 3 may possess flippase activity.[56] The NH_2-terminus is the target for binding by hemichromes, which are generated by denaturation or oxidation of hemoglobin. Finally, band 3 contains important binding sites for interaction with peripheral membrane proteins, binding to ankyrin, protein 4.1, protein 4.2, and possibly spectrin.

Binding of the 43 kDa cytoplasmic domain of band 3 to ankyrin is a critical mechanism for attachment of the cytoskeleton to the plasma membrane and the inter-domain hinge at this attachment point may be a crucial determinant of the flexibility or rigidity of erythrocytes.[53, 57] Binding of band 3 by hemichromes appears to stimulate aggregation into "patches," which are uniquely recognized by a red cell senescence isoantibody, leading to opsonization of the cell and its removal from the circulation by the reticuloendothe-

lial system.[33] Increasing evidence supports the notion that this is a major mechanism by which aging red cells are sequestered. Biogenesis of the red cell membrane in erythroblasts in vitro depends on the use of the cytoplasmic domain of band 3 as the nidus for stable assembly of the multimolecular complexes forming the spectrin latticework.[58] Recent findings using knock-out mice have contested this assertion, as band 3-/- mice have stably assembled membrane skeletons.[58, 59] Band 3 is thus potentially crucial for biogenesis of the membrane, modulation of elasticity or rigidity, anion transport, and immune marking of aging red cells for removal. Band 3 carries the Diego, Wright, ELO, Van Vugt, BOW, Moen, Wulfsberg, Hughes, and Bishop blood groups.[60]

Band 3 is a member of a gene family of anion ex-

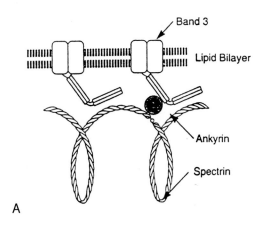

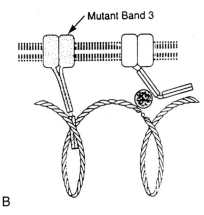

Figure 8–7. Diagrammatic representation of the functional configuration of band 3 in association with the membrane and cytoskeletal lattice. *A* shows how the "interdomain hinge" in the cytoplasmic domain of band 3 permits it to interact flexibly and non-obstructively with ankyrin and spectrin. Mutations in band 3 that abolish the hinge, shown in *B*, cause the cytoplasmic domain to become entangled in the latticework. The importance of this arrangement is discussed in more detail in the section on hereditary ovalocytosis. (Adapted from the Journal of Clinical Investigation, 1992, Vol. 89, pp. 686–692, by copyright permission of the American Society for Clinical Investigation.)

changers expressed in many tissues.[61] The nonerythroid isoforms (AE2 and AE3) that have been well characterized exhibit specialized patterns of expression, transport of anions or organic acids, and may also key organizing centers for membrane and cytoskeletal structures. These family members share significant, but localized regional homology with AE1. The hydrophobic channel domains of the proteins tend to be conserved, but the cytoplasmic domains are more divergent, implying conservation of anion exchange properties but specialization of the domains that bind to the cytoskeleton. These binding functions may be adapted to particular cell types. Additional diversity is provided to this family of proteins by alternate splicing or translation pathways. A truncated isoform of AE1 is expressed outside the red cell in the intercalated cells in the collecting ducts of the kidney. This isoform, generated by alternate splicing, lacks the NH$_2$-terminal binding sites for glycolytic enzymes, ankyrin, and protein 4.1.[62–64]

The Glycophorins

The glycophorins were originally identified as the most abundant integral membrane glycoproteins in erythrocytes.[65–67] Because of their high sialic acid content, they account for more than 95% of the periodic acid-Schiff (PAS)-staining capacity of erythrocytes. In the aggregate, these proteins are highly abundant; glycophorin A is the major component, $5–9 \times 10^6$ copies per cell, with glycophorins B, C, and D accounting for $0.8–3 \times 10^5$, $0.5–1 \times 10^5$, and $0.1–0.2 \times 10^5$ copies per cell, respectively.[32, 65] Characterization of cDNA and genomic clones encoding the glycophorins has revealed that they fall into two distinct subgroups.[66–71] Glycophorins A and B are homologous to each other and are encoded by two closely linked genes. Glycophorins C and D arise from a single locus bearing no particular homology to the genes for glycophorins A and B. Glycophorin D differs from glycophorin C by use of an alternate translation start site created by alternative messenger RNA splicing. Another gene linked in tandem with those for glycophorins A and B has been isolated; it would encode a putative fifth glycophorin, glycophorin E, which seems to have evolved from glycophorin A by homologous recombination at *Alu* repeats.[72, 73] No protein product of this gene has been identified. The glycophorins are 0-glycosylated[66, 67] and have a single extracellular hydrophilic NH$_2$-terminal domain, a single membrane-spanning domain, and a COOH-terminal cytoplasmic tail.

Glycophorins A and B are nearly identical except for their cytoplasmic tails. After posttranslational cleavage of a leader peptide, the first domain is composed of 70 exoplasmic amino acids, followed by the membrane-spanning domain, and a COOH-terminal cytoplasmic domain. Amino acids 90 to 93 of the membrane-spanning domain appear to be particularly important for the formation of glycophorin A dimers, the predominant form encountered in the membrane.[74] Recently, determination of the solution NMR structure of the transmembrane domain of a GPA dimer revealed a small, well-packed interface between the molecules, and demonstrated that van der Waals interactions alone can mediate stable and specific associations between transmembrane helices.[75] Glycophorin B is quite similar, except that exon 3, which encodes residues 27 to 55 in the glycophorin A gene, is not retained in fully processed mRNA of GPB.[65] The cytoplasmic domain is also shortened, containing only three amino acids in addition to the three amino acid hinge region.

The genes for glycophorins A, B, and E are located on chromosome 4q28-q31, in the order A>B>E.[76] The genomic structure and promoters of all three genes are highly conserved[76, 77] and all 3 contain cleavable leader peptides. The major differences between the three isoforms are due to variations in the exoplasmic domains and in the COOH-terminal regions. The three genes are so closely linked and homologous that unequal crossover events occur, yielding fused gene products, analogous to hemoglobin Lepore.[74]

The precise biological functions of the glycophorins are incompletely characterized. Because of their high sialic acid content, the glycophorins, constitute more than 60% of the net negative surface charge of red cells, suggesting that they are important for modulating red cell-red cell and red cell-endothelial interactions. For example, removal of sialic acids causes red cell clumping.[74] Glycophorins A and B are relevant to clinical immunohematology; blood groups M and N reside on glycophorin A (reviewed in ref. 78). Group M differs from group N by polymorphic changes in amino acid residues 1 and 5. Similarly, the Ss phenotype results from a polymorphism at amino acid 29 (methionine and threonine, respectively). Certain rare variant blood groups, such as Miltenberger V, En(a⁻), and M^{K}M^k, are glycophorin variants. Miltenberger V arises by a gene fusion event, whereas some forms of En(a⁻) result from deletion of the glycophorin A gene. Some "glycophorin-deficient" states, defined by lack of immunochemical reactivity, are actually due to unequal crossing over events that yield fusion genes giving rise to novel glycophorin immunotypes unreactive with established antisera.

No biological function has been assigned to glycophorin B other than its association with the Ss blood group. Like glycophorin A, it is found only in erythroid cells. GPA and GPB are expressed only during terminal erythroid maturation, appearing for the first time at the proerythroblast stage.[65] Most information about the function of glycophorins A and B has come from studies of glycophorin A. Glycophorin A-deficient red cells exhibit increased glycosylation of band 3, owing to the addition of extra sialic acid.[79] The quantitative increase almost exactly counterbalances the normal contribution expected from GPA. This suggests that maintenance of total surface charge density is important for red cell survival. GPA-deficient red cells exhibit no abnormalities of shape or deformability, suggesting that these glycophorins are not critical for maintaining mechanical stability, deformability, or shape of the membrane.[80, 81] Binding of immunologically non-specific ligands to red cells, such as wheat germ agglutinin, causes aggregation of glycophorin and decreased red cell deformability, but the clinical relevance of this alteration is not known.[65] Also poorly understood is the observation that glycophorin-deficient red cells are considerably more resistant to invasion by malaria parasites than are normal cells.[65, 82] Interestingly, band 3-/- mice have complete deficiency of GPA in their red cells.[83]

Glycophorins C and D are encoded by a single gene located on chromosome 2ql4-q2l. They differ in their use of alternative translation start sites; when translation is initiated at the first AUG, glycophorin C is produced. When initiation occurs at the AUG encoding methionine at position 20, a truncated protein, glycophorin D, is generated. Residues 21 to 128 of the two proteins are identical. GPC does not express a cleavable signal peptide.[84–86] The extracellular NH$_2$-terminal domain is 57 amino acids long, containing 1 N-glycosylation and 12 0-glycosylation sites, a 24 amino acid membrane-spanning segment, and a 47 residue COOH-terminal cytoplasmic domain. Residues 41 to 50 encode the Gerbich (Ge:3) blood group antigens.[87] Variants of glycophorin C give rise to unusual immunohematological phenotypes,[65, 87] including Gerbich YUS and WEPB. These appear to arise by intragenic crossing over between the highly homologous exons 2 and 3, resulting in the deletion of exons or the generation of hybrid exons encoding novel epitopes.

Glycophorin C is expressed in multiple nonerythroid tissues, but the level of expression is far higher during erythropoiesis.[88] This feature may result from the use of different transcription start sites. Posttranslational modification of GPC may change during erythropoiesis, as evidenced by the differential reactivity of early and later progenitors with different monoclonal antibodies raised against the protein. GPC plays a critical role in regulating the stability, deformability, and shape of the membrane. Deficiency is associated with elliptocytic red cells without hemolytic anemia; these cells are less stable and less deformable than are normal red cells.[89–91] Naturally occurring mutations in the exoplasmic domain appear to have no effect on these properties, suggesting that the abnormalities of deficient cells arise from absence of the cytoplasmic domain. The cytoplasmic tail of GPC interacts in a ternary complex with protein 4.1 and p55.[92–94] Protein 4.1 deficiency leads to increased detergent extractability of GPC in vitro and GPC deficiency in vivo.[90, 91] Reconstitution of these membranes with protein 4.1 restores the resistance of GPC to detergent extraction. Thus, the cytoplasmic tail of GPC, like that of band 3, serves as an important anchoring site for attachment to the cytoskeleton.

Other Embedded Membrane Proteins

The red cell membrane contains small amounts (fewer than 10,000 copies per cell) of numerous ion pumps and channels, including Na$^+$K$^+$ATPase and the recently cloned, calcium-dependent potassium (Gardos) channel.[95–97] The activities of these proteins are often altered in response to primary abnormalities of membrane or cytoskeleton, but disease states originating with mutations in these proteins have not yet been described. Therefore, they will not be considered further. Similarly, knowledge is rapidly emerging about the structure and about the structure-function and structure-epitope relationships within the protein constituting the core determinant of the Rh antigen blood system, the Rh D peptide. The gene encoding this protein has been cloned and characterized.[98] Some Rh immunotypes arise as the result of the alternative splicing of Rh gene products. The molecular basis for the so-called Rh (null phenotype), a state associated with absence of Rh antigen activity and chronic hemolysis, is discussed below.

The aquaporins are membrane channel proteins that serve as selective pores through which water crosses the plasma membranes of many cell types.[99] Aquaporin-1, AQP1, is expressed in many tissues, including erythrocytes, and may contribute to the ability of the red cell to adjust rapidly to changes in osmolality. The extracellular surface of AQP1 contains the epitope for the Colton blood group system.[100] In one patient, the genetic basis of the rare Colton null phenotype has been identified as a mutation of the highly conserved NPA motif of AQP1 essential for channel function.[99, 101] Colton null individuals exhibit no obvious clinical phenotype, although mice with targeted inactivation of AQP1 become hyperosmolar after fluid restriction.[103] Recently, evidence for the presence of AQP3 in erythrocytes has been presented.[104]

▼ CYTOSKELETAL PROTEINS THAT ATTACH TO THE MEMBRANE

The major proteins of the erythrocyte cortical cytoskeleton are spectrin, ankyrin, short filaments of F-actin, proteins 4.1, 4.2, and 4.9, p55, and the adducins. As noted earlier, these form an interlocking network or lattice that attaches to the membrane largely by binding to the cytoplasmic domains of the glycophorins and band 3. Spectrin, ankyrin, protein 4.1, and protein 4.2 are considered in more detail because of their known roles in hereditary hemolytic anemias.

The Spectrin Protein Family

Spectrin is the major constituent of the erythrocyte membrane skeleton, constituting 75% of its mass, and it is present at a concentration of 200,000 molecules per cell.[1, 105] The fundamental structure of the spectrin molecule is that of a heterodimer, consisting of two highly homologous chains, the α and β chains. The α chain has a molecular mass of 280 kDa and the β chain 240 kDa (Fig. 8–8). The chains align and intertwine with each other in antiparallel fashion with respect to their NH_2-termini to form flexible, rod-like heterodimers (see Fig. 8–8). These dimers further self-associate to form tetramers and higher order oligomers. From a physiological perspective, the critical functional unit is probably the tetramer, resulting from head-to-head linkages of the heterodimers. Tetramers have a contour length of approximately 200 nm.

The α and β subunits of spectrin are highly homologous. Each consists of a series of 106 amino acid tandem repeats, 21 in α spectrin, 17 in β spectrin, characterized by an invariant tryptophan residue surrounded by a short consensus sequence.[1, 106–109] At some points along the subunit chains, some of the repeats exhibit more divergence from the canonical structure than others, particularly in the NH_2- and COOH-termini. The essential structural feature of each repeat is the formation of three amphipathic α helices, linked to one another by short sequences exhibiting less highly ordered structure; the linkage between adjacent repeats is also by relatively short random coil sequences. The crystal structure of one of these spectrin repeats has been determined (Fig. 8–9),[110] allowing the phasing of the repeats.[111] Thus the spectrin molecule is often portrayed as "links of sausage on a chain," as depicted in Figure 8–8. Each "link" is composed of three helical segments. The somewhat more open structures present at the termini give the rod-like structure a barbell appearance.

The NH_2- and COOH-termini appear to be the key regions of dimer-dimer self-association and for interaction with actin, ankyrin, and protein 4.1.[1, 112–115] The NH_2-terminus of β spectrin contains the binding site for protein 4.1; ankyrin binding occurs in repeats β15 and β16[115] near the COOH-terminus. More moderately divergent repeats along the chain are utilized as recognition sites for binding to other modifiers, including kinases and calmodulin.[116, 117] The

overall effect of this repeating structure is to provide for a strong, elastic, rod-like filament that can associate into complex multi-molecular assemblies capable of lending shape and resiliency to the overlying plasma membrane via formation of a meshwork able to link to integral membrane proteins. Direct interactions of a weaker nature may also occur between the spectrin filament and the lipid bilayer itself.

The genes encoding erythroid α and β spectrin have been cloned and characterized at both the cDNA and the genomic levels.[108, 109, 118, 119] Analysis of genomic DNA, RNA expression, and immunologically cross-reactive molecules from a variety of tissues and organisms has revealed that the erythroid spectrin chains are prototypical members of a multigene family that includes fodrin (brain spectrin), dystrophin, and α actinin.[120] Each of these proteins contains multiple helical repeats separated by short regions of random coil, forming rod-like filaments capped at each end by looser "barbell-like" structures that interact with other molecules. NH_2- and COOH-terminal "membrane association domains" (MADs), pleckstrin homology domains, SH3 domains, and calcium-binding EF hand structures are also characteristic of several family members. Thus the spectrin family may well represent the fundamental motif utilized by cells for the formation of intracellular scaffolds and matrices. The binding partners and functional roles of these domains in both erythroid and nonerythroid cells are beginning to be revealed. For example, repeat 10 of α spectrin contains an SH3 domain for which a candidate binding protein belonging to a family of tyrosine-kinase binding proteins has recently been identified.[121]

Heterodimer formation between α and β chains appears to depend on appropriate alignment and intercalation of helical coils from one chain, with grooves provided by gaps in the helical array on the other chains, i.e., there appears to be helix-helix interaction along most of the chains. Tetramer formation may depend on the fact that the usual three-coil helix motif is not well preserved near the ends of the α and β chains. Rather, the α chain has a one-coil repeat and the β chain has a two-coil repeat. It is postulated that these combine to form the apparently more stable three-helix structure, thereby linking two heterodimers together (see Fig. 8–8).[122–125] The exact physical description of these interactions is still being established; their importance is illustrated

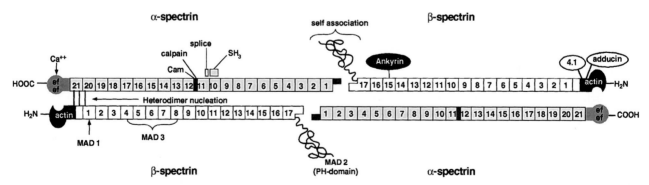

Figure 8–8. Spectrin typically is a multifunctional heterodimer that self-associates. The functional unit is most often an αβ-heterodimer. Each subunit contains non-homologous NH_2- and COOH-terminal domains (domains I and III, respectively), joined by a central domain (domain II) composed of multiple homologous repeats of ≈106 residues each. Within the molecules are many sites that interact with other proteins or regulator molecules. (From Morrow, J.S., Rimm, D.L., Kennedy, S.P., Cianci, C.D., Sinard, J.H., Weed, S.A.: Of membranes stability and mosaics: the spectrin cytoskeleton. *In* Hoffman, J., and Jamieson, J. [eds.]: Handbook of Physiology. London, Oxford, 1997, pp. 485–540.)

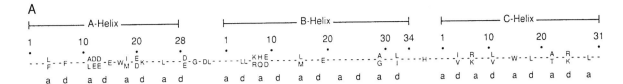

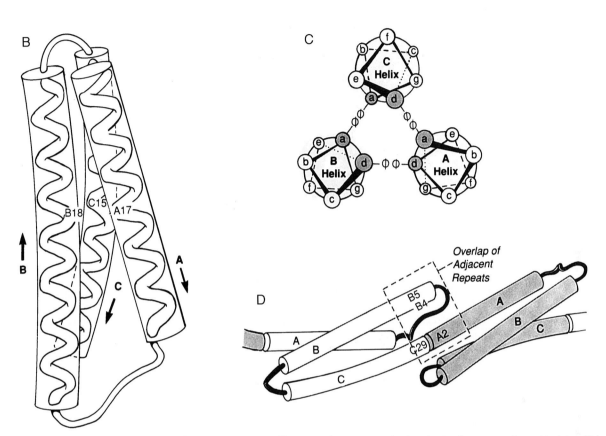

Figure 8–9. Structure of spectrin repeats. *A.* Consensus sequence of human erythrocyte spectrin phased according to crystallographic data, which defines three α helices that encompass the amino acids shown. Less conserved residues are marked with a dash. Residues a and d are the major contact points between helices. They tend to be hydrophobic and are conserved in most spectrins. *B.* Model of a single repeat based on the crystal structure of *Drosophila* α-fodrin. The positions of the nearly invariant tryptophans at A17 and C15 are shown. They interact with surrounding residues, including B18, at the central junction where the A helix crosses over from B to C. *C.* Cross section of a typical repeat. The A, B, and C helices are in a triangular array, and the a and d residues lie on one face of each helix. The side chains of these amino acids are usually hydrophobic (φ) and interact with each other to stabilize the triple helical configuration. Salt bonds between the typically polar amino acids at positions e and g also help attach the B and C and A and C helices to each other. *D.* Interconnection of two adjacent repeats. The A and C helices are directly connected, forming one long helix. The distal repeat of each pair is rotated 60 degrees (right-handed). The B helix of the proximal repeat (black and white) overlaps the A helix of the following repeat (shaded). Interactions in the overlap region among conserved hydrophobic residues such as C29, B4, and B5 and the mostly hydrophobic residues at A2 probably stabilize the connection and limit mobility at the repeat junction. (From Lux, S.E., and Palek, J.: Disorders of the red cell membrane. *In* Handin, R.J., Lux, S.E., and Stossel, T.P. [eds.]: Blood: Principles and Practice of Hematology. Philadelphia, W.B. Saunders Co., 1995, pp. 1701–1818.)

by the fact that, as discussed later, some hereditary hemolytic anemias arise as a result of defective heterodimer or tetramer formation.

The side to side assembly of α and β spectrin chains in a zipper-like fashion begins at a defined nucleation site composed of four repeats from each chain, α19 to α22 and β1 to β4, respectively. It is proposed that after tight association of complementary nucleation sites, a conformational change is initiated the promotes pairing of the remainder of the two chains[122–124] A common α-spectrin polymorphism, α[LELY], interferes with normal nucleation and decreases the synthesis of functionally-competent α-spectrin chains.[124, 125] This may influence clinical expression of spectrin mutations (see below).

Mild proteolytic cleavage of spectrin subdivides the protein into a reproducible pattern of domains of the α (αI through αV, in order of decreasing size) and β (βI through βV) chains, 20 to 80 kDa in size. These patterns provide useful fingerprints of the normal molecule that are changed by many mutations altering spectrin function. Mild tryptic or chymotryptic digestion is thus used to localize and partially characterize mutations of these very large proteins (see below).[1, 7, 130]

The gene for erythrocyte α spectrin is located on chromosome 1[131] and that for erythroid β spectrin is found on chromosome 14.[132] Although these genes exhibit similar intron/exon structures, the exons do not correspond exactly to the 106 amino acid repeats.[118,119] The mechanisms responsible for tissue-specific expression of these genes are rapidly being characterized. Of particular note is the fact that spectrin, like several other cytoskeletal proteins, appears to utilize alternative mRNA splicing as a favored mechanism for the establishment of unique tissue-specific isoforms. For example, a muscle isoform of β spectrin appears to result from alternative mRNA splicing of the mRNA transcript of the erythroid β spectrin gene.[133] The splice alters translation termination near the COOH-terminus, leading to elongation of the COOH-terminus of the muscle form.

The immediate family of spectrin isoforms have been classified by their sequence and functional homology to the α and β isoforms.[1, 134] Thus 2 α-spectrin and 3 β-spectrin isoforms have been identified to date. A βIII isoform localized to the Golgi apparatus of many cell types has recently been described.[135, 136]

Proteins That Bind to Spectrin

Protein 4.1. In erythrocytes, protein 4.1 is an 80 kDa phosphoprotein present in ~80,000 copies per erythrocyte.[32, 137] It and its recently discovered close family members share a mosaic of sequence homologies with other protein families.[138] Especially striking is the 20–45% homology seen at the NH₂-terminus within which the "FERM" domain ("*Four*.1 Protein," *Ezrin, Radixin, Moesin*) defines a family of proteins linking the actin cytoskeleton to membranes in many cell types.[139, 140] This grouping has also been called the "ERM" or "MERM" family of actin binding proteins (moesin, ezrin, radixin, merlin). Interestingly, this family is

homologous to coraclin, a *Drosophila* protein that interacts with a large disc protein (Dlg) that is homologous to tumor suppressor proteins (e.g., APC, hDlg1) in mammals.[141] It is intriguing that merlin itself is a tumor suppressor protein whose mutation is associated with neurofibromatosis-2.[138] More recently, it has become clear that erythrocyte protein 4.1 (4.1R) is the prototype of a much more closely related family of at least four members that are generally distributed (4.1G), confined to brain (4.1B), or expressed predominantly in neurons (4.1N). These forms have no defined functions at present but share 60–95% homology across most domains of the molecule.[142, 143]

Protein 4.1 can be subdivided by mild chymotryptic digestion into four domains of apparent molecular mass of 30 kDa, 16 kDa, 10 kDa, and 22 to 24 kDa, proceeding from NH₂-terminus to COOH-terminus (Fig. 8–10). Of these, the 16 kDa domain of protein 4.1R is not particularly closely related to the other 4.1 family members. 4.1R is variably but highly phosphorylated; other distinctive features are clustering of cysteine residues near the NH₂-terminus, O-linked glycosylation in the 10 kDa domain, a markedly acidic COOH-terminus, and a markedly basic NH₂-terminus.[1] Phosphorylation sites are located near the COOH-terminal extremity of the 30 kDa domain and in the middle of the 10 kDa domain.[144, 145] The latter appears to be cyclic AMP (cAMP) dependent, whereas the others may be modulated by protein kinase C. At least one site appears to be a substrate for cdc2 kinase. Protein 4.1 is the prototype of non-membrane proteins that are glycosylated by an 0-linked N-acetylglucosamine mechanism, a feature that contributes

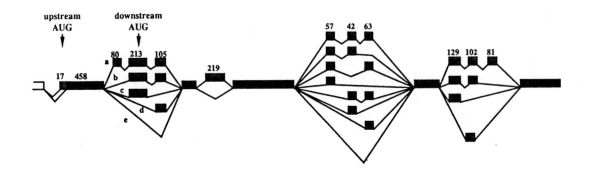

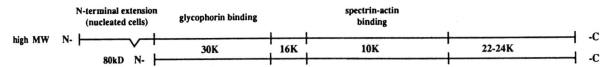

Figure 8–10. Model of protein 4.1 and alternative splicing of protein 4.1 mRNAs. *Below.* The five domains generated by chymotryptic digestion are shown in the lower half of the figure. The amino-terminal 30 kDa domain is thought to be necessary for binding to the cytoplasmic domain of glycophorin in the presence of phospholipids. The central 10 kDa domain has been shown to be necessary and sufficient for binding to spectrin-actin. The 24 kDa domain, present in protein 4.1a, and the 22 kDa present in its place in protein 4.1b are now known to differ only by deamidation of asparagine residues at positions 478 and 502. *Above.* Portions of the protein 4.1 mRNA transcribed into mRNA in all tissues are drawn on the central line of the diagram. Exons expressed selectively in certain tissues are drawn above or below the central line with thin lines indicating the pattern of exons retained in certain tissues, with length in nucleotides indicated. One exon, 80 nucleotides in length, does not code for a protein because it contains translation termination codons in all three reading frames. For simplicity, some exons expressed at extremely low levels in many tissues have been omitted from the diagram. The key exons described in the text are the 17 nucleotide and 213 nucleotide exons containing AUG translation start codons and the 63 nucleotide exon important for spectrin-actin binding. The latter is expressed in large amounts predominantly in red cells and to a lesser extent in muscle and testes. The 17 nucleotide "exon," which inserts an upstream AUG, permitting synthesis of a high molecular weight isoform with an N-terminal extension, is called exon 2 in the text. The 213 nucleotide exon containing the downstream AUG must be expressed for synthesis of the 80 kDa isoform in red cells, which do not express the 17 nucleotide exon 2. The 63 nucleotide exon, described as exon 16 in the text, is essential for spectrin-actin binding.

to its higher apparent molecular weight on acrylamide gels than predicted on the basis of known amino acid sequence.[146] In red cells, two molecular weight forms, protein 4.1a and protein 4.1b, are consistently seen.[147] Protein 4.1a, which is of higher molecular weight, increases as red cells age; it is barely apparent in young red cells. Protein 4.1a results from the deamidation of two Asn residues (478 and 502) in a non-enzymatic, age-dependent fashion[128] that lowers the mobility of the protein in gels.[147] The functional significance of glycosylation and deamidation, if any, is unknown, but the latter provides a useful marker of red cell age.

Protein 4.1 links the spectrin-actin framework to the lipid bilayer (see Fig. 8–4) by facilitating complex formation between spectrin-actin fibers, the cytoplasmic domain of band 3, and p55/glycophorin C. Protein 4.1 is thus critical for the strength of the membrane. Abnormalities and deficiencies produce hereditary elliptocytosis.[7]

Protein 4.1 was originally thought to be expressed only in red cells. It is now known to be widely expressed in a variety of tissues, identifiable as immunologically cross-reactive forms that are heterogeneous with respect to molecular weight, abundance, and intracellular localization.[148, 149] Protein 4.1R isoforms arise from a single genomic locus, positioned near the Rh locus at chromosome 1q32-9ter.[150] The gene is 250–300 kb long. Its primary mRNA transcript is subjected to extensive alternative splicing, giving rise to a family of mRNAs 6.5 to 7.0 kb long.[150–155] There are at least 12 alternately spliced exons, as well as an important cryptic acceptor site, that lead to the production of a diverse protein family from a single gene (see Fig. 8–10). Mature mRNA transcripts representing many of the over 2000 possible mRNA spliceoforms have been identified by cDNA cloning or polymerase chain reaction (PCR) analysis. Splicing events in only two regions have been shown to have functional relevance in red cells: that encoding the spectrin-actin-binding domain and that encoding the 5′ untranslated region.

Three alternatively spliced exons are located in the region encoding the NH$_2$-terminal end of the 10 kDa domain.[154, 155] This domain is known to encompass the spectrin-actin-binding activity of the protein.[156] In particular, the NH$_2$-terminal end of the 10 kDa fragment was tentatively implicated as the binding site on the basis of competition assays and analysis with peptide-specific antibodies. One of the three exons, exon 16, is 63 nucleotides long and codes for 21 amino acids found at the NH$_2$-terminus of the red cell form (see Fig. 8–10). This sequence is present in mature erythroid mRNA and protein but absent from most nonerythroid forms. The erythroid mRNA splicing pattern depends on tissue-specific and differentiation stage-specific alternative splicing that is induced late in the course of terminal erythroid maturation.[151, 152, 155, 157] Recombinant isoforms containing these 21 amino acids bind to spectrin-actin complexes efficiently.[158] Otherwise identical recombinant proteins lacking the sequence fail to bind. Thus, alternative splicing of this exon during late erythropoiesis is essential to generate a functioning protein isoform.

Muscle and testes (and, to a lesser degree, brain) are the only non-erythroid tissues that express exon 16 in significant amounts.[153, 155] The relevance of the erythroid splicing pattern to testicular and muscle cell function remains unknown; however, it is intriguing that a major isoform of β spectrin expressed in muscle is the erythroid form. This spectrin isoform is also abundant in brain, in which small to moderate amounts of protein 4.1 mRNA containing exon 16 can be found.[114, 133]

Two additional exons are adjacent to the one responsible for binding to erythroid spectrin-actin. There are thus eight possible variants of the 10 kDa spectrin-actin-binding domain arising from combinatorial splicing of three consecutive exons.[153, 155] In lymphocytes, none of the exons are retained in the majority of the mRNA transcripts. In brain, multiple isoforms containing various combinations of the exons are encountered, including a uniquely expressed form retaining all three exons, whereas in erythrocytes, nearly all of the protein 4.1 mRNA contains exon 16, but not 14 or 15.[153] This multiplicity of isoforms may be important for interaction with spectrin isoforms in different cell types.

The biochemical role of protein 4.1 in linking spectrin to the membrane is complex. Spectrin binds actin weakly, as does protein 4.1. Protein 4.1 greatly facilitates and stabilizes spectrin-actin interaction and the formation of a ternary complex that can bind to glycophorin or protein 3. This binding is weakened by phosphorylation of protein 4.1. Much less is known about the structural requirements for binding of protein 4.1 to the cytoplasmic domains of transmembrane proteins or to lipids. Lipid binding may facilitate binding to the proteins. Alternatively spliced exons located near the COOH-terminus of the 30 kDa domain are expressed differentially to significant degrees in some tissues.[152–156] Even though no clear functional significance has been attached to these splicing patterns, it is now clear that the 30kd domain is involved in attaching 4.1R and its homologues to proteins like p55, glycophorin C, band 3, and other embedded moieties such as the chloride channel pIcln.

As illustrated in Figure 8–10, two splicing events that modify the structure of the 5′ untranslated region of erythroid protein 4.1 can generate, in nonerythroid tissues, a high molecular weight isoform resulting from initiation of mRNA translation at an upstream initiation codon inserted by use of a cryptic acceptor splice site in exon 2.[152–154] The high molecular weight isoform (apparent molecular mass of 120 kDa) has been identified immunochemically in cells by the use of antibodies generated against the novel upstream peptides.

In most nonerythroid tissues the higher molecular weight isoforms (120–150 kDa) and low molecular weight isoforms (60–90 kDa) coexist in varying ratios. These presumably represent two different families of protein spliceoforms translated from the upstream (high molecular weight) or downstream (low molecular weight) translation start site. The relative amounts of each family produced could depend on the relative amounts of alternative mRNA splicing or the preferential use of one or the other translation start sites. Recent work has shown that the upstream translation start site, when present, is used almost exclusively, thus greatly reducing the likelihood of translational regulation.[159] These studies indirectly, but strongly, implicate the regulated use of a cryptic splice site in exon 2 as the determinant of high and low molecular weight isoform distribution.

The functional importance of the high molecular weight isoforms remains unknown. The COOH-terminal 80 kDa of these isoforms is identical to their low molecular weight analogues. It is possible that the additional amino acid residues form a "headpiece" that alters the behavior of the 30 kDa membrane-binding domain or causes localization of the protein to other regions of the cell. Preliminary data suggest that the spectrin-actin binding is not affected, provided that exon is expressed.[156] Multiple alternative mRNA splicing events might generate isoforms with different affinities for membrane and intracellular structures. There is now persuasive evidence that high molecular weight isoforms associate with NuMa, a major organizing protein of the mitotic apparatus,[160–162] ZO-2, a component of the tight junctions in epithelial and endothelial cells, and other "membrane associated guanylate kinase" (MAGUK) family proteins in addition to p55.[162–164] The diverse array of spliceoforms is thus likely to provide for the multiple locations (perinuclear regions, stress fibers, cytoplasmic filaments of unknown significance, and centrioles) in which protein 4.1 isoforms are found, in addition to its erythroid localization underneath the plasma membrane. The "headpiece" is unique to 4.1R; it can be distinguished from the other family members, allowing verification that 4.1R is actually involved in these other sites. In view of their widespread expression and interaction with key components of mitotic spindles and tight junctions, it is surprising that the recently reported protein 4.1R gene knock-out mouse exhibits only anemia and subtle neurologic abnormalities.[165]

The alternate splicing events leading to the production of high molecular weight isoforms of protein 4.1 are highly relevant to the pathophysiology of certain protein 4.1 deficiency states, even though the normal functional significance of adding a headpiece to protein 4.1 remains unknown. The high molecular weight isoforms are completely absent from mature red cells. Indeed, mRNA containing the 17 amino acid extension of exon 2 needed for the synthesis of high molecular weight forms is essentially absent from erythroid cells, at least from the proerythroblast stage forward.[152–155] Thus, only the downstream translation initiation site is available for protein 4.1 biosynthesis during erythropoiesis. Mutations abolishing this site will lead to protein 4.1 deficiency in red cells, but deficiency of only the low molecular weight family of isoforms in nonerythroid cells as the upstream methionine will be available for synthesis of high molecular weight forms. Erythropoiesis is marked by the induction of splicing events leading to retention of the spectrin-actin-

binding sequence motif in the 10 kDa domain, but exclusion of the sequences containing the upstream translation initiator codon needed for production of high molecular weight isoforms. Mutations altering either of these events can thus cause selective deficiencies or abnormalities in red cells.

Ankyrin. Ankyrin, or protein 2.1, is a 210 kDa sulfhydryl-rich molecule containing three defined domains: an NH$_2$-terminal 89 kDa domain that contains sites for binding to band 3, a 62 kDa domain containing spectrin-binding sites, and a 55 kDa regulatory domain at the COOH-terminus (Fig. 8–11).[1, 7, 166] It is present in 100,000 copies per cell. Ankyrin is globular but, like protein 4.1, is highly asymmetrical.[167–169] The band 3-binding domain is basic; the central spectrin-binding domain is neutral, but heavily phosphorylated; and the regulatory domain is highly acidic, at least in the predominant erythroid form.[169] Phosphorylation occurs by casein kinase and cAMP-independent protein kinase.[170, 171]

The NH$_2$-terminal 90 kDa domain contains a complex repeated internal structure that gives rise to multiple protein binding sites. There are 24 consecutive, highly conserved tandem repeats called cdc10 or ankyrin repeats. Ankyrin repeats have been found throughout nature in proteins with a diverse array of functions.[172–174] In erythrocyte ankyrin, these repeats are subdivided into 6 folding units. Folding units 2 and 3 + 4 form distinct, cooperative binding sites for band 3.[175, 176] Determination of the crystal structure of ankyrin repeats in the 53BP2, GABPα/β, p19^{Ink4d}, and IκBα proteins reveals that ankyrin repeats are L-shaped structures composed of a pair of α helices that form an antiparallel coiled-coil, followed by an extended loop perpendicular to the helices and a β hairpin.[177–181]

Like other membrane cytoskeletal proteins, erythrocyte ankyrin has proven to be the prototype for a diverse family of closely related but distinct proteins arising from at least three distinct genes, and from complex patterns of alternative pre-mRNA splicing, polyadenylation,[182–192] and the use of alternate promoters.[184, 193] Erythrocyte ankyrin (also called ankyrin$_R$, or ANK1) is expressed not only in red cells, but also in brain and spinal cord. An ankyrin isoform expressed largely in brain is called ankyrin$_B$, or ANK2, and ankyrin$_G$ or ANK3, has a broad tissue distribution, but it is especially abundant in kidney. The nonerythroid ankyrins also bind to cytoplasmic domains of embedded membrane proteins and

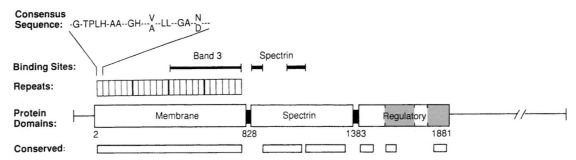

Figure 8–11. Structure of erythrocyte ankyrin, ANK1. The 89 kDa membrane domain contains 24 repeats grouped in folding units of six. Their consensus sequence is shown at the top left in single-letter amino acid code. Dashes indicate less conserved residues. Repeats 7–12 (folding unit 2) and repeats 13–24 (folding units 3 and 4) form two distinct but cooperative binding sites for band 3. The 62 kDa spectrin domain contains the binding site(s) for spectrin. The 55 kDa regulatory domain is thought to modulate the binding functions of the other two domains. In the middle of the domain, a highly acidic inhibitory region in exon 38 is spliced out of full-length ankyrin (ANK2.1) to make ANK2.2. At least eight isoforms of the last three exons exist. The last three isoforms contain a basic sequence (open area) that is common in brain ANK1 but rare in the red cell protein. In addition, isoforms lacking exons 38 and 39, 36 through 39, and 36 through 41 have been detected. (From Lux, S.E., and Palek, J.: Disorders of the red cell membrane. *In* Handin, R.J., Lux, S.E., and Stossel, T.P. [eds.]: Blood: Principles and Practice of Hematology. Philadelphia, W.B. Saunders Co., 1995, pp. 1701–1818.)

appear to be important for their dynamic spatial organization, as well as the integrity of supramolecular structures, e.g., the Nodes of Ranvier, to which they contribute. Representative binding partners include the Na$^+$K$^+$ATPase, band 3 homologues such as AE3 in kidney, certain sodium channels, and adhesion molecules such as L1 and neurofascin.[1, 7, 166] Even though the 3 ankyrin genes exhibit distinctive patterns of expression, their patterns overlap. For example, ANK1 and ANK3 are both found in brain, a fact that may account for the observation that mice lacking ANK1[194] or ANK3[195] exhibit neurological abnormalities including Purkinje cell degeneration and ataxia. Mice with targeted disruption of ANK2 exhibit brain defects as well, but with more clear cut abnormalities in brain development.[196]

Multiple erythroid-specific isoforms arise by alternative mRNA splicing and polyadenylation events that generate diversity of the COOH-terminal regulatory domain. Use of alternative promoters has recently been shown to generate a muscle-tissue specific, truncated isoform of ANK1.[184-186] An important erythroid isoform of ANK1 is protein 2.2, which has been truncated near the COOH-terminus by removal of the 162 amino acids that render the regulatory domain of protein 2.1 highly acidic. This alternatively spliced isoform has a higher affinity for both the cytoplasmic domain of band 3 and spectrin, suggesting that the acidic portion of the regulatory domain exerts an inhibitory effect on ankyrin binding.

Ankyrin is multivalent, binding to the COOH-terminal region of the spectrin β chain with its 55 kDa central domain and to the cytoplasmic tail of the anion exchanger via repeated sequences in the amino-terminal 90 kDa domain. Binding creates a tight association between spectrin and protein 3, but the strength of binding can be modified by phosphorylation. The stoichiometry of the abundance of spectrin and ankyrin suggests strongly that one ankyrin molecule is available to link each spectrin tetramer to the membrane. Moreover, the binding interactions are cooperative. Attachment of ankyrin to band 3 greatly facilitates the ability of the molecule to organize the spectrin to which it is attached into tetramers. Conversely, spectrin binding enhances the affinity for protein 3. Ankyrin thus functions both as an attachment point for the spectrin-actin latticework and, with band 3, as a nidus for organization of the lattice itself. The importance of these functions to red cell integrity is illustrated by naturally occurring deficiency states in the mouse (the normoblastosis or *nb/nb* mouse)[194] and humans with ankyrin-associated hereditary spherocytosis (see below).

The p55 Protein. p55 has recently been recognized as an important component of the red cell cytoskeleton.[162] Originally discovered as a subband in the protein 4.9 region on Fairbanks gels, p55 is a 55 kDa membrane-associated phosphoprotein. It is related to a family of MAGUK homologues that also include one or more "PDZ" domains, and an SH3 domain embedded in the MAGUK domain. The homologues of p55 include signal transduction proteins (e.g., LIN-2 in *C. elegans*) tumor suppressor gene products such as the *Drosophila* large disc protein that interacts with the protein 4.1 analogue, coracle, and proteins vital for cell-cell interactions, such as ZO-1 and ZO-2.

P55 binds to the 30 kDa protein 4.1 through a 39 amino acid binding motif embedded in the carboxyl-terminal MAGUK domain, and to the cytoplasmic tail of glycophorin C by means of its single PDZ motif.[93] Deficiencies of either glycophorin or protein 4.1R cause concomitant deficiency of p55 in the cytoskeleton. A primary deficiency state for p55 has not been delineated, possibly because p55 is widely expressed and found in critical interactions with brain proteins, cell-cell junctions, etc. Even though the its actual role in erythrocyte membrane function is still not clear, p55 is clearly intriguing because its obligate association with protein 4.1 and glycophorin. Its relationship to signal transduction and tumor suppressor proteins offer new mechanisms whereby the cytoskeleton might influence cellular metabolism.

Protein 4.2. Protein 4.2, 72 kDa, is present at about 200,000 copies per erythrocyte.[1] It is encoded by a gene located on chromosome 15q15-q2l and gives rise to a principal isoform, protein 4.2 "long" (p4.2L), and a minor short isoform (p4.2S) by alternative mRNA splicing.[198-200] Its amino acid sequence places it, surprisingly, in a protein family including factor XIII and guinea pig transglutaminase. Protein 4.2 shows strong conservation with many transglutaminase genes. However, it cannot catalyze cross-linking of proteins like other transglutaminases because there is an alanine, instead of the essential cysteine, in its potential active site.[201]

Protein 4.2 binds to several proteins, including band 3, protein 4.1, ankyrin, and ankyrin-protein 3 complexes.[202, 203] The major function of protein 4.2 is probably to stabilize the spectrin-actin-ankyrin association with band 3.[204] It has also been proposed that protein 4.2 protects the cytoskeleton from premature aging by binding calcium and other cofactors that normally activate red cell transglutaminases. Since these transglutaminases would otherwise cross-link proteins, possibly leading to their inactivation in an age dependent manner, protein 4.2 has been postulated to act as a false agonist. Protein 4.2, which has multiple isoforms, is expressed late in erythropoiesis.[205] As discussed later, the importance of protein 4.2 to cytoskeletal integrity is supported by the existence of hereditary hemolytic anemias due to deficiency states. Protein 4.2 and dematin (see below) share an 11 amino acid ATP binding motif of unknown significance.[206]

Adducin. This calcium/calmodulin binding phosphoprotein composed of αβ adducin heterodimers is located at spectrin-actin junctions in erythrocytes.[1, 7, 12] α and β adducin are structurally similar but they are encoded by separate genes. Adducin contains a "MARCKS" phosphorylation domain that seems to regulate at least one defined biochemical function, calcium/calmodulin regulated capping and bundling of actin filaments.[207-209] Adducin enhances spectrin-actin via beta spectrin binding; it also binds to actin and bundles actin filaments.[210-212]

Adducin is expressed early in erythroid differentiation and is present at about 30,000 copies per cell. The mechanism and extent of its contribution to red cell membrane function are not yet clear. However, mice with targeted inactivation of β adducin suffer from compensated spherocytic anemia and neurologic abnormalities,[213] suggesting a previously unassigned role for these proteins in disease pathogenesis.

Other Proteins That Associate With Spectrin-Actin Complexes. Dematin (protein 4.9), tropomyosin, proteins related to troponin, and other proteins known to be associated with actin in nonerythroid cells are found in variable amounts in red cells. The functional role of these proteins are now being defined, as is their potential relevance to hereditary anemias. For example, dematin declines in amount during erythroid maturation; it may be more important for red cell development than for life in the circulation.

Biogenesis and Assembly of the Membrane During Red Cell Development

A great deal of information has been gathered about red cell membrane biogenesis, but no clear picture of the sequence of steps involved has emerged. Several issues have confounded mechanistic analysis. First, it has been difficult to obtain synchronized erythroid precursors representing each stage of erythropoiesis from BFUE/CFUE through reticulocytes in sufficient amounts and purity. Second, knowledge of the diversity of protein isoforms and isoform switching occurring during erythropoiesis is still emerging. The presence of multiple alternatively spliced or translated isoforms complicates interpretation of earlier studies of the erythrocyte membrane biogenesis; these studies detected only entire proteins, or mRNA transcripts, which are actually composites of several isoforms increasing or decreasing in amount during various stages of erythropoiesis. Third, reliance on inducible transformed cell lines, such as the mouse erythroleukemia cell (MEL-C), as an alternative source of pure synchronized cells has been compromised by the fact that these lines appear to support an imperfect and incomplete mode of membrane development during erythroblast maturation. Despite these limitations, some features of red cell membrane biogenesis are beginning to emerge. Most of this information has been gathered by use of murine or avian cells obtained during early embryonic or fetal life, when partial synchronization can be achieved by purifying cells from yolk sac or fetal liver as a function of time after gestation or by the use of cells undergoing stress erythropoiesis in response to a pharmacological or hormonal (erythropoietin) manipulation.

Only a few studies have attempted to provide point-by-point temporal correlations of mRNA levels, protein biosynthetic rates, steady-state accumulation of protein in the cell, and stable quantitative incorporation of the protein products into the membrane. When those correlative measurements have been made, mRNA and protein biosynthetic levels have correlated well.[214] Therefore, the discussion that follows refers to mRNA and protein biosynthetic levels interchangeably. In contrast, the primary rates of protein biosynthesis often do not correlate well with stable incorporation into the membrane.[214] One consistent principle of membrane protein biosynthesis appears to be that some proteins are synthesized in excess of the others. The proteins synthesized in lesser amounts thus become rate limiting for the assembly of macromolecular complexes. The unused excess amounts of the proteins synthesized in higher initial abundance tend to be catabolized.

Only small pools of unincorporated membrane proteins exist, particularly during the later stages of erythropoiesis. This feature has great implications for the molecular pathogenesis of hereditary membrane defects. Clearly, a mutation diminishing production of a rate limiting protein will have far more profound functional effects than a mutation diminishing production of a protein produced in relative excess. Similarly, co-inheritance of an allele with altered function and an allele with diminished output will accentuate the impact of the allele with altered function on membrane formation. These considerations complicate the interpretation of the phenotypes of individuals with compound heterozygous states for mutant alleles of the same gene.

Membrane protein biosynthesis occurs asynchronously during erythropoiesis. There is no evidence to support the idea of a coordinate simultaneous induction of the genes encoding the red cell membrane proteins.[215–221] Rather, biosynthesis of different components peaks at different stages of erythropoiesis. Those components expressed in the earlier stages could direct assembly of the cytoskeleton as additional components are produced in the later stages. In some cases, modification of the multiple mRNA products of a single gene proceeds in temporally separated stages. In the case of protein 4.1 gene expression, the mRNA splicing event that excludes the upstream translation start codon (used for biosynthesis of high molecular weight forms in nonerythroid cells) occurs at very early stages, probably well before the proerythroblast stage. In contrast, the splicing event that leads to inclusion of the 63 nucleotide exon 16 encoding the erythroid spectrin-actin-binding domain does not occur until the mid to late stages of erythroblast maturation (see above).

Early studies in avian erythroblasts, corroborated in part by studies of murine and human cells, provided evidence for the notion that the early steps of red cell membrane assembly are directed by production of the erythroid form of protein3.[216, 218] Band 3, once inserted into the membrane, directs the assembly of stable macromolecular complexes from presynthesized pools of the other proteins. There are also complicated switches in the predominance of the 9.0 kb and 7.0 kb mRNA transcripts arising from the ankyrin gene in mice and humans.[222] Although both transcripts are found at all stages of erythropoiesis, the 9.0 kb transcript predominates in early cells, the 7.5 kb transcript is more abundant in later cells. Ankyrin also appears to be synthesized at relatively high levels during early stages of erythropoiesis, suggesting that it, too, is an important element for assembly by virtue of its direct interaction with band 3.[216, 218]

This view has been challenged by two observations that demonstrate the need for more detailed analysis of membrane biogenesis in nontransformed erythroblasts from wild type and knock-out models. First, the abrupt organization of preformed pools of cytoskeletal elements induced by the induction of band 3 synthesis is not seen in nontransformed cells. Second, band 3 knock-out mice exhibit normal membrane biogenesis even though their red cell membranes are unstable in the circulation.[58, 59]

The biosynthesis and assembly of spectrin subunits is complex. β spectrin biosynthesis exceeds that of α spectrin in the early erythroblasts derived from both embryonic (yolk sac) and fetal/adult (liver/spleen) origins. This ratio is preserved during later stages of erythropoiesis in embryonic cells, but not in fetal/adult-derived late erythroblasts and reticulocytes. In these latter cells, α-spectrin gene expression increases, whereas β-spectrin gene expression remains constant, resulting in a predominance of α mRNA and protein during the late stages, when active assembly of the actual membrane is occurring most rapidly. To some degree, these changing ratios may reflect differential sensitivity to erythropoietin or other stimulants of stress erythropoiesis; β-spectrin gene expression has been shown to increase selectively in erythropoietin-stimulated Friend leukemia virus-infected spleen cells, induced MEL-C, and human ankyrin-deficient erythroblasts. α-spectrin gene expression predominates in late human erythroid precursors.

The feature of spectrin biosynthesis relevant to the analysis of hereditary hemolytic anemias is that spectrin subunits are incorporated into the membrane in a 1:1 stoichiometric ratio, regardless of their primary rates of biosynthesis on polyribosomes.[221-223] Chains not incorporated must be unstable, since large pools do not accumulate. Human α spectrin synthesis exceeds that of β spectrin by a factor of nearly 2:1 during the later stages of erythropoiesis, when, presumably, membrane assembly is proceeding rapidly. The availability of β spectrin subunits thus determines the maximum rate and amount of stable spectrin assembly. Therefore, mutations reducing steady-state levels of newly synthesized β spectrin should have a far greater phenotypic impact than do mutations causing comparable decreases in α spectrin biosynthesis. Analyses of patients with hereditary hemolytic anemias support this prediction.[7]

Considerable remodeling and maturation of the red cell membrane occurs after enucleation of late erythroblasts. Some biosynthesis of spectrin, protein 3, protein 4.1 and glycophorin C continues in the newly enucleated reticulocyte, but most membrane remodeling occurs posttranslationally. The reticulocyte is multi-lobular and motile; it possesses mitochondria, polyribosomes, and numerous membrane proteins that are either absent or much less abundant in mature red cells. In addition, phospholipid composition and inside-outside lipid distribution are different. Reticulocytes are far less deformable and considerably more unstable mechanically than are mature erythrocytes. Maturation begins in the bone marrow and lasts for 2 or 3 days. It is completed in the circulation and perhaps in the spleen (splenic polishing). Reticulocytes first become cup shaped before acquiring their final biconcave disc shape. This process involves major reorganization of both membrane phospholipids and cytoskeletal and embedded proteins, as well as the loss of lipids and numerous proteins, including transferrin receptors, insulin receptors, and fibronectin receptors. At the end of this process, deformability is close to that of the mature red cell.

The differences between the membranes of reticulocytes and mature erythrocytes are relevant to studies of membrane abnormalities in various forms of anemia, such as sickle cell anemia. Clearly, an elevated reticulocyte count will confound analysis of changes, such as the altered lipid asymmetry or adherence properties of red cells in sickle cell anemia. Distinguishing perturbations attributable to the effect of the primary abnormality (e.g., sickling of hemoglobin S), from effects due to the altered distribution of red cell ages in such patients presents a formidable challenge.

Understanding of membrane protein gene regulation during erythropoiesis will require reexamination in the light of new knowledge concerning tissue- and differentiation-specific isoforms, as well as the role of alternative mRNA splicing in generating these isoforms. The primary rates of production of these proteins are probably not major determinants. Rather, posttranslational events, including stabilization of newly synthesized proteins by assembly processes, may be the key regulatory foci. These considerations greatly complicate attempts to relate mutations of membrane proteins to particular clinical syndromes. A single mutation can have pleiotropic effects on synthesis, assembly, remodeling, and/or biochemical function in the mature cell. The fact that particular morphological abnormalities, degrees of clinical severity, and patterns of inheritance in particular kindreds do not always correlate in a straightforward way with the nature or location of a particular mutation is more understandable in view of these complexities.

Disorders of the Red Cell Membrane Lipids

Inherited and acquired abnormalities of the red cell membrane manifest as morphological abnormalities accompanied by shortened red cell life spans and hemolytic anemias of varying degree. Only a few are severe enough to require therapeutic intervention. Most of the acquired abnormalities are in fact important primarily as stigmata of non-hematologic diseases or of disease progression in other organ systems. We first focus on a very brief survey of disorders attributable to abnormal membrane lipids and then devote more detailed attention to disorders of the membrane proteins, about which far more molecular information is available. (Note: The material in this section is reviewed in references 1, 7, and 33).

▼ TARGET CELLS

Target cells result from an increase in surface-to-volume ratio, due either to increased membrane surface areas or to decreased intracellular volume. The latter occurs when cells are poorly hemoglobinized, in part because the negative charge of hemoglobin tends to draw sodium and, thereby, water into cells. Thus, microcytic target cells are encountered with variable frequency in iron deficiency and the thalassemia syndromes. Hemoglobin C, which crystallizes in red cells and thus lowers its effective intracellular concentration, is also characterized by the presence of target cells.

An increase in the membrane surface area is most commonly the result of a net increase in erythrocyte membrane lipids seen in patients with liver disease and intrahepatic cholestasis. Net uptake of free plasma cholesterol and phospholipids by the membrane is increased because the cholesterol/phospholipid/protein ratios of low density lipoproteins are abnormal in these conditions, resulting in redistribution. Target cells in these patients have an increased surface area with normal or only slightly increased cell volumes.

Target cells are also encountered in a rare autosomal recessive condition called lecithin cholesterol acyltransferase (LCAT) deficiency. LCAT deficiency is characterized by hyperlipidemia, premature atherosclerosis, corneal opacities, chronic nephritis, proteinuria and anemia (reviewed in 224). The normal function of LCAT is to transfer fatty acids from phosphatidylcholine to cholesterol. LCAT is normally complexed to high density lipoproteins in the plasma. Deficient patients have increased cholesterol and phospholipid content in their membranes and large numbers of target cells on the peripheral smear. There is mild anemia due to a mildly shortened RBC lifespan and ineffective erythropoiesis. Bone marrow aspiration and biopsy reveals characteristic sea blue histiocytes and abnormal marrow storage cells. The most severe consequence of LCAT deficiency is premature atherosclerosis. Target cells and the mild anemia are useful diagnostic manifestations.

▼ ACANTHOCYTOSIS AND SPUR CELL ANEMIA

Acanthocytes, so named because of the thorn-like projections of the membrane protruding from the body of the red cell, arise from several conditions, many of which are associated with abnormal membrane lipid composition and altered distribution of lipids between the outer and inner leaflets of the bilayer. These include severe liver disease, abetalipoproteinemia, and the chorea-acanthocytosis syndrome. Acanthocytes also appear to be associated with the inheritance of certain polymorphisms of red cell antigens, such as the McLeod blood group. The molecular pathophysiology of acanthocytosis has been most thoroughly examined in the acquired condition of severe end-stage liver disease. Only a small percentage of patients with liver disease acquire the syndrome of spur cell hemolytic anemia, but the prevalence of liver disease is so high that these individuals account for the majority of cases of acanthocytosis encountered clinically.

Acanthocytes, like target cells, result from increased acquisition of free cholesterol from the plasma due to abnormal cholesterol/lipoprotein ratios. In severe liver disease, an extraordinarily high ratio of free cholesterol to phospholipids is found in lipoproteins; the free cholesterol readily partitions into the membrane, where it preferentially associates with the outer leaflet. The outer leaflet becomes less fluid; attempts to remodel the membrane are made by the spleen, producing rigid spherical cells possessing the characteristic spiculated projections. On subsequent passes through the spleen, these poorly deformable cells have difficulty negotiating the narrow sinusoids of the splenic circulation and are hemolyzed.

Spur cell anemia is an ominous clinical marker of the terminal stages of liver disease. It is primarily important as a sign of worsening liver function; the anemia itself is not usually a major clinical problem, but it can aggravate preexisting anemias (e.g., due to gastrointestinal bleeding) to the point that transfusion therapy is needed. Prior to the availability of liver transplantation, patients reaching this stage rarely lived for more than a few weeks. Spur cell anemia is sometimes confused with Zieve's syndrome, a transient, relatively mild spherocytic hemolytic anemia that occurs during acute fatty metamorphosis accompanied by hyperglycemia. The molecular basis of this membrane abnormality remains unknown.

Numerous conditions are also associated with cells having *regular* projections from the red cell membrane, called echinocytes, or burr cells. These include malnutrition and renal disease. Essentially nothing is known about the molecular basis of burr cell formation. ATP depletion, abnormal calcium loading, and the binding of certain drugs have all been implicated. Like acanthocytes, burr cells seem to result from asymmetry in the lipid content of the outer and inner leaflets of the membrane. In experimental models, overloading of the outer leaflet results in spiculated cells, like acanthocytes and echinocytes, whereas overloading of the inner leaflet results in stomatocytic cells.

▼ ABETALIPOPROTEINEMIA

Abetalipoproteinemia (Bassen-Kornzweig syndrome) is an autosomal recessive disorder characterized by the complete absence of apolipoprotein B (reviewed in 225). Affected patients have mild anemia with dramatic acanthocytosis, retinitis pigmentosa, progressive ataxic neurologic disease, celiac syndrome and other multisystem defects. Abetalipoproteinemia is caused by failure to synthesize or secrete products of the apolipoprotein B gene into the plasma.

Acanthocytes in abetalipoproteinemia are characterized by overloading of the outer leaflet with sphingomyelin. Indeed, the discoid shape can be restored by mild extraction of lipids from the outer leaflet or by incubation of red cells with chlorpromazine, which binds to the inner leaflet, restoring the balance of inner and outer leaflet mass. These acanthocytes are not as rigid as in liver disease; consequently, the hemolytic diathesis is not as severe.

Less impressive degrees of acanthocytosis are seen in the related syndrome hypobetalipoproteinemia and in the chorea-acanthocytosis syndrome, an autosomal recessive disorder characterized primarily by neurological movement disorders and high levels of unsaturated fatty acids in the red cell membrane, but no anemia.

Disorders of Red Cell Cytoskeletal Proteins

Clinically relevant derangements of the red cell membrane proteins include the following: (1) hereditary hemolytic anemias due to genetic defects of these proteins; (2) acquired abnormalities of membrane proteins due to derangement of other red cell components, especially abnormal hemoglobins or hemoglobin-derived products; (3) alterations in membrane proteins, notably band 3, that occur with advancing red cell age and lead to eventual sequestration and destruction; and (4) incompletely understood hemolytic states associated with abnormal membrane antigens. The final common pathway characterizing these disorders appears to be altered amounts or function, or both, of cytoskeletal proteins, leading to reduced deformability or reduced mechanical stability, or both. The focus of this discussion is on the genetic defects and the molecular basis of the pathophysiology of the disorders. For detailed discussion of natural history, clinical diagnosis, management, and genetic counseling, the reader is referred to several recent reviews.[7, 226–228] To conserve space, individual literature citations are not provided for the well-established clinical principles outlined in this section. The reader is referred to the aforementioned references for access to this vast literature.

▼ INHERITED DEFECTS OF THE RED CELL CYTOSKELETON

Inherited red cell abnormalities attributable to primary genetic defects in red cell membrane proteins were originally classified by their morphological presentation. They include hereditary spherocytosis (HS), hereditary elliptocytosis (HE), hereditary pyropoikilocytosis (HPP), and southeast Asian ovalocytosis (SAO). Less common conditions, such as hereditary xerocytosis and hereditary stomatocytosis, are also thought to arise from red cell membrane protein abnormalities, but their etiology is less clear. We shall focus on the better characterized disorders: HS, HE, HPP, and SAO.

Each of the inherited disorders of red cell membrane proteins is extremely heterogeneous, both clinically and in terms of the primary molecular defect. There is also considerable overlap, both morphologically and genetically. For example, in some patients with HPP, elliptocytes are common. In some kindreds only HE is encountered, whereas in others both HE and HPP are found in different family members. These facts, coupled with rapidly expanding knowledge of the structure, function, biogenesis, and molecular pathology of the membrane proteins, make a simple classification of these disorders difficult. One cannot correlate a particular abnormality, such as HS, strictly with a particular pattern of inheritance or membrane protein defect. For example, spectrin mutations can participate in the pathogenesis of HE, HPP, and HS. Conversely, HS can arise from defects in spectrin, protein 4.2, ankyrin, or protein 3. Therefore, the discussion that follows attempts to organize knowledge about these disorders in two tiers. First, we consider the traditional nosology of HS, HE, HPP, and SAO. Second, molecular defects of the individual membrane proteins and the diverse disorders produced by these mutations are surveyed.

Hereditary Spherocytosis (HS)

Hereditary spherocytosis is characterized by the predominance of spherocytic erythrocytes on the peripheral smear. The most common form is an autosomal dominant hemolytic

anemia of variable severity. Autosomal recessive forms, which are usually quite severe in their clinical presentation, and very mild forms that present late in life are also common. HS occurs sporadically in all ethnic groups but tends to be more frequent in the Western world, notably in northern Europeans. However, this apparent preponderance may reflect observer bias because cases may go unnoticed or undiagnosed.

Pathogenesis. The common feature of HS red cells is a marked decrease in surface area due to reduced amounts of all lipid components of the membrane (Fig. 8–12). Loss of redundant surface area makes these cells less capable of distention in hypoosmolar solutions, leading to increased susceptibility to rupture (osmotic fragility). This phenomenon is the basis for a clinical test in which the ability of normal red cells and the ability of test red cells to resist lysis under conditions of progressively decreasing tonicity are compared (osmotic fragility test). The osmotic fragility test is regarded as a standard maneuver during the diagnostic evaluation of hereditary hemolytic anemias.

Red cells in HS are also less deformable because of the loss of the redundant surface area needed for the flexible disc shape. They tend to become entrapped in the fenestrations in the wall of splenic sinuses. This leads to engorgement of the spleen and an increased time of residency in contact with splenic macrophages. Further damage and loss of membrane and increased osmotic fragility occur. Damage occurs cumulatively, resulting in eventual premature sequestration and destruction by macrophages in the spleen, liver, or perhaps other tissues; hemolytic anemia results.

Most HS red cells exhibit quantitative reductions of 20–50% in spectrin content. Spectrin deficiency is a hallmark of HS cells; this defect probably accounts for the reduced surface area of the overlying membrane (see Fig. 8–12). Even in normal red cells, the lipid bilayer fragments or sheds

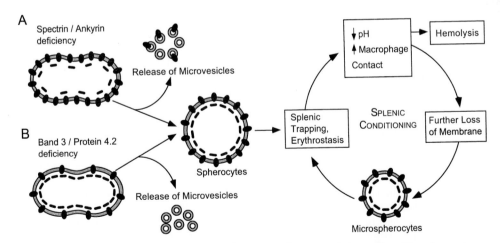

Figure 8–12. Pathobiology of the erythrocyte lesion in hereditary spherocytosis. The principal abnormality of hereditary spherocytes is the deficiency of membrane surface area, leading to microspherocytosis. Three distinct pathways produce surface area deficiency. A partial deficiency of spectrin, resulting either from a primary defect of spectrin or a primary defect of ankyrin, leads to a reduced density of the skeletal monolayer. As a result, the lipid bilayer is destabilized, as manifested by a release of membrane lipids in the form of microvesicles. The second pathway involves a primary defect of band 3, which leads to band 3 protein deficiency and, consequently, a decrease in the number of band 3-containing intramembrane particles. As a result, particle-free lipid regions are formed that subsequently bleb off in the form of microvesicles. In the third pathway, a primary defect of band 3 protein (or possibly of ankyrin) leads to a loss from the cells of band 3 together with lipids that surround this protein (boundary lipids). Each of the three pathways ultimately results in the loss of membrane material and, hence, in surface area deficiency. The resulting decrease in whole red cell deformability predisposes red cells to splenic entrapment. Subsequent splenic conditioning of hereditary spherocytes inflicts additional damage, thereby amplifying the vicious circle of red cell injury. (From Gallagher, P.G., and Jarolim, P.: Disorders of the erythrocyte membrane. *In* Hoffman, R., Benz, E. J., Jr., Shattil, S., Furie, B., and Cohen, H. [eds.]: Hematology: Basic Principles and Practice. New York, Churchill Livingstone, 1999, In press; with permission.)

microvesicles when subjected to severe shear stress, leading to loss of surface area. This tendency is counteracted by the dense hexagonal network of spectrin filaments attached to the membrane. Spectrin deficiency leads to a decrease in the amount of lipids that are anchored and stabilized by this mechanism. Thus in response to the normal mechanical and biochemical stresses of the circulation, microvesiculation and fragmentation occur. Mechanical fragility can be demonstrated by ektacytometry;[33] susceptibility to biochemically induced fragmentation can be induced by allowing red cells to incubate in the absence of glucose, which leads to ATP depletion, membrane fragmentation, and, ultimately, hemolysis.[226] HS cells are far more susceptible to hemolysis under these conditions than are normal cells. This phenomenon formed the basis for the autohemolysis test, which is rarely used today because other defects can mimic the results seen with HS cells. Micro-vesicles released as the result of these stresses contain integral membrane proteins, but no cytoskeletal proteins, suggesting that they do indeed result from a failure to be anchored to the cytoskeleton.

Many secondary abnormalities of red cell membrane function have been described, including increased sodium influx, associated with a paradoxical *dehydration*, possibly due to secondary over-activity of the $Na^+K^+ATPase$.[97, 228, 229] Since the sodium pump extrudes three sodium ions for every two potassium ions entering the cell, the net effect of uncompensated over-activity is net loss of cations and cellular dehydration. Protein 4.2-deficient HS erythrocytes exhibit increased anion transport, whereas HS erythrocytes deficient in spectrin, ankyrin, or band 3 have normal or decreased anion transport.[229]

Clinical Manifestations. The clinical manifestations of HS are extremely variable. The most common form is inherited as an autosomal dominant disorder associated with minimal, mild, or moderate hemolysis. Anemia is rarely severe and the blood count is often normal due to compensatory marrow erythropoiesis. In the mildest cases, spherocytes are seen on the peripheral smear, but hemolytic stigmata (anemia, reticulocytosis, hepatosplenomegaly, jaundice due to hyperbilirubinemia, bilirubin gallstones leading to premature gallbladder disease, or leg ulcers) are minimal. Patients with moderate HS have reticulocytosis and/or anemia. Occasionally, these patients present in adult life with secondary complications of chronic hemolysis, such as biliary tract disease, acute onset of anemia due to failure of compensatory erythroid hyperplasia (aplastic or hypoplastic crises caused by suppression of erythropoiesis by viral infections, cytotoxic drugs, etc.), or superimposition of a second hemolytic diathesis, such as conditions predisposing to hypersplenism. It is the exceptional patient, often one with the rare autosomal recessive or compound heterozygous forms of the disease, who exhibits a lifetime of severe chronic hemolytic anemia with all of the associated stigmata. These patients may develop leg ulcers, dermatitis and paravertebral masses due to extramedullary erythropoiesis. A number of cases of hematologic malignancy, including myeloproliferative disorders and leukemia, developing late in life in moderate to severe HS patients have been described. It is unknown if long-term hematopoietic stress predisposes to the development of these disorders.

In most HS cases, the clinical manifestations are confined to the erythroid lineage. However, in some HS kindreds, cosegregating neurologic or muscular abnormalities have been described. Ankyrin and β spectrin are not only expressed in red cells but also in muscle, brain, and spinal cord, raising the possibility that a defect of these proteins may be responsible for both abnormalities. Studies of a mouse model of HS, ankyrin-deficient *nb/nb* mice, develop a neurologic syndrome that coincides with the degeneration of Purkinjie cells in the cerebellum.[194] Two kindreds with cosegregating HS, renal acidification defects, and RNA processing mutations of the band 3 gene have been described.[230, 231] In an ever growing number of patients with distal renal tubular acidosis *without HS*, missense mutations of band 3 have been found.[232–235] The precise pathogenesis of the renal tubular acidosis in these cases is unknown, but it is thought to relate to the function of band 3 isoforms in the kidney.

Inheritance. The patterns of inheritance of HS are complex.[7, 226, 227] In most HS patients, inheritance is autosomal dominant and the defect resides in the gene for ankyrin, β spectrin or band 3. In approximately one quarter of kindreds, inheritance is autosomal recessive. In these cases, the defect is in the gene for α spectrin or protein 4.2. Homozygosity for the typical autosomal dominant form of HS is rare and may be lethal or associated with severe, transfusion-dependent anemia.

HS patients with varying degrees of clinical symptomatology may coexist within the same kindred. This is due to coexistence in the same kindred of: heterozygosity for silent, mild, or more severe alleles; homozygosity for alleles that may be clinically silent in the simple heterozygous state; or compound heterozygosity for mild (silent carrier) and more severe alleles. Other explanations for variations in clinical severity include variable penetrance of the genetic defect, the presence of modifier alleles that influence the expression of a membrane protein, or tissue-specific mosaicism of the defect. Interestingly, molecular studies of HS have demonstrated that there is an unusually high occurrence of spontaneous mutations in the genes responsible for HS (see below)

As discussed later in more detail, HS can arise from mutations in the genes for ankyrin, α spectrin, β spectrin, protein 4.2, and band 3.[226, 227, 236, 237] In all cases, the biochemical abnormalities arising from these mutations lead, as a final common pathway, to instability of the association of the cytoskeleton with the lipid bilayer. Membrane cytoskeletal proteins, including spectrin, that are not stabilized by this association tend to be catabolized. Instability of membrane association thus leads to a net spectrin deficiency. Quantitative measurements of membrane-associated spectrin can be a useful adjunct to diagnosis.

Although spectrin deficiency is a hallmark of HS, it is not a finding exclusively associated with HS. Spectrin deficiency can also occur as part of the pathogenesis of acquired membrane defects resulting from oxidation of the cytoskeleton by hemichromes or binding to certain structurally abnormal hemoglobins or free globin chains.

Diagnosis. Clinical diagnosis of HS is usually based on the characteristic spherocytic appearance of the red cells. In contrast to many other conditions accompanied by the presence of spherocytes, such as immune hemolytic anemia and hypersplenism, the peripheral blood smear of most HS patients shows a relatively uniform population of spherocytes. The mean corpuscular hemoglobin concentration

(MCHC) value is usually increased in HS patients, reflecting the secondary defects that generate dehydrated red cells. These changes are far less dramatic in other conditions associated with spherocytosis. Histogram analysis of MCHC as determined by the Technicon H1 counter and its successors (Tarrytown, NY) has been claimed to identify nearly all HS patients.[238] Additional morphologic features have been correlated with the underlying molecular defect in some HS patients. Band 3 deficient patients have been described to have pincered erythrocytes on peripheral blood smear, while patients with β spectrin defects have been associated with spiculated or acanthocytic spherocytes. The Japanese patients with protein 4.2-deficient HS have been described to have sphero-ovalocytes and sphero-stomatocytes on their peripheral blood films.

Osmotic fragility testing remains the gold standard in the diagnosis of HS. Subtle but useful and reproducible differences in measurements of osmotic fragility may be helpful in diagnosis of difficult cases. Other tests, such as the autohemolysis test, the glycerol lysis test, etc., suffer from lack of sensitivity, specificity, or both.

Therapy. Most patients with HS require no therapeutic intervention besides folate supplementation and careful observation for development of complications such as aplastic crises and biliary tract disease. In cases where splenectomy is warranted, the response to splenectomy is generally good, leading to amelioration or elimination of the anemia. Hemolysis may persist in more severe forms of the disease, particularly in the autosomal recessive form. In the most severe forms of the disease, individuals may require prolonged transfusion support.

Hereditary Elliptocytosis and Hereditary Pyropoikilocytosis

Hereditary elliptocytosis and hereditary pyropoikilocytosis are distinct but interrelated disorders often found within a single kindred. The morphological hallmark of HE is the predominance of elliptical or cigar-shaped red cells on the peripheral blood smear. In HPP, red cell morphology is extremely bizarre, consisting of fragmented red cells, spiculated cells, microspherocytes, and elliptocytes. HE and HPP erythrocytes may be thermally unstable, acquiring bizarre morphology and undergoing fragmentation at lower temperatures than normal cells. HPP tends to be inherited in a complex fashion, often in kindreds with HE, and is usually associated with significant clinical hemolytic anemia. In contrast, HE is extremely variable in terms of clinical severity and inheritance, although it is typically asymptomatic and inherited in a dominant fashion. HE erythrocytes exhibit resistance to malarial invasion, a fact that may account for the somewhat higher frequency of HE in equatorial African populations.

Pathogenesis. The molecular basis of HE is heterogeneous. Several major categories have been identified: spectrin defects involving abnormal self-association of spectrin heterodimers to tetramers; defects resulting in abnormal binding of spectrin to protein 4.1 or ankyrin; deficiencies or abnormal functions of protein 4.1; or deficiency of glycophorin C.

The common feature uniting these diverse defects is that each weakens the formation of the junctional complexes important for structural integrity of the spectrin latticework. Thus, the spectrin abnormalities underlying HE tend to be those disrupting spectrin self-association or β spectrin mutations affecting binding to protein 4.1. Glycophorin C deficiency leads to secondary protein 4.1 deficiency, which, like defects of protein 4.1 itself, removes the essential component necessary for forming the spectrin/actin/protein 4.1/protein 4.2/p55 junctional complex. Protein 4.2 and p55 defects are predicted to have the same impact. Thus, defects of spectrin self-association or spectrin association with other components of the junctional complex are the molecular hallmarks of these disorders, resulting in spectrin deficiencies, producing fragile, nondeformable, physically unstable membranes. In HE, the quantity of spectrin in the latticework appears to be nearly normal. Qualitative defects disrupt the junctional complexes. The net effect is a membrane that is less tolerant of shear stress. These membranes are more susceptible to permanent plastic deformation in the circulation because of the loss of resiliency. This may be the reason that they acquire the elliptocytic shape, although the molecular basis for acquisition of this shape remains unknown.

Hereditary pyropoikilocytosis appears, in those cases that have been studied, to represent a compound heterozygous state in which clinical manifestations are more severe because there is coinheritance of a mutation that results in qualitative deficiency of normal spectrin and a mutation that leads to spectrin deficiency. Cells from these patients exhibit features of both decreased deformability and resiliency as well as increased membrane fragmentation, resulting in a syndrome with morphology different from that of either HE or HS. In this regard, it is interesting to note that some of the more severe forms of HE are associated with poikilocytosis. The thermal instability that is highly characteristic of HPP can also be encountered in some HE patients carrying a similar spectrin mutation.

The exact pathophysiology responsible for the formation of elliptocytes and poikilocytes in HE and HPP is not yet clear. Bone marrow precursor cells have normal morphology, suggesting that the shapes are acquired in the circulation. The elliptical shapes of HE cells are retained by the membrane skeleton and membrane ghosts after detergent extraction in vitro, a situation similar to that observed when normal red cells are subjected to enough mechanical stress to induce plastic deformation. The weakened complexes thought to arise from mutations producing HE may lead to this plastic deformation under normal shear stress. Poikilocytes occur in patients with severely defective spectrin self-association. The spectrin latticework in these patients is disrupted by fixation into an extended state by mild to moderate shear stress. Indeed, HPP might represent the biochemically extreme form of defective self-association present in moderately severe forms of HE. The disruption of the latticework adds the element of mechanical instability to that of lost resiliency.

Clinical Manifestations. Typical HE is usually either asymptomatic or associated with a very mild hemolytic anemia. Superimposition of other hemolytic diatheses, such as disseminated intravascular coagulation (DIC), can result in sporadic periods of more severe hemolytic anemia. Occasionally, neonates with HE have been found to exhibit poikilocytosis, hemolysis, and anemia in the first few months of life. These symptoms tend to resolve during the first postnatal year as fetal hemoglobin in the circulation is replaced by adult hemoglobin.[239] This phenotypic switch results from the fact that fetal hemoglobin binds 2,3-diphosphoglycerate (2,3-DPG) much more poorly than adult hemoglobin. 2,3-DPG, like other phosphorylated compounds, tends to weaken the formation of junctional complexes. The higher free 2,3-DPG levels in cells with high hemoglobin F content accentuate the defective behavior of the mutant spectrin.

Inheritance. HE is usually inherited as an autosomal dominant trait. Homozygosity or compound heterozygosity for spectrin or protein 4.1 mutations produce variable degrees of hemolysis, depending on the severity of the functional defect encoded by the mutation. At the extreme end, these patients resemble those with HPP as much as those with severe HE, because of the appearance of substantial numbers of poikilocytes and microspherocytes on peripheral blood smear. One unusual kindred with X-linked HE, Alport syndrome, and mental retardation associated with a deletion of the X chromosome has been reported.[240]

As noted above, HPP often results from co-inheritance of a mutation that impairs spectrin self-association and a mutation that causes a quantitative deficiency of spectrin. Parents of the propositus have HE or are asymptomatic. In some families, the self-association mutant is coinherited with an apparent thalassemia-like allele that results in quantitative spectrin deficiency. In others, the second allele carries a mutation that results in spectrin instability. The net effect is to combine quantitative deficiency of normal spectrin with dysfunction of the small amount of spectrin that is incorporated. The characteristic poikilocytosis and thermal instability of cells at 49°C are observed.

Diagnosis and Therapy. Diagnosis is usually appreciated by the presence of abnormal morphology on the blood film, anemia, or, in severe cases, stigmata of both anemia and chronic hemolysis. In typical HE, the erythrocyte indices and osmotic fragility are normal. In HPP, the combination of a characteristic blood smear, microcytosis and an abnormal incubated osmotic fragility are diagnostic. Because elliptocytes and poikilocytes, like spherocytes, tend to be sequestered in the spleen, splenectomy can relieve symptoms in severe cases. Rare forms of HE in which there are also defects in erythropoiesis (ineffective erythropoiesis) and mild to moderate defects in platelet function have been reported. Otherwise, to date, no involvement of nonerythroid tissues has been reported in patients with these red cell disorders.

Hereditary Ovalocytosis

Two major subtypes of hereditary ovalocytosis have been defined. The first, also called *spherocytic HE,* is characterized by clear evidence of hemolytic anemia accompanied by a blood film showing somewhat rounded elliptical cells, but no poikilocytes or fragmented forms. Osmotic fragility is increased into the range found in patients with HS. In one case, complete protein 4.1 deficiency was detected. In others, mutations of β spectrin in the region of spectrin self-association have been identified. The other major subtype of hereditary ovalocytosis is southeast Asian ovalocytosis.

Southeast Asian Ovalocytosis (SAO) is characterized by erythrocytes with a distinctive oval cup shape reminiscent of stomatocytes. SAO is extraordinarily common in some South Asian populations, particularly in regions where malaria is endemic.[241–242] It has been estimated that 5 to 25 per cent of the population in some regions of Malaysia and Papua New Guinea have SAO. In vivo, SAO provides some protection against malaria, particularly against heavy infections and cerebral malaria.[243–245] The prevalence of SAO increases with age in populations where malaria is endemic, suggesting that SAO individuals enjoy a selective advantage. In vitro, SAO erythrocytes are resistant to invasion by malarial parasites apparently because the membrane is 10 to 20 times more rigid than normal.[246, 247]

The molecular basis of this increased rigidity is a 9 amino acid deletion in the inter-domain hinge region of band 3 that enhances the tightness of association between band 3, ankyrin, and the spectrin lattice (see Fig. 8–7).[247–252] It is interesting that the treatment of normal red cells with cross-linking agents also generates rigid ovalocytes with tightened associations among cytoskeletal components. SAO has only been described in heterozygotes; the homozygous state has been hypothesized to lead to embryonic or fetal lethality.

▼ HEREDITARY STOMATOCYTOSIS

Stomatocytes, like ovalocytes, have a cup or bowl shape with a transverse slit or stoma. Stomatocytes are seen in a variety of hereditary and acquired disorders. The inherited disorders are a heterogeneous group of autosomal dominant disorders characterized by varying degrees of anemia and stomatocytes on peripheral blood smear. Erythrocytes exhibit abnormal cation permeability leading to increased (hydrocytosis), decreased (xerocytosis), or in some cases, normal, red cell volume. Currently, there is no unifying theory to explain the morphologic abnormality seen in this group of disorders.

Hereditary Hydrocytosis

Patients with classic hereditary stomatocytosis, or hydrocytosis, suffer from moderate to severe hemolytic anemia. There is a predominance of stomatocytes on the peripheral blood smear. The osmotic fragility is markedly increased in patients with hereditary stomatocytosis; the cells look and behave like "swollen" red cells. Membrane lipids and surface area are increased. Cells from patients with stomatocytosis exhibit a marked increase in intracellular sodium and water due to a vastly increased sodium leak into the cells. $Na^+K^+ATPase$ pump activity is much higher than normal but inadequate to compensate for the leak, resulting in engorged, distended cells. The precise molecular defect is unknown. Various abnormalities in membrane proteins have been reported but have been found to be unrelated to the primary defect upon follow-up study. Early evidence that protein 7.2b (stomatin) might be involved have not been substantiated[253–256] Indeed, mice with targeted disruption of the band 7.2b gene have normal erythrocytes.[257]

Hereditary Xerocytosis

Patients with hereditary xerocytosis (HX) suffer from mild to moderate hemolytic anemia. Hydrops fetalis with fetal and neonatal anemia have been reported in several HX kindreds. On peripheral blood smear, stomatocytes are not always present; target cells and dessicocytes are frequently seen. Because the erythrocytes are dehydrated, the osmotic fragility is markedly decreased and the MCHC is increased. Paradoxically, the MCV is frequently increased. In Coulter-type electronic counters, the conversion of pulse height (from the resistance of a cell passing through an electronic field) to a cellular volume is dependent on cell shape. Xerocytes do not deform to the same degree as normal cells, which causes the MCV to be estimated about 10 per cent too high.

Dehydration appears to result from a loss of potassium that is uncompensated by sodium intake. The molecular basis of HX is not understood. Interestingly, HX has recently been shown to be allelic with pseudohyperkalemia, and to map to chromosome 16q23.[258]

Intermediate Syndromes

Some patients exhibit features of both hydrocytosis and xerocytosis and have been described as having "intermediate syndromes."[226] These patients characteristically have both stomatocytes and target cells on peripheral blood smear. Cation permeability is increased, but the intracellular cation content is either normal or slightly reduced. The precise biochemical and molecular defects are unknown.

Stomatocytes are also encountered in a variety of acquired conditions, such as cardiovascular and hepatobiliary disease, alcoholism, and therapy with drugs, some of which are known to be stomatocytogenic in vitro. In some of these conditions, the percentage of stomatocytes on peripheral blood smear approaches 100 per cent. The molecular basis of these findings is unclear; the condition rarely causes significant hematological abnormalities.

Rh Deficiency Syndromes

Rh deficiency syndrome designates individuals whose erythrocytes have either absent (Rh_{null}) or markedly reduced (Rh_{mod}) Rh antigen expression. Rh deficient erythrocytes demonstrate increased cation permeability, elevated ATPase activity and altered lipid organization. This recessively inherited syndrome is clinically and genetically heterogeneous. Typically, there is a mild to moderate hemolytic anemia with stomatocytes and spherocytes on peripheral smear.[226, 259]

Genetically, two groups have been defined, the *amorph* type due to mutations at the Rh locus itself, and the *regulator* type due to mutations in the Rh50, a modulator of Rh expression.[260–267] Most Rh_{null} patients studied to date have mutations of the Rh50 gene including missense, deletion, and splicing mutations. Studies of these rare patients have provided direct evidence that both the Rh locus and Rh50 are required for the expression and function of the Rh structures as a multimeric complex in the erythrocyte membrane.

The McLeod Phenotype

McLeod syndrome is an X-linked abnormality of the Kell blood group system in which erythrocytes and/or leukocytes react poorly with Kell antisera.[268] Clinically, it is characterized by mild anemia with varying degrees of acanthocytosis. The Kell antigen consists of two components.[269, 270] One, Kx,

is a 37 kDa protein integral membrane transporter that carries the Kx antigen and serves as a precursor necessary for Kell antigen expression. The other is a 93 kDa protein that carries the Kell blood group antigen. As expected, in McLeod syndrome, Kx is defective. Thus McLeod red cells lack Kx expression and have significant deficiency of the 93 kDa protein. Phosphorylation of some proteins and lipids, water permeability, and the density of intramembrane particles are abnormal in McLeod erythrocytes; however, it is unclear why acanthocytes form under these circumstances. In vitro exposure of McCleod cells to agents (e.g., chlorpromazine) that expand the inner leaflet correct the acanthocytic shape. Therefore, the loss of the Kx protein, the reduced amounts of the 93kDa protein, or both may lead to either expansion of the outer leaflet or contraction of the inner leaflet, thereby generating acanthocytes.

Chronic granulomatous disease, retinitis pigmentosa, and Duchenne muscular dystrophy have been associated with the McLeod syndrome, because of the close proximity of the genes responsible for these disorders to the genes for the Kell antigen system on chromosome Xp2l.[271] Early reports that attempted to associate red cell morphological abnormalities with Duchenne muscular dystrophy may in fact simply have reflected simultaneous loss of the Kell and Duchenne loci from the X chromosome as part of a contiguous gene syndrome.

▼ RED CELL CYTOSKELETAL PROTEINS AND NORMAL RED CELL SENESCENCE

The survival of normal red cells in the circulation is remarkably long (120 days) and remarkably uniform. Erythrocytes experience progressive loss of vital constituents as they age in the circulation, yet their morphology and biochemistry remain nearly normal until they are abruptly sequestered from the circulation. Many theories have been advanced to explain this abrupt senescence and destruction.[7, 31] The *geometric theory* is based on the supposition that red cells progressively lose small amounts of membrane as they pass through the spleen, resulting eventually in the formation of rigid spherocytes that are sequestered. The *metabolic* theory states that progressive loss of red cell enzymes causes diminished glycolysis, decreased membrane pump function, and loss of reducing capacity, with consequent oxidation of hemoglobin and membrane protein damage. Neither of these theories satisfactorily explains the uniform appearance and biochemical behavior of erythrocytes that are heterogeneous with respect to age.

Low and coworkers[272–277] have presented evidence that immune clearance of senescent red cells contributes significantly to normal red cell destruction. Acceleration of the conditions leading to immune clearance may also explain premature destruction of red cells bearing abnormal hemoglobins, enzyme defects, and/or dysfunctional membrane components.[272] In this model, metabolic aging results in oxidation of intracellular hemoglobin, followed by the generation of hemichromes from the denatured hemoglobin. Hemichromes have a high affinity for the cytoplasmic domain of band 3. Upon binding, they promote the aggregation of protein 3 into localized membrane clusters or patches.[272, 273] Thus hemoglobin denaturation due to any cause results directly in alteration of the external topology of the red cell. Humans possess an autologous immunoglobulin G (IgG) antibody that recognizes band 3 clusters, but not normally configured band 3.[273, 274] This polyvalent IgG binds to the erythrocyte, and the immune complex is cleared by macrophages.

From a clinical perspective, delineation of this clearance mechanism is of fundamental importance for understanding the hemolytic component of many inherited and acquired red cell abnormalities, including the hemoglobinopathies and enzymopathies. A final common pathway in these conditions may well be hemoglobin denaturation with release of hemichromes. Thus, hemoglobin sickling, denaturation of unstable hemoglobins, or hemoglobins oxidized because of red cell enzyme deficiencies could result in sufficient hemichrome formation to accelerate protein 3 clustering and lead to premature clearance (i.e., hemolysis) of the affected red cells. Acceleration of this type of immune clearance has been demonstrated in sickle cell anemia and thalassemia.[275–277]

▼ RED CELL MEMBRANE PROTEINS IN PATIENTS WITH HEMOGLOBINOPATHIES

Changes in the membrane cytoskeleton have been implicated in the hemolytic diathesis accompanying sickle cell anemia and the thalassemia syndromes. Spectrin deficiency reminiscent of that encountered in HS has been documented in these patients.[278] Controversy exists regarding the exact mechanism by which spectrin deficiencies develop. Binding of denatured hemoglobin, hemichromes, or free globin chains to the cytoskeleton, probably directly to spectrin, has been reported.[279] Spectrin deficiency may contribute to the shape changes seen in these diseases as well as to the hemolytic diathesis.

In sickle cell erythrocytes, defective ankyrin-spectrin and ankyrin-band 3 interactions have been described.[280] In thalassemic erythroid progenitors, spectrin and ankyrin were seen to interact with α-globin accumulations and both proerythroblasts and basophilic erythroblasts were deficient in band 3.[281] The mechanisms and pathologic effects of these observations are unknown.

Molecular Defects Underlying Red Cell Membrane Protein Disorders

The foregoing discussion has emphasized the fact that different defects in the same cytoskeletal protein can give rise to different forms of hereditary hemolytic anemia; conversely, a single clinical syndrome can arise from defects in many different proteins. Thus, HS, which results from abnormalities in the band 3/spectrin/ankyrin association, could conceivably arise from abnormalities of any of those proteins (see Fig. 8–12). HE, which involves abnormal spectrin self-association and weakened junctional complexes, could arise from defects in α spectrin, β spectrin, protein 4.1, protein 4.2, or glycophorin C. These predictions have been verified by direct analysis of the genes and mRNAs encoding abnormal proteins in patients with HS, HE, HPP, and SAO. In general, the characterization of these mutations has utilized a common approach. Membrane abnormalities were first correlated with biochemical deficiencies or abnormalities of individual proteins in a given patient or kindred. The abnormality was then characterized at the genetic level, usually by use of PCR amplified segments of the genes or mRNAs predicted to be abnormal by protein analyses. Mutations in the genes encoding α spectrin, β spectrin, ankyrin, protein 4.1, glycophorin C, protein 4.2 and band 3 have all been implicated as the cause of HE, HS, HPP, and/or SAO. In this section, we examine the defects in each gene, noting the syndromes associated with particular defects.

▼ SPECTRIN DEFECTS

Spectrin defects constitute the most complex and thoroughly analyzed group of mutations. Because of the large size of the spectrin α and β chains, their mRNAs, and their genomic loci, it was important to have preliminary methods for "scanning" the spectrin chains for the likely location of the mutation. This scanning would then allow analysis of a limited region along the mRNA sequence by the use of PCR technology. Fortunately, spectrin can be subdivided into reproducible domains by limited proteolytic digestion at 0°C followed by one-dimensional or two-dimensional electrophoresis.[1, 282–284] This yields a fingerprint of normal spectrin domains (Fig. 8–13) that can be compared with comparable fingerprints from patients. The fragments are named according to their chain of origin, T = tryptic fragment, size order (I = largest, II = next largest, and so on), and apparent molecular weight (see Fig. 8–12B). Thus, T$\alpha^{I/80}$ refers to the largest tryptic peptide domain of the spectrin α chain, having a molecular weight of approximately 80 kDa; T$\alpha^{I/74}$ refers to an abnormal tryptic peptide of 74 kDa, rather than 80 kDa, found in some patients with spectrin mutations.[282–284] Domains of particular interest in which spectrin mutations have been identified are αI, αII, and βIV; mutations have also been identified at the extreme COOH-terminus of the spectrin β chain.

α Spectrin Mutations

The location of mutations in the α-spectrin molecule can be correlated to the resulting phenotype. Mutations of the NH$_2$-terminal αI domain (Fig. 8–14), the region involved in spectrin dimer-dimer self-association to tetramers and oligomers, are found in patients with HE and HPP. Mutations outside the αI domain, when inherited in a homozygous or compound heterozygous fashion, may be associated with elliptocytic, poikilocytic or spherocytic phenotypes. αI domain mutations presumably alter the native conformation of spectrin, thereby exposing normally inaccessible recognition sequences to protease and altering the tryptic digestion pattern, as discussed above. Mutations have been subclassified by the size of the abnormal peptide produced. The most common and important mutations are those producing the $\alpha^{I/74}$ peptide, the $\alpha^{I/50}$ peptide, and the $\alpha^{I/65-68}$ peptide.[226, 285]

The interaction of a single helix from the NH$_2$-terminus of α spectrin interacts with two helices of the COOH-terminus of β spectrin at the dimer self-association site (see Fig. 8–8). It is not surprising that mutations in these helices

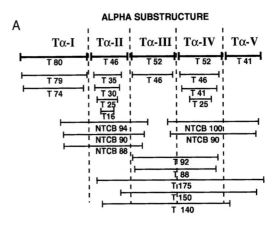

ALPHA SUBSTRUCTURE

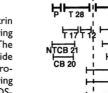

BETA SUBSTRUCTURE

Figure 8–13. Domain maps of spectrin generated by trypsin digestion. αI/βI spectrin extracted from erythrocytes was subjected to mild trypsin digestion at 0°C, cleaving the protein into a reproducible number of well-characterized large fragments. *A.* The alignment of the various tryptic fragments, as determined by high-resolution peptide mapping. Also shown is the alignment of some of the fragments generated by 2-nitro-5-thiocyanobenzoic acid (NTCB) digestion of αI/βI spectrin. *B.* The pattern following limited trypsin digestion. Peptide fragments are resolved by two-dimensional IEF-SDS-PAGE analysis, and visualized by Coomassie blue. The pattern that results is of limited complexity, facilitating the identification of the sites of functional domains, posttranslational modifications, and inherited mutations in this very large protein. (From Morrow, J.S., Rimm, D.L., Kennedy, S.P., Cianci, C.D., Sinard, J.H., and Weed, S.A.: Of membrane stability and mosaics: the spectrin cytoskeleton. *In* Hoffman, J., and Jamieson, J. [eds.]: Handbook of Physiology. London, Oxford, 1997, pp. 485–540.)

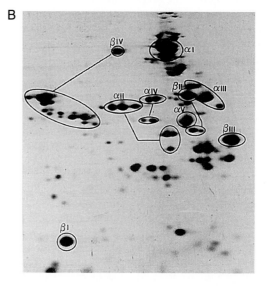

of the α and β spectrin chains are the most common and most widespread cause of defective self-association. These mutations lead to the spectrin T[αI74] phenotype on spectrin tryptic digests. Amino acid 28, a particularly common site of T[αI74] HE/HPP mutations, is probably a critical contact site of αβ spectrin self-association.[285, 286]

Less common mutations cleave the αI domain to 65, 50, or 78 kDa tryptic peptides. These mutations share certain features: They are base substitutions producing single amino acid changes that affect the ability of spectrin dimers to form tetramers. The positions of these mutations localize specific amino acids that are critical for self association,

such as amino acids 41 to 49, amino acid 28, and regions around amino acid 260 and 471. Most of these changes cause mild to moderately severe HE. The α[I/74] and α[I/50α] mutations can produce HPP in the doubly heterozygous or homozygous state. α[I/65] homozygotes have mild to moderate HE. Recently, a patient who is a compound heterozygote for mutations in the self-association site of both α and β spectrin has been described.[287]

Variants of the αII domain have been identified in several kindreds. Because α spectrin is synthesized in excess, these variants are asymptomatic in the heterozygous state, but lead to mild to severe anemia in the homozygous state.[1]

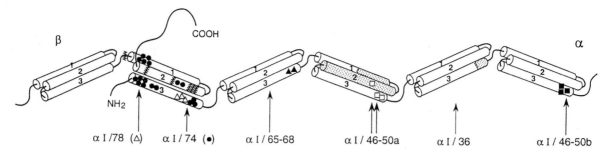

Figure 8–14. A model of mutations of the spectrin self-association site. A triple helical model of the spectrin repeats that constitute the spectrin self-association site is shown. The symbols denote positions of various genetic defects identified in patients with hereditary elliptocytosis or hereditary pyropoikilocytosis. Limited tryptic digestion of spectrin followed by two-dimensional gel electrophoresis identifies abnormal cleavage sites in spectrin associated with different mutations. These cleavage sites are denoted by arrows. (From Current Opinion in Hematology, 1997, Vol. 4, pp. 128–135, by copyright permission of Rapid Science Publishers.)

[7, 226, 286, 288] These mutants may have varying degrees of long-range effect on spectrin self-association.[289]

A low expression allele of α spectrin, α^{LELY}, is characterized by an amino acid substitution, Leu1857Val, and partial skipping of exon 46. These abnormalities are located in the spectrin nucleation site; α-spectrin chains lacking exon 46 are poorly assembled into αβ heterodimers and are rapidly degraded. By itself, the α^{LELY} allele is clinically silent. When it is present *in trans* to an α-spectrin mutation, it has the effect of increasing the concentration of mutant spectrin in the cytoskeleton and worsening the severity of the disease. Conversely, when the α^{LELY} allele is *in cis* to an α-spectrin mutation, it mutes the elliptocytic phenotype.[124, 125, 285]

In nondominantly inherited HS, the degree of spectrin deficiency has been correlated with the spheroidicity of the HS erythrocytes, the severity of hemolysis, and the response to splenectomy. Heterozygotes for α-spectrin defects produce enough normal α spectrin to pair with all, or nearly all, of the available β-spectrin chains. Thus spectrin deficiency should be obvious only in HS patients who are homozygotes or compound heterozygotes for α-spectrin defects. Approximately half the patients with nondominantly inherited HS and marked spectrin deficiency have a mutation in intron 29 that leads to an aberrantly spliced α-spectrin mRNA.[290] This mutant allele, α^{LEPRA} (low-expression Prague), produces 6 times less of the correctly spliced α-spectrin transcript than the normal allele. The combination of the α^{LEPRA} allele with other α-spectrin defects *in trans*, such as a truncated α-spectrin chain, leads to severe spectrin deficiency and spherocytic hemolytic anemia.[291] Patients who are homozygotes for the α^{LEPRA} allele have a less severe clinical phenotype than those with α^{LEPRA} and another α-spectrin defect. The α^{LEPRA} allele is in linkage equilibrium with a polymorphism of the αII domain of spectin, $\alpha^{Bug\ Hill}$, formerly known as αIIa.[292]

β Spectrin Mutations

Mutations of β spectrin associated with HS, HE, and HPP phenotypes have been described.[285, 286] Like α-spectrin gene mutations, the location of the abnormality correlates well with the clinical phenotype. Mutations of the COOH-terminal β spectrin repeat 17, the region involved in αβ spectrin self-association, (see Fig. 8–14), are typically associated with elliptocytic and/or poikilocytic phenotypes. As ex-

pected, mutations in this region of β spectrin produce effects similar to those of the NH$_2$-terminal αI domain of spectrin. However, compared to αI domain mutations which are predominantly due to amino acid substitutions, these β spectrin variants are primarily COOH-terminal truncations due to mutations that disrupt splicing, lead to frameshifts, or both.

Some β spectrin mutations, such as Ala2053 Pro, are particularly instructive. Initially, spectrin tryptic digests from individuals with this mutation demonstrated an abnormal $T^{\alpha I/74}$ phenotype; however no abnormalities of the corresponding α-spectrin sequence were found.[293] Later, the defect was identified in β spectrin, and the concept of the disruptive effects of an abnormal β spectrin on the conformation of αβ spectrin self-association developed. Thus, mutations in one spectrin chain can clearly alter the conformation and, presumably, the function or stability of the other chain. In a few cases, homozygosity for COOH-terminal β-spectrin gene mutations has been associated with severe fetal and neonatal anemia and nonimmune hydrops fetalis.[293, 294]

A number of dominantly-inherited, heterozygous β-spectrin gene mutations associated with HS have been described.[237, 294–297] These mutations occur outside the spectrin self-association site and are frequently associated with decreased β-spectrin mRNA accumulation. With one exception, these are private mutations, i.e, unique to a kindred. One interesting HS-associated NH$_2$-terminal mutation of β spectrin results from the substitution of an arginine for a tryptophan in the region involved in β spectrin-protein 4.1 interaction.[296] For unknown reasons, this mutation results in a secondary spectrin deficiency, possibly due to the weakened formation of junctional complexes. The reciprocal mutation of protein 4.1 that weakens the junctions does not, interestingly, cause HS; rather, mild to moderate HE results.

Intermediate phenotypes due to β-spectin gene mutations have been described. For example, the erythrocytes from a kindred with spherocytic elliptocytosis exhibited spectrin deficiency and impaired spectrin dimer self-association. These findings were due to a truncated β-spectrin chain that lacked both the ankyrin-binding site and the self-association site.[298]

▼ BAND 3 DEFECTS

Defects of band 3 have been associated with HS and the much less common disorders southeast Asian ovalocytosis and acanthocytosis. The HS patients are a subset of those with typical, dominant HS who generally suffer from mild to moderate HS. Their erythrocytes are deficient in band 3 and protein 4.2 but contain a normal amount of spectrin. A large number of HS-associated band 3 mutations have been reported including missense, nonsense, duplication, insertion, deletion, and RNA processing mutations.[226, 236] These mutations are spread throughout the band 3 molecule in both the cytoplasmic and membrane spanning domains. Homozygous mutations in band 3 may be lethal.[299, 230]

HS-associated missense variants include a group of mutations clustered in the transmembrane domain that replace highly conserved arginines.[301] These arginines, all located at the cytoplasmic end of a predicted transmembrane helix, are thought to aid in maintaining the orientation of transmembrane spanning segments. It is thought that these mutant band 3 molecules do not fold or insert into the endoplasmic reticulum, and, ultimately, into the erythrocyte membrane. The nonsense mutations are thought to lead to decreased mRNA accumulation, presumably due to mRNA instability.[302] Band 3 alleles that influence band 3 expression have been identified. When these alleles are inherited *in trans* to an HS-associated band 3 mutation, they aggravate band 3 deficiency and worsen the clinical severity of the disease.[303, 304]

Another consequence of a band 3 defect is southeast Asian ovalocytosis. Molecular analysis of the common form has identified an intron/exon deletion that results in loss of amino acids 400 to 408; this is the inter-domain hinge region that may be important for the flexibility of the cytoskeleton at the point of the protein 3 ankyrin/spectrin association. A tightly linked polymorphism at codon 56 is coinherited with the most common of these defects.[230] This mutation of the hinge region produces marked reductions in lateral mobility, increased phosphorylation, tightening and rigidification of the vertical association of band 3 with the cytoskeleton, and rigid red cells. The anion transport function of band 3 may also be abnormal, since binding to the specific inhibitor of the protein, DIDS, and actual anion transport have both been shown to be altered.

Finally, a missense mutation in band 3, Pro868Leu, was discovered in a kindred with chorea-acanthocytosis. Affected members had mild anemia with reticulocytosis, 20–25% acanthocytosis, and increased rates of ion transport in erythrocyte membranes.[305]

Recent studies of band 3 in animals has yielded important insight into its function. Targeted disruption of the murine band 3 gene leads to severe spherocytic hemolytic anemia in homozygous mice.[58, 59] Erythrocytes from homozygous mice shed membrane vesicles and tubules and exhibit a tendency to become depleted in band 3-anchored membrane complexes. However, these erythrocytes have near normal levels of the major erythrocyte membrane skeleton proteins with a normally assembled membrane skeleton. These studies suggest that band 3 is critical for membrane stability, but not for membrane biogenesis as previously hypothesized. Band 3-deficient mice will serve as valuable tools in the investigation of the role of band 3 in membrane-skeleton interactions, malarial invasion of the erythrocyte, acid-base physiology, and red cell senescence.

▼ ANKYRIN MUTATIONS

The most common abnormality observed in the erythrocyte membranes from HS patients is combined deficiency of spectrin and ankyrin. Concomitant spectrin and ankyrin deficiency is not unexpected; decreased ankyrin synthesis, decreased ankyrin assembly on the membrane, or assembly of an abnormal ankyrin could lead to decreased assembly of spectrin on the membrane because spectrin binding sites on ankyrin may be absent or defective. It is not unexpected then that the most common cause of typical dominant HS is a defect in erythrocyte ankyrin.

Genetic evidence implicating ankyrin in the pathogenesis of HS was first suggested by cytogenetic study of ankyrin-deficient HS patients with dysmorphic features, including mental retardation, typical facies and hypogonadism with cytogenetic abnormalities around 8p11.2, later discovered to be the erythrocyte ankyrin gene locus.[308, 309] Later, linkage of HS to the ankyrin gene[310] and the discovery that approximately one third of HS patients with combined spectrin and ankyrin deficiency only express one of their two ankyrin alleles in reticulocyte RNA[311] added further evidence to support the role of ankyrin in the pathogenesis of HS.

Genetic screening has now identified a number of ankyrin mutations in individuals with HS, including missense, nonsense, and frameshift mutations.[237, 213] The majority of the mutations discovered are either frameshift or nonsense mutations which may lead to a defective ankyrin molecule, ankyrin deficiency, or both. One missense mutation, ankyrin Waldsrode, has been shown to lead to a decrease in ankyrin affinity for band 3.[313] Like HS-associated β-spectrin gene mutations, ankyrin gene mutations are private. The one exception to this observation, ankyrin Florianopolis, is a frameshift mutation identified from 3 HS kindreds from different genetic backgrounds.[314] Analysis of ankyrin gene polymorphisms in members of these kindreds demonstrated that this mutation is on different ankyrin alleles, suggesting that the ankyrin Florianopolis mutation has occurred more than once on different genetic backgrounds.

Genetic variations have been identified in the promoter of the erythrocyte ankyrin gene in a number of patients with recessively inherited HS.[312, 315] Whether these are disease causing mutations or are merely polymorphisms in linkage dysequilibrium with the as yet unidentified mutation is unknown.

▼ PROTEIN 4.1 DEFECTS

Two major classes of molecular abnormality of protein 4.1 have been reported: those producing selective deficiency of protein 4.1 from red cells and those disrupting the erythroid-specific spectrin-actin-binding domain (exon 16).[7, 226] Both categories are associated with mild HE in the simple heterozygous state. Homozygous protein 4.1 deficiency is associated with severe HE and is common in North Africa.[316]

Two abnormalities of the spectrin-actin-binding domain of protein 4.1 have been identified.[317, 318] One produces an elongated protein, 95 kDa long, resulting from duplication of three exons encoding the spectrin-actin domain, with consequent duplication of amino acids 407 to 529. Duplication causes a mild abnormality of junctional complex formation. A truncated form of protein 4.1, protein 4.1[68/65], lacks the spectrin-actin-binding domain because of deletion of the exons encoding the spectrin-actin-binding site and amino acids 407 to 486, with consequent weakened interaction with spectrin and actin.

In the forms of protein 4.1 deficiency studied thus far, the deficiency occurs selectively in red cells, because of the complex regulation of tissue-specific alternative mRNA splicing that occurs during erythropoiesis. As shown in Figure 8–9, and discussed in an earlier section, nonerythroid cells synthesize considerable amounts of a high molecular weight isoform of protein 4.1, owing to splicing events at the 5' end of the gene that convert a portion of the 5' untranslated region into translatable sequence. The high molecular weight isoform thus contains the entire 80 kDa segment found in erythroid protein 4.1, plus a 209 amino acid "headpiece" added to the amino-terminus. These splicing events are totally suppressed at an early stage of erythropoiesis, so that virtually no high molecular weight isoform is present in mature red cells. Rather, the translation of the protein is initiated at an internal methionine codon. One form of selective erythroid protein 4.1 deficiency has been shown to arise by deletion and/or gene rearrangement that removes the exon containing this internal translation initiation site. Thus, erythroid cells, lacking the ability to translate from the upstream start site, cannot produce protein 4.1 from the mutant allele. Nonerythroid cells, possessing the upstream start site, synthesize the high molecular weight form. A form of protein 4.1 deficiency encountered in Spaniards has been shown to result from an analogous mechanism, a point mutation that abolishes the downstream initiator methionine.

Targeted disruption of 4.1R in mice leads to a moderately severe spherocytic, hemolytic anemia. Erythrocytes from 4.1R-/- mice exhibited lowered membrane stability and dramatic reductions in p55 and GPC, as well as unexpected decreases in spectrin and ankyrin content.[165] The full extent of fine neurologic abnormalities in these mice continues to be explored.

▼ GLYCOPHORIN DEFECTS

As noted earlier, mutations resulting in the production of abnormal or deficient glycophorin A and B have been documented.[7, 226] None of these result in phenotypic abnormalities of red cells, other than alteration of blood group phenotypes and increased resistance to malarial invasion. Elliptocytes have been noted in the smears of patients with the Leach phenotype. These erythrocytes lack GPC, GPD, and presumably p55 and protein 4.1. The Leach phenotype is usually due to a genomic deletion that includes GPC exons 3 and 4; in one case, the phenotype was due to a nucleotide deletion.[319] In both instances, frameshift and premature chain termination results. An interesting aspect of these mutations is the fact that protein 4.1 deficiency occurs concomitantly in these cells, suggesting once again that protein stability after translation depends on successful incorporation into the cytoskeleton.

▼ PROTEIN 4.2 DEFECTS

Recessively inherited HS due to protein 4.2 mutations is relatively common in Japan.[7, 226] Erythrocytes from these patients exhibit nearly complete absence of protein 4.2; they are frequently deficient in band 3 and ankyrin. Ankyrin appears to be required for the normal association of protein 4.2 to the erythrocyte membrane. One common HS-associated variant, protein 4.2[Nippon], is due to a point mutation that presumably affects mRNA processing.[306] Other variants are due to frameshift, missense, or mRNA processing mutations of the protein 4.2 gene.

Protein 4.2 deficiency has also been described in patients with mutations in the cytoplasmic domain of band 3. These mutations presumably involve sites of band 3-protein 4.2 interactions. Mice with targeted disruption of the protein 4.2 gene exhibit spherocytosis with intact membrane skeletons, mild band 3 deficiency and abnormalities of cation transport.[307]

▼ IMPACT OF THE CYTOSKELETAL PROTEIN MUTATIONS ON NONERYTHROID TISSUES

For the most part, hereditary hemolytic anemias due to abnormal cytoskeletal proteins exhibit clinical abnormalities confined to the red cells, despite the fact that many of these cytoskeletal proteins are widely expressed. In some cases, the selectivity of clinical abnormalities can be attributed to the fact that the defects occur only in erythroid-specific genes or isoforms. Most nonerythroid tissues rely, for example, on a different gene for production of the α spectrin isoform, fodrin; similarly, abnormal or deficient protein 4.1 in some forms of hereditary elliptocytosis is due to abnormalities that affect only the erythroid specific spliceoforms. This explanation alone is not completely satisfying, however, because "erythroid specific" forms of some of these proteins are in fact expressed selectively in some other tissues. For instance, the erythroid form of β spectrin and the exon associated with the erythroid spectrin-actin-binding domain of protein 4.1 both appear to be expressed abundantly in muscle. Although homozygosity for the β spectrin self-association site mutation spectrin[Providence] leads to a lethal anemia, it does not appear to impact the function of β spectrin in skeletal muscle.[320] Erythroid ankyrin may be expressed in muscle, kidney, and some parts of the central nervous system, even though a brain-specific isoform of ankyrin clearly exists. Indeed, as already noted, ankyrin deficiency in mice and in some forms of HS has been associated with mental retardation, neuronal degeneration, ataxia, and spinal cord abnormalities, as has loss of protein 4.1R via gene knockout. Band 3-deficient patients and knockout mice have recently been shown to suffer from distal renal tubular acidosis.[58, 59, 230–235] Yet, the vast majority of patients with cytoskeletal protein defects are phenotypically normal except for their red cells. In those cases where other organ systems seem to be involved, the central nervous system or kidney is the most frequent site of additional pathology. This pattern is also seen in knock-out mice for the relevant genes.

These findings demand explanation. Why should quantitative or qualitative defects of cytoskeletal proteins disrupt erythroid homeostasis without always deranging function more dramatically in at least some other tissue? A mutation producing an abnormal cytoskeletal protein might impair red cell function without causing significant abnormalities in nonerythroid cells because of the unique mechanical and biochemical demands placed on the membrane and cytoskeleton of erythrocytes. For the most part, the mutations that cause hereditary hemolytic anemia are those that alter the ability of the membrane to withstand shear stress. Indeed, in the most commonly encountered forms of these diseases, these abnormalities are relatively mild. They are detected more often by a distinctive morphology or abnormality in a routine blood count than by major clinical symptomatology. Comparably mild defects in other organ systems may not come to clinical attention. Indeed, mutations that primarily affect mechanical stability under conditions of shear stress may not produce any deleterious effects on the cytoskeletons of noncirculating cells. Conversely, mutations severely disrupting function could be embryonic lethal defects.

Red cells are unique in that they must survive for long periods, even though they cannot repair or replenish their proteins. A final pathway common to forms of hereditary spherocytosis and elliptocytosis is quantitative deficiency of one or more proteins, resulting in shortening of red cell survival. In other tissues, it is possible, even likely, that these deficiencies can be overcome by the continual biosynthesis of new proteins, or utilization of functionally redundant isoforms. As noted in an earlier section, actual assembly of most cytoskeletal components appears to be limited more by posttranslational incorporations of these proteins into the cytoskeleton than by the rates of *de novo* biosynthesis. Deficiencies in red cells result largely because the erythrocyte is released into the circulation with only the amount of protein that is already incorporated into the cytoskeleton. Once lost from the cytoskeleton, these proteins cannot be replaced. This is probably not the case for nucleated cells. Red cell membrane protein defects are instructive for understanding the complex relationships that can exist between a mutation and its ultimate phenotypic expression in different tissues.

Summary and Conclusions

Membranes form the boundaries of cells, defining their interface with the external environment and protecting them from noxious materials in that environment, while at the same time permitting communication and selective molecular exchange with it. Membranes also provide hydrophobic sites for sequestration, compartmentalization, and regulation of intracellular metabolic events. The ability of membranes to serve these fundamental biological functions is, as outlined in this chapter, dependent on the precise assembly and noncovalent interaction of a complex array of lipids, integral proteins, and the attached proteins that form the cytoskeleton. In particular, membranes can survive and function only because of their interaction with cytoskeletal protein frameworks that confer shape and mechanical stability on the lipid bilayer. Abnormalities of the membrane-cytoskeletal unit that lead to human disease have been best exemplified by defects of the red cell membrane that produce hereditary hemolytic anemias or morphologic abnormalities. Recent

progress in identifying the molecular basis of these disorders has been useful in that it has validated the basic model discussed in this chapter, revealed the refinements needed in the model, and illuminated by analogy the types of protein-membrane complexes that are important throughout nature. Indeed, spectrin, ankyrin, band 3, protein 4.1, p55, and adducin have been enlightening as prototypes of gene families coding for diverse isoforms that subserve analogous, but diverse functions in almost all cell types. Yet, the red cell remains for many purposes the best and most accommodating system for detailed functional analysis. In the near future, crystal structures for several red cell isoforms of these proteins are likely to become available. These data will be most useful for defining the actual chemical behavior of these proteins in normal and perturbed environments, and should guide the way to infer intelligently the detailed behavior of homologues in more complex cells and physiological circumstances.

As recently as a decade ago, the notion of the cell membrane as a dynamic structure was taken to be largely reflective of its role in organizing and compartmentalizing cells and maintaining the integrity of intracellular and extracellular boundaries. The discovery that key cytoplasmic (i.e., reversibly attached) cytoskeletal protein families such as those for protein 4.1, ankyrin, adducin, and p55 are homologous to, or interact with signal transduction molecules, adhesion molecules, key channels and pumps, and receptors, and that some, such as several p55 homologues, are tumor suppressor genes, is opening an entirely new dimension for their study. It seems clear already that these proteins are key players in signal transduction, cell differentiation, organogenesis, and apoptosis, as well as their long appreciated roles in topology and trans-membrane trafficking. Further study of the cytoskeleton is likely to point to a need to develop experimental strategies to study the dynamic formation and trafficking of reversibly formed multicomponent complexes in real time, and the means by which altering the organization of such entities alters metabolism.

Finally, the roles played by nonerythroid homologues imply that the red cell cytoskeleton may be more dynamic and complicated than the models described in this chapter suggest. There is already preliminary evidence suggesting that signal transduction pathways do function in red cells, and that they could, for example amplify the generation of platelet agonist compounds at the site of a wound. The implications of this type of behavior are enormous, since red cells might then participate in processes such as thrombosis, endothelial cell responses to injury, or inflammation in ways not previously conceived. Even if these effects seem negligible in individual red cells, the sheer mass of erythrocytes in the blood could render them physiologically relevant. Pursuit of these new avenues of red cell research could thus alter fundamentally our notions of both the scope and the importance of red cells in many areas for which they were previously not considered relevant. An obvious corollary of these assertions is that they would alter our views about the clinical importance of anemia or erythrocytosis in various clinical settings. These properties might also present opportunities for using engineered red cells for therapeutic purposes extending beyond the support of oxygen transport to tissues.

REFERENCES

1. Morrow, J.S., Rimm, D.L., Kennedy, S.P., Cianci, C.D., Sinard, J.H., and Weed, S.A.: Of membrane stability and mosaics: The spectrin cytoskeleton. *In* Hoffman, J., Jamieson, J. (eds.): Handbook of Physiology. London, Oxford, 1997, p. 485.
2. Stryer, L.: Biochemistry. 4th ed. New York, W.H. Freeman, 1995.
3. Alberts, B., Bray, D., Lewis, J., Raff, M., Roberts, K., and Watson, J.D.: Molecular Biology of the Cell. 3rd ed. New York, Garland, 1994.
4. Tanford, C. The Hydrophobic Effect: Formation of Micelles and Biological Membranes. 2nd ed. New York, Wiley-Interscience, 1980.
5. Fairbanks, G., Steck, T.L., and Wallach, D.F.H.: Electrophoretic analysis of the major polypeptides of the human erythrocyte membrane. Biochemistry 10:2606, 1971.
6. Steck, T.L., Fairbanks, G., and Wallach, D.F.H.: Disposition of the major proteins in the isolated erythrocyte membrane. Proteolytic dissection. Biochemistry 10:2617, 1971.
7. Lux, S.E., and Palek, J.: Disorders of the red cell membrane. *In* Handin, R.I., Lux, S.E., Stossel, T.P. (eds.): Blood: Principles and Practice of Hematology. Philadelphia, JB Lippincott. 1995, pp. 1701.
8. Skene, J.H. and Virag, I.: Posttranslational membrane attachment and dynamic fatty acylation of a neuronal growth cone protein, GAP-43. J. Cell Biol. 108:613, 1989.
9. Rosse, W.F.: The glycolipid anchor of membrane surface proteins. Semin. Hematol. 30:219, 1993.
10. Marchesi, V.T.: Functional adaptations of transbilayer proteins. *In* Dhindsu, D.S., and Bahl, O.P. (eds.): Molecular and Cellular Aspects of Reproduction. New York, Plenum, 1986, p. 107.
11. Kleffel, B., Garavito, R.M., Baumeister, W., and Rosenbusch, J.P.: Secondary structure of a channel-forming protein: Porin from *E. coli* outer membranes. EMBO J. 4:1589, 985.
12. Bennett, V.: The spectrin actin junction of erythrocyte membrane skeletons. Biochim. Biophys. Acta 988:107,1989.
13. Vaz, W.K.C., Derzko, Z.I., and Jacobson, K.A.: Photobleaching measurements of the lateral diffusion of lipids and proteins in artificial phospholipid bilayer membranes. Cell Surf. Rev. 8:83, 1982.
14. Kornberg, R.D., and MacConnell, H.M.: Inside-outside transitions of phospholipids in vesicle membranes. Biochemistry 10:1111, 1971.
15. Bevers, E.M., Comfurius, P., Dekkers, D.W.C., Harmsma, M., and Zwaal, R.F.A.: Transmembrane phospholipid distribution in blood cells—control mechanisms and pathophysiological significance. J. Biol. Chem. 379:973, 1998.
16. Tang, X., Halleck, M.S., Schlegel, R.A., and Williamson, P.: A subfamily of P-type ATPases with aminophospholipid transporting activity. Science 272:1495, 1996.
17. Kamp, D., and Haest, C.W.: Evidence for a role of the multidrug resistance protein (MRP) in the outward translocation of NBD-phospholipids in the erythrocyte membrane. Biochim. Biophys. Acta 1372:91, 1998.
18. Dekkers, D.W., Comfurius, P., Schroit, A.J., Bevers, E.M., and Zwaal, R.F.: Transbilayer movement of NBD-labeled phospholipids in red blood cell membranes: outward-directed transport by the multidrug resistance protein 1 (MRP1). Biochemistry 37:14833, 1998.
19. Basse, F., Stout, J.G., Sims, P.J., and Wiedmer, T.: Isolation of an erythrocyte membrane protein that mediates Ca2+-dependent transbilayer movement of phospholipid. J. Biol. Chem. 271:17205, 1996.
20. Zhou, Q., Zhao, J., Stout, J.G., Luhm, R.A., Wiedmer, T., and Sims, P.J.: Molecular cloning of human plasma membrane phospholipid scramblase. A protein mediating transbilayer movement of plasma membrane phospholipids. J. Biol. Chem. 272:18240, 1997.
21. Zhao, J., Zhou, Q., Wiedmer, T., and Sims, P.J.: Level of expression of phospholipid scramblase regulates induced movement of phosphatidylserine to the cell surface. J. Biol. Chem. 273:6603, 1998.
22. Zhou, Q., Sims, P.J., and Wiedmer, T.: Identity of a conserved motif in phospholipid scramblase that is required for Ca2+-accelerated transbilayer movement of membrane phospholipids. Biochemistry 37:2356, 1998.
23. Stout, J.G., Zhou, Q., Wiedmer, T., and Sims, P.J.: Change in conformation of plasma membrane phospholipid scramblase induced by occupancy of its Ca2+ binding site. Biochemistry 37:14860, 1998.
24. Stout, J.G., Basse, F., Luhm, R.A., Weiss, H.J., Wiedmer, T., and Sims, P.J.: Scott syndrome erythrocytes contain a membrane protein capable of mediating Ca2+-dependent transbilayer migration of membrane phospholipids. J. Clin. Invest. 99:2232, 1997.
25. Dekkers, D.W., Comfurius, P., Vuist, W.M., Billheimer, J.T., Dicker, I., Weiss, H.J., Zwaal, R.F., and Bevers, E.M.: Impaired Ca2+-induced tyrosine phosphorylation and defective lipid scrambling in erythrocytes from a patient with Scott syndrome: a study using an inhibitor for scramblase that mimics the defect in Scott syndrome. Blood 91:2133, 1998.
26. Golan, D.E.: Red blood cell membrane proteins and lipid diffusion: *In* Agre, P., and Parker, J.C. (eds.): Red Blood Cell Membranes: Structure, Function, Clinical Implications. New York, Marcel Dekker, 1989, p. 367.
27. Buck, C.A., and Horwitz, A.F.: Cell surface receptors for extracellular matrix molecules. Annu. Rev. Cell Biol. 3:179, 1987.
28. Anderson, R.A., and Marchesi, V.T.: Regulation of the association of membrane skeletal protein 4.1 with glycophorin by a polyphosphoinositide. Nature 318:295, 1985.
29. Sato, S.B., and Ohnishi, S.: Interaction of a peripheral protein of the erythrocyte membrane, band 4.1, with phosphatidylserine-containing liposomes and erythrocyte inside-out vesicles. Eur. J. Biochem. 130:19, 1983.
30. Cohen, C.M., and Gascard, P.: Regulation and post-translational modification of erythrocyte membrane and membrane-skeletal proteins. Semin. Hematol. 29:244, 1992.
31. Nelson, W.J., and Veshnock, P.J.: Ankyrin binding to (Na + K)ATPase and implications for the organization of membrane domains in polarized cells. Nature 328:533, 1987.
32. Becker, P.S., and Benz, E.J., Jr.: Molecular biology of the red cell membrane proteins. *In* Chien, S. (ed.): Molecular Biology of the Cardiovascular System. Philadelphia, Lea and Febiger, 1990, p. 155.
33. Narla, M.: The red cell membrane. *In* Hoffman, R., Benz, E.J., Jr., Shattil, S., Furie, B., and Cohen, H. (eds.): Hematology: Basic Principles and Practice. New York, Churchill Livingstone, 1991, p. 264.
34. Kannan, R., Yuan J., and Low P.S.: Isolation and partial characterization of antibody and globin-enriched complexes from membranes of dense human erythrocytes. Biochem. J. 278:57, 1991.
35. Waugh, S.M., and Low, P.S.: Hemochrome binding to band 3: Nucleation of Heinz bodies on the erthrocyte membrane. Biochemistry 24:34, 1985.
36. Chien, S.: Red cell deformability and its relevance to blood flow. Annu. Rev. Physiol. 49:177, 1987.
37. Narla, M., Chasis, J.A., and Shohet, S.B.: The influence of membrane skeleton on red cell deformability, membrane material properties, and shape. Semin. Hematol. 20:225, 1983.
38. Narla, M., Phillips, W.M., and Bessis, M.: Red blood cell deformability and hemolytic anemias. Semin. Hematol. 16:95, 1979.
39. Chasis, J.A., Agre, P., and Narla, M.: Decreased membrane mechanical stability and *in vivo* loss of surface area reflect spectrin deficiencies in hereditary spherocytosis. J. Clin. Invest. 82:617, 1988.
40. Evans, E.A., and La Celle, P.L.: Intrinsic material properties of erythrocyte membrane indicated by mechanical analysis of deformation. Blood 45:29, 1975.
41. Hochmuth, R.M., and Waugh, R.E.: Erythrocyte membrane elasticity and viscosity. Annu. Rev. Physiol. 49:209, 1987.
42. Liu, S.C., Derick, L.H., and Palek, J.: Visualization of the hexagonal lattice in the erythrocyte membrane skeleton. J. Cell Biol. 104:527, 1987.
43. Fowler, V., and Taylor, D.L.: Spectrin plus band 4.1 crosslink actin: Regulation by micromolar calcium. J. Cell Biol. 85:361, 1980.
44. Ways, P., and Hanahan, D.J.: Characterization and quantitation of red cell lipids in normal man. J. Lipid Res. 5:318, 1964.
45. Verkleij, A.J., Zwaal, R.F.A., Roelofsen, B., et al.: The asymmetric distribution of phospholipids in the human red cell membrane. A combined study using phospholipases and freeze-etch electron microscopy. Biochim. Biophys. Acta 323:178, 1973.
46. Lux, S.E., John, K.M., Kopito, R.R., and Lodish, H.F.: Cloning and characterization of band 3, the human erythrocyte anion exchange protein (AE1). Proc. Natl. Acad. Sci. USA 86:9089, 1989.
47. Tanner, M.J.A., Wainwright, S.D., and Martin, P.G.: The structure and molecular genetics of the human erythrocyte anion transport protein. *In* Hamasaki, N., and Jennings, M. J. (eds.): Anion Transport Proteins of the Red Cell Membrane. Amsterdam, Elsevier, 1989, p. 121.
48. Low, P.S.: Structure and function of the cytoplasmic domain of band 3: Center of erythrocyte membrane-peripheral protein interactions. Biochim. Biophys. Acta 864:145, 1986.
49. Low, P.S., Willardson, B. M., Thevenin, B., Kannan, R., Mahler, E., Geahlen, R.L., and Harrison, M.: The other functions of erythrocyte membrane band 3. *In* Hamasaki, N., and Jennings, M.J. (eds.): Anion

Transport Proteins of the Red Cell Membrane. Amsterdam, Elsevier, 1989, p. 103.

50. Hargreaves, W.R., Giedd, K.N., Verleij, A., and Branton, D.: Reassociation of ankyrin with band 3 in erythrocyte membranes and lipid vesicles. J. Biol. Chem. 225:11965, 1980.

51. Bennet, V., and Stenbuck, P.J.: Association between ankyrin and the cytoplasmic domain of band 3 isolated from the human erythrocyte membrane. J. Biol. Chem. 225:6426, 1980.

52. Kopito, R.R., Anderson, M., and Lodish, H.F.: Structure and organization of the murine band 3 gene. J. Biol. Chem. 262:8035, 1987.

53. Narla, M., Winardi, R., Knowles, D., Leung, A., Parra, M., George, E., Conboy, J., and Chasis, J.: Molecular basis for membrane rigidity of hereditary ovalocytosis: A novel mechanism involving the cytoplasmic domain of band 3. J. Clin. Invest. 89:686, 1992.

54. Van Dort, H.M., Moriyama, R., and Low, P.S.: Effect of band 3 subunit equilibrium on the kinetics and affinity of ankyrin binding to erythrocyte membrane vesicles. J. Biol. Chem. 273:14819, 1998.

55. Vince, J.W., and Reithmeier, R.A.: Carbonic anhydrase II binds to the carboxyl terminus of human band 3, the erythrocyte Cl^-/HCO_3^- exchanger. J. Biol. Chem. 273:28430, 1998.

56. Ortwein, R., Oslender-Kohnen, A., and Deuticke, B.: Band 3, the anion exchanger of the erythrocyte membrane, is also a flippase. Biochim. Biophys. Acta 1191:317, 1994.

57. Liu, S.C., Zhai, S., Palek, J., Golan, D.E., Amato, D., Hassan, K., Nurse, G.T., Babona, T., Koetzer, T., Jarolim, P., Zaik, M., and Borwein, S.: Molecular defect of the band 3 protein in Southeast Asian ovalocytosis. N. Engl. J. Med. 323:1530, 1990.

58. Peters, L.L., Shivdasani, R.A., Liu, S.C., John, K.M., Gonzalez, J.M., Brugnara, C., Gwynn, B., Mohandas, N., Alper, S.L., Orkin, S.H., and Lux, S.E.: Anion exchanger 1 (band 3) is required to prevent erythrocyte membrane surface loss but not to form the membrane skeleton. Cell 86:917, 1996.

59. Southgate, C.D., Chishti, A.H., Mitchell, B., Yi, S.J., and Palek, J.: Targeted disruption of the murine erythroid band 3 gene results in spherocytosis and severe haemolytic anaemia despite a normal membrane skeleton. Nature Genet. 14:227, 1996.

60. Jarolim, P., Rubin, H.L., Zakova, D., Storry, J., and Reid, M.E.: Characterization of seven low incidence blood group antigens carried by erythrocyte band 3 protein. Blood 92:4836, 1998.

61. Alper, S.L.: The band 3-related anion exchanger (AE) gene family. Annu. Rev. Physiol. 53:549, 1991.

62. Brosius, F.C.D., Alper, S.L., Garcia, A.M., and Lodish, H.F.: The major kidney band 3 gene transcript predicts an amino-terminal truncated band 3 polypeptide. J. Biol. Chem. 264:7784, 1989.

63. Ding, Y., Casey, J.R., and Kopito, R.R.: The major kidney AE1 isoform does not bind ankyrin (Ank1) in vitro. An essential role for the 79 NH2-terminal amino acid residues of band 3. J. Biol. Chem. 269:32201, 1994.

64. Wang, C.C., Moriyama, R., Lombardo, C.R., and Low, P.S.: Partial characterization of the cytoplasmic domain of human kidney band 3. J. Biol. Chem. 270:17892, 1995.

65. Chasis, J.A., and Narla, M.: Red cell glycophorins. Blood 80:1869, 1992.

66. Tomita, M., Furthmayr, H., and Marchesi, V.T.: Amino-acid sequence and oligosaccharide attachment sites of human erythrocyte glycophorin. Proc. Natl. Acad. Sci. USA 72:2964, 1975.

67. Tomita, M., Furthmayr, H., and Marchesi, V.T.: Primary structure of human erythrocyte glycophorin-A. Isolation and characterization of peptides and complete amino acid sequence. Biochemistry 17:4756, 1987.

68. Siebert, P.D., and Fukuda, M.: Isolation and characterization of human glycophorin A cDNA clones by a synthetic oligonucleotide approach: Nucleotide sequence and mRNA structure. Proc. Natl. Acad. Sci. USA 83:1665, 1986.

69. Siebert, P.D., and Fukuda, M.: Molecular cloning of human glycophorin-B cDNA: Nucleotide sequence and relationship to glycophorin-A. Proc. Natl. Acad. Sci. USA 85:421, 1987.

70. Colin, Y., Rahuel, C., London, J., Romeo, P.H., d'Auriol, L., Galibert, F., and Cartron, J.P.: Isolation of cDNA clones for human erythrocyte glycophorin C. J. Biol. Chem. 261:229, 1986.

71. Blanchard, D., Dahr, W., Hunnel, M., Latron, F., Beyreuther, K., and Cartron, J.P.: Glycophorin-B and C from human erythrocyte membranes: Purification and sequence analysis. J. Biol. Chem. 262:5808, 1987.

72. Kudo, S., and Fukuda, M.: Identification of a novel human glycopho-

rin, glycophorin E, by isolation of genomic clones and complementary DNA clones utilizing polymerase chain reaction. J. Biol. Chem. 265:1102, 1990.

73. Vignal, A., Rahuel, C., London, J., Cherif-Zahar, B., Schaff, S., Hattab, C., Okubo, Y., and Cartron, J.P.: A novel member of the glycophorin A and B family. Molecular cloning and expression. Eur. J. Biochem. 191:619, 1990.

74. Welsh, E.J., and Thom, D.: Molecular organization of glycophorin A: Implications for molecular interactions. Biopolymers 24:2301, 1985.

75. MacKenzie, K.R., Prestegard, J.H., and Engelman, D.M.: A transmembrane helix dimer: structure and implications. Science 276:131, 1997.

76. Vignal, A., London, J., Rahuel, C., and Cartron, J.P.: Promoter sequence and chromosomal organization of the genes encoding glycophorins A, B and E. Gene 95:289, 1990.

77. Onda, M., and Fukuda, M.: Detailed physical mapping of the genes encoding glycophorins A, B and E, as revealed by P1 plasmids containing human genomic DNA. Gene 159:225, 1995.

78. Blumenfeld, O.O., and Huang, C.H.: Molecular genetics of glycophorin MNS variants. Transfus. Clin. Biol. 4:357, 1997.

79. Reid, M.E., Anstee, D.J., Jensen, R.H., and Narla, M.: Normal membrane function of abnormal β-related erythrocyte sialoglycoproteins. Br. J. Haematol. 67:467, 1987.

80. Tanner, M.J.A., and Anstee, D.J.: The membrane change in En(AB) human erythrocytes. Absence of the major erythrocyte sialoglycoprotein. Biochem. J. 153:271, 1976.

81. Tokunaga, E., Sasakawa, S., Tamaka, K., Kawamata, H., Giles, C.M., Ikin, E.W., Poole, J., Anstee, D.J., Mawby, W., and Tanner, M.J.A.: Two apparently healthy Japanese individuals to type MᵏMᵏ have erythrocytes which lack both the blood group MN and Ss-active sialoglycoproteins. J. Immunogenet. 6:383, 1979.

82. Chishti, A.H., Palek, J., Fisher, D., Maalouf, G.J., and Liu, S.C.: Reduced invasion and growth of Plasmodium falciparum into elliptocytic red blood cells with a combined deficiency of protein 4.1, glycophorin C, and p55. Blood 87:3462, 1996.

83. Hassoun, H., Hanada, T., Lutchman, M., Sahr, K.E., Palek, J., Hanspal, M., and Chishti, A.H.: Complete deficiency glycophorin A in red blood cells from mice with targeted inactivation of the band 3 (AE1) gene. Blood 91:2146, 1998.

84. El-Maliki, B., Blanchard, D., Dahr, W., Beyreuther, K., and Cartron, J.P.: Structural homology between glycophorins C and D of human erythrocytes. Eur. J. Biochem. 183:639, 1989.

85. Colin, Y., Le Van Kim, C., Tsapis, A., Clerget, M., d'Auriol, L., London, J., and Cartron, J.P.: Human erythrocyte glycophorin-C. Gene structure and rearrangement in genetic variants. J. Biol. Chem. 264:3773, 1989.

86. High, S., and Tanner, M.J.A.: Human erythrocyte membrane sialoglycoprotein-B. The cDNA sequence suggests the absence of a cleaved N-terminal signal sequence. Biochem. J. 243:277, 1987.

87. Dahr, W., Kiedrowski, S., Blanchard, D., Hermand P., Moulds, J.J., and Cartron, J.P.: High frequency of human erythrocyte membrane sialoglycoproteins. V. Characterization of the Gerbich blood group antigens. Ge2 and Ge3. Biol. Chem. Hoppe-Seyler, 368:1375, 1987.

88. Villeval, J.L., LeVan Kim, C., Bettaieb, A., Debili, N., Colin, Y., El Maliki, B., Blanchard, D., Vainchenker, W., and Cartron, J.P.: Early expression of glycophorin-C during normal and leukemic human erythrocyte differentiation. Cancer Res. 49:2626, 1989.

89. Telen, M.J., LeVan Kim, C., Chung, A., Cartron, J.P., and Colin, Y.: Molecular basis for elliptocytosis associated with glycophorin C and D deficiency in Leach phenotype. Blood 78:1603, 1991.

90. Allosio, N., Morle, L., Bachir, D., Guetarni, D., Colonna, D., and Delaunay, J.: Red cell membrane sialoglycoprotein in homozygous and heterozygous 4.1 (B) hereditary elliptocytosis. Biochem. Biophys. Acta 816:57, 1985.

91. Reid, M.E., Takakuwa, Y., Conboy, J., Tchernia, G., and Narla, M.: Glycophorin-C content of human erythrocyte membrane is regulated by protein 4.1. Blood 75:2229, 1990.

92. Marfatia, S.M., Leu, R.A., Branton, D., and Chishti, A.H.: Identification of the protein 4.1 binding interface on glycophorin C and p55, a homologue of the Drosophila discs-large tumor suppressor protein. J. Biol. Chem. 270:715, 1995.

93. Marfatia, S.M., Morais-Cabral, J.H., Kim, A.C., Byron, O., and Chishti, A.H.: The PDZ domain of human erythrocyte p55 mediates its binding to the cytoplasmic carboxyl terminus of glycophorin C. Analysis of the binding interface by in vitro mutagenesis. J. Biol. Chem. 272:24191, 1997.

94. Hemming, N.J., Anstee, D.J., Staricoff, M.A., Tanner, M.J., and Mohandas, N.: Identification of the membrane attachment sites for protein 4.1 in the human erythrocyte. J. Biol. Chem. 270:5360, 1995.

95. Ishii, T.M., Silvia, C., Hirschberg, B., Bond, C.T., Adelman, J.P., and Maylie, J.: A human intermediate conductance calcium-activated potassium channel. Proc. Natl. Acad. Sci. USA 94:11651, 1997.

96. Vandorpe, D.H., Shmukler, B.E., Jiang, L., Lim, B., Maylie, J., Adelman, J.P., de Franceschi, L., Cappellini, M.D., Brugnara, C., and Alper, S.L.: cDNA cloning and functional characterization of the mouse Ca₂⁺-gated K⁺ channel, mIK1. Roles in regulatory volume decrease and erythroid differentiation. J. Biol. Chem. 273:21542, 1998.

97. Brugnara, C.: Erythrocyte membrane transport physiology. Curr. Opin. Hematol. 4:122, 1997.

98. Cartron, J.P., and Agre, P.: Rh blood group antigens: protein and gene structure. Semin. Hematol. 30:193, 1993.

99. Agre, P., Bonhivers, M., and Borgnia, M.J.: The aquaporins, blueprints for cellular plumbing systems. J. Biol. Chem. 273:14659, 1998.

100. Lee, M.D., King, L.S., and Agre, P.: The aquaporin family of water channel proteins in clinical medicine. Medicine (Baltimore) 76:141, 1997.

101. Chretien, S., de Figueiredo, M., and Cartron, J.P.: A single mutation inside the NPA motif of aquaporin 1 found in a Colton-null phenotype. Blood 92:5a, 1998.

102. Mathai, J.C., Mori, S., Smith, B.L., Preston, G.M., Mohandas, N., Collins, M., van Zijl, P.C., Zeidel, M.L., and Agre, P.: Functional analysis of aquaporin-1 deficient red cells. The Colton-null phenotype. J. Biol. Chem. 271:1309, 1996.

103. Ma, T.H., Yang, B.X., Gillespie, A., Carlson, E.J., Epstein, C.J., and Verkman, A.S.: Severely impaired urinary concentrating ability in transgenic mice lacking aquaporin-1 water channels. J. Biol. Chem. 273:4296, 1998.

104. Roudier, N., Verbavatz, J.M., Maurel, C., Ripoche, P., and Tacnet, F.: Evidence for the presence of aquaporin-3 in human red blood cells. J. Biol. Chem. 273:8407, 1998.

105. Winkelman, J.C., and Forget, B.G.: Erythroid and nonerythroid spectrins. Blood 81:373, 1993.

106. Bennett, V., and Lambert, S.: The spectrin skeleton: From red cells to brain. J. Clin. Invest. 87:1483, 1991.

107. Speicher, D.W., and Marchesi, V.T.: Erythrocyte spectrin is comprised of many homologous triple helical segments. Nature 311:177, 1984.

108. Sahr, K.E., Laurila, P., Kotula, L., Scarpa, A.l., Coupal, E., Leto, T.L., Linnenbach, A.J., Winkelmann, J.C., Speicher, D.W., Marchesi, V.T., Curtis, P.J., and Forget, B.G.: The complete cDNA and polypeptide sequences of human erythroid α-spectrin. J. Biol. Chem. 265:4434, 1990.

109. Winkelmann, J.C., Chang, J.G., Tse, W.T., Scarpa, A.L., Marchesi, V.T., and Forget, B.G.: Full-length sequence of the cDNA for human erythroid beta-spectrin. J. Biol. Chem. 265:11827, 1990.

110. Yan, Y., Winograd, E., Viel, A., Cronin, T., Harrison, S.C., and Branton, D.: Crystal structure of the repetitive segments of spectrin. Science 262:2027, 1993.

111. Winograd, E., Hume, D., and Branton, D.: Phasing the conformational unit of spectrin. Proc. Natl. Acad. Sci. USA 88:10788, 1991.

112. Tanaka, T., Kadowski, K., Lazarides, E., and Sobue, K.: Ca₂⁺-dependent regulation of the spectrin actin interaction by calmodulin and protein 4.1. J. Biol. Chem. 266:1134, 1991.

113. Cohen, C.M., and Langley, R.C., Jr.: Functional characterization of human erythrocyte spectrin alpha and beta chains: Association with actin and erythrocyte protein 4.1. Biochemistry 23:4488, 1984.

114. Becker, P.S., Schwartz, M.A., Morrow, J.S., and Lux, S.E.: Radiolabel-transfer cross-linking demonstrates that protein 4.1 binds to the N-terminal region of beta spectrin and to actin in binary interactions. Eur. J. Biochem. 193:827, 1990.

115. Kennedy, S.P., Warren, S.L., Forget, B.G., and Morrow, J.S.: Ankyrin binds to the 15th repetitive unit of erythroid and nonerythroid β-spectrin. J. Cell Biol. 115:267, 1991.

116. Harris, H.W., Jr., and Lux, S.E.: Structural characterzationof the phosphorylation sites of human erythrocyte spectrin. J. Biol. Chem. 225:11512, 1980.

117. Mische, S.M., and Morrow, J.S.: Multiple kinases phosphorylate spectrin. In Cohen, C.M. and Palek, J. (eds.): Molecular and Cellular Biology of Normal and Abnormal Erythrocyte Membranes. New York, Alan R. Liss, 1990, p. 113.

118. Kotula, L., Laury-Kleintop, L.D., Showe, L., Sahr, K., Linnenbach, A.J., Forget, B.G., and Curtis, P.J.: The exon-intron organization of the human erythrocyte α spectrin gene. Genomics 9:131, 1991.

119. Amin, K.M., Scarpa, A.L., Winkelmann, J.C., Curtis, P.J., and Forget, B.G.: The exon-intron organization of the human erythroid beta-spectrin gene. Genomics 18:118, 1993.

120. Gallagher, P.G., and Forget, B.G.: Spectrin genes in health and disease. Semin. Hematol. 30:4, 1993.

121. Ziemnicka-Kotula, D., Xu, J., Gu, H., Potempska, A., Kim, K.S., Jenkins, E.C., Trenkner, E., and Kotula, L.: Identification of a candidate human spectrin Src homology 3 domain-binding protein suggests a general mechanism of association of tyrosine kinases with the spectrin-based membrane skeleton. J. Biol. Chem. 273:13681, 1998.

122. Speicher, D.W., DeSilva, T.M., Speicher, K.D., Ursitti, J.A., Hembach, P., and Weglarz, L.: Location of the human red cell spectrin tetramer binding site and detection of a related "closed" hairpin loop dimer using proteolytic footprinting. J. Biol. Chem. 268:4227, 1993.

123. Morris, S.A., Eber, S.W., and Gratzer, W.B.: Structural basis for the high activation energy of spectrin self-association. FEBS Lett. 244:68, 1989.

124. Ursitti, J.A., Kotula, L., DeSilva, T.M., Curtis, P.J., and Speicher, D.W.: Mapping the human erythrocyte beta-spectrin dimer initiation site using recominant peptides and correlation of its phasing with the alpha-actinin dimer site. J. Biol. Chem. 271:6636, 1996.

125. Tse, W.T., Lecomte, M.C., Costa, F.F., Garbarz, M., Feo, C., Boivin, P., Dhermy, D., and Forget, B.: Point mutation in the β-spectrin gene associated with αᴵ/74 hereditary elliptocytosis. J. Clin. Invest. 86:909, 1990.

126. Wilmotte, R., Harper, S.L., Ursitti, J.A., Marechal, J., Delaunay, J., and Speicher, D.W.: The exon 46 encoded sequence is essential for stability of human erythroid alpha-spectrin and heterodimer formation. Blood 90:4188, 1996.

127. Viel, A., Gee, M.S., Tomooka, L., and Branton, D.: Motifs involved in interchain binding at the tail-end of spectrin. Biochim. Biophys. Acta 1384:396, 1998.

128. Alloisio, N., Morlé, L., Maréchal, J., Roux, A.F., Ducluzeau, M.T., Guetarni, D., Pothier, B., Baklouti, F., Ghanem, A., Kastally, R., and Delaunay, J.: Sp αⱽ/⁴¹: A common spectrin polymorphism at the αᴵⱽ-αⱽ domain junction. Relevance to the expression level of hereditary elliptocytosis due to a-spectrin variants located in trans. J. Clin. Invest. 87:2169, 1991.

129. Speicher, D.W., Weglarz, L., and DeSilva, T.M.: Properties of human red cell spectrin heterodimer (side-to-side) assembly and identification of an essential nucleation site. J. Biol. Chem. 267:14775, 1992.

130. Marchesi, S.L., Letsinger, J.T., Speicher, D.W., Marchesi, V.T., Agre, P., Hyun. B., and Gulati, G.: Mutant forms of spectrin α-subunits in hereditary elliptocytosis. J. Clin. Invest. 80:191, 1987.

131. Huebner, K., Palumbo, A.P., Isobe, M., Kozak, C.A., Monaco, S., Rovera, G., Croce, C.M., and Curtis, P.J.: The α-spectrin gene is on chromosome 1 in mouse and man. Proc. Natl. Acad. Sci. USA 82:3790, 1985.

132. Fukushima, Y., Byers, M.G., Watkins, P.C., Winkelmann, J.C., Forget, B.G., and Shows, T.B.: Assignment of the gene for β-spectrin (SPTB) to chromosome 14q23-q24.2 by in situ hybridization. Cytogenet. Cell Genet. 53:232, 1990.

133. Winkelmann, J.C., Costa, F.F., Linzie, B.L., and Forget, B.G.: β spectrin in human skeletal muscle: Tissue-specific diffferential processing of 3′ β-spectrin pre-mRNA generates a β-spectrin isoform with a unique carboxyl terminus. J. Biol. Chem. 265:20449, 1990.

134. Leto, T.L., Fortugno-Erikson, D., Barton, B.E., Yang-Feng, T.L., Francke, U., Morrow, J.S., Marchesi, V.T., and Benz, E.J., Jr.: Comparison of nonerythroid α-spectrin genes reveals strict homology among diverse species. Mol. Cell Biol. 8:1, 1988.

135. Ohara, O., Ohara, R., Yamakawa, H., Nakajima, D., and Nakayama, M.: Characterization of a new beta-spectrin gene which is predominantly expressed in brain. Brain Res. Mol. Brain Res. 57:181, 1998.

136. Stankewich, M.C., Tse, W.T., Peters, L.L., Chng, Y., John, K.M., Stabach, P.R., Devarajan, P., Morrow, J.S., and Lux, S.E.: A widely expressed beta-III spectrin associated with Golgi and cytoplasmic vesicles. Proc. Natl. Acad. Sci. USA 95:14158, 1998.

137. Leto, T.L. and Marchesi, V.T.: A structural model of human erythrocyte protein 4.1. J. Biol. Chem. 259:4603, 1984.

138. Turunen, O., Sainio, M., Jaaskelainen, J., Carpen, O., and Vaheri, A.: Structure-function relationships in the ezrin family and the effect of tumor-associated point mutations in neurofibromatosis 2 protein. Biochim. Biophys. Acta 1387:1, 1998.

139. Tsukita, S., and Yonemura, S.: ERM (ezrin/radixin/moesin) family: from cytoskeleton to signal transduction. Curr. Opin. Cell Biol. 9:70, 1997.

140. Bretscher, A., Reczek, D., and Berryman, M.: Ezrin: a protein requiring conformational activation to link microfilaments to the plasma membrane in the assembly of cell surface structures. J. Cell Sci. 110:3011, 1997.

141. Ward, R.E., Lamb, R.S., and Fehon, R.G.: A conserved functional domain of *Drosophila* coracle is required for localization at the septate junction and has membrane-organizing activity. J. Cell Biol. 140:1463, 1998.

142. Parra, M., Gascard, P., Walensky, L.D., Snyder, S.H., Mohandas, N., and Conboy, J.G.: Cloning and characterization of 4.1G (EPB41L2), a new member of the skeletal protein 4.1 (EPB41) gene family. Genomics 49:298, 1998.

143. Walensky, L.D., Gascard, P., Fields, M.E., Blackshaw, S., Conboy, J.G., Mohandas, N., and Snyder, S.H.: The 13-kD FK506 binding protein, FKBP13, interacts with a novel homologue of the erythrocyte membrane cytoskeletal protein 4.1. J. Cell Biol. 141:143, 1998.

144. Wolfe, L.C., Lux, S.E., and Ohanian, V.: Regulation of spectrin-actin binding by protein 4.1 and polyphosphates. J. Cell Biol. 87:203a, 1980.

145. Cohen, C.M., Liu, S.C., Lawler, J., and Palek, J.: Identification of the protein 4.1 binding site to phosphatidylserine vesicles. Biochemistry 27:614, 1988.

146. Miller, J.A., Gravallese, E., and Bunn, H.F.: Nonenzymatic glycosylation of erythrocyte membrane proteins. J. Clin. Invest. 65:896, 1980.

147. Inaba, N., Gupta, K.C., Kuwabara, M., Takahashi, I., Benz, E.J., Jr., and Maeda, Y.: Deamidation of human erythrocyte protein 4.1: Possible role in aging. Blood. 79:3355, 1992.

148. Tang, K.T., Qin, Z., Leto, T., Marchesi, V.T., and Benz, E.J., Jr.: Membrane skeletal protein 4.1 of human erythroid and non-erythroid cells is composed of multiple isoforms with novel sizes, functions and tissue specific expression. *In* Cohen, C.M., and Palek, J. (eds.): Cellular and Molecular Biology of Normal and Abnormal Erythroid Membranes. New York, Alan R. Liss, 1990, p. 43.

149. Conboy, J.: The role of alternative pre-mRNA splicing in regulating the structure and function of skeletal protein 4.1. Proc. Soc. Exper. Biol. Med. 220:73, 1999.

150. Conboy, J., Kan, Y.W., Shobet, S.B., and Narla, M.: Molecular cloning of protein 4.1: A major structural element of the human erythrocyte membrane cytoskeleton. Proc. Natl. Acad. Sci. USA 83:9512, 1986.

151. Tang, T.K., Leto, T.L., Correas, I., Alonso, M., Marchesi, V.T., and Benz, E.J., Jr.: Selective expression of an erythroid-specific isoform of protein 4.1. Proc. Natl. Acad. Sci. USA 85:3713, 1988.

152. Tang, T.K., Qin, Z., Leto, T.L., Marchesi, V.T., and Benz, E.J., Jr.: Heterogeneity of mRNA and protein products arising from the protein 4.1 gene in erythroid and nonerythroid tissues. J. Cell Biol. 110:617, 1990.

153. Huang, J.P., Tang, C.J., Kou, G.H., Marchesi, V.T., Benz, E.J., Jr., Tang, T.K.: Genomic structure of the locus encoding protein 4.1. Structural basis for complex combination patterns of tissue-specific alternative RNA splicing. J. Biol. Chem. 268:3758, 1993.

154. Ngai, J., Stack, J.W., Moon, R.T., and Lazarides, E.: Regulated expression of multiple chicken erythroid membrane skeleton protein 4.1 variants is governed by differential RNA processing and translation control. Proc. Natl. Acad. Sci. USA 84:4432, 1987.

155. Conboy, J.G., Chan, J.Y., Chasis, J.A., Kan, Y.W., and Narla, M.: Tissue and development-specific alternative RNA splicing regulates expression of multiple isoforms of erythroid membrane protein 4.1. J. Biol. Chem. 266:8273, 1991.

156. Correas, I., Leto, T.L., Speicher, D.W., and Marchesi, V.T.: Identification of the functional site of erythrocyte protein 4.1 involved in spectrin actin binding. J. Biol. Chem. 261:3310, 1986.

157. Gascard, P., Lee, G., Coulombel, L., Auffray, I., Lum, M., Parra, M., Conboy, J.G., Mohandas, N., and Chasis, J.A.: Characterization of multiple isoforms of protein 4.1R expressed during erythroid terminal differentiation. Blood 92:4404, 1998.

158. Horne, W.C., Huang S.C., Becker, P.S., Tang, T.K., and Benz, E.J., Jr.: Tissue-specific alternative splicing of protein 4.1 inserts an exon necessary for formation of the ternary complex with erythrocyte spectrin and F-actin. Blood 82:2558, 1993.

159. Chasis, J.A., Coulombel, L., Conboy, J., McGee, S., Andrews, K., Kan, Y.W., and Mohandas, N.: Differentiation-associated switches in protein 4.1 expression. Synthesis of multiple structural isoforms during normal human erythropoiesis. J. Clin. Invest. 91:329, 1993.

160. Lallena, M.J., Martinez, C., Valcarcel, J., and Correas, I.: Functional association of nuclear protein 4.1 with pre-mRNA splicing factors. J. Cell Sci. 111:1963, 1998.

161. Mattagajasingh, S.N., Huang, S.C., Hartenstein, J.S., Snyder, M., Marchesi, V.T., and Benz, E.J.: A nonerythroid isoform of protein 4.1R interacts with the nuclear mitotic apparatus (NuMA) protein. J. Cell Biol. 145:29, 1999.

162. Chishti, A.H.: Function of p55 and its nonerythroid homologues. Curr. Opin. Hematol. 5:116, 1998.

163. Cohen, A.R., Woods, D.F., Marfatia, S.M., Walther, Z., Chishti, A.H., Anderson, J.M., and Woods, D.F.: Human CASK/LIN-2 binds syndecan-2 and protein 4.1 and localizes to the basolateral membrane of epithelial cells. J. Cell Biol. 142:129, 1998.

164. Wu, H., Reuver, S.M., Kuhlendahl, S., Chung, W.J., and Garner, C.C.: Subcellular targeting and cytoskeletal attachment of SAP97 to the epithelial lateral membrane. J. Cell Sci. 111:2365, 1998.

165. Shi, Z.T., Afzal, V., Coller, B., et al.: Protein 4.1R-deficient mice are viable but have erythroid membrane skeleton abnormalities. J. Clin. Inv. 103:331, 1999.

166. Bennett, V.: Ankyrins. Adaptors between diverse plasma membrane proteins and the cytoplasm. J. Biol. Chem. 267:8703, 1992.

167. Davis, J.Q., and Bennett, V.: Brain ankyrin purification of a 72,000 M$_r$ spectrin binding domain. J. Biol. Chem. 259:1874, 1984.

168. Wallin, R., Culp, E.N., and Coleman, D.B.: A structural model of human erythrocyte band 2.1: Alignment of chemical and functional domains. Proc. Natl. Acad. Sci. USA 81:4095, 1984.

169. Weaver, D.C., and Marchesi, V.T.: The structural basis of ankyrin function, Parts I and II. J. Biol. Chem. 259:6165; 6170, 1984.

170. Cianci, C.D., Giorgi, M., and Morrow, J.S.: Phosphorylation of ankyrin downregulates its cooperative interaction with spectrin and protein 3. J. Cell Biochem. 37:301, 1988.

171. Lu, P.-W., Soong, C.F., and Tao, M.: Phosphorylation of ankyrin decreases its affinity for spectrin tetramer. J. Biol. Chem. 262:14958, 1985.

172. Lux, S.E., John, K.M., and Bennett, V.: Analysis of cDNA for human erythrocyte ankyrin indicates a repeated structure with homology to tissue-differentiation and cell-cycle control proteins. Nature 344:36, 1990.

173. Lambert, S., Yu, H., Prchal, J.T., Lawler, J., Ruff, P., Speicher, D., Cheung, M.C., Kan, Y.W., and Palek, J.: cDNA sequence for human erythrocyte ankyrin. Proc. Natl. Acad. Sci. USA 87:1730, 1990.

174. Bork, P.: Hundreds of ankyrin-like repeats in functionally diverse proteins: mobile modules that cross phyla horizontally? Proteins 17:363, 1993.

175. Michaely, P., and Bennett, V.: The membrane-binding domain of ankyrin contains four independently folded subdomains, each comprised of six ankyrin repeats. J. Biol. Chem. 268:22703, 1993.

176. Michaely, P., and Bennett, V.: The ANK repeats of erythrocyte ankyrin form two distinct but cooperative binding sites for the erythrocyte anion exchanger. J. Biol. Chem. 270:22050, 1995.

177. Gorina, S., and Pavletich, N.: Structure of the p53 tumor suppressor bound to the ankyrin and SH3 domains of 53BP2. Science 274:1001, 1996.

178. Jacobs, M.D., and Harrison, S.C.: Structure of an I kappa B alpha/NF-kappa B complex. Cell 95:749, 1998.

179. Huxford, T., Huang, D.B., Malek, S., and Ghosh, G.: The crystal structure of the I kappa B alpha/NF-kappa B complex reveals mechanisms of NF-kappa B inactivation. Cell 95:759, 1998.

180. Batchelor, A.H., Piper, D.E., de la Brousse, F.C., McKnight, S.L., and Wolberger, C.: The structure of GABPalpha/beta: an ETS domain-ankyrin repeat heterodimer bound to DNA. Science 279:1037, 1998.

181. Luh, F.Y., Archer, S.J., Domaille, P.J., Smith, B.O., Owen, D., Brotherton, D.H., Raine, A.R., Xu, X., Brizuela, L., Brenner, S.L., and Laue, E.D.: Structure of the cyclin-dependent kinase inhibitor p19Ink4d. Nature 389:999, 1997.

182. Davis, L.H., Davis, J.Q., and Bennett, V.: Ankyrin regulation: an alternatively spliced segment of the regulatory domain functions as an intramolecular modulator. J. Biol. Chem. 267:18966, 1992.

183. Gallagher, P.G., Tse, W.T., Scarpa, A.L., Lux, S.E., and Forget, B.G.: Structure and organization of the human ankyrin-1 gene: basis for complexity of pre-mRNA processing. J. Biol. Chem. 272:19220, 1997

184. Gallagher, P.G., and Forget, B.G.: An alternate promoter directs expression of a truncated, muscle-specific isoform of the human ankyrin 1 gene. J. Biol. Chem. 273:1339, 1998.

185. Birkenmeier, C.S., Sharp, J.J., Gifford, E.J., Deveau, S.A., and Barker,

J.E.: An alternative first exon in the distal end of the erythroid ankyrin gene leads to production of a small isoform containing an NH2-terminal membrane anchor. Genomics 50:79, 1998.

186. Zhou, D., Birkenmeier, C.S., Williams, M.W., Sharp, J.J., Barker, J.E., and Bloch, R.J.: Small, membrane-bound, alternatively spliced forms of ankyrin 1 associated with the sarcoplasmic reticulum of mammalian skeletal muscle. J. Cell Biol. 136:621, 1997.

187. Otto, E., Kunimoto, M., McLaughlin, T., and Bennett, V.: Isolation and characterization of cDNAs encoding human brain ankyrins reveal a family of alternatively spliced genes. J. Cell Biol. 114:241, 1991.

188. Peters, L.L., John, K.M., Lu, F.M., Eicher, E.M., Higgins, A., Yialamas, M., Turtzo, L.C., Otsuka, A.J., and Lux, S.E.: Ank3 (epithelial ankyrin), a widely distributed new member of the ankyrin gene family and the major ankyrin in kidney, is expressed in alternatively spliced forms, including forms that lack the repeat domain. J. Cell Biol. 130:313, 1995.

189. Kordeli, E., Lambert, S., and Bennett, V.: AnkyrinG. A new ankyrin gene with neural-specific isoforms localized at the axonal initial segment and node of Ranvier. J. Biol. Chem. 270:2352, 1995.

190. Lambert, S., and Bennett, V.: Postmitotic expression of ankyrinR and beta R-spectrin in discrete neuronal populations of the rat brain. J. Neurosci. 13:3725, 1993.

191. Lux, S.C., John, K.M., and Bennett, V.: Analysis of cDNA for human erythrocyte ankyrin indicates a repeated structure with homology to tissue-differentiation and cell-cycle control proteins. Nature 344:36, 1990.

192. Lambert, S., Yu, H., Prchal, J.T., and Palek, J.: The cDNA sequence for human erythrocyte ankyrin. Proc. Natl. Acad. Sci. USA 87:1730, 1990.

193. Gallagher, P.G., Sabatino, D.E., Garrett, L.J., Bodine, D.M., and Forget, B.G.: Erythroid-specific expression of the human ankyrin 1 (Ank1) gene in vitro and in vivo is mediated by a promoter that requires GATA-1 and CACCC-binding proteins for its activity. Blood 90:7a, 1998

194. Peters, L.L., and Barker, J.E.: Spontaneous and targeted mutations in erythrocyte membrane skeleton genes: mouse models of hereditary spherocytosis. In press, 1999.

195. Zhou, D., Lambert, S., Malen, P.L., Carpenter, S., Boland, L.M., and Bennett, V.: Ankyrin G is required for clustering of voltage-gated Na channels at axon initial segments and for normal action potential firing. Mol. Biol. Cell 9:37a, 1998.

196. Tuvia, S., Buhusi, M., Reedy, M., and Bennett, V.: Ankyrin-B: a candidate for sorting and organization of sarcoplasmic reticulum proteins involved in Ca_2^+ homeostasis. Mol. Biol. Cell 9:411a, 1998.

197. Korsgren, C., Lawler, J., Lambert, S., Speicher, P., and Cohen, C.M.: Complete amino acid sequence and homologies of human erythrocyte membrane protein band 4.2. Proc. Natl. Acad. Sci. USA 87:613, 1990.

198. Korsgren, C., and Cohen, C.M.: Association of human erythrocyte band 4.2 binding to ankyrin and to the cytoplasmic domain of band 3. J. Biol. Chem. 263:10212, 1988.

199. Sung, L.A., Chien, S., Chang, L.S., Lambert, K., Bliss, S.A., Bouhassira, E.E., Nagel, R.L., Schwartz, R.S., and Rybicki, A.C.: Molecular cloning of human protein 4.2: A major component of the erythrocyte membrane. Proc. Natl. Acad. Sci. USA 87:955, 1990.

200. Sung, L.A., Chien, S., Fan, Y.S., Lin, C.C., Lambert, K., Zhu, L., Lam, J.S., and Chang, L.S.: Human erythrocyte protein 4.2: Isoform expression, differential splicing, and chromosomal assignment. Blood 79:2763, 1992.

201. Folk, J.G.: Transglutaminases. Ann. Rev. Biochem. 49:517, 1980.

202. Yawata, Y.: Red cell membrane protein band 4.2: phenotypic, genetic and electron microscopic aspects. Biochim. Biophys. Acta 1204:131, 1994.

203. Rybicki, A.C., Heath, R., Wolf, J.S., Lubin, B., and Schwartz, R.S.: Deficiency of protein 4.2 in erythrocytes from a patient with a Coombs negative hemolytic anemia: Evidence for a role of protein 4.2 in stabilizing ankyrin on the membrane. J. Clin. Invest. 81:898, 1988.

204. Rybicki, A.C., Schwartz, R.S., Hustedt, E.J., and Cobb, C.E.: Increased rotational mobility and extractability of band 3 from protein 4.2-deficient erythrocyte membranes: evidence of a role for protein 4.2 in strengthening the band 3-cytoskeleton linkage. Blood 88:2745, 1996.

205. Wada, H., Kanzaki, A., Yawata, A., Inoue, T., Kaku, M., Takezono, M., Sugihara, T., Yamada, O., and Yawata, Y.: Late expression of red cell membrane protein 4.2 in normal human erythroid maturation with seven isoforms of the protein 4.2 gene. Exper. Hematol. 27:54, 1999.

206. Azim, A.C., Marfatia, S.M., Korsgren, C., Dotimas, E., Cohen, C.M., and Chishti, A.H.: Human erythrocyte dematin and protein 4.2 (pallidin) are ATP binding proteins. Biochemistry 35:3001, 1996.

207. Matsuoka, Y., Hughes, C.A., and Bennett, V.: Adducin regulation. Definition of the calmodulin-binding domain and sites of phosphorylation by protein kinases A and C. J. Biol. Chem. 271:25157, 1996.

208. Kuhlman, P.A., Hughes, C.A., Bennett, V., and Fowler, V.M.: A new function for adducin. Calcium/calmodulin-regulated capping of the barbed ends of actin filaments. J. Biol. Chem. 271:7986, 1996.

209. Kuhlman, P.A., and Fowler, V.M.: Purification and characterization of an alpha 1 beta 2 isoform of CapZ from human erythrocytes: cytosolic location and inability to bind to Mg_2^+ ghosts suggest that erythrocyte actin filaments are capped by adducin. Biochemistry 36:13461, 1997.

210. Li, X., and Bennett, V.: Identification of the spectrin subunit and domains required for formation of spectrin/adducin/actin complexes. J. Biol. Chem. 271:15695, 1996.

211. Li, X., Matsuoka, Y., and Bennett, V.: Adducin preferentially recruits spectrin to the fast growing ends of actin filaments in a complex requiring the MARCKS-related domain and a newly defined oligomerization domain. J. Biol. Chem. 273:19329, 1998.

212. Matsuoka, Y., Li, X., and Bennett, V.: Adducin is an in vivo substrate for protein kinase C: phosphorylation in the MARCKS-related domain inhibits activity in promoting spectrin-actin complexes and occurs in many cells, including dendritic spines of neurons. J. Cell Biol. 142:485, 1998.

213. Gilligan, D.M., Lozovatsky, L., Gwynn, B., Brugrara, C., Mohandas, N., and Peters, L.L.: Targeted disruption of the beta-adducin gene (Add2) causes red blood cell spherocytosis in mice. Proc. Natl. Acad. Sci., in press, 1999.

214. Palek, J., and Lambert, S.: Genetics of the red cell membrane skeleton. Semin. Hematol. 27:290, 1990.

215. Koury, M.J., Bondurant, M.C., and Rana, S.S.: Changes in erythroid membrane proteins during erythropoietin-mediated terminal differentiation. J. Cell. Physiol. 133:438, 1987.

216. Lazarides, E.: From genes to structural morphogenesis: The genesis and epigenesis of a red blood cell. Cell 51:345, 1987.

217. Cox, J.V., Stack, J.H., and Lazarides, E.: Erythroid anion transporter assembly is mediated by a development regulated recruitment onto a preassembled membrane cytoskeleton. J. Cell Biol. 105:1405, 1987.

218. Woods, C.M., Boyer, B., Vogt, P.K., and Lazarides, E.: Control of erythroid differentiation: Asynchronous expression of the anion transporter and the peripheral components of the membrane skeleton in AEV- and S13-transformed cells. J. Cell Biol. 103:1789, 1986.

219. Moon, R.T., and Lazarides, E.: Biogenesis of the avian erythroid membrane skeleton: Receptor-mediated assembly and stabilization of ankyrin (globin) and spectrin. J. Cell Biol. 98:1899, 1984.

220. Blikstad, I., Nelson, W.J., Moon R.T., and Lazarides, E.: Synthesis and assembly of spectrin during avian erythropoiesis: Stoichiometric assembly, but unequal synthesis of α and β spectrin. Cell 32:1081, 1983.

221. Hanspal, M., and Palek, J.: Synthesis and assembly of membrane skeletal proteins in mammalian red cell precursors. J. Cell Biol. 105:147, 1987.

222. Peters, L.L., White R.A., Birkenmeier, C.S., Bloom ML, Lux, S.E., and Barker, J.E.: Changing in cytoskeletal mRNA expression and protein synthesis patterns during murine erythropoiesis in vivo. Proc. Natl. Acad. Sci. USA 89:5749, 1992.

223. Bodine, D.M., Birkenmeier, C.S., and Barker, J.E.: Spectrin deficient inherited hemolytic anemias in the mouse: Characterization by spectrin synthesis and mRNA activity in reticulocytes. Cell 37:721, 1984.

224. Glomset, J., Assmann, G., Gjone, E., et al.: Lecithin: cholesterol acyltransferase deficiency and fish eye disease. In Scriver, C., Beaudet, A., Sly, W. (eds.): The Metabolic and Molecular Bases of Inherited Disease. 7th. New York, McGraw-Hill, 1995, p. 1933.

225. Kane, J., and Havel, R.: Disorders of the biogenesis and secretion of lipoproteins containing the B apolipoproteins. In Scriver, C., Beaudet, A., Sly, W. (eds.): The Metabolic and Molecular Bases of Inherited Disease. 7th. New York, McGraw-Hill, 1995, p. 1853.

226. Gallagher, P.G., Forget, B.G., and Lux, S.E.: Disorders of the Erythrocyte Membrane. In Nathan, D.G., Orkin, S.H. (eds.): Hematology of Infancy and Childhood. 5th. Philadelphia, W.B. Saunders, 1997, p. 544.

227. Gallagher, P.G., and Ferriera, J.D.: Molecular basis of erythrocyte membrane disorders. Curr. Opin. Hematol. 4:128, 1997.

228. Joiner, C.H., Franco, R.S., Jiang, M., Franco, M.S., Barker, J.E., and

Lux, S.E.: Increased cation permeability in mutant mouse red blood cells with defective membrane skeletons. Blood 86:4307, 1995.

229. De Franceschi, L., Olivieri, O., Miraglia del Giudice, E., Perrotta, S., Sabato, V., Corrocher, R., and Iolascon, A.: Membrane cation and anion transport activities in erythrocytes of hereditary spherocytosis: effects of different membrane protein defects. Am. J. Hematol. 55:121, 1997.

230. Jarolim, P., Brabec, V., Tesar, V., and Rysava, R.: Association of a band 3 gene mutation with renal tubular acidosis. Blood 88:4a, 1996.

231. Lima, P.R.M., Gontijo, J.A.R., Lopes de Faria, J.B., Costa, F.F., and Saad, S.T.O.: Band 3 Campinas: a novel splicing mutation in the band 3 gene (AE1) associated with hereditary spherocytosis, hyperactivity of Na^+/Li^+ countertransport and an abnormal renal bicarbonate handling. Blood 90:2810, 1997.

232. Bruce, L.J., Cope, D.L., Jones, G.K., Schofield, A.E., Burley, M., Povey, S., Unwin, R.J., Wrong, O., and Tanner, M.J.: Familial distal renal tubular acidosis is associated with mutations in the red cell anion exchanger (Band 3, AE1) gene. J. Clin. Invest. 100:1693, 1997.

233. Jarolim, P., Shayakul, C., Prabakaran, D., et al.: Autosomal dominant distal renal tubular acidosis in three families with heterozygosity for the R589H mutaton in the AE1 (Band 3) Cl^-/HCO_3^- exchanger. J. Biol. Chem. 273:6380, 1998.

234. Tanphaichitr, V.S., Sumboonnanonda, A., Ideguchi, H., Shayakul, C., Brugnara, C., Takao, M., Veerakul, G., and Alper, S.L.: Novel AE1 mutations in recessive distal renal tubular acidosis—Loss-of-function is rescued by glycophorin A. J. Clin. Invest. 102:2173, 1998.

235. Karet, F.E., Gainza, F.J., Gyory, A.Z., et al.: Mutations in the chloride-bicarbonate exchanger gene AE1 cause autosomal dominant but not autosomal recessive distal renal tubular acidosis. Proc. Natl. Acad. Sci. USA 95:6337, 1998.

236. Gallagher, P.G., and Forget, B.G.: Hematologically important mutations—Band 3 and Protein 4.2 variants in hereditary spherocytosis. Blood Cells Mol. Dis. 23:417, 1997.

237. Gallagher, P.G., and Forget, B.G.: Hematologically important mutations: Spectrin and ankyrin variants in hereditary spherocytosis. Blood Cells Mol. Dis. 24:539, 1998.

238. Gilsanz, F., Ricard, M.P., and Millan, I.: Diagnosis of hereditary spherocytosis with dual-angle differential light scattering. Am. J. Clin. Pathol. 100:119, 1993.

239. Mentzer, W.C., Jr., Iarocci, T.A., and Narla, M.: Modulation of erythrocyte membrane mechanical fragility by 2,3 diphosphoglycerate in neonatal poikilocytosis/elliptocytosis syndrome. J. Clin. Invest. 79:943, 1987.

240. Jonsson, J.J., Renieri, A., Gallagher, P.G., Kashtan, C.E., Merill, E., Bruttini, M., Piccini, M., Ballabio, A., and Pober, B.R.: Alport syndrome, mental retardation, midface hypoplasia, and elliptocytosis: a new X-linked contiguous gene deletion syndrome. Am. J. Med. Genet. 35:273, 1997.

241. Cattani, J.A., Gibson, F.D., Alpers, M.P., and Crane, G.G.: Hereditary ovalocytosis and reduced susceptibility to malaria in Papua New Guinea. Trans. R. Soc. Trop. Med. Hyg. 81:705, 1987.

242. Fix, A.G., Baer, A.S., and Lie-Injo, L.E.: The mode of inheritance of ovalocytosis/elliptocytosis in Malaysian Orang Asli families. Hum. Genet. 61:250, 1982.

243. Serjeantson, S., Bryson, K., Amato, D., and Babona, D.: Malaria and hereditary ovalocytosis. Hum. Genet. 37:161, 1977.

244. Foo, L.C., Rekhraj, V., Chiang, G.L., and Mak, J.W.: Ovalocytosis protects against severe malaria parasitemia in the Malayan aborigines. Am. J. Trop. Med. Hyg. 47:271, 1992.

245. Genton, B., al-Yaman, F., Mgone, C.S., Alexander, N., Paniu, M.M., Alpers, M.P., and Mokela, D.: Ovalocytosis and cerebral malaria. Nature 378:564, 1995.

246. Hadley, T., Saul, A., Lamont, G., Hudson, D.E., Miller, L.H., and Kidson, C.: Resistance of Melanesian elliptocytes (ovalocytes) to invasion by Plasmodium knowlesi and Plasmodium falciparum malaria parasites in vitro. J. Clin. Invest. 71:780, 1983.

247. Liu, S.C., Zhai, S., Palek, J., et al.: Molecular defect of the band 3 protein in southeast Asian ovalocytosis. N. Engl. J. Med. 323:1530, 1990.

248. Saul, A., Lamont, G., Sawyer, W.H., and Kidson, C.: Decreased membrane deformability in Melanesian ovalocytes from Papua New Guinea. J. Cell Biol. 98:1348, 1984.

249. Mohandas, N., Lie-Injo, L.E., Friedman, M., and Mak, J.W.: Rigid membranes of Malayan ovalocytes: a likely genetic barrier against malaria. Blood 63:1385, 1984.

250. Mohandas, N., Winardi, R., Knowles, D., Leung, A., Parra, M., George, E., Conboy, J., and Chasis, J.: Molecular basis for membrane rigidity of hereditary ovalocytosis. A novel mechanism involving the cytoplasmic domain of band 3. J Clin. Invest. 89:686, 1992.

251. Schofield, A.E., Tanner, M.J., Pinder, J.C., Clough, B., Bayley, P.M., Nash, G.B., Dluzewski, A.R., Reardon, D.M., Cox, T.M., Wilson, R.J., and Gratzer, W.B.: Basis of unique red cell membrane properties in hereditary ovalocytosis. J. Mol. Biol. 223:949, 1992.

252. Jarolim, P., Palek, J., Amato, D., Hassan, K., Sapak, P., Nurse, G.T., Rubin, H.L., Zhai, S., Sahr, K.E., and Liu, S.C.: Deletion in erythrocyte band 3 gene in malaria-resistant Southeast Asian ovalocytosis. Proc. Natl. Acad. Sci. USA 88:11022, 1991.

253. Lande, W.M., Thiemann, P.V., and Mentzer, W.C., Jr.: Missing band 7 membrane protein in two patients with high Na, low K erythrocytes. J. Clin. Invest. 70:1273, 1982.

254. Morle, L., Pothier, B., Alloisio, N., Feo, C., Garay, R., Bost, M., and Delaunay, J.: Reduction of membrane band 7 and activation of volume simulated (K^+, Cl^-)-cotransport in a case of congenital stomatocytosis. Br. J. Haematol. 71:141, 1989.

255. Eber, S.W., Lande, W.M., Iarocci, T.A., Mentzer, W.C., Hohn, P., Wiley, J.S., and Schroter, W.: Hereditary stomatocytosis: Consistent association with an integral membrane protein deficiency. Br. J. Haematol. 72:452, 1989.

256. Stewart, G.W., Hepworth-Jones, B.E., Keen, J.N., Dash, B.C., Argent, A.C., and Casimir, C.M.: Isolation of cDNA coding for an ubiquitous membrane protein deficient in high Na^+, low K^+ stomatocytic erythrocytes. Blood 79:1593, 1992.

257. Zhu, Y., Pastzy, C., Turetsky, T., Tsai, S., Kuypers, F.A., Lee, G., Cooper, P., Gallagher, P., Stevens, M., Rubin, E., Mohandas, N., and Mentzer, W.C. Stomatocytosis is absent in "stomatin" deficient red cells. Blood 93:2404, 1999.

258. Carella, M., Stewart, G., Ajetunmobi, J.F., Perrotta, S., Grootenboer, S., Tchernia, G., Delaunay, J., Totaro, A., Zelante, L., Gasparini, P., and Iolascon, A.: Genomewide search for dehydrated hereditary stomatocytosis (hereditary xerocytosis): mapping of locus to chromosome 16 (16q23-qter). Am. J. Hum. Genet. 63:810, 1998.

259. Nash, R., and Shojania, A.M.: Hematological aspects of Rh deficiency syndrome: A case report and a review of the literature. Am. J. Hematol. 24:267, 1987.

260. Cherif-Zahar, B., Matassi, G., Raynal, V., Gane, P., Delaunay, J., Arrizabalaga, B., and Cartron, J.P.: Rh-deficiency of the regulator type caused by splicing mutations in the human RH50 gene. Blood 92:2535, 1998.

261. Huang, C.H., Cheng, G.J., Liu, Z., Chen, Y., Reid, M.E., and Okubo, Y.: Identification of novel missense mutations of the RhAG (Rh50) gene in Rh^{null} cases of the regulator type. Blood 92:5a, 1998.

262. Huang, C.H., Cheng, G.J., Reid, M.E., and Chen, Y.: Rh mod syndrome: A family study of the translation-initiator mutation in the Rh50 glycoprotein gene. Am. J. Hum. Genet. 64:108, 1999.

263. Cherif-Zahar, B., Raynal, V., Gane, P., Mattei, M.G., Bailly, P., Gibbs, B., Colin, Y., and Cartron, J.P.: Candidate gene acting as a suppressor of the Rh locus in most cases of Rh-deficiency. Nat. Genet. 12:168, 1996.

264. Cherif-Zahar, B., Matassi, G., Raynal, V., Gane, P., Mempel, W., Perex, C., and Cartron, J.P.: Molecular defects of the RhCe gene in Rh-deficient individuals of the amorph type. Blood 92:639, 1998.

265. Huang, C.H.: The human Rh50 glycoprotein gene. Structural organization and associated splicing defect resulting in Rh^{null} disease. J. Biol. Chem. 273:2207, 1998.

266. Huang, C.H., Chen, Y., Reid, M.E., and Seidl, C.: Rh^{null} disease: the amorph type results from a novel double mutation in RhCe gene on D-negative background. Blood 92:664, 1998.

267. Huang, C.H., Liu, Z., Cheng, G., and Chen, Y.: Rh50 glycoprotein gene and Rh^{null} disease: a silent splice donor in trans to a $Gly^{279}->Glu$ missense mutation in the conserved transmembrane segment. Blood 92:1776, 1998.

268. Redman, C.M., and Marsh, W.L.: The Kell blood group system and the McLeod phenotype. Semin. Hematol. 30:209, 1993.

269. Ho, M., Chelly, J., Carter, N., Danek, A., Crocker, P., and Monaco, A.P.: Isolation of the gene for McLeod syndrome that encodes a novel membrane transport protein. Cell 77:869, 1994.

270. Khamlichi, S., Bailly, P., Blanchard, D., Goossens, D., Cartron, J.P., and Bertrand, O.: Purification and partial characterization of the erythrocyte Kx protein deficient in McLeod patients. Eur. J. Biochem. 228:931, 1995.

271. Francke, U., Ochs, H.D., de Martinville, B., Giacalone, J., Lindgren, V., Disteche, C., Pagon, R.A., Hofker, M.H., van Ommen, G.J., Pearson, P.L., et al.: Minor Xp21 chromosome deletion in a male associated with expression of Duchenne muscular dystrophy, chronic granulomatous disease, retinitis pigmentosa, and McLeod syndrome. Am. J. Hum. Genet. 37:250, 1985.

272. Low, P.S., Waugh, S.M., Zinke, K., and Drenckhahn, D.: The role of hemoglobin denaturation and band 3 clustering in red blood cell aging. Science 227:531, 1985.

273. Turrini, F., Arese, P., Yuan, J., and Low, P.S.: Clustering of integral membrane proteins of the human erythrocyte membrane stimulates autologous IgG binding, complement deposition and phagocytosis. J. Biol. Chem. 266:23611, 1991.

274. Low, P.S., and Kannan, R.: Effect of hemoglobin denaturation on membrane structure and IgG binding: Role in red cell aging. In Brewer, G. (ed.): The Red Cell. Seventh Ann Arbor Conference. New York, Alan R. Liss, 1989, p. 525.

275. Kannan, R., Labotka, R., and Low, P.S.: Isolation and characterization of the hemochrome-stabilized membrane protein aggregates from sickle erythrocytes: Major site of autologous antibody binding. J. Biol. Chem. 263:13766, 1988.

276. Yuan, J., Kannan, R., Shinar, E., Rachmilewitz, E.A., and Low, P.S.: Isolation, characterization and immunoprecipitation studies of immune complexes from membranes of β-thalassemic erythrocytes. Blood 79:3007, 1992.

277. Waugh, S.M., Willardson, B.M., Kannan, R., Labotka, R.J., and Low, P.S.: Heinz bodies induce clustering of band 3, glycophorin and ankyrin in sickle cell erythrocytes. J. Clin. Invest. 78:1155, 1986.

278. Yuan, J., Bunyaratvej, A., Fucharoen, S., Fung, C., Shinar, E., and Schrier, S.L.: The instability of the membrane skeleton in thalassemic red blood cells. Blood 86:3945, 1995.

279. Shinar, E., Shaley, O., Rachmilewitz, E.A., and Schreier, S.L.: Erythrocyte membrane skeleton abnormalities in severe beta thalassemia. Blood 70:158, 1987.

280. Platt, O.S., and Falcone, J.F.: Membrane protein interactions in sickle red blood cells: evidence of abnormal protein 3 function. Blood 86:1992, 1995.

281. Aljurf, M., Ma, L., Angelucci, E., Lucarelli, G., Snyder, L.M., Kiefer, C.R., Yuan, J., and Schrier, S.L.: Abnormal assembly of membrane proteins in erythroid progenitors of patients with beta-thalassemia major. Blood 87:2049, 1996.

282. Speicher, D.W., Morrow, J.S., Knowles, W.J., and Marchesi, V.T.: A structural model of human erythrocyte spectrin. Alignment of chemical and functional domains. J. Biol. Chem. 257:9093, 1982.

283. Speicher, D.W., Morrow, J.S., Knowles, W.J., and Marchesi, V.T.: Identification of proteolytically resistant domains of human erythrocyte spectrin. Proc. Natl. Acad. Sci. USA 77:5673, 1980.

284. Morrow, J.S., Speicher, D.W., Knowles, W.J., Hsu, J., and Marchesi, V.T.: Identification of functional domains of human erythrocyte spectrin. Proc. Natl. Acad. Sci. USA 77:6592, 1980.

285. Delaunay, J., and Dhermy, D.: Mutations involving the spectrin heterodimer contact site: clinical expression and alterations in specific function. Semin. Hematol. 30:21, 1993.

286. Gallagher, P.G., and Forget, B.G.: Hematologically important mutations: spectrin variants in hereditary elliptocytosis and hereditary pyropoikilocytosis. Blood Cells Mol. Dis. 22:254, 1996.

287. Dhermy, D., Galand, C., Bournier, O., King, M.J., Cynober, T., Roberts, I., Kanyike, F., and Adekile, A.: Coinheritance of alpha- and beta-spectrin gene mutations in a case of hereditary elliptocytosis. Blood 92:4481, 1998.

288. Fournier, C.M., Nicolas, G., Gallagher, P.G., Dhermy, D., Grandchamp, B., and Lecomte, M.C.: Spectrin St Claude, a splicing mutation of the human alpha-spectrin gene associated with severe poikilocytic anemia. Blood 89:4584, 1997.

289. Cherry, L., Menhart, N., and Fung, L.W.: Interactions of the α-spectrin N-terminal region with β-spectrin. J. Biol. Chem. 274:2077, 1999.

290. Jarolim P, Wichterle H, Palek J, Gallagher PG, Forget BG: The low expression α spectrin lepra is frequently associated with autosomal recessive/non-dominant hereditary spherocytosis. Blood 88:4a, 1996

291. Wichterle, H., Hanspal, M., Palek, J., and Jarolim, P.: Combination of two mutant alpha spectrin alleles underlies a severe spherocytic hemolytic anemia. J. Clin. Invest. 98:2300, 1996.

292. Tse, W.T., Gallagher, P.G., Jenkins, P.B., Wang, Y., Benoit, L., Speicher, D., Winkelmann, J.C., Agre, P., Forget, B.G., and Marchesi, S.L.: Amino acid substitution in α-spectrin commonly coinherited

293. Tse, W.T., Lecompte, M.C., Costa, F.F., Garbarz, M., Feo, C., Boivin, P., Dhermy, D., and Forget, B.G.: Point mutation in β-spectrin gene associated with α$^{I/74}$ hereditary elliptocytosis. J. Clin. Invest. 86:909, 1985.

294. Gallagher, P.G., Weed, S.A., Tse, W.T., Benoit, L., Morrow, J.S., Marchesi, S.L., Mohandas, N., and Forget, B.G.: Recurrent fatal hydrops fetalis associated with a nucleotide substitution in the erythrocyte beta-spectrin gene. J. Clin. Invest. 95:1174, 1995.

295. Gallagher, P.G., Petruzzi, M.J., Weed, S.A., Zhang, Z., Marchesi, S.L., Mohandas, N., Morrow, J.S., and Forget, B.G.: Mutation of a highly conserved residue of βI spectrin associated with fatal and near-fatal neonatal hemolytic anemia. J. Clin. Invest. 99:267, 1997.

296. Becker, P.S., Tse, W.T., Lux, S.E., and Forget, B.G.: Beta spectrin kissimmee: a spectrin variant associated with autosomal dominant hereditary spherocytosis and defective binding to protein 4.1. J. Clin. Invest. 92:612, 1993.

297. Hassoun, H., Vassiliadis, J.N., Murray, J., Schaffer, F., Jarolim, P., Ballas, S.K., Brabec, V., and Palek, J.: Characterization of the underlying molecular defect in hereditary spherocytosis associated with spectrin deficiency. Blood 90:398, 1997.

298. Jarolim, P., Wichterle, H., Hanspal, M., Murray, J., Rubin, H.L., and Palek, J.: β spectrin^{PRAGUE}: a truncated β spectrin producing spectrin deficiency, defective spectrin heterodimer self-association and a phenotype of spherocytic elliptocytosis. Brit. J. Haematol. 91:502, 1995.

299. Alloisio, N., Texier, P., Forissier, A., Ribeiro, M.L., Morle, L., Bozon, M., Bursaux, E., Maillet, P., Tanner, M.J.A., Tamagnini, G., and Delaunay, J.: Band 3 Coimbra: A variant associated with dominant hereditary spherocytosis and band 3 deficiency. Blood 82:4a, 1993.

300. Perrotta, S., Nigro, V., Iolascon, A., Nobili, B., d'Urzo, G., Conte, M.L., Poggi, V., Cutillo, S., and Miraglia del Giudice, E.: Dominant hereditary spherocytosis due to band 3 Neapolis produces a life-threatening anemia at the homozygous state. Blood 92:9a, 1998.

301. Jarolim, P., Rubin, H.L., Brabec, V., Chrobak, L., Zolotarev, A.S., Alper, S.L., Brugnara, C., Wichterle, H., and Palek, J.: Mutations of conserved arginines in the membrane domain of erythroid band 3 lead to a decrease in membrane-associated band 3 and to the phenotype of hereditary spherocytosis. Blood 85:634, 1995.

302. Jenkins, P.B., Abou-Alfa, G.K., Dhermy, D., Bursaux, E., Feo, C., Scarpa, A.L., Lux, S.E., Garbarz, M., Forget, B.G., and Gallagher, P.G.: A nonsense mutation in the erythrocyte band 3 gene associated with decreased mRNA accumulation in a kindred with dominant hereditary spherocytosis. J. Clin. Invest. 97:373, 1996.

303. Alloisio, N., Maillet, P., Carre, G., Texier, P., Vallier, A., Baklouti, F., Philippe, N., and Delaunay, J.: Hereditary spherocytosis with band 3 deficiency. Association with a nonsense mutation of the band 3 gene (allele Lyon), and aggravation by a low-expression allele occurring in trans (allele Genas). Blood 88:1062, 1996.

304. Coetzer, T.L., Lawler, J., Liu, S.C., Prchal, J.T., Gualtieri, R.J., Brain, M.C., Dacie, J.V., and Palek, J.: Partial ankyrin and spectrin deficiency in severe, atypical hereditary spherocytosis. N. Engl. J. Med. 318:230, 1988.

305. Bruce, L.J., Kay, M.M., Lawrence, C., and Tanner, M.J.: Band 3 HT, a human red-cell variant associated with acanthocytosis and increased anion transport, carries the mutation Pro-868→Leu in the membrane domain of band 3. Biochem. J. 293:317, 1993.

306. Bouhassira, E.E., Schwartz, R.S., Yawata, Y., Ata, K., Kanzaki, A., Qiu, J.J., Nagel, R.L., and Rybicki, A.C.: An alanine-to-threonine substitution in protein 4.2 cDNA is associated with a Japanese form of hereditary hemolytic anemia (protein 4.2^{NIPPON}). Blood 79:1846, 1992.

307. Peters, L.L., Jindel, H.K., Gwynn, B., Korsgren, C., John, K.M., Lux, S.E., Mohandas, N., Cohen, C.M., Cho, M.R., Golan, D.E., and Brugnara, C.: Mild spherocytosis and altered red cell ion transport in mice with a targeted deletion of the erythrocyte protein 4.2 gene (Epb4.2). J. Clin. Invest. 103:1527, 1999.

308. Lux, S.E., Tse, W.T., Menninger, J.C., John, K.M., Harris, P., Shalev, O., Chilcote, R.R., Marchesi, S.L., Watkins, P.C., Bennett, V., McIntosh, S., Collins, F.S., Francke, U., Ward, D.C., and Forget, B.G.: Hereditary spherocytosis associated with deletion of human erythrocyte ankyrin gene on chromosome 8. Nature 345:736, 1990.

309. Cohen, H., Walker, H., Delhanty, J.D.A., Lucus, S.B., and Huehns, E.R.: Congenital spherocytosis, B19 parovirus infection and inherited interstitial deletion of the short arm of chromosome 8. Br. J. Haematol. 78:251, 1991.

with nondominant hereditary spherocytosis. Am. J. Hematol. 54:233, 1997.

310. Costa, F.F., Agre, P., Watkins, P.C., Winkelmann, J.C., Tang, T.K., John K.M., Lux, S.E., and Forget, B.G.: Linkage of dominant hereditary spherocytosis to the gene for the erythrocyte membrane skeleton protein ankyrin. N. Engl. J. Med. 323:1046, 1990.

311. Jarolim, P., Rubin, H.L., Brabec, V., and Palek, J.: Comparison of the ankyrin (AC)n microsatellites in genomic DNA and mRNA reveals absence of one ankyrin mRNA allele in 20% of patients with hereditary spherocytosis. Blood 85:3278, 1995.

312. Eber, S.W., Gonzalez, J.M., Lux, M.L., et al.: Ankyrin-1 mutations are a major cause of dominant and recessive hereditary spherocytosis. Nature Genet. 13:214, 1996.

313. Eber, S.W., Pekrun, A., Reinhardt, D., Schroter, W., and Lux, S.E.: Hereditary spherocytosis with ankyrin Walsrode, a variant ankyrin with decreased affinity for band 3. Blood 84:362a, 1994.

314. Gallagher, P.G., Ferreira, J.D.S., Saad, S.T.O., Kerbally, J., Costa, F.F., and Forget, B.: A recurring frameshift mutation of the ankyrin-1 gene associated with severe hereditary spherocytosis in Brazil. Blood 88:6a, 1996.

315. Basseres, D., Bordin, S., Costa, F., Gallagher, P., and Saad, S.: A novel ankyrin promoter mutation associated with hereditary spherocytosis. Blood 92:8a, 1998.

316. Venezia, N.D., Gilsanz, F., Alloisio, N., Ducluzeau, M.T., Benz, E.J., Jr., and Delaunay, J.: Homozygous 4.1 (B) hereditary elliptocytosis associated with point mutation in downstream initiation codon of protein 4.1 gene. J. Clin. Invest. 90:1713, 1992.

317. Marchesi, S.L., Conboy, J., Agre, P., Letsinger, J.T., Marchesi, V.T., Speicher, D.W., and Narla, M.: Molecular analysis of insertion/deletion mutations in protein 4.1 elliptocytosis. I. Biochemical identification of rearrangements in the spectrin/actin binding and functional characterizations. J. Clin. Invest. 86:516, 1990.

318. Conboy, J., Marchesi, S., Kim, R., Agre, P., Kan, Y.W., and Narla, M.: Molecular analysis of insertion/deletion mutations in protein 4.1 in elliptocytosis. II. Determination of molecular genetic origins or rearrangements. J. Clin. Invest. 86:524, 1990.

319. Winardi, R., Reid, M., Conboy, J., and Mohandas, N.: Molecular analysis of glycophorin C deficiency in human erythrocytes. Blood 81:2799, 1993.

320. Weed, S.A., Stabach, P.R., Oyer, C.E., Gallagher, P.G., and Morrow, J.S.: The lethal hemolytic mutation in $\beta I\epsilon 2$ Spectrin Providence yields a null phenotype in neonatal skeletal muscle. Lab. Invest. 74:1117, 1996.

9 Red Cell Membrane Antigens

▼▼▼▼ John B. Lowe

▼ ▼

The human erythrocyte represents a therapeutic entity when it is used to replenish oxygen-carrying capacity lost through hemorrhage. In this respect, the red cell transfusion represents an organ transplantation procedure. As in other transplantation procedures, it is to be expected that the recipient's immune system will identify non-self molecules on the transfused red cells and will thus mount an immune response. It was appreciated early on that infusion of red cells obtained from one individual could provoke either immediate or delayed untoward reactions in the recipient.[1, 2] Laboratory and clinical investigation of red cell "incompatibility" in the context of transfusion has led to the identification of "blood groups" whose expression is genetically determined. Subsequent studies have assigned distinct erythrocyte surface molecules to many of these blood group antigens. As discussed below, inherited structural polymorphisms in these molecules, and interindividual (genetic) differences in the ability to express them, are in many instances responsible for red cell incompatibility. It is also clear that many of these molecules are expressed both by red cells and by other tissues in the body.

Some compilations of blood group antigens have listed as many as 243 different determinants, belonging to one of 19 distinct blood group systems or "collections" of antigenic determinants that exhibit allelism.[3, 4] However, there have been efforts to unify and simplify these systems, aided by many studies that have defined the molecular basis for nearly all of the genetically polymorphic blood group antigens.[5–7] This chapter summarizes the clinical relevance of many of these antigens, together with current information about their biochemical and genetic properties, and the molecular basis for the inherited polymorphisms in these molecules (Table 9–1). Polypeptide antigen systems are discussed first, followed by the polymorphic systems whose component antigens are composed of complex carbohydrate molecules. The clinical significance of these molecules is discussed only briefly; readers desiring additional detailed diagnostic and therapeutic information related to blood group determinants are urged to consult texts and literature reviews relevant to transfusion medicine.[8–11] Few blood group systems have not yet been assigned a corresponding molecular antigen, and virtually all of these may be considered minor from a clinical or physiological perspective. Readers interested in the details regarding these systems are referred to references 4 to 8.

The RH Blood Group System

The RH blood group system was discovered in the context of a case of erythroblastosis fetalis or hemolytic disease of the newborn.[12–14] The pathogenesis of this disorder involves maternal alloimmunization by Rh antigens encoded by paternal genes and displayed on the surface of the fetal red cells. Alloimmunization generates antibodies that can cross the placenta and destroy fetal red cells.

The term Rh or Rhesus derives from studies performed simultaneously by Landsteiner and Wiener[15] involving the

Table 9–1. Major Human Blood Group Systems

ISBT No.	System Name/Symbol	Gene Name	Antigen Type	Antigen Copy No. per Red Cell	Number of Alleles	Chromosome
001	ABO/ABO	ABO	Oligosaccharide	$8 \times 10^5 - 2 \times 10^6$	3 major (cis-AB, subgroups) Several minor	9q34.1–q34.2
002	MNS/MNS MN (glycophorin A)	GYPA, (GYPE)	Glycoproteins	$\sim 1 \times 10^6$	2 major (M or N) Multiple minor	4q28–q31
	S (glycophorin B)	GYPB		$\sim 1.5 \times 10^5$	2 major (S or s) Multiple minor	4q28–q31
003	P/P1	P1	Oligosaccharide	$\sim 10^3$	Complex	22q11.2–qter
004	Rh/RH		Protein complex		~48 haplotypes Includes minor C/c and E/e alleles	1p34.3–p36.1
	D	RHD		$\sim 2 \times 10^4$	2 major (D+ or D−)	
	C/c, E/e	RHCE		$\sim 2 \times 10^4$	2 major (C or c, and E or e)	
005	Lutheran/LU	LU	Glycoprotein	$\sim 1600–4100$	3 major (Lu^a, Lu^b, recessive null)	19q12–q13
006	Kell/KEL	KEL	Glycoprotein	$\sim 5 \times 10^3$	2 major (KEL1, KEL2) Several minor	7q33
007	Lewis/LE	FUT3	Oligosaccharide	4500–7300	2 major	19p13.3
008	Duffy/FY	FY	Glycoprotein	$\sim 12,000–17,000$	2 major (Fy^a and Fy^b)	1q22–q23
009	Kidd/JK	JK	Glycoprotein	$\sim 14,000$	2 major (Jk^a, Jk^b)	18q11–q12
010	Diego/DI	AE1	Glycoprotein (band 3)	$\sim 15,000$	Several Di^a, Di^b Wr^a, Wr^b Other high-frequency antigens	17q12–q21
011	Cartwright/YT	ACHE	Glycoprotein (acetylcholinesterase)	Not determined	1 major (Yt^a) 1 minor (Yt^b)	7q22
012	XG/XG	XG	Glycoprotein	~ 9000	1 major (Xg^a) 1 minor (Xg, a hypothetical null)	Xp22.32
013	Scianna/SC	SC	Glycoprotein	Not determined	3; Sc1, Sc2, and Sc3	1p36.2–p22.2
014	Dombrock/DO	DO	Glycoprotein (GPI-linked)	Not determined	1 major (Do^a) 1 minor (Do^b)	unknown
015	Colton/CO	AQP1	Glycoprotein (aquaporin-1)	Not determined	2 major (Co^a and Co^b)	7p14
016	Landsteiner-Weiner/LW	LW	Glycoprotein (ICAM-4)	~ 4400 (on D+ cells)	2 major (LW^a, LW^b)	19p13.3
017	Chido-Rogers/CH/RG	C4A, C4B	Glycoprotein (4th component of complement; C4A and C4B)	2835–3620 (on D− cells)	Rare nulls Ch (1 major, several minor) Rg (1 major, several minor)	6p21.3
018	Hh/H	FUT1	Oligosaccharide	see ABO	1 major	19q13
019	Kx/XK	XK	Protein	Not determined	Several minor (Bombay, para-Bombay) 1 major (K^x)	Xp21.1
020	Gerbich/GE (glycophorins C and D)	GYPC, GYPD	Glycoproteins	$\sim 1 \times 10^5$ (glycophorin C) $\sim 2 \times 10^4$ (glycophorin D)	1 major (Ge: 1, 2, 3, 4) Multiple minor	2q14–q21
021	Cromer/CROM	DAF	Glycoprotein (decay-accelerating factor)	$\sim 10^3$	2 major (Cr^a, Cr^b) Several minor	1q32
022	Knops/KN	CR1	Glycoprotein (complement receptor CR1)	Not determined	Several major (Kn^a, Kn^b, Mc^a, Mc^b, Yk^a, Sl^a)	1q32
023	Indian/IN	CD44	Glycoprotein	Not determined	2 major (In^a, In^b)	11p13
Not applicable	Secretor/Se	FUT2	Oligosaccharide	see Lewis	2 major (Secretor, non-Secretor)	19q13
Not applicable	Ii		Oligosaccharide	see ABO	1 major (I), at least 1 minor	9q21

ISBT, International Society of Blood Transfusion.

315

Table 9–2. Common Rh Gene Complexes in Whites

Haplotype	Frequency	Antigens Produced	Haplotype	Frequency	Antigens Produced
CDe	0.40	C, D, e	cdE	0.013	c, E
cde	0.38	c, e	Cde	0.009	C, e
cDE	0.14	c, D, E	CDE	Rare	C, D, E
cDE	0.025	c, D, E	CdE	Very rare	C, E

generation of heteroantisera. In these studies, guinea pigs and rabbits were immunized with red cells taken from *Macaca* rhesus monkeys. Antisera taken from these immunized animals, after appropriate absorption and dilution, were found to detect one or more antigens on the red cells of roughly 85 per cent of humans. This new antigen was termed Rhesus or Rh.

At the time, it was proposed that the specificities of the human alloantibody and the heteroantibody were similar or identical,[13, 15] although virtually contemporaneous studies implied a substantial distinction between the two.[16] Some 20 years later, it was demonstrated that these antibodies detect different molecules.[17, 18] The heteroantibody was renamed LW after the investigators who discovered that antigenic system. The human alloantibody continued to be called Rh. It is now known that RH and LW are antigenic systems determined by distinct gene complexes found, respectively, on chromosome 1 and chromosome 19. There is, however, a relationship between the expression of antigens determined by the *RH* and *LW* loci in that rare persons whose red cells do not express Rh antigens (Rh$_{null}$) are also deficient in LW antigen expression (reviewed in reference 19). As discussed later in this section, there is evidence that LW and the Rh antigen complex associate in the membrane and that LW expression requires Rh polypeptide expression.

▼ SEROLOGY

Approximately 85 per cent of whites are termed Rh "positive," whereas roughly 15 per cent are classified as Rh "negative." These terms refer, respectively, to whether the red cells display the Rh D antigen (Rh positive) or do not display that determinant (Rh negative). The RH blood group system is made complex by the fact that there are other antigens (the C/c and E/e antigens) in this system, whose expression is determined by a second locus distinct from but extraordinarily tightly linked to the locus that determines D antigen expression. Alleles at these two loci are inherited together in a group termed a haplotype (Table 9–2). Numerous antigens in the C/c and E/e groups have been defined, whereas it has been found that virtually all red cells are either D positive or lack D expression (Rh negative) (reviewed in reference 20). Three distinct nomenclatures have evolved to describe the various antigens (Table 9–3). In contrast to the C/c and E/e groups, there is no product of the hypothetical *d* allele of the *D* gene, hence the absence of the d antigen in this system.

In whites, there are eight relatively common Rh gene complexes (see Table 9–2) considering only *D*, *C*, *c*, *E*, and *e* alleles. Wiener[21] suggested that these three groups of Rh antigens (D, C/c, E/e) are localized to a single protein

encoded by a single gene. By contrast, Fisher[22] proposed that these three Rh antigens correspond to three distinct polypeptides encoded by three closely linked genes. As discussed below, however, analyses of the genes encoding these antigens demonstrate that the C/c and E/e antigens are displayed on a single polypeptide encoded by a single locus. These analyses also demonstrate that the D antigen is expressed on a protein that is strikingly similar in its primary sequence to the C/c and E/e molecule but that is encoded by a second locus tightly linked to the *C/c-E/e* locus and is partially or completely deleted in many individuals of the Rh-negative phenotype (i.e., deficient in D antigen expression). A two-locus model that corresponds to these observations was predicted on the basis of serological and genetic data before a molecular definition of these antigens.[23]

▼ CLINICAL RELEVANCE

The Rh antigens are among the most antigenic of the polymorphic red cell surface polypeptide molecules (reviewed in references 8, 20, and 24). Consequently, these antigens have been implicated in immune hemolytic transfusion reactions, but they are of primary clinical significance in the context of hemolytic disease of the newborn. The D determinant is a highly immunogenic alloantigen. Nearly 80 per cent of Rh-negative persons will generate anti-D reactivity after immunization with D-positive red cells (reviewed in reference 8). Formation of anti-C and anti-E antibodies in conjunction with immunization against D determinants has been described, but formation of these antibodies in subjects who are D positive and do not form anti-D antibodies is uncommon.[8] Antibodies directed against Rh determinants are typically of the immunoglobulin (Ig) G class. Formation of such alloantibodies consequently may lead to extravascular hemolysis, and a delayed hemolytic transfusion reaction, if antigen-positive red cells are subsequently transfused. Likewise, Rh antigen–negative mothers sensitized to Rh antigens as a consequence of pregnancy, or transfusion, may generate IgG anti-D antibodies that can cross the placenta, bind to Rh antigen–positive fetal red cells, and mediate destruction

Table 9–3. Nomenclature of Rh Antigens

Fisher-Race	Wiener	Rosenfield (Numerical)
D	Rh$_0$	RH1
C	rh'	RH2
E	rh''	RH3
c	hr'	RH4
e	hr''	RH5

of fetal erythrocytes. This disorder now occurs relatively infrequently because Rh immune globulin, routinely given to Rh D-negative mothers giving birth to D-positive infants, eliminates circulating and potentially immunogenic fetal red cells before they are recognized by the maternal immune system.[9]

▼ BIOCHEMICAL AND MOLECULAR CHARACTERISTICS

Early biochemical analyses indicated that the red cell polypeptides corresponding to the Rh antigens represent a complex of possibly distinct, non-glycosylated polypeptides tightly associated with the red cell membrane.[25–32] This has been confirmed by more recent molecular cloning studies. The C/c and E/e antigens correspond to a single, non-glycosylated, 417 amino acid–long polypeptide termed RhCE, encoded by the *RHCE* locus.[33, 34] This 33,100 dalton polypeptide is predicted to maintain a topology with 12 membrane-spanning domains[33–38] (reviewed in reference 39) (Fig. 9–1). The *RHCE* gene is composed of 10 exons dispersed among approximately 70 kb of genomic DNA.[40] The D antigen corresponds to a distinct non-glycosylated protein, also 417 amino acids long, with a predicted size of M_r 33,100.[25, 41] This protein, termed RhD, is encoded by the *RHD* locus. The RhD protein shares approximately 90 per cent primary amino acid sequence identity with the RhCE protein (differing at 35 or 36 positions only) and is also predicted to maintain a multimembrane-spanning topology[32, 33, 42, 43] (reviewed in reference 39) (see Fig. 9–1). The *RHD* locus maintains an intron/exon boundary structure virtually identical to that defined for the *RHCE* locus, at least through the regions where this work has been completed for the *RHD* locus.[40] The *RHD* locus and the *RHCE* locus are closely linked on human chromosome 1p34–36.[44] The Rh blood group locus had been previously assigned to this chromosome position by genetic mapping studies.[45, 46]

A third polypeptide, known as Rh50, has been biochemically associated with the Rh antigen system. Molecular cloning studies demonstrate that Rh50 is a 409 amino acid–long glycoprotein that shares approximately 36 per cent primary amino acid sequence identity with the Rh30 polypeptides RhD and RhCE.[47, 48] Rh50 is also predicted to assume a 12-pass membrane-spanning topology (see Fig. 9–1). This protein is encoded by the *RH50* locus, which is localized to human chromosome 6p11–21.1.[47] The sizes of the 10 exons of the 32 kb *RH50* locus, and the positions of its intron/exon boundaries, are similar to those defined for the *RHD* and *RHCE* loci, indicating that these three loci can be considered members of the same gene family.[49, 50] As discussed in detail below, biochemical, serological, and genetic studies indicate that the Rh50 protein does not itself display Rh antigens. However, Rh50 physically interacts in the membrane with the Rh30 polypeptides and is apparently required for the formation of a heterotetrameric complex, Rh50:Rh50:Rh30(RhD):Rh30(RhCE), essential to normal cell surface expression of the Rh30-encoded Rh antigens.

The RhD and RhCE polypeptides are post-translationally modified by fatty acylation[51] and are palmitylated through a thioester linkage to free sulfhydryls on cysteine residues, by analogy to other palmitylated polypeptides. The

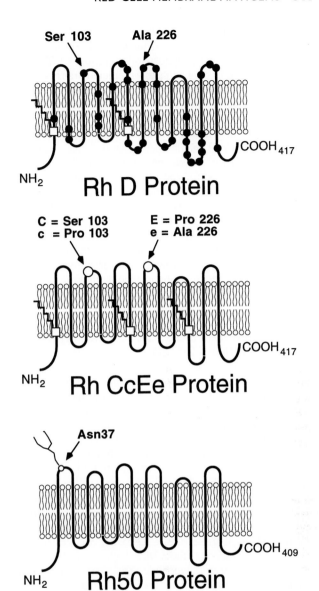

Figure 9–1. Predicted transmembrane topologies of Rh polypeptides and relative positions of amino acid sequence polymorphisms between the RhD and RhCcEe positions. The RhD, RhCcEe, and Rh50 proteins are predicted to maintain multiple membrane-spanning segments. The approximate relative positions of the 35 amino acid sequence differences between the 417 amino acid–long RhD and RhCcEe proteins[43] are predicted by the solid circles on the RhD schematic. The predicted positions of palmitylation of the RhD protein (two sites) and the RhCcEe protein (three sites), based on a consensus tripeptide motif Cys-Leu-Pro,[33] are indicated by the short wavy lines attached to open square boxes on the RhD and RhCcEe schematics. The approximate relative positions, and nature, of the amino acid sequence polymorphisms accounting for C/c and E/e antigenic polymorphism are indicated on the RhCcEe schematic. The serine and alanine residues on the RhD protein at positions 103 and 226, respectively, do not yield C or e reactivity on this protein, because these are apparently conformation-dependent antigens that form in the context of the RhCcEe protein but not in the context of the RhD protein. The Rh50 protein is 409 amino acids long and is glycosylated at asparagine residue 37. The Rh50 protein shares approximately 36 per cent amino acid sequence identity with the RhD and RhCcEe proteins.

positions of palmitylation are predicted to occur at cysteine residues within a consensus tripeptide (Cys-Leu-Pro) found with the RhD and RhCE polypeptides (see Fig. 9–1). The functional significance of this modification is not yet known.

Rh antigenic reactivity is influenced by the lipid composition of the membrane environment, including alterations in red cell membrane cholesterol/phospholipid ratios.[52, 53] These observations are consistent with the predicted transmembrane orientation of the Rh30 and Rh50 proteins and indicate that alterations of the plasma membrane lipid concentration can modulate the display or conformation of the Rh determinants. There is also evidence that the Rh polypeptides interact with the red cell membrane skeleton. Under conditions in which the major protein components of the membrane skeleton (spectrin, actin, and other associated proteins) remain insoluble (low concentrations of non-ionic detergents), the Rh polypeptides may be found in association with these proteins.[54–56] There is evidence that the Rh proteins maintain a physical association with other membrane polypeptides.[26, 57, 58] These include the glycophorins and the glycoprotein corresponding to the Landsteiner-Wiener antigen (the LW antigen), an antigenically polymorphic membrane-associated molecule discussed in the major section that follows.

▼ THE MOLECULAR BASIS FOR POLYMORPHISM IN THE Rh ANTIGEN SYSTEM

Serological, biochemical, genetic, and molecular studies have illuminated the molecular basis for many polymorphisms in the Rh antigen system. Much of this information has been reviewed elsewhere[5, 7, 39]; it is summarized here and supplemented with more recent information. This information can be divided into studies that define the basis for the Rh D-negative phenotype, for Rh partial D variants, for polymorphism in the C/c and E/e antigens, and for rare Rh_{null} and Rh_{mod} phenotypes. As discussed above, molecular analyses indicate that Rh D-positive persons maintain two tightly linked and homologous genes termed *RHD* and *RHCE*.[5, 39] One of these (the *RHD* locus) encodes the RhD protein, and the second (the *RHCE* locus) encodes a single C/c and E/e–reactive polypeptide. The third protein in this system, Rh50, associates in the membrane with, and is thought to be required for expression by, the two Rh30 proteins. These considerations imply that the wide variety of polymorphisms in the Rh system will be accounted for by deletion of, missense and nonsense mutations within, and aberrance of expression of the *RHD*, *RHCE*, or *RH50* loci.

The Rh D-negative phenotype is characterized by an absence of detectable erythrocyte RhD protein with generally normal amounts of the Rh C/c and E/e antigens. In analyses completed on a largely white population, in which Rh D-negative individuals are found with a frequency of approximately 17 per cent, nearly all Rh D-negative individuals have been shown to be homozygous for partial or complete deletions of the *RHD* locus.[42, 43, 46, 59] In a rare exception, a grossly intact *RHD* locus in an Rh D-negative individual was shown to be non-functional owing to a 4 bp deletion in a coding exon of the locus.[60] By contrast, in a Japanese population, in which the Rh D-negative phenotype is rare (0.5 per cent), an analysis of a series of Rh D-negative individuals disclosed that the *RHD* locus was grossly intact in approximately 27 per cent of the individuals analyzed.[61] The molecular basis for absence of RhD protein expression in such persons remains to be defined.

A large number of antigenic variants of the RhD poly-

peptide also exist. These have been defined serologically, with use of sera from Rh D-positive individuals that contain anti-D reactivity and with monoclonal anti-D antibodies. These D variants, or "partial D's," are separated into categories D_{II} through D_{VII}.[62] The phenotype of a given D variant category is defined by the lack of expression of one or more of a series of more than 30 D antigenic epitopes, termed epD1 through epD30 and higher.[63, 64] Most variants maintain multiple epitopic changes. Sequence analysis of the genomic DNA corresponding to several such partial D variants indicates that the "missing" epitopes are essentially "replaced" by a new epitope that corresponds to the amino acid sequences present at identical positions in the RhCE protein. Molecular analyses indicate that in most instances, gene conversion events can account for the generally localized "conversion" of RhD-specific amino acid sequence to RhCE-specific amino acid sequence. Such gene conversion events will be relatively favored by the close physical proximity of the *RHD* and *RHCE* loci, by the striking degree of DNA sequence similarity between the two genes, and by the presence of interspersed repetitive DNA sequence elements within the two loci. Partial D variants also occur through events that generate point mutations, in a manner distinct from the gene conversion mechanism.[65] A review summarizes the molecular details of many of these variants.[5]

In most individuals who do not express antigens of the C/c or E/e complex, the *Cc/Ee* gene remains largely intact but has apparently suffered mutations that render it unable to generate its polypeptide products.[46] The generation of C and E determinants by the *Cc/Ee* gene has been defined by sequencing of Rh cDNAs and corresponding genomic DNA from Rh D-negative individuals with informative C/c and E/e phenotypes[59] (see Fig. 9–1). These analyses indicate that the C/c and E/e phenotypes can be accounted for by amino acid sequence polymorphisms at residues 103 (C = Ser, c = Pro) and 226 (E = Pro, e = Ala). An early model[66] proposing an alternative splicing mechanism to account for C/c and E/e antigenic polymorphism is no longer considered to be correct.[67]

Molecular analyses are under way to define the basis for the wide variety of other relatively rare antigenic polymorphisms in the Rh system (reviewed in reference 5). For example, such analyses indicate that the low-frequency antigens C^W and C^X derive, respectively, from a glutamine to arginine change at codon 41 and from an alanine to threonine change at codon 36, in the *RHCE* locus.[68] The VS antigen has been shown to correspond to a leucine to valine change at codon 245 in the *RHCE* locus.[69] Finally, the weak D (Du) phenotype, characterized by low but detectable levels of D antigen, has been shown in at least three instances to be a consequence of expression of abnormally low amounts of a qualitatively normal RhD transcript.[70] The mechanism responsible for diminished amounts of the RhD transcript in these weak D (Du) patients is not yet known. Conversely, in patients with the RN phenotype characterized by low expression of the C/e antigen, molecular analyses identified abnormal RhC and Rhe transcripts that generate hybrid RhCe-D-Ce peptides with apparently reduced expression efficiency.[70]

▼ Rh_{null} AND Rh_{mod} PHENOTYPES

Rh_{null} cells are completely deficient in Rh antigens and exhibit stomatocytosis, spherocytosis, and increased in vitro osmotic fragility. The rare individuals with the Rh$_{null}$ phenotype typically suffer from a chronic, mild to moderate non-immune hemolytic anemia (reviewed in reference 71). These cells also exhibit abnormalities in ion transport, ATPase activity, and water content[72, 73]; their membranes are relatively deficient in cholesterol content,[73] and they maintain an abnormal membrane phospholipid distribution.[74] A similar phenotype, known as Rh$_{mod}$, has also been described.[75] Rh$_{mod}$ red cells express low levels of Rh antigen, and like individuals with the Rh$_{null}$ phenotype, persons with the Rh$_{mod}$ phenotype suffer from a mild compensated hemolytic anemia.

Rh$_{null}$ (and Rh$_{mod}$) red cells also have diminished or absent expression of other blood group determinants,[76] including glycophorin B (the Ss antigens[77]) and Duffy determinants (reviewed in reference 19). These cells are also deficient in the expression of other membrane-associated molecules, including the Rh50 protein,[5] the LW glycoprotein to be discussed below,[30, 32, 37, 58, 78, 79] and others defined by monoclonal antibodies.[80, 81]

Genetic considerations reviewed in references 71 and 76 have predicted that the Rh$_{null}$ phenotype will be accounted for either by homozygosity for silent alleles at the *RH* locus (the less common "amorph type" Rh$_{null}$) or by homozygosity for an allele (termed X^{O}r) at an autosomal locus that is genetically independent of the *RH* locus (the more common "regulator type" of Rh$_{null}$). The Rh$_{mod}$ phenotype has been predicted to be a consequence of homozygosity for an allele (termed X^Q) at an autosomal locus distinct from the *RH* locus.[75] It is not known whether the X^{O}r and X^Q may correspond to alleles at the same locus.

Recent molecular analyses confirm some of these predictions and implicate mutant *RH50* alleles in the regulator-type Rh$_{null}$ phenotypes. Defects in the *RH50* locus that have been identified in several individuals with the regulator-type Rh$_{null}$ include frameshift[48] and missense[82] leading to disrupted RH50 protein expression and a splice donor site mutation yielding an aberrantly spliced *RH50* transcript with an altered, prematurely terminated, and apparently non-functional Rh50 polypeptide.[49] In each of these instances, the identified mutation is accompanied by transcriptionally silent *RH50* alleles in compound heterozygote individuals. By contrast, homozygosity for splice donor or splice acceptor site mutations within the *RH50* locus accounts for some cases of the regulator-type Rh$_{null}$ phenotype.[83] When considered together with biochemical results supporting a role for the Rh50 protein in the assembly of red cell membrane protein complexes, these results confirm a pathogenic role for dysfunctional *RH50* alleles in patients with the regulator type of Rh$_{null}$ phenotype.

Defects in the *RH30* locus have been assigned a causative role in the amorph Rh$_{null}$ phenotype and satisfy the prediction that this phenotype is the consequence of deficiency within the *Rh* locus proper. In one study, small nucleotide sequence mutations were identified within the *RhCe* gene that predict a translational frameshift leading to a truncated RhCe polypeptide. These mutations exist in the context of deletion of the *RhD* gene (i.e., in Rh D-negative individuals) and lead, presumably, to deficient expression of all members of the Rh30:Rh50 complex.[84] Frameshift and splicing mutations identified in the *RHCE* locus have also been associated with the amorph type of Rh$_{null}$ phenotype.[85] These observations lend support to other studies suggesting

that the Rh30 and Rh50 peptides are both required for normal expression of the large red cell membrane complexes that include the Rh, LW, and glycophorin molecules.

Molecular defects that account for the modifier type of the Rh$_{null}$ phenotype remain to be defined.

▼ FUNCTION OF THE Rh PROTEINS

The genetic and biochemical abnormalities associated with the Rh$_{null}$ and Rh$_{mod}$ cells and biochemical evidence for the presence of Rh proteins in multiprotein red cell membrane complexes imply that these molecules, including especially the Rh50 protein, play an essential role in facilitating red cell membrane/protein complex assembly and expression. By physically associating with these molecules, the Rh peptides may fix them within the membrane or otherwise stabilize their conformations, possibly through association with proteins of the membrane skeleton.

The proposed multimembrane-spanning topology of the three Rh proteins suggests that they may represent components of a membrane transporter complex. Amino acid sequence comparisons have led some to propose that the Rh proteins maintain structural similarity to NH4$^+$ transporters,[86] but a functional correlate to this suggestion, or any other, remains to be demonstrated. Several groups have proposed that the Rh polypeptides may participate in a process that maintains the asymmetrical distribution of phospholipids in red cell membranes (reviewed in reference 87). This process requires an enzyme termed ATP-dependent phosphatidylserine translocase, or PS flippase. It seems unlikely, however, that the Rh polypeptides participate in these events because the PS flippase activities in Rh$_{null}$ cells and in normal red cells are virtually identical.[88]

Remaining work in this blood group system is likely to focus on completing the understanding of the basis for polymorphisms in the structure and expression of these antigens, on defining the physical relationships between the Rh polypeptides and the other red cell polypeptides that associate with them, and on determining the functions of the Rh complex.

The LW Blood Group System

As noted above, the antigens of the LW (Landsteiner-Wiener) blood group were discovered through experiments involving antisera developed by guinea pigs in response to immunization with rhesus monkey red cells.[15] Subsequent work demonstrated an immunological distinction between the Rh and LW antigens.[16–18] There are two major allelic antigens with the LW blood group, termed LW^a and LW^b.[89] The *LW^a* allele predominates in most populations, leaving the LW^b antigen to be detected in less than 1 per cent of most individuals. The two alleles yield the common phenotype LW(a+b−) and the much less common phenotypes LW(a−b+) and LW(a+b+). Rare individuals without detectable LW antigens [LW(a−b−)] are homozygous for null alleles at the LW locus. As noted earlier, expression of the LW polypeptides is quantitatively dependent on expression of the Rh polypeptides. This accounts for the observation that anti-LW antibodies react more strongly with D-positive red cells (with approximately 4400 LW molecules per red cell[84]) than with D-negative red cells (expressing between approximately 2835 and 3620 LW molecules per red cell[84]) and not at all with Rh$_{null}$ red cells. Clinically relevant anti-LW alloantibodies are observed infrequently, largely because most individuals share the same LW phenotype.

The LW antigen corresponds to a 42 kDa red cell glycoprotein with a deglycosylated molecular mass of 25,000 daltons.[30, 37, 78] The COOH-terminal portion of the LW glycoprotein is displayed at the surface of the red cell and contributes to epitopes recognized by anti-LW antibodies (Fig. 9–2). Two structurally distinct cDNAs encoding the LW protein have been defined.[90] One predicts a type I transmembrane protein with a short cytoplasmic tail, whereas the other predicts a molecule without the membrane-spanning and cytoplasmic segments of the longer form. The predicted protein sequence shares approximately 30 per cent identity with three members of the intracellular adhesion molecule (ICAM) family,[90] ICAM-1, ICAM-2, and ICAM-3.[91] The LW glycoprotein has been designated ICAM-4,[92] because of the primary sequence relationship among the four molecules and because the LW glycoprotein can engage in adhesive interactions with the ICAM ligands CD11/CD18.[92] Physiological correlates of these observations remain to be confirmed.

The *LW* locus corresponds to three exons that span 2.65 kb on human chromosome 19.[93] The *LW^a* and *LW^b* alleles differ at a single base pair, in a codon corresponding to one amino acid residue (LW^a = Gln 70, LW^b = Arg 70).[94] One LW null allele has been found to maintain a 10 bp deletion

that truncates the protein at a position proximal to its transmembrane and cytosolic domains, but defects that account for other molecularly distinct LW null alleles have not yet been defined.[93]

Glycophorins A, B, and E and the MNSs Blood Group Locus

The red cell antigens M and N were first discovered by Landsteiner and Levine,[95] using antisera prepared from rabbits immunized with human red cells. The S and s antigens were later defined with human antisera.[96–98] Detailed discussions of MNSs blood group system serology may be found in references 19 and 20.

Early genetic and immunological studies indicated that the M and N determinants represent allelic products of a single gene closely linked to another gene that gives rise to the allelic S and s determinants. Four common haplotypes at these two loci exist, with frequencies that depend on the population examined. Northern European populations, for example, maintain haplotype frequencies of approximately 0.38 for *Ns*, 0.30 for *Ms*, 0.24 for *MS*, and 0.07 for *NS*. There are other phenotypes within the MNSs system that also deserve mention. The U antigen, first described in 1953 by Wiener and coworkers,[99] is expressed by the red cells of most white people but is absent from the red cells of approximately 1 per cent of black individuals. Among S-negative and s-negative blacks, approximately 84 per cent also have red cells that are deficient in the U determinant, whereas the remainder express low levels of the U determinant.

Two other high-frequency antigens have been described in whites. The En^a antigen is absent from red cells taken from individuals with the En(a−) phenotype. As discussed later in this section, En(a−) red cells are deficient in part or all of the glycophorin A protein. Another high-frequency antigen, known as the Wr^b determinant, is also absent from some individuals whose red cells are deficient in glycophorin A and glycophorin B. The molecular basis for its absence in rare individuals is poorly understood.

In addition to these high-frequency determinants, there are a large number of MN and Ss variants encoded by alleles at the corresponding loci. These have typically been identified by investigating alloantibodies generated during transfusion or in pregnancy. These variants include those of the Miltenberger (Mi) class, Henshaw (He), and St^a, for example.

The clinical significance of the MNSs blood group system is relatively minor.[8, 9, 19] Many anti-M and anti-N antibodies are found as "naturally occurring" antibodies. These antibodies may often be heterogeneous mixtures of IgM and IgG molecules that display enhanced binding at low temperatures (i.e., cold-reactive). They are generally of little clinical significance. Examples of alloantibodies directed against the M and N determinants are rare. Anti-S and anti-s antibodies may be generated after exposure to antigen-positive red cells, through transfusion or pregnancy, although this is also a relatively infrequent occurrence. These antibodies are typically of the IgG class and have been known to be responsible for transfusion reactions and hemolytic disease of the newborn.[8, 9, 19]

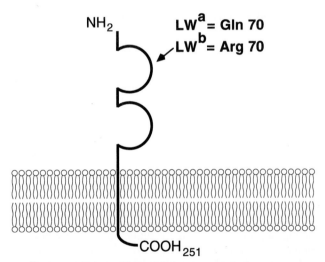

NH$_2$

LW^a = Gln 70
LW^b = Arg 70

COOH$_{251}$

Figure 9–2. The Landsteiner-Wiener (LW, ICAM-4) blood group polypeptide. The LW blood group antigens are found on a 251 amino acid–long type I transmembrane glycoprotein. This protein shares approximately 30 per cent identity with the three members of the intracellular adhesion molecule family ICAM-1, ICAM-2, and ICAM-3. Like these molecules, the LW glycoprotein, also termed ICAM-4, is predicted to maintain immunoglobulin superfamily domains (two) capable of engaging adhesive interactions with ICAM ligands CD11/CD18. Each of the immunoglobulin superfamily domains of the LW glycoprotein maintains two consensus asparagine-linked glycosylation sites (not shown), accounting for the difference between the 42,000 dalton molecular mass observed for the native LW glycoprotein and the 25,000 dalton molecular mass observed for its deglycosylated form. The two major allelic antigens of the LW blood group system, termed LW^a and LW^b, are determined by a single amino acid polymorphism at residue 70.

▼ GLYCOPHORINS

Biochemical and immunological methods have assigned the MN antigens to the glycophorin A (GPA, encoded by the *GYPA* locus) red cell surface sialoglycoprotein, and the Ss antigens to glycophorin B (GPB, encoded by the *GYPB* locus) (reviewed in references 100 and 101).

The *GYPA* locus (Fig. 9–3) gives rise to three transcripts of 2.8, 1.7, and 1.0 kb.[102–105] The 5' ends of these transcripts are virtually identical; transcript length heterogeneity is dictated by the use of alternative polyadenylation sites.[105, 106] GPA is synthesized with a cleavable leader peptide that ultimately yields a type I transmembrane protein 131 amino acids long. The protein is heavily glycosylated, carrying a single asparagine-linked glycan and 15 serine-threonine–linked oligosaccharide units. Carbohydrate composes approximately 60 per cent of the mass of GPA. The M and N antigens on GPA are determined by amino acid polymorphism at positions 1 and 5 of the mature polypeptide. The M antigen is defined by a serine at amino acid position 1 and a glycine at position 5, whereas the N antigen is defined by a leucine at position 1 and a glutamine at position 5. Anti-M and anti-N antibodies can recognize these peptide determinants exclusively but may also exhibit carbohydrate-dependent recognition properties.[107, 108]

GPB is a structurally similar type I transmembrane protein derived from a gene consisting of five exons (see Fig. 9–3). This gene yields a single 0.5 kb transcript.[103–105, 109] GPB is synthesized with a cleavable signal sequence to yield a type I transmembrane protein 72 amino acids in length. There are no asparagine-linked carbohydrate chains on this molecule, whereas there are approximately 11 serine-threonine–linked oligosaccharide chains. Approximately 50 per cent of the mass of GPB consists of oligosaccharide. The peptide sequence that determines N antigen reactivity on GPA is also found on GPB. This antigen, termed N, is relatively weakly expressed, probably because substantially fewer copies of the GPB molecule are expressed at the surface of the red cell (0.15×10^6 copies per cell), relative to GPA copy number (approximately 1×10^6 copies per cell). The blood group S and s antigens are specified by a methionine and a threonine, respectively, at amino acid residue 29.[110]

Molecular cloning studies have been used to identify a gene homologous to *GYPA* and *GYPB*, termed *GYPE*.[111, 112] Its sequence predicts a mature glycophorin E protein 59 amino acids long, with residues 1 and 5 occupied by serine and glycine, respectively (i.e., corresponding to the blood group M determinant). The *GYPE* locus lacks DNA sequences corresponding to amino acid residues 27 to 39 of GPB, encompassing the position of the Ss amino acid sequence polymorphism in GPB. *GYPE* also contains a DNA sequence insertion, relative to *GYPA* and *GYPE*, at a position corresponding to exon 5 of *GYPA*. This insertion is predicted to encode eight amino acids not present in GPA or GPB. Efforts to identify a polypeptide product corresponding to the *GYPE* locus have been largely unsuccessful, although immunoblotting studies using a murine anti-M monoclonal antibody suggest that a product of *GYPE* can be identified as a 20,000 dalton molecule (reviewed in reference 113). *GYPA*, *GYPB*, and *GYPE* are tandemly oriented in a gene cluster (Fig. 9–4).

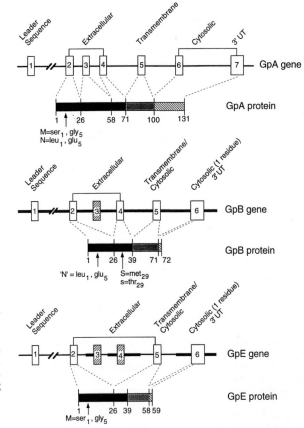

Figure 9–3. Glycophorins A, B, and E gene and protein structures. The glycophorin A (GPA) gene is composed of seven exons. Exon 1 yields a leader peptide, whereas the extracellular domain is encoded by exons 2, 3, and 4. Exon 5 encodes the transmembrane domain. Exons 6 and 7 generate the cytosolic domain and 3' untranslated region. Positions of amino acid residues corresponding to domain boundaries are indicated below the GPA protein. Amino acid sequence polymorphisms encoded by exon 2 yield either an M-specific GPA molecule (serine at position 1 and glycine at residue 5) or an N-specific molecule (leucine at residue 1 and glutamine at residue 5).

The glycophorin B (GPB) gene is composed of five functional exons (numbers 1, 2, 4, 5, and 6); sequences corresponding to exon 3 are designated a pseudoexon, because they are not present in GPB transcripts as a consequence of a non-functional splice acceptor sequence at its 3' border. Exon 1 yields a leader peptide. The extracellular domain is encoded by exons 2 and 4, and exon 5 encodes the transmembrane and short cytosolic segment. Exon 6 generates the 3' untranslated region. Positions of amino acid residues corresponding to domain boundaries are indicated below the GPB protein. Amino acid sequence polymorphisms encoded by exon 4 yield either an S-specific GPB molecule (methionine at position 29) or an s-specific molecule (threonine at residue 29). The amino acid sequence encoded by exon 2 yields the N antigen, with leucine at position 1 and glutamine at position 5.

The glycophorin E (GpE) gene is predicted to be composed of four functional exons (numbers 1, 2, 5, and 6) and two non-utilized pseudoexons (numbers 3 and 4). Exon 1 yields a leader peptide, exon 2 encodes the putative extracellular domain, and exon 5 encodes the predicted transmembrane segment. Exon 6 generates the 3' untranslated region. Positions of amino acid residues corresponding to domain boundaries are indicated below the GpE protein. The extracellular domain is predicted to display M antigenic specificity. Thick lines correspond to segments of the GpE gene most similar to corresponding segments in the GPB gene; thin lines denote regions most similar to corresponding locations in the GPA gene.

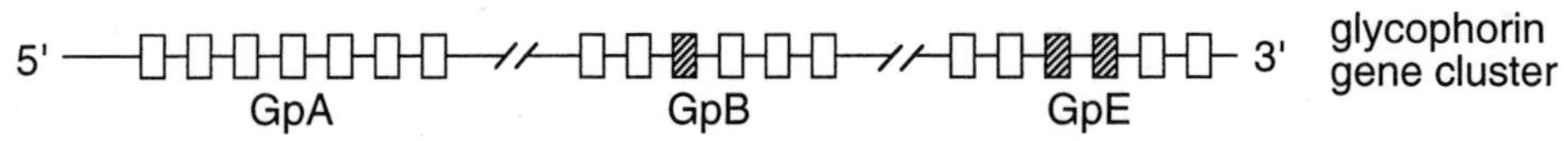

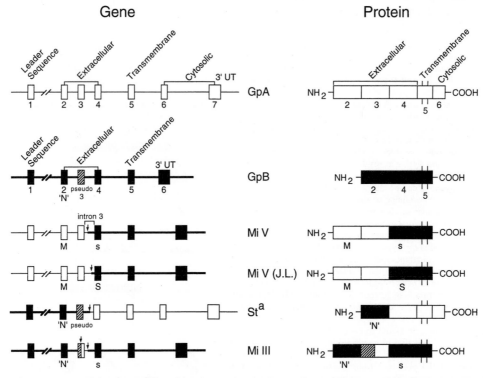

Figure 9–4. Genomic organization of the glycophorin ABE gene cluster. Exons are indicated by the open boxes. Pseudoexons in the GPB and GpE genes are denoted by hatched boxes.

▼ MOLECULAR BASIS OF ANTIGENIC VARIATION

The molecular basis has been determined for a variety of variant phenotypes of the MNSs blood group system (reviewed in references 101 and 114) (Fig. 9–5). These variants may be grouped into sets, according to the apparent mechanisms that generated them. Members of one of these sets appear to have been derived as a consequence of genetic cross-over events between intron 3 of *GYPA* and intron 3 of *GYPB* (Fig. 9–6). Members of a second group of variants appear to have been generated by gene replacement events (either double cross-over events or gene conversion) that have substituted a portion of *GYPB* pseudoexon 3 and intron 3 with a corresponding segment of *GYPA* derived from exon 3 and intron 3. A third group consists of members derived by structurally significant deletions of *GYPA* or *GYPB*. Last, variants have been described whose antigenic properties are different from the wild-type versions by virtue of alterations in the serine-threonine–linked glycans attached to otherwise normal GPA and GPB polypeptides.

Examples of variants produced by unequal cross-over include the MiV, MiV (J.L.), and St[a] phenotypes (reviewed in reference 115) (see Figs. 9–4 and 9–5). The cross-over events that have engendered these phenotypes yield chimeric glycophorin protein products derived from the donor genes. In the case of the MiV and MiV (J.L.) phenotypes, this yields hybrid glycophorin molecules derived from the first three exons of *GYPA* and the last three exons of *GYPB*. These two phenotypes differ by virtue of the particular Ss allele derived from the donor *GYPB* locus (see Fig. 9–5). By contrast, the St[a] phenotype is derived from a hybrid glycophorin molecule encoded by a chimeric gene constructed from the first two exons of *GYPB* and the last three exons of *GYPA* (see Figs. 9–4 and 9–5).

Examples of variants produced by sequence replacement mechanisms include the MiIII, MiX, and MiVI variants.[115] In these variants, a segment of *GYPB* between the 3' portion of pseudoexon 3 and a position within intron 3 has been replaced by a corresponding segment of *GYPA* (see Fig. 9–5). In each instance, the replacement events have occurred at different positions and are of different sizes. Nonetheless, the GPA insert always composes the 3' end of exon 3 from

Figure 9–5. Genomic structures and polypeptides of representative variant glycophorins A and B. The structures of the wild-type GPA (open boxes and thin lines) and GPB (solid boxes and thick lines) genes *(left)* and their corresponding proteins *(right)* are displayed at the top. Variant glycophorin genes and their protein products are displayed below the wild-type sequences. The MiV and MiV (J.L.) variant glycophorins arise as a consequence of recombination events (see Fig. 9–6) that have juxtaposed 5' segments of the GPA gene with 3' segments of the GPB gene, with the cross-overs (denoted by an arrow) occurring within the intron 3' to GPA exon 3 and the intron 5' to GPB exon 4. These hybrid molecules will display M and S, or M and s, determinants, depending on the Ss genotype of the donor GPB segment. A reciprocal cross-over event is apparently responsible for generating the St[a] variant glycophorin. Double cross-over events, or gene conversion events, are apparently responsible for replacing a segment of the GPB gene with a corresponding portion of the GPA gene (denoted by paired vertical arrows) to generate the MiIII glycophorin variant.

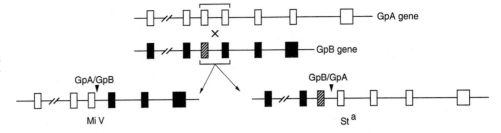

Figure 9–6. Recombination events predicted to yield variant glycophorin A and B genes and proteins.

GYPA as well as sequences corresponding to the 5′ end of intron 3 of *GYPA*. This segment thus incorporates a functional 5′ splice junction derived from *GYPA* intron 3 and therefore replaces the non-functional corresponding splice site at the distal end of *GYPB* pseudoexon 3. Consequently, the chimeric molecules contain a peptide sequence encoded by portions of *GYPB* pseudoexon 3 as well as a peptide sequence derived from the distal end of *GYPA* exon 3.

Variants derived from partial or complete deletion of *GYPA* or *GYPB* naturally are detected as red cells with deficiencies of the GPA or GPB proteins. Red cells with no detectable MN antigens fall into the En(a−) class of such variants. Two types of En(a−) variant are known. In an extensively studied Finnish pedigree, Southern blot analyses indicate that substantial portions of *GYPA* are absent, whereas *GYPB* locus is virtually intact.[116] These observations, and biochemical studies, indicate that absence of GPA in En(a−) individuals in this pedigree is due to a homozygous deletion of the *GYPA* locus. By contrast, in an En(a−) pedigree studied in the United Kingdom, genomic studies indicate that this En(UK) gene is a hybrid consisting of the 5′ end of *GYPA* linked to the 3′ portion of the *GYPA* locus.[117] This chimeric gene presumably gives rise to a hybrid glycophorin molecule composed of the NH$_2$-terminal portion of an M-specific GPA linked to the COOH-terminal portion of a GPB molecule with S specificity.[116–118]

Red cells deficient for the Ss and U determinants are found rarely among North American populations but are present at low to moderate levels in certain regions of Africa.[119] Biochemical analyses indicate that S− s− U− red cells are deficient in GPB or express a non-glycosylated, defective form of this protein.[120, 121] Southern blot hybridization analyses on DNA from S− s− U− persons indicate that in most instances, absence of red cell GPB expression correlates with large deletions of the *GYPB* locus.[122, 123] Rare individuals of the S− s− U− phenotype have been identified who maintain partial deletions of *GYPB*[122] or an apparently normal *GYPB* structure.[124] In these instances, it is probable that expression of the GPB polypeptide is deficient as a consequence of the partial deletions observed on Southern blots or as a consequence of point mutations or small deletions not detectable by Southern blot analyses.

Finally, phenotypes have been described that are apparently due to deletion of the *GYPA* and *GYPB* loci.[112, 124] In heterozygotes of the Mk variant,[125] red cell MN and Ss antigens are present at 50 per cent of the wild-type levels. In homozygotes,[126] red cells lack detectable GPA and GPB proteins as well as all MN and Ss antigens, Wr^b determinants, and the En^a antigen.[19, 20, 127] Southern blot analyses have confirmed that *GYPA* and *GYPB* are deleted in one such homozygous Mk individual.[112, 124] Interestingly, homozygous

individuals exhibit no obvious detrimental phenotype associated with complete deficiency of the GPA and GPB proteins. There are no red cell morphological abnormalities, and red cell function and survival are essentially normal. These observations suggest that the GPA and GPB polypeptides exhibit no essential function (reviewed in references 100, 101, and 128). Thus, the functions of the human glycophorins A, B, and E, if any, are not yet known.

Glycophorins C and D and the Gerbich Blood Group Locus

Antigens of the Gerbich (Ge or GE) blood group were first described by Rosenfield and colleagues[129] in 1960. Excepting rare variants, these antigens are found on the red cells from nearly all individuals. Consequently, generation of alloantibodies directed against Gerbich blood group determinants in the context of transfusion or pregnancy is an exceedingly rare event.[8] Four high-frequency antigens within the Gerbich blood group have been defined by human antisera and Gerbich variant red cells.[130, 131] These are denoted Ge:1, Ge:2, Ge:3, and Ge:4. These determinants define four phenotypes, including the most common phenotype, Ge:1, 2, 3, 4, and three variants that lack one or more of these determinants. These variants are known as the Melanesian type, which lacks the Ge:1 determinant (Ge:−1, 2, 3, 4); the Yussef type, Ge:−1, −2, 3, 4; and the Gerbich type, Ge:−1, −2, −3, 4. There is, in addition, a rare variant known as the Leach phenotype (Ge:−1, −2, −3, −4).[131–135]

Red cells taken from individuals of the Leach phenotype are elliptocytotic and are deficient in red cell membrane proteins glycophorin C (GPC, encoded by the *GYPC* locus) and glycophorin D (GPD, a truncated form of GPC, also encoded by the *GYPC* locus; see below).[134, 135] This observation demonstrated that the Gerbich antigens correspond to determinants on GPC or GPD. Biochemical and immunological analyses indicate that the Ge:3 determinant may be destroyed by neuraminidase treatment, or trypsin digestion, and that it is expressed on GPC and GPD.[136–138] By contrast, the Ge:2 determinant, although neuraminidase and trypsin sensitive, is found only on GPD.[137, 138] The positions of the Ge:1 and Ge:2 determinants remain to be defined.

Cloned cDNAs encoding GPC have been obtained from a human reticulocyte cDNA library with use of peptide sequence information.[139–142] The cDNA sequence predicts a 128 amino acid protein with a molecular mass of 14,000 daltons (Fig. 9–7A). This size predicted for the primary translation product is substantially smaller than the size of the GPC protein observed on SDS–polyacrylamide gel electrophoresis (32,000 daltons).[140, 143] This discrepancy can

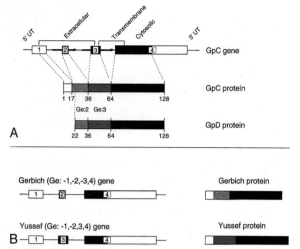

Figure 9–7. Glycophorin C gene and variants. A, Wild-type glycophorin C (GPC) gene and derived protein products. The GPC gene is composed of four exons. The extracellular domain of GPC is encoded by exons 1 and 2. Its transmembrane segment is encoded by exons 3 and 4, and the cytosolic portion by exon 4. Arrows encompassing exons 2 and 3 represent repeat sequences believed to be involved in recombination events that have deleted exon 2 or 3 in some GPC variants (see B). Glycophorin D (GPD) is believed to be derived from the same transcript that yields GPC, through translation initiation at an internal methionine residue corresponding to residue 22 of GPC. Positions of amino acid residues corresponding to exon boundaries are indicated below the GPC and GPD proteins. The Ge:2 and Ge:3 determinants have been localized to positions corresponding to exons 2 and 3, respectively. B, Variant GPC proteins. The Gerbich-type variant GPC gene lacks sequences corresponding to exon 3, through a postulated recombination event occurring between repeated sequences depicted in A. This variant gene encodes a shortened GPC molecule deficient in amino acid residues corresponding to exon 3. The Yussef-type variant GPC gene lacks sequences corresponding to exon 2, by a similar mechanism, and is predicted to express a shortened protein deficient in amino acid residues corresponding to exon 2.

be accounted for by extensive post-translational modification by glycosylation at the single predicted asparagine-linked glycosylation site and the multiple potential serine-threonine–linked glycosylation sites. These positions are located within a 57 amino acid–long domain at the NH_2 terminus that is predicted to be displayed at the surface of the red cell. A 24 amino acid–long hydrophobic segment is appended to this extracellular domain and is predicted to constitute a membrane-spanning segment, whereas the COOH-terminal portion presumably resides in the cytosolic compartment.

Protein sequencing studies indicate that GPD represents a molecular variant of the GPC molecule, corresponding to residues 22 to 128 of GPC.[144] This hypothesis is supported by immunochemical studies indicating that the COOH-terminal domain of GPD cross-reacts immunologically with GPC, whereas the monoclonal antibodies specific for an NH_2-terminal segment of GPC do not react with GPD.[145] These considerations are also consistent with the observation that GPC (32,000 daltons) is approximately 9000 daltons larger than GPC (23,000 daltons). Inspection of the cDNA sequence encoding GPC suggests that the same transcript yields both GPC and GPD through a mechanism involving translation initiation at an internal ATG codon corresponding to the methionine residue at amino acid 22 in the GPD protein sequence.

GPC is encoded by the *GYPC* gene, which is composed of four exons[101, 146–148] (Fig. 9–7A). The extracellular portion of GPC is encoded by exons 1 and 2 and a large part of exon 3, whereas the transmembrane segment and COOH-terminal cytosolic domains are encoded by exon 4. This gene represents a single-copy sequence located on chromosome 2q14–q21.[149, 150] The fact that this represents a single-copy sequence that yields a single 1.1 kb transcript in the erythroid lineage provides additional support for the notion that a single transcript yields both GPC and GPD proteins.

The molecular basis has been determined for several of the variants of the Gerbich blood group antigens. As noted previously, Leach variant red cells exhibit elliptocytosis and are deficient in the GPC and GPD cell surface sialoglycoproteins. Four unrelated individuals with the Leach phenotype have been examined by Southern blot analyses with use of segments of *GYPC*.[151, 152] These studies indicate that three of these individuals are homozygous for a deletion of *GYPC* encompassing exons 3 and 4, whereas exons 1 and 2 are grossly intact.[151] These reports did not provide information on whether these aberrant genes were transcribed, although it would be predicted that this would yield aberrant GPC and GPD molecules deficient in the membrane-spanning and cytoplasmic segments. Molecular analyses of a fourth individual of the Leach phenotype identified a grossly normal *GYPC* locus by Southern blotting that also generated an apparently normal transcript. Nonetheless, sequence analysis of this transcript identified DNA sequence alterations at a position corresponding to codons 44 and 45.[152] These alterations change the tryptophan codon at position 44 to a leucine codon and also delete a single nucleotide in the adjacent codon. The frameshift mutation yields a termination codon at a position corresponding to residue 56 of the native protein, and the resulting predicted protein would thus consist of 43 residues derived from the native sequence followed by 12 new amino acids. This aberrant polypeptide, if expressed, would presumably not be displayed at the cell surface because it would not contain a transmembrane segment.

Red cells of the Yussef-type and Gerbich-type variants lack membrane GPC and GPD molecules but display instead a single structurally related glycoprotein with a molecular weight intermediate between that displayed by GPC and GPD. Structural analysis of *GYPC* in Yussef-type individuals indicates that it has suffered a deletion of exon 2[149, 151] (Fig. 9–7B). Similarly, the *GYPC* locus in Gerbich-type individuals has suffered a deletion of sequences corresponding to exon 3[149, 151] (Fig. 9–7B). It has been hypothesized that these deletions occur as a consequence of recombination between direct repeats within *GYPC*[147, 148] (Fig. 9–7A and B).

The deletion in the Yussef-type variant yields a transcript derived from exons 1 and 3 that is in turn translated into a 109 amino acid–long protein deficient in the 19 residues encoded by exon 2. By contrast, a deletion in the Gerbich-type individuals yields a transcript that is translated into a 100 amino acid–long protein deficient in the 28 amino acids encoded by exon 3. These aberrant GPC molecules thus retain a transmembrane and COOH-terminal cytosolic domain but display truncated forms of the extracellular domain. Alternative splicing of exon 2 of the wild-type *GYPC* locus may occur normally in some tissues to yield a truncated polypeptide identical to that expressed by the Yussef-type variant.[153] It is predicted that variant GPD molecules will also be synthesized by these molecular variants through the internal initiation mechanism outlined above, although these molecules have yet to be described.

Other variants of the Gerbich blood group have been described, including the Ls[a] phenotype, in which the red cells display a larger GPC and GPD variant molecules as a consequence of duplicated exon 3.[154, 155] The Webb (Wb) variant is a trypsin-sensitive antigen displayed by an aberrant GPC molecule.[156–158] Sequence analysis of a Wb allele identified a single base pair sequence difference within the codon corresponding to the asparagine residue at amino acid 8. This alteration changes the asparagine codon to a serine codon and thus removes the single asparagine-linked glycosylation site found on wild-type GPC. Thus, absence of the asparagine-linked glycan chain at this position accounts for the smaller size observed for Wb GPC.[158] Other point mutations in the *GYPC* locus define the basis for the An[a] and Dh[a] antigens.[159, 160]

The elliptocytotic morphology exhibited by Leach erythrocytes (deficient in GPC and GPD molecules) suggests that these proteins function to maintain the normal shape of the red cell by interactions with the erythrocytes of skeletal proteins.[132, 133, 161–165] Biochemical analyses indicate that GPC and GPD remain associated with red cell membrane skeleton proteins after extraction with non-ionic detergent.[133, 162] Similarly, patients who are genetically deficient in red cell protein 4.1 are concomitantly deficient in GPC and GPD molecules and Gerbich blood group determinants.[166, 167] These observations imply that surface expression of GPC and GPD requires an interaction with protein 4.1, shown experimentally.[168]

The Kell Blood Group System

The Kell blood group system was discovered in 1945 and named for the individual who made antibodies leading to its discovery.[8] At least 24 alloantigens have been described, most of which fall into one of seven sets of antithetical antigens (see Table 9–4 for the most common representatives; reviewed in references 8 and 169). Historically, these alloantigens have been referred to by a complex nomenclature, now substantially simplified to one based on a straightforward numbering system (see Table 9–4).

The KEL1 antigen is highly immunogenic, relative to other human blood group alloantigens; it is second only to the RhD determinant in its immunogenicity. Approximately 5 per cent of KEL1-deficient recipients will mount an alloantibody response to the KEL1-determinant after transfusion with a single unit of KEL1-positive red cells.[170] Thus, anti-KEL1 antibodies are frequently represented among the alloantibodies found in association with both immediate and delayed hemolytic transfusion reactions and in hemolytic disease of the newborn (reviewed in reference 8). Indeed, anti-KEL1 accounts for approximately two thirds of non-Rh immune red cell alloantibodies.[8] Alloantibodies directed against other Kell determinants have been implicated in transfusion reactions and hemolytic disease of the newborn. These antibodies are substantially less common, largely because most represent high-frequency antigens. In most instances, anti-KEL1 antibodies are IgG; it has been estimated that approximately 17 per cent of these antibodies can activate complement when bound to KEL1-positive red cells.[171]

Red cells express approximately 5000 Kell determi-

Table 9–4. Nomenclature and Amino Acid Polymorphisms of Representative Kell Blood Group Antigens

NAME	LETTER	NUMBER	ISBT NUMBER	Antigen Frequency (Percentage)	Polymorphism
Kell	K	K1	KEL1	9.0	Met 193
Cellano	k	K2	KEL2	99.8	Thr 193
Penny	Kp[a]	K3	KEL3	2.0	Trp 281
Rautenberg	Kp[b]	K4	KEL4	>99.9	Arg 281
	Kp[c]	K21	KEL21	1.0	Gln 281
Peltz (K₀)	Ku	K5	KEL5	>99.9	—
Sutter	Js[a]	K6	KEL6	<1.0 in whites 19.5 in blacks	Pro 597
Matthews	Js[b]	K7	KEL7	>99.9 in whites 99.9 in blacks	Leu 597
Karhula	Ula+	K10	KEL10	<0.1; 2.6 in Finns	Glu 494 → Val
Cote		K11	KEL11	>99.9	Val 302
Weeks	Wka	K17	KEL17	0.3	Ala 302
Bockman		K12	KEL12	>99.9	His 548
			KEL:−12	<0.1	Arg 548
Sublett		K19	KEL19	>99.9	Arg 492
			KEL:−19	<0.1	Gln 492
Santini		K14	KEL14	>99.9	Arg 180
Callois	Cls	K24	KEL24	<2.0	Pro 180
	Kx	K15	KEL15	>99.9	—

ISBT, International Society of Blood Transfusion.

nants.[172, 173] Immunoprecipitation studies using monospecific anti-Kell antibodies identify a single 93,000 dalton red cell membrane protein that displays two different Kell epitopes.[174] This molecule may exist as part of a larger complex under non-reducing conditions, migrating with sizes ranging from 115,000 daltons to above 200,000 daltons. Immunoblotting experiments suggest that the Kell glycoprotein may exist as a homodimer in the membrane.[175, 176] The 93,000 dalton Kell-reactive polypeptide was not detectable on red cells taken from individuals of the K_0 (K_{null}) phenotype, which are known to be deficient in all Kell determinants.[174-176]

Sequence of a cDNA encoding the Kell protein[177] predicts a 732 amino acid–long, 83,000 dalton polypeptide. This protein is predicted to maintain a topology consisting of a cytosolic NH_2-terminal segment, a single hydrophobic membrane-spanning segment, and a large COOH-terminal extracellular domain (Fig. 9–8). Six potential asparagine-

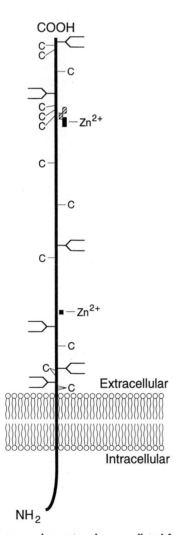

Figure 9–8. Transmembrane topology predicted for the Kell protein. Molecular cloning and biochemical studies outlined in the text predict that the Kell protein maintains a single transmembrane segment, with a large COOH-terminal extracellular domain. Positions of potential asparagine-linked glycosylation sites are indicated by the small branched structure. Locations of extracellular cysteine residues are indicated by C. Putative leucine zipper motifs are depicted by the small patterned boxes. Potential zinc coordination sites are shown by the small solid boxes.

linked glycosylation sites and 15 cysteine residues are located in the extracellular domain. The Kell protein displays two heptad arrays of leucine residues, with clustered cysteine residues, in a leucine zipper motif that may be involved in protein/protein interactions. The Kell glycoprotein shares primary sequence similarity with the neprilysin family of zinc-binding neutral endopeptidases that includes polypeptides like bradykinin, neurotensin, enkephalin, oxytocin, and angiotensins I and II.[177] It is not yet known whether the Kell glycoprotein functions as an endopeptidase.

Experiments involving the expression of the Kell cDNA in transfected cultured cells[178] and sequence analysis of Kell locus exons[179] in individuals with defined Kell phenotypes show that polymorphisms at single codons in the *Kell* locus account for simple amino acid substitutions that dictate the common Kell system antigenic polymorphisms[180-184] (see Table 9–4).

Two unusual Kell phenotypes have been described. The first, known as K_0 or K_{null} phenotype, refers to the absence of the Kell glycoprotein from red cells[185] (reviewed in reference 169). Red cells of persons homozygous for the K_{null} allele are deficient in all known Kell antigens. K_{mod} is a rare, genetically heterogeneous phenotype in which the red cells display extraordinarily weak Kell antigen reactivity (reviewed in reference 171). Kell$_{null}$ and Kell$_{mod}$ red cells display a normal morphology and survive normally in vivo. The molecular defects responsible for these phenotypes remain undefined.

The second unusual Kell phenotype is termed the McLeod syndrome, an X-linked disorder with a defect at a locus termed *Xk*.[186] Red cells of patients with the McLeod syndrome express markedly reduced levels of the 93,000 dalton Kell protein and are relatively or absolutely deficient in an antigen termed Kx, or KEL15. These abnormalities are associated with an acanthocytic red cell morphology as well as reduced in vivo red cell survival.[187] Female carriers of a defective *Xk* locus maintain two populations of red cells as a consequence of X chromosome lyonization. One red cell population maintains a normal shape and displays a quantitatively normal amount of Kell determinants. The second population displays acanthocytosis and is presumably derived from an erythroid progenitor clone wherein the wild-type *Xk* allele has been inactivated.

The *McLeod syndrome* locus is closely linked to the loci that are defective in chronic granulomatous disease and in Duchenne muscular dystrophy.[188, 189] The Kx or Kel15 determinant absent from McLeod red cells is carried on a 37,000 dalton polypeptide.[190] Molecular cloning studies predict that this 444 amino acid–long polypeptide maintains 10 membrane-spanning segments.[191] Deficiency of the Kx protein corresponds to splice site mutations in the locus in some patients, whereas large deletions that encompass part or all of this locus account for the defect in other individuals.[191] Although the predicted multimembrane-spanning topology of this protein suggests a transport function, this remains to be demonstrated. The functional significance of the apparent association between the Kx and Kell proteins is also unknown.

The Kidd Blood Group System

The Kidd blood group system was first described in 1951, in the context of a case of hemolytic disease of the newborn.[192] The pathological IgG antibody here was directed against an antigen termed Jk^a. An antibody against a distinct *Kidd* allele, termed *Jk^b*, was described in 1953.[193] These two antigenic determinants (Jk^a and Jk^b) represent the only common alleles in most populations. The gene frequency in whites is 0.514 for the *Jk^a* allele and 0.486 for the *Jk^b* allele. Thus, approximately 26 per cent of such individuals have red cells with the phenotype Jk(a+b−), corresponding to the genotype *Jk^aJk^a*. Roughly 50 per cent of individuals have red cells with the phenotype Jk(a+b+), corresponding to the genotype *Jk^aJk^b*, whereas 24 per cent of such individuals are of the genotype *Jk^bJk^b*, with red cells of the phenotype Jk(a−b+). Rare individuals have been described with the Jk(a−b−) phenotype.[194–196] Anti-Jk^a and anti-Jk^b antibodies are typically generated in the context of pregnancy or transfusion and are most often IgG class antibodies, although IgM antibodies have also been described. Anti-Jk^a and anti-Jk^b antibodies have been implicated in hemolytic transfusion reactions and are among the more common types of antibodies implicated in delayed hemolytic transfusion reactions.[8]

Some Jk(a−b−) individuals generate antibodies capable of reacting with both Jk^a and Jk^b determinants.[194] Transfused or multiparous Jk(a−b−) individuals may generate an antibody termed Jk3 that recognizes Kidd blood group determinants distinct from the Jk^a and Jk^b determinants.[195, 196] By analogy to null phenotypes in other blood group systems (i.e., K_null, Rh negative), these observations imply that some Jk(a−b−) individuals are genetically deficient in the ability to express meaningful amounts of the Kidd molecule.

There are approximately 14,000 Kidd molecules expressed at the surface of the red cell.[197] The Kidd determinants reside on a 46,000 to 60,000 dalton protein.[198] Early studies implicated this protein in the transport of urea or other solutes, because Kidd null red cells [Jk(a−b−)] resist hemolysis in the presence of 2M urea[199–201] and because Jk(a−b−) individuals exhibit a defective ability to concentrate their urine.[202] These observations also suggested that Kidd blood group determinants may be expressed on a urea transporter molecule also expressed in the kidney (reviewed in references 203 and 204). cDNA cloning studies have defined the primary sequence of a human red cell urea transporter and have demonstrated that this molecule corresponds to the Kidd antigen.[205] This molecule is immunoreactive with anti-Kidd antisera and corresponds to an antigen that is present on all red cells except those of the Jk(a−b−) phenotype.[205, 206] A single amino acid polymorphism in this protein accounts for the difference between Jk^a (Asp 280) and Jk^b (Asn 280).[207] Mutations in the *Kidd* locus that lead to aberrant splicing account for the Kidd null phenotype in some individuals.[208]

The Duffy (Fy) Blood Group System

In whites, there are two major alleles in the Duffy blood group system, *Fy^a* and *Fy^b*, with roughly equivalent frequencies (0.425 and 0.557, respectively) (reviewed in reference 209). Two other alleles also exist; *Fy^x* determines the expression of a weakly reactive version of Fy^b, whereas a null allele termed *Fy* generates neither Fy^a nor Fy^b determinants. In most populations, the *Fy^x* and *Fy* alleles are found with frequencies substantially less than 0.02. By contrast, the *Fy* allele is common in blacks with African ancestry, and all endogenous inhabitants in certain regions in Africa are homozygous for this null allele.

Anti-Fy^a typically represents an IgG-type immune antibody; it has been implicated in hemolytic transfusion reactions and in hemolytic disease of the newborn. Anti-Fy^b is typically an anti-IgG antibody, although it is detected much less frequently than is anti-Fy^a.

The Fy^a and Fy^b determinants are localized on a glycoprotein that migrates as a broad band with a molecular mass between 38,000 and 90,000 daltons.[210, 211] A significant amount of the mass of this molecule corresponds to asparagine-linked oligosaccharides, which probably accounts for its heterogeneous migration properties in its native state.[212] Molecular cloning studies indicate that this Duffy antigen–reactive molecule is a 338 amino acid–long polypeptide predicted to maintain seven membrane-spanning segments[213] (Fig. 9–9). This protein maintains strong primary sequence similarity to a growing family of seven-pass transmembrane receptors for chemokines.[214] Functional expression studies confirm that this protein corresponds to the red cell chemokine receptor.[215, 216] This property accounts for the emerging use of the term DARC (Duffy antigen receptor for chemokines) to describe this polypeptide.[217] DARC is proposed to remove excess chemokines from the blood and tissues, although this hypothesis is not yet well supported by experimental evidence.

Duffy antigens are essential for invasion of human red cells by *Plasmodium vivax*, an agent of human malaria, and also by *Plasmodium knowlesi*, a parasite that affects Old World monkeys but that is also capable of invading human red cells (reviewed in reference 218). Merozoites derived from these parasites are competent to attach to both Duffy-positive human erythrocytes and Duffy-negative

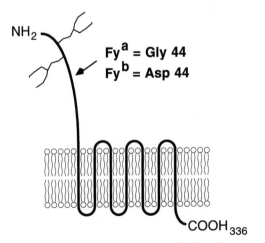

Figure 9–9. The Duffy blood group polypeptide. The Duffy blood group antigens localize to a 336 amino acid–long glycoprotein and to a quantitatively minor splice variant that is shorter by two amino acids at its amino terminus (not shown). The protein is highly glycosylated and is predicted to maintain at least two asparagine-linked sites near its amino terminus. The Duffy protein shares primary sequence similarity with members of the G protein–coupled, seven-pass transmembrane receptors for chemokines. The Duffy protein is therefore also termed DARC, for Duffy antigen receptor for chemokines. The Fy^a and Fy^b antigens correspond to a single amino acid sequence polymorphism at residue 44. This polymorphism has no apparent effect on chemokine binding by the Duffy protein.

[Fy(a − b −)] human red cells. After binding, the merozoite reorients (on both types of red cells) so that its apical end contacts the erythrocyte surface. Successful entry of the merozoite into the red cell requires the subsequent formation of a junction between the apex of the merozoite and the red cell.[219] Formation of this junction and penetration of the merozoite into the erythrocyte only occur on Duffy-positive red cells. Consequently, humans who lack Duffy blood group antigens are resistant to infection by *P. vivax*. This accounts for the observation that infection with this parasite is rarely seen in West Africa where the frequency of the Duffy locus null allele *(Fy)* is nearly 1.0.

Study of the tissue-specific expression patterns of DARC and molecular analysis of the Duffy locus in West African Fy(a − b −) individuals demonstrate that these Duffy null alleles suffer from a mutation that alters the normal expression pattern of the locus.[220] In patients with an *Fyᵃ* or *Fyᵇ* allele, DARC is normally expressed by red cell precursors in the marrow and elsewhere, including by postcapillary endothelium in the kidney.[220] By contrast, in individuals who are homozygous for the *Fy* allele, marrow DARC expression is defective, although extramarrow expression of DARC remains intact. This heritable polymorphism in the tissue-specific expression of DARC is accounted for by a single base pair difference between the *Fy* allele and the *Fyᵃ* or *Fyᵇ* alleles. The sequence change localizes to the promoter region of the *DARC* gene, and in the *Fy* allele, this change disrupts a binding site for the erythroid lineage–specific transcription factor GATA-1. This change accounts for lack of DARC expression in the red cells of *Fy* homozygotes.[220] By contrast, a translational frameshift caused by a 14 bp deletion in the *DARC* locus accounts for absence of Duffy antigen expression by an *Fy* allele in a white individual.[221] Similar molecular analyses indicate that the *Fyᵃ* and *Fyᵇ* alleles differ only at codon 44, yielding a glycine residue at this position in the Fyᵃ polypeptide versus an aspartic acid at this position in the Fyᵇ protein.[221–224]

The Lutheran Blood Group System

The Lutheran blood group system[19, 225] was first described during an investigation of an antibody formed in a patient who had received two blood transfusions.[226] Four major phenotypes are observed in this system (see Table 9–5 for nomenclature; International Society of Blood Transfusion nomenclature is used here, except for the brief discussion that cites older literature dealing with two types of inhibitors of Lutheran antigen expression). Approximately 90 per cent of individuals maintain the phenotype LU: − 1, 2 [Lu(a − b +)], and nearly all have the genotype *LU2/2*. Most

of the remaining 10 per cent of individuals exhibit the phenotype LU:1, 2 [Lu(a + b +)], with the genotype *LU1/2*. The phenotype LU:1, −2 [Lu(a + b −)] with the genotype *LU1/1* is relatively infrequent, owing to the low frequency of the *LU1* allele in most populations. Rare individuals display no detectable Lutheran determinants (phenotype LU:0). This Lutheran null phenotype is a consequence of three known genetic backgrounds. One represents homozygosity for null alleles at the *LU* locus.[19, 225] A second corresponds to inheritance of a rare, autosomal dominant inhibitor gene termed *In(Lu)*, which is not linked to the Lutheran locus.[227, 228] *In(Lu)* also suppresses expression of antigens from other blood group systems, including the P₁ and i antigens,[229] and the CD44 epitope.[230, 231] Because two of these antigens are composed of oligosaccharide determinants (P₁, i) and the others represent glycoproteins (LU and CD44), it is possible that the *In(Lu)* gene encodes a glycosyltransferase that masks or otherwise alters these determinants by glycosylation. Third, an X-linked dominantly acting inhibitor gene termed *XS2* can also suppress Lutheran antigen expression.[232] In homozygotes for the null alleles, Lutheran antigens are not detectable, whereas in persons who have inherited an inhibitor gene, Lutheran antigens are expressed at low levels.

Anti-LU1 or anti-LU2 antibodies are rarely encountered, virtually always in the context of transfusion or prior pregnancy. Immune anti-LU1 or anti-LU2 antibodies have typically not been associated with transfusion reactions or hemolytic disease of the newborn.[19, 225] In blood, the Lutheran blood group proteins are restricted in their expression to erythrocytes and, as noted below, to B lymphocytes. The Lutheran locus is also expressed in fetal hepatic epithelia, in the placenta, and within the walls of arteries in many tissues.[233] Lutheran blood group proteins, or antigenically related ones, have also been described in kidney endothelial cells and in hepatocytes.[234]

The Lutheran determinants are expressed on a pair of membrane glycoproteins with molecular weights of 78,000 and 83,000.[235] Other allelic antigens encoded by the Lutheran locus (Lu6 and Lu9, Lu8 and Lu14) and the so-called para-Lutheran antigens (Lu4, Lu12, and Lu17, for example) also appear to be displayed by these two polypeptides.[236] The Auberger blood group determinants Auᵃ and Auᵇ are also located on the Lutheran glycoproteins.[237, 238]

Molecular cloning efforts have defined the primary sequences of the polypeptides corresponding to the Lutheran blood group antigens and have illuminated the molecular basis for antigenic polymorphism in this blood group system.[233, 239–241] The Lutheran blood group antigens are displayed on a 597 amino acid–long type I transmembrane protein. The extracellular domain contains five potential *N*-glycosylation sites and five peptide segments that share primary sequence similarity with members of the immunoglobulin superfamily (Fig. 9–10). Its structural organization is similar to the melanoma-associated, mucin-like protein MUC18 and related neural cell adhesion molecules. The extracellular domain is associated with the cell membrane through a single membrane-spanning segment and has the potential to communicate with the cell interior through an Src homology 3 domain within its 59 amino acid–long intracellular segment. The gene encoding this protein yields a pair of alternatively spliced transcripts. These account for

Table 9–5. Lutheran Blood Group System Nomenclature

Traditional Phenotype	ISBT Phenotype	Traditional Genotype	ISBT Genotype
Lu (a − b +)	LU: − 1,2	*Luᵇ Luᵇ*	*LU2/2*
Lu (a + b +)	LU:1,2	*Luᵃ Luᵇ*	*LU1/2*
Lu (a + b −)	LU:1, − 2	*Luᵃ Luᵃ*	*LU1/1*
Lu (a − b −)	LU:0	*Lu Lu*	*LU0/0*

ISBT, International Society of Blood Transfusion.

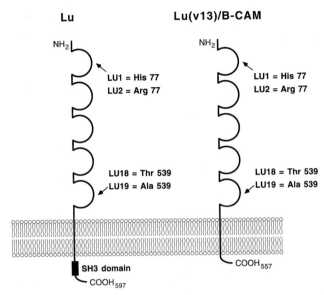

Figure 9–10. The Lutheran blood group polypeptides. The Lutheran blood group antigens localize to a pair of type I transmembrane proteins of 597 and 557 amino residues in length. Each maintains five extracellular domains with primary sequence similarity to members of the immunoglobulin superfamily. The two proteins derive from the *Lutheran* blood group locus through alternative splicing processes that retain (Lu) or delete (Lu(v13)), a segment of the cytosolic domain encoded by exon 13. The splice variant that is deleted for this segment is identical to a previously identified glycoprotein expressed on basal cell carcinoma cells, termed basal cell adhesion molecule (B-CAM). Each splice variant maintains five potential asparagine-linked glycosylation sites on the extracellular domain (not shown). The cytosolic segment in the Lutheran protein maintains an Src homology 3 domain (SH3 domain). The LU1 (Lu^a) and LU2 (Lu^b) polymorphism and the LU18 (Au^a) and LU19 (Au^b) polymorphism correspond to single amino acid sequence polymorphisms at residues 77 and 539, respectively.

the presence of two molecular weight isoforms of the protein that differ in the lengths of their cytosolic domains. One isoform of the Lutheran polypeptide is identical to a previously characterized basal cell carcinoma/epithelial cancer adhesion molecule termed B-CAM.[242]

The Lutheran blood group locus corresponds to a 12.5 kb gene composed of 15 exons.[240] Molecular analysis of this locus in individuals informative for Lutheran blood group antigens identifies a single antigenically relevant nucleotide polymorphism in exon 3 at base pair 229 of the coding sequence.[240] In Lutheran (a + b −) individuals (LU: −1, 2), the nucleotide at this position (A) contributes to a histidine codon corresponding to residue 77 of the Lutheran polypeptide. In Lutheran (a − b +) individuals (LU:1, −2), the nucleotide at this position is G and contributes to an arginine codon at residue 77 of the Lutheran polypeptide. Expression of cDNAs corresponding to these two polymorphic forms of the polypeptide confirms that 229 A and its cognate histidine residue contribute to the epitope recognized by anti-Lu1 antibodies, whereas 229 G and its cognate arginine residue form an anti-Lu2–reactive epitope. Analogous studies[241] demonstrate that the Auberger antigen Au^a (Lu18) corresponds to an epitope defined by a threonine at residue 539, derived from a codon that includes a polymorphic nucleotide (A) at base pair 1637 in exon 12. By contrast, the Au^b (Lu19 antigen) is defined by an alanine at the same position, corresponding to a G residue at base pair 1637.[241] These

studies also localize the domain positions of the epitopes that account for polymorphism at the allelic antigens Lu6 or Lu9 and Lu8 or Lu14, although confirmatory molecular analyses to assign these to discrete amino acid residues remain to be completed.[241]

Complement System Proteins as Blood Group Determinants; The Chido/Rodgers Antigens and the Cromer-Related Antigens

The Chido (Ch) and Rodgers (Rg) blood group determinants were identified by corresponding alloantibodies appearing in transfused patients.[243, 244] Ch or Rg determinants also circulate in plasma.[243–245] Antibodies directed against these determinants are typically of the IgG class and are generated only in transfused patients who lack Ch or Rg determinants. Ch or Rg alloantibodies are encountered relatively infrequently, because more than 95 per cent of random donors are Ch positive[245, 246] and more than 95 per cent are Rg positive.[244] Except in rare circumstances,[247] these antibodies are not clinically significant,[248, 249] most probably because the circulating forms of the corresponding antigens neutralize the antibody reactivities in vivo. Nonetheless, these antibodies can present difficulties during crossmatching procedures.

The Chido and Rodgers determinants are displayed by the two isotypes of the fourth component of complement, C4A and C4B (reviewed in reference 250). The human C4 molecules are glycoproteins with molecular weight of approximately 210,000.[250] They are synthesized as single-chain precursors (pro-C4A and pro-C4B), which are converted to mature forms consisting of three disulfide bond–linked polypeptide chains. Complement activation cleaves the C4 molecules into specific fragments. The α chain of the mature form ultimately yields a fragment, termed C4d, that remains stably associated with the red cell membrane. Biochemical studies have demonstrated that the Ch and Rg determinants localize to the C4d fragment.[251] These molecules thus represent antigens that are acquired from plasma. It is believed that in vivo, the C4 proteins are subject to a constant, low-level fluid-phase activation. This ultimately yields red cell–associated C4d molecules (reviewed in reference 252). Genetic, biochemical, and serological studies indicate that in most instances, the Rodgers determinant corresponds to rare amino acid sequence polymorphisms within a region of the C4d fragment derived from the C4A isotype, within a region between amino acid residues 1054 and 1191 (summarized in reference 250). Similarly, Chido antigenic determinants generally correlate with rare amino acid sequence polymorphisms within the same region of the C4d fragment derived from the C4B isotype.[250] Rare exceptions to these assignments have been described in which variants of the C4A and C4B molecules (i.e., C4A1 and C4B5) express the Chido and Rodgers determinants typically assigned to the other C4 isotype.[253, 254]

The complement regulatory protein decay-accelerating factor (DAF) also displays polymorphic antigens that associate with the red cell membrane (reviewed in references 255 and 256). DAF is a 347 amino acid–long protein that associates with cell membranes through a glycophosphatidylinositol (GPI) moiety (a GPI anchor).[256] DAF-associated antigens have been termed Cromer-related antigens, after the patient who made the alloantibody used to discover the Cromer-related system. Antibodies against these determinants have been described independently numerous times. In addition to being termed Cromer (Cr^a), the locus that determines the expression of these antigens has been independently termed *Tc*, *Dr*, *WES*, *Es*, and *UMC*.[255] The rare Inab phenotype corresponds to a complete deficiency in Cromer-related antigens.[257]

Antibodies directed against Cromer-related antigens normally are not clinically significant,[258] although exceptions have been described in which these antibodies diminish red cell survival.[259] Biochemical and immunochemical approaches have been used to demonstrate that the Cromer-related antigens are carried on DAF.[260, 261] This assignment is further supported by the observation that red cells in individuals with the Inab phenotype are deficient in DAF expression,[262] which can be accounted for, in some such individuals, by a nonsense mutation in codon 53 of the DAF gene that truncates the protein near its amino terminus.[263] Other point mutations in the DAF locus that delete DAF expression in Inab individuals have been described subsequently.[264]

Molecular characterization of polymorphisms in the DAF locus also define the basis for antigenic variation in the Cromer system. A specific amino acid sequence polymorphism in DAF (Ser 165 → Leu) leads to loss of expression of the Dr^a epitope [the Dr(a−) phenotype] and defines the *Dr^b* allele within the Cromer system.[266] The reduced expression of DAF observed in patients with the Dr(a−) phenotype has been shown to be a consequence of a reduction in the amount of transcripts corresponding to the Leu 165 DAF variant.[263] This reduction is accompanied by an increase in the amount of an aberrantly spliced DAF transcript containing a frameshifted reading frame incapable of elaborating a normal, membrane-anchored DAF molecule. Aberrant splicing in this context is a consequence of the creation of a cryptic splicing branch point by the point mutation responsible for the Ser 165 → Leu change. This leads, in turn, to utilization of a downstream cryptic acceptor splice site and the generation of the non-productive mutant DAF transcript. Missense mutations within the DAF locus have also been correlated with Cromer-related epitopes Cra [Cr(a−); Ala 193 → Pro] and Tca [Tc(a−b+); Arg 18 → Leu].[264, 265]

The Complement Receptor I Protein and the Knops Blood Group Antigens

The Knops family of red cell antigens are expressed by the complement receptor 1 protein (CR1).[267–269] These include antigens defined by the alloantisera Knops (Kn^a), McCoy (McC^a), Swain-Langley (Sl^a), and York (Yk^a). These antigens are expressed by more than 90 per cent of most individuals; the antigens Kn^b and McC^b, allelic to Kn^a and McC^a, respectively, are found at low frequency in most populations. Whereas antibodies to antigens within the Knops family have been observed in transfused patients, they are not generally associated with hemolytic transfusion reactions or delayed red cell survival, but they can be clinically relevant because of the problems they can cause with crossmatching procedures. Rare individuals with an apparent Knops null

phenotype (the Hegelson phenotype) express low but detectable levels of CR1.[268, 269] Red cell expression of CR1 is quantitatively variable, which apparently accounts for serological difficulties that can be typical of this system.[269] The antigenic differences in this system are not yet defined at the molecular level.

Polymorphism in Red Cell Acetylcholinesterase; The Cartwright Blood Group System

The Cartwright blood group system is defined by the allelic antigens Yt^a and Yt^b. The Yt^b allele is rare in most populations (8 per cent of white individuals, for example), and anti-Yt antibodies are variably associated with diminished red cell survival.[8] The Yt antigens are borne by red cell acetylcholinesterase, a GPI-linked membrane protein.[270] A nucleotide sequence polymorphism in codon 322 of the YT locus yields histidine at residue 322 in the Yt^a antigen and asparagine in the Yt^b antigen.[271] The genetic deficiency in the synthesis of GPI anchors observed in patients with paroxysmal nocturnal hemoglobinuria type III accounts for the Cartwright null phenotype in these individuals.[270]

Polymorphism in Red Cell CD44; The Indian Blood Group System

The Indian blood group system is composed of the allelic antigens In^a and In^b. Most individuals in most populations express the *In^b* allele and maintain the phenotype In(a−b+) or, rarely, In(a+b+). In^b-negative individuals are rare [In(a+b−)], except in some Indian and Arabic populations, where the *In^a* allele can be found in approximately 3 to 10 per cent of individuals. These persons can develop clinically significant anti-In^a alloantibodies in the context of transfusion. The In antigens are expressed on the red cell isoform of the hyaluronan-binding protein CD44.[230, 272] Antigenic polymorphism within the Indian blood group is accounted for by an arginine at residue 46 of In^b versus a proline at this position in the In^a molecule.[273] A complete deficiency of the Indian antigens is observed in individuals harboring the dominantly acting product of an unknown gene, *In(Lu)*, that inhibits expression of red cell CD44 and the Lutheran blood group antigens.[230, 274]

Polymorphism in the Red Cell Water Channel Aquaporin-I; The Colton Blood Group System

The allelic antigens of the Colton blood group are termed Co^a and Co^b; the *Co^a* allele is exceedingly more frequent than the *Co^b* allele in most populations (the frequency of the *Co^a* allele exceeds 99 per cent in white individuals, for example).[8] Alloantibodies directed toward Colton antigens have been associated with both immediate and delayed-type hemolytic transfusion reactions and with hemolytic disease of the newborn. The Colton antigens are carried on a red cell glycoprotein termed aquaporin-1.[275] Aquaporin-1 is a channel-forming protein that participates in the disposition of water across the red cell membrane.[276] Analysis of the aquaporin gene in individuals informative for Colton blood group polymorphisms assigns alanine to residue 45 of the Co^a antigen and valine to this residue in the Co^b antigen.[275] Homozygosity for aquaporin-1 null alleles in humans is associated with absence of Colton antigen expression [the Co(a−b−) phenotype] and low red cell osmotic water permeabilities but no other clinical abnormality.[277]

Peptide Sequence Polymorphisms on Band 3, the Red Cell Anion Exchange Protein, and the Diego Blood Group System

The red cell anion exchange protein termed AE1 (also known as band 3) bears several polymorphic peptide epitopes that have been assigned to the Diego blood group system.[4, 7, 8] These include allelic Diego (Di^a and Di^b) and Wright (Wr^a and Wr^b) antigens and several other low-frequency antigens. None of these many antigenic variants has any apparent consequence for band 3 function.

The *Diego* (*Di^a*) allele is exceedingly rare in most white populations but has been observed at variable frequencies in some South American and Central Asian populations. Anti-Di^a and anti-Di^b antibodies have been associated with hemolytic disease of the newborn and, rarely, transfusion reactions. Di^a and Di^b antigens correspond to a proline or a leucine residue, respectively, at position 854 of the 911 amino acid–long AE1 glycoprotein.[278, 279]

The *Wright* alleles correspond to the antigens Wr^a and Wr^b. The *Wr^a* allele is rare; in the few populations examined, the *Wr^b* allele is found at a frequency that exceeds 99 per cent. Anti-Wr antibodies have been associated with hemolytic transfusion reactions and hemolytic disease of the newborn. Wr^a and Wr^b antigens correspond to a lysine or a glutamine residue, respectively, encoded by codon 658 of the AE1 locus.[280] Wr^b expression is suppressed in individuals who are deficient in GPA.[280] Whereas this observation implies an important molecular interaction between GPA and band 3, the mechanism that accounts for suppression of Wr^b expression in GPA-null individuals is unknown.

Band 3 also carries several antigens that are found at low frequency in most populations.[4, 7] These antigens are termed Waldner (Wd^a), Redelberger (Rb^a), Traversu (Tr^a), Wulfsberg (Wu), Moen (Mo^a), ELO, and Warrior (WARR). WARR and Wu correspond to Thr 552 → Ile and Gly 565 → Ala substitutions, respectively, in the band 3 polypeptide.[281, 282] ELO, Rb(a+), Tr(a+), and Wd(a+) correspond to Arg 432 → Trp, Pro 548 → Leu, Lys 551 → Asn, and Val 557 → Met substitutions, respectively.[283-285]

Antigens on Uncharacterized Proteins

The Scianna antigen system is composed of Sc1, a high-frequency antigen; Sc2, a low-frequency antigen; and Sc3, which is absent only from red cells of the rare Scianna null phenotype.[4, 8] Alloantibodies corresponding to this system are uncommon, do not fix complement, and therefore are of clinical importance largely in the context of laboratory efforts to identify crossmatch-compatible blood. These anti-

gens correspond to a red cell glycoprotein with a molecular mass of 60 to 68 kDa but whose molecular identity is unknown.[286] The molecular basis for polymorphism in this system and the physiological relevance of this molecule are also not known.

The Dombrock antigen system includes the allelic antigens Do^a and Do^b and the high-frequency antigens Holley (Hy), Gregory (Gya), and Joa.[4, 8] The Dombrock antigens are carried on a GPI-linked glycoprotein of molecular mass 50 kDa.[287] Alloantibodies that recognize antigens within the Dombrock system have been implicated in immediate and delayed transfusion reactions. The molecular nature of the glycoprotein that carries these antigens is not yet defined, nor is there information yet about the function of this protein or molecular basis for polymorphism in this system.

The Xg system is composed of the Xg^a antigen, a 22,500 to 28,000 M_r glycoprotein encoded by a gene on the X chromosome.[288] Anti-Xg^a antibodies are rare and typically without clinical consequence. This gene is not subject to lyonization because the majority of the locus lies within the pseudoautosomal region of the X chromosome. Molecular cloning of the *Xg* locus predicts a 149 amino acid–long protein that shares approximately 48 per cent primary sequence identity with CD99, a molecule that functions in T-lymphocyte trafficking.[289] The protein is predicted to maintain a type I transmembrane topology with an O-glycosylated amino-terminal extracellular domain, a single transmembrane segment, and a short cytoplasmic domain. A hypothetical null allele has yet to be defined molecularly. The function of Xg^a is unknown.

The *ABO* Blood Group Locus

At the beginning of this century, Landsteiner and associates, and other investigators, discovered a system of genetically polymorphic erythrocyte surface molecules that came to be known as the ABO blood group system.[290, 291] Humans could be grouped into distinct classes depending on the presence or absence of substances in the serum that would agglutinate red cells from humans of other classes. These early results quickly found practical use in the field of blood transfusion.[8, 9, 292] The antigens of the ABO system, known as A, B, and H determinants, are expressed by the erythrocyte and by many other tissues, including the epithelium that lines glands and internal organs and the vascular endothelium.[293] The cells of some human tissues can elaborate water-soluble forms of these molecules as components of the glycans on secreted and soluble glycoproteins, on glycosphingolipids, and on free oligosaccharides. The ability to elaborate soluble ABH-active blood group molecules is a genetically inherited trait determined by the *Secretor* or *Se* locus.

▼ OLIGOSACCHARIDE STRUCTURE

The polymorphic and immunoreactive portions of the ABO blood group determinant are displayed at the termini of structurally heterogeneous oligosaccharides (Fig. 9–11). The membrane-associated A, B, and H determinants are components of integral membrane proteins and membrane-associated glycolipids (reviewed in references 293 to 296). A, B,

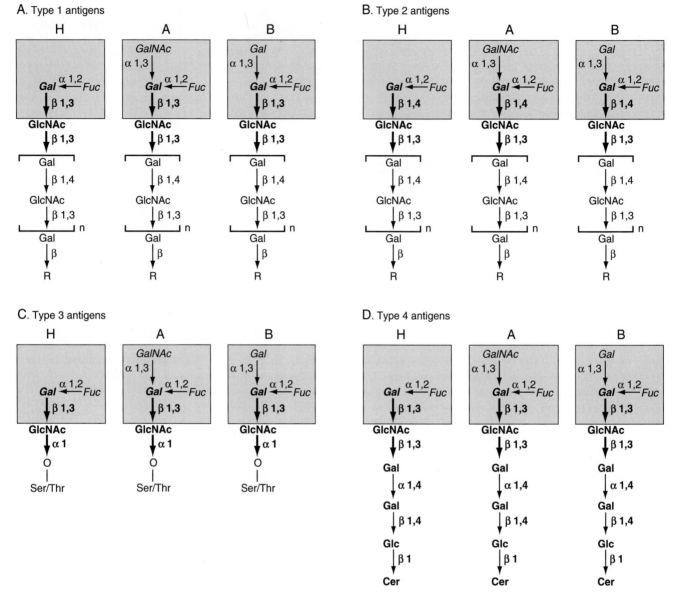

Figure 9–11. Oligosaccharide structures that display red cell ABH blood group determinants. The immunodominant part of each antigen is enclosed within a shaded box, and its monosaccharide components are circled. Component monosaccharides displayed in bold type determine whether the oligosaccharide may be classified as type 1, 2, 3, or 4. *A* and *B,* Type 1 and type 2 determinants, respectively. R represents the asparagine-linked, serine-threonine–linked, or lipid-linked glycoconjugate backbone (see Fig. 9–13). Single lactosamine units are bracketed; this unit may be represented many times as a component of a linear polymer, where n may be 1 to more than 5, or it may not be found at all (n = 0). Not shown are β1,6-linked *N*-acetylgalactosamine residues that yield I antigenic determinants (see Fig. 9–22) and multiple A, B, and H determinants on a branched oligosaccharide. *C,* Type 3 A, B, and H determinants. These oligosaccharides are attached to some serines (Ser) or threonines (Thr) by an α-linked *N*-acetylgalactosamine moiety. *D,* Type 4 A, B, and H determinants. Monosaccharide components of the globo-series backbone shown here are indicated by bold type. These molecules associate with the erythrocyte membrane through their ceramide (Cer) moiety. Similar oligosaccharides based on ganglio-series glycolipid precursors (Galβ1,3GalNAcβ1,3Galβ1,4Glcβ1-Cer) also exist in human tissues (reviewed in reference 297).

and H blood group molecules are constructed by sequential action of distinct glycosyltransferases that are in turn each encoded by a distinct genetic locus (Fig. 9–12). These enzymes operate on one of four structurally distinct oligosaccharide precursor types known to be synthesized in human cells (see Fig. 9–11). Type 1 and type 2 precursors are found at the termini of linear and branched chain oligosaccharides that are themselves linked to proteins (see Fig. 9–11) by some asparagine residues (asparagine-linked oligosaccharides; Fig. 9–13A) or by some serine or threonine residues (serine-threonine–linked oligosaccharides; Fig. 9–13B). Type

1 and type 2 chains may also be displayed as components of lipid-linked oligosaccharides (Fig. 9–13C; see also Fig. 9–11). Type 3 chains are found exclusively as components of serine-threonine–linked oligosaccharides (see Fig. 9–11), whereas type 4 chains are restricted to lipids (see Fig. 9–11). Type 1 oligosaccharide precursors are in general synthesized only by the epithelia lining the digestive, respiratory, urinary, and reproductive tracts as well as by some exocrine glandular epithelium.[293] ABH determinants displayed by proteins and lipids in body fluids and secretions generally derive from these sources and thus are largely represented by type

Figure 9–12. Biosynthesis of type 2 H, A, and B antigens. An α(1,2)fucosyltransferase (encoded either by the *H* locus or by the *Secretor* locus) operates on the type 2 precursor oligosaccharide to form an H determinant. The H determinant may in turn be used by the α(1,3)*N*-acetylgalactosaminyltransferase activity encoded by the *A* blood group locus or by the α(1,3)galactosyltransferase encoded by the *B* blood group locus to form, respectively, the A or B blood group antigen. The *A* transferase requires UDP-*N*-acetylgalactosamine (UDP-GalNAc) as its sugar nucleotide donor, whereas the *B* transferase uses UDP-galactose (UDP-Gal). Types 1, 3, and 4 A, B, and H determinants are constructed in a manner virtually identical to the reactions shown here. R represents the asparagine-linked, serine-threonine–linked, or lipid-linked glycoconjugate backbone.

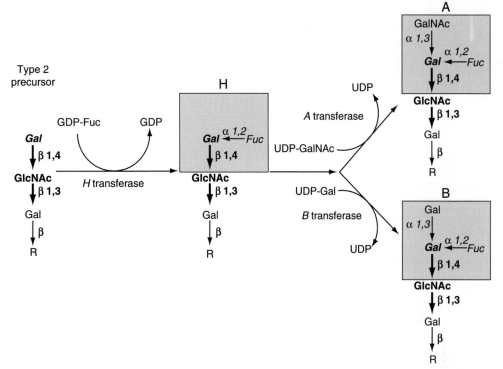

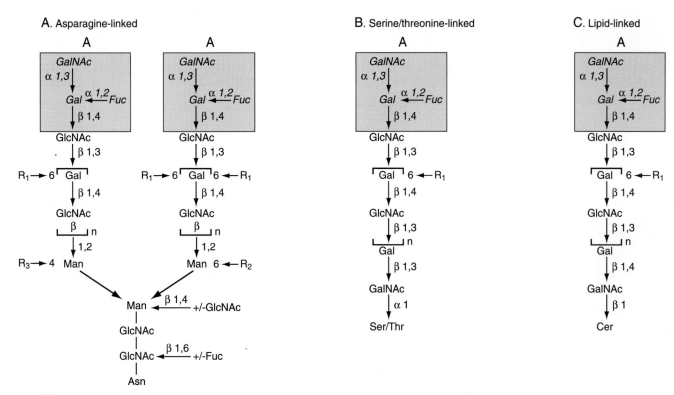

Figure 9–13. Glycoconjugate substructures that display the ABH blood group determinants. An A-active asparagine-linked oligosaccharide is shown in *A*, a serine-threonine–linked A determinant is displayed in *B*, and *C* shows a lipid-linked A-active oligosaccharide molecule. R_1 denotes branching oligosaccharide chains linked by β1→6-linked *N*-acetylglucosamine (GlcNac) residues that form portions of I determinants (see Fig. 9–22). R_2 and R_3 indicate positions where other GlcNAc residues may be added to form tri- and tetra-antennary oligosaccharides.[341] Lactosamine units that may be polymerized (n = 0 to 5 or more) are enclosed in brackets.

1 molecules. By contrast, the ABH determinants displayed by erythrocytes, and the epidermis, are based largely on type 2 precursor chains.[294, 296, 297] Type 3 A, B, and H antigens are relatively abundant components of mucins that are elaborated by the gastric mucosa or by the cells that line ovarian cysts (reviewed in references 297 and 298). The mucin-based type 3 ABH determinants are not found on human erythrocytes.[299] A variant of type 3 ABH-active chains, however, known as the A-associated type 3 chain (Fig. 9–14), has been shown to be present in the glycolipids isolated from blood group A red cells.[299, 300] Human red cell glycolipids also contain A, B, and H determinants based on type 4 chains.[301, 302]

▼ GLYCOSYLTRANSFERASES

During the formation of the ABO blood group determinants, oligosaccharide precursors are first modified in a transglycosylation reaction catalyzed by $\alpha(1,2)$fucosyltransferases (see Fig. 9–12). These enzymes utilize the nucleotide sugar substrate GDP-fucose and transfer the fucose moiety to carbon 2 of the galactose molecule at the oligosaccharide precursor's non-reducing terminus. The fucose is attached in alpha anomeric linkage and forms the blood group H determinant, represented by the disaccharide unit Fucα(1,2)Galβ- (reviewed in references 293 and 294). Genetic and biochemical evidence to be summarized below indicates that the human genome encodes at least two different $\alpha(1,2)$fucosyltransferases, which correspond to the products of the *H* and the *Se* blood group loci. The $\alpha(1,2)$fucosyltransferases encoded by the two loci exhibit characteristic tissue-specific expression patterns (reviewed in reference 303) and display different affinities for the various ABH blood group precursor types. For example, the *H* locus–encoded enzyme, expressed in erythrocyte precursors, uses type 2[304] and type 4[305] precursors

to form type 2 (see Figs. 9–11 and 9–12) and type 4 H determinants (see Fig. 9–11). By contrast, the *Se* $\alpha(1,2)$fucosyltransferase, expressed in endodermally derived epithelia,[303] operates on type 1[304] and type 3[300] precursors to form the corresponding type 1 and type 3 H determinants (see Fig. 9–11).

Codominant glycosyltransferases encoded by the *ABO* blood group locus in turn use type 1, 2, 3, or 4 H determinants to form A or B blood group determinants (reviewed in references 293 to 295). The *A* allele at the *ABO* locus encodes an $\alpha(1,3)N$-acetylgalactosaminyltransferase that uses H molecules to form the blood group A molecule (see Fig. 9–12). The blood group *B* allele, by contrast, encodes an $\alpha(1,3)$galactosyltransferase that operates on H-active oligosaccharide precursors to form the blood group B determinant (see Fig. 9–12). The *O* allele represents a null allele incapable of encoding a functional glycosyltransferase that will further modify H-active precursors. Thus, an individual's complement of alleles at the *ABO* locus determines whether that individual is capable of constructing A molecule exclusively (genotype *AA* or *AO*), only B determinants (genotype *BB* or *BO*), or both A and B determinants (genotype *AB*). Individuals who maintain two null alleles at the *ABO* locus (genotype *OO*) do not modify their H-active precursors, and their red cells and tissues thus do not construct A or B determinants.

▼ EXPRESSION IN THE RED BLOOD CELL

Most of the ABH determinants expressed on human erythrocytes are components of membrane-associated glycoproteins. Roughly 80 per cent of the red cell ABH determinants (1 to 2 million molecules per red cell)[306] are displayed by the anion transport protein, also known as band 3.[307] The red cell glucose transport protein (band 4.5) also displays a

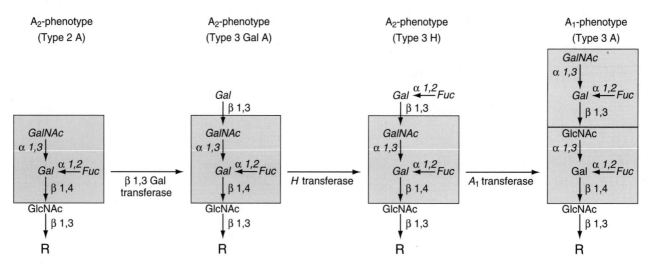

Figure 9–14. Model for structural differences between antigens constructed by the A$_1$ and A$_2$ subgroup transferases.[297, 299, 305] Type 2 A determinants representative of the A$_2$ phenotype (far left) are constructed by both A$_1$ and A$_2$ subgroup transferases. These determinants are then modified by a $\beta(1,3)$galactosyltransferase (β1,3Gal transferase) to form a type 3 precursor (type 3 Gal A, or "A-associated" determinant) also typical of the A$_2$ phenotype. This precursor is then fucosylated by the *H* locus–encoded $\alpha(1,2)$fucosyltransferase to yield a type 3 H determinant. Type 3 H determinants are efficiently used by the A$_1$ transferase to form a repetitive A-reactive unit that terminates with a type 3 A structure. These moieties are proposed to be responsible for the A$_1$ phenotype.[297, 299] By contrast, the A$_2$ transferase is unable to efficiently complete this reaction.[305] R represents the underlying glycosphingolipid substructure, as shown in Figure 9–13C. A-reactive portions of the molecule are circled, and the component monosaccharides of these moieties are italicized.

significant number of ABH determinants (roughly 5×10^5 molecules).[308, 309] These two polypeptides are integral membrane proteins, and each displays ABH determinants on a single asparagine-linked oligosaccharide molecule.[309, 310] This asparagine-linked oligosaccharide is a branched poly-*N*-acetylgalactosaminoglycan, whose terminal branches may display several ABH determinants[311] (see Fig. 9–13). Other red cell glycoproteins, including the Rh-related proteins and the aquaporin-1 glycoprotein,[312] also display ABH determinants, albeit in smaller numbers.[313] The precise structures of the A-, B-, and H-active glycans attached to these proteins are not yet well defined. Red cell membrane-associated glycolipids account for the rest of the red cell ABH molecules (approximately 5×10^5 determinants per red cell). These molecules are also poly-*N*-acetylgalactosaminoglycan based and have been termed polyglycosylceramides, or macroglycolipids[314, 315] (see Fig. 9–13).

▼ ANTI-A AND ANTI-B ANTIBODIES

The structural polymorphisms in these erythrocyte surface-localized oligosaccharides, determined by the *ABO* locus, are clinically important entities under some circumstances.[8, 9] During infancy, the human immune system elaborates IgM antibodies specific for ABO oligosaccharide determinants that are *not* displayed by that person's erythrocytes or by other cells or tissues. It is believed that this immune response is a consequence of exposure to microbial oligosaccharide antigens that are structurally similar to, or identical to, the A and B blood group molecules. For example, type O persons lack A and B determinants and consequently maintain substantial titers of naturally occurring IgM antibodies, or isoagglutinins, reactive with A and B blood group molecules. Likewise, blood group B individuals maintain anti-A IgM-type isoagglutinins but not anti-B isoagglutinins. Similarly, sera taken from blood group A individuals contain IgM-type anti-B antibodies but not anti-A antibodies. Finally, blood group AB persons make neither anti-A nor anti-B IgM-type isoagglutinins. In most individuals, antibodies directed against H determinants are not formed because a substantial number of the blood group H precursors are not enzymatically converted to A or B determinants, even in persons with a functional *A* or *B* allele. However, as discussed below, individuals exist whose cells and tissues are relatively or completely deficient in H determinants. These persons, with the Bombay or para-Bombay phenotype, do typically generate anti-H antibodies, and also anti-A and anti-B antibodies, because they cannot construct A or B determinants in their red cell precursors, regardless of their genotype at the *ABO* locus (see Fig. 9–12).

The naturally occurring IgM isoagglutinins fix complement with efficiency and are present in sufficiently high titer to allow them to rapidly lyse transfused erythrocytes that display the corresponding antigen. This event is typically accompanied by the other clinical manifestations of an immediate or acute transfusion reaction and is normally avoided by the now-routine ABO blood group typing and crossmatching procedures that were implemented earlier in this century.[8, 9] These procedures ensure compatibility between the ABO phenotype of transfused red cells and recipient plasma or, conversely, compatibility between transfused plasma and a recipient's red cells. Similar ABO compatibility issues are of concern in heart, liver, kidney, and marrow transplantation procedures (reviewed in reference 316).

▼ A AND B SUBGROUPS

Routine ABO blood group typing and crossmatching procedures identify variants of blood group A determinants, termed A subgroups.[8, 317, 318] For example, blood group A individuals may be subgrouped according to whether their red cells will be agglutinated with an appropriately diluted solution of a carbohydrate-binding protein, or lectin, termed *Dolichos biflorus*.[319] Red cells that are agglutinated with this procedure are termed A_1 cells, whereas the red cells that are not agglutinated are termed A_2 cells. Antibody specific for A_1 cells may be prepared from group O or group B sera by prior adsorption with A_2 cells. In contrast, antibody specific for A_2 cells cannot be prepared by the converse procedure, adsorption with A_1 cells.[8] As discussed below, A_1 and A_2 phenotypes correspond to different alleles at the *ABO* locus.[294, 295] Their frequency varies among different ethnic groups,[320] although the A^1 allele is substantially more frequent than the A^2 allele in most populations. The enzymes corresponding to the A^1 and A^2 alleles, and those of other A subgroups, differ in their isoelectric points, metal ion requirements, pH activity profiles, and glycan precursors and nucleotide sugar substrate affinities (reviewed in references 294 and 295). The absolute number of immunodominant molecules is greater on A_1 cells than it is on A_2 cells.[321, 322] The A_1 and A_2 subgroup antigens also differ in their molecular structure in a way that can be accounted for by the more active catalytic activity of the A^1 transferase[321, 323–325] (see Fig. 9–14). Several other relatively rare subgroups of A also exist (reviewed in references 317 and 318) and represent the products of biochemically distinct $\alpha(1,3)N$-acetylgalactosaminyltransferase activities that lead to weakly positive red cell A-active structures with distinct antigenic properties. Unusual, weakly reactive blood group B antigens also exist.[8, 317, 318] The serological properties that allow an assignment of a given individual's red cell ABO phenotype to the various A and B subgroups are treated in detail in reference 318. The molecular polymorphisms that correspond to the *A* and *B* subgroup alleles are discussed below.

The cis-AB phenotype has been described in rare pedigrees in which the ability to express both A and B determinants is inherited on a single chromosome transmitted from one parent.[326–328] In most such pedigrees, the cis-AB phenotype is characterized by a weakly reactive A antigen, similar in reactivity to A_2 cell reactivity. Typically, red cells from individuals with the cis-AB phenotype also display only weak B antigen reactivity. The relatively weak A and B reactivities are similar to those observed in the A_2B_3 phenotype.[318]

Two genetic models, supported by family studies and molecular analyses described below, account for the cis-AB phenotype.[329–331] In one model, now supported by molecular analyses,[332] a wild-type *A* or *B* transferase allele has evolved to yield a single polypeptide capable of using both UDP-*N*-acetylgalactosamine and UDP-galactose and thus also capable of synthesizing both A and B determinants. In a second model, the cis-AB phenotype is determined by two closely linked loci that each encode separate transferases, one with A-like activity and one with B-like activity. Such duplicated alleles could have arisen through an intrachromosomal duplication of an *A* (or *B*) allele to first yield a pair of tandemly repeated but otherwise identical transferase loci, followed by mutation of one locus to a *B*-like (or *A*-like) configuration. This mechanism has not yet been observed in any individuals with the cis-AB phenotype.

A related rare phenotype, termed B$_{(A)}$, is characterized by red cells with abundant B antigen activity and small but detectable amounts of A reactivity. In some families, this trait is inherited on a single chromosome and is accounted for by an *ABO* allele encoding a single enzyme capable of robust B antigen synthesis and residual A antigen synthesis.[333]

▼ MOLECULAR GENETICS

The human A transferase cDNA has been cloned and sequenced,[334, 335] and the structure of the corresponding locus has been defined.[336, 337] The cDNA sequence predicts a 353 amino acid–long protein with a 15 residue NH$_2$-terminal segment, a 24 residue hydrophobic segment, and a 314 residue COOH-terminal domain. The hydrophobic segment functions as a signal anchor sequence to yield a protein with a type II transmembrane orientation (Fig. 9–15). This topology is typical for mammalian glycosyltransferases (reviewed in references 338 and 339) and places the enzyme's COOH-terminal catalytic domain within the membrane-delimited compartments of the Golgi and the *trans*-Golgi network,[340] where terminal glycosylation reactions occur.[341] The peptide sequence predicts a single potential site for aspara-

gine-linked glycosylation, suggesting the possibility that this enzyme is itself synthesized as a glycoprotein, as are other mammalian glycosyltransferases.[338, 339] The enzyme shares substantial primary amino acid sequence similarity to murine and bovine α(1,3)galactosyltransferases,[342, 343] with sequences predicted by a pair of human α(1,3)galactosyltransferase pseudogenes[344, 345] and a glycosyltransferase that can construct the Forssman antigen,[346] but not to other previously described proteins.

Whereas the cDNA sequence predicts a transmembrane enzyme, the A transferase was purified as a soluble, catalytically active polypeptide from human lung.[334] The NH$_2$ terminus of the soluble enzyme corresponds to the alanine residue encoded by codon 54 of the cDNA sequence, indicating that the soluble, catalytically active form of the A transferase is derived from its transmembrane precursor by one or more specific proteolytic events (see Fig. 9–15). Similar processes have been described for other mammalian glycosyltransferases known to exist in both membrane-associated and soluble, catalytically active forms.[338, 339] It is presumed that such proteolytic events also generate the soluble A and B transferase activities found in human serum (reviewed in reference 294).

The molecular basis for polymorphism at the *ABO* locus has been defined[347] (Fig. 9–16; Table 9–6). In the first of what is now a large number of studies that have explored this issue, the blood group O phenotype was shown to be due to a single base pair deletion of one nucleotide in the codon for amino acid 87 of the A transferase.[347] This frameshift mutation generates a protein whose amino acid sequence differs completely from that of the A transferase at residues distal to amino acid residue 86 (see Fig. 9–16). The frameshifted reading frame ends at a termination codon corresponding to amino acid residue 117 of the A transferase. This single base pair deletion in the O allele thus predicts the synthesis of an altered and shortened polypeptide lacking a functional catalytic domain. The truncated protein is consequently unable to modify the H antigen to form A or B structures. These results explain why no detectable A or B transferase activity is found in the sera taken from blood group O individuals (genotype *OO*) and why the erythrocytes of these individuals are devoid of A or B determinants.

Comparisons of the sequences of the cDNAs isolated from cultured human cell lines that express the A or B phenotype identified seven nucleotide sequence differences within their protein-coding segments.[347] Three of these represent functionally neutral polymorphisms. The other four generate amino acid sequence differences between the A and B transferases expressed by these cell lines (see Fig. 9–16). The four amino acid sequence polymorphisms are located at residues 176 (arginine, A; glycine, B), 235 (glycine, A; serine, B), 266 (leucine, A; methionine, B), and 268 (glycine, A; alanine, B). The polymorphisms at positions 266 and 268 exert a strong influence on the enzyme's ability to discriminate between UDP–*N*-acetylgalactosamine and UDP-galactose.[348] Thus, leucine at 266 and glycine at 268 generate an A phenotype, independent of the polypeptide sequence at the other two polymorphic positions; similarly, a B transferase phenotype is observed whenever B transferase residues are placed at these positions (methionine at 266, alanine at 268), irrespective of the residues at positions 176 and 235. The

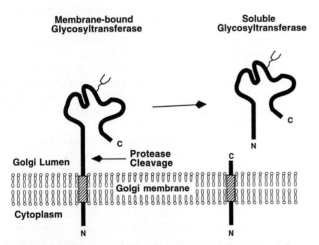

Figure 9–15. Topology and biosynthesis of type II transmembrane-oriented mammalian glycosyltransferases. The enzyme's NH$_2$ terminus (N) of the full-length enzyme orients to the cytosolic face of the Golgi membrane, whereas its larger COOH-terminal catalytic domain (C) resides within the lumen of the Golgi apparatus. A short, hydrophobic transmembrane segment *(hatched box)* anchors the enzyme within the Golgi membrane. The A, B, H, and Lewis blood group transferases are each predicted to contain one or more asparagine-linked glycosylation sites (oligosaccharide is represented by the branched structure attached to the protein backbone). Soluble, catalytically active forms of mammalian glycosyltransferases *(right)* derive from their membrane-bound precursors by one or more proteolytic events that release the catalytic domain from its membrane-associated NH$_2$ terminus.

Figure 9–16. Molecular basis for polymorphism at the ABO locus. The polypeptide products of representative *ABO* alleles are displayed as boxes. NH_2-terminal transmembrane segments are denoted by the hatched portion within each box. The *A¹* allele encodes a 353 amino acid–long α(1,3)N-acetylgalactosaminyltransferase. An *A²* subgroup allele differs from the *A¹* allele by a leucine for proline substitution at amino acid residue 156 and by a single base pair deletion at nucleotide position 1059. This deletion leads to a translational frameshift that elongates the protein by 21 amino acids. The α(1,3)galactosyltransferase encoded by the *B* locus is identical in length to the A α(1,3)N-acetylgalactosaminyltransferase. The *A¹* and *B* transferases differ at the four amino acid positions indicated by the numbered arrows above the boxes. The *cis-AB* allele–encoded transferase maintains amino acid sequence residues that help determine nucleotide sugar substrate specificity both for the A transferase (glycine at position 235 and leucine at position 266) and for the B transferase (alanine at position 268). The sequence of the *O¹* allele–encoded protein is identical to the sequences of A and B transferases up to a valine residue at amino acid position 86. It is different at the 30 subsequent positions (indicated by the fine hatched lines at the COOH terminus of the box depicting the *O¹* allele–encoded protein) because of a frameshifting single base deletion within codon 87. A termination codon within the altered reading frame truncates the resulting protein at 116 residues and yields a non-functional protein. Another common *O* allele *(O²)* is predicted to encode a protein with a length identical to the A and B transferases but is enzymatically inactive because of the presence of an arginine substitution at amino acid position 268.

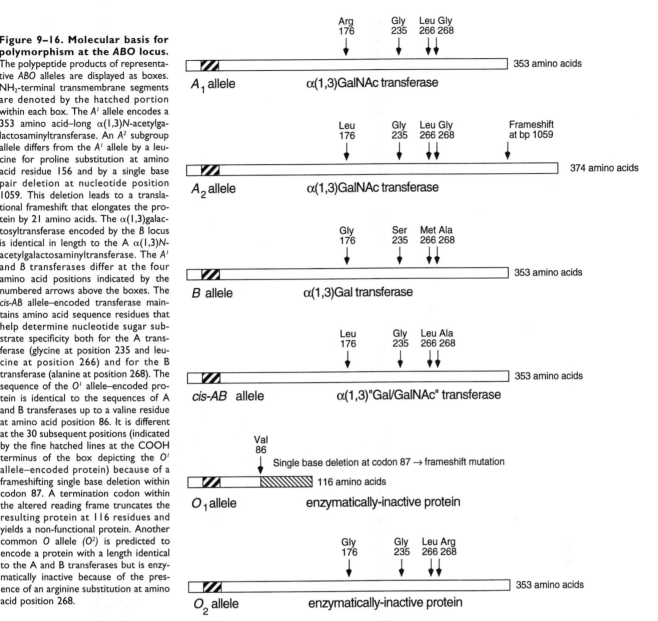

polymorphism at position 176 has virtually no detectable influence on substrate discrimination.

These initial observations have now been expanded to define a large degree of polymorphism within the *ABO* locus (see Table 9–6). This includes DNA and corresponding amino acid sequence polymorphisms that account for alleles representative of most A and B subgroups as well as multiple alleles within some specific subgroups.[333, 349–356] These polymorphisms are characterized by single or multiple amino acid substitutions, sometimes occurring in combination with a single nucleotide deletion (one example of an *A²* allele[349]) or a single nucleotide insertion (two examples of an *A^el* allele[353, 354]). These insertions or deletions yield an altered polypeptide sequence distal to the resulting translational frameshift (see Table 9–6). In most cases, these A and B subgroup enzymes have not been characterized with respect to their catalytic properties, but limited information implies a direct correlation between the catalytic efficiency of a given enzyme and the relative immunoreactivity of the cor-

responding subgroup antigen.[295, 318] Many of these studies have explored the basis for A and B subgroup phenotype by characterizing polymorphisms within the two exons of the *ABO* locus that correspond to amino acids between residue 80 and the COOH terminus of the protein (exons 6 and 7). This approach may neglect to identify functionally relevant polymorphisms in exon 5, corresponding to the amino-terminal 80 amino acids. The amino-terminal location of these 80 residues, proximal to the catalytic domain of the transferase,[338] implies that they will have little, if any, effect on catalytic activity and will thus merit less consideration in the evaluation of polymorphisms that can account for subgroup phenotypes. Nonetheless, *A³* and *B³* alleles have been described in which the sequences of exons 6 and 7 do not predict amino acid sequence differences, relative to an *A¹* allele.[333, 350] It is not yet known whether the A₃ or B₃ phenotype in these individuals can be assigned to alterations elsewhere in the *ABO* locus (in exon 5, for example) or whether these phenotypes are a consequence of alterations in other loci.

Table 9–6. Representative Sequence Polymorphisms Corresponding to Variant A, B, and O Alleles of the ABO Blood Group Locus

Allele	156 (467)	176 (526)	214 (641)	216 (646)	223 (669)	235 (703)	266 (796)	268 (803)	277 (829)	291 (871)	352 (1054)	Note	References
					Amino Acid (Nucleotide) Position								
A^1	Pro	Arg	Met	Phe	Glu	Gly	Leu	Gly	Val	Asp	Arg		347
A^1	**Leu**	Arg	Met	Phe	Glu	Gly	Leu	Gly	Val	Asp	Arg	Elongated fusion protein[1]	354
A^2	**Leu**	Arg	Met	Phe	Glu	Gly	Leu	Gly	Val	Asp	Arg		349
A^2	Pro	Arg	Met	Phe	Glu	Gly	Leu	Gly	Val	Asp	**Trp**		354
A^2	Pro	Arg	Met	Phe	Glu	Gly	Leu	Gly	Val	Asp	**Gly**		354
A^3	Pro	**Gly**	Met	Phe	Glu	**Ser**	Leu	Gly	**Met**	**Asn**	Arg		350
A^el	Pro	Arg	Met	Phe	Glu	Gly	Leu	Gly	Val	Asp	—	Elongated fusion protein[2]	353, 354
A^el	**Leu**	Arg	Met	**Ile**	Glu	Gly	Leu	Gly	Val	Asp	Arg		354
A^x	Pro	Arg	Met	**Ile**	Glu	Gly	Leu	Gly	Val	Asp	Arg		333
B	Pro	**Gly**	Met	Phe	Glu	**Ser**	**Met**	**Ala**	Val	Asp	Arg		347
B^3	Pro	**Gly**	Met	Phe	Glu	**Ser**	**Met**	**Ala**	Val	Asp	**Trp**		350
B^x	Pro	**Gly**	**Arg**	Phe	Glu	**Ser**	**Met**	**Ala**	Val	**Asn**	Arg		354
B^el	Pro	**Gly**	Met	Phe	Glu	**Ser**	**Met**	**Ala**	Val	Asp	Arg		354
B^el	Pro	**Gly**	Met	Phe	**Asp**	**Ser**	**Met**	**Ala**	Val	Asp	Arg		354
cis-AB	**Leu**	Arg	Met	Phe	Glu	Gly	Leu	**Ala**	Val	Asp	Arg		332
B^(A)	Pro	**Gly**	Met	Phe	Glu	Gly	**Met**	**Ala**	Val	Asp	Arg		333
O^1	—	—	—	—	—	—	—	—	—	—	—	Truncated fusion protein[3]	347
O^1var	Pro	—	Met	Phe	Glu	Gly	Leu	**Arg**	Val	Asp	—	Truncated fusion protein[4]	347, 355
O^2	Pro	**Gly**	Met	Phe	Glu	Gly	Leu	**Arg**	Val	Asp	Arg		351, 352
O^3	**Leu**	Arg	Met	Phe	Glu	Gly	Leu	Gly	—	—	—	Elongated fusion protein[5]	356

[1] Also contains a single nucleotide deletion at bp 1059, leading to a translational frameshift that adds 21 amino acids to the COOH terminus.
[2] Contains a single nucleotide insertion in a stretch of seven consecutive Gs in the A^1 allele at bp 798 to 804, leading to a translational frameshift that adds amino acids to the COOH terminus.
[3] Contains a single nucleotide deletion at bp 261, leading to a translational frameshift that truncates the protein at 117 amino acids in length.
[4] Same single nucleotide deletion at bp 261 found in O^1 allele, but additional DNA sequence differences elsewhere.
[5] Also has the same single nucleotide insertional frameshift between bp 798 and 804 found in an A^el allele.

Examples of alleles encoding enzymes with the ability to construct both A and B antigens (in individuals with the cis-AB and B$_{(A)}$ phenotypes) have been characterized.[332, 333] As might be expected, these alleles predict the expression of chimeric enzymes that include amino acid residues important both to UDP-galactose utilization (the B-specific alanine residue at position 268, for example)[357] and to UDP-N-acetylgalactosamine utilization (the A-specific glycine residue at position 235, for example)[357] (see Table 9–6).

O alleles distinct from the one originally defined (O^1) have also been described (see Table 9–6). These include the relatively common O^{1var} allele, which, like the originally described O allele (O^1), predicts a truncated polypeptide but differs from the DNA sequence of the O^1 allele at several positions.[347, 355] The O^{1var} allele is estimated to account for 40 to 50 per cent of the O alleles in several different populations.[354, 355] There is evidence that the transcript corresponding to the O^1 allele is unstable,[358] implying reduced or absent expression of the truncated fusion protein predicted by these alleles. The relatively rare O^2 allele predicts glycine and arginine substitutions at amino acid residues 176 and 268, respectively. The latter substitution is presumed to be catalytically inactivating.[351, 352] The rare O^3 allele maintains a leucine residue at position 156 characteristic of an A^1 allele and the single G insertion characteristic of an A^{el} allele (see Table 9–6). The combination of these two alterations is presumed to yield a catalytically inactive protein. The relative stability of the O^2 and O^3 transcripts has not been examined.

▼ FUNCTIONS

The functions of the ABO blood group oligosaccharides remain unknown, as do the processes that may account for polymorphism in the ABO locus. Numerous associations between ABO blood group phenotype and relative risk for a number of diseases have been reported (reviewed in references 359 to 362). These associations remain substantially imperfect and generally without an identifiable causal relationship, with two possible exceptions.

The first possible exception concerns the long-standing observation that plasma levels of the factor VIII/von Willebrand factor complex correlate with an individual's ABO phenotype (reviewed in reference 363). The biochemical basis for these observations is not understood, although studies in the mouse suggest that polymorphisms in glycosyltransferase loci that modify von Willebrand factor glycans can have a profound effect on the circulating half-life of this glycoprotein.[364] Specifically, these observations demonstrate that in a mouse strain with a von Willebrand disease phenotype, low plasma levels of von Willebrand factor can be accounted for by a dominantly inherited trait that directs expression of a β(1,4)N-acetylgalactosaminyltransferase to vascular endothelial cells, a major site of von Willebrand factor synthesis. Endothelial cell expression of this enzyme decorates von Willebrand factor glycans with the corresponding β(1,4)N-acetylgalactosamine modification, leading, in turn, to rapid clearance of this von Willebrand factor glycoform through the hepatic asialoglycoprotein receptor.[364] Similar mechanisms may account for generally lower von Willebrand factor levels in persons of the O phenotype, because von Willebrand factor is modified by the ABO blood group antigens in humans and because the A, B, and H blood group structures may be recognized with different affinities by lectins in humans.

A second possible exception is the proposed role for ABO and Lewis blood group structures in the pathogenesis of *Helicobacter pylori* infection and the pathophysiological consequences thereof (reviewed in reference 365; discussed in additional detail below). Examples relevant to this possibility include the association between group A phenotype and slight increase in the relative risk for stomach cancer (relative risk of approximately 1.2)[366] and the association between blood group O phenotype and a mildly increased propensity to develop peptic ulcers (relative risk of roughly 1.3).[367] Selective advantage, such as protection from various infectious agents, has been invoked to explain the establishment of the ABO blood group frequencies in human populations (reviewed in reference 368). However, no evidence from population or other studies has been provided in support of this notion, including more recent studies that have used molecular genotyping to define ABO allele frequencies in various races. It remains possible that environmental pressures once selected for, or against, expression of A or B determinants and that such pressures are no longer widely operative (discussed in reference 368). The nature of such pressures remains a subject for speculation.

The *H* and *Se* Blood Group Loci

H blood group oligosaccharide precursors represent essential substrates for the transferases encoded by the *ABO* locus (see Fig. 9–12). H-active precursors display terminal Fucα(1,2)Galβ linkages, which are also an integral part of the A and B antigenic determinants (see Figs. 9–11 and 9–12). H-active Fucα(1,2)Galβ linkages are synthesized by α(1,2)fucosyltransferases (GDP-fucose:Galβ 2-α-L-fucosyltransferase, E.C. 2.4.1.69) (see Fig. 9–12). These transferases can use types 1, 2, 3, and 4 glycoprotein or glycolipid substrates (reviewed in reference 294) as well as low molecular weight β-D-galactosides.[369]

In humans, the ability to synthesize H-active blood group substances, and thus also A- or B-active substances (depending on the *ABO* locus genotype), is determined by at least two discrete genetic loci. These loci are termed the *H* locus and the *Secretor* (*Se*) locus (reviewed in references 293 and 294). The *Se* locus determines expression of an α(1,2)fucosyltransferase activity, and also membrane-associated and soluble H-active blood group substances, in epithelial cells that line the digestive, respiratory, and urinary tracts, for example, and in the acinar cells of the salivary glands. In secretor-positive individuals, it is possible to detect such soluble group-active substances by testing saliva for their presence, with use of hemagglutination-inhibition methods.[8] Nearly all of this soluble blood group–active substance is constructed from type 1 precursors[293] and is elaborated largely by the sublingual and submaxillary glands and to a lesser extent by the parotid gland.[370, 371] If the tested individual also maintains a functional *A* or *B* allele, the saliva will contain soluble A- or B-active blood group molecules in addition to H-active blood group substance, because the *ABO* locus is also expressed in these tissues. By contrast, the saliva taken from non-secretor individuals does not contain H-active blood group substance or significant levels of $\alpha(1,2)$fucosyltransferase activity. Moreover, because H determinants represent essential precursors for the synthesis of A and B determinants, their absence precludes synthesis of A- and B-active molecules, regardless of the non-secretor's *ABO* locus genotype.

By contrast, erythrocytes taken from both secretors and non-secretors maintain an essentially identical complement of H determinants and also A or B determinants, depending on the *ABO* locus genotype. This is because the synthesis of $\alpha(1,2)$fucosyltransferase activity, and thus H determinants, in erythrocyte precursors, is directed by the *H* locus.[293, 294] Rare individuals have been described, however, whose red cells are deficient in H (and also A and B) determinants. These individuals are homozygous for null alleles at the *H* locus. The first description of such individuals termed this the Bombay (O_h) blood group phenotype,[372] after the city of origin of the pedigree. The saliva and other secretions taken from individuals with the Bombay phenotype in this pedigree, and from similar such individuals in other subsequently described Bombay pedigrees, are also deficient in H determinants and also A and B determinants. Consequently, individuals with the Bombay phenotype maintain high titers of naturally occurring isoagglutinins that react with H determinants (and with A and B antigens as well). As with A and B isoagglutinins in O phenotype individuals, it is again presumed that these IgM-type anti-H antibodies develop in response to H antigens elaborated by microbes. These anti-H isoagglutinins render these individuals crossmatch incompatible with all blood group donors, except other Bombay donors whose red cells do not display H determinants.[8, 9]

Subsequent studies have identified a related phenotype, termed the para-Bombay phenotype.[373] Red cells taken from these individuals are relatively deficient in H, A, and B determinants, but their saliva contains an essentially normal amount of H blood group substance. These individuals often maintain low-titer circulating antibodies reactive with H antigens.

▼ GENETIC MODELS

A model accounting for each of the four phenotypes described above (Fig. 9–17) proposes that the *H* and *Se* loci

correspond to distinct genes encoding different $\alpha(1,2)$fucosyltransferases with disparate tissue-specific expression patterns.[374] This model proposes that the *H* locus is expressed predominantly by cells of the erythroid lineage, by keratinocytes in the epidermis, and by primary sensory neurons within the peripheral nervous system.[293, 297, 375] By contrast, the *Se* locus represents a second $\alpha(1,2)$fucosyltransferase locus whose expression is generally restricted to the epithelia lining the respiratory, digestive, biliary, and urinary tracts and to the acinar cells of salivary glands.[376, 377] Individuals with the common secretor phenotype (roughly 80 per cent of most populations[378]) are thus believed to maintain at least one functional allele at both the *H* locus and the *Se* locus. Individuals with the non-secretor phenotype (nearly all of the remaining 20 per cent of individuals) maintain two null alleles at the *Se* locus but at least one functional *H* allele. The model proposes that the rare Bombay phenotype is the consequence of homozygosity for null alleles at the *H* locus and also at the *Se* locus, whereas the equally rare para-Bombay phenotype results from a state of homozygosity for null alleles at the *H* locus in the context of at least one functional *Se* allele (see Fig. 9–17).

▼ MOLECULAR GENETICS

The two-locus model is supported by biochemical, genetic, and molecular evidence. Careful analysis of the catalytic activities of the $\alpha(1,2)$fucosyltransferase determined by the *H* locus, and the corresponding enzyme determined by the *Se* locus, indicate that the *Se*-determined $\alpha(1,2)$fucosyltransferase maintains a significantly higher affinity for type 1 precursors than does the *H*-determined enzyme.[379–381] These observations are additionally consistent with the finding that blood group–active substances elaborated by secretory epithelia (where the *Se* locus is expressed) are constructed mainly from type 1 precursors, whereas erythrocyte H determinants, synthesized by the *H*-encoded $\alpha(1,2)$fucosyltransferase, are based largely on type 2 precursors (reviewed in references 293 and 303). These observations also support a hypothesis that optimal utilization of the stereochemically distinct type 1 and type 2 precursors should require structurally and enzymatically distinct $\alpha(1,2)$fucosyltransferases (reviewed in reference 382). Furthermore, early genetic and biochemical studies of several H-deficient pedigrees indicate

Phenotype	Phenotype (trivial name)	Genotype
H (A&B) on red cells		*HH* or *Hh*
	Secretor	
H (A&B) in secretions		*Sese* or *SeSe*
H (A&B) on red cells		*HH* or *Hh*
	Non-Secretor	
H (A&B) absent from secretions		*sese*
weak or absent H (A&B) on red cells (antigens adsorbed from plasma)		*hh*
	para-Bombay	
H (A&B) in secretions		*Sese* or *SeSe*
H (A&B) absent from red cells		*hh*
	Bombay, or O_h	
H (A&B) absent from secretions		*sese*

Figure 9–17. The two-locus model for H and Se phenotypes. The *H* and *Se* loci correspond to distinct, chromosome 19–localized $\alpha(1,2)$fucosyltransferase genes with different tissue-specific expression patterns. The table displays the red cell and secretion antigenic phenotypes predicted for various genotypes at the two loci. A and B antigens are included in parentheses to indicate that they will be displayed also only if the individual maintains a functional A or B transferase allele. Red cells of para-Bombay individuals display H (and A or B) antigens weakly, or not at all, because they are acquired in low amounts from glycosphingolipid-based antigens circulating in the plasma.

that although the *H* and *Se* loci are closely linked on chromosome 19 (lod score of 12.9 at 1 per cent recombination[374]), they nonetheless determine expression of α(1,2)fucosyltransferases with distinctly different catalytic properties.

Molecular cloning studies have defined the structures of the human *H* and *Se* loci (also known as *FUT1* and *FUT2*, respectively).[380, 383–387] The human *H* locus (Fig. 9–18) encodes a 365 amino acid–long polypeptide with the type II transmembrane topology characteristic of mammalian glycosyltransferases. The amino acid sequence predicts an 8 amino acid–long NH$_2$-terminal cytosolic domain, a 17 residue hydrophobic domain that presumably spans the Golgi membrane, and a 340 amino acid–long COOH-terminal domain corresponding to a Golgi-localized catalytic domain (see Figs. 9–15 and 9–18). Two potential asparagine-linked glycosylation sites are located within the COOH-terminal domain, suggesting that the fucosyltransferase is synthesized as a glycoprotein. Gene fusion experiments have directly confirmed that this polypeptide is an α(1,2)fucosyltransferase.[384] This enzyme exhibits affinities for acceptor and donor substrates that are essentially identical to those previously ascribed to the human *H* α(1,2)fucosyltransferase.[379, 388] The properties of this enzyme are significantly different, however, from those attributed to the *Se* α(1,2)fucosyltransferase activity.[381] This gene localizes to the position on human chromosome 19[384] to which the human *H* locus maps.[389]

The human *Se* locus (see Fig. 9–18) has been cloned on the basis of DNA sequence homology to the human *H* locus.[386] This locus encodes a polypeptide predicted to share 68 per cent amino acid sequence identity with the COOH-terminal 292 residues of the human *H* blood group α(1,2)fu-

cosyltransferase.[387] Two potential initiator codons predict proteins of 332 or 343 amino acids in length. The polypeptides are also predicted to maintain a type II topology, with a 3 or 14 residue–long cytosolic domain, a 14 residue hydrophobic membrane-spanning domain, and a 315 amino acid–long COOH-terminal domain predicted to localize to the Golgi lumen (see Fig. 9–18). Three potential asparagine-linked glycosylation sites are predicted by the sequence, suggesting that the enzyme is a glycoprotein. Gene transfer experiments confirm that this protein is an α(1,2)fucosyltransferase and demonstrate that the enzyme exhibits substrate affinities characteristic of the *Se* α(1,2)fucosyltransferase but distinct from those of the *H* α(1,2)fucosyltransferase.[387] This gene also localizes to human chromosome 19 and is separated from the *H* locus by 35 kb of genomic DNA.[386] As discussed below, genetic analysis confirms that this gene corresponds to the *Secretor* locus. The extremely close physical proximity of these two α(1,2)fucosyltransferase genes is entirely consistent with prior genetic studies demonstrating close linkage between the *H* and *Se* loci.[374] The *Secretor* locus occupies a position between the *H* locus and an α(1,2)fucosyltransferase pseudogene termed the *Sec1* locus, which is separated from the *Secretor* locus by a distance of 12 kb.[386]

▼ MOLECULAR BASIS FOR THE SECRETOR, NON-SECRETOR, BOMBAY, AND PARA-BOMBAY PHENOTYPES

The structure and function of these loci have been examined in H-positive pedigrees and individuals informative for secretor status and in H-deficient Bombay and para-Bombay pedigrees[385, 387] (reviewed in reference 390). Initial analysis of the *H* locus (see Fig. 9–18) in a Bombay pedigree identified a termination codon corresponding to a tyrosine at amino acid residue 316 (Tyr 316 → ter)[385] (see Fig. 9–18). Gene transfer experiments confirmed that the mutation inactivates this allele. The Bombay propositus was found to be homozygous for this null allele, whereas the parents were shown to be heterozygous. In a para-Bombay pedigree (secretor positive, erythroid H deficient),[373] the propositus was found to be a compound heterozygote for two functionally significant mutations that segregate separately in the family. One mutant allele contains a missense mutation in the DNA sequence corresponding to amino acid residue 164; the other allele contains a mutation that creates a termination codon corresponding to amino acid residue 276 (Glu 276 → ter) (see Fig. 9–18). Gene transfer experiments indicate that the nonsense mutation and the missense mutation each yield an inactive α(1,2)fucosyltransferase gene. These studies demonstrated that the cloned α(1,2)fucosyltransferase gene determines expression of H blood group antigen on red cells and thus corresponds to the *H* locus. They also implied that the human genome must contain a second functional α(1,2)fucosyltransferase gene distinct from the *H* locus, because the para-Bombay individual who contains the two inactivated α(1,2)fucosyltransferase alleles is still capable of expressing wild-type, *Se* locus–determined α(1,2)fucosyltransferase activity. This hypothesis was confirmed by the isolation of a candidate for the *Secretor* locus and analysis of this α(1,2)fu-

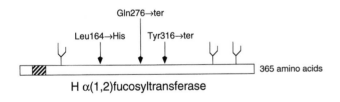

Gln276→ter
Leu164→His   Tyr316→ter

H α(1,2)fucosyltransferase   365 amino acids

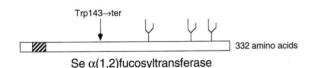

Trp143→ter

Se α(1,2)fucosyltransferase   332 amino acids

Figure 9–18. Structure of, and polymorphism in, the *H* and *Se* locus blood group α(1,2)fucosyltransferases. The *H* locus encodes a protein that is 365 amino acids long. The *Se* locus encodes proteins predicted to be 332 amino acids long (shown) or a 343 amino acid–long polypeptide (not shown), depending on which of two predicted initiator methionine codons is used. The H and the Se polypeptides are predicted to be a type II transmembrane protein. NH$_2$-terminal transmembrane domains are indicated by the hatched segments. The sequences of the H and Se α(1,2)fucosyltransferases predict three potential asparagine-linked glycosylation sites, indicated by the branched structures attached to each protein's backbone. The approximate relative positions of inactivating amino acid sequence changes in the H α(1,2)fucosyltransferase in a representative Bombay individual (Tyr 316 → ter) and in a representative para-Bombay individual (Leu 164 → His; Glu 276 → ter) are displayed above the schematic of the α(1,2)fucosyltransferase. The approximate relative position of an inactivating amino acid sequence change that accounts for a large fraction of se alleles in some populations (Tyr 143 → ter) is displayed above the schematic of the Se α(1,2)fucosyltransferase.

Table 9–7. Representative Sequence Polymorphisms Corresponding to *H (FUT1)* Null Alleles

Amino Acid Sequence Change	Nucleotide Sequence Change	References
His 117 → Tyr	C 349 → T	391
Asp 148 → Tyr	G 442 → T	392
Tyr 154 → His	T 460 → C	392–394
Tyr 154 → Cys	A 461 → G	395
Leu 164 → His	T 491 → A	385
Trp 171 → Cys	G 513 → C	395
182 frameshift	AG deletion 547	394
Arg 220 → Cys	C 658 → T	394
Trp 232 → ter	G 695 → A	392
Tyr 241 → His	T 721 → C	392
Leu 242 → Arg	T 725 → G	391
Val 259 → Glu	T 776 → A	395
Trp 267 → Cys	G 801 → C/T	396
Ser 276 → ter	C 826 → T	385
Asp 278 → Asn	G 832 → A	396
294 frameshift	TT deletion 880	394
Ala 315 → Val	C 944 → T	395
Tyr 316 → ter	GC 948 → G	385
323 frameshift	C deletion 969	395
Asn 327 → Thr	A 980 → C	394
330 frameshift	G deletion 990	392, 396
Glu 348 → Lys	G 1042 → A	392, 393
Trp 349 → Cys	G 1047 → C	395

cosyltransferase gene in secretor and non-secretor individuals.[387] These studies identified an enzyme-inactivating nonsense allele (Trp 143 → ter) at this locus in approximately 20 per cent of randomly selected individuals (see Fig. 9–18). The frequency of this null allele is in close correspondence to the frequency of the non-secretor phenotype in most human populations. In addition, each of six unrelated non-secretor individuals were also found to be homozygous for this null allele. These observations confirmed the identify of this α(1,2)fucosyltransferase gene as the *Secretor* locus and suggested that homozygosity for a common nonsense allele is responsible for the non-secretor phenotype in many non-secretor individuals.

Subsequent studies have defined a number of allelic variants of the *H* (reviewed in references 390 and 391) (Table 9–7) and *Se* loci (Table 9–8). Molecular analyses of Bombay and para-Bombay individuals define numerous different null alleles in the *H* locus (see Table 9–7). All

Table 9–8. Representative Sequence Polymorphisms Corresponding to *Se (FUT2)* Null Alleles

Amino Acid Sequence Change	Nucleotide Sequence Change	References
Ile 129 → Phe	A 385 → T	398–401
Trp 143 → ter	G 428 → A	387, 397
Arg 191 → ter	C 571 → T	403–405
Arg 210 → ter	C 628 → T	404
260 frameshift	C deletion 778	397
Trp 283 → ter	G 849 → A	405
Large deletion encompassing the Se locus Sec1 pseudogene/Se locus recombination		391, 402 404

correspond to point mutations or deletions of one or two nucleotides.[391–396] By contrast, non-secretors are most commonly found to harbor one of two relatively frequent null alleles (see Table 9–8). These include the Trp 143 → ter allele described in the original analysis of a predominantly white population[387] and in some African populations[397] and an Ile 129 → Phe allele yielding a partially active α(1,2)fucosyltransferase and the so-called weak secretor phenotype predominant in Asian and Polynesian populations.[398–401] Deletion of the *Se* locus,[391, 402] other less common point mutations,[398, 403–405] and a structurally aberrant *Se* locus derived from a recombination event with the adjacent *Sec1* pseudogene[404] can also account for the non-secretor phenotype (see Table 9–8).

▼ FUNCTION

As is the case with the *ABO* locus, no clear functions have been assigned to the oligosaccharides whose synthesis is determined by the *H* and *Se* loci. Many associations between secretor status and predilection for various illnesses have been reported.[359, 360, 368] These include an increased relative risk for peptic ulceration exhibited by non-secretors[406] and an increased relative risk for recurrent urinary tract infection in non-secretor females.[407] These observations may reflect influences exerted by soluble blood group substances on the binding of bacterial pathogens to oligosaccharide receptors displayed by urothelial surfaces.[408, 409] Indeed, as discussed below in the context of the Lewis blood group system, this notion is supported to some extent by the observation that Lewis b-active glycans, and related H-type structures synthesized in part through the action of the Se α(1,2)fucosyltransferase, can support adhesion of some strains of the ulcerogenic spirochete *H. pylori*.[365, 410] Most other such reported associations have had no obvious causal relationship demonstrated, however. The apparently normal phenotype of Bombay subjects suggests that oligosaccharides containing terminal, H-active Fucα(1,2)Galβ moieties determined by the *H* and *Se*α(1,2)fucosyltransferases are not essential molecules, unless one invokes the existence of still other α(1,2)fucosyltransferase genes (proposed in reference 411) with important (if as yet unidentified) functions during embryogenesis (discussed in references 368 and 412).

The *Lewis* Blood Group Locus

The first description of the human Lewis blood group system was reported after an investigation into two cases of hemolytic disease of the newborn.[413] The term Lewis is derived from the last name of one of the women with anti-Lewis antibodies. The antigenic portions of the Lewis blood group–active molecules are composed of carbohydrates[414–416] (Fig. 9–19).

Expression of Lewis a (Le^a) or Lewis b (Le^b) antigens, or of no Lewis antigens at all, by human red cells is a function of an individual's *Se* and Lewis (*Le*) genotypes. Le^a and Le^b antigens displayed by red cells are not themselves synthesized by red cell precursors. They are instead adsorbed by the erythrocyte membrane through an apparently passive process that uses Lewis-active glycosphingolipid molecules

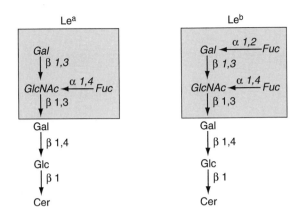

Figure 9–19. Structures of Le^a and Le^b blood group glycosphingolipids. The immunodominant portion of each molecule is highlighted by a shaded rectangle. Component monosaccharides are italicized. The molecule associates with the erythrocyte membrane by the ceramide moiety (Cer).

(see Fig. 9–19) circulating in plasma.[417] These Le^a- and Le^b-active glycosphingolipid molecules[415, 416] (see Fig. 9–19) are found in the plasma as complexes with low- and high-density lipoproteins and as aqueous dispersions.[417] It has been estimated that there are between approximately 4500 and 7300 Le^a molecules per red cell.[418]

Antibodies directed against Lewis determinants are relatively common entities and in most cases are naturally occurring (reviewed in reference 8). High-titer anti-Le^a antibodies have in some cases played causative roles in clinically significant hemolytic transfusion reactions, whereas anti-Le^b antibodies typically are not associated with clinical problems.[8, 9] Circulating anti-Lewis antibodies are effectively neutralized in most cases by transfused plasma,[8, 9] which contains soluble Le^a or Le^b substances.[419] In addition, transfused Lewis antigen–positive erythrocytes can rapidly become Lewis antigen negative after transfusion, through reversal of the passive absorptive process by which they acquire these antigens in the donor.[8, 9] Red cells taken from newborns are typically deficient in Lewis antigens. These determinants appear at approximately 10 days after birth and are displayed first as Le^a activity in Lewis-positive infants.[420] The full complement of red cell Lewis antigens is realized at approximately 24 months of age.[421]

Synthesis of the Le^a and Le^b antigens is catalyzed by two distinct fucosyltransferases whose expression is independently controlled by the *Le* blood group locus and the *Se* blood group locus (reviewed in references 293, 294, and 390) (Fig. 9–20; see also Fig. 9–19). Strong biochemical and genetic evidence indicates that the *Le* locus corresponds to an α(1,3/1,4)fucosyltransferase gene also known as the *Fuc-TIII* or *FUT3* locus[422–425] (reviewed in reference 390). The enzyme encoded by this gene can use a structurally diverse group of oligosaccharide precursors, including unsubstituted type 1 oligosaccharide precursors to form the Le^a determinant and type 1 H determinants to construct Le^b determinants.[422, 423, 425] Histochemical and biochemical procedures identify *Le* locus–dependent expression of Le^a and Le^b molecules by epithelia lining the respiratory tract, urinary tract, and digestive tract, salivary glands, and bile ducts, for

example (reviewed in references 293, 294, 303, and 390). These tissues correspond almost perfectly to the tissue types capable of expression of type 1 H molecules, whose synthesis is determined by the *Se* locus.

Because the *Lewis* α(1,3/1,4)fucosyltransferase can use the oligosaccharide products formed by the *Se*-determined α(1,2)fucosyltransferase, and because the *Se* and *Le* fucosyltransferases are expressed in many of the same tissues, it follows that the genotype at these two loci will determine which, if any, of the Lewis-active oligosaccharide molecules will be constructed (see Fig. 9–20). In secretor-positive individuals, type 1 oligosaccharide precursors initially are converted to type 1 H molecules.[294, 390] These in turn represent substrates for the action of the *Lewis* locus–encoded α(1,3/1,4)fucosyltransferase, which converts these to Le^b-active molecules [Le(a−b+) phenotype] (Fig. 9–20A). By contrast, non-secretors are incapable of constructing type 1 H determinants in secretory epithelia, and these unsubstituted type 1 molecules are thus converted into Le^a-active oligosaccharides by the action of the *Le*-encoded α(1,3/1,4)fucosyltransferase [Le(a+b−) phenotype] (Fig. 9–20B). In individuals homozygous for null alleles at the *Le* locus, two possible outcomes are observed. In secretor-positive, Lewis-negative individuals, type 1 H determinants are constructed but remain unconverted to Le^b determinants (Fig. 9–20C). Alternatively, in Lewis-negative, secretor-negative persons, the type 1 precursors remain unsubstituted by the action of either blood group fucosyltransferase (Fig. 9–20D). In either of the last two circumstances, the individual's phenotype is denoted Le(a−b−).

▼ MOLECULAR GENETICS

A cloned cDNA assigned to the human *Lewis* blood group locus has been isolated,[425] the corresponding gene has been characterized,[426] and the molecular basis for null alleles at the locus has been defined. Sequence analysis of the Lewis blood group α(1,3/1,4)fucosyltransferase (FUT3) cDNA predicts a 363 amino acid–long type II transmembrane glycoprotein with a 15 amino acid–long NH$_2$-terminal cytosolic segment, a 19 residue transmembrane segment, and a 320 amino acid–long COOH-terminal, Golgi-localized catalytic domain. The enzyme encoded by this cDNA is capable of efficiently constructing several types of α(1,3)- and α(1,4)fucosylated oligosaccharides. These include Le^a, Le^b, Le^x (SSEA-1), and Le^y molecules and sialylated forms of the Le^a and Le^x determinants[424, 425] (Fig. 9–21; see also Fig. 9–20).

The *FUT3* locus maps to chromosome 19 and is a member of an α(1,3)fucosyltransferase gene family, whose members maintain substantial primary sequence similarity and overlapping catalytic activities. These include a pair of human α(1,3)fucosyltransferase genes (*FUT5*[427] and *FUT6*[428]) that maintain more than 85 per cent DNA primary sequence similarity to the *FUT3* locus and that exist in close and tandem linkage to the *FUT3* locus on chromosome 19p13.3.[426] Three other α(1,3)fucosyltransferase genes have also been described (*FUT4*,[429–431] *FUT7*,[432, 433] and *FUT9*[434]). These genes are less similar to each other and to the three fucosyltransferase genes on chromosome 19. *FUT4* and *FUT7* localize to human chromosomes 11q21 and 9, respec-

A. Lewis-positive, Secretor-positive

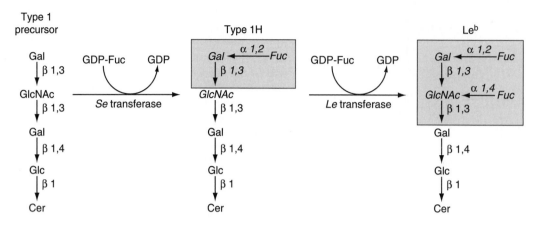

B. Lewis-positive, Non-secretor

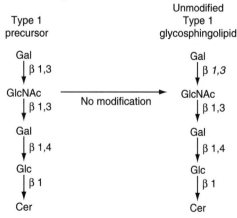

C. Lewis-positive, Secretor-positive

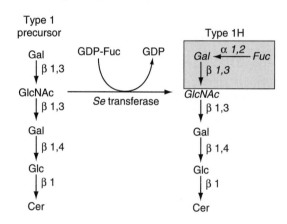

D. Lewis-negative, Non-secretor

Figure 9–20. Biosynthesis of the Le^a and Le^b determinants. The α(1,3/1,4)fucosyltransferase encoded by the *Lewis* locus (*Le* fucosyltransferase) and the α(1,2)fucosyltransferase determined by the *Secretor* locus (*Se* transferase) operate singly, or sequentially, on type 1 glycosphingolipid precursors. The final product depends on the genotype at both loci (see text for details). The oligosaccharide products of each of the four possible phenotypes are indicated in panels *A* through *D*. The immunodominant portion of each antigen is highlighted by a shaded rectangle. Component monosaccharides are italicized.

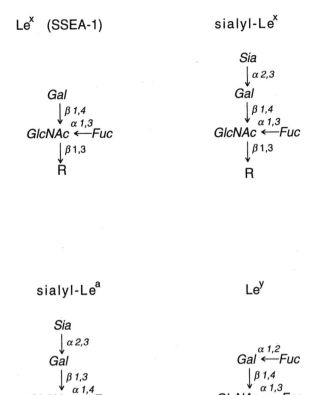

Figure 9–21. Le^x, sialyl-Le^x, sialyl-Le^a, and Le^y structures. The Lewis x determinant (CD15) has also been described as a murine stage-specific embryonic antigen, termed SSEA-1.[412] R denotes the underlying glycoconjugate, which may be represented by a protein- or lipid-linked oligosaccharide or free oligosaccharide. Monosaccharide components of each epitope are italicized.

tively. A human chromosomal assignment for *FUT9* is not yet available.

▼ MOLECULAR BASIS FOR THE LEWIS NEGATIVE PHENOTYPE

Expression of the Lewis blood group determinants in humans is believed to be determined exclusively by the *FUT3* locus. This conclusion is supported by the enzyme's catalytic properties (discussed in reference 425) and by analysis of this locus in individuals and pedigrees informative for different Lewis blood group phenotypes.[435–443] These analyses identify eight different *FUT3* haplotypes that cosegregate with the Lewis negative phenotype. Seven of these contain missense mutations leading to one or two amino acid sequence changes that disable the enzyme (*le^2* through *le^8*; Table 9–9). An additional null allele, *le^1*, corresponds to a Leu 20 → Arg amino acid sequence polymorphism that localizes to the enzyme's transmembrane segment. The Leu 20 → Arg polymorphism does not significantly diminish the enzyme's inherent catalytic activity, as assayed in vitro, but it disables expression of surface-localized Lewis antigens when expressed in cultured cells.[436] These observations imply that the Leu 20 → Arg polymorphism interferes with

membrane association processes required for access to intracellular substrates.

▼ FUNCTION

As with the *ABO* locus, a variety of associations between Lewis phenotype and disease susceptibility have been reported. Most of these associations are weak and remain without demonstrated mechanistic relationship (reviewed in references 360 to 362). There are two possible exceptions that merit discussion because of experimental evidence for a mechanistic basis. These include the relevance of Lewis blood group antigen variants to leukocyte and tumor cell adhesion processes mediated by the selectin family of cell adhesion molecules and the possible relevance of the Lewis antigens to *H. pylori* infection and pathogenesis.

The first of these exceptions concerns two of the six human α(1,3)fucosyltransferase genes (*FUT4*[444] and *FUT7*[445] but not *FUT3*) and members of the Lewis family of oligosaccharides that have been implicated in oligosaccharide-dependent cell adhesion mechanisms relevant to leukocyte trafficking in inflammation (reviewed in reference 446). Early and essential events in this process involve the binding of neutrophils, monocytes, and subsets of T lymphocytes to vascular endothelium. Initial binding is a prerequisite for leukocyte transmigration through the endothelial barrier and subsequent participation in an extravascular locus of inflammation. The initial, low-affinity binding of leukocytes to the interior of the vessel wall is mediated by endothelial leukocyte adhesion molecule-1,[447] now termed E-selectin,[448] and by P-selectin (reviewed in reference 446). Both selectins are expressed by activated vascular endothelial cells, and each exhibits structural similarity to members of the family of C-type carbohydrate-binding proteins (lectins).[449] Leukocyte adhesion to E- or P-selectin is mediated by interactions involving the sialyl-Le^x determinant (see Fig. 9–21) and its structural variants (see Fig. 9–21), which are abundantly expressed at the surface of myeloid cells.[424, 450–452] Sulfated variants of the sialyl-Le^x structure containing 3-*O*-sulfate on the subterminal *N*-acetylglucosamine (6-sulfo sialyl–Lewis x) have also been implicated as essential components of the counterreceptors for L-selectin, the third member of the selectin family of cell adhesion molecules. These sulfated sialyl-Le^x variants are expressed by the cuboidal endothelial cells that line the high postcapillary venules within secondary lymphoid organs, are recognized by lymphocyte-borne L-selectin, and facilitate lymphocyte adhesive interactions required for normal lymphocyte homing to lymph nodes (reviewed in reference 446). It is now clear that the authentic E-, P-, and L-selectin counterreceptors include monofucosylated and polyfucosylated forms of the prototypical sialyl-Le^x–type glycans,[453] that these glycans decorate specific membrane-associated protein and lipid moieties on the leukocyte (for E-, P-, and L-selectin–dependent adhesion) and high endothelial venular endothelium in lymph nodes (for L-selectin), and that protein and glycan sulfation also contribute to selectin-dependent adhesive mechanisms (reviewed in reference 446).

The importance of the sialyl-Le^x determinant in the normal human inflammatory response is well illustrated by the phenotype of individuals with the recently described

Table 9–9. Representative Sequence Polymorphisms Corresponding to Null Alleles of the Lewis Blood Group Locus (*FUT3*)

FUT3 Allele	Amino Acid (Nucleotide) Position							References
	20 (59)	**68 (202)**	**105 (314)**	**146 (445)**	**170 (508)**	**336 (1007)**	**356 (1067)**	
Le	Leu	Trp	Thr	Leu	Gly	Asp	Ile	425, 438
le¹	**Arg***	Trp	Thr	Leu	Gly	Asp	Ile	436, 438
le²	Leu	Trp	Thr	Leu	Gly	Asp	<u>**Lys**</u>	438, 442
le³	**Arg***	Trp	Thr	Leu	Gly	Asp	<u>**Lys**</u>	435, 437, 438, 442
le⁴	**Arg***	Trp	Thr	Leu	<u>**Ser**</u>	Asp	Ile	435, 438, 441, 442
le⁵	Leu	<u>**Arg**</u>	**Met**	Leu	Gly	Asp	Ile	437, 438, 440, 443
le⁶	**Arg***	<u>**Arg**</u>	Thr	Leu	Gly	Asp	<u>**Lys**</u>	436, 438
le⁷	**Arg***	Trp	Thr	**Met**	Gly	Asp	Ile	438
le⁸	**Arg***	Trp	Thr	Leu	Gly	Asp	<u>**Ala**</u>	439

Nomenclature for *FUT3* haplotypes is according to reference 438. Numbering is according to the sequence published in reference 425. Amino acid sequence differences within each haplotype, relative to the wild-type FUT3 sequence, are indicated in bold. Amino acid sequence changes known to be catalytically inactivating are underlined. The Leu 20 → Arg polymorphism indicated by the asterisk alters the ability of the enzyme to direct Lewis antigen synthesis within the cell but does not alter the enzyme's inherent catalytic properties. The Thr 105 → Met substitution does not inactivate the enzyme, whereas the Leu 146 → Met substitution has not been tested.

leukocyte adhesion deficiency type II.[454] These patients are unusually susceptible to bacterial infections and exhibit a variety of other abnormalities.[454] The immune deficiency in these patients is a consequence of defective expression of cell surface sialyl-Le^x determinants by their neutrophils and monocytes and a corresponding inability to complete normal and E- and P-selectin–dependent endothelial adhesion and transmigration in response to inflammatory insult.[455] The cells of these patients express the normal complement of leukocyte fucosyltransferase activities[456] but are incapable of synthesizing fucosylated oligosaccharides under normal circumstances. Defective synthesis of fucosylated glycans in these patients' cells is a consequence of a still undefined defect in the ability to synthesize normal amounts of intracellular GDP-fucose,[456, 457] an essential substrate for all known human fucosyltransferases. As might be expected, these patients also exhibit a Lewis-negative Bombay phenotype because they are incapable of constructing the H or Lewis blood group molecules.[454]

The sialyl-Le^a determinant (see Fig. 9–21) can also mediate adhesive interactions with E-selectin,[452, 458, 459] with P-selectin,[460, 461] and with L-selectin.[462] Because the sialyl-Le^a determinant is not normally expressed by leukocytes, nor by high endothelial venular endothelial cells in secondary lymphoid organs, it follows that the sialyl-Le^a moiety does not represent a physiologically relevant contributor to selectin-dependent leukocyte trafficking. Nonetheless, whereas sialyl-Le^x and sialyl-Le^a type glycans are also not normally found on erythrocytes, both epitopes are often "aberrantly" expressed by a variety of malignant neoplasms.[463] Aberrant expression of these determinants may occur as a consequence of aberrant expression of the *FUT3* locus, and of other α(1,3)fucosyltransferase genes, and may facilitate E-, P-, or L-selectin–dependent spread of malignant cells.[424, 459, 464, 465]

A second proposed functional role for the Lewis blood group antigens concerns the human spirochetal pathogen *H. pylori*. This organism is a major causative agent in chronic active gastritis, and infestation of the organism is strongly associated with duodenal ulcer, hypertrophic gastropathy, gastric adenocarcinoma, and lymphoma of the mucosa-associated lymphoid tissue (reviewed in references 365 and 466

to 469). *H. pylori* colonization of the stomach most probably requires adhesion of the organism to the gastric mucosal epithelium and to the mucus elaborated by such cells. The Lewis b blood group antigen can mediate adhesion of this organism to gastric epithelium, suggesting that this glycan represents a pathophysiologically relevant receptor for the organism.[410] This hypothesis is supported by the observation that individuals with the blood group O phenotype express more receptors for the organism than do A or B subjects (and more Lewis b antigenic sites, because the A and B transferases compete with the Lewis transferase for H-active glycan precursors) and by the observation that the organism does not adhere to Lewis b-negative gastric tissue (in nonsecretors or in Lewis blood group–negative individuals).[410] Clinical studies have tested this hypothesis by characterizing the relationship, in vivo, between gastric colonization by *H. pylori* and ABO, Lewis, and secretor status (see references 470 and 471, for example). These studies find no correlation between Lewis b phenotype and *H. pylori* infection, little[471] or no[470] correlation between *H. pylori* infection and ABO and secretor phenotype, and only a modest association between ABO or secretor status and lymphocytic infiltration in *H. pylori* infection.[471] Furthermore, recent observations indicate that fucosyltransferases encoded by the genome of some strains of *H. pylori* can direct expression of Lewis b antigen by the organism itself.[472] These observations imply that the relationship between *H. pylori* pathobiology and the antigens synthesized by the enzymes of the human host *Lewis*, *Secretor*, and *ABO* blood group loci cannot necessarily be explained by a straightforward interaction between host-derived Lewis b antigen and *H. pylori* adhesins.

The Ii Blood Group System

The Ii blood group system was discovered during an investigation of a cold hemagglutinating antibody in a patient with acquired hemolytic anemia.[473] To find unreactive cells for transfusion into this patient, several thousand blood donors were screened for crossmatch compatibility. The antigen identified by the cold agglutinin antibody was found to be absent from the red cells of just 5 of some 22,000 tested individuals. The commonly expressed antigen was called I, and its absence was denoted i. Subsequent studies identified cold agglutinins with relative specificity for i-type cells.[474] Later studies demonstrated that red cell expression of these antigens is developmentally regulated.[475] Red cells taken from the embryo, or from umbilical cord blood, are relatively deficient in I determinants but are strongly reactive with anti-i antibodies. During the first 18 months of infancy, this relationship is reversed to yield red cells with robust anti-I reactivity and diminished i reactivity, as is observed in most adults.

The Ii antigens are carbohydrate molecules and correspond to portions of the oligosaccharide chains that function as precursors to the ABO and H blood group determinants (reviewed in references 476 and 477). Molecules with i reactivity correspond to oligosaccharide chains containing at least two repeating N-acetylgalactosamine units (Fig. 9–22). By contrast, I activity corresponds to branched oligosaccharide structures formed by an N-acetylgalactosamine unit attached in β1,6 linkage to a galactose residue within linear lactosamine polymers[478, 479] (see Fig. 9–19). These structural results are consistent with the studies demonstrating that neonatal erythrocyte oligosaccharide chains are largely unbranched, whereas those in adult red cells are highly branched,[480, 481] and suggest that the increase in the I reactivity, with a corresponding decrease in i reactivity, during early infancy corresponds to the elaboration and display of increasing numbers of β1,6-linked lactosamine units. These observations are also consistent with the notion that I reactivity is determined by a locus encoding an N-acetylglucosaminyltransferase that is expressed in a developmentally regulated fashion in most individuals, except rare individuals (i phenotype) who are homozygous for null alleles at this locus.[482] This particular β(1,6)N-acetylglucosaminyltransferase activity and a chain-elongating β(1,3)N-acetylglucosaminyltransferase activity (see Fig. 9–22) have been described in human serum[483, 484] or in animal cells and tissues.[485, 486] A candidate for the human I transferase locus has been isolated[487, 488]; it has not been examined in i individuals or in families informative for this phenotype.

Ii-reactive oligosaccharide chains are ubiquitous entities displayed at the surfaces of many human cell lines and tissues,[486, 489–492] including those of the erythroid lineage.[493, 494] Ii determinants are also displayed as developmentally regulated cell surface molecules during murine embryogenesis[495] and as tissue-specific entities in the adult mouse.[488] The functions of these molecules remain to be defined.

The P Blood Group System

The P blood group system was discovered during experiments designed to uncover new human red cell alloantigens by immunizing rabbits with human red cells.[496] The nomenclature, biochemistry, and genetics of this system are complex, largely because so little is known about the corresponding enzymes and genes (reviewed in references 476 and 497). The system is perhaps best understood by first considering the chemical structures and biosynthesis of its antigens. The P antigens are displayed virtually exclusively on red cell membrane-associated glycosphingolipids[498] (Fig. 9–23). Like the antigens of the *ABO*, *H*, and *Lewis* blood group loci, P molecules are constructed by the sequential action of a series of distinct glycosyltransferases.

Biosynthesis of the P system molecules[497] may be divided into two distinct pathways; lactosylceramide serves as a common precursor for both (Fig. 9–23A). P antigen biosynthesis is initiated by the action of an α(1,4)galactosyltransferase (Pᵏ transferase) that creates the Pᵏ antigen. The Pᵏ antigen in turn serves as a precursor for the action of a β(1,3)-N-acetylgalactosaminyltransferase, termed the *P* transferase, which forms the P antigen. Polymorphisms are observed in the ability to express each of these two glycosyltransferase activities, as will be discussed below, which in turn can lead to polymorphism in P and Pᵏ antigen expression.

In the parallel pathway that directs the synthesis of the P₁ antigen, lactosylceramide serves as a precursor for the synthesis of paragloboside, through two of the enzymatic glycosylations that are apparently not polymorphic (Fig.

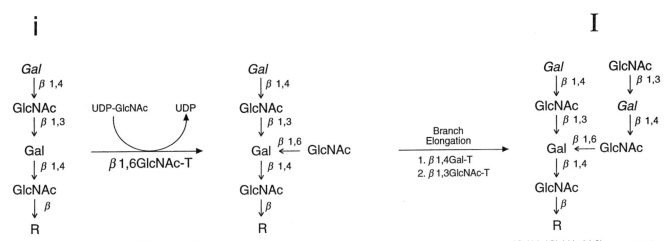

Figure 9–22. Antigens and biosynthesis of the Ii blood group system. Linear polymers of lactosamine units (Galβ1,4GlcNAcβ1,3) represent i-reactive oligosaccharide antigens. These molecules are used by a β(1,6)GlcNAc transferase (whose expression is determined by the *I* locus), which attaches N-acetylglucosamine in β1,6 linkage to internal galactose residues. These β1,6-linked N-acetylglucosamine moieties are then modified by two sequentially acting elongating enzymes, forming branched oligosaccharide determinants with I reactivity. (These positions are also indicated in Fig. 9–13.) R denotes the underlying glycoconjugate, which may be represented by a protein- or lipid-linked oligosaccharide or free oligosaccharide.

P antigen biosynthesis

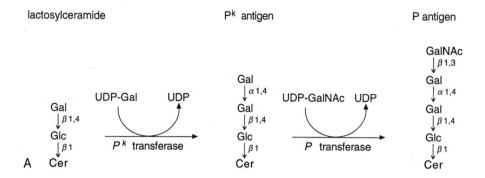

P$_1$ antigen biosynthesis

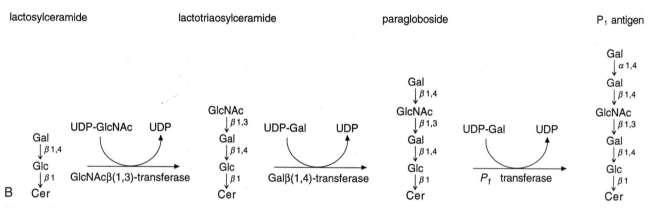

Figure 9–23. Antigens and biosynthesis of the P blood group system. Two distinct and polymorphic enzymes operate to construct the P^k and P antigens (A). The P$_1$ antigen is constructed (B) from lactosylceramide through the action of two apparently non-polymorphic enzymes (yielding the precursor paragloboside), followed by the action of the polymorphic P$_1$ transferase.

9–23B). Paragloboside in turn serves as a substrate for the action of P_1 transferase, which forms the P$_1$ molecule. Polymorphisms are often observed in the ability to express P_1 transferase activity and thus in P$_1$ antigen expression.

▼ PHENOTYPES AND GENOTYPES OF THE P SYSTEM

A consideration of these pathways and antigens, and of the functional polymorphisms in the three enzyme activities that determine their synthesis, can account for the observed red cell phenotypes in virtually all individuals. The most common phenotype, termed P$_1$, is the result of full activity of each of the polymorphic enzymes (Table 9–10). Consequently, P$_1$ red cells display normal amounts of both P and P$_1$ antigens. Small amounts of P^k determinants are also detectable because the P transferase is apparently incapable of completely converting all P^k precursor determinants into P determinants.

The P$_2$ phenotype represents the other most common

phenotype (see Table 9–10). These persons presumably maintain two null alleles at the P_1 transferase locus. Their red cells consequently do not display a normal complement of P$_1$ determinants but do express levels of the P and P^k antigens similar to those found on P$_1$ cells.

Three rare phenotypes have also been described. Individuals with the P$_1$^{k} phenotype are deficient in P transferase activity and thus presumably maintain two null alleles at this locus.[499–501] These persons therefore do not convert their P^k molecules into P determinants and thus express supranormal amounts of P^k determinants. The parallel pathway for P$_1$ synthesis is intact and yields normal amounts of P$_1$ determinants.

Persons with the rare P$_2$^{k} phenotype are presumably homozygous for null alleles at the P transferase and the P_1 transferase loci.[499, 500] Neither pathway is completed, leading to deficiencies in both P and P$_1$ antigen expression, but with increased expression of P^k molecules.

Red cells of the p phenotype are deficient in all three P antigens (P, P$_1$, and P^k).[20, 499, 502] Homozygosity for null alleles at the P^k transferase and P_1 transferase loci can account for

Table 9–10. Common and Rare P Blood Group System Phenotypes

Phenotype	Frequency	Red Cell Antigens	Possible Genotypes	Serum Antibodies
P_1	75%	P, P_1, (weak P^k)	$P^k/- \ P/- \ P_1/-$	None
P_2	25%	P, (weak P^k)	$P^k/- \ P/- \ p_1/p_1$	anti-P_1
$P_1^{\ k}$	Rare	P_1, p^k	$P^k/- \ p/p \ P_1/-$	anti-P
$P_2^{\ k}$	Rare	p^k	$P^k/- \ p/p \ p_1/p_1$	anti-P
p	Rare	(weak P)	$p^k/p^k \ -/- \ p_1/p_1$	anti-PP$_1$P^k (or anti-Tj^a)

Phenotype frequencies are those observed in white populations. Predicted genotypes are based on the three–glycosyltransferase locus model discussed in the text. Dashes indicate that a functional or a null allele will yield the same phenotype. Antigens expressed at low levels are preceded by the term "weak" and are enclosed within parentheses.

this phenotype.[502–504] Normal levels of P antigen are not synthesized, regardless of *P* transferase activity, because the P precursor (P^k) is not available. Nonetheless, red cells of the p phenotype typically display low levels of P reactivity because the *P* transferase can attach a galactose moiety in $\alpha(1,4)$ linkage to paragloboside, formed in the other pathway, which yields a molecule with P antigen reactivity (see Fig. 9–23).

The preceding discussion assumes that the *P*, *P_1*, and *P^k* transferases represent distinct enzymes, encoded by three different loci. However, at least two alternative biochemically and genetically consistent models may be proposed to explain the p phenotype and the others (discussed in reference 497). One such model[505] proposes that the *P_1* transferase and the *P^k* transferase "activities" in fact correspond to a single transferase locus that in most instances encodes one enzyme capable of constructing both P^k and P_1 determinants (P_1 phenotype). A second model proposes that the *P_1* locus encodes a regulatory molecule capable of modulating the substrate specificity of an $\alpha(1,4)$galactosyltransferase encoded by the *p^k* locus.[497] Which, if any, of these three models is correct remains to be determined, because their cognate genes have not yet been isolated.

▼ FUNCTIONS

Functions for these oligosaccharides remain unknown. Two significant associations have been made between pathological states and P blood group phenotype, however. One centers on the observation that some uropathogenic strains of *Escherichia coli* express adhesins that recognize the Gal$\alpha(1,4)$Gal moiety of the P^k and P_1 antigens (references 408 and 506 to 509, for example). This determinant is relatively more abundant on the urothelium of P_1 persons and may facilitate bacterial attachment to, and invasion of, the urinary tract lining, including the kidney proper. This possibility is consistent with reports that individuals with the P_1 blood group are at a slightly increased risk, relative to persons with the P_2 phenotype, for urinary tract infection and for pyelonephritis.[409, 510, 511] It is also consistent with the observation that a Gal$\alpha(1,4)$Gal-specific PapG adhesin expressed by a pyelonephritic strain of *E. coli* is required for adhesion to renal tissues, and deficiency of this adhesin eliminates the ability of the strain to cause pyelonephritis in primates.[512]

A second strong association concerns the P blood group antigens and infection with the human parvovirus B19 (see also Chapter 28). This virus is the etiological agent in erythema infectiosum and has been implicated in transient aplastic crisis in patients with hemolytic anemia, in cases of pure red cell aplasia and chronic anemia in immunocompromised individuals, and in congenital anemia and hydrops fetalis after infection in utero (reviewed in reference 513). Parvovirus B19 replication is restricted to erythroid progenitor cells, and it infects such cells through an adhesive interaction with P antigen–active glycolipids.[514, 515] Individuals with the p blood group phenotype are apparently resistant to infection with this virus.[515]

Antibodies directed against the P_1 antigen are often found in persons of the P_2 phenotype.[8, 20] These are typically naturally occurring, cold-agglutinating IgM molecules and have only rarely been associated with red cell destruction. Antibodies against P, P_1, and P^k determinants (anti-PP$_1$P^k, or anti-Tj^a, reference 8) are found in individuals with the p phenotype. These antibodies have been implicated in hemolytic transfusion reactions and in hemolytic disease of the newborn, and they may play causative roles in some women who experience spontaneous abortion early in pregnancy.[516] Anti-P antibodies with similar characteristics have also been described in $P_1^{\ k}$ and $P_2^{\ k}$ individuals. Cold, complement-fixing Donath-Landsteiner antibodies responsible for intravascular hemolysis in paroxysmal cold hemoglobinuria display anti-P specificity.[8]

REFERENCES

1. Landsteiner, K., Levine, P., and Janes, M.L.: On the development of isoagglutinins following transfusions. Proc. Soc. Exp. Biol. (N.Y.) 25:672, 1928.
2. Landsteiner, K.: Individual differences in human blood. Science 73:405, 1931.
3. Lewis, M., Anstee, D.J., and Bird, G.W.G.: Blood group terminology. Vox Sang. 58:152, 1990.
4. Daniels, G.L., Anstee, D.J., Cartron, J.P., Dahr, W., Issitt, P.D., Jorgensen, J., Kornstad, L., Levene, C., Lomas-Francis, C., Lubenko, A., et al.: Blood group terminology 1995. ISBT Working Party on terminology for red cell surface antigens. Vox Sang. 69:265, 1995.
5. Cartron, J.P., Bailly, P., Le Van Kim, C., Cherif-Zahar, B., Matassi, G., Bertrand, O., and Colin, Y.: Insights into the structure and function of membrane polypeptides carrying blood group antigens. Vox Sang. 4(suppl. 2):29, 1998.
6. Reid, M.E., McManus, K., and Zelinski, T.: Chromosome location of genes encoding human blood groups. Transfus. Med. Rev. 12:151, 1998.
7. Avent, N.: Human erythrocyte antigen expression: its molecular basis. Br. J. Biomed. Sci. 54:16, 1997.
8. Mollison, P.L., Engelfriet, C.P., and Contreras, M. (eds.): Blood Transfusion in Clinical Medicine. 10th ed. Oxford, Blackwell, 1997.
9. Rossie, E.C., Simon, T.L., and Moss, G.S. (eds.): Principles of Transfusion Medicine. 2nd ed. Baltimore, Williams & Wilkins, 1996.
10. Garratty, G.: Problems associated with passively transfused blood group alloantibodies. Am. J. Clin. Pathol. 109:769, 1998.
11. Capon, S.M., and Goldfinger, D.: Acute hemolytic transfusion reac-

tion, a paradigm of the systemic inflammatory response: new insights into pathophysiology and treatment. Transfusion 35:513, 1995.

12. Levine, P., and Stetson, R.E.: An unusual case of intragroup agglutination. J.A.M.A. 113:126, 1939.

13. Levine, P., Burnham, L., Katzin, E.M., and Vogel, P.: The role of isoimmunization in the pathogenesis of erythroblastosis fetalis. Am. J. Obstet. Gynecol. 42:925, 1941.

14. Levine, P., Katzin, E.M., and Burnham, L.: Isoimmunization in pregnancy, its possible bearing on etiology of erythroblastosis fetalis. J.A.M.A. 116:822, 1941.

15. Landsteiner, K., and Wiener, A.S.: An agglutinable factor in human blood recognized by immune sera for rhesus blood. Proc. Soc. Exp. Biol. Med. 43:223, 1940.

16. Fisk, R.T., and Foord, A.G. Observations on the Rh agglutinogen of human blood. Am. J. Clin. Pathol. 12:545, 1942.

17. Levine, P., Cellano, M., Fenichel, R.: A 'D-like' antigen in rhesus monkey, human Rh positive and human Rh negative red blood cells. J. Immunol. 87:6, 1961.

18. Levine, P., Cellano, M.J., Wallace, J., and Sanger, R.: A human 'D-like' antibody. Nature 198:596, 1963.

19. Issitt, P.D.: Applied Blood Group Serology. 3rd ed. Miami, Montgomery Scientific Publications, 1985.

20. Race, R.R., and Sanger, R.: Blood Groups in Man. 6th ed. Oxford, Blackwell, 1975.

21. Wiener, A.S.: The Rh series of allelic genes. Science 100:595, 1944.

22. Fisher, R.A.; cited in Race, R.R.: An 'incomplete' antibody in human serum. Nature 153:771, 1944.

23. Tippett, P.: A speculative model for the Rh blood groups. Ann. Hum. Genet. 50(pt 3):241, 1986.

24. Siegel, D.L.: The human immune response to red blood cell antigens as revealed by repertoire cloning. Immunol. Res. 17:239, 1998.

25. Gahmberg, C.G.: Molecular characterization of the human red-cell Rho(D) antigen. EMBO J. 2:223, 1983.

26. Moore, S., and Green, C.: The identification of specific Rhesus polypeptide blood group ABH active glycoprotein complexes in the human red cell membrane. Biochem. J. 244:735, 1987.

27. Agre, P., Saboori, A.M., Asimos, A., and Smith, B.L.: Purification and partial characterization of the M_r 30,000 integral membrane protein associated with the erythrocyte Rh(D) antigen. J. Biol. Chem. 262:17497, 1987.

28. Bloy, C., Blanchard, D., Lambin, P., Goossens, D., Rouger, P., Salmon, C., and Cartron, J.P.: Human monoclonal antibody against Rh(D) antigen: partial characterization of rh Rh(D) polypeptide from human erythrocytes. Blood 69:1491, 1987.

29. Blanchard, D., Bloy, C., Hermand, P., Cartron, J.P., Saboori, A.M., Smith, B.L., and Agre, P.: Two-dimensional iodopeptide mapping demonstrates erythrocyte RhD, c, and E polypeptides are structurally homologous but nonidentical. Blood 72:1424, 1988.

30. Bloy, C., Hermand, P., Chérif-Zahar, B., Sonneborn, H.H., and Cartron, J.P.: Comparative analysis by two-dimensional iodopeptide mapping of the RhD protein and LW glycoprotein. Blood 75:2245, 1990.

31. Saboori, A.M., Smith, B.L., and Agre, P.: Polymorphism in the M_r 32,000 Rh protein purified from Rh(D) positive and negative erythrocytes. Proc. Natl. Acad. Sci. USA 85:4042, 1988.

32. Avent, N.D., Ridgwell, K., Mawby, W.J., Tanner, M.J., Anstee, D.J., and Kumpel, B.: Protein-sequence studies of Rh-related polypeptides suggest the presence of at least two groups of proteins which associated in the human red-cell membrane. Biochem. J. 256:1043, 1988.

33. Avent, N.D., Ridgwell, K., Tanner, M.J.A., and Anstee, D.J.: cDNA cloning of a 30 kDa erythrocyte membrane protein associated with Rh (Rhesus)-blood-group-antigen expression. Biochem. J. 271:821, 1990.

34. Chérif-Zahar, B., Bloy, C., Le Van Kim, C., Blanchard, D., Bailly, P., Hermand, P., Salmon, C., Cartron, J.P., and Colin, Y.: Molecular cloning and protein structure of a human blood group Rh polypeptide. Proc. Natl. Acad. Sci. USA 87:6243, 1990.

35. Avent, N.D., Butcher, S.K., Liu, W., Mawby, W.J., Mallison, G., Parsons, S.F., Anstee, D.J., and Tanner, M.J.A.: Localization of the C termini of the Rh (Rhesus) polypeptides to the cytosolic face of the human erythrocyte membrane. J. Biol. Chem. 267: 15134, 1992.

36. Suyama, K., and Goldstein, J.: Membrane orientation of Rh(D) polypeptide and partial localization of its epitope-containing domain. Blood 79:808, 1992.

37. Bloy, C., Hermand, P., Blanchard, D., Chérif-Zahar, B., Goosens, D., and Cartron, J-P.: Surface orientation and antigen properties of Rh and Lw polypeptides of the human erythrocyte. J. Biol. Chem. 265:21482, 1990.

38. Hartmann, E., Rapoport, T.A., and Lodish, H.F.: Predicting the orientation of eukaryotic membrane-spanning proteins. Proc. Natl. Acad. Sci. USA 86:5786, 1989.

39. Huang, C.H.: Molecular insights into the Rh protein family and associated antigens. Curr. Opin. Hematol. 4:94, 1997.

40. Chérif-Zahar, B., Le Van Kim, C., Rouillac, C., Raynal, V., Cartron, J.P., and Colin, Y.: Organization of the gene (RHCE) encoding the human blood group RhCcEe antigens and characterization of the promoter region. Genomics 19:68, 1994.

41. Smythe, J.S., Avent, N.D., Judson, P.A., Parsons, S.F., Martin, P.G., and Anstee, D.J.: Expression of RHD and RHCE gene products using retroviral transduction of K562 cells establishes the molecular basis of Rh blood group antigens. Blood 87:2968, 1996.

42. Le Van Kim, C., Mouro, I., Chérif-Zahar, B., Raynal, V., Cherrier, C., Cartron, J.P., and Colin, Y.: Molecular cloning and primary structure of the human blood group RhD polypeptide. Proc. Natl. Acad. Sci. USA 89:10925, 1992.

43. Arce, M.A., Thompson, E.S., Wagner, S., Coyne, K.E., Ferdman, B.A., and Lublin, D.M.: Molecular cloning of RhD cDNA derived from a gene present in RhD-positive, but not RhD-negative individuals. Blood 82:651, 1993.

44. Chérif-Zahar, B., Mattei, M.G., Le Van Kim, C., Bailly, P., Cartron, J.P., and Colin, Y.: Localization of the human Rh blood group gene structure to chromosome 1p34.3–1p36.1 region by in situ hybridization. Hum. Genet. 86:398, 1991.

45. Bruns, G.A.P., and Sherman, S.L.: Report of the committee on genetic constitution of chromosome I. Cytogenet. Cell Genet. 51:67, 1989.

46. Colin, Y., Chérif-Zahar, B., Le Van Kim, C., Raynal, V., Van Huffel, V., and Cartron, J.P.: Genetic basis of the RhD-positive and RhD-negative blood group polymorphism as determined by Southern analysis. Blood 78:2747, 1991.

47. Ridgwell, K., Spurr, N.K., Laguda, B., MacGeoch, C., Avent, N.D., and Tanner, M.J.: Isolation of cDNA clones for a 50 kDa glycoprotein of the human erythrocyte membrane associated with Rh (rhesus) blood-group antigen expression. Biochem. J. 287(pt 1):223, 1992.

48. Chérif-Zahar, B., Raynal, V., Gane, P., Mattei, M.G., Bailly, P., Gibbs, B., Colin, Y., and Cartron, J.P.: Candidate gene acting as a suppressor of the RH locus in most cases of Rh-deficiency. Nat. Genet. 12:168, 1996.

49. Huang, C.H.: The human Rh50 glycoprotein gene. Structural organization and associated splicing defect resulting in Rh(null) disease. J. Biol. Chem. 273:2207, 1998.

50. Matassi, G., Chérif-Zahar, B., Raynal, V., Rouger, P., and Cartron, J.P.: Organization of the human RH50A gene (RHAG) and evolution of base composition of the RH gene family. Genomics 47:286, 1998.

51. deVetten, M.P., and Agre, P.: The Rh polypeptide is a major fatty acid acylated erythrocyte membrane protein. J. Biol. Chem. 263:18193, 1988.

52. Shinitzky, M., and Souroujon, M.: Passive modulation of blood group antigens. Proc. Natl. Acad. Sci. USA 76:4438, 1979.

53. Basu, M.K., Flamm, M., Schacter, D., Bertles, J.F., and Maniatis, A.: Effects of modulating erythrocyte membrane cholesterol on Rho(D) antigen expression. Biochem. Biophys. Res. Commun. 95:887, 1980.

54. Gahmberg, C.G., and Karhi, K.K.: Association of Rho(D) polypeptides with the membrane skeleton in Rho(D)-positive human red cells. J. Immunol. 133:334, 1984.

55. Ridgwell, K., Tanner, M.J.A., and Anstee, D.J.: The Rhesus(D) polypeptide is linked to the human erythrocyte cytoskeleton. FEBS Lett. 174:7, 1984.

56. Moore, S., Woodrow, C.F., and McClelland, D.B.: Isolation of membrane components associated with human red cell antigens Rho(D), (c), (E), and Fyᵃ. Nature 295:529, 1982.

57. von dem Borne, A.E., Bos, M.J., Lomas, C., Tippett, P., Bloy, C., Hermand, P., Cartron, J.P., Admiraal, L.G., van de Graaf, J., and Overbeeke, M.A.: Murine monoclonal antibodies against a unique determinant of erythrocytes related to Rh and U antigens. Br. J. Haematol. 75:254, 1990.

58. Avent, N.D., Judson, P.A., Parsons, S.F., Mollison, G., Anstee, D.J., Tanner, M.J., Evans, P.R., Hodges, E., Maciver, A.G., and Holmes, C.: Monoclonal antibodies that recognize different membrane proteins that are deficient in Rh-Rh$_{null}$ human erythrocytes. Biochem. J. 251:499, 1988.

59. Mouro, I., Colin, Y., Chérif-Zahar, B., Cartron, J.P., and Le Van Kim, C.: Molecular genetic basis of the human Rhesus blood group system. Nat. Genet. 5:62, 1993.

60. Andrews, K.T., Wolter, L.C., Saul, A., and Hyland, C.A.: The RhD-trait in a white patient with the RhCCee phenotype attributed to a four-nucleotide deletion in the RHD gene. Blood 92:1839, 1998.

61. Okuda, H., Kawano, M., Iwamoto, S., Tanaka, M., Seno, T., Okubo, Y., and Kajii, E.: The RHD gene is highly detectable in RhD-negative Japanese donors. J. Clin. Invest. 100:373, 1997.

62. Tippett, P., Lomas-Francis, C., and Wallace, M.: The Rh antigen D: partial D antigens and associated low incidence antigens. Vox Sang. 70:123, 1996.

63. Lomas, C., McColl, K., and Tippett, P.: Further complexities of the Rh antigen D disclosed by testing category DII cells with monoclonal anti-D. Transfus. Med. 3:67, 1993.

64. Jones, J., Scott, M.L., and Voak, D.: Monoclonal anti-D specificity and Rh D structure: criteria for selection of monoclonal anti-D reagents for routine typing of patients and donors. Transfus. Med. 5:171, 1995.

65. Avent, N.D., Jones, J.W., Liu, W., Scott, M.L., Voak, D., Flegel, W.A., Wagner, F.F., and Green, C.: Molecular basis of the D variant phenotypes DNU and DII allows localization of critical amino acids required for expression of Rh D epitopes epD3, 4 and 9 to the sixth external domain of the Rh D protein. Br. J. Haematol. 97:366, 1997.

66. Le Van Kim, C., Chérif-Zahat, B., Raynal, V., Mouro, I., Lopez, M., Cartron, J-P., and Colin, Y.: Multiple Rh messenger RNA isoforms are produced by alternative splicing. Blood 80:1074, 1992.

67. Avent, N.D., Liu, W., Warner, K.M., Mawby, W.J., Jones, J.W., Ridgwell, K., and Tanner, M.J.: Immunochemical analysis of the human erythrocyte Rh polypeptides. J. Biol. Chem. 271:14233, 1996.

68. Mouro, I., Colin, Y., Sistonen, P., Le Pennec, P.Y., Cartron, J.P., and Le Van Kim, C.: Molecular basis of the RhCW (Rh8) and RhCX (Rh9) blood group specificities. Blood 86:1196, 1995.

69. Blunt, T., Daniels, D., and Carrit, B.: Serotype switching in a partially deleted RHD gene. Vox Sang. 67:397, 1994.

70. Rouillac, C., Gane, P., Cartron, J., Le Pennec, P.Y., Cartron, J.P., and Colin, Y.: Molecular basis of the altered antigenic expression of RhD in weak D(Du) and RhC/e in RN phenotypes. Blood 87:4853, 1996.

71. Nash, R., and Shojania, A.M.: Hematological aspect of Rh deficiency syndrome: a case report and review of the literature. Am. J. Hematol. 24:267, 1987.

72. Lauf, P.K., and Joiner, C.H.: Increased potassium transport and ouabain binding in human Rh$_{null}$ red blood cells. Blood 48:457, 1976.

73. Ballas, S., Clark, M.R., Mohandas, N., Colfer, H.F., Caswell, M.S., Bergen, M.O., Paerkins, H.A., and Shohet, S.B.: Red cell membranes and cation deficiency in Rh$_{null}$ syndrome. Blood 63:1046, 1984.

74. Kuypers, F., van Linde-Sibenius-Trip, M., Roelofsen, B., Tanner, M.J., Anstee, D.J., and Op den Kamp, J.A.: Rh-Rh$_{null}$ human erythrocytes have an abnormal membrane phospholipid organization. Biochem. J. 221:931, 1984.

75. Chown, B., Lewis, M., Kaita, H., and Lowen, B.: An unlinked modifier of Rh blood groups: effect when heterozygous and homozygous. Am. J. Hum. Genet. 24:623, 1972.

76. Tippett, P.: Regulator genes affecting red cell antigens. Transfus. Med. Rev. 4:56, 1990.

77. Dahr, W., Kordowicz, M., Moulds, J., Gielen, W., Lebeck, L., and Kruger, J.: Characterization of the Ss sialoglycoprotein and its antigens in Rh-Rh$_{null}$ erythrocytes. Blut 54:13, 1987.

78. Bloy, C., Blanchard, D., Hermand, P., Kardowicz, M., Sonneborn, H.H., and Cartron, J.P.: Properties of the blood group LW glycoprotein and preliminary comparison with Rh proteins. Mol. Immunol. 26:1013, 1989.

79. Mallinson, G., Martin, P.G., Anstee, D.J., Tanner, M.J., Merry, A.H., Tills, D., and Sonneborn, H.H.: Identification and partial characterization of the human erythrocyte membrane component(s) which express the antigens of the LW blood group system. Biochem. J. 234:649, 1986.

80. Miller, Y.E., Daniels, G.L., Jones, C., and Palmer, D.K.: Identification of a cell-surface antigen produced by a gene on human chromosome 3 (cenq22) and not expressed by Rh-Rh$_{null}$ cells. Am. J. Hum. Genet. 41:1061, 1987.

81. Sonneborn, H.H., Ernst, M., Tills, D., Lomas, C.G., Gorick, B.D., and Hughes-Jones, N.C.: Comparison of the reactions of the Rh-related murine monoclonal antibodies BS58 and R6A. Vox Sang. 58:219, 1990.

82. Hyland, C.A., Chérif-Zahar, B., Cowley, N., Raynal, V., Parkes, J., Saul, A., and Cartron, J.P.: A novel single missense mutation identified along the RH50 gene in a composite heterozygous Rh$_{null}$ blood donor of the regulator type. Blood 91:1458, 1998.

83. Chérif-Zahar, B., Matassi, G., Raynal, V., Gane, P., Delaunay, J., Arrizabalaga, B., and Cartron, J.P.: Rh-deficiency of the regulator type caused by splicing mutations in the human RH50 gene. Blood 92:2535, 1998.

84. Huang, C.H., Chen, Y., Reid, M.E., and Seidl, C.: Rh$_{null}$ disease: the amorph type results from a novel double mutation in RhCe gene on D-negative background. Blood 92:664, 1998.

85. Chérif-Zahar, B., Matassi, G., Raynal, V., Gane, P., Mempel, W., Perez, C., and Cartron, J.P.: Molecular defects of the *RHCE* gene in Rh-deficient individuals of the amorph type. Blood 92:639, 1998.

86. Marini, A.M., Urrestarazu, A., Beauwens, R., and Andre, B.: The Rh (rhesus) blood group polypeptides are related to NH4$^+$ transporters. Trends Biochem. Sci. 22:460, 1997.

87. Zachowski, A., and Devaux, P.F.: Transmembrane movements of lipids. Experientia 46:644, 1990.

88. Smith, R.E., and Daleke, D.L.: Phosphatidylserine transport in Rh$_{null}$ erythrocytes. Blood 76:1021, 1990.

89. Storry, JR.: The LW blood group system. Immunohematology 8:87, 1992.

90. Hayflick, J.S., Kilgannon, P., and Gallatin, W.M.: The intercellular adhesion molecule (ICAM) family of proteins. New members and novel functions. Immunol. Res. 17:313, 1998.

91. Bailly, P., Hermand, P., Callebaut, I., Sonneborn, H.H., Khamlichi, S., Mornon, J.-P., and Cartron, J.-P.: The LW blood group glycoprotein is homologous to intercellular adhesion molecules. Proc. Natl. Acad. Sci. USA 91:5306, 1994.

92. Bailly, P., Tontti, E., Hermand, P., Cartron, J.P., and Gahmberg, C.G.: The red cell LW blood group protein is an intercellular adhesion molecule which binds to CD11/CD18 leukocyte integrins. Eur. J. Immunol. 25:3316, 1995.

93. Hermand, P., Le Pennec, P.Y., Rouger, P., Cartron, J.P., and Bailly, P.: Characterization of the gene encoding the human LW blood group protein in LW+ and LW− phenotypes. Blood 87:2962, 1996.

94. Hermand, P., Gane, P., Mattei, M.G., Sistonen, J.-P., Cartron, J.-P., and Bailly, P.: Molecular basis and expression of the LWa/LWb blood group polymorphism. Blood 86:1590, 1995.

95. Landsteiner, K., and Levine, P.: A new agglutinable factor differentiating individual human bloods. Proc. Soc. Exp. Biol. 24:600, 1927.

96. Sanger, R., and Race, R.R.: Subdivisions of the MN blood groups in man. Nature 160:55, 1947.

97. Sanger, R., Race, R.R., Walsh, R.J., and Montgomery, C.: An antibody which subdivides the human MN blood groups. Heredity 2:131, 1948.

98. Levine, P., Kuhmichel, A.B., Wigod, M., and Koch, E.: A new blood factor, s allelic to S. Proc. Soc. Exp. Biol. 78:218, 1951.

99. Wiener, A.S., Unger, L.J., and Gordon, E.B.: Fatal hemolytic transfusion reaction caused by sensitization to a new blood factor U. J.A.M.A. 153:1444, 1953.

100. Blanchard, D.: Human red cell glycophorins: biochemical and antigenic properties. Transfus. Med. Rev. 4:170, 1990.

101. Cartron, J.P., Colin, Y., Kudo, S., and Fukuda, M.: Molecular genetics of human erythrocyte sialoglycoproteins, glycophorins A, B, C, and D. *In* Harris, J.R. (ed.): Blood Cell Biochemistry. Vol. 1. New York, Plenum Press, 1990, pp. 299–335.

102. Siebert, P.D., and Fukuda, M.: Molecular cloning of human glycophorin B cDNA: nucleotide sequence and genomic relationship to glycoprotein A. Proc. Natl. Acad. Sci. USA 84:6735, 1987.

103. Tate, C.G., and Tanner, M.J.A.: Isolation of cDNA clones for human erythrocyte membrane sialoglycoproteins a and d. Biochem. J. 254:743, 1988.

104. Siebert, P.D., and Fukuda, M.: Isolation and characterization of human glycophorin A cDNA clones by a synthetic oligonucleotide approach: nucleotide sequence and mRNA structure. Proc. Natl. Acad. Sci. USA 83:1665, 1986.

105. Rahuel, C., Vignal, A., London, J., Hamel, S., Romeo, P.H., Colin, Y., and Cartron, J.P.: Structure of the 5′ flanking region of the glycophorin A gene and analysis of its multiple transcripts. Gene 85:471, 1989.

106. Hamid, J., and Burness, A.T.H.: The mechanism of production of multiple mRNAs for human glycophorin A. Nucleic Acids Res. 18:5829, 1990.

107. Judd, W.J., Issitt, P.D., Pavone, B.G., Anderson, J., and Aminoff, D.: Antibodies that define NANA-independent MN-system antigens. Transfusion 19:12, 1979.

108. Lisowska, E.: Antigenic properties of human erythrocyte glycophorins. *In* Wu, A.M. (ed.): Molecular Immunology of Complex Carbohydrates. New York, Plenum Press, 1988, pp. 265–317.

109. Le Van Kim, C., Colin, Y., Mitjavila, M.T., Clerget, M., Dubart, A., Nakazawa, M., Vainchenker, W., and Cartron, J.P.: Structure of the promoter region and tissue specificity of the human glycophorin C. J. Biol. Chem. 264:20407, 1989.

110. Dahr, W., Beyreuther, K., Steinbach, H., Gielen, W., and Kruger, J.: Structure of the Ss blood group antigens. II. A methionine/threonine polymorphism within the N-terminal sequence of Ss glycoprotein. Hoppe Seylers Z. Physiol. Chem. 361:895, 1980.

111. Kudo, S., and Fukuda, M.: Identification of a novel human glycophorin, glycophorin E, by isolation of genomic clones and complementary DNA clones utilizing polymerase chain reaction. J. Biol. Chem. 265:1102, 1990.

112. Vignal, A., Rahuel, C., London, J., Chérif-Zahar, B., Schaff, S., Hattab, C., Okubo, Y., and Cartron, J.P.: A novel gene member of the human glycophorin A and B gene family. Molecular cloning and expression. Eur. J. Biochem. 191:619, 1990.

113. Anstee, D.J.: The nature and abundance of human red cell surface glycoproteins. J. Immunogenet. 17:219, 1990.

114. Huang, C.-H., Johe, K.K., Seifter, S., and Blumenfeld, O.O.: Biochemistry and molecular biology of MNSs blood group antigens. Baillieres Clin. Haematol. 4:821, 1992.

115. Huang, C.H., and Blumenfeld, O.O.: Molecular genetics of human erythrocyte MiIII and MiVI glycophorins. J. Biol. Chem. 266:7248, 1991.

116. Dahr, W., Uhlenbruck, G., Leikola, J., and Wagstaff, W.: Studies on the membrane glycoprotein defect of En(a−) erythrocytes. III. N-terminal amino acids of sialoglycoproteins from normal and En(a−) red cells. J. Immunogenet. 5:117, 1978.

117. Rahuel, C., London, J., Vignal, A., Chérif-Zahar, B., Colin, Y., Siebert, P., Fukuda, M., and Cartron, J.P.: Alteration of the genes for glycophorin A and B in glycophorin A deficient individuals. Eur. J. Biochem. 177:605, 1988.

118. Bigbee, W.L., Langlois, R.G., Vanderlaan, M., and Jensen, R.H.: Binding specificities of eight monoclonal antibodies to human glycophorin A. Studies with M^{c}M and M^{k}En(UK) variant erythrocytes and M- and MN^v-type chimpanzee erythrocytes. J. Immunol. 133:3149, 1984.

119. Lowe, R.F., and Moores, P.P.: Red cell factor in Africans of Rhodhesia, Malawi, Mozambique and Natal. Hum. Hered. 22:344, 1972.

120. Dahr, W., Uhlenbruck, G., Issitt, P., and Allen, F.H.: SDS-polyacrylamide gel electrophoretic analysis of the membrane glycoproteins from S− s− U− erythrocytes. J. Immunogenet. 2:249, 1975.

121. Tanner, M.J.A., Anstee, D., and Judon, P.A.: A carbohydrate-deficient membrane glycoprotein in human erythrocytes of phenotype S− s−. Biochem. J. 165:157, 1977.

122. Huang, C.H., Lu, W.M., Boots, M.E., Guizzo, M.L., and Blumenfeld, O.O.: Two types of d glycophorin gene alterations in S− s− U− individuals. Transfusion 29:35S, 1989.

123. Rahuel, C., London, J., Vignal, A., Ballas, S.K., and Cartron, J.P.: Erythrocyte glycophorin B deficiency may occur by two distinct gene alterations. J. Am. Haematol. 37:57, 1991.

124. Tate, C.G., Tanner, M.J.A., Judson, P.A., and Anstee, D.J.: Studies on human red-cell membrane glycophorin A and glycophorin B genes in glycophorin-deficient individuals. Biochem. J. 263:993, 1989.

125. Metaxas, N.N., and Metaxas-Buhler, M.: An apparently silent allele at the MN locus. Nature 202:1123, 1964.

126. Tokunaga, E., Sasakama, S., Tamaka, K., Kawamata, H., Giles, C.M., Ikin, E.W., Poole, J., Anstee, D.J., Mawby, W., and Tanner, M.J.: Two apparently healthy Japanese individuals of type Mk/Mk have erythrocytes which lack both the blood group MN and Ss active sialoglycoproteins. J. Immunogenet. 6:383, 1979.

127. Issitt, P.D.: The MN Blood Group System. Miami, Montgomery Scientific Publications, 1981.

128. Furthmayr, H.: Structural comparison of glycophorins and immunochemical analysis of genetic variants. Nature 271:519, 1978.

129. Rosenfield, R.E., Haber, G.V., Kissmeyer-Nielson, J.A., Jack, J.A., Sanger, R., and Race, R.R.: Ge, a very common red cell antigen. Br. J. Haematol. 6:344, 1960.

130. Booth, P.B., and McLoughlin, K.: The Gerbich blood group system especially in Melanesians. Vox Sang. 22:73, 1972.

131. McShane, K., and Chung, A.: A novel human allo antibody in the Gerbich system. Vox Sang. 57:205, 1989.

132. Anstee, D.J., Parsons, S.F., Ridgwell, K., Tanner, M.J.A., Merry, A.H., Thomson, E.E., Judson, P.A., Johnson, P., Bates, S., and Fraser, I.D.: Two individuals with elliptocytic red cells lack three minor erythrocyte membrane sialoglycoproteins. Biochem. J. 218:615, 1984.

133. Anstee, D.J., Ridgwell, K., Tanner, M.J.A., Daniels, G.L., and Parsons, S.F.: Individuals lacking the Gerbich blood-group antigen have alterations in the human erythrocyte membrane sialoglycoproteins b and g. Biochem. J. 221:97, 1984.

134. Rountree, J., Chen, J., Moulds, M.K., Moulds, J.J., Green, A.M., and Telen, M.J.: A second family demonstrating inheritance of the Leach phenotype. Transfusion 29(suppl.):15S, 1989.

135. Daniels, G.L., Reid, M.E., Anstee, D.J., Beattie, K.M., and Judd, W.J.: Transient reduction in erythrocyte membrane sialoglycoprotein b associated with the presence of elliptocytes. Br. J. Haematol. 70:971, 1988.

136. Dahr, W., Moulds, J., Baumeister, G., Moulds, M., Kiedrowski, S., and Hummel, M.: Altered membrane sialoglycoproteins in human erythrocytes lacking the Gerbich blood group antigens. Biol. Chem. Hoppe Seyler 366:201, 1985.

137. Dahr, W., Kiedrowski, S., Blanchard, D., Hermand, P., Moulds, J.J., and Cartron, J.P.: High frequency of human erythrocyte membrane sialoglycoproteins. V. Characterization of the Gerbich blood group antigens: Ge2 and Ge3. Biol. Chem. Hoppe Seyler 368:1375, 1987.

138. Reid, E.M., Anstee, D.J., Tanner, M.J.A., Ridgwell, K., and Nurse, C.T.: Structural relationships between human erythrocyte sialoglycoproteins b and g and abnormal sialoglycoproteins found in certain rare human erythrocyte variants lacking the Gerbich blood-group antigen(s). Biochem. J. 244:123, 1987.

139. Furthmayr, H.: Glycophorins A, B, C: a family of sialoglycoproteins. Isolation and preliminary characterization of trypsin-derived peptides. J. Supramol. Struct. 9:79, 1978.

140. Colin, Y., Rahuel, C., London, J., Romeo, P.H., d'Auriol, L., Galibert, F., and Cartron, J.P.: Isolation of cDNA clones for human erythrocyte glycophorin C. J. Biol. Chem. 261:229, 1986.

141. Dahr, W., Beyreuther, K., Kordowicz, M., and Kruger, J.: N-terminal amino acid sequence of sialoglycoprotein D (glycophorin C) from human erythrocyte membranes. Eur. J. Biochem. 125:57, 1982.

142. Blanchard, D., Dahr, W., Hummal, M., Latron, F., Beyreuther, K., and Cartron, J.P.: Glycophorins B and C from human erythrocyte membranes: purification and sequence analysis. J. Biol. Chem. 262:5808, 1987.

143. High, S., and Tanner, M.J.A.: Human erythrocyte membrane sialoglycoprotein b. The cDNA sequence suggests the absence of a cleaved N-terminal signal sequence. Biochem. J. 243:277, 1987.

144. El-Maliki, B., Blanchard, D., Dahr, W., Beyreuther, K., and Cartron, J.P.: Structural homology between glycophorins C and D of human erythrocytes. Eur. J. Biochem. 183:639, 1989.

145. Dahr, W., Blanchard, D., Kiedrowski, S., Poschmann, A., Cartron, J.P., and Moulds, J.: High frequency antigens of human erythrocyte membrane sialoglycoproteins. VI. Monoclonal antibodies reacting with the N-terminal domain of glycophorin C. Biol. Chem. Hoppe Seyler 370:849, 1989.

146. Colin, Y., Le Van Kim, C., Tsapis, A., Clerget, M., d'Auriol, L., London, J., Galibert, F., and Cartron, J.P.: Human erythrocyte glycophorin C gene structure and rearrangement in genetic variants. J. Biol. Chem. 264:3773, 1989.

147. High, S., Tanner, M.J.A., Macdonald, E.B., and Anstee, D.J.: Rearrangements of the red cell membrane glycophorin C (sialoglycoprotein b) gene. Biochem. J. 262:47, 1989.

148. Le Van Kim, C., Colin, Y., Blanchard, D., Dahr, W., London, J., and Cartron, J.P.: Gerbich group deficiency of the Ge:1, −2, −3 and Ge:−1, −2, 3 types. Eur. J. Biochem. 165:571, 1987.

149. Mattei, M.G., Colin, Y., Le Van Kim, C., Mattei, J.F., and Cartron, J.P.: Localization of the gene for human erythrocyte glycophorin C to chromosome 2q14–q21. Hum. Genet. 74:420, 1986.

150. Tanner, M.J.A., High, S., Martin, P.G., Anstee, D.J., Judson, P.A., and Jones, T.J.: Genetic variants of human red cell membrane sialoglycoprotein b. Study of the alterations occurring in the sialoglycoprotein b gene. Biochem. J. 250:407, 1988.

151. High, S., Tanner, M.J., Macdonald, E.B., and Anstee, D.J.: Rearrangements of the red-cell membrane glycophorin C (sialoglycoprotein beta) gene. A further study of alterations in the glycophorin C gene. Biochem. J. 262:47, 1989.

152. Telen, M.J., Le Van Kim, C., Chung, A., Cartron, J.P., and Colin, Y.: Molecular basis for elliptocytosis associated with glycophorin C and D deletions in the Leach phenotype. Blood 78:1603, 1991.

153. Le Van Kim, C., Mitjavila, M.-T., Clerget, M., Cartron, J.P., and Colin, Y.: An ubiquitous isoform of glycophorin C is produced by alternative splicing. Nucleic Acids Res. 18:3076, 1990.

154. Macdonald, E.B., Condon, J., Ford, D., Fisher, B., and Gerns, L.M.: Abnormal beta and gamma sialoglycoprotein associated with the low-frequency antigen Ls^a. Vox Sang. 58:300, 1990.

155. Reid, M.E., Mawby, W., King, M.J., and Sistonen, P.: Duplication of exon 3 in the glycophorin C gene gives rise to the Lsa blood group antigen. Transfusion 34:966, 1994.

156. Macdonald, E.B., and Gerns, L.M.: An unusual sialoglycoprotein associated with the Webb-positive phenotype. Vox Sang. 50:112, 1986.

157. Reid, M.E., Shaw, M.A., Rowe, G., Anstee, D.J., and Tanner, M.J.A.: Abnormal minor human erythrocyte membrane sialoglycoprotein b in association with the rare blood-group antigen Webb (Wb). Biochem. J. 232:289, 1985.

158. Telen, M.J., Le Van Kim, C., Guizzo, M.L., Cartron, J.P., and Colin, Y.: Erythrocyte Webb-type glycophorin C variant lacks N-glycosylation due to an asparagine to serine substitution. Am. J. Hematol. 37:51, 1991.

159. Daniels, G.L., King, M.J., Avent, N.D., Khalid, G., Reid, M., Mallinson, G., Symthe, J., and Cedergren, B.: A point mutation in the *GYPC* gene results in the expression of the blood group Ana antigen on glycophorin D but not on glycophorin C. Further evidence that glycophorin D is a product of the *GYPC* gene. Blood 82:3198, 1993.

160. King, M.J., Avent, N.D., Mallinson, D., and Reid, M.E.: Point mutation in the glycophorin C gene results in the expression of the blood group antigen Dha. Vox Sang. 63:56, 1992.

161. Nash, G.B., Parmar, J., and Reid, M.E.: Effects of deficiencies of glycophorins C and D on the physical properties of the red cell. Br. J. Haematol. 76:282, 1990.

162. Mueller, T.J., and Morrison, M.: Glycoconnectin (PAS 2), a membrane attachment site for the human erythrocyte cytoskeleton. *In* Kruckenberg, W.C., Eaton, J.W., and Brewer, G.J. (eds.): Erythrocyte Membrane 2: Recent Clinical and Experimental Advances. New York, Alan R. Liss, 1981, pp. 95–112.

163. Bennett, V.: Spectrin-based membrane skeleton: a multipotential adaptor between plasma membrane and cytoplasm. Physiol. Rev. 70:1029, 1990.

164. Chasis, J.A., and Mohandas, N.: Erythrocyte membrane deformability and stability: two distinct membrane properties that are independently regulated by skeletal protein associations. J. Cell Biol. 103:343, 1986.

165. Reid, E.M., Chasis, J.A., and Mohandas, N.: Identification of a functional role for human erythrocyte sialoglycoproteins b and g. Blood 69:1068, 1987.

166. Alloisio, N., Morle, L., Bachir, D., Guetarni, D., Colonna, P., and Dulaunay, J.: Red cell membrane sialoglycoprotein in homozygous and heterozygous 4.1(−) hereditary elliptocytosis. Biochem. Biophys. Acta 816:57, 1985.

167. Sondag, D., Alloisio, N., Blanchard, D., Ducluzeau, M.T., Colonna, P., Bachir, D., Bloy, C., Cartron, J.P., and Delaunay, J.: Gerbich reactivity in 4.1(−) hereditary elliptocytosis and protein 4.1 level in blood group Gerbich deficiency. Br. J. Haematol. 65:43, 1987.

168. Reid, M.E., Takakuwa, Y., Conboy, J., Tchernia, G., and Mohandas, N.: Glycophorin C content of human erythrocytes membrane is regulated by protein 4.1. Blood 75:2229, 1990.

169. Marsh, W.L., and Redmund, C.M.: The Kell blood group system: a review. Transfusion 30:158, 1990.

170. Giblett, E.R.: A critique of the theoretical hazard of inter vs. intraracial transfusion. Transfusion 1:233, 1961.

171. Marsh, W.L., and Redman, C.M.: Recent developments in the Kell blood group system. Transfus. Med. Rev. 1:4, 1987.

172. Masouredis, S.P., Sudora, E., Mahan, L.C., and Victoria, E.J.: Immunoelectron microscopy of Kell and Cellano antigens on red cell ghosts. Haematologia (Budap) 13:59, 1980.

173. Hughes-Jones, N.L., and Gardner, B.: The Kell system studied with radioactively-labelled anti-K. Vox Sang. 21:154, 1971.

174. Redman, C.M., Avellino, G., and Pfeffer, S.R.: Kell blood group antigens are part of a 93,000-dalton red cell membrane protein. J Biol. Chem. 261:9521, 1987.

175. Jaber, A., Blanchard, D., Goossens, D., Bloy, C., Lambin, P., Rouger, P., Salmon, C., and Cartron, J.-P.: Characterization of the blood group Kell (K1) antigen with a human monoclonal antibody. Blood 73:1597, 1989.

176. Wallas, C., Simon, R., Sharpe, M.A., and Byler, C.: Isolation of a Kell-reactive protein from red cell membranes. Transfusion 26:173, 1986.

177. Lee, S., Zambas, E.D., Marsh, W.L., and Redman, C.M.: Molecular cloning and primary structure of Kell blood group protein. Proc. Natl. Acad. Sci. USA 88:6353, 1991.

178. Russo, D.C.W., Lee, S., Reid, M., and Redman, C.M.: Topology of Kell blood group protein and the expression of multiple antigens by transfected cells. Blood 84:3518, 1994.

179. Lee, S., Zambas, E.D., Greed, E.D., and Redman, C.M.: Organization of the gene encoding the human blood group Kell protein. Blood 85:1364, 1995.

180. Lee, S., Wu, X., Reid, M.E., Zelinski, T., and Redman, C.M.: Molecular basis of the Kell (K1) phenotype. Blood 85:912, 1995.

181. Lee, S., Wu, X., Reid, M.E., Zelinski, T., and Redman, C.M.: Molecular basis of the K-6–7 [Js(a + b +)] phenotype in the Kell blood group system. Transfusion 35:822, 1995.

182. Lee, S., Wu, X., Son, D., Naime, D., Reid, M., Okubo, Y., Sistonen, P., and Redman, C.: Point mutations characterize KEL10, the KEL3 and KEL4 and KEL21 alleles, and the KEL17 and KEL11 alleles. Transfusion 36:490, 1996.

183. Lee, S., Naime, D.S., Reid, M.E., and Redman, C.M.: Molecular basis for the high-incidence antigens of the Kell blood group system. Transfusion 37:1117, 1997.

184. Lee, S., Naime, S.D., Reid, M.E., and Redman, C.M.: The KEL24 and KEL14 alleles of the Kell blood group system. Transfusion 37:1035, 1997.

185. Chown, B., Lewis, M., Kaita, K.: A "new" Kell blood-group phenotype [letter]. Nature 180:7111, 1957.

186. Allen, F.H., Crabbe, S.M.R., and Corcoran, P.A.: A new phenotype (McLeod) in the Kell blood-group system. Vox Sang. 6:555, 1961.

187. Wimer, B., Marsh, W.L., Taswell, H.F., and Galey, W.R.: Haematological changes associated with the McLeod phenotype of the Kell blood group system. Br. J. Haematol. 36:219, 1977.

188. Bertelson, C.J., Pogo, A.O., and Chaudhuri, A.: Localization of the McLeod locus (Xk) within Xp21 by deletion analysis. Am. J. Hum. Genet. 42:703, 1988.

189. Franke, U., Ochs, H.D., and de Martinville, B.: Minor Xp21 chromosome deletion in a male associated with expression of Duchenne muscular dystrophy, chronic granulomatous disease, retinitis pigmentosa, and the McLeod syndrome. Am. J. Hum. Genet. 37:250, 1985.

190. Redman, C.M., Marsh, W.L., Scarborough, A., Johnson, C.L., Rabin, B.I., and Overbeeke, M.: Biochemical studies on McLeod phenotype red cells and isolation of Kx antigen. Br. J. Haematol. 68:131, 1988.

191. Ho, M., Chelly, J., Carter, N., Danek, A., Crocker, P., and Monaco, A.P.: Isolation of the gene for McLeod syndrome that encodes a novel membrane transport protein. Cell 77:869, 1994.

192. Allen, F.H., Jr., Diamond, L.K., and Niedziela, B.: A new blood group antigen. Nature 167:482, 1951.

193. Plaut, G., Irkin, E.W., Mourant, A.E., Sanger, R., and Race, R.R.: A new blood-group antibody, anti Jk^b. Nature 171:431, 1953.

194. Pinkerton, F.J., Mermod, L.E., Liles, B.A., Jack, J. Jr., and Noades, J.: The phenotype of Jk(a − b −) in the Kidd blood group system. Vox Sang. 4:155, 1959.

195. Woodfield, D.G., Douglas, R., Smith, J., Simpson, A., Pinder, L., and Staveley, J.M.: The Jk(a − b −) phenotype in New Zealand Polynesians. Transfusion 22:276, 1982.

196. Okubo, Y.H., Yamaguchi, H., Nagao, N., Tomita, T., Seno, T., and Tanaka, M.: Heterogeneity of the phenotype Jk(a − b −) found in Japanese. Transfusion 26:237, 1986.

197. Masouredis, S.P., Sudora, E., Mahan, L., and Victoria, E.J.: Quantitative immunoferratin microassay of Fy^a, Fy^b, Jk^a, U and Di^b antigen site numbers on human red cells. Blood 56:969, 1980.

198. Sinor, L.T., Eastwood, K.L., and Plapp, F.V.: Dot blot purification of the Kidd blood group antigen. Med. Lab. Sci. 44:294, 1987.

199. Heaton, D.C., and McLaughlin, K.: Jk(a − b −) red blood cells resist urea lysis. Transfusion 22:70, 1982.

200. Edwards-Moulds, J., and Kasschau, M.: The effect of 2M urea on Jk(a − b −) red cells. Vox Sang. 55:181, 1988.

201. Froelich, O., Macy, R.I., Edwards-Moulds, J., Gargas, J.J., and Gunn, R.B.: Urea transport deficiency in Jk(a − b −) erythrocytes. Am. J. Physiol. 260:C778, 1991.

202. Sands, J.M., Gargus, J.J., Frohlich, O., Gunn, R.B., and Kokko, J.P.: Importance of carrier-mediated urea transport to urine concentrating ability in patients with the Jk(a − b −) blood type. J. Am. Soc. Nephrol. 1:678, 1990.

203. Gargus, J.J., and Mitas, M.: Physiological processes revealed through analysis of inborn errors. J. Am. Physiol. Soc. 255:F1047, 1988.

204. Gunn, R.B., Gargus, J.J., and Fröhlich, O.: Kidd antigens and urea transport. *In* Agre, P., and Cartron, J.P. (eds.): Protein blood group

antigens of the human red cell: structure, function, and clinical significance. Baltimore, Johns Hopkins University Press, 1992, pp. 88–100.

205. Olives, B., Neau, P., Bailly, P., Hediger, M.A., Rousselet, G., Cartron, J.P., and Ripoche, P.: Cloning and functional expression of a urea transporter from human bone marrow cells. J. Biol. Chem. 269:31649, 1994.

206. Olives, B., Mattei, M.G., Huet, M., Neau, P., Martial, S., Cartron, J.P., and Bailly, P.: Kidd blood group and urea transport function of human erythrocytes are carried by the same protein. J. Biol. Chem. 270:15607, 1995.

207. Olives, B., Merriman, M., Bailly, P., Bain, S., Barnett, A., Todd, J., Cartron, J.P., and Merriman, T.: The molecular basis of the Kidd blood group polymorphism and its lack of association with type 1 diabetes susceptibility. Hum. Mol. Genet. 6:1017, 1997.

208. Lucien, N., Sidoux-Walter, F., Olives, B., Moulds, J., Le Pennec, P.Y., Cartron, J.P., and Bailly, P.: Characterization of the gene encoding the human Kidd blood group/urea transporter protein. Evidence for splice site mutations in Jk$_{null}$ individuals. J. Biol. Chem. 273:12973, 1998.

209. Issitt, P.D., and Issitt, C.H.: The Duffy blood group system. In Issitt, P.D. (ed.): Applied Blood Group Serology. 3rd ed. Miami, Montgomery Scientific Publications, 1985, pp. 278–288.

210. Moore, S., Woodrow, C.F., and McClelland, D.B.L.: Isolation of membrane components associated with human red cell antigens Rh (D), (c), (E) and Fy^a. Nature 295:429, 1982.

211. Hadley, T.J., David, P.H., and McGinniss, M.H.: Identification of an erythrocyte component carrying the Duffy blood group Fy^a antigen. Science 223:597, 1984.

212. Tanner, M.J.A., Anstee, D.J., and Mallinson, G.: Effect of endoglycosidase F preparations on the surface components of the human erythrocyte. Carbohydr. Res. 178:203, 1988.

213. Chaudhuri, A., Polyakova, J., Zbrzezna, V., Williams, K., Gulati, S., and Pogo, A.O.: Cloning of glycoprotein D cDNA, which encodes the major subunit of the Duffy blood group system and the receptor for the Plasmodium vivax malaria parasite. Proc. Natl. Acad. Sci. USA 90:10793, 1993.

214. Hadley, T.J., and Peiper, S.C.: From malaria to chemokine receptor: the emerging physiologic role of the Duffy blood group antigen. Blood 89:3077, 1997.

215. Neote, K., Mak, J.Y., Kolakowski, L.F., and Schall, T.J.: Functional and biochemical analysis of the cloned Duffy antigen: identity with the red blood cell chemokine receptor. Blood 84:44, 1994.

216. Chaudhuri, A., Zbrzezna, V., Polyakova, J., Pogo, A.O., Hesselgesser, J., and Horuk, R.: Expression of the Duffy antigen in K562 cells: evidence that it is the human erythrocyte chemokine receptor. J. Biol. Chem. 269:7835, 1994.

217. Hadley, T.J., Lu, Z.H., Wasniowska, K., Martin, A.W., Peiper, S.C., Hesselgesser, J., and Horuk, R.: Postcapillary venule endothelial cells in kidney express a multispecific chemokine receptor that is structurally and functionally identical to the erythroid isoform, which is the Duffy blood group antigen. J. Clin. Invest. 94:985, 1994.

218. Barnwell, J. W., and Wertheimer, S.P.: Plasmodium vivax: merozoite antigens, the Duffy blood group, and erythrocyte invasion. Prog. Clin. Biol. Res. 313:1, 1989.

219. Miller, L.H., Alkawa, M., Johnson, J.G., and Shiroishi, T.: Interaction between cytochalasin B–treated malarial parasites and erythrocytes. Attachment and junction formation. J. Exp. Med. 149:172, 1979.

220. Tournamille, C., Colin, Y., Cartron, J.-P., and Le Van Kim, C.: Disruption of a GATA motif in the Duffy gene promoter abolishes erythroid gene expression in Duffy-negative individuals. Nat. Genet. 10:224, 1995.

221. Mallinson, G., Soo, K.S., Schall, T.J., Pisacka, M., and Anstee, D.J.: Mutations in the erythrocyte chemokine receptor (Duffy) gene: the molecular basis of the Fya/Fyb antigens and identification of a deletion in the Duffy gene of an apparently healthy individual with the Fy(a−b−) phenotype. Br. J. Haematol. 90:823, 1995.

222. Chaudhuri, A., Polyakova, J., Zbrzezna, V., and Pogo, A.O.: The coding sequence of Duffy blood group gene in humans and simians: restriction fragment length polymorphism, antibody and malarial parasite specificities, and expression in nonerythroid tissues in Duffy-negative individuals. Blood 85:615, 1995.

223. Iwamoto, S., Omi, T., Kajii, E., and Ikemoto, S.: Genomic organization of the glycoprotein D gene: Duffy blood group Fya/Fyb alloantigen system is associated with a polymorphism at the 44-amino acid residue. Blood 85:622, 1995.

224. Tournamille, C., Le Van Kim, C., Gane, P., Cartron, J.P., and Colin, Y.: Molecular basis and PCR-DNA typing of the Fya/fyb blood group polymorphism. Hum. Genet. 95:407, 1995.

225. Crawford, M.N.: The Lutheran blood group systems: serology and genetics. In Pierce, S.R., and MacPherson, C.R. (eds.): Blood Group Systems: Duffy, Kidd, and Lutheran. Arlington, VA, American Association of Blood Banks, 1988.

226. Callendar, S., Race, R.R., and Paykoc, Z.V.: Hypersensitivity to transfused blood. Br. Med. J. 2:83, 1945.

227. Shaw, M.-A., Leak, M.R., Daniels, G.L., and Tippett, P.: The rare Lutheran blood group phenotype Lu(a−b−): a genetic study. Ann. Hum. Genet. 48:229, 1984.

228. Marsh, W.L., Brown, P.J., and DiNapoli, J.: Anti-Wj: an autoantibody that defines a high-incidence antigen modified by the In(Lu) gene. Transfusion 23:128, 1983.

229. Norman, P.C., Tippett, P., and Beal, R.W.: An Lu(a−b−) phenotype caused by an X-linked recessive gene. Vox Sang. 51:49, 1986.

230. Spring, F.A., Dalchau, R., Daniels, G.L., Mallinson, G., Judson, P.A., Parson, S.F., Fabre, J.W., and Anstee, D.J.: The In^a and In^b blood group antigens are located on a glycoprotein of 80,000 MW (the CD44 glycoprotein) whose expression is influenced by the In(Lu) gene. Immunology 64:37, 1988.

231. Picker, L.J., de los Toyos, J., Telen, M.J., Haynes, B.F., and Butcher, E.C.: Identity of CD44 [In(Lu)-related p80], Pgp-1, and the Hermes class of lymphocyte homing receptors. J. Immunol. 142:2046, 1989.

232. Norman, P.C., Tippett, P., and Beal, R.W.: An Lu(a−b−) phenotype caused by an X-linked recessive gene. Vox Sang. 51:49, 1986.

233. Parsons, S.F., Mallinson, G., Holmes, C.H., Houlihan, J.M., Simpson, K.L., Mawby, W.J., Spurr, N.K., Warne, D., Barclay, A.N., and Anstee, D.J.: The Lutheran blood group glycoprotein, another member of the immunoglobulin superfamily, is widely expressed in human tissues and is developmentally regulated in human liver. Proc. Natl. Acad. Sci. USA 92:5496, 1995.

234. Anstee, D.J., Mallinson, G., and Yendle, J.E.: Evidence for the occurrence of Lu^b-active glycoproteins in human erythrocytes, kidney and liver [abstract]. Proceedings of the XXth Congress of the International Society of Blood Transfusion. Manchester, British Blood Transfusion Society, 1988, p. 263.

235. Parsons, S.F., Mallinson, G., Judson, P.A., Anstee, D.J., Tanner, M.J.A., and Daniels, G.L.: Evidence that the Lu^b blood group antigen is located on red cell membrane glycoproteins of 85 and 78 kd. Transfusion 27:61, 1987.

236. Daniels, G., and Khalid, G.: Identification, by immunoblotting, of the structures carrying Lutheran and para-Lutheran blood group antigens. Vox Sang. 57:137, 1989.

237. Daniels, G.: Evidence that the Auberger blood group antigens are located on the Lutheran glycoproteins. Vox Sang. 58:56, 1990.

238. Daniels, G.L., Le Pennec, P.Y., Rouger, P., Salmon, C., and Tippett, P.: The red cell antigens Au^a and Au^b belong to the Lutheran system. Vox Sang. 60:191, 1991.

239. Rahuel, C., Le Van Kim, C., Mattei, M.G., Cartron, J.P., and Colin, Y.: A unique gene encodes spliceoforms of the B-cell adhesion molecule cell surface glycoprotein of epithelial cancer and of the Lutheran blood group glycoprotein. Blood 88:1865, 1996.

240. El Nemer, W., Rahuel, C., Colin, Y., Gane, P., Cartron, J.P., and Le Van Kim, C.: Organization of the human LU gene and molecular basis of the Lu(a)/Lu(b) blood group polymorphism. Blood 89:4608, 1997.

241. Parsons, S.F., Mallinson, G., Daniels, G.L., Green, C.A., Smythe, J.S., and Anstee, D.J.: Use of domain-deletion mutants to locate Lutheran blood group antigens to each of the five immunoglobulin superfamily domains of the Lutheran glycoprotein: elucidation of the molecular basis of the Lu(a)/Lu(b) and the Au(a)/Au(b) polymorphisms. Blood 89:4219, 1997.

242. Campbell, I.G., Foulkes, W.D., Senger, G., Trowsdale, J., Garin-Chesa, P., and Rettig, W.J.: Molecular cloning of the B-CAM cell surface glycoprotein of epithelial cancers: a novel member of the immunoglobulin superfamily. Cancer Res. 54:5761, 1994.

243. Harris, J.P., Tegoli, J., Swanson, J., Fisher, N., Gavin, J., and Noades, J.: A nebulous antibody responsible for cross-matching difficulties (Chido). Vox Sang. 12:140, 1967.

244. Longster, G., and Giles, C.M.: A new antibody specificity, anti-Rg^a, reacting with a red cell and serum antigen. Vox Sang. 30:175, 1976.

245. Middleton, J., and Crookston, M.C.: Chido-substance in plasma. Vox Sang. 23:256, 1972.

246. Humphreys, J., Stout, T.D., Middleton, J., and Crookston, M.C.: The

identification of Chido-negative donors by a plasma-inhibition test [abstract]. Transfusion Congress, Washington, DC, 1972, p. 57.

247. Westhoff, C.M., Sipherd, B.D., Wylie, D.E., and Toalson, L.D.: Severe anaphylactic reactions following transfusions of platelets to a patient with anti-Ch. Transfusion 32:576, 1992.

248. Moore, H.C., Issitt, P.D., and Pavone, B.G.: Successful transfusion of Chido-positive blood to two patients with anti-Chido. Transfusion 15:266, 1975.

249. Tilley, C.A., Crookston, M.C., Haddad, S.A., and Shumak, K.H.: Red blood cell survival studies in patients with anti-Chᵃ, anti-Ykᵃ, anti-Ge, and anti-Vel. Transfusion 17:171, 1977.

250. Yu, C.Y., Campbell, R.D., and Porter, R.R.: A structural model for the location of the Rodgers and the Chido antigenic determinants and their correlation with the human complement component C4A/C4B isotypes. Immunogenetics 27:399, 1988.

251. Tilley, C.A., Romans, D.G., and Crookston, M.C.: Localisation of Chido and Rodgers determinants to the C4d fragment of human C4. Nature 276:713, 1978.

252. Atkinson, J.P., Chan, A.C., Karp, D.R., Killion, C.C., Brown, R., Spinella, D., Schreffler, D.C., and Levine, R.P.: Origin of the fourth component of complement related Chido and Rodgers blood group antigens. Complement 5:65, 1988.

253. Rittner, C., Giles, C.M., Roos, M.H., Demant, P., and Mollenhauer, E.: Genetics of human C4 polymorphism: detection and segregation of rare and duplicated haplotypes. Immunogenetics 19:321, 1984.

254. Roos, M.H., Giles, C.M., Demant, P., Mollenhauer, E., and Rittner, C.: Rodgers (Rg) and Chido (Ch) determinants on human C4; characterisation of two C4 B5 subtypes, one of which contains Rg and Ch determinants. J. Immunol. 133:2634, 1984.

255. Daniels, G.: Cromer-related antigens—blood group determinants on decay-accelerating factor. Vox Sang. 56:205, 1989.

256. Telen, M.J.: Glycosyl phosphatidylinositol–linked blood group antigens and paroxysmal nocturnal hemoglobinuria. Transfus. Clin. Biol. 2:277,1995.

257. Daniels, G.L., Tohyama, H., and Uchikawa, M.: A possible null phenotype in the Cromer blood group complex. Transfusion 22:362, 1982.

258. Smith, K.J., Coonce, L.S., and South, S.F.: Anti-Crᵃ: family study and survival of chromium-labeled incompatible red cells in a Spanish-American patient. Transfusion 23:167, 1983.

259. McSwain, B., and Robins, C.: A clinically significant anti-Crᵃ. Transfusion 28:289, 1988.

260. Telen, M.J., Hall, S.E., and Green A.M.: Identification of human erythrocyte blood group antigens on decay accelerating factor (DAF) and an erythrocyte phenotype negative for DAF. J. Exp. Med. 167:93, 1988.

261. Parsons, S.F., Spring, F.A., and Merry, A.H.: Evidence that Cromer-related blood group antigens are carried on decay accelerating factor (DAF) suggests that the Inab phenotype is a novel form of DAF deficiency [abstract]. Proceedings of the XXth Congress of the International Society of Blood Transfusion. Manchester, British Blood Transfusion Society, 1988, p. 116.

262. Telen, M.J., and Green, A.M.: The Inab phenotype: characterization of the membrane protein and complement regulatory defect. Blood 74:437, 1989.

263. Lublin, D.M., Mallinson, G., Poole, J., Reid, M.E., Thompson, E.S., Ferdman, B.R., Telen, M.J., Anstee, D.J., and Tanner, M.J.: Molecular basis of reduced or absent expression of decay-accelerating factor in Cromer blood group phenotypes. Blood 84:1276, 1994.

264. Wang, L., Uchikawa, M., Tsuneyama, H., Tokunaga, K., Tadokoro, K., and Juji, T.: Molecular cloning and characterization of decay-accelerating factor deficiency in Cromer blood group Inab phenotype. Blood 91:680, 1998.

265. Lublin, D.M., Thompson, E.S., Green, A.M., Levene, C., and Telen, M.J.: Dr(a−) polymorphism of decay accelerating factor. Biochemical, functional, and molecular characterization and production of allele-specific transfectants. J. Clin. Invest. 87:1945, 1991.

266. Telen, M.J., Rao, N., Udani, M., Thompson, E.S., Kaufman, R.M., and Lublin, D.M.: Molecular mapping of the Cromer blood group Cra and Tca epitopes of decay accelerating factor: toward the use of recombinant antigens in immunohematology. Blood 84:3205, 1994.

267. Rao, N., Ferguson, D.J., Lee, S.F., and Telen, M.J.: Identification of human erythrocyte blood group antigens on the C3b/C4b receptor. J. Immunol. 146:3502, 1991.

268. Moulds, J.M., Nickells, M.W., Moulds, J.J., Brown, M.C., and Atkin-

son, J.P.: The C3b/C4b receptor is recognized by the Knops, McCoy, Swain-Langley, and York blood group antisera. J. Exp. Med. 173:1159, 1991.

269. Moulds, J.M., Moulds J.J., Brown, M., and Atkinson, J.P.: Antiglobulin testing for CR1-related (Knops/McCoy/Swain-Langley/York) blood group antigens: negative and weak reactions are caused by variable expression of CR1. Vox Sang. 62:230, 1992.

270. Rao, N., Whitsett, C.F., Oxendine, S.M., and Telen, M.J.: Human erythrocyte acetylcholinesterase bears the Ytᵃ blood group antigen and is reduced or absent in the Yt(a−b−) phenotype. Blood 81:815, 1993.

271. Bartels, C.F., Zelinski, T., and Lockridge. O.: Mutation at codon 322 in the human acetylcholinesterase (ACHE) gene accounts for YT blood group polymorphism. Am. J. Hum. Genet. 52:928, 1993.

272. Lesley, J., and Hyman, R.: CD44 structure and function. Front. Biosci. 3:D616, 1998.

273. Telen, M.J., Udani, M., Washington, M.K., Levesque, M.C., Lloyd, E., and Rao, N.: A blood group–related polymorphism of CD44 abolishes a hyaluronan-binding consensus sequence without preventing hyaluronan binding. J. Biol. Chem. 271:7147, 1996.

274. Telen, M.J.: Lutheran antigens, CD44-related antigens, and Lutheran regulatory genes. Transfus. Clin. Biol. 2:291, 1995.

275. Smith, B.L., Preston, G.M., Spring, F.A., Anstee, D.J., and Agre, P.: Human red cell aquaporin CHIP. I. Molecular characterization of ABH and Colton blood group antigens. J. Clin. Invest. 94:1043, 1994.

276. Lee, M.D., King, L.S., and Agre, P.: The aquaporin family of water channel proteins in clinical medicine. Medicine (Baltimore) 76:141, 1997.

277. Preston, G.M., Smith, B.L., Zeidel, M.L., Moulds, J.J., and Agre, P.: Mutations in aquaporin-1 in phenotypically normal humans without functional CHIP water channels. Science 265:1585, 1994.

278. Spring, F.A., Bruce, L.J., Anstee, D.J., and Tanner, M.J.A.: A red cell band 3 variant with altered stilbene disulfonate binding and the Diego (Diᵃ) blood group antigen. Biochem. J. 288:713, 1992.

279. Bruce, L.J., Anstee, D.J., Spring, F.A., and Tanner, M.J.A.: Band 3 Memphis variant II: Altered stilbene disulfonate binding and the Diego (Diᵃ) blood group antigen are associated with the human erythrocyte band 3 mutation Pro⁸⁵⁴-Leu. J. Biol. Chem. 269:16155, 1994.

280. Bruce, L.J., Ring, S.M., Anstee, D.J., Reid, M.E., Wilkinson, S., and Tanner, M.J.: Changes in the blood group Wright antigens are associated with a mutation at amino acid 658 in human erythrocyte band 3: a site of interaction between band 3 and glycophorin A under certain conditions. Blood 85:541, 1995.

281. Jarolim, P., Murray, J.L., Rubin, H.L., Coghlan, G., and Zelinski, T.: A Thr552→Ile substitution in erythroid band 3 gives rise to the Warrior blood group antigen. Transfusion 37:398, 1997.

282. Zelinski, T., McManus, K., Punter, F., Moulds, M., and Coghlan, G.: A Gly565→Ala substitution in human erythroid band 3 accounts for the Wu blood group polymorphism. Transfusion 38:745, 1998.

283. Jarolim, P., Murray, J.L., Rubin, H.L., Smart, E., and Moulds, J.M.: Blood group antigens Rb(a), Tr(a), and Wd(a) are located in the third ectoplasmic loop of erythroid band 3. Transfusion 37:607, 1997.

284. Zelinski, T., Punter, F., McManus, K., and Coghlan, G.: The ELO blood group polymorphism is located in the putative first extracellular loop of human erythrocyte band 3. Vox Sang. 75:63, 1998.

285. Bruce, L.J., Zelinski, T., Ridgwell, K., and Tanner, M.J.: The low-incidence blood group antigen, Wda, is associated with the substitution Val557→Met in human erythrocyte band 3 (AE1). Vox Sang. 71:118, 1996.

286. Spring, F.A., Herron, R., and Rowe, G.: An erythrocyte glycoprotein of apparent Mᵣ 60,000 expresses the Sc1 and Sc2 antigens. Vox Sang. 58:122, 1993.

287. Banks, J.A., Parker, N., and Poole, J.: Evidence that the Gyᵃ, Hy, and Joᵃ antigens belong to the Dombrock blood group system. Vox Sang. 68:177, 1995.

288. Ellis, N.A., Ye, T.-Z., Patton, S., German, J., Goodfellow, P.N., and Weller, P.: Cloning of PBDX, an MIC2-related gene that spans the pseudoautosomal boundary on chromosome Xp. Nat. Genet. 6:394, 1994.

289. Ellis, N.A., Tippett, P., Petty, A., Reid, M., Weller, P.A., Ye, T.Z., German, J., Goodfellow, P.N., Thomas, S., and Banting, G.: PBDX is the XG blood group gene. Nat. Genet. 8:285, 1994.

290. Landsteiner, K.: Zur Kenntnis der antifermentativen, lytischen und agglutinierenden Wirkungen des Blutserums und der Lymphe. Zentralbl. Batk. 27:357, 1900.

291. Landsteiner, K.: Über Agglutinationserscheinungen normalen menschlichen Blutes. Wien. Klin. Wochenschr. 14:1132, 1901.

292. Walker, R.H. (ed.): American Association of Blood Banks Technical Manual. Arlington, VA, American Association of Blood Banks, 1990.

293. Oriol, R., Le Pendu, J., and Mollicone, R.: Genetics of ABO, H, Lewis, X and Related Antigens. Vox Sang. 51:161, 1986.

294. Watkins, W.M.: Biochemistry and Genetics of the ABO, Lewis, and P blood group systems. Adv. Hum. Genet. 10:1, 1980.

295. Yamamoto, F.: Molecular genetics of the ABO histo-blood group system. Vox Sang. 69:1, 1995.

296. Hakomori, S.: Blood group ABH and Ii antigens of human erythrocytes: chemistry, polymorphism, and their developmental change. Semin. Hematol. 18:39, 1981.

297. Clausen, H., and Hakomori, S.: ABH and related histo-blood group antigens: immunochemical differences in carrier isotypes and their distribution. Vox Sang. 46:1, 1989.

298. Sadler, J.E.: Biosynthesis of glycoproteins: formation of O-linked oligosaccharides. In Ginsburg, V., and Robbins, P.W. (eds.): Biology of Carbohydrates. Vol. 2. New York, John Wiley, 1984, pp. 199–288.

299. Clausen, H., Levery, S.B., Nudelman, E., Tsuchiya, S., and Hakomori, S.: Repetitive A epitope (type 3 chain A) defined by blood group A_1–specific monoclonal antibody TH-1: Chemical basis of qualitiative A_1 and A_2 distinction. Proc. Natl. Acad. Sci. USA 82:1199, 1985.

300. Le Pendu, J., Lambert, F., Samuelsson, B.E., Breimer, M.E., Seitz, R.C., Urdaniz, M.P., Suesa, N., Ratcliffe, M., Francoise, A., Poschmann, A., Vinas, J., and Oriol, R.: Monoclonal antibodies specific for type 3 and type 4 chain-based blood group determinants: relationship to the A1 and A2 subgroups. Glycoconj. J. 3:255, 1986.

301. Clausen, H., Levery, S.B., Nudelman, E., Baldwin, M., and Hakomori, S.: Further characterization of type 2 and type 3 chain blood group A glycosphingolipids from human erythrocyte membranes. Biochemistry 25:7075, 1986.

302. Kannagi, R., Levery, S.B., and Hakomori, S.: Blood group H antigen with globo-series structure: isolation and characterization from human blood group O erythrocytes. FEBS Lett. 175:397, 1984.

303. Oriol, R.: Genetic control of the fucosylation of ABH precursor chains. Evidence for new epistatic interactions in different cells and tissues. J. Immunogenet. 17:235, 1990.

304. Betteridge, A., and Watkins, W.M.: Acceptor substrate specificities of human α-2-L-fucosyltransferases from different tissues. Biochem. Soc. Trans. 13:1126, 1986.

305. Clausen, H., Holmes, E., and Hakomori, S.: Novel blood group H glycolipid antigens exclusively expressed in blood group A and AB erythrocytes (type 3 chain H). II. Differential conversion of different H substrates by A_1 and A_2 enzymes, and type 3 chain H expression in relation to secretor status. J. Biol. Chem. 261:1388, 1986.

306. Laine, R.A., and Rush, J.S.: Chemistry of human erythrocyte polylactosamine glycopeptides (erythroglycans) as related to ABH blood group antigenic determinants. Adv. Exp. Med. Biol. 228:331, 1988.

307. Steck, T.L.: The organisation of proteins in the human red blood cell membrane. J. Cell Biol. 62:1, 1974.

308. Allard, W.J., and Lienhard, G.E.: Monoclonal antibodies to the glucose transporter from human erythrocytes. J. Biol. Chem. 160:668, 1985.

309. Tanner, M.J.A., Martin, P.G., and High, S.: The complete amino acid sequence of the human erythrocyte membrane anion-transport protein deduced from the cDNA sequence. Biochem. J. 256:703, 1988.

310. Mueckler, M., Caruso, C., and Baldwin, S.A.: Sequence and structure of a human glucose transporter. Science 229:941, 1985.

311. Fukuda, M., and Fukuda, M.N.: Changes in cell surface glycoproteins and carbohydrate structures during the development and differentiation of human erythroid cells. J. Supramol. Struct. 17:313, 1974.

312. Smith, B.L., Preston, G.M., Spring, F.A., Anstee, D.J., and Agre, P.: Human red cell aquaporin CHIP. I. Molecular characterization of ABH and Colton blood group antigens. J. Clin. Invest. 94:1043, 1994.

313. Moore, S.J., and Green, C.: The identification of Rhesus polypeptide–blood group ABH–active glycoprotein complex in the human red cell membrane. Biochem. J. 244:735, 1987.

314. Dejter-Juszynski, M., Harpaz, N., Flowers, H.M., and Sharon, N.: Blood-group ABH–specific macroglycolipids of human erythrocytes: isolation in high yield from a crude membrane glycoprotein fraction. Eur. J. Biochem. 83:363, 1978.

315. Koscielak, J., Miller-Podraza, H., Krauze, R., and Piasek, A.: Isolation and characterization of poly(glycosyl)ceramides (megaloglycolipids) with A, H, and I blood-group activities. Eur. J. Biochem. 71:9, 1976.

316. Eastlund, T. The histo-blood group ABO system and tissue transplantation. Transfusion 38:975, 1998.

317. Salmon, C.H., and Cartron, J.P.: ABO phenotypes. In Greenwalt, T.J., and Steane, E.A. (eds.): CRC Handbook Series in Clinical Laboratory Science. Section D: Blood Banking. Vol. 1. Cleveland, OH, CRC Press, 1977, p. 71.

318. Daniels, G.: Human Blood Groups. Oxford, Blackwell, 1995.

319. Bird, G.W.G.: Haemagglutinins in seeds. Br. Med. Bull. 15:165, 1959.

320. Mourant, A.E., Kopèc, A.C., and Domaniewska-Sobczak, K.: The Distribution of the Human Blood Groups and Other Biochemical Polymorphisms. 2nd ed. London, Oxford University Press, 1976.

321. Economidou, J., Hughes-Jones, N.C., and Gardner, B.: Quantitative measurements concerning A and B antigen sites. Vox Sang. 12:321, 1967.

322. Mäkela, O., Ruoslahti, E., and Ehnholm, C.: Subtypes of human ABO blood groups and subtype-specific antibodies. J. Immunol. 10:763, 1969.

323. Kisailus, E.C., and Kabat, E.A.: Immunochemical studies on blood groups. LXVI. Competitive binding assays of A_1 and A_2 blood group substances with insolubilized anti-A serum and insolubilized A agglutinine from Dolichos biflorus. J. Exp. Med. 147:830, 1978.

324. Mohn, J.F., Cunningham, R.K., and Bates, J.F.: Qualitative distinctions between subgroups A_1 and A_2. In Mohn, J.F., Plunkett, R., Cunningham, R.K., and Lambert, R. (eds.): Human Blood Groups. New York, Karger, 1977, pp. 316–325.

325. Moreno, C., Lundblad, A., and Kabat, E.A.: Immunochemical studies on blood groups. LI. A comparative study of the reaction of A_1 and A_2 blood group glycoproteins with human anti-A. J. Exp. Med. 134:439, 1971.

326. Yamaguchi, H., Okubo, Y., and Hazama, F.: Another Japanese A_2B_3 blood-group family with the propositus having O-group father. Proc. Jpn. Acad. 42:417, 1966.

327. Seyfried, H., Walewska, I., and Verblinska, B.: Unusual inheritance of ABO group in a family with weak B antigens. Vox Sang. 9:268, 1964.

328. Lopez, M., Liberge, G., Gerbal, A., Brocteur, J., and Salmon, C.: Cis AB blood groups. Immunologic, thermodynamic and quantitative studies of ABH antigens. Biomedicine 24:265, 1976.

329. Yoshida, A., Yamaguchi, H., and Okubo, Y.: Genetic mechanism of cis-AB inheritance. I. A case associated with unequal chromosomal crossing over. Am. J. Hum. Genet. 32:332, 1980.

330. Yoshida, A., Yamaguchi, H., Okubo, Y.: Genetic mechanism of cis-AB inheritance. II. Cases associated with structural mutation of blood group glycosyltransferases. Am. J. Hum. Genet. 32:645, 1980.

331. Watkins, W.M., Greenwell, P., and Yates, A.D.: The genetic and enzymatic regulation of the synthesis of the A and B determinants in the ABO blood group system. Immunol. Commun. 10:83, 1981.

332. Yamamoto, F., McNeill, P.D., Kominato, Y., Yamamoto, M., Hakomori, S., Ishimoto, S., Nishida, S., Shima, M., and Fujimura, Y.: Molecular genetic analysis of the ABO blood group system: 2. Cis-AB alleles. Vox Sang. 64:120, 1993.

333. Yamamoto, F., McNeill, P.D., Yamamoto, M., Hakomori, S., and Harris, T.: Molecular genetic analysis of the ABO blood group system: 3. A(X) and B(A) alleles. Vox Sang. 64:171, 1993.

334. Clausen, H., White, T., Takio, K., Titani, K., Stroud, M., Holmes, E., Karkov, J., Thim, L., and Hakomori, S.: Isolation to homogeneity and partial characterization of a histo-blood group A defined Fuc α1→2-Gal α1→3-N-acetylgalactosaminyltransferase from human lung tissue. J. Biol. Chem. 265:1139, 1990.

335. Yamamoto, F.-I., Marken, J., Tsuji, T., White, T., Clausen, H., and Hakomori, S.-I.: Cloning and characterization of DNA complementary to human UDP-GalNAc:Fucα1→2Gal α1→3GalNAc transferase (histo-blood group A transferase) mRNA. J. Biol. Chem. 264:1146, 1990.

336. Yamamoto, F., McNeill, P.D., and Hakomori, S.: Genomic organization of human histo-blood group ABO genes. Glycobiology 5:51, 1995.

337. Bennett, E.P., Steffensen, R., Clausen, H., Weghuis, D.O., and Geurts van Kessel, A.: Genomic cloning of the human histo-blood group ABO locus. Biochem. Biophys. Res. Commun. 211:347, 1995.

338. Lowe, J.B.: Molecular cloning, expression, and uses of mammalian glycosyltransferases. Semin. Cell Biol. 2:289, 1991.

339. Joziasse, D.H.: Mammalian glycosyltransferases: genomic organization and protein structure. Glycobiology 2:271, 1992.

340. Griffiths, G., and Simons, K.: The trans Golgi network: sorting at the exit site of the Golgi complex. Science 234:438, 1986.

341. Kornfeld, R., and Kornfeld, S.: Assembly of asparagine-linked oligosaccharides. Annu. Rev. Biochem. 54:631, 1985.

342. Larsen, R.D., Rajan, V.P., Ruff, M.M., Kukowska-Latallo, J., Cum-

mings, R.D., and Lowe, J.B.: Isolation of a cDNA encoding a murine UDPgalactose:β-D-galactosyl-1,4-N-acetyl-D-glucosaminide α-1,3-galactosyltransferase: expression cloning by gene transfer. Proc. Natl. Acad. Sci. USA 86:8227, 1989.

343. Joziasse, D.H., Shaper, J.H., van den Eijnden, D.H., Van Tunen, A.J., and Shaper, N.L.: Bovine α1→3-galactosyltransferase: isolation and characterization of a cDNA clone. Identification of homologous sequences in human genomic DNA. J. Biol. Chem. 264:14290, 1989.

344. Larsen, R.D., Rivera-Marrero, C.A., Ernst, L.K., Cummings, R.D., and Lowe, J.B.: Frameshift and nonsense mutations in a human genomic sequence homologous to a murine UDP-Gal:β-D-Gal(1,4)-D-GlcNAc α(1,3)-galactosyltransferase cDNA. J. Biol. Chem. 265:7055, 1990.

345. Joziasse, D.H., Shaper, J.H., Jabs, E.W., and Shaper, N.L.: Characterization of an alpha 1→3-galactosyltransferase homologue on human chromosome 12 that is organized as a processed pseudogene. J. Biol. Chem. 266:6991, 1991.

346. Haslam, D.B., and Baenziger, J.U.: Expression cloning of Forssman glycolipid synthetase: a novel member of the histo-blood group ABO gene family. Proc. Natl. Acad. Sci. USA 93:10697, 1996.

347. Yamamoto, F.-I., Clausen, H., White, T., Marken, J., and Hakomori, S.-I.: Molecular genetic basis of the histo-blood group ABO system. Nature 345:229, 1990.

348. Yamamoto, F.-I., and Hakomori, S.-I.: Sugar-nucleotide donor specificity of histo-blood group A and B transferases is based on amino acid substitutions. J. Biol. Chem. 265:19257, 1990.

349. Yamamoto, F., McNeill, P.D., and Hakomori, S.: Human histo-blood group A2 transferase coded by A2 allele, one of the A subtypes, is characterized by a single base deletion in the coding sequence, which results in an additional domain at the carboxyl terminal. Biochem. Biophys. Res. Commun. 187:366, 1992.

350. Yamamoto, F., McNeill, P.D., Yamamoto, M., Hakomori, S., Harris, T., Judd, W.J., and Davenport, R.D.: Molecular genetic analysis of the ABO blood group system: 1. Weak subgroups: A3 and B3 alleles. Vox Sang. 64:116, 1993.

351. Yamamoto, F., McNeill, P.D., Yamamoto, M., Hakomori, S., Bromilow, I.M., and Duguid, J.K.: Molecular genetic analysis of the ABO blood group system: 4. Another type of O allele. Vox Sang. 64:175, 1993.

352. Grunnet, N., Steffensen, R., Bennett, E.P., and Clausen, H.: Evaluation of histo-blood group ABO genotyping in a Danish population: frequency of a novel O allele defined as O2. Vox Sang. 67:210, 1994.

353. Olsson, M.L., Thuresson, B., and Chester, M.A.: An Ael allele-specific nucleotide insertion at the blood group ABO locus and its detection using a sequence-specific polymerase chain reaction. Biochem. Biophys. Res. Commun. 216:642, 1995.

354. Ogasawara, K., Bannai, M., Saitou, N., Yabe, R., Nakata, K., Takenaka, M., Fujisawa, K., Uchikawa, M., Ishikawa, Y., Juji, T., and Tokunaga, K.: Extensive polymorphism of ABO blood group gene: three major lineages of the alleles for the common ABO phenotypes. Hum. Genet. 97:777, 1996.

355. Olsson, M.L., and Chester, M.A.: Frequent occurrence of a variant O1 gene at the blood group ABO locus. Vox Sang. 70:26, 1996.

356. Olsson, M.L., and Chester, M.A.: Evidence for a new type of O allele at the ABO locus, due to a combination of the A2 nucleotide deletion and the Ael nucleotide insertion. Vox Sang. 71:113, 1996.

357. Seto, N.O., Palcic, M.M., Compston, C.A., Li, H., Bundle, D.R., and Narang, S.A.: Sequential interchange of four amino acids from blood group B to blood group A glycosyltransferase boosts catalytic activity and progressively modifies substrate recognition in human recombinant enzymes. J. Biol. Chem. 272:14133, 1997.

358. O'Keefe, D.S., and Dobrovic, A.: Decreased stability of the O allele mRNA transcript of the ABO gene. Blood 87:3061, 1996.

359. Roberts, J.A. Fraser: Blood groups and suceptibility to disease. Brit. J. Prev. Soc. Med. 11:107, 1957.

360. Mourant, A.E.: Blood groups and diseases. A Study of Associations of Diseases with Blood Groups and Other Polymorphisms. Oxford, Oxford University Press, 1978.

361. Garratty, G.: Blood group antigens as tumor markers, parasitic/bacterial/viral receptors, and their association with immunologically important proteins. Immunol. Invest. 24:213, 1995.

362. Greenwell, P.: Blood group antigens: molecules seeking a function? Glycoconj. J. 14:159, 1997.

363. Phillips, M.D., and Santhouse, A.: von Willebrand disease: recent advances in pathophysiology and treatment. Am. J. Med. Sci. 316:77, 1998.

364. Mohlke, K.L., Purkayastha, A.A., Westrick, R.J., Smith, P.L., Petryniak, B., Lowe, J.B., and Ginsburg, D.: Mvwf, a dominant modifier of murine von Willebrand factor, results from altered lineage-specific expression of a glycosyltransferase. Cell 96:111, 1999.

365. Boren, T., Normark, S., and Falk, P.: *Helicobacter pylori:* molecular basis for host recognition and bacterial adherence. Trends Microbiol. 2:221, 1994.

366. Aird, I., and Bentall, H.H.: A relationship between cancer of the stomach and the ABO blood groups. Br. Med. J. 1:799, 1953.

367. Aird, I., Bentall, H.H., Mehigan, J.A., and Roberts, J.A. Fraser: The blood groups in relation to peptic ulceration and carcinoma of colon, rectum, breast, and bronchus: an association between the ABO groups and peptic ulceration. Br. Med. J. 2:315, 1954.

368. Le Pendu, J.: A hypothesis on the dual significance of the ABH, Lewis, and related antigens. J. Immunogenet. 16:53, 1989.

369. Chester, M.A., Yates, A.D., and Watkins, W.M.: Phenyl-β-D-galactopyranoside as an acceptor substrate for the blood-group H gene associated guanosine diphosphate L-fucose:β-D-galactosyl α-2-L-fucosyltransferase. Eur. J. Biochem. 69:583, 1976.

370. Wolf, R.O., and Taylor, L.L.: The concentration of blood-group substances in the parotid, sublingual and submaxillary salivas. J. Dent. Res. 43:272, 1964.

371. Milne, R.W., and Dawes, C.: The relative contributions of different salivary glands to the blood group activity of whole saliva in humans. Vox Sang. 25:298, 1973.

372. Levine, P., Robinson, E., Celano, M., Briggs, O., and Falkinburg, L.: Gene interaction resulting in suppression of blood group substance B. Blood 10:1100, 1955.

373. Solomon, J., Waggoner, R., and Leyshon, W.C.: A quantitative immunogenetic study of gene suppression invoking A1 and H antigens of erythrocyte without affecting secreted blood group substance. The Ahm and Ohm. Blood 25:470, 1965.

374. Oriol, R., Danilovs, J., and Hawkins, B.R.: A new genetic model proposing that the Se gene is a structural gene closely linked to the H gene. Am. J. Hum. Genet. 33:421, 1981.

375. Mollicone, R., Davies, D.R., Evans, B., Dalix, A.M., and Oriol, R.: Cellular expression and genetic control of ABH antigens in primary sensory neurons of marmoset, baboon and man. J. Neuroimmunol. 10:255, 1986.

376. Szulman, A.E.: The ABH and Lewis antigens of human tissues during prenatal and postnatal life. *In* Mohn, J.F., Plunkett, R., Cunningham, R.K., Lambert, R. (eds.): Human Blood Groups. New York, Karger, 1977, pp. 426–436.

377. Rouger, P., Poupon, R., Gane, P., Mallissen, B., Darnis, F., and Salmon, C.: Expression of blood group antigens including HLA markers in human adult liver. Tissue Antigens 27:78, 1986.

378. Gaensslen, R.E., Bell, S.C., and Lee, H.C.: Distribution of genetic markers in United States populations: I. Blood group and secretor systems. J. Forensic Sci. 32:1016, 1987.

379. Le Pendu, J., Cartron, J.P., Lemieux, R.U., and Oriol, R.: The presence of at least two different H-blood-group–related β-D-Gal α-2-L-fucosyltransferases in human serum and the genetics of blood group H substances. Am. J. Hum. Genet. 37:749, 1985.

380. Rajan, V.P., Larsen, R.D., Ajmera, S., Ernst, L.K., and Lowe, J.B.: A cloned human DNA restriction fragment determines expression of a GDP-L-fucose:β-D-galactoside 2-α-L-fucosyltransferase in transfected cells. J. Biol. Chem. 24:11158, 1991.

381. Sarnesto, A., Kohlin, T., Hindsgaul, O., Thurin, J., and Blaszczyk-Thurin, M.: Purification of the secretor-type beta-galactoside alpha 1→2-fucosyltransferase from human serum. J. Biol. Chem. 267:2737, 1992.

382. Lemieux, R.U.: Human blood groups and carbohydrate chemistry. Chem. Soc. Rev. 7:423, 1978.

383. Ernst, L.K., Rajan, V.P., Larsen, R.D., Ruff, M.M., and Lowe, J.B.: Stable expression of blood group H determinants and GDP-L-fucose:β-D-galactoside 2-α-L-fucosyltransferase in mouse cells after transfection with human DNA. J. Biol. Chem. 264:3436, 1989.

384. Larsen, R.D., Ernst, L.K., Nair, R.P., and Lowe, J.P.: Molecular cloning, sequence, and expression of human GDP-L-fucose:β-D-galactoside 2-α-L-fucosyltransferase cDNA that can form the H blood group antigen. Proc. Natl. Acad. Sci. USA 87:6674, 1990.

385. Kelly, R.J., Ernst, L.K., Larsen, R.D., Bryant, J.G., Robinson, J.S., and Lowe, J.B.: Molecular basis for H blood group deficiency in Bombay (Oh) and para-Bombay individuals. Proc. Natl. Acad. Sci. USA 91:5843, 1994.

386. Rouquier, S., Lowe, J.B., Kelly, R.J., Fertitta, A.L., Lennon, G.G., and Giorgi, D.: Molecular cloning of a human genomic region containing the H blood group alpha(1,2)fucosyltransferase gene and two H locus–related DNA restriction fragments. Isolation of a candidate for the human Secretor blood group locus. J. Biol. Chem. 270:4632, 1995.

387. Kelly, R.J., Rouquier, S., Giorgi, D., Lennon, G.G., and Lowe, J.B.: Sequence and expression of a candidate for the human Secretor blood group alpha(1,2)fucosyltransferase gene (FUT2). Homozygosity for an enzyme-inactivating nonsense mutation commonly correlates with the non-secretor phenotype. J. Biol. Chem. 270:4640, 1995.

388. Sarnesto, A., Kohlin, T., Thurin, J., and Blaszczyk-Thurin, M.: Purification of H gene–encoded β-galactoside α1→2 fucosyltransferase from human serum. J. Biol. Chem. 265:15067, 1990.

389. Ball, S.P., Tongue, N., Gibaud, A., Le Pendu, J., Mollicone, R., Gerard, G., and Oriol, R.: The human chromosome 19 linkage group FUT1 (H), FUT2 (SE), LE, LU, PEPD, C3, APOC2, D19S7, and D19S9. Ann. Hum. Genet. 55(pt 3):225, 1991.

390. Costache, M., Cailleau, A., Fernandez-Mateos, P., Oriol, R., and Mollicone, R.: Advances in molecular genetics of alpha-2- and alpha-3/4-fucosyltransferases. Transfus. Clin. Biol. 4:367, 1997.

391. Fernandez-Mateos, P., Cailleau, A., Henry, S., Costache, M., Elmgren, A., Svensson, L., Larson, G., Samuelsson, B.E., Oriol, R., and Mollicone, R.: Point mutations and deletion responsible for the Bombay H null and the Reunion H weak blood groups. Vox Sang. 75:37, 1998.

392. Kaneko, M., Nishihara, S., Shinya, N., Kudo, T., Iwasaki, H., Seno, T., Okubo, Y., and Narimatsu, H.: Wide variety of point mutations in the H gene of Bombay and para-Bombay individuals that inactivate H enzyme. Blood 90:839, 1997

393. Wang, B., Koda, Y., Soejima, M., and Kimura, H.: Two missense mutations of H type alpha(1,2)fucosyltransferase gene (FUT1) responsible for para-Bombay phenotype. Vox Sang. 72:31, 1997.

394. Yu, L.C., Yang, Y.H., Broadberry, R.E., Chen, Y.H., and Lin, M.: Heterogeneity of the human H blood group alpha(1,2)fucosyltransferase gene among para-Bombay individuals. Vox Sang. 72:36, 1997.

395. Wagner, F.F., and Flegel, W.A.: Polymorphism of the h allele and the population frequency of sporadic nonfunctional alleles. Transfusion 37:284, 1997.

396. Johnson, P.H., Mak, M.K., Leong, S., Broadberry, R., Duraisamy, G., Gooch, A., Lin, C.M., Makar, I., Okubo, Y., Smart, E., Koepsall, E., and Ewers, M.: Analysis of mutations in the blood group H gene in donors with H-deficient phenotypes [abstract]. Vox Sang. 67(suppl. 2):25, 1994.

397. Liu, Y., Koda, Y., Soejima, M., Pang, H., Schlaphoff, T., du Toit, E.D., and Kimura, H.: Extensive polymorphism of the FUT2 gene in an African (Xhosa) population of South Africa. Hum. Genet. 103:204, 1998.

398. Henry, S., Mollicone, R., Fernandez, P., Samuelsson, B., Oriol, R., and Larson, G.: Molecular basis for erythrocyte Le(a+b+) and salivary ABH partial-secretor phenotypes: expression of a FUT2 secretor allele with an A→T mutation at nucleotide 385 correlates with reduced alpha(1,2) fucosyltransferase activity. Glycoconj. J. 13:985, 1996.

399. Henry, S., Mollicone, R., Fernandez, P., Samuelsson, B., Oriol, R., and Larson, G.: Homozygous expression of a missense mutation at nucleotide 385 in the FUT2 gene associates with the Le(a+b+) partial-secretor phenotype in an Indonesian family. Biochem. Biophys. Res. Commun. 219:675, 1996.

400. Yu, L.C., Yang, Y.H., Broadberry, R.E., Chen, Y.H., Chan, Y.S., and Lin, M.: Correlation of a missense mutation in the human Secretor alpha 1,2-fucosyltransferase gene with the Lewis(a+b+) phenotype: a potential molecular basis for the weak Secretor allele (Sew). Biochem. J. 312(pt 2):329, 1995.

401. Kudo, T., Iwasaki, H., Nishihara, S., Shinya, N., Ando, T., Narimatsu, I., and Narimatsu, H.: Molecular genetic analysis of the human Lewis histo-blood group system. II. Secretor gene inactivation by a novel single missense mutation A385T in Japanese nonsecretor individuals. J. Biol. Chem. 271:9830, 1996.

402. Koda, Y., Soejima, M., Johnson, P.H., Smart, E., and Kimura, H.: Missense mutation of FUT1 and deletion of FUT2 are responsible for Indian Bombay phenotype of ABO blood group system. Biochem. Biophys. Res. Commun. 238:21, 1997.

403. Henry, S., Mollicone, R., Lowe, J.B., Samuelsson, B., and Larson, G.: A second nonsecretor allele of the blood group alpha(1,2)fucosyl-transferase gene (FUT2). Vox Sang. 70:21, 1996.

404. Koda, Y., Soejima, M., Liu, Y., and Kimura, H.: Molecular basis for secretor type alpha(1,2)-fucosyltransferase gene deficiency in a Japanese population: a fusion gene generated by unequal crossover responsible for the enzyme deficiency. Am. J. Hum. Genet. 59:343, 1996.

405. Yu, L.C., Broadberry, R.E., Yang, Y.H., Chen, Y.H., and Lin, M.: Heterogeneity of the human secretor α(1,2)fucosyltransferase gene among Lewis (a+b−) non-secretors. Biochem. Biophys. Res. Commun. 222:390, 1996.

406. Clarke, C.A., Edwards, J. Wyn, Haddock, D.R.W., Howel-Evans, A.W., McConnell, R.B., and Sheppard, P.M.: ABO blood groups and secretor character in duodenal ulcer. Br. Med. J. 2:725, 1956.

407. Sheinfeld, J., Schaeffer, A.J., Cordon-Cardo, C., Rogatko, A., and Fair, W.R.: Association of the Lewis blood group phenotype with recurrent urinary tract infections in women. N. Engl. J. Med. 320:773, 1989.

408. Lund, B., Lindberg, F.P., Baga, M., and Normark, S.: Globoside-specific adhesions of uropathogenic Escherichia coli are encoded by similar trans-complementable gene clusters. J. Bacteriol. 162:1293, 1985.

409. Lomberg, H., and Eden, C.S.: Influence of P blood group phenotype on susceptibility to urinary tract infection. FEMS Microbiol. Immunol. 1:363, 1989.

410. Boren, T., Falk, P., Roth, K.A., Larson, G., and Normark, S.: Attachment of Helicobacter pylori to human gastric epithelium mediated by blood group antigens. Science 262:1892, 1993.

411. Blaszczyk-Thurin, M., Sarnesto, A., Thurin, J., Hindsgaul, O., and Koprowski, H.: Biosynthetic pathways for the Leb and Y glycolipids in the gastric carcinoma cell line KATO III as analyzed by a novel assay. Biochem. Biophys. Res. Commun. 151:100, 1988.

412. Feizi, T.: Demonstration by monoclonal antibodies that carbohydrate structures of glycoproteins and glycolipids are onco-developmental antigens. Nature 314:53, 1985.

413. Mourant, A.E.: A 'new' human blood group antigen of frequent occurrence. Nature 158:237, 1946.

414. Rege, V.P., Painter, T.J., Watkins, W.M., and Morgan, W.T.J.: Isolation of a serologically active fucose containing trisaccharide from human blood group Le^a substrate. Nature 240:740, 1964.

415. Hanfland, P., and Graham, H.: Immunochemistry of the Lewis blood group system: partial characterization of Le^a, Le^b and H type 1 (Le^{dh}) blood group active glycosphingolipids from human plasma. Arch. Biochem. Biophys. 220:383, 1981.

416. Hanfland, P., Kardowicz, M., Peter-Katalinic, J., Pfannschmidt, G., Crawford, R.J., Graham, H.A., and Egge, H.: Immunochemistry of the Lewis blood group system: isolation and structures of the Lewis c active and related glycosphingolipids from the plasma of blood-group OLe(a−b−) nonsecretors. Arch. Biochem. Biophys. 246:655, 1986.

417. Marcus, D.M., and Cass, L.E.: Glycosphingolipids with Lewis blood group activity: uptake by human erythrocytes. Science 164:553, 1969.

418. Holburn, A.M.: Quantitative studies with [125I]IgM anti-Le^a. Immunology 24:1019, 1973.

419. Mollison, P.L., and Polley, M.J.: Temporary suppression of the Lewis blood-group antibodies to permit incompatible transfusion. Lancet 1:909, 1963.

420. Cutbush, M., Giblett, E.R., and Mollison, P.L.: Demonstration of the phenotype Le(a+b+) in infants and adults. Br. J. Haematol. 2:210, 1956.

421. Grubb, R., and Morgan, W.T.J.: The 'Lewis' blood group characters of erythrocytes and body fluids. Br. J. Exp. Pathol. 30:198, 1949.

422. Johnson, P.H., Yates, A.D., and Watkins, W.M.: Human salivary fucosyltransferases: evidence for two distinct α-3-L-fucosyltransferase activities one of which is associated with the Lewis blood group Le gene. Biochem. Biophys. Res. Commun. 100:1611, 1981.

423. Prieels, J.P., Monnom, D., Dolmans, M., Beyer, T.A., and Hill, R.L.: Copurification of the Lewis blood group N-acetylglucosaminide α1→4 fucosyltransferase and an N-acetylglucosaminide α1→3 fucosyltransferase from human milk. J. Biol. Chem. 256:10456, 1981.

424. Lowe, J.B., Stooolman, L.M., Nair, R.P., Larsen, R.D., Berhend, T.L., and Marks, R.M.: ELAM-1–dependent cell adhesion to vascular endothelium determined by a transfected human fucosyltransferase cDNA. Cell 63:475, 1990.

425. Kukowska-Latallo, J.F., Larsen, R.D., Nair, R.P., and Lowe, J.B.: A cloned human cDNA determines expression of a mouse stage-specific embryonic antigen and the Lewis blood group α(1,3/1,4)fucosyltransferase. Genes Dev. 4:1288, 1990.

426. McCurley, R.S., Recinos, A., 3rd, Olsen, A.S., Gingrich, J.C., Szczepaniak, D., Cameron, H.S., Krauss, R., and Weston, B.W.: Physical maps of human alpha (1,3)fucosyltransferase genes *FUT3–FUT6* on chromosomes 19p13.3 and 11q21. Genomics 26:142, 1995.

427. Weston, B.W., Nair, R.P., Larsen, R.D., and Lowe, J.B.: Isolation of a novel human α(1,3)fucosyltransferase gene and molecular comparison to the human Lewis blood group α(1,3/1,4)fucosyltransferase gene. J. Biol. Chem. 267:4152, 1992.

428. Weston, B.W., Smith, P.L., Kelly, R.J., and Lowe, J.B.: Molecular cloning of a fourth member of a human α(1,3)fucosyltransferase gene family: multiple homologous sequences that determine expression of the Lewis x, sialyl Lewis x, and difucosyl sialyl Lewis x epitopes. J. Biol. Chem. 267:24575, 1992.

429. Goelz, S.E., Hession, C., Goff, D., Griffiths, B., Tizard, R., Newman, B., Chi-Rosso, G., and Lobb, R.: *ELFT:* a gene that directs the expression of an ELAM-1 ligand. Cell 63:1349, 1990.

430. Lowe, J.B., Kukowska-Latallo, J.F., Nair, R.P., Larsen, R.D., Marks, R.M., Macher, B.A., Kelly, R.J., and Ernst, L.K.: Molecular cloning of a human fucosyltransferase gene that determines expression of the Lewis x and VIM-2 epitopes but not ELAM-1–dependent cell adhesion. J. Biol. Chem. 266:17467, 1991.

431. Kumar, R., Potvin, B., Muller, W.A., and Stanley, P.: Cloning of a human α(429,3)fucosyltransferase gene that encodes *ELFT* but does not confer ELAM-1 recognition on CHO transfections. J. Biol. Chem. 266:21777, 1991.

432. Sasaki, K., Kurata, K., Funayama, K., Nagata, M., Watanabe, E., Ohta, S., Hanai, N., and Nishi, T.: Expression cloning of a novel alpha 1,3-fucosyltransferase that is involved in biosynthesis of the sialyl Lewis x carbohydrate determinants in leukocytes. J. Biol. Chem. 269:14730, 1994.

433. Natsuka, S., Gersten, K.M., Zenita, K., Kannagi, R., and Lowe, J.B.: Molecular cloning of a cDNA novel human leukocyte alpha(1,3)fucosyltransferase capable of synthesizing the sialyl Lewis x determinant. J. Biol. Chem. 269:16789, 1994.

434. Kudo, T., Ikehara, Y., Togayachi, A., Kaneko, M., Hiraga, T., Sasaki, K., and Narimatsu, H.: Expression cloning and characterization of a novel murine alpha1,3-fucosyltransferase, mFuc-TIX, that synthesizes the lewis x (CD15) epitope in brain and kidney. J. Biol. Chem. 273:26729, 1998.

435. Nishihara, S., Narimatsu, H., Iwasaki, H., Yazawa, S., Akamatsu, S., Ando, T., Seno, T., and Narimatsu, I.: Molecular genetic analysis of the human Lewis histo-blood group system. J. Biol. Chem. 269:29271, 1994.

436. Mollicone, R., Reguigne, I., Kelly, R.J., Fletcher, A., Watt, J., Chatfield, S., Aziz, A., Cameron, H.S., Weston, B.W., Lowe, J.B., and Oriol, R.: Molecular basis for Lewis alpha (1,3/1,4)-fucosyltransferase gene deficiency (*FUT3*) found in Lewis-negative Indonesian pedigrees. J. Biol. Chem. 269:20987, 1994.

437. Elmgren, A., Borjeson, C., Svensson, L., Rydberg, L., and Larson, G.: DNA sequencing and screening for point mutations in the human Lewis (*FUT3*) gene enables molecular genotyping of the human Lewis blood group system. Vox Sang. 70:97, 1996.

438. Orntoft, T.F., Vestergaard, E.M., Holmes, E., Jakobsen, J.S. Grunnet, N., Mortensen, M., Johnson, P., Bross, P., Gregersen, N., Skorstengaard, K., Jensen, U.B., Bolund, L., and Wolf, H.: Influence of human alpha 1-3/4-L-fucosyltransferase (*FUT3*) gene mutations on enzyme activity, erythrocyte phenotyping, and circulating tumor marker sialyl-Lewis a levels. J. Biol. Chem. 271:32260, 1996.

439. Nishihara, S., Yazawa, S., Iwasaki, H., Nakazato, M., Kudo, T., Ando, T., and Narimatsu, H.: Alpha (1,3/1,4)fucosyltransferase (FucT-III) gene is inactivated by a single amino acid substitution in Lewis histo-blood type negative individuals. Biochem. Biophys. Res. Commun. 196:624, 1993.

440. Elmgren, A., Rydberg, L., and Larson, G.: Genotypic heterogeneity among Lewis negative individuals. Biochem. Biophys. Res. Commun. 196:515, 1993.

441. Koda, Y., Kimura, H., and Mekada, E.: Analysis of Lewis fucosyltransferase genes from the human gastric mucosa of Lewis-positive and -negative individuals. Blood 82:2915, 1993.

442. Liu, Y., Koda, Y., Soejima, M., Uchida, N., and Kimura, H.: PCR analysis of Lewis-negative gene mutations and the distribution of Lewis alleles in a Japanese population. J. Forensic Sci. 41:1018, 1996.

443. Elmgren, A., Mollicone, R., Costache, M., Borjeson, C., Oriol, R., Harrington, J., and Larson, G.: Significance of individual point mutations, T202C and C314T, in the human Lewis (*FUT3*) gene for

expression of Lewis antigens by the human alpha(1,3/1,4)-fucosyltransferase, Fuc-TIII. J. Biol. Chem. 272:21994, 1997.

444. Thall, A.D., Maly, P., and Lowe, J.B.: Unpublished data.

445. Maly, P., Thall, A., Petryniak, B., Rogers, C.E., Smith, P.L., Marks, R.M., Kelly, R.J., Gersten, K.M., Cheng, G., Saunders, T.L., Camper, S.A., Camphausen, R.T., Sullivan, F.X., Isogai, Y., Hindsgaul, O., von Andrian, U.H., and Lowe, J.B.: The alpha(1,3)fucosyltransferase Fuc-TVII controls leukocyte trafficking through an essential role in L-, E-, and P-selectin ligand biosynthesis. Cell 86:643, 1996.

446. Kansas, G.S.: Selectins and their ligands: current concepts and controversies. Blood 88:3259, 1996.

447. Bevilacqua, M.P., Stengelin, S., Gimbrone, M.A., and Seed, B.: Endothelial leukocyte adhesion molecule 1: an inducible receptor for neutrophils related to complement regulatory proteins and lectins. Science 243:1160, 1989.

448. Bevilacqua, M., Butcher, E., Furie, B., Furie, B., Gallatin, M., Gimbrone, M., Harlan, J., Kishimoto, K., Lasky, L., McEver, R., et al.: Selectins: a family of adhesion receptors. Cell 67:233, 1991.

449. Weis, W.I., and Drickame, K.: Structural basis of lectin-carbohydrate recognition. Annu. Rev. Biochem. 65:441, 1996.

450. Phillips, M.L., Nudelman, E., Gaeta, F.C., Perez, M., Singhal, A.K., Hakomori, S., and Paulson, J.C.: ELAM-1 mediates cell adhesion by recognition of a carbohydrate ligand, sialyl-Lex. Science 250:1130, 1990.

451. Walz, G., Aruffo, A., Kolanus, W., Bevilacqua, M., and Seed, B.: Recognition by ELAM-1 of the sialyl-Lex determinant on myeloid and tumor cells. Science 250:1132, 1990.

452. Tyrrel, D., Pames, P., Rao, N., Foxall, C., Abbas, S., Dasgupta, F., Nashed, M., Hasegawa, A., Kiso, M., Asa, D., Kidd, J., and Brandley, B.K.: Structural requirements for the carbohydrate ligand of E-selectin. Proc. Natl. Acad. Sci. USA 88:10372, 1991.

453. Wilkins, P.P., McEver, R.P., and Cummings, R.D.: Structures of the O-glycans on P-selectin glycoprotein ligand-1 from HL-60 cells. J. Biol. Chem. 271:18732, 1996.

454. Etzioni, A., Frydman, M., Pollack, S., Avidor, I., Phillips, M.L., Paulson, J.C., and Gershoni-Baruch, R.: Brief report: recurrent severe infections caused by a novel leukocyte adhesion deficiency. N. Engl. J. Med. 327:1789, 1992.

455. Phillips, M.L., Schwartz, B.R., Etzioni, A., Bayer, R., Ochs, H.D., Paulson, J.C., and Harlan, J.M.: Neutrophil adhesion in leukocyte adhesion deficiency syndrome type 2. J. Clin. Invest. 96:2898, 1995.

456. Smith, P.L., Paulson, J.C., and Lowe, J.B.: Unpublished data.

457. Sturla, L., Etzioni, A., Bisso, A., Zanardi, D., De Flora, G., Silengo, L., De Flora, A., and Tonetti, M.: Defective intracellular activity of GDP-D-mannose-4,6-dehydratase in leukocyte adhesion deficiency type II syndrome. FEBS Lett. 429:274, 1998.

458. Berg, E.L., Robinson, M.K., Mansson, O., Butcher, E.C., and Magnani, J.L.: A carbohydrate domain common to both sialyl Lea and sialyl Lex is recognized by the endothelial cell leukocyte adhesion molecule ELAM-1. J. Biol. Chem. 266:14869, 1991.

459. Takada, A., Ohmori, K., Takahashi, N., Tsuyuoka, K., Yago, A., Zenita, K., Hasegawa, A., and Kannagi, R.: Adhesion of human cancer cells to vascular endothelium mediated by a carbohydrate antigen, sialyl Lewis A. Biochem. Biophys. Res. Commun. 179:713, 1991.

460. Zhou, Q., Moore, K.L., Smith, D.F., Varki, A., McEver, R.P., and Cummings, R.D.: The selectin GMP-140 binds to sialylated, fucosylated lactosaminoglycans on both myeloid and nonmyeloid cells. J. Cell Biol. 115:557, 1991.

461. Polley, M.J., Phillips, M.L., Wayner, E., Nudelman, E., Singhal, A.K., Hakomori, S.-I., and Paulson, J.C.: CD62 and endothelial cell–leukocyte adhesion molecule 1 (ELAM-1) recognize the same carbohydrate ligand, sialyl-Lewis x. Proc. Natl. Acad. Sci. USA 88:6224, 1991.

462. Brandley, B.K., Watson, S.R., Dowbenko, D., Fennie, C., Lasky, L.A., Hasegawa, A., Kiso, M., and Foxall, C.: The sialyl Lewis x oligosaccharide is a ligand for L-selectin. FASEB J. 6:1890, 1992.

463. Kim, Y.S., and Itzkowitz, S.: Carbohydrate antigen expression in the adenoma-carcinoma sequence. Prog. Clin. Biol. Res. 279:241, 1988.

464. Mannori, G., Crottet, P., Cecconi, O., Hanasaki, K., Aruffo, A., Nelson, R.M., Varki, A., and Bevilacqua, M.P.: Differential colon cancer cell adhesion to E-, P-, and L-selectin: role of mucin-type glycoproteins. Cancer Res. 55:4425, 1995.

465. Kim, Y.J., Borsig, L., Varki, N.M., and Varki, A.: P-selectin deficiency attenuates tumor growth and metastasis. Proc. Natl. Acad. Sci. USA 95:9325, 1998.

466. Forman, D.: *Helicobacter pylori* infection and cancer. Br. Med. Bull. 54:71, 1998.

467. Wotherspoon, A.C.: *Helicobacter pylori* infection and gastric lymphoma. Br. Med. Bull. 54:79, 1998.

468. Atherton, J.C.: *H. pylori* virulence factors. Br. Med. Bull. 54:105, 1998.

469. Bodger, K., and Crabtree, J.E.: *Helicobacter pylori* and gastric inflammation. Br. Med. Bull. 54:139, 1998.

470. Oberhuber, G., Kranz, A., Dejaco, C., Dragosics, B., Mosberger, I., Mayr, W., and Radaszkiewicz, T.: Blood groups Lewis(b) and ABH expression in gastric mucosa: lack of inter-relation with *Helicobacter pylori* colonisation and occurrence of gastric MALT lymphoma. Gut 41:37, 1997.

471. Heneghan, M.A., Moran, A.P., Feeley, K.M., Egan, E.L., Goulding, J., Connolly, C.E., and McCarthy, C.F.: Effect of host Lewis and ABO blood group antigen expression on *Helicobacter pylori* colonisation density and the consequent inflammatory response. FEMS Immunol. Med. Microbiol. 20:257, 1998.

472. Monteiro, M.A., Chan, K.H., Rasko, D.A., Taylor, D.E., Zheng, P.Y., Appelmelk, B.J., Wirth, H.P., Yang, M., Blaser, M.J., Hynes, S.O., Moran, A.P., and Perry, M.B.: Simultaneous expression of type 1 and type 2 Lewis blood group antigens by *Helicobacter pylori* lipopolysaccharides. Molecular mimicry between *H. pylori* lipopolysaccharides and human gastric epithelial cell surface glycoforms. J. Biol. Chem. 273:11533, 1998.

473. Wiener, A.S., Unger, L.T., and Cohen, L.: Type-specific cold autoantibodies as a cause of acquired hemolytic anemia and hemolytic transfusion reactions: biologic test with bovine red cells. Ann. Intern. Med. 44:221, 1956.

474. Marsh, W.L., and Jenkins, W.J.: Anti-i: a new cold antibody. Nature 188:753, 1960.

475. Marsh, W.L.: Anti-i: a cold antibody defining the Ii relationship in human red cells. Br. J. Haematol. 7:200, 1961.

476. Hakomori, S.-I.: Blood group ABH and Ii antigens of human erythrocytes: chemistry, polymorphism, and their developmental change. Semin. Hematol. 18:39, 1981.

477. Feizi, T.: The blood group Ii system: a carbohydrate antigen system defined by naturally monoclonal or oligoclonal autoantibodies of man. Immunol. Commun. 10:127, 1981.

478. Niemann, H., Watanabe, K., Hakomori, S., Childs, R.A., and Feizi, T.: Blood group i and I activities of "lacto-*N*-norhexaosyl-ceramide" and its analogues: the structural requirements for i-specificities. Biochem. Biophys. Res. Commun. 81: 1286, 1978.

479. Watanabe, K., Hakomori, S., Childs, R.A., and Feizi, T.: Characterization of a blood group I-active ganglioside: structural requirements for I and i specificities. J. Biol. Chem. 254:3221, 1979.

480. Koscielak, J., Zdebska, E., Wileznska, Z., Miller-Podraza, H., and Dzierzkowa-Borodej, W.: Immunochemistry of Ii-active glycosphingolipids of erythrocytes. Eur. J. Biochem. 96:331, 1979.

481. Watanabe, K., and Hakomori, S.: Status of blood group carbohydrate chains in ontogenesis and in oncogenesis. J. Exp. Med. 144:644, 1976.

482. Koscielak, J., Zdebska, E., Wilczynska, Z., Miller-Podraza, H., and Dzierzkowa-Borodej, W.: Immunochemistry of Ii-active glycosphingolipids of erythrocytes. Eur. J. Biochem. 96:331, 1979.

483. Yates, A.D., and Watkins, W.M.: Enzymes involved in the biosynthesis of glycoconjugates. A UDP-2-acetamido-2-deoxy-D-glucose: beta-D-galactopyranosyl-(1→4)-saccharide (1→3)-2-acetamido-2-deoxy-beta-D-glucopyranosyltransferase in human serum. Carbohydr. Res. 120:251, 1983.

484. Piller, F., and Cartron, J.P.: UDP-GlcNAc:Galβ1→4Glc (NAc)β1→3*N*-acetylglucosaminyltransferase. Identification and characterization in human serum. J. Biol. Chem. 258:12293, 1983.

485. Van den Eijnden, D.H., Winterwerp, H., Smeeman, P., and Schiphorst, W.E.: Novikoff ascites tumor cells contain *N*-acetyllactosaminide β1→3 and β1→6 *N*-acetylglucosaminyltransferase activity. J. Biol. Chem. 258:3435, 1983.

486. Gu, J., Nishikawa, A., Fujii, S., Gasa, S., and Taniguchi, N.: Biosynthesis of blood group I and i antigens in rat tissues. Identification of a novel β1-6-*N*-acetylglucosaminyltransferase. J. Biol. Chem. 267:2994, 1992.

487. Bierhuizen, M.F., Mattei, M.G., and Fukuda, M.: Expression of the developmental I antigen by a cloned human cDNA encoding a member of a beta-1,6-*N*-acetylglucosaminyltransferase gene family. Genes Dev. 7:468, 1993.

488. Bierhuizen, M.F., Maemura, K., Kudo, S., and Fukuda, M.: Genomic organization of core 2 and I branching beta-1,6-*N*-acetylglucosaminyltransferases. Implication for evolution of the beta-1,6-*N*-acetylglucosaminyltransferase gene family. Glycobiology 5:417, 1995.

489. Childs, R.A., Kapadia, A., and Feizi, T.: Blood group I and i antigens as common surface antigens on a variety of human and animal cell lines. *In* Schauer, R., Boer, P., Buddecke, E., Karamer, M.F., Vliegenthart, J.F.G., and Wiegandt, H. (eds.): Glycoconjugates. Stuttgart, Georg Thieme, 1979, pp. 518–519.

490. Childs, R.A., Kapadia, A., and Feizi, T.: Expression of blood group I and i active carbohydrate sequences on cultured human and animal cell lines assessed by radioimmunoassays with monoclonal cold agglutinins. Eur. J. Immunol. 10:379, 1980.

491. Shumak, K.H., Rachkewich, R.A., Crookston, M.C., and Crookston, J.H.: Antigens of the Ii system on lymphocytes. Nature New Biol. 231:148, 1971.

492. Thomas, D.B.: The i antigen complex: a new specificity unique to dividing human cells. Eur. J. Immunol. 4:819, 1974.

493. Fukuda, M.: K562 human leukaemic cells express fetal type (i) antigen on different glycoproteins from circulating erythrocytes. Nature 285:405, 1980.

494. Papayannopoulou, T., Chen, P., Maniatis, A., and Stamatoyannopoulos, G.: Simultaneous assessment of i-antigenic expression and fetal hemoglobin in single red cells by immuno-fluorescence. Blood 55:221, 1980.

495. Kapadia, A., Feizi, T., and Evans, M.J.: Changes in expression and polarization of blood group I and i antigens in post-implantation embryos and teratocarcinomas of mouse associated with cell differentiation. Exp. Cell Res. 131:185, 1981.

496. Landsteiner, K., and Levine, P.: Further observations on individual differences of human blood. Proc. Soc. Exp. Biol. Med. 24:941, 1927.

497. Marcus, D.M., Kundu, S.K., and Suzuki, A.: The P blood group system: recent progress in immunochemistry and genetics. Semin. Hematol. 18:63, 1981.

498. Yang, Z., Bergstrom, J., and Karlsson, K.A.: Glycoproteins with Gal alpha 4Gal are absent from human erythrocyte membranes, indicating that glycolipids are the sole carriers of blood group P activities. J. Biol. Chem. 269:14620, 1994.

499. Kortekangas, A.E., Kaarsalo, E., and Melartin, L.: The red cell antigen P^k and its relationship to the P system. The evidence of three more Pk families. Vox Sang. 10:385, 1965.

500. Matson, G.A., Swandon, J., and Noades, J.: A 'new' antigen and antibody belonging to the P blood group system. Am. J. Hum. Genet. 11:26, 1959.

501. Kijimoto-Ochiai, S., Naiki, M., and Makita, A.: Defects of glycosyltransferase activities in human fibroblast of P^k and p blood group phenotypes. Proc. Natl. Acad. Sci. USA 74:5407, 1973.

502. Marcus, D.M., Naiki, M., and Kundu, S.K.: Abnormalities in the glycosphingolipids content of human P^k and p erythrocytes. Proc. Natl. Acad. Sci. USA 73:3262, 1976.

503. Fellous, M., Gerbal, A., and Tessier, C.: Studies on the biosynthetic pathway of human P erythrocyte antigens using somatic cells in culture. Vox Sang. 26:518, 1974.

504. Fellous, M., Gerbal, A., and Nobillot, G.: Studies on the biosynthetic pathway of human P erythrocyte antigens using genetic complementation tests between fibroblasts from rare p and P^k phenotype donors. Vox Sang. 32:262, 1977.

505. Graham, H.A., and Williams, A.N.: A genetic model for the inheritance of the P₁P₁ and P^k antigens. Transfusion 18:638, 1978.

506. Leffler, H., and Svanborg, E.C.: Chemical identification of a glycosphingolipid receptor for *Escherichia coli* attaching to human urinary epithelial cells and agglutinating human erythrocytes. FEMS Microbiol. Lett. 8:127, 1980.

507. Wold, A.E., Thorssen, M., Hull, S., and Svanborg, E.C.: Attachment of *Escherichia coli* to mannose or Galα1→4Galβ–containing receptors in human colonic epithelial cells. Infect. Immun. 56:2531, 1988.

508. Stapleton, A.E., Stroud, M.R., Hakomori, S.I., and Stamm, W.E.: The globoseries glycosphingolipid sialosyl galactosyl globoside is found in urinary tract tissues and is a preferred binding receptor in vitro for uropathogenic *Escherichia coli* expressing pap-encoded adhesins. Infect. Immun. 66:3856, 1998.

509. Striker, R., Nilsson, U., Stonecipher, A., Magnusson, G., and Hultgren, S.J.: Structural requirements for the glycolipid receptor of human uropathogenic *Escherichia coli*. Mol. Microbiol. 16:1021, 1995.

510. Lomberg, H., Hanson, L.A., Jacobsson, B., Jodal, U., Leffler, H., and Svanborg, E.C.: Correlation of P blood group, vesicoureteral reflux,

and bacterial attachment in patients with recurrent pyelonephritis. N. Engl. J. Med. 308:1189, 1983.

511. Tomisawa, S., Kogure, T., Kuroume, T., Leffler, H., Lomberg, H., Shimabukoro, N., Terao, K., and Svanborg Eden, C.: P blood group and proneness to urinary tract infection in Japanese children. Scand. J. Infect. Dis. 21:403, 1989.

512. Roberts, J.A., Marklund, B.I., Ilver, D., Haslam, D., Kaack, M.B., Baskin, G., Louis, M., Mollby, R., Winberg, J., and Normark, S.: The Gal(alpha 1→4)Gal–specific tip adhesin of *Escherichia coli* P-fimbriae is needed for pyelonephritis to occur in the normal urinary tract. Proc. Natl. Acad. Sci. USA 91:11889, 1994.

513. Brown, K.E., and Young, N.S.: Parvovirus B19 in human disease. Annu. Rev. Med. 48:59, 1997.

514. Brown, K.E., Anderson, S.M., and Young, N.S.: Erythrocyte P antigen: cellular receptor for B19 parvovirus. Science 262:114,1993.

515. Brown, K.E., Hibbs, J.R., Gallinella, G., Anderson, S.M., Lehman, E.D., McCarthy, P., and Young, N.S.: Resistance to parvovirus B19 infection due to lack of virus receptor (erythrocyte P antigen). N. Engl. J. Med. 330:1192,1994.

516. Levine, P., and Koch, E.A.: The rare human isoagglutinin anti-Tj[a] and habitual abortion. Science 120:239, 1954.

10 Molecular Basis of Iron Metabolism

Tracey A. Rouault and Richard D. Klausner

Introduction

Iron is a critical component of numerous enzymes and is an essential nutrient for virtually all life forms. Enzymes contain iron either in the porphyrin ring structure of heme or in a variety of non-heme forms, such as iron-sulfur clusters. The heme (iron protoporphyrin) prosthetic group is associated with enzymes required for oxidative phosphorylation and detoxification of chemical agents or drugs and also serves as a functional group for the binding of oxygen by hemoglobin and myoglobin, which together represent the repository of most of the body's total iron. Iron-sulfur clusters are contained in a number of critical enzymes, particularly in mitochondrial enzymes important in respiration.

A variety of mechanisms exist to allow organisms to obtain sufficient iron from the environment and to sequester excess iron in a non-reactive form. The ability of iron to interact with oxygen species to produce damaging free radicals underlies the considerable toxicity of iron. As a consequence of that toxicity, iron uptake and distribution are regulated, and the study of iron metabolism in diverse organisms has resulted in the discovery of a rich variety of sensing and regulatory mechanisms.[1-5]

Iron Acquisition by Microorganisms

Although iron is the fourth most abundant element and the second most abundant metal in the earth's crust, it exists virtually entirely in the highly insoluble, oxidized ferric form rather than in the more soluble, reduced ferrous form. Many plants and certain unicellular organisms synthesize and secrete iron-binding proteins derived from either phenol catechols or hydroxamic acid known as siderophores.[4,5] The high affinity of siderophores for ferric iron facilitates formation of iron-chelate complexes despite the very low concentration of soluble ferric iron in the extracellular milieu. Iron-siderophore complexes are generally taken up by a specific membrane receptor, and after internalization, the complex is me-

tabolized and iron is released for utilization by the organism. Desferrioxamine is a siderophore released by the fungus *Streptomyces pilous* that binds ferric iron with high affinity and has been used extensively as an iron chelator in humans (Fig. 10–1).[6] In *Escherichia coli*, the genes involved in iron uptake are part of a single operon that is under the control of a regulatory molecule called "fur" that represses transcription when iron is bound to the fur molecule.[7] Under conditions of low intracellular iron, the repressor is relatively inactive, and expression of the operon leads to synthesis of both the siderophore (known as aerobactin) and the siderophore receptor. As the iron level is increased, active repressor accumulates, and the operon is turned off.

An alternative strategy for iron solubilization and acquisition is used by the yeast *Saccharomyces cerevisiae*. Yeast

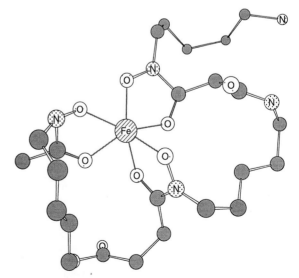

Figure 10–1. Structure of the fungal iron chelator desferrioxamine. Desferrioxamine (Df) is a trihydroxamate siderophore. A stable metal-chelate complex is formed when the hydroxamate functional groups fully saturate the complexing valencies of the ferric ion.

lack siderophores, but reductases on the surface contribute to solubilization of ferric iron. Uptake of iron in *S. cerevisiae* is accomplished by an iron transport complex composed of a multicopper oxidase known as FET3 and a permease known as FTR1 (for Fe transporter).[8] Expression of both genes in yeast is transcriptionally activated by a regulatory protein, AFT1 (for activator of ferrous transport), in yeasts that are deprived of iron.[9] The FET3 oxidase of yeast is similar in sequence to ceruloplasmin, a mammalian multicopper oxidase that plays a role in mammalian iron homeostasis.[10] Thus far, mammalian homologues to FTR1 have not been identified.

As will become evident, higher eukaryotes utilize mechanisms for iron acquisition that are variations on the two strategies for iron acquisition by microorganisms outlined above. Plasma transferrin (Tf) serves as the functional equivalent of a siderophore in that it binds and solubilizes extracellular ferric iron. Transferrin differs from siderophores in that it is a large protein rather than a small organic compound. Similarly to the siderophores, Tf is recognized by a specific cell surface receptor and internalized. Once inside the cell, iron is released for utilization. Analogous to the ferrous transporter of yeast, higher eukaryotes also encode an iron transporter, DCT1 or Nramp2, which transports iron across endosomal and plasma membranes (see below).

Overview of Human Iron Economy

In humans, the amount of iron in the body is regulated by control of iron absorption.[11] Factors that determine the level of iron absorption include the amount of iron in the diet, the content of the diet, and the dietary form of iron (heme versus non-heme).[12] The average American diet contains 15 mg of iron per day, of which approximately 3 mg is taken into cells of the duodenum and proximal jejunum, with about 1 mg finding its way into the plasma (Fig. 10–2). The daily requirement for iron increases dramatically during pregnancy, with approximately 5 mg/day being transferred to the fetus via the placenta.[13] Regulation of the intestinal transfer of iron to the plasma depends on the existing level of iron stores and the rate of erythropoiesis (iron absorption is enhanced in certain disease states characterized by ineffective erythropoiesis).[14–16] Iron excretion is limited to obligatory losses occurring as a consequence of the shedding of epithelial cells from the intestinal and urinary tracts and from the skin and small amounts of intestinal bleeding. No regulatory mechanism seems to exist for the excretion of iron in mammals.

Essential to the economy of iron is a recycling process in which erythrocyte iron is reutilized for synthesis of new hemoglobin[16] (Fig. 10–3). Tf, a serum protein to which iron is bound in the ferric form, has a central role in this cycling process. Although only 3 to 5 mg of iron is associated with Tf in the plasma of a normal adult individual, the flux through this pool is 30 to 35 mg/day, of which approximately 1 mg is acquired through intestinal absorption and the remainder from macrophages that have phagocytosed senescent erythrocytes and metabolized and released the red cell heme.

Cellular uptake of iron in dividing cells of higher eukaryotes is mediated largely by the interaction of Tf with a membrane receptor protein, the TfR. The ligand-receptor complex is endocytosed, and iron is transported from the endosome into the cytosol. Iron enters a soluble "chelatable" pool in which it is partitioned between utilization for synthe-

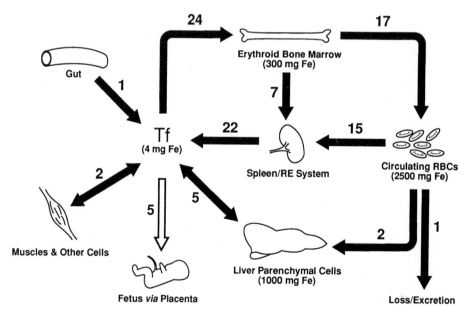

Figure 10–2. Pathways of human iron exchange. Dietary iron enters from the gut and is incorporated into plasma transferrin (Tf). Tf iron is the source of iron for the erythroid bone marrow and other dividing cells (and is delivered to the fetus via the placenta). Effete red blood cells (RBCs) are catabolized by the reticuloendothelial (RE) system. Some RBC iron is processed as free hemoglobin by the liver, and the liver is the primary source of Tf synthesis. Iron is lost from the body by incidental bleeding as well as through loss of skin cells and hair. Numbers on the arrows of the figure represent amounts of iron, in milligrams per day, involved in the traffic in iron. Numbers in parentheses are the approximate total iron stores of the indicated tissues. Iron that is taken into gut mucosal cells but lost via sloughing of these cells without making it into the plasma is not considered absorbed iron. (Adapted from Bothwell, T. H., Charlton, R. W., Cook, J. D., and Finch, C. A.: Iron Metabolism in Man. Oxford, Blackwell Scientific Publications, 1979; with permission.)

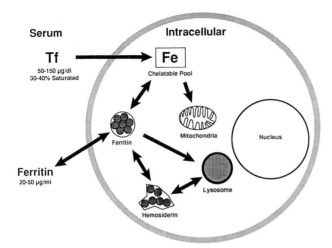

Figure 10–3. Cellular iron pools in normal individuals. From serum, transferrin (Tf) iron enters the cell via the transferrin receptor (see Fig. 10–7) and is transferred to a chelatable intracellular pool. Iron in the intracellular pool is utilized for the metabolic needs of cells (e.g., mitochondrial cytochromes) or incorporated into ferritin. Iron can be remobilized from ferritin, or the ferritin can be partially degraded to form hemosiderin, some of which may be seen in lysosomes. Serum ferritin released by macrophages may be a mechanism for redistribution of iron in the body, but the role of serum ferritin in iron physiological processes remains unclear.

sis of essential cellular iron-containing constituents and deposition in ferritin as a non-toxic form (Fig. 10–4). Another form of intracellular iron is hemosiderin, an amorphous, insoluble aggregate of iron oxide and organic constituents that is thought to be a partially degraded form of ferritin.

Some insight into the physiological and pathophysiological characteristics of iron exchange is provided by the analysis of the distribution of iron stores. In the normal adult, about two thirds of reserve iron is in reticuloendothelial (RE) cells and about one third is in hepatocytes. RE cells play a prominent role in iron homeostasis, supplying perhaps two thirds of iron passing through the plasma. Within the RE cell, there is a constantly changing distribution of iron processed from effete red cells between storage and return of iron to Tf.[17–21] When more iron is required for red cell production, an increased amount of iron is returned to Tf, and, in addition, storage iron is mobilized.

In addition to the reticuloendothelial system, the liver represents another major repository of body iron. Although the Tf-TfR cycle is important in iron uptake, the hepatocyte also possesses several alternative mechanisms for iron uptake. Heme bound to hemopexin appears to be internalized via a specific receptor, after which hemopexin is recycled to the circulation.[22] Similarly, uptake of a hemoglobin-haptoglobin complex has been reported to result in release of heme iron and degradation of both globin and haptoglobin.[23–26] There also appears to be a receptor for ferritin on hepatocytes,[27] although under normal circumstances it is thought that very little iron reaches the liver by this mechanism. Both hepatocytes and macrophages can donate iron to plasma Tf. If plasma iron levels decrease, the hepatocyte releases iron, whereas with an increase in plasma Tf saturation, there is an increased net flow into hepatocyte ferritin and hemosiderin stores.[28–30] One other notable aspect of hepatocyte-iron exchange is the facility with which hepato-

cytes take up non-Tf bound iron from the plasma. Iron citrate or ascorbate that is injected intravenously in an organism that already has fully saturated Tf is nevertheless rapidly removed from circulation by the hepatocytes.[31] Thus, by virtue of its large number of TfRs and additional mechanisms of iron uptake, the hepatocyte is often the immediate repository of excess iron.

Historically, consideration of human iron metabolism has focused on the critical roles of Tf, the TfR, and ferritin. Much is known about the genes and structure of these proteins and how they interact to make iron available to the cell while protecting the cell from iron toxicity. More recently, the genes that encode iron-sensing regulatory proteins that regulate expression of ferritin and the TfR have been characterized and cloned; two ribonucleic acid (RNA)-binding proteins, iron-regulatory proteins 1 and 2 (IRP1, IRP2), sense changes in the availability of iron in cells and accordingly modify expression of many other genes of iron metabolism by binding to messenger RNA (mRNA) sequence elements known as iron-responsive elements (IREs). Additionally, within the last several years, two genes important in mammalian iron homeostasis have been cloned, including the iron transporter of the duodenal mucosa, termed either DCT1 or Nramp2, and the disease gene for hereditary hemochromatosis, HFE. Each of these genes is discussed in detail in later sections of this chapter.

Transferrin

Human serum Tf is a single polypeptide chain glycoprotein with a molecular weight of 75,000 to 80,000 that binds ferric iron with high affinity. Transferrin is part of a larger protein

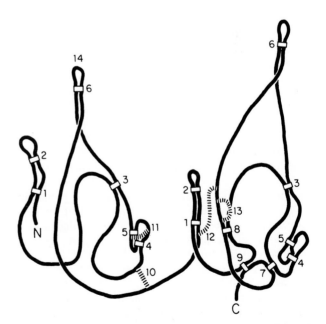

Figure 10–4. The disulfide bridges of plasma transferrin (Tf) molecules. In this string model of the Tf protein, the positions of disulfide bonds that are common to human and chicken Tf molecules are shown as open boxes. The four disulfide bridges found in human Tf that are not in the chicken molecule are indicated by the hatched lines. (Adapted from Williams, J.: The evolution of transferrin. Trends Biol. Sci. 2:394, 1982; with permission.)

family that includes ovotransferrin; lactoferrin, which is present in extracellular secretions; and p97, a membrane protein discovered on human melanoma cells.[32] A likely reason that mammals utilize a macromolecular binder of iron rather than a low molecular weight siderophore is that the size of Tf is sufficient to allow retention in the circulation rather than loss in urine via glomerular filtration. Tf consists of two domains, each of which has an iron-binding site.

▼ THE TRANSFERRIN GENE

Complementary DNAs (cDNAs) for human Tf have been identified and sequenced,[33, 34] verifying the protein's structure as determined by biochemical techniques.[30] These cDNA clones have been used to identify genomic clones containing the human Tf gene.[35, 36] Fifteen exons have been characterized; two additional exons are thought to exist on the basis of protein structure and analogy to the ovotransferrin gene. The 15 exons are distributed over 30 kilobases (kb) of genomic DNA.

Analysis of gene structure has provided strong support for a gene duplication event in the evolution of Tf. Seven pairs of homologous exons can be identified from the N-terminal and C-terminal domains. These exons resemble each other by a 50 to 56 per cent sequence identity at both the amino acid and the nucleotide levels and by virtue of very similar size and preservation of splicing junctions. Mutations arising subsequent to the proposed duplication are thought to have produced the alterations in exon structure and intron length that are characteristic of the two halves of the human Tf gene. The Tf gene has been mapped to the distal portion of the long arm of chromosome 3 (3q21) (3qter).[37]

▼ TRANSFERRIN STRUCTURE AND FUNCTION

The Tf polypeptide has 679 amino acids.[31, 33, 34, 38] By weight it consists of 6 per cent carbohydrate[29, 30] present as branched structures joined by *N*-glycosidic linkages to asparagine residues 415 and 608, both of which are in the C-terminal domain of the protein.[30] X-ray crystallographic studies have verified that the protein folds into two domains, each of which contains an iron-binding site. There are 19 disulfide bridges in human Tf, 8 in the N-terminal domain and 11 in the C-terminal domain. Several of the disulfide bridges are positioned identically in the two domains of the protein and are also phylogenetically invariant.[39] A model of the three-dimensional structure showing the disulfide bridges and the two domains of the protein is shown in Figure 10–4. Although several genetic variants of human Tf have been characterized[29, 40] no functional significance of these substitutions has been established.

The sites of interaction of iron with the protein have been deduced from spectroscopic studies, chemical modification, and sequence data.[41] Binding of iron to Tf is accompanied by binding of an anion, carbonate, or bicarbonate. The three-dimensional structure provides a pocket in which the metal- and anion-binding residues reside (Fig. 10–5). X-ray crystallographic studies indicate that the iron is coordinated by four residues: the phenolate oxygens of tyrosine

residues 185 and 188, an imidazole of a histidine, and a carboxylate of an aspartic acid residue. The anion is thought to interact with arginine 124 and to occupy one of the six coordination sites of the iron. Conformational changes in transferrin may be induced as a consequence of iron binding, and binding of iron is associated with the release of several protons.

Although Tf has a very high affinity for ferric iron (K_a ~10^{-20} M), its affinity for ferrous iron is much lower.[42] Release of ferric iron from Tf occurs predominantly, if not exclusively, in the intracellular environment. At least five mechanisms have been proposed to participate in the release of ferric iron from the protein: (1) protonation of the protein's iron-binding ligands, (2) reduction of bound ferric iron to ferrous iron, (3) a primary attack on the anion, (4) competition between Tf and a strong chelator, and (5) an influence on iron binding by the binding of ferric Tf to the TfR.

The presence of two iron-binding sites on Tf has led to the proposal that the two sites function differently.[43] Occupancy of the two sites of transferrin significantly influences the affinity with which transferrin is bound. Diferric Tf is bound with fourfold higher affinity than monoferric Tf by the TfR at the cell surface, whereas the affinity measured in cells for the binding of apotransferrin Tf (apoTf) by the TfR is extremely low.[44] Release of iron from free diferric Tf does not take place unless pH levels are below pH 4.6. However,

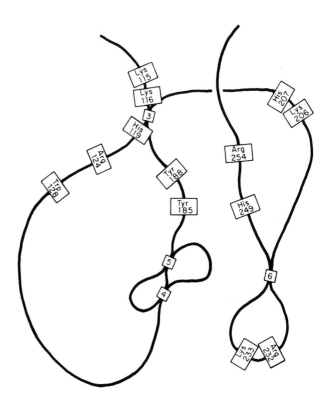

Figure 10–5. Proposed iron- and anion-binding sites in the N-terminal domain of human plasma transferrin (Tf). Iron is thought to bind to tyrosines 185 and 188 and to two of the three histidines found at 119, 206, and 207. Arginine 124 represents the probable site of anion binding. Four disulfide bonds (boxes 3 to 6) are similarly indicated in Figure 10–4. (Adapted from Chasteen, N. D.: The identification of the probable locus of iron and anion binding in the transferrins. Trends Biol. Sci. 2:272, 1983; with permission.)

iron release from transferrin is nearly complete upon acidification of endosomes in cells, even though the endosomal pH does not drop below 5.4. The answer to this apparent paradox lies in the role of the TfR itself. In cells, association of Tf with the TfR facilitates release of iron at a less acidic pH than is required for release from free Tf, and this difference may be important in permitting the release of iron at pH levels that are achieved within endosomes.[45–47]

▼ SYNTHESIS AND DEGRADATION OF TRANSFERRIN

Most serum Tf is synthesized in the liver.[48] Lymphocytes, Sertoli cells, and cells in the muscle, heart, brain, and mammary gland also have the capacity for Tf synthesis.[49–51] Local synthesis of transferrin is probably functionally important in the brain and testis, as access to these areas by serum transferrin is prevented by the blood-brain barrier and a similar type of barrier in the testis. The rate of Tf synthesis may be modulated by iron levels.[52, 53] Although variations in Tf concentration are observed in disease states such as iron deficiency or various inflammatory conditions, the molecular basis of these variations has not been elucidated. The Tf protein has a half-life of 7 to 10 days,[54] in contrast to the half-life of Tf-bound iron, which is only 2 hours, indicating that Tf may be used to deliver iron about 100 times in its lifetime. Clearance and degradation of desialated Tf molecules can occur via the asialoglycoprotein receptor of hepatocytes,[55, 56] although it is not known whether this is a physiologically relevant degradative pathway.

The Transferrin Receptor

The polypeptide that forms the TfR is a 760 amino acid glycoprotein of molecular weight approximately 90,000.[57–64] Carbohydrate represents 5 per cent by weight and is distributed in three N-linked oligosaccharide chains. The functional TfR is composed of two identical disulfide-linked polypeptides (Fig. 10–6). Each chain has an N-terminal cytoplasmic domain of 61 amino acids and an extracellular segment of 671 residues. The transmembrane domain of the TfR is composed of 28 amino acids spanning residues 62 to 89. The TfR polypeptide lacks an N-terminal leader sequence.[59–61] It resembles the asialoglycoprotein receptor in having the majority of its C-terminal segment as an external domain. Integration into the membrane is thought to occur via insertion of a hydrophobic transmembrane segment that functions as an internal signal peptide.[65] The mature receptor contains covalently bound fatty acid,[66] which might also have a role in its integration into the membrane. Serine residues within the N-terminal segment may be phosphorylated.[57] It is not yet clear what functional significance, if any, is associated with post-translational modifications of the TfR.[64] Analysis of the cDNA sequence has indicated that the TfR lacks similarity to other proteins involved in iron metabolism, including Tf.[59, 61] Limited sequence similarity exists between the TfR and the mouse epidermal growth factor (EGF) precursor. The region of relatedness within the EGF precursor overlaps with a region of similarity to the low density lipoprotein (LDL) receptor.[67] The respective regions of simi-

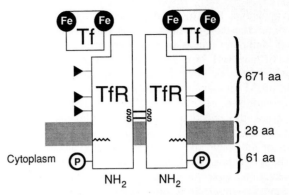

Figure 10–6. Structure and orientation in the plasma membrane of the transferrin receptor (TfR). The TfR is depicted as a disulfide-linked homodimer with two molecules of diferric plasma transferrin (Tf) bound. The amino-terminus of each polypeptide is oriented toward the cytoplasm. The intracellular domain contains a site for phosphorylation by protein kinase C. There is also a site for covalently bound fatty acid (depicted as a squiggle in the membrane-spanning domain). In addition to the ligand-binding domain, the extracellular portion of each polypeptide contains sites for the addition of three N-linked carbohydrate chains (depicted as triangles). (Adapted from Harford, J. B., Casey, J. L., Koeller, D. M., and Klausner, R. D.: Structure, function, and regulation of the transferrin receptor: Insights from molecular biology. *In* Steer, C. J., and Hanover, J. A. [eds.]: Intracellular Trafficking of Proteins. Cambridge, Cambridge University Press, 1991; with permission.)

larity to the EGF precursor within the TfR and the LDL receptor lie just outside their membrane-spanning domains.

The gene for the TfR is found in 19 exons distributed over 31 kb of genomic DNA and maps to the distal portion of the long arm of chromosome 3 (3q26) (3qter)[68, 69] in the same region where the genes for Tf[37] and the p97 antigen[70] have been mapped. Transcriptional control sequences for the TfR gene have been localized in the immediate 5′ flanking region.[71] These sequences may be involved in induction of gene expression in response to iron deprivation or in response to various growth factors. Two nuclear proteins (termed TREF-1 and TREF-2 [transferrin receptor enhancer factor]) have been identified as binding to the transcriptional control region of the TfR gene.[72]

▼ CELLULAR UPTAKE OF IRON: THE TRANSFERRIN CYCLE

The existence of a specific receptor for Tf was proposed in 1963,[54] but the purification and detailed characterization of the TfR did not begin until more than a decade later.[62, 63] It was initially observed in 1969 by electron microscopy that Tf entered reticulocytes in endocytic vesicles.[73, 74] These fundamental observations that Tf first interacts with its specific high-affinity receptor and is subsequently internalized by the cell provided the basis for understanding the iron delivery process (see Fig. 10–6). The TfR is thus placed in that large group of receptors that mediate internalization of their specific ligands, and the Tf cycle can be understood in terms of the general pathway of receptor-mediated endocytosis.[75, 76]

Most cells possess, on their surface, numerous different receptors, each having a high affinity for a specific ligand. These receptors mediate the action of hormones, neurotransmitters, growth factors, differentiation factors, and chemotactic factors. They also provide for the specific recognition of serum transport proteins, such as Tf, LDL, and transcobalamin, and other important molecules, such as immunoglobulin G (IgG), IgE, IgA, and lysosomal enzymes. Microscopy and, in particular, electron microscopy allowed the visualization of the interaction of both specific and nonspecific proteins within the cell. In the late 1950s, Bessis and coworkers observed the uptake of single molecules of ferritin into pinocytotic vesicles.[77] Their striking observation was that the sites of entry into the cell were definable as small indentations in the plasma membrane. By the early 1960s, these indentations were identified as coated pits because of the appearance in electron micrographs of a fuzzy electron-dense coat beneath the invagination.[78] Coated pits have been observed in virtually all cells (except mature enucleated erythrocytes) and serve as the site of entry of receptors and their ligands.

Although many of the molecular events underlying the endocytic pathway remain obscure, studies using a wide variety of receptors and ligands in many cell types have elucidated a general process. The first event in the endocytosis of a ligand is the binding to the surface receptor. Dissociation constants for a wide array of ligand-receptor interactions range from 10^{-7} M to 10^{-10} M. Most receptors, in the absence of ligand, are found randomly distributed in the plane of the plasma membrane. Some, including the TfR, are preferentially clustered into coated pits even in the apparent absence of ligand.[79] The coat itself is composed of a polygonal structure reminiscent of geodesic domes formed by a mixture of hexagons and pentagons that are made up of a 180,000 dalton protein called clathrin and several smaller proteins.[80, 81]

The coated pit regions of cells are constantly invaginating, with the coat most likely closing into a completed polygonal cage around a cytoplasmic vesicle referred to as a coated vesicle. Receptor-ligand complexes contained within the invaginating pit are thus internalized. These coated vesicles are short lived, and the newly formed vesicle most likely loses its coat. This smooth-walled vesicle containing newly internalized material is referred to as an endocytotic vesicle, or endosome.[82] In the TfR, the sequence YTRF in the N-terminal cytosolic tail is a binding site for adaptor proteins that target the receptor to endosomes.[75] The endosome compartment comprises a highly polymorphic set of vesicles and tubules found in the cell periphery. After 15 to 45 minutes, the evolving endosome (or some vesicular structure derived from the endosome) fuses with a lysosome, thereby delivering the internalized contents for hydrolytic degradation. It is important to note that endocytosis defines a pathway of vesicular transfer of external molecules to lysosomes. This pathway per se does not provide a route for the transfer of molecules from outside the cell (or from inside the endosome) into the cytoplasm.

The one-way pathway from the cell surface to the lysosome is taken by the vast majority of ligands. The fate of most receptors is quite different from that of their ligands, and one of the most striking aspects of this general pathway is the recycling of receptors.[83] Thus, many receptors mediate the internalization and degradation of scores of ligand molecules, but the receptors are not themselves degraded. These receptors can be recycled to the plasma membrane and reutilized repeatedly for the internalization of new ligand molecules. At some point subsequent to internalization, the

ligand and receptor take different physical paths, the former going to lysosomes and the latter returning intact to the plasma membrane. The prerequisite for this divergence is a physicochemical mechanism for the intravesicular dissociation of the ligand from the receptor. Endosomes are acidified by an adenosine triphosphate (ATP)-dependent proton pump present in the membrane of these organelles that is similar, if not identical, to that found in lysosomal membranes.[84–86] The majority of endocytic receptor-ligand interactions are highly pH dependent, with the ligand rapidly dissociating at pHs below 5.5. Once the ligand is released into the fluid phase of the lumen of the endocytotic vesicle, the freed ligand is sorted to enter a vesicular pathway that leads to fusion with lysosomes, whereas the membrane receptor is recycled to the cell surface.

Studies over a number of years have clarified the somewhat unusual endocytotic pathway taken by Tf,[87–91] referred to as the Tf cycle. Monoferric or diferric Tf binds to the cell surface TfR and is rapidly internalized via coated pits. Shortly after internalization, the transferrin is detected in acidified endocytic vesicles.[92] Up to this point, Tf endocytosis is indistinguishable from the generalized pathway taken by other ligands. However, in contrast to these other ligands, the Tf is not delivered to lysosomes and is therefore not degraded. Rather, the Tf is rapidly released from the cell. In a single cycle through the cell, the vast majority of diferric Tf is released as apotransferrin after about a 5 to 15 minute transit. The efficiency of this recycling is greater than 95 per cent. As with many other receptor systems, the TfR recycles and is reutilized. The rates of cycling of the TfR and its ligand Tf are the same.

How does Tf avoid delivery to and degradation in the lysosome? The answer lies in the interesting details of the pH dependence of the ligand-receptor interaction.[92–94] Soon after internalization, the vesicle that contains the Tf-TfR complex is acidified. The acidity of the environment is an absolute requirement for the release of iron.[95–97] At neutral pH, the release of iron from the Tf-TfR complex would result in a rapid dissociation of apotransferrin from the TfR. However, the dissociation constant of the apotransferrin-receptor interaction is much lower at acidic pH, so that apotransferrin, in contrast to other ligands, remains bound to its receptor in the acidic endosome (Fig. 10–7). The relative affinities of apotransferrin for the TfR at neutral and acidic pH are also observed when affinities of recombinant proteins are measured in vitro, indicating that contributions from other interacting proteins are not required in the observed affinity changes.[98] The normally recycling receptor carries the apotransferrin back to the cell surface, where, upon encountering the neutral pH of the outside environment, the apotransferrin rapidly dissociates and is released from the membrane. This cycle allows for the reutilization of both ligand and receptor, the former to be reloaded with ferric iron and the latter to engage in additional rounds of endocytosis. The acidic endosome in this and other systems provides the mechanism for sorting components of endocytotic systems (Fig. 10–8). During the uptake of ligands such as LDL and asialoglycoproteins, the pH-dependent dissociation allows the ligand to be delivered without its receptor to lysosomes. During iron uptake, acidification allows the iron to dissociate from Tf and be transported across the endosomal membrane into the cytosol, whereas Tf is returned to the cell surface.

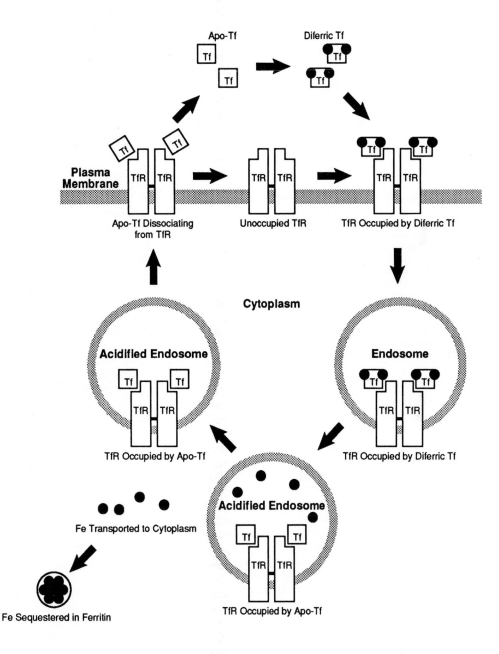

Figure 10–7. The plasma transferrin (Tf) cycle for iron uptake. Tf and the transferrin receptor (TfR) are depicted as in Figure 10–6. The Tf cycle involves binding of diferric Tf by the TfR, internalization of the TfR-Tf complex, endosome acidification, transfer of iron to the cytoplasm, externalization of the TfR-apotransferrin complex, and release of apotransferrin upon encounter with the neutral pH of the extracellular milieu. Details of the transfer of iron from the endosome are given in Figure 10–8. Cytoplasmic iron is either utilized or incorporated into ferritin (see Fig. 10–3). (Adapted from Harford, J. B., and Klausner, R. D.: Coordinate post-transcriptional regulation of ferritin and transferrin receptor expression: The role of regulated RNA-protein interaction. Enzyme 44:28, 1991; with permission of S. Karger AG, Basel.)

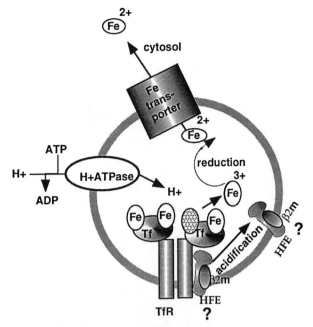

Figure 10–8. Iron release within the endocytotic vesicle and transfer to the cytoplasm. Iron release from plasma transferrin (Tf) depends on the acidic pH of the endosome. Vesicle acidification depends on a proton-pumping adenosine triphosphatase (ATPase). In addition to the lowered pH, other factors may participate in the release of iron from Tf, including the interaction of the Tf with the transferrin receptor (TfR). HFE binds to the TfR at the plasma membrane. Although it is not yet established, it is likely that HFE internalizes into endosomes along with the TfR but is released from the TfR when the endosome is acidified. Once released, ferric iron must be reduced to ferrous iron, using an electron-transporting reductase with electrons coming from cytoplasmic reducing equivalents (reduced nicotinamide-adenine dinucleotide [NADH] or reduced nicotinamide-adenine dinucleotide phosphate [NADHP]) and transported to the cytoplasm by a ferrous transporter such as DCT1/Nramp2.

The acidic environment of the endosome, although necessary, is likely insufficient to account for iron unloading of Tf, since even at pH 5, release of iron from recombinant Tf is much slower than release from Tf bound to TfR in the endosome. The interaction of Tf with the TfR also appears to facilitate release of iron from Tf,[46, 47] and an intraendosomal chelator may also participate. The recently identified gene for the disease hereditary hemochromatosis, HFE, binds to the transferrin receptor at neutral pH but is released from the TfR at acidic pH; it is possible that HFE somehow contributes to the efficiency of iron release from the TfR, although there are few data on the exact role of HFE at present (see below).[98] The molecular details of the transfer of iron from the endosome to the cytoplasm were obscure until recently, but it is now established that a recently cloned iron transporter, DCT1 or Nramp2, transports iron from within the endosome to the cytosol in some settings. The iron transporter is discussed in detail in a later section of this chapter.

▼ CONTROL OF TRANSFERRIN RECEPTOR SYNTHESIS

Iron has several roles in cellular metabolic processes. Iron is required for the synthesis of ribonucleotide reductase,

which is in turn required for DNA synthesis and cell division.[99] Hence, the availability of iron may influence the rate of cell proliferation, and the number of receptors is highest on proliferating cells. Iron is also required for the synthesis of many other cellular proteins, such as the cytochromes involved in oxidative metabolism, and for certain specialized functions, such as hemoglobin synthesis in erythroid cells. Clearly, control of iron acquisition and utilization must be modulated to meet these varied and diverse demands.

Rapidly dividing cells require more iron than quiescent cells. Moreover, growth arrest occurs upon removal of Tf from cell culture medium. This growth arrest can be explained by the requirement for iron to synthesize essential enzymes such as ribonucleotide reductase.[99] The fact that the growth requirement for Tf is related to the iron it carries is evidenced by the fact that the addition of iron in a chelated form that passes through the cell membrane results in reinitiation of cell proliferation independently of the presence of Tf.[100, 101] Conversely, the addition of strong chelators such as desferrioxamine produces an arrest in cell growth independent of the presence of Tf.[102, 103] The level of TfR expression is related to the proliferative state of the cells[104–106] as well as to the induction of differentiation.[107–109] Resting lymphocytes express almost no surface TfR, but a rapid and dramatic increase in TfR expression follows lymphocyte activation.[110–112] The transcription rate of the TfR gene has also been assessed by nuclear runoff experiments in activated T cells[108] and in HL60 cells induced to differentiate with dibutyryl cyclic adenosine monophosphate (AMP) (cAMP).[109] Activation of T cells leads to increased TfR expression, whereas cAMP treatment of HL60 results in decreased TfR expression. The corresponding changes in nuclear runoffs that were observed in both instances are consistent with a transcriptional contribution to TfR gene expression.

Receptor number may also be modulated by the redistribution of receptor molecules between the surface and internal membranes.[113–116] Fluctuations that occur during the cell cycle may reflect such partitioning. Many more receptors are found on the surface during the S phase of the cell cycle than during the G_1 phase.[106, 117, 118] Treatment of human fibroblasts with EGF results in a rapid increase in the ability of the cell membrane to bind Tf by accelerating the return of internalized receptors, retarding their internalization, or doing both.[113] Exposure of human erythroleukemia cells to a monoclonal antibody with specificity for the TfR results in internalization of the antibody-receptor complex.[114] An increased fraction of the receptor is directed to lysosomes for degradation compared with internalization initiated by Tf binding, leading to a decrease in surface receptor number. Furthermore, rapid, short-term changes in receptor number that accompany activation of erythroleukemia cells by phorbol esters have been shown to reflect receptor redistribution from an intracellular pool.[115, 116] The TfR persists on maturing erythroblasts even after nuclear extrusion, as reflected by its presence in large numbers on reticulocytes. This feature ensures availability of iron for hemoglobin synthesis. After maturation of reticulocytes to red cells, the receptors appear to be shed.[119, 120] The mechanisms by which specialized cells control receptor number during maturation are largely unknown.

Within populations of proliferating cells, the expression

of TfR is modulated by iron availability in a manner that resembles feedback regulation, such that fewer receptors are expressed when iron is abundant and more receptors are expressed when iron is scarce.[121–125] The predominant locus of iron regulation of TfR expression lies not in the promoter but in sequences corresponding to the 3′UTR of the TfR messenger RNA (mRNA).[126–129] The regulation of the TfR is discussed in detail in the section on cellular iron homeostasis later in this chapter.

Ferritin

Protection from the harmful effects of iron is in large measure accomplished by the sequestration of excess iron in cells. The best-characterized protein that serves this function is ferritin, a highly conserved protein found in all vertebrates.[130, 131] Ferritin-like sequestration compounds have been reported in bacteria as well as in simple eukaryotes. Vertebrate ferritin subunits assemble into a well-characterized structure containing a total of 24 subunits that form a spherical shell into which as many as 4500 atoms of iron can be sequestered and detoxified as a ferric oxyhydroxide micelle. How iron that has entered ferritin can be remobilized for metabolic uses is still unclear.[38, 131–136] Two types of apoferritin subunits have been identified. The human L chain contains 174 residues and has a molecular weight of 19,700, whereas the human H chain has 182 residues with a molecular weight of 21,100. The H chain is four amino acids longer on either end than the L chain. Despite only 55 per cent identity at the protein sequence level, the secondary and tertiary conformations of the H and L chains are quite similar.

▼ FERRITIN GENES

Both the H and the L genes are part of relatively large multigene families.[134–144] There are at least 10 genes in the H chain gene family and more than a dozen in the L chain gene family. Most or all of these are on separate chromosomes. A functional gene for the H chain has been molecularly cloned and mapped to chromosome 11.[144] It is a relatively compact gene, having four exons and three introns, with a total size of only 3 kb. An L chain gene with similar organization has also been cloned.[142] A functional L chain gene was mapped to chromosome 19 by immunological analyses using somatic cell hybrids.[145] Several of the H chain–related genes have been shown to be processed intronless pseudogenes both by heteroduplex mapping of cloned DNA fragments, which revealed the absence of introns, and by DNA sequence analysis, which revealed inactivating mutations.[134, 135, 143]

▼ FERRITIN STRUCTURE

Each ferritin subunit is folded into a roughly cylindrical molecule containing four long and nearly parallel right-handed helices (A, B, C, D), a shorter helix (E), a helical turn (P), a long extended chain (L), and some irregular regions (Fig. 10–9A).[132, 133] The relative orientation of the

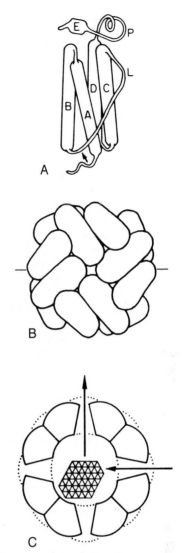

Figure 10–9. The structure of ferritin. *A,* Three-dimensional representation of an apoferritin subunit. The segments labeled A to E and P are helical in nature, whereas L is a non-helical loop. The numbers of amino acids in each helical segment are as follows: A, 27; B, 25; C, 28; D, 20; P, 7; and E, 10; this is the order of the helical segments, starting with the amino-terminus. *B,* Quaternary structure of the apoferritin shell viewed down one axis of its fourfold axis of symmetry. The central opening represents a channel through which iron enters the ferritin core. *C,* A cross-sectional view of the ferritin shell after oxidation of ferrous iron to ferric iron as it enters. As many as 4500 atoms of iron may be sequestered within the ferritin shell, although typically the number is lower. (Adapted with permission from Clegg, G. A., Fitton, J. E., Harrison, P. M., and Treffry, A.: Ferritin: Molecular structure and iron-storage mechanisms. Prog. Biophys. Mol. Biol. 36:56, 1980; with permission of Pergamon Press.)

various subunits to one another in the assembly of the 24 subunit shell is illustrated in Figure 10–9B. An interesting feature of this quaternary structure is the presence of six channels with a fourfold axis of symmetry that passes through the shell (Fig. 10–9C). These channels may allow iron and other molecules necessary for its storage and mobilization to enter or to leave the central cavity.

Isoelectric focusing of ferritin molecules extracted from a variety of tissues revealed a very complex pattern with multiple bands.[132, 133, 146–149] This heterogeneity reflects, at least in part, the assembly of ferritin shells having variable numbers of H and L subunits in the cytosol. Indeed, variable expression of H and L chain genes occurs in different tissues. For example, the human liver contains predominantly L chains, whereas the heart contains predominantly H chains.[147, 148] The H chain subunit appears to be important in facilitating rapid iron uptake by the heteropolymer.[150] The multiplicity of isoferritins detected could also reflect expression of more than the ferritin genes of the H and L types, but only two functional ferritin genes have been identified in humans. Three distinct ferritin cDNAs have been characterized in frog red cells.[151] Post-translational modification of the ferritin polypeptides may also introduce heterogeneity into ferritin subunits[152–155] and contribute to the multiplicity of isoferritins demonstrable in various tissues.

Ferritin is found not only within parenchymal cells but also in the serum. The serum form is glycosylated and less loaded with iron than are tissue ferritins.[152] The observation that serum ferritin is glycosylated is consistent with the possibility that ferritin is actively secreted by cells, acquiring sugar modifications in its passage through the secretory pathway. For that reason, a third gene of the ferritin family that encodes a secretory form of ferritin has long been sought. Variations in serum ferritin levels quite often reflect cellular iron status, as serum ferritin levels increase in patients who are iron overloaded.

Recently, description of a rare genetic disease has raised questions about whether secreted ferritin is encoded by a third expressed ferritin gene. In the hereditary hyperferritinemia bilateral cataract syndrome, serum levels of ferritin are markedly elevated, and yet the causal mutations are clearly present in the ferritin L chain gene (see below). Although ferritin L chain is known to coassemble with ferritin H chain subunits in the cytosol, it is possible that some portion of newly synthesized ferritin L chain is targeted to the endoplasmic reticulum and actively secreted. A hydrophobic sequence near the N-terminus of the protein could potentially act as a cryptic targeting sequence, and the sequence NYS present within the sequence could act as a glycosylation site, the consensus sequence of which is NxS/T. If a portion of ferritin L is actively secreted, then it is possible that iron within serum ferritin is acquired in the endoplasmic reticulum (ER). Little is known about iron concentrations in the ER, but heme oxygenase-1, the enzyme that catalyzes formation of biliverdin, CO, and iron from heme, is associated with the ER (see below), and heme could potentially represent a source of iron in the ER.

▼ UPTAKE AND RELEASE OF IRON FROM FERRITIN

Incorporation of iron is thought to follow assembly of the apoferritin subunit shell. Relatively soluble ferrous iron is oxidized by ferroxidase sites within the H chain, and oxidized iron is precipitated on the inner surface of the subunits.[156] Ultimately, as many as 4500 iron atoms may be accomodated within each protein shell, although ferritin molecules having many fewer iron atoms are common.

Release of iron from ferritin shells can be readily demonstrated in vitro. Various flavins or other reducing agents, such as cysteine, glutathione, or ascorbic acid, or chelators, can facilitate such release.[132, 156–158] These substances are

thought to be able to pass through the channels in the ferritin shell. Iron may be released within cells by similar mechanisms. Alternatively, ferritin shells may undergo degradation, either within lysosomes to form hemosiderin or within cytoplasm.[159] Iron exposed to cytoplasmic constituents after degradation of the ferritin subunit shell may be more readily mobilized.

Ferritin and hemosiderin iron are storage forms of iron. The absence of storage iron in iron deficiency states and the mobilization of excess iron stores during phlebotomy of patients with hemochromatosis document the gradual flux from these storage forms into a metabolically active pool.[16] However, rapidly proliferating cells may depend exclusively on external Tf as a source of iron. Indeed, cells deprived of Tf or treated with chelators such as desferrioxamine experience growth arrest and altered expression of the TfR and ferritin despite having intracellular stores in the form of ferritin.[100, 103]

▼ FERRITIN SYNTHESIS

Ferritin genes are expressed in all cells, but the differential expression of the H and L chain genes in different tissues suggests tight regulation of ferritin gene expression. In addition to the cell type–specific expression of ferritins, cells possess the ability to respond quickly to increased exposure to iron by modulation of ferritin biosynthesis. Accelerated biosynthesis and assembly of apoferritin shells can be demonstrated within minutes of increasing intracellular iron concentration.[160–163] The increase in ferritin biosynthesis occurs by a post-transcriptional mechanism, as was established initially by the observation that treatment with actinomycin D, an inhibitor of RNA synthesis, did not prevent the increase in response to iron treatment.[164, 165] This iron-dependent modulation of ferritin biosynthesis is now known to occur at the level of mRNA translation (see below).

Cellular Iron Homeostasis

▼ IRON-RESPONSIVE ELEMENTS

Cells respond to iron deprivation by increasing synthesis of the TfR and decreasing synthesis of the iron sequestration protein, ferritin. The coordinate regulation of expression of ferritin and TfR is achieved post-transcriptionally through the binding of iron-sensing proteins known as iron-regulatory proteins (IRPs) to stem loops within transcripts known as iron-responsive elements (IREs). IREs are RNA stem loops in which a stable base-paired stem contains an unpaired cytosine 5 base pairs removed from a six-membered loop. The sequence CAGUG is conserved in the first five nucleotides of the loop, and the sixth position can be any nucleotide but G (Fig. 10–10).

IREs were initially identified within ferritin transcripts; cloning and expression of ferritin H and L chains revealed that the information required for regulation of ferritin biosynthesis according to cellular iron homeostasis was contained within the 5'UTR of the ferritin transcripts.[165, 166] Although overall sequence homology within the transcripts was not impressive, comparison of human ferritin transcripts to ferri-

Figure 10–10. The structure of an iron-responsive element (IRE). All known ferritin messenger ribonucleic acids (mRNAs) contain a single IRE within their 5' untranslated region. All known plasma transferrin receptor (TfR) mRNAs contain five IREs within their 3' untranslated region. The consensus IRE shown is derived from the sequences and possible secondary structures of IREs from ferritin and TfR mRNAs. (Adapted from Harford, J. B., and Klausner, R. D.: Coordinate post-transcriptional regulation of ferritin and transferrin receptor expression: The role of regulated RNA-protein interaction. Enzyme 44:28, 1991; with permission of S. Karger AG, Basel.)

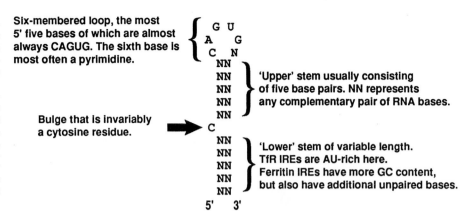

Six-membered loop, the most 5' five bases of which are almost always CAGUG. The sixth base is most often a pyrimidine.

Bulge that is invariably a cytosine residue.

'Upper' stem usually consisting of five base pairs. NN represents any complementary pair of RNA bases.

'Lower' stem of variable length. TfR IREs are AU-rich here. Ferritin IREs have more GC content, but also have additional unpaired bases.

tin transcripts of other species revealed that the IRE sequence was conserved in ferritin transcripts.[167] Deletional analysis demonstrated that the IRE sequence was indispensable in iron-dependent regulation of ferritin biosynthesis. Furthermore, the IRE sequence could be introduced into the 5'UTR of reporter genes, where it was sufficient to confer the capacity for iron-dependent regulation upon these unrelated genes.[168]

The role of IREs in post-transcriptional gene regulation was extended when analysis of the regulation of TfR expression led to the insight that a regulatory element within the 3'UTR contained IREs. Iron-dependent regulation of TfR biosynthesis was post-transcriptional and was based on a decrease in stability of the TfR transcript within iron-depleted cells.[169, 170] Portions of the TfR cDNA corresponding to the 3'UTR of the TfR mRNA were shown to be sufficient to confer iron regulation on the expression of a chimeric transcript encoding heterologous genes.[126, 127] A fragment of 678 nucleotides within the 3'UTR of the TfR mRNA was identified as the predominant locus of iron regulation, and within this fragment, five consensus IREs were identified.[127] RNA folding programs revealed that a secondary structure similar to that predicted for the human TfR was predicted to form in a corresponding sequence within the 3'UTR of the chicken TfR mRNA.[128, 129] Structural studies of the regulatory region performed with ribonuclease H (RNase H) and other ribonucleases verified that the structure of the regulatory region contained IREs and was relatively static.[171]

The structure of an IRE is generally represented as containing an unstructured six-membered loop, as indicated in Figure 10–10. However, binding studies of mutagenized IREs indicate that there is base pairing between nucleotides in positions 1 and 5 of the loop,[172–174] and these findings have been verified in nuclear magnetic resonance (NMR) structures of the IRE.[175, 176]

▼ IRON-REGULATORY PROTEINS

Iron-regulatory proteins are iron-sensing proteins that bind with high affinity to IREs in cells that are depleted of iron. These proteins were initially identified as proteins that bound with high affinity to radiolabeled IRE sequences and caused a mobility shift of the IRE in non-denaturing gels.[177, 178] Binding activity increased in lysates from iron-depleted cells,

and these proteins, initially termed IRE-binding proteins (IRE-BPs), ferritin repressor protein, or iron-regulatory factor, were purified and cloned.[179–184]

Although the mechanisms of iron sensing differ for the two identified IRE-binding proteins, which are now referred to as iron-regulatory proteins (IRPs) 1 and 2, binding of each of the proteins to IREs is markedly decreased in iron-replete cells. High-affinity binding of IRPs to transcripts that contain IREs results in iron-dependent regulation of expression of these genes (Fig. 10–11). When the IRE is close to the site of translational initiation, translation is repressed. In the case of ferritin transcripts and other mRNAs that contain IREs near the 5' end of the mRNA, binding of IRPs causes a decrease in the rate of new biosynthesis. Thus, the synthesis of new ferritin appropriately decreases in the iron-depleted cell, since the role of ferritin in the cells is to sequester excess iron. The mechanism of translational repression is likely to depend on simple steric hindrance in which IRPs prevent binding of initiation factors to the 5' cap of the transcript.[185]

In the TfR, an endonucleolytic cleavage site is contained within this regulatory region of the transcript, and the cleavage site is flanked by IREs; it is thought that the cleavage and rapid degradation of the transcript are prevented in iron-depleted cells when IRPs are bound to the transcript, and that IRPs bound to IREs sterically prevent endonucleases from gaining access to the endonucleolytic cleavage site.[186] When IREs in the regulatory region contain point mutations that destroy high-affinity binding by IRPs, the transcript is unstable and is constitutively degraded in a non–iron-dependent fashion.[187]

Insights into how IRPs sense iron and accordingly modify ferritin translation and turnover of the TfR transcript came from the recognition that these proteins are members of a larger gene family. IRP1 is homologous to mitochondrial aconitase, a mitochondrial iron-sulfur protein that interconverts citrate and isocitrate in the citric acid cycle.[188] When IRP1 was cloned, mitochondrial aconitase had already been crystallized[189] and extensively biochemically characterized,[190] and this information guided studies on IRP1; IRP1 was discovered to contain a cubane iron-sulfur cluster bound to cysteines within the enzymatic active site cleft and to function as a fully active aconitase in the cytoplasm of iron-replete mammalian cells.[191] Further studies demonstrated that IRP1 purified from iron-depleted cells lacked an iron-sulfur cluster, and that the apoprotein present in iron-depleted cells

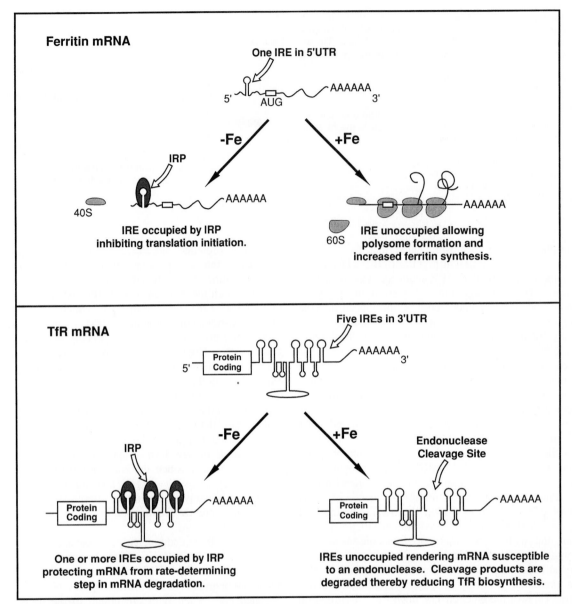

Figure 10–11. Coordinate regulation of the expression of ferritin and the plasma transferrin receptor (TfR). The 5′ untranslated region (UTR) of ferritin messenger ribonucleic acid (mRNA) contains a single iron-responsive element (IRE). The 3′ untranslated region of the TfR mRNA contains five similar elements (see Fig. 10–11). When iron is scarce, cytoplasmic, high-affinity IRE-binding proteins (IRPs) interact with the IREs of these mRNAs. In the case of the ferritin mRNA and other transcripts that contain IREs at the 5′ end, this interaction serves to reduce the translation of the mRNA and results in reduced synthesis with no alteration in the level of the mRNA. In the case of the TfR, the interaction of IRE-binding proteins, IRP$_1$ and IRP$_2$, with the IREs results in protection of the mRNA from degradation. This in turn leads to more TfR synthesis as a result of the elevated level of its mRNA. (Adapted from Harford, J. B., and Klausner, R. D.: Coordinate post-transcriptional regulation of ferritin and transferrin receptor expression: The role of regulated RNA-protein interaction. Enzyme 44:28; 1991; with permission of S. Karger AG, Basel.)

was the form of the protein that bound IREs with high affinity.[192, 193] Cross-linking studies revealed that the IRE was bound to the active site cleft of the protein[194–196] and that arginines within the active site contributed significantly to high-affinity binding of IREs.[197]

The fact that the IRE-binding site overlaps with the enzymatic active site explains why the two activities of the protein, aconitase activity and IRE-binding activity, are mutually exclusive. Although the half-life of IRP1 is long (approximately 24 hours) relative to the observable time frame of iron regulation of target transcripts within cells (approximately 3 hours),[198] it is likely that the turnover of

the iron-sulfur cluster is rapid, in part because of inherent instability of iron-sulfur prosthetic groups in oxidizing environments,[199, 200] or perhaps because of more complex signaling pathways.[201] Thus, the key to regulation of IRP1 appears to depend on the continuous resynthesis of iron-sulfur clusters, which would in turn depend on the availability of sufficient inorganic sulfur and iron.

A second protein that binds IREs with high affinity, IRP2, is present within all cells and tissues that have been examined and is highly homologous to IRP1.[202] Similar to that of IRP1, IRE-binding activity of IRP2 increases markedly in iron-depleted cells. However, in contrast to IRP1,

IRP2 is not detectable on Western blots in iron-replete cells.[183, 184] IRP2 is degraded in iron-replete cells, and the feature of iron-dependent degradation depends upon the insertion of 73 amino acids into the coding sequence of IRP2. When the 73 amino acid sequence is deleted from IRP2, IRP2 is no longer degraded in iron-replete cells. When this sequence is inserted into an analogous position in IRP1, the chimeric protein is degraded in iron-replete cells, indicating that the 73 amino acid domain can confer the phenotype of iron-dependent degradation on another protein.[203] Thus, an insert of 73 amino acids in IRP2 functions as an iron-dependent degradation domain and IRP2 levels are regulated by degradation in iron-replete cells.[203, 204]

Analysis of the degradation pathway of IRP2 has revealed that IRP2 in cells is degraded by large multisubunit cytosolic protease complexes known as proteasomes. Most proteins degraded by proteasomes are tagged for degradation by the conjugation of multiple chains of ubiquitin, a 76 amino acid protein, to the protein. Specific features of proteins, such as phosphorylated residues, can serve as the targets for enzymes known as ubiquitin ligases that covalently link ubiquitin to proteins.[205, 206] In many systems, the use of inhibitors of proteasome function has allowed characterization of the protein modifications that predispose to degradation. In iron-replete cells treated with proteasome inhibitors, IRP2 is oxidatively modified, as revealed in a carbonyl assay that detects certain types of oxidized amino acid side chains.[207] Also, IRP2 in cells treated with iron and proteasome inhibitors is ubiquitinated, and in vitro assays reveal that oxidative modification of IRP2 predisposes to ubiquitination.[208]

Several observations indicate that the degradation domain is likely to be an iron-binding site. When several cysteines within the degradation domain are simultaneously mutagenized to serines, iron-dependent degradation is abolished.[203] Since cysteine residues often participate in ligation of iron, this observation is consistent with the possibility that direct binding of iron is important in IRP2 degradation. Also, IRP2 is exquisitely sensitive to oxidation and cleavage reactions when iron and reductants are added in vitro.[208] The efficiency of this metal-catalyzed oxidation reaction is high, again consistent with the possibility that an iron-binding site is present within the degradation domain of IRP2.

Taken together, these observations permit a description of the steps involved in the iron-dependent degradation of IRP2: Initially, the degradation domain is proposed to bind iron that is readily available in iron-replete cells. Because the degradation domain is predicted to be on the surface of the protein, the bound iron could readily interact with soluble oxygen species, generating hydroxyl radicals in situ. The hydroxyl radicals are highly reactive and would be expected to oxidize residues in close proximity to the site at which the radicals are formed, most likely within the degradation domain of IRP2. These oxidized residues could then act as a target for a specific ubiquitin ligase, which would target the modified protein for degradation by tagging it with ubiquitin multimers. Thus, the appropriate iron-dependent degradation of IRP2 depends not only on iron, but also on the presence of soluble oxygen species that can interact with iron, generate free radicals, and oxidize IRP2. Unlike IRP1, IRP2 does not appear to assemble an iron-sulfur cluster in

the RNA-binding cleft, and elimination of IRE-binding activity is achieved through degradation of the protein.[183]

Functional IREs have now been described in the 5'UTR of several other transcripts, including erythroid 5-aminolevulinate (eALA) synthase,[209, 210] the rate-limiting step in heme biosynthesis, mammalian mitochondrial aconitase,[211–213] and succinate dehydrogenase of *Drosophila melanogaster*.[214] Both mitochondrial aconitase and succinate dehydrogenase are mitochondrial enzymes that require iron-sulfur prosthetic groups for function, and the presence of IREs in these transcripts could help prevent synthesis of non-functional apoproteins. In the heme biosynthetic pathway, accumulation of the heme precursor protoporphyrin IX is toxic, and this may explain why an early step in the biosynthetic pathway is repressed in iron-depleted erythroid cells. Recently, an IRE has been described in the 3'UTR of the mammalian ferrous transporter (see below), and it is possible that the ferrous transporter will be regulated similarly to the TfR. Constant refinement of regulation in the course of evolution may mean that many more IRE-containing transcripts remain to be discovered.

It is not yet clear what advantages are gained by cells and organisms from the apparent redundancy in IRP function. IRP2 is 58 per cent identical to IRP1 but differs in that the genomic sequence contains the extra exon that confers the property of iron-dependent degradation on IRP2, which is likely to have been inserted into a duplicated gene by exon shuffling.[203] Although gene duplication offers the possibility of subsequent divergence and specialization of gene products, there are as yet few insights into how variations in expression, mechanism of regulation, or specificity are important in regulation of iron metabolism. Both IRPs are expressed in all tissues and cell lines that have been examined to date, and although the relative levels of expression vary from tissue to tissue, it is not clear whether these differences are important in regulation.[183, 184, 215] However, the differing mechanisms of regulation of the two IRPs may prove to be important in some physiological settings; in hypoxic cells, IRP1 binding activity might be expected to decrease because of decreased turnover of the oxygen-sensitive iron-sulfur cluster, whereas the binding activity of IRP2 would be expected to increase because of decreased iron-dependent oxidation and degradation by the ubiquitin-proteasome system. Another important difference between the two proteins that could be physiologically relevant involves differences in the RNA-binding sites of the two IRPs; each IRP can bind with measurable affinity to an RNA stem loop that differs from an IRE, and these non-IRE stem loops are different for the two proteins.[172–174] Incorporation of several of these sequences into transcripts reveals that both IRP1 and IRP2 can independently function as translational repressors in cells.[216] It is therefore theoretically possible that transcripts that do not contain consensus IREs are targets for regulation by only one of the two IRPs, although such endogenous transcripts have not as yet been discovered.

Mammalian Iron Physiology

Thus far, the focus of this chapter has been on the role of specific gene products in the maintenance of iron homeostasis in individual cells. However, in mammals, appropriate regulation of total body iron stores results from a complex interplay of regulatory events. Macrophages and duodenal mucosal cells are important sites for regulation of total body iron homeostasis, and therefore, these cells must be discussed in greater detail. In addition, a number of human disease states and mammalian genetic diseases cause dysregulation of iron homeostasis, and therefore each of these diseases will be discussed so that themes that are central in iron homeostasis may emerge.

▼ IDENTIFICATION OF THE DUODENAL MUCOSAL IRON TRANSPORTER

Recently, the gene that encodes an iron transporter in the duodenal mucosa was cloned in both rat and mouse. The rat gene was cloned by expression cloning of rat cDNAs in *Xenopus* oocytes. A cDNA was identified that encoded a multispanning membrane protein capable of facilitating uptake of divalent cations, including ferrous iron, cadmium, cobalt, manganese, and lead, into the oocyte.[217] The same gene was simultaneously identified by using a positional cloning strategy to identify the disease gene in the *mk* mouse, a strain that develops severe microcytic anemia and generally dies before weaning.[218] A single mutation in which a glycine in the fourth transmembrane motif was substituted by an arginine accounted for inability to absorb iron in *mk* mice, and the same mutation was identified independently in a second strain of mice with the *mk* phenotype. Interestingly, a second rodent model that is also characterized by severe microcytic hypochromic anemia, the Belgrade rat, carries exactly the same G-R mutation,[219] and although a CpG dinucleotide at the mutation site could predispose to the G-to-A transition observed in both *mk* alleles, a TpG dinucleotide, which is not unusually prone to mutation, is present at the same site in the rat. The fact that the same mutation has arisen independently twice in mice and once in rats implies that insertion of a bulky charged residue in this transmembrane domain is particularly deleterious to function.

Another rodent disease gene mutation underscores the importance of residues in transmembrane domain 4 in function. In mice prone to development of disease with intracellular parasite infections, positional cloning identified a mutation in a gene that was named Nramp1 (for natural resistance–associated macrophage protein).[220] Nramp1 is expressed only in macrophages and polymorphonuclear leukocytes and is approximately 75 per cent similar in sequence to Nramp2.[221] Although the function of Nramp1 was initially not known, the high degree of sequence similarity to the subsequently cloned iron transporter Nramp2 is consistent with the possibility that Nramp1 transports iron out of the phagosome, thereby enhancing resistance to intracellular parasite infections by depriving the parasites within phagosomes of available iron. In the Nramp1 disease gene, a single substitution of glycine 169 with an aspartic acid (G169D) is present; notably, G169 is immediately adjacent in sequence alignments to the glycine mutated in *mk* mice and the Belgrade rat, in which a glycine-to-arginine mutation is identified, and these adjacent glycines in transmembrane 4 are conserved in Nramp sequences of many species. Nramp1 protein is detected in late endosomes and is observed to fuse with phagosomes in the course of phagocytosis.[221] In mice

that carry the G169D mutation, the mature protein is not detectable, a finding that is consistent with the possibility that insertion of a bulky charged residue into this region of transmembrane domain 4, which already contains a highly conserved aspartic acid and two polar threonines, may be sufficient to cause gross misfolding of the protein and degradation.

Charged amino acids within transmembrane domains are unusual because of the hydrophobic environment of the membrane, and when present they are generally functionally important. In addition to the conserved aspartic acid in transmembrane domain 4, two other transmembrane domains in the Nramp proteins also contain negative charges, and the positioning of these negative charges may be important in transport of positively charged ions. In the ferrous transporter of yeast, the amino acid sequence REGLE is present within the transmembrane domain, and mutation of the glutamic acids to alanines abolishes iron transport.[8] It is not yet reported whether the abnormal Nramp2/DCT1 protein is present in the endosomes of *mk* mice or Belgrade rats. Another potential feature of importance that is lost in transmembrane 4 when the glycines are mutated is that in addition to introducing an extra charge to a region of the transmembrane helix, the amino acid substitutions would introduce side chains with greater bulk into this region of the membrane-spanning sequence.

In Belgrade rats, a role for the product of the disease gene in endosomal iron transport was established before positional cloning identified the disease gene as Nramp2. In the reticulocytes of Belgrade rats, iron that is internalized in endosomes inappropriately recycles to the extracellular space, even though dissociation from the Tf-TfR complex is normal,[222] and DCT1/Nramp2 is therefore unexpectedly implicated in endosomal iron transport. DCT1/Nramp2 is expressed at a low level in many tissues, many of which are able to take up iron by a non-transferrin-dependent route. The ability of cells to absorb iron that is not bound by transferrin is important in pathophysiological processes, and although it has been often assumed that such uptake is carried out by non-specific transporters, it is possible that DCT1/Nramp2 expressed on the surface of cells mediates the uptake of non–transferrin-bound iron by cells other than intestinal mucosal cells.[219] Other iron transporters may also be important in this process.[223] Abnormalities of DCT1/Nramp2 are not likely to explain the anemia of hemoglobin-deficient mice (*hbd/hbt*).[224]

Once iron is taken up by the intestinal mucosal cell, it must be exported from the cell across the basolateral membrane. The basolateral iron transporter has not yet been cloned, but its existence is strongly supported by the abnormalities described in the *sla* mouse[225, 226] described in a later section of this chapter.

The expression of DCT1/Nramp2 is regulated by iron at the mRNA level over a 50-fold range, with mRNA levels increasing in iron-depleted animals, similar to the TfR.[227] Interestingly, an IRE sequence is present in the 3′UTR of the rat gene, the human gene,[228] and an alternatively spliced form of the mouse gene.[219] Thus, there is a possibility that DCT1/Nramp2 transcript will be subject to IRP binding and iron-dependent regulation of mRNA turnover, similar to the TfR.[186]

▼ IRON REDISTRIBUTION AND THE RETICULOENDOTHELIAL CELL

In normal individuals, about 30 mg of iron passes through the plasma iron pool each day, and the iron is almost entirely derived from phagocytosis of senescent red cells and retrieval of iron from hemoglobin in macrophages. Despite the central role of macrophages in iron homeostasis, the mechanisms by which iron retrieved from red cells is returned to the circulation from macrophages remain unclear. Careful studies of uptake of red cells in which ^{59}Fe was incorporated into the animal have revealed that about half of the iron released from macrophages is carried by a protein that is the appropriate size for ferritin and that can be precipitated with antiferritin antibodies.[227, 228] Monitoring for release of hemoglobin as an indicator of cell lysis supports the conclusion that rupture of the cells is not required for the release of ferritin. The remainder of the macrophage iron is released in a form that can be readily bound by extracellular transferrin. It is not yet clear how much the secretion of iron in ferritin contributes to the redistribution of mammalian iron stores.[229] There is evidence to suggest that ferritin receptors are present in hepatocytes and erythroid precursors.[230] It is also not clear how the iron that is bound by transferrin upon release by macrophages is exported. An iron exporter similar to the basolateral transporter of intestinal mucosal cells is likely to be involved, particularly since iron exported at both sites is bound by serum transferrin upon release.

▼ DISORDERS IN HUMANS AND ANIMAL MODELS THAT LEAD TO ABNORMALITIES OF TOTAL BODY IRON HOMEOSTASIS

Hereditary Hemochromatosis and Iron Overload

Several human disease states are known that predispose to parenchymal iron overload and toxicity. The best-known of these diseases is hereditary hemochromatosis, an iron overload disease of insidious onset in which parenchymal iron overload predisposes to a variety of complications, the most common of which are cirrhosis of the liver, diabetes, arthritis, and cardiomyopathy. Hemochromatosis is common in whites of Northern European descent, and it is estimated that 1 in 200 to 400 individuals is an affected homozygote.[231] Hemochromatosis is frequently not diagnosed, in part because onset of symptoms is insidious and manifestations are protean but also because the best diagnostic tests include the serum transferrin saturation,[232] which is not included in most screening panels, and Prussian blue staining for iron in liver biopsy tissue, a procedure that is generally performed only when there is already diagnostic suspicion. Genetic iron overload likely contributes significantly to the incidence of cirrhosis of the liver and cardiomyopathies much more than is commonly recognized.[233]

Although the hemochromatosis gene was known to be linked to the human leukocyte antigen A (HLA-A) locus of chromosome 6 as early as 1977, the gene itself was not successfully cloned until 1996.[234] Cloning efforts based on traditional positional cloning methods were particularly difficult because the recombination frequency in the vicinity of the disease gene was unusually low, and informative recombination events within pedigrees were not available. The group that successfully cloned the hemochromatosis gene used the low recombination frequency to define genetic markers near the disease gene that were linked with the mutant allele at the time when the original mutation is thought to have arisen, approximately 5000 years ago. Even though recombination events in this region of chromosome 6 are rare, enough recombinations occurred over a 5000-year time span so that borders of the region containing the founder mutation could be defined. Sequencing of the entire region defined as carrying the disease gene led to identification of 14 open reading frames, 12 of which encoded histones, and 2 of which were candidate genes. Sequencing of affected individuals revealed that all affected individuals had a mutation in a gene that encoded an atypical major histocompatibility class (MHC) class I protein, initially termed HLA-H, and renamed HFE, in which a mutation at amino acid 282 replaced a cysteine with a tyrosine. Cys-282 is one of four cysteines in the extracellular domain of MHC proteins that form two extracellular disulfide bonds and are important in maintenance of the correct tertiary structure of the protein. Interestingly, the C282Y mutation is one of only two mutations that have been identified in HFE. A second missense mutation, His-63-Asp (H63D), has been identified in hemochromatosis patients who are heterozygous for the C282Y mutation,[234, 235] but it also remains possible that H63D is a common polymorphism that does not contribute to disease.[236, 237]

The effect of the C282Y mutation has been studied in cells in which the mutant allele is expressed. Normal HFE associates with β_2-microglobulin in the endoplasmic reticulum similarly to other MHC class I molecules, and the majority of the mature HFE-β_2m complex is at the plasma membrane. The mutation C282Y eliminates the ability of HFE to bind β_2m, and the misfolded protein accumulates in the ER.[238, 239] Thus, the C282Y mutation results in absence of functional HFE at the plasma membrane.

Although the exact role of HFE remains a mystery, recent observations indicate that HFE binds to the transferrin receptor. In cells in which HFE is overexpressed, HFE can be coprecipitated with the TfR, and conversely, TfR can be coprecipitated with antibodies to HFE.[240–242] Furthermore, the presence of associated HFE leads to a decrease in the affinity of the TfR for diferric transferrin.[240] The C282Y protein does not interfere with Tf binding, as expected, since C282Y is not expressed at the plasma membrane. Interestingly, the H63D protein that associates with TfR does not decrease the affinity of TfR for Tf.[240] Assessment of the effect of overexpressed HFE on the affinity of the TfR for Tf is the first assay to reveal a possible functional difference between the H63D protein and wild-type HFE. These results provide some support for the possibility that H63D contributes to disease in the compound heterozygotes. It remains unclear whether H63D homozygotes are prone to iron overload, and more information will be needed to determine the role of H63D in pathophysiology.

It is somewhat difficult to envision how the observed effect of HFE on affinity of the TfR for Tf would lead to the iron overload observed in hemochromatosis. However, the HFE-dependent decrease in affinity of the TfR for Tf was observed in cells in which overexpression of HFE permits the expression levels of HFE to approach those of the

TfR. Endogenous HFE protein and mRNA are difficult to detect, consistent with the possibility that HFE is of low abundance in cells and tissues. From a functional standpoint, it seems unlikely that there is enough HFE in most tissues to bind the majority of TfR in a bimolecular complex at the cell surface. HFE lacks an identifiable C-terminal endosomal targeting sequence, and binding to the TfR may be important in part because it would result in sorting of HFE to endosomes along with the TfR. Binding of HFE to the TfR is pH dependent; binding affinity of the TfR for HFE is as high as binding affinity for Tf at neutral pH, but at pH 6.0, HFE and TfR no longer form a complex.[98] Therefore, if HFE internalizes with the TfR, it might be expected to dissociate from TfR upon acidification of the endosome (see Fig. 10–8). In the endosome, HFE released from the TfR could become free to engage in other interactions, perhaps binding other endosomal proteins or a ligand such as iron.

The crystal structure of the HFE-β_2m heterodimer has been identified, and important structural features have been identified.[98] Unlike classical class I MHC molecules, HFE lacks a functional peptide-binding groove. The mutation H63D may cause local loop rearrangement in the $\alpha 1$ domain because of potential charge repulsion. A prominent patch of histidines, consisting of four histidines in proximity to a tyrosine, could be important in mediating the highly pH-dependent binding of HFE to TfR. Gel-filtration assays have established that HFE, TfR, and Tf can bind simultaneously to form a ternary complex, with a stoichiometry of 1:2:2 in vitro, thus indicating that HFE does not directly interfere with the Tf-binding sites of the TfR.[98]

Hereditary hemochromatosis will not be understood until more is known about the mechanisms that maintain normal iron homeostasis in the body. The cells of the duodenal mucosa are key in this process, since these cells modulate iron uptake according to total body iron stores, and iron uptake that is inappropriately high relative to total body iron stores is a hallmark of hereditary hemochromatosis. Whereas normal individuals absorb approximately 1 mg of iron per day into the plasma, absorption may be increased to as much as 3.5 mg/day in normal individuals under conditions of iron deficiency or in patients with hemochromatosis or other iron overload diseases and may be decreased to 0.5 mg/day in normal individuals in the presence of iron overload. Another distinctive feature of the disease is the abnormal saturation level of serum transferrin. Serum transferrin saturation is generally about 30 per cent, whereas levels of transferrin saturation in hemochromatosis patients are frequently much higher, often as high as 100 per cent in older patients with advanced disease. Tf saturation levels rarely exceed 62 per cent except in genetic hemochromatosis, and, as a result, abnormal Tf saturation is an excellent marker for genetic hemochromatosis.[232] In hemochromatosis, excess iron absorption leads to complete saturation of serum transferrin, and consequently, non–transferrin-bound iron (NTBI) is present in the serum (Fig. 10–12). The presence of other routes through which non–transferrin-bound iron can enter cells permits bypass of the TfR and the protection afforded by its regulation. Consequently, iron overload and toxicity can develop in cells that might otherwise protect against iron overload by decreasing TfR expression.

Another unusual feature of hemochromatosis is that macrophages are relatively depleted of iron.[1] Although the pathway by which macrophages return iron to the circulation is not molecularly characterized, it is clear that this pathway is important in maintaining iron homeostasis because the release of iron from macrophages appears to be regulated according to body iron stores. In heavily transfused and iron overloaded patients, the macrophages are loaded with iron. Remarkably, the macrophages in hemochromatosis patients are very low in iron, raising the question of whether the macrophages independently contribute to the disease by failing to sequester iron. If iron release from macrophages is regulated according to total body iron stores, then it is impressive to note that both macrophages and intestinal mucosal cells of hemochromatotics are responding as though they have sensed that total body iron stores are low: Both

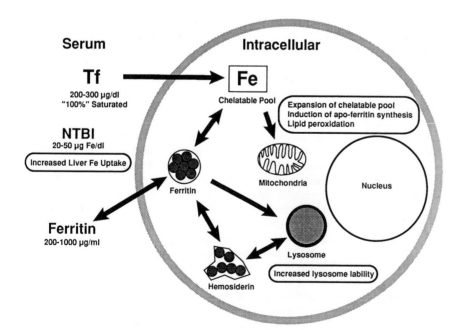

Figure 10–12. Cellular iron pools in an individual with human leukocyte antigen (HLA)-linked hemochromatosis. Because of increased gut absorption of dietary iron, the serum plasma transferrin (Tf) of the patient with hemochromatosis becomes saturated. With no unoccupied Tf to bind incoming iron, the level of non–Tf-bound iron (NTBI) is elevated. Although the molecular nature of this NTBI is unknown, it is taken up by the parenchymal cells (primarily of liver and heart), which become severely iron overloaded. Increased intracellular iron acquired through elevated uptake either via the transferrin receptor (TfR) or via NTBI will lead to increased ferritin synthesis. In iron-overloaded individuals with hemochromatosis, serum ferritin levels are elevated. Increased Tf saturation, increased serum ferritin levels, and increased iron deposition in liver parenchymal cells are the most common indices of hemochromatosis. Excess intracellular iron can engage in oxidative reactions leading to lipid peroxidation, which in turn might be responsible for increased lysosome lability. In liver, the oxidative damage induced by excess iron is thought to cause fibrosis and to lead to an increased incidence of hepatocellular carcinoma in individuals with hemochromatosis.

cell types are acting to increase circulating iron levels, either by releasing iron in the case of the macrophage or by excessively absorbing iron from the intestinal lumen in the case of duodenal mucosal cells.

At present, the C282Y mutation in HFE accounts for approximately 85 per cent of cases of hereditary hemochromatosis.[231, 243] Targeted disruption of the murine homologue of HFE produces a mouse model for hemochromatosis, verifying that the C282Y mutation produces a loss of function of HFE rather than a gain of function.[244] It is possible that the remaining 15 per cent of cases will be attributable to abnormalities of other proteins that function in the same pathway as HFE. Even though all hemochromatosis patients cannot be identified by sequencing of HFE, a simple diagnostic test using polymerase chain reaction (PCR) from DNA in a blood sample or a buccal smear can be used in screening,[245] thus sparing patients a liver biopsy, in which detection of parenchymal iron staining is often used to verify a diagnosis of hemochromatosis.

β₂m Knockout Mice

Even before the disease gene for hereditary hemochromatosis was discovered and recognized to be an atypical class I gene, it was clear that β_2m was a likely participant in a protein complex important in regulation of iron metabolism. Mice engineered to lack β_2m expression developed significant iron overload similar in distribution to the iron overload of hereditary hemochromatosis in that parenchymal cells are observed to be overloaded with iron whereas Kupffer cells are not.[246, 247] However, when β_2m$(-/-)$ animals were reconstituted with normal bone marrow, Kupffer cells became iron overloaded. These observations indicate that primary abnormalities are present both in the cells of the intestinal mucosa and in macrophages of the β_2m$(-/-)$ animals, but that the macrophages derived from the transplanted marrow function normally to sequester iron in animals that are iron overloaded as a result of intestinal misregulation.[82]

African Iron Overload

Iron overload is prevalent in Africa in Bantu populations who consume a form of traditional beer that is brewed in steel drums. Genetic predisposition to iron overload, which was initially thought to be entirely attributable to environmental factors, has been shown to be present in these patients.[248, 249] Mutations in the HFE gene have not been identified in affected Africans, a finding that is somewhat expected since the pattern of iron distribution in these patients is markedly different from that of hereditary hemochromatosis.[249a] The most noteworthy distinguishing characteristic is that macrophages are iron loaded in African iron overload, and parenchymal iron overload does not occur until later in the course of disease.[84] Case reports in the United States indicate that iron overload similar to African iron overload affects African-Americans.[250, 251] In several of these patients, presence of the C292Y and H63D HFE mutations has been excluded, indicating that the iron overload is not attributable to white gene admixture. Another iron homeostasis gene may be abnormal in these patients, and it will be important to continue to evaluate candidate genes as

new genes involved in iron homeostasis are cloned. Since iron overload can lead to cardiovascular disease, diabetes, and cancer, it will be important in the future to determine whether iron overload contributes to the prevalence of these disorders in the African-American population.

Aceruloplasminemia

Ceruloplasmin (Cp) is a 130 kD serum protein that catalyzes oxidation of ferrous to ferric iron (ferroxidase activity).[252] Six Cu^{2+} ions are bound per protein, and copper incorporation is necessary for ferroxidase function. By oxidizing ferrous iron, ceruloplasmin accelerates incorporation of iron into apotransferrin. Copper-deficient swine develop hypoferremia, which is thought to arise from impaired ability of the duodenal mucosa, the reticuloendothelial cell, and hepatocytes to release iron to the plasma.[253] Iron release from cells may be facilitated by the formation of a negative concentration gradient created by ceruloplasmin-mediated oxidation of ferrous iron and binding of ferric iron to transferrin. Thus, absence of functional ceruloplasmin might be expected to result in iron overload in tissues that export elemental iron, such as duodenal mucosal cells and reticuloendothelial cells.

A mutation in the ceruloplasmin gene leads to systemic hemosiderosis in humans, with particularly impressive accumulations of iron occurring in the brain, liver, heart, kidney, spleen, and thyroid gland. Clinically, these patients develop cerebellar ataxia, choreoathetosis, diabetes mellitus, and retinal degeneration. In the brain, prominent neuronal loss is observed in the striatum and dentate nucleus.[254] The mechanism of iron accumulation in these tissues is not clear since the accumulation of iron occurs in many tissues that are not recognized to have specific pathways for excretion of elemental iron. In conjunction with an uncharacterized transporter protein synthesized in response to iron depletion, Cp also appears to facilitate transferrin receptor–independent iron uptake in cells.[255] Because this process appears to be iron regulated, it also does not explain the development of iron overload in the tissues affected in aceruloplasminemia. However, the absence of plasma ferroxidase activity may mean that ferrous iron remains in the circulation and can be taken up by cells by a route that is not subject to regulation, such as ion channels on plasma membranes. Analogous to the role of non–transferrin-bound iron in hemochromatosis, aceruloplasminemia could result in accumulation of NTBI that would differ from the NTBI pool of hemochromatotics and atransferrinemic mice in that it would contain more ferrous iron, which is oxidized slowly in serum in the absence of ceruloplasmin. When ferrous iron is injected in copper-deficient swine that lack functional ceruloplasmin, the iron is rapidly cleared from the circulation, whereas in normal animals, much more iron is retained in the plasma 10 minutes after injection because it has been oxidized and bound to serum transferrin.[252]

Congenital Hypotransferrinemia

In both humans and mice, a syndrome has been described in which a marked decrease in serum transferrin levels leads to parenchymal iron overload.[256, 257] In mice, hypotransferrinemia results from a splicing abnormality in which the mature transferrin transcript retains several introns and does not give rise to normal transferrin protein.[258] These mice have less than 2 per cent normal transferrin levels, and survival is markedly compromised without treatment. However, these mice can remain viable if they receive weekly doses of normal transferrin from serum injections. Measurements of uptake of iron from the gut lumen into the duodenal mucosa and the whole animal reveal that iron uptake is markedly increased in hypotransferrinemic mice. Since transferrin levels are extremely low, the newly absorbed iron is not bound to transferrin, and it is taken up by tissues that have a non–transferrin-dependent iron uptake system. Hepatic cells can take up iron that is not bound to transferrin; in animals lacking transferrin, the majority of a dose of intravenously injected ^{59}Fe is taken up by the liver within 30 seconds, whereas Tf-bound iron has a half-life in the circulation of 50 minutes.[259] Thus, the marked deposition of parenchymal iron in hepatic cells in these mice reflects the presence of an uptake system for non–transferrin-bound iron in hepatic cells, although the molecular basis of uptake of non–transferrin-bound iron is not yet established. The fact that duodenal absorption of iron is abnormally increased in hypotransferrinemic mice implies that transferrin is required for the correct sensing of total body iron stores by mucosal cells. Atransferrinemic mice develop severe microcytic anemia, a fact that has been taken as evidence that erythroid precursors obtain iron solely from serum transferrin.[260]

Hypoxia

Duodenal absorption of iron is also markedly increased in hypoxic animals. The timing of increased iron uptake is biphasic; within 6 hours of onset of hypoxia, large increases in uptake into the cells of the duodenal mucosa are measured, but transfer from mucosal cells into the circulation is delayed, with no substantial movement of iron into the plasma until 20 hours after onset of hypoxia.[261] The temporal distinction between iron uptake into the intestinal mucosa versus transfer into the serum is consistent with a long-held belief that the process of initial uptake into the mucosal cell is mediated by a process that is regulated differently from that involved in the transfer of iron across the basolateral membrane into the serum. Changes in duodenal iron uptake under hypoxic conditions occur independently of changes in erythropoiesis and appear to depend on a direct local effect on the intestinal mucosa. Until recently, it was impossible to speculate on the nature of the direct effect because the mechanism of intestinal iron uptake was not understood. However, since the intestinal iron transporter has now been cloned and characterized, the presence of an IRE in the 3′UTR raises the question of whether stabilization of IRP2 in hypoxic cells may contribute to stabilization of the intestinal transporter transcript and increased expression.

Ineffective Erythropoiesis

The ineffective erythropoiesis associated with thalassemia leads to parenchymal iron overload, even when transfusions have not been received. Animals subjected to exchange transfusion with blood high in reticulocyte content experience a rapid increase in iron absorption,[262] but increased erythropoiesis alone is not a sufficient stimulus to increase intestinal iron uptake.[263] Increased iron uptake is seen when erythropoiesis is ineffective, raising the question as to whether the gut mucosa is sensing another variable associated with ineffective erythropoiesis such as hypoxia.

Portacaval Shunts

Creation of portacaval shunts in cirrhotic patients has been reported to lead to profound iron overload within a relatively short time frame,[264, 265] but the mechanism of iron overload is not understood.

Heme Oxygenase-I Deficiency

When heme oxygenase-1 (HO1) function is knocked out in mice, iron overload develops prominently in Kupffer cells, the tissue macrophages of the liver, and to a lesser extent parenchymal cells of the liver and renal cortex.[266, 267] The pathophysiological characteristics of iron overload in these mice are not yet understood.

SLA Mice

In the cells of the polarized epithelium of the duodenal mucosa, the gene responsible for iron uptake from the intestinal lumen, DCT1 or Nramp2, has been unequivocally identified. Another gene product that can transport iron from within the cell to the extracellular space must be present at the basolateral membrane. A disease gene that produces severe X-linked anemia in mice, the sex-linked anemia gene (sla), is likely to carry a mutation in this gene,[255, 256] but positional cloning efforts have not yet led to its identification. Not only does this gene have an important role in iron transport across the basolateral membrane, but it also appears to play an important role in transfer of iron across the placenta to the fetus.[256] Numerous studies have shown that iron accumulates abnormally in the intestinal mucosal cells in sla mice while the mice develop marked iron deficiency. Tracer iron that is injected intravenously is also abnormally retained by the mucosal cells of sla mice, indicating that intestinal mucosal cells normally take up iron from serum transferrin and then recycle the iron back to the serum.

Mitochondrial Iron Homeostasis

Recently, a gene that can lead to mitochondrial iron overload in yeast was identified in a genetic screen that selected for multicopy suppressors of mutants unable to grow on iron-limited medium. The yeast gene that corrected the low-iron growth defect was found to be homologous to the gene for Friedreich's ataxia, which had been identified by positional cloning but for which there was no known function. The human homologue, termed frataxin, localizes to the mitochondria and appears to be important in protecting mitochondria from iron overload.[268] In Friedreich's ataxia, levels of frataxin mRNA decrease in 98 per cent of affected patients as a result of expansion of a GAA repeat in the first intron, and loss of functional protein results in marked mitochondrial iron overload.[269] Deletions in mitochondrial DNA are found, presumably as a result of damage to DNA from iron-catalyzed Fenton chemical processes. Affected tissues, including the heart, spinal cord, and dorsal root ganglia, are tissues in which frataxin transcription is highest. Deficiencies of a number of iron-sulfur enzymes of the mitochondria have been detected, leading to a suggestion that increased oxidative stress associated with mitochondrial iron overload leads to disassembly of iron-sulfur clusters and decreases in activity of critical enzymes.[269]

Ringed sideroblasts in sideroblastic anemia are now recognized to represent iron-loaded mitochondria that are perinuclear in distribution.[270] Little else is presently understood about why the mitochondria become iron overloaded in sideroblastic anemias, but the role of the mitochondria in causing sideroblastic anemia has been supported by the discovery of deletions of the mitochondrial genome in Pearson's syndrome, a multisystem mitochondrial disorder in which refractory sideroblastic anemia is found.[271]

Hereditary Hyperferritinemia and Bilateral Cataract Syndrome

Recently, a genetic syndrome has been described in which mutations in the IRE for the ferritin L chain lead to high ferritin L chain synthesis and bilateral cataract formation.[272, 273] Affected individuals were initially identified because high serum ferritin levels led to clinical suspicion of iron overload, but further testing indicated that these individuals were not iron overloaded; patients became rapidly iron depleted while undergoing a therapeutic phlebotomy program. Different IRE mutations impair binding of IRPs to differing degrees, leading to a range in the severity of cataracts and magnitude of hyperferritinemia (Fig. 10–13).[274, 275] The high serum ferritin levels in this syndrome are consistent with the conclusion that serum ferritin is derived from ferritin L chain expression. The pathophysiological mechanism of cataract formation is not yet understood in these patients, but it is intriguing to speculate that high secretion of a protein into the poorly perfused lens may result in lens clouding because there may be few mechanisms for removal of the secreted protein.

Mechanisms of Tissue Damage by Iron

Although many hypotheses have been advanced to explain specific features of tissue iron toxicity, there is general agreement that the fundamental problems in iron toxicity relate to the harmful effects of hydroxyl radicals generated in the reaction of ferrous iron with oxygen species.[276] Highly reactive free radicals abstract electrons from lipids, proteins, and nucleic acids, leading to loss of integrity of complex molecules and membranes. Lysosomal membranes are thought to be among the membranes damaged by iron overload, and a consequence of lysosomal damage could be release of hydrolytic enzymes to the cytosol. Little is known about the exact composition of the hemosiderin in iron-overloaded cells or the mechanisms by which it is resorbed over time. Improvements in techniques used in measuring free iron, free radicals, and oxidized lipids and proteins will likely provide further insights into iron toxicity in the future.

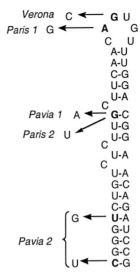

Figure 10–13. Mutations of the ferritin light (L) chain iron-responsive element (IRE) found in the hereditary hyperferritinemia–bilateral cataract syndrome. Mutations in the IRE of ferritin L chain lead to hyperferritinemia because of decreased affinity for binding of iron regulatory proteins (IRPs). The mutations in the loop, Verona[109] and Paris 1,[108] are likely to represent sites of contact of the protein, whereas the mutations in the stem (Pavia 1, Pavia 2,[111] and Paris 2[109]) are more likely to interfere with IRP recognition by interfering with correct folding and secondary structure of the IRE. (From Allerson, C. R., Cazzola, M., and Rouault, T. A.: Clinical severity and thermodynamic effects of iron-responsive element mutations in hereditary hyperferritinemia-cataract syndrome. J. Biol. Chem. 274(37):26439, 1999.)

Perspectives and Future Directions

Although much progress has been made in understanding the molecular details of iron metabolism, description of iron metabolism in molecular terms remains far from complete. In particular, the genes that are responsible for export of elemental iron from the cells of the intestinal mucosa and the macrophage have not yet been cloned, and therefore the regulation of these proteins cannot yet be studied. The mechanisms that explain iron uptake in the placenta, brain, and testis are also not yet understood, and much remains to be learned about the processes involved in sequestration and export of iron from macrophages. Mitochondrial iron homeostasis is clearly an area that will be important in the future, particularly since deposition of iron in mitochondria is associated with numerous human diseases. It is quite likely that the insights into iron metabolism that will be gained in the years ahead will significantly improve understanding and treatment of many human diseases.

REFERENCES

1. Bothwell, T. H., Charlton, R. W., Cook, J. D., and Finch, C. A.: Iron Metabolism in Man. Oxford, Blackwell Scientific Publications, 1979.
2. Emmery, T.: Iron metabolism in humans and plants. Am. Sci. 70:626, 1982.
3. London, I.: Iron and heme: Crucial carriers and catalysts. *In* Wintrobe, M. M. (ed.): Blood, Pure and Eloquent. New York, McGraw-Hill Book Co., 1980.
4. Lewin, R.: How micro-organisms transport iron. Science 225:401, 1984.

5. Crichton, R. R.: Inorganic Biochemistry of Iron Metabolism. New York, Ellis Horwood, 1991.
6. Singh, S., Hider, R. C., and Porter, J. B.: Separation and identification of desferrioxamine and its iron chelating metabolites by high-performance liquid chromatography and fast atom bombardment mass spectrometry: Choice of complexing agent and application to biological fluids. Anal. Biochem. 187:212, 1990.
7. Neilands, J. B., Bindereif, A., and Montgomerie, J. Z.: Genetic basis of iron assimilation in pathogenic *Escherichia coli*. Curr. Top. Microbiol. Immunol. 118:179, 1985.
8. Stearman, R. D. S., Yuan, T., Yamaguchi-Iwai Y., Klausner, R. D., and Dancis, A.: A permease-oxidase complex involved in high-affinity iron uptake in yeast [see comments]. Science 271:1552, 1996.
9. Yamaguchi-Iwai, Y., Stearman, R., Dancis, A., and Klausner, R. D.: Iron-regulated DNA binding by the AFT1 protein controls the iron regulon in yeast. EMBO J. 15:3377, 1996.
10. Askwith, C., Eide, D., Van Ho, A., Bernard, P. S., Li, L., Davis-Kaplan, S., Sipe, D. M., and Kaplan, J.: The FET3 gene of S. cerevisiae encodes a multicopper oxidase required for ferrous iron uptake. Cell 76:403, 1994.
11. Finch, C. A., and Huebers, H. A.: Iron metabolism. Clin. Physiol. Biochem. 4:5, 1986.
12. Hallberg, L.: Bioavailability of dietary iron in man. Annu. Rev. Nutr. 1:123, 1981.
13. Van Dijk, J. P.: Regulatory aspects of placental iron transfer: A comparative study. Placenta 9:315, 1988.
14. Finch, C. A., and Huebers, H.: Perspectives in iron metabolism. N. Engl. J. Med. 306:1520, 1982.
15. Weintraub, L. R., Conrad, M. E., and Crosby, W. H.: Regulation of the intestinal absorption of iron by the rate of erythropoiesis. Br. J. Haematol. 11:432, 1965.
16. Finch, C. A., Deubelbeiss, K., Cook, J. D., Eachbach, J. W., Harker, L. A., Funk, D. D., Marsaglia, G., Hilman, R. S., Slichter, S., Adamson, J. W., Ganzoni, A., and Biblett, E. R.: Ferrokinetics in man. Medicine 49:17, 1970.
17. Morgan, E. H.: Transferrin: Biochemistry, physiology and clinical significance. Mol. Aspects Med. 4:1, 1981.
18. Garby, L., and Noyes, W. D.: Studies on hemoglobin metabolism. II. Pathways of hemoglobin iron metabolism in normal man. J. Clin. Invest. 38:1484, 1959.
19. Hershko, C., Cook, J. D., and Finch, C. A.: Storage iron kinetics. II. The uptake of hemoglobin iron by hepatic parenchymal cells. J. Lab. Clin. Med. 80:624, 1972.
20. Deiss, A.: Iron metabolism in reticuloendothelial cells. Semin. Hematol. 20:81, 1983.
21. Uchida, T., Akitsuki, T., Kimura, H., Tanaka, T., Matsuda, S., and Kariyone, S.: Relationship among plasma iron, plasma iron turnover, and reticuloendothelial iron release. Blood 61:799, 1983.
22. Smith, A., and Morgan, W. T.: Hemopexin-mediated heme transport to the liver: Evidence for a heme-binding protein in liver plasma membranes. J. Biol. Chem. 260:8325, 1985.
23. Kino, K., Tsunoo, H., Higa, Y., Takami, M., Hamaguchi, H., and Nakajima, H.: Hemoglobin receptor in rat liver plasma membrane. J. Biol. Chem. 255:9161, 1980.
24. Kino, K., Tsunoo, H., Higa, Y., Takami, H., and Nakajima, H.: Kinetic aspects of hemoglobin: Haptoglobin-receptor interaction in rat liver plasma membranes, isolated liver cells, and liver cells in primary culture. J. Biol. Chem. 257:4828, 1982.
25. Lowe, M. E., and Ashwell, G.: Solubilization and assay of an hepatic receptor for the haptoglobin-hemoglobin complex. Arch. Biochem. Biophys. 216:704, 1982.
26. Mack, U., Powell, L. W., and Halliday, J. W.: Detection and isolation of a hepatic membrane receptor for ferritin. J. Biol. Chem. 258:4672, 1983.
27. Bacon, B. R., and Tavill, A. S.: Role of the liver in normal iron metabolism. Semin. Liver Dis. 4:181, 1984.
28. Aisen, P.: Transferrin metabolism and the liver. Semin. Liver Dis. 4:193, 1984.
29. Aisen, P.: Transferrin and the alcoholic liver. Hepatology 5:902, 1985.
30. Fawwaz, R. A., Winchell, H. S., Pollycove, M., and Sargent, T.: Hepatic iron deposition in humans. I. First-pass hepatic deposition of intestinally absorbed iron in patients with low plasma latent iron-binding capacity. Blood 30:417, 1967.
31. Aisen, P., and Brown, E. B.: Structure and function of transferrin. *In* Brown, E. B. (ed.): Progress in Hematology. New York, Grune & Stratton, 1975.
32. Williams, J.: The structure of transferrins. *In* Spik, G., Montreuil, J., Crichton, R. R., and Mazurier, J. (eds.): Proteins of Iron Storage and Transport. New York, Elsevier Science Publishing Co., 1985.
33. Uzan, G., Frain, M., Park, I., Besmond, C., Maessen, G., Triepat, J. S., Zakin, M. M., and Kahn, A.: Molecular cloning and sequence analysis of cDNA for human transferrin. Biochem. Biophys. Res. Commun. 119:273, 1984.
34. Yang, F., Lum, J. B., McGill, J. R., Moore, C. M., Naylor, S. L., van Bragt, P. H., Baldwin, W. D., and Bowman, B. H.: Human transferrin: cDNA characterization and chromosomal localization. Proc. Natl. Acad. Sci. USA 81:2752, 1984.
35. Park, I., Schaeffer, E., Sidoli, A., Baralle, F. E., Cohen, G. N., and Zakin, M. M.: Organization of the human transferrin gene: Direct evidence that it originated by gene duplication. Proc. Natl. Acad. Sci. USA 82:3149, 1985.
36. Schaeffer, E., Park, I., Cohen, G. N., and Zakin, M. M.: Organization of the human serum transferrin gene. *In* Spik, G., Montreuil, J., Crichton, R. R., and Mazurier, J. (eds.): Structure and Function of Transferrins. New York, Elsevier Science Publishing Co., 1985, p. 361.
37. Huerre, C., Uzan, G., Grzeschik, K. H., Weil, D., Levin, M., Hors-Cayla, M. C., Boue, J., Kahn, A., and Junien, C.: The structural gene for transferrin (TF) maps to 3q21m3qter. Ann. Genet. (Paris) 27:5, 1984.
38. Aisen, P., and Listowski, I.: Iron transport and storage proteins. Annu. Rev. Biochem. 49:357, 1980.
39. Williams, J.: The evolution of transferrin. Trends Biol. Sci. 2:394, 1982.
40. Wang, A. C., and Sutton, H. E.: Human transferrins C and D1: Chemical differences in a peptide. Science 149:435, 1965.
41. Richardson, D. R., and Ponka, P.: The molecular mechanisms of the metabolism and transport of iron in normal and neoplastic cells. Biochim. Biophys. Acta 1331:1, 1997.
42. Aisen, P., Leibman, A., and Zweier, J.: Stoichiometric and site characteristics of the binding of iron to human transferrin. J. Biol. Chem. 253:1930, 1978.
43. Huebers, H. A., Huebers, E., Csiba, E., and Finch, C. A.: Heterogeneity of the plasma iron pool: Explanation of the Fletcher-Huehns phenomenon. Am. J. Physiol. 247:R280, 1984.
44. Huebers, H., Csiba, E., Huebers, E., and Finch, C. A.: Molecular advantage of diferric transferrin in delivering iron to reticulocytes: A comparative study. Proc. Soc. Exp. Biol. Med. 179:222, 1985.
45. Bali, P. K., Zak, O., and Aisen, P.: A new role for the transferrin receptor in release of iron from transferrin. Biochemistry 30:324, 1991.
46. Bali, P. K., and Aisen, P.: Receptor-modulated iron release from transferrin: Differential effects on the N- and C-terminal sites. Biochemistry 30:9947, 1991.
47. Mason, A. B., Tam, B. M., Woodworth, R. C., Oliver, R. W., Green, B. N., Lin, L. N., Brandts, J. F., Savage, K. J., Lineback, J. A., and MacGillivray, R. T.: Receptor recognition sites reside in both lobes of human serum transferrin. Biochem J 326:77, 1997.
48. Morgan, E. H., and Peters, T., Jr.: The biosynthesis of rat transferrin: Evidence for rapid glycosylation, disulfide bond formation, and tertiary folding. J. Biol. Chem. 260:14793, 1985.
49. Bloch, B., Popovici, T., Levin, M. J., Tuil, D., and Kahn, A.: Transferrin gene expression visualized in oligodendrocytes of the rat brain by using in situ hybridization and immunohistochemistry. Proc. Natl. Acad. Sci. USA 82:6706, 1985.
50. Levin, M. J., Tuil, D., Uzan, G., Dreyfus, J. C., and Kahn, A.: Expression of the transferrin gene during development of non-hepatic tissues: High level of transferrin mRNA in fetal muscle and adult brain. Biochem. Biophys. Res. Commun. 122:212, 1984.
51. Skinner, M. K., Cosand, W. L., and Griswold, M. D.: Purification and characterization of testicular transferrin secreted by rat Sertoli cells. Biochem. J. 218:313, 1984.
52. McKnight, G. S., Lee, D. C., Hemmaplardh, D., Finch, C. A., and Palmiter, R. D.: Transferrin gene expression: Effects of nutritional iron deficiency. J. Biol. Chem. 255:144, 1980.
53. Idzerda, R. L., Huebers, H., Finch, C. A., and McKnight, G. S.: Rat transferrin gene expression: Tissue-specific regulation by iron deficiency. Proc. Natl. Acad. Sci. USA 83:3723, 1986.
54. Jandl, J. H., and Katz, J. H.: The plasma to cell cycle of transferrin. J. Clin. Invest. 42:314, 1963.
55. Debanne, M. T., Chindemi, P. A., and Regoeczi, E.: Binding of

asialotransferrins by purified rat liver plasma membranes. J. Biol. Chem. 256:4929, 1981.

56. Young, S. P., Bomford, A., and Williams, R.: Dual pathways for the uptake of rat asialotransferrin by rat hepatocytes. J. Biol. Chem. 258:4972, 1983.

57. Schneider, C., Sutherland, R., Newman, R., and Greaves, M.: Structural features of the cell surface receptor for transferrin that is recognized by the monoclonal antibody OKT9. J. Biol. Chem. 257:8516, 1982.

58. Omary, M. B., and Trowbridge, I. S.: Biosynthesis of the human transferrin receptor in cultured cells. J. Biol. Chem. 256:12888, 1981.

59. Schneider, C., Owen, M. J., Banville, D., and Williams, J. G.: Primary structure of human transferrin receptor deduced from the mRNA sequence. Nature 311:675, 1984.

60. Kuhn, L. C., McClelland, A., and Ruddle, F. H.: Gene transfer, expression, and molecular cloning of the human transferrin receptor gene. Cell 37:95, 1984.

61. McClelland, A., Kuhn, L. C., and Ruddle, F. H.: The human transferrin receptor gene: Genomic organization, and the complete primary structure of the receptor deduced for a cDNA sequence. Cell 39:267, 1984.

62. Seligman, P. A., Schleicher, R. B., and Allen, R. H.: Isolation and characterization of the transferrin receptor from human placenta. J. Biol. Chem. 254:9943, 1979.

63. Enns, C. A., and Sussman, H. H.: Physical characterization of the transferrin receptor in human placentae. J. Biol. Chem. 256:9820, 1980.

64. Harford, J. B., Casey, J. L., Koeller, D. M., and Klausner, R. D.: Structure, function and regulation of the transferrin receptor: Insights from molecular biology. *In* Steer, C. J., and Hanover, J. A. (eds.): Intracellular Trafficking of Proteins. Cambridge, Cambridge University Press, 1991.

65. Zerial, M., Melancon, P. M., Schneider, C., and Garoff, H.: The transmembrane sequence of the transferrin receptor functions as a signal peptide. EMBO J. 5:1543, 1986.

66. Omary, M. B., and Trowbridge, I. S.: Covalent binding of fatty acid to the transferrin receptor in cultured human cells. J. Biol. Chem. 256:4715, 1981.

67. Gray, A., Dull, T. J., and Ullrich, A.: Nucleotide sequence of epidermal growth factor cDNA predicts a 128,000-molecular weight protein precursor. Nature 303:722, 1983.

68. Miller, Y. E., Jones, C., Scoggin, C., Morse, H., and Seligman, P.: Chromosome 3q (22-ter) encodes the human transferrin receptor. Am. J. Hum. Genet. 35:573, 1983.

69. Rabin, M., McClelland, A., Kuhn, L., and Ruddle, F. H.: Regional localization of the human transferrin receptor gene to 3q26mqter. Am. J. Hum. Genet. 37:1112, 1985.

70. Plowman, G. D., Brown, J. P., Enns, C. A., Schroder, J., Nikinmaa, B., Sussman, H. H., and Hellstrom, K. E.: Assignment of the gene for human melanoma-associated antigen to chromosome 3. Nature 303:70, 1983.

71. Casey, J. L., Di Jeso, B., Rao, K., Klausner, R. D., and Harford, J. B.: Deletional analysis of the promoter region of the transferrin receptor. Nucleic Acids Res. 16:629, 1988.

72. Roberts, M. R., Miskimins, W. K., and Ruddle, F. H.: Nuclear proteins TREF-1 and TREF-2 bind to the transcriptional control element of the transferrin receptor gene and appear to be associated as a heterodimer. Cell Regul. 1:151, 1989.

73. Morgan, E. H., and Appleton, T. C.: Autoradiographic location of ^{125}I-labeled transferrin in rabbit reticulocytes. Nature 223:1371, 1969.

74. Sullivan, A. L., Grasso, J. A., and Weintraub, L. R.: Micropinocytosis of transferrin by developing red cells: An electron microscopic study utilizing ferritin-conjugates antibodies to transferrin. Blood 47:133, 1976.

75. Sandoval I. V., Bakke O. 1994. Targeting of membrane proteins to endosomes and lysosomes. Trends Cell Biol. 4:292–297.

76. Trowbridge, I. S., Collawn, J. F., and Hopkins, C. R.: Signal-dependent membrane protein trafficking in the endocytic pathway. Annu. Rev. Cell Biol. 9:129, 1993.

77. Bessis, M.: Cytologic aspects of hemoglobin production. Harvey Lect. 58:125, 1963.

78. Roth, T. F., and Porter, K. R.: Yolk protein uptake in the oocyte of the mosquito *Aedes aegypti*. L. J. Cell Biol. 20:313, 1964.

79. Pastan, I., and Willingham, M. C.: The pathway of endocytosis. *In* Pastan, I., and Willingham, M. D. (eds.): Endocytosis. New York, Plenum Press, 1985.

80. Pearse, B. M. F.: On the structural and functional components of coated vesicles. J. Mol. Biol. 126:803, 1978.

81. Steer, C. J., and Heuser, J.: Clathrin and coated vesicles: Critical determinants of intracellular trafficking. *In* Steer, C. J., and Hanover, J. A. (eds.): Intracellular Trafficking of Proteins. Cambridge, Cambridge University Press, 1991.

82. Helenius, A., Mellman, I. L., Wall, D., and Hubbard, A.: Endosomes. Trends Biochem. Sci. 8:245, 1983.

83. Brown, M. S., Anderson, R. G. W., and Goldstein, J. L.: Recycling receptors: The round-trip itinerary of migrant membrane proteins. Cell 32:663, 1983.

84. Tycko, B., and Maxfield, F. R.: Rapid acidification of endocytic vesicles containing alpha-macroglobulin. Cell 28:643, 1982.

85. Harford, J., Wolkoff, A., Ashwell, G., and Klausner, R. D.: Intracellular dissociation of receptor-bound asialoglycoproteins in cultured hepatocytes. J. Cell Biol. 258:3191, 1983.

86. Galloway, C. J., Dean, G. E., Marsh, M., Rudnick, G., and Mellman, I.: Acidification of macrophage and fibroblast endocytic vesicles *in vitro*. Proc. Natl. Acad. Sci. USA 80:3343, 1983.

87. Karin, M., and Minz, B.: Receptor-mediated endocytosis of transferrin developmentally totipotent mouse teratocarcinoma cells. J. Biol. Chem. 256:3245, 1981.

88. Bleil, J. D., and Bretscher, M. S.: Transferrin receptor and its recycling in HeLa cells. EMBO J. 1:351, 1982.

89. Klausner, R. D., van Renswoude, J., Ashwell, G., Kempf, C., Schreichter, A. N., Dean, A., and Bridges, K. R.: Receptor-mediated endocytosis of transferrin K562 cells. J. Biol. Chem. 258:4715, 1983.

90. Lacopetta, B. J., Morgan, E. H., and Yeoh, G. C. T.: Receptor-mediated endocytosis of transferrin by developing erythroid cells from the fetal rat liver. J. Histochem. Cytochem. 31:336, 1983.

91. Ciechanover, A., Schwartz, A. L., Dautry-Varsat, A., and Lodish, H. F.: Kinetics of internalization and recycling of transferrin and the transferrin receptor in a human hepatoma cell line. J. Biol. Chem. 258:9681, 1983.

92. Van Renswoude, J. K., Bridges, K. R., Harford, J. B., and Klausner, R. D.: Receptor-mediated endocytosis of transferrin and the uptake of Fe in K562 cells: Identification of a non-lysosomal acidic compartment. Proc. Natl. Acad. Sci. USA 79:6186, 1982.

93. Klausner, R. D., Ashwell, G., van Renswoude, J., Harford, J. B., and Bridges, K. R.: Binding of apotransferrin to K562 cells: Explanation of the transferrin cycle. Proc. Natl. Acad. Sci. USA 80:2263, 1983.

94. Duatry-Varsat, A., Ciechanover, A., and Lodish, H. F.: pH and the recycling of transferrin during receptor-mediated endocytosis. Proc. Natl. Acad. Sci. USA 80:2258, 1983.

95. Morgan, E. H.: Inhibition of reticulocyte iron uptake by NH_4Cl and CH_3NH_2. Biochim. Biophys. Acta 642:119, 1981.

96. Rao, K., van Renswoude, J., Kempf, C., and Klausner, R. D.: Separation of Fe^{3+} from transferrin in endocytosis: Role of the acidic endosome. FEBS Lett. 160:213, 1983.

97. Klausner, R. D., van Renswoude, J., Kempf, C., Rao, K., Bateman, J. L., and Robbins, A. R.: Failure to release iron from transferrin in a Chinese hamster ovary cell mutant pleiotropically defective in endocytosis. J. Cell Biol. 98:1098, 1984.

98. Lebron, J. A., Bennett, M. J., Vaughn, D. E., Chirino, A. J., Snow, P. M., Mintier, G. A., Feder, J. N., and Bjorkman, P. J.: Crystal structure of the hemochromatosis protein HFE and characterization of its interaction with the transferrin receptor. Cell 93:111, 1998.

99. Graslund, A., Ehrenberg, A., and Thelander, L.: Characterization of the free radical mammalian ribonucleotide reductase. J. Biol. Chem. 257:5711, 1982.

100. Robbins, E., and Pederson, T.: Iron: Its intracellular localization and possible role in cell division. Proc. Natl. Acad. Sci. USA 66:1244, 1970.

101. Stragand, J. J., and Hagemann, R. F.: An iron requirement for the synchronous progression of colonic cells following fasting and refeeding. Cell Tissue Kinet. 11:513, 1978.

102. Soyano, A., Chinea, M., and Romano, E. L.: The effect of desferrioxamine on the proliferative response of rat lymphocytes stimulated with various mitogens *in vitro*. Immunopharmacology 8:163, 1984.

103. Lederman, H. M., Cohen, A., Lee, J. W., Freedman, M. H., and Gelfand, E. W.: Deferoxamine: A reversible S-phase inhibitor of human lymphocyte proliferation. Blood 64:748, 1984.

104. Larrick, J. W., and Creswell, P.: Modulation of cell surface iron transferrin receptors by cellular density and state of activation. J. Supramol. Struct. 11:579, 1979.

105. Trowbridge, I. S., and Omary, M. B.: Human cell surface glycoprotein related to cell proliferation is the receptor for transferrin. Proc. Natl. Acad. Sci. USA 78:3039, 1981.

106. Chitambar, C. R., Massey, E. J., and Seligman, P. A.: Regulation of transferrin receptor expression on human leukemic cells during proliferation and induction of differentiation: Effects of gallium and dimethylsulfoxide. J. Clin. Invest. 72:1314, 1983.

107. Hu, H. Y., Gardner, J., and Aisen, P.: Inducibility of transferrin receptors on friend leukemia cells. Science 197:559, 1977.

108. Kronke, M., Leonard, W. J., Depper, J. M., and Greene, W. C.: Sequential expression of genes involved in human T lymphocyte growth and differentiation. J. Exp. Med. 161:1593, 1985.

109. Trepel, J. B., Colamonici, O. R., Kelly, K., Schwab, G., Watt, R. A., Sausville, E. A., Jaffe, E. S., and Neckers, L. M.: Transcriptional inactivation of c-myc and the transferrin receptor in dibutyryl cyclic-AMP–treated HL60 cells. Mol. Cell. Biol. 7:2644, 1987.

110. Sutherland, R., Delia, D., Schneider, C., Newman, R., Keurhead, J., and Greaves, M.: Ubiquitous cell-surface glycoprotein on tumor cells is proliferation associated receptor for transferrin. Proc. Natl. Acad. Sci. USA 78:4515, 1981.

111. Galbraith, R. M., and Galbraith, G. M.: Expression of transferrin receptors on mitogen-stimulated human peripheral blood lymphocytes: Relation to cellular activation and related metabolic events. Immunology 44:703, 1981.

112. Hamilton, T. A.: Regulation of transferrin receptor expression in concanavalin A stimulated and gross virus transformed rat lymphoblasts. J. Cell. Physiol. 113:40, 1982.

113. Wiley, H. S., and Kaplan, J.: Epidermal growth factor rapidly induces a redistribution of transferrin receptor pools in human fibroblasts. Proc. Natl. Acad. Sci. USA 81:7456, 1984.

114. Weissman, A., Rao, K., Klausner, R. D., and Harford, J. B.: Exposure of K562 cells to anti-receptor monoclonal antibody OKT9 results in rapid redistribution and enhanced degradation of the transferrin receptor. J. Cell Biol. 102:951, 1986.

115. May, W. S., Jacobs, S., and Cuatrecasas, P.: Association of phorbol ester-induced hyperphosphorylation and reversible regulation of transferrin membrane receptors in HL60 cells. Proc. Natl. Acad. Sci. USA 81:2016, 1984.

116. Klausner, R. D., Harford, J., and van Renswoude, J.: Rapid internalization of the transferrin receptor in K562 cells is triggered by ligand binding or treatment with a phorbol ester. Proc. Natl. Acad. Sci. USA 81:3005, 1984.

117. Musgrove, E., Rugg, C., Taylor, I., and Hedley, D.: Transferrin receptor expression during exponential and plateau phase growth of human tumor cells in culture. J. Cell. Physiol. 118:6, 1984.

118. Sager, P. R., Brown, P. A., and Berlin, R. D.: Analysis of transferrin recycling in mitotic and interphase HeLa cells by quantitative fluorescence microscopy. 39:275, 1984.

119. Pan, B. T., Teng, K., Wu, C., Adam, M., and Johnstone, R. M.: Electron microscopic evidence for externalization of the transferrin receptor in vesicular form in sheep reticulocytes. J. Cell Biol. 101:942, 1985.

120. Harding, C., Heuser, J., and Stahl, P.: Endocytosis and intracellular processing of transferrin and colloidal gold–transferrin in rat reticulocytes: Demonstration of a pathway for receptor shedding. Eur. J. Cell Biol. 35:256, 1984.

121. Ward, J. H., Kushner, J. P., and Kaplan, J.: Regulation of HeLa cell transferrin receptors. J. Biol. Chem. 257:10317, 1982.

122. Pelicci, P. G., Tabillio, A., Thomopoulos, P., Titieux, M., Vainchenker, W., Rochant, H., and Testa, U.: Hemin regulates the expression of transferrin receptors in human hematopoietic cell lines. FEBS Lett. 145:350, 1982.

123. Mattia, E., Rao, K., Shapiro, D. S., Sussman, H. H., and Klausner, R. D.: Biosynthetic regulation of the human transferrin receptor by desferrioxamine in K562 cells. J. Biol. Chem. 529:2689, 1984.

124. Rao, D., Harford, J. B., Rouault, T., McClelland, A., Ruddle, F. H., and Klausner, R. D.: Transcriptional regulation by iron of the gene for the transferrin receptor. Mol. Cell. Biol. 6:236, 1986.

125. Rouault, T., Rao, K., Harford, J., Mattia, E., and Klausner, R. D.: Hemin, chelatable iron and the regulation of transferrin receptor biosynthesis. J. Biol. Chem. 260:14862, 1985.

126. Owen, D., and Kühn, L. C.: Noncoding 3′ sequences of the transferrin receptor gene are required for mRNA regulation by iron. EMBO J. 6:1287, 1987.

127. Casey, J. L., Hentze, M. W., Koeller, D. M., Caughman, S. W., Rouault, T. A., Klausner, R. D., and Harford, J. B.: Iron-responsive elements: Regulatory RNA sequences that control mRNA levels and translation. Science 240:924, 1988.

128. Koeller, D. M., Casey, J. L., Hentze, E. M., Chan, L.-N. L., Klausner, R. D., and Harford, J. B.: A cytosolic protein binds to structural elements within the iron regulatory region of the transferrin receptor mRNA. Proc. Natl. Acad. Sci. USA 86:3574, 1989.

129. Chan, L.-N. L., Grammatikakis, N., Banks, J. M., and Gerhardt, E. M.: Chicken transferrin receptor gene: Conservation of the 3′ noncoding sequences and expression in erythroid cells. Nucleic Acids Res. 17:3763, 1989.

130. Munro, H. N., and Linder, M. C.: Ferritin: Structure, biosynthesis, and role in iron metabolism. Physiol. Rev. 58:317, 1978.

131. Theil, E. C.: Ferritin: Structure, gene regulation, and cellular function in animals, plants, and microorganisms. Annu. Rev. Biochem. 56:289, 1987.

132. Clegg, G. A., Fitton, J. E., Harrison, P. M., and Treffry, A.: Ferritin: Molecular structure and iron-storage mechanisms. Prog. Biophys. Mol. Biol. 36:56, 1980.

133. Ford, G. C., Harrison, P. M., Rice, D. W., Smith, J. M., Treffry, A., White, J. L., and Yariv, J.: Ferritin: Design and formation of an iron-storage molecule. Philos. Trans. R. Soc. Lond. 304:551, 1984.

134. Munro, H. N., Leibold, E. A., Vass, J. K., Aziz, N., Roges, J., Murray, M., and White, K.: Ferritin gene structure and expression. In Spik, G., Montreuil, J., Crichton, R. R., and Mazurier, J. (eds.): Proteins of Iron Storage and Transport. New York, Elsevier Science Publishing Co., 1985.

135. Drysdale, J., Jain, S. K., Boyd, D., Barrett, K. J., Vecoli, C., Belcher, D. M., Beaumont, C., Worwood, M., Lebo, R., McGill, J., and Crampton, J.: Human ferritins: Genes and proteins. In Spik, G., Montreuil, J., Crichton, R. R., and Mazurier, J. (eds.): Proteins of Iron Storage and Transport. New York, Elsevier Science Publishing Co., 1985.

136. Lebo, R. V., Kan, Y. W., Cheung, M. C., Jain, S. K., and Drysdale, J. H.: Human ferritin light chain gene sequences mapped to several sorted chromosomes. Hum. Genet. 71:325, 1985.

137. Jain, S. K., Barrett, K. J., Boyd, D., Favreau, M. F., Crampton, J., and Drysdale, J. W.: Ferritin H and L chains are derived from different multigene families. J. Biol. Chem. 260:11762, 1985.

138. Boyd, D., Vecoli, C., Belcher, D. M., Jain, S. K., and Drysdale, J. W.: Structural and functional relationships of human ferritin H and L chains deduced from cDNA clones. J. Biol. Chem. 260:11755, 1985.

139. Boyd, D., Jain, S. K., Crampton, J., Barrett, K. J., and Drysdale, J.: Isolation and characterization of a cDNA clone for human ferritin heavy chain. Proc. Natl. Acad. Sci. USA 81:4751, 1984.

140. Dorner, M. H., Salfeld, J., Will, H., Leibold, E. W., Vass, J. K., and Munro, H. N.: Structure of human ferritin light subunit messenger RNA: Comparison with heavy subunit message and functional implications. Proc. Natl. Acad. Sci. USA 82:3139, 1985.

141. Leibold, E. A., Azia, N., Brown, A. J., and Munro, H. N.: Conservation in rat liver of light and heavy subunit sequences of mammalian ferritin: Presence of unique octopeptide in the light subunit. J. Biol. Chem. 259:4327, 1984.

142. Santoro, C., Marone, M., Ferrone, M., Costanzo, F., Colombo, M., Mingvanti, C., Cortese, R., and Silengo, L.: Cloning of the gene coding for human L apoferritin. Nucleic Acids Res. 11:2863, 1986.

143. Costanzo, F., Columbo, M., Staempfli, S., Santoro, C., Marone, M., Mingvanti, C., Cortese, R., and Silengo, L.: Structure of gene and pseudogenes of human apoferritin H. Nucleic Acids Res. 11:2863, 1986.

144. Hentze, M. W., Keim, S., Papadopoulos, P., O'Brien, S., Modi, W., Drysdale, J., Leonard, W. J., Harford, J. B., and Klausner, R. D.: Cloning, characterization, expression and chromosomal localization of a human ferritin heavy chain gene. Proc. Natl. Acad. Sci. USA 83:7226, 1986.

145. Caskey, J. H., Jones, C., Miller, Y. E., and Seligman, P. A.: Human ferritin gene is assigned to chromosome 19. Proc. Natl. Acad. Sci. USA 80:482, 1983.

146. Harrison, P. M., White, J. L., Smith, J. M. A., Farrants, G. W., Ford, G. C., Rice, D. W., Addison, J. M., and Treffry, A.: Comparative aspects of ferritin structure, metal-binding and immunochemistry. In Spik, G., Montreuil, J., Crichton, R. R., and Mazurier, J. (eds.): Proteins of Iron Storage and Transport. New York, Elsevier Science Publishing Co., 1985.

147. Arosio, P., Adelman, T. G., and Drysdale, J. W.: On ferritin heterogeneity: Further evidence for heteropolymers. J. Biol. Chem. 253:4451, 1978.

148. Drysdale, J. W., Adelman, T. G., Arosio, P., Casareale, D., Fitzpatrick, P., Hazard, J. T., and Yokota, M.: Human isoferritins in normal and disease states. Semin. Hematol. 14:71, 1977.
149. Hazard, J. T., Yokota, M., Arosio, P., and Drysdale, J. W.: Immunologic differences in human isoferritins: Implications for immunologic quantitation of serum ferritin. Blood 49:139, 1977.
150. Rucker, P., Torti, F. M., and Torti, S. V.: Role of H and L subunits in Mouse Ferritin. J. Biol. Chem. 271:33352, 1996.
151. Didsbury, J. R., Theil, E. C., Kaufman, R. E., and Dickey, L. F.: Multiple red cell ferritin mRNAs, which code for an abundant protein in the embryonic cell type, analyzed by cDNA sequence and by primer extension of the 5′-untranslated regions. J. Biol. Chem. 261:949, 1986.
152. Worwood, M.: Ferritin. Blood Rev. 4:250, 1990.
153. Bomford, A., Conlon-Hollingshead, C., and Munro, H. M.: Adaptive responses of rat tissue isoferritins to iron administration: Changes in subunit synthesis, isoferritin abundance, and capacity for iron storage. J. Biol. Chem. 256:948, 1981.
154. Mertz, J. R., and Theil, E. C.: Subunit dimers in sheep spleen apoferritin: The effect on iron storage. J. Biol. Chem. 258:11719, 1983.
155. Treffry, A., Lee, P. J., and Harrison, P. M.: Iron-induced changes in rat liver isoferritins. Biochem. J. 220:717, 1984.
156. Treffry, A., Zhao, Z., Quail, M. A., Guest, J. R., and Harrison, P. M.: Dinuclear center of ferritin: Studies of iron binding and oxidation show differences in the two iron sites. Biochemistry 36:432, 1997.
157. Funk, F., Lenders, J. P., Crichton, R. R., and Schneider, W.: Reductive mobilization of ferritin iron. Eur. J. Biochem. 152:167, 1985.
158. Pape, L., Multani, J. S., Stitt, C., and Saltman, P.: The mobilization of iron from ferritin by chelating agents. Biochemistry 7:613, 1968.
159. Weir, M. P., Gibson, J. F., and Peters, T. J.: Biochemical studies on the isolation and characterization of human spleen haemosiderin. Biochem. J. 223:31, 1984.
160. Aziz, N., and Munro, H. N.: Both subunits of rat liver ferritin are regulated at a translational level by iron induction. Nucleic Acids Res. 14:915, 1986.
161. Zahringer, J., Baliga, B. S., and Munro, H. N.: Novel mechanism for translational control in regulation of ferritin synthesis by iron. Proc. Natl. Acad. Sci. USA 73:857, 1976.
162. Shull, G. E., and Theil, E. C.: Translational control of ferritin synthesis by iron in embryonic reticulocytes of the bullfrog. J. Biol. Chem. 257:14187, 1982.
163. Schaefer, F. V., and Theil, E. C.: The effect of iron on the synthesis and amount of ferritin in red blood cells during ontogeny. J. Biol. Chem. 256:1711, 1981.
164. Rouault, T. A., Hentze, M. W., Dancis, A., Caughman, S. W., Harford, J. B., and Klausner, R. D.: Influence of altered transcription on the translational control of human ferritin expression. Proc. Natl. Acad. Sci. USA 84:6335, 1987.
165. Aziz, N., and Munro, H. N.: Both subunits of rat liver ferritin are regulated at a translational level by iron induction. Nucleic Acids Res. 14:915, 1986.
166. Hentze, M. W., Rouault, T. A., Caughman, S. W., Dancis, A., Harford, J. B., and Klausner, R. D.: A cis-acting element is necessary and sufficient for translational regulation of human ferritin expression in response to iron. Proc. Natl. Acad. Sci. USA 84:6730, 1987.
167. Hentze, M. W., Caughman, S. W., Rouault, T. A., Barriocanal, J. G., Dancis, A., Harford, J. B., and Klausner, R. D. Identification of the iron-responsive element for the translational regulation of human ferritin mRNA. Science 238, 1570, 1987.
168. Caughman, S. W., Hentze, M. W., Rouault, T. A., Harford, J. B., and Klausner, R. D.: The iron-responsive element is the single element responsible for iron-dependent translational regulation of ferritin biosynthesis: Evidence for function as the binding site for a translational repressor. J. Biol. Chem. 263:19048, 1988.
169. Owen, D., and Kuhn, L. C.: Noncoding 3′ sequences of the transferrin receptor gene are required for mRNA regulation by iron. EMBO J. 6:1287, 1987.
170. Casey, J. L., Di Jeso, B., Rao, K., Klausner, R. D., and Harford, J. B.: Two genetic loci participate in the regulation by iron of the gene for the human transferrin receptor. Proc. Natl. Acad. Sci. USA 85:1787, 1988.
171. Horowitz, J. A., and Harford, J. B.: The secondary structure of the regulatory region of the transferrin receptor mRNA deduced by enzymatic cleavage. New Biol. 4:330, 1992.
172. Henderson, B. R., Menotti, E., Bonnard, C., and Kuhn, L. C.: Optimal sequence and structure of iron-responsive elements-selection of RNA stem-loops with high-affinity for iron regulatory factor. J. Biol. Chem. 269:17481, 1994.
173. Henderson, B. R., Menotti, E., and Kuhn, L. C.: Iron regulatory proteins 1 and 2 bind distinct sets of RNA target sequences. J. Biol. Chem. 271:4900, 1996.
174. Butt, J., Kim, H. Y., Basilion, J. P., Cohen, S., Iwai, K., Philpott, C. C., Altschul, S., Klausner, R. D., and Rouault, T. A.: Differences in the RNA binding sites of iron regulatory proteins and potential target diversity. Proc. Natl. Acad. Sci. USA 93:4345, 1996.
175. Addess, K. J., Basilion, J. P., Klausner, R. D., Rouault, T. A., and Pardi, A. J.: Structure and dynamics of the iron responsive element RNA: Implications for binding of the RNA by iron regulatory proteins. J. Mol. Biol. 274:72, 1997.
176. Sierzputowska-Gracz, H., McKenzie, R. A., and Theil, E. C.: The importance of a single G in the hairpin loop of the iron responsive element (IRE) in ferritin mRNA for structure: an NMR spectroscopy study. Nucleic Acids Res. 23:146, 1995.
177. Leibold, E. A., and Munro, H. N.: Cytoplasmic protein binds in vitro to a highly conserved sequence in the 5′ untranslated region of ferritin heavy- and light-subunit mRNAs. Proc. Natl. Acad. Sci. USA 85:2171, 1988.
178. Rouault, T. A., Hentze, M. W., Caughman, S. W., Harford, J. B., and Klausner, R. D.: Binding of a cytosolic protein to the iron-responsive element of human ferritin messenger RNA. Science 241:1207, 1988.
179. Rouault, T. A., Tang, C. K., Kaptain, S., Burgess, W. H., Haile, D. J., Samaniego, F., McBride, O. W., Harford, J. B., and Klausner, R. D.: Cloning of the cDNA encoding an RNA regulatory protein—the human iron-responsive element–binding protein. Proc. Natl. Acad. Sci. USA 87:7958, 1990.
180. Hirling, H., Emery-Goodman, A., Thompson, N., Neupert, B., Seiser, C., and Kuhn, L. C.: Expression of active iron regulatory factor from a full-length human cDNA by in vitro transcription/translation. Nucleic Acids Res. 20:33, 1992.
181. Patino, M. M., and Walden, W. E.: Cloning of a functional cDNA for the rabbit ferritin mRNA repressor protein: Demonstration of a tissue specific pattern of expression. J. Biol. Chem. 267:19011, 1992.
182. Yu, Y., Radisky, E., and Leibold, E. A.: The iron-responsive element binding protein: Purification, cloning and regulation in rat liver. J. Biol. Chem. 267:19005, 1992.
183. Samaniego, F., Chin, J., Iwai, K., Rouault, T. A., and Klausner, R. D.: Molecular characterization of a second iron responsive element binding protein, iron regulatory protein 2 (IRP2): Structure, function and post-translational regulation. J. Biol. Chem. 269:30904, 1994.
184. Guo, B., Yu, Y., and Leibold, E. A.: Iron regulates cytoplasmic levels of a novel iron-responsive element–binding protein without aconitase activity. J. Biol. Chem. 269:24252, 1994.
185. Stripecke, R., Oliveira, C. C., McCarthy, J. E., and Hentze, M. W.: Proteins binding to 5′ untranslated region sites: A general mechanism for translational regulation of mRNAs in human and yeast cells. Mol. Cell. Biol. 14:5898, 1994.
186. Binder, R., Horowitz, J. A., Basilion, J. P., Koeller, D. M., Klausner, R. D., and Harford, J. B.: Evidence that the pathway of transferrin receptor mRNA degradation involves an endonucleolytic cleavage within the 3′ UTR and does not involve poly(A) tail shortening. EMBO J. 13:1969, 1994.
187. Casey, J. L., Koeller, D. M., Ramin, V. C., Klausner, R. D., and Harford, J. B.: Iron regulation of transferrin receptor mRNA levels requires iron-responsive elements and a rapid turnover determinant in the 3′ untranslated region of the mRNA. EMBO J. 8:3693, 1989.
188. Rouault, T. A., Stout, C. D., Kaptain, S., Harford, J. B., and Klausner, R. D.: Structural relationship between an iron-regulated RNA-binding protein (IRE-BP) and aconitase: Functional implications. Cell 64:881, 1991.
189. Robbins, A. H., and Stout, C. D.: The structure of aconitase. Proteins 5:289, 1989.
190. Kennedy, M. C., and Beinert, H.: The state of cluster SH and S2- of aconitase during cluster interconversions and removal. J. Biol. Chem. 263:8194, 1988.
191. Kennedy, M. C., Mende-Mueller, L., Blondin, G. A., and Beinert, H.: Purification and characterization of cytosolic aconitase from beef liver and its relationship to the iron-responsive element binding protein (IRE-BP). Proc. Natl. Acad. Sci. USA 89:11730, 1992.
192. Haile, D. J., Rouault, T. A., Tang, C. K., Chin, J., Harford, J. B., and Klausner, R. D.: Reciprocal control of RNA binding and aconitase activity in the regulation of the iron responsive element binding

protein: Role of the iron-sulfur cluster. Proc. Natl. Acad. Sci. USA 89:7536, 1992.

193. Haile, D. J., Rouault, T. A., Harford, J. B., Kennedy, M. C., Blondin, G. A., Beinert, H., and Klausner, R. D.: Cellular regulation of the iron-responsive element binding protein: Disassembly of the cubane iron-sulfur cluster results in high affinity RNA binding. Proc. Natl. Acad. Sci. USA 89:11735, 1992.

194. Basilion, J. P., Rouault, T. A., Massinople, C. M., Klausner, R. D., and Burgess, W. H.: The iron-responsive element-binding protein: Localization of the RNA binding site to the aconitase active-site cleft Proc. Natl. Acad. Sci. USA 91:574, 1994.

195. Swenson, G. R., and Walden, W. E.: Localization of an RNA binding element of the iron responsive element binding protein within a proteolytic fragment containing iron coordination ligands. Nucleic Acids Res. 22:2627, 1994.

196. Neupert, B., Menotti, E., and Kuhn, L. C.: A novel method to identify nucleic acid binding sites in proteins by scanning mutagenesis: Application to iron regulatory protein. Nucleic Acids Res. 23:2579, 1995.

197. Philpott, C. C., Klausner, R. D., and Rouault, T. A.: The bifunctional iron-responsive element binding protein/cytosolic aconitase: The role of active-site residues in ligand binding and regulation. Proc. Natl. Acad. Sci. USA 91:7321, 1994.

198. Tang, C. K., Chin, J., Harford, J. B., Klausner, R. D., and Rouault, T. A.: Iron regulates the activity of the iron-responsive element binding protein without changing its rate of synthesis or degradation. J. Biol. Chem. 267:24466, 1992.

199. Rouault, T. A., and Klausner, R. D.: Iron-sulfur clusters as biosensors of oxidants and iron. Trends Biochem. Sci. 21:174, 1996.

200. Beinert, H., and Kiley, P.: Redox control of gene expression involving iron-sulfur proteins: Change of oxidation-state or assembly/disassembly of Fe-S clusters? FEBS Lett. 382:218, 1996.

201. Pantopoulos, K., and Hentze, M. W.: Rapid responses to oxidative stress mediated by iron regulatory protein. EMBO J. 14:2917, 1995.

202. Rouault, T. A., Haile, D. H., Downey, W. E., Philpott, C. C., Tang, C., Samaniego, F., Chin, J., Paul, I., Orloff, D., Harford, J. B., and Klausner, R. D.: An iron-sulfur cluster plays a novel regulatory role in the iron-responsive element binding protein. Biometals 5:131, 1992.

203. Iwai, K., Klausner, R. D., and Rouault, T. A.: Requirements for iron-regulated degradation of the RNA binding protein, iron regulatory protein 2. EMBO J. 14:5350, 1995.

204. Guo, B., Phillips, J. D., Yu, Y., and Leibold, E. A.: Iron regulates the intracellular degradation of iron regulatory protein 2 by the proteasome. J. Biol. Chem. 270:21645, 1995.

205. Hochstrasser, M.: Ubiquitin, proteasomes, and the regulation of intracellular protein degradation. Curr. Opin. Cell. Biol. 7:215, 1995.

206. Rubin, D. M., and Finley, D.: Proteolysis: The proteasome: A protein-degrading organelle? Curr. Biol. 5:854, 1995.

207. Levine, R. L., Williams, J. A., Stadtman, E. R., and Shacter, E.: Carbonyl assays for determination of oxidatively modified proteins. Methods Enzymol. 233:346, 1994.

208. Iwai, K., Drake, S. K., Wehr, N. B., Weissman, A. M., LaVaute, T., Minato, M., Klausner, R. D., Levine, R. L., and Rouault, T. A.: Iron-dependent oxidation, ubiquitination and degradation of iron regulatory protein 2: Implications for degradation of oxidized proteins. Proc. Natl. Acad. Sci. USA 95:4924, 1998.

209. Cox, T. C., Bawden, M. J., Martin, A., and May, B. K.: Human erythroid 5-aminolevulinate synthase: Promoter analysis and identification of an iron-responsive element in the mRNA. EMBO J. 10:1891, 1991.

210. Melefors, O., Goossen, B., Johansson, H. E., Stripecke, R., Gray, N. K., and Hentze, M. W.: Translational control of 5-aminolevulinate synthase mRNA by iron-responsive elements in erythroid cells. J. Biol. Chem. 268:5974, 1993.

211. Gray, N. K., Pantopoulos, K., Dandekar, T., Ackrell, B. A. C., and Hentze, M. W.: Translational regulation of mammalian and drosophila citric-acid cycle enzymes via iron-responsive elements. Proc. Natl. Acad. Sci. USA 93:4925, 1996.

212. Kim, H. Y., LaVaute, T., Iwai, K., Klausner, R. D., and Rouault, T. A.: Identification of a conserved and functional iron-responsive element in the 5′UTR of mammalian mitochondrial aconitase. J. Biol. Chem. 271:24226, 1996.

213. Zheng, L., Kennedy, M. C., Blondin, G. A., Beinert, H., and Zalkin, H.: Binding of cytosolic aconitase to the iron responsive element of porcine mitochondrial aconitase mRNA. Arch. Biochem. Biophys. 299:356, 1992.

214. Kohler, S. A., Henderson, B. R., and Kuhn, L. C.: Succinate dehydrogenase b mRNA of *Drosophila melanogaster* has a functional iron-responsive element in its 5′-untranslated region. J. Biol. Chem. 270:30781, 1995.

215. Henderson, B. R., Seiser, C., and Kuhn, L. C.: Characterization of a second RNA-binding protein in rodents with specificity for iron-responsive elements. J. Biol. Chem. 268:27327, 1993.

216. Menotti, E., Henderson, B. R., and Kuhn, L. C.: Translational regulation of mRNAs with distinct IRE sequences by iron regulatory proteins 1 and 2. J. Biol. Chem. 273:1821, 1998.

217. Gunshin, H., Mackenzie, B., Berger, U. V., Gunshin, Y., Romero, M. F., Boron, W. F., Nussberger, S., Gollan, J. L., and Hediger, M. A.: Cloning and characterization of a mammalian proton-coupled metal-ion transporter. Nature 388:482, 1997.

218. Fleming, M. D., Trenor, C. C. R., Su, M. A., Foernzler, D., Beier, D. R., Dietrich, W. F., and Andrews, N. C.: Microcytic anaemia mice have a mutation in Nramp2, a candidate iron transporter gene. Nat. Genet. 16:383, 1997.

219. Fleming, M. D., Romano, M. A., Su, M. A., Garrick, L. M., and Andrews, N. C.: Nramp2 is mutated in the anemic Belgrade (b) rat: Evidence of a role for Nramp2 in endosomal iron transport. Proc. Natl. Acad. Sci. USA 95:1148, 1998.

220. Vidal, S. M., Malo, D., Vogan, K., Skamene, E., and Gros, P.: Natural resistance to infection with intracellular parasites: Isolation of a candidate for BCG. Cell 73:469, 1993.

221. Gruenheid, S., Pinner, E., Desjardins, M., and Gros, P.: Natural resistance to infection with intracellular pathogens: The Nramp1 protein is recruited to the membrane of the phagosome. J. Exp. Med. 185:717, 1997.

222. Garrick, M. D., Gniecko, K., Liu, Y., Cohan, D. S., and Garrick, L. M.: Transferrin and the transferrin cycle in Belgrade rat reticulocytes. J. Biol. Chem. 268:14867, 1993.

223. Gutierrez, J. A., Yu, J., Rivera, S., and Wessling-Resnick, M.: Functional expression cloning and characterization of SFT, a stimulator of Fe transport. J. Cell. Biol. 139:895, 1997.

224. Bannerman, R. M., Garrick, L. M., Rusnak-Smalley, P., Hoke, J. E., and Edwards, J. A.: Hemoglobin deficit: An inherited hypochromic anemia in the mouse. Proc. Soc. Exp. Biol. Med. 182:52, 1986.

225. Bannerman, R. M.: Genetic defects of iron transport. Fed. Proc. 35:2281, 1976.

226. Kingston, P. J., Bannerman, C. E., and Bannerman, R. M.: Iron deficiency anaemia in newborn sla mice: A genetic defect of placental iron transport. Br. J. Haematol. 40:265, 1978.

227. Kondo, H., Saito, K., Grasso, J. P., and Aisen, P.: Iron metabolism in the erythrophagocytosing Kupffer cell. Hepatology 8:32, 1988.

228. Saito, K., Nishisato, T., Grasso, J. A., and Aisen, P.: Interaction of transferrin with iron-loaded rat peritoneal macrophages. Br. J. Haematol. 62:275, 1986.

229. Siimes, M. A., and Dallman, P. R.: New kinetic role for serum ferritin in iron metabolism. Br. J. Haematol. 28:7, 1974.

230. Gelvan, D., Fibach, E., Meyron-Holtz, E. G., and Konijn, A. M.: Ferritin uptake by human erythroid precursors is a regulated iron uptake pathway. Blood 88:3200, 1996.

231. Cuthbert, J. A.: Iron, HFE, and hemochromatosis update. J. Invest. Med. 45:518, 1997.

232. McLaren, C. E., McLachlan, G. J., Halliday, J. W., Webb, S. I., Leggett, B. A., Jazwinska, E. C., Crawford, D. H., Gordeuk, V. R., McLaren, G. D., and Powell, L. W.: Distribution of transferrin saturation in an Australian population: Relevance to the early diagnosis of hemochromatosis. Gastroenterology 114:543, 1998.

233. George, D. K., Goldwurm, S., MacDonald, G. A., Cowley, L. L., Walker, N. I., Ward, P. J., Jazwinska, E. C., and Powell, L. W.: Increased hepatic iron concentration in nonalcoholic steatohepatitis is associated with increased fibrosis. Gastroenterology 114:311, 1998.

234. Feder, J. N., Gnirke, A., Thomas, W., Tsuchihashi, Z., Ruddy, D. A., Basava, A., Dormishian, F., Domingo, R. J., Ellis, M. C., Fullan, A., Hinton, L. M., Jones, N. L., Kimmel, B. E., Kronmal, G. S., Lauer, P., Lee, V. K., Loeb, D. B., Mapa, F. A., McClelland, E., Meyer, N. C., Mintier, G. A., Moeller, N., Moore, T., Morikang, E., Wolff, R. K., et al.: A novel MHC class I-like gene is mutated in patients with hereditary haemochromatosis. Nat. Genet. 13:399, 1996.

235. Beuler, E.: The significance of the 187G (H63D) mutation in hemochromatosis (letter). Am. J. Hum. Genet. 61:762, 1997.

236. Jouanolle, A. M., Gandon, G., Jezequel, P., Blayau, M., Campion, M. L., Yaouanq, J., Mosser, J., Fergelot, P., Chauvel, B., Bouric, P.,

Carn, G., Andrieux, N., Gicquel, I., Le Gall, J. Y., and David, V.: Haemochromatosis and HLA-H (letter). Nat. Genet. 14:251, 1996.

237. Jazwinska, E. C., Cullen, L. M., Busfield, F., Pyper, W. R., Webb, S. I., Powell, L. W., Morris, C. P., and Walsh, T. P.: Haemochromatosis and HLA-H (letter). Nat. Genet. 14:249, 1996.

238. Feder, J. N., Tsuchihashi, Z., Irrinki, A., Lee, V. K., Mapa, F. A., Morikang, E., Prass, C. E., Starnes, S. M., Wolff, R. K., Parkkila, S., Sly, W. S., and Schatzman, R. C.: The hemochromatosis founder mutation in HLA-H disrupts beta2-microglobulin interaction and cell surface expression. J. Biol. Chem. 272:14025, 1997.

239. Waheed, A., Parkkila, S., Zhou, X. Y., Tomatsu, S., Tsuchihashi, Z., Feder, J. N., Schatzman, R. C., Britton, R. S., Bacon, B. R., and Sly, W. S.: Hereditary hemochromatosis: Effects of C282Y and H63D mutations on association with beta2-microglobulin, intracellular processing, and cell surface expression of the HFE protein in COS-7 cells. Proc. Natl. Acad. Sci. USA 94:12384, 1997.

240. Feder, J. N., Penny, D. M., Irrinki, A., Lee, V. K., Lebrón, J. A., Watson, N., Tsuchihashi, Z., Sigal, E., Bjorkman, P. J., and Schatzman, R. C.: The hemochromatosis gene product complexes with the transferrin receptor and lowers its affinity for ligand binding. Proc. Natl. Acad. Sci. USA 95:1472, 1998.

241. Parkkila, S., Waheed, A., Britton, R. S., Bacon, B. R., Zhou, X. Y., Tomatsu, S., Fleming, R. E., and Sly, W. S.: Association of the transferrin receptor in human placenta with HFE, the protein defective in hereditary hemochromatosis. Proc. Natl. Acad. Sci. USA 94:13198, 1997.

242. Gross, C. N., Irrinki, A., Feder, J. N., and Enns, C. A.: Co-trafficking of HFE, a nonclassical major histocompatibility complex class I protein, with the transferrin receptor implies a role in intracellular iron regulation. J. Biol. Chem. 273:22068, 1998.

243. Merryweather-Clarke, A. T., Pointon, J. J., Shearman, J. D., and Robson, K. J.: Global prevalence of putative haemochromatosis mutations. J. Med. Genet. 34:275, 1997.

244. Zhou, X. Y., Tomatsu, S., Fleming, R. E., Parkkila, S., Waheed, A., Jiang, J., Fei, Y., Brunt, E. M., Ruddy, D. A., Prass, C. E., Schatzman, R. C., O'Neill, R., Britton, R. S., Bacon, B. R., and Sly, W. S.: HFE gene knockout produces mouse model of hereditary hemochromatosis. Proc. Natl. Acad. Sci. USA 95:2492, 1998.

245. Merryweather-Clarke, A. T., Liu, Y. T., Shearman, J. D., Pointon, J. J., and Robson, K. J.: A rapid non-invasive method for the detection of the haemochromatosis C282Y mutation. Br. J. Haematol. 99:460, 1997.

246. Santos, M., Schilham, M. W., Rademakers, L. H., Marx, J. J., de Sousa, M., and Clevers, H.: Defective iron homeostasis in beta 2-microglobulin knockout mice recapitulates hereditary hemochromatosis in man. J. Exp. Med. 184:1975, 1996.

247. Rothenberg, B. E., and Voland, J. R.: Beta2 knockout mice develop parenchymal iron overload: A putative role for class I genes of the major histocompatibility complex in iron metabolism. Proc. Natl. Acad. Sci. USA 93:1529, 1996.

248. Gordeuk, V., Mukiibi, J., Hasstedt, S. J., Samowitz, W., Edwards, C. Q., West, G., Ndambire, S., Emmanual, J., Nkanza, N., Chapanduka, Z., et al.: Iron overload in Africa. Interaction between a gene and dietary iron content. N. Engl. J. Med. 326:95, 1992.

249. Moyo, V. M., Mandishona, E., Hasstedt, S. J., Gangaidzo, I. T., Gomo, A., Khumalo, H., Saungweme, T., Kiire, C. F., Paterson, A. C., Bloom, P., MacPhail, A. P., Rouault, T., and Gordeuk, V. R.: Evidence of genetic transmission in African iron overload. Blood 91:1076, 1998.

249a. McNamara, L., MacPhail, A. P., Gordeuk, V. R., Hasstedt, S. J., and Rouault, T.: Is there a link between African iron overload and the described mutations of the hereditary haemochromatosis gene? Br. J. Haematol. 102:1176, 1998.

250. Barton, J. C., Edwards, C. Q., Bertoli, L. F., Shroyer, T. W., and Hudson, S. L.: Iron overload in African Americans. Am. J. Med. 99:616, 1995.

251. Wurapa, R. K., Gordeuk, V. R., Brittenham, G. M., Khiyami, A., Schechter, G. P., and Edwards, C. Q.: Primary iron overload in African Americans. Am. J. Med. 101:9, 1996.

252. Roeser, H. P., Lee, G. R., Nacht, S., and Cartwright, G. E.: The role of ceruloplasmin in iron metabolism. J. Clin. Invest. 49:2408, 1970.

253. Lee, G. R., Nacht, S., Lukens, J. N., and Cartwright, G. E.: Iron metabolism in copper-deficient swine. J. Clin. Invest. 47:2058, 1968.

254. Yoshida, K., Furihata, K., Takeda, S., Nakamura, A., Yamamoto, K., Morita, H., Hiyamuta, S., Ikeda, S., Shimizu, N., and Yanagisawa, N.: A mutation in the ceruloplasmin gene is associated with systemic hemosiderosis in humans. Nat. Genet. 9:267, 1995.

255. Mukhopadhyay, C. K., Attieh, Z. K., and Fox, P. L.: Role of ceruloplasmin in cellular iron uptake. Science 279:714, 1998.

256. Hamill, R. L., Woods, J. C., and Cook, B. A.: Congenital atransferrinemia: A case report and review of the literature. Am. J. Clin. Pathol. 96:215, 1991.

257. Bernstein, S. E.: Hereditary hypotransferrinemia with hemosiderosis, a murine disorder resembling human atransferrinemia. J. Lab. Clin. Med. 110:690, 1987.

258. Huggenvik, J. I., Craven, C. M., Idzerda, R. L., Bernstein, S., Kaplan, J., and McKnight, G. S.: A splicing defect in the mouse transferrin gene leads to congenital atransferrinemia. Blood 74:482, 1989.

259. Kaplan, J., Craven, C., Alexander, J., Kushner, J., Lamb, J., and Bernstein, S.: Regulation of the distribution of tissue iron: Lessons learned from the hypotransferrinemic mouse. Ann. NY Acad. Sci. 526:124, 1988.

260. Ponka, P.: Tissue-specific regulation of iron metabolism and heme synthesis: Distinct control mechanisms in erythroid cells. Blood 89:1, 1997.

261. Raja, K. B., Simpson, R. J., Pippard, M. J., and Peters, T. J.: In vivo studies on the relationship between intestinal iron (Fe^{3+}) absorption, hypoxia and erythropoiesis in the mouse. Br. J. Haematol. 68:373, 1988.

262. Finch, C. A., Huebers, H., Eng, M., and Miller, L.: Effect of transfused reticulocytes on iron exchange. Blood 59:364, 1982.

263. Pootrakul, P., Kitcharoen, K., Yansukon, P., Wasi, P., Fucharoen, S., Charoenlarp, P., Brittenham, G., Pippard, M. J., and Finch, C. A.: The effect of erythroid hyperplasia on iron balance. Blood 71:1124, 1988.

264. Sabesin, S. M., and Thomas, L. B.: Parenchymal siderosis in patients with preexisting portal cirrhosis. Gastroenterology 46:477, 1964.

265. Tisdale, W. A.: Parenchymal siderosis in patients with cirrhosis after portasystemic-shunt surgery. N. Engl. J. Med. 265:928, 1961.

266. Poss, K. D., and Tonegawa, S.: Reduced stress defense in heme oxygenase 1-deficient cells. Proc. Natl. Acad. Sci. USA 94:10925, 1997.

267. Poss, K. D., and Tonegawa, S.: Heme oxygenase 1 is required for mammalian iron reutilization. Proc. Natl. Acad. Sci. USA 94:10919, 1997.

268. Babcock, M., de Silva, D., Oaks, R., Davis-Kaplan, S., Jiralerspong, S., Montermini, L., Pandolfo, M., and Kaplan, J.: Regulation of mitochondrial iron accumulation by Yfh1p, a putative homolog of frataxin. Science 276:1709, 1997.

269. Rotig, A., de Lonlay, P., Chretien, D., Foury, F., Koenig, M., Sidi, D., Munnich, A., and Rustin, P.: Aconitase and mitochondrial iron-sulphur protein deficiency in Friedreich ataxia. Nat. Genet. 17:215, 1997.

270. Fitzsimons, E. J., and May, A.: The molecular basis of the sideroblastic anemias. Curr. Opin. Hematol. 3:167, 1996.

271. Rotig, A., Bourgeron, T., Chretien, D., Rustin, P., and Munnich, A.: Spectrum of mitochondrial DNA rearrangements in the Pearson marrow-pancreas syndrome. Hum. Mol. Genet. 4:1327, 1995.

272. Beaumont, C., Leneuve, P., Devaux, I., Scoazec, J. Y., Berthier, M., Loiseau, M. N., Grandchamp, B., and Bonneau, D.: Mutation in the iron responsive element of the L ferritin mRNA in a family with dominant hyperferritinaemia and cataract. Nat. Genet. 11:444, 1995.

273. Girelli, D., Corrocher, R., Bisceglia, L., Olivieri, O., De Franceschi, L., Zelante, L., and Gasparini, P.: Molecular basis for the recently described hereditary hyperferritinemia-cataract syndrome: a mutation in the iron-responsive element of ferritin L-subunit gene (the Verona mutation). Blood 86:4050, 1995.

274. Martin, M. E., Fargion, S., Brissot, P., Pellat, B., and Beaumont, C.: A point mutation in the bulge of the iron-responsive element of the L ferritin gene in two families with the hereditary hyperferritinemia-cataract syndrome. Blood 91:319, 1998.

275. Cazzola, M., Bergamaschi, G., Tonon, L., Arbustini, E., Grasso, M., Vercesi, E., Barosi, G., Bianchi, P. E., Cairo, G., and Arosio, P.: Hereditary hyperferritinemia-cataract syndrome: Relationship between phenotypes and specific mutations in the iron-responsive element of ferritin light-chain mRNA. Blood 90:814, 1997.

276. Gutteridge, J. M.: Hydroxyl radicals, iron, oxidative stress, and neurodegeneration. Ann. NY Acad. Sci. 738:201, 1994.

▼▼▼▼ Part III
LYMPHOPOIESIS

11 Gene Rearrangements in Lymphoid Cells
▼▼▼▼ Ilan R. Kirsch and W. Michael Kuehl

▼ ▼

Introduction

The elucidation of the structure and organization of the genetic loci that encode the immunoglobulin and T-cell antigen receptor genes is one of the earliest and currently most important successes of the use of recombinant DNA technology. In terms of our understanding of cell growth, development, and differentiation there are critical lessons to be learned from a molecular genetic analysis of the necessary and sufficient factors required for the generation of a humoral or cell-mediated immune response. Since the mid-1980s this work has not only solved the riddle of immune diversity but has demonstrated a particularly profound example of the fundamental principle of genomic instability (see below). In terms of societal impact, the cloning and characterization of the immunoglobulin and T-cell antigen receptor genes have provided a set of extremely diverse, powerful, and specific reagents that can be applied to a variety of biomedical concerns from the diagnosis, staging, and treatment of cancer,[1, 2] to the synthesis of new kinds of "designer" catalytic enzymes.[3, 4]

Immunoglobulins became an early target of recombinant DNA research for two basic reasons. The mystery of how a higher organism was capable of responding specifically to the myriad "foreign" antigenic stimuli with which it might or might not come into contact during its lifetime was an obviously important question that had been explored and debated for the previous century. Required, however, to approach this problem at the outset of DNA cloning technology was a model system in which abundant immunoglobulin messenger RNA (mRNA) could be obtained for the commencement of cloning studies. Today, essentially any gene or piece of DNA can be cloned, but initially there was a critical requirement for mRNA abundance as a prerequisite to practical consideration of gene cloning. Such a model system existed for the immunoglobulin genes through the in vivo propagation and in vitro expansion in cell culture of murine plasmacytomas,[5] plasma cell tumors in which as much as 10 per cent of the total mRNA encoded a particular immunoglobulin molecule. With this resource at hand the full force of a new technology could be brought to bear on the problem. The rest is history and the result can now be delineated in textbook form.

The Question of Immune Diversity

A species becomes a species because, over time, it can safeguard the integrity of its genetic material. Bacteria maintain this ability in part through the restriction-modification system exploited in recombinant DNA technology.[6] In higher organisms it is not just the integrity of the DNA of the population, but also the protection (at least until reproductive age is achieved) of the viability of the cells that the individual organism comprises that provide a selective advantage for a particular species. Thus higher organisms have developed a variety of mechanisms, for example, the mechanical barrier of the skin, or the neuromuscular capacity of fight or flight, or the immune response, that protect them from discernible or microbial threats within their environment. Inherent in the ability to perceive a threat is the ability to distinguish between oneself and the rest of the world. Our neurological system fulfills this function for the discernible world. Our immunological system serves this function with regard to the viruses, bacteria, fungi, and protozoa (or transformed cells) that we cannot "see" but that can invade the "sanctity" of our bodies.

The immune system serves two defensive functions: (1) the recognition of a microbial agent or cell as "foreign" and (2) the processing/elimination of this foreign entity (the "effector" function). We are situated in the midst of a sea of foreign substances, many of which are capable of invading and infecting us. We are capable of responding with great specificity to the majority of these substances via the recognition of specific "antigenic" determinants that these foreign molecules carry. This recognition is carried out by the immune receptors (immunoglobulins and T-cell antigen receptors) expressed by our lymphocytes. We have the capability of responding to myriad antigens only some of which can we count on being exposed to in our lifetime. What gives us this ability of being able to respond to this diversity of "foreignness"? How is this capability encoded in our DNA? This was a question that challenged immunologists for most of this century, stimulated by the work of Landsteiner establishing that the repertoire of the immune response was essentially infinite.[7]

This issue became the focus for the elucidation of immune diversity, an issue summarized by the question, How

can an essentially infinite repertoire of immune responsiveness be encoded in a finite amount of DNA? One possible solution to this question envisioned an expansive array of potentially functional immune receptor genes spread across and occupying a large proportion of germline DNA, one gene for each possible antigen with which the organism might come in contact. A diametrically opposed view suggested the existence of a single "platonic" immune receptor gene that, upon antigenic stimulation, would mutate until it developed the capacity to recognize and interact with the antigen. The answer to this question, partially predicted by Dreyer and Bennett,[8] exists between the two extreme possibilities described. These investigators suggested that the key to immune receptor diversity might reside in a structural reconfiguration of primary genetic material so as to associate one of multiple segments of variable sequence with a single segment of constant sequence. The implication of their suggestion was that the DNA of a functional mature lymphocyte would, therefore, structurally no longer be the same as that of other cells. This was a novel and radical concept at the time of its suggestion and has been proved to be absolutely true.

The Basis of Immune Diversity—a Generic Overview

▼ IMMUNE RECEPTOR PROTEINS—STRUCTURE AND TERMINOLOGY

The proteins that combine to form the immunoglobulin and T-cell antigen receptors share common amino acid motifs (see Figs. 11–1 and 11–2). Each of these proteins has domains that are more or less constant among all members of a particular immune receptor class. This "constancy" in fact defines a protein as a member of a particular class. In some cases variations in these domains divide members of a class into subclasses. The immunoglobulins kappa (Igκ) and lambda (Igλ), and the T-cell antigen receptor alpha (TCRα), beta (TCRβ), gamma (TCRγ), and delta (TCRδ) classes all have a single such domain. The immunoglobulin heavy chain genes mu (Igμ), delta (Igδ), gamma (Igγ), epsilon (Igε), and alpha (Igα) comprise three or four constant domains and a "hinge" sequence found between the first two constant domains.[9] An additional "constant" domain is associated with these immunoglobulin proteins when they are membrane bound (see below). Constant domains define the "effector" functions of these molecules, functions that are described fully in other chapters of this text.

The antigen recognition function of immune receptors is primarily handled by the amino terminal domain of the molecule, which shows marked amino acid variability among all members of a particular class or subclass. Within this variable domain are regions that are "hypervariable," the complementarity determining regions (CDRs), which have been shown by X-ray crystallography (at least for immunoglobulins) to be the parts of the protein that directly interact with antigen.[10–12]

Immunoglobulins have a basic four chain structure consisting of two identical heavy chain peptides of the μ, δ, γ, ε, or α class (corresponding to IgM, IgD, IgG, IgE, and IgA antibodies, respectively) and two identical light chain

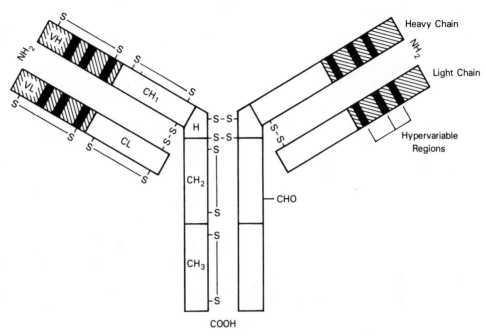

Figure 11–1. A schematic representation of an antibody molecule. The basic immunoglobulin consists of two identical heavy (H) chains and two identical light (L) chains. Each chain is divided into an amino (NH₂) terminal region, which is variable (V), and a carboxy- (COOH) terminal region, which is constant (C) among all members of that H or L chain subclass. Within the V regions are regions that show hypervariability from one chain to another. The hypervariable regions are predominantly responsible for the antigen-binding function of the molecule, and the C regions mediate the molecule's "effector" function(s). The chains are glycosylated (CHO) and contain intra- and interchain disulfide bonds (-S-S-). H chain C regions comprise three or four C domains (e.g., CH1); L chains have a single C segment. Some H chain classes have a separate "hinge" domain (designated H in Fig. 11–1) between CH1 and CH2.

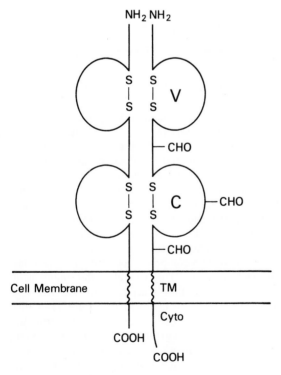

Figure 11–2. The T-cell antigen receptor heterodimer. The fundamental antigen recognition component of the T-cell antigen receptor consists of a heterodimeric molecule formed from an α and a β chain or a γ and δ chain. Similar to immunoglobulins these chains are divided into portions that are variable (V) and constant (C) among all members of the particular class. The amino (NH₂) portion of the molecule is extracellular, and the carboxy-terminus is within the cellular cytoplasm (cyto) with the two segments connected by a transmembrane (TM) domain. Like the membrane-associated immunoglobulin molecules, the T-cell antigen receptors are part of a macromolecular complex of proteins that confer stability and coordinate effector function (see text). The αβ heterodimer is interchain disulfide linked, but one type of γδ heterodimer is not.

peptides of the κ or λ class. For some classes of immunoglobulin this basic structure undergoes oligomerization to form pentameric (e.g., IgM) or dimeric (e.g., IgA) proteins. T-cell antigen receptors form a basic two chain structure consisting of an αβ or γδ heterodimer, although many other membrane proteins become associated with this primary structure.

▼ THE GERMLINE STRUCTURE OF IMMUNE RECEPTOR GENES[13–16]

The genes that eventually encode the peptide chains of functional immune receptor proteins initially reside in germline DNA as a number of discrete discontinuous segments (Fig. 11–3). For a given immune receptor these segments can be found spread out across hundreds of thousands of nucleotides at a particular chromosomal location. There are variations among these receptors in terms of the actual number and configurations of the segments (see below for a detailed description of each immune receptor locus), but a general structural theme is shared by all these genes. There are multiple (sometimes hundreds of) variable or "V" segments, each with its own leader sequence and promoter region. For some of the loci (immunoglobulin H [IgH], T-cell antigen receptor beta [TCRβ], T-cell antigen receptor delta [TCRδ]) there are diversity or "D" segments. For all the loci one finds joining or "J" segments a few thousand nucleotides upstream from constant or "C" segments. These constant segments are the nucleic acid counterpart of the constant portion of the immune receptor polypeptide. The constant segment thus "defines" the locus. Sequences that are capable of enhancing the transcription of the locus are often found in proximity to these C regions.

As a prerequisite to the formation of a functional immunoglobulin or T-cell antigen receptor one of the V segments undergoes a site-specific recombination event with a D, J, or previously site-specifically rearranged D-D or D-J segment. This forms a now contiguous VJ or VDJ continuous coding region still a few thousand nucleotides upstream of the constant segment. The now contiguous VJ or VDJ region of DNA corresponds to the variable domain of the immune receptor polypeptide described above. The rearranged gene is transcribed into RNA and, after appropriate splicing out of intervening sequences, translated into protein. The recombination event is mediated by a set of enzymes that cause a DNA breakage and rejoining event that appears to commence with the recognition of specific "signal" sequences (recombination signal sequences [RSSs], 3′ of V segments, 5′ of J segments, and flanking the interposed D segments. The signal sequences are shown schematically as triangles in Figure 11–3 (for a more complete description of this recombination event see The Mechanism of V(D)J Recombination, page 396). The end result of this recombination is the irreversible structural reconfiguration of the DNA in the lymphocyte that has undergone the recombination event. Depending on the orientation of the various recombining segments, the recombination event can occur via either deletion or inversion of the DNA between the segments to be joined. Both deletions and inversions have been, in fact, demonstrated as part of V(D)J recombination.[17, 18] As classically envisioned, V(D)J recombination occurs within a given immunoglobulin or T-cell antigen receptor locus, but it can occur between loci as well, via either sister chromatid exchange[19] or frank interchromosomal translocation or inversion.[20, 21]

Immune receptor diversity is achieved by the sum of five features of the structure and activation of these loci: (1) germline diversity, (2) combinatorial joining, (3) junctional diversity, (4) combinatorial association, and (5) somatic mutation.

▼ GERMLINE DIVERSITY

The germline element of diversity arises from the proliferation over evolutionary time of V, D, and J segments within immune receptor loci. Some loci contain hundreds of potential V segments. Most contain at least a handful of J segments (the T-cell antigen receptor alpha [TCRα] locus contains dozens; see below). A few of the loci contain D segments as well.

▼ COMBINATORIAL JOINING

Theoretically, any V segment can combine with any D and any J. Thus diversity arises in this case simply from the number of distinctive segments that are available to participate in the process. For example, if any one of 100 V segments can recombine with any of 10 D and 5 J segments, 5000 distinct variable regions can be formed from these 115 discrete segments.

▼ JUNCTIONAL DIVERSITY

Variation at the Point of Recombination/Nucleotide Deletion

Although site specific, the V(D)J recombination event is not absolutely precise to a specific nucleotide. In fact there is flexibility at the point of alignment of V, D, and J segments. The simplest example of this can be seen in studies of VJ rearrangement in the Ig light chain genes. The germline kappa V segment can potentially encode amino acids 1–95 of the mature kappa polypeptide. The amino acid sequence continues with amino acid 96 at the start of the J segment. This sequence is indeed formed if recombination occurs precisely between the end of codon 95 of the V segment and the beginning of codon 96 of the J segment, but that is not always the case. The rearrangement can occur within codon 95 or 96 to create a composite codon with nucleotides provided by each segment. This can alter the amino acid encoded by that codon and thus generate additional diversity as a result of the joining event itself. In Figure 11–4 this feature is illustrated for the TCRγ locus, using one particular Vγ and one particular Jγ segment for the demonstration. The figure raises several issues for consideration. It should be noted that the heptamer signal sequences are not always exactly flush or in-frame with the known V or J coding segments. Next, the point needs to be made that the "flexibility" of point of joining is actually a reflection of variable deletion of nucleotides from one, the other, or both partners in the rearrangement event. Initially, this flexibility was

Figure 11–3. V(D)J recombination. A generalized schematic illustrating the structural reconfigurations of immune receptor loci that are a prerequisite to the formation of a functional polypeptide and therefore to the generation of immune diversity. The gene that eventually constitutes the immune receptor exists initially in germline DNA as a set of discrete non-contiguous segments. There are multiple variable (V) segments with their upstream leader (L) exons that mediate transport of the polypeptide into or through a membrane. For certain of the immune receptor loci (IgH, TCRβ, TCRδ) there are diversity (D) segments. For all the loci one finds joining (J) segments upstream from constant (C) segments. Prior to gene rearrangement, "sterile" transcription (solid and dashed arrows over the first line of the schematic) of the loci about to be rearranged occurs, probably indicative of a change in the status and "accessibility" of the chromatin at these sites (see text). Structural and irreversible rearrangement of the DNA occurs either by deletion of the DNA between the rearranging segments or by inversion. The reaction is essentially site specific, mediated by a recombinase enzyme complex that recognizes heterologous recombination signal sequences (RSS) (denoted by solid and open triangles) that flank the rearranging segments. After recombination, a now contiguous V(D)J region is formed, still upstream of a C region. Transcription of the rearranged gene can begin from the promoter located 5′ of the rearranged V segment, with transcriptional activity "enhanced" by enhancer elements (En) that are found around the DNA flanking the C segment. A precursor RNA is transcribed up to the point where addition of a run of adenosine residues (An) is sited. RNA intervening between coding segments is spliced out, yielding the mature messenger RNA (mRNA). The mRNA is translated into protein and transported to its position in the membrane. The mature polypeptide is finished after additional processing, which includes cleavage of the leader peptide and possible glycosylation (CHO) of certain sites within the peptide. (From Kirsch, I.R.: Genetics of pediatric tumors: The causes and consequences of chromosomal aberrations. In Pizzo, P., and Poplack, D. (eds.): Principles and Practice of Pediatric Oncology. 2nd ed. Philadelphia, J.B. Lippincott Co., 1993; with permission.)

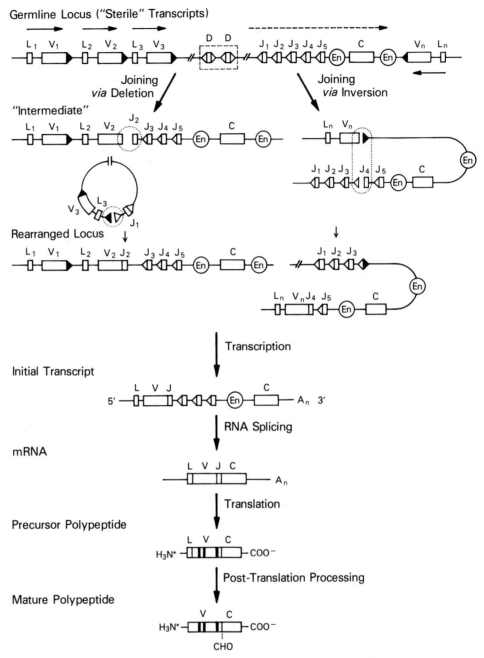

viewed as variability in the cross-over point of recombination, but now it is recognized as being instead an example of the more general theme of exonucleolytic "nibbling" of the coding ends involved in V(D)J recombination. This realization has arisen because of the finding that the signal sequences from the two opposing segments are almost always joined in a precise and flush fashion without any loss of nucleotides.[22] The implication of this finding is that first a cut is made at the signal sequence-coding sequence border. The signal sequences are then joined directly. The coding sequences, however, can be subjected to loss of nucleotides before ligation to each other. It should also be noted at this point that this "flexibility" of VJ joining need not always

result in a recombination event that maintains a continuous reading frame from V segment through J segment. Indeed in the characterization of these rearrangements such "out of frame" non-functional recombinants are frequently noted.[23, 24] The system is built so that absolute precision (and indeed guaranteed functionality) is sacrificed in order to enhance diversity. In one model system that has been studied extensively, one or the other of the rearranged coding ends (V, D, or J) shows nucleotide loss about 75 per cent of the time when compared to its germline sequence. Thus, these rearrangements are accompanied by nucleotide loss from one or both coding ends (usually fewer than five nucleotides from each end) more than 90 per cent of the time.[22]

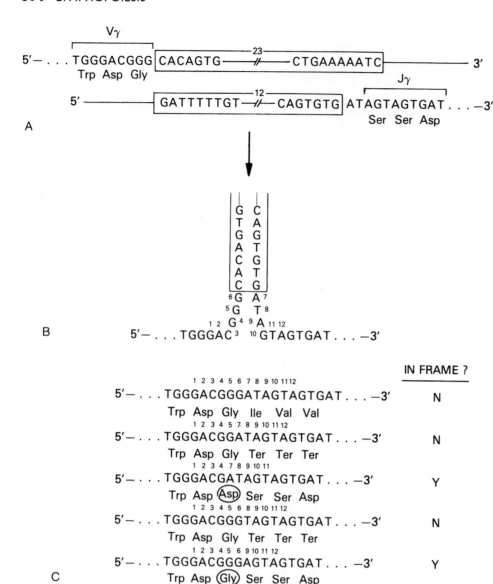

A, B, C

Figure 11–4. V(D)J recombination, signal sequences, "nibbling" of coding ends. A, The nucleotide sequence at the 3' border of a V segment and 5' border of a J segment is shown, using segments from the TCRγ locus in this example. The signal heptamer and nonamer sequences are boxed. There is a "spacer" of 23 nucleotides separating heptamer from nonamer 3' of a Vγ coding segment. A 12 nucleotide spacer is found 5' of a Jγ segment. A signal sequence abuts the V coding segment but is separated from the J coding segment by two nucleotides. The amino acids encoded at the border of these segments in their germline state are shown. B, The coding segments are approximated by the V(D)J recombinase complex, possibly aided by potential hydrogen bonding between complementary nucleotides of the opposing signal sequences. A DNA break occurs at the border of the signal sequences, which are then ligated to each other (see Fig. 11–3). C, Variable nucleotide deletion occurs at the ends of the coding segments prior to ligation. Depending on the extent of deletion the resolved contiguous V-J region can maintain a single reading frame and be translatable into a functional TCRγ polypeptide or become contiguous but out-of-frame and nonfunctional (see examples). For in-frame structures, additional variability can occur at the amino acid encoded at the V-J junction (in the example shown, Asp or Gly), depending on the deletion.

Insertion

Nucleotide addition also occurs at the coding segment junctions in about 75 per cent of rearrangements (Fig. 11–5). The addition of these nucleotides appears to be of at least two types. The first type of nucleotide addition is related to the specific sequences found at the end of the coding segments that are joined and involves the creation of a 1–3 base pair inverted repeat of one and/or the other coding segment end. These inverted repeats are called P nucleotides and are postulated to occur through a sequence of cleavage, hairpin formation, endonucleolytic activity, and ligation.[25] P nucleotides are only found when there has been no nucleotide loss from the coding strands, suggesting that the generation of these additional nucleotides occurs early in the process of V(D)J recombination and can be "erased" by subsequent exonucleolytic "nibbling" of the coding ends. The second type of nucleotide addition seen at the boundary of V, D, or J coding segment rearrangements appears to be DNA template independent. Usually fewer than five non-templated nucleotides are found at these junctions. The non-templated nucleotides often show a predisposition to addition of G and C

residues. This is consistent with the preference for G and C residues by the enzyme terminal deoxynucleotidyl transferase (TdT), and indeed the presence of these non-templated nucleotides, N regions, correlates with the presence and level of TdT activity.[26–28] Rearrangements of the Ig heavy chain locus are almost invariably accompanied by N sequence addition, in contrast to Ig light chain rearrangements, in which N sequences are a rarity. This supports the observation that TdT is much more active at the time of IgH than IgL V(D)J recombination. Putative N sequences can be found with regularity in TCR gene rearrangements. There may be an additional requirement for complementary bases to exist at the ends of the two coding ends in order for a successful resolution and ligation of the ends to be achieved.[29]

Depending on (1) the relationship of the signal sequences to the V, D, and J coding segments; (2) the ability of the ends of the segments to form complementary base pairs with each other; (3) the stringency and universality of postulated "hairpin" (see Fig. 11–5) formation and reopening; and (4) the presence or absence of "nibbling" exonucleases and N sequences added by TdT, certain combi-

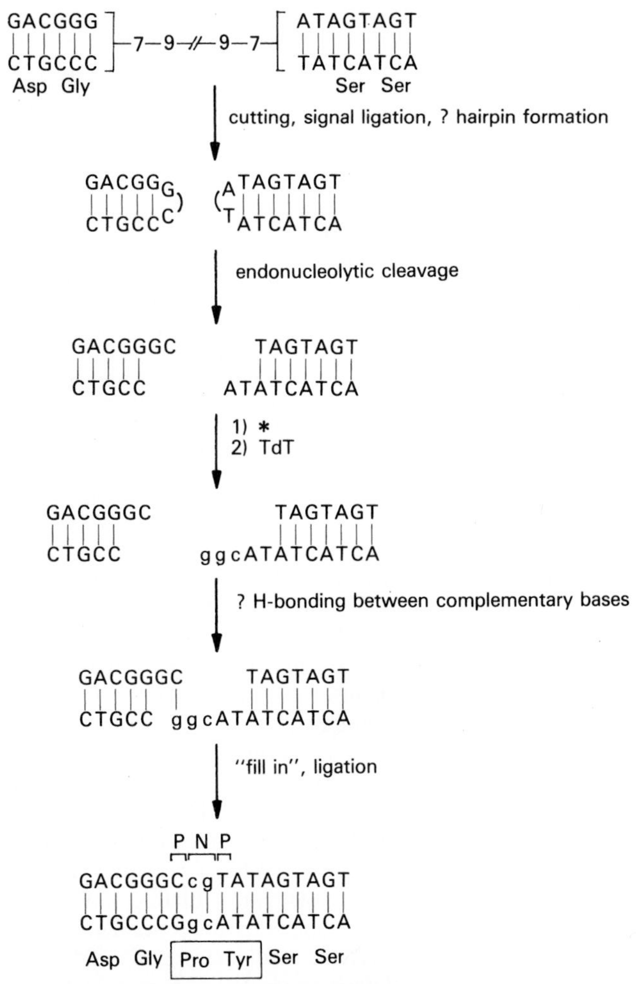

Figure 11–5. V(D)J recombination, nucleotide insertion, P and N nucleotides. An abbreviated and still speculative model is shown, using (as in Fig. 11–4) a Vγ-Jγ juxtaposition. After approximation of the signal ends, endonucleolytic cleavage occurs, generating short single strands at the ends of the coding segments (via a postulated hairpin intermediate). (*It is at this point where exonucleolytic nibbling might, but need not occur. The consequent occurrence of nucleotide deletions is shown in Fig. 11–4.) Terminal deoxynucleotidyl transferase (TdT) adds non-templated nucleotides to the junctional coding ends. Complementarity of terminal nucleotides aids in aligning the two coding ends, and after double-stranded repair mechanisms and ligation a contiguous V-J segment is formed. The P nucleotides are the short, single-nucleotide, inverted repeats resulting from the endonucleolytic cleavage and repair. (They can be longer than single nucleotides, depending on the point of endonucleolytic cleavage.) The N sequences, shown in lowercase, are the result of TdT activity. In this example these two processes have combined to create additional diversity at the V-J junction. Two additional amino acids, proline and tyrosine, are now part of the TCRγ polypeptide. A more refined and extensive discussion of models like this one is available in the text and elsewhere.[25, 114]

nations of Vs, Ds, and Js may be favored at different times of development. For example (although there is no evidence that this example is true), if a rearrangement were to occur at a time when the exonuclease was not active, then only those V and J segments whose distance from the heptamer signals resulted in in-frame recombination would be functional. Thus there would be a selection for certain Vs to recombine with certain Js, Ds, and so on. This example is complicated and possibly made irrelevant if the formation of 1–3 P nucleotides at the ends of the coding segments is

a stochastic process since that would alter the reading frame randomly. Whether these or other factors do exert a selective effect on immune receptor expression is not yet established, but it does appear that in embryonic development, there may be a more restricted repertoire of immune receptors than during later development[30] (Table 11–1).

▼ COMBINATORIAL ASSOCIATION

There is no evidence that the particular rearrangement of one receptor biases the choice of V or J utilized by its dimerizing partner. Thus additional diversity is generated by the possibility that (at least theoretically) any IgH chain can dimerize with any Ig light chain, any TCRα with any TCRβ, or any TCRγ with any TCRδ. Once a functional immune receptor has been formed via V(D)J recombination there appears to be a shutdown of further recombinational activity on the other allele of that immune receptor. This results in the production of only a single functional immune receptor chain of any given type by a single cell (this is called *allelic exclusion* and will be dealt with more extensively later in this chapter).

▼ SOMATIC MUTATION[31]

Early on in this chapter we contrasted two extreme views of the generation of immune receptor diversity, one in which all potential antigen binding possibilities were encoded in place in germline DNA, the other in which a single gene became subject to a mechanism of hypermutation on antigenic stimulation. We have seen that germline diversity does indeed exist, although it is not as extensive as in the extreme example. Similarly, at least for the immunoglobulin heavy and light chain loci, a mechanism of somatic hypermutation of the V(D)J regions formed by site-specific recombination has been amply demonstrated. Numerous cases have been described in which the V region sequence in a functionally rearranged immunoglobulin produced by a B lymphocyte differs from the germline V segment from which it arose, not just in junctional sequences but in the body of the segment as well. Most of these examples are found in B cells that have "switched" (see below) from a "primary" IgM response to an IgG or IgA "secondary" response. The conceptual framework in which somatic mutation is viewed postulates that such mutation acts to increase the binding affinity of antibody for antigen, and that those cells that have mutated their initial immunoglobulins to those of higher affinity for a particular antigen are more selectively stimulated by antigenic challenge.

The rate of somatic mutation within the V segments of immunoglobulin genes has been estimated to be remarkably high; some investigators estimate it to be as high as 10^{-3} per base pair per cell generation.[29] This process can continue during several cycles of cell division.[32] Remarkably, this mutational mechanism appears to be restricted mainly to the variable regions of rearranged immunoglobulins in B cells. In fact, the rest of the immunoglobulin locus appears to be unaffected, with the 5′ boundary of mutational activity found near the promoter of the rearranged V segment and the 3′ boundary about 1000 nucleotides distal to the rearranged J

Table 11–1. Potential Diversity of Human Immunoglobulin (IG) and T-Cell Antigen Receptor (TCR) Variable Region Domains*

	IG			TCRαβ		TCRγδ	
	H	**κ**	**λ**	**α**	**β**	**γ**	**δ**
V segments	50	25	30	60	46	8	10
D segments	24	0	0	0	2	0	3
J segments	6	5	4	50	12	5	3
V(D)J combinations	10^4	125	120	3000	2000	40	200
N regions	2	0	0	1	2	1	4
V domains	10^{10}	10^3	10^3	3×10^6	2×10^9	4×10^4	2×10^{14}
V domain pairs	10^{13}			10^{16}		10^{19}	

*The approximate number of V, C, and J segments is indicated for each locus. The number of N regions corresponds to the number of joining events except for IgL chains (κ and λ), which rarely have N sequences. The approximate number of potential V domains for each locus is calculated as the number of V, (D), and J segment combinations multiplied by the potential extent of junctional diversity as a result of one or more joining events. As a rough estimate, joints lacking N sequences are assumed to have 10 possible amino acid sequences as a result of exonuclease nibbling and P sequences, whereas joints containing N sequences are assumed to have 1000 possible template independent amino acid sequences. Additional variability of Ig V domains results from antigen driven somatic hypermutation. Potential variability is decreased early in ontogeny by lack of N regions; preferential joining of specific V, D, and J segments; and so on, as indicated in the text. A more complex discussion of the potential variability at sites of joining can be found elsewhere.[114]

segment.[33] Thus, there appears to be a mutational system activated in B lymphocytes that because of a combination of structural information and transcriptional activity targets the rearranged V(D)J region in antigen selected cells. This process does not appear to be active in T cells. Perhaps the different "recognition" requirements of T cells make a hypermutation mechanism a disadvantage in this lineage. (See Chapter 13.)

The five mechanisms of generation of immune receptor diversity just described are responsible for the almost infinite variety of binding sites that allow a response to essentially any antigenic challenge (see Table 11–1).

The Mechanism of V(D)J Recombination

▼ THE RECOMBINASE COMPLEX

In the above section we have provided an overview of the process of the generation of immune receptor diversity, a process that relies largely, though not totally, on a structural, irreversible reconfiguration of the DNA encoding the immune receptor genes. In this section we will describe in greater detail some of the components and the mechanism of action of the "recombinase complex" that mediates V(D)J rearrangement. The development of cell free systems for analysis of V(D)J recombination has greatly aided in the dissection and elucidation of the various components of this process.[33a–33c] It seems that there are probably a number of enzymes whose concerted action leads to the recognition and juxtaposition of V, D, and J segments. Included among these are likely to be those discussed in the following sections.

Recombination Activating Genes 1 and 2

The recombination activating genes 1 and 2 (RAG-1) and (RAG-2) were discovered because of their ability to induce measurable V(D)J recombination activity (on an exogenously introduced substrate) synergistically when transfected into fibroblasts, cells that normally have no "recombinase" activity.[34, 35] These genes are tightly linked on human chromosome 11 and, remarkably, may represent the legacy of an

evolutionarily distant event with a transposable element (see below). Although it was formally possible that the protein products of these genes regulate the expression of the actual recombinase, in vitro experiments have demonstrated that these two proteins by themselves are capable of cleaving exogenously supplied recombination-signal containing substrates.[36, 37] The reaction is, however, enhanced and made more efficient by the presence of the DNA-bending high mobility group proteins, HMG1 and HMG2.[38] The genes are conserved in those species that are known to carry out V(D)J recombination. When transfected into fibroblasts they initiate V(D)J recombination activity without initiating any other evidence of a lymphoid developmental program. Their dual expression is closely correlated with those lymphoid cells and cell lines that have demonstrated V(D)J recombinational activity and not with those that do not.

Double-stranded DNA Break/Repair Enzymes

In the mouse there is a mutation, *scid*, which, when present in the homozygous form, abrogates normal B- and T-cell mediated immunity.[39] It was demonstrated[40] that these mice were incapable of generating functionally V(D)J rearranged immune receptor genes. More refined molecular analysis revealed that recognition of signal sequences and DNA breakage were taking place in these animals, but the ends of the V, D, or J coding segments were not being ligated back together. The signal ends, however, were ligated without apparent problem.[41–43] Without this reaction no functional immunoglobulins or T-cell antigen receptors could be formed, and no antigen driven stimulation and proliferation of lymphocytes achieved. Thus the product of this *scid* locus appears to be an integral part of the complex that mediates the site-specific V(D)J recombinational mechanism. Elucidation of the *scid* gene product was aided by the parallel study of genes that effected a response to DNA damaging agents. In particular a series of complementing mutations were characterized in hamster cell lines that demonstrated increased sensitivity to ionizing radiation and other agents capable of generating double-stranded (DS) DNA breaks. These mutations were charaterized as X-ray cross complementation (XRCC) groups 4, 5, and 7.[44, 45] Cells from *scid* mice were unable to complement the XRCC 7 mutation.[46] Previous work had identified a protein serine-threonine kinase (DNA-PK) that required the presence of and binding to DNA to manifest its activity.[47–49] Biochemical studies using the purified catalytic subunit (CS) of DNA-PK to complement extracts from *scid* cells and cellular transfection using the cloned DNA-PK gene to restore DS-DNA break repair and V(D)J recombination in scid cells demonstrated that the *scid* gene itself was DNA-PKCS.[50–52] The category of severe combined immunodeficiency (SCID) in humans covers a broad range of genetic defects including adenosine deaminase deficiency, purine nucleoside phosphorylase deficiency, and x-linked immunodeficiency.[53–56] Among those SCID patients whose defect has not yet been characterized there may be individuals who manifest a syndrome analogous to that seen in the *scid* mice.

The binding of DNA-PK to the ends of double-stranded DNA is stabilized by a heterodimeric protein complex called Ku.[57] The 70 and 86 kDa Ku proteins (Ku70 and Ku86, [sometimes referred to as Ku80], respectively) bind to DS-DNA, stem-loop, or double strand–single strand transitions and have DNA-dependent adenosine triphosphatase (ATPase) activities.[58] The Ku complex was originally identified as an autoantigen present in patients with the scleroderma-polymyositis syndrome.[59] Ku86 corresponds to the *XRCC5* gene and Ku70 is believed to represent the *XRCC6* gene activity.[60–62] A complementary DNA (cDNA) designated XRCC4 was cloned because of its ability to restore double strand break repair and V(D)J recombination to a defective cell line.[63] The cell line had been noted to be capable of initiating V(D)J recombination but incapable of completing the reaction with the formation of coding and signal joints, and therefore a role for XRCC4 in strand ligation was postulated. Indeed, XRCC4 has been found to associate with and stimulate ligation activity of DNA ligase IV.[64] XRCC4 is also both a substrate for and facilitator of DNA binding by DNA-PK via its association with the Ku complex.[65]

Terminal Deoxynucleotidyl Transferase

As noted above, the appearance of N sequences at the junction of V(D)J rearrangements is consistent with the known pattern of expression and demonstrated activity of the enzyme terminal deoxynucleotidyl transferase (TdT). Terminal transferase is a DNA polymerase that does not require a DNA template but does require a DNA primer, preferably a protruding 3' hydroxyl terminus.[66] TdT is capable of adding any of the four nucleoside triphosphates to this 3' end of the molecule. The level of N sequence addition directly correlates with the level of TdT function as validated experimentally in TdT "null" or overexpressing model systems.[26, 67–69] In a transgenic mouse model that constitutively expressed TdT, it could be demonstrated that the normal restriction on N sequence addition within Ig loci during early development and beyond heavy chain rearrangement was lifted without obvious ill effect. This suggests that expression of TdT during fetal development is not by itself deleterious and that it may be sufficient for the addition of N sequences at any Ig locus.[70] It has been noted, however, that in the rare recombination products that occur in Ku86 "null" mice no N sequences are found, suggesting a role

or required interaction of Ku with TdT for N sequence addition.[71]

Recombination Signal Sequence Binding Proteins

A number of investigators have used oligonucleotides based on the signal sequences that flank the recombining segments (see below) as a tool for dissecting out protein elements that may play a role in the process of recombination.[72–78] So far no gene identified in this way has been shown to be either necessary or sufficient for V(D)J recombination; nor has an immunologically distinctive phenotype yet been associated with its loss or mutation. Nevertheless, one or more of these genes may indeed be components of the recombinase complex mediating one or another aspect of the recognition or breakage and rejoining reaction.

▼ SIGNAL SEQUENCE RECOGNITION

The activity of the recombinase complex is focused on certain sites in the genome where a specific nucleotide signal sequence occurs. This signal sequence is conserved in all species known to rearrange immune receptors via a recombinase complex. It consists of a heptamer with a consensus sequence CACA/TGTG separated by 12 or 23 random nucleotides from a consensus nonamer sequence ACAAAAACC (or GGTTTTTGT, depending on the orientation). These sequences are found 3' of the V segments, 5' of the J segments, and flanking the D segments. The heptamer is always flush to the coding segments of the nonamer up- or downstream of it, in the direction of the segment with which potential rearrangement can occur (see Fig. 11–4). For the recombinase complex to be able to join any two coding segments it appears that one heptamer/nonamer must enclose a random spacer of 12 base pairs and the other heptamer/nonamer a spacer of 23 base pairs. This spacing corresponds roughly to one or two turns of a DNA double helix, suggesting a potential three-dimensional structure recognized by the recombinase complex.

A refined analysis of these signal sequences[79] has suggested that the heptamer sequence is more crucial for recombination than the nonamer. Indeed V(D)J recombination can occur (though with less efficiency) even in the absence of the nonamer from one or the other side of the rearranging segments. The four bases of the heptamer closest to the coding segments are the most crucial nucleotides for signal recognition. Alterations of the sequence in this area can lower by over 100-fold the efficiency of recombination of experimentally designed constructs introduced into cells in which the recombinase complex is known to be active. The efficiency of recombination is also markedly lowered if more than two base pairs are added or deleted from the spacer between the heptamer and nonamer.

▼ ACCESSIBILITY

The presence of appropriate signal sequences and active recombinase enzymes is probably not sufficient to cause structural reconfiguration of a particular immune receptor locus. Introduction of RAG-1 and RAG-2 into fibroblasts was sufficient to cause V(D)J-like rearrangement of exogenously introduced (and actively transcribed) substrates, but not of the immune receptor genes in the endogenous DNA of the fibroblast.[34, 35] This finding supported the concept that in addition to the enzymes and signal sequences, a locus must be "accessible" to the recombinase complex in order for recombination to occur. In a fibroblast, the immune receptor genes are inactive and transcriptionally silent. Thus there is no evidence that a recombinase enzyme complex could gain access to them. Earlier work[80] had demonstrated that transcriptional activity can be detected from V segments prior to their rearrangement (see Fig. 11–3). Although it is possible that the "sterile" (not coding for a functional protein) transcript itself might play a role in the recombinational mechanism, it is perhaps equally likely that it is simply a marker of a change in the status of the chromatin in which the V segments reside. This latter argument would suggest that if a segment of DNA were accessible to an RNA polymerase it might be similarly accessible to the recombinase complex. In lymphocytes in which IgH but not the endogenous Ig light chains or TCR loci are transcribed or subject to rearrangement, exogenously introduced substrates carrying Ig light chain genes or *TCR* genes are ready targets for V(D)J recombination as long as they are provided on a transcriptionally active vector.[81, 82] These experiments also provided evidence that the same recombinase system was capable of rearranging Ig and TCR loci. In other words, the regulation of rearrangement of these loci does not occur at the level of V(D)J recombinase recognition, but more likely is decided by which loci are accessible to the recombinase complex at a point in lymphocyte development and lineage determination. If signal sequences are present within two given loci, and if the recombinase complex is active, those two loci are at risk of being rearranged if they are transcriptionally active, even if neither encodes an immune receptor.[83] Thus the V(D)J recombinase complex can be an important factor in increasing genomic instability in lymphocytes, instability that can cause chromosomal aberrations and, in so doing, contribute to malignant transformation by disrupting or dysregulating genes that control cell growth or development (this will be discussed in greater detail later in this chapter). The concept that chromatin must be in an accessible conformation in order for breakage and rejoining events to occur may, indeed, transcend a discussion of V(D)J recombination and be generally relevant to the generation of most chromosomal aberrations.[84, 85]

Regulation of Transcription[86–106]

There are at least five kinds of *cis-* elements that regulate transcription in mammalian cells: promoters, enhancers, silencers, enhancer blocking boundary elements, and locus control regions (LCRs). *Promoters*, which are the minimal element necessary for RNA polymerase to initiate transcription, are located immediately upstream from transcription initiation sites and generally function in a distance- and orientation-dependent manner. *Enhancers* increase transcription from promoters when present in either orientation and can be located either upstream or downstream of the transcription initiation site; in addition they can be active over relatively long distances (up to 10 kb or more). *Silencers* repress transcription independently of the orientation or distance from a promoter or enhancer and can also be located either upstream or downstream of the promoter or enhancer. *Enhancer blocking boundary elements* block transcription activity from being propagated distal to the element but do not repress the transcriptional activity of either a promoter or an enhancer proximal to the boundary defined by this element and thus is different from a silencer. *Locus control regions*, which have been best studied in the β globin locus, are defined as elements that confer copy dependent, integration-site independent, tissue specific expression of a heterologous gene and can act in either orientation over very long distances (hundreds of kilobases). It is thought that the function of an LCR is mediated, at least in part, by establishing open chromatin domains over long distances.

In fact, the five kinds of elements described above often occur in combinations. For example, promoters or LCRs can contain enhancer elements, and enhancers can contain silencers. Each kind of element is often associated with multiple DNA binding motifs, with several motifs contributing to generate a particular effect on transcription in a given cell type. There is often redundancy of function so that removal of several DNA binding motifs from a regulatory element, or even removal of the entire regulatory element, may have no effect on transcription in a particular setting. For example, removal of an IgH Eμ intronic enhancer has little effect on transcription of IgH chain in a myeloma cell, presumably because of the redundant effect of the Eα 3′ enhancer in this setting. Each DNA binding motif might bind a variety of *trans-* acting transcription factors, and the presence of these factors, or an active form of these factors, may depend on the cell type or the physiological state of the cell.

For example, all Ig promoters and many Ig enhancers contain an octamer motif, which can interact with transcription factors called Oct-1 and Oct-2. Most cells express Oct-1, whereas Oct-2 is restricted primarily to all stages of B-cell development but only a limited number of other cell types. It appears that Oct-1 can partially substitute for Oct-2 in mice lacking the *Oct2* gene. In addition, the specificity of Oct-2 and Oct-1 for specific octamer sites in B cells is provided by their interaction with a B-cell-specific coactivater called OCA-B. Other factors that are expressed in most tissues contribute to increased Ig transcription by binding to additional (nonoctamer) motifs present in Ig promoters or enhancers. Another well-studied example of a B-cell tissue specific transcriptional activator is NF-κB, which binds a 10 bp motif in the JCκ intronic enhancer and is present in an active form in virtually all cells in the B-cell lineage except pre-B cells. In fact, NF-κB is present in an inactive form in most kinds of cells (including pre-B cells) and can be converted to an active form, even in the presence of protein synthesis inhibitors, by stimulating the cells through a variety of signaling pathways. In some cases transcription factors interact with other proteins or each other, and thereby alter their DNA binding specificity or the effect of DNA binding.

As a result of the complex interplay of distinct DNA binding motifs and multiple transcription factors, any of the five regulatory elements described above may be active in one kind of cell but inactive in another kind. One complex example in T cells is particularly instructive. The TCRαδ locus, which contains the δ locus nested within the α locus, contains each of the five kinds of elements described above (Fig. 11–6). Regulation is thought to occur in the following manner: The downstream locus control regionαδ (LCRαδ) is active in cells that express TCRαβ or TCRγδ and presumably "opens" the chromatin to permit function of both the Eδ enhancer and the Eα enhancer (the latter is located immediately 5′ of the LCR). However, a silencer element (Sα in Fig. 11–6) immediately upstream of Eα specifically blocks activity of Eα in γδ T cells or non-T cells, so that only the δ region is active for gene rearrangements and transcription in γδ T cells (positive effect of Eδ), and neither TCR locus is active in non-T cells (the Eδ is not active in non-T cells). In this situation, an enhancer blocking boundary element (*B* in Fig. 11–6) prevents spread of transcription from the δ region to the immediately downstream TEA promoter that initiates transcripts just upstream of the 5′-most Jα segment (it is thought that transcription from the TEA promoter is associated with accessibility of the Jα segments for VJα joining). Upon entry into the TCRαβ pathway, the Sα silencer is inactive. The LCR competition hypothesis suggests that competition between the proximal Eα and distal Eδ results in an active Eα at the expense of an inactive Eδ. The active Eα enhances transcription from the TEA promoter, VJα joining, and then VJα transcription.

Despite progress in the past few years, we have only a fragmentary knowledge of how transcription of the Ig and TCR loci is regulated in B and T lymphoid cells. Nonetheless, it is worthwhile summarizing a few general features of transcription regulation of the Ig and TCR loci. There is a strong association of transcriptional activity and "accessibility" of sequences for the unique recombinational processes that occur in lymphoid cells. In addition, it should be noted that transcriptional regulation of the Ig and TCR loci is unique in that gene rearrangements lead to important changes in the distances over which transcriptional regulatory elements are separated from one another at different times in the maturation of lymphocytes. To illustrate these ideas, we will focus on Ig loci in B cells.

Depending on the state of B-cell maturation, there are a variety of transcripts that can be expressed from rearranged or unrearranged loci. For example, pro-B cells can express germline V_H segment transcripts, germline Cμ transcripts initiating about 1 kb upstream from a germline Cμ gene, DJC transcripts initiating upstream of DJ rearranged genes, and VDJC (IgH chain) transcripts after completion of rearrangements. Pre-B cells can express germline V_κ and germline JC_κ transcripts, as well as VJC_κ (Igκ chain) transcripts after completion of rearrangements, but probably not germline V_H transcripts. Beyond the pre-B cell stage germline VL transcripts are not expressed. In fact, the B-cell developmental stage at which these germline or partially rearranged loci (e.g., DJ) are transcribed coincides with the time that these loci are involved in VDJ rearrangements (see below). Many of the transcripts from unrearranged loci appear to be *"sterile"* transcripts (i.e., transcripts that do not seem to encode a protein). However, in some cases, it appears that transcripts from an unrearranged locus do encode a protein; for example, a protein of uncertain significance is translated from the incompletely rearranged DJC_H sequence. Highly differentiated B cells continue to express rearranged H and L genes but prior to switching can express sterile transcripts that initiate upstream of switch regions associated with C regions that are programmed to be involved in the IgH switch recombination process (see below). Plasma cells transcribe IgH and IgL chain genes at significantly higher rates and have higher steady-state levels of the corresponding messenger RNAs (mRNAs) than less mature B or pre-B cells (it should be noted that the higher levels of Ig heavy and light chain mRNAs in plasma cells are a consequence of both transcriptional and post-transcriptional mechanisms).

There is a continuing, but as yet incomplete, accumulation of information regarding the function of promoters in the Ig loci. Intronic enhancers located between the J segments and the constant regions have been well defined for the IgH and Igκ loci, whereas 3′ enhancers have been defined downstream of the IgH, Igκ, and Igλ loci (see Fig. 11–9). The IgH intronic enhancer (Eμ) seems to be active in all B cells. In pro-B cells, there is a promoter/enhancer element upstream of the most proximal D that enhances DJ transcription and D/J joining, with the Eμ enhancer contributing somewhat. The Eμ enhancer has a major positive effect on V/DJ joining. The 3′ IgH enhancer(s) seem to have only a small effect in transcription and VDJ joining in early B cells but is exremely active in plasma cells and has

Figure 11–6. The human T-cell antigen receptor loci. The chromosomal localization and genetic organization of the three TCR loci are shown in schematic form although not to scale. The orientation from left to right is centromeric (c) to telomeric (t). V segments, each containing two exons, are indicated by dark boxes. D segments and J segments are indicated by thin and thick lines, respectively. Constant region genes, each of which contains a number of exons, are indicated by open boxes. The arrows over Vβ14 and Vδ5 segments indicate transcription toward the centromere, whereas all other segments are transcribed away from the centromere. Regulatory elements are as follows: large gray circles (E, enhancers; LCR, locus control regions); diagonal dark boxes (S, silencers); B, open arrow (enhancer blocking boundary element); TEA promoter (arrow) upstream of the Jα segments. See text for further details.

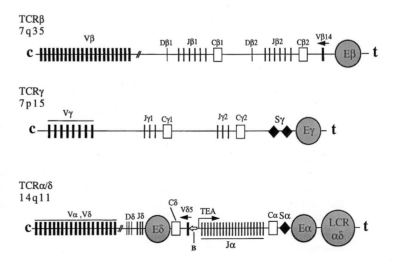

a very strong effect on regulating IgH switch recombination and somatic hypermutation. There is some evidence that the 3′IgH enhancer may include an LCR function. The Igκ intronic (Eκ) and 3′ IgL (3′Eκ and 3′Eλ) enhancers are active in B cells and plasma cells but have little or no activity in pro-B cells. In pre-B cells, deletion of either iEκ or 3′Eκ causes a decreased efficiency of VJκ rearrangements and increased numbers of cells expressing Igλ, but Igκ transcription is decreased only when the 3′Eκ is deleted, and not when iEκ is deleted. Although these and other data provide some insights, many questions remain to be answered regarding the *cis-* elements and *trans-* factors that regulate transcription and rearrangement of Ig loci: (1) What are the regulatory elements that turn specific germline V_H or V_L transcripts on and then off as B lymphoid cells progress along the developmental pathway? (2) Are there LCR regions in the Ig loci, and, if so, are the 3′ enhancers part of an LCR region? (3) Are the 3′ enhancers responsible for the dysregulation of translocated oncogenes that can be located hundreds of kilobases from translocation breakpoints in the Ig loci (see description of translocations in a latter section)? (4) Is transcription necessary for, or merely associated with, recombination?

T-Cell Antigen Receptors

▼ STRUCTURE AND FUNCTION[107–111]

There are two basic kinds of T-cell antigen receptors (TCRs), each comprising a pair of disulfide linked heterodimeric glycoproteins (i.e., α/β and γ/δ) with a composite molecular weight of about 90 kDa (see Fig. 11–2). All four types of TCR chains (α, β, δ, γ) have a similar size (30–40 kDa of amino acids) and structural organization, with a large extracellular region, a transmembrane domain of about 20 amino acids that includes a conserved lysine (as well as an arginine for α and β chains), and a very small cytoplasmic domain containing fewer than 20 amino acids. Starting at the amino-terminus, the extracellular region is divided into three domains, a variable region with an intradomain disulfide bond, a constant region with an intradomain disulfide bond, as well as several N-linked oligosaccharides, and a hinge or connecting domain containing a cysteine residue that can form an interchain disulfide bond with the other member of the heterodimer. In addition, there is a pre-T α chain (which has a structure that is similar to that of the α chain except for the lack of a variable domain) that can form heterodimers with a β chain.

Both kinds of TCR are non-covalently associated with a number of non-polymorphic glycopeptides that collectively are designated as the CD3 complex. The CD3 complexes include four kinds of polypeptides, CD3-γ, CD3-δ, CD3-ε, and CD3-ζ chains, with similar structural features. Each chain includes an extracellular domain, a transmembrane domain containing a negatively charged amino acid, and an intracellular domain that contains conserved serine and tyrosine residues. It is thought that the negative charges on the transmembrane domains of CD3 chains interact with the positive charges in the transmembrane domains of the TCR chains, thus ensuring cell surface expression of a functional TCR-CD3 membrane complex. The TCR-CD3 complex includes two copies of α/β or δ/λ heterodimers, two copies of CD3-ε, two copies of disulfide linked CD3-ζ, and two copies of either CD3-δ or CD3-γ. Importantly, the CD3 complex transduces the antigen/TCR binding signal to the interior of the cell by a process involving a change in the phosphorylation status of the serine and/or tyrosine residues on the cytoplasmic portions of the CD3 chains.

Although α/β TCRs appear later in ontogeny than γ/δ TCRs, the former represent 95 per cent or more of T cells in peripheral blood and secondary lymphoid tissues. An α/β TCR cannot recognize free antigen but instead recognizes antigen expressed on a cell surface. More specifically, the α/β TCR is thought to recognize an antigenic determinant primarily as a breakdown product (derived from either an intra- or an extracellular antigen) that is non-covalently complexed either to a major histocompatibility class (MHC) class I (i.e., human leukocyte antigen [HLA] A, B, or C antigens) or to an MHC class II (i.e., HLA-DR, DS, or SB) molecule on the surface of an appropriate cell. In fact, a functional TCR response requires simultaneous corecognition of the antigenic determinant and the MHC product by the TCR. The ability of T lymphocytes to recognize a complex that comprises an antigenic determinant and an MHC class I or class II molecule is enhanced by the additional interaction of T-cell receptors (CD4 and CD8) for the two respective MHC products. CD4 and CD8 receptors are glycopeptides, each of which is a member of the immunoglobulin supergene family that also includes Ig, TCR, MHC class I, and MHC class II genes. Thus the functional interaction of antigen with an α/β TCR receptor includes not only an association of an antigen/MHC complex and the CD3 complex with TCR, but also an interaction of CD8 with MHC class I or CD4 with MHC class II molecules on the antigen presenting cell. In general, cytotoxic T cells express CD8 so that they can recognize antigen-MH class I complexes on essentially any cell. In contrast, helper T cells generally express CD4 so that they can efficiently recognize antigen/MHC class II complexes on macrophages or B lymphocytes.

In contrast to α/β TCRs, γ/δ TCRs may not require MHC interaction to bind antigen and recognize not only cell surface antigens but also polyvalent soluble antigens, including non-peptide antigens. The physiological significance of differences between TCRs that comprise α/β versus γ/δ heterodimers is not entirely clear, although a consistent difference in pattern of expression has been well established. T cells expressing γ/δ TCR heterodimers occur earlier in ontogeny, as supported by expression on CD4-8-cells and also appear to be relatively more abundant in some sites, such as epidermis and intestinal epithelium. Most T cells with γ/δ TCR receptors are CD4-8-, with a small fraction CD4-8+, and an even smaller fraction CD4+8-.

▼ CHROMOSOMAL LOCALIZATION AND GENETIC ORGANIZATION[87, 90, 106–109, 112, 113]

A knowledge of the chromosomal localization and genetic organization of the four TCR loci is critical for understanding the pattern and significance of normal and abnormal (e.g., chromosomal translocations) TCR gene rearrangements in normal and malignant cells. The overall organization of the four TCR loci is highly conserved for the extensively studied human and murine systems, although we will focus on the human system as much as possible.

T-Cell Antigen Receptor Beta Locus

The TCRβ locus has been localized at chromosome band 7q35 and includes nearly 700 kb of DNA, all of which has been sequenced (see Fig. 11–6).

At the centromeric end of the locus, there are 46 functional V segments, each with the same orientation as the J and C segments, so that intrachromosomal joining of V to DJ results in deletion of intervening sequences (cf. Fig. 11–3). One additional functional V gene (Vβ14) is present near the telomeric end of the locus and has an inverse orientation so that rearrangement with D1 or D2 results in an inversion and not loss of intervening sequences. Each V segment contains two exons organized as for Cκ (cf. Fig. 11–3). In an approximately 20 kb region at the telomeric end of the locus, there is a single D segment (D1) followed by one non-functional pseudo J and 6 functional J segments (J1.1–1.6) and a C gene (C1); then another D segment (D2) followed by 6 J segments (J2.1–2.6) and another C gene (C2). The two C genes, each of which includes four exons, are highly homologous, with only six amino acid substitutions distinguishing them and no known functional difference. Although the number and organization of C gene exons are not identical for all TCR C genes, collectively the C gene exons, including the Cβ gene exons, encode the constant region domain, a short connecting or hinge-like region containing the cysteine involved in the disulfide bond to the TCR heterodimeric partner, the transmembrane domain, the cytoplasmic domain, and the 3′ untranslated region. The Cβ genes are unique among TCR genes in that there is a fourth cysteine of unknown significance located between the cysteines that form the intradomain disulfide bridge in the constant region. The initial rearrangement event in this locus is D to J, and at a later time V to DJ. Position and orientation dictate that D1 can join to any of the 12 functional J segments, but D2 can join only to J2.1–2.7. Important regulatory elements include promoters upstream of each V segment and an enhancer at the telomeric end of the locus, beyond Vβ14.

T-Cell Antigen Receptor Gamma Locus

The TCRγ locus, which has been localized to human chromosomal band 7p15, includes 160 kb of DNA (see Fig. 11–6).

At the centromeric end of the locus there are 10 functional V segments, each in the same orientation as the C genes. By sequence homology, there are six subfamilies, with five subfamilies containing one sequence. There are no D regions. In an approximately 30 kb region at the telomeric end of the locus, there are three J segments (J1.1–1.3) followed by a C gene (C1), and then 2 more J segments (J2.1–2.2) followed by another C gene (C2). The C1 gene has 3 exons, whereas the highly homologous C2 gene is represented by alleles with 4 or 5 exons, resulting from a duplication or triplication, respectively, of the second exon. In addition, the C2 gene lacks the cysteine residue that forms an interchain disulfide bridge for all other TCR heterodimeric pairs. Thus γ chains of subtype 2 (i.e., γ2 chains) are

larger than γ chains of subtype 1 and other TCR chains and provide the only example of human or mouse TCR that cannot be disulfide linked to its heterodimeric partner. It should be noted that Cβ and Cγ chains are structurally more similar to each other than to either Cα or Cδ chains. Regulatory elements appear to include an enhancer and a silencer downstream of Cγ2.

T-Cell Antigen Receptor Alpha Locus

The TCRα locus, which has been localized to human band 14q11, includes about 1.1 mb of DNA (see Fig. 11–6).

At the centromeric end of the locus there are approximately 60 known V segments, mostly if not only in the same orientation as the C genes. By sequence homology there are 22 V segment subfamilies, with 15 subfamilies containing only one member. Members of the same V subfamily can be adjacent or widely dispersed over more than 600 kb. There are no known D segments, but there are about 50 J segments covering an 80 kb region separated by about 100 kb from the 3′-most V segment. This pattern of numerous and broadly distributed J segments diverges markedly from the J clusters associated with other immune receptors. Approximately 5 kb from the 3′-most Jα segment is a single Cα gene. Regulatory elements downstream of C include silencers (Sα in Fig. 11–6), an enhancer (Eα), and then a locus control region (LCRαδ).

T-Cell Antigen Receptor Delta Locus

The TCRδ locus is localized within and has the same transcriptional orientation as the TCRα locus (see Fig. 11–6). The Dδ, Jδ, and Cδ sequences are localized between the most telomeric Vα and the most centromeric Jα gene segments. The interspersion of these two structurally and functionally related loci is consistent with the notion that one locus evolved from the other by gene duplication. Moreover, this unusual organization of these two loci results in deletion of the δ locus upon rearrangement of Vα and Jα segments. The single Cδ gene, which contains 4 exons, is located about 80 kb upstream from the Cα gene. There are 3 Dδ segments (Dδ1–3) within a 10 kb sequence, with the most 3′ Dδ segment about 1 kb from the 5′ Jδ segment. There are also 3 Jδ segments (Jδ1–3) within a 10 kb sequence, with the most 3′ J about 3 kb from the 5′ end of the first Cδ exon. There are approximately 10 Vδ gene segments, 9 of which are interspersed within the Vα segments and also have the same orientation as Cα and Cδ. In principle, the interspersed Vα and Vδ segments could be joined with either Dδ or Jα. In fact, there are several examples demonstrating that the same V segment can be rearranged to either a Jα or a Dδ gene segment, but it seems that most V segments join mainly with only one of the two loci. A single Vδ gene segment (Vδ5) is localized about 3 kb 3′ of the 3′ exon of the Cδ gene and is oriented in an opposite transcriptional orientation, so that an inversion rather than a deletion occurs when this V gene segment is rearranged to a D segment. Interestingly, the TCRδ locus provides the only example of a TCR locus in which there is DD joining in addition to VD or DJ joining. In fact, it appears that a functionally rearranged human delta gene can include all 3 D segments and 4 sets of N sequences corresponding to the 4 joining events, suggesting that this chain has the most potential diversity (see Table 11–1). Unlike the rearrangement of TCRβ genes, which first join a D segment to a J segment and then a V segment to a DJ segment, there is initial VD and DD joining, and then VD/J joining in the δlocus. Finally, there is an enhancer element (Eδ in Fig. 11–6) between Jδ and Cδ, and an enhancer blocking boundary element downstream of Cδ (designated B in Fig. 11–6).

▼ T-CELL RECEPTOR GENE REARRANGEMENT AND DIVERSITY[107–109, 111, 114]

The structural organization of TCR genes and signal sequences for joining dictates how these genes can be rearranged to generate the vast number of different V regions to recognize the diverse antigenic determinants that are encountered by an individual. As described above, the heptamer/nonamer signals for joining are located so that the heptamer is adjacent to the structural sequence that is to be joined. Also, the two structural gene segments (i.e., V, D, J) to be joined are constrained in that the signal sequence adjacent to one segment must have a separation of 11 or 12 bp (about one turn of the DNA helix) between the heptamer and nonamer sequences, whereas the other segment must have a separation of 22 or 23 bp (about two turns of the DNA helix) between the heptamer and nonamer sequences (i.e., 12/23 bp rule). On the basis of the organization of signal sequences for joining as shown in Figure 11–7, one can predict which segments (V, D, J) can be joined for each of the TCR genes, although not all possibilities occur at a detectable frequency. For all four TCR loci, the heptamer/nonamer separation is 23 bp downstream of the V gene segment and 12 bp upstream of the J gene segment. Yet a V segment is directly joined to a J segment only in the α and γ loci. Similarly, since the heptamer and nonamer sequences are separated by 12 and 23 bp, respectively, for the joining signals upstream and downstream of D segments, it should be possible to join two D segments in either the β or δ loci. Although the joining of two or three D segments can occur in the δ locus as described above, the two D segments in the β locus have not been observed to join to one another. It is not clear why VJ joining does not occur in either the β or δ locus, and also why there is not DD joining in the β locus.

For all four TCR loci, the various mechanisms described above (with the exception of somatic hypermutation) can be used to generate an incredible diversity of V regions. The relative contribution of different mechanisms is not identical for each locus, and there is also a striking difference in how a similar extent of potential diversity can be achieved for the α/β receptor compared to the γ/δ receptor. As summarized in Table 11–1, there are many more potential combinations of V, D, and J segments for TCR α/β receptors than for TCR γ/δ receptors. For each type of receptor, however, the relative contribution of junctional mechanisms would seem to outweigh greatly the contribution of the number of V, D, and J germline segments in generating TCR diversity. As a rationale for this finding, it has been hypothesized that the junctional region is critically involved in recognizing the vast number of antigenic determinants, whereas the remainder of the V region is important for recognizing the more limited number of MHC molecules. For each kind of receptor, one of the two chains (β or δ) has D segments, which mostly can be read in three frames. Among all TCR and Ig loci, the powerful diversity mechanism of D to D joining apparently occurs only in the δ locus. For all loci and kinds of joints (VD, DD, DJ, VJ) there is a marked degree of flexibility (i.e., exonuclease nibbling as described above) in the precise nucleotides that are used to join two segments. Similarly, for each of these instances there can be addition of as many as five or more N nucleotides since TdT is expressed in all T cells undergoing VDJ recombination. Thus, one can predict the possibility of 10^{15} or more heterodimeric combinations for all three kinds of Ig and TCR receptors (Table 11–1).

Despite the incredible potential diversity of heterodi-

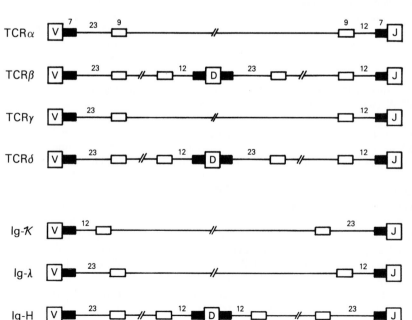

Figure 11–7. Organization of heptamer/nonamer sequences for V, D, and J segments located in the four TCR and three Ig loci. The V, D, and J segments are indicated by large open boxes, the heptamer by closed boxes, and the nonamers by small open boxes. The heptamer and nonamer sequences are separated by 12 or 23 bp, creating two kinds of joining signals. Intra- or, rarely, interlocus joining can occur between segments that have different joining signals, e.g., VH to D or D to JH but not VH to JH or D to D in the IgH locus. See text for details.

mers, the actual diversity achieved may be considerably less, depending on the type of receptor, the age of the individual, and so on. For example, whereas δ chains in adult mice demonstrate DD joining and addition of N regions at all joints, the δ chains in fetal mice contain only one D and have few if any N regions. Also, there seems to be a preferential rearrangement of some Vγ gene segments, so that Vγ genes located most 3' are rearranged preferentially early in murine development, but more random use of Vγ segments occurs at a later time in development. In addition, for γδ TCR bearing T cells, a different predominant V region is expressed in fetal murine thymocytes compared to peripheral T cells. Moreover, T cells associated with various kinds of epithelium express a different but highly restricted set of TCRγ/δ variable regions. Finally, there is not enough evidence, particularly in humans, to assess whether these and other constraints limit the actual extent of heterodimeric TCR diversity for different circumstances.

▼ ONTOGENY OF T-CELL ANTIGEN RECEPTOR EXPRESSION[107, 109, 115–120]

The pattern and anatomical locations of T lymphocyte development are similar in mice and men. A simplified version of the developmental pathways thought to be involved in this process is shown in Figure 11–8. Depending on the age of the individual, pluripotent hematopoietic stem cells in the yolk sac, fetal liver, or bone marrow give rise to pro-T cells that express CD7, as well as cytoplasmic TdT and possibly some components of the CD3 complex also localized in the cytoplasm. The pro-T cells migrate to the thymus, where they continue the developmental process as pre-T cells in

the cortex of the thymus. In addition to CD7 and TdT, the earliest pre-T cells in the thymic cortex express CD1, CD2, and interleukin-2R (IL-2R) but do not express surface CD3, CD4, or CD8. It appears that a small fraction of these CD3-4-8- pre-T cells productively rearrange and express functional γ and δ genes, generating a population of CD3+4-8- cells that express low levels of a γ/δ TCR; the surface expression of CD3 and TCR apparently requires the expression of both complexes. A much larger fraction of the CD3-4-8- pre-T cells begin to express CD8 and then CD4. The CD3-4+8+ pre-T cells rearrange and express β and then α TCR genes, generating a population of CD3+4+8+ cells that express very low levels of an α/β TCR. Late in ontogeny, the vast majority of cells in the thymus are CD4+8+, with a significant portion also expressing CD3 and low levels of α/β TCR but a substantial portion expressing neither CD3 nor any kind of TCR. This latter CD3-4+8+ TCR population includes cells that have not completed α and β TCR rearrangements, as well as cells that have made incorrect rearrangements and thus are no longer capable of generating a functional α/β TCR receptor. A small fraction of cells in the thymic cortex are CD3+4+8-TCRα/β or CD3+4-8+TCRα/β, although most of the cells with these two phenotypes are found in the thymic medulla.

On the basis of a variety of evidence, it appears that CD3+4+8+TCRα/β cells (as well as CD3-4+8+TCR- negative cells that have been unable to generate a functional TCR receptor by functionally rearranging both α and β TCR genes) pass through a selection process involving the thymic epithelium in which more than 98 per cent of thymocytes die within the thymus. A negative selection process apparently eliminates cells expressing a functional TCR receptor that is reactive against self-antigen/MHC complexes. A positive

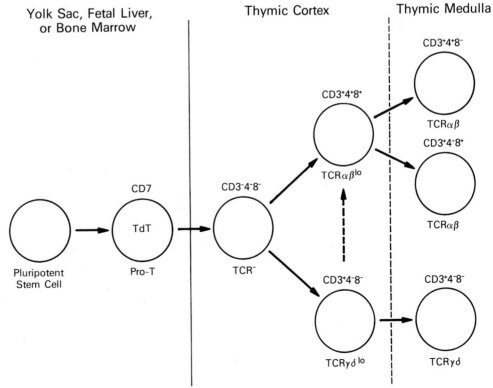

Figure 11–8. T-cell developmental pathway. This simplified scheme shows a limited number of intermediates in the developmental process, and only a few of the known markers. It should be noted that terminal deoxynucleotidyl transferase (TDT), which is first expressed in pro-T cells, continues to be expressed in pre-T cells in the thymic cortex. The early pre-T cells generate more mature pre-T cells that express either TCRαβ or TCRγδ. The dashed arrow indicates that TCRγδ cells can turn off expression of TCRγδ and proceed to express TCRαβ as well as CD4 and CD8. The TCR receptor is subjected to a combination of positive and negative selection, resulting in a limited fraction of T cells that up-regulate TCR expression and turn off VDJ recombinase as they progress to the thymic medulla. See text for additional details.

Yolk Sac, Fetal Liver, or Bone Marrow

Thymic Cortex

Thymic Medulla

selection process generates a subset of cells with functionally useful receptors (e.g., having the ability to interact productively with MHC molecules), which results in elimination of cells that do not express a functionally useful receptor, including cells that express no receptor as a result of aberrant rearrangements. In any case, after these positive and negative selection processes, the selected cells present in the thymic medulla are mainly functional CD3+4+8-TCRα/β or CD3+4-8+TCRα/β thymocytes, which express much higher levels of the α/β TCR and also generate the various kinds of cytoxic and helper T cells, respectively, that are found in the peripheral blood and secondary lymphoid organs. Although less well worked out, it appears that CD3+4-8- thymocytes with γ/δ TCR go through a poorly defined selection process that presumably does not involve CD4 or CD8 or positive selection for interaction with MHC molecules. As described below for B cells, in some instances a receptor that interacts with self-antigens can be altered by a process called *receptor editing* so that it no longer interacts with self-antigen. It has been suggested that this process occurs also during central T-cell development in the thymus, but the evidence to support this idea is not convincing at present.

▼ REGULATION OF T-CELL ANTIGEN RECEPTOR GENE FORMATION[90, 91, 102-104, 106, 107, 109, 119-126]

For the most part, individual T cells express a single species of functional TCR receptor. This may be important because of the stringent positive and negative selection processes involved in generating functional T cells, and the advantage of producing a T cell having a TCR that recognizes only one kind of antigen/MHC interaction. Since the formation of variable regions by gene rearrangements, as described above, is not a precise process, the rearrangement and expression of TCR genes must be regulated to achieve this goal of mostly expressing only one kind of functional TCR receptor per cell. What are the results of this regulatory process? First, since V and J segments can be read in only one reading frame, the flexible joining process probably results in an in-frame V(D)J one out of three times (the efficiency would be even lower if TdT did not show a bias of adding Gs or Cs in N regions, or if D regions could be read in only one or two frames). The actual efficiency of forming an in-frame V(D)J sequence at a given locus might be somewhat higher than 33 per cent since secondary rearrangements involving, for example, an upstream V and a downstream J are possible. Second, only one of the two kinds of TCR receptors (α/β TCR or γ/δ TCR) is expressed on a particular cell. Third, for at least some kinds of TCR chains expressed in a functional receptor, only one parental allele is used to encode that chain and the other parental allele is excluded from encoding a chain that contributes to a functional receptor (*allelic exclusion* phenomenon).

This process is not regulated by changes in the VDJ recombinase that are common to all Ig and TCR rearrangements. All of the enzymes involved in VDJ joining are turned on and remain on throughout the time that VDJ recombination is occurring. For example, TdT is present before pro-T cells enter the thymic cortex and begin to express RAG-1 and RAG-2. The timing of rearrangements seems to be determined by the accessibility of the various loci, which is controlled by the various transcription regulatory elements described above. Sterile transcripts in the various loci provide one measure of accessibility. It remains to be determined, however, whether sterile transcripts are directly involved in the recombination process.

In any case, the earliest rearrangements in ontogeny apparently occur in the δ locus, although VJ joining in the γ locus and DJ joining in the β locus also occur at a relatively early time. A variety of evidence, most notably γ/δ transgenic mice that express normal levels of α/β receptors, indicates that most thymocytes are destined to become cells that express α/β receptors, and that this decision process involves the turning off of accessibility and expression at germline or functionally rearranged γ loci through *cis*-silencer sequences associated with this locus (see Fig. 11–6). In addition the δ locus is deleted and/or silenced when the TCR α locus becomes activated and rearranges. Since much, although not all, extrachromosmal circular DNA generated by Vα-Jα joinings retains the δ gene segments in the germline configuration, the decision to follow the α/β TCR pathway is often made before δ rearrangements. If cells are not determined to enter the α/β pathway, it remains unclear how cells in the γ/δ pathway regulate γ and δ rearrangements and expression to ensure expression of only one kind of TCR γ/δ receptor.

We have a better understanding of the regulation of rearrangements in the α/β pathway. After earlier DJβ rearrangements, thymocytes in the α/β receptor pathway begin to express the pre-Tα chain. They then rearrange a Vβ gene segment to a previously rearranged and transcribed DβJβ gene segment, forming a VDJβ sequence that is transcribed and translated as a β chain. Unlike normal mice, in which most T cells express a single functional β chain, mice lacking the pre-Tα gene have a high fraction of T cells that express two functional β chains. Thus, it is hypothesized that if the β chain can form a functional complex (pTCR) with the pre-Tα chain, there is a signal to stop additional TCRβ rearrangements, and possibly additional TCRγ and TCRδ rearrangements as well. In normal individuals, approximately 1 per cent of cells express two apparently functional TCRβ chains, thus providing some indication of the effectiveness of allelic exclusion for TCRβ expression. The functional TCRβ/ pre-Tα complex also appears to provide a signal to initiate rearrangements in the TCRα locus (perhaps by alleviating the effect of a silencer located 3' of the Cα gene), and also to enhance expression of CD4 and CD8. Despite the highly efficient allelic exclusion for the TCRβ locus, there seems to be no allelic exclusion for the TCRα locus: That is, in both αβ transgenic mice and normal individuals a significant fraction of cells that contain TCRαβ receptors express two in-frame TCRα chains. This stands in marked contrast to efficient allelic exclusion of both IgH and IgL B cells (see below). Allelic exclusion may be less important for TCRαβ receptors than for Ig receptors for the following reasons: Assuming that the efficiency of forming an in-frame VJα joint is 33 per cent, about 20 per cent of cells that have at least one in-frame joint will have two in-frame joints. Perhaps not all αβ combinations pair well so that one α TCR chain will outcompete the other chain. Perhaps even more important is the probability that only a small fraction of αβ pairs are able to interact with an MHC molecule and thus be positively selected. Thus even if there are two productive TCRα chains, it would be unusual if both are functional. Of course, this does not explain why there is a quite efficient allelic exclusion mechanism for TCRβ.

The VDJ recombinase does not seem to be turned off when a functional receptor is made, but only after it has gone through the positive and negative selection processes. Studies on human thymocytes demonstrated that RAG-1 and RAG-2 are expressed in TCR-CD3- thymocytes and also in TCR+CD3+4+8+ thymocytes but not in TCR+CD3+4+8- or TCR+CD3+4-8+ thymocytes, regardless of whether the latter were present in the cortex or medulla of the thymus. Cross-linking of the CD3-TCR complex causes a rapid loss of expression of RAG-1 and RAG-2. Thus it appears that the positive and/or negative selection processes that act on the CD3-TCR complex may serve to shut down the enzymatic machinery required for TCR gene rearrangements. Recently it has been suggested that VDJ recombinase can be reactivated to cause *receptor editing* in peripheral T lymphocytes, a phenomenon well documented for germinal center B lymphocytes (see below). However, there is only one report thus far, so that it is unclear whether this is the correct explanation, and if so, how often, where, and how significant receptor editing is in peripheral T cells.

Finally, it is important to note that approximately 10 per cent of peripheral T cells have undergone DJ rearrangements in the IgH locus, but rarely, if ever, have VDJH rearrangements or rearrangements in the Ig light chain loci. Usually, however, the rearranged DJ genes are not transcribed efficiently in T cells. Since the TCR and Ig loci are thought to share identical enzymatic machinery for rearrangements, the rearrangements of IgH loci in T cells suggest that there is a significant chance that the IgH locus becomes transiently accessible for rearrangement during the period when there is recombinase activity in T cells.

Immunoglobulins

▼ STRUCTURE AND FUNCTION[15, 127–130]

Immunoglobulins are similar in structure and function to T-cell antigen receptors but pose some specialized problems and unique solutions to these problems. First, although immunoglobulin can function as a B-cell surface receptor for antigen, most immunoglobulin is secreted from the cells to circulate in extracellular fluids. This problem is solved by generating distinct membrane and secreted forms of heavy chain mRNA by alternative processing of RNA generated from a single transcription unit. Second, different classes and subclasses of secreted immunoglobulin are able to mediate different effector functions depending on carboxy-terminal constant region domains present in the heavy chains. To preserve the same antigen binding site but different classes of immunoglobulin in progeny of a B-cell clone, B cells are able alternatively to process RNA (IgD) or rearrange DNA (all isotypes except μ) so that the heavy chain variable region (VDJ) is juxtaposed immediately upstream from the appropriate heavy chain constant region. Finally, immunoglobulins are able to hypermutate both VDJH and VL variable regions somatically to generate binding sites with higher affinity for antigen. The somatic hypermutation process oc-

curs at a restricted time and in a particular site (germinal centers) after antigenic stimulation, with mutation rates as high as 10^{-3}/nucleotide/generation (see below).

As indicated above, immunoglobulins have a basic four chain monomeric structure consisting of two identical heavy chains and two identical light chains that are held together by interchain disulfide bonds (see Fig. 11–1). There are two light chain isotypes, κ and λ. The light chains contain an amino-terminal variable region domain (V_L) and a carboxy-terminal constant region domain (C_L), with each domain having a single intradomain disulfide bond. There are five heavy chain classes (α, δ, γ, ε, and α), with four γ subclasses (γ1–4) and two α subclasses (α1–2). Starting at the amino-terminal end of the heavy chain, there is a variable region domain (V_H), followed by the CH1, hinge region (except μ and ε), CH2, CH3, and CH4 (μ and ε only) domains. The V domain and the four CH domains contain intradomain disulfide bonds. The paired V_H/V_L domains constitute an antigen recognition site, so that each Ig monomer has two identical antigen recognition sites. Both the V_L and the V_H domains can be divided into alternating framework (FR1, FR2, FR3, and FR4) and complementarity (to antigen) determining regions (CDR1, CDR2, CDR3). The CDR regions are more variable in structure than framework regions, particularly the CDR3 region, which is encoded by the VJ junctional region (light chain) or the D region plus the VD and DJ junctional regions (heavy chain). The paired C_L/CH1 domains are called the immunoglobulin CH1 domain. The paired CH2, CH3, and CH4 domains are responsible for the unique biological effector functions (e.g., complement fixation, histamine release by mast cells, binding to Fc receptors on monocytes) of different classes or subclasses of immunoglobulin. The secreted forms of IgM and IgA contain, respectively, five and two monomeric units that are disulfide bonded to each other and to a single J chain (J chain is a 15.5 kDa cysteine-rich protein that is expressed in activated B cells and all plasma cells but not at earlier stages of B-cell development).

The membrane form of immunoglobulin differs only in that each class of heavy chain has two additional carboxy-terminal domains, a transmembrane domain and a short cytoplasmic domain, but otherwise the same light chain and the same basic structure. For most classes of immunoglobulin, expression of the membrane form of immunoglobulin on the cell surface requires that the immunoglobulin interact with a disulfide complex of two glycoproteins called Igα and Igβ. The Igα/Igβ heterodimer is analogous to the proteins composing the CD3 complex on T cells. These two proteins not only are required to anchor the immunoglobulin on the cell surface, but are also involved in transduction of an antigenic signal from the outside to the inside of a B cell.

▼ CHROMOSOMAL LOCALIZATION AND GENETIC ORGANIZATION[9, 15, 88, 98, 131–135]

As for TCR, a knowledge of the chromosomal localization and genetic organization of the three Ig loci is critical for understanding the pattern and significance of normal and abnormal Ig gene rearrangements in normal and malignant cells. Although the overall organization of these three loci is similar to that of the four TCR loci, there are important differences, particularly for the IgH locus. In general the overall organization of the three Ig loci is highly conserved for the human and murine systems.

Immunoglobulin Kappa Locus

The Igκ locus has been localized at chromosome band 2p11.2 and includes about 1.6 Mb (Fig. 11–9).

At the centromeric end of the locus there are 76 Vκ segments, which are organized into a pair of duplicated 0.4 Mb regions separated by a 0.8 Mb region apparently devoid of V segments. The V segments are divided into 6 subgroups that, in contrast to those in the mouse, are not clustered but are interspersed among V segments from other subgroups. Although 50 V segments have apparent open reading frames, only 25 have been shown to rearrange with a J segment. Nearly 95 per cent of rearranged V segments are present in the proximal repeat unit. Generally, the V segments in the proximal repeat unit have the same transcriptional orientation as the J and C segments, whereas the V segments in the distal repeat unit have the opposite orientation. In addition to the V segments in this locus, there are about 25 V_κ-like gene segments dispersed to other chromosomes, including 1, 2q near the centromere; 15; and 22; with those on chromosome 22 localized at band 22q11, centromeric to the Vλ segments.

In a 5 kb region at the telomeric end of the locus there are five functional J segments, separated from one another by about 300 bp, and a single C exon that encodes the entire constant region domain and the 3′ untranslated region. The J1 segment is about 25 kb from the most proximal V, and the J5 segment is separated by 2.5 kb from C. Critical regulatory elements include the intronic enhancer (iEκ) about 0.7 kb centromeric to C and a 3′ enhancer (3′ Eκ) about 12 kb telomeric to C. Approximately 24 kb telomeric to C, there is a conserved region called the 3′ kappa deleting element (3′ kde), with a joining signal that comprises a heptamer separated by 23 bp from the more centromeric nonamer. In addition, there is an isolated heptamer (h) located in the JCκ intron about 1 kb centromeric to iEκ. The significance of h and 3′ kde will be discussed below.

Immunoglobulin Lambda Locus

The Igλ locus has been localized to chromosome band 22q11.22 and includes about 1.1 Mb, all of which has been sequenced (Fig. 11–9).

The V segments are located at the centromeric end of the locus. There are 10 subgroups that appear to include 30 functional V segments, all with the same transcriptional orientation as the C genes. About 14 kb telomeric to the most proximal V are 7 C genes, each with an associated J segment, uniformly distributed within an approximately 40 kb region. There are 4 highly homologous functional C genes (C1, C2, C3, and C7), and 3 pseudogenes (C4, C5, and C6). There are individuals with duplications of the C2/C3 genes, so that chromosomal loci from different individuals can contain a total of 7 to 10 C genes. There is a 3′ enhancer (3′ Eλ) about 30 kb telomeric to C7, but no intronic enhancer.

In addition to these conventional V, J, and C sequences, there are four related genes that are present on chromosome 22. One gene, which is called V-pre-B, is homologous to a V segment. However, it is expressed uniquely in pre-B cells without gene rearrangement and encodes an approximately 16 kDa protein (see below). The V-pre-B gene is localized near the centromeric end of the V segments. The precise chromosomal location of the other three genes, each of which is homologous to λ C genes, is unclear. One of these genes (the equivalent of λ5 in the mouse), which is called 14.1 and is telomeric of C7, is expressed uniquely in pre-B cells without gene rearrangement. It encodes an approximately 22 kDa protein that contains sequences homologous to J as well as C sequences (see below). A second gene, called 16.1, is similar to 14.1, although its expression pattern and full coding sequence have not been clearly established. The third gene, called 18.1, is a pseudogene, which contains sequences homologous to C genes but not to J segments. Finally, there is a processed pseudogene (i.e., a pseudogene lacking intronic sequences, suggesting that it is derived from a processed RNA transcript) that is not present on chromosome 22.

Immunoglobulin Heavy Chain Locus

The Ig heavy chain locus is located on human chromosomal band 14q32.33, immediately adjacent to the 14q telomere, and includes about 1.1 Mb of DNA (Fig. 11–9).

In contrast to all of the other TCR and Ig loci, the VH segments are localized at the telomeric end of the locus. There are approximately 50 functional VH segments, and a

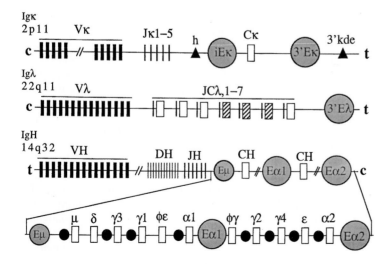

Figure 11–9. The human immunoglobulin loci. The chromosomal localization and genetic organization of the three Ig loci are shown in schematic form although not to scale. Except for the IgH locus, the orientation from left to right is centromeric (c) to telomeric (t). The positions of V segments are depicted by dark boxes, D segments by thin lines, J segments by thick lines, and functional C region genes by open boxes (Cλ genes with diagonal stripes are non-functional). Each V segment contains two exons and each C gene contains multiple exons as described in the text. With the exception of the δC gene and the φε and φγ C genes, each H chain C region is preceded by a functional switch region, which is depicted by a dark circle. Regulatory elements are shown as large gray circles. The dark triangles in the Igκ locus represent an isolated intronic heptamer (h) and a nonamer/heptamer pair (3′kde), which can be involved in developmentally regulated rearrangement events that specifically delete the Cκ region. See text for additional details.

similar number of non-functional VH segments (including approximately 20 that map to chromosomes 15 and 16). By sequence homology, there are 6 V segment subgroups, which are interspersed throughout the locus. Unlike Vκ segments, all VH segments appear to have the same transcriptional orientation as the C genes.

Toward the centromeric end of the locus, there is an approximately 50 kb region containing 3 pseudo D segments and 24 functional D segments. Immediately adjacent to the 3'-most D segment, there are 6 functional J segments (J1–6), with 3 pseudo J segments interspersed among the functional J segments. Approximately 8 kb downstream from the J6 segment is the first C gene (Cμ).

Unlike any of the other TCR or Ig loci, the IgH locus contains multiple C genes, with only the Cμ gene immediately juxtaposed to a J segment. There are 11 IgH C genes, including 2 pseudogenes, which occur in a region of about 250 kb: JH-8-μ-δ-60-γ3-26-γ1-19-φε-13-α1-35-φγ-40-γ2-18-γ4-23-ε-10-α2. Compared with that of the mouse there is a γγεα duplication, with the downstream γ2-γ4-ε-α2 region corresponding to the upstream γ3-γ1-φε-α1 region. Each C gene contains multiple exons that generally correspond to functional domains in the corresponding H chain: CH1, hinge, CH2, CH3, and CH4. In addition, for each C gene there are 2 downstream exons (M1 and M2) that together encode the transmembrane domain, the short cytoplasmic tail, and the 3' untranslated portion of the membrane form of the corresponding mRNA (see below). Each functional C gene (except the delta and two pseudo C genes) has a repetitive switch region sequence (see below) located immediately upstream of the CH1 exon. The unique organization of the IgH C genes reflects the need for expression of different heavy chain constant region sequences with the same VDJ sequence (see below) at different times in the lifetime of a B cell and its progeny. Critical regulatory elements include the μ intronic enhancer (Eμ) located about 2 kb upstream of switch μ and a pair of strong 3' enhancers (possible locus control regions) about 5 kb downstream of each Cα gene, that is, Eα1 and Eα2. In addition, immediately upstream of each functional switch region there is a promoter that initiates transcription within I exons (Iμ, Iγ3, Iα1, etc.) that lack an open reading frame (see below).

▼ IMMUNOGLOBULIN GENE REARRANGEMENT AND DIVERSITY[15, 29, 30, 32, 86, 114, 127]

Depending on the transcriptional orientation of the V segment relative to the C gene, intrachromosomal gene rearrangement results in release of an extrachromosomal circle (same orientation of V and C) or a chromosomal inversion (see Fig. 11–3), with rearrangements between sister chromatids or homologous chromosomes occurring rarely. The structural relationship of the V, D, and J segments to their corresponding signal sequence(s) is shown in Figure 11–7. It is significant that the separation of heptamer/nonamer joining signals from each other is the same on each side of the IgH D segments. Thus, in contrast to TCR receptors, D segments cannot be joined to one another, so that all functional IgH rearrangements result in a VDJ sequence. Also, in contrast to the TCR loci, IgH D segments usually can be read in only one frame. Immunoglobulin loci are similar to

TCR loci in that secondary rearrangements involving an upstream segment (V) and a downstream segment (DH or JL) are possible if appropriate joining signals remain available. For example, this is true for primary IgL VJ or IgH DJ joints but not primary IgH VDJ joints (in this latter case all D segments have been deleted and the joining signals are not appropriate for the direct joining of an IgH V segment to a J segment).

Uniquely in the IgH locus, *V region replacement* (another kind of secondary rearrangement) can result in replacement of the V segment portion of a rearranged IgH VDJ sequence with an upstream V segment. This IgH V segment replacement is possible since there is a heptamer signal (but no nonamer signal) within the coding region at the 3' end of many IgH V segments. It is not clear whether there is distinct regulation of joining directed by a pair of heptamer-nonamer sequences versus joining directed by a heptamer-nonomer sequence and an isolated heptamer sequence, as occurs in VH replacements. Gene conversion of V segments, in which one V segment (V1) replaces a second V segment (V2) by a recombination mechanism that retains the original copy of V1 but replaces V2 with V1, is clearly an important mechanism in generating diversity of avian Ig genes. However, this mechanism does not seem to occur at a significant rate in diversification of murine or human Ig genes.

The potential diversity of Ig variable regions involves all of the mechanisms described above (including somatic hypermutation of IgH and IgL chain variable regions), although IgL chains rarely have N sequences. Table 11–1 summarizes the extent of potential diversity of Ig variable regions prior to somatic hypermutation. Since somatic hypermutation can occur within any portion of the IgH or IgL variable regions after antigenic stimulation, the potential diversity of Ig variable regions is essentially infinite.

As is true for TCR, the actual diversity achieved may be much more restricted, depending on the age of the animal, type and situation of antigen exposure, and so forth. For example, IgH VDJ sequences from fetal or young individuals show few N regions. Also, early in ontogeny, there may be a preferential rearrangement of certain V, D, and J segments (e.g., 3'-most V segments with 5'-most J segments or V segments and J segments that share a few nucleotides of homology at their joining ends). Currently, however, we have limited evidence in humans to assess the constraints that bias or limit Ig variable region diversity.

▼ ONTOGENY OF IMMUNOGLOBULIN REARRANGEMENTS[94, 102, 104, 119, 120, 122, 129, 136–140]

The anatomical locations and patterns of B lymphocyte development are similar in mice and men. Depending on the age of the individual, pluripotent hematopoietic stem cells in the yolk sac, fetal liver, and finally spleen and bone marrow give rise to progenitor B cells that progress through an ordered process of Ig gene rearrangements. These various stages of B-cell differentiation have been determined in humans and/or mice by analysis of normal tissues; laboratory generated "knockout" (hetero- or homozygous genome deletions), "knock-in" (replacement of one gene sequence with another), or transgenic (insertion of a normal or altered gene at an unspecified site); hybridomas involving normal B-cell

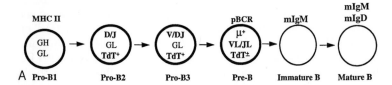

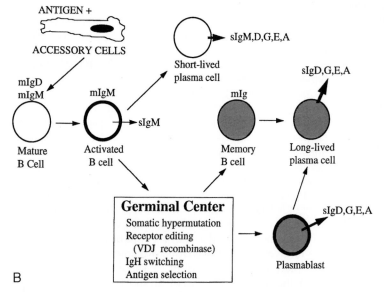

Figure 11–10. B-cell developmental pathway. This simplified scheme depicts a limited number of intermediates in the developmental process, and only a few of the known markers. *A*, Antigen independent maturation events from pro-B to mature B cells. *B*, Antigen dependent maturation, which occurs principally in secondary lymphoid organs, usually requires both antigen presenting cells and helper T cells (accessory cells) in addition to antigen (Ag). Proliferating cells have bold outlines, whereas quiescent cells do not. Cells that have been selected after passage through the germinal center are shaded. GH and GL, germline IgH and IgL genes; TdT, terminal deoxynucleotidyl transferase; mIg and sIg, membrane and secreted Ig, respectively. For additional details, see text.

precursors, and various B-cell tumors. This process is divided into antigen independent (Fig. 11–10*A*) and antigen dependent phases (Fig. 11–10*B*) even though antigen can, in fact, influence the late phases in "antigen independent" B-cell development (see below).

The process is initiated when a lymphoid progenitor cell gives rise to a pro-B cell that is committed to the B-cell lineage. The pro-B1 cell expresses specific B-cell markers, including MHC class II antigens and CD43 but has all Ig loci in an unrearranged germline state. A pro-B1 cell progresses to a pro-B2 cell, which expresses TdT, RAG-1, RAG-2, and *surrogate L chain* (i.e., V-pre-B, and 14.1) and proceeds to join D segments to J segments at both IgH loci; secondary D to J rearrangements can also occur at this stage of development. Subsequently, the cells begin to express germline V gene transcripts that correlate with cells at a developmental stage (pro-B3) that join V segments to DJ segments generated during the pro-B2 stage. Pro-B3 cells that generate a functional VDJ sequence can express a functional μ heavy chain that assembles with a surrogate IgL chain complex (see below) to express a *pre-B-cell receptor (pBCR)*, resulting in differentiation to a pre-B cell. If the pro-B3 cell does not generate a functional pBCR, additional primary and secondary rearrangements occur. The pre-B cell with a functional pBCR stops further IgH rearrangements, downregulates TdT to low or absent levels, initiates expression of sterile germline transcripts from IgL V and J/C regions, and then begins to join VL and JL segments.

If the pre-B cell generates a functional VLJL sequence so that a functional mIgM is produced, the pre-B cell stops dividing and develops into an immature B cell that downregulates VDJ recombinase (RAG-1 and RAG-2). If the mIgM on the pre-B cell or new immature B cell encounters a self-

antigen, VDJ recombinase is upregulated to activate *receptor editing*, that is, secondary VJ rearrangements of the functional or non-functional IgL alleles, de novo VJ rearrangements of germline IgL alleles, and, much less frequently, V replacement of VDJ sequences. After receptor editing, the generation of a functional mIgM permits differentiation to an immature B cell. When an older immature B cell encounters a self-antigen, clonal deletion (apoptosis) or clonal anergy occurs instead of receptor editing. By analogy to the T-cell developmental pathway (see above), immature B cells that express a functional mIgM are positively selected to turn off VDJ recombinase and differentiate into mIgM+mIgD+ mature B cells that migrate into the blood en route to peripheral lymphoid tissues. Cells that express no mIgM or a non-functional IgM die for lack of a positive signal. Mature B cells that interact with self-antigen in secondary lymphoid tissues may still become tolerant by clonal anergy.

Antigen dependent B cell development (Fig. 11–10*B*) begins when a quiescent mature B cell has a productive interaction with antigen, accessory cells, and cytokines. The resultant activated B cell proliferates and differentiates into a short-lived (3 day life span) quiescent plasma cell that can secrete IgM or undergo switching to secrete another IgH isotype. Late in a primary response or in a secondary response, when germinal centers are available, the activated B cell can enter a germinal center where it undergoes multiple cycles of somatic hypermutation of IgH and IgL variable regions followed by antigen selection of cells with high affinity receptors to abrogate apoptosis. Perhaps some cells with low affinity for antigen can be rescued by germinal center *receptor editing* as a consequence of reactivation of VDJ recombinase, providing another chance for selection by antigen. In addition, cells frequently undergo IgH switching in the germinal center. Cells that ultimately avoid apoptosis can become memory B cells that express mIgM or other isotypes. Alternatively the selected cells that have switched to another IgH isotype generate plasmablasts that migrate to other sites (e.g., bone marrow or mucosal regions) and terminally differentiate into long-lived, quiescent plasma cells that secrete high levels of IgD, G, E, or A and survive for 30 days or more.

▼ REGULATION OF IMMUNOGLOBULIN GENE FORMATION: ALLELIC AND ISOTYPE EXCLUSION[15, 24, 94, 102, 104, 122, 135, 136, 139, 141–146]

With rare exceptions, individual B cells express a single species of functional Ig. The Ig expressed by a cell contains *either* Igκ or Igλ L chains and thus requires *isotypic exclusion* of one of the IgL isotypes. In addition, individual B cells express a functional IgH encoded by a rearranged gene located in *either* the maternal or paternal IgH locus, plus a single functional IgL encoded by a rearranged gene located in *either* the maternal or the paternal Igκ (or Igλ) locus. Thus there is *allelic exclusion* involving both IgH and IgL loci that together encode a functional Ig. Rearrangement is an inefficient process, succeeding perhaps in 1/3 and 1/9 primary attempts to generate in-frame VJ light chain and VDJ heavy chain genes, respectively (it should be noted that in-frame joining may not be sufficient to ensure functionality; for instance, there may be mutations in one of the coding regions, such as a pseudo V, or some combinations of IgH and IgL may not interact efficiently). If all primary rearrangements to generate a functional IgH or IgL chain are unsuccessful, the cell must either proceed to attempt secondary rearrangements or replacements or be eliminated since B cells that do not express Ig are found only rarely in peripheral lymphoid tissues. On the basis of limited information regarding the coexistence of functional and non-functional Ig rearrangements in single B cells, it was initially proposed that allelic and isotype exclusion is actively regulated and is mediated by the products of the rearrangement process. Although non-regulated, stochastic models have been proposed, most available evidence supports the hypothesis that allelic and isotypic exclusion is mediated by the protein products that are encoded by the rearranged Ig or TCR genes.

An attractive model that suggests how Ig gene formation is regulated in B cells is described below. The data for this model come from studies on normal and malignant B cells from humans and mice, as well as from studies of "knockout" mice lacking specific Ig regulatory elements and transgenic mice that contain a rearranged and functional IgH and/or IgL gene. A fundamental assumption underlying this model is that the formation of VJ or VDJ sequences by gene rearrangement is immediately followed by transcription and translation of the newly rearranged gene. If a rearranged IgH (Fig. 11–10A, stage pro-B cell 3) is "functional," the cell stops additional V to DJ joining events. Correspondingly, if a rearranged IgL (Fig. 11–10, pre-B cell) is "functional," the cell stops additional V to J joining events at all IgL chain loci. In fact, a similar hypothesis may apply to β, and possibly δ or γ TCR gene rearrangements (see above). The

key question is, How does a cell determine whether an individual chain is functional? Since IgH rearrangements occur before IgL rearrangements, it was possible to propose that the "functionality" of a light chain is determined by the ability of the IgL to form a functional complex with a functional IgH that was generated at an earlier stage. From studies of transgenic mice that received a rearranged and functional H chain, it was shown that the membrane form of H chain can mediate this kind of regulation whereas the secreted form of H chain cannot. Thus the functionality of the IgH-IgL complex requires cell surface expression of this complex.

A tougher problem was to explain how the "functionality" of a newly rearranged IgH can be determined since the cells express no IgL at the pro-B3 stage of differentiation. If no L chain is available, the CH1 domain of the heavy chain binds to heavy chain binding protein (BiP), which prevents secretion or surface expression of the heavy chain. Parenthetically, the heavy chain in "heavy chain disease" (see below) usually has deleted the CH1 domain so that it does not bind to BiP and can then be expressed on the membrane or secreted. The apparent answer is that pre-B cells express a surrogate light chain that comprises two polypeptides, which are encoded by the V-pre-B and λ14.1 genes (see above). A variety of evidence indicates that V-pre-B encodes a 16,000 dalton polypeptide called iota that is homologous to a λV region but contains about 20 additional amino acids, having a significant net negative charge, at its carboxy-terminal end. Correspondingly, the λ14.1 gene encodes a 22,000 dalton polypeptide called omega that is homologous to a λC region at its carboxy-terminal end but contains approximately 100 additional amino acids, with a substantial net positive charge, at its amino-terminus. In addition, the following have been shown: (1) Iota and omega form a non-covalent complex, perhaps involving the non-Ig-like sequences at the carboxy-terminal and amino-terminal ends, respectively; (2) a ternary complex composed of a disulfide linked heterodimer of H chain and omega plus a non-covalently associated iota chain has been identified in pre-B cells; and (3) the expression of iota plus omega can substitute for L chain in enabling a H chain to be secreted or expressed on the cell surface.

To summarize this model, after D to J joining events at both IgH loci, the cells progress from stage pro-B2 to stage pro-B3, in which they begin to make V to DJ rearrangements. It is not clear whether there is a positive signal to move from stage pro-B2 to stage pro-B3. When an in-frame VDJ rearrangement results in expression of a functional H chain, the H chain associates with Igα, Igβ, iota, and omega polypeptides to generate a pBCR complex that is expressed on the cell surface (Fig. 11–10A). It is presumed that the surface expression of this functional complex somehow generates a signal that results in differentiation to the pre-B stage, which must then include (1) an inhibition of further V to DJ joining events (perhaps by decreasing accessibility of unrearranged VH genes for transcription and rearrangements); (2) a turn-off of TdT expression; and (3) a turn-on of VL to JL joining. When joining of V to J generates a functional L chain, it is hypothesized that the functional L chain associates with a functional H chain so that a functional mIgM receptor is expressed on the cell surface. It is presumed that the surface expression of this functional complex generates a signal that prevents additional joining events and turns off expression of the surrogate L chain. The signal generated by the presence of a functional mIgM might decrease accessibility of unrearranged V segments in both IgL loci or might result in a shut-off of recombinase activity. Cells that do not express a functional mIgM presumably continue to make additional gene rearrangements, but if unsuccessful eventually die for lack of positive selection.

It is unclear how and when a decision is made to rearrange and express Igλ genes. Consistent with the model above, Igλ and Igκ transgenic mice show a marked inhibition of rearrangement of endogenous κ and λ genes. However, it is well established that B cells expressing a κ chain almost always have germline Cλ genes, whereas B cells expressing a λ chain have deleted or non-functionally rearranged both κC region genes. Deletion of κC genes occurs by VDJ recombinase-mediated joining of either a Vκ segment or a JCκ intronic heptamer element (h) to the 3' kde (Fig. 11–9). Mainly on the basis of these data, it has been argued that rearrangements occur in the λ locus only when rearrangements in the κ locus have failed to generate a functional κ chain. Alternatively, it is possible that a cell begins to rearrange either κ or λ genes, and that the decision to rearrange λ genes or the rearrangement process per se somehow activates the κC region deleting mechanism. Three observations support this alternative model. First, the fraction of B cells expressing λ is about 5 per cent in mice and 40 per cent in humans, similar to the fraction of functional VL that is Vλ in each species. Second, deletion of either iEk or 3' Ek results in a marked increase in the fraction of cells that rearrange and express Igλ (see above). Third, *receptor editing* in pre-B/immature B cells or germinal center B cells raises a significant problem for maintaining allelic exclusion, since VJ recombination (or the much less frequent VH replacement) could, in principle, occur on functional or non-functional alleles, but it has been shown that receptor editing in early B cells is associated with deletion of one Cκ allele even if the editing process affects Cκ instead of Cλ. These observations are consistent with the following hypothesis: Perhaps the kappa deleting mechanism is normally inoperative during primary Igκ rearrangements and becomes operative when secondary rearrangements and receptor editing occur either centrally or in germinal centers but also becomes operative when Igλ rearrangements are initiated. Much remains to be done before we have a full understanding of mechanisms that ensure *IgL isotypic exclusion* and *allelic exlusion* at all Ig loci.

▼ EXPRESSION OF SECRETED AND MEMBRANE IMMUNOGLOBULIN H CHAINS BY ALTERNATIVE POLYADENYLATION AND RIBONUCLEIC ACID PROCESSING[15, 127, 147]

As indicated above, all classes and subclasses of immunoglobulin can be expressed as a membrane associated receptor or in a secreted form. In each case, the membrane form of H chain contains additional carboxy-terminal sequences that encode a transmembrane domain and a short cytoplasmic tail. The membrane and secreted forms of H chain are encoded by membrane and secreted forms of H chain mRNA that are generated by alternative polyadenylation and then joining of all adjacent splice donor/splice acceptor pairs. The differential expression of the membrane and secreted forms of H chain mRNA is developmentally regulated. For example, pre-B cells and resting B cells (immature, mature, and memory B cells as shown in Fig. 11–10) express similar levels of the membrane and secreted forms of H chain mRNA. In contrast, activated B cells and terminally differentiated plasma cells express much higher levels of the secreted form than of the membrane form of H chain mRNA.

It is important to note that the presence of the membrane or secreted form of H chain mRNA does not ensure that the corresponding protein will be expressed, respectively, on the cell surface or in extracellular secretions. The site of expression of the membrane or secreted form of H chain (or immunoglobulin) is determined by developmentally regulated post-translational mechanisms. For example, expression of the membrane form of heavy chain on the cell surface generally does not occur in plasma cells since plasma cells usually do not express a protein (Igα) that is necessary for cell surface expression (see above). Similarly, the secreted form of heavy chain is not secreted from immature or mature B cells. The lack of secretion of the secreted form of immunoglobulin from these early B cells is poorly understood but is not likely due to the absence of J chain expression at this time in B cell development.

▼ COEXPRESSION OF IMMUNOGLOBULIN M AND IMMUNOGLOBULIN D BY ALTERNATIVE RNA PROCESSING[15, 127, 136, 148]

Up to the immature B cell stage of development (Fig. 11–10), B cells express μ chain as a pBCR and ultimately as a cell surface IgM receptor when there is a functional pair of H and L chains. As the cells progress to the mature B cell stage (i.e., the major kind of B cell in peripheral lymphoid tissues), they coexpress cell surface IgM and IgD receptors (but at a later developmental stage express only IgM again). Parenthetically, the function of IgD in B cells remains enigmatic. In any case, the IgM and IgD share the same L chain and the same VDJ sequence but differ in the H chain C region associated with the VDJ sequence. As indicated above, the μ constant region gene is immediately downstream from the J segments and the δ constant region gene is immediately downstream of the μ constant region (Fig. 11–9). Since cells that coexpress μ and δ H chains have no DNA rearrangement involving the μ or δ H chain C region genes and can progress to a developmental stage in which they express only IgM again, it is hypothesized that a single transcription unit can generate μ and δ mRNAs by alternative RNA processing. The developmentally regulated mechanism for this process is unclear. However, it differs from the mechanism for generating the membrane and secreted forms of H chain mRNA since the decision to generate a δ mRNA requires that the VDJ splice donor site bypass all splice acceptor sites on μ exons to use the splice acceptor site on the CH1 δ exon.

▼ EXPRESSION OF OTHER H CHAIN CLASSES BY SWITCH RECOMBINATION[15, 131, 136, 149–159]

The stable expression of all classes of immunoglobulin except μ (the regulated expression of δ as described above is an exception) involves a switch recombination event that replaces the Cμ gene with another C region gene. This developmentally regulated, antigen dependent recombination event most often occurs in germinal centers but can occur outside germinal centers (Fig. 11–10*B*). Recombination generally occurs within or near isotype specific repetitive switch sequences (Sμ, Sγ1, etc., as in Figs. 11–9 and 11–11) that are located upstream of all heavy chain constant regions except δ (Fig. 11–11). Curiously, stable switching to δ, which occurs infrequently but selectively in germinal center cells that express λ L chain, can occur by two mechanisms: (1) recombination between Sμ and a 2 kb region that is located about 4 kb upstream of δ and (2) less frequent homologous recombination between a pair of 440 bp repeats that are located immediately upstream of Sμ (σμ sequence) and about 2 kb upstream of δ (Σμ sequence). There are two clear structural consequences of the IgH switch recombination event. First, the VDJ segment and the IgH intronic enhancer (Eμ) are positioned immediately upstream of the appropriate constant region gene. Second, there is formation of a hybrid switch region (e.g., Sμγ2 in Fig. 11–11).

Repetitive switch sequences, which usually are about 1–3 kb in length in humans, comprise tandem repeats of unique nucleotide sequences containing about 10–100 nucleotides per repeat, depending on the particular switch region. The switch regions associated with different constant region genes share limited homology to one another, including the presence of GAGCT and GGGGT or TGGGG pentanucleotide sequences in each kind of repeat. However, they differ substantially in the lengths, sequences, and organization of the repeats. The human and mouse switch sequences are highly homologous. The precise point at which heterologous switch sequences join is highly variable and can occur essentially anywhere within (and in some cases near) the switch sequences. There may be insertion, deletion, or substitutions of a limited number of nucleotides at or near the site of joining. The nature of the switch sequences and the hybrid switch joint indicates that recombination is a non-homologous and non-site-specific type of recombination, even though it has been suggested that there might be limited homologous pairing of heterologous switch sequences. In contrast to VDJ recombination, the imprecision of the switch recombination does not have a functional consequence since recombination occurs in intervening, non-coding sequences.

Switch recombination is similar to VDJ recombination in that most recombination events appear to be intrachromasomal. The excised intervening sequences form an episomal covalent switch recombination circle (Fig. 11–11) that appears to be eliminated from the cell. Switch recombination generally occurs from Sμ directly to another H chain switch region, although sequential switching (e.g., μ > γ1 > ε) is not unusual. Rarely the intervening sequences reintegrate at the same site but in an inverted orientation, which would result in a non-functional transcription unit. Even more rarely, the deleted sequences can reintegrate at another site, potentially resulting in insertion of the Eα1 and some gene at another site (see below and Figs. 11–11 and 11–17). Interchromosomal switching events as a result of sister chromatid exchange or switch recombination involving IgH loci on homologous chromosomes occurs at a low but significant frequency (perhaps a small percentage of switch recombination events). During interchromosomal switching, one chromosome loses sequences and the other chromosome gains the same sequences, with the chromosomal partners segregated at the next cell division. Interchromosomal switching would explain the rare occurrence of back-switching (e.g., α2 to ε or γ1). It is of interest that a transgenic μ gene can undergo switch recombination with an endogenous IgH locus, which provides a situation analogous to chromosomal translocations mediated by IgH switch recombinase.

The mechanism and regulation of switch recombination are poorly understood. Switch recombination is not a random process involving two switch regions but can be regulated to target specific switch regions. First, switching often affects the same isotype of constant region at both IgH loci, even though only one IgH locus expresses a functional heavy chain. Second, tumor cell lines can reproducibly switch from μ to one or a limited number of specific switch regions. Third, addition of T helper cell cytokines (e.g. IL-4, transforming growth factor β [TGFβ]) can promote or inhibit switch recombination to specific switch regions (these cytokines are elaborated by different types of helper T cells, supporting the concept that the context in which antigen, T cells, and B cells interact directs switching to specific IgH C regions). The mechanism by which switch recombination is directed to specific IgH chain switch regions is thought to be mediated by accessibility of the target region. The increased accessibility of a particular switch region has been associated with the following events: (1) decreased DNA methylation and/or increased deoxyribonuclease (DNase) I

Figure 11–11. Intrachromosomal IgH switch recombination. The top line depicts an IgH locus after VDJ recombination (open box), with IgC genes (vertical dark boxes); repetitive switch regions (open circles except μ, which is a dark circle); sigma repeats (smaller circles with vertical lines); enhancer elements (large shaded circles); transcribed regions (constitutive, solid arrow and induced, dashed arrow); t and c, telomeric and centromeric ends of IgH locus. The bottom line shows a covalent hybrid μγ2 switch region after switching from μ to γ2. The excised intervening sequences ultimately form a covalent circle that also has the reciprocal hybrid μγ2 switch region. Note that if recombination occurs between Sμ and a switch sequence downstream of Sα1, the switch circle includes the Eα1 regulatory element.

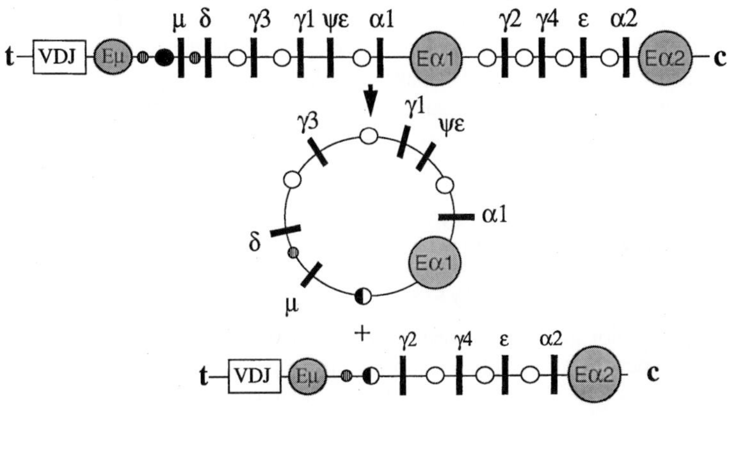

hypersensitivity, (2) deletions within the recipient switch region due to homologous recombination (or switch recombination within a switch region), and (3) sterile RNA transcripts that can be initiated in ca. 500 bp non-coding "I" exons that are present upstream of each switch region (Figs. 11–11 and 11–16). The cytokines that enhance or inhibit switch recombination to specific switch regions enhance or inhibit transcription from the corresponding I region promoter. Although much evidence indicates that this transcription process is important in regulating switching, it is not known whether the sterile I transcripts, which splice to the corresponding constant regions, have a direct role in switch recombination. Efficient transcription from the I regions and IgH switching are clearly dependent on the 3′ Eα enhancer in the mouse, and it is presumed that Eα1 and Eα2 are critical in regulating IgH switching in humans. In addition to antigen and cytokines, switching is facilitated by the interaction of CD40 on B cells and CD40L on activated T-helper cells. Individuals with X-linked hyper-IgM syndrome have a defective *CD40L* gene, providing an explanation for the extremely low levels of other Ig isotypes in their serum. Little is known about switch recombinase although transfection experiments with model switch recombination substrates demonstrate that switch recombination can occur in an appropriate B cell line but not in a fibroblast line. Switch recombinase is clearly different from VDJ recombinase in that RAG-2 is required only for the latter. On the other hand, at least one component (the DNA dependent serine threonine protein kinase composed of Ku70 and Ku86 elements) is essential for both IgH switching and VDJ recombination.

Immune Receptor Gene Rearrangements as Markers of Clonal Proliferation

In a previous section we described the foundation for immune receptor diversity. In that section it was emphasized that fundamental and irreversible structural reconfigurations of DNA accompany the formation of functional immune receptor genes. These gene rearrangements are not abstractions of strictly academic interest. They are real changes in the DNA of a lymphocyte that can be visualized and applied to answer questions posed in basic research and clinical patient care. At the basis of studies that utilize the study of gene rearrangements (genotyping) is the realization that these rearrangements distinguish one lymphocyte from any other not derived from it or a common parent. The structural diversity inherent and necessary to immune responsiveness creates a situation in which each rearranged lymphocyte carries within its DNA a unique "molecular fingerprint" based on its utilization of a particular V, D, and J segment with or without P and N region addition and somatic mutation.

▼ THE RECOGNITION OF IMMUNE RECEPTOR GENE REARRANGEMENTS

Southern Blot Analysis

Southern blot analysis of restriction enzyme digested DNA that comes from peripheral blood lymphocytes of normal individuals reveals only the germline pattern of immune

receptor loci. The complete diversity of rearrangements present in the population cannot be appreciated by Southern blot analysis because the level of sensitivity is at best 1 per cent. That is, a particular pattern of gene rearrangement must be present in at least 1 of every 100 cells in order to be appreciated when using this technique. If, however, one particular lymphocyte or clone of lymphocytes begins to proliferate selectively so that it comprises 1 per cent or more of the population, its unique pattern of gene rearrangement begins to emerge through the background "haze" of all the other rearrangements present in the population (Figs. 11–12 and 11–13). Thus, this assay has found general use as a means of characterizing and establishing a tumor specific marker for lymphoid malignancies. It is also valuable in the assessment of whether a proliferation of lymphocytes represents a polyclonal reaction, as might occur in a variety of inflammatory situations, or a monoclonal proliferation, most often associated with malignant transformation.[126, 160] For example, a study of patients with *Mycosis fungoides* infection at the plaque stage of the disease was able to demonstrate clonal TCR gene rearrangement even in circumstances in which histological and immunological assays were non-diagnostic.[161]

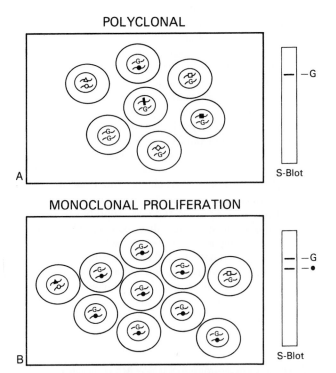

Figure 11–12. *A,* Polyclonal immune receptor gene rearrangements. In the schematic "G" represents a germline, unrearranged allele of a particular immune receptor. The various other shapes represent different rearrangements of the same locus. Some cells have no rearrangements (they could be stem cells, granulocytes, or the majority of T cells if one were considering Ig gene rearrangements). Other cells have one or both alleles rearranged. If a Southern blot analysis is performed (see earlier chapter and Fig. 11–13) the sensitivity of the technique is such that only the germline band is recognizable. *B,* If, however, one particular cell begins to predominate in the population (for example, through transformation, growth stimulation, or abrogation of programmed cell death), its unique pattern of gene rearrangement begins to emerge through the background of all the other rearrangements present in the sample. In most laboratories the sensitivity of detection of this predominant clone occurs at the 1–5 per cent level.

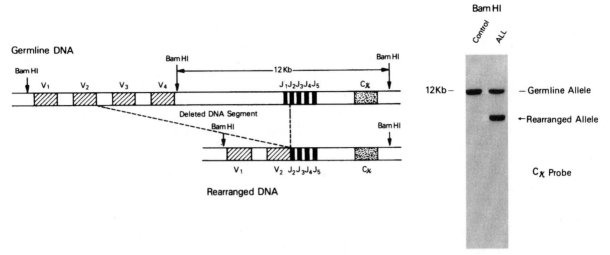

Figure 11–13. Recognition of an Igκ V-J rearrangement in a leukemia by Southern blot analysis. If germline DNA is digested with the restriction endonuclease *Bam*HI, size fractionated on an agarose gel, denatured, and transferred to a solid matrix (e.g., nitrocellulose), hybridized to a probe homologous to the Cκ segment, and autoradiographed, a single band of 12,000 base pairs (12 kb) is identified. In this example the same analysis is performed on DNA extracted from the malignant cells of a patient with B-cell precursor acute lymphoblastic leukemia (ALL). Presumably as part of its normal development the transformed cell had undergone V-J rearrangement in which a Vκ segment had recombined in a site-specific fashion with a Jκ segment. This resulted in a deletion of DNA between the V and J and therefore, by definition, the introduction of a different 5′ *Bam*HI site vis-à-vis the Cκ probe. This can be appreciated as a novel hybridizing band on the Southern blot lane to the right of the control (germline) DNA. The germline fragment is also present in the leukemic cells because only one of the two kappa encoding alleles has rearranged. Despite the fact that the rearrangement of the κ gene most likely had no direct relation to the leukemic transformation, it provides a "molecular fingerprint" of the leukemic clone.

The identification of immunoglobulin and T-cell antigen receptor gene rearrangements provides tumor-specific markers despite the fact that in most cases the particular gene rearrangements themselves had nothing to do with the event(s) that led to malignant transformation. Although this is generally assumed to be the case it need not be universally true. For example, a particular immune receptor might provide a target for the binding of a particular transforming virus. A particular prolonged or substantial antigenic challenge may cause cells bearing a particular immune receptor to receive such a stimulus to further growth and expansion that this particular clone becomes a more likely target for additional random growth affecting events that contribute incrementally to malignant transformation. Despite these possible exceptions, most immune receptor gene rearrangements are probably incidental to the transforming cause of the malignant clone in which they are found. The cell was engaged in its normal differentiated activity, which involved the structural rearrangement and elaboration of an immune receptor at the time it was transformed.

In many cases, a study of immune receptor gene rearrangements offers a glimpse into the status of cellular development at the time transformation occurred.[144, 162] Classification of lymphoid neoplasms on the basis of immune receptor genotypic analyses should be viewed as an addition to and not a replacement of immunophenotypic analyses. Each technique has its limitations, ambiguities, and instructive insights.[163, 164] A telling example of this comes from a retrospective study of the malignant lymphocytes from 70 patients with immunophenotypic B-cell precursor acute lymphoblastic leukemia of childhood.[165] These lymphoblasts were analyzed for rearrangements of all their immune receptor genes. All but three cases had a rearranged IgH locus, certainly consistent with their phenotypic lineage. However, 80 per cent had a rearrangement of TCRδ. In addition,

rearrangements of TCRγ and TCRβ were each seen in about 50 per cent of the cases (Table 11–2). One question that arises from such a study is the issue of what it means to call something a "B-cell" when it has a germline IgH locus but a rearranged TCRδ gene. The safest answer to such a prob-

Table 11–2. Immunoglobulin and T-Cell Antigen Receptor Gene Rearrangements in Acute Leukemias

	B-Cell Precursor ALL (%)	T-Cell ALL (%)	AML (%)	ALL of Infancy (%)
IgH				
R	98	14	14	64
Igκ				
R	28	0	2	18
D	17	0	0	0
	45			
Igλ				
R	20	0	0	0
TCRβ				
R	33	89	7	9
TCRγ				
R	55	91	5	0
TCRδ				
R	54	68	8	NA
D	26	28	1	NA
	80	96	9	

*ALL, acute lymphoblastic leukemia; AML, acute myeloblastic leukemia; Ig, immunoglobulin; TCR, T-cell antigen receptor; R, rearranged; D, deleted.

Data derived from Felix, C.A., Poplack, D.G., Reaman, G.H., et al: Characterizations of immunoglobulin and T-cell receptor gene patterns in B-cell precursor acute lymphoblastic leukemia of childhood. J. Clin. Oncol. 8:431, 1990; Van Dongen, J.J.M., Breitz, T.M., Adriaansen, H.J., Beishuizen, A., and Hooijkaas, H.: Detection of minimal residual disease in acute leukemia by immunological marker analysis and polymerase chain reaction. Leukemia 6(Suppl.):47, 1992; Felix, C.A., Reaman, G.H., Korsmeyer, S.J., et al: Immunoglobulin and T-cell receptor gene configuration in acute lymphoblastic leukemia of infancy. Blood 70:536, 1987.

lem is not to become constrained by forcing a cell into one or another lineage if it does not quite fit. Instead it should be considered simply as a composite of its phenotypic, genotypic, and functional attributes. The second issue raised by studies such as this deals with the designation of these cells as "B-cell precursors." More "mature" B-cell or T-cell malignancies or Epstein-Barr virus transformed B-lymphoblastoid cell lines do not show nearly this level of simultaneous Ig and TCR locus rearrangement.[166–170] So one is left to ponder what these cells are the precursors of since their more mature successors are not readily apparent. This leads to the speculation that the target cell population in B-cell precursor acute lymphoblastic leukemia (ALL) of childhood may represent a temporally or physiologically distinct entity. For example, it could be that the increased incidence of multiple immune receptor gene rearrangements could reflect a clone that as a population of cells spends more time at a stage where the V(D)J recombinase complex is active.

▼ THE USE OF IMMUNE RECEPTOR GENE REARRANGEMENTS FOR THE DETERMINATION OF MINIMAL RESIDUAL DISEASE

The sensitivity of Southern blot analysis for the detection of clonal proliferation is not distinctly greater than that offered by morphological diagnosis (e.g., bone marrow examination) for following the course of treatment and response of a patient with a lymphoid malignancy. Recently, however, molecular genetic techniques have been developed that greatly increase the sensitivity with which a particular leukemic cell can be identified and thus provided the opportunity to determine minimal residual disease at the level of 1 cell per 10^5–10^6 as opposed to the 1 in 100 offered by Southern blot analysis.

The kinds of assays described in this section all make use of the polymerase chain reaction (PCR)[171] to amplify the unique rearrangement(s) that forms a molecular "fingerprint" of a particular leukemic cell. The amplification proceeds to the point that evidence of the presence of the leukemic cell is unequivocal and easily visualized. The specificity of this technique can be made essentially absolute.

PCR analysis should be seen as part of the continuum of remarkable advances of recombinant DNA technology that have occurred since 1980 and that have brought a new era to biomedical endeavors. The underlying principle of PCR technology is beautifully simple: It is controlled and focused DNA replication. DNA polymerase requires a primer that starts it off on its synthesis of a complementary strand. In PCR a specific segment of DNA is repeatedly replicated through the judicious choice of opposing primers, one specific for each complementary strand and oriented so that the direction of replication will be such as to replicate the region between the two primers. Repeated rounds of primer annealing, replication, denaturation, reannealing to the index and newly synthesized DNA, replication, and so on, are accomplished via a thermal cycling machine and a heat resistant DNA polymerase. Thirty-five such cycles could theoretically amplify a single segment of DNA 2^{35} times. It is also possible to amplify a specific mRNA by this process after an initial step in which the RNA is converted

into complementary DNA (cDNA). This assay is fast, relatively inexpensive, automated, and amenable to the development of quality control standards in the hands of experienced personnel.[172] With appropriate resource allocation the use of molecular genetics in the determination of minimal residual disease could be incorporated into protocols covering the care of almost every patient with acute lymphoblastic leukemia (ALL). Whether this increased sensitivity of detection of minimal residual disease will translate into better therapy and increased survival rate remains to be determined.

We have noted that malignant lymphocytes often have rearrangements of their immune receptor genes that can be used to identify the specific leukemic clone. In addition to these rearrangements, malignant lymphocytes, and hematopoietic malignancies in general often carry a variety of disease specific chromosomal rearrangements (see below, as well as the Chapters 25 and 26 on oncogenes and neoplasia) whose structure and unique configurations also make them available as tumor-specific markers. Either of these markers can theoretically provide the basis of minimal residual disease determination. The use of immunoglobulin or T-cell antigen receptor gene rearrangements offers an advantage with regard to their being the most universally applicable to lymphoid malignancies since over 95 per cent of lymphoid leukemias or lymphomas involve lymphocytes that have rearranged either one or more Ig or TCR loci. The disadvantages of this approach include (1) the need to individualize the assay for each patient (see below); (2) the fact that the assay itself is slightly more complicated than just screening for a chromosomal aberration; (3) the fact that, in some cases, the focus of the assay (the specific Ig or TCR) may somatically mutate so as to become invisible and therefore lead to a falsely negative result; and (4) that the genetic sequence being assayed is not related (in most cases) to the cause of the transformation; as discussed earlier, it is an epiphenomenon. Assaying specific chromosomal breaks eliminates these four disadvantages but at present is not as universally applicable because the majority of leukemia-/lymphoma-associated chromosomal aberrations have not been identified or characterized to the point where they are amenable to PCR-based assay. Furthermore, certain characterized chromosomal aberrations (e.g. myc-Ig) may have breakpoints too diverse and scattered for different patients to be amenable to PCR analysis using a single panel of primers.

The key to the use of Ig and TCR rearrangements for determination of minimal residual disease is the junctional diversity described earlier in this chapter. There are four basic steps to the use of Ig and TCR gene rearrangements in this assay:

1. Identification (of locus rearrangement).
2. Characterization (of the unique junctional sequence).
3. Determination (of the presence of leukemic cells in "remission" samples).
4. Quantitation (of the number of leukemic cells present).

Identification

On presentation of a patient with the clinical and morphological diagnosis of lymphoid malignancy, a determination must be made of whether there is a clonal immune receptor rearrangement carried by the malignant cells. Classically, this is accomplished by Southern blot analysis.

Denaturing Gradient Gel Electrophoresis

One way to speed up this process may be through the use of denaturing gradient gel electrophoresis (DGGE).[173] DGGE technology in this particular application begins with the fundamental PCR assay for junctional diversity. In this assay one PCR primer (or group of primers) is synthesized so that it will be complementary to part of the variable segment of the immune receptor being studied. The part of the variable segment that is chosen for this primer is ideally the *least* variable part of the segment, for example, the 5′ end of the V segment or in some cases framework region (FR) 3. This allows for the construction of a "consensus" V primer that can be utilized successfully to prime DNA replication from every or practically every V segment in that particular immune receptor locus. The downstream primer is related to the J segments, either a consensus J sequence or, if the structure of the locus is suitable, a primer from just 3′ of the most 3′ J segment. It is possible to use this exact 3′ sequence as a primer in those cases in which the J segments are few in number and not spread out over more than 1000 nucleotides of DNA. If this is the case the amplified product of a V(D)J rearrangement is less than 2000 base pairs. Products larger than 2000 base pairs cannot be amplified with an efficiency that makes them reasonable substrates for this analysis.

When the appropriate primer pairs are developed they are then used to amplify V(D)J rearranged DNA in the sample to be analyzed. The vastly predominant clone in a sample population (as would be the case in a newly diagnosed lymphoid malignancy) is the predominant amplified product. A consensus primer works in most cases because (1) it only need bind to a particular sequence well enough and long enough to initiate replication, and (2) after the first cycle of replication it is identical to one end of all the newly synthesized DNA fragments. When placed on a denaturing gradient gel the amplified fragment migrates until it begins to undergo regional denaturation[174] (the point at which this occurs is sequence specific), at which time migration is markedly slowed. After gel staining the fragment(s) associated with the clone appears as a notable band that emerges from the background haze caused by the migratory patterns of the other polyclonal rearrangements, which are below the level of detection in this particular kind of gel visualization. Without the use of DGGE one could not distinguish a monoclonal proliferation from a polyclonal one because the size of the amplified fragments would be the same in either case. DGGE is sensitive to DNA sequence.

Which immune receptor should be studied for which disease? Depending on the type of lymphoid malignancy it is more or less likely that a particular immune receptor gene will be rearranged. With regard to minimal residual disease determination, rather than screen every malignancy for rearrangement of every immune receptor it is possible to play the percentages and only screen for those rearrangements that are the most likely and most usable in a PCR based assay. Table 11–2 provides a general sense of the frequency of immune receptor gene rearrangements in acute leukemia.

Clearly, study of immune receptor rearrangements is more or less applicable depending on the leukemic type. For example, for B-cell precursor ALL, rearrangement of the IgH locus is most applicable and has indeed been used in preliminary studies.[175, 176] However, the use of IgH PCR amplification can present problems because the great diversity of V segments in the IgH locus complicates the preparation of a "consensus" V_H segment. Furthermore, as noted above, the IgH locus is subject to continued somatic mutation, which can occasionally change the unique molecular "fingerprint" and thus defeat the characterization and determination steps to be described next. The TCRγ and δ loci are almost always rearranged in T-ALL and each is rearranged in over 50 per cent of B-cell precursor ALLs. The repertoire of V segments for these loci is much more restricted than for the IgH locus, and these loci are not subject to somatic hypermutation. Thus, in situations in which such TCR rearrangements can be identified, they may be logistically simpler to work with and interpret.[177, 178] For example, identifying both a TCRδ and an IgH rearrangement in the ALL cells of a patient with B-cell precursor ALL may be advantageous in terms of the more homologous (less "degenerate" in order to achieve "consensus") primers that can be used for TCRδ. Having both of these loci available for the analysis of this patient would also provide a comforting and useful "backup" for pinpointing the minimal residual disease clone.

Characterization

The next step, characterization, requires PCR amplification of the hypervariable, junctional part of the V(D)J rearranged region. Once amplified the unique molecular fingerprint, which is the precise DNA sequence of this junction, must be determined. The most straightforward way to do this is by sequencing this region, which can either be accomplished by cloning and sequencing of the PCR product or by newer sequencing techniques that may not give quite as much resolution but are accomplished directly at the time of PCR amplification. "Nested" PCR analysis is an alternative to actually sequencing the junction. In nested PCR, primers from inside the originally amplified fragment are used to amplify a shorter stretch of DNA that is almost pure hypervariable region. This fragment is then used as a probe of subsequent amplifications of the same patient's "remission" DNAs. The premise is that at very high stringency of hybridization, only the absolutely identical sequence hybridizes (here one is not asking only for an oligonucleotide to prime a polymerization reaction transiently but rather for it to bind with high energy and stay bound). Thus, a hybridization signal from a study performed using a "clonospecific" probe (derived at patient presentation) on a DNA sample from that patient would be indicative of residual leukemic cells even if morphological and clinical remission had been achieved. Actual sequencing of the junction provides a more controlled way of generating a smaller and completely specific oligonucleotide probe that can be utilized for such hybridization studies.

Determination

As just described, the determination step involves the preparation of DNA (or cDNA) from patient samples obtained at various times during a course of treatment. The appropriate consensus primers are used to amplify the V(D)J re-arrangements present in the sample. A probe, prepared either from known sequence of the leukemic clone or by nested PCR, is then applied to the products of the amplification reaction. Positive hybridization indicates the presence of DNA that carries a molecular fingerprint identical to that of the probe, and (the presumption is) therefore of residual leukemic cells. Obviously, crucial attention must be paid to making the conditions of the hybridization reaction high enough to be absolutely specific but still allow formation of double-stranded DNA (in this case one strand is the probe and the other the target DNA).

Quantitation

It may not be sufficient to know simply whether residual leukemic cells exist in a sample. It may be important to be able to quantitate at least roughly how many such cells remain. A variety of strategies exist for this quantitation. One strategy involves the cloning of products of a PCR amplification into bacteriophage and plating out the phage on a bacterial lawn. Duplicate lifts of phage DNA are then made, one lift hybridized to a clonospecific probe, the other to a probe that will recognize every V(D)J rearrangement of the particular immune receptor being analyzed in the sample. The ratio of clonospecific phage to total hybridizing phage provides one kind of quantitation when combined with morphological/immunophenotypic data concerning the proportion of lymphoid, erythroid, and myeloid cells in the sample.[176] Another means of quantitation involves making a standard titration curve by diluting known amounts of clonospecific cells in a background of miscellaneous cells. The signal generated from the sample containing an unknown amount of clonospecific DNA is then plotted on a standard curve (prepared as an internal control by mixing known quantities of clonal and polyclonal DNAs together) to provide a rough estimate of the number of leukemic cells in the sample.[175]

Some Results

Enough pilot studies[175, 177–181] have been performed by these methods to begin to produce a rough picture of the dynamics of leukemic cell kill during current accepted therapy for ALL. Different studies yield varying results, but a consensus pattern seems to be emerging at present. Induction therapy results in a three- to five-fold log reduction in the number of leukemic cells (down to as few as 0.001 per cent of cells in a given sample). This level of cells may plateau for a while (usually measured in many months), often corresponding to the maintenance therapy phase of treatment. Whether these cells are viable and capable of cell division and "rekindling" of the leukemia is not known at this time. However, it is clear that the majority of children who complete a full 2 to 3 year course of therapy for ALL test negative for residual leukemic cells by these pilot assays. In at least one study,[177] differences in the duration of minimal residual disease were not associated with any particular clinical or hematological parameter of the underlying disease. In another example, a different and possibly more sensitive study[182] reported that patients ($n = 22$) with $<2 \times 10^{-5}$

leukemic cells per bone marrow cell after induction remained in complete remission at a median duration of 63 months from diagnosis, whereas patients ($n = 4$) with a higher leukemic cell burden all relapsed after a median duration of 21 months from diagnosis. A larger study[183] demonstrated that the presence of 1 per cent ($>10^{-2}$) or more residual bone marrow leukemic blasts after induction therapy or 0.1 per cent or more residual leukemic blasts at any subsequent point during therapy was associated with a markedly poorer outcome. Reappearance of the leukemic clone either during or after therapy is a bad prognostic sign and can precede clinical evidence of relapse by several months. Whether such information obtained a few months before clinical relapse would help rescue certain patients if acted upon by a physician is an issue that needs to be tested in prospective protocols.

Immune Receptors as Participants in the Generation of Chromosomal Aberrations
(Table 11–3)

▼ THE BURKITT'S LYMPHOMA PRECEDENT

It could be said that the study of gene rearrangements in lymphoid cells gave birth to the entire field of molecular genetic analysis of cancer-associated chromosomal aberrations. In 1982 the chromosomal localization of the murine and human immunoglobulin genes had been established. It was striking that the chromosomal bands to which these genes had been localized were precisely those bands disrupted by the consistent translocations associated with the development of Burkitt's lymphoma in humans and plasmacytoma in *Balb/c* mice. One group of investigators studying the c-*myc* gene in plasmacytomas came across its structural juxtaposition to the IgH locus.[184] Two other groups approached the translocation breakpoint in Burkitt's lymphoma and murine plasmacytomas by the cloning and characterization of "peculiar," uncharacteristic rearrangements of the immunoglobulin genes in these malignant cells and similarly found that the IgH locus had rearranged with the c-*myc* proto-oncogene.[185, 186] This was the first time the genes that precisely flanked a cancer-associated chromosomal aberration had been identified. It was not only the simple fact of their identification but the fact of precisely what genes they were that made the finding so compelling. In Burkitt's lymphoma, a B-cell tumor, the characteristic translocation carried by the malignant cells juxtaposed the primary differentiated product of those cells, immunoglobulins, with a gene, c-*myc*, whose dysregulation was associated with malignant transformation. It was impossible not to speculate that the translocated c-*myc* gene might now be inappropriately controlled by those factors that promoted transcription of the immunoglobulin genes, and that the net effect of this dysregulation would be qualitatively and possibly quantitatively inappropriate expression of a gene with known growth effecting properties. Although complete elucidation of the mechanism by which this translocation contributes to malignant transformation has not yet been achieved, the basic speculative premise just described is firmly established. Studies of many examples of sporadically occurring Burkitt's lymphoma suggested that in the approximately 80 per cent

Table 11–3. Immune Receptors in the Generation of Chromosomal Aberrations

Translocation	Cancer	Loci
Involvement of Ig Genes in Human B-Cell Malignancy		
t(5;14)(q31;q32)	ALL with hypereosinophilia	IL3-IgH
t(8;14)(q24;q32.3)	(Burkitt's lymphoma, MM advanced lymphomas)	c-Myc-IgH
t(2;8)(p12;q24)*		Igκ-c-Myc
t(8;22)(q24;q11)		c-Myc-Igλ
t(3;14)(q27;q32.3)	DLCL	Bcl6-IgH
t(2;3)(p12;q27)		Igκ-Bcl6
t(3;22)(q27;q11)		Bcl6-Igλ
t(10;14)(q24;q32)	High and low grade lymphoma	LYT10-IgH
t(11;14)(q13;q32.3)	MCL, MM, CLL	CCND1-IgH
t(11;22)(q13;q11)		Igκ-CCND1
t(14;18)(q32.3;q21)	FL, MM, CLL	IgH-Bcl2
t(2;18)(p12;q21)	DLCL	Igκ-Bcl2
t(14;19)(q32;q11.3)	CLL	IgH-Bcl3
t(4;14)(p16.3;q32.3)†	MM	FGFR3 and MMSET-IgH
t(14;16)(q32.3;q23)†	MM	IgH-c-maf
t(16;22)(q23;q11)		c-maf-Igλ
t(6;14)(p25;q32)†	MM	IRF4(MUM1)-IgH
t(9;14)(p13;q32)	LPL, MM	PAX5-IgH
t(1;14)(q21;q32)	B-ALL, ?MM	Bcl9-IgH
t((14;15)(q32;q11–13)	DLCL	IgH-Bcl8
t(1;14)(p22;q32)	Malt B lymphoma	Bcl10-IgH
Involvement of TCR Genes in Human T-Cell Malignancy		
t(1;7)(p34;q35)	T-ALL	Lck-TCRβ
t(1;14)(p33;q11.2)	Stem cell leukemia, T-ALL	Scl(Tall)-TCRα/δ
t(7;9)(q35;q34.2)	T-ALL	TCRβ-Ta12
t(7;9)(q35;q34)	T-ALL	TCRβ-Tan1
t(7;10)(q35;q24)	T-ALL	TCRβ-HOX11
t(7;19)(q35;p13)	T-ALL	TCRβ-Lyl-1
t(8;14)(q24;q11)	T-ALL, T-CLL	c-Myc-TCRα/δ
t(10;14)(q23;q11)	T-ALL	HOX11-TCRα/δ
t(11;14)(q13;q11)	T-ALL	LMO2-TCRα/δ
t(11;14)(p15;q11)	T-ALL	LMO1-TCRα/δ
inv(14)(q11.2;q32.1)	T-PLL	TCRα/δ-TCL1
t(14;14)(q11.2;q32.1)	T-CLL	TCRα/δ-TCL1
Involvement of TCR Genes in Clonal Proliferation/Malignancy in Ataxia-telangiectasia		
t(7;14)(q35;32.1)		TCRβ-TCL1
inv(14)(q11.2q32.1)		TCRα/δ-TCL1
t(14;14)(q11.2;q32.1)		TCRα/δ-TCL1
t(X;14)(q28;q11.2)		MTCP-TCRα/δ
Involvement of the Ig and TCR Loci in Chromosomal Aberration in Normal Individuals		
t(2;14)(p12;q32.3)‡		Igκ-IgH
inv(7)(p13q35)		TCRγ-TCRβ
t(7;7)(p13;p35)		TCRγ-TCRβ
t(7;14)(p13;q11.2)		TCRγ-TCRα/δ
t(7;14)(q35;q11.2)		TCRβ-TCRα/δ
inv(14)(2q11.2;q32.2)‡		TCRα-IgH
t(14;14)(q11.2;q32.3)		TCRα-IgH
V(D)J Recombinase Mediated Rearrangement of Other Genes		
del(1p33)	T-ALL	Sil-Scl
Involvement of Other Immune-Related Genes		
t(1;19)(q23;p13)	Pre-B-ALL	E2A-Pbx1

*Variant (IgL) translocations, with no apparent preference for kappa vs. lambda, are associated with most of the same partners as IgH translocations.
†Chromosomal partner not identifiable by routine cytogenetic analysis.
‡Also seen in rare malignancies.
ALL, acute lymphoblastic leukemia; CLL, chronic lymphocytic leukemia; B-CLL, B-cell CLL; T-ALL, T-cell ALL; ATL, adult T-cell leukemia; PLL, prolymphocytic leukemia; MM, multiple myeloma; LPL, lymphoplasmacytic lymphoma; DLCL, diffuse large cell lymphoma; MCL, mantle cell lymphoma; FL, follicular lymphoma.

that involved the IgH locus (as opposed to the Igκ or Igλ locus) the heavy chain "switch" region had been targeted in the breakage and rejoining event.[187] Thus, not only was the immunoglobulin locus involved in the translocation, its involvement seemed to be selected by one of its cell-type specific recombinational processes. The switch region of the IgH locus is similarly involved by the t(14;19) (q32;q13.1) translocation associated with the development of some cases of B-cell chronic lymphocytic leukemia (B-CLL). The translocation juxtaposes the IgH locus with a putative cell-cycle control related gene, BCL3.[188] It is not known what enzymes and structural signals and conformations are necessary for these chromosomal breakage and rejoining events that involve these IgH switch regions.

▼ V(D)J RECOMBINASE-MEDIATED CHROMOSOMAL ABERRATIONS

A large and diverse number of chromosomal aberrations that occur within the immune receptor loci seem to implicate the V(D)J recombinase complex as playing some role in their occurrence. Characterization of the chromosomal regions involved in these aberrations often suggests that the deletion, inversion, or translocation occurred at the time that the immune receptor locus was undergoing its normal physiological segment rearrangements (Fig. 11–14). Instead of completing the process within the locus, material from a different part of the genome becomes interposed. In many cases the results of the aberration are essentially balanced. For example, a V segment for an immune receptor locus becomes contiguous with nucleotide x from another chromosome, and the J segment to which that V might have rearranged becomes contiguous with nucleotide x+1 on the other chromosome. The material between that V and J is deleted as it might have been in normal intralocus VJ rearrangement. The structure of such chromosomal aberrations has strong implications for their mechanism of occurrence. Such balanced structures are not consistent with temporally unrelated times of breakage of the two involved regions. One cannot easily imagine a V and J segment becoming dislodged from each other and floating around in the nucleus of the cell until they encounter two new chromosomal regions to which to ligate or why those two new chromosomal regions should have any relationship to each other. It is conceptually simpler to visualize (see Fig. 11–15) all of the participants in the generation of a chromosomal aberration being present at the same time. If chromosomal aberrations do indeed occur at one point in time (as seems most consistent with the data), then they almost certainly occur at a point in space where relevant recombinase enzyme complexes can function and interact. The likely temporal and spatial localization for the

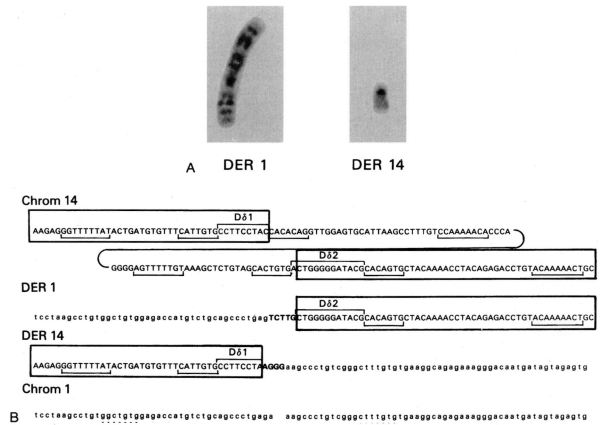

Figure 11–14. Analysis of the breakpoint in a t(1;14) translocation associated with the development of a stem cell leukemia. A, The reciprocal chromosome partners of the translocation, the derivative chromosome 1 (which maintains the chromosome 1 centromere) and the derivative 14 (maintaining the chromosome 14 centromere), are shown in a G-banded partial karyotype. B, Sequence analysis of a reciprocal t(1;14) translocation. The uppermost sequence is the germline chromosome 14 sequence (uppercase letters). Note the two Dδ segments flanked by heptamer and nonamer signal sequences (underlined) and the intervening DNA (interrupted line) between these segments. Derivative chromosome 1 (DER [1]) shows the germline chromosome 14 sequence at the 3′ end and the germline chromosome 1 sequence (lowercase letters) at the 5′ end. Five nucleotides attributed to N region diversity are shown in boldface. DER(14) shows 3′ germline chromosome 1 sequence, N nucleotides, and 5′ chromosome 14 sequence. Note that the intervening DNA between the Dδ segments has been deleted from the translocated chromosomes, suggesting that the translocation may have taken place during physiological D-D rearrangement, which would have normally deleted this intervening DNA (see Fig. 11–15). The bottom line shows the germline chromosome 1 sequence with two possible heptamer signal sequences (dashed underline). A gap that corresponds to the area involved in N region addition has been introduced into the germline chromosome 1 sequence to allow alignment of nucleotides on der(1) and der(14). Data and figure modified from the original research report (reference 189).

occurrence of chromosomal aberrations in which the V(D)J recombinase plays a role suggests an inherent organization of the interphase nucleus and may provide as well a key to understanding the requirement of chromatin accessibility discussed in an earlier section of this chapter.

▼ A MODEL

The speculative model depicted in Figure 11–15 attempts to suggest a temporal and spatial focus for one kind of V(D)J recombinase mediated translocation. In this example, on the basis of the cloning and characterization of a t(1;14) translocation associated with the development of a stem cell leukemia,[189] breaks occur at precise signal sequences flanking two diversity segments from the TCRδ locus (see Fig. 11–14A and B). The chromosomal breaks within the 3′ SCL gene on chromosome 1 do not clearly focus on immune receptor–like signal sequences. (This 3′ SCL breakpoint should be contrasted with the 5′ SCL breakpoints seen in the interstitial deletion of part of chromosome 1, to be described in a moment; the 5′ breakpoints are proximate to clear heptamer/nonamer signal sequences.) This raises the question of whether the V(D)J recombinase is necessary but not sufficient for the occurrence of such translocations. Other structures that have been suggested as facilitating recombinase mediated aberrations (or, for that matter, chromosomal aberrations in general) include alternating stretches of purine and pyrimidine residues forming Z DNA configurations[84] and sequences with homology to the prokaryotic recombinogenic signal, chi.[190, 191] Insight into this issue has now been derived by analysis of recombinase-mediated DNA transposition in a cell-free system.[192, 193] In this system it has been demonstrated that the RAG proteins, in the presence of the non-specific DNA-binding protein high mobility group 1 (HMG1), generate a blunt ended "signal" end and a hairpin "coding" end. The signal end is capable of insertion into non–recombination signal sequence (RSS) containing DNA by strand transfer. The intermediates that follow in this reaction are capable of being resolved in a manner consistent with the known mechanics of V(D)J joining. Thus the data suggest that the recombinase complex alone and the DNA by-products of its action can explain the occurrence of potentially oncogenic (as well as immune response required) structural DNA rearrangements. The genomic structure and activity of the RAG1 and RAG2 genes are consistent with an origin of these genes as a transposable element that became fortuitously and vitally incorporated into an early vertebrate genome and led to the logistic underpinning of the generation of immune diversity by structural DNA rearrangements.

▼ IMMUNOGLOBULIN TRANSLOCATIONS IN B-CELL TUMORS: AN OVERVIEW[85, 194–215]

Nearly 80 per cent of hematopoietic tumors involve some kind of lymphoid cell, the vast majority of which are derived from the B lymphoid lineage. One of the probable explanations for the predominance of B lymphoid tumors is the fact that two kinds of error-prone developmentally regulated Ig gene rearrangements occur during normal B lymphocyte development: (1)VDJ recombinase mediated IgH and IgL

gene formation in pro- and pre-B cells plus receptor editing in pre-B/immature B cells and germinal center lymphocytes and (2) IgH switch recombination, principally in germinal centers late in B-cell development. In addition, germinal center B lymphocytes undergo somatic hypermutation that is largely restricted to IgL and IgH V regions but apparently can also affect other genes. For example, the promoter region of the human bcl-6 proto-oncogene seems to be susceptible to somatic hypermutation in germinal center B lymphocytes undergoing repeated rounds of somatic hypermutation.

The frequency with which somatic hypermutation contributes to B lymphocyte oncogenesis remains uncertain. However, dysregulation of oncogenes by translocation with an Ig locus represents a critical oncogenic event in a high proportion of most B-cell tumors. Chronic lymphocytic leukemia represents the most notable exception at present, since only about 10 per cent of these tumors have a detectable Ig translocation. There are two principal types of breakpoints involving an Ig locus. The first kind, which affects IgH and IgL loci (and TCR loci in T lymphocytes), occurs near—often immediately adjacent to—sites of D or J recombination involved in receptor formation. These are presumed to result from rare errors mediated by VDJ recombinase during receptor formation or editing in early B cells or during receptor editing in germinal center cells. However, recently it was suggested that the frequent insertions, deletions, and duplications that occur during somatic hypermutation may generate breaks that serve as substrates for translocations. It is noteworthy that pregerminal center (e.g., mantle cell lymphoma) and some germinal center (e.g., follicular lymphoma) tumors mostly have breakpoints immediately adjacent to the site of normal J recombination, whereas most germinal center (e.g., Burkitt's lymphoma, diffuse large cell lymphoma) and post–germinal center (multiple myeloma) tumors have breakpoints relatively distant from the normal site of normal J recombination. The breakpoints on the diverse partners involved in translocations near the IgJ regions sometimes have RSS but usually do not. The second kind of breakpoint occurs within or near IgH repetitive switch regions and is presumed to result from rare errors mediated by IgH switch recombinase. The breakpoints on the partner chromosomes do not have switch-like sequences or any other obvious sequence characteristics. Infrequently other sites, such as V regions or C region exons, may be involved.

From an analysis of translocation breakpoints, it appears that dysregulation of the corresponding oncogene is caused by the proximity with one of the known IgH or IgL enhancer elements. Figure 11–16A shows illustrative examples of several kinds of reciprocal translocations involving an IgH locus. Translocations near a JH region generate a derivative 14 (der [14]) that contains the centromere of 14 plus the Eμ enhancer and both Eα enhancers. The oncogene dysregulated by this translocation must reside on der(14) but can be located up to at least 400 kb from the breakpoint (e.g., cyclin D1 dysregulated by the t[11;14] in mantle cell lymphoma). Dysregulation of the bcl2 gene in follicular lymphoma is similar, although a rare variant breakpoint in the downstream non-coding region can result in hybrid transcripts (but not a hybrid protein) that include Ig sequences. In contrast, translocation into a switch region results in segregation of Eμ (and Eα1 if the breakpoint involves a switch region

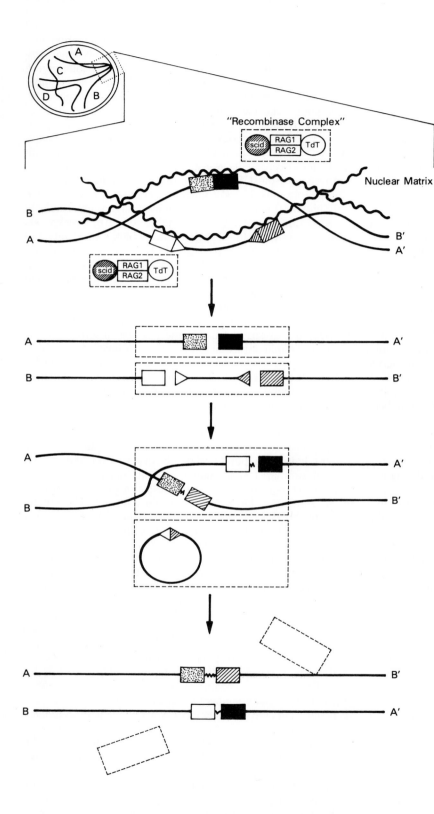

Figure 11–15. Postulated nuclear localization of the recombinase complex and targets of recombinase mediated translocation. The circle at the top of the figure represents a cell, for example, a lymphocyte, in which a part of chromosomes A′ and B′ is sequestered in a part of the nucleus, perhaps attached to the nuclear matrix (wavy line) because of their particular structure, function, chromatin status, or accessibility or chance. The recombinase complexes are operative in this part of the nucleus and act on the two chromosomes to cause breakage and rejoining events. The complex (dashed line box) consists of targeting, nucleolytic, and repair enzymes including RAG1, RAG2, the scid gene product and TdT. The hatched and open boxes delineate "coding" segments, the triangle "signal" sequences. The structure shown on chromosome B′ in the upper part of the figure is consistent with an immune receptor locus, for example, the TCRDδ locus shown in Fig. 11–14. Part of the recombination reaction proceeds normally; the intervening sequence carrying the signal segments is joined together in an extrachromosomal circle. However, the topographical and topological characteristics of chromosomes A′ and B′ cause an interchromosomal rather than an intrachromosomal rearrangement, which results in a chromosomal translocation. (From Kirsch, I.R.: Genetics of pediatric tumors: The causes and consequences of chromosomal aberrations. In Pizzo, P., and Poplack, D. (eds.): Principles and Practice of Pediatric Oncology, 2nd ed. Philadelphia, J. B. Lippincott Co., 1993; with permission.)

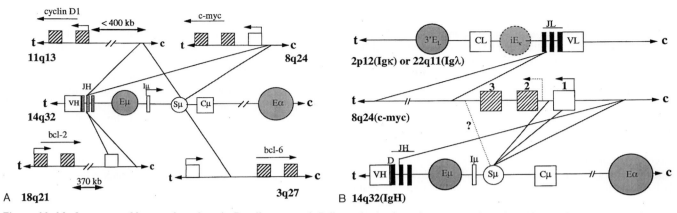

Figure 11–16. Anatomy of Ig translocations in B-cell tumors. *A,* Different kinds of translocations involving the IgH locus. Boxes represent Ig gene segments as identified, or exons of other genes (diagonal stripes indicate the presence of coding sequences). Open circles indicate μ switch region and larger shaded circles indicate Ig enhancers, with the circle enclosed by a dashed line representing an enhancer (iEκ) present in the Igκ but not the Igλ locus. Vertical lines with horizontal arrows indicate position of conventional (solid) or cryptic (dotted) promoters. All sequences are shown with the telomere (t) to centromere (c) orientation from left to right. Lines connecting two different sequences indicate established (solid) or potential (dotted) translocation breakpoints. The derivative reciprocal chromosomes can be determined by starting at the centromeric (or, respectively) telomeric end of the Ig locus and then following the connecting lines from either J or switch sequences to the telomeric (or, respectively, centromeric) end of the other chromosome. The derivative chromosome is named by the origin of the centromere; e.g., in the reciprocal t(3;14)(q27;q32) translocation, der(14) has the centromere of 14, and der(3) has the centromere of 3. *B,* Translocation of c-*myc* to an IgH versus an IgL locus. See *A* and text for additional details.

downstream of Sα1; see Figs. 11–9 or 11–11) to the other (der) chromosome, but segregation of Eα2 (and Eα1 if the breakpoint involves Sα1 or an upstream switch region) to der(14). Thus for translocations into switch regions, the dysregulated oncogene may be on either der(14) (e.g., cyclin D1 up to at least 300 kb from the breakpoint with t [11;14] in myeloma); or the recombinant partner chromosome (e.g., bcl6 with t[3;14] in diffuse large cell lymphoma). In the latter case, Eμ provides an enhancer and Iμ provides a substitute promoter to generate dysregulated Iμ/bcl6 hybrid transcripts (but a normal bcl6 protein). It remains to be determined over what distance the Eμ enhancer is capable of dysregulating downstream oncogenes.

Figure 11–16*B* compares IgH with variant IgL translocations that result in dysregulation of the c-*myc* oncogene. The t(8;14) translocations can involve either JH or IgH switch regions, and in both cases (but illustrated only for IgH switch breakpoints) breakpoints on 8q24 can occur upstream (centromeric) of exon 1, within exon 1, or in intron 1 so that c-*myc* is on the der(14). Breakpoints that occur upstream of exon 1 of c-*myc* generate c-*myc* transcripts from an endogenous c-*myc* promoter, whereas breakpoints in exon 1 or in intron 1 generate c-*myc* transcripts from cryptic promoters. A translocation involving a switch region and a site downstream of exon 3 of c-*myc* would put Eμ and c-*myc* on the der(8) and could, in principle, generate dysregulated c-*myc* transcripts from the endogenous c-*myc* promoter under the influence of Eμ. Although this model predicts that such a structural variant IgH translocation should dysregulate c-*myc*, this particular reconfiguration of the loci has not yet been identified. Analogous variant IgL c-*myc* translocations have been identified. These have breakpoints near JL and downstream of exon 3 of c-*myc* so that the c-*myc* and IgL enhancers are present on the der(8), resulting in initiation of dysregulated transcripts at the endogenous c-*myc* promoter. The variant breakpoints occur up to 300 kb downstream of c-*myc*, often into the Pvt-1 locus, which expresses a non-coding transcript and is thought to influence the expression

of c-*myc*. Generally, then, IgH and variant IgL translocations bracket the critical oncogene dysregulated by the translocation.

There is mainly one translocation partner (and corresponding oncogene) associated with an Ig locus for many tumors, for example, 8q24.1(c-*myc*) in Burkitt's lymphoma, 18q21 (bcl2) in follicular lymphoma, and 11q13 (cyclin D1) in mantle cell lymphoma. For other tumors there are several non-random partners. For example, in myeloma, at least 18 different chromosomal partners have been identified, although 3 partners are quite frequent (each accounting for about 20 per cent of tumors), 6 other partners are recurrent but with a lower frequency, and the remainder have been identified only once thus far. Although most tumor cells probably have a single translocation involving an Ig locus, some have two or even three different translocations involving IgH and IgL loci. The t(4;14) translocation in myeloma seems simultaneously to dysregulate two potential oncogenes, one localized on the der(14) and the other generating a hybrid transcript from the der(4). Given that genes localized within 400 kb of an Eα can be dysregulated, it seems likely that there will be other translocations in which two oncogenes are dysregulated by a single translocation event.

The technology for identifying and characterizing translocations involving an Ig locus has advanced substantially in the past few years. In the past many translocations were not detected by conventional karyotypes, particularly if breakpoints occurred near the telomeres of each chromosome, the tumor cells had a low-mitotic index, or the tumor cells had numerous karyotypic abnormalities. The development of fluorescent in situ hybridization (FISH) techniques that utilize chromosome painting probes and probes specific for different parts of an Ig locus, different chromosomal regions, and various oncogenes has largely solved this problem by permitting analyses of either metaphase chromosomes or interphase nuclei (see Plate 11–1 for examples). Even with karyotypic identification of a translocation into an Ig locus, a significant challenge remains in cloning the translocation breakpoint, identifying genes that are dysregulated (selective expression in tumors containing the translocation, or selective expression of the translocated allele) or altered as a result of the translocation, and then determining which dysregulated or altered genes can function as oncogenes in the tumor of interest.

▼ HYBRID IMMUNE RECEPTOR GENES

Invoking more complex mechanisms is not a problem when both partners in reciprocal chromosomal exchanges have reasonable heptamer sequences at their site of recombination. Such is the case in many aberrations associated with lymphoid malignancies. One common type would be a chromosomal aberration involving V(D)J recombination that occurs between two immune receptor loci instead of within one or the other locus. All humans carry within a subset of their peripheral blood lymphocytes chromosomal translocations or inversions that are formed by site specific V(D)J recombination between two immune receptor loci. The result of these aberrations is to form hybrid genes with a V segment from one receptor and a J and a C segment from another. The most common such abnormality appears to be a hybrid IgH variable–TCRα constant segment that occurs at a frequency as high as 0.1 per cent of a normal individual's peripheral blood T-cell population.[216, 217] Other such hybrids that have been extensively characterized include TCRγ-TCRα hybrids caused by V(D)J mediated t(7;14) (p13;q11.2) translocation[21] and TCRγ-TCRβ hybrids caused by V(D)J mediated inv(7) (p13;q35).[20] In general these hybrid genes are found at low frequency, although their structures and expression suggest that they may make some contribution of their own to immune receptor diversity or stimulation of cellular proliferation. Although approximately 50 per cent of such hybrid junctions are in-frame at the DNA level there is a selection for the expression of in-frame recombinants such that over 90 per cent of such hybrid mRNAs are in-frame,[20] a phenomenon that could be related to antigenic selection or mRNA stability.[218] The same phenomenon has been observed for normal intralocus V(D)J recombinants and suggests that hybrid immune receptors can be expressed, translated, placed in the membrane of a host lymphocyte, and selected by antigenic stimulation. This has been confirmed in human T lymphocytes in which hybrid TCRγ V/TCRβ (D)J chains have been shown to form pairwise associations with TCRα polypeptides. Such cells bearing these dimers can be shown to express either CD4 or CD8 and frequently be alloreactive.[219] Given the apparent diversity of effector functions and lineage determination based on what immune receptor is expressed on a cell, the implications of having a TCRγ V segment expressed on a TCRβ constant segment could be significant, although as yet, no particular function or phenotype has been associated with this or any other hybrid.

What has been observed with these hybrids is that their frequency is increased about 100-fold in patients suffering from the disease ataxia-telangiectasia (AT).[20] Ataxia-telangiectasia is a disease of protean manifestations including progressive cerebellar degeneration; oculocutaneous telangiectasia; radiosensitivity; immunodeficiency; predisposition to the development of certain malignancies, particularly lymphoid; and, as noted, increase in cell-type specific chromosomal

aberrations. This increase of hybrid gene formation reflects multiple independent events. Although as much as 10 per cent of an AT patient's peripheral T-cell population may carry an inversion of chromosome 7, this population, when analyzed at the level of the DNA, demonstrates an array of distinct Vγ recombined with any one of a number of Jβ segments. So the picture in the peripheral blood of an AT patient represents an exaggeration of the normal polyclonal population of hybrid genes found in everyone's normal peripheral blood T-cell population.

What is the relationship of this finding in AT to other aspects of the phenotype of this complex disease? There is no evidence at present that the increase in hybrid gene formation is caused by an overexpression or overactivity of the V(D)J recombinase complex. One possibility might be that part of the AT phenotype is caused by an inappropriate "accessibility" of the genome to the activity of DNA interactive factors, such as the recombinase complex. This might explain why loci that are only rarely simultaneously accessible in normal lymphocytes (such as the TCRγ and β loci) are more frequently capable of forming interlocus hybrids in AT lymphocytes. The exaggeration of hybrid gene formation in AT is not restricted to T cells. There is also an increase of Igκ-IgH hybrids (corresponding to t[2;14] translocations[220] in the B-cell population of these patients.[85] This "exaggeration" in AT of V(D)J recombinase mediated chromosomal aberration extends from hybrid gene formation to formation of translocations and inversions frankly associated with abnormal proliferation and malignancy. Over time in AT patients a clonal proliferation can develop within the T-cell population associated with the formation of an inversion or translocation of chromosome 14, inv(14) (q11.2;q32.1), t(14;14) (q11.2;q32.1). Much more rarely this clonal proliferation is associated with a t(X;14) translocation. Carrying one or another of these aberrations a particular T-cell clone can persist or proliferate in the peripheral blood of an AT patient to the point where it constitutes essentially 100 per cent of the peripheral T-cell population.[221] At this point the overall white blood cell count of the individual can still be within a normal range and there can be no evidence or stigmata of lymphoid malignancy. However, in a percentage of such patients with these clonal proliferations a T-cell malignancy subsequently develops in which the malignant cell contains the marker inv(14) or t(14;14). Cloning of the chromosomal breakpoints in these cells revealed site-specific recombination between TCRα J segments and a region within chromosomal band 14q32.1 in which a growth-affecting gene was presumed to reside.[222, 223] A cytogenetically identical aberration is associated with the development of T-cell prolymphocytic leukemia, a relatively virulent malignancy that is seen most commonly in older males.[224] Cloning studies of these malignancies in non-AT patients have revealed an identical V(D)J contributory mechanism.[225, 226] Two genes have now been identified residing at 14q32.1 and Xq28 and are implicated in these T-cell clonal proliferations. The gene at Xq28, 224-232MTCP (c6.1B),[227, 228] and the gene at 14q32.1, TCL-1[229] share some homology and may define a distinct family of proteins that are capable of binding small hydrophobic ligands.[230] Furthermore, in studies relying on transgenic animal model systems both TCL-1[231] and MTCP1[232] cause the development of T-cell leukemias.

▼ OTHER TARGETS FOR THE V(D)J RECOMBINASE

The V(D)J recombinase is a powerful mechanism for rearranging DNA. In the presence of this enzyme complex accessible signal sequences are targeted for structural reconfiguration. The usual targets are the immune receptor loci, but any accessible signal sequence is "at risk" for rearrangement. Thus, two loci, *Sil* and *Scl*, which either fortuitously or for reasons yet to be discovered carry within appropriate signal recognition signals, have been shown to be rearranged with each other by the V(D)J recombinase although neither is an immune receptor locus.[83] The *Sil* locus encodes a product that is not easily fit into current families of structurally similar proteins.[233] *Sil* is an "immediate early" gene expressed in all proliferative tissues although possibly exerting cell-lineage specific effects.[234] *Scl* is a basic domain helix-loop-helix transcription factor that likely functions at a nodal point in hematopoietic differentiation.[235–237] The V(D)J recombinase mediated interstitial deletions that unites these two loci is seen in the malignant cells of 20–30 per cent of all patients with T-ALL.[238, 239]

▼ REFINED CYTOGENETIC TECHNOLOGY FOR DELINEATION OF CHROMOSOMAL ABERRATIONS

A major advance in the elucidation of chromosomal aberrations in hematopoietic malignancies (or, for that matter, cancers in general) was the ability simultaneously to label and identify each distinct pair of chromosomes in a metaphase spread by a unique "color."[240] This technique allows an investigator to complement an analysis of chromosomal banding patterns and quickly identify major structural alterations as juxtapositions of the distinct colors of two chromosomes brought together by insertion or translocation. Such analyses have already made significant progress in reducing the number of ill-defined chromosomal aberrations heretofore simply categorized as "markers" of a particular tumor or cell line. In hematopoietic malignancies these analyses have allowed for the identification of these "markers," increased the sensitivity and resolution of detection of aberrations, and allowed more accurate identification and delineation of "complex" translocations (see Plate 11–2).[241]

▼ TIMING OF GENE REARRANGEMENT, TRANSLOCATIONS, AND SOMATIC HYPERMUTATION IN LYMPHOID CELLS[122, 138, 187, 198, 205]

As indicated above there is a sequential pattern of VDJ rearrangements to generate functional TCR or Ig variable regions in lymphoid cells. This process is occurring in pre-T or pre-B cells but can also occur by receptor editing in immature B cells and germinal center B cells (discussed previously) (see Figs. 11–8 and 11–10). In central lymphoid tissues, TCRα genes and IgL genes rearrange later than their respective counterparts. In addition, IgL genes rarely contain N sequences since TdT is not expressed when J/VL rearrangements are occurring in pre-B cells. In addition to other markers, a normal or malignant lymphoid tumor can be classified as having progressed to a certain stage of differentiation on the basis of the genotype as defined by the

nature of these gene rearrangements. Similarly, lymphocyte-associated translocations can be classified as to the time of occurrence by the nature of the breakpoint. For example, a translocation to one of the IgL loci probably occurred at a later time in development than a VDJ-mediated translocation to an IgH locus. Switch recombination in the IgH locus generally occurs after antigen stimulation (Fig. 11–10). Thus rearrangements involving IgH switch regions, including translocations involving switch regions, provide a genotypic marker for the stage of differentiation through which a B cell has passed. Somatic hypermutation occurs after antigen and helper T-cell stimulation and during a limited period in germinal centers, with the selected progeny of this process generating memory cells and/or plasma cells (Fig. 11–10). The presence or absence of somatic hypermutation of rearranged IgH or IgL V regions also provides a genotypic marker of whether or not a cell (plasmacytoma or B lymphoma or B cells from a patient with combined variable immunodeficiency, for example) has progressed through the stage of B-cell development in which somatic hypermutation occurs. If somatic hypermutation has not occurred, translocations mediated by VDJ recombinase must have occurred centrally during primary V(D)J rearrangements in pro- or pre-B cells or during receptor editing in pre-B/immature B cells. However, the presence of somatic hypermutation in IgH or IgL V regions means that the translocation could have occurred early or could have occurred during receptor editing in the germinal center.

For example, mantle cell lymphoma is a pre–germinal center B-cell tumor that does not have somatic hypermutation of IgH or IgL V regions, so that the t(11;14) into JH or JL must have occurred centrally in early B cells (see Table 11–3). Alternatively, both sporadic and endemic Burkitt's lymphoma cells have IgH and IgL genes with extensive somatic hypermutation, indicating that they are germinal center or post–germinal center B-cell tumors. The most common kind of translocation in sporadic Burkitt's lymphoma involves switch regions, consistent with the fact that physiological IgH switch recombination occurs principally in germinal center B cells. By contrast, in endemic Burkitt's lymphoma tumors, the translocation breakpoints usually are near JH or JL regions, suggesting that they have occurred as a result of an error in VDJ recombination. Until recently, when receptor editing in germinal center B cells was discovered, it was assumed that endemic translocations into or near J regions occurred early in B-cell development. However, it now seems likely that both endemic and sporadic Burkitt's lymphoma are associated with t(8;14) translocations (see Table 11–3) that occur in germinal center B cells.

▼ SUMMARY

The immune receptor loci are the most characteristic targets of the chromosomal aberrations associated with the development of lymphoid malignancies. In the usual case a chromosomal aberration juxtaposes one or another growth-effecting gene with an immune receptor that is being highly expressed in the particular lymphocyte. The current view is that such juxtaposition places the control of the growth-affecting gene under those factors driving immune receptor expression. This leads to inappropriate, dysregulated, and often increased expression of the growth-effecting gene that results in abnormal growth and contributes to malignant translocation. The entire process could be viewed as random. In that view chromosomes would be presumed to be constantly breaking and rejoining, but only when the particular growth-effecting gene–immune receptor juxtaposition was achieved would that particular cell have a selective growth advantage and thus emerge from the general population of all cells undergoing chromosomal reconfigurations. This view is probably too simplistic and may be frankly incorrect. The cell type specificity of particular chromosomal aberrations suggests that not all genes and not all parts of the genome are equally susceptible in a particular type of cell to participation in a chromosomal aberration and transforming event. There may be a strong influence of chromatin structure and DNA accessibility on predisposition to gene rearrangement. Furthermore, lymphocytes elaborate a powerful system for rearranging DNA, namely the "switch" and V(D)J recombinase complexes. Those parts of the genome that are accessible and that contain recognition signals for these complexes are likely to be at much greater risk for rearrangement.

The Use of Polymerase Chain Reaction to Follow Chromosomal Aberrations

Earlier in this chapter we described the use of PCR analysis for Ig and TCR rearrangements to follow minimal residual disease in patients with leukemia or lymphoma. All of the steps described then could be applied in the analysis of chromosomal aberrations, but often they are not all necessary. Thus the assay can sometimes be made simpler. Part of the reason for this is that there are a group of leukemia-associated chromosomal aberrations that are leukemic type but *not* patient specific, so that a single set of primers can be applied to every patient whose cells carry the aberration and there is not always a need to develop a clonogenic probe unique for each patient. The very presence of an amplified product is indicative of the presence of chromosomal aberration. The primers must be oriented so that at the genomic DNA or cDNA level an amplified product of between 200 and 2000 base pairs is generated. One primer comes from one side of the aberration, the other from the other side. By definition, normally the two primers are far enough apart (or even on two different chromosomes) that amplification of a DNA segment that lies between them is impossible. Only when the aberration has occurred is an amplified product generated. The premise for the use of this assay in minimal residual disease determination is that the juxtaposition of the two chromosomal regions that makes amplification possible *only occurs in the leukemic cells*. Although this appears to be generally true (and, indeed, is part of the basis for the study of cancer-associated chromosomal aberrations as a means of identifying genes that can contribute to malignant transformation), it may not be correct in every case. For example, it is now known that the t(14;18) translocation associated with adult follicular lymphoma can be identified in the reactive tonsils or lymph nodes of a significant number (20–40 per cent) of normal children.[242] In fact, it may be possible to find evidence of B-lymphocytes' carrying this translocation in everyone if one looks hard enough, and the frequency of this translocation may increase with age.[243]

Immune Receptor Gene Deletions/ Alterations and Disease

▼ HEAVY CHAIN DISEASES

The heavy chain class of diseases is characterized by lymphoproliferation of varying degree and severity in which the proliferative clone produces an aberrant, usually truncated IgH chain *unlinked* to an Ig light chain. The truncated chain can be of any heavy chain subclass.[244] An analysis of a case of μ heavy chain disease revealed that a DNA insertion/ deletion had removed a $_{JH}$ splice donor site from the rearranged J segment, leading to splicing of the leader sequence to the constant segment.[245] It has been speculated that continued synthesis of Ig might be important for optimal viability of the cell, but that absence of V segment peptides might allow the cell to escape idiotypic control.[246] It is also possible that this truncated IgH segment, lacking a V segment and therefore unresponsive to antigen, but theoretically capable of membrane emplacement, might provide an aberrant stimulus to proliferation of the lymphocyte on which it was anchored. It might be that an analogy could be drawn between this effect and the presumed proliferative effect on fibroblasts of a truncated epidermal growth factor, erbB.[247] Cases of α heavy chain disease have been observed in which the cells bear surface α chain but do not secrete it.[248] Cases of α and γ heavy chain disease have been associated with deletions within the variable and part of the constant segments.[248–250]

▼ IMMUNODEFICIENCY

The majority of immunodeficiency syndromes defined to date do not appear to have as their root cause deletion of the immune receptor loci. Although rare individuals who lacked immunoglobulin subclasses have been identified on the basis of deletions of a part of the IgH locus,[251] most such immunodeficiencies appear to have a regulatory rather than a structural basis.[252, 253] Studies of individuals heterozygous for alleles that carry IgH deletions have revealed that the level of Ig subclass production from the remaining genes was variable. One such study of individuals heterozygous for a large deletion stretching from φγ-α2 revealed essentially normal IgG production but below normal IgA2 levels. This was postulated to reflect a dosage and switching defect.[254]

Summary

Genomic DNA is unstable and dynamic, not static and immutable. This ability of primary genetic material to undergo reconfiguration is one of the keys to the rapidity of evolutionary development. Structural realignments of DNA also provide the fundamental basis for our ability to mount an almost infinitely diverse immune response. The mechanism that causes "innocent" or malignant lymphocyte-specific chromosomal aberrations is often just a variation on the physiological mechanism of V(D)J or "switch" recombination. The elucidation of this mechanism was one of the early successes of recombinant DNA research. The fine mechanistic details of the recombination events are now being elucidated. Understanding recombination at this refined level will not only give us crucial insight into the necessary and sufficient features for immune responsiveness, but provide a conceptual basis for viewing all mutation and rearrangement of DNA, thus gaining insight into development, cancer and carcinogenesis, and aging. In the meantime, techniques based on recognition of DNA alterations from the germline pattern are expanding our knowledge and pinpointing steps of lymphocyte-lineage differentiation. They are also providing a basis for the diagnosis, classification, staging, and tracking of a variety of hematological diseases.

REFERENCES

1. Suresh, M. R., Cuello, A. C., and Milstein, C.: Advantages of bispecific hybridomas in one-step immunocytochemistry and immunoassays. Proc. Natl. Acad. Sci. USA 83:7989, 1986.
2. Vitetta, E. S., Fulton, R. J., May, R. D., Till, M., and Uhr, J. W.: Redesigning nature's poisons to create anti-tumor reagents. Science 238:1098, 1987.
3. Tramontano, A., Janda, K. D., and Lerner, R. A.: Catalytic antibodies. Science 234:1566, 1986.
4. Pollack, S. J., Jacobs, J. W., and Schultz, P. G.: Selective chemical catalysis by an antibody. Science 234:1570, 1986.
5. Potter, M.: Immunoglobulin-producing tumors and myeloma proteins of mice. Physiol. Rev. 62:631, 1972.
6. Nathans, D., and Smith, H.: Restriction endonucleases in the analysis and restructuring of DNA molecules. Annu. Rev. Biochem. 46:273, 1975.
7. Landsteiner, K.: The Specificity of Serologic Reactions. Cambridge, Mass., Harvard University Press, 1945.
8. Dreyer, W. J., and Bennett, J. C.: The molecular basis of antibody formation. Proc. Natl. Acad. Sci. USA 54:864, 1965.
9. Kabat, E. A., Wu, T. T., Perry, H. M., Gottesman, K. S., and Foeller, C.: Sequences of Proteins of Immunological Interest. 5th ed. Washington, D.C., DHHS, U.S. Public Health Service, 1991.
10. Amit, A. G., Mariuzza, R. A., Phillips, S.E.V., and Poljack, R. J.: Three-dimensional structure of antigen-antibody complex at 2.8 Angstrom resolution. Science 233:747, 1986.
11. Capra, J. D., and Edmondson, A. B.: The antibody combining site. Sci. Am. 236:50, 1977.
12. Davies, D. R., and Metzger, H.: Structural basis of antibody function. Annu. Rev. Immunol. 1:87, 1983.
13. Lewin, B.: Genes IV. Cambridge, Cell Press, 1997.
14. Lodish, H., Baltimore, D., Berk, A., Zipursky, S. L., Matsudaira, P., Darnell, J.: Chapter 27, In: Molecular Cell Biology. 3rd ed. New York, W. H. Freeman & Co., 1995.
15. Max, E. E.: Immunoglobulins: Molecular genetics. In Paul W. E. (eds). Fundamental Immunology. 4th ed. Philadelphia, Lipincott-Raven Press, 1999.
16. Watson, J. D., Hopkins, N. H., Roberts, J. W., Steitz, J. A., and Weiner, A. M.: The generation of immunological specificity. Molecular Biology of the Gene. 4th ed. Menlo Park, Calif., Benjamin/Cummings, 1987.
17. Malissen, M., McCoy, C., Blanc, D., et al.: Direct evidence for chromosomal inversion during T-cell receptor beta-gene rearrangements. Nature 319:28, 1986.
18. Okazaki, K., Davis, D. D., and Sakano, H.: Cell receptor beta gene sequences in the circular DNA of thymocyte nuclei: Direct evidence for intramolecular DNA deletion in V-D-J joining. Cell 49:47, 1987.
19. Kronenberg, M., Goverman, J., Haars, R., Malissen, M., Kraig, E., Phillips, L., Delovitch, T., Suciu-Foca, N., and Hood, L.: Rearrangement and transcription of the beta-chain genes of the T-cell antigen receptor in different types of murine lymphocytes. Nature 313:647, 1985.
20. Lipkowitz, S., Stern, M. H., and Kirsh, I. R.: Hybrid T cell receptor genes formed by interlocus recombination in normal and ataxia-telangiectasia lymphocytes. J. Exp. Med. 172:409, 1990.
21. Tycko, B., Palmer, J. D., and Sklar, J.: T-cell receptor gene transrearrangements: Chimeric γ–δ genes in normal lymphoid tissues. Science 245:1242, 1989.
22. Lieber, M. R., Hesse, J., Mizuuchi, K., and Gellert, M.: Lymphoid V(D)J recombination: Nucleotide insertion at signal joints as well as coding joints. Proc. Natl. Acad. Sci. USA 85:8588, 1988.
23. Altenburger, W., Steinmetz, M., and Sachau, H. G.: Functional and nonfunctional joining in immunoglobulin light chain gene of a mouse myeloma. Nature 287:603, 1980.
24. Bernard, O., Gough, N. M., and Adams, J. M.: Plasmacytomas with more than one immunoglobulin kappa mRNA: Implications for allelic exclusion. Proc. Natl. Acad. Sci. USA 78:5812, 1981.
25. Lafaille, J. J., DeCloux, A., Bonneville, M., Takagaki, Y., and Tonegawa, S.: Junctional sequences of T cell receptor γδ T cell lineages and for a novel intermediate of V-(D)-J joining. Cell 59:859, 1989.
26. Landau, N. R., Schatz, D. G., Rosa, M., and Baltimore, D.: Increased frequency of N-region insertion in a murine pre-B-cell line infected with a terminal deoxynucleotidyl transferase retroviral expression vector. Mol. Cell. Biol. 7:3237, 1987.
27. Alt, F., and Baltimore, D.: Joining of immunoglobulin heavy chain gene segments: Implications from a chromosome with evidence of three D-JH fusions. Proc. Natl. Acad. Sci. USA 79:4118, 1982.
28. Blackwell, T. K., and Alt, F. W.: Molecular characterization of the lymphoid V(D)J recombination activity. J. Biol. Chem. 264:10327, 1989.
29. Levy, N. S., Malipero, U. V., Lebecque, S. G., and Gearhart, P. J.: Early onset of somatic mutation in immunoglobulin VH genes during the primary immune response. J. Exp. Med. 169:2007, 1989.
30. Gu, H., Foster, I., and Rajewsky, K.: Sequence homologies, N sequence insertion and JH gene utilization in VDJ joining: Implications for the joining mechanism and the ontogenetic timing of Ly1 B cell and B-CLL progenitor generation. EMBO J. 9:2133, 1990.
31. Berek, C.: Affinity maturation. In Paul, W. E. (ed): Fundamental Immunology. 4th ed. Philadelphia, Lippincott-Raven Press, 1999.
32. McKean, D., Huppi, K., Bell, M., Staudt, L., Gerhard, W., and Weigert, M.: Generation of antibody diversity in the immune response of BALB/c mice to influenza virus hemagglutinin. Proc. Natl. Acad. Sci. USA 81:3180, 1984.
33. Lebecque, S. G., and Gearhart, P. J.: Boundaries of somatic mutation in rearranged immunoglobulin genes: 5' boundary is near the promoter, and 3' boundary is 1 kb from V(D)J gene. J. Exp. Med. 172:1717, 1990.
33a. Shatz, D. G.: V(D)J recombination moves in vitro. Semin. Immunol. 9:149, 1997.
33b. Gellert, M.: Recent advances in understanding V(D)J recombination. Adv. Immunol. 64:39, 1997.
33c. Lieber, M. R.: Warner-Lambert/Parke-Davis Award Lecture. Pathological and physiological double-strand breaks: Roles in cancer, aging, and the immune system. Am. J. Pathol. 153:1323, 1998.
34. Oettinger, M. A., Schatz, D. G., Gorka, C., and Baltimore, D.: RAG-1 and RAG-2, adjacent genes that synergistically activate V(D)J recombination. Science 248:1517, 1990.
35. Schatz, D. G., Oettinger, M. A., and Baltimore, D.: The V(D)J recombination activating gene, RAG-1. Cell 59:1035, 1989.
36. McBlane, J. F. et al.: Cleavage at a V(D)J recombination signal requires only RAG1 and RAG2 proteins and occurs in two steps. Cell 83:387, 1995.
37. Ramsden, D. A., Paull, T. T., and Gellert, M.: Cell-free V(D)J recombination. Nature 388:488, 1997.
38. van Gent, D. C., Hiom, K., Paull, T. T., and Gellert, M.: Stimulation of V(D)J cleavage by high mobility group proteins. EMBO J. 16:2665, 1997.
39. Bosma, G. C., Custer, R. P., and Bosma, M. J.: A severe combined immunodeficiency mutation in the mouse. Nature 301:527, 1983.
40. Schuler, W., Weiler, I. J., Schuler, A. et al.: Rearrangement of antigen receptor genes is defective in mice with severe combined immune deficiency. Cell 46:963, 1986.
41. Lieber, M. R., Hesse, J. E., Lewis S., et al.: The defect in murine severe combined immune deficiency: Joining of signal sequences but not coding segments in V(D)J recombination. Cell 55:7, 1988.
42. Malynn, B. A., Blackwell, T. K., Fulop, G. M. Rathbun, G. A., Furley, A. J., Ferrier, P., Heinke, L. B., Phillips, R. A., Yancopoulos, G. D., and Alt, F. W.: The scid defect affects the final step of the immunoglobulin VDJ recombinase mechanism. Cell 54:453, 1988.
43. Okazaki, K., Nishikawa, S., and Sakano, H.: Aberrant immunoglobulin gene rearrangement in scid mouse bone marrow cells. J. Immunol. 141:1348, 1988.
44. Zdzienicka, M. Z.: Mammalian mutants defective in the response to ionizing radiation-induced DNA damage. Mutat. Res. 336:203, 1995.

45. Jeggo, P. A., Taccioli, G. E. and Jackson, S. P.: Menage a trois: Double strand break repair, V(D)J recombination, and DNA-PK. Bioessays 17:949, 1995.

46. Zdzienicka, M. Z., Jongsmans, W., Oshimura, M., Priestly, A., Whitmore, G. F., and Jeggo, P. A.: Complementation analysis of the murine scid cell line. Radiat. Res. 143:238, 1995.

47. Walker, A. I., Hunt, T., Jackson, R. J., and Anderson, C. W.: Double-stranded DNA induces the phosphorylation of several proteins including the 90,000 mol. wt. heat-shock protein in animal cell extracts. EMBO J. 4:139, 1985.

48. Lees-Miller, S. P., Chen, Y.-R., and Anderson, C. S.: Human cells contain a DNA-activated protein kinase that phosphorylates simian virus 40 T antigen, mouse TP53, and the human Ku autoantigen. Mol. Cell Biol. 10:6472, 1990.

49. Gottlieb, T. M., and Jackson, S. P.:The DNA-dependent protein kinase: Requirement for DNA ends and association with Ku antigen. Cell 72:131, 1993.

50. Kirshgessner, C. U., Patil, C. K., Evans, J. W., Carter, T., and Brown, J. M.: DNA dependent kinase (p350) is a candidate gene for murine scid defect. Science 267:1178, 1995.

51. Sipley, J. D., Mennenger, J., Harley, K. O., Ward, D., Jackson, S. P., and Anderson, C. W.: The gene for the catalytic subunit of the human DNA-activated protein kinase maps to the site of the XRCC7 gene on chromosome 8. Proc. Natl. Acad. Sci. USA 92:7515, 1995.

52. Blunt, T., Finnie, N. J., Taccioli, G. E., Smith, G., Demengeot, J., Gottlieb, T., Mizuta, R., Varghese, A., Alt, F. W., Jeggo, P. A.: Defective DNA-dependent protein kinase activity is linked to V(D)J recombination and DNA repair defects associated with the murine scid mutation. Cell 80:813, 1995.

53. Gelfand, E. W., and Dosch, H. M.: Diagnosis and classification of severe combined immunodeficiency disease. Birth Defects 19:65, 1983.

54. Giblett, E. R., Anderson, J. E., Cohen, I., Pollara, B., and Mewissen, J. H.: Adenosine-deaminase deficiency in two patients with severely impaired cellular immunity. Lancet 2:1067, 1972.

55. Giblett, E. R., Ammann, A. J., Wara, D. W., Sandman, R., and Diamond, L. K.: Nucleoside-phosphorylase deficiency in a child with severely defective T-cell immunity and normal B-cell immunity. Lancet 1:1010, 1974.

56. Rosen, F. S., Gitlin, D., and Janeway, C. A.: Alymphocytosis agammaglobulinemia, homografts, and delayed hypersensitivity: Study of a case. Lancet 2:380, 1962.

57. Hammarsten, O., and Chu, G.: DNA-dependent protein kinase: DNA binding and activation in the absence of Ku. Proc. Natl. Acad. Sci. USA 95:525, 1998.

58. Cao, Q., Pitt, S., Leszyk, J., and Baril, E.: DNA-dependent ATPase from HeLa cells is related to human Ku autoantigen. Biochemistry 33:8548, 1994.

59. Reeves, W.: Antibodies to the p70/p80 (Ku) antigens in systemic lupus erythematosus. Rheum. Dis. Clin. North Am. 18:391, 1992.

60. Taccioli, G., Gottlieb, T. M., Blunt, T., Priestly, A., Demengeot, J., Mizuta, R., Lehmann, A., Alt, F., Jackson, S., and Jeggo, P.: Ku 80: Product of the SRCC5 gene and its role in DNA repair and V(D)J recombination. Science 265:1442, 1994.

61. Smider, V., Rathmell, W. K., Lieber, M., and Chu, G.: Restoration of X-ray resistance and V(D)J recombination in mutant cells by Ku cDNA. Science 266:288, 1994.

62. Gu, Y., Jin, S., Weaver, D., and Alt, F.: Ku70-deficient embryonic stem cells have increased ionizing radiosensitivity, defective DNA end-binding activity, and inability to support V(D)J recombination. Proc. Natl. Acad. Sci. USA 94:8076, 1997.

63. Li, Z., Otevrel, T., Gao, Y., Cheng, H. L., Seed, B., Stamato, T. D., Taccioli, G. E., and Alt, F. W.: The XRCC4 gene encodes a novel protein involved in DNA double-strand break repair and V(D)J recombination. Cell 83:1079, 1995.

64. Grawunder, U., Wilm, M., Wu, X., Kulesza, P., Wilson, T. E., Mann, M., and Lieber, M. R.: Activity of DNA ligase IV stimulated by complex formation with XRCC4 protein in mammalian cells. Nature 388:492, 1997.

65. Leber, R., Wise, T. W., Mizuta, R., and Meek, K.: The XRCC4 gene product is a target for and interacts with the DNA-dependent protein kinase. J. Biol. Chem. 273:1794, 1998.

66. Chang, L.M.S., and Bollum, F. J.: Molecular biology of terminal transferase. Crit. Rev. Biochem. 21:27, 1986.

67. Gilfillan, S., Dierich, A., Lemeur, M., Benoist, C., and Mathis, D.: Mice lacking TdT: Mature animals with an immature lymphocyte repertoire. Science 261:1175, 1993.

68. Komori, T., Okada, A., Stewart, V., and Alt, F.: Lack of N regions in antigen receptor variable region genes of TdT-deficient lymphocytes. Science 261:1171, 1993.

69. Kallenbach, S., Doyen, N., Fanton d'Andon, M., and Rougeon, F.: Three lymphoid-specific factors account for all junctional diversity characteristics of somatic assembly of T-cell receptor and immunoglobulin genes. Proc. Natl. Acad. Sci. USA 89:2799, 1992.

70. Bentolila, L., Wu, G., Nourrit, F., Fanton d'Andon, M., Rougeon, F., and Doyen, N.: Constitutive expression of terminal deoxynucleotidyl transferase in transgenic mice is sufficient for N region diversity to occur at any Ig locus throughout B cell differentiation. J. Immunol. 158:715, 1997.

71. Bogue, M., Wang, C., Zhu, C., and Roth, D.: V(D)J recombination in Ku86-deficient mice: Distinct effects on coding, signal, and hybrid joint formation. Immunity 7:31, 1997.

72. Aguilera, R., Akira, S., Okazaki, K., and Sakano, H.: A pre-B cell nuclear protein that specifically interacts with the immunoglobulin V-J recombination sequences. Cell 51:909, 1987.

73. Matsunami, N., Hamaguchi, Y., Yamamoto, Y., Kuze, K., Kangawa, K., Matsuo, H., Kawaichi, M., and Honjo, T.: A protein binding to the Jκ recombination sequence of immunoglobulin genes contains a sequence related to the integrase motif. Nature 342:934, 1989.

74. Li, M., Morzycka, W., and Desiderio, S.: NBP, a protein that specifically binds an enhancer of immunoglobulin gene rearrangement: Purification and characterization. Genes Dev. 3:1801, 1989.

75. Miyake, S., Sugiyama, H., Tani, Y., Fukuda, T., and Kishimoto, S.: Identification of a recombinational signal sequence-specific DNA-binding protein(s) of Mr 115,000 in the nuclear extracts from immature lymphoid cell lines. J. Immunogenet. 17:67, 1990.

76. Shirakata, M., Huppi, K., Usuda, S., Okazaki, K., Yoshida, K., and Sakano, H.: HMG1-related DNA-binding protein isolated with V-(D)-J recombination signal probes. Mol. Cell. Biol. 11:4528, 1991.

77. Muegge, K., West, M., and Durum, S.: Recombination sequence-binding protein in thymocytes undergoing T-cell receptor gene rearrangement. Proc. Natl. Acad. Sci. USA 90:4151, 1993.

78. Wu, L., Mak, C., Dear, N., Boehm, T., Foroni, L., and Rabbitts, T.: Molecular cloning of a zinc finger protein which binds to the heptamer of the signal sequence for V(D)J recombination. Nucleic Acids Res. 22:383, 1993.

79. Hesse, J. E., Lieber, M. R., Mizuuchi, K., and Gellert, M.: V(D)J recombination: A functional definition of the joining signals. Genes Dev. 3:1053, 1989.

80. Yancopolous, G. D., and Alt, F. W.: Developmentally controlled and tissue specific expression of unrearranged VH gene segments. Cell 40:271, 1985.

81. Yancopoulos, G. D., Blackwell, T. K., Suh, H., Hood, L., and Alt, F.: Introduced T cell receptor variable region gene segments recombine in pre-B cells: Evidence that B and T cells use a common recombinase. Cell 44:251, 1986.

82. Blackwell, T. K., Moore, M. W., Yancopoulos, G. D., Suh, H., Lutzker, S., Selsing, E., and Alt, F. W.: Recombination between immunoglobulin variable region segments is enhanced by transcription. Nature 324:585, 1986.

83. Aplan, P. D., Lombardi, D. P., Ginsberg, A. M., Cossman, J., Bertness, V. L., and Kirsch, I. R.: Disruption of the human SCL locus by "illegitimate" V(D)J recombinase activity. Science 250:1426, 1990.

84. Boehm, T., Mengle-Gaw, L., Kees, U. R., Spurr, N., Lavenir, I., Forster, A., and Rabbitts, T. H.: Alternating purine-pyrimidine tracts may promote chromosomal translocations seen in a variety of human lymphoid tumors. EMBO J. 8:2621, 1989.

85. Kirsch, I. R., Brown, J. A., Lawrence, J., Korsmeyer, S., and Morton, C. C.: Translocations that highlight chromosomal regions of differentiated activity. Cancer Genet. Cytogenet. 18:159, 1985.

86. McCormack, W. T., Tjoelker, L. W., and Thompson, C. B.: Avian B-cell development: Generation of an immunoglobulin repertoire by gene conversion. Annu. Rev. Immunol. 9:219, 1991.

87. Arden, B., Clark, S. P., Kabelitz, D., and Mak, T. W.: Human T-cell receptor variable gene segment families. Immunogenetics 42:455, 1995.

88. Chen, C., and Birshtein, B. K.: Virtually identical enhancers containing a segment of homology to murine 3'IgH-E(hs1,2) lie downstream of human Ig C alpha 1 and C alpha 2 genes. J. Immunol. 159(3):1310, 1997.

89. Chung, J. H., Bell, A. C., and Felsenfeld, G.: Characterization of the chicken beta-globin insulator. Proc. Natl. Acad. Sci. USA 94(2):575, 1997.

90. Diaz, P., Cado, D., and Winoto, A.: A locus control region in the T cell receptor α/δ locus. Immunity. 1:207, 1994.

91. Goldman, J. P., Spencer, D. M., and Raulet, D. H.: Ordered rearrangement of variable region genes of the T cell receptor γ locus correlates with transcription of the unrearranged genes. J. Exp. Med. 177:729, 1993.

92. Gu, H., Kitamura, D., and Rajewsky, K.: B cell development regulated by gene rearrangement: Arrest of maturation by membrane-bound Dμ protein and selection of DH element reading frames. Cell 65:47, 1991.

93. Halle, J.-P., Haus-Seuffert, P., Woltering, C., and Meisterernst, M. A.: A conserved tissue-specific structure at a human T-cell receptor β-chain core promoter. Mol. Cell. Biol. 17:4220, 1997.

94. Henderson, A., and Calame, K.: Transcriptional regulation during B cell development. Annu. Rev. Immunol. 16:163, 1998.

95. Leiden, J. M.: Transcriptional regulation of T cell receptor genes. Annu. Rev. Immunol. 11:539, 1993.

96. Li, Q., Zhou, B., Powers, P., Enver, T., Stamatoyannopoulos, G.: β-globin locus activation regions: Conservation of organization, structure, and function. Proc. Natl. Acad. Sci. USA 87:8207, 1990.

97. Madisen, L., Krumm, A., Hebbes, T. R., and Groudine, M.: The immunoglobulin heavy chain locus control region increases histone acetylation along linked c-myc genes. Mol. Cell. Biol. 18:6281, 1998.

98. Mills, F. C., Harindranath, N., Mitchell, M., Max, E. E.: Enhancer complexes located downstream of both human immunoglobulin C alpha genes. J. Exp. Med. 186(6):845, 1997.

99. Raynal, M., Liu, Z., Hirano, T., Mayer, L., Kishimoto, T., and Chen-Kiang, S.: Interleukin 6 induces secretion of IgG1 by coordinated transcriptional activation and differential mRNA accumulation. Proc. Natl. Acad. Sci. USA 86:8024, 1989.

100. Schlissel, M. S., Corcoran, L. M., and Baltimore, D.: Virus-transformed pre-B cells show ordered activation but not inactivation of immunoglobulin gene rearrangement and transcription. J. Exp. Med. 173:711, 1991.

101. Staudt, L. M., and Lenardo, M. J.: Immunoglobulin gene transcription. Annu. Rev. Immunol. 9:373, 1991.

102. Sleckman, B. P., Gorman, J. R., and Alt, F. W.: Accessibility control of Antigen-receptor variable-region gene assembly: Role of cis-acting elements. Annu. Rev. Immunol. 14:459, 1996.

103. Sleckman, B. P., Bardon, C. G., Ferrini, R., Davidson, L., and Alt, F. W.: Function of the TCRα Enhancer in αβ and γδ T cells. Immunity 7:505, 1997.

104. Willerford, D. M., Swat, W., and Alt, F. W.: Developmental regulation of V(D)J recombination and lymphocyte differentiation. Curr. Opin. Genet. Develop. 6:603, 1996.

105. Winoto, A., and Baltimore, D.: αβ Lineage-specific expression of the α T cell receptor gene by nearby silencers. Cell 59:649, 1989.

106. Zhong, X.-P., and Krangel, M. S.: An enhancer-blocking element between α and δ gene segments within the human T cell receptor αδ locus. Proc. Natl. Acad. Sci. USA 94:5219, 1997.

107. Davis, M. M., and Chien Y.-H.: T-Cell Antigen Receptors. In Paul W. E. (ed.): Fundamental Immunology. 4th ed. Philadelphia, Lippincott-Raven Press, 1999.

108. Davis, M. M.: T cell receptor gene diversity and selection. Annu. Rev. Biochem. 59:475, 1990.

109. Benoist, C., and Mathis, D.: T-lymphocyte differentiation and biology. In Paul, W. E. (ed.): Fundamental Immunology. 4th ed. New York, Lippincott-Raven Press, 1999.

110. Ashwell, J. D., and Klausner, R. D.: Genetic and mutational analysis of the T-cell antigen receptor. Annu. Rev. Immunol. 8:139, 1990.

111. Allison, J. P., and Havran, W. L.: The immunobiology of T cells with invariant γδ antigen receptors. Annu. Rev. Immunol. 9:679, 1991.

112. Boysen, C., Simon, M. I., and Hood, L.: Analysis of the 1.1-Mb human alpha/delta T-cell receptor locus with bacterial artificial chromosomes. Genome Res. 4:330, 1997.

113. Rowen, L., Koop, B. F., and Hood, L.: The complete 685-kilobase DNA sequence of the human β T cell receptor locus. Science 272:1755, 1996.

114. Lieber, M. R.: Site-specific recombination in the immune system. FASEB J. 5:2934, 1991.

115. Bonneville, M., Ishida, I., Itohara, S., Verbeek, S., Berns, A., Kanaagawa, O., Haas, W., and Tonegawa, S.: Self-tolerance to transgenic γδ T cells by intrathymic inactivation. Nature 344:163, 1990.

116. Dent, A. L., Matis, L. A., Hooshmand, F., Widacki, S. M., Bluestone, J. A., and Hedrick, S. M.: Self-reactive γδ T cells are eliminated in the thymus. Nature 343:714, 1990.

117. Fowlkes, B. J., and Pardoll, D. M.: Molecular and cellular events of T cell development. Adv. Immunol. 44:207, 1989.

118. Wells, F. B., Gahm, S., Hedfick, S. M., Bluestone J. A., Dent, A., and Matis, L. A.: Requirement for positive selection of γδ receptor-bearing T cells. Science 253:903, 1991.

119. Fischer, A., and Malissen, B.: Natural and engineered disorders of lymphocyte development. Science 280:237, 1998.

120. Van Parijs, L., and Abbas, A. K.: Homeostasis and self-tolerance in the Immune system: Turning lymphocytes off. Science 280:243, 1998.

121. Ishida, I., Verbeek, S., Bonneville, M., Itohara, S., Berns, A., and Tonegawa, S.: T-cell receptor γδ and γ transgenic mice suggests a role of a γ gene silencer in the generation of the αβ T cells. Proc. Natl. Acad. Sci. USA 87:3067, 1990.

122. Nussenzweig, M. C.: Immune receptor editing: Revise and select. Cell 95:875, 1998.

123. Turka, L. A., Schatz, D. G., Oettinger, M. A., Chun, J. J. M., Gorka, C., Lee, K., McCormack, W. T., and Thompson, C. B.: Thyomcyte expression of RAG-1 and RAG-2: Termination by T cell receptor cross-linking. Science 253:778, 1991.

124. Takeshita, S., Toda, M., and Yamagishi, H.: Excision products of the T cell receptor gene support a progressive rearrangement model of the αδ locus. EMBO J. 8:3261, 1989.

125. von Boehmer, H., and Fehling, H. J.: Structure and function of the pre-T cell receptor. Annu. Rev. Immunol. 15:433, 1997.

126. Weiss, L. M., Wood, G. S., Nickoloff, B. J., and Sklar, J.: Gene rearrangement studies in lymphoproliferative disorders of skin. Adv. Dermatol. 3:141, 1988.

127. Frazer, J. K., and Capra, J. D.: Immunoglobulins: Structure and Function. In Paul, W. E. (ed.): Fundamental Immunology. 4th ed. Philadelphia, Lippincott-Raven Press, 1999.

128. Koshland, M. E.: The immunoglobulin helper: The J chain. In Honjo, T., Alt, F. W., and Rabbitts, T. H. (eds.): Immunoglobulin Genes. New York, Academic Press, 1989, p. 345.

129. Rolink, A., and Melchers, F.: Molecular and cellular origins of B lymphocyte diversity. Cell 66:1081, 1991.

130. Venkitaraman, A.R.J., Williams, G. T., Dariavach, P., and Neuberger, M. S.: The B-cell antigen receptor of the five immunoglobulin classes. Nature 352: 777, 1991.

131. Arpin, C., de Bouteiller, O., Razanajaona, D., Fugier-Vivier, I., Briere, F., Banchereau, J., Levecque, S., and Liu, Y.-J.: The normal counterpart of IgD myeloma cells in germinal center displays extensively mutated IgVH gene, Cμ-Cδ Switch, and λ Light Chain Expression. J. Exp. Med. 187:1169, 1998.

132. Cook, G. P., Tomlinson, I. M., Walter, G., Riethman, H., Carter, N. P., Buluwela, L., Winter, G., and Rabbitts, T. H.: A map of the human immunoglobulin VH locus completed by analysis of the telomeric region of chromosome 14q. Nature Genet. 7:162, 1994.

133. Ermert, K., Itlohner, H., Schempp, W., and Zachau, H. G.: The Immunoglobulin kappa locus of primates. Genomics 25:623, 1995.

134. Kawasaki, K., Minoshima, S., Nakato, E., Shibuya, K., Shintani, A., Schmeits, J. L., Wang, J., and Shimizu, N.: One-megabase sequence analysis of the human immunoglobulin lambda gene locus. Genome Res. 7:250, 1997.

135. Klobeck, H. G., and Zachau, H. G.: The Human CK gene segment and the kappa deleting element are closely linked. Nucleic Acids Res. 14:4591, 1986.

136. Melchers, F., and Rolink, A.: Immunoglobulins: B-lymphocyte development and biology. In Paul W. E. (ed.): Fundamental Immunology. 4th ed. Philadelphia, Raven Press, 1999.

137. MacLennan, I.C.M.: The centre of hypermutation. Nature 354:352, 1991.

138. MacLennan, I.C.M.: Germinal centers. Annu. Rev. Immunol. 12:117, 1994.

139. Pelanda, R., Schwers, S., Sonoda, E., Torres, R. M., Nemazee, D., and Rajewsky, K.: Receptor editing in a transgenic mouse model: Site, efficiency, and role in B cell tolerance and antibody diversification. Immunity 7:765, 1997.

140. Okun, F. M.: Regulation of human B-cell ontogeny. Blood 76:1908, 1990.

141. Melchers, F., Haasner, D., Grawunder, U., Kalberer, C., Karasuyama, H., Winkler, T., and Rolink, A. G.: Roles of IgH and L chains and of surrogate H and L chains in the development of cells of the B lymphocyte lineage. Annu. Rev. Immunol. 12:209, 1994.

142. Alt, F. W., Rosenberg, N., Lewis, S., Thomas, E., and Baltimore, D.: Organization and reorganization of immunoglobulin genes in A-MuLV-transformed cells: Rearrangement of heavy but not light chain genes. Cell 27:381, 1981.

143. Hendershot, L., Bole, D., Kohler, G., and Kearney, J. F.: Assembly and secretion of heavy chains that do not associate posttranslationally with immunoglobulin heavy chain-binding protein. J. Cell Biol. 104:761, 1987.

144. Korsmeyer, S. J., Hieter, P. A., Ravetch, J. V., Poplack, D. G., Waldmann, T. A., and Leder P.: Developmental hierarchy of immunoglobulin gene rearrangements in human leukemic pre-B-cells. Proc. Natl. Acad. Sci. USA 78:7096, 1981.

145. Karasuyama, H., Kudo, A., and Melchers, F.: The proteins encoded by the VpreB and λ5 pre-B cell-specific genes can associate with each other and with μ heavy chain. J. Exp. Med. 172:969, 1990.

146. Rose, S. M., Smith, G. P., and Kuehl, W. M.: Cloned MPC 11 myeloma cells express two kappa genes: A gene for a complete light chain and a gene for a constant region polypeptide. Cell 12:453, 1977.

147. Wall, R., and Kuehl, M.: Biosynthesis and regulation of immunoglobulins. Annu. Rev. Immunol. 1:393, 1983.

148. Guise, J. W., Galli, G., Nevins, J. R., and Tucker, P. W.: Developmental regulation of secreted and membrane forms of immunoglobulin μ chain. In Honjo, T., Alt, F. W., and Rabbitts, T. H. (eds.): Immunoglobulin Genes. New York, Academic Press, 1989, p. 275.

149. Durda, J., Gerstien, R. M., Rath, S., Robbins, P. F., Nisnoff, and Selsing, E.: Isotype switching by a microinjected μ immunoglobulin heavy chain gene in transgenic mice. Proc. Natl. Acad. Sci. USA 86:2346, 1989.

150. Esser, C., and Radbruch, A.: Immunoglobulin class switching: Molecular and cellular analysis. Annu. Rev. Immunol. 8:717, 1990.

151. Gritzmacher, C. A.: Molecular aspects of heavy-chain class switching. Crit. Rev. Immunol. 9:173, 1989.

152. Harriman, W., Volk, H., Defranoux, N., and Wabl, M.: Immunoglobulin class switch recombination. Annu. Rev. Immunol. 11:361, 1993.

153. Matsuoka, M., Yoshida, K., Maeda, T., Usuda, S., and Sakano, H.: Switch circular DNA formed in cytokine-treated mouse splenocytes: Evidence for intramolecular DNA deletion in immunoglobulin class switching. Cell 62:135, 1990.

154. Snapper, C. M., and Finkelman, F. D.: Immunoglobulin class switching. In Paul, W. E. (ed.): Fundamental Immunology. 4th ed. Philadelphia, Lippincott-Raven Press, 1999.

155. Stavnezer, J.: Antibody class switching. Adv. Immunol. 61:79, 1996.

156. Zhang, K., Mills, F. C., and Saxon, A.: Switch circles from IL-4-directed epsilon class switching from human B lymphocytes: Evidence for direct, sequential, and multiple step sequential switch from mu to epsilon Ig heavy chain gene. J. Immunol. 152(7):3427, 1994.

157. Allen, R. C., Armitage, R. J., Conley, M. E., Rosenblatt, H., Jenkins, N. A., Copeland, N. G., Bedell, M. A., Edelhoff, S., Disteche, C. M., Simoneaux, D. K., Fanslow, W. C., Belmont, J., and Spriggs, M. K.: CD40 ligand gene defects responsible for X-linked hyper-IgM syndrome. Science 250:990, 1993.

158. Daniels, G. A., and Lieber, M. R.: Strand specificity in the transcriptional targeting of recombination at immunoglobulin switch sequences. Proc. Natl. Acad. Sci. USA 92:5625, 1995.

159. Rolink, A., Melchers, F., Andersson, J.: The SCID but not the RAG-2 gene product is required for Sμ-Sε heavy chain class switching. Immunity 5:319, 1996.

160. Cleary, M. I., Warnke, R., and Sklar, J.: Monoclonality of lymphoproliferative lesions in cardiac transplant recipients. N. Engl. J. Med. 310:477, 1984.

161. Weiss, L. M., Hu, E., Wood, G. S., Moulds, C., Cleary, M. L., Warnke, R., and Sklar, J.: Clonal rearrangements of the T cell receptor gene in mycosis fungoides and dermatopathic lymphadenopathy. N. Engl. J. Med. 313:539, 1985.

162. Sklar, J., Cleary, M. L., Thielemans, K., Gralow, J., Warnke, R., and Levy, R.: Biclonal B-cell lymphoma. N. Engl. J. Med. 311:20, 1984.

163. Korsmeyer, S. J., Arnold, A., Bakhshi, A., Ravetch, J. V., Siebenlist, U., Hieter, P. A., Sharrow, S. O., LeBein, T. W., Kersey, J. H., Poplack, D. G., Leder, P., and Waldmann, T. A.: Immunoglobulin gene rearrangement and cell surface antigen expression in acute lymphocytic leukemias of T cell and B cell precursor origins. J. Clin. Invest. 71:301, 1983.

164. Waldmann, T. A., Korsmeyer, S. J., Bakhshi, A., Arnold, A., and Kirsch, I. R.: Molecular genetic analyses of human lymphoid neoplasms: Immunoglobulin genes and c-myc oncogene. A combined clinical staff conference. Ann. Intern. Med. 102:497, 1985.

165. Felix, C. A., Poplack, D. G., Reaman, G. H., Steinberg, S. M., Cole, D. E., Taylor, B. J., Begley, C. G., and Kirsch, I. R.: Characterization of immunoglobulin and T-cell receptor gene patterns in B-cell precursor acute lymphoblastic leukemia of childhood. J. Clin. Oncol. 8:431, 1990.

166. Bertness, V., Kirsch, I., Hollis, G., Johnson, B., and Bunn, P. A.: T-cell receptor gene rearrangements as clinical markers of human T-cell lymphomas. N. Engl. J. Med. 313:534, 1985.

167. Flug, F., Pelicci, P. G., Bonetti, R., Knowles, D. M., and Dalla-Favera, R.: T-cell receptor gene rearrangements as markers of lineage and clonality in T-cell neoplasms. Proc. Natl. Acad. Sci. USA 82:3460, 1985.

168. Kitchingman, G. R., Rovigatti, U., Mauer, A. M., Melvin, S., Murphy, S. B., and Stass, S.: Rearrangement of immunoglobulin heavy chain genes in T cell acute lymphoblastic leukemia. Blood 65:725, 1985.

169. Pelicci, P. G., Knowles, D. M., and Dalla-Favera, R.: Lymphoid tumors displaying rearrangements of both immunoglobulin and T cell receptor genes. J. Exp. Med. 162:1015, 1985.

170. Siegelman, M., Cleary, M. L., Warnke, R., and Sklar, J.: Frequent biclonality and immunoglobulin gene alterations among B cell lymphomas that show histologic forms. J. Exp. Med. 161:850, 1985.

171. Erlich, H. A. (ed.): PCR Technology. New York, Stockton Press, 1989.

172. Sasavage, N.: Are clinical labs ready for PCR? J. NIH Res. 3:47, 1991.

173. Bourguin, A., Tung, R., Galili, N., and Sklar, J.: Rapid, nonradioactive detection of clonal T-cell receptor gene rearrangements in lymphoid neoplasms. Proc. Natl. Acad Sci. USA 87:8536, 1990.

174. Myers, R. M., Maniatis, T., and Lerman, L. S.: Detection and localization of single base changes by denaturing gradient gel electrophoresis. Methods Enzymol. 155:501, 1986.

175. Billadeau, D., Blackstadt, M., Griepp, P., Kyle, R. A., Oken, M. M., Kay, N., and Van Ness, B.: Analysis of B-lymphoid malignancies using allele-specific polymerase chain reaction: A technique for sequential quantitation of residual disease. Blood 78:3021, 1991.

176. Yamada, M., Wasserman, R., Lange, B., Reichard, B., Womer, R., and Rovera, G.: Minimal residual disease in childhood B-lineage lymphoblastic leukemia. N. Engl. J. Med. 323:448, 1990.

177. Yokota, S., Hansen-Hagge, T. E., Ludwig, W. D., Reiter, A., Raghavachar, A., Kleihauer, E., and Bartram, C. R.: Use of polymerase chain reaction to monitor minimal residual disease in acute lymphoblastic leukemia patients. Blood 77:331, 1991.

178. MacIntyre E.D., Auriol, L., Duparc, N., Leverger, G., Galibert, F., and Siguax, F.: Use of oligonucleotide probes directed against T cell antigen receptor gamma delta variable-(diversity)-joining junctional sequences as a general method for detecting minimal residual disease in acute lymphoblastic leukemias. J. Clin. Invest. 86:2125, 1990.

179. Van Dongen, J.J.M., Breit, T. M., Adriaansen, H. J., Beishuizen, A., and Hooijkaas, H.: Detection of minimal residual disease in acute leukemia by immunological marker analysis and polymerase chain reaction. Leukemia 6(suppl):47, 1992.

180. Szczepanski, T., Langerak, A. W., Wolvers-Tettero, I. L., Ossenkoppele, G. J., Verhoef, G., Stul, M., Petersen, E. J., de Bruijn, M. A., van't Veer, M. B., and van Dongen, J.J.M.: Immunoglobulin and T cell receptor gene rearrangement patterns in acute lymphoblastic leukemia are less mature in adults than in children: Implications for selection of PCR targets for detection of minimal residual disease. Leukemia 12:1081, 1998.

181. Beishuizen, A., de Bruijn, M. A., Pongers-Willemse, M. J., Verhoeven, M. A., van Wering, E. R., Hahlen, K., Breit, T. M., de Bruin-Versteeg, S., Hooijkaas, H., and van Dongen, J.J.M.: Heterogeneity in junctional regions of immunoglobulin kappa deleting element rearrangements in B cell leukemias: A new molecular target for detection of minimal residual disease. Leukemia 11:2200, 1997.

182. Gruhn, B., Hongeng, S., Yi, H., Hancock, M. L., Rubnitz, J. E., Neale, G. A., and Kitchingman, G. R.: Minimal residual disease after intensive induction therapy in childhood acute lymphoblastic leukemia predicts outcome. Leukemia 12:675, 1998.

183. Cave, H., van der Werff ten Bosch, J., Suciu, S., Guidal, C., Waterkeyn, C., Otten, J., Bakkus, M., Thielemans, K., Grandchamp, B., and Vilmer, E.: Clinical significance of minimal residual disease in childhood acute lymphoblastic leukemia. N. Engl. J. Med. 339:591, 1998.

184. Shen-Ong, G.L.C., Keath, E. J., Piccoli, S. P., and Cole, M. D.: Novel c-myc oncogene RNA from abortive immunoglobulin gene recombination in mouse plasmacytomas. Cell 31:443, 1982.

185. Taub, R., Kirsch, I., Morton, C., Lenoir, G., Swan, D., Tronick, S.,

Aaronson, S., and Leder, P.: Translocation of the c-*myc* gene into the immunoglobulin heavy chain locus in human Burkitt lymphoma and murine plastacytoma cells. Proc. Natl. Acad. Sci. USA 79:7837, 1982.

186. Dalla-Favera, R., Bregni, M., Erikson, J., Patterson, D., Gallo, R. C., and Croce, C. M.: Human c-*myc* oncogene is located on the region of chromosome 8 that is translocated in Burkitt lymphoma cells. Proc. Natl. Acad. Sci. USA 79:7824, 1982.

187. Magrath, I.: The pathogenesis of Burkitt's lymphoma. Adv. Cancer Res. 55:133, 1990.

188. Ohno, H., Takimoto, G., and McKeithan T. W.: The candidate proto-oncogene *bcl*-3 is related to genes implicated in cell lineage determination and cell cycle control. Cell 60:991, 1990.

189. Begley, C. G., Aplan, P. D., Davey, M. P., Nakahara, K., Tchorz, K., Kurtzberg, J., Hershfield, M. S., Haynes, B. F., Cohen, D. I., Waldmann, T. A., and Kirsch, I. R.: Chromosomal translocation in a human leukemic stem cell line disrupts the TCR δ region and results in a previously unreported fusion transcript. Proc. Natl. Acad. Sci. USA 86:2031, 1989.

190. Krowczynska, A. M., Rudders, R. A., and Krontiris, T. G.: The human minisatellite consensus at breakpoints of oncogene translocations. Nucleic Acids Res. 18:1121, 1989.

191. Smith, G. R.: Chi hotspots of generalized recombination. Cell 34:709, 1983.

192. Agrawal, A., Eastman, Q. M., and Schatz, D. G.: Transposition mediated by RAG1 And RAG2 and its implications for the evolution of the immune system. Nature 394:744, 1998.

193. Hiom, K., Melek, M., and Gellert, M.: DNA transposition by the RAG1 and RAG2 proteins: A possible source of oncogenic translocations. Cell 94:415, 1998.

194. Adachi, M., Cossman, J., Longo, D., Croce, C. M., and Tsujimoto, Y.: Variant translocation of the bcl-2 gene to immunoglobulin lambda light chain gene in chronic lymphocytic leukemia. Proc. Natl. Acad. Sci. USA 86(8):2771, 1989.

195. Bergsagel, P. L., Chesi, M., Nardini, E., Brents, L. A., Kirby, S. L., and Kuehl, W. M.: Promiscuous translocations into immunoglobulin heavy chain switch regions in multiple myeloma. Proc. Natl. Acad. Sci. USA 93(24):13931, 1996.

196. Chesi, M., Bergsagel, P. L., Shonukan, O. O., Martelli, M. L., Brents, L. A., Chen, T., Schrock, E., Ried, T., and Kuehl, W. M.: Frequent dysregulation of the c-maf proto-oncogene at 16q23 by translocation to an Ig locus in multiple myeloma. Blood 91(12):4457, 1998.

197. Chesi, M., Nardini, E., Lim, R.S.C., Smith, K. D., Kuehl, W. M., and Bergsagel, P. L.: The t(4;14) translocation in myeloma dysregulates both FGFR3 and a novel gene, MMSET, resulting in IgH/MMSET hybrid transcripts. Blood 92(12):3025, 1998.

198. Dalla-Favera, R.: Chromosomal translocations involving the c-myc oncogene in lymphoid neoplasia. *In* Kirsch, I. R. (ed.): The Causes and Consequences of Chromosomal Aberrations. New York, CRC Press, 1993.

199. Dyomin, V. G., Rao, P. H., Dalla-Favera, R., and Chaganti, R.S.K.: BCL8, a novel gene involved in translocations affecting band 15q11-13 in diffuse large-cell lymphoma. Proc. Natl. Acad. Sci. USA 94:5728, 1997.

200. Iida, S., Rao, P. H., Nallasivam, P., Hibshoosh, H., Butler, M., Louie D. C., Dyomin, V., Ohno, H., Chaganti, R. S. K., and Dalla-Favera, R.: The t(9;14)(p13;q32) chromosomal translocation associated with lymphoplasmacytoid lymphoma involves the PAX-5 gene. Blood 88:4110, 1996.

201. Iida, S., Rao, P. H., Butler, M., Corradini, P., Boccadoro, M., Klein, B., Chaganti, R. S., and Dalla-Favera, R.: Deregulation of MUM1/IRF4 by chromosomal translocation in multiple myeloma. Nature Genet. 17(2):226, 1997.

202. Korsmeyer, S. J.: Chromosomal translocations in lymphoid malignancies reveal novel proto-oncogenes. Annu. Rev. Immunol. 10:785, 1992.

203. Komatsu, H., Iida, S., Yamamoto, K., Mikuni, C., Nitta, M., Takahashi, T., Ueda, R., and Seto, M.: A variant chromosome translocation at 11q13 identifying PRAD1/cyclin D1 as the BCL-1 gene. Blood 84(4):1226, 1994.

204. Kirsch, I. R.: The Causes and Consequences of Chromosomal Aberrations. Boca Raton, Fla., CRC Press, 1993.

205. Goossens, T., Klein, U., and Kuppers, R.: Frequent occurrence of deletions and duplications during somatic hypermutation: Implications for oncogene translocations and heavy chain disease. Proc. Natl. Acad. Sci. USA 95:2463, 1998.

206. Popescu, N. C., and Zimonjic, D. B.: New genetic techniques in cancer analysis: Molecular cytogenetic characterization of cancer cell alterations. Cancer Genet. Cytogenet. 93:10, 1997.

207. Shen, H. M., Peters, A., Baron, B., Zhu, X., and Storb, U.: Mutation of BCL-6 gene in normal B cells by the process of somatic hypermutation of Ig genes. Science 280:1750, 1998.

208. Vaandrager, J. W., Kluin, P., and Schuuring, E.: The t(11;14) (q13;q32) in multiple myeloma cell line KMS12 has its 11q13 breakpoint 330 kb centromeric from the cyclin D1 gene (letter). Blood 89:349, 1997.

209. Willis, T. G., Zalcberg, I. R., Coignet, L. J., Wlodarska, I., Stul, M., Jadayel, D. M., Bastard, C., Treleaven, J. G., Catovsky, D., Silva, M. L., and Dyer, M. J.: Molecular cloning of translocation t(1;14)(q21;q32) defines a novel gene (:BCL9) at chromosome lq21. Blood 91:1873, 1998.

210. Willis, T. G., Jadayel, D. M., Du, M.-Q., Peng, H., Perry, A. R., Abdul-Rauf, M., Price, H., Karran, L, Majekodunmi, O., Wlodarska, I., Pan, L., Crook, T., Hamoudi, R., Isaacson, P. G., and Dyer, M.J.S.: Bcl10 is involved in t(1;14)(p22;q32) of MALT B cell lymphoma and mutated in multiple tumor types. Cell 96:35, 1999.

211. Ye, B. H., Changanti, S., Changg, C. C., Niu, H., Corradini, P., Chaganti, R. S., and Dalla-Favera, R.: Chromosomal translocations cause deregulated BCL6 expression by promoter substitution in B cell lymphoma. EMBO J. 14:6209, 1995.

212. Gabrea, A., Bergsagel, P. L., Chesi, M., Shou, Y., and Kuehl, W. M.: Insertion of excised IgH switch sequences causes overexpression of cyclin D1 in a myeloma tumor cell. Mol. Cell Biol. 3:1, 1999.

213. Pasqualucci, L., Migliazza, A., Fracchiolla, N., William, C., Neri, A., Baldini, L., Chaganti, R. S., Klein, U., Kuppers, R., Rajewsky, K., and Dalla-Favera, R.: BCL-6 mutations in normal germinal center B cells: Evidence of somatic hypermutation acting outside Ig loci. Proc. Natl. Acad. Sci. USA 95:11816, 1998.

214. DeVita, V. T., Hellman S., and Rosenberg, S. A.: Cancer: Principles and Practice of Oncology. 5th ed. Philadelphia, Lippincott-Raven, 1997.

215. Takashima, T., Itoh, M., Ueda, Y., Nishida, K., Tamaki, T., Misawa, S., Abe, T., Seto, M., Machii, T., and Taniwaki, M.: Detection of 14q32.33 translocation and t(11;14) in interphase nuclei of chronic B-cell leukemia/lymphomas by in situ hybridization. Int. J. Cancer 72:31, 1997.

216. Aurias, A., Couturier, J., Dutrillaux, A. M., Dutrillaux, B., Herpin, F., Lamoliatte, E., Lombard, M., Muleris, M., Paravatou, M., Prieur, M., Prod'homme, M., Sportes, M., Viegas-Péquignot, E., and Volobouev, V.: Inversion 14 (q12qter) or (q11.2q32.3): The most frequently acquired rearrangement in lymphocytes. Hum. Genet. 71:19, 1985.

217. Denny, C. T., Hollis, G. F., Hecht, F., et al.: Common mechanism of chromosomal inversion in B and T cell tumors: Relevance to lymphocyte development. Science 234:197, 1986.

218. Jack, H. M., Berg, J., and Wabl, M.: Translation affects immunoglobulin mRNA stability. Eur. J. Immunol. 19:843, 1989.

219. Davodeau, F., Peyrat, M., Gaschet, J., Hallet, M., Triebel, F., Vie, Kabelitz, D., and Bonneville, M.: Surface expression of functional T cell receptor chains formed by interlocus recombination on human T lymphocytes. J. Exp. Med. 180:1685, 1994.

220. Sonnier, J. A., Buchanan, G. R., Howard-Peebles, P. N., Rutledge, J., and Smith, R. G.: Chromosomal translocation involving the immunoglobulin kappa-chain and heavy-chain loci in a child with chronic lympocytic leukemia. N. Engl. J. Med. 309:590, 1983.

221. Aurias, A., Croquette, M. F., Nuyts, V. P., Griscelli, C., and Dutrillaux, B.: New data on clonal anomalies of chromosome 14 in ataxia-telangiectasia: tct(14;14) and inv(14). Hum. Genet. 72:22, 1986.

222. Davey, M. P., Bertness, V., Nakahara, K., Johnson, J. P., McBride, O. W., Waldmann, T. A., and Kirsch, I. R.: Juxtaposition of the T-cell receptor α-chain locus (14q11) and a region (14q32) of potential importance in leukemogenesis by 14;14 translocation in a patient with T-cell chronic lymphocytic leukemia and ataxia-telangiectasia. Proc. Natl. Acad. Sci. USA 85:9287, 1988.

223. Russo, G. M., Isobe, M., Gatti, R., Finan, J., Batuman, O., Huebner, K., Nowell, P. C., and Croce, C.M.: Molecular analysis of a t(14;14) translocation in leukemic T-cells of an ataxia-telangiectasia patient. Proc. Natl. Acad. Sci. USA 86:602, 1989.

224. Brito-Babapulle, V., Pomfret, M., Matutes, E., and Catovsky, D.: Cytogenetic studies on prolymphocytic leukemia. II. T cell prolymphocytic leukemia. Blood 70:926, 1987.

225. Baer, R., Heppell, A., Taylor, A.M.R., Rabbitts, P. H., Boullier, B., and Rabbitts, T. H.: The breakpoint of an inversion chromosome 14

in a T cell leukemia: Sequence downstream of the immunoglobulin heavy chain locus implicated in tumorigenesis. Proc. Natl. Acad. Sci. USA 84:9069, 1987.

226. Bertness, V., Felix, C. A., McBride, O. W., Morgan, R., Smith, S. D., Sandberg, A. A., and Kirsch, I. R.: Characterization of the breakpoint of a t(14;14) (q11.22) from the leukemic cells of a patient with T-cell acute lymphoblastic leukemia. Cancer Genet. Cytogenet. 44:47, 1990.

227. Thick, J., Mak, Y. F., Metcalfe, J., Beatty, D., and Taylor, A. M.: A gene on chromosome Xq28 associated with T-cell prolymphocytic leukemia in two patients with ataxia telangiectasia. Leukemia 8:564, 1994.

228. Stern, M. H., Soulier, J., Rosenzwajg, M., Nakahara, K., Canki-Klain, N., Aurias, A., Sigaux, F., and Kirsch, I. R.: MTCP-1: A novel gene on the human chromosome Xq28 translocated to the T cell receptor alpha/delta locus in mature T cell proliferations. Oncogene 8:2475, 1993.

229. Virgilio, L., Narducci, M. G., Isobe, M., Billips, L. G., Cooper, M. C., Croce, C. M., and Russo, G.: Identification of the TCL1 gene involved in T-cell malignancies. Proc. Natl. Acad. Sci. USA 91:12530, 1994.

230. Fu, Z. Q., Du Bois, G. C., Song, S. P., Kulikovskaya, I., Virgilio, L., Rothstein, J. L., Croce, C. M., Weber, I. T., and Harrison, R. W.: Crystal structure of MTCP-1: Implications for role of TCL-1 and MTCP-1 in T cell malignancies. Proc. Natl. Acad. Sci. USA 95:3413, 1998.

231. Virgilio, L., Lazzeri, C., Bichi, R., Nibu, K., Narducci, M. G., Russo, G., Rothstein, J. L., and Croce, C. M.: Deregulated expression of TCL1 causes T cell leukemia in mice. Proc. Natl. Acad. Sci. USA 95:3885, 1998.

232. Gritti, C., Dastot, H., Soulier, J., Janin, A., Daniel, M.-T., Madani, A., Grimber, G., Biand, P., Sigaux, F., and Stern, M. H.: Transgenic mice for MTCP1 develop T-cell prolymphocytic leukemia. Blood 92:368, 1998.

233. Aplan, P. D., Lombardi, D. P., and Kirsch, I. R.: Structural characterization of SIL, a gene frequently disrupted in T-cell acute lymphoblastic leukemia. Mol. Cell Biol. 11:5462, 1991.

234. Izraeli, S., Colaizzo-Anas, T., Bertness, V. L., Mani, K., Aplan, P. D., and Kirsch, I. R.: Expression of the SIL gene is correlated with growth induction and cellular proliferation. Cell Growth Differ. 8:1171, 1997.

235. Porcher, C., Swat, W., Rockwell, K., Fujiwara, Y., Alt, F. W., and Orkin, S. H.: The T cell leukemia oncoprotein SCL/tal-1 is essential for development of all hematopoietic lineages. Cell 86:47, 1996.

236. Robb, L., Elwood, N. J., Elefanty, A. G., Kontgen, F., Li, R., Barnett, L. D., and Begley, C. G.: The scl gene product is required for the generation of all hematopoietic lineages in the adult mouse. EMBO J. 15:4123, 1996.

237. Aplan, P. D., Begley, C. G., Bertness, V., Nussmeier, M., Ezquerra, A., Coligan, J., and Kirsch, I. R.: The SCL gene is formed from a transcriptionally complex locus. Mol. Cell Biol. 10:6426, 1990.

238. Aplan, P. D., Lombardi, D. P., Reaman, G. H., Sather, H. N., Hammond, G. D., and Kirsch, I. R.: Involvement of the putative hematopoietic transcription factor SCL in T-cell acute lymphoblastic leukemia. Blood 79:1327, 1992.

239. Brown, L., Cheng, J. T., Chen, Q., Siciliano, M. J., Crist, W. Buchanan, G., and Baer, R.: Site-specific recombination of the *tal*-1 gene is a common occurrence in human T cell leukemia. EMBO J. 9:3343, 1990.

240. Schrock, E., du Manoir, S., Veldman, T., Schoell, B., Wienberg, J., Ferguson-Smith, M. A., Ning, Y., Ledbetter, D. H., Bar-Am, I., Soenksen, D., Garini, Y., and Ried, T.: Multicolor spectral karyotyping of human chromosomes. Science 273:494, 1996.

241. Veldman, T., Vignon, C., Schrock, E., Rowley, J. D., and Ried, T.: Hidden chromosome abnormalities in haematological malignancies detected by multicolour spectral karyotyping. Nature Genet. 15:406, 1997.

242. Limpens, J., de Jong, D., van Krieken, J. H., Price, C. G., Young, B. D., Van Ommen, G. J., and Kluin, P. M.: Bcl-2/JH rearrangements in benign lymphoid tissues with follicular hyperplasia. Oncogene 6:2271, 1991.

243. Liu, Y., Hernandez, A. M., Shibata, D., and Cortopassi, G. A.: BCL2 translocation frequency rises with age in humans. Proc. Natl. Acad. Sci. USA 91:8910, 1994.

244. Seligmann, M., Mihaesco, E., Preud'homme, J. L., Danao, F., and Brouet, J. C.: Heavy chain disease: Current findings and concepts. Immunol. Rev. 48:145, 1979.

245. Bakhshi, A., Guglielmi, P., Siebenlist, U., Ravetch, J. V., Jensen, J. P., and Korsmeyer, S. J.: A DNA insertion/deletion necessitates an aberrant RNA splice accounting for human μ heavy chain disease protein. Proc. Natl. Acad. Sci. USA 83:2689, 1986.

246. Cogne, M., Preud'homme, J.-L., and Guglielmi, P.: Immunoglobulin gene alterations in human heavy chain diseases. Res. Immunol. 140:487, 1989.

247. Downward, J., Yarden, Y., Mayes, E., Scrace, G., Totty, N., Stockwell, P., Ullrich, A., Schlessinger, J., and Waterfield, M. D.: Close similarity of epidermal growth factor receptor and v-*erb*-B oncogene protein sequences. Nature 307:521, 1984.

248. Brouet, J. C., Mason, D. Y., Danon F., Preud'homme, J. L., Seligmann, M., Reyes, F., Navab, F., Galian, A., Rene, E., and Rambaud, J. C.: Alpha-chain disease: Evidence for a common clonal origin of intestinal immunoblastic lymphoma and plasmacytic proliferation. Lancet 1:861, 1977.

249. Alexander, A., Steinmetz, M., Barritault, D., Frangione, B., Franklin, E. C., Hood, L., and Buxbaum, J. N.: γ heavy chain disease in man: cDNA sequence supports partial gene deletion model. Proc. Natl. Acad. Sci. USA 79:3260, 1982.

250. Guglielmi, P., Bakhshi, A., Miahesco, E., Broudet, J., Waldmann, T. A., and Korsmeyer, S. J.: DNA deletion in human gamma heavy chain disease. Clin. Res. 32:348A, 1984.

251. LeFranc, M. P., LeFranc, G., and Rabbitts, T. H.: Inherited deletion of immunoglobulin heavy chain constant region genes in normal human individuals. Nature 300:760, 1982.

252. Keyeux, G., LeFranc, M. P., Chevailler, A., and LeFranc, G.: Molecular analysis of the IgHA and MHC class III region genes in one family with IgA and C4 deficiencies. Exp. Clin. Immunogenet. 7:170, 1990.

253. Rosen, F. S.: Genetic deficiencies in specific immune responses. Semin. Hematol. 27:333, 1990.

254. Hendricks, R. W., vanTol, M. J., deLange, G. G., and Schuurman, R. K.: Inheritance of a large deletion within the human immunoglobulin heavy chain constant region gene complex and immunological implications. Scand. J. Immunol. 29:535, 1989.

255. Felix, C. A., Reaman, G. H., Korsmeyer, S. J., Hollis, G. F., Dinndorf, P. A., Wright, J. J., and Kirsch, I. R.: Immunoglobulin and T-cell receptor gene configuration in acute lymphoblastic leukemia of infancy. Blood 70:536, 1987.

12 Lymphocyte Development
Gerald Siu

▼ ▼

Principles of Lymphocyte Development

The proper maturation of lymphocytes is critical for the generation and maintenance of the human immune response. Like most cells, lymphocytes develop from multipotent precursors that respond to environmental cues affecting their course of development. The cell receives a developmental signal from the external environment, which is then transmitted through the cytoplasm to the nucleus. Fate determination is mediated through the alteration of the program of gene expression of the precursor cell in response to these signals. The resulting differentiated lymphocyte thus expresses the appropriate genes that enable it to assume its proper role in the mature immune response.

Lymphocytes have several special developmental requirements, unlike most other somatic cells. To avoid autoimmunity, lymphocytes must be able to distinguish self molecules from non-self molecules. This problem is especially acute for T cells. As discussed in Chapter 13, T cells can recognize only antigen bound to self-encoded major histocompatibility complex (MHC) molecules, in a process referred to as MHC restriction. Thus, the T cell must be able to recognize self MHC molecules but not react unless the MHC molecule is binding a foreign antigen. To complicate matters even further, lymphocytes must be able to recognize a seemingly infinite number of different foreign antigens and thus must express a wide variety of different antigen-specific receptors. To generate the sequence diversity necessary to encode these different receptors, the genes that encode the antigen-recognition portion undergo somatic rearrangement during lymphocyte development. This process generates a wide variety of different genes that can encode receptors of all sorts of specificities, most of which are either useless in an immune response or potentially autoreactive. The lymphocyte development process is designed both to select out lymphocytes that express receptors likely to be useful, in a process referred to as positive selection, and to delete potentially harmful lymphocytes, in a process referred to as negative selection. Another developmental requirement unique to lymphocytes is the need to acquire specific effector functions that correlate with the specificity of its particular antigen receptor. Once again, this requirement is especially important for T cells; as described in Chapter 13, expression of the CD4 and CD8 coreceptors correlates with the MHC specificity of the T-cell antigen receptor (TCR) and to a large extent with T-cell functional subclass. Finally, the immune system must establish functional memory. Exposure of the immune system to a foreign antigen enhances its subsequent ability to respond again to that antigen. These subsequent responses, referred to as secondary responses, are qualitatively different from the initial immune response in that they are greater in magnitude and occur more rapidly. The ability of the immune system to remember exposure to antigens and to enhance subsequent responses to those same antigens is referred to as immunological memory.

Proper lymphoid development therefore requires an intricate maturation and selection process to ensure a functioning immune system. Unfortunately, studying human lymphocyte development is complicated by the facts that much of the defining work was conducted in mouse systems, the defining cell surface markers often differ between mouse and man, and different laboratories use different nomenclatures and occasionally different markers to define each class. Because of this, reviews of the immunological literature can often be extremely confusing at first glance. In sorting it all out, it is important to keep three unifying principles in mind.

1. *Lymphocyte development occurs in discrete functional steps that are defined by the onset of expression of specific molecules.* Predictably, many of these defining factors are required for proper development. Staging of lymphopoiesis is thus done primarily by determining the expression or lack of expression of different stage-specific molecules. With the advent of multiparameter flow cytometry, this method is widely used in both basic research and clinical diagnosis.
2. *The early developmental stages are defined by the gene rearrangements required to generate a functional antigen receptor gene.* As discussed in Chapter 11, genes that encode the lymphocyte antigen receptors rearrange at precise times in lymphopoiesis. Early stages of lymphocyte development can be identified by the lack of receptor gene rearrangements

and the onset of expression of the factors required for the rearrangement process. Intermediate stages can be defined by identifying which of the receptor genes have rearranged and which of the receptor chains are expressed on the surface of the immature lymphocyte. Later stages can be defined by the surface expression of the antigen receptors and the loss of expression of the factors important in gene rearrangement.

3. *There are many underlying parallels between B-cell and T-cell development.* B and T cells face similar fate decisions. In early lymphocyte development, survival of the precursor is dependent on the successful rearrangement and expression of an antigen receptor that has an appropriate antigenic specificity. Rearrangements occur in a stepwise fashion; successful rearrangement of an antigen receptor gene induces the cell to progress to the next stage. The elimination of lymphocytes that express antigen receptors of inappropriate specificities begins as soon as the antigen receptor is expressed on the surface and continues throughout the life of the cell. Late in development, on being presented with its appropriate antigen, the mature lymphocyte must determine whether it will undergo terminal differentiation to become a short-lived effector cell, whose responsibility is to eliminate the pathogen, or a long-lived memory cell, whose responsibility is to remember the exposure to the pathogen and to enhance future responses to the same pathogen.

In this chapter, I describe each of these developmental steps in detail for both T and B lymphocytes.

Architecture of the Immune System

The lymph organs are anatomically defined sites that are designed to provide microenvironments for the maturation of lymphocytes as well as to regulate the interactions of different classes of lymphocytes and antigen-presenting cells

(APCs) during the mature immune response. Lymphoid tissue is classified into two major groups: primary lymph organs, such as the bone marrow and the thymus; and secondary or peripheral lymph organs, including the spleen, lymph nodes, and Peyer patches in the ileum. In general, early development of functionally competent lymphocytes from precursors occurs in the primary lymph organs, whereas the secondary lymph organs are the sites where the mature lymphocyte responds to foreign antigen. However, as we shall see, development and maturation of lymphocytes is a continuous process that occurs in virtually all lymph organs.

Bone Marrow. Fetal hematopoiesis occurs sequentially in the blood islands of the yolk sac, the liver, and the spleen. After birth, the site of hematopoiesis begins to shift to the bone marrow; by puberty, hematopoiesis occurs primarily in the bone marrow of the flat bones, including the sternum, vertebrae, ribs, and pelvic bones. The marrow consists of a sponge-like reticular framework filled with fat cells, blood cell precursors, mature B cells, and antibody-secreting plasma cells that develop in peripheral lymphoid tissue and migrate back to the marrow. In adults, the bone marrow is the source of the pluripotent stem cell that is capable of repopulating all hematopoietic cell types. As discussed below, for T cells, the pluripotent precursor migrates to the thymus for further development. Most of the early and intermediate steps in B-lymphocyte development, however, occur in the bone marrow.

Thymus. The thymus is an anterior mediastinal organ consisting of two lobes. Each lobe is further divided into lobules, each consisting of an outer cortex and an inner medulla (Fig. 12–1). The cortex is densely packed with T lymphocytes at various stages of maturation, whereas the medulla is more sparsely populated with T cells of mostly mature phenotypes. Non-lymphoid epithelial cells and bone marrow–derived dendritic cells are scattered throughout the thymus; however, well above 90 per cent of the cells found in the thymus are of T-cell origin. T-cell precursors enter the thymic cortex through blood vessels and migrate slowly toward the medulla, in the process interacting with epithelial

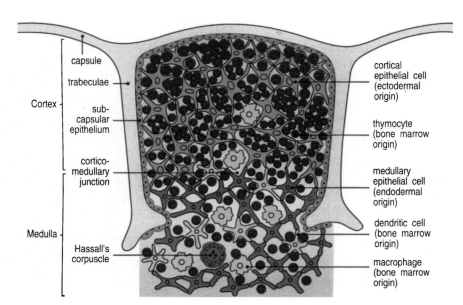

Figure 12–1. Organization of the thymus. The thymus is made up of several lobules, each containing an outer cortical region and an inner medullary region. The cortex contains mostly immature double-positive thymocytes (dark blue), cortical epithelial cells (pale blue), and macrophages (yellow). The medulla consists of the more mature single-positive thymocytes (dark blue), medullary epithelial cells (orange), dendritic cells, and macrophages (yellow). Hassall's corpuscles, found in the medulla, are probably also sites of cell destruction. (From Janeway, C.A., and Travers, P.: Immunobiology, 3rd ed. New York, Current Biology Limited/Garland Publishing, 1997, p. 6:4.)

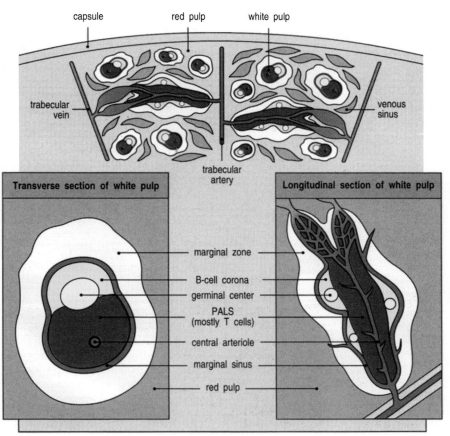

capsule   red pulp   white pulp

trabecular vein

venous sinus

trabecular artery

Transverse section of white pulp

Longitudinal section of white pulp

marginal zone

B-cell corona

germinal center

PALS (mostly T cells)

central arteriole

marginal sinus

red pulp

Figure 12–2. Organization of the spleen. The spleen consists of red pulp (pink area) interspersed with white pulp (yellow and blue areas). The center panel shows general organization of the spleen; most white pulp areas are shown in transverse section, with one in longitudinal section. Smaller diagrams show enlargements of a transverse section *(left)* and a longitudinal section *(right)* of the white pulp. Blood carrying lymphocyte and antigen flows from a trabecular artery into a central arteriole in the white pulp. Cells and antigen then pass into a marginal sinus and eventually drain into a trabecular vein. The marginal sinus is surrounded by the marginal zone; the central arteriole is surrounded by the periarteriolar lymphoid sheath (PALS). The follicles (yellow) consist mainly of B cells, including germinal centers (white). (From Janeway, C.A., and Travers, P.: Immunobiology, 3rd ed. New York, Current Biology Limited/Garland Publishing, 1997, p. 1:9.)

cells, dendritic cells, and macrophages. These interactions are important for the T-cell repertoire selection processes described below; survivors of these processes enter the medulla, acquire the mature T-cell phenotype, and emigrate to the peripheral lymph organs. Thus, the thymus is an important site of early T-cell development.

Spleen. The spleen is a large organ in the upper left quadrant of the abdomen. It is supplied by the splenic artery, which on entering the spleen divides progressively into smaller arterioles and sinusoid structures. The arterioles are surrounded by periarteriolar lymphoid sheaths that contain aggregates of cells called lymphoid follicles, which in turn often contain central areas referred to as germinal centers (Fig. 12–2). The germinal centers are densely packed with lymphocytes undergoing late stages of development. Both the periarteriolar lymphoid sheaths and the follicles are surrounded by the marginal zone, a region containing both lymphocytes and APCs. Taken together, the periarteriolar lymphoid sheaths, follicles, and marginal zones are referred to as the white pulp region of the spleen. The lymphocytes and APCs are anatomically segregated in the white pulp: the periarteriolar lymphoid sheath region contains mostly T cells, the follicles and germinal centers contain mostly B cells, and the marginal zone contains both B and T cells. As we will see later in this chapter, this segregation reflects the functions of these cells in the mature immune response. The arterioles eventually end in vascular sinusoids containing erythrocytes, macrophages, and dendritic cells; this region is called the red pulp. The sinusoids end in venules that eventu-

ally drain into the splenic vein, which carries blood out of the spleen into the portal circulation.

The spleen is a major site for the collection of antigen from peripheral sites and the initiation of the immune response to blood-borne antigens. Antigens enter the spleen through the vascular sinusoids and encounter lymphocytes in the marginal zones; activated B cells then migrate to the germinal centers, where they proliferate and give rise to progeny B cells that produce antibodies with high affinities for antigen (see below). Thus, the spleen is an important site for late stages of B-lymphocyte development.

Lymph Nodes. Lymph nodes are small anatomical structures distributed throughout the lymphatic channels of the body. Draining lymph from the epithelia and mucosa is brought into the cortex of the lymph node by the afferent lymphatics. Much like the spleen, the cortex of the lymph node contains B cell–rich follicles, many of which contain germinal centers (Fig. 12–3). T cells are located between the follicles and in the deep cortex, referred to as the parafollicular areas. Naive T cells that first arrive from the thymus enter the lymph node through endothelial venules. Here the T cells first encounter foreign antigen; T cells that are stimulated by their cognate antigen then develop into mature T effector or memory cells. The lymph node is therefore an important site for late stages of T-cell development.

The Gut-Associated Lymphoid Tissue. Many important pathogens enter the body through mucosal surfaces, such as rhinoviruses, influenza viruses, and enteroinvasive bacteria. The mucosal immune response is critical in recog-

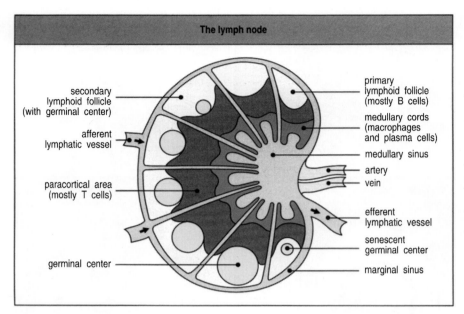

The lymph node

secondary
lymphoid follicle
(with germinal center)

afferent
lymphatic vessel

paracortical area
(mostly T cells)

germinal center

primary
lymphoid follicle
(mostly B cells)

medullary cords
(macrophages
and plasma cells)

medullary sinus

artery

vein

efferent
lymphatic vessel

senescent
germinal center

marginal sinus

Figure 12–3. Organization of the lymph node. The lymph node consists of an outer cortex and an inner medulla. The cortex itself is composed of an outer cortex consisting mainly of follicles containing B cells and a deep or paracortical area consisting of T cells and dendritic cells. The medulla consists of strings of macrophages and plasma cells. Antigen is transported to the lymph node through the afferent lymphatics. Naive lymphocytes enter the lymph node from the blood stream through the postcapillary venules (not shown) and leave with the lymph through the efferent lymphatics. (From Janeway, C.A., and Travers, P.: Immunobiology, 3rd ed. New York, Current Biology Limited/Garland Publishing, 1997, p. 1:8.)

nizing and eliminating these pathogens. For example, immunity to poliovirus and other picornaviruses is mediated primarily by intraepithelial lymphocytes that reside in the small intestine. Lymphocytes in most of the mucosal tissues are conventional lymphocytes, originating from the thymus and bone marrow. The lymphocytes present in the human digestive tract (principally the small intestine) appear to develop independently from the lymphocytes originating in the thymus, bone marrow, and spleen. A subset of bone marrow hematopoietic precursors homes directly to the intestines, where these cells undergo all of the developmental and selection steps that occur with the lymphocytes of the conventional immune system in the bone marrow and thymus. Because of the relative independence of the gut-associated lymphoid tissue (GALT), the GALT immune system is often considered separately from the immune system of the rest of the body. Because the GALT lymphocytes undergo the same developmental processes as other lymphocytes do, in the interests of brevity I will not consider them as a special case in this review.

Defining Lymphocytes by Cell Surface Molecule Expression

Because lymphocytes are morphologically indistinguishable, immunologists determine the pattern of expression of cell surface molecules on individual cells to classify them. Monoclonal antibodies and flow cytometry have enabled scientists and clinicians not only to easily separate B and T cells but to define precise developmental and functional lymphocyte populations. The different combinations of cell surface antigens expressed at different developmental stages as well as the hodgepodge of names that different groups give to the same molecule can often drive the uninitiated to distraction. However, the differential expression of cell surface antigens is used to track all lymphocyte developmental pathways and to mark crucial stages of this process. In addition, aberrant cell types in disease states can be classified

with respect to both cell type and developmental stage by use of this approach. Cell surface marker analysis, for example, has proved invaluable in the identification and staging of lymphomas and leukemias. Thus, a basic knowledge of how these stages are defined is important to the clinician. Table 12–1 summarizes some well-defined cell surface markers that are used to identify developmental stages in human lymphocyte development and are discussed in this chapter; Table 12–2 summarizes markers that are useful in defining murine lymphocyte development but have not yet been characterized in humans. More inclusive lists of all CD molecules are available in the literature.[1]

Predictably, most of these molecules play important roles in each developmental process, and their initial expression often correlates with the stage of development in which they play an important role. As we will see, because different groups working in mouse and human systems generated and used different antibodies, several of the developmental stages have not been precisely correlated between the two species. Of course, the overall progression is basically the same, and we can obtain a fairly clear picture of how lymphocytes develop by comparing the defined stages in the two systems.

Thymopoiesis

The thymus produces, selects, and exports functional T lymphocytes to the periphery.[2, 3] The T-cell precursor originates from the pluripotent hematopoietic stem cell (HSC) that seeds the thymus from the bone marrow.[4] Once it is within the thymus, the precursor commits to the T-cell lineage and undergoes a series of complicated molecular and biochemical events that result in its immunocompetency or death, including the rearrangement and expression of the TCR genes, selection on the basis of TCR specificity, and acquisition of mature effector T-cell function.[5–7] The survivors of this complicated process emigrate from the thymus to the peripheral lymph organs. In strict cost-benefit terms, this process is extremely inefficient. The thymus of a young

Table 12–1. Human Lymphocyte Cell Surface Markers

CD Name	Other Names	Structure	Tissue/Lineage	Function
CD2	T11	Ig superfamily	T cells, NK cells	Transduces signal to T cell
CD3	T3, Leu4	Multicomponents	Mature T cells	Transduces TCR signal
CD4	T4, Leu3a	Ig superfamily	T_H cells, monocytes, microglial cells	Binds HLA class II, transduces signal to T cell via Lck
CD7	3A1, Leu9	Ig superfamily	T cells, NK cells, precursors	??
CD8	T8, Leu2a	Two chains: α, β; Ig superfamily	T_C cells	Binds HLA class I, transduces signal to T cell via Lck
CD10	Common acute lymphoblastic leukemia antigen (CALLA)	Integrin	B-cell progenitors	Peptide cleavage
CD19	B4	Ig superfamily	B cells	Amplifies signal from B-cell receptor
CD20	B1, Bp35	—	B cells	Mediates B-cell activation
CD21	CR2, B2	Complement regulatory protein family	B cells	Amplifies signal from B-cell receptor
Cd22	Bgp135	Ig superfamily	B cells	Mitogenic for B-cell activation, receptor for CD45RO
CD23	Low-affinity receptor for IgE, FcεRII	Lectin-like	Activated B cells, macrophages, eosinophils, platelets	Receptor for IgE
CD24	Heat-stable antigen (HSA), BA-1	—	B cells, polymorphonuclear leukocytes	??Signaling
CD25	TAC, IL-2R α chain	—	Activated T and B cells, monocytes	Low-affinity receptor for IL-2
CD28	TP44	Ig superfamily	T cells, activated B cells	Costimulatory molecule for T cells; regulates cytokine stability and expression; receptor for B7
CD34	MY10	—	T cells, stem cells	??Marker for the pluripotent HSC
CD35	CR1, C3b receptor	—	B cells, NK cells, polymorphonuclear leukocytes, monocytes, red blood cells	Binds immune complexes
CD38	OKT10, T10		Activated lymphocytes, immature B cells	
CD39	gp80	—	Activated B cells, T cells	B-cell adhesion
CD40	gp50	Homology to tumor necrosis factor receptor, Fas	B cells, macrophages, follicular dendritic cells	B-cell activation
CD43	Leukosialin	—	Lymphocytes, NK cells, monocytes	Leukocyte activation
CD44	Pgp-1, Hermes extracellular matrix receptor type III	—	Lymphocytes of different developmental stages, NK cells, monocytes, red blood cells	Homing, activation
CD45	Leukocyte common antigen, T200	Multiple isoforms generated by splicing (see below)	Leukocytes	Regulation of lymphocyte activation
	CD45RA	220 kDa form	B cells, monocytes, CD8 SP T cells, naive T cells	
	CD45RB	220, 205, 190 kDa forms	B cells, monocytes, macrophages, subsets of memory T cells	
	CD45RO	180 kDa form	Monocytes, thymocytes, activated T cells, memory T cells	
CD54	ICAM-1	Ig superfamily	Activated lymphocytes, endothelial cells	Ligand for LFA-1, rhinoviruses
CD73	Ecto 5′-nucleotidase	—	Lymphocyte subsets	Regulates uptake of nucleotides
CD80	B7-1	Ig superfamily	Activated B cells, monocytes, macrophages, dendritic cells	Ligand for CD28, costimulation
CD86	B7-2	Ig superfamily	Activated lymphocytes, macrophages, dendritic cells, monocytes	Ligand for CD152, costimulation
CD152	CTLA-4, Ly56	Ig superfamily	Activated T cells	Negative signaling during immune responses
CD154	CD40 ligand, CD40L, gp39	—	Activated T cells	Receptor for CD40

Table 12–2. Additional Mouse Lymphocyte Cell Surface Markers

CD Name	Other Names	Structure	Tissue/Lineage	Function
Sca-1	Ly6 A/E	—	Lymphocytes, myeloid cells, early stem cells	??
Sca-2	TSA-1, Ly97	—	Subclasses of thymocytes, myeloid cells, B cells	??
CD45R	B220	Unspliced form of CD45	B cells	Regulation of lymphocyte activation
CD90	Thy-1		All T cells, stem cells	??Signaling
CF117	c-Kit		Hematopoietic stem cells	Receptor for steel factor
IL-7R			Early lymphocytes, mature T cells	Receptor for interleukin-7
CD62L	L-selectin, LECAM-1		Lymphocyte subsets, NK cells, neutrophils, monocytes	Homing receptor for lymph node high endothelial venules

adult mouse contains 1 to 2×10^8 thymocytes and generates 5×10^7 new thymocytes per day, either by proliferation of thymocytes or by immigration of bone marrow precursors.[8–11] However, only 10^6 cells will emigrate from the thymus as mature T cells during the same time period.[12] These observations indicate that most developing T cells in the thymus are destined to die without gaining immunocompetency and led to the hypothesis that cell death in the thymus is the result of selection processes required to delete autoreactive T lymphocytes.[13] Much progress has been made in the past 15 years to characterize these complex processes in both humans and mice. In this section, I discuss the molecular and cellular mechanisms by which T cells acquire appropriate antigen and MHC specificity and mature effector function in the thymus.

▼ αβ VERSUS γδ T-CELL DEVELOPMENT: ONE LINEAGE OR TWO?

As discussed in Chapter 11, there are two major types of TCR: the αβ TCR, which is expressed by most functional mature T cells, and the γδ TCR, which is expressed on a variably sized but small subset of mature T cells and thymocytes. The role of γδ T cells in the mammalian immune system has remained murky since the discovery of the γ chain by Tonegawa and colleagues[14] in 1984. The developmental relationship between the αβ and γδ T cells is no clearer and for years has been the source of considerable discussion.[15] The simplest model is that αβ and γδ T cells originate from a common thymocyte lineage and are fated to take either developmental pathway before commitment to TCR gene rearrangement. However, virtually all αβ TCR–bearing T cells contain rearrangements in the γ gene locus, implying a common relationship between T-cell precursors that rearrange the γ and αβ genes.[16] Supporters of a second hypothesis propose that functional rearrangement of the γ genes leads to γδ TCR–bearing T cells, whereas non-functional γ gene rearrangements lead to subsequent β chain gene rearrangement and the αβ lineage. However, some αβ T cells have functional γ gene rearrangements and express the γ chain.[14–17] Attempts to delineate the relationship between these two lineages by studying the rearrangement of the δ chain gene locus vis-à-vis the α chain gene locus in developing T cells have yielded diametrically opposing answers.[18, 19] Using fetal thymic repopulation culture studies, several groups have shown that early thymocyte stages are capable of repopulating both αβ and γδ T lineages, thus

indicating that they do have a common thymic precursor.[15] Because the majority of mature T cells in most organisms are of the αβ lineage and most immune responses are mediated primarily by αβ T cells, to simplify matters I restrict the discussion to the development of the αβ lineage.

▼ THYMUS SEEDING BY HEMATOPOIETIC STEM CELLS

In young mice, the thymus contains up to 5×10^8 thymocytes; typically, thymuses from older adult mice are 100- to 1000-fold smaller.[10, 11] Despite this age-dependent decrease in thymus size and activity, seeding of the thymus by HSCs occurs throughout life. Indeed, continued thymic education is critical for the bone marrow transplant patient to regenerate a functional mature T-cell population. Most estimates suggest that the rate of seeding of the thymus by bone marrow precursors is extremely low, perhaps 100 to 1000 cells per day.[20–22] Because of the enormous proliferative and differentiative potential of the HSC, this rate is nonetheless sufficient to maintain the levels of peripheral mature T cells, even in adults (Fig. 12–4).

What is the nature of the bone marrow prothymocyte? The earliest stem cell precursor that seeds the thymus is

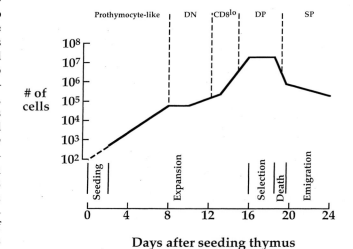

Figure 12–4. Cell surface marker expression and expansion of cell numbers in the thymus. The illustration depicts the development of a cohort of stem cells injected into a thymus of a young adult mouse; cell production (y-axis) is estimated on a daily basis.

capable of regenerating the hematopoietic system of an irradiated animal and thus is considered to be a pluripotent HSC.[23-26] In the mouse, this cell expresses low levels of heat-stable antigen (HSA) and Thy-1 and higher levels of CD44, Sca-1, c-Kit, and interleukin (IL)–7R.[27-36] The expression of c-Kit and IL-7R is functionally relevant, because the early precursor requires the c-Kit ligand and IL-7 to survive and proliferate[37]; the precise function of the other cell surface markers is unknown. This HSA^{low} Thy-1^{low} CD44$^+$ Sca-1$^+$ c-Kit$^+$ IL-7R$^+$ population also does not express cell surface molecules that are characteristic of the different mature hematopoietic lineages, such as CD3 and CD8 (T cells; see below), B220 (B cells; see below), Mac-1 (macrophages), Gr-1 (granulocytes), and ter-119 (reticulocytes); and thus are considered to be "lineage negative," or lin$^-$.[29, 38] Interestingly, CD4 expression can be detected on certain subclasses of HSCs and is considered by some groups to be a marker for more differentiated, proliferating HSCs.[39, 40] The HSC that seeds the murine thymus maintains the HSA^{low} Thy-1^{low} CD44$^+$ Sca-1$^+$ phenotype and in addition becomes Sca-2$^+$ CD4^{low}.[24, 39] This cell is also capable of generating B-cell, natural killer (NK) cell, and dendritic cell precursors in in vitro systems; this cell is probably committed to the T-cell lineage as the result of cell/cell interactions in the thymic microenvironment.[23, 24]

In humans, the homologous early prothymocyte is less well defined and is difficult to distinguish from the pluripotent HSC.[41-43] Experiments by several groups have demonstrated that the earliest human lymphocyte precursor is CD34$^+$ CD45RA$^+$ CD44$^+$ CD10$^+$ CD38$^+$ HLA$^-$ DR$^+$ lin$^-$ and, in contrast with mice, does not express Thy-1 or c-Kit.[6, 44-51] This stem cell is capable of generating the lymphocyte, NK cell, and dendritic cell populations and thus is not yet completely committed to the lymphocyte lineage. In addition to these markers, the earliest prothymocyte precursor also expresses the γ, δ, and ε chains of the CD3 complex in the cytoplasm.[50] Experiments by Toribio and colleagues[52] demonstrated that a CD34$^+$ CD44^{int} population within the human thymus is capable of differentiating into either T cells or monocytes and dendritic cells on culturing with IL-7, and thus this population may be the human homologue for the murine HSA^{low} Thy-1^{low} CD44$^+$ Sca-1$^+$ Sca-2$^+$ CD4^{low} c-Kit$^+$ IL-7R$^+$ population. Once in the thymus, the early thymocyte proliferates at a moderate rate for several days before continuing development.

▼ EARLY STEPS IN THYMOCYTE DEVELOPMENT: THE CD4$^-$ CD8$^-$ THYMOCYTE

The earliest subsequent stage of thymocyte development is often referred to as the double-negative (DN) population, which refers to the fact that this population does not express the CD4 or CD8 coreceptor molecules[53] (Fig. 12–5). To separate the true pre-T cell population from other, more mature DN thymocytes, this population is also called the triple-negative (TN) population, which refers to the lack of expression of CD4, CD8, and TCR/CD3. This population is found primarily in the subcortical region of the thymus.[54, 55] Like the prothymocytes, the DN pre-T cell population can be subdivided into distinct developmental subclasses on the basis of cell surface molecule expression.[35, 36, 50] Unlike with

markers of the later stages of development, the functional relationship between the expression of these markers and the developmental stages has not been defined; however, because important molecular and developmental events occur at each of these stages, the classification of thymocytes on the basis of their expression is nonetheless useful.

In mice, the earliest DN population is the CD44$^+$ CD25$^-$ HSA$^+$ Thy-1$^+$ c-Kit$^+$ IL-7R$^+$ thymocyte.[36] This population is difficult to distinguish from the earlier prothymocyte-like population discussed above and in fact may be the same population.[27-36] This population then begins to express surface CD25 and completely downregulates CD4; this CD44$^+$ CD25$^+$ HSA$^+$ Thy-1$^+$ c-Kit$^+$ IL-7R$^+$ population expresses the recombination-activating gene (RAG) proteins and thus is the first to begin to rearrange the TCR genes.[35, 56] As discussed in Chapter 11, the thymocyte first rearranges the genes encoding the γ and β chains. Using transgenic and targeted-disruption techniques in murine systems, several groups have determined that the successful rearrangement of the β chain gene of the TCR leads to several important developmental steps.[57-61] First, additional rearrangement at the β chain locus stops, thus ensuring that the T cell will express only one functional β chain.[62, 63] The mechanism by which this process, referred to as allelic exclusion, occurs is not completely understood. Second, the thymocyte downregulates CD25, CD44, and c-Kit expression to become the CD4$^-$ CD8$^-$ CD3$^-$ HSA$^+$ Thy-1$^+$ population.[34, 35] Third, the β chain is expressed at low levels on the surface of the thymocyte with the CD3 complex and a surrogate TCR α chain referred to as pre-Tα.[64, 65] This population proliferates rapidly and begins to express CD8. The CD4$^-$ CD8^{low} CD3$^-$ HSA$^+$ Thy-1$^+$ thymocyte population continues to proliferate rapidly; indeed, this is the highest proliferating population in the thymus. Finally, the successful rearrangement and expression of the β chain gene permits the thymocyte to progress to the next stage of development. Targeted disruptions of the β chain locus or the RAG genes in mice, both of which would prohibit successful endogenous β chain gene rearrangement and expression, result in mice whose thymuses consist primarily of cells blocked at this stage of development[58, 60]; breeding these mice to mice that are transgenic for a rearranged TCR β chain gene releases this block and permits further development.[61]

For many years, the lack of a good in vitro model system to study early thymopoiesis hindered the analysis of the DN population in humans. The SCID-hu mouse system[41] and the human fetal thymus organ culture system[64] have proved useful in overcoming these handicaps. Comparing human DN thymocyte development with that of the mouse is also complicated by the lack of expression of CD25 at this stage in humans. Nonetheless, a developmental pathway for human DN thymocytes has been delineated by use of the expression of the CD34, CD44, CD2, CD45RO, and CD45RA molecules and cytoplasmic expression of the individual chains of the CD3 complex. The earliest intrathymic precursor is believed to be the CD34$^+$ CD44^{int} lin$^-$ population.[45, 49, 50, 52, 65] This population then upregulates CD7 expression and maintains cytoplasmic expression of the CD3 chains.[45, 50, 65] Although it has been argued that CD7 is an early T lineage marker even in the bone marrow prothymocyte, this CD34$^+$ CD7$^+$ population may represent mostly NK cell precursors.[66] This CD34$^+$ CD44^{int} CD7$^+$ cCD3$^+$

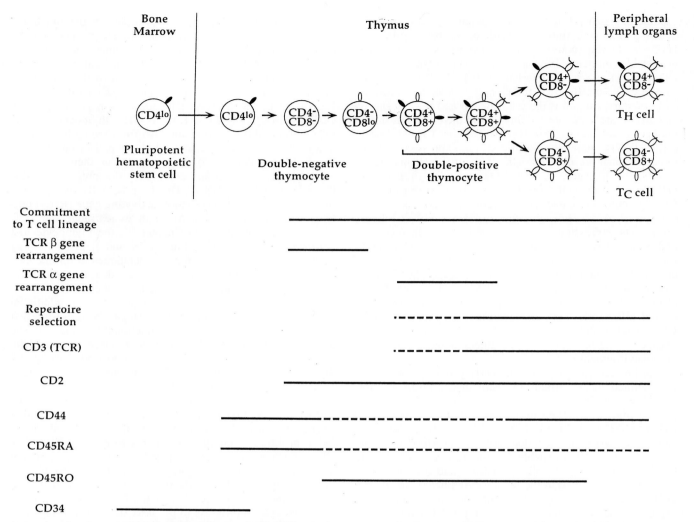

Figure 12–5. Stages of human thymocyte development. Surface expression of CD4 (black ovals), CD8 (white ovals), and the T-cell antigen receptor are indicated above. Onset and duration of important developmental events and expression of different cell surface molecules are indicated below. For cell surface marker expression, dotted line indicates low-level expression and solid line indicates high-level expression.

lin⁻ population then downregulates CD34 expression and upregulates the expression of CD44, CD2, and the 220 kDa isoform of CD45, CD45RA.[49, 52, 67–69] Unlike in the mouse, however, the precise correlation of these DN thymocyte markers with the molecular events involved in TCR gene rearrangement is not known.

Molecular Mechanisms That Drive Early Thymopoiesis

The factors and signaling pathways that control DN thymocyte development have not been characterized extensively. The cytokine IL-7 plays an important role in the maintenance of viability of the DN population, which in turn permits the DN thymocyte to proliferate and mature.[70, 71] Mice with homozygous targeted disruptions of the IL-7 and IL-7R genes have significant reductions in thymus and peripheral lymphoid tissue cellularity, consistent with this hypothesis.[72, 73] Two non-receptor protein tyrosine kinases, p50ᶜˢᵏ and p56ˡᶜᵏ, also play important roles in DN development; targeted disruptions of the genes encoding both Csk and Lck lead to

a profound developmental block in the DN compartment after commitment to the T-cell lineage.[74, 75] Furthermore, genetic experiments have demonstrated that Lck, in addition to its role in mature T-cell activation (see Chapter 13), also plays an important role in late DN thymocyte development in the control of β chain gene rearrangement.[76–79] Because progression of the DN thymocyte to the double-positive (DP) cell requires TCR β chain gene rearrangement, any factors that induce gene rearrangement are required for progression of the committed DN thymocyte to the DP stage; for example, the proper expression and function of the RAG proteins required for gene rearrangement are required for proper DP development.

As in all developmental signaling pathways, the ultimate targets of signaling molecules are transcription factors that alter the gene expression program in the precursor thymocyte, thus enabling it to express genes characteristic of the more mature phenotype. Targeted disruptions and RAG blastocyst chimera experiments have indicated a role for three transcription factors at different stages of early T-lymphocyte development. Ikaros is important for the development of the earliest lymphocyte precursor[80, 81] and GATA-3 for development of the T-cell precursor,[82] although as discussed in Chapter 3, both of these factors mediate development of the precursor before it seeds the thymus. Interestingly, experiments using c-Myb$^{-/-}$/RAG-1$^{-/-}$ chimeric mice have demonstrated that c-Myb is required for the commitment of the oligopotent stem cell in the thymus to the T-cell lineage, indicating that this factor may be playing a critical role in the actual T-cell fate determination process.[83] Genetic experiments have also determined that the loss of both T-cell factor-1 (TCF-1) and leukocyte enhancer factor-1 (LEF-1) in combination leads to a developmental block at the immature CD3$^-$ CD4$^-$ CD8^{low} stage, the immediate precursor to the DP population; TCR gene rearrangement was detected, indicating that these factors are not mediating the rearrangement process per se but are in and of themselves important for this stage of development.[83a]

▼ CELL EXPANSION AND DEATH IN THE CD4$^+$ CD8$^+$ POPULATION

Once the murine thymocyte has successfully rearranged and expressed the TCR β chain, it immediately begins expression first of CD8, becoming the CD4$^-$ CD8^{low} CD3$^-$ thymocyte, and then of CD4, becoming the CD4$^+$ CD8$^+$ CD3$^-$ thymocyte[84] (see Fig. 12–5). Thymocytes expressing both CD4 and CD8 are DP cells. These cells make up 80 to 90 per cent of all thymocytes and are found primarily in the cortex of the thymus.[54, 55] The DP thymocyte then rearranges the α chain genes of the TCR and, should the rearrangement be successful, expresses the complete TCR on its surface for the first time.[85, 86] Thus, the DP population within the thymus is actually heterogeneous, including, for example, cells that can be distinguished by their levels of expression of TCR/CD3. CD3$^{-/low}$ DP cells constitute the majority of the DP thymocytes; the remainder are CD4$^+$ CD8$^+$ CD3$^+$ thymocytes.[53, 86] About a quarter of the DP thymocytes are large, dividing cells. Although these cells represent only the last few divisions in a long period of expansion starting in the DN stage (see Fig. 12–4), they are by far the most numerous dividing cells in the thymus.[11] The remaining three quarters of the DP thymocytes are small G$_0$ cell products of these terminal divisions and do not divide further.[87] Using kinetic labeling experiments, Shortman and colleagues[11] have determined that there is a 50-fold expansion of the DP thymocyte population above the input from the DN population. Most of these cells have a 3-day life span after the last division; because the emigration rate of mature T cells from the thymus corresponds to only 1 to 5 per cent of thymocyte production,[12] these data indicate that the majority of the DP thymocytes are fated to die at the end of their 3-day life span.

What is the nature of this cell death? Remember that one of the most critical roles of the thymus is selectively to expand thymocyte precursors that express TCRs of appropriate MHC and antigen specificities and to delete all useless thymocytes. The rearrangement process that generates the sequence diversity in the genes that encode the TCR is essentially random. Thus, at the start of the selection process, the thymus is confronted with immature DP thymocytes expressing TCRs with a wide variety of antigenic specificities, most of which are either useless or autoreactive. The

process whereby the right T cells are selected to grow and the wrong T cells are killed off is called repertoire selection.[88, 89] During this period, thymocytes that can recognize peptides bound to MHC molecules are permitted to survive, in a process referred to as positive selection[90]; however, thymocytes that recognize self antigens are deleted, in a process referred to as negative selection.[91] Finally, there are selection processes that somehow correlate coreceptor molecule expression with the specificity of the TCR, that is, all T cells that recognize antigen presented on MHC class II molecules must also express CD4, whereas all T cells that recognize antigen presented on MHC class I molecules must also express CD8.[92, 93] Because of the randomness of the gene rearrangement process, most of the DP thymocytes contain unsuccessfully rearranged α chain genes or fail the selection process. It is therefore not surprising that this extensive screening process is reflected in massive thymic cell death.

Interestingly, most thymic lymphomas originate in cells of either the CD4$^-$ CD8^{low} CD3$^-$ or the CD4$^+$ CD8$^+$ CD3$^-$ developmental stages. Although the actual surface phenotype of the lymphomas is generally CD4$^-$ CD8$^-$, TCR gene rearrangement analysis as well as expression of other markers usually identifies these cells as being from these more mature stages. The reasons for the predominance of tumors from these populations are unknown. However, a significant number of selection events occur at these stages, the majority of which will result in the induction of death in the thymocyte. In addition, genomic rearrangements to generate the TCR are an integral part of these stages of development. Although both of these processes are strictly controlled, owing to their fundamental nature, it is perhaps not surprising that when they go awry, transformation can result.

▼ THE TCR-MEDIATED REPERTOIRE SELECTION PROCESS

Selection of the TCR repertoire has always been puzzling from a conceptual viewpoint because of its contradictory nature.[89] Because of the dual requirements of TCR specificity, thymocytes attempting to navigate the shoals of selection must steer between the Scylla of the loss of self MHC restriction and the Charybdis of autoreactivity. Genes encoding MHC molecules are polymorphic, and T cells are capable of making fine distinctions between self MHC molecules and closely related non-self MHC molecules. The thymus nurtures only those T cells that can recognize antigen bound to self MHC molecules.[92] However, surviving thymocytes that have high affinity for self MHC are likely to be autoreactive and therefore must be eliminated. To achieve this balance, the thymocytes are believed to undergo a TCR-based selection process based on the affinity of the TCR for self peptide/MHC complexes expressed by thymic APCs.[89, 94–96] Positive selection permits all thymocytes that express TCRs that recognize MHC and self peptide to develop. T cells that express TCRs that do not recognize MHC molecules will die of neglect. Thymocytes that express TCRs that have high affinity for self MHC are then deleted during negative selection. The surviving T cells express TCRs that weakly recognize self MHC/peptide combinations. This model for T-cell selection has several attractive aspects.

First, it provides a mechanism whereby T cells can be selected to recognize yet not react to self MHC/peptide complexes. In addition, it provides a mechanism through which the immune system can select for T cells expressing TCRs that recognize only antigen bound to self MHC molecules. Once in the periphery, the T cell recognizes its cognate antigen bound to self MHC; the differences between the antigenic peptide and the self peptide used for thymic selection presumably are sufficient to increase the affinity of the T cell for the MHC/peptide complex, thus leading to activation.

Expression of cell surface molecules on both the T cell and the APC is also important for the selection process. On the T cell, in addition to the TCR, signaling from the CD4 and CD8 coreceptors affects the selection process in several ways.[53, 91, 97] First, signaling from the coreceptor is an integral part of the selection signal that is transmitted from the TCR complex.[98] For example, increased signaling from CD8 increases the overall signal from the TCR complex, resulting in the deletion of thymocytes bearing self MHC–restricted TCRs that normally pass negative selection.[99, 100] In addition, the coreceptors are required to convey the appropriate MHC class specificity of the TCR[101]; deletion of CD4 in the germline leads to a mature T-cell population devoid of MHC class II–restricted T cells,[102] whereas deletion of CD8 leads to a similar lack of MHC class I–restricted T cells.[103] On the APC, the MHC is of course critical. Germline deletion of MHC class II molecules leads to defective development of the CD4 single-positive (SP) T_H population.[104, 105] For example, in patients with bare lymphocyte syndrome, a mutation in a transcription factor inhibits the expression of MHC class II molecules on all APCs, resulting in decreased numbers of CD4 SP T_H cells in the periphery and profound immunosuppression.[106] Similarly, deletion of MHC class I molecules leads to defective development of CD8 SP T_C cells.[107, 108] Thus, the expression of the appropriate MHC molecules on thymic APCs is required for proper development of mature SP T-cell populations.

Molecular Events That Drive Thymic Selection

Much work has been done to characterize the molecular pathways that are used by the thymocyte to transmit signals during the selection process.[76] Interestingly, most of the signaling pathways identified in determining T-cell lineage fate in the thymus are the homologous pathways to those initially identified in cell fate determination in lower eukaryotes. As expected, the tyrosine kinase Lck plays an important role in transmitting signals from the CD4 and CD8 coreceptor molecules during selection.[74, 77, 109, 110] Mouse genetic experiments have also demonstrated a critical role for the Ras-mediated signaling pathway in the thymic selection process. Different branches of the Ras-mediated signaling pathway appear to be critical for positive and negative selection.[111] Transcription factors that are targets of the mitogen-activated protein kinase pathway, such as the Ets family proteins, are known to bind to the transcriptional control elements of genes that encode proteins important in T-cell development, including the CD4, TCRα, and TCRβ genes,[112–114] supporting the hypothesis that this pathway plays an important role in T-cell fate decisions. Mouse genetic

experiments have also implicated the Notch signaling pathway in thymopoiesis.[115] Indeed, the human homologue of *Notch-1*, referred to as *TAN1*, was first identified as a common chromosomal breakpoint in T-cell leukemias.[116] Although a transcription factor target of the Notch pathway is one of several factors to bind to and mediate the function of a critical transcriptional silencer required for proper CD4 gene expression,[117–119] the precise role of this pathway in T-cell lineage decisions is much less clear and awaits the results of further experiments.

Few transcription factors have been demonstrated to be important for mediating the thymic selection signaling processes. However, a novel transcription factor has been identified that is localized in different subcellular compartments during thymopoiesis.[119] This factor, referred to as silencer-associated factor (SAF), was initially described as being important in the repression of CD4 transcription. In DP thymocytes, SAF is localized primarily in the cytoplasm, whereas in CD8 SP T cells, SAF is localized to the nucleus. These data led to the hypothesis that the translocation of SAF from the cytoplasm to the nucleus during the DP to CD8 SP thymocyte transition may help mediate the differentiation of the pluripotent DP thymocyte to the CD8 SP T-cell lineage.[119] Further delineation of the function of SAF is therefore likely to be important in the characterization of the signaling events that mediate thymic selection.

▼ T-CELL LINEAGE FATE DECISIONS AND THE ACQUISITION OF MATURE T-CELL FUNCTION

The mechanism through which the specificity of the TCR on the thymocyte is correlated with coreceptor expression and, to a significant extent, mature T-cell function is one of the most debated questions in the thymic development field.[93] As discussed above, the exclusive expression of the CD4 or CD8 coreceptor on mature T cells correlates with T-cell specificity and function. Thus, $CD4^+$ $CD8^-$ T cells recognize only antigen bound to MHC class II molecules and are primarily T_H cells, whereas $CD4^-$ $CD8^+$ T cells recognize only antigen bound to MHC class I molecules and are primarily T_C cells. Three general models have been proposed to explain this correlation (Fig. 12–6). The instructional hypothesis proposes that the specificity of the TCR expressed on the DP thymocyte directly determines the fate of that cell.[120] A DP thymocyte that expresses a TCR capable of recognizing MHC class II receives a signal on TCR/CD4-MHC interaction, causing it to downregulate CD8 and differentiate toward the CD4 SP lineage. Similarly, thymocytes expressing TCRs that recognize MHC class I, on TCR/CD8-MHC interaction, transmit a signal that causes the downregulation of CD4 and commitment to the CD8 SP lineage pathway. Thus, positive selection is directly linked to the T-cell lineage decision, and no mature SP T cell will express an inappropriately restricted "mismatched" TCR. A second model proposes that downregulation of the CD4 or CD8 coreceptor molecule and subsequent differentiation to either SP lineage is a random event that occurs just before and independently of selection and irrespective of the MHC class specificity of the TCR.[121, 122] This model, referred to as the stochastic or selection model, predicts that the DP thymocyte will randomly cease expression of either CD4 or CD8.

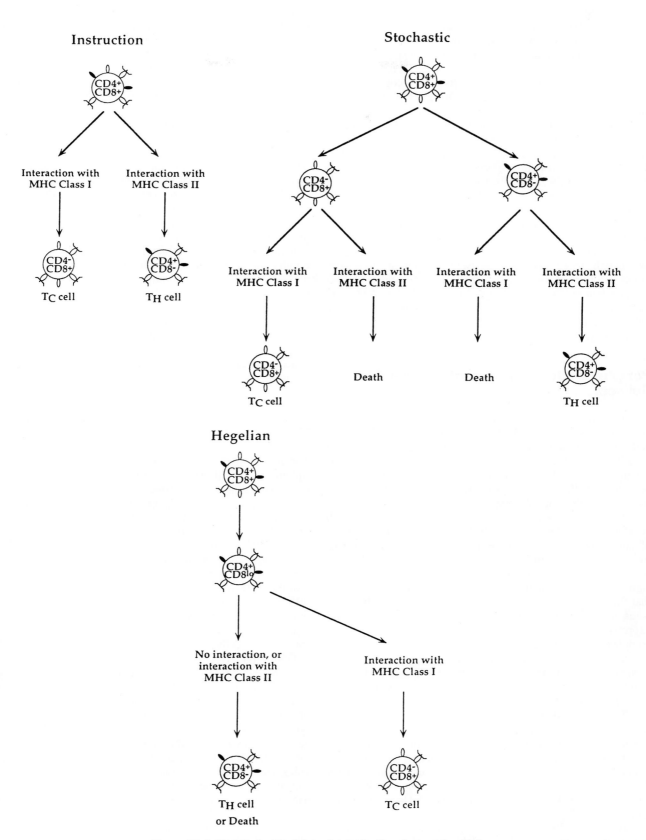

Figure 12–6. Models for T-cell fate determination. See text for details.

Resulting SP thymocytes that fortuitously bear TCRs that recognize MHC class II molecules and coexpress CD4 or TCRs that recognize MHC class I molecules and coexpress CD8 will receive a survival signal during positive selection and will differentiate to become mature SP T cells. Alternatively, SP thymocytes that bear TCRs that recognize MHC class II molecules and coexpress CD8 or TCRs that recognize MHC class I molecules and coexpress CD4, that is, mismatched receptors, will not receive the survival signal and will thus die in the thymus. Proponents of a third model took a Hegelian approach by developing a new synthesis that incorporates major aspects of each of the first two models.[123–125] In the default/instructive model, the DP thymocyte commits to a CD4+ CD8low stage. At this point, the thymocyte may receive a signal directing the cell to differentiate to the CD8 SP lineage or receive no signal, whereupon the thymocyte will continue to develop as a CD4 SP cell.

Although many experiments have been conducted to distinguish between these models, the issues are still very much in doubt. Until full details of the molecular mechanisms whereby TCR-based signaling is linked to CD4 and CD8 gene expression and to mature T-cell fate decisions are delineated, this topic will continue to generate significant controversy.

Peripheral Development of Mature T-Cell Subsets

The thymic selection and development process outlined above results in the production of CD4 SP and CD8 SP T cells that emigrate from the thymus to seed the peripheral lymph organs. These T cells must continue to undergo critical developmental and selective processes in the periphery both to gain their ultimate effector functions and to refine their role in the immune response.

The newly developed peripheral CD4 or CD8 SP T cell is referred to as the naive T cell. In mice, this cell is capable of surviving for at least several months in the absence of overt antigen exposure.[126, 127] Because the average life span of a mouse is approximately 18 months, this represents a significant portion of the life span of the animal, indicating that there are large reserves of mature long-lived T lymphocytes available in the peripheral lymph organs. This cell expresses on its cell surface, in addition to the TCR/CD3 complex and either the CD4 or CD8 coreceptor molecules, several molecules that are important for the naive T cell to home to tissues in the periphery. These molecules include the lymph node homing receptor CD62L, CD45RA, CD45RB, CD45RC, and, at lower levels, the integrin very late antigen-4 (VLA-4), CD44, and CD43.[128] After recognizing its cognate antigen, the naive T cell develops into mature effector T cells, which are more specialized functionally and thus better able to respond to antigenic challenge. For activated T cells, the pattern of cell surface molecule expression for the homing molecules reverses: these cells downregulate CD62L and CD45 and upregulate CD44, CD43, and VLA-4 expression.[128–132]

Helper T cells can be further subdivided into two functional subclasses: T$_H$1 cells, which respond to intracellular pathogens by activating the macrophage/monocyte response, and T$_H$2 cells, which respond to ingested extracellular antigens by activating naive antigen-specific B cells and thus initiating the humoral immune response.[133, 134] These functional subclasses are distinguishable phenotypically by the patterns of lymphokines that they secrete. T$_H$1 cells release interferon-γ (IFN-γ), IL-2, and lymphotoxin; as discussed below, these lymphokines are important in recruiting and stimulating macrophages and monocytes. Thus, T$_H$1 cells play an important role in all cell-mediated immune responses, such as delayed-type hypersensitivity, graft rejection, and direct cytoxicity. In contrast, T$_H$2 cells release IL-4, IL-5, IL-10, and IL-13; these lymphokines are important in stimulating B cells, and thus these cells play an important role in the generation of the humoral immune response.

The first encounter of naive T cells with their cognate antigen results in two major effector responses.[135] First, this encounter results in the primary immune response, that is, the initial development of a pool of lymphocytes that specifically recognize the antigen and are capable of responding rapidly and effectively. This causes the rapid proliferation of naive T$_H$ cells and their subsequent development into the two specialized functional subclasses. Second, the initial encounter generates immunological memory, which provides protection from subsequent challenge by the same pathogen. I discuss immunological memory in a later section; here, I discuss how naive T cells further develop into functional subclasses, each of which plays a distinct and critical role in the immune response.

▼ MOLECULAR EVENTS IN THE ACTIVATION OF NAIVE T CELLS

The initiation of adaptive immune responses occurs in peripheral lymphoid tissues, where migrating naive T cells first recognize antigen.[136] As discussed in greater detail in Chapter 13, T cells must be exposed to two types of stimulus to become activated. First, the TCR and the appropriate CD4 or CD8 coreceptor molecule must recognize its cognate antigen/MHC complex. The second signal required for T-cell activation includes costimulators and cytokines that promote clonal expansion of the specific T cells and their differentiation into effector and memory cells.[137–139] This second signal differs between naive and effector cells; naive T cells require the ligation of cell surface receptors with their cognate ligands on the APCs.[140] The best-characterized costimulators for naive T cells are the members of the B7 family: B7-1 (CD80) and B7-2 (CD86).[141] The CD28 receptors on T cells recognize the B7-1 molecule during T-cell antigen recognition and deliver critical regulatory signals to the T cell.[138, 142] This leads to the expression in activated T cells of antiapoptotic factors of the Bcl family as well as of lymphokines such as IL-2. Differentiation from the naive T-cell pool thus requires that the T cell integrate signals from the TCR/CD3 complex, the CD4 or CD8 coreceptor molecules, and the CD28 accessory molecule. This second signal can also play a role in the deletion of mature T cells. For example, the presentation of antigen bound to MHC in the absence of the CD28/B7-1 (CD80) interaction results in anergy and, ultimately, apoptosis of the naive T cell. As mentioned above, B7-1 is a member of a family of ligands, one of which, B7-2 (CD86), is the ligand for the cytotoxic T lymphocyte–associated antigen-4 (CTLA-4) receptor.[141]

Unlike CD28, however, CTLA-4 transmits a negative signal to the T cell and is thus believed to be an important signaling pathway in inducing tolerance in potentially autoreactive mature T cells.[143]

The receptor/ligand interactions that occur when the naive T cell recognizes antigen activate a series of different signaling pathways in the T cell that ultimately result, as in thymic development, in the activation and function of transcription factors that alter its program of gene expression.[144-146] Because model systems for T-cell activation are more accessible than those for development, activation signaling pathways are far better characterized. For example, the activation of transcription of the IL-2 gene and the subsequent release of IL-2 is an important initial response when a T cell recognizes antigen. This is accomplished by use of several distinct signaling pathways. Activation of the TCR/coreceptor by antigen/MHC complexes leads to protein phosphorylation–mediated signaling through a Ras-dependent[147, 148] and a Ca^{2+}-dependent pathway.[146] These signaling events eventually lead to the activation of the nuclear factor of activated T cells (NF-AT), which binds to the promoter of the IL-2 gene and stimulates its transcription.[149] Signaling from the CD28 accessory molecule leads to the activation of the AP-1 and NF-κB transcription factors, which also bind to the IL-2 gene promoter.[150] The combined effect of all of these signals is to increase dramatically the synthesis and release of IL-2 by newly activated T cells.[151] Although similar effects are observed with the transcription of other genes important for T-cell activation, including the IL-2R itself, TCR-mediated induction of the IL-2 gene is one of the most important events in early T-cell activation, because the release of IL-2 by the T cell plays a critical role in mobilizing the immune response. The importance of IL-2 gene activation is underscored by the common clinical use of immunosuppressive drugs that target this specific pathway. For example, both cyclosporin A and FK-506 inhibit IL-2 production by blocking the TCR-mediated Ca^{2+}-dependent signaling pathway, preventing the activation of NF-AT.[152-154] Of course, these drugs inhibit the activation of all T cells, regardless of antigenic specificity, and thus, despite their success and common current usage, much work is being conducted to develop drugs that act specifically to inhibit antigen-specific T-cell responses.

▼ DEVELOPMENT OF HETEROGENEOUS T_H CELL SUBSETS

Activation of the naive T cell by antigen thus induces the cell to secrete IL-2 as well as to express the IL-2 receptor on its surface. This results in the autostimulation of the naive T cell and subsequent clonal expansion; after a few days of rapid growth, the progeny cells differentiate into effector cells that are able to synthesize all of the proteins required for their specialized functions.[155, 156] In addition, all effector cells undergo changes that distinguish them from naive T cells. For example, the initial activation requirements for the effector T cell differ significantly from those of a naive T cell. Once a T cell is differentiated into an effector cell, its activation becomes less dependent on CD28/B7-1 interactions. In addition, the T cell alters its expression of cell surface adhesion molecules that are used to target the T cell

to specific tissues; instead of expressing adhesion molecules that permit circulation to lymph nodes for antigen presentation, the effector T cell will express adhesion molecules that allow it to bind to vascular epithelium to enhance its migration to sites of infection (see Table 12–1).

The mechanisms through which a naive T cell develops into either a T_H1 or a T_H2 cell are not fully understood.[157, 158] Because the decision to differentiate into functional subclasses occurs early after antigenic challenge, the ability of pathogens to stimulate particular cytokine responses from T cells plays an important role in shaping the adaptive response.[159] It has been proposed that the precise nature of the peptide/MHC complex and the costimulatory molecules used to drive the response contribute to the development of the different T_H subclasses.[159-163] In addition, experiments in vitro have shown that CD4 cells initially stimulated in the presence of IL-12 and IFN-γ develop into T_H1 cells, in part because IL-12 enhances T_H1 development and IFN-γ inhibits T_H2 development[158, 164-171] (Fig. 12–7). Because IL-12 and IFN-γ are produced by macrophages and NK cells in the early responses to intracellular parasites, these responses tend to be dominated by T_H1 cells.[171] In contrast, CD4 T cells activated in the presence of IL-4 and IL-6 tend to differentiate toward T_H2 cells; these lymphokines stimulate T_H2 development and, in conjunction with IL-10, tend to inhibit T_H1 development[172-174] (see Fig. 12–7). Interestingly, IFN-γ and IL-2 are released by T_H1 cells in response to antigenic challenge, whereas IL-4, IL-5, and IL-10 are released by T_H2 cells. It is thus apparent that the factors that mediate a particular response will also stimulate the T cell that induces and augments that particular response and repress development of T cells that mediate other responses. This makes teleological sense—after all, if you are infected with an intracellular pathogen, mobilizing your response to serum-borne pathogens would not make much sense, and thus activation of T_H1 responses inhibits the development of the T_H2 response to prevent the body from wasting resources

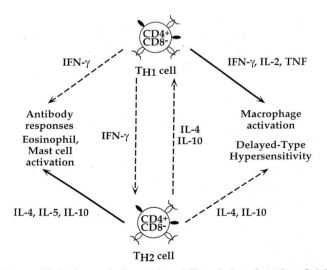

Figure 12–7. Control of peripheral T_H subclass function. Solid arrows indicate that the factors shown are stimulating a response; dotted arrows indicate inhibition of the response. Factors secreted by T_H1 cells inhibit the development and function of T_H2 cells, whereas factors secreted by T_H2 cells inhibit the development and function of T_H1 cells. See text for details.

and indirectly weakening the response against the known infecting pathogen.

▼ DEVELOPMENT OF THE CD8 SP T$_C$ CELL

Mosmann and colleagues[175, 176] have characterized two different functional subsets of cytotoxic T cells by stimulating naive T$_C$ cells in vitro: the T$_C$1 subset, which secretes IL-2 and IFN-γ; and the T$_C$2 subset, which secretes IL-4, IL-5, and IL-10. However, neither of these T$_C$ subclasses could provide cognate help for B-cell antibody production, and both induced similar inflammatory reactions in vivo.[177] It is thus unclear whether the T$_C$1 versus T$_C$2 distinction is a relevant in vivo phenomenon, and for this review I consider all mature T$_C$ cells to have the same function and phenotype. Nonetheless, like T$_H$ cells, T$_C$ cells emigrate from the thymus as naive T cells and require specific stimulatory signals to mature into functional T$_C$ cells. This initial activation step for naive CD8 SP T cells can be done in two ways. First, the naive CD8 SP T cell can be activated by an APC presenting antigen alone; the high density of costimulatory molecules on the APC can stimulate the CD8 SP T cell to secrete sufficient IL-2 to drive its own proliferation and differentiation.[178] Alternatively, the presence of CD4 SP T$_H$1 cells that have the same antigen specificity as the naive CD8 SP T cell can also drive its development to effector cytotoxic status. In this case, the T$_H$1 cell can compensate for the inadequate costimulation of the naive CD8 SP T cell by the APC.[175] This is done in several ways. First, on activation with antigen, the T$_H$1 cells secrete IL-2, which stimulates the naive CD8 SP T cell to proliferate and differentiate. Second, activated T$_H$1 cells release cytokines that stimulate APCs to increase their surface expression of costimulatory molecules.[179] Thus, development and function of the effector CD8 SP T$_C$ cell essentially require T$_H$1 function.

B-Cell Development

As for T lymphocytes, the stages of B-cell differentiation in mice and humans are marked by successive steps in the rearrangement and expression of the immunoglobulin genes as well as by changes in the expression of both cell surface and intracellular molecules. B-cell development can be divided into two phases. The first is the formation of the pre-immune B-cell repertoire, defined by successive steps of the immunoglobulin gene rearrangement process (Fig. 12–8). As discussed in Chapter 11, each mature B cell expresses only one immunoglobulin heavy chain and one light chain and thus bears receptors of only one antigenic specificity. This involves two series of gene rearrangements, the success of which determines whether further development can occur. The second phase is the subsequent formation of the mature B-cell repertoire in response to antigenic challenge. As we shall see, this process involves the collaboration of mature, activated T and B cells in specialized structures within the peripheral lymph organs.

▼ B-CELL DEVELOPMENT IN THE BONE MARROW

Immature B cells are generated initially in the fetal liver and, in the adult, almost exclusively in the bone marrow.[180]

Early B-cell precursors first contact stromal cells in the subendosteum of the bone marrow, directly adjacent to the bone surface.[181–183] As maturation proceeds, the precursor B cell migrates toward the center of the marrow cavity. Later stages of B-cell development are less dependent on contact with the bone marrow stroma and can occur in either the bone marrow or the peripheral lymph organs (see below). Much like T-cell development, early B-cell development requires the interaction of a pluripotent precursor with non-lymphoid stromal cells.[184–187] The bone marrow stroma provides two essential stimuli to the developing B cell. First, adhesion molecules on the stroma interact with their ligands on the B-cell precursor, providing important adhesion contacts as well as sending differentiation signals to the precursor. For example, CD44 and the integrin VLA-4 expressed on B-cell progenitors bind to hyaluronate and fibronectin on the stromal cell, respectively[188–192]; blocking this interaction with antibodies to either CD44 or VLA-4 leads to the inhibition of early B-cell progenitor development.[189, 191, 193] Second, the bone marrow stroma expresses important growth factors required for precursor growth and development, such as the c-Kit ligand and IL-7.[37, 194–196]

As discussed before for T cells, the common lymphocyte precursor found in the bone marrow is the HSA^{low} Thy-1^{low} CD44$^+$ Sca-1$^+$ c-Kit$^+$ IL-7R$^+$ population in mice and the CD34$^+$ CD45RA$^+$ CD10$^+$ CD38$^+$ HLA$^-$ DR$^+$ lin$^-$ population in humans. The subsequent commitment of this cell to the B-cell lineage is marked by the expression of both novel cell surface molecules and intracellular proteins. The earliest stage of B-cell development is the early pro-B cell stage; in mice, this population is also referred to as the A fraction.[197, 198] These cells begin to express the RAG-1 and RAG-2 proteins and terminal deoxynucleotidyl transferase (TdT),[199, 200] which are required for proper immunoglobulin gene rearrangement. Because the pro-B cells are just beginning to express RAG-1 and RAG-2, their immunoglobulin gene loci are mostly unrearranged, although some partial D$_H$-J$_H$ rearrangements are detectable. The pro-B cell also begins to express the λ5, VpreB, Igα, and Igβ proteins,[199, 200] which are required for surface expression of the immunoglobulin heavy chain at later stages of development. In mice, the earliest pro-B cells can also be distinguished by their expression of B220 and CD43 and the lack of immunoglobulin on their surfaces[197, 199]; in humans, early pro-B cells are identified by the expression of CD10 and by the IL-7 and IL-3 receptors.[194, 201–204] The early pro-B cell then matures into a pro-B cell, which differs from the early pro-B cell in that D$_H$-J$_H$ rearrangements are detectable at the heavy chain gene loci and V$_H$-D$_H$-J$_H$ rearrangements are beginning to occur.[205, 206] In addition, the pro-B cell expresses high levels of the λ5, VpreB, Igα, and Igβ proteins as well as the RAG-1 and RAG-2 proteins and TdT. In the mouse, this population is often referred to as the B and C fractions.[182, 197, 198] The A, B, and C fractions are large, proliferating cells and thus are actively generating a large pool of precursor B cells.[197, 198] As in mice, the human pro-B cell has D$_H$-J$_H$ and some V$_H$-D$_H$-J$_H$ rearrangements and expresses high levels of the rearrangement enzymes.[205, 206] In addition, the human pro-B cell maintains expression of CD34, CD10, IL-3R, and IL-7R and begins to express CD19 and CD40 and, eventually, CD73, CD22, CD24, and CD38.[203, 204, 207–210]

Successful rearrangement and expression of the immunoglobulin heavy chain genes permits the pro-B cell to

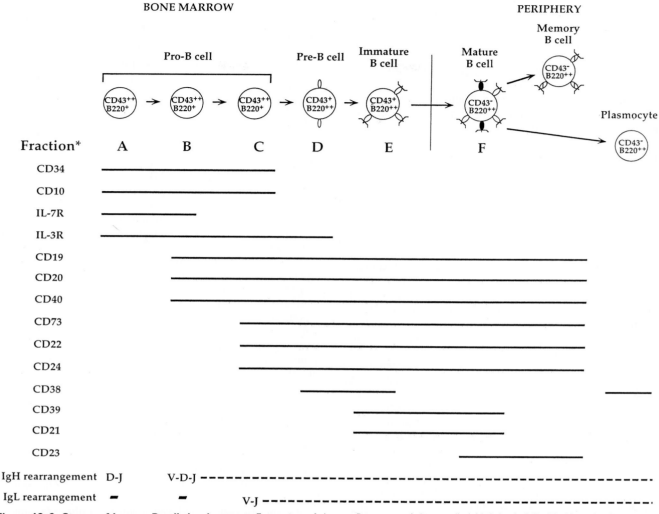

Figure 12–8. Stages of human B-cell development. Expression of the pre-B receptor (white oval), IgM (white), IgD (black), and other isotypes (striped) is indicated above. The B-cell fraction is based on CD43 and B220 surface expression and is defined in the mouse; the pro-B and pre-B cell stages shown are believed to be the homologous human B-cell populations. One set of immunoglobulin heavy chain (IgH) and light chain (IgL) gene rearrangement is indicated; dotted line indicates that the locus is fully rearranged after the indicated step and is not meant to indicate ongoing rearrangement of the locus.

mature further into the pre-B cell. Several important developmental events occur at this stage. First, the complete immunoglobulin heavy chain (IgH) is expressed in the endoplasmic reticulum and, at low levels, on the cell surface associated with the λ5, VpreB, Igα, and Igβ proteins as the pre-B cell receptor.[199, 211, 212] The surface expression of the pre-B cell receptor complex is essential for further development. In mice, mutations that prevent the expression of the pre-B cell receptor on the cell surface or inhibit its ability to transmit signals lead to significant impairment of B-cell development and loss of heavy chain allelic exclusion.[213–216] Second, as noted in Chapter 11, light chain gene rearrangement begins and TdT expression decreases. The successful rearrangement of the immunoglobulin light chain is required for the pre-B cell both to express immunoglobulin and to develop further. In the mouse, surface CD43 expression drops significantly, as does surface expression of c-Kit[195, 197]; in humans, pre-B cells downregulate expression of CD34 and CD10 and upregulate expression of CD21.[203,]

[204, 209] Third, the pre-B cell stops proliferating, and thus it is much smaller than the pro-B cells. In the mouse, this fraction is referred to as fraction D.[182, 197]

Once successful light chain rearrangement occurs, the pre-B cell expresses the complete immunoglobulin on its surface and becomes the immature B cell.[217] The surface immunoglobulin at this stage is of the μ isotype; all other heavy chain isotypes are expressed only on the surface of more mature B cells.[217] The immature B cell downregulates expression of IL-7R and CD43 as well as of the λ5 and VpreB proteins. Interestingly, RAG-2 expression is still maintained in these cells, indicating that this population may still be able to rearrange immunoglobulin genes.[200] This population is referred to as fraction E.[182, 197] In humans, the immature B cell downregulates CD38 but maintains expression of all other pre-B cell markers.[203, 204, 209] At this point, the developing B cell migrates to the peripheral lymph organs, where it first expresses surface Igδ and becomes fully immunocompetent.

Molecular Events in B-Cell Development

Predictably, many of the molecules that are important for T-cell development are also important in B-cell development; and, as for T cells, most of the identified factors affect either very early or very late stages of development. Many of these factors are required for the proper assembly of the B-cell receptor. For example, as for the T-cell receptor genes, the deficiencies in factors required for generating the immunoglobulin genes inhibit the development of pre-B cells.[58, 60] Deficiencies of the pre-B cell receptor components lead to failure of the transport of the rearranged immunoglobulin to the cell surface, which in turn also leads to a block just before the pre-B cell stage.[213] In addition, IL-7 and the IL-7R are both required for early pro-pre-B cell development; as for T cells, IL-7 is likely to be serving a survival and maintenance role to keep the precursor alive for subsequent developmental events.[72] The Ras signaling pathway also appears to be critical in generating pro-pre-B cells, leading to the hypothesis that components of the IL-7R signaling pathway may intersect with Ras-mediated pathways.[218] In addition, the receptor tyrosine kinases c-Kit and Flk2/Flt3 have been shown to act with IL-7 to induce pro-B cell growth.[71, 219] However, as for T cells, how these different molecules interact to mediate B-cell development is still a topic of much research.

Much is known about the factors and molecules that drive B lymphopoiesis. Pax-5/BSAP is essential for the development of the pre-B cell lineage. Interestingly, although full V_H-D-J_H rearrangements do not occur, partial D_H-J_H rearrangements are detectable, indicating that as for TCF-1 and LEF-1 in T-cell development, Pax-5/BSAP is important in mediating this specific stage of development instead of the gene rearrangement process. In addition, transcription factors of the basic helix-loop-helix (bHLH) family play an important role in both B-cell development and oncogenesis. Targeted disruption of the E2A locus, which encodes the E box–binding factors, leads to an early block at the pro-B cell stage[220, 221]; indeed, the gene products from this locus bias precursor cells to the B-cell lineage.[222] However, transgenic mice that overexpress dominant negative inhibitors of bHLH proteins also lead to the inhibition of B-cell as well as T-cell development,[223, 224] indicating that the balance of bHLH protein levels as opposed to the absolute level of any one bHLH protein may be critical in maintaining B-cell homeostasis.

▼ PERIPHERAL B-CELL DEVELOPMENT: GENERATION OF THE ANTIBODY RESPONSE

In the mouse, there are approximately 1×10^8 B cells in the peripheral immune system, most of which are mature B cells that express both IgM and IgD on their surfaces.[183, 195, 198] Mature IgM$^+$ IgD$^+$ B cells are constantly circulating between the lymph, the blood, and the peripheral lymph organs, in the process screening the body for the presence of antigen. In the peripheral lymph organs, the mature B cells are found primarily in follicles and the splenic marginal zone. Marginal zone B cells are predominantly long-lived, non-dividing cells that express complement receptors 1 and 2 (CR1/CR2; CD21/CD35). Although some marginal zone B cells are memory B cells, others are formed in the absence of immuni-

zation and are thus likely to be part of the preimmune repertoire. Altogether, marginal zone B cells represent 5 to 10 per cent of all splenic B cells. The follicular B cells consist mainly of small IgM$^+$ IgD$^+$ B220$^+$ CD23$^+$(CD21/CD35)$^+$ B cells[225]; for humans, this B-cell population is CD19$^+$ CD40$^+$ CD73$^+$ CD22$^+$ CD24$^+$ CD21$^+$ CD23$^+$ CD38$^+$ (see Fig. 12–8).[182, 209, 226] Once the immune system has detected the presence of foreign antigens, lymphocytes that are best suited to eliminate infecting pathogens that express those antigens are activated. For the B-lymphocyte population, the appropriate B cell is expanded selectively on the basis of the affinity of its immunoglobulin for the specific antigen. Subsequent stages of B-cell development are therefore initiated when the small mature B cell recognizes its cognate antigen and receives stimuli from T$_H$ cells.

Sequencing of complete immunoglobulins and the genes that encode them revealed that many immunoglobulins had point mutations in the V region encoding portions of their genes.[227–230] Subsequent studies identified a correlation between the increased number of these mutations and higher antigen-binding affinities of the resulting variable region[231, 232] (Fig. 12–9). Taken together, these observations led to the hypothesis that there is a process that induces point mutations in immunoglobulin variable region genes during the antigen-dependent phase of development of the immune response. This mutation process, referred to as somatic hypermutation, generates a wide variety of different variants of the same variable region. The extent of mutation and the speed at which these mutations accumulate can be extensive. Mutated immunoglobulins are first detected 7 to 10 days after the initiation of a primary immune response and continue to accumulate at least until day 18 by the stepwise introduction of one to three nucleotide substitutions, resulting in clonal genealogies that recapitulate the repeated rounds of intraclonal mutation, selection, and proliferation.[232] The advantages of this process are immense. As discussed below, the B cell is induced both to proliferate and to undergo somatic hypermutation when it is presented with antigen. This enables the body to generate many progeny B cells that express antigen-specific immunoglobulins, each with different minor sequence variations in the antigen-binding regions. B cells that express mutated immunoglobulins that are either self-reactive or less efficient at binding antigen than the original unmutated parent immunoglobulin will die. However, those B cells that express mutated immunoglobulins that bind to antigen with increased affinity are selectively expanded. This process results in the continuing generation of B cells that are progressively more efficient in the elimination of the infecting pathogen—a "fine-tuning" of the immune response, if you will. This stage of development occurs in specialized structures within the peripheral lymph organs referred to as germinal centers.[233, 234]

▼ STRUCTURE AND FUNCTION OF THE GERMINAL CENTER

The germinal center is an important site for the development of both end-stage effector and memory lymphocytes.[225, 235] The germinal center is where antigen-specific lymphocytes are driven to proliferate at high levels and, for the B cell, generate and secrete large amounts of high-affinity antibody. Mistakes at this stage have profound consequences; for ex-

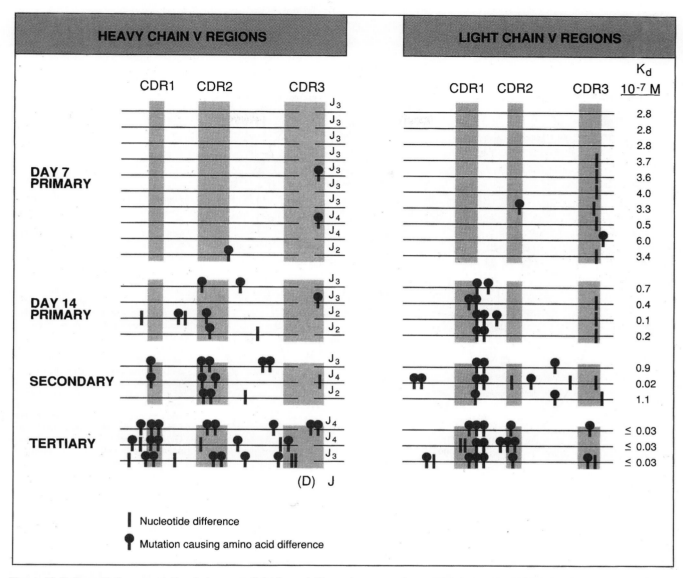

Figure 12–9. Somatic hypermutation in immunoglobulin variable region genes. Immunoglobulins were isolated and sequenced from the spleen cells of mice immunized 7 or 14 days after injection with antigen or from spleen cells obtained after secondary and tertiary immunizations with the same antigen. Affinity of the individual immunoglobulins to the antigen is indicated on the right as K_d (dissociation constant); low K_d indicates higher affinity. Note concomitant increases of the number of amino acid replacement mutations in the V gene and affinity of the immunoglobulin for antigen as the immune response matures. CDR, complementarity-determining regions (or hypervariable regions), the antigen contact region of the immunoglobulins. (From Abbas, A.K., Lichtman, A.H., and Pober, J.S.: Cellular and Molecular Immunology, 2nd ed. Philadelphia, W.B. Saunders, 1994, p. 88.)

ample, an unstimulated immature autoreactive B cell is not likely to cause much trouble, but the situation could turn critical if this B cell is stimulated to produce large quantities of autoreactive antibody in the germinal center. Thus, the germinal center is important both in activating the immune response and in providing a final selection step to delete autoreactive lymphocytes.

The germinal center begins to form when the B cell first encounters antigen and its cognate T cell in the periarteriolar lymphoid sheaths of the peripheral lymphoid tissues[235, 236] (Fig. 12–10). Once activated, the mature B cell proliferates and subsequently either develops locally into a focus of antibody-secreting B cells or migrates to a pre-existing follicle. Once established in a follicle, progeny from the dividing B cell accumulate within an extensive network consisting of the processes of follicular dendritic cells (FDCs). The germi-

nal center reaction is initiated when the antigen-primed B cell comes into contact with FDCs that bear antigen/antibody and antigen/complement complexes.[237] These FDCs are capable of retaining these antigen-containing complexes on their surfaces for a long time and thus act as reservoirs of antigen that sustain both the germinal center reaction and B-cell memory.[238] The B cell rapidly proliferates and acquires new phenotypic characteristics, including the binding of peanut agglutinin and the expression of an epitope recognized by the GL-7 antibody.[239] This early phase of the germinal center reaction compresses the surrounding uninvolved follicular cells to form a mantle zone surrounding the new germinal center, also known as a secondary follicle.

Immediately after its formation, the germinal center polarizes to form a dark zone proximal to the T-cell area and a more distal light zone.[240] The dark zone contains

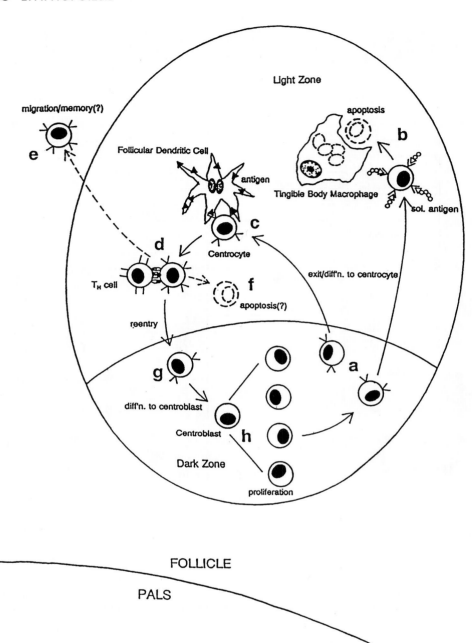

Light Zone

migration/memory(?)

e

apoptosis

b

Follicular Dendritic Cell

antigen

Tingible Body Macrophage

sol. antigen

c

Centrocyte

d

exit/diff'n. to centrocyte

T$_H$ cell

f

apoptosis(?)

reentry

g

a

diff'n. to centroblast

Centroblast

h

Dark Zone

proliferation

Figure 12–10. The germinal center reaction. The reaction is initiated with the migration of dark zone B cells to the light zone (a). These non-dividing mIg$^+$ B cells, now referred to as centrocytes, undergo apoptosis on binding soluble antigen (b) and are removed by macrophages. Centrocytes expressing high-affinity antibodies that recognize antigen bound to FDCs internalize the antigen (c) and present it to T$_H$ cells, where contact-dependent signals necessary for survival and differentiation are interchanged (d). Failed T/B interactions result in apoptosis and removal of the dead cells (f); successful T/B collaboration leads to either the peripheral migration of memory B cells (e) or a return to the dark zone for another round of proliferation as mIg$^-$ centroblasts. (From Han, S.H., Zheng, B., Takahashi, Y., and Kelsoe, G.: Distinctive characteristics of germinal center B cells. Semin. Immunol. 9:255–260, 1997.)

FOLLICLE

PALS

rapidly dividing B cells that provide most of the cells in the dark zone. The light zone consists of non-dividing B cells, the bulk of the FDC network, and T$_H$ cells. Cell labeling studies have shown that newly replicated B cells originate in the dark zone of the germinal center and migrate to the light zone. Conversely, B cells in the light zone can also re-enter the dark zone and resume proliferation; these cyclic migrations stimulate repeated rounds of replication of the B cell, leading to the development of the memory B cell (see below) as well as to the induction of somatic hypermutation.[241–244] As described above, this leads to the steady accumulation of mutations in the immunoglobulin variable regions and to the concomitant proliferation of those B cells that express mutant variants of the original immunoglobulin

that bind to antigen with increasing affinity.[245] Although the precise mechanism of this process is still unclear, the most likely model is based on the hypothesis that the B cell is stimulated by its cognate antigen on the FDC in the dark zone of the germinal center and is stimulated both to grow and to collect mutations in its V gene. Those few progeny B-cell clones that sustain mutations that increase the affinity of their immunoglobulin for antigen proliferate faster and ultimately migrate to the light zone, where they are induced to secrete immunoglobulin by T$_H$ cells; the remaining progeny of the original B-cell clone die in the dark zone.[246] The light zone B cells then re-enter the dark zone, and the process is repeated. Thus, with repeated cycles, a hierarchy of mutations accumulates in the variable region gene, each of which serves to increase the affinity of the immunoglobulin for its antigen, until a single variant that binds to antigen at an extremely high affinity is obtained. In addition to the somatic hypermutation process, the activated mature B cell undergoes isotype switch recombination.[217, 228] In this process, a DNA recombination event juxtaposes the gene encoding different constant region isotypes to the rearranged variable region gene, deleting the intervening DNA. Because the different constant regions are capable of different effector functions, this process enables the body to generate antigen-specific immunoglobulins that are capable of performing specialized functions. For example, because of its multivalency, IgM is efficient at fixing complement, whereas IgE binds to FcE receptors on mast cells and basophils, thus providing an important component of allergic responses.

The germinal center/antigen-affinity model for B-cell development correlates well with what is known about the nature of the antibody response to antigen and the physiology of germinal center formation. First, many antibody responses are dominated by immunoglobulins that are encoded by variants of only one variable region gene.[247] This is predicted by the somatic hypermutation model, because one would expect that only a fraction of the mutations would increase the affinity of the variable region for antigen sufficiently such that the B cell will initiate the germinal center process and predominate after repeated cycles of mutation and selection.[230] Second, sequencing studies of hypermutations in immunoglobulin genes have demonstrated that these mutations accumulate gradually, concomitant with the formation and growth of the germinal center.[245, 248, 249] Specific B-cell clones that contain somatic mutations can be identified in the dark zones of germinal centers, and at later stages of the immune response, B-cell clones in the dark zone of the germinal center have increased amounts of mutations in their variable region genes.[245] These observations are thus consistent with the hypothesis that the germinal center plays an important role in the generation of a high-affinity immunoglobulin response to antigen.

▼ TOLERANCE INDUCTION DURING B-CELL DEVELOPMENT

Much the same as for T cells, the developing B-cell population undergoes ligand-mediated negative selection to delete B cells that express autoreactive antibodies. Complete B-cell tolerance is the result of a series of selection events that occur at different stages of development. The earliest selection event occurs in the bone marrow, where the deletion of autoreactive B cells is accomplished by at least two different mechanisms, depending on the nature of the antigen and the intensity and duration of antigenic exposure.[250–252] High-valency self antigens, that is, antigens that have many epitopes, induce the immature autoreactive B cell to stop differentiating. The autoreactive B cell then undergoes immediate cell death in a process referred to as clonal deletion.[251–253] The molecular mechanism for clonal deletion is still unclear; experiments in vivo and in vitro have implicated a role for the antiapoptotic factor Bcl-2 in this process.[254–259] Immature B cells in the bone marrow can also be rendered inactive when they encounter soluble antigen of low valency. Although these non-responsive cells still express IgM, much

of it is retained in the cytoplasm and not transported to the cell surface. In addition, signal transduction through surface immunoglobulin is blocked such that the remaining surface immunoglobulin is incapable of transmitting a full signal to the B cell. This state of non-reactivity is referred to as anergy.[252] Ultimately, these anergic B cells migrate to the peripheral lymph organs, where they eventually are eliminated during competition for antigen with other B cells.

A second major B-cell tolerance checkpoint occurs during the initiation of the mature B-cell response in the secondary lymph organ. Naive B cells compete for entry into the follicle during the initial stages of the germinal center reaction.[260] B cells that successfully compete for a niche in the follicle undergo the FDC-dependent activation and proliferation process; those that are excluded fail to proliferate and eventually die owing to either the lack of stimulation or the removal of extracellular signals required for continued survival. As discussed above, the activated B cell in the germinal center reaction requires cell/cell contact with both cognate T_H cells in the light zone and FDCs in the dark zone to continue development.[237] Loss of either of these interactions leads to inactivation of the B cell. For example, should a mature B cell escape the bone marrow selection process expressing an immunoglobulin that cross-reacts with a self-antigen, it would still require interaction with the antigen on the FDC as well as stimulation by an activated T_H cell that reacts to the same antigen. The lack of either the antigen-charged FDC or the activated T_H cell can therefore also lead to the deletion of autoreactive B cells.

In addition to competition for follicular entry, the mature B cell can be deleted during the germinal center formation process itself.[261–264] Several groups have proposed that Fas-dependent apoptosis of germinal center B cells is the major mechanism for this selection step.[265–269] B cells that are activated normally by foreign antigen are induced to express many different costimulatory molecules on their surfaces. Signals mediated by these costimulatory molecules are believed to suppress the concomitant apoptosis signals mediated by the expression of Fas ligand on the B cell. Autoreactive B cells, however, are chronically exposed to antigen, and thus normal signaling through the antigen receptor is depressed. Under these circumstances, activation stimuli are inadequate to suppress Fas-induced apoptosis.[264, 268–272]

These observations indicate that despite the intricate selective mechanisms in the bone marrow, mature autoreactive B cells still exist in the periphery and must be eliminated to maintain self-tolerance. This is perhaps not surprising given the fact that B cells undergo somatic hypermutation in the periphery. Because somatic hypermutation generates B cells with altered specificities, it is entirely possible that novel autoreactive B cells could be generated in the germinal center reaction, and thus some mechanism for deleting these cells must exist.

Immunological Memory

Immune responses are generally followed by a state of long-lived memory during which subsequent contact with antigen leads to a more effective response than the initial primary response.[273, 274] This phenomenon, referred to as memory, is mediated by both T and B cells and is the result of both increased precursor frequency of antigen-specific lymphocytes and increased sensitivity to antigen. The proper development of memory cells is crucial for the success of vaccinations as a method for providing long-lived immunity against infections. Despite much effort, however, the mechanisms that determine and control immunological memory are still a mystery. The phenomenon of memory has been described for centuries and is not controversial. For example, Jenner's use of cowpox vaccinations to provide immunity against smallpox depended—although of course he did not know it—on the long-lived memory of his patients' immune systems. Whether memory is mediated by specific cell types that develop when a naive lymphocyte encounters antigen or by continual stimulation of short-lived effector cells by leakage of minute amounts of antigen from storage depots is yet another highly disputed topic in immunology.[275-277] Because of the significant medical implications of immunological memory, however, a discussion of this topic is warranted despite the uncertainty.

▼ NAIVE VERSUS MEMORY T-CELL CLASSES

Antigen-activated lymphocytes express a wide variety of different cell surface markers that differ from those expressed by naive lymphocytes. These include those molecules that are important for homing the lymphocyte to the correct tissues and those important for adhesion (see Table 12–1). Several of these markers are expressed on the lymphocyte for long periods after antigen activation and are thus believed to be markers for memory lymphocytes.[128-131, 134, 273, 275, 278-280] One of the more useful markers in defining mature T-cell classes is the leukocyte common antigen, or CD45.[281-284] CD45 is a highly abundant cell surface tyrosine phosphatase; as the result of alternative splicing, it comes in at least four different isoforms of 220, 205, 190, and 180 kDa.[285] The most common isoforms are defined by antibodies. In man, CD45RA antibodies immunoprecipitate the 220 kDa isoform; CD45RB antibodies immunoprecipitate the 220, 205, and 190 kDa isoforms; and the CD45RO antibodies immunoprecipitate only the 180 kDa isoform.[286] Human CD4 SP T cells were originally subdivided into two broad categories by use of the CD45RA and CD45RO antibodies.[287] CD45RA$^+$ CD4$^+$ T cells are required for the suppression of mitogen-induced CD8 SP T-cell responses and were thus termed suppresser/inducer T cells. In contrast, CD45RO$^+$ CD4$^+$ T cells respond strongly to specific recall antigens and are capable of providing help for both mitogen-driven and antigen-specific antibody responses; these cells were referred to as helper/inducer cells. Subsequent studies showed that the poor response of the CD45RA$^+$ CD4$^+$ T cells was actually the result of a low frequency of responder cells; similarly, the CD45RO$^+$ CD4$^+$ T-cell population had a much higher frequency of responders.[288] Later work demonstrated that this difference in function can be correlated to cytokine production: both populations release IL-2, but only the CD45RO$^+$ CD4$^+$ T-cell population is capable of secreting high levels of the other cytokines, including IL-4, IFN-γ, tumor necrosis factor-α, and granulocyte-monocyte colony-stimulating factor.[280, 289-291] Thus, the cytokine profiles of the two populations were consistent with the hypothesis that the CD45RA$^+$ CD4$^+$ T-cell population represented the

naive T$_H$ cells, whereas the CD45RO$^+$ CD4$^+$ T-cell population represented the memory T$_H$ cells.[292, 293] Data that cord blood contains CD45RA$^+$ CD4$^+$ T cells almost exclusively and that there is a gradual increase in the proportion of CD45RO$^+$ CD4$^+$ T cells by about 20 years of age are also consistent with this hypothesis.[294]

Although this distinction is still widely used, it is not as straightforward as was originally thought. For example, the CD45RA$^+$ CD4$^+$ and the CD45RO$^+$ CD4$^+$ T cells do not represent two stable populations; under many culture conditions, CD45RA$^+$ CD4$^+$ can be induced to alter CD45 expression to the CD45RO isoform, and vice versa.[293, 295, 296] This phenomenon has also been observed in vivo.[297, 298] It is possible that effector T cells are not end-stage cells but are capable of returning to a "memory state" after the immune system clears the antigen; however, this hypothesis flatly contradicts the concept of two functionally distinct effector and memory classes. Thus, despite data from animal systems that on balance support a functional distinction, the human in vitro data do not clearly demonstrate a precise relationship between the CD45RA$^+$ and the CD45RO$^+$ T-cell subsets.

▼ B-CELL MEMORY

The relationship between effector B cells and memory B cells is much clearer. Memory B cells differ from the activated mature B cell in many important ways.[273, 274] First, memory and effector B cells differ in expression of cell surface markers (see Fig. 12–8); for example, in humans, memory cells are CD38$^-$ CD39$^+$ CD20$^+$,[211, 294] whereas plasma cells are CD38$^+$ CD23$^-$ CD22$^-$ CD19$^-$ HLA$^-$.[209, 299-302] As discussed above, generation of the memory B cell requires multiple antigenic stimulations; this results in prolonged antibody responses that are of increased magnitude and are generated with rapid kinetics.[303] In addition, memory B cells accumulate somatic hypermutations in their variable region genes and often express immunoglobulins that have constant region isotypes other than IgM and IgD.[304-306] Finally, there are significant differences in homing and circulation patterns as well as in the longevity of the B cell itself.[307, 308] In contrast, effector B cells are end-stage plasma cells.[303] These cells do not express cell surface immunoglobulin, are much larger in size than other lymphocytes, and secrete significantly greater amounts of immunoglobulin than other classes of B cells. Plasma cells are short-lived, lasting no longer than 4 weeks, thus limiting the time in which a large amount of high-affinity immunoglobulin is secreted into the blood stream.

Memory and effector B cells are generated from the activated mature B-cell precursor during the germinal center reaction.[235, 248, 309-311] As discussed above, the activated mature B cell requires cell/cell contact both with FDCs and with T$_H$ cells to continue to proliferate and differentiate. B cells that express immunoglobulins with higher affinities are more successful in competing for antigen on the FDC; these B cells in turn present antigen to cognate T$_H$ cells in the T cell–rich marginal zone. During this T$_H$/B cell interaction, the CD40 molecule on the surface of the B cell binds to its ligand (CD40L, or CD154) on the surface of the T cell.[263] This molecule is a critical signaling molecule in the activation, expansion, and survival of B cells participating in T-dependent responses. Signaling along the CD40 pathway in germinal center B cells blocks B-cell differentiation before plasma cell formation; on withdrawal of CD40L, these cells differentiate into plasma cells.[312] These observations led several groups to hypothesize that the CD40/CD40L interaction between the germinal center B cell and the T_H cell during antigen presentation is critical in determining whether the B cell will differentiate along the memory or effector pathway.[313–316] The distinction between memory and effector B cells has important functional consequences. The effector B cell will begin to secrete large amounts of high-affinity antibody to combat the infection; because it is short-lived, the maintenance of a high-affinity antibody response requires the constant generation of effector B cells. Memory B cells undergo the cyclic migration described above for the germinal center reaction; at the end of an immune response, the memory B cell migrates to the marginal zones of the spleen, the reservoir to augment subsequent immune responses to the same antigen.[308] On rechallenge with antigen, the memory B cell will migrate into the primary follicle and reinitiate the germinal center reaction as described before, thus reestablishing the affinity maturation process as well as generating new effector B cells.

Conclusions

For many reasons, lymphocyte development has long been a major field of research for basic and clinical scientists. The multispecific nature of the lymphocyte population and its ability to recognize self versus non-self put elaborate constraints on the developmental process. The study of lymphocyte development has therefore led to significant insights concerning not only the biology of lymphocytes but also the general issue of developmental cell fate decisions. Perhaps more apropos for a practicing clinician, however, is that many autoimmune and immunodeficiency diseases are the result of inadequate lymphocyte antigen receptor repertoire selection. In addition, many of the common laboratory tests conducted to diagnose lymphomas and leukemias are designed to determine their developmental stage, which is a significant factor in treatment and prognosis. Therefore, the knowledge gained from the basic research has made a significant impact on modern medicine. However, from a philosophical viewpoint, there is another reason for appreciating lymphocyte development: despite the confusing collection of developmental stages and processes, the concept is actually simple: keep all that is useful, and delete all that is harmful.

REFERENCES

1. Lai, L., Alaverdi, N., Chen, Z., Kroese, F.G.M., Bos, N.A., and Huang, E.C.: Monoclonal antibodies to human, mouse, and rat cluster of differentiation (CD) antigens. *In* Herzenberg, L.A., Weir, D.M., Herzenberg, L.A., and Blackwell, C. (eds.): Handbook of Experimental Immunology. New York, Blackwell Science, 1997, pp. 61.1–61.37.
2. Moore, M.A., and Owen, J.J.: Experimental studies on the development of the thymus. J. Exp. Med. 126:715, 1967.
3. Kadish, J.L., and Basch, R.S.: Hematopoietic thymocyte precursors. I. Assay and kinetics of the appearance of progeny. J. Exp. Med. 143:1082, 1976.
4. Kadish, J.L., and Basch, R.S.: Hematopoietic thymocyte precursors. III. A population of thymocytes with the capacity to return ("home") to the thymus. Cell. Immunol. 30:12, 1977.
5. Marrack, P., Kushnir, E., Born, W., McDuffie, M., and Kappler, J.: The development of helper T cell precursors in mouse thymus. J. Immunol. 140:2508, 1988.
6. Shortman, K., and Wu, L.: Early T lymphocyte progenitors. Annu. Rev. Immunol. 14:29, 1996.
7. Shortman, K., Egerton, M., Spangrude, G.J., and Scollay, R.: The generation and fate of thymocytes. Semin. Immunol. 2:3, 1990.
8. Penit, C., and Vasseur, F.: Cell proliferation and differentiation in the fetal and early postnatal mouse thymus. J. Immunol. 142:3369, 1989.
9. Scollay, R., and Shortman, K.: Thymocyte subpopulations: an experimental review, including flow cytometric cross-correlations between the major murine thymocyte markers. Thymus 5:245, 1983.
10. Egerton, M., Scollay, R., and Shortman, K.: Kinetics of mature T-cell development in the thymus. Proc. Natl. Acad. Sci. USA 87:2579, 1990.
11. Egerton, M., Shortman, K., and Scollay, R.: The kinetics of immature murine thymocyte development in vivo. Int. Immunol. 2:501, 1990.
12. Scollay, R., Butcher, E., and Weissman, I.: Thymus migration: quantitative studies on the rate of migration of cells from the thymus to the periphery in mice. Eur. J. Immunol. 10:210, 1980.
13. Bevan, M., and Fink, P.: The influence of thymus H-2 antigens on the specificity of maturing killer and helper cells. Immunol. Rev. 42:3, 1978.
14. Saito, H., Kranz, D.M., Takagaki, Y., Hayday, A.C., Eisen, H.N., and Tonegawa, S.: Complete primary structure of a heterodimeric T-cell receptor deduced from cDNA sequences. Nature 309:757, 1984.
15. Kang, J.S., and Raulet, D.H.: Events that regulate differentiation of $\alpha\beta$ TCR^+ and $\gamma\delta$ TCR^+ T cells from a common precursor. Semin. Immunol. 9:171, 1997.
16. Traunecker, A., Oliveri, F., Allen, N., and Karjalainen, K.: Normal T cell development is possible without 'functional' gamma chain genes. EMBO J. 5:1589, 1986.
17. Burtrum, D.B., Kim, S., Dudley, E.C., Hayday, A.C., and Petrie, H.T.: TCR gene recombination and alpha beta–gamma delta lineage divergence: productive TCR-beta rearrangement is neither exclusive nor preclusive of gamma delta cell development. J. Immunol. 157:4293, 1996.
18. Winoto, A., and Baltimore, D.: Separate lineages of T cells expressing the alpha beta and gamma delta receptors. Nature 338:430, 1989.
19. Livak, F., Petrie, H.T., Crispe, I.N., and Schatz, D.G.: In-frame TCR delta gene rearrangements play a critical role in the alpha beta/gamma delta T cell lineage decision. Immunity 2:617, 1995.
20. Wallis, V.J., Leuchars, E., Chawlinski, S., and Davies, A.J.S.: On the sparse seeding of bone marrow and thymus in radiation chimaeras. Transplantation 19:2, 1975.
21. Scollay, R., Smith, J., and Stauffer, V.: Dynamics of early T cells: prothymocyte migration and proliferation in the adult mouse thymus. Immunol. Rev. 91:129, 1986.
22. Penit, C., Vasseur, F., and Papiernik, M.: In vivo dynamics of CD4$^-$8$^-$ thymocytes. Proliferation, renewal and differentiation of different cell subsets studied by DNA biosynthetic labeling and surface antigen detection. Eur. J. Immunol. 18:1343, 1988.
23. Wu, L., Antica, M., Johnson, G.R., Scollay, R., and Shortman, K.: Developmental potential of the earliest precursor cells from the adult mouse thymus. J. Exp. Med. 174:1617, 1991.
24. Wu, L., Scollay, R., Egerton, M., Pearse, M., Spangrude, G.J., and Shortman, K.: CD4 expressed on earliest T-lineage precursor cells in the adult murine thymus. Nature 349:71, 1991.
25. Kimoto, H., Kitamura, K., Sudo, T., Suda, T., Ogawa, Y., Kitagawa, H., Taniguchi, M., and Takemori, T.: The fetal thymus stores immature hemopoietic cells capable of differentiating into non–T lineage cells constituting the thymus stromal element. Int. Immunol. 5:1535, 1993.
26. Peault, B., Khazaal, I., and Weissman, I.L.: In vitro development of B cells and macrophages from early mouse fetal thymocytes. Eur. J. Immunol. 24:781, 1994.
27. Lesley, J., Trotter, J., and Hyman, R.: The Pgp-1 antigen is expressed on early fetal thymocytes. Immunogenetics 22:149, 1985.
28. Crispe, I.N., and Bevan, M.J.: Expression and functional significance of the J11d marker on mouse thymocytes. J. Immunol. 138:2013, 1987.
29. Spangrude, G.J., Heimfeld, S., and Weissman, I.L.: Purification and characterization of mouse hematopoietic stem cells. Science 241:58, 1988.

30. Spangrude, G.J., Klein, J., Heimfeld, S., Aihara, Y., and Weissman, I.L.: Two monoclonal antibodies identify thymic-repopulating cells in mouse bone marrow. J. Immunol. 142:425, 1989.

31. Hyman, R., Lesley, J., Schulte, R., and Trotter, J.: Progenitor cells in the thymus: most thymus-homing progenitor cells in the adult mouse thymus bear Pgp-1 glycoprotein but not interleukin-2 receptor on their cell surface. Cell. Immunol. 101:320, 1986.

32. Lesley, J., Schulte, R., Trotter, J., and Hyman, R.: Qualitative and quantitative heterogeneity in Pgp-1 expression among murine thymocytes. Cell. Immunol. 112:40, 1988.

33. Lesley, J., Schulte, R., and Hyman, R.: Kinetics of thymus repopulation by intrathymic progenitors after intravenous injection: evidence for successive repopulation by an IL-2R+, Pgp-1− and by an IL-2R−, Pgp-1+ progenitor. Cell. Immunol. 117:378, 1988.

34. Godfrey, D.I., Zlotnik, A., and Suda, T.: Phenotypic and functional characterization of c-kit expression during intrathymic T cell development. J. Immunol. 149:2281, 1992.

35. Godfrey, D.I., Kennedy, J., Suda, T., and Zlotnik, A.: A developmental pathway involving four phenotypically and functionally distinct subsets of CD3−CD4−CD8− triple-negative adult mouse thymocytes defined by CD44 and CD25 expression. J. Immunol. 150:4244, 1993.

36. Godfrey, D.I., and Zlotnik, A.: Control points in early T-cell development. Immunol. Today 14:547, 1993.

37. Fleming, W.H., Alpern, E.J., Uchida, N., Ikuta, K., and Weissman, I.L.: Steel factor influences the distribution and activity of murine hematopoietic stem cells in vivo. Proc. Natl. Acad. Sci. USA 90:3760, 1993.

38. Jordan, C.T., McKearn, J.P., and Lemischka, I.R.: Cellular and developmental properties of fetal hematopoietic stem cells. Cell 61:953, 1990.

39. Chervenak, R., Dempsey, D., Soloff, R., Wolcott, R.M., and Jennings, S.R.: The expression of CD4 by T cell precursors resident in both the thymus and the bone marrow. J. Immunol. 151:4486, 1993.

40. Onishi, M., Nagayoshi, K., Kitamura, K., Hirai, H., Takaku, F., and Nakauchi, H.: CD4dull+ hematopoietic progenitor cells in murine bone marrow. Blood 81:3217, 1993.

41. Peault, B., Weissman, I.L., Baum, C., McCune, J.M., and Tsukamoto, A.: Lymphoid reconstitution of the human fetal thymus in SCID mice with CD34+ precursor cells. J. Exp. Med. 174:1283, 1991.

42. Peault, B., Weissman, I.L., Buckle, A.M., Tsukamoto, A., and Baum, C.: Thy-1–expressing CD34+ human cells express multiple hematopoietic potentialities in vitro and in SCID-hu mice. Nouv. Rev. Fr. Hematol. 35:91, 1993.

43. Galy, A.H., Cen, D., Travis, M., Chen, S., and Chen, B.P.: Delineation of T-progenitor cell activity within the CD34+ compartment of adult bone marrow. Blood 85:2770, 1995.

44. Egerton, M., Pruski, E., and Pilarski, L.M.: Cell generation within human thymic subsets defined by selective expression of CD45 (T200) isoforms. Hum. Immunol. 27:333, 1990.

45. Terstappen, L.W., Huang, S., and Picker, L.J.: Flow cytometric assessment of human T-cell differentiation in thymus and bone marrow. Blood 79:666, 1992.

46. Sanchez, M.J., Spits, H., Lanier, L.L., and Phillips, J.H.: Human natural killer cell committed thymocytes and their relation to the T cell lineage. J. Exp. Med. 178:1857, 1993.

47. Spits, H., Barcena, A., Hori, T., Sanchez, M.J., Phillips, J.H., and Galy, A.: Early events in human intrathymic T-cell development. Res. Immunol. 145:128; discussion 155, 1994.

48. Sanchez, M.J., Muench, M.O., Roncarolo, M.G., Lanier, L.L., and Phillips, J.H.: Identification of a common T/natural killer cell progenitor in human fetal thymus. J. Exp. Med. 180:569, 1994.

49. Galy, A., Verma, S., Barcena, A., and Spits, H.: Precursors of CD3+CD4+CD8+ cells in the human thymus are defined by expression of CD34. Delineation of early events in human thymic development. J. Exp. Med. 178:391, 1993.

50. Haynes, B.F., Denning, S.M., Singer, K.H., and Kurtzberg, J.: Ontogeny of T-cell precursors: a model for the initial stages of human T-cell development. Immunol. Today 10:87, 1989.

51. Haynes, B.F., and Heinly, C.S.: Early human T cell development: analysis of the human thymus at the time of initial entry of hematopoietic stem cells into the fetal thymic microenvironment. J. Exp. Med. 181:1445, 1995.

52. Marquez, C., Trigueros, C., Fernandez, E., and Toribio, M.L.: The development of T and non-T cell lineages from CD34+ human thymic precursors can be traced by the differential expression of CD44. J. Exp. Med. 181:475, 1995.

53. Fowlkes, B.J., and Pardoll, D.: Molecular and cellular events of T cell development. Adv. Immunol. 44:207, 1989.

54. Scollay, R., and Shortman, K.: Identification of early stages of T lymphocyte development in the thymus cortex and medulla. J. Immunol. 134:3632, 1985.

55. Butcher, E.C., and Weissman, I.L.: Lymphoid tissues and organs. In Paul, W. (ed.): Fundamental Immunology. New York, Raven Press, 1989, pp. 117–137.

56. Godfrey, D.I., Kennedy, J., Mombaerts, P., Tonegawa, S., and Zlotnik, A.: Onset of TCR-beta gene rearrangement and role of TCR-beta expression during CD3−CD4−CD8− thymocyte differentiation. J. Immunol. 152:4783, 1994.

57. Borgulya, P., Kishi, H., Uematsu, Y., and Boehmer, H.V.: Exclusion and inclusion of α and β T cell receptor alleles. Cell 69:529, 1992.

58. Mombaerts, P., Iacomini, J., Johnson, R.S., Herrup, K., Tonegawa, S., and Papaioannou, V.E.: RAG-1–deficient mice have no mature B and T lymphocytes. Cell 68:869, 1992.

59. Mombaerts, P., Clarke, A.R., Rudnicki, M.A., Iacomini, J., Itohara, S., Lafaille, J.J., Wang, L., Ichikawa, Y., Jaenisch, R., Hooper, M.L., and Tonegawa, S.: Mutations in T-cell antigen receptor genes alpha and beta block thymocyte development at different stages. Nature 360:225, 1992.

60. Shinkai, Y., Rathbun, G., Lam, K.P., Oltz, E.M., Stewart, V., Mendelsohn, M., Charron, J., Datta, M., Young, F., Stall, A.M., and Alt, F.W.: RAG-2–deficient mice lack mature lymphocytes owing to inability to initiate V(D)J rearrangement. Cell 68:855, 1992.

61. Shinkai, Y., Koyasu, S., Nakayama, K., Murphy, K.M., Loh, D.Y., Reinherz, E.L., and Alt, F.W.: Restoration of T cell development in RAG-2–deficient mice by functional TCR transgenes. Science 259:822, 1993.

62. Bluthmann, H., Kisielow, P., Uematsu, Y., Malissen, M., Krimpenfort, P., Berns, A., von Boehmer, H., and Steinmetz, M.: T-cell–specific deletion of T-cell receptor transgenes allows functional rearrangement of endogenous alpha- and beta-genes. Nature 334:156, 1988.

63. Uematsu, Y., Ryser, S., Dembic, Z., Borgulya, P., Krimpenfort, P., Berns, A., von Boehmer, H., and Steinmetz, M.: In transgenic mice the introduced functional T cell receptor beta gene prevents expression of endogenous beta genes. Cell 52:831, 1988.

64. Fisher, A.G., Larsson, L., Goff, L.K., Restall, D.E., Happerfield, L., and Merkenschlager, M.: Human thymocyte development in mouse organ cultures. Int. Immunol. 2:571, 1990.

65. Sotzik, F., Rosenberg, Y., Boyd, A.W., Honeyman, M., Metcalf, D., Scollay, R., Wu, L., and Shortman, K.: Assessment of CD4 expression by early T precursor cells and by dendritic cells in the human thymus. J. Immunol. 152:3370, 1994.

66. Barcena, A., Muench, M.O., Galy, A.H., Cupp, J., Roncarolo, M.G., Phillips, J.H., and Spits, H.: Phenotypic and functional analysis of T-cell precursors in the human fetal liver and thymus: CD7 expression in the early stages of T- and myeloid-cell development. Blood 82:3401, 1993.

67. Pilarski, L.M., and Deans, J.P.: Selective expression of CD45 isoforms and of maturation antigens during human thymocyte differentiation: observations and hypothesis. Immunol. Lett. 21:187, 1989.

68. Pilarski, L.M., Gillitzer, R., Zola, H., Shortman, K., and Scollay, R.: Definition of the thymic generative lineage by selective expression of high molecular weight isoforms of CD45 (T200). Eur. J. Immunol. 19:589, 1989.

69. Wallace, V.A., Fung-Leung, W.P., Timms, E., Gray, D., Kishihara, K., Loh, D.Y., Penninger, J., and Mak, T.W.: CD45RA and CD45RBhigh expression induced by thymic selection events. J. Exp. Med. 176:1657, 1992.

70. Suda, T., and Zlotnik, A.: IL-7 maintains the T cell precursor potential of CD3−CD4−CD8− thymocytes. J. Immunol. 146:3068, 1991.

71. Rodewald, H.R., Ogawa, M., Haller, C., Waskow, C., and DiSanto, J.P.: Pro-thymocyte expansion by c-kit and the common cytokine receptor gamma chain is essential for repertoire formation. Immunity 6:265, 1997.

72. Peschon, J.J., Morrissey, P.J., Grabstein, K.H., Ramsdell, F.J., Maraskovsky, E., Gliniak, B.C., Park, L.S., Ziegler, S.F., Williams, D.E., Ware, C.B., et al.: Early lymphocyte expansion is severely impaired in interleukin 7 receptor–deficient mice. J. Exp. Med. 180:1955, 1994.

73. von Freeden-Jeffry, U., Solvason, N., Howard, M., and Murray, R.: The earliest T lineage–committed cells depend on IL-7 for Bcl-2 expression and normal cell cycle progression. Immunity 7:147, 1997.

74. Levin, S.D., Abraham, K.M., Anderson, S.J., Forbush, K.A., and

Perlmutter, R.M.: The protein tyrosine kinase p56lck regulates thymocyte development independently of its interaction with CD4 and CD8 coreceptors. J. Exp. Med. 178:245, 1993.

75. Gross, J.A., Appleby, M.W., Chien, S., Nada, S., Bartelmez, S.H., Okada, M., Aizawa, S., and Perlmutter, R.M.: Control of lymphopoiesis by p50csk, a regulatory protein tyrosine kinase. J. Exp. Med. 181:463, 1995.

76. Perlmutter, R.M.: In vivo dissection of lymphocyte signaling pathways. Clin. Immunol. Immunopathol. 67:S44, 1993.

77. Levin, S.D., Anderson, S.J., Forbush, K.A., and Perlmutter, R.M.: A dominant-negative transgene defines a role for p56lck in thymopoiesis. EMBO J 12:1671, 1993.

78. Anderson, S.J., Levin, S.D., and Perlmutter, R.M.: Protein tyrosine kinase p56lck controls allelic exclusion of T-cell receptor β-chain genes. Nature 365:552, 1993.

79. Mombaerts, P., Anderson, S.J., Perlmutter, R.M., Mak, T.W., and Tonegawa, S.: An activated lck transgene promotes thymocyte development in RAG-1 mutant mice. Immunity 1:261, 1994.

80. Georgopoulos, K., Moore, D.D., and Derfler, B.: Ikaros, an early lymphoid-specific transcription factor and a putative mediator for T cell commitment. Science 258:808, 1992.

81. Georgopoulos, K., Bigby, M., Wang, J.H., Molnar, A., Wu, P., Winandy, S., and Sharpe, A.: The Ikaros gene is required for the development of all lymphoid lineages. Cell 79:143, 1994.

82. Ting, C.N., Olson, M.C., Barton, K.P., and Leiden, J.M.: Transcription factor GATA-3 is required for development of the T-cell lineage. Nature 384:474, 1996.

83. Allen, R.D., Bender, T.P., and Siu, G.: c-Myb is essential for T cell lineage commitment. Genes Dev. 13:1073, 1999.

83a. Okamura, R.M., Sigvardssen, M., Galceran, J, Verbeck, S., Clevers, H., and Grosschedl, R.: Redundant regulation of T cell differentiation and TCR alpha gene expression by the transcription factors LEF and TCF-1. Immunity 8:11, 1998.

84. Guidos, C.J., Weissman, I.L., and Adkins, B.: Intrathymic maturation of murine T lymphocytes from CD8+ precursors. Proc. Natl. Acad. Sci. USA 86:7542, 1989.

85. Havran, W.L., Poenie, M., Kimura, J., Tsien, R., Weiss, A., and Allison, J.P.: Expression and function of the CD3-antigen receptor on murine CD4+CD8+ thymocytes. Nature 330:170, 1987.

86. Hugo, P., Boyd, R.L., Waanders, G.A., and Scollay, R.: CD4+CD8+CD3high thymocytes appear transiently during ontogeny: evidence from phenotypic and functional studies. Eur. J. Immunol. 21:2655, 1991.

87. Borum, K.: Cell kinetics in mouse thymus studied by simultaneous use of 3H-thymidine and colchicine. Cell Tissue Kinet. 6:545, 1973.

88. von Boehmer, H.: The developmental biology of T lymphocytes. Annu. Rev. Immunol. 6:309, 1988.

89. Bevan, M.J., Hogquist, K.A., and Jameson, S.C.: Selecting the T cell receptor repertoire. Science 264:796, 1994.

90. Fink, P.J., and Bevan, M.J.: Positive selection of thymocytes. Adv. Immunol. 59:99, 1995.

91. Nossal, G.J.V.: Negative selection of lymphocytes. Cell 76:229, 1994.

92. Fink, P.J., and Bevan, M.J.: H-2 antigens of the thymus determine lymphocyte specificity. J. Exp. Med. 148:766, 1978.

93. Robey, E., and Fowlkes, B.J.: Selective events in T cell development. Annu. Rev. Immunol. 12:675, 1994.

94. Jameson, S.C., Hogquist, K.A., and Bevan, M.J.: Positive selection of thymocytes. Annu. Rev. Immunol. 13:93, 1995.

95. Janeway, C.A., Jr.: Ligands for the T-cell receptor: hard times for avidity models. Immunol. Today 16:223, 1995.

96. McKeithan, T.W.: Kinetic proofreading in T-cell receptor signal transduction. Proc. Natl. Acad. Sci. USA 92:5042, 1995.

97. von Boehmer, H.: Positive selection of lymphocytes. Cell 76:219, 1994.

98. Perlmutter, R.M., Marth, J.D., Ziegler, S.F., Garvin, A.M., Pawar, S., Cooke, M.P., and Abraham, K.M.: Specialized protein tyrosine kinase proto-oncogenes in hematopoietic cells. Biochim. Biophys. Acta 948:245, 1988.

99. Robey, E.A., Ramsdell, F., Kioussis, D., Sha, W., Loh, D., Axel, R., and Fowlkes, B.J.: The level of CD8 expression can determine the outcome of thymic selection. Cell 69:1089, 1992.

100. Lee, N.A., Loh, D.Y., and Lacy, E.: CD8 surface levels alter the fate of alpha/beta T cell receptor–expressing thymocytes in transgenic mice. J. Exp. Med. 175:1013, 1992.

101. Berg, L.J., Pullen, A.M., Groth, B.F.d.S., Mathis, D., Benoist, C., and Davis, M.M.: Antigen/MHC-specific T cells are preferentially exported from the thymus in the presence of their MHC ligand. Cell 58:1035, 1989.

102. Rahemtulla, A., Fung-Leung, W.P., Schillham, M.W., Kundig, T.M., Sambhara, S.R., Narendran, A., Arabian, A., Wakeham, A., Paige, C.J., Zinkernagal, R.M., Miller, R.G., and Mak, T.W.: Normal development and function of CD8+ cells but markedly decreased helper cell activity in mice lacking CD4. Nature 353:180, 1991.

103. Bachmann, M.F., Oxenius, A., Mak, T.W., and Zinkernagel, R.M.: T cell development in CD8−/− mice. Thymic positive selection is biased toward the helper phenotype. J. Immunol. 155:3727, 1995.

104. Cosgrove, D., Gray, D., Dierich, A., Kaufman, J., Lemeur, M., Benoist, C., and Mathis., D.: Mice lacking MHC class II molecules. Cell 66:1051, 1991.

105. Grusby, M.J., Johnson, R.S., Papaionnou, V.E., and Glimcher., L.H.: Depletion of CD4+ T cells in major histocompatibility complex class II–deficient mice. Science 253:1417, 1991.

106. Kara, C.J., and Glimcher, L.H.: In vivo footprinting of MHC class II genes: bare promoter in the bare lymphocyte syndrome. Science 252:709, 1991.

107. Koller, B.H., and Smithies, O.: Inactivating the beta 2-microglobulin locus in mouse embryonic stem cells by homologous recombination. Proc. Natl. Acad. Sci. USA 86:8932, 1989.

108. Zijlstra, M., Li, E., Sajjadi, F., Subramani, S., and Jaenisch, R.: Germ-line transmission of a disrupted beta 2-microglobulin gene produced by homologous recombination in embryonic stem cells. Nature 342:435, 1989.

109. Abraham, K.M., Levin, S.D., Marth, J.D., Forbush, K.A., and Perlmutter, R.M.: Delayed thymocyte development induced by augmented expression of p56lck. J. Exp. Med. 173:1421, 1991.

110. Anderson, S.J., Levin, S.D., and Perlmutter, R.M.: Involvement of the protein tyrosine kinase p56lck in T cell signaling and thymocyte development. Adv. Immunol. 56:151, 1994.

111. Alberola-Ila, J., Forbush, K.A., Seger, R., Krebs, E.G., and Perlmutter, R.M.: Selective requirement for MAP kinase activation in thymocyte differentiation. Nature 373:620, 1995.

112. Wotton, D., Prosser, H.M., and Owen, M.J.: Regulation of human T cell receptor beta gene expression by Ets-1. Leukemia 7:S55, 1993.

113. Sarafova, S.D., and Siu, G.: A potential role for Elf-1 in CD4 promoter function. J. Biol. Chem. 274:16126, 1999.

114. Bassuk, A.G., and Leiden, J.M.: The role of Ets transcription factors in the development and function of the mammalian immune system. Adv. Immunol. 64:65, 1997.

115. Robey, E., Chang, D., Itano, A., Cado, D., Alexander, H., Lane, D., Weinmaster, G., and Salmon, P.: An activated form of Notch influences the choice between CD4 and CD8 T cell lineages. Cell 87:483, 1996.

116. Ellisen, L.W., Bird, J., West, D.C., Soreng, A.L., Reynolds, T.C., Smith, S.D., and Sklar, J.: TAN-1, the human homolog of the *Drosophila* notch gene, is broken by chromosomal translocations in T lymphoblastic neoplasms. Cell 66:649, 1991.

117. Duncan, D.D., Adlam, M., and Siu, G.: Asymmetric redundancy in CD4 silencer function. Immunity 4:301, 1996.

118. Kim, H.K., and Siu, G.: The Notch pathway intermediate HES-1 silences CD4 gene expression. Mol. Cell. Biol. 18:7166, 1998.

119. Kim, W.W.S., and Siu, G.: Subclass-specific nuclear localization of a novel CD4 silencer-binding factor. J. Exp. Med. 190:281, 1999.

120. Robey, E.A., Fowlkes, B.J., Gordon, J.W., Kioussis, D., Boehmer, H.v., Ramsdell, F., and Axel, R.: Thymic selection in CD8 transgenic mice supports an instructive model for commitment to a CD4 or CD8 lineage. Cell 64:99, 1991.

121. Chan, S.H., Cosgrove, D., Waltzinger, C., Benoist, C., and Mathis, D.: Another view of the selective model of thymocyte selection. Cell 73:225, 1993.

122. Davis, C.B., Killeen, N., Crooks, M.E.C., Raulet, D., and Littman, D.R.: Evidence for a stochastic mechanism of the differentiation of mature subsets of T lymphocytes. Cell 73:237, 1993.

123. Lucas, B., Vasseur, F., and Penit, C.: Stochastic coreceptor shut-off is restricted to the CD4 lineage maturation pathway. J. Exp. Med. 181:1623, 1995.

124. Suzuki, H., Punt, J.A., Granger, L.G., and Singer, A.: Asymmetric signaling requirements for thymocyte commitment to the CD4+ versus CD8+ T cell lineages: a new perspective on thymic commitment and selection. Immunity 2:413, 1995.

125. Lucas, B., and Germain, R.N.: Unexpectedly complex regulation of

CD4/CD8 coreceptor expression supports a revised model for CD4[+] CD8[+] thymocyte differentiation. Immunity 5:461, 1996.

126. Sprent, J., Schaefer, M., Hurd, M., Surh, C.D., and Ron, Y.: Mature murine B and T cells transferred to SCID mice can survive indefinitely and many maintain a virgin phenotype. J. Exp. Med. 174:717, 1991.

127. von Boehmer, H., and Hafen, K.: The life span of naive alpha/beta T cells in secondary lymphoid organs. J. Exp. Med. 177:891, 1993.

128. Butcher, E.C., and Picker, L.J.: Lymphocyte homing and homeostasis. Science 272:60, 1996.

129. Christensen, J.P., Ropke, C., and Thomsen, A.R.: Virus-induced poly-clonal T cell activation is followed by apoptosis: partitioning of CD8[+] T cells based on alpha 4 integrin expression. Int. Immunol. 8:707, 1996.

130. Andrew, D.P., Rott, L.S., Kilshaw, P.J., and Butcher, E.C.: Distribution of alpha 4 beta 7 and alpha E beta 7 integrins on thymocytes, intestinal epithelial lymphocytes and peripheral lymphocytes. Eur. J. Immunol. 26:897, 1996.

131. Rott, L.S., Briskin, M.J., Andrew, D.P., Berg, E.L., and Butcher, E.C.: A fundamental subdivision of circulating lymphocytes defined by adhesion to mucosal addressin cell adhesion molecule-1. Comparison with vascular cell adhesion molecule-1 and correlation with beta 7 integrins and memory differentiation. J. Immunol. 156:3727, 1996.

132. Youseffi-Etemad, R., and Axelsson, B.: Parallel pattern of expression of CD43 and of LFA-1 on the CD45RA[+] (naive) and CD45RO[+] (memory) subsets of human CD4[+] and CD8[+] cells. Correlation with the aggregative response of the cells to CD43 monoclonal antibodies. Immunology 87:439, 1996.

133. Sprent, J., and Webb, S.R.: Function and specificity of T cell subsets in the mouse. Adv. Immunol. 41:39, 1987.

134. Swain, S.L., Bradley, L.M., Croft, M., Tonkonogy, S., Atkins, G., Weinberg, A.D., Duncan, D.D., Hedrick, S.M., Dutton, R.W., and Huston, G.: Helper T-cell subsets: phenotype, function and the role of lymphokines in regulating their development. Immunol. Rev. 123:115, 1991.

135. Sprent, J.: T Lymphocytes and the thymus. In Paul, W. (ed.): Funda-mental Immunology. New York, Raven Press, 1989, pp. 69–93.

136. Sprent, J.: Circulating T and B lymphocytes of the mouse. I. Migratory properties. Cell. Immunol. 7:10, 1973.

137. Schwartz, R.H.: Costimulation of T lymphocytes: the role of CD28, CTLA-4, and B7/BB1 in interleukin-2 production and immunotherapy. Cell 71:1065, 1992.

138. Janeway, C.A., Jr., and Bottomly, K.: Signals and signs for lymphocyte responses. Cell 76:275, 1994.

139. Guerder, S., and Flavell, R.A.: T-cell activation. Two for T. Curr. Biol. 5:866, 1995.

140. Sprent, J., and Schaefer, M.: Antigen-presenting cells for unprimed T cells. Immunol. Today 10:17, 1989.

141. Linsley, P.S., Greene, J.L., Brady, W., Bajorath, J., Ledbetter, J.A., and Peach, R.: Human B7-1 (CD80) and B7-2 (CD86) bind with similar avidities but distinct kinetics to CD28 and CTLA-4 receptors. Immunity 1:793, 1994.

142. June, C.H., Ledbetter, J.A., Linsley, P.S., and Thompson, C.B.: Role of the CD28 receptor in T cell activation. Immunol. Today 11:211, 1990.

143. Walunas, T.L., Lenschow, D.J., Bakker, C.Y., Linsley, P.S., Freeman, G.J., Green, J.M., Thompson, C.B., and Bluestone, J.A.: CTLA-4 can function as a negative regulator of T cell activation. Immunity 1:405, 1994.

144. Rao, A.: Signaling mechanisms in T cells. Crit. Rev. Immunol. 10:495, 1991.

145. Ullman, K.S., Northrup, J.P., Verweij, C.L., and Crabtree, G.R.: Trans-mission of signals from the T lymphocyte antigen receptor to the genes responsible for cell proliferation and immune function: the missing link. Annu. Rev. Immunol. 8:421, 1990.

146. Weiss, A., and Littman, D.R.: Signal transduction by lymphocyte antigen receptors. Cell 76:263, 1994.

147. Rayter, S.I., Woodrow, M., Lucas, S.C., Cantrell, D.A., and Down-ward, J.: p21ras mediates control of IL-2 gene promoter function in T cell activation. EMBO J. 11:4549, 1992.

148. Woodrow, M.A., Rayter, S., Downward, J., and Cantrell, D.A.: p21ras function is important for T cell antigen receptor and protein kinase C regulation of nuclear factor of activated T cells. J. Immunol. 150:3853, 1993.

149. Rao, A.: NF-ATp: a transcription factor required for the co-ordinate induction of several cytokine genes. Immunol. Today 15:274, 1994.

150. Jain, J., Valge-Archer, V.E., and Rao, A.: Analysis of the AP-1 sites in the IL-2 promoter. J. Immunol. 148:1240, 1992.

151. Umlauf, S.W., Beverly, B., Kang, S.M., Brorson, K., Tran, A.C., and Schwartz, R.H.: Molecular regulation of the IL-2 gene: rheostatic control of the immune system. Immunol. Rev. 133:177, 1993.

152. Schreiber, S.L., and Crabtree, G.R.: The mechanism of action of cyclosporin A and FK506. Immunol. Today 13:136, 1992.

153. Jain, J., McCaffrey, P.G., Miner, Z., Kerppola, T.K., Lambert, J.N., Verdine, G.L., Curran, T., and Rao, A.: The T-cell transcription factor NFATp is a substrate for calcineurin and interacts with Fos and Jun. Nature 365:352, 1993.

154. McCaffrey, P.G., Perrino, B.A., Soderling, T.R., and Rao, A.: NF-ATp, a T lymphocyte DNA-binding protein that is a target for cal-cineurin and immunosuppressive drugs. J. Biol. Chem. 268:3747, 1993.

155. Le Gros, G., Ben-Sasson, S.Z., Seder, R., Finkelman, F.D., and Paul, W.E.: Generation of interleukin 4 (IL-4)–producing cells in vivo and in vitro: IL-2 and IL-4 are required for in vitro generation of IL-4–producing cells. J. Exp. Med. 172:921, 1990.

156. Ehlers, S., and Smith, K.A.: Differentiation of T cell lymphokine gene expression: the in vitro acquisition of T cell memory. J. Exp. Med. 173:25, 1991.

157. Bottomly, K.: A functional dichotomy in CD4[+] T lymphocytes. Immu-nol. Today 9:268, 1988.

158. Mosmann, T.R., and Coffman, R.L.: TH1 and TH2 cells: different patterns of lymphokine secretion lead to different functional proper-ties. Annu. Rev. Immunol. 7:145, 1989.

159. Murray, J.S., Madri, J., Tite, J., Carding, S.R., and Bottomly, K.: MHC control of CD4[+] T cell subset activation. J. Exp. Med. 170:2135, 1989.

160. Duncan, D.D., and Swain, S.L.: Role of antigen-presenting cells in the polarized development of helper T cell subsets: evidence for differential cytokine production by ThO cells in response to antigen presentation by B cells and macrophages. Eur. J. Immunol. 24:2506, 1994.

161. Constant, S., Pfeiffer, C., Woodard, A., Pasqualini, T., and Bottomly, K.: Extent of T cell receptor ligation can determine the functional differentiation of naive CD4[+] T cells. J. Exp. Med. 182:1591, 1995.

162. Constant, S.L., and Bottomly, K.: Induction of Th1 and Th2 CD4[+] T cell responses: the alternative approaches. Annu. Rev. Immunol. 15:297, 1997.

163. Sedlik, C., Deriaud, E., and Leclerc, C.: Lack of Th1 or Th2 polariza-tion of CD4[+] T cell response induced by particulate antigen targeted to phagocytic cells. Int. Immunol. 9:91, 1997.

164. Manetti, R., Parronchi, P., Giudizi, M.G., Piccinni, M.P., Maggi, E., Trinchieri, G., and Romagnani, S.: Natural killer cell stimulatory factor (interleukin 12 [IL-12]) induces T helper type 1 (Th1)-specific immune responses and inhibits the development of IL-4–producing Th cells. J. Exp. Med. 177:1199, 1993.

165. Manetti, R., Gerosa, F., Giudizi, M.G., Biagiotti, R., Parronchi, P., Piccinni, M.P., Sampognaro, S., Maggi, E., Romagnani, S., Trinchieri, G., et al.: Interleukin 12 induces stable priming for interferon gamma (IFN-gamma) production during differentiation of human T helper (Th) cells and transient IFN-gamma production in established Th2 cell clones. J. Exp. Med. 179:1273, 1994.

166. Hsieh, C.S., Macatonia, S.E., Tripp, C.S., Wolf, S.F., O'Garra, A., and Murphy, K.M.: Development of TH1 CD4[+] T cells through IL-12 produced by Listeria-induced macrophages. Science 260:547, 1993.

167. Gerosa, F., Paganin, C., Peritt, D., Paiola, F., Scupoli, M.T., Aste-Amezaga, M., Frank, I., and Trinchieri, G.: Interleukin-12 primes human CD4 and CD8 T cell clones for high production of both interferon-gamma and interleukin-10. J. Exp. Med. 183:2559, 1996.

168. Kaplan, M.H., Sun, Y.L., Hoey, T., and Grusby, M.J.: Impaired IL-12 responses and enhanced development of Th2 cells in Stat4-deficient mice. Nature 382:174, 1996.

169. Palm, N., Germann, T., Goedert, S., Hoehn, P., Koelsch, S., Rude, E., and Schmitt, E.: Co-development of naive CD4[+] cells towards T helper type 1 or T helper type 2 cells induced by a combination of IL-12 and IL-4. Immunobiology 196:475, 1996.

170. Jacobson, N.G., Szabo, S.J., Guler, M.L., Gorham, J.D., and Murphy, K.M.: Regulation of interleukin-12 signaling during T helper pheno-type development. Adv. Exp. Med. Biol. 409:61, 1996.

171. Trinchieri, G.: Proinflammatory and immunoregulatory functions of interleukin-12. Int. Rev. Immunol. 16:365, 1998.

172. Fiorentino, D.F., Bond, M.W., and Mosmann, T.R.: Two types of mouse T helper cell. IV. Th2 clones secrete a factor that inhibits cytokine production by Th1 clones. J. Exp. Med. 170:2081, 1989.

173. Rincon, M., Anguita, J., Nakamura, T., Fikrig, E., and Flavell, R.A.: Interleukin (IL)–6 directs the differentiation of IL-4–producing CD4+ T cells. J. Exp. Med. 185:461, 1997.

174. Kopf, M., Le Gros, G., Bachmann, M., Lamers, M.C., Bluethmann, H., and Kohler, G.: Disruption of the murine IL-4 gene blocks Th2 cytokine responses. Nature 362:245, 1993.

175. Sad, S., Marcotte, R., and Mosmann, T.R.: Cytokine-induced differentiation of precursor mouse CD8+ T cells into cytotoxic CD8+ T cells secreting Th1 or Th2 cytokines. Immunity 2:271, 1995.

176. Mosmann, T.R., Li, L., and Sad, S.: Functions of CD8 T-cell subsets secreting different cytokine patterns. Semin. Immunol. 9:87, 1997.

177. Li, L., Sad, S., Kagi, D., and Mosmann, T.R.: CD8Tc1 and Tc2 cells secrete distinct cytokine patterns in vitro and in vivo but induce similar inflammatory reactions. J. Immunol. 158:4152, 1997.

178. Guerder, S., Carding, S.R., and Flavell, R.A.: B7 costimulation is necessary for the activation of the lytic function in cytotoxic T lymphocyte precursors. J. Immunol. 155:5167, 1995.

179. Schoenberger, S.P., Toes, R.E., van der Voort, E.I., Offringa, R., and Melief, C.J.: T-cell help for cytotoxic T lymphocytes is mediated by CD40-CD40L interactions. Nature 393:480, 1998.

180. Kincaide, P.W., and Gimble, J.M.: B Lymphocytes. In Paul, W. (ed.): Fundamental Immunology. New York, Raven Press, 1989, pp. 41–67.

181. Jacobsen, K., Tepper, J., and Osmond, D.G.: Early B-lymphocyte precursor cells in mouse bone marrow: subosteal localization of B220+ cells during postirradiation regeneration. Exp. Hematol. 18:304, 1990.

182. Osmond, D.G.: B cell development in the bone marrow. Semin. Immunol. 2:173, 1990.

183. Melchers, F., Haasner, D., Karasuyama, H., Reininger, L., and Rolink, A.: Progenitor and precursor B lymphocytes of mice. Proliferation and differentiation in vitro and population, differentiation and turnover in SCID mice in vivo of normal and abnormal cells. Curr. Top. Microbiol. Immunol. 182:3, 1992.

184. Trentin, J.J.: Hemopoietic microenvironments. Transplant. Proc. 10:77, 1978.

185. Witte, P.L., Kincade, P.W., and Vetvicka, V.: Interculture variation and evolution of B lineage lymphocytes in long-term bone marrow culture. Eur. J. Immunol. 16:779, 1986.

186. Dorshkind, K., Schouest, L., and Fletcher, W.H.: Morphologic analysis of long-term bone marrow cultures that support B-lymphopoiesis or myelopoiesis. Cell Tissue Res. 239:375, 1985.

187. Jacobsen, K., and Osmond, D.G.: Microenvironmental organization and stromal cell associations of B lymphocyte precursor cells in mouse bone marrow. Eur. J. Immunol. 20:2395, 1990.

188. Aruffo, A., Stamenkovic, I., Melnick, M., Underhill, C.B., and Seed, B.: CD44 is the principal cell surface receptor for hyaluronate. Cell 61:1303, 1990.

189. Miyake, K., Underhill, C.B., Lesley, J., and Kincade, P.W.: Hyaluronate can function as a cell adhesion molecule and CD44 participates in hyaluronate recognition. J. Exp. Med. 172:69, 1990.

190. Lewinsohn, D.M., Nagler, A., Ginzton, N., Greenberg, P., and Butcher, E.C.: Hematopoietic progenitor cell expression of the H-CAM (CD44) homing-associated adhesion molecule. Blood 75:589, 1990.

191. Miyake, K., Weissman, I.L., Greenberger, J.S., and Kincade, P.W.: Evidence for a role of the integrin VLA-4 in lympho-hemopoiesis. J. Exp. Med. 173:599, 1991.

192. Kina, T., Majumdar, A.S., Heimfeld, S., Kaneshima, H., Holzmann, B., Katsura, Y., and Weissman, I.L.: Identification of a 107-kD glycoprotein that mediates adhesion between stromal cells and hematolymphoid cells. J. Exp. Med. 173:373, 1991.

193. Williams, D.A., Rios, M., Stephens, C., and Patel, V.P.: Fibronectin and VLA-4 in haematopoietic stem cell–microenvironment interactions. Nature 352:438, 1991.

194. Melchers, F., Haasner, D., Streb, M., and Rolink, A.: B-lymphocyte lineage–committed, IL-7 and stroma cell–reactive progenitors and precursors, and their differentiation to B cells. Adv. Exp. Med. Biol. 323:111, 1992.

195. Rolink, A., Haasner, D., Nishikawa, S., and Melchers, F.: Changes in frequencies of clonable pre B cells during life in different lymphoid organs of mice. Blood 81:2290, 1993.

196. Rico-Vargas, S.A., Weiskopf, B., Nishikawa, S., and Osmond, D.G.: c-kit expression by B cell precursors in mouse bone marrow. Stimulation of B cell genesis by in vivo treatment with anti–c-kit antibody. J. Immunol. 152:2845, 1994.

197. Hardy, R.R., Carmack, C.E., Shinton, S.A., Kemp, J.D., and Hayakawa, K.: Resolution and characterization of pro-B and pre-pro-B cell stages in normal mouse bone marrow. J. Exp. Med. 173:1213, 1991.

198. Osmond, D.G.: Proliferation kinetics and the lifespan of B cells in central and peripheral lymphoid organs. Curr. Opin. Immunol. 3:179, 1991.

199. Burrows, P.D., and Cooper, M.D.: Regulated expression of cell surface antigens during B cell development. Semin. Immunol. 2:189, 1990.

200. Li, Y.S., Hayakawa, K., and Hardy, R.R.: The regulated expression of B lineage associated genes during B cell differentiation in bone marrow and fetal liver. J. Exp. Med. 178:951, 1993.

201. Anderson, K.C., Bates, M.P., Slaughenhoupt, B.L., Pinkus, G.S., Schlossman, S.F., and Nadler, L.M.: Expression of human B cell–associated antigens on leukemias and lymphomas: a model of human B cell differentiation. Blood 63:1424, 1984.

202. Nadler, L.M., Korsmeyer, S.J., Anderson, K.C., Boyd, A.W., Slaughenhoupt, B., Park, E., Jensen, J., Coral, F., Mayer, R.J., Sallan, S.E., et al.: B cell origin of non–T cell acute lymphoblastic leukemia. A model for discrete stages of neoplastic and normal pre-B cell differentiation. J. Clin. Invest. 74:332, 1984.

203. Loken, M.R., Shah, V.O., Dattilio, K.L., and Civin, C.I.: Flow cytometric analysis of human bone marrow. II. Normal B lymphocyte development. Blood 70:1316, 1987.

204. Loken, M.R., Shah, V.O., Hollander, Z., and Civin, C.I.: Flow cytometric analysis of normal B lymphoid development. Pathol. Immunopathol. Res. 7:357, 1988.

205. Korsmeyer, S.J., Hieter, P.A., Ravetch, J.V., Poplack, D.G., Waldmann, T.A., and Leder, P.: Developmental hierarchy of immunoglobulin gene rearrangements in human leukemic pre-B-cells. Proc. Natl. Acad. Sci. USA 78:7096, 1981.

206. Korsmeyer, S.J., Arnold, A., Bakhshi, A., Ravetch, J.V., Siebenlist, U., Hieter, P.A., Sharrow, S.O., LeBien, T.W., Kersey, J.H., Poplack, D.G., Leder, P., and Waldmann, T.A.: Immunoglobulin gene rearrangement and cell surface antigen expression in acute lymphocytic leukemias of T cell and B cell precursor origins. J. Clin. Invest. 71:301, 1983.

207. Ryan, D., Kossover, S., Mitchell, S., Frantz, C., Hennessy, L., and Cohen, H.: Subpopulations of common acute lymphoblastic leukemia antigen-positive lymphoid cells in normal bone marrow identified by hematopoietic differentiation antigens. Blood 68:417, 1986.

208. Uckun, F.M., and Ledbetter, J.A.: Immunobiologic differences between normal and leukemic human B-cell precursors. Proc. Natl. Acad. Sci. USA 85:8603, 1988.

209. Uckun, F.M.: Regulation of human B-cell ontogeny. Blood 76:1908, 1990.

210. LeBien, T.W., Elstrom, R.L., Moseley, M., Kersey, J.H., and Griesinger, F.: Analysis of immunoglobulin and T-cell receptor gene rearrangements in human fetal bone marrow B lineage cells. Blood 76:1196, 1990.

211. Nishimoto, N., Kubagawa, H., Ohno, T., Gartland, G.L., Stankovic, A.K., and Cooper, M.D.: Normal pre-B cells express a receptor complex of mu heavy chains and surrogate light-chain proteins. Proc. Natl. Acad. Sci. USA 88:6284, 1991.

212. Reth, M.: Antigen receptors on B lymphocytes. Annu. Rev. Immunol. 10:97, 1992.

213. Kitamura, D., Kudo, A., Schaal, S., Muller, W., Melchers, F., and Rajewsky, K.: A critical role of lambda 5 protein in B cell development. Cell 69:823, 1992.

214. Ehlich, A., Schaal, S., Gu, H., Kitamura, D., Muller, W., and Rajewsky, K.: Immunoglobulin heavy and light chain genes rearrange independently at early stages of B cell development. Cell 72:695, 1993.

215. Papavasiliou, F., Misulovin, Z., Suh, H., and Nussenzweig, M.C.: The role of Ig beta in precursor B cell transition and allelic exclusion. Science 268:408, 1995.

216. Loffert, D., Ehlich, A., Muller, W., and Rajewsky, K.: Surrogate light chain expression is required to establish immunoglobulin heavy chain allelic exclusion during early B cell development. Immunity 4:133, 1996.

217. Rajewsky, K.: Clonal selection and learning in the antibody system. Nature 381:751, 1996.

218. Iritani, B.M., Forbush, K.A., Farrar, M.A., and Perlmutter, R.M.: Control of B cell development by Ras-mediated activation of Raf. EMBO J. 16:7019, 1997.

219. Hunte, B.E., Hudak, S., Campbell, D., Xu, Y., and Rennick, D.: flk2/flt3 ligand is a potent cofactor for the growth of primitive B cell progenitors. J. Immunol. 156:489, 1995.

220. Bain, G., Maandag, E.C., Izon, D.J., Amsen, D., Kruisbeek, A.M., Weintraub, B.C., Krop, I., Schlissel, M.S., Feeney, A.J., van Roon, M., van der Valk, M., te Reile, H.P.J., Berns, A., and Murre, C.: E2A proteins are required for proper B cell development and initiation of immunoglobulin gene rearrangements. Cell 79:885, 1994.

221. Zhuang, Y., Soriano, P., and Weintraub, H.: The helix-loop-helix gene E2A is required for B cell formation. Cell 79:875, 1994.

222. Bain, G., Maandag, E.C., te Riele, H.P., Feeney, A.J., Sheehy, A., Schlissel, M., Shinton, S.A., Hardy, R.R., and Murre, C.: Both E12 and E47 allow commitment to the B cell lineage. Immunity 6:145, 1997.

223. Sun, X.-H.: Constitutive expression of the Id1 gene impairs mouse B cell development. Cell 79:893, 1994.

224. Morrow, M.A., Mayer, E.W., Perez, C.A., Adlam, M., and Siu, G.: Overexpression of the helix-loop-helix protein Id2 blocks T cell development at multiple stages. Mol. Immunol. 36:491, 1999.

225. Liu, Y.J., de Bouteiller, O., and Fugier-Vivier, I.: Mechanisms of selection and differentiation in germinal centers. Curr. Opin. Immunol. 9:256, 1997.

226. Lebecque, S., de Bouteiller, O., Arpin, C., Banchereau, J., and Liu, Y.J.: Germinal center founder cells display propensity for apoptosis before onset of somatic mutation. J. Exp. Med. 185:563, 1997.

227. Gearhart, P.J., Johnson, N.D., Douglas, R., and Hood, L.: IgG antibodies to phosphorylcholine exhibit more diversity than their IgM counterparts. Nature 291:29, 1981.

228. Crews, S., Griffin, J., Huang, H., Calame, K., and Hood, L.: A single VH gene segment encodes the immune response to phosphorylcholine: somatic mutation is correlated with the class of the antibody. Cell 25:59, 1981.

229. Kim, S., Davis, M., Sinn, E., Patten, P., and Hood, L.: Antibody diversity: somatic hypermutation of rearranged VH genes. Cell 27:573, 1981.

230. Perlmutter, R.M., Crews, S.T., Douglas, R., Sorensen, G., Johnson, N., Nivera, N., Gearhart, P.J., and Hood, L.: The generation of diversity in phosphorylcholine-binding antibodies. Adv. Immunol. 35:1, 1984.

231. Griffiths, G.M., Berek, C., Kaartinen, M., and Milstein, C.: Somatic mutation and the maturation of immune response to 2-phenyl oxazolone. Nature 312:271, 1984.

232. Berek, C., and Milstein, C.: Mutation drift and repertoire shift in the maturation of the immune response. Immunol. Rev. 96:23, 1987.

233. Grouard, G., de Bouteiller, O., Barthelemy, C., Lebecque, S., Banchereau, J., and Liu, Y.J.: Regulation of human B cell activation by follicular dendritic cell and T cell signals. Curr. Top. Microbiol. Immunol. 201:105, 1995.

234. Liu, Y.J., Arpin, C., de Bouteiller, O., Guret, C., Banchereau, J., Martinez-Valdez, H., and Lebecque, S.: Sequential triggering of apoptosis, somatic mutation and isotype switch during germinal center development. Semin. Immunol. 8:169, 1996.

235. Przylepa, J., Himes, C., and Kelsoe, G.: Lymphocyte development and selection in germinal centers. Curr. Top. Microbiol. Immunol. 229:85, 1998.

236. McHeyzer-Williams, M.G.: Visualizing immune responses in vivo. Curr. Opin. Immunol. 8:321, 1996.

237. Kosco-Vilbois, M.H., Gray, D., Scheidegger, D., and Julius, M.: Follicular dendritic cells help resting B cells to become effective antigen-presenting cells: induction of B7/BB1 and upregulation of major histocompatibility complex class II molecules. J. Exp. Med. 178:2055, 1993.

238. Tew, J.G., Burton, G.F., Kupp, L.I., and Szakal, A.: Follicular dendritic cells in germinal center reactions. Adv. Exp. Med. Biol. 329:461, 1993.

239. Han, S., Zheng, B., Takahashi, Y., and Kelsoe, G.: Distinctive characteristics of germinal center B cells. Semin. Immunol. 9:255, 1997.

240. Kelsoe, G.: The germinal center: a crucible for lymphocyte selection. Semin. Immunol. 8:179, 1996.

241. Liu, Y.J., Zhang, J., Lane, P.J., Chan, E.Y., and MacLennan, I.C.: Sites of specific B cell activation in primary and secondary responses to T cell-dependent and T cell-independent antigens [published erratum appears in Eur J Immunol 22:615, 1992]. Eur. J. Immunol. 21:2951, 1991.

242. Han, S., Zheng, B., Dal Porto, J., and Kelsoe, G.: In situ studies of the primary immune response to (4-hydroxy-3-nitrophenyl)acetyl. IV. Affinity-dependent, antigen-driven B cell apoptosis in germinal centers as a mechanism for maintaining self-tolerance. J. Exp. Med. 182:1635, 1995.

243. Liu, Y.J., Joshua, D.E., Williams, G.T., Smith, C.A., Gordon, J., and MacLennan, I.C.: Mechanism of antigen-driven selection in germinal centres. Nature 342:929, 1989.

244. Berek, C., Berger, A., and Apel, M.: Maturation of the immune response in germinal centers. Cell 67:1121, 1991.

245. Kuppers, R., Zhao, M., Hansmann, M.L., and Rajewsky, K.: Tracing B cell development in human germinal centres by molecular analysis of single cells picked from histological sections. EMBO J. 12:4955, 1993.

246. MacLennan, I.C., Gulbranson-Judge, A., Toellner, K.M., Casamayor-Palleja, M., Chan, E., Sze, D.M., Luther, S.A., and Orbea, H.A.: The changing preference of T and B cells for partners as T-dependent antibody responses develop. Immunol. Rev. 156:53, 1997.

247. Rajewsky, K.: Immunology. The power of clonal selection. Nature 363:208, 1993.

248. Jacob, J., Kelsoe, G., Rajewsky, K., and Weiss, U.: Intraclonal generation of antibody mutants in germinal centres. Nature 354:389, 1991.

249. Liu, Y.J., de Bouteiller, O., Arpin, C., Briere, F., Galibert, L., Ho, S., Martinez-Valdez, H., Banchereau, J., and Lebecque, S.: Normal human IgD+IgM− germinal center B cells can express up to 80 mutations in the variable region of their IgD transcripts. Immunity 4:603, 1996.

250. Goodnow, C.C.: Transgenic mice and analysis of B-cell tolerance. Annu. Rev. Immunol. 10:489, 1992.

251. Hartley, S.B., Crosbie, J., Brink, R., Kantor, A.B., Basten, A., and Goodnow, C.C.: Elimination from peripheral lymphoid tissues of self-reactive B lymphocytes recognizing membrane-bound antigens. Nature 353:765, 1991.

252. Hartley, S.B., Cooke, M.P., Fulcher, D.A., Harris, A.W., Cory, S., Basten, A., and Goodnow, C.C.: Elimination of self-reactive B lymphocytes proceeds in two stages: arrested development and cell death. Cell 72:325, 1993.

253. Nemazee, D., and Buerki, K.: Clonal deletion of autoreactive B lymphocytes in bone marrow chimeras. Proc. Natl. Acad. Sci. USA 86:8039, 1989.

254. Martinez-Valdez, H., Guret, C., de Bouteiller, O., Fugier, I., Banchereau, J., and Liu, Y.J.: Human germinal center B cells express the apoptosis-inducing genes Fas, c-myc, p53, and Bax, but not the survival gene Bcl-2. J. Exp. Med. 183:971, 1996.

255. McDonnell, T.J., Deane, N., Platt, F.M., Nunez, G., Jaeger, U., McKearn, J.P., and Korsmeyer, S.J.: bcl-2–immunoglobulin transgenic mice demonstrate extended B cell survival and follicular lymphoproliferation. Cell 57:79, 1989.

256. Vaux, D.L., Cory, S., and Adams, J.M.: Bcl-2 gene promotes haemopoietic cell survival and cooperates with c-myc to immortalize pre-B cells. Nature 335:440, 1988.

257. Strasser, A., Harris, A.W., Corcoran, L.M., and Cory, S.: Bcl-2 expression promotes B- but not T-lymphoid development in scid mice. Nature 368:457, 1994.

258. Strasser, A., Whittingham, S., Vaux, D.L., Bath, M.L., Adams, J.M., Cory, S., and Harris, A.W.: Enforced BCL2 expression in B-lymphoid cells prolongs antibody responses and elicits autoimmune disease. Proc. Natl. Acad. Sci. USA 88:8661, 1991.

259. Smith, K.G., Weiss, U., Rajewsky, K., Nossal, G.J., and Tarlinton, D.M.: Bcl-2 increases memory B cell recruitment but does not perturb selection in germinal centers. Immunity 1:803, 1994.

260. Cyster, J.G., Hartley, S.B., and Goodnow, C.C.: Competition for follicular niches excludes self-reactive cells from the recirculating B-cell repertoire. Nature 371:389, 1994.

261. Shokat, K.M., and Goodnow, C.C.: Antigen-induced B-cell death and elimination during germinal-centre immune responses. Nature 375:334, 1995.

262. Pulendran, B., Kannourakis, G., Nouri, S., Smith, K.G., and Nossal, G.J.: Soluble antigen can cause enhanced apoptosis of germinal-centre B cells. Nature 375:331, 1995.

263. Han, S., Hathcock, K., Zheng, B., Kepler, T.B., Hodes, R., and Kelsoe, G.: Cellular interaction in germinal centers. Roles of CD40 ligand and B7-2 in established germinal centers. J. Immunol. 155:556, 1995.

264. Galibert, L., Burdin, N., Barthelemy, C., Meffre, G., Durand, I., Garcia, E., Garrone, P., Rousset, F., Banchereau, J., and Liu, Y.J.: Negative selection of human germinal center B cells by prolonged BCR cross-linking. J. Exp. Med. 183:2075, 1996.

265. Ju, S.T., Cui, H., Panka, D.J., Ettinger, R., and Marshak-Rothstein, A.: Participation of target Fas protein in apoptosis pathway induced by CD4+ Th1 and CD8+ cytotoxic T cells. Proc. Natl. Acad. Sci. USA 91:4185, 1994.

266. Singer, G.G., Carrera, A.C., Marshak-Rothstein, A., Martinez, C., and Abbas, A.K.: Apoptosis, Fas and systemic autoimmunity: the MRL-lpr/lpr model. Curr. Opin. Immunol. 6:913, 1994.

267. Vignaux, F., and Golstein, P.: Fas-based lymphocyte-mediated cytotoxicity against syngeneic activated lymphocytes: a regulatory pathway? Eur. J. Immunol. 24:923, 1994.

268. Rathmell, J.C., Cooke, M.P., Ho, W.Y., Grein, J., Townsend, S.E., Davis, M.M., and Goodnow, C.C.: CD95 (Fas)–dependent elimination of self-reactive B cells upon interaction with CD4+ T cells. Nature 376:181, 1995.

269. Rathmell, J.C., Townsend, S.E., Xu, J.C., Flavell, R.A., and Goodnow, C.C.: Expansion or elimination of B cells in vivo: dual roles for CD40- and Fas (CD95)–ligands modulated by the B cell antigen receptor. Cell 87:319, 1996.

270. Adams, E., Basten, A., and Goodnow, C.C.: Intrinsic B-cell hyporesponsiveness accounts for self-tolerance in lysozyme/anti-lysozyme double-transgenic mice. Immunology 87:5687, 1990.

271. Rothstein, T.L., Wang, J.K., Panka, D.J., Foote, L.C., Wang, Z., Stanger, B., Cui, H., Ju, S.T., and Marshak-Rothstein, A.: Protection against Fas-dependent Th1-mediated apoptosis by antigen receptor engagement in B cells. Nature 374:163, 1995.

272. Garrone, P., Neidhardt, E.M., Garcia, E., Galibert, L., van Kooten, C., and Banchereau, J.: Fas ligation induces apoptosis of CD40-activated human B lymphocytes. J. Exp. Med. 182:1265, 1995.

273. Sprent, J.: T and B memory cells. Cell 76:315, 1994.

274. Zinkernagel, R.M., Bachmann, M.F., Kundig, T.M., Oehen, S., Pirchet, H., and Hengartner, H.: On immunological memory. Annu. Rev. Immunol. 14:333, 1996.

275. Sprent, J., and Tough, D.F.: Lymphocyte life-span and memory. Science 265:1395, 1994.

276. Gray, D., and Matzinger, P.: T cell memory is short-lived in the absence of antigen. J. Exp. Med. 174:969, 1991.

277. Gray, D.: Immunological memory: a function of antigen persistence. Trends Microbiol. 1:39; discussion 41, 1993.

278. Picker, L.J., Terstappen, L.W., Rott, L.S., Streeter, P.R., Stein, H., and Butcher, E.C.: Differential expression of homing-associated adhesion molecules by T cell subsets in man. J. Immunol. 145:3247, 1990.

279. McHeyzer-Williams, M.G., Altman, J.D., and Davis, M.M.: Enumeration and characterization of memory cells in the TH compartment. Immunol. Rev. 150:5, 1996.

280. Sanders, M.E., Makgoba, M.W., Sharrow, S.O., Stephany, D., Springer, T.A., Young, H.A., and Shaw, S.: Human memory T lymphocytes express increased levels of three cell adhesion molecules (LFA-3, CD2, and LFA-1) and three other molecules (UCHL1, CDw29, and Pgp-1) and have enhanced IFN-gamma production. J. Immunol. 140:1401, 1988.

281. Morimoto, C., Letvin, N.L., Distaso, J.A., Aldrich, W.R., and Schlossman, S.F.: The isolation and characterization of the human suppressor inducer T cell subset. J. Immunol. 134:1508, 1985.

282. Smith, S.H., Brown, M.H., Rowe, D., Callard, R.E., and Beverley, P.C.: Functional subsets of human helper-inducer cells defined by a new monoclonal antibody, UCHL1. Immunology 58:63, 1986.

283. Bottomly, K., Luqman, M., Greenbaum, L., Carding, S., West, J., Pasqualini, T., and Murphy, D.B.: A monoclonal antibody to murine CD45R distinguishes CD4 T cell populations that produce different cytokines. Eur. J. Immunol. 19:617, 1989.

284. Morimoto, C., Matsuyama, T., Rudd, C.E., Forsgren, A., Letvin, N.L., and Schlossman, S.F.: Role of the 2H4 molecule in the activation of suppressor inducer function. Eur. J. Immunol. 18:731, 1988.

285. Rudd, C.E., Morimoto, C., Wong, L.L., and Schlossman, S.F.: The subdivision of the T4 (CD4) subset on the basis of the differential expression of L-C/T200 antigens. J. Exp. Med. 166:1758, 1987.

286. Thomas, M.L.: The leukocyte common antigen family. Annu. Rev. Immunol. 7:339, 1989.

287. Sanders, M.E., Makgoba, M.W., and Shaw, S.: Human naive and memory T cells: reinterpretation of helper-inducer and suppressor-inducer subsets. Immunol. Today 9:195, 1988.

288. Merkenschlager, M., Terry, L., Edwards, R., and Beverley, P.C.: Limiting dilution analysis of proliferative responses in human lymphocyte populations defined by the monoclonal antibody UCHL1: implications for differential CD45 expression in T cell memory formation. Eur. J. Immunol. 18:1653, 1988.

289. Bettens, F., Walker, C., Gauchat, J.F., Gauchat, D., Wyss, T., and Pichler, W.J.: Lymphokine gene expression related to CD4 T cell subset (CD45R/CDw29) phenotype conversion. Eur. J. Immunol. 19:1569, 1989.

290. Salmon, M., Kitas, G.D., and Bacon, P.A.: Production of lymphokine mRNA by CD45R+ and CD45R− helper T cells from human peripheral blood and by human CD4+ T cell clones. J. Immunol. 143:907, 1989.

291. Hirohata, S., and Lipsky, P.E.: T cell regulation of human B cell proliferation and differentiation. Regulatory influences of CD45R+ and CD45R− T4 cell subsets. J. Immunol. 142:2597, 1989.

292. Tedder, T.F., Cooper, M.D., and Clement, L.T.: Human lymphocyte differentiation antigens HB-10 and HB-11. II. Differential production of B cell growth and differentiation factors by distinct helper T cell subpopulations. J. Immunol. 134:2989, 1985.

293. Rothstein, D.M., Sohen, S., Daley, J.F., Schlossman, S.F., and Morimoto, C.: CD4+CD45RA+ and CD4+CD45RA− T cell subsets in man maintain distinct function and CD45RA expression persists on a subpopulation of CD45RA+ cells after activation with Con A. Cell. Immunol. 129:449, 1990.

294. Hayward, A.R., Lee, J., and Beverley, P.C.: Ontogeny of expression of UCHL1 antigen on TcR-1+ (CD4/8) and TcR delta+ T cells. Eur. J. Immunol. 19:771, 1989.

295. Warren, H.S., and Skipsey, L.J.: Loss of activation-induced CD45RO with maintenance of CD45RA expression during prolonged culture of T cells and NK cells. Immunology 74:78, 1991.

296. Rothstein, D.M., Yamada, A., Schlossman, S.F., and Morimoto, C.: Cyclic regulation of CD45 isoform expression in a long term human CD4+CD45RA+ T cell line. J. Immunol. 146:1175, 1991.

297. Bell, E.B., and Sparshott, S.M.: Interconversion of CD45R subsets of CD4 T cells in vivo. Nature 348:163, 1990.

298. Sparshott, S.M., and Bell, E.B.: Membrane CD45R isoform exchange on CD4 T cells is rapid, frequent and dynamic in vivo. Eur. J. Immunol. 24:2573, 1994.

299. Ruzek, M.C., and Mathur, A.: Plasma cell tumors decrease CD23 mRNA expression in vivo in murine splenic B cells. Eur. J. Immunol. 25:2228, 1995.

300. Tedder, T.F., Tuscano, J., Sato, S., and Kehrl, J.H.: CD22, a B lymphocyte–specific adhesion molecule that regulates antigen receptor signaling. Annu. Rev. Immunol. 15:481, 1997.

301. Scheuermann, R.H., and Racila, E.: CD19 antigen in leukemia and lymphoma diagnosis and immunotherapy. Leuk. Lymphoma 18:385, 1995.

302. Silacci, P., Mottet, A., Steimle, V., Reith, W., and Mach, B.: Developmental extinction of major histocompatibility complex class II gene expression in plasmocytes is mediated by silencing of the transactivator gene CIITA. J. Exp. Med. 180:1329, 1994.

303. MacLennan, I.C., and Gray, D.: Antigen-driven selection of virgin and memory B cells. Immunol. Rev. 91:61, 1986.

304. Zhang, J., MacLennan, I.C., Liu, Y.J., and Lane, P.J.: Is rapid proliferation in B centroblasts linked to somatic mutation in memory B cell clones? Immunol. Lett. 18:297, 1988.

305. McHeyzer-Williams, M.G., Nossal, G.J., and Lalor, P.A.: Molecular characterization of single memory B cells. Nature 350:502, 1991.

306. McHeyzer-Williams, M.G., McLean, M.J., Lalor, P.A., and Nossal, G.J.: Antigen-driven B cell differentiation in vivo. J. Exp. Med. 178:295, 1993.

307. MacLennan, I.C., Bazin, H., Chassoux, D., Gray, D., and Lortan, J.: Comparative analysis of the development of B cells in marginal zones and follicles. Adv. Exp. Med. Biol. 186:139, 1985.

308. Liu, Y.J., Oldfield, S., and MacLennan, I.C.: Memory B cells in T cell–dependent antibody responses colonize the splenic marginal zones. Eur. J. Immunol. 18:355, 1988.

309. Weiss, U., and Rajewsky, K.: The repertoire of somatic antibody mutants accumulating in the memory compartment after primary immunization is restricted through affinity maturation and mirrors that expressed in the secondary response. J. Exp. Med. 172:1681, 1990.

310. Schittek, B., and Rajewsky, K.: Maintenance of B-cell memory by long-lived cells generated from proliferating precursors. Nature 346:749, 1990.

311. Schittek, B., and Rajewsky, K.: Natural occurrence and origin of somatically mutated memory B cells in mice. J. Exp. Med. 176:427, 1992.

312. Randall, T.D., Heath, A.W., Santos-Argumendo, L., Howard, M.C., Weissman, I.L., and Lund, F.E.: Arrest of B lymphocyte terminal differentiation by CD40 signaling: mechanism for lack of antibody-secreting cells germinal centers. Immunity 8:733, 1998.

313. Gray, D., Dullforce, P., and Jainandunsing, S.: Memory B cell development but not germinal center formation is impaired by in vivo blockade of CD40–CD40 ligand interaction. J. Exp. Med. 180:141, 1994.

314. Arpin, C., Dechanet, J., Van Kooten, C., Merville, P., Grouard, G., Briere, F., Banchereau, J., and Liu, Y.J.: Generation of memory B cells and plasma cells in vitro. Science 268:720, 1995.

315. Lane, P., Burdet, C., McConnell, F., Lanzavecchia, A., and Padovan, E.: CD40 ligand-independent B cell activation revealed by CD40 ligand-deficient T cell clones: evidence for distinct activation requirements for antibody formation and B cell proliferation. Eur. J. Immunol. 25:1788, 1995.

316. Callard, R.E., Herbert, J., Smith, S.H., Armitage, R.J., and Costelloe, K.E.: CD40 cross-linking inhibits specific antibody production by human B cells. Int. Immunol. 7:1809, 1995.

13 Antigen Processing and T-Cell Effector Mechanisms

▼▼▼▼ Roger M. Perlmutter

ANTIGEN PROCESSING AND PRESENTATION
- ▼ T Lymphocytes Recognize Peptides Associated With Major Histocompatibility Complex–Encoded Proteins
- ▼ Differential Processing of Exogenous and Endogenous Antigens
- ▼ Specialization of T Cells for Recognition of Major Histocompatibility Complex Class I or Class II Structures

MOLECULAR BIOLOGY OF THE HUMAN LEUKOCYTE ANTIGEN COMPLEX
- ▼ Class I Genes Encode Classical Transplantation Antigens
- ▼ Atypical Class I Genes Subserve Multiple Functions
- ▼ Class II Genes Encode Regulators of Immune Responsiveness
- ▼ Regulation of Class II Gene Expression

ANTIGEN PROCESSING: PRESENTATION OF ENDOGENOUSLY SYNTHESIZED PROTEINS

ALLELIC VARIATION IN MAJOR HISTOCOMPATIBILITY COMPLEX GENES
- ▼ Polymorphism in Peptide Transporters
- ▼ The Class III Region

RECOGNITION OF ANTIGEN BY T LYMPHOCYTES

ARCHITECTURE OF THE T-CELL RECEPTOR
- ▼ Structure of the CD3 Molecules and the Genes That Encode Them
- ▼ Binding of the T-Cell Receptor to Antigen-Presentation Structures
- ▼ Coreceptor Structures Contributing to T-Cell Activation

THE BIOCHEMISTRY OF T-CELL SIGNALING
- ▼ Protein Tyrosine Kinases Mediating Lymphocyte Activation
- ▼ Control of T-Cell Activation by Phosphotyrosine Phosphatases
- ▼ Adaptor Proteins in T-Cell Signaling
- ▼ Insights into T-Cell Signaling Derived from the Study of Immunophilin Ligands
- ▼ Alternative Outcomes of T-Cell Stimulation: Activation, Anergy, and Apoptosis

T-CELL EFFECTOR MECHANISMS
- ▼ Types of Responses
- ▼ Effector Properties of CD8[+] Cells

SUMMARY

▼ ▼

White blood cells exist to provide broad protection from parasitism. The effector mechanisms that constitute host defense operate with considerable vigor. This fact requires that strategies must also exist to permit satisfactory discrimination of potential pathogens from normal host cells. Not surprisingly, the cellular and molecular processes that permit this exquisitely subtle identification of nonself structures are highly sophisticated.

The pathway underlying an immune response to a typical protein antigen can be schematized as follows (Fig. 13–1). The primary B-cell repertoire is sufficiently large (>10⁸ different species at a minimum) to permit binding of most proteins with some measurable affinity (see Chapter 11.)

Foreign proteins, bound to the surface immunoglobulins of a B lymphocyte or ingested by a macrophage, are then internalized and digested in an endosomal compartment, yielding peptide fragments, some of which can bind to class II antigen presentation molecules. Peptide/class II complexes appear on the B-cell or macrophage surface, permitting recognition by T-cell antigen receptors. This recognition event stimulates elaboration of lymphokines and T-cell replication. In this way, additional cells bearing receptors for the peptide/class II complex antigen are produced. B-cell replication and antibody production are also enhanced. Moreover, lymphokine expression by helper T lymphocytes encourages migration of additional inflammatory cells to the site of antigen contact. The process is maintained until all stimulatory antigen has been consumed and degraded.

Three simple lessons may be deduced from considering

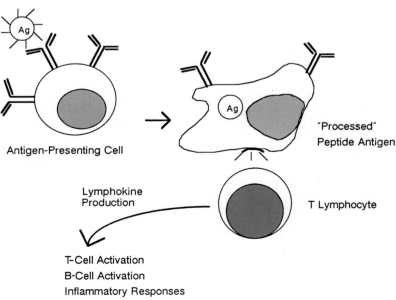

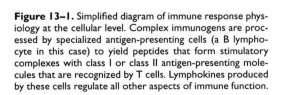

Figure 13–1. Simplified diagram of immune response physiology at the cellular level. Complex immunogens are processed by specialized antigen-presenting cells (a B lymphocyte in this case) to yield peptides that form stimulatory complexes with class I or class II antigen-presenting molecules that are recognized by T cells. Lymphokines produced by these cells regulate all other aspects of immune function.

Antigen-Presenting Cell

"Processed" Peptide Antigen

Lymphokine Production

T Lymphocyte

T-Cell Activation
B-Cell Activation
Inflammatory Responses

immune function in this schematic way. First, T lymphocytes regulate all immune responses. Antigen recognition by T cells permits elaboration of potent lymphokines that regulate the activity of phagocytic cells, B lymphocytes, and other T cells. Second, T lymphocytes recognize peptide antigens derived from the digestion of proteins within antigen-presenting cells. This means of recognition provides fundamental safeguards against the propagation of autoimmune responses and directly underlies self/nonself discrimination. Third, there exist cellular (principally involving cytotoxic T cells and phagocytic cells) and humoral (principally involving antibodies and complement components) immune effector mechanisms, both types of which are required for satisfactory host defense against parasitism.

In the following discussion, the cellular effector mechanisms that mediate immune function are considered in detail, beginning with a description of the molecular features of antigen processing and presentation, proceeding to examine the biochemistry of lymphocyte activation, and finally evaluating the molecules elaborated by T cells that coordinate immune attack. Each of these areas has experienced dramatic advances in understanding during the past few years, resulting in a fairly comprehensive view of mammalian host defense mechanisms. Moreover, abnormalities in the recognition and effector functions of T-cell immunity contribute to the pathogenesis of many inflammatory diseases.

Antigen Processing and Presentation

▼ T LYMPHOCYTES RECOGNIZE PEPTIDES ASSOCIATED WITH MAJOR HISTOCOMPATIBILITY COMPLEX–ENCODED PROTEINS

Early studies of humoral immunity permitted identification of B lymphocytes as antibody-secreting cells that also bear cell surface antibody molecules.[1] In these cells, the recognition element (surface antibody) differs from the effector molecule simply by the presence of a membrane-spanning region at the carboxy-terminal end of two constituent polypeptides (the antibody heavy chains). Not surprisingly, binding of cognate antigen by B cells can be demonstrated directly.[2, 3]

This situation contrasts with that observed in the case of T lymphocytes. Such cells do not recognize polypeptide antigens in soluble form. Moreover, no binding of antigen to immune T cells can be demonstrated. Careful experiments conducted over a period of years revealed that T-cell recognition of protein antigens requires degradation of the antigen by a presenting cell, which then displays fragments of the protein in association with specialized dimeric glycoproteins, the class I and class II molecules. It is this complex of peptide fragment and cell surface presentation molecules that commands the attention of the T-cell antigen receptor, which must distinguish between self-polypeptides and foreign polypeptides that are presented simultaneously. The biochemical pathway that converts proteins to appropriate T-cell antigens is called *antigen processing*.

▼ DIFFERENTIAL PROCESSING OF EXOGENOUS AND ENDOGENOUS ANTIGENS

Although pulsing of antigen-presenting cells with antigen is required to permit generation of a substrate capable of stimulating T cells, the antigenic molecule may be synthesized endogenously in some circumstances. This occurs, for example, in virally infected cells, in which viral proteins synthesized on host ribosomes nevertheless yield antigenic determinants that can be recognized by T lymphocytes interacting with cell surface structures. Moreover, a variety of self-antigens are routinely presented to T cells and provide a mechanism for deleting or neutralizing clones of cells that potentially mediate autoimmune responses.[4] Comprehensive studies over many years demonstrate that the distinction between exogenous antigens, acquired by phagocytosis, and endogenous antigens, which are synthesized directly by the presenting cell itself, is quite rigorous. They are processed in distinct compartments and are presented by different cell surface glycoproteins. Exogenous antigens for the most part appear on the cell surface in association with class II molecules, whereas endogenous antigens are typically presented in association with class I molecules. These two types of peptide-presenting proteins are structurally related and are encoded by linked genes.

▼ SPECIALIZATION OF T CELLS FOR RECOGNITION OF MAJOR HISTOCOMPATIBILITY COMPLEX CLASS I OR CLASS II STRUCTURES

The restriction of antigen presentation to class I or class II pathways is mirrored by a similar specialization of T cells themselves. Although all T cells bear similar antigen receptors on their surfaces, they differ with respect to the synthesis of two coreceptor structures. In healthy adults, about two thirds of peripheral T cells express the CD4 coreceptor molecule. These T cells are specialized to recognize exogenous antigens and to respond to antigen interaction by elaborating potent lymphokines. The remaining one third of circulating T cells instead express the CD8 coreceptor, and these cells usually recognize endogenous antigens. The response of CD8+ T cells to endogenous antigens presented in association with class I molecules also results in the production of lymphokines and can stimulate the maturation of cytolytic pathways that permit the CD8-bearing cell to specifically lyse target cells bearing appropriate antigens.

In normal adult T cells, CD4 expression and CD8 expression are mutually exclusive, reflecting the subspecialization of T cells bearing these structures (Fig. 13–2). However, T cells of both types must be presented with a processed antigen. Many of the enzymes required for this processing to take place, as well as the class I and class II presentation molecules themselves, are encoded within a multigene complex, the human leukocyte antigen region.

Molecular Biology of the Human Leukocyte Antigen Complex

Classic experiments performed more than 50 years ago by Owen and by Medawar and colleagues defined a set of simple rules that govern the fate of tissue grafts exchanged between individuals.[5] A rapid, immune-mediated rejection is observed for virtually all such allografts (i.e., performed between members of the same species) unless identity exists in a genetic region that came to be called the *major histo-*

CD4+ T Cell

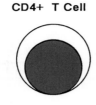

* Recognize peptide/class II complexes
* Produce IL-2, IL-3, IL-4, IL-5, IL-6, GM-CSF
* Regulate antibody production by B cells
* Regulate maturation of cytotoxic T cells

CD8+ T Cell

* Recognize peptide/class I complexes
* Produce interferon-gamma and IL-2
* Stimulate antigen presentation
* Activate inflammatory cells
* Directly mediate cytotoxicity

Figure 13–2. Subspecialization in the T-cell compartment. Mature T cells can be divided into two distinct populations, those that bear CD4 surface coreceptors and those that bear analogous CD8 polypeptides. The main functions of these two classes of cells are tabulated.

compatibility complex (MHC). Defined in all vertebrates, the MHC includes a set of codominantly inherited genes that function to permit appropriate antigen presentation to T lymphocytes. In humans, the genes of the MHC were first identified using serological reagents that detect white blood cell antigens. The MHC gene complex came to be known as the *human leukocyte antigen* (HLA) locus.[6] During the past decade, energetic application of molecular analysis has resulted in the nearly complete dissection of genes that reside within the HLA complex and its mouse analogue, the H-2 complex. Included within the fully sequenced 3.84 million base pairs (bp) that encompass the HLA complex are more than 200 genes, most of which exert direct effects on immune responsiveness.[7, 8] Up-to-the-minute information on MHC genes and gene functions can be found on the World-wide Web (http://www.sanger.ac.uk/HGP/Chr6/MHC.shtml).

▼ CLASS I GENES ENCODE CLASSICAL TRANSPLANTATION ANTIGENS

Traditionally, genes positioned within the HLA complex are divided into three classes. Class I genes are expressed in all nucleated cells and encode proteins that present peptide antigens to CD8-bearing T cells. The HLA-A, HLA-B, and HLA-C subregions include genes that encode human class I molecules. The class II molecules are structurally related and are encoded within the HLA-D region. A third set of molecules, encoded within the class III region, includes the complement components C2, C4, and factor B. Additional genes have been identified that encode components of the intracellular antigen-processing machinery. Figure 13–3 presents a diagram of the human HLA locus, indicating the approximate positions of the various genetic elements and the subregions into which these are grouped. Determination

of the complete sequence of the HLA region has yielded substantial new information on the organization and evolution of coding and regulatory regions that govern immune function.[9]

The class I molecules define targets for recognition by cytotoxic T lymphocytes (CTLs) and hence are often called classical transplantation antigens. Typical representatives of the extended family of immunoglobulin-like cell surface molecules, the class I proteins exist on the surfaces of all nucleated cells as non-covalently linked heterodimers of a 44-kDa heavy chain, the HLA-A, -B, or -C product, and a 12-kDa polypeptide, β_2-microglobulin, encoded separately on chromosome 15. Each class I heavy chain consists of three extracellular domains, $\alpha1$, $\alpha2$, and $\alpha3$, fused to a membrane-spanning region and a short intracytoplasmic extension (Fig. 13–4). The $\alpha1$ and $\alpha2$ domains, each about 90 amino acids long, fold to yield two parallel helical segments that form the boundaries of a groove that ordinarily accommodates peptide antigens.[10, 11] The floor of the groove is formed by an eight-stranded antiparallel α-pleated sheet to which both the $\alpha1$ and the $\alpha2$ domains contribute. The $\alpha3$ domain assumes a more conventional β-barrel structure, like that of other immunoglobulin superfamily members, and forms a stable interaction with β_2-microglobulin, itself similarly configured.[10] The $\alpha3$ domain also includes a site that interacts with the CD8 coreceptor glycoprotein expressed on most T lymphocytes that recognize class I–presented antigens.[12, 13] Figure 13–5 provides two views of the class I crystal structure first determined by Wiley and colleagues for an HLA-A molecule.[10] These investigators found that positioned within the outward-facing groove was additional electron density, representing processed peptide antigens that copurify with class I proteins.[11] Persuasive evidence supports the view that stable assembly of class I proteins at physiological temperatures usually requires additional peptides that

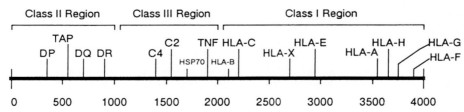

| | Class II Region | | | Class III Region | | | Class I Region | | |

Figure 13–3. Genetic structure of the HLA locus. Some of the more than 200 known genes that reside within this genetic region that spans 3.8 million base pairs on chromosome 6 are indicated. The positions of these genes are indicated along a scale calibrated in kilobase pairs. The centromere is at the left. The complete data set is available at http://www.sanger.ac.uk and is summarized in reference 8. TNF, tumor necrosis factor; HLA, human leukocyte antigen.

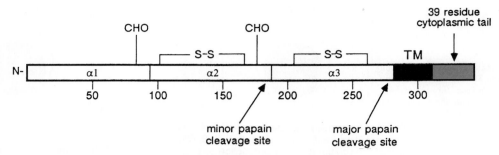

Figure 13–4. Structure of a class I molecule. Three extracellular domains are juxtaposed to a single transmembrane sequence and a short cytoplasmic tail. The presence of a dominant papain cleavage site near the outer membrane boundary has facilitated purification and crystallization of this molecule (see Fig. 13–5). The $\alpha2$ and $\alpha3$ domains contain typical immunoglobulin homology units with centrally placed disulfide bonds. The positions of carbohydrate residues are indicated. Data used to generate this diagram were derived from the structure of a murine class I molecule (H-2K^b); the structures of all class I molecules are closely related (see reference 10 for details).

interact non-covalently and that result from intracellular proteolysis of autologous proteins.[14] It should be apparent from Figure 13–5 that variations in the structure of HLA class I proteins between individuals could potentially influence the efficiency with which certain peptides are bound. Such differences almost certainly account for some variations in immune responses to infections in the human population and also contribute to susceptibility to numerous autoimmune diseases.

▼ ATYPICAL CLASS I GENES SUBSERVE MULTIPLE FUNCTIONS

The similar HLA-A, -B, and -C proteins are encoded by closely related genes (Fig. 13–6). In each case, the organization of exons parallels to a large extent the structure of the protein itself; each exon defines a distinct protein domain. Control of HLA class I expression depends primarily on transcriptional regulatory mechanisms that direct the synthesis of HLA-A, -B, and -C transcripts simultaneously in virtually all cells.[15] Defects in this transcriptional regulation may in part explain certain cases of bare lymphocyte syndrome in which the class I gene products are absent.[16, 17]

Analysis of the complete HLA sequence coupled with sequencing of ESTs has permitted identification of three additional classes of class I molecules. The class IB genes include those encoding HLA-E, -F and -G sequences. HLA-E presents a peptide derived from the leader sequence of other class I heavy chains to inhibitory receptors found on natural killer (NK) cells.[18–20] This interaction is believed to promote the destruction of cells that fail to express traditional class I molecules. The class IC genes include MICA and MICB (MHC class I-related peptide sequences A and B[21]), which interact with T cells of an unusual type, the $V_\delta1^+$ subset of those expressing the $\gamma\delta$ form of the T cell antigen receptor,[22] that appears prominently among intraepithelial lymphocytes of the intestine. Within this group is the *Hfe* gene, which encodes a class I–like protein that associates with the transferrin receptor, defects in which are responsible for hereditary hemochromatosis.[23]

The analysis of atypical class I proteins remains an active field of inquiry, providing many novel insights into immune function. Some atypical class I heavy chains are encoded outside the HLA locus. These polypeptides share overall organization with conventional HLA-A, -B, and -C molecules, and they associate with β_2-microglobulin.[21] Included in this group are the CD1 heavy chains CD1A, CD1B, CD1C, and CD1D, all of which are distinguished by their ability to present glycolypid antigens.[24] The human CD1D molecule, in common with the mouse mCD1 protein, can present the glycosphingolipid α-galactosylceramide to NK T cells,[25, 26] resulting in NK cell activation. These proteins, like their more conventional HLA-encoded counterparts, assist in coordinating immune recognition. The human neonatal Fc receptor, which assists in directing antibody secretion across epithelia, consists of a class ID heavy chain interacting with β_2-microglobulin.[27]

▼ CLASS II GENES ENCODE REGULATORS OF IMMUNE RESPONSIVENESS

Genetically determined differences in immune responsiveness between individuals of the same species frequently result from sequence variability in genes encoding class II molecules.[28, 29] Early studies in inbred animals established that the immune response (IR) loci mapped coordinately with class II specificities defined using lymphocyte proliferation assays.[29] In most cases, MHC-linked genetically determined nonresponsiveness displays recessive inheritance, although exceptions, apparent instances of MHC-encoded immunosuppression, have been widely described.[30] Biochemical studies provide a firm basis for understanding the immune response differences determined by class II genes. These elements encode cell surface proteins that present peptide antigens, derived from catabolism of ingested proteins, to CD4-bearing T lymphocytes.[31, 32] Allelic differences in class II gene structure almost certainly correspond directly to differences in the ability to present certain protein antigens properly.

Figure 13–7 shows the structure of class II molecules derived from analysis of the crystal structure of HLA-DR1.[33] Each consists of two approximately 30-kDa glycoproteins, the α and β chains, which are both encoded within the HLA complex.[7] In humans, three sets of functional α and β chain genes have been directly identified by DNA sequencing the HLA-DP, -DQ, and -DR families (Fig. 13–8). All class II molecules share the same general structure, reflecting their common antigen presentation function and a common evolu-

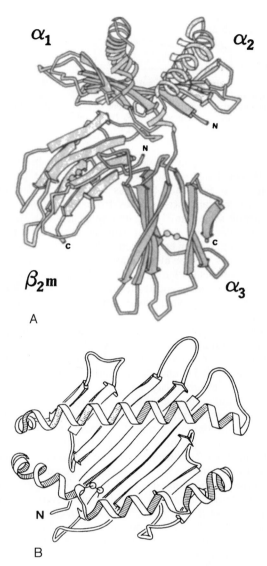

molecules. During intracellular assembly, class II molecules are associated with a non-MHC-encoded *invariant chain* (Ii), which assists in regulating intracellular transport of class II complexes.[35]

▼ REGULATION OF CLASS II GENE EXPRESSION

The class II proteins are expressed on the surfaces of specialized antigen-presenting cells: B lymphocytes, macrophages, dendritic cells, thymic epithelia, and some other stromal cell types. This restricted expression of class II molecules in inflammatory cells provides a mechanism whereby immune function can be triggered most effectively at sites of inflammation. In humans, class II gene expression can also be induced in activated T lymphocytes.[36, 37]

As in the case of class I genes, expression of the HLA class II genes is coordinately regulated (Fig. 13–9).[15] Transcriptional control regions for the class II genes have been determined,[38] and nuclear factors that participate in regulating the expression of class II transcripts have been rigorously identified. Restriction of class II protein expression to specialized antigen-presenting cells appears to be important. For example, evidence supports the view that inappropriate class II expression in certain cell types stimulates a focused autoimmune response. For example, enhanced expression of class II molecules in the β cells of pancreatic islets may precipitate the development of diabetes in some cases.[39] Similarly, class II expression on thyroid follicular cells in autoimmune thyroiditis has been occasionally observed. However, these results may reflect the action of inflammatory cytokines that act to increase class II gene transcription in many cell types.[40–43]

Although controversy exists regarding the deleterious effects of inappropriate class II gene expression, the failure to transcribe class II genes produces unambiguous immune deficits.[44–49] Because the class II genes are coordinately expressed, individuals lacking class II proteins were believed to have sustained mutations in a critical *trans*-acting factor that regulates all class II genes simultaneously. This hypothesis was borne out by somatic cell hybridization studies demonstrating that B cells from patients with bare lymphocyte syndrome, type II (a form in which class II gene expression is selectively abrogated, leaving class I gene expression intact), reacquire expression of all class II proteins simultaneously after fusion with B cells from a normal individual.[44, 45] Such studies defined four distinct complementation groups of genes regulating basal class II protein expression,[46] and all four yielded to molecular analysis, permitting definition of the class II transactivator *(CIITA)* gene and a complex set of polypeptides called RFX, which is believed to assist in permitting formation of transcription complexes for class I and class II genes but which does not exhibit independent transactivating properties.[16, 50] All forms of bare lymphocyte syndrome, including those in which class I gene expression is also affected, appear to result from defects in these two sets of proteins.

Although class I protein expression can be adjusted to only a limited degree in most normal cells, class II expression is highly responsive to the presence of certain lymphokines, notably interferon-γ (IFN-γ) and interleukin-4 (IL-4).[40–43] In both cases, expression is regulated at the level of

Figure 13–5. The three-dimensional structure of a class I molecule. The ribbon diagrams illustrate the structure of HLA-A2. *A,* Complete structure of the two-chain molecule seen from an axis perpendicular to the cell membrane. The free amino- and carboxy-termini of both the heavy chain and β2-microglobulin are indicated. The α strands appear as thick arrows in the amino- to carboxy-terminal direction. Loops and helical regions are depicted as thin lines and ribbons, respectively. Disulfide bonds are indicated by small circles. The carboxy-terminus of the heavy chain has been truncated at a papain cleavage site (see Fig. 13–4) near the membrane. Processed peptides bind within the helical groove defined at the top of the figure. The CD8 molecule on T cells interacts with class I heavy chains via sequences on both faces of the β barrel of the α3 domain. *B,* A second view of the HLA-A2 molecule locking down on the peptide-binding groove. This is the perspective that we imagine confronts a T-cell receptor molecule bent on antigen recognition. The T-cell receptor appears to make contacts with both the peptide and the class I molecule. (From Bjorkman, P.J., Saper, M.A., Samaroui, B., Bennett, W.S., Strominger, J.L., and Wiley, D.C.: Structure of the human class I histocompatibility antigen, HLA-A2. Nature 329:506, 1987; with permission.)

tionary origin that they share with class I molecules.[34] The class II polypeptides consist of two extracellular domains linked to the cell surface by a transmembrane helix and a short cytoplasmic tail. Interaction between the α1 and β1 chains yields an antigen-binding cleft like that in class I

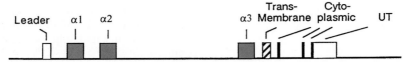

Figure 13-6. Organization of genes encoding class I molecules. The domain organization of these proteins is mirrored in the exon structures of the genes that encode them. Open boxes designate exons encoding the leader or the 3' untranslated region. Three distinct exons *(filled areas)* contribute to the synthesis of the 39 residue cytoplasmic domain. The sizes of the intervening sequences vary somewhat from element to element. (Data from Hood, L., Steinmetz, M., and Malissen, B.: Genes of the major histocompatibility complex of the mouse. Annu. Rev. Immunol. 1:529, 1988.)

transcription initiation. In most cell types, including several that do not ordinarily participate in antigen presentation, the addition of IFN-γ results in significant expression of class II molecules.[40] Because there is reason to believe that the proteolytic machinery responsible for antigen processing is widely distributed, the induction of class II transcription can suffice to promote effective antigen presentation by a variety of cells. An outline of the known transcriptional regulatory elements in typical class II genes is presented in Figure 13–10; notice especially the presence of IFN-γ regulatory sequences.

Antigen Processing: Presentation of Endogenously Synthesized Proteins

Two fundamental types of antigens must gain access to antigen-presentation molecules: products of intracellular synthesis and materials ingested through phagocytosis. Until recently, the mechanisms that permit catabolism of protein antigens and those that direct interactions between peptides and MHC-encoded presentation molecules were enigmatic. Remarkably, several crucial components of the antigen-processing apparatus (i.e., the HLA) are themselves encoded within the MHC complex.[51, 52] Moreover, refinements in microscale protein chemistry have led to the purification and characterization of processed peptides eluted from class I and class II molecules.[53–56] With this information, it has become possible to distill a satisfactory working model of antigen-processing pathways.

Proteins encoded by most chromosomal genes and those that are synthesized on cellular ribosomes using viral RNA templates are presented in peptide form to CD8-bearing T lymphocytes by class I molecules. The basic steps in this process involve digestion by endogenous proteases, transport of peptides to an appropriate site for interaction with class I proteins, and movement of the class I/peptide complex to the cell surface. Because the class I heavy chain and β2-microglobulin are glycoproteins synthesized on membrane-bound polysomes, peptide binding to the nascent class I protein must occur within the lumen of the endoplasmic

reticulum or in the Golgi complex. However, because peptides derived from proteins synthesized on free polysomes are effectively presented by class I molecules, mechanisms must exist to transport peptides from the cytosol into the endoplasmic reticulum.[56] Elegant experiments by Bevan and colleagues demonstrated that soluble proteins, introduced into the cytoplasm of cells through hypotonic lysis of pinocytotic vesicles, can be cleaved to yield peptides that become associated with class I molecules. The transport mechanism must act to "pump" peptides from the cytoplasm into secretory compartments, where assembly of class I molecules is achieved.[57]

Components of the proteolytic apparatus and the peptide pump are encoded within the class II region of the HLA complex. Two subunits of multifunctional protease structures (LMP2 and LMP7), known generally as proteasomes, that are expressed ubiquitously and have been highly conserved throughout eukaryotic evolution are found here (Fig. 13–11).[58] The proteasome is a 20S hydrolase possessing an active site threonine residue.[59, 60] Treatment of cells with proteasome inhibitors blocks the generation of peptides associated with class I molecules, and hence lowers the density of class I molecules at the cell surface.[61] In addition to these proteasome components, the TAP-1 and TAP-2 genes, which encode proteins that act as peptide transporters, also reside within the class II subregion.[62] These transporters are members of a larger "ABC" family of ATP-binding transmembrane pumps, but they function in this case to bring peptides from the cytoplasm to the lumen of the endoplasmic reticulum.

Studies of mutant mouse and human cell lines that cannot present peptides in association with class I molecules strongly suggest that proper assembly of these structures requires association with peptides generated in situ.[63, 64] This finding is reflected in heightened thermal instability of the "empty" class I structures. Intact class I molecules appear when such mutant cells are cultivated at low temperature, but they separate into constituent heavy and light chains when the temperature is raised to 37°C.[64] The peptide-free class I structures can be stabilized by adding exogenous peptide. Proper folding of the class I molecule with peptides

Class I heavy chain

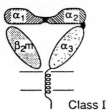

Class II α chain   Class II β chain

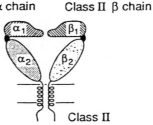

Figure 13–7. Class I and class II MHC proteins share a common structure. Comparison of the schematic organization of class I and class II proteins shows how β2-microglobulin, interacting with the α3 and α1 domains of the class I heavy chain, could have come to take the place of the α2 domain of the class II protein. (Adapted from Lawlor, D.A., Zemmour, J., Ennis, P.D., and Parham, P.: Evolution of class-I MHC genes and proteins: from natural selection to thymic selection. Annu. Rev. Immunol. 8:23, 1990; with permission.)

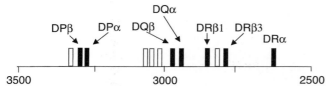

Figure 13–8. Structure of the class II region of the HLA locus. The HLA-D subregions span approximately 1000 kb. Filled boxes denote functional genes; the open boxes are pseudogenes in the completed sequence. Substantial polymorphism in HLA-D region organization exists in the human population. For example, individuals with as few as one DRβ gene element or as many as four (with two central pseudogenes) have been identified. (Adapted from MHC Sequencing Consortium. Nature 401:921, 1999; with permission.)

Table 13–1. Consensus Motifs in Peptides Eluted From MHC Class I Molecules*

Species	Class I Allele	\multicolumn{9}{c}{Peptide Sequence at Position}
		1	2	3	4	5	6	7	8	9
Mouse	D^b	X	M L P V	I E Q V	K	**N** F	L	X	X	**M** I
Mouse	K^d	X	**Y** I L	N	P	M	K F	T N	X	I L
Mouse	K^b	X	X	Y	X	F Y	X	X	**L** M	
Human	HLA-A2	X	**L** M	X	E K	X	V	X	K	**V**
Human	HLA-B27	R K G	**R**	X	X	X	X	X	X	K R

*Shown are consensus sequences, in single-letter code, with X denoting any amino acid, of peptides eluted from immunoprecipitates containing the indicated class I molecule. In each case, multiple different peptides were purified by high-performance liquid chromatography, and alignment was achieved with reference to the few highly conserved residues. Assignments noted in boldface are those believed to be critical for binding to the indicated class I protein. The class I protein encoded by the mouse K^b gene binds octamer sequences that differ dramatically from those nonamers found associated with the allelic K^d class I protein. See Falk et al.[59] and Jardetzky et al.[62] for additional information.

is probably facilitated by molecular chaperones, and two members of the heat shock protein (hsp 70) family, believed to assist in this process, are encoded within the HLA complex.[65]

From a biochemical perspective, it is difficult to imagine that three major class I proteins, the HLA-A, -B, and -C molecules, can satisfactorily present the full range of viral peptides that may be necessary for immune defense. Similarly, it is difficult to imagine how satisfactory antigen presentation can be achieved when peptides derived by catabolism of host proteins must certainly outnumber to a very large extent those encoded by intracellular parasites. Purification of the peptides associated with class I proteins from humans and mice provides a sense of the overall capabilities of the class I antigen presentation system.[4, 53, 54] This strategy, first pursued by Rammensee and colleagues, has proved to be extraordinarily revealing. In general, papain-solubilized class I molecules are purified and the peptide components eluted using organic acid. These peptide products can be fractionated and characterized. Several general conclusions emerge from this analysis. First, class I proteins bind peptides of quite specific length; only peptides composed of

eight or nine amino acids are acceptable. X-ray crystallographic evidence supports the view that nonamer peptides bind to class I molecules in an expanded conformation in which both the amino- and the carboxy-termini of the peptide fit within small pockets in the class I molecule-binding surface.[66, 67] Moreover, each class I molecule exhibits a distinct preference for peptides with certain primary structures.[68] This observation applies even to allelic class I proteins. Table 13–1 lists sets of peptides that have been found

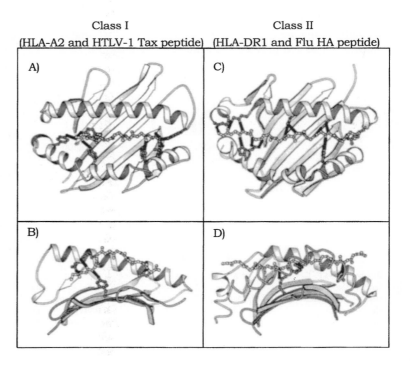

Class I
(HLA-A2 and HTLV-1 Tax peptide)

Class II
(HLA-DR1 and Flu HA peptide)

Figure 13–9. Class II and class I molecules have similar overall structures. The structure of HLA-A2 binding to a peptide from the human T cell leukemia virus *Tax* gene (HTLV-1 Tax), (*A* and *B*) is compared with that of the HLA-DR1 protein presenting an influenza hemagglutinin peptide (Flu HA) (*C* and *D*). A and C show the perspective looking down on the antigen presenting surface, and B and D show the features of peptide binding as viewed from the side. The peptide is shown in each case as a string of open circles. (Adapted from Madden, D.R.: The three-dimensional structure of peptide-MHC complexes. Annu. Rev. Immunol. 13:587, 1995; with permission.)

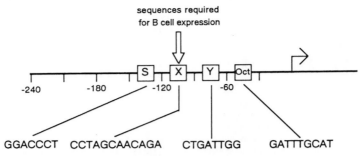

sequences required
for B cell expression

GGACCCT   CCTAGCAACAGA   CTGATTGG   GATTTGCAT

Figure 13–10. Sequences involved in regulating class II gene expression. The positions of regulatory elements within the DRα gene are indicated schematically, with the transcription start site (conventionally defined as +1) designated with an arrow at the right. Base pairs in the 5′ direction are preceded by a minus sign. A set of critical regulatory "boxes," representing the sequences indicated at the bottom, determines class II gene expression and responsiveness to extracellular stimuli. In DRα, 5′ truncation to the X box depresses expression in B cells but not in T cells or fibroblasts. Similarly, deletion of the X box markedly reduces B-cell expression. The X box also appears to be involved in the response to interferon-γ and is affected by the S and Y regions. (Data on transcriptional regulation of class II genes from references 38, 190, 193, and 194.)

to be bound to representative class I molecules and distills a consensus sequence for binding based on these results. By using the sequence rules inferred from such studies, it has been possible to correctly assign class I–presented peptides in whole-protein immunogens[69] and in proteins derived from parasites that reside intracellularly, such as *Listeria monocytogenes*.[70] The weight of evidence supports the view that endogenously synthesized proteins are in part degraded by a proteasome-based proteolytic mechanism, yielding peptides that in aggregate can be transported to the lumen of the endoplasmic reticulum, and that simple affinity mechanisms select those peptides that bear appropriate residues and that fit within the class I peptide–binding groove. The entire process is illustrated schematically in Figure 13–12.

Can class I molecules bind sufficient peptides to permit recognition of the entire universe of potential pathogens? Determination of the permissible binding sequences for HLA-B27 (an allele of HLA-B) allows some inferences. Tabulating all of the identified amino acid residues at each of the eight variable sequence positions (position 2 is an invariant arginine) and assuming that all amino acid combinations are acceptable (an untested assumption), we find that 13 million unique peptide sequences could be accommodated. This should provide an adequate mechanism for sam-

pling and presenting the majority of significant protein antigens. Perhaps not surprisingly, most of those peptides that have been characterized in HLA-B27 eluates derive from very abundant cellular proteins, such as histones and ribosomal proteins.[71] Peptide abundance in part determines the efficacy of expression; however, many studies suggest that there also exists a hierarchy for peptide binding.[72] This observation has prompted a search for high-affinity binding peptides that could be used to block presentation of self-antigens, thereby interdicting immune activation in autoimmune diseases.[73, 74] Such "masking" peptides would have the potential to serve as broad-spectrum immunosuppressants.

Similar concepts apply in understanding the mechanisms responsible for presentation of peptide antigens in association with class II proteins (reviewed by Watts[75]). In this case, exogenous proteins are ingested and degraded within

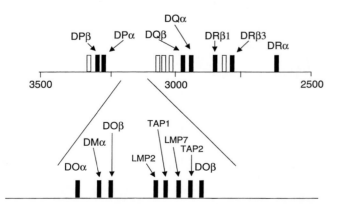

Figure 13–11. Components of a peptide-processing system are encoded within the HLA class II region. The positions of the TAP-1 and TAP-2 transporter genes and the LMP2 and LMP7 genes encoding components of the proteasome are indicated with respect to the DP and DQ subregions of the HLA complex. The DM and DO genes encode class II–like proteins that assist in regulating peptide loading within endosomal compartments. (Data from references 8 and 243.)

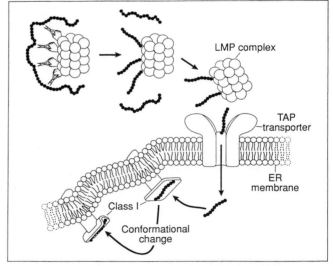

Figure 13–12. A model of class I antigen processing. Cytoplasmic proteins are degraded by the low-molecular-mass polypeptide (LMP) complex, which represents a subset of the cellular pool of proteasomes. Multiple peptides, believed to be confined primarily to nine residue segments, can be generated from each polypeptide targeted for degradation. Peptides are delivered to the TAP transporter, composed of both TAP-1– and TAP-2–encoded proteins. Once within the lumen of the endoplasmic reticulum, peptides bind to class I molecules, precipitating a change in class I conformation. (Adapted from Monaco, J. J.: A molecular model of MHC class-I–restricted antigen processing. Immunol. Today 13:173, 1992; with permission.)

membrane-bound vesicles, either endosomes or lysosomes. During synthesis, class II polypeptides extrude within the lumen of the endoplasmic reticulum and become associated with the invariant chain. This 30-kDa protein, another immunoglobulin-like molecule, binds to class II proteins in the endoplasmic reticulum but becomes cleaved and dissociates when these molecules transit the Golgi apparatus.[76] The invariant chain, the gene for which is coordinately regulated with class II genes,[77] prevents binding of peptides to class II molecules until Golgi-derived vesicles fuse with endosomes. This process is diagrammed in Figure 13–13. The invariant chain also helps to sort newly synthesized class II polypeptides to the endocytic compartment.[35] Although the precise timing of the interaction of class II molecules with catabolyzed ingested protein is unknown, the association is favored at low pH, a condition like that which occurs in phagocytic vesicles.[78] This association between class II molecules and their cognate peptides is remarkably stable, even in vivo.[79] The peptide may be thought of as an integral component of the surface-expressed class II molecule. Mutant cell lines bearing intact class II genes that nevertheless fail to assemble class II/peptide complexes permitted isolation of the *DM* gene within the HLA locus.[80] The DM protein serves as a chaperone for class II molecules and accelerates the loading of peptides on to the class II structure, in this way replacing the invariant chain, by a factor of 10^4.[81] The release of invariant chain is assisted by a proteolytic process that yields

a dominant peptide called CLIP.[82] Proteolytic cleavage of invariant chain is required for optimal antigen presentation and is mediated at least in part by cathepsins L and S, acting differentially in a tissue-specific fashion.[83–85]

As in the case of class I proteins, peptides that normally associate with class II molecules can be eluted from immunopurified class II structures and characterized directly.[55, 86, 87] Not surprisingly, most of these peptides derive from processing of self molecules.[83, 88] In this case, however, no simple consensus sequence can be derived by inspection of the amino acid sequences represented in the purified peptides (Table 13–2). In contrast to the situation described for class I molecules, class II protein–associated peptides vary dramatically in length and amino acid content.[87] It has also been possible to generate class II molecule–binding peptides that specifically block T-cell responses in an antigen-specific fashion.[89] These antigen antagonists may prove useful as pharmacological agents in that they offer the potential to block self-directed immune responses manifesting limited clonal heterogeneity.[90]

Allelic Variation in Major Histocompatibility Complex Genes

One of the most striking features of class I and class II genes is their extraordinary degree of sequence polymorphism. The

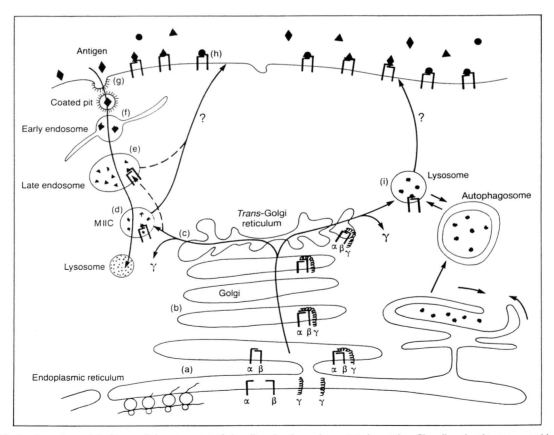

Figure 13–13. A schematic model of intracellular transport of class II molecules and associated peptides. Class II molecules are assembled from α and β chains, along with the invariant (denoted as γ) chain, shown at step *a* in the endoplasmic reticulum. These are transported through the endoplasmic reticulum to the *trans*-Golgi as a complex. The invariant chain assists in directing transport to the endocytic vesicle, where processed peptides arrive from coated pit-mediated internalization (steps *d* through *g*). Cytosolic proteins can enter the class II pathway through autophagosomes. In either case, the resulting class II–peptide complex, lacking the invariant chain that has been degraded, is transported to the surface. (Adapted from Neefjes, J. J., and Ploegh, H. L.: Intracellular transport of MHC class II molecules. Immunol. Today 13:174, 1992; with permission.)

Table 13–2. Heterogeneous Sequences Eluted from the Mouse I-A^d Class II Molecules*

Peptide	Sequence	Length	Source
1	W A N L M E K I Q A S V A T N P I	17	APO-E
2	D A Y H S R A I Q V V R A R K Q	16	CYS-C
3	A S F E A Q G A L A N I A V D K A	17	I-E^d-α
4	E E Q T Q Q I R L Q A E I F Q A R	17	APO-E
5	K P V S Q M R M A T P L L M R P M	17	Ii
6	V P Q L N Q M V R T A A E V A G Q X	18	TF RCP

*Shown are sequences of six peptides eluted in good yield from a mouse class II molecule. Compared with class I–associated peptides (Table 13–1), these peptides vary in length from 16 to 18 residues and vary dramatically in sequence. Perhaps not surprisingly, the most abundant peptides are derived from abundant cell surface molecules that have been internalized after expression or processed coordinately with expression of the class II molecule. The sources, deduced by comparison with all known proteins, are as follows: APO-E, mouse apolipoprotein-E; CYS-C, rat cystatin-C; I-E^d-α, mouse class II protein; Ii, mouse class I invariant chain; TF RCP, rat transferrin receptor. Peptides derived from processing of a different class II protein (I-E^d) can associate with the I-A^d molecule. See Hunt et al.[215] for additional discussion.

unusually large number of MHC alleles and the fact that no single allele predominates in most human populations stimulated early interest in the MHC on the part of human geneticists. Assignment of this allelic variation to specific substitutions in gene sequences has provided a fairly comprehensive view of variability within the class I and class II genes.

In considering only the class I genes, no special constraints dictate the precise number of such elements that exist in mammals. The rat MHC includes more than 60 classical and non-classical class I genes, whereas the pig SLA locus includes perhaps as few as 6 such elements.[91, 92] Examination of the allelic differences among human HLA-A, -B, and -C genes, defined from complementary DNA (cDNA) cloning studies, shows that most variability is concentrated within the α1 and α2 domains that figure prominently in defining the peptide-binding site. Virtually all of the residues exhibiting high variability between alleles are believed to participate in peptide binding.[67, 92, 93] These are residues located within the groove-flanking α helices or the β-pleated sheet floor that display inwardly directed side chains (Fig. 13–14). Polymorphism of the MHC genes contributes directly to variations in the antigen presentation repertoire in humans, as previously suggested based on peptide elution analyses.[68] This type of variation almost certainly provides an important substrate for environmental selection. Of the 50 known alleles at the HLA-B locus, the HLA-Bw53 allele is uniquely associated with a decreased risk of severe infection with *Plasmodium falciparum* malaria in West Africa.[94] Similarly, inheritance of a particular set of class II genes confers some protection from malarial disease. The HLA-Bw53 allele and the malaria-resistant class II haplotype are present at 10- to 15-fold increased frequency in West Africans compared with other ethnic groups, and the geographical distribution of these alleles follows that of the classically protective hemoglobin mutation Hb S.[94]

Polymorphisms in class I and class II sequences also contribute dramatically to susceptibilities to certain autoimmune diseases. Included among these are insulin-dependent diabetes mellitus, ankylosing spondylitis, and juvenile rheumatoid arthritis.[95] Table 13–3 shows the proportion of affected individuals who inherit specific MHC alleles can be quite high. Although the mechanism responsible for disease susceptibility in these cases remains enigmatic, it is attractive to postulate that certain class I or class II binding specifici-

ties present a peptide that stimulates T cells capable of interacting with a self-antigen.[96–98]

Regardless of the precise mechanism involved, sequence variations in MHC genes can profoundly affect disease susceptibility. This observation suggests that strong environmental selection, acting locally, is responsible for maintaining the high degree of polymorphism of MHC genes. How does this sequence variation arise? Studies in mice suggest intriguing possibilities. Experimental selection of mutant mice that no longer accept skin grafts from isogenic donors or that can no longer donate grafts capable of surviving without rejection led to the isolation of a series of class I gene mutations generated by an unusual mechanism of intergenic gene conversion.[99] For example, the bm3, bm4, bm10, and bm11 mutations in the mouse H-2K class I gene result from a non-reciprocal genetic exchange process that substitutes short segments derived from different class I genes in place of the analogous segment in the H-2K gene.[100] Segmental intergenic gene conversion appears to predomi-

Table 13–3. A Sampling of Diseases for Which Susceptibility Has Been Linked to Certain HLA Alleles*

Disease	Susceptible Allele	Approximate Relative Risk
Ankylosing spondylitis	B27	210
Anterior uveitis	B27	8
Behçet's disease	B5	5
Celiac disease	DR3	12
Dermatitis herpetiformis	DR3	17
Goodpasture's syndrome	DR2	14
Hemochromatosis	A3	7
Narcolepsy	DR2	130
Psoriasis	B37	8
Reiter's syndrome	B27	37
Rheumatoid arthritis	DR4	5
Sjögren's syndrome	DW5	6

*Susceptibility to more than 500 different diseases is associated with inheritance of certain HLA alleles or haplotypes. Some of the more significant examples are tabulated here. The mechanisms responsible for these disease associations almost certainly vary, but many diseases for which the relative risk to individuals at least heterozygous for an HLA allele is very high are believed to be autoimmune in nature. The most dramatic association remains one of the first to be discovered, that of HLA-B27 with susceptibility to ankylosing spondylitis. Different susceptibility patterns emerge in various racial backgrounds. In the case of narcolepsy, for example, susceptibility of individuals at least heterozygous for the HLA-DR2 allele is especially profound in Asians (relative risk >350). A comprehensive tabulation of these disease association data is presented in reference 216.

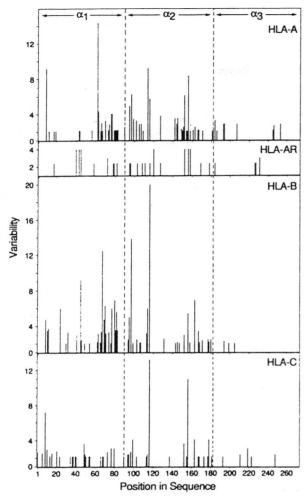

Figure 13–14. Polymorphisms are concentrated in the $\alpha 1$ and $\alpha 2$ domains of class I heavy chains. Deduced sequences of a series of 23 HLA-A, 6 HLA-AR, 30 HLA-B, and 11 HLA-C genes were aligned, and variability was plotted in each case as the quotient of the number of amino acids found at the indicated sequence position divided by the frequency of the most common amino acid. Relative "hot spots," indicating sites that presumably define differences in the ability to present peptide antigens, are readily discernible. (Adapted from Lawlor, D.A., Zemmour, J., Ennis, P.D., and Parham, P.: Evolution of class-I MHC genes and proteins: from natural selection to thymic selection. Annu. Rev. Immunol. 8:23, 1990; with permission.)

An intriguing example of the rapidity with which sequence heterogeneity can become fixed in the human class I genes has emerged through study of Native-American populations. These peoples are believed to be descended from Asian immigrants who arrived relatively recently, certainly during the past 40,000 years. Remarkably, the HLA-B alleles of South American Indians are both novel and highly diverse, reflecting a pattern of interallelic segmental exchange that has occurred at very high frequency.[101–103] These data suggest that gene conversion contributes more to allelic variation in human class I sequences than does point mutation.

▼ POLYMORPHISM IN PEPTIDE TRANSPORTERS

Although polymorphisms in the side-chain–binding pockets of class I molecules alter the characteristics of peptide binding and promote allelic differences in the efficacy of presentation of some antigens, other genes undoubtedly influence this process. For example, there is reason to believe that the peptide transporters responsible for conveying products of proteolysis from the cytoplasm to the lumen of the endoplasmic reticulum may preferentially select certain peptide sequences. In one study, an allelic difference in a putative peptide transporter gene positioned within the class II locus of the rat (i.e., the mtp-2 gene, which is the TAP-2 gene in this species) proved responsible for variations in the representation of class I peptide complexes obtained when identical class I genes were present.[104] Similarly, variations in the efficacy of HLA-B27–restricted peptide presentation by different cell lines have been mapped to genes that reside in the human class II region, presumably TAP-1 or TAP-2.[105] Some data support the view that polymorphisms in peptide transporters contribute to variations in susceptibility to autoimmune diseases, notably insulin-dependent diabetes mellitus,[106] but in most cases, these observations reflect linkage disequilibrium with class II alleles that themselves affect disease susceptibility.[7]

▼ THE CLASS III REGION

The human MHC class III region comprises more than 1 million base pairs of DNA, within which at least 36 transcriptional units have been described.[6, 8] Included among these are the genes encoding steroid 21-hydroxylase (a P-450 enzyme[107]), hsp 70,[108] tumor necrosis factor (TNF)–α and –β,[109] and the complement components C2, C4A, C4B, and factor B[110–112] (Fig. 13–15). Allelic variations in the structures of some class III genes have been defined, and evidence suggests that this genetic variation may influence susceptibility to some diseases. The C4A and C4B genes provide good examples. These two genes are 99 per cent similar, differing by only 14 nucleotides, and encode classical pathway components involved in the formation of the C3 convertase.[113] Probably as a result of one amino acid difference, the C4A protein is most effective in interacting with antigen-antibody complexes, via the formation of an amide bond between C4A and free NH_2 groups on immune complex polypeptides, whereas the C4B protein forms ester bonds with carbohydrate moieties.[114] Approximately 35 per

nate in generating sequence substitutions in the H-2K gene. Similar mechanisms may help to explain some examples of variation in the HLA-A, -B, and -C genes; however, most observed variations in these elements occur intragenically. The HLA-A, -B, and -C loci thereby retain their independent identities over evolutionary time. For example, some HLA-A alleles can be recognized within the background of variation observed in the chimpanzee,[92] an organism that shared a common ancestor with humans at most 15 million years ago. These observations suggest two principal conclusions: first, that evolutionary selection, presumably reflecting susceptibility to childhood infectious diseases, acts on the accumulated allelic variation in the human population to maintain a high degree of polymorphism, and second, that from the perspective of the species, the presence of a large repertoire of MHC class I and class II specificities is highly desirable.

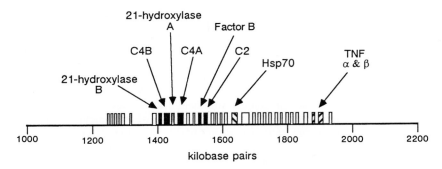

Figure 13–15. Gene organization in the HLA class III region. The positions of defined open reading frames (see Table 13–1) are indicated in a magnified view of Figure 13–3. Genes encoding components of the complement pathway (C4B, C4A, and factor B) are juxtaposed with those encoding enzymes of steroid biosynthesis (21-hydroxylase), elements that regulate protein folding (the heat shock protein Hsp70), and potent cytokines (tumor necrosis factors [TNF]–α and –β). It is perhaps unsurprising that polymorphisms in genes that reside in this region may be in linkage disequilibrium with others that potently affect immune function.

cent of individuals in most populations, irrespective of race, have at least one nonfunctional C4 allele. Persons inheriting MHC haplotypes that lack a full set of functional C4 genes are at considerably increased risk for a variety of autoimmune diseases. For example, the frequency of individuals with at least one C4A^{null} allele is greatly increased in populations of those afflicted with systemic lupus erythematosus. Moreover, almost all patients with complete C4 deficiency manifest systemic or discoid lupus erythematosus,[115] presumably resulting from a decreased ability to clear immune complexes. Deficiency of the C4A gene may occur in as much as 8 per cent of some populations and may be associated with a variety of immunodeficiency states. An intriguing report suggests that other genes within the class III complex may influence susceptibility to immunoglobulin A deficiency (the most common primary immunodeficiency disease) or common variable immunodeficiency.[116] Details of the functions of and sequence variation in immune-associated molecules can be found on the Internet at (http://imgt.cnvsc.fr).

Recognition of Antigen by T Lymphocytes

The response of T lymphocytes to appropriate antigen-presenting cells determines in a fundamental way all subsequent features of the immune response. T-cell–derived lymphokines regulate the influx of inflammatory cells, the maturation of antigen-specific B cells, and the recruitment of cytotoxic effector cells. The response of CD4-bearing helper T cells is especially important, because these cells are the principal sources of lymphokines.

Mature peripheral T lymphocytes provide a highly mobile surveillance system, passing through the interstitial spaces of all organs and into secondary lymphoid sites. Throughout these migrations, T cells make frequent contacts with potential antigen-presenting cells. Adhesion molecules expressed on the T-cell surface provide a molecular basis for interactions between cells bearing class I and class II proteins and circulating T cells. Included among these cell surface proteins are specialized integrins, adhesion molecules of the immunoglobulin superfamily (e.g., N-CAM, L-CAM), and the lectin-like molecules called *selectins*. Descriptions of these adhesion molecules are provided in Chapter 12.

Two key points regarding the interactions between T cells and antigen-presenting cells deserve special emphasis. First, variations in the expression of the adhesion structures can fundamentally alter the consequences of interaction between antigen-presenting cells and T lymphocytes. For ex-

ample, loss of the β_1 integrin LFA-1, a feature of patients with leukocyte adhesion deficiency, dramatically reduces T-cell responses.[117–120] Second, T-cell activation, usually stimulated by cross-linking of the T-cell antigen receptor, improves the avidity of the interaction between T cells and antigen-presenting cells. This phenomenon is well-illustrated in the case of LFA-1/ICAM-1 interactions, in which high-affinity binding results from productive stimulation of the T-cell antigen receptor.[121] Weak interactions between cell adhesion molecules on the T lymphocyte and its cognate presenting cell initially serve to juxtapose the antigen receptor with appropriate antigen presentation molecules. If the T-cell activation sequence is not initiated through this juxtaposition, de-adhesion permits dissociation of the two cells. In contrast, if antigen receptor stimulation occurs, the avidity of the cell interaction rapidly increases through post-translational changes in the affinity of adhesion molecule pairs and through enhanced synthesis of new adhesion molecules (e.g., the α_4 integrin VLA-4).

These mechanisms presumably ensure an adequate and prolonged T-cell response.[122, 123] Simple cross-linking of the T-cell antigen receptor by cognate antigen is not sufficient in most cases to direct the full T-cell activation response. Improved adhesion resulting from T-cell receptor cross-linking probably serves to increase the likelihood that accessory stimuli, crucial for T-cell responses, are provided. Included among the latter are signals from the CD28 molecule.[124] The T-cell activation responses reflect the result of a protracted molecular "dialogue" between T cells and antigen-presenting cells, wherein interactions among cognate ligands regulate responsiveness.[125, 126] The principal structure mediating T-cell activation is the T-cell antigen receptor itself.

Architecture of the T-Cell Receptor

As discussed in Chapter 11, the T-cell antigen receptor is a cell surface glycoprotein formed from two distinct polypeptide chains: α and β. A second isoform of T-cell receptor, composed of γ and δ chains, forms the antigen-binding structure on a small minority (<5 per cent) of circulating T lymphocytes.[127] The α and β chains (also γ and δ) are encoded by gene segments positioned discontinuously in germline DNA that become juxtaposed during intrathymic development. Combinatorial mechanisms permit the generation of an astonishingly large number (>10^8) of T-cell receptors from a relatively small set of germline gene segments. The nature of these combinatorial strategies, coupled with an active feedback regulatory mechanism, ensures that each

T lymphocyte expresses on its surface only a single type of receptor—the product of functional gene rearrangements driven to completion on only one allelic T-cell receptor gene copy.[128, 129]

Each T-cell receptor polypeptide is a glycoprotein composed of two immunoglobulin-like extracellular domains linked to a transmembrane sequence that terminates in a quite short (about six amino acids) cytoplasmic tail. The T-cell receptor membrane-spanning domains are unusual in that they contain a single negatively charged residue positioned within an otherwise hydrophobic sequence. It is widely believed that this charge is masked through interaction with other cell surface proteins bearing positively charged transmembrane residues. The T-cell receptor heterodimer ordinarily associates with just such structures, the γ, δ, and ϵ chains of the CD3 complex.[130]

▼ STRUCTURE OF THE CD3 MOLECULES AND THE GENES THAT ENCODE THEM

The CD3γ, CD3δ, and CD3ϵ components were originally detected by using monoclonal antibodies that identified a surface structure capable of transmitting activation signals to naive T lymphocytes. Each is an immunoglobulin-like, membrane-spanning, single-chain glycoprotein with a basic residue positioned within the putative membrane-spanning helix. All three proteins are encoded by closely linked genes positioned on chromosome 11 (11q23) in man.[131] The CD3γ and δ genes reside within 2 kb of each other. The human and mouse CD3 proteins are closely related and are expressed according to a similar developmental hierarchy. (See Chapter 12.) Compared with the T-cell receptor heterodimer, the CD3 chains boast comparatively long cytoplasmic extensions. These cytoplasmic domains constitute part of the signal transduction apparatus that links antigen recognition to the cell interior. Moreover, CD3 expression is absolutely required for appropriate assembly of the T-cell receptor protein complex.[130, 132] Immunoprecipitation of T-cell surface molecules with anti-CD3 reagents led to the discovery of a disulfide-linked homodimer, the ζ chain, which also forms part of the T-cell receptor complex.[133] Like the CD3 components, the ζ homodimer must be present to permit efficient intracellular assembly of the T-cell receptor. Only 6 residues of the mature ζ polypeptide are displayed extracellularly, whereas the comparatively long (113 residues) cytoplasmic portion contributes to the machinery of T-cell receptor signal transduction.[134, 135]

Figure 13–1 provides a schematic diagram of the structure of the T-cell receptor complex, indicating molecules that interact directly at the cell surface and depicting several of the coreceptor and signal transduction components that contribute to T-cell signaling. The enormous complexity of this cell surface receptor oligomer probably reflects a need to permit multiple different signal transduction responses to be activated selectively, depending on the nature of the stimulating cell. Evidence supports the view that a short sequence segment (minimally consisting of 18 amino acids), which exists in three copies in the ζ chain and in analogous forms in the CD3γ, δ, and ϵ chains, provides the link between the surface features of these signaling molecules and the signal transduction machinery at the cytoplasmic

face of the cell membrane[136, 137] by providing a substance for phosphorylation. Each of these repeat elements is called an ITAM motif, and there is reason to believe that the related but distinct coupling motifs of these different CD3 polypeptides provide a means to deliver subtly different signals following antigen recognition.[138] Another related sequence element, the ITIM motif, appears to coordinate inhibitory responses, such as those delivered from surface Fc receptors.[138, 139]

▼ BINDING OF THE T-CELL RECEPTOR TO ANTIGEN-PRESENTATION STRUCTURES

The T-cell receptor heterodimer recognizes peptide antigens presented in the context of class I or class II HLA-encoded structures. With the use of highly purified class II molecules and a soluble form of the T-cell receptor (generated by producing a phosphatidylinositol-linked form of the $\alpha\beta$ heterodimer and cleaving it from the surfaces of transfected cells by using phospholipases), it has been possible to study the characteristics of antigen recognition by T cells. These studies demonstrate that the T-cell receptor binds the class II/peptide complex and recognizes all three components (the peptide and both class II chains) together. In this manner, the specificity of antigen recognition is conferred by the T-cell receptor. However, the binding affinity for this interaction is quite low, at least an order of magnitude below that which characterizes antigen-antibody binding.[140] Several features of this binding reaction merit attention. First, under normal circumstances, T cells are multivalent structures, and antigen receptor binding may well exhibit cooperative characteristics. Second, other accessory molecules help to stabilize the interaction between the T-cell receptor and its cognate antigen presentation structure. Included among these are the adhesion molecules, the accessory signaling molecules, and the coreceptor structures CD4 and CD8. These coreceptors play especially important roles in thymocyte development. (See Chapter 12.)

Studies of antigen recognition by T lymphocytes led to the development of reagents composed of soluble peptide/MHC complexes, expressed in such a way that multimeric structures capable of binding directly to T cells in an antigen-specific fashion could be produced.[141] These tetramers (usually assembled using streptavidin to bind to biotinylated proteins) provide a means for directly visualizing those T cells that are active in an immune response.[142]

▼ CORECEPTOR STRUCTURES CONTRIBUTING TO T-CELL ACTIVATION

Although most thymocytes simultaneously express CD4 and CD8 surface glycoproteins, mature T lymphocytes express these genes in a mutually exclusive fashion, reflecting two distinct developmental programs. CD4$^+$ cells recognize peptide antigens presented by class II proteins and, when activated, respond by elaborating lymphokines. CD8$^+$ cells recognize peptide antigens presented in association with class I antigen presentation molecules and respond to stimulation primarily by maturing into cytolytic effector cells (although some cytokines, particularly interferon-γ, are produced by these cells as well). The CD4 and CD8 coreceptor structures themselves are superficially similar products of unlinked genes that conform to the general outline of immunoglobulin superfamily members. The CD4 protein is a monomer that recognizes monomorphic determinants present on all class II molecules.[143] It boasts a simple membrane-spanning domain and a short (28 residues) cytoplasmic tail. The CD8 structure is composed of two polypeptides, CD8α and CD8β, that are most often expressed as heterodimers but that can exist as homodimers as well.[144] Both forms of CD8 recognize determinants in the β3 domains of class I molecules.[12] Crystal structures defining this interaction have been determined.[75]

Despite the easily documented recognition of class I and class II proteins by CD8 and CD4, respectively, the structure of the T-cell receptor heterodimer by determines the recognition specificity of the T cell on which it is expressed. Experiments performed in hybridomas demonstrated persuasively that nominal peptide antigen specificity and specificity for either class I or class II presentation molecules were discretely defined by the presence of the α and β T-cell receptor chains.[145] In subsequent years, the crystal structures of several soluble T-cell antigen receptors were determined in association with class I molecules, and the nature of the antigen recognition complex has been more carefully defined.[129] Color plate 13–1 presents the structure of a mouse αβ T-cell receptor specific for an ovalbumin peptide presented in the context of the H-2K^b class I gene. Complementarity between the variable region loops of the T cell receptor and the peptide/class I complex can be readily appreciated.[146]

Although it was initially proposed that CD4 and CD8 might act to improve the affinity of interaction between T cells and antigen-presenting cells,[144] the CD4 molecule becomes incorporated into the antigen-receptor complex during cognate recognition of appropriate ligands by T cells.[147] A similar situation applies in the case of CD8. Antibodies directed against these coreceptor structures usually block T-cell receptor–mediated activation. Nevertheless, the CD4 and CD8 coreceptors are not required for T-cell signaling, because there exist T lymphocytes, particularly those bearing γδ T-cell receptors, that do not express either coreceptor structure. Experiments performed using gene transfection methods to direct coreceptor expression in T-cell lines that lack CD4 and CD8 indicate that, given a T-cell receptor with complementary specificity, the presence of coreceptor structures dramatically improves the efficiency of T-cell activation in response to a minimal antigen dose.[143] Possible mechanisms for this effect are described below.

The Biochemistry of T-Cell Signaling

Ligand occupancy of the T-cell antigen receptor leads to a series of readily measured biochemical changes that evolve over a period of hours and culminate in cell replication. Experiments performed using antibodies to the T-cell receptor complex as surrogate activators suggest that, as in the case of B-cell immunoglobulin, cross-linking of the receptor is absolutely required to permit a full activation response. Monovalent T-cell receptor ligands are ineffective.[148] Studies performed using purified MHC class I molecules embedded in artificial membranes support the view that as few as 50

to 300 class I protein molecules can efficiently trigger a T-cell–bearing receptor of the appropriate specificity.[149, 150] Similar estimates derive from analyses of antigen-presenting cells themselves.[151, 152] Although in most cases antigen-presenting cells display more than 10,000 class I or class II molecules per cell, only a small fraction of these, perhaps less than 1 per cent, can be expected to contain a given processed peptide. There is reason to believe that nonspecific adhesive interactions linking stimulator/responder cell pairs are necessary to permit the juxtaposition of sufficient T-cell receptor structures with appropriate cognate antigen presentation molecules.

Within seconds after T-cell receptor stimulation, it is possible to observe the accumulation of protein substrates that have become phosphorylated on tyrosine.[153, 154] Although the complete range of phosphotyrosine-containing substrates is unknown, several potentially important signaling molecules have been identified among the newly appearing phosphoproteins (Fig. 13–16), and in general, the pathways that become activated through kinase activation closely resemble those that participate in other growth factor–elicited signaling systems. The molecules involved in mediating T-cell activation are known in considerable detail (see below).

Within 30 seconds after cross-linking of T-cell antigen receptors, mobilization of intracellular calcium stores is observed. As a result, cytosolic free calcium levels rise from mean basal concentrations of 100 nM to values exceeding 500 nM.[155, 156] After the initial rise in intracellular free calcium concentrations, there follows a series of contingent regulatory events, including the accumulation of p21ras in its GTP-bound form,[157] augmented transcription of the IL-2 receptor α chain gene,[158] augmented translation of ornithine decarboxylase transcripts,[159] and the synthesis of IL-2 itself.[160] DNA synthesis commences after about 24 hours, and replication occurs within 48 hours.[161]

Figure 13–17 outlines the biochemical events associated with T-cell receptor–stimulated T-cell activation, placing these along an arbitrary time line. In most cases, T-cell activation can be fully achieved via artificial treatment with a calcium ionophore and an activator of protein kinase C. This observation suggested a two-signal model of T-cell activation in which T-cell receptor stimulation would stimulate membrane phospholipid breakdown, leading to production of inositol phosphate second messengers that could trigger the release of calcium from intracellular stores.[162] Simultaneously, activation of protein kinase C would strongly promote alterations in transcriptional regulatory molecules. Later studies have focused on the protein tyrosine phosphorylation events that occur at the beginning of the lymphocyte activation sequence.[163] These changes in the activity of protein tyrosine kinases and phosphotyrosine phosphatases lie at the very heart of the lymphocyte response to antigen.

▼ PROTEIN TYROSINE KINASES MEDIATING LYMPHOCYTE ACTIVATION

Through a combination of molecular genetics and traditional biochemistry, a fairly comprehensive description of the early events in T-cell activation has been achieved. Binding of the T-cell receptor to cognate ligand stimulates the activity of

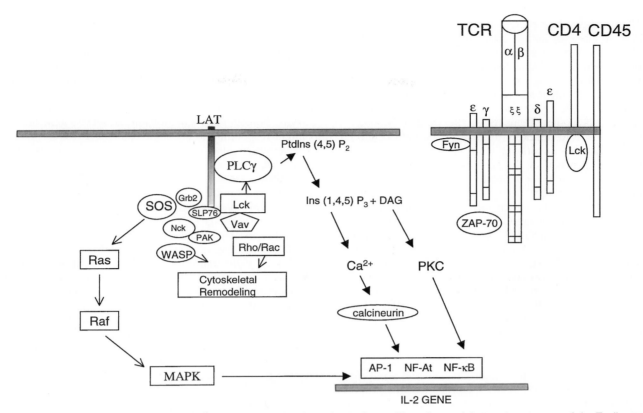

Figure 13–16. A schematic representation of T-cell receptor–reduced signaling pathways. The right panel depicts the structure of the T-cell receptor complex, noting the CD3γ, CD3δ, and CD3ε polypeptides, as well as the TCR ζ homodimer. The horizontal crossbars denote the presence of ITAM motifs, which can be phosphorylated by protein tyrosine kinases, most probably Lck and Fyn. This permits binding and activation of the ZAP-70 protein tyrosine kinase, which triggers a variety of metabolic changes depicted in the left panel. The biochemical details of this process are facilitated by a set of adaptor proteins, including the membrane-associated LAT molecule, which coordinates the binding of SLP-76, Grb2, Vav, and Nck. Assembly of Grb2 triggers GTP exchange on Ras, which ultimately results in MAP kinase activation. The Vav adaptor mediates cytoskeletal changes through the traditional action of the Rho/Rac small GTPases and the WASP protein, which is defective in patients with Wiscott-Aldrich syndrome.[244] Activation of Lck assists in the stimulation of phospholipase Cγ, which results in phosphatidylinositol breakdown, the mobilization of intracellular free calcium, and the activation of protein kinase C (PKC). Transmission of the calcium-derived signal is mediated in part by calcineurin, which is the target of cyclosporin A and tacrolimus (FK506). The signaling pathways converge on transcription factors that regulate cytokine expression. More detailed explications of these signaling events are available in references 178, 216, 245, and 246.

Figure 13–17. The biochemistry of T-cell activation. A sequence of biochemical changes is induced in a hypothetical T cell after antigen activation. In most cells, the first hour of ligand occupancy of the receptor induces an irreversible commitment to the subsequent activation sequence. Effects are represented on an approximate time line, with the magnitude of the effect graded in per cent on the ordinate. (Adapted from Ullman, K.S., Northrop, J.P., Verweij, C.L., and Crabtree, G.R.: Transmission of signals from the T lymphocyte antigen receptor to the genes responsible for cell proliferation and immune function: the missing link. Annu. Rev. Immunol. 8:421, 1990; with permission.)

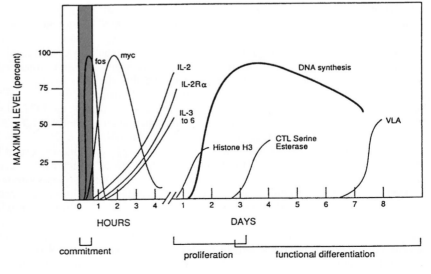

p56[164], a non-receptor protein tyrosine kinase that was first defined by virtue of its involvement in some cases of Moloney leukemia virus–induced transformation.[164] The *lck* gene encodes a lymphocyte-specific, membrane-associated protein tyrosine kinase that is expressed in T lymphocytes at all stages of development and at much lower levels in some B-lineage cells. NK cells also contain high levels of p56[lck] protein.[165] Like other members of the *src* family, p56[lck] is myristoylated at its amino-terminus and boasts three discrete sequence domains: a carboxy-terminal kinase domain occupying more than half of the 509 residues, a central domain containing so-called *src* homology motifs (SH2 and SH3 regions), and a unique amino-terminal domain, spanning about 70 amino acids, which differs for each of the eight well-characterized *src* family kinases but is conserved between species when analogous kinase genes are examined.[166] This amino-terminal segment, in the case of p56[lck], directs the interaction of the kinase with the carboxy-terminal cytoplasmic tails of the CD4 and CD8 coreceptor molecules.[167, 168]
Immunoprecipitation of either CD4 or CD8 from lymphocyte membranes results in coprecipitation of p56[lck] kinase activity.[169] Two pairs of cysteine residues surrounded by seemingly complementary basic (in CD4 and CD8) or acidic (in p56[lck]) amino acids form the highly specific binding sites that link coreceptor and kinase together. Because the association can be disrupted by certain chelating agents (e.g., orthophenanthroline) and because elimination of any of the four cysteine residues also prevents association,[167] it is possible that the interaction between these two molecules requires tetravalent coordination of a metal ion, probably Zn^{2+}.[170] Whatever the mechanism, antibody-mediated cross-linking of CD4 provokes readily observable increases in p56[lck] kinase activity.[169] These observations suggest a straightforward model for T-cell activation in which interaction of T-cell receptors with antigen-presenting molecules results in juxtaposition of the T-cell receptor complex with CD4 or CD8 coreceptors and hence the intracellular apposition of the T-cell receptor CD3 components with the p56[lck] protein tyrosine kinase, now in an activated form (see color plate 16–1).
Evidence supporting this model was derived from two types of experiments. First, in a T-cell line that absolutely requires CD4 coreceptor expression to sustain a signaling response, mutations in this coreceptor that compromise the interaction with p56[lck] also compromise antigen-induced activation.[143] Second, introduction of an artificially activated form of p56[lck], bearing a mutation in a regulatory phosphorylation site (Tyr505) positioned near the carboxy-terminus into some T-cell lines yields cells that respond more vigorously to antigenic challenge.[171] It is also intriguing that the *lck* gene is rearranged in at least two examples of human acute lymphocytic leukemia[172] and that overexpression of the *lck* gene in transgenic mice induces rapid lymphomagenesis.[173] Mutations in the *lck* gene were first identified in screen for variant T-lymphoma cells that were incapable of mobilizing intracellular calcium.[174] Subsequently, mice lacking functional Lck[175] or expressing a dominant-negative version of the Lck protein[176] were shown to manifest a profound block in T-cell development, corresponding to the inability to deliver signals from the pre-T-cell receptor. One report demonstrates that *lck* mutations are a rare cause of severe combined immunodeficiency disease in humans.[177] Strong data support the view that p56[lck] plays a pivotal role in signal generation after ligand occupancy of the T-cell antigen receptor.

Subsequent steps in this signaling process consist of phosphorylation of ITAM motif tyrosine residues in the CD3γ, CD3δ, CD3ε, and CDζ.[138] This permits docking of another protein tyrosine kinase, ZAP-70, through its phosphotyrosine-binding SH2 domains.[178] T cells from infants carrying homozygous mutations in the *ZAP70* gene are incapable of responding to antigenic challenge. Not surprisingly, these children also manifest a form of severe combined immunodeficiency.[179–181]
Another kinase that assists in coupling T-cell receptor–derived signals to the cell is p59[fyn]. The *fyn* gene is expressed at high levels in neuronal cells[182] and in T lymphocytes and directs the synthesis of slightly different proteins in these two cell types. This situation results from mutually exclusive alternative splicing of a single pair of *fyn* exons (exons 7A and 7B) to yield transcripts differing only in a central 150 nucleotide sequence.[183] In human[184] and murine developing thymocytes, p59[fyn] expression correlates with the acquisition of signal transduction capability by the T-cell antigen receptor.[185] Moreover, overexpression of p59[fyn] in the thymocytes of transgenic mice yields cells that exhibit hyperstimulable phenotypes when exposed to T-cell receptor–specific triggering events.[185] The T-cell form of p59[fyn] proved especially capable of mediating this effect when expressed in an insulin-reactive T-cell line.[186] These results provide evidence favoring a functional coupling of p59[fyn] with the T-cell receptor complex. A small fraction of total cellular p59[fyn] protein associates with the T-cell antigen receptor complex itself.[187] Overexpression of a catalytically inactive form of p59[fyn] blocks T-cell receptor–induced proliferation of mature thymocytes,[185] suggesting that p59[fyn] activity is required for antigen-stimulated responses in these cells. This result was confirmed in mice that lack a functional *fyn* gene, which were produced through gene targeting methods.[188] It appears that Lck and Fyn can transduce similar signals, because simultaneous disruption of both *fyn* and *lck* genes yields a more profound block in thymopoiesis than does either mutation by itself.[189] No human immunodeficiency diseases have been ascribed to *FYN* mutations.
Almost certainly, other protein tyrosine kinases participate in controlling T-cell receptor signaling. These include the Csk kinase, which acts in part by phosphorylating a regulatory site on Lck and Fyn,[190, 191] and the Itk kinase, which assists in modulating calcium entry.[192] In addition, the *syk* kinase, which is structurally related to ZAP-70, may be active in some T-cell subsets.

▼ CONTROL OF T-CELL ACTIVATION BY PHOSPHOTYROSINE PHOSPHATASES

One important feature of the protein tyrosine kinases is that they often receive critical regulatory input from other protein tyrosine kinases. For example, the *src*-like protein tyrosine kinases all possess tyrosine residues near their carboxy-termini that, when phosphorylated, act as negative regulators of kinase activity. Protein phosphorylation is achieved in the context of a regulatory cascade. Not surprisingly, dephosphorylation plays a critical role in the control of kinase signaling pathways. The importance of phosphotyrosine phosphatases in T-cell signaling became apparent with the discovery that the leukocyte common antigen CD45 contains two intracellular phosphotyrosine phosphatase domains.[193] The CD45 molecule is an extremely abundant protein on most leukocytes (>100,000 molecules per cell) and can be found in multiple different forms as a result of alternative splicing of exons that encode extracellular portions of the molecule.[194] Although some evidence favors the view that the CD22 molecule can serve as a ligand for at least one form of CD45 (CD45RO), definitive identification of ligands for other CD45 extracellular structures has not been achieved.[195] Remarkably, CD45 function is required for normal T-cell activation. Mutant T-cell lines lacking CD45 expression no longer sustain activation signals from the T-cell antigen receptor.[196, 197] Moreover, CD45 can dephosphorylate the carboxy-terminal phosphotyrosine (Tyr505) of p56^{lck} in a relatively specific fashion.[198, 199] Dephosphorylation of this carboxy-terminal site proceeds more efficiently than does dephosphorylation of a second, internally positioned phosphotyrosine. These observations further refine models for the control of T-cell activation through T-cell receptor signaling. If, as has been proposed, antigen recognition induces coaggregation of T-cell receptors, coreceptor structures, and CD45, activation of the p56^{lck} and p59^{fyn} protein tyrosine kinases might result from dephosphorylation of their carboxy-termini. They could phosphorylate and presumably activate phospholipases and other protein kinases that would provide the necessary signals to permit activation to proceed.

▼ ADAPTOR PROTEINS IN T-CELL SIGNALING

The activation of Lck, ZAP-70, and Fyn after T-cell receptor stimulation leads ultimately to changes in transcription of a variety of important genes and to cell replication. Linking these events are common signaling pathways that have been identified in cells responding to growth-promoting stimuli. These include the activation of phosphatidylinositol-specific phospholipase Cγ, leading to the accumulation of inositol 1,4,5-trisphosphate, the mobilization of intracellular free calcium, the release of diacylglycerol, and the activation of protein kinase C (reviewed by Dai and Lakkis[200]). A second major signaling pathway involves the accumulation of GRP-bound RAS, which binds and activates the Raf kinase, thereby stimulating the MAP kinase cascade.[201] Together these two pathways converge on important transcription factors, notably the AP-1 and NF-κB systems. How are the activities of these signaling pathways coordinated? Studies emphasize the importance of adaptor proteins in linking signaling modules within each T lymphocyte.

The adaptor proteins include a variety of cytosolic and membrane-bound structures that lack intrinsic enzymatic activity but that contain numerous motifs capable of binding other signaling proteins and often other adaptor proteins. Some of these proteins (e.g., LAT, SLP-76, FYB/SLAP, Gads, 3BP2) are expressed in a tissue-specific fashion, but others (e.g., Grb-2, Nck, c-Cbl) are relatively ubiquitous.[202, 203] The importance of the adaptor proteins was derived from analysis of their phosphorylation after T-cell activation and from direct binding experiments in which the interactions among the adaptors and their ligands were viewed by immunoprecipitation. There is no complete catalog of these molecules, much less of the importance of each in the signaling process. However, through the introduction of targeted gene disruptions in the mouse, it has become apparent that LAT,[204] an integral membrane protein with ten potential tyrosine phosphorylation sites, and SLP-76,[205] a cytosolic protein containing an SH2 domain, are absolutely required for T-cell receptor signaling.

Figure 13–16 presents a schematic view of the circuitry linking the T-cell antigen receptor to intracellular regulatory mechanisms. The broad array of adaptor molecules involved in the signaling cascade provides ample opportunity for variations in responsiveness, reflecting the integration of signals from accessory molecules. One of the most important features of T-cell receptor signaling is that the cellular responses to these signals vary enormously, ranging from proliferation to apoptosis to the imposition of a state of relative refractoriness to subsequent signals. Understanding how such diverse responses can be generated from the T-cell receptor complex remains the single most important challenge faced by those studying signal transduction in immune cells.

▼ INSIGHTS INTO T-CELL SIGNALING DERIVED FROM THE STUDY OF IMMUNOPHILIN LIGANDS

Additional features of the signal transduction pathways regulating T-cell activation have emerged through study of a set of clinically useful drugs that suppress allograft rejection. The first of these, cyclosporine, is a fungal product that binds an abundant intracellular protein called cyclophilin.[206] A structurally unrelated compound called FK506 (Fig. 13–18) exhibits a similar spectrum of activities but binds a different target, one or more of a group of FK506-binding proteins (FKBPs). Cyclosporine and FK506 act early in the T-cell activation process (within the first few hours) and block subsequent proliferation in large part by preventing transcription of lymphokine genes, particularly IL-2.[207] This effect results from the failure to correctly assemble critical transcription factors required for IL-2 expression.[208]

Remarkably, cyclophilin and the FKBPs behave as *cis-trans* prolyl isomerases.[206] These relatively abundant proteins appear to participate in regulating protein folding in various cellular compartments. Cyclophilin and FK506 block the isomerase activities of their respective ligands, which naturally suggested that the isomerization process was in some fashion crucial to T-cell activation. Instead it was learned that the drug/protein complexes form the active principles that abrogate signaling from the T-cell antigen receptor. For example, structural analogues of FK506 that retain the ability to inhibit prolyl isomerization by their respective ligands, but that no longer block T-cell activation, have been generated.[209] Moreover, the amount of drug required to inhibit T-cell function falls far below that required to saturate even 50 per cent of the cellular binding sites for each.[206] These observations prompted several groups to attempt to define additional signaling molecules that interact with the complex of cyclosporine plus cyclophilin. One such protein is the calcium-sensitive phosphoserine-specific phosphatase calcineurin.[210–212] Calcineurin-induced activation of IL-2 gene transcription is mediated by a set of transcription factors called NFAT (nuclear factor of activated T cells[213]), which

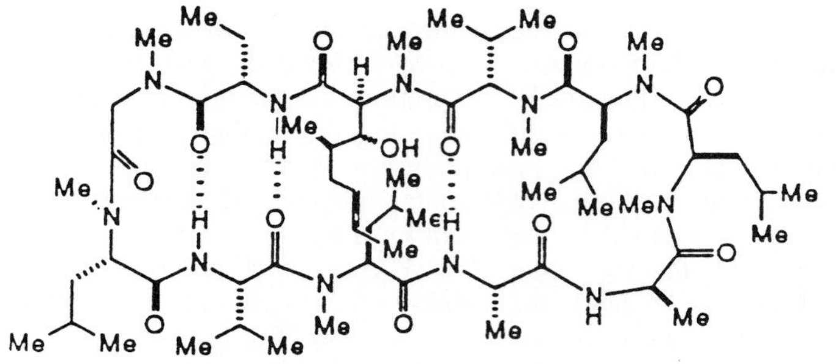

Cyclosporin A (CsA)

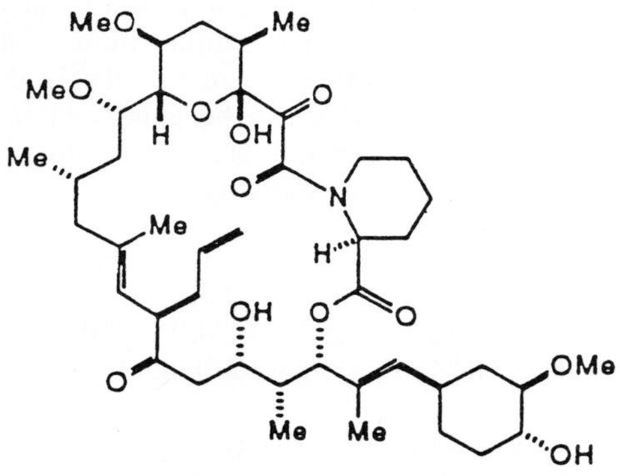

FK506

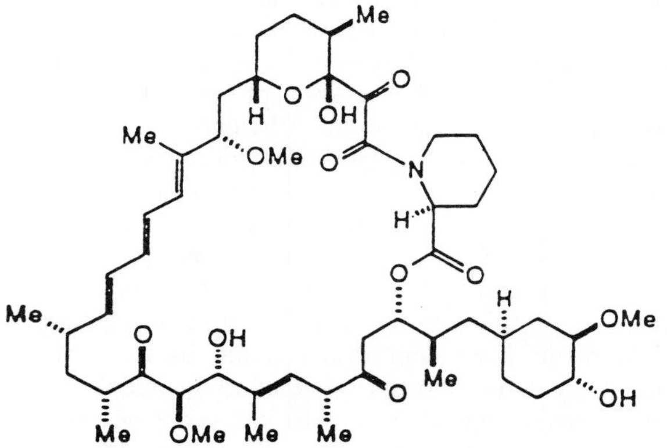

Rapamycin

Figure 13–18. Structures of three potent immunosuppressants that bind *cis-trans* prolyl isomerases. (Adapted from Schreiber, S. L.: Chemistry and biology of the immunophilins and their immunosuppressive ligands. Science 251:283, 1991; with permission.)

when dephosphorylated, translocate to the nucleus. This process is blocked by FK506 binding to FKBP.[214]

One interesting feature of cyclosporine and FK506 is that, although they effectively block T-cell activation stimulated from the T-cell antigen receptor, signaling from some other cell surface structures (notably CD28) remains intact. This observation emphasizes the underlying complexity of T-cell signaling pathways. Similarly, the macrolide rapamycin, which closely resembles FK506 in structure (see Fig. 13–18), fails to block T-cell receptor–mediated signaling but instead acts to prevent proliferation by binding to the TOR protein,[215] a member of the phosphatidylinositol kinase (PIK) family whose activity is inhibited by rapamycin binding.[216] In budding yeast, Tor activity controls aspects of the starvation response, but the precise role of TOR in human lymphocytes remains enigmatic. The immunophilin ligands provide remarkably specific tools with which to dissect the circuitry of lymphocyte signaling.

▼ ALTERNATIVE OUTCOMES OF T-CELL STIMULATION: ACTIVATION, ANERGY, AND APOPTOSIS

Not all interactions between T-cell receptor and cognate antigen-presenting molecules stimulate mitogenesis. Under some circumstances, signaling from the T-cell antigen receptor fails to deliver an activation signal and induces a state of relative refractoriness to subsequent antigenic challenge.[217] This phenomenon, called *clonal anergy*, can be readily demonstrated in transgenic mouse models in which a self-reactive T-cell antigen receptor is deliberately expressed in all developing T lymphocytes.[218] Depending on the nature of the receptor genes used, two distinct outcomes have been observed. First, self-reactive thymocytes may be deleted during development through apoptosis.[219–221] In some cases, however, thymocytes bearing a self-reactive receptor survive to populate secondary lymphoid organs, where they remain for the most part unresponsive to signals from their antigen receptors.[222] This phenomenon reflects a kind of fail-safe mechanism that ordinarily prevents T-cell activation in the absence of accessory signals normally provided by antigen-presenting cells.

In vitro systems that model the clonal anergy phenomenon suggest that a single signal derived from the T-cell antigen receptor in isolation probably produces a refractory state in most cases.[223] Appropriate second signals can be provided using fresh accessory cells and appear to result from cell-to-cell contact.[224] Although numerous candidates exist for relaying second signals, evidence supporting such a role for the CD28 molecule is especially strong. Expressed on virtually all T cells, CD28 interacts effectively with the B7/BB1 molecule on B lymphocytes.[225] B cells, which are extremely efficient antigen-presenting cells, can supply a second signal through CD28 that prevents anergy induction and permits proliferative responses.[202] The activity of CD28 is balanced by a related receptor, CTLA-4, which appears to play a blocking or inhibitory role.[200, 202]

In summary, T-cell interactions with antigen-presenting cells are initiated through relatively nonspecific adhesion events that are stabilized as activation proceeds. The T-cell stimulation pathway requires recognition of cognate antigen by the T-cell antigen receptor, which results in the activation of intracellular protein tyrosine kinases and a series of subsequent biochemical events leading ultimately to lymphokine secretion and proliferation. Satisfactory propagation of a T-cell receptor–derived stimulus requires additional signals that ordinarily result from interactions between surface structures present on the antigen-presenting cell and the responding T lymphocyte. In the absence of such accessory signals, an anergic state may result. It is easy to predict that a more detailed understanding of these signaling processes should permit the therapeutic manipulation of immune responses to reduce the risk of allograft rejection or autoimmune disease activity.

T-Cell Effector Mechanisms

▼ TYPES OF RESPONSES

Antigen recognition by mature CD4$^+$ T cells results in the elaboration of lymphokines that regulate all other immune phenomena. For example, TNF and the related molecule lymphotoxin (LT) help to stimulate inflammatory cells and epithelial cells. Similarly, IL-4 and IL-2 can act on B lymphocytes and on T cells. Products of activated CD4$^+$ T cells stimulate specific and nonspecific immunity. However, within the CD4$^+$ T-cell population there exist subsets of more specialized cells that differ with respect to cytokine repertoire. Initially defined in the mouse, it is now apparent that human T cells exhibit similar specialization. Among CD4$^+$ T cells, the Th1 cells secrete primarily IL-2 and IFN-γ when activated and stimulate cellular immune responses.[226] IFN-γ stimulates macrophage phagocytic activity and augments expression of class I and class II molecules. In contrast, Th2 cells secrete primarily IL-4, IL-5, and IL-6 and are potent regulators of B-cell responses to antigen.[227] Variations in the representation of Th1 and Th2 subsets may be responsible for different manifestations of common infectious syndromes. For example, lepromatous and tuberculoid responses to infection with *Mycobacterium leprae* result from a relative preponderance of Th2 and Th1 cells, respectively.[228]

Similar distinctions exist in the variable response to *Leishmania* infection in humans and mice.[229] Infection of most inbred mouse strains with *L. major* produces a cutaneous lesion that heals spontaneously, whereas progressive fatal infection is observed in a few strains. This difference in outcome appears to reflect the action of either Th1 or Th2 CD4+ cells in strains that respectively recover or succumb to the infectious process.[230] Differential outcomes of infection with *Plasmodium* and with various helminths have also been reported to depend on the relative extent to which Th1 versus Th2 cells are activated.[231] The mechanisms responsible for the preponderance of one response compared with another are unknown; however, the cytokines released by each subset are mutually inhibitory for cytokine production in cells of the other subset.[232] This observation may explain the phenomenon of conditioning of immune responses,

whereby a previously established Th1 response, for example, renders subsequent Th2 responses less likely.

▼ EFFECTOR PROPERTIES OF CD8$^+$ CELLS

Like CD4$^+$ T lymphocytes, mature CD8-bearing T cells exert part of their effector function through the release of cytokine molecules that activate other cell populations. Stimulated CD8$^+$ T cells in particular release IFN-γ, which stimulates phagocytic cells and promotes the expansion of B cells secreting certain immunoglobulin (IgG) isotypes and TNF. CD8$^+$ T lymphocytes also participate directly in the destruction of foreign targets through a contact-dependent, cell-mediated cytolysis mechanism. In general, cytolytic effector cells are CD8$^+$ T cells that specifically lyse membrane-enclosed targets after stimulation of their antigen receptors. The lytic process has been resolved into three steps involving Mg^{2+}-dependent binding; delivery of a "lethal hit," a calcium- and temperature-dependent phenomenon; and disintegration of the target. The precise molecular features of CTL-mediated cell lysis remain controversial; however, there exists a coherent model, supported by much experimental evidence, linking target cell destruction to the release of specific toxins from CTL granules by a calcium-requiring exocytotic process.[233] CTLs also can kill target cells by virtue of their expression of Fas-ligand, which binds and activates the death domain-containing Fas receptor on target cells, stimulating apoptosis.[234]

The potential importance of granules in CD8$^+$ T cells first became apparent when ultrastructural studies revealed the presence of pore-like structures in CTL targets undergoing lysis. These pores resembled those produced by the membrane attack complex, the terminal components in the complement cascade.[235] Systematic evaluation of the contents of CTL granules provided a candidate molecule that may mediate pore formation. This protein, perforin, shares sequence similarity with complement components C6 to C9.[236, 237] Purified perforin is a 65 to 70 kDa protein that readily polymerizes to form polyperforin. Perforin also directly lyses target cells when applied in solution, presumably by polymerizing to form pore structures.[238] In addition to perforin, the granules of CD8$^+$ CTLs and of NK cells contain serine esterases and lysosomal enzymes that assist in disrupting the integrity of target cells. A pivotal feature of this process is the activation of the caspase cascade of the target cell through the activity of granzyme B.[221, 239] Table 13–4 provides an updated list of those enzymes known to reside in the granules of CTLs.

Summary

Application of microscale biochemical and molecular biological methods has resulted in assembly of a fairly comprehensive view of immune function. Mechanisms that permit processing and presentation of foreign antigens, recognition by T lymphocytes, activation of these T cells, and the subsequent elaboration of potent effector molecules acting to stimulate or in some cases to eliminate target cells are now understood in considerable molecular detail. The impact of these discoveries is just being felt in the clinical setting. The

Table 13–4. Components of Cytoplasmic Granules in Cytotoxic T Lymphocytes

Molecule	Function
Perforin	Pore formation
Granzyme A	Trypsin-like protease
Granzyme B	Protease (cleaves after methionines)
Granzyme C	Protease
Granzyme D	Protease
Granzyme E	Protease
Granzyme F	Protease
Granzyme G	Protease
Chondroitin sulfate A	Carrier molecule
Leukolexin	Lymphokine (resembles TNF)
Cathepsin D	Lysosomal enzyme
Arylsulfatase	Lysosomal enzyme
α-Glucuronidase	Lysosomal enzyme
β-Hexosaminidase	Lysosomal enzyme
Granulysin	Saposin-like protein

A discussion of the potential importance of granulysin can be found in reference 247.

Adapted from Tschopp, J., and Nabholz, M.: Perforin-mediated target cell lysis by cytolytic T lymphocytes. Annu. Rev. Immunol. 8:279, 1990; with permission.

biochemical basis of disease susceptibility for autoimmune processes and for decreased resistance to infectious agents has become apparent in many cases. Successful defense against the universe of all potential pathogens requires a recognition mechanism capable of extraordinarily subtle discrimination and effector mechanisms of substantial power. In the future, improved understanding of both processes will permit design of novel therapeutic strategies. The immunophilin ligands, which capably interdict lymphocyte signaling pathways, will soon share clinical duties with potent inhibitors of lymphocyte signaling, which act through extracellular blockade of costimulatory signals or through interdiction of protein phosphorylation.[126]

An especially bright future can be predicted for antagonists of T-cell–derived cytokines, particularly with the clinical success of anti-TNF antibodies and soluble receptors in inflammatory bowel disease[240] and rheumatoid arthritis.[241] Modulation of the regulatory circuitry that dictates release of and response to these molecules holds special promise for immune intervention. Careful manipulation of these various strategies should permit substantial improvement in the prevention and treatment of autoimmune diseases without global compromise of immune responsiveness. Moreover, a detailed understanding of immune function should someday permit much more effective implementation of tissue transplantation. Advances in understanding of immune recognition and effector mechanisms have already had a profound effect on the design of vaccines, which in many cases provide the most cost-effective means of protecting human health. The successful eradication of human immunodeficiency virus–mediated diseases and of the parasitic diseases of underdeveloped countries depends on progress in each of these areas of immune system physiology.

ACKNOWLEDGMENTS

I thank Laura Peterson and Kimberly Doria for help in preparing this manuscript.

REFERENCES

1. Nossal, G.J.V., Szenberg, A., Ada, G.L., and Austin, C.M.: Single cell studies on 19S antibody production. J. Exp. Med. 119:485, 1964.
2. Naor, D., and Sulitzeanu, D.: Binding of radioiodinated bovine serum albumin to mouse spleen cells. Nature 214:687, 1967.
3. Davie, J.M., and Paul, W.E.: Receptors on immunocompetent cells. IV. Direct measurement of avidity of cell receptors and cooperative binding of multivalent ligands. J. Exp. Med. 135:643, 1972.
4. Udaka, K., Tsomides, T.J., and Eisen, H.N.: A naturally occurring peptide recognized by alloreactive CD8⁺ cytotoxic T lymphocytes in association with a class I MHC protein. Cell 69:989, 1992.
5. Medawar, P.B.: The behavior and fate of skin autografts and skin homografts in rabbits. J. Anat. 78:176, 1947.
6. Dausset, J.: Iso-leuco-anticorps. Acta Haematol. 20:156, 1958.
7. Beck, S., and Trowsdale, J.: Sequence organization of the class II region of the human MHC. Immunol. Rev. 167:201, 1999.
8. The MHC Sequencing Consortium: Complete sequence and gene map of a human major histocompatibility complex. Nature 401:921, 1999.
9. Moss, D.J., and Khanna, R.: Major histocompatibility complex: from genes to function. Immunol. Today 20:165, 1999.
10. Bjorkman, P.J., Saper, M.A., Samraoui, B., Bennett, W.S., Strominger, J.L., and Wiley, D.C.: Structure of the human class I histocompatibility antigen, HLA-A2. Nature 329:506, 1987.
11. Bjorkman, P.J., Saper, M.A., Samraoui, B., Bennett, W.S., Strominger, J.L., and Wiley, D.C.: The foreign antigen binding site and T cell recognition regions of class I histocompatibility antigens. Nature 329:512, 1987.
12. Salter, R.D., Benjamin, R.J., Wesley, P.K., Buxton, S.E., Garrett, T.P., Clayberger, C., Krensky, A. M., Norment, A.M., Littman, D.R., and Parham, P.: A binding site for the T-cell coreceptor CD8 on the alpha 3 domain of HLA-A2. Nature 345:41, 1990.
13. Kern, P.S., Teng, M., Smolyar, A., Liu, J., Hussey, R., Spoert, R., Chang, H.S., Reinherz, E.L., and Wang, J.: Structural basis of CD8 coreceptor function revealed by crystallographic analysis of a murine CDα ectodomain fragment in complex with H-2K. Immunity 9:519, 1999.
14. Ljunggren, H.G., Stam, N.J., Ohlen, C., Neefjes, J.J., Hoglund, P., Heemels, M.T., Bastin, J., Schumacher, T.N., Townsend, A., and Karre, K.: Empty MHC class I molecules come out in the cold. Nature 346:476, 1990.
15. van den Elsen, P.J., Gobin, S.J.P., van Eggermond, M.C.J.A., and Peijnenburg, A.: Regulation of MHC class I and class II gene transcription: differences and similarities. Immunogenetics 48:208, 1998.
16. DeSandro, A., Nagarajan, U.M., and Boss, J.M.: The bare lymphocyte syndrome: molecular clues to the transcriptional regulation of major histocompatibility complex class II genes. Immunogenetics 65:279, 1999.
17. Fischer, A., Cavazzana-Calvo, G., Basile, G.D.S., DeVillartay, J.P., Di Santo, J.P., Hivroz, C., Rieux-Laucat, F., and LeDeist, F.: Naturally occurring primary deficiencies of the immune system. Annu. Rev. Immunol. 15:93, 1997.
18. Borrego, F., Ulbrecht, M., Weiss, E.H., Coligan, J.E., and Brooks, A.G.: Recognition of human histocompatibility leukocyte antigen (HLA)-E complexed with HLA class I signal sequence-derived peptides by CD94/NKG2 confers protection from natural killer cell-mediated lysis. J. Exp. Med. 187:813, 1998.
19. Braud, V.M., Allan, D.S., O'Callaghan, C.A., Soderstrom, K., D'Andrea, A., Ogg, G.S., Lazetic, S., Young, N.T., Bell, J.I., Phillips, J.H., Lanier, L.L., and McMichael, A.J.: HLA-E binds to natural killer cell receptors CD94/NKG2A, B and C. Nature 391:795, 1998.
20. O'Callaghan, C.A., Tormo, J., Wilcox, B.E., Braud, V.M., Jakobsen, B.K., Stuart, D.I., McMichael, A.J., Bell, J.I., and Jones, E.Y.: Structural features impose tight peptide binding specificity in the nonclassical MHC molecule HLA-E. Mol. Cell 1:531, 1998.
21. Hughes, A.L., Yeager, M., Ten Elshof, A.E., and Chorney, M.J.: A new taxonomy of mammalian MHC class I molecules. Immunol. Today 20:22, 1999.
22. Groh, V., Steinle, A., Bauer, S., and Spies, T.: Recognition of stress-induced MHC molecules by intestinal epithelial γδ T cells. Science 279:1737, 1998.
23. Lebron, J.A., Bennett, M.J., Vaughn, D.E., Chirino, A.J., Snow, P.M., Mintier, G.A., Feder, J.N., and Bjorkman, P.J.: Crystal structure of the hemochromatosis protein HFE and characterization of its interaction with transferrin receptor. Cell 93:111, 1998.

24. Zeng, Z.-H., Castaño, A.R., Segelke, B.W., Stura, E.A., Peterson, P.A., and Wilson, I.A.: Crystal structure of mouse CD1: an MHC-like fold with a large hydrophobic binding groove. Science 277:339, 1997.

25. Brossay, L., Naidenko, O., Burdin, N., Matsuda, J., Sakai, T., and Kronenberg, M.: Structural requirements for galactosylceramide recognition by CD1-restricted NK T cells. J. Immunol. 161:5124, 1998.

26. Brossay, L., Chioda, M., Burdin, N., Koezuka, Y., Casorati, G., Dellabona, P., and Kronenberg, M.: CD1d-mediated recognition of an alpha-galactosylceramide by natural killer T cells is highly conserved through mammalian evolution. J. Exp. Med. 188:1521, 1998.

27. Burmeister, W.P., Gastinel, L.N., Simister, N.E., Blum, M.L., and Bjorkman, P.J.: Crystal structure at 2.2 A resolution of the MHC-related neonatal Fc receptor. Nature 372:336, 1994.

28. Klein, J., Figueroa, F., and Nagy, Z.A.: Genetics of the major histocompatibility complex: the final act. Annu. Rev. Immunol. 1:119, 1982.

29. McDevitt, H.O., Deak, B.D., Shreffler, D.C., Klein, J., Stimpfling, J.H., and Snell, G.D.: Genetic control of the immune response. Mapping of the Ir-1 locus. J. Exp. Med. 135:1259, 1972.

30. Watanabe, H., Matsushita, S., Kamikawaji, N., Hirayama, K., Okumura, M., and Sasazuki, T.: Immune suppression gene on HLA-Bw54-DR4-DRw53 haplotype controls nonresponsiveness in humans to hepatitis B surface antigen via CD8$^+$ suppressor T cells. Hum. Immunol. 22:9, 1988.

31. Harding, C.V., Leyva Cobian, F., and Unanue, E.R.: Mechanisms of antigen processing. Immunol. Rev. 106:77, 1988.

32. Buus, S., Sette, A., and Grey, H.M.: The interaction between protein-derived immunogenic peptides and Ia. Immunol. Today 98:115, 1987.

33. Stern, L.J., Brown, J.H., Jardetzky, T.S., Gorgo, J.C., Urban, R.G., Strominger, J.L., and Wiley, D. C.: Crystal structure of the human class II MHC protein HLA-DR1 complexed with an influenza virus peptide. Nature 368:215, 1994.

34. Hood, L., Steinmetz, M., and Malissen, B.: Genes of the major histocompatibility complex of the mouse. Annu. Rev. Immunol. 1:529, 1983.

35. Lotteau, V., Teyton, L., Peleraux, A., Nilsson, T., Karlsson, L., Schmid, S.L., Quaranta, V., and Peterson, P.A.: Intracellular transport of class II MHC molecules directed by invariant chain. Nature 348:600, 1990.

36. Benoist, C., and Mathis, D.: Regulation of major histocompatibility complex genes: X,Y, and other letters of the alphabet. Annu. Rev. Immunol 8:681, 1990.

37. Glimcher, L.H., and Kara, C.J.: Sequences and factors: a guide to MHC class-II transcription. Annu. Rev. Immunol. 10:13, 1992.

38. Boss, J.M.: Regulation of transcription of MHC class II genes. Curr. Opin. Immunol. 9:107, 1997.

39. Bottazzo, G.F., Dean, B.M., McNally, J.M., MacKay, E.H., Swift, P.G.F., and Gamble, D.R.: In situ characterization of autoimmune phenomena and expression of HLA molecules in the pancreas in diabetic insulitis. N. Engl. J. Med. 313:353, 1985.

40. Blanar, M.A., Boettger, E.C., and Flavell, R.A.: Transcriptional activation of HLA-DRa by interferon-γ requires a *trans*-acting protein. Proc. Natl. Acad. Sci. USA 85:4672, 1988.

41. Amaldi, I., Reither, W., Berte, C., and Mach, B.: Induction of HLA class II genes by IFN-γ is transcriptional and requires *trans*-acting protein. J. Immunol. 142:999, 1989.

42. Boothby, M., Gravallese, E., Liou, H.C., and Glimcher, L.H.: A DNA binding protein regulated by IL-4 and by differentiation in B cells. Science 242:1559, 1988.

43. Rosa, F.M., and Fellous, M.: Regulation of HLA-DR gene by IFN-γ. J. Immunol. 140:1660, 1988.

44. Hume, C.R., and Lee, J.S.: Congenital immunodeficiencies associated with absence of HLA class II antigens on lymphocytes result from distinct mutations in *trans*-acting factors. Hum. Immunol. 26:288, 1989.

45. Yang, Z., Accolla, R.S., Pious, D., Zegers, B.J.M., and Strominger, J.L.: Two distinct genetic loci regulating class II gene expression are defective in human mutant and patient cell lines. EMBO J. 7:1965, 1988.

46. Benichou, B., and Strominger, J.L.: Class II-antigen-negative patient and mutant B-cell lines represent at least three, and probably four, distinct genetic defects defined by complementation analysis. Proc. Natl. Acad. Sci. USA 88:4285, 1991.

47. Reith, W., Satola, S., Herrero Sanchez, C., Amaldi, I., Lisowska-Grospierre, B., Griscelli, C., Hadam, M.R., and Mach, B.: Congenital immunodeficiency with a regulatory defect in MHC class II gene expression lacks a specific HLA-DR promoter binding protein, RF-X. Cell 53:897, 1988.

48. Cosgrove, D., Gray, D., Dierich, A., Kaufman, J., Lemeur, M., Benoist, C., and Mathis, D.: Mice lacking MHC class II molecules. Cell 66:1051, 1991.

49. Grusby, M.J., Johnson, R.S., Papaioannou, V.E., and Glimcher, L.H.: Depletion of CD4$^+$ T cells in major histocompatibility complex class I deficient mice. Science 253:1417, 1991.

50. Gobin, S., Peijnenburg, A., Eggermond, M., Zutphen, M., van den Berg, R., and van den Elsen, P.J.: The RFX complex is crucial for the constitutive and CIITA-mediated transactivation of MHC class I and b2 microglobulin genes. Immunity 9:531, 1999.

51. Bahram, S., Arnold, D., Bresnahan, M., Strominger, J.L., and Spies, T.: Two putative subunits of a peptide pump encoded in the human major histocompatibility complex class II region. Proc. Natl. Acad. Sci. USA 88:10094, 1991.

52. Trowsdale, J., Hanson, I., Mockridge, I., Beck, S., Townsend, A., and Kelly, A.: Sequences encoded in the class II region of the MHC related to the "ABC" superfamily of transporters. Nature 348:741, 1990.

53. Rötzschke, O., Falk, K., Deres, K., Schild, H., Norda, M., Metzger, J., Jung, G., and Rammensee, H. G.: Isolation and analysis of naturally processed viral peptides as recognized by cytotoxic T cells. Nature 348:252, 1990.

54. Falk, K., Rötzschke, O., and Rammensee, H.G.: Cellular peptide composition governed by major histocompatibility complex class I molecules. Nature 348:248, 1990.

55. Rudensky, A.Y., Preston-Hurlburt, P., Murphy, D.B., and Janeway, C.A., Jr.: On the complexity of self. Nature 353:660, 1991.

56. Bevan, M.J.: Class discrimination in the world of immunology. Nature 325:192, 1987.

57. Moore, M.W., Carbone, F.R., and Bevan, M.J.: Introduction of soluble protein into the class I pathway of antigen processing and presentation. Cell 54:777, 1988.

58. Martinez, C.K., and Monaco, J.J.: Homology of proteasome subunits to a major histocompatibility complex-linked LMP gene. Nature 353:664, 1991.

59. Seemuller, E., Lupus, A., Stock, D., Lowe, J., Huber, R., and Baumeister, W.: Proteasome from thermoplasma acidophilum: a threonine protease. Science 268:579, 1995.

60. Coux, O., Tanaka, K., and Goldberg, A.L.: Structure and functions of the 20S and 26S proteasomes. Annu. Rev. Biochem. 65:801, 1996.

61. Rock, K.L., Gramm, C., Rothstein, L., Clark, K., Stein, R., Dick, L., Hwang, D., and Goldberg, A.L.: Inhibitors of the proteasome block the degradation of most cell proteins and the generation of peptides presented on MHC class I molecules. Cell 78:761, 1994.

62. Spies, T., Cerundolo, V., Colonna, M., Cresswell, P., Townsend, A., and DeMars, R.: Presentation of viral antigen by MHC class I molecules is dependent on a putative peptide transporter heterodimer. Nature 355:644, 1992.

63. Machold, R.P., Andree, S., Van Kaer, L., Ljunggren, H.G., and Ploegh, H.L.: Peptide influences the folding and intracellular transport of free major histocompatibility complex class I heavy chains. J. Exp. Med. 181:1111, 1995.

64. Elliott, T., Cerundolo, V., Elvin, J., and Townsend, A.: Peptide-induced conformational change of the class I heavy chain. Nature 351:402, 1991.

65. Spies, T., Bresnahan, M., and Strominger, J.L.: Human major histocompatibility complex contains a minimum of 19 genes between the complement cluster and HLA-B. Proc. Natl. Acad. Sci. USA 86:8955, 1989.

66. Madden, D.R., Gorga, J.C., Strominger, J.L., and Wiley, D.C.: The structure of HLA-B27 reveals nonamer self-peptides bound in an extended conformation. Nature 353:321, 1991.

67. Garrett, T.P., Super, M.A., Bjorkman, P.J., Strominger, J.L., and Wiley, D.C.: Specificity pockets for the side chains of peptide antigens in HLA-Aw68. Nature 342:692, 1989.

68. Falk, K., Rötzschke, O., Stevanovic, S., Jung, G., and Rammensee, H.G.: Allele-specific motifs revealed by sequencing of self-peptides eluted from MHC molecules. Nature 351:290, 1991.

69. Rötzschke, O., Falk, K., Stevanovic, S., Jung, G., Walden, P., and Rammensee, H.G.: Exact prediction of a natural T cell epitope. Eur. J. Immunol. 21:2891, 1991.

70. Pamer, E.G., Harty, J.T., and Bevan, M.J.: Precise prediction of a dominant class I MHC–restricted epitope of *Listeria monocytogenes*. Nature 353:852, 1991.

71. Jardetzky, T.S., Lane, W.S., Robinson, R.A., Madden, D.R., and Wiley, D.C.: Identification of self peptides bound to purified HLA-B27. Nature 353:326, 1991.

72. Smith, K., Pyrdol J., Gauthier, L., Wiley, D.C., and Wucherpfennig, K.W.: Crystal structure of HLA-DR2 (DRA*0101, DRb1*1501) complexed with a peptide from human myelin basic protein. J. Exp. Med. 188:1511, 1999.

73. Smilik, D.E., Lock, C.B., and McDevitt, H.O.: Antigen recognition and peptide-mediated immunotherapy in autoimmune disease. Immunol. Rev. 118:37, 1990.

74. Sinha, A.A., Lopez, M.T., and McDevitt, H.O.: Autoimmune diseases: the failure of self tolerance. Science 248:1380, 1990.

75. Watts, C.: Capture and processing of exogenous antigens for presentation on MHC molecules. Annu. Rev. Immunol. 15:821, 1997.

76. Roche, P.A., and Cresswell, P.: Invariant chain association with HLA-DR molecules inhibits immunogenic peptide binding. Nature 345:615, 1990.

77. Rahmsdorf, H.J., Harth, N., Eades, A.M., Litfin, M., Steinmetz, M., Forni, L., and Herrlich, P.: Interferon-γ, mitomycin C, and cycloheximide as regulatory agents of MHC class II–associated invariant chain expression. J. Immunol. 136:2293, 1986.

78. Wettstein, D.A., Boniface, J.J., Reay, P.A., Schild, H., and Davis, M.M.: Expression of a class II major histocompatibility complex (MHC) heterodimer in a lipid-linked form with enhanced peptide/soluble MHC complex formation at low pH. J. Exp. Med. 174:219, 1991.

79. Lanzavecchia, A., Reid, P.A., and Watts, C.: Irreversible association of peptides with class II MHC molecules in living cells. Nature 357:249, 1992.

80. Mellins, E., Kempin, S., Smith, L., Monji, T., and Pious, D.: A gene required for class II–restricted antigen presentation maps to the major histocompatibility complex. J. Exp. Med. 174:1607, 1991.

81. Mosyak, L., Zaller, D., and Wiley, D.C.: The structure of HLA-DM, the peptide exchange catalyst that loads antigen onto class II MHC molecules during antigen presentation. Immunity 9:377, 1999.

82. Ghosh, P., Amaya, M., Mellins, E., and Wiley, D.C.: The structure of an intermediate in class II MHC maturation: CLIP bound to HLA-DR3. Nature 378:457, 1995.

83. Rudensky, A.Y.: Endogenous peptides associated with MHC class II and selection of CD4 T cells. Semin Immunol 7:399, 1995.

84. Nakagawa, T., Roth, W., Wong, P., Nelson, A., Farr, A., Deussing, J., Villadangos, J.A., Ploegh, H., Peters, C., and Rudensky, A.Y.: Cathepsin L: critical role in Ii degredation and CD4 T cell selection in the thymus. Science 280:450, 1999.

85. Nakagawa, T., Brissett, W.H., Lira, P.D., Griffiths, R.J., Petrushova, N., Stock, J., McNeish, J.D., Eastman, S.E., Howard, E.D., Clarke, S.R., Rosloniec, E.F., Elliot, E.A., and Rudensky, A.Y.: Impaired invariant chain degradation and antigen presentation and diminished collagen-induced arthritis in cathepsin S null nice. Immunity 10:207, 1999.

86. Rudensky, A.Y., Preston-Hurlburt, P., Hong, S.C., Barlow, A., and Janeway, C.A., Jr.: Sequence analysis of peptides bound to MHC class II molecules. Nature 353:622, 1991.

87. Sette, A., Buus, S., Colon, S., Miles, C., and Grey, H.M.: Structural analysis of peptides capable of binding to more than one Ia antigen. J. Immunol. 142:35, 1989.

88. Hunt, D.F., Michel, H., Dickinson, T.A., Shabanowitz, J., Cox, A.L., Sakaguchi, K., Appella, E., Grey, H.M., and Sette, A.: Peptides presented to the immune system by the murine class II major histocompatibility complex molecule 1-A^d. Science 256:1817, 1992.

89. DeMagistris, M.T., Alexander, J., Coggeshall, M., Altman, A., Gaeta, F.C.A., Grey, H.M., and Sette, A.: Antigen analog–major histocompatibility complexes act as antagonists of the T cell receptor. Cell 68:625, 1992.

90. Rabinowitz, J.D., Beeson, C., Wulfing, C., Tate, K., Allen, P.M., Davis, M.M., and McConnell, H.M.: Altered T cell receptor ligands trigger a subset of early T cell signals. Immunity 5:125, 1996.

91. Rogers, J.H.: Mouse histocompatibility-related genes are not conserved in other mammals. EMBO J. 4:749, 1985.

92. Lawlor, D.A., Zemmour, J., Ennis, P.D., and Parham, P.: Evolution of class-I MHC genes and proteins: from natural selection to thymic selection. Annu. Rev. Immunol. 8:23, 1990.

93. Bjorkman, P.J., Strominger, J.L., and Wiley, D.C.: Crystallization and x-ray diffraction studies on the histocompatibility antigens HLA-A2 and HLA-A28 from human cell membranes. J. Mol. Biol. 186:205, 1985.

94. Hill, A.V.S., Allsopp, C.E.M., Kwiatkowski, D., Anstey, N.M., Twumasi, P., Rowe, P.A., Bennett, S., Brewster, D., McMichael, A.J., and Greenwood, B.M.: Common West African HLA antigens are associated with protection from severe malaria. Nature 352:595, 1991.

95. Tiwari, J.L., and Terasaki, P.I.: HLA and disease associations.

96. Wraith, D.C., Smilek, D.E., Mitchell, D.J., Steinman, L., and McDevitt, H.O.: Antigen recognition in autoimmune encephalomyelitis and the potential for peptide-mediated immunotherapy. Cell 59:247, 1989.

97. Todd, J.A., Bell, J.I., and McDevitt, H.O.: HLA antigens and insulin-dependent diabetes. Nature 333:710, 1988.

98. Todd, J.A., Bell, J.I., and McDevitt, H.O.: HLA-DQ beta gene contributes to susceptibility and resistance to insulin-dependent diabetes mellitus. Nature 329:599, 1987.

99. Hemmi, S., Geliebter, J., Zeff, R.A., Melvold, R.W., and Nathenson, S.G.: Three spontaneous H-2Db mutants are generated by genetic micro-recombination (gene conversion) events. Impact on the H-2-restricted immune responsiveness. J. Exp. Med. 168:2319, 1988.

100. Geliebter, J., and Nathenson, S.G.: Microrecombinations generate sequence diversity in the murine major histocompatibility complex: analysis of the Kbm3, Kbm4, Kbm10, and Kbm11 mutants. Mol. Cell. Biol. 8:4342, 1988.

101. Watkins, D.I., McAdam, S.N., Liu, Z., Strang, C.R., Milford, E.L., Levine, C.G., Garber, T.L., Dogon, A.L., Lord, C.I., Ghim, S.H., Troup, G.M., Hughes, A.L., and Letvin, N.L.: New recombinant HLA-B alleles in a tribe of South American Amerindians indicate rapid evolution of MHC class I loci. Nature 357:329, 1992.

102. Belich, M.P., Madrigal, J.A., Hildebrand, W.H., Zemmour, J., Williams, R.C., Luz, R., Petzl-Erler, M.L., and Parham, P.: Unusual HLA-B alleles in two tribes of Brazilian Indians. Nature 357:326, 1992.

103. Howard, J.: Fast forward in the MHC. Nature 357:284, 1992.

104. Powis, S.J., Deverson, E.V., Coadwell, W.J., Ciruela, A., Huskisson, N.S., Smith, H., Butcher, G. W., and Howard, J.C.: Effect of polymorphism of an MHC-linked transporter on the peptides assembled in a class I molecule. Nature 357:211, 1992.

105. Pazmany, L., Rowland-Jones, S., Huet, S., Hill, A., Sutton, J., Murray, R., Brooks, J., and McMichael, A.: Genetic modulation of antigen presentation by HLA-B27 molecules. J. Exp. Med. 175:361, 1992.

106. Faustman, D., Li, X., Lin, H.Y., Fu, Y., Eisenbarth, G., Avruch, J., and Guo, J.: Linkage of faulty major histocompatibility complex class I to autoimmune diabetes. Science 254:1756, 1991.

107. White, P.C., Grossberger, D., Onufer, B.J., Chaplin, D.D., New, M.I., Dupont, B., and Strominger, J.L.: Two genes encoding steroid 21-hydroxylase are located near the genes encoding the fourth component of complement in man. Proc. Natl. Acad. Sci. USA 82:1089, 1985.

108. Spies, T., Blanck, G., Bresnahan, M., Sands, J., and Strominger, J.L.: A new cluster of genes within the human major histocompatibility complex. Science 243:214, 1989.

109. Spies, T., Morton, C.C., Nedospasov, S.A., Fiers, W., Pious, D., and Strominger, J.L.: Genes for the tumor necrosis factors alpha and beta are linked to the human major histocompatibility complex. Proc. Natl. Acad. Sci. USA 83:8699, 1986.

110. Carroll, M.C., Palsdottir, A., Belt, K.T., and Porter, R.R.: Deletion of complement C4 and steroid 21-hydroxylast genes in the HLA class III region. EMBO J. 4:2547, 1985.

111. Woods, D.E., Edge, M.D., and Colten, H.R.: Isolation of a complementary DNA clone for the human complement protein C2 and its use in the identification of a restriction fragment length polymorphism. J. Clin. Invest. 74:634, 1984.

112. Morley, B.J., and Campbell, R.D.: Internal homologies of the Ba fragment from human complement component factor B, a class III MHC antigen. EMBO J. 3:153, 1984.

113. Yu, C.Y., Belt, K.T., Giles, C.M., Campbell, R.D., and Porter, R.R.: Structural basis of the polymorphism of human complement components C4A and C4B: gene size, reactivity and antigenicity. EMBO J. 35:2873, 1986.

114. Isenman, D.E., and Young, J.R.: The molecular basis for the difference in immune hemolysis activity of the Chido and Rodgers isotypes of human complement C4. J. Immunol. 132:3019, 1984.

115. Colten, H.R., and Rosen, F.S.: Complement deficiencies. Annu. Rev. Immunol 10:809, 1992.

116. Volanakis, J.E., Zhu, Z.-B., Schaffer, F.M., Macon, K.J., Palermos, J., Barger, B.O., Go, R., Campbell, R.D., and Schroeder, H.W., Jr.: Major histocompatibility complex class III genes and susceptibility to immunoglobulin A deficiency and common variable immunodeficiency. J. Clin. Invest. 89:1914, 1992.

117. Hibbs, M.L., Wardlaw, A.J., Stacker, S.A., Anderson, D.C., Lee, A., Roberts, T.M., and Springer, T.A.: Transfection of cells from patients with leukocyte adhesion deficiency with an integrin beta subunit (CD18) restores lymphocyte function-associated antigen-1 expression and function. J. Clin. Invest. 85:674, 1990.

118. Kishimoto, T.K., Larson, R.S., Corbi, A.L., Dustin, M.L., Staunton, D.E., and Springer, T.A.: The leukocyte integrins. Adv. Immunol. 46:149, 1989.

119. Kishimoto, T.K., and Springer, T.A.: Human leukocyte adhesion deficiency: molecular basis for a defective immune response to infections of the skin. Curr. Probl. Dermatol. 18:106, 1989.

120. Voss, L.M., Abraham, R.T., Rhodes, K.H., Schoon, R.A., and Leibson, P.J.: Defective T-lymphocyte signal transduction and function in leukocyte adhesion deficiency. J. Clin. Immunol. 11:175, 1991.

121. Dustin, M.L., and Springer, T.A.: T-cell receptor cross-linking transiently stimulates adhesiveness through LFA-1. Nature 341:619, 1989.

122. Hibbs, M.L., Xu, H., Stacker, S.A., and Springer, T.A.: Regulation of adhesion of ICAM-1 by the cytoplasmic domain of LFA-1 integrin beta subunit. Science 251:1611, 1991.

123. Larson, R.S., and Springer, T.A.: Structure and function of leukocyte integrins. Immunol. Rev. 114:181, 1990.

124. Harding, F.A., McArthur, J.G., Gross, J.A., Raulet, D.H., and Allison, J.P.: CD28-mediated signalling co-stimulates murine T cells and prevents induction of energy in T-cell clones. Nature 356:607, 1992.

125. Clark, E.A., and Brugge, J.S.: Integrins and signal transduction pathways: the road taken. Science 268:233, 1995.

126. Bolen, J.B., and Brugge, J.S.: Leukocyte protein tyrosine kinases: potential targets for drug discover. Annu. Rev. Immunol. 15:371, 1999.

127. Groh, V., Porcelli, S., Fabbi, M., Lanier, L.L., Picker, L.J., Anderson, T., Warnke, R.A., Bhan, A.K., Strominger, J.L., and Brenner, M.B.: Human lymphocytes bearing T cell receptor gamma/delta are phenotypically diverse and evenly distributed throughout the lymphoid system. J. Exp. Med. 169:1277, 1989.

128. Kronenberg, M., Siu, G., and Hood, L.E.: The molecular genetics of the T-cell antigen receptor and T-cell antigen recognition. Annu. Rev. Immunol 4:529, 1986.

129. Davis, M.M., Boniface, J.J., Reich, Z., Lyons, D., Hampl, J., Arden, B., and Chien, Y.: Ligand recognition by alpha beta T cell receptors. Annu. Rev. Immunol. 16:523, 1998.

130. Ashwell, J.D., and Klausner, R.D.: Genetic and mutational analysis of the T-cell antigen receptor. Annu. Rev. Immunol 8:139, 1990.

131. Tunnacliffe, A., Buluwela, L., and Rabbitts, T.H.: Physical linkage of three CD3 genes on human chromosone 11. EMBO J. 6:2953, 1987.

132. Berkhout, B., Alarcon, B., and Terhorst, C.: Transfection of genes encoding the T cell receptor-associated CD3 complex into COS cells results in assembly of the macromolecular structure. J. Biol. Chem. 263:8528, 1988.

133. Weissman, A.M., Baniyash, M., Hou, D., Samelson, L.E., Burgess, W.H., and Klausner, R.D.: Molecular cloning of the zeta chain of the T cell antigen receptor. Science 239:1018, 1988.

134. Irving, B.A., and Weiss, A.: The cytoplasmic domain of the T cell receptor a chain is sufficient to couple to receptor-associated signal transduction pathways. Cell 64:891, 1991.

135. Letourneur, F., and Klausner, R.D.: Activation of T cells by a tyrosine kinase activation domain in the cytoplasmic tail of CD3. Science 255:79, 1992.

136. Wegener, A.-M.K., Letourneur, F., Hoeveler, A., Brocker, T., Luton, F., and Malissen, B.: The T cell receptor/CD3 complex is composed of at least two autonomous transduction modules. Cell 68:83, 1992.

137. Romeo, C., and Seed, B.: Cellular immunity to HIV activated by CD4 fused to T cell or Fc receptor polypeptides. Cell 64:1037, 1991.

138. Healy, J.I., and Goodnow, C.C.: Positive versus negative signaling by lymphocyte antigen receptors. Annu. Rev. Immunol 16:645, 1999.

139. Ravetch, J.V., and Clynes, R.A.: Divergent roles for Fc receptors and complement in vivo. Annu. Rev. Immunol 16:421, 1999.

140. Matsui, K., Boniface, J.J., Reay, P.A., Schild, H., Fazekas de St. Groth, B., and Davis, M.M.: Low affinity interaction of peptide-MHC complexes with T cell receptors. Science 254:1788, 1991.

141. Altman, J.D., Moss, P.A.H., Goulder, P.J.R., Barouch, D.H., McHeyzer-Williams, M.G., Bell, J.I., McMichael, A.J., and Davis, M.M.: Phenotypic analysis of antigen-specific T lymphocytes. Science 274:94, 1996.

142. He, X.S., Rehermann, B., Lopez-Labrador, F.X., Boisvert, J., Cheung, R., Mumm, J., Wedemeyer, H., Berenguer, M., Wright, T.L., Davis, M.M., and Greenberg, H.B.: Quantitative analysis of hepatitis C virus-specific CD8(+) T cells in peripheral blood and liver using peptide-MHC tetramers. Proc. Natl. Acad. Sci. USA 96:5692, 1991.

143. Glaichenhaus, N., Shastri, N., Littman, D.R., and Turner, J.M.: Requirement for association of p56^{lck} with CD4 in antigen-specific signal transduction in T cells. Cell 64:511, 1991.

144. Norment, A.M., and Littman, D.R.: A second subunit of CD8 is expressed in human T cells. EMBO J. 7:3433, 1988.

145. Kappler, J.W., Skidmore, B., White, J., and Marrack, P.: Antigen-inducible, H-2 restricted interleukin-2–producing T cell hybridomas: lack of independent antigen and H-2 recognition. J. Exp. Med. 153:1198, 1981.

146. Garcia, K.C., Degano, M., Stanfield, R.L., Brunmark, A., Jackson, M.R., Peterson, P.A., Teyton, L., and Wilson, I.A.: An αβ T cell receptor structure at 2.5 Å and its orientation in the TCR-MHC complex. Science 274:209, 1996.

147. Rojo, J.M., Saizawa, K., and Janeway, C.A., Jr.: Physical association of CD4 and the T cell receptor can be induced by anti-T cell receptor antibodies. Proc. Natl. Acad. Sci. USA 86:3311, 1989.

148. Janeway, C.A., Jr.: The T cell receptor as a multicomponent signalling machine: CD4/CD8 coreceptors and CD45 in T cell activation. Annu. Rev. Immunol 10:645, 1992.

149. Brian, A.A., and McConnell, H.M.: Allogeneic stimulation of cytotoxic T cells by supported planar membranes. Proc. Natl. Acad. Sci. USA 81:6159, 1984.

150. Watts, T.H., and McConnell, H.M.: Biophysical aspects of antigen recognition by T cells. Annu. Rev. Immunol 5:461, 1987.

151. Harding, C.V., and Unanue, E.R.: Quantitation of antigen-presenting cell MHC class II/peptide complexes necessary for T-cell stimulation. Nature 346:574, 1990.

152. Demotz, S., Grey, H.M., and Sette, A.: The minimal number of class II MHC-antigen complexes needed for T cell activation. Science 249:1028, 1990.

153. Samelson, L.E., Patel, M.D., Weissman, A.M., Harford, J.B., and Klausner, R.D.: Antigen activation of murine T cells induces tyrosine phosphorylation of a polypeptide associated with the T cell antigen receptor. Cell 46:1083, 1986.

154. June, C.H., Fletcher, M.C., Ledbetter, J.A., and Samelson, L.E.: Increases in tyrosine phosphorylation are detectable before phospholipase C activation after T cell receptor stimulation. J. Immunol. 144:1591, 1990.

155. Imboden, J., Weiss, A., and Stobo, J.D.: The antigen receptor on a human T cell line initiates activation by increasing cytoplasmic free calcium. J. Immunol. 134:663, 1985.

156. Lewis, R.S., and Cahalan, M.D.: Ion channels and signal transduction in lymphocytes. Annu. Rev. Physiol. 52:415, 1990.

157. Downward, J., Graves, J.D., Warne, P.H., Rayter, S., and Cantrell, D.A.: Stimulation of p21ras upon T-cell activation. Nature 346:719, 1990.

158. Kronke, M., Leonard, W.J., Depper, J.M., and Green, W.C.: Sequential expression of genes involved in human T lymphocyte growth and differentiation. J. Exp. Med. 161:1593, 1985.

159. Abrahamsen, M.S., and Morris, D.R.: Cell type-specific mechanisms of regulating expression of the ornithine decarboxylase gene after growth stimulation. Mol. Cell. Biol. 10:5525, 1990.

160. Shaw, J.P., Utz, P., Durand, D.B., Toole, J.J., Emmel, E.A., and Crabtree, G.R.: Identification of a putative regulator of early T cell activation genes. Science 241:202, 1988.

161. Ullman, K.S., Northrop, J.P., Verweij, C.L., and Crabtree, G.R.: Transmission of signals from the T lymphocyte antigen receptor to the genes responsible for cell proliferation and immune function: the missing link. Annu. Rev. Immunol 8:421, 1990.

162. Wiskocil, R., Weiss, A., Imboden, J., Kamin-Lewis, R., and Stobo, J.: Activation of a human T cell line: a two stimulus requirement in the pretranslational events involved in the coordinate expression of IL-2 and gamma interferon gene. J. Immunol. 134:1599, 1985.

163. Altman, A., Coggeshall, K.M., and Mustelin, T.: Molecular events mediating T cell activation. Adv. Immunol. 48:227, 1990.

164. Marth, J.D., Peet, R., Krebs, E.G., and Perlmutter, R.M.: A lymphocyte-specific protein-tyrosine kinase is rearranged and overexpressed in the murine T cell lymphoma LSTRA. Cell 43:393, 1985.

165. Biondi, A., Paganin, C., Rossi, V., Benvestito, S., Perlmutter, R.M., Mantovani, A., and Allavena, P.: Expression of lineage-restricted protein tyrosine kinase genes in human natural killer cells. Eur. J. Immunol. 21:843, 1991.

166. Perlmutter, R.M., Marth, J.D., Ziegler, S.F., Garvin, A.M., Pawar, S.,

Cooke, M.P., and Abraham, K.M.: Specialized protein tyrosine kinase proto-oncogenes in hematopoietic cells. Biochem. Biophys. Acta 948:245, 1988.

167. Turner, J.M., Brodsky, M.H., Irving, B.A., Levin, S.D., Perlmutter, R.M., and Littman, D.R.: Interaction of the unique N-terminal region of the tyrosine kinase p56lck with the cytoplasmic domains of CD4 and CD8 is mediated by cysteine motifs. Cell 60:755, 1990.

168. Veillette, A., Bookman, M.A., Horak, E.M., Samelson, L.E., and Bolen, J.B.: The CD4 and CD8 T cell surface antigens are associated with the internal membrane tyrosine protein kinase p56lck. Cell 55:301, 1988.

169. Veillette, A., Bookman, M.A., Horak, E.M., Samelson, L.E., and Bolen, J.B.: Signal transduction through the CD4 receptor involves the activation of the internal membrane tyrosine-protein kinase p56lck. Nature 338:257, 1989.

170. Lin, R.S., Rodriguez, C, Veillette, A., and Lodish, H.F.: Zinc is essential for binding of p56(lck) to CD4 and CD8alpha. J. Biol. Chem. 273:32878, 1998.

171. Abraham, N., Miceli,M.C., Parnes, J.R., and Veillette, A.: Enhancement of T cell responsiveness by the lymphocyte-specific tyrosine protein kinase p56lck. Nature 305:62, 1991.

172. Tycko, B., Smith, S.D., and Sklar, J.: Chromosomal translocation joining LCK and TCRB loci in human T cell leukemia. J. Exp. Med. 174:867, 1991.

173. Abraham, K.M., Levin, S.D., Marth, J.D., Forbush, K.A., and Perlmutter, R.M.: Thymic tumorigenesis induced by overexpression of p56lck. Proc. Natl. Acad. Sci. USA 88:3977, 1991.

174. Strauss, D.B., and Weiss, A.: Genetic evidence for the involvement of the lck tyrosine kinase in signal transduction through the T cell antigen receptor. Cell 70:585, 1992.

175. Molina, T.J., Kishihara, K., Siderovski, D.P., van Ewijk, W., Narendran, A., Timms, E., Wakeham, A., Paige, C.J., Hartmann, K.U., and Veillette, A.: Profound block in thymocyte development in mice lacking p56lck. Nature 357:161, 1992.

176. Levin, S.D., Anderson, S.J., Forbush, K.A., and Perlmutter, R.M.: A dominant-negative transgene defines a role for p56lck in thymopoiesis. EMBO J. 12:1671, 1993.

177. Goldman, F.D., Ballas, Z.K., Schutte, B.C., Kemp, J., Hollenback, C., Noraz, N., and Taylor, N.: Defective expression of p56lck in an infance with severe combined immunodeficiency. J. Clin. Invest. 102:421, 1998.

178. Chu, D.H., Morita, C.T., and Weiss, A.: The Syk family of protein tyrosine kinases in T-cell activation and development. Immunol. Rev. 165:167, 1999.

179. Elder, M. E.: ZAP-70 and defects of T-cell receptor signaling. Semin. Hematol. 35:310, 1998.

180. Arpaia, E., Shahar, M., Dadi, H., Cohen, A., and Roifman, C.M.: Defective T cell receptor signaling and CD8+ thymic selection in humans lacking zap-70 kinase. Cell 76:947, 1994.

181. Elder, M.E., Lin, D., Clever, J., Chan, A.C., Hope, T.J., Weiss, A., and Parslow, T.G.: Human severe combined immunodeficiency due to a defect in ZAP-70, a T cell tyrosine kinase. Science 264:1596, 1994.

182. Ingraham, C.A., Cooke, M.P., Chuang, Y.-N., Perlmutter, R.M., and Maness, P.F.: Cell type and developmental regulation of the fyn proto-oncogene in neural retina. Oncogene 7:95, 1992.

183. Cooke, M.P., and Perlmutter, R.M.: Expression of a novel form of the fyn proto-oncogene in hematopoietic cells. New Biologist 1:66, 1989.

184. Sancho, J., Silverman, L.B., Castigli, E., Ahern, D., Laudano, A.P., Tarhorst, C., Geha, R.S., and Chatila, T.A.: Developmental regulation of transmembrane signaling via the T cell antigen receptor/CD3 complex in human T lymphocytes. J. Immunol. 148:1315, 1992.

185. Cooke, M.P., Abraham, K.M., Forbush, K.A., and Perlmutter, R.M.: Regulation of T cell receptor signalling by a src family protein-tyrosine kinase (p59fyn). Cell 65:281, 1991.

186. Davidson, D., Chow, L.M., Fournel, M., and Veillette, A.: Differential regulation of T cell antigen responsiveness by isoforms of the src-related tyrosine protein kinase p59fyn. J. Exp. Med. 175:1483, 1992.

187. Samelson, L.E., Phillips, A.F., Luong, E.T., and Klausner, R.D.: Association of the fyn protein tyrosine kinase with the T cell antigen receptor. Proc. Natl. Acad. Sci. USA 87:4358, 1990.

188. Appleby, M.W., Gross, J.A., Cooke, M.P., Levin, S.D., Qian, X., and Perlmutter, M.D.: Defective T cell receptor signaling in mice lacking the thymic isoform of p59fyn. Cell 70:751, 1993.

189. Groves, T., Smiley, P., Cooke, M.P., Forbush, K.A., Perlmutter, R.M., and Guidos, C.J.: Fyn can partially substitute for Lck in T lymphocyte development. Immunity 5:417, 1996.

190. Nada, S., Okada, M., MacAuley, A., Cooper, J., and Nakagawa, H.: Cloning of a complementary DNA for a protein-tyrosine kinase that specifically phosphorylates a negative regulatory site of p60c-src. Nature 351:69, 1991.

191. Schmedt, C., Saijo, K., Niidome, T., Kuhn, R., Aizawa, S., and Tarakhovsky, A.: Csk controls antigen receptor-mediated development and selection of T-lineage cells. Nature 394:901, 1998.

192. Liu, K.-Q., Bunnell, S.C., Gurniak, C.B., and Berg, L.J.: T cell receptor-initiated calcium release is uncoupled from capacitative calcium entry in Itk-deficient T cells. J. Exp. Med. 187:1721, 1999.

193. Fischer, E.H., Charbonneau, H., and Tonks, N.K.: Protein tyrosine phosphatases: a diverse family of intracellular and transmembrane enzymes. Science 253:401, 1991.

194. Fernandez Luna, J.L., Matthews, R.J., Brownstein, B.H., Schreiber, R.D., and Thomas, M.L.: Characterization and expression of the human leukocyte-common antigen (CD45) gene contained in yeast artificial chromosomes. Genomics 10:756, 1991.

195. Stamenkovic, I., Sgroi, D., Aruffo, A., Sy, M.S., and Anderson, T.: The B lymphocyte adhesion molecule CD22 interacts with leukocyte common antigen CD45RO on T cells and α2–6 sialyltransferase, CD75, on B cells. Cell 66:1133, 1991.

196. Koretzky, G.A., Picus, J., Thomas, M.L., and Weiss, A.: Tyrosine phosphatase CD45 is essential for coupling T-cell antigen receptor to the phosphatidyl inositol pathway. Nature 346:66, 1990.

197. Weaver, C.T., Pingel, J.T., Nelson, J.O., and Thomas, M.L.: CD8+ T-cell clones deficient in the expression of the CD45 protein tyrosine phosphatase have impaired responses to T-cell receptor stimuli. Mol. Cell. Biol. 11:4415, 1991.

198. Mustelin, T., and Altman, A.: Dephosphorylation and activation of the T cell tyrosine kinase pp56lck by the leukocyte common antigen (CD45). Oncogene 5:809, 1990.

199. Seavitt, J.R., White, L.S., Murphy, K.M., Loh, D.Y., Perlmutter, R.M., and Thomas, M.L.: Expression of the p56(Lck) Y505F mutation in CD45-deficient mice rescues thymocyte development. Mol. Cell. Biol. 19:4200, 1999.

200. Dai, Z., and Lakkis, F.G.: The role of cytokines, CTLA-4 and costimulation in transplant tolerance and rejection. Curr. Opin. Immunol. 5:504, 1999.

201. Tan, P.B., and Kim, S.K.: Signaling specificity: the RTK/RAS/MAP kinase pathway in metazoans. Trends Genet. 15:145, 1999.

202. Chambers, C.A., and Allison, J.P.: Costimulatory regulation of T cell function. Curr. Opin. Cell Biol. 2:203, 1999.

203. Clements, J.L., Boerth, N.J., Lee, J.R., and Koretzky, G.A.: Integration of T cell receptor–dependent signaling pathways by adaptor proteins. Annu. Rev. Immunol. 17:89, 1999.

204. Zhang, W., Sommers, C.L., Burshtyn, D.N., Stebbins, C.C., DeJarnette, J.B., Trible, R.P., Grinberg, A., Tsay, H.C., Jacobs, H.M., Kessler, C.M., Long, E.O., Love, P.E., and Samelson, L.E.: Essential role of LAT in T cell development. Immunity 10:323, 1999.

205. Pivniouk, V., Tsitsikov, E., Swinton, P., Rathbun, G., Alt, F.W., and Geha, R.S.: Impaired viability and profound block in thymocyte development in mice lacking the adaptor protein SLP-76. Cell 94:229, 1998.

206. Schreiber, S.L.: Chemistry and biology of the immunophilins and their immunosuppressive ligands. Science 251:283, 1991.

207. Tocci, M.J., Matkovich, D.A., Collier, K.A., Kwok, P., Dumont, F., Lin, S., Degudicibus, S., Siekierka, J.J., Chin, J., and Hutchinson, N.I.: The immunosuppressant FK506 selectively inhibits expression of early T cell activation genes. J. Immunol. 143:718, 1989.

208. Emmel, E.A., Verweij, C.L., Durand, D.B., Higgins, K.M., Lacy, E., and Crabtree, G.R.: Cyclosporin A specifically inhibits function of nuclear proteins involved in T cell activation. Science 246:1617, 1989.

209. Bierer, B.E., Somers, P.K., Wandless, T.J., Burakoff, S.J., and Schreiber, S.L.: Probing immunosuppressant action with a nonnatural immunophilin ligand. Science 250:556, 1990.

210. Liu, J., Farmer, J.D., Jr., Lane, W.S., Friedman, J., Weissman, I., and Schreiber, S.L.: Calcineurin is a common target of cyclophilin-cyclosporin A and FKBP-FK506 complexes. Cell 66:807, 1991.

211. O'Keefe, S.J., Tamura, J., Kincaid, R.L., Tocci, M.J., and O'Neill, E.A.: FK-506- and CsA-sensitive activation of the interleukin-2 promotor by calcineurin. Nature 357:692, 1992.

212. Clipstone, N.A., and Crabtree, G.R.: Identification of calcineurin as a key signalling enzyme in T-lymphocyte activation. Nature 357:695, 1992.

213. Rao, A., Luo, C., and Hogan, P.G.: Transcription factors of the NFAT family: regulation and function. Annu. Rev. Immunol. 15:707, 1997.

214. Aramburu, J., Yaffe, M.B., Lopez-Rodriguez, C., Cantley, L.C., Hogan, P.G., and Rao, A.: Affinity-driven peptide selection of an NFAT inhibitor more selective than cyclosporin A. Science 285:2129, 1999.

215. Brown, E.J., Albers, M.W., Shin, T.B., Ichikawa, K., Keith, C.T., Lane, W.S., and Schreiber, S.L.: A mammalian protein targeted by G1-arresting rapamycin-receptor complex. Nature 369:756, 1994.

216. Rudd, C.E.: Adaptors and molecular scaffolds in immune cell signaling. Cell 96:5, 1999.

217. Schwartz, R.H.: A cell culture model for T lymphocyte clonal energy. Science 248:1349, 1990.

218. Blackman, M.A., Gerhard-Burgert, H., Woodland, D.L., Palmer, E., Kappler, J.W., and Marrack, P.: A role for clonal inactivation in T cell tolerance to M1s-1a. Nature 345:540, 1990.

219. Von Boehmer, H., and Kisielow, P.: Self-nonself discrimination by T cells. Science 248:1369, 1990.

220. Blackman, M.A., Kappler, J., and Marrack, P.: The role of the T cell receptor in positive and negative selection of developing T cells. Science 248:1335, 1990.

221. Nicholson, D.W., and Thornberry, N.A.: Caspases: killer proteases. Trends Biochem. Sci. 22:299, 1997.

222. Swat, W., Ignatowicz, L., Von Boehmer, H., and Kisielow, P.: Clonal deletion of immature CD4$^+$8$^+$ thymocytes in suspension culture by extrathymic antigen-presenting cells. Nature 351:150, 1991.

223. Jenkins, M.K., and Schwartz, R.H.: Antigen presentation by chemically modified splenocytes induces antigen specific T cell unresponsiveness in vitro and in vivo. J. Exp. Med. 165:302, 1987.

224. Jenkins, M.K., Ashwell, J.D., and Schwartz, R.H.: Allogeneic non-T spleen cells restore the responsiveness of normal T cell clones stimulated with antigen and chemically modified antigen-presenting cells. J. Immunol. 140:3324, 1988.

225. Linsley, P.S., Clark, E.A., and Ledbetter, J.A.: T-cell antigen CD28 mediates adhesion with B cells by interacting with activation antigen B7/BB-1. Proc. Natl. Acad. Sci. USA 87:5031, 1990.

226. Swain, S.L., Bradley, L.M., Croft, M., Tonkonogy, S., Atkins, G., Weinberg, A.D., Duncan, D.D., Hedrick, S.M., Dutton, R.W., and Huston, G.: Helper T-cell subsets: phenotype, function and the role of lymphokines in regulating their development. Immunol. Rev. 123:115, 1991.

227. Finkelman, F.D., Holmes, J., Katona, I.M., Urban, J.F., Jr., Beckmann, M.P., Park, L.S., Schooley, K.A., Coffman, R.L., Mossman, T.R., and Paul, W.E.: Lymphokine control of in vivo immunoglobulin isotype selection. Annu. Rev. Immunol. 8:303, 1990.

228. Yamamura, M., Uyemura, K., Deans, R.J., Weinberg, K., Rea, T.H., Bloom, B.R., and Modlin, R.L.: Defining protective responses to pathogens: cytokine profiles in leprosy lesions. Science 254:277, 1991.

229. Liew, F.Y.: Functional heterogeneity of CD4$^+$ T cells in leishmaniasis. Immunol. Today 10:40, 1989.

230. Heinzel, F.P., Sadick, M.D., Mutha, S.S., and Locksley, R.M.: Production of IFN-gamma, IL-2, IL-4 and IL-10 by CD4$^+$ lymphocytes in vivo during healing and progressive murine leishmaniasis. Proc. Natl. Acad. Sci. USA 88:7011, 1991.

231. Sher, A., and Coffman, R.L.: Regulation of immunity to parasites by T cells and T cell–derived cytokines. Annu. Rev. Immunol. 10:385, 1992.

232. Coffman, R.L., Mocci, S., and O'Garra, A.: The stability and reversibility of Th1 and Th2 populations. Curr. Top. Microbiol. 238:1 1999.

233. Tschopp, J., and Nabholz, M.: Perforin-mediated target cell lysis by cytolytic T lymphocytes. Annu. Rev. Immunol 8:279, 1990.

234. Nagata, S.: Fas-mediated apoptosis. Adv. Exp. Med. Biol. 406:119, 1996.

235. Podack, E.R., and Dennert, G.: Assembly of two types of tubules with putative cytolytic function by cloned natural killer cells. Nature 302:442, 1983.

236. Podack, E.R., Young, J.D.E., and Cohn, Z.A.: Isolation and biochemical and functional characterization of perforin 1 from cytolytic T-cell granules. Proc. Natl. Acad. Sci. USA 82:8629, 1985.

237. Zalman, L.S., Martin, D.E., Jung, G., and Müller-Eberhard, H.J.: The cytolytic protein of human lymphocytes related to the ninth component (C9) of human complement: isolation from anti-CD3–activated peripheral blood mononuclear cells. Proc. Natl. Acad. Sci. USA 84:2426, 1987.

238. Young, J.D.E., Hengartner, H., Podack, E.R., and Cohn, Z.A.: Purification and characterization of a cytolytic pore-forming protein from granules of cloned lymphocytes with natural killer activity. Cell 44:849, 1986.

239. Trapani, J.A., Sutton, V.R., and Smyth, M.J.: CTL granules: evolution of vesicles essential for combating virus infections. Immunol. Today 20:351, 1999.

240. Mouser, J.F., and Hyams, J.S.: Infliximab: a novel chimeric monoclonal antibody for the treatment of Crohn's disease. Clin. Ther. 21:932, 1999.

241. Jones, R.E., and Moreland, L.W.: Tumor necrosis factor inhibitors for rheumatoid arthritis. Bull. Rheum. Dis. 48:1, 1999.

242. Madden, D.R.: The three-dimensional structure of peptide-MHC complexes. Annu. Rev. Immunol. 13:587, 1995.

243. Kropshofer, H., Vogt, A.B., Thery, C., Armandolar, E.A., Li, B.C., Moldenhauer, G., Amigorena, S., and Hammerling, G.J.: A role of HLA-DO as a co-chaperone of HLA-DM in peptide loading of MHC class II molecules. EMBO J. 17:2971, 1998.

244. Snapper, S.B., and Rosen, F.S.: The Wiskott-Aldrich syndrome protein (WASP): roles in signaling and cytoskeletal organization. Annu. Rev. Immunol. :905, 1999.

245. Schraven, B., Cardine, A.M., Hubener, C., Bruyns, E., and Ding, I.: Integration of receptor-mediated signals in T cells by transmembrane adaptor proteins. Immunol. Today 10:431, 1999.

246. Lupher, M.L., Rao, N., Eck, M.J., and Band, H.: The Cbl protooncoprotein: a negative regulator of immune receptor signal transduction. Immunol. Today 20:375, 1999.

247. Stenger, S., Rosat, J.P., Bloom, B.R., Krensky, A.M., and Modlin, R.: Granulysin: a lethal weapon of cytolytic T cells. Immunol. Today 20:390, 1999.

Part IV

MYELOPOIESIS/ WHITE BLOOD CELLS

14 Integrins in Hematology
▼▼▼▼ Roy Zent, David M. Rose, and Mark H. Ginsberg

▼ ▼

Adhesion and migration are essential activities for normal development and function of the hematological system. Structural and functional aberrations of adhesion molecules result in abnormal hematopoiesis as well as platelet and leukocyte dysfunction. These disorders manifest primarily as immunological diseases, bleeding disorders, and neoplasia.

Leukocytes circulate in the vascular system and move into tissues in response to antigen presentation or injury. This migration is dependent on tightly coordinated cell/cell and cell/extracellular matrix interactions mediated through integrins, a specialized group of ligand-binding receptors. Integrin ligands include extracellular matrix proteins, cell surface immunoglobulin superfamily receptors, and certain plasma proteins. In addition to facilitating adhesion and migration by multivalent ligands, integrins are also important signaling molecules. When integrins are bound by clustered ligand, they transmit signals into cells that coordinate with other plasma membrane receptor signals and result in anchorage-dependent cellular function, so-called outside-in signaling. Furthermore, integrin affinity for ligand can be dynamically regulated as a result of inside-out signaling. Both signaling mechanisms are crucial for cell migration and adhesion and are also important in controlling cell differentiation and critical decisions specifying cell proliferation and programmed cell death. This chapter describes the general principles of integrin structure, their ability to recognize ligand, cellular regulation of integrin function, their contribution to normal development and function of blood cells, and their role in some hematological diseases.

Integrins of Blood Cells

Integrins are heterodimeric molecules composed of an α and β subunit, both of which are type I transmembrane glycoproteins. In humans, there are 17 α and 8 β subunits that combine in a restricted manner to form different dimers, each of which exhibits different ligand-binding properties. The subunits are products of separate genes[1-4] and are generally interdependent for biosynthetic processing and surface expression.[5] The α subunits appear to have evolved independently of β subunits,[6] and several α subunits have multiple β partners.[7-9]

Most of the more than 20 known mammalian integrins are expressed on one or more of the cell types found in the developing and mature hematological system. β_1, β_2, and β_3 heterodimers have been identified on hematopoietic progenitor cells. Although mature red blood cells do not express integrins, $\alpha_4\beta_1$ (very late antigen [VLA]–4) and $\alpha_5\beta_1$ (VLA-5) integrins are expressed by their precursors until they mature into reticulocytes.[10] Leukocyte and platelet progenitor cells have $\alpha_4\beta_1$ (VLA-4), $\alpha_5\beta_1$ (VLA-5), and $\alpha_L\beta_2$ (lymphocyte function–associated antigen-1 [LFA-1]) integrins.[11, 12] $\alpha_{IIb}\beta_3$ is expressed on megakaryocytes. Integrin expression on leukocytes is heterogeneous and depends on cell type. Integrins $\alpha_E\beta_7$, $\alpha_L\beta_2$, $\alpha_M\beta_2$, $\alpha_x\beta_2$, $\alpha_D\beta_2$, $\alpha_4\beta_1$, $\alpha_5\beta_1$, $\alpha_v\beta_3$, and $\alpha_4\beta_7$ have been found on white blood cells. Platelets express $\alpha_2\beta_1$ (VLA-2), $\alpha_5\beta_1$ (VLA-5), $\alpha_{IIb}\beta_3$ (glycoprotein IIb/IIIa), $\alpha_v\beta_3$, and $\alpha_6\beta_1$ (VLA-6).

Integrin Structure

The major part of most integrins, including the NH_2 terminus of the molecule, is the extracellular domain. The α and β subunits usually contain approximately 1000 and 750 amino acid residues, respectively, and have a single transmembrane segment. Except for the β_4 cytoplasmic C-terminal tail, which contains more than 1000 amino acid residues,[13–15] integrin tails range in size from about 20 to 70 residues.[16–18]

Electron microscopy suggests that integrins are composed of a globular, approximately 10 nm ligand-binding head[19–21] and two extended tails that contain carboxyl-terminal portions of α and β subunits[19, 22] and their transmembrane domains.[23] The molecules are asymmetrical as determined by biophysical analyses of integrins in detergent solutions.[24, 25] In addition, disulfide bond arrangements and intersubunit contacts have been proposed in proteolytic fragments of integrin $\alpha_{IIb}\beta_3$.[26–31] Integrins are conformationally labile[32–35] and are subject to disulfide bond exchange.[36]

▼ LIGAND-BINDING SITES OF INTEGRINS

The N-terminal half of both α and β integrin subunits is necessary for ligand binding,[37, 38] and the ligand recognition sites also reside in this portion of both subunits.[39–42] In addition, high-affinity ligand recognition usually requires both subunits[43–48] and consequently may involve multiple ligand contact points. Several potential contact points have now been identified.

A conserved sequence in the integrin β chains (D109 to E171 in β_3) is proximal to a bound peptide ligand[42, 41] and is probably involved in ligand recognition because (1) point mutations here abrogate ligand-binding function,[49] (2) select antibodies directed against this region inhibit ligand binding,[50–53] (3) mutations here cause ligand-binding function to increase,[54] and (4) an isolated peptide from this region binds ligand.[53] This region is highly conserved between integrin classes, and mutations at similar residues in other β integrins suggest that this is a common ligand contact site.[49, 55–60]

This highly conserved region of the β integrin subunit is rich in oxygenated residues whose linear spacing approximates that of the oxygenated residues in the calcium-binding loop of EF-hand proteins.[61] Mutation of these oxygenated residues blocks ligand binding[49, 55, 56, 58–60] and can alter divalent cation–dependent conformation,[62] which suggests that these residues may provide coordinating ligands for divalent cations. A synthetic peptide from this region directly binds ligands and terbium, a luminescent calcium analogue.[53] These data support the hypothesis that ligands interact with divalent cations bound to this highly conserved site in the β subunit.[49] Critical oxygenated residues found in integrin ligands provide additional support for this idea.[63–71] In addition

to this conserved site, other non-conserved sites appear to contribute to ligand recognition specificity by different β subunits.[72, 73]

At least eight integrin α subunits contain an approximately 200 residue sequence in their amino-terminal third[74–76] that is inserted by exon shuffling.[77–80] This region is referred to as the I (inserted) domain, and it is homologous to the A domains of von Willebrand factor (vWF).[81–85] Five of these integrin subunits ($\alpha_E\beta_7$, $\alpha_L\beta_2$, $\alpha_M\beta_2$, $\alpha_x\beta_2$, $\alpha_D\beta_2$) are found on mature leukocytes, and $\alpha_2\beta_1$ is present on platelets. This domain is functionally important in ligand binding. There are striking similarities between the ligand-binding region of the β subunit and the ligand-binding region of I domains (of the α subunit). These include a conserved motif of D $(\phi)_5$DXSXSϕ, where ϕ is any hydrophobic residue and X is any residue.[86] The similarity in hydropathy of the two regions suggests a similar global fold[87] (see below), which has led to the proposal of hypothetical molecular models.[60, 88] These models predict the role of sequentially dispersed oxygenated residues in cation coordination and ligand binding. The ligand-binding residues that have an impact on ligand binding have been identified by site-directed[59, 60, 88] and random mutagenesis.[89] Validation of the proposed molecular models and resolution of their differences await a high-resolution structure of the region. Studies indicate that this region's folding depends on its association with the α subunit.[90] Consequently, structural analysis of an $\alpha\beta$ heterodimer or of proteolytic[37, 91] or recombinant[92] "mini-dimers" will probably be required to resolve this issue.

Ligands also bind proximal to the N-terminal region of the α subunit.[93, 40] Moreover, antibodies against this region block ligand binding, and synthetic peptides and fragments that contain this region reportedly bind ligands.[94–96] The most decisive studies have been a combination of epitope mapping, point mutagenesis, and domain exchange experiments, which strongly argue that repeats two to five of the seven N-terminal repeats of integrin α subunits are involved in ligand binding.[97–100] An *ab initio* prediction proposed that each of the seven N-terminal integrin α subunit repeats folds into four stranded β sheets arranged in a torus around an axis of pseudosymmetry, the β propeller model.[101] This model predicted the ligand site to be on the upper surface of the propeller. Mutational and immunochemical analyses support the prediction,[98, 102] and the lower surface, containing cation-binding repeats, can interface with the predicted I domain–like structure present in the β subunit. The remarkable similarity of this predicted protein/protein interaction to that between α and β subunits of G proteins is appealing.[103] High-resolution structural studies of this region are awaited to confirm this insightful model. Because this region's folding seems to depend on β subunit interactions,[76] structural studies will probably require analyses of either intact heterodimers or fragment dimers.

As noted above, at least eight integrin subunits contain an approximately 200 residue I domain that participates in ligand binding. Function-altering antibodies map to I domains of $\alpha_M\beta_2$ (macrophage-1 antigen [Mac-1], CD11b/CD18, complement receptor type 3),[104, 105] $\alpha_1\beta_1$ (VLA-1),[106] $\alpha_L\beta_2$ (LFA-1, CD11a/CD18),[107] and $\alpha_2\beta_1$ (VLA-2).[108] Moreover, mutations in these domains block ligand-binding function.[105, 106, 108] Because these domains are protein modules,[77–80] they fold autonomously[87, 109] as isolated proteins or in the intact α subunits[76, 110] and bind ligands.[105, 107, 108, 111] The I domain also binds cations,[105] and cations are important in its ligand-binding function.[105, 112] Crystal structures of several I domains have been solved,[87, 113, 114] and they confirm the role of the DXSXS motif in coordinating bound cation. Two other coordination positions are filled by oxygenated residues near the DXSXS motif in the folded protein, but more than 50 residues distant in the primary sequence. These residues thus form the novel metal ion–dependent adhesion site (MIDAS).[87] The overall structure is a dinucleotide-binding fold with a central parallel β sheet surrounded by α helices. The MIDAS motif lies at the C-terminal end of the β sheet. Mutational analyses show that the I domain ligand-binding residues cluster about the MIDAS face.[115, 116] A striking exception is the binding site for echovirus in α_2, which maps to one edge of the β sheet.[113, 117]

The relative ligand-binding roles of the three contact sites described above remains unresolved. Clearly, in I domain–containing integrins, that domain is involved. Nevertheless, Bajt and colleagues[56] showed that mutations of the DXSXS motif in β_2 impairs ligand recognition by both $\alpha_M\beta_2$ and $\alpha_L\beta_2$. These effects are not likely to be due to alterations of the autonomously folded I domain conformation. Nor do these mutations appear to block accessibility of the I domain to certain ligands.[118] Furthermore, other studies implicate sites from the putative propeller motif of the subunit in ligand binding to $\alpha_L\beta_2$[96] and $\alpha_2\beta_1$.[119] Thus, in I domain integrins, other sites are probably involved in ligand recognition.

In integrins lacking the I domain, the picture is less clear. One idea proposes that ligands can interact independently with spatially discrete sites in both α and β subunits. Studies using fibrinogen and fibronectin-derived ligands support this hypothesis. Peptides derived from fibrinogen γ chain C terminus cross-link preferentially to α_{IIb}, whereas RGD peptides cross-link to the β_3 subunit.[39] Furthermore, differential cross-competition occurs between fibronectin-derived ligands lacking either the RGD sequence or the "synergy" sites and antibodies against the integrin α_5 or β_1 subunit.[120] However, the interdependence of the folding and function of α and β subunit ligand-binding sites[43–48, 90, 110, 121] suggests that both sites participate in the formation of a common ligand-binding pocket. Indeed, there is cross-inhibition between fibrinogen γ chain and RGD peptides for binding to $\alpha_{IIb}\beta_3$.[122] The binding of the isolated synergy site to $\alpha_{IIb}\beta_3$ is inhibited by RGD peptides (R. D. Bowditch and M. H. Ginsberg, unpublished observations). Visualizing structure of ligand-bound integrin heterodimer will probably be required to decipher the topology of the ligand-binding site.

▼ THE CYTOPLASMIC DOMAIN

Although integrin cytoplasmic tails are relatively short, their distinctive sequences allow them to interact with a number of cytoskeletal proteins and signaling molecules. The membrane-proximal regions of the α and β cytoplasmic domains have a similar organization of sequential polar and apolar amino acids. In the α chain, this is reflected by a highly conserved GFFKR sequence and a LLXXXHDR sequence in the β chain.[123] Other than the proximally conserved se-

quence, the varying degrees of similarity between the subunits allow subunit-specific interactions with different α cytoskeletal and signaling proteins.[2] In contrast to the chains, the β_1, β_2, β_3, β_5, β_6, and β_7 tails are reasonably similar to each other (30 to 60 per cent).[78] The β_1 and β_3 tails share the highest degree of homology and are functionally interchangeable in many assays.[124]

Integrin Signaling

▼ INTEGRIN ACTIVATION (INSIDE-OUT SIGNALING)

Although integrin tails (excepting β_4) are short, they are able to mediate cell anchorage and initiate elaborate signaling cascades. They regulate the functional state of integrins by changing ligand-binding affinity (affinity activation) and by receptor clustering (avidity modulation). Structural changes responsible for the switch between low- and high-affinity forms are not known. Possible mechanisms for this altered conformational state are discussed below.

Integrin Cytoplasmic Domains Modulate Integrin Activation

Chimeric and deletion mutants have been used to identify important tail sequences necessary for activating integrins from a resting low-affinity to a high-affinity state. Deletion of α or β subunit conserved sequences activates integrins to a high-affinity state that is independent of cell type and physiological signaling pathways.[125, 126] This suggests that these sequences normally lock integrins into a low-affinity conformation through a structural constraint, sometimes referred to as the membrane-proximal hinge.[127] This constraint appears to form from a combination of hydrophobic and ionic interactions between the conserved membrane-proximal motifs of the integrin α and β subunits.[126, 127]

Sequences distal to these membrane-proximal motifs in both α and β subunit cytoplasmic domains play a crucial role in integrin activation; for example, deletions of motifs COOH-terminal to the GFFKR motif of the α_2, α_4 and α_6 tails inhibit cell adhesion, suggesting that these sequences are required for integrin activation.[128–130] The α subunit cytoplasmic domain may also play a role in cell type–specific integrin activation.[126] Deletions of amino acids from the COOH terminus of β_2 integrin cytoplasmic domains result in alterations of integrin activation. For example, there is loss of constitutive adhesion and phorbol ester–stimulated function of $\alpha_L\beta_2$ in lymphoblastoid cells.[131] In addition, there is a well-conserved NPXY motif in β integrins essential for integrin activation.[126]

Direct Interactions of Integrins With Cellular Proteins

To understand how integrin affinity is modulated, a vast effort has been made to identify proteins that bind to integrins and thereby activate them. A large number of these proteins have been isolated by use of different techniques; however, their physiological relevance and mechanisms of action are incompletely understood (Fig. 14–1). Integrin-

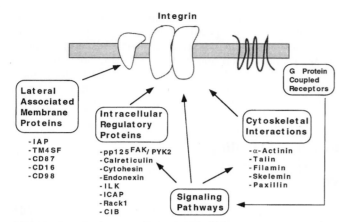

Figure 14–1. Factors implicated in integrin affinity modulation. The affinity state of integrins is a complex function of multiple parameters, each of which can influence ligand-binding affinity. Proteins that directly interact with cytoplasmic tails are obvious potential regulators of activation. Activating signaling pathways regulate activation by targeting these proteins and alter their ability to bind to the cytoplasmic tails. Lateral associations with other transmembrane proteins such as IAP might modulate integrin affinity. IAP, integrin-associated protein; TMS4, tetraspanin transmembrane protein; pp[125FAK], focal adhesion kinase; ILK, integrin-linked kinase; ICAP, integrin cytoplasmic domain–associated protein; RACK-1, receptor for activated protein kinase C; CIB, calcium- and integrin-binding protein.

binding proteins that may interact with integrins expressed on blood cells are discussed in this section.

The cytoskeletal proteins talin (an actin-binding protein) and α-actinin (an actin-bundling protein) bind to β integrin tails.[132–136] Talin binds to β_1 (both the β_{1A} and β_{1D} splice variants) and β_3, and α-actinin to β_1 and β_2 tails. These interactions appear to be functionally relevant because mutations in the cytoskeletal protein-binding sites result in decreased formation of stress fibers and focal adhesions.[137–139] Filamin, another actin-binding protein, binds to β_{1A}, β_3, and β_7 integrin tail mimics[133] and to β_2 integrin subunits as shown by co-immunoprecipitation experiments.[140] The physiological relevance of this binding is as yet unclear. Paxillin binds to mimics of both β_1 and α_4 integrin tails[141] (S. Liu and M. H. Ginsberg, unpublished data). Disruption of paxillin binding to α_4 results in increased cell spreading and decreased cell migration (S. Liu and M. H. Ginsberg, unpublished data). Actin associates with β_2 integrins in vitro[142]; however, this interaction needs to be demonstrated in a more physiological system. β_1 and β_3 integrin tails interact with the cytoskeletal protein skelemin, which regulates the organization of myosin filaments in muscle.[143] It is postulated that skelemin may mediate integrin interactions with myosin.

Integrin cytoplasmic tails interact with intracellular signaling proteins. Cytohesin-1 associates with the cytoplasmic domain of β_2 but not β_1 integrins, as shown by yeast two-hybrid assays,[144] and may play a role in phosphatidylinositol 3' kinase (PI3 kinase)–dependent activation of β_2 integrins. In vitro peptide-binding studies suggest that focal adhesion kinase (pp125[FAK]) binds to β_1 integrin tail protein mimics.[141] However, deletions of the tail binding site in pp125[FAK] do not reduce focal adhesion recruitment of pp125[FAK].[138] Pyk2, a protein related to pp125[FAK], is expressed in hematopoietic cells. It is slightly smaller than pp125[FAK], appears to be indirectly regulated by integrin clustering, and co-localizes with vinculin in megakaryocyte focal adhesion contact

sites.[145] Pyk2 is also phosphorylated when β_1 integrins on B cells are engaged.[146] The serine-threonine kinase, integrin-linked kinase (ILK), binds to β_1, β_2, and β_3 and regulates numerous cellular functions, such as cell adhesion, cell growth, and fibronectin matrix assembly.[147–149]

Integrin tails bind to an assortment of other proteins. Integrin β_3 tails associate specifically with β_3-endonexin, resulting in increased integrin $\alpha_{IIb}\beta_3$ affinity.[150–152] Integrin cytoplasmic domain–associated protein-1 (ICAP-1) binds directly to the β_1 integrin cytoplasmic tail, and the protein is phosphorylated when cells adhere to fibronectin. The functional relevance of this interaction is as yet undetermined.[153] The receptor for activated protein kinase C (RACK-1) interacts with the membrane-proximal region of β_1, β_2, and β_5 integrin tails.[154] This association appears to be dependent on prior stimulation with phorbol esters, suggesting that RACK-1 may act as a link between protein kinase C (PKC) and integrins. Integrin α_{IIb} interacts with calcium- and integrin-binding protein (CIB).[155] The α cytoplasmic tails associate with the chaperone protein calreticulin, which binds to the highly conserved GFFKR motif and is reported to increase ligand adhesion.[156, 157] The amino acid transporter CD98 interacts with β_1 integrin tails, and this interaction is associated with increased integrin affinity for ligand (R. Zent, C. A. Fenczik, and M. H. Ginsberg, unpublished data).

Integrin function can also be modulated by *cis*-forming associations with other receptors on the same cell to form multireceptor complexes.[158] Integrin-associated protein (IAP, CD47) is a widely expressed protein consisting of an extracellular immunoglobulin domain, five putative transmembrane domains, and a short cytoplasmic tail.[159, 160] It associates with $\alpha_v\beta_3$, $\alpha_{IIb}\beta_3$, and $\alpha_2\beta_1$ integrins through its immunoglobulin domain[159, 161] and is important in myeloid cell activation and migration across endothelial and epithelial monolayers.[158] It is proposed that leukocyte platelet-endothelial cell adhesion molecule-1 (CD31) engages the IAP/$\alpha_v\beta_3$ complex on endothelial cells, causing an influx of Ca^{2+}, which leads to endothelial retraction and loosening of tight junctions to allow leukocyte migration.[158] When leukocytes bind IAP/$\alpha_v\beta_3$, $\alpha_4\beta_1$-mediated adhesion to the endothelial ligand vascular cell adhesion molecule-1 (VCAM-1) is inhibited, thereby increasing the speed of cell mobility.[162] The role of IAP in neutrophil activity is emphasized by the fact that IAP knockout mice are more susceptible to *Escherichia coli* challenge because of neutrophil recruitment and activation failure.[163]

A subset of integrins associate with the transmembrane-4 superfamily (TM4SF) of proteins, also called tetraspanins. Members of this family have four membrane-spanning domains that result in two extracellular loops and an intracellular N and C terminus.[164] Co-immunoprecipitation experiments have revealed almost all the associations of TM4SF proteins, which include CD9, CD53, CD63, CD81, CD82, CD151/PETA-3, and NAG-2, with integrins.[158] The integrins that form complexes with tetraspanins include $\alpha_3\beta_1$, $\alpha_4\beta_1$, $\alpha_6\beta_1$, $\alpha_4\beta_7$, and $\alpha_{IIb}\beta_3$.[164] TM4SF are implicated in controlling cell adhesion, motility, metastasis, and growth and are thought to recruit signaling enzymes, such as PI4 kinase and PKC, into complexes with integrins.[165] The specificity of TM4SF and integrin associations is dependent on the extracellular domain of the integrin chain. This introduces an interesting paradigm in integrin signaling whereby an integrin extracellular domain interacts with the TM4SF extracellular domain, thus specifying the recruitment of intracellular enzymes.[165]

The leukocyte-specific integrin $\alpha_M\beta_2$ associates with glycophosphatidylinositol (GPI)–linked membrane glycoproteins. These proteins lack intracellular domains and signal through transmembrane partners. Examples of these proteins include the urokinase plasminogen activator (uPAR, CD87), which mediates binding to vitronectin; FcγRIIIb (CD16), which binds with $\alpha_M\beta_2$ to promote antibody-dependent phagocytosis[166]; and CD14, which binds with $\alpha_M\beta_2$ to form a polysaccharide and binding protein complex that generates proinflammatory mediators.[166] GPI-linked receptors form their interactions with $\alpha_M\beta_2$ by binding to a lectin site on the subunit extracellular domain.

Non–Integrin-Related Receptors and Signal Transduction Pathways

Cell surface receptors that couple through non-receptor tyrosine kinases or heterotrimeric G proteins can regulate integrin function (see Fig. 14–1). One way these receptors control integrin function is by modulating phospholipases that result in phosphatidylinositol lipid breakdown, Ca^{2+} mobilization, and PKC activation.[167] For example, integrin activation in leukocytes is increased by activation of PKC with phorbol esters and, in most cases, inhibited by PKC inhibitors like staurosporine and calphostin C. Although there is little doubt that PKC is an upstream regulator of β_1, β_2, and β_3 integrin activation, the direct targets of PKC in integrin pathways are not clear.

The lipid kinases, in particular PI3 kinase, play significant roles in leukocyte and platelet integrin activation. Cell receptors such as CD2, CD28, and CD7 associate with and activate PI3 kinase, which in turn triggers $\alpha_4\beta_1$ adhesion to fibronectin.[168] Stimulation of G protein–coupled receptors by substances like N-formyl-methionyl-leucyl-phenylalanine (FMLP), thrombin, RANTES, and monocyte chemoattractant protein-1 (MIP-1), also increases adhesiveness of β_1 and β_2 integrins by activating PI3 kinase.[168] Furthermore, wortmannin, a PI3 kinase inhibitor, can partially block the activation of $\alpha_{IIb}\beta_3$ in platelets.[169]

The Ras family of small guanosine triphosphate (GTP)–binding proteins and their effectors play a critical role in regulating integrin affinity[170] (see Fig. 14–1). H-Ras and its kinase effector Raf-1 decrease ligand binding to an otherwise constitutively high-affinity chimeric integrin, containing an $\alpha_{IIb}\beta_3$ extracellular domain and $\alpha_6\beta_1$ cytoplasmic domain, in Chinese hamster ovary (CHO) cells. The suppressive effect correlates with activation of the extracellular signal-regulated kinase/mitogen-activated protein (MAP) kinase pathway.[171] Subsequent studies have shown that H-Ras is involved in T-cell receptor–mediated $\alpha_L\beta_2$ integrin activation in T lymphocytes,[172] indicating that the effects of H-Ras signaling on integrin activation are cell type or integrin specific. R-Ras, which is highly homologous to H-Ras except for 24 NH_2-terminal amino acids, also modulates integrin affinity. This protein reverses H-Ras suppression of integrin activity and stimulates integrin (ERK)/ligand binding affinity.[173] Thus, H-Ras and R-Ras act in concert to modulate integrin affinity. Both proteins have a highly conserved binding domain that allows them to bind common effectors like Raf, Ral-GDS,

and PI3 kinase.[174-177] R-Ras fails to stimulate Raf and Ral-GDS activity. This suggests that R-Ras and H-Ras mediate their opposing effects through competition of the common effectors Raf and Ral-GDS. R-Ras can stimulate PI3 kinase, and this could explain the effects of R-Ras on integrin activation.[123]

▼ OUTSIDE-IN SIGNALING

The clustering and occupancy of integrins by multivalent ligands promote changes in cytoskeletal organization (e.g., microfilament bundles) and preferential gene expression. In this section, we outline major signaling pathways involved in outside-in integrin signaling.

Protein Tyrosine Kinases

Integrin cross-linking by antibodies[178] and integrin-mediated adhesion to extracellular matrix result in cellular protein tyrosine phosphorylation.[179, 180] This process is dependent on intact integrin cytoplasmic domains.[179] A major substrate for integrin-induced tyrosine phosphorylation is pp125[FAK]. The mechanism whereby pp125[FAK] is activated is unknown; however, β integrins may bind indirectly to pp125[FAK] through the intermediary cytoskeletal protein talin. In this case, integrin ligation may induce talin-linked cytoskeletal kinase clustering, resulting in transphosphorylation of pp125[FAK] on Tyr 397.[181] This autophosphorylation of Tyr 397 recruits Src family members (such as c-Src and Fyn) through their SH2 domains, and these kinases result in further phosphorylation of pp125[FAK].[181] Once it is fully phosphorylated, pp125[FAK] can associate with the growth factor receptor–bound protein-2 (GRB2) adaptor protein. GRB2 recruits the guanine nucleotide exchange factor Sos, resulting in MAP kinase activation through the Ras pathway[182] (Fig. 14–2). Although this is a

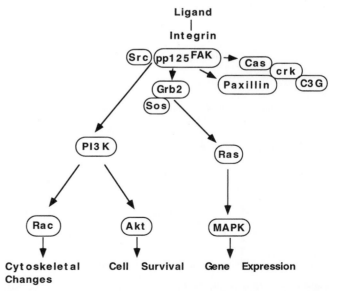

Figure 14–2. Integrin signaling pathways through pp[125FAK]. Ligand binding to integrins leads to activation of pp[125FAK] and its subsequent association with Src. Activated pp[125FAK] triggers several pathways that lead to alterations in the cytoskeleton, gene expression, and cell survival.

cogent mechanism whereby integrins activate the Ras–MAP kinase pathway, other experiments suggest that $\alpha_6\beta_4$, $\alpha_1\beta_1$, $\alpha_5\beta_1$, and $\alpha_v\beta_3$ activate MAP kinase by an alternative pathway, involving the adaptor protein Shc and the Fyn tyrosine kinase.[183]

There are a number of other downstream targets of pp125[FAK] that include cytoskeletal proteins tensin, paxillin, and p130[cas]. Tensin is an actin-binding protein with an SH2 domain[184] that, when pp125[FAK] phosphorylated, may change its actin-capping ability and regulate microfilament assembly.[185] Paxillin and p130[cas] bind pp125[FAK] directly[186, 187] (see Fig. 14–2). pp125[FAK] phosphorylates paxillin, and this complex may regulate the actin cytoskeleton as paxillin binds to the cytoskeletal protein vinculin.[188] In addition to the effects on cytoskeletal regulation, tyrosine phosphorylation of paxillin and p130[cas] by pp125[FAK] can generate binding sites for SH2 domain–containing proteins. Phosphorylated p130[cas] and paxillin bind the adaptor protein Crk,[189] which in turn binds to the guanine nucleotide exchange factor C3G.[190] C3G activates the Ras family member Rap1 but not any other isoforms of Ras.[191] pp125[FAK] also associates with the p85 subunit of PI3 kinase on integrin activation[192] in fibroblasts and platelets[193] (see Fig. 14–2).

Rho Family of Proteins and Lipids

Rho, Rac, and Cdc42, members of the Ras-related GTP-binding protein family, are important regulators of the actin cytoskeleton.[194] Fibroblast microinjection studies demonstrate that Rho stimulates actin stress fiber organization, Rac causes formation of lamellipodia and membrane ruffles, and Cdc42 regulates filopodia formation.[195] There appears to be a hierarchical organization of these proteins, wherein Cdc42 activates Rac, which in turn activates Rho. Ras can also activate Rho[196] (Fig. 14–3). Rac and Cdc42 can be activated by G-coupled serpentine and tyrosine kinase receptors. For example, platelet-derived growth factor (PDGF)– and insulin-induced membrane ruffling are blocked by dominant negative Rac,[197] and lysophosphatidic acid (LPA) induces

stress fiber formation through Rho.[196] Rac activation by growth factors and RasV12-dependent cell ruffling (in some cell types) appear to be dependent on PI3 kinase.[195, 198, 199]

Rho family members are necessary for focal adhesion formation[200]; however, their role in focal adhesion assembly is not known. Integrin activation stimulates phosphatidylinositol 4,5-bisphosphate (PIP$_2$) production,[201] which probably occurs through the interaction of Rho and Rac with phosphatidylinositol 4-phosphate 5-kinase (PIP4,5K).[202] This PIP$_2$ production may explain some of the effects of Rho on the cytoskeleton as PIP$_2$ promotes actin polymerization by binding to and releasing actin-capping proteins such as gelsolin and profilin.[203] In addition, PIP$_2$ binds and unfolds vinculin, which unmasks talin- and actin-binding sites in focal adhesions[204] (see Fig. 14–3).

There are effector targets of Rho, other than PIP4,5K, that result in changes to the cytoskeleton. Rho binds to serine-threonine kinases that include ROKα/Rho kinase.[205] Injection of ROKα into HeLa cells causes stress fiber and focal adhesion formation.[206] Another mechanism whereby Rho may contribute to focal adhesion formation is through Rho kinase activation of actin stress fibers.[207, 208] Rho kinase is a positive regulator of myosin light chain kinase (MLCK) and a negative regulator of myosin phosphatase.[209] By these mechanisms, Rho kinase increases phosphorylation of myosin light chains, which induces a conformational change in myosin and increases its actin binding.

A number of targets for Cdc42 and Rac have been described. The well-known family of serine-threonine kinases known as PAKs (p21-activated kinases) bind to both Cdc42 and Rac through a 18 amino acid motif referred to as CRIB (Cdc42/Rac interactive binding). Although PAKs may alter cytoskeletal organization, they are not required for Rac-elicited membrane ruffling and lamellipodia or for Cdc42-triggered filopodia formation.[210, 211] PAK's main function is to link MAP kinases such as JNK and p38 to Cdc42 and Rac. Rac binds to WASP, the Wiskott-Aldrich syndrome protein, through CRIB in a GTP-dependent manner. This protein may link Cdc42 to actin in hematopoietic cells[212]; however, its function is unknown. Another protein that binds to Rac through CRIB is the 34 kDa protein POR1 (partner of Rac), which plays a role in Rac-mediated ruffling.[213] As with Rho, a potential link of Rac to the cytoskeleton might be through phospholipid metabolism. In platelets, Rac-induced PIP$_2$ generation, possibly through PIP4,5K, leads to enhanced actin filament polymerization by inducing uncapping of actin filaments.[214]

Integrin signaling by the PI3 kinase pathway plays a role in protecting cells from programmed cell death, or apoptosis. Integrin-induced cellular adhesion results in PI3 kinase activation that provides a protective signal, acting through the serine-threonine kinase protein kinase B (PKB)/Akt, in a Rac-dependent manner.[215] When non-transformed cells are detached from their extracellular matrix, PI3 kinase and PKB/Akt become inactive even in the presence of serum factors, and an apoptotic pathway is engaged. An inability to inhibit this pathway is implicated as a key mediator of the aberrant survival of unattached Ras-transformed epithelial cells.[216] The mechanism whereby integrin attachment leads to activation of PI3 kinase in normal cells is unknown. One mechanism could be through pp125[FAK], because this protein associates with the SH2 domain of PI3 kinase and may

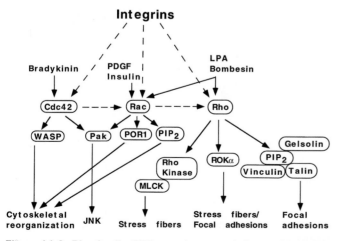

Figure 14–3. Rho family GTPases alter cytoskeleton. Cdc42, Rac, and Rho are stimulated by various extracellular stimuli. There appears to be a direct link between the GTPases in which Cdc42 activates Rac, which in turn activates Rho. Multiple targets of the small GTPases resulting in cytoskeletal alterations are present.

contribute to the constitutive activation of PI3 kinase[192] (see Fig. 14–2). In addition, PI3 kinase is a major Ras target effector that is activated by integrin occupancy and growth factor receptor activation[217] (see Fig. 14–2). The exact mechanism whereby PKB/Akt is activated is unknown. It is postulated that the 85 kDa regulatory subunit of PI3 kinase associates with its effector through its SH2 domain and is activated. This in turn localizes the p110 catalytic domain to the plasma membrane, where it produces PIP$_2$ and PIP$_3$. These phosphoinositides attract PKB/Akt and the serine-threonine kinases PDK1 and PDK2, resulting in formation of a phosphorylated PKB/Akt complex.[218] This new complex alters the effects of downstream controllers of cell growth and proliferation, for example, E2F.[218]

Integrin engagement stimulates inositol-lipid synthesis and inositol 1,4,5-triphosphate (IP$_3$) generation.[219] This leads to IP$_3$-dependent Ca^{2+} release, diacylglycerol formation, and PKC activation because of the stimulation of phospholipase C.[220, 221] Inhibition of PKC activation inhibits pp125^{FAK} phosphorylation as well as cell spreading, suggesting that arachidonic acid and diacylglycerol production are early steps in the signaling pathway leading to cell spreading and pp125^{FAK} activation.[222] Vascular smooth muscle cell binding to fibronectin induces a rapid translocation of PKCα to the cell nucleus and PKCα and PKCε to focal adhesions.[223] The role of the various PKC isoforms on integrin-induced outside-in signaling is being pursued.

Integrin Ligands in Hematology

The ligands to which integrins bind provide the structural scaffolding for cell adhesion, motility, and counterreceptors for integrin-mediated signal transduction.[2, 224] The major integrin ligands are extracellular matrix proteins,[225–227] immunoglobulin superfamily members,[228] microorganisms,[229, 230] and certain plasma proteins.[231–233] Integrin/ligand interaction is often divalent cation dependent and invariably involves short peptide sequences with an important acidic residue.[63, 64, 66, 67,] [69, 71] These sequences are usually on extended loops containing β turns,[234–236] but other protein ligand regions provide secondary interactive sites. A subset of integrin ligands has a primary role in hematology:

1. The immunoglobulin family members are important in hematopoiesis and leukocyte trafficking. These ligands include intercellular adhesion molecules (ICAMs, ligands for β$_2$ integrins), VCAM-1 (a ligand for α$_4$β$_1$ and α$_4$β7), and mucosal addressin cell adhesion molecule-1 (MAdCAM-1, a ligand for α$_4$β$_7$).
2. Three plasma proteins play important roles in hemostasis: vWf (a ligand for α$_{IIb}$β$_3$), fibrinogen (a ligand for α$_{IIb}$β$_3$), and factor X (a ligand for α$_M$β$_2$).

We focus on the structure and distribution of these ligands. For ligands having a more general role in integrin biology, such as the extracellular matrix proteins fibronectin, collagen, and laminin, the reader is referred to several excellent reviews.[224, 237, 238]

▼ STRUCTURE OF INTEGRIN LIGANDS

In general, many of the integrin ligands involved in cell/cell interactions in hematology contain immunoglobulin domains consisting of a sandwich of antiparallel β sheets (reviewed in reference 239). Usually, the N-terminal immunoglobulin domain (domain 1) is most critical for integrin binding[240–243] (Fig. 14–4). An exception is the interaction of α$_M$β$_2$ with domain 3 of ICAM-1.[244] The N-terminal immunoglobulin domain 1 of ICAM-1 is important for binding to non-integrin ligands, such as rhinovirus and *Plasmodium falciparum*, that bind to distinct sites on domain 1 that only partially overlap with the integrin-binding site.[240]

VCAM-1 contains two immunoglobulin domains that bind to integrins. The seven-domain form of VCAM-1 has α$_4$ integrin–binding sites located in immunoglobulin domains 1 and 4,[245] whereas the alternatively spliced six-domain form lacks domain 4. Domain 1 and domain 4 can support cell

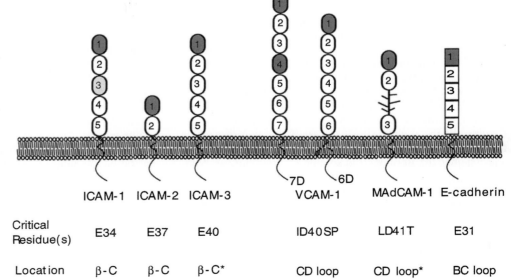

Figure 14–4. Integrin ligands of the immunoglobulin superfamily. Schematic structures of immunoglobulin family members are illustrated. Immunoglobulin domains are numbered, and domains important in integrin binding are shaded. The critical residues for integrin binding are listed, and location of the residues within the domains, as determined by X-ray crystal structure, is also shown (asterisks denote predicted location based on homology modeling).

	ICAM-1	ICAM-2	ICAM-3	VCAM-1	MAdCAM-1	E-cadherin
Critical Residue(s)	E34	E37	E40	ID40SP	LD41T	E31
Location	β-C	β-C	β-C*	CD loop	CD loop*	BC loop

adhesion independently,[245] but differences exist in cellular activation requirements for recognition of these domains.[246] Integrins $\alpha_4\beta_1$ and $\alpha_4\beta_7$ are differentially regulated with respect to binding to domain 1 and domain 4 in static[247] and flowing[248] systems. Differing recognition of domain 1 and domain 4 by α_4 integrins suggests that alternative splicing can be used to regulate cell adhesion in the immune response.

Mutational and structural analyses have defined integrin-binding amino acid motifs. In fibronectin, a prototype ligand, integrins $\alpha_{IIb}\beta_3$ and $\alpha_5\beta_1$ use two spatially separated sites, the RGD site in the type III repeat 10[64] and the synergy site in repeat 9.[249–253] Both sites are present within loops between β strands.[254] A similar theme has emerged in some immunoglobulin superfamily ligands. In VCAM-1, the amino acid motif IDSP is critical for α_4 integrin binding[69, 70] to both domain 1 and domain 4. In domain 1, the motif is located on a loop projecting between β strands.[255] A similar motif in MAdCAM-1, LDT, involved in $\alpha_4\beta_7$ binding,[256] is found on a loop between β strands.[257] Synergy sites occur in these α_4 ligands as well.[257, 258]

Critical acidic Glu residues are important for ICAM binding to integrins. Glu 34 in immunoglobulin domain 1 of ICAM-1[240] and homologous residues in ICAM-2 and ICAM-3 are necessary for this interaction to occur.[241, 242] Crystal structures of ICAM-1 and ICAM-2 established that the critical Glu residue is on a flat recognition surface[259, 260] on a β strand. Furthermore, the $\alpha_E\beta_7$ binding site on E-cadherin also contains a critical Glu that resides on a quasi-helix connecting β strands, rather than on a projecting loop.[243] Thus, the integrin I domain surface may form extended contacts with a "flat" surface structure on the ligand. In contrast, as noted above, I domain–lacking integrins such as $\alpha_{IIb}\beta_3$, $\alpha_5\beta_1$, and $\alpha_4\beta_1$ recognize critical residues that are within loops.[255] These loops may dock into and form limited contacts within a binding pocket on the integrin. High-affinity small ligands have been readily identified for integrins that lack I domains.[261–267] This structural difference in ligand recognition could account for the inhibitory peptide's low affinity for I domain integrins.[268–270] Furthermore, this difference could explain why small molecule competitive antagonists of I domain integrins might be difficult to identify.

The soluble plasma molecules fibrinogen, vWf, and factor X are not immunoglobulin superfamily members, but they also have short peptide sequences involved in integrin binding. Fibrinogen contains three sites that can potentially interact with $\alpha_{IIb}\beta_3$. An RGDF sequence (amino acids 95 to 98) is located on the A chain, as is an RGDS motif (amino acids 572 to 575). A dodecapeptide sequence HHLGGAK-QAGDV (amino acids 400 to 411) is located on the carboxyl terminus of the γ chain.[271, 272] The $\alpha_{IIb}\beta_3$ binding of each of these sites is dependent on the affinity state of the integrin and whether the fibrinogen is soluble or immobilized. Nonstimulated platelets do not bind soluble fibrinogen, but they do adhere to immobilized fibrinogen through $\alpha_{IIb}\beta_3$.[273, 274] This is primarily mediated by the dodecapeptide γ chain 400–411 sequence, although other sequences also contribute to platelet adhesion, especially under flow conditions.[274, 275] High-affinity $\alpha_{IIb}\beta_3$ can bind soluble fibrinogen, and this largely involves the γ chain 400–411 sequence.[276, 277] Platelets expressing high-affinity $\alpha_{IIb}\beta_3$ can adhere to all three

regions of immobilized fibrinogen.[122, 274, 278] The RGDS sequence can compete with the γ chain 400–411 sequence for $\alpha_{IIb}\beta_3$ binding, suggesting overlapping or adjacent binding sites.[122, 279] However, direct cross-linking studies suggest that the RGDS sequence primarily binds the β subunit, whereas the γ chain 400–411 sequence primarily binds the α subunit.[39]

vWF is another $\alpha_{IIb}\beta_3$ ligand.[232] It also contains a critical RGDS motif located in the C1 repeat.[280, 281] This is the primary binding site for $\alpha_{IIb}\beta_3$, but other regions may contribute to ligand binding.[282, 283] Like fibrinogen, $\alpha_{IIb}\beta_3$ interacts with the RGDS site on vWF when it is in the high-affinity state.

The coagulation molecule factor X can bind to high-affinity $\alpha_M\beta_2$ expressed on activated monocytes.[231, 284] Mapping studies reveal three short peptide sequences of factor X responsible for integrin binding.[285] These sequences are spatially distant, non-homologous, and located on surface loops of factor X.[285] In contrast to fibrinogen and ICAM-1, the I domain of $\alpha_M\beta_2$ does not appear to play a prominent role in factor X binding.[286] Recently, however, one region of factor X (GL[238]YQAKRFKV[246]G) has been shown to interact with a region of the I domain involved in ICAM-1 binding.[287] This peptide fragment of factor X blocks full-length factor X binding to $\alpha_M\beta_2$ by indirectly modulating unidentified integrin binding sites for factor X.[287]

▼ LOCALIZATION OF INTEGRIN LIGANDS

The spatial localization of integrin ligands provides positional landmarks that guide hematological cells, for example, in leukocyte trafficking. In addition, integrin ligands provide signals involved in development and function of these cells. Vascular endothelium, lymphoid tissues, leukocytes, and circulating plasma are major loci for important hematological integrin ligands.

On peripheral vascular endothelium, VCAM-1 and ICAM-1 are minimally expressed, but their expression is markedly upregulated at sites of inflammation.[288–291] This increased expression is due in part to the effects of cytokines, such as tumor necrosis factor-α and interleukin-1.[289, 290, 292] Induction of these integrin ligands plays a major role in the leukocyte recruitment to sites of inflammation.[293, 294] In contrast to ICAM-1, ICAM-2 is constitutively expressed on vascular endothelium, and inflammatory stimuli do not significantly increase expression.[295] The constitutive expression on endothelium may play a role in leukocyte migration into early inflammatory sites before the induced expression of ICAM-1 and VCAM-1 as well as in normal lymphocyte recirculation. ICAM-3 is not normally expressed on vascular endothelium either constitutively or at sites of inflammation.[296, 297] However, like ICAM-2, its expression is upregulated on endothelium at tumor sites.[296, 297] Thus, ICAM-3 is not thought to play a major role in leukocyte influx during inflammation but may be involved in tumor development. ICAM-3 is also expressed at high levels on lymphocytes, neutrophils, and monocytes,[298, 299] and ICAM-3 engagement by $\alpha_L\beta_2$ plays a role in leukocyte responses.[300, 301]

In contrast to its expression in peripheral endothelial cells, VCAM-1 is constitutively expressed in primary and secondary lymphoid tissue and on reticular cells in the bone marrow.[302] It participates in adhesion, proliferation, survival, and differentiation of hematological cells at these sites. VCAM-1/$\alpha_4\beta_1$ interactions are involved in the lymphoid cell adhesion to bone marrow stroma[303] and the formation of erythroblastic islands.[304, 305] In germinal centers, adhesion through VCAM-1 is implicated in the prevention of B-cell apoptosis.[306] VCAM-1 is also expressed on thymic cortical epithelial cells. Here it may play a role in thymocyte adhesion and development. Blocking studies suggest that $\alpha_4\beta_1$ integrins and VCAM-1 are involved in T-cell proliferation and survival.[307, 308] However, α_4-null cells exhibit normal short-term T-cell development in the thymus.[303]

ICAM-1 is also constitutively expressed in various cell types in primary and secondary lymphoid organs.[292] Lymph node high endothelial venules (HEVs) express 5 to 30 times the level of ICAM-1 compared with other vessels.[309] This high level of ligand expression aids recruitment of lymphocytes into the lymph node. ICAM-1 is also highly expressed on dendritic cells, but its role is unclear. The clustering of B cells and dendritic cells is blocked by antibodies to $\alpha_L\beta_2$ but not by anti–ICAM-1 antibodies.[310] Dendritic cells express ICAM-3, which may be the major ligand for $\alpha_L\beta_2$ in T-cell costimulation. ICAM-1 is also important in the development of normal intestinal immunity. ICAM-1–deficient mice have reduced T-cell number in the Peyer patches, lamina propria, and intraepithelial region of the intestinal mucosa.[311] This is speculated to be due to a defect in in situ T-cell activation and expansion.

MAdCAM-1 and E-cadherin are two other integrin ligands that play key roles in the mucosal immune system. MAdCAM-1, a specific ligand for integrin $\alpha_4\beta_7$, is expressed on HEV in Peyer patches and mesenteric lymph nodes and in venules in the lamina propria.[312] During inflammation, MAdCAM-1 expression is upregulated in the gut, the choroid plexus,[313] and the pancreatic endothelium.[314] The $\alpha_4\beta_7$-bearing lymphocytes are selectively directed to the sites of MAdCAM-1 expression.[315] The MAdCAM-1/$\alpha_4\beta_7$ interaction plays a key role in development and maintenance of the gut immune system and in inflammation at this site. It may also participate in inflammation of the pancreas and brain.

The primary role of E-cadherin is adhesion of epithelial cells during epithelial sheet development as cadherins interact with adjacent cadherins on opposing cells in a homotypic nature.[316] In addition, E-cadherin is a specific ligand for $\alpha_E\beta_7$ integrin.[317, 318] In contrast to MAdCAM-1, E-cadherin does not function as a homing ligand for lymphocytes to the gut but instead facilitates adhesion between lymphocytes and gut epithelial cells.[319] This cellular interaction could be involved in the retention of intraepithelial lymphocytes, immune surveillance, and the general health of the gut mucosa.

Integrins in Hematopoiesis

Hematopoiesis is the ordered process by which populations of erythrocytes, platelets, and leukocytes are generated from a common pluripotent progenitor cell. The interaction of hematopoietic cells with their extracellular environments influences this process. Integrins play important roles in hematopoiesis, both in adhesion and in signaling, and act in concert with cytokines/growth factors to regulate hematopoietic cell differentiation.[320]

▼ EMBRYONIC/FETAL HEMATOPOIESIS

The yolk sac is the earliest hematopoietic organ. Around embryonic day 10 in the mouse, stem cells migrate to the fetal liver and take over major hematopoietic function until birth.[321] Chimeric mice embryos generated from β_1-null embryonic stem cells have β_1-null hematopoietic cells in their yolk sac and blood, and these cells differentiate properly in in vitro colony-forming assays.[322] Thus, early hematopoiesis is β_1 independent. However, no β_1-null hematopoietic cells are found in the fetal liver or in the blood of newborn mice.[322] These results suggest that β_1 integrins play a critical role in the seeding of the fetal liver with stem cells. The α integrin partner involved in this process is not known. The α_4 integrin subunit does not appear to be involved because chimeric mice generated from $\alpha_4\beta_1$-null stem cells have normal fetal hematopoiesis; however, α_4 integrins play a critical role in lymphopoiesis in the adult bone marrow.[303] Similarly, anti-$\alpha_4\beta_1$ antibody administration in utero to pregnant mice did not effect lymphopoiesis or myelopoiesis, but fetal mice were born anemic, suggesting that $\alpha_4\beta_1$ may play a role in embryonic erythropoiesis.[323] The role of other β_1 integrins such as $\alpha_5\beta_1$ and $\alpha_6\beta_1$ in hematopoiesis has not been analyzed with genetic knockouts.

Hematopoiesis is grossly normal in β_2-deficient[324] and β_7-deficient mice,[325] suggesting that these integrins do not play a prominent role in hematopoiesis. However, Mebius and colleagues[326] suggested that $\alpha_4\beta_7$ may play a special role in the seeding of embryonic lymph nodes with $\gamma\delta$ T cells. Similarly, α_v gene ablation, although lethal in mice, is not reported to impair hematopoiesis.[327] Whereas β_3-deficient mice have an expected Glanzmann thrombasthenia, hematopoiesis is normal.[328]

▼ HEMATOPOIESIS IN THE ADULT

After birth, the bone marrow takes over as the major hematopoietic organ. Bone marrow progenitors express the integrins $\alpha_4\beta_1$, $\alpha_5\beta_1$, and $\alpha_L\beta_2$, and under in vitro conditions, these cells can adhere to the respective integrin ligands.[329] Integrin $\alpha_4\beta_1$ and its ligand VCAM-1 are implicated in playing a prominent role in bone marrow hematopoiesis.[330, 331] The homing of hematopoietic progenitors to the bone marrow is blocked by antibodies to α_4 but not to α_5.[332, 333] Furthermore, anti–VCAM-1, but not connecting segment-1–containing fragments of fibronectin, block early implantation of progenitors in the bone marrow.[332, 333] Of note, although these antibodies blocked localization of progenitors to the bone marrow, they did not block splenic engraftment, which suggests that the effect is not from selective destruction or loss of these cells.[332] In addition, anti-α_4 and anti–VCAM-1 antibodies cause mobilization of stem cells from the bone marrow, whereas an anti-β_2 antibody failed to induce this.[334] Interestingly, a report by Papayannopoulou and colleagues[335] suggests that anti-α_4–induced mobilization not only is due to blockade of $\alpha_4\beta_1$-mediated adhesion but may involve complex signaling events affecting other integrins and molecules regulating cell migration.

Integrin $\alpha_4\beta_1$ is also critical in normal lymphopoiesis in adult bone marrow. α_4-null chimeric mice have greatly reduced numbers of B cells in their adult bone marrow, blood, and lymphoid organs.[303] It is unclear whether the requirement for $\alpha_4\beta_1$ in B-cell development is simply an adhesive one or whether biochemical signaling through integrins is involved. T-cell numbers are initially normal in α_4-null chimeric mice at birth, but with time, these numbers decline and the thymus atrophies. Thus, embryonic T-cell precursor development in the fetal liver and migration and development in the thymus are α_4 independent. However, after birth, T-cell precursor development in bone marrow is α_4 dependent. The intravenous administration of bone marrow precursor cells reconstitutes the thymus of these animals, which suggests that α_4 is not involved in thymus engraftment. The α_6 integrins appear to be necessary in thymus seeding with pro-T cells.[336] Monocyte and NK cell development is normal in α_4-null chimeric mice, suggesting that there is a lymphocyte-specific requirement for α_4 integrins in hematopoiesis in the bone marrow.[303]

▼ INTEGRIN SIGNALING IN HEMATOPOIESIS

Outside-in signaling appears to play a role in normal hematopoiesis. For example, primitive hematopoietic progenitor cell adhesion to stroma inhibits their replication,[337] and $\alpha_4\beta_1$ integrin cross-linking prevents G_1 to S phase transition in progenitor cell cycle progression.[338] The molecular mechanism for this induction of quiescence is not known, but it could be through regulation of signaling pathways such as Ras/Raf-mediated MAP kinase, Akt/PKB, and cyclin-dependent kinases. Another example in which integrin signaling regulates hematopoiesis is in B-cell development. B cells adhere to follicular dendritic cells through $\alpha_L\beta_2$/ICAM-1 and $\alpha_4\beta_1$/VCAM-1, and disruption of such interactions triggers B-cell apoptosis.[306, 339] It is unclear whether the molecular mechanisms defined for detachment-induced apoptosis in mesenchymal cells also apply to B cells.[216, 340–342]

Integrins in Leukocyte Trafficking

The primary function of leukocytes is surveying tissues for pathogens and mounting an appropriate effector response. This requires leukocytes to leave the circulation at appropriate times and locations. The trafficking of leukocytes through vessel walls occurs by a remarkably stereotypic sequence of adhesion events.[288, 343] The steps in the cascade (Fig. 14–5) are as follows:

1. Initial tethering and rolling of the leukocyte on the endothelial surface. This is usually mediated by selectins and their glycosylated counterreceptors, but α_4 integrins also participate in rolling.[344]
2. Leukocytes then undergo a stimulation of integrin-mediated adhesive function. This stimulation usually involves peptide chemokines, bacterial chemoattractants, or lipid mediators. These agents typically interact with heterotrimeric G protein–coupled receptors on the leukocyte surface. This receptor/ligand interaction results in an intercellular signal that "activates" integrins. This takes the form of an increase in integrin affinity for ligand or changes in integrin mobility/clustering within the membrane plane.[345]
3. Integrin activation and interaction with ligands on the endothelium (usually immunoglobulin family members such as VCAM-1 or ICAMs) result in stable leukocyte arrest on the vessel wall.
4. The leukocyte then migrates through the vessel wall. This complex process, potentially involving β_1 and β_2 integrins, requires spatial and temporal regulation of integrin ligand binding, motive force generation, and detachment.[346] The rate of migration is dependent on integrin density, ligand density, and affinity of ligand binding.[346]

Specificity is added to this general scheme of leukocyte trafficking by the combinatorial inputs determined by (1) the adhesion molecule repertoires expressed on both the leukocyte and the endothelial cell and (2) site-specific expression of integrin-activator molecules.[288, 347] In this section, we focus on lymphocyte trafficking as a general model for how integrins and their ligands modulate leukocyte trafficking.

▼ LYMPHOCYTE RECIRCULATION

Naive T cells circulate through the body and selectively migrate into lymph nodes and secondary lymphoid organs

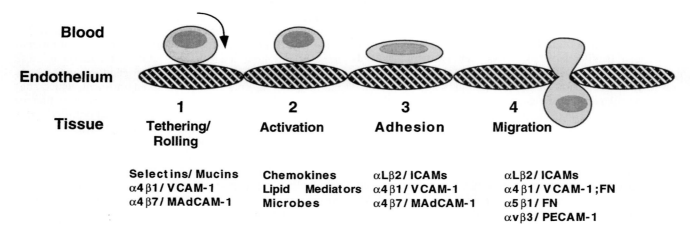

Figure 14–5. Model of leukocyte trafficking through blood vessel wall. This process involves four sequential steps: (1) initial tethering and rolling of the leukocyte on the endothelial surface; (2) leukocyte activation through agents such as chemokines, lipid mediators, and microbial chemoattractants; (3) integrin-mediated firm adhesion and arrest on the vessel wall; and (4) migration through the vessel wall. Examples of adhesion molecules mediating each step are indicated in the diagram.

in search of T-cell receptor–restricted antigens. These cells enter lymph nodes through interactions with specialized HEVs.[348, 349] Tethering and rolling of lymphocytes on HEVs are primarily mediated by L-selectins.[350, 351] HEVs express two mucin molecules, glycosylation-dependent cell adhesion molecule-1 (GlyCAM-1) and CD34, which serve as the principal ligands for L-selectins.[352, 353] The signal that stimulates stable arrest of naive T cells is unclear, but recent work implicates the chemokine 6Ckine, also known as secondary lymphoid tissue chemokine. This chemokine has a restricted expression on the HEVs of lymph nodes and Peyer patches, and it activates β_2 integrins on naive T cells.[354] Integrin $\alpha_L\beta_2$ is the primary β_2 integrin responsible for lymphocyte migration into peripheral lymph nodes, and ICAM-1 and ICAM-2 serve as ligands.[295, 355]

After naive T cells encounter appropriate antigen stimulation, they undergo proliferation and differentiation into "memory" T-cell phenotypes.[356] In contrast to naive cells, memory T cells have a marked heterogeneity in integrin expression.[357, 358] This is thought to facilitate tissue-specific redistribution. Evidence suggests that memory T cells may preferentially localize to tissue types in which the original antigen stimulation occurred.[359] This would allow a quicker response should the antigen be encountered again. In general, memory T cells express higher levels of β_1 and β_2 integrins.[360, 361] Three broad populations of memory cells have been classified on the basis of integrin expression and trafficking (Fig. 14–6). The $\alpha_4\beta_1{}^{high}/\beta_7{}^{low}$ memory T cells are typically excluded from trafficking to mucosal sites and often migrate into non-mucosal inflammatory sites such as the skin.[349, 362] In contrast, $\alpha_4\beta_7{}^{high}$ memory T cells preferentially migrate to gut-associated lymphoid tissue (GALT), which includes Peyer patches, lamina propria lymphocytes, and intestinal intraepithelial lymphocytes.[363–365] A small subgroup of memory T cells expressing $\alpha_E\beta_7$ make up the intraepithelial lymphocyte compartment.[357]

Enteric pathogens stimulate the generation of $\alpha_4\beta_7{}^{high}$ memory T cells, and this integrin plays a critical role in the GALT homing of these cells.[359] In vivo studies show a direct relationship between $\alpha_4\beta_7$ integrin expression and homing to Peyer patches.[363] Furthermore, β_7-deficient and α_4-null chimeric mice have a markedly reduced size and cellularity of their Peyer patches.[303, 325] As in the migration of naive T cells into peripheral lymph nodes, memory T-cell migration through the HEVs of Peyer patches also involves L-selectin and $\alpha_L\beta_2$.[366] However, $\alpha_4\beta_7$ can function in overlapping concert with these adhesion molecules to mediate both rolling and stable arrest.[366] As previously mentioned, the major ligand for $\alpha_4\beta_7$ in the GALT is MAdCAM-1. As for other integrins, differing activation states of $\alpha_4\beta_7$ exist and dictate its relative contribution to cell migration.[125, 366] Activated cells expressing high levels of $\alpha_4\beta_7$ can arrest on Peyer patch HEVs in an L-selectin–independent fashion.[366]

Integrin $\alpha_E\beta_7$ also plays a special role in mucosal immunity. This integrin is found on a unique population of memory T cells that reside in the intestinal epithelium.[367, 368] These cells are primarily CD8$^+$ and express either the $\alpha\beta$ or the $\gamma\delta$ T-cell receptor. The cells have an unusually small T-cell receptor repertoire that appears to develop outside the thymus. The expression of $\alpha_E\beta_7$ on intraepithelial lymphocytes can be upregulated by transforming growth factor-β, which is expressed by intestinal epithelium.[369] E-cadherin,

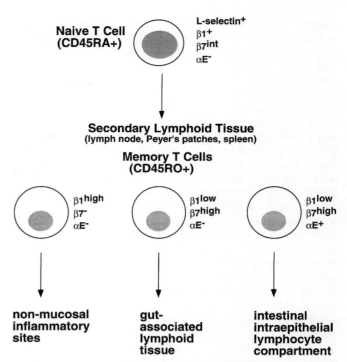

Figure 14–6. T-lymphocyte recirculation and integrin expression. Naive T cells (CD45RA$^+$) express a uniform pattern of L-selectin and β_1, β_2, and β_7 integrins; they recirculate primarily through secondary lymphoid tissue such as peripheral lymph nodes, Peyer patches, and spleen. Naive T cells that encounter antigen at these sites expand and differentiate into memory T cells (CD45RO$^+$). Memory T cells are heterogeneous in integrin expression and recirculation patterns. The $\beta_1{}^{high}/\beta_7{}^-$ memory cells effectively migrate through non-mucosal sites of inflammation by an interaction of $\alpha_4\beta_1$ with endothelial VCAM-1. The $\beta_7{}^{high}/\alpha_E{}^-$ memory cells efficiently traffic to gut-associated lymphoid tissue such as Peyer patches and lamina propria by the interaction of $\alpha_4\beta_7$ with MAdCAM-1. A small population of $\alpha_E{}^+$ memory T cells localizes to the intraepithelial compartment of the gut.

which is also expressed on intestinal epithelium, is the counterreceptor for $\alpha_E\beta_7$.[317, 318, 370, 371] The physiological function mediated by $\alpha_E\beta_7$/E-cadherin interactions is unclear. Unlike the interaction of $\alpha_4\beta_7$ with MAdCAM-1, the interaction of $\alpha_E\beta_7$ with E-cadherin does not appear to mediate cell homing to the intestinal epithelium.[319] The binding of $\alpha_E\beta_7$ to E-cadherin may aid in the retention of intraepithelial lymphocytes in the intestines. A reduction in the number of intraepithelial lymphocytes in α_E-deficient mice supports this hypothesis.[318] In addition, $\alpha_E\beta_7$-mediated adhesion may play a role in regulating intraepithelial lymphocyte effector function. Integrin $\alpha_E\beta_7$ has been reported to provide a signal that enhances T-cell activation.[368, 372, 373] Integrin $\alpha_E\beta_7$ is not solely responsible for intraepithelial lymphocyte function, because mice with deficient expression of β_2 and ICAM-1 also have defects in lamina propria lymphocyte and intraepithelial lymphocyte function.[311] Thus, like the role of $\alpha_4\beta_7$ in the recruitment of memory T cells to Peyer patches, multiple integrin/ligand interactions are required for normal mucosal T-cell immunity.

Integrins play a key role in leukocyte infiltration to inflammatory sites. This is exemplified by the inherited genetic defect leukocyte adhesion deficiency type 1, in which β_2 integrin expression is decreased.[374] These patients have a profound impairment in the influx of leukocytes to inflammatory sites and suffer from recurrent non-suppurative bacterial and fungal infections and impaired wound healing. Because the general paradigms of leukocyte and T-lymphocyte influx into sites of inflammation are similar, we focus only on the role of integrins in T-cell trafficking.

During inflammation, T cells migrate through vascular endothelium as opposed to specialized structures like HEVs. To facilitate recruitment, inflamed vascular endothelium typically expresses increased levels of ICAM-1 and VCAM-1.[288–290] Upregulation of MAdCAM-1 is restricted to select inflammatory sites, such as gut, choroid plexus of the central nervous system, and pancreas during diabetes.[313, 314] T cells recruited to sites of inflammation are typically memory cells, on the basis of CD45RO or CD44 expression, and have increased levels of α_4 and β_2 integrins.[357, 375, 376] Expression of β_1 and β_7 is heterogeneous. Cells recruited to the central nervous system in experimental autoimmune encephalomyelitis and the joints in rheumatoid arthritis are $\beta_1^{high}/\beta_7^{low}$, whereas cells recruited to the gut in inflammatory bowel disease and to the pancreas in non-obese diabetic mice are $\beta_7^{high}/\beta_1^{low}$.[377–380] This correlates with prominent α_4 integrin/ligand expression at these sites. As previously mentioned, α_4 integrins can mediate both tethering and rolling as well as the firm adhesion of lymphocytes under flow conditions.[344, 381] Furthermore, these adhesive events can be mediated by α_4 integrins in the absence of exogenous activation with chemokines, although chemokines can trigger α_4 integrin activation.[344, 381, 382] The α_4 integrins can exist in different activation states that influence cell adhesion events.[125, 383] Chen and coworkers[384] have reported that both high- and low-affinity $\alpha_4\beta_1$ integrins can mediate tethering and rolling on VCAM-1 but that high-affinity $\alpha_4\beta_1$ plays a prominent role in the establishment of firm adhesion. We have found that high-affinity $\alpha_4\beta_1$ integrins are stimulated preferentially on memory T cells compared with naive cells, and this may contribute to the preferential recruitment of memory T cells to sites of inflammation.[385]

Function-blocking antibodies to integrins and their ligands have been used to delineate important adhesion molecules involved in various inflammatory/immune diseases mediated by T lymphocytes. These studies demonstrate that different integrin/ligand pairs play dramatically different roles in different diseases. The development of experimental autoimmune encephalomyelitis, a mouse model of multiple sclerosis, is effectively blocked by antibodies to $\alpha_4\beta_1$ and VCAM-1, whereas antibodies to $\alpha_4\beta_7$, β_2, MAdCAM-1, and ICAM-1 have little effect on the pathogenesis.[386–388] In contrast, whereas anti-$\alpha_4\beta_1$ or anti-β_2 antibodies alone only partially block T-cell migration and the clinical development of adjuvant-induced arthritis in rats, a combination of two antibodies is more effective.[389, 390] This suggests that a combination of both $\alpha_4\beta_1$ and β_2 integrins is involved in the development of arthritis in these animals. The development of diabetes in non-obese diabetic mice is dramatically inhibited by antibodies against $\alpha_4\beta_7$ and MAdCAM-1, partially inhibited by anti–VCAM-1, and poorly inhibited with anti–ICAM-1.[380, 391] Thus, a prominent role for $\alpha_4\beta_7$/MAdCAM-1 and $\alpha_4\beta_1$/VCAM-1 in the pathogenesis of diabetes in non-obese diabetic mice is suggested. Furthermore, in both primates and mice, anti-$\alpha_4\beta_7$ inhibited the development of inflammatory bowel disease.[379, 392] In these studies, it is unclear whether the antibodies are acting solely by inhibiting

leukocyte recruitment or by other means, such as inhibition of lymphocyte activation. For example, antibodies specific to β_2 integrins and ICAM promote cardiac allograft acceptance in mouse models, perhaps by inducing immunological tolerance.[393] It is clear, however, that different lymphocyte integrin/ligand pairs are important in different diseases, and selected disruption of these interactions may be an effective therapy.

Integrins in Platelet Function

Circulating platelets are in a resting non-adherent state; however, after exposure and adherence to subendothelial matrix at sites of vascular injury, they become activated. These activated platelets adhere firmly and spread onto the subendothelial matrix and aggregate into a primary thrombus. Platelet aggregation leads to secondary platelet responses, which include secretion of granule contents, further platelet aggregation, and clot retraction. Platelet adhesion and aggregation are mediated by the interaction of platelet adhesive molecules and their respective ligands. These adhesive molecules are divided into two primary categories. One group mediates initial platelet adhesion and activation, and a second group functions primarily in response to platelet activation.

When the endothelium is injured, subendothelial components that are not normally exposed to platelets, including collagen, subendothelial matrix-bound vWF, fibronectin, and other matrix components, are exposed. Platelet receptors capable of binding these ligands are constitutively active, and they mediate initial platelet adhesion. They include glycoprotein Ib/IX complex, which functions as a vWF receptor; glycoprotein IV and glycoprotein VI, which function as collagen receptors; and $\alpha_2\beta_1$, $\alpha_6\beta_1$, and $\alpha_5\beta_1$ integrins, which function respectively as collagen, laminin, and fibronectin receptors.[394] The most important and abundant adhesion receptor on activated platelets is $\alpha_{IIb}\beta_3$. It mediates platelet aggregation, firm adhesion, and spreading and binds to fibrinogen, fibronectin, vitronectin, vWF, and thrombospondin. Another important receptor is P-selectin, which binds a glycoprotein, PSGL-1, and mediates adhesion of activated platelets to leukocytes.[395] The ligands for both $\alpha_{IIb}\beta_3$ and P-selectin are always available, and the interactions of the receptors are modulated by altering receptor affinity in the case of $\alpha_{IIb}\beta_3$ or by translocating the receptor to the platelet surface in the case of P-selectin.

The $\alpha_2\beta_1$ integrin and its ligand, collagen, have a significant role in platelet function. At high shear forces, collagen plays an indirect role in regulating platelet adhesion and activation as it binds vWF. However, at low shear rates, collagen can support platelet adhesion in the absence of vWF.[396] Binding of $\alpha_2\beta_1$ is the major interaction supporting platelet adhesion to most forms of collagen.[397] This interaction is strongly dependent on Mg^{2+} and inhibited by Ca^{2+}.[398] The collagen binding site of the integrin is on the I domain of α_2.[108] Even though the $\alpha_2\beta_1$ receptor provides the initial platelet attachment site to collagen, it is not sufficient to activate platelets.[399] It is postulated that platelet binding to an initial site on collagen brings a second site of the collagen molecule into the vicinity of a low-affinity platelet activation receptor. This receptor may be a number of molecules, including $\alpha_{IIb}\beta_3$, glycoprotein IV, the C1q receptor, or the uncloned glycoprotein VI, which appears to be a likely candidate.[396] When platelets bind to collagen, glycoprotein VI forms a multimeric structure with the platelet surface receptor for immune complexes, FcγRIIa. FcγRIIa contains an immune receptor tyrosine activation motif in its cytoplasmic tail. The two tyrosines on the motif are phosphorylated by a Src family tyrosine kinase, resulting in tyrosine phosphorylation of Syk and activation of phospholipase Cγ2 (the predominant form of phospholipase Cγ in platelets), which activates platelets.[396]

Resting platelets have about 40,000 to 80,000 copies of the $\alpha_{IIb}\beta_3$ integrin on their surface in the resting state, and this can increase up to 100 per cent after activation. Each integrin is capable of binding a single fibrinogen molecule. The α_{IIb} subunit consists of a 125 kDa heavy chain (glycoprotein IIbα) and a 25 kDa light chain (glycoprotein IIbβ) linked by a disulfide bond.[36] These chains are generated by proteolytic cleavage of a single polypeptide.[400] The heavy chain has 871 residues, and the light chain has 137 residues. The predicted transmembrane and 26 amino acid cytoplasmic domains are located in the light chain.[401] The 95 kDa β_3 subunit has 762 amino acid residues; 692 are extracellular, 25 form the transmembrane domain, and 45 form the cytoplasmic region.[402, 403] Both the α_{IIb} and β_3 cytoplasmic domains, with a GFFKR motif and two NPXY motifs, respectively, share these domains with other integrins. Four calpain cleavage sites flank the two NXPY motifs of the β_3 tail.[404] The ligands and their binding sites were discussed previously.

Integrin $\alpha_{IIb}\beta_3$ does not bind soluble ligands unless platelets are activated by appropriate agonists, which include adenosine diphosphate (ADP), arachidonate and its metabolites, serotonin, and platelet-activating factor. These agonists are released from platelets, thereby enabling stimulated cells to recruit additional platelets. Collagen is a potent agonist, as are thrombin, which links platelets to the coagulation system, and epinephrine, which permits hormonal control of platelets. Platelet agonists act through specific receptors, resulting in a number of intracellular reactions that lead to a final common step allowing the cells to aggregate. Activation of the $\alpha_{IIb}\beta_3$ integrins is rapid, occurring within seconds of platelets' encountering agonists.[394]

The mechanism whereby agonists modulate affinity and avidity of $\alpha_{IIb}\beta_3$ is not fully understood. Thrombin, ADP, epinephrine, and thromboxane A$_2$ bind to heptahelical receptors coupled to $(\alpha\beta\gamma)$ heterotrimeric G proteins.[405, 406] The α subunit of the receptor activates phospholipase Cβ, resulting in hydrolysis of phosphatidylinositol and diacylglycerol and IP$_3$ production.[214] Mouse platelets rendered null for the Gq are unable to aggregate in response to thrombin, ADP, epinephrine, and thromboxane A$_2$, suggesting a role for this pathway.[407] IP$_3$ stimulates an increase in Ca^{2+}; however, this alone is not sufficient to activate $\alpha_{IIb}\beta_3$.[408] Like other integrins, $\alpha_{IIb}\beta_3$ is activated by phorbol esters, and PKC inhibitors can block this activation.[409]

G protein–coupled receptors activate a number of nonreceptor protein tyrosine kinases, including Src, Syk, and Pyk2,[410] which in turn tyrosine phosphorylate a number of other proteins, including phospholipase Cγ, Vav (a guanine nucleotide exchange factor for Rac), and the cortical actin-binding protein cortactin.[411–413] Evidence that tyrosine phos-

phorylation plays a role in platelet activation is suggested by tyrosine kinase inhibitors blocking fibrinogen binding and phosphatase inhibitors inducing platelet aggregation.[410, 414] In addition, Syk null mouse platelets show reduced binding to fibrinogen in response to ADP and epinephrine.[214]

The small GTPases and phosphoinositides appear to play a role in $\alpha_{IIb}\beta_3$ activation and aggregate formation. Thrombin-induced release of PIP$_2$ and PIP$_3$ is thought to be important in stabilization but not in primary platelet aggregation initiation. When Rho is inhibited in platelets, there is no effect on affinity modulation of $\alpha_{IIb}\beta_3$; however, focal adhesion and stress fiber formation are blocked when platelets spread on fibrinogen.[415] This suggests that Rho regulates cytoskeletal organization rather than integrin affinity. As in other cells, Rac in platelets modulates thrombin-induced actin polymerization.[203]

Activation of $\alpha_{IIb}\beta_3$ can be inhibited by a number of substances predominantly secreted by the endothelial lining of blood vessels. Prostaglandin I$_2$ binds to G protein–coupled receptors that activate cyclic adenosine monophosphate–dependent protein kinase A and thus inhibit platelet aggregation. Another potent platelet aggregation inhibitor is nitric oxide synthesized by both endothelium and platelets.[416] It activates soluble guanylate cyclase, which together with protein kinase A has a common substrate in the form of the 50 kDa vasodilator-stimulated phosphoprotein (VASP). VASP localizes to focal adhesions and interacts with the actin-binding protein profilin.[417] Phosphorylation of VASP by either guanylate cyclase or protein kinase A inhibits platelet aggregation.

Integrins and Hematological Diseases

▼ LEUKOCYTE ADHESION DEFICIENCY

Leukocyte adhesion deficiency type 1 (LAD-1) is a rare autosomal recessive disease characterized by recurrent bacterial and occasional fungal infection, without pus formation, despite leukocytosis. It is caused by mutations in the β_2 integrin gene found on chromosome 22q21. The lesion presents as either absence or markedly decreased expression of β_2 on the cell surface. The syndrome's spectrum ranges from complete absence to 20 to 30 per cent of normal expression.[374] Severity of the disease correlates with expression level, and patients with less than 1 per cent expression suffer from life-threatening infections requiring bone marrow transplantation for survival.[418] Patients who express 1 to 10 per cent of β_2 have defects in leukocyte mobility, adherence, and endocytosis that manifest as periodontitis, skin infections, and retarded wound healing. Heterozygous relatives express 60 to 80 per cent of normal β_2 levels and are clinically normal.[419] The reasons for the lack of β_2 can vary and may be due to lack of expression of β_2 mRNA, expression of mRNA for protein of aberrant sizes, or failure to process normal-sized protein precursors to the mature product.[419, 420] At the molecular level, the syndrome is due to either point mutations leading to biosynthesis of defective proteins with single amino acid substitutions or splicing defects resulting in abnormal protein production.[421, 422] In other cases, deletions of the coding sequence have been reported.[423]

Until recently, all the clinical cases of LAD-1 were reported in association with decreased expression of β_2. However, a patient has been described who presented with all the clinical signs of LAD-1 but expressed β_2 at 50 per cent of normal levels, which is the same as heterozygotes who are clinically normal.[424] This patient has a Ser 138 → Pro and a Gly 273 → Arg mutation, both of which lie in the putative I domain of the integrin β_2 subunit. The Ser 138 → Pro mutation is the first reported mutation in the MIDAS motif, which is the key Mg^{2+}/Mn^{2+} integrin-binding site on which the ligand binding depends.[425] A case of LAD-1 with normal expression of wild-type β_2 has been described. This disease is probably due to a mutation in a gene involved in β_2 integrin activation. Furthermore, bleeding abnormalities due to reduced platelet aggregation later developed despite normal expression levels of $\alpha_{IIb}\beta_3$. The normal β_2 integrin structure and presence of a bleeding diathesis make this a clinically distinct variant of leukocyte adhesion deficiency.[426]

▼ GLANZMANN THROMBASTHENIA

Glanzmann thrombasthenia (GT) is a hereditary bleeding disorder caused by a qualitative defect in platelets. Platelet count and morphological features are normal, but aggregation induced by physiological agonists including ADP, collagen, thrombin, and epinephrine is absent or significantly decreased. GT is usually caused by mutations in the gene encoding either α_{IIb} or β_3 with a resultant deficiency or functional defect of $\alpha_{IIb}\beta_3$.[427] The genes for both α_{IIb} and β_3 are located within 4 cM at the chromosome region of 17q21–22.[403, 428] GT is an autosomal recessive trait, and heterozygotes are asymptomatic.[429] A β_3-deficient mouse displays many of the features of GT.[328]

GT is classified into three types[430]:

1. Primary GT is a mutation of either α_{IIb} or β_3. This is further subdivided into pre-Golgi defects, which result in decreased mRNA; post-translational defects, which result in degradation of misfolded or unstable complex in the Golgi; and post-Golgi defects, in which functionally abnormal $\alpha_{IIb}\beta_3$ is degraded in the endoplasmic reticulum or by lysosomes.
2. Secondary GT is an acquired functional impairment of $\alpha_{IIb}\beta_3$.
3. PseudoGT is a mutation of unknown genes leading to heterogeneous $\alpha_{IIb}\beta_3$ functional defects, including the distribution of the integrin.

More than 26 causative mutations of GT have been described, 14 in the α_{IIb} gene and 12 in the β_3 gene. The mutations include large-scale deletions, a large-scale inversion with a deletion, small-scale deletions, and point mutations.

Although this condition is rare, it has helped us determine important residues and domains within $\alpha_{IIb}\beta_3$ that alter integrin affinity for ligand. A good example is that position 752 in β_3 integrin tails is involved in activation of the $\alpha_{IIb}\beta_3$ integrin and results in a variety of Glanzmann thrombasthenia when the normal serine is mutated to proline.[431] There are numerous other point mutations in both the extracellular and intracellular integrin domains that result in decreased binding of $\alpha_{IIb}\beta_3$ to fibrinogen.

▼ ANTIPLATELET DRUGS

Thrombosis in the cardiovascular system, particularly in coronary and cerebral arteries, is a major cause of mortality. Therefore, strategies have been developed to inhibit platelet aggregation by interfering with fibrinogen binding to $\alpha_{IIb}\beta_3$. This approach should be successful because it affects the final common pathway of platelet aggregation. Several $\alpha_{IIb}\beta_3$ antagonists have been developed, including monoclonal antibodies and a variety of peptide and non-peptide antagonists. The peptide antagonists include RGD-containing snake venoms called disintegrins, synthetic linear RGD-containing peptides, and cyclic RGD or KGD peptides.[432] The Fab fragment of a monoclonal antibody to $\alpha_{IIb}\beta_3$, termed 7E3, was produced and joined with the constant regions of human immunoglobulin to create a chimeric compound called abciximab.[433] This monoclonal antibody is used clinically and is effective in reducing early reocclusion of percutaneous transluminal coronary angioplasty (PTCA).[434]

Peptide antagonists have been produced to compete with the RGD-binding site of integrins in the form of conformationally constrained cyclic peptides. They are more stable and potent than linear RGD-containing peptides. One such compound is the cyclic hectapeptide eptifibatide, which contains a KGD rather than the RGD sequence. The substitution of the single lysine for arginine makes this inhibitor $\alpha_{IIb}\beta_3$ specific. Inhibition of platelet aggregation with eptifibatide reduces the incidence of the composite end point of death or non-fatal myocardial infarction in patients with acute coronary syndromes.[435] In addition, the speed of reperfusion after PTCA is enhanced when eptifibatide is combined with accelerated alteplase, aspirin, and intravenous heparin.[436]

Non-peptide mimetics mimic the shape and charge characteristics of the RGD sequence and thereby inhibit platelet aggregation.[432] One of these inhibitors, tirofiban, a synthetic, short-acting, highly selective non-peptide inhibitor of fibrinogen binding to the $\alpha_{IIb}\beta_3$, has been shown to reduce the risk of death, myocardial infarction, and repeated revascularization procedure at 2 and 7 days after PTCA; however, the risk is not reduced significantly at 30 days.[437] Oral non-peptide mimetics have been developed and are currently being tested as a form of chronic antiplatelet therapy.

ACKNOWLEDGMENTS

R. Z. is a fellow of the National Kidney Foundation of the United States of America. D. M. R. was supported by funds from the California Breast Cancer Research Program of the University of California, grant 3FB-01640. Research for the Ginsberg laboratory was supported by National Institutes of Health grants HL31950, HL48728, AR27214, and HL59007. This is publication 12294-VB for the Scripps Research Institute.

REFERENCES

1. Ginsberg, M.H., O'Toole, T.E., Loftus, J.C., and Plow, E.F.: Ligand binding to integrins: dynamic regulation and common mechanisms. Cold Spring Harb. Symp. Quant. Biol. 57:221, 1992.
2. Hynes, R.O.: Integrins: versatility, modulation, and signalling in cell adhesion. Cell 69:11, 1992.
3. Akiyama, S.K., Nagata, K., and Yamada, K.M.: Cell surface receptors

for extracellular matrix components. Biochim. Biophys. Acta 1031:91, 1990.

4. Albelda, S.M., and Buck, C.A.: Integrins and other cell adhesion molecules. FASEB J. 4:2868, 1990.

5. O'Toole, T.E., Loftus, J.C., Plow, E.F., Glass, A., Harper, J.R., and Ginsberg, M.H.: Efficient surface expression of platelet GPIIb-IIIa requires both subunits. Blood 74:14, 1989.

6. Takada, Y., and Hemler, M.E.: The primary structure of the VLA-2/collagen receptor α_2 subunit (platelet GPIa): homology to other integrins and the presence of a possible collagen-binding domain. J. Cell Biol. 109:397, 1989.

7. Kajiji, S., Tamura, R.N., and Quaranta, V.: A novel integrin ($\alpha_E\beta_4$) from human epithelial cells suggests a fourth family of integrin adhesion receptors. EMBO J. 8:673, 1989.

8. Cheresh, D.A., Smith, J.W., Cooper, H.M., and Quaranta, V.: A novel vitronectin receptor integrin ($\alpha_v\beta_x$) is responsible for distinct adhesive properties of carcinoma cells. Cell 57:59, 1989.

9. Hemler, M.E., Crouse, C., and Sonnenberg, A.: Association of the VLA alpha 6 subunit with a novel protein. A possible alternative to the common VLA beta 1 subunit of certain cell lines. J. Biol. Chem. 264:6529, 1989.

10. Coulombel, L., Auffray, I., Gaugler, M.H., and Rosemblatt, M.: Expression and function of integrins on hematopoietic progenitor cells. Acta Haematol. 97:13, 1997.

11. Papayannopoulou, T., and Brice, M.: Integrin expression profiles during erythroid differentiation. Blood 79:1686, 1992.

12. Kansas, G.S., Muirhead, M.J., and Dailey, M.O.: Expression of the CD11/CD18, leukocyte adhesion molecule 1, and CD44 adhesion molecules during normal myeloid and erythroid differentiation in humans. Blood 76:2483, 1990.

13. Hogervorst, F., Kuikman, I., Von dem Borne, A.E.G., and Sonnenberg, A.: Cloning and sequence analysis of beta-4 cDNA: an integrin subunit that contains a unique 118 kd cytoplasmic domain. EMBO J. 9:765, 1990.

14. Suzuki, S., and Naitoh, Y.: Amino acid sequence of a novel integrin β_4 subunit and primary expression of the mRNA in epithelial cells. EMBO J. 9:757, 1990.

15. Tamura, R.N., Rozzo, C., Starr, L., Chambers, J., Reichardt, L.F., Cooper, H.M., and Quaranta, V.: Epithelial integrin alpha 6 beta 4: complete primary structure of alpha 6 and variant forms of beta 4. J. Cell Biol. 111:1593, 1990.

16. Sastry, S.K., and Horwitz, A.F.: Integrin cytoplasmic domains: mediators of cytoskeletal linkages and extra- and intracellular initiated transmembrane signaling. Curr. Opin. Cell Biol. 5:819, 1993.

17. Hemler, M.E., Weitzman, J.B., Pasqualini, R., Kawaguchi, S., Kassner, P.D., and Berdichevsky, F.B.: Structure, biochemical properties, and biological functions of integrin cytoplasmic domains. In Takada, Y. (ed.): Integrins: The Biological Problem. Boca Raton, FL, CRC Press, 1994, p. 1.

18. Williams, M.J., Hughes, P.E., O'Toole, T.E., and Ginsberg, M.H.: The inner world of cell adhesion: integrin cytoplasmic domains. Trends Cell Biol. 4:109, 1994.

19. Weisel, J.W., Nagaswami, C., Vilaire, G., and Bennett, J.S.: Examination of the platelet membrane glycoprotein IIb-IIIa complex and its interaction with fibrinogen and other ligands by electron microscopy. J. Biol. Chem. 267:16637, 1992.

20. Nermut, M.V., Green, N.M., Eason, P., Yamada, S.S., and Yamada, K.M.: Electron microscopy and structural model of human fibronectin receptor. EMBO J. 7:4093, 1988.

21. Carrell, N.A., Fitzgerald, L.A., Steiner, B., Erickson, H.P., and Phillips, D.R.: Structure of human platelet membrane glycoproteins IIb and IIIa as determined by electron microscopy. J. Biol. Chem. 260:1743, 1985.

22. Du, X., Gu, M., Weisel, J.W., Nagaswami, C., Bennett, J.S., Bowditch, R.D., and Ginsberg, M.H.: Long range propagation of conformational changes in integrin $\alpha_{IIb}\beta_3$. J. Biol. Chem. 268:23087, 1993.

23. Parise, L.V., and Phillips, D.R.: Platelet membrane glycoprotein IIb-IIIa complex incorporated into phospholipid vesicles. Preparation and morphology. J. Biol. Chem. 260:1750, 1985.

24. Jennings, L.K., and Phillips, D.R.: Purification of glycoproteins IIb and III from human platelet plasma membranes and characterization of a calcium-dependent glycoprotein IIb-III complex. J. Biol. Chem. 257:10458, 1982.

25. Hantgan, R.R., Braaten, J.V., and Rocco, M.: Dynamic light scattering studies of $\alpha IIb\beta 3$ solution conformation. Biochemistry 32:3935, 1993.

26. Calvete, J.J., Henschen, A., and Gonzalez-Rodriguez, J.: Assignment of disulfide bonds in human platelet GPIIIa. A disulfide pattern for the beta-subunits of the integrin family. Biochem. J. 274:63, 1991.

27. Calvete, J.J., Henschen, A., and Gonzalez-Rodriguez, J.: Complete localization of the intrachain disulphide bonds and the N-glycosylation points in the alpha-subunit of human platelet glycoprotein IIb. Biochem. J. 261:561, 1989.

28. Calvete, J.J., Arias, J., Alvarez, M.V., Lopez, M.M., Henschen, A., and Gonzalez-Rodriguez, J.: Further studies on the topography of the N-terminal region of human platelet glycoprotein IIIa. Localization of monoclonal antibody epitopes and the putative fibrinogen-binding sites. Biochem. J. 274:457, 1991.

29. Calvete, J.J., Alvarez, M.V., Rivas, G., Hew, C.L., Henschen, A., and Gonzalez-Rodriguez, J.: Interchain and intrachain disulphide bonds in human platelet glycoprotein IIb. Localization of the epitopes for several monoclonal antibodies. Biochem. J. 261:551, 1989.

30. Calvete, J.J., Mann, K., Alvarez, M.V., Lopez, M.M., and Gonzalez-Rodriguez, J.: Proteolytic dissection of the isolated platelet fibrinogen receptor, integrin GPIIb/IIIa. Biochem. J. 282:523, 1992.

31. Calvete, J.J., Mann, K., Schafer, W., Fernandez-Lafuente, R., and Guisan, J.M.: Proteolytic degradation of the RGD-binding and non–RGD-binding conformers of human platelet integrin glycoprotein IIb/IIIa: clues for identification of regions involved in the receptor's activation. Biochem. J. 298:1, 1994.

32. Parise, L.V., Helgerson, S.L., Steiner, B., Nannizzi, L., and Phillips, D.R.: Synthetic peptides derived from fibrinogen and fibronectin change the conformation of purified platelet glycoprotein IIb-IIIa. J. Biol. Chem. 262:12597, 1987.

33. Steiner, B., Parise, L.V., Leung, B., and Phillips, D.R.: Ca^{2+}-dependent structural transitions of the platelet glycoprotein IIb-IIIa complex. J. Biol. Chem. 266:14986, 1991.

34. Frelinger, A.L., III, Lam, S.C.-T., Plow, E.F., Smith, M.A., Loftus, J.C., and Ginsberg, M.H.: Occupancy of an adhesive glycoprotein receptor modulates expression of an antigenic site involved in cell adhesion. J. Biol. Chem. 263:12397, 1988.

35. Frelinger, A.L., III, Cohen, I., Plow, E.F., Smith, M.A., Roberts, J., Lam, S.C.T., and Ginsberg, M.H.: Selective inhibition of integrin function by antibodies specific for ligand-occupied receptor conformers. J. Biol. Chem. 265:6346, 1990.

36. Phillips, D.R., and Agin, P.P.: Platelet plasma membrane glycoproteins. Evidence for the presence of non-equivalent disulfide bonds using non-reduced–reduced two-dimensional gel electrophoresis. J. Biol. Chem. 252:2121, 1977.

37. Lam, S.C.T.: Isolation and characterization of a chymotryptic fragment of platelet glycoprotein IIb-IIIa retaining Arg-Gly-Asp binding activity. J. Biol. Chem. 267:5649, 1992.

38. Wippler, J., Kouns, W.C., Schlaeger, E.J., Kuhn, H., Hadvary, P., and Steiner, B.: The integrin $\alpha_{IIb}\beta_3$, platelet glycoprotein IIb-IIIa, can form a functionally active heterodimer complex without the cysteine-rich repeats of the β_3 subunit. J. Biol. Chem. 269:8754, 1994.

39. Santoro, S.A., and Lawing, W.J., Jr.: Competition for related but nonidentical binding sites on the glycoprotein IIb-IIIa complex by peptides derived from platelet adhesive proteins. Cell 48:867, 1987.

40. Smith, J.W., and Cheresh, D.A.: Integrin ($\alpha_v\beta_3$)–ligand interaction. Identification of a heterodimeric RGD binding site on the vitronectin receptor. J. Biol. Chem. 265:2168, 1990.

41. Smith, J.W., and Cheresh, D.A.: The Arg-Gly-Asp binding domain of the vitronectin receptor. Photoaffinity cross-linking implicates amino acid residues 61–203 of the β subunit. J. Biol. Chem. 263:18726, 1988.

42. D'Souza, S.E., Ginsberg, M.H., Burke, T.A., Lam, S.C.-T., and Plow, E.F.: Localization of an Arg-Gly-Asp recognition site within an integrin adhesion receptor. Science 242:91, 1988.

43. Fitzgerald, L.A., and Phillips, D.R.: Calcium regulation of the platelet membrane glycoprotein IIb-IIIa complex. J. Biol. Chem. 260:11366, 1985.

44. Pidard, D., Didry, D., Kunicki, T.J., and Nurden, A.T.: Temperature-dependent effects of EDTA on the membrane glycoprotein IIb-IIIa complex and platelet aggregability. Blood 67:604, 1986.

45. Brass, L.F., Shattil, S.J., Kunicki, T.J., and Bennett, J.S.: Effect of calcium on the stability of the platelet membrane glycoprotein IIb-IIIa complex. J. Biol. Chem. 260:7875, 1985.

46. Kunicki, T.J., Pidard, D., Rosa, J.-P., and Nurden, A.T.: The formation of Ca^{++}-dependent complexes of platelet membrane glycoproteins IIb and IIIa in solution as determined by crossed immunoelectrophoresis. Blood 58:268, 1981.

47. Shattil, S.J., Brass, L.F., Bennett, J.S., and Pandhi, P.: Biochemical and functional consequences of dissociation of the platelet membrane glycoprotein IIb-IIIa complex. Blood 66:92, 1985.

48. Buck, C.A., Shea, E., Duggan, K., and Horwitz, A.F.: Integrin (the CSAT antigen): functionality requires oligomeric integrity. J. Cell Biol. 103:2421, 1986.

49. Loftus, J.C., O'Toole, T.E., Plow, E.F., Glass, A., Frelinger, A.L., III, and Ginsberg, M.H.: A β_3 integrin mutation abolishes ligand binding and alters divalent cation-dependent conformation. Science 249:915, 1990.

50. Andrieux, A., Rabiet, M.J., Chapel, A., Concord, E., and Marguerie, G.: A highly conserved sequence of the Arg-Gly-Asp–binding domain of the integrin beta 3 subunit is sensitive to stimulation. J. Biol. Chem. 266:14202, 1991.

51. Calvete, J.J., Arias, J., Alvarez, M.V., Lopez, M.M., Henschen, A., and Gonzalez-Rodriguez, J.: Further studies on the topography of human platelet glycoprotein IIb. Biochem. J. 273:767, 1991.

52. Wang, R., Furihata, K., McFarland, J.G., Friedman, K., Aster, R.H., and Newman, P.J.: An amino acid polymorphism within the RGD binding domain of platelet membrane glycoprotein IIIa is responsible for the formation of the pen-a/pen-b alloantigen system. J. Clin. Invest. 90:2038, 1992.

53. D'Souza, S.E., Haas, T.A., Piotrowicz, R.S., Byers-Ward, V., McGrath, D.E., Soule, H.R., Cierniewski, C., Plow, E.F., and Smith, J.W.: Ligand and cation binding are dual functions of a discrete segment of the integrin β_3 subunit: cation displacement is involved in ligand binding. Cell 79:659, 1994.

54. Bajt, M.L., Loftus, J.C., Gawaz, M.P., and Ginsberg, M.H.: Characterization of a gain of function mutation of integrin αIIbβ3 (platelet GPIIb-IIIa). J. Biol. Chem. 267:22211, 1992.

55. Takada, Y., Ylanne, J., Mandelman, D., Puzon, W., and Ginsberg, M.H.: A point mutation of integrin β_1 subunit blocks binding of $\alpha_5\beta_1$ to fibronectin and invasin but not recruitment to adhesion plaques. J. Cell Biol. 119:913, 1992.

56. Bajt, M.L., Goodman, T., and McGuire, S.L.: $\beta2$ (CD18) is involved in ligand recognition by I domain integrins, LFA-1 (α L β 2, CD11a/CD18) and MAC-1 (α M β 2, CD11b/CD18). J. Biol. Chem. 270:94, 1995.

57. Huang, X.-Z., Chen, A., Agrez, M., and Sheppard, D.: A point mutation in the integrin β_6 subunit abolishes both $\alpha_v\beta_6$ binding to fibronectin and receptor localization to focal adhesion plaques [abstract]. Mol. Biol. Cell 4:283a, 1993.

58. Bajt, M.L., and Loftus, J.C.: Mutation of a ligand binding domain of β_3 integrin. Integral role of oxygenated residues in $\alpha_{IIb}\beta_3$ (GPIIb-IIIa) receptor function. J. Biol. Chem. 269:20913, 1994.

59. Puzon-McLaughlin, W., and Takada, Y.: Critical residues for ligand binding in an I domain–like structure of the integrin $\beta1$ subunit. J. Biol. Chem. 271:1996.

60. Lin, E.C.K., Ratnikov, B.I., Tsai, P.M., Gonzalez, E.R., McDonald, S., Pelletier, A.J., and Smith, J.W.: Evidence that the integrin beta3 and beta5 subunits contain a metal ion–dependent adhesion site–like motif but lack an I domain. J. Biol. Chem. 272:14236, 1997.

61. Kretsinger, R.H.: Structure and evolution of calcium-modulated proteins. Crit. Rev. Biochem. 8:119, 1980.

62. Ginsberg, M.H., Lightsey, A., Kunicki, T.J., Kaufman, A., Marguerie, G.A., and Plow, E.F.: Divalent cation regulation of the surface orientation of platelet membrane glycoprotein IIb: correlation with fibrinogen binding function and definition of a novel variant of Glanzmann thrombasthenia. J. Clin. Invest. 78:1103, 1986.

63. Ginsberg, M.H., Pierschbacher, M.D., Ruoslahti, E., Marguerie, G.A., and Plow, E.F.: Inhibition of fibronectin binding to platelets by proteolytic fragments and synthetic peptides which support fibroblast adhesion. J. Biol. Chem. 260:3931, 1985.

64. Pierschbacher, M.D., and Ruoslahti, E.: Cell attachment activity of fibronectin can be duplicated by small synthetic fragments of the molecule. Nature 309:30, 1984.

65. Pierschbacher, M.D., and Ruoslahti, E.: Variants of the cell recognition site of fibronectin that retain attachment-promoting activity (cell adhesion/extracellular matrices/collagen/synthetic peptides). Proc. Natl. Acad. Sci. USA 81:5985, 1984.

66. Ruggeri, Z.M., Houghten, R.A., Russell, S.R., and Zimmerman, T.S.: Inhibition of platelet function with synthetic peptides designed to be high-affinity antagonists of fibrinogen binding to platelets (platelet receptors/platelet aggregation/thrombosis). Proc. Natl. Acad. Sci. USA 83:5708, 1986.

67. Humphries, M.J., Akiyama, S.K., Komoriya, A., Olden, K., and Yamada, K.M.: Identification of an alternatively spliced site in human plasma fibronectin that mediates cell type–specific adhesion. J. Cell Biol. 103:2637, 1986.

68. Komoriya, A., Green, L.J., Mervic, M., Yamada, S.S., Yamada, K.M., and Humphries, M.J.: The minimal essential sequence for a major cell type–specific adhesion site (CS1) within the alternatively spliced type III connecting segment domain of fibronectin is leucine–aspartic acid–valine. J. Biol. Chem. 266:15075, 1991.

69. Vonderheide, R.H., Tedder, T.F., Springer, T.A., and Staunton, D.E.: Residues within a conserved amino acid motif of domains 1 and 4 of VCAM-1 are required for binding to VLA-4. J. Cell Biol. 125:215, 1994.

70. Osborn, L., Vassallo, C., Browning, B.G., Tizard, R., Haskard, D.O., Benjamin, C.D., Dougas, I., and Kirchhausen, T.: Arrangement of domains, and amino acid residues required for binding of vascular cell adhesion molecule-1 to its counter-receptor VLA-4(α4β1). J. Cell Biol. 124:601, 1994.

71. Berendt, A.R., McDowall, A., Craig, A.G., Bates, P.A., Sternberg, M.J.E., Marsh, K., Newbold, C.I., and Hogg, N.: The binding site on ICAM-1 for *Plasmodium falciparum*–infected erythrocytes overlaps, but is distinct from, the LFA-1–binding site. Cell 68:71, 1992.

72. Lin, E.C.K., Ratnikov, B.I., Tsai, P.M., Carron, C.P., Myers, D.M., Barbas, C.F., and Smith, J.W.: Identification of a region in the integrin beta3 subunit that confers ligand binding specificity. J. Biol. Chem. 272:23912, 1997.

73. Takagi, J., Kamata, T., Meredith, J.E., Jr., Puzon-McLaughlin, W., and Takada, Y.: Changing ligand specificities of alpha v beta 1 and alpha v beta 3 integrins by swapping a short diverse sequence of the beta subunit. J. Biol. Chem. 272:19794, 1997.

74. Hemler, M.E.: VLA proteins in the integrin family: structures, functions, and their role on leukocytes. Annu. Rev. Immunol. 8:365, 1990.

75. Shaw, S.K., Cepek, K.L., Murphy, E.A., Russell, G.J., Brenner, M.B., and Parker, C.M.: Molecular cloning of the human mucosal lymphocyte integrin α_E subunit. Unusual structure and restricted RNA distribution. J. Biol. Chem. 269:6016, 1994.

76. Camper, L., Hellman, U., and Lundgren-Akerlund, E.: Isolation, cloning and sequence analysis of the integrin subunit alpha 10, a beta 1–associated collagen binding integrin expressed on chondrocytes. J. Biol. Chem. 273:20383, 1998.

77. Fleming, J.C., Pahl, H.L., Gonzalez, D.A., Smith, T.F., and Tenen, D.G.: Structural analysis of the CD11b gene and phylogenetic analysis of the X alpha-integrin gene family demonstrate remarkable conservation of genomic X organization and suggest early diversification during evolution. J. Immunol. 150:480, 1993.

78. Hughes, A.L.: Coevolution of the vertebrate integrin alpha- and beta-chain genes. Mol. Biol. Evol. 9:216, 1992.

79. Larson, R.S., Corbi, A.L., Berman, L., and Springer, T.A.: Primary structure of the leukocyte function–associated molecule-1 α subunit: an integrin with an embedded domain defining a protein superfamily. J. Cell Biol. 108:703, 1989.

80. Springer, T.A.: Adhesion receptors of the immune system. Nature 346:425, 1990.

81. Bonthron, D., Orr, E.C., Mitsock, L.M., Ginsburg, D., Handin, R.I., and Orkin, S.H.: Nucleotide sequence of pre-pro-von Willebrand factor cDNA. Nucleic Acids Res. 14:7125, 1986.

82. Shelton-Inloes, B.B., Titani, K., and Sadler, J.E.: cDNA sequences for human von Willebrand factor reveal five types of repeated domains and five possible protein sequence polymorphisms. Biochemistry 25:3164, 1986.

83. Titani, K., Kumar, S., Takio, K., Ericsson, L.H., Wade, R.D., Ashida, K., Walsh, K.A., Chopek, M.W., Sadler, J.E., and Fujikawa, K.: Amino acid sequence of human von Willebrand factor. Biochemistry 25:3171, 1986.

84. Verweij, C.L., Diergaarde, P.J., Hart, M., and Pannekoek, H.: Full-length von Willebrand factor (vWF) cDNA encodes a highly repetitive protein considerably larger than the mature vWF subunit. EMBO J. 5:1839, 1986.

85. Corbi, A.L., Kishimoto, T.K., Miller, L.J., and Springer, T.A.: The human leukocyte adhesion glycoprotein Mac-1 (complement receptor type 3, CD11b) α subunit: cloning, primary structure, and relation to the integrins, von Willebrand factor and factor B. J. Biol. Chem. 263:12403, 1988.

86. Loftus, J.C., Smith, J.W., and Ginsberg, M.H.: Integrin-mediated cell adhesion: the extracellular face. J. Biol. Chem. 269:25235, 1994.

87. Lee, J.-O., Rieu, P., Arnaout, M.A., and Liddington, R.: Crystal structure of the A domain from the α subunit of integrin CR3 (CD11b/CD18). Cell 80:631, 1995.

88. Tozer, E.C., Liddington, R.C., Sutcliffe, M.J., Smeeton, A.H., and Loftus, J.C.: Ligand binding to integrin $\alpha_{IIb}\beta_3$ is dependent on a MIDAS-like domain in the β3 subunit. J. Biol. Chem. 271:21978, 1996.

89. Baker, E.K., Tozer, E.C., Pfaff, M., Shattil, S.J., Loftus, J.C., and Ginsberg, M.H.: A genetic analysis of integrin function: Glanzmann thrombasthenia in vitro. Proc. Natl. Acad. Sci. USA 94:1973, 1997.

90. Huang, S., Jiang, Y., Li, Z., Nishida, E., Mathias, P., Lin, S., Ulevitch, R.J., Nemerow, G.R., and Han, J.: Apoptosis signaling pathway in T cells is composed of ICE/Ced 3 family proteases and MAP kinase kinase 6b. Immunity 6:739, 1997.

91. Lam, S.C.-T., Plow, E.F., and Ginsberg, M.H.: Platelet membrane glycoprotein IIb heavy chain forms a complex with glycoprotein IIIa that binds Arg-Gly-Asp peptides. Blood 73:1513, 1989.

92. McKay, B.S., Annis, D.S., Honda, S., Christie, D., and Kunicki, T.J.: Molecular requirements for assembly and function of a minimized human integrin alpha IIb beta 3. J. Biol. Chem. 271:30544, 1996.

93. D'Souza, S.E., Ginsberg, M.H., Burke, T.A., and Plow, E.F.: The ligand binding site of the platelet integrin receptor GPIIb-IIIa is proximal to the second calcium binding domain of its alpha subunit. J. Biol. Chem. 265:3440, 1990.

94. D'Souza, S.E., Ginsberg, M.H., Matsueda, G.R., and Plow, E.F.: A discrete sequence in a platelet integrin is involved in ligand recognition. Nature 350:66, 1991.

95. Gulino, D., Boudignon, C., Zhang, L.Y., Concord, E., Rabiet, M.J., and Marguerie, G.: Ca^{2+}-binding properties of the platelet glycoprotein IIb ligand-interacting domain. J. Biol. Chem. 267:1001, 1992.

96. Stanley, P., Bates, P.A., Harvey, J., Bennett, R.I., and Hogg, N.: Integrin LFA-1 α contains an ICAM-1 binding site in domains V and VI. EMBO J. 13:1790, 1994.

97. Loftus, J.C., Halloran, C.E., Ginsberg, M.H., Feigen, L.P., Zablocki, J.A., and Smith, J.W.: The amino-terminal one-third of α_{IIb} defines the ligand recognition specificity of integrin $\alpha_{IIb}\beta_3$. J. Biol. Chem. 271:2033, 1996.

98. Irie, A., Kamata, T., and Takada, Y.: Multiple loop structures critical for ligand binding of the integrin alpha4 subunit in the upper face of the beta-propeller mode 1. Proc. Natl. Acad. Sci. USA 94:7198, 1997.

99. Kamata, T., Irie, A., Tokuhira, M., and Takada, Y.: Critical residues of integrin αIIb subunit for binding of αIIbβ3 (glycoprotein IIb-IIIa) to fibrinogen and ligand-mimetic antibodies (PAC-1, OP-G2, and LJ-CP3). J. Biol. Chem. 271:18610, 1996.

100. Kamata, T., Puzon, W., and Takada, Y.: Identification of putative ligand-binding sites of the integrin α4β1 (VLA-4, CD49d/CD29). Biochem. J. 305:945, 1995.

101. Springer, T.A.: Folding of the N-terminal, ligand-binding region of integrin alpha-subunits into a beta-propeller domain. Proc. Natl. Acad. Sci. USA 94:65, 1997.

102. Oxvig, C., and Springer, T.A.: Experimental support for a beta-propellor domain in integrin alpha-subunits and a calcium binding site on its lower surface. Proc. Natl. Acad. Sci. USA 95:4870, 1998.

103. Hamm, H.E.: The many faces of G-protein signaling. J. Biol. Chem. 273:669, 1998.

104. Diamond, M.S., and Springer, T.A.: A subpopulation of Mac-1 (CD11b/CD18) molecules mediates neutrophil adhesion to ICAM-1 and fibrinogen. J. Cell Biol. 120:545, 1993.

105. Michishita, M., Videm, V., and Arnaout, M.A.: A novel divalent cation-binding site in the A domain of the β2 integrin CR3 (Cd11b/CD18) is essential for ligand binding. Cell 72:857, 1993.

106. Kern, A., Briesewitz, R., Bank, I., and Marcantonio, E.E.: The role of the I domain in ligand binding of the human integrin α1β1. J. Biol. Chem. 269:22811, 1994.

107. Randi, A.M., and Hogg, N.: I domain of beta 2 integrin lymphocyte function–associated antigen-1 contains a binding site for ligand intercellular adhesion molecule-1. J. Biol. Chem. 269:12395, 1994.

108. Kamata, T., Puzon, W., and Takada, Y.: Identification of putative ligand binding sites within I domain of integrin α2β1 (VLA-2, CD49b/CD29). J. Biol. Chem. 269:9659, 1994.

109. Perkins, S.J., Smith, K.F., Williams, S.C., Haris, P.I., Chapman, D., and Sim, R.B.: The secondary structure of the von Willebrand factor type A domain in factor B of human complement by Fourier transform infrared spectroscopy. Its occurrence in collagen types VI, VII, XII and XIV, the integrins and other proteins by averaged structure predictions. J. Mol. Biol. 238:104, 1994.

110. Huang, C., and Springer, T.A.: Folding of the beta-propellor domain of the integrin alpha L subunit is independent of the I domain and dependent on the beta 2 subunit. Proc. Natl. Acad. Sci. USA 94:3162, 1997.

111. Kamata, T., and Takada, Y.: Direct binding of collagen to the I domain of integrin alpha 2 beta 1 (VLA-2, CD49b/CD29) in a divalent cation-independent manner. J. Biol. Chem. 269:26006, 1994.

112. Muchowski, P.J., Zhang, L., Chang, E.R., Soule, H.R., Plow, E.F., and Moyle, M.: Functional interaction between the integrin antagonist neutrophil inhibitory factor and the I domain of CD11b/CD18. J. Biol. Chem. 269:26419, 1994.

113. Emsley, J., King, S.L., Bergelson, J.M., and Liddington, R.C.: Crystal structure of the I domain from integrin alpha2beta1. J. Biol. Chem. 272:28512, 1997.

114. Qu, A., and Leahy, D.J.: Crystal structure of the I-domain from the CD11a/CD18 (LFA-1, $\alpha_L\beta_2$) integrin. Proc. Natl. Acad. Sci. USA 92:10277, 1995.

115. Zhang, L., and Plow, E.F.: Identification and reconstruction of the binding site within alphaMbeta2 for a specific and high affinity ligand, NIF. J. Biol. Chem. 272:17558, 1997.

116. van Kooyk, Y., Binnerts, M.E., Edwards, C.P., Champe, M., and Berman, P.W.: Critical amino acids in the lymphocyte function–associated antigen-1 I domain mediate intercellular adhesion molecule 3 binding and immune function. J. Exp. Med 183:1247, 1996.

117. King, S.L., Kamata, T., Cunningham, J.A., Emsley, J., Liddington, R.C., Takada, Y., and Bergelson, J.M.: Echovirus 1 interaction with the human very late antigen-2 (integrin alpha2beta1) I domain. Identification of two independent virus contact sites distinct from the metal ion–dependent adhesion site. J. Biol. Chem. 272:28518, 1997.

118. Zhang, L., and Plow, E.F.: A discrete site modulates activation of I domains. Application to integrin alphaMbeta2. J. Biol. Chem. 271:29953, 1996.

119. Dickenson, S.K., Walsh, J.J., and Santoro, S.A.: Contributions of the I and EF hand domains to the divalent cation–dependent collagen binding activity of the alpha 2 beta 1 integrin. J. Biol. Chem. 272:7661, 1997.

120. Mould, A.P., Askari, J.A., Aota, S., Yamada, K.M., Irie, A., Takada, Y., Mardon, H.J., and Humphries, M.J.: Defining the topology of integrin alpha5beta1-fibronectin interactions using inhibitory anti-alpha5 and anti-beta1 monoclonal antibodies. Evidence that the synergy sequence of fibronectin is recognized by the amino-terminal repeats of the alpha5 subunit. J. Biol. Chem. 272:17283, 1997.

121. Cheresh, D.A., and Harper, J.H.: Arg-Gly-Asp recognition by a cell adhesion receptor requires its 130-kDa α subunit. J. Biol. Chem. 262:1434, 1987.

122. Lam, S.C.-T., Plow, E.F., Smith, M.A., Andrieux, A., Ryckwaert, J.-J., Marguerie, G.A., and Ginsberg, M.H.: Evidence that arginyl-glycyl-aspartate peptides and fibrinogen gamma chain peptides share a common binding site on platelets. J. Biol. Chem. 262:947, 1987.

123. Hughes, P.E., and Pfaff, M.: Integrin affinity modulation. Trends Cell Biol. 8:359, 1998.

124. Solowska, J., Edelman, J.M., Albelda, S.M., and Buck, C.A.: Cytoplasmic and transmembrane domains of integrin β1 and β3 subunits are functionally interchangeable. J. Cell Biol. 114:1079, 1991.

125. Crowe, D.T., Chiu, H., Fong, S., and Weissman, I.L.: Regulation of the avidity of integrin α4β7 by the β7 cytoplasmic domain. J. Biol. Chem. 269:14411, 1994.

126. O'Toole, T.E., Katagiri, Y., Faull, R.J., Peter, K., Tamura, R.N., Quaranta, V., Loftus, J.C., Shattil, S.J., and Ginsberg, M.H.: Integrin cytoplasmic domains mediate inside-out signal transduction. J. Cell Biol. 124:1047, 1994.

127. Hughes, P.E., Diaz-Gonzalez, F., Leong, L., Wu, C., McDonald, J.A., Shattil, S.J., and Ginsberg, M.H.: Breaking the integrin hinge: a defined structural constraint regulates integrin signaling. J. Biol. Chem. 271:6571, 1996.

128. Kassner, P.D., and Hemler, M.E.: Interchangeable chain cytoplasmic domains play a positive role in control of cell adhesion mediated by VLA-4, a β1 integrin. J. Exp. Med. 178:649, 1993.

129. Kawaguchi, S., and Hemler, M.E.: Role of the subunit cytoplasmic domain in regulation of adhesive activity mediated by the integrin VLA-2. J. Biol. Chem. 268:16279, 1993.

130. Shaw, L.M., and Mercurio, A.M.: Regulation of alpha 6 beta 1 integrin laminin receptor function by the cytoplasmic domain of the alpha 6 subunit. J. Cell Biol. 123:1017, 1993.

131. Hibbs, M.L., Xu, H., Stacker, S.A., and Springer, T.A.: Regulation of

adhesion to ICAM-1 by the cytoplasmic domain of LFA-1 integrin beta subunit. Science 251:1611, 1991.

132. Horwitz, A., Duggan, K., Buck, C.A., Beckerle, M.C., and Burridge, K.: Interaction of plasma membrane fibronectin receptor with talin—a transmembrane linkage. Nature 320:531, 1986.

133. Pfaff, M., Liu, S., Erle, D.J., and Ginsberg, M.H.: Integrin β cytoplasmic domains differentially bind to cytoskeletal proteins. J. Biol. Chem. 273:6104, 1998.

134. Knezevic, I., Leisner, T., and Lam, S.: Direct binding of the platelet integrin $\alpha_{IIb}\beta_3$ (GPIIb-IIIa) to talin. J. Biol. Chem. 271:16416, 1996.

135. Otey, C.A., Pavalko, F.M., and Burridge, K.: An interaction between alpha actinin and the beta 1 integrin subunit in vitro. J. Cell Biol. 111:721, 1990.

136. Pavalko, F.M., and LaRoche, S.M.: Activation of human neutrophils induces an interaction between the integrin β2-subunit (CD18) and the actin binding protein α-actinin. J. Immunol. 151:3795, 1993.

137. Otey, C.A., Vasquez, G.B., Burridge, K., and Erickson, B.W.: Mapping of the α-actinin binding site within the β1 integrin cytoplasmic domain. J. Biol. Chem. 268:21193, 1993.

138. Lyman, S., Gilmore, A., Burridge, K., Gidwitz, S., and White, G.C., 2nd: Integrin-mediated activation of focal adhesion kinase is independent of focal adhesion formation or integrin activation. Studies with activated and inhibitory beta3 cytoplasmic domain mutants. J. Biol. Chem. 272:22538, 1997.

139. Reszka, A.A., Hayashi, Y., and Horwitz, A.F.: Identification of amino acid sequences in the integrin β1 cytoplasmic domain implicated in cytoskeletal association. J. Cell Biol. 117:1321, 1992.

140. Sharma, C.P., Ezzell, R.M., and Arnaout, M.A.: Direct interaction of filamin (ABP-280) with the β2-integrin subunit CD18. J. Immunol. 154:3461, 1995.

141. Schaller, M.D., Otey, C.A., Hildebrand, J.D., and Parsons, J.T.: Focal adhesion kinase and paxillin bind to peptides mimicking β integrin cytoplasmic domains. J. Cell Biol. 130:1181, 1995.

142. Kieffer, J.D., Plopper, G., Ingber, D.E., Hartwig, J.H., and Kupper, T.S.: Direct binding of F actin to the cytoplasmic domain of the α2 integrin chain in vitro. Biochem. Biophys. Res. Commun. 217:466, 1995.

143. Reddy, K.B., Gascard, P., Price, M.G., Negrescu, E.V., and Fox, J.E.B.: Identification of an interaction between the M-band protein skelemin and β-integrin subunits. Colocalization of a skelemin-like protein with beta 1 and beta 3 integrins in non-muscle cells. J. Biol. Chem. 273:1998.

144. Kolanus, W., Nagel, W., Schiller, B., Zeitlmann, L., Godar, S., Stockinger, H., and Seed, B.: αLβ2 integrin/LFA-1 binding to ICAM-1 induced by cytohesin-1, a cytoplasmic regulatory molecule. Cell 86:233, 1996.

145. Li, J., Avraham, H., Rogers, R.A., Raja, S., and Avraham, S.: Characterization of RAFTK, a novel focal adhesion kinase, and its integrin-dependent phosphorylation and activation in megakaryocytes. Blood 88:417, 1996.

146. Astier, A., Avraham, H., Manie, S.N., Groopman, J.E., Canty, T., Avraham, S., and Freedman, A.S.: The related adhesion focal tyrosine kinase is tyrosine-phosphorylated after beta 1–integrin stimulation in B cells and binds to p130 Cas. J. Biol. Chem. 272:228, 1997.

147. Hannigan, G.E., Leung-Hagesteijn, C., Fitz-Gibbon, L., Coppolino, M.G., Radeva, G., Filmus, J., Bell, J.C., and Dedhar, S.: Regulation of cell adhesion and anchorage-dependent growth by a novel β1 integrin–linked protein kinase. Nature 379:91, 1995.

148. Radeva, G., Petrocelli, T., Behrend, E.I., Leung-Hagesteijn, C., Filmus, J., Slingerland, J., and Dedhar, S.: Overexpression of the integrin-linked kinase promotes anchorage-independent cell cycle progression. J. Biol. Chem. 272:13937, 1997.

149. Wu, C., Keightley, S.Y., Leung-Hagesteijn, C., Radeva, G., Coppolino, M., Goicoechea, S., McDonald, J.A., and Dedhar, S.: Integrin-linked protein kinase regulates fibronectin matrix assembly, E-cadherin expression, and tumorigenicity. J. Biol. Chem. 273:528, 1998.

150. Shattil, S.J., O'Toole, T.E., Eigenthaler, M., Thon, V., Williams, M.J., Babior, B., and Ginsberg, M.H.: β3 endonexin, a novel polypeptide that interacts specifically with the cytoplasmic tail of the integrin β3 subunit. J. Cell Biol. 131:807, 1995.

151. Eigenthaler, M., Hofferer, L., Shattil, S.J., and Ginsberg, M.H.: A conserved sequence motif in the integrin β3 cytoplasmic domain is required for its specific interaction with β3-endonexin. J. Biol. Chem. 272:7693, 1997.

152. Kashiwagi, H., Schwartz, M.A., Eigenthaler, M., Davis, K.A., Ginsberg, M.H., and Shattil, S.J.: Affinity modulation of platelet integrin alphaIIbbeta3 by beta3-endonexin, a selective binding partner of the beta3 integrin cytoplasmic tail. J. Cell Biol. 137:1433, 1997.

153. Chang, D.D., Wong, C., Smith, H., and Liu, J.: ICAP-1, a novel beta1 integrin cytoplasmic domain–associated protein, binds to a conserved and functionally important NPXY sequence motif of β1 integrin. J. Cell Biol. 138:1149, 1997.

154. Liliental, J., and Chang, D.D.: Rack1, a receptor for activated protein kinase C, interacts with integrin beta subunit. J. Biol. Chem. 273:2379, 1998.

155. Naik, U.P., Patel, P.M., and Parise, L.V.: Identification of a novel calcium-binding protein that interacts with the integrin alpha IIb cytoplasmic domain. J. Biol. Chem. 272:4651, 1997.

156. Roijani, M.V., Finlay, B.B., Gray, V., and Dedhar, S.: In vitro interaction of a polypeptide homologous to human Ro/SS-A antigen (calreticulin) with a highly conserved amino acid sequence in the cytoplasmic domain of integrin alpha subunits. Biochemistry 30:9859, 1991.

157. Coppolino, M.G., Woodside, M.J., Demaurex, N., Grinstein, S., St-Arnaud, R., and Dedhar, S.: Calreticulin is essential for integrin-mediated calcium signalling and cell adhesion. Nature 386:843, 1997.

158. Porter, J.C., and Hogg, N.: Integrins take partners: cross-talk between integrins and other membrane receptors. Trends Cell Biol. 8:390, 1998.

159. Lindberg, F.P., Gresham, H.D., Schwarz, E., and Brown, E.J.: Molecular cloning of integrin-associated protein: an immunoglobulin family member with multiple membrane-spanning domains implicated in $\alpha_v\beta_3$-dependent ligand binding. J. Cell Biol. 123:485, 1993.

160. Chung, J., Gao, A.G., and Frazier, W.A.: Thrombospondin acts via integrin-associated protein to activate the platelet integrin alphaIIb-beta3. J. Biol. Chem. 272:14740, 1997.

161. Wang, X.Q., and Frazier, W.A.: The thrombospondin receptor CD47 (IAP) modulates and associates with alpha2 beta1 integrin in vascular smooth muscle cells. Mol. Biol. Cell 9:865, 1998.

162. Imhof, B.A., Weerasinghe, D., Brown, E.J., Linberg, F.P., Hammel, P., Piali, L., Dessing, M., and Gisler, R.: Cross talk between alpha(v)beta3 and alpha4beta1 integrins regulates lymphocyte migration on vascular cell adhesion molecule 1. Eur. J. Immunol. 27:3242, 1997.

163. Lindberg, F.P., Bullard, D., Caver, T.E., Gresham, H.D., Beaudet, A.L., and Brown, E.J.: Decreased resistance to bacterial infection and granulocyte defects in IAP-deficient mice. Science 274:795, 1996.

164. Hemler, M.E., Mannion, B.A., and Berdichevsky, F.B.: Association of TM4SF proteins with integrins: relevance to cancer. Biochim. Biophys. Acta 1287:67, 1996.

165. Hemler, M.E.: Integrin associated proteins. Curr. Opin. Cell Biol. 10:578, 1998.

166. Todd, R.F., III, and Petty, H.R.: Beta 2 (CD11/CD18) integrins can serve as signaling partners for other leukocyte receptors. J. Lab. Clin. Med. 129:492, 1997.

167. Lub, M., van Kooyk, Y., and Figdor, C.G.: Ins and outs of LFA-1. Immunol. Today 16:479, 1995.

168. Shimizu, Y., and Hunt, S.W.: Regulating integrin-mediated adhesion: one more function for PI3-kinase? Immunol. Today 13:106, 1996.

169. Zhang, J., Shattil, S.J., Cunningham, M.C., and Rittenhouse, S.E.: Phosphoinositide 3–kinase and p85/phosphoinositide 3–kinase in platelets. J. Biol. Chem. 271:6265, 1996.

170. Keely, P.J., Parise, L.V., and Juliano, R.: Integrins and GTPases in tumour cell growth, motility and invasion. Trends Cell Biol. 8:101, 1998.

171. Hughes, P.E., Renshaw, M.W., Pfaff, M., Forsyth, J., Keivens, V.M., Schwartz, M.A., and Ginsberg, M.H.: Suppression of integrin activation: a novel function of a Ras/Raf-initiated MAP kinase pathway. Cell 88:521, 1997.

172. O'Rourke, A.M., Shao, H., and Kaye, J.: Cutting edge: a role for p21ras/MAP kinase in TCR-mediated activation of LFA-1. J. Immunol. 161:5800, 1998.

173. Zhang, Z., Vuori, K., Wang, H.-G., Reed, J.C., and Ruoslahti, E.: Integrin activation by R-ras. Cell 85:61, 1996.

174. Marte, B.M., Rodriguez-Viciana, P., Wennstrom, S., Warne, P.H., and Downward, J.: R-Ras can activate the phosphoinositide 3–kinase but not the MAP kinase arm of the Ras effector pathways. Curr. Biol. 7:63, 1997.

175. Urano, T., Emkey, R., and Feig, L.A.: Ral-GTPases mediate a distinct downstream signaling pathway from Ras that facilitates cellular transformation. EMBO J. 15:810, 1996.

176. Marte, B.M., Rodriguez-Viciana, P., Wennstrom, S., Warne, P.H., and Downward, J.: R-Ras can activate the phosphoinositide 3–kinase but not the MAP kinase arm of the Ras effector pathways. Curr. Biol. 7:197, 1997.

177. Marte, B.M., and Downward, J.: PKB/Akt: connecting phosphoinositide 3–kinase to cell survival and beyond. Trends Biochem. Sci. 22:355, 1997.

178. Kornberg, L.J., Earp, H.S., Turner, C.E., Prockop, C., and Juliano, R.L.: Signal transduction by integrins: increased protein tyrosine phosphorylation caused by clustering of β_1 integrins. Proc. Natl. Acad. Sci. USA 88:8392, 1991.

179. Guan, J.-L., Trevithick, J.E., and Hynes, R.O.: Fibronectin/integrin interaction induces tyrosine phosphorylation of a 120-kDa protein. Cell Regul. 2:951, 1991.

180. Burridge, K., Turner, C.E., and Romer, L.H.: Tyrosine phosphorylation of paxillin and pp125FAK accompanies cell adhesion to extracellular matrix: a role in cytoskeletal assembly. J. Cell Biol. 119:193, 1992.

181. Schlaepfer, D.D., and Hunter, T.: Integrin signalling and tyrosine phosphorylation: just the FAKs? Trends Cell Biol. 8:151, 1998.

182. Schlaepfer, D.D., Hanks, S.K., Hunter, T., and van der Geer, P.: Integrin-mediated signal transduction linked to Ras pathway by GRB2 binding to focal adhesion kinase. Nature 372:786, 1994.

183. Wary, K.K., Mainiero, F., Isakoff, S.J., Marcantonio, E.E., and Giancotti, F.G.: The adaptor protein Shc couples a class of integrins to the control of cell cycle progression. Cell 87:733, 1996.

184. Davis, S., Lu, M.L., Lo, S.H., Lin, S., Butler, J.A., Druker, B.J., Roberts, T.M., An, Q., and Chen, L.B.: Presence of an SH2 domain in the actin-binding protein tensin. Science 252:712, 1991.

185. Guan, J.-L.: Role of focal adhesion kinase in integrin signaling. Int. J. Biochem. Cell Biol. 29:1623, 1997.

186. Turner, C.E., and Miller, J.T.: Primary sequence of paxillin contains putative SH2 and SH3 domain binding motifs and multiple LIM domains: identification of a vinculin and pp125Fak-binding region. J. Cell Sci. 107:1583, 1994.

187. Polte, T.R., and Hanks, S.K.: Interaction between focal adhesion kinase and Crk-associated tyrosine kinase substrate p130Cas. Proc. Natl. Acad. Sci. USA 92:10678, 1995.

188. Turner, C.E., Glenney, J.R.J., and Burridge, K.: Paxillin: a new vinculin-binding protein present in focal adhesions. J. Cell Biol. 111:1059, 1990.

189. Songyang, Z., Shoelson, S.E., Chaudhuri, M., Gish, G., Pawson, T., Haser, W.G., King, F., Roberts, T., Ratnofsky, S., Lechleider, J., Neel, B.G., Birge, R.B., Fajardo, J.E., Chou, M.M., Hanafusa, H., Schaffhausen, B., and Cantley, L.C.: SH2 domains recognize specific phosphopeptide sequences. Cell 72:767, 1993.

190. Matsuda, M., Hashimoto, Y., Muroyo, K., Hasegawa, H., Kurata, T., Tanaka, S., and Hattori, S.: CRK protein binds to two guanine nucleotide–releasing proteins for the Ras family and modulates nerve growth factor–induced activation of Ras in PC12 cells. Mol. Cell. Biol. 14:5495, 1994.

191. Gotoh, T., Hattori, S., Nakamura, S., Noda, M., Takai, Y., Kaibuchi, K., Matsui, H., and Takahashi, H.: Identification of Rap1 as a target for the Crk SH3 domain–binding guanine nucleotide–releasing factor C3G. Mol. Cell. Biol. 15:6746, 1995.

192. Chen, H.-C., and Guan, J.-L.: Association of focal adhesion kinase with its potential substrate phosphatidylinositol 3–kinase. Proc. Natl. Acad. Sci. USA 91:10148, 1994.

193. Guinebault, C., Payrastre, B., Racaud-Sultan, C., Mazarguil, H., Breton, M., Mauco, G., Plantavid, M., and Chap, H.: Integrin-dependent translocation of phosphoinositide 3–kinase to the cytoskeleton of thrombin-activated platelets involves specific interactions of p85 alpha with actin filaments and focal adhesion kinase. J. Cell Biol. 129:831, 1995.

194. Hall, A.: Rho GTPases and the actin cytoskeleton. Science 23:509, 1998.

195. Nobes, C.D., and Hall, A.: Rho, Rac and Cdc42 GTPases regulate the assembly of multimolecular focal complexes associated with actin stress fibers, lamellipodia and filopodia. Cell 81:53, 1995.

196. Ridley, A.J., and Hall, A.: The small GTP-binding protein rho regulates the assembly of focal adhesions and actin stress fibers in response to growth factors. Cell 70:389, 1992.

197. Ridley, A.J., Paterson, H.F., Johnston, C.L., Diekmann, C., and Hall, A.: The small GTP-binding protein rac regulates growth factor–induced membrane ruffling. Cell 70:401, 1992.

198. Wennstrom, S., Hawkins, P., Cooke, F., Hara, K., Yonezawa, K., Kasuga, M., Jackson, T., Claesson-Welsh, L., and Stephens, L.: Activation of phosphoinositide 3–kinase is required for PDGF-stimulated membrane ruffling. Curr. Biol. 4:385, 1994.

199. Rodriguez-Viciana, P., Warne, P.H., Khwaja, A., Marte, B.M., Pappin, D., Das, P., Waterfield, M.D., Ridley, A., and Downward, J.: Role of phosphoinositide 3–OH kinase in cell transformation and control of the actin cytoskeleton by Ras. Cell 89:457, 1997.

200. Hotchin, N.A., and Hall, A.: The assembly of integrin adhesion complexes requires both extracellular matrix and intracellular rho/rac GTPases. J. Cell Biol. 131:1857, 1995.

201. Chong, L.D., Kaplan, A.T., Bokoch, G.M., and Schwartz, M.A.: The small GTP binding protein Rho regulates a phosphatidylinositol 4-phosphate 5-kinase in mammalian cells. Cell 79:507, 1994.

202. Ren, X.D., Bokoch, G.M., Traynor-Kaplan, A., Jenkins, G.H., Anderson, R.A., and Schwartz, M.A.: Physical association of the small GTPase Rho with a 68-kDa phosphatidylinositol 4-phosphate 5-kinase in Swiss 3T3 cells. Mol. Biol. Cell 7:435, 1996.

203. Hartwig, J., Bokoch, G., Carpenter, C., Janmey, P., Taylor, L., Toker, A., and Stossel, T.: Thrombin receptor ligation and activated Rac uncap actin filament barbed ends through phosphoinositide synthesis in permeabilized human platelets. Cell 82:643, 1995.

204. Gilmore, A.P., and Burridge, K.: Regulation of vinculin binding to talin and actin by phosphatidyl-inositol-4-5-bisphosphate. Nature 381:531, 1996.

205. Leung, T., Manser, E., Tan, L., and Lim, L.: A novel serine/threonine kinase binding the Ras-related RhoA GTPase which translocates the kinase to peripheral membranes. J. Biol. Chem. 270:29051, 1995.

206. Leung, T., Chen, X.Q., Manser, E., and Lim, L.: The p160 RhoA-binding kinase ROK alpha is a member of a kinase family and is involved in the reorganization of the cytoskeleton. Mol. Cell. Biol. 16:5313, 1996.

207. Lauffenburger, D.A., and Horowitz, A.F.: Cell migration: a physically integrated molecular process. Cell 84:359, 1996.

208. Amano, M., Chihara, K., Kimura, K., Fukata, Y., Nakamura, N., Matsuura, Y., and Kaibuchi, K.: Formation of actin stress fibers and focal adhesions enhanced by Rho-kinase. Science 275:1308, 1997.

209. Kureishi, Y., Kobayashi, S., Amano, M., Kimura, K., Kanaide, H., Nakanao, T., Kaibuchi, K., and Ito, M.: Rho-associated kinase directly induces smooth muscle contraction through myosin light chain phosphorylation. J. Biol. Chem. 272:12257, 1997.

210. Lamarche, N., Tapon, N., Stowers, L., Burbelo, P.D., Aspenstrom, P., Bridges, T., Chant, J., and Hall, A.: Rac and Cdc42 induce actin polymerization and G1 cell cycle progression independently of p65 PAK and the JNK/SAPK MAP kinase cascade. Cell 87:519, 1996.

211. Joneson, T., McDonough, M., Bar-Sagi, D., and Van Aelst, L.: RAC regulation of actin polymerization and proliferation by a pathway distinct from Jun kinase. Science 274:1374, 1996.

212. Symons, M., Derry, J.M.J., Karlsen, K., Jiang, S., Lemahieu, V., McCormick, F., Francke, U., and Abo, A.: Wiskott-Aldrich syndrome protein, a novel effector for the GTPase CDC42Hs, is implicated in actin polymerization. Cell 84:723, 1996.

213. Van Aelst, L., Joneson, T., and Bar-Sagi, D.: Identification of a novel Rac1-interacting protein involved in membrane ruffling. EMBO J. 15:3778, 1996.

214. Shattil, S.J., Kashiwagi, H., and Pampori, N.: Integrin signaling: the platelet paradigm. Blood 91:2645, 1998.

215. Reif, K., Nobes, C.D., Thomas, G., Hall, A., and Cantrell, D.A.: Phosphatidylinositol 3–kinase signals activate a selective subset of Rac/Rho-dependent effector pathways. Curr. Biol. 6:1445, 1996.

216. Khwaja, A., Rodriguez-Viciana, P., Wennstrom, S., Warne, P.H., and Downward, J.: Matrix adhesion and Ras transformation both activate a phosphoinositide 3–OH kinase and protein kinase B/Akt cellular survival pathway. EMBO J. 16:2783, 1997.

217. Rodriguez-Viciana, P., Warne, P.H., Dhand, R., Vanhaesebroeck, B., Gout, I., Fry, M.J., and Downward, J.: Phosphatidylinositol-3-OH kinase as a direct target of Ras. Nature 370:527, 1994.

218. Coffer, P.J., Jin, J., and Woodgett, J.R.: Protein kinase B (c-Akt): a multifunctional mediator of phosphatidylinositol 3–kinase activation. Biochem. J. 335:1, 1998.

219. McNamee, H.P., Ingber, D., and Schwartz, M.A.: Adhesion to fibronectin stimulates inositol lipid synthesis and enhances PDGF-induced inositol lipid breakdown. J. Cell Biol. 121:673, 1993.

220. Chun, J.-S., and Jacobson, B.S.: Spreading of HeLa cells on a collagen substratum requires a second messenger formed by the lipoxygenase metabolism of arachidonic acid released by collagen receptor clustering. Mol. Biol. Cell 3:481, 1992.

221. Cybulsky, A.V., Stewart, D.J., and Cybulsky, M.I.: Glomerular epithelial cells produce endothelin-1. J. Am. Soc. Nephrol. 3:1398, 1993.

222. Vuori, K., and Ruoslahti, E.: Activation of protein kinase C precedes alpha 5 beta 1 integrin–mediated cell spreading on fibronectin. J. Biol. Chem. 268:21459, 1993.

223. Haller, H., Lindschau, C., Maasch, C., Olthoff, H., Kuscheid, D., and Luft, F.C.: Integrin-induced protein kinase C and C translocation to focal adhesions mediates vascular smooth muscle cell spreading. Circ. Res. 82:157, 1998.

224. Schwartz, M.A., Schaller, M.D., and Ginsberg, M.H.: Integrins: emerging paradigms of signal transduction. Annu. Rev. Cell Dev. Biol. 11:549, 1995.

225. Ginsberg, M.H., Forsyth, J., Lightsey, A., Chediak, J., and Plow, E.F.: Reduced surface expression and binding of fibronectin by thrombin-stimulated thrombasthenic platelets. J. Clin. Invest. 71:619, 1983.

226. Pytela, R., Pierschbacher, M.D., and Ruoslahti, E.: Identification and isolation of a 140 kd cell surface glycoprotein with properties expected of a fibronectin receptor. Cell 40:191, 1985.

227. Parise, L.V., and Phillips, D.R.: Fibronectin-binding properties of the purified platelet glycoprotein IIb-IIIa complex. J. Biol. Chem. 261:14011, 1986.

228. Marlin, S.D., and Springer, T.A.: Purified intercellular adhesion molecule-1 (ICAM-1) is a ligand for lymphocyte function–associated antigen 1 (LFA-1). Cell 51:813, 1987.

229. Isberg, R.R., and Leong, J.M.: Multiple β1 chain integrins are receptors for invasin, a protein that promotes bacterial penetration into mammalian cells. Cell 60:861, 1990.

230. Relman, D., Tuomanen, E., Falkow, S., Golenbock, D.T., Saukkonen, K., and Wright, S.D.: Recognition of a bacterial adhesin by an integrin: macrophage CR3 (alpha M beta 2, CD11b/CD18) binds filamentous hemagglutinin of *Bordetella pertussis*. Cell 61:1375, 1990.

231. Altieri, D.C., and Edgington, T.S.: The saturable high affinity association of factor X to ADP-stimulated monocytes defines a novel function of the Mac-1 receptor. J. Biol. Chem. 263:7007, 1988.

232. Ruggeri, Z.M.: von Willebrand factor. J. Clin. Invest. 99:559, 1997.

233. Bennett, J.S., Vilaire, G., and Cines, D.B.: Identification of the fibrinogen receptor on human platelets by photoaffinity labeling. J. Biol. Chem. 257:8049, 1982.

234. Leahy, D.J., Hendrickson, W.A., Aukhil, I., and Erickson, H.P.: Structure of a fibronectin type III domain from tenascin phased by MAD analysis of the selenomethionyl protein. Science 258:987, 1992.

235. Main, A.L., Harvey, T.S., Baron, M., Boyd, J., and Campbell, I.D.: The three-dimensional structure of the tenth type III module of fibronectin: an insight into RGD-mediated interactions. Cell 71:671, 1992.

236. Tomiyama, Y., Brojer, E., Ruggeri, Z.M., Shattil, S.J., Smiltneck, J., Gorski, J., Kumar, A., Kieber-Emmons, T., and Kunicki, T.J.: A molecular model of RGD ligands: antibody D gene segments that direct specificity for the integrin IIb3. J. Biol. Chem. 267:18085, 1992.

237. Hemler, M., and Lobb, R.: The leukocyte beta 1 integrin. Curr. Opin. Hematol. 2:61, 1995.

238. Wei, J., Shaw, L.M., and Mercurio, A.M.: Integrin signaling in leukocytes: lessons from the alpha6beta1 integrin. J. Leukoc. Biol. 61:397, 1997.

239. Leahy, D.J.: Implications of atomic-resolution structures for cell adhesion. Annu. Rev. Cell Dev. Biol. 13:363, 1997.

240. Staunton, D.E., Dustin, M.L., Erickson, H.P., and Springer, T.A.: The arrangement of immunoglobulin-like domains of ICAM-1 and the binding sites of LFA-1 and rhinovirus. Cell 61:243, 1990.

241. Li, R., Xie, Y., Kantor, C., Koistinen, V., Altieri, D.C., Nortamo, P., and Gahmberg, C.G.: A peptide derived from the intercellular adhesion molecule-2 regulates the avidity of the leukocyte integrin CD11b/CD18 and CD11c/CD18. J. Cell Biol. 129:1143, 1995.

242. Klickstein, L.B., York, M.R., Fougerolles, A.R., and Springer, T.A.: Localization of the binding site on intercellular adhesion molecule-3 (ICAM-3) for lymphocyte function–associated antigen 1 (LFA-1). J. Biol. Chem. 271:23920, 1996.

243. Karecla, P.I., Green, S.J., Bowden, S.J., Coadwell, J., and Kilshaw, P.J.: Identification of a binding site for integrin alphaEbeta7 in the N-terminal domain of E-cadherin. J. Biol. Chem. 271:30909, 1996.

244. Diamond, M.S., Staunton, D.E., Marlin, S.D., and Springer, T.A.: Binding of the integrin Mac-1 (CD11b/CD18) to the third immunoglobulin-like domain of ICAM-1 (CD54) and its regulation by glycosylation. Cell 65:961, 1991.

245. Osborn, L., Vassallo, C., and Benjamin, C.D.: Activated endothelium binds lymphocytes through a novel binding site in the alternately spliced domain of vascular cell adhesion molecule-1. J. Exp. Med. 176:99, 1992.

246. Needham, L.A., Van Dijk, S., Pigott, R., Edwards, R.M., Shepherd, M., Hemingway, I., Jack, L., and Clements, J.M.: Activation dependent and independent VLA-4 binding sites on vascular cell adhesion molecule-1. Cell Adhes. Commun. 2:87, 1994.

247. Kilger, G., Needham, L.A., Nielsen, P.J., Clements, J., Vestweber, D., and Holzmann, B.: Differential regulation of α_4 integrin–dependent binding to domains 1 and 4 of vascular cell adhesion molecule-1. J. Biol. Chem. 270:5979, 1995.

248. Abe, Y., Ballantyne, C.M., and Smith, C.W.: Functions of domains 1 and 4 of vascular cell adhesion molecule-1 in alpha4 integrin dependent adhesion under static and flow conditions are differentially regulated. J. Immunol. 157:5061, 1996.

249. Bowditch, R.D., Halloran, C.E., Aota, S., Obara, M., Plow, E.F., Yamada, K.M., and Ginsberg, M.H.: Integrin $\alpha_{IIb}\beta_3$ (platelet GPIIb-IIIa) recognizes multiple sites in fibronectin. J. Biol. Chem. 266:23323, 1991.

250. Bowditch, R.D., Hariharan, M., Tominna, E.F., Smith, J.W., Yamada, K.M., Getzoff, E.D., and Ginsberg, M.H.: Identification of a novel integrin binding site in fibronectin: differential utilization by β3 integrins. J. Biol. Chem. 269:10856, 1994.

251. Aota, S., Nagai, T., and Yamada, K.M.: Characterization of regions of fibronectin besides the Arg-Gly-Asp sequence required for adhesive function of the cell-binding domain using site-directed mutagenesis. J. Biol. Chem. 266:15938, 1991.

252. Aota, S., Nomizu, M., and Yamada, K.M.: The short amino acid sequence pro-his-ser-arg-asn in human fibronectin enhances cell-adhesive function. J. Biol. Chem. 269:24756, 1994.

253. Danen, E.H.J., Aota, S.-I., van Kraats, A.A., Yamada, K.M., Ruiter, D.J., and van Muijen, G.N.P.: Requirement for the synergy site for cell adhesion to fibronectin depends on the activation state of integrin α5β1. J. Biol. Chem. 270:21612, 1995.

254. Leahy, D.J., Aukhil, I., and Erickson, H.P.: 2.0 A crystal structure of a four-domain segment of human fibronectin encompassing the RGD loop and synergy region. Cell 84:155, 1996.

255. Wang, J., Pepinsky, R.B., Stehle, T., Liu, J., Karpusas, M., Browning, B., and Osborn, L.: The crystal structure of an N-terminal two-domain fragment of vascular cell adhesion molecule 1 (VCAM-1); a cyclic peptide based on domain 1 C-D loop can inhibit VCAM-1–alpha4 integrin interaction. Proc. Natl. Acad. Sci. USA 92:5714, 1995.

256. Viney, J.L., Jones, S., Chiu, H.H., Lagrimas, B., Renz, M.E., Presta, L.G., Jackson, D., Hillan, K.J., Lew, S., and Fong, S.: Mucosal addressin cell adhesion molecule-1. A structural and functional analysis demarcates the integrin binding motif. J. Immunol. 157:2488, 1996.

257. Tan, K., Casasnovas, J.M., Liu, J., Briskin, M.J., Springer, T.A., and Wang, J.: The structure of immunoglobulin superfamily domains 1 and 2 of MAdCAM-1 reveals novel features important for integrin recognition. Structure 6:793, 1998.

258. Newham, P., Craig, S.E., Seddon, G.N., Schofield, N.R., Rees, A., Edwards, R.M., Jones, E.Y., and Humphries, M.J.: Alpha4 integrin binding interfaces on VCAM-1 and MAdCAM-1. Integrin binding footprints identify accessory binding sites that play a role in integrin specificity. J. Biol. Chem. 272:19429, 1997.

259. Casasnovas, J.M., Springer, T.A., Liu, J.-H., Harrison, S.C., and Wang, J.-H.: Crystal structure of ICAM-2 reveals a distinctive integrin recognition surface. Nature 387:312, 1997.

260. Casasnovas, J.M., Stehle, T., Liu, J.-H., Wang, J.-H., and Springer, T.A.: A dimeric crystal structure for the N-terminal two domains of intercellular adhesion molecule-1. Proc. Natl. Acad. Sci. USA 95:4134, 1998.

261. Cheng, S., Craig, W.S., Mullen, D., Tschopp, J.F., Dixon, D., and Pierschbacher, M.D.: Design and synthesis of novel cyclic RGD-containing peptides as highly potent and selective integrin $\alpha_{IIb}\beta_3$ antagonists. J. Med. Chem. 37:1, 1994.

262. Barbas, C.F., Languino, L.R., and Smith, J.W.: High-affinity self-reactive human antibodies by design and selection: targeting the integrin ligand binding site. Proc. Natl. Acad. Sci. USA 90:10003, 1993.

263. Greenspoon, N., Hershkoviz, R., Alon, R., Varon, D., Shenkman, B., Marx, G., Federman, S., Kapustina, G., and Lider, O.: Structural analysis of integrin recognition and the inhibition of integrin-mediated cell functions by novel nonpeptidic surrogates of the Arg-Gly-Asp sequence. Biochemistry 32:1001, 1993.

264. Horton, M.A., Dorey, E.L., Nesbitt, S.A., Samanen, J., Ali, F.E., Stadel, J.M., Nichols, A., Greig, R., and Helfrich, M.H.: Modulation

of vitronectin receptor–mediated osteoclast adhesion by Arg-Gly-Asp peptide analogs: a structure-function analysis. J. Bone Miner. Res. 8:239, 1993.

265. Koivunen, E., Gay, D.A., and Ruoslahti, E.: Selection of peptides binding of the $\alpha_5\beta_1$ integrin from phage display library. J. Biol. Chem. 268:20205, 1993.

266. Nowlin, D.M., Gorcsan, F., Moscinski, M., Chiang, S.L., Lobl, T.J., and Cardarelli, P.M.: A novel cyclic pentapeptide inhibits alpha 4 beta 1 and alpha 5 beta 1 integrin–mediated cell adhesion. J. Biol. Chem. 268:20352, 1993.

267. Alig, L., Edenhofer, A., Hadvary, P., Hurzeler, M., Knopp, D., Muller, M., Steiner, B., Trzeciak, A., and Weller, T.: Low molecular weight, non-peptide fibrinogen receptor antagonists. J. Med. Chem. 35:4393, 1992.

268. Li, R., Nortamo, P., Kantor, C., Kovanen, P., Timonen, T., and Gahmberg, C.G.: A leukocyte integrin binding peptide from intercellular adhesion molecule-2 stimulates T cell adhesion and natural killer cell activity. J. Biol. Chem. 268:21474, 1993.

269. Ross, L., Hassman, F., and Molony, L.: Inhibition of molt-4-endothelial adherence by synthetic peptides from the sequence of ICAM-1. J. Biol. Chem. 267:8537, 1992.

270. Staatz, W.D., Fok, K.F., Zutter, M.M., Adams, S.P., Rodriguez, B.A., and Santoro, S.A.: Identification of a tetrapeptide recognition sequence for the alpha-2 beta-1 integrin in collagen. J. Biol. Chem. 266:7363, 1991.

271. Hawiger, J., Timmons, S., Kloczewiak, M., Strong, D.D., and Doolittle, R.F.: Alpha and beta chains of human fibrinogen possess sites reactive with human receptors. Proc. Natl. Acad. Sci. USA 79:2068, 1982.

272. Kloczewiak, M., Timmons, S., Lukas, T.J., and Hawiger, J.: Platelet receptor recognition site on human fibrinogen. Synthesis and structure-function relationship of peptides corresponding to the carboxy-terminal segment of the gamma chain. Biochemistry 23:1767, 1984.

273. Marguerie, G.A., Plow, E.F., and Edgington, T.S.: Human platelets possess an inducible and saturable receptor specific for fibrinogen. J. Biol. Chem. 254:5357, 1979.

274. Savage, B., Bottini, E., and Ruggeri, Z.M.: Interaction of integrin alphaIIbbeta3 with multiple fibrinogen domains during platelet adhesion. J. Biol. Chem. 270:28812, 1995.

275. Gartner, T.K., Amrani, D.L., Derrick, J.M., Kirschbaum, N.E., Matsueda, G.R., and Taylor, D.B.: Characterization of adhesion of "resting" and stimulated platelets to fibrinogen and its fragments. Thromb. Res. 71:47, 1993.

276. Farrell, D.H., Thiagarajan, P., Chung, D.W., and Davie, E.W.: Role of fibrinogen alpha and gamma chain sites in platelet aggregation. Proc. Natl. Acad. Sci. USA 89:10729, 1992.

277. Farrell, D.H., and Thiagarajan, P.: Binding of recombinant fibrinogen mutants to platelets. J. Biol. Chem. 269:226, 1994.

278. Pytela, R.P., Pierschbacher, M.D., Ginsberg, M.H., Plow, E.F., and Ruoslahti, E.: Platelet membrane glycoprotein IIb/IIIa: member of a family of Arg-Gly-Asp–specific adhesion receptors. Science 231:1559, 1986.

279. Bennett, J.S., Shattil, S.J., Power, J.W., and Gartner, T.K.: Interaction of fibrinogen with its platelet receptor. Differential effects of α and gamma chain fibrinogen peptides on the glycoprotein IIb-IIIa complex. J. Biol. Chem. 263:12948, 1988.

280. Ruoslahti, E., and Pierschbacher, M.D.: New perspectives in cell adhesion: RGD and integrins. Science 238:491, 1987.

281. Berliner, S., Niiya, K., Roberts, J.R., Houghten, R.A., and Ruggeri, Z.M.: Generation and characterization of peptide-specific antibodies that inhibit von Willebrand factor binding to glycoprotein IIb-IIIa without interacting with other adhesive molecules. Selectivity is conferred by Pro and other amino acid residues adjacent to the sequence Arg-Gly-Asp. J. Biol. Chem. 263:7500, 1988.

282. Girma, J.-P., Kalafatis, M., Pietu, G., Lavergne, J.-M., Chopek, M.W., Edgington, T.S., and Meyer, D.: Mapping of distinct von Willebrand factor domains interacting with platelet GPIb/GPIIIa and with collagen using monoclonal antibodies. Blood 67:1356, 1986.

283. Trapani, L.V., Hodson, E., Roberts, J.R., Kunicki, T.J., Zimmerman, T.S., and Ruggeri, Z.M.: Independent modulation of von Willebrand factor and fibrinogen binding to the platelet membrane glycoprotein IIb/IIa complex as demonstrated by monoclonal antibody. J. Clin. Invest. 76:1950, 1985.

284. Altieri, D.C., Morrissey, J.H., and Edgington, T.S.: Adhesive receptor Mac-1 coordinates the activation of factor X on stimulated cells of monocytic and myeloid differentiation: an alternative initiation of the coagulation protease cascade. Proc. Natl. Acad. Sci. USA 85:7462, 1988.

285. Altieri, D.C., Etingin, O.R., Fair, D.S., Brunck, T.K., Geltosky, J.E., Hajjar, D.P., and Edgington, T.S.: Structurally homologous ligand binding of integrin Mac-1 and viral glycoprotein C receptors. Science 254:1200, 1991.

286. Zhou, L., Lee, D.H., Plescia, J., Lau, C.Y., and Altieri, D.C.: Differential ligand binding specificities of recombinant CD11b/CD18 integrin I-domain. J. Biol. Chem. 269:17075, 1994.

287. Mesri, M., Plescia, J., and Altieri, D.C.: Dual regulation of ligand binding by CD11b I domain. Inhibition of intercellular adhesion and monocyte procoagulant activity by a factor X–derived peptide. J. Biol. Chem. 273:744, 1998.

288. Springer, T.A.: Traffic signals on endothelium for lymphocyte recirculation and leukocyte emigration. Annu. Rev. Physiol. 57:827, 1995.

289. Bevilacqua, M.P.: Endothelial-leukocyte adhesion molecules. Annu. Rev. Immunol. 11:767, 1993.

290. Schleimer, R.P., Sterbinsky, S.A., Kaiser, J., Bickel, C.A., Klunk, D.A., Tomioka, K., Newman, W., Luscinskas, F.W., Gimbrone, M.A.J., McIntyre, B.W., and Bochner, B.S.: IL-4 induces adherence of human eosinophils and basophils but not neutrophils to endothelium. Association with expression of VCAM-1. J. Immunol. 148:1086, 1992.

291. Gahmberg, C.G., Tolvanen, M., and Kotovuori, P.: Leukocyte adhesion. Structure and function of human leukocyte beta2-integrins and their cellular ligands. Eur. J. Biochem. 245:215, 1997.

292. Dustin, M.L., Rothlein, R., Bhan, A.K., Dinarello, C.A., and Springer, T.A.: Induction by IL 1 and interferon-γ: tissue distribution, biochemistry, and function of a natural adherence molecule (ICAM-1). J. Immunol. 137:245, 1986.

293. Cornejo, C.J., Winn, R.K., and Harlan, J.M.: Anti-adhesion therapy. Adv. Pharmacol. 39:99, 1997.

294. Sligh, J.E., Ballantyne, C.M., Rich, S.S., Hawkins, H.K., Smith, C.W., Bradley, A., and Beaudet, A.L.: Inflammatory and immune responses are impaired in mice deficient in intracellular adhesion molecule 1. Proc. Natl. Acad. Sci. USA 90:8529, 1993.

295. de Fougerolles, A.R., Stacker, S.A., Schwarting, R., and Springer, T.A.: Characterization of ICAM-2 and evidence for a third counter-receptor for LFA-1. J. Exp. Med 174:253, 1991.

296. Doussis-Anagnostopoulou, I., Kaklamanis, L., Cordell, J.L., Jones, M., Turley, H., Pulford, K., Simmons, D., Mason, D., and Gatter, K.: ICAM-3 expression on endothelium in lymphoid malignancy. Am. J. Pathol. 143:1040, 1993.

297. Patey, N., Vazeux, R., Canioni, D., Potter, T., Gallatin, W.M., and Brousse, N.: Intercellular adhesion molecule-3 on endothelial cells. Expression in tumors but not in inflammatory responses. Am. J. Pathol. 148:465, 1996.

298. de Fougerolles, A.R., and Springer, T.A.: Intercellular adhesion molecule 3, a third adhesion counter-receptor for lymphocyte function associated molecule 1 on resting lymphocytes. J. Exp. Med 175:185, 1992.

299. Fawcett, J., Holness, C.L., Needham, L.A., Turley, E.A., Gatter, K.C., Mason, D.Y., and Simmons, D.L.: Molecular cloning of ICAM-3, a third ligand for LFA-1, constitutively expressed on resting leukocytes. Nature 360:481, 1992.

300. de Fougerolles, A.R., Qin, X., and Springer, T.A.: Characterization of the function of intercellular adhesion molecule (ICAM)-3 and comparison with ICAM-1 and ICAM-2 in immune response. J. Exp. Med. 179:619, 1994.

301. Cid, M.C., Esparza, J., Juan, M., Miralles, A., Ordi, J., Vilella, R., Urbano-Marquez, A., Gaya, A., Vives, J., and Yague, J.: Signaling through CD50 (ICAM-3) stimulates T lymphocyte binding to human umbilical vein endothelial cells and extracellular matrix proteins via an increase in beta1 and beta2 integrin function. Eur. J. Immunol. 24:1377, 1994.

302. Jacobsen, K., Kravitz, J., Kincade, P.W., and Osmond, D.G.: Adhesion receptors on bone marrow stromal cells: in vivo expression of vascular cell adhesion molecule-1 by reticular cells and sinusoidal endothelium in normal and gamma-irradiated mice. Blood 87:73, 1996.

303. Arroyo, A.G., Yang, J.T., Rayburn, H., and Hynes, R.O.: Differential requirements for α4 integrins in hematopoiesis. Cell 85:997, 1996.

304. Yanai, N., Sekine, C., Yagita, H., and Obinata, M.: Roles for integrin very late activation antigen-4 in stroma-dependent erythropoiesis. Blood 83:2844, 1994.

305. Sadahira, Y., Yoshino, T., and Monobe, Y.: Very late activation antigen

4–vascular cell adhesion molecule 1 interaction is involved in the formation of erythroblastic islands. J. Exp. Med 181:411, 1995.

306. Koopman, G., Keehnen, R.M.J., Lindhout, E., Newman, W., Shimizu, Y., VanSeventer, G.A., deGroot, C., and Pals, S.T.: Adhesion through the LFA-1 (CD11a/CD18)–ICAM-1 (CD54) and VLA-4(CD49d)–VCAM-1(CD106) pathways prevents apoptosis of germinal center B cells. J. Immunol. 152:3760, 1994.

307. Damle, N.K., Klussman, K., Leytze, G., Aruffo, A., Linsley, P.S., and Ledbetter, J.A.: Costimulation with integrin ligands intercellular adhesion molecule-1 or vascular cell adhesion molecule-1 augments activation-induced death of antigen specific CD4+ T-lymphocytes. J. Immunol. 151:2368, 1993.

308. Udagwa, T., Woodside, D.G., and McIntyre, B.W.: Alpha4beta1 (CD49d/CD29) integrin costimulation of human T cells enhances transcription factor and cytokine induction in absence of altered sensitivity to anti-CD3 stimulation. J. Immunol. 157:1965, 1996.

309. Sasaki, K., Okouchi, Y., Rothkotter, H.J., and Pabst, R.: Ultrastructural localization of the intercellular adhesion molecule (ICAM-1) on the cell surface of high endothelial venules in lymph nodes. Anat. Rec. 244:105, 1996.

310. Kushnir, N., Liu, L., and MacPherson, G.G.: Dendritic cells and resting B cells form clusters in vitro and in vivo: T cell independence, partial LFA-1 dependence, and regulation by cross-linking surface molecules. J. Immunol. 160:1774, 1998.

311. Huleatt, J.W., and Lefrancois, L.: Beta 2 integrins and ICAM-1 are involved in establishment of intestinal mucosal T cell compartment. Immunity 5:263, 1996.

312. Nakache, M., Berg, E.L., Streeter, P.R., and Butcher, E.C.: The mucosal vascular addressin is a tissue-specific endothelial cell adhesion molecule for circulating lymphocytes. Nature 337:179, 1989.

313. Steffen, P.J., Breier, G., Butcher, E.C., Schulz, M., and Engelhardt, B.: ICAM-1, VCAM-1, and MAdCAM-1 are expressed on choroid plexus epithelium but not endothelium and mediates binding of lymphocytes in vitro. Am. J. Pathol. 148:1819, 1996.

314. Hanninen, A., Taylor, C., Streeter, P.R., Stark, L.S., Sarte, J.M., and Shizuru, J.A.: Vascular addressins are involved on islet vessels during insulitis in nonobese diabetic mice and are involved in lymphoid cell binding to islet endothelium. J. Clin. Invest. 92:2509, 1993.

315. Berlin, C., Berg, E.L., Briskin, M.J., Andrew, D.P., Kilshaw, P.J., Holzmann, B., Weissman, I.L., Hamann, A., and Butcher, E.C.: α4β7 Integrin mediates lymphocyte binding to the mucosal vascular addressin MAdCAM-1. Cell 74:185, 1993.

316. Yaps, A.S., Brieher, W.M., and Gumbiner, B.M.: Molecular and functional analysis of cadherin-based adherens junction. Annu. Rev. Cell Dev. Biol. 13:119, 1997.

317. Cepek, K.L., Shaw, S.K., Parker, C.M., Russell, G.J., Morrow, J.S., Rimm, D.L., and Brenner, M.B.: Adhesion between epithelial cells and T-lymphocytes mediated by E-cadherin and the alpha E beta 7 integrin. Nature 372:190, 1994.

318. Higgins, J.M., Mandlebrot, D.A., Shaw, S.K., Russell, G.L., Murphy, E.A., Chen, Y.T., Nelson, W.J., Parker, C.M., and Brenner, M.B.: Direct and regulated interaction of integrin alphaEbeta7 with E-cadherin. J. Cell Biol. 140:197, 1998.

319. Austrup, F., Rebstock, S., Kilshaw, P.J., and Hamann, A.: Transforming growth factor-beta1–induction expression of the mucosa-related integrin alpha E on lymphocytes is not associated with mucosa-specific homing. Eur. J. Immunol. 25:1487, 1995.

320. Verfaillie, C.M.: Adhesion receptors as regulators of the hematopoietic process. Blood 92:2609, 1998.

321. Johnson, G.R., and Moore, M.A.: Role of stem cell migration in initiation of mouse foetal liver haemopoiesis. Nature 258:726, 1975.

322. Hirsch, E., Iglesias, A., Potocnik, A.J., Hartmann, U., and Fassler, R.: Impaired migration but not differentiation of haematopoietic stem cells in the absence of β1 integrins. Nature 380:171, 1996.

323. Hamamura, K., Matsuda, H., Takeuchi, Y., Habu, S., Yagita, H., and Okumura, K.: A critical role of VLA-4 in erythropoiesis in vivo. Blood 87:2513, 1996.

324. Schmits, R., Kundig, T.M., Baker, D.M., Shumaker, G., Simard, J.J.L., Duncan, G., Wakeham, A., Shahinian, A., van der Heiden, A., Bachmann, M.F., Ohashi, P.S., Mak, T.W., and Hickstein, D.D.: LFA-1–deficient mice show normal CTL responses to virus but fail to reject immunogenic tumor. J. Exp. Med. 183:1415, 1996.

325. Wagner, N., Lohler, J., Kunkel, E., Ley, K., Leung, E., Krissansen, G., Rajewsky, K., and Muller, W.: Critical role for beta7 integrins in formation of the gut-associated lymphoid tissue. Nature 382:366, 1996.

326. Mebius, R.E., Streeter, P.R., Michie, S., Butcher, E.C., and Waeissman, I.L.: A developmental switch in lymphocyte homing receptor and endothelial vascular addressin expression regulates lymphocyte homing and permits CD4+CD3− cells to colonize lymph nodes. Proc. Natl. Acad. Sci. USA 93:11019, 1996.

327. Bader, B., Rayburn, H., Crowley, D., and Hynes, R.O.: Extensive vasculogenesis, angiogenesis, and organogenesis precede lethality in mice lacking all alpha v integrins. Cell 95:507, 1998.

328. Hodivala-Dilke, K.M., McHugh, K.P., Tsakiris, D.A., Rayburn, H., Crowley, D., Ullman-Cullere, M., Ross, F.P., Coller, B.S., Teitelbaum, S., and Hynes, R.O.: Beta-3-integrin–deficient mice are a model for Glanzmann thrombasthenia showing placental defects and reduced survival. J. Clin. Invest. 103:229, 1999.

329. Liesveld, J.L., Winslow, J.M., Frediani, K.E., Ryan, D.H., and Abboud, C.N.: Expression of integrins and examination of their adhesive function in normal and leukemic hematopoietic cells. Blood 81:112, 1993.

330. Oostendorp, R.A.J., and Dormer, P.: VLA-4 mediated interactions between normal human hematopoietic progenitors and stromal cells. Leuk. Lymphoma 24:423, 1997.

331. Papayannopoulou, T., and Craddock, C.: Homing and trafficking of hemopoietic progenitor cells. Acta Haematol. 97:97, 1997.

332. Papayannopoulou, T., Craddock, C., Nakamoto, B., Priestley, G.V., and Wolf, N.S.: The VLA4/VCAM-1 adhesion pathway defines contrasting mechanisms of lodgement of transplanted murine hemopoietic progenitors between bone marrow and spleen. Proc. Natl. Acad. Sci. USA 92:9647, 1995.

333. Craddock, C., Nakamoto, B., and Papayannopoulou, T.: The VLA4/CS-1 pathway does not actively participate in VLA4 mediated hematopoietic progenitor trafficking in vivo. Blood 86:975, 1995.

334. Papayannopoulou, T., and Nakamoto, B.: Peripheralization of hemopoietic progenitors in primates treated with anti-VLA4 integrins. Proc. Natl. Acad. Sci. USA 90:9374, 1993.

335. Papayannopoulou, T., Priestley, G.V., and Nakamoto, B.: Anti-VLA4/VCAM-1–induced mobilization requires cooperative signaling through the kit/mkit ligand pathway. Blood 91:2231, 1998.

336. Ruiz, P., Wiles, M.V., and Imhof, B.A.: Alpha6 integrins participate in pro-T cell homing to the thymus. Eur. J. Immunol. 25:2034, 1995.

337. Cashman, J., Eaves, A.C., and Eaves, C.J.: Regulated proliferation of primitive hematopoietic progenitor cells in longterm human marrow cultures. Blood 66:1002, 1985.

338. Hurley, R.W., McCarthy, J.B., Wayner, E.A., and Verfaillie, C.M.: Monoclonal antibody crosslinking of the alpha 4 or beta 1 integrin inhibits committed clonogenic hematopoietic progenitor proliferation. Exp. Hematol. 25:321, 1997.

339. Koopman, G., Parmentier, H.K., Schuurman, W., Newman, W., Shimizu, Y., VanSeventer, G.A., deGroot, C., and Pals, S.T.: Adhesion of human B-cells to follicular dendritic cells involves both lymphocyte function–associated antigen-1/intercellular adhesion molecule 1 and very late activation antigen 4/vascular cell adhesion molecule 1 pathways. J. Exp. Med. 173:1297, 1991.

340. Frisch, S.M., and Francis, H.: Disruption of epithelial cell–matrix interactions induces apoptosis. J. Cell Biol. 124:619, 1994.

341. Cardone, M., Salvesen, G.S., Widmann, C., Johnson, G., and Frisch, S.M.: The regulation of anoikis: MEKK-1 activation requires cleavage by caspases. Cell 90:315, 1997.

342. Nakamura, H., Oda, T., Hamada, K., Shimizu, N., and Utiyama, H.: Survival by Mac-1–mediated adherence and anoikis in phorbol ester–treated HL-60 cells. J. Biol. Chem. 273:15345, 1998.

343. Carlos, T.M., and Harlan, J.M.: Leukocyte-endothelial adhesion molecules. Blood 84:2068, 1994.

344. Berlin, C., Bargatze, R.F., Campbell, J.J., von Andrian, U.H., Szabo, M.C., Hasslen, S.R., Nelson, R.D., Berg, E.L., Erlandsen, S.L., and Butcher, E.C.: α4 integrins mediate lymphocyte attachment and rolling under physiologic flow. Cell 80:413, 1995.

345. Stewart, M., and Hogg, N.: Regulation of leukocyte integrin function: affinity vs. avidity. J. Cell. Biochem. 61:554, 1996.

346. Palecek, S.P., Schmidt, C.E., Lauffenburger, D.A., and Horwitz, A.F.: Integrin dynamics on the tail region of migrating fibroblasts. J. Cell Sci. 109:941, 1996.

347. Butcher, E.C., and Picker, L.J.: Lymphocyte homing and homeostasis. Science 272:60, 1996.

348. Mackay, C.R., Marston, W.L., and Dudler, L.: Naive and memory T cells show distinct pathways of lymphocyte recirculation. J. Exp. Med. 171:801, 1990.

349. Springer, T.A.: Traffic signals for lymphocyte recirculation and leukocyte emigration: the multistep paradigm. Cell 76:301, 1994.

350. Gallatin, W.M., Weissman, I.L., and Butcher, E.C.: A cell-surface molecule involved in organ-specific homing of lymphocytes. Nature 304:30, 1983.

351. Arbones, M.L., Ord, D.C., Ley, K., Ratech, H., Maynard-Curry, C., Otten, G., Capon, D.J., and Tedder, T.F.: Lymphocyte homing and leukocyte rolling and migration are impaired in L-selectin–deficient mice. Immunity 1:247, 1994.

352. Lasky, L.A.: Selectins: interpreters of cell-specific carbohydrate information during inflammation. Science 258:964, 1992.

353. Baumhueter, S., Singer, M.S., Henzel, W.J., Hemmerich, S., Renz, M., Rosen, S.D., and Lasky, L.A.: Binding of L-selectin to the vascular sialomucin, CD34. Science 262:436, 1993.

354. Gunn, M.D., Tangemann, K., Tam, C., Cyster, J.G., Rosen, S.D., and Williams, L.T.: A chemokine expressed in lymphoid high endothelial venules promotes the adhesion and chemotaxis of naive T lymphocytes. Proc. Natl. Acad. Sci. USA 95:258, 1998.

355. Warnock, R.A., Askari, S., Butcher, E.C., and von Andrian, U.H.: Molecular mechanisms of lymphocyte homing to peripheral lymph nodes. J. Exp. Med 187:205, 1998.

356. Bell, E.B., Sparshott, S.M., and Bunce, C.: CD4+ T-cell memory, CD45R subsets and persistence of antigen-A unifying concept. Immunol. Today 19:60, 1998.

357. Rott, L.S., Briskin, M.J., Andrew, D.P., Berg, E.L., and Butcher, E.C.: A fundamental subdivision of circulating lymphocytes defined by adhesion to mucosal addressin cell adhesion molecule-1. Comparison with vascular cell adhesion molecule-1 and correlation with beta 7 integrins and memory differentiation. J. Immunol. 156:3727, 1996.

358. Abitorabi, M.A., Mackay, C.R., Jerome, E.H., Osorio, O., Butcher, E.C., and Erle, D.J.: Differential expression of homing molecules on recirculating lymphocytes from sheep gut, peripheral, and lung lymph. J. Immunol. 156:3111, 1996.

359. Rott, L.S., Rose, J.S., Bass, D., Williams, M.B., Greenberg, H.B., and Butcher, E.C.: Expression of mucosal homing receptor alpha4beta7 by circulating CD4+ cells with memory for intestinal rotavirus. J. Clin. Invest. 100:1204, 1997.

360. Sanders, M.E., Makgoba, M.W., Sharrow, S.O., Stephany, D., Springer, T.A., Young, H.A., and Shaw, S.: Human memory T lymphocytes express increased levels of three cell adhesion molecules (LFA-3, CD2, and LFA-1) and three other molecules (UCHL1, CDw29, and Pgp-1) and have enhanced IFN-gamma production. J. Immunol. 140:1401, 1988.

361. Shimizu, Y., VanSeventer, G.A., Horgan, K.J., and Shaw, S.: Regulated expression and binding of three VLA (B1) integrin receptors on T cells. Nature 345:250, 1990.

362. Mackay, C.R., Marston, W.L., Dudler, L., Spertini, O., Tedder, T.F., and Hein, W.R.: Tissue-specific migration pathways by phenotypically distinct subpopulations of memory T cells. Eur. J. Immunol. 22:887, 1992.

363. Williams, M.B., and Butcher, E.C.: Homing of naive and memory T lymphocyte subsets to Peyer's patches, lymph nodes, and spleen. J. Immunol. 159:1746, 1997.

364. Holzmann, B., McIntyre, B.W., and Weissman, I.L.: Identification of a murine Peyer's patch–specific lymphocyte homing receptor as an integrin molecule with an α chain homologous to human VLA-4α. Cell 56:37, 1989.

365. Kraehenbuhl, J.P., and Neutra, M.R.: Molecular and cellular basis of immune protection of mucosal surfaces. Physiol. Rev. 72:853, 1992.

366. Bargatze, R.F., Jutila, M.A., and Butcher, E.C.: Distinct roles of L-selectin and integrins alpha4beta7 and LFA-1 in lymphocyte homing to Peyer's patches–HEV in situ: the multistep model confirmed and refined. Immunity 3:99, 1995.

367. Goodman, T., and Lefrancois, L.: Intraepithelial lymphocytes. Anatomical site, not T cell receptor form, dictates phenotype and function. J. Exp. Med 170:1569, 1989.

368. Kilshaw, P.J., and Karecla, P.I.: Structure and function of the mucosal T-cell integrin alphaEbeta7. Biochem. Soc. Trans. 25:433, 1997.

369. Barnard, J.A., Warwick, G.J., and Gold, L.I.: Localization of transforming growth factor-beta isoforms in the normal murine small intestine and colon. Gastroenterology 105:67, 1993.

370. Cepek, K.L., Parker, C.M., Madara, J.L., and Brenner, M.B.: Integrin alphaEbeta7 mediates adhesion of T lymphocytes to epithelial cells. J. Immunol. 150:3459, 1993.

371. Karecla, P.I., Bowden, S.J., Green, S.J., and Kilshaw, P.J.: Recognition of E-cadherin on epithelial cells by mucosal T cell integrin alpha M290 beta 7 (alpha E beta 7). Eur. J. Immunol. 25:852, 1995.

372. Sarnacki, S., Begue, B., Buc, H., Le Deist, F., and Cerf-Bensussan, N.: Enhancement of CD3-induced activation of human intestinal intraepithelial lymphocytes by stimulation of the beta7-containing integrin defined by HML-1 monoclonal antibody. Eur. J. Immunol. 22:2887, 1992.

373. Begue, B., Sarnacki, S., Le Deist, F., Buc, H., Gagnon, J., Meo, T., and Cerf-Bensussan, N.: HML-1, a novel integrin made of the beta7 chain and a distinctive alpha chain, exerts an accessory function in the activation of human IEL via the CD3-TCR pathway. Adv. Exp. Med. Biol. 371A:67, 1995.

374. Anderson, D.C., and Springer, T.A.: Leukocyte adhesion deficiency: an inherited defect in the Mac-1, LFA-1, and p150-95 glycoproteins. Annu. Rev. Med. 38:175, 1987.

375. Mackay, C.R., Andrew, D.P., Briskin, M., Ringler, D.J., and Butcher, E.C.: Phenotype and migration properties of three major subsets of tissue-homing T cells in sheep. Eur. J. Immunol. 26:1892, 1996.

376. Shimizu, Y., Rose, D.M., and Ginsberg, M.H.: Integrins in the immune system. Adv. Immunol. 72:325, 1999.

377. Engelhardt, B., Conley, F.C., Kilshaw, P.J., and Butcher, E.C.: Lymphocytes infiltrating the CNS during inflammation display a distinctive phenotype and bind VCAM-1 but not MAdCAM-1. Int. Immunol. 7:481, 1995.

378. Postigo, A.A., Rosario, G.A., Laffon, A., and Sanchez-Madrid, F.: The role of adhesion molecules in the pathogenesis of rheumatoid arthritis. Autoimmunity 16:69, 1993.

379. Picarella, D., Hurlbut, P., Rottman, J., Shi, X., Butcher, E., and Ringler, D.J.: Monoclonal antibodies specific for beta 7 integrin and mucosal addressin cell adhesion molecule-1 (MAdCAM-1) reduce inflammation in the colon of scid mice reconstituted with CD45RDhigh CD4+ T cells. J. Immunol. 158:2099, 1997.

380. Baron, J.L., Reich, E.P., Visintin, I., and Janeway, C.A.J.: The pathogenesis of adoptive murine autoimmune diabetes requires an interaction between α4-integrins and vascular cell adhesion molecule-1. J. Clin. Invest. 93:1700, 1994.

381. Alon, R., Kassner, P.D., Carr, M.W., Finger, E.B., Hemler, M., and Springer, T.A.: The integrin VLA-4 supports tethering and rolling in flow on VCAM-1. J. Cell Biol. 127:1485, 1995.

382. Campbell, J.J., Qin, S., Bacon, K.B., Mackay, C.R., and Butcher, E.C.: Biology of chemokine and classical chemoattractant receptors: differential requirements for adhesion-triggering versus chemotactic responses in lymphoid cells. J. Cell Biol. 134:255, 1996.

383. Yednock, T.A., Cannon, C., Vandevert, C., Goldbach, E.C., Shaw, G., Ellis, D.K., Liaw, C., Fritz, L.C., and Tanner, L.I.: α4β1 Integrin–dependent cell adhesion is regulated by a low affinity receptor pool that is conformationally responsive to ligand. J. Biol. Chem. 270:28740, 1995.

384. Chen, C., Mobley, J.L., Dwir, O., Shimron, F., Grabovsky, V., Lobb, R., Shimizu, Y., and Alon, R.: High affinity very late antigen-4 subsets expressed on T cells are mandatory for spontaneous adhesion strengthening but not for rolling on VCAM-1 in shear flow. J. Immunol. 162:1084, 1999.

385. Rose, D.M., Cardarelli, P.M., Cobb, R.R., and Ginsberg, M.H.: Soluble VCAM-1 binding to alpha4 integrins is cell-type specific, activation-dependent, and disrupted during apoptosis in T cells. Submitted for publication, 1999.

386. Yednock, T.A., Cannon, C., Fritz, L.C., Sanchez-Madrid, F., Steinman, L., and Karin, N.: Prevention of experimental autoimmune encephalomyelitis by antibodies against alpha 4 beta 1 integrin. Nature 356:63, 1992.

387. Engelhardt, B., Laschinger, M., Schulz, M., Samulowitz, U., Vestweber, D., and Hoch, G.: The development of experimental autoimmune encephalomyelitis in the mouse requires alpha4-integrin but not alpha4beta7-integrin. J. Clin. Invest. 102:2096, 1998.

388. Cannella, B., Cross, A.H., and Raines, C.S.: Anti-adhesion molecule therapy in experimental autoimmune encephalomyelitis. J. Neuroimmunol. 46:43, 1993.

389. Issekutz, A.C., and Issekutz, T.B.: Monocyte migration to arthritis in the rat utilizes both CD11/CD18 and very late antigen 4 integrin mechanisms. J. Exp. Med 181:1197, 1995.

390. Issekutz, A.C., Ayer, L., Miyasaka, M., and Issekutz, T.B.: Treatment of established adjuvant arthritis in rats with monoclonal antibody to CD18 and very late activation antigen-4 integrins suppresses neutrophil and T-lymphocyte migration to the joints and improves clinical disease. Immunology 88:569, 1996.

391. Michie, S.A., Sytwu, H.K., McDevitt, J.O., and Yang, X.D.: The roles of alpha 4-integrins in the development of insulin-dependent diabetes mellitus. Curr. Top. Microbiol. Immunol. 231:65, 1998.

392. Hesterberg, P.E., Winsor-Hines, D., Briskin, M.J., Soler-Ferran, D., Merrill, C., Mackay, C.R., Newman, W., and Ringler, D.J.: Rapid resolution of chronic colitis in the cotton-top tamarin with an antibody to a gut-homing integrin alpha4beta7. Gastroenterology 111:1373, 1996.

393. Isobe, M., Yagita, H., Okumura, K., and Ihara, A.: Specific acceptance of cardiac allograft after treatment with antibodies to ICAM-1 and LFA-1. Science 255:1125, 1992.

394. Ginsberg, M.H., Du, X., O'Toole, T.E., and Loftus, J.C.: Platelet integrins. Thromb. Haemost. 74:352, 1995.

395. Furie, B., and Furie, B.C.: The molecular basis of platelet and endothelial cell interaction with neutrophils and monocytes: role of P-selectin and the P-selectin ligand, PSGL-1. Thromb. Haemost. 74:224, 1995.

396. Watson, S.P., and Gibbins, J.M.: Collagen receptor signalling in platelets: extending the role of ITAM. Immunol. Today 19:260, 1998.

397. Saelman, E.U., Nieuwenhuis, H.K., Hese, K.M., De Groot, P.G., Heijnen, H.F., Sage, E.H., McKeown, L., Gralnick, H.R., and Sixma, J.J.: Platelet adhesion to collagen types I through VIII under conditions of stasis and flow is mediated by GPIa/IIa ($\alpha_2\beta_1$-integrin). Blood 83:1244, 1994.

398. Staatz, W.D., Rajpara, S.M., Wayner, E.A., Carter, W.G., and Santoro, S.A.: The membrane glycoprotein Ia-IIa (VLA-2) complex mediates the Mg^{++}-dependent adhesion of platelets to collagen. J. Cell Biol. 108:1917, 1989.

399. Santoro, S.A., Walsh, J.J., Staatz, W.D., and Baranski, K.J.: Distinct determinants on collagen support alpha 2 beta 1 integrin–mediated platelet adhesion and platelet activation. Cell Regul. 2:905, 1991.

400. Loftus, J.C., Plow, E.F., Jennings, L., and Ginsberg, M.H.: Alternative proteolytic processing of platelet membrane glycoprotein IIb. J. Biol. Chem. 263:11025, 1988.

401. Poncz, M., Eisman, R., Heidenreich, R., Silver, S.M., Vilaire, G., Surrey, S., Schwartz, E., and Bennett, J.S.: Structure of the platelet membrane glycoprotein IIb. J. Biol. Chem. 262:8476, 1987.

402. Fitzgerald, L.A., Steiner, B., Rall, S.C., Jr., Lo, S.-S., and Phillips, D.R.: Protein sequence of endothelial glycoprotein IIIa derived from a cDNA clone. Identity with platelet glycoprotein IIIa and similarity to "integrin." J. Biol. Chem. 262:3936, 1987.

403. Rosa, J.-P., Bray, P.F., Gayet, O., Johnston, G.I., Cook, R.G., Jackson, K.W., Shuman, M.A., and McEver, R.P.: Cloning of glycoprotein IIIa cDNA from human erythroleukemia cells and localization of the gene to chromosome 17. Blood 72:593, 1988.

404. Du, X., Saido, T.C., Tsubuki, S., Indig, F.E., Williams, M.J., and Ginsberg, M.H.: Calpain cleavage of the cytoplasmic domain of the integrin β_3 subunit. J. Biol. Chem. 270:26146, 1995.

405. Brass, L.F., Manning, D.R., Cichowski, K., and Abrams, C.S.: Signaling through G proteins in platelets: to the integrins and beyond. Thromb. Haemost. 78:581, 1997.

406. Gachet, C., Hechler, B., Leon, C., Vial, C., Leray, C., Ohlmann, P., and Cazenave, J.-P.: Activation of ADP receptors and platelet function. Thromb. Haemost. 78:271, 1997.

407. Offermanns, S., Toombs, C.F., Hu, Y.H., and Simon, M.I.: Defective platelet activation in G alpha(q)-deficient mice. Nature 389:183, 1997.

408. Shattil, S.J., and Brass, L.F.: Induction of the fibrinogen receptor on human platelets by intracellular mediators. J. Biol. Chem. 262:992, 1987.

409. Shattil, S.J., Cunningham, M., Wiedmer, T., Zhao, J., Sims, P.J., and Brass, L.F.: Regulation of glycoprotein IIb-IIIa receptor function studied with platelets permeabilized by the pore-forming complement proteins C5b-9. J. Biol. Chem. 267:18424, 1992.

410. Jackson, S.P., Schoenwaelder, S.M., Yuam, Y., Salem, H.H., and Cooray, P.: Non-receptor protein tyrosine kinases and phosphatases in human platelets. Thromb. Haemost. 76:640, 1996.

411. Tate, B.F., and Rittenhous, S.E.: Thrombin activation of human platelets causes tyrosine phosphorylation of PLC-gamma 2. Biochim. Biophys. Acta 1178:282, 1993.

412. Cichowski, K., Brugge, J.S., and Brass, L.F.: Thrombin receptor activation and integrin engagement stimulate tyrosine phosphorylation of the proto-oncogene product, p95[vav], in platelets. J. Biol. Chem. 271:7544, 1996.

413. Rosa, J.P., Artcanuthurry, V., Grelac, F., Maclouf, J., Caen, J.P., and Levy-Toledano, S.: Reassessment of protein tyrosine phosphorylation in thrombasthenic platelets: evidence that phosphorylation of cortactin and a 64-kD protein is dependent on thrombin activation and integrin alphaIIb beta3. Blood 89:4385, 1997.

414. Lerea, K.M., Tonks, N.K., Krebs, E.G., Fischer, E.H., and Glomset, J.A.: Vanadate and molybdate increase tyrosine phosphorylation in a 50-kilodalton protein and stimulate secretion in electropermeabilized platelets. Biochemistry 28:9286, 1989.

415. Morii, N., Teru-uchi, T., Tominaga, T., Kumagai, N., Kozaki, S., Ushikubi, F., and Narumiya, S.: A rho gene product in human blood platelets. II. Effects of the ADP-ribosylation by botulinum C3 ADP-ribosyltransferase on platelet aggregation. J. Biol. Chem. 267:20921, 1992.

416. Freedman, J.E., Loscalzo, J., Barnard, M.R., Alpert, C., Kearney, J.F., and Michelson, A.D.: Nitric oxide released from activated platelets inhibits platelet recruitment. J. Clin. Invest. 100:350, 1997.

417. Haffner, C., Jarchau, T., Reinhard, M., Hoppe, J., Lohmann, S.M., and Walter, U.: Molecular cloning, structural analysis and functional expression of the proline-rich focal adhesion and microfilament-associated protein VASP. EMBO J. 14:19, 1995.

418. Fischer, A., Trung, P.H., Descamps-Latscha, B., Lisowska-Grospierre, B., Gerota, I., Perez, N., Scheinmetzler, C., Durandy, A., Virelizier, J.L., and Griscelli, C.: Bone-marrow transplantation for inborn error of phagocytic cells associated with defective adherence, chemotaxis, and oxidative response during opsonised particle phagocytosis. Lancet 2:473, 1983.

419. Anderson, D.C., Schmalstieg, F.C., Finegold, M.J., Hughes, B.J., Rothlein, R., Miller, L.J., Kohl, S., Tosi, M.F., Jacobs, R.L., and Waldrop, E.A.: The severe and moderate phenotypes of heritable Mac-1, LFA-1 deficiency: their quantitative definition and relation to leukocyte dysfunction and clinical features. J. Infect. Dis. 152:668, 1985.

420. Kishimoto, T.K., Hollander, N., Roberts, T.M., Anderson, D.C., and Springer, T.A.: Heterogeneous mutations in the beta subunit common to the LFA-1, Mac-1, and p150,95 glycoproteins cause leukocyte adhesion deficiency. Cell 50:193, 1987.

421. Kishimoto, T.K., O'Connor, K., and Springer, T.A.: Leukocyte adhesion deficiency. Aberrant splicing of a conserved integrin sequence causes a moderate deficiency phenotype. J. Biol. Chem. 264:3588, 1989.

422. Arnaout, M.A., Dana, N., Gupta, S.K., Tenen, D.G., and Fathallah, D.M.: Point mutations impairing cell surface expression of the common B subunit (CD18) in a patient with leukocyte adhesion molecule (Leu-CAM) deficiency. J. Clin. Invest. 85:977, 1990.

423. Nelson, C., Rabb, H., and Arnaout, M.A.: Genetic cause of leukocyte adhesion molecule deficiency. Abnormal splicing and a missense mutation in a conserved region of CD18 impair cell surface expression of beta 2 integrins. J. Biol. Chem. 267:3351, 1992.

424. Hogg, N., Stewart, M.P., Scarth, S.L., Newton, R., Shaw, J.M., Alex Law, S.K., and Klein, N.: A novel leukocyte adhesion deficiency caused by expressed but nonfunctional $\beta2$ integrins Mac-1 and LFA-1. J. Clin. Invest. 103:97, 1999.

425. Lee, J., Rieu, P., Arnaout, M.A., and Liddington, R.: Crystal structure of the A domain from the α subunit of integrin CR3 (CD11b/CD18). Cell 80:631, 1995.

426. Kuijpers, T.W., Van Lier, R.A.W., Hamann, D., de Boer, M., Yin, T.L., Weening, R.S., Verhoeven, A.J., and Roos, D.: Leukocyte adhesion deficiency type 1 (LAD-1)/variant. A novel immunodeficiency syndrome characterized by dysfunctional beta 2 integrins. J. Clin. Invest. 100:1725, 1997.

427. Phillips, D.R., and Agin, P.P.: Platelet membrane defects in Glanzmann's thrombasthenia. J. Clin. Invest. 60:535, 1977.

428. Bray, P.F., Rosa, J.-P., Johnston, G.I., Shiu, D.T., Cook, R.G., Lau, C., Kan, Y.W., McEver, R.P., and Shuman, M.A.: Platelet glycoprotein IIb. Chromosomal localization and tissue expression. J. Clin. Invest. 80:1812, 1987.

429. Stormorken, H., Brosstad, F., and Seim, H.: Diagnosis of heterozygotes in Glanzmann's thrombasthenia. Thromb. Haemost. 49:120, 1982.

430. Kato, A.: The biologic and clinical spectrum of Glanzmann's thrombasthenia: implications of integrin alpha IIb beta 3 for its pathogenesis. Crit. Rev. Oncog. 26:1, 1997.

431. Chen, Y.-P., Djaffar, I., Pidard, D., Steiner, B., Cieutat, A.M., Caen, J.P., and Rosa, J.P.: Ser-752–Pro mutation in the cytoplasmic domain of integrin $\beta3$ subunit and defective activation of platelet integrin αIIb$\beta3$ (glycoprotein IIb-IIIa) in a variant of Glanzmann thrombasthenia. Proc. Natl. Acad. Sci. USA 89:10169, 1992.

432. Schafer, A.I.: Antiplatelet therapy with glycoprotein IIb/IIIa receptor inhibitors and other novel agents. Tex. Heart Inst. J. 24:90, 1997.

433. Faulds, D., and Sorkin, E.M.: Abciximab (c7E3 Fab). A review of its pharmacology and therapeutic potential in ischaemic heart disease. Drugs 48:583, 1994.

434. Brener, S.J., Barr, L.A., Burchenal, J.E., Katz, S., George, B.S., Jones, A.A., Cohen, E.D., Gainey, P.C., White, H.J., Cheek, H.B., Moses, J.W., Moliterno, D.J., Effron, M.B., and Topol, E.J.: Randomized, placebo-controlled trial of platelet glycoprotein IIb/IIIa blockade with primary angioplasty for acute myocardial infarction. ReoPro and Primary PTCA Organization and Randomized Trial (RAPPORT) Investigators. Circulation 98:734, 1998.

435. The PURSUIT trial investigators: Inhibition of platelet glycoprotein IIb/IIIa with Eptifibatide in patients with acute coronary syndromes. N. Engl. J. Med 339:436, 1998.

436. Ohman, E.M., Kleiman, N.S., Gacioch, G., Worley, S.J., Navetta, F.I., Talley, J.D., Anderson, H.V., Ellis, S.G., Cohen, M.D., Spriggs, D., Miller, M., Kereiakes, D., Yakubov, S., Kitt, M.M., Sigmon, K.N., Califf, R.M., Krucoff, M.W., and Topol, E.J.: Combined accelerated tissue-plasminogen activator and platelet glycoprotein IIb/IIIa integrin receptor blockade with Integrilin in acute myocardial infarction: results of a randomized, placebo-controlled, dose-ranging trial. Circulation 95:854, 1997.

437. Gibson, C.M., Goel, M., Cohen, D.J., Piana, R.N., Deckelbaum, L.I., Harris, K.E., and King, S.B.: Six-month angiographic and clinical follow-up of patients prospectively randomized to receive either tirofiban or placebo during angioplasty in the RESTORE trial. J. Am. Coll. Cardiol. 32:28, 1998.

15 ▼▼▼▼ Chemokines and Their Receptors

David I. Jarmin and Craig Gerard

▼ ▼

Critical processes in the host response to infection, trauma, or inflammation are the migration and basal trafficking of leukocytes. It is now evident that these processes are controlled in part by a class of small cytokines known as the chemokines. The chemokines have recently become the focus of considerable interest, after the discovery of the critical role certain chemokines and their receptors play in the pathogenesis of human immunodeficiency virus (HIV) infection. Indeed, it is becoming clear that the chemokines play a far greater role than merely controlling leukocyte movement and are in fact involved in a wide variety of functions ranging from inflammation, hematopoiesis, infectious disease, cancer, and developmental aspects.

This chapter provides an overview of chemokine biology as we understand it today, discussing the role of chemokines and their receptors both in normal physiology and in a number of disease states. In addition, the importance of animal models in understanding the extreme complexity of chemokine function is discussed, together with the exciting potential of chemokines as novel targets for therapy against a number of diseases.

Overview of the Chemokine Superfamily

The first *chemo*tactic cyto*kine*, or chemokine, was described in 1977.[1, 2] A decade later, it was apparent that chemokines were a new gene family.[3, 4] Since then, this family has grown rapidly to now number in excess of 40 members (reviewed in reference 5). This expansion has been particularly marked in the last few years, and novel members are still being isolated. Much of this progress is due to advances in genomics and the ability to access and search data bases containing novel DNA sequences (so-called bioinformatics).[6] On the basis of the current pace, it has been estimated that as many as 50 to 100 unique chemokines may eventually be identified. Table 15–1 lists those chemokines identified to date, together with their abbreviations. The complexity of chemokine nomenclature stems from their historical identification by individual groups of researchers. Many were initially isolated as proteins with particular properties and thus named, for example, IP-10 (interferon-inducible protein of 10 kDa).[7] This has resulted in a system with multiple names, acronyms, and idiosyncrasies that often appears confusing to those outside the field of chemokine research. The chemokine genes cluster at specific chromosome loci, suggesting that chemokines evolved from a common primordial chemokine by divergent evolution. For instance, most CC chemokines map to human chromosome 17q11.2–12 (chromosome 11 in the mouse), whereas most CXC chemokines map to human chromosome 4q13 (chromosome 5 in the mouse); however, there are some individual exceptions. A similar clustering has been observed for several genes encoding chemokine receptors; several CC chemokine receptors map to chromosome 3p21 (chromosome 9 in the mouse), whereas many human CXC chemokine receptors map to chromosome 2q33–36 (chromosome 1 in the mouse).

The chemokines are all small inducible heparin-binding

Table 15–1. The Chemokine Superfamily

Name (Abbreviation)	Other Names
CC	
Macrophage inflammatory protein-1α (MIP-1α)	LD78, SCI
Macrophage inflammatory protein-1β (MIP-1β)	Act-2
Reactivated and normal T-cell expressed and secreted (RANTES)	
Monocyte chemoattractant protein-1 (MCP-1)	JE, MCAF
Monocyte chemoattractant protein-2 (MCP-2)	
Monocyte chemoattractant protein-3 (MCP-3)	MARC, *fic*
Monocyte chemoattractant protein-4 (MCP-4)	NCC-1, CKβ-10
Monocyte chemoattractant protein-5 (MCP-5)*	
I-309	TCA-3 (mouse)
Eotaxin	
Hemofiltrate CC chemokine-1 (HCC-1)	NCC-2
Hemofiltrate CC chemokine-4 (HCC-4)	NCC-4, liver-expressed chemokine (LEC)
	Lymphocyte and monocyte chemoattractant (LMC)
Thymus and activation-regulated chemokine (TARC)	
DC-CK1	Pulmonary and activation-regulated chemokine (PARC), MIP-4
	Alternative macrophage activation-associated CC chemokine-1 (AMAC-1)
Macrophage inflammatory protein-3α (MIP-3α)	Liver and activation-regulated chemokine (LARC), exodus
Macrophage inflammatory protein-3β (MIP-3β)	EBI1-ligand chemokine (ELC), exodus-3, CKβ-11
Macrophage-derived chemokine (MDC)	Stimulated T-cell chemoattractant protein-1 (STCP-1)
Myeloid progenitor inhibitory factor-2 (MPIF-2)	Eotaxin-2, CKβ-6
Thymus-expressed chemokine (TECK)	
Secondary lymphoid tissue chemokine (SLC)	6Ckine, exodus-2, TCA-4
C-10*	MIP-related protein-1 (MRP-1)
Macrophage inflammatory protein-1γ (MIP-1γ)*	CCF18
MIP-related protein-2 (MRP-2)	MIP-1δ
Leukotactin-1 (Lkn-1)	HCC-2, NCC-3, MIP-5
CKβ-8 and CKβ-8-1	MIP-3, MPIF-1
ABCD-1*	
ESkine	ALP
CXC	
Interleukin-8 (IL-8)	Neutrophil-activating peptide-1 (NAP-1)
Neutrophil-activating peptide-2 (NAP-2)	
Platelet factor-4 (PF-4)	
Growth-regulated oncogene (GRO)–α	Melanocyte growth-stimulating activity-α (MGSA-α), KC
Growth-regulated oncogene (GRO)–β	MGSA-β, MIP-2α
Growth-regulated oncogene (GRO)–γ	MIP-2β
Interferon-inducible protein-10 (IP–10)	Crg-2
Monokine induced by interferon-γ (MIG)	Crg-10
Neutrophil-activating peptide-78 (ENA-78)	LPS-induced CXC chemokine (LIX)
Granulocyte chemotactic protein (GCP-2)	
Stromal cell–derived factor-1α (SDF-1α)	Pre-B cell–stimulating factor (PBSF)
Stromal cell–derived factor-1β (SDF-1β)	
Interferon-inducible T-cell alpha chemoattractant (I-TAC)	
C	
Lymphotactin	Single C motif-1 (SCM-1), ATAC
CX₃C	
Fractalkine	Neurotactin

* Mouse only, to date.

In addition, a number of unpublished novel chemokines also exist in the sequence data bases.

Shown on the left are the most commonly used names, and when these are also known by other names, they are listed on the right. Abbreviations for the various chemokines are given in brackets where appropriate.

proteins, 8 to 18 kDa in size. They are related to each other on the basis of sequence homology and the presence of a characteristic cysteine motif in their N terminus (Fig. 15–1). Their N terminus is anchored to the rest of the molecule by disulfide bonds that form between the two N-terminal cysteines. The N-terminal domain is involved in receptor interaction and specificity. Following the N-terminal domain, there is an extended loop that leads into three antiparallel β sheets. The C-terminal regions form an α helix, which extends over the three β sheets. The C-terminal domain appears important for full biological activity and this is due, at least

in part, to the high affinity of the C-terminal region for proteoglycans. Chemokines are able to multimerize, and the question as to whether chemokines are functionally active as monomers or as dimers is still controversial (see reference 5 and references therein).

The family was originally subdivided into two classes on the basis of the spacing of the first two N-terminal cysteine residues. Thus, in the CC or β subfamily, these two cysteines are adjacent to each other; in the CXC or α subfamily, they are separated by a single residue. More recently, this designation has been expanded to include

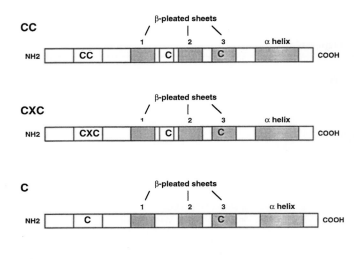

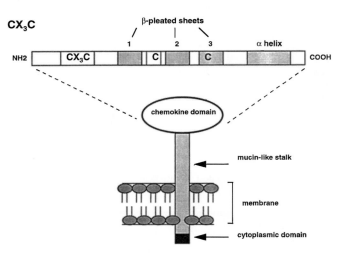

Figure 15–1. Schematic drawing illustrating the structure of the CC, CXC, C, and CX₃C chemokine subfamilies. The Cs represent conserved cysteines.

unique members of two novel chemokine subfamilies. The C subfamily, with a sole member, lymphotactin, has only a single N-terminal cysteine identified to date.[8] The fourth family, the CX₃C subfamily, with its sole member fractalkine or neurotactin, has two amino-terminal cysteines separated by three amino acid residues, with the chemokine domain atop a mucin-like stalk embedded in the plasma membrane[9, 10] (see Fig. 15–1).

Historically, the CXC chemokines were considered to be mainly neutrophil agonists, and the CC chemokines were in general thought to act not on neutrophils but rather on lymphoid cells. Monocytes and macrophages are targets for both subfamilies. Whereas this statement is in broad terms still true, particularly with regard to the CC chemokines, it is clearly not so straightforward as was originally believed. Basal trafficking with activation by chemokines is not restricted to leukocytes but extends to neurons and epithelial cells as well.

CXC Chemokines

The CXC family of chemokines numbers more than a dozen members to date (see Table 15–1). It is possible to further

subdivide the CXC chemokines on the basis of the presence or absence of the sequence glutamic acid–leucine–arginine (so-called ELR motif), located in the N-terminal region just before the CXC motif. The ELR chemokines, such as interleukin-8 (IL-8) and epithelial cell–derived neutrophil attractant-78 (ENA-78), are potent neutrophil chemoattractants; the non-ELR chemokines, such as platelet factor-4 (PF-4) and IP-10, show little or no neutrophil activities. Modification of these ELR residues prevents receptor binding and thus also neutrophil chemotaxis.[11, 12] Insertion of an ELR motif into the N terminus of non-ELR chemokines enables them to become neutrophil chemoattractants.[12]

▼ INTERLEUKIN-8

IL-8 (originally called neutrophil-activating protein [NAP]–1), is considered to be the prototypic CXC chemokine and is the most extensively studied. To date, no rat or murine homologue of IL-8 has been identified. Human IL-8 is produced by a wide variety of cell types, including monocytes, neutrophils, fibroblasts, endothelial cells, epithelial cells, and T lymphocytes, and it can be induced by a number of inflammatory stimuli, such as IL-1, tumor necrosis factor (TNF), and lipopolysaccharide (LPS) (reviewed in references 4 and 13). IL-8 was originally identified as an activity that was directed toward neutrophils but not monocytes and that may also chemoattract T lymphocytes.[14–16] In addition to chemoattraction of neutrophils, IL-8 induces granule exocytosis and stimulates the respiratory burst.[17] IL-8 has also been suggested to play a role in angiogenesis.[18, 19] There is some evidence that IL-8 may also contribute to the control of some aspects of hematopoietic stem cell proliferation (see later section on hematopoiesis).

▼ STROMAL CELL–DERIVED FACTOR-1

The chemokine stromal cell–derived factor-1 (SDF-1) was originally cloned from a "signal sequence trap library" (designed to enrich for proteins containing a signal peptide sequence).[20] It was also cloned from a stromal cell line as pre-B cell growth-stimulating factor, and as the name suggests, it stimulates the growth of B-cell progenitors in vitro.[21] Unusually for a chemokine, it is constitutively expressed in a broad range of tissues. Although SDF-1 is grouped with the CXC chemokines, it is distantly related to both CC and CXC chemokines. Furthermore, it has a unique degree of conservation; the murine and human homologues share 99 per cent amino acid identity, suggesting that of all the chemokines to date, SDF-1 is the least diverged from any prospective primordial ancestor. Unlike most CXC chemokines, which map to human chromosome 4, SDF-1 maps to chromosome 10.

An insight into the probable role of SDF-1 in vivo has come from the generation of mice in which the gene for SDF-1 has been disrupted.[22] These SDF-1⁻/⁻ mice die perinatally, showing a severe reduction in the number of B-cell progenitors in both the fetal liver and bone marrow and a reduction in myelopoietic progenitors in the bone marrow (but not in the fetal liver), thus suggesting that SDF-1 is a regulator of B-cell lymphopoiesis and bone marrow myelopoiesis. These SDF-1$^{-/-}$ mice also exhibit a defect in the development of the cardiac ventricular septum and vascular remodeling in the developing gut. SDF-1 is a low-potency, high-efficacy lymphocyte and monocyte chemoattractant in vitro. As a non-ELR chemokine, neutrophil-directed activities are not observed.[23] The important role of SDF-1 in HIV infection pathogenesis is discussed in a later section.

▼ IP-10 AND MIG

Interferon-inducible protein-10 (IP-10) was originally isolated in 1985 as a product induced by interferon-γ (IFN-γ) from a monocytic cell line.[7] IP-10 is expressed by a variety of cell types, including monocytes, keratinocytes, fibroblasts, endothelial cells, and T lymphocytes.[7] IP-10 is a non-ELR chemokine, and this is in keeping with its poor neutrophil activity, but it does appear to be chemotactic for monocytes, smooth muscle cells, T lymphocytes, and natural killer cells (NK cells).[24–26] In addition to chemotactic functions, IP-10 appears to be an inhibitor of angiogenesis, in contrast to IL-8, which appears to stimulate angiogenesis.[19, 27]

Monokine induced by IFN-γ (MIG) is a recently identified chemokine, and like IP-10, it is also an IFN-γ–inducible protein that was isolated from macrophages. MIG is a chemoattractant in vitro for tumor-infiltrating lymphocytes and for peripheral blood lymphocytes.[28]

MIG and IP-10 can cross-desensitize each other in receptor activation, and in fact they share the same receptor, CXCR3, along with another novel CXC chemokine, interferon-inducible T-cell alpha chemoattractant (I-TAC).[29, 30] Like IL-8, both MIG and IP-10 have been reported to act in vitro as inhibitors of hematopoietic progenitor cell proliferation.[31–33] The fact that only a single receptor for IP-10/MIG has been identified to date coupled with its limited expression on activated T cells suggests that IP-10 and MIG are crucial to the trafficking of T lymphocytes in T-helper type 1 (T$_H$1) host defenses against viral or parasitic organisms in which cell-mediated immunity predominates.

▼ OTHER CXC CHEMOKINES

The early study of PF-4 as an immunoregulator has been well documented (reviewed in reference 13). PF-4 inhibits megakaryocytopoiesis, and it has been proposed that PF-4, as well as IL-8 and NAP-2, supports the viability and survival of normal (but not leukemic) progenitor cells.[34–37] A more detailed discussion of the role of PF-4 and other chemokines in the control of stem cell proliferation and angiogenesis can be found in a later section. Relatively little is known about the functions of other CXC chemokines like ENA-78 or LIX (LPS-induced CXC chemokine, which may be the murine orthologue of ENA-78) or some of the more recently identified members, such as granulocyte chemotactic protein-2 (GCP-2), beyond the initial reports of their isolation and characterization.[38–40]

CC Chemokines

The CC chemokines appear to be much larger in number than the CXC chemokine subfamily, and their effects are more diverse. There are now more than 20 known, distinct CC chemokines. Many of these have only recently been discovered and are poorly characterized to date. The following discussion is limited to a handful of CC chemokines whose functions have been relatively well characterized.

Although many members were initially characterized as monocyte/macrophage chemoattractants, it is now evident that they act on an extremely wide range of cell types, including basophils, mast cells, eosinophils, B and T lymphocytes, and NK cells (reviewed in reference 5). In general, they do not exert neutrophil-directed effects, although there are a few examples of specific chemokines that may be exceptions to this, such as macrophage inflammatory protein (MIP)–1α and CCR1 on some neutrophil populations.

▼ THE MONOCYTE CHEMOATTRACTANT PROTEINS

MCP-1/JE

Human monocyte chemoattractant protein-1 (MCP-1) was first isolated in 1989 from monocytic cell lines and activated monocytes, and its amino acid sequence was found to be identical to that of the previously cloned human homologue of the mouse *JE* gene.[41–43] *JE* was originally reported as a gene that was highly inducible by platelet-derived growth factor (PDGF) in the 3T3 fibroblast cell line.[43] It is now generally assumed that *JE* is the murine homologue of the human MCP-1 gene, and *JE* is therefore often commonly also referred to as MCP-1.

MCP-1 is an extremely potent monocyte chemoattractant but has also been reported to function in vitro as a chemoattractant for activated T lymphocytes and NK cells.[41, 44, 45] In an eloquent study, Weber and colleagues[46] demonstrated that MCP-1 could be converted from a potent inducer of mediator release from basophils to an eosinophil chemoattractant by deletion of the N-terminal amino acid residue from full-length mature MCP-1. They also demonstrated that deletion of another residue led to inactivity with both basophils and eosinophils, whereas deletion of three or four additional residues resulted in mutants that gained function on both cell types. This strongly suggests that N-terminal processing is a potential mechanism for regulating MCP-1 cell selectivity and function.

Several laboratories are currently trying to address the in vivo role of MCP-1 through the generation and study of MCP-1 transgenic and "knockout" mice. In one report, the murine MCP-1 gene was coupled to the strong mouse mammary tumor virus (MMTV) promoter, resulting in transgenic mice (MMTV–MCP-1) with a high level of MCP-1 expression that correlated with an increased susceptibility to intracellular pathogens, presumably due to monocyte desensitization.[47] No monocyte infiltrates were observed in any of these transgenic mice, and this was proposed to be the result of monocyte unresponsiveness to locally produced MCP-1 due to either receptor desensitization or disruption of monocyte chemoattractant gradients. In a second study by this same group, transgenic mice expressing MCP-1 under the control of the rat insulin promoter (RIP) were reported to elicit monocyte recruitment into pancreatic islets without the development of diabetes.[48] When these RIP–MCP-1 transgenic mice were crossed with the MMTV–MCP-1 mice (thus generating mice expressing both transgenes), the resulting mice did develop less monocyte infiltration in the pancreas. This suggests that high systemic levels of MCP-1 prevent monocytes from responding to local MCP-1, and therefore the ability of MCP-1 to elicit monocyte infiltration will be dependent on its expression at low levels and on its being restricted to the appropriate site. These studies raise interesting points relevant to other chemokines concerning the importance of chemokine gradients for their correct functioning in vivo. The role of chemokine gradients in the process of leukocyte trafficking is addressed elsewhere in this chapter.

There is increasing evidence that MCP-1 and other chemokines may be critically important mediators of inflammation in the central nervous system (CNS). Chemokine expression, particularly of MCP-1 and MIP-1α, has been reported in many animal models of CNS inflammation[49] (reviewed in reference 50).

MCP-2 and MCP-3

MCP-2 and MCP-3 are part of a small subgroup of CC chemokines with extensive sequence homology to MCP-1 (>60 per cent). In comparison to MCP-1 and MCP-3, MCP-2 is still poorly understood. MCP-2 and MCP-3 were both identified through their monocyte chemoattractant abilities, and they are both as effective as MCP-1 in this respect.[51] Like MCP-1, they function as T-lymphocyte chemoattractants. It appears that the biological effects of MCP-2 and MCP-3 partially overlap those of MCP-1, yet others are clearly distinct. They often appear to be less effective, however, and are produced at lower levels than MCP-1 (reviewed in reference 52). Whereas all three MCPs chemoattract basophils, MCP-3 is a particularly effective stimulator of basophil chemotaxis and release.[53]

MCP-4 and MCP-5

MCP-4 and MCP-5 are the two most recently described MCPs. MCP-4 shares closest homology to MCP-3 and another CC chemokine, eotaxin. In fact, MCP-4 appears to share functional properties similar to those of MCP-3 and eotaxin. Like MCP-3 and eotaxin, it is a strong chemoattractant for eosinophils as well as for monocytes and T lymphocytes, and it is also reported to stimulate histamine release from basophils.[54, 55]

To date, only murine MCP-5 has been identified, and it appears to share greatest homology with human MCP-1 (66 per cent amino acid identity).[56, 57] MCP-5 attracts monocytes, eosinophils, and T lymphocytes.

▼ RANTES

RANTES (regulated on activation normal T-cell expressed and secreted) was identified by Schall and colleagues[58] as a gene inducible by antigenic or mitogenic stimulation in a variety of T-cell lines and circulating T lymphocytes. RANTES is produced by a variety of cell types including platelets and eosinophils.[59, 60] RANTES is a potent chemoattractant of monocytes and subsets of T lymphocytes, particularly of the CD4+, CD45RO+ memory phenotype, but it is also a potent chemoattractant of CD8+ T cells.[61, 62] RANTES has also been reported to chemoattract and activate eosinophils and basophils as well as NK cells.[45, 63, 64]

▼ MIP-1α AND MIP-1β

MIP-1α and MIP-1β are clearly distinct molecules. However, they do share some striking similarities in their functions, barring a few specific exceptions. Therefore, the following discussion is largely limited to MIP-1α, unless stated otherwise. MIP-1α and MIP-1β were originally isolated as MIP-1 from the macrophage cell line RAW264.7, stimulated by LPS.[65] MIP-1 was subsequently found to comprise two distinct proteins, which were renamed MIP-1α and MIP-1β.[66] The cDNA previously cloned as MIP-1 corresponded to that of MIP-1α.[67] The amino acid sequences of MIP-1α and MIP-1β are 59.8 per cent identical. The human homologues of MIP-1α and MIP-1β were previously identified as LD78 and Act-2, respectively.[68, 69] The MIP-1 proteins are encoded by distinct genes clustered on chromosome 17 in humans, and on chromosome 11 in mice, along with most other CC chemokines.

One of the original observations made during the isolation of MIP-1 was its propensity to undergo self-aggregation.[65] In fact, this self-aggregation is a phenomenon noted for both human and murine MIP-1α and MIP-1β. The aggregation results from non-covalent and electrostatic interactions between molecules and occurs to such an extent that multimers may result with molecular masses in excess of 100 kDa in physiological buffers in vitro, and even greater aggregation occurs at higher concentrations (>10^6 kDa).[70] Further understanding of this aggregation has been achieved through the derivation of three MIP-1α mutants, in which the C-terminal acidic amino acids have been sequentially neutralized, resulting in the generation of non-aggregating forms of MIP-1α.[71] These three mutants formed tetramers, dimers, and monomers, which were equipotent to each other and to wild-type MIP-1α, both in stem cell inhibition assays and monocyte shape-change assays. This suggests that aggregation is not necessary for the function of MIP-1α in these assays and implies that the aggregated forms spontaneously disaggregate and are ultimately functional as monomers.[71]

MIP-1α mRNA has been reported to be expressed by a wide variety of hematopoietic cell types, including monocytes and macrophages, T lymphocytes, mast cells, basophils, eosinophils, neutrophils, NK cells, and epidermal Langerhans cells.[68, 72–77] Elevated MIP-1α expression has been observed in a number of disorders and disease states, and some of these are detailed further in later sections.

▼ EOTAXIN

Eotaxin is an eosinophil-attracting chemokine, originally isolated from the bronchoalveolar fluid of allergic guinea pigs.[78, 79] Guinea pig, human, and murine homologues were subsequently cloned.[80–85] Eotaxin is unusual in its specificity for eosinophils and is inactive on both monocytes and neutrophils, but it also appears to show some chemotactic activity toward IL-2–conditioned lymphocytes as well as basophils and mast cells.[54] As with many other chemokines, control of cell responsiveness occurs at the level of receptor expression. The specific and only receptor for eotaxin is CCR3, whose expression is mostly limited to those cells involved in allergic responses, such as eosinophils, basophils, and T-helper type 2 (T_H2) cells.[84, 85] Eotaxin message is found constitutively in a variety of tissues and organs including small intestine, colon, heart, kidney, and pancreas and is hypothesized to control basal trafficking to these tissues.[86] Other studies have shown that eotaxin may play a role in myelopoiesis and mast cell development and that eotaxin may be involved in the mobilization of eosinophils and their progenitors from the bone marrow.[87, 88]

▼ I-309

I-309 and its putative murine homologue, TCA-3, are produced by activated mast cells and T cells and are unusual in having an extra pair of cysteines.[89, 90] TCA-3 is activated in a wide variety of cell types, including neutrophils. The receptor for I-309 is CCR8, which is expressed on activated T_H2-type T cells but not on T_H1-type cells.[91] Thus, a communication between mast cells and T cells is implied.

The C Subfamily

To date, lymphotactin is the only member of the so-called C subfamily. The two cysteinyl residues correspond to cysteines 2 and 4 in the CXC and CC chemokines. Lymphotactin was originally cloned from activated pro-T cells, and a human orthologue, single C motif-1 (SCM-1), was subsequently isolated.[8, 92] Lymphotactin was demonstrated to be a T-cell chemoattractant. More recently, lymphotactin has also been identified as an agonist for NK cells both in vitro and in vivo.[93] Curiously, lymphotactin may act as an autocrine factor for NK cells as well as for immunoglobulin E plus antigen-stimulated mast cells.[93, 94]

The CX$_3$C Subfamily

The identification of a fourth chemokine subfamily has caused considerable interest. This is because fractalkine, the only member identified to date, appears unique in being the only known membrane-anchored chemokine. Fractalkine was cloned from non-hematopoietic cells and shown to be a 373 amino acid glycoprotein that displays a chemokine domain on a long extended mucin-like stalk[9, 10] (see Fig. 15–1). Fractalkine exists either in a membrane-bound form or as a secreted protein. The secreted form attracts T cells and monocytes, and the anchored form acts as a leukocyte adhesion molecule.[95] The expression of fractalkine is also unique among chemokines. Little or no expression is detectable in peripheral blood leukocytes; rather, fractalkine is expressed on tissue cells including cytokine-activated endothelial cells, particularly in the CNS. The precise function of fractalkine/neurotactin is still uncertain, but it appears to bridge roles both as a chemotactic factor and an adhesion molecule.

Interspecies Homology and Function

Several chemokines have been identified only in the mouse, leading to questions as to the identity of human orthologues. Examples include MCP-5, MIP-1γ, C10, and CCF18/MIP-related protein-2 (MRP-2).[56, 57, 96–99] Given the shared sequence homology between different chemokines and the clustering of chemokine genes on specific chromosomes, the system is likely to have evolved to serve specific functions for the host species. Thus, there is not a straight "one-for-one" homology relationship among species. For instance, rodents and humans clearly exhibit unique physiologies and habitats. The selective pressures in each mammal have selected chemokines and receptors accordingly. IL-8 may be one such example in that no rodent homologue of IL-8 has been identified to date. Many characteristics of IL-8 and CXCR1 (a receptor for IL-8) appear to be subserved by MIP-1α and CCR1 (a receptor for MIP-1α).

Chemokine Receptors

▼ EARLY CHARACTERIZATION OF RECEPTORS

A great deal of research has been directed at trying to understand how various chemokines interact with their cognate receptors on the extracellular surface of cells. It is now evident that the receptors for the various members of the chemokine superfamily all belong to the seven transmembrane–spanning G protein–coupled receptor (7TMGPCR or GPCR) superfamily, and a multitude of chemokine receptors have now been cloned and characterized.

The first chemokine receptors to be identified were those for IL-8 and were named IL-8R$_A$ and IL-8R$_B$.[100, 101] IL-8 binds to both with high affinity, but IL-8R$_A$ is specific for IL-8, whereas IL-8R$_B$ binds other CXC chemokines (Table 15–2). With the cloning of these receptors, it became possible to clone additional receptors by polymerase chain reaction, using primers based on conserved sequences within the IL-8 receptors and other GPCRs. Subsequently, a receptor called CC-CKR1 was cloned from myeloid/monocytic cell lines, which bound the CC chemokines MIP-1α, MIP-1β, and RANTES.[102, 103] Receptors are now prefixed with CXCR, CCR, XCR, or CX$_3$CR, depending on whether they bind CXC, CC, C, or CX$_3$C chemokines. Thus, IL-8R$_A$ and IL-8R$_B$ became CXCR1 and CXCR2, respectively; CC-CKR1 became CCR1. The known human CC and CXC chemokine receptors and their known ligands are summarized in Table 15–2.

The overlapping ligand/receptor pairings are a confusing aspect of the chemokine system. For example, MIP-1α is an agonist at CCR1, CCR4, and CCR5. On the other side, CCR1 recognizes RANTES, MCP-3, and MCP-4 as well as MIP-1α. Several interpretations have been proposed for this phenomenon.

First, the apparent redundancies may afford a means of control in vivo. Kinetics of induction, cell type of origin, and the half-life of the chemokine itself may differ. At the receptor level, affinities, off-rates, and desensitization properties may allow a responding cell to discriminate between chemokines.

Second, whereas a given receptor may recognize a num-

Table 15–2. The Chemokine Receptor Superfamily

	Receptor Name	Known Ligand(s)
CC receptors	CCR1	MIP-1α, RANTES, MCP-1, MCP-3, Lkn-1, CKβ-8
	CCR2	MCP-1, MCP-2, MCP-3
	CCR3	Eotaxin, RANTES, MCP-3, (MCP-2, MCP-4)
	CCR4	TARC, MDC
	CCR5	MIP-1α, MIP-1β, RANTES
	CCR6	MIP-3α = LARC = exodus
	CCR7	MIP-3β = exodus-3 = CKβ-11
	CCR8	I-309, TARC
	CCR9	TECK
	D6	MIP-1α, MIP-1β, RANTES, MCPs 1–4, eotaxin, HCC-1
CXC receptors	CXCR1	IL-8 (GCP-2)
	CXCR2	IL-8, KC, NAP-2, GRO-α, GRO-β, GRO-γ, ENA-78, GCP-2
	CXCR3	IP-10, MIG, I-TAC
	CXCR4	SDF-1
	CXCR5	BLC = BCA-1
XC receptors	XCR1	Lymphotactin
CX₃C receptors	CX₃CR1	Fractalkine = neurotactin
Others	DARC	Binds CC and CXC chemokines (except MIP-1α)
Viral homologues		
Human cytomegalovirus (hCMV)	US28	MIP-1α, MIP-1β, RANTES, MCP-1, MCP-3
Herpesvirus saimiri	ECRF3	IL-8, GRO, NAP-2
Kaposi sarcoma–associated herpesvirus (KSHV)	KSHV GPCR	IL-8, NAP-2, I-309, GRO, RANTES
Myxoma virus	M-T7	Binds CC and CXC chemokines through their GAG domains
Human herpesvirus 6 (HHV6)	U12	MIP-1α, MIP-1β, RANTES, MCP-1

ber of chemokines, the receptor has been "optimized" for a given ligand. For example, CCR2 recognizes MCPs 1, 2, 3, 4, and 5; yet the gene knockouts of CCR2 and MCP-1 have a phenotype in common, suggesting that MCPs 2, 3, 4, and 5 are less important in vivo as CCR2 agonists.

Finally, it has become appreciated that the receptors may exist in a number of affinity states that isomerize. Some of these conformational isomers are coupled to activate the heterotrimeric G protein–coupled pathway, whereas others are not. Thus, as a cell migrates up a concentration gradient, it must adapt to increasing levels of receptor occupancy. In vivo, as a cell migrates in response to a given chemokine and receptor coupling, encountering a "new" chemokine may be part of the signal to arrest movement or to continue, or perhaps to recruit a different signal transduction pathway leading to the exocytosis of granule contents.

▼ OVERVIEW OF CHEMOKINE RECEPTOR BIOLOGY: THE SEVEN TRANSMEMBRANE–SPANNING G PROTEIN–COUPLED RECEPTOR SUPERFAMILY

The chemokine receptors identified to date are all members of the GPCR superfamily that also includes receptors for other proinflammatory mediators such as C5a and the β₂-adrenergic receptors. The proposed topology of one such chemokine receptor, CCR1, is shown in Figure 15–2. The structure consists of an NH₂-terminal segment that projects from the extracellular surface and seven transmembrane domains that result in extracellular transmembrane and intracellular domains. The most conserved regions are located in the transmembrane segments. In addition, all chemokine receptors appear to have two conserved cysteines, located in

the NH₂ terminus and the third extracellular loop, and these are believed to form a disulfide bond that is important in maintaining the correct conformational arrangement of the regions that form the ligand-binding domain (reviewed in reference 104). These are in addition to the ubiquitous cysteinyl residues that link extracellular loops 1 and 2.

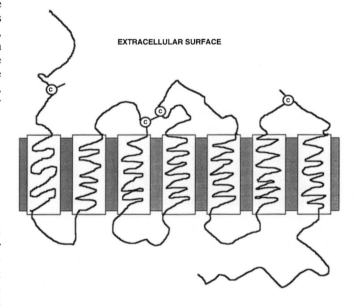

Figure 15–2. The proposed structure of a seven transmembrane–spanning G protein–coupled chemokine receptor (human CCR1). The Cs represent conserved cysteines.

Binding of the cognate ligand results in activation of heterotrimeric guanosine triphosphate–binding protein complexes, followed by dissociation of the α subunit from the $\beta\gamma$ subunit. Many different forms of G protein subunit exist and fall into several classes. The $G_{\alpha i}$ proteins are pertussis toxin sensitive; the $G_{\alpha q}$ class are pertussis toxin resistant. The $G_{\alpha s}$ class of proteins stimulate adenylate cyclase, whereas both $G_{\alpha i}$ and $G_{\alpha q}$ proteins are inhibitory to adenylate cyclase. After receptor activation, the receptor becomes desensitized (i.e., decreased responsiveness to the presence of cognate ligand). Figure 15–3 and references 105 to 107 summarize some of what is known about the downstream signaling pathways that may be activated after binding of a ligand to its cognate GPCR.

Several different signal transduction pathways may be activated, depending on the chemokine and receptor. These include adenylate cyclase; protein kinase C; phospholipases A, C, and D; and the tyrosine and mitogen-activated protein kinases. For example, the activated $G_{\alpha q}$ proteins are believed to activate phospholipase C β_1 and β_2. Phospholipase C activation then results in the generation of the second mes-

sengers diacylglycerol and inositol 1,4,5-triphosphate (IP_3). These secondary messengers then trigger a signaling cascade in which diacylglycerol activates protein kinase C; IP_3 mobilizes calcium from intracellular stores in the cytoplasm. Evidence is now also emerging from the study of other GPCR systems of a role for the dissociated $\beta\gamma$ subunit in activating GPCR signal transduction pathways through $p21^{ras}$-dependent and Rac/Rho-dependent pathways.[105] However, it is unclear as yet whether this also occurs in chemokine GPCR systems. The various activated pathways converge in the nucleus where they act on a variety of transcription factors that mediate the regulation of gene expression. It is these changes in gene expression that ultimately regulate a variety of cellular processes, such as chemotaxis, degranulation, and the respiratory burst. Not all the pathways summarized in Figure 15–3 are activated by all chemokine receptors. The precise signal transduction pathways activated differ according to the chemokine/receptor pairing involved and may even differ between different cell types. Research is currently ongoing in many laboratories to further understand these pathways.

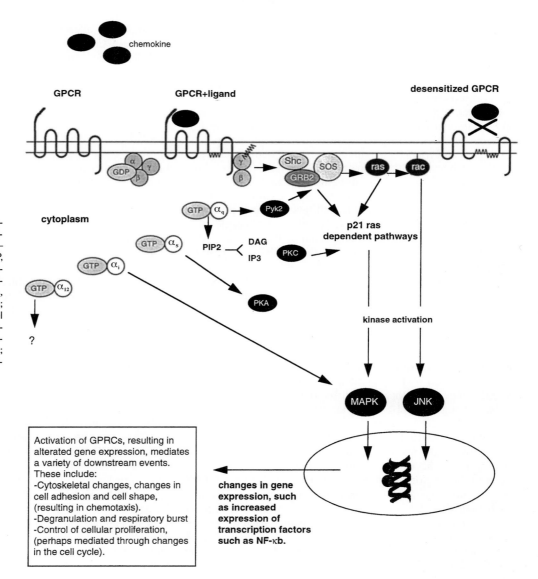

Figure 15–3. Signaling cascade pathways that may be involved after binding of a chemokine to a G protein–coupled receptor (GPCR). GTP, guanosine triphosphate; GDP, guanosine diphosphate; PKA, protein kinase A; PKC, protein kinase C; PIP_2, phosphatidylinositol bisphosphate; DAG, diacylglycerol; IP_3, inositol 1,4,5-triphosphate; SOS, son of sevenless protein; GRB2, adapter protein GBR2; Shc, adapter protein Shc; MAPK, mitogen-activated protein kinase; JNK, Jun kinases.

Activation of GPRCs, resulting in altered gene expression, mediates a variety of downstream events. These include:
-Cytoskeletal changes, changes in cell adhesion and cell shape, (resulting in chemotaxis).
-Degranulation and respiratory burst
-Control of cellular proliferation, (perhaps mediated through changes in the cell cycle).

changes in gene expression, such as increased expression of transcription factors such as NF-κb.

▼ RECEPTORS FOR THE CC CHEMOKINES

CCR1

As can be seen from Table 15–2, CCR1 is a receptor for multiple chemokines. It was initially reported to recognize MIP-1α and RANTES, although MCP-2 and MCP-3 were later demonstrated to be functional ligands as well.[102, 103, 108] CCR1 appears to be expressed on a wide variety of cell types, including primary monocytes/macrophages and cell lines, neutrophils, B and T lymphocytes, eosinophils, and astrocytes.[102, 103, 108–110] Investigators have attempted to address the in vivo function of CCR1 through generation of CCR1 homozygous null mice. On gross evaluation, these CCR1$^{-/-}$ mice are phenotypically normal.[111] These mice have normal numbers of leukocytes and are healthy when raised under pathogen-free conditions, suggesting that CCR1 is not necessary for normal development. However, closer investigation reveals a non-redundant role for CCR1 in immune responses under inflammatory stress. After challenge of mice with LPS, myeloid progenitors from CCR1$^{-/-}$ mice show disordered trafficking from the bone marrow to the spleen and blood as well as reduced proliferation. Furthermore, mature neutrophils from CCR1$^{-/-}$ mice fail to exhibit chemotaxis in vitro in response to MIP-1α and fail to mobilize into the peripheral blood in response to MIP-1α. CCR1$^{-/-}$ mice are also more susceptible than wild-type mice to infection with *Aspergillus fumigatus*, a fungal infection that is particularly infectious when low neutrophil numbers are present.

Taken together, these results suggest that CCR1 has a non-redundant role in hematopoiesis and in mouse neutrophil-mediated host responses in vivo. The phenotypes of CCR1$^{-/-}$ and MIP-1α$^{-/-}$ mice share some common aspects in that neither CCR1$^{-/-}$ mice nor MIP-1α$^{-/-}$ mice show overt abnormalities in basal hematopoiesis.[112] Studies by Graham and colleagues[113] suggest that CCR1 is not the receptor through which MIP-1α inhibits stem cell proliferation. In another study using CCR1-deficient mice, deletion of CCR1 was associated with protection from pancreatitis-associated lung injury, suggesting that CCR1 is important for progression of inflammation.[114] CCR1 was reported to be a receptor for the novel CC chemokines leukotactin-1 (Lkn-1) and Ckβ-8.[115, 116]

CCR2

The CCR2 receptor was first cloned from the MonoMac6 cell line.[117] The receptor appears to exist in two forms, CCR2A and CCR2B, generated by alternative splicing of a single gene. They appear to differ only in their C-terminal tails, although CCR2A is not as well expressed on the cell surface. CCR2B is an MCP-specific receptor and does not bind MIP-1α, MIP-1β, or RANTES.[118]

Through the use of truncation mutants and site-directed mutagenesis, the Charo group[119–122] has been productive in determining regions involved in interactions between CCR2 and in particular MCP-1. Targeted disruption of CCR2 and its ligand MCP-1 has revealed a non-redundant role in macrophage recruitment and host defense against bacterial pathogens in vivo, and it may also be involved in the initiation of atherosclerosis.[123–125] Compelling evidence supporting a role for CCR2/MCP-1 in the inflammatory aspects of atheroma formation was gathered by crossing CCR2/MCP-1–deficient mice with strains deficient in apolipoprotein B and the low-density lipoprotein receptor. The size of lesions in models of atherosclerosis was significantly decreased in the absence of the monocyte/macrophage chemokine systems.[125, 126]

CCR3

CCR3, a receptor with a restricted expression pattern, is highly expressed on eosinophils and basophils.[85, 127, 128] Limited expression has also been reported on elicited macrophages and neutrophils, although the functional relevance of this is questionable.[129] Human CCR3 is specific in binding only eotaxin, MCP-3, MCP-4, and RANTES, all of which are eosinophil chemoattractants. This further reinforces the notion that CCR3 is an eosinophil/basophil-specific receptor. However, a study suggests a wider role in the allergic response in that CCR3 appears to be expressed on T$_H$2 cells; moreover, eotaxin was able to stimulate increases in intracellular calcium and chemotaxis of CCR3$^+$ T cells.[130] This finding is particularly interesting because it suggests that eotaxin can attract eosinophils, basophils, and T$_H$2 cells, three of the most important cells for development of an inflammatory allergic response. CCR3 is also a receptor for the novel CC chemokine Lkn-1.[115] A non-redundant role for CCR3 in basal eosinophil trafficking is inferred from targeted disruption of the CCR3 ligand eotaxin. Mice deficient in eotaxin have reduced numbers of eosinophils in the jejunum and thymus.[86]

CCR4

Human CCR4 was originally cloned from a human immature basophilic cell line and is expressed strongly in the thymus as well as in T and B lymphocytes, peripheral blood monocytes, and IL-5–stimulated basophils.[131] Originally, human CCR4 was reported to be a functional receptor for MIP-1α, RANTES, and MCP-1; however, it is now uncertain whether this is indeed true. The murine homologue was subsequently cloned and shown to have binding characteristics and tissue expression similar to those of its human homologue.[132] Imai and colleagues[133] have demonstrated that the T cell–directed CC chemokine thymus and activation-regulated chemokine (TARC) is a specific ligand for CCR4. Macrophage-derived chemokine (MDC) is also a functional ligand for CCR4.[134] Both TARC and MDC are chemotactic for T$_H$2-type cells, suggesting that CCR4 is likely to be involved in polarized T$_H$2 lymphocyte responses.

CCR5

CCR5 is abundantly expressed on macrophages and T cells and appears to be a relatively specific receptor, binding only MIP-1α, MIP-1β, and RANTES.[135–137] A region within the second extracellular loop of CCR5 is critical for high-affinity binding of these ligands and subsequent functional response.[138] In contrast to CCR3 and CCR4, which appear to be associated with a T$_H$2-type response, CCR5 (along with CXCR3) appears to be associated with T$_H$0 and T$_H$1 lymphocytes.[130, 139–142] CCR5 is now also the focus of intense study as a result of its identification as a cofactor for HIV entry, and this is discussed further in a later section.

Other CC Receptors

CCRs 1 to 5 are the most studied CC chemokine receptors to date, but several other novel receptors have been identified. CCR6 appears to show relatively restricted expression on B and T lymphocytes (particularly on memory T cells positive for the marker CD26).[143] It is also strongly expressed in CD34+-derived dendritic cells, but not on monocyte-derived dendritic cells, nor on monocytes, granulocytes, or NK cells.[144, 145]

CCR7 is a receptor for the novel chemokines MIP-3β/ELC and 6Ckine/SLC and is strongly expressed on B and T lymphocytes.[146, 147] The role of this receptor and its ligands in lymphocyte homing to secondary organs is discussed in a later section.

CCR8 is a receptor for I-309 and for TARC.[148, 149] Interestingly, CCR8 is also strongly expressed on T_H2 lymphocytes, and its expression is upregulated on these cells after activation.[91, 150]

D6, a recently characterized receptor, is unusual in having an altered DRYLAIV motif in the second intracellular loop, which is normally highly conserved and appears critical for signaling.[151, 152] D6 is a high-affinity receptor for MIP-1α and also binds MIP-1β, MCPs 1 to 4, eotaxin, and hemofiltrate CC chemokine-1 (HCC-1). However, D6 does not appear to flux calcium in transfected HEK293 cells, and the functional significance of this and the other unusual characteristics of D6, such as strong placental expression, is unclear at present.

▼ RECEPTORS FOR THE CXC CHEMOKINES

CXCR1 and CXCR2

Early studies demonstrated the presence of two classes of IL-8–binding receptors on human neutrophilic granulocytes. These two types of IL-8 receptors differ in their respective ability to bind particular CXC chemokines. The IL-8R_A receptor, now referred to as CXCR1, is highly specific for IL-8, and most evidence to date suggests that it does not bind any other ligands, with the exception of GCP-2.[100, 101, 153] IL-8R_B, or CXCR2, also binds IL-8 with high affinity, but in contrast to CXCR1, it can also bind NAP-2, KC, growth-regulated oncogene (GRO)–α, GRO-β, GRO-γ, ENA-78/LIX, and GCP-2.[154, 155]

Expression of CXCR1 and CXCR2 is mostly restricted to neutrophils but is also found at lower levels on subsets of T lymphocytes, basophils, keratinocytes, mast cells, and eosinophils (although this last one is controversial).[156–159] CXCR2 has also been shown to be expressed on subsets of neurons within the CNS and appears to be overexpressed in the epidermis of human psoriatic tissue.[160, 161]

It is postulated that CXCR1 and CXCR2 play different roles during inflammation because of different specificities and affinities for their ligands. This is further supported by the observation that only CXCR1 stimulation results in the activation of phospholipase D and the respiratory burst, whereas CXCR2 is associated with granule exocytosis.[157]

Although no murine homologue of IL-8 has been identified to date, a murine CXCR2 receptor homologue (mIL-8Rh) has been characterized. This receptor recognizes the murine chemokines KC and MIP-2, which are orthologous to the human GRO-α, GRO-β, and GRO-γ genes. Mice deficient in this receptor have been generated and under barrier isolation show a profound neutrophilic leukocytosis. This suggests a negative role for the mIL-8Rh in regulating neutrophil numbers.[162, 163] In addition, these mice also show an increased number of B cells in their lymph nodes; enlarged spleens are due to enhanced proliferation of specific myeloid elements and megakaryocytes. There is also enhanced myelopoiesis in the bone marrow. Additional data suggest the involvement of the IL-8Rh in the negative regulation of myeloid progenitor cells. Strikingly, mice deficient in mIL-8Rh (mIL-8Rh$^{-/-}$) that are raised in a gnotobiotic environment are virtually indistinguishable from wild-type mice. These data suggest a role for CCR2 in surveillance of environmental pathogens as well as normal flora.

There is increasing evidence that the functions of IL-8 and CXCR1 in humans (namely, on neutrophils) are in fact subserved by CCR1 and MIP-1α in the mouse.[111, 114]

CXCR3

One of the most interesting CXC receptors to be characterized to date is CXCR3. It is of particular interest because its expression is restricted solely to activated T cells and NK cells. It is a receptor specific for IP-10, MIG, and I-TAC, and it does not bind to any of the other known CXC chemokines.[29, 30] I-TAC binds to CXCR3 with a much higher affinity than does either IP-10 or MIG and is more potent and efficacious, suggesting that I-TAC is likely to be the principal ligand for CXCR3.[30] CXCR3, like CCR5, seems to be associated with a polarized T_H1-type response.[140] Indeed, this is further supported by the fact that all three CXCR3 ligands are induced by interferons and that expression of IP-10 has been observed in diseases associated with a T_H1-type response. CXCR3 is therefore likely to be a key player in T-cell recruitment in cell-mediated immunity.

CXCR4

Interest in chemokine receptors was sparked by the observation that an "orphan" receptor, previously known as LESTR (leukocyte-expressed seven-transmembrane receptor), functioned as a coreceptor for HIV entry into T cells.[164, 165] This coreceptor was given the name fusin. Subsequent to these observations, SDF-1 was shown to be the ligand for this receptor.[166, 167] This receptor is now known more commonly as CXCR4. The role of CXCR4 and other chemokine receptors in HIV entry is discussed in greater detail in a later section.

Mouse CXCR4, like CCR2, appears to be expressed in two forms (CXCR4A and B) derived from a single gene by alternative splicing, although only a single form of human CXCR4 has been reported to date.[168, 169] In addition to its role as a cofactor for HIV entry, it is now evident that CXCR4 and its ligand, SDF-1, have important roles in development and hematopoiesis. As mentioned previously in the section on SDF-1, mice lacking SDF-1 (SDF-1$^{-/-}$) exhibit hematopoietic defects in B-cell lymphopoiesis and bone marrow myelopoiesis as well as a cardiac ventricular septum defect.[22] Subsequent to this report, several groups also derived mice that were deficient for the SDF-1 receptor CXCR4. These studies confirm the defects observed for SDF-1$^{-/-}$ mice, but in addition, these CXCR4$^{-/-}$ mice also show defects in fetal cerebellar development.[170, 171] Another study also showed that CXCR4 was essential for vascularization of the gastrointestinal tract.[172] Taken together, these suggest that in addition to roles in normal immune function, SDF-1 and CXCR4 appear to have wide-ranging roles in aspects of hematopoiesis and development.

CXCR5/BLR-1

Identification of the CXCR5 receptor followed characterization of an orphan receptor known as Burkitt lymphoma receptor 1 (BLR-1). Mice with a targeted disruption of BLR-1 show an unusual phenotype in that these BLR$^{-/-}$ mice lack inguinal lymph nodes and show a defective formation of the primary follicles and germinal centers of the spleen and Peyer patches.[173] This suggests a role for the BLR-1 receptor and its ligands in B-cell homing to lymphoid organs. The ligand for CXCR5 is B-cell chemoattracting chemokine (BCA)–1, also known as B-lymphocyte chemoattractant (BLC).[174, 175]

▼ THE DUFFY ANTIGEN RECEPTOR FOR CHEMOKINES

One of the most unusual identified chemokine receptors is the Duffy antigen receptor for chemokines (DARC). The Duffy antigen is an erythrocyte cell surface receptor for the malarial parasite *Plasmodium vivax* (reviewed in reference 176). Surprisingly, a promiscuous chemokine receptor that bound both CXC and CC chemokines (with the exception of MIP-1α) was also identified on erythrocytes and subsequently shown to be identical to the Duffy antigen.[177, 178] DARC, as it was named, is also expressed on the endothelial cells lining some postcapillary venules and on Purkinje cells in the cerebellum of the brain.[179] The precise function of DARC in vivo is still unclear, because it does not appear to present chemokines in an active form to receptors, nor does it appear to signal. It may instead function as a "chemokine sink"—to remove excess chemokines from the circulation. Its strong conservation between species and the observation that Duffy blood group–negative individuals (who are malaria resistant) do still express Duffy on endothelial cells of postcapillary venules suggest that it does serve a critical role in vivo. It was recently shown that IL-8 is actually internalized by venular endothelial cells and transcytosed to the luminal surface, where it is presented to adherent leukocytes on the membrane of the endothelial cell.[180] It is possible that DARC plays a role in this chemokine transcytosis and presentation.

Role of Chemokines in Normal Leukocyte Trafficking

For systemic immune responses to occur effectively, the various subsets of leukocytes must traffic in a highly regulated fashion. Lymphocytes continually circulate as a form of surveillance. They travel from the blood, through the tissues, into the lymphatic system, and thence back into the blood to recirculate. Other cells, such as neutrophilic granulocytes and monocytes, cannot recirculate; they emigrate from the blood stream constitutively and in response

to signals resulting from infection or injury. It is the nature of this signal that ultimately determines the type of response and therefore the particular leukocyte subsets that will participate. It is believed that chemokines play a crucial role in the basal migration of all leukocyte subsets.

One widely accepted model of leukocyte trafficking is outlined in Figure 15–4 (reviewed in reference 181). This model hypothesizes that leukocytes in blood roll in a controlled manner along the endothelium, lightly tethered through interactions with a particular class of adhesion molecules called selectins.[181, 182] L-selectin is expressed on almost all circulating lymphocytes; P-selectin and E-selectin are expressed on endothelial cells. In response to inflammatory mediators, endothelial cell surface expression of P-selectin and E-selectin is increased. This occurs by mobilization from preformed stores in the case of P-selectin or through de novo synthesis of E-selectin. The cognate ligands for P-selectin and L-selectin contain mucins attached by O-linked glycosylation. The ligands for L-selectin are glycosylation-dependent cell adhesion molecule-1 (GlyCAM-1), which is secreted, and CD34 on the cell surface. P-selectin binds to the mucin-like P-selectin glycoprotein ligand (PSGL-1), which is disulfide-linked dimer.[181] The interactions between the endothelial cells and the leukocytes are of relatively low affinity and occur in a coordinated fashion of association and dissociation in a matter of milliseconds, such that the leukocytes tumble in the direction of the blood flow, a process therefore known as rolling. The leukocyte rolls along the endothelium until it encounters a local concentration of chemoattractant, such as a chemokine. The chemokines are believed to be held in this localized concentration on the cell surface and extracellular matrix, through interaction with heparan sulfate proteoglycan molecules.[183] Binding of a chemokine to its GPCR transduces a signal that increases the adhesion of the leukocyte to the endothelium by upregulating the affinity or expression of another type of adhesion molecule, the integrins, on the leukocyte cell surface that then interact with intracellular adhesion molecules on the surface of the endothelium.[181] After this activation-dependent firm adherence, the leukocyte ceases rolling and undergoes diapedesis and extravasates—passing from the lumen, through the endothelium, and into the tissues. The recruited leukocyte may then become further activated by other proinflammatory triggers and may in turn lead to the production of additional cytokines and chemokines in an amplification process.

If one accepts this model as being correct, then it is simple to extend it to explain the homing of particular lymphocyte subsets to secondary lymphoid organs. Control for circulation and homing would involve specific upregulation and downregulation of receptors and a constitutive localized concentration of chemokines in the target tissue. For instance, as discussed in an earlier section, the CXCR5 receptor and its ligand BCA-1 (BLC) appear to be involved in the homing of B cells to the lymph nodes, spleen, and Peyer patches.[173] Naive T lymphocytes will recirculate through the secondary lymphoid tissues, such as the lymph nodes, Peyer patches, and spleen, and thence into the lymphatic system and back into the blood. Strong evidence for the role of chemokines in T-cell homing is also now mounting. For example, study of mice that are naturally defective in the expression of the CC chemokine SLC has revealed

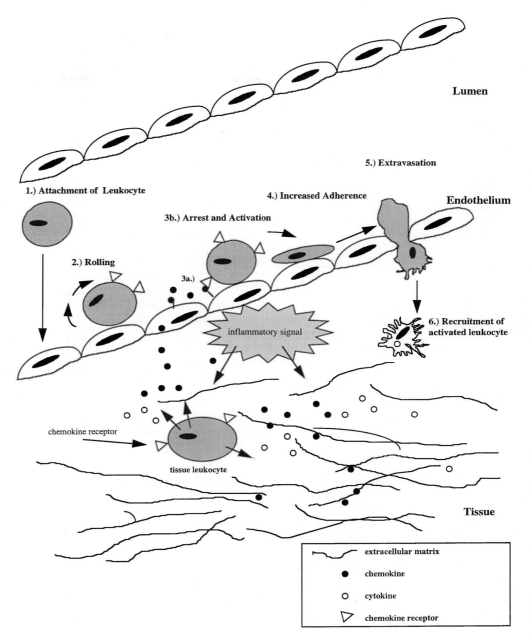

Figure 15–4. Proposed model of leukocyte trafficking. After an inflammatory signal, chemokines are released by resident or recruited leukocytes. These chemokines are held in the localized environment and concentration gradients through interactions with heparan sulfate proteoglycans in the extracellular matrix. Some chemokine is presented on the extracellular surface of the endothelium, perhaps through the actions of DARC and heparan sulfate proteoglycans (3a). Leukocytes passing through the lumen tether to the endothelium through selectins and roll along the endothelium (1 and 2). Chemokine binding results in activation of cell surface integrins, increased adherence, diapedesis, and extravasation (3–5). The recruited activated leukocyte may in turn recruit additional cells.

that SLC is necessary for proper homing of naive T cells to secondary lymphoid organs and for the homing of dendritic cells to the T-cell zones of the spleen and lymph nodes.[184]

Regulatory Control of the Expression of Chemokines and Their Receptors

Some researchers speculate that a large number of chemokines share overlapping effects and may therefore be redundant. The fact that every knockout for a chemokine or chemokine receptor generated so far has a unique phenotype would argue against this (see later section). An answer to this question must await the further analysis of additional chemokine and chemokine receptor knockouts. However, it is possible to offer another explanation. For example, although MCP-1 and MIP-1α display overlap in their ability to attract monocytes/macrophages, it is clear from studies of MCP-1 and CCR2 knockout mice that MCP-1 is indispensable for monocyte/macrophage function in vivo and that MIP-1α is unable to subserve its role.[123, 124, 185] Other examples exist, such as the effects of eotaxin, MCP-3 and MCP-4, and RANTES on eosinophils and basophils.[186]

We and others have postulated that chemokines and their receptors are expressed in a highly temporal and spatial fashion, in response to a wide variety of stimuli. Indeed, it is clear that in some inflammatory responses, certain leukocyte subsets are recruited before others, and a similar temporal pattern of gene expression can be seen for many chemokines. For example, evidence of an ordered, temporal pattern of particular chemokines and leukocyte subsets in a rodent model of multiple sclerosis is well documented.[50]

Many of the chemokines were initially characterized as immediate early genes that were inducible (e.g., PDGF stimulation of *JE*).[42] With the exception of SDF-1, which is constitutively expressed in most tissues, most chemokines are not expressed at high levels constitutively and are instead expressed on selective cells and tissues. The expression of many receptors appears even more selective; for example, CXCR3 is expressed only on activated T cells.[29] Table 15–3 summarizes the expression patterns for the chemokines and some of the regulators of this expression; Table 15–4 shows a similar summary for the various chemokine receptors. For example, treatment of CD45RO⁺ T lymphocytes with IL-2 will induce expression of CCR1 and CCR2. If IL-2 treatment is withdrawn, their expression is rapidly downregulated, but if IL-2 is again added, expression is restored fully.[187] As can be seen from Tables 15–3 and 15–4, most of these characterized regulators are cytokines or components of bacterial cell walls (LPS). Many are generally inducers of chemokine gene expression; however, a select few have been characterized as downregulators of chemokine gene expression (although not always). These downregulators include IL-10 and transforming growth factor-β (TGF-β). In addition to the obvious cytokines and LPS, other mechanisms exist to enable cells to respond to inflammatory stimuli. These include glucocorticoids, trauma, adhesion events, and components of the extracellular matrix.[188–190] For example, low-density lipoprotein and shear stress both induce MCP-1 expression.[191, 192]

Although the regulation of chemokine expression has been intensely studied for many years, the complexity of the numerous regulatory networks has made interpretation difficult. The downstream signaling pathways that control the expression of chemokine and chemokine receptor genes are only just beginning to be understood in any detail. The elements of some chemokine promoters, such as RANTES and IP-10, are better understood than others.[193, 194] However, it is clear that certain gene regulatory elements and transcription factors are particularly involved in the control of chemokine and chemokine receptor gene expression. For instance, in mouse mast cells, immunoglobulin E plus antigen stimulation results in the activation of FcεRI, which feeds through the p21ʳᵃˢ pathway, causing the AP-3/NF-AT transcription factor to induce the expression of both MCP-3 and IL-5.[195, 196] Table 15–5 summarizes some of the regulatory elements and factors known to be involved. The response of a cell in a particular tissue to a particular chemokine will ultimately depend on several factors, namely, (1) the expression of the appropriate receptor, (2) the expression of the chemokine in the local environment, and (3) the receptor's actually seeing that chemokine, which may involve active presentation. Therefore, to better understand the role of chemokines in vivo, it is necessary to further understand the temporal and spatial kinetics of chemokine and chemokine receptor expression as it actually occurs in vivo.

Inflammatory Disease

Given this basic, general mechanism of leukocyte trafficking outlined in the preceding sections, it is possible to view inflammatory disease as an extension of basal trafficking

Table 15–3. Cellular Expression and Some of the Known Regulators of Chemokine Gene Expression

Chemokine	Cell Expressed By	Upregulated By	Downregulated by
MIP-1α	Monocytes, macrophages, T cells, B cells, mast cells, eosinophils, basophils, neutrophils, NK cells, fibroblasts, microglia, astrocytes, epidermal Langerhans cells	LPS, TNF-α, IL-6, IFN-γ, GM-CSF, IL-3	TGF-β, IL-10, IFN-γ
MIP-1β	Monocytes, macrophages, T cells, B cells, mast cells, NK cells, astrocytes, microglia	LPS, TNF-α, GM-CSF	TGF-β, IL-10
RANTES	T cells, smooth muscle cells, NK cells, platelets, eosinophils	TNF-α plus IFN-γ, PMA + ionomycin	IL-4, IL-10, IL-13
MCP-1	Monocytes, macrophages, endothelial cells, astrocytes, fibroblasts	LPS, PDGF, TNF-α, IL-6, IFN-γ, trauma	TGF-β
MCP-3	Monocytes, macrophages, mast cells, fibroblasts	IgE plus antigen, PMA + ionomycin	TGF-β
I-309	Activated T cells, monocytes, neutrophils	Concanavalin A, IgG plus Fc, LPS, IL-1α	
Eotaxin	Fibroblasts, epithelial cells	IL-13, IL-4, TNF-α, IL-1α, IFN-γ	
HCC-1	Stimulated monocytes	IL-10	
DC-CK1/PARC	Dendritic cells	IL-4, IL-10, IL-13	IFN-γ
MDC/STCP-1	Monocytes, macrophages, B cells, dendritic cells	IL-4, IL-13	
C-10/MRP-1	Macrophages	IL-4, GM-CSF, IL-3	
IL-8	Monocytes, neutrophils, endothelial cells, fibroblasts, epithelial cells, T lymphocytes	GM-GSF, adhesion, cholesterol loading, LPS, IL-1	IFN-γ, IFN-α
KC	Macrophages, fibroblasts, astrocytes, hepatic cells	LPS, PDGF, IL-1α	IL-10
IP-10	Macrophages, keratinocyte, monocytes, lymphocytes, endothelial cells	IFN-γ	IL-4
MIG	Macrophages	IFN-γ	
I-TAC	Monocytes, stimulated astrocytes	IFN-α, IFN-β, IFN-γ, IL-1	
ENA-78	Monocytes, epithelial cells, endothelial cells, mast cells, platelets	LPS, IL-1β, TNF-α	IFN-γ
GCP-2	Osteosarcoma cells, fibroblasts	LPS, IL-1, TNF-α	IFN-γ
SDF-1	Stromal cells, constitutively expressed		
Lymphotactin	CD8⁺ T cells, NK cells, mast cells, glomerular mesangial cells, vascular endothelial cells	TCR stimulation, IL-1β	CD28
Fractalkine	Endothelial cells, astrocytes, neuronal cells	LPS, TNF-α, IL-1	

LPS, lipopolysaccharide; TNF, tumor necrosis factor, IL, interleukin; IFN, interferon; GM-CSF, granulocyte-macrophage colony-stimulating factor; TGF, transforming growth factor; Ig, immunoglobulin; PDGF, platelet-derived growth factor; PMA, phorbol 12-myrisate 13-acetate; TCR, T-cell receptor.

Table 15–4. Cellular Expression and Some of the Known Regulators of Chemokine Receptor Gene Expression

Receptor	Cell Expressed By	Upregulated By	Downregulated By
CCR1	Neutrophils, macrophages, monocytes, activated T cells, NK cells, basophils, mast cells, myeloid progenitors, astrocytes, neurons	IL-2	IFN-γ, phytohemagglutinin
CCR2	Monocytes, activated T cells, basophils	IL-2	IFN-γ, phytohemagglutinin
CCR3	Eosinophils, basophils, dendritic cells, neuronal cells, microglia	IFN-γ, IL-5	
CCR4	Thymocytes, basophils, T$_H$2-type T cells, platelets		
CCR5	Monocytes, macrophages, microglia, dendritic cells, activated T cells	IFN-γ	
CCR6	B cells, CD8⁻ splenic dendritic cells, CD34⁺-derived dendritic cells, CD4⁺ T cells, memory T cells		
CCR7	Activated B and T lymphocytes, Epstein-Barr virus–infected B cells, human herpesvirus 6 and 7–infected T cells	LPS, IL-1, TNF-α	
CCR8	Thymocytes, T$_H$2-type T cells		
CCR9	Placenta, fetal liver, spleen		
CXCR1	Monocytes, neutrophils, basophils, T lymphocytes, mast cells, NK cells		
CXCR2	Neutrophils, mast cells, activated T cells, neurons, astrocytes, myeloid progenitors		TNF-α
CXCR3	Activated T lymphocytes	IL-2	
CXCR4	CD34⁺ cells, B cells, microglia, resting T cells, neuronal cells, megakaryocytes, platelets		
CXCR5	B lymphocytes, Burkitt lymphoma cells, (memory T cells?)		
XCR1	Placenta		
CX₃CR1	Microglia, NK cells, T cells	IL-2, phytohemagglutinin	

See Table 15–3 for abbreviations.

driven by the localized de novo synthesis of chemokines. As discussed throughout this review, the various chemokines are crucial to the trafficking of leukocytes in response to signals indicating the presence of foreign antigen and injury. It is now clear that chemokines are present in a large number of disease states. Table 15–6 summarizes some of these observations.

Different pathological processes are often characterized by an infiltration of particular inflammatory cells. For instance, allergies and parasitic infections are associated with eosinophilia, leading to the suggestion that CCR3 and its ligands are likely to be downstream of IL-5 in causing emigration of eosinophils from the blood to the tissue spaces. Likewise, a link between MCP-1 and atherosclerosis has been proposed because of the expression of MCP-1 and macrophages in atherosclerotic plaques.[197] The expression of several chemokines, most notably MCP-1 and IL-8, also

appears to be upregulated in various forms of inflammatory bowel disease.[198, 199]

A number of chemokines have been implicated in the recruitment of leukocytes in rheumatoid arthritis, one of these being MIP-1α.[200] Rheumatoid arthritis is characterized by elicitation and activation of various leukocyte populations within the synovial space and in joint tissue. These recruited leukocytes are known to be critical participants in the resulting pathological process (reviewed in reference 201).

Aberrant chemokine expression has also been documented by many researchers in a variety of inflammatory neurological disease states. One of the most intensively studied has been multiple sclerosis (MS), characterized by focal T-cell and macrophage infiltration into white matter and resulting demyelination. Significant elevation of MIP-1α has been reported in MS patients undergoing relapse.[202] Experimental allergic encephalomyelitis (EAE) is a rodent model frequently used to study MS. Investigation of EAE has revealed that the kinetics of MIP-1α expression (and

Table 15–5. Elements and Factors Involved in the Transcriptional Regulation of Chemokine and Chemokine Receptor Gene Expression

	Transcription Factors and Regulatory Elements
Chemokines	
MIP-1α	NF-κb, C/EBP, c-Ets
MCP-1	NF-κb
MCP-3/MARC	AP-3–like/NF-AT
RANTES	NF-κb
KC	NF-κb
GRO	NF-κb, Sp1, HMGI(Y)
IP-10	NF-κb
MIG	NF-κb
Receptors	
CXCR1	PU.1
CXCR5	Oct-2, Bob1, NF-κb

Table 15–6. Chemokines Involved in Inflammatory Disease

Disease	Chemokines Involved
Asthma	Eotaxin, MCP-1, MCP-4, MIP-1α, RANTES
Sinusitis and rhinitis	Eotaxin
Sarcoidosis	IP-10
Interstitial lung	MIP-1α
Bacterial pneumonia	IL-8, ENA-78
Psoriasis	IL-8, GRO-α, MIG, IP-10, MCP-1
Atherosclerosis	MCP-1, MCP-4, IP-10, IL-8
Inflammatory bowel disease	MCP-1, MIP-1α, IL-8, ENA-78
Glomerulonephritis	MCP-1, RANTES, IP-10
Rheumatoid arthritis	MIP-1α, MCP-1, IL-8, ENA-78, RANTES, MIP-1β
Multiple sclerosis	MCP-1, MIP-1α, RANTES, IP-10, MIG
Bacterial meningitis	IL-8, GRO-α, MCP-1, MIP-1α, MIP-1β
Viral meningitis	IP-10, MCP-1

certain other chemokines) parallels that of leukocyte recruitment and disease severity.[203] MIP-1α is produced by microglial cells within the CNS and by glial and neuronal cells within the brain.[204, 205] Perhaps the most suggestive evidence for chemokine involvement comes from the observation that administration of anti–MIP-1α antibodies prevents the development of EAE.[206] Taken together, these studies strongly implicate MIP-1α (and other chemokines) as important mediators of inflammation within the CNS.

Infectious Diseases

Immunity may be divided into two classes, namely, innate and acquired. Innate immunity is relatively non-specific and is mounted by "pattern recognition."[206a] For example, nonself isomers of carbohydrate structures, LPS, and bacterial or fungal cell membranes are recognized by mannose-binding protein (an opsonin), LPS receptors such as Toll, and complement, respectively. Acquired immunity to a pathogen is a complex process that involves antigen presentation through major histocompatibility complex molecules, T-cell and B-cell recognition, and the development of either cellular (cytotoxic T lymphocytes, for example) or humoral (immunoglobulin) responses. Because of their dominant role in cellular recruitment and trafficking, chemokines are believed to be intimately involved in bridging innate and acquired immune responses.

Consider a bacterial infection, as an example. Recognition of the pathogen by phagocytic cells leads to the production of cytokines such as TNF-α and IL-1 (innate immunity). These cytokines activate the expression of genes for local chemokine generation (for example, IL-8 and MCP-1). IL-8 recruits neutrophils to clear bacteria; MCP-1 recruits monocytes, macrophages, and dendritic cells, which may begin to present antigen. T-cell and B-cell responses then lead to the production of specific immunity through immunoglobulins. It is now apparent that certain pathogens have evolved to exploit such responses in an attempt to evade the immune response. Two such examples include the use of chemokine receptors by HIV as cofactors for viral entry and the observation that many viruses have evolved chemokine and chemokine receptor homologues.

▼ CHEMOKINES, THEIR RECEPTORS, AND SIGNIFICANCE TO HIV PATHOGENESIS

The fields of chemokine biology and virology have surprisingly merged. This has arisen through many outstanding contributions and resulted in the identification of an essential role for chemokines and chemokine receptors in the pathogenesis of HIV infection and one of the most significant breakthroughs in acquired immunodeficiency syndrome (AIDS) research during the last 15 years. The review by D'Souza and Harden[207] provides an excellent summary of this. The following section briefly reviews some of the reports that led to the discovery of the critical role of chemokines and their receptors in HIV infection pathogenesis.

Until recently, one of the unsolved questions in AIDS research was the identity of the cofactor/receptor required for entry of HIV-1 into cells in addition to the previously identified CD4 molecule.[208] The first clues to solving this puzzle followed the identification of MIP-1α, MIP-1β, and RANTES as three soluble factors released by CD8+ T cells that suppressed the entry of primary strains of HIV-1.[209] In 1996, Berger and colleagues[165] made a seminal discovery and identified the second receptor necessary for HIV-1 entry into T-cell lines, so-called T-tropic viruses. They named this protein fusin, because it aided HIV fusion. Fusin is identical to CXCR4, the receptor for SDF-1, and is permissive only for entry of T-tropic strains, not for macrophage-tropic (M-tropic) viruses.[166, 167] Subsequently, five groups simultaneously reported that the cofactor for M-tropic viruses was the CCR5 receptor and that CCR2B and CCR3 also functioned as cofactors, although less effectively.[210–213] It is now clear that during infection, some viruses evolve to become dually tropic and can use both CC and CXC receptors, whereas some strains of HIV-2 appear to be able to use CXCR4 in a CD4-independent fashion.[214, 215] Intense study is now directed at determining critical interactions between different regions of CD4, HIV, and various receptors. After attachment of the HIV virion to a target cell by high-affinity interactions between the envelope (env) gp120 protein and CD4, a conformational change in gp120 is induced that exposes a chemokine receptor binding site. Binding of discrete regions of CCR5 or CXCR4 leads to the exposure of the fusion peptide gp41, which is shielded until chemokine receptor recognition.[216, 217] The V3 domain of HIV gp120 appears critical for this interaction but may be indirectly involved in tropism by interacting or not interacting with the chemokine receptor.[218] Figure 15–5 summarizes the current knowledge of the role of chemokines and their receptors in HIV entry.

Receptor signaling and internalization do not appear to be required for CCR5 to function as an HIV-1 entry cofactor.[219–221] It has been demonstrated, however, that recombinant M-tropic HIV and simian immunodeficiency virus envelope proteins can induce a signal through CCR5 on CD4+ T cells, which mediates T-cell chemotaxis.[222] Recent data suggest that chemokines and HIV-1 envelope glycoproteins induce tyrosine phosphorylation of the protein tyrosine kinase Pyk2.[223] This response requires CXCR4 and CCR5 to be accessible at the cell surface. The significance of these intracellular signaling events is unclear at present, but they may be integral to both pathogenesis and CNS disease.

A series of "experiments in nature" confirm the obligate role of the chemokine system in HIV disease. The CD8+ T cells of individuals who remained uninfected, despite multiple high-risk exposures, have greater antiviral activity than those of unexposed control subjects.[224] Their CD4+ T cells also appear less susceptible to M-tropic viral infection. This protection appears to relate to the activity of the suppressive factors MIP-1α, MIP-1β, and RANTES. Several groups have demonstrated a genetic basis for protection of multiply exposed high-risk individuals against HIV-1 infection. Some exposed, uninfected individuals lack CCR5 expression. This is due to a 32 bp deletion in the CCR5 allele, resulting in expression of a truncated CCR5 protein, which is not expressed on the cell surface.[225, 226] A heterozygous allelic defect may or may not provide a limited protective effect.[227, 228] It is clear, however, that the protective role of the CCR5 deletion allele is not absolute. Although rare, individuals who are homozygous for this defect can be infected, perhaps if the original infecting virus evolves to use CXCR4.[229, 230]

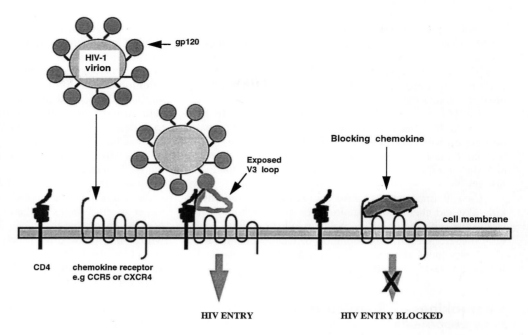

Figure 15–5. Summary of interaction between HIV-1 and the CCR5/CXCR4 coreceptors. Interaction of the virion, CD4, and the coreceptor results in exposure of the previously concealed V3 loop of gp120 and ultimately enables virus entry (shown in left two parts of figure). These interactions can be prevented by the addition of suppressive chemokines, resulting in a block in HIV entry (right-hand side of figure).

Reports have also identified allelic variants of CCR2, although the existence of any protective role is less pronounced.[231, 232]

In addition to genetic variants in cofactor receptors (coreceptors), the role of endogenous suppressive chemokines in protection against HIV infection is crucial. Unfortunately, determination of their roles is not so simple. Whereas it is clear that SDF-1 can suppress T-tropic infection through CXCR4, and the CC chemokines MIP-1α, MIP-1β, and RANTES suppress M-tropic infection, it is unlikely that these are the only suppressive chemokines.[166, 167, 209, 233] Indeed, another CC chemokine, macrophage-derived chemokine (MDC), also appears to have the ability to suppress HIV entry.[234] A rare genetic variant of SDF-1 has also been identified.[235] This polymorphism (SDF-1 3′A) is in the 3′ untranslated region of SDF-1, and the homozygous variant provides a protective effect against the onset of AIDS; the heterozygous variant is also protective, particularly during the later stages of disease progression. This protective effect is even more effective than that conferred by the heterozygous CCR5 (CCR5 del32) and CCR2 (CCR2-641) receptor variants discussed previously in this section. It has been speculated that this protective effect may be due to an enhanced level of SDF-1 production.

Although CCR5 and CXCR4 appear to be the primary coreceptors along with CCR2B, and CCR3 in the CNS, other chemokine receptors also function as coreceptors for HIV entry.[236] These include CCR8 and CXC$_3$R1 as well as the orphan receptors STRL33/Bonzo/TYMSTR, BOB/GPR15, GPR1, APJ, and the cytomegalovirus (CMV) receptor homologue US28.[237–245] Unusually, STRL33 appears to function as a fusion cofactor for both M-tropic and T-tropic HIV-1.[240]

The field of HIV-related chemokine biology is clearly in its infancy, but already chemokine antagonists and other strategies are being developed in attempts to produce therapeutic solutions for intervention and perhaps ultimately a cure for HIV infection.

▼ VIRALLY ENCODED CHEMOKINE AND CHEMOKINE RECEPTOR HOMOLOGUES

Independent of the interest in chemokines and viral pathogenesis, it has now emerged that many viruses encode homologues of chemokine and chemokine receptor–like genes. The first evidence for this was reported in 1994, with the identification of a chemokine receptor–like gene in the US28 open reading frame of the human CMV. The US28 gene encodes a receptor that is functional in response to MIP-1α, MIP-1β, RANTES, MCP-1, and MCP-3.[246] It is proposed that this receptor homologue may function to sequester chemokines from the environment, perhaps by internalization, and thus allow evasion of host immune surveillance by hCMV infected cells.[247] Alternatively, it may allow CMV-infected cells to carry virus to secondary lymphoid organs to propagate infection. A viral homologue of the CXCR2 receptor is also encoded by the *ECRF3* gene of herpesvirus saimiri.[248]

More recently, human herpesvirus 8 or Kaposi sarcoma–associated herpesvirus (KSHV) has been shown to encode several viral homologues. vMIP-I and vMIP-II have homology to MIP-1α, in addition to a viral form of IL-6, vIL-6.[249] A KSHV-encoded G protein–coupled receptor-like gene, with homology to the IL-8 receptors and *ECRF3* gene, has also been identified.[250] This receptor-like protein appears to bind both CC and CXC chemokines. Unusually, this homologue appears to be constitutively active and stimulates cell proliferation, suggesting that it could be a potential viral oncogene. This oncogenic potential was confirmed by demonstration that signaling through this G protein–coupled KSHV-encoded receptor results in cell transformation, tumorigenicity, and a switch to an angiogenic phenotype mediated by vascular endothelial growth factor.[251] vMIP-II also functions as a broad-spectrum antagonist and inhibits HIV-1 entry through CCR3, CCR5, and CXCR4 as well as being a chemoattractant for CCR3$^+$ eosinophils.[252, 253]

Molluscum contagiosum virus types I and II also encode a chemokine-like gene. The products are able to block the chemotactic responses of monocytes to MIP-1α but are not chemotactic themselves. These proteins are also active as inhibitors of human progenitor cell proliferation, with even greater potency than human MIP-1α.[254]

An IFN-γ receptor homologue, M-T7, encoded by myxoma virus has been shown to interact with the heparin-binding domains of both CC and CXC chemokines. M-T7 has no homology with any known chemokine receptors, and the significance of its apparent abilities is unclear at present.[255]

Clearly, many viruses have evolved or acquired chemokine-like and chemokine receptor–like genes, which demonstrates the critical role of chemokines in host defense against viral disease. Genetic manipulation of these elements and in vivo assessment are under way in a number of laboratories for the above-mentioned systems.

Chemokines as Regulators of Hematopoiesis

The role of chemokines as regulators of hematopoietic stem cell proliferation was first indicated by Broxmeyer and colleagues.[256] They used purified MIP-1, containing both MIP-1α and MIP-1β, and observed that addition of MIP-1 to in vitro model assays of hematopoiesis led to enhanced proliferation of macrophage or granulocyte-macrophage (GM) colony-stimulating factor (CSF)–stimulated committed progenitors (so-called GM colony-forming cells [GM-CFC]). MIP-1 had no effect on granulocyte CSF–stimulated colony formation. Graham and colleagues,[257] who were trying to purify a stem cell inhibitory factor from bone marrow, subsequently demonstrated that this inhibitory activity was identical to MIP-1α and called this factor stem cell inhibitor (SCI). MIP-1α inhibits colony formation from colony-forming unit (CFU)–A type stem cells and its in vivo correlate, splenic colony-forming unit (CFU-S), but not that from more committed GM-CFC progenitors. Neutralizing polyclonal serum raised against MIP-1 blocks the inhibitory activity of both SCI and recombinant MIP-1α. MIP-1β, however, was unable to inhibit stem cell proliferation at the concentrations used in these studies. The inhibitory action of MIP-1α, and the inability of MIP-1β to function as an inhibitor were subsequently confirmed.[258] MIP-1β is in fact able to block the suppressive effects of MIP-1α on BFU-E (burst-forming unit erythrocyte), CFU-GEMM (granulocytes, erythroid cells, macrophages, and megakaryocytes), and CFU-GM colony formation.[259] However, this block occurred only when MIP-1β was added in an excess to MIP-1α; a 1:1 ratio did not result in a block of MIP-1α inhibition (explaining why MIP-1, composed of a 1:1 ratio of MIP-1α and MIP-1β, was active as an inhibitor in earlier studies).[258, 259]

The ability of MIP-1α to function in vivo as an inhibitor of stem cell proliferation has also been addressed in several studies. Human MIP-1α is active in a dose-dependent manner in vitro on day 12 CFU-S cells and to a lesser extent on more mature day 8 CFU-S cells.[260] Administration of multiple doses of MIP-1α is also sufficient to protect the CFU-A/S compartment after treatment with the cytotoxic drug cytosine arabinoside (ara-C).[260] MIP-1α will also protect CFU-S cells against the cytotoxic effects of hydroxyurea.[261] However, a subsequent study showed that more primitive stem cells were not protected by human MIP-1α.[262] In this model, a primary injection of 5-fluorouracil (5-FU) was used to eliminate late progenitors and cause the more primitive, and normally quiescent, long-term repopulating (LTR) stem cells to enter the cell cycle and therefore become sensitive to administration of a second dose of 5-FU. MIP-1α did not prevent the depletion of LTR stem cells after the second 5-FU injection, suggesting that it does not prevent cycling of the LTR stem cells. MIP-1α is able to inhibit the formation of more mature hematopoietic progenitors, however. Cytotoxic drugs (such as ara-C, hydroxyurea, and 5-FU) that target specific stages of the cell cycle are not the only drugs used in chemotherapy. They are often used in combination with non–S phase drugs, such as cyclophosphamide. Studies are currently being undertaken to address whether MIP-1α is a potentially useful myeloprotective agent against therapeutic regimens that are more applicable to current clinical settings.[263]

The therapeutic value of MIP-1α against leukemic cells is also being investigated. MIP-1α does not inhibit the cycling of primitive chronic myeloid leukemia (CML) cells supported in long-term cultures.[264] MIP-1α does, however, inhibit the activation of normal primitive progenitors (but not more mature ones) in similar long-term cultures. This provides hope that MIP-1α could prove useful in a therapeutic role by providing protection of normal primitive stem cells against any cytotoxic agents, such as those used in chemotherapy, while simultaneously leaving CML cells susceptible. CML cells are relatively refractory to inhibition by MIP-1α; moreover, these CML cells express levels of MIP-1α receptors similar to those of normal CD34+ cells.[265] This suggests that the inability of MIP-1α to inhibit CML cells may lie in a downstream signaling event. MIP-1α can inhibit the proliferation of subsets of acute myelogenous leukemia (AML) progenitors.[266] However, contradictory data also show that some subsets of AML cells are not inhibited by MIP-1α.[267] It is possible nevertheless that in addition to CML cells, some subsets of AML cells may be potential targets for therapeutic regimens, in conjunction with MIP-1α as a protective agent.

In addition to its inhibition of bone marrow hematopoiesis, MIP-1α functions in vitro as a potent, reversible inhibitor of both human and murine epidermal keratinocyte proliferation.[268] MIP-1α mRNA is produced by epidermal Langerhans cells, and it is proposed that within the skin, epidermal stem cells are held quiescent by MIP-1α derived from Langerhans cells located within the same epidermal proliferative unit.[77, 269]

Inhibition by MIP-1α seems to occur on a relatively restricted subset of hematopoietic stem cells, represented by the CFU-A/S compartment. MIP-1α will not inhibit the most primitive stem cells or more mature ones. In fact, it appears to function as a stimulator of more mature progenitors. In this respect, MIP-1α shares many similarities with TGF-β. Indeed, MIP-1α and TGF-β show overlapping as well as distinct functions on hematopoietic stem cells.[270] MIP-1α and MIP-1β have extensive homology to each other, but MIP-1α is more effective as an inhibitor than TGF-β. However, the question of whether MIP-1α actually plays a role in vivo in regulating hematopoietic stem cell proliferation is still open to question. MIP-1α–deficient mice have been generated and exhibit normal hematopoiesis, although it is possible that so-called redundancy exists and another chemokine may fulfill the hematopoietic functions of MIP-1α.[112] However, regardless of whether MIP-1α actually plays a role in vivo in regulating hematopoietic stem cell proliferation, MIP-1α may nevertheless be of potential benefit in the development of better stem cell transplantation therapies. For a more detailed understanding of hematopoietic stem cells and the role of MIP-1α and other regulators in controlling their proliferation, the reader is referred to the reviews in references 271 and 272.

In addition to MIP-1α, other chemokines such as PF-4, IL-8, and MCP-1 have been reported to function as inhibitors of colony formation from cytokine-stimulated progenitor cells.[273] There is increasing evidence that IL-8 may also function as a regulator of hematopoietic stem cell proliferation. A single injection of IL-8 rapidly mobilizes hematopoietic progenitors, and stem cell factor augments this mobilization.[274–276] Further evidence comes from the study of mice deficient in the putative murine IL-8 receptor homologue (see earlier section on CXCR1 and CXCR2).

The exact mechanisms by which chemokines are able to inhibit or stimulate hematopoietic stem cell proliferation are at present unknown. For instance, current evidence suggests that the inhibitory effects of MIP-1α are not mediated through any currently identified GPCR and instead may occur through an as yet unidentified receptor. It is also possible that inhibition occurs through known receptors, but in a manner that is undetermined. The first clues as to how this inhibition may occur are just becoming evident. Recent data provide evidence that PF-4 may prevent the downregulation of the cyclin-dependent kinase inhibitor p21[Cip1/WAF1], although this study investigated the inhibition of human endothelial cell proliferation (human umbilical vein endothelial cell proliferation) rather than inhibition of stem cells.[277] Nevertheless, this is the first evidence that a chemokine is able to disrupt the function of components involved in the control of the cell cycle.

SDF-1 is also a chemoattractant for human CD34+ progenitor cells.[278] These progenitors consist of moderately primitive and more lineage committed CD34+ cells. This suggests that SDF-1 may be important in the migration and homing of bone marrow CD34+ progenitors to different organs during development and to different niches during the differentiation and maturation of hematopoietic progenitor cells. Such a role would certainly provide a feasible explanation for the myelopoietic defects observed in SDF-1$^{-/-}$ mice.[22, 170, 171] Indeed, data from several studies provide yet more support for a crucial role for CXCR4 and SDF-1 in the homing of stem cells. Overexpression of CD4 and CXCR4 receptors on murine CD4+ cells leads to the enhanced homing of these cells to the murine bone marrow.[279] SDF-1 and CXCR4 are critical for the engraftment of human severe combined immunodeficient (SCID) repopulating cells in murine bone marrow.[280] Furthermore, antibodies against CXCR4 prevent engraftment of these human cells in murine bone marrow. Stem cells expressing high levels of CXCR4 (CD38$^-$/CXCR4$^+$) appear to represent a population of stem cells with the potential to migrate and repopulate. This suggests that increasing the expression of CXCR4 on transplanted stem cells could help to increase the engraftment and repopulating potential of such transplantation procedures.

It is impossible to detail within this review all the chemokines that have been reported to have hematopoietic effects. In addition to those chemokines that have been well characterized in hematopoiesis and therefore mentioned previously in this review, many other novel chemokines may also function in aspects of hematopoiesis.[97, 281–284] Table 15–7 shows a summary of those chemokines reported to exert effects on hematopoietic progenitors and stem cells.

Angiogenesis, Cancer, and Chemokines

▼ ANGIOGENESIS

Angiogenesis is critical for tumor growth, and there are postulated to be both inhibitors and inducers of angiogenesis

Table 15–7. Chemokines With Hematopoietic Effects

Reported Effects on Hematopoiesis	
CC Chemokines	
MIP-1α	Suppression of immature myeloid progenitors in vitro and in vivo
	Enhanced proliferation of more mature myeloid progenitors in vitro
	Inhibition of megakaryocytopoiesis in vitro
	Mobilizes hematopoietic progenitors in vivo
MIP-1β	Enhanced proliferation of more mature myeloid progenitors in vitro
	Inhibition of megakaryocytopoiesis in vitro
MCP-1	Suppression of GM-SCF/SCF-stimulated myeloid progenitors in vitro
	Cooperates with TGF-β to inhibit cycling of primitive progenitors in vitro
Eotaxin	Mobilization of eosinophil progenitors
	Synergizes with SCF to accelerate mast cell differentiation from fetal progenitors
	Synergizes with SCF to promote Mac-1+ myeloid cells from embryonic progenitors
MIP-3α	Inhibition of myeloid progenitors in vitro
MIP-3β	Chemoattraction of granulocyte-macrophage progenitors in vitro
MPIF-2	Inhibition of myeloid progenitors in vitro
MRP-2	Inhibition of myeloid progenitors in vitro.
CKβ-8	Inhibition of myeloid progenitors in vitro
LMC	Inhibition of myeloid progenitors in vitro
Lkn-1	Inhibition of myeloid progenitors in vitro
C-10	Inhibition of megakaryocytopoiesis in vitro
	Inhibition of myeloid progenitors in vitro
CXC Chemokines	
IL-8	Mobilizes hematopoietic progenitors and pluripotent stem cells in vivo
	Inhibition of megakaryocytopoiesis in vitro
GRO-β	Suppression of GM-SCF/SCF-stimulated myeloid progenitors in vitro
NAP-2	Inhibition of megakaryocytopoiesis in vitro
PF-4	Inhibition of megakaryocytopoiesis in vitro
IP-10	Inhibition of early progenitors in vitro
SDF-1	Chemoattraction of CD34+ progenitors in vitro
	SDF-1$^{-/-}$ mice show defects in B-cell lymphopoiesis and myelopoiesis

(reviewed in reference 285). As mentioned previously, some CXC chemokines appear to play a role in promoting angiogenesis. These angiogenic CXC chemokines appear to be only of the ELR type. Of these, IL-8 and PF-4 are perhaps the best characterized, but ENA-78, GCP-2, and the GRO proteins are all active as chemoattractants for endothelial cells.[18, 286, 287] They are also angiogenic in an in vitro model of angiogenesis, the rat cornea vascularization assay. Other non-ELR CXC chemokines such as PF-4, IP-10, and MIG appear to be non-angiogenic and may even act to inhibit the effects of the angiogenic ELR chemokines.[288, 289] A brief discussion follows of two chemokines, IL-8 and PF-4, reported to function, respectively, as a mediator and as an inhibitor of angiogenesis (angiostasis).

The role of IL-8 in angiogenesis was initially investigated because of its heparin-binding properties, a characteristic of many other angiogenic cytokines. Recombinant human IL-8 was shown to be potently angiogenic when implanted into the avascular cornea of rats.[18] IL-8 also induced the proliferation and chemotaxis of human umbilical vein endothelial cells. The angiogenic activity appears to be macrophage derived.[18] Increased IL-8 expression is observed in many tumor cell lines and in lung tumor tissue.[19, 290] IL-8 inhibition also attenuates angiogenesis in in vivo corneal vascularization assays and tumorigenesis of human non–small cell lung cancer.[291] Expression of IL-8 is proposed to be initiated early in human astrocytoma development and subsequently during tumor progression, and expression of the IL-8 receptors CXCR1, CXCR2, and DARC occurs in astrocytomas.[292] The observation that DARC expression is observed in human astrocytomas is particularly interesting, suggesting that DARC may well function as an endothelial cell receptor and have a role in chemokine function beyond its currently postulated role as a non-specific chemokine sink. Taken together, these and other data provide strong evidence that inhibition of IL-8 may be a potential target for therapies against the progression of particular forms of cancer.

PF-4 inhibits both angiogenesis and hematopoietic stem cell proliferation, and the processes by which these inhibitory effects are mediated are still unknown. PF-4 and derivatives of it were originally reported to inhibit angiogenesis in an in vitro assay.[288] PF-4 may also undergo proteolytic cleavage, resulting in more potent variants. One such variant has been reported to be 30 to 50 times more potent than PF-4 itself.[293]

▼ CANCER

In addition to their angiogenic or angiostatic effects (and therefore their potential role in the development of human cancers), chemokines are being intensively studied for their potential to enhance host antitumor responses. Several chemokines have been reported to show antitumor effects when they are expressed in tumor cells injected in vivo, including MCP-1, IP-10, TCA-3, and lymphotactin.[294–297] Exactly how these antitumor responses occur is unclear, but they probably occur through mononuclear, T cell, and NK cell–dependent mechanisms.

Chemokines with inhibitory effects on hematopoietic stem cell proliferation, such as MIP-1α, are of potential interest to the treatment of human leukemias. Current chemotherapeutic regimens are extremely toxic and may result in extensive hematopoietic damage to the bone marrow. Protection of the stem cell compartment by inhibitors such as MIP-1α may enable higher doses of chemotherapy to be used and thus increase the response and even survival. Indeed, genetically engineered variants are currently undergoing clinical trials.[298–301]

Animal Studies

Despite all the evidence supporting a non-redundant role for individual chemokines in leukocyte trafficking and other processes, confirmation that these events actually occur in vivo is only just beginning to emerge. The best evidence to date for in vivo roles for chemokines and their receptors has come from the derivation and analysis of genetically altered mouse models. These models fall into two basic forms: (1) generation of transgenic mice, in which the gene of interest is overexpressed by placing it under the control of a particular promoter; and (2) generation of knockout mice, in which the gene of interest is actually mutated by genetic targeting, leading to a complete absence of its expression. Each of these approaches has proved productive to defining in vivo roles for specific chemokines (see reference 302 for a review on the theory behind genetic approaches to studying chemokine function). The analysis of MCP-1 transgenic mice is one such example, and these have already been discussed in the earlier section on monocyte chemotactic proteins.[47, 48]

The first chemokine to be knocked out, MIP-1α, clearly showed a subtle but unique phenotype.[112] Whereas these mice had no overt hematopoietic abnormalities (suggesting that MIP-1α either is dispensable for normal hematopoiesis or is functionally redundant and its actions are replaced by another factor in these MIP-1α$^{-/-}$ mice), MIP-1α was required for generation of an inflammatory response to viral infection. Homozygous null mice were resistant to coxsackievirus-induced myocarditis compared with infected wild-type mice, which did develop myocarditis. A reduced pneumonitis and delayed viral clearance were also observed in influenza virus–infected MIP-1α$^{-/-}$ mice compared with infected wild-type mice. Thus, MIP-1α is involved in the inflammatory response associated with viral infection in vivo.

To date, various reports have been published on chemokine and receptor knockouts, including those for MIP-1α, MCP-1, eotaxin, SDF-1, CCR1, CCR2, CCR5, mIL-8Rh, CXCR4, and CXCR5 (see Table 15–8 for a list of chemokine and chemokine receptor knockouts). Each of these has different phenotypic defects; in some cases these are striking, whereas others are more subtle. Studies are currently ongoing to generate knockout mice for many of the chemokines and most of their receptors.

Conclusions and Future Directions

As the data from more in vivo studies become available, it is likely that further evidence for unique, non-redundant roles for individual chemokines will become apparent, and thus it may become possible to target individual chemokines

Table 15–8. Summary of Chemokine and Chemokine Receptor Mouse Knockouts

Phenotype of Mouse Knockout		Reference
CC Chemokines		
MIP-1α	Normal hematopoiesis; resistant to coxsackievirus and influenza A infection	112
MCP-1	Normal number of leukocytes and resident macrophages; decreased secondary pulmonary granulomas in response to *Schistosoma mansoni* infection; decreased levels of splenocyte IL-4, IL-5, and IFN-γ production; normal response to *Mycobacterium tuberculosis* infection	185
	Low-density lipoprotein receptor–deficient model for atherosclerosis: decreased lipid deposition, and fewer macrophages in aortic wall	126
Eotaxin	Reduced number of resident eosinophils in jejunum and thymus	86
CXC Chemokines		
SDF-1	Mice die perinatally; defects in B-cell lymphopoiesis and myelopoiesis; defect in cardiac ventricular septum formation	22
mIL-8Rh	Increased neutrophil and B-cell numbers	162
	Progenitor cells non-responsive to human IL-8 and mouse MIP-2; expansion of numbers of myeloid progenitors in bone marrow, spleen, and blood under normal/non–germ free conditions (i.e., may be inducible)	163
CC Receptors		
CCR1	Normal distribution of mature leukocytes; abnormal steady-state and induced trafficking and proliferation of myeloid progenitors; neutrophil chemotaxis and mobilization disrupted; decreased granulomas in response to *Schistosoma mansoni* infection; decreased levels of IL-4 and IL-5 and increased level of IFN-γ production, suggesting role for CCR1 in controlling balance between T_H1 and T_H2 responses	111
	Protection from pulmonary inflammation secondary to acute pancreatitis; decreased levels of TNF-α	114
CCR2	Decreased leukocyte adhesion to and reduced extravasation of monocytes	123
	Defects in macrophage recruitment and host defense	124
	Decreased lesion formation in apoE$^{-/-}$ mice, suggesting role for MCP-1 in atherosclerosis	125
	Enhanced myeloid progenitor cell cycling and apoptosis	303
CCR5	Impaired macrophage function and enhanced T cell–dependent immune responses	304
CXC Receptors		
CXCR4	Fetal lethality; defects in B-cell lymphopoiesis and myelopoiesis; defect in cardiac ventricular septum formation; fetal cerebellar development also disrupted	170, 171
	As above, but also reported to have defective formation of the large vessels supplying the gastrointestinal tract	172
CXCR5	Mice lack inguinal lymph nodes and possess no or few Peyer patches; impaired migration of lymphocytes into splenic follicles, resulting in morphologically altered primary lymphoid follicles; activated B cells also fail to migrate from T cell–rich zone into the B-cell follicles of the spleen, resulting in absence of functional B-cell germinal centers	173

or their receptors as the basis for therapies in a wide variety of human diseases. The identification of chemokine receptors as HIV entry cofactors and of the ability of certain chemokines to suppress HIV infection has given great impetus to such strategies. Indeed, a multitude of agonists, antagonists, analogues, and small molecule compounds are being tested for their ability to provide therapeutic benefits.[305–307] Whereas much focus is directed against HIV infection, some successes have already been obtained against other targets. Indeed, an antagonist of the CCR2 receptor MCP-1 (9–76), an MCP-1 analogue derived by deletions in the N terminus, was shown to inhibit arthritis in the MRL-*lpr* model, a murine model in which mice spontaneously develop a chronic inflammatory arthritis similar to human rheumatoid arthritis.[308]

A little more than 10 years ago, the chemokines were unknown. Today they are recognized as critical regulators of a wide variety of functions including normal leukocyte trafficking, inflammation, hematopoiesis, infectious disease, cancer, and development. As such, they continue to present an exciting area for further research and the development of novel therapies targeted against many human diseases.

REFERENCES

1. Walz, D.A., Wu, V.Y., Delano, R., and McCoy, L.E.: Primary structure of human platelet factor 4. Thromb. Res. 11:833, 1977.
2. Deuel, T.F., Keim, P.S., Farmer, M., and Henrikson. R.L.: Amino acid sequence of human platelet factor 4. Proc. Natl. Acad. Sci. USA 74:2256, 1977.
3. Schall, T.J.: Biology of the RANTES/SIS cytokine family. Cytokine 3:165, 1991.
4. Oppenheim, J.J., Zachariae, C.O.C., Mukaida, N., and Matsushima, K.: Properties of the novel proinflammatory supergene "intercrine" cytokine family. Annu. Rev. Immunol. 9:617, 1991.
5. Rollins, B.J.: Chemokines. Blood 90:909, 1997.
6. Wells, T.C.: The chemokine information source: identification and characterization of novel chemokines using the WorldWideWeb and expressed sequence tag databases. J. Leukoc. Biol. 61:545, 1997.
7. Luster, A.D., Unkeless, J.C., and Ravech, J.V.: γ-Interferon transcriptionally regulates an early-response gene containing homology to platelet proteins. Nature 315:672, 1985.
8. Kelner, G.S., Kennedy, J., Bacon, K.B., Kleyensteuber, S., Largaespada, D.A., Jenkins, N.A., Copeland, N.G., Bazan, J.F., Moore, K.W., Schall, T.J., and Zlotnik, A.: Lymphotactin: a cytokine that represents a new class of chemokine. Science 266:1395, 1994.
9. Bazan, J.F., Bacon, K.B., Hardiman, G., Wang, W., Soo, K., Rossi, D., Greaves, D.R., Zlotnik, A., and Schall, T.J.: A new class of membrane-bound chemokine with a CX_3C motif. Nature 385:640, 1997.

10. Pan, Y., Lloyd, C., Zhou, H., Dolich, S., Deeds, J., Gonzalo, J.-A., Vath, J., Gosselin, M., Ma, J., Dussault, B., Woolf, E., Alperin, G., Culpepper, J., Gutierrez-Ramos, J.C., and Gearing, D.: Neurotactin, a membrane-anchored chemokine upregulated in brain inflammation. Nature 387:611, 1997.

11. Beall, C.J., Mahajan, S., and Kolattukudy, P.E.: Conversion of monocyte chemoattractant protein-1 into a neutrophil attractant by substitution of two amino acids. J. Biol. Chem. 267:3455, 1992.

12. Clark-Lewis, I., Dewald, B., Geiser, T., Moser, B., and Baggiolini, M.: Platelet factor 4 binds to interleukin 8 receptors and activates neutrophils when its N terminus is modified with Glu-Leu-Arg. Proc. Natl. Acad. Sci. USA 90:3574, 1993.

13. Stoeckle, M.Y., and Barker, K.A.: Two burgeoning families of platelet factor 4–related proteins: mediators of the inflammatory response. New Biol. 2:313, 1990.

14. Yoshimura, T., Matsushima, K., Tanaka, S., Robinson, E.A., Appella, E., Oppenheim, J.J., and Leonard, E.J.: Purification of a human monocyte-derived neutrophil chemotactic factor that has peptide sequence similarity to other host-defence cytokines. Proc. Natl. Acad. Sci. USA 84:9233, 1987.

15. Schroeder, J.-M., Mrowietz, U., Morita, E., and Christophers, E.: Purification and partial biochemical characterization of a human monocyte-derived, neutrophil-activating peptide that lacks interleukin 1 activity. J. Immunol. 139:3474, 1987.

16. Larsen, C.G., Anderson, A.O., Appella, E., Oppenheim, J.J., and Matsushima, K.: Neutrophil activating protein (NAP-1) is also chemotactic for T lymphocytes. Science 243:1464, 1989.

17. Walz, A., Peveri, P., Aschauer, H., and Baggiolini, M.: Purification and amino acid sequencing of NAF, a novel neutrophil-activating factor produced by monocytes. Biochem. Biophys. Res. Commun. 149:755, 1987.

18. Koch, A.E., Polverini, P.J., Kunkel, S.L., Harlow, L.A., DiPietro, L.A., Elner, V.M., and Strieter, R.M.: Interleukin-8 as a macrophage-derived mediator of angiogenesis. Science 258:1798, 1992.

19. Smith, D.R., Polverini, P.J., Kunkel, S.L., Orringer, M.B., Whyte, R.I., Burdick, M.D., Wilke, C.A., and Strieter, R.M.: Inhibition of interleukin 8 attenuates angiogenesis in human bronchogenic carcinoma. J. Exp. Med. 179:1409, 1994.

20. Tashiro, K., Tada, H., Heilker, R., Shirozu, M., Nakano, T., and Honjo, T.: Signal sequence trap: a cloning strategy for secreted proteins and type I membrane proteins. Science 261:600, 1993.

21. Nagasawa, T., Kikutani, H., and Kishimoto, T.: Molecular cloning and structure of a pre-B-cell growth-stimulating factor. Proc. Natl. Acad. Sci. USA 91:2305, 1994.

22. Nagasawa, T., Hirota, S., Tachibana, K., Takakura, N., Nishikawa, S., Kitamura, Y., Yoshida, N., Kikutani, H., and Kishimoto, T.: Defects of B-cell lymphopoiesis and bone marrow myelopoiesis in mice lacking the CXC chemokine PBSF/SDF-1. Nature 382:635, 1996.

23. Bleul, C.C., Fuhlbrigge, R.C., Casasnovas, J.M., Aiuti, A., and Springer, T.A.: A highly efficacious lymphocyte chemoattractant, stromal cell–derived factor 1 (SDF-1). J. Exp. Med. 184:1101, 1996.

24. Dewald, B., Moser, B., Barella, L., Schumacher, C., Baggiolini, M., and Clark-Lewis, I.: IP-10, a γ-interferon–inducible protein related to interleukin-8, lacks neutrophil activating properties. Immunol. Lett. 32:81, 1992.

25. Taub, D.D., Longo, D.L., and Murphy, W.J.: Human interferon-inducible protein-10 induces mononuclear cell infiltration in mice and promotes the migration of human T lymphocytes into the peripheral tissues of human peripheral blood lymphocytes-SCID mice. Blood 87:1423, 1996.

26. Wang, X., Yue, T.-L., Ohlstein, E.H., Sung, C.-P., and Feuerstein, G.Z.: Interferon-inducible protein-10 involves vascular smooth muscle cell migration, proliferation, and inflammatory response. J. Biol. Chem. 271:24286, 1996.

27. Angiolillo, A.L., Sgadari, C., Taub, D.D., Liao, F., Farber, J.M., Maheshwari, S., Kleinman, H.K., Reaman, G.H., and Tosato, G.: Human interferon-inducible protein 10 is a potent inhibitor of angiogenesis in vivo. J. Exp. Med. 182:155, 1995.

28. Liao, F., Rabin, R.L., Yannelli, J.R., Koniaris, L.G., Vanguri, P., and Farber, J.M.: Human Mig chemokine: biochemical and functional characterization. J. Exp. Med. 182:1301, 1995.

29. Loetscher, M., Gerber, B., Loetscher, P., Jones, S.A., Piali, L., Clark-Lewis, I., Baggiolini, M., and Moser, B.: Chemokine receptor specific for IP-10 and Mig: structure, function, and expression in activated T-lymphocytes. J. Exp. Med. 184:963, 1996.

30. Cole, K.E., Strick, C.A., Paradis, T.J., Ogborne, K.T., Loetscher, M., Gladue, R.P., Lin, W., Boyd, J.G., Moser, B., Wood, D.E., Sahagan, B.G., and Neote, K.: Interferon-inducible T cell chemoattractant (I-TAC): a novel non-ELR CXC chemokine with potent activity on activated T cells through selective high affinity binding to CXCR3. J. Exp. Med. 187:2009, 1998.

31. Sarris, A.H., Broxmeyer, H.E., Wirthmueller, U., Karasavvas, N., Cooper, S., Lu, L., Drueger, J., and Ravetch, J.C.: Human interferon-inducible protein 10: expression and purification of recombinant protein demonstrate inhibition of early human hematopoietic progenitors. J. Exp. Med. 178:1127, 1993.

32. Sarris, A.H., Talpaz, M., Deisseroth, A.B., and Estrov, Z.: Human recombinant interferon-inducible protein-10 inhibits the proliferation of normal and acute myelogenous leukemia. Leukemia 10:757, 1996.

33. Schwartz, G.N., Liao, F., Gress, R.E., and Farber, J.M.: Suppressive effects of recombinant human monokine induced by IFN-γ (rHuMig) chemokine on the number of committed and primitive hemopoietic progenitors in liquid cultures of CD34+ human bone marrow cells. J. Immunol. 159:895, 1997.

34. Gewirtz, A.M., Calabretta, B., Rucinski, B., Niewiarowski, S., and Xu, W.Y.: Inhibition of human megakaryocytopoiesis in vitro by platelet factor 4 (PF4) and a synthetic COOH-terminal PF4 peptide. J. Clin. Invest. 83:1477, 1989.

35. Han, Z.C., Sensebe, L., Abgrall, J.F., and Briere, J.: Platelet factor 4 inhibits human megakaryocytopoiesis in vitro. Blood 75:1234, 1990.

36. Gewirtz, A.M., Zhang, J., Ratajczak, J., Ratajczak, M., Park, K.S., Li, C.Q., Yan, Z., and Poncz, M.: Chemokine regulation of human megakaryocytopoiesis. Blood 86:2559, 1995.

37. Han, Z.C., Lu, M., Li, J., Defard, M., Boval, B., Schlegel, N., and Caen, J.P.: Platelet factor 4 and other CXC chemokines support the survival of normal hematopoietic cells and reduce the chemosensitivity of cells to cytotoxic agents. Blood 89:2328, 1997.

38. Walz, A., Burgener, R., Car, B., Baggiolini, M., Kunkel, S.L., and Strieter, R.M.: Structure and neutrophil-activating properties of a novel inflammatory peptide (ENA-78) with homology to interleukin 8. J. Exp. Med. 174:1355, 1991.

39. Smith, J.B., and Herschman, H.R.: Glucocorticoid-attenuated response genes encode intercellular mediators, including a new C-X-C chemokine. J. Biol. Chem. 270:16756, 1995.

40. Proost, P., de Wolf-Peeters, C., Connings, R., Opdenakker, G., Billiau, A., and Van Damme, J.: Identification of a novel granulocyte chemotactic protein (GCP-2) from human tumor cells: in vitro and in vivo comparison with natural forms of GRO, IP-10, and IL-8. J. Immunol. 150:1000, 1993.

41. Yoshimura, T.K., Robinson, E.A., Tanaka, S., Appella, E., and Leonard, E.J.: Purification and amino acid analysis of two human monocyte chemoattractants produced by phytohemagglutinin-stimulated human blood mononuclear leukocytes. J. Immunol. 142:1956, 1989.

42. Rollins, B.J., Morrison, E.D., and Stiles, C.D.: Cloning and expression of JE, a gene inducible by platelet-derived growth factor and whose product has cytokine-like properties. Proc. Natl. Acad. Sci. USA 85:3738, 1988.

43. Rollins, B.J., Stier, P., Ernst, T.E., and Wong, G.G.: The human homologue of the JE gene encodes a monocyte secretory protein. Mol. Cell. Biol. 9:4687, 1989.

44. Carr, M.W., Roth, S.J., Luther, E., Rose, S.S., and Springer, T.A.: Monocyte chemoattractant protein 1 acts as a T-lymphocyte chemoattractant. Proc. Natl. Acad. Sci. USA 91:3652, 1994.

45. Taub, D.D., Sayers, T.J., Carter, C.R.D., and Ortaldo, J.R.: α and β chemokines induce NK cell migration and enhance NK-mediated cytolysis. J. Immunol. 155:3877, 1995.

46. Weber, M., Uguccioni, M., Baggiolini, M., Clark-Lewis, I., and Dahinden, C.A.: Deletion of the NH₂-terminal residue converts monocyte chemotactic protein 1 from an activator of basophil mediator release to an eosinophil chemoattractant. J. Exp. Med. 183:681, 1996.

47. Rutledge, B.J., Rayburn, H., Rosenberg, R., North, R.J., Gladue, R.P., Corless, C.L., and Rollins, B.J.: High level monocyte chemoattractant protein-1 expression transgenic mice increases their susceptibility to intracellular pathogens. J. Immunol. 155:4838, 1995.

48. Grewal, I.S., Rutledge, B.J., Fiorillo, J.A., Gu, L., Gladue, R.P., Flavell, R.A., and Rollins, B.J.: Transgenic monocyte chemoattractant protein-1 (MCP-1) in pancreatic islets produces monocyte-rich insulitis without diabetes. J. Immunol. 159:401, 1997.

49. Berman, J.W., Guida, M.P., Warren, J., Amat, J., and Brosnan, C.F.: Localization of monocyte chemoattractant peptide-1 expression in the

central nervous system in experimental autoimmune encephalomyelitis and trauma in the rat. J. Immunol. 156:3017, 1996.

50. Ransohoff, R.M., Glabinski, A., and Tani, M.: Chemokines in immune-mediated inflammation of the central nervous system. Cytokine Growth Factor Rev. 7:35, 1996.

51. Van Damme, J., Proost, P., Lenaerts, J.P., and Opdenakker, G.: Structural and functional identification of two human, tumor-derived monocyte chemotactic proteins (MCP-2 and MCP-3) belonging to the chemokine family. J. Exp. Med. 176:59, 1992.

52. Proost, P., Wuyts, A., and Van Damme, J.: Human monocyte chemotactic proteins-2 and -3: structural and functional comparison with MCP-1. J. Leukoc. Biol. 59:67, 1996.

53. Alam, R., Forsythe, P., Stafford, S., Heinrich, J., Bravo, R., Proost, P., and Van Damme, J.: Monocyte chemotactic protein-2, monocyte chemotactic protein-3, and fibrobalst-induced cytokine. J. Immunol. 153:3155, 1994.

54. Uguccioni, M., Loetscher, P., Forssmann, U., Dewald, B., Li, H., Lima, S.H., Li, Y., Kreider, B., Garotta, G., Thelen, M., and Baggiolini, M.: Monocyte chemotactic protein 4 (MCP-4), a novel structural and functional analogue of MCP-3 and eotaxin. J. Exp. Med. 183:2379, 1996.

55. Garcia-Zepeda, E.A., Combadiere, C., Rothenberg, M.E., Sarafi, M.N., Lavigne, F., Hamid, Q., Murphy, P.M., and Luster, A.D.: Human monocyte chemoattractant protein (MCP)-4 is a novel CC chemokine with activities on monocytes, eosinophils, and basophils induced in allergic and nonallergic inflammation that signals through the CC chemokine receptors (CCR)-2 and -3. J. Immunol. 157:5613, 1996.

56. Jia, G.-Q., Gonzalo, J.A., Lloyd, C., Kremer, L., Lu, L., Martinez-A, C., Wershil, B.K., and Gutierrez-Ramos, J.C.: Distinct expression and function of the novel mouse chemokine monocyte chemotactic protein-5 in lung allergic inflammation. J. Exp. Med. 184:1939, 1996.

57. Sarafi, M.N., Garcia-Zepeda, E.A., MacLean, J.A., Charo, I.F., and Luster, A.D.: Murine monocyte chemoattractant protein (MCP)-5: A novel CC chemokine that is a structural and functional homologue of human MCP-1. J. Exp. Med. 185:99, 1997.

58. Schall, T.J., Jongstra, J., Dryer, B.J., Jorgensen, J., Clayberger, C., Davis, M.M., and Krensky, A.M.: A human T-cell specific molecule is a member of a new gene family. J. Immunol. 141:1018, 1988.

59. Kameyoshi, Y., Dorschner, A., Mallet, A.I., Christophers, E., and Schroder, J.-M.: Cytokine RANTES released by thrombin-stimulated platelets is a potent attractant for human eosinophils. J. Exp. Med. 176:587, 1992.

60. Lim, K.G., Wan, H.C., Bozza, P.T., Resnick, M.B., Wong, D.T.W., Cruickshank, W.W., Kornfeld, H., Center, D.M., and Weller, P.F.: Human eosinophils elaborate the lymphocyte chemoattractants IL-16 (lymphocyte chemoattractant factor) and RANTES. J. Immunol. 156:2566, 1996.

61. Schall, T.J., Bacon, K., Toy, K.J., and Goeddel, D.V.: Selective attraction of monocytes and T lymphocytes of the memory phenotype by cytokine RANTES. Nature 347:669, 1990.

62. Roth, S.J., Carr, M.W., and Springer, T.A.: C-C chemokines, but not the C-X-C chemokines interleukin-8 and interferon-γ inducible protein-10, stimulate transendothelial chemotaxis of T lymphocytes. Eur. J. Immunol. 25:3482, 1995.

63. Rot, A., Kreiger, M., Brunner, T., Bischoff, S.C., Schall, T.J., and Dahinden, C.A.: RANTES and macrophage inflammatory protein 1α induce the migration and activation of normal human eosinophil granulocytes. J. Exp. Med. 176:1489, 1992.

64. Bischoff, S.C., Krieger, M., Brunner, T., Rot, A., Tscharner, V., Baggiolini, M., and Dahinden, C.A.: RANTES and related chemokines activate human basophil granulocytes through different G protein–coupled receptors. Eur. J. Immunol. 23:761, 1993.

65. Wolpe, S.D., Davatelis, G., Sherry, B., Beutler, B., Hesse, D.G., Nguyen, H.T., Moldawer, L., Nathan, C.F., Lowry, S.F., and Cerami, A.: Macrophages secrete a novel heparin-binding protein with inflammatory and neutrophil chemokinetic properties. J. Exp. Med. 167:570, 1988.

66. Sherry, B., Tekamp-Olson, P., Gallegos, C., Bauer, D., Davatelis, G., Wolpe, S.D., Masiarz, K., Coit, D., and Cerami, A.: Resolution of the two components of macrophage inflammatory protein 1, and cloning and characterization of one of those components, macrophage inflammatory protein 1β. J. Exp. Med. 168:2251, 1988.

67. Davatelis, G., Tekamp-Olson, P., Wolpe, S.D., Hermsen, K., Luedke, C., Gallegos, C., Coit, D., Merryweather, J., and Cerami, A.: Cloning and characterization of a cDNA for murine macrophage inflammatory

68. Obaru, K., Fukuda, M., Maeda, S., and Shimada, K.: A cDNA clone used to study mRNA inducible in human tonsillar lymphocytes by a tumour promoter. J. Biochem. 99:885, 1986.

69. Lipes, M.A., Napolitano, M., Jeang, K.-T., Chang, N.T., and Leonard, W.J.: Identification, cloning, and characterization of an immune activation gene. Proc. Natl. Acad. Sci. USA 85:9704, 1988.

70. Graham, G.J., Freshney, M.G., Donaldson, D., and Pragnell, I.B.: Purification and biochemical characterisation of human and murine stem cell inhibitors (SCI). Growth Factors 7:151, 1992.

71. Graham, G.J., MacKenzie, J., Lowe, S., Tsang, M.L.-S., Weatherbee, J.A., Issacson, A., Medicherla, J., Fang, F., Wilkinson, P.C., and Pragnell, I.B.: Aggregation of the chemokine MIP-1α is a dynamic and reversible phenomenon. J. Biol. Chem. 269:4974, 1994.

72. Burd, P.R., Rodgers, H.W., Gordon, J.R., Martin, C.A., Jayaraman, S., Wilson, S.D., Dvorak, A.M., Galli, S.J., and Dorf, M.E.: Interleukin 3–dependent and -independent mast cells stimulated with IgE and antigen express multiple cytokines. J. Exp. Med. 170:245, 1989.

73. Costa, J.J., Matossian, K., Resnick, M.B., Beil, W.J., Wong, D.T.W., Gordon, J.R., Dvorak, A.M., Weller, P.E., and Galli, S.J.: Human eosinophils can express the cytokines tumour necrosis factor-α and macrophage inflammatory protein-1α. J. Clin. Invest. 91:2673, 1993.

74. Li, H., Sim, T.C., Grant, J.A., and Alam, R.: The production of macrophage inflammatory protein-1α by human basophils. J. Immunol. 157:1207, 1996.

75. Kasama, T., Strieter, R.M., Standiford, T.J., Burdick, M.D., and Kunkel, S.J.: Expression and regulation of human neutrophil-derived macrophage inflammatory protein 1α. J. Exp. Med. 178:63, 1993.

76. Bluman, E.M., Bartynski, K.J., Avalos, B.R., and Caligiuri, M.A.: Human natural killer cells produce abundant macrophage inflammatory protein-1α in response to monocyte-derived cytokines. J. Clin. Invest. 97:2722, 1996.

77. Heufler, C., Topar, G., Koch, F., Trockenbacher, B., Kampgen, E., Romani, N., and Schuler, G.: Cytokine gene expression in murine epidermal cell suspensions: interleukin 1β and macrophage inflammatory protein 1α are selectively expressed in Langerhans cells but are differentially regulated in culture. J. Exp. Med. 176:1221, 1992.

78. Griffiths-Johnson, D.A., Collins, P.D., Rossi, A.G., Jose, P.J., and Williams, T.J.: The chemokine, eotaxin, activates guinea-pig eosinophils in vitro, and causes their accumulation into the lung in vivo. Biochem. Biophys. Res. Commun. 197:1176, 1993.

79. Jose, P.J., Griffiths-Johnson, D.A., Collins, P.D., Walsh, D.T., Moqbel, R., Totty, N.F., Truong, O., Hsuan, J.J., and Williams, T.J.: Eotaxin: a potent eosinophil chemoattractant cytokine detected in a guinea pig model of allergic airways inflammation. J. Exp. Med. 179:881, 1994.

80. Jose, P.J., Adcock, I.M., Griffiths-Johnson, D.A., Berkman, N., Wells, T.N.C., Williams, T.J., and Power, C.A.: Eotaxin: cloning of an eosinophil chemoattractant cytokine and increased mRNA expression in allergen-challenged guinea-pig lungs. Biochem. Biophys. Res. Commun. 205:788, 1995.

81. Rothenburg, M.E., Luster, A.D., and Leder, P.: Murine eotaxin: an eosinophil chemoattractant inducible in endothelial cells and in interleukin 4–induced tumour suppression. Proc. Natl. Acad. Sci. USA 92:8960, 1995.

82. Gonzalo, J., Jia, G., Aguirre, V., Friend, D., Coyle, A.J., Jenkins, N.A., Lin, G., Katz, H., Lichtman, A., Copeland, N., Kopf, M., and Gutierrez-Ramos, J.: Mouse eotaxin expression parallels eosinophil accumulation during lung allergic inflammation, but it is not restricted to a Th2-type response. Immunity 4:1, 1996.

83. Ponath, P.D., Qin, S.X., Ringler, D.J., Clark-Lewis, I., Wang, J., Kassam, N., Smith, H., Shi, X., Gonzalo, J., Newman, W., Gutierrez-Ramos, J., and Mackay, C.R.: Cloning of the human eosinophil chemoattractant, eotaxin. Expression, receptor binding and functional properties suggest a mechanism for the selective recruitment of eosinophils. J. Clin. Invest. 97:604, 1996.

84. Garcia-Zepeda, E.A., Rothenburg, M.E., Ownbey, R.T., Celestin, J., Leder, P., and Luster, A.D.: Human eotaxin is a specific chemoattractant for eosinophil cells and provides a new mechanism to explain tissue eosinophilia. Nat. Med. 2:449, 1996.

85. Ponath, P.D., Qin, S.X., Post, T.W. Wang, J., Wu, L., Gerard, N.P., Newman, W., Gerard, C., and Mackay, C.R.: Molecular cloning and characterization of a human eotaxin receptor expressed selectively on eosinophils. J. Exp. Med. 183:2437, 1996.

86. Matthews, A.N., Friend, D.S., Zimmermann, N., Sarafi, M.N., Luster,

A.D., Pearlman, E., Wert, S.E., and Rothenberg, M.E.: Eotaxin is required for the baseline level of tissue eosinophils. Proc. Natl. Acad. Sci. USA 95:6273, 1998.

87. Quackenbush, E.J., Wershil, B.K., Aguirre, V., and Gutierrez-Ramos, J.-C. Eotaxin modulates myelopoiesis and mast cell development from embryonic hematopoietic progenitors. Blood 92:1887, 1998.

88. Palframan, R.T., Collins, P.D., Williams, T.J., and Rankin, S.A.: Eotaxin induces a rapid release of eosinophils and their progenitors from the bone marrow. Blood 91:2240, 1998.

89. Miller, M.D., Hata, S., DeWaal Malefyt, R., and Krangel, M.S.: A novel polypeptide secreted by activated human T lymphocytes. J. Immunol. 143:2907, 1989.

90. Burd, P.R., Freeman, G.J., Wilson, S.D., Berman, M., DeKruyff, R., Billings, P.R., and Dorf, M.E.: Cloning and characterization of a novel T cell activation gene. J. Immunol. 139:3126, 1987.

91. Zingoni, A., Soto, H., Hedrick, J.A., Stoppacciaro, A., Storlazzi, C.T., Sinigaglia, F., D'Ambrosio, D., O'Garra, A., Robinson, D., Rocchi, M., Santoni, A., Zlotnik, A., and Napolitano, M.: The chemokine receptor CCR8 is preferentially expressed in Th2 but not Th1 cells. J. Immunol. 161:547, 1998.

92. Yoshida, T., Imai, T., Kakizaki, M., Nishimura, M., and Yoshie, O.: Molecular cloning of a novel C or γ type chemokine, SCM-1. FEBS Lett. 360:155, 1995.

93. Hedrick, J.A., Saylor, V., Figueroa, D., Mizoue, L., Xu, Y., Menon, S., Abrams, J., Handel, T., and Zlotnik, A.: Lymphotactin is produced by NK cells and attracts both NK cells and T cells in vivo. J. Immunol. 158:1533, 1997.

94. Rumsaeng, V., Vliagoftis, H., Oh, C.K., and Metcalf, D.D.: Lymphotactin gene expression in mast cells following Fcε receptor I aggregation. J. Immunol. 158:1353, 1997.

95. Fong, A.M., Robinson, L.A., Steeber, D.A., Tedder, T.F., Yoshie, O., Imai, T., and Patel, D.D.: Fractalkine and CXC₃R1 mediate a novel mechanism of leukocyte capture, firm adhesion, and activation under physiolgic flow. J. Exp. Med. 188:1413,1998.

96. Mohamadzadeh, M., Poltorak, A.N., Bergstresser, P.R., Beutler, B., and Takashima, A.: Dendritic cells produce macrophage inflammatory protein-1γ, a new member of the CC chemokine family. J. Immunol. 156:3102, 1996.

97. Orlofsky, A., Berger, M.S., and Prystowsky, M.B.: Novel expression pattern of a new member of the MIP-1 family of cytokine-like genes. Cell Regul. 2:403, 1991.

98. Youn, B.S., Jang, I.-K., Broxmeyer, H.E., Cooper, S., Jenkins, N.A., Gilbert, D.J., Copeland, N.G., Elick, T.A., Fraser, M.J., Jr., and Kwon, B.S.: A novel chemokine, macrophage inflammatory protein-related protein-2, inhibits colony formation of bone marrow myeloid progenitors. J. Immunol. 155:2661, 1995.

99. Hara, T., Bacon, K.B., Cho, L.C., Yoshimura, A., Morikawa, Y., Copeland, N.G., Gilbert, D.J., Jenkins, N.A., Schall, T.J., and Miyajima, A.: Molecular cloning and functional characterization of a novel member of the C-C chemokine family. J. Immunol. 155:5352, 1995.

100. Holmes, W.E., Lee, J., Kuang, W.-J., Rice, G.C., and Wood, W.I.: Structure and functional expression of a human interleukin-8 receptor. Science 253:1278, 1991.

101. Murphy, P.M., and Tiffany, H.L.: Cloning of complementary DNA encoding a functional human interleukin-8 receptor. Science 253:1280, 1991.

102. Neote, K., DiGregorio, D., Mak, J.Y., Horuk, R., and Schall, T.J.: Molecular cloning, functional expression and signalling characteristics of a C-C chemokine receptor. Cell 72:415, 1993.

103. Gao, J.-L., Kuhns, D.B., Tiffany, H.L., McDermott, D., Li, X., Francke, U., and Murphy, P.M.: Structure and functional expression of the human macrophage inflammatory protein 1α/RANTES receptor. J. Exp. Med. 177:1421, 1993.

104. Murphy, P.M.: Chemokine receptors: structure, function, and role in microbial pathogenesis. Cytokine Growth Factors Rev. 7:47, 1996.

105. Gutkind, J.S.: The pathways connecting G protein–coupled receptors to the nucleus through divergent mitogen-activated protein kinase cascades. J. Biol. Chem. 273:1839, 1998.

106. Nardelli, B., Tiffany, H.L., Bong, G.W., Yourey, P.A., Morahan, D.K., Li, Y., Murphy, P.M., and Alderson, R.F.: Characterization of the signal transduction pathway activated in human monocytes and dendritic cells by MPIF-1, a specific ligand for CC chemokine receptor 1. J. Immunol. 162:435, 1999.

107. Ganju, R.K., Brubaker, S.A., Meyer, J., Dutt, P., Yang, Y., Qin, X., Newman, W., and Groopman, J.E.: The α-chemokine, stromal cell–derived factor-1α, binds to the transmembrane G-protein-coupled CXCR-4 receptor and activates multiple signal transduction pathways. J. Biol. Chem. 273:23169, 1998.

108. Ben-Baruch, A., Xu, L., Young, P.R., Bengali, K., Oppenheim, J.J., and Wang, J.M.: Monocyte chemotactic protein-3 (MCP3) interacts with multiple leukocyte receptors. J. Biol. Chem. 270:22123, 1995.

109. Post, T.W., Bozic, C.R., Rothenberg, M.E., Luster, A.D., Gerard, N.P., and Gerard, C.: Molecular characterization of two murine eosinophil β chemokine receptors. J. Immunol. 155:5299, 1995.

110. Tanabe, S., Heesen, M., Berman, M.A., Fischer, M.B., Yoshizawa, I., Luo, Y., and Dorf, M.E.: Murine astrocytes express a functional chemokine receptor. J. Neurosci. 17:6522, 1997.

111. Gao, J.-L., Wynn, T.A., Chang, Y., Lee, E.J., Broxmeyer, H.E., Cooper, S., Tiffany, H.L., Westphal, H., Kwon-Chung, J., and Murphy, P.M.: Impaired host defence, hematopoiesis, granulomatous inflammation and type 1–type 2 cytokine balance in mice lacking CC chemokine receptor 1. J. Exp. Med. 185:1959, 1997.

112. Cook, D.N., Beck, M.A., Coffman, T.M., Kirby, S.L., Sheridan, J.F., Pragnell, I.B., and Smithies, O.: Requirement of MIP-1α for an inflammatory response to viral infection. Science 269:1583, 1995.

113. Graham, G.J., Wilkinson, P.C., Nibbs, R.J.B., Lowe, S., Kolset, S.O., Parker, A., Freshney, M.G., Tsang, M.L.-S., and Pragnell, I.B.: Uncoupling of stem cell inhibition from monocyte chemoattraction in MIP-1α by mutagenesis of the proteoglycan binding site. EMBO J. 15:101, 1996.

114. Gerard, C., Frossard, J.-L., Bahtia, M., Saluja, A., Gerard, N.P., Lu, B., and Steer, M.: Targeted disruption of the β-chemokine receptor CCR1 protects against pancreatitis-associated lung injury. J. Clin. Invest. 100:2022, 1997.

115. Youn, B.S., Zhang, S.M., Lee, E.K., Park, D.H., Broxmeyer, H.E., Murphy, P.M., Locati, M., Pease, J.E., Kim, K.K., Antol, K., and Kwon, B.S.: Molecular cloning of leuktactin-1: a novel human β-chemokine, a chemoattractant for neutrophils, monocytes, and lymphocytes, and a potent agonist at CC chemokine receptors 1 and 3. J. Immunol. 159:5201, 1998.

116. Youn, B.S., Zhang, S.M., Cooper, S., Broxmeyer, H.E., Antol, K., Fraser, M., Jr., and Kwon, B.S.: Characterization of Ckβ8 and Ckβ8-1: two alternatively spliced forms of human β -chemokine, chemoattractants for neutrophils, monocytes, and lymphocytes, and potent agonists at CC chemokine receptor 1. Blood 91:3118, 1998.

117. Charo, I.F., Myers, S.J., Herman, A., Franci, C., Connolly, A.J., and Coughlin, S.R.: Molecular cloning and functional expression of two monocyte chemoattractant protein 1 receptors reveals alternative splicing of the carboxyl-terminal tails. Proc. Natl. Acad. Sci. USA 91:2752, 1994.

118. Myers, S.J., Wong, L.M., and Charo, I.F.: Signal transduction and ligand specificity of the human monocyte chemoattractant protein-1 receptor in transfected embryonic kidney cells. J. Biol. Chem. 270:5786, 1995.

119. Monteclaro, F.S., and Charo, I.F.: The amino-terminal extracellular domain of the MCP-1 receptor but not the RANTES/MIP-1α receptor, confers chemokine selectivity. J. Biol. Chem. 271:19084, 1996.

120. Monteclaro, F.S., and Charo, I.F.: The amino-terminal domain of CCR2 is both necessary and sufficient for high affinity binding of monocyte chemoattractant protein 1. J. Biol. Chem. 272:23186, 1997.

121. Wong, L.-M., Myers, S.J., Tsou, C.-L., Gosling, J., Arai, H., and Charo, I.F.: Organization and differential expression of the human monocyte chemoattractant protein 1 receptor gene. J. Biol. Chem. 272:1038, 1997.

122. Arai, H., Monteclaro, F.S., Tsou, C.-L., Franci, C., and Charo, I.F.: Dissociation of chemotaxis from agonist-induced receptor internalization in a lymphocyte cell line transfected with CCR2B. J. Biol. Chem. 272:25037, 1997.

123. Kurihara, T., Warr, G., Loy, J., and Bravo, R.: Defects in macrophage recruitment and host defence in mice lacking the CCR2 chemokine receptor. J. Exp. Med. 186:1757, 1997.

124. Kuziel, W.A., Morgan, S.J., Dawson, T.C., Griffin, S., Smithies, O., Ley, K., and Maeda, N.: Severe reduction in leukocyte adhesion and monocyte extravasation in mice deficient in CC chemokine receptor 2. Proc. Natl. Acad. Sci. USA 94:12053, 1997.

125. Boring, L., Gosling, J., Cleary, M., and Charo, I.F.: Decreased lesion formation in CCR2−/− mice reveals a role for chemokines in the initiation of atherosclerosis. Nature 394:894, 1998.

126. Gu., L., Okada, Y., Clinton, S.K., Gerard, C., Sukhova, G.K., Libby, P., and Rollins, B.J.: Absence of monocyte chemoattaractant protein-

1 reduces atherosclerosis in low density lipoprotein receptor-deficient mice. Mol. Cell 2:275, 1998.

127. Kitaura, M., Nakajima, T., Imai, T., Harada, S., Combadiere, C., Tiffany, H.L., Murphy, P.M., and Yoshie, O.: Molecular cloning of human eotaxin, an eosinophil-selective CC chemokine, and identification of a specific eosinophil eotaxin receptor, CC chemokine receptor 3. J. Biol. Chem. 271:7725, 1996.

128. Uguccioni, M., Mackay, C.R., Ochensberger, B., Loetscher, P., Rhis, S., LaRosa, G.J., Rao, P., Ponath, P.D., Baggiolini, M., and Dahinden, C: High expression of the chemokine receptor CCR3 in human blood basophils. J. Clin. Invest. 100:1137, 1997.

129. Gao, J.-L., Sen, A.I., Kitaura, M., Yoshie, O., Rothenberg, M.E., Murphy, P.M., and Luster, A.D.: Identification of a mouse eosinophil receptor for the CC chemokine eotaxin. Biochem. Biophys. Res. Commun. 223:679, 1996.

130. Sallusto, F., Mackay, C.R., and Lanzavechhia, A.: Selective expression of the eotaxin receptor CCR3 by human T helper 2 cells. Science 277:2005, 1997.

131. Power, C.A., Meyer, A., Nemeth, K., Bacon, K.B., Hoogewerf, A.J., Proudfoot, A.E.I., and Wells, T.N.C.: Molecular cloning and functional expression of a novel CC chemokine receptor cDNA from a human basophilic cell line. J. Biol. Chem. 270:19495, 1995.

132. Hoogewerf, A.J., Black, D., Proudfoot, A.E.I., Wells, T.N.C., and Power, C.A.: Molecular cloning of murine CC CKR-4 and high affinity binding of chemokines to murine and human CC CKR-4. Biochem. Biophys. Res. Commun. 218:337, 1996.

133. Imai, T., Baba, M., Nishimura, M., Kakizaki, M., Takagi, S., and Yoshie, O.: The T cell–directed CC chemokine TARC is a highly specific biological ligand for CC chemokine receptor 4. J. Biol. Chem. 272:15036, 1997.

134. Imai, T., Chantry, D., Raport, C.J., Wood, C.L., Nishimura, M., Godiska, R., Yoshie, O., and Gray, P.W.: Macrophage-derived chemokine is a functional ligand for the CC chemokine receptor 4. J. Biol. Chem. 273:1764, 1998.

135. Samson, M., Labbe, O., Mollereau, C., Vassart, G., and Parmentier, M.: Molecular cloning and functional expression of a new human CC-chemokine receptor gene. Biochemistry 35:3362, 1996.

136. Raport, C.J., Gosling, J., Schweickart, V.L., Gray, P.W., and Charo, I.F.: Molecular cloning and functional characterization of a novel human CC chemokine receptor (CCR5) for RANTES, MIP-1β, and MIP-1α. J. Biol. Chem. 271:17161, 1996.

137. Combadiere, C., Ahuja, S.K., Tiffany, H.L., and Murphy, P.M.: Cloning and functional expression of CC CKR5, a human monocyte CC chemokine receptor selective for MIP-1α, MIP-1β, and RANTES. J. Leukoc. Biol. 60:147, 1996.

138. Samson, M., LaRosa, G., Libert, F., Paindavoine, P., Detheux, M., Vassart, G., and Parmentier, M.: The second extracellular loop of CCR5 is the major determinant of ligand specificity. J. Biol. Chem. 272:24934, 1997.

139. Sallusto, F., Lenig, D., Mackay, C.R., and Lanzavecchia, A.: Flexible programs of chemokine receptor expression on human polarized T helper 1 and 2 lymphocytes. J. Exp. Med. 187:875, 1998.

140. Bonecchi, R., Bianchi, G., Bordignon, P.P., D'Ambrosio, D., Lang, R., Borsatti, A., Sozzani, S., Allavena, P., Gray, P.W., Mantovani, A., and Sinigaglia, F.: Differential expression of chemokine receptors and chemotactic responsiveness of type 1 T helper cells (Th1s) and Th2s. J. Exp. Med. 187:129, 1998.

141. Loetscher, P., Uguccioni, M., Bordoli, L., Baggiolini, M., Moser, B., Chizzolini, C., and Dayer, J.-M.: CCR5 is characteristic of Th1 lymphocytes. Nature 391:344, 1998.

142. Qin, S.X., Rottman, J.B., Myers, P., Kassam, N., Weinblatt, M., Loetscher, M., Koch, A.E., Moser, B., and Mackay, C.R.: The chemokine receptors CXCR3 and CCR5 mark subsets of T cells associated with certain inflammatory reactions. J. Clin. Invest. 101:746, 1998.

143. Liao, F., Rabin, R.L., Smith, C.G., Sharma, G., Nutman, T.B., and Farber, J.M.: CC-chemokine receptor 6 is expressed on diverse memory subsets of T cells and determines responsiveness to macrophage inflammatory protein 3α. J. Immunol. 162:186, 1999.

144. Baba, M., Imai, T., Nishimura, M., Kakizaki, M., Takagi, S., Hieshima, K., Nomiyama, H., and Yoshie, O.: Identification of CCR6, the specific receptor for a novel lymphocyte-directed CC chemokine LARC. J. Biol. Chem. 272:14893, 1997.

145. Greaves, D.R., Wang, W., Dairaghi, D.J., Dieu, M.C., de Saint-Vis, B., Franz-Bacon, K., Rossi, D., Caux, C., McClanahan, T., Gordon, S., Zlotnik, A., and Schall, T.J.: CCR6, a CC chemokine receptor that interacts with macrophage inflammatory protein 3α and is highly expressed in human dendritic cells. J. Exp. Med. 186:837, 1997.

146. Yoshida, R., Imai, T., Hieshima, K., Kusuda, J., Baba, M., Kitaura, M., Nishimura, M., Kakizaki, M., Nomiyama, H., and Yoshie, O.: Molecular cloning of a novel human CC chemokine EBI1-ligand chemokine that is a specific functional ligand for EBI1, CCR7. J. Biol. Chem. 272:13803, 1997.

147. Birchenbach, M., Josefsen, K., Yalamanchili, R., Lenoir, G., and Kieff, E.: Epstein-Barr virus–induced genes: first lymphocyte-specific G protein–coupled peptide receptors. J. Virol. 67:2209, 1993.

148. Tiffany, H.L., Lautens, L.L., Gao, J.-L., Pease, J., Locati, M., Combadiere, C., Modi, W., Bonner, T.I., and Murphy, P.M.: Identification of CCR8: a monocyte and thymus receptor for the CC chemokine I-309. J. Exp. Med. 186:165, 1997.

149. Stuber-Roos, R., Loetscher, M., Legler, D.F., Clark-Lewis, I., Baggiolini, M., and Moser, B.: Identification of CCR8, the receptor for the human CC chemokine I-309. J. Biol. Chem. 272:17251, 1997.

150. D'Ambrosio, D., Iellem, I., Bonecchi, R., Mazzeo, D., Sozzani, S., Mantovani, A., and Sinigaglia, F.: Selective up-regulation of chemokine receptors CCR4 and CCR8 upon activation of polarized human type 2 Th cells. J. Immunol. 161:5111, 1998.

151. Nibbs, R.J.B., Wylie, S.M., Pragnell, I.B., and Graham, G.J.: Cloning and characterization of a novel murine β chemokine receptor, D6. J. Biol. Chem. 272:12495, 1997.

152. Nibbs, R.J.B., Wylie, S.M., Yang, J., Landau, N.R., and Graham, G.J.: Cloning and characterization of a novel promiscuous human β-chemokine receptor D6. J. Biol. Chem. 272:32078, 1998.

153. Wuyts, A., Van Osselaer, N., Haelens, A., Samson, I., Herdewijn, P., Proost, P., Ben-Baruch, A., Oppenheim, J.J., and Van Damme, J.: Characterization of synthetic human granulocyte chemotactic protein-2: usage of chemokine receptors CXCR1 and CXCR2 and in vivo inflammatory properties. Biochemistry 36:2716, 1997.

154. Ahuja, S.K., and Murphy, P.M.: The CXC chemokines growth regulated oncogene (GRO) α, GROβ, GROγ, neutrophil-activating peptide-2, and epithelial-cell-derived neutrophil attractant-78 are potent agonists for the type B, but not the type A, human interleukin-8 receptor. J. Biol. Chem. 271:20545, 1996.

155. Wuyts, A., Proost, P., Lenaerts, J.-P., Ben-Baruch, A., Van Damme, J., and Wang, J.M.: Differential usage of the CXC chemokine receptors 1 and 2 by interleukin-8, granulocyte chemotactic protein-2 and epithelial-cell-derived neutrophil attractant-78. Eur. J. Biochem. 255:67, 1998.

156. Baggiolini, M., Dewald, B., and Moser, B.: Interleukin-8 and related chemotactic cytokines—CXC and CC chemokines. Adv. Immunol. 55:97-179, 1994.

157. Oin, S., LaRosa, G., Campbell, J.J., Smith-Heath, H., Kassam, N., Shi, X., Zeng, L., Butcher, E.C., and Mackay, C.R.: Expression of monocyte chemoattractant protein-1 and interleukin-8 receptors on subsets of T cells: correlation with transendothelial chemotactic potential. Eur. J. Immunol. 26:640, 1996.

158. Lippert, U., Artuc, M., Grutzkau, A., Moller, A., Kenderessy-Szabo, A., Schadendorf, D., Norgauer, J., Hartmann, K., Schweitzer-Stenner, R., Zuberbier, T., Henz, B.M., and Kruger-Krasagakes, S.: Expression and functional activity of the IL-8 receptor type CXCR1 and CXCR2 on human mast cells. J. Immunol. 161:2600, 1998.

159. Petering, H., Gotze, O., Kimmig, D., Smolarski, R., Kapp, A., and Elsner, J.: The biologic role of interleukin-8: functional analysis and expression of CXCR1 and CXCR2 on human eosinophils. J. Immunol. 93:694, 1999.

160. Horuk, R., Martin, A.W., Wang, Z., Schweitzer, L., Gerassimides, A., Guo, H., Lu, Z., Hesselgesser, J., Perez, H.D., Kim, J., Parker, J., Hadley, T.J., and Peiper, S.C.: Expression of chemokine receptors by subsets of neurons in the central nervous system. J. Immunol. 158:2882, 1997.

161. Kulke, R., Bornscheuer, E., Schluter, C., Bartels, J., Rowert, J., Sticherling, M., and Christophers, E.: The CXC receptor 2 is overexpressed in psoriatic epidermis. J. Invest. Dermatol. 110:90, 1998.

162. Cacalano, G., Lee, J., Kikly, K., Ryan, A.M., Pitts-Meek, S., Hultgren, B., Wood, W.I., and Moore, M.W.: Neutrophil and B cell expansion in mice that lack the murine IL-8 receptor homolog. Science 265:682, 1994.

163. Broxmeyer, H.E., Cooper, S., Cacalano, G., Hague, N.L., Bailish, E., and Moore, M.W.: Involvement of interleukin (IL) 8 receptor in negative regulation of myeloid progenitor cells in vivo: evidence from mice lacking the murine IL-8 receptor homologue. J. Exp. Med. 184:1825, 1996.

164. Loetscher, M., Geiser, T., O'Reilly, T., Zwahlen, R., Baggiolini, M., and Moser, B.: Cloning of a human seven-transmembrane domain receptor, LESTR, that is highly expressed in leukocytes. J. Exp. Med. 269:232, 1994.

165. Feng, Y., Broder, C.C., Kennedy, P.E., and Berger, E.A.: HIV-1 entry cofactor: functional cDNA cloning of a seven-transmembrane, G protein–coupled receptor. Science 272:872, 1996.

166. Bleul, C.C., Farzan, M., Choe, H., Parolin, C., Clark-Lewis, I., Sodroski, J., and Springer, T.A.: The lymphocyte chemoattractant SDF-1 is a ligand for LESTR/fusin and blocks HIV-1 entry. Nature 382:829, 1996.

167. Oberlin, E., Amara, A., Bacherlie, F., Bessia, C., Virelizier, J.L., Arenzana-Seisdedos, F., Schwartz, O., Heard, J.M., Clark-Lewis, I., Legler, D.F., Loetscher, M., Baggiolini, M., and Moser, B.: The CXC chemokine SDF-1 is the ligand for LESTR/fusin and prevents infection by T-cell-line-adapted HIV-1. Nature 382:833, 1996.

168. Heesen, M., Berman, M.A., Benson, J.D., Gerard, C., and Dorf, M.E.: Cloning of the mouse fusin gene, homologue to a human HIV-1 cofactor. J. Immunol. 157:5455, 1996.

169. Frodl, R., Gierschik, P., and Moepps, B.: Genomic organization and expression of the CXCR4 gene in mouse and man: absence of a splice variant corresponding to mouse CXCR4-B in human tissues. J. Recept. Signal Transduct. Res. 18:321, 1998.

170. Zou, Y.-R., Kottmann, A.H., Kuroda, M., Taniuchi, I., and Littman, D.R.: Function of the chemokine receptor CXCR4 in haematopoiesis and in cerebellar development. Nature 393:595, 1998.

171. Ma, Q., Borghesani, P.R., Segal, R.A., Nagasawa, T., Kishimoto, T., Bronson, R.T., and Springer, T.A.: Impaired B-lymphopoiesis, myelopoiesis, and derailed cerebellar neuron migration in CXCR4- and SDF-1 deficient mice. Proc. Natl. Acad. Sci. USA 95:9448, 1998.

172. Tachibana, K., Hirota, S., Iizasa, H., Yoshida, H., Kawabata, K., Kataoka, Y., Kitamura, Y., Matsushima, K., Yoshida, N., Nishikawa, S., Kishimoto, T., and Nagasawa, T.: The chemokine receptor CXCR4 is esential for vascularization of the gastrointestinal tract. Nature 393:591, 1998.

173. Forster, R., Mattis, A.E., Kremmer, E., Wolf, E., Brem, G., and Lipp, M.: A putative chemokine receptor, BLR1, directs B cell migration to defined lymphoid organs and specific anatomic compartments of the spleen. Cell 87:1037, 1996.

174. Legler, D.F., Loetscher, M., Roos, R.S., Clark-Lewis, I., Baggiolini, M., and Moser, B.: B cell–attracting chemokine 1, a human CXC chemokine expressed in lymphoid tissues, selectively attracts B lymphocytes via BLR1/CXCR5. J. Exp. Med. 187:655, 1998.

175. Gunn, M.D., Ngo, V.N., Ansel, K.M., Ekland, E.H., Cyster, J.G., and Williams, L.T.: A B-cell homing chemokine made in lymphoid follicles activates Burkitt's lymphoma receptor-1. Nature 391:799, 1998.

176. Hadley, T.J., and Peiper, S.C.: From malaria to chemokine receptor: the emerging physiologic role of the Duffy blood group antigen. Blood 89:3077, 1997.

177. Neote, K., Darbonne, W., Ogez, J., Horuk, R., and Schall, T.J.: Identification of a promiscuous inflammatory peptide receptor on the surface of red blood cells. J. Biol. Chem. 268:12247, 1993.

178. Horuk, R., Chitnis, C.E., Darbonne, W.C., Colby, T.J., Rybicki, A., Hadley, T.J., and Miller, L.H.: A receptor for the malarial parasite *Plasmodium vivax*: the erythrocyte chemokine receptor. Science 261:1182, 1993.

179. Horuk, R., Martin, A., Hesselgesser, J., Hadley, T., Lu, Z., Wang, Z., and Peiper, S.C.: The Duffy antigen receptor for chemokines: structural analysis and expression in the brain. J. Leukoc. Biol. 59:29, 1996.

180. Middleton, J., Neil, S., Wintle, J., Clark-Lewis, I., Moore, H., Lam, C., Auer, M., Hub, E., and Rot, A.: Transcytosis and surface presentation of IL-8 by venular endothelial cells. Cell 91:385, 1997.

181. Springer, T.A.: Traffic signals for lymphocyte recirculation and leukocyte emigration: the multistep paradigm. Cell 76:301, 1994.

182. Lawrence, M.B., and Springer, T.A.: Leukocytes roll on a selectin at physiologic flow rates: distinction from and prerequisite for adhesion through integrins. Cell 65:859, 1991.

183. Tanaka, Y., Adams, D.H., Hubscher, S., Hirano, H., Siebenlist, U., and Shaw, S.: T-cell adhesion induced by proteoglycan-immobilized cytokine MIP-1β. Nature 361:79, 1993.

184. Gunn, M.D., Kyuwa, S., Tam, C., Kakiuchi, T., Matsuzawa, A., Williams, L.T., and Nakano, H.: Mice lacking expression of secondary lymphoid organ chemokine have defects in lymphocyte homing and dendritic cell localization. J. Exp. Med. 189:451, 1999.

185. Lu, B., Rutledge, B.J., Gu, L., Fiorillo, J., Lukacs, N.W., Kunkel, S.L., North, R., Gerard, C., and Rollins, B.J.: Abnormalities in monocyte recruitment and cytokine expression in monocyte chemoattractant protein-1 deficient mice. J. Exp. Med. 187:601, 1998.

186. Uguccioni, M., Mackay, C.R., Ochensberger, B., Loetscher, P., Rhis, S., LaRosa, G.J., Rao, P., Ponath, P.D., Baggiolini, M., and Dahinden, C.A.: High expression of the chemokine receptor CCR3 in human blood basophils. Role in activation by eotaxin, MCP-4, and other chemokines. J. Clin. Invest. 100:1137, 1997.

187. Loetscher, P., Seitz, M., Baggiolini, M., and Moser, B.: Interleukin-2 regulates CC chemokine expression and chemotactic responsiveness in T lymphocytes. J. Exp. Med. 184:569, 1996.

188. Rovai, L.E., Herschman, H.R., and Smith, J.B.: The murine neutrophil-chemoattractant chemokines LIX, KC, and MIP-2 have distinct induction kinetics, tissue distributions, and tissue-specific sensitivities to glucocorticoid regulation in endotoxemia. J. Leukoc. Biol. 64:494, 1998.

189. Wang, N., Tabas, I., Winchester, R., Ravalli, S., Rabbani, L.E., and Tall, A.: Interleukin 8 is induced by cholesterol loading of macrophages and expressed by macrophage foam cells in human atheroma. J. Biol. Chem. 271:8837, 1996.

190. Glabinski, A.R., Balasingam, V., Tani, M., Kunkel, S.L., Strieter, R.M., Yong, V.W., and Ransohoff, R.M.: Chemokine monocyte chemoattractant protein-1 is expressed by astrocytes after mechanical injury to the brain. J. Immunol. 156:4363, 1996.

191. Shyy, Y.J., Hsieh, H.J., Usami, S., and Chien, S.: Fluid shear stress induces a biphasic response of human monocyte chemoattractant protein 1 gene expression in vascular endothelium. Proc. Natl. Acad. Sci. USA 91:4678, 1994.

192. Berliner, J.A., Territo, M.C., Sevanian, A., Ramin, S., Kim, J.A., Bamshad, B., Esterson, M., and Fogelman, A.M.: Minimally modified low density lipoprotein stimulates monocyte endothelial interactions. J. Clin. Invest. 85:1260, 1990.

193. Nelson, P.J., Kim, H.T., Manning, W.C., Goralski, T.J., and Krensky, A.M.: Genomic organization and transcriptional regulation of the RANTES chemokine gene. J. Immunol. 151:2601, 1993.

194. Ohmori, Y., and Hamilton, T.A.: Cooperative interaction between interferon (IFN) stimulus response element and kappa B sequence motifs controls IFN gamma- and lipopolysaccharide-stimulated transcription from the murine IP-10 promoter. J. Biol. Chem. 268:6677, 1993.

195. Jarmin, D.I., Kulmburg, P.A., Huber, N.E., Baumann, G., Prieschl-Strassmayr, E.E., and Baumruker, T.: A transcription factor with AP3-like binding specificity mediates gene regulation after an allergic triggering with IgE and Ag in mouse mast cells. J. Immunol. 153:5720, 1994.

196. Prieschl, E.E., Pendl, G.G., Harrer, N.E., and Baumruker, T.: p21ras links FcεRI to NF-AT family member in mast cells. The AP3-like factor in this cell type is an NF-AT family member. J. Immunol. 155:4963, 1995.

197. Yla-Herttuala, S., Lipton, B.A., Rosenfeld, M.E., Sarkioja, T., Yoshimura, T., Leonard, E.J., Witztum, J.L., and Steinberg, D.: Expression of monocyte chemoattractant protein 1 in macrophage-rich areas of human and rabbit atherosclerotic lesions. Proc. Natl. Acad. Sci. USA 88:5252, 1991.

198. Macdermott, R.P., Sanderson, I.R., and Reinecker, H.-C.: The central role of chemokines (chemotactic cytokines) in the immunopathogenesis of ulcerative colitis and Crohn's disease. Inflammatory Bowel Dis. 4:54, 1998.

199. Mazzucchelli, L., Hauser, C., Z'graggen, K., Wagner, J., Hess, M., Laissue, J.A., and Mueller, C.: Expression of interleukin-8 gene in inflammatory bowel disease is related to the histological grade of active inflammation. Am. J. Pathol. 144:997, 1994.

200. Koch, A.E., Kunkel, S.L., Harlow, L.A., Mazarakis, D.D., Haines, G.K., Burdick, M.D., Pope, R.M., and Strieter, R.M.: Macrophage inflammatory protein-1α. A novel chemotactic cytokine for macrophages in rheumatoid arthritis. J. Clin. Invest. 93:921, 1994.

201. Kunkel, S.L., Lukacs, N., Kasama, T., and Strieter, R.M.: The role of chemokines in inflammatory joint disease. J. Leukoc. Biol. 59:6, 1996.

202. Miyagishi, R., Kikuchi, S., Fukazawa, T., and Tashiro, K.: Macrophage inflammatory protein-1α in the cerebrospinal fluid of patients with multiple sclerosis and other inflammatory neurological diseases. J. Neurol. Sci. 129:223, 1995.

203. Miyagishi, R., Kikuchi, S., Takayama, C., Inoue, Y., and Tashiro, K.: Identification of cell types producing RANTES, MIP-1α and MIP-1β in rat experimental autoimmune encephalomyelitis by in situ hybridization. J. Neuroimmunol. 77:17, 1997.

204. Hayashi, M., Luo, Y., Laning, J., Strieter, R.M., and Dorf, M.E.: Production and function of monocyte chemoattractant protein-1 and other β-chemokines in murine glial cells. J. Neuroimmunol. 60:143, 1995.

205. Ishizuka, K., Igata-Yi, R., Kimura, T., Hieshima, K., Kukita, T., Kin, Y., Misumi, Y., Yamamoto, M., Nomiyama, H., Miura, R., Takamatsu, J., Katsuragi, S., and Miyakawa, T.: Expression and distribution of CC chemokine macrophage inflammatory protein-1α/LD78 in the human brain. Neuroreport 8:1215, 1997.

206. Karpus, W.J., Lukacs, N.W., McRae, B.L., Strieter, R.M., Kunkel, S.J., and Miller, S.D.: An important role for the chemokine macrophage inflammatory protein-1α in the pathogenesis of the T cell–mediated autoimmune disease, experimental autoimmune encephalomyelitis. J. Immunol. 155:5003, 1995.

206a. Medzhitov, R., and Janeway, C.A., Jr.: Innate immunity: the virtues of a nonclonal system of recognition. Cell 91:295, 1997.

207. D'Souza, M.P., and Harden, V.A.: Chemokines and HIV-1 second receptors. Nat. Med. 2:1293, 1996.

208. Dalgleish, A.G., Beverly, P.C.L., Clapham, P.R., Crawford, D.H., Greaves, M.F., and Weiss, R.A.: The CD4 (T4) antigen is an essential component of the receptor for the AIDS retrovirus. Nature 312:763, 1984.

209. Cocchi, F., DeVico, A.L., Garzino-Demo, A., Arya, S.K., Gallo, R.C., and Lusso, P.: Identification of RANTES, MIP-1α, and MIP-1β as the major HIV-suppressive factors produced by CD8⁺ T cells. Science 270:1811, 1995.

210. Dragic, T., Litwin, V., Allaway, G.P., Martin, S.R., Huang, Y., Nagashima, K.A., Cayanan, C., Maddon, P.J., Koup, R.A., Moore, J.P., and Paxton, W.A.: HIV-1 entry into CD4⁺ cells is mediated by the chemokine receptor CC-CKR-5. Nature 381:667, 1996.

211. Deng, H., Lui, R., Ellmeier, W., Choe, S., Unutmaz, D., Burkhart, M., Di Marzio, P., Marmon, S., Sutton, R.E., Hill, C.M., Davis, C.B., Peiper, S.C., Schall, T.J., Littman, D.R., and Landau, N.R.: Identification of a major co-receptor for primary isolates of HIV-1. Nature 381:661, 1996.

212. Alkhatib, G., Combadiere, C., Broder, C.C., Feng, Y., Kennedy, P.E., Murphy, P.M., Berger, E.A.: CC CKR5: a RANTES, MIP-1α, MIP-1β receptor as a fusion cofactor for macrophage-tropic HIV-1. Science 272:1955, 1996.

213. Doranz, B.J., Rucker, J., Yi, Y., Smyth, R.J., Samson, M., Peiper, S.C., Parmentier, M., Collman, R.G., and Doms, R.W.: A dual-tropic primary HIV-1 isolate that uses fusin and the β-chemokine receptors CKR-5, CKR-3, and CKR-2b as fusion cofactors. Cell 85:1149, 1996.

214. Choe, H., Farzan, M., Sun, Y., Sullivan, N., Rollins, B., Ponath, P.D., Wu, L., Mackay, C.R., LaRosa, G., Newman, W., Gerard, N., Gerard, C., and Sodroski, J.: The β-chemokine receptors CCR3 and CCR5 facilitate infection by primary HIV-1 isolates. Cell 85:1135, 1996.

215. Endres, M.J., Clapham, P.R., Marsh, M., Ahuja, M., Davis Turner, J., McKnight, A., Thomas, J.F., Stoebenau-Haggarty, B., Choe, S., Vance, P.J., Wells, T.N.C., Power, C.A., Sutterwala, S.S., Doms, R.W., Landau, N.R., and Hoxie, J.A.: CD4-independent infection by HIV-2 is mediated by fusin/CXCR4. Cell 87:745, 1996.

216. Lapham, C.K., Ouyang, J., Chandrasekhar, B., Nguyen, N.Y., Dimitrov, D.S., and Golding, H.: Evidence for cell-surface association between fusin and the CD4-gp120 complex in human cell lines. Science 274:602, 1996.

217. Wu, L., Gerard, N.P., Wyatt, R., Choe, H., Parolin, C., Ruffing, N., Borsetti, A., Cardoso, A., Desjardin, E., Newman, W., Gerard, C., and Sodroski, J.: CD4-induced interaction of primary HIV-1 gp120 glycoproteins with the chemokine receptor CCR-5. Nature 384:179, 1996.

218. Cocchi, F., DeVico, A.L., Garzino-Demo, A., Cara, A., Gallo, R.C., and Lusso, P.: The V3 domain of the HIV-1 gp120 envelope glycoprotein is critical for chemokine-mediated blockade of infection. Nat. Med. 2:1244, 1996.

219. Gosling, J., Monteclaro, F.S., Atchison, R.E., Arai, H., Tsou, C.-L., Goldsmith, M.A., and Charo, I.F.: Molecular uncoupling of C-C chemokine receptor 5-induced chemotaxis and signal transduction from HIV-1 coreceptor activity. Proc. Natl. Acad. Sci. USA 94:5061, 1997.

220. Aramori, I., Zhang, J., Ferguson, S.S.G., Bieniasz, P.D., Cullen, B.R., Caron, M.G.: Molecular mechanism of desensitization of the chemokine receptor CCR-5: receptor signaling and internalization are dissociable from its role as an HIV-1 co-receptor. EMBO J. 16:4606, 1997.

221. Farzan, M., Choe, H., Martin, K.A., Sun, Y., Sidelko, M., Mackay, C.R., Gerard, N.P., Sodroski, J., and Gerard, C.: HIV-1 entry and macrophage inflammatory protein-1β–mediated signaling are independent functions of the chemokine receptor CCR5. J. Biol. Chem. 272:6854, 1997.

222. Weissman, D., Rabin, R.L., Arthos, J., Rubbert, A., Dybul, M., Swofford, R., Venkatesan, S., Farber, J.M., and Fauci, A.S.: Macrophage-tropic HIV and SIV envelope proteins induce a signal through the CCR5 chemokine receptor. Nature 389:981, 1997.

223. Davis, C.B., Dikic, I., Unutmaz, D., Hill, C.M., Arthos, J., Siani, M.A., Thompson, D.A., Schlessinger, J., and Littman, D.R.: Signal transduction due to HIV envelope interactions with chemokine receptors CXCR4 or CCR5. J. Exp. Med. 186:1793, 1997.

224. Paxton, W.A., Martin, S.R., Tse, D., O'Brien, T.R., Skurnick, J., VanDevanter, N.L., Padian, N., Braun, J.F., Kotler, D.P., Wolinsky, S.M., and Koup, R.A.: Relative resistance to HIV-1 infection of CD4 lymphocytes from persons who remain uninfected despite multiple high-risk sexual exposures. Nat. Med. 2:412, 1996.

225. Samson, M., Libert, F., Doranz, B.J., Rucker, J., Liesnard, C., Farber, J.M., Saragosti, S., Lapoumeroulie, C., Cognaux, J., Forceille, C., Muyldermans, G., Verhofstede, C., Burtonboy, G., Georges, M., Imai, T., Rana, S., Yi, Y., Smyth, R.J., Collman, R.G., Doms, R.W., Vassart, G., and Parmentier, M.: Resistance to HIV-1 infection in Caucasian individuals bearing mutant alleles of the CCR-5 chemokine receptor gene. Nature 382:722, 1996.

226. Liu, R., Paxton, W.A., Choe, S., Ceradini, D., Martin, S.R., Horuk, R., MacDonald, M.E., Stuhlmann, H., Koup, R., and Landau, N.R.: Homozygous defect in HIV-1 coreceptor accounts for resistance of some multiply-exposed individuals to HIV-1 infection. Cell 86:367, 1996.

227. Dean, M., Carrington, M., Winkler, C., Huttley, G.A., Smith, M.W., Allikmets, R., Goedert, J.J., Buchbinder, S.P., Vittinghoff, E., Gomperts, E., Donfield, S., Vlahov, D., Kaslow, R., Saah, A., Rinaldo, C., Detels, R., and O'Brien, S. J.: Genetic resolution of HIV-1 infection and progression to AIDS by a deletion allele of the CKR5 structural gene. Hemophilia Growth and Development Study, Multicenter AIDS Cohort Study, Multicenter Hemophilia Cohort Study, San Francisco City Cohort, ALIVE Study. Science 273:1856, 1996.

228. Huang, Y., Paxton, W.A., Wolinsky, S.M., Neumann, A.U., Zhang, L., He, T., Kang, S., Ceradini, D., Jin, Z., Yazdanbakhsh, K., Kunstman, K., Erickson, D., Dragon, E., Landau, N.R., Phair, J., Ho, D.D., and Koup, R.A.: The role of a mutant CCR5 allele in HIV-1 transmission and disease progression. Nat. Med. 2:1240, 1996.

229. Biti, R., Ffrench, R., Young, J., Bennetts, B., Stewart, G., and Liang, T.: HIV-1 infection in an individual homozygous for the CCR5 deletion allele. Nat. Med. 3:252, 1997.

230. Michael, N.L., Chang, G., Louie, L.G., Mascola, J.R., Dondero, D., Birx, D.H., and Sheppard, H.W.: The role of viral phenotype and CCR5 gene defects in HIV-1 transmission and disease progression. Nat. Med. 3:338, 1997.

231. Michael, N.L., Louie, L.G., Rohrbaugh, A.L., Schultz, K.A., Dayhoff, D.E., Wang, E., and Sheppard, H.W.: The role of CCR5 and CCR2 polymorphisms in HIV-1 transmission and disease progression. Nat. Med. 3:1160, 1997.

232. Smith, M.W., Dean, M., Carrington, M., Winkler, C., Huttley, G.A., Lomb, D.A., Goedert, J.J., O'Brien, T.R., Jacobson, L.P., Kaslow, R., Buchbinder, S., Vittinghoff, E., Vlahov, D., Hoots, K., Hilgartner, M.W., and O'Brien, S.J.: Contrasting genetic influences of CCR2 and CCR5 variants on HIV-1 infection and disease progression. Hemophilia Growth and Development Study (HGDS), Multicenter AIDS Cohort Study (MACS), Multicenter Hemophilia Cohort Study (MHCS), San Francisco City Cohort (SFCC), ALIVE Study. Science 277:959, 1997.

233. Moriuchi, H., Moriuchi, M., Combadiere, C., Murphy, P.M., and Fauci, A.S.: CD8⁺ T-cell-derived soluble factors(s), but not β-chemokines RANTES, MIP-1α, and MIP-1β, suppress HIV-1 replication in monocyte/macrophages. Proc. Natl. Acad. Sci. USA 93:15341, 1996.

234. Pal, R., Garzino-Demo, A., Markham, P.D., Burns, J., Brown, M., Gallo, R.C., and DeVico, A.L.: Inhibition of HIV-1 infection by the β-chemokine MDC. Science 278:695, 1997.

235. Winkler, C., Modi, W., Smith, M.W., Nelson, G.W., Wu, X., Carrington, M., Dean, M., Honjo, T., Tashiro, K., Yabe, D., Buchbinder, S., Vittinghoff, E., Goedert, J., O'Brien, T.R., Jacobson, L.P., Detels, R., Donfield, S., Willoughby, A., Gomperts, E., Vlahov, D., Phair, J., and O'Brien, S.J.: Genetic restriction of AIDS pathogenesis by an SDF-1 chemokine gene variant. ALIVE Study, Hemophilia Growth and

Development Study (HGDS), Multicenter AIDS Cohort Study (MACS), Multicenter Hemophilia Cohort Study (MHCS), San Francisco City Cohort (SFCC). Science 279:389, 1998.

236. He, J., Chen, Y., Farzan, M., Choe, H., Ohagen, A., Gartner, S., Busciglio, J., Yang, X., Hofmann, W., Newman, W., Mackay, C.R., Sodroski, J., and Gabuzda. D.: CCR3 and CCR5 are co-receptors for HIV-1 infection of microglia. Nature 385:645, 1997.

237. Horuk, R., Hesselgesser, J., Zhou, Y., Faulds, D., Halks-Miller, M., Harvey, S., Taub, D., Samson, M., Parmentier, M., Rucker, J., Doranz, B.J., and Doms, R.W.: The CC chemokine I-309 inhibits CCR8-dependent infection by diverse HIV-1 strains. J. Biol. Chem. 273:386, 1998.

238. Reeves, J.D., McKnight, A., Potempa, S., Simmons, G., Gray, P.W., Power, C.A., Wells, T., Weiss, R.A., and Talbot, S.J.: CD4-independent infection by HIV-2 (ROD/B): use of the 7-transmembrane receptors CXCR-4, CCR-3, and V28 for entry. Virology 231:130, 1997.

239. Rucker, J., Edinger, A.L., Sharron, M., Samson, M., Lee, B., Berson, J.F., Li, Y., Margulies, B., Collman, R.G., Doranz, B.J., Parmentier, M., and Doms, R.W: Utilization of chemokine receptors, orphan receptors, and herpesvirus-encoded receptors by diverse human and simian immunodeficiency viruses. J. Virol. 71:8999, 1997.

240. Liao, F., Alkhatib, G., Peden, K.W.C., Sharma, G., Berger, E.A., and Farber, J.M.: STRL33, a novel chemokine receptor–like protein, functions as a fusion cofactor for both macrophage-tropic and T cell line–tropic HIV-1. J. Exp. Med. 185:2015, 1997.

241. Loetscher, M., Amara, A., Oberlin, E., Brass., N., Legler, D.F., Loetscher, P., D'Apuzzo, M., Meese, E., Rousset, D., Virelizier, J.-L., Baggiolini, M., Arenzana-Seisdedos, F., and Moser, B.: TYMSTR, a putative chemokine receptor selectively expressed in activated T cells, exhibits HIV-1 coreceptor function. Curr. Biol. 7:652, 1997.

242. Farzan, M., Choe, H., Martin, K., Marcon, L., Hofmann, W., Karlsson, G., Sun, Y., Barrett, P., Marchand, N., Sullivan, N., Gerard, N., Gerard, C., and Sodroski, J.: Two orphan seven-transmembrane segment receptors which are expressed in CD4-positive cells support simian immunodeficiency virus infection. J. Exp. Med. 186:405, 1997.

243. Choe, H., Farzan, M., Konkel, M., Martin, K., Sun, Y., Marcon, L., Cayabyab, M., Berman, M., Dorf, M.E., Gerard, N., Gerard, C., and Sodroski, J.: The ophan seven-transmembrane receptor Apj supports the entry of primary T-cell-line-tropic and dualtropic human immunodeficiency virus type 1. J. Virol. 72:6113, 1998.

244. Edinger, A.L., Hoffman, T.L., Sharron, M., Lee, B., Yi, Y., Choe, W., Kolson, D.L., Mitrovic, B., Zhou, Y., Faulds, D., Collman, R.G., Hesselgesser, J., Horuk, R., and Doms, R.W.: An orphan seven-transmembrane domain receptor expressed widely in the brain functions as a co-receptor for human immunodeficiency virus type 1 and simian immunodeficiency virus. J. Virol. 72:7934, 1998.

245. Pleskoff, O., Treboute, C., Brelot, A., Heveker, N., Seman, M., and Alizon, M.: Identification of a chemokine receptor encoded by human cytomegalovirus as a cofactor for HIV-1 entry. Science 276:1874, 1997.

246. Gao, J.-L., and Murphy, P.M.: Human cytomegalovirus open reading frame *US28* encodes a functional β chemokine receptor. J. Biol. Chem. 269:28539, 1994.

247. Bodaghi, B., Jones, T.R., Zipeto, D., Vita, C., Sun, L., Laurent, L., Arenzana-Seisdedos, F., Virelizier, J.-L., and Michelson, S.: Chemokine sequestration by viral chemoreceptors as a novel viral escape strategy: withdrawal of chemokines from the environment of cytomegalovirus-infected cells. J. Exp. Med. 188:855, 1998.

248. Ahuja, S.K., and Murphy, P.M.: Molecular piracy of mammalian interleukin-8 receptor type B by Herpesvirus saimiri. J. Biol. Chem. 268:20691, 1993.

249. Moore, P.S., Boshoff, C., Weiss, R.A., and Chang, Y.: Molecular mimicry of human cytokine and cytokine response pathway genes by KSHV. Science 274:1739, 1996.

250. Arvanitakis, L., Geras-Raaka, E., Varma, A., Gershengorn, M.C., and Cesarman, E.: Human herpesvirus KSHV encodes a constitutively active G-protein-coupled receptor linked to cell proliferation. Nature 385:347, 1997.

251. Bais, C., Santomasso, B., Coso, O., Avaranitakis, L., Raaka, E.G., Gutkind, J.S., Asch, A.S., Cesarman, E., Gerhengorn, M.C., and Mesri, E. A.: G-protein-coupled receptor of Kaposi's sarcoma–associated herpesvirus is a viral oncogene and angiogenesis activator. Nature 391:86, 1998.

252. Kledal, T.N., Rosenkilde, M.M., Coulin, F., Simmons, G., Johnsen, A.H., Alouani, S., Power, C.A., Luttichau, H.R., Gerstoft, J., Clapham,

P.R., Clark-Lewis, I., Wells, T.N.C., and Schwartz, T.W.: A broad-spectrum chemokine antagonist encoded by Kaposi's sarcoma-associated herpes virus. Science 277:1656, 1997.

253. Boshoff, C., Endo, Y., Collins, P.D., Takeuchi, Y., Reeves, J.D., Schweickart, V.L., Siani, M.A., Sasaki, T., Williams, T.J., Gray, P.W., Moore, P.S., Chang, Y., and Weiss, R.A.: Angiogenic and HIV-inhibitory functions of KSHV-encoded chemokines. Science 278:290, 1997.

254. Krathwohl, M.D., Hromas, R., Brown, D.R., and Broxmeyer, H.E.: Functional characterization of the C-C chemokine–like molecules encoded by molluscum contagiosum virus types 1 and 2. Proc. Natl. Acad. Sci. USA 94:9875, 1997.

255. Lalani, A.S., Graham, K., Mossman, K., Rajarathnam, K., Clark-Lewis, I., Kelvin, D., and McFadden, G.: The purified myxoma virus gamma interferon receptor homolog M-T7 interacts with the heparin-binding domains of chemokines. J. Virol. 71:4356, 1997.

256. Broxmeyer, H.E., Sherry, B., Lu, L., Cooper, S., Carow, C., Wolpe, S.D., and Cerami, A.: Myelopoietic enhancing effects of murine macrophage inflammatory proteins 1 and 2 on colony formation in vitro by murine and human bone marrow granulocyte/macrophage progenitor cells. J. Exp. Med. 170:1583, 1989.

257. Graham, G.J., Wright, E.G., Hewick, R., Wolpe, S.D., Wilkie, N.M., Donaldson, D., Lorimore, S., and Pragnell, I.B.: Identification and characterization of an inhibitor of haemopoietic stem cell proliferation. Nature 344:442, 1990.

258. Broxmeyer, H.E., Sherry, B., Lu, L., Cooper, S., Oh, K.-O., Tekamp-Olson, P., Kwon, B.S., and Cerami, A.: Enhancing and suppressing effects of recombinant murine macrophage inflammatory proteins on colony formation in vitro by bone marrow myeloid progenitor cells. Blood 76:1110, 1990.

259. Broxmeyer, H.E., Sherry, B., Cooper, S., Ruscetti, F.W., Williams, D.E., Arosio, P., Kwon, B.S., and Cerami, A.: Macrophage inflammatory protein (MIP)-1β abrogates the capacity of MIP-1α to suppress myeloid progenitor cell growth. J. Immunol. 147:2586, 1991.

260. Dunlop, D., Wright, E.G., Lorimore, S., Graham, G.J., Holyoake, T., Kerr, D.J., Wolpe, S.D., and Pragnell, I.B.: Demonstration of stem cell inhibition and myeloprotective effects of SCI/rhMIP-1α in vivo. Blood 79:2221, 1992.

261. Lord, B.I., Dexter, T.M., Clements, J.M., Hunter, M.G., and Gearing, A.J.H.: Macrophage-inflammatory protein protects multipotent hematopoietic cells from the cytotoxic effects of hydroxyurea in vivo. Blood 79:2605, 1992.

262. Quesniaux, V.F.J., Graham, G.J., Pragnell, I., Donaldson, D., Wolpe, S.D., Iscove, N.N., and Fagg, B.: Use of 5-fluorouracil to analyze the effect of macrophage inflammatory protein-1α on long-term reconstituting stem cells in vivo. Blood 81:1497, 1993.

263. Marshall, E., Woolford, L.B., and Lord, B.I.: Continuous infusion of macrophage inflammatory protein MIP-1α enhances leucocyte recovery and haemopoietic progenitor cell mobilization after cyclophosphamide. Br. J. Cancer 75:1715, 1997.

264. Eaves, C.J., Cashman, J.D., Wolpe, S.D., and Eaves, A.C.: Unresponsiveness of primitive chronic myeloid leukemia cells to macrophage inflammatory protein 1α, an inhibitor of primitive normal hematopoietic cells. Proc. Natl. Acad. Sci. USA 90:12015, 1993.

265. Chasty, R.C., Lucas, G.S., Owen-Lynch, P.J., Pierce, A., and Whetton, A.D.: Macrophage inflammatory protein-1α receptors are present on cells enriched for CD34 expression from patients with chronic myeloid leukemia. Blood 86:4270, 1995.

266. Ferrajoli, A., Talpaz, M., Zipf, T.F., Hirsch-Ginsberg, C., Estey, E., Wolpe, S.D., and Estrov, Z.: Inhibition of acute myelogenous leukemia progenitor proliferation by macrophage inflammatory protein 1-α. Leukemia 8:798, 1994.

267. Owen-Lynch, P.J., Adams, J.A., Brereton, M.L., Czaplewski, L.G., Whetton, A.D., and Liu Yin, J.A.: The effect of the chemokine rhMIP-1α, and a non-aggregating variant BB-10010, on blast cells from patients with acute myeloid leukaemia. Br. J. Haematol. 95:77, 1996.

268. Parkinson, E.K., Graham, G.J., Daubersies, P., Burns, J.E., Heufler, C., Plumb, M., Schuler, G., and Pragnell, I.B.: Hemopoietic stem cell inhibitor (SCI/MIP-1α) also inhibits clonogenic epidermal keratinocyte proliferation. J. Invest. Dermatol. 101:113, 1993.

269. Graham, G.J., and Pragnell, I.B.: SCI/MIP-1α: a potent stem cell inhibitor with potential roles in development. Dev. Biol. 151:377, 1992.

270. Keller, J.R., Bartelmez, S.H., Sitnicka, E., Ruscetti, F.W., Ortiz, M., Gooya, J.M., and Jacobsen, S.E.W.: Distinct and overlapping direct effects of macrophage inflammatory protein-1α and transforming

growth factor β on hematopoietic progenitor/stem cell growth. Blood 84:2175, 1994.

271. Graham, G.J.: Growth inhibitors in haemopoiesis and leukaemogenesis. Baillieres Clin. Haematol. 10:539, 1997.

272. Graham, G.J., and Wright, E.G.: Haemopoietic stem cells: their heterogeneity and regulation. Int. J. Exp. Pathol. 78:197, 1997.

273. Broxmeyer, H.E., Sherry, B., Cooper, S., Lu, L., Maze, R., Beckmann, M.P., Cerami, A., and Ralph, P.: Comparative analysis of the human macrophage inflammatory protein family of cytokines (chemokines) on proliferation of human myeloid progenitor cells. J. Immunol. 150:3448, 1993.

274. Laterveer, L., Lindley, I.J.D., Hamilton, M.S., Willemze, R., and Fibbe, W.E.: Interleukin-8 induces rapid mobilization of hematopoietic stem cells with radioprotective capacity and long-term myelolymphoid repopulating ability. Blood 85:2269, 1995.

275. Laterveer, L., Lindley, I.J.D., Heemskerk, D.P.M., Camps, J.A.J., Pauwels, E.K.J., Willemze, R., and Fibbe, W.E.: Rapid mobilization of hematopoietic progenitor cells in rhesus monkeys by a single intravenous injection of interleukin-8. Blood 87:781, 1996.

276. Laterveer, L., Zijlmans, J.M., Lindley, I.J.D., Hamilton, M.S., Willemze, R., and Fibbe, W.E.: Improved survival of lethally irradiated recipient mice transplanted with circulating progenitor cells mobilized by IL-8 after pretreatment with stem cell factor. Exp. Hematol. 24:1387, 1996.

277. Gentilini, G., Kirschbaum, N.E., Augustine, J.A., Aster, R.H., and Visentin, G.P.: Inhibition of human umbilical vein endothelial cell proliferation by the CXC chemokine, platelet factor 4 (PF4), is associated with impaired downregulation of p21$^{Cip1/WAF1}$. Blood 93:25, 1999.

278. Aiuti, A., Webb, I.J., Bleul, C., Springer, T., and Gutierrez-Ramos, J.C.: The chemokine SDF-1 is a chemoattractant for human CD34$^+$ hematopoietic progenitor cells and provides a new mechanism to explain the mobilization of CD34$^+$ progenitors to peripheral blood. J. Exp. Med. 185:111, 1997.

279. Sawada, S., Gowrishankar, K., Kitamura, R., Suzuki, M., Tahara, S., and Koito, A.: Disturbed CD4$^+$ T cell homeostasis and in vitro HIV-1 susceptibility in transgenic mice expressing T cell–line tropic HIV-1 receptors. J. Exp. Med. 187:1439, 1998.

280. Peled, A., Petit, I., Kollet, O., Magid, M., Ponomaryov, T., Byk, T., Nagler, A., Ben-Hur, H., Many, A., Shultz, L., Lider, O., Alon, R., Zipori, D., and Lapidot, T.: Dependence of human stem cell engraftment and repopulation of NOD/SCID mice on CXCR4. Science 283:845, 1999.

281. Hromas, R., Gray, P.W., Chantry, D., Godiska, R., Krathwohl, M., Fife, K., Bell, G.I., Takeda, J., Aronica, S., Gordon, M., Cooper, S., Broxmeyer, H.E., and Klemsz, M.J.: Cloning and characterization of Exodus, a novel β-chemokine. Blood 89:3315, 1997.

282. Hromas, R., Kim, C.H., Klemsz, M., Krathwohl, M., Fife, K., Cooper, S., Schnizlein-Bick, C., and Broxmeyer, H.E.: Isolation and characterization of Exodus-2, a novel C-C chemokine with a unique 37–amino acid carboxyl-terminal extension. J. Immunol. 159:2554, 1997.

283. Patel, V.P., Kreider, B.L., Li, Y., Li, H., Leung, K., Salcedo, T., Nardelli, B., Pippalla, V., Gentz, S., Thotakura, R., Parmelee, D., Gentz, R., and Garotta, G.: Molecular and functional characterization of two novel human C-C chemokines as inhibitors of two distinct classes of myeloid progenitors. J. Exp. Med. 185:1163, 1997.

284. Kim, C.H., Pelus, L.M., White, J.R., and Broxmeyer, H.E.: Macrophage-inflammatory protein-3β/EBI1-ligand chemokine/CKβ-11, a CC chemokine, is a chemoattractant with a specificity for macrophage progenitors among myeloid progenitor cells. J. Immunol. 161:2580, 1998.

285. Hanahan, D., and Folkman, J.: Patterns and emerging mechanisms of the angiogenic switch during tumorigenesis. Cell 86:353, 1996.

286. Strieter, R.M., Polverini, P.J., Kunkel, S.L., Arenberg, D.A., Burdick, M.D., Kasper, J., Dzuiba, J., Van, D.J., Walz, A., Marriott, D., Chan, S.Y., Roczniak, S., Shanafelt, A.B.: The functional role of the ELR motif in CXC chemokine–mediated angiogenesis. J. Biol. Chem. 270:27348, 1995.

287. Strieter, R.M., Polverini, P.J., Arenberg, D.A., Walz, A., Opdenakker, G., Van Damme, J., and Kunkel, S.L.: Role of C-X-C chemokines as regulators of angiogenesis in lung cancer. J. Leukoc. Biol. 57:752, 1995.

288. Maione, T.E., Gray, G.S., Petro, J., Hunt, A.J., Donner, A.L., Bauer, S.I., Carson, H.F., and Sharpe, R.J.: Inhibition of angiogenesis by recombinant human platelet factor-4 and related peptides. Science 247:77, 1990.

289. Angiolillo, A.L., Sgadari, C., Taub, D.D., Liao, F., Farber, J.M., Maheshwari, S., Kleinman, H.K., Reaman, G.H., and Tosato, G.: Human interferon-inducible protein 10 is a potent inhibitor of angiogenesis in vivo. J. Exp. Med. 182:155, 1995.

290. Van Meir, E., Ceska, F., Effenberger, F., Walz, A., Grouzmann, E., Desbaillets, I., Frei, K., Fontana, A., and deTribolet, N.: Interleukin-8 is produced in neoplastic and infectious disease of the human central nervous system. Cancer Res. 52:4297, 1992.

291. Arenberg, D.A., Kunkel, S.L., Polverini, P.J., Glass, M., Burdick, M.D., and Steiter R.M.: Inhibition of interleukin-8 reduces tumorigenesis of human non-small cell lung cancer in SCID mice. J. Clin. Invest. 97:2792, 1996.

292. Desbaillets, I., Diserens, A.-C., deTribolet, N., Hamou, M.-F., and Van Meir, E.G.: Upregulation of interleukin 8 by oxygen-deprived cells in glioblastoma suggests a role in leukocyte activation, chemotaxis, and angiogenesis. J. Exp. Med. 186:1201, 1997.

293. Gupta, S.K., Hassel, T., and Singh, J.P.: A potent inhibitor of endothelial cell proliferation is generated by proteolytic cleavage of the chemokine platelet factor 4. Proc. Natl. Acad. Sci. USA 92:7799, 1995.

294. Rollins, B.J., and Sunday, M.E.: Suppression of tumor formation in vivo by expression of the JE gene in malignant cells. Mol. Cell. Biol. 11:3125, 1991.

295. Luster, A.D., and Leder, P.: IP-10, a -C-X-C- chemokine, elicits a potent thymus-dependent anti-tumor response in vivo. J. Exp. Med. 178:1057, 1993.

296. Laning, J., Kawasaki, H., Tanaka, E., Luo, Y., and Dorf, M.E.: Inhibition of in vivo tumor growth by the beta chemokine TCA3. J. Immunol. 153:4625, 1994.

297. Dilloo, D., Bacon, K., Holden, W., Zhong, W., Burdach, S., Zlotnik, A., and Brenner, M.: Combined chemokine and cytokine gene transfer enhances antitumor immunity. Nat. Med. 2:1090, 1996.

298. Hunter, M.G., Bawden, L., Brotherton, D., Craig, S., Cribbes, S., Czaplewski, L.G., Dexter, T.M., Drummond, A.H., Gearing, A.H., Heyworth, C.M., Lord, B.I., McCourt, M., Varley, P.G., Wood, L.M., Edwards, R.M., and Lewis, P.J.: BB-10010: an active variant of human macrophage inflammatory protein-1 alpha with improved pharmaceutical properties. Blood 12:4400, 1995.

299. Lord, B.I., Marshall, E., Woolford, L.B., and Hunter, M.G.: BB-10010/MIP-1α in vivo maintains haemopoietic recovery following repeated cycles of sublethal irradiation. Br. J. Cancer 75:1715, 1997.

300. Clemons, M.J., Marshall, E., Durig, J., Wanatabe, K., Howell, A., Miles., D., Earl, H., Kiernan, J., Griffiths, A., Towlson, K., DeTakats, P., Testa, N.G., Dougal, M., Hunter, M.G., Wood, L.M., Czaplewski, L., Millar, A., Dexter, T.M., and Lord, B.I.: A randomised phase-II study of BB-10010 (macrophage inflammatory protein-1α) in patients with advanced breast cancer receiving 5-fluorouracil, adriamycin, and cyclophosphamide chemotherapy. Blood 92:1532, 1997.

301. Marshall, E., Howell, A.H., Powles, R., Hunter, M.G., Edwards, M., Wood, L.M., Czaplewski, L., Puttick, R., Warrington, S., Boyce, M., Testa, N., Dexter, T.M., Lord, B.I., and Millar, A.: Clinical effects of human macrophage inflammatory protein-1 alpha MIP-1 alpha (LD78) administration to humans: a phase I study in cancer patients and normal healthy volunteers with the genetically engineered variant, BB-10010. Eur. J. Cancer 34:1023, 1998.

302. Lira, S.: Genetic approaches to study chemokine function. J. Leukoc. Biol. 59:45, 1996.

303. Reid, S., Ritchie, A., Boring, L., Gosling, J., Cooper, S., Hangoc, G., Charo, I.F., and Broxmeyer, H.E.: Enhanced myeloid progenitor cell cycling and apoptosis in mice lacking the chemokine receptor CCR2. Blood 93:1524, 1999.

304. Zhou, Y., Kurihara, T., Ryseck, R.P., Yang, Y., Ryan, C., Loy, J., Warr, G., and Bravo, R.: Impaired macrophage function and enhanced T-cell dependent immune response in mice lacking CCR5, the mouse homologue of the major HIV-1 coreceptor. J. Immunol. 160:4018, 1998.

305. Baggiolini, M., and Moser, B.: Blocking chemokine receptors. J. Exp. Med. 186:1189, 1998.

306. Damon, I., Murphy, P.M., and Moss, B.: Broad spectrum chemokine antagonistic activity of a human poxvirus chemokine homolog. Proc. Natl. Acad. Sci. USA 95:6403, 1998.

307. Simmons, G., Clapham, P.R., Picard, L., Offord, R.E., Rosenkilde, M.M., Schwartz, T.W., Ruser, R., Wells, T.N.C., and Proudfoot, A.E.I.: Potent inhibition of HIV-1 infectivity in macrophages and lymphocytes by a novel CCR5 antagonist. Science 276:276, 1997.

308. Gong, J.-H., Ratkay, L.R., Waterfield, J.D., and Clark-Lewis, I.: An antagonist of monocyte chemoattractant protein 1 (MCP-1) inhibits arthritis in the MRL-*lpr* mouse model. J. Exp. Med. 186:131, 1997.

16 Genetic Disorders of Phagocyte Killing

John T. Curnutte and Mary C. Dinauer

▼ ▼

Phagocytes serve as major effector cells of the innate immune system that provides a first line of defense against invading bacteria, fungi, and parasites. This subset of marrow-derived cells is equipped with specialized machinery enabling them to seek out, ingest, and kill microorganisms. The phagocyte system has two principal limbs, granulocytes (neutrophils, eosinophils, and basophils) and mononuclear phagocytes (monocytes and tissue macrophages). Granulocytes circulate in the blood stream until they encounter specific chemotactic signals that promote adhesion to the vascular endothelium, diapedesis, and migration to sites of microbial invasion. In contrast, mononuclear phagocytes spend only a brief time in the intravascular compartment and function primarily as resident cells in certain tissues, such as lung, liver, spleen, and peritoneum. At those sites, they perform a surveillance role in antimicrobial protection and also interact closely with lymphocytes in the immune response. Both groups of phagocytes destroy appropriately opsonized targets by engulfing and sequestering them within intracellular vacuoles. Destruction of the target is mediated by the release of hydrolytic enzymes and bactericidal antibiotic proteins from storage granules as well as by the generation of highly reactive oxygen derivatives from the respiratory burst pathway.

Clinical disorders in which phagocyte dysfunction leads to a propensity for infection are relatively rare, which probably reflects a redundancy within the pathways that operate in each step of phagocyte antimicrobial activity. This chapter reviews inherited disorders that impair microbial killing, with a particular focus on chronic granulomatous disease (CGD). Although phagocyte adhesion, chemotaxis, and phagocytosis are normal in this disease, defects in the respiratory burst result in a distinctive clinical syndrome with recurrent, often life-threatening bacterial and fungal infections. The investigation of the cellular and molecular basis of CGD has made major contributions to our understanding of normal phagocyte function.

Microbicidal Pathways in Phagocytes

Ingested microorganisms are sequestered within intracellular vacuoles (phagosomes), where they are destroyed by the release of digestive lysosomal enzymes and bactericidal antibiotic proteins from storage granules, along with highly reactive oxidants generated by the respiratory burst. The existence of multiple and complementary microbicidal pathways is not surprising, given the crucial importance of this aspect of host defense. This section summarizes the basic features of oxidative and non-oxidative mechanisms of microbial killing and their associated genetic disorders. The two following sections then focus in detail on the respiratory burst oxidase and inherited defects in CGD.

▼ OXYGEN-DEPENDENT MECHANISMS

The unstimulated neutrophil relies primarily on glycolysis for energy and hence consumes relatively little oxygen.[1] Within seconds after contacting appropriately opsonized microorganisms or certain soluble factors, oxygen consumption increases dramatically, often by more than 100-fold. This phenomenon, referred to as the respiratory burst, represents the non-mitochondrial conversion of oxygen to the superoxide radical (O_2^-) by the transfer of a single electron from NADPH[1, 2] (Fig. 16–1, reaction 1). This reaction and related pathways are summarized in Figure 16–1.

The production of superoxide is mediated by a phagocyte-specific NADPH oxidase, also referred to as the respiratory burst oxidase, that is associated with the plasma membrane and phagocytic vacuoles.[3] As detailed in the following section, the active oxidase complex is formed by both cytosolic and membrane proteins and includes a membrane-bound flavocytochrome *b* that mediates the transfer of electrons from NADPH to molecular oxygen.[2, 4–6] Superoxide, although not an important microbicidal agent by itself, is the precursor to a family of potent oxidants.[1, 2] The O_2^- radical is first converted, either spontaneously or by means of superoxide dismutase, into hydrogen peroxide (H_2O_2) (Fig. 16–1, reaction 2). Myeloperoxidase (MPO), in the presence of halides, catalyzes the conversion of hydrogen peroxide to hypochlorous acid (HOCl) (Fig. 16–1, reaction 4). Hydrogen peroxide may also be converted into the hydroxyl radical (OH·) in a non-enzymatic reaction with superoxide catalyzed by either iron or copper ions[7] (Fig. 16–1, reaction 3). Hydrogen peroxide, hypochlorous acid, and the hydroxyl radical are all strong oxidants[8] that are important for effective microbial killing within the phagocytic vacuole.[9] In addition, reactive oxidants modulate phagocyte proteolytic activity by activating latent phagocyte metalloproteinases (such as collagenase and gelatinase) and inactivating plasma antiproteinases.[10] Enhanced phagocyte proteolytic activity at localized

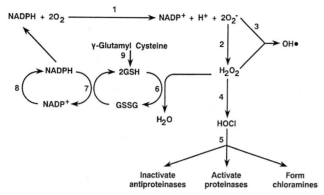

Figure 16–1. Reactions of the respiratory burst pathway. The enzymes responsible for reactions 1 to 9 are as follows: (1) the respiratory burst oxidase (NADPH oxidase); (2) superoxide dismutase or spontaneous; (3) non-enzymatic, Fe^{2+}-catalyzed; (4) myeloperoxidase; (5) spontaneous; (6) glutathione peroxidase; (7) glutathione reductase; (8) glucose-6-phosphate dehydrogenase; (9) glutathione synthetase. (Adapted from Curnutte, J.T.: Disorders of phagocyte function. *In* Hoffman, R., Benz, E.J., Jr., Shattil, S.J., Furie, B., and Cohen, H.J. [eds.]: Hematology: Basic Principles and Practice. New York, Churchill Livingstone, 1991, pp. 571–589; with permission.)

sites may be important for facilitating cellular migration from the blood stream into tissues, removal of cellular debris, and destruction of microbes.

Other enzymatic reactions related to the production of oxidants include the detoxification of excess hydrogen peroxide by glutathione peroxidase and reductase (Fig. 16–1, reactions 6 and 7). Glutathione is produced from γ-glutamylcysteine by the enzyme glutathione synthetase[1, 8] (Fig. 16–1, reaction 9). Other important antioxidant systems present in phagocytes and other tissues include catalase (which catalyzes the conversion of hydrogen peroxide into oxygen and water), ascorbic acid, and α-tocopherol (vitamin E).[8] The generation of NADPH is important in providing a source of reducing equivalents for the glutathione detoxification pathway as well as the respiratory burst oxidase itself. NADPH is replenished from $NADP^+$ by the action of leukocyte glucose-6-phosphate dehydrogenase (G6PD) (Fig. 16–1, reaction 8) in the hexose monophosphate shunt.

The production of nitric oxide (NO) from the oxidation of L-arginine to L-citrulline is another oxygen-dependent pathway that may be of importance for human host defense. This reaction is catalyzed by nitric oxide synthase (NOS), with molecular oxygen supplying the oxygen in NO.[11–13] There are three different nitric oxide synthases, each encoded by a different gene. Two are constitutively expressed in a variety of tissues, including endothelium, brain, and neutrophils. Expression of a third form, known as iNOS, can be induced by inflammatory stimuli in a variety of cells, including macrophages and neutrophils, where it has a wide spectrum of antimicrobial activity against bacteria, parasites, helminths, and viruses.[11, 14] Mice with genetic absence of iNOS, generated by targeted disruption of the iNOS gene in murine embryonic stem cells, have increased susceptibility to infection with *Listeria monocytogenes*.[15] High levels of iNOS-catalyzed NO production are easily elicited in wild-type mouse macrophages by exposure, for example, to endotoxin or interferon-γ (IFN-γ). However, it had been difficult to consistently document a similar phenomenon in human

phagocytes, casting doubt for many years. Nevertheless, evidence for the induction of NOS in human phagocytes and consequent production of nitrated derivatives has been accumulating.[16–19] The formation of NO–derived inflammatory oxidants by neutrophil MPO has also been reported.[20] It is likely that phagocyte production of NO and derivatives plays an adjunctive role to oxidants produced through the respiratory burst.

▼ OXYGEN-INDEPENDENT MECHANISMS

Oxidant-mediated destruction by phagocytes is supplemented by non-oxidative antimicrobial systems.[21–23] In addition to providing another avenue of attack, oxygen-independent mechanisms enable effective killing under the adverse conditions of hypoxia and acidosis often encountered locally at the site of infection. Neutrophils store an array of degradative enzymes and antimicrobial proteins within both the primary (azurophil) and secondary (specific) granules.[22, 24, 25] The best-characterized "antibiotic" proteins are listed in Table 16–1.[26] Lysozyme hydrolyzes the cell wall of saprophytic gram-positive organisms and may also assist in the non-lytic killing of other microbes.[21, 27] The iron-binding glycoprotein lactoferrin has bactericidal properties both related and unrelated to the chelation of iron compounds required for bacterial metabolism. In addition, lactoferrin may participate in the non-enzymatic formation of hydroxyl radicals during the respiratory burst (Fig. 16–1, reaction 3).[28] Bactericidal/permeability-increasing factor (BPI), cathepsin G, the serpocidins, and the defensins[23] are an important group of microbicidal polypeptides localized to azurophilic granules. BPI (identical to a cationic antimicrobial protein of 57 kDa [CAP57]) is specific for gram-negative bacteria, binding avidly to lipopolysaccharide to damage the bacterial membrane and to neutralize endotoxin in serum and bacterial cell walls.[29, 30] The serpocidins are members of the serine protease superfamily and include cathepsin G, a 37 kDa cationic antimicrobial protein termed CAP37 or azurocidin, elastase, and proteinase 3.[21, 24, 25, 31, 32] The genes for the last three proteins are found in a cluster on chromosome 19pter.[33] Serpocidin microbial activity can proceed in vitro in the presence of proteolytic inhibitors, suggesting a non-enzymatic mechanism of action; gram-negative bacteria are particularly susceptible. Cathepsin G has a broader spectrum of activity and is even more active against gram-positive bacteria and fungi. Defensins are small (25 to 29 residues) basic peptides, which constitute more than 5 per cent of the total cellular protein of human neutrophils.[34, 35] These cationic, amphipathic proteins kill susceptible bacteria, fungi, and viruses by damaging microbial cytoplasmic membranes and forming voltage-regulated channels.[21] Defensin-like peptides have also been found in small intestinal Paneth cells and in tracheal epithelium.[34]

▼ REGULATION OF ANTIMICROBIAL ACTIVITY

Although critical for effective killing of pathogens, the toxic antimicrobial molecules produced by phagocytic cells have the potential for causing damage to normal tissues.[36] The cellular release of microbicidal products is therefore coupled

Table 16–1. Neutrophil Granule Microbicides

Neutrophil Antimicrobial Granule Components	Molecular Mass (kDa)	Chromosome Location	Granule Distribution
Lysozyme	14.4	12	Azurophil and specific granules
Lactoferrin	80		Specific granules
Bactericidal/permeability-increasing factor (BPI, CAP57)	58	20q11–q12	Azurophil granules
Cathepsin G	25–29	14q11.2	Azurophil granules
Cationic antimicrobial protein (CAP37, azurocidin)	37	19pter	Azurophil granules
Proteinase 3	29	19pter	Azurophil granules
Elastase	28	19pter	Azurophil granules
Defensins	3.6–4.0	8p23	Azurophil granules

See text for details and references.

to specific receptor-mediated events and largely confined to protected intracellular compartments. Receptor-mediated signal transduction in phagocytes is mediated by a molecular cascade of second messengers, which regulate chemotaxis, phagocytosis, and subsequent degranulation and activation of the respiratory burst.

The biochemical pathways involved in phagocyte signal transduction are overlapping and complex. A common early downstream event of receptor binding is the activation of membrane phospholipid metabolism to generate two important second messengers, diacylglycerol and inositol 1,4,5-triphosphate,[37, 38] which in turn cause release of calcium from intracellular stores and activate protein kinase C. Neutrophil activation is also accompanied by alterations in the phosphorylation status of intracellular proteins, as regulated by protein kinase C,[39, 40] receptor-coupled tyrosine kinases,[41–43] and serine and threonine kinases of the mitogen-activated kinase family.[44–46] Guanine nucleotide–binding proteins also play important roles in phagocyte signal transduction. These include the heterotrimeric guanosine triphosphate (GTP)–binding proteins that are coupled to the seven transmembrane–spanning domain receptors for chemokines and other chemoattractants[47, 48] as well as the low molecular weight GTPases of the Ras p21 superfamily.[39, 49]

The respiratory burst oxidase is quiescent in the resting phagocyte. Oxidase activation involves the translocation of a complex of cytosolic proteins to the plasma membrane, which contains the redox carrier flavocytochrome *b* (see next section). The physical separation of various oxidase components in the resting cell may be an important "failsafe" means of preventing inappropriate oxidase activity. Oxidase assembly can be triggered by receptor-mediated binding of many soluble chemotactic agents, such as N-formylated peptides secreted by bacteria, interleukin-8, and C5 complement fragments.[39, 49] Note that stimulation of the respiratory burst requires higher concentrations of these molecules compared with initiation of chemotaxis. The binding of opsonized microorganisms to phagocyte Fcγ[50–53] and C3bi[54–56] receptors is another major physiological trigger of the respiratory burst that can be activated at localized sites of microbial contact.[57]

Another mechanism by which phagocyte antimicrobial products are restricted to sites of infection or inflammation is their localization to specific subcellular compartments. Degradative lysosomal enzymes and antibiotic peptides are sequestered within azurophil granules until phagocytosis triggers degranulation. The contents of the azurophil gran-

ules are carefully delivered into the phagocytic vacuole with minimal extracellular release.[21, 22] The activated oxidase, assembled in the plasma membrane, is also incorporated into phagolysosomes during ingestion. Because release of superoxide occurs largely at the extracellular side of the membrane[2, 3] (but see also reference 58), oxidants are restricted to the extracellular space at sites of microbial contact or within the phagocytic vacuole. Indeed, the interaction of granule contents and respiratory burst products within the phagosome potentiates their microbicidal effects. For example, azurophil granules provide MPO for catalysis of hypochlorous acid production.[59, 60] The degranulation and membrane fusion of specific granules, which contain the majority of flavocytochrome *b* in the neutrophil,[61] may contribute to a sustained respiratory burst.

▼ GENETIC DEFECTS IN PHAGOCYTE ANTIMICROBIAL PATHWAYS

MPO deficiency is the most common inherited disorder of phagocytes; complete deficiency is seen in approximately 1 in 4000 individuals, partial deficiency in approximately 1 in 2000.[59, 62] The *MPO* gene is located on chromosome 17 at q22–23, and a variety of specific gene defects associated with MPO deficiency are now being identified. One patient has been reported with a likely pretranslational defect,[63] but most patients studied to date have immunochemical evidence of MPO precursors and therefore presumably have defects in post-translational processing. Three genotypes have been reported thus far.[64–67] Biosynthetic processing of MPO has been studied for a missense mutation at codon 569, in which an arginine is replaced by a tryptophan, which appears to impair the ability of the apoprotein to incorporate heme.[67] Despite the pivotal role of MPO in the production of hypochlorous acid, affected persons are notable for the lack of symptoms. In vitro neutrophil killing is slower than normal but eventually complete.[59] A more active and sustained respiratory burst, coupled with the toxic effects of other oxidants and non-oxidative killing mechanisms, may account for the lack of clinical manifestations in the majority of cases of MPO deficiency. Disseminated fungal infections, however, have been described in patients who suffer from both MPO deficiency and diabetes mellitus.

CGD occurs at a frequency of approximately 1 in 500,000[1] and is characterized by the deficient production of superoxide. This disorder results from inherited defects in any of four different genes that encode components of the respiratory burst oxidase[4, 5] and is discussed in detail in the following section. The rare condition of severe X-linked G6PD deficiency, in which extremely low steady-state levels of NADPH are associated with hemolytic anemia even in the absence of redox stress, exhibits a similar clinical pattern because NADPH is the required substrate for the respiratory burst oxidase.[1] It is distinguished by the presence of low levels of G6PD and congenital hemolytic anemia. A few cases of autosomal recessive inheritance of severe deficiencies in glutathione reductase or glutathione synthetase have been reported that can be associated with a CGD-like syndrome[68, 69] (see Fig. 16–1). The oxidase can be activated in the absence of glutathione but is soon damaged by oxidants, resulting in premature termination of the respiratory burst.[70]

Two inherited disorders of granule function that affect primarily non-oxidative killing have also been described. Chédiak-Higashi syndrome is an uncommon autosomal recessive disorder characterized by giant cytoplasmic granules in multiple tissues and cells throughout the body.[22, 71–74] The abnormal granules are associated with defects in phagocyte and platelet function, and partial oculocutaneous albinism results from uneven pigment distribution by giant melanosomes. The underlying etiology is unknown but may be related to abnormal granule morphogenesis. The recent cloning of the Chédiak-Higashi gene, whose murine homologue is affected in *beige* mice, should help shed light on the underlying molecular defect.[75] A variety of functional neutrophil defects have been noted in this disorder and contribute to an enhanced susceptibility to bacterial infections of the skin, mucous membranes, and respiratory tract. These include abnormal adherence and chemotaxis, delayed degranulation, and slow killing of ingested microorganisms. Specific granule deficiency is another exceedingly rare disorder affecting phagocyte granule function and has been described in only 5 patients.[22, 76] It is presumed to be autosomal recessive, and the underlying gene involved is unknown. Affected patients have suffered from recurrent infections, primarily involving the skin and lungs. Normal-appearing specific granules are absent, and deficiencies in proteins of both azurophil (defensins) and specific granules (lactoferrin, cobalamin-binding protein, gelatinase) have been observed.[74, 77, 78] The underlying defect may be specific to the regulation of granule protein synthesis in the myeloid lineage, because lactoferrin was secreted normally in glandular epithelium in these patients.[78] Circulating neutrophils commonly have bilobed nuclei similar to those seen in the Pelger-Huët anomaly; how this relates to granule defects is unknown.

The Respiratory Burst Oxidase

▼ OVERVIEW

The "extra respiration of phagocytosis" was first observed in 1933,[79] but not until more than 20 years later was it appreciated that this process is insensitive to mitochondrial poisons and hence not directly related to increased energy demands.[80] Subsequent enzymological studies established that NADPH oxidase (alternatively referred to as the respiratory burst oxidase) is associated with the plasma and phago-

lysosomal membranes and catalyzes the transfer of electrons from NADPH to molecular oxygen, thereby forming superoxide.[1, 81, 82] As described in the preceding section, superoxide is the precursor to a family of toxic oxidants important for efficient microbial killing. The importance of this pathway to normal host defense was underscored by the discovery that phagocytes obtained from patients with "fatal granulomatosus of childhood" (CGD), first described in 1957,[83, 84] lack detectable respiratory burst oxidase activity.[85, 86] In the initial reports of CGD, affected patients were males who appeared to inherit the disorder in an X-linked recessive manner. Subsequently, females with an identical clinical syndrome and pedigree consistent with autosomal recessive inheritance were described.[1, 87] That at least three different gene products were required for intact oxidase function was elegantly demonstrated by the functional analysis of monocyte heterokaryons derived from different patients with CGD.[88, 89] This genetic heterogeneity hinted at the complexity of the active oxidase, which was originally viewed as a single "enzyme."

In the past decade, a convergence of biochemical and molecular genetic approaches has revealed that the active respiratory burst oxidase is a complex, multisubunit enzyme containing both membrane-bound and soluble subunits (Fig. 16–2). The emerging picture of this superoxide-generating enzyme has benefited greatly from the analysis of patients with CGD. This disorder results from genetic mutations in any one of four polypeptides that are essential for respiratory burst function, whose corresponding genes have all been identified and cloned (Table 16–2). The oxidase subunits have been given the designation *phox* (abbreviated from *ph*agocyte *ox*idase) and are referred to by the apparent molecular mass of the component (in kilodaltons) and a letter indicating whether it is a protein (p) or glycoprotein (gp). A phagocyte-specific b-type flavocytochrome *b* heterodimer, formed by the gp91-*phox* and p22-*phox* polypeptides,[90, 91] is located in the plasma and specific granule membranes and is the terminal electron carrier of the oxidase.[2, 3, 92, 93] Two other oxidase components that can be affected in CGD, p47-*phox* and p67-*phox*,[94–96] are located in the cytosol of unstimulated cells but translocate to the membrane with oxidase activation.[97, 98] A fifth *phox* protein, p40-*phox*, is associated with p67-*phox* in resting neutrophils and plays an unknown but dispensable role in superoxide production. Finally, regulation of superoxide formation involves the small GTP-binding proteins Rac and Rap1a; Rac is required for respiratory burst oxidase activity.[99–102]

▼ FLAVOCYTOCHROME *b*

An unusual low-potential b-type cytochrome was first described in horse neutrophils[2, 103] and subsequently identified in membranes of human neutrophils, monocytes, macrophages, and eosinophils.[104, 105] Because the wavelength of the alpha band of light absorption is at 558 nm, this cytochrome has often been referred to as cytochrome b_{558}. It has also been called cytochrome b_{245}, in reference to its midpoint potential of -245 mV, which is among the lowest reported for any mammalian cytochrome.[3, 106] Its redox properties suggested that this cytochrome might be the terminal elec-

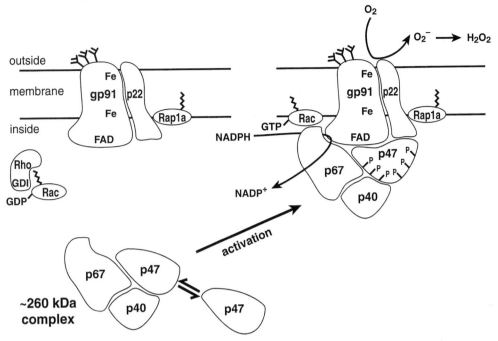

Figure 16–2. Model of NADPH oxidase activation. Current knowledge of the oxidase suggests that in its dormant state *(left),* it is composed of both membrane-bound and cytosolic components. Membrane-bound components include gp91-*phox* and p22-*phox,* which together form the flavocytochrome *b* heterodimer that also contains the redox centers of the enzyme: FAD and two heme groups (Fe). Rap1A, a low molecular weight GTP-binding protein, is also present in the membrane and may functionally associate with the flavocytochrome. The cytosolic components include p40-*phox,* p47-*phox,* and p67-*phox,* which exist in a complex of 260 kDa. A pool of free, monomeric p47-*phox* is also present in the cytosol prepared from resting neutrophils. In its inactive GDP-bound state, the small GTP-binding protein Rac (Rac2 in human neutrophils) is also cytosolic and is bound to RhoGDP-dissociation inhibitor (GDI). On stimulation *(right),* p47-*phox,* p67-*phox,* and p40-*phox* become associated with the plasma membrane primarily through interactions between p47-*phox* and the subunits of the flavocytochrome. This translocation process is accompanied by and perhaps requires (1) the release of Rac from RhoGDI, its conversion to an active (GTP-bound) state, and its association with the plasma membrane and (2) the multisite phosphorylation of p47-*phox.* By a mechanism that is not fully understood, binding of the cytosolic components activates the flavocytochrome to catalyze the transfer of electrons from NADPH to oxygen through the FAD and heme redox centers. The compartment labeled "inside" is the cytoplasmic space; "outside" refers to either the extracellular or phagosomal space. (From Heyworth, P.G., Curnutte, J.T., and Badwey, J.A.: Structure and regulation of NADPH oxidase of phagocytic leukocytes. Insights from chronic granulomatous disease. *In* Serhan, C.N., and Ward, P.A. [eds.]: Molecular and Cellular Basis of Inflammation. Totowa, NJ, Humana Press, 1999, pp. 165–191; with permission.)

tron carrier in respiratory burst oxidase, according to the following scheme[2]:

$$NADPH \rightarrow Flavin \rightarrow Heme \rightarrow O_2 \rightarrow O_2^-$$

$$-330\ mV \quad -256\ mV \quad -245\ mV \quad -160\ mV$$

Further suspicion that cytochrome *b* might be a component of the respiratory burst oxidase resulted from the discovery that its characteristic heme spectrum was absent in neutrophils obtained from patients with X-linked CGD, whereas normal levels were detected in those with the autosomal recessive disease.[107] However, a few X-linked CGD patients had detectable neutrophil cytochrome *b,*[1, 108] and certain autosomal recessive patients did not.[89, 109, 110] Furthermore, additional biochemical abnormalities in X-linked CGD neutrophils had also been observed. For example, membrane flavoprotein concentrations were consistently about half that of normal neutrophils.[3, 93, 111] Indeed, whether the cytochrome actually was part of the respiratory burst complex at all was controversial.[1] Hence, it was uncertain whether the absence of the cytochrome *b* spectrum represented the primary genetic defect in X-linked CGD.

Two independent experimental approaches finally established that the product of the gene encoding X-linked CGD was in fact a subunit of cytochrome *b* and, as such, an essential component of the respiratory burst oxidase. One

approach relied on a genetic strategy, whereby the gene mutated in X-linked CGD was identified and cloned on the basis of its chromosome location at Xp21.1.[112, 113] Antibodies raised to the predicted polypeptide sequence reacted with the 91 kDa glycoprotein (gp91-*phox*) subunit of cytochrome *b,*[114] which on conventional purification appeared to be a complex of two tightly associated integral membrane polypeptides.[90, 91] This approach represented the first example in which the protein defect responsible for a human disease was identified by "reverse genetics" (positional cloning), a strategy that has since been applied with notable success to an ever increasing number of inherited diseases. The other approach was biochemical; the cytochrome was purified by chromatographic methods, and the N-terminal amino acid sequence of its heavily glycosylated larger subunit (gp91-*phox*) was found to correspond to that predicted by the cDNA derived from the identified locus at Xp21.1.[115]

The identification of cytochrome *b* as an oligomer composed of 91 kDa and 22 kDa subunits provided an explanation for the observation that neutrophil cytochrome *b* is also absent in some cases of autosomal recessive CGD. The hypothesis that mutations in the gene for p22-*phox* lead to this form of CGD proved correct on the basis of DNA sequence analysis of affected patients.[116] Subsequent analyses of purified cytochrome *b* have indicated that it also bears

Table 16–2. Properties of the Phagocyte Respiratory Burst Oxidase (*phox*) Components

Property	gp91-*phox*	p22-*phox*	p47-*phox*	p67-*phox*	p40-*phox*
Synonyms	β-Chain Heavy chain	α-Chain Light chain	NCF-1 SOC II C4	NCF-2 SOC III C2	NCF-4
Amino acids	570	195	390	526	339
Molecular mass (kDa)					
Predicted	65.0	20.9	44.6	60.9	39.0
As seen by PAGE	91	22	47	67	40
Glycosylation	Yes (N-linked)	No	No	No	No
Phosphorylation	No	No	Yes	No	?
pI	9.7	10.0	9.5	5.8	6.4
mRNA	4.7 kb	0.8 kb	1.4 kb	2.4 kb	
Gene locus	CYBB Xp21.1	CYBA 16q24	NCF1 7q11.23	NCF2 1q25	NCF4 22q.13.1
Exons/span	13/30 kb	6/8.5 kb	11/15 kb	16/40 kb	10/18 kb
Cellular location in resting neutrophil	Specific granule membrane Plasma membrane	Specific granule membrane Plasma membrane	Cytosol Cytoskeleton	Cytosol Cytoskeleton	Cytosol Cytoskeleton
Level in neutrophil (pmol/10^6 cells)	3.3–5.3	3.3–5.3	3.3	1.2	?
Tissue specificity	Myeloid, B lymphocytes	mRNA in all cells tested; protein only in myeloid cells	Myeloid, B lymphocytes	Myeloid, B lymphocytes	Myeloid, other hematopoietic cells
Functional domains	Binding sites for heme, FAD, and NADPH; binding sites for cytosolic oxidase components	Proline-rich domain in carboxyl terminus that binds p47-*phox*	9 potential serine phosphorylation sites; SH3 domains, proline-rich domains	SH3 domains	SH3 domains
Homologies	Ferredoxin-NADP⁺ reductase (FNR)*	Polypeptide I of cytochrome *c* oxidase (weak homology)	SH3 domain of *src*	SH3 domain of *src*	SH3 domain of *src*, homology to p47-*phox* amino terminus
GenBank accession	X04011†	M21186, J03774	M25665, M26193	M32011	U5070–U50729

*phox, ph*agocyte *ox*idase component; NCF, neutrophil cytosol factor; SOC, soluble oxidase component; C, component; PAGE, polyacrylamide gel electrophoresis; SH3, *src* homology domain 3.

  * Weak homology to both the NADPH- and FAD-binding domains in the FNR family.

  † GenBank accession number refers to sequence as originally published. The complete corrected sequence (encoding an additional 64 amino acids) has not been deposited in GenBank but is available in Orkin.[252]

  Adapted from Curnutte, J.T.: Molecular basis of the autosomal recessive forms of chronic granulomatous disease. Immunodefic. Rev. 3:149, 1992.

a flavin group (see below), and hence, the respiratory burst oxidase cytochrome is now referred to as flavocytochrome *b*.

Expression of the gp91-*phox* gene is restricted almost exclusively to mature phagocytic cells of the myeloid lineage[113] (see Table 16–2). RNA transcripts for gp91-*phox* have been seen in Epstein-Barr virus–transformed B-lymphocyte cell lines in which at least a subpopulation appears to be capable of mounting a respiratory burst[117, 118]; gp91-*phox* (or a form of it) was also detected in renal mesangial cells, in which low rates of superoxide production have been detected.[119] In contrast to this relative tissue specificity, p22-*phox* mRNA is constitutively expressed in a wide variety of cell types.[120] However, it appears that coordinate synthesis of both subunits is required for normal intracellular stability of each polypeptide chain. Only trace amounts of the p22-*phox* subunit are detectable in non-phagocytic cells, which lack the gp91-*phox* transcript,[120] or in neutrophils obtained from patients with X-linked CGD who are genetically deficient in gp91-*phox*.[90, 91, 120, 121] Conversely, gp91-*phox* is absent in neutrophils from patients with autosomal recessive CGD who are genetically deficient in p22-*phox*.[116, 121] These observations are reminiscent of those made for the leukocyte adhesion β₂ integrins and other oligomeric membrane protein complexes, in which steady-state levels of each sub-

unit are dependent on interchain association during biosynthesis.[122, 123]

The flavocytochrome *b* is an integral membrane protein complex in which its gp91-*phox* and p22-*phox* subunits are present in a 1:1 stoichiometry.[124, 125] The hydrodynamic mass of the cross-linked cytochrome is most consistent with a heterodimer,[126] and each unit contains two heme moieties[127] with slightly different midpoint potentials[127] and one flavin adenine dinucleotide (FAD) group.[92, 93] The actual location of the protoporphyrin IX heme rings[128] had been in doubt, but evidence indicates that the gp91-*phox* subunit contains both heme groups.[129] Current data support a model in which the two heme prosthetic groups are embedded within the membrane[130] where they are ligated by histidine residues[128, 131, 132] in the gp91-*phox* subunit.[129] The heme groups are likely to reside in the amino terminus of gp91-*phox*, which contains multiple hydrophobic segments that probably span the membrane at least several times. The flavin- and NADPH-binding sites also appear to reside in gp91-*phox*. Regions in the hydrophilic carboxyl terminus of gp91-*phox* contain homology with the ferredoxin-NADH⁺ reductase family of flavoproteins,[92, 93, 133, 134] and the level of FAD is diminished by half or more in membranes from neutrophils in patients with X-linked CGD.[135–138] Several structural models for gp91-*phox* incorporating these features and the sites of N-linked glycosylation have been proposed[129, 139–141] (see Fig. 16–3, for example). A protein similar to gp91-*phox*, with homologies in both the putative heme- and flavin-binding domains, has also been identified in yeast, in which it acts as a ferric iron reductase involved in transmembrane iron transport,[142] and in plants,[143] in which it has an unknown function but may be involved in generation of oxidative signals important for cellular regulation and host defense.[144]

The role of the p22-*phox* subunit in the superoxide production is less clear. It is also an integral membrane protein and is tightly associated with gp91-*phox*.[91] The amino-terminal half of p22-*phox* contains multiple hydrophobic regions, whereas its intracellular carboxyl terminus is hydrophilic and proline rich.[145] Heterodimer formation appears to be important for the intracellular stability of each subunit, particularly in phagocytic cells.[121, 146] One region in p22-*phox* has some resemblance to heme-binding domains in other heme-bearing polypeptides,[120] and indirect evidence had suggested that p22-*phox* may participate in coordination of at least one of the heme prosthetic groups.[147, 148] Recent experiments, however, have disproved this hypothesis.[129] The proline-rich carboxyl terminus of p22-*phox* includes at least one binding site for an SH3 (*src* homology domain 3) domain in p47-*phox* that is critical for assembly of the oxidase complex, acting as a docking site for p47-*phox*.[145, 149–151]

In resting neutrophils, the majority (up to 80 per cent) of flavocytochrome *b* resides in specific granules; the remainder is in the plasma membrane.[1, 61] The specific granule

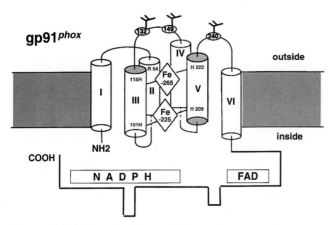

Figure 16–3. Model of gp91-*phox*. The model shows gp91-*phox* with both the NH₂- and COOH-terminal tails oriented in the cytoplasm of the phagocyte, which contains both the FAD- and NADPH-binding sites. Three asparagine residues in two extracellular loops are shown glycosylated (Asn 132, 149, and 240). Six transmembranous helices, all in the NH₂ half of the polypeptide, are represented. Substantial spectral data suggest that the flavocytochrome contains two low-spin, bis-histidinyl hemes that have midpoint potentials of −225 mV and −265 mV. The model shows the heme with the Em of −225 mV close to the inner face of the membrane, coordinated by His 101 and 209 and positioned to accept electrons from the FAD in the cytoplasmic domain. The lower potential heme is situated toward the outer face of the membrane coordinated by His 115 and 222 where it can transfer electrons from the −225 mV heme to molecular O_2 to form O_2^-. Arg 54 in helix II is shown in proximity to the −265 mV heme, consistent with a report of a CGD patient with an Arg 54 Ser mutation and a defective flavocytochrome *b* characterized by a shift in the Em of the −265 mV heme to −300 mV. (From Yu, L., Quinn, M.T., Cross, A.R., and Dinauer, M.C.: Gp91(phox) is the heme binding subunit of the superoxide-generating NADPH oxidase. Proc. Natl. Acad. Sci. USA 95:7993, 1998; with permission.)

pool may serve as a reservoir to maintain sustained respiratory burst activity. Flavocytochrome *b* is also incorporated into the phagosomal membrane during phagocytosis.[104, 152]

▼ CYTOSOLIC *phox* SUBUNITS

The development of a cell-free assay of oxidase activity in the mid-1980s was a major breakthrough that led directly to the recognition that cytosol-derived proteins were absolutely required for catalytic activity of the membrane-associated, activated oxidase.[153–156] In this assay, the addition of certain anionic amphophiles (such as sodium dodecyl sulfate or arachidonic acid) to mixtures of membrane and cytosol fractions isolated from resting neutrophils elicits oxidase activity at rates comparable to those observed in intact cells. The capacity to reconstitute the oxidase in this manner has proved to be a powerful tool for the analysis of specific oxidase components.

The identification of two cytosol-derived oxidase components was greatly facilitated by the discovery that neutrophil cytosol obtained from autosomal recessive CGD patients with normal flavocytochrome *b* levels could not reconstitute the oxidase in the presence of normal membranes.[157] Subsequent complementation studies using cytosols from different cytochrome-positive autosomal recessive CGD patients indicated that there were at least two distinct cytosolic defects, each involving a different oxidase component.[95, 96] One proved to be a highly basic 47 kDa phosphoprotein (p47-*phox*) (see Table 16–2)[94–96] that was already a suspected oxidase component because of the absence of its phosphorylation pattern in cytochrome-positive autosomal recessive CGD patients.[3, 158] The other complementing cytosolic oxidase component was identified as a 67 kDa species (p67-*phox*) that is slightly acidic.[94–96] The corresponding cDNAs for both p47-*phox* and p67-*phox* were subsequently cloned, and the recombinant proteins were shown to restore oxidase activity to cytosol deficient in either p47-*phox* or p67-*phox*, respectively.[159–161] More recently, a 40 kDa protein, p40-*phox*, has been identified in immunoprecipitates of p67-*phox*,[162, 163] although its function in the oxidase complex, if any, remains to be determined. The expression of p47-*phox*, p67-*phox*, and p40-*phox* is restricted to mature myelomonocytic cells and B lymphocytes,[164] similar to what is observed for gp91-*phox*.

The p47-*phox*, p67-*phox*, and p40-*phox* polypeptides have multiple regions with homology to SH3 domains and their target proline-rich binding sites.[159–163, 165, 166] The C terminus of p47-*phox* is rich in basic residues and in serines, which lie in a favorable context for phosphorylation by protein kinase C and other protein kinases.[159, 160] Oxidase activation is accompanied by the stepwise phosphorylation of up to nine serines on p47-*phox*.[167–171] Phosphorylation at serines 303 and 304 appears to be of particular importance for oxidase activation in intact neutrophils.[171] The initial modifications occur in the cytosol, but complete phosphorylation is dependent on membrane binding and requires flavocytochrome *b*. The kinases responsible for phosphorylation of p47-*phox* have not been conclusively identified. However, p47-*phox* phosphorylation is not required for oxidase activity per se, because superoxide production in the cell-free assay is independent of phosphorylation.[110, 172, 173]

Low-level phosphorylation of p67-*phox* has also been reported but is of doubtful significance.[174, 175]

In resting neutrophils, p47-*phox,* p67-*phox,* and p40-*phox* polypeptides can be isolated as a complex, with additional p47-*phox* (representing one half to one third of the cellular content) existing in a monomeric form.[110, 176, 177] Stabilization of this complex is likely to be mediated in part by interactions between SH3 and proline-rich domains within these proteins.[159–163, 165, 166] Phagocyte activation results in translocation of this complex to the membrane to assemble the active oxidase complex (see below). There is also indirect evidence that p67-*phox* and p40-*phox* are associated with the cytoskeleton in both resting and activated cells and, for p47-*phox,* after cellular activation.[178, 179]

Neither p47-*phox* nor p67-*phox* appears to function enzymatically in the respiratory burst oxidase and more likely serves a regulatory role, perhaps modulating some aspect of flavocytochrome b_{558} function at the plasma membrane. Studies using cell-free oxidase systems have shown that substantial amounts of superoxide can be generated from neutrophil membranes in the absence of p47-*phox,* provided that high concentrations of p67-*phox* and the small G protein Rac (see below) are supplied.[180, 181] Hence, it has been postulated that p67-*phox* may participate in the catalytically active complex, whereas p47-*phox* functions as a docking protein to bring p67-*phox* to the membrane. It has been proposed that p67-*phox* may also be involved in NADPH binding,[182] but this is difficult to reconcile with evidence indicating that this function is mediated by gp91-*phox.* As previously mentioned, p40-*phox* is not required for NADPH oxidase activity.[92, 183]

▼ SMALL GTP-BINDING PROTEINS

A large number of small GTP-binding proteins with homology to Ras have been identified in recent years.[184–186] All share common features of size (approximately 21 to 26 kDa), slow spontaneous exchange of guanosine diphosphate (GDP) and GTP, and intrinsic GTPase activity. Most small GTP-binding proteins also undergo a post-translational attachment of polyisoprenoid units at the carboxyl terminus that results in localization to the membrane. Like other guanine nucleotide–binding proteins, small GTP-binding proteins are thought to serve as molecular "switches" through changes in conformation as the protein cycles between inactive GDP- and active GTP-bound forms.[165] The relative levels of the two forms are modulated by other proteins that regulate guanine nucleotide exchange or GTP hydrolysis (GTPase-activating protein).[165, 187] Different subfamilies have been implicated in receptor-mediated signal transduction, cytoskeletal organization, intracellular vesicle transport, and secretion.[184, 188–191] It is now clear that one or more small GTP-binding proteins also play a direct role in regulating respiratory burst oxidase activity.[99–102, 183, 192–196] The involvement of small GTP-binding proteins in regulation of oxidase activity provides an attractive explanation for the observation that the oxidase has an absolute requirement for GTP.[172, 173, 197]

Investigators in three laboratories have demonstrated that a small GTPase is a third essential cytosolic factor in the oxidase, in addition to p47-*phox* and p67-*phox.* Attempts

to isolate cytosolic proteins that stimulate the oxidase consistently yielded a fraction distinct from those containing p47-*phox* and p67-*phox.*[95, 96, 198, 199] The active component of this fraction subsequently proved to be either Rac1 or Rac2, two closely related (92 per cent homologous at the amino acid level) proteins that are members of the Rho family of small GTP-binding proteins that have been implicated in controlling cytoskeletal organization.[184, 188, 189] Rac2 is expressed almost exclusively in myeloid cells, whereas Rac1 appears to have a ubiquitous distribution.[200]

Disagreement exists as to whether Rac1 or Rac2 is the specific G protein involved in vivo in regulation of oxidase activity; sound experimental evidence supports a role for each.[100, 183, 193] In resting neutrophils, isoprenylated Rac is complexed with a GDP dissociation inhibitor (GDI), a regulatory protein that interacts with GDP-bound forms of Rho proteins,[201] and thereby the Rac remains cytosolic. With activation, the GTP-bound form of Rac releases GDI and interacts with the other oxidase components at the plasma membrane. Translocation of Rac2 is decreased in CGD neutrophils lacking flavocytochrome b_{558}, suggesting a direct interaction with the cytochrome.[202] Rac has also been shown to bind to p67-*phox.*[60, 203] Full oxidase activity can be reconstituted with recombinant p47-*phox,* recombinant p67-*phox,* GTP-bound recombinant Rac1 or Rac2, a detergent, and a source of flavocytochrome *b.*[183, 204] It thus appears that either Rac1 or Rac2 can support oxidase activity. However, interaction with additional small GTPase regulatory proteins is important for GDP/GTP nucleotide exchange. Further evidence for the key role of these G proteins in NADPH oxidase function is the finding that the superoxide-generating activity of stimulated Epstein-Barr virus–transformed B lymphocytes is inhibited by introduction of antisense oligonucleotides encoding regions shared by Rac1 and Rac2.[205]

The generation of Rac2-deficient mice by gene targeting has shed some light on the relative roles of Rac1 and Rac2 in neutrophil function in vivo.[206] Neutrophils from Rac2$^{-/-}$ mice had profound defects in actin remodeling and chemotaxis as induced by chemoattractants or ligation of cell surface adhesion molecules, consistent with the recognized importance of the Rho family in cytoskeletal regulation. Phorbol ester–activated NADPH oxidase activity was also substantially reduced in Rac2$^{-/-}$ bone marrow neutrophils but nearly normal in exudate neutrophils and after exposure of marrow neutrophils to tumor necrosis factor-α. Hence, although Rac2 plays an important role in regulating NADPH oxidase in vivo, this function can partially be replaced by Rac1.

Flavocytochrome *b* purified from solubilized neutrophil membranes by either conventional column chromatography or immunoaffinity matrices is associated with approximately equimolar amounts of a 22 kDa polypeptide identified as Rap1 (or Krev-1), a GTP-binding protein that is roughly 55 per cent homologous to Ras.[102] Rap1 is a ubiquitously expressed protein with two closely related forms, Rap1A and Rap1B, that are 95 per cent identical at the amino acid level.[207, 208] Rap1A appears to be the predominant form in neutrophils,[209] and its stoichiometric association with flavocytochrome *b* is inhibited by Rap1A phosphorylation by cyclic adenosine monophosphate (cAMP)–dependent protein kinase.[194] This observation is intriguing in light of the inhibition of neutrophil activation and superoxide production by hormones that increase the intracellular concentration of cAMP.[210] However, the specific role played by Rap1A in respiratory burst function remains to be clarified. It has been reported that immunodepletion of Rap1 in the cell-free system abolishes oxidase activity, which is reversed by the addition of a truncated form of recombinant Rap1A.[101] However, others have found that full-length recombinant Rap1A does not stimulate oxidase activity under similar conditions (see reference 100).

▼ ASSEMBLY OF THE ACTIVE OXIDASE COMPLEX

With the identification of the proteins that compose the respiratory burst oxidase complex, current research is focused on defining how these polypeptides interact to achieve the regulated production of superoxide in phagocytes (for reviews, see references 211 to 213). Multiple potential interactions have been identified in vitro by use of recombinant proteins or the yeast two-hybrid system, although how these relate to assembly and function of the oxidase complex in intact neutrophils remains to be clearly defined. The translocation of the soluble oxidase components to the membrane is triggered in response to chemotactic factors or binding of opsonized microbes, as already discussed. The specific second messenger signals that interface receptor-mediated events at the cell surface with assembly of the catalytically active oxidase complex are not known with certainty but are likely to involve activation of Rac1/2 and phosphorylation of p47-*phox*. Changes in the association of flavocytochrome *b*, p47-*phox*, and p67-*phox* with the submembranous cytoskeleton have also been observed with oxidase assembly.[178, 179]

Kinetic analysis has suggested that cytosolic factors are incorporated as subunits into the oxidase complex.[214] Cytosolic factors are believed to modify flavocytochrome *b* so that electron flow can proceed efficiently from NADPH through its flavin and heme centers to reduce molecular oxygen to superoxide. The observation that respiratory burst activation can result in low levels of intracellular oxidants in CGD patients deficient in p47-*phox* supports this regulatory role.[58] The role of small GTP-binding proteins in oxidase function is also likely to involve modulation of oxidase assembly or activity rather than a direct role in electron transport.

Although p47-*phox* and p67-*phox* are present in the cytosol of resting neutrophils as a complex that also includes p40-*phox*,[110, 162, 163, 215] these subunits become associated with the membrane on oxidase activation (see Fig. 16–2). In studies performed with CGD neutrophils deficient in either p47-*phox* or p67-*phox*, p47-*phox* appeared to be essential for the translocation process.[98] Thus, although p47-*phox* could associate with the membrane in the absence of p67-*phox*, p67-*phox* translocation failed to occur in p47-*phox*–deficient cells. Translocation is also dependent on the presence of flavocytochrome *b*, because it fails to occur in neutrophils obtained from cytochrome-negative CGD patients.[98, 216] There is good evidence for a critical interaction between an SH3 domain in p47-*phox* (residues 151 to 160) and a target proline-rich sequence in p22-*phox*.[145, 149, 150, 217] Multiple potential contact points between p47-*phox* and gp91-*phox* have also been identified.[211, 212, 218–220] Interactions between p67-

phox and flavocytochrome *b* are less well characterized, although a small region in p67-*phox* proximal to its proline-rich and SH3 domains has been proposed as a candidate.[221]

Oxidase activation is also associated with phosphorylation of p47-*phox* at multiple serine residues, which has been postulated to expose SH3 and proline-rich domains that are otherwise inaccessible in resting cells and that control key steps in oxidase assembly.[166, 211–213] In studies performed on intact neutrophils activated by phorbol myristate acetate (a direct activator of protein kinase C), inhibition of p47-*phox* phosphorylation by staurosporine blocked p47-*phox* and p67-*phox* translocation to neutrophil membranes. This suggests that phosphorylation by protein kinase C or another staurosporine-sensitive kinase may be an important regulatory signal for translocation and oxidase activation under these conditions.[178] As already mentioned, however, p47-*phox* phosphorylation is not directly required for oxidase activity, because superoxide production in cell-free assays is independent of phosphorylation.[110, 172, 173]

On neutrophil activation, Rac dissociates from GDI in the cytosol to bind to the membrane (see Fig. 16–2). Rac has also been shown to bind to p67-*phox* subunit through an effector domain encompassed within amino acids 30 to 40 in Rac.[60, 203, 222, 223] Conflicting results have been obtained for the interdependence of Rac translocation and that of p47-*phox* and p67-*phox*.[202, 224–226] Translocation of Rac is decreased in CGD neutrophils lacking flavocytochrome *b*, suggesting that its stable association with the membrane of activated neutrophils is influenced by an interaction with the flavocytochrome.[202, 220] A current model proposes that the Rac binds to p67-*phox* through its effector domain; to a different subunit, possibly flavocytochrome *b*, through a more carboxyl-terminal domain; and to the membrane through its isoprenylated carboxyl terminus.[60, 213, 227]

Many phagocytic antimicrobial functions can be potentiated or "primed" by prior exposure to various agents that include lipopolysaccharide, chemotactic peptides, and cytokines (e.g., granulocyte-macrophage colony-stimulating factor, interleukin-1, IFN-γ) (reviewed in references 228 to 231; see also reference 232). Priming of the respiratory burst is a complex phenomenon that is poorly understood. Depending on the agent and duration of exposure, effects on both the rapidity of oxidase activation and rate of superoxide production can be observed. The underlying molecular mechanisms may involve changes in transcription of oxidase subunit mRNAs[228] as well modifications in the signaling pathways that activate oxidase assembly.[229–231]

Chronic Granulomatous Disease

▼ CLINICAL FEATURES

CGD is a rare, genetically heterogeneous disorder that occurs in approximately 1 in 500,000 individuals according to estimates from large urban areas. On the basis of data from the United States CGD Registry encompassing 368 registered patients, the birth rate between 1980 and 1990 was 1 in 200,000. CGD is caused by inherited defects in the phagocyte NADPH oxidase and is typically manifested as a complete absence of respiratory burst activity.[1, 62, 233–235] A respiratory burst of 1 to 10 per cent of normal is detectable in

Table 16–3. Infections in Chronic Granulomatous Disease

Infections	Percentage of Infections	Infecting Organisms
Pneumonia	70–80	*Aspergillus, Staphylococcus, Burkholderia cepacia, Pseudomonas, Nocardia, Mycobacterium* (including atypical), *Serratia, Candida, Klebsiella, Paecilomyces*
Lymphadenitis	50–60	*Staphylococcus, Serratia, Candida, Klebsiella, Nocardia*
Cutaneous infections/impetigo	50–60	*Staphylococcus, Serratia, Aspergillus, Klebsiella, Candida*
Hepatic/perihepatic abscesses	20–30	*Staphylococcus, Serratia, Streptococcus viridans, Nocardia, Aspergillus*
Osteomyelitis	20–30	*Serratia, Aspergillus, Paecilomyces, Staphylococcus, B. cepacia, Pseudomonas, Nocardia*
Perirectal abscesses/fistulas	15–30	Enteric gram-negative organisms, *Staphylococcus*
Septicemia	10–20	*B. cepacia, Salmonella, Staphylococcus, Candida, Serratia, Klebsiella, Pseudomonas*
Urinary tract infections/pyelonephritis	5–15	Enteric gram-negative organisms
Brain abscesses	<5	*Aspergillus, Staphylococcus*
Meningitis	<5	*Candida lusitania, Haemophilus influenzae, B. cepacia*

The relative frequencies of different types of infections in CGD are estimated from data pooled from several large series of patients in the United States, Europe, and Japan.[238-245] These series encompass approximately 550 patients with CGD after accounting for overlap between reports. Unpublished data from the United States CGD Registry encompassing 368 patients were also used to estimate the relative frequencies of infections and the responsible organisms. The infecting organisms are arranged in approximate order of frequency for each type of infection.

approximately 5 per cent of all patients, who are said to have "variant" CGD.[4, 5, 236, 237] In all cases of CGD studied at the molecular level to date, genetic defects have been identified in one of four oxidase components summarized in Table 16–2.

The CGD phenotype provides direct evidence for the in vivo importance of the phagocyte respiratory burst pathway. Affected patients develop severe, recurrent bacterial and fungal infections, often by organisms not ordinarily considered pathogens.[238, 239] The majority of patients with CGD manifest symptoms within the first year of life. Table 16–3 summarizes the types of infections and infecting organisms associated with CGD according to data from more than 800 patients derived from several published series of patients, literature reviews, and data from the United States CGD Registry.[238-245] Pneumonia, lymphadenitis, and cutaneous infections are the most frequently encountered events. Hepatic abscesses, osteomyelitis, rectal abscesses, and septicemia are also seen fairly frequently. The most common pathogens include *Staphylococcus aureus*, *Aspergillus* species, and a variety of gram-negative bacilli including *Serratia marcescens*, *Burkholderia (Pseudomonas) cepacia*, and various *Salmonella* species. It has long been recognized that CGD patients are particularly susceptible to organisms that contain catalase, which prevents the CGD phagocyte from scavenging microbe-generated H_2O_2 for phagosomal killing.[1] Some of the pathogens encountered in CGD have also been shown to be resistant to phagocyte oxygen-independent killing mechanisms that are vital to the remaining microbicidal potency of the CGD neutrophil and monocyte.[246, 247]

Chronic conditions associated with CGD (Table 16–4) are responsible for many of the major complications of CGD. These include the formation of granulomas, another hallmark of this disorder, which is believed to reflect a chronic inflammatory response to inadequate phagocytic killing or digestion. These lesions contain lymphocytes and pigmented, lipid-containing macrophages.[84, 248] Granuloma formation can lead to obstructive symptoms in the upper gastrointestinal tract and urinary tract as well as a chronic ileocolitis syndrome resembling Crohn's disease.[249, 250]

▼ MOLECULAR BASIS OF CHRONIC GRANULOMATOUS DISEASE

A modern classification of CGD is by type according to the oxidase component affected (Table 16–5). Nomenclature has also been adopted for an abbreviated designation within each major group and includes the mode of inheritance, oxidase component by molecular weight, and level of *phox* protein expression. Overall, defects in the X-linked gene for gp91-*phox* subunit of flavocytochrome *b* account for approximately 74 per cent of CGD, whereas autosomal recessive defects in the p22-*phox* flavocytochrome subunit are rare (4 per cent).[141, 235, 236, 251] Autosomal recessive deficiencies in

Table 16–4. Chronic Conditions Associated With Chronic Granulomatous Disease

Condition	Relative Frequency (%)
Lymphadenopathy	98
Hypergammaglobulinemia	60–90
Hepatomegaly	50–90
Splenomegaly	60–80
Anemia of chronic disease	Common*
Underweight	70
Chronic diarrhea	20–60
Short stature	50
Gingivitis	50
Dermatitis	35
Hydronephrosis	10–25
Granulomatous ileocolitis	10–15
Gastric antral narrowing	10–15
Ulcerative stomatitis	5–15
Granulomatous cystitis	5–10*
Pulmonary fibrosis	<10*
Esophagitis	<10*
Granulomatous cystitis	<10
Chorioretinitis	<10
Glomerulonephritis	<10
Discoid lupus erythematosus	<10

The relative frequencies of the chronic conditions associated with CGD were estimated from the series of reports listed in Table 16–3. In some instances (asterisks), the incidence is estimated from a series of 50 cases followed at Scripps Clinic and Research Foundation and Stanford University (unpublished data).

Table 16–5. Classification of Chronic Granulomatous Disease

Component Affected	Gene Locus	Inheritance	Subtype Designation*	NBT Score (% Positive)	O_2^- Production (% Normal)	Cytochrome *b* Spectrum (% Normal)	Defect in Cell-Free System	Families Evaluated		Frequency (% of Cases)
								SCRIPPS†	EUROPE‡	
gp91-phox	Xp21.1	X	$X91^0$	0	0	0	Membrane	147	36	68
			$X91^-$	80–100 (weak)	3–30	3–30	Membrane	11	2	5
			$X91^-$	5–10	5–10	5–10	Membrane	2	0	<1
			$X91^+$	0	0	100	Membrane	4	0	1
p22-phox	16p24	AR	$A22^0$	0	0	0	Membrane	7	3	4
			$A22^+$	0	0	100	Membrane	1	0	<1
p47-phox	7q11.23	AR	$A47^0$	0	0–1	100	Cytosol	31	13	17
p67-phox	1q25	AR	$A67^0$	0	0	100	Cytosol	9	3	5

X, X-linked; AR (or A), autosomal recessive; NBT, nitroblue tetrazolium.

*In this nomenclature, the first letter represents the mode of inheritance (X-linked [X] or autosomal recessive [A]); the number indicates the *phox* component that is genetically affected. The superscript symbols indicate whether the level of protein of the affected component is undetectable (^{0}), diminished ($^-$), or normal ($^+$) as measured by immunoblot analysis.

†This group represents 209 kindreds evaluated at the Scripps Clinic/Stanford University CGD Clinic.

‡Cooperative study reported in 1992[236] represents 57 kindreds and 63 patients.

Modified from Curnutte, J.T.: Chronic granulomatous disease: the solving of a clinical riddle at the molecular level. Clin. Immunol. Immunopathol. 67:S2, 1993.

Table 16–6. Summary of Mutations in the *CYBB* Gene Encoding gp91-*phox* in 261 Kindreds With X-Linked CGD

Type of Mutation	Number of Kindreds	Frequency (%)	Phenotype
Deletions	63	24.2	X91⁰
Insertions	27	10.3	X91⁰
Splice site mutations	42	16.1	X91⁰
Missense mutations	59	22.6	X91⁰, X91⁻, X91⁺
Nonsense mutations	70	26.8	X91⁰

Data are from a multicenter data base.[257]

the cytosolic factors p47-*phox* and p67-*phox* represent approximately 17 per cent and 5 per cent of cases, respectively.[235, 236, 251]

Mutations in Flavocytochrome *b*

The gp91-*phox* gene (termed *CYBB*) that encodes the large subunit of flavocytochrome *b* contains 13 exons and spans approximately 30 kb in the Xp21.1 region of the X chromosome.[112, 113, 252–255] Defects in the gene are heterogeneous and mostly family specific as demonstrated in two large series of X-linked CGD patients analyzed at the molecular genetic level[141, 256] and summarized in two published data bases.[257–259] Table 16–6 shows a summary from one of these multicenter data bases of the mutations identified in *CYBB* in 261 kindreds with X-linked CGD.[257] Nonsense mutations, deletions, and missense mutations each account for approximately 25 per cent of the mutations seen. The bulk of the remaining 25 per cent are either insertions (10 per cent) or splice site mutations (16 per cent). Whereas all of these mutations are in the coding or splice regions of the gene, it is of note that four regulatory region mutations have also been reported to

date, all clustered in a small area of the *CYBB* promoter between nucleotides -52 and -57.[255, 260] As shown in Figure 16–4, the distribution of the mutations in the gp91-*phox* gene are heterogeneous and apparently random without any obvious mutational hot spots.[141] More than 90 per cent of these mutations result in undetectable levels of flavocytochrome *b* and complete absence of phagocyte respiratory burst activity (the X91⁰ subtype; see Table 16–5). In most cases, this is caused by marked instability of the mRNA or the mutant protein (or both). The rarity of recognized polymorphisms in gp91-*phox* and the paucity of restriction fragment length polymorphisms (RFLPs) in *CYBB* point to the extreme sensitivity of this protein to minor alterations in structure. Also of interest in this regard are the *CYBB* nonsense mutations. The gp91-*phox* protein is undetectable even in those patients whose mutations are near the 3' end of the gene and would permit the synthesis of minimally truncated forms of gp91-*phox*.

In approximately 5 per cent of X-linked CGD patients, relatively large deletions (>30 kb) in Xp21.1 encompassing all of *CYBB* have been described.[112, 113, 141, 256, 261–265] Depending on the size of the deletion and the number of flanking genes affected, these individuals can have complex phenotypes that include not only X91⁰ CGD but also McLeod syndrome (a mild hemolytic anemia associated with depressed levels of Kell antigens due to defects in the red cell antigen Kx encoded by the *XK* gene), Duchenne muscular dystrophy (*DMD* gene), X-linked retinitis pigmentosa (*RP3* gene), and ornithine transcarbamoylase deficiency (*OTC* gene). The map of Xp21.1–p21.2 places the genes in the following order from centromere to pter: *OTC, RP3, CYBB, XK,* and *DMD*.[266] The *CYBB* and *XK* genes are relatively close to each other (~500 kb), consistent with the frequent finding of McLeod syndrome in those X-linked CGD patients with large interstitial deletions. Partial gp91-*phox* gene deletions ranging from 1 to 10 kb have been found in several other patients.[113, 141, 267]

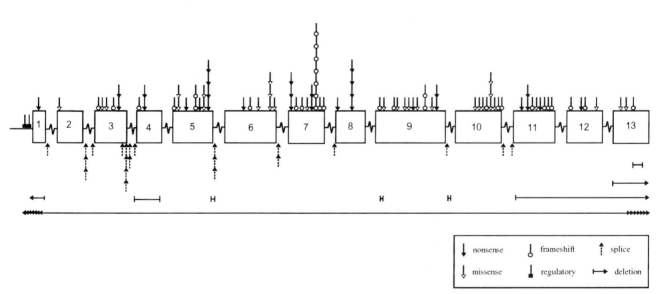

Figure 16–4. Heterogeneity in the positions of *CYBB* mutations causing X-linked CGD. Each arrow represents a single kindred; the type of arrowhead indicates the type of mutation (as defined by the inset box within the figure). Stacked vertical arrows represent multiple unrelated kindreds with mutations at the same location. Solid horizontal lines indicate deletion mutations, their lengths corresponding to the size of the deletion. Arrowheads on the horizontal lines represent unknown deletion length in the direction of the arrow. (From Rae, J., Newburger, P.E., Dinauer, M.C., Noack, D., Hopkins, P.J., Kuruto, R., and Curnutte, J.T.: X-linked chronic granulomatous disease: mutations in the *CYBB* gene encoding the gp91-phox component of respiratory-burst oxidase. Am. J. Hum. Genet. 62:1320, 1998; with permission.)

Of particular interest are mutations identified in the subgroup of variant patients with residual oxidase function associated with small amounts of flavocytochrome *b* (X91⁻ CGD; see Table 16–5). This type of CGD is caused almost exclusively by a small subset of the *CYBB* missense and splicing mutations. For example, the missense mutation Glu 309 → Lys results in normal levels of gp91-*phox* mRNA and low but detectable levels of flavocytochrome *b,* which permits a residual level of oxidase activity that is about 5 per cent of normal[141] (shown at amino acid residue 309 in Fig. 16–5). The two affected cousins have enjoyed a relatively mild clinical course. The Glu 309 → Lys mutation must reduce the stability of gp91-*phox* in some manner distinguishable from other missense mutations associated with X91⁰ CGD (e.g., the patients with amino acid substitutions at residues 20 and 516 in Fig. 16–5). Figure 16–5 also shows three other examples of X91 variant CGD with missense mutations involving amino acids 156 (Ala → Thr), 325 (Ile → Phe), and 339 (Pro → His). Variant CGD can also be seen in patients with splicing mutations. This type of mutation usually results in undetectable levels of flavocytochrome *b* and X91⁰ CGD, particularly if it occurs in the intronic splice donor (5′) or acceptor (3′) site. X91⁻ CGD can arise, however, by nucleotide substitutions at the intron/exon border that lead to alternatively spliced forms of mRNA, including the normally spliced species. When appreciable levels of the normal message are present, sufficient gp91-*phox* can be present to permit low levels of respiratory burst activity.[141] Another mechanism by which a splice mutation can lead to variant CGD is through a cryptic splice site. One such example is a kindred in which abnormal mRNA

splicing is due to an A → G mutation in the acceptor splice site at the 3′ end of intron 11.[268] A cryptic splice site in exon 12 leads to the in-frame deletion of 30 nucleotides in this exon and the loss of 10 amino acids (Ala 488–Glu 497) in the middle of the large intracytoplasmic carboxyl-terminal domain of gp91-*phox* (see model in Fig. 16–5). Whereas the level and spectral characteristics of flavocytochrome *b* are unaffected as a result of this deletion, rates of superoxide production are only 6 per cent of normal. This may reflect an impaired ability of gp91-*phox* to interact with cytosolic oxidase subunits.[268] This patient had no history of significant infections until the age of 69; however, his grandson died at the age of 5 years of *B. cepacia* sepsis. Finally, one kindred with X91⁻ CGD was found to have an intronic mutation six nucleotides in from the 5′ donor site in intron 1 (GTAAGT → GTAAGC).[141] The affected brothers have low levels of normal transcripts. Interestingly, these patients are unique in their responsiveness to recombinant IFN-γ (rIFN-γ) in that their phagocytes have complete restoration of respiratory burst function with either in vitro or in vivo exposure to the interferon.[269, 270] Presumably, the steady-state level of the normal transcript increases in the presence of rIFN-γ.

Patients with X91⁺ CGD (see Table 16–5) are of particular interest because they have normal levels of a dysfunctional flavocytochrome *b* and as such provide important information regarding the properties of the different domains of gp91-*phox*. Most of these rare patients have missense mutations, three examples of which are shown in Figure 16–5: Arg 54 → Ser, Pro 415 → His, and Cys 537 → Arg.[141, 271] The first of these mutations has been studied in detail and provides an example of the insights that can be

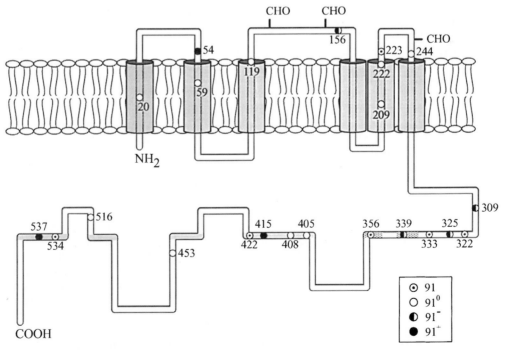

Figure 16–5. Sites of gp91-*phox* missense mutations in X-linked CGD. Sites of missense mutations are identified by the number of the affected amino acid and the type of mutation as indicated by the symbols defined in the inset. The shaded regions between amino acids 403 and 546 are part of the putative NADPH-binding site; the stippled sections between amino acids 335 and 360 represent the likely FAD-binding domain (see also Fig. 16–3). Glycosylation sites are indicated by CHO. (From Rae, J., Newburger, P.E., Dinauer, M.C., Noack, D., Hopkins, P.J., Kuruto, R., and Curnutte, J.T.: X-linked chronic granulomatous disease: mutations in the *CYBB* gene encoding the gp91-phox component of respiratory-burst oxidase. Am. J. Hum. Genet. 62:1320, 1998; with permission.)

gained regarding the function of flavocytochrome *b* as well as the molecular basis of the CGD in the patient.[127, 272] The Arg 54 → Ser mutation results in a nonfunctional heme that is unable to accept electrons from the reduced flavin center and generate superoxide. It has an abnormal visible spectrum with a slightly shifted Soret band. In contrast, the flavin group is fully functional; it is able to become reduced by NADPH and pass the electrons onto an artificial dye acceptor (iodonitrotetrazolium violet) at rates similar to normal flavocytochrome *b*. After stimulation, intact neutrophils from the patient also show low levels of nitroblue tetrazolium (NBT) staining in the NBT slide test. Potentiometric titrations of the cytochrome revealed that the effect of the Arg 54 → Ser mutation is to reduce the midpoint potential of one of the two heme centers by 35 mV (possibly through altered interactions with a heme propionate side chain) and thereby impede the flow of electrons from FAD to the heme (see above and Fig. 16–3).

Mutations in the regulatory region of the gp91-*phox* gene have been reported in four unrelated kindreds and are associated with a highly unusual CGD phenotype. In the three affected males in the first two kindreds identified, approximately 5 per cent of the circulating granulocytes generate a normal respiratory burst after stimulation and appear to contain normal levels of flavocytochrome *b*.[273] The remaining 95 per cent of cells are devoid of activity and have the X91^0 phenotype. Remarkably, similar mutations were identified in the two families: an A → C substitution at nucleotide −57 in the 5′ flanking region in one and a T → C change at position −55 in the other.[260] Subsequently, two other kindreds have been reported with a similar cellular phenotype and mutations strikingly similar to the first two kindreds: C → T at position −53 and C → T at nucleotide −52.[255, 274] In these two kindreds, only the eosinophils were found to have respiratory burst activity, raising the intriguing hypothesis that the −53/−52 region is not necessary to control transcription in eosinophils but is critical for gp91-*phox* expression in all other phagocytes. It is not known whether the functional granulocytes in the first two kindreds might, in fact, be eosinophils. If not, then the possibility remains that positions −57 and −55 affect gene expression in a different manner. Two transcription activators have been found to bind to the −57 to −52 region: PU.1[255] and hematopoiesis-associated factor (HAF-1).[254] Their relative roles in regulating *CYBB* transcription are under investigation.

Mutations in the gene for the p22-*phox* subunit of flavocytochrome *b* are an uncommon cause of CGD and account for approximately 5 per cent of all cases[116] (see Table 16–5). The p22-*phox* gene (termed *CYBA*) resides at 16q24 and contains 6 exons that span 8.5 kb (see Table 16–2). The genetic defects that have been identified are heterogeneous and range from a large interstitial gene deletion[116, 275] to point mutations associated with missense, frameshift, and RNA splicing defects.[116, 145, 168, 276–279] Because of consanguinity, all but two of nine reported cases are homozygous for the specific mutation. A gene defect associated with normal levels of flavocytochrome *b* and a dysfunctional oxidase, analogous to the cases of X91$^+$ CGD described above, has been reported.[145] The Pro 156 → His mutation occurs in the intracytoplasmic carboxyl terminus of p22-*phox* in a proline-rich domain that normally serves as a docking site for one of the SH3 domains of p47-*phox* as discussed before.[149–151, 217] The replacement of Pro 156 by His at this critical position completely disrupts the binding of p47-*phox* to p22-*phox* and probably prevents the activation of the oxidase.[149–151]

Mutations in the p47-*phox* and p67-*phox* Subunits

The gene for p67-*phox*, termed *NCF2*, is located on the long arm of chromosome 1 at position q25[280] and contains 16 exons spanning 40 kb[281] (see Table 16–2). Approximately 5 per cent of all cases of CGD are caused by mutations in *NCF2*, the large majority of which result in the A67^0 phenotype in which the levels of p67-*phox* in phagocytes are undetectable (see Table 16–5). In most but not all cases, the p67-*phox* mRNA is undetectable as well.[282] As with the X91 and A22 forms of CGD, there is a marked heterogeneity in the mutations encountered in 12 patients with A67 CGD,[282–289] many of which appear to be family specific. A total of 14 different mutant alleles have been reported that contain deletions (36 per cent), missense mutations (28 per cent), splicing defects (21 per cent), insertions (7 per cent), and nonsense mutations (7 per cent). In 8 of 12 of the kindreds, the patients were homozygous for the mutation, although in only half of these cases was there known consanguinity in the parents. One case of A67$^-$ CGD has been identified in which the neutrophils contain approximately half the normal levels of p67-*phox*.[286] The patient is a compound heterozygote; one of the alleles contains an 11 to 13 kb deletion that precludes the production of any protein. The other allele, however, has an in-frame deletion of three nucleotides that predicts the loss of a single amino acid, Lys 58, that must be compatible with roughly normal protein expression. This mutant p67-*phox* is nonfunctional and fails to translocate to the membrane on activation of the phagocyte.[286]

The gene for p47-*phox*, termed *NCF1*, resides on chromosome 7 at q11.23[280] and contains 11 exons spanning 15 kb[290] (see Table 16–2). Mutations at this locus are associated with one fifth of all cases of CGD (see Table 16–5). This form of CGD stands in stark contrast to the other three subtypes in that a single common mutation has been reported in each of the 35 patients characterized to date.[291–295] All but four of these patients are homozygous for the mutation, a dinucleotide deletion (ΔGT) at a GTGT repeat at the beginning of exon 2 that results in a frameshift and premature translational termination after the synthesis of a 50 residue protein. One other mutation has been identified in one of the apparent heterozygotes—a single nucleotide deletion involving G 502.[293] All 35 patients have undetectable levels of p47-*phox* (hence A47^0 CGD), a finding consistent with the ΔGT mutation and the G 502 deletion. Despite the fact that 31 of 35 of these patients are homozygous for the ΔGT mutation, none is reported to arise from parental consanguinity.

An important clue that helped to solve the mystery of the unusual genetics of A47^0 CGD was the finding that each of 34 normal individuals appeared to be heterozygous for the ΔGT mutation.[295] This pointed to the possibility of a highly homologous *NCF1* pseudogene containing the ΔGT sequence that was coamplified and sequenced along with the wild-type p47-*phox* gene in these normal individuals. This was, in fact, the case; the pseudogene was cloned from three different human genomic libraries and found to contain the GT mutation in all cases.[295] Both the wild-type gene and the pseudogene colocalize to chromosome 7q11.23.[295] This proximity suggests that the high frequency of the GT mutation in the CGD population is due to recombination events between the two genes.[292, 295] In addition, there are more than 30 potential recombination hot spots in *NCF1* that have been identified and that could serve to facilitate the introduction of pseudogene sequences into the wild-type gene.[295]

Defects in the other polypeptides involved in oxidase function, such as Rac1, Rac2, p40-*phox*, and Rap1A, have not been reported. On the basis of the large number of CGD patients who have been characterized at the molecular level, the prevalence of a mutation causing clinically apparent CGD in any one of these proteins would be less than 1 per cent.

Molecular Basis of Clinical Heterogeneity

The classification of CGD according to specific gene defects provides an explanation for many of the previously confusing aspects of this disorder. Identification of specific mutations by DNA sequence analysis is also helping to clarify the basis for some of the variability in clinical severity. Variant X-linked CGD patients with low but detectable respiratory burst activity usually, but not always, have a milder clinical course. Many of these patients have mutations associated with a residual level of flavocytochrome *b*. Molecular analysis has not yet been reported for members of another rare subset of variant X-linked CGD who have undetectable levels of neutrophil flavocytochrome *b* yet some residual oxidase activity (reviewed in reference 1; see also references 296 to 299). The K_m of the oxidase complex for NADPH has been studied in broken cell preparations obtained from such patients and found to be 20 to 70 times higher than the normal level of 40 μM. Whether an alternative pathway is used for electron transport in the absence of flavocytochrome *b* or whether a tiny amount of flavocytochrome *b* is able to maintain some oxidase function is unknown.

Patients with defects in cytosolic oxidase components have often been noted to exhibit milder disease than patients with X-linked CGD, particularly those with a deficiency of p47-*phox*.[239, 300–302] One possible reason for this less severe phenotype is that stimulated neutrophils from A47⁰ patients have low levels of intracellular oxidant production[58, 303] that can be quantitated on a flow cytometer by use of a sensitive intracellular fluorescent probe that detects hydrogen peroxide (e.g., dichlorofluorescein or dihydrorhodamine 123).[304–306] In contrast, patients with X91⁰ CGD have undetectable or trace levels of fluorescence in this assay.[58, 303] The biochemical basis for this residual oxidative activity appears to be the different roles the various cytosolic oxidase components play in regulating electron flow through the flavocytochrome *b*. Even in the absence of p47-*phox*, NADPH can transfer electrons to FAD, which in turn can auto-oxidize to generate hydrogen peroxide.[307, 308]

It is likely that other factors affecting the clinical severity of CGD are related to the ability of auxiliary microbicidal systems to maintain an effective host defense. These disease-modifying factors may be either environmental (e.g., diet) or genetic. There is now evidence that polymorphisms in host defense molecules influence the risk for immune-mediated complications of CGD, such as colitis, gastric outlet obstruction, and perirectal abscesses.[309] In this study of 129 CGD patients, for example, genotypes of MPO and FcγRIIIb were strongly associated with an increased risk for gastrointestinal complications.

▼ DIAGNOSIS AND TREATMENT

The diagnosis of CGD is suggested by the characteristic clinical features or by a family history of the disease. In light of the variable severity of symptoms among different patients, the diagnosis of CGD should still be considered in adolescents and adults who present with an unusual infection typical of CGD (see Tables 16–3 and 16–4). The diagnostic feature of CGD is an absent or greatly diminished neutrophil respiratory burst. Numerous assays have been used to quantitate respiratory burst activity (reviewed in reference 310; see also references 304 to 306). The simplest and most commonly used is the NBT test, in which the water-soluble yellow tetrazolium dye is reduced into a blue insoluble formazan pigment by O_2^- generated by the activated oxidase complex.[1, 4] A typical example is shown in Figure 16–6. Figure 16–6A shows the normal positive heavy staining of a group of seven peripheral blood neutrophils and one monocyte; the staining is absent in cells obtained from a patient with X91⁰ CGD as shown in Figure 16–6B. The NBT test is also helpful in diagnosing the female carrier state in X-linked CGD, in which cells will stain positively or negatively, depending on random X-chromosome inactivation. This is demonstrated in an obligate carrier female in Figure 16–6C. Because X-linked CGD may arise by a de novo germline mutation in a parent, NBT-negative cells are not always seen in the mother of a child with X-linked CGD.[311] One study of 131 consecutive unrelated X-linked CGD kindreds found that 10 of 87 mothers were not carriers. The NBT test result is normal in carriers of autosomal recessive forms of CGD. Light staining with formazan deposits in an NBT test may suggest the presence of variant forms of CGD with low levels of respiratory burst function.[4]

With the exception of cases with unequivocal X-linked inheritance in a CGD male, identification of the specific oxidase protein component affected in an individual CGD patient generally requires immunoblot analysis of neutrophil extracts or, alternatively, spectral assay in the case of flavocytochrome *b*. In a male with absent flavocytochrome *b*[310] without clear evidence for a maternal carrier, it would be necessary to identify the mutation directly by DNA sequencing or other analysis of the gp91-*phox* and p22-*phox* genes. The diagnosis of most cases of A47⁰ CGD can be established by demonstrating homozygosity for the ΔGT mutation with use of genomic DNA or cDNA. In the rare case in which all four known oxidase components are present at the protein level, functional analysis of membrane and cytosol fractions can be helpful[310] (e.g., the A22⁺ and X91⁺ forms of CGD in Table 16–5[145, 271]).

Until somatic genetic therapy becomes a realistic therapeutic option, classification of the specific CGD subgroup is useful primarily for purposes of genetic counseling and pre-

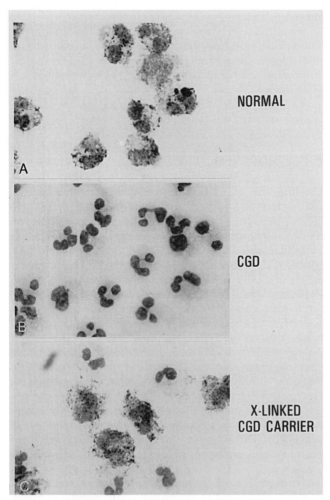

NORMAL

CGD

X-LINKED
CGD CARRIER

Figure 16–6. NBT slide test. Peripheral blood neutrophils and mono-cytes from a drop of fresh whole blood were made adherent to glass slides and stimulated with phorbol myristate acetate in the presence of NBT. *A,* Normal neutrophils and monocytes, all of which are NBT positive. *B,* Neutrophils and monocytes from an X-linked CGD patient, which are all NBT negative. *C,* A mixture of NBT-positive and NBT-negative neutrophils from the X-linked carrier mother of the patient in *B.* (From Curnutte, J.T.: Disorders of phagocyte function. *In* Hoffman, R., Benz, E.J., Jr., Shattil, S.J., Furie, B., and Cohen, H.J. [eds.]: Hematology: Basic Principles and Practice. New York, Churchill Livingstone, 1991, pp. 571–589; with permission.)

natal diagnosis. In utero fetal blood sampling and NBT slide test analysis of fetal blood neutrophils have been used for prenatal diagnosis (reviewed in reference 312) but have been replaced in recent years by DNA analysis of amniocytes or chorionic villus biopsy tissue. Results of Southern blot analysis of gene structure will be normal in most cases, because the majority of CGD-associated alleles appear to have point mutations. RFLPs have been identified for gp91-*phox*[264, 313, 314] and p67-*phox*[281, 315] and can be useful for diagnosis in informative families. The gene for gp91-*phox* also contains at least two highly polymorphic (GT/AC)$_n$ repeats, which can be diagnostic in informative families in a manner analogous to RFLPs.[316] Alleles differing in the number of (GT/AC)$_n$ repeats can be identified by amplification with the polymerase chain reaction using nanogram quantities of DNA.

The most specific approach to prenatal diagnosis is to first determine the family-specific mutation and then analyze

fetal DNA for the specific mutation. Polymerase chain reaction amplification of individual exons from genomic DNA followed by single-stranded conformation polymorphism analysis on denaturing gels has proved to be a rapid way of identifying point mutations in families seeking genetic counseling.[141, 312] The majority of prenatal diagnoses are now made by direct sequencing of chorionic villus or amniocyte DNA.[141, 317, 318]

The prognosis for patients with CGD has continued to improve during the years since the disorder was first described in the 1950s, at which time the majority of patients died in childhood. The most recent mortality rates for CGD are between 1 and 2 per cent per year.[62] With newer treatment strategies, a large majority of patients should survive well into their adult years, particularly those with the A47^0 and A67^0 forms of the disease. The key elements in current management of CGD include (1) prevention and early treatment of infections; (2) aggressive use of parenteral antibiotics, augmented by surgical drainage or resection of recalcitrant infections; (3) use of prophylactic trimethoprim-sulfamethoxazole or dicloxacillin; (4) use of prophylactic rIFN-γ.[301, 319, 320] Corticosteroids should be avoided except in severe asthma or in the management of refractory granulomatous lesions in the gastrointestinal or urinary tract.[321]

Recombinant human IFN-γ has been shown to be an effective and well-tolerated treatment that reduces the incidence of serious infections in patients in all four genetic subgroups of CGD.[301] IFN-γ enhances many aspects of normal phagocyte function, including microbial killing, FcγRI expression, phagocytosis, and rates of hydrogen peroxide production.[322–324] Augmentation of oxidant production appears, in part, related to increased levels of gp91-*phox* mRNA[269] and prompted attempts to correct the functional deficiency in CGD phagocytes with rIFN-γ. Initial studies demonstrated that rIFN-γ led to some improvement in O_2^- production and bacterial killing by CGD neutrophils both in vitro and in vivo.[269, 270, 325] This effect was most dramatic in patients with variant X-linked CGD. These encouraging results prompted a double-blind, placebo-controlled Phase III trial to evaluate whether prophylactic rIFN-γ could reduce the incidence of serious infections in different genetic forms of CGD.[301] The key results of this study are summarized in the first two columns of Table 16–7. The group receiving rIFN-γ had significantly fewer patients who developed at least one serious infection (14 versus 30), and the total number of serious infections (20 versus 56) was also markedly reduced in the rIFN-γ cohort. Put another way, the placebo group had 1.1 serious infections per patient-year compared with 0.38 in the treatment group—a 2.8-fold decrease. The beneficial effects were independent of age, mode of inheritance, and concomitant use of prophylactic antibiotics. Treatment (50 μg/m^2 three times a week subcutaneously) was well tolerated and easy to administer. Surprisingly, there was no difference in neutrophil superoxide production and *S. aureus* killing between the rIFN-γ and placebo groups.[301, 326] This suggests that the beneficial effect of rIFN-γ in most CGD patients is achieved by enhancing non-oxidative microbicidal mechanisms or other aspects of phagocyte function. This observation raises the possibility of a more general role for rIFN-γ as an adjunct to conventional antimicrobial therapy in other clinical settings.

Two longer term follow-up studies have also been re-

Table 16–7. Efficacy of IFN-γ in Preventing Serious Infections in CGD

Variable	Clinical Study			
	PHASE III PLACEBO*	PHASE III IFN-γ*	PHASE IV (U.S.) IFN-γ†	PHASE IV (EUROPE) IFN-γ‡
Number of patients	65	63	30	28
Average duration of therapy on study (years)	0	0.83	1.03	2.4
Patient-years on study	50.9	52.1	31.0	67.2
Serious infections per patient-year	1.10	0.38	0.13	0.25
Number of hospital days per patient-year	28.2	8.6	2.2	15.0

*Results from The International Chronic Granulomatous Disease Cooperative Study Group.[301]
†Results from The Scripps Research Institute CGD Clinic.[319]
‡Results from Weening et al.[320]

ported and are shown in Table 16–7 as well.[319, 320] Although these Phase IV studies do not have a placebo control arm, they nonetheless show a sustained lower number of serious infections per patient-year comparable to that seen in the Phase III study.

▼ FUTURE DIRECTIONS

Allogeneic bone marrow stem cell transplantation can be used to treat CGD and has been successfully employed in a number of cases.[327–334] However, because of the risks associated with this procedure and difficulties often encountered in finding a suitable donor, stem cell transplantation in the management of CGD is not routine and generally considered only for those individuals who have frequent and severe infections despite aggressive medical management. Exciting developments in pretransplantation conditioning regimens could lead to the more ready use of allogeneic transplantation for treatment of CGD and other genetic blood diseases. Success has been reported with non-myeloablative regimens using fludarabine, anti–T-lymphocyte globulin, and low-dose busulfan for pretransplantation conditioning in both hematological malignant neoplasms and inherited blood cell disorders. These regimens were much better tolerated than intensive cytoreduction based on irradiation and also appear to greatly reduce the incidence of significant graft-versus-host disease.[335, 336]

Because CGD results from genetic defects in specific phagocyte oxidase proteins whose cDNAs have been cloned, the disorder should in principle be correctable by gene transfer into bone marrow hematopoietic stem cells. Female carriers of X-linked CGD can have few or no symptoms even with as little as 5 to 10 per cent oxidase-positive neutrophils,[273, 337–339] which suggests that long-term correction of only a minority of phagocytes could provide substantial clinical benefit. Retroviral vectors have been successfully used to transfer a functional copy of the affected gene in CGD myeloid cell lines and primary hematopoietic cells in vitro.[340–344] At least for the X-linked gene product, gp91-phox, it appears that expression of even modest amounts of recombinant protein can lead to considerable reconstitution of superoxide-generating capacity.[342, 345] Mouse models for both the X-linked (gp91-phox$^{-/-}$) and the p47-phox–deficient (p47-phox$^{-/-}$) forms of CGD have been developed by use of gene targeting technology.[346, 347] Retrovirus-mediated gene transfer of the corresponding cDNA into bone marrow cells

corrected the neutrophil respiratory burst in vivo and improved the defect in host defense against bacterial and fungal pathogens.[337, 342]

A Phase I clinical trial for gene therapy of p47-phox–deficient CGD has been conducted in which autologous peripheral blood CD34$^+$ cells collected by apheresis were transduced with a p47-phox–containing retroviral vector and then reinfused.[348] Peripheral blood neutrophils with respiratory burst oxidase activity were seen for up to 3 to 6 months in all five patients studied, although their frequency was only 0.02 to 0.005 per cent of neutrophils. This low percentage most likely reflects the relative inefficiency of current methods for retrovirus-mediated gene transfer into human hematopoietic cells capable of engraftment and the fact that patients received no myeloablative conditioning before infusion of transduced cells. However, ongoing research in human hematopoietic stem cell biology and the development of more effective approaches for introducing genes into bone marrow stem cells are likely to make gene replacement therapy a future option for treatment of CGD and other inherited blood disorders.

REFERENCES

1. Curnutte, J.T., and Babior, B.M.: Chronic granulomatous disease. *In* Harris, H., and Hirschhorn, K. (eds.): Advances in Human Genetics. New York, Plenum Publishing, 1987, pp. 229–297.
2. Cross, A.R., and Jones, O.T.G.: Enzymic mechanisms of superoxide production. Biochim. Biophys. Acta 1057:281, 1991.
3. Segal, A.W.: The electron transport chain of the microbicidal oxidase of phagocytic cells and its involvement in the molecular pathology of chronic granulomatous disease. J. Clin. Invest. 83:1785, 1989.
4. Smith, R.M., and Curnutte, J.T.: Molecular basis of chronic granulomatous disease. Blood 77:673, 1991.
5. Curnutte, J.T.: Molecular basis of the autosomal recessive forms of chronic granulomatous disease. Immunodefic. Rev. 3:149, 1992.
6. Jesaitis, A.J.: Structure of human phagocyte cytochrome *b* and its relationship to microbicidal superoxide production. J. Immunol. 155:3286, 1995.
7. Halliwell, B.: Reactive oxygen species in living systems: source, biochemistry, and role in human disease. Am. J. Med. 91(suppl. 3C):14S, 1991.
8. Bast, A., Haenen, G.R.M.M., and Doelman, C.J.A.: Oxidants and antioxidants: state of the art. Am. J. Med. 91(suppl. 3C):2S, 1991.
9. Hampton, M.B., Kettle, A.J., and Winterbourn, C.C.: Inside the neutrophil phagosome: oxidants, myeloperoxidase, and bacterial killing. Blood 92:3007, 1998.
10. Weiss, S.J.: Mechanisms of disease. Tissue destruction by neutrophils. N. Engl. J. Med. 320:365, 1989.
11. Nathan, C.: Nitric oxide as a secretory product of mammalian cells. FASEB J. 6:3051, 1992.

12. Prince, R.C., and Gunson, D.E.: Rising interest in nitric oxide synthase. Trends Biochem. Sci. 18:35, 1993.

13. Marletta, M.A.: Nitric oxide synthase: aspects concerning structure and catalysis. Cell 78:927, 1994.

14. Nathan, C.: Inducible nitric oxide synthase: what difference does it make? J. Clin. Invest. 100:2417, 1997.

15. MacMicking, J.D., Nathan, C., Hom, G., Chartrain, N., Fletcher, D.S., Trumbauer, M., Stevens, K., Xie, Q.W., Sokol, K., and Hutchinson, N.: Altered responses to bacterial infection and endotoxic shock in mice lacking inducible nitric oxide synthase [published erratum appears in Cell 81:following 1170, 1995]. Cell 81:641, 1995.

16. Wheeler, M.A., Smith, S.D., Garcia-Cardena, G., Nathan, C.F., Weiss, R.M., and Sessa, W.C.: Bacterial infection induces nitric oxide synthase in human neutrophils. J. Clin. Invest. 99:110, 1997.

17. Evans, T.J., Buttery, L.D., Carpenter, A., Springall, D.R., Polak, J.M., and Cohen, J.: Cytokine-treated human neutrophils contain inducible nitric oxide synthase that produces nitration of ingested bacteria. Proc. Natl. Acad. Sci. USA 93:9553, 1996.

18. Weinberg, J.B., Misukonis, M.A., Shami, P.J., Mason, S.N., Sauls, D.L., Dittman, W.A., Wood, E.R., Smith, G.K., McDonald, B., and Bachus, K.E.: Human mononuclear phagocyte inducible nitric oxide synthase (iNOS): analysis of iNOS mRNA, iNOS protein, biopterin, and nitric oxide production by blood monocytes and peritoneal macrophages. Blood 86:1184, 1995.

19. Malawista, S.E., Montgomery, R.R., and Van Blaricom, G.: Evidence for reactive nitrogen intermediates in killing of staphylococci by human neutrophil cytoplasts. A new microbicidal pathway for polymorphonuclear leukocytes. J. Clin. Invest. 90:631, 1992.

20. Eiserich, J.P., Hristova, M., Cross, C.E., Jones, A.D., Freeman, B.A., Halliwell, B., and van der Vliet, A.: Formation of nitric oxide–derived inflammatory oxidants by myeloperoxidase in neutrophils. Nature 391:393, 1998.

21. Spitznagel, J.K.: Antibiotic proteins of human neutrophils. J. Clin. Invest. 86:1381, 1990.

22. Boxer, L.A., and Smolen, J.E.: Neutrophil granule constituents and their release in health and disease. Hematol. Oncol. Clin. North Am. 2:101, 1988.

23. Lehrer, R.I., and Ganz, T.: Antimicrobial polypeptides of human neutrophils. Blood 76:2169, 1990.

24. Gabay, J.E., and Almeida, R.P.: Antibiotic peptides and serine protease homologs in human polymorphonuclear leukocytes: defensins and azurocidin. Curr. Opin. Immunol. 5:97, 1993.

25. Weiss, J.: Leukocyte-derived antimicrobial proteins. Curr. Opin. Hematol. 1:78, 1994.

26. Lehrer, R.I., Ganz, T., Selsted, M.E., Babior, B.M., and Curnutte, J.T.: Neutrophils and host defense. Ann. Intern. Med. 109:127, 1988.

27. Peters, C.W., Kruse, U., Pollwein, R., Grzeschik, K.H., and Sippel, A.E.: The human lysozyme gene. Sequence organization and chromosomal localization. Eur. J. Biochem. 182:507, 1989.

28. Ambruso, D.R., and Johnston, R.B., Jr.: Lactoferrin enhances hydroxyl radical production by human neutrophils, neutrophil particulate fractions, and an enzymatic generating system. J. Clin. Invest. 67:352, 1981.

29. Elsbach, P.: The bactericidal/permeability-increasing protein (BPI) in antibacterial host defense. J. Leukoc. Biol. 64:14, 1998.

30. Gray, P.W., Corcorran, A.E., Eddy, R.L.J., Byers, M.G., and Shows, T.B.: The genes for the lipopolysaccharide binding protein (LBP) and the bactericidal permeability increasing protein (BPI) are encoded in the same region of human chromosome 20. Genomics 15:188, 1993.

31. Morgan, J.G., Sukiennicki, T., Pereira, H.A., Spitznagel, J.K., Guerra, M.E., and Larrick, J.W.: Cloning of the cDNA for the serine protease homolog CAP37/azurocidin, a microbicidal and chemotactic protein from human granulocytes. J. Immunol. 147:3210, 1991.

32. Hohn, P.A., Popescu, N.C., Hanson, R.D., Salvesen, G., and Ley, T.J.: Genomic organization and chromosomal localization of the human cathepsin G gene. J. Biol. Chem. 264:13412, 1989.

33. Zimmer, M., Medcalf, R.L., Fink, T.M., Mattmann, C., Lichter, P., and Jenne, D.E.: Three human elastase-like genes coordinately expressed in the myelomonocyte lineage are organized as a single genetic locus on 19pter. Proc. Natl. Acad. Sci. USA 89:8215, 1992.

34. Ganz, T., and Weiss, J.: Antimicrobial peptides of phagocytes and epithelia. Semin. Hematol. 34:343, 1997.

35. Sparkes, R.S., Kronenberg, M., Heinzmann, C., Daher, K.A., Klisak, I., Ganz, T., and Mohandas, T.: Assignment of defensin gene(s) to human chromosome 8p23. Genomics 5:240, 1989.

36. Cochrane, C.G.: Cellular injury by oxidants. Am. J. Med. 91(suppl. 3C):23S, 1991.

37. Toker, A., and Cantley, L.C.: Signalling through the lipid products of phosphoinositide-3-OH kinase. Nature 387:673, 1997.

38. Cockcroft, S.: Phospholipid signaling in leukocytes. Curr. Opin. Hematol. 3:48, 1996.

39. Downey, G.P., Fukushima, T., and Fialkow, L.: Signaling mechanisms in human neutrophils. Curr. Opin. Hematol. 2:76, 1995.

40. Oancea, E., and Meyer, T.: Protein kinase C as a molecular machine for decoding calcium and diacylglycerol signals. Cell 95:307, 1998.

41. Ptasznik, A., Prossnitz, E.R., Yoshikawa, D., Smrcka, A., Traynor-Kaplan, A.E., and Bokoch, G.M.: A tyrosine kinase signaling pathway accounts for the majority of phosphatidylinositol 3,4,5-trisphosphate formation in chemoattractant-stimulated human neutrophils. J. Biol. Chem. 271:25204, 1996.

42. Rollet, E., Caon, A.C., Roberge, C.J., Liao, N.W., Malawista, S.E., McColl, S.R., and Naccache, P.H.: Tyrosine phosphorylation in activated human neutrophils. Comparison of the effects of different classes of agonists and identification of the signaling pathways involved. J. Immunol. 153:353, 1994.

43. Kiefer, F., Brumell, J., Al-Alawi, N., Latour, S., Cheng, A., Veillette, A., Grinstein, S., and Pawson, T.: The Syk protein tyrosine kinase is essential for Fcgamma receptor signaling in macrophages and neutrophils. Mol. Cell. Biol. 18:4209, 1998.

44. Grinstein, S., Furuya, W., Butler, J.R., and Tseng, J.: Receptor-mediated activation of multiple serine/threonine kinases in human leukocytes. J. Biol. Chem. 268:20223, 1993.

45. Ding, J., and Badwey, J.A.: Stimulation of neutrophils with a chemoattractant activates several novel protein kinases that can catalyze the phosphorylation of peptides derived from the 47-kDa protein component of the phagocyte oxidase and myristoylated alanine-rich C kinase substrate. J. Biol. Chem. 268:17326, 1993.

46. Nick, J.A., Avdi, N.J., Young, S.K., Knall, C., Gerwins, P., Johnson, G.L., and Worthen, G.S.: Common and distinct intracellular signaling pathways in human neutrophils utilized by platelet activating factor and FMLP. J. Clin. Invest. 99:975, 1997.

47. Perez, H.D.: Chemoattractant receptors. Curr. Opin. Hematol. 1:40, 1994.

48. Murphy, P.M.: Neutrophil receptors for interleukin-8 and related CXC chemokines. Semin. Hematol. 34:311, 1997.

49. Bokoch, G.M.: Chemoattractant signaling and leukocyte activation. Blood 86:1649, 1995.

50. Unkeless, J.C.: Function and heterogeneity of human Fc receptors for immunoglobulin G. J. Clin. Invest. 83:355, 1989.

51. Sanchez-Mejorada, G., and Rosales, C.: Signal transduction by immunoglobulin Fc receptors. J. Leukoc. Biol. 63:521, 1998.

52. Ravetch, J.V., and Clynes, R.A.: Divergent roles for Fc receptors and complement in vivo. Annu. Rev. Immunol. 16:421, 1998.

53. Ravetch, J.V.: Fc receptors. Curr. Opin. Immunol. 9:121, 1997.

54. Todd, R.F., III, and Freyer, D.R.: The CD11/CD18 leukocyte glycoprotein deficiency. Hematol. Oncol. Clin. North Am. 2:13, 1988.

55. Larson, R.S., and Springer, T.A.: Structure and function of leukocyte integrins. Immunol. Rev. 114:181, 1990.

56. Fearon, D.T.: The complement system and adaptive immunity. Semin. Immunol. 10:355, 1998.

57. Ohno, Y.I., Hirai, K.I., Kanoh, T., Uchino, H., and Ogawa, K.: Subcellular localization of hydrogen peroxide production in human polymorphonuclear leukocytes stimulated with lectins, phorbol myristate acetate, and digitonin: an electron microscope study using CeCl3. Blood 60:1195, 1982.

58. Bemiller, L.S., Rost, J.R., Ku-Balai, T.L., and Curnutte, J.T.: The production of intracellular oxidants by stimulated neutrophils correlates with the clinical severity of chronic granulomatous disease (CGD). Blood 78:377a, 1991.

59. Nauseef, W.M.: Myeloperoxidase deficiency. Hematol. Oncol. Clin. North Am. 2:135, 1988.

60. Nisimoto, Y., Freeman, J.R., Motalebi, S.A., Hirshberg, M., and Lambeth, J.D.: Rac binding to p67(phox). Structural basis for interactions of the Rac1 effector region and insert region with components of the respiratory burst oxidase. J. Biol. Chem. 272:18834, 1997.

61. Borregaard, N., Heiple, J.M., Simons, E.R., and Clark, R.A.: Subcellular localization of the b-cytochrome component of the human neutrophil microbicidal oxidase: translocation during activation. J. Cell Biol. 97:52, 1983.

62. Malech, H.L., and Nauseef, W.M.: Primary inherited defects in neutrophil function: etiology and treatment. Semin. Hematol. 34:279, 1997.

63. Tobler, A., Selsted, M.E., Miller, C.W., Johnson, K.R., Novotny, M.J., Rovera, G., and Koeffler, H.P.: Evidence for a pretranslational defect in hereditary and acquired myeloperoxidase deficiency. Blood 73:1980, 1989.

64. Nauseef, W.M., Brigham, S., and Cogley, M.: Hereditary myeloperoxidase deficiency due to a missense mutation of arginine 569 to tryptophan. J. Biol. Chem. 269:1212, 1994.

65. DeLeo, F.R., Goedken, M., McCormick, S.J., and Nauseef, W.M.: A novel form of hereditary myeloperoxidase deficiency linked to endoplasmic reticulum/proteasome degradation. J. Clin. Invest. 101:2900, 1998.

66. Romano, M., Dri, P., Dadalt, L., Patriarca, P., and Baralle, F.E.: Biochemical and molecular characterization of hereditary myeloperoxidase deficiency. Blood 90:4126, 1997.

67. Nauseef, W.M., Cogley, M., and McCormick, S.: Effect of the R569W missense mutation on the biosynthesis of myeloperoxidase. J. Biol. Chem. 271:9546, 1996.

68. Roos, D., Weening, R.S., Voetman, A.A., van Schaik, M.L.J., Bot, A.A.M., Meerhof, L.J., and Loos, J.A.: Protection of phagocytic leukocytes by endogenous glutathione: studies in a family with glutathione reductase deficiency. Blood 53:851, 1979.

69. Spielberg, S.P., Garrick, M.D., Corash, L.M., Butler, J.D., Tietze, F., Rogers, L., and Schulman, J.D.: Biochemical heterogeneity in glutathione synthetase deficiency. J. Clin. Invest. 61:1417, 1978.

70. Whitin, J.C., and Cohen, H.J.: Disorders of respiratory burst termination. Hematol. Oncol. Clin. North Am. 2:289, 1988.

71. Blume, R.S., and Wolff, S.M.: The Chédiak-Higashi syndrome: studies in four patients and a review of the literature. Medicine (Baltimore) 51:247, 1972.

72. Wolff, S.M., Dale, D.C., Clark, R.A., Root, R.K., and Kimball, H.R.: The Chédiak-Higashi syndrome: studies of host defenses. Ann. Intern. Med. 76:293, 1972.

73. Witkop, C.J., Jr., Quevedo, W.C., Jr., Fitzpatrick, T.B., and King, R.A.: Albinism. In Scriver, C.R., Beaudet, A.L., Sly, W.S., and Valle, D. (eds.): The Metabolic Basis of Inherited Disease. 6th ed. New York, McGraw-Hill, 1989, pp. 2905–2947.

74. Ganz, T., Metcalf, J.A., Gallin, J.I., Boxer, L.A., and Lehrer, R.I.: Microbicidal/cytotoxic proteins of neutrophils are deficient in two disorders: Chédiak-Higashi syndrome and "specific" granule deficiency. J. Clin. Invest. 82:552, 1988.

75. Barbosa, M.D., Nguyen, Q.A., Tchernev, V.T., Ashley, J.A., Detter, J.C., Blaydes, S.M., Brandt, S.J., Chotai, D., Hodgman, C., Solari, R.C., Lovett, M., and Kingsmore, S.F.: Identification of the homologous beige and Chédiak-Higashi syndrome genes [published erratum appears in Nature 385:97, 1997]. Nature 382:262, 1996.

76. Gallin, J.I.: Neutrophil specific granule deficiency. Annu. Rev. Med. 36:263, 1985.

77. Boxer, L.A., Coates, T.D., Haak, R.A., Wolach, J.B., Hoffstein, S., and Baehner, R.L.: Lactoferrin deficiency associated with altered granulocyte function. N. Engl. J. Med. 307:404, 1982.

78. Lomax, K.J., Gallin, J.I., Rotrosen, D., Raphael, G.D., Kaliner, M.A., Benz, E.J., Jr., Boxer, L.A., and Malech, H.L.: Selective defect in myeloid cell lactoferrin gene expression in neutrophil specific granule deficiency. J. Clin. Invest. 83:514, 1989.

79. Baldridge, C.W., and Gerard, R.W.: The extra respiration of phagocytosis. Am. J. Physiol. 103:235, 1933.

80. Sbarra, A.J., and Karnovsky, M.L.: The biochemical basis of phagocytosis. I. Metabolic changes during the ingestion of particles by polymorphonuclear leukocytes. J. Biol. Chem. 234:1355, 1959.

81. Babior, B.M.: Oxygen-dependent microbial killing by phagocytes. N. Engl. J. Med. 298:659, 1978.

82. Babior, B.M., Kipnes, R.S., and Curnutte, J.T.: Biological defense mechanisms: the production by leukocytes of superoxide, a potential bactericidal agent. J. Clin. Invest. 52:741, 1973.

83. Berendes, H., Bridges, R.A., and Good, R.A.: Fatal granulomatosus of childhood: clinical study of new syndrome. Minn. Med. 40:309, 1957.

84. Landing, B.H., and Shirkey, H.S.: A syndrome of recurrent infection and infiltration of viscera by pigmented lipid histiocytes. Pediatrics 20:431, 1957.

85. Quie, P.G., White, J.G., Holmes, B., and Good, R.A.: In vitro bactericidal capacity of human polymorphonuclear leukocytes: diminished activity in chronic granulomatous disease of childhood. J. Clin. Invest. 46:668, 1967.

86. Curnutte, J.T., Whitten, D.M., and Babior, B.M.: Defective superoxide production by granulocytes from patients with chronic granulomatous disease. N. Engl. J. Med. 290:593, 1974.

87. Azimi, P.H., Bodenbender, J.G., Hintz, R.L., and Kontras, S.B.: Chronic granulomatous disease in three female siblings. JAMA 206:2865, 1968.

88. Hamers, M.N., de Boer, M., Meerhof, L.J., Weening, R.S., and Roos, D.: Complementation in monocyte hybrids revealing genetic heterogeneity in chronic granulomatous disease. Nature 307:553, 1984.

89. Weening, R.S., Corbeel, L., de Boer, M., Lutter, R., van Zwieten, R., Hamers, M.N., and Roos, D.: Cytochrome *b* deficiency in an autosomal form of chronic granulomatous disease. A third form of chronic granulomatous disease recognized by monocyte hybridization. J. Clin. Invest. 75:915, 1985.

90. Segal, A.W.: Absence of both cytochrome b_{245} subunits from neutrophils in X-linked chronic granulomatous disease. Nature 326:88, 1987.

91. Parkos, C.A., Allen, R.A., Cochrane, C.G., and Jesaitis, A.J.: Purified cytochrome *b* from human granulocyte plasma membrane is comprised of two polypeptides with relative molecular weights of 91,000 and 22,000. J. Clin. Invest. 80:732, 1987.

92. Rotrosen, D., Yeung, C.L., Leto, T.L., Malech, H.L., and Kwong, C.H.: Cytochrome b_{558}: the flavin-binding component of the phagocyte NADPH oxidase. Science 256:1459, 1992.

93. Segal, A.W., West, I., Wientjes, F., Nugent, J.H.A., Chavan, A.J., Haley, B., Garcia, R.C., Rosen, H., and Scrace, G.: Cytochrome b_{245} is a flavocytochrome containing FAD and the NADPH-binding site of the microbicidal oxidase of phagocytes. Biochem. J. 284:781, 1992.

94. Volpp, B.D., Nauseef, W.M., and Clark, R.A.: Two cytosolic neutrophil oxidase components absent in autosomal chronic granulomatous disease. Science 242:1295, 1988.

95. Nunoi, H., Rotrosen, D., Gallin, J.I., and Malech, H.L.: Two forms of autosomal chronic granulomatous disease lack distinct neutrophil cytosol factors. Science 242:1298, 1988.

96. Curnutte, J.T., Scott, P.J., and Mayo, L.A.: Cytosolic components of the respiratory burst oxidase: resolution of four components, two of which are missing in complementing types of chronic granulomatous disease. Proc. Natl. Acad. Sci. USA 86:825, 1989.

97. Clark, R.A., Volpp, B.D., Leidal, K.G., and Nauseef, W.M.: Two cytosolic components of the human neutrophil respiratory burst oxidase translocate to the plasma membrane during cell activation. J. Clin. Invest. 85:714, 1990.

98. Heyworth, P.G., Curnutte, J.T., Nauseef, W.M., Volpp, B.D., Pearson, D.W., Rosen, H., and Clark, R.A.: Neutrophil nicotinamide adenine dinucleotide phosphate oxidase assembly. Translocation of p47-*phox* and p67-*phox* requires interaction between p47-*phox* and cytochrome b_{558}. J. Clin. Invest. 87:352, 1991.

99. Abo, A., Pick, E., Hall, A., Totty, N., Teahan, C.G., and Segal, A.W.: Activation of the NADPH oxidase involves the small GTP-binding protein p21[rac1]. Nature 353:668, 1991.

100. Knaus, U.G., Heyworth, P.G., Evans, T., Curnutte, J.T., and Bokoch, G.M.: Regulation of phagocyte oxygen radical production by the GTP-binding protein Rac 2. Science 254:1512, 1991.

101. Eklund, E.A., Marshall, M., Gibbs, J.B., Crean, C.D., and Gabig, T.G.: Resolution of a low molecular weight G protein in neutrophil cytosol required for NADPH oxidase activation and reconstitution by recombinant Krev-1 protein. J. Biol. Chem. 266:13964, 1991.

102. Quinn, M.T., Parkos, C.A., Walker, L., Orkin, S.H., Dinauer, M.C., and Jesaitis, A.J.: Association of a Ras-related protein with cytochrome *b* of human neutrophils. Nature 342:198, 1989.

103. Hattori, H.: Studies on the labile, stable NADI oxidase and peroxidase staining reactions in the isolated particles of horse granulocyte. Nagoya J. Med. Sci. 23:362, 1961.

104. Segal, A.W., and Jones, O.T.: Novel cytochrome *b* system in phagocytic vacuoles of human granulocytes. Nature 30:515, 1978.

105. Segal, A.W., Garcia, R., Goldstone, A.H., Cross, A.R., and Jones, O.T.G.: Cytochrome b_{245} of neutrophils is also present in human monocytes, macrophages, and eosinophils. Biochem. J. 196:363, 1981.

106. Cross, A.R., Jones, O.T.G., Harper, A.M., and Segal, A.W.: Oxidation-reduction properties of the cytochrome *b* found in the plasma-membrane fraction of human neutrophils. Biochem. J. 194:599, 1981.

107. Segal, A.W., Cross, A.R., Garcia, R.C., Borregaard, N., Valerius, N.H., Soothill, J.F., and Jones, O.T.G.: Absence of cytochrome b_{245} in chronic granulomatous disease: a multicenter European evaluation of its incidence and relevance. N. Engl. J. Med. 308:245, 1983.

108. Borregaard, N., Staehr-Johansen, K., Taudorff, E., and Wandall, J.H.: Cytochrome *b* is present in neutrophils from patients with chronic granulomatous disease. Lancet 1:949, 1979.

109. Ohno, Y., Buescher, E.S., Roberts, R., Metcalf, J.A., and Gallin, J.I.:

Reevaluation of cytochrome *b* and flavin adenine dinucleotide in neutrophils from patients with chronic granulomatous disease and description of a family with probable autosomal recessive inheritance of cytochrome *b* deficiency. Blood 67:1132, 1986.

110. Curnutte, J.T., Kuver, R., and Scott, P.J.: Activation of neutrophil NADPH oxidase in a cell-free system. Partial purification of components and characterization of the activation process. J. Biol. Chem. 262:5563, 1987.

111. Cross, A.R., Jones, O.T.G., Garcia, R., and Segal, A.W.: The association of FAD with the cytochrome b_{245} of human neutrophils. Biochem. J. 208:759, 1982.

112. Baehner, R.L., Kunkel, L.M., Monaco, A.P., Haines, J.L., Conneally, P.M., Palmer, C., Heerema, N., and Orkin, S.H.: DNA linkage analysis of X chromosome–linked chronic granulomatous disease. Proc. Natl. Acad. Sci. USA 83:3398, 1986.

113. Royer-Pokora, B., Kunkel, L.M., Monaco, A.P., Goff, S.C., Newburger, P.E., Baehner, R.L., Cole, F.S., Curnutte, J.T., and Orkin, S.H.: Cloning the gene for an inherited human disorder—chronic granulomatous disease—on the basis of its chromosomal location. Nature 322:32, 1986.

114. Dinauer, M.C., Orkin, S.H., Brown, R., Jesaitis, A.J., and Parkos, C.A.: The glycoprotein encoded by the X-linked chronic granulomatous disease locus is a component of the neutrophil cytochrome *b* complex. Nature 327:717, 1987.

115. Teahan, C., Rowe, P., Parker, P., Totty, N., and Segal, A.W.: The X-linked chronic granulomatous disease gene codes for the beta-chain of cytochrome b_{245}. Nature 327:720, 1987.

116. Dinauer, M.C., Pierce, E.A., Bruns, G.A.P., Curnutte, J.T., and Orkin, S.H.: Human neutrophil cytochrome *b* light chain (p22-*phox*): gene structure, chromosomal location, and mutations in cytochrome-negative autosomal recessive chronic granulomatous disease. J. Clin. Invest. 86:1729, 1990.

117. Volkman, D.J., Buescher, E.S., Gallin, J.I., and Fauci, A.S.: B cell lines as models for inherited phagocytic diseases: abnormal superoxide generation in chronic granulomatous disease and giant granules in Chédiak-Higashi syndrome. J. Immunol. 133:3006, 1984.

118. Maly, F.E., Cross, A.R., Jones, O.T.G., Wolf-Vorbeck, G., Walker, C., Dahinden, C.A., and DeWeck, A.L.: The superoxide generating system of B cell lines: structural homology with the phagocytic oxidase and triggering via surface Ig. J. Immunol. 140:2334, 1988.

119. Radeke, H.H., Cross, A.R., Hancock, J.T., Jones, O.T.G., Nakamura, M., Kaever, V., and Resch, K.: Functional expression of NADPH oxidase components (alpha and beta subunits of cytochrome b_{558} and 45-kDa flavoprotein) by intrinsic human glomerular mesangial cells. J. Biol. Chem. 266:21025, 1991.

120. Parkos, C.A., Dinauer, M.C., Walker, L.E., Allen, R.A., Jesaitis, A.J., and Orkin, S.H.: Primary structure and unique expression of the 22-kilodalton light chain of human neutrophil cytochrome *b*. Proc. Natl. Acad. Sci. USA 85:3319, 1988.

121. Parkos, C.A., Dinauer, M.C., Jesaitis, A.J., Orkin, S.H., and Curnutte, J.T.: Absence of both the 91kD and 22kD subunits of human neutrophil cytochrome *b* in two genetic forms of chronic granulomatous disease. Blood 73:1416, 1989.

122. Kishimoto, T.K., O'Connor, K., Lee, A., Roberts, T.M., and Springer, T.A.: Cloning of the β subunit of the leukocyte adhesion proteins: homology to an extracellular matrix receptor defines a novel supergene family. Cell 48:681, 1987.

123. Minami, Y., Weissman, A.M., Samelson, L.E., and Klausner, R.D.: Building a multichain receptor: synthesis, degradation, and assembly of the T-cell antigen receptor. Proc. Natl. Acad. Sci. USA 84:2688, 1987.

124. Wallach, T.M., and Segal, A.W.: Stoichiometry of the subunits of flavocytochrome b_{558} of the NADPH oxidase of phagocytes. Biochem. J. 320:33, 1996.

125. Huang, J., Hitt, N.D., and Kleinberg, M.E.: Stoichiometry of p22-*phox* and gp91-*phox* in phagocyte cytochrome b_{558}. Biochemistry 34:16753, 1995.

126. Parkos, C.A., Allen, R.A., Cochrane, C.G., and Jesaitis, A.J.: The quaternary structure of the plasma membrane b-type cytochrome of human granulocytes. Biochim. Biophys. Acta 932:71, 1988.

127. Cross, A.R., Rae, J., and Curnutte, J.T.: Cytochrome b_{245} of the neutrophil superoxide-generating system contains two nonidentical hemes. Potentiometric studies of a mutant form of gp91phox. J. Biol. Chem. 270:17075, 1995.

128. Hurst, J.K., Loehr, T.M., Curnutte, J.T., and Rosen, H.: Resonance

Raman and electron paramagnetic resonance structural investigations of neutrophil cytochrome b_{558}. J. Biol. Chem. 266:1627, 1991.

129. Yu, L., Quinn, M.T., Cross, A.R., and Dinauer, M.C.: Gp91(phox) is the heme binding subunit of the superoxide-generating NADPH oxidase. Proc. Natl. Acad. Sci. USA 95:7993, 1998.

130. Quinn, M.T., Mullen, M.L., and Jesaitis, A.J.: Human neutrophil cytochrome *b* contains multiple hemes. Evidence for heme associated with both subunits. J. Biol. Chem. 267:7303, 1992.

131. Ueno, I., Fujii, S., Ohya-Nishiguchi, H., Iizuka, T., and Kanegasaki, S.: Characterization of neutrophil b-type cytochrome in situ by electron paramagnetic resonance spectroscopy. FEBS Lett. 281:130, 1991.

132. Miki, T., Fujii, H., and Kakinuma, K.: EPR signals of cytochrome b_{558} purified from porcine neutrophils. J. Biol. Chem. 267:19673, 1992.

133. Karplus, P.A., Daniels, M.J., and Herriott, J.R.: Atomic structure of ferredoxin-NADP$^+$ reductase: prototype for a structurally novel flavoenzyme family. Science 251:60, 1991.

134. Sumimoto, H., Sakamoto, N., Nozaki, M., Sakaki, Y., Takeshige, K., and Minakami, S.: Cytochrome b_{558}, a component of the phagocyte NADPH oxidase, is a flavoprotein. Biochem. Biophys. Res. Commun. 186:1368, 1992.

135. Cross, A.R., Jones, O.T., Garcia, R., and Segal, A.W.: The association of FAD with the cytochrome b_{245} of human neutrophils. Biochem. J. 208:759, 1982.

136. Gabig, T.G.: The NADPH-dependent O_2-generating oxidase from human neutrophils. Identification of a flavoprotein component that is deficient in a patient with chronic granulomatous disease. J. Biol. Chem. 258:6352, 1983.

137. Bohler, M.-C., Seger, R.A., Mouy, R., Vilmer, E., Fischer, A., and Griscelli, C.: A study of 25 patients with chronic granulomatous disease: a new classification by correlating respiratory burst, cytochrome *b*, and flavoprotein. J. Clin. Immunol. 6:136, 1986.

138. Segal, A.W., West, I., Wientjes, F., Nugent, J.H.A., Chavan, A.J., Haley, B., Garcia, R.C., Rosen, H., and Scrace, G.: Cytochrome b_{245} is a flavocytochrome containing FAD and the NADPH-binding site of the microbicidal oxidase of phagocytes. Biochem. J. 284:781, 1993.

139. Wallach, T.M., and Segal, A.W.: Analysis of glycosylation sites on gp91phox, the flavocytochrome of the NADPH oxidase, by site-directed mutagenesis and translation in vitro. Biochem. J. 321:583, 1997.

140. Taylor, W.R., Jones, D.T., and Segal, A.W.: A structural model for the nucleotide binding domains of the flavocytochrome b_{245} beta-chain. Protein Sci. 2:1675, 1993.

141. Rae, J., Newburger, P.E., Dinauer, M.C., Noack, D., Hopkins, P.J., Kuruto, R., and Curnutte, J.T.: X-Linked chronic granulomatous disease: mutations in the CYBB gene encoding the gp91-phox component of respiratory-burst oxidase. Am. J. Hum. Genet. 62:1320, 1998.

142. Shatwell, K.P., Dancis, A., Cross, A.R., Klausner, R.D., and Segal, A.W.: The FRE1 ferric reductase of *Saccharomyces cerevisiae* is a cytochrome *b* similar to that of NADPH oxidase. J. Biol. Chem. 271:14240, 1996.

143. Keller, T., Damude, H.G., Werner, D., Doerner, P., Dixon, R.A., and Lamb, C.: A plant homolog of the neutrophil NADPH oxidase gp91phox subunit gene encodes a plasma membrane protein with Ca^{2+} binding motifs. Plant Cell 10:255, 1998.

144. Lamb, C.J.: Plant disease resistance genes in signal perception and transduction. Cell 76:419, 1994.

145. Dinauer, M.C., Pierce, E.A., Erickson, R.W., Muhlebach, T.J., Messner, H., Orkin, S.H., Seger, R.A., and Curnutte, J.T.: Point mutation in the cytoplasmic domain of the neutrophil p22-*phox* cytochrome *b* subunit is associated with a nonfunctional NADPH oxidase and chronic granulomatous disease. Proc. Natl. Acad. Sci. USA 88:11231, 1991.

146. Yu, L., Zhen, L., and Dinauer, M.C.: Biosynthesis of the phagocyte NADPH oxidase cytochrome b558. Role of heme incorporation and heterodimer formation in maturation and stability of gp91phox and p22phox subunits. J. Biol. Chem. 272:27288, 1997.

147. Nugent, J.H.A., Gratzer, W., and Segal, W.: Identification of the haem-binding subunit of cytochrome b_{245}. Biochem. J. 264:921, 1989.

148. Yamaguchi, T., Hayakawa, T., Kaneda, M., Kakinuma, K., and Yoshikawa, A.: Purification and some properties of the small subunit of cytochrome b_{558} from human neutrophils. J. Biol. Chem. 264:112, 1989.

149. Leusen, J.H., Bolscher, B.G., Hilarius, P.M., Weening, R.S., Kaulfersch, W., Seger, R.A., Roos, D., and Verhoeven, A.J.: 156Pro→Gln substitution in the light chain of cytochrome b558 of the human

NADPH oxidase (p22-phox) leads to defective translocation of the cytosolic proteins p47-phox and p67-phox [see comments]. J. Exp. Med. 180:2329, 1994.

150. Leto, T.L., Adams, A.G., and De Mendez, I.: Assembly of the phagocyte NADPH oxidase: binding of Src homology 3 domains to proline-rich targets. Proc. Natl. Acad. Sci. USA 91:10650, 1994.

151. Sumimoto, H., Kage, Y., Nunoi, H., Sasaki, H., Nose, T., Fukumaki, Y., Ohno, M., Minakami, S., and Takeshige, K.: Role of Src homology 3 domains in assembly and activation of the phagocyte NADPH oxidase. Proc. Natl. Acad. Sci. USA 91:5345, 1994.

152. Jesaitis, A.J., Buescher, E.S., Harrison, D., Quinn, M.T., Parkos, C.A., Livesey, S., and Linner, J.: Ultrastructural localization of cytochrome *b* in the membranes of resting and phagocytosing human granulocytes. J. Clin. Invest. 85:821, 1990.

153. Bromberg, Y., and Pick, E.: Unsaturated fatty acids stimulate NADPH-dependent superoxide production by cell-free system derived from macrophages. Cell. Immunol. 88:213, 1984.

154. Heyneman, R.A., and Vercauteren, R.E.: Activation of a NADPH oxidase from horse polymorphonuclear leukocytes in a cell-free system. J. Leukoc. Biol. 36:751, 1984.

155. Curnutte, J.T.: Activation of human neutrophil nicotinamide adenine dinucleotide phosphate, reduced (triphosphopyridine nucleotide, reduced) oxidase by arachidonic acid in a cell-free system. J. Clin. Invest. 75:1740, 1985.

156. McPhail, L.C., Shirley, P.S., Clayton, C.C., and Snyderman, R.: Activation of the respiratory burst enzyme from human neutrophils in a cell-free system. J. Clin. Invest. 75:1735, 1985.

157. Curnutte, J.T., Berkow, R.L., Roberts, R.L., Shurin, S.B., and Scott, P.J.: Chronic granulomatous disease due to a defect in the cytosolic factor required for nicotinamide adenine dinucleotide phosphate oxidase activation. J. Clin. Invest. 81:606, 1988.

158. Segal, A.W., Heyworth, P.G., Cockcroft, S., and Barrowman, M.M.: Stimulated neutrophils from patients with autosomal recessive chronic granulomatous disease fail to phosphorylate a Mr-44,000 protein. Nature 316:547, 1985.

159. Lomax, K.J., Leto, T.L., Nunoi, H., Gallin, J.I., and Malech, H.L.: Recombinant 47 kD cytosol factor restores NADPH oxidase in chronic granulomatous disease. Science 245:409, 1989.

160. Volpp, B.D., Nauseef, W.M., Donelson, J.E., Moser, D.R., and Clark, R.A.: Cloning of the cDNA and functional expression of the 47-kilodalton cytosolic component of human neutrophil respiratory burst oxidase [published erratum appears in Proc. Natl. Acad. Sci. USA 86:9563, 1989]. Proc. Natl. Acad. Sci. USA 86:7195, 1989.

161. Leto, T.L., Lomax, K.J., Volpp, B.D., Nunoi, H., Sechler, J.M.G., Nauseef, W.M., Clark, R.A., Gallin, J.I., and Malech, H.L.: Cloning of a 67-kD neutrophil oxidase factor with similarity to a noncatalytic region of p60[c-src]. Science 248:727, 1990.

162. Wientjes, F.B., Hsuan, J.J., Totty, N.F., and Segal, A.W.: p40phox, a third cytosolic component of the activation complex of the NADPH oxidase to contain src homology 3 domains. Biochem. J. 296:557, 1993.

163. Tsunawaki, S., Mizunari, H., Nagata, M., Tatsuzawa, O., and Kuratsuji, T.: A novel cytosolic component, p40phox, of respiratory burst oxidase associates with p67phox and is absent in patients with chronic granulomatous disease who lack p67phox. Biochem. Biophys. Res. Commun. 199:1378, 1994.

164. Rodaway, A.R., Teahan, C.G., Casimir, C.M., Segal, A.W., and Bentley, D.L.: Characterization of the 47-kilodalton autosomal chronic granulomatous disease protein: tissue-specific expression and transcriptional control by retinoic acid. Mol. Cell. Biol. 10:5388, 1990.

165. Heyworth, P.G., Peveri, P., and Curnutte, J.T.: Cytosolic components of NADPH oxidase: identity, function and role in regulation of oxidase activity. *In* Cochrane, C.G., and Gimbrone, M.A., Jr. (eds.): Cellular and Molecular Mechanisms of Inflammation. Vol. 4. Biological Oxidants: Generation and Injurious Consequences, 1. San Diego, Academic Press, 1992, pp. 43–81.

166. McPhail, L.C.: SH3-dependent assembly of the phagocyte NADPH oxidase [comment]. J. Exp. Med. 180:2011, 1994.

167. Okamura, N., Curnutte, J.T., Roberts, R.L., and Babior, B.M.: Relationship of protein phosphorylation to the activation of the respiratory burst in human neutrophils. Defects in the phosphorylation of a group of closely related 48-kDa proteins in two forms of chronic granulomatous disease. J. Biol. Chem. 263:6777, 1988.

168. Okamura, N., Malawista, S.E., Roberts, R.L., Rosen, H., Ochs, H.D., Babior, B.M., and Curnutte, J.T.: Phosphorylation of the oxidase-

related 48K phosphoprotein family in the unusual autosomal cytochrome-negative and X-linked cytochrome-positive types of chronic granulomatous disease. Blood 72:811, 1988.

169. Rotrosen, D., and Leto, T.L.: Phosphorylation of neutrophil 47-kDa cytosolic oxidase factor: translocation to membrane is associated with distinct phosphorylation events. J. Biol. Chem. 265:19910, 1990.

170. El Benna, J., Faust, L.P., and Babior, B.M.: The phosphorylation of the respiratory burst oxidase component p47phox during neutrophil activation. Phosphorylation of sites recognized by protein kinase C and by proline-directed kinases. J. Biol. Chem. 269:23431, 1994.

171. Faust, L.R., El Benna, J., Babior, B.M., and Chanock, S.J.: The phosphorylation targets of p47phox, a subunit of the respiratory burst oxidase. Functions of the individual target serines as evaluated by site-directed mutagenesis. J. Clin. Invest. 96:1499, 1995.

172. Peveri, P., Heyworth, P.G., and Curnutte, J.T.: Absolute requirement for GTP in the activation of the human neutrophil NADPH oxidase in a cell-free system. Role of ATP in regenerating GTP. Proc. Natl. Acad. Sci. USA 89:2494, 1992.

173. Uhlinger, D.J., Burnham, D.N., and Lambeth, J.D.: Nucleoside triphosphate requirements for superoxide generation and phosphorylation in a cell-free system from human neutrophils. Sodium dodecyl sulfate and diacylglycerol activate independently of protein kinase C. J. Biol. Chem. 266:20990, 1991.

174. Dusi, S., and Rossi, F.: Activation of NADPH oxidase of human neutrophils involves the phosphorylation and the translocation of cytosolic p67phox. Biochem. J. 296:367, 1993.

175. Heyworth, P.G., Ding, J., Erickson, R.W., Lu, D.J., Curnutte, J.T., and Badwey, J.A.: Protein phosphorylation in neutrophils from patients with p67-phox–deficient chronic granulomatous disease. Blood 87:4404, 1996.

176. Park, J.-W., Ma, M., Ruedi, J.M., Smith, R.M., and Babior, B.M.: The cytosolic components of the respiratory burst oxidase exist as a M_r ~240,000 complex that acquires a membrane-binding site during activation of the oxidase in a cell-free system. J. Biol. Chem. 267:17327, 1992.

177. Someya, A., Nagaoka, I., and Yamashita, T.: Purification of the 260 kDa cytosolic complex involved in the superoxide production of guinea pig neutrophils. FEBS Lett. 330:215, 1993.

178. Nauseef, W.M., Volpp, B.D., McCormick, S., Leidal, K.G., and Clark, R.A.: Assembly of the neutrophil respiratory burst oxidase: protein kinase C promotes cytoskeletal and membrane association of cytosolic oxidase components. J. Biol. Chem. 266:5911, 1991.

179. Woodman, R.C., Ruedi, J.M., Jesaitis, A.J., Okamura, N., Quinn, M.T., Smith, R.M., Curnutte, J.T., and Babior, B.M.: Respiratory burst oxidase and three of four oxidase-related polypeptides are associated with the cytoskeleton of human neutrophils. J. Clin. Invest. 87:1345, 1991.

180. Freeman, J.L., and Lambeth, J.D.: NADPH oxidase activity is independent of p47phox in vitro. J. Biol. Chem. 271:22578, 1996.

181. Koshkin, V., Lotan, O., and Pick, E.: The cytosolic component p47(phox) is not a sine qua non participant in the activation of NADPH oxidase but is required for optimal superoxide production. J. Biol. Chem. 271:30326, 1996.

182. Smith, R.M., Connor, J.A., Chen, L.M., and Babior, B.M.: The cytosolic subunit p67phox contains an NADPH-binding site that participates in catalysis by the leukocyte NADPH oxidase. J. Clin. Invest. 98:977, 1996.

183. Abo, A., Boyhan, A., West, I., Thrasher, A.J., and Segal, A.W.: Reconstitution of neutrophil NADPH oxidase activity in the cell-free system by four components: p67-*phox*, p47-*phox*, p21*rac*1, and cytochrome b_{245}. J. Biol. Chem. 267:16767, 1992.

184. Hall, A.: The cellular functions of small GTP-binding proteins. Science 249:635, 1990.

185. Bokoch, G.M., and Der, C.J.: Emerging concepts in the Ras superfamily of GTP-binding proteins. FASEB J. 7:750, 1993.

186. Lobell, R.B.: Prenylation of Ras GTPase superfamily proteins and their function in immunobiology. Adv. Immunol. 68:145, 1998.

187. Hall, A.: Signal transduction through small GTPases—a tale of two GAPs. Cell 69:389, 1992.

188. Ridley, A.J., and Hall, A.: The small GTP-binding protein rho regulates the assembly of focal adhesions and actin stress fibers in response to growth factors. Cell 70:389, 1992.

189. Ridley, A.J., Peterson, H.F., Johnston, C.L., Diekmann, D., and Hall, A.: The small GTP-binding protein rac regulates growth factor–induced membrane ruffling. Cell 70:401, 1992.

190. Bourne, H.R., Sanders, D.A., and McCormick, F.: The GTPase super-family: conserved structure and molecular mechanism. Nature 349:117, 1991.

191. Haubruck, H., and McCormick, F.: Ras p21: effects and regulation. Biochim. Biophys. Acta 1072:215, 1991.

192. Quinn, M.T., Mullen, M.L., Jesaitis, A.J., and Linner, J.G.: Subcellular distribution of the Rap1A protein in human neutrophils: colocalization and cotranslocation with cytochrome b_{559}. Blood 79:1563, 1992.

193. Mizuno, T., Kaibuchi, K., Ando, S., Musha, T., Hiraoka, K., Takaishi, K., Asada, M., Nunoi, H., Matsuda, I., and Takai, Y.: Regulation of the superoxide-generating NADPH oxidase by a small GTP-binding protein and its stimulatory and inhibitory GDP/GTP exchange proteins. J. Biol. Chem. 267:10215, 1992.

194. Bokoch, G.M., Quilliam, L.A., Bohl, B.P., Jesaitis, A.J., and Quinn, M.T.: Inhibition of Rap1A binding to cytochrome b_{558} of NADPH oxidase by phosphorylation of Rap1A. Science 254:1794, 1991.

195. Bokoch, G.M., and Prossnitz, V.: Isoprenoid metabolism is required for stimulation of the respiratory burst oxidase of HL-60 cells. J. Clin. Invest. 89:402, 1992.

196. Knaus, U.G., Heyworth, P.G., Kinsella, B.T., Curnutte, J.T., and Bokoch, G.M.: Purification and characterization of Rac 2: a cytosolic GTP-binding protein that regulates human neutrophil NADPH oxidase. J. Biol. Chem. 267:23575, 1992.

197. Gabig, T.G., English, D., Akard, L.P., and Schell, M.J.: Regulation of neutrophil NADPH oxidase activation in a cell-free system by guanine nucleotides and fluoride. Evidence for participation of a pertussis and cholera toxin–insensitive G protein. J. Biol. Chem. 262:1685, 1987.

198. Bolscher, B.G.J.M., Denis, S.W., Verhoeven, A.J., and Roos, D.: The activity of one soluble component of the cell-free NADPH: O_2 oxidoreductase of human neutrophils depends on guanosine 5'-O-(3-thio) triphosphate. J. Biol. Chem. 265:15782, 1990.

199. Pick, E., Kroizman, T., and Abo, A.: Activation of the superoxide-forming NADPH oxidase of macrophages requires two cytosolic components—one of them is also present in certain nonphagocytic cells. J. Immunol. 143:4180, 1989.

200. Didsbury, J., Weber, R.F., Bokoch, G.M., Evans, T., and Snyderman, R.: *rac*, a novel *ras*-related family of proteins that are botulinum toxin substrates. J. Biol. Chem. 264:16378, 1989.

201. Ueda, T., Kikuchi, A., Ohga, N., Yamamoto, J., and Takai, Y.: Purification and characterization from bovine brain cytosol of a novel regulatory protein inhibiting the dissociation of GDP from and the subsequent binding of GTP or rhoB p20, a ras p21-like GTP-binding protein. J. Biol. Chem. 265:9373, 1990.

202. Heyworth, P.G., Bohl, B.P., Bokoch, G.M., and Curnutte, J.T.: Rac translocates independently of the neutrophil NADPH oxidase components p47phox and p67phox. Evidence for its interaction with flavocytochrome b558. J. Biol. Chem. 269:30749, 1994.

203. Diekmann, D., Abo, A., Johnston, C., Segal, A.W., and Hall, A.: Interaction of Rac with p67-*phox* and regulation of phagocytic NADPH oxidase activity. Science 267:531, 1994.

204. Heyworth, P.G., Knaus, U.G., Xu, X., Uhlinger, D.J., Conroy, L., Bokoch, G.M., and Curnutte, J.T.: Requirement for posttranslational processing of rac GTP-binding proteins for activation of human neutrophil NADPH oxidase. Mol. Biol. Cell 4:261, 1993.

205. Dorseuil, O., Vazquez, A., Lang, P., Bertoglio, J., Gacon, G., and Leca, G.: Inhibition of superoxide production in B lymphocytes by rac antisense oligonucleotides. J. Biol. Chem. 267:20540, 1992.

206. Roberts, A.W., Kim, C., Zhen, L., Lowe, J.B., Kapur, R., Petryniak, B., Spaetti, A., Pollock, J.D., Borneo, J.B., Bradford, G.B., Atkinson, S.J., Dinauer, M.C., and Williams, D.A.: Deficiency of the hematopoietic cell–specific Rho family GTPase Rac2 is characterized by abnormalities in neutrophil function and host defense [in process citation]. Immunity 10:183, 1999.

207. Pizon, V., Chardin, P., Lerosey, I., Olofsson, B., and Tavitian, A.: Human cDNAs rap1 and rap2 homologous to the *Drosophila* gene Dras3 encode proteins closely related to ras in the 'effector' region. Oncogene 3:201, 1988.

208. Pizon, V., Lerosey, I., Chardin, P., and Tavitian, A.: Nucleotide sequence of a human cDNA encoding a ras-related protein (rap1B). Nucleic Acids Res. 16:7719, 1988.

209. Quilliam, L.A., Mueller, H., Bohl, B.P., Prossnitz, V., Sklar, L.A., Der, C.J., and Bokoch, G.M.: Rap1A is a substrate for cyclic AMP–dependent protein kinase in human neutrophils. J. Immunol. 147:1628, 1991.

210. Mueller, H., Motulsky, H.J., and Sklar, L.A.: The potency and kinetics of the beta-adrenergic receptors on human neutrophils. Mol. Pharmacol. 34:347, 1988.

211. DeLeo, F.R., and Quinn, M.T.: Assembly of the phagocyte NADPH oxidase: molecular interaction of oxidase proteins. J. Leukoc. Biol. 60:677, 1996.

212. Leusen, J.H., Verhoeven, A.J., and Roos, D.: Interactions between the components of the human NADPH oxidase: intrigues in the phox family. J. Lab. Clin. Med. 128:461, 1996.

213. Heyworth, P.G., Curnutte, J.T., and Badwey, J.A.: Structure and regulation of NADPH oxidase of phagocytic leukocytes. Insights from chronic granulomatous disease. *In* Serhan, C.N., and Ward, P.A. (eds.): Molecular and Cellular Basis of Inflammation. Totowa, NJ, Humana Press, 1999, pp. 165–191.

214. Babior, B.M., Kuver, R., and Curnutte, J.T.: Kinetics of activation of the respiratory burst oxidase in a fully soluble system from human neutrophils. J. Biol. Chem. 263:1713, 1988.

215. Heyworth, P.G., Tolley, J.O., Smith, R.M., and Curnutte, J.T.: The cytosolic components of the NADPH oxidase system exist as two complexes in the unstimulated neutrophil. Blood 76:183a, 1990.

216. Heyworth, P.G., Shrimpton, C.F., and Segal, A.W.: Localization of the 47 kDa phosphoprotein involved in the respiratory-burst NADPH oxidase of phagocytic cells. Biochem. J. 260:243, 1989.

217. Sumimoto, H., Hata, K., Mizuki, K., Ito, T., Kage, Y., Sakaki, Y., Fukumaki, Y., Nakamura, M., and Takeshige, K.: Assembly and activation of the phagocyte NADPH oxidase. Specific interaction of the N-terminal Src homology 3 domain of p47phox with p22phox is required for activation of the NADPH oxidase. J. Biol. Chem. 271:22152, 1996.

218. DeLeo, F.R., Yu, L., Burritt, J.B., Loetterle, L.R., Bon, C.W., Jesaitis, A.J., and Quinn, M.T.: Mapping sites of interaction of p47-*phox* and flavocytochrome b with random-sequence peptide phage display libraries. Proc. Natl. Acad. Sci. USA 92:7110, 1995.

219. DeLeo, F.R., Nauseef, W.M., Jesaitis, A.J., Burritt, J.B., Clark, R.A., and Quinn, M.T.: A domain of p47-*phox* that interacts with human neutrophil flavocytochrome b_{558}. J. Biol. Chem. 270:26246, 1995.

220. Biberstine-Kinkade, K.J., Yu, L., and Dinauer, M.C.: Mutagenesis of an arginine- and lysine-rich domain in the gp91(phox) subunit of the phagocyte NADPH-oxidase flavocytochrome b558. J. Biol. Chem. 274:10451, 1999.

221. Han, C.H., Freeman, J.L., Lee, T., Motalebi, S.A., and Lambeth, J.D.: Regulation of the neutrophil respiratory burst oxidase. Identification of an activation domain in p67(phox). J. Biol. Chem. 273:16663, 1998.

222. Dorseuil, O., Reibel, L., Bokoch, G.M., Camonis, J., and Gacon, G.: The Rac target NADPH oxidase p67phox interacts preferentially with Rac2 rather than Rac1. J. Biol. Chem. 271:83, 1996.

223. Kwong, C.H., Adams, A.G., and Leto, T.L.: Characterization of the effector-specifying domain of Rac involved in NADPH oxidase activation. J. Biol. Chem. 270:19868, 1995.

224. Dusi, S., Donini, M., and Rossi, F.: Mechanisms of NADPH oxidase activation: translocation of p40-*phox* Rac1 and Rac2 from the cytosol to the membranes in human neutrophils lacking p47-*phox* or p67-*phox*. Biochem. J. 314:409, 1996.

225. Dusi, S., Donini, M., and Rossi, F.: Mechanisms of NADPH oxidase activation in human neutrophils: p67phox is required for the translocation of rac 1 but not of rac 2 from cytosol to the membranes. Biochem. J. 308:991, 1995.

226. Dorseuil, O., Quinn, M.T., and Bokoch, G.M.: Dissociation of Rac translocation from p47phox/p67phox movements in human neutrophils by tyrosine kinase inhibitors. J. Leukoc. Biol. 58:108, 1995.

227. Kreck, M.L., Freeman, J.L., Abo, A., and Lambeth, J.D.: Membrane association of Rac is required for high activity of the respiratory burst oxidase. Biochemistry 35:15683, 1996.

228. Newburger, P.E., Dai, Q., and Whitney, C.: In vitro regulation of human phagocyte cytochrome b heavy chain and light chain gene expression by bacterial lipopolysaccharide and recombinant human cytokines. J. Biol. Chem. 266:16171, 1991.

229. Downey, G.P., Fukushima, T., Fialkow, L., and Waddell, T.K.: Intracellular signaling in neutrophil priming and activation. Semin. Cell Biol. 6:345, 1995.

230. Edwards, S.W.: Cell signalling by integrins and immunoglobulin receptors in primed neutrophils. Trends Biochem. Sci. 20:362, 1995.

231. Hallett, M.B., and Lloyds, D.: Neutrophil priming: the cellular signals that say 'amber' but not 'green.' Immunol. Today 16:264, 1995.

232. Green, S.P., Chuntharapai, A., and Curnutte, J.T.: Interleukin-8 (IL-8), melanoma growth-stimulatory activity, and neutrophil-activating

peptide selectively mediate priming of the neutrophil NADPH oxidase through the type A or type B IL-8 receptor. J. Biol. Chem. 271:25400, 1996.

233. Curnutte, J.T.: Molecular basis of the autosomal recessive forms of chronic granulomatous disease. Immunodefic. Rev. 3:149, 1992.
234. Curnutte, J.T.: Chronic granulomatous disease: the solving of a clinical riddle at the molecular level. Clin. Immunol. Immunopathol. 67:S2, 1993.
235. Roos, D., and Curnutte, J.T.: Chronic granulomatous disease. *In* Ochs, H.D., Smith, C.I.E., and Puck, J.M. (eds.): The Genetics of Primary Immunodeficiency Diseases. New York, Oxford University Press, 1999, pp. 353–374.
236. Casimir, C., Chetty, M., Bohler, M.-C., Garcia, R., Fischer, A., Griscelli, C., Johnson, B., and Segal, A.W.: Identification of the defective NADPH-oxidase component in chronic granulomatous disease: a study of 57 European families. Eur. J. Clin. Invest. 22:403, 1992.
237. Roos, D., de Boer, M., Borregaard, N., Bjerrum, O.W., Valerius, N.H., Seger, R.A., Muhlebach, T., Belohradsky, B.H., and Weening, R.S.: Chronic granulomatous disease with partial deficiency of cytochrome b_{558} and incomplete respiratory burst: variants of the X-linked, cytochrome b_{558}-negative form of the disease. J. Leukoc. Biol. 51:164, 1992.
238. Tauber, A.I., Borregaard, N., Simons, E., and Wright, J.: Chronic granulomatous disease: a syndrome of phagocyte oxidase deficiencies. Medicine (Baltimore) 62:286, 1983.
239. Forrest, C.B., Forehand, J.R., Axtell, R.A., Roberts, R.L., and Johnston, R.B., Jr.: Clinical features and current management of chronic granulomatous disease. Hematol. Oncol. Clin. North Am. 2:253, 1988.
240. Johnston, R.B., Jr., and Newman, S.L.: Chronic granulomatous disease. Pediatr. Clin. North Am. 24:365, 1977.
241. Hitzig, W.H., and Seger, R.A.: Chronic granulomatous disease, a heterogeneous syndrome. Hum. Genet. 64:207, 1983.
242. Mouy, R., Fischer, A., Vilmer, E., Seger, R., and Griscelli, C.: Incidence, severity, and prevention of infections in chronic granulomatous disease. J. Pediatr. 114:555, 1989.
243. Hayakawa, H., Kobayashi, N., and Yata, J.: Chronic granulomatous disease in Japan: a summary of the clinical features of 84 registered patients. Acta Paediatr. Jpn. 27:501, 1985.
244. Gallin, J.I., Buescher, E.S., Seligmann, B.E., Nath, J., Gaither, T., and Katz, P.: Recent advances in chronic granulomatous disease. Ann. Intern. Med. 99:657, 1983.
245. Cohen, M.S., Isturiz, R.E., Malech, H.L., Root, R.K., Wilfert, C.M., Gutman, L., and Buckley, R.H.: Fungal infection in chronic granulomatous disease. The importance of the phagocyte in defense against fungi. Am. J. Med. 71:59, 1981.
246. Odell, E.W., and Segal, A.W.: Killing of pathogens associated with chronic granulomatous disease by the non-oxidative microbicidal mechanisms of human neutrophils. J. Med. Microbiol. 34:129, 1991.
247. Speert, D.P., Bond, M., Woodman, R.C., and Curnutte, J.T.: Infection with *Pseudomonas cepacia* in chronic granulomatous disease: role of nonoxidative killing by neutrophils in host defense. J. Infect. Dis. 170:1524, 1994.
248. Curnutte, J.T.: Disorders of granulocyte function and granulopoiesis. *In* Nathan, D.G., and Oski, F.A. (eds.): Hematology of Infancy and Childhood. 4th ed. Philadelphia, W.B. Saunders, 1992, pp. 904–977.
249. Mulholland, M.W., Delaney, J.P., and Simmons, R.L.: Gastrointestinal complications of chronic granulomatous disease: surgical implications. Surgery 94:569, 1983.
250. Isaacs, D., Wright, V.M., Shaw, D.G., Raafat, F., and Walker-Smith, J.A.: Case report: chronic granulomatous disease mimicking Crohn's disease. J. Pediatr. Gastroenterol. Nutr. 4:498, 1985.
251. Clark, R.A., Malech, H.L., Gallin, J.I., Nunoi, H., Volpp, B.D., Pearson, D.W., Nauseef, W.M., and Curnutte, J.T.: Genetic variants of chronic granulomatous disease: prevalence of deficiencies of two cytosolic components of the NADPH oxidase system. N. Engl. J. Med. 321:647, 1989.
252. Orkin, S.H.: Molecular genetics of chronic granulomatous disease. Annu. Rev. Immunol. 7:277, 1989.
253. Skalnik, D.G., Strauss, E.C., and Orkin, S.H.: CCAAT displacement protein as a repressor of the myelomonocytic-specific gp91-*phox* gene promoter. J. Biol. Chem. 266:16736, 1991.
254. Eklund, E.A., and Skalnik, D.G.: Characterization of a gp91-phox promoter element that is required for interferon gamma–induced transcription. J. Biol. Chem. 270:8267, 1995.
255. Suzuki, S., Kumatori, A., Haagen, I.A., Fujii, Y., Sadat, M.A., Jun,

H.L., Tsuji, Y., Roos, D., and Nakamura, M.: PU.1 as an essential activator for the expression of gp91(phox) gene in human peripheral neutrophils, monocytes, and B lymphocytes. Proc. Natl. Acad. Sci. USA 95:6085, 1998.
256. Roos, D., de Boer, M., Kuribayashi, F., Meischl, C., Weening, R.S., Segal, A.W., Ahlin, A., Nemet, K., Hossle, J.P., Bernatowska-Matuszkiewicz, E., and Middleton-Price, H.: Mutations in the X-linked and autosomal recessive forms of chronic granulomatous disease. Blood 87:1663, 1996.
257. Roos, D.: X-CGDbase: a database of X-CGD–causing mutations. Immunol. Today 17:517, 1996.
258. Cross, A.R., Curnutte, J.T., Rae, J., and Heyworth, P.G.: Hematologically important mutations: X-linked chronic granulomatous disease. Blood Cells Mol. Dis. 22:90, 1996.
259. Heyworth, P.G., Curnutte, J.T., Noack, D., and Cross, A.R.: Hematologically important mutations: X-linked chronic granulomatous disease—an update. Blood Cells Mol. Dis. 23:443, 1997.
260. Newburger, P.E., Skalnik, D.G., Hopkins, P.J., Eklund, E.A., and Curnutte, J.T.: Mutations in the promoter region of the gene for gp91-phox in X-linked chronic granulomatous disease with decreased expression of cytochrome b558. J. Clin. Invest. 94:1205, 1994.
261. Francke, U., Ochs, H.D., De Martinville, B., Giacalone, J., Lindgren, V., Disteche, C., Pagon, R.A., Hofker, M.H., van Ommen, G.J., and Pearson, P.L.: Minor Xp21 chromosome deletion in a male associated with expression of Duchenne muscular dystrophy, chronic granulomatous disease, retinitis pigmentosa, and McLeod syndrome. Am. J. Hum. Genet. 37:250, 1985.
262. Kousseff, B.: Linkage between chronic granulomatous disease and Duchenne's muscular dystrophy? Am. J. Dis. Child. 135:1149, 1981.
263. Frey, D., Machler, M., Seger, R., Schmid, W., and Orkin, S.H.: Gene deletion in a patient with chronic granulomatous disease and McLeod syndrome: fine mapping of the Xk gene locus. Blood 71:252, 1988.
264. Pelham, A., O'Reilly, M.-A.J., Malcolm, S., Levinsky, R.J., and Kinnon, C.: RFLP and deletion analysis for X-linked chronic granulomatous disease using the cDNA probe: potential for improved prenatal diagnosis and carrier determination. Blood 76:820, 1990.
265. Brown, J., Dry, K.L., Edgar, A.J., Pryde, F.E., Hardwick, L.J., Aldred, M.A., Lester, D.H., Boyle, S., Kaplan, J., Dufier, J.L., Ho, M.F., Monaco, A.M., Musarella, M.A., and Wright, A.F.: Analysis of three deletion breakpoints in Xp21.1 and the further localization of RP3. Genomics 37:200, 1996.
266. Ho, M.F., Monaco, A.P., Blonden, L.A., van Ommen, G.J., Affara, N.A., Ferguson-Smith, M.A., and Lehrach, H.: Fine mapping of the McLeod locus (XK) to a 150–380-kb region in Xp21. Am. J. Hum. Genet. 50:317, 1992.
267. de Saint-Basile, G., Bohler, M.C., Fischer, A., Cartron, J., Dufier, J.L., Griscelli, C., and Orkin, S.H.: Xp21 DNA microdeletion in a patient with chronic granulomatous disease, retinitis pigmentosa, and McLeod phenotype. Hum. Genet. 80:85, 1988.
268. Schapiro, B.L., Newburger, P.E., Klempner, M.S., and Dinauer, M.C.: Chronic granulomatous disease presenting in a 69-year-old man. N. Engl. J. Med. 325:1786, 1991.
269. Ezekowitz, R.A.B., Orkin, S.H., and Newburger, P.E.: Recombinant interferon gamma augments phagocyte superoxide production and X-chronic granulomatous disease gene expression in X-linked variant chronic granulomatous disease. J. Clin. Invest. 80:1009, 1987.
270. Ezekowitz, R.A.B., Dinauer, M.C., Jaffe, H.S., Orkin, S.H., and Newburger, P.E.: Partial correction of the phagocyte defect in patients with X-linked chronic granulomatous disease by subcutaneous interferon gamma. N. Engl. J. Med. 319:146, 1988.
271. Dinauer, M.C., Curnutte, J.T., Rosen, H., and Orkin, S.H.: A missense mutation in the neutrophil cytochrome *b* heavy chain in cytochrome-positive X-linked chronic granulomatous disease. J. Clin. Invest. 84:2012, 1989.
272. Cross, A.R., Heyworth, P.G., Rae, J., and Curnutte, J.T.: A variant X-linked chronic granulomatous disease patient (X91+) with partially functional cytochrome *b* [published erratum appears in J. Biol. Chem. 270:17056, 1995]. J. Biol. Chem. 270:8194, 1995.
273. Woodman, R.C., Newburger, P.E., Anklesaria, P., Erickson, R.W., Rae, J., Cohen, M.S., and Curnutte, J.T.: A new X-linked variant of chronic granulomatous disease characterized by the existence of a normal clone of respiratory burst–competent phagocytic cells. Blood 85:231, 1995.
274. Kuribayashi, F., Kumatori, A., Suzuki, S., Nakamura, M., Matsumoto, T., and Tsuji, Y.: Human peripheral eosinophils have a specific mecha-

nism to express gp91-phox, the large subunit of cytochrome b558. Biochem. Biophys. Res. Commun. 209:146, 1995.

275. Baehner, R.L., and Nathan, D.G.: Quantitative nitroblue tetrazolium test in chronic granulomatous disease. N. Engl. J. Med. 278:971, 1968.

276. Quie, P.G., Kaplan, E.L., Page, A.R., Gruskay, F.L., and Malawista, S.E.: Defective polymorphonuclear-leukocyte function and chronic granulomatous disease in two female children. N. Engl. J. Med. 278:976, 1968.

277. de Boer, M., de Klein, A., Hossle, J.-P., Seger, R., Corbeel, L., Weening, R.S., and Roos, D.: Cytochrome b_{558}-negative, autosomal recessive chronic granulomatous disease: two new mutations in the cytochrome b_{558} light chain of the NADPH oxidase (p22-*phox*). Am. J. Hum. Genet. 51:1127, 1992.

278. Porter, C.D., Parkar, M.H., and Kinnon, C.: Identification of a donor splice site mutation leading to loss of p22-phox exon 5 in autosomal chronic granulomatous disease. Hum. Mutat. 7:374, 1996.

279. Hossle, J.P., de Boer, M., Seger, R.A., and Roos, D.: Identification of allele-specific p22-phox mutations in a compound heterozygous patient with chronic granulomatous disease by mismatch PCR and restriction enzyme analysis. Hum. Genet. 93:437, 1994.

280. Francke, U., Hsieh, C.-L., Foellmer, B.E., Lomax, K.J., Malech, H.L., and Leto, T.L.: Genes for two autosomal recessive forms of chronic granulomatous disease assigned to 1q25 (NCF2) and 7q11.23 (NCF1). Am. J. Hum. Genet. 47:483, 1990.

281. Kenney, R.T., Malech, H.L., Epstein, N.D., Roberts, R.L., and Leto, T.L.: Characterization of the p67phox gene: genomic organization and restriction fragment length polymorphism analysis for prenatal diagnosis in chronic granulomatous disease. Blood 82:3739, 1993.

282. Patino, P., Rae, J., Noack, D., Erickson, R., Ding, J., Garcia de Olarte, D., and Curnutte, J.T.: Molecular characterization of autosomal recessive chronic granulomatous disease caused by a defect in the NADPH oxidase component p67-*phox*. Blood (in press).

283. de Boer, M., Hilarius-Stokman, P.M., Hossle, J.P., Verhoeven, A.J., Graf, N., Kenney, R.T., Seger, R., and Roos, D.: Autosomal recessive chronic granulomatous disease with absence of the 67-kD cytosolic NADPH oxidase component: identification of mutation and detection of carriers. Blood 83:531, 1994.

284. Tanugi-Cholley, L.C., Issartel, J.P., Lunardi, J., Freycon, F., Morel, F., and Vignais, P.V.: A mutation located at the 5' splice junction sequence of intron 3 in the p67phox gene causes the lack of p67phox mRNA in a patient with chronic granulomatous disease. Blood 85:242, 1995.

285. Nunoi, H., Iwata, M., Tatsuzawa, S., Onoe, Y., Shimizu, S., Kanegasaki, S., and Matsuda, I.: AG dinucleotide insertion in a patient with chronic granulomatous disease lacking cytosolic 67-kD protein. Blood 86:329, 1995.

286. Leusen, J.H.W., de Klein, A., Hilarius, P.M., Ahlin, A., Palmblad, J., Smith, C.I.E., Diekmann, D., Hall, A., Verhoeven, A.J., and Roos, D.: Disturbed interaction of p21-*rac* with mutated p67-*phox* causes chronic granulomatous disease. J. Exp. Med. 184:1243, 1996.

287. Aoshima, M., Nunoi, H., Shimazu, M., Shimizu, S., Tatsuzawa, O., Kenney, R.T., and Kanegasaki, S.: Two-exon skipping due to a point mutation in p67-phox–deficient chronic granulomatous disease. Blood 88:1841, 1996.

288. Bonizzato, A., Russo, M.P., Donini, M., and Dusi, S.: Identification of a double mutation (D160V-K161E) in the p67phox gene of a chronic granulomatous disease patient. Biochem. Biophys. Res. Commun. 231:861, 1997.

289. Cross, A.R., Curnutte, J.T., and Heyworth, P.G.: Hematologically important mutations: the autosomal recessive forms of chronic granulomatous disease. Blood Cells Mol. Dis. 22:268, 1996.

290. Chanock, S.J., Barrett, D.M., Curnutte, J.T., and Orkin, S.H.: Gene structure of the cytosolic component, *phox*-47 and mutations in autosomal recessive chronic granulomatous disease. Blood 78:165a, 1991.

291. Casimir, C.M., Bu-Ghanim, H.N., Rodaway, A.R.F., Bentley, D.L., Rowe, P., and Segal, A.W.: Autosomal recessive chronic granulomatous disease caused by deletion at a dinucleotide repeat. Proc. Natl. Acad. Sci. USA 88:2753, 1991.

292. Roesler, J., Gorlach, A., Rae, J., Hopkins, P.J., Lee, P., Curnutte, J.T., and Chanock, S.J.: Recombination events between the normal p47-*phox* gene and a highly homologous pseudogene are the main cause of autosomal recessive chronic granulomatous disease (CGD). Blood 86:260a, 1995.

293. Volpp, B.D., and Lin, Y.: In vitro molecular reconstitution of the respiratory burst in B lymphoblasts from p47-phox–deficient chronic granulomatous disease. J. Clin. Invest. 91:201, 1993.

294. Iwata, M., Nunoi, H., Yamazaki, H., Nakano, T., Niwa, H., Tsuruta, S., Ohga, S., Ohmi, S., Kanegasaki, S., and Matsuda, I.: Homologous dinucleotide (GT or TG) deletion in Japanese patients with chronic granulomatous disease with p47-phox deficiency. Biochem. Biophys. Res. Commun. 199:1372, 1994.

295. Gorlach, A., Lee, P.L., Roesler, J., Hopkins, P.J., Christensen, B., Green, E.D., Chanock, S.J., and Curnutte, J.T.: A p47-phox pseudogene carries the most common mutation causing p47-phox–deficient chronic granulomatous disease. J. Clin. Invest. 100:1907, 1997.

296. Lew, P.D., Southwick, F.S., Stossel, T.P., Whitin, J.C., Simons, E., and Cohen, H.J.: A variant of chronic granulomatous disease: deficient oxidative metabolism due to a low-affinity NADPH oxidase. N. Engl. J. Med. 305:1329, 1981.

297. Seger, R.A., Tiefenauer, L., Matsunaga, T., Wildfeuer, A., and Newburger, P.E.: Chronic granulomatous disease due to granulocytes with abnormal NADPH oxidase activity and deficient cytochrome-*b*. Blood 61:423, 1983.

298. Styrt, B., and Klempner, M.S.: Late-presenting variant of chronic granulomatous disease. Pediatr. Infect. Dis. J. 3:556, 1984.

299. Newburger, P.E., Luscinskas, F.W., Ryan, T., Beard, C.J., Wright, J., Platt, O.S., Simons, E.R., and Tauber, A.I.: Variant chronic granulomatous disease: modulation of the neutrophil defect by severe infection. Blood 68:914, 1986.

300. Weening, R.S., Adriaansz, L.H., Weemaes, C.M.R., Lutter, R., and Roos, D.: Clinical differences in chronic granulomatous disease in patients with cytochrome *b*–negative or cytochrome *b*–positive neutrophils. J. Pediatr. 107:102, 1985.

301. Gallin, J.I., Malech, H.L., Weening, R.S., Curnutte, J.T., Quie, P.G., Ezekowitz, R.A.B., et al.: A controlled trial of interferon gamma to prevent infection in chronic granulomatous disease. N. Engl. J. Med. 324:509, 1991.

302. Margolis, D.M., Melnick, D.A., Alling, D.W., and Gallin, J.I.: Trimethoprim-sulfamethoxazole prophylaxis in the management of chronic granulomatous disease. J. Infect. Dis. 162:723, 1990.

303. Vowells, S.J., Fleisher, T.A., Sekhsaria, S., Alling, D.W., Maguire, T.E., and Malech, H.L.: Genotype-dependent variability in flow cytometric evaluation of reduced nicotinamide adenine dinucleotide phosphate oxidase function in patients with chronic granulomatous disease. J. Pediatr. 128:104, 1996.

304. Bass, D.A., Parce, J.W., Dechatelet, L.R., Szejda, P., Seeds, M.C., and Thomas, M.: Flow cytometric studies of oxidative product formation by neutrophils: a graded response to membrane stimulation. J. Immunol. 130:1910, 1983.

305. Roesler, J., Hecht, M., Freihorst, J., Lohmann-Matthes, M.L., and Emmendorffer, A.: Diagnosis of chronic granulomatous disease and of its mode of inheritance by dihydrorhodamine 123 and flow microcytofluorometry. Eur. J. Pediatr. 150:161, 1991.

306. Vowells, S.J., Sekhsaria, S., Malech, H.L., Shalit, M., and Fleisher, T.A.: Flow cytometric analysis of the granulocyte respiratory burst: a comparison study of fluorescent probes. J. Immunol. Methods 178:89, 1995.

307. Cross, A.R., Yarchover, J.L., and Curnutte, J.T.: The superoxide-generating system of human neutrophils possesses a novel diaphorase activity. Evidence for distinct regulation of electron flow within NADPH oxidase by p67-phox and p47-phox. J. Biol. Chem. 269:21448, 1994.

308. Cross, A.R., and Curnutte, J.T.: The cytosolic activating factors p47phox and p67phox have distinct roles in the regulation of electron flow in NADPH oxidase. J. Biol. Chem. 270:6543, 1995.

309. Foster, C.B., Lehrnbecher, T., Mol, F., Steinberg, S.M., Venzon, D.J., Walsh, T.J., Noack, D., Rae, J., Winkelstein, J.A., Curnutte, J.T., and Chanock, S.J.: Host defense molecule polymorphisms influence the risk for immune-mediated complications in chronic granulomatous disease. J. Clin. Invest. 102:2146, 1998.

310. Curnutte, J.T.: Classification of chronic granulomatous disease. Hematol. Oncol. Clin. North Am. 20:241, 1988.

311. Curnutte, J.T., Hopkins, P.J., Kuhl, W., and Beutler, E.: Studying X inactivation. Lancet 339:749, 1992.

312. Hopkins, P.J., Bemiller, L.S., and Curnutte, J.T.: Chronic granulomatous disease: diagnosis and classification at the molecular level. Clin. Lab. Med. 12:277, 1992.

313. Battat, L., and Francke, U.: Nsi I RFLP at the X-linked chronic granulomatous disease locus (CYBB). Nucleic Acids Res. 17:3619, 1989.

314. Muhlebach, T.J., Robinson, W., Seger, R.A., and Machler, M.: A

second NsiI RFLP at the CYBB locus. Nucleic Acids Res. 18:4966, 1990.

315. Kenney, R.T., and Leto, T.L.: A *Hind*III polymorphism in the human *NCF2* gene. Nucleic Acids Res. 18:7193, 1990.

316. Gorlin, J.B.: Identification of (CA/GT)$_n$ polymorphisms within the X-linked chronic granulomatous disease (X-CGD) gene: utility for prenatal diagnosis. J. Pediatr. Hematol. Oncol. 20:112, 1998.

317. de Boer, M., Bolscher, B.G., Sijmons, R.H., Scheffer, H., Weening, R.S., and Roos, D.: Prenatal diagnosis in a family with X-linked chronic granulomatous disease with the use of the polymerase chain reaction. Prenat. Diagn. 12:773, 1992.

318. Roos, D., de Boer, M., de Klein, A., Bolscher, B.G., and Weening, R.S.: Chronic granulomatous disease: mutations in cytochrome b558. Immunodeficiency 4:289, 1993.

319. Bemiller, L.S., Roberts, D.H., Starko, K.M., and Curnutte, J.T.: Safety and effectiveness of long-term interferon gamma therapy in patients with chronic granulomatous disease. Blood Cells Mol. Dis. 21:239, 1995.

320. Weening, R.S., Leitz, G.J., and Seger, R.A.: Recombinant human interferon-gamma in patients with chronic granulomatous disease—European follow up study. Eur. J. Pediatr. 154:295, 1995.

321. Quie, P.G., and Belani, K.K.: Corticosteroids for chronic granulomatous disease. J. Pediatr. 111:393, 1987.

322. Nathan, C.F., Murray, H.W., Wiebe, M.E., and Rubin, B.Y.: Identification of interferon gamma as the lymphokine that activates human macrophage oxidative metabolism and antimicrobial activity. J. Exp. Med. 158:670, 1983.

323. Murray, H.W.: Interferon-gamma, the activated macrophage, and host defense against microbial challenge. Ann. Intern. Med. 108:595, 1988.

324. Schiff, D.E., Rae, J., Martin, T.R., Davis, B.H., and Curnutte, J.T.: Increased phagocyte Fc gammaRI expression and improved Fc gamma-receptor–mediated phagocytosis after in vivo recombinant human interferon-gamma treatment of normal human subjects. Blood 90:3187, 1997.

325. Sechler, J.M.G., Malech, H.L., White, C.J., and Gallin, J.I.: Recombinant human interferon-gamma reconstitutes defective phagocyte function in patients with chronic granulomatous disease of childhood. Proc. Natl. Acad. Sci. USA 85:4874, 1988.

326. Woodman, R.C., Erickson, R.W., Rae, J., Jaffe, H.S., and Curnutte, J.T.: Prolonged recombinant interferon-gamma therapy in chronic granulomatous disease: evidence against enhanced neutrophil oxidase activity. Blood 79:1558, 1992.

327. Rappeport, J.M., Newburger, P.E., Goldblum, R.M., Goldman, A.S., Nathan, D.G., and Parkman, R.: Allogeneic bone marrow transplantation for chronic granulomatous disease. J. Pediatr. 101:952, 1982.

328. Kamani, N., August, C.S., Douglas, S.D., Burkey, E., Etzioni, A., and Lischner, H.W.: Bone marrow transplantation in chronic granulomatous disease. J. Pediatr. 105:42, 1984.

329. Kamani, N.: Marrow transplantation in pediatric hematologic disorders. Pediatr. Ann. 14:661, 1985.

330. Di Bartolomeo, P., Di Girolamo, G., Angrilli, F., Schettini, F., De Mattia, D., Manzionna, M.M., Dragani, A., Iacone, A., and Torlontano, G.: Reconstitution of normal neutrophil function in chronic granulomatous disease by bone marrow transplantation. Bone Marrow Transplant. 4:695, 1989.

331. Hobbs, J.R., Monteil, M., McCluskey, D.R., Jurges, E., and el Tumi, M.: Chronic granulomatous disease 100% corrected by displacement bone marrow transplantation from a volunteer unrelated donor. Eur. J. Pediatr. 151:806, 1992.

332. Kamani, N., August, C.S., Campbell, D.E., Hassan, N.F., and Douglas, S.D.: Marrow transplantation in chronic granulomatous disease: an update, with 6-year follow-up [see comments]. J. Pediatr. 113:697, 1988.

333. Calvino, M.C., Maldonado, M.S., Otheo, E., Munoz, A., Couselo, J.M., and Burgaleta, C.: Bone marrow transplantation in chronic granulomatous disease. Eur. J. Pediatr. 155:877, 1996.

334. Ho, C.M., Vowels, M.R., Lockwood, L., and Ziegler, J.B.: Successful bone marrow transplantation in a child with X-linked chronic granulomatous disease. Bone Marrow Transplant. 18:213, 1996.

335. Slavin, S., Nagler, A., Naparstek, E., Kapelushnik, Y., Aker, M., Cividalli, G., Varadi, G., Kirschbaum, M., Ackerstein, A., Samuel, S., Amar, A., Brautbar, C., Ben-Tal, O., Eldor, A., and Or, R.: Nonmyeloablative stem cell transplantation and cell therapy as an alternative to conventional bone marrow transplantation with lethal cytoreduction for the treatment of malignant and nonmalignant hematologic diseases. Blood 91:756, 1998.

336. Khouri, I.F., Keating, M., Korbling, M., Przepiorka, D., Anderlini, P., O'Brien, S., Giralt, S., Ippoliti, C., von Wolff, B., Gajewski, J., Donato, M., Claxton, D., Ueno, N., Andersson, B., Gee, A., and Champlin, R.: Transplant-lite: induction of graft-versus-malignancy using fludarabine-based nonablative chemotherapy and allogeneic blood progenitor-cell transplantation as treatment for lymphoid malignancies. J. Clin. Oncol. 16:2817, 1998.

337. Mardiney, M., Jackson, S.H., Spratt, S.K., Li, F., Holland, S.M., and Malech, H.L.: Enhanced host defense after gene transfer in the murine p47phox-deficient model of chronic granulomatous disease. Blood 89:2268, 1997.

338. Mills, E.L., Rholl, K.S., and Quie, P.G.: X-linked inheritance in females with chronic granulomatous disease. J. Clin. Invest. 66:332, 1980.

339. Johnston, R.B., Harbeck, R.J., and Johnston, R.B., Jr.: Recurrent severe infections in a girl with apparently variable expression of mosaicism for chronic granulomatous disease. J. Pediatr. 106:50, 1985.

340. Li, F., Linton, G.F., Sekhsaria, S., Whiting-Theobald, N., Katkin, J.P., Gallin, J.I., and Malech, H.L.: CD34$^+$ peripheral blood progenitors as a target for genetic correction of the two flavocytochrome b558 defective forms of chronic granulomatous disease. Blood 84:53, 1994.

341. Sekhsaria, S., Gallin, J.I., Linton, G.F., Mallory, R.M., Mulligan, R.C., and Malech, H.L.: Peripheral blood progenitors as a target for genetic correction of p47phox-deficient chronic granulomatous disease. Proc. Natl. Acad. Sci. USA 90:7446, 1993.

342. Bjorgvinsdottir, H., Ding, C., Pech, N., Gifford, M.A., Li, L.L., and Dinauer, M.C.: Retroviral-mediated gene transfer of gp91phox into bone marrow cells rescues defect in host defense against *Aspergillus fumigatus* in murine X-linked chronic granulomatous disease. Blood 89:41, 1997.

343. Porter, C.D., Parkar, M.H., Levinsky, R.J., Collins, M.K., and Kinnon, C.: X-linked chronic granulomatous disease: correction of NADPH oxidase defect by retrovirus-mediated expression of gp91-phox. Blood 82:2196, 1993.

344. Ding, C., Kume, A., Bjorgvinsdottir, H., Hawley, R.G., Pech, N., and Dinauer, M.C.: High-level reconstitution of respiratory burst activity in a human X-linked chronic granulomatous disease (X-CGD) cell line and correction of murine X-CGD bone marrow cells by retroviral-mediated gene transfer of human gp91phox. Blood 88:1834, 1996.

345. Zhen, L., King, A.A., Xiao, Y., Chanock, S.J., Orkin, S.H., and Dinauer, M.C.: Gene targeting of X chromosome–linked chronic granulomatous disease locus in a human myeloid leukemia cell line and rescue by expression of recombinant gp91phox. Proc. Natl. Acad. Sci. USA 90:9832, 1993.

346. Pollock, J.D., Williams, D.A., Gifford, M.A., Li, L.L., Du, X., Fisherman, J., Orkin, S.H., Doerschuk, C.M., and Dinauer, M.C.: Mouse model of X-linked chronic granulomatous disease, an inherited defect in phagocyte superoxide production. Nat. Genet. 9:202, 1995.

347. Jackson, S.H., Gallin, J.I., and Holland, S.M.: The p47phox mouse knock-out model of chronic granulomatous disease. J. Exp. Med. 182:751, 1995.

348. Malech, H.L., Maples, P.B., Whiting-Theobald, N., Linton, G.F., Sekhsaria, S., Vowells, S.J., Li, F., Miller, J.A., DeCarlo, E., Holland, S.M., Leitman, S.F., Carter, C.S., Butz, R.E., Read, E.J., Fleisher, T.A., Schneiderman, R.D., Van Epps, D.E., Spratt, S.K., Maack, C.A., Rokovich, J.A., Cohen, L.K., and Gallin, J.I.: Prolonged production of NADPH oxidase-corrected granulocytes after gene therapy of chronic granulomatous disease. Proc. Natl. Acad. Sci. USA 94:12133, 1997.

17 Paroxysmal Nocturnal Hemoglobinuria

▼▼▼▼ Monica Bessler and John P. Atkinson

▼ ▼

In recounting the history of the development of knowledge about paroxysmal nocturnal hemoglobinuria, the roles of the clinician, the basic scientist, and the clinician-investigator are apparent. Without the observations of the clinicians, the problem could not be posed. Without the contributions from basic science (the biochemistry of complement, the biology of glycosylphosphatidylinositol anchors, etc.), the information necessary to the solution of the problem would not be available. Without the synthesis of the clinician-investigator, the two elements would not be fused to result in knowledge about the disease.[1]

In this chapter, we discuss the remarkable biochemical and molecular developments of the past decade that have increased our understanding of a clinical syndrome featuring paroxysms of nighttime intravascular hemolysis followed by morning hemoglobinuria. The pathogenesis of paroxysmal nocturnal hemoglobinuria (PNH) provides important insights into the function of the complement cascade.

PNH is a chronic hemolytic anemia resulting from an intrinsic defect in the red blood cell (RBC) membrane that renders affected erythrocytes highly susceptible to complement-mediated lysis.[2, 3] PNH is an acquired disease, unlike most other hemolytic anemias caused by abnormalities of the erythrocyte membrane, which are commonly inherited.

PNH is rare. The estimated annual incidence is two to six cases per million persons. Both genders are equally affected. The median age at diagnosis is about 35 years old, although PNH has been reported at both extremes of life.[4–7] The incidence of PNH is higher in Southeast Asia, probably reflecting the higher frequency of aplastic anemia (AA) in these areas[8, 9] (see below).

The three cardinal symptoms of PNH are chronic intravascular hemolysis with acute exacerbations, cytopenia of varying severity, and an increased frequency of venous thrombosis.[10] The natural history of PNH is that of a chronic disorder, with a median survival of 10 to 15 years. The most common causes of death are venous thrombosis and complications from progressive pancytopenia.[4–7]

The only curative therapy for PNH is bone marrow transplantation. Because it is frequently associated with a significant risk of morbidity and mortality, treatment is often restricted to supportive therapy. Five per cent of patients with PNH develop acute myelogenous leukemia.[10, 11] Between 10 and 15 per cent of patients experience spontaneous remissions of PNH,[5, 10] which is of interest with respect to the pathogenesis of the disease and must be taken into account in the choice of a treatment regimen.

Diagnosis

The characteristic feature of blood cells in patients with PNH is that they are deficient in all proteins that are linked to the membrane by a glycosylphosphatidylinositol (GPI) anchor.[12, 13] Table 17–1 lists the proteins missing on blood cells of patients with PNH. Two of the missing proteins are complement regulatory molecules. The deficiency of these proteins explains the increased sensitivity of erythrocytes toward activated complement and thus complement-mediated intravascular hemolysis in patients with PNH. The presence of erythrocytes with increased sensitivity to lysis by activated complement was used for the diagnosis of PNH for many years (Table 17–2).

The deficiency of GPI-linked molecules is measured by flow cytometry using monoclonal antibodies.[14] In contrast to erythrocytes, which have a reduced half-life because of lysis, the half-life of PNH granulocytes is normal.[15] Consequently, the measurement of GPI-linked molecules on granulocytes may be employed to increase the sensitivity of the analysis.[16] The deficiency of at least two different GPI-linked molecules on the cell surface is specific for the diagnosis and excludes the possibility of an isolated protein deficiency. By definition, PNH type III cells lack GPI-linked molecules, PNH type II cells exhibit decreased expression, and PNH type I cells normally express GPI-linked surface molecules[17] (Table 17–3). The size of the affected clonal cell population and the degree of protein deficiency are variable and are important determinants of clinical symptoms.

Hemolysis of Erythrocytes

How does a deficiency of GPI-linked proteins lead to hemolysis by the complement system? Because two such proteins are known to be complement inhibitors, compared with just a few years ago, this pathophysiological discussion is much more straightforward.

▼ CLINICAL CHARACTERISTICS OF HEMOLYSIS

The dominant clinical hallmark of PNH is chronic hemolysis with occasional acute exacerbations—hence the name of the

Table 17–1. Surface Proteins Missing on PNH Blood Cells

Antigen	Expression Pattern
Enzymes	
Acetylcholinesterase (AchE)	Red blood cells
Ecto-5'-nucleotidase (CD73)	Some B and T lymphocytes
Neutrophil alkaline phosphatase (NAP)	Neutrophils
ADP-ribosyl transerase	Some T lymphocytes, neutrophils
Adhesion Molecules	
Blast-1/CD48	Lymphocytes
Lymphocyte function–associated antigen-3 (LFA-3 or CD58)	All blood cells*
CD67	Neutrophils, eosinophils
CD66	Neutrophils, eosinophils
Complement Regulating Surface Proteins	
Decay accelerating factor (DAF or CD55)	All blood cells†
Membrane inhibitor of reactive lysis (MIRL or CD59)	All blood cells
Receptors	
Fcγ receptor III (FcγRIII or CD16)	Neutrophils, NK-cells,‡ macrophages,‡ some T lymphocytes‡
Monocyte differentiation antigen (CD14)	Monocytes, macrophages, granulocytes
Urokinase-type plasminogen activator receptor (u-PAR, CD87)	Monocytes, granulocytes
Blood Group Antigens	
Cromer antigens (DAF)	Red blood cells
Yt antigens (AchE)	Red blood cells
Holley Gregory antigen	Red blood cells
John Milton Hagen antigen (JMH)	Red blood cells, lymphocytes
Dombrock reside	Red blood cells
Neutrophil Antigens	
NA1/NA2 (CD16) neutrophils	Neutrophils
NB1/NB2	Neutrophils
Other Surface Proteins of Unknown Functions	
CAMPATH-1 antigen (Cdw52)	Lymphocytes, monocytes
CD24	B lymphocytes, neutrophils, eosinophils
p50-80	Neutrophils
GP500	Platelets
GP175	Platelets

*On lymphocytes expressed in GPI-linked and transmembrane form.
†Level of expression on T lymphocytes varies.
‡Expressed in a transmembrane form.

disease and the characteristic occurrence in some patients of nocturnal hemolysis followed by morning hemoglobinuria.[5, 6, 10, 18–22] The hemolytic anemia is mediated solely by the complement system, and as the symptoms and signs indicate, the RBCs are destroyed intravascularly. About one half of these patients have prominent paroxysmal exacerbations of hemolysis superimposed on the chronic condition. In many of these patients, flares tend to occur at night, and infectious illnesses can accelerate the hemolysis. Biochemical correlates of this hemolytic picture include a macrocytic and normochromic anemia, although iron deficiency anemia often is superimposed on this condition because of urinary iron loss (i.e., perpetual hemosiduria). Lactate dehydrogenase levels are typically elevated, reticulocyte counts are increased, haptoglobin levels are negligible, and the antiglobulin test is negative. Antibodies do not play a role.

Table 17–2. Tests Designed to Demonstrate Erythrocyte Abnormalities Relative to the Complement System in PNH

Date	Procedure*	Investigator	Reference
1911	Carbonic acid	Van den Burgh	111
1937	Ham's test (acidified serum)	Ham and colleagues	2, 112, 113
1966	Sugar water or sucrose hemolysis test (low ionic strength)	Hartmann and Jenkins	114
1966	Complement lysis sensitivity test (complement-fixing antibody)	Ross and Dacie	115
1973	Acidified serum combined with optimal magnesium concentrations	May and Frank	116
1985	Cobra venom factor–induced reactive lysis	Hu and Nicholson-Weller	117
1990	FACS analysis of GPI-anchored proteins	Multiple groups	14, 118–121

*The procedures developed between 1911 and 1985 reflect means of triggering the complement system. The underlying premise is that paroxysmal nocturnal hemoglobinuria (PNH) red blood cells (RBCs) are more sensitive to complement-mediated lysis than normal RBCs. In that sense, these tests are indirect measures of the functional consequences of a lack of complement regulatory proteins. Fluorescence-activated cell sorter (FACS) analysis directly identifies the deficient expression of glycosylphosphatidylinositol (GP)-anchored proteins on RBCs or other hematopoietic cells.

Table 17–3. Types of Erythrocytes in Patients with Paroxysmal Nocturnal Hemoglobinuria

Type	DAF	CD59	Complement Sensitivity	Erythrocyte Survival (t½ in days)	Derivation
Type I	Normal	Normal	Normal	120	Normal stem cell clone
Type II	10–50% of normal*	10–50% of normal*	Intermediate (⅓ to 1/15)†	30–60	Defective clone with some ability to make GPT anchor
Type III	Absent	Absent	Very sensitive (1/15 to 1/25)†	4–6	Clone unable to synthesize anchor

*The expression levels of decay-accelerating factor (DAF) and CD59 are variable but congruous for a given patient's clone.
†It requires ⅓ to ⅕ (intermediate) or 1/15 to 1/25 (very sensitive) as much complement to lyse these cells compared with normal red blood cells.

Circulating cells have only a modest increase in C3 fragment deposition, suggesting that cells accumulating C3 fragments are rapidly lysed (see below).

▼ COMPLEMENT DEPENDENCY OF HEMOLYSIS

It was first clearly demonstrated in 1937 by Ham and colleagues[2] that the complement system mediates lysis of PNH RBCs (see Table 17–2). Subsequently, the alternative pathway was shown to be responsible, consistent with the antibody-independent nature of the hemolytic process mediated by this pathway.[23] The alternative pathway is an ancient, innate system of host defense against infection[24] and is present in jawless fishes that lack immunoglobulins and probably in invertebrate species as well.[25] Acidification, low ionic strength, and increased magnesium concentrations all increase the efficiency of activation of the alternative pathway. Infectious diseases may be associated with endotoxemia and other alterations that enhance complement activation.

Activation of the alternative pathway is of relevance to the PNH hemolytic syndrome (Figs. 17–1 through 17–3). Native C3 possesses a remarkable post-translational modification known as an internal thioester bond (see Fig. 17–1). Two other plasma proteins, C4 and α₂-macroglobulin, also demonstrate this structure. Over a four amino acid stretch, a γ-COOH group of glutamic acid is linked to a sulfhydryl of cysteine.[26] This bond is inherently unstable, and 1 to 2 per cent per hour of plasma C3 is turned over (the so-called spontaneous tickover of C3).[27] *Turnover* refers to the break-

ing of the thioester bond. This process results in a highly but transiently (<1.0 second) reactive species that forms an ester linkage with nearby hydroxyl groups. If this reaction takes place with self-tissue, the bound C3b is almost always immediately inactivated by the ubiquitously expressed complement membrane regulatory proteins. If this occurs in the fluid phase (plasma), activated C3 usually forms an adduct with water, and this species is rapidly inactivated by plasma complement regulatory proteins. If the activated C3 deposits on microbes, most of which lack complement regulatory proteins (like PNH cells), the feedback loop of the alternative pathway is triggered. This cascade can deposit a large quantity of C3b molecules on target cells quickly, such as several million molecules on a single bacterium in less than 5 minutes.[28, 29]

The self-amplifying loop of the alternative pathway requires two proteases.[28] The first is factor D, which cleaves the zymogen factor B. The second is the fragment of factor B (Bb), which carries the catalytic domain of the C3 and C5 convertases (see Fig. 17–2). Properdin increases the half-life of a convertase from a few seconds to a few minutes. It is

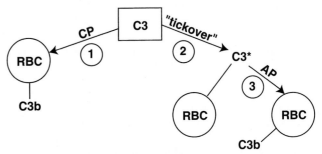

Figure 17–2. The covalent attachment of C3 through an ester linkage is both the trigger and initiation site for the alternative pathway. Three possibilities for how this first C3 fragment becomes bound are illustrated. Red blood cells (RBCs) were chosen as the target to represent what would happen in paroxysmal nocturnal hemoglobinuria (PNH). C3b could be deposited by the classical pathway (Step 1 in figure), but there is no evidence for autoantibodies in PNH or for another means of classical pathway activation. The thioester bond of C3 is unstable and, on cleavage, the activated C3* can directly attach to an RBC (Step 2 in figure) or form a fluid phase alternative pathway C3 convertase (Step 3 in figure). The latter cleaves C3 to C3b, which attaches to an RBC. Chaplin and colleagues[124] demonstrated that RBCs of normal individuals have several hundred covalently bound C3d molecules. C3d is the thioester-containing 40 kDa fragment that remains attached to the target after C3b cleavage by factor I and cofactor proteins. These "immunologic scars" accumulate over the life span of an RBC and reflect the events outlined previously. Such C3 deposition occurs in all individuals. Amplification (see Fig. 17–3) is blocked by complement regulatory proteins, but the PNH RBCs, lacking these regulators, are susceptible to alternative pathway activation.

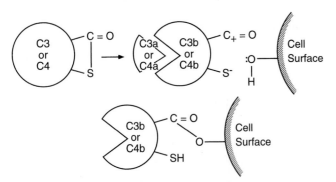

Figure 17–1. Activation of the thioester bond in C3 and C4 and its condensation with a hydroxyl group (formation of an ester bond) are shown. Amino groups on the target can also be engaged producing an amide linkage. (From Hughes-Jones, N.E.: *In* Ross, G.D., ed.: Immunobiology of the Complement System. Orlando, Academic Press, 1986; with permission.)

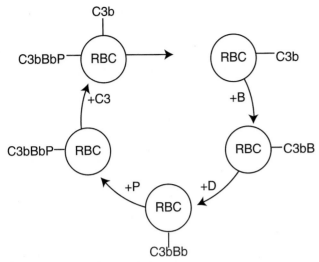

Figure 17–3. Amplification and feedback loop design of the alternative pathway. In the diagram of the amplification scheme of the alternative pathway, the target is a red blood cell (RBC), as occurs in paroxysmal nocturnal hemoglobinuria. The source of the initial C3b is discussed in the text and diagrammed in Figure 17–2. This illustration focuses on what happens next—the amplification of C3b deposition. The target-bound C3b combines with factor B. C3bB is a substrate for the plasma serine protease factor D. It cleaves factor B to Ba (leaves in fluid phase) and Bb (remains bound to the C3b). C3bBb is the C3 convertase of the alternative pathway. Properdin (P) increases the half-life of this enzyme. The C3 convertase cleaves C3 to C3b and C3a. C3a is liberated in the surrounding milieu. C3b binds to the same RBC on which the initial convertase is located, and it can then form another convertase. Each convertase molecule can cleave hundreds of C3s, but only one is shown for simplicity.

required for meaningful activation, and once initiated, the feedback loop is highly efficient. C3b, once deposited, is an opsonin for complement receptors and an important few per cent of immobilized C3b becomes part of a C5 convertase. The C5b produced by the C5 convertase (C5 → C5a + C5b) then begins to assemble the terminal membrane attack complex (MAC) (Fig. 17–4). C5b, in a series of protein-protein interactions not requiring proteolysis, interacts sequentially with C6, C7, C8, and multiple C9s. The fully formed MAC readily lyses RBCs, but it is less efficient at lysing nucleated cells. Some cells and bacteria, such as most gram-positive organisms, are highly resistant to complement-mediated lysis.

The same tickover of C3 that occurs in normal individuals takes place in persons with PNH, but because PNH

Formation of the Membrane Attack Complex (MAC)

$$C5b + C6 + C7 \rightarrow C5b67$$

$$C5b67 + C8 + poly\ C9 \rightarrow C5b6789_{(n)}$$

Figure 17–4. Assembly of the membrane attack complex (MAC) of complement. After C5b is formed by the C5 convertase, no further proteolytic reactions occur in the complement cascade. The MAC is formed by protein-protein interactions. C5b67 can insert into biologic membranes by a poorly understood mechanism. A cell can be lysed (slowly) by C8, but efficient lysis requires multiple (5 to 15) C9 molecules bound to the MAC.

cells lack the GPI-linked complement regulatory proteins, immobilized C3b is not rapidly inactivated. Paroxysms of hemolysis may be related to subtle alterations in pH and cations that facilitate the tickover of C3 (see Fig. 17–2), the efficiency of formation of the feedback loop, or both (see Fig. 17–3).

▼ MECHANISMS OF ACTION OF COMPLEMENT REGULATORY PROTEINS

The C3 and C5 convertases are bimolecular and trimolecular complexes, respectively. They consist of one protein attached covalently to a target, which is C3b in the case of the alternative pathway (Figs. 17–2 and 17–5). The second component, factor B, is non-covalently bound to the C3b and contains a serine protease catalytic domain. The alternative pathway C5 convertase represents a modification of the C3 convertase in which a second C3b is attached to the first C3b. The catalytic domain is the same as for the C3 convertase but the substrate specificity has changed.

Decay-accelerating activity refers to the ability of a regulatory protein to disassociate (or accelerate decay of) the catalytic domains from the C3 and C5 convertases (Fig. 17–6). Normal erythrocytes express approximately 3000 molecules of the CD55 complement regulatory protein called

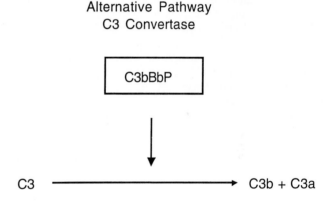

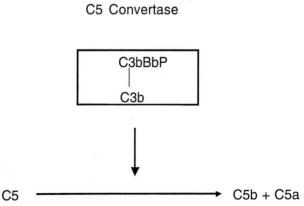

Figure 17–5. Alternative pathway C3 and C5 convertases. C3a and C5a are anaphylatoxins and are liberated into the milieu.

A. C3 Convertase Decay

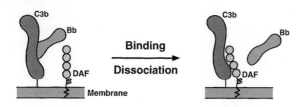

B. C5 Convertase Decay

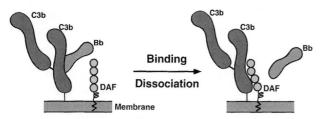

Figure 17–6. Regulation of complement activation by decay-accelerating activity. After Bb has been released, it cannot reattach. Because the affinity of decay-accelerating factor (DAF) is much lower for C3b than the convertases, it becomes available to bind to another convertase.

decay-accelerating factor (DAF). To lyse an erythrocyte through activation of the classical or alternative pathway requires overriding the activity of these DAF molecules.[18–22, 30–32] On normal erythrocytes, the alternative pathway rarely has the capacity to accomplish such a feat. The initially deposited C3b may never become associated with factor B. Moreover, even if a C3b were successful in capturing a factor B, the C3 convertase subsequently formed would be disassociated by DAF.

The second deficient GPI-anchored complement regulatory protein on PNH erythrocytes is CD59, the membrane inhibitor of the MAC.[18–22, 33–35] This protein binds to the forming MAC, thereby preventing C8 and C9 from properly inserting into the complex (Fig. 17–7). Ordinarily, C5b binds C6 and C7, and then C8 and C9 are engaged by the C5bC6C7 complex to form a MAC. A single completed MAC site appears to be sufficient to lyse an RBC (i.e., one-hit theory).[36, 37] The complete absence of the usual several thousand copies of CD59 on PNH type III cells allows the assembly of MACs to proceed unchecked.

▼ PRINCIPLES OF COMPLEMENT REGULATION

The complement system comprises an efficient, proteolytic cascade that undergoes rapid activation in response to extrinsic stimuli.[24, 28, 29, 38] Not surprisingly, the activation of these protein cascades is highly focused in space and time, preventing the formation of destructive complexes in the fluid phase (i.e., no target) or on self-tissue (i.e., wrong target). Control of the fraction of complement proteins that become activated and of the period over which activation is sustained is achieved through the influence of plasma and membrane proteins with overlapping regulatory activity for the C3/C5 cleavage step and for the lytic step.[38]

▼ DEFICIENT COMPLEMENT REGULATORY PROTEINS

DAF and CD59 are GPI-anchored molecules and are deficient on erythrocytes and other hematopoietic cells in patients with PNH. Only erythrocytes are lysed in PNH, although other blood cells can be shown in vitro to be more sensitive to complement-mediated lysis than normal cells. One reason why platelets, neutrophils, monocytes, and lymphocytes are more resistant to complement-mediated lysis is that they all express an additional complement regulatory protein known as membrane cofactor protein (MCP, CD46).[38–41] This protein inhibits deposited C4b and C3b by serving as a cofactor for their degradation by the plasma serine protease factor I. MCP is not expressed on human erythrocytes, although it does appear on the RBCs of most other primates. A second reason is that it takes substantially more MAC complexes to lyse a leukocyte than to lyse an erythrocyte. Several factors, including intrinsic susceptibility to lysis, deficiency of two GPI-anchored complement regulatory proteins, and failure to express another important membrane regulatory protein, combine to make the PNH erythrocyte particularly susceptible to complement-mediated lysis.

▼ STRUCTURAL AND FUNCTIONAL FEATURES OF DAF AND CD59

The cDNA for human DAF encodes a 34 amino acid signal peptide followed by a 347 amino acid sequence.[30, 31, 42] The amino-terminus of the protein consists of four independently folding complement control protein repeats (CCP), also known as short consensus repeats or sushi domains, and each one is approximately 60 amino acids long and contains two disulfide bridges. This region is followed by a 67 amino acid module composed of 43 per cent serine and threonine residues. This domain is heavily modified by O-linked glycosylation.

The human DAF gene spans 40 kb in the "regulators of complement-activation" gene cluster on the long arm of chromosome 1. There are 10 exons, with CCP modules 1, 2, and 4 encoded by a single exon, and CCP 3 is encoded by two exons (Figs. 17–8 and 17–9).

DAF contains one N-linked, complex-type oligosaccharide unit that is attached to the aspartic acid at residue 61. The protein is extensively modified by O-linked oligosaccharides, which are all attached to the serine/threonine-rich

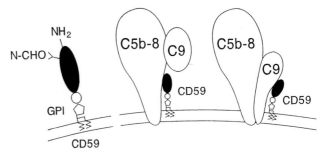

Figure 17–7. Schematic representation of CD59 function. CD59 binds C8 and C9 to inhibit the further assembly of the membrane attack complex on host cells.

DAF

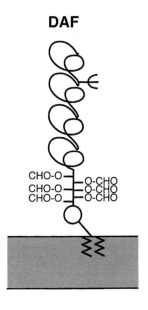

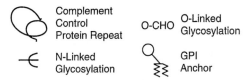

Figure 17–8. Structure of decay-accelerating factor (DAF). DAF is composed of four control protein repeats (CCPs), one of which is *N*-glycosylated. This is followed by a serine/threonine/proline (STP)–rich domain segment, which is a site for *O*-glycosylation. DAF is tethered to the cell membrane by a glycosylphosphatidylinositol (GPI) anchor that is added post-translationally.

region. DAF is initially synthesized as a precursor of 46,000 M_r that gives rise to the mature DAF on the cell surface with an M_r of 70,000 to 80,000. Heterogeneity in glycosylation accounts for the modest size variation of DAF among different cell types. Its GPI anchor is added as an early post-translational modification in the endoplasmic reticulum, with removal of the 28 carboxy-terminal amino acids and their replacement with the preformed GPI anchor, which is attached to serine 319.[43]

DAF was initially purified based on its ability to accelerate the decay of the classical pathway C3 convertase.[31] It carries out the same function with respect to the alternative pathway C3 convertase, C3bBb (see Fig. 17–6). The binding

site for DAF on the convertase is not clear. DAF does not inhibit the initial binding of factor B to a cell with deposited C3b. DAF does lead to the rapid release of the Bb fragment of B from its binding site on C3b, thereby dissociating the C3 convertase.[44] An endogenous association of DAF with C3b on the cell surface has been shown.[45] The binding of DAF, however, to the C3 convertase is much greater than to C3b alone.[46] Because there are a limited number of DAF molecules on the cell surface, it would be advantageous if the binding of DAF to the C3 convertase was lowered after dissociation of Bb. In this way, the DAF would be released and become available to dissociate another C3 convertase.

The binding site on DAF for its decay-accelerating activity has been localized to CCP 2, 3, and 4.[47] CCP 1 can be deleted without altering activity. The *O*-linked carbohydrate region functions in part as a spacer, because DAF lacking this region loses activity but a non-glycosylated peptide of similar length restores activity.

The complement protective function of membrane DAF on cells is only exerted intrinsically (i.e., on C3 and C5 convertases assembled on the same cell as DAF).[48] DAF on normal cells therefore does not help in regulating complement on a DAF-deficient PNH erythrocyte. Soluble DAF, which is found in body fluids, can be produced in vitro by treatment of cells with phosphatidylinositol-specific phospholipase C (PIPLC).[49] It cannot, however, then reincorporate into cell membranes. Soluble DAF has a much lower efficiency than membrane DAF for inhibiting complement activation on cell surfaces. Normal amounts of soluble DAF precursor are produced by PNH cells, but the protein is secreted or destroyed intracellularly because no GPI tail can be assembled (see below).[50]

CD59 is an 18 to 20 kDa, GPI-linked membrane protein (see Fig. 17–7) that is widely expressed on host cells and is an inhibitor of MAC formation on the same cell on which it is tethered (i.e., intrinsic activity).[32–35, 51–54] Like DAF, CD59 on a normal cell can provide no protection for a CD59-deficient PNH cell. Because it was simultaneously identified by several groups, it bears a number of names, such as MAC inhibitory factor (MACIF), membrane inhibitor of reactive lysis (MIRL), protectin, homologous restriction factor 20 (HRF20), and p18.

The precursor to CD59 consists of 128 amino acids, containing a 25-residue signal peptide. A hydrophobic sequence of 26 amino acids at the carboxy-terminus provides the signal for the GPI substitution that occurs at Asn 77.[55] There is a single *N*-linked glycosylation site at Asn 18 and

Figure 17–9. Organization of the decay-accelerating factor (DAF) gene. 5'UT/SP, 5'-untranslated region/signal peptide; CCP, complement control protein repeat; STP, serine/threonine/proline-rich domain; Alu, Alu family sequence (in a minor class of mRNA); H/3'UT, hydrophobic carboxy-terminal domain/3' untranslated DAF. Carboxy-terminal amino acids are replaced post-translationally with a glycosylphosphatidylinositol (GPI) anchor.

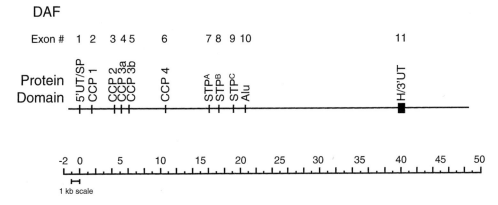

extensive intrachain disulfide bonding by the 10 cysteine residues. Nuclear magnetic resonance spectroscopy has determined that CD59 is folded into a disc-shaped domain, with the disulfide bonds clustered in the hydrophobic center and with four looped extensions protruding from the disc.[56, 57]

The CD59 gene is located on chromosome 11 at position 11p13.[58, 59] The gene encompasses more than 20 kb and contains four exons. Expression of CD59 may be upregulated by cytokines, phorbol myristate acetate, and calcium ionophores.[60–63] There is evidence that CD59 expression is regulated at the level of transcription[63] and that some cells possess intracellular pools that can be rapidly mobilized.[62]

CD59 binds C8 and C9, inhibiting formation of the MAC on host cells (see Fig. 17–7). CD59 blocks MAC extension after the stage of C5b-7 insertion into a cell membrane. CD59 possesses binding sites for the α chain of C8 and the b domain of C9.[64] Deletion of *N*-linked carbohydrate reduces the ability of CD59 to bind C8 and C9.[65]

▼ CD59 DEFICIENCY UNDERLIES CLINICAL FEATURES OF PAROXYSMAL NOCTURNAL HEMOGLOBINURIA

Considerable insight into the pathogenesis of the erythrocyte lysis in PNH came through the study of a Japanese patient deficient in only CD59 with normal DAF levels who presented with the PNH syndrome.[66] This clinical observation is consistent with function-blocking experiments employing monoclonal antibodies. For example, antibodies directed against CD59 on normal erythrocytes produce much greater susceptibility to lysis than DAF-blocking antibodies.[54] Lysis of PNH type III cells is therefore largely related to CD59 deficiency. These data are consistent with reports of individuals with isolated deficiency of DAF. They do not present with the PNH syndrome[67] or other evidence of a hemolytic anemia.[67, 68] Despite increased C3 deposition because of DAF deficiency, CD59 is able to prevent lysis.

The fact that a patient selectively deficient in CD59 presented with the PNH syndrome raises several questions. One relates to how the MAC complex is triggered when DAF is present. The presence of DAF should prevent C3 and C5 convertases from forming. Perhaps this "protection" is only partially effective and is overcome by alterations favoring C3 activation in plasma. The other possibility is that reactive lysis is responsible for providing a MAC.[33] *Reactive lysis* refers to insertion of a C5b67 complex into a cell membrane that is near a complement activation site (i.e., the C5b67 is liberated and it binds to a nearby membrane). Moreover, transfer of C5b-7 and C5b-9 from the membrane of the cell undergoing complement activation to a neighboring cell occurs in vitro and may account for several puzzling clinical and experimental lytic phenomena.

In the case of PNH type II cells, there is a less severe clinical hemolytic state.[18–22, 32–35] The deficiency of DAF also plays a role. DAF occurs at 10 to 50 per cent of normal levels, and CD59 is expressed at comparably reduced levels in such patients. It appears that this reduced quantity of CD59 is unable to inhibit the increased quantity of MAC that forms because of the relative DAF deficiency. The heightened susceptibility to lysis of type II cells can be largely abrogated by incorporation of additional DAF and by additional CD59.

The preceding facts indicate that replacing CD59 would ameliorate the hemolytic anemia of the PNH syndrome. Specific CD59 gene transfer to a hematopoietic stem cell population is an attractive but not yet technically feasible possibility. On the other hand, bone marrow transplantation has been successfully accomplished in patients with PNH (see below). A second approach would be to produce large quantities of CD59 protein bearing the GPI anchor and incubate this protein with PNH cells. Sufficient CD59 would become incorporated into the RBCs, and they would be much less susceptible to lysis. However, the logistics and expense of this type of a procedure are prohibitive. Transfusion therefore remains the mainstay of therapy in crisis situations.

The Glycosylphosphatidylinositol Anchor

GPI anchors are complex glycolipid structures that have been highly conserved in all eukaryotic cells. Comparison of GPI anchors from yeast, protozoa, and mammalian cells reveals a common core region consisting of a phosphatidylinositol-glucosamine-[mannose]₃ phosphoethanolamine molecule.[69, 70] A diagram of the structure of the GPI anchor of human erythrocyte acetylcholinesterase is shown in Figure 17–10.

GPI anchor biosynthesis starts on the cytoplasmic side of the rough endoplasmic reticulum and consists of the sequential addition of sugar molecules and phosphoethanolamine to phosphatidylinositol.[70] The amidine linkage between the ethanolamine and the carboxy-terminus of the protein occurs on the luminal side.[71, 72] The actual step at which the GPI-precursor is transferred from the cytoplasmic side to the luminal side is controversial.[71, 73] Most of the mammalian genes involved in GPI anchor biosynthesis have been cloned.[73–79] A more detailed diagram of the biosynthesis of GPI anchors is shown in Figure 17–11. The protein that is destined to be GPI linked is transferred en bloc to the preformed GPI precursor after 17 to 31 amino acids have been removed from its carboxy-terminus. The protein with its GPI anchor is then transported to the cell membrane.

PNH blood cells are unable to synthesize the mature GPI anchor precursors.[80] Analysis of lymphoblastoid cell lines obtained from patients with PNH has revealed that the block always occurs at the step when *N*-acetylglucosamine is transferred from UDP-*N*-acetylglucosamine to phosphatidylinositol.[80] This is the first identifiable step of the pathway and is catalyzed by the α1,6-*N*-acetylglucosaminyltransferase, which is an unusual quaternary enzyme complex formed by four different gene products: PIGA, PIGC, PIGH, and the human homologue of the yeast protein GPI1 (hGP1).[79]

The *PIGA* Gene

The *PIGA* cDNA was cloned by Miyata and his colleagues by expression cloning, using its ability to restore the expression of GPI-linked proteins in a mutant cell line that belonged to the same complementation group as the lymphoblastoid cell lines derived from patients with PNH.[74] The

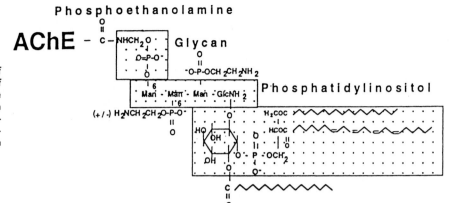

Figure 17–10. Diagram of the structure of the glycosylphosphatidylinositol (GPI) anchor of human erythrocyte acetylcholinesterase (AChE).[125] Analyzed GPI anchors have a common core structure *(hatched)* that is a phosphatidylinositol molecule linked to a phosphoethanolamine molecule through an intervening glycan structure.

candidate cDNA isolated was named *PIGA*, which stands for phosphatidylinositol glycan complementation group A; *PIGA* refers to the human gene, *Piga* to the murine gene, and PIGA to either gene product.[81] Transfection experiments revealed that the candidate cDNA was able to restore the expression of GPI-linked proteins in lymphoblastoid cells with the PNH abnormality derived from PNH patients.[82, 83]

The *PIGA* gene consists of six exons and encodes a putative protein of 484 amino acids.[84, 85] The molecular

identity of the gene is shown in Table 17–4. *PIGA* maps to the X chromosome.[82, 84]

▼ *PIGA* MUTATIONS AND FUNCTIONAL CONSEQUENCES

More than 100 mutations have been reported in the *PIGA* gene of blood cells from patients with PNH.[86–88] Most muta-

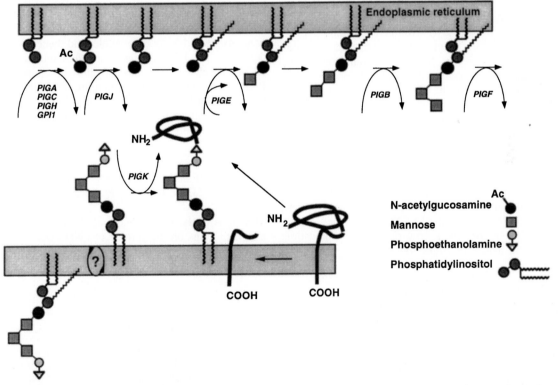

Figure 17–11. Biosynthetic pathway of glycosylphosphatidylinositol (GPI) anchors and the formation of the protein-anchor complex in the endoplasmic reticulum (ER). Initial steps occur on the cytoplasmic side of the ER. *N*-Acetylglucosamine is transferred to a phosphatidylinositol acceptor. The product is deacetylated to form glucosamidyl phosphatidylinositol. After acylation of inositol, the first mannose is donated from dolichol-phosphate-mannose, which is also the direct donor of the two other mannose residues. The phosphoethanolamine is then added. Addition of the GPI anchor precursor to the carboxy-terminus of the protein, from which a block of 17 to 31 amino acids has been cleaved, occurs on the luminal side of the ER. At what step the GPI anchor precursor is transferred to the luminal side is controversial, and the details are unknown. In some proteins, the inositol is finally deacylated. Several human and mouse cell lines deficient in GPI-linked proteins have been described and have been assigned to different complementation groups (PIGA to PIGK). The block in the biosynthetic pathway of GPI anchors for each individual complementation group is shown.

Table 17–4. Molecular Identity of *PIGA*

Genome

PIGA maps to Xp22.1
Consists of 6 exons, spans 17 kb
Pseudo PIGA maps to 12q21, is a processed pseudogene*

Complementary DNA

Open reading frame of 1455 bp

Protein

Putative protein of 484 amino acids
Approximately 60 kDa
Located in the rough endoplasmic reticulum
The amino-terminus is facing the cytoplasmic side
Part of the α1,6,-*N*-acetylglucosaminyl transferase complex

*The general structural characteristics of processed pseudogenes include the complete lack of intervening sequences found in the functional counterparts, a poly A tract at the 3′ end, and direct repeats flanking the pseudogene sequence. In all the cases studied, these pseudogenes have been on a different chromosome from that of their functional counterparts.[122]

tions are small deletions or insertions or a combination of both, causing a shift of the open reading frame and an early stop codon. This change yields an unstable *PIGA* mRNA transcript that produces a truncated, catalytically inactive protein. Early stop codons due to nonsense mutations, also frequently found, have a similar effect on the α1,6-*N*-acetylglucosaminyltransferase.

Mutations affecting the splice sites and causing exon skipping or leading to a shift in the open reading frame also occur. Missense mutations producing a single amino acid change tend to be clustered over exon 2, suggesting that this exon is important for the formation of the enzyme complex or encodes catalytic sites of the glycosyltransferase. Missense mutations shown to cause a partial deficiency of GPI-linked proteins are located in exon 2[89, 90] or exon 3[91] and encode *PIGA* proteins that form α1,6-*N*-acetylglucosaminyltransferases with some residual activity. Large deletions or duplications in the *PIGA* gene are rare. These mutations, when they occur, are present only in PNH cells, not in patients' normal cells, and hence are somatic mutations. One exception is a missense mutation that replaces an arginine with a tryptophan residue at amino acid position 19.[90, 92] This particular mutation shows a mendelian inheritance pattern and on its own does not produce a PNH phenotype.

Localization of the *PIGA* gene on the X chromosome and the somatic nature of *PIGA* mutations have important

clinical implications. A single mutation can cause a PNH phenotype, although GPI anchor deficiency was recessive in somatic cell hybrid experiments.[93] Moreover, as a result of X-chromosome inactivation, the frequency of PNH is equal in males and females because both are haploid with respect to their X-linked genes (with the exception of those that escape X-chromosome inactivation) (Fig. 17–12).

Table 17–5 illustrates examples of the genotype-phenotype correlations in four patients with PNH. All mutations in the *PIGA* gene (with the exception of the inherited *PIGA* mutation mentioned previously) abolish or severely impair the function of the glycosyltransferase. This may mean that only a significant reduction of one or several GPI-linked proteins provides the growth advantage that leads to the expansion of the PNH clone. Alternatively, to cause the disease (hemolysis), the deficiency of GPI-linked proteins (CD59) must be severe. *PIGA* mutations ascertained through analysis of PNH patients probably represent a biased sample of *PIGA* mutations that markedly impair the function of the glycosyl transferase.

▼ CLONAL EVOLUTION

PNH results from the expansion of an abnormal hematopoietic stem cell bearing a somatic mutation in the *PIGA* gene.[94] This conclusion was first supported by the finding that the erythrocytes of a woman with PNH who was heterozygous for two electrophoretically distinguishable alleles of the X chromosome–linked glucose-6-phosphate dehydrogenase gene expressed only one allele and hence were clonally derived.[95] The fact that the same *PIGA* mutation is found in all blood cell lineages demonstrates the clonal evolution of PNH. However, often more than one PNH clone is found in patients with PNH, coexisting with clones supporting some normal hematopoiesis.[92, 96, 97] This finding places certain constraints on hypotheses explaining the pathogenesis of PNH.[98]

▼ ROLES OF SOMATIC MUTATION AND CELLULAR SELECTION IN PATHOGENESIS

Mutations of the *PIGA* gene underlie the deficiency of GPI-linked proteins on the surface of PNH cells, and the lack of these proteins explains some of the clinical symptoms, such

Somatic mutation in the *PIGA* gene

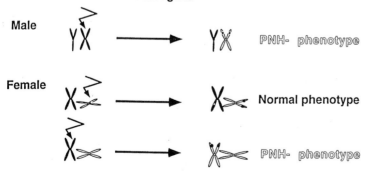

Figure 17–12. Somatic cells are functionally haploid with respect to X-linked genes. The *PIGA* gene is on the X chromosome and is subject to X-chromosome inactivation. Because males have only one X chromosome, a single inactivating mutation in the *PIGA* gene abrogates *PIGA* function and leads to the paroxysmal nocturnal hemoglobinuria (PNH) phenotype of the affected cell. Females have two X chromosomes. If the mutation occurs on the inactive X (horizontal X), the expression of glycosylphosphatidylinositol-linked proteins remains unaltered. If the mutation occurs on the *PIGA* gene on the active X chromosome (upright X), as in men, a single mutation leads to the PNH phenotype in the affected cell and all its progeny.

Table 17–5. Examples of Genotype-Phenotype Correlations in Four Patients With Paroxysmal Nocturnal Hemoglobinuria

UPN HH5[83]

Clinical type	Transfusion-dependent hemolytic PNH with thrombotic complications
PNH phenotype of red cells	84% type I, 0% type II, 6% type III
Granulocytes with the PNH phenotype	94%
PIGA mutation	Nucleotide change: 634 insertion TAGAT;
	Amino acid change: 209 aa protein
Conclusion	Frameshift mutation wth an early stop codon
	Unstable PIGA mRNA
	No residual functional activity of the glycosyl transferase

UPN HH12[90]

Clinical type	Transfusion independent hemolytic PNH after AA
PNH phenotype of red cells	6% type I, 94% type II, 0% type III
Granulocytes with the PNH phenotype	96%
PIGA mutation	Nucleotide change: 548 G→T;
	Amino acid change: 183 Cys→Phe
Conclusion	Missense mutation
	Conservative amino acid change (neutral-polar→neutral-polar)
	Some residual functional activity of the mutated *PIGA* protein

UPN Leeds[123]

Clinical type	Transfusion indepenedent hemolytic PNH after AA
Phenotype of red cells	64% type I, 0% type II, 36% type III
Granulocytes with the PNH phenotype	90%
PIGA mutation	Nucleotide change: 549 T→G;
	Amino acid change: 183 Cys→Tryp
Conclusion	Missense mutation
	Non-conservative amino acid change (neutral-polar→neutral-nonpolar)
	No residual functional activity of the glycosyl transferase

UPN HH8[83, 96]

Clinical type	Transfusion dependent hemolytic PNH with thrombotic complication
PNH phenotype of red cells	77% type I, 0% type II, 23% type III
Granulocytes with the PNH phenotype	36%
PIGA mutation I	Nucleotide change: 336 GC→T
	Amino acid change: 123 aa protein
PIGA mutation 2	Nucleotide change: 1309 C deletion
	Amino acid change: 414 aa protein
Conclusion	Two independent frameshift mutations
	Mutation 1: unstable PIGA mRNA
	Mutation 2: mislocalization of the truncated protein[79]
	No residual functional activity of either glycosyl transferase

AA, aplastic anemia; aa, amino acid; UPN, unique patient number.

as intravascular hemolysis. It remains unclear why a mutant hematopoietic stem cell, which might be expected to be at a substantial disadvantage compared with a normal stem cell, is able to expand and contribute significantly to hematopoiesis in PNH patients.

Two possibilities may account for the seeming accumulation of blood cells devoid of GPI-linked proteins: blood cells lacking GPI-linked proteins have the intrinsic capability to grow abnormally quickly, or additional external environmental factors exert a selective pressure in favor of the expansion of blood cells deficient in GPI anchors. Clinical and experimental data strongly support the latter conclusion.

Clinical observations show that there is a close association between PNH and AA, which is pancytopenia resulting from non-functioning bone marrow.[99] Cytopenia of one or all blood cell lineages is also a common feature in PNH. Conversely, it appears that patients with AA and up to 23 per cent of patients with myelodysplasia (MDS) frequently develop clinical PNH or have laboratory evidence of blood cells with the PNH abnormality in their peripheral blood or bone marrow or MDS.[100, 100a, 100b] Clinical studies using flow cytometry for the detection of PNH cells demonstrated that up to 52 per cent of patients with AA have GPI-deficient blood cells at some stage of their disease.[100a, 101]

Analysis of the mutations in the *PIGA* gene in peripheral blood cells or bone marrow cells of PNH patients reveals that more than one mutation often is present in the same patient and that these mutations typically occur independently.[96, 97, 102] This observation strongly suggests that in PNH there is selection for cells lacking GPI-linked proteins. Nevertheless, although patients with PNH have a decreased number of hematopoietic progenitor cells, no difference in growth was observed between normal progenitors or progenitors with the PNH phenotype in in vitro bone marrow culture studies.[103, 104] Mice chimeric for a non-functional *PIGA* gene, obtained by targeted disruption of the *Piga* locus in murine embryonic stem cells, followed by injection into C57BL/6 blastocysts, show that embryonic stem cells lacking GPI-linked proteins are able to contribute to hematopoiesis and to differentiate into mature blood cells with the PNH phenotype. However, no growth advantage can be demonstrated when normal hematopoiesis in the same mouse is compared with hematopoiesis from progenitors lacking GPI anchors.[105, 106]

What is the nature of the additional factor that confers a growth advantage to the PNH clone? The close association between PNH and AA suggests that this second factor may be whatever causes or maintains the bone marrow failure in AA.[103] There is evidence that the decreased number of hematopoietic stem cells in AA results from apoptosis.[104] Apoptosis of hematopoietic stem cells is thought to be immune mediated, most likely by cytotoxic T cells, directly through cell-cell contact, or indirectly by the release of cytokines. A possible explanation for the evolution of PNH is that hematopoietic stem cells with the PNH phenotype are less affected by the impairment of the bone marrow than their normal counterparts; they are more resistant to whatever triggers apoptosis of the normal hematopoietic cells in AA. If PNH cells are spared this insult because of their lack of GPI-linked proteins, they would be able to grow in favor of their normal counterparts.[103]

To develop the disease of PNH, two components are required: a somatic mutation in the *PIGA* gene occurring in a hematopoietic stem cell and an injury to normal hematopoiesis. *PIGA* mutations may occur in normal bone marrow[107a, 107b] but do not cause the disease without suppression of the normal hematopoietic stem cell compartment. Only the somatic mutation plus bone marrow impairment of AA could result in the expansion of the PNH clone that leads to the disease of PNH.[98]

Future Directions

The *PIGA* mutation in PNH cells can be considered as nature's own gene therapy that maintains hematopoiesis in patients with AA.[98] This phenomenon is not unique to PNH. Similar "rescuing mutations" have been described in hereditary disorders of blood.[108–110] However, in these reported instances, the inherited genetic abnormality resulting in the growth defect is usually corrected by spontaneous mutation of the mutated gene (i.e., somatic reversion). In contrast, to rescue hematopoiesis in AA, the somatic mutation in PNH occurs in an unrelated gene (*PIGA*), and the result is a loss of function rather than a reversion to normality. PNH is unique in that the development of an abnormal clone ameliorates the phenotype of another disorder unrelated to the rescuing gene. It therefore seems hazardous to reverse this process of natural selection. However, we may be able to learn from nature to develop strategies to treat patients with bone marrow failure. It may become possible to inactivate the *PIGA* gene or imitate the cause conferring the growth advantage of PNH cells in AA.

The center of scientific interest in PNH and AA and the current focus of research investigations are on the identification of the specific GPI-linked proteins that, when missing the GPI anchor, result in the PNH cells' ability to escape the aplastic process. Studies designed to permit characterization of these proteins will provide the foundation for the development of new therapeutic modalities for PNH and possibly for AA.

REFERENCES

1. Rosse, W.F.: Evolution of clinical understanding: paroxysmal nocturnal hemoglobinuria as a paradigm. Am. J. Hematol. 42:122, 1993.

2. Ham, T.H.: Chronic hemolytic anemia with paroxysmal nocturnal haemoglobinuria: study of the mechanism of hemolysis in relation to acid-base equilibrium. N. Engl. J. Med. 217:915, 1937.

3. Dacie, J.V., Israels, M.C.G., and Wilkinson, J.F.: Paroxysmal nocturnal haemoglobinuria of the Marchiafava type. Lancet 1:479, 1938.

4. Ware, R.E., Hall, S.E., and Rosse, W.F.: Paroxysmal nocturnal haemoglobinuria with onset in childhood and adolescence. N. Engl. J. Med. 325:991, 1992.

5. Hillmen, P., Lewis, M.S., Bessler, M., Luzzatto, L., and Dacie, J.V.: Natural history of paroxysmal nocturnal haemoglobinuria. N. Engl. J. Med. 333:1253, 1995.

6. Socie, G., Mary, J.Y., deGramont, A., Rio, B., Leporrier, M., Rose, C., Heudier, P., Rochant, H., Cahn, J.Y., and Gluckman, E.: Paroxysmal nocturnal haemoglobinuria: long-term follow-up and prognostic factors. Lancet 348:573, 1996.

7. Spath-Schwalbe, E., Schrezenmeier, H., and Heimpel, S.H.: Paroxysmale nachtliche Hamoglobinurie. Dtsch. Med. Wochenschr. 120:1027, 1995.

8. Young, N.S., Issaragrisil, S., Chen, W.C., and Takaku, F.: Aplastic anemia in the Orient. Br. J. Haematol. 62:1, 1986.

9. Kruatrachue, M., Wasi, P., and NA-Nakorn, S.: Paroxysmal nocturnal haemoglobinuria in Thailand with special reference to an association with aplastic anaemia. Br. J. Haematol. 39:267, 1978.

10. Dacie, J.V., and Lewis, S.M.: Paroxysmal nocturnal haemoglobinuria: clinical manifestations, haematology and nature of disease. Ser. Haematol. 5:3, 1972.

11. Dameshek, W.: Riddle: What do aplastic anaemia, paroxysmal nocturnal haemoglobinuria (PNH) and hypoplastic anaemia have in common? Blood 30:251, 1967.

12. Davitz, M.A., Low, M.G., and Nussenzweig, V.: Release of decay-accelerating factor (DAF) from the cell membrane by phosphatidylinositol-specific phospholipase C (PIPLC). J. Exp. Med. 163:1150, 1986.

13. Rosse, W.F.: Phosphatidylinositol-linked proteins and paroxysmal nocturnal haemoglobinuria. Blood 75:1595, 1990.

14. Hall, S.E., and Rosse, W.F.: The use of monoclonal antibodies and flow cytometry in the diagnosis of paroxysmal nocturnal haemoglobinuria. Blood 87:5332, 1996.

15. Aster, R.H., and Enright, S.E.: A platelet and granulocyte membrane defect in paroxysmal nocturnal haemoglobinuria: usefulness for the detection of platelet antibodies. J. Clin. Invest. 48:1199, 1969.

16. Bessler, M., and Fehr, J.: Fcγ-receptors (FcγRIII) on granulocytes: a new specific and sensitive diagnostic test for paroxysmal nocturnal haemoglobinuria. Eur. J. Haematol. 47:179, 1991.

17. Rosse, W.F.: Variations in the red cells in paroxysmal nocturnal haemoglobinuria. Br. J. Haematol. 24:327, 1973.

18. Rosse, W.F.: Paroxysmal nocturnal hemoglobinuria. Curr. Top. Microbiol. Immunol. 178:163, 1992.

19. Socie, G.: Recent advances in paroxysmal nocturnal hemoglobinuria: from the biology to the clinic. Hematol. Cell Ther. 39:175, 1997.

20. Nakakuma, H., and Kawaguchi, T.: Paroxysmal nocturnal hemoglobinuria (PNH): mechanism of intravascular hemolysis. Crit. Rev. Oncol. Hematol. 24:213, 1996.

21. Rosse, W.F.: Paroxysmal nocturnal hemoglobinuria as a molecular disease. Medicine (Baltimore) 76:63, 1997.

22. Packman, C.H.: Pathogenesis and management of paroxysmal nocturnal haemaglobinuria. Blood Rev. 12:1, 1998.

23. Hinz, C.J., Jr., Jordan, W.S., Jr., and Pillemer, L.: The properdin system and immunity. IV. The hemolysis of erythrocytes from patients with paroxysmal nocturnal hemoglobinuria. J. Clin. Invest. 35:453, 1956.

24. Farries, T.C., and Atkinson, J.P.: Evolution of the complement system. Immunol. Today 12:295, 1991.

25. Al-Sharif, W.Z., Sunyer, J.O., Lambris, J.D., and Smith, L.C.: Sea urchin coelomocytes specifically express a homologue of the complement component C3. J. Immunol. 160:2983, 1998.

26. Lambris J.D., Sahu A., and Wetsel R.A.: The chemistry and biology of C3, C4 and C5. *In* Volanakis J.E., and Frank M.M., eds.: The Human Complement System in Health and Disease. New York, Marcel Dekker, 1998, pp. 83–118.

27. Lachmann, P.J., and Nichol, P.A.E. Reaction mechanism of the alternative pathway of complement fixation. Lancet 1:465, 1973.

28. Pangburn, M.K., and Muller-Eberhard, H.J.: The alternative pathway of complement. Springer Semin. Immunopathol. 7:163, 1984.

29. Schreiber, R.D., Morrison, D.C., Podack, E.R., and Muller-Eberhard, H.J.: Bactericidal activity of the alternative complement pathway

generated from eleven isolated plasma proteins. J. Exp. Med. 149:870, 1979.

30. Lublin, D.M., and Atkinson, J.P.: Decay accelerating factor: biochemistry, molecular biology, and function. Annu. Rev. Immunol. 7:35, 1989.

31. Nicholson-Weller, A.: Decay accelerating factor (CD55). Curr. Top. Microbiol. Immunol. 178:10, 1992.

32. Kinoshita, T., Inoue, N., and Takeda, J.: Defective glycosyl phosphatidylinositol anchor synthesis and paroxysmal nocturnal hemoglobinuria. Adv. Immunol. 60:57, 1995.

33. Holguin, M.H., and Parker, C.J.: Membrane inhibitor of reactive lysis. Curr. Top. Microbiol. Immunol. 178:61, 1992.

34. Nakakuma, H.: Mechanism of intravascular hemolysis in paroxysmal nocturnal hemoglobinuria (PNH). Am. J. Hematol. 53:22, 1996.

35. Parker, C.J.: Molecular basis of paroxysmal nocturnal hemoglobinuria. Stem Cells 14:396, 1996.

36. Mayer MM: Development of a one-hit theory of immune hemolysis. *In* Heidelberger, M., and Plescia D.J., eds.: Approaches to Problems in Microbiology. New Brunswick, Rutgers University Press, 1961, pp. 268–279.

37. Muller-Eberhard, H.J.: Molecular organization and function of the complement system. Annu. Rev. Biochem. 57:321, 1988.

38. Liszewski, M.K., Farries, T., Lublin, D., Rooney, I., and Atkinson, J.P.: Control of the complement system. Adv. Immunol. 61:201, 1996.

39. Liszewski, M.K., and Atkinson, J.P.: Membrane cofactor protein. Curr. Top. Microbiol. Immunol. 178:45, 1992.

40. Liszewski, M.K., Post, T.W., and Atkinson, J.P.: Membrane cofactor protein (MCP or CD46): newest member of the regulators of complement activation gene cluster. Annu. Rev. Immunol. 9:431, 1991.

41. Dorig, R.E., Marcil, A., and Richardson, C.D.: CD46, a primate-specific receptor for measles virus. Trends Microbiol. 2:312, 1994.

42. Caras, I.W., Davitz, M.A., Rhee, L., Weddell, G., Martin, D.W., Jr., and Nussenzweig, V.: Cloning of decay-accelerating factor suggests novel use of splicing to generate two proteins. Nature 325:545, 1987.

43. Moran, P., Raab, H., Kohr, W.J., and Caras, I.W.: Glycophospholipid membrane anchor attachment. Molecular analysis of the cleavage/attachment site. J. Biol. Chem. 266:1250, 1991.

44. Fujita, T., Inoue, T., Ogawa, K., Iida, K., and Tamura, N.: The mechanism of action of decay-accelerating factor (DAF). DAF inhibits the assembly of C3 convertases by dissociating C2a and Bb. J. Exp. Med. 166:1221, 1987.

45. Kinoshita, T., Medof, M.E., and Nussenzweig, V.: Endogenous association of decay-accelerating factor (DAF) with C4b and C3b on cell membranes. J. Immunol. 136:3390, 1986.

46. Pangburn, M.K.: Differences between the binding sites of the complement regulatory proteins DAF, CR1, and factor H on C3 convertases. J. Immunol. 136:2216, 1986.

47. Coyne, K.E., Hall, S.E., Thompson, E.S., Arce, M.A., Kinoshita, T., Fujita, T., Anstee, D.J., Rosse, W., and Lublin, D.M.: Mapping of epitopes, glycosylation sites, and complement regulatory domains in human decay accelerating factor. J. Immunol. 149:2906, 1992.

48. Medof, M.E., Kinoshita, T., and Nussenzweig, V.: Inhibition of complement activation on the surface of cells after incorporation of decay-accelerating factor (DAF) into their membranes. J. Exp. Med. 160:1558, 1984.

49. Medof, M.E., Walter, E.I., Rutgers, J.L., Knowles, D.M., and Nussenzweig, V.: Identification of the complement decay-accelerating factor (DAF) on epithelium and glandular cells and in body fluids. J. Exp. Med. 165:848, 1987.

50. Stafford, H.A., Tykocinski, M.L., Lublin, D.M., Holers, V.M., Rosse, W.F., Atkinson, J.P., and Medof, M.E.: Normal polymorphic variations and transcription of the decay accelerating factor gene in paroxysmal nocturnal hemoglobinuria cells. Proc. Natl. Acad. Sci. USA 85:880, 1988.

51. Okada, N., Harada, R., Fujita, T., and Okada, H.: Monoclonal antibodies capable of causing hemolysis of neuraminidase treated erythrocytes by homologous complement. J. Immunol. 143:2262, 1989.

52. Sugita, Y., Tobe, T., Oda, E., Tomita, M., Yasukawa, K., Yami, N., Takemoto, K., Furuichi, K., Takayama, M., and Yano, S.: Molecular cloning and characterization of MACIF, an inhibitor of membrane channel formation of complement. J. Biochem. (Tokyo) 106:555, 1989.

53. Holguin, M.H., Fredrick, L.R., Bernshaw, N.J., Wilcox, L.A., and Parker, C.J.: Isolation and characterization of a membrane protein from normal human erythrocytes that inhibits reactive lysis of the

erythrocytes of paroxysmal nocturnal hemoglobinuria. J. Clin. Invest. 84:7, 1989.

54. Avies, A., Simmons, D.L., Hale, G., Harrison, R.A., Tighe, H., Lachman, P.J., and Waldmann, H.: CD59- and LY6-like protein expressed in human lymphoid cells, regulates the action of the complement membrane attack complex on homologous cells. J. Exp. Med. 170:637, 1989.

55. Sugita, Y., Nakano, Y., Oda, E., Noda, K., Tobe, T., Miura, N.H., and Tomita, M.: Determination of carboxy-terminal residue and disulfide bonds of MACIF (CD59), a glycosylphosphatidylinositol anchored membrane protein. J. Biochem. 114:473, 1993.

56. Fletcher, C.M., Harrison, R.A., Lachmann, P.J., and Neuhaus, D.: Structure of a soluble, glycosylated form of the complement regulatory protein CD59. Structure 2:185, 1994.

57. Kieffer, B., Driscoll, P.C., Campbell, I.D., Willis, A.C., van der Merwe, P.A., and Davis, S.J.: Three dimensional solution structure of the extracellular region of the complement regulatory protein CD59, a new cell-surface protein domain related to snake venom neurotoxins. Biochemistry 33:4471, 1994.

58. Hekhl-Ostreicher, B., Ragg, S., Drechsler, M., Scherthan, H., and Royer-Pokora, B.: Localization of the human CD59 gene by fluorescence in situ hybridization and pulsed-field gel electrophoresis. Cytogenet. Cell Genet. 63:144, 1993.

59. Tone, M., Walsh, L.A., and Waldmann, H.: Gene structure of human CD59 and demonstration that discrete mRNAs are generated by alternative polyadenylation. J. Mol. Biol. 227:971, 1992.

60. Moutabarrik, A., Nakanishi, I., Namiki, M., Hara, T., Matsumoto, M., Ishibashi, M., Okuyama, A., Zaid, D., and Seya, T.: Cytokine-mediated regulation of the surface expression of complement regulatory proteins CD46 (MCP), CD55 (DAF) and CD59 on human vascular endothelial cells. Lymphokine Cytokine Res. 12:167, 1993.

61. Meri, S., Nattila, P., and Renkonken, R.: Regulation of CD59 expression on the human endothelial cell line EAhy 926. Eur. J. Immunol. 23:2511, 1993.

62. Gordon, D.L., Papazaharoudakis, H., Sadlon, T.A., Arellano, A., and Okada, N.: Upregulation of human neutrophil CD59, a regulator of the membrane attack complex of complement, following cell activation. Immunol. Cell Biol. 72:222, 1994.

63. Holguin, M.H., Martin, C.B., Weis, J.H., and Parker, C.J.: Enhanced expression of the complement regulatory protein membrane inhibitor of reactive lysis (CD59) is regulated at the level of transcription. Blood 82:968, 1993.

64. Ninoyima, H., and Sims, P.J.: The human complement regulatory protein CD59 binds to the alpha chain of C8 and to the "b" domain of C9. J. Biol. Chem. 267:13675, 1992.

65. Ninoyimi, H., Stewart, B.H., Rollins, S.A., Zhao, J., Bothwell, L.M., and Sim, P.J.: Contribution of the *N*-linked carbohydrate of erythrocyte antigen CD59 to its complement inhibitory activity. J. Biol. Chem. 267:8404, 1992.

66. Yamashina, M., Ueda, T., Kinoshita, T., Takami, T., Ojima, A., Ono, H., Tanaka, H., Kondo, N., Orii, T., Okada, N., Okada, H., Inoue, K., and Kitani, T.: Inherited complete deficiency of 20-kilodalton homologous restriction factor (CD59) as a cause of paroxysmal nocturnal hemoglobinuria. N. Engl. J. Med. 323:1184, 1990.

67. Telen, M.J., and Green, A.M.: The Inab phenotype: characterization of the membrane protein and complement regulatory defect. Blood 74:437, 1989.

68. Daniels, G.L., Green, C.A., Mallinson, G., Okubo, Y., Hori, Y., Kataoka, A., and Kaihara, M.: Decay-accelerating factor (CD55) deficiency phenotypes in Japanese. Transfusion Med. 8:141, 1998.

69. Low, M.G., Ferguson, M.A.J., Futerman, A.H., and Silman, I.: Covalent attached phosphoinositol as a hydrophobic anchor for membrane proteins. Trends Biochem. Sci. 11:212, 1986.

70. Ferguson, M.A.J.: Glycosyl-phosphatidylinositol membrane anchor: the tale of a tail. Biochem. Soc. Trans. 20:243, 1992.

71. Vidugiriene, J., and Menon, A.: The GPI-anchor of cell surface proteins is synthesized on the cytoplasmic face of the endoplasmic reticulum. J. Cell Biol. 127:333, 1994.

72. Vidugiriene, J., and Menon, A.: Biosynthesis of glycosyl-phosphatidylinositol anchors. Methods Enzymol. 250:513, 1995.

73. Takahashi, M., Inoue, N., Ohishi, K., Maeda, Y., Nakamura, N., Endo, Y., Fujita, T., Takeda, J., and Kinoshita, T.L.: PIG-B, a membrane protein of the endoplasmic reticulum with a large luminal domain, is involved in transferring the third mannose of the GPI-anchor. EMBO J. 15:4254, 1996.

74. Miyata, T., Takeda, J., Iida, Y., Yamada, N., Inoue, N., Takahashi, M., Maeda, K., Kitani, T., and Kinoshita, T.: The cloning of PIG-A, a component in the early step of GPI-anchor biosynthesis. Science 259:1318, 1993.
75. Inoue, N., Kinoshita, T., Orii, T., and Takeda, J.: Cloning of a human gene PIG-F, a component of glycosyl-phosphatidylinositol-anchor biosynthesis, by novel expression cloning. J. Biol. Chem. 268:6882, 1993.
76. Inoue, N., Watanabe, R., Takeda, J., and Kinoshita, T.: PIG-C, one of the three human genes involved in the first step of glycosyl-phosphatidylinositol biosynthesis is a homologue of *Saccharomyces cerevisiae* GP12. Biochem. Biophys. Res. Commun. 226:193, 1996.
77. Kamitani, T., Chang, H-M., Rollins, C., Waneck, G.L., and Yeh, E.T.H.: Correction of the class H defect in glycosyl-phosphatidylinositol anchor biosynthesis in Ltk⁻ cells by a human cDNA clone. J. Biol. Chem. 268:20733, 1993.
78. Nakamura, N., Inoue, N., Wantanabe, R., Takahashi, M., Takeda, J., Stevens, V.L., and Kinoshita, T.: Expression cloning of PIG-L, a candidate N-acetylglucosaminyl-phosphatidylinositol deacetylase. J. Biol. Chem. 272:15834, 1997.
79. Watanabe, R., Inoue, N., Westfall, B., Taron, C.H., Orlean, P., Takeda, J., and Kinoshita, T.: The first step of glycosylphosphatidylinositol biosynthesis is mediated by a complex of PIG-A, PIG-H, PIG-C and GPI1. EMBO J. 17:877, 1998.
80. Armstrong, C., Schubert, J., Veda, E., Knez, J.J., Gelperin, D., Hirose, S., Silber, R., Hollan, S., Schmidt, R.E., and Medof, M.E.: Affected paroxysmal nocturnal hemoglobinuria T lymphocytes harbour a common defect in assembly of N-acetyl-D-glucosamine inositol phospholipid corresponding to that in class A Thy-1-murine lymphoma mutants. J. Biol. Chem. 267:25347, 1992.
81. Davisson, M.T.: Rules and guidelines for genetic nomenclature in mice: excerpted version. Committee on standardized genetic nomenclature for mice. Transgenic Res. 6:309, 1997.
82. Takeda, J., Miyata, T., Kawagoe, K., Iida, Y., Endo, Y., Fujita, T., Takahashi, M., Kitani, T., and Kinoshita, T.: Deficiency of the GPI anchor caused by a somatic mutation of the PIG-A gene in paroxysmal nocturnal haemoglobinuria. Cell 73:703, 1993.
83. Bessler, M.: Paroxysmal nocturnal haemoglobinuria (PNH) is caused by somatic mutations in the PIG-A gene. EMBO J. 13:110, 1994.
84. Bessler, M., Hillman, P., Longo, L., Luzzatto, L., and Mason, P.J.: Genomic organization of the X-linked gene (PIG-A) that is mutated in paroxysmal nocturnal haemoglobinura and of a related pseudogene mapped to 12q21. Hum. Mol. Genet. 3:751, 1994.
85. Iida, Y., Takeda, J., Miyata, T., Inoue, N., Mishimura, J., Kitani, T., Maeda, K., and Kinoshita, T.: Characterization of genomic PIG-A gene: a gene for glycosyl-phosphatidylinositol-anchor biosynthesis and paroxysmal nocturnal haemoglobinuria. Blood 83:3126, 1994.
86. Kinoshita, T., Inoue, N., and Takeda, J.: Role of phosphatidylinositol-linked proteins in paroxysmal nocturnal haemoglobinuria pathogenesis. Annu. Rev. Med. 47:1, 1996.
87. Luzzatto, L., and Bessler, M.: The dual pathogenesis of paroxysmal nocturnal haemoglobinuria. Curr. Opin. Hematol. 3:101, 1996.
88. Rosse, W., and Ware, R.E.: The molecular basis of paroxysmal nocturnal haemoglobinuria. Blood 86:3277, 1995.
89. Bessler, M., Mason, P.J., Hillmen, P., and Luzzatto, L.: Mutations in the PIG-A gene causing partial deficiency of GPI-linked surface proteins (PNH II) in patients with paroxysmal nocturnal haemoglobinuria. Br. J. Haematol. 87:863, 1994.
90. Nafa, K., Mason, P., Hillmen, P., Luzzatto, L., and Bessler, M.: Mutations in the PIG-A gene causing paroxysmal nocturnal haemoglobinuria (PNH) are mainly of the frameshift type. Blood 86:4650, 1995.
91. Ware, R.E., Rosse, W.F., and Howard, T.A.: Mutations within the PIG-A gene in patients with paroxysmal nocturnal haemoglobinuria. Blood 83:2418, 1994.
92. Endo, M., Ware, R.E., Vreeke, T.M., Howard, T.A., and Parker, C.J.: Identification and characterization of an inherited mutation of PIG-A in a patient with paroxysmal nocturnal haemoglobinuria. Br. J. Haematol. 93:590, 1996.
93. Hillmen, P., Bessler, M., Bungey, J., and Luzzatto, L.: Paroxysmal nocturnal haemoglobinuria: correction of the abnormal phenotype by somatic cell hybridisation. Somat. Cell Mol. Genet. 19:123, 1993.
94. Dacie, J.V.: Paroxysmal nocturnal haemoglobinuria. Proc. R. Soc. Med. 56:587, 1963.
95. Oni, S.B., Osunkoya, B.O., and Luzzatto, L.: Paroxysmal nocturnal haemoglobinuria: evidence for monoclonal origin of abnormal red cells. Blood 36:145, 1970.
96. Bessler, M., Mason, P.J., Hillmen, P., and Luzzatto, L.: Somatic mutations and cellular selection in paroxysmal nocturnal haemoglobinuria. Lancet 343:951, 1994.
97. Nishimura, J., Inoue, N., Wada, H., Ueda, E., Pramoonjago, P., Hirota, T., Machii, T., Kageyama, T., Kanamaru, A., Takeda, J., Kinoshita, T., and Kitani, T.: A patient with paroxysmal nocturnal haemoglobinuria bearing four independent PIG-A mutant clones. Blood 89:3470, 1997.
98. Luzzatto, L., Bessler, M., and Rotoli, B.: Somatic mutation in paroxysmal nocturnal hemoglobinuria: a blessing in disguise? Cell 88:1, 1997.
99. Young, N.S.: Aplastic anemia. Lancet 346:228, 1995.
100. Dacie, J.V., and Lewis, S.M.: Paroxysmal nocturnal haemoglobinuria: variation in clinical severity and association with bone marrow hypoplasia. Br. J. Haematol. 7:442, 1961.
100a. Dunn, D.E., Tanawattanacharoen, P., Boccuni, P., Nagakura, S., Green, S.W., Kirby, M.R., Kumar, M.S.A., Rosenfeld, S., and Young, N.S.: Paroxysmal nocturnal hemoglobinuria cells in patients with bone marrow failure syndromes. Ann. Int. Med. 131:401, 1999.
100b. Benz, E.J., Jr.: Clonal variation, autoimmunity, and neoplasia: An ecology lesson from paroxysmal nocturnal hemoglobinuria. Ann. Intern. Med. 131:467, 1999.
101. Schrezenmeier, H., Hertenstin, B., Wagner, B., Raghavachar, A., and Heimpel, H.: A pathogenetic link between aplastic anemia and paroxysmal nocturnal haemoglobinuria is suggested by a high frequency of aplastic anemia patients with a deficiency of phosphatidylinositol glycan anchored proteins. Exp. Hematol. 23:81, 1995.
102. Endo, M., Ware, R.E., Vreeke, T.M., Singh, S.P., Howard, T.A., Tomita, A., Holguin, M.H., and Parker, C.J.: Molecular basis of the heterogeneity of expression of glycosyl phosphatidylinositol anchored proteins in paroxysmal nocturnal haemoglobinuria. Blood 87:2546, 1996.
103. Rotoli, B., and Luzzatto, L.: Paroxysmal nocturnal haemoglobinuria. Baillieres Clin. Haematol. 2:113, 1989.
104. Maciejewski, J., Selleri, C., and Young, N.S.: Fas antigen expression on CD34⁺ human bone marrow cells is induced by interferon gamma and tumor necrosis factor alpha and potentiates hematopoietic suppression in vitro. Blood 85:3183, 1995.
105. Kawagoe, K., Kitamura, D., Okabe, M., Taniuchi, I., Ikawa, M., Watanabe, T., Kinoshita, T., and Takeda, J.: Glycosyl-phosphatidylinositol-anchor–deficient mice: implications for clonal dominance of mutant cells in paroxysmal nocturnal haemoglobinura. Blood 87:3600, 1996.
106. Rosti, V., Tremml, G., Soares, V., Pandolfi, P.P., Luzzatto, L., and Bessler, M.: Embryonic stem cells without PIG-A gene activity are competent for hematopoiesis with the PNH phenotype but not for clonal expansion. J. Clin. Invest. 100:1028, 1997.
107a. Araten, D.J., Nafa, K., Pakdeesuwan, K., and Luzzatto, L.: Clonal populations of hematopoietic cells with paroxysmal nocturnal hemoglobinuria genotype and phenotype are present in normal individuals. Proc. Natl. Acad. Sci. USA 96:5209, 1999.
107b. Rawstrom, A.C., Rollinson, S.J., Richards, S., Short, M.A., English, A., Morgan, G.J., Hale, G., and Hillmen, P.: The PNH phenotype cells that emerge in most patients after CAMPATH-1H therapy are present prior to treatment. Br. J. Haematol. 107:148, 1999.
108. Ellis, N.A., Lennon, D.J., Proytcheva, M., Alhadeff, B., Henderson, E.E., and German, J.: Somatic intragenic recombination within the mutated locus BLM can correct the high sister-chromatid exchange phenotype of Bloom syndrome cells. Am. J. Hum. Genet. 57:1019, 1995.
109. Hirschhorn, R., Yang, D.R., Puck, J.M., Huie, M.L., Jiang, C.K., and Kurlandsky, L.E.: Spontaneous in vivo reversion to normal of an inherited mutation in a patient with adenosine deaminase deficiency. Nat. Genet. 13:290, 1996.
110. Lo Ten Foe, J., Kwee, M.L., Rooimens, M.A., Oostra, A.B., Veerman, A.J., van Weel, M., Pauli, R.M., Shahidi, N.T., Dokal, I., Roberts, I., Altay, C., Gluckman, E., Gibson, R.A., Mathew, C.G., Arwert, F., and Joenje, H.: Somatic mutation in Fanconi anemia: molecular basis and clinical significance. Eur. J. Hum. Genet. 5:137, 1997.
111. Hijmans van den Bergh, A.A.: Ictere hemolytique avec crises hemoglobinuriques. Fragilite globulaire. Rev. Med. 31:63, 1911.
112. Ham, T.H., and Dingle, J.H.: Studies on destruction of red blood cells. II. Chronic hemolytic anemia with paroxysmal nocturnal hemoglobinuria: certain immunological aspects of the hemolytic mechanism with special reference to serum complement. J. Clin. Invest. 18:657, 1939.
113. Ham, T.H.: Studies on the destruction of red blood cells. I. Chronic hemolytic anemia with paroxysmal nocturnal hemoglobinuria: an in-

vestigation of the mechanism of hemolysis with observations on five cases. Arch. Intern. Med. 64:1271, 1939.

114. Hartmann, R.C., Jenkins, D.E., Jr., and Arnold, A.B.: Diagnostic specificity of sucrose hemolysis test for paroxysmal nocturnal hemoglobinuria. Blood 35:462, 1970.

115. Rosse, W.F., and Davie, J.V.: Immune lysis of normal human and paroxysmal nocturnal hemoglobinuria red blood cells. I. The sensitivity of PNH red cells to lysis by complement and specific antibody. J. Clin. Invest. 45:736, 1966.

116. May, J.E., Frank, M.M., and Rosse, W.F.: Alternate complement-pathway–mediated lysis induced by magnesium. N. Engl. J. Med. 298:705, 1973.

117. Hu, V.W., and Nicholson-Weller, A.: Enhanced complement–mediated lysis of type III paroxysmal nocturnal hemoglobinuria erythrocytes involves increased C9 binding and polymerization. Proc. Natl. Acad. Sci. USA 82:5520, 1985.

118. Plesner, T., Hansen, N.E., and Carlsen, K.: Estimation of PI-bound proteins on blood cells from PNH patients by quantitative flow cytometry. Br. J. Haematol. 75:585, 1990.

119. Schubert, J., Alvarada, M., Uciechowski, P., Zielinka-Skowroner, M., Freund, M., Vogt, H., and Schmidt, R.E.: Diagnosis of paroxysmal nocturnal haemoglobinuria using immunophenotyping of peripheral blood cells. Br. J. Haematol. 79:487, 1991.

120. Schichishima, T., Terssawa, T., Saitoh, Y., Hashimoto, C., Ohto, H., and Maruyama, T.: Diagnosis of paroxysmal nocturnal haemoglobinuria by phenotypic analysis of erythrocytes using two-colour flow cytometry with monoclonal antibodies to DAF and CD59/MACIF. Br. J. Haematol. 85:378, 1993.

121. vanderSchoot, E., Huizinga, W.J., van't Veer-Korthof, E.T., Wijmans, R., Pinkster, J., and vondem Borne, A.E.G.K.: Deficiency of glycosyl-phosphatidylinositol–linked membrane glycoproteins of leukocytes in paroxysmal nocturnal hemoglobinuria, description of a new diagnostic cytofluorometric assay. Blood 76:1853, 1990.

122. Vanin, E.F.: Processed pseudogenes: characteristics and evolution. Annu. Rev. Genet. 19:253, 1985.

123. Rollinson, S., Richards, S., Norfolk, B., Bibi, K., Morgan, G., and Hillmen, P.: Both paroxysmal nocturnal hemoglobinuria (PNH) type II cells and PNH type III cells can arise from different point mutations involving the same codon of the PIG-A gene. Blood 89:3069, 1997.

124. Chaplin, H., Nasongkla, M., and Monroe, M.D.: Quantitation of red blood cell–bound C3d in normal subjects and random hospitalized patients. Br. J. Haematol. 48:69, 1981.

125. Roberts, W.L., Myher, J.J., Kukis, A., Low, M.G., and Rosenberry, T.L.: Lipid analysis of the glycoinositol phospholipid membrane anchor of human erythrocyte acetylcholinesterase: palmitoylation of inositol results in resistance to phosphatidylinositol-specific phospholipase. J. Biol. Chem. 263:18766, 1988.

Part V

HEMOSTASIS

18 Vitamin K–Dependent Proteins in Blood
▼▼▼▼ Coagulation

Johan Stenflo and Björn Dahlbäck

▼ ▼

Introduction

Prothrombin activation is the final step in a series of zymogen activations resulting in precisely regulated generation of thrombin at the site of injury.[1–7] This sequence of reactions can proceed by either the *intrinsic* or the *extrinsic* pathway. In the intrinsic pathway, factor XI is activated by contact phase factors (factor XII, prekallikrein, and high molecular weight kininogen). Active factor XI (factor XIa) then activates factor IX by limited proteolysis, and factor IXa activates factor X (Fig. 18–1). Although the contact phase factors initiate coagulation in vitro, when blood is exposed to negatively charged surfaces, they are of little or no significance for the initiation of blood coagulation in vivo. However, a thrombin-mediated positive feed-back loop, leading to the activation of factor IX, appears to be important to maintain fibrin formation once the coagulation cascade is activated.[8–10] Initiation of blood coagulation results from activation of the extrinsic pathway, also referred to as the *tissue factor* (TF) pathway, a set of reactions triggered by the interaction of factor VII/VIIa with TF.[5, 11] This insight, largely gained during the past decade, is founded on an abundance of biochemical and clinical evidence. The critical event in the TF pathway is the exposure of TF to the blood as a result of vascular damage or activation of monocytes. Factor VII bound to TF is activated either by trace amounts of factors VIIa, IXa, or Xa or thrombin, or by some enzyme released from damaged cells.[12] About 0.8 per cent of factor VII in plasma is active.[13–15] Circulating factor VIIa is very slowly if at all inactivated by antithrombin, and has a half-

life in plasma of about 2 hours. The physiological substrates of factor VIIa are factors IX and X. The intrinsic and extrinsic pathways are thus intimately related. Factors IXa and Xa formed on activated monocytes/macrophages seem to have distinct physiological functions.[16] The factor X initially activated by FVIIa-TF catalyzes a small initial burst of prothrombin activation followed by thrombin-mediated activation of platelets (the thrombin concentration required to activate platelets is much lower than that required to cleave fibrinogen). The factor IXa formed by factor VIIa-TF generates substantial amounts of factor Xa on the surface of the activated platelets with subsequent formation of prothrombinase (a macromolecular membrane–bound enzymatically active complex that consists of factor Xa, factor Va, phospholipid and calcium). In the final step of the blood coagulation cascade, the prothrombinase complex activates prothrombin to thrombin, which then cleaves soluble fibrinogen with the formation of fibrin that polymerizes to a delicate network surrounding the blood cells in the thrombus.

Among the proteins involved in blood coagulation, factors VII, IX, and X, prothrombin, and protein C are zymogens of serine proteases, which require vitamin K for normal biosynthesis and hence contain α-carboxyglutamic acid (Gla).[4] Protein S is a vitamin K–dependent cofactor of activated protein C (see Chapter 19). Some properties of these proteins, collectively referred to as the vitamin K–dependent coagulation factors, are shown in Table 18–1. Protein Z is a homologue of factors VII, IX, X, and protein C that is enzymatically inactive.[17, 18] Its function is unknown. A recently discovered growth arrest protein, Gas 6, is a homo-

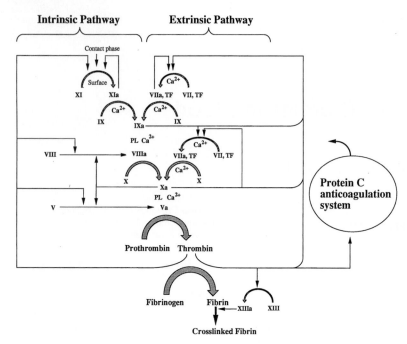

Figure 18–1. Schematic diagram of the intrinsic and extrinsic pathways of blood coagulation. The coagulation cascade is initiated via the extrinsic pathway as a result of tissue damage and the exposure of blood to tissue factor (TF). The two pathways converge when factor X is activated. The active forms of the serine proteases and of the two cofactors V and VIII are indicated by a lower case a; for example, X denotes the zymogen factor X, and Xa the active enzyme factor Xa. The activation of factors V and VIII by thrombin and by factor Xa is denoted, as well as the initiation of the *intrinsic* pathway by thrombin-mediated activation of factor XI. Thrombin also activates factor XIII and protein C of the protein C anticoagulant system. PL = phospholipid.

logue of protein S.[19] In addition, mineralized tissues have Gla-containing proteins; the so-called bone Gla protein and the matrix Gla protein.[20] It has now been demonstrated that vitamin K and Gla have functions extending well beyond blood coagulation and mineralized tissues. Recently, two human cDNAs were identified that encode putative Gla-containing proteins.[21] Unlike blood coagulation proteins, these two messages were expressed in a variety of extrahepatic tissues such as the spinal cord and the thyroid. Finally, certain peptide toxins isolated from the venom of molluscs of the genus *Conus* contain Gla residues that are essential for the function of the toxin.[22]

A characteristic property of the vitamin K–dependent serine proteases, in the absence of their respective cofactors, is the very weak activity against the physiological substrates.[3, 6, 23] The cofactors of factors IXa and Xa are factors VIIIa and Va, respectively. The two homologous cofactors are high molecular weight proteins present as inactive precursors in plasma. They are activated by trace amounts of thrombin or factor Xa.[23, 24] Activation results in the assembly of biologically active macromolecular complexes, the factor Xase complex, and the prothrombinase complex. The factor Xase complex consists of factors IXa and VIIIa, negatively charged phospholipid, and calcium ions; the prothrombinase complex consists of factors Xa and Va, negatively charged phospholipid, and calcium ions. Factor Xa is 10^5- to 10^6-fold more active against prothrombin when it is part of the prothrombinase complex than in the absence of phospholipid and factor Va, whereas its amidolytic activity against low molecular weight substrates is unaffected.[3] Factor IXa is about 10^9-fold more active against factor X when in the Xase complex than in absence of cofactor and phospholipid.[25] Factors VIIIa and Va are substrates of activated protein C and are biologically inactive after cleavage.[26] Protein C is activated by thrombin in complex with the endothelial cell cofactor thrombomodulin (TM). This set of reactions is a regulatory, anticoagulant counterpart of the blood coagulation cascade, and is known as the protein C anticoagulant pathway (see Chapter 19).

It is noteworthy that the cofactors of factor VIIa and thrombin, i.e., TF and TM, are integral membrane proteins.[5, 27] Neither of them requires proteolytic activation to be biologically active. However, whereas TM is expressed on the surface of endothelial cells, TF is normally inaccessible to blood, as it is located on fibroblasts in the adventitia of blood vessels, and is exposed to blood only as a result of tissue damage. Recently, a receptor that links the blood coagulation process and the inflammatory response was iden-

Table 18–1. Vitamin K–Dependent Plasma Proteins

Protein	Plasma Concentration (mg/l)	Molecular Weight	Amino Acids	Size of Gene	Exons	Reference
Prothrombin	100	72,000	579	21 kb	14	59
Factor VII	0.5	48,000	406	13 kb	8	60
Factor IX	4	57,000	415	38 kb	8	61
Factor X	8	59,000	448	22 kb	8	62
Protein C	4	56,000	417	11 kb	9	63, 64
Protein S	20	75,000	635	>80 kb	15	65, 66, 67
Protein Z	2	62,000	360	?	?	18

tified.[28] The receptor, an integral membrane protein, which is designated effector cell protease receptor-1 (EPR-1) binds factor Xa with high affinity. By binding to EPR-1, factor Xa appears to function as a mediator of inflammation in vivo.[29] An endothelial cell protein C receptor has also been identified.[30, 31] This receptor, also an integral membrane protein, seems to act in concert with TM. It is involved in the regulation of hemostasis and perhaps in the regulation of vascular injury in response to inflammation.

Findings in recent studies of the assembly of the enzymatically active macromolecular complexes that constitute the blood coagulation cascade,[3, 5–7] and the protein C anticoagulant system, dovetail with those of structural studies and studies of naturally occurring point mutations in these coagulation factors, and with those of site directed mutagenesis studies of recombinant proteins. The three-dimensional structures of prothrombin fragment 1, consisting of a γ-carboxyglutamic acid (Gla) containing module (*Note*: Rather than domain, the term *module,* suggested by Patthy[32] and by Baron and colleagues,[33] is used throughout this chapter) and a kringle module, has been determined with X-ray diffraction methods using both crystals grown in the presence of calcium and crystals grown in its absence.[34, 35] Determination of the structure of thrombin provided the impetus for a large number of site-directed mutagenesis studies aimed at understanding the structural basis for the pro- as well as anticoagulant properties of this enzyme.[36, 37] More recently, the structures of factors Xa, IXa, and of factor VIIa in complex with TF have been determined and so has the structure of activated protein C.[38–41] NMR spectroscopy has been used to study the structure of isolated modules and pairs of modules, calcium-induced conformational transitions, and module-module interactions. The structure of the Gla module from factor IX has been determined both in the presence and in the absence of Ca^{2+},[42, 43] and the structure of that from factor X has been determined when linked to the first EGF-like module.[44, 45] Modules homologous to the epidermal growth factor (EGF) have been identified in all but one of the vitamin K–dependent clotting factors.[46–48] The structure of the isolated NH_2-terminal EGF module in factor X has been determined by NMR spectroscopy,[49, 50] as has the corresponding module of factor IX.[51, 52] Both EGF modules and kringle modules have been found in many non-vitamin K–dependent proteins with diverse functions.[32, 48, 53]

A rational approach to the diagnosis and treatment of hemorrhagic and thrombotic diseases presupposes an understanding in molecular detail of the biochemical properties and metabolism not only of the traditional blood clotting factors but also of several cell surface receptors and complex polysaccharides. Elucidating structure-function relationships of proteins involved in blood clotting thus poses a formidable but worthwhile challenge. In this chapter we describe structural features that characterize the vitamin K–dependent proteins involved in blood coagulation, with emphasis on the modular design of the proteins and on some structure-function relationships. Only a few mutations are discussed, and only inasmuch as they shed light on an issue under consideration. For more penetrating discussions of factor IX and protein C, the reader is referred to Chapters 19 and 21. X-ray crystallography determination of the structures of several of the proteins involved in the blood coagulation cascade in conjunction with studies of naturally occurring

mutant proteins with functional defects, primarily factor IX, and site-directed mutagenesis studies has yielded a wealth of detailed information that cannot be covered here. The reader is referred to relevant publications for information on the structures[34–44] and for compilations of mutations in factor IX, protein C, and protein S.[54–56]

Modular Organization of Vitamin K–Dependent Plasma Proteins

Seven plasma proteins require vitamin K for normal biosynthesis.[57, 58] They contain 406 to 635 amino acids, and the size of their genes ranges from 11 to more than 80 kilobases (kb; see Table 18–1).[59–67] Accordingly, the exons are short, as in most other extracellular proteins, and are separated by introns of variable length.[68–70] On the basis of their modular structure, three types of vitamin K–dependent coagulation factors can be discerned (Fig. 18–2). Factors VII, IX, and X and protein C form one group, whereas prothrombin and protein S have unique modular structures.[2] Gas 6, a homologue of protein S, is not involved in blood coagulation.[19, 71] The NH_2-terminal module in all of these proteins contains 9 to 12 Gla residues, formed by vitamin K–dependent carboxylation of Glu residues.[2, 57, 58, 72–74] A characteristic feature of the first group is that the Gla module is followed by two modules that are homologous to the EGF precursor and by a C-terminal serine protease module. Protein Z, a vitamin K–dependent plasma protein of unknown function, should also belong to this group, as it is similar in structure to factors VII, IX, and X and protein C.[75] However, it has no amidolytic activity, as two of the residues in the catalytic triad have been mutated. In prothrombin there is a tetradeca-peptide, encoded by a separate exon, with a disulfide loop C-terminal of the Gla module.[59, 70] This region is followed by the two kringle modules, and the C-terminal half of the protein is occupied by the serine protease module. In protein S, the Gla module is followed by a thrombin-sensitive region, a short peptide stretch with an internal disulfide bond and two arginyl bonds, which are susceptible to cleavage by thrombin. The thrombin-sensitive module is followed by four EGF-like modules.[76–78] The C-terminal part of protein S is not homologous to the serine proteases, but to the sex hormone–binding globulin (SHBG) of human plasma and to the androgen-binding protein in rat testis.[79, 80]

The family of vitamin K–dependent plasma proteins is representative of the view that complex genes in eukaryotes have been assembled via intron-mediated recombinations of exons.[47, 81, 82] The exons encode intact functional units, modules, or smaller structural elements. A module in the protein may thus be coded for by one or more exons, such as the kringle modules in prothrombin.[70] According to this view, the exons are remnants of primordial genes that in the course of evolution have been shuffled between genes and duplicated, giving rise to proteins of complex modular design. In this scenario, the coagulation proteins are derived from simple primordial serine proteases that contained a signal peptide required for secretion and a C-terminal serine protease module. The recruitment of exons and exon duplications resulted in an increase in size of the N-terminal, non-catalytic region that accounts for approximately half of each of the vitamin K–dependent serine protease zymogens. These

Factor X

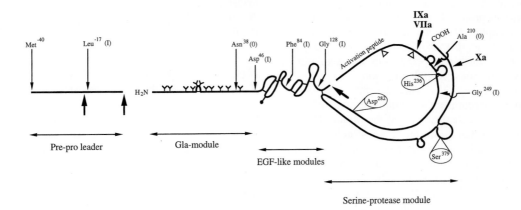

Prothrombin

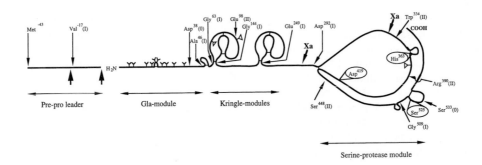

Protein S

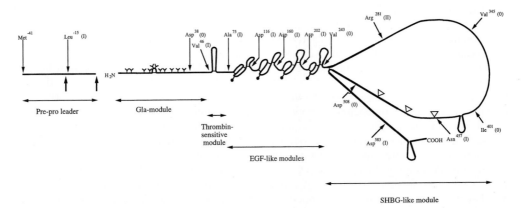

Figure 18–2. Modular structure of the vitamin K–dependent plasma proteins. The structure of factor X also represents the closely related factors VII and IX, protein C, and protein Z. The pre-pro leader sequences are shown to the left. Open triangles denote carbohydrate side chains. Cleavages in factor X and prothrombin that are mediated by factor VIIa or IXa and by factor Xa, respectively, are denoted by arrows. The remaining bold arrows denote, from left to right, cleavages that release the pre or signal sequence; the pro sequence; and, in factor X, the four residues that connect the light and heavy chains in the factor X precursor. Thin arrows denote the location of introns and the corresponding amino acid. The type of splice junction is given in brackets. The residues in the active site of factor X and prothrombin are shown within ovals. The symbol Y denotes γ-carboxyglutamic acid, whereas a "lollipop" symbol on an EGF-like module denotes a β-hydroxyaspartic acid or β-hydroxyasparagine residue. EGF = epidermal growth factor; SHBG = sex hormone–binding globulin.

non-catalytic modules have important functions relating to protein secretion, to interaction with biological membranes and cofactors, and thus to the regulation of the coagulation response at the site of injury.

A characteristic feature of the non-catalytic modules is that the exons encoding separate modules are symmetrical in the sense that they have introns of the same phase class on either side.[83] The exons that have been shuffled in the vitamin K–dependent proteins, as well as in related proteins, are surrounded by introns of phase class 1 (i.e., the intron is between the first and second nucleotide of a codon).[70] Symmetry of the exons with respect to phase class is a prerequisite for exon shuffling, since otherwise insertion or duplication of an exon would result in disruption of the reading frame. It has been suggested that the preference for phase 1 introns between modules, in the proteins of the blood coagulation, fibrinolysis, and complement systems, has its origin in a separation of the exon encoding the signal peptide and the exon encoding the serine protease module in an ancestral protease by a phase 1 intron that has since served as the recipient for exons with class 1 splice junctions on either side.[32]

In the precursors of the vitamin K–dependent proteins, the propeptide and the Gla module constitute a functional unit that is encoded by two exons.[59–67, 70] The intron separates the exon encoding the propeptide and the N-terminal part of the Gla module from the exon encoding the C-terminal α-helical part of the Gla module (often referred to as the α-helical stack region; see Figs. 18–2 and 18–13, and Plate 18–1). The exon encoding the α-helical region has a type 0 splice junction in its 5′ end and a type 1 splice junction in its 3′ end. Thus, the two exons encoding the Gla module appear to have been recruited en bloc to the gene of an ancestral protease prior to the divergence of the vitamin K–dependent blood coagulation zymogens. It should be emphasized that the α-helical stack region is part of the Gla module (or Gla domain). The exon on the 5′ end of the propeptide encodes the signal peptide and exons on the 3′ end relative to the DNA that encodes the Gla module encode a small disulfide loop peptide in prothrombin; EGF modules in factors VII, IX, and X and protein C; and the thrombin-sensitive region in protein S. The propeptide region is recognized by the vitamin K–dependent carboxylase and is removed by proteolytic cleavage *after* carboxylation of appropriate Glu residues but *prior to* or concomitant with secretion (see below). The first kringle module in prothrombin is encoded by two exons, and the second by one exon.[59, 70] Again, the phase of the splice junctions suggests that the two exons encoding the first kringle module have been recruited en bloc. However, it is also possible that introns

have been inserted into the exons encoding the Gla and kringle modules after they were recruited to an ancestor of the vitamin K–dependent proteins. It is assumed that two kringle modules were recruited from a plasminogen ancestor to prothrombin in separate events, rather than a single kringle module that was subsequently duplicated.

It is noteworthy that the locations of introns are conserved in vitamin K–dependent proteins of comparable modular structure. For instance, the first three introns in factors VII, IX, and X and prothrombin are located at precisely the same positions, whereas in protein C the first intron is moved 6 base pairs upstream, probably as a result of an intron sliding mechanism.[59–64] Each of the EGF-like modules is encoded by a single exon. The first exon of the serine protease part of each of these proteins has a type 1 splice junction in its 5′ end, allowing recombination by exon shuffling. In prothrombin, the serine protease part is encoded by six exons, with the residues of the catalytic triad, His 43, Asp 99, and Ser 205 (numbering as in reference 459), on different exons as in most other serine proteases. The positioning of the introns in the prothrombin gene is unique and has no counterpart in any other serine protease. In the serine protease parts of factors VII, IX, and X and protein C, the positions of the two introns are conserved. The large exon that encodes the C-terminal part contains both the active site Asp and Ser residues. The intron-exon organization of factors VII, IX, and X and protein C is compatible with an evolutionary process whereby the archetype of these proteins developed by gene duplication and point mutations.

Gla-Containing Modules

▼ STRUCTURE OF Gla-CONTAINING MODULES

The Gla modules of the vitamin K–dependent proteins contain approximately 47 amino acids (Fig. 18–3). They are homologues with a pronounced sequence similarity. In this region, all 9 to 12 Glu residues are carboxylated to Gla in vitamin K–dependent reactions.[2, 58, 72, 84–86] The 10–12 C-terminal residues of each Gla module form an α-helical portion (residues 35 to 45 in prothrombin). There is one Gla residue in this region in factors IX and X and protein Z, but not in factor VII, prothrombin, protein C, or protein S. The remaining 9 to 11 Gla residues are located between residues 6 and 39. Three pairs of Gla residues are conserved in all proteins, as are the Gla residues corresponding to positions 14, 16, and 29 in prothrombin. The Gla residues occur singly and in pairs, and can be surrounded both by charged and by hydrophobic residues, a feature that has long focused atten-

				10			**20**			**30**		O↓		**40**	I↓
Prothrombin	A N T - F L γ γ	V R K G N L γ R γ C	V γ γ T C S Y γ γ A F	γ A L γ S - S T A T	D V F W A K Y T
Factor VII	A N A - F L γ γ	L R P G S L γ R γ C	K γ γ Q C S F γ γ A R	γ I F K D - A γ R T K	L F W I S Y S
Factor IX	Y N S G K L γ γ	F V Q G N L γ R γ C	M γ γ K C S F γ γ A R	γ V F γ N - T γ R T T	γ F W K Q Y V
Factor X	A N S - F L γ γ	M K K G H L γ R γ C	M γ γ T C S Y γ γ A R	γ V F γ D - S D K T N	γ F W N K Y K
Protein C	A N S - F L γ γ	L R H S S L γ R γ C	I γ γ I C D F γ γ A K	γ I F Q N - V D D T L	A F W S K H V
Protein S	A N S - L L γ γ	T K Q G N L γ R γ C	I γ γ L C N K γ γ A R	γ V F γ N D P γ - T D	Y F Y P K Y L
Protein Z	A G S Y L L γ γ	L F γ G N L γ K T C	Y γ γ I C V Y γ γ A R	γ γ F γ N - γ V V T D	γ F W R R Y K

Figure 18–3. Amino acid sequences in the Gla modules of the human vitamin K–dependent plasma proteins. The numbering is that of human prothrombin. O denotes the position (and type of splice junction) of the intron separating the two exons that encode the Gla module. The aromatic cluster is formed by Phe 40, Trp 41, and Tyr 44. Residues are shaded when at least three of seven are identical.

tion on the substrate recognition mechanism of the carboxylase.

The involvement of Gla in Ca^{2+} binding became evident when it was demonstrated that normal prothrombin contains Gla and binds Ca^{2+}, whereas abnormal prothrombin, synthesized in the presence of such vitamin K antagonistic drugs as warfarin, contains Glu in the corresponding positions, does not bind Ca^{2+}, has no phospholipid affinity, and lacks biological activity.[57, 87–93] In factor Xa-mediated prothrombin activation, the addition of negatively charged phospholipid in the presence of Ca^{2+} results in a reduction of the K_m for prothrombin by more than two orders of magnitude.[3, 23, 94] This effect is not obtained with uncarboxylated prothrombin. Warfarin administration also results in the synthesis of forms of prothrombin with intermediate degrees of carboxylation.[95] A marked reduction in phospholipid binding and activation is observed already with the loss of 3 or 4 of the 10 Gla residues in prothrombin. Similar results have been obtained with prothrombin from patients with hereditary vitamin K–dependent carboxylation abnormalities.[96]

X-ray crystallography determination of the three-dimensional structure of bovine prothrombin fragment 1 represents an important step toward an understanding of the function of the Gla module in Ca^{2+} binding, and provides a structural basis for future studies aimed at elucidation of the interactions of vitamin K–dependent plasma proteins with biological membranes and protein cofactors.[34, 35] Fragment 1, formed during limited proteolysis of bovine or human prothrombin by thrombin, consists of the N-terminal 156 or 155 amino acids, respectively.[97, 98] It contains the Gla module, the tetradecapeptide disulfide loop, and the N-terminal kringle module. Residue numbers in the following refer to human fragment 1.[59] The α-helical part of the Gla module, residues 35 to 45, forms three turns of α-helix, such that the side chains of Phe 40, Trp 41, and Tyr 44 form an aromatic cluster that is adjacent to the disulfide bond connecting Cys 17 and Cys 22. In crystals of fragment 1, obtained in the absence of Ca^{2+}, the part of the Gla module N-terminal to the α-helical segment does not diffract X-rays, presumably because of a high degree of mobility.[34, 35] When the crystallization was performed in the presence of Ca^{2+}, the structure of the entire Gla module could be solved at 2.25 Å resolution (Fig. 18–4).[35] The gross structure of the module is discoid. Calcium ions interact with the carboxylate groups of Gla residues and seem to cross-link parts of the module that are fairly remote in the linear sequence. The carboxylate groups of Gla residues 16, 25, 26, and 29 form a negatively charged surface within the module in apposition to another negatively charged surface formed by the carboxylate groups of Gla residues 6 and 7. Four or five calcium ions are interposed between the two negatively charged surfaces. Each ion interacts with at least two carboxylate groups. Gla residues 14, 19, and 20 form a negatively charged cluster adjacent to the tetradecapeptide disulfide loop peptide. Two calcium ions have been identified in this region. Of the seven calcium ions identified, three seem to be inaccessible to solvent. Only six carboxylate groups are exposed on the surface of the module. The N-terminal residues in the Gla module are folded in an Ω-like fashion, such that the amino group of Ala 1 is buried and makes ion pair interactions with Gla residues, thus rendering it inaccessible to chemical modification.[99] Recently, the structure of prothrombin fragment 1 crystallized in the presence of strontium rather than calcium was determined.[100] The structure of Sr-prothrombin fragment 1 was found to be very similar to that of the calcium form.

Owing to the pronounced sequence similarity, it has long been assumed that the Gla modules in the vitamin K–dependent plasma proteins have a fold similar to that of the Gla module in prothrombin fragment 1. And indeed the Gla module of factor VIIa, in complex with tissue factor, has the same fold as the Gla module of prothrombin fragment 1.[41] In factors IX and X and protein C, all studied by X-ray crystallography, the Gla module was either lost by proteolytic cleavage during crystallization (factor X and protein C),[40, 101] or did not diffract well for other reasons (factor IX).[39] However, a synthetic Gla module from factor IX has been studied by NMR spectroscopy and demonstrated to have a fold that appears to be essentially identical to that of prothrombin fragment 1 and that of factor VII.[43] The Mg^{2+} form of the Gla module of factor IX has a structure for residues 12–46 that is similar to that of the Ca^{2+} form, whereas the 11 N-terminal residues lacked defined structure.[102] Similarity of structure in the Gla modules of several vitamin K–dependent clotting factors has also been inferred from studies with a monoclonal antibody that binds to a common epitope in all these proteins in a metal ion and conformation-dependent manner.[103] Finally, the calcium ion-induced spectroscopic perturbations observed in Gla module-containing proteins and in fragments of these proteins are quite similar, further attesting to the structural similarity of the Gla modules.[104–107] To attain a native structure the entire Gla module is required, that is including the C-terminal α-helical stack region. The Gla modules of factor IX and protein C have been chemically synthesized.[108, 109] Determination of the structure of the calcium-form of the factor IX module demonstrated that it was folded to a native conformation.[43] However, in the absence of calcium this module, as well as the corresponding module from factor X, is less structured than that of the Gla module of factor X linked to the EGF module (see below). Gla modules, produced by proteolytic cleavage in the aromatic cluster of the α-helical connecting peptide but otherwise intact, can be isolated from factors VII, IX, and X and protein C.[107, 110–113] The isolated cleaved Gla modules from factor X (residues 1 to 44), factor IX (residues 1 to 43), and prothrombin (residues 1 to 45) bind Ca^{2+} with lower affinity than does the Gla module in the intact protein.[107, 109, 112, 114, 115] Nevertheless,

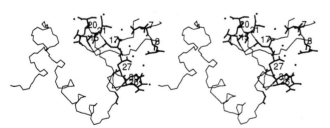

Figure 18–4. Structure of Gla module. Stereoview of the structure of the Gla module in bovine prothrombin fragment 1. The polypeptide backbone is shown, as well as the side chains of the Gla residues. The filled circles denote calcium ions. Bovine prothrombin has a Gly residue in position 4 that has no counterpart in human prothrombin. Gla 7 and 8 in the figure thus correspond to Gla 6 and 7 in human prothrombin. (From Tulinsky, A.: The structures of domains of blood proteins. Thromb. Haemost. 66:16, 1991; with permission.)

they bind to negatively charged phospholipid vesicles, albeit at higher Ca^{2+} concentrations than those required to mediate binding (for instance) of prothrombin fragment 1.[114] It appears as if the C-terminal, α-helical, part of the Gla modules is a nucleation site for folding in the presence of Ca^{2+}. Moreover, the adjacent EGF-like module appears to be a scaffold for the Gla module.[44, 116, 117]

▼ CALCIUM- AND PHOSPHOLIPID-BINDING PROPERTIES OF Gla MODULES

The conversion of 9 to 12 Glu residues to Gla in each of the vitamin K–dependent plasma proteins endows them with Ca^{2+}-binding properties at physiological Ca^{2+} concentrations (≈ 1.2 mM free Ca^{2+}). A monocarboxylic acid such as acetic acid binds Ca^{2+} with $K_d \approx 300$ mM, whereas malonic acid (a dicarboxylic acid similar to Gla) binds Ca^{2+} with higher affinity, $K_d \approx 30$ mM, but still far above the concentration of Ca^{2+} in plasma.[106] Binding of Ca^{2+} to prothrombin and prothrombin fragment 1, as well as to the other vitamin K–dependent plasma proteins, is characterized by a pronounced positive cooperativity in the binding of the first two or three Ca^{2+}, which was originally observed as a characteristic bell-shaped binding curve in Scatchard plots (Fig. 18–5).[91, 93, 106, 118, 119] The drastic conformational change that is induced by Ca^{2+}-binding to Gla modules is also evident from the Ca^{2+}-induced quenching of the intrinsic protein fluorescence.[104–107] Typically the half-maximum quenching is observed at about 0.5 mM Ca^{2+}, i.e., not far from the physiological Ca^{2+} concentration in blood plasma. The cooperative Ca^{2+} binding is consistent with the complex structure of the Gla module and the involvement of Ca^{2+} in its folding to a native conformation. Although metal ion-binding studies provided clear evidence of Ca^{2+}-induced

conformational changes, interpretation of the binding data was initially confounded by metal ion-induced dimerization in (for instance) prothrombin fragment 1.[106] The Ca^{2+}-binding properties of these proteins are particularly interesting in the light of the three-dimensional structure of the Gla module of prothrombin fragment 1 and of factors VII, and IX, in which Ca^{2+} serves to cross-link Gla residues that are remote in the linear sequence, thus illustrating the part played by the metal ion in the folding of Gla modules to their native conformation. For instance, the Ω-like fold of the NH_2-terminal residues in the Gla module with the amino group of Ala 1 buried and making an ion pair with Gla residues, renders it inaccessible to chemical modification in the presence of calcium ions.[120] In the absence of calcium, the amino group of Ala 1 is readily modfied, for instance, by reductive methylation. The membrane binding of the modified protein is greatly impaired. A similar observation was made when the amino-terminal residues of factors IX and X were modified.[114]

The vitamin K–dependent plasma proteins also bind other divalent cations, such as Mg^{2+}, Mn^{2+}, and Sr^{2+}, that do not, however, substitute for Ca^{2+} in blood coagulation.[106, 119, 121, 122] The Sr^{2+} form of prothrombin fragment 1 has a structure that is very similar to the Ca^{2+} form.[100] On the other hand, the Mg^{2+} form of the factor IX Gla module is not structured in the N-terminal part.[102] The metal ion-induced conformational transition in the Gla domain can be divided into at least two stages. Binding of the first two or three cations induces a conformational change that can be discerned by the drastic quenching of the intrinsic protein fluorescence from the Trp residue in postion 41,[112, 123] or by the interaction with conformation-specific monoclonal antibodies [124] or fractionated polyclonal antisera.[122, 125] This first step is relatively nonspecific with respect to the cation in that it is induced by Ca^{2+} but can also be induced by Mg^{2+} and other divalent cations. The second class of binding sites is specific for Ca^{2+} and is required for the structural transition necessary for membrane binding. It should be borne in mind that the free Ca^{2+} concentration in plasma is about 1.2 mM, whereas the free Mg^{2+} concentration is about 0.5 mM. In all K–dependent proteins but factor IX, both conformational transitions are induced by Ca^{2+}.

In factor IX there is at least one site in the Gla module that requires Mg^{2+} and that does not appear to have a counterpart in Gla modules of the other K–dependent coagulation factors.[126–128] This is reflected by the fact that, at saturating Ca^{2+} concentrations, Mg^{2+} enhances the rate of activation of factor IX by factor XIa. Moreover, the factor IXa-mediated rate of factor X activation is also enhanced by Mg^{2+}, apparently by a Mg^{2+}-induced increase in the affinity of factor IXa for factor VIIIa. As the Gla module interacts with phospholipid, these findings illustrate another, as yet rather poorly understood aspect of the function of these proteins, i.e., the importance of module-module interactions. Interaction between the Gla module and the adjacent modules was also inferred from studies of the Ca^{2+}-binding properties of protein S in which the thrombin-sensitive bond had been cleaved. In cleaved protein S, the Gla module is linked to the remainder of the molecule by a disulfide bond. The Gla module in the cleaved protein appears to have lower Ca^{2+} affinity than that in intact protein S, and the cleaved molecule has no biological activity.[78]

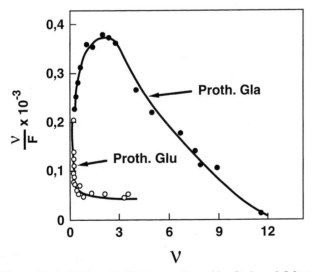

Figure 18–5. Calcium-binding to prothrombin. Binding of Ca^{2+} to normal (solid circles) and uncarboxylated (open circles) prothrombin. The data have been plotted according to Scatchard, and {nu} is (mol Ca^{2+}/mol prothrombin) and F is the molar concentration of free Ca^{2+}. The upward convexity denotes a positive cooperativity in the binding of Ca^{2+}. (Modified from Stenflo, J., and Ganrot, P.: Binding of Ca^{2+} to normal and dicoumarol-induced prothrombin. Biochem. Biophys. Res. Commun. 50:98, 1974; with permission.)

New insight into the folding mechanism of Gla modules was obtained in studies of the structure of a fragment from bovine factor X using 2D NMR.[44] The fragment contained the Gla module linked to the N-terminal EGF-like module. In the X-ray structures of prothrombin fragment 1, performed in the absence of Ca^{2+}, no diffraction was observed N-terminal of the α-helical stack region of the Gla module, either because the module was very mobile or simply because it lacked an ordered structure.[34] In the factor X fragment the EGF module had a structure that was almost identical to that previously determined for the isolated module.[49, 50] More important, the Gla module was found to have a structure that was rather well defined, also in the absence of Ca^{2+}, except for the nine N-terminal residues (see Fig. 18–4). All three α-helices were preserved, but were less well defined than in the Ca^{2+}-form (modeled on the Ca^{2+}-form of prothrombin fragment 1), and apparently assembled in a more dynamic manner, which may explain the difficulties encountered in attempts to determine the structure by X-ray crystallography. The interesting feature of the structure is that the nine to ten most N-terminal residues of the Gla module adopt an entirely different fold. In the Ca^{2+}-free form of the module, this part of the structure is poorly defined but it is evident that the hydrophobic residues Phe 4, Leu 5, and Val 8, residues that surround the first pair of Gla residues, form a hydrophobic cluster that faces the interior of the module. In the Ca^{2+} form of the module, these three residues are exposed to solvent. There is a concurrent change in the orientation of Gla residues. In the Ca^{2+}-free form, they are exposed to the solvent and provide a negatively charge surface. When Ca^{2+} is bound, Gla residues 6, 7, 16, 20, and 29 fold into the core of the module to ligate calcium ions in the space previously occupied by the hydrophobic residues. Comparison of the Ca^{2+}-free and Ca^{2+}-loaded forms of this part of the Gla module sheds light on the cooperativity of the Ca^{2+}-binding. Each Gla residue is a ligand to one or more Ca^{2+}. It is apparent that binding one Ca^{2+} recruits one or more Gla residues to bind the next Ca^{2+}. Intermediates will be highly disfavored due to strong uncompensated electrostatic repulsion between neighboring Gla residues, which promotes cooperative binding. The all or nothing nature of binding is reflected by the effects of mutation of Gla residues 7, 16, 26, and 29 in protein C and prothrombin. Mutation of any of these residues results in loss of Ca^{2+} binding and membrane binding and loss of biological activity.[129, 130] It can be envisioned that in the Ca^{2+}-free form the negatively charged Gla residues, that are exposed to solvent, generate a very negative electrostatic potential surface that cannot interact with the negative head groups present on the surface of procoagulant cell membranes. Moreover, the hydrophobic side-chains, thought to be inserted into the membrane, are now hidden in the interior of the module.

The data accumulated thus far indicate that the isolated intact Gla module (with the α-helical stack region) has little structure in the absence of calcium but attains a native structure in the presence of saturating calcium (both in factor IX and factor X). The C-terminal α-helical stack region of the Gla module functions as a nucleation site for the folding of the module and is essential for normal structure. When attached to the the adjacent EGF module, the calcium-free form of the Gla module is considerably more structured and has an essentially normal, although more dynamic fold than that of the calcium form, except for the 11 N-terminal residues that are poorly defined.[44] This structure resembles the structure of the Mg^{2+} form of the factor IX module.[102] The adjacent EGF module thus appears to function as a scaffold for the Gla module, particularly in the absence of calcium.

The interaction of vitamin K–dependent proteins with negatively charged phospholipid membranes is crucial to biological activity of this group of proteins. Typical artificial membranes contain 25 per cent phosphatidyl serine and 75 per cent phosphatidylcholine. It is now known that phosphatidyl serine is crucially important as it promotes the membrane-bound enzymatic reactions much more effectively than do other equally charged lipids.[3, 131, 132] There is a wide span in the affinity of the K–dependent proteins for biological membranes. Yet, the sequence similarity between the modules is very high (see Fig. 18–3). For instance, bovine factor X binds with a Kd of ≈ 40 nM, whereas bovine protein C binds with a Kd > 15000 nM[133] despite the fact that there are only five significant amino acid differences between the amino-terminal 34 residues involved in binding. In vivo suitable membranes are provided by activated platelets (see Chapter 24) and by cells damaged such that the phosphatidylserine-containing inner bilayer is exposed. The biological membranes can promote the enzymatic reactions in at least three ways. Interaction with the membrane promotes the assembly of the macromolecular, enzymatically active complex (e.g. the prothrombinase complex). The membrane can also induce a conformational transition in enzyme and/or substrate; and finally, the membrane reduces the dimensionality of the reactions involved, i.e., blood coagulation becomes a series of reactions occurring in two dimensions.

The interaction between K-dependent proteins and biological membranes has been difficult to study, and there is still no consensus as to the mode of interaction. It was long generally assumed that the interaction was mediated by calcium ions bridging between Gla residues in the proteins and negatively charged groups on the phospholipid surface. This notion derived support from experimental results demonstrating that high calcium ion concentrations tend to dissociate the proteins from the membrane surfaces.[114] More recent experiments have demonstrated the importance of the hydrophobic component to the binding energy.[134, 135] Support for the hydrophobic component comes from site-directed mutagenesis experiments that have demonstrated that mutation of Leu 5 and Leu 8, surrounding the first pair of Gla residues, in protein C reduces the phospholipid affinity of the mutant protein considerably.[136–138] This effect should be regarded in light of the dramatic calcium-induced conformational transition in the N-terminal part of the Gla module that has been described above. The mutated hydrophobic residues surrounding the N-terminal Gla residues are hidden in the interior of the module in the absence of calcium, but are exposed on the surface of the membrane-binding calcium form of the module. The model predicts insertion of the side chain of one or more of the three hydrophobic amino acids surrounding the first pair of Gla residues into the hydrocarbon region of the membrane, thereby allowing bound calcium ions and positively charged amino acids to interact with phosphate head groups in the membrane. Experimental support for the model has also been provided by the observation that a photoactivatable amino acid in position 6 or 9 in the factor IX Gla module crosslinks specifically to the phospholipid membrane.[102] The model is attractive as it links calcium binding to the conformational change that is a prerequisite for membrane interaction. Moreover, it also accommodates the observation that the interaction is not only hydrophobic in nature but has an ionic component. Weaknesses of the theory are that the membrane affinity differs very much betweeen the Gla-containing proteins, yet the sequence similarity and the fold of the domains are very similar.[139] Furthermore, mutation of one of the hydrophobic residues implicated in the interaction was found to have surprisingly little impact on the affinity of the protein for the membrane.[137] This has led to the advancement of an alternative theory based on the structure and membrane-binding properties of these proteins.[139] A central feature of this theory, that is currently undergoing testing, is the formation of an isolated protein-lipid ion pair, similar to that which characterizes the interaction of phospholipase A2 with biological membranes.[140] The theory gains support from the recent identification of a specific phosphatidylserine-binding site on factor Xa, identified using a soluble form of the phospholipid.[141] The site has not been localized, but binding of the soluble phospholipid has been demonstrated to enhance the factor Xa–mediated prothrombin activation rate about 60-fold, i.e., about 20 per cent of the optimal rate observed with phospholipid membranes with optimal composition.

In addition to binding to phospholipid surfaces, factor IX binds to endothelial cells in a saturable and reversible manner. The binding is characterized by a Kd of about 2 nM.[142] It is calcium-dependent and is mediated by residues 3–11 in the Gla module.[143, 144] Factor IX bound to endothelial cells treated with phorbol esters and expressing tissue factor could be activated by factor VIIa.[145] The binding has now been shown to be mediated by collagen 4 on the cells.[146, 147] The physiological implications of this binding are not yet known.

▼ MUTATIONS IN Gla MODULES

Numerous mutations have been identified in the vitamin K-dependent proteins, and they have also been extensively studied by site-directed mutagenesis. Databases of mutations in factor IX and protein C and protein S have been compiled.[54–56, 148, 149] Several mutations that give rise to hemophilia B have been identified in the Gla module of factor IX. Only a few are point mutations that result in the synthesis of an abnormal protein with low biological activity (see Chapter 21). However, some properties of the factor IX mutant Oxford b1 (Cys 23 ->Tyr; see Fig. 18–3) have been studied. The mutant factor IX appears in plasma at 19 per cent of the normal concentration, whereas its biological activity is below 1 per cent.[150] Defective adsorption of the mutant factor IX to alumina and its weak interaction with a monoclonal antibody that recognizes a Ca^{2+}-dependent epitope suggest that Ca^{2+} binding to the mutant molecule is impaired. Factor IX Zutphen (Cys 18 ->Arg) has a normal plasma concentration, but its biological activity is below 1 per cent.[54, 151, 152] It does not bind Ca^{2+} normally. Moreover, Cys 18 appears to be linked to another polypeptide by a

disulfide bridge. Both these mutants preclude formation of the disulfide bond between Cys 18 and Cys 23, which is required for the structural integrity of the hexapeptide disulfide loop in the Gla module, and thus for normal biological activity and Ca^{2+} binding to the module. These results are consistent with the observation that reduction and alkylation of the Cys residues in this disulfide loop result in reduced Ca^{2+} affinity.[118]

There are two point mutations of Gla 27 in factor IX. Factor IX Seattle 3 is Gla 27 ->Lys, and factor IX Chongqing is Gla 27 -> Val.[153, 154] Both mutations result in severe hemophilia B. Substitution of Gla 15 or Gla 20 by Asp has been shown to result in only a slight reduction of the clotting activity, whereas the mutant with Asp instead of Gla in position 7 was reported to be almost completely inactive.[155] Recently, it was found that, in recombinant factor IX, Gla 36 and Gla 40 are not required for biological activity in factor IX.[156] A factor IX species with Glu in both these positions was fully active. The factor IX mutant, Gly 12-> Arg is particularly interesting.[157] The mutant protein had almost normal phospholipid binding, but had very low biological activity in the presence of factor VIIIa. It was demonstrated that the affinity of the mutant factor IXa for factor VIIIa was reduced approximately 170-fold, as compared to the wild type protein. Presumably there is no direct contact between the Gla module and factor VIIIa. Instead it was assumed that the mutated Gly residue was critical for normal inter-module contact, which when broken results in defective interaction with factor VIIIa.

In factor X Voralberg, Gla 14 is mutated to Lys.[158] The rate of activation of mutant factor X was only 15 per cent of that of normal factor X on activation by factor VIIa/TF, but 75 per cent of normal on activation with factor IXa/ factor VIIIa. On activation with the factor X activator from Russell's viper venom, it was fully active. The reason for the different activation rates is unknown. Factor Xa Voralberg activated prothrombin at a normal rate, although a higher than normal concentration of Ca^{2+} was required. Site-specific mutagenesis has been used to alter the Gla residues in recombinant protein C (see Chapter 19). A mutant in which both Gla 6 and Gla 7 were replaced with Asp possessed less than 5 per cent of the activity of wild-type recombinant activated protein C toward its substrate, factor VIIIa.[129] Two other recombinant protein C species have been characterized: one in which Gla 19 and Gla 20 were mutated to Asp, and one in which Cys 22 was mutated to Ser.[159] Both activated protein C species manifested less than 1 per cent of the activity of recombinant wild-type activated protein C in the activated partial thromboplastin assay and in the inactivation of purified factor VIIIa. In prothrombin a systematic study of the importance of individual Gla residues has been made by site-directed mutagenesis.[160] Mutation of other residues than Gla and Cys can of course have detrimental effects on the biological activity of these proteins. For instance, mutation of the conserved Arg residue in position 15 of protein C results in defective phospholipid binding and less than 10 per cent of the normal biological activity.[161]

The functional defects of proteins with point mutations in the Gla modules (naturally occurring or recombinant mutant proteins) clearly demonstrate that the Gla residues are not functionally equivalent. Certain Gla residues can be mutated and yet the structure of the domain appears to be retained as judged from a normal biological activity. In contrast, other mutants have very low activity.

Other types of recombinant mutant Gla-containing proteins are chimeras in which, for instance, the Gla module (residues 1–46 or 47) of protein C is replaced with the corresponding module from factor IX.[162] To study which parts of factor VII/VIIa that interact with tissue factor, chimeras have been made of factors VII and IX, in which entire modules have been exchanged.[163, 164] These studies demonstrated the importance of the EGF module in the interaction between factor VIIa and tissue factor whereas the Gla module contributed less to binding. These chimeric proteins have corroborated the notion that the Gla module is an independently folded unit. Moreover, they have demonstrated that the functions of the Gla modules in these proteins are often sufficiently general in nature to be switched between the proteins without major loss of biological activity in systems so far tested.

▼ FUNCTION OF Gla IN THE SECRETION OF VITAMIN K–DEPENDENT PROTEINS

The post-translational carboxylation of Glu to Gla is required not only for normal Ca^{2+} binding and membrane interaction of the proteins but also for normal transport of the vitamin K–dependent proteins from the rough endoplasmic reticulum of the hepatocytes to the blood plasma.[57, 58] Treatment of patients with vitamin K antagonistic coumarin anticoagulants such as warfarin results in an approximately 50 per cent reduction of the plasma prothrombin concentration.[87, 92] The abnormal prothrombin in plasma, either uncarboxylated or undercarboxylated, manifests defective Ca^{2+} binding and membrane interaction. The coupling of carboxylation to secretion is particularly striking in the rat, in which uncarboxylated vitamin K–dependent proteins accumulate in the rough endoplasmic reticulum of the liver in vitamin K deficiency, with a concomitant reduction of the plasma concentration to very low values.[165, 166] The same effect is observed with such vitamin K antagonistic drugs as warfarin. This finding suggests the presence of a microsomal transport protein capable of distinguishing between carboxylated and uncarboxylated proteins.

Warfarin treatment of rats results in the accumulation of several isoelectric forms of the prothrombin precursor in the endoplasmic reticulum of the liver. The precursors are rich in mannose and are susceptible to cleavage by endoglycosidase H.[167, 168] However, glycosylation is not coupled to carboxylation, as tunicamycin, which inhibits core glycosylation, does not affect the degree of carboxylation. Recently, it was suggested that there are different binding proteins for prothrombin and factor X in the microsomal membrane.[169] For detailed information on the effects of glycosylation on the secretion of vitamin K–dependent proteins the reader is referred to specialized articles.[170–173] There is no evidence to suggest that the effect of glycosylation in the K–dependent proteins differs from that of this type of modification in other plasma proteins.

▼ PROPEPTIDES: STRUCTURES RECOGNIZED BY THE CARBOXYLASE

N-terminal of the propeptide, the vitamin K–dependent proteins, like other extracellular and membrane proteins, have a so-called signal peptide. The signal peptide, which is usually 30 to 60 amino acid residues long, mediates association of the nascent peptide chain with the cytosolic part of the endoplasmic reticulum.[174] Insertion of the signal peptide into the endoplasmic reticulum initiates translocation of the peptide chain across the membrane. The signal peptide is removed by a signal peptidase that appears to recognize amino acids with small side-chains, such as Ala or Gly in positions -3 and -1.[175] Removal of the signal peptide, a cotranslational event in the endoplasmic reticulum, exposes the N-terminus of the propeptide.

In the Gla module, 9 to 12 Glu residues are carboxylated to Gla (see Fig. 18–3). It is noteworthy that there are no obvious sequences in the Gla modules that can constitute carboxylase recognition sites. There are three Gla-Gla sequences as well as Gla residues that occur singly, sometimes with adjacent hydrophobic residues and sometimes with a neighboring Arg residue. This suggests the presence of a substrate recognition mechanism of the vitamin K–dependent carboxylase that is fundamentally different from those of other enzymes that carry out postribosomal modifications, such as prolyl-4-hydroxylase, which recognizes proline in the sequence Gly-Xxx-Pro,[176] and N-glycosylating enzymes that recognize Asn in the sequence Asn-Xxx-Ser/Thr.[177] The existence of an intricate substrate recognition mechanism was also inferred from early experiments that demonstrated uncarboxylated prothrombin to be a poor substrate for the carboxylase, whether it has been synthesized in vivo under the influence of such vitamin K antagonistic drugs as warfarin or formed by heat decarboxylation of normal plasma prothrombin.[178] The synthetic peptide Phe-Leu-Glu-Glu-Leu and similar synthetic peptides have been used as substrates in many studies of the carboxylase.[58] However, these peptides are poor substrates, with K_m values in the millimolar range, that is, far higher than can be obtained with the uncarboxylated forms of prothrombin and related proteins that are substrates in vivo. In contrast to the synthetic peptides and the uncarboxylated prothrombin, the prothrombin precursor purified from rat liver is an excellent substrate for the carboxylase and has a K_m value in the low micromolar range.[58, 72]

Determination of the complementary DNA (cDNA) sequences of vitamin K–dependent plasma proteins and the use of synthetic peptides as substrates for the carboxylase have provided insight into the mechanism by which the enzyme recognizes its substrates.[179–181] The vitamin K–dependent proteins were found to contain an N_2-terminal extension of the Gla module, located between the signal peptide and the mature protein.[2] In the propeptides, several residues are conserved between the vitamin K–dependent proteins, whereas others have been changed by conservative mutations (Fig. 18–6). Two Gla-containing proteins from mineralized tissues are particularly interesting in this respect: osteocalcin, or bone Gla protein that contains three Gla residues, and matrix Gla protein that contains five Gla residues.[20, 182] There is no apparent sequence similarity between the mature Gla-containing proteins from mineralized tissue and the vitamin K–dependent plasma proteins. However, osteocalcin contains an N-terminal propeptide with a sequence that is clearly related to corresponding regions of the vitamin K–dependent plasma proteins (see Fig. 18–6).[20, 183] Moreover, in the matrix Gla-containing protein, a sequence

```
                    -25           -20           -15           -10           -5            -1
Prothrombin         L C S L V H S Q H V  F  L A P Q Q  A  R S  L  L  Q R V R  R
FVII                M P W K P G P H R V  F  V T Q E E  A  H G V  L  H R R R  R
FIX                 G Y L L S A E C T V  F  L D H E N  A  N K I  L  N R P K  R
FX                  A G L L L L G E S L  F  I R R E Q  A  N N I  L  A R V T  R
Protein C           S G T P A P L D S V  F  S S S E R  A  H Q V  L  R I R K  R
Protein S           L L V L P V S E A N  F  L S K Q Q  A  S Q V  L  V R K R  R
Bone Gla protein    K P S G A E S S K A  F  V S K Q E     S E V     K R P R  R
Matrix Gla protein  E S M E S Y E L N P  F  I N R R N  A  N T F     S P Q Q  R
```

Figure 18–6. Sequence similarity in the propeptide regions of the vitamin K–dependent plasma proteins and the two vitamin K–dependent bone proteins osteocalcin and matrix Gla protein. Residues are shaded when at least six of the eight residues are identical. In factor IX, the signal peptidase cleavage site (arrowhead) is between residues -19 and -18; in factor X, it is between residues -18 and -17; and in protein C, it is between residues -25 and -24.

segment containing residues 15 to 30 appears to be homologous to the propeptides of the vitamin K–dependent plasma proteins.[182] It is noteworthy that this sequence in the matrix Gla protein is not removed by proteolytic cleavage prior to secretion. In addition, there is one Gla residue N-terminal to this propeptide-related peptide segment in the matrix Gla protein. These results have established that not only the Gla residues but also the propeptides are common structural denominators of vitamin K–dependent proteins, whether in blood plasma or in bone. It should also be emphasized that the propeptides are encoded on the same exon as the Gla module; they are indeed a functional unit.

The function of the propeptides as structural elements recognized by the vitamin K–dependent carboxylase has been amply documented by the expression of recombinant vitamin K–dependent proteins.[184–188] The proteins are secreted by eukaryotic cells and are carboxylated if the messenger RNA encodes the propeptide region and vitamin K is present, whereas no carboxylation occurs in the absence of the propeptide. Moreover, synthetic peptides that contain the propeptide region and the N-terminal amino acids of the mature protein (residues -18 to +10) are excellent substrates for the carboxylase in in vitro carboxylation assays, with K_m values between 1 and 10 μM, whereas the corresponding peptides lacking the propeptide region are poor substrates, with K_m values three orders of magnitude greater.[58, 179, 188] It is also noteworthy that the isolated propeptide stimulates carboxylation of small peptides containing glutamic acid, such as Phe-Leu-Glu-Glu-Leu. This observation has recently been followed up using recombinant carboxylase (see below).

The propeptides can be exchanged between the proteins. For instance, the propeptide of factor IX can direct carboxylation of protein C and vice versa.[189] Moreover, in a recombinant prothrombin fragment with the Gla and kringle regions deleted and with the propeptide attached to a glutamate-rich region of the C-terminal part of prothrombin (residues 249–530), the propeptide directed carboxylation of at least seven out of eight Glu residues within the first 40 residues.[190] It should be emphasized that this region has no sequence similarity to a Gla domain. It is thus obvious that the propeptide is the sole recognition site for the vitamin K-dependent carboxylase. Nonetheless, recombinant factor X with the first EGF-like domain replaced by the first EGF-like domain from factor IX is only about 15 per cent carboxylated. This is presumably due to interactions between adjacent modules that are known to occur but that are still poorly understood.

Mechanistically the propeptide binds the substrate to the enzyme and in addition activates the enzyme. Thus a high substrate concentration is obtained adjacent to the active site of the enzyme. It has now been demonstrated that in incubation mixtures containing recombinant carboxylase and substrate/product there will be essentially fully carboxylated product and uncarboxylated substrate with few molecules with intermediate degrees of carboxylation.[191] It was also shown that this results from multiple carboxylation events occurring with one substrate molecule bound to the enzyme. This processive type of carboxylation is unique among post-ribosomal modifications, but is a characteristic of the replication and modification of DNA and RNA. Recently it was reported that the vitamin K–dependent carboxylase also carboxylates itself in a vitamin K–dependent reaction.[192]

Comparison of the sequences of propeptides of vitamin K–dependent proteins shows certain residues to be conserved.[2] The Phe residue in position -16 is present in all propeptides; Ala in position -10 is found in the plasma proteins, whereas bone Gla protein has Gly in this position. The hydrophobic amino acids in positions -6, -7, and -17 are conserved in most cases or replaced by other hydrophobic amino acids. Site-directed mutagenesis of factor IX and prothrombin, as well as studies using synthetic peptides as substrates for the carboxylase in vitro, indicate residues -10, -15, -16, -17, and -18 to be crucial for substrate recognition by the carboxylase.[2, 184] In contrast, mutation of the residues in positions -14, -8, and -1 in factor IX does not affect the degree of carboxylation. Site-directed mutagenesis studies suggest that some differences exist between the vitamin K–dependent proteins. In factor IX, mutation of Ala at -10 completely abolished γ-carboxylation, whereas in protein C deletion of residues -1 to -12 had relatively little effect on γ-carboxylation.[184, 193] It has been proposed that the propeptide region in the coagulation factors forms an α-helix in solution with the residues that appear to be crucial for recognition by the carboxylase on one side of the helix.[194]

The signal peptidase cleavage site has been localized in factors IX and X and protein C.[186, 195–197] In factor IX, cleavage is between residues -19 and -18; in protein C, between residues -25 and -24; and in factor X, between residues -18 and -17. The four residues in the propeptide that immediately precede the mature protein (residues -1 to -4) constitute the recognition site for the propeptide-processing enzyme (see Fig. 18–6). In all vitamin K–dependent plasma proteins, at least two of the four residues are Arg, and in factor VII all four are Arg. Position P1 is always Arg, whereas position

P4 is Arg except in protein C. In the matrix Gla protein where the P4 position is Pro, the propeptide occupies residues 15–30 and is not removed by proteolytic cleavage.[182] Protein C and factor X, which are both two chain-proteins, have the sequences SerHisLeuLysArgAsp (corresponding to positions 153 to 158) and GluArgArgLysArgSer (corresponding to positions 138 to 143), respectively. Cleavage occurs between the ArgAsp and ArgSer residues and is presumably mediated by the same enzyme. It is noteworty that protein C, which has a His residue in the P4 position, processing to the two-chain form is incomplete. Propeptide processing at basic amino acids occurs not only in the Gla-containing coagulation factors and bone proteins but also (for instance) in the von Willebrand factor, in complement proteins C3, C4, and C5, and in serum albumin.

Enzymes that are candidates for removal of the propeptides in vivo have been identified.[198] The first well characterized enzyme was called Kex2 and isolated from *Saccharomyces cerevisiae*.[199, 200] It is a calcium-dependent subtilisin-like endopeptidase. This so called PACE/furin group of enzymes can process peptides with Arg in the P1 and P4 positions. A human homologue of Kex2 has been identified and shown to be able to cleave, for instance, proalbumin and profactor IX.[201] This has been shown in cotransfection experiments where a PACE expression vector and a factor IX expression vector have yielded complete processing of the proform of factor IX. An unrelated propeptide processing enzyme, purified from liver microsomes, appears to have the same specificity as PACE/furin but it is structurally unrelated, being a cobalt-dependent metalloproteinase.[202, 203]

The processing of these coagulation factors can be summarized as follows. After cotranslational removal of the signal peptide, the protein precursor is carboxylated and glycosylated in the endoplasmic reticulum.[204–206] After transport to the Golgi complex, and trimming of the N-linked carbohydrate side chains the propeptide is removed by limited proteolysis immediately before secretion.[206] Removal of the propeptide allows the carboxylated Gla module to bind calcium fully and attain its native conformation with affinity for biological membranes.[206]

▼ MUTATIONS IN PROPEPTIDES

Several mutations have been identified in the propeptide region of factors IX and X, and protein C and protein S.[54–56, 148, 149, 207] In factor IX Oxford [195] and in factor IX San Dimas, [197] Arg -4 is mutated to Gln; and in factor IX Cambridge, Arg -1 is mutated to Ser.[208] In protein C the mutation Arg -1 to His results in aberrant propeptide processing.[209] In neither case is the propeptide cleaved, and accordingly the mature proteins are secreted with an approximately 18 residue long N-terminal extension. The mutant proteins are fully carboxylated but have very low biological activity.[209, 210] Synthetic peptides with these point mutations have also been demonstrated to be equally good substrates for the carboxylase as a peptide with the wild-type sequence, indicating that the basic residue region is not involved in the substrate recognition of the carboxylase.[180] When the propeptide is retained, the residue that is N-terminal in the mature protein cannot make an ion pair interaction with a Gla

residue as it does in prothrombin fragment 1 (see Fig. 18–4). It has also been experimentally demonstrated that the propeptide precludes normal membrane binding of these proteins.[210]

A factor X mutation called factor X Santo Domingo (Gly20 ->Arg) has been described. When the mutant factor X was expressed, no protein was produced despite normal mRNA levels in the cells. Since signal peptidase cleaves between residues -18 and -17 in factor X, it was suggested that the mutation prevented this cleavage, resulting in defective secretion of the mutant protein.[196]

▼ VITAMIN K–DEPENDENT CARBOXYLASE

Vitamin K–dependent carboxylase activity, first identified in rat liver microsomes,[57, 58, 211, 212] has now been found in many tissues. Yet Gla was long assumed to be confined to coagulation factor in blood plasma and certain proteins in mineralized tissues.[20, 58] The finding of Gas 6, a Gla-containing protein S homologue that functions as a ligand to a tyrosine kinase receptor, demonstrated that vitamin K might be involved in other processes than those related to blood coagulation and bone mineralization.[19] With the identification of Gla and of vitamin K–dependent carboxylase in the venom of molluscs of the genus *Conus,* it became evident that the biological function of Gla is much more extensive and diversified than hitherto assumed.[213–217] The recent cloning of two novel putative Gla-containing membrane proteins seems to corroborate this.[21] Most of the early studies of the carboxylase were performed on crude fractions obtained from either rat or bovine liver.[57, 58, 211, 212] Rat liver was particularly useful, as the uncarboxylated vitamin K–dependent proteins accumulate in the rough endoplasmic reticulum, forming a pool of endogenous substrate.[165] The vitamin K–dependent carboxylase is an integral microsomal membrane protein that catalyzes the incorporation of CO_2 from HCO_3^- into glutamate residues (Fig. 18–7).[58, 72–74, 218, 219] When exogenous substrates such as synthetic peptides are used rather than the endogenous precursors of the vitamin K–dependent proteins, the endoplasmic reticulum has to be solubilized with detergents. For reasons already discussed, peptides such as the commonly used pentapeptide Phe-Leu-Glu-Glu-Leu are characterized by high K_m values. Enzyme activity is readily quantified by measuring the incorporation of $^{14}CO_2$ into glutamate residues in the endogenous microsomal precursor, or into the appropriate synthetic peptide.[211, 220] The product of the reaction, γ-carboxyglutamic acid, has been chemically characterized in detail. A characteristic feature of Gla is that, like malonic acid, it is decarboxylated when heated under acidic conditions, forming glutamic acid.[84] Standard conditions of acid hydrolysis of Gla-containing proteins thus result in the conversion of Gla to Glu; and if the Gla-containing peptide has been formed, for instance by in vitro carboxylation with incorporation of $^{14}CO_2$, 50 per cent of the radioactivity is lost. Gla is stable in alkali, however, and is measured after base hydrolysis of the proteins.

The vitamin K–dependent carboxylase requires molecular oxygen and uses CO_2 rather than HCO_3^- in the carboxylation reaction.[221, 222] ATP is not involved in the reaction, nor is biotin. The biologically active form of vitamin K in the

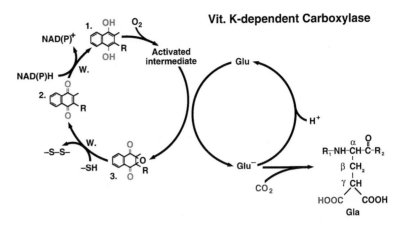

Figure 18–7. Gla formation and the vitamin K cycle. The vitamin K–dependent cleavage of a CH bond in peptide-bound glutamate and the addition of a carboxyl group at the γ position are shown to the right in the figure. In the absence of CO_2, Glu is regenerated. To the left, vitamin K (2) is reduced by a quinone reductase to vitamin KH_2 (1), the active form of the vitamin. Vitamin KH_2 and O_2 form an activated intermediate, the nature of which is uncertain, that abstracts a proton from the γ-carbon atom of Glu. Carboxylation is coupled to the formation of the 2,3-epoxide of vitamin K. Vitamin K is then regenerated in a reaction catalyzed by a vitamin K epoxide reductase. W = the two reactions that are inhibited by warfarin and related anticoagulants.

carboxylation is the reduced, hydroquinone form, which is oxidized to 2,3-epoxide in the reaction (see Fig. 18–7).[223, 224] In crude microsomal preparations, the hydroquinone form of the vitamin is regenerated by microsomal reductases if they are supplied with NAD(P)H or dithiols. Alternatively, the chemically reduced, hydroquinone form of the vitamin can be used. The enzymatic epoxide reduction occurs in two steps. First, the vitamin K epoxide is reduced to the corresponding quinone, and in a second step the quinone is reduced to the biologically active hydroquinone form of vitamin K. Both reductase activities are strongly inhibited by 4-hydroxy-coumarin derivatives, such as the widely used anticoagulant warfarin.[58, 219] It is not yet known whether the two reductions are carried out by the same reductase or by two different ones. Anticoagulant drugs thus inhibit the recycling of the vitamin in the liver rather than the carboxylase itself.

The vitamin K–dependent carboxylase has been purified to homogeneity, cloned and expressed both from the human and bovine species.[225–229] In its purification, advantage was taken of the affinity of the carboxylase for the propeptide that was immobilized and used in affinity chromatography. The overall recovery of carboxylase activity was 34 per cent and the purification 7000-fold.[226] The purified carboxylase consists of a single polypeptide chain with a molecular weight of approximately 94,000. The human carboxylase has 758 amino acids, but no amino-terminal signal peptide. In the N-terminal part of the molecule, there are three hydrophobic putative transmembrane structural motifs. Comparison of the carboxylase sequence with that of soybean lipoxygenase revealed 19 per cent identity. The carboxylase gene is about 13 kb and contains 15 exons.[230] Interestingly, of five patients with a very rare combined deficiency of factors II, VII, IX, and X, one had a mutation in the carboxylase gene.[74] Moreover, three of the other patients appeared to have mutations in the epoxide reductase gene.

The reaction mechanism for the vitamin K–dependent carboxylase has not yet been completely elucidated. In early studies, crude microsomal preparations from rat liver were used, or partially purified preparations in which the active carboxylase is still a very minor part of the total protein. The vitamin K–dependent step in the carboxylation reaction is the removal of a hydrogen atom from the γ-carbon of glutamic acid.[231] This step was deduced from experiments in which the peptide Phe-Leu-Glu-Glu-Leu (FLEEL) with ^{3}H in the γ-carbon of each glutamic acid residue was used as a substrate for the enzyme. In the absence of CO_2, the enzyme

catalyzed an O_2^- and vitamin K hydroquinone-dependent abstraction of [3]H. If the carboxylation reaction cannot proceed, for instance when the bicarbonate concentration is severely depleted, the activated glutamic acid residue will again be protonated in the γ position rather than form adducts with other components in the reaction mixture. Accordingly, in the presence of the hydroquinone form of vitamin K, the carboxylase catalyzed an O_2-dependent exchange of ^{3}H from [3]H_2O into the γ position of glutamic acid in a peptide substrate.[232, 233] The vitamin K epoxide formation is coupled to the carboxylation.[232] Using recombinant enzyme it has been demonstrated that carboxylation of Glu and epoxidation of the vitamin are associated with a single enzyme.[234] Under reaction conditions in which the glutamyl substrate concentration is high, the ratio of vitamin K epoxide to Gla formed approaches unity. Using recombinant enzyme it has also been possible to demonstrate that the propeptide and Glu-containing peptides stimulate the epoxidation activity; i.e., in the absence of these components the enzyme lacks epoxidase activity.[235] The currently favored hypothesis regarding the mode of action of vitamin K assumes that an oxygenated intermediate of vitamin K, such as a 2- or 3-hydroperoxide, provides the energy for the cleavage of the bond between the γ carbon and the hydrogen atom, and that this intermediate is on the pathway of epoxide formation (see Fig. 18–7).[58] Mechanisms involving either free radical abstraction from the γ-carbon atom of Glu or formation of a carbon ion at the γ-carbon have been proposed.[231, 232, 236–238] A 'base strength amplification mechanism' has also been proposed to explain the conversion of the hydroquinone form of the vitamin into an oxygenated intermediate that is basic enough to abstract a proton from the γ-carbon of a Glu residue.[239] This mechanism also allows epoxidation of the vitamin without carboxylation of Glu.

Recently, with the availability of recombinant carboxylase, studies of the mechanism of action of the carboxylase have progressed rapidly.[73, 74] The carboxylase molecule has been mapped to clarify, for instance, which part has carboxylase activity and which part has epoxidase activity. Accordingly, both the glutamate binding and the propeptide binding regions of the carboxylase have now been found to be located in the N-terminal half of the molecule.[73] It has also been clarified beyond doubt that carboxylation and epoxidation are carried out by the same molecule. The propeptide has been found to exert a sophisticated regulation of the carboxylase.

To sum up: the propeptide tethers the substrate to the enzyme and also activates the enzyme, resulting in a processive reaction with carboxylation of 9–12 Glu residues without release of the substrate. After the carboxylation is complete there is presumably a conformational transition in the substrate that results in its release from the enzyme. Following removal of the propeptide in the Golgi stack, the N-terminal part of the Gla module binds calcium ions and attains its biologically active phospholipid-binding conformation.

Epidermal Growth Factor–Like Modules

Epidermal growth factor is a small protein (53 amino acids) with six Cys residues linked by disulfide bonds in a characteristic pattern.[240, 241] EGF and the structurally related growth factor, transforming growth factor α (TGF-α), are released from membrane-bound precursor molecules by limited proteolysis.[242] The EGF receptor is a transmembrane protein to which EGF and TGF-α bind with similar affinity. The ligands endow the receptor with protein tyrosine kinase activity. Activation of the receptor elicits a host of proliferative and developmental responses.

Modules homologous to EGF have been found in many extracellular proteins and membrane proteins.[48, 53, 241] These proteins include the vitamin K–dependent plasma proteins, which all, except prothrombin, contain EGF-like modules. There are two EGF modules in factors VII, IX, and X, and protein C, whereas protein S and Gas 6 contain four. Each of the EGF modules is encoded by a separate exon.

▼ STRUCTURE OF EPIDERMAL GROWTH FACTOR–LIKE MODULES IN VITAMIN K–DEPENDENT PROTEINS

In EGF-like modules from nonvitamin K–dependent proteins, the pairing of disulfide bonds is identical to that in EGF itself, i.e., 1–3, 2–4, and 5–6, as demonstrated by sequence determination[243] and X-ray crystallography[38–41, 244] and NMR spectroscopy.[49, 50, 245] The structures are dominated by β sheets and turns (Fig. 18–8).

The EGF-like modules in the vitamin K–dependent proteins contain four types of postribosomal amino acid modifications; hydroxylation of Asp or Asn residues to *erythro*-β-hydroxyaspartic acid and *erythro*-β-hydroxyasparagine, respectively, was identified in protein C, factor X, and protein S (see below).[246, 247] In the C-terminal EGF module of protein C, there is a carbohydrate chain linked by an *N*-glycosidic bond. Recently, disaccharide and trisaccharide units linked by *O*-glycosidic bonds were identified in human and bovine factors VII and IX and protein Z.[248–250] The disaccharide units were found in the human proteins and the trisaccharide units in the bovine proteins. The structure of the trisaccharide unit in bovine factor IX is D-Xyl*p*a 1-3-D-Xyl*p*a 1-3-D-Glc b1-*O*-Ser-53.[250] The disaccharide units in the human proteins lack the terminal Xyl residue.[249] The Ser residue, to which the carbohydrate side chain is attached, is located between the first and second Cys where the consensus sequence Cys-Xxx-Ser-Xxx-Pro-Cys (corresponding to residues 51 to 56 in bovine factor IX; see Plate 18–2) has

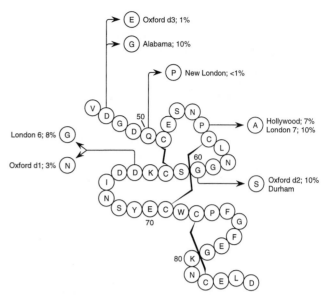

Figure 18–8. The N-terminal EGF module of factor IX. A few mutations causing hemophilia B and the clotting activity of the mutant factor IX molecules are denoted. For details, see text.

been identified. Factor X and protein C do not have the corresponding Ser residue and lack the carbohydrate chain. The consensus sequence has also been found in EGF modules of many non-vitamin K–dependent plasma proteins. In this context, it is noteworthy that the disaccharide chain has been isolated from human urine in amounts that are larger than can be accounted for by the vitamin K–dependent plasma proteins, thus suggesting that at least some of these proteins have the carbohydrate side chain.[251] The glycosylating enzyme (or enzymes) has not yet been identified, and the function of the carbohydrate moiety is unknown.

EGF-like modules from several proteins, e.g., factors IX and X, have been chemically synthesized and expressed in yeast and shown to fold spontaneously to their respective native conformations.[252, 253] Intact EGF-like modules have been isolated in a preparative scale from proteolytic digests of factors IX and X, protein C, and, in smaller amounts, protein S.[107, 254–257] The structure of the N-terminal EGF module from factors IX and X (corresponding to residues 45 to 86 in bovine factor X) have been determined by two-dimensional NMR spectroscopy.[50, 51] The EGF-like module from factor X was isolated from an enzymatic digest of intact factor X, and accordingly Asp 63 had been hydroxylated to β-hydroxyaspartic acid. The overall structure was found to be similar to those of human and murine EGF,[240, 258] which is noteworthy as only 11 residues (including 6 Cys residues) of 42 are identical between factor X and EGF. The structure is dominated by β sheets. The largest one is antiparallel and encompasses residues 59 to 64 and 67 to 72, which are linked by β-turn, residues 64 to 67. In murine and human EGF, the amino acids N-terminal to the first Cys residue form a triple-stranded β sheet with the major antiparallel β sheet at least part of the time. In the factor X module, this part of the molecule appears to be freely mobile in the absence of Ca^{2+}. There is no evidence of triple-stranded sheet formation, perhaps because of electrostatic repulsion caused by the two Asp residues (positions

46 and 48 in factor X) that are conserved in factors VII, IX, and X and in protein C.[49, 259] The pleated sheet structures and β turns in the C-terminal part of the module occur in the same positions as in human and in murine EGF. The N-terminal EGF module from factor X and factor IX, and three of the EGF modules in protein S, bind Ca^{2+}.[50, 245, 254, 256, 260, 261] The structure of the N-terminal EGF module from factor IX has now also been determined by X-ray crystallography.[262] It is very similar to that of the N-terminal EGF module of bovine factor X, as expected from the sequence similarity.

▼ β-HYDROXYASPARTIC ACID AND β-HYDROXYASPARAGINE

Erythro-β-hydroxyaspartic acid (Hya) was described as a constituent of the N-terminal EGF module of human and bovine vitamin K–dependent coagulation factors.[246, 247, 263] In human factor IX, the hydroxylation is partial (about 30 per cent), whereas bovine factor IX is fully hydroxylated in this position. Human factor VII has no Hya. *Erythro*-β-hydroxyasparagine (Hyn) was identified in the second, third, and fourth EGF modules of protein S.[247] Free Hya and Hyn, also in the *erythro* form, have been isolated from urine in amounts larger than can be accounted for by the turnover of vitamin K–dependent coagulation factors,[264] which may be explained by the fact that both postribosomal modifications are present in many non-vitamin K–dependent proteins and extracellular proteins, as well as integral membrane proteins such as the complement proteins C1r and C1s.[265] Among these proteins are also thrombomodulin,[27] fibrillin,[266–268] and the Notch protein.[269–271] The two amino acids have been found only in EGF modules. They are positioned between the third and fourth Cys residues in the module (corresponding to residues 62 to 69 in bovine factor X; see Fig. 18–8) where the consensus sequence Cys-Xxx-Asp*/Asn*-Xxx-Xxx-Xxx-Xxx-Tyr/Phe-Xxx-Cys has been identified (the hydroxylated residues are denoted with an asterisk).[247, 272] This part constitutes the major antiparallel β sheet in the EGF module, the size of which appears to be crucial for recognition by the hydroxylase, as there are always eight residues between the two Cys residues. The hydroxylated Asp/Asn residue is in juxtaposition to the Tyr/Phe residue. The lack of Hya in human factor VII, that has the consensus sequence and the partial hydroxylation of human factor IX, indicates that the β sheet structure and the consensus sequence do not constitute a sufficient structural requirement for the hydroxylase.

▼ Asp/Asn-β-HYDROXYLASE

Asp/Asn-β-hydroxylase is a 2-oxoglutarate–dependent dioxygenase.[46, 273, 274] It thus belongs to the same group of enzymes as prolyl-4-hydroxylase, prolyl-3-hydroxylase, lysyl hydroxylase, and γ-butyrobetaine hydroxylase.[176] The N-terminal EGF-like module in factors IX and X, protein C, protein S, and protein Z is substrate for the enzyme.[46, 274] In the reaction, one hydroxyl group is attached to the β-carbon atom of Asp, forming Hya. The oxygen atom in the hydroxyl group derives from O_2. The other oxygen atom of O_2

Asp/Asn-β-hydroxylase

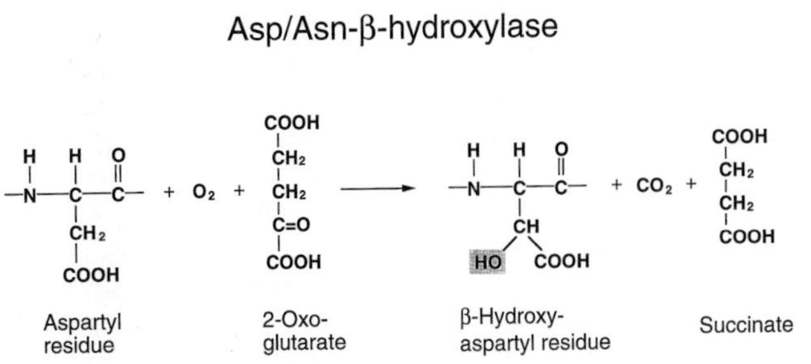

Figure 18–9. Hydroxylation of an aspartyl residue by Asp/Asn-β-hydroxylase to form *erythro*-β-hydroxyaspartic acid. The enzyme is a dioxygenase that requires molecular oxygen and a cosubstrate, 2-oxoglutarate (α-ketoglutarate). The cosubstrate is decarboxylated to succinate.

emerges in succinate, which is formed from the cosubstrate 2-oxoglutarate, hence the term dioxygenase (Fig. 18–9). In addition to succinate, CO_2 is formed from the 2-oxoglutarate. Structural analysis of a hydroxylated EGF module has established that the Hya residue is localized to the position predicted by the consensus sequence (see Fig. 18–9).[247, 272, 274] The three-dimensional structure of the EGF module appears to be crucial for substrate recognition by the enzyme, as linear peptides with the appropriate sequence do not stimulate 2-oxoglutarate decarboxylation.[46] The metal ion requirement of both prolyl-4-hydroxylase and Asp/Asn-β-hydroxylase is satisfied by Fe^{2+}.[176, 275]

Of the 2-oxoglutarate–dependent dioxygenases, prolyl-4-hydroxylase has been studied in the greatest detail.[176] Analogues of 2-oxoglutarate, such as 2,4-dicarboxypyridine, which inhibit prolyl-4-hydroxylase, also inhibit Asp-β-hydroxylase. This compound (2,4-dicarboxypyridine) also inhibits hydroxylation of the appropriate Asp residue in recombinant factor IX expressed in mammalian tissue culture.[273] Unlike prolyl-4-hydroxylase, the Asp/Asn-β-hydroxylase does not require ascorbate or other reducing agents in vitro. It has also been demonstrated that the Hya content of the vitamin K–dependent proteins purified from severely scorbutic guinea pigs is normal.[276] Asp/Asn hydroxylation does not require vitamin K.[277]

Asp/Asn-β-hydroxylase has been purified to homogeneity from bovine liver microsomes.[275, 278] The predominant form of the enzyme is a monomer with an apparent molecular weight of 52,000. It appears to hydroxylate both Asp- and Asn-containing substrates. The cDNA encodes a protein of 754 amino acid residues.[279] A fully active catalytic domain of bovine Asp/Asn-β-hydroxylase has been expressed, and the active site region and the Fe^{2+}-binding region have been identified.[280, 281]

▼ CALCIUM BINDING TO EPIDERMAL GROWTH FACTOR–LIKE MODULES

In attempts to elucidate structure-function relationships in the EGF modules of vitamin K–dependent serine proteins, including studies of the Ca^{2+}-binding properties, the modular organization of the non-catalytic parts of the proteins has been exploited in four ways. First, modules have been isolated from limited proteolytic digests of the proteins. This approach was introduced when the Gla module in factor X was removed after careful chymotryptic cleavage of the intact protein.[282, 283] The products of the reaction were the Gla module cleaved in the aromatic cluster (C-terminal of Tyr 44) and the intact C-terminal remainder of the protein, known as Gla-domainless factor X. After activation, the latter had full amidolytic activity against low molecular weight substrates. The Gla module can now easily be removed from factors VII, IX, and X, protein C and protein Z.[111, 113, 284, 285] Subsequently, methods were developed to isolate one or two intact EGF modules with or without the Gla module attached.[107, 254, 255, 286] This approach has the advantage that the modules presumably are native and contain postribosomal modifications. In the second approach, individual recombinant modules or pairs of modules have been expressed in yeast and bacteria and then folded to a native conformation[287–289] or chemically synthesized.[260, 290, 291] In either case, the Hya residue has been replaced with an Asp residue. In the third approach, EGF modules have been exchanged between recombinant proteins.[164, 292–294] For instance, recombinant factor IX, with the N-terminal EGF modules exchanged for the corresponding module in factor X, has been expressed in mammalian tissue culture and shown to have essentially normal clotting activity. Finally, recombinant factor IX and protein C with point mutations have been expressed in mammalian tissue culture, purified to homogeneity and used to study the function of individual amino acids, for instance in Ca^{2+} binding.[295, 296] Analysis of factor IX from hemophilia B patients with point mutations in the EGF modules has served the same purpose (see below).

The Gla-domainless forms of factors VII, IX, and X and protein C have two metal ion-binding sites that bind Ca^{2+} with apparent dissociation constants of 40 to 200 μM.[111, 113, 297–299] Ca^{2+} binding to these sites seems to induce global conformational changes in the proteins.[111, 113] The functional significance of Gla-independent Ca^{2+} binding became evident when it was demonstrated that Gla-domainless protein C was much more rapidly activated by thrombin-thrombomodulin in the presence of Ca^{2+} than in its absence.[113, 297]

One of the Gla-independent Ca^{2+} sites is located in the N-terminal EGF module in factors VII, IX, and X, and in protein C.[50, 254, 287, 288, 296, 300] The dissociation constant for Ca^{2+} binding to this site varies from 200 μM to 2 mM, depending on which module is studied, the pH, and the ionic strength. The COOH-terminal EGF-like module in factors VII, IX, and X, and in protein C does not have the consensus sequence for Asp/Asn-β-hydroxylation and Ca^{2+}-binding and it does not bind Ca^{2+}. In factor X, the N-terminal EGF-like module binds Ca^{2+} with a Kd ≈ 0.8 mM at physiological pH and ionic strength.[254] In a factor X fragment containing both the Gla module and the N-terminal EGF-like module, K_d for Ca^{2+} binding to this site was approximately 0.1 mM.[301] This presumably reflects the Ca^{2+}-affinity of this site in the intact protein. At physiological extracellular Ca^{2+}, the site is thus essentially saturated. The N-terminal EGF-like module from factors VII, IX, and X have similar Ca^{2+}-binding properties. The β-carboxyl group of the Asp residue that is hydroxylated is a Ca^{2+}-ligand, but the β-hydroxyl group is not a ligand; neither in factor X, nor in factor IX.[50, 262] Accordingly, the N-terminal EGF-like module from factor X binds Ca^{2+} with the same affinity irrespective of whether it is hydroxylated or not.[290]

Epidermal growth factor–like modules that bind Ca^{2+}

have two conserved Asp residues, corresponding to positions 46 and 48 in factor X, that are located opposite to the conserved Hya/Asp residue in the major pleated sheet.[50, 254] Studies, using site-directed mutagenesis to change the residues in the N-terminal EGF module of factor IX, have shed light on the nature of the Ca^{2+}-binding site. The mutant factor IX species (Asp 47 ->Lys or Gly; Asp 49 ->Glu; and Asp/Hya 64 ->Lys, Val, or Gly) were secreted by the eukaryotic cell line and shown to have biological activities of 1 to 8 per cent in factor IX clotting assays (see Fig. 18–8).[295] These residues are conserved in factors VII, IX and X, and protein C. Although the amounts of protein produced did not allow direct Ca^{2+} binding measurements, the results support the notion that these residues ligate Ca^{2+}. It was also found that mutation of the Gln residue in position 50 to Glu resulted in an increased affinity for Ca^{2+}.[288] In protein C, the Asp residue that becomes hydroxylated has been mutated to Glu, which resulted in a reduction of the biological activity to 10 per cent of normal.[302] Moreover, the mutant protein was not recognized by a monoclonal antibody that recognizes a Ca^{2+}-dependent epitope in the N-terminal EGF module, suggesting an involvement of the Hya residue in Ca^{2+} binding.

Two-dimensional NMR studies of the Ca^{2+}-saturated form of the N-terminal EGF module of factor X have demonstrated that the chemical shifts corresponding to residues in the major β sheet and the residues NH_2-terminal to the first Cys (residues 45 to 49) are influenced by the metal ion (see Fig. 18–8).[50, 254] The backbone carbonyls of Gly 47 and Gly 64 are well-defined ligands to the Ca^{2+}, as well as the side-chain carbonyl of Gln 49 and one of the carboxyl oxygens of Hya 63. In contrast, the residues in the COOH-terminal part of the module appear not to be involved in the metal ion binding. These results were corroborated when the structure of the Ca^{2+}-saturated form of the first EGF-like module of factor IX was determined by X-ray crystallography.[262] The Ca^{2+} seems to have six ligands, whereas most Ca^{2+} ions have been found to have seven.

On determination of the structure of the Gla EGF module pair from factor X, in the absence of Ca^{2+}, with NMR it was observed that the Gla module was structured (see above) and that the structure of the EGF module was almost identical to that of the isolated EGF module.[44, 49] Although the individual modules were well defined, their relative orientation was very poorly defined, indicating that they are joined by a flexible hinge region (see Plate 18–3). On saturation of the single Ca^{2+} site in the EGF module in the pair (Kd ≈ 0.1 mM as opposed to ≈0.8 mM in the isolated EGF module) the two modules fold towards each other using the Ca^{2+} as a hinge.[117] It was recently proposed that the Ca^{2+} site in the EGF module of factor VIIa has a similar function, and that it promotes the interaction between the factor VIIa and TF.[303]

In protein S, the N-terminal EGF module has one Hya residue, whereas the three following modules have partially hydroxylated Asn residues. Acid hydrolysates of human protein S contain an average of 2.2 mol of Hya per mole of protein.[77] Bovine protein S has four sites with very high Ca^{2+} affinity, the dissociation constants being 10^{-8} M to 10^{-6} M.[256] At least two of these sites seemed to be located in the EGF-like modules.[261] Calcium-binding studies performed on recombinant EGF modules in tandem have demonstrated that EGF modules 3–4 have very high Ca^{2+} affinity, Kd 10^{-8} to Kd 10^{-6} M at physiological salt concentration, whereas the affinity of module 2 is much lower (Kd $\approx 10^{-5}$ M). The N-terminal module does not appear to bind Ca^{2+}. It is noteworthy that the synthetic isolated EGF modules 3 and 4 both have a Kd for Ca^{2+} of about 1 mM, i.e., similar to the modules in factors VII, IX, and X, and protein C. It is thus obvious that in protein S the neighboring modules have a profound influence on the Ca^{2+} affinity.[291] It should be mentioned that EGF modules 3 and 4 in protein S have the sequence Asp-Val/Ile-Asp-Glu-Cys, corresponding to residues 46 to 50 in factor X; i.e., they have Glu where the other EGF modules have Gln, and Ile/Val where the others have Gly. Moreover, modules 2–4 have Hyn rather than Hya. These modules are more similar to other EGF-like modules such as those in fibrillin, the TGF-β-binding protein and the EGF precursor than to those in factors VII, IX and X, and protein C.[266, 267, 304, 305] The structure of a pair of similar Ca^{2+}-binding EGF modules (from fibrillin) was recently determined.[306]

The structural reason for the very high affinity calcium-binding of EGF modules 3 and 4 in protein S is still unknown. Although many of the non-vitamin K–dependent proteins that have EGF modules containing the consensus sequence recognized by the Asp/Asn hydroxylase have been characterized only at the cDNA level, it seems safe to infer that many of them have Ca^{2+}-binding sites with high affinity. This consensus is phylogenetically coupled to conservation of the calcium ligands immediately before the first Cys residue in these EGF modules (see Fig. 18–8).[50]

▼ MUTATIONS IN EPIDERMAL GROWTH FACTOR–LIKE MODULES

Mutations in the EGF modules have been found in factor IX in several patients with hemophilia B and in one patient with protein C deficiency. For detailed information, the appropriate database should be consulted.[54–56, 148, 149, 207] In this chapter, only point mutations that result in the secretion of a functionally defective molecule are considered. Almost all of these mutations are in the N-terminal EGF module. Positions of some mutations and biological activities of the mutant factor IX are shown in Figure 18–8. Mutations involving amino acids that have been implicated in Ca^{2+} binding are factor IX Alabama (Asp 47 ->Gly),[307, 308] factor IX Oxford d3 (Asp 47 ->Glu),[150] factor IX Oxford d1 (Asp/Hya 64 ->Asn),[150] and factor IX London 6 (Asp/Hya 64 ->Gly).[309] The biological activity of the defective factor IX molecules varies between less than 1 per cent and 10 per cent. Of the mutant factor IX molecules, factor IX Alabama has been studied in the greatest detail. Metal ion-binding studies with factor IX Alabama have been interpreted as suggesting that Asp 47 in normal factor IX coordinates with the bound Ca^{2+} ion, inducing a conformational change in the molecule. Factor IX New London (Gln 50 ->Pro) causes severe hemophilia B.[310] Its Ca^{2+}-binding properties have not been studied. In general, the results of these studies corroborate those obtained by means of site-directed mutagenesis. The amino acids in factor X that correspond to Asp 47, Gln 50, and Asp/Hya 64 in factor IX have now been shown to be Ca^{2+} ligands.[50] The Pro 55 - >Ala and Gly 60 - >Ser

mutations presumably cause a reduction in the biological activity of factor IX by affecting the tertiary structure of the EGF-like module.

Factor IX Fukuoka (Asn 92 -> His) is a mutation in the second EGF module.[311] The factor IX antigen concentration is 64 per cent of normal, and the coagulant activity 3 per cent of normal. Although factor IX Fukuoka has normal amidolytic activity against low molecular weight substrates, V_{max} for the activation of factor X is 10-fold lower than normal. It was suggested that this is due to defective interaction of the second EGF module with factor VIIIa or factor X or both.

▼ FUNCTION OF EPIDERMAL GROWTH FACTOR–LIKE MODULES

The EGF modules of the vitamin K–dependent proteins do not bind to the EGF receptor and have no growth factor activity.[260] They also lack the residues identified in EGF and TGF-α as necessary for binding to the EGF receptor.[240, 312] In urokinase, the single EGF module mediates binding to a cell surface receptor, and in thrombomodulin it has been demonstrated that the EGF modules bind thrombin.[26, 313–315] The affinities of these interactions are similar to that of EGF for its receptor ($K_d = 10^{-9}$ to 10^{-10} M). Many other non-vitamin K–dependent proteins, for instance the low density lipoprotein receptor, contain EGF-like modules, often several in tandem. In most instances the function of these modules is not known. Many are presumably involved in protein-protein interactions, whereas others may function as spacers. In those modules that bind Ca^{2+} the metal ion-binding may be a means of orienting an adjacent module such that it is biologically active. Fibrillin is a striking example of a protein with numerous calcium-binding EGF-like modules in tandem.[266, 267] Certain mutations in fibrillin have been shown to cause Marfan's syndrome.

One function of the EGF modules in the vitamin K–dependent proteins is to function as a spacer between the Gla modules and the serine protease parts. The distance between the active site of factor Xa and the phospholipid surface that is in direct contact with the Gla module has been estimated to be 61 Å in the absence of Ca^{2+} and 69 Å in the presence of Ca^{2+}.[316] This distance is crucial as the enzyme is part of a membrane-bound macromolecular complex with a substrate that is moving in the plane of the surface. We now know that in factors VII, IX and X, and protein C the binding of Ca^{2+} to the EGF module orients the Gla module in a well-defined position that appears to be a prerequisite for biological activity.[44, 117] Without Ca^{2+} in the EGF module, the two modules appear to be freely mobile relative to each other. This suggests that those factor IX mutants, e.g., factor IX Alabama (Asp 47 -> Gly), where a ligand to the Ca^{2+} in the EGF module is lost, are biologically inactive (activity between 1 and 10 per cent of normal in the mutant proteins) because the Gla and EGF modules are either mobile relative to each other or perhaps fixed in a position that does not allow biological activity (see above).[307, 308] In factor IX Alabama, a small difference was found between mutant and normal factor IXa in the ability to activate factor X in the presence of phospholipid. In the presence of factor VIIIa and phospholipid, normal factor IXa activated factor X much more rapidly than did the mutant factor IXa. These effects are due to a defective Ca^{2+}-binding, affecting the interaction between the EGF module and the Gla module, but the mutation may also cause a defective interaction with the cofactor, either directly or by inducing a conformational change in a distant part of the molecule, presumably the serine protease module. Recently, recombinant factor IX with mutation of Asp/Hya 64 to Glu, Lys, or Val has been expressed and characterized.[317] The mutations destroyed the Ca^{2+} binding site and resulted in a reduction of amidolytic activity and in impaired interaction with factor VIIIa. Moreover, the clotting activity was reduced. The low amidolytic activity indicates the importance of long-range interactions in these molecules ('module crosstalk'). Whether the impaired interaction with factor VIIIa is due to a local effect or to a remote effect in the serine protease module remains unclear. However, subsequent experiments showing Glu 78 in the N-terminal EGF module to interact with Arg 94 in the C-terminal module are compatible with the idea that mutations in the N-terminal EGF module indeed influence the function of the serine protease module.[44, 117, 318] The two residues may 'relay' the conformational transition from the first module to the serine protease module via the second EGF module. The fact that X-ray crystallography has demonstrated an extended area of contact between the C-terminal EGF module and the serine protease module in all these proteins is consistent with these observations.[38, 40, 319]

A direct interaction between the EGF modules of factor IXa and the substrate factor X has been proposed based on the observation that a fragment containing the two EGF modules from factor IX inhibits the factor IXa-mediated activation of factor X in the absence of both phospholipid and factor VIIIa as well as in their presence.[320] The interaction between the EGF module and the substrate or cofactor, albeit weak, may be significant on the phospholipid surface.

Hybrids between factor IX and factor X have been expressed in mammalian tissue culture to gain insight into the function of these modules.[163, 164, 292, 294, 321, 322] In factor IX, either the N-terminal EGF module was exchanged for the corresponding module in factor X, or both EGF modules were exchanged. Factor IXa with only the N-terminal EGF module from factor X manifested near-normal biological activity in clotting assays. However, a hybrid in which both EGF modules in factor IX had been exchanged for the modules in factor X had only 4 per cent of the normal clotting activity. The C-terminal EGF-like module is presumably indispensable because of the close contact with the serine protease module, which cannot be maintained by the corresponding factor X module. The COOH-terminal EGF module may simply be required for normal folding of the serine protease part. Recently, chimeric proteins composed of modules from factors VII and IX have been prepared and tested for their ability to bind to human TF.[163, 164] The results indicate the high-affinity interaction to occur between the N-terminal EGF-like module in factor VII(a) and TF. Detailed information is now available about this interaction as the three-dimensional structure of the TF-factor VIIa complex has now been determined by X-ray crystallography.[41] An interesting observation with possible practical implications is that factor IX in which the first EGF-like module has been replaced with the corresponding module from factor VII

manifests enhanced biological activity both in vivo and in vitro.[294]

In protein S the first EGF-like module interacts with activated protein C, apparently with its first EGF module—as a proteolytic fragment consisting of the Gla and the first EGF module of protein C is known to interact with protein S.[323–325] This interaction is discussed in more detail in Chapter 19.

Kringle Modules

Determination of the amino acid sequence of prothrombin and elucidation of the pairing of its cysteine residues established the presence of two regions within the molecule, which manifest a high degree of sequence similarity and identical disulfide bond pairing (see Fig. 18–2).[326] Each region encompasses 80 to 85 amino acids and has 6 Cys residues that are paired 1–6, 2–4, and 3–5. The sequence identity between the two regions is approximately 35 per cent. The structure is reminiscent of a Danish pastry called a *kringle*, hence its name.[326] The identification of the two kringle modules in prothrombin demonstrated that the immunoglobulins were not unique in being composed of structural motifs judged to be homologous owing to pronounced sequence similarity. Moreover, from the structure of prothrombin, it was evident that a protein could be composed of modules of different type; that is, in addition to the two kringle modules, prothrombin contains an N-terminal Gla module and a C-terminal serine protease module.

Although prothrombin is the only vitamin K–dependent protein that contains kringle modules,[2, 32] kringles have been found in several other plasma proteins. Plasminogen contains five kringles, urokinase and factor XII contain one each, tissue-type plasminogen activator contains two, and the hepatocyte growth factor four.[32, 327, 328] Apolipoprotein-a is remarkable in that it contains 38 kringles in tandem.[329] Like the first kringle in prothrombin, the kringles in urokinase, tissue-type plasminogen activator, and factor XII all contain an internal intron localized at a conserved position, attesting to their phylogenetic relationship.[2, 32, 59, 70, 83]

The structure of isolated kringle modules from plasminogen has been determined by X-ray crystallography and NMR spectroscopy, and the structure of prothrombin fragment 1, which contains one kringle, has been ascertained by X-ray crystallography.[35, 330–332] In all the kringles studied so far, the backbone is folded in much the same way, despite considerable differences in amino acid sequence.[330] The overall shape of a kringle is discoid, the approximate dimensions beeing 15 × 30 × 30 Å. It contains three disulfide bonds, the first of which links Cys 1 and Cys 6, keeping the N- and C-termini in close proximity, whereas the disulfide bonds that link Cys 2 and 4 and 3 and 5 are buried in the interior of the kringle, apparently inaccessible to solvent. The disulfide-linked peptide segments protrude from the center as antiparallel β strands connected by β turns (for details of the structure, the reader is referred to appropriate sources).[330–333]

Kringles 1 and 4 in plasminogen and kringle 2 in tissue-type plasminogen activator have physiologically important fibrin-binding sites that also bind lysine, ε-aminocaproic acid, and similar ω-carboxylic acids.[330–332] The kringles in prothrombin do not bind ε-aminocaproic acid with measurable affinity. The N-terminal kringle in prothrombin contains a single low affinity calcium-binding site.[334, 335] Fragment 2, the second kringle, has been reported to bind four calcium ions with comparatively low affinity.[336] However, the kringles do not influence the phospholipid-binding properties of the Gla domain of prothrombin.[337] Determinants in kringle 2 interact with factor Va in the prothrombinase complex and increase the rate of substrate turnover substantially.[338, 339] Kringle 2 also interacts with α-thrombin with a K_d of 7.7–10^{-10} M and with prethrombin 2 with a $K_d = 1.3 \times 10^{-10}$ M, suggesting fragment 2 to be associated with α-thrombin in vivo.[340] The structure of the noncovalent complex between fragment 2 and thrombin has been solved by X-ray crystallography.[341] The fragment has no effect on the clotting activity of α-thrombin.

Recently, using hybrids of human and rat prothrombin, it was demonstrated that the kringles, particularly the N-terminal one, determine the intracellular degradation of under-γ-carboxylated prothrombin.[342] Uncarboxylated human prothrombin is well secreted, also in tissue culture, whereas uncarboxylated rat prothrombin is almost quantitatively retained and degraded in the liver.[342] The protein in the endoplasmic reticulum that identifies the undercarboxylated protein and destines it for degradation has not yet been identified.

A Module in Protein S With Thrombin-Sensitive Bonds

Protein S contains a unique module with two thrombin-sensitive bonds located between the Gla module and the four EGF modules (see Fig. 18–2). It is 29 amino acids long (Val 46 to Asn 74), and is encoded by a separate exon. There is no apparent sequence similarity with the peptide in prothrombin (residues 47 to 63) that links the Gla module and the NH₂-terminal kringle module. Thrombin cleaves the bovine protein S module at Arg 70.[343] A second cleavage at Arg 52 results in the release of a peptide, 18 amino acids long. The thrombin cleavage sites are conserved in human protein S.[77] The module contains two Cys residues (positions 47 and 72) linked by a disulfide bond. The Gla module thus remains attached to the remainder of the molecule after cleavage. The peptide bond at Arg 70 is much more accessible to thrombin cleavage in the absence of Ca^{2+} than in its presence.[344]

Compared with intact protein S, the Gla module in the thrombin-cleaved molecule appears to have a lower affinity for Ca^{2+}.[344] Moreover, its affinity for negatively charged phospholipid vesicles is low at 1 to 2 mM Ca^{2+}, suggesting that the Gla module in the cleaved molecule cannot attain the native conformation.[114] Thrombin-cleaved protein S does not function as a cofactor to activated protein C.[345, 346] It is thus apparent that Ca^{2+} has a profound effect upon the structure of this part of the protein S molecule, and that thrombin cleavage at Arg 70 results in structural alterations in the protein S molecule that preclude normal Ca^{2+} binding and cofactor activity. Protein S is discussed in detail in Chapter 19.

Serine Protease Modules

The vitamin K–dependent serine proteases and the proteases of the fibrinolytic and complement systems are similar in that each has a large N-terminal non-catalytic assemblage with modular organization.[2] The non-catalytic modules are regulatory elements; they bind Ca^{2+} and interact with phospholipid and with their respective cofactors, receptors, and substrates. At the molecular level, regulation of the coagulation system stems from the finely tuned assembly and the subsequent inactivation of enzymatically active macromolecular complexes, such as the factor Xase and prothrombinase complexes, the factor VIIa–tissue factor complex, and the thrombin-thrombomodulin complex.[1–7] The substrate specificities of the active enzymes, which are much narrower than those of the archetype serine proteases chymotrypsin and trypsin, also contribute to the precise regulation of each step in the coagulation cascade. In addition, extended substrate-binding regions, so called exosites, mediate interaction with macromolecular substrates and cofactors, e.g., fibrinogen and thrombomodulin. The coagulation enzymes are with few exceptions specific for Arg in the P1 position (nomenclature of Schechter and Berger) of the substrate.[347] Of the many arginyl bonds, only one or two are cleaved during zymogen activation. In contrast, trypsin cleaves most peptide bonds with Arg or Lys in the P1 position (except Arg/Lys-Pro and Arg/Lys-Gla), and accordingly cleaves several arginyl and lysyl bonds in the serine protease zymogens. The substrates of factor VIIa are factors VII, IX, and X; the substrates of factor IXa are factors VII and X; the substrates of factor Xa are factor VII, prothrombin, and factors V and VIII, whereas the substrates of activated protein C are factors Va and VIIIa. Although the specificities of the enzymes overlap to some extent, no other substrates of physiological significance have been found for these enzymes. In addition to initiating the fibrinogen to fibrin conversion, thrombin cleaves certain peptide bonds in other substrates. The discrete cleavages in factors V, VIII and XI are important to initiate and maintain the coagulation cascade,[9, 23, 348, 349] whereas activation of factor XIII is a prerequisite for the covalent cross-linking of fibrin.[4, 350] Thrombin also downregulates the coagulation cascade by activating protein C (see Chapter 19). Finally, thrombin is a potent cellular stimulator and elicits secretion and arachidonic acid metabolism in platelets and endothelial cells.[351–354] The recently elucidated thrombin-mediated cleavage of the platelet thrombin receptor has revealed an interesting novel mechanism of receptor/substrate activation of possible future therapeutic significance.[354–356] Most mammalian cell types (except erythrocytes) respond to thrombin. The structural basis of the narrow substrate specificity of thrombin and of the active forms of the other coagulation enzymes is now beginning to be unraveled. Determination of the three-dimensional structure of thrombin by X-ray crystallography represents a crucial step in this direction.[36, 37, 357]

All the vitamin K–dependent serine proteases are synthesized as single-chain molecules, but the plasma forms of factor X and protein C have been processed to two chain forms prior to secretion (although approximately 15 per cent of single-chain protein C remains in plasma). On activation by limited proteolysis, full amidolytic and clotting activity is obtained after cleavage of one or two polypeptide bonds in prothrombin and factors VII, IX and X, and protein C.

Although the serine proteases are homologous, profound structural differences exist between factors VIIa, IXa, and Xa and activated protein C on the one hand, and thrombin on the other. In the former enzymes, the non-catalytic N-terminal parts remain bound to the active serine protease modules by a disulfide bond, which ensures that factors VIIa, IXa, and Xa and activated protein C all retain their phospholipid affinity. On activation of prothrombin, however, the non-catalytic N-terminal modules are released as activation peptides or remain non-covalently associated with thrombin.[4, 94, 340] The 36 residue thrombin A chain is linked to the serine protease B chain by a disulfide bond.[36, 59, 326] During prothrombin activation, intermediates possessing an active site are formed. Thrombin lacks affinity for the phospholipid and factors Va and VIIIa, and leaves the prothrombinase complex by diffusion. This is reflected by the fact that thrombin, in addition to the cleavage of four peptide bonds in the soluble fibrinogen molecule, has several other seemingly diverse effects that are central to hemostasis.[351–354]

▼ THE SERINE PROTEASE MODULES OF FACTORS IXa AND Xa INTERACT WITH FACTORS VIIIa AND Va

The factor Xase and prothrombinase complexes are the result of binary protein-protein, protein-Ca^{2+}, and protein-phospholipid interactions. Factors V and VIII, the inactive precursors of factors Va and VIIIa, can be regarded as circulating precursors that upon activation by limited proteolysis are inserted into anionic phospholipid, thus forming complex receptors for factors Xa and IXa, respectively.[3, 4, 23] Since the K_d for the binding of factor Xa to factor Va is approximately 1×10^{-6} M (the stoichiometry is 1:1), the interaction between the two proteins is too weak to promote complex formation in solution at physiological concentrations.[358] However, factor Va interacts with phospholipid having a K_d of approximately 3×10^{-9} M,[359] and factor Xa interacts with phospholipid having a K_d of approximately 4×10^{-8} M.[139] In the presence of Ca^{2+}, the interaction of factor IXa with factor VIIIa-phospholipid is characterized by a K_d of approximately 0.5×10^{-9} M,[25, 360] and the interaction of factor Xa with factor Va-phospholipid by a K_d of approximately 0.7×10^{-9} M.[94, 361] It is noteworthy that the affinity of factor Va for phospholipid is not influenced by factor Xa.[359] Although the part played by the phospholipid surface in the assembly of the prothrombinase and factor Xase complexes is multifaceted, one of the effects is that the concentrations of the reactants adjacent to or on the surface are high enough to promote complex formation between enzyme and cofactor.[132, 141]

The Gla modules of factors IXa and Xa bind Ca^{2+} and interact with phospholipid, but do not interact with their cofactors, factors VIIIa and Va, with high affinity. Whether the EGF modules contribute to the interactions between enzymes and cofactors is still controversial.[317] However, several lines of evidence suggest that most of the binding energy is accounted for by interactions between the serine protease parts of factors IXa and Xa and their respective cofactors.[3, 94] This has been inferred, for instance, from the fact that factor Xa interacts with a platelet receptor (factor Va) with high affinity, whereas the affinity between the

zymogen and the receptor is not measurable and accordingly several orders of magnitude lower.[362–364] The specificity is explained by the major conformational change in the serine protease parts that results from the activation of zymogens of serine proteases.[365] The conformational changes in the Gla and EGF modules of factor X that accompany activation appear negligible. Furthermore, a monoclonal antibody with the epitope in the serine protease part of factor IXa inhibits the interaction between enzyme and cofactor.[366] Similarly, several peptides corresponding to the serine protease part of factor Xa inhibit the interaction between factor Xa and factor Va.[367]

▼ INTERMEDIATES IN THE ACTIVATION OF PROTHROMBIN TO THROMBIN

In the activation of prothrombin to thrombin by factor Xa, two or three peptide bonds are cleaved, Arg271-Thr272, and/or Arg284-Thr285, and Arg320-Ile321 (in bovine prothrombin the cleaved bonds are Arg274-Thr275 and Arg323-Ile324).[94, 368–371] If the Arg320-Ile321 bond is cleaved first, meizothrombin is formed (Fig. 18–10). In a subsequent step, meizothrombin is cleaved at the bond between Arg 271-Thr272, resulting in the formation of α-thrombin and fragment 1–2. If the initial factor Xa-mediated cleavage is between Arg271-Thr272, fragment 1–2 and prethrombin 2 are intermediates. Subsequent cleavage of prethrombin 2 by factor Xa generates α-thrombin. Activation can proceed by either pathway, depending on the reaction conditions. The pathway with meizothrombin as an intermediate is favored when the reaction is catalyzed by the intact prothrombinase complex.[204, 369, 372] In the absence of factor Va, large amounts of prethrombin 2 accumulate. Cleavage of the Arg320-Ile321 bond appears to facilitate subsequent cleavage of the Arg271-Thr272 bond. In addition to the Arg271-Thr272 bond, the nearby Arg284-Thr285 bond in human prothrombin is susceptible to cleavage by factor Xa.[371, 372] The factor Xa-mediated cleavage at Arg284 results in the formation of fragment 1-2-3, which can subsequently be cleaved by factor Xa or thrombin to fragment 1–2.[371] The Arg155-Ser156 bond in fragment 1–2 can be cleaved by meizothrombin or thrombin. Cleavage of meizothrombin at Arg 155 yields meizothrombin (des fragment 1) and fragment 1; cleavage of fragment 1–2 yields fragment 1 and fragment 2; cleavage of prothrombin yields prethrombin 1 and fragment 1.

The high-affinity interaction of bovine fragment 2 with thrombin ($K_d = 7.7 \times 10^{-10}$ M) suggests that the product of either activation pathway is to a large extent a non-covalent complex of α-thrombin and fragment 1–2.[340] The complex probably remains reversibly associated with the phospholipid surface. Subsequent cleavage at Arg155-Ser156 would release fragment 2 in complex with α-thrombin from the membrane surface. In studies of the activation of prethrombin 1 by factor Xa alone, both the prethrombin 2-fragment 2 and the meizothrombin (des fragment 1) pathways were observed.[204] Recently, it was been demonstrated that factor Va enhances the rate of cleavage of the Arg323-Ile324 bond 100-fold more rapidly than the Arg274-Thr275 bond.[373] Moreover, it has now been demonstrated that phosphatidylserine itself upregulates factor Xa and alters its activity such that it preferentially cleaves the Arg323-Ile324

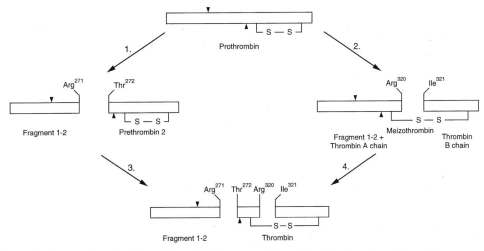

Figure 18–10. Schematic diagram showing the pathways for human prothrombin activation. Factor Xa catalyzes two peptide bond cleavages in prothrombin: between Arg 271 and Thr 272 and between Arg 320 and Ile 321. Pathway 1 yields fragment 1–2 and prethrombin 2, whereas pathway 2 yields meizothrombin. Prethrombin 2 can be cleaved to yield thrombin (3), and meizothrombin is cleaved to yield fragment 1–2 and thrombin (4). The thrombin-mediated cleavage that can separate fragment 1 from fragment 2 (between residues Arg 155 and Ser 156) is denoted by an arrowhead pointing downward. When prothrombin is cleaved, the products are fragment 1 and prethrombin 1; when fragment 1–2 is cleaved, the products are fragment 1 and fragment 2. The thrombin/factor Xa mediated cleavage between Arg 284 and Thr 285 is denoted by an arrowhead pointing upward.

bond, i.e., promotes the meizothrombin pathway.[374] Overall, there is a strong preference to channel prothrombin the meizothrombin pathway with only little accumulation of prethrombin 2. The relative importance of the two pathways of prothrombin activation under physiological conditions has not yet been definitively resolved. Studies of blood clotting in general and prothrombin activation in particular are now beeing made in whole blood in order to evaluate the relative importance of the various zymogen activation pathways under as physiological conditions as possible.[375]

The amidolytic activities of meizothrombin and meizothrombin des fragment 1 against chromogenic substrates are identical to that of α-thrombin, whereas their proteolytic activities against fibrinogen, factor V, and the platelet thrombin receptor are only about 1 per cent and 10 per cent, respectively, of that of α-thrombin.[376] The activation of factor V to Va by meizothrombin in solution is slow, as compared to the thrombin-mediated activation (0.06×10^6 M^{-1}s^{-1} and 4×10^6 M^{-1}s^{-1}).[377] However, in the presence of phospholipid, activation mediated by meizothrombin, that retains the Gla module, is dramatically enhanced (18×10^6 M^{-1}s^{-1}) and presumably physiologally significant. Like thrombin, meizothrombin activates protein C.[376, 378] This is discussed in detail in Chapter 19.

Prothrombin can be activated not only by factor Xa but also by a bacterial protein, *staphylocoagulase*.[379, 380] Staphylocoagulase forms complex with prothrombin and induces a conformational change in prothrombin, exposing its active site, which thus expresses amidolytic and clotting activity without prior cleavage of any peptide bond. The complex is therefore an 'active zymogen.' The Gla module is not involved in complex formation between staphylocoagulase and prothrombin. Prothrombin is also activated by enzymes from the venom of the snakes *Echis carinatus*[381] and *Oxyuranus scutellatus*,[382] whereas factors IX and X and protein C are activated by the venom from *Vipera russelli*.[94, 383] The venom from *O. scutellatus* also activates human factor VII.[384]

▼ STRUCTURE OF THROMBIN

Human α-thrombin is a glycoprotein that consists of two disulfide-linked polypeptide chains, an A chain of 36 amino acids (49 amino acids if there has been no autocatalytic cleavage at Arg284) and a B chain of 259 residues.[36, 37, 59, 351, 357, 385] The thrombin molecule has an isoelectric point of approximately 7.4 and thus has no net charge at physiological pH. It is sparingly soluble and readily adheres to negatively charged and apolar surfaces.[386] The B chain of thrombin is closely related to chymotrypsin, the archetype serine protease, with a sequence identity of approximately 65 per cent.[36, 387] A remarkable feature is that, although thrombin has no net charge at physiological pH, it has an unusually large number of charged residues (twice as many as trypsin and chymotrypsin), many of which are located on the surface of the molecule.[36]

The structure of active site-inhibited human α-thrombin has been determined by X-ray crystallography to a resolution of 1.9 Å,[36, 37] and that of the complex between the leech anticoagulant hirudin and thrombin complex to 2.3 Å.[388, 389] (For more penetrating discussion of these structures and for illustrations that shed light on detail, the reader is recommended to consult these references.) Knowledge of the atomic structure of thrombin constitutes a wealth of important information and provided a strong impetus to pursue incisive site-directed mutagenesis studies designed, for instance, to modify the activity of thrombin such that it becomes primarily a protein C activator. The thrombin molecule is almost spherical, with the dimensions 45 × 45 × 50 Å. The B chain carries the active site residues and epitopes that interact with the substrates, e.g., fibrinogen. It is folded in the manner characteristic of trypsin, chymotrypsin, and other serine proteases. Two six-stranded β barrels of similar structure are packed together in an asymmetrical manner and accommodate the active site residues at the interface (see Plate 18–4). The A chain, a disulfide-bonded activation peptide of unknown function, is linked to the B chain on the side of the molecule opposite the active site. The major difference between the α-thrombin B chain and chymotrypsin is the insertion of several loops in thrombin that change the surface topography of the molecule. Certain of these loops restrict access to the active site and make it resemble an elongated canyon.

The active site residues of the so-called charge-relay system are arranged as in trypsin and chymotrypsin.[36] However, this region, together with the substrate-binding region, has a most conspicuous elongated and kinked cleft, which accommodates residues both N- and C-terminal to the substrate's cleavage site. In trypsin, the active site cleft is less well demarcated and appears to be more easily accessible. Trypsin also has a much broader substrate specificity than thrombin and the other serine proteases involved in blood coagulation. The sides of the cleft in thrombin are lined primarily with hydrophobic residues, whereas its bottom contains several charged residues. One conspicuous loop, that defines the upper rim of the active site canyon is formed by residues that surround Trp60d (for nomenclature and to be able to appreciate the detailed topology of the thrombin molecule, the reader is recommended to consult appropriate references[36, 37]). The lower side of the active site canyon is defined by residues 145–150 with the indole side chain of Trp148 in a very exposed position. Between the two insertion loops, Glu192 (with an uncompensated negative charge) discriminates against substrates with acidic groups near the scissile bond. Trypsin and several other serine proteases have Gln in this position. In the Aα chain of fibrinogen, a hydrophobic motif, Phe 8, Leu 9, Val 15, preceding the scissile peptide bond (Arg 16 Gly 17) probably interacts with the hydrophobic active site region in thrombin. This would also explain why it is favorable to have a tosyl group N-terminal to Gly in the P3 position in substrates such as Tos-Gly-Pro-Arg-pNA. The active site groove in thrombin extends far beyond the active site adjoining P' subsites. It is coated with positively charged amino acids, including Lys 21 Lys 52, Arg 62, Arg 70, and Arg 73, and is commonly referred to as the anion-binding exosite or exosite 1 (see reference 21 and Plate 18–4). The positive charges provide electrostatic guidance for the docking of fibrinogen, thrombomodulin and hirudin. Exosite 1 is clearly the dominant factor in the recognition of fibrinogen,[390, 391] thrombomodulin,[392, 393] hirudin,[388] and the thrombin receptors.[352, 354, 394] Thrombomodulin and hirudin compete with fibrinogen for binding to exosite 1.[330, 387, 395] The binding sites for fibrinogen and hirudin overlap almost completely,[396] but there is only a partial overlap of the sites for fibrinogen and thrombomodulin. Competition between fibrinogen and thrombomodulin is noteworthy in view of the modulation of thrombin from a procoagulant to an anticoagulant enzyme upon binding of thrombomodulin. On the other side of the enzyme, a C-terminal α-helix hosts several positive charges, anion binding exosite 2. This site interacts with polyanionic compounds such as heparin and chondroitin sulfate.[36, 397]

Recently, a Na$^+$-binding site that has important regulatory functions has been identified in thrombin.[357, 398] Enzymes that are activated/regulated by monovalent cations have been known for some time.[399] Most of these enzymes are intracellular and depend on K$^+$ for activity, and many of them catalyze phosphoryl transfer. In view of the intra- and extra-

cellular concentrations of K$^+$ and Na$^+$, it is not surprising that certain extracellular proteins such as several serine proteases of the blood coagulation system depend on Na$^+$.[357] The Kd for Na$^+$-binding to thrombin is 100–200 mM, i.e., the site is partially saturated at physiological extracellular Na$^+$ ($\approx$140 mM). The site is in a loop consisting of residues 215 to 227 in thrombin (see Plate 18–4). The Na$^+$ is coordinated by two carbonyl oxygen atoms and by three water molecules.[385] Na$^+$ is a functionally important allosteric regulator of thrombin.[400] The slow ->fast transition induced by Na$^+$ increases the activity against physiological substrates such as fibrinogen and also against low molecular weight chromogenic substrates, whereas the Na$^+$-free form is more active as a protein C activator (in the absence of thrombomodulin). As fibrinogen binds to the fast form with higher affinity, it promotes the slow -> fast transition and Na$^+$-binding. Likewise, hirudin binds with approximately 30-fold higher affinity to the fast form than does thrombomodulin (see Chapter 19). In addition to thrombin factors VII, IX, X, and protein C have the Na$^+$-binding site, as well as a few serine proteases involved in the complement system. These proteases, all with highly specialized functions, have a conserved Tyr at position 225.[400] Interestingly, other proteases that do not bind Na$^+$ have Pro in the corresponding position. It is also of phylogenetic interest that correlation exists between Tyr 225 and the codon used for the active site Ser residue.

Hirudin consists of 65 amino acids and has three disulfide bonds. Its solution structure has been determined with two-dimensional NMR techniques, which also revealed that the 18 C-terminal residues have no defined structure.[401, 402] In the complex between thrombin and hirudin, the NH$_2$-terminal disulfide bridge-containing part of hirudin interacts with the catalytic site region of thrombin, whereas the C-terminal 18 residue tail adopts an extended conformation, which wraps around the thrombin molecule within the anion-binding exosite 1.[388, 403] This tail region makes more electrostatic and hydrophobic interactions with the thrombin molecule than occur in other protease-inhibitor complexes. In the complex between trypsin and bovine pancreatic trypsin inhibitor, the area of contact has been estimated to be 475 Å^2, whereas in the complex between thrombin and hirudin, the contact area is approximately 1400 Å^2.[403] The large contact area presumably contributes to the extraordinarily high affinity of hirudin for thrombin (K$_d \approx 10^{-14}$ M). In this context, it is noteworthy that the platelet receptor for thrombin contains a structural motif that resembles the C-terminal tail of hirudin and is thought to interact with the anion-binding exosite on thrombin.[352, 355, 404]

Cleavage at the exposed Arg73 in thrombin results in the formation of β-thrombin with greatly reduced clotting activity. It is assumed that this cleavage renders the fibrinogen-binding exosite more flexible and non-functional thus accounting for the loss of clotting activity.[37, 405] The surface loop formed by residues Ala 150 to Lys 154 in thrombin corresponds to the 'autolysis loop' of α-chymotrypsin and harbors residues susceptible to proteolytic cleavage. Cleavage of β-thrombin by trypsin at the lysyl residue in position 154 yields γ-thrombin with clotting activity less than 0.1 per cent of that of thrombin itself. Although both β-thrombin and γ-thrombin have lost clotting activity, they have full amidolytic activity.[387, 395] Pancreatic elastase and elastase from neutrophil granulocytes both cleave thrombin at a single site. Hydrolysis by elastase following Ala 150 yields ε-thrombin,[387, 395, 405] and cathepsin-G cleavage at the adjacent Trp 148 yields ζ-thrombin.[406] There is only a partial loss of fibrinogen clotting activity in both ε-thrombin and ζ-thrombin, with retention of amidolytic activity. During blood coagulation, α-thrombin is incorporated into the clot owing to its fibrin(ogen) affinity, which is mediated by the anionic exosite, whereas γ-thrombin, lacking the exosite, is not incorporated, nor is the α-thrombin/hirudin complex.[387] It is conceivable that α-thrombin in the clot is degraded by granulocyte elastase, and that the elastase-degraded forms, with low clotting activity, retain other activities and may provide a potent stimulus for fibrinolysis by releasing tissue-type plasminogen activator from the endothelial cells.

▼ FACTORS VII, IX AND X, AND PROTEIN C

Since the determination of the three-dimensional structure of thrombin,[36, 37, 407] the structure of factor VIIa in complex with TF,[41] and the structures of factors IX,[39] and X[38, 408] and protein C[40] have been reported. These studies constitute a milestone in blood coagulation research by providing detailed structural information and thereby a solid basis for a rational approach to site-directed mutagenesis studies and to efforts directed at tailoring inhibitors of potential medical interest (for detailed discussions of these structures, and for detailed figures, the reader is recommended to consult the original references; see also Chapters 19 and 21). Thus far, the structure of the factor VIIa–TF complex appears to be unique. Attempts at crystallizing complexes between the other enzymes and their cofactors have hitherto been fraught with difficulty, presumably because of the size and extreme lability of factors Va and VIIIa and their high content of N- and O-linked carbohydrate side chains. Factors VII, IX and X and protein C are elongated molecules (factor IXa ≈130 Å). In factors VII, and IX and X, it is obvious that the C-terminal EGF module is in intimate contact with the serine protease module, which explains why the serine protease module cannot be expressed and folded to a native conformation without the C-terminal EGF module. Likewise, attempts at selective reduction of the disulfide bond that links the serine protease part to the light chain, even when sucessful, result in aggregation of the serine protease module and loss of activity.[116] In contrast, the serine protease module linked to the C-terminal EGF module can be expressed, also in prokaryotes, and folded to a native conformation.[409, 410] Whereas the second EGF module is fixed relative to the serine protease module and the Gla module seems to be fixed relative to the first EGF module, although it can be altered upon interaction with the cofactor, the orientation of the first and second EGF modules is ambiguous. For instance, in factor X there are two residues more between the first and second EGF modules, which presumably allows greater mobility. In certain crystal forms of factor X, a compact globular fold of the molecule has been observed.[408] It is thus uncertain whether factor X assumes a rigid elongated structure in solution. It may well be that module-module orientation of the molecule is altered upon interaction with phospholipid and/or with its cofactor, factor Va. Owing to the interaction between modules and the perhaps variable

fold of the modules, it is difficult to evaluate results of site-directed mutagenesis studies or of studies where modules have been exchanged between the proteins. For instance, mutation of a calcium ligand in the first EGF module of factor IX results in a defective interaction with factor VIIIa.[295, 317] Does this indicate that the EGF module interacts directly with factor VIIIa? The mutation presumably alters the orientation of the Gla module and if so, is this the reason for the defective interaction with factor VIIIa? Perhaps the mutation instead results in a defective interaction between the first and second EGF-like modules transmitting a signal to the serine protease module. Secondary to this, there may be a defective interaction between the serine protease module and factor VIIIa.

The active site regions of factor IX and X and protein C resemble each other and have the characteristic features of trypsin class enzymes. However, compared to that of thrombin, the active sites of these molecules have a less canyon-like surrounding and appear slightly more accessible. The active site regions of factors IXa and Xa are particularly similar. Yet, the specificity constant for factor Xa for preferred synthetic substrates is three to four orders of magnitude higher than that for factor IXa. Knowledge of the structure around the active site of the two molecules, including loops that are characteristic for each enzyme, has made possible mutagenesis studies in which single residues and entire loops have been exchanged between the mutant proteins.[410] These studies allowed the construction of a mutant factor IX with 130-fold higher amidolytic activity than that of the wild-type enzyme.

Factors VII, IX and X and protein C each have a calcium-binding site in the serine protease module. The corresponding region in thrombin (exosite 1) does not bind calcium. The archetype of this site was identified in trypsin and trypsinogen, which bind a single Ca^{2+} ($K_d \approx 400$ mM).[411] Determination of the trypsin structure with X-ray crystallography allowed identification of the ligands to the metal ion.[411, 412] The side chains of Glu 70 and Glu 80 (chymotrypsin numbering[413]) are ligands, whereas the side chain of Glu 77 seems to interact with the Ca^{2+} by means of an H_2O molecule that is sandwiched between the side-chain carboxylate group and the metal ion (Fig. 18–11; amino acids are numbered beginning with the residue that is N-terminal in the serine protease module after activation). The backbone carbonyls of Asn72 and Val75 are also ligands to the Ca^{2+}. This Ca^{2+}, which is 21 Å from the active site

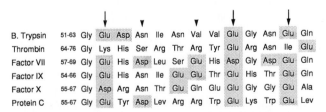

Figure 18–11. Amino acid sequence in the Ca^{2+}-binding region of bovine trypsin and the vitamin K–dependent serine proteases. Glu and Asp residues are shaded. Residues with backbone carbonyl oxygens that are ligands in trypsin are denoted with arrowheads, and residues with side-chain carboxyl groups that are ligands are denoted with arrows. Amino acids are numbered beginning with the residue that is N-terminal in the serine protease module *after* activation.

Ser residue in trypsin, stabilizes the molecule and inhibits its degradation by autodigestion.

As shown in Figure 18–11, the residues contributing side-chain ligands to the Ca^{2+} in trypsin are conserved. Factors VII,[414] IX,[415, 416] and X,[417, 418] and protein C[419] all bind a single Ca^{2+} with a Kd of approximately 200 µM. This site in protein C is crucial for its activation by thrombin (see Chapter 19). However, thrombin itself does not have this Ca^{2+}-binding site and has Lys in position 70 rather than Glu. Presumably the Lys stabilizes the loop (exosite 1) by forming a salt bridge with the Glu residue in position 80.[419]

▼ MUTATIONS IN SERINE PROTEASE MODULES

Genetic defects that affect the serine protease regions range from complete gene deletions to point mutations that result in the secretion of mutant proteins having low specific activity. The databases on factor IX and protein C mutations contain a vast amount of detailed information.[54, 55, 148, 149, 207] Most of these mutations have been identified in factor IX and cause hemophilia B (see Chapter 21).[420] A few point mutations that shed light on the function of these proteins are discussed here.

One group of mutations involve the activation cleavage sites. In prothrombin Barcelona/Madrid (Arg 271–>Cys; numbering begins with the first residue in the intact protein),[59] the factor Xa-mediated cleavage of meizothrombin to fragment 1–2 and thrombin is prevented (see Plate 18–3).[371] However, subsequent factor Xa/thrombin-mediated cleavage at Arg284 may yield thrombin, explaining the modest bleeding tendency associated with the defect.

Single-chain factor IX is activated either by factor XIa and Ca^{2+} or by a factor VIIa-TF-mediated cleavage of the Arg145-Ala146 bond yielding factor IXα that has neither amidolytic nor proteolytic activity. In a second rate-limiting step, the Arg180-Val181 bond is cleaved, yielding factor IXaβ[61] (see Chapter 21). The factor X activator from Russell's viper venom cleaves only the Arg180-Val181 bond, yielding factor IXaα. Factor IXaα and factor IXaβ have similar amidolytic activity against low molecular weight substrates, though the clotting activity of factor IXaα is much lower.[422] Two mutations of Arg 145 have been described; in factor IX Chapel Hill, the Arg residue is replaced by His (mild hemophilia B),[423] and in factor IX Cardiff, it is replaced by Cys (moderate hemophilia B).[424] Since the Arg 145 Ala 146 cleavage normally occurs before the Arg180-Val181 cleavage, the low specific activity of the two mutant factor IX species may be due to slow cleavage of the Arg180-Val181 bond in the single-chain factor IX mutants. There are also two mutations of Arg180, both causing severe hemophilia B. Factor IX B_m Nagoya is an Arg180 ->Trp mutation, and factor IX Hilo is an Arg180 ->Gln mutation[425, 426]; neither of these factor IX mutants is activated by factor XIa, but factor IX B_m Nagoya can be activated by chymotrypsin. In the factor IX mutant designated Kashihara, there is a Val 182 -> Phe mutation (position 2 in the active enzyme)[427]; this mutant factor IX is not activated by factor XIa Ca^{2+} or the factor X activator from Russell's viper venom. Mutations around position 180 are usually associated with a normal plasma concentration of factor IX with low biological activity.

Factor IX B_M Lake Elsinore is an Ala 390 -> Val mutation (numbering begins with the first residue in the heavy chain of the active enzyme), that is, occurring immediately C-terminal of the last Cys residue in factor IX.[428] Factor IX Vancouver, identified in several patients with hemophilia B, is an Ile397 -> Thr mutation.[429, 430] In both these types of mutation, the amidolytic activity of the mutant factor IXa is normal, whereas factor X activation is slow, suggesting that the mutations disrupt secondary binding sites for the substrate, factor X. Another mutation in this region, Gly396 -> Arg (factor IX Angers), gives rise to severe hemophilia B.[431] This mutation, like the other mutations in this region, is associated with an approximately normal concentration of a dysfunctional protein. Considered together with the three-dimensonal structure of factor IXa, these and similar mutations help characterize the enzyme-cofactor interactions in the Xase complex and its interaction with the substrate, factor X.

By contrast with factor IX, there are few mutations of factor X. In factor X Friuli, a Pro 149 -> Ser mutation in the serine protease module, the mutant protein has low activity against both low molecular weight substrates and its physiological substrate prothrombin.[432]

Recent studies using site-directed mutagenesis of residues in the anion-binding exosite in thrombin have demonstrated that it is possible, at least to some extent, to dissociate the fibrinogen-clotting and thrombomodulin-binding activities of thrombin. These developments are discussed in Chapter 19.

Three amino acid substitutions have been identified in congenitally mutant thrombins: thrombin Quick I, thrombin Quick II, and thrombin Tokushima. Thrombin Quick I, Arg 62 -> Cys, has very low fibrinogen-clotting activity but almost normal activity against low molecular weight substrates.[433] The k_{cat}/K_m for release of fibrinopeptide A by thrombin Quick I is 100-fold lower than that for thrombin. In this context, it is noteworthy that Arg 62 is one of the positively charged residues in the anion-binding exosite that is thought to interact with fibrinogen. Thrombin Quick I also has a markedly reduced affinity for thrombomodulin, which also interacts with the anion-binding exosite.[434] Thrombin Quick II results from a Gly238 -> Val mutation. Gly238 is a conserved residue within the primary substrate-binding pocket. This mutant lacks catalytic activity toward thrombin substrates but binds diisopropyl fluorophosphate (DFP) stoichiometrically.[435] Thrombin Tokushima is an Arg 98 -> Trp mutation.[436] This residue is adjacent to the Asp of the catalytic triad, and its mutation results in reduced activity against both low molecular weight substrates and the physiological substrate fibrinogen.

A Module in Protein S Resembling Sex Hormone–Binding Globulin

The C-terminal half of protein S (residues 245 to 635) is homologous to SHBG[79] and to rat androgen-binding protein (see Fig. 18–2).[437] Gas 6, a homologue of protein S, also has a SHBG-like module.[71] SHBG consists of two identical noncovalently linked subunits and binds a single steroid hormone molecule.[438, 439] SHBG with bound hormone interacts with a cell surface receptor.[439] Intron/exon boundaries in protein S and SHBG are in homologous positions.[440] The Cys residues in the SHBG-like part of protein S are paired as in SHBG, that is, Cys 247 to Cys 527, Cys 408 to Cys 434, and Cys 598 to Cys 625.[76, 77] It is noteworthy, however, that the part of SHBG that has been implicated in steroid hormone binding, a hydrophobic region with alternating leucine residues, is not found in protein S. There is no evidence of dimer formation in protein S. The SHBG-like module of protein S has been implicated in the binding of protein S to C4b-binding protein (see Chapter 19).

ACKNOWLEDGMENT

The authors want to thank Dr. Bruno Villoutreix for critically reading the manuscript and for help with Plates 18–1, 18–2, and 18–4.

REFERENCES

1. Nemerson, Y. 1988. Tissue factor and hemostasis. Blood 71:1–8.
2. Furie, B., and B. C. Furie. 1988. The molecular basis of blood coagulation. Cell 53:505–518.
3. Mann, K. G., M. E. Nesheim, W. R. Church, P. Haley, and S. Krishnaswamy. 1990. Surface-dependent reactions of the vitamin K–dependent enzyme complexes. Blood 76:1–16.
4. Davie, E. W., K. Fujikawa, and W. Kisiel. 1991. The coagulation cascade: Initiation, maintainance, and regulation. Biochemistry 30:10363–10370.
5. Rapaport, S. I., and L. V. Rao. 1995. The tissue factor pathway: How it has become a "prima ballerina." Thromb. Haemost. 74(1):7–17.
6. Mann, K. G., and L. Lorand. 1993. Introduction: Blood coagulation. Methods Enzymol. 222:1–10.
7. Edgington, T. S., C. D. Dickinson, and W. Ruf. 1997. The structural basis of function of the TF. VIIa complex in the cellular initiation of coagulation. Thromb. Haemost. 78(1):401–5.
8. Naito, K., and K. Fujikawa. 1991. Activation of human blood coagulation factor XI independent of factor XII. Factor XI is activated by thrombin and factor XIa in the presence of negatively charged surfaces. J. Biol. Chem. 266:7353–7358.
9. Gailani, D., and G. J. J. Broze. 1991. Factor XI activation in a revised model of blood coagulation. Science 253:909–912.
10. Broze, G. J., Jr., and D. Gailani. 1993. The role of factor XI in coagulation. Thromb. Haemost. 70(1):72–4.
11. Broze, G. J., Jr. 1995. Tissue factor pathway inhibitor and the revised theory of coagulation. Annu Rev. Med. 46:103–12.
12. Morrissey, J. H., P. F. Neuenschwander, Q. Huang, C. D. McCallum, B. Su, and A. E. Johnson. 1997. Factor VIIa–tissue factor: Functional importance of protein-membrane interactions. Thromb. Haemost. 78(1):112–6.
13. Wildgoose, P., Y. Nemerson, L. L. Hansen, F. E. Nielsen, S. Glazer, and U. Hedner. 1992. Measurement of basal levels of factor VIIa in hemophilia A and B patients [see comments]. Blood 80(1):25–8.
14. Morrissey, J. H., B. G. Macik, P. F. Neuenschwander, and P. C. Comp. 1993. Quantitation of activated factor VII levels in plasma using a tissue factor mutant selectively deficient in promoting factor VII activation. Acta Chem. Scand. 81:734–744.
15. Morrissey, J. H. 1995. Tissue factor modulation of factor VIIa activity: Use in measuring trace levels of factor VIIa in plasma. Thromb. Haemost. 74(1):185–8.
16. Hoffman, M., D. M. Monroe, J. A. Oliver, and H. R. Roberts. 1995. Factors IXa and Xa play distinct roles in tissue factor–dependent initiation of coagulation. Blood 86(5):1794–801.
17. Prowse, C. W., and M. P. Esnouf. 1977. The isolation of a new warfarin-sensitive protein from bovine plasma. Biochem. Soc. Trans. 5:255–256.
18. Hojrup, P., M. S. Jensen, and T. E. Petersen. 1985. Amino acid sequence of bovine protein Z: A vitamin K–dependent serine protease homolog. FEBS Lett. 184(2):333–8.
19. Manfioletti, G., C. Brancolini, G. Avanzi, and C. Schneider. 1993. The protein encoded by a growth arrest–specific gene (gas6) is a new member of the vitamin K–dependent proteins related to protein S, a negative coregulator in the blood coagulation cascade. Mol. Cell Biol. 13(8):4976–85.
20. Hauschka, P. A., J. B. Lian, D. E. C. Cole, and C. M. Gendberg. 1989. Osteocalcin and Matrix Gla protein: Vitamin K–dependent proteins in bone. Physiol. Rev. 69:990–1047.
21. Kulman, J. D., J. E. Harris, B. A. Haldeman, and E. W. Davie. 1997. Primary structure and tissue distribution of two novel proline-rich gamma-carboxyglutamic acid proteins. Proc. Natl. Acad. Sci. U.S.A. 94(17):9058–62.
22. Olivera, B. M., J. Rivier, C. Clark, C. A. Ramillo, G. P. Corpuz, F. C. Abogadie, E. E. Mena, S. R. Woodward, D. R. Hillyard, and L. J. Cruz. 1990. Diversity of Conus neuropeptides. Science 249:257–263.
23. Rosing, J., and G. Tans. 1997. Coagulation factor V: An old star shines again. Thromb. Haemost. 78(1):427–33.
24. Regan, L. M., and P. J. Fay. 1995. Cleavage of factor VIII light chain is required for maximal generation of factor VIIIa activity. J. Biol. Chem. 270(15):8546–52.
25. van Dieijen, G., G. Tans, J. Rosing, and H. C. Hemker. 1981. The role of phospholipid and factor VIIIa in the activation of bovine factor X. J. Biol. Chem. 256:3433–3442.
26. Esmon, C. T. 1989. The roles of protein C and thrombomodulin in the regulation of blood coagulation. J. Biol. Chem. 264:4743–4746.
27. Esmon, C. T. 1995. Thrombomodulin as a model of molecular mechanisms that modulate protease specificity and function at the vessel surface. FASEB J. 9(10):946–55.
28. Altieri, D. C. 1995. Xa receptor EPR-1. FASEB J. 9(10):860–5.
29. Cirino, G., C. Cicala, M. Bucci, L. Sorrentino, G. Ambrosini, G. DeDominicis, and D. C. Altieri. 1997. Factor Xa as an interface between coagulation and inflammation. Molecular mimicry of factor Xa association with effector cell protease receptor–1 induces acute inflammation in vivo [see comments]. J. Clin. Invest. 99(10):2446–51.
30. Fukudome, K., Esmon, C.T. 1994. Identification, cloning, and regulation of a novel endothelial cell protein C/activated protein C receptor*. J. Biol. Chem. 269:26486–26491.
31. Esmon, C. T., W. Ding, K. Yasuhiro, J. M. Gu, G. Ferrell, L. M. Regan, D. J. Stearns Kurosawa, S. Kurosawa, T. Mather, Z. Laszik, and N. L. Esmon. 1997. The protein C pathway: New insights. Thromb. Haemost. 78(1):70–4.
32. Patthy, L. 1985. Evolution of the proteases of blood coagulation and fibrinolysis by assembly from modules. Cell 41:657–663.
33. Baron, M., D. G. Norman, and I. D. Campbell. 1991. Protein modules. Trends Biochem. Sci. 16:13–17.
34. Tulinsky, A., C. H. Park, and E. Skrzypczak-Jankun. 1988. Structure of prothrombin fragment 1 refined at 2.8 Å resolution. J. Mol. Biol. 202:885–901.
35. Soriano Garcia, M. W., K. Padmanabhan, A. M. deVos, and A. Tulinsky. 1992. The Ca2+ ion and membrane binding structure of the Gla-domain of Ca2+-prothrombin fragment 1. Biochemistry 31:2554–2566.
36. Bode, W., I. Mayr, Y. Bauman, R. Huber, S. R. Stone, and J. Hofsteenge. 1989. The refined 1.9 Å crystal structure of human α-thrombin: Interaction with D-Phe-Pro-Arg chloromethylketone and significance of the Tyr-Pro-Pro-Trp insertion segment. EMBO J. 88:3467–3475.
37. Bode, W., D. Turk, and A. Karshikov. 1992. The refined 1.9-Å X-ray crystal structure of D-Phe-Pro-Arg chloromethylketone-inhibited human α-thrombin: Structure analysis, overall structure, electrostatic properties, detailed active-site geometry, and structure-function relationships. Protein Sci. 1:426–471.
38. Padmanabhan, K., K. P. Padmanabhan, A. Tulinsky, C. H. Park, W. Bode, R. Huber, D. T. Blankenship, A. D. Cardin, and W. Kisiel. 1993. Structure of human Des(1–45) factor Xa at 2.2 Å resolution. J. Mol. Biol. 232:947–966.
39. Brandstetter, H., M. Bauer, R. Huber, P. Lollar, and W. Bode. 1995. X-ray structure of clotting factor IXa: active site and module structure related to Xase activity and hemophilia B. Proc. Natl. Acad. Sci. U.S.A. 92(21):9796–800.
40. Mather, T., V. Oganessyan, P. Hof, R. Huber, S. Foundling, C. Esmon, and W. Bode. 1996. The 2.8 Å crystal structure of Gla-domainless activated protein C. EMBO J. 15(24):6822–31.
41. Banner, D. W., A. D'Arcy, C. Chene, F. K. Winkler, A. Guha, W. H. Konigsberg, Y. Nemerson, and D. Kirchhofer. 1996. The crystal structure of the complex of blood coagulation factor VIIa with soluble tissue factor. Nature 380(6569):41–6.

42. Freedman, S. J., B. C. Furie, B. Furie, and J. D. Baleja. 1995. Structure of the metal-free γ-carboxyglutamic acid–rich membrane binding region of Factor IX by two-dimensional NMR spectroscopy. J. Biol. Chem. 270:7980–7987.

43. Freedman, S. J., B. C. Furie, B. Furie, and J. D. Baleja. 1995. Structure of the calcium ion–bound γ-carboxyglutamic acid–rich domain of Factor IX. Biochemistry 34:12126–12137.

44. Sunnerhagen, M., S. Forsen, A. M. Hoffren, T. Drakenberg, O. Teleman, and J. Stenflo. 1995. Structure of the Ca^{2+}-free Gla domain sheds light on membrane binding of blood coagulation proteins. Nat. Struct. Biol. 2(6):504–9.

45. Sunnerhagen, M., G. A. Olah, J. Stenflo, S. Forsen, T. Drakenberg, and J. Trewhella. 1996. The relative orientation of Gla and EGF domains in coagulation factor X is altered by Ca2 + binding to the first EGF domain. A combined NMR–small angle X-ray scattering study. Biochemistry 35(36):11547–59.

46. Stenflo, J., E. Holme, S. Lindstedt, N. Chandramouli, L. H. Tsai Huang, J. Tam, and R. B. Merrifield. 1989. Hydroxylation of aspartic acid in domains homologous to the epidermal growth factor precursor is catalyzed by a 2-oxoglutarate–dependent dioxygenase. Proc. Natl. Acad. Sci. U.S.A. 86:444–447.

47. Patthy, L. 1993. Modular design of proteases of coagulation, fibrinolysis, and complement activation: Implications for protein engineering and structure-function studies. Methods Enzymol. 222:10–21.

48. Bork, P., A. K. Downing, B. Kieffer, and I. D. Campbell. 1996. Structure and distribution of modules in extracellular proteins. Q. Rev. Biophys. 29(2):119–67.

49. Ullner, M., M. Selander, E. Persson, J. Stenflo, T. Drakenberg, and O. Teleman. 1992. Three-dimensional structure of the apo form of the N-terminal EGF-like module of blood coagulation factor X as determined by NMR spectroscopy and simulated folding. Biochemistry 31(26):5974–83.

50. Selander-Sunnerhagen, M., M. Ullner, E. Persson, O. Teleman, J. Stenflo, and T. Drakenberg. 1992. How an epidermal growth factor (EGF)–like domain binds calcium. High resolution NMR structure of the calcium form of the NH2-terminal EGF-like domain in coagulation factor X. J. Biol. Chem. 267:19642–19649.

51. Baron, M., D. G. Norman, T. S. Harvey, P. A. Handford, M. Mayhew, A. G. Tse, G. G. Brownlee, and I. D. Campbell. 1992. The three-dimensional structure of the first EGF-like module of human factor IX: Comparison with EGF and TGF-alpha. Protein Sci. 1(1):81–90.

52. Mayhew, M., P. Handford, M. Baron, A. G. Tse, I. D. Campbell, and G. G. Brownlee. 1992. Ligand requirements for Ca2 + binding to EGF-like domains. Protein Eng. 5(6):489–94.

53. Campbell, I. D., and P. Bork. 1993. Epidermal growth factor–like modules. Curr. Op. Struct. Biol. 3:385–392.

54. Giannelli, F., P. M. Green, S. S. Sommer, M. C. Poon, M. Ludwig, R. Schwaab, P. H. Reitsma, M. Goossens, A. Yoshioka, M. S. Figueiredo, and G. G. Brownlee. 1997. Haemophilia B: Database of point mutations and short additions and deletions, 7th edition. Nucleic Acids Res. 25(1):133–5.

55. Reitsma, P. H. 1996. Protein C deficiency: Summary of the 1995 database update. Nucleic Acids Res. 24:157–9.

56. Gandrille, S., D. Borgel, H. Ireland, D. A. Lane, R. Simmonds, P. H. Reitsma, C. Mannhalter, I. Pabinger, H. Saito, K. Suzuki, C. Formstone, D. N. Cooper, Y. Espinosa, N. Sala, F. Bernardi, and M. Aiach. 1997. Protein S deficiency: A database of mutations. For the Plasma Coagulation Inhibitors Subcommittee of the Scientific and Standardization Committee of the International Society on Thrombosis and Haemostasis. Thromb. Haemost. 77(6):1201–14.

57. Stenflo, J., and J. W. Suttie. 1977. Vitamin K–dependent formation of gamma-carboxyglutamic acid. Annu. Rev. Biochem. 46:157–172.

58. Suttie, J. 1985. Vitamin K–dependent carboxylase. Annu. Rev. Biochem. 54:459–477.

59. Friezner-Degen, S. J., and E. W. Davie. 1987. Nucleotide sequence of the gene for human prothrombin. Biochemistry 26:6165–6177.

60. O'Hara, P. J., F. Grant, J., B. A. Haldeman, C. I. Gray, M. Y. Insley, F. S. Hagen, and M. J. Murray. 1987. Nucleotide sequence of the gene coding for human factor VII, a vitamin K–dependent protein participating in blood coagulation. Proc. Natl. Acad. Sci. U.S.A. 84:5158–5162.

61. Yoshitake, S., G. Schach, D. C. Foster, E. W. Davie, and K. Kurachi. 1985. Nucleotide sequence of the gene for human factor IX. Biochemistry 24:3736–3750.

62. Leytus, S. P., D. C. Foster, K. Kurachi, and E. W. Davie. 1986.

63. Gene for human factor X: A blood coagulation factor whose gene organization is essentially identical with that of factor IX and protein C. Biochemistry 25:5098–5102.

63. Foster, D. C., S. Yoshitake, and E. W. Davie. 1985. The nucleotide sequence of the gene for human protein C. Proc. Natl. Acad. Sci. U.S.A. 82:4673–4677.

64. Plutzky, J., J. A. Hoskins, G. L. Long, and G. R. Crabtree. 1987. Evolution and organization of the human protein C gene. Proc. Natl. Acad. Sci. U.S.A. 83:546–550.

65. Schmidel, D. K., A. V. Tatro, L. G. Phelps, J. A. Tomczak, and G. L. Long. 1990. Organization of the human protein S gene. Biochemistry 29:7845.

66. Edenbrandt, C. M., Å. Lundwall, R. M. Wydro, and J. Stenflo. 1990. Molecular analysis of the gene for vitamin K–dependent protein S and its pseudogene. Cloning and partial gene organization. Biochemistry 29:7861.

67. Ploos van Amstel, H. K., P. H. Reitsma, P. E. van der Logt, and R. M. Bertina. 1990. Intro-exon organization of the active human protein S gene PSa and its pseudogene PSb: Duplication and silencing during primate evolution. Biochemistry 29:7853.

68. Gilbert, W. 1978. Why genes in pieces? Nature 271:501.

69. Traut, T. W. 1988. Do exons code for structural or functional units in proteins. Proc. Natl. Acad. Sci. U.S.A. 85:2944–2948.

70. Irwin, D. M., K. A. Robertson, and R. T. A. MacGillivray. 1988. Structure and evolution of the bovine prothrombin gene. J. Mol. Biol. 200:31–45.

71. Matsubara, N., Y. Takahashi, Y. Nishina, Y. Mukouyama, M. Yanagisawa, T. Watanabe, T. Nakano, K. Nomura, H. Arita, Y. Nishimune, M. Obinata, and Y. Matsui. 1996. A receptor tyrosine kinase, Sky, and its ligand Gas 6 are expressed in gonads and support primordial germ cell growth or survival in culture. Dev. Biol. 180(2):499–510.

72. Vermeer, C. 1990. Gamma-carboxyglutamate–containing proteins and the vitamin K–dependent carboxylase. Biochem. J. 266:625.

73. Furie, B. C., and B. Furie. 1997. Structure and mechanism of action of the vitamin K–dependent gamma-glutamyl carboxylase: Recent advances from mutagenesis studies. Thromb. Haemost. 78(1):595–8.

74. Wu, S. M., T. B. Stanley, V. P. Mutucumarana, and D. W. Stafford. 1997. Characterization of the gamma-glutamyl carboxylase. Thromb. Haemost. 78(1):599–604.

75. Höjrup, P., M. S. Jensen, and T. E. Petersen. 1985. Amino acid sequence of bovine protein Z: A vitamin K–dependent serine protease homolog. FEBS. Lett. 184:333.

76. Dahlbäck, B., Å. Lundwall, and J. Stenflo. 1986. Primary structure of bovine vitamin K–dependent protein S. Proc. Natl. Acad. Sci. U.S.A. 83:4199–4203.

77. Lundwall, Å., W. Dackowski, E. H. Cohen, M. Shaffer, A. Mahr, B. Dahlbäck, J. Stenflo, and R. M. Wydro. 1986. Isolation and sequence of the cDNA for human protein S, a regulator of blood coagulation. Proc. Natl. Acad. Sci. U.S.A. 83:6716–6720.

78. Dahlbäck, B. 1991. Protein S and C4b-binding protein: Components involved in the regulation of the protein C anticoagulant system. Thromb. Haemost. 66:49–61.

79. Gershagen, S., P. Fernlund, and Å. Lundwall. 1987. A cDNA coding for human sex hormone binding globulin. Homology to vitamin K–dependent protein S. FEBS. Lett. 220:129–135.

80. Baker, M. E., F. S. French, and D. R. Joseph. 1987. Vitamin K–dependent protein S is similar to rat androgen-binding protein. Biochem. J. 243:293–296.

81. Patthy, L. 1991. Modular exchange principles in proteins. Curr. Op. Struct. Biol. 1:351–361.

82. Patthy, L. 1994. Introns and exons. Curr. Op. Struct. Biol. 4:383–392.

83. Patthy, L. 1987. Intron-dependent evolution: Preferred types of exons and introns. FEBS. Lett. 214:1–7.

84. Stenflo, J., P. Fernlund, W. Egan, and P. Roepstorff. 1974. Vitamin K–dependent modifications of glutamic acid residues. Proc. Natl. Acad. Sci. U.S.A. 71:2730–2733.

85. Nelsestuen, G. L., T. H. Zytkovicz, and J. B. Howard. 1974. The mode of action of vitamin K. Identification of γ-carboxyglutamic acid as a component of prothrombin. J. Biol. Chem. 249:6347–6350.

86. Magnusson, S., L. Sottrup Jensen, T. E. Petersen, H. R. Morris, and A. Dell. 1974. Primary structure of the vitamin K–dependent part of prothrombin. FEBS. Lett. 44:189–193.

87. Ganrot, P. O., and J. E. Niléhn. 1968. Plasma prothrombin during treatment with dicoumarol. Scand. J. Clin. Lab. Invest. 22:23–28.

88. Stenflo, J. 1970. Dicoumarol-induced prothrombin in bovine plasma. Acta Chem. Scand. 24:3762–3763.

89. Stenflo, J., and P. Ganrot. 1972. Vitamin K and the biosynthesis of prothrombin. 1. Identification and purification of a dicumarol-induced abnormal prothrombin from bovine plasma. J. Biol. Chem. 247:8160–8166.

90. Nelsestuen, G. L., and J. W. Suttie. 1972. The purification and properties of an abnormal prothrombin protein produced by dicoumarol-treated cows. Comparison to normal prothrombin. J. Biol. Chem. 247:8176–8182.

91. Nelsestuen, G. L., and J. W. Suttie. 1972. Mode of action of vitamin K. Calcium binding properties of bovine prothrombin. Biochemistry 11:4961–4964.

92. Reekers, P. P. M., M. J. Lindhout, B. H. M. Kop Klaassen, and H. C. Hemker. 1973. Demonstration of three anomalous plasma proteins induced by a vitamin K-antagonist. Biochim. Biophys. Acta 317:559–562.

93. Stenflo, J., and P. Ganrot. 1973. Binding of Ca^{2+} to normal and dicoumarol-induced prothrombin. Biochem. Biophys. Res. Commun. 50:98–104.

94. Mann, K. G., R. J. Jenny, and S. Krishnaswamy. 1988. Cofactor proteins in the assembly and expression of blood clotting enzyme complexes. Annu. Rev. Biochem. 57:915–956.

95. Malhotra, O. P., M. E. Nesheim, and K. G. Mann. 1985. The kinetics of activation of normal and γ-carboxyglutamic acid–deficient prothrombins. J. Biol. Chem. 260:279–287.

96. Borowski, B., B. C. Furie, G. H. Goldsmith, and B. Furie. 1985. Metal and phospholipid binding properties of partially carboxylated human prothrombin variants. J. Biol. Chem. 260:9258–9264.

97. Gitel, S. N., W. G. Owen, C. T. Esmon, and C. M. Jackson. 1973. A polypeptide region of bovine prothrombin specific for binding to phospholipids. Proc. Natl. Acad. Sci. U.S.A. 70:1344–1348.

98. Morita, T., S. Iwanaga, T. Suzuki, and K. Fujikawa. 1973. Characterization of amino-terminal fragment liberated from prothrombin by activated factor X. FEBS. Lett. 36:313–317.

99. Welsch, D. J., and G. L. Nelsestuen. 1988. Amino-terminal alanine functions in a calcium-specific process essential for membrane binding by prothrombin fragment 1. Biochemistry 27:4939–4945.

100. Seshadri, T. P., E. Skrzypczak Jankun, M. Yin, and A. Tulinsky. 1994. Differences in the metal ion structure between Sr- and Ca-prothrombin fragment 1. Biochemistry 33(5):1087–92.

101. Padmanabhan, K., K. P. Padmanabhan, A. Tulinsky, C. H. Park, W. Bode, R. Huber, D. T. Blankenship, A. D. Cardin, and W. Kisiel. 1993. Structure of human des(1–45) factor Xa at 2.2 A resolution. J. Mol. Biol. 232(3):947–66.

102. Freedman, S. J., M. D. Blostein, J. D. Baleja, M. Jacobs, B. C. Furie, and B. Furie. 1996. Identification of the phospholipid binding site in the vitamin K–dependent blood coagulation protein factor IX. J. Biol. Chem. 271(27):16227–36.

103. Church, W. R., L. L. Boulanger, T. L. Meissier, and K. G. Mann. 1989. Evidence for a common metal ion-dependent transition in the 4-carboxyglutamic acid domains of several vitamin K–dependent proteins. J. Biol. Chem. 264:17882–17887.

104. Nelsestuen, G. L. 1976. Role of γ-carboxyglutamic acid. An unusual protein transition required for the calcium-dependent binding of prothrombin to phospholipid. J. Biol. Chem. 25:5648–5656.

105. Bloom, J. W., and K. G. Mann. 1978. Metal ion induced conformational transitions of prothrombin and prothrombin fragment 1. Biochemistry 17:4430–4438.

106. Jackson, C. M. 1988. Calcium ion binding to gamma-carboxyglutamic acid-containing proteins from the blood clotting system: What we still don't understand. J. W. Suttie, editor. Current Advances in Vitamin K Research, New York, Elsevier, 305–324.

107. Persson, E., I. Björk, and J. Stenflo. 1991. Protein structural requirements for Ca^{2+}-binding to the light chain of factor X. Studies using isolated intact fragments containing the gamma-carboxyglutamic acid region and/or the epidermal growth factor-like domains. J. Biol. Chem. 266:2444.

108. Jacobs, M., S. J. Freedman, B. C. Furie, and B. Furie. 1994. Membrane binding properties of the factor IX gamma-carboxyglutamic acid-rich domain prepared by chemical synthesis. J. Biol. Chem. 269(41):25494–501.

109. Colpitts, T. L., and F. J. Castellino. 1994. Calcium and phospholipid binding properties of synthetic gamma-carboxyglutamic acid-containing peptides with sequence counterparts in human protein C. Biochemistry 33:3501–3508.

110. Nicolaisen, E. M., L. Thim, J. K. Jacobsen, P. F. Nielsen, I. Mollerup, T. Jorgensen, and U. Hedner. 1993. FVIIa derivatives obtained by autolytic and controlled cathepsin G mediated cleavage. FEBS Lett. 317(3):245–9.

111. Morita, T., B. S. Isaacs, C. T. Esmon, and A. E. Johnson. 1984. Derivative of blood coagulation factor IX containing a high affinity Ca^{2+}-binding site that lacks gamma-carboxyglutamic acid. J. Biol. Chem. 259:5698.

112. Astermark, J., I. Björk, A. K. Öhlin, and J. Stenflo. 1991. Structural requirements for Ca2+-binding to the gamma-carboxyglutamic acid and epidermal growth factor-like regions of factor IX. Studies using intact domains isolated from controlled proteolytic digests of bovine factor X. J. Biol. Chem. 266:2430.

113. Esmon, N. L., L. E. DeBault, and C. Y. Esmon. 1983. Proteolytic formation and properties of γ-carboxyglutamic acid domainless protein C. J. Biol. Chem. 258:5548–5553.

114. Schwalbe, R. A., J. Ryan, D. M. Stern, W. Kisiel, B. Dahlbäck, and G. L. Nelsestuen. 1989. Protein structural requirements and properties of membrane binding by γ-carboxyglutamic acid-containing plasma proteins and peptides. J. Biol. Chem. 264:20288–20296.

115. Pollock, J. S., A. J. Shephard, D. J. Weber, D. L. Olson, D. G. Klapper, L. G. Pedersen, and R. G. Hiskey. 1988. Phospholipid binding properties of bovine prothrombin peptide residues 1–45. J. Biol. Chem. 263:14216–14223.

116. Valcarce, C., A. Holmgren, and J. Stenflo. 1994. Calcium-dependent interaction between Gla-containing and N-terminal EGF-like modules in factor X. J. Biol. Chem. In press.:26011–26016.

117. Sunnerhagen, M., A. O. Glenn, J. Stenflo, S. Forsén, T. Drakenberg, and J. Trewhella. 1996. The relative orientation of Gla and EGF domains in coagulation factor X is altered by Ca^{2+} binding to the first EGF domain: A combined NMR-small angle X-ray scattering study. Biochemistry 35:11547–11559.

118. Henriksen, R. A., and C. M. Jackson. 1975. Cooperative calcium binding by the phospholipid binding region of bovine prothrombin: A requirement for intact disulfide bridges. Arch. Biochem. Biophys. 170:149–159.

119. Prendergast, F. G., and K. G. Mann. 1977. Differentiaton of metal ion-induced transitions of prothrombin fragment 1. J. Biol. Chem. 252:840–850.

120. Welsch, D. J., C. H. Pletcher, and G. L. Nelsestuen. 1988. Chemical modification of prothrombin fragment 1: Documentation of sequential, two-stage loss of protein function. Biochemistry 27:4933–4938.

121. Deerfield, D. W., D. L. Olson, P. Berkowitz, P. A. Byrd, K. A. Koehler, L. G. Pedersen, and R. G. Hiskey. 1987. Mg(II) binding by bovine prothrombin fragment 1 via equilibrium dialysis and the relative roles of Mg(II) and(CaII) in blood coagulation. J. Biol. Chem. 262:4017–4023.

122. Borowski, M., B. C. Furie, S. Bauminger, and B. Furie. 1986. Prothrombin requires two sequential metal-dependent conformational transitions to bind phospholipid. Conformation-specific antibodies directed against the phospholipid-binding site on prothrombin. J. Biol. Chem. 261:14969–14975.

123. Jacobs, M., S. J. Freedman, B. C. Furie, and B. Furie. 1994. Membrane binding properties of the factor IX gamma-carboxyglutamic acid-rich domain prepared by chemical synthesis. J. Biol. Chem. 269:25494–25501.

124. Geng, J. P., and F. J. Castellino. 1997. Properties of a recombinant chimeric protein in which the gamma-carboxyglutamic acid and helical stack domains of human anticoagulant protein C are replaced by those of human coagulation factor VII. Thromb. Haemost. 77(5):926–933.

125. Liebman, H. A., Furie, B.C., Furie, B. 1987. The fctor IX phospholipid-binding site is required for calcium-dependent activation of factor IX by factor XIa. J Biol. Chem. 262:7605–7612.

126. Sekiya, F., Yamashita, T., Atoda, H., Komiyama, Y., Morita, T. 1995. Regulation of the tertiary structure and function of coagulation factor IX by magnesium (II) ions. J. Biol. Chem. 270:14325–14331.

127. Sekiya, F., Yoshida, M., Yamashita, T., Morita, T. 1996. Magnesium(II) is a crucial constitent of the blood coagulation cascade. J. Biol. Chem. 271:8541–8544.

128. Sekiya, F., M. Yoshida, T. Yamashita, and T. Morita. 1996. Localization of the specific binding site for magnesium (II) ions in factor IX. FEBS Lett. 392(3):205–208.

129. Zhang, L., and F. Castellino. 1990. A gamma-carboxyglutamic acid (gamma) variant (gamma6D, gamma7D) of human activated protein C displays greatly reduced activity as an anticoagulant. Biochemistry 29:10828–10834.

130. Ratcliff, J. V., B. Furie, and B. C. Furie. 1993. The importance of specific γ-carboxyglutamic acid residues in prothrombin. J. Biol. Chem. 268:24339–24345.

131. Gerads, I., J. W. P. Govers-Riemslag, G. Tans, R. F. A. Zwaal, and J. Rosing. 1990. Prothrombin activation on membranes with anionic lipids containing phosphate, sulfate, and/or carboxyl groups. Biochemistry 29:7967–7974.

132. Pei, G., D. D. Powers, and B. R. Lentz. 1993. Specific contribution of different phospholipid surfaces to the activation of prothrombin by the fully assembled prothrombinase. J. Biol. Chem. 268:3226–3233.

133. McDonald, J. F., and G. L. Nelsestuen. 1997. Potent inhibition of terminal complement assembly by clusterin: Characterization of its impact on C9 polymerization. Biochemistry 36(24):7464–73.

134. Atkins, J., and P. Ganz. 1992. The association of human coagulation factors VIII, IXa and X with phospholipid vesicles involves both electrostatic and hydrophobic interactions. Mol. Cell. Biochem. 112:61–71.

135. Govers Riemslag, J. W., M. P. Janssen, R. F. Zwaal, and J. Rosing. 1992. Effect of membrane fluidity and fatty acid composition on the prothrombin-converting activity of phospholipid vesicles. Biochemistry 31(41):10000–8.

136. Zhang, L., and F. J. Castellino. 1994. The binding energy of human coagulation protein C to acidic phospholipid vesicles contains a major contribution from leucine 5 in the gamma-carboxyglutamic acid domain. J.. Biol. Chem. 269(5):3590–5.

137. Christiansen, W. T., L. R. Jalbert, R. M. Robertson, A. Jhingan, M. Prorok, and F. J. Castellino. 1995. Hydrophobic amino acid residues of human anticoagulation protein C that contribute to its functional binding to phospholipid vesicles. Biochemistry 34(33):10376–82.

138. Jalbert, L. R., J. C. Chan, W. T. Christiansen, and F. J. Castellino. 1996. The hydrophobic nature of residue-5 of human protein C is a major determinant of its functional interactions with acidic phospholipid vesicles. Biochemistry 35(22):7093–9.

139. McDonald, J. F., A. M. Shah, R. A. Schwalbe, W. Kisiel, B. Dahlback, and G. L. Nelsestuen. 1997. Comparison of naturally occurring vitamin K–dependent proteins: Correlation of amino acid sequences and membrane binding properties suggests a membrane contact site. Biochemistry 36(17):5120–7.

140. Scott, D. L., S. P. White, J. L. Browning, J. J. Rosa, M. H. Gelb, and P. B. Sigler. 1991. Structures of free and inhibited human secretory phospholipase A2 from inflammatory exudate. Science 254(5034):1007–10.

141. Koppaka, V., J. Wang, M. Banerjee, and B. R. Lentz. 1996. Soluble phospholipids enhance factor Xa-catalyzed prothrombin activation in solution. Biochemistry 35(23):7482–91.

142. Stern, D. M., M. Drillings, H. L. Nossel, A. Hurlet Jensen, K. S. LaGamma, and J. Owen. 1983. Binding of factors IX and IXa to cultured vascular endothelial cells. Proc. Natl. Acad. Sci. U.S.A. 80(13):4119–23.

143. Toomey, J. R., K. J. Smith, H. R. Roberts, and D. W. Stafford. 1992. The endothelial cell binding determinant of human factor IX resides in the gamma-carboxyglutamic acid domain. Biochemistry 31:1806–1808.

144. Cheung, W.-F., N. Hamaguchi, K. J. Smith, and D. W. Stafford. 1992. The binding of human factor IX to endothelial cells is mediated by residues 3–11. J. Biol. Chem. 267:20529–20531.

145. Stern, D. M., M. Drillings, W. Kisiel, P. Nawroth, H. L. Nossel, and K. S. LaGamma. 1984. Activation of factor IX bound to cultured bovine aortic endothelial cells. Proc. Natl. Acad. Sci. U.S.A. 81(3):913–7.

146. Cheung, W. F., J. van den Born, K. Kuhn, L. Kjellen, B. G. Hudson, and D. W. Stafford. 1996. Identification of the endothelial cell binding site for factor IX. Proc. Natl. Acad. Sci. U.S.A. 93(20):11068–73.

147. Wolberg, A. S., D. W. Stafford, and D. A. Erie. 1997. Human factor IX binds to specific sites on the collagenous domain of collagen IV. J. Biol. Chem. 272(27):16717–20.

148. Reitsma, P. H., S. R. Poort, F. Bernardi, S. Gandrille, G. L. Long, N. Sala, and D. N. Cooper. 1993. Protein C deficiency: A database of mutations. Thromb. Haemost. 69:77–84.

149. Reitsma, P. H., F. Bernardi, R. G. Doig, S. Gandrille, J. S. Greengard, H. Ireland, M. Krawczak, B. Lind, G. L. Long, S. R. Poort, et al. 1995. Protein C deficiency: A database of mutations, 1995 update. On behalf of the Subcommittee on Plasma Coagulation Inhibitors of the Scientific and Standardization Committee of the ISTH. Thromb. Haemost. 73(5):876–89.

150. Winship, P. R., and A. C. Dragon. 1991. Identification of haemophilia B patients with mutations in the two calcium binding domains of factor IX: Importance of a β-OH Asp 64 Asn change. Br. J. Haematol. 1991:102–109.

151. Bertina, R. M., and I. K. Van Der Linden. 1982. Factor IX Zutphen. A genetic variant of blood coagulation factor IX with an abnormally high molecular weight. J. Lab. Clin. Med. 100:695–704.

152. Bertina, R. M., and J. J. Veltkamp. 1979. A genetic variant of factor IX with decreased capacity for Ca^{2+} binding. Br. J. Haematol. 42:623–635.

153. Chen, S. H., A. R. Thompson, M. Zhang, and R. C. Scott. 1989. Three point mutations in the factor IX genes of five hemophilia B patients. Identification strategy using localization by altered epitopes and their hemophilic proteins. J. Clin. Invest. 84:113–118.

154. Wang, N. S., M. Zhang, A. R. Thompson, and S. H. Chen. 1990. Factor IX Chongqing: A new mutation in the calcium-binding domain of factor IX resulting in severe hemophilia B. Thromb. Haemost. 63:24–26.

155. Berkner, K. L., K. Walker, J. King, and A. A. Kumar. 1989. Individual residues within the Gla domain of factor IX have different effects upon coagulant activity and upon overall gamma-carboxylation. Thromb. Haemost. 62:1074.

156. Gillis, S., B. C. Furie, B. Furie, H. Patel, M. C. Huberty, M. Switzer, W. B. Foster, H. A. Scoble, and M. D. Bond. 1997. Gamma-carboxyglutamic acids 36 and 40 do not contribute to human factor IX function. Protein Sci. 6(1):185–196.

157. Larson, P. J., S. A. Stanfield Oakley, W. J. VanDusen, C. K. Kasper, K. J. Smith, D. M. Monroe, and K. A. High. 1996. Structural integrity of the gamma-carboxyglutamic acid domain of human blood coagulation factor IXa is required for its binding to cofactor VIIIa. J. Biol.. Chem. 271(7):3869–3876.

158. Watzke, H. H., K. Lechner, H. R. Roberts, S. V. Reddy, D. J. Welch, P. Friedman, G. Mahr, P. Jagadeeswaran, D. M. Monroe, and K. A. High. 1990. Molecular defect (Gla + 14 Lys) and its functional consequences in a hereditary factor X deficiency (factor X "Voralberg"). J. Biol. Chem. 265:11982–11989.

159. Zhang, L., and F. Castellino. 1991. Role of the hexapeptide disulfide loop present in the gamma-carboxyglutamic acid domain of human protein X in its activation properties and in the in vitro anticoagulant activity of activated protein C. Biochemistry 30:6696–6704.

160. Ratcliffe, J. V., B. Furie, and B. C. Furie. 1993. The importance of specific gamma-carboxyglutamic acid residues in prothrombin. Evaluation by site-specific mutagenesis. J. Biol. Chem. 268(32):24339–45.

161. Thariath, A., and F. J. Castellino. 1997. Highly conserved residue arginine-15 is required for the Ca2 + -dependent properties of the gamma-carboxyglutamic acid domain of human anticoagulation protein C and activated protein C. Biochem. J. 322(Pt 1):309–15.

162. Christiansen, W. T., and F. J. Castellino. 1994. Properties of recombinant chimeric human protein C and activated protein C containing the gamma-carboxyglutamic acid and trailing helical stack domains of protein C replaced by those of human coagulation factor IX. Biochemistry 33(19):5901–11.

163. Toomey, J. R., K. J. Smith, and D. W. Stafford. 1991. Localization of the human tissue factor recognition determinant of human factor VIIa. J. Biol. Chem. 266:19198–19202.

164. Chang, J.-Y., D. W. Stafford, and D. L. Straight. 1995. The roles of factor VII's structural domains in tissue factor binding. Biochemistry 34:12227–12232.

165. Suttie, J. W. 1973. Mechanism of action of vitamin K: Demonstration of a liver precursor of prothrombin. Science 179:192–194.

166. Shah, D. V., J. C. Swanson, and J. W. Suttie. 1984. Abnormal prothrombin in the vitamin K–deficient rat. Thromb. Res. 35:451-458.

167. Swanson, J. C. 1985. Prothrombin biosynthesis: Characterization of processing events in rat liver microsomes. Biochemistry 24:3890–3897.

168. Graves, C. B., G. G. Grabau, R. E. Olson, and T. W. Munns. 1980. Immunochemical isolation and electrophoretic characterization of precursor prothrombins in H-35 rat hepatoma cells. Biochemistry 19:266–272.

169. Wallin, R., and L. F. Martin. 1988. Early processing of prothrombin and factor X by the vitamin K–dependent carboxylase. J. Biol. Chem. 263:9994–10001.

170. Helenius, A. 1994. How N-linked oligosaccharides affect glycoprotein folding in the endoplasmatic reticulum. Mol. Biol. Cell. 5:253–265.

171. Dorner, A. J., D. G. Bole, and R. J. Kaufman. 1987. The relationship

of N-linked glycosylation and heavy chain-binding protein associationb with the secretion of glycoproteins. J. Cell. Biol. 105:2665–2674.

172. McClure, D. B., J. D. Walls, and B. W. Grinnell. 1992. Post-translational processing events in the secretion pathway of human protein C, a complex vitamin K–dependent antithrombotic factor. J. Biol. Chem. 267:19710–19717.

173. Dorner, A. J., and R. J. Kaufman. 1990. Analysis of synthesis, processing, and secretion of proteins expressed in mammalian cells. Methods Enzymol. 185:577–596.

174. Martoglio, B., M. W. Hofmann, J. Brunner, and B. Dobberstein. 1995. The protein-conducting channel in the membrane of the endoplasmic reticulum is open laterally toward the lipid bilayer. Cell 81:207–214.

175. Nielsen, H., J. Engelbrecht, S. Brunak, and G. von Heijne. 1997. Identification of prokaryotic and eukaryotic signal peptides and prediction of their cleavage sites. Protein Eng. 10:1–6.

176. Kivirikko, K. I., and R. Myllylä. 1987. Recent developments in post-translational modification: Intracellular processing. Methods Enzymol. 144:96–114.

177. Kornfeld, R., and S. Kornfeld. 1985. Assembly of asparagine-linked oligosaccharides. Annu. Rev. Biochem. 54:631–664.

178. Shah, D. V., J. C. Swanson, and J. W. Suttie. 1983. Vitamin K–dependent carboxylase: Effect of detergent concentrations, vitamin K status, and added protein precursor on activity. Arch. Biochem. Biophys. 222:216–221.

179. Knobloch, J. E., and J. W. Suttie. 1987. Vitamin K–dependent carboxylase: Control of enzyme activity by the propeptide region of factor X. J. Biol. Chem. 262:15334–15337.

180. Ulrich, M. M. M., B. Furie, C. Vermeer, and B. B. Furie. 1988. Vitamin K–dependent carboxylation: A synthetic peptide based upon the gamma-carboxylation recognition site sequence of the prothrombin propeptide is an active substrate for the carboxylase in vitro. J. Biol. Chem. 263:9697–9702.

181. Hubbard, B. R., M. Jacobs, M. M. W. Ulrich, B. Furie, and B. C. Furie. 1989. Vitamin K–dependent carboxylation: In vitro modification of synthetic peptides containing the gamma-carboxylation recognition site. J. Biol. Chem. 264:14145–14150.

182. Price, P. A., J. D. Fraser, and G. Metz-Virca. 1987. Molecular cloning of matrix Gla protein: Implications for substrate recognition by the vitamin K–dependent gamma-carboxylase. Proc. Natl. Acad. Sci. U.S.A. 84:8335–8389.

183. Pan, L. C., and P. A. Price. 1985. The propeptide of rat bone gamma-carboxyglutamic acid proteins shares homology with other vitamin K–dependent protein precursors. Proc. Natl. Acad. Sci. U.S.A. 82:6109–6113.

184. Rabiet, M.-J., M. J. Jorgensen, B. Furie, and B. C. Furie. 1987. Effect of propeptide mutations on posttranslational processing of factor IX: Evidence that beta-hydroxylation and gamma-carboxylation are independent events. J. Biol. Chem. 262:14895–14898.

185. Suttie, J. W., J. A. Hoskins, J. Engelke, A. Hopfgartner, H. Ehrlich, N. U. Bang, R. M. Belagaje, B. Schoner, and G. L. Long. 1987. Vitamin K–dependent carboxylase: Possible role of the substrate "Propeptide" as an intracellular recognition site. Proc. Natl. Acad. Sci. U.S.A. 84:634–637.

186. Foster, D. C., M. S. Rudinski, B. G. Schach, K. L. Berkner, A. A. Kumar, F. S. Hagen, C. A. Sprecher, M. Y. Insley, and E. W. Davie. 1987. Propeptide of human protein C is necessary for gamma-carboxylation. Biochemistry 26:7003–7011.

187. Yamada, M., A. Kuliopulos, N. P. Nelson, D. A. Roth, B. Furie, B. C. Furie, C. T. Walsh. 1995. Localization of the factor IX propeptide binding site on recombinant vitamin K–dependent carboxylase using benzoylphenylaline photoaffinity peptide inactivators. Biochemistry 34:481–489.

188. Jorgensen, M. J., A. B. Cantor, B. C. Furie, C. L. Brown, C. B. Shoemaker, and B. Furie. 1987. Recognition site directing vitamin K–dependent gamma-carboxylation resides on the propeptide of factor IX. Cell 48:185–191.

189. Geng, J. P., and F. J. Castellino. 1996. The propeptides of human protein C, factor VII, and factor IX are exchangeable with regard to directing gamma-carboxylation of these proteins. Thromb. Haemost. 76(2):205–7.

190. Furie, B. C., J. Ratcliff, J. Tward, M. J. Jorgensen, L. Blaszkowsky, D. DiMichele, and B. Furie. 1997. The γ-carboxylation recognition site is sufficient to direct vitamin K–dependent carboxylation on an adjacent glutamate-rich region of thrombin in a propeptide-thrombin chimera. J. Biol. Chem. 272:28258–28262.

191. Morris, D. P., R. D. Stevens, D. J. Wright, and D. W. Stafford. 1995. Processive post-translational modification. Vitamin K–dependent carboxylation of a peptide substrate. J. Biol. Chem. 270(51):30491–8.

192. Berkner, K. L., and B. N. Pudota. 1998. Vitamin K–dependent carboxylation of the carboxylase. Proc. Natl. Acad. Sci. U.S.A. 95:466–471.

193. Wu, M., B. A. M. Soute, C. Vermeer, and D. W. Stafford. 1990. In vitro-carboxylation of a 59-residue recombinant peptide including the propeptide and the gamma-carboxyglutamic acid domain of coagulation factor IX. Effect of mutation near the propeptide cleavage site. J. Biol. Chem. 265:13124–13129.

194. Sanford, D. G., C. Kanagy, J. L. Sudmeier, B. C. Furie, B. Furie, and W. W. Bachovchin. 1991. Structure of the propeptide of prothrombin containing the gamma-carboxylation recognition site determined by two-dimensional NMR spectroscopy. Biochemistry 30:9835–9841.

195. Bentley, A. K., D. J. G. Rees, C. Rizza, and G. G. Brownlee. 1986. Defective propeptide processing of blood clotting factor IX caused by mutation of arginine to glutamine in position -4. Cell 45:343–348.

196. Watzke, H. H., A. Wallmark, N. Hamaguchi, P. Giardina, D. W. Stafford, and K. A. High. 1991. Factor X Santo Domingo. Evidence that the severe clinical phenotype arises from a mutation blocking secretion. J. Clin. Invest. 88:1685–1689.

197. Ware, J., D. L. Diuguid, H. L. Liebman, M.-J. Rabiet, C. K. Kasper, B. C. Furie, B. Furie, and D. W. Stafford. 1989. Factor IX San Dimas: Substitution of glutamine for Arginine-4 in the propeptide leads to incomplete gamma-carboxylation and altered phospholipid binding properties. J. Biol. Chem. 264:11401–11406.

198. Rehemtulla, A., and R. J. Kaufman. 1992. Protein processing within the secretory pathway. Curr. Opin. Biotechnol. 3(5):560–5.

199. Julius, D., A. Brake, L. Blair, R. Kunisawa, and J. Thorner. 1984. Isolation of the putative structural gene for the lysine-arginine-cleaving endopeptidase required for processing of yeast prepro-alpha-factor. Cell 37:1075–1089.

200. Bathurst, I. C., S. O. Brennan, R. W. Carrell, L. S. Cousens, A. J. Brake, and P. J. Barr. 1987. Yeast KEX3 protease has the properties of a human proalbumin converting enzyme. Science 235:348–350.

201. Wasley, L. C., A. Rehemtulla, J. A. Bristol, and R. J. Kaufman. 1993. PACE/Furin processes the vitamin K–dependent pro-factor IX precursor within the secretory pathway. J. Biol. Chem. 268:8458–8465.

202. Kawabata, S., and E. W. Davie. 1992. A microsomal endopeptidase from liver with substrate specificity for processing proproteins such as the vitamin K–dependent proteins of plasma. J. Biol. Chem. 267(15):10331–6.

203. Kawabata, S., K. Nakagawa, T. Muta, S. Iwanaga, and E. W. Davie. 1993. Rabbit liver microsomal endopeptidase with substrate specificity for processing proproteins is structurally related to rat testes metal-loendopeptidase 24.15. J. Biol. Chem. 268(17):12498–503.

204. Carlisle, T. L., P. E. Bock, and C. M. Jackson. 1990. Kinetic intermediates in prothrombin activation. Bovine prothrombin 1 conversion to thrombin by factor X. J. Biol. Chem. 265:22044–22055.

205. Wallin, R., C. Stanton, and S. M. Hutson. 1993. Intracellular maturation of the gamma-carboxyglutamic acid (Gla) region in prothrombin coincides with release of the propeptide. Biochem. J. 291(Pt 3):723–7.

206. Bristol, J. A., J. V. Ratcliffe, D. A. Roth, M. A. Jacobs, B. C. Furie, B. Furie. 1996. Biosynthesis of prothrombin: Intracellular localzation of the vitamin K–dependent carboxylase and the sites of γ-carboxylation. Blood 88:2585–2593.

207. Giannelli, F., P. M. Green, S. S. Sommer, M. C. Poon, M. Ludwig, R. Schwaab, P. H. Reitsma, M. Goossens, A. Yoshioka, and G. G. Brownlee. 1996. Haemophilia B (sixth edition): A database of point mutations and short additions and deletions. Nucleic Acids Res. 24(1):103–18.

208. Diuguid, D. L., M. J. Rabiet, B. C. Furie, H. A. Liebman, and B. Furie. 1986. Molecular basis of hemophilia B: A defective enzyme due to an unprocessed propeptide is caused by a point mutation in the factor IX precursor. Proc. Natl. Acad. Sci. U.S.A. 83:5803–5807.

209. Lind, B., A. H. Johnsen, and S. Thorsen. 1997. Naturally occurring Arg(-1) to His mutation in human protein C leads to aberrant propeptide processing and secretion of dysfunctional protein C. Blood 89(8):2807–16.

210. Bristol, J. A., S. J. Freedman, B. C. Furie, and B. Furie. 1994. Profactor IX: The propeptide inhibits binding to membrane surfaces and activation by factor XIa. Biochemistry 33(47):14136–14143.

211. Esmon, C. T., J. A. Sadowski, and J. W. Suttie. 1975. A new carboxylation reaction. The vitamin K–dependent incorporation of H14CO3 into prothrombin. J. Biol. Chem. 250:4744–4748.

212. Sadowski, J. A., C. T. Esmon, and J. W. Suttie. 1976. Vitamin K–dependent carboxylase. Requirements of the rat liver microsomal enzyme system. J. Biol. Chem. 251:2770–2776.

213. Olivera, B. M., W. R. Gray, R. Zeikus, J. M. McIntosh, J. Varga, J. Rivier, V. de Santos, and L. J. Cruz. 1985. Peptide neurotoxins from fish-hunting cone snails. Science 230(4732):1338–43.

214. Olivera, B. M., J. Rivier, C. Clark, C. A. Ramilo, G. P. Corpuz, F. C. Abogadie, E. E. Mena, S. R. Woodward, D. R. Hillyard, and L. J. Cruz. 1990. Diversity of Conus neuropeptides. Science 249(4966):257–63.

215. Prorok, M., S. E. Warder, T. Blandl, and F. J. Castellino. 1996. Calcium binding properties of synthetic gamma-carboxyglutamic acid–containing marine cone snail "sleeper" peptides, conantokin-G and conantokin-T. Biochemistry 35(51):16528–34.

216. Rigby, A. C., J. D. Baleja, B. C. Furie, and B. Furie. 1997. Three-dimensional structure of a gamma-carboxyglutamic acid-containing conotoxin, conantokin G, from the marine snail *Conus geographus*: the metal-free conformer. Biochemistry 36(23):6906–14.

217. Stanley, T. B., D. W. Stafford, B. M. Olivera, and P. K. Bandyopadhyay. 1997. Identification of a vitamin K–dependent carboxylase in the venom duct of a Conus snail. FEBS Lett. 407(1):85–8.

218. Friedman, P. A., and C. T. Przysiecki. 1987. Vitamin K–dependent carboxylation. Int. J. Biochem. 19:1–7.

219. Suttie, J. 1993. Synthesis of vitamin K–dependent proteins. FASEB J. 7:445–452.

220. Suttie, J. W., J. M. Hageman, S. R. Lehrman, and D. H. Rich. 1976. Vitamin K–dependent carboxylase. Development of a peptide substrate. J. Biol. Chem. 251:5827–5830.

221. Suttie, J. W., P. C. Preusch, and J. J. McTigue. 1983. Vitamin K–dependent carboxylase: Recent studies of the rat liver enzyme system. *In* Posttranslational Covalent Modification of Proteins. B. Johnson, editor. Academic Press, New York. 253–279.

222. Jones, J. P., E. J. Gardner, T. G. Cooper, and R. E. Olson. 1977. Vitamin K–dependent carboxylation of peptide-bound glutamate: The active species of CO2 utilized by the membrane-bound preprothrombin carboxylase. J. Biol. Chem. 252:7738–7742.

223. Bell, R. G. 1978. Metabolism of vitamin K and prothrombin synthesis: Anticoagulants and the vitamin K-epoxide cycle. Fed. Proc. 37:599–604.

224. Larsson, A. E., P. E. Friedman, and J. W. Suttie. 1981. Vitamin K–dependent carboxylase: Stoichiometry of carboxylation and vitamin K 2,3-epoxide formation. J. Biol. Chem. 256:11032–11035.

225. Hubbard, B. R., M. M. Ulrich, M. Jacobs, C. Vermeer, C. Walsh, B. Furie, and B. C. Furie. 1989. Vitamin K–dependent carboxylase: Affinity purification from bovine liver by using a synthetic propeptide containing the gamma-carboxylation recognition site. Proc. Natl. Acad. Sci. U.S.A. 86(18):6893–7.

226. Wu, S. M., D. P. Morris, and D. W. Stafford. 1991. Identification and purification to near homogeneity of the vitamin K–dependent carboxylase. Proc. Natl. Acad. Sci. U.S.A. 88:2236–2240.

227. Wu, S. M., W. F. Cheung, D. Frazier, and D. W. Stafford. 1991. Cloning and expression of the cDNA for human gamma-glutamyl carboxylase. Science 254:1634–1636.

228. Rehemtulla, A., D. A. Roth, L. C. Wasley, A. Kuliopulos, C. T. Walsh, B. Furie, B. C. Furie, and R. J. Kaufman. 1993. In vitro and in vivo functional characterization of bovine vitamin K–dependent gamma-carboxylase expressed in Chinese hamster ovary cells. Proc. Natl. Acad. Sci. U.S.A. 90(10):4611–5.

229. Lingenfelter, S. E., and K. L. Berkner. 1996. Isolation of the human gamma-carboxylase and a gamma-carboxylase–associated protein from factor IX-expressing mammalian cells. Biochemistry 35(25):8234–43.

230. Wu, S. M., D. W. Stafford, L. D. Frazier, Y. Y. Fu, K. A. High, K. Chu, B. Sanchez Vega, and J. Solera. 1997. Genomic sequence and transcription start site for the human gamma-glutamyl carboxylase. Blood 89(11):4058–62.

231. Friedman, P. A., M. A. Shia, P. M. Gallop, and A. E. Griep. 1979. Vitamin K–dependent gamma-carbon-hydrogen bond cleavage and nonmandatory concurrent carboxylation of peptide-bound glutamic acid residues. Proc. Natl. Acad. Sci. U.S.A. 76:3126–3129.

232. McTigue, J. J., and J. W. Suttie. 1983. Vitamin K–dependent carboxylase: Demonstration of a vitamin K and O₂-dependent exchange of 3H from ³H2O into glutamic acid residues. J. Biol. Chem. 258:12129–12131.

233. Anton, D. L., and P. A. Friedman. 1983. Fate of the activated gamma-carbon-hydrogen bond in the uncoupled vitamin K–dependent gamma-glutamyl carboxylation reaction. J. Biol. Chem. 258:14084–14087.

234. Morris, D. P., B. A. Soute, C. Vermeer, and D. W. Stafford. 1993. Characterization of the purified vitamin K–dependent gamma-glutamyl carboxylase. J. Biol. Chem. 268(12):8735–42.

235. Sugiura, I., B. Furie, C. T. Walsh, and B. C. Furie. 1997. Propeptide and glutamate-containing substrates bound to the vitamin K–dependent carboxylase convert its vitamin K epoxidase function from an inactive to an active state. Proc. Natl. Acad. Sci. U.S.A. 94(17):9069–74.

236. Suttie, J. W., A. E. Larson, L. M. Canfield, and T. L. Carlisle. 1978. Relationship between vitamin K–dependent carboxylation and vitamin K epoxidation. Fed. Proc. 37:2605–2609.

237. de Metz, M., B. A. Soute, H. C. Hemker, R. Fokkens, J. Lugtenburg, and C. Vermeer. 1982. Studies on the mechanism of the vitamin K–dependent carboxylation reaction. Carboxylation without the concurrent formation of vitamin K 2,3-epoxide. J. Biol. Chem. 257(10):5326–9.

238. Dubois, J., M. Gaudry, S. Bory, R. Azerad, and A. Marquet. 1983. Vitamin K–dependent carboxylation. Study of the hydrogen abstraction stereochemistry with gamma-fluoroglutamic acid-containing peptides. J. Biol. Chem. 258(13):7897–9.

239. Dowd, P., R. Hershline, S. W. Ham, and S. Naganathan. 1995. Vitamin K and energy transduction: A base strength amplification mechanism. Science 269(5231):1684–91.

240. Carpenter, G., and S. Cohen. 1990. Epidermal growth factor. J. Biol. Chem. 265:7709–7712.

241. Stenflo, J. 1991. Structure-function relationships of epidermal growth factor modules in vitamin K–dependent clotting factors. Blood 78:1637–1651.

242. Massagué, J. 1990. Transforming growth factor-β. A model for membrane-anchored growth factors. J. Biol. Chem. 265:21393–21396.

243. Höjrup, P., and S. Magnusson. 1987. Disulphide bridges of bovine factor X. Biochem. J. 245:887–892.

244. Rao, Z., P. Handford, M. Mayhew, V. Knott, G. G. Brownlee, and D. Stuart. 1995. The structure of a Ca²⁺-binding epidermal growth factor–like domain: Its role in protein-protein interactions. Cell 82(1):131–41.

245. Baron, M., D. G. Norman, T. S. Harvey, P. A. Handford, M. Mayhew, A. G. D. Tse, G. G. Brownlee, and I. D. Campbell. 1992. The three-dimensional structure of the first EGF-like module of human factor IX: Comparison with EGF and TGF-a. Protein Sci. 1:81–90.

246. Drakenberg, T., P. Fernlund, P. Roepstorff, and J. Stenflo. 1983. Beta-hydroxyaspartic acid in vitamin K–dependent protein C. Proc. Natl. Acad. Sci. U.S.A. 80:1802–1806.

247. Stenflo, J., Å. Lundwall, and B. Dahlbäck. 1987. Beta-hydroxyasparagine in domains homologous to the epidermal growth factor precursor in vitamin K–dependent protein S. Proc. Natl. Acad. Sci. U.S.A. 84:368–372.

248. Hase, S., S.-I. Kawabata, H. Nishimura, H. Takeya, T. Sueyoshi, T. Miyata, S. Iwanaga, T. Takao, Y. Shimonishi, and T. Ikenaka. 1988. A new trisaccharide sugar chain linked to a serine residue in bovine coagulation factors VII and IX. J. Biochem. 104:867–868.

249. Nishimura, H., S.-I. Kawabata, W. Kisiel, S. Hase, T. Ikenaka, T. Takao, Y. Shimonishi, and S. Iwanaga. 1989. Identification of a disaccharide (Xyl2-Glc) and a trisaccharide (Xyl2-Glc) O-glycosidically linked to a serine residue in the first epidermal growth factor-like domain of human factors VII and IX and protein Z and bovine protein Z. J. Biol. Chem. 264:20320–20325.

250. Hase, S., H. Nishimura, S.-I. Kawabata, S. Iwanaga, and T. Ikenaka. 1990. The structure of (xylose)2 glucose-O-serine 53 found in the first epidermal growth factor–like domain of bovine blood clotting factor IX. J. Biol. Chem. 265:1858–1861.

251. Lundblad, A., and S. Svensson. 1973. Isolation and characterization of 3-O-†-D-xylopyranosyl-D-glucose and 2-O-†-L-fucopyranosyl-D-glucose from normal human urine. Biochemistry 12:306–309.

252. Handford, P. A., M. Baron, M. Mayhew, A. Willis, T. Beesley, G. G. Brownlee, and I. D. Campbell. 1990. The first EGF-like domain from human factor IX contains a high-affinity calcium binding site. EMBO J. 9(2):475–480.

253. Sunnerhagen, M. S., E. Persson, I. Dahlqvist, T. Drakenberg, J. Stenflo, M. Mayhew, M. Robin, P. Handford, J. W. Tilley, I. D. Campbell, et al. 1993. The effect of aspartate hydroxylation on calcium binding to epidermal growth factor-like modules in coagulation factors IX and X. J. Biol. Chem. 268(31):23339–44.

254. Persson, E., M. Selander, T. Drakenberg, A. K. Öhlin, and J. Stenflo.

1989. Calcium binding to the isolated β-hydroxyaspartic acid-containing epidermal growth factor containing domain of bovine factor X. J. Biol. Chem. 264:16897–16904.

255. Öhlin, A. K., I. Björk, and J. Stenflo. 1990. Proteolytic formation and properties of a fragment of protein C containing the gamma-carboxyglutamic acid rich region and the EGF-like region. Biochemistry 29:644–651.

256. Dahlback, B., B. Hildebrand, and S. Linse. 1990. Novel type of very high affinity calcium-binding sites in beta-hydroxyasparagine-containing epidermal growth factor-like domains in vitamin K–dependent protein S. J. Biol. Chem. 265(30):18481-18489.

257. Sekiya, F., M. Yoshida, T. Yamashita, and T. Morita. 1996. Localization of the specific binding site for magnesium (II) ions in factor IX. FEBS Lett. 392:205–208.

258. Kline, T. P., F. K. Brown, S. C. Brown, P. W. Jeffs, K. D. Kopple, and L. Mueller. 1990. Solution structure of human transforming growth factor † derived from 1H NMR data. Biochemistry 29:7805–7813.

259. Selander, M., E. Persson, J. Stenflo, and T. Drakenberg. 1990. 1H NMR assignment and secondary structure of the Ca²⁺-free form of the amino-terminal epidermal growth factor like domain in coagulation factor X. Biochemistry 29:8111–8118.

260. Huang, L. H., X.-H. Ke, W. Sweeny, and J. P. Tam. 1989. Calcium binding and putative activity of the epidermal growth factor domain of blood coagulation factor IX. Biochem. Biophys. Res. Commun. 60:133–139.

261. Stenberg, Y., S. Linse, T. Drakenberg, and J. Stenflo. 1997. The high affinity calcium-binding sites in the epidermal growth factor module region of vitamin K–dependent protein S. J. Biol. Chem. 272:23255–60.

262. Rao, Z., P. Handford, M. Mayhew, V. Knott, G. G. Brownlee, and D. Stuart. 1995. The structure of a Ca²⁺-binding epidermal growth factor-like domain: Its role in protein-protein interactions. Cell 82:131–141.

263. Fernlund, P., and J. Stenflo. 1983. Beta-hydroxyaspartic acid in vitamin K–dependent proteins. J. Biol. Chem. 258:12509–12512.

264. Ikegami, T. 1975. Studies on the metabolism of β-hydroxyaspartic acid. Acta Med. Okayama 29:241–247.

265. Przysiecki, C. T., J. E. Staggers, H. G. Rajmit, D. G. Musson, A. M. Stern, C. D. Bennet, and P. A. Friedman. 1987. Occurence of beta-hydroxylated asparagine residues in non-vitamin K–dependent proteins containing epidermal growth factor-like domains. Proc. Natl. Acad. Sci. U.S.A. 84:7856–7860.

266. Lee, B., M. Godfrey, E. Vitale, H. Hori, M. G. Mattei, M. Sarfarazi, P. Tsipouras, F. Ramirez, and D. W. Hollister. 1991. Linkage of Marfan syndrome and a phenotypically related disorder to two different fibrillin genes. Nature 352:330–334.

267. Maslen, C. L., G. M. Corson, B. K. Maddox, R. W. Glanville, and L. Y. Sakai. 1991. Partial sequence of a candidate gene for the Marfan syndrome. Nature 352:334–337.

268. Downing, A. K., V. Knott, J. M. Werner, C. M. Cardy, I. D. Campbell, and P. A. Handford. 1996. Solution structure of a pair of calcium-binding epidermal growth factor-like domains: Implications for the Marfan syndrome and other genetic disorders. Cell 85:597–605.

269. Ellison, L. W., J. Bird, D. C. West, A. L. Soreng, T. C. Reynolds, S. D. Smith, and J. Sklar. 1991. TAN-1, the human homolog of Drosophila notch gene, is broken by chromosomal translocations in T lymphoblastic neoplasms. Cell 66:649–661.

270. Muskavitch, M. A. T. 1994. Delta-notch signaling and Drosophila cell fate choice. Dev. Biol. 166:415.

271. Joutel, A., C. Corpechot, A. Ducros, K. Vahedi, H. Chabriat, P. Mouton, S. Alamowitch, V. Domenga, M. Cecillion, E. Marechal, J. Maciazek, C. Vayssiere, C. Cruaud, E. A. Cabanis, M. M. Ruchoux, J. Weissenbach, J. F. Bach, M. G. Bousser, and E. Tournier Lasserve. 1996. Notch3 mutations in CADASIL, a hereditary adult-onset condition causing stroke and dementia. Nature 383(6602):707–10.

272. Stenflo, J., A. K. Öhlin, W. G. Owen, and W. J. Schneider. 1988. beta-hydroxyaspartic acid or beta-hydroxyasparagine in bovine low density lipoprotein receptor and in bovine thrombomodulin. J. Biol. Chem. 263:21–24.

273. Derian, C. K., W. VanDusen, C. T. Przysieck, P. N. Walsh, K. L. Berkner, R. J. Kaufman, and P. A. Friedman. 1989. Inhibitors of 2-ketoglutarate-dependent dioxygenases block aspartyl beta-hydroxylation of recombinant human factor IX in several mammalian expression systems. J. Biol. Chem. 264:6615–6618.

274. Gronke, R. S., W. J. VanDusen, V. M. Garsky, J. W. Jacobs, M. K. Saranda, A. M. Stern, and P. A. Friedman. 1989. Aspartyl beta-hydroxylase: In vitro hydroxylation of a synthetic peptide based on the structure of the first growth factor-like domain of human factor IX. Proc. Natl. Acad. Sci. U.S.A. 86:3609–3613.

275. Wang, Q., W. J. VanDusen, C. J. Petroski, V. M. Garsky, A. M. Stern, and P. A. Friedman. 1991. Bovine liver aspartyl beta-hydroxylase. Purification and characterization. J. Biol. Chem. 266:14004–14010.

276. Stenflo, J., and P. Fernlund. 1984. Beta-hydroxyaspartic acid in vitamin K–dependent plasma proteins from scorbutic and warfarin-treated guinea pigs. FEBS Lett. 168:287–292.

277. Sugo, T., U. Persson, and J. Stenflo. 1985. Protein C in bovine plasma after warfarin treatment. Purification, partial characterization, and beta-hydroxyaspartic acid content. J. Biol. Chem. 260:10453.

278. Gronke, R. S., D. J. Welsh, W. J. VanDusen, V. M. Garsky, M. Sardana, A. M. Stern, and P. A. Friedman. 1990. Partial purification and characterization of bovine liver aspartyl beta-hydroxylase. J. Biol. Chem. 265:8558–8565.

279. Jia, S., W. J. VanDusen, R. E. Diehl, N. E. Kohl, R. A. Dixon, K. O. Elliston, A. M. Stern, and P. A. Friedman. 1992. cDNA cloning and expression of bovine aspartyl(asparaginyl) beta-hydroxylase. J. Biol. Chem. 267(20):14322–7.

280. Jia, S., K. McGinnis, W. J. VanDusen, C. J. Burke, A. Kuo, P. R. Griffin, M. K. Sardana, K. O. Elliston, A. M. Stern, and P. A. Friedman. 1994. A fully active catalytic domain of bovine aspartyl (asparaginyl) beta-hydroxylase expressed in Escherichia coli: Characterization and evidence for the identification of an active-site region in vertebrate alpha-ketoglutarate–dependent dioxygenases. Proc. Natl. Acad. Sci. U.S.A. 91:7227–7231.

281. McGinnis, K., G. M. Ku, W. J. VanDusen, J. Fu, V. Garsky, A. M. Stern, and P. A. Friedman. 1996. Site-directed mutagenesis of residues in a conserved region of bovine aspartyl(asparaginyl) beta-hydroxylase: Evidence that histidine 675 has a role in binding Fe2 + . Biochemistry 35(13):3957–62.

282. Morita, T., and C. M. Jackson. 1980. Structural and functional characteristics of a proteolytically modified, "Gla domain-less" bovine Factor X and Xa (des light chain residues 1–144). In Suttie J.W (ed): Vitamin K Metabolism and Vitamin K–Dependent Proteins. University Park Press, Baltimore, 124–128.

283. Morita, T., and C. M. Jackson. 1986. Preparation and properties of derivatives of bovine factor X and factor Xa from which the γ-carboxyglutamic acid containing domain has been removed. J. Biol. Chem. 261:4015–4023.

284. Sakai, T., T. Lund Hansen, L. Thim, and W. Kisiel. 1990. The γ-carboxyglutamic acid domain of human factor VIIa is essential for its interaction with cell surface tissue factor. J. Biol. Chem. 265:1890–1894.

285. Morita, T., H. Kaetsu, J. Mizuguchi, S. I. Kawabata, and S. Iwanaga. 1988. A characteristic property of vitamin K–dependent plasma protein Z. J. Biochem. 104:368–374.

286. Valcarce, C., E. Persson, J. Astermark, A. K. Ohlin, and J. Stenflo. 1993. Isolation of intact modules from noncatalytic parts of vitamin K–dependent coagulation factors IX and X and protein C. Methods Enzymol. 222:416–35.

287. Handford, P. A., M. Baron, M. Mayhew, A. Wills, T. Beesley, G. G. Brownlee, and I. D. Campbell. 1990. The first EGF-like domain from human factor IX contains a high-affinity calcium binding site. EMBO J. 9:475–480.

288. Handford, P. A., M. Mayhew, M. Baron, P. R. Winship, I. D. Campbell, and G. G. Brownlee. 1991. Key residues involved in calcium-binding motifs in EGF-like domains. Nature 351:164–167.

289. Knott, V., K. Downing, C. M. Cardy, and P. Handford. 1996. Calcium binding properties of an epidermal growth factor–like domain pair from human fibrillin-1. J. Mol. Biol. 255:22–27.

290. Selander Sunnerhagen, M., E. Persson, I. Dahlqvist, T. Drakenberg, J. Stenflo, M. Mayhew, M. Robin, P. Handford, J. W. Tilley, I. D. Campbell, and G. G. Brownlee. 1993. The effect of aspartate hydroxylation on calcium binding to epidermal growth factor-like modules in coagulation factors IX and X. J. Biol. Chem. 268:23339–23344.

291. Stenberg, Y., K. Julenius, I. Dahlqvist, T. Drakenberg, and J. Stenflo. 1997. Calcium-binding properties of the third and fourth epidermal-growth-factor-like modules in vitamin-K–dependent protein S. Eur. J. Biochem. 248:163–170.

292. Lin, S. W., K. J. Smith, D. Welsch, and D. W. Stafford. 1990. Expression and characterization of human factor IX and factor IX–factor X chimeras in mouse C127 cells. J. Biol. Chem. 265:144–150.

293. Hertzberg, M. S., O. Ben-Tal, B. Furie, and B. C. Furie. 1992. Construction, expression, and characterization of a chimera of factor IX and factor X. The role of the second epidermal growth factor domain and serine protease domain in factor Va binding. J. Biol. Chem. 267:14759–14766.

294. Chang, J. Y., D. M. Monroe, D. W. Stafford, K. M. Brinkhous, and H. R. Roberts. 1997. Replacing the first epidermal growth factor-like domain of factor IX with that of factor VII enhances activity in vitro and in canine hemophilia B. J. Clin. Invest. 100(4):886–92.

295. Rees, D. J. G., I. M. Jones, P. A. Handford, S. J. Walter, M. P. Esnouf, K. J. Smith, and G. G. Brownlee. 1988. The role of beta-hydroxyaspartate and adjacent carboxylate residues in the first EGF domain of human factor IX. EMBO J. 7:2053–2061.

296. Öhlin, A. K., G. Landes, P. Bourdon, C. Oppenheimer, R. M. Wydro, and J. Stenflo. 1988. beta-hydroxyaspartic acid in the first epidermal growth factor–like domain of protein C. Its role in Ca2 + binding and biological activity. J. Biol. Chem. 263:19240–19248.

297. Johnson, A. E., N. L. Esmon, T. M. Laue, and C. T. Esmon. 1983. Structural changes required for activation of protein C are induced by Ca2 + binding to a high affinity site that does not contain γ-carboxyglutamic acid. J. Biol. Chem. 258:5554–5560.

298. Sugo, T., I. Björk, A. Holmgren, and J. Stenflo. 1984. Calcium-binding properties of bovine factor X lacking the gamma-carboxyglutamic acid-containing region. J. Biol. Chem. 259:5705–5710.

299. Morita, T., and W. Kisiel. 1985. Calcium binding to a human factor IXa derivative lacking gamma-carboxyglutamic acid: Evidence for two high-affinity sites that do not involve beta-hydroxyaspartic acid. Biochem. Biophys. Res. Commun. 130:841–847.

300. Persson, E., O. H. Olsen, A. Östergaard, and L. S. Nielsen. 1997. Calcium-binding to the first epidermal growth factor–like domain of Factor VIIa increases amidolytic activity and tissue factor affinity. J. Biol. Chem. 272:19919–19924.

301. Valcarce, C., M. Selander-Sunnerhagen, A.-M. Tämlitz, T. Drakenberg, I. Björk, and J. Stenflo. 1993. Calcium affinity of the NH2-terminal epidermal growth factor-like module of factor X. Effect of the gamma-carboxyglutamic acid-containing module. J. Biol. Chem. 268:26673–26678.

302. Ohlin, A. K., G. Landes, P. Bourdon, C. Oppenheimer, R. Wydro, and J. Stenflo. 1988. Beta-hydroxyaspartic acid in the first epidermal growth factor-like domain of protein C. Its role in Ca2 + binding and biological activity. J. Biol. Chem. 263(35):19240–8.

303. Kelly, C. R., C. D. Dickinson, and W. Ruf. 1997. Calcium binding to the first epidermal growth factor module of coagulation Factor VIIa is important for cofactor interaction and porteolytic function. J. Biol. Chem. 272:17467–17472.

304. Kanazaki, T., A. Olofsson, A. Morén, C. Wernstedt, U. Hellman, K. Miyazono, L. Claesson Welsh, and C. H. Heldin. 1990. TGF-beta1 binding protein: A component of the large latent complex of TGT-beta1 with multiple repeat sequences. Cell 61:1051.

305. Gray, A., T. J. Dull, and A. Ullrich. 1983. Nucleotide sequence of epidermal growth factor cDNA predicts a 128,000-molecular weight protein precursor. Nature 303:722–725.

306. Downing, A. K., V. Knott, J. M. Werner, C. M. Cardy, I. D. Campbell. 1996. Solution structure of a pair of calcium-binding epidermal growth factor-like domains: Implications for the marfan syndrome and other genetic disorders. Cell 85:597–605.

307. Davis, L. M., R. A. McGraw, J. L. Ware, H. Roberts, and D. W. Stafford. 1987. Factor IX Alabama: A point mutation in a clotting protein results in hemophilia B. Acta Chem. Scand. 69:140–143.

308. McCord, D. M., D. M. Monroe, K. J. Smith, and H. R. Roberts. 1990. Characterization of the functional defect in factor IX Alabama. Evidence for a conformational change due to high affinity calcium binding in the first epidermal growth factor domain. J. Biol. Chem. 265:10250–10254.

309. Green, P. M., A. J. Montandon, R. Ljung, D. R. Bentley, I. M. Nilsson, S. Kling, and F. Giannelli. 1991. Haemophilia B mutations in a complete Swedish population sample: A test of new strategy for the genetic counselling of diseases with high mutational heterogeneity. Br. J. Haematol. 78:390–397.

310. Lozier, J. N., D. M. Monroe, and S. A. Stanfield Oakley. 1990. Factor IX New London: Substitution of proline for glutamine at position 50 causes severe hemophilia B. Blood 75:1097–1104.

311. Miyata, T., H. Nishimura, K. Suehiro, H. Takeya, T. Okamura, M. Murakawa, Y. Niho, and S. Iwanaga. 1991. The 2nd EGF-like domain in factor IX is required for interaction with factor VIII. Thromb. Haemost. 65:471.

312. Carpenter, G., and M. I. Wahl. 1990. The epidermal growth factor family. In Handbook of Experimental Pharmacology, Vol. 95. M. B. Sporn, and A. B. Roberts, editors, Springer. 69–171.

313. Blasi, F., J. D. Vassalli, and J. Danö. 1987. Urokinase-type plasminogen activator: Proenzyme, receptor, and inhibitors. J. Cell. Biol. 104:801–804.

314. Zushi, M., K. Gomi, S. Yamamoto, I. Maruyama, T. Hayashi, and K. Suzuki. 1989. The last three consecutive epidermal growth factor–like structures of human thrombomodulin comprise the minimum functional domain for protein C-activating cofactor activity and anticoagulant activity. J. Biol. Chem. 264:10351–10353.

315. Hrabal, R., E. A. Komives, F. Ni. 1996. Structural resiliency of an EGF-like subdomain bound to its target protein, thrombin. Protein Sci. 5:195–203.

316. Husten, E. J., C. T. Esmon, and A. E. Johnson. 1987. The active site of blood coagulation factor Xa. Its distance from the phospholipid surface and its conformational sensitivity to components of the prothrombinase complex. J. Biol. Chem. 262:12953–12961.

317. Lenting, P. J., H. ter Maat, O. D. Christophe, D. J. G. Rees, K. Mertens. 1996. Calcium binding to the first epidermal growth factor–like domain of human blood coagulation factor IX promotes enzyme activity and factor VIII light chain binding. J. Biol. Chem. 271:25332–25337.

318. Christophe, O. D., P. J. Lenting, J. A. Kolkman, G. L. Brownlee, and K. Mertens. 1998. Blood coagulation Factor IX residues Glu78 and Arg94 provide a link between both epidermal growth factor–like domains that is crucial in the interaction with Factor VIII light chain. J. Biol. Chem. 273:222–227.

319. Brandstetter, H., D. Turk, H. W. Hoeffken, D. Grosse, J. Sturzebecher, P. D. Martin, B. F. Edwards, and W. Bode. 1992. Refined 2.3 An X-ray crystal structure of bovine thrombin complexes formed with the benzamidine and arginine-based thrombin inhibitors NAPAP, 4-TA-PAP and MQPA. A starting point for improving antithrombotics. J. Mol. Biol. 226(4):1085–99.

320. Astermark, J., P. W. Hogg, I. Björk, and J. Stenflo. 1992. Effects of gamma-carboxyglutamic acid and epidermal growth factor-like modules of factor IX on factor X activation. Studies using proteolytic fragments of bovine factor IX. J. Biol. Chem. 267:3249–3256.

321. Cheung, W. F., D. L. Straight, K. J. Smith, S. W. Lin, H. Roberts, and D. W. Stafford. 1991. The role of the epidermal growth factor–1 and hydrophobic stack domains of human factor IX in binding to endothelial cells. J. Biol. Chem. 266:8797–8800.

322. Hertzberg, M. S., O. Ben Tal, B. Furie, and B. C. Furie. 1992. Construction, expression, and characterization of a chimera of factor IX and factor X. The role of the second epidermal growth factor domain and serine protease domain in factor Va binding. J. Biol. Chem. 267(21):14759–66.

323. Dahlbäck, B., B. Hildebrand, and J. Malm. 1990. Characterization of functionally important domains in human vitamin K–dependent protein S using monoclonal antibodies. J. Biol. Chem. 265:8127–8135.

324. He, X., L. Shen, and B. Dahlbäck. 1995. Expression and functional characterization of chimeras between human and bovine vitamin K–dependent protein S defining modules important for the species-specificity of the activated protein C cofactor activity. Eur. J. Biochem. 227:433–440.

325. Hogg, P. J., A. K. Öhlin, and J. Stenflo. 1992. Identification of structural domains in protein C involved in its interaction with thrombin-thrombomodulin on the surface of endothelial cells. J. Biol. Chem. 267:703–706.

326. Magnusson, S., T. E. Petersen, L. Sottrup-Jensen, and H. Claeys. 1975. Complete Primary Structure of Prothrombin: Structure and Reactivity of Ten Carboxylated Glutamic Acid Residues and Regulation of Prothrombin Activation by Thrombin. In Proteases and Biological Control. E. Reich, D. B. Rifkin, and E. Shaw, editors. Cold Spring Harbor Laboratory., Cold Spring Harbor, N.Y. 123–149.

327. Gardell, S. J., L. T. Duong, R. E. Diehl, J. D. York, T. R. Hare, B. R. Register, J. W. Jacobs, R. A. F. Dixon, and P. A. Friedman. 1989. Isolation, characterization and cDNA cloning of vampire bat salivary plasminogen activator. J. Biol. Chem. 264:17947–17952.

328. Nakamura, T., T. Nishizawa, M. Hagiya, T. Seki, M. Shimonishi, A. Sugimura, K. Tashiro, and S. Shimizu. 1989. Molecular cloning and expression of human hepatocyte growth factor. Nature 342:440–443.

329. McLean, J. M., J. E. Tomlinson, W. J. Kuang, D. L. Eaton, E. Y. Chen, G. M. Fless, A. M. Scanu, and R. M. Lawn. 1987. cDna sequence of human apolipoprotein(a) is homologous to plasminogen. Nature 300:132–137.

330. Tulinsky, A. 1991. The structures of domains of blood proteins. Thromb. Haemost. 66:16–31.

331. Mulichak, A. M., and A. Tulinsky. 1990. Structure of the lysine-fibrin binding subsite of human plasminogen Kringle 4. Blood Coagul. Fibrinol. 1:673–679.

332. Seshadri, T. P., A. Tulinsky, E. Skrzypczak Jankun, and C. H. Park. 1991. Structure of bovine prothrombin fragment 1 refined at 2.25 Å resolution. J. Mol. Biol. 220:481–494.

333. Williams, R. J. P. 1989. NMR studies of mobility within protein structure. Eur. J. Biochem. 183:479–497.

334. Welsch, D. J., Nelsestuen, G.L. 1988. Carbohydrate-linked asparagine-101 of prothrombin contains a metal ion protected acetylation site. Acetylation of this site causes loss of metal ion induced protein fluorescence change. Biochemistry 27:4946–4952.

335. Berkowitz, P., N. W. Huh, K. E. Brostrom, M. G. Panek, D. J. Weber, A. Tulinsky, L. G. Pedersen, and R. G. Hiskey. 1992. A metal ion-binding site in the kringle region of bovine prothrombin fragment 1. J. Biol. Chem. 267(7):4570–4.

336. Bajaj, S. P., R. L. Butkowski, and K. G. Mann. 1975. Prothrombin fragments. Ca²⁺ binding and activation kinetics. J. Biol. Chem. 250:2150–2156.

337. Kotkow, K. J., B. Furie, and B. C. Furie. 1993. The interaction of prothrombin with phospholipid membranes is independent of either kringle domain. J. Biol. Chem. 268(21):15633–9.

338. Esmon, C. T., and C. M. Jackson. 1974. The conversion of prothrombin to thrombin. IV. The function of the fragment 2 region during activation in the presence of factor V. J. Biol. Chem. 249:7791–7797.

339. Kotkow, K. J., S. R. Deitcher, B. Furie, and B. C. Furie. 1995. The second kringle domain of prothrombin promotes factor Va–mediated prothrombin activation by prothrombinase. J. Biol. Chem. 270(9):4551–4557.

340. Myrmel, K. H., R. L. Lundblad, and K. G. Mann. 1976. Characteristics of the association between prothrombin fragment 2 and alpha-thrombin. Biochemistry 15:1767–1773.

341. Arni, R. K., K. Padmanabhan, K. P. Padmanabhan, T. P. Wu, and A. Tulinsky. 1993. Structures of the noncovalent complexes of human and bovine prothrombin fragment 2 with human PPACK-thrombin. Biochemistry 32(18):4727–4737.

342. Wu, W., J. D. Bancroft, and J. W. Suttie. 1997. Structural features of the kringle domain determine the intracellular degradation of under-γ-carboxylated prothrombin: Studies of chimeric rat/human prothrombin. Proc. Natl. Acad. Sci. U.S.A. 94:13654–13660.

343. Dahlback, B., A. Lundwall, and J. Stenflo. 1986. Localization of thrombin cleavage sites in the amino-terminal region of bovine protein S. J. Biol. Chem. 261(11):5111-5.

344. Dahlbäck, B. 1983. Purification of human vitamin K–dependent protein S and its limited proteolysis by thrombin. Biochem. J. 209:837–846.

345. Suzuki, K., J. Nishioka, and S. Hashimoto. 1983. Regulation of activated protein C by thrombin-modified protein S. J. Biochem. 94:699–705.

346. Walker, F. J. 1984. Regulation of vitamin K–dependent protein S. Inactivation with thrombin. J. Biol. Chem. 259:10335–10339.

347. Schechter, I., and A. Berger. 1967. On the size of the active site in proteases. I. Papain. Biochem. Biophys. Res. Commun. 27:157–162.

348. Kane, W. H., and E. W. Davie. 1988. Blood coagulation factors V and VIII: Structural and functional similarities and their relationship to hemorrhagic and trombotic disorders. Blood 71:539–555.

349. Gailani, D., and G. J. Broze, Jr. 1993. Factor XI activation by thrombin and factor XIa. Semin. Thromb. Hemost. 19(4):396–404.

350. Lorand, L. 1986. Activation of blood coagulation factor XIII. Ann. N.Y. Acad. Sci. 485:144–158.

351. Walz, D. E., I. J. W. Fenton, and M. A. Shuman. 1986. Bioregulatory functions of thrombin. Ann. N.Y. Acad. Sci. 485:1986.

352. Vu, T. K. H., V. I. Wheaton, D. T. Hung, I. F. Charo, and S. R. Coughlin. 1991. Domains specifying thrombin-receptor interaction. Nature 353:674–677.

353. Grand, R. J. A., A. S. Turnell, and P. W. Grabham. 1996. Cellular consequences of thrombin-receptor activation. Biochem. J. 313:353–368.

354. Ishihara, H., A. J. Connolly, D. Zeng, M. L. Kahn, Y. W. Zheng, C. Timmons, T. Tram, and S. R. Coughlin. 1997. Protease-activated receptor 3 is a second thrombin receptor in humans. Nature 386(6624):502–6.

355. Vu, T. K. H., D. T. Hung, V. I. Wheaton, and S. R. Coughlin. 1991. Molecular cloning of a functional thrombin receptor reveals a novel proteolytic mechanism of receptor activation. Cell 64:1057–1068.

356. Coughlin, S. R., T. K. Vu, D. T. Hung, and V. I. Wheaton. 1992. Characterization of a functional thrombin receptor. Issues and opportunities. J. Clin. Invest. 89(2):351–5.

357. Di Cera, E., Q. D. Dang, and Y. M. Ayala. 1997. Molecular mechanisms of thrombin function. CMLS, Cell. Mol. Life. Sci. 53:701–730.

358. Pryzdial, E. L. G., and K. G. Mann. 1991. The association of coagulation factor Xa and factor Va. J. Biol. Chem. 266:8969–8977.

359. Krishnaswamy, S., and K. G. Mann. 1988. The binding of factor Va to phospholipid vesicles. J. Biol. Chem. 263:5714–5723.

360. Ahmed, S. S., R. Rawala Sheikh, and P. N. Walsh. 1992. Comparative interactions of factor IX and factor IXa with human platelets. J. Biol. Chem. 264:3244–3251.

361. Krishnaswamy, S. 1990. Prothrombin complex assembly. Contributions of protein-protein and protein-membrane interactions toward complex formation. J. Biol. Chem. 265:3708–3718.

362. Miletich, J. P., C. M. Jackson, and P. W. Majerus. 1977. Interaction of coagulation factor Xa with human platelets. Proc. Natl. Acad. Sci. U.S.A. 74:4033–4036.

363. Miletich, J. P., C. M. Jackson, and P. W. Majerus. 1978. Properties of the factor Xa binding site on human platelets. J. Biol. Chem. 253:6908–6916.

364. Dahlbäck, B., and J. Stenflo. 1978. Binding of bovine coagulation factor Xa to platelets. Biochemistry 17:4938–4945.

365. Keyt, B., B. C. Furie, and B. Furie. 1982. Structural transitions in bovine factor X associated with metal binding and zymogen activation. Studies using conformation-specific antibodies. J. Biol. Chem. 257:8687–8695.

366. Bajaj, S. P., S. I. Rapaport, and S. L. Maki. 1985. A monoclonal antibody to factor IX that inhibits the factor VIII:Ca potentiation of factor X activation. J. Biol. Chem. 260:11574–11580.

367. Chattopadhya, A., and D. S. Fair. 1989. A limited number of regions on factor Xa are involved in prothrombin activation. Acta Chem. Scand. P 1102.

368. Jackson, C. M., and Y. Nemerson. 1980. Blood coagulation. Annu. Rev. Biochem. 49:765–811.

369. Rosing, J., R. F. A. Zwaal, and G. Tans. 1986. Formation of meizothrombin as intermediate in factor Xa–catalyzed prothrombin activation. J. Biol. Chem. 261:4224–4228.

370. Krishnaswamy, S., K. G. Mann, and M. E. Nesheim. 1986. The prothrombinase-catalyzed activation of prothrombin proceeds through the intermediate meizothrombin in an ordered, sequential reaction. J. Biol. Chem. 261:8997–8984.

371. Rabiet, M. J., A. Blashill, B. Furie, and B. C. Furie. 1986. Prothrombin fragment 1.2.3, a major product of prothrombin activation in human plasma. J. Biol. Chem. 261:13210–13215.

372. Krishnaswamy, S., W. R. Church, M. E. Nesheim, and K. G. Mann. 1987. Activation of human prothrombin by human prothrombinase. Influence of factor Va on the reaction mechanism. J. Biol. Chem. 262:3291–3299.

373. Wu, J. R., J. F. Wang, C. Zhou, and B. R. Lentz. 1998. Role of procoagulant lipids in human prothrombin activation 3: Analysis of multiple data sets in terms of a parallel/sequential kinetic model modified by membrane-mediated intermediate channeling. Manuscript.

374. Koppaka, V., J. Wang, M. Banerjee, and B. R. Lentz. 1996. Soluble phospholipids enhance factor Xa-catalyzed prothrombin activation in solution. Biochemistry. 35:7482.

375. Rand, M. D., J. B. Lock, C. van't Veer, D. P. Gaffney, and K. G. Mann. 1996. Blood clotting in minimally altered whole blood. Blood 88(9):3432–45.

376. Doyle, M. F., and K. G. Mann. 1990. Multiple active forms of thrombin. IV. Relative activities of meizothrombins. J. Biol. Chem. 265:10693–10701.

377. Tans, G., G. A. Nicolaes, M. C. L. G. D. Thomassen, H. C. Hemker, A. J. van Zonneveld, H. Pannekoek, and J. Rosing. 1994. Activation of human factor V by meizothrombin. J. Biol. Chem. 269:15969–15972.

378. Wu, Q., M. Tsiang, S. R. Lentz, and J. E. Sadler. 1992. Ligand specificity of human thrombomodulin. Equilibrium binding of human thrombin, meizothrombin, and factor Xa to recombinant thrombomodulin. J. Biol. Chem. 267(10):7083–8.

379. Kawabata, S. I., T. Morita, S. Iwanaga, and H. Igarashi. 1985. Staphylocoagulase-binding region in human prothrombin. J. Biochem. 97:325–331.

380. Kawabata, S. I., T. Morita, S. Iwanaga, and H. Igarashi. 1985. Differ-

ence in enzymatic properties between α-thrombin-staphylocoagulase complex and free α-thrombin. J. Biochem. 97:1073–1078.

381. Morita, T., and S. Iwanaga. 1981. Prothrombin activator from echis carinatus venom. Methods Enzymol. 80:303–311.

382. Spijer, H., J. W. P. Govers Riemslag, R. F. A. Zwaal, and J. Rosing. 1986. Prothrombin activation by an activator from the venom of *Oxyuranus scutellatus* (Taipan snake). J. Biol. Chem. 261:13258–13267.

383. Kisiel, W., M. A. Hermodson, and E. W. Davie. 1976. Factor X activating enzyme from Russell's viper venom: Isolation and characterization. Biochemistry 15:4901–4906.

384. Nakagaki, T., P. Lin, and W. Kisiel. 1992. Activation of human factor VII by the prothrombin activator from the venom of *Oxyuranus scutellatus* (Taipan snake). Thromb. Res. 65(1):105–16.

385. Di Cera, E., E. R. Guinto, A. Vindigni, Q. D. Dang, Y. M. Ayala, M. Wuyi, and A. Tulinsky. 1995. The Na+ binding site of thrombin. J. Biol. Chem. 270(38):22089–92.

386. Fenton, I. J. W., M. J. Fasco, A. B. Stackrow, D. L. Aronson, A. M. Young, and J. S. Finlayson. 1977. Human thrombins. Production, evaluation, and properties of α-thrombin. J. Biol. Chem. 252:3587–3598.

387. Fenton, J. W. 1986. Thrombin. Ann. N.Y. Acad. Sci. 485:5–15.

388. Rydel, T. J., K. G. Ravichandran, A. Tulinsky, W. Bode, R. Huber, C. Roitsch, and I. J. W. Fenton. 1990. The structure of a complex of recombinant hirudin and human α-thrombin. Science 249:277–280.

389. Skrzypczak-Jankun, E., V. E. Carperos, K. G. Ravichandran, A. Tulinsky, M. Westbrook, and J. M. Maraganore. 1991. Structure of the hirugen and hirulog 1 complexes of alpha-thrombin. J. Mol. Biol. 221(4):1379–93.

390. Fenton, J. 1988. Thrombin specificity. Ann. N.Y. Acad. Sci. 370:468–495.

391. Hopfner, K. P., and E. DiCera. 1992. Energetics of thrombin-fibrinogen interactions. Biochemistry 31:11567–11571.

392. Mathews, I. I., K. P. Padmanabhan, A. Tulinsky. 1994. Structure of a nonadecapeptide of the fifth EGF domain of thrombomodulin complexed with thrombin. Biochemistry 33:13547–13552.

393. Srinivasan, J., S. Hu, R. Hrabal, Y. Zhu, E.A. Komives, and F. Ni. 1994. Thrombin-bound structure of an EGF subdomain from human thrombomodulin determined by transferred nuclear overhauser effect. Biochemistry 33:13553–13560.

394. Mathews, II, K. P. Padmanabhan, V. Ganesh, A. Tulinsky, M. Ishii, J. Chen, C. W. Turck, S. R. Coughlin, and J. W. N. Fenton. 1994. Crystallographic structures of thrombin complexed with thrombin receptor peptides: existence of expected and novel binding modes. Biochemistry 33(11):3266–79.

395. Hofsteenge, J., P. J. Braun, and S. R. Stone. 1988. Enzymatic properties of proteolytic derivatives of human α-thrombin. Biochemistry 27:2144–2151.

396. Guintor, E. R., A. Vindigni, Y. M. Ayala, Q. D. Dang, E. Di Cera. 1995. Identification of residues linked to the slow -> fast transition of thrombin. Proc. Natl. Acad. Sci. U.S.A. 92:11185–11189.

397. Church, F. C., C. W. Pratt, C. M. Noyes, T. Kalayanamit, G. B. Sherrill, R. B. Tobin, and J. B. Meade. 1989. Structural and functional properties of human α-thrombin, phosphopyridoxylated α-thrombin, and gammaT-thrombin. J. Biol. Chem. 264:18419–18425.

398. Wells, C. M., and E. Di Cera. 1992. Thrombin is a Na(+)-activated enzyme. Biochemistry 31(47):11721–30.

399. Suelter, C. H. 1970. Enzymes activated by monovalent cations. Science 168:789–795.

400. Dang, O. D., A. Vindigni, and E. Di Cera. 1995. An allosteric switch controls the procoagulant and anticoagulant activities of thrombin. Proc. Natl. Acad. Sci. U.S.A. 92(13):5977–81.

401. Folkers, P. J. M., G. Clore, D. C. Friscol, J. Dodt, S. Kohler, and A. M. Gronenborn. 1989. Solution structure of recombinant Hirudin and the Lys 47-Glu mutant: A nuclear magnetic resonance and hybrid geometry-dynamical stimulated annealing study. Biochemistry 28:2601–2617.

402. Haruyama, H., and K. Wuthrich. 1989. Conformation of recombinant desulfatohirudin in aqueous solution determined by nuclear magnetic resonance. Biochemistry 28(10):4301–12.

403. Grütter, M. G., J. P. Priestle, J. Rahuel, H. Grossenbacher, W. Bode, J. Hofstenge, and R. S. Stone. 1990. Crystal structure of the thrombin-Hirudin complex: A novel mode of serine protease inhibition. EMBO J. 9:2361–2365.

404. Blackhart, B. D., G. Cuenco, T. Toda, R. M. Scarborough, D. L. Wolf, and V. Ramakrishnan. 1994. The anion-binding exosite is critical for the high affinity binding of thrombin to the human thrombin receptor. Growth Factors 11(1):17–28.

405. Fenton, I. J. W., and D. H. Bing. 1986. Thrombin active-site regions. Semin. Thromb. Hemost. 12:200–208.

406. Brezniak, D. V., M. S. Brown, J. I. Witting, D. A. Walz, and I. J. W. Fenton. 1990. Human α-to EPSILON-thrombin cleavage occurs with neutrophil cathepsin g or chymotrypsin while fibrinogen clotting activity is retained. Biochemistry 29:3536–3542.

407. Bode, W., H. Brandstetter, T. Mather, and M. T. Stubbs. 1997. Comparative analysis of haemostatic proteinases: Structural aspects of thrombin, factor Xa, factor IXa and protein C. Thromb. Haemost. 78(1):501–11.

408. Brandstetter, H., A. Kühne, W. Bode, R. Huber, W. von der Saal, K. Wirthensohn, and R. A. Engh. 1996. X-ray structure of active site-inhibited clotting factor Xa. Implications for drug design and substrate recognition. J. Biol. Chem. 271:29988–29992.

409. Rezaie, A. R., P. F. Neuenschwander, J. M. Morrissey, and C. T. Esmon. 1993. Analysis of the functions of the first epidermal growth factor–like domain of factor X. J. Biol. Chem. 268:8176–8180.

410. Hopfner, K. P., H. Brandsetter, A. Karcher, E. Kopetzki, R. Huber, R. A. Engh, and W. Bode. 1997. Converting blood coagulation factor IXa into factor Xa: Dramatic increase in amidolytic activity identifies important active site determinants. EMBO J. 16:6626–6635.

411. Bode, W., and P. Schwager. 1975. The single calcium-binding site of crystalline bovine beta-Trypsin. FEBS Lett. 56:139–143.

412. Bode, W., and P. Schwager. 1975. The refined crystal structure of bovine beta-Trypsin at 1.8 Å resolution. II. Crystallographic refinement, calcium binding site, benzamidine binding site and active site at pH 7.0. J. Mol. Biol. 98:693–717.

413. Bode, W., I. Mayr, U. Baumann, R. Huber, S. R. Stone, and J. Hofsteenge. 1989. The refined 1.9 Å crystal structure of human alpha-thrombin: Interaction with D-Phe-Pro-Arg chloromethylketone and significance of the Tyr-Pro-Pro-Trp insertion segment. EMBO J. 8(11):3467–75.

414. Sabharwal, A. K., J. J. Birktoft, J. Gorka, P. Wildgoose, L. C. Petersen, and S. P. Bajaj. 1995. High affinity Ca²⁺-binding site in the serine protease domain of human factor VIIa and its role in tissue factor binding and development of catalytic activity. J. Biol. Chem. 270:15523–15530.

415. Bajaj, S. P., A. K. Sabharwal, J. Gorka, and J. J. Birktoft. 1991. Use of antibodies and factor IX variants in probing conformational transitions in the protease domain of factor IX. Thromb. Haemost. 65:293.

416. Bajaj, S. P., A. K. Sabharwal, J. Gorka, and J. J. Birktoft. 1992. Antibody-probed conformational transitions in the protease domain of human factor IX upon calcium binding and zymogen activation: Putative high affinity Ca²⁺-binding site in the protease domain. Proc. Natl. Acad. Sci. U.S.A. 89:152–156.

417. Rezaie, A. R., P. F. Neuenschwander, J. H. Morrissey, and C. T. Esmon. 1993. Analysis of the functions of the first epidermal growth factor-like domain of factor X. J. Biol. Chem. 268(11):8176–80.

418. Rezaie, A. R., Esmon, C.T. 1994. Asp-70→lys mutant of factor X lacks high affinity Ca²⁺ binding site yet retains function. J. Biol. Chem. 269:21495–21499.

419. Rezaie, A. R., T. Mather, F. Sussman, and C. T. Esmon. 1994. Mutation of Glu 80 to Lys results in a protein C mutant that no longer requires Ca²⁺ for rapid activation by the thrombin-thrombomodulin complex. J. Biol. Chem. 269:3151–3154.

420. Roberts, H. R. 1993. Molecular biology of hemophilia B. Thromb. Haemost. 70(1):1–9.

421. Reiner, A. P., and E. W. Davie. 1994. The Physiology and Biochemistry of Factor IX. Churchill Livingstone. pp. 309–331.

422. Link, R. P., and F. J. Castellino. 1983. Kinetic comparison of bovine blood coagulation factors IXa alpha and IXa beta toward bovine factor X. Biochemistry 22:4033–4041.

423. Noyes, C. M., M. J. Griffith, H. R. Roberts, and R. L. Lundblad. 1983. Identification of the molecular defect in factor IX Chapel Hill: Substitution of histidine for arginine at position 145. Proc. Natl. Acad. Sci. U.S.A. 80:4200–4202.

424. Liddell, M. B., I. R. Peake, S. A. M. Taylor, D. P. Lillicrap, J. C. Giddings, and A. L. Bloom. 1989. Factor IX Cardiff: A variant factor IX protein that shows abnormal activation is caused by an arginine to cysteine substitution at position 145. Br. Med. J. 72:556–560.

425. Suehiro, K., S. I. Kawabata, T. Miyata, H. Takeya, J. Takamutsu, K.

Ogata, T. Kamiya, H. Saito, Y. Niho, and S. Iwanaga. 1989. Blood clotting factor IX BM Nagoya. Substitution of arginine 180 by tryptophan and its activation by α-chymotrypsin and rat mast cell chymase. J. Biol. Chem. 264:21257–21265.

426. Huang, M. N., C. K. Kasper, H. R. Roberts, D. W. Stafford, and K. A. High. 1989. Molecular defect in factor IX Hilo, a hemophilia Bm variant: Arg–>Gln at the carboxyterminal clevage site of the activation peptide. Acta Chem. Scand. 73:718–721.

427. Sakai, T., A. Yoshioka, K. Yamamono, K. Niinomi, Y. Fujimura, H. Fukui, T. Miyata, and S. Iwanaga. 1989. Blood clotting factor IX Kashihara: Amino acid substitution of Valine-182 by Phenylalanine. J. Biochem. 105:756–759.

428. Spitzer, S. G., U. R. Pendurti, C. K. Kasper, and S. P. Bajaj. 1988. Molecular defect in factor IXBm Lake Elsinore. Substitution of Ala 390 by Val in the datalytic domain. J. Biol. Chem. 263:10545–10548.

429. Ware, J., L. Davis, D. Frazier, P. S. Bajaj, and D. W. Stafford. 1988. Genetic defect responsible for the dysfunctional protein: Factor IX Long Beach. Blood 72:820–822.

430. Spitzer, S. G., B. J. Warner Cramer, C. K. Kasper, and S. P. Bajaj. 1990. Replacement of Isoleucine-397 by Threonine in the clotting proteinase factor IXa (Los Angeles and Long Beach variants) affects macromolecular catalysis but not L-Tosylarginine Methyl Ester Hydrolysis. Biochem. J. 265:219–225.

431. Attree, O., D. Vidaud, M. Vidaud, S. Amselm, J. M. Lavergne, and M. Goossens. 1989. Mutations in the catalytic domain of human coagulation factor IX: Rapid characterization by direct genomic sequencing of DNA fragments displaying an altered melting behavior. Genomics 4:266–272.

432. James, H. L., A. Girolami, and D. S. Fair. 1991. Moleculara defect in coagulation factor X Friuli results from a substitution of serine for Proline at position 343. Blood 77:317–323.

433. Henriksen, R. A., and K. G. Mann. 1988. Identification of the primary structure defect in the dysthrombin thrombin quick I: Substitution of cysteine for Arginine-392. Biochemistry 27:9160–9165.

434. Jakubowski, H. V., and W. G. Owen. 1989. Macromolecular specificity determinants on thrombin for fibrinogen and thrombomodulin. J. Biol. Chem. 264:11117–11121.

435. Henriksen, R. A., and K. G. Mann. 1989. Substitution of valine for glycine-558 in the congenital dysthrombin thrombin quick II alters primary substrate specificy. Biochemistry 28:2078–2082.

436. Miyata, T., T. Morita, T. Inomoto, S. Kawauchi, A. Shirakami, and S. Iwanaga. 1987. Prothrombin Tokushima, a replacement of Arginine-418 by tryptophan that imparis the fibrinogen clotting activity of derived thrombin Tokushima. Biochemistry 26:1117–1122.

437. Joseph, D. R., S. H. Hall, and F. S. French. 1987. Rat androgen-binding protein: Evidence for identical subunits and amino acid sequence homology with human sex hormone-binding globulin. Proc. Natl. Acad. Sci. U.S.A. 84:339–343.

438. Petra, P. H., S. Kumar, R. Hayes, L. H. Ericsson, and K. Titani. 1986. Molecular organization of the sex steroid-binding protein(SBP) of human plasma. J. Steroid. Biochem. 24:45–49.

439. Hryb, D. J., M. S. Kahn, N. A. Romas, and W. Rosner. 1990. The control of the interaction of sex hormone-binding globulin with its receptor by steroid hormones. J. Biol. Chem. 265:6048–6054.

440. Gershagen, S., P. Fernlund, and C. M. Edenbrandt. 1991. The genes for SHBG/ABP and the SHBG-like region of vitamin K–dependent protein S have evolved from a common ancestral gene. J. Steroid Biochem. Molec. Biol. 40:763–769.

19 The Protein C Anticoagulant System

▼▼▼▼ Björn Dahlbäck and Johan Stenflo

▼ ▼

Introduction

Blood coagulation is rapidly activated in response to vascular injury. A cascade of zymogen activations results in the formation of thrombin, a multifunctional serine protease which activates platelets and converts soluble fibrinogen to a fibrin network.[1–5] Thrombin also stimulates the coagulation cascade by feed-back activation of the two regulatory proteins, factor V (FV) and factor VIII (FVIII) (Fig. 19–1). The multiple zymogen activations of the coagulation cascade provide the potential for explosive amplification resulting in local generation of high thrombin concentrations and coagulation. In vivo, the coagulation system is carefully regulated to ensure precise delivery of thrombin at the site of lesion, without clot propagation resulting in occlusion of the circulatory system. Under normal conditions, the balance between pro- and anticoagulant activities is shifted in favor of anticoagulation. The endothelial cells are crucial for the inhibition of clot formation, e.g., they synthesize and secrete prostacyclin, several potent vessel wall relaxing factors, and tissue type plasminogen activator.[6, 7] Two other anticoagulant mechanisms involve close interactions between plasma proteins and the endothelial cell surface. One depends on the presence of heparin-like molecules on the endothelial cell surface which accelerate antithrombin (AT)-dependent inactivation of coagulation proteases.[8, 9] The other involves the endothelial cell membrane protein, thrombomodulin (TM), which binds thrombin with high affinity and changes its substrate specificity. When thrombin binds to TM, its procoagulant properties are lost and it is converted into a potent activator of protein C, which is the key component in a physiologically important anticoagulant system, commonly referred to as the protein C anticoagulant system.[10–13]

Protein C

Protein C was purified from bovine plasma in 1976 and described as a previously unknown vitamin K–dependent

protein.[14] It was soon found to be a zymogen of a serine protease with anticoagulant properties.[15, 16] A few years later, protein C was also isolated from human plasma.[17] The rapid elucidation of the functions of activated protein C (APC) was facilitated by the discovery that it was identical to autoprothrombin II-A, an anticoagulant factor described already in 1960.[18] Autoprothrombin II-A activity was formed upon incubation of 'prothrombin complex' with thrombin and was originally believed to be derived from the prothrombin molecule. In the early 1970s it was shown that the precursor protein of autoprothrombin II-A was distinct from prothrombin.[19]

After its activation on the surface of endothelial cells by the thrombin-TM complex, APC catalyzes the proteolytic degradation of the membrane-bound thrombin-activated forms of FV and FVIII (FVa and FVIIIa) (see Fig. 19–1). This mechanism is of crucial importance for the regulation of blood coagulation in vivo. The anticoagulant activity of APC is stimulated by two synergistic cofactors, protein S and FV. In human plasma, approximately 40 per cent of protein S is free, the remaining 60 per cent circulating bound to C4b-binding protein (C4BP), an inhibitor of the classical complement pathway.[20, 21] Only free protein S has APC cofactor activity, whereas both forms of protein S have been found to express an anticoagulant activity which is independent of APC.[22–24] FV serves as APC cofactor in the inhibition of FVIIIa, whereas it is not known if FV is also an APC cofactor in the inhibition of FVa.[25–28] APC is slowly neutralized in vivo by at least three protease inhibitors, the protein C inhibitor (PCI), α_1-antitrypsin, and α_2-macroglobulin.[29–34]

The physiological importance of the protein C anticoagulant system is most clearly demonstrated by the massive thrombotic complications occurring in infants with homozygous protein C or S deficiency.[35] Recent gene knock-out experiments in mice confirmed the importance of protein C for regulation of blood coagulation, as mice deficient in

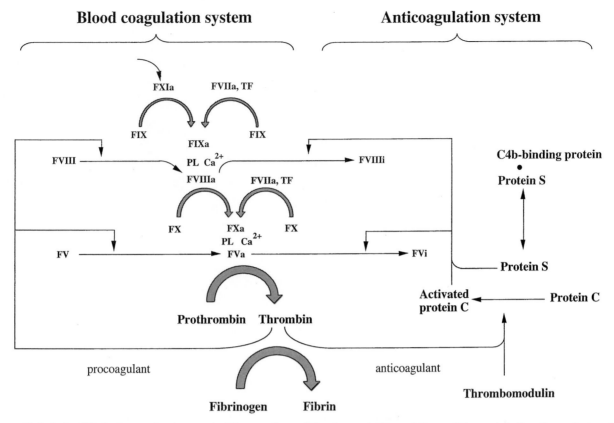

Figure 19–1. A simplified scheme showing most of the reactions of blood coagulation and those of the protein C anticoagulant system. The reactions resulting in the formation of FXIa have not been included in the coagulation cascade, nor are the feed-back activations of FV, FVII, and FVIII by FXa shown. The scheme emphasizes the balance between the pro- and anticoagulant mechanisms of thrombin and the specificity of APC. APC degrades FVa and FVIIIa when they are bound to phospholipid (PL). The synergistic APC cofactor function of protein S and FV is not indicated in the figure. The binding of protein S to C4b-binding protein results in inhibition of its anticoagulant properties. TF denotes tissue factor which triggers the reactions involving FVII.

protein C have a severe thrombotic phenotype.[36] In many patients with venous thrombosis, genetic defects affecting the function of the protein C system, either causing heterozygous deficiencies of protein C and protein S or activated protein C resistance due to a common $R^{506}Q$ mutation in the FV gene, are risk factors for the disease.[37–43]

▼ FACTOR Va AND FACTOR VIIIa, SUBSTRATES FOR ACTIVATED PROTEIN C

The two substrates for APC, FVa and FVIIIa, are homologous high molecular weight plasma glycoproteins.[44–46] The inactive procofactors FV and FVIII are converted to FVa and FVIIIa through limited proteolysis by thrombin or FXa (Fig. 19–2). FVIII is described in detail elsewhere in this book. (See Chapter 21.) FV is a single-chain high molecular weight glycoprotein ($M_r = 330,000$), occurring in human plasma at a concentration of approximately 7 mg/l. In addition, platelets contain approximately 30 per cent of the FV in human blood. After its activation by thrombin or FXa, FVa together with negatively charged phospholipid and Ca^{2+} functions as a high affinity receptor for FXa (K_d approximately 1×10^{-10} M).[45–48] This membrane-bound macromolecular complex, the so-called prothrombinase complex, can be assembled on the surface of activated platelets, platelet microparticles, macrophages, and endothelial cells. The in-

tact prothrombinase complex activates prothrombin 10^5–10^6-fold more rapidly than does FXa alone. The rate enhancement has two causes: (1) a lowering of the K_m for prothrombin mediated by phospholipid; and (2) an increase in the V_{max} for prothrombin activation mediated by FVa.[46, 48] The latter effect accounts for an approximately 10^3-fold increase in the rate of prothrombin activation. The potent anticoagulant activity of APC is in part mediated by the degradation of FVa, resulting in inhibition of the prothrombinase activity. FVIIIa has a function analogous to that of FVa in the FXase complex (FVIIIa, phospholipid, Ca^{2+}, and FIXa), and its activity is regulated in a similar fashion by APC.[1, 2, 47, 49]

FV (comprising 2196 amino acid residues) and FVIII (2332 amino acid residues long) have evolved from a common ancestral protein.[45, 49–52] Both contain two types of internal repeats, three A-domains and two C-domains (see Fig. 19–2). Three A-domains also appear in ceruloplasmin, a copper-binding protein in plasma. The amino acid sequences of the A-domains in FV, FVIII, and ceruloplasmin are approximately 40 per cent identical. The 3-D structure of ceruloplasmin, determined with X-ray crystallography, has been used to create molecular models of the three A-domains in FV and FVIII.[53–55] In ceruloplasmin the three A-domains are arranged in a triangular fashion and it is reasonable to suppose the A-domains of FV and FVIII to have similar molecular arrangements (see Fig. 19–2). FV contains one copper ion, the function of which is unknown.[56] In FV,

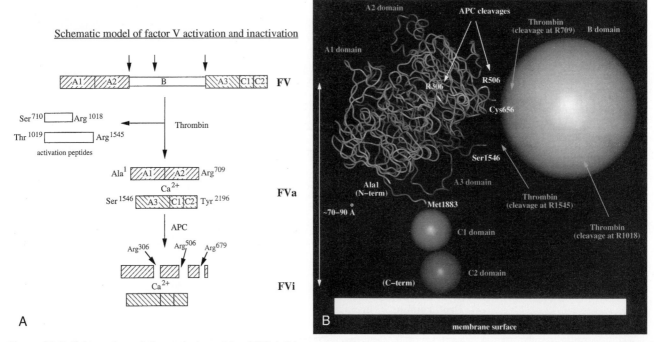

Schematic model of factor V activation and inactivation

Figure 19–2. Schematic and theoretical models of FV. *A*, Schematic model demonstrating the multiple domains of FV (A1-A2-B-A3-C1-C2) and the proteolytic activation and inactivation events. Thrombin cleaves three peptide bonds, as indicated by the arrows. The heavy (residues 1–709) and light (residues 1546–2196) chains form a calcium-dependent complex, constituting FVa, whereas the activation fragments from the B-domain have no known function. APC inactivates FVa by cleavage of the heavy chain at Arg306, Arg506, and Arg679. *B*, A theoretical model of the three A domains of FV.[55] Arg306 and Arg506 (cleavage sites for APC) are shown as spheres; the N-term of the A1 domain and the N-term and C-term of the A3 domain are labeled for orientation. The B-domain has no known 3-D structure. The three thrombin cleavage sites within this domain are indicated. The C2 and possibly A3 domains have been reported to be important for membrane binding (see text). (Fig. 19–2*B* was kindly prepared by Dr Bruno Villoutreix.)

two A-domains occupy the aminoterminal region (residues 1–709), whereas the third A-domain and the two C-domains constitute the carboxy-terminal part of the molecule (residues 1546–2196). The two C-domains in FV and those in FVIII manifest approximately 35 to 50 per cent amino acids sequence identity, and share approximately 20 per cent amino acid sequence identity with the first 150 amino acids of discoidin I, a tetrameric galactose binding lectin essential for cell adhesion in the slime mold *Dictyostelium discoidium*.[52, 57] FV is very rich in carbohydrate and contains both N- and O-linked sugars. The central portion of FV, the B-domain, contains many potential N-linked carbohydrate attachment sites and has been found to be highly glycosylated. The B-domain of FVIII is also rich in carbohydrate, but manifests no significant amino acid sequence similarity with the B-domain of FV.

During thrombin activation of FV, three peptide bonds are cleaved, Arg709–Ser710, Arg1018–Thr1019, and Arg1545–Ser1546, yielding four major fragments.[44, 45, 50–52, 58–62] The same three sites can also be cleaved by FXa, resulting in the activation of FV.[63] The heavy chain (residues 1–709) forms a noncovalent complex with the light chain (residues 1546–2196), and together they constitute FVa. The two fragments that are derived from the B-domain are activation peptides with no known function. Two phospholipid binding regions have been localized to the light chain of FVa, one in the A3-domain and the other in the C2-domain.[64–67] Both chains support the interaction with FXa, whereas only the heavy chain appears to interact with prothrombin.[48, 68–72] A peptide corresponding to residues 493–506 of FV has been found to inhibit the interaction between

FXa and FVa, suggesting this region of FV to contain a binding site for FXa.[73] The carboxyl-terminal Asp683–Arg709 part of the heavy chain is required for optimal interaction of FVa with FXa and prothrombin.[74]

APC efficiently degrades phospholipid-bound FVa and FVIIIa, but is also able to cleave intact FV and FVIII.[10, 45, 75–78] In vivo, the specificity of APC for the membrane-bound forms of the cofactors is illustrated by the observation that the plasma concentrations of FV and FVIII are unaffected by APC infusion.[79–81] APC cleaves three peptide bonds in the heavy chain of FVIIIa, Arg336–Met337, Arg562–Gly563, and Arg740–Ser741.[77]

In phospholipid bound human FVa, APC cleaves the heavy chain at Arg306, Arg506, and Arg679.[78] Cleavage at Arg506 precedes the cleavages at Arg306 and Arg679. Two explanations have been put forward to account for the apparently sequential cleavage at Arg506, Arg306, and Arg679. One is that the Arg506 cleavage facilitates subsequent cleavages at Arg306 and Arg679.[78] The other explanation is that the Arg506 site is kinetically preferred over the Arg306 and Arg679 sites but that the cleavages occur independently of each other.[82] Owing to the difference in kinetics between the two most important sites at Arg306 and Arg506, inactivation of FVa by APC on phospholipid proceeds via a biphasic reaction consisting of a rapid (k = 4.3 × 10⁷ M⁻¹ s⁻¹) and a slow phase (k = 2.3 × 10⁶ M⁻¹ s⁻¹). The rapid phase correlates to the Arg506 cleavage and yields an intermediate with reduced FVa activity. The slow phase is the result of the Arg306 cleavage. After cleavage at Arg506, FVa manifests 40 per cent cofactor activity in a prothrombin activation system that contains a high FXa concentration (5 nM) but has virtually no cofactor activity at low FXa concentration (0.3 nM). Thus, FVa which is cleaved at Arg506 is impaired in its ability to interact with FXa. The cleavage at Arg506 in membrane-bound FVa is characterized by a low K_m for FVa (20 nM) and by a k_{cat} of 0.96 s^{-1}, whereas the cleavage at Arg306 has a K_m of 196 nM and a k_{cat} of 0.37 s^{-1}.[82] In FVa, the Arg506 site can be cleaved also in the absence of phospholipid membranes, though the cleavage reaction is quite inefficient. In human FVa, the light chain is not cleaved by APC. Intact human FV bound to negatively charged phospholipid vesicles can be cleaved by APC at Arg306, Arg506, Arg679, and Lys994.[78] In the absence of a membrane surface, there is no cleavage of FV by APC.

As FXa and APC compete for binding sites on FVa, the binding of FXa to FVa is associated with protection of FVa from degradation by APC.[75, 76, 83] Only the Arg506 site in FVa is protected by FXa, which is consistent with the suggestion that the binding site on FVa for FXa involves residues 493–506.[73, 84] As a consequence of the interaction between FXa and FVa, FVa is optimally protected from inactivation by APC when incorporated in the prothrombinase complex. FVa residues 493–506 also contribute a binding site for protein S, thus accounting for the observed ability of protein S to counteract the protective effect of FXa toward APC cleavage of FVa.[73, 85] Protein S functions as a cofactor to APC in the degradation of FVa by promoting the cleavage at Arg306 about 20-fold, whereas the Arg506 site is unaffected by the APC cofactor activity of protein S.[84]

The mechanism by which protein S selectively promotes the Arg306 cleavage in FVa is beginning to be unraveled. Protein S is involved in multiple protein–protein interactions on the surface of negatively charged phospholipid vesicles, including interactions with APC, FV/FVa, and possibly also with FXa. Protein S affects the binding of APC to negatively charged phospholipid, which in the absence of protein S is characterized by a K_d of approximately 7 × 10^{-8} M.[86] The presence of protein S on the phospholipid membrane enhances the affinity of APC for the membrane approximately 10-fold.[87] In a system with purified components, FVa has a similar effect and increases the affinity of active-site inhibited APC for the membrane approximately 10-fold.[86] Intact FV gives a fivefold increase in the affinity of active-site inhibited APC for the membrane, suggesting that APC may interact with both FVa and FV. The interaction between APC and FV may be physiologically important because FV functions as a synergistic APC cofactor with protein S in the inactivation of the membrane-bound FVIIIa.[25, 26, 28, 88]

The interaction between APC and protein S on the membrane surface affects the orientation of the active site of APC. In a study using the fluorescence resonance energy transfer technique, it was estimated that the distance of the active site of APC from the phospholipid membrane in the absence of protein S was around 94 Å, a distance which decreased to 84 Å in the presence of protein S.[89] The relocation of the active site of APC relative to the membrane surface may be the structural explanation of the specific stimulation by protein S of the APC-mediated cleavage at Arg306 in FVa. The activity of APC is not only influenced by protein components such as protein S and FV, but also by the phospholipid composition of the membrane and by heparin. Thus, although phosphatidylserine is required for expression of anticoagulant APC activity, the concomitant

presence of phosphatidylethanolamine in the membrane results in a 10-fold increase in APC anticoagulant activity.[90] Heparin, on the other hand, appears to specifically stimulate APC-mediated cleavage of intact FV, but not to affect the degradation of FVa.[91]

▼ STRUCTURE-FUNCTION RELATIONSHIPS OF PROTEIN C

Protein C is a zymogen of a serine protease with a plasma concentration of 3–5 mg/l.[14, 15, 17, 92] It is synthesized in the liver as a 461 amino acid single-chain precursor which contains a signal peptide and a propeptide.[93–95] Prior to secretion, the 42 amino acid preproleader sequence is removed by two proteolytic cleavages, first by a signal peptidase at Gly-25 and then by the propeptide processing enzyme at Arg-1.[96] The propeptide in protein C is similar to propeptides in the other vitamin K–dependent proteins and is recognized by the vitamin K–dependent carboxylase (see Chapter 18). Single-chain protein C is cleaved between Arg157 and Thr158 by an enzyme with trypsin-like specificity, in the Golgi apparatus. In a subsequent step, presumably in plasma, Arg157 and Lys156 (numbering from the NH$_2$-terminus of the mature single chain protein) are removed by an unidentified enzyme with carboxypeptidase B–like specificity.[97] In human plasma, approximately 85 per cent of protein C consists of two polypeptide chains linked by a single disulfide bridge, whereas the remaining 15 per cent is single-chain protein C.[98] Single- and two-chain protein C appear to have equal biological activity after activation. The light and heavy chains of protein C in plasma contain 155 and 262 amino acids, respectively, and the apparent molecular weight of the mature protein is approximately 62,000. The molecular weight calculated from the amino acid sequence of the apoprotein is 47,456. Protein C contains four N-linked carbohydrate side chains, one in the light chain and three in the heavy chain, which together account for approximately 23 per cent of the molecular weight. The amino acid sequence identity between human and bovine protein C is 74 per cent, and the identity between the two species at the nucleotide level is 82 per cent.[93–95, 99, 100] cDNA sequences of mouse and rat protein C have been reported.[101, 102] In addition, partial nucleotide sequences for the catalytic domain of protein C from rhesus monkey, dog, cat, goat, and horse are known.[103] The mature protein C molecule contains a Gla-domain, two EGF-like domains, and a serine protease domain (Fig. 19–3). The three-dimensional (3-D) structure of the Gla-less form of active site-inhibited human APC has been determined at 2.8 Å resolution.[104]

Gla-domain

The Gla-domain in human protein C contains nine Gla-residues, and that of bovine protein C eleven.[93–95, 99] The 3-D structure of the Gla-domain has not been determined, but the pronounced sequence similarity with the Gla-domain of prothrombin suggests that both the 3-D structure and the Ca^{2+}-binding properties of the protein C Gla-domain are similar to those of prothrombin fragment 1.[105] In its calcium-saturated conformation, the Gla-domain interacts with negatively charged phospholipid containing phosphatidylserine

Protein C

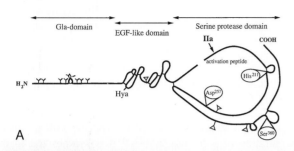

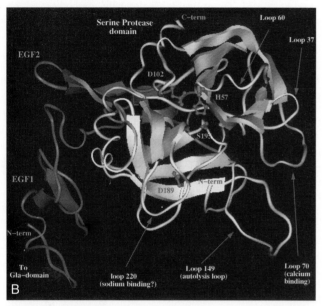

Figure 19–3. Human protein C. *A,* Schematic model demonstrating the modular composition of protein C. The arrow indicates the thrombin (IIa) cleavage site, a cleavage resulting in activation of protein C. The amino acid residues in the catalytic triad are enclosed in the ovals. Human protein C contains nine Gla-residues (Y) and four potential sites for N-linked glycosylation (Y). *B,* Richardson drawing of the X-ray structure of the Gla-domain-less activated protein C with a view down the active site.[104] Residues belonging to the active site triad are displayed. This triad involves the nucleophilic Ser360 (S195; chymotrypsin numbering), the nearby His211 (H57; chymotrypsin numbering) and the negatively charged Asp257 (D102; chymotrypsin numbering). Also shown is the residue at the bottom of the specificity pocket, Asp354 (D189; chymotrypsin numbering). Some loops of functional importance surrounding the active site cleft are labeled (see text). (Fig. 19–3B was kindly prepared by Dr Bruno Villoutreix.)

and/or phosphatidylethanolamine. The presence of phosphatidylethanolamine in the membrane enhances both protein C activation and the anticoagulant activity of APC[90, 106]

The mechanism of interaction of the Gla-domain of protein C and the phospholipid membrane is not fully understood. There are two hypotheses about the location of the phospholipid binding site in Gla-domains and the mode of interaction between Gla-domains and the membrane. According to one model, a small hydrophobic cluster present in the Gla-domain of all vitamin K–dependent clotting factors (Phe4, Leu5, and Leu8 in human protein C) inserts into the hydrocarbon region of the membrane to a depth that allows simultaneous bridging of the protein-bound calcium ions to the phospholipid head groups.[107–110] The importance of Leu5 in protein C for anticoagulant activity and for

phospholipid binding has been demonstrated by site-directed mutagenesis. Replacement of Leu5 with Gln, Ala, Val, Ile, or Trp yielded protein C mutants expressing anticoagulant activities of approximately 2 per cent, 28 per cent, 51 per cent, 98 per cent, and 105 per cent, respectively.[108, 109] Using a similar approach, Phe4 and Leu8 have been shown to be functionally important.[111] The low level of activity was interpreted as being related to loss of phospholipid binding ability. However, the insertion mechanism does not explain a number of earlier observations regarding the interaction between the phospholipid membrane and Gla-domains, e.g., it does not explain the 1000-fold range of membrane affinities observed with different naturally occurring vitamin K–dependent proteins.[112] This suggests electrostatic interactions between the Gla-domain and the phospholipid membrane to be important determinants for the binding characteristics. The membrane-binding properties of the Gla-domain-containing proteins appear to correlate best with amino acid residue differences at positions 11, 33, and 34 (numbers in prothrombin which correlate to positions 10, 32, and 33 in protein C), residues which are clustered on the Gla-domain surface near a calcium-lined pore in the Gla-domain. To accommodate such observations and earlier results, an alternative binding mechanism was proposed which consists of membrane attachment through an ion pair that is formed between one phospholipid head group and the calcium-lined pore, in addition to protein-membrane interactions involving amino acid residues at positions 32 and 33 in protein C.[112] Site-directed mutagenesis of recombinant human and bovine protein C has yielded results in support of this hypothesis.[113] The background to these experiments is that bovine protein C has 10-fold less affinity than human protein C for negatively charged phospholipid membranes. This was hypothesized to be due to a Pro at position 10 in bovine protein C, versus a His at the corresponding locus in human protein C. Replacement of Pro10 in bovine protein C with His and the reverse change in human protein C resulted in a 10-fold increase in membrane affinity for bovine protein C (and increased anticoagulant activity), and a fivefold decrease in affinity of human protein C for phospholipid membranes (plus decreased activity).[113]

A systematic in vitro mutagenesis approach has been taken to elucidate the importance of individual Gla-residues for Ca^{2+}- and phospholipid binding, as well as for anticoagulant activity.[114–121] This demonstrated that the function of the different Gla-residues is not equivalent. Some Gla-residues are buried and are mainly important for the folding of the domain, whereas others are surface exposed. Certain mutations (Gla to Asp mutations at positions 7, 16, 20, and 26) severely affected Ca^{2+}- and phospholipid binding as well as anticoagulant activity, whereas others had little (Gla to Asp mutations at positions 6, 14, and 19) or moderate effects (Gla to Asp mutations at positions 25 and 29). High affinity Ca^{2+}-binding was related to Gla-residues at positions 6, 16, 25, and 26, whereas Gla-residues at positions 7, 14, 19, 20, and 29 bound Ca^{2+} more weakly.[121] Gla16 and Gla26 were found to be more important than Gla14 and Gla19 for the induction of conformational changes.[117]

The importance of Gla20 and Gla26 is further demonstrated by the defective function of naturally occurring protein C mutants in patients with thrombosis; Gla20 to Ala in protein C Vermont and Gla26 to Lys in protein C Mie.[122–125]

Other amino acid residues of the Gla-domain have also been shown to be crucial for Ca^{2+}- and phospholipid binding. The highly conserved Arg at position 15 was mutated to His, Leu, and Trp, and these mutants all expressed very low anticoagulant activity as well as impaired Ca^{2+}-induced conformational change and phospholipid binding. It was speculated that hydrogen bonds between the side chain of Arg15 and Gla16 and the carbonyl oxygen in the peptide bond of His10 are critical for adoption of a proper conformation.[126] Several naturally occurring mutations in protein C–deficient patients have been found to affect Arg15.[127] Thus, there is no doubt that the Gla-domain is crucial for proper interaction with phospholipid membranes containing phosphatidylserine and phosphatidylethanolamine but it is also apparent that the Gla-domain contributes relatively little specificity in functional activity. Thus, replacement of the Gla-domain and the helical stack with corresponding domains from FVII resulted in a molecule with full protein C anticoagulant activity.[128]

EGF-domains

The first EGF-domain (EGF1) of protein C, like the corresponding domains of FVII, FIX, and FX, contains a Ca^{2+} binding site.[129–133] (See Chapter 18.) The Asp residue in position 71 of protein C, i.e., in the second loop of EGF1, is hydroxylated to erythro-β-hydroxyaspartic acid (Hya).[134] Mutations of the Hya residue to Glu or to Ala result in functionally defective molecules with low Ca^{2+}-affinity and low biological activity.[130, 135] Site directed mutagenesis of Asp46, and Asp48 to Ala also resulted in diminished Ca^{2+}-binding ability, but had no effect on protein C activation or anticoagulant activity.[135] EGF1 of protein C is unique in that it contains a seven amino acid residues long insert, and one disulfide loop (Cys59–Cys64) more than the other EGF-like domains. The domain contains the three typical loops of an EGF-domain, but the seven residue insert creates a lateral bulge of bilobate appearance.[104] The first EGF-domain appears to contain structural determinants which are important for the expression of protein S–stimulated anticoagulant activity, as suggested by the observation that a Gla-EGF-1 fragment inhibits the activity of APC in the presence of protein S.[132] Moreover, Fab′ fragments of a monoclonal antibody against a Ca^{2+}-binding epitope of the first EGF-domain were found to inhibit protein S–potentiation of APC anticoagulant activity.[130]

The peptide connecting the two EGF-domains in protein C is three residues longer than corresponding peptide in FIX and FX, and the path taken by the peptide is more tortuous in APC than in these proteins.[104] The peptide forms a short antiparallel pleated sheet structure with parts of EGF-1. The long link and the lack of contact between EGF-1 and EGF-2 allow more flexibility between these two EGF-domains than between corresponding domains in FIXa and FXa.

The 3-D structure of the second EGF-domain is typical of its class.[104] In the second EGF-like domain, there is an N-linked carbohydrate at Asn97 immediately N-terminal of the first cysteine residue. In vitro mutation of this residue to Gln has shown the glycosylation at Asn97 to be critical for efficient secretion of protein C, and to affect the degree of glycosylation at Asn329.[136] Inhibition studies of protein C activation on endothelial cells by thrombin-TM using fragments composed of either the Gla-domain, of the two EGF

domain or a Gla-EGF1-EGF2 fragment suggested the light chain region of protein C to contain most of the binding energy of protein C for the thrombin-TM complex.[137] However, more recent site-directed mutagenesis experiments of positively charged amino acid residues (Lys174, Arg177, Arg178 and Lys191, Lys192, Lys193) in the catalytic domain of protein C also suggest that amino acids in this part of the molecule are important for optimal interaction with TM.[138, 139] Synthetic peptide inhibition studies have demonstrated that two peptide regions in the light chain inhibit the anticoagulant activity of APC: Arg81–Phe95 occupying the inner surface of the EGF-1–EGF-2 contact regions and Gly142-Leu155 constituting the C-terminal portion of the light chain.[140]

Thrombin activates human protein C by cleavage of the peptide bond between Arg169 and Leu170. The 12 amino acid residues long activation peptide (residues 158–169 of the intact molecule) is rapidly eliminated from the circulation.[141] An interesting recombinant protein C mutant has been expressed, in which the activation peptide was replaced by an octapeptide derived from the insulin receptor precursor protein: Pro-Arg-Pro-Ser-Arg-Lys-Arg-Arg.[142] This peptide is cleaved C-terminal of the four basic residues when the insulin receptor precursor is converted to the two chain form. The expected processing on the C-terminal end of the four basic residues also occurred in protein C, resulting in the secretion of activated protein C.

Serine Protease Domain

The heavy chain of protein C constitutes the catalytic domain of protein C. The recent elucidation of the 3-D structure of APC provides the basis for a better understanding of the structure-function relationships of this domain of APC.[104] In the following discussion, two amino acid numbering systems are used. The number following the amino acid code refers to the position in the mature single chain protein C, whereas the number in brackets corresponds to the chymotrypsinogen (c) nomenclature, which is often used to facilitate comparisons of the 3-D structures of different serine protease domains.[143]

The protease domain of APC contains two six-stranded antiparallel β barrel domains, and the overall fold is typical of a serine protease of the trypsin class.[104] The domain manifests sequence identities ranging from 60 to 70 per cent vis-à-vis chymotrypsin, trypsin, and FIX and FX.[100] There are three conserved disulfide bridges between Cys196 (c42) and Cys212 (c58), Cys331 (c168) and Cys345 (c182), and Cys356 (c191) and Cys384 (c220), positions conserved among the serine proteases. There are two prominent insertions resulting in a helix between Asp280 (c125) and Gln290 (c131) and a loop between Ser305 (c146) and Thr315 (c152). The heavy chain of human protein C contains three N-linked carbohydrate side chains at positions Asn248 (c93), Asn313 (c150), and Asn329 (c166).[94, 95] The glycosylation site at Asn329 is unusual in that it appears in the sequence Asn-X-Cys rather than the commonly encountered Asn-X-Ser/Thr.[100] A similar glycosylation pattern has been found in von Willebrand factor.[144] Approximately 30 per cent of protein C in human plasma is not glycosylated at Asn329.[145] This so-called β form of protein C is of lower molecular weight than fully glycosylated protein C, and its biological activity is normal. It has been suggested that the degree of glycosylation of Asn329 is partly determined by the rate of disulfide bond formation during protein folding. The N-linked glycosylation sites at Asn248 and Asn313 are conserved in different species. Mutagenesis of Asn248 or Asn313 to Gln, which results in loss of the carbohydrate attachment sites, yielded a protein C which after its activation expressed approximately twofold increased anticoagulant activity.[136] The mechanism underlying the higher anticoagulant activity of these mutants is not clear. The Asn313 -> Gln mutant also manifested a two- to threefold increased activation rate by thrombin-TM, due to a lower Km.

The catalytic domain of APC resembles that of thrombin with the active site located in a deep cleft (see Fig. 19–3). The catalytic triad in human protein C comprises His211 (c57), Asp257 (c102), and Ser360 (c195).[94, 95] After activation, Leu170 (c16) occupies the N-terminus of the heavy chain, and it forms a buried ion pair with Asp359 (c194). Protein C is unusual in this respect as all other serine proteases have Val or Ile in the N-terminal position of the activate enzyme. By analogy with other serine proteases,[146] Asp354 (c189) is located at the bottom of the S1 specificity pocket (nomenclature as in Ref. 147). APC cleaves substrates with Arg in the P1 position. The S2 pocket is much more polar and open than the corresponding area in FXa or thrombin. This may explain why APC prefers residues with large side chains at the P2 position. The natural substrates, FVa and FVIIIa, have either Arg, Glu, Leu, or Pro in the P2 position, but either Gln, Asp, or Glu in the P3 position.[45, 49, 78] FVa and FVIIIa are the only known physiologically important substrates for APC. It is not known which structural features account for this narrow specificity of APC, but it probably involves an interaction between the substrate and a secondary binding site on APC located outside the catalytic center, as in FIXa and thrombin. Mutagenesis studies have also shown Glu357 (c192) located at the rim of the active site to be a major determinant of substrate/inhibitor specificity.[148] An activated protein C mutant in which Glu357 was replaced with Gln was inhibited by antitrypsin, antithrombin, and TFPI > 100 times more efficiently than was wild-type APC. In addition, the mutant APC inhibited FVa threefold faster than did wild-type APC, even though it had lower anticoagulant activity in plasma. Thus, even though Glu is not an optimal residue for catalyzing FVa inactivation, it represents an evolutionary adaptation to reduce the slow inhibition by its main serpin inhibitor.

On the surface of the catalytic domain of APC, close to the active site cleft, there is a cluster of positively charged amino acid residues similar to that found in the anion exosite 1 of thrombin. By analogy with thrombin, this cluster may form a secondary binding region for the substrates FVa and FVIIIa. Many residues in the c37-loop, the c60-loop, the Ca²⁺-binding loop (c70–c80), and the c148-loop contribute to the positive charge in the exosite 1-like region, including Lys191 (c37), Lys192 (c38), Lys193 (c39), Arg222 (c67), Arg229 (c74), Arg230 (c75), Lys233 (c78), Lys308 (c149), Lys311 (c149C), and Arg314 (c151). These positively charged amino acid residues may be important for interactions with substrates, inhibitors, and also with TM. That areas outside the active site cleft are important for interaction with the substrates is suggested by peptide inhibition studies. A synthetic peptide corresponding to residues Lys311–

Val325 (c149C–c162) of protein C was found to inhibit APC-mediated degradation of Va, suggesting that this region in APC provides a binding site for FVa.[149] Another peptide corresponding to residues Tyr390–His404 (c225–c239) had similar activity, suggesting also this region to be important for the anticoagulant activity of APC.[150] Site-directed mutagenesis of Lys191 (c37), Lys192 (c38), Lys193 (c39) to either Glu (all three), Asp (all three), or Gly (all three) demonstrated this positively charged cluster to be important for activation by thrombin-TM.[139] Another positively charged area closer to the activation peptide has also been found to be important for thrombin and thrombin-TM activation. A protein C mutant in which Lys174 (c20), Arg177 (c23), and Arg178 (c24) (P5′, P7′, and P8′ postions) were replaced by Glu (all positions) was found to be activated 12-fold more efficiently by thrombin alone, though the activation was not at all stimulated by TM.[138] It was suggested that the cluster of positively charged amino acids in protein C interacts directly with TM, resulting in optimal presentation of the activation peptide to the thrombin-TM complex.

The surface charge distribution of APC is asymmetric, one side of the catalytic domain being mainly positively charged (25 basic residues compared with 18 acidic residues), whereas the other side of the molecule is negative (17 acidic residues and 12 basic). This gives a surface polarity with a positively charged N-terminal half and a negatively charged C-terminal half.[104]

Monovalent cations stimulate the amidolytic activity of activated protein C, indicating that, like thrombin APC is an enzyme allosterically modulated by the binding of monovalent cations.[151–159] Cs⁺ is a more effective stimulator than Li⁺ or Na⁺, suggesting the stimulatory effect to increase with increasing ionic radius.[151, 155] Recently, the Na⁺-binding site in thrombin was localized to the loop corresponding to the c222-loop which in protein C would be around Leu387 (c222). It remains to be determined whether the Na⁺-binding site in protein C is located in this loop. Also Ca²⁺ has a moderate stimulatory effect on the amidolytic activity of protein C.[160] The effect of Ca²⁺ is due to a high affinity binding site in the catalytic domain in the loop between Glu225 (c70) and Glu235 (c80) at a position corresponding to similar Ca²⁺ binding sites in trypsin, FIX, and FX.[146, 161, 162]

▼ GENE STRUCTURE AND BIOSYNTHETIC PROCESSING

Protein C is synthesized in the liver and in the male reproductive system, in cells such as in Leydig cells, in the excretory epithelium of epididymis, and in some of the epithelial glands of the prostate.[93–95, 163] Protein C undergoes several post-translational modifications, including γ-carboxylation, Asp-β-hydroxylation, N-linked glycosylation, and internal proteolytic processing. γ-Carboxylation is required both for efficient secretion and for anticoagulant activity, but this post-translational modification is not rate-limiting for secretion under conditions optimal for vitamin K–dependent carboxylation. The nonglycosylated protein C is secreted inefficiently, and processing of the N-linked core in the endoplasmic reticulum, but not in the Golgi, is required for secretion. Proteolytic processing of the internal Lys-Arg dipeptide occurs late in the secretion pathway, and this cleavage is calcium dependent but not required for efficient secretion.[164] The mRNA of human protein C is 1800–1850 nucleotides long with a minor species (<10 per cent) which is approximately 200 nucleotides shorter.[94] The protein C mRNA contains a short 5′ untranslated region of 75 nucleotides. The 461 amino acid precursor protein is encoded by 1383 nucleotides, and the 3′-non-coding region contains 296 nucleotides. The polyadenylation signal AATAAA is 19 nucleotides upstream of the polyadenylation segment. An alternative polyadenylation recognition sequence (ATTAAA) is located 229 nucleotides upstream of this region. The smaller mRNA species may result from utilization of the latter polyadenylation signal.[94]

The protein C gene is located on chromosome 2, position q14–q21, and is approximately 11 kilobases long.[165–170] The transcription start site has been identified 10,772 nucleotides upstream of the polyadenylation site.[169] Regulatory elements of the human protein C gene promotor located between nucleotides −418 and +45 (relative to transcription start) confer liver specificity, whereas nucleotides −88 to +45 are sufficient for basal promotor activity.[171] Five cis-elements corresponding to binding sites for liver-specific transcription factors HNF-1, HNF-3, and NF-I/CTF, which play critical parts in the transcriptional regulation, are present in the promotor. In patients with protein C deficiency, four heterozygous mutations have been shown to disrupt HNF-3 binding [mutants of A(-32)G and T(-27)A] and HNF-1 [T(-14)C and C(-10)T].[171, 172] Mutations in the HNF-I-binding site also significantly impair the promotor activity.

The protein C gene is composed of nine exons and eight introns.[169] All the intron-exon boundaries follow the GT/AG rule. In protein C, as in factors VII, IX, and X, the domains in the non-catalytic part of the protein are encoded by separate exons. Exon 1 encodes the 5′ untranslated segment, and exon 2 the signal peptide (Met-42 to Gly-25) and six amino acids of the propeptide. Exon 3 encodes the rest of the propeptide and the first part of the Gla-domain (Asp-19 to Thr37) whereas the remaining helical stack of the Gla-domain is encoded by exon 4, and the two EGF-domains are encoded by exons 5 and 6. The serine protease part is encoded by three exons corresponding to those observed in factors VII, IX, and X. The splice-junction types are also conserved between the four genes. Exon 7 encodes the C-terminal part of the light chain, the activation peptide and the first 27 amino acids of the heavy chain. Exon 8 encodes Val185 to Leu223 in the heavy chain, and exon 9 the COOH-terminal part of the heavy chain. Sequence similarities of 35 to 40 per cent between protein C and factors VII, IX, and X, and the conservation of intron locations and splice-junction types attest to the common evolutionary origin of these proteins. However, there are no similarities in sequence or size between the introns of the four genes.[169, 170]

▼ ACTIVATED PROTEIN C AND FIBRINOLYSIS

Several early reports suggested APC to possess profibrinolytic activity, but until recently the underlying mechanism remained an enigma because APC does not significantly influence the activity of fibrinolytic components.[173–176] Instead it was shown that the profibrinolytic effect of protein C is indirect and depends on the anticoagulant activity of

APC, i.e., that APC stimulates fibrinolysis by decreasing thrombin generation.[176, 177] Subsequently, a thrombin-activatable fibrinolysis inhibitor (TAFI) was purified from plasma and found to be identical to a known carboxypeptidase B.[178] After activation by thrombin, TAFI inhibits fibrinolysis by removing C-terminal Lys residues from the fibrin clot, which results in impaired interaction between fibrin and the lysine binding sites on plasminogen. As a result of the APC-mediated inhibition of thrombin generation, less TAFI is activated and consequently APC appears to have profibrinolytic effects. The profibrinolytic properties of protein C have been shown to be entirely dependent on TAFI.[179] Not only protein C but also other components of the protein C system are important for the generation of active TAFI. Thus, TM gives a 1250-fold stimulation of thrombin-mediated TAFI activation, suggesting that thrombin bound to TM has both anticoagulant and antifibrinolytic properties.[180] The relative importance of these properties in vivo is not known.

▼ INHIBITION OF ACTIVATED PROTEIN C

APC is slowly neutralized in plasma and its half-life in the circulation is 15 to 20 minutes.[79, 80, 181, 182] In plasma, several serpins such as PCI and α_1-antitrypsin can inhibit APC, PCI being the prime inhibitor in vivo.[29–31] In addition, APC is inhibited by plasma α_2-macroglobulin, a non-serpin macromolecular 'trap.'[33, 34] Protease nexin 1, which is not normally present in plasma, and platelet PAI 1 can also inhibit APC.[183, 184] The APC-PCI interaction is stimulated by heparin, whereas the inhibition of APC by α_1-antitrypsin is heparin-independent. α_1-Antitrypsin and α_2-macroglobulin are major protease inhibitors in blood, circulating at concentrations of approximately 1.4 g/l (25 μM) and 2 g/l (2.5 μM), respectively. The plasma concentration of PCI, a single-chain glycoprotein with a molecular weight of 57,000, is much lower, 5 mg/l (90 nM).[29] APC is not the only enzyme in the protein C system which is inhibited by PCI, which also inhibits thrombin bound to TM.[185] Thus, PCI has the capacity to inhibit the protein C anticoagulant system at the level of both zymogen activation and enzyme inhibition. The concentration of PCI is about 40-fold higher in seminal plasma than in blood plasma. PCI is an important inhibitor of serine proteases from the prostatic gland, and also of the sperm-associated serine protease acrosin.[186–188] cDNA cloning showed the mature PCI molecule to contain 387 amino acid residues, and the reactive site sequence for APC to be Arg354–Ser355.[29] The sequence identities with both α_1-antitrypsin and α_1-antichymotrypsin are approximately 42 per cent. Once complexes between APC and PCI are formed, they are rapidly cleared from the circulation. The complexes between APC and α_1-antitrypsin have a much longer in vivo half-life than the APC-PCI complexes.[181, 189] The long half-life of APC and its specificity for the activated forms of FV and FVIII are prerequisites for the proper function of APC as a circulating anticoagulant in vivo.

Thrombomodulin

Thrombin itself is a poor activator of protein C, and it was not until the discovery of TM that thrombin's physiological involvement in the activation of protein C was fully appreciated, and the concept of a protein C anticoagulant system emerged. In the experiments that led to the discovery of TM, the coronary circulation in a so-called Langendorff heart preparation (an isolated rabbit heart) was simultaneously perfused with thrombin and protein C.[190] During its passage through the capillary system, when the endothelial cell surface to blood volume ratio increases dramatically, protein C was rapidly activated by thrombin reversibly bound to a high affinity receptor on the endothelium. This receptor was named thrombomodulin (TM) since binding of thrombin to TM is associated with a dramatic change in the specificity of thrombin. Bound thrombin is a potent activator of protein C, but has lost its procoagulant properties, including the ability to coagulate fibrinogen, activate platelets and factors V, VIII, and XIII.[191–195] Soon after the initial description, TM was solubilized with detergents and isolated from rabbit lung endothelium by means of thrombin-affinity chromatography.[196] It was later purified from human placenta, and from bovine and mouse lung.[194, 197, 198] The primary structures of bovine, human, and mouse TM are highly conserved; the amino acid sequence of mouse TM, for instance, is 68 per cent identitical to that of its human counterpart.[199–203]

TM has been found to be identical to fetomodulin (FM), a glycoprotein which has been postulated to be involved in organogenesis via quantitative modulation mediated by alterations in intracellular cAMP levels.[204] That TM indeed is important for embryonic development has been further demonstrated by gene knock-out experiments. Mice which are heterozygous for the TM deletion are healthy even though their endothelial TM is half the normal level. In contrast, homozygous TM deficient embryos were found to die in utero by embryonic day 9.5, the lethal phenotype being due to an overall growth retardation secondary to a defect in the parietal yolk sac.[205] The lethal phenotype may be caused by the loss of a TM-dependent function unrelated to the protein C system, because a 'knock in' of a functionally defective mutation (Glu387Pro which leads to loss of the TM-mediated stimulation of protein C activation) in the TM locus was found to bypass the developmental block.[206] Homozygous Glu387Pro mice manifested less than 0.2 per cent of the protein C cofactor activity of wild type mice, suggesting that the embryonic lethality may not primarily be associated with a defective thrombin cofactor function but rather with an unknown function affecting the developmental process.

▼ STRUCTURE-FUNCTION RELATIONSHIPS

TM is a multimodular membrane-spanning protein, with an extracellular amino-terminus (Fig. 19–4). After proteolytic removal of an 18 amino acid residues long signal peptide, the mature single chain human glycoprotein contains 557 amino acids.[199–201] The molecular weight of the apoprotein is 60,300. From its N-terminus, TM contains a lectin-like domain (residues 1–154), a hydrophobic region (residues 155–222), six EGF-like domains (residues 223–462), a Ser/Thr-rich region (residues 463–497), a 23 amino acid residues long transmembrane part (residues 498–521), and a 35 amino acid residues long cytoplasmic tail (residues 522–557). Human TM contains five potential sites for N-linked carbohy-

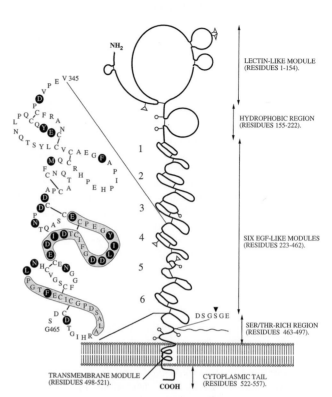

THROMBOMODULIN

Figure 19–4. Schematic model of thrombomodulin. TM is a single chain membrane protein composed of different domains as indicated in the figure. The organization of the disulfide bonds is tentative and based on homology with other proteins, in which disulfide bond locations have been experimentally determined (see the text). The amino acid sequences of the fourth to sixth EGF-like domains are shown, as these EGFs are crucial for thrombin binding and protein C activation. The 23 amino acid residues which are in indicated in black circles are important for cofactor activity because substitution of any of these residues results in <25 per cent activity, as compared with wild-type TM.[225–227] The disulfide bridging of EGF4 and EGF5 is that determined experimentally for TM fragments expressed in P. pastoris.[232] Shaded areas denote peptides that inhibit thrombin binding to TM.[213, 218] The wavy line in the Ser/Thr-rich region symbolizes the chondroitin sulfate chain. The probable site for its attachment at Ser474 is indicated by the arrow head. The positions of the potential O- (φ) and N-linked (Y) carbohydrate side chains are indicated.

drate side chain attachment (three in the lectin domain and one in each of EGF domains 4 and 5), and multiple potential O-glycosylation sites (Ser/Thr-X-X-Pro sequence). Five of the O-glycosylation sites are in the Ser-Thr rich region,[207] two in the hydrophobic region (residues 155–222), and two in the EGF-domains.[200]

The amino-terminal 154 residues of TM are homologous to the lectin-domains in the hepatic asialoglycoprotein receptor, the IgE receptor, and members of the selectin family.[208, 209] It is not known whether TM has any lectin-like properties. It has been proposed that the lectin-like domain of human TM serves to regulate cell surface expression of TM via the endocytic route, because recombinant TM in which the lectin domain was deleted failed to support internalization of thrombin-TM complexes.[210] The lectin-domain of TM contains eight cysteines, and the pairing of three disulfide bridges is suggested from the lectin homology: Cys12–Cys17, Cys34–Cys149, and Cys119–Cys140.[209]

Cys78 is probably linked to Cys115, as most other lectins lack cysteines in corresponding positions, but it can not be excluded that these cysteines form disulfide bridges with Cys157 and Cys206. Whether the two cysteines which are located in the 68 residues long hydrophobic region form a disulfide bridge, as we propose in Figure 19–4, is not known.

The six tandem EGF-domains contain sites for thrombin binding and protein C interaction. The importance of the EGF-like domains for the function of TM was demonstrated when a proteolytic fragment (formed after elastase digestion), which consisted of the six EGF-like domains, was found to catalyze thrombin activation of protein C.[211] A 10 kDa cyanogen bromide fragment (designated CB3), composed of the fifth and sixth EGF-like domains (residues 389–468), was later found to bind thrombin with high affinity, but had no cofactor activity.[212] It functioned as an inhibitor in protein C activation by the thrombin-TM complex by competing with TM for binding to thrombin. The CB3 fragment also lowered the rate of thrombin-catalyzed fibrinopeptide release from fibrinogen, indicating that the fifth and sixth EGF-domains contain enough structural information to alter the substrate specificity of thrombin. Thrombin binding to TM is inhibited by two linear peptides derived from the sequence of the C-terminal half of the fifth EGF-like domain, suggesting the thrombin binding site to be located on this domain.[213, 214] In human, mouse and bovine TM, the fifth EGF-like domain contains an N-linked carbohydrate side chain (Asn391 in mature human TM).[207] It does not influence thrombin binding, and its function is unknown. The observation that a fragment (CB23), containing the third to the sixth EGF-domains (residues 292–468), not only bound thrombin but also accelerated protein C activation suggested that the third or fourth EGF-like domain interacts with protein C.[215]

Experiments using recombinant TM have corroborated that thrombin binds to the fifth EGF-domain, and that the site for protein C interaction is on the fourth EGF-domain.[213, 216–220] Moreover, the region 333–350 in EGF34 was found to be critical for protein C activation, and the region 447–462 in EGF6 for thrombin binding.[220] Recombinant TM containing EGF4-6 expressed full cofactor activity in thrombin-catalyzed protein C activation, whereas EGF56 had no cofactor activity and EGF45 had about one-tenth of the cofactor activity of EGF4-6.[213, 219] A recombinant TM expressed in Pichia Pastoris containing EGF4-6 interacted with thrombin with slightly lower affinity (K_m 12 nM)[219] than cell-associated full-length TM (K_d 1.3–3.1 nM)[218]. When TM-fragments or recombinant deletion mutants of TM were used as cofactors to thrombin, intact protein C was found to be activated more rapidly than protein C lacking the Gla-domain.[211, 213, 216, 217, 221] This indicates that the Gla-domain of protein C may be involved in a calcium-dependent interaction with EGF-like domains in TM or with the bound thrombin.

The structure-function relationships for EGF4-6 have been further elucidated with peptide inhibition experiments and site-directed mutagenesis. Two peptides, Glu408–Glu426 of EGF5 and Pro441–Cys462 of EGF6, were found to inhibit thrombin binding to TM with K_i of 85–95 μM and 117 μM, respectively.[213, 218] A more constrained cyclic peptide analog of the Glu408–Glu426 peptide in which Ile420 was deleted was found to be more potent in inhibiting the thrombin-TM interaction (K_i of 26 μM).[222] The interaction

between this peptide analog and thrombin has also been studied with NMR which demonstrated a potential thrombin binding surface between Tyr413 and Phe419.[223] Two regions of EGF4 were identified as being essential for cofactor activity using loop swapping mutagenesis.[224] The two sequences were Glu357–Gln359 and Glu374–Phe376, suggesting that amino acids critical for thrombomodulin cofactor activity are located near the junction between the two subdomains of the fourth EGF-like domain. Alanine scanning mutagenesis was used to further identify amino acid side chains which are important for thrombin binding and cofactor activity.[225-227] In recombinant TM, 77 alanine point mutants were made between Cys-333 and Cys-462 by site-directed mutagenesis (all residues except Ala, Cys, Gly, and Pro). In EGF4, particularly important residues were Asp349, Glu357, Tyr358, and Phe376 (see Fig. 19–4). In EGF5, critical residues within a proposed acidic thrombin-binding region were Glu408, Tyr413 to Asp417, Asp423 to Glu426. In EGF5, Asp398, Asp400, Asn402, and Asn429 were important, as well as Asp461 in the C-loop of EGF6. The short loop between EGF4 and EGF5 has also been found to be critical for TM function.[227] A large number of substitutions were made in this loop, and most of them (38/57) resulted in a greater than 50 per cent decrease in TM cofactor activity, while changes in the length of the loop resulted in a greater than 90 per cent loss of activity. A Met388 –> Leu substitution resulted in a twofold increase in activity. Oxidation of Met388 destroys 75 to 90 per cent of TM activity, and this reaction may be physiologically important because in inflamed tissues activated neutrophils may oxidize Met388 in TM.[228] The inhibition of thrombin binding by a peptide Pro441–Cys462 of EGF6 indicated EGF6 also to be important for thrombin binding.[218] A similar conclusion was based on deletion mutants which demonstrated the presence of an intact EGF6 to be crucial for the expression of maximum TM activity.[218, 229]

The 3-D structures of a recombinant fourth EGF-like domain of TM, comprising Glu346 to Phe389, and of a 19 amino acid residues long C-terminal fragment of EGF4, have been elucidated with NMR and the results provide a basis for the interpretation of structure-function studies.[230, 231] The EGF4 structure resembles the structure of other EGF-like domains. Residues Asp349, Glu357, and Glu374, which are critical for cofactor activity, lie in a patch near the C-terminal loop, and are accessible to solvent. The other critical residues, Tyr358 and Phe376, are buried and probably play a structural part.

Studies of the disulfide bridge pattern of both recombinant and chemically synthesized EGF5 of TM yielded surprising results. The three disulfide bonds in EGF-like domains previously characterized have been arranged 1–3, 2–4, 5–6, but the pattern in the EGF5 was found to be 1–2, 3–4, 5–6.[232, 233] An EGF5 isomer with the traditional 1–3, 2–4, 5–6 pattern was synthesized and found to bind thrombin with 7-fold lower affinity than the 1–2, 3–4, 5–6 EGF5 isoform. The unusual disulfide bonding pattern may be physiologically important to provide a TM with high affinity for thrombin, but it remains to be determined whether this disulfide structure is present in natural thrombomodulin.

The thrombin-bound structures of various cyclic EGF5 fragments comprising the Glu408–Glu426 region of TM have also been studied with NMR and transferred NOE spectroscopy[223, 234] and by X-ray crystallography.[235] In the crystallographic structure, the key contacts with thrombin were hydrophobic interactions between the side chains of Tyr413, Ile414, and Leu415 and a hydrophobic pocket on thrombin formed by residues Phe19, Leu60, Tyr71, and Ile78. The NMR studies yielded similar results, although the predictions for certain side chain interactions were slightly different. In the NMR structure, primarily the side chains of Ile414 and Ile424 of TM were found to interact with a hydrophobic pocket on the thrombin surface.[234]

The 34 amino acid residues long Ser/Thr-rich segment, located between the EGF-domains and the membrane spanning region, contains five O-linked carbohydrate chains, at Ser474, Ser480, Thr482, Thr486, and Thr488.[207] A sulfated glycosaminoglycan, important for the expression of full anticoagulant activity is located in the Ser/Thr-rich region in some TM molecules.[236–244] The glycosaminoglycan has been isolated from rabbit TM and chemically characterized as a chondroitin sulfate.[240, 245] Its attachment site is primarily Ser474, a residue which is conserved in mouse and bovine thrombomodulin, and which lies within a sequence (Ser-Gly-Ser474-Gly-Glu-Pro) that is similar to chondroitin sulfate attachment sites in other proteoglycans. The chondroitin sulfate chain is approximately 25 disaccharide units long.[246] In studies of recombinant TM, it was found that some cell lines do not attach any chondroitin sulfate chains to TM, whereas others were more efficient in this respect.[244] Ser474 is the major acceptor site for the chondroitin sulfate chain, but mutagenesis of Ser474 to Ala revealed that Ser472 also has the capacity to be an acceptor site for the chondroitin sulfate chain. Only a fraction of TM molecules in human endothelium contain the condroitin sulfate chain. Thus, approximately 18 per cent of TM molecules expressed on human umbilical vein endothelial cells contained chondroitin sulfate, whereas the corresponding proportion in endothelial cells from aorta was 34 per cent.[244]

The importance of the chondroitin sulfate chain in TM for expression of full anticoagulant activity was first demonstrated in rabbit TM, and then in recombinant human TM.[221, 236, 237, 239, 242, 243] When the chondroitin sulfate chain is released from TM, e.g., by chondroitin ABC-lyase digestion, the molecular weight of TM decreases and its affinity for thrombin is reduced by a factor of 2 to 3.[221, 239, 247] The glycosaminoglycan moiety thus contributes to the binding of thrombin to TM. The site on thrombin which interacts with the chondroitin sulfate has been located to Arg93, Arg97, and Arg101 in exosite 2, which is the site also known to interact with heparin.[248, 249] Under certain experimental conditions, the chondroitin sulfate can itself bind a thrombin molecule, and each TM thus has the capacity to bind two distinct thrombin molecules.[250, 251] The chondroitin sulfate chain of TM has indirect anticoagulant effects, as it stimulates the inhibition of thrombin by AT. It also appears to be important for the direct (AT-independent) anticoagulant activity of TM, because recombinant soluble TM lacking the chondroitin sulfate moiety has relatively small inhibitory effect on thrombin-induced platelet activation and fibrinogen clotting.[221, 247, 252] The chondroitin sulfate is not directly involved in protein C activation, but affects the calcium-dependence of the reaction (see below). The chondroitin sulfate in TM is important for expression of full anticoagulant activity on the cell surface. Thus, endothelial cells treated with β-D-xyloside (which inhibits glycosaminoglycan attachment) manifest a thrombin-TM interaction with 3- to 5-fold lower affinity than that of untreated cells, paralleled by a reduction in the rate of protein C activation on the cell surface.[253] The distance of the thrombin-binding site on TM above the membrane surface is important because substitutions of the Ser/Thr-rich region with segments of decreasing length progessively decreased both thrombin affinity and cofactor function.[218] The chondroitin sulfate chain may have an important biological activity outside the protein C system, because it was recently shown that it functions as cell-surface receptor for the malarial parasite, Plasmodium falciparum.[254, 255]

The transmembrane part of TM is the region where sequence conservation between species is most pronounced.[199–202] The cytoplasmic tail is short and has potential phoshorylation sites. Mouse TM is phosphorylated in hemangioma cells after treatment with phorbol myristate acetate (*PMA*) or dimethyl sulfoxide.[202] The phosphorylation event is associated with increased endocytosis and degradation of TM. However, recent studies showing TM lacking the cytoplasmic tail to also efficiently undergo endocytosis raise the question how important the cytoplasmic tail really is for the endocytosis process.[256, 257]

▼ LOCATION OF THROMBOMODULIN

TM is present on the vascular surface of endothelial cells of arteries, veins, capillaries, and lymphatic vessels.[258, 259] In humans, it is present in all blood vessels with the notable exception of vessels in the central nervous system where only a regional distribution of TM is found.[260, 261] Hepatic sinusoids and postcapillary venules of lymph nodes do not appear to contain TM.[258] TM is present at low levels in platelets, approximately 60 molecules per platelet.[262] It has been found in keratinocytes in epidermis, on a variety of malignant and cultured cells, and on endothelial cell neoplasms.[263–266] Soluble forms of TM which presumably are proteolytic products have been identified in human plasma at approximately 20 µg/l and in urine.[267, 268] Although the physiological function of soluble TM is not known, the level of circulating TM may be useful as a clinical marker of vascular injury and certain malignancies.[269, 270]

There are $0.3–1 \times 10^5$ TM molecules per endothelial cell.[271] Within the circulation, the endothelial cell surface area per unit blood volume increases as the blood passes from the larger vessels to the capillaries. The endothelial cell surface area per unit blood volume is dramatically greater in the microcirculation than in the major vessels.[272] Assuming the number of TM molecules/endothelial cell to be independent of vessel diameter, the concentration of solid phase TM is more than 1000-fold higher in the microcirculation than in the major vessels, ensuring that thrombin will be bound to endothelial TM, even at thrombin concentrations that are nonthrombogenic. In larger vessels, thrombin will be free, but as soon as the blood enters the microcirculation it will encounter TM and protein C will be activated. Owing to the possible accumulation of thrombin in the microvasculature, the TM-mediated modulation of thrombin from a procoagulant to an anticoagulant enzyme is crucially important. In vivo, thrombin bound to TM will be eliminated either through inhibition by AT or by endocytosis of the thrombin-

TM complex and the half-life of the thrombin-TM complex on the cell membrane is less than 15 s.[10]

▼ ACTIVATION OF PROTEIN C BY THE THROMBIN-THROMBOMODULIN COMPLEX

Thrombin binds to TM on the surface of endothelial cells with high affinity ($K_d = 0.2–0.5 \times 10^{-9}$ M) (Fig. 19–5).[273] The formation of the thrombin-TM complex results in a 20,000-fold increase in the rate of thrombin-mediated activation of protein C.[190, 273] The K_m for protein C in this system is approximately 0.5 μM. When thrombin is bound to TM, the active site of the thrombin molecule is approximately 65 Å away from the membrane surface, as estimated with a fluorescence energy transfer technique.[274] Even though soluble TM efficiently supports thrombin-mediated protein C activation, the phospholipid membrane in which TM is located presumably also has an important and possibly modulatory function. Thus, incorporation of rabbit TM into neutral phosphatidyl choline phospholipid vesicles reduced the K_m for protein C from 7.6 μM to 0.7 μM, but membrane incorporation had no effect on the activation of protein C lacking the Gla-domain.[275] The K_m for protein C on phosphatidyl choline vesicles was similar to that observed on endothelial cells. Although most data tend to support the concept that the Gla-domain of protein C interacts with the phospholipid membrane during the activation process, it has been proposed that the Gla-domain does not interact with the phospholipid but rather with TM. According to this hypothesis, incorporation of TM into neutral phospholipid results in the exposure of a binding site for the Gla-domain of protein C on the TM molecule, a binding site which is also exposed on soluble TM fragments.[213, 215–217, 226, 275]

The observation that the activation of protein C does not require the exposure of negatively charged phospholipid may be physiologically important, as TM is present on intact endothelial cells of the vessel wall surface, where negatively charged phospholipid is not normally exposed. However, it should be borne in mind that rabbit and human TM may differ in the acidic phospholipid requirement, as in phospholipid reconstitution experiments using human TM protein C was found to be more rapidly activated on acidic phospholipid vesicles containing phosphatidylserine than on neutral vesicles.[275, 276] Recently, vesicles containing phosphatidylethanolamine were shown to be superior to those containing phosphatidylserine and/or phosphatidylcholine in supporting protein C activation.[106] The fatty acid composition of the phosphatidylethanolamine was also found to be important, as unsaturated fatty acids gave more efficient protein C activation than did saturated fatty acids. Thus, the level of thrombin-dependent protein C activation by TM reconstituted in dilinolenoyl phosphatidylethanolamine/distearoyl phosphatidylcholine mixture was 14.6 times higher than that obtained by TM reconstituted in vesicles with distearoyl phosphatidylethanolamine/distearoyl phosphatidylcholine. The enhanced protein C activation was the result of a decrease in both the K_d for thrombin and the K_m for protein C. This may be of physiological importance because phosphatidylethanolamine is exposed on the outside phospholipid surface of cultured human umbilical vein endothelial cells after thrombin stimulation.

Bovine meizothrombin (a prothrombin activation intermediate) binds TM and is able to activate protein C efficiently.[277] As meizothrombin has poor procoagulant properties, its function has been suggested to be anticoagulative. However, this conclusion was questioned by results obtained in a study using a human prothrombin mutant, S205A, in which the active site serine was replaced by alanine. The mutant prothrombin was used to generate stable but catalytically inactive human thrombin and meizothrombin. Meizothrombin S205A did not manifest any affinity for TM, whereas thrombin S205A was found to bind to recombinant human TM with the same affinity as did normal thrombin.[278] These results argue against human meizothrombin being an important TM-dependent protein C activator. However, two more recent reports provide evidence in favor of the hypothesis that meizothrombin-TM in fact is a better protein C activator than thrombin-TM.[279, 280] Thus, to date most reports have been consistent with meizothrombin-TM being a potentially important activator of protein C. Meizothrombin bound to TM can also function as an effective activator of TAFI.[280]

FXa bound to negatively charged phospholipid vesicles can activate protein C.[281, 282] This reaction is not potentiated by TM but is stimulated by sulfated polysaccharides.[282] In the presence of dextran sulfate, the activation rate of protein C by FXa on vesicles containing 40 per cent phosphatidylethanolamine has been found to be almost comparable to that observed using the thrombin-TM complex. These results suggest the existence of a template mechanism where the

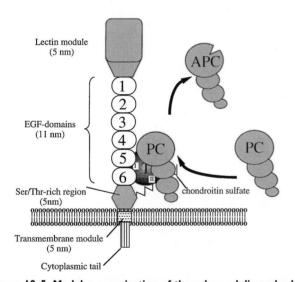

Figure 19–5. Modular organization of thrombomodulin and schematic representation of the molecular interactions occurring during protein C activation. The single high affinity thrombin (T) binding site in TM is located in the fifth-sixth EGF-like domains and interacts with exosite I, marked (I), in thrombin. The fourth EGF-domain is important for the interaction between TM and protein C (presumably mainly with the serine protease domain of protein C). The chondroitin sulfate chain of TM appears to interact with exosite 2 (marked with II) on the bound thrombin. The chondroitin sulfate chain is important for expression of full anticoagulant activity of TM, and is also required for stimulation of AT-dependent inhibition of bound thrombin. TM has been examined with electronmicroscopy which demonstrated TM to be an elongated molecule with a globular head consisting of the lectin domain. The dimensions of the different domains that were estimated from the electron microscopy studies are given.[251]

dextran sulfate chain serves as a bridge between FXa and protein C.[283]

TM may not be the only cofactor to thrombin in the activation of protein C, because human FVa and its isolated light chain have been shown to function as cofactors in thrombin-mediated activation of protein C.[284–287] The activity of the FVa light chain as thrombin cofactor was approximately 1/20 of that of TM, and the functional significance of this activity in vivo is unknown.

On binding to TM, thrombin loses its ability to clot fibrinogen, and to activate factors V, VIII, and XIII and platelets.[191–195] These effects have been demonstrated with rabbit and bovine TM, but have not been found with human TM purified from placenta.[288, 289] However, purified human TM is often contaminated with the multifunctional plasma protein vitronectin, which may bind to the glycosaminoglycan and affect the anticoagulant activity of TM.[290] Consistent with this interpretation, a soluble recombinant form of human TM, which contained the glycosaminoglycan chain but no contaminating vitronectin, was found to inhibit the procoagulant and platelet activating activities of thrombin.[221, 247, 252] Thrombin bound to rabbit TM can be inactivated by AT, a reaction catalyzed by the glycosaminoglycan present on TM. This effect, which it has not been possible to demonstrate with TM isolated from bovine[194, 198] or human sources,[197, 288, 289, 291] is obtained with recombinant human TM.[247, 252] The reason for this discrepancy between species is not known.

The activation of protein C by thrombin-TM can be influenced by proteins which are secreted from eosinophil granulocytes and platelets. The eosinophil specific granule protein, major basic protein (MBP), binds to TM and inhibits protein C activation. The inhibition is reversed by polyanions such as chondroitin sulfate E and heparin. Only TM containing the chondroitin sulfate chain is inhibited by MBP, indicating that MBP binds to this part of TM.[292] The cationic platelet alpha-granule protein platelet factor 4 (PF4) has the opposite effect on protein C activation, i.e., it induces a four- to 25-fold stimulation of TM cofactor activity. No such stimulation occurs when protein C lacking its Gla-domain is the substrate. Heparin and chondroitin sulfates A and E reverse PF4 stimulation. PF4 affects the K_d for thrombin only minimally, but induces a 30-fold decrease (from 8.3 to 0.3 μM) in the K_m for the activation of protein C by TM containing chondroitin sulfate. PF4 also transforms the Ca^{2+}-dependence profile of rabbit and chondroitin sulfate containing TM to resemble that of TM without chondroitin sulfate. PF4 may stimulate TM function by interacting electrostatically with both the chondroitin sulfate chain of TM and with the protein C Gla domain which would results in enhanced affinity of the thrombin-TM complex for protein C. Through such a mechanism, PF4 may play a part in the physiologic regulation of clotting.[293]

The Function of Calcium in the Activation of Protein C

The part played by Ca^{2+} in the activation of protein C by thrombin is complex and remains to be fully elucidated. On one hand, Ca^{2+} inhibits activation by thrombin alone, and on the other it is required for activation of protein C by the thrombin-TM complex.[190, 196, 273, 294] Although protein C

activation by the thrombin-TM complex is Ca^{2+}-dependent, *binding* neither of thrombin nor of protein C to TM requires calcium.[196, 295]

Protein C contains at least three different types of Ca^{2+}-binding sites, some of which appear to be important for protein C activation. The multiple Ca^{2+}-binding sites in protein C contribute to the complexity of the part played by Ca^{2+} in the activation process. Binding of Ca^{2+} to an intact Gla-domain of protein C is required for optimal activation of protein C, not only by phospholipid bound thrombin-TM complex, but also for activation by thrombin bound either to soluble TM fragments or to recombinant deletion mutants of TM containing the EGF-like domains 4–6.[211, 216, 217, 275, 296, 297] The Gla-domain of protein C is required for rapid activation by thrombin bound to the soluble TM derivatives but the molecular explanation for this is not known. One possibility is that the Gla-domain of protein C interacts directly with the EGF-like domains of soluble TM.[216, 217] Direct interaction between the Gla-domain of protein C and a fragment of TM formed by elastase digestion has been demonstrated in experiments using ultracentrifugation.[295] Another possibility is that the Gla-domain of protein C interacts with the thrombin that is bound to TM.

Activation of protein C on intact endothelium, or on phospholipid vesicles with reconstituted TM, is optimal at 2 mM Ca^{2+}. In contrast, soluble TM-fragments lacking the chondroitin sulfate chain yield bell-shaped Ca^{2+}-titration curves with peak activation at 0.1–0.3 mM Ca^{2+}.[211, 221, 275, 276] This type of Ca^{2+}-titration curve is obtained only when intact protein C and TM lacking chondroitin sulfate are used.[211, 216, 217, 221] Exosite 2 on thrombin may affect the calcium-dependence, because the Ca^{2+}-titration curve was not bell shaped when meizothrombin des-fragment 1 (exosite 2 is covered by the fragment 2 region) was used.[249] Liu and coworkers also showed that, at a low calcium level (0.27 mM Ca^{2+}), thrombin bound with 45 times higher affinity (K_d = 0.3 nM) to TM containing chondroitin sulfate than did the meizothrombin des-fragment 1 (K_d = 14 nM). In contrast, thrombin bound to TM lacking chondroitin-sulfate with only four times higher affinity (K_d = 2.4 nM) than did the meizothrombin des-fragment 1 (K_d = 9.4 nM). The authors concluded that occupancy of exosite 2 by either chondroitin sulfate or fragment 2 affected the Ca^{2+}-dependence of the protein C activation.

Saturation of high affinity Gla-independent Ca^{2+}-binding sites in protein C is also important for its rapid activation.[296, 297] Although the NH_2-terminal EGF-like domain of protein C binds Ca^{2+},[131] this Ca^{2+}-binding does not affect protein C activation.[298] The conformation of the activation peptide close to the thrombin cleavage site is by unknown mechanisms affected by Ca^{2+}, a calcium dependence altered by site directed mutagenesis of Asp167 in protein C (P3 position in the thrombin cleavage site) to either Gly or Phe.[299] In the presence of Ca^{2+}, the activation rates of these mutants by thrombin alone were five- to eightfold higher than that of wild type protein C. Mutant protein C was also more rapidly activated by the thrombin-TM complex. A similar but extended mutagenesis study, including both Asp167 -> Gly (P3-position) and Asp172 -> Gly (P3′ position) of protein C, demonstrated the importance of both these Asp residues for the calcium-dependence of the activation process.[300] In contrast to the Gly mutations, it was found that Asp -> Asn mutation at the P3 and P3′ positions did not significantly alter the calcium-dependence of the protein C activation.[301] A Pro168 -> Val mutation in the P2 position (P2 in fibrinogen is Val) was found to affect the Ca^{2+}-dependence of the thrombin-TM mediated activation of protein C.[302] Wild-type protein C demonstrated half-maximum rate of activation at 50 μM Ca^{2+}, as compared with 5 mM Ca^{2+} for mutant protein C. Thus, Pro168 is a determinant of the Ca^{2+}-dependent conformational changes in protein C that control activation.

Combined mutagenesis of Asp167 -> Phe and Asp172 -> Asn yielded a protein C which was activated 30-fold more efficiently by thrombin alone than was wild-type protein C. When this double mutation was combined with a genetically altered glycoform (Asn313 -> Gln), the resulting protein C (denoted FLIN-Q3) manifested a 60-fold increased activation rate by thrombin alone. The mutant protein C was found to be activated by the amount of thrombin that was generated during coagulation of plasma, i.e., in the absence of TM.[303] In a guinea pig thrombosis model, FLIN-Q3 was compared with protein C and APC. The infusion doses for APC, FLIN-Q3, and the protein C zymogen required to yield 50 per cent reduction of thrombus mass were 2.7, 24, and 250 mg/kg/h, respectively. The 'hyper-activatable' protein C molecule FLIN-Q3 represents a potentially interesting molecule for anticoagulant therapy.[304]

The importance of calcium for protein-protein interactions involving the activation peptide has also been illustrated by results obtained with a monoclonal antibody (HPC4) against protein C, which reacts with an epitope spanning residues Glu163–Lys174. The interaction between this epitope and the antibody is calcium-dependent, even though neither the antibody, nor the peptide alone binds calcium. Thus, both protein C and the antibody appear to contribute ligands to the calcium ion.[305]

Another high affinity calcium-binding site located in the heavy chain has been shown to be important for protein C to attain the proper conformation for rapid activation by thrombin-TM. This high affinity calcium-binding site is homologous to similar sites found in trypsin, FVII, FIX, and FX but missing in thrombin.[161] It involves a loop structure between Glu225 (c70) and Glu235 (c80), and the calcium site comprises Glu225, Glu232, and Glu235.[162] In thrombin, Glu-70 (chymotrypsinogen numbering) is replaced by Lys, creating an internal salt bridge with Glu-80, yielding the stabilization of this loop without the requirement of a calcium ion. The activation of a protein C mutant, in which Glu235 (c80) was replaced with Lys, was accelerated by TM in a Ca^{2+}-independent fashion. Moreover, Ca^{2+} did not inhibit activation of the mutant by free thrombin, and both the Ca^{2+}-stimulation of chromogenic activity and the Ca^{2+}-dependent quenching of intrinsic fluorescence were absent. Thus it appears that the high affinity Ca^{2+}-binding site in protein C, which is critical for zymogen activation, involves the loop between Glu225 and Glu235.[161]

Thrombomodulin Modulates the Substrate Specificity of Thrombin and Makes Protein C a Better Substrate

Binding of thrombin to TM induces an anticoagulant shift in thrombin substrate specificity.[10, 212, 214, 306] This is due to steric hindrance restricting the accessibility to the active site of thrombin, to allosteric conformational changes in the active site of thrombin, and to the ability of TM to make protein C a better substrate. The TM binding site on thrombin overlaps with the anion binding exosite 1, which also interacts with fibrinogen, hirudin, factors V, VIII, and XIII, and the platelet receptor for thrombin.[214, 307–309] The steric hindrance caused by the overlapping binding sites explains why thrombin bound to TM is less efficient as a procoagulant enzyme. An allosteric conformational change in the active site of thrombin induced by the binding of thrombin to TM has been demonstrated using spin-labeled active site inhibitors to thrombin.[306, 310, 311] This allosteric change is not specific for the thrombin-TM interaction because similar changes are induced by acidic synthetic peptides corresponding to segments of several nonhomologous thrombin inhibitors.[312] An alternative hypothesis has been proposed according to which the enhanced proteolysis of protein C mediated by thrombin-TM, as compared to thrombin alone, is due to an effect of TM on the bound protein C in the ternary complex. Thus, according to this hypothesis, TM would exert its physiological effect by making protein C a better substrate for thrombin, rather than making thrombin a better enzyme for protein C.[313]

Localization of the Thrombomodulin Binding Site on Thrombin

The binding site for TM on thrombin appears to be discontinuous, involving at least two different regions. A monoclonal antibody against an epitope located between Thr147 and Asp175 (amino acid position in linear sequence of the B-chain of thrombin) of thrombin was found to block the thrombin-TM interaction, and a synthetic peptide corresponding to Thr147 to Ser158 inhibited the binding of thrombin to TM.[314, 315] The synthetic peptide also inhibited the procoagulant activities of thrombin.[315] Another peptide corresponding to Arg89–Asn95 was subsequently reported to inhibit the thrombin-TM interaction.[316] Other investigators have suggested that the region comprising residues Arg62 to Arg73 of the B-chain of thrombin, which is part of the anion-binding exosite 1, interacts not only with fibrinogen and hirudin but also with TM.[317, 318] The 3-D structure of thrombin is similar to that of trypsin-like proteases, but is characterized by several insertion loops protruding around the active site and narrowing the substrate binding cleft.[308, 319–322] In particular, two pronounced loops that border the active site cleft play a major part in thrombin's restricted specificity, the 'c60-insertion loop' and the 'c149-insertion loop' which correspond to residues Tyr47–Ile55 and Thr147–Gly153, respectively, in the linear sequence of the B-chain. [Thrombin is discussed in detail in Chapter 18.]

Site-directed mutagenesis studies revealed that mutation of either Arg68 or Arg70 in thrombin to Glu compromises TM binding and reduces the rate of protein C activation, whereas a Lys52 to Glu mutation results in a 2.5-fold increase in protein C activating capacity and a major loss of fibrinogen-clotting activity.[323] Both Arg68 and Arg70 contribute to the positive character of the anion binding exosite 1 of thrombin.[319–322] Interestingly, the Arg68 -> Glu mutation lost the ability to clot fibrinogen and activate platelets, whereas the Arg70 -> Glu mutant was normal in both respects. The results suggest that the TM- and fibrinogen-binding sites on thrombin overlap, but are not identical.[323] A systematic site-directed mutagenesis approach was used to identify additional residues involved in the various functions of thrombin.[324] A total of 77 surface exposed charged and polar residues were substituted with alanine. Residues were identified that are required for the recognition and cleavage of protein C (Lys21, Trp50, Lys65, His66, Arg68, Tyr71, Arg73, Lys77, Lys106, Lys107, Glu229, Arg233) and interactions with the cofactor thrombomodulin (Gln24, Arg70). Although there was considerable overlap between the functional epitopes, distinct and specific residues with unique functions were identified. Functional residues were located on a single hemisphere of thrombin that included both the active site cleft and the highly basic exosite 1. Residues with procoagulant or anticoagulant functions were not spatially separated but interdigitated with residues of opposite or shared function. Thus thrombin utilizes the same general surface for substrate recognition, regardless of substrate although the critical contact residues may vary.[324]

In a followup study of the alanine scanning mutagenesis of thrombin, residues Trp50, Lys52, Glu229, and Arg233 were each substituted with all 19 naturally occurring amino acids. A single mutation, Glu229 -> Lys was found to shift the substrate specificity of thrombin 130-fold in favor of the activation of protein C over fibrinogen. This mutation was characterized by a number of other noteworthy features. It was less effective in activating platelets (18-fold), was more resistant to inhibition by antithrombin (33-fold and 22-fold in the presence and absence of heparin), and manifested a prolonged half-life in plasma (26-fold). Thus this mutant manifested an optimal phenotype, functioning as a potent and specific activator of endogenous protein C and as an anticoagulant in vivo. Subsequent infusion of the mutant in monkeys caused an anticoagulant effect through the activation of endogenous protein C without concomitantly stimulating fibrinogen clotting and platelet activation as observed with wild-type thrombin.[324]

Another approach used to obtain thrombin mutants with unique properties has been described. It was based on the discovery of a Na$^+$-dependent allosteric regulation of the two states of thrombin, the 'slow' and 'fast' forms, the activities of which are balanced in anticoagulant and procoagulant direction, respectively.[325] The slow -> fast transition is induced by Na$^+$ binding to a site contained within a cylindrical cavity formed by three antiparallel beta-strands of the B-chain (Met185–Tyr190, Lys236–Tyr240, and Val225–Gly228) diagonally crossed by the Glu194–Glu202 strand. (See Chapter 18.) Mutation of two Asp residues flanking Arg233 (Asp232 to Ala and Asp234 to Lys) almost abolishes the allosteric properties of thrombin and shows the Na$^+$ binding loop to be involved in direct recognition of protein C. Thus, site-directed mutagenesis of residues controlling Na$^+$ binding can profoundly alter the properties of thrombin. By suppressing Na$^+$ binding to thrombin, the balance between procoagulant and anticoagulant activities of the enzyme can be shifted. Compared to wild-type thrombin, such mutants are characterized by reduced activity toward fibrinogen, but enhanced or slightly reduced activity toward protein C.

The autolysis loop of thrombin comprising nine residues, from Glu147 to Lys155 has also been the target for mutagenesis experiments. Deletion of the insertion Ala151–Lys155 caused no significant change in the properties of the enzyme, except for a slight enhancement of protein C activation, whereas deletion of the entire Glu147–Lys155 loop reduced fibrinogen clotting 240-fold, but decreased protein C activation only twofold.[326]

Protein C has Asp-residues both in positions 167 and 172, which correspond to the P3 and P'3 positions in relation to the thrombin cleavage site. Unlike trypsin, thrombin is a poor enzyme for cleavage of peptides with acidic residues in these positions. This was demonstrated to be at least partly due to Glu202 (c192) in thrombin, which is located three residues distant from the active site Ser205 (c195) and close to Glu25 (c39).[327, 328] Most trypsin-like proteases have Gln in the position corresponding to Glu202 of thrombin, and site-directed mutagenesis of Glu202 to Gln yielded a thrombin which was more efficient in activating protein C.[327] The increase in efficiency was more pronounced in the absence of TM than in its presence (22-fold vs. twofold). The thrombin-catalyzed release of fibrinopeptide A was unaffected. It was concluded that Glu202 in thrombin is important in restricting its substrate specificity, and that TM binding to thrombin alters the enzyme-substrate interaction near this residue. The Asp residues in the P3 and P'3 positions appear to contribute to the slow activation of protein C by thrombin in the absence of TM, as the rate of thrombin cleavage of a peptide which corresponded to P7–P'5 in protein C (residues 163–174) was 30 times lower than the cleavage rate of a similar peptide with Gly residues replacing the Asp residues at P3 and P'3.[328] A Glu25 (c39) -> Lys mutation in thrombin showed this residue to be involved in the restriction of P3' residues to a nonacidic amino acids.[328]

A pharmacologically interesting way of modulating thrombin function was recently proposed when a low molecular weight modulator of the enzymatic activity of thrombin was found which enhanced the thrombin-catalyzed activation of protein C and concomitantly inhibited thrombin-dependent fibrinogen clotting.[329] The change in enzymatic substrate specificity of thrombin was believed to be mediated through an alteration in thrombin's S3 substrate recognition site, a mechanism that appeared to be independent of allosteric changes induced either by sodium ions or by TM. A compound with such properties may represent the prototype of a class of agents that are able to specifically modulate the balance between the procoagulant and anticoagulant functions of thrombin.

▼ THE STRUCTURE OF THE GENE OF THROMBOMODULIN AND ITS REGULATION OF EXPRESSION

There is a single TM gene in the human genome located on chromosome 20, position p12-cen.[201, 330–332] The gene is unusual in that it contains no introns. Northern blotting of human endothelial and placenta RNA revealed a single 3.7 kilobases long mRNA species.[201] Human full-length cDNA clones contain an approximately 150 nucleotides long 5' untranslated segment, a coding region of 1725 base pairs, and a 1779 base pair long 3' untranslated segment.[200, 201] The

3′ untranslated region is highly conserved between mouse, human and bovine TM.[199–202, 330]

TM is one of several important anticoagulant activities expressed on the surface of endothelial cells, and the level of TM expression is regulated by a variety of mechanisms. It has been proposed that the TM level on endothelium is regulated by internalization and degradation, and that internalization is induced by the binding of thrombin.[271] The lectin domain of TM is crucial for internalization whereas the cytoplasmic tail is not required.[210, 256, 257] Thrombin in complex with TM is believed to be transported to the lysosomes where it is released and degraded, whereas the TM is recirculated to the cell surface. This endocytosis has been found to be inhibited by protein C.[333] A similar recycling of TM has been found on A549 lung cancer cells, whereas no internalization and recycling of TM was found when endothelial cells from human saphenous veins or an endothelial cell line EA,hy 926 were studied.[334]

Inflammatory mediators such as endotoxin, interleukin 1 (IL-1) and tumor necrosis factor (TNF) decrease the expression of TM.[335–339] TNF inhibits transcription of the TM gene in endothelial cells, resulting in decreased mRNA levels and TM synthesis.[339–341] A decrease in the surface concentration of TM has also been observed after exposure of cultured endothelial cells to hypoxia and in association with a viral infection (Herpes simplex) of endothelial cell cultures.[342, 343] Parallel to the decreasing TM expression, inflammatory mediators, hypoxia, and herpes simplex infections increased the surface activity of tissue factor (TF). In an in vivo situation, such a shift in the balance between pro- and anti-coagulant mechanisms would favor coagulation and might contribute to the pathogenesis of disseminated intravascular coagulation in gram-negative septicemia. Interleukin-4, a product of activated T-cells which exerts anti-inflammatory effects on endothelial cells, has been shown to neutralize the downregulation of TM by IL-1, TNF, and endotoxin.[344] Another potentially physiologically important downregulation of TM on endothelial cells results from exposure of the cells to oxidized LDL. This effect is mediated through inhibition of TM gene transcription by lysosomal degradation of oxidized LDL, and a lipid component in the LDL may be an active species in this process. A decrease in TM expression on the surface of endothelial cells may contribute to promote thrombosis in atherosclerotic lesions.[345]

In vivo, mouse TM was found to be phosphorylated on serine residues, though this is believed not to be the result of protein kinase C activity but rather due to the action of another phosphorylating enzyme, possibly protein kinase A.[203, 346, 347] Phorbol myristate acetate (PMA) is a potent activator of protein kinase C. In hemangioma cells, it was found to induce endocytosis and degradation of TM after short term incubation (<6 hours).[202] Under these conditions TM was not phosphorylated. Longer incubations with PMA (>6 hours) reversed the down-regulatory effect by increasing mRNA levels for TM and enhancing surface expression.[347] In cultured human umbilical endothelial cells, okadaic acid, a potent specific inhibitor of phosphatases 1 and 2A, significantly increases TM levels, thus supporting the idea that kinases and phosphatases are involved in the cell regulatory mechanisms for TM expression.[348]

TM expression in human umbilical vein endothelial cells, in a human megakaryoblastic leukemia cell line and in mouse hemangioma cells, is upregulated by different agents that increase the intracellular cAMP levels.[346, 347, 349] Such agents include dibuturic cAMP, pentoxifylline, forskolin and isobutylmethylxanthine. Increased mRNA levels accompanied the increased surface expression, suggesting that cAMP regulates TM gene transcription. The effect of cAMP is inhibited by cyclohexamide, suggesting the enhanced TM gene transcription to be dependent on de novo protein synthesis.[350] A cAMP responsive element is located at position 2092 in the 3′ untranslated part of the TM gene.[351] Other cAMP responsive elements are found upstream of the transcription start site.[352, 353] Agents that upregulate TM transcription counteract the effects of IL-1 and TNF. Upregulation of TM expression by activation of histamine H_1-receptors in human umbilical vein endothelial cells in vitro has been demonstrated not to be mediated by increased cAMP.[354]

TM gene expression is affected by retinoic acid, and a retinoic acid response element is present in the 5′ region of the TM gene.[352, 355–362] It is noteworthy that the effect of retinoic acid on TM expression is more pronounced in keratinocytes and leukemia/carcinoma cells than in endothelial cells. On the other hand, inhibition of TM gene expression by TNF is less pronounced in keratinocytes than in endothelial cells, suggesting TM gene expression to be differently regulated in these two cell types.[356]

Transcription of the TM gene has been shown to increase after treatment of mouse hemangioma cells with cyclohexamide and thrombin.[363] Cyclohexamide, an inhibitor of protein synthesis, enhanced TM transcription approximately fourfold. Between two- and sevenfold increased transcription was induced by thrombin, but the effects of thrombin and cyclohexamide were not additive. Thrombin treatment of the cells increased the mRNA levels by approximately 50 per cent, accompanied by a concomitant 50 per cent increase in TM synthesis. The increased transcription in response to cyclohexamide has been interpreted as an indication of the existence of a labile protein repressor of TM transcription. The stimulatory effect of thrombin may be mediated by inhibition of such a repressor. In contrast to the results obtained with hemangioma cells, there was no effect of thrombin on TM expression on human saphenous vein endothelial cells even though thrombin treatment induced an increase in the TM mRNA level.[337, 364]

Cell surface TM in cultured human umbilical vein endothelial cells (HUVEC) and A549 cells was found to increase 3.2- and 6.7-fold, respectively, in response to 24 h of continuous 42°C heat shock stress.[365] The predominant mechanism of augmentation was transcriptional, and the heat shock-induced up-regulation of TM in HUVEC abrogated the suppressive effect of TNF. In the 5′ region of the TM gene there are six highly conserved tandem copies of the five base pair recognition unit that is the consensus sequence for a heat shock element. The biological function of the stress-induced augmentation of TM gene transcription may be to protect the vascular endothelium during a variety of stresses such as inflammation.

▼ THROMBOMODULIN IN CLINICAL MEDICINE

Complete TM deficiency is incompatible with life, as illustrated by the lethal phenotype in mice lacking a functional

TM gene.[205] However, heterozygous TM deficiency in mice is not associated with a disease phenotype. It is therefore likely that TM mutations are present in humans, but it remains to be determined whether such mutations are associated with disease. It is not even known whether heterozygous deficiency of TM in humans is associated with an increased risk of thrombosis. However, it is noteworthy that a number of point mutations resulting in amino acid replacements (Ala25 ->Thr, Gly61 -> Ala, Asp468 -> Tyr, and Pro483 -> Leu) have been identified in patients with venous thrombosis.[366, 367] However, it should be noted that not one of these mutations has been shown to be a risk factor for thrombosis. Mutations in the TM promotor might be risk factors for myocardial infarction.[368] Among 104 patients with diagnosed myocardial infarction, five mutations (three distinct) were identified (GG-9/-10 -> AT, G-33 -> A, and C-133 ->A). The GG-9/-10 -> AT mutation was identified in 3 individuals (2 heterozygous, 1 homozygous). One of the mutations was also identified in a control subject (G-33 -> A). These mutations are located close to transcription control elements. A C/T dimorphism predicting an Ala455 to Val replacement in the sixth EGF domain is present in the TM gene.[369] The allelic frequencies were found to be 82 per cent (Ala) and 18 per cent (Val) in a normal population. In an unexplained thrombophilia series, the allelic frequencies were found to be the same as in the normal population, indicating that the dimorphism is neutral with respect to thrombophilia. With respect to myocardial infarction, published results are conflicting with respect to differences in allelic frequencies between patients and controls; i.e., a significant difference between patients and controls was found in one study,[370] but not in another.[368]

Lupus anticoagulants, which are antibodies directed against epitopes exposed on certain protein-phospholipid complexes (usually the protein is β2-glycoprotein 1, but it can also be prothrombin or a protein in the protein C system) have occasionally been found to inhibit TM function in vitro.[371–375] Lupus anticoagulants are more often associated with thrombosis than with bleeding, and inhibition of protein C activation may contribute to the thrombotic tendency in these patients. Lupus anticoagulants can also inhibit other reactions in the protein C anticoagulant system, and it has been reported that they may inhibit the function of APC and/or protein S.[376, 377]

Methods have been devised for measuring soluble TM in blood and in urine.[267, 270, 378, 379] It may be useful to measure the plasma concentration of soluble TM as a marker of endothelial cell damage, but its value in routine clinical medicine is not yet established. Recombinant soluble TM or TM derivatives may become useful therapeutic anticoagulant agents. TM has been used successfully to inhibit thrombin-induced thromboembolism, disseminated intravascular coagulation (DIC), and endotoxin induced pulmonary damage in mice and rats.[380–385]

Cell Surface Receptors for Protein C and Activated Protein C

The presence of an endothelial cell surface receptor for APC was predicted, based on findings in binding experiments.[386] A noteworthy observation was that active site-inhibited APC and the protein C zymogen bound with similar characteristics as APC, whereas removal of the Gla-domain of protein C abolished binding. The binding of APC was also found to be independent of protein S. Shortly after the initial report, a protein C binding protein, designated endothelial cell protein C receptor (EPCR), was cloned from endothelial cells.[387] The expression cloning yielded a 1.3-kb cDNA that coded for a transmembrane glycoprotein found to be a member of the CD1/major histocompatibility complex superfamily. Even greater sequence identity (62 per cent identity) was detected with the murine protein, CCD41, which had previously been characterized as a centrosome-associated, cell cycle-dependent protein. Subsequently it was shown that murine ECPR is identical to murine CCD41 and, like its human counterpart, it is expressed on endothelial cells and binds both protein C and APC.[388] The centrosomal localization of mEPCR/CCD1 as determined by immunohistochemistry raised questions about the location of the EPCR gene product and its involvement in protein C binding. Subsequent studies have demonstrated EPCR to be present on the cell surface of endothelial cells and transfected cells.[388] Protein C and APC bind EPCR in a Ca^{2+}-dependent manner with a K_d of 30 nM. Approximately 7000 EPCR molecules are expressed on the surface of cultured endothelial cells and in vivo EPCR is mainly present on the endothelium of larger vessels and not on that of capillaries, in contrast to TM which is present on all vascular endothelium.[389, 390] The EPCR protein and mRNA are down-regulated by exposure of endothelium to TNF. A possible function of EPCR is to augment the activation of protein C by thrombin-TM.[391] This was suggested after the observation that monoclonal antibodies against EPCR that blocked protein C binding reduced the rate of protein C activation by the thrombin-TM complex on endothelium, whereas antibodies that bound to EPCR without blocking protein C binding had no such effect. The blocking of the EPCR-protein C interaction increased the K_m for protein C without altering the affinity of thrombin for thrombomodulin. Activation rates of Gla-domain-less protein C (the Gla-domain is required for binding to EPCR) were not altered by the anti-EPCR antibodies.[391] Even though EPCR appears to augment protein C activation, soluble EPCR has been shown to inhibit the anticoagulant activity of APC. EPCR does not alter the inactivation of APC by α_1-antitrypsin or PCI, and does not influence the catalytic activity of APC.[392] A soluble form of EPCR (43 kDa) is present at low concentrations (100 µg/l) in normal human plasma. The physiological function of plasma EPCR is uncertain.[393] Even though a large body of data is accumulating about EPCR, its true functional significance remains unclear.

On macrophages, APC has been found to inhibit the production of TNF-alpha and to prevent down-regulation of certain membrane proteins such as CD11b, CD14, and CD18.[394] The effect of APC may be related to APC-binding to a specific receptor on mononuclear phagocytes, a receptor site which is distinct from EPCR.[395] The functional significance of the APC binding to macrophages is not known at present.

A possible mechanism by means of which protein C exerts its anti-ischemic and anti-inflammatory effects is inhibition of E-selectin-mediated cell adhesion. This effect is not mediated through the serine protease activity of protein

C, but through its carbohydrates which are found to be more potent ligands for E-selectin than the sialylated Lewis X antigen.[396]

Protein S

▼ A COFACTOR TO ACTIVATED PROTEIN C

The total concentration of protein S in plasma is 20–25 mg/l (0.26–0.30 μM). The free fraction corresponds to 30 to 40 per cent of the total protein S, the remainder being bound to C4BP.[20, 397] Protein S functions as an APC cofactor in the degradation of both FVa and FVIIIa.[87, 398, 399] Although several mechanisms have been proposed, its mode of action is still not fully understood. Of the vitamin K–dependent proteins, protein S has the highest affinity for negatively charged phospholipids, and it has been shown to increase the affinity of APC for negatively charged phospholipid approximately 10-fold.[87, 400, 401] Although it has not been possible to demonstrate an interaction betwen protein S and APC in fluid phase, they appear to form complex on this type of surface.[87, 400] In vivo, the phospholipid surface for the protein S-APC interaction may be provided by platelets, platelet microparticles and endothelial cells, cells on which a protein S-dependent increased binding of APC has been observed.[402–406]

FXa has been found to protect FVa from degradation by APC.[75, 76, 83] The protective effect of FXa is specific for the Arg506 site in phospholipid bound FVa.[84] Protein S has been suggested to abrogate the protective effect of FXa on FVa.[85] In addition, protein S functions as an APC cofactor for the cleavage at Arg306 but not for the cleavage at Arg506. The cleavage at Arg506 thus mainly occurs in FVa which is not in complex with FXa. This cleavage results in only partial loss of FVa activity, whereas cleavage at Arg306 is required for complete FVa inactivation.[84, 407] Thus, protein S increases the APC-mediated cleavage at the Arg306 site, whereas the site at Arg506 is unaffected by protein S. This argues against increased phospholipid binding of APC as being the only mechanism by means of which protein S functions as an APC cofactor. A more specific role of protein S was proposed when it was shown that the distance of the active site of APC from the phospholipid membrane is reduced 10 Å in the presence of protein S.[89] As a result of this protein S–induced change in the localization of the serine protease domain of membrane bound APC, the active site of APC could be more favorably oriented to the Arg306 site than to the Arg506 site. A similar mechanism may be involved in the degradation of FVIIIa because the Xase complex is similar to the prothrombinase complex in that FIXa protects the Arg562 site in FVIIIa from degradation by APC.[408]

In APC-mediated degradation of FVIIIa complexed to FIXa on the membrane surface, protein S is not the only APC cofactor of importance because FV has been found to enhance the APC-mediated FVIIIa degradation.[26–28, 88] The mechanism by which protein S and FV function as synergistic cofactors is not clear. It is not yet known whether FV and protein S function as synergistic APC cofactors also in the degradation of FVa.

Protein S also expresses APC-independent anticoagulant activity, which originally was believed to be due to direct interactions of protein S with FVa and FXa.[23, 24, 409] A similar interaction between protein S and FVIIIa resulting in inhibition of the intrinsic Xase complex has also been suggested.[410, 411] Subsequent studies have demonstrated the APC-independent anticoagulant activity of protein S to be mainly related to the ability of protein S to interact with phospholipid membranes.[412] This may be a particularly important anticoagulant function of protein S under conditions where limited amounts of negatively charged phospholipid are available. Support for the phospholipid-blocking hypothesis was derived from results obtained in a flow system using endothelial cells where protein S depleted plasma gave considerably higher prothrombin activation than plasma containing protein S.[413]

Protein S may be involved in the regulation of the classical pathway of the complement system, because approximately 60 per cent of protein S in human plasma is present in a high molecular weight, non-covalent complex with C4BP.[20, 414] Only the free form of protein S functions as an APC cofactor, whereas both free and complexed protein S have APC-independent anticoagulant activity.[22, 410, 412, 415, 416] Bovine and rabbit plasmas differ from their human counterpart in not containing the complexed form of protein S.[417, 418] In bovine plasma, this is due to a deletion of the protein S binding N-terminal domain of the C4BP β-chain gene, whereas in rabbits no β-chain gene appears to be expressed.[419] In the mouse, the C4BP β-chain gene has evolved into a pseudogene.[420] In contrast, rat plasma contains a complex between protein S and C4BP, and a rat β-chain gene is expressed.[421]

▼ THE PROTEIN S MOLECULE

Protein S was discovered as a vitamin K–dependent plasma protein of unknown function.[422–424] Human protein S is known to be synthesized in the liver, in endothelial cells, by testicular Leydig cells, and by osteoblasts.[425–428] In an extensive study in rabbits, protein S expression was found in several organs including liver, lung, testis, epididymis, ovary, uterus, and brain.[429] Protein S synthesis is up-regulated by IL-6 and down-regulated by TNF.[430–433] In addition, it is inducible by IL-4 in T-cells.[434] Protein S is present at low concentrations in platelets, and it is synthesized by megakaryocytic cell lines and by neural tumor cells.[435–437] The primary structures of human, monkey, bovine, porcine, rat, and mouse protein S have been determined by protein sequencing and/or cDNA cloning.[438–445] Bovine liver contains an mRNA species of approximately 2.4 kb, whereas its human counterpart is 3.5 kb.[438, 439] The difference between human and bovine mRNA resides in the 3′-untranslated region, which is 826 bp longer in human mRNA. Human protein S is synthesized as a precursor protein with 676 amino acids, of which 41 form a leader sequence that is cleaved off before secretion. Mature human protein S is a single-chain glycoprotein (7–8 per cent carbohydrate) of 635 amino acids, the bovine counterpart being one amino acid shorter. The molecular weight of human protein S, calculated from the amino acid composition, is 70,690. Three types of modified amino acids are found in human protein S, namely Gla-, Hya-, and Hyn-residues, as well as three N-linked carbohydrate side chains.

The human genome contains two protein S genes (PSα and PSβ).[446-448] Chimpanzee and gorilla also have two protein S genes, whereas orangutan, rhesus monkey and African green monkey have one.[447] It has been concluded that the gene duplication event occurred after the branching of the orangutan from the African apes. The PSα gene is expressed, whereas the PSβ gene is a pseudogene. Both protein S genes are located on chromosome 3 close to the centromer (band q11.2).[166, 449, 450] The sequence identity between the exons of the two genes is 96.5 per cent. The PSα gene is more than 80 kb long and contains 15 exons and 14 introns.

Mature protein S is a mosaic protein composed of multiple domains (Fig. 19–6).[438, 439] Starting from the N-terminus, it contains a Gla-domain, a thrombin-sensitive region, four EGF-like domains, and a carboxy-terminal region which is unrelated to the serine proteases but homologous to sex hormone binding globulin (SHBG) and to rat androgen binding protein (ABP).[451, 452] The modular structure of protein S correlates with the intron/exon organization of the gene, and suggests that it has evolved through a combination of exon shuffling and gene duplication events.[446-448] The regions in protein S that are encoded by exons I–VIII (except the exon encoding the thrombin-sensitive domain) are homologous to corresponding regions in the other vitamin K–dependent coagulation proteins. (See Chapter 18.) Residues -41 to -18 constitute the hydrophobic signal peptide responsible for transport across the endoplasmic reticulum. The signal peptide cleavage site between Ala-18 and Asn-17 is tentative. The 17 amino acid long propeptide (residues Asn-17 to Arg-1) contains the recognition site for the vitamin K–dependent carboxylase and is homologous to corresponding structures in the other vitamin K–dependent proteins. Both the signal peptide and the propeptide are removed by proteolytic cleavage before secretion of protein S from the cell. The 5′ untranslated region and the signal peptide are encoded by the first exon.

The second exon encodes the propeptide and the Gla-domain. Residues Ala1 to Thr37 constitute the Gla-domain which contains 11 Gla-residues. It binds multiple Ca^{2+}-ions, and the Ca^{2+}-stabilized structure has high affinity for negatively charged phospholipid membranes. The Gla-domain includes a short connecting aromatic segment (residues 38–46), which is encoded by a separate exon. The thrombin-sensitive region (exon IV; residues 46–75) contains two cysteines, forming a disulfide bridge. In bovine protein S, two peptide bonds in this region are sensitive to proteolysis by thrombin: Arg52–Ala53 and Arg70–Ser71.[453] Human protein S has similar thrombin-sensitivity and Arg70 is conserved, whereas the human equivalent to the Arg52–Ala53 cleaveage site is Arg49–Ser50.[454] After cleavage by thrombin, the Gla-domain remains attached to the rest of protein S via the disulfide bond (Cys47–Cys72). However, in thrombin-cleaved protein S, the Ca^{2+}-mediated conformational change of the Gla-domain required for biological activity does not occur at physiological Ca^{2+}, suggesting the thrombin-sensitive region (TSR) to be intimately involved in the folding of the Gla-domain.[397] At physiological free Ca^{2+}-concentrations (around 1.2 mM), thrombin-cleaved protein S does not bind negatively charged phospholipid membranes, whereas at a fivefold higher Ca^{2+} concentration, cleaved protein S binds to the phospholipid with the same affinity as the uncleaved protein S molecule.[455] This suggests that the Gla-domain in thrombin-cleaved protein S attains a correct conformation at higher Ca^{2+} concentration. The APC cofactor function of protein S is lost in the thrombin-cleaved form.[456, 457] This suggests the TSR to interact with APC on the phospholid surface, an interpretation deriving support from findings in experiments using monoclonal antibodies.[458] The function of protein S is partly species-specific because human protein S does not work as a cofactor to bovine APC.[22, 399] Differences in the amino acid sequence of TSR and EGF1 between human and bovine protein S explain the species-specificity and a recombinant human protein S in which these two domains are replaced by corresponding domains from bovine protein S was found to function like bovine protein S, i.e., it stimulated the activity of bovine APC.[459] A computer model of the 3-D structure of Gla-, TSR-, and EGF1 domains was recently presented, which will facilitate further structure-function investigations of this region of protein S (see Fig. 19–6).[460]

Protein S

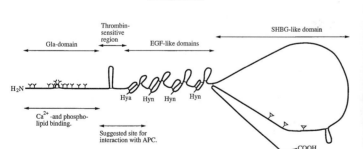

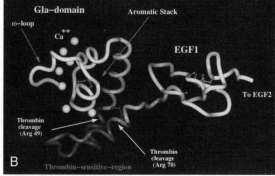

Figure 19–6. Models of human protein S. *A,* Schematic model of human protein S which is a single chain, 635 amino acids long, molecule composed of different domains. The positions of the Hya and the three Hyn-residues are shown. Human protein S contains eleven Gla-residues (Y), and three potential N-linked glycosylation sites (Ψ). *B,* Ribbon diagram of the protein S model showing the Gla, TSR, and EGF-1 regions. The spheres represent the calcium ions, and the side chains of cysteines involved in disulfide bridge are shown as ball and stick symbols. The ω-loop at the beginning of the Gla-domain is important for membrane binding. The two thrombin cleavage sites are labeled. This theoretical model, although still speculative, helps in the understanding of the functions of this region of protein S and allows structural investigation of point mutations resulting in type I or II deficiency.[460] (Fig. 19–6B was kindly prepared by Dr Bruno Villoutreix.)

Protein S is unique among the vitamin K–dependent proteins in containing four EGF-like domains (positions 76–242), each encoded by a separate exon (exons V–VIII). The phase of the splice junctions (predominantly phase I) in this part of the protein S gene supports the idea of the gene being formed by exon shuffling with the notable exception of the exon encoding the fourth EGF-like domain, which does not have the same splice junction type in the 3′ end as the others have. The first EGF-like domain contains a Hya and the three following Hyn.[461] Recombinant human protein S synthesized under conditions that inhibited the hydroxylation still expressed full cofactor function and C4BP binding.[462] To date, the importance of the hydroxylation of Asp/Asn in protein S is not known. Several lines of evidence suggest EGF1 in protein S to be important for the APC-cofactor function.[458, 459, 463] The Hyn-containing EGF-like domains in protein S, in particular EGF4, contain very high affinity Ca^{2+}-binding sites (K_d down to nM).[464-466] The Ca^{2+} binding is important for protein S to attain protease resistance and a native conformation.

Exons IX–XV encode the carboxy-terminal half of protein S (amino acids 243–635), which is homologous to SHBG and ABP.[446-448, 451, 452] The SHBG-domain of protein S seems to be composed of two repeats each of which is distantly related to the laminin G-type repeats, and contains about 2 per cent α-helix and 30 to 50 per cent β-strand.[467] The three-dimensional structure of the SHBG domain of protein S is not known but the observation that the G-type laminin repeats are distantly related to the subunits of the pentraxin family will facilitate development of theoretical models.[468] The intron/exon organization of this region of protein S is very similar to that of SHBG, including the positions of the introns and their splice/junction phases.[469] This domain contains two small disulfide loops formed by internal disulfide bridges (Cys408–Cys434 and Cys 597 to Cys625),[438] each of which is encoded by a separate exon. In human protein S, there are three N-linked glycosylation sites in the SHBG-like domain, at Asn458, Asn468, and Asn489, each of which contains a carbohydrate side chain. Mutagenesis of these sites resulting in loss of glycosylation failed to identify a specific functional role of the carbohydrate side chains.[470] Although the SHBG-like domain is homologous to the steroid-hormone binding proteins, it does not appear to bind steroids.[427]

A modular organization very similar to that of protein S is also found in another vitamin K–dependent protein designated growth arrest specific protein number 6 (Gas6). This name was chosen because the Gas6 gene is induced by growth arrest (e.g., by serum starvation) in cultured cells.[471] Gas6 is widely expressed, but unlike protein S, the level of its expression in the liver is low. The plasma level of Gas6 is also low, and the major function of Gas6 is outside the protein C and coagulation systems. Gas6 binds to a family of membrane-bound tyrosine kinase receptors, the Axl/Sky-family, and induces tyrosine phosphorylation and an intracellular signal.[472-474] Several biological responses have been assigned to Gas6 including inhibition of apoptosis, mitogenic activity and growth stimulation.[475, 476] An early suggestion that protein S also functions as a ligand for the Axl/Sky receptor family,[477] was challenged when it was found that only protein S from certain species stimulated the tyrosine kinase receptors.[478] Thus, bovine protein S was found to stimulate the human Sky receptor whereas human protein S manifested no such activity. The structural difference between human and bovine protein S accounting for this species specificity is located in the SHBG region of protein S. This was demonstrated when a human-bovine recombinant protein S hybrid with the SHBG from bovine protein S was found to stimulate the human Sky receptor.[479]

▼ BINDING SITE IN PROTEIN S FOR C4b-BINDING PROTEIN

Protein S and C4BP form a 1:1 noncovalent complex, in which protein S has no anticoagulant cofactor function.[20, 22, 414, 415, 480] The K_d is approximately 10^{-7} M in the absence of calcium, and around 5×10^{-10} M in its presence.[481-483] The effect of calcium is a combination of association rate acceleration and dissociation rate reduction.[483]

The binding site for C4BP is fully contained within the SHBG domain of protein S.[483] Three different regions, encompassing residues 605–614, 413–433, and 447–460 have been suggested to be of importance for the binding of protein S to C4BP.[484-486] The 605–614 and 414–433 regions were identified because peptides corresponding to the two sequences were found to inhibit the interaction between protein S and C4BP. Identification of the more recently suggested 447–460 sequence was based on findings in phage display experiments and peptide inhibition studies.[486] The very different regions suggested may indicate that the interaction between the two proteins involves multiple sites on the protein S molecule. No 3-D structure has been determined for the SHBG-region of protein S which might help ascertain whether or not the three identifed regions are in close proximity to each other. A mutant in which the region Asp583-Ser635 (corresponding to exon XV) was deleted still bound C4BP, albeit with 3 orders of magnitude lower affinity than native protein S.[487] Point mutations in this region also resulted in reduced affinity for C4BP.[488] These results are inconsistent with the notion that the full binding site for C4BP is located within the Cys597–Cys625 region, but suggest that binding may be complex and involve more than one site on the protein S molecule.

C4b-Binding Protein
▼ STRUCTURE-FUNCTION RELATIONSHIPS

C4BP (plasma concentration approximately 300 nM) is important for the regulation of the classical complement pathway.[489-496] It binds the activated complement protein C4b which is formed during complement activation. C4b bound to C4BP is a substrate for the serine protease factor I, and the proteolytic degradation of C4b results in loss of C4b functional activity. In addition, C4BP regulates the classical complement pathway by accelerating the natural decay of C2a from the C4bC2a complex (the classical pathway C3 convertase). The high molecular weight C4BP (M_r approximately 570 kDa) is composed of seven identical 70 kDa α-chains and a single 45 kDa β-chain.[497-499] The C4BP molecule is spider or octopus shaped, as revealed by high resolution electron microscopy (Fig. 19–7).[497, 500] Detailed

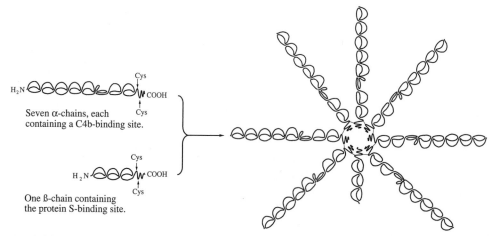

Figure 19–7. Subunit composition and assembly of C4b-binding protein. Electron microscopy of C4BP reveals an octopus-like structure with multiple long tentacles.[497] The distance from the center of the molecule to the peripheral end of an extended tentacle is 330 Å, and the diameter of a tentacle is 30 Å. C4BP contains two types of subunits, seven α-chains and one β-chain. Each of the α-chains contains a C4b-binding site and a site for the streptococcal surface protein Arp, whereas the protein S binding site is located in the β-chain. The subunits are linked by disulfide bridges, involving cysteine residues located in the COOH-terminal ends of both α- and β-chains. The major form of C4BP contains seven α-chains and one β-chain.

molecular models of the C4BP α- and β-chains based on homology modeling are also available.[501, 502] Each α-chain forms a thin (30 Å) extended (300 Å) tentacle that radiates from a central body. The β-chain is considerably shorter than the α-chains. The α- and the β-chains contain 549 and 235 amino acids, respectively.[499, 503] Both chains are composed of internally homologous repeats, known as short consensus repeats (SCRs), complement control protein repeats (CPs) or Suchi domains.[504, 505] They will be referred to as CP domains, in accordance with published nomenclature recommendations.[505] Each α-chain contains eight CPs, and the β-chain three. The carboxy-terminal regions of the α- and β-chains contain two cysteines that are involved in interchain disulfide bridging, and the formation of the central C4BP body. The sequence identity between the three β-chain CPs ranges from 26 to 34 per cent, and that between the α- and β-chain CPs from 17 to 35 per cent. The β-chain has presumably evolved from the α-chain during evolution through gene-duplication.[499, 506] The β-chain sequence contains five potential N-linked glycosylation sites, and all or most of them contain complex carbohydrate side chains.[499]

A CP is approximately 60 amino acid residues long and contains a framework of conserved amino acid residues including four cysteines, two prolines, one tryptophane, and several other partially conserved glycines and hydrophobic residues. A large number of complement reglatory proteins contain one or more CPs.[504] These proteins include factor H, the complement receptors 1 (CR1) and 2 (CR2), membrane cofactor protein (MCP), and decay accelerating factor (DAF). Other complement proteins with CPs are C1r, C1s, C2, factor B, C6, and C7. Each CP constitutes a distinct protein domain; and the cysteines form two disulfide bridges linked 1–3 and 2–4, and with few exceptions each CP is encoded by a separate exon. The 3-D structures of individual and paired CPs from factor H and a Vaccinia virus encoded complement regulatory protein have been resolved with NMR.[507–509] CPs have a compact structure based on a β-sandwich arrangement; one face made up of three β-strands and the other face formed from two separate β-strands. The genes for MCP, CR1, CR2, DAF, C4BP (α- and β-chains),

and factor H are closely linked in a cluster of genes known as the regulator of complement activation (RCA) gene cluster, which is located on the long arm of chromosome 1, band q32.[510, 511] The α- and β-chain genes of C4BP are very close, only approximately 4 kb apart, in a head to tail orientation.[512, 513]

C4BP is an acute-phase protein, and in certain inflammatory disorders its concentration increases to 400 per cent of normal.[514, 515] During inflammation, the α-chain synthesis increases more than the β-chain synthesis due to differential regulation of the α- and β-chain genes by cytokines, which results in C4BP molecules being formed of α-chains only.[516–518] Such molecules do not bind protein S because the protein S binding site is located on the β-chain, whereas each of the α-chains contains a C4b-binding site. This differential regulation ensures stable levels of free protein S also during inflammatory states even though the plasma C4BP level may be several times higher than normal.[516] In normal plasma at least 80 per cent of the C4BP molecules contain the β-chain (C4BPβ +).[519] The normal C4BPβ + concentration is on a molar basis approximately 30 to 40 per cent lower than that of total protein S. The interaction between protein S and C4BP is of very high affinity, and the level of free protein S is equivalent to the molar surplus of protein S over the C4BPβ +.[520]

The β-chain is required for protein S binding, but not for the polymerization of the C4BP chains during assembly of the molecule.[498, 521] As the binding sites for protein S and C4b on the C4BP molecule are distinct, the protein S binding does not affect the function of C4BP as a regulator of the classical C3 convertase.[522] The protein S binding site is fully contained within the first CP domain of the β-chain.[523–525] Available data suggest the C4b-binding site to be complex, involving at least the first three CP domains of the α-chains.[497, 526–528] This region of the C4BP α-chain has also been shown to bind to Arp and Sir, which are surface proteins on *Streptococcus pyogenes*.[502, 528, 529] The binding of C4BP to the bacterial surface may provide complement regulatory activity there.

The high affinity binding of serum amyloid P (SAP)

component to C4BP is an interaction of unknown biological significance.[530] SAP, which is homologous to the acute phase protein CRP, is a normal constituent in plasma and extravascular tissues and also present in amyloid deposits.[531] It is a so-called pentraxin, composed of five identical subunits (molecular weight of 25,000) linked by non-covalent bonds. The biological function of SAP is not known. The stoichiometry of the SAP–C4BP interaction is 1:1, and it is optimal at 0.4 mM calcium. The self-association of SAP and its interactions with phospholipid or C4BP are mutually exclusive, its binding to C4BP being favored over self-association or its binding to phospholipid membranes. SAP binds to the central core of C4BP but the binding sites for protein S and SAP on C4BP are independent.[532, 533] Although the binding sites for SAP and C4b are distinct, SAP binding is (by unknown mechanisms) associated with inhibition of factor I cofactor activity in the degradation of C4b.[532] The macromolecular complex of C4BP, SAP, protein S and C4b can bind to phospholipid membranes in the presence of calcium. The vitamin K–dependent part of protein S is required for membrane interaction of the complex.[530]

C4BP is unique in the group of CP-containing proteins in being composed of two distinct CP-containing subunits with different binding specificities, and the protein S binding to the β-chain of C4BP is the only example of a vitamin K–dependent protein binding to a CP-containing protein. The binding of protein S to C4BP suggests linkage between the regulations of the coagulation and complement systems. C4BP regulates the expression of protein S anticoagulant activity, as binding of C4BP to protein S results in a loss of protein S cofactor activity. Protein S may affect the function of C4BP as a regulator of the classical complement pathway, because the C4BP-protein S complex binds to anionic phospholipid surfaces where blood coagulation may be ongoing and this could provide local regulation of the complement system.[481, 530, 534] Other CP-containing proteins are known to regulate the complement system on cell membranes, i.e., DAF is covalently linked to a glycolipid, whereas CR1, CR2, and MCP are integral membrane proteins with phospholipid spanning regions.[489] Activation of complement results in a local inflammatory reaction, partly due to the release of anaphylatoxins and the attraction of leukocytes. Inhibition of the complement system where blood coagulation occurs may be beneficial, as an inflammatory reaction at the same site may result in impaired regulation of coagulation (e.g., due to the release of leukocyte proteases).

The Protein C Anticoagulant System, an Important Regulator of Blood Coagulation in Vivo

The importance of the protein C anticoagulant system in vivo is most clearly illustrated by the severe thromboembolic disease that affects individuals with homozygous deficiency of either protein C or protein S.[35] Moreover, the increased risk of thrombosis in people with heterozygous deficiency of either protein C or protein S or APC resistance due to the Arg506Gln mutation in the FV gene supports the notion that this anticoagulant system is important for the regulation of blood coagulation in vivo. Under normal conditions, protein C appears to be slowly activated, as the protein C activation

peptide can be detected in blood, albeit at very low concentration.[141] Moreover, low levels of circulating activated protein C (approximately 40 pM) are also found under normal circumstances.[535] Activation of protein C is the result of a low grade activation of coagulation with a constant slow generation of thrombin or possibly meizothrombin.[13, 279, 280] Dramatically increased levels of protein C activation peptides were found in patients with disseminated intravascular coagulation, deep vein thrombosis or pulmonary embolism.[536] In addition to these clinical findings, studies in experimental animals have shed light on the function of the protein C anticoagulant system in vivo, and have suggested that this system may be involved in the host-defense reactions occurring during such intravascular inflammatory challenges as sepsis.[537–539]

In vivo experiments using rabbits, dogs or monkeys have shown protein C to be activated in response to infusion of thrombin or a mixture of FXa and acidic phospholipid vesicles.[79, 80, 182, 540] In a coronary artery occlusion model, using porcine hearts, ischemic insult induced rapid protein C activation in the coronary microcirculation, and recovery was impaired when protein C activation was blocked.[541] In humans, it has been shown that protein C is activated in response to thromboembolic events and during intravascular coagulation and that complexes between APC and either PCI or α1-antitrypsin inhibitor circulate, during these conditions.[542–545]

Infusion of APC in experimental animals prolongs the activated partial thromboplastin time.[79, 81, 546–550] However, the bleeding time is unaffected and the plasma levels of FV and FVIII remain normal during and after the infusion. This is due to the high specificity of APC, i.e., it degrades the phospholipid-bound forms of FV/FVa and FVIIIa, but does not cleave the circulating procofactors. When administered in a baboon arterial thrombosis model, APC was found to inhibit platelet-dependent thrombus formation.[546] In a rabbit model of microarterial thrombosis, APC manifested potent antithrombotic effects.[548] In this model, the antithrombotic effect of APC was found to be potentiated by protein S.[549, 550] Activated protein C has also been shown to prevent thrombin-induced thromboembolism in mice.[551] Other components of the protein C system are also powerful anticoagulants, e.g., purified natural or recombinant TM has antithrombotic effects on thrombin-induced thromboembolism in vivo.[380, 381, 384, 552–554] This is mainly due to stimulation of protein C activation, but direct anticoagulant functions of TM due to modulation of thrombin activity may also be involved. It is possible that therapeutic uses will be found for protein C, APC, and/or TM in the future.

In addition to its important anticoagulant functions, the protein C system appears to play a major protective part in limiting tissue damage due to gram negative septicemia.[539] In a baboon model, APC infusions prevented the coagulopathy and the E. coli-induced shock that was fatal in untreated animals.[555] Active site inhibited FXa (DEGR-Xa) blocked the disseminated intravascular coagulation initiated by E. coli, but in contrast to APC, did not prevent shock and organ damage.[556] This suggested that in addition to blocking the formation of thrombin, APC has other protective, anti-inflammatory functions. This hypothesis is consistent with findings in other in vivo experiments where inhibition of the intravascular coagulation response observed after E. coli infusion was obtained with heparin or with antibodies to tissue factor. However, these components failed to protect the animals from shock.[539, 540] Protein C concentrates have potential as useful therapeutic agents in certain septic conditions, e.g., in meningococcemia, a life-threatening septic condition with mortality rates greater than 50 per cent. Meningococcemia is associated with purpura fulminans, hemodynamic deterioration, and acquired protein C deficiency which contributes to the thrombotic necrotic lesions in the skin and other organs. Infusion of protein C concentrates in severe cases has been shown to reverse the condition and improved mortality rates considerably.[557]

Activation of protein C is critical in host defense against infection by *E. coli*, as borne out by the observation that inhibition of protein C activation by a monoclonal antibody, exacerbated the shock response after infusion of sublethal doses of *E. coli*. The APC cofactor function of protein S is also crucial for the APC-mediated protection. Thus, when baboons were first given a monoclonal antibody against protein S, a lethal response was obtained after an otherwise sublethal dose of *E. coli*.[539, 558] Monoclonal antibodies against protein S that blocked the APC cofactor activity produced the lethal response, whereas non-inhibitory antibodies did not. The functional importance of the free form of protein S was obvious since infusion of C4BP prior to administration of the sublethal E. coli dose exacerbated the inflammatory response and made the outcome fatal. This did not happen when C4BP was given together with a slight excess of protein S.[558, 559] These in vivo experiments clearly demonstrated the protein C anticoagulant system to play an important protective part in host defense inflammatory reactions induced by septicemia, although the basic biochemical mechanisms remain unclear.

Molecular Genetics of Venous Thromboembolism

The annual incidence of venous thrombosis in industrialized countries of the Western world is approximately 1–2/1000.[560, 561] Although genetic defects are frequently involved in the pathogenesis as risk factors, thrombotic episodes tend to occur in conjunction with surgery, fractures, pregnancy, oral contraceptive usage, and immobilization. Thus, the pathogenesis of venous thrombosis is multifactorial, including combinations of circumstantial (acquired) and genetic risk factors. Up to 40 per cent of patients with thrombosis have family histories of thrombotic disease, thus demonstrating the importance of genetic factors.[562] Genetic defects known to predispose to thrombosis include inherited APC-resistance due to the Arg506Gln mutation in the FV gene, and deficiencies of protein C, protein S, or antithrombin. There is a general consensus that inherited APC resistance is the most frequent genetic risk factor for familial thrombophilia yet described.[563, 564]

A point mutation in the prothrombin gene (nucleotide 20210 G -> A) has been identified as the second most common independent risk factor for venous thrombosis.[565] The mutation is located in the 3′ untranslated region, and the mechanism by means of which this mutation results in an increased risk of thrombosis is not fully understood, even though the mutation has been shown to be associated with

increased plasma levels of prothrombin. The prevalence of the mutation in the general population is 1 to 2 per cent, and the mutation is associated with an approximately threefold increased risk of thrombosis.[565–568]

▼ APC RESISTANCE (FV:Q506)

In 1993, APC resistance was described as a previously unrecognized cause of inherited thrombophilia.[569] It was soon demonstrated that APC resistance is highly prevalent (20–60 per cent) among thrombosis patients.[570–573] In the APC-resistant patient, the addition of APC to plasma does not result in the expected prolongation of the clotting time (Fig. 19–8). In more than 95 per cent of cases, the molecular background to inherited APC resistance is a single point mutation in the FV gene.[574–578] The mutation is a G to A substitution at nucleotide position 1691 in the FV gene, which predicts replacement of Arg506 (in one of the three APC cleavage sites) with a Gln. The mutant FV is usually referred to as FVR506Q, FV Leiden, or FV:Q506 (R and Q are one letter codes for Arg and Gln, respectively).

The FV:Q506 allele is only present in individuals of European ancestry (Caucasians), and in the Western world the prevalence of the mutant FV:Q506 allele in the general population is characterized by considerable international variation. The highest prevalence (15 per cent) has been reported from southern Sweden in an area noted for its high incidence of thrombosis.[579] The prevalence has also been found to be high in Germany and Greece,[580–582] as well as in Israel (both Arabs and Jews but with great variation among Jews depending on their ethnic background),[583, 584] and 3 to 5 per cent in the Netherlands, the UK, and the United States,[574, 582, 585, 586] but lower (around 2 per cent) among Hispanic Americans and in Italy and Spain.[586, 587] The mutation is not present among Japanese or Chinese.[588–593] It is noteworthy that large differences may even exist within the same country, e.g., in France prevalences ranging from 1 per

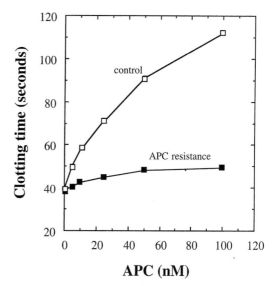

Figure 19–8. APC resistance in a thrombosis patient. In APC resistance, the addition of APC to an APTT reaction mixture does not result in the normal anticoagulant response. Filled squares = APC resistance; open squares = control plasma.[569]

cent (Lille) to 10 per cent (Strasbourg) have been found.[594] The prevalence in a given society depends on a number of factors including the prevalence of the mutation in the founder population. The high prevalence of the FV:Q506 allele in certain populations suggests a possible survival advantage to be associated with the mutation. A low bleeding tendency after delivery among women carrying the mutation may be one such survival advantage.[595] In the human history, the slightly increased thrombosis risk associated with the FV:Q506 allele has presumably not been a negative survival factor, because thrombosis developed relatively late in life and does not affect fertility. Moreover, our forebears were not exposed to many of the circumstantial risk factors for thrombosis such as surgery, oral contraceptive usage or the relatively sedentary nature of modern life.

The high prevalence of the FV:Q506 allele in Western societies is the result of a founder effect.[596–598] It is suggested that the mutation occurred around 30,000 years ago, i.e., after the migration from Africa which took place 100,000 years ago, and also after the segregation of Asians from Europeans.[598] This would explain why the mutation is common in European populations but is not found in Japanese or Chinese, or in the original populations of Africa, Australia, or America.

The occasional occurrence of inherited APC resistance in thrombosis patients not carrying the FV:Q506 allele suggests that APC resistance may also be caused by other mechanisms yet to be identified.[575, 599] Two different mutations affecting the Arg306 site have been found in thrombosis cases, but such mutations appear to be extremely rare and it is uncertain whether they result in APC resistance and whether they constitute risk factors for thrombosis. An Arg306Thr mutation (FV Cambridge) was found in a single individual among a group of 17 thrombosis patients with unexplained APC resistance.[600] Although the individual carrying the mutation had APC resistance, no causal link was established. The Arg306Thr mutation, which can be detected by a changed restriction enzyme cleavage pattern using BstNI, was not present in any of a cohort of 601 thrombosis patients, thus demonstrating the mutation not to be a common risk factor for thrombosis. In a study of a cohort of Hong Kong Chinese with thrombosis, an Arg306Gly mutation (FV Hong Kong) was found in 4.7 per cent (2/43) of the patients and in 2.4 per cent (1/42) of their controls, though the APC resistance phenotype was expressed in none of these three individuals, as determined with the APTT-based APC resistance test.[601]

Mechanisms of APC Resistance Associated With FV:Q506

There are two mechanisms by means of which the presence of the FV:Q506 allele results in a hypercoagulability and an increased risk of thrombosis. One is that a natural APC cleavage site in FVa is lost which affects the normal degradation of FVa by APC.[82, 407, 602, 603] The other is association of the mutation with a defect in the expression of APC-cofactor activity of FV in the degradation of FVIIIa.[25, 28, 46] In FVa, the APC cleavage at Arg506 is associated with favorable kinetics, as compared to cleavage at Arg306 or Arg679.[78, 82, 407] Thus, the K_m for the 506 site is approximately 10-fold lower than the K_m for the 306 site, whereas the V_{max} values

of the two sites are similar. Thus, the rate at which the two sites are cleaved depends on the concentration of FVa. At physiological concentrations of FVa, cleavage at Arg506 is approximately 10-fold faster than cleavage at Arg306, and the activity of FVa:Q506 is inhibited at approximately 10-fold lower rate than that of FVa:R506. Generated FVa persists longer, and can form active prothrombinase complexes with FXa. This results in increased thrombin generation and hypercoagulability, which is reflected by increased levels of prothrombin activation fragments in plasma of individuals with inherited APC resistance.[604, 605] The FVR506Q mutation does not affect the activation of FV to FVa, and FVa:Q506 is associated with normal procoagulant activity.

Degradation of 'free FVa' (i.e., FVa not bound to FXa) differs from that of FVa which is part of the prothrombinase complex. In the prothrombinase complex, the Arg506 site is protected by FXa from degradation by APC.[46, 84] In addition, protein S functions as an APC cofactor primarily for the Arg306 cleavage but not for cleavage at Arg506.[46, 84] Accordingly, FVa which is part of the prothrombinase complex differs from free FVa in the pathway of APC-mediated degradation. Thus, when they are components of corresponding prothrombinase complex, FVa:R506 and FVa:Q506 do not differ significantly in the rate of their degradation by APC plus protein S. This may explain why FVa:Q506 is inhibited at almost the same rate as FVa:R506 when coagulation is initiated by FXa or the tissue factor pathway.[46, 84, 569] It may also explain the relatively mild phenotype which is associated with inherited APC resistance. The second way in which the FV mutation gives rise to hypercoagulability is related to the poor anticoagulant activity of FV:Q506 which was demonstrated in a FVIIIa degradation system using FV isolated from an individual with homozygous APC resistance.[28, 46]

Laboratory Investigation of APC Resistance

Laboratory investigation of inherited APC resistance due to the FV mutation can be done with a functional APC resistance test and with molecular biology assays.[38] A modified APC resistance test involving dilution of the patient plasma in FV-deficient plasma has been shown to be highly sensitive and specific for the presence of the FV:Q506 allele.[606–608] It should be borne in mind that the modified test is specific for the FV mutation and will not detect APC resistance due to other causes, such as acquired APC resistance. However, the clinical significance of acquired APC resistance remains unclear. If in the investigation of patients it is also desired to detect acquired APC resistance and inherited APC resistance not caused by the FV mutation, it is recommended that both the original and the modified APC resistance tests be performed.[38]

The most commonly used molecular biology assay for FV:Q506 is based on PCR amplification and cleavage with Mnl I, because the mutation results in the loss of an Mnl 1 site.[574] Other assays used for genotyping involve amplification from RNA, DNA sequencing, SSCP, DGGE, capillary electrophoresis, allele-specific hybridization techniques, or oligonucleotide ligation assays (for list of references see Ref. 37).

Epidemiology of APC Resistance

Since the first report of inherited APC resistance in 1993, a large number of studies have demonstrated relationship to exist between the presence of the APC resistance phenotype, and/or the FV:Q506 allele, and an increased risk of venous thrombosis.[570–572, 574, 585, 609, 610] In all likelihood, discrepancies in reported results are largely attributable to differences in selection criteria—e.g., higher prevalences of APC resistance in conjunction with thrombosis have been reported for familial thrombosis series than for consecutive series.[571, 572, 610] Nonetheless, the prevalence of inherited APC resistance was found to be about 20 per cent among consecutive Dutch outpatients with thrombosis, but 28 per cent among consecutive thrombosis patients in southern Sweden,[574, 610] an area characterized by a high prevalence of the FV mutation in the population. In the Physicians Health Study, apparently healthy men were followed for a mean duration of 8.6 years and the prevalence of the FV:Q506 allele in the thrombotic subgroup was only 11.6 per cent.[609] Nevertheless, it was concluded that APC resistance due to the FV mutation was an important risk factor for thrombosis. Indeed, there is a general consensus that inherited APC resistance caused by the FV mutation is the most common genetic risk factor for venous thrombosis yet discovered. In terms of the odds ratio, the increased risk of thrombosis in individuals with APC resistance due to the FV mutation has been calculated to be six to eightfold among heterozygotes but 30–140-fold among homozygotes.[38, 611] The FV:Q506 allele does not appear to be a strong risk factor for arterial thrombosis, such as myocardial infarction.[609, 612] However, the FV mutation may nonetheless be a risk factor for myocardial infarction in the presence of certain circumstantial risk factors—e.g., presence of the FV mutation has been found to be associated with an increased risk of myocardial infarction in young female smokers.[613]

▼ DEFICIENCY OF PROTEIN C OR PROTEIN S AND VENOUS THROMBOSIS

Heterozygous deficiency of protein C or protein S is a risk factor for venous thromboembolic disease, and each of these deficiencies is found in 2 to 5 per cent of thrombosis patients.[562, 614–616] The prevalence of protein C deficiency in the population is estimated to be approximately 1/300.[617, 618] The 10-fold higher prevalence of protein C deficiency in thrombosis cohorts suggests carriership of this genetic defect to be associated with an approximately 10-fold increased risk of venous thrombosis, a figure consistent with results on record.[619, 620] Protein C deficiency is not a risk factor for arterial thrombosis. The prevalence of AT deficiency in the population is approximately 10-fold lower than that of protein C deficiency, which taken together with its 1 to 2 per cent prevalence among thrombosis patients suggests the risk of venous thrombosis associated with AT deficiency to be higher than that associated with protein C deficiency.[621] The prevalence of protein S deficiency in the population is not known, but findings in family studies suggest the associated risk of venous thrombosis to be similar to that associated with protein C deficiency and APC resistance.[622, 623]

Protein C Deficiency

The diagnosis of protein C deficiency is based on results obtained with immunological or functional (amidolytic or coagulation) assays, possibly combined with family data and identification of a mutation in the protein C gene. It is often difficult to diagnose protein C deficiency based on results of protein C assays alone, because there is an overlap in protein concentrations between those with and those without the genetic trait.[624] Moreover, it should be borne in mind that many functional assays do not fully evaluate all functional aspects of the protein C molecule. For example, many commercial amidolytic assays are based on activation with snake venoms and detection of amidolytic activity with a synthetic substrate which means that most functional properties of protein C such as phospholipid membrane binding, activation by the thrombin-TM complex, and interactions with natural substrates are not tested.

Two types of protein C deficiency have been described (reviewed in[42]). In type I, there is a parallel reduction in protein C antigen and functional activity. Type II is characterized by a functional defect in the protein, and its plasma concentration may be normal. The majority (approximately 90 per cent) of reported cases of protein C deficiency belong to type I. The prevalence of heterozygous protein C deficiency is approximately 1/300 whereas homozygous or compound heterozygous protein C deficiency is a rare condition (1/200,000–1/400,000).[35, 625, 626] It causes severe and fatal thrombosis in the neonatal period. The clinical picture is that of purpura fulminans, and the symptoms include necrotic skin lesions due to microvascular thrombosis. Other major symptoms are thrombosis in the brain and disseminated intravascular coagulation. Several cases have been successfully treated with fresh frozen plasma or with protein C concentrates.[626]

Rarely, skin necrosis develops after initiation of anticoagulant therapy with such vitamin K–antagonists as warfarin, and this condition has been found to be associated with protein C deficiency.[627, 628] Four of 118 Dutch or French patients with protein C deficiency developed skin necrosis during anticoagulant therapy.[629] It is believed that skin necrosis develops as a result of transient severe protein C deficiency due to the short biological half-life of the protein.[630–632] During the induction phase of anticoagulant therapy, functional protein C levels decline more rapidly ($t\frac{1}{2} \approx 8$ hours) than those of FIX, FX and prothrombin ($t\frac{1}{2} > 40$ hours). Accordingly, functional protein C levels can be very low during the first days of anticoagulant therapy, particularly in protein C deficient patients, which increases the risk of microvascular thrombosis and skin necrosis. However, the occurrence of skin necrosis is not restricted to patients with protein C deficiency.[628, 633]

In a large number of cases of protein C deficiency, genetic analysis has been performed and a published database comprises 160 different mutations.[40, 127, 634] New mutations are continuously reported and up-dated databases are available on internet. The majority of entries in the database are missense mutations located within the region coding for the mature protein, which result in single amino acid substitutions and type I deficiency. Mutations in the promotor region of the gene which affect the plasma protein concentration and mutations affecting the RNA splicing have also been found. Other mutations predict premature stopcodons as the mechanism for the deficiency.

In a minority of cases with known mutations, the genetic defect results in a type II deficiency. Any of the functions of protein C can be affected, and mutations resulting in type II deficiency have been found in almost all the domains of protein C, including the propeptide, the Gla-domain, EGF1, the activation peptide, and the serine protease domain.[40, 42, 127, 634] Mutations in the propeptide (Arg-5 to Trp; Arg-1 to His, Ser, or Cys) result in defective cleavage of the propeptide. Gla-domain mutations (Glu7 to Asp; Glu20 to Ala; Glu26 to Lys) affect γ-carboxylation and calcium- and phospholipid-binding. The importance of Arg15 is demonstrated by the type II protein C deficiency affecting patients with an Arg15 to Trp mutation. Type II mutations in EGF1 (Arg87 to His; His66 to Asn creating a potential carbohydrate attachment site) demonstrate the functional importance of this domain. An Arg169 to Trp mutation destroys the activation cleavage site yielding a molecule which can not be activated. This molecular defect has been found in at least two independent families, in protein C Tochigi and in Protein C London 1.[635, 636] Several mutations resulting in type II deficiency have been found in the serine protease domain. An Asp359 to Asn mutation occurs in an amino acid that is located next to the active site Ser360. Asp359 has been predicted to form an ion pair with the carbonyl of Leu170 after activation, and the mutation resulting in an Asn probably affects this interaction.[637] The His211 to Gln mutation affects the catalytic triad. An Arg229 to Gln mutation which is located in the Ca^{2+}-binding loop causes impaired activation of protein C by the thrombin-TM complex.[42] A Ser252 to Asn mutation creates a new potential carbohydrate attachment site. Several type II mutations such as Arg147 to Trp, Arg157 to Gln, Arg229 to Gln, and Arg352 to Trp are clustered in a positively charged area which presumably is an important exosite for substrate interaction.

Protein S Deficiency

Family studies have clearly demonstrated protein S deficiency due to a mutation in the protein S gene to be a risk factor for thrombosis.[622, 623, 638] In contrast, a recent case-control study failed to identify protein S as a risk factor for thrombosis.[619] Analysis of free protein S discriminates better between those with and those without protein S deficiency, than does analysis of total protein S.[623, 638, 639] The concentrations of protein S and C4BPβ+ are approximately equimolar in protein S-deficient individuals, which taken together with the high affinity of the protein S-C4BP interaction explains the low plasma levels of free protein S which characterize the disease.[639] The C4BPβ+ level in plasma correlates with that of protein S and, depending on the severity of the protein S deficiency, the plasma concentration of total protein S may be low or in the low normal range. Protein S deficiency with low levels of both free and total protein S has been referred to as type I, whereas protein S deficiency with low free protein S and normal total protein S has been suggested to constitute a separate genetic type (referred to as either type IIa or type III). However, demonstration of the coexistence of the two types in many protein S deficient families suggested that they represent different phenotypic variants of the same genetic disease.[638, 639] The

plasma levels of protein S and C4BPβ+ increase slightly with age, which may explain why the total protein S level can be within the lower normal range in affected individuals. Mutations in the protein S that result in functionally defective molecules are referred to as type II deficiency. To date, very few type II deficiencies have been found, presumably due to the poor diagnostic performance of available functional protein S assays. Homozygous protein S deficiency is extremely rare, but appears to be associated with a clinical picture similar to that of homozygous protein C deficiency with purpura fulminans in the neonatal period.[35, 640–643]

The clinical manifestations of hereditary protein S deficiency are similar to those of protein C deficiency.[622, 639, 644] Protein S deficiency may also predispose to arterial thrombotic disease.[620] However, protein S deficiency appears to be a very mild risk factor for arterial disease as it is found only very rarely. A possible gene-gene interaction between protein S deficiency and a 4G polymorphism in the PAI 1 promotor increasing the risk of arterial disease has been suggested by findings in studies of large protein S deficient families.[645] In this study, only individuals carrying both protein S deficiency and homozygosity for the 4G allele manifested an increased risk of arterial thrombosis and pulmonary embolism. A few cases of warfarin-induced skin necrosis associated with protein S deficiency have been described.[646–648]

Acquired protein S deficiency is associated with oral anticoagulation, nephrotic syndrome, disseminated intravascular coagulation and pregnancy.[649] In nephrotic syndrome, the concentration of C4BP is high, since its molecular weight does not allow glomerular filtration. Accordingly, the concentration of the complexed form of protein S is increased.[650] Free protein S is lost in the urine resulting in a decreased level of functionally active protein S. During normal pregnancy, the concentrations of both total and free protein S in plasma drop and reach levels found in heterozygous protein S deficient patients.[651, 652] In particular, the levels of free protein S decrease. Whether this contributes to the thrombotic tendency during pregnancy is unknown. Acquired protein S deficiency may also be the result of immunological mechanisms (e.g., in patients with autoimmune disease or HIV).[653–662] It is noteworthy that several children have been described with thrombosis and autoantibodies to protein S after varicella infections.[656, 663, 664]

To date, approximately seventy defects in the protein S gene have been reported (reviewed in Refs. 42 and 43). Most (67 per cent) of the gene defects are missense or nonsense mutations, and mutations affecting splicing or insertion/deletion defects are less common. Most characterized defects cause type I/III protein S deficiency, and only few mutations have been found to be associated with type II deficiency. Two mutations in the Gla-domain (Lys9 to Glu and Gla26 to Ala) result in defects in γ-carboxylation, and presumably to folding problems and instability as well as poor Ca^{2+}- and phospholipid binding.[460] A Thr103 to Asn mutation in EGF1 causes type II deficiency by unknown mechanisms. A Lys155 to Glu mutation in EGF2 results in a functional defect in protein S, protein S Tokushima. Protein S Tokushima has poor APC cofactor activity, and has been shown to interact poorly with APC suggesting that EGF2 in protein S is important for expression of APC cofactor activity.[665]

▼ SEVERE THROMBOPHILIA IS A MULTIGENETIC DISEASE

It is now generally accepted that venous thrombosis is a typical multigenetic disease. Thus, the FV:Q506 allele causing APC resistance has been shown to be an additional genetic risk factor in families with deficiency of protein C,[666–668] protein S,[578, 622, 669] or antithrombin,[670] as well as in cases of the prothrombin mutation (G20210 to A).[671] The penetrance of clinical manifestations is lower in those individuals having a single gene defect than among those with two or more defects (Fig. 19–9). Deficiencies of protein C or protein S and inherited APC resistance (FV:Q506) are essentially equally severe risk factors for thrombosis and should be managed in a similar way, whereas the prothrombin mutation is possibly associated with a somewhat lower thrombosis risk.

In the general population of Western societies, many individuals carry more than one genetic risk factor for thrombosis, because the prevalence of the FV:Q506 allele is high. By contrast, in countries where the FV mutation is rare, the prevalence of individuals carrying more than one genetic defect is much lower. This probably explains the lower incidence of thromboembolic disease in Japan and China, as compared to Europe and the United States. The frequency of individuals carrying two or more defects can be calculated on the basis of the prevalence in the general population of the individual genetic defects. Protein C deficiency has been determined to be present in 0.1 to 0.3 per cent.[617] In a country where the prevalence of FV:Q506 is 10 per cent, combinations of protein C deficiency and FV:Q506 are consequently expected to be present in 1/3000–1/10,000 individuals. A similar calculation for the combination of the pro-

thrombin mutation and FV:Q506 suggests the prevalence of the combined defects to be 1–2/1000 individuals. This indicates that a large number of people carry more than one genetic defect and such individuals are at considerably increased risk of thrombosis.

The penetrance of thrombosis in individuals with inherited genetic defects is highly variable, and some individuals never get thrombosis, whereas others develop recurrent severe thrombotic events at an early age. The severity of the thrombotic tendency is dependent on the genotype, the coexistence of other genetic defects and the presence of environmental risk factors. Risk factors commonly seen in association with thrombosis include oral contraceptive usage, trauma, surgery and pregnancy. Thus, among women using oral contraceptives, the increase in risk of thrombosis has been estimated to be 35–50-fold among heterozygotes for the FV:Q506 allele, but several hundred-fold among homozygotes.[672]

REFERENCES

1. Davie, E. W., Fujikawa, K., and Kisiel, W.: The coagulation cascade: initiation, maintenance, and regulation. Biochemistry 30:10363, 1991
2. Davie, E. W.: Biochemical and molecular aspects of the coagulation cascade. Thromb Haemost 74:1, 1995
3. Furie, B., and Furie, B. C.: Molecular and cellular biology of blood coagulation. N Engl J Med 326:800, 1992
4. Nemerson, Y.: The tissue factor pathway of blood coagulation. Semin Hematol 29:170, 1992
5. Mann, K. G., and Lorand, L.: Introduction: blood coagulation. Methods Enzymol 222:1, 1993
6. Wu, K. K., and Thiagarajan, P.: Role of endothelium in thrombosis and hemostasis. Annu Rev Med 47:315, 1996
7. Bombeli, T., Mueller, M., and Haeberli, A.: Anticoagulant properties of the vascular endothelium. Thromb Haemost 77:408, 1997
8. Bauer, K. A., and Rosenberg, R. D.: Role of antithrombin III as a regulator of in vivo coagulation. Semin Hematol 28:10, 1991
9. Lindahl, U., Lidholt, K., Spillmann, D., and Kjellen, L.: More to "heparin" than anticoagulation. Thromb Res 75:1, 1994
10. Esmon, C. T.: The roles of protein C and thrombomodulin in the regulation of blood coagulation. J Biol Chem 264:4743, 1989
11. Dahlbäck, B.: The protein C anticoagulant system: inherited defects as basis for venous thrombosis. Thromb Res 77:1, 1995
12. Esmon, C. T.: Molecular events that control the protein C anticoagulant pathway. Thromb Haemost 70:29, 1993
13. Esmon, C. T., Esmon, N. L., Le Bonniec, B. F., and Johnson, A. E.: Protein C activation. Methods Enzymol 222:359, 1993
14. Stenflo, J.: A new vitamin K–dependent protein. Purification from bovine plasma and preliminary characterization. J Biol Chem 251:355, 1976
15. Kisiel, W., Ericsson, L. H., and Davie, E. W.: Proteolytic activation of protein C from bovine plasma. Biochemistry 15:4893, 1976
16. Kisiel, W., Canfield, W. M., Ericsson, L. H., and Davie, E. W.: Anticoagulant properties of bovine plasma protein C following activation by thrombin. Biochemistry 16:5824, 1977
17. Kisiel, W.: Human plasma protein C. Isolation, characterization and mechanism of activation by α-thrombin. J Clin Invest 64:761, 1979
18. Seegers, W. H., Novoa, E., Henry, R. L., and Hassouna, H. I.: Relationship of 'new' vitamin K–dependent protein C and 'old' autoprothrombin II-A. Thromb Res 8:543, 1976
19. Marciniak, E.: Inhibitor of human blood coagulation elicited by thrombin. J Lab Clin Med 79:921, 1972
20. Dahlbäck, B., and Stenflo, J.: High molecular weight complex in human plasma between vitamin K–dependent protein S and complement component C4b-binding protein. Proc Natl Acad Sci USA 78:2512, 1981
21. Dahlbäck, B.: Protein S and C4b-binding protein: components involved in the regulation of the protein C anticoagulant system. Thromb Haemost 66:49, 1991
22. Dahlbäck, B.: Inhibition of protein Ca cofactor function of human and

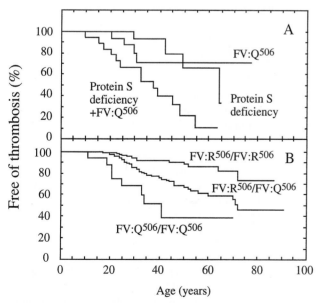

Figure 19–9. Thrombosis-free survival curves in relation to genetic defects. *A*, Thrombosis-free survival curves in families with both hereditary protein S deficiency and APC resistance (FV:Q506 allele). Twenty-one family members had isolated protein S deficiency, 21 APC resistance (FV:Q506) only, and 18 both defects.[622] *B*, In families with inherited APC resistance, the differences in survival curves between normals (FV:R506/FV:R506) and heterozygotes (FV:R506/FV:Q506), and between heterozygotes and homozygotes (FV:Q506/FV:Q506), were highly significant.[575]

bovine protein S by C4b-binding protein. J Biol Chem 261:12022, 1986

23. Heeb, M. J., Mesters, R. M., Tans, G., Rosing, J., and Griffin, J. H.: Binding of protein S to factor Va associated with inhibition of prothrombinase that is independent of activated protein C. J Biol Chem 268:2872, 1993

24. Hackeng, T. M., van't Veer, C., Meijers, J. C., and Bouma, B. N.: Human protein S inhibits prothrombinase complex activity on endothelial cells and platelets via direct interactions with factors Va and Xa. J Biol Chem 269:21051, 1994

25. Dahlbäck, B., and Hildebrand, B.: Inherited resistance to activated protein C is corrected by anticoagulant cofactor activity found to be a property of factor V. Proc Natl Acad Sci USA 91:1396, 1994

26. Shen, L., and Dahlbäck, B.: Factor V and protein S as synergistic cofactors to activated protein C in degradation of factor VIIIa. J Biol Chem 269:18735, 1994

27. Shen, L., He, X., and Dahlbäck, B.: Synergistic cofactor function of factor V and protein S to activated protein C in inactivation of factor VIIIa. Thromb Haemost 78:1030, 1997

28. Varadi, K., Rosing, J., Tans, G., Pabinger, I., Keil, B., and Schwarz, H. P.: Factor V enhances the cofactor function of protein S in the APC-mediated inactivation of factor VIII: influence of the factor VR506Q mutation. Thromb Haemost 76:208, 1996

29. Suzuki, K., Deyashiki, Y., Nishioka, J., and Toma, K.: Protein C inhibitor: structure and function. Thromb Haemost 61:337, 1989

30. van der Meer, F. J., van Tilburg, N. H., van Wijngaarden, A., van der Linden, I. K., Briet, E., and Bertina, R. M.: A second plasma inhibitor of activated protein C: alpha 1-antitrypsin. Thromb Haemost 62:756, 1989

31. Heeb, M. J., and Griffin, J. H.: Physiologic inhibition of human activated protein C by alpha 1-antitrypsin. J Biol Chem 263:11613, 1988

32. Heeb, M. J., Espana, F., and Griffin, J. H.: Inhibition and complexation of activated protein C by two major inhibitors in plasma. Blood 73:446, 1989

33. Heeb, M. J., Gruber, A., and Griffin, J. H.: Identification of divalent metal ion-dependent inhibition of activated protein C by alpha 2-macroglobulin and alpha 2-antiplasmin in blood and comparisons to inhibition of factor Xa, thrombin, and plasmin. J Biol Chem 266:17606, 1991

34. Hoogendoorn, H., Toh, C. H., Nesheim, M. E., and Giles, A. R.: Alpha 2-macroglobulin binds and inhibits activated protein C. Blood 78:2283, 1991

35. Marlar, R. A., and Neumann, A.: Neonatal purpura fulminans due to homozygous protein C or protein S deficiencies. Semin Thromb Hemost 16:299, 1990

36. Jalbert, L. R., Rosen, E. D., Carmeliet, P., Castelina, F. J., and Collen, D.: Characterization of the anticoagulant protein C by targeted inactivation in mice. Blood 90 suppl. 1:258a, 1997

37. Dahlbäck, B., Hillarp, A., Rosen, S., and Zoller, B.: Resistance to activated protein C, the FV:Q506 allele, and venous thrombosis. Ann Hematol 72:166, 1996

38. Dahlbäck, B.: Resistance to activated protein C as risk factor for thrombosis: molecular mechanisms, laboratory investigation, and clinical management. Semin Hematol 34:217, 1997

39. Dahlbäck, B.: Resistance to activated protein C caused by the factor VR506Q mutation is a common risk factor for venous thrombosis. Thromb Haemost 78:483, 1997

40. Reitsma, P. H.: Protein C deficiency: from gene defects to disease. Thromb Haemost 78:344, 1997

41. Bertina, R. M.: Introduction: hypercoagulable states. Semin-Hematol 34:167, 1997

42. Aiach, M., Borgel, D., Gaussem, P., Emmerich, J., Alhenc Gelas, M., and Gandrille, S.: Protein C and protein S deficiencies. Semin Hematol 34:205, 1997

43. Borgel, D., Gandrille, S., and Aiach, M.: Protein S deficiency. Thromb Haemost 78:351, 1997

44. Kalafatis, M., Krishnaswamy, S., Rand, M. D., and Mann, K. G.: Factor V. Methods Enzymol 222:224, 1993

45. Kane, W. H., and Davie, E. W.: Blood coagulation factors V and VIII: structural and functional similarities and their relationship to hemorrhagic and thrombotic disorders. Blood 71:539, 1988

46. Rosing, J., and Tans, G.: Coagulation factor V: an old star shines again. Thromb Haemost 78:427, 1997

47. Mann, K. G., Krishnaswamy, S., and Lawson, J. H.: Surface-dependent hemostasis. Semin-Hematol 29:213, 1992

48. Mann, K. G., Nesheim, M. E., Church, W. R., Haley, P., and Krishnaswamy, S.: Surface-dependent reactions of the vitamin K–dependent enzyme complexes. Blood 76:1, 1990

49. Fay, P. J.: Factor VIII structure and function. Thromb Haemost 70:63, 1993

50. Kane, W. H., and Davie, E. W.: Cloning of a cDNA coding for human factor V, a blood coagulation factor homologous to factor VIII and ceruloplasmin. Proc Natl Acad Sci USA 83:6800, 1986

51. Kane, W. H., Ichinose, A., Hagen, F. S., and Davie, E. W.: Cloning of cDNAs coding for the heavy chain region and connecting region of human factor V, a blood coagulation factor with four types of internal repeats. Biochemistry 26:6508, 1987

52. Jenny, R. J., Pittman, D. D., Toole, J. J., Kriz, R. W., Aldape, R. A., Hewick, R. M., Kaufman, R. J., and Mann, K. G.: Complete cDNA and derived amino acid sequence of human factor V. Proc Natl Acad Sci USA 84:4846, 1987

53. Pemberton, S., Lindley, P., Zaitsev, V., Card, G., Tuddenham, E. G. D., and Kemball-Cook, G.: A molecular model for the triplicated A-domains of human factor VIII based on the crystal structure of human ceruloplasmin. Blood 89:2413, 1997

54. Zaitseva, I., Zaitsev, V., Card, G., Moshkov, K., Bax, B., Ralph, A., and Lindley, P.: The X-ray structure of human serum ceruloplasmin at 3.1 Å: nature of the copper centres. J Biol Inorg Chem 1:15, 1996

55. Villoutreix, B. O., and Dahlbäck, B.: Structural investigation of the A domains of human blood coagulation factor V by molecular modeling. Protein Sci in press, 1998

56. Mann, K. G., Lawler, C. M., Vehar, G. A., and Church, W. R.: Coagulation Factor V contains copper ion. J Biol Chem 259:12949, 1984

57. Baumgartner, S., Hofmann, K., Chiquet-Ehrismann, R., and Bucher, P.: The discoidin domain family revisited: New members from prokaryotes and a homology-based prediction. Protein Science in press, 1998

58. Nesheim, M. E., and Mann, K. G.: Thrombin-catalyzed activation of single chain bovine factor V. J Biol Chem 254:1326, 1979

59. Esmon, C. T.: The subunit structure of thrombin-activated factor V. Isolation of activated factor V, separation of subunits, and reconstitution of biological activity. J Biol Chem 254:964, 1979

60. Dahlbäck, B.: Human coagulation factor V purification and thrombin-catalyzed activation. J Clin Invest 66:583, 1980

61. Kane, W. H., and Majerus, P. W.: Purification and characterization of human coagulation factor V. J Biol Chem 256:1002, 1981

62. Suzuki, K., Dahlbäck, B., and Stenflo, J.: Thrombin-catalyzed activation of human coagulation factor V. J Biol Chem 257:6556, 1982

63. Thorelli, E., Kaufman, R. J., and Dahlbäck, B.: Cleavage requirements for activation of factor V by factor Xa. Eur J Biochem 247:12, 1997

64. Kalafatis, M., Jenny, R. J., and Mann, K. G.: Identification and characterization of a phospholipid-binding site of bovine factor Va. J Biol Chem 265:21580, 1990

65. Ortel, T. L., Devore Carter, D., Quinn Allen, M., and Kane, W. H.: Deletion analysis of recombinant human factor V. Evidence for a phosphatidylserine binding site in the second C-type domain. J Biol Chem 267:4189, 1992

66. Ortel, T. L., Quinn Allen, M. A., Keller, F. G., Peterson, J. A., Larocca, D., and Kane, W. H.: Localization of functionally important epitopes within the second C-type domain of coagulation factor V using recombinant chimeras. J Biol Chem 269:15898, 1994

67. Kalafatis, M., Rand, M. D., and Mann, K. G.: Factor Va-membrane interaction is mediated by two regions located on the light chain of the cofactor. Biochemistry 33:486, 1994

68. Annamalai, A. E., Rao, A. K., Chiu, H. C., Wang, D., Dutta Roy, A. K., Walsh, P. N., and Colman, R. W.: Epitope mapping of functional domains of human factor Va with human and murine monoclonal antibodies. Evidence for the interaction of heavy chain with factor Xa and calcium. Blood 70:139, 1987

69. Guinto, E. R., and Esmon, C. T.: Loss of prothrombin and of factor Xa-factor Va interactions upon inactivation of factor Va by activated protein C. J Biol Chem 259:13986, 1984

70. Kalafatis, M., Xue, J., Lawler, C. M., and Mann, K. G.: Contribution of the heavy and light chains of factor Va to the interaction with factor Xa. Biochemistry 33:6538, 1994

71. Tucker, M. M., Foster, W. B., Katzmann, J. A., and Mann, K. G.: A monoclonal antibody which inhibits the factor Va:factor Xa interaction. J Biol Chem 258:1210, 1983

72. Luckow, E. A., Lyons, D. A., Ridgeway, T. M., Esmon, C. T., and

Laue, T. M.: Interaction of clotting factor V heavy chain with pro-thrombin and prethrombin 1 and role of activated protein C in regulating this interaction: analysis by analytical ultracentrifugation. Biochemistry 28:2348, 1989

73. Heeb, M. J., Kojima, Y., Hackeng, T. M., and Griffin, J. H.: Binding sites for blood coagulation factor Xa and protein S involving residues 493–506 in factor Va. Protein Sci 5:1883, 1996

74. Bakker, H. M., Tans, G., Thomassen, M. C., Yukelson, L. Y., Ebberink, R., Hemker, H. C., and Rosing, J.: Functional properties of human factor Va lacking the Asp683-Arg709 domain of the heavy chain. J Biol Chem 269:20662, 1994

75. Walker, F. J., Sexton, P. W., and Esmon, C. T.: The inhibition of blood coagulation by activated Protein C through the selective inactivation of activated Factor V. Biochim Biophys Acta 571:333, 1979

76. Suzuki, K., Stenflo, J., Dahlbäck, B., and Teodorsson, B.: Inactivation of human coagulation factor V by activated protein C. J Biol Chem 258:1914, 1983

77. Fay, P. J., Smudzin, T. M., and Walker, F. J.: Activated protein C-catalyzed inactivation of human factor VIII and factor VIIIa. Identification of cleavage sites and correlation of proteolysis with cofactor activity. J Biol Chem 266:20139, 1991

78. Kalafatis, M., Rand, M. D., and Mann, K. G.: The mechanism of inactivation of human factor V and human factor Va by activated protein C. J Biol Chem 269:31869, 1994

79. Comp, P. C.: Animal studies of protein C physiology. Thromb Haemost 10:149, 1984

80. Comp, P. C., Jacocks, R. M., Ferrell, G. L., and Esmon, C. T.: Activation of protein C in vivo. J Clin Invest 70:127, 1982

81. Gruber, A., Hanson, S. R., Kelly, A. B., Yan, B. S., Bang, N., Griffin, J. H., and Harker, L. A.: Inhibition of thrombus formation by activated recombinant protein C in a primate model of arterial thrombosis [see comments]. Circulation 82:578, 1990

82. Nicolaes, G. A., Tans, G., Thomassen, M. C., Hemker, H. C., Pabinger, I., Varadi, K., Schwarz, H. P., and Rosing, J.: Peptide bond cleavages and loss of functional activity during inactivation of factor Va and factor VaR506Q by activated protein C. J Biol Chem 270:21158, 1995

83. Nesheim, M. E., Canfield, W. M., Kisiel, W., and Mann, K. G.: Studies of the capacity of factor Xa to protect factor Va from inactivation by activated protein C. J Biol Chem 257:1443, 1982

84. Rosing, J., Hoekema, L., Nicolaes, G. A., Thomassen, M. C., Hemker, H. C., Varadi, K., Schwarz, H. P., and Tans, G.: Effects of protein S and factor Xa on peptide bond cleavages during inactivation of factor Va and factor VaR506Q by activated protein C. J Biol Chem 270:27852, 1995

85. Solymoss, S., Tucker, M. M., and Tracy, P. B.: Kinetics of inactivation of membrane-bound factor Va by activated protein C. Protein S modulates factor Xa protection. J Biol Chem 263:14884, 1988

86. Krishnaswamy, S., Williams, E. B., and Mann, K. G.: The binding of activated protein C to factors V and Va [published erratum appears in J Biol Chem 1987 Feb 5;262(4):1926]. J Biol Chem 261:9684, 1986

87. Walker, F. J.: Regulation of activated protein C by protein S. The role of phospholipid in factor Va inactivation. J Biol Chem 256:11128, 1981

88. Lu, D., Kalafatis, M., Mann, K. G., and Long, G. L.: Comparison of activated protein C/protein S-mediated inactivation of human factor VIII and factor V. Blood 87:4708, 1996

89. Yegneswaran, S., Wood, G. M., Esmon, C. T., and Johnson, A. E.: Protein S alters the active site location of activated protein C above the membrane surface. A fluorescence resonance energy transfer study of topography. J Biol Chem 272:25013, 1997

90. Smirnov, M. D., and Esmon, C. T.: Phosphatidylethanolamine incorporation into vesicles selectively enhances factor Va inactivation by activated protein C. J Biol Chem 269:816, 1994

91. Petaja, J., Fernandez, J. A., Gruber, A., and Griffin, J. H.: Anticoagulant synergism of heparin and activated protein C in vitro. Role of a novel anticoagulant mechanism of heparin, enhancement of inactivation of factor V by activated protein C. J Clin Invest 99:2655, 1997

92. Esmon, C. T., Stenflo, J., and Suttie, J. W.: A new vitamin K–dependent protein. A phospholipid-binding zymogen of a serine esterase. J Biol Chem 251:3052, 1976

93. Long, G. L., Belagaje, R. M., and MacGillivray, R. T.: Cloning and sequencing of liver cDNA coding for bovine protein C. Proc Natl Acad Sci USA 81:5653, 1984

94. Beckmann, R. J., Schmidt, R. J., Santerre, R. F., Plutzky, J., Crabtree, G. R., and Long, G. L.: The structure and evolution of a 461 amino acid human protein C precursor and its messenger RNA, based upon the DNA sequence of cloned human liver cDNAs. Nucleic Acids Res 13:5233, 1985

95. Foster, D., and Davie, E. W.: Characterization of a cDNA coding for human protein C. Proc Natl Acad Sci USA 81:4766, 1984

96. Foster, D. C., Rudinski, M. S., Schach, B. G., Berkner, K. L., Kumar, A. A., Hagen, F. S., Sprecher, C. A., Insley, M. Y., and Davie, E. W.: Propeptide of human protein C is necessary for gamma-carboxylation. Biochemistry 26:7003, 1987

97. Foster, D. C., Holly, R. D., Sprecher, C. A., Walker, K. M., and Kumar, A. A.: Endoproteolytic processing of the human protein C precursor by the yeast Kex2 endopeptidase coexpressed in mammalian cells. Biochemistry 30:367, 1991

98. Miletich, J. P., Leykam, J. F., and Broze Jr, G. J.: Detection of single chain protein C in plasma. Blood (suppl. 1) 62:306a, 1983

99. Fernlund, P., and Stenflo, J.: Amino acid sequence of the light chain of bovine protein C. J Biol Chem 257:12170, 1982

100. Stenflo, J., and Fernlund, P.: Amino acid sequence of the heavy chain of bovine protein C. J Biol Chem 257:12180, 1982

101. Okafuji, T., Maekawa, K., Nawa, K., and Marumoto, Y.: The cDNA cloning and mRNA expression of rat protein C. Biochim Biophys Acta 1131:329, 1992

102. Tada, N., Sato, M., Tsujimura, A., Iwase, R., and Hashimoto Gotoh, T.: Isolation and characterization of a mouse protein C cDNA. J Biochem Tokyo 111:491, 1992

103. Murakawa, M., Okamura, T., Kamura, T., Kuroiwa, M., Harada, M., and Niho, Y.: A comparative study of partial primary structures of the catalytic region of mammalian protein C. Br J Haematol 86:590, 1994

104. Mather, T., Oganessyan, V., Hof, P., Huber, R., Foundling, S., Esmon, C., and Bode, W.: The 2.8 A crystal structure of Gla-domainless activated protein C. EMBO J 15:6822, 1996

105. Tulinsky, A.: The structures of domains of blood proteins. Thromb Haemost 66:16, 1991

106. Horie, S., Ishii, H., Hara, H., and Kazama, M.: Enhancement of thrombin-thrombomodulin-catalysed protein C activation by phosphatidylethanolamine containing unsaturated fatty acids: possible physiological significance of phosphatidylethanolamine in anticoagulant activity of thrombomodulin. Biochem J 301:683, 1994

107. Soriano Garcia, M., Padmanabhan, K., de Vos, A. M., and Tulinsky, A.: The Ca2+ ion and membrane binding structure of the Gla domain of Ca-prothrombin fragment 1. Biochemistry 31:2554, 1992

108. Zhang, L., and Castellino, F. J.: The binding energy of human coagulation protein C to acidic phospholipid vesicles contains a major contribution from leucine 5 in the gamma-carboxyglutamic acid domain. J Biol Chem 269:3590, 1994

109. Jalbert, L. R., Chan, J. C., Christiansen, W. T., and Castellino, F. J.: The hydrophobic nature of residue-5 of human protein C is a major determinant of its functional interactions with acidic phospholipid vesicles. Biochemistry 35:7093, 1996

110. Sunnerhagen, M., Forsen, S., Hoffren, A. M., Drakenberg, T., Teleman, O., and Stenflo, J.: Structure of the Ca²⁺-free Gla domain sheds light on membrane binding of blood coagulation proteins. Nat Struct Biol 2:504, 1995

111. Christiansen, W. T., Jalbert, L. R., Robertson, R. M., Jhingan, A., Prorok, M., and Castellino, F. J.: Hydrophobic amino acid residues of human anticoagulation protein C that contribute to its functional binding to phospholipid Vesicles. Biochemistry 34:10376, 1995

112. McDonald, J. F., Shah, A. M., Schwalbe, R. A., Kisiel, W., Dahlbäck, B., and Nelsestuen, G. L.: Comparison of naturally occurring vitamin K–dependent proteins: correlation of amino acid sequences and membrane binding properties suggests a membrane contact site. Biochemistry 36:5120, 1997

113. Shen, L., Shah, A. M., Dahlbäck, B., and Nelsestuen, G.: Enhancing the activity of protein C by mutagenesis to improve the membrane-binding site: studies related to proline-10. Biochemistry 36, 1997

114. Zhang, L., and Castellino, F. J.: A gamma-carboxyglutamic acid (gamma) variant (gamma 6D, gamma 7D) of human activated protein C displays greatly reduced activity as an anticoagulant. Biochemistry 29:10828, 1990

115. Zhang, L., and Castellino, F. J.: Role of the hexapeptide disulfide loop present in the gamma-carboxyglutamic acid domain of human protein C in its activation properties and in the in vitro anticoagulant activity of activated protein C. Biochemistry 30:6696, 1991

116. Zhang, L., Jhingan, A., and Castellino, F. J.: Role of individual gamma-carboxyglutamic acid residues of activated human protein C in defining its in vitro anticoagulant activity. Blood 80:942, 1992

117. Zhang, L., and Castellino, F. J.: Influence of specific gamma-carboxy-glutamic acid residues on the integrity of the calcium-dependent conformation of human protein C. J Biol Chem 267:26078, 1992

118. Zhang, L., and Castellino, F. J.: The contributions of individual gamma-carboxyglutamic acid residues in the calcium-dependent binding of recombinant human protein C to acidic phospholipid vesicles. J Biol Chem 268:12040, 1993

119. Christiansen, W. T., Tulinsky, A., and Castellino, F. J.: Functions of individual gamma-carboxyglutamic acid (Gla) residues of human protein c. Determination of functionally nonessential Gla residues and correlations with their mode of binding to calcium. Biochemistry 33:14993, 1994

120. Jhingan, A., Zhang, L., Christiansen, W. T., and Castellino, F. J.: The activities of recombinant gamma-carboxyglutamic-acid-deficient mutants of activated human protein C toward human coagulation factor Va and factor VIII in purified systems and in plasma. Biochemistry 33:1869, 1994

121. Colpitts, T. L., Prorok, M., and Castellino, F. J.: Binding of calcium to individual gamma-carboxyglutamic acid residues of human protein C. Biochemistry 34:2424, 1995

122. Bovill, E. G., Tomczak, J. A., Grant, B., Bhushan, F., Pillemer, E., Rainville, I. R., and Long, G. L.: Protein CVermont: symptomatic type II protein C deficiency associated with two GLA domain mutations. Blood 79:1456, 1992

123. Lu, D., Bovill, E. G., and Long, G. L.: Molecular mechanism for familial protein C deficiency and thrombosis in protein CVermont (Glu20->Ala and Val34->Met). J Biol Chem 269:29032, 1994

124. Lu, D., Kalafatis, M., Mann, K. G., and Long, G. L.: Loss of membrane-dependent factor Va cleavage: a mechanistic interpretation of the pathology of protein CVermont. Blood 84:687, 1994

125. Nishioka, J., Ido, M., Hayashi, T., and Suzuki, K.: The Gla26 residue of protein C is required for the binding of protein C to thrombomodulin and endothelial cell protein C receptor, but not to protein S and factor Va. Thromb Haemost 75:275, 1996

126. Thariath, A., and Castellino, F. J.: Highly conserved residue arginine-15 is required for the Ca2+-dependent properties of the gamma-carboxyglutamic acid domain of human anticoagulation protein C and activated protein C. Biochem J 322:309, 1997

127. Reitsma, P. H., Bernardi, F., Doig, R. G., Gandrille, S., Greengard, J. S., Ireland, H., Krawczak, M., Lind, B., Long, G. L., Poort, S. R., and et al.: Protein C deficiency: a database of mutations, 1995 update. On behalf of the Subcommittee on Plasma Coagulation Inhibitors of the Scientific and Standardization Committee of the ISTH. Thromb Haemost 73:876, 1995

128. Geng, J. P., and Castellino, F. J.: Properties of a recombinant chimeric protein in which the gamma-carboxyglutamic acid and helical stack domains of human anticoagulant protein C are replaced by those of human coagulation factor VII. Thromb Haemost 77:926, 1997

129. Ohlin, A. K., and Stenflo, J.: Calcium-dependent interaction between the epidermal growth factor precursor-like region of human protein C and a monoclonal antibody. J Biol Chem 262:13798, 1987

130. Ohlin, A. K., Landes, G., Bourdon, P., Oppenheimer, C., Wydro, R., and Stenflo, J.: Beta-hydroxyaspartic acid in the first epidermal growth factor-like domain of protein C. Its role in Ca²⁺ binding and biological activity. J Biol Chem 263:19240, 1988

131. Ohlin, A. K., Linse, S., and Stenflo, J.: Calcium binding to the epidermal growth factor homology region of bovine protein C. J Biol Chem 263:7411, 1988

132. Ohlin, A. K., Bjork, I., and Stenflo, J.: Proteolytic formation and properties of a fragment of protein C containing the gamma-carboxyglutamic acid rich domain and the EGF-like region. Biochemistry 29:644, 1990

133. Sunnerhagen, M., Olah, G. A., Stenflo, J., Forsen, S., Drakenberg, T., and Trewhella, J.: The relative orientation of Gla and EGF domains in coagulation factor X is altered by Ca²⁺ binding to the first EGF domain. A combined NMR-small angle X-ray scattering study. Biochemistry 35:11547, 1996

134. Drakenberg, T., Fernlund, P., Roepstorff, P., and Stenflo, J.: beta-Hydroxyaspartic acid in vitamin K–dependent protein C. Proc Natl Acad Sci USA 80:1802, 1983

135. Geng, J. P., Cheng, C. H., and Castellino, F. J.: Functional consequences of mutations in amino acid residues that stabilize calcium binding to the first epidermal growth factor homology domain of human protein C. Thromb Haemost 76:720, 1996

136. Grinnell, B. W., Walls, J. D., and Gerlitz, B.: Glycosylation of human

137. Hogg, P. J., Ohlin, A. K., and Stenflo, J.: Identification of structural domains in protein C involved in its interaction with thrombin-thrombomodulin on the surface of endothelial cells. J Biol Chem 267:703, 1992

138. Grinnell, B. W., Gerlitz, B., and Berg, D. T.: Identification of a region in protein C involved in thrombomodulin-stimulated activation by thrombin: potential repulsion at anion-binding site I in thrombin. Biochem J 303:929, 1994

139. Gerlitz, B., and Grinnell, B. W.: Mutation of protease domain residues Lys37–39 in human protein C inhibits activation by the thrombomodulin-thrombin complex without affecting activation by free thrombin. J Biol Chem 271:22285, 1996

140. Mesters, R. M., Heeb, M. J., and Griffin, J. H.: A novel exosite in the light chain of human activated protein C essential for interaction with blood coagulation factor Va. Biochemistry 32:12656, 1993

141. Bauer, K. A., Kass, B. L., Beeler, D. L., and Rosenberg, R. D.: Detection of protein C activation in humans. J Clin Invest 74:2033, 1984

142. Ehrlich, H. J., Jaskunas, S. R., Grinnell, B. W., Yan, S. B., and Bang, N. U.: Direct expression of recombinant activated human protein C, a serine protease. J Biol Chem 264:14298, 1989

143. Bode, W., and Stubbs, M. T.: Spatial structure of thrombin as a guide to its multiple sites of interaction. Semin Thromb Hemost 19:321, 1993

144. Titani, K., Kumar, S., Takio, K., Ericsson, L. H., Wade, R. D., Ashida, K., Walsh, K. A., Chopek, M. W., Sadler, J. E., and Fujikawa, K.: Amino acid sequence of human von Willebrand factor. Biochemistry 25:3171, 1986

145. Miletich, J. P., and Broze, G. J., Jr.: Beta protein C is not glycosylated at asparagine 329. The rate of translation may influence the frequency of usage at asparagine-X-cysteine sites. J Biol Chem 265:11397, 1990

146. Bode, W., and Schwager, P.: The refined crystal structure of bovine beta-trypsin at 1.8 A resolution. II. Crystallographic refinement, calcium binding site, benzamidine binding site and active site at pH 7.0. J Mol Biol 98:693, 1975

147. Schechter, I., and Berger, A.: On the size of the active site in proteases. I, Papain. Biochem Biophys Res Commun 27:157, 1967

148. Rezaie, A. R., and Esmon, C. T.: Conversion of glutamic acid 192 to glutamine in activated protein C changes the substrate specificity and increases reactivity toward macromolecular inhibitors. J Biol Chem 268:19943, 1993

149. Mesters, R. M., Heeb, M. J., and Griffin, J. H.: Interactions and inhibition of blood coagulation factor Va involving residues 311–325 of activated protein C. Protein Sci 2:1482, 1993

150. Mesters, R. M., Houghten, R. A., and Griffin, J. H.: Identification of a sequence of human activated protein C (residues 390–404) essential for its anticoagulant activity. J Biol Chem 266:24514, 1991

151. Steiner, S. A., Amphlett, G. W., and Castellino, F. J.: Stimulation of the amidase and esterase activity of activated bovine plasma protein C by monovalent cations. Biochem Biophys Res Commun 94:340, 1980

152. Steiner, S. A., and Castellino, F. J.: Kinetic studies of the role of monovalent cations in the amidolytic activity of activated bovine plasma protein C. Biochemistry 21:4609, 1982

153. Steiner, S. A., and Castellino, F. J.: Kinetic mechanism for stimulation by monovalent cations of the amidase activity of the plasma protease bovine activated protein C. Biochemistry 24:609, 1985

154. Steiner, S. A., and Castellino, F. J.: Effect of monovalent cations on the pre-steady-state kinetic parameters of the plasma protease bovine activated protein C. Biochemistry 24:1136, 1985

155. Hill, K. A., and Castellino, F. J.: The stimulation by monovalent cations of the amidase activity of bovine des-1-41 light chain activated protein C. J Biol Chem 261:14741, 1986

156. Hill, K. A., and Castellino, F. J.: The effect of monovalent cations on the pre-steady state reaction kinetics of bovine activated plasma protein C and des-1-41-light chain activated plasma protein C. J Biol Chem 262:140, 1987

157. Hill, K. A., and Castellino, F. J.: Topographical relationships between the monovalent and divalent cation binding sites of des-1-41-light chain bovine plasma protein C and des-1-41-light chain-activated bovine plasma protein C. J Biol Chem 262:7105, 1987

158. Hill, K. A., Steiner, S. A., and Castellino, F. J.: Estimation of the distance between the divalent cation binding site of des-1-41-light chain-activated bovine plasma protein C and a nitroxide spin label attached to the active-site serine residue. Biochem J 251:229, 1988

159. Di Cera, E., Hopfner, K. P., and Dang, Q. D.: Theory of allosteric effects in serine proteases. Biophys-J 70:174, 1996

160. Hill, K. A., Kroon, L. M., and Castellino, F. J.: The effect of divalent cations on the amidolytic activity of bovine plasma activated protein C and des-1-41-light chain activated protein C. J Biol Chem 262:9581, 1987

161. Rezaie, A. R., Mather, T., Sussman, F., and Esmon, C. T.: Mutation of Glu-80–<Lys results in a protein C mutant that no longer requires Ca^{2+} for rapid activation by the thrombin-thrombomodulin complex. J Biol Chem 269:3151, 1994

162. Rezaie, A. R., and Esmon, C. T.: Tryptophans 231 and 234 in protein C report the Ca^{2+}-dependent conformational change required for activation by the thrombin-thrombomodulin complex. Biochemistry 34:12221, 1995

163. He, X., Shen, L., Bjartell, A., Malm, J., Lilja, H., and Dahlbäck, B.: The gene encoding vitamin K–dependent anticoagulant protein C is expressed in human male reproductive tissues. J Histochem Cytochem 43:563, 1995

164. McClure, D. B., Walls, J. D., and Grinnell, B. W.: Post-translational processing events in the secretion pathway of human protein C, a complex vitamin K–dependent antithrombotic factor. J Biol Chem 267:19710, 1992

165. Rocchi, M., Roncuzzi, L., Santamaria, R., Archidiacono, N., Dente, L., and Romeo, G.: Mapping through somatic cell hybrids and cDNA probes of protein C to chromosome 2, factor X to chromosome 13, and alpha 1-acid glycoprotein to chromosome 9. Hum Genet 74:30, 1986

166. Long, G. L., Marshall, A., Gardner, J. C., and Naylor, S. L.: Genes for human vitamin K–dependent plasma proteins C and S are located on chromosomes 2 and 3, respectively. Somat Cell Mol Genet 14:93, 1988

167. Kato, A., Miura, O., Sumi, Y., and Aoki, N.: Assignment of the human protein C gene (PROC) to chromosome region 2q14–q21 by in situ hybridization. Cytogenet Cell Genet 47:46, 1988

168. Patracchini, P., Aiello, V., Palazzi, P., Calzolari, E., and Bernardi, F.: Sublocalization of the human protein C gene on chromosome 2q13-q14. Hum Genet 81:191, 1989

169. Plutzky, J., Hoskins, J. A., Long, G. L., and Crabtree, G. R.: Evolution and organization of the human protein C gene. Proc Natl Acad Sci USA 83:546, 1986

170. Foster, D. C., Yoshitake, S., and Davie, E. W.: The nucleotide sequence of the gene for human protein C. Proc Natl Acad Sci USA 82:4673, 1985

171. Tsay, W., Lee, Y. M., Lee, S. C., Shen, M. C., and Chen, P. J.: Characterization of human protein C gene promoter: insights from natural human mutants. DNA Cell Biol 15:907, 1996

172. Tsay, W., Lee, Y. M., Lee, S. C., Shen, M. C., and Chen, P. J.: Synergistic transactivation of HNF-1alpha, HNF-3, and NF-I contributes to the activation of the liver-specific protein C gene. DNA Cell Biol 16:569, 1997

173. Comp, P. C., and Esmon, C. T.: Generation of fibrinolytic activity by infusion of activated protein C into dogs. J Clin Invest 68:1221, 1981

174. Taylor, F. B. J., and Lockhart, M. S.: Whole blood clot lysis: in vivo modulation by activated protein C. Thromb Res 37:639, 1985

175. Bajzar, L., Fredenburgh, J. C., and Nesheim, M.: The activated protein C-mediated enhancement of tissue-type plasminogen activator-induced fibrinolysis in a cell-free system. J Biol Chem 265:16948, 1990

176. Bajzar, L., and Nesheim, M.: The effect of activated protein C on fibrinolysis in cell-free plasma can be attributed specifically to attenuation of prothrombin activation. J Biol Chem 268:8608, 1993

177. de Fouw, N. J., van Tilburg, N. H., Haverkate, F., and Bertina, R. M.: Activated protein C accelerates clot lysis by virtue of its anticoagulant activity. Blood Coagul Fibrinolysis 4:201, 1993

178. Bajzar, L., Manuel, R., and Nesheim, M. E.: Purification and characterization of TAFI, a thrombin-activable fibrinolysis inhibitor. J Biol Chem 270:14477, 1995

179. Bajzar, L., Nesheim, M. E., and Tracy, P. B.: The profibrinolytic effect of activated protein C in clots formed from plasma is TAFI-dependent. Blood 88:2093, 1996

180. Bajzar, L., Morser, J., and Nesheim, M.: TAFI, or plasma procarboxypeptidase B, couples the coagulation and fibrinolytic cascades through the thrombin-thrombomodulin complex. J Biol Chem 271:16603, 1996

181. Espana, F., Gruber, A., Heeb, M. J., Hanson, S. R., Harker, L. A., and Griffin, J. H.: In vivo and in vitro complexes of activated protein C with two inhibitors in baboons. Blood 77:1754, 1991

182. Hoogendoorn, H., Nesheim, M. E., and Giles, A. R.: A qualitative and quantitative analysis of the activation and inactivation of protein C in vivo in a primate model. Blood 75:2164, 1990

183. Hermans, J. M., and Stone, S. R.: Interaction of activated protein C with serpins. Biochem J 295:239, 1993

184. Fay, W. P., and Owen, W. G.: Platelet plasminogen activator inhibitor: Purification and characterization of interaction with plasminogen activators and activated protein C. Biochemistry 28:5773, 1989

185. Rezaie, A. R., Cooper, S. T., Church, F. C., and Esmon, C. T.: Protein C inhibitor is a potent inhibitor of the thrombin-thrombomodulin complex. J Biol Chem 270:25336, 1995

186. Laurell, M., Christensson, A., Abrahamsson, P. A., Stenflo, J., and Lilja, H.: Protein C inhibitor in human body fluids. Seminal plasma is rich in inhibitor antigen deriving from cells throughout the male reproductive system. J Clin Invest 89:1094, 1992

187. Espana, F., Gilabert, J., Estelles, A., Romeu, A., Aznar, J., and Cabo, A.: Functionally active protein C inhibitor/plasminogen activator inhibitor-3 (PCI/PAI-3) is secreted in seminal vesicles, occurs at high concentrations in human seminal plasma and complexes with prostate-specific antigen. Thromb Res 64:309, 1991

188. Hermans, J. M., Jones, R., and Stone, S. R.: Rapid inhibition of the sperm protease acrosin by protein C inhibitor. Biochemistry 33:5440, 1994

189. Laurell, M., Stenflo, J., and Carlson, T. H.: Turnover of ^{125}I-protein C inhibitor and *I-alpha 1-antitrypsin and their complexes with activated protein C. Blood 76:2290, 1990

190. Esmon, C. T., and Owen, W. G.: Identification of an endothelial cell cofactor for thrombin-catalyzed activation of protein C. Proc Natl Acad Sci USA 78:2249, 1981

191. Esmon, C. T., Esmon, N. L., and Harris, K. W.: Complex formation between thrombin and thrombomodulin inhibits both thrombin-catalyzed fibrin formation and factor V activation. J Biol Chem 257:7944, 1982

192. Esmon, N. L., Carroll, R. C., and Esmon, C. T.: Thrombomodulin blocks the ability of thrombin to activate platelets. J Biol Chem 258:12238, 1983

193. Hofsteenge, J., and Stone, S.: The effect of thrombomodulin on the cleavage of fibrinogen and fibrinogen fragments by thrombin. Eur J Biochem 168:49, 1987

194. Jakubowski, H. V., Kline, M. D., and Owen, W. G.: The effect of bovine thrombomodulin on the specificity of bovine thrombin. J Biol Chem 261:3876, 1986

195. Polgar, J., Lerant, I., Muszbek, L., and Machovich, R.: Thrombomodulin inhibits the activation of factor XIII by thrombin. Thromb Res 43:685, 1986

196. Esmon, N. L., Owen, W. G., and Esmon, C. T.: Isolation of a membrane-bound cofactor for thrombin-catalyzed activation of protein C. J Biol Chem 257:859, 1982

197. Salem, H. H., Maruyama, I., Ishii, H., and Majerus, P. W.: Isolation and characterization of thrombomodulin from human placenta. J Biol Chem 259:12246, 1984

198. Suzuki, K., Kusumoto, H., and Hashimoto, S.: Isolation and characterization of thrombomodulin from bovine lung. Biochim Biophys Acta 882:343, 1986

199. Jackman, R. W., Beeler, D. L., VanDeWater, L., and Rosenberg, R. D.: Characterization of a thrombomodulin cDNA reveals structural similarity to the low density lipoprotein receptor. Proc Natl Acad Sci U S A 83:8834, 1986

200. Suzuki, K., Kusumoto, H., Deyashiki, Y., Nishioka, J., Maruyama, I., Zushi, M., Kawahara, S., Honda, G., Yamamoto, S., and Horiguchi, S.: Structure and expression of human thrombomodulin, a thrombin receptor on endothelium acting as a cofactor for protein C activation. EMBO J 6:1891, 1987

201. Wen, D. Z., Dittman, W. A., Ye, R. D., Deaven, L. L., Majerus, P. W., and Sadler, J. E.: Human thrombomodulin: complete cDNA sequence and chromosome localization of the gene. Biochemistry 26:4350, 1987

202. Dittman, W. A., Kumada, T., Sadler, J. E., and Majerus, P. W.: The structure and function of mouse thrombomodulin. Phorbol myristate acetate stimulates degradation and synthesis of thrombomodulin without affecting mRNA levels in hemangioma cells. J Biol Chem 263:15815, 1988

203. Dittman, W. A., and Majerus, P. W.: Structure and function of thrombomodulin: a natural anticoagulant. Blood 75:329, 1990

204. Imada, S., Yamaguchi, H., Nagumo, M., Katayanagi, S., Iwasaki, H.,

and Imada, M.: Identification of fetomodulin, a surface marker protein of fetal development, as thrombomodulin by gene cloning and functional assays. Dev Biol 140:113, 1990

205. Healy, A. M., Rayburn, H. B., Rosenberg, R. D., and Weiler, H.: Absence of the blood-clotting regulator thrombomodulin causes embryonic lethality in mice before development of a functional cardiovascular system. Proc Natl Acad Sci U S A 92:850, 1995

206. Rosenberg, R. D.: Thrombomodulin gene disruption and mutation in mice. Thromb Haemost 78:705, 1997

207. Parkinson, J. F., Vlahos, C. J., Yan, S. C., and Bang, N. U.: Recombinant human thrombomodulin. Regulation of cofactor activity and anticoagulant function by a glycosaminoglycan side chain. Biochem J 283:151, 1992

208. Petersen, T. E.: The amino-terminal domain of thrombomodulin and pancreatic stone protein homologous with lectins. FEBS Lett 231:51, 1988

209. Patthy, L.: Detecting distant homologies of mosaic proteins. Analysis of the sequences of thrombomodulin, thrombospondin complement components C9, C8 alpha and beta, vitronectin and plasma cell membrane glycoprotein PC-1. J Mol Biol 202:689, 1988

210. Conway, E. M., Pollefeyt, S., Collen, D., and Steiner Mosonyi, M.: The amino terminal lectin-like domain of thrombomodulin is required for constitutive endocytosis. Blood 89:652, 1997

211. Kurosawa, S., Galvin, J. B., Esmon, N. L., and Esmon, C. T.: Proteolytic formation and properties of functional domains of thrombomodulin. J Biol Chem 262:2206, 1987

212. Kurosawa, S., Stearns, D. J., Jackson, K. W., and Esmon, C. T.: A 10-kDa cyanogen bromide fragment from the epidermal growth factor homology domain of rabbit thrombomodulin contains the primary thrombin binding site. J Biol Chem 263:5993, 1988

213. Hayashi, T., Zushi, M., Yamamoto, S., and Suzuki, K.: Further localization of binding sites for thrombin and protein C in human thrombomodulin. J Biol Chem 265:20156, 1990

214. Tsiang, M., Lentz, S. R., Dittman, W. A., Wen, D., Scarpati, E. M., and Sadler, J. E.: Equilibrium binding of thrombin to recombinant human thrombomodulin: effect of hirudin, fibrinogen, factor Va, and peptide analogues. Biochemistry 29:10602, 1990

215. Stearns, D. J., Kurosawa, S., and Esmon, C. T.: Microthrombomodulin. Residues 310–486 from the epidermal growth factor precursor homology domain of thrombomodulin will accelerate protein C activation. J Biol Chem 264:3352, 1989

216. Suzuki, K., Hayashi, T., Nishioka, J., Kosaka, Y., Zushi, M., Honda, G., and Yamamoto, S.: A domain composed of epidermal growth factor-like structures of human thrombomodulin is essential for thrombin binding and for protein C activation. J Biol Chem 264:4872, 1989

217. Zushi, M., Gomi, K., Yamamoto, S., Maruyama, I., Hayashi, T., and Suzuki, K.: The last three consecutive epidermal growth factor-like structures of human thrombomodulin comprise the minimum functional domain for protein C-activating cofactor activity and anticoagulant activity. J Biol Chem 264:10351, 1989

218. Tsiang, M., Lentz, S. R., and Sadler, J. E.: Functional domains of membrane-bound human thrombomodulin. EGF-like domains four to six and the serine/threonine-rich domain are required for cofactor activity. J Biol Chem 267:6164, 1992

219. White, C. E., Hunter, M. J., Meininger, D. P., White, L. R., and Komives, E. A.: Large-scale expression, purification and characterization of small fragments of thrombomodulin: the roles of the sixth domain and of methionine 388. Protein-Eng 8:1177, 1995

220. Parkinson, J. F., Nagashima, M., Kuhn, I., Leonard, J., and Morser, J.: Structure-function studies of the epidermal growth factor domains of human thrombomodulin. Biochem Biophys Res Commun 185:567, 1992

221. Parkinson, J. F., Grinnell, B. W., Moore, R. E., Hoskins, J., Vlahos, C. J., and Bang, N. U.: Stable expression of a secretable deletion mutant of recombinant human thrombomodulin in mammalian cells. J Biol Chem 265:12602, 1990

222. Lougheed, J. C., Bowman, C. L., Meininger, D. P., and Komives, E. A.: Thrombin inhibition by cyclic peptides from thrombomodulin. Protein Sci 4:773, 1995

223. Srinivasan, J., Hu, S., Hrabal, R., Zhu, Y., Komives, E. A., and Ni, F.: Thrombin-bound structure of an EGF subdomain from human thrombomodulin determined by transferred nuclear Overhauser effects. Biochemistry 33:13553, 1994

224. Lentz, S. R., Chen, Y., and Sadler, J. E.: Sequences required for thrombomodulin cofactor activity within the fourth epidermal growth

factor-like domain of human thrombomodulin. J Biol Chem 268:15312, 1993

225. Nagashima, M., Lundh, E., Leonard, J. C., Morser, J., and Parkinson, J. F.: Alanine-scanning mutagenesis of the epidermal growth factor-like domains of human thrombomodulin identifies critical residues for its cofactor activity. J Biol Chem 268:2888, 1993

226. Zushi, M., Gomi, K., Honda, G., Kondo, S., Yamamoto, S., Hayashi, T., and Suzuki, K.: Aspartic acid 349 in the fourth epidermal growth factor-like structure of human thrombomodulin plays a role in its Ca(2+)-mediated binding to protein C. J Biol Chem 266:19886, 1991

227. Clarke, J. H., Light, D. R., Blasko, E., Parkinson, J. F., Nagashima, M., McLean, K., Vilander, L., Andrews, W. H., Morser, J., and Glaser, C. B.: The short loop between epidermal growth factor-like domains 4 and 5 is critical for human thrombomodulin function. J Biol Chem 268:6309, 1993

228. Glaser, C. B., Morser, J., Clarke, J. H., Blasko, E., McLean, K., Kuhn, I., Chang, R. J., Lin, J. H., Vilander, L., Andrews, W. H., and Light, D. R.: Oxidation of a specific methionine in thrombomodulin by activated neutrophil products blocks cofactor activity. A potential rapid mechanism for modulation of coagulation. J Clin Invest 90:2565, 1992

229. Honda, G., Masaki, C., Zushi, M., Tsuruta, K., and Sata, M.: The roles played by the D2 and D3 domains of recombinant human thrombomodulin in its function. J Biochem Tokyo 118:1030, 1995

230. Meininger, D. P., Hunter, M. J., and Komives, E. A.: Synthesis, activity, and preliminary structure of the fourth EGF-like domain of thrombomodulin. Protein Sci 4:1683, 1995

231. Adler, M., Seto, M. H., Nitecki, D. E., Lin, J. H., Light, D. R., and Morser, J.: The structure of a 19-residue fragment from the C-loop of the fourth epidermal growth factor-like domain of thrombomodulin. J Biol Chem 270:23366, 1995

232. White, C. E., Hunter, M. J., Meininger, D. P., Garrod, S., and Komives, E. A.: The fifth epidermal growth factor-like domain of thrombomodulin does not have an epidermal growth factor-like disulfide bonding pattern. Proc Natl Acad Sci USA 93:10177, 1996

233. Hunter, M. J., and Komives, E. A.: Thrombin-binding affinities of different disulfide-bonded isomers of the fifth EGF-like domain of thrombomodulin. Protein Sci 4:2129, 1995

234. Hrabal, R., Komives, E. A., and Ni, F.: Structural resiliency of an EGF-like subdomain bound to its target protein, thrombin. Protein Sci 5:195, 1996

235. Mathews, II, Padmanabhan, K. P., Tulinsky, A., and Sadler, J. E.: Structure of a nonadecapeptide of the fifth EGF domain of thrombomodulin complexed with thrombin. Biochemistry 33:13547, 1994

236. Preissner, K. T., Delvos, U., and Müller-Berghaus, G.: Binding of thrombin to thrombomodulin accelerates inhibition of the enzyme by antithrombin III. Evidence for a heparin-independent mechanism. Biochemistry. 26:2521, 1987

237. Bourin, M. C., Boffa, M. C., Björk, I., and Lindahl, U.: Functional domains of rabbit thrombomodulin. Proc Natl Acad Sci USA 83:5924, 1986

238. Hofsteenge, J., Taguchi, H., and Stone, S. R.: Effect of thrombomodulin on the kinetics of the interaction of thrombin with substrates and inhibitors. Biochem J 237:243, 1986

239. Preissner, K. T., Koyama, T., Müller, D., Tschopp, J., and Müller-Berghaus, G.: Domain structure of the endothelial cell receptor thrombomodulin as deduced from modulation of its anticoagulant functions. J Biol Chem 265:4915, 1990

240. Bourin, M. C., Lundgren-Åkderlund, E., and Lindahl, U.: Isolation and characterization of the glycosaminoglycan component of rabbit thrombomodulin proteoglycan. J Biol Chem 265:15424, 1990

241. Bourin, M. C., and Lindahl, U.: Functional role of the polysaccharide component of rabbit thrombomodulin proteoglycan. Effects on inactivation of thrombin by antithrombin, cleavage of fibrinogen by thrombin and thrombin-catalysed activation of factor V. Biochem J 270:419, 1990

242. Bourin, M. C.: Effect of rabbit thrombomodulin on thrombin inhibition by antithrombin in the presence of heparin. Thromb Res 54:27, 1989

243. Bourin, M. C., Ohlin, A. K., Lane, D. A., Stenflo, J., and Lindahl, U.: Relationship between anticoagulant activities and polyanionic properties of rabbit thrombomodulin. J Biol Chem 263:8044, 1988

244. Lin, J. H., McLean, K., Morser, J., Young, T. A., Wydro, R. M., Andrews, W. H., and Light, D. R.: Modulation of glycosaminoglycan addition in naturally expressed and recombinant human thrombomodulin. J Biol Chem 269:25021, 1994

245. Nawa, K., Sakano, K., Fujiwara, H., Sato, Y., Sugiyama, N., Ternuchi, T., Iwamoto, M., and Murimoto, Y.: Presence and function of chondroitin-4-sulfate on recombinant human soluble thrombomodulin. Biochem Biophys Res Commun 171:729, 1990

246. Gerlitz, B., Hassell, T., Vlahos, C. J., Parkinson, J. F., Bang, N. U., and Grinnell, B. W.: Identification of the predominant glycosaminoglycan-attachment site in soluble recombinant human thrombomodulin: potential regulation of functionality by glycosyltransferase competition for serine474. Biochem J 295:131, 1993

247. Koyama, T., Parkinson, J. F., Sie, P., Bang, N. U., Muller Berghaus, G., and Preissner, K. T.: Different glycoforms of human thrombomodulin. Their glycosaminoglycan-dependent modulatory effects on thrombin inactivation by heparin cofactor II and antithrombin III. Eur J Biochem 198:563, 1991

248. Ye, J., Rezaie, A. R., and Esmon, C. T.: Glycosaminoglycan contributions to both protein C activation and thrombin inhibition involve a common arginine-rich site in thrombin that includes residues arginine 93, 97, and 101. J Biol Chem 269:17965, 1994

249. Liu, L. W., Rezaie, A. R., Carson, C. W., Esmon, N. L., and Esmon, C. T.: Occupancy of anion binding exosite 2 on thrombin determines Ca2+ dependence of protein C activation. J Biol Chem 269:11807, 1994

250. Ye, J., Esmon, C. T., and Johnson, A. E.: The chondroitin sulfate moiety of thrombomodulin binds a second molecule of thrombin. J Biol Chem 268:2373, 1993

251. Weisel, J. W., Nagaswami, C., Young, T. A., and Light, D. R.: The shape of thrombomodulin and interactions with thrombin as determined by electron microscopy. J Biol Chem 271:31485, 1996

252. Koyama, T., Parkinson, J. F., Aoki, N., Bang, N. U., Muller Berghaus, G., and Preissner, K. T.: Relationship between post-translational glycosylation and anticoagulant function of secretable recombinant mutants of human thrombomodulin. Br J Haematol 78:515, 1991

253. Parkinson, J. F., Garcia, J. G., and Bang, N. U.: Decreased thrombin affinity of cell-surface thrombomodulin following treatment of cultured endothelial cells with beta-D-xyloside. Biochem Biophys Res Commun 169:177, 1990

254. Rogerson, S. J., Novakovic, S., Cooke, B. M., and Brown, G. V.: Plasmodium falciparum-infected erythrocytes adhere to the proteoglycan thrombomodulin in static and flow-based systems. Exp Parasitol 86:8, 1997

255. Gysin, J., Pouvelle, B., Le Tonqueze, M., Edelman, L., and Boffa, M. C.: Chondroitin sulfate of thrombomodulin is an adhesion receptor for Plasmodium falciparum-infected erythrocytes. Mol Biochem Parasitol 88:267, 1997

256. Conway, E. M., Nowakowski, B., and Steiner Mosonyi, M.: Thrombomodulin lacking the cytoplasmic domain efficiently internalizes thrombin via nonclathrin-coated, pit-mediated endocytosis. J Cell Physiol 158:285, 1994

257. Teasdale, M. S., Bird, C. H., and Bird, P.: Internalization of the anticoagulant thrombomodulin is constitutive and does not require a signal in the cytoplasmic domain. Immunol Cell Biol 72:480, 1994

258. Maruyama, I., Bell, C. E., and Majerus, P. W.: Thrombomodulin is found on endothelium of arteries, veins, capillaries, and lymphatics, and on syncytiotrophoblast of human placenta. J Cell Biol 101:363, 1985

259. DeBault, L. E., Esmon, N. L., Smith, G. P., and Esmon, C. T.: Localization of thrombomodulin antigen in rabbit endothelial cells in culture. An immunofluorescence and immunoelectron microscope study. Lab Invest 54:179, 1986

260. Ishii, H., Salem, H. H., Bell, C. E., Laposata, E. A., and Majerus, P. W.: Thrombomodulin, an endothelial anticoagulant protein, is absent from the human brain. Blood 67:362, 1986

261. Wong, V. L. Y., Hofman, F. M., Ishii, H., and Fisher, M.: Regional distribution of thrombomodulin in human brain. Brain Res 556:1, 1991

262. Suzuki, K., Nishioka, J., Hayashi, T., and Kosaka, Y.: Functionally active thrombomodulin is present in human platelets. J Biochem Tokyo 104:628, 1988

263. Yonezawa, S., Maruyama, I., Tanaka, S., Nakamura, T., and Sato, E.: Immunohistochemical localization of thrombomodulin in chorionic diseases of the uterus and choriocarcinoma of the stomach. A comparative study with the distribution of human chorionic gonadotropin. Cancer 62:569, 1988

264. Yonezawa, S., Maruyama, I., Sakae, K., Igata, A., Majerus, P. W., and Sato, E.: Thrombomodulin as a marker for vascular tumors. Comparative study with factor VIII and Ulex europaeus I lectin. Am J Clin Pathol 88:405, 1987

265. Jackson, D. E., Mitchell, C. A., Bird, P., Salem, H. H., and Hayman, J. A.: Immunohistochemical localization of thrombomodulin in normal human skin and skin tumours. J Pathol 175:421, 1995

266. Jackson, D. E., Mitchell, C. A., Mason, G., Salem, H. H., and Hayman, J. A.: Altered thrombomodulin staining in blistering dermatoses. Pathology 28:225, 1996

267. Ishii, H., and Majerus, P. W.: Thrombomodulin is Present in Human Plasma and Urine. J Clin Invest 76:2178, 1985

268. Jackson, D. E., Tetaz, T. J., Salem, H. H., and Mitchell, C. A.: Purification and characterization of two forms of soluble thrombomodulin from human urine. Eur J Biochem 221:1079, 1994

269. Blann, A., and Seigneur, M.: Soluble markers of endothelial cell function. Clin Hemorheol Microcirc 17:3, 1997

270. Blann, A. D., and Taberner, D. A.: A reliable marker of endothelial cell dysfunction: does it exist? Br J Haematol 90:244, 1995

271. Maruyama, I., and Majerus, P. W.: The turnover of thrombin-thrombomodulin complex in cultured human umbilical vein endothelial cells and A549 lung cancer cells. Endocytosis and degradation of thrombin. J Biol Chem 260:15432, 1985

272. Busch, C., Cancilla, P., DeBault, L. E., Goldsmith, J. C., and Owen, W. G.: Use of endothelium cultured on microcarriers as a model for the microcirculation. Lab Invest 47:498, 1982

273. Owen, W. G., and Esmon, C. T.: Functional properties of an endothelial cell cofactor for thrombin-catalyzed activation of protein C. J Biol Chem 256:5532, 1981

274. Lu, R. L., Esmon, N. L., Esmon, C. T., and Johnson, A. E.: The active site of the thrombin-thrombomodulin complex. A fluorescence energy transfer measurement of its distance above the membrane surface. J Biol Chem 264:12956, 1989

275. Galvin, J. B., Kurosawa, S., Moore, K., Esmon, C. T., and Esmon, N. L.: Reconstitution of rabbit thrombomodulin into phospholipid vesicles. J Biol Chem 262:2199, 1987

276. Freyssinet, J. M., Gauchy, J., and Cazenave, J. P.: The effect of phospholipids on the activation of protein C by the human thrombin-thrombomodulin complex. Biochem J 238:151, 1986

277. Doyle, M. F., and Mann, K. G.: Multiple active forms of thrombin. IV. Relative activities of meizothrombins. J Biol Chem 265:10693, 1990

278. Wu, Q., Tsiang, M., Lentz, S. R., and Sadler, J. E.: Ligand specificity of human thrombomodulin. Equilibrium binding of human thrombin, meizothrombin, and factor Xa to recombinant thrombomodulin. J Biol Chem 267:7083, 1992

279. Hackeng, T. M., Tans, G., Koppelman, S. J., de Groot, P. G., Rosing, J., and Bouma, B. N.: Protein C activation on endothelial cells by prothrombin activation products generated in situ: meizothrombin is a better protein C activator than alpha-thrombin. Biochem J 319:399, 1996

280. Cote, H. C., Bajzar, L., Stevens, W. K., Samis, J. A., Morser, J., MacGillivray, R. T., and Nesheim, M. E.: Functional characterization of recombinant human meizothrombin and meizothrombin(desF1). Thrombomodulin-dependent activation of protein C and thrombin-activatable fibrinolysis inhibitor (TAFI), platelet aggregation, antithrombin-III inhibition. J Biol Chem 272:6194, 1997

281. Haley, P. E., Doyle, M. F., and Mann, K. G.: The activation of bovine protein C by factor Xa. J Biol Chem 264:16303, 1989

282. Freyssinet, J. M., Wiesel, M. L., Grunebaum, L., Pereillo, J. M., Gauchy, J., Schuhler, S., Freund, G., and Cazenave, J. P.: Activation of human protein C by blood coagulation factor Xa in the presence of anionic phospholipids. Enhancement by sulphated polysaccharides. Biochem J 261:341, 1989

283. Rezaie, A. R.: Rapid activation of protein C by thrombin and factor Xa in the presence of polyanionic compounds. Blood 90:144a, 1997

284. Salem, H. H., Broze, G. J., Miletich, J. P., and Majerus, P. W.: Human coagulation factor Va is a cofactor for the activation of protein C. Proc Natl Acad Sci USA 80:1584, 1983

285. Salem, H. H., Broze, G. J., Miletich, J. P., and Majerus, P. W.: The light chain of factor Va contains the activity of factor Va that accelerates protein C activation by thrombin. J Biol Chem 258:8531, 1983

286. Salem, H. H., Esmon, N. L., Esmon, C. T., and Majerus, P. W.: Effects of thrombomodulin and coagulation Factor Va-light chain on protein C activation in vitro. J Clin Invest 73:968, 1984

287. Maruyama, I., Salem, H. H., and Majerus, P. W.: Coagulation factor Va binds to human umbilical vein endothelial cells and accelerates protein C activation. J Clin Invest 74:224, 1984

288. Maruyama, I., Salem, H. H., Ishii, H., and Majerus, P. W.: Human thrombomodulin is not an efficient inhibitor of the procoagulant activity of thrombin. J Clin Invest 75:987, 1985

289. Kurosawa, S., and Aoki, N.: Preparation of thrombomodulin from human placenta. Thromb Res 37:353, 1985
290. Preissner, K. T.: Specific binding of plasminogen to vitronectin. Evidence for a modulatory role of vitronectin on fibrin(ogen)-induced plasmin formation by tissue plasminogen activator. Biochem Biophys Res Commun 168:966, 1990
291. Hirahara, K., Koyama, M., Matsuishi, T., and Kurata, M.: The effect of human thrombomodulin on the inactivation of thrombin by human antithrombin III. Thromb Res 57:117, 1990
292. Slungaard, A., Vercellotti, G. M., Tran, T., Gleich, G. J., and Key, N. S.: Eosinophil cationic granule proteins impair thrombomodulin function. A potential mechanism for thromboembolism in hypereosinophilic heart disease. J Clin Invest 91:1721, 1993
293. Slungaard, A., and Key, N. S.: Platelet factor 4 stimulates thrombomodulin protein C-activating cofactor activity. A structure-function analysis. J Biol Chem 269:25549, 1994
294. Esmon, C. T., and Esmon, N. L.: Protein C activation. Semin Thromb Hemost 10:122, 1984
295. Olsen, P. H., Esmon, N. L., Esmon, C. T., and Laue, T. M.: Ca2+ dependence of the interactions between protein C, thrombin, and the elastase fragment of thrombomodulin. Analysis by ultracentrifugation. Biochemistry 31:746, 1992
296. Johnson, A. E., Esmon, N. L., Laue, T. M., and Esmon, C. T.: Structural changes required for activation of protein C are induced by Ca2+ binding to a high affinity site that does not contain gamma-carboxyglutamic acid. J Biol Chem 258:5554, 1983
297. Esmon, N. L., DeBault, L. E., and Esmon, C. T.: Proteolytic formation and properties of gamma-carboxyglutamic acid-domainless protein C. J Biol Chem 258:5548, 1983
298. Rezaie, A. R., Esmon, N. L., and Esmon, C. T.: The high affinity calcium-binding site involved in protein C activation is outside the first epidermal growth factor homology domain. J Biol Chem 267:11701, 1992
299. Ehrlich, H. J., Grinnell, B. W., Jaskunas, S. R., Esmon, C. T., Yan, S. B., and Bang, N. U.: Recombinant human protein C derivatives: altered response to calcium resulting in enhanced activation by thrombin. EMBO J 9:2367, 1990
300. Rezaie, A. R., and Esmon, C. T.: The function of calcium in protein C activation by thrombin and the thrombin-thrombomodulin complex can be distinguished by mutational analysis of protein C derivatives. J Biol Chem 267:26104, 1992
301. Rezaie, A. R., and Esmon, C. T.: Calcium inhibition of the activation of protein C by thrombin. Role of the P3 and P3' residues. Eur J Biochem 223:575, 1994
302. Rezaie, A. R., and Esmon, C. T.: Proline at the P2 position in protein C is important for calcium-mediated regulation of protein C activation and secretion. Blood 83:2526, 1994
303. Richardson, M. A., Gerlitz, B., and Grinnell, B. W.: Enhancing protein C interaction with thrombin results in a clot-activated anticoagulant. Nature 360:261, 1992
304. Kurz, K. D., Smith, T., Wilson, A., Gerlitz, B., Richardson, M. A., and Grinnell, B. W.: Antithrombotic efficacy in the guinea pig of a derivative of human protein C with enhanced activation by thrombin. Blood 89:534, 1997
305. Stearns, D. J., Kurosawa, S., Sims, P. J., Esmon, N. L., and Esmon, C. T.: The interaction of a Ca2+-dependent monoclonal antibody with the protein C activation peptide region. Evidence for obligatory Ca2+ binding to both antigen and antibody. J Biol Chem 263:826, 1988
306. Musci, G., Berliner, L. J., and Esmon, C. T.: Evidence for multiple conformational changes in the active center of thrombin induced by complex formation with thrombomodulin: an analysis employing nitroxide spin-labels. Biochemistry 27:769, 1988
307. Bode, W., Brandstetter, H., Mather, T., and Stubbs, M. T.: Comparative analysis of haemostatic proteinases: structural aspects of thrombin, factor Xa, factor IXa and protein C. Thromb Haemost 78:501, 1997
308. Stubbs, M. T., and Bode, W.: A player of many parts: the spotlight falls on thrombin's structure. Thromb Res 69:1, 1993
309. Stubbs, M. T., and Bode, W.: The clot thickens: clues provided by thrombin structure [published erratum appears in Trends Biochem Sci 1995 Mar;20(3):131]. Trends Biochem Sci 20:23, 1995
310. Ye, J., Esmon, N. L., Esmon, C. T., and Johnson, A. E.: The active site of thrombin is altered upon binding to thrombomodulin. Two distinct structural changes are detected by fluorescence, but only one correlates with protein C activation. J Biol Chem 266:23016, 1991
311. Ye, J., Liu, L. W., Esmon, C. T., and Johnson, A. E.: The fifth and sixth growth factor-like domains of thrombomodulin bind to the anion-binding exosite of thrombin and alter its specificity. J Biol Chem 267:11023, 1992
312. Hortin, G. L., and Trimpe, B. L.: Allosteric changes in thrombin's activity produced by peptides corresponding to segments of natural inhibitors and substrates. J Biol Chem 266:6866, 1991
313. Vindigni, A., White, C. E., Komives, E. A., and Di Cera, E.: Energetics of thrombin-thrombomodulin interaction. Biochemistry 36:6674, 1997
314. Suzuki, K., Nishioka, J., and Hayashi, T.: Localization of thrombomodulin-binding site within human thrombin. J Biol Chem 265:13263, 1990
315. Suzuki, K., and Nishioka, J.: A thrombin-based peptide corresponding to the sequence of the thrombomodulin-binding site blocks the procoagulant activities of thrombin. J Biol Chem 266:18498, 1991
316. Nishioka, J., Taneda, H., and Suzuki, K.: Estimation of the possible recognition sites for thrombomodulin, procoagulant, and anticoagulant proteins around the active center of alpha-thrombin. J Biochem Tokyo 114:148, 1993
317. Noe, G., Hofsteenge, J., Rovelli, G., and Stone, S. R.: The use of sequence-specific antibodies to identify a secondary binding site in thrombin. J Biol Chem 263:11729, 1988
318. Hofsteenge, J., Braun, P. J., and Stone, S. R.: Enzymatic properties of proteolytic derivatives of human alpha-thrombin. Biochemistry. 27:2144, 1988
319. Bode, W., Mayr, I., Baumann, U., Huber, R., Stone, S. R., and Hofsteenge, J.: The refined 1.9 A crystal structure of human alpha-thrombin: interaction with D-Phe-Pro-Arg chloromethylketone and significance of the Tyr-Pro-Pro-Trp insertion segment. EMBO J 8:3467, 1989
320. Grutter, M. G., Priestle, J. P., Rahuel, J., Grossenbacher, H., Bode, W., Hofsteenge, J., and Stone, S. R.: Crystal structure of the thrombin-hirudin complex: a novel mode of serine protease inhibition. EMBO J 9:2361, 1990
321. Rydel, T. J., Tulinsky, A., Bode, W., and Huber, R.: Refined structure of the hirudin-thrombin complex. J Mol Biol 221:583, 1991
322. Rydel, T. J., Ravichandran, K. G., Tulinsky, A., Bode, W., Huber, R., Roitsch, C., and Fenton, J. W. d.: The structure of a complex of recombinant hirudin and human alpha-thrombin. Science 249:277, 1990
323. Wu, Q. Y., Sheehan, J. P., Tsiang, M., Lentz, S. R., Birktoft, J. J., and Sadler, J. E.: Single amino acid substitutions dissociate fibrinogen-clotting and thrombomodulin-binding activities of human thrombin. Proc Natl Acad Sci USA 88:6775, 1991
324. Tsiang, M., Jain, A. K., Dunn, K. E., Rojas, M. E., Leung, L. L., and Gibbs, C. S.: Functional mapping of the surface residues of human thrombin. J Biol Chem 270:16854, 1995
325. Di Cera, E., Dang, Q. D., Ayala, Y., and Vindigni, A.: Linkage at steady state: allosteric transitions of thrombin. Methods Enzymol 259:127, 1995
326. Dang, Q. D., Sabetta, M., and Di Cera, E.: Selective loss of fibrinogen clotting in a loop-less thrombin. J Biol Chem 272:19649, 1997
327. Le Bonniec, B. F., and Esmon, C. T.: Glu-192–Gln substitution in thrombin mimics the catalytic switch induced by thrombomodulin. Proc Natl Acad Sci USA 88:7371, 1991
328. Le Bonniec, B. F., MacGillivray, R. T., and Esmon, C. T.: Thrombin Glu-39 restricts the P'3 specificity to nonacidic residues. J Biol Chem 266:13796, 1991
329. Berg, D. T., Wiley, M. R., and Grinnell, B. W.: Enhanced protein C activation and inhibition of fibrinogen cleavage by a thrombin modulator. Science 273:1389, 1996
330. Jackman, R. W., Beeler, D. L., Fritze, L., Soff, G., and Rosenberg, R. D.: Human thrombomodulin gene is intron depleted: nucleic acid sequences of the cDNA and gene predict protein structure and suggest sites of regulatory control. Proc Natl Acad Sci USA 84:6425, 1987
331. Shirai, T., Shiojiri, S., Ito, H., Yamamoto, S., Kusumoto, H., Deyashiki, Y., Maruyama, I., and Suzuki, K.: Gene structure of human thrombomodulin, a cofactor for thrombin-catalyzed activation of protein C. J Biochem Tokyo 103:281, 1988
332. Espinosa, R. d., Sadler, J. E., and Le Beau, M. M.: Regional localization of the human thrombomodulin gene to 20p12-cen. Genomics 5:649, 1989
333. Maruyama, I., and Majerus, P. W.: Protein C inhibits endocytosis of thrombin-thrombomodulin complexes in A549 lung cancer cells and human umbilical vein endothelial cells. Blood 69:1481, 1987

334. Beretz, A., Freyssinet, J. M., Gauchy, J., Schmitt, D. A., Klein Soyer, C., Edgell, C. J., and Cazenave, J. P.: Stability of the thrombin-thrombomodulin complex on the surface of endothelial cells from human saphenous vein or from the cell line EA.hy 926. Biochem J 259:35, 1989

335. Moore, K. L., Andreoli, S. P., Esmon, N. L., Esmon, C. T., and Bang, N. U.: Endotoxin enhances tissue factor and suppresses thrombomodulin expression of human vascular endothelium in vitro. J Clin Invest 79:124, 1987

336. Nawroth, P. P., Handley, D. A., Esmon, C. T., and Stern, D. M.: Interleukin 1 induces endothelial cell procoagulant while suppressing cell-surface anticoagulant activity. Proc Natl Acad Sci USA 83:3460, 1986

337. Archipoff, G., Beretz, A., Freyssinet, J. M., Klein-Soyer, C., Brisson, C., and Cazenave, J. P.: Heterogeneous regulation of constitutive thrombomodulin or inducible tissue-factor activities on the surface of human saphenous-vein endothelial cells in culture following stimulation by interleukin-1, tumor necrosis factor, thrombin or phorbol ester. Biochem J 272:679, 1991

338. Nawroth, P. P., and Stern, D. M.: Modulation of endothelial cell hemostatic properties by tumor necrosis factor. J-Exp-Med 163:740, 1986

339. Conway, E. M., and Rosenberg, R. D.: Tumor necrosis factor suppresses transcription of the thrombomodulin gene in endothelial cells. Mol Cell Biol 8:5588, 1988

340. Scarpati, E. M., and Sadler, J. E.: Regulation of endothelial cell coagulant properties. Modulation of tissue factor, plasminogen activator inhibitors, and thrombomodulin by phorbol 12-myristate 13-acetate and tumor necrosis factor [published erratum appears in J Biol Chem 1990 Aug 25;265(24):14696]. J Biol Chem 264:20705, 1989

341. Lentz, S. R., Tsiang, M., and Sadler, J. E.: Regulation of thrombomodulin by tumor necrosis factor-alpha: comparison of transcriptional and posttranscriptional mechanisms. Blood 77:542, 1991

342. Ogawa, S., Gerlach, H., Esposito, C., Pasagiau-Macaulay, A., Brett, J., and Stern, D. M.: Hypoxia modulates the barrier and coagulant function of cultured bovine endothelium. J Clin Invest 85:1090, 1990

343. Key, N. S., Vercellotti, G. M., Winkelmann, J. C., Moldow, C. F., Goodman, J. L., Esmon, N. L., Esmon, C. T., and Jacob, H. S.: Infection of vascular endothelial cells with herpes simplex virus enhances tissue factor activity and reduces thrombomodulin expression. Proc Natl Acad Sci USA 87:7095, 1990

344. Kapotis, S., Besemer, J., Bevec, D., Valent, P., Bettelheim, P., Lechner, K., and Speiser, W.: Interleukin-4 counteracts pyrogen-induced down-regulation of thrombomodulin in cultured human vascular endothelial cells. Blood 78:410, 1991

345. Ishii, H., Kizaki, K., Horie, S., and Kazama, M.: Oxidized low density lipoprotein reduces thrombomodulin transcription in cultured human endothelial cells through degradation of the lipoprotein in lysosomes. J Biol Chem 271:8458, 1996

346. Ohdama, S., Tahano, S., Ohashi, K., Miyake, S., and Aoki, N.: Pentoxifylline prevents tumor necrosis factor induced suppression of endothelial cell surface thrombomodulin. Thromb Res 62:745, 1991

347. Hirokawa, K., and Aoki, N.: Up-regulation of thrombomodulin in human umbilical vein endothelial cells in vitro. J.Biochem. 108:839, 1990

348. Oida, K., Maeda, H., Kohno, M., Nakai, T., Horie, S., and Ishii, H.: Effect of a protein phosphatase inhibitor, okadaic acid, on thrombomodulin expression in cultured human umbilical vein endothelial cells. Thromb Res 85:169, 1997

349. Maruyama, I., Soejima, Y., Osame, M., Ito, T., Ogawa, K., Yamamoto, S., Dittman, W. A., and Saito, H.: Increased expression of thrombomodulin on the cultured human umbilical vein endothelial cells and mouse hemangioma cells by cyclic AMP. Thromb Res 61:301, 1991

350. Traynor, A. E., Cundiff, D. L., and Soff, G. A.: cAMP influence on transcription of thrombomodulin is dependent on de novo synthesis of a protein intermediate: evidence for cohesive regulation of myogenic proteins in vascular smooth muscle. J Lab Clin Med 126:316, 1995

351. Tazawa, R., Yamamoto, K., Suzuki, K., Hirokawa, K., Hirosawa, S., and Aoki, N.: Presence of functional cyclic AMP responsive element in the 3'-untranslated region of the human thrombomodulin gene. Biochem Biophys Res Commun 200:1391, 1994

352. Niforas, P., Chu, M. D., and Bird, P.: A retinoic acid/cAMP-responsive enhancer containing a cAMP responsive element is required for the activation of the mouse thrombomodulin-encoding gene in differentiating F9 cells. Gene 176:139, 1996

353. Shirayoshi, Y., Imada, S., Katayanagi, S., Uyeno, M., and Imada, M.: Cyclic AMP-mediated augmentation of thrombomodulin gene expression: cell type-dependent usage of control regions. Exp Cell Res 208:75, 1993

354. Hirokawa, K., and Aoki, N.: Up-regulation of thrombomodulin by activation of histamine H1-receptors in human umbilical-vein endothelial cells in vitro. Biochem J 276:739, 1991

355. Dittman, W. A., Nelson, S. C., Greer, P. K., Horton, E. T., Palomba, M. L., and McCachren, S. S.: Characterization of thrombomodulin expression in response to retinoic acid and identification of a retinoic acid response element in the human thrombomodulin gene. J Biol Chem 269:16925, 1994

356. Raife, T. J., Demetroulis, E. M., and Lentz, S. R.: Regulation of thrombomodulin expression by all-trans retinoic acid and tumor necrosis factor-alpha: differential responses in keratinocytes and endothelial cells. Blood 88:2043, 1996

357. Senet, P., Peyri, N., Berard, M., Dubertret, L., and Boffa, M. C.: Thrombomodulin, a functional surface protein on human keratinocytes, is regulated by retinoic acid. Arch Dermatol Res 289:151, 1997

358. Kizaki, K., Ishii, H., Horie, S., and Kazama, M.: Thrombomodulin induction by all-trans retinoic acid is independent of HL-60 cells differentiation to neutrophilic cells. Thromb Haemost 72:573, 1994

359. Koyama, T., Hirosawa, S., Kawamata, N., Tohda, S., and Aoki, N.: All-trans retinoic acid upregulates thrombomodulin and downregulates tissue-factor expression in acute promyelocytic leukemia cells: distinct expression of thrombomodulin and tissue factor in human leukemic cells. Blood 84:3001, 1994

360. Miyake, S., Ohdama, S., Tazawa, R., and Aoki, N.: Retinoic acid prevents cytokine-induced suppression of thrombomodulin expression on surface of human umbilical vascular endothelial cells in vitro. Thromb Res 68:483, 1992

361. Weiler Guettler, H., Yu, K., Soff, G., Gudas, L. J., and Rosenberg, R. D.: Thrombomodulin gene regulation by cAMP and retinoic acid in F9 embryonal carcinoma cells. Proc Natl Acad Sci U S A 89:2155, 1992

362. Horie, S., Kizaki, K., Ishii, H., and Kazama, M.: Retinoic acid stimulates expression of thrombomodulin, a cell surface anticoagulant glycoprotein, on human endothelial cells. Differences between up-regulation of thrombomodulin by retinoic acid and cyclic AMP. Biochem J 281:149, 1992

363. Dittman, W. A., Kumada, T., and Majerus, P. W.: Transcription of thrombomodulin mRNA in mouse hemangioma cells is increased by cycloheximide and thrombin. Proc Natl Acad Sci USA 86:7179, 1989

364. Bartha, K., Brisson, C., Archipoff, G., de la Salle, C., Lanza, F., Cazenave, J., P., and Beretz, A.: Thrombin regulates tissue factor and thrombomodulin mRNA levels and activities in human saphenous vein endothelial cells by distinct mechanisms. J Biol Chem 268:421, 1993

365. Conway, E. M., Liu, L., Nowakowski, B., Steiner Mosonyi, M., and Jackman, R. W.: Heat shock of vascular endothelial cells induces an up-regulatory transcriptional response of the thrombomodulin gene that is delayed in onset and does not attenuate. J Biol Chem 269:22804, 1994

366. Ohlin, A. K., and Marlar, R. A.: The first mutation identified in the thrombomodulin gene in a 45-year-old man presenting with thromboembolic disease. Blood 85:330, 1995

367. Ohlin, A. K., Norlund, L., and Marlar, R. A.: Thrombomodulin gene variations and thromboembolic disease. Thromb Haemost 78:396, 1997

368. Ireland, H., Kunz, G., Kyriakoulis, K., Stubbs, P. J., and Lane, D. A.: Thrombomodulin gene mutations associated with myocardial infarction [see comments]. Circulation 96:15, 1997

369. van der Velden, P. A., Krommenhoek Van Es, T., Allaart, C. F., Bertina, R. M., and Reitsma, P. H.: A frequent thrombomodulin amino acid dimorphism is not associated with thrombophilia. Thromb Haemost 65:511, 1991

370. Norlund, L., Holm, J., Zoller, B., and Ohlin, A. K.: A common thrombomodulin amino acid dimorphism is associated with myocardial infarction. Thromb Haemost 77:248, 1997

371. Comp, P. C., DeBault, L. E., Esmon, N. L., and Esmon, C. T.: Human thrombomodulin is inhibited by IgG from two patients with nonspecific anticoagulants. Blood 62:299, 1983

372. Freyssinet, J. M., and Cazenave, J. P.: Lupus-like anticoagulants, modulation of the protein C pathway and thrombosis. Thromb Haemost 58:679, 1987

373. Cariou, R., Tobelem, G., Bellucci, S., Soria, J., Soria, C., Maclouf, J., and Caen, J.: Effect of lupus anticoagulant on antithrombogenic prop-

erties of endothelial cells—inhibition of thrombomodulin-dependent protein C activation. Thromb Haemost 60:54, 1988

374. Ruiz Arguelles, G. J., Ruiz Arguelles, A., Deleze, M., and Alarcon Segovia, D.: Acquired protein C deficiency in a patient with primary antiphospholipid syndrome. Relationship to reactivity of anticardiolipin antibody with thrombomodulin. J Rheumatol 16:381, 1989

375. Tsakiris, D. A., Settas, L., Makris, P. E., and Marbet, G. A.: Lupus anticoagulant-antiphospholipid antibodies and thrombophilia. Relation to protein C-protein S-thrombomodulin. J Rheumatol 17:785, 1990

376. Marciniak, E., and Romond, E. H.: Impaired catalytic function of activated protein C: a new in vitro manifestation of lupus anticoagulant. Blood 74:2426, 1989

377. Malia, R. G., Kitchen, S., Greaves, M., and Preston, F. E.: Inhibition of activated protein C and its cofactor protein S by antiphospholipid antibodies. Br J Haematol 76:101, 1990

378. Yoshida, M., Kozaki, M., Ioya, N., Kaji, N., Tamaki, T., Hiraishi, S., Ishii, H., Kazama, M., Fukutomi, K., and Nagasawa, T.: Plasma thrombomodurine levels as an indicator of vascular injury caused by cyclosporine nephrotoxicity. Transplant 50:1066, 1990

379. Amiral, J., Adam, M., Mimilla, F., Larrivaz, I., Chambrette, B., and Boffa, M. C.: Design and validation of a new immunoassay for soluble forms of thrombomodulin and studies on plasma. Hybridoma 13:205, 1994

380. Kumada, T., Dittman, W. A., and Majerus, P. W.: A role for thrombomodulin in the pathogenesis of thrombin-induced thromboembolism in mice. Blood 71:728, 1987

381. Gomi, K., Zushi, M., Honda, G., Kawahara, S., Matsuzaki, O., Kanabayashi, T., Yamamoto, S., Maruyama, I., and Suzuki, K.: Antithrombotic effect of recombinant human thrombomodulin on thrombin-induced thromboembolism in mice. Blood 75:1396, 1990

382. Solis, M. M., Vitti, M., Cook, J., Young, D., Glaser, C., Light, D., Morser, J., Wydro, R., Yu, S., Fink, L., and et al.: Recombinant soluble human thrombomodulin: a randomized, blinded assessment of prevention of venous thrombosis and effects on hemostatic parameters in a rat model. Thromb Res 73:385, 1994

383. Mohri, M., Oka, M., Aoki, Y., Gonda, Y., Hirata, S., Gomi, K., Kiyota, T., Sugihara, T., Yamamoto, S., Ishida, T., and et al.: Intravenous extended infusion of recombinant human soluble thrombomodulin prevented tissue factor-induced disseminated intravascular coagulation in rats. Am J Hematol 45:298, 1994

384. Mohri, M., Gonda, Y., Oka, M., Aoki, Y., Gomi, K., Kiyota, T., Sugihara, T., Yamamoto, S., Ishida, T., and Maruyama, I.: The antithrombotic effects of recombinant human soluble thrombomodulin (rhsTM) on tissue factor-induced disseminated intravascular coagulation in crab-eating monkeys (Macaca fascicularis). Blood Coagul Fibrinolysis 8:274, 1997

385. Uchiba, M., Okajima, K., Murakami, K., Nawa, K., Okabe, H., and Takatsuki, K.: Recombinant human soluble thrombomodulin reduces endotoxin-induced pulmonary vascular injury via protein C activation in rats. Thromb Haemost 74:1265, 1995

386. Bangalore, N., Drohan, W. N., and Orthner, C. L.: High affinity binding sites for activated protein C and protein C on cultured human umbilical vein endothelial cells. Independent of protein S and distinct from known ligands. Thromb Haemost 72:465, 1994

387. Fukudome, K., and Esmon, C. T.: Identification, cloning, and regulation of a novel endothelial cell protein C/activated protein C receptor. J Biol Chem 269:26486, 1994

388. Fukudome, K., and Esmon, C. T.: Molecular cloning and expression of murine and bovine endothelial cell protein C/activated protein C receptor (EPCR). The structural and functional conservation in human, bovine, and murine EPCR. J Biol Chem 270:5571, 1995

389. Laszik, Z., Mitro, A., Taylor, F. B. J., Ferrell, G., and Esmon, C. T.: Human protein C receptor is present primarily on endothelium of large blood vessels: implications for the control of the protein C pathway. Circulation 96:3633, 1997

390. Esmon, C. T., Ding, W., Yasuhiro, K., Gu, J. M., Ferrell, G., Regan, L. M., Stearns Kurosawa, D. J., Kurosawa, S., Mather, T., Laszik, Z., and Esmon, N. L.: The protein C pathway: new insights. Thromb Haemost 78:70, 1997

391. Stearns Kurosawa, D. J., Kurosawa, S., Mollica, J. S., Ferrell, G. L., and Esmon, C. T.: The endothelial cell protein C receptor augments protein C activation by the thrombin-thrombomodulin complex. Proc Natl Acad Sci USA 93:10212, 1996

392. Regan, L. M., Stearns Kurosawa, D. J., Kurosawa, S., Mollica, J., Fukudome, K., and Esmon, C. T.: The endothelial cell protein C receptor. Inhibition of activated protein C anticoagulant function without modulation of reaction with proteinase inhibitors. J Biol Chem 271:17499, 1996

393. Kurosawa, S., Stearns Kurosawa, D. J., Hidari, N., and Esmon, C. T.: Identification of functional endothelial protein C receptor in human plasma. J Clin Invest 100:411, 1997

394. Grey, S. T., Tsuchida, A., Hau, H., Orthner, C. L., Salem, H. H., and Hancock, W. W.: Selective inhibitory effects of the anticoagulant activated protein C on the responses of human mononuclear phagocytes to LPS, IFN-gamma, or phorbol ester. J Immunol 153:3664, 1994

395. Hancock, W. W., Grey, S. T., Hau, L., Akalin, E., Orthner, C., Sayegh, M. H., and Salem, H. H.: Binding of activated protein C to a specific receptor on human mononuclear phagocytes inhibits intracellular calcium signaling and monocyte-dependent proliferative responses. Transplantation 60:1525, 1995

396. Grinnell, B. W., Hermann, R. B., and Yan, S. B.: Human protein C inhibits selectin-mediated cell adhesion: role of unique fucosylated oligosaccharide. Glycobiology 4:221, 1994

397. Dahlbäck, B.: Purification of human vitamin K–dependent protein S and its limited proteolysis by thrombin. Biochem J 209:837, 1983

398. Walker, F. J.: Regulation of activated protein C by a new protein. A possible function for bovine protein S. J Biol Chem 255:5521, 1980

399. Walker, F. J.: Regulation of bovine activated protein C by protein S: the role of the cofactor protein in species specificity. Thromb Res 22:321, 1981

400. Walker, F. J.: Interactions of protein S with membranes. Semin Thromb Hemost 14:216, 1988

401. Nelsestuen, G. L., Kisiel, W., and Di Scipio, R. G.: Interaction of vitamin K dependent proteins with membranes. Biochemistry 17:2134, 1978

402. Suzuki, K., Nishioka, J., Matsuda, M., Murayama, H., and Hashimoto, S.: Protein S is essential for the activated protein C-catalyzed inactivation of platelet-associated factor Va. J Biochem 96:455, 1984

403. Harris, K. W., and Esmon, C. T.: Protein S is required for bovine platelets to support activated protein C binding and activity. J Biol Chem 260:2007, 1985

404. Stern, D. M., Nawroth, P. P., Harris, K., and Esmon, C. T.: Cultured bovine aortic endothelial cells promote activated protein C-protein S-mediated inactivation of factor Va. J Biol Chem 261:713, 1986

405. Hackeng, T. M., Hessing, M., van't Veer, C., Meijer Huizinga, F., Meijers, J. C., de Groot, P. G., van Mourik, J. A., and Bouma, B. N.: Protein S binding to human endothelial cells is required for expression of cofactor activity for activated protein C. J Biol Chem 268:3993, 1993

406. Dahlbäck, B., Wiedmer, T., and Sims, P. J.: Binding of anticoagulant vitamin K–dependent protein S to platelet-derived microparticles. Biochemistry 31:12769, 1992

407. Kalafatis, M., Bertina, R. M., Rand, M. D., and Mann, K. G.: Characterization of the molecular defect in factor VR506Q. J Biol Chem 270:4053, 1995

408. Regan, L. M., Lamphear, B. J., Huggins, C. F., Walker, F. J., and Fay, P. J.: Factor IXa protects factor VIIIa from activated protein C. Factor IXa inhibits activated protein C-catalyzed cleavage of factor VIIIa at Arg562. J Biol Chem 269:9445, 1994

409. Heeb, M. J., Rosing, J., Bakker, H. M., Fernandez, J. A., Tans, G., and Griffin, J. H.: Protein S binds to and inhibits factor Xa. Proc Natl Acad Sci USA 91:2728, 1994

410. Koppelman, S. J., van't Veer, C., Sixma, J. J., and Bouma, B. N.: Synergistic inhibition of the intrinsic factor X activation by protein S and C4b-binding protein. Blood 86:2653, 1995

411. Koppelman, S. J., Hackeng, T. M., Sixma, J. J., and Bouma, B. N.: Inhibition of the intrinsic factor X activating complex by protein S: evidence for a specific binding of protein S to factor VIII. Blood 86:1062, 1995

412. van Wijnen, M., Stam, J. G., van't Veer, C., Meijers, J. C., Reitsma, P. H., Bertina, R. M., and Bouma, B. N.: The interaction of protein S with the phospholipid surface is essential for the activated protein C-independent activity of protein S. Thromb Haemost 76:397, 1996

413. van't Veer, C., Hackeng, T. M., Biesbroeck, D., Sixma, J. J., and Bouma, B. N.: Increased prothrombin activation in protein S-deficient plasma under flow conditions on endothelial cell matrix: an independent anticoagulant function of protein S in plasma. Blood 85:1815, 1995

414. Dahlbäck, B.: Purification of human C4b-binding protein and forma-

tion of its complex with vitamin K–dependent protein S. Biochem J 209:847, 1983

415. Comp, P. C., Nixon, R. R., Cooper, M. R., and Esmon, C. T.: Familial protein S deficiency is associated with recurrent thrombosis. J Clin Invest 74:2082, 1984

416. Bertina, R. M., van Wijngaarden, A., Reinalda Poot, J., Poort, S. R., and Bom, V. J.: Determination of plasma protein S—the protein cofactor of activated protein C. Thromb Haemost 53:268, 1985

417. He, X., and Dahlbäck, B.: Rabbit plasma, unlike its human counterpart, contains no complex between protein S and C4b-binding protein. Thromb Haemost 71:446, 1994

418. Hillarp, A., Thern, A., and Dahlbäck, B.: Bovine C4b binding protein. Molecular cloning of the alpha- and beta-chains provides structural background for lack of complex formation with protein S. J Immunol 153:4190, 1994

419. Garcia de Frutos, P., and Dahlbäck, B.: cDNA structure of rabbit C4b-binding protein alpha-chain. Preserved sequence motive in complement regulatory protein modules which bind C4b. Biochim Biophys Acta 1261:285, 1995

420. Rodriguez de Cordoba, S., Perez Blas, M., Ramos Ruiz, R., Sanchez Corral, P., Pardo Manuel de Villena, F., and Rey Campos, J.: The gene coding for the beta-chain of C4b-binding protein (C4BPB) has become a pseudogene in the mouse. Genomics 21:501, 1994

421. Hillarp, A., Wiklund, H., Thern, A., and Dahlbäck, B.: Molecular cloning of rat C4b binding protein alpha- and beta-chains: structural and functional relationships among human, bovine, rabbit, mouse, and rat proteins. J Immunol 158:1315, 1997

422. Di Scipio, R. G., Hermodson, M. A., Yates, S. G., and Davie, E. W.: A comparison of human prothrombin, factor IX (Christmas factor), factor X (Stuart factor), and protein S. Biochemistry 16:698, 1977

423. DiScipio, R. G., and Davie, E. W.: Characterization of protein S, a gamma-carboxyglutamic acid containing protein from bovine and human plasma. Biochemistry 18:899, 1979

424. Stenflo, J., and Jonsson, M.: Protein S, a new vitamin K–dependent protein from bovine plasma. FEBS Lett 101:377, 1979

425. Fair, D. S., Marlar, R. A., and Levin, E. G.: Human endothelial cells synthesize protein S. Blood 67:1168, 1986

426. Fair, D. S., and Marlar, R. A.: Biosynthesis and secretion of factor VII, protein C, protein S, and the protein C inhibitor from a human hepatoma cell line. Blood 67:64, 1986

427. Malm, J., He, X. H., Bjartell, A., Shen, L., Abrahamsson, P. A., and Dahlbäck, B.: Vitamin K–dependent protein S in Leydig cells of human testis. Biochem J 302:845, 1994

428. Maillard, C., Berruyer, M., Serre, C. M., Dechavanne, M., and Delmas, P. D.: Protein-S, a vitamin K–dependent protein, is a bone matrix component synthesized and secreted by osteoblasts. Endocrinology 130:1599, 1992

429. He, X., Shen, L., Bjartell, A., and Dahlbäck, B.: The gene encoding vitamin K–dependent anticoagulant protein S is expressed in multiple rabbit organs as demonstrated by northern blotting, in situ hybridization, and immunohistochemistry. J Histochem Cytochem 43:85, 1995

430. Hooper, W. C., Phillips, D. J., Ribeiro, M. J., Benson, J. M., George, V. G., Ades, E. W., and Evatt, B. L.: Tumor necrosis factor-alpha downregulates protein S secretion in human microvascular and umbilical vein endothelial cells but not in the HepG-2 hepatoma cell line. Blood 84:483, 1994

431. Hooper, W. C., Phillips, D. J., Ribeiro, M., Benson, J., and Evatt, B. L.: IL-6 upregulates protein S expression in the HepG-2 hepatoma cells. Thromb Haemost 73:819, 1995

432. Hooper, W. C., Phillips, D. J., and Evatt, B. L.: TNF-alpha suppresses IL-6 upregulation of protein S in HepG-2 hepatoma cells. Thromb Res 81:315, 1996

433. Hooper, W. C., Phillips, D. J., and Evatt, B. L.: Endothelial cell protein S synthesis is upregulated by the complex of IL-6 and soluble IL-6 receptor. Thromb Haemost 77:1014, 1997

434. Smiley, S. T., Boyer, S. N., Heeb, M. J., Griffin, J. H., and Grusby, M. J.: Protein S is inducible by interleukin 4 in T cells and inhibits lymphoid cell procoagulant activity. Proc Natl Acad Sci USA 94:11484, 1997

435. Schwarz, H. P., Heeb, M. J., Wencel Drake, J. D., and Griffin, J. H.: Identification and quantitation of protein S in human platelets. Blood 66:1452, 1985

436. Ogura, M., Tanabe, N., Nishioka, J., Suzuki, K., and Saito, H.: Biosynthesis and secretion of functional protein S by a human megakaryoblastic cell line (MEG-01). Blood 70:301, 1987

437. Phillips, D. J., Greengard, J. S., Fernandez, J. A., Ribeiro, M., Evatt, B. L., Griffin, J. H., and Hooper, W. C.: Protein S, an antithrombotic factor, is synthesized and released by neural tumor cells. J Neurochem 61:344, 1993

438. Dahlbäck, B., Lundwall, A., and Stenflo, J.: Primary structure of bovine vitamin K–dependent protein S. Proc Natl Acad Sci USA 83:4199, 1986

439. Lundwall, A., Dackowski, W., Cohen, E., Shaffer, M., Mahr, A., Dahlbäck, B., Stenflo, J., and Wydro, R.: Isolation and sequence of the cDNA for human protein S, a regulator of blood coagulation. Proc Natl Acad Sci USA 83:6716, 1986

440. Hoskins, J., Norman, D. K., Beckmann, R. J., and Long, G. L.: Cloning and characterization of human liver cDNA encoding a protein S precursor. Proc Natl Acad Sci USA 84:349, 1987

441. Ploos van Amstel, H. K., van der Zanden, A. L., Reitsma, P. H., and Bertina, R. M.: Human protein S cDNA encodes Phe-16 and Tyr 222 in consensus sequences for the post-translational processing. FEBS Lett 222:186, 1987

442. Greengard, J. S., Fernandez, J. A., Radtke, K. P., and Griffin, J. H.: Identification of candidate residues for interaction of protein S with C4b binding protein and activated protein C. Biochem J 305:397, 1995

443. Lu, D., Schmidel, D. K., and Long, G. L.: Structure of mouse protein S as determined by PCR amplification and DNA sequencing of cDNA. Thromb Res 74:135, 1994

444. Chu, M. D., Sun, J., and Bird, P.: Cloning and sequencing of a cDNA encoding the murine vitamin K–dependent protein S. Biochim Biophys Acta 1217:325, 1994

445. Yasuda, F., Hayashi, T., Tanitame, K., Nishioka, J., and Suzuki, K.: Molecular cloning and functional characterization of rat plasma protein S. J Biochem 117:374, 1995

446. Edenbrandt, C. M., Lundwall, A., Wydro, R., and Stenflo, J.: Molecular analysis of the gene for vitamin K dependent protein S and its pseudogene. Cloning and partial gene organization. Biochemistry 29:7861, 1990

447. Ploos van Amstel, H. K., Reitsma, P. H., van der Logt, C. P., and Bertina, R. M.: Intron-exon organization of the active human protein S gene PS alpha and its pseudogene PS beta: duplication and silencing during primate evolution. Biochemistry 29:7853, 1990

448. Schmidel, D. K., Tatro, A. V., Phelps, L. G., Tomczak, J. A., and Long, G. L.: Organization of the human protein S genes. Biochemistry 29:7845, 1990

449. Ploos van Amstel, J. K., van der Zanden, A. L., Bakker, E., Reitsma, P. H., and Bertina, R. M.: Two genes homologous with human protein S cDNA are located on chromosome 3. Thromb Haemost 58:982, 1987

450. Watkins, P. C., Eddy, R., Fukushima, Y., Byers, M. G., Cohen, E. H., Dackowski, W. R., Wydro, R. M., and Shows, T. B.: The gene for protein S maps near the centromere of human chromosome 3. Blood 71:238, 1988

451. Gershagen, S., Fernlund, P., and Lundwall, A.: A cDNA coding for human sex hormone binding globulin. Homology to vitamin K–dependent protein S. FEBS Lett 220:129, 1987

452. Baker, M. E., French, F. S., and Joseph, D. R.: Vitamin K–dependent protein S is similar to rat androgen-binding protein. Biochem J 243:293, 1987

453. Dahlbäck, B., Lundwall, A., and Stenflo, J.: Localization of thrombin cleavage sites in the amino-terminal region of bovine protein S. J Biol Chem 261:5111, 1986

454. Chang, G. T., Aaldering, L., Hackeng, T. M., Reitsma, P. H., Bertina, R. M., and Bouma, B. N.: Construction and characterization of thrombin-resistant variants of recombinant human protein S. Thromb Haemost 72:693, 1994

455. Schwalbe, R. A., Ryan, J., Stern, D. M., Kisiel, W., Dahlbäck, B., and Nelsestuen, G. L.: Protein structural requirements and properties of membrane binding by gamma-carboxyglutamic acid-containing plasma proteins and peptides. J Biol Chem 264:20288, 1989

456. Suzuki, K., Nishioka, J., and Hashimoto, S.: Regulation of activated protein C by thrombin-modified protein S. J Biochem 94:699, 1983

457. Walker, F. J.: Regulation of vitamin K–dependent protein S. Inactivation by thrombin. J Biol Chem 259:10335, 1984

458. Dahlbäck, B., Hildebrand, B., and Malm, J.: Characterization of functionally important domains in human vitamin K–dependent protein S using monoclonal antibodies. J Biol Chem 265:8127, 1990

459. He, X., Shen, L., and Dahlbäck, B.: Expression and functional characterization of chimeras between human and bovine vitamin-K-dependent protein-S-defining modules important for the species speci-

ficity of the activated protein C cofactor activity. Eur J Biochem 227:433, 1995

460. Villoutreix, B. O., Teleman, O., and Dahlbäck, B.: A theoretical model for the Gla-TSR-EGF-1 region of the anticoagulant cofactor protein S: from biostructural pathology to species-specific cofactor activity. J Comput Aided Mol Des 11:293, 1997

461. Stenflo, J., Lundwall, A., and Dahlbäck, B.: beta-Hydroxyasparagine in domains homologous to the epidermal growth factor precursor in vitamin K–dependent protein S. Proc Natl Acad Sci USA 84:368, 1987

462. Nelson, R. M., VanDusen, W. J., Friedman, P. A., and Long, G. L.: beta-Hydroxyaspartic acid and beta-hydroxyasparagine residues in recombinant human protein S are not required for anticoagulant cofactor activity or for binding to C4b-binding protein. J Biol Chem 266:20586, 1991

463. Stenberg, Y., Dahlbäck, B., and Stenflo, J.: Characterization of recombinant EGF modules from vitamin K–dependent protein S expressed in *Spodoptera* cells. The cofactor activtiy depends on the N-terminal EGF module in human protein S. Eur J Biochem 251:558, 1998

464. Dahlbäck, B., Hildebrand, B., and Linse, S.: Novel type of very high affinity calcium-binding sites in beta-hydroxyasparagine-containing epidermal growth factor-like domains in vitamin K–dependent protein S. J Biol Chem 265:18481, 1990

465. Stenberg, Y., Linse, S., Drakenberg, T., and Stenflo, J.: The high affinity calcium-binding sites in the epidermal growth factor module region of vitamin K–dependent protein S. J Biol Chem 272:23255, 1997

466. Stenberg, Y., Julenius, K., Dahlqvist, I., Drakenberg, T., and Stenflo, J.: Calcium-binding properties of the third and fourth epidermal-growth-factor-like modules in vitamin-K–dependent protein S. Eur J Biochem 248:163, 1997

467. Villoutreix, B., Garcia de Frutos, P., Lövenklev, M., Linse, S., Fernlund, P., and Dahlbäck, B.: The SHBG region of the anticoagulant cofactor protein S: secondary structure prediction circular dichroism spectroscopy and analysis of naturally occurring mutations. Proteins Structure Function and Genetic 29:1, 1997

468. Beckmann, G., Hanke, J., Bork, P., and Reich, J. G.: Mergin extracellular domains: Fold prediction for laminin G-like and aminoterminal thrombospondin-like modules based on homology to pentraxins. J Mol Biol 275:725, 1998

469. Gershagen, S., Fernlund, P., and Edenbrandt, C. M.: The genes for SHBG/ABP and the SHBG-like region of vitamin K–dependent protein S have evolved from a common ancestral gene. J Steroid Biochem Mol Biol 40:763, 1991

470. Lu, D., Xie, R. L., Rydzewski, A., and Long, G. L.: The effect of N-linked glycosylation on molecular weight, thrombin cleavage, and functional activity of human protein S. Thromb Haemost 77:1156, 1997

471. Manfioletti, G., Brancolini, C., Avanzi, G., and Schneider, C.: The protein encoded by a growth arrest-specific gene (gas6) is a new member of the vitamin K–dependent proteins related to protein S, a negative coregulator in the blood coagulation cascade. Mol Cell Biol 13:4976, 1993

472. Varnum, B. C., Young, C., Elliott, G., Garcia, A., Bartley, T. D., Fridell, Y. W., Hunt, R. W., Trail, G., Clogston, C., Toso, R. J., Yanagihara, D., Bennett, L., Sylber, M., Merewether, L. A., Tseng, A., Escobar, E., Liu, E. T., and Yamane, H. K.: Axl receptor tyrosine kinase stimulated by the vitamin K–dependent protein encoded by growth-arrest-specific gene 6. Nature 373:623, 1995

473. Mark, M. R., Chen, J., Hammonds, R. G., Sadick, M., and Godowsk, P. J.: Characterization of Gas6, a member of the superfamily of G domain-containing proteins, as a ligand for Rse and Axl. J Biol Chem 271:9785, 1996

474. Ohashi, K., Nagata, K., Toshima, J., Nakano, T., Arita, H., Tsuda, H., Suzuki, K., and Mizuno, K.: Stimulation of sky receptor tyrosine kinase by the product of growth arrest-specific gene 6. J Biol Chem 270:22681, 1995

475. Nakano, T., Kawamoto, K., Higashino, K., and Arita, H.: Prevention of growth arrest-induced cell death of vascular smooth muscle cells by a product of growth arrest-specific gene, gas6. FEBS Lett 387:78, 1996

476. Goruppi, S., Ruaro, E., and Schneider, C.: Gas6, the ligand of Axl tyrosine kinase receptor, has mitogenic and survival activities for serum starved NIH3T3 fibroblasts. Oncogene 12:471, 1996

477. Stitt, T. N., Conn, G., Gore, M., Lai, C., Bruno, J., Radziejewski, C., Mattsson, K., Fisher, J., Gies, D. R., Jones, P. F., and et al.: The

478. Godowski, P. J., Mark, M. R., Chen, J., Sadick, M. D., Raab, H., and Hammonds, R. G.: Reevaluation of the roles of protein S and Gas6 as ligands for the receptor tyrosine kinase Rse/Tyro 3. Cell 82:355, 1995

479. Nyberg, P., He, X., Hardig, Y., Dahlbäck, B., and Garcia de Frutos, P.: Stimulation of Sky tyrosine phosphorylation by bovine protein S—domains involved in the receptor-ligand interaction. Eur J Biochem 246:147, 1997

480. Bertina, R. M., van Wijngaarden, A., Reinalda-Poot, J., Poort, S. R., and Bom, V. J.: Determination of plasma protein S—the protein cofactor of activated protein C. Thromb Haemost 53:268, 1985

481. Schwalbe, R., Dahlbäck, B., Hillarp, A., and Nelsestuen, G.: Assembly of protein S and C4b-binding protein on membranes. J Biol Chem 265:16074, 1990

482. Nelson, R. M., and Long, G. L.: Solution-phase equilibrium binding interaction of human protein S with C4b-binding protein. Biochemistry 30:2384, 1991

483. He, X., Shen, L., Malmborg, A. C., Smith, K. J., Dahlbäck, B., and Linse, S.: Binding site for C4b-binding protein in vitamin K–dependent protein S fully contained in carboxy-terminal laminin-G-type repeats. A study using recombinant factor IX-protein S chimeras and surface plasmon resonance. Biochemistry 36:3745, 1997

484. Walker, F. J.: Characterization of a synthetic peptide that inhibits the interaction between protein S and C4b-binding protein. J Biol Chem 264:17645, 1989

485. Fernandez, J. A., Heeb, M. J., and Griffin, J. H.: Identification of residues 413–433 of plasma protein S as essential for binding to C4b-binding protein. J Biol Chem 268:16788, 1993

486. Linse, S., Hardig, Y., Schultz, D. A., and Dahlbäck, B.: A region of vitamin K–dependent protein S that binds to C4b binding protein (C4BP) identified using bacteriophage peptide display libraries. J Biol Chem 272:14658, 1997

487. Chang, G. T., Maas, B. H., Ploos van Amstel, H. K., Reitsma, P. H., Bertina, R. M., and Bouma, B. N.: Studies of the interaction between human protein S and human C4b-binding protein using deletion variants of recombinant human protein S. Thromb Haemost 71:461, 1994

488. Nelson, R. M., and Long, G. L.: Binding of protein S to C4b-binding protein. Mutagenesis of protein S. J Biol Chem 267:8140, 1992

489. Law, S. K. A., and Reid, K. B. M.: Complement. Oxford, UK, IRL Press, 1995

490. Scharfstein, J., Ferreira, A., Gigli, I., and Nussenzweig, V.: Human C4b-binding protein. I. Isolation and characterization. J Exp Med 148:207, 1978

491. Scharfstein, J., Correa, E. B., Gallo, G. R., and Nussenzweig, V.: Human C4-binding protein. Association with immune complexes in vitro and in vivo. J Clin Invest 63:437, 1979

492. Fujita, T., Gigli, I., and Nussenzweig, V.: Human C4b-binding protein. II. Role of proteolysis of C4b by C3b-inactivator. J Exp Med 148:1044, 1978

493. Fujita, T., and Nussenzweig, V.: The role of C4-binding protein and beta1H in proteolysis of C4b and C3b. J Exp Med 150:267, 1979

494. Gigli, I., Fujita, T., and Nussenzweig, V.: Modulation of the classical pathway C3 convertase by plasma proteins C4 binding protein and C3b inactivator. Proc Natl Acad Sci USA 76:6596, 1979

495. Nagasawa, S., Ichihara, C., and Stroud, R.: Cleavage of C4b by C3b inactivator: Production of a nicked form of C4b, C4b', as an intermediate cleavage product of C4b and C3b inactivator. J Immunol 125:578, 1980

496. Barnum, S. R.: C4b-binding protein, a regulatory protein of complement. Immunol Res 10:28, 1991

497. Dahlbäck, B., Smith, C. A., and Muller Eberhard, H. J.: Visualization of human C4b-binding protein and its complexes with vitamin K–dependent protein S and complement protein C4b. Proc Natl Acad Sci USA 80:3461, 1983

498. Hillarp, A., and Dahlbäck, B.: Novel subunit in C4b-binding protein required for protein S binding. J Biol Chem 263:12759, 1988

499. Hillarp, A., and Dahlbäck, B.: Cloning of cDNA coding for the beta chain of human complement component C4b-binding protein: sequence homology with the alpha chain. Proc Natl Acad Sci USA 87:1183, 1990

500. Dahlbäck, B., and Muller Eberhard, H. J.: Ultrastructure of C4b-binding protein fragments formed by limited proteolysis using chymotrypsin. J Biol Chem 259:11631, 1984

501. Villoutreix, B. O., Fernandez, J. A., Teleman, O., and Griffin, J. H.:

Comparative modeling of the three CP modules of the beta-chain of C4BP and evaluation of potential sites of interaction with protein S. Protein Eng 8:1253, 1995

502. Villoutreix, B. O., Hardig, Y., Wallqvist, A., Covell, D. G., García de Frutos, P., and Dahlbäck, B.: Structural investigation of C4b-binding protein by molecular modeling: localization of putative binding sites. Proteins Struct Funct and Genet in press, 1998

503. Chung, L. P., Bentley, D. R., and Reid, K. B. M.: Molecular cloning and characterization of the cDNA coding for C4b-binding protein, a regulatory protein of the classical pathway of the human complement system. Biochem J 230:133, 1985

504. Baron, M., Norman, D. G., and Campbell, I. D.: Protein modules. Trends Biochem Sci 16:13, 1991

505. Bork, P., and Koonin, E. V.: Protein sequence motifs. Curr Opin Struct Biol 6:366, 1996

506. Henikoff, S., Greene, E. A., Pietrokovski, S., Bork, P., Attwood, T. K., and Hood, L.: Gene families: the taxonomy of protein paralogs and chimeras. Science 278:609, 1997

507. Wiles, A. P., Shaw, G., Bright, J., Perczel, A., Campbell, I. D., and Barlow, P. N.: NMR studies of a viral protein that mimics the regulators of complement activation. J Mol Biol 19:253, 1997

508. Barlow, P. N., Steinkasserer, A., Norman, D. G., Kieffer, B., Wiles, A. P., Sim, R. B., and Campbell, I. D.: Solution structure of a pair of complement modules by nuclear magnetic resonance. J Mol Biol 232:268, 1993

509. Norman, D. G., Barlow, P. N., Baron, M., Day, A. J., Sim, R. B., and Campbell, I. D.: Three-dimensional structure of a complement control protein module in solution. J Mol Biol 219:717, 1991

510. Rey Campos, J., Rubinstein, P., and Rodriguez de Cordoba, S.: A physical map of the human regulator of complement activation gene cluster linking the complement genes CR1, CR2, DAF, and C4BP. J Exp Med 167:664, 1988

511. Carroll, M. C., Alicot, E. M., Katzman, P. J., Klickstein, L. B., Smith, J. A., and Fearon, D. T.: Organization of the genes encoding complement receptors type 1 and 2, decay accelerating factor and C4b-binding protein in the RCA locus on human chromosome 1. J Exp Med 167:1271, 1988

512. Andersson, A., Dahlbäck, B., Hanson, C., Hillarp, A., Levan, G., Szpirer, J., and Szpirer, C.: Genes for C4b-binding protein alpha- and beta-chains (C4BPA and C4BPB) are located on chromosome 1, band 1q32, in humans and on chromosome 13 in rats. Somat Cell Mol Genet 16:493, 1990

513. Padro-Manuel, F., Rey-Campos, J., Hillarp, A., Dahlbäck, B., and Rodriguez de Cordoba, S.: Human genes for the alpha and beta-chains of complement C4b-binding protein are closely linked in a head-to-tail arrangement. Proc Natl Acad Sci USA 87:4529, 1990

514. Saeki, T., Hirose, S., Nukatsuka, M., Kusunoki, Y., and Nagasawa, S.: Evidence that C4b-binding protein is an acute phase protein. Biochem Biophys Res Commun 164:1446, 1989

515. Barnum, S. R., and Dahlbäck, B.: C4b-binding protein, a regulatory component of the classical pathway of complement, is an acute-phase protein and is elevated in systemic lupus erythematosus. Complement Inflamm 7:71, 1990

516. Garcia de Frutos, P., Alim, R. I., Hardig, Y., Zoller, B., and Dahlbäck, B.: Differential regulation of alpha and beta chains of C4b-binding protein during acute-phase response resulting in stable plasma levels of free anticoagulant protein S. Blood 84:815, 1994

517. Criado Garcia, O., Sanchez Corral, P., and Rodriguez de Cordoba, S.: Isoforms of human C4b-binding protein. II. Differential modulation of the C4BPA and C4BPB genes by acute phase cytokines. J Immunol 155:4037, 1995

518. Sanchez Corral, P., Criado Garcia, O., and Rodriguez de Cordoba, S.: Isoforms of human C4b-binding protein. I. Molecular basis for the C4BP isoform pattern and its variations in human plasma. J Immunol 155:4030, 1995

519. Hillarp, A., Hessing, M., and Dahlbäck, B.: Protein S binding in relation to the subunit composition of human C4b-binding protein. FEBS Lett 259:53, 1989

520. Griffin, J. H., Gruber, A., and Fernandez, J. A.: Reevaluation of total, free, and bound protein S and C4b-binding protein levels in plasma anticoagulated with citrate or hirudin. Blood 79:3203, 1992

521. Hardig, Y., Garcia de Frutos, P., and Dahlbäck, B.: Expression and characterization of a recombinant C4b-binding protein lacking the beta-chain. Biochem J 308:795, 1995

522. Dahlbäck, B., and Hildebrand, B.: Degradation of human complement component C4b in the presence of the C4b-binding protein-protein S complex. Biochem J 209:857, 1983

523. Hardig, Y., Rezaie, A., and Dahlbäck, B.: High affinity binding of human vitamin K–dependent protein S to a truncated recombinant beta-chain of C4b-binding protein expressed in Escherichia coli. J Biol Chem 268:3033, 1993

524. Hardig, Y., and Dahlbäck, B.: The amino-terminal module of the C4b-binding protein beta-chain contains the protein S-binding site. J Biol Chem 271:20861, 1996

525. Fernandez, J. A., and Griffin, J. H.: A protein S binding site on C4b-binding protein involves beta chain residues 31–45. J Biol Chem 269:2535, 1994

526. Ogata, R. T., Mathias, P., Bradt, B. M., and Cooper, N. R.: Murine C4b-binding protein. Mapping of the ligand binding site and the N-terminus of the pre-protein. J Immunol 150:2273, 1993

527. Hardig, Y., Hillarp, A., and Dahlbäck, B.: The amino-terminal module of the C4b-binding protein alpha-chain is crucial for C4b binding and factor I-cofactor function. Biochem J 323:469, 1997

528. Accardo, P., Sanchez Corral, P., Criado, O., Garcia, E., and Rodriguez de Cordoba, S.: Binding of human complement component C4b-binding protein (C4BP) to Streptococcus pyogenes involves the C4b-binding site. J Immunol 157:4935, 1996

529. Thern, A., Stenberg, L., Dahlbäck, B., and Lindahl, G.: Ig-binding surface proteins of Streptococcus pyogenes also bind human C4b-binding protein (C4BP), a regulatory component of the complement system. J Immunol 154:375, 1995

530. Schwalbe, R. A., Dahlbäck, B., and Nelsestuen, G. L.: Independent association of serum amyloid P component, protein S, and complement C4b with complement C4b-binding protein and subsequent association of the complex with membranes. J Biol Chem 265:21749, 1990

531. Skinner, M., and Cohen, A. S.: Amyloid P component. Methods Enzymol 163:523, 1988

532. Garcia de Frutos, P., and Dahlbäck, B.: Interaction between serum amyloid P component and C4b-binding protein associated with inhibition of factor I-mediated C4b degradation. J Immunol 152:2430, 1994

533. Garcia de Frutos, P., Hardig, Y., and Dahlbäck, B.: Serum amyloid P component binding to C4b-binding protein. J Biol Chem 270:26950, 1995

534. Furmaniak Kazmierczak, E., Hu, C. Y., and Esmon, C. T.: Protein S enhances C4b binding protein interaction with neutrophils. Blood 81:405, 1993

535. Gruber, A., and Griffin, J. H.: Direct detection of activated protein C in blood from human subjects. Blood 79:2340, 1992

536. Rosenberg, R. D.: Regulation of the hemostatic mechanism. In Stamatoyannopoulos, G., Nienhuis, A. W., Leder, P., and Majerus, P. W. (eds): The Molecular Basis of Blood Diseases, 1st Ed. Philadelphia, W. B. Saunders, 1986, p. 534

537. Esmon, C. T.: Inflammation. They're not just for clots anymore. Curr Biol 5:743, 1995

538. Esmon, C. T.: Inflammation and thrombosis: the impact of inflammation on the protein C anticoagulant pathway. Haematologica 80:49, 1995

539. Esmon, C. T., Taylor, F. B., Jr., and Snow, T. R.: Inflammation and coagulation: linked processes potentially regulated through a common pathway mediated by protein C. Thromb Haemost 66:160, 1991

540. Taylor, F. B., Jr.: Studies on the inflammatory-coagulant axis in the baboon response to E. coli: regulatory roles of proteins C, S, C4bBP and of inhibitors of tissue factor. Prog Clin Biol Res 388:175, 1994

541. Snow, T. R., Deal, M. T., Dickey, D. T., and Esmon, C. T.: Protein C activation following coronary artery occlusion in the in situ porcine heart [see comments]. Circulation 84:293, 1991

542. Marlar, R. A., Endres-Brooks, J., and Miller, C.: Serial studies of protein C and its plasma inhibitor in patients with disseminated intravascular coagulation. Blood 66:59, 1985

543. Espana, F., Vicente, V., Tabernero, D., Scharrer, I., and Griffin, J. H.: Determination of plasma protein C inhibitor and of two activated protein C-inhibitor complexes in normals and in patients with intravascular coagulation and thrombotic disease. Thromb Res 59:593, 1990

544. Tabernero, D., Espana, F., Vicente, V., Estelles, A., Gilabert, J., and Aznar, J.: Protein C inhibitor and other components of the protein C pathway in patients with acute deep vein thrombosis during heparin treatment. Thromb Haemost 63:380, 1990

545. Vicente, V., Espana, F., Tabernero, D., Estelles, A., Aznar, J., Hendl,

S., and Griffin, J. H.: Evidence of activation of the protein C pathway during acute vascular damage induced by Mediterranean spotted fever. Blood 78:416, 1991

546. Gruber, A., Griffin, J. H., Harker, L. A., and Hanson, S. R.: Inhibition of platelet-dependent thrombus formation by human activated protein C in a primate model. Blood 73:639, 1989

547. Colucci, M., Triggiani, R., Cavallo, L. G., and Semeraro, N.: Thrombin infusion in endotoxin-treated rabbits reduces the plasma levels of plasminogen activator inhibitor: evidence for a protein-C-mediated mechanism [see comments]. Blood 74:1976, 1989

548. Arnljots, B., Bergqvist, D., and Dahlbäck, B.: Inhibition of microarterial thrombosis by activated protein C in a rabbit model. Thromb Haemost 72:415, 1994

549. Arnljots, B., and Dahlbäck, B.: Antithrombotic effects of activated protein C and protein S in a rabbit model of microarterial thrombosis. Arterioscler Thromb Vasc Biol 15:937, 1995

550. Arnljots, B., and Dahlbäck, B.: Protein S as an in vivo cofactor to activated protein C in prevention of microarterial thrombosis in rabbits. J Clin Invest 95:1987, 1995

551. Gresele, P., Momi, S., Berrettini, M., Nenci, G. G., Schwarz, H. P., Semeraro, N., and Colucci, M.: Activated human protein C prevents thrombin-induced thromboembolism in mice. Evidence that activated protein C reduces intravascular fibrin accumulation through the inhibition of additional thrombin generation. J Clin Invest 101:667, 1998

552. Kishida, A., Akatsuka, Y., Yanagi, M., Aikou, T., Maruyama, I., and Akashi, M.: In vivo and ex vivo evaluation of the antithrombogenicity of human thrombomodulin immobilized biomaterials. ASAIO J 41:M369, 1995

553. Aoki, Y., Takei, R., Mohri, M., Gonda, Y., Gomi, K., Sugihara, T., Kiyota, T., Yamamoto, S., Ishida, T., and Maruyama, I.: Antithrombotic effects of recombinant human soluble thrombomodulin (rhs-TM) on arteriovenous shunt thrombosis in rats. Am J Hematol 47:162, 1994

554. Ohishi, R., Watanabe, N., Aritomi, M., Gomi, K., Kiyota, T., Yamamoto, S., Ishida, T., and Maruyama, I.: Evidence that the protein C activation pathway amplifies the inhibition of thrombin generation by recombinant human thrombomodulin in plasma. Thromb Haemost 70:423, 1993

555. Taylor, F. B., Jr., Chang, A., Esmon, C. T., D'Angelo, A., Vigano, D. A. S., and Blick, K. E.: Protein C prevents the coagulopathic and lethal effects of Escherichia coli infusion in the baboon. J Clin Invest 79:918, 1987

556. Taylor, F. B., Jr., Chang, A. C., Peer, G. T., Mather, T., Blick, K., Catlett, R., Lockhart, M. S., and Esmon, C. T.: DEGR-factor Xa blocks disseminated intravascular coagulation initiated by Escherichia coli without preventing shock or organ damage. Blood 78:364, 1991

557. Smith, O. P., White, B., Vaughan, D., Rafferty, M., Claffey, L., Lyons, B., and Casey, W.: Use of protein-C concentrate, heparin, and haemodiafiltration in meningococcus-induced pupura fulminans. Lancet 350:1590, 1997

558. Taylor, F. B., Jr., Dahlbäck, B., Chang, A. C., Lockhart, M. S., Hatanaka, K., Peer, G., and Esmon, C. T.: Role of free protein S and C4b binding protein in regulating the coagulant response to Escherichia coli. Blood 86:2642, 1995

559. Taylor, F., Chang, A., Ferrell, G., Mather, T., Catlett, R., Blick, K., and Esmon, C. T.: C4b-binding protein exacerbates the host response to Escherichia coli. Blood 78:357, 1991

560. Nordstrom, M., Lindblad, B., Bergqvist, D., and Kjellstrom, T.: A prospective study of the incidence of deep-vein thrombosis within a defined urban population. J Intern Med 232:155, 1992

561. Anderson, F. A. J., Wheeler, H. B., Goldberg, R. J., Hosmer, D. W., Patwardhan, N. A., Jovanovic, B., Forcier, A., and Dalen, J. E.: A population-based perspective of the hospital incidence and case-fatality rates of deep vein thrombosis and pulmonary embolism. The Worcester DVT Study. Arch Intern Med 151:933, 1991

562. Malm, J., Laurell, M., Nilsson, I. M., and Dahlbäck, B.: Thromboembolic disease—critical evaluation of laboratory investigation [see comments]. Thromb Haemost 68:7, 1992

563. Lane, D. A., Mannucci, P. M., Bauer, K. A., Bertina, R. M., Bochkov, N. P., Boulyjenkov, V., Chandy, M., Dahlbäck, B., Ginter, E. K., Miletich, J. P., Rosendaal, F. R., and Seligsohn, U.: Inherited thrombophilia: Part 2. Thromb Haemost 76:824, 1996

564. Lane, D. A., Mannucci, P. M., Bauer, K. A., Bertina, R. M., Bochkov, N. P., Boulyjenkov, V., Chandy, M., Dahlbäck, B., Ginter, E. K., Miletich, J. P., Rosendaal, F. R., and Seligsohn, U.: Inherited thrombophilia: Part 1. Thromb Haemost 76:651, 1996

565. Poort, S. R., Rosendaal, F. R., Reitsma, P. H., and Bertina, R. M.: A common genetic variation in the 3′-untranslated region of the prothrombin gene is associated with elevated plasma prothrombin levels and an increase in venous thrombosis. Blood 88:3698, 1996

566. Hillarp, A., Zoller, B., Svensson, P. J., and Dahlbäck, B.: The 20210 A allele of the prothrombin gene is a common risk factor among Swedish outpatients with verified deep venous thrombosis. Thromb Haemost 78:990, 1997

567. Brown, K., Luddington, R., Williamson, D., Baker, P., and Baglin, T.: Risk of venous thromboembolism associated with a G to A transition at position 20210 in the 3′-untranslated region of the prothrombin gene. Br J Haematol 98:907, 1997

568. Cumming, A. M., Keeney, S., Salden, A., Bhavnani, M., Shwe, K. H., and Hay, C. R.: The prothrombin gene G20210A variant: prevalence in a U.K. anticoagulant clinic population. Br J Haematol 98:353, 1997

569. Dahlbäck, B., Carlsson, M., and Svensson, P. J.: Familial thrombophilia due to a previously unrecognized mechanism characterized by poor anticoagulant response to activated protein C: prediction of a cofactor to activated protein C [see comments]. Proc Natl Acad Sci USA 90:1004, 1993

570. Griffin, J. H., Evatt, B., Wideman, C., and Fernandez, J. A.: Anticoagulant protein C pathway defective in majority of thrombophilic patients [see comments]. Blood 82:1989, 1993

571. Koster, T., Rosendaal, F. R., de Ronde, H., Briet, E., Vandenbroucke, J. P., and Bertina, R. M.: Venous thrombosis due to poor anticoagulant response to activated protein C: Leiden Thrombophilia Study [see comments]. Lancet 342:1503, 1993

572. Svensson, P. J., and Dahlbäck, B.: Resistance to activated protein C as a basis for venous thrombosis [see comments]. N Engl J Med 330:517, 1994

573. Halbmayer, W. M., Haushofer, A., Schon, R., and Fischer, M.: The prevalence of poor anticoagulant response to activated protein C (APC-resistance) among patients suffering from stroke or venous thrombosis and among healthy subjects [see comments]. Blood Coagul Fibrinolysis 5:51, 1994

574. Bertina, R. M., Koeleman, B. P., Koster, T., Rosendaal, F. R., Dirven, R. J., de Ronde, H., van der Velden, P. A., and Reitsma, P. H.: Mutation in blood coagulation factor V associated with resistance to activated protein C [see comments]. Nature 369:64, 1994

575. Zoller, B., Svensson, P. J., He, X., and Dahlbäck, B.: Identification of the same factor V gene mutation in 47 out of 50 thrombosis-prone families with inherited resistance to activated protein C. J Clin Invest 94:2521, 1994

576. Voorberg, J., Roelse, J., Koopman, R., Buller, H., Berends, F., ten Cate, J. W., Mertens, K., and van Mourik, J. A.: Association of idiopathic venous thromboembolism with single point-mutation at Arg506 of factor V [see comments]. Lancet 343:1535, 1994

577. Greengard, J. S., Sun, X., Xu, X., Fernandez, J. A., Griffin, J. H., and Evatt, B.: Activated protein C resistance caused by Arg506Gln mutation in factor Va [letter]. Lancet 343:1361, 1994

578. Zoller, B., and Dahlbäck, B.: Linkage between inherited resistance to activated protein C and factor V gene mutation in venous thrombosis [see comments]. Lancet 343:1536, 1994

579. Zoller, B., Norlund, L., Leksell, H., Nilsson, J. E., von Schenck, H., Rosen, U., Jepsson, J. O., and Dahlbäck, B.: High prevalence of the FVR506Q mutation causing APC-resistance in a region of southern Sweden with a high incidence of venous thrombosis [letter]. Thromb Res 83:475, 1996

580. Schroder, W., Koesling, M., Wulff, K., Wehnert, M., and Herrmann, F. H.: Large-scale screening for factor V Leiden mutation in a northeastern German population. Haemostasis 26:233, 1996

581. Chaida, C., Gialeraki, A., Tsoukala, C., and Mandalaki, T.: Prevalence of the FVQ506 mutation in the Hellenic population [letter]. Thromb Haemost 76:127, 1996

582. Rees, D. C., Cox, M., and Clegg, J. B.: World distribution of factor V Leiden [see comments]. Lancet 346:1133, 1995

583. Seligsohn, U., and Zivelin, A.: Thrombophilia as a multigenic disorder. Thromb Haemost 78:297, 1997

584. Dzimiri, N., and Meyer, B.: World distribution of factor V Leiden [letter; comment]. Lancet 347:481, 1996

585. Beauchamp, N. J., Daly, M. E., Hampton, K. K., Cooper, P. C., Preston, F. E., and Peake, I. R.: High prevalence of a mutation in the factor V gene within the U.K. population: relationship to activated protein C resistance and familial thrombosis. Br J Haematol 88:219, 1994

586. Ridker, P. M., Miletich, J. P., Hennekens, C. H., and Buring, J. E.: Ethnic distribution of factor V Leiden in 4047 men and women. Implications for venous thromboembolism screening. JAMA 277:1305, 1997

587. Mari, D., Mannucci, P. M., Duca, F., Bertolini, S., and Franceschi, C.: Mutant factor V (Arg506Gln) in healthy centenarians [letter]. Lancet 347:1044, 1996

588. Pepe, G., Rickards, O., Vanegas, O. C., Brunelli, T., Gori, A. M., Giusti, B., Attanasio, M., Prisco, D., Gensini, G. F., and Abbate, R.: Prevalence of factor V Leiden mutation in non-European populations. Thromb Haemost 77:329, 1997

589. Ko, Y. L., Hsu, T. S., Wu, S. M., Ko, Y. S., Chang, C. J., Wang, S. M., Chen, W. J., Cheng, N. J., Kuo, C. T., Chiang, C. W., and Lee, Y. S.: The G1691A mutation of the coagulation factor V gene (factor V Leiden) is rare in Chinese: an analysis of 618 individuals. Hum Genet 98:176, 1996

590. Chan, L. C., Bourke, C., Lam, C. K., Liu, H. W., Brookes, S., Jenkins, V., and Pasi, J.: Lack of activated protein C resistance in healthy Hong Kong Chinese blood donors—correlation with absence of Arg506-Gln mutation of factor V gene [letter]. Thromb Haemost 75:522, 1996

591. Shen, M. C., Lin, J. S., and Tsay, W.: High prevalence of antithrombin III, protein C and protein S deficiency, but no factor V Leiden mutation in venous thrombophilic Chinese patients in Taiwan. Thromb Res 87:377, 1997

592. Zama, T., Murata, M., Ono, F., Watanabe, K., Watanabe, R., Moriki, T., Yokoyama, K., Tokuhira, M., and Ikeda, Y.: Low prevalence of activated protein C resistance and coagulation factor V Arg506 to Gln mutation among Japanese patients with various forms of thrombosis, and normal individuals. Int J Hematol 65:71, 1996

593. Kodaira, H., Ishida, F., Shimodaira, S., Takamiya, O., Furihata, K., and Kitano, K.: Resistance to activated protein C and Arg 506 Gln factor V mutation are uncommon in eastern Asian populations. Acta Haematol 98:22, 1997

594. Soubrier, F., Fery, I., Verdy, E., Rene, M. N., Varsat, B., Visvikis, S., and Siest, G.: The frequency of the factor V gene R506Q mutation varies between regions of France [letter]. Nouv Rev Fr Hematol 37:175, 1995

595. Lindqvist, P. G., Svensson, P. J., Dahlbäck, B., and Marsal, K.: Factor V R506Q mutation (activated protein C resistance) associated with reduced intrapartum blood loss—a possible evolutionary selection mechanism. Thromb Haemost 79:69, 1998

596. Cox, M. J., Rees, D. C., Martinson, J. J., and Clegg, J. B.: Evidence for a single origin of factor V Leiden. Br J Haematol 92:1022, 1996

597. Zoller, B., Hillarp, A., and Dahlbäck, B.: Activated protein C resistance caused by a common factor V mutation has a single origin. Thromb Res 85:237, 1997

598. Zivelin, A., Griffin, J. H., Xu, X., Pabinger, I., Samama, M., Conard, J., Brenner, B., Eldor, A., and Seligsohn, U.: A single genetic origin for a common Caucasian risk factor for venous thrombosis. Blood 89:397, 1997

599. Inbal, A., Griffin, J. H., Xu, X., Fernandez, J. A., Zivelin, A., Gitel, S., Martinowitz, U., Halkin, H., and Seligsohn, U.: Extensive venous and arterial thrombosis in a patient with familial APC-resistance without R506Q mutation. Blood 90(Suppl. 1):150a, 1997

600. Williamson, D., Brown, K., Luddington, R., Baglin, C., and Baglin, T.: Factor V Cambridge: A new mutation (Arg306 ->Thr) associated with resistance to activated protein C. Blood 91:1140, 1998

601. Chan, W. P., Lee, C. K., Kwong, Y. L., Lam, C. K., and Liang, R.: A novel mutation of Arg306 of factor V gene in Hong Kong Chinese. Blood 91:1135, 1998

602. Aparicio, C., and Dahlbäck, B.: Molecular mechanisms of activated protein C resistance. Properties of factor V isolated from an individual with homozygosity for the Arg506 to Gln mutation in the factor V gene. Biochem J 313:467, 1996

603. Heeb, M. J., Kojima, Y., Greengard, J. S., and Griffin, J. H.: Activated protein C resistance: molecular mechanisms based on studies using purified Gln506-factor V. Blood 85:3405, 1995

604. Simioni, P., Scarano, L., Gavasso, S., Sardella, C., Girolami, B., Scudeller, A., and Girolami, A.: Prothrombin fragment 1+2 and thrombin-antithrombin complex levels in patients with inherited APC-resistance due to factor V Leiden mutation. Br J Haematol 92:435, 1996

605. Zoller, B., Holm, J., Svensson, P., and Dahlbäck, B.: Elevated levels of prothrombin activation fragment 1 + 2 in plasma from patients with heterozygous Arg506 to Gln mutation in the factor V gene (APC-resistance) and/or inherited protein S deficiency. Thromb Haemost 75:270, 1996

606. Jorquera, J. I., Montoro, J. M., Fernandez, M. A., Aznar, J. A., and Aznar, J.: Modified test for activated protein C resistance [letter] [see comments]. Lancet 344:1162, 1994

607. Trossaert, M., Conard, J., Horellou, M. H., Samama, M. M., Ireland, H., Bayston, T. A., and Lane, D. A.: Modified APC-resistance assay for patients on oral anticoagulants [letter; comment]. Lancet 344:1709, 1994

608. Svensson, P. J., Zoller, B., and Dahlbäck, B.: Evaluation of original and modified APC-resistance tests in unselected outpatients with clinically suspected thrombosis and in healthy controls. Thromb Haemost 77:332, 1997

609. Ridker, P. M., Hennekens, C. H., Lindpaintner, K., Stampfer, M. J., Eisenberg, P. R., and Miletich, J. P.: Mutation in the gene coding for coagulation factor V and the risk of myocardial infarction, stroke, and venous thrombosis in apparently healthy men [see comments]. N Engl J Med 332:912, 1995

610. Svensson, P. J., Zoller, B., Mattiasson, I., and Dahlbäck, B.: The factor VR506Q mutation causing APC-resistance is highly prevalent amongst unselected outpatients with clinically suspected deep venous thrombosis. J Intern Med 241:379, 1997

611. Rosendaal, F. R.: Risk factors for venous thrombosis: prevalence, risk and interaction. Semin Hematol 34:171, 1997

612. Holm, J., Zoller, B., Berntorp, E., Erhardt, L., and Dahlbäck, B.: Prevalence of factor V gene mutation amongst myocardial infarction patients and healthy controls is higher in Sweden than in other countries. J Intern Med 239:221, 1996

613. Rosendaal, F. R., Siscovick, D. S., Schwartz, S. M., Beverly, R. K., Psaty, B. M., Longstreth, W. T., Jr., Raghunathan, T. E., Koepsell, T. D., and Reitsma, P. H.: Factor V Leiden (resistance to activated protein C) increases the risk of myocardial infarction in young women. Blood 89:2817, 1997

614. Tabernero, M. D., Tomas, J. F., Alberca, I., Orfao, A., Lopez Borrasca, A., and Vicente, V.: Incidence and clinical characteristics of hereditary disorders associated with venous thrombosis. Am J Hematol 36:249, 1991

615. Heijboer, H., Brandjes, D. P., Buller, H. R., Sturk, A., and ten Cate, J. W.: Deficiencies of coagulation-inhibiting and fibrinolytic proteins in outpatients with deep-vein thrombosis [see comments]. N Engl J Med 323:1512, 1990

616. Pabinger, I., Brucker, S., Kyrle, P. A., Schneider, B., Korninger, H. C., Niessner, H., and Lechner, K.: Hereditary deficiency of antithrombin III, protein C and protein S: prevalence in patients with a history of venous thrombosis and criteria for rational patient screening. Blood Coagul Fibrinolysis 3:547, 1992

617. Miletich, J., Sherman, L., and Broze, G., Jr.: Absence of thrombosis in subjects with heterozygous protein C deficiency. N Engl J Med 317:991, 1987

618. Tait, R. C., Walker, I. D., Reitsma, P. H., Islam, S. I., McCall, F., Poort, S. R., Conkie, J. A., and Bertina, R. M.: Prevalence of protein C deficiency in the healthy population. Thromb Haemost 73:87, 1995

619. Koster, T., Rosendaal, F. R., Briet, E., van der Meer, F. J., Colly, L. P., Trienekens, P. H., Poort, S. R., Reitsma, P. H., and Vandenbroucke, J. P.: Protein C deficiency in a controlled series of unselected outpatients: an infrequent but clear risk factor for venous thrombosis (Leiden Thrombophilia Study) [see comments]. Blood 85:2756, 1995

620. Allaart, C. F., Aronson, D. C., Ruys, T., Rosendaal, F. R., van Bockel, J. H., Bertina, R. M., and Briet, E.: Hereditary protein S deficiency in young adults with arterial occlusive disease. Thromb Haemost 64:206, 1990

621. van Boven, H. H., and Lane, D. A.: Antithrombin and its inherited deficiency states. Semin Hematol 34:188, 1997

622. Zoller, B., Berntsdotter, A., Garcia de Frutos, P., and Dahlbäck, B.: Resistance to activated protein C as an additional genetic risk factor in hereditary deficiency of protein S. Blood 85:3518, 1995

623. Simmonds, R. E., Ireland, H., Lane, D. A., Zoller, B., de Frutos, P. G., and Dahlbäck, B.: Clarification of the risk for venous thrombosis associated with hereditary protein S deficiency by investigation of a large kindred with a characterized gene defect. Ann Intern Med 128:8, 1998

624. Allaart, C. F., Poort, S. R., Rosendaal, F. R., Reitsma, P. H., Bertina, R. M., and Briet, E.: Increased risk of venous thrombosis in carriers

of hereditary protein C deficiency defect [see comments]. Lancet 341:134, 1993

625. Seligsohn, U., Berger, A., Abend, A., Rubin, L., Attias, D., Zivelin, A., and Rapaport, S. I.: Homozygous protein C deficiency manifested by massive thrombosis in the newborn. N Engl J Med 310:559, 1984

626. Dreyfus, M., Masterson, M., David, M., Rivard, G. E., Muller, F. M., Kreuz, W., Beeg, T., Minford, A., Allgrove, J., Cohen, J. D., and et al.: Replacement therapy with a monoclonal antibody purified protein C concentrate in newborns with severe congenital protein C deficiency. Semin Thromb Hemost 21:371, 1995

627. Broekmans, A. W., Bertina, R. M., Loeliger, E. A., Hofmann, V., and Klingemann, H. G.: Protein C and the development of skin necrosis during anticoagulant therapy [letter]. Thromb Haemost 49:251 *LHM: This title is owned by this library *LHC: 35(1976), 1983

628. Rose, V. L., Kwaan, H. C., Williamson, K., Hoppensteadt, D., Walenga, J., and Fareed, J.: Protein C antigen deficiency and warfarin necrosis. Am J Clin Pathol 86:653, 1986

629. Broekmans, A. W., and Conard, J.: Hereditary protein C deficiency. In Bertina, R.M. (ed.): Protein C and Related Proteins. Churchill Livingstone Longman Group UK, 1988, p. 160

630. Vigano, S., Mannucci, P. M., Solinas, S., Bottasso, B., and Mariani, G.: Decrease in protein C antigen and formation of an abnormal protein soon after starting oral anticoagulant therapy. Br J Haematol 57:213, 1984

631. Epstein, D. J., Bergum, P. W., Bajaj, P., and Rapaport, S. I.: Radioimmunoassays for protein C and factor X. Plasma antigen levels in abnormal hemostatic states. Am J Clin Pathol 82:573, 1984

632. Weiss, P., Soff, G. A., Halkin, H., and Seligsohn, U.: Decline of proteins C and S and factors II, VII, IX and X during the initiation of warfarin therapy. Thromb Res 45:783, 1987

633. Rowbotham, B., Clouston, W., Kime, N., Rowell, J., and Exner, T.: Coumarin skin necrosis without protein C deficiency [letter]. Aust N Z J Med 16:513, 1986

634. Reitsma, P. H.: Protein C deficiency: summary of the 1995 database update. Nucleic Acids Res 24:157, 1996

635. Matsuda, M., Sugo, T., Sakata, Y., Murayama, H., Mimuro, J., Tanabe, S., and Yoshitake, S.: A thrombotic state due to an abnormal protein C. N Engl J Med 319:1265, 1988

636. Grundy, C., Chitolie, A., Talbot, S., Bevan, D., Kakkar, V., and Cooper, D. N.: Protein C London 1: recurrent mutation at Arg 169 (CGG–TGG) in the protein C gene causing thrombosis. Nucleic Acids Res 17:10513, 1989

637. Greengard, J. S., Fisher, C. L., Villoutreix, B., and Griffin, J. H.: Structural basis for type I and type II deficiencies of antithrombotic plasma protein C: patterns revealed by three-dimensional molecular modelling of mutations of the protease domain. Proteins 18:367, 1994

638. Simmonds, R. E., Zoller, B., Ireland, H., Thompson, E., de Frutos, P. G., Dahlbäck, B., and Lane, D. A.: Genetic and phenotypic analysis of a large (122-member) protein S-deficient kindred provides an explanation for the familial coexistence of type I and type III plasma phenotypes. Blood 89:4364, 1997

639. Zoller, B., Garcia de Frutos, P., and Dahlbäck, B.: Evaluation of the relationship between protein S and C4b-binding protein isoforms in hereditary protein S deficiency demonstrating type I and type III deficiencies to be phenotypic variants of the same genetic disease. Blood 85:3524, 1995

640. Mahasandana, C., Suvatte, V., Marlar, R. A., Manco Johnson, M. J., Jacobson, L. J., and Hathaway, W. E.: Neonatal purpura fulminans associated with homozygous protein S deficiency [letter]. Lancet 335:61, 1990

641. Mahasandana, C., Suvatte, V., Chuansumrit, A., Marlar, R. A., Manco Johnson, M. J., Jacobson, L. J., and Hathaway, W. E.: Homozygous protein S deficiency in an infant with purpura fulminans. J Pediatr 117:750, 1990

642. Mahasandana, C., Veerakul, G., Tanphaichitr, V. S., Suvatte, V., Opartkiattikul, N., and Hathaway, W. E.: Homozygous protein S deficiency: 7-year follow-up [letter]. Thromb Haemost 76:1122, 1996

643. Gomez, E., Ledford, M. R., Pegelow, C. H., Reitsma, P. H., and Bertina, R. M.: Homozygous protein S deficiency due to a one base pair deletion that leads to a stop codon in exon III of the protein S gene. Thromb Haemost 71:723, 1994

644. Engesser, L., Broekmans, A. W., Briet, E., Brommer, E. J., and Bertina, R. M.: Hereditary protein S deficiency: clinical manifestations. Ann Intern Med 106:677, 1987

645. Zöller, B., García de Frutos, P., and Dahlbäck, B.: A common 4G allele in the promotor of the plasminogen activator inhibitor-1 (PAI-1) gene is a risk factor for pulmonary embolism and arterial thrombosis in hereditary protein S deficiency. Thromb Haemost 79:802, 1998

646. Craig, A., Taberner, D. A., Fisher, A. H., Foster, D. N., and Mitra, J.: Type I protein S deficiency and skin necrosis. Postgrad Med J 66:389, 1990

647. Grimaudo, V., Gueissaz, F., Hauert, J., Sarraj, A., Kruithof, E. K., and Bachmann, F.: Necrosis of skin induced by coumarin in a patient deficient in protein S. BMJ 298:233, 1989

648. Goldberg, S. L., Orthner, C. L., Yalisove, B. L., Elgart, M. L., and Kessler, C. M.: Skin necrosis following prolonged administration of coumarin in a patient with inherited protein S deficiency. Am J Hematol 38:64, 1991

649. D'Angelo, A., Vigano, D. A. S., Esmon, C. T., and Comp, P. C.: Acquired deficiencies of protein S. Protein S activity during oral anticoagulation, in liver disease, and in disseminated intravascular coagulation. J Clin Invest 81:1445, 1988

650. Vigano, D. A. S., D'Angelo, A., Kaufman, C. E., Jr., Sholer, C., Esmon, C. T., and Comp, P. C.: Protein S deficiency occurs in the nephrotic syndrome. Ann Intern Med 107:42, 1987

651. Comp, P. C., Thurnau, G. R., Welsh, J., and Esmon, C. T.: Functional and immunologic protein S levels are decreased during pregnancy. Blood 68:881, 1986

652. Malm, J., Laurell, M., and Dahlbäck, B.: Changes in the plasma levels of vitamin K–dependent proteins C and S and of C4b-binding protein during pregnancy and oral contraception. Br J Haematol 68:437, 1988

653. Sorice, M., Arcieri, P., Griggi, T., Circella, A., Misasi, R., Lenti, L., Di Nucci, G. D., and Mariani, G.: Inhibition of protein S by autoantibodies in patients with acquired protein S deficiency. Thromb Haemost 75:555, 1996

654. Sugerman, R. W., Church, J. A., Goldsmith, J. C., and Ens, G. E.: Acquired protein S deficiency in children infected with human immunodeficiency virus. Pediatr Infect Dis J 15:106, 1996

655. Deitcher, S. R., Erban, J. K., and Limentani, S. A.: Acquired free protein S deficiency associated with multiple myeloma: a case report. Am J Hematol 51:319, 1996

656. Manco Johnson, M. J., Nuss, R., Key, N., Moertel, C., Jacobson, L., Meech, S., Weinberg, A., and Lefkowitz, J.: Lupus anticoagulant and protein S deficiency in children with postvaricella purpura fulminans or thrombosis. J Pediatr 128:319, 1996

657. Ginsberg, J. S., Demers, C., Brill Edwards, P., Bona, R., Johnston, M., Wong, A., and Denburg, J. A.: Acquired free protein S deficiency is associated with antiphospholipid antibodies and increased thrombin generation in patients with systemic lupus erythematosus. Am J Med 98:379, 1995

658. Prince, H. M., Thurlow, P. J., Buchanan, R. C., Ibrahim, K. M., and Neeson, P. J.: Acquired protein S deficiency in a patient with systemic lupus erythematosus causing central retinal vein thrombosis. J Clin Pathol 48:387, 1995

659. Vaezi, M. F., Rustagi, P. K., and Elson, C. O.: Transient protein S deficiency associated with cerebral venous thrombosis in active ulcerative colitis. Am-J-Gastroenterol 90:313, 1995

660. Bergmann, F., Hoyer, P. F., D'Angelo, S. V., Mazzola, G., Oestereich, C., Barthels, M., and D'Angelo, A.: Severe autoimmune protein S deficiency in a boy with idiopathic purpura fulminans. Br J Haematol 89:610, 1995

661. Bissuel, F., Berruyer, M., Causse, X., Dechavanne, M., and Trepo, C.: Acquired protein S deficiency: correlation with advanced disease in HIV-1-infected patients [see comments]. J Acquir Immune Defic Syndr 5:484, 1992

662. Kemkes Matthes, B.: Acquired protein S deficiency. Clin Investig 70:529, 1992

663. D'Angelo, A., Della Valle, P., Crippa, L., Pattarini, E., Grimaldi, L. M., and Vigano, D. A. S.: Brief report: autoimmune protein S deficiency in a boy with severe thromboembolic disease [see comments]. N Engl J Med 328:1753, 1993

664. D'Angelo, A., Mazzola, G., Bergmann, F., Safa, O., Della Valle, P., and D'Angelo, S. V.: Autoimmune protein S deficiency: a disorder predisposing to thrombosis. Haematologica 80:114, 1995

665. Hayashi, T., Nishioka, J., and Suzuki, K.: Molecular mechanism of the dysfunction of protein S(Tokushima) (Lys155->Glu) for the regulation of the blood coagulation system. Biochim Biophys Acta 1272:159, 1995

666. Koeleman, B. P., Reitsma, P. H., Allaart, C. F., and Bertina, R. M.: Activated protein C resistance as an additional risk factor for thrombosis in protein C-deficient families. Blood 84:1031, 1994

667. Gandrille, S., Greengard, J. S., Alhenc Gelas, M., Juhan Vague, I., Abgrall, J. F., Jude, B., Griffin, J. H., and Aiach, M.: Incidence of activated protein C resistance caused by the ARG 506 GLN mutation in factor V in 113 unrelated symptomatic protein C-deficient patients. The French Network on the behalf of INSERM. Blood 86:219, 1995

668. Hallam, P. J., Millar, D. S., Krawczak, M., Kakkar, V. V., and Cooper, D. N.: Population differences in the frequency of the factor V Leiden variant among people with clinically symptomatic protein C deficiency. J Med Genet 32:543, 1995

669. Koeleman, B. P., van Rumpt, D., Hamulyak, K., Reitsma, P. H., and Bertina, R. M.: Factor V Leiden: an additional risk factor for thrombosis in protein S deficient families? Thromb Haemost 74:580, 1995

670. van Boven, H. H., Reitsma, P. H., Rosendaal, F. R., Bayston, T. A., Chowdhury, V., Bauer, K. A., Scharrer, I., Conard, J., and Lane, D. A.: Factor V Leiden (FV R506Q) in families with inherited antithrombin deficiency. Thromb Haemost 75:417, 1996

671. Zoller, B., Svensson, P. J., Dahlbäck, B., and Hillarp, A.: The A20210 allele of the prothrombin gene is frequently associated with the factor V Arg 506 to Gln mutation but not with protein S deficiency in thrombophilic families. Blood 91:2210, 1998

672. Vandenbroucke, J. P., Koster, T., Briet, E., Reitsma, P. H., Bertina, R. M., and Rosendaal, F. R.: Increased risk of venous thrombosis in oral-contraceptive users who are carriers of factor V Leiden mutation [see comments]. Lancet 344:1453, 1994

20 Regulation of Blood Coagulation by Protease Inhibitors

George J. Broze, Jr., and
Douglas M. Tollefsen

▼ ▼

Blood coagulation is part of the hemostatic response to injury and serves to maintain the integrity of the vascular system. Coagulation involves a complex series of interactions between protease zymogens, enzymes, and cofactors that leads to the generation of thrombin and a fibrin clot (see Chapter 18). This process is regulated to limit the extent of coagulation to the site of injury and to allow the eventual dissolution of fibrin concomitant with the healing process. The endogenous mechanisms for the regulation of coagulation include the inhibition of coagulation enzymes, the inactivation of coagulation cofactors (the protein C, protein S, thrombomodulin pathway; see Chapter 19), and fibrinolysis (see Chapter 23). Abnormalities in any of these control mechanisms may be associated with bleeding or thrombosis. This chapter describes the control of the initiation of coagulation by tissue factor pathway inhibitor (TFPI) and the regulation of thrombin by antithrombin and heparin cofactor II.

Tissue Factor Pathway Inhibitor

In the current concept, coagulation is initiated when damage to blood vessels at the site of a wound allows the exposure of blood to the tissue factor produced constitutively by cells beneath the endothelium. The factor VII or VIIa present in plasma binds to this tissue factor, and the factor VIIa/tissue factor catalytic complex activates limited quantities of factor X and factor IX. TFPI regulates this initiation of coagulation by producing factor Xa–dependent feedback inhibition of the factor VIIa/tissue factor complex.

▼ HISTORY

In 1947, Thomas[1] and Schneider[2] independently showed that the preincubation of crude tissue thromboplastin (containing tissue factor) with serum prevented the lethal disseminated intravascular coagulation that occurs after thromboplastin infusion in animals. Thomas also noted that this inhibitory effect of serum required the presence of calcium ions, that the inhibitor appeared to bind to the thromboplastin, and that the inhibition could be reversed by calcium ion chelators. Later, Hjort[3] showed that the serum inhibitor recognized the factor VIIa/Ca^{2+}/tissue factor complex, which he called convertin, rather than factor VIIa or tissue factor alone. About the same time, Biggs and her colleagues[4, 5] reported that coagulation was delayed and incomplete after the addition of low concentrations of tissue factor to hemophilic plasma, lacking either factor VIII or IX.

More than 20 years later, Marlar and colleagues[6] showed that when coagulation was induced by small amounts of tissue factor, much less factor X was activated in hemophilic plasma than in normal plasma. Subsequently, Morrison and Jesty[7] noted that this apparent inhibition of factor VIIa/tissue factor enzymatic activity was directly related to the presence of factor X or to brief pretreatment of the plasma with factor Xa. In 1985, Sanders and associates[8] demonstrated that the presence of not only factor X but also an inhibitor present in the total lipoprotein fraction of plasma after density centrifugation was required for this apparent inhibition of tissue factor–initiated coagulation. Additional studies from several groups confirmed these results and went on to show that the inhibition was reversed by chelation of calcium ions with ethylenediaminetetraacetic acid (EDTA), with the release of functionally active factor VIIa and tissue factor.[9–11] Thus, the rediscovered inhibitor appears to be identical to the anticonvertin studied by Hjort in 1957.[3] Previously referred to as lipoprotein-associated coagulation inhibitor and extrinsic pathway inhibitor, the inhibitor was renamed tissue factor pathway inhibitor in 1991 by a subcommittee of the Scientific and Standardization Committee of the International Society on Thrombosis and Haemostasis.

The inhibitor was initially purified from the conditioned media of HepG2 (human hepatoma) cells[12, 13] by use of factor Xa affinity chromatography, and TFPI from human plasma[14, 15] was also isolated later. Complementary DNAs for human,[16, 17] rhesus monkey,[18] canine,[19] rabbit,[20, 21] rat,[22] and mouse[23] have been isolated and cloned, and the organization of the human gene encoding TFPI has been determined.[24, 25]

▼ MOLECULAR BIOLOGY

The gene encoding TFPI spans 70 kb on the long arm of chromosome 2 (q32) and contains nine exons and eight

657

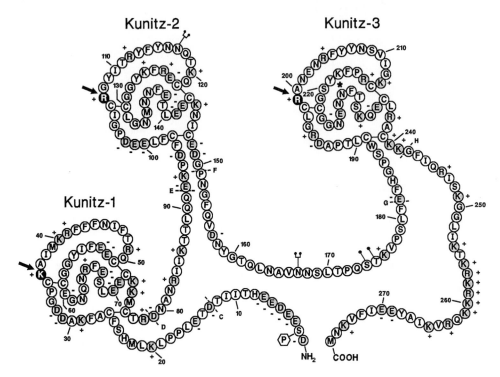

Figure 20–1. Primary structure of TFPI. The three Kunitz-type inhibitory domains of TFPI are labeled, and arrows indicate the location of the respective active site inhibitory clefts. The P1 residue of each Kunitz domain is shown in bold. Charged residues are stippled. *N*-linked glycosylation is denoted as ⵋ; *O*-linked glycosylation is denoted as ⵑ; a site for potential *N*-linked glycosylation in the Kunitz-3 domain that is apparently not used is labeled with an asterisk. Potential phosphorylation at Ser 2 is also shown. Sites of introns in the TFPI gene are labeled with capital letters.

introns.[24–26] Exons 1 and 2 encode a 5′ untranslated region; exon 3 encodes the signal peptide, which is removed during processing of the protein, and the amino terminus of the mature TFPI. The TFPI molecule contains three tandem Kunitz-type proteinase inhibitor domains that are encoded by separate exons (4, 6, and 8). The intervening peptides between Kunitz domains are encoded by exons 5 and 7 (Fig. 20–1). The carboxyl terminus of the TFPI protein and an extensive 3′ untranslated region are encoded by exon 9. All the splice junctions between exons are of the same type (type 1), suggesting that the TFPI gene was assembled during evolution through a process of gene duplication and exon shuffling.[27] A *Pst*I restriction fragment length polymorphism has been described in the TFPI gene.[28]

The putative promoter region of the TFPI gene contains one NF-1 sequence[29] and two imperfect AP-1 sequences.[30] AP-1–binding sites have been shown to act as phorbol ester–responsive elements in several other genes,[31] and the induction of TFPI expression in cultured monocytic cells (U937) after phorbol myristate acetate treatment has been reported.[32] A GATA consensus element lies approximately 400 bp upstream of the transcription initiation sites.[33] This DNA motif appears essential for the expression of certain genes by erythroid, megakaryocytic, and endothelial cells.[34–36] The 5′ flanking region of the gene, however, does not contain a TATA box or CAAT sequence, which may account for the apparent use of multiple, alternative transcription start sites.[24, 25] Alternative splicing of the short exon 2 in the 5′ untranslated region of the TFPI message occurs, but its significance is unclear. Cells that constitutively express TFPI produce TFPI mRNA of two sizes, 1.4 and 4.0 kb, that arise through the use of alternative polyadenylation signals.[17] The 3′ untranslated region of the 4.0 kb message contains many AUUU motifs and two UAAUUUAU sequences, which have been associated with mRNA instability in other messages.[37, 38]

Preliminary evidence, however, suggests that both the 1.4 and 4.0 kb TFPI mRNAs are relatively stable.[17]

▼ BIOCHEMISTRY

The primary structure of TFPI, as predicted by cDNA sequencing, is unique.[16, 17] After a 24 or 28 amino acid signal peptide, the mature protein has 276 residues (32 kDa) and contains an acidic amino-terminal region followed by three tandem Kunitz-type protease inhibitory domains and a basic carboxyl-terminal region (see Fig. 20–1). The molecule contains N-linked carbohydrate at Asn 117 and Asn 167 and O-linked carbohydrate at Ser 174 and Thr 175.[39] The oligosaccharides in TFPI expressed by certain cells in vitro (e.g., endothelial and kidney cells) are sulfated.[40, 41] Ser 2 is partially phosphorylated in the TFPI expressed by some cells in tissue culture, but similar phosphorylation has not been detected in TFPI circulating in plasma.[42] These post-translational modifications do not appear to affect the known functional properties of TFPI.[42–44]

Kunitz-type inhibitors appear to act by the standard mechanism[45] in which the inhibitor feigns to be a good substrate, but after the enzyme binds, the subsequent cleavage between the P1 and P1′ amino acid residues at the active site cleft of the inhibitor occurs only slowly or not at all. The P1 residue is an important determinant of the specificity of these inhibitors, and alterations of the residue in the P1 position can profoundly affect their inhibitory activity. In kinetic terms, Kunitz-type inhibitors typically produce slow, tight-binding, competitive, and reversible enzyme inhibition. Slow implies that the final degree of inhibition does not occur immediately, and tight-binding refers to the fact that these inhibitors produce significant inhibition at a concentration near that of the enzyme being inhibited. On the basis of the known structure of the prototype Kunitz-type inhibitor, bovine basic pancreatic trypsin inhibitor (aprotinin, Trasylol), and its interaction with trypsin, the disulfide bonds, the active site cleft, and the P1 residue are depicted in Figure 20–1 for each of the three Kunitz modules of the TFPI molecule.[46]

Experiments in which the P1 residue of each Kunitz domain in TFPI was individually altered have shown that the second Kunitz domain of TFPI mediates factor Xa binding and inhibition, whereas the first Kunitz domain is necessary for the inhibition of the factor VIIa/tissue factor complex.[47] Alteration of the P1 residue in the third Kunitz domain does not affect either of these functions of TFPI. Studies examining the inhibitory properties of the isolated Kunitz domains of TFPI have reached the same conclusions.[48] The Kunitz-3 domain appears to lack proteinase inhibitory activity,[48] and the physiological role of this domain is not known. TFPI also inhibits trypsin and chymotrypsin reasonably well, and cathepsin G, plasmin, and activated protein C poorly.[48–50] The physiological significance of these inhibitory reactions is doubtful, however.

▼ INHIBITION OF FACTOR Xa BY TFPI

TFPI not only inhibits the factor VIIa/tissue factor enzymatic complex in a factor Xa–dependent manner but also produces direct inhibition of factor Xa by binding at or near its catalytic serine site.[51] The factor Xa/TFPI complex demonstrates 1:1 stoichiometry, and its formation does not require the presence of calcium ions; it is reversed by treatment with sodium dodecyl sulfate or high concentrations of the serine protease inhibitor benzamidine, which binds to the active site of factor Xa.[13, 51]

Other parts of the TFPI molecule besides the Kunitz-2 domain are involved in its interaction with factor Xa. The basic carboxyl-terminal region of TFPI is required for rapid, efficient factor Xa inhibition, and carboxyl-terminal–truncated forms of TFPI are considerably less potent inhibitors of factor Xa.[48, 52–54] Further, neutrophil elastase–mediated cleavage of TFPI between Kunitz domains 1 and 2 dramatically reduces the ability of TFPI to inhibit factor Xa.[50, 55]

The inhibition of factor Xa by TFPI in the presence of physiological calcium ion concentrations is enhanced by procoagulant phospholipids,[56] and the carboxyl-terminal region of the TFPI molecule is important for this effect.[53, 54] TFPI at physiological concentrations, however, does not effectively inhibit prothrombin activation by factor Xa in a preformed prothrombinase complex.[57, 58]

Heparin and other polyanions accelerate TFPI-mediated inhibition of factor Xa.[53] The heparin dose-response for this effect exhibits optima suggesting that the polyanion forms a "template" to which factor Xa and TFPI simultaneously bind.[53, 56] Basic residues within the carboxyl-terminal region of TFPI are required for optimal heparin binding, and progressive carboxyl-terminal truncation of the TFPI molecule produces proteins with decreasing affinity for heparin.[53] The Kunitz-3 domain contains a heparin-binding site, but whether this site is important for TFPI function above and beyond separate heparin-binding sites located more distally in the molecule is not clear.[53, 59] Charge density, rather than a specific binding epitope, on the glycosaminoglycan appears most important for TFPI binding.[60]

▼ INHIBITION OF THE FACTOR VIIa/TISSUE FACTOR COMPLEX BY TFPI

Factor Xa–dependent inhibition of factor VIIa/tissue factor involves the formation of a quaternary factor Xa/TFPI–factor VIIa/tissue factor complex[51] (Fig. 20–2). This inhibitory complex can result from the initial binding of factor Xa to TFPI in fluid phase, with subsequent binding of the factor Xa/TFPI complex to factor VIIa/tissue factor. The rate of factor VIIa/tissue factor inhibition produced by TFPI during the activation of factor X to factor Xa, however, is dramatically faster than that produced by a preformed factor Xa/TFPI complex.[61] Thus, the predominant pathway for the formation of the quaternary inhibitory complex may involve the interaction of TFPI with factor Xa either bound or remaining in proximity to the factor VIIa/tissue factor complex assembled on the phospholipid surface. The Gla domain of factor Xa and Lys 165–Lys 166 of tissue factor, structures required for the optimal recognition of factor X by factor

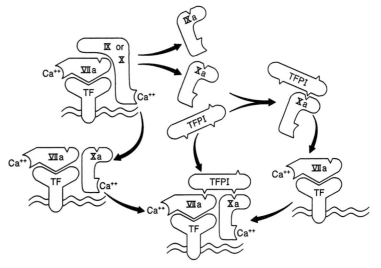

Figure 20–2. Inhibition of factor Xa and the factor VIIa/ tissue factor complex by TFPI. The indentations represent the active sites of factor VIIa and factor Xa; the protrusions represent the three Kunitz-type inhibitory domains of TFPI. In the factor Xa/TFPI complex, the active site of factor Xa is bound to the second Kunitz domain of TFPI. In the final quaternary factor Xa/TFPI–factor VIIa/tissue factor complex, factor Xa is bound at its active site to Kunitz-2 of TFPI and factor VIIa is bound at its active site to Kunitz-1 of TFPI. Two potential pathways for the formation of the final quaternary inhibitory complex are depicted: on the right, TFPI binds to factor Xa and the factor Xa/TFPI complex then binds to factor VIIa/tissue factor; on the left, TFPI binds to factor Xa, which remains associated with or in proximity to the factor VIIa/tissue factor complex. In vitro studies suggest that the pathway on the left predominates.

VIIa/tissue factor, are also important for the inhibition of factor VIIa/tissue factor by factor Xa/TFPI.[51, 62, 63] Studies of the effects of heparin on factor Xa–dependent factor VIIa/tissue factor inhibition by TFPI have produced conflicting results.[64, 65]

Some investigators report that the inhibition of factor X activation by factor VIIa/tissue factor is much more rapid (10-fold) with full-length TFPI than with carboxyl-terminal–truncated forms of TFPI and relate this difference to the relative rates at which the TFPI forms bind factor Xa.[54] Others have found full-length and carboxyl-truncated TFPI to produce comparable rates of factor VIIa/tissue factor inhibition.[65, 66] The ultimate affinity of the quaternary inhibitory complex formed with full-length TFPI, however, is clearly greater than that of complexes formed with truncated TFPI, and the latter inhibitory complexes dissociate more rapidly.[66, 67] In one-stage plasma coagulation assays, the anticoagulant effect of exogenously added full-length TFPI is considerably greater than that of carboxyl-truncated TFPI.[52, 53, 68] When plasma coagulation is induced by factor Xa or the factor X–coagulant protein (XCP) from Russell's viper venom, the disparity in anticoagulant effect between the TFPI forms reflects their ability to inhibit factor Xa. The difference seen when tissue factor is used to induce coagulation (prothrombin time) presumably represents the combination of anti–factor Xa and anti–factor VIIa/tissue factor activities.

The requirement of factor Xa for the inhibition of factor VIIa/tissue factor by TFPI is not absolute, and high concentrations of TFPI will inhibit factor VIIa/tissue factor in the absence of factor Xa.[48, 69–71] This factor Xa–independent inhibition of factor VIIa/tissue factor by TFPI is of uncertain physiological relevance but could be important when TFPI is used as a therapeutic agent and the plasma level of TFPI is more than 50-fold that of normal plasma.[72–74]

▼ CELL BIOLOGY AND CATABOLISM

The endothelium is presumed to be the major source of TFPI in vivo. Immunohistochemical studies of normal tissues have detected TFPI in the endothelium of the microvasculature, megakaryocytes, macrophages, and the microglia of the brain.[75, 76] A range of TFPI mRNA levels is detected by Northern analysis of tissues: highest in placenta and lung, lowest in brain.[77] In tissue culture, cell lines derived from a wide variety of tissues synthesize TFPI. The production of TFPI by these cells in tissue culture, however, may not reflect sites of TFPI expression in vivo. For example, several hepatoma cell lines express TFPI in culture, yet TFPI is not detected in hepatocytes in primary culture or by immunohistochemical staining of liver sections.[75, 78]

Cultured endothelial cells and adherent monocytes/macrophages express TFPI, a significant fraction of which appears to remain membrane associated.[32, 78–80] A report suggests that TFPI is stored in granules distinct from Weibel-Palade bodies in cultured endothelial cells and is redistributed to the cell surface and released into the media after thrombin treatment.[81] Others report that more than 90 per cent of the cell-associated TFPI in a endothelial cell line stimulated with tumor necrosis factor is on the cell surface.[82] Heparin as well as thrombin treatment appears to increase the release of TFPI from cells in culture.[81, 83] Whereas the stimulation of endothelial cells and adherent monocytes with inflammatory mediators induces a dramatic induction of tissue factor synthesis, such treatment produces minimal changes in TFPI expression.[33, 84] Megakaryocytes synthesize TFPI, and the TFPI carried by circulating blood platelets is released after their stimulation with thrombin or other agonists.[85]

After its infusion in animals, full-length TFPI is cleared rapidly from plasma (α phase t½, $\approx$2 minutes; β phase t½, $\approx$80 minutes) and is predominantly taken up by the liver and kidney.[86, 87] At least two separate processes appear to contribute to this phenomenon: (1) reversible binding of TFPI at cell surfaces, presumably including the endothelium in vivo, and (2) cellular endocytosis and degradation of TFPI mediated by the low-density lipoprotein (LDL) receptor–related protein/α_2-macroglobulin receptor (LRP).

TFPI binds to a wide variety of cells in vitro. Most of this binding is mediated by relatively low affinity sites that require the basic carboxyl terminus of TFPI for binding and whose interaction with TFPI is inhibited by heparin or protamine.[70, 88–90] Whether these TFPI-binding sites involve phospholipids,[91] heparan sulfate glycosaminoglycans,[92] specific cell surface proteins, or a combination of these elements has not been established. Nevertheless, the characteristics of the cell surface TFPI binding in vitro appear to explain the markedly lower recovery of full-length versus carboxyl-terminal–truncated forms of TFPI after their infusion in animals and the inhibition of full-length TFPI clearance produced by concomitant heparin or protamine infusion.[87, 93, 94]

LRP functions as an endocytosis receptor for several proteins, including α_2-macroglobulin/protease complexes, free plasminogen activators as well as plasminogen activators complexed with their inhibitors, lipoprotein lipase, and β-migrating very low density lipoproteins enriched with apolipoprotein E.[95] A 39 kDa protein that copurifies with LRP (receptor-associated protein, RAP) competes with all known LRP ligands for binding. LRP is particularly abundant in liver, brain, and placenta, and a closely related receptor, glycoprotein 330, that binds many of the same ligands is produced predominantly in the kidney.[95, 96] In rats, the combination of high levels of protamine to prevent presumed cell surface binding at the endothelium and high levels of the 39 kDa protein to inhibit LRP-mediated endocytosis dramatically slows the clearance of infused TFPI from plasma.[94]

An additional pathway for the endocytosis and degradation of TFPI has been identified.[97] In vitro studies show that the uptake and degradation of factor Xa by hepatoma cells and embryonic fibroblasts require cell surface TFPI and, further, that the uptake and degradation of surface-bound TFPI are also markedly stimulated in response to factor Xa binding. The cellular kinetics of factor Xa and TFPI internalization/degradation are similar, suggesting that factor Xa and surface-bound TFPI are taken up as a bimolecular complex. This TFPI/factor Xa endocytic pathway is independent of LRP and does not require tissue factor. Indirect studies in rabbits suggest that a similar process is operational in vivo, because the clearance of heparin-releasable, presumably endothelial cell surface–bound, TFPI/factor Xa complexes is faster than that of TFPI alone.[98]

TFPI also apparently participates in the downregulation of factor VIIa/tissue factor complexes at the surface of stimulated endothelial cells.[82] This process requires the formation of the quaternary factor Xa/TFPI–factor VIIa/tissue factor inhibitory complex and involves translocation of the complex into caveolae. Differential detergent solubility and the effect of phosphatidylinositol-specific phospholipase C strongly suggest that a glycophosphatidylinositol-anchored membrane protein, which may represent a cell surface TFPI-binding site, is involved in the internalization mechanism. Whether staurosporine, which inhibits the phosphorylation of the cytoplasmic domain of tissue factor and blocks downregulation of tissue factor in stimulated monocytes, effects this translocation process in endothelial cells has not been tested.[99] The relationship between this pathway and the factor Xa/TFPI degradation pathway described above is not clear.

▼ PHYSIOLOGY

There is a broad range of plasma TFPI concentrations in normal individuals (mean, ≈2.5 nmol/l or ≈100 ng/ml).[100–102] Much of the circulating TFPI is bound to lipoproteins, predominantly LDL and high-density lipoproteins (HDL), but also very low density lipoproteins and Lp(a) lipoprotein.[14, 103, 104] Because LDL is a major carrier, plasma concentrations of TFPI are related to LDL levels, increasing with diet-induced hypercholesterolemia in animals and decreasing in response to drug therapy in patients with familial hypercholesterolemia.[105–109] Individuals with abetalipoproteinemia, who lack LDL, have low levels of TFPI in plasma.[101]

Predominant forms of TFPI in plasma have molecular masses of 34 and 41 kDa, and less abundant forms of higher molecular mass are also present.[14, 110, 111] This size heterogeneity of plasma TFPI at least in part reflects the apparent carboxyl-terminal truncation of the molecule and the formation of mixed disulfide complexes with apolipoprotein A-II, itself, and potentially other proteins.[110, 111] The major form of TFPI bound to LDL has a molecular mass of 34 kDa and lacks the distal portion of full-length TFPI, including at least a large portion of the Kunitz-3 domain. The 41 kDa form of TFPI that circulates with HDL is apparently a similar carboxyl-truncated form of TFPI that is disulfide linked to monomeric apolipoprotein A-II. Additional forms with less extensive carboxyl-terminal truncation and full-length TFPI (43 kDa) also circulate in plasma. The mechanism underlying the association of the 34 kDa carboxyl-truncated form of TFPI with LDL is not clear, because the carboxyl terminus of TFPI is reportedly required for the binding of TFPI to plasma lipoproteins in vitro and after its infusion in vivo.[93] Proteolytic processing by as yet unidentified proteinases is most likely responsible for the circulating forms of TFPI with modest truncation of the carboxyl-terminal tail.[68] Additional or alternative modifications may be involved in the production of the 34 kDa form of TFPI that is bound tightly in LDL. Oxidation of LDL in vitro reportedly reduces its associated TFPI activity.[112]

Estimates of the proportion of total plasma TFPI that circulates "free" of lipoproteins range from 10 to 60 per cent.[15, 113, 114] The in vitro manipulations required to separate lipoprotein-bound TFPI from free TFPI (e.g., gel filtration, density gradient lipoprotein isolation) result in poor recovery of free TFPI[93, 113] and, conversely, may separate loosely bound TFPI from the lipoproteins. A TFPI immunoassay based on an antibody against the Kunitz-3 domain, which reportedly does not recognize lipoprotein-bound TFPI,[114] detected 19.2 ± 4.0 ng/ml of free TFPI in nine normal individuals.[115] The concentration of full-length TFPI normally circulating in plasma has not been established.

The parenteral administration of heparin, low molecular weight heparin, and other polyanions increases the circulating levels of TFPI in plasma.[100, 101, 116] It is presumed, but not proved, that the source of this additional TFPI is the endothelium. The mechanism underlying the heparin-induced release phenomenon is not known but may involve the displacement of TFPI from binding sites (perhaps glycosaminoglycans) at the endothelial cell surface. After the intravenous infusion of a heparin bolus, the plasma TFPI level peaks at 3 to 5 minutes and then returns to the pretreatment level with a half-life that mirrors that of the administered heparin. Protamine treatment during this time causes the TFPI level to immediately return to the baseline level.[116, 117] Heparin-releasable TFPI is not associated with lipoproteins; on the basis of its molecular weight, tight binding to heparin-agarose, and potent anticoagulant activity, it is thought to represent full-length or a nearly full-length form of TFPI.[15] The extent of TFPI release reportedly decreases with repeated (every 4 hours) and continuous heparin infusion.[115]

Quantitative assessment of the heparin-induced increase in plasma TFPI levels is hampered by discrepancies between the results of functional and antigenic assays.[118] Two-stage (endpoint) functional assays based on factor VIIa/tissue factor inhibition show a post-heparin increase in plasma TFPI levels of approximately twofold to threefold, whereas antigen-based assays typically suggest a considerably greater increase. This discrepancy may be due to the fact that lipoprotein-bound, carboxyl-terminal–truncated forms of TFPI are underrepresented in antigen assays, whereas their contribution to factor VIIa/tissue factor inhibition is detected by functional assay. The substantial extraplasma reservoir of TFPI defined by heparin releasability is probably physiologically important. Although patients with abetalipoproteinemia have low baseline plasma levels of TFPI (<25 per cent of normal), they have normal levels of heparin-releasable TFPI and do not have an increased risk of thrombosis.[101] Whether TFPI contributes to the antithrombotic effect of heparin therapy is not known.

Plasma TFPI concentrations in normal individuals are stable, with little variation during the day, after meals, and during at least many months' time.[102] There is a modest increase in TFPI levels with age in adults, which probably reflects, in part, plasma lipoprotein levels[102, 119, 120]; low levels are present in midgestation fetuses (≈30 per cent) and newborn infants (≈55 per cent).[121] Unlike levels of tissue plasminogen activator and von Willebrand factor, which are also synthesized by endothelial cells, TFPI levels in plasma are not increased by infusion of DDAVP or venous occlusion.[100–102] TFPI is not elevated in patients with pneumonia and does not increase postoperatively, suggesting that TFPI does not behave like an acute phase reactant.[102, 122–124] Increased levels of TFPI have been noted with advanced cancer,[125] with uremia and regular hemodialysis,[126] and in late pregnancy[101, 102, 127]; decreased levels have been reported in thrombotic thrombocytopenic purpura.[128] Levels of TFPI are normal in patients with the lupus anticoagulant and those treated with warfarin.[100–102] Although low levels of plasma TFPI are occasionally seen in septicemia and disseminated intravascular coagulation, more often the TFPI concentrations are normal or elevated.[101, 124, 129–134] Clinical studies thus far have failed to demonstrate a clear relationship between TFPI levels and arterial or venous thrombotic disease.[101, 135–138]

Animal studies have shown that the depletion of endogenous TFPI sensitizes rabbits to the disseminated intravascular coagulation induced by tissue factor or endotoxin infusion.[139, 140] Similar depletion of endogenous TFPI does not affect the coagulopathy produced by the infusion of a complex of factor Xa and phospholipids, suggesting that the major physiological role of TFPI is the regulation of factor VIIa/tissue factor activity.[141]

The murine TFPI gene has been disrupted by gene targeting. Because of alternative mRNA splicing, the disrupted allele in these mice produces a TFPI lacking the first Kunitz-type domain (responsible for factor VIIa/tissue factor binding) at 40 per cent of the expected expression level.[142] TFPI$_{K1}$-heterozygotic animals have a normal phenotype, whereas TFPI$_{K1}$-null mice suffer embryonic hemorrhage and intrauterine lethality. Sixty per cent of the TFPI$_{K1}$ mice die at midgestation (embryonic day E9.5 to E11.5) with signs of yolk sac hemorrhage. Organogenesis, including cardiac and vascular development, appears normal in the 40 per cent of TFPI$_{K1}$-null embryos surviving to later gestational dates. Thus, TFPI does not appear to be essential for the development of a specific tissue. Intraembryonic hemorrhage, particularly in the brain, spinal canal, and tail, is the predominant feature of these older TFPI$_{K1}$-deficient embryos. TFPI is a potent inhibitor of factor VIIa/tissue factor–initiated coagulation in vitro, and the hemorrhagic phenotype of the TFPI$_{K1}$ animals is likely to be related to unrestrained tissue factor action and the development of a consumptive coagulopathy. Indeed, the detection of intravascular thrombi and hepatic fibrin(ogen) deposition in the older TFPI$_{K1}$-null embryos (>E12.5) is consistent with disseminated intravascular coagulation.[142] Because fibrinogen-deficient mice do not develop embryonic hemorrhage,[143] it is conceivable that the consumption of specific coagulation factors (e.g., thrombin) or toxic effects of the generated coagulation enzymes may produce effects on vascular integrity in the TFPI$_{K1}$ mice that are not directly related to hemostasis. The absence of TFPI may produce a similar fate in humans because an individual with TFPI deficiency has not been identified.

Antithrombin

▼ FUNCTIONS OF THROMBIN IN HEMOSTASIS

Thrombin promotes hemostasis by cleaving the following substrates:

1. the platelet thrombin receptor, which is cleaved to release a tethered peptide ligand that stimulates platelet aggregation and secretion[144];
2. factors V and VIII, which are activated to Va and VIIIa and serve as nonenzymatic cofactors for factors Xa and IXa, respectively;

3. factor XI, which is converted to XIa[145, 146];
4. fibrinogen, which is cleaved near the amino-terminal ends of the Aα and Bβ chains to produce fibrin monomers that polymerize to form the clot;
5. factor XIII, a transglutaminase that cross-links polymerized fibrin to stabilize the clot; and
6. a thrombin-activatable plasma carboxypeptidase that inhibits fibrinolysis.[147]

The first three reactions provide positive feedback loops that are presumed to accelerate thrombin generation at the site of a wound. If normal vascular endothelial cells are present, thrombin binds to the integral membrane protein thrombomodulin and activates protein C, which produces an anticoagulant effect by proteolytically inactivating factors Va and VIIIa.[148] Thrombin also has mitogenic[149–151] and chemotactic[152] activities that may be important in wound healing.

Factor Xa converts prothrombin to thrombin by cleavage of the peptide bonds after Arg 271 and Arg 320. When factor Xa and its cofactor, factor Va, are assembled on a membrane surface in the presence of Ca^{2+}, factor Xa first cleaves at Arg 320, producing meizothrombin.[153] Subsequent cleavage at Arg 271 in meizothrombin yields thrombin. Although meizothrombin hydrolyzes synthetic peptide substrates at a rate comparable with that of thrombin, meizothrombin is much less active with respect to fibrinogen clotting, platelet activation, and activation of the thrombin-activatable fibrinolysis inhibitor.[154–156] However, meizothrombin activates protein C faster than thrombin does in the presence of thrombomodulin, which suggests that meizothrombin may function as an anticoagulant protease.[156, 157]

Thrombin is inhibited by antithrombin, heparin cofactor II, and protein C inhibitor, whereas meizothrombin is inhibited preferentially by heparin cofactor II.[158] Antithrombin and heparin cofactor II require the presence of a glycosaminoglycan such as heparin for maximal activity. Protein C inhibitor rapidly inactivates thrombin bound to thrombomodulin.[159] The association between antithrombin deficiency and recurrent venous thromboembolism,[160, 161] first reported by Egeberg in 1965,[162] established the idea that antithrombin plays a critical role in regulating hemostasis. Heparan sulfate synthesized by vascular endothelial cells appears to constitutively activate antithrombin to prevent thrombosis within normal blood vessels.[163] The physiological roles of heparin cofactor II and protein C inhibitor are unknown.

▼ BIOCHEMISTRY AND MOLECULAR BIOLOGY OF ANTITHROMBIN

Antithrombin is a 58 kDa glycoprotein that belongs to the serpin superfamily.[164] The amino acid sequence of antithrombin, determined directly[165] and by cDNA sequencing,[166–168] is about 30 per cent identical to other serpins.[164] Antithrombin contains three disulfide bonds, one of which (Cys 8 to Cys 128) is required for heparin cofactor activity.[169] In addition, it contains glycosylation sites at Asn 96, Asn 135, Asn 155, and Asn 192 that are occupied by three or four N-linked biantennary oligosaccharides.[170] No other post-translational modifications have been reported.

Two forms of antithrombin that differ in their carbohydrate content have been isolated from normal human plasma by heparin-agarose affinity chromatography.[171] The major form (α-antithrombin), composing approximately 90 per cent of the total antithrombin, is eluted from the affinity matrix with 1M NaCl and appears to be fully glycosylated. The minor form (β-antithrombin) is eluted at a higher salt concentration and lacks the oligosaccharide unit linked to Asn 135, which lies near the proposed heparin-binding site.[172, 173] Both α- and β-antithrombin inhibit thrombin rapidly in the presence of heparin. However, β-antithrombin requires a lower concentration of heparin for full activity, consistent with its higher heparin affinity.

The antithrombin gene on human chromosome 1q23–25[174] contains seven exons distributed over about 13.5 kb of DNA.[175] The introns contain 10 *Alu* repeats, which are present at a greater density than average for the human genome. Homologous recombination among these repetitive elements appears to be an important mechanism by which deletions producing type I deficiency occur. The mRNA for antithrombin is about 1500 nucleotides in length. It encodes a signal peptide of 32 residues followed by the mature protein of 432 residues.[166–168] Antithrombin mRNA is present in the liver, and synthesis of antithrombin has been demonstrated in cultured human hepatoma cells.[176] Alternative splicing of the antithrombin mRNA has been demonstrated in the liver.[177] The alternative splicing event introduces a 42-base segment between codons -19 and -18 of the signal peptide. This segment of mRNA contains an in-frame termination codon such that the predicted protein product encoded by the alternatively spliced mRNA would be only 19 amino acids long. Although the alternatively spliced mRNA accounts for 20 to 40 per cent of the antithrombin mRNA in human liver, it is not known whether translation occurs. In the adult rat, antithrombin mRNA was detected in the kidney at a level approximately 20 per cent of that found in the liver.[178]

Little is known about the regulation of antithrombin biosynthesis. The 5' flanking sequence of the antithrombin gene lacks a TATA-like sequence at the expected location 25 to 30 bases upstream from the transcription initiation site.[177] A DNA length polymorphism, resulting from insertion of either 32 or 108 bp of DNA at the position 345 bases upstream from the translation initiation codon, has been identified.[179] This polymorphism does not appear to affect the level of expression of antithrombin in human plasma.[180] The 5' flanking region of the antithrombin gene also contains short sequences that are similar to an enhancer element found in the immunoglobulin Jκ-Cκ gene.[181] When the antithrombin enhancer element was ligated to the chloramphenicol acetyltransferase gene and transfected into cells, expression of chloramphenicol acetyltransferase activity was increased preferentially in Alexander hepatoma (liver) and Cos-1 (kidney) cells. Thus, the enhancer may be involved in tissue-specific expression of the antithrombin gene. More recently, a 700 bp fragment of the human antithrombin promoter was shown to confer a high level of tissue-specific expression in the liver and kidney of transgenic mice,[182] and several transcription factors that bind to regions flanking exon 1 of the antithrombin gene were identified.[183] Biosynthesis of antithrombin by isolated rat hepatocytes is unaffected by the presence of protease/antithrombin complexes or by the supernatant medium of macrophages incubated with these complexes.[184] However, antithrombin biosynthesis is stimulated by the supernatant medium of macrophages incubated with endotoxin or fibrinogen fragment D. Under these conditions, fibrinogen and α_1-antitrypsin biosynthesis is stimulated concurrently.

▼ PROTEASE INHIBITION BY ANTITHROMBIN

Antithrombin inhibits the coagulation proteases thrombin, factor Xa, factor IXa, factor XIa, factor XIIa, and kallikrein.[185] It also inhibits the fibrinolytic protease plasmin.[186] In vitro experiments suggest that antithrombin is the major inhibitor of factor IXa, factor Xa, and thrombin in plasma.[187–189] By contrast, factor XIa appears to be inhibited primarily by α_1-antitrypsin,[190] factor XIIa by C1 inhibitor,[191] and plasmin by α_2-antiplasmin.[192] Antithrombin inhibits factor VIIa bound to tissue factor and dissociates the factor VIIa/tissue factor complex.[193, 194] Antithrombin does not inhibit activated protein C.[195]

Antithrombin forms an essentially irreversible, equimolar complex with each of its target proteases.[196] The serine residue at the active site of the protease is required for complex formation but thereafter becomes inaccessible to substrates. Furthermore, a small peptide is cleaved from the carboxyl terminus of antithrombin during complex formation.[197] Thrombin, factor Xa, and factor IXa cleave the same peptide bond in antithrombin (Arg 393–Ser 394), which is termed the reactive site.[198] The antithrombin/protease complex resists dissociation in denaturing agents, suggesting that a covalent bond is formed between the two proteins. The complex can be dissociated by treatment with nucleophiles, which release the protease along with the cleaved form of antithrombin from the complex.[197, 199] These properties are consistent with the presence of an ester linkage between the active center serine hydroxyl group of thrombin and the α-carbonyl group of Arg 393 in the reactive site of antithrombin.

Antithrombin and other serpins undergo a striking conformational change after proteolytic cleavage at the reactive site. X-ray crystallography of intact ovalbumin suggests that the P1 to P12 residues amino-terminal to the cleavage site form an exposed loop on the surface of the molecule[200] (Fig. 20–3). This structure is consistent with the finding that the region immediately upstream from the reactive site in many serpins is susceptible to proteolytic cleavage by enzymes other than the target protease, resulting in loss of the serpin's inhibitory activity.[201] In α_1-antitrypsin cleaved at P1 to P1', movement of the exposed loop about a "hinge" located near P12 allows residues P1 to P12 to become the fourth strand of a six-membered β sheet (termed β sheet A), separating the P1 and P1' amino acids by 69 Å.[202] This conformational change results in greater thermal stability of the cleaved ("relaxed") form in comparison to the intact ("stressed") form of the serpin. Mutations of the hinge region (e.g., P10 Ala $\rightarrow$ Pro or P12 Ala $\rightarrow$ Thr) appear to interfere with intercalation of the exposed reactive site loop into β sheet A, prevent the stressed to relaxed conformational change, and convert antithrombin from an inhibitor to a substrate for thrombin and factor Xa.[203, 204] Antithrombin is also converted from an inhibitor to a substrate by a monoclonal antibody that recognizes the P8 to P12 sequence[205] or by a synthetic

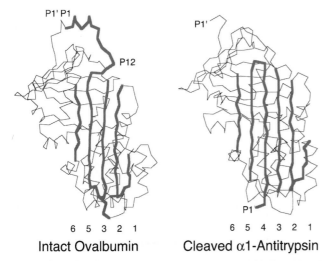

P1' P1

P12

6 5 3 2 1
Intact Ovalbumin

P1'

P1

6 5 4 3 2 1
Cleaved α1-Antitrypsin

Figure 20–3. Structures of serpins. The structures of uncleaved oval-bumin and cleaved α₁-antitrypsin were determined by X-ray crystallography. The α carbon tracing of the polypeptide backbone is shown for each protein. The P1 to P12 residues of ovalbumin form an exposed loop on the surface of the protein that is susceptible to proteolytic attack. After cleavage, the P1 and P1′ amino acid residues of α₁-antitrypsin are separated by 69 Å, and residues P1 to P12 are incorporated into β sheet A *(thick lines).*

peptide that corresponds to P1 to P14,[206, 207] reagents that are assumed to prevent insertion of the reactive site loop into β sheet A. Thus, the ability of the reactive site loop to become inserted into β sheet A appears to be critical for the inhibitory activity of a serpin. X-ray crystallographic studies demonstrated partial insertion of the reactive site loop into β sheet A of the uncleaved, inhibitory form of antithrombin.[208–211]

▼ STIMULATION OF ANTITHROMBIN BY HEPARIN

The concentration of antithrombin in plasma ($\approx$2.6 μmol/l, 150 μg/ml) greatly exceeds that of any of the target proteases generated during coagulation. Under these conditions, protease inhibition follows pseudo–first-order kinetics. In the absence of heparin, thrombin and factor Xa are inhibited by antithrombin in plasma with t½ values of 0.5 to 1.5 minutes, whereas factor IXa is inhibited about 10 times more slowly.[212] Addition of heparin to plasma increases the rate of inhibition of thrombin, factor Xa, and factor IXa by antithrombin at least 1000-fold. As a result, inhibition of these proteases becomes essentially instantaneous (t½ = 10 to 60 msec).[212] Heparin also stimulates inhibition of XIa, XIIa, kallikrein, and plasmin, but the magnitude of the effect is much less.[185]

Heparin is found in the secretory granules of mast cells. It is synthesized from uridine diphosphate (UDP)–sugar precursors as a polymer of alternating D-glucuronic acid (linked β1→4) and N-acetyl-D-glucosamine (linked α1→4)[213] (Fig. 20–4). The glycosaminoglycan chains are built on a core structure consisting of one xylose and two galactose residues covalently attached to serine in a polypeptide backbone. About 10 to 15 glycosaminoglycan chains, each containing 200 to 300 monosaccharide units, are attached to a single core protein to yield a proteoglycan with a mass of 750 to 1000 kDa. As the glycosaminoglycan chains are being synthesized, they rapidly undergo a series of modification

reactions that include the following[213, 214]: (1) N-deacetylation of glucosamine residues, followed by sulfation of virtually all the free amino groups to yield N-sulfo-D-glucosamine; (2) epimerization at the C5 position of D-glucuronic acid to yield L-iduronic acid; (3) O-sulfation of iduronic acid residues at the C2 position; and (4) O-sulfation of glucosamine residues at the C6 position. In addition, several minor but important reactions occur, including O-sulfation of glucuronic acid at C2 and C3 and of glucosamine at C3. The reactions that modify the glycosaminoglycan chain appear to be catalyzed by membrane-bound enzymes in the endoplasmic reticulum or Golgi apparatus of the mast cell and are completed within minutes of synthesis of the core protein. Many of these reactions are regulated by modifications that have occurred on neighboring sugar residues. Furthermore, all the reactions, with the exception of N-sulfation, are incomplete, yielding heterogeneous oligosaccharide structures within the glycosaminoglycan chain. After the heparin proteoglycan has been transported to the mast cell secretory granules, an endo-β-D-glucuronidase catalyzes partial degradation of the glycosaminoglycan chains to 5 to 10 kDa fragments during a period of hours.

Two other glycosaminoglycans, heparan sulfate and dermatan sulfate, possess anticoagulant activity in vitro.[215] Heparan sulfate is closely related to heparin and is found on the surface of most eukaryotic cells and in the extracellular matrix. Heparan sulfate proteoglycans vary considerably in structure. In general, they are smaller than the heparin proteoglycan, containing fewer glycosaminoglycan chains linked to a larger and more complex core protein. In some cases, the core protein has a hydrophobic domain that anchors the proteoglycan to the cell membrane. Heparan sulfate is synthesized from the same repeating disaccharide precursor (D-glucuronic acid linked to N-acetyl-D-glucosamine) as heparin.[216] However, heparan sulfate undergoes less polymer modification than heparin and, therefore, contains higher proportions of glucuronic acid and N-acetylglucosamine and fewer sulfate groups. Dermatan sulfate is a repeating polymer of L-iduronic acid and N-acetyl-D-galactosamine (instead of glucosamine).[216] O-Sulfation of iduronic acid residues at the C2 position and of galactosamine residues at the C4 and C6 positions occurs to a variable extent. Like heparan sulfate, dermatan sulfate is a component of proteoglycans on the cell surface and in the extracellular matrix.

Heparin can be fractionated according to its ability to bind to antithrombin. About 30 per cent of heparin extracted from porcine intestinal mucosa binds to antithrombin with high affinity.[217–219] The high-affinity molecules account for virtually all the anticoagulant activity of the starting material; the low-affinity molecules are inactive. Antithrombin binds to heparin with a dissociation constant of approximately 20 nmol/l.[220, 221] The binding is disrupted at high ionic strength, which implies that electrostatic interactions occur between basic amino acid residues on antithrombin and sulfate groups on the heparin molecule. The smallest fragment of heparin that binds to antithrombin with high affinity is the pentasaccharide shown in Figure 20–5.[222–224] This structure contains a 3-O-sulfate group that is predominantly found in the high-affinity binding site. Several of the sulfate groups within the pentasaccharide are essential for binding to antithrombin, whereas others do not appear to be required. In commercial heparin preparations, about 30 per

Figure 20–4. Biosynthesis of heparin. *N*-Acetyl-D-glucosamine and D-glucuronic acid are transferred from UDP-sugar precursors to a trisaccharide structure linked to a serine residue in the core protein *(A)*, forming the unmodified glycosaminoglycan chain *(B)*. *N*-Deacetylation of some of the *N*-acetyl-D-glucosamine residues then occurs, followed by *N*-sulfation of the free amino groups *(C)*. Epimerization of D-glucuronic acid to L-iduronic acid and *O*-sulfation occur to a limited extent to yield the final product *(D)*, which is then transported to the mast cell secretory granule. The structure of the antithrombin-binding site is shown in Figure 20–5. (Modified from Lindahl, U., Kusche, M., Lidholt, K., and Oscarsson, L.-G.: Biosynthesis of heparin and heparan sulfate. Ann. N. Y. Acad. Sci. 556:36, 1989; with permission.)

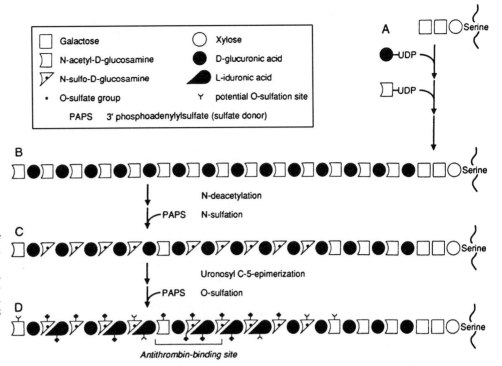

cent of the molecules contain this structure and bind to antithrombin with high affinity. An identical structure is thought to arise during the biosynthesis of heparan sulfate chains, although at a much lower frequency. Heparan sulfate chains that contain this structure bind to antithrombin and stimulate protease inhibition. Other glycosaminoglycans that lack the specific pentasaccharide structure (e.g., dermatan sulfate, chondroitin 4-sulfate, or chondroitin 6-sulfate) do not interact with antithrombin.[225]

The heparin-binding site in antithrombin has been studied by chemical modification, analysis of natural and site-directed mutants, and X-ray crystallography. For example, chemical modification of several lysine residues, including Lys 107, Lys 114, Lys 125, and Lys 136, blocks heparin binding and stimulation of antithrombin activity without affecting the inhibitory activity in the absence of heparin.[226, 227] These results are consistent with the observation that the presence of an oligosaccharide linked to Asn 135 decreases the affinity of α-antithrombin for heparin relative to that of β-antithrombin.[172, 228] Chemical modification of a single tryptophan residue, identified as Trp 49, also blocks heparin binding to antithrombin.[229] Furthermore, structural analyses of inherited antithrombin variants that react normally with thrombin but lack the ability to bind heparin have revealed mutations of

Arg 47 and Pro 41.[230–232] These studies suggest that Pro 41, Arg 47, and Trp 49 lie within or near the heparin-binding site of antithrombin. Carrell and coworkers[211] succeeded in crystallizing antithrombin complexed with the high-affinity heparin pentasaccharide. X-ray diffraction analysis suggested that hydrogen bonds occur between sulfate and carboxylate groups on the pentasaccharide and the side chains of Arg 46, Arg 47, Lys 114, Lys 125, and Arg 129, in general agreement with the previous studies.

Rapid kinetic analyses indicate that heparin binding induces a conformational change in antithrombin that locks the heparin molecule into place on the surface of the inhibitor.[221] The heparin/antithrombin complex can then react rapidly with a target protease. Binding of a protease to antithrombin reduces the affinity of antithrombin for heparin, allowing the antithrombin/protease complex to dissociate from the heparin molecule.[233] Thus, heparin is able to function in a catalytic manner in the reaction.

The mechanism by which heparin catalyzes the inhibition of proteases by antithrombin involves both allosteric and template effects:

1. Heparin binding induces a conformational change that affects the reactive site of antithrombin, allowing

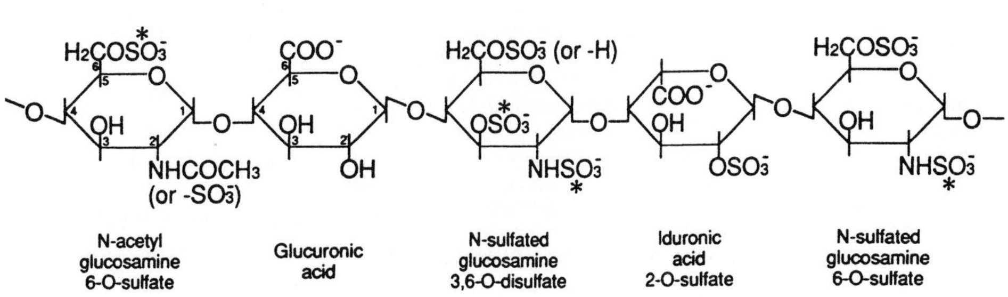

Figure 20–5. Structure of the antithrombin-binding pentasaccharide of heparin. Sulfate groups marked with asterisks are essential for high-affinity binding to antithrombin. The first residue may be either *N*-sulfated or *N*-acetylated, and the C6 position of the third residue may or may not be sulfated.

target proteases to interact more rapidly with this site. This model is supported by the fact that changes in antithrombin as a consequence of heparin binding can be detected by ultraviolet absorbance,[234] fluorescence,[235, 236] circular dichroism,[234, 237] and proton nuclear magnetic resonance.[238] Additional evidence for a conformational linkage between the heparin binding site and the reactive site has been obtained by use of a fluorescence probe covalently attached to the reactive site P1 residue[239] and a monoclonal antibody that binds to the 1C/4B region adjacent to the reactive site loop.[240] Comparison of the structures of antithrombin crystallized with and without the pentasaccharide suggests that binding of heparin induces elongation of α helix D, which in turn causes closure of β sheet A with expulsion of the partially inserted reactive site loop[211, 241] (Fig. 20–6). As a result, the orientation of the P1 arginine residue may change so that it becomes accessible to attack by a proteolytic enzyme.[242]

2. Heparin can also function as a template to which both antithrombin and the target protease bind. Thus, catalysis occurs mainly by an approximation effect. This model is supported by the fact that heparin molecules containing 18 or more sugar residues are required to catalyze the reaction of antithrombin with thrombin, even though smaller molecules bind with high affinity and induce a conformational change.[223, 243] Formation of ternary complexes that contain antithrombin, heparin, and thrombin is supported also by physical evidence.[244, 245]

The balance between the allosteric and template effects may explain differences in the rate enhancement for inhibition of thrombin and factor Xa produced by heparin chains of varying length. For example, the synthetic pentasaccharide that contains only the antithrombin-binding site of heparin increases the rate of inhibition of factor Xa 270-fold but has relatively little effect on the rate of inhibition of thrombin (less than twofold increase).[246] Because an oligosaccharide of this size is unlikely to function as a template, induction of a conformational change in antithrombin may be sufficient to catalyze inhibition of factor Xa. Longer heparin chains produce an additional twofold increase in the rate of factor Xa inhibition, which may represent the contribution of the template mechanism. Stimulation of the thrombin/antithrombin reaction (4300-fold) requires heparin molecules that contain at least 18 sugar residues, which are the smallest chains able to form a ternary complex with thrombin and antithrombin.[245] At low heparin concentrations, the rate of inhibition of thrombin or factor Xa is proportional to the concentration of heparin/antithrombin complexes present in the incubation.[212, 220] The rate of inhibition plateaus at a concentration of heparin (usually in the micromolar range) that is sufficient to saturate the antithrombin. Higher concentrations of heparin decrease the rate of inhibition of thrombin, presumably by favoring the binding of thrombin and antithrombin to separate heparin chains, but do not decrease the rate of inhibition of factor Xa.[212, 220] These observations are consistent with predominance of the template effect in catalysis of the thrombin/antithrombin reaction.[247]

▼ ACTIVITY OF ANTITHROMBIN IN VIVO

Radiolabeled thrombin rapidly forms complexes with antithrombin after intravenous injection in rabbits.[248] Furthermore, low concentrations of thrombin/antithrombin complex (20 to 100 pmol/l) can be detected in plasma from healthy human subjects and may reflect the basal rate of generation of thrombin under normal circumstances.[249] The concentration of the thrombin/antithrombin complex is increased in certain pathological conditions such as disseminated intravascular coagulation.[249, 250]

Formation of factor IXa/antithrombin complexes also occurs rapidly in vivo.[188] By contrast, factor Xa mainly forms complexes with α2-macroglobulin after intravenous injection in the mouse, although the major inhibitors of factor Xa incubated with murine plasma in vitro are α1-antitrypsin and antithrombin.[251] Factor Xa is protected from inhibition by antithrombin in vitro when the protease is bound to platelets[252] or to the prothrombinase complex that contains factor Va, prothrombin, and phospholipids.[253] Because the factor Xa/antithrombin complex (20 to 50 pmol/l) can be detected at low concentrations in normal subjects,[254] it is uncertain to what extent these mechanisms may protect factor Xa from inhibition by antithrombin in vivo.

Antithrombin/protease complexes are cleared from the circulation by hepatocytes with a half-life of 2 to 3 minutes,[188, 255] which is considerably more rapid than the rate of clearance of free antithrombin ($t\frac{1}{2} \approx 3$ days).[256] The hepatocyte uptake mechanism is saturable both in vivo and in vitro.[257] Cross-competition experiments indicate that the receptor for hepatic uptake also recognizes complexes of prote-

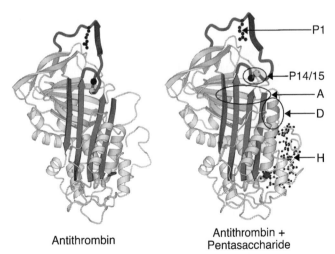

Figure 20–6. Conformational changes in antithrombin induced by heparin. Shown are the structures of native inhibitory antithrombin and the antithrombin/pentasaccharide complex determined by X-ray crystallography. Binding of heparin (H) is associated with elongation of α helix D (D), closure of the upper portion of β sheet A (A), and expulsion of residues P14 and P15 of the reactive site loop (P14/15). As a result of heparin binding, the orientation of the P1 arginine residue (P1) may change so that it becomes accessible to attack by a target protease. However, this change is not apparent on comparison of the two structures, because the P1 residue in both crystals was constrained by contact with an adjacent antithrombin molecule. (Modified from Jin, L., Abrahams, J.P., Skinner, R., Petitou, M., Pike, R.N., and Carrell, R.W.: The anticoagulant activation of antithrombin by heparin. Proc. Natl. Acad. Sci. USA 94:14683, 1997; with permission.)

ases with α_1-antitrypsin, α_1-antichymotrypsin, and heparin cofactor II.[258] The LDL receptor–related protein (LRP) was shown to be responsible for endocytosis and degradation of thrombin/antithrombin complexes by human hepatoma (HepG2) cells and for the in vivo clearance of ^{125}I-thrombin/antithrombin complexes in rats.[259] In human serum, the thrombin/antithrombin complex is associated with vitronectin.[260] Vitronectin mediates binding of the thrombin/antithrombin complex to endothelial cells in vitro,[261] and internalization of the thrombin/antithrombin complex by cultured human umbilical vein endothelial cells has been demonstrated.[262] Whether these processes contribute to the clearance of thrombin/antithrombin complexes from the circulation or serve some other function remains to be determined.

▼ ACTIVATION OF ANTITHROMBIN BY VASCULAR HEPARAN SULFATE

Because of the dramatic effect of heparin on the activity of antithrombin in vitro, it has been assumed that an endogenous heparin-like substance must stimulate antithrombin in vivo. Under normal circumstances, heparin is not released from mast cells into the circulation and cannot be detected in plasma. However, a small amount of heparin may appear in the circulation of patients with systemic mastocytosis and produce mild prolongation of the activated partial thromboplastin time.[263] Circulating heparan sulfate, apparently released from damaged tissues, has been reported to cause marked prolongation of the activated partial thromboplastin time and bleeding in a few severely ill patients.[264–267]

Current evidence suggests that heparan sulfate proteoglycans anchored in the vessel wall interact with circulating antithrombin to produce an antithrombotic effect. Glycosaminoglycans extracted from cloned endothelial cells possess anticoagulant activity.[268] Treatment of the extracts with heparinase abolishes the activity, indicating that the active moiety is heparin-like. De novo biosynthesis of heparan sulfate proteoglycans has been demonstrated by culturing endothelial cells in the presence of [35S]sulfate.[269] Approximately 1 to 10 per cent of the labeled heparan sulfate from endothelial cells binds to immobilized antithrombin with high affinity, and this fraction possesses essentially all the anticoagulant activity of the cell extract. Structural analysis of the high-affinity heparan sulfate has revealed the presence of the 3-O-sulfated glucosamine residue that is characteristic of the antithrombin-binding structure of heparin.[269]

Direct binding of antithrombin to endothelial cells cloned from bovine aorta has been demonstrated. The inhibitor binds to approximately 60,000 sites per cell with a dissociation constant of 12 nmol/l.[269] Binding is diminished by pretreatment of the cells with heparinase. Similar results have been obtained with intact segments of bovine aorta.[270] However, the binding of antithrombin to intact rabbit aortic endothelium is weak, whereas antithrombin appears to bind more avidly to heparinase-sensitive components beneath the endothelial cell layer.[271] Electron microscopic autoradiography of ^{125}I-labeled antithrombin bound to endothelial cells in culture or after perfusion of segments of rat aorta ex vivo indicates that more than 90 per cent of the antithrombin is associated with the extracellular matrix located in the subendothelium.[272] Binding to the subendothelial matrix is greatly increased after crush injury of the aorta, which removes most of the endothelial cells. Because the intact endothelium may be permeable to proteins, interaction of coagulation proteases with antithrombin bound to subendothelial heparan sulfate proteoglycans may inhibit thrombosis.[272] Inhibition of thrombin in the subendothelium appears to be mediated primarily by β-antithrombin.[273]

Rosenberg and coworkers[274] used a rodent hind limb preparation to obtain evidence for stimulation of antithrombin by vascular heparan sulfate in vivo. The hind limb was perfused with thrombin until a constant concentration of the protease was present in the venous effluent. Then antithrombin was perfused through the preparation, and the amount of thrombin/antithrombin complex that formed was determined in comparison to the amount that formed during a similar period in vitro. A 15- to 19-fold increase in the rate of complex formation appeared to occur within the microvasculature compared with in vitro incubations in the absence of heparin. The rate enhancement was diminished by prior perfusion of the hind limb preparation with heparinase or when Trp 49–modified antithrombin was used, suggesting that interaction of antithrombin with microvascular heparan sulfate was responsible for the effect.

A different process may occur when only a trace amount of thrombin is injected into the circulation. Under these circumstances, thrombin may become bound initially to thrombomodulin on the endothelial cell surface.[248] A modest (approximately threefold) increase in the rate of thrombin inhibition by circulating antithrombin may then occur because of the altered substrate specificity of thrombin when it is bound to thrombomodulin.[275] In comparison with free thrombin, thrombin bound to thrombomodulin in vitro reacts less rapidly with fibrinogen and heparin cofactor II, more rapidly with protein C, and at about the same rate with antithrombin. The net effect of these changes in substrate specificity is postulated to be a small increase in the rate of the thrombin/antithrombin reaction because of diminished competition from other substrates. According to this hypothesis, only when thrombomodulin becomes saturated with thrombin will the excess thrombin interact with antithrombin in a heparan sulfate–catalyzed reaction.

Thrombomodulin may have different effects on the thrombin/antithrombin reaction, depending on the tissue or species of origin. Rabbit lung thrombomodulin is a proteoglycan that bears a single chondroitin sulfate chain. It accelerates the thrombin/antithrombin reaction fourfold to eightfold by a mechanism that depends on the presence of both the protein and glycosaminoglycan components.[276, 277] Expression of recombinant human thrombomodulin in human embryonal kidney cells yields two forms of the protein; the higher molecular weight form contains a chondroitin sulfate chain and stimulates the thrombin/antithrombin reaction.[278] By contrast, thrombomodulin purified from human placenta or bovine lung does not have these properties.[275, 279]

Several proteins competitively inhibit antithrombin binding to heparin. They include histidine-rich glycoprotein[280] and vitronectin,[281] both of which are present in plasma at micromolar concentrations. Whether these proteins regulate hemostasis remains to be determined. Platelet factor-4 is released from the α granules during platelet aggregation and binds tightly to heparin.[280] It is likely to promote local clot formation at the site of hemostasis by blocking the binding of antithrombin to heparan sulfate.

▼ ANTITHROMBIN DEFICIENCY

Antithrombin deficiency was the first inherited abnormality to be associated with a thrombotic tendency.[162] The diagnosis is usually made in patients who experience the onset of recurrent thromboembolic disease at an early age or in whom a positive family history of thromboembolic disease is obtained. The concentration of antithrombin in adult plasma is approximately 150 μg/ml (2.6 μmol/l).[282] The range of antithrombin activity determined in 9669 healthy individuals 17 to 65 years of age was 105.6 ± 11.2 IU/dl (mean ± SD).[283] Small differences in antithrombin levels have been noted depending on age, sex, hormonal status, and cardiovascular risk factors.[283, 284] Healthy, full-term newborn infants have antithrombin antigen concentrations of 39 to 87 per cent of adult values.[285] The level gradually increases to the normal adult range by 3 months of age.

Classical (type I) antithrombin deficiency is inherited as an autosomal dominant trait. Affected heterozygotes have approximately 50 per cent of the normal plasma levels of both antithrombin activity and antigen.[286] Total absence of antithrombin has not been reported and may be lethal in utero. Type I antithrombin deficiency can result from deletion of one of the two antithrombin genes; from a dysfunctional gene; or from missense, nonsense, or frameshift mutations in the coding sequence. Approximately 80 point mutations and 12 large deletions have been reported to cause type I deficiency.[287] The catabolic rate of infused radiolabeled antithrombin is normal in patients with inherited antithrombin deficiency, implying that the decreased plasma concentration is not caused by accelerated clearance of normal antithrombin.[288, 289]

Patients who have a low level of antithrombin activity but approximately normal antithrombin antigen have type II deficiencies. The occurrence of variant forms of the inhibitor with impaired activity has provided important insights into the mechanism of action of antithrombin.[290, 291] Approximately 35 such variants have been identified and can be grouped into several categories[287]:

1. Type II RS (reactive site) mutations interfere with the ability of antithrombin to inhibit proteases. These mutations generally have been found at the P2, P1, or P1′ residue of the reactive site or at the hinge region (P10 or P12). Another type II RS mutation (Asn 187 → Asp) is associated with formation of inactive polymers of antithrombin at 41°C, which may explain the occurrence of thrombosis during febrile episodes in patients with this abnormality.[292]
2. Type II HBS (heparin-binding site) mutations occur in residues that appear to bind directly to heparin (e.g., Arg 47 or Arg 129) or at nearby locations where mutations may distort the structure of the heparin-binding site (e.g., Pro 41 and Leu 99). The Ile 7 → Asn mutation creates a new glycosylation site, and the presence of an oligosaccharide at this site may sterically interfere with heparin binding.
3. Type II PE (pleiotropic effect) mutations affect both the reactive site and the heparin-binding site. Most of these mutations occur in the region P9′ to P14′, which is thought to be involved in the conformational linkage between the reactive site and the heparin-binding site.

Although some type II mutations may impair the intracellular processing and secretion of antithrombin,[293] type II variants generally appear to be synthesized at a normal rate and have a normal half-life in the circulation. Therefore, in most instances, the plasma of an affected heterozygote has approximately equimolar amounts of normal and variant antithrombin. In contrast to type I antithrombin deficiency, several homozygous patients with type II HBS deficiency have been identified,[230, 294, 295] and individuals with heterozygous type II HBS deficiency are generally asymptomatic.[296]

With the exception of decreased plasma antithrombin activity, no laboratory abnormalities are associated consistently with antithrombin deficiency. Immunoassays of plasma for prothrombin activation fragment 1 + 2 and fibrinopeptide A, which are indicative of factor Xa and thrombin activity, respectively, have been used to assess the degree of activation of the coagulation system in vivo. A report that fragment 1 + 2 levels are elevated twofold to threefold in patients with antithrombin deficiency was later found to be incorrect owing to an artifact of sample collection.[297, 298] A later study found a small but statistically significant increase in mean plasma fragment 1 + 2 concentration in deficient adults not receiving warfarin (0.87 ± 0.26 nmol/l), in comparison with nondeficient adults (0.70 ± 0.21 nmol/l, p = .03).[299] However, most of the fragment 1 + 2 values in the deficient adults were within the normal range. No increase in fibrinopeptide A has been found in antithrombin-deficient subjects.[297, 299]

The prevalence of inherited antithrombin deficiency in the general population has been estimated to range from 1 per 2000 to 1 per 5000, on the basis of the number of symptomatic patients identified in large referral populations.[300, 301] However, a study of 4189 healthy blood donors 18 to 65 years of age in Scotland identified 16 unrelated individuals with antithrombin deficiency (1 type I, 2 type II RS, and 13 type II HBS), suggesting that the prevalence may be closer to 1 per 250.[302] Only one of the deficient individuals in this series had a history of thrombosis, which is consistent with previous estimates for the prevalence of symptomatic antithrombin deficiency.

The prevalence of antithrombin deficiency in patients with thrombosis has been estimated to range from 2 to 6 per cent,[296] although a Spanish study found a prevalence of only 0.5 per cent.[303] In a series of 752 patients with thromboembolic disease, inherited antithrombin deficiency was established in 13 (1.7 per cent) by family studies.[304] Only 1 of the 13 deficient patients in this series had a type II abnormality, in contrast to the much more frequent occurrence of type II abnormalities in asymptomatic individuals.[302] The observation that antithrombin deficiency is more common in patients with thromboembolism than in asymptomatic individuals suggests that antithrombin deficiency increases the risk for development of the disease.

The prevalence of thromboembolic complications in patients with inherited antithrombin deficiency has been estimated from retrospective reviews of published case reports.[160, 161, 296] Clinical data from 62 families with antithrombin deficiency, excluding 14 families with type II HBS deficiency, have been summarized.[305] About half of the 964 individuals studied had low plasma antithrombin activities and were apparently heterozygous. The mean prevalence of venous thromboembolism was 50.8 per cent in the deficient subjects, in comparison with 1.5 per cent in the nondeficient subjects. However, the prevalence of venous thromboembolism in the deficient members of different families ranged from 15 to 100 per cent. Thrombosis occurred with approximately equal frequency in male and female patients and included deep venous thrombosis of the lower extremities or pulmonary embolism (89.9 per cent), mesenteric vein thrombosis (3.1 per cent), and cerebral vein thrombosis (0.9 per cent). Arterial occlusion was rare. Risk factors such as pregnancy or surgery were associated with 32 per cent of the thrombotic episodes and were absent in 16 per cent; however, information about risk factors was not included in the majority of case reports. In some families, coinheritance of antithrombin deficiency and factor V Leiden (which maps to chromosome 1q21–25 and is 3 to 11 cM from the antithrombin gene) appears to result in a more severe thromboembolic phenotype in comparison with individuals who have only one of these molecular abnormalities.[306–308]

Thrombosis has been reported rarely in antithrombin-deficient patients before 15 years of age. It has been suggested that the high levels of α_2-macroglobulin present during childhood (two to three times the adult level) protect antithrombin-deficient children from thrombosis.[309] The incidence of thrombosis in the reported cases was greatest between 15 and 35 years of age and decreased thereafter, presumably because the majority of individuals who became symptomatic were given long-term oral anticoagulant therapy. By 30 years of age, about 60 per cent of the antithrombin-deficient subjects had at least one thromboembolic episode.[305] Despite the high incidence of thrombosis, the mortality of patients with antithrombin deficiency, many of whom are anticoagulated indefinitely after their first thromboembolic episode, appears to be no different from that of the general population.[310–312] It is uncertain whether less aggressive treatment of patients with antithrombin deficiency would result in increased mortality.

Most reported cases of antithrombin deficiency have been discovered by laboratory investigation of patients with recurrent thromboembolic disease. The bias of ascertainment inherent in such reports may lead to overestimation of the frequency of complications in patients with antithrombin deficiency. Furthermore, the diagnosis of thromboembolism was established by objective tests in only 17 per cent of reported cases.[305] Because the clinical manifestations of deep venous thrombosis and pulmonary embolism are nonspecific, thromboembolism has probably been misdiagnosed in at least some individuals with antithrombin deficiency. In a large Canadian family, type II RS antithrombin deficiency was established in 31 of 67 individuals by analysis of genomic DNA.[305] Only six episodes of venous thromboembolism, five of which were associated with known risk factors, were documented by objective tests in the 31 deficient subjects (mean age, 36 years), whereas none occurred in the 36 nondeficient subjects. This study suggests that idiopathic

thrombosis may occur less frequently than previously estimated in antithrombin-deficient patients.

The clinical manifestations of patients with type II HBS antithrombin deficiency, in which abnormalities are limited to the heparin-binding site, are distinguishable from those of patients with the other types of deficiencies. Only three episodes of thrombosis have been reported among 51 individuals with inherited type II HBS antithrombin deficiency[296]; all three of these episodes occurred in homozygous patients. For example, one family included a child born to consanguineous parents, both of whom had asymptomatic antithrombin deficiency.[295] The child had undetectable heparin cofactor activity and died at 3 years of age of massive intracardiac thrombosis while receiving oral anticoagulant therapy.

Heparin Cofactor II

▼ STRUCTURE AND PROTEASE SPECIFICITY OF HEPARIN COFACTOR II

Heparin cofactor II is a 66 kDa glycoprotein that consists of a single polypeptide chain.[313] The gene for heparin cofactor II on human chromosome 22q11 contains five exons distributed over approximately 16 kb of DNA.[314, 315] The positions of the introns are similar to those of the α_1-antitrypsin and angiotensinogen genes but differ from those of the antithrombin, plasminogen activator inhibitor-1, plasminogen activator inhibitor-2, and ovalbumin genes. No TATA or CAAT sequences (nor a variety of other proposed regulatory elements) have been identified at the 5′ end of the gene, and transcription may initiate at several positions.[314] A 2200 nucleotide mRNA for heparin cofactor II was isolated from human liver,[316] and biosynthesis was demonstrated in cultured human hepatoma cells (HepG2).[317, 318] The amino acid sequence of heparin cofactor II has been determined by cDNA cloning.[316, 319] The protein contains 480 amino acid residues preceded by a signal peptide 19 residues in length, three potential N-linked glycosylation sites, and two tyrosine residues near the amino terminus that become O-sulfated during biosynthesis.[318] Three cysteine residues are present that apparently do not form disulfide bonds.[320] Heparin cofactor II is about 30 per cent identical in sequence to other members of the serpin family, with the greatest similarity occurring in the carboxyl-terminal two thirds of the protein. Heparin cofactor II contains an amino-terminal extension of about 80 amino acid residues that shares no homology with other serpins.

The reactive site of heparin cofactor II contains the peptide bond Leu 444–Ser 445.[321] In part because of the leucine residue in the P1 position, heparin cofactor II differs from antithrombin with respect to its protease specificity. In the absence of a glycosaminoglycan, heparin cofactor II inhibits chymotrypsin more rapidly than it inhibits thrombin.[322] Furthermore, heparin cofactor II does not inhibit other proteases involved in coagulation or fibrinolysis that preferentially cleave substrates following basic amino acid residues.[323] Cleavage of the Leu 444–Ser 445 bond occurs during inhibition of both thrombin and chymotrypsin.[322] Mutation of Leu 444 to arginine increases the basal rate of inhibition of thrombin in the absence of glycosaminoglycan approximately 100-fold and decreases the ability of heparin cofactor II to inhibit chymotrypsin.[324] These results emphasize the importance of the P1 residue in determining the rate of protease inhibition and suggest that heparin cofactor II has evolved to be essentially inactive toward thrombin in the absence of a glycosaminoglycan.

▼ STIMULATION OF HEPARIN COFACTOR II BY GLYCOSAMINOGLYCANS

The rate of inhibition of thrombin by heparin cofactor II is increased approximately 1000-fold by heparin, heparan sulfate, or dermatan sulfate.[225] The affinity of heparin cofactor II for heparin is lower than that of antithrombin, and heparin cofactor II does not require the specific pentasaccharide structure shown in Figure 20–5 for stimulation by heparin.[325, 326] Heparin cofactor II is unique among serpins with regard to its ability to be stimulated by dermatan sulfate. The binding site for heparin cofactor II in mammalian dermatan sulfate is a tandem repeat of three iduronic acid 2-sulfate→N-acetylgalactosamine 4-sulfate disaccharide subunits, which appear to be clustered within the polymer.[327] This hexasaccharide increases the rate of inhibition of thrombin by heparin cofactor II 50-fold, although dermatan sulfate chains containing 14 or more monosaccharide units are required for maximal stimulation.[328] Invertebrate dermatan sulfate, composed predominantly of iduronic acid 2-sulfate→N-acetylgalactosamine 6-sulfate disaccharide subunits, is 100-fold less active than mammalian dermatan sulfate, indicating that 4-O-sulfation of galactosamine is essential for activity with heparin cofactor II.[329] Addition of dermatan sulfate to plasma in vitro causes prolongation of the thrombin time and the activated partial thromboplastin time,[215] and intravenous infusion of dermatan sulfate produces an antithrombotic effect in experimental animals[330–333] and humans.[334–336] These effects appear to be mediated primarily by heparin cofactor II.[225, 337, 338]

Analysis of the natural variant heparin cofactor II Oslo (Arg 189 → His) established that heparin and dermatan sulfate interact with different amino acid residues on the surface of the inhibitor.[339] This mutation causes a marked decrease (≈60-fold) in the affinity of heparin cofactor II for dermatan sulfate but does not affect the affinity of the inhibitor for heparin. Arg 189 occurs within a cluster of basic amino acid residues that can be aligned with basic residues in the heparin-binding site of antithrombin but are poorly conserved in other serpins. Mutations of Lys 173, Arg 184, and Arg 185 in recombinant heparin cofactor II affect heparin binding, whereas mutations of Arg 184, Arg 185, Arg 189, Arg 192, and Arg 193 affect dermatan sulfate binding.[340–343] These results indicate that the binding sites for heparin and dermatan sulfate overlap but are not identical.

The stimulatory effect of heparin and dermatan sulfate on thrombin inhibition depends on the presence of an acidic polypeptide domain near the amino terminus of heparin cofactor II.[344] The acidic domain contains a tandem repeat of two nearly identical sequences, each of which is similar to the carboxyl-terminal sequence of hirudin, a potent thrombin inhibitor in the saliva of the medicinal leech. The carboxyl-terminal portion of hirudin binds with high affinity to anion-binding exosite I of thrombin; the amino-terminal domain of hirudin occupies the catalytic site.[345, 346] A synthetic peptide corresponding to the acidic domain of heparin cofactor II competes with hirudin for binding to thrombin but does not affect the ability of thrombin to hydrolyze a tripeptide p-nitroanilide substrate.[347] Thus, binding of thrombin to the acidic domain of heparin cofactor II could facilitate covalent complex formation by bringing the active site of thrombin into approximation with the reactive site of heparin cofactor II.

Experiments with recombinant heparin cofactor II have established the importance of the amino-terminal acidic domain.[341, 342, 344] Although deletion of both acidic repeats does not affect the rate of inhibition of thrombin or chymotrypsin in the absence of a glycosaminoglycan, deletion of the first acidic repeat greatly diminishes the ability of dermatan sulfate or heparin to stimulate the inhibition of thrombin.[344] The deletion mutants bind heparin more tightly, which suggests that the acidic domain occupies the glycosaminoglycan binding site in native heparin cofactor II. These findings are consistent with a model in which heparin or dermatan sulfate displaces the amino-terminal acidic domain from the glycosaminoglycan binding site of heparin cofactor II, thus enabling the acidic domain to interact with exosite I of thrombin (Fig. 20–7).

In addition to anion-binding exosite I, thrombin contains a distinct site (termed anion-binding exosite II) that binds glycosaminoglycans, including heparin and dermatan sulfate. Studies with thrombin variants have clarified the roles these

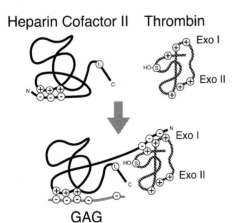

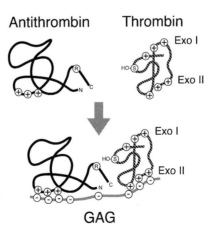

Figure 20–7. Proposed mechanisms of inhibition of thrombin by antithrombin and heparin cofactor II. The catalytic serine hydroxyl group of thrombin (S–OH) and the reactive site P1 residues of antithrombin (R) and heparin cofactor II (L) are indicated. The + symbols represent positively charged residues in the glycosaminoglycan (GAG)-binding sites of antithrombin and heparin cofactor II as well as in anion-binding exosite I (Exo I) and anion-binding exosite II (Exo II) of thrombin. The − symbols represent negatively charged residues in the glycosaminoglycan chain.

exosites play in inhibition by heparin cofactor II and antithrombin.[348-353] Mutations in exosite I do not affect the rate of inhibition of thrombin by antithrombin in the presence of heparin, whereas exosite II mutations decrease the rate approximately 100-fold. Conversely, mutations in exosite I decrease the rate of inhibition of thrombin by heparin cofactor II in the presence of heparin or dermatan sulfate approximately 100-fold, whereas exosite II mutations have little or no effect. These observations suggest that antithrombin and heparin cofactor II inhibit thrombin by different mechanisms as shown schematically in Figure 20–7. In meizothrombin, exosite II is blocked by the fragment 2 domain of prothrombin.[354] Because of this, meizothrombin is preferentially inhibited by heparin cofactor II.[156, 158]

▼ PHYSIOLOGY OF HEPARIN COFACTOR II

The concentration of heparin cofactor II in normal human plasma is 1.2 ± 0.4 μmol/l (mean $\pm$ 2 SD).[355] Several individuals with inherited partial deficiency of heparin cofactor II (50 per cent of normal) were reported to have histories of thrombotic disease.[356, 357] In one series, however, 4 of 379 apparently healthy individuals had heparin cofactor II levels below 60 per cent.[358] Because heterozygous deficiency of heparin cofactor II may be a coincidental finding in about 1 per cent of patients with thrombosis, it is premature to conclude that heparin cofactor II deficiency is a risk factor for development of the disease.[359] No individuals with homozygous deficiency of heparin cofactor II have been identified.

Cultured fibroblasts and vascular smooth muscle cells accelerate inhibition of thrombin by heparin cofactor II, whereas endothelial cells do not.[360, 361] In the case of fibroblasts, a dermatan sulfate proteoglycan was demonstrated to be responsible for this effect.[360] By contrast, a heparan sulfate proteoglycan has been implicated in the case of arterial smooth muscle cells.[361] These results suggest that heparin cofactor II may inhibit thrombin in the connective tissues rather than within the blood vessels and perhaps modulate wound healing or inflammation. Theoretically, heparin cofactor II could promote coagulation by inhibiting the activation of protein C by meizothrombin.[158]

During pregnancy, both the maternal plasma and the fetal plasma contain a dermatan sulfate proteoglycan that stimulates inhibition of thrombin by plasma heparin cofactor II approximately twofold,[362] and elevated levels of the thrombin/heparin cofactor II complex are present.[363] The placenta is rich in dermatan sulfate[364] and may be the source of this proteoglycan. Thus, heparin cofactor II could be activated locally to inhibit coagulation within the placenta.

REFERENCES

1. Thomas, L.: Studies on the intravascular thromboplastin effect of tissue suspensions in mice: II. A factor in normal rabbit serum which inhibits the thromboplastin effect of the sedimentable tissue component. Bull Johns Hopkins Hosp. 81:26, 1947.
2. Schneider, C.L.: The active principle of placental toxin: thromboplastin; its inactivator in blood: antithromboplastin. Am. J. Physiol. 149:123, 1947.
3. Hjort, P.F.: Intermediate reactions in the coagulation of blood with tissue thromboplastin. Scand. J. Clin. Lab. Invest. 9(suppl. 27):1, 1957.
4. Biggs, R., and MacFarlane, R.G.: The reaction of hemophiliac plasma to thromboplastin. J. Clin. Invest. 4:445, 1951.
5. Biggs, R., and Nossel, H.L.: Tissue extract and the contact reaction in blood coagulation. Thromb. Diath. Haemorrh. 6:1, 1961.
6. Marlar, R.A., Kleiss, A.J., and Griffin, J.H.: An alternative extrinsic pathway of human blood coagulation. Blood 60:1353, 1982.
7. Morrison, S.A., and Jesty, J.: Tissue factor–dependent activation of tritium-labeled factor IX and factor X in human plasma. Blood 63:1338, 1984.
8. Sanders, N.L., Bajaj, S.P., Zivelin, A., and Rapaport, S.I.: Inhibition of tissue factor/factor VIIa activity in plasma requires factor X and an additional plasma component. Blood 66:204, 1985.
9. Hubbard, A.R., and Jennings, C.A.: Inhibition of tissue thromboplastin-mediated blood coagulation. Thromb. Res. 42:489, 1986.
10. Broze, G.J., Jr., and Miletich, J.P.: Characterization of the inhibition of tissue factor in serum. Blood 69:150, 1987.
11. Rao, L.V.M., and Rapaport, S.I.: Studies of a mechanism inhibiting the initiation of the extrinsic pathway of coagulation. Blood 69:645, 1987.
12. Broze, G.J., Jr., and Miletich, J.P.: Isolation of the tissue factor inhibitor produced by HepG2 hepatoma cells. Proc. Natl. Acad. Sci. USA 84:1886, 1987.
13. Broze, G.J., Jr., Warren, L.A., Girard, J.J., and Miletich, J.P.: Isolation of the lipoprotein associated coagulation inhibitor produced by HepG2 (human hepatoma) cells using bovine factor Xa affinity chromatography. Throm. Res. 48:253, 1987.
14. Novotny, W.F., Girard, T.J., Miletich, J.P., and Broze, G.J. Jr.: Purification and characterization of the lipoprotein-associated coagulation inhibitor from human plasma. J. Biol. Chem. 264:18832, 1989.
15. Novotny, W.F., Palmier, M., Wun, T.C., Broze, G.J., Jr., and Miletich, J.P.: Purification and properties of heparin-releasable lipoprotein-associated coagulation inhibitor. Blood 78:394, 1991.
16. Wun, T.C., Kretzmer, K.K., Girard, T.J., Miletich, J.P. and Broze, G.J., Jr.: Cloning and characterization of a cDNA coding for the lipoprotein-associated coagulation inhibitor shows that it consists of three tandem Kunitz-type inhibitory domains. J. Biol. Chem. 263:6001, 1988.
17. Girard, T.J., Warren, L.A., Novotny, W.F., Bejcek, B.E., Miletich, J.P., and Broze, G.J., Jr.: Identification of the 1.4 kb and 4.0 kb messages for the lipoprotein associated coagulation inhibitor and expression of the encoded protein. Thromb. Res. 55:37, 1989.
18. Kamei, S., Kamikubo, Y., Hamuro, T., Fujimoto, H., Ishihara, M., Yonemura, H., Miyamoto, S., Funatsu, A., Enjyoji, K., and Abumiya, T.: Amino acid sequence and inhibitory activity of rhesus monkey tissue factor pathway inhibitor (TFPI): comparison with human TFPI. J. Biochem. 115:708, 1994.
19. Girard, T.J., Gailani, D., and Broze, G.J., Jr.: Complementary DNA sequencing of canine tissue factor pathway inhibitor reveals a unique nanomeric repetitive sequence between the second and third Kunitz domains. Biochem. J. 303:923, 1994.
20. Wesselschmidt, R.L., Girard, T.J., and Broze, G.J., Jr.: cDNA sequence of rabbit lipoprotein-associated coagulation inhibitor [published erratum appears in Nucleic Acids Res. 20:3548, 1992]. Nucleic Acids Res. 18:6440, 1990.
21. Belaaouaj, A., Kuppuswamy, M.N., Birktoft, J.J., and Bajaj, S.P.: Revised cDNA sequence of rabbit tissue factor pathway inhibitor. Thromb. Res. 69:547, 1993.
22. Enjyoji, K., Emi, M., Mukai, T., and Kato, H.: cDNA cloning and expression of rat tissue factor pathway inhibitor (TFPI). J. Biochem. 111:681, 1992.
23. Chang, J.-Y., Monroe, D.M., Oliver, J.A., Liles, D.K., and Roberts, H.R.: Cloning, expression, and characterization of mouse tissue factor pathway inhibitor (TFPI). Thromb. Haemost. 79:306, 1998.
24. van der Logt, C.P., Reitsma, P.H., and Bertina, R.M.: Intron-exon organization of the human gene coding for the lipoprotein-associated coagulation inhibitor: the factor Xa dependent inhibitor of the extrinsic pathway of coagulation. Biochemistry 30:1571, 1991.
25. Girard, T.J., Eddy, R., Wesselschmidt, R.L., MacPhail, L.A., Likert, K.M., Byers, M.G., Shows, T.B., and Broze, G.J., Jr.: Structure of the human lipoprotein-associated coagulation inhibitor gene. Intro/exon gene organization and localization of the gene to chromosome 2. J. Biol. Chem. 266:5036, 1991.
26. van der Logt, C.P., Kluck, P.M., Wiegant, J., Landegent, J.E., and Reitsma, P.H.: Refined regional assignment of the human tissue factor pathway inhibitor (TFPI) gene to chromosome band 2q32 by nonisotopic in situ hybridization. Hum. Genet. 89:577, 1992.

27. Patthy, L.: Intron-dependent evolution: preferred types of exons and introns. FEBS Lett. 214:1, 1987.

28. van der Logt, C.P.E., Reitsma, P.H., and Bertina, R.M.: A *Pst*I RFLP of the *LACI* gene. Nucleic Acids Res. 18:5920, 1990.

29. Gronostajski, R.M.: Site-specific DNA binding of nuclear factor I: effect of the spacer region. Nucleic Acids Res. 15:5545, 1987.

30. Lee, W., Haslinger, A., Karin, M., and Tjian, R.: Activation of transcription by two factors that bind promoter and enhancer sequences of the human metallothionein gene and SV40. Nature 325:368, 1987.

31. Angel, P., Baumann, I., Stein, B., Delius, H., Rahmsdorf, H.J., and Herrlich, P.: 12-*O*-tetradecanoyl-phorbol-13-acetate induction of the human collagenase gene is mediated by an inducible enhancer element located in the 5′-flanking region. Mol. Cell. Biol. 7:2256, 1987.

32. Rana, S.V., Reimers, H.J., Pathikonda, M.S., and Bajaj, S.P.: Expression of tissue factor and factor VIIa/tissue factor inhibitor activity in endotoxin or phorbol ester stimulated U937 monocyte-like cells. Blood 71:259, 1988.

33. Ameri, A., Kuppuswamy, M.N., Basu, S., and Bajaj, S.P.: Expression of tissue factor pathway inhibitor by cultured endothelial cells in response to inflammatory mediators. Blood 79:3219, 1992.

34. Martin, D.I., Zon, L.I., Mutter, G., and Orkin, S.H.: Expression of an erythroid transcription factor in megakaryocytic and mast cell lineages. Nature 344:444, 1990.

35. Wilson, D.B., Dorfman, D.M., and Orkin, S.H.: A nonerythroid GATA-binding protein is required for function of the human preproendothelin-1 promoter in endothelial cells. Mol. Cell. Biol. 10:4854, 1990.

36. Lee, M.E., Temizer, D.H., Clifford, J.A., and Quertermous, T.: Cloning of the GATA-binding protein that regulates endothelin-1 gene expression in endothelial cells. J. Biol. Chem. 266:16188, 1991.

37. Caput, D., Beutler, B., Hartog, K., Thayer, R., Brown, S.S., and Cerami, A.: Identification of a common nucleotide sequence in the 3′-untranslated region of mRNA molecules specifying inflammatory mediators. Proc. Natl. Acad. Sci. USA 83:1670, 1986.

38. Shaw, G., and Kamen, R.: A conserved AU sequence from the 3′ untranslated region of GM-CSF mRNA mediates selective mRNA degradation. Cell 46:659, 1986.

39. Nakahara, Y., Miyata, T., Hamuro, T., Funatsu, A., Miyagi, M., Tsunasawa, S., and Kato, H.: Amino acid sequence and carbohydrate structure of a recombinant human tissue factor pathway inhibitor expressed in Chinese hamster ovary cells: One N- and two O-linked carbohydrate chains are located between Kunitz domains 2 and 3 and one N-linked carbohydrate is in Kunitz domain 2. Biochemistry 35:233, 1996.

40. Colburn, P., and Buonassisi, V.: Identification of an endothelial cell product as an inhibitor of tissue factor activity. In Vitro Cell. Dev. Biol. Animal 24:1133, 1988.

41. Smith, P.L., Skelton, T.P., Fiete, D., Dharmesh, S.M., Beranek, M.C., MacPhail, L., Broze, G.J., Jr., and Baenziger, J.U.: The asparagine-linked oligosaccharides on tissue factor pathway inhibitor terminate with SO4-4GalNAc beta 1, 4GlcNAc beta 1,2 Mana alpha. J. Biol. Chem. 267:19140, 1992.

42. Girard, T.J., McCourt, D., Novotny, W.F., MacPhail, L.A., Likert, K.M., and Broze, G.J., Jr.: Endogenous phosphorylation of the lipoprotein-associated coagulation inhibitor at serine-2. Biochem. J. 270:621, 1990.

43. Gustafson, M.E., Junger, K.D., Wun, T.C., Foy, B.A., Diaz-Collier, J.A., Welsch, D.J., Obukowicz, M.G., Bishop, B.F., Bild, G.S., and Leimgruber, R.M.: Renaturation and purification of human tissue factor pathway inhibitor expressed in recombinant *E. coli*. Protein Expr. Purif. 5:233, 1994.

44. Holst, J., Lindblad, B., Nordfang, O., Ostergaard, P.B., and Hedner, U.: Does glycosylation influence the experimental antithrombotic effect of a two-domain tissue factor pathway inhibitor? Haemostasis 26:23, 1996.

45. Laskowski, M., Jr., and Kato, I.: Protein inhibitors of proteinases [review]. Annu. Rev. Biochem. 49:593, 1980.

46. Gebhard, W., Tschesche, H., and Fritz, H.: Biochemistry of aprotinin and aprotinin-like inhibitors. *In* Barrett, A.J., and Salvesen, G.: Protease Inhibitors. Amsterdam, Elsevier Science, 1986, pp. 375–388.

47. Girard, T.J., Warren, L.A., Novotny, W.F., Likert, K.M., Brown, S.G., Miletich, J.P., and Broze, G.J., Jr.: Functional significance of the Kunitz-type inhibitory domains of lipoprotein-associated coagulation inhibitor. Nature 338:518, 1989.

48. Petersen, L.C., Bjorn, S.E., Olsen, O.H., Nordfang, O., Norris, F., and Norris, K.: Inhibitory properties of separate recombinant Kunitz-type-inhibitor domains from tissue factor pathway inhibitor. Eur. J. Biochem. 235:310, 1996.

49. Hamamoto, T., and Kisiel, W.: Full-length human tissue factor pathway inhibitor inhibits human activated protein C in the presence of heparin. Thromb. Res. 80:291, 1995.

50. Petersen, L.C., Bjorn, S.E., and Nordfang, O.: Effect of leukocyte proteinases on tissue factor pathway inhibitor. Thromb. Haemost. 67:537, 1992.

51. Broze, G.J., Jr., Warren, L.A., Novotny, W.F., Higuchi, D.A., Girard, J.J., and Miletich, J.P.: The lipoprotein-associated coagulation inhibitor that inhibits the factor VII–tissue factor complex also inhibits factor Xa: insight into its possible mechanism of action. Blood 71:335, 1988.

52. Wesselschmidt, R., Likert, K., Girard, T., Wun, T.C., and Broze, G.J., Jr.: Tissue factor pathway inhibitor: the carboxy-terminus is required for optimal inhibition of factor Xa. Blood 79:2004, 1992.

53. Wesselschmidt, R.I., Likert, K.M., Huang, Z.-F., MacPhail, L., and Broze, G.J., Jr.: Structural requirements for tissue factor pathway inhibitor interactions with factor Xa and heparin. Blood Coagul. Fibrinolysis 4:661, 1993.

54. Lindhout, T., Franssen, J., and Willems, G.: Kinetics of the inhibition of tissue factor–factor VIIa by tissue factor pathway inhibitor. Thromb. Haemost. 74:910, 1995.

55. Higuchi, D.A., Wun, T.C., Likert, K.M., and Broze, G.J., Jr.: The effect of leukocyte elastase on tissue factor pathway inhibitor. Blood 79:1712, 1992.

56. Huang, Z.-F., Wun, T.-C., Likert, K.M., and Broze, G.J., Jr.: Kinetics of factor Xa inhibition by tissue factor pathway inhibitor. J. Biol. Chem. 268:26950, 1993.

57. van't Veer, C., Hackeng, T.M., Delahaye, C., Sixma, J.J., and Bouma, B.N.: Activated factor Xa and thrombin formation triggered by tissue factor on endothelial cell matrix in a flow model: effect of the tissue factor pathway inhibitor. Blood 84:1132, 1994.

58. Mast, A.E., and Broze, G.J., Jr.: Physiological concentrations of tissue factor pathway inhibitor do not inhibit prothrombinase. Blood 87:1845, 1996.

59. Enjyoji, K., Miyata, T., Kamikubo, Y., and Kato, H.: Effect of heparin on the inhibition of factor Xa by tissue factor pathway inhibitor. A segment, Gly$_{212}$-Phe$_{243}$, in the third Kunitz domain is a heparin binding site. Biochem. 34:5725, 1995.

60. Valentin, S., Larnkjaer, A., Ostergaard, P., Nielsen, J.I., and Nordfang, O.: Characterization of the binding between tissue factor pathway inhibitor and glycosaminoglycans. Thomb. Res. 75:173, 1994.

61. Baugh, R.J., Broze, G.J., Jr., and Krishnaswamy, S.: Regulation of extrinsic pathway factor Xa formation by tissue factor pathway inhibitor. J. Biol. Chem. 273:4378, 1998.

62. Warn-Cramer, B.J., Rao, L.V., Maki, S.L., and Rapaport, S.I.: Modifications of extrinsic pathway inhibitor (EPI) and factor Xa that affect their ability to interact and to inhibit factor VIIa/tissue factor: evidence for a two-step model of inhibition. Thromb. Haemost. 60:453, 1988.

63. Rao, L.V.M., and Ruf, W.: Tissue factor residues Lys^{165} and Lys^{166} are essential for rapid formation of the quaternary complex of tissue factor–VIIa with Xa–tissue factor pathway inhibitor. Biochemistry 34:10867, 1995.

64. Jesty, J., Wun, T.-C., and Lorenz, A.: Kinetics of the inhibition of factor Xa and the tissue factor–factor VIIa complex by the tissue factor pathway inhibitor in the presence and absence of heparin. Biochemistry 33:12686, 1994.

65. Hamamoto, T., and Kisiel, W.: The effect of heparin on the regulation of factor VIIa–tissue factor activity by tissue factor pathway inhibitor. Blood Coagul. Fibrinolysis 7:470, 1996.

66. Valentin, S., Retlingsperger, C.P.M., Nordfang, O., and Lindhout, T.: Inhibition of factor X activation at extracellular matrix of fibroblasts during flow conditions: a comparison between tissue factor pathway inhibitor and inactive factor VIIa. Thromb. Haemost. 74:1478, 1995.

67. Petersen, L.C., Valentin, S., and Hedner, U.: Regulation of the extrinsic pathway system of health and disease: the role of factor VIIa and tissue factor pathway inhibitor. Thromb. Res. 79:1, 1995.

68. Nordfang, O., Bjorn, S.E., Valentin, S., Nielsen, L.S., Wildgoose, P., Beck, T.C., and Hedner, U.: The C-terminus of tissue factor pathway inhibitor is essential to its anticoagulant activity. Biochemistry 30:10371, 1991.

69. Pedersen, A.H., Nordfang, O., Norris, F., Wiberg, F.C., Christensen, P.M., Moeller, K.B., Meidahl, P.J., Beck, T.C., Norris, K., and Hedner, U.: Recombinant human extrinsic pathway inhibitor. Production, isolation, and characterization of its inhibitory activity on tissue factor-initiated coagulation reactions. J. Biol. Chem. 265:16786, 1990.

70. Callander, N.S., Rao, L.V., Nordfang, O., Sandset, P.M., Warn-Cramer, B., and Rapaport, S.I.: Mechanisms of binding of recombinant extrinsic pathway inhibitor (rEPI) to cultured cell surfaces. Evidence that rEPI can bind to and inhibit factor VIIa–tissue factor complexes in the absence of factor Xa. J. Biol. Chem. 267:876, 1992.

71. Girard, T.J., and Broze, G.J., Jr.: Tissue factor pathway inhibitor. Meth. Enzymol. 222:195, 1993.

72. Day, K.C., Hoffman, L.C., Palmier, M.O., Kretzmer, K.K., Huang, M.D., Pyla, E.Y., Spokas, E., Broze, G.J., Jr., Warren, T.G., and Wun, T.C.: Recombinant lipoprotein-associated coagulation inhibitor inhibits tissue thromboplastin-induced intravascular coagulation in the rabbit. Blood 76:1538, 1990.

73. Haskel, E.J., Torr, S.R., Day, K.C., Palmier, M.O., Wun, T.C., Sobel, B.E., and Abendschein, D.R.: Prevention of arterial reocclusion after thrombolysis with recombinant lipoprotein-associated coagulation inhibitor [see comments]. Circulation 84:821, 1991.

74. Creasey, A.A., Chang, A.C., Feigen, L., Wun, T.C., Taylor, F.B., Jr., and Hinshaw, L.B.: Tissue factor pathway inhibitor reduces mortality from *Escherichia coli* septic shock. J. Clin. Invest. 91:2850, 1993.

75. Werling, R.W., Zacharski, L.R., Kisiel, W., Bajaj, S.P., Memoli, V.A., and Rousseau, S.M.: Distribution of tissue factor pathway inhibitor in normal and malignant human tissues. Thromb. Haemost. 69:366, 1993.

76. Hollister, R.D., Kisiel, W., and Hyman, B.T.: Immunohistochemical localization of tissue factor pathway inhibitor-1 (TFPI-1), a Kunitz proteinase inhibitor, in Alzheimer's disease. Brain Res. 728:13, 1996.

77. Bajaj, M.S., Kuppuswamy, M.N., Leingang, K., and Bajaj, P.: Transcriptional expression of tissue factor pathway inhibitor in normal human tissues [abstract 1071]. Blood 82(suppl. 1):271a, 1993.

78. Bajaj, M.S., Kuppuswamy, M.N., Saito, H., Spitzer, S.G., and Bajaj, S.P.: Cultured normal human hepatocytes do not synthesize lipoprotein-associated coagulation inhibitor: evidence that endothelium is the principal site of its synthesis. Proc. Natl. Acad. Sci. USA 87:8869, 1990.

79. McGee, M.P., Foster, S., and Wang, X.: Simultaneous expression of tissue factor and tissue factor pathway inhibitor by human monocytes. J. Exp. Med. 179:1847, 1994.

80. Bajaj, M.S., Ameri, A., Kuppuswamy, M.N., and Bajaj, S.P.: Expression of tissue factor pathway inhibitor (TFPI) and GATA-2 transcription factor by activated human monocytes [abstract 1355]. Blood 82(suppl. 1):343a, 1993.

81. Lupu, C., Lupu, F., Dennehy, U., Kakkar, V.V., and Scully, M.F.: Thrombin induces the redistribution and acute release of tissue factor pathway inhibitor from specific granules within human endothelial cells in culture. Arterioscler. Thromb. 15:2055, 1995.

82. Sevinsky, J.R., Rao, L.V.M., and Ruf, W.: Ligand induced protease receptor translocation into caveolae: a mechanism for regulating cell surface proteolysis of the tissue factor–dependent coagulation pathway. J. Cell Biol. 133:293, 1996.

83. Yamabe, H., Osawa, H., Inuma, H., Kaizuka, M., Tamura, N., Tseunoda, S., Fujita, Y., Shirato, K., and Onodera, K.: Tissue factor pathway inhibitor production by human mesangial cells in culture. Thromb. Haemost. 76:215, 1996.

84. van der Logt, C.P.E., Dirven, R.J., Reitsma, P.H., and Bertina, R.M.: Expression of tissue factor and tissue factor pathway inhibitor in response to bacterial lipopolysaccharide and phorbol ester. Blood Coagul. Fibrinolysis 5:211, 1994.

85. Novotny, W.F., Girard, T.J., Miletich, J.P., and Broze, G.J., Jr.: Platelets secrete a coagulation inhibitor functionally and antigenically similar to the lipoprotein associated coagulation inhibitor. Blood 72:2020, 1988.

86. Palmier, M.O., Hall, L.J., Reisch, C.M., Baldwin, M.K., Wilson, A.G., and Wun, T.C.: Clearance of recombinant tissue factor pathway inhibitor (TFPI) in rabbits. Thromb. Haemost. 68:33, 1992.

87. Bregengaard, C., Nordfang, O., Ostergaard, P., Petersen, J.G.L., Meyn, G., Biness, V., Svendsen, O., and Hedner, U.: Pharmacokinetics of full-length and two-domain tissue factor pathway inhibitor in combination with heparin in rabbits. Thromb. Haemost. 70:454, 1993.

88. Warshawsky, I., Broze, G.J., Jr., and Schwartz, A.L.: The low density lipoprotein receptor-related protein mediates the cellular degradation of tissue factor pathway inhibitor. Proc. Natl. Acad. Sci. USA 91:6664, 1994.

89. Warshawsky, I., Bu, G., Mast, A., Saffitz, J.E., Broze, G.J., Jr., and Schwartz, A.L.: The carboxy-terminus of tissue factor pathway inhibitor is required for interacting with hepatoma cells in vitro and in vivo. J. Clin. Invest. 95:1773, 1995.

90. Warshawsky, I., Herz, J., Broze, G.J., Jr., and Schwartz, A.L.: The low density lipoprotein receptor-related protein can function independently from heparan sulfate proteoglycans in tissue factor pathway inhibitor endocytosis. J. Biol. Chem. 271:25873, 1996.

91. Valentin, S., and Schousboe, I.: Factor Xa enhances the binding of tissue factor pathway inhibitor to acidic phospholipids. Thromb. Haemost. 75:796, 1996.

92. Kojima, T., Ksumi, A., Yamazaki, T., Muramatsu, T., Nagasaka, T., Ohsumi, K., and Saito, H.: Human ryudocan from endothelium-like cells binds basic fibroblast growth factor, midkine, and tissue factor pathway inhibitor. J. Biol. Chem. 271:5914, 1996.

93. Valentin, S., Nordfang, O., Bregengard, C., and Wildgoose, P.: Evidence that the C-terminus of tissue factor pathway inhibitor (TFPI) is essential for its in vitro and in vivo interaction with lipoproteins. Blood Coagul. Fibrinolysis 4:713, 1993.

94. Narita, M., Bu, G., Olins, G.M., Higuchi, D.A., Herz, J., Broze, G.J., Jr., and Schwartz, A.: Two receptor systems are involved in the plasma clearance of tissue factor pathway inhibitor in vivo. J. Biol. Chem. 270:24800, 1995.

95. Kreiger, M., and Herz, J.: Structures and functions of multiligand lipoprotein receptors: macrophage scavenger receptors and LDL receptor-related protein (LRP). Annu. Rev. Biochem. 63:601, 1994.

96. Willnow, T.E., Goldstein, J.L., Orth, K., Brown, M.S., and Herz, L.: Low density lipoprotein receptor-related protein and gp330 bind similar ligands, including plasminogen activator-inhibitor complexes and lactoferrin, an inhibitor of chylomicron remnant clearance. J. Biol. Chem. 267:26172, 1992.

97. Ho, G., Toomey, J.R., Broze, G.J., Jr., and Schwartz, A.: Receptor-mediated endocytosis of coagulation factor Xa requires cell surface-bound tissue factor pathway inhibitor. J. Biol. Chem. 271:9497, 1996.

98. Kamikubo, Y., Hamuro, T., Matsuda, J., Kamei, S., Jyu-ri, K., Miyamoto, S., Funatsu, A., and Kato, H.: The clearance of proteoglycan-associated human recombinant tissue factor pathway inhibitor (h-rTFPI) in rabbits: a complex formation of h-rTFPI with factor Xa promotes a clearance rate of h-rTFPI. Thromb. Res. 83:161, 1996.

99. Brozna, J.P., Forman, M., and Carson, S.D.: Staurosporine blocks down-regulation of monocyte-associated tissue factor. Blood Coagul. Fibrinolysis 5:929, 1994.

100. Sandset, P.M., Abildgaard, U., and Larsen, M.L.: Heparin induces release of extrinsic coagulation pathway inhibitor (EPI). Thromb. Res. 50:803, 1988.

101. Novotny, W.F., Brown, S.G., Miletich, J.P., Rader, D.J., and Broze, G.J., Jr.: Plasma antigen levels of the lipoprotein-associated coagulation inhibitor in patient samples. Blood 78:387, 1991.

102. Warr, T.A., Warn-Cramer, B.J., Rao, L.V., and Rapaport, S.I.: Human plasma extrinsic pathway inhibitor activity: I. Standardization of assay and evaluation of physiologic variables. Blood 74:201, 1989.

103. Hubbard, A.R., and Jennings, C.A.: Inhibition of the tissue factor–factor VII complex: involvement of factor Xa and lipoproteins. Thromb. Res. 46:527, 1987.

104. Lesnik, P., Vonica, A., Guerin, M., Moreau, M., and Chapman, M.J.: Anticoagulant activity of tissue factor pathway inhibitor in human plasma is preferentially associated with dense subspecies of LDL and HDL and with Lp(a). Arterioscler. Thromb. 13:1066, 1993.

105. Sandset, P.M., Lund, H., Norseth, J., Abildgaard, U., and Ose, L.: Treatment with hydroxymethylglutaryl-coenzyme A reductase inhibitors in hypercholesterolemia induces changes in the components of the extrinsic coagulation system. Arterioscler. Thromb. 11:138, 1991.

106. Hansen, J.-B., Huseby, N.-E., Sandset, P.M., Svensson, B., Lyngmo, V., and Nordoy, A.: Tissue factor pathway inhibitor and lipoproteins. Evidence for association with and regulation by LDL in human plasma. Arterioscler. Thromb. 14:223, 1994.

107. Abumiya, T., Nakamura, S., Takenaka, A., Takenaka, O., Yoshikuni, Y., Miyamoto, S., Kimura, T., Enjoyoji, D., and Kato, H.: Response of plasma tissue factor pathway inhibitor to diet-induced hypercholesterolemia in crab-eating monkeys. Arterioscler. Thromb. 14:483, 1994.

108. Hansen, J.-B., Huseby, K.R., Huseby, N.E., Sandset, P.M., Hanssen, T.-A., and Nordoy, A.: Effect of cholesterol lowering on intravascular pools of TFPI and its anticoagulant potential in type II hyperlipoproteinemia. Arterioscler. Thromb. Vasc. Biol. 15:879, 1995.

109. Moor, E., Hamsten, A., Karpe, F., Bavenholm, P., Blomback, M., and Silveira, A.: Relationship of tissue factor pathway inhibitor activity to plasma lipoproteins and myocardial infarction at a young age. Thromb. Haemost. 71:707, 1994.

110. Warn-Cramer, B.J., Maki, S.L., Zivelin, A., and Rapaport, S.I.: Partial

purification and characterization of extrinsic pathway inhibitor (the factor Xa–dependent plasma inhibitor of factor VIIa/tissue factor). Thromb. Res. 48:11, 1987.

111. Broze, G.J., Jr., Lange, G.W., Duffin, K.L., and MacPhail, L.: Heterogeneity of plasma tissue factor pathway inhibitor. Blood Coagul. Fibrinolysis 5:551, 1994.

112. Lesnik, P., Dentan, C., Vonica, A., Moreau, M., and Chapman, M.J.: Tissue factor pathway inhibitor activity associated with LDL is inactivated by cell- and copper-mediated oxidation. Arterioscler. Thromb. Vasc. Biol. 15:1121, 1995.

113. Kokawa, T., Abumiya, T., Kimura, T., Harada-Shiba, M., Koh, H., Tsushima, M., Yamamoto, A., and Kato, H.: Tissue factor pathway inhibitor activity in human plasma. Measurement of lipoprotein-associated and free forms in hyperlipidemia. Arterioscler. Thromb. 15:504, 1995.

114. Abumiya, T., Enjyoji, K., Kokawa, T., Kamikubo, Y., and Kato, H.: An anti-tissue factor pathway inhibitor (TFPI) monoclonal antibody recognized the third Kunitz domain (K3) of free-form TFPI but not lipoprotein-associated forms in plasma. J. Biochem. 118:178, 1995.

115. Hansen, J.B., Sandset, P.M., Huseby, K.R., Huseby, N.E., and Nordoy, A.: Depletion of intravascular pools of tissue factor pathway inhibitor (TFPI) during repeated or continuous intravenous infusion of heparin in man. Thromb. Haemost. 76:703, 1996.

116. Holst, J., Lindblad, B., Bergqvist, D., Hedner, U., Garre, K., Nordfang, O., and Ostergaard, P.: Effect of protamine sulfate on tissue factor pathway inhibitor released by iv or sc standard or low molecular weight heparin. Thromb. Haemost. 69:1114, 1993.

117. Harenberg, J., Siegele, M., Dempfle, C.-E., Stehle, G., and Heene, D.L.: Protamine neutralization of the release of tissue factor pathway inhibitor activity by heparins. Thromb. Haemost. 70:942, 1993.

118. Hubbard, A.R., Weller, I.J., and Gray, E.: Measurement of tissue factor pathway inhibitor in normal and post-heparin plasma. Blood Coagul. Fibrinolysis 5:819, 1994.

119. Ariens, R.A.S., Coppola, R., Potenza, I., and Mannucci, P.M.: The increase with age of the components of the tissue factor coagulation pathway is gender-dependent. Blood Coagul. Fibrinolysis 6:433, 1995.

120. Sandset, P.M., Larsen, M.L., Abildgaard, U., Lindahl, A.K., and Odegaard, O.R.: Chromogenic substrate assay of extrinsic pathway inhibitor (EPI): levels in the normal population and relation to cholesterol. Blood Coagul. Fibrinolysis 2:425, 1991.

121. Reverdiau-Moalic, P., Delahousse, B., Body, G., Bardos, P., Leroy, J., and Gruel, Y.: Evolution of blood coagulation activators and inhibitors in the healthy human fetus. Blood 88:900, 1996.

122. Sandset, P.M., and Andersson, T.R.: Coagulation inhibitor levels in pneumonia and stroke: changes due to consumption and acute phase reaction. J. Intern. Med. 225:311, 1989.

123. Sandset, P.M., Hellgren, M., Uvebrandt, M., and Bergstrom, H.: Extrinsic coagulation pathway inhibitor and heparin cofactor II during normal and hypertensive pregnancy. Thromb. Res. 55:6645, 1989.

124. Abildgaard, U., Sandset, P.M., Andersson, T.R., Odegaard, O.R., and Rosen, S.: The inhibitor of TF VIIa in plasma measured with a sensitive chromogenic substrate assay: comparison with antithrombin, protein C and heparin cofactor II in a clinical material. Folia Haematol. Int. Magazin Klin. Morphol. Blutforsch. 115:274, 1988.

125. Lindahl, A.K., Sandset, P.M., Abildgaard, U., Andersson, T.R., and Harbitz, T.B.: High plasma levels of extrinsic pathway inhibitor and low levels of other coagulation inhibitors in advanced cancer. Acta Chirurg. Scand. 155:389, 1989.

126. Kario, K., Matsuo, T., Yamada, T., and Matsuo, M.: Increased tissue factor pathway inhibitor levels in uremic patients on regular hemodialysis. Thromb. Haemost. 71:275, 1994.

127. Sandset, P.M., Hellgren, U., Uvebrandt, M., and Bergstrom, H.: Extrinsic pathway inhibitor and heparin cofactor II during normal and hypertension pregnancy. Thromb. Res. 55:6645, 1989.

128. Kobayashi, M., Wada, H., Wakita, Y., Shimura, M., Nakase, T., Hiyoyama, K., Nagaya, S., Minami, N., Nakano, T., and Shiku, H.: Decreased plasma tissue factor pathway inhibitor levels in patients with thrombotic thrombocytopenic purpura. Thromb. Haemost. 73:10, 1995.

129. Rapaport, S.I.: The extrinsic pathway inhibitor: a regulator of tissue factor–dependent blood coagulation [review]. Thromb. Haemost. 66:6, 1991.

130. Bajaj, M.S., Rana, S.V., Wysolmerski, R.B., and Bajaj, S.P.: Inhibitor of the factor VIIa–tissue factor complex is reduced in patients with disseminated intravascular coagulation but not in patients with severe hepatocellular disease. J. Clin. Invest. 79:1874, 1987.

131. Warr, T.A., Rao, L.V., and Rapaport, S.I.: Human plasma extrinsic pathway inhibitor activity: II. Plasma levels in disseminated intravascular coagulation and hepatocellular disease. Blood 74:994, 1989.

132. Brandtzaeg, P., Sandset, P.M., Joo, G.B., Ovstebo, R., Abildgaard, U., and Kierulf, P.: The quantitative association of plasma endotoxin, antithrombin, protein C, extrinsic pathway inhibitor and fibrinopeptide A in systemic meningococcal disease. Thromb. Res. 55:459, 1989.

133. Yakahashi, H., Sato, N., and Shibata, A.: Plasma tissue factor pathway inhibitor in disseminated intravascular coagulation: comparison of its behavior with plasma tissue factor. Thromb. Res. 80:339, 1995.

134. Sandset, P.M., Rosio, O., Aasen, A.O., and Abildgaard, U.: Extrinsic pathway inhibitor in postoperative/posttraumatic septicemia: increased levels in fatal cases. Haemostasis 19:189, 1989.

135. Sandset, P.M., Sirnes, P.A., and Abildgaard, U.: Factor VII and extrinsic pathway inhibitor in acute coronary disease. Br. J. Haematol. 72:391, 1989.

136. Abumiya, T., Yamaguchi, T., Terasaki, T., Kokawa, T., Kario, K., and Kato, H.: Decreased plasma tissue factor pathway inhibitor activity in ischemic stroke patients. Thromb. Haemost. 74:1050, 1995.

137. Holst, J., Lindblad, B., Wedeberg, E., Bergqvist, D., Nordfang, O., Ostergaard, P.B., and Hedner, U.: Tissue factor pathway inhibitor (TFPI) and its response to heparin in patients with spontaneous deep vein thrombosis. Thromb. Res. 72:467, 1993.

138. Llobet, D., Falkon, L., Mateo, J., Vallve, C., Martinez, E., Fontcuberta, J., and Borrell, M.: Low levels of tissue factor pathway inhibitor (TFPI) in two out of three members of a family with thrombophilia. Thromb. Res. 80:413, 1995.

139. Sandset, P.M., Warn-Cramer, B.J., Rao, L.V., Maki, S.L., and Rapaport, S.I.: Depletion of extrinsic pathway inhibitor (EPI) sensitizes rabbits to disseminated intravascular coagulation induced with tissue factor: evidence supporting a physiologic role for EPI as a natural anticoagulant. Proc. Natl. Acad. Sci. USA 88:708, 1991.

140. Sandset, P.M., Warn-Cramer, B.J., Maki, S.L., and Rapaport, S.I.: Immunodepletion of extrinsic pathway inhibitor sensitizes rabbits to endotoxin-induced intravascular coagulation and the generalized Shwartzman reaction. Blood 78:1496, 1991.

141. Warn-Cramer, B.J., and Rapaport, S.I.: Studies of factor Xa/phospholipid induced intravascular coagulation in rabbits. Effects of immunodepletion of tissue factor pathway inhibitor. Arterioscler. Thromb. 13:1551, 1993.

142. Huang, Z.-F., Higuchi, D.A., Lasky, N.M., and Broze, G.J., Jr.: Tissue-factor pathway inhibitor (TFPI) gene-deletion in mice produces intrauterine lethality. Blood 88(suppl.):470a, 1996.

143. Suh, T.T., Holmback, K., Jensen, N.J., Daugherty, C.C., Small, K., Simon, D.I., Potter, S., and Degen, J.L.: Resolution of spontaneous bleeding events but failure of pregnancy in fibrinogen-deficient mice. Genes Dev. 9:2020, 1995.

144. Vu, T.K., Hung, D.T., Wheaton, V.I., and Coughlin, S.R.: Molecular cloning of a functional thrombin receptor reveals a novel proteolytic mechanism of receptor activation. Cell 64:1057, 1991.

145. Naito, K., and Fujikawa, K.: Activation of human blood coagulation factor XI independent of factor XII. Factor XI is activated by thrombin and factor XIa in the presence of negatively charged surfaces. J. Biol. Chem. 266:7353, 1991.

146. Gailani, D., and Broze, G.J., Jr.: Factor XI activation in a revised model of blood coagulation. Science 253:909, 1991.

147. Bajzar, L., Manuel, R., and Nesheim, M.E.: Purification and characterization of TAFI, a thrombin-activatable fibrinolysis inhibitor. J. Biol. Chem. 270:14477, 1995.

148. Esmon, C.T., and Fukudome, K.: Cellular regulation of the protein C pathway. Semin. Cell Biol. 6:259, 1995.

149. Chen, L.B., and Buchanan, J.M.: Mitogenic activity of blood components. I. Thrombin and prothrombin. Proc. Natl. Acad. Sci. USA 72:131, 1975.

150. Glenn, K.C., Carney, D.H., Fenton, J.W., II, and Cunningham, D.D.: Thrombin active site regions required for fibroblast receptor binding and initiation of cell division. J. Biol. Chem. 255:6609, 1980.

151. Bar-Shavit, R., Kahn, A.J., Mann, K.G., and Wilner, G.D.: Identification of a thrombin sequence with growth factor activity on macrophages. Proc. Natl. Acad. Sci. USA 83:976, 1986.

152. Bar-Shavit, R., Kahn, A., Wilner, G.D., and Fenton, J.W., II: Monocyte chemotaxis: stimulation by specific exosite region in thrombin. Science 220:728, 1983.

153. Krishnaswamy, S., Church, W.R., Nesheim, M.E., and Mann, K.G.: Activation of human prothrombin by human prothrombinase. Influence

of factor Va on the reaction mechanism. J. Biol. Chem. 262:3291, 1987.

154. Doyle, M.F., and Mann, K.G.: Multiple active forms of thrombin. IV. Relative activities of meizothrombins. J. Biol. Chem. 265:10693, 1990.

155. Stevens, W.K., Côté, H.C.F., MacGillivray, R.T.A., and Neisheim, M.E.: Calcium ion modulation of meizothrombin autolysis at Arg55-Asp56 and catalytic activity. J. Biol. Chem. 271:8062, 1996.

156. Côté, H.C.F., Bajzar, L., Stevens, W.K., Samis, J.A., Morser, J., MacGillivray, R.T.A., and Nesheim, M.E.: Functional characterization of recombinant human meizothrombin and meizothrombin(desF1). Thrombomodulin-dependent activation of protein C and thrombin-activatable fibrinolysis inhibitor (TAFI), platelet aggregation, anti-thrombin-III inhibition. J. Biol. Chem. 272:6194, 1997.

157. Hackeng, T.M., Tans, G., Koppelman, S.J., de Groot, P.G., Rosing, J., and Bouma, B.N.: Protein C activation on endothelial cells by pro-thrombin activation products generated in situ: meizothrombin is a better protein C activator than α-thrombin. Biochem. J. 319:399, 1996.

158. Han, J.-H., Côté, H.C.F., and Tollefsen, D.M.: Inhibition of mei-zothrombin and meizothrombin(desF1) by heparin cofactor II. J. Biol. Chem. 272:28660, 1997.

159. Rezaie, A.R., Cooper, S.T., Church, F.C., and Esmon, C.T.: Protein C inhibitor is a potent inhibitor of the thrombin-thrombomodulin complex. J. Biol. Chem. 270:25336, 1995.

160. Thaler, E., and Lechner, K.: Antithrombin III deficiency and thrombo-embolism. Clin. Haematol. 10:369, 1981.

161. Cosgriff, T.M., Bishop, D.T., Hershgold, E.J., Skolnick, M.H., Martin, B.A., Baty, B.J., and Carlson, K.S.: Familial antithrombin III defi-ciency: its natural history, genetics, diagnosis and treatment. Medicine (Baltimore) 62:209, 1983.

162. Egeberg, O.: Inherited antithrombin deficiency causing thrombophilia. Thromb. Diath. Haemorrh. 13:516, 1965.

163. Rosenberg, R.D.: Regulation of the hemostatic mechanism. In Stama-toyannopoulos, G., et al.: The Molecular Basis of Blood Diseases. Philadelphia, W.B. Saunders Co., 1987, pp. 534–574.

164. Carrell, R.W., and Boswell, D.R.: Serpins: the superfamily of plasma serine proteinase inhibitors. In Barrett, A.J., and Salveson, G.: Protein-ase Inhibitors. Amsterdam, Elsevier Science, 1986, pp. 403–420.

165. Petersen, T.E., Dudek-Wojciechowska, G., Sottrup-Jensen, L., and Magnusson, S.: Primary structure of antithrombin-III (heparin cofac-tor). Partial homology between α₁-antitrypsin and antithrombin-III. In Collen, D., Wiman, B., and Verstraete, M.: The Physiological Inhibi-tors of Coagulation and Fibrinolysis. Amsterdam, Elsevier/North Hol-land, 1979, pp. 43–54.

166. Bock, S.C., Wion, K.L., Vehar, G.A., and Lawn, R.M.: Cloning and expression of the cDNA for human antithrombin III. Nucleic Acids Res. 10:8113, 1982.

167. Prochownik, E.V., Markham, A.F., and Orkin, S.H.: Isolation of a cDNA clone for human antithrombin III. J. Biol. Chem. 258:8389, 1983.

168. Stackhouse, R., Chandra, T., Robson, K.J., and Woo, S.L.: Purification of antithrombin III mRNA and cloning of its cDNA. J. Biol. Chem. 258:703, 1983.

169. Sun, X.J., and Chang, J.Y.: Heparin binding domain of human anti-thrombin III inferred from the sequential reduction of its three disul-fide linkages. An efficient method for structural analysis of partially reduced proteins. J. Biol. Chem. 264:11288, 1989.

170. Franzén, L.-E., Svensson, S., and Larm, O.: Structural studies on the carbohydrate portion of human antithrombin III. J. Biol. Chem. 255:5090, 1980.

171. Peterson, C.B., and Blackburn, M.N.: Isolation and characterization of an antithrombin III variant with reduced carbohydrate content and enhanced heparin binding. J. Biol. Chem. 260:610, 1985.

172. Brennan, S.O., George, P.M., and Jordan, R.E.: Physiological variant of antithrombin-III lacks carbohydrate sidechain at Asn 135. FEBS Lett. 219:431, 1987.

173. Picard, V., Ersdal-Badju, E., and Bock, S.C.: Partial glycosylation of antithrombin III asparagine-135 is caused by the serine in the third position of its N-glycosylation consensus sequence and is responsible for production of the β-antithrombin III isoform with enhanced hepa-rin affinity. Biochemistry 34:8433, 1995.

174. Bock, S.C., Harris, J.F., Balazs, I., and Trent, J.M.: Assignment of the human antithrombin III structural gene to chromosome 1q23–25. Cytogenet. Cell Genet. 39:67, 1985.

175. Olds, R.J., Lane, D.A., Chowdury, V., De Stefano, V., Leone, G., and

Thein, S.L.: Complete nucleotide sequence of the antithrombin gene. Evidence for homologous recombination causing thrombophilia. Bio-chemistry 32:4216, 1993.

176. Fair, D.S., and Bahnak, B.R.: Human hepatoma cells secrete single chain factor X, prothrombin, and antithrombin III. Blood 64:194, 1984.

177. Prochownik, E.V., and Orkin, S.H.: In vivo transcription of a human antithrombin III "minigene." J. Biol. Chem. 259:15386, 1984.

178. D'Souza, S.E., and Mercer, J.F.: Antithrombin III mRNA in adult rat liver and kidney and in rat liver during development. Biochem. Bio-phys. Res. Commun. 142:417, 1987.

179. Bock, S.C., and Levitan, D.J.: Characterization of an unusual DNA length polymorphism 5' to the human antithrombin III gene. Nucleic Acids Res. 11:8569, 1983.

180. Winter, P.C., Scopes, D.A., Berg, L.-P., Millar, D.S., Kakkar, V.V., Mayne, E.E., Krawczak, M., and Cooper, D.N.: Functional analysis of an unusual length polymorphism in the human antithrombin III (AT3) gene promoter. Blood Coagul. Fibrinolysis 6:659, 1995.

181. Prochownik, E.V.: Relationship between an enhancer element in the human antithrombin III gene and an immunoglobulin light-chain gene enhancer. Nature 316:845, 1985.

182. Tremp, G.L., Duchange, N., Branellec, D., Cereghini, S., Tailleux, A., Berthou, L., Fievet, C., Touchet, N., Schombert, B., Fruchart, J.-C., et al.: A 700-bp fragment of the human antithrombin III promoter is sufficient to confer high, tissue-specific expression on human apolipo-protein A-II in transgenic mice. Gene 156:199, 1995.

183. Fernandez-Rachubinski, F.A., Weiner, J.H., and Blajchman, M.A.: Regions flanking exon 1 regulate constitutive expression of the human antithrombin gene. J. Biol. Chem. 271:29502, 1996.

184. Hoffman, M., Fuchs, H.E., and Pizzo, S.V.: The macrophage-mediated regulation of hepatocyte synthesis of antithrombin III and alpha 1-proteinase inhibitor. Thromb. Res. 41:707, 1986.

185. Rosenberg, R.D.: Biologic actions of heparin. Semin. Hematol. 14:427, 1977.

186. Highsmith, R.F., and Rosenberg, R.D.: The inhibition of human plas-min by human antithrombin-heparin cofactor. J. Biol. Chem. 249:4335, 1974.

187. Downing, M.R., Bloom, J.W., and Mann, K.G.: Comparison of the inhibition of thrombin by three plasma protease inhibitors. Biochemis-try 17:2649, 1978.

188. Fuchs, H.E., Trapp, H.G., Griffith, M.J., Roberts, H.R., and Pizzo, S.V.: Regulation of factor IXa in vitro in human and mouse plasma and in vivo in the mouse. Role of the endothelium and the plasma proteinase inhibitors. J. Clin. Invest. 73:1696, 1984.

189. Gitel, S.N., Medina, V.M., and Wessler, S.: Inhibition of human activated factor X by antithrombin III and alpha 1-proteinase inhibitor in human plasma. J. Biol. Chem. 259:6890, 1984.

190. Scott, C.F., Schapira, M., James, H.L., Cohen, A.B., and Colman, R.W.: Inactivation of factor XIa by plasma protease inhibitors: pre-dominant role of alpha 1-protease inhibitor and protective effect of high molecular weight kininogen. J. Clin. Invest. 69:844, 1982.

191. de Agostini, A., Lijnen, H.R., Pixley, R.A., Colman, R.W., and Schap-ira, M.: Inactivation of factor XII active fragment in normal plasma. Predominant role of C1-inhibitor. J. Clin. Invest. 73:1542, 1984.

192. Wiman, B., and Collen, D.: On the kinetics of the reaction between human antiplasmin and plasmin. Eur. J. Biochem. 84:573, 1978.

193. Rao, L.V.M., Rapaport, S.I., and Hoang, A.D.: Binding of factor VIIa to tissue factor permits rapid antithrombin III/heparin inhibition of factor VIIa. Blood 81:2600, 1993.

194. Rao, L.V.M., Nordfang, O., Hoang, A.D., and Pendurthi, U.R.: Mecha-nism of antithrombin III inhibition of factor Xa/tissue factor activity on cell surfaces. Comparison with tissue factor pathway inhibitor/factor Xa–induced inhibition of factor VIIa/tissue factor activity. Blood 85:121, 1995.

195. Suzuki, K., Nishioka, J., and Hashimoto, S.: Protein C inhibitor: purification from human plasma and characterization. J. Biol. Chem. 258:163, 1983.

196. Rosenberg, R.D., and Damus, P.S.: The purification and mechanism of action of human antithrombin-heparin cofactor. J. Biol. Chem. 248:6490, 1973.

197. Fish, W.W., and Björk, I.: Release of a two-chain form of antithrombin from the antithombin-thrombin complex. Eur. J. Biochem. 101:31, 1979.

198. Björk, I., Jackson, C.M., Jörnvall, H., Lavine, K.K., Nordling, K., and Salsgiver, W.J.: The active site of antithrombin. Release of the same

proteolytically cleaved form of the inhibitor from complexes with factor IXa, factor Xa, and thrombin. J. Biol. Chem. 257:2406, 1982.

199. Owen, W.G.: Evidence for the formation of an ester between thrombin and heparin cofactor. Biochim. Biophys. Acta 405:380, 1975.

200. Stein, P.E., Leslie, A.G.W., Finch, J.T., Turnell, W.G., McLaughlin, P.J., and Carrell, R.W.: Crystal structure of ovalbumin as a model for the reactive centre of serpins. Nature 347:99, 1990.

201. Carrell, R.W., and Owen, M.C.: Plakalbumin, α_1-antitrypsin, antithrombin and the mechanism of inflammatory thrombosis. Nature 317:730, 1985.

202. Huber, R., and Carrell, R.W.: Implications of the three-dimensional structure of α_1-antitrypsin for structure and function of serpins. Biochemistry 28:8951, 1989.

203. Perry, P.J., Harper, P.L., Fairham, S., Daly, M., and Carrell, R.W.: Antithrombin Cambridge, 384 Ala to Pro: a new variant identified using the polymerase chain reaction. FEBS Lett. 254:174, 1989.

204. Austin, R.C., Rachubinski, R.A., Ofosu, F.A., and Blajchman, M.A.: Antithrombin-III-Hamilton, Ala 382 to Thr: an antithrombin-III variant that acts as a substrate but not an inhibitor of α-thrombin and factor Xa. Blood 77:2185, 1991.

205. Asakura, S., Hirata, H., Okazaki, H., Hashimoto-Gotoh, T., and Matsuda, M.: Hydrophobic residues 382–386 of antithrombin III, Ala-Ala-Ala-Ser-Thr, serve as the epitope for an antibody which facilitates hydrolysis of the inhibitor by thrombin. J. Biol. Chem. 265:5135, 1990.

206. Carrell, R.W., Evans, D.L., and Stein, P.E.: Mobile reactive centre of serpins and the control of thrombosis. Nature 353:576, 1991.

207. Björk, I., Ylinenjärvi, K., Olson, S.T., and Bock, P.E.: Conversion of antithrombin from an inhibitor of thrombin to a substrate with reduced heparin affinity and enhanced conformational stability by binding of a tetradecapeptide corresponding to the P1 to P14 region of the putative reactive bond loop of the inhibitor. J. Biol. Chem. 267:1976, 1992.

208. Schreuder, H.A., de Boer, B., Dijkema, R., Mulders, J., Theunissen, H.J., Grootenhuis, P.D., and Hol, W.G.: The intact and cleaved human antithrombin III complex as a model for serpin-proteinase interactions. Nat. Struct. Biol. 1:48, 1994.

209. Carrell, R.W., Stein, P.E., Fermi, G., and Wardell, M.R.: Biological implications of a 3 Å structure of dimeric antithrombin. Structure 2:257, 1994.

210. Skinner, R., Abrahams, J.-P., Whisstock, J.C., Lesk, A.M., Carrell, R.W., and Wardell, M.R.: The 2.6 Å structure of antithrombin indicates a conformational change at the heparin binding site. J. Mol. Biol. 266:601, 1997.

211. Jin, L., Abrahams, J.P., Skinner, R., Petitou, M., Pike, R.N., and Carrell, R.W.: The anticoagulant activation of antithrombin by heparin. Proc. Natl. Acad. Sci. USA 94:14683, 1997.

212. Jordan, R.E., Oosta, G.M., Gardner, W.T., and Rosenberg, R.D.: The kinetics of hemostatic enzyme-antithrombin interactions in the presence of low molecular weight heparin. J. Biol. Chem. 255:10081, 1980.

213. Lindahl, U., Kusche, M., Lidholt, K., and Oscarsson, L.-G.: Biosynthesis of heparin and heparan sulfate. Ann. N. Y. Acad. Sci. 556:36, 1989.

214. Conrad, H.E.: Heparin-Binding Proteins. San Diego, Academic Press, 1998, pp. 22–47.

215. Teien, A.N., Abildgaard, U., and Höök, M.: The anticoagulant effect of heparan sulfate and dermatan sulfate. Thromb. Res. 8:859, 1976.

216. Conrad, H.E.: Structure of heparan sulfate and dermatan sulfate. Ann. N. Y. Acad. Sci. 556:18, 1989.

217. Höök, M., Björk, I., Hopwood, J., and Lindahl, U.: Anticoagulant activity of heparin: separation of high-activity and low-activity species by affinity chromatography on immobilized antithrombin. FEBS Lett. 66:90, 1976.

218. Andersson, L.-O., Barrowcliffe, T.W., Holmer, E., Johnson, E.A., and Sims, G.E.C.: Anticoagulant properties of heparin fractionated by affinity chromatography on matrix-bound antithrombin III and by gel filtration. Thromb. Res. 9:575, 1976.

219. Lam, L.H., Silbert, J.E., and Rosenberg, R.D.: The separation of active and inactive forms of heparin. Biochem. Biophys. Res. Commun. 69:570, 1976.

220. Jordan, R., Beeler, D., and Rosenberg, R.: Fractionation of low molecular weight heparin species and their interaction with antithrombin. J. Biol. Chem. 254:2902, 1979.

221. Olson, S.T., Srinivasan, K.R., Björk, I., and Shore, J.D.: Binding of high affinity heparin to antithrombin III. Stopped flow kinetic studies of the binding interaction. J. Biol. Chem. 256:11073, 1981.

222. Choay, J., Petitou, M., Lormeau, J.C., Sinay, P., Casu, B., and Gatti, G.: Structure-activity relationship in heparin: a synthetic pentasaccharide with high affinity for antithrombin III and eliciting high anti-factor Xa activity. Biochem. Biophys. Res. Commun. 116:492, 1983.

223. Lindahl, U., Thunberg, L., Bäckström, G., Riesenfeld, J., Nordling, K., and Björk, I.: Extension and structural variability of the antithrombin-binding sequence in heparin. J. Biol. Chem. 259:12368, 1984.

224. Atha, D.H., Lormeau, J.C., Petitou, M., Rosenberg, R.D., and Choay, J.: Contribution of monosaccharide residues in heparin binding to antithrombin III. Biochemistry 24:6723, 1985.

225. Tollefsen, D.M., Pestka, C.A., and Monafo, W.J.: Activation of heparin cofactor II by dermatan sulfate. J. Biol. Chem. 258:6713, 1983.

226. Pecon, J.M., and Blackburn, M.N.: Pyridoxylation of essential lysines in the heparin-binding site of antithrombin III. J. Biol. Chem. 259:935, 1984.

227. Peterson, C.B., Noyes, C.M., Pecon, J.M., Church, F.C., and Blackburn, M.N.: Identification of a lysyl residue in antithrombin which is essential for heparin binding. J. Biol. Chem. 262:8061, 1987.

228. Turk, B., Brieditis, I., Bock, S.C., Olson, S.T., and Bjork, I.: The oligosaccharide side chain on Asn-135 of alpha-antithrombin, absent in beta-antithrombin, decreases the heparin affinity of the inhibitor by affecting the heparin-induced conformational change. Biochemistry 36:6682, 1997.

229. Blackburn, M.N., Smith, R.L., Carson, J., and Sibley, C.C.: The heparin-binding site of antithrombin III. Identification of a critical tryptophan in the amino acid sequence. J. Biol. Chem. 259:939, 1984.

230. Koide, T., Odani, S., Takahashi, K., Ono, T., and Sakuragawa, N.: Antithrombin III Toyama: replacement of arginine-47 by cysteine in hereditary abnormal antithrombin III that lacks heparin-binding ability. Proc. Natl. Acad. Sci. USA 81:289, 1984.

231. Owen, M.C., Borg, J.Y., Soria, C., Soria, J., Caen, J., and Carrell, R.W.: Heparin binding defect in a new antithrombin III variant: Rouen, 47 Arg to His. Blood 69:1275, 1987.

232. Chang, J.Y., and Tran, T.H.: Antithrombin III Basel. Identification of a Pro-Leu substitution in a hereditary abnormal antithrombin with impaired heparin cofactor activity. J. Biol. Chem. 261:1174, 1986.

233. Olson, S.T., and Shore, J.D.: Transient kinetics of heparin-catalyzed protease inactivation by antithrombin III. The reaction step limiting heparin turnover in thrombin neutralization. J. Biol. Chem. 261:13151, 1986.

234. Nordenman, B., and Björk, I.: Binding of low-affinity and high-affinity heparin to antithrombin. Ultraviolet difference spectroscopy and circular dichroism studies. Biochemistry 17:3339, 1978.

235. Einarsson, R., and Andersson, L.-O.: Binding of heparin to human antithrombin III as studied by measurements of tryptophan fluorescence. Biochim. Biophys. Acta 490:104, 1977.

236. Olson, S.T., and Shore, J.D.: Binding of high affinity heparin to antithrombin III. Characterization of the protein fluorescence enhancement. J. Biol. Chem. 256:11065, 1981.

237. Stone, A.L., Beeler, D., Oosta, G., and Rosenberg, R.D.: Circular dichroism spectroscopy of heparin-antithrombin interactions. Proc. Natl. Acad. Sci. USA 79:7190, 1982.

238. Horne, A.P., and Gettins, P.: ^{1}H NMR spectroscopic studies on the interactions between human plasma antithrombin III and defined low molecular weight heparin fragments. Biochemistry 31:2286, 1992.

239. Gettins, P.G.W., Fan, B., Crews, B.C., Turko, I.V., Olson, S.T., and Streusand, V.J.: Transmission of conformational change from the heparin binding site to the reactive center of antithrombin. Biochemistry 32:8385, 1993.

240. Dawes, J., James, K., and Lane, D.A.: Conformational change in antithrombin induced by heparin, probed with a monoclonal antibody against the 1C/4B region. Biochemistry 33:4375, 1994.

241. Huntington, J.A., Olson, S.T., Fan, B., and Gettins, P.G.: Mechanism of heparin activation of antithrombin. Evidence for reactive center loop preinsertion with expulsion upon heparin binding. Biochemistry 35:8495, 1996.

242. Pike, R.N., Potempa, J., Skinner, R., Fitton, H.L., McGraw, W.T., Travis, J., Owen, M., Jin, L., and Carrell, R.W.: Heparin-dependent modification of the reactive center arginine of antithrombin and consequent increase in heparin binding affinity. J. Biol. Chem. 272:19652, 1997.

243. Oosta, G.M., Gardner, W.T., Beeler, D.L., and Rosenberg, R.D.: Multiple functional domains of the heparin molecule. Proc. Natl. Acad. Sci. USA 78:829, 1981.

244. Pomerantz, M.W., and Owen, W.G.: A catalytic role for heparin. Evidence for a ternary complex of heparin cofactor, thrombin and heparin. Biochim. Biophys. Acta 535:66, 1978.

245. Danielsson, Å., Raub, E., Lindahl, U., and Björk, I.: Role of ternary complexes, in which heparin binds both antithrombin and proteinase, in the acceleration of the reactions between antithrombin and thrombin or factor Xa. J. Biol. Chem. 261:15467, 1986.

246. Olson, S.T., Björk, I., Sheffer, R., Craig, P.A., Shore, J.D., and Choay, J.: Role of the antithrombin-binding pentasaccharide in heparin acceleration of antithrombin-proteinase reactions. Resolution of the antithrombin conformational change contribution to heparin rate enhancement. J. Biol. Chem. 267:12528, 1992.

247. Olson, S.T., and Björk, I.: Predominant contribution of surface approximation to the mechanism of heparin acceleration of the antithrombin-thrombin reaction. Elucidation from salt concentration effects. J. Biol. Chem. 266:6353, 1991.

248. Lollar, P., and Owen, W.G.: Clearance of thrombin from the circulation in rabbits by high-affinity binding sites on the endothelium. Possible role in the inactivation of thrombin by antithrombin III. J. Clin. Invest. 66:1222, 1980.

249. Boisclair, M.D., Lane, D.A., Wilde, J.T., Ireland, H., Preston, F.E., and Ofosu, F.A.: A comparative evaluation of assays for markers of activated coagulation and/or fibrinolysis: thrombin-antithrombin complex, D-dimer and fibrinogen/fibrin fragment E antigen. Br. J. Haematol. 74:471, 1990.

250. Deguchi, K., Noguchi, M., Yuwasaki, E., Endou, T., Deguchi, A., Wada, H., Murashima, S., Nishikawa, M., Shirakawa, S., Tanaka, K., et al.: Dynamic fluctuations in blood of thrombin/antithrombin III complex (TAT). Am. J. Hematol. 38:86, 1991.

251. Fuchs, H.E., and Pizzo, S.V.: Regulation of factor Xa in vitro in human and mouse plasma and in vivo in mouse. Role of the endothelium and plasma proteinase inhibitors. J. Clin. Invest. 72:2041, 1983.

252. Miletich, J.P., Jackson, C.M., and Majerus, P.W.: Properties of the factor Xa binding site on human platelets. J. Biol. Chem. 253:6908, 1978.

253. Lindhout, T., Baruch, D., Schoen, P., Franssen, J., and Hemker, H.C.: Thrombin generation and inactivation in the presence of antithrombin III and heparin. Biochemistry 25:5962, 1986.

254. Gouin-Thibault, I., Dewar, L., Kulczycky, M., Sternbach, M., and Ofosu, F.A.: Measurement of factor Xa–antithrombin III in plasma: relationship to prothrombin activation in vivo. Br. J. Haematol. 90:669, 1995.

255. Shifman, M.A., and Pizzo, S.V.: The in vivo metabolism of antithrombin III and antithrombin III complexes. J. Biol. Chem. 257:3243, 1982.

256. Collen, D., de Cock, F., and Verstraete, M.: Quantitation of thrombin–antithrombin III complexes in human blood. Eur. J. Clin. Invest. 7:407, 1977.

257. Fuchs, H.E., Shifman, M.A., Michalopoulos, G., and Pizzo, S.V.: Hepatocyte receptors for antithrombin III–proteinase complexes. J. Cell. Biochem. 24:197, 1984.

258. Pizzo, S.V., Mast, A.E., Feldman, S.R., and Salvesen, G.: In vivo catabolism of a₁-antichymotrypsin is mediated by the serpin receptor which binds a₁-proteinase inhibitor, antithrombin III and heparin cofactor II. Biochim. Biophys. Acta 967:158, 1988.

259. Kounnas, M.Z., Church, F.C., Argraves, W.S., and Strickland, D.K.: Cellular internalization and degradation of antithrombin III–thrombin, heparin cofactor II–thrombin, and α₁-antitrypsin–trypsin complexes is mediated by the low density lipoprotein receptor-related protein. J. Biol. Chem. 271:6523, 1996.

260. Ill, C.R., and Ruoslahti, E.: Association of thrombin–antithrombin III complex with vitronectin in serum. J. Biol. Chem. 260:15610, 1985.

261. de Boer, H.C., Preissner, K.T., Bouma, B.N., and de Groot, P.G.: Binding of vitronectin–thrombin–antithrombin III complex to human endothelial cells is mediated by the heparin binding site of vitronectin. J. Biol. Chem. 267:2264, 1992.

262. van Iwaarden, F., Acton, D.S., Sixma, J.J., Meijers, J.C.M., de Groot, P.G., and Bouma, B.N.: Internalization of antithrombin III by cultured human endothelial cells and its subcellular localization. J. Lab. Clin. Med. 113:717, 1989.

263. Nenci, G.G., Berrettini, M., Parise, P., and Agnelli, G.: Persistent spontaneous heparinaemia in systemic mastocytosis. Folia Haematol. (Leipz.) 109:453, 1982.

264. Khoory, M.S., Nesheim, M.E., Bowie, E.J.W., and Mann, K.G.: Circulating heparan sulfate proteoglycan anticoagulant from a patient with a plasma cell disorder. J. Clin. Invest. 65:666, 1980.

265. Bussel, J.B., Steinherz, P.G., Miller, D.R., and Hilgartner, M.W.: A heparin-like anticoagulant in an 8-month-old boy with acute monoblastic leukemia. Am. J. Hematol. 16:83, 1984.

266. Palmer, R.N., Rick, M.E., Rick, P.D., Zeller, J.A., and Gralnick, H.R.: Circulating heparan sulfate anticoagulant in a patient with a fatal bleeding disorder. N. Engl. J. Med. 310:1696, 1984.

267. Tefferi, A., Nichols, W.L., and Bowie, E.J.W.: Circulating heparin-like anticoagulants: report of five consecutive cases and a review. Am. J. Med. 88:184, 1990.

268. Marcum, J.A., and Rosenberg, R.D.: Heparin-like molecules with anticoagulant activity are synthesized by cultured endothelial cells. Biochem. Biophys. Res. Commun. 126:365, 1985.

269. Marcum, J.A., Atha, D.H., Fritze, L.M., Nawroth, P., Stern, D., and Rosenberg, R.D.: Cloned bovine aortic endothelial cells synthesize anticoagulantly active heparan sulfate proteoglycan. J. Biol. Chem. 261:7507, 1986.

270. Stern, D., Nawroth, P., Marcum, J., Handley, D., Kisiel, W., Rosenberg, R., and Stern, K.: Interaction of antithrombin III with bovine aortic segments. Role of heparin in binding and enhanced anticoagulant activity. J. Clin. Invest. 75:272, 1985.

271. Hatton, M.W., Moar, S.L., and Richardson, M.: On the interaction of rabbit antithrombin III with the luminal surface of the normal and deendothelialized rabbit thoracic aorta in vitro. Blood 67:878, 1986.

272. de Agostini, A.I., Watkins, S.C., Slayter, H.S., Youssoufian, H., and Rosenberg, R.D.: Localization of anticoagulantly active heparan sulfate proteoglycans in vascular endothelium: antithrombin binding on cultured endothelial cells and perfused rat aorta. J. Cell Biol. 111:1293, 1990.

273. Frebelius, S., Isaksson, S., and Swedenborg, J.: Thrombin inhibition by antithrombin III on the subendothelium is explained by the isoform AT beta. Arterioscler. Thromb. Vasc. Biol. 16:1292, 1996.

274. Marcum, J.A., McKenney, J.B., and Rosenberg, R.D.: Acceleration of thrombin-antithrombin complex formation in rat hindquarters via heparinlike molecules bound to the endothelium. J. Clin. Invest. 74:341, 1984.

275. Jakubowski, H.V., Kline, M.D., and Owen, W.G.: The effect of bovine thrombomodulin on the specificity of bovine thrombin. J. Biol. Chem. 261:3876, 1986.

276. Bourin, M.-C., Lundgren-Åkerlund, E., and Lindahl, U.: Isolation and characterization of the glycosaminoglycan component of rabbit thrombomodulin proteoglycan. J. Biol. Chem. 265:15424, 1990.

277. He, X., Ye, J., Esmon, C.T., and Rezaie, A.R.: Influence of arginines 93, 97, and 101 of thrombin to its functional specificity. Biochemistry 36:8969, 1997.

278. Koyama, T., Parkinson, J.F., Sié, P., Bang, N.U., Müller-Berghaus, G., and Preissner, K.T.: Different glycoforms of human thrombomodulin. Their glycosaminoglycan-dependent modulatory effects on thrombin inactivation by heparin cofactor II and antithrombin III. Eur. J. Biochem. 198:563, 1991.

279. Preissner, K.T., Koyama, T., Müller, D., Tschopp, J., and Müller-Berghaus, G.: Domain structure of the endothelial cell receptor thrombomodulin as deduced from modulation of its anticoagulant functions. Evidence for a glycosaminoglycan-dependent secondary binding site for thrombin. J. Biol. Chem. 265:4915, 1990.

280. Lane, D.A., Pejler, G., Flynn, A.M., Thompson, E.A., and Lindahl, U.: Neutralization of heparin-related saccharides by histidine-rich glycoprotein and platelet factor 4. J. Biol. Chem. 261:3980, 1986.

281. Preissner, K.T., and Muller-Berghaus, G.: S protein modulates the heparin-catalyzed inhibition of thrombin by antithrombin III. Evidence for a direct interaction of S protein with heparin. Eur. J. Biochem. 156:645, 1986.

282. Conard, J., Brosstad, F., Lie-Larsen, M., Samama, M., and Abildgaard, U.: Molar antithrombin concentration in normal human plasma. Haemostasis 13:363, 1983.

283. Tait, R.C., Walker, I.D., Islam, S.I.A.M., McCall, F., Conkie, J.A., Mitchell, R., and Davidson, J.F.: Influence of demographic factors on antithrombin III activity in a healthy population. Br. J. Haematol 84:476, 1993.

284. Conlan, M.G., Folsom, A.R., Finch, A., Davis, C.E., Marcucci, G., Sorlie, P., and Wu, K.K.: Antithrombin III: associations with age, race, sex and cardiovascular risk factors. Thromb. Haemost. 72:551, 1994.

285. Andrew, M., Paes, B., Milner, R., Johnston, M., Mitchell, L., Tollefsen, D.M., and Powers, P.: Development of the human coagulation system in the full-term infant. Blood 70:165, 1987.

286. van Boven, H.H., and Lane, D.A.: Antithrombin and its inherited deficiency states. Semin. Hematol. 34:188, 1997.

287. Lane, D.A., Bayston, T., Olds, R.J., Fitches, A.C., Cooper, D.N., Millar, D.S., Jochmans, K., Perry, D.J., Okajima, K., Thein, S.L., et al.: Antithrombin mutation database: 2nd (1997) update. Thromb. Haemost. 77:197, 1997.

288. Ambruso, D.R., Leonard, B.D., Bies, R.D., Jacobson, L., Hathaway, W.E., and Reeve, E.B.: Antithrombin III deficiency: decreased synthesis of a biochemically normal molecule. Blood 60:78, 1982.

289. Knot, E.A., de Jong, E., ten Cate, J.W., Iburg, A.H., Henny, C.P., Bruin, T., and Stibbe, J.: Purified radiolabeled antithrombin III metabolism in three families with hereditary AT III deficiency: application of a three-compartment model. Blood 67:93, 1986.

290. Perry, D.J., and Carrell, R.W.: Molecular genetics of human antithrombin deficiency [review]. Hum. Mutat. 7:7, 1996.

291. Bayston, T.A., and Lane, D.A.: Antithrombin: molecular basis of deficiency. Thromb. Haemost. 78:339, 1997.

292. Bruce, D., Perry, D.J., Borg, J.Y., Carrell, R.W., and Wardell, M.R.: Thromboembolic disease due to thermolabile conformational changes of antithrombin Rouen-VI (187 Asn→Asp). J. Clin. Invest. 94:2265, 1994.

293. Sheffield, W.P., Castillo, J.E., and Blajchman, M.A.: Intracellular events determine the fate of antithrombin Utah. Blood 86:3461, 1995.

294. Fischer, A.M., Cornu, P., Sternberg, C., Meriane, F., Dautzenberg, M.D., Chafa, O., Beguin, S., and Desnos, M.: Antithrombin III Alger: a new homozygous AT III variant. Thromb. Haemost. 55:218, 1986.

295. Boyer, C., Wolf, M., Vedrenne, J., Meyer, D., and Larrieu, M.J.: Homozygous variant of antithrombin III: AT III Fontainebleau. Thromb. Haemost. 56:18, 1986.

296. Hirsh, J., Piovella, F., and Pini, M.: Congenital antithrombin III deficiency. Incidence and clinical features. Am. J. Med. 87:34s, 1989.

297. Bauer, K.A., Goodman, T.L., Kass, B.L., and Rosenberg, R.D.: Elevated factor Xa activity in the blood of asymptomatic patients with congenital antithrombin deficiency. J. Clin. Invest. 76:826, 1985.

298. Bauer, K.A., Barzegar, S., and Rosenberg, R.D.: Influence of anticoagulants used for blood collection on plasma prothrombin fragment F1 + 2 measurements. Thromb. Res. 63:617, 1991.

299. Demers, C., Ginsberg, J.S., Henderson, P., Ofosu, F.A., Weitz, J.I., and Blajchman, M.A.: Measurement of markers of activated coagulation in antithrombin III deficient subjects. Thromb. Haemost. 67:542, 1992.

300. Ødegård, O.R., and Abildgaard, U.: Antithrombin III: critical review of assay methods. Significance of variations in health and disease. Haemostasis 7:127, 1978.

301. Rosenberg, R.D.: Actions and interactions of antithrombin and heparin. N. Engl. J. Med. 292:146, 1975.

302. Tait, R.C., Walker, I.D., Perry, D.J., Carrell, R.W., Islam, S.I.A., McCall, F., Mitchell, R., and Davidson, J.F.: Prevalence of antithrombin III deficiency subtypes in 4000 healthy blood donors [abstract]. Thromb. Haemost. 65:839, 1991.

303. Mateo, J., Oliver, A., Borrell, M., Sala, N., and Fontcuberta, J.: Laboratory evaluation and clinical characteristics of 2,132 consecutive unselected patients with venous thromboembolism—results of the Spanish Multicentric Study on Thrombophilia (EMET-Study). Thromb. Haemost. 77:444, 1997.

304. Vikydal, R., Korninger, C., Kyrle, P.A., Niessner, H., Pabinger, I., Thaler, E., and Lechner, K.: The prevalence of hereditary antithrombin-III deficiency in patients with a history of venous thromboembolism. Thromb. Haemost. 54:744, 1985.

305. Demers, C., Ginsberg, J.S., Hirsh, J., Henderson, P., and Blajchman, M.A.: Thrombosis in antithrombin-III–deficient persons. Report of a large kindred and literature review. Ann. Intern. Med. 116:754, 1992.

306. McColl, M., Tait, R.C., Walker, I.D., Perry, D.J., McCall, F., and Conkie, J.A.: Low thrombosis rate seen in blood donors and their relatives with inherited deficiencies of antithrombin and protein C: correlation with type of defect, family history, and absence of the factor V Leiden mutation. Blood Coagul. Fibrinolysis 7:689, 1996.

307. van Boven, H.H., Reitsma, P.H., Rosendaal, F.R., Bayston, T.A., Chowdhury, V., Bauer, K.A., Scharrer, I., Conard, J., and Lane, D.A.: Factor V Leiden (FV R506Q) in families with inherited antithrombin deficiency. Thromb. Haemost. 75:417, 1996.

308. Martinelli, I., Magatelli, R., Cattaneo, M., and Mannucci, P.M.: Prevalence of mutant factor V in Italian patients with hereditary deficiencies of antithrombin, protein C or protein S. Thromb. Haemost. 75:694, 1996.

309. Mitchell, L., Piovella, F., Ofosu, F., and Andrew, M.: α_2-Macroglobulin may provide protection from thromboembolic events in antithrombin III–deficient children. Blood 78:2299, 1991.

310. Rosendaal, F.R., Heijboer, H., Briët, E., Büller, H.R., Brandjes, D.P.M., de Bruin, K., Hommes, D.W., and Vandenbroucke, J.P.: Mortality in hereditary antithrombin-III deficiency—1830 to 1989. Lancet 337:260, 1991.

311. Rosendaal, F.R., and Heijboer, H.: Mortality related to thrombosis in congenital antithrombin III deficiency [letter]. Lancet 337:1545, 1991.

312. van Boven, H.H., Vandenbroucke, J.P., Westendorp, R.G., and Rosendaal, F.R.: Mortality and causes of death in inherited antithrombin deficiency. Thromb. Haemost. 77:452, 1997.

313. Tollefsen, D.M., Majerus, D.W., and Blank, M.K.: Heparin cofactor II. Purification and properties of a heparin-dependent inhibitor of thrombin in human plasma. J. Biol. Chem. 257:2162, 1982.

314. Ragg, H., and Preibisch, G.: Structure and expression of the gene coding for the human serpin hLS2. J. Biol. Chem. 263:12129, 1988.

315. Herzog, R., Lutz, S., Blin, N., Marasa, J.C., Blinder, M.A., and Tollefsen, D.M.: Complete nucleotide sequence of the gene for human heparin cofactor II and mapping to chromosomal band 22q11. Biochemistry 30:1350, 1991.

316. Ragg, H.: A new member of the plasma protease inhibitor gene family. Nucleic Acids Res. 14:1073, 1986.

317. Jaffe, E.A., Armellino, D., and Tollefsen, D.M.: Biosynthesis of functionally active heparin cofactor II by a human hepatoma-derived cell line. Biochem. Biophys. Res. Commun. 132:368, 1985.

318. Hortin, G., Tollefsen, D.M., and Strauss, A.W.: Identification of two sites of sulfation of human heparin cofactor II. J. Biol. Chem. 261:15827, 1986.

319. Blinder, M.A., Marasa, J.C., Reynolds, C.H., Deaven, L.L., and Tollefsen, D.M.: Heparin cofactor II: cDNA sequence, chromosome localization, restriction fragment length polymorphism, and expression in *Escherichia coli*. Biochemistry 27:752, 1988.

320. Church, F.C., Meade, J.B., and Pratt, C.W.: Structure-function relationships in heparin cofactor II: spectral analysis of aromatic residues and absence of a role for sulfhydryl groups in thrombin inhibition. Arch. Biochem. Biophys. 259:331, 1987.

321. Griffith, M.J., Noyes, C.M., Tyndall, J.A., and Church, F.C.: Structural evidence for leucine at the reactive site of heparin cofactor II. Biochemistry 24:6777, 1985.

322. Church, F.C., Noyes, C.M., and Griffith, M.J.: Inhibition of chymotrypsin by heparin cofactor II. Proc. Natl. Acad. Sci. USA 82:6431, 1985.

323. Parker, K.A., and Tollefsen, D.M.: The protease specificity of heparin cofactor II. Inhibition of thrombin generated during coagulation. J. Biol. Chem. 260:3501, 1985.

324. Derechin, V.M., Blinder, M.A., and Tollefsen, D.M.: Substitution of arginine for Leu444 in the reactive site of heparin cofactor II enhances the rate of thrombin inhibition. J. Biol. Chem. 265:5623, 1990.

325. Hurst, R.E., Poon, M.-C., and Griffith, M.J.: Structure-activity relationships of heparin. Independence of heparin charge density and antithrombin-binding domains in thrombin inhibition by antithrombin and heparin cofactor II. J. Clin. Invest. 72:1042, 1983.

326. Maimone, M.M., and Tollefsen, D.M.: Activation of heparin cofactor II by heparin oligosaccharides. Biochem. Biophys. Res. Commun. 152:1056, 1988.

327. Maimone, M.M., and Tollefsen, D.M.: Structure of a dermatan sulfate hexasaccharide that binds to heparin cofactor II with high affinity. J. Biol. Chem. 265:18263, 1990.

328. Tollefsen, D.M., Peacock, M.E., and Monafo, W.J.: Molecular size of dermatan sulfate oligosaccharides required to bind and activate heparin cofactor II. J. Biol. Chem. 261:8854, 1986.

329. Pavão, M.S.G., Mourão, P.A.S., Mulloy, B., and Tollefsen, D.M.: A unique dermatan sulfate–like glycosaminoglycan from ascidian: its structure and the effect of its unusual sulfation pattern on anticoagulant activity. J. Biol. Chem. 270:31027, 1995.

330. Fernandez, F., van Ryn, J., Ofosu, F.A., Hirsh, J., and Buchanan, M.R.: The haemorrhagic and antithrombotic effects of dermatan sulfate. Br. J. Haematol. 64:309, 1986.

331. Maggi, A., Abbadini, M., Pagella, P.G., Borowska, A., Pangrazzi, J., and Donati, M.B.: Antithrombotic properties of dermatan sulphate in a rat venous thrombosis model. Haemostasis 17:329, 1987.

332. Merton, R.E., and Thomas, D.P.: Experimental studies on the relative efficacy of dermatan sulphate and heparin as antithrombotic agents. Thromb. Haemost. 58:839, 1987.

333. Van Ryn-McKenna, J., Gray, E., Weber, E., Ofosu, F.A., and Buchanan, M.R.: Effects of sulfated polysaccharides on inhibition of thrombus formation initiated by different stimuli. Thromb. Haemost. 61:7, 1989.

334. Agnelli, G., Cosmi, B., Di Filippo, P., Ranucci, V., Veschi, F., Longetti, M., Renga, C., Barzi, F., Gianese, F., Lupattelli, L., et al.: A randomised, double-blind, placebo-controlled trial of dermatan sulphate for prevention of deep vein thrombosis in hip fracture. Thromb. Haemost. 67:203, 1992.

335. Lane, D.A., Ryan, K., Ireland, H., Curtis, J.R., Nurmohamed, M.T., Krediet, R.T., Roggekamp, M.C., Stevens, P., and ten Cate, J.W.: Dermatan sulphate in haemodialysis. Lancet 339:334, 1992.

336. Cofrancesco, E., Boschetti, C., Leonardi, P., and Cortellaro, M.: Dermatan sulphate in acute leukaemia. Lancet 339:1177, 1992.

337. Ofosu, F.A., Modi, G.J., Smith, L.M., Cerskus, A.L., Hirsh, J., and Blajchman, M.A.: Heparan sulfate and dermatan sulfate inhibit the generation of thrombin activity in plasma by complementary pathways. Blood 64:742, 1984.

338. Sié, P., Ofosu, F., Fernandez, F., Buchanan, M.R., Petitou, M., and Boneu, B.: Respective role of antithrombin III and heparin cofactor II in the in vitro anticoagulant effect of heparin and of various sulphated polysaccharides. Br. J. Haematol. 64:707, 1986.

339. Blinder, M.A., Andersson, T.R., Abildgaard, U., and Tollefsen, D.M.: Heparin cofactor II Oslo. Mutation of Arg-189 to His decreases the affinity for dermatan sulfate. J. Biol. Chem. 264:5128, 1989.

340. Blinder, M.A., and Tollefsen, D.M.: Site-directed mutagenesis of arginine 103 and lysine 185 in the proposed glycosaminoglycan-binding site of heparin cofactor II. J. Biol. Chem. 265:286, 1990.

341. Ragg, H., Ulshöfer, T., and Gerewitz, J.: On the activation of human leuserpin-2, a thrombin inhibitor, by glycosaminoglycans. J. Biol. Chem. 265:5211, 1990.

342. Ragg, H., Ulshöfer, T., and Gerewitz, J.: Glycosaminoglycan-mediated leuserpin-2/thrombin interaction. Structure-function relationships. J. Biol. Chem. 265:22386, 1990.

343. Whinna, H.C., Blinder, M.A., Szewczyk, M., Tollefsen, D.M., and Church, F.C.: Role of lysine 173 in heparin binding to heparin cofactor II. J. Biol. Chem. 266:8129, 1991.

344. Van Deerlin, V.M.D., and Tollefsen, D.M.: The N-terminal acidic domain of heparin cofactor II mediates the inhibition of α-thrombin in the presence of glycosaminoglycans. J. Biol. Chem. 266:20223, 1991.

345. Grutter, M.G., Priestle, J.P., Rahuel, J., Grossenbacher, H., Bode, W., Hofsteenge, J., and Stone, S.R.: Crystal structure of the thrombin-hirudin complex: a novel mode of serine protease inhibition. EMBO J. 9:2361, 1990.

346. Rydel, T.J., Ravichandran, K.G., Tulinsky, A., Bode, W., Huber, R., Roitsch, C., and Fenton, J.W., II: The structure of a complex of recombinant hirudin and human α-thrombin. Science 249:277, 1990.

347. Hortin, G.L., Tollefsen, D.M., and Benutto, B.M.: Antithrombin activity of a peptide corresponding to residues 54–75 of heparin cofactor II. J. Biol. Chem. 264:13979, 1989.

348. Rogers, S.J., Pratt, C.W., Whinna, H.C., and Church, F.C.: Role of thrombin exosites in inhibition by heparin cofactor II. J. Biol. Chem. 267:3613, 1992.

349. Phillips, J.E., Shirk, R.A., Whinna, H.C., Henriksen, R.A., and Church, F.C.: Inhibition of dysthrombins Quick I and II by heparin cofactor II and antithrombin. J. Biol. Chem. 268:3321, 1993.

350. Sheehan, J.P., Wu, Q., Tollefsen, D.M., and Sadler, J.E.: Mutagenesis of thrombin selectively modulates inhibition by serpins heparin cofactor II and antithrombin III. Interaction with the anion-binding exosite determines heparin cofactor II specificity. J. Biol. Chem. 268:3639, 1993.

351. Sheehan, J.P., and Sadler, J.E.: Molecular mapping of the heparin-binding exosite of thrombin. Proc. Natl. Acad. Sci. USA 91:5518, 1994.

352. Sheehan, J.P., Tollefsen, D.M., and Sadler, J.E.: Heparin cofactor II is regulated allosterically and not primarily by template effects. Studies with mutant thrombins and glycosaminoglycans. J. Biol. Chem. 269:32747, 1994.

353. Tsiang, M., Jain, A.K., and Gibbs, C.S.: Functional requirements for inhibition of thrombin by antithrombin III in the presence and absence of heparin. J. Biol. Chem. 272:12024, 1997.

354. Arni, R.K., Padmanabhan, K., Padmanabhan, K.P., Wu, T.-P., and Tulinsky, A.: Structures of the noncovalent complexes of human and bovine prothrombin fragment 2 with human PPACK-thrombin. Biochemistry 32:4727, 1993.

355. Tollefsen, D.M., and Pestka, C.A.: Heparin cofactor II activity in patients with disseminated intravascular coagulation and hepatic failure. Blood 66:769, 1985.

356. Sié, P., Dupouy, D., Pichon, J., and Boneu, B.: Constitutional heparin co-factor II deficiency associated with recurrent thrombosis. Lancet 2:414, 1985.

357. Tran, T.H., Marbet, G.A., and Duckert, F.: Association of hereditary heparin co-factor II deficiency with thrombosis. Lancet 2:413, 1985.

358. Andersson, T.R., Larsen, M.L., Handeland, G.F., and Abildgaard, U.: Heparin cofactor II activity in plasma: application of an automated assay method to the study of a normal adult population. Scand. J. Haematol. 36:96, 1986.

359. Bertina, R.M., van der Linden, I.K., Engesser, L., Muller, H.P., and Brommer, E.J.P.: Hereditary heparin cofactor II deficiency and the risk of development of thrombosis. Thromb. Haemost. 57:196, 1987.

360. McGuire, E.A., and Tollefsen, D.M.: Activation of heparin cofactor II by fibroblasts and vascular smooth muscle cells. J. Biol. Chem. 262:169, 1987.

361. Shirk, R.A., Church, F.C., and Wagner, W.D.: Arterial smooth muscle cell heparan sulfate proteoglycans accelerate thrombin inhibition by heparin cofactor II. Arterioscler. Thromb. Vasc. Biol. 16:1138, 1996.

362. Andrew, M., Mitchell, L., Berry, L., Paes, B., Delorme, M., Ofosu, F., Burrows, R., and Khambalia, B.: An anticoagulant dermatan sulfate proteoglycan circulates in the pregnant woman and her fetus. J. Clin. Invest. 89:321, 1992.

363. Liu, L., Dewar, L., Song, Y., Kulczycky, M., Blajchman, M.A., Fenton, J.W., II, Andrew, M., Delorme, M., Ginsberg, J., Preissner, K.T., et al.: Inhibition of thrombin by antithrombin III and heparin cofactor II in vivo. Thromb. Haemost. 73:405, 1995.

364. Brennan, M.J., Oldberg, A., Pierschbacher, M.D., and Ruoslahti, E.: Chondroitin/dermatan sulfate proteoglycan in human fetal membranes: demonstration of an antigenically similar proteoglycan in fibroblasts. J. Biol. Chem. 259:13742, 1984.

21 ▼▼▼▼ Hemophilia A, Hemophilia B, and von Willebrand Disease

J. Evan Sadler and Earl W. Davie

▼ ▼

Most of our knowledge of the mechanism of hereditary bleeding disorders has been acquired only recently. What we know as hemophilia A apparently was recognized more than 1700 years ago, as documented in the Talmud,[1] and the genetics of the disease was described in detail by 1800.[2] However, the first correct description of the role of antihemophilic factor (factor VIII) in hemostasis was not published until 1937,[3] and the resolution of hemophilia into two distinct disorders, hemophilia A (factor VIII deficiency) and hemophilia B (factor IX deficiency), did not occur until 1952.[4, 5] The relationship between hereditary factor VIII deficiency and von Willebrand disease was once controversial because a deficiency of von Willebrand factor, which is autosomally inherited, is usually associated with some degree of factor VIII deficiency. Furthermore, factor VIII and von Willebrand factor tend to copurify. Classical hemophilia A, however, is an X chromosome–linked disease. Consequently, for almost four decades, factor VIII (with varying suffixes) has been the term used to designate the protein that is defective in either hemophilia A or von Willebrand disease, or both, depending on the context.

In this chapter, *factor VIII* refers to the protein, specified by an X chromosome–linked gene, that is defective in hemophilia A and accelerates the activation of factor X by factor IXa in the presence of calcium ions and phospholipid. Similarly, *von Willebrand factor* (VWF) refers to the protein, specified by an autosomal gene, that is defective in severe von Willebrand disease (VWD) and participates in normal platelet function as measured by the bleeding time. The complex of these proteins that occurs in vivo is referred to as the *factor VIII/VWF complex*.

Factor VIII and Hemophilia A

▼ PURIFICATION AND STRUCTURAL CHARACTERIZATION OF FACTOR VIII

Assays for Factor VIII

Antihemophilic factor (factor VIII) was first assayed as an activity that corrects the clotting defect in hemophilic plasma.[3] Assays based on this principle are still widely used. Factor VIII has no intrinsic enzyme activity but acts as a cofactor in a multicomponent reaction; furthermore, thrombin converts the cofactor to a much more active form that subsequently decays into an inactive form. The complex kinetics of activation and inactivation makes the measurement of factor VIII cofactor activity highly dependent on specific assay conditions. *One unit* of factor VIII is that amount of activity in 1 ml of pooled normal plasma, usually measured as shortening of the clotting time of hemophilia A plasma. Local and national standard plasmas can be calibrated against an international reference plasma standard established by the World Health Organization.

When greater precision is necessary, methods based on the specific cofactor activity of factor VIII in a purified system can be employed. For example, the ability of factor

VIII to accelerate the activation of factor X may be measured by mixing factor VIII with factor IXa, phospholipid, and calcium ions. The resultant factor Xa activity generated in this reaction can be determined by a plasma clotting assay,[6] by measurement of the cleavage of a chromogenic peptide substrate for factor Xa (S-2222),[7] or by direct measurement of the factor IXa–mediated release of radiolabeled activation peptide from factor X.[8] The characteristics of these reactions are discussed under Biological Function of Factor VIII.

Factor VIII protein can be measured by standard immunological methods with sufficient sensitivity to detect less than 0.1 per cent of normal factor VIII antigen levels.[9, 10]

Purification of Factor VIII

In blood, factor VIII is bound non-covalently to VWF. The plasma concentration of factor VIII is 100 to 200 ng/ml, or approximately 0.7 nmol/l, assuming an average M_r of 280,000. This corresponds to about 2 per cent of the mass of circulating VWF. The VWF moiety of the factor VIII/VWF complex is polymeric and extremely large, with molecular weights ranging from 500,000 to more than 10,000,000. By exploiting this peculiarity of VWF, human factor VIII can be extensively purified 7000-fold to 10,000-fold as part of the factor VIII/VWF complex.[11, 12]

Further purification of factor VIII is achieved after dissociation of the factor VIII/VWF complex in solutions of high ionic strength, such as approximately 1M NaCl[13] or approximately 0.25 to 0.5M $CaCl_2$.[14] Once dissociated, factor VIII can be resolved from VWF by a variety of chromatographic methods. The highest specific activities obtained for factor VIII purified from plasma are in the range of 2300 to 6000 U/mg for the human,[15, 16] bovine,[17] and porcine pro-

teins.[18, 19] These values, however, may not correspond precisely to the specific activity of intact factor VIII, because factor VIII preparations are often a mixture of inactive precursor and activated and inactivated proteins.

Structure of Factor VIII

Factor VIII is derived from a primary translation product of 2351 amino acids.[20–23] After removal of a signal peptide of 19 amino acids, single-chain factor VIII consists of 2332 amino acids and has a calculated M_r of 264,763. Although factor VIII is synthesized as a single polypeptide chain, almost all of the factor VIII in plasma is a heterodimer. During biosynthesis or in the circulation, factor VIII is cleaved after Arg 1648 to generate the amino terminus of the light chain of approximately M_r 80,000. Additional cleavages within the connecting peptide region generate several species of heavy chain with M_r of 90,000 to 210,000.[15, 16, 20, 21, 24, 25] The proteases responsible for these reactions have not been identified, although thrombin can cleave after Arg 740 to give the smallest heavy chain fragment with M_r of 90,000.[20] Similar patterns have been described for bovine[17] and porcine[18, 19] factor VIII.

Factor VIII contains a total of 25 potential asparagine-linked carbohydrate binding sites (Fig. 21–1). If all these asparagine residues were glycosylated, the M_r for the glycoprotein would be approximately 330,000 ($\pm 20,000$). Both the heavy and light chains of human factor VIII contain N-linked[16, 26] and O-linked[27] carbohydrate chains. The N-linked oligosaccharides on the heavy chain appear to be mainly of the hybrid or complex type, whereas some oligosaccharides on the light chain are of the high-mannose type.[27]

Factor VIII contains two types of repeated homologous

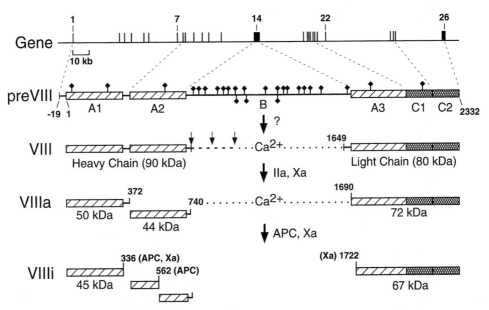

Figure 21–1. Structure of human factor VIII gene and protein. *Gene:* The region of the X chromosome containing the factor VIII gene is represented. Selected exons are numbered, and the scale in kilobases of DNA is shown. The relationship among segments of the gene and repeated domains of the protein is indicated by the dotted lines connecting the gene to pre-VIII. *Pre-VIII:* The primary translation product consists of a signal peptide (amino acid residues −19 to 1) and single-chain precursor (amino acid residues 1 to 2332). Sites of N-linked glycosylation are indicated (♦), and structural domains of the protein are labeled. *VIII:* Factor VIII in plasma consists of one heavy chain and one light chain, stabilized by calcium ions. Unknown proteases (?) are responsible for generating the amino terminus of the light chain and the carboxyl-terminal heterogeneity of the heavy chain. *VIIIa:* Thrombin (IIa) or factor Xa (Xa) can activate factor VIII by cleaving at the indicated amino acid residues. *VIIIi:* Activated protein C (APC) or factor Xa (Xa) can cleave and inactivate factor VIIIa at the sites that are indicated.

domains (see Fig. 21–1). Two A domains occur in the amino-terminal region of the molecule (residues 1 to 329 and 380 to 711), and one is present in the carboxyl-terminal region of the molecule (residues 1649 to 2019). The second and third A domains are separated by a large 980 amino acid connecting peptide (B domain). The other repeated domain (C domain) occurs in tandem repeats of approximately 150 amino acids, in the carboxyl-terminal region of the molecule. The A domains are about 30 per cent identical in amino acid sequence, whereas the C domains are about 40 per cent identical.[20, 21]

Factor VIII is homologous to factor V.[28–30] Both proteins share a similar organization into domains (A1-A2-B-A3-C1-C2), and corresponding A and C domains of factor VIII and factor V are about 40 per cent identical in amino acid sequence. In contrast, the connecting regions (B domains) show no significant sequence similarity. The evolutionary and structural similarities of factor V and factor VIII are reflected in their biological functions, which involve similar mechanisms as cofactors.

The A domains of factor VIII (and factor V) are homologous to each of three similar domains of ceruloplasmin[28] and other related copper-oxidases. The degree of sequence conservation is sufficiently high to permit molecular modeling of the factor VIII A domains based on the crystallographic structures of these oxidases[31, 32] (see Plate 21–1).

The C domains of factor VIII are about 20 per cent identical to the first 150 amino acids of discoidin I, a galactose-binding and phospholipid-binding protein of slime mold.[33] The C domains of factor VIII are also about 54 per cent identical in sequence to an approximately 300 amino acid segment of a mouse milk fat globule protein that contains two tandemly repeated C-like domains.[34]

The heavy and light chains of human factor VIII contain a total of 19 cysteine residues, but none of these residues is involved in intersubunit disulfide bonds. Each A domain has two intradomain disulfide bonds and one free cysteine; each C domain contains one intradomain disulfide bond. The positions of most of the disulfide bonds are conserved with factor V and ceruloplasmin.[35–38]

Like two-chain factor Va, the polypeptides of factor VIII are dissociated by high concentrations of EDTA, with loss of procoagulant activity,[19, 39] suggesting that metal ions are required for structural integrity. As might be predicted on the basis of its homology to ceruloplasmin, factor VIII contains one copper ion, apparently in the reduced Cu(I) state.[40] Calcium ions are also required for optimal reconstitution of activity from the isolated chains and to maintain the normal association between the heavy and light chains.[41]

Human factor VIII contains six sulfated tyrosine residues at positions 346, 718, 719, 723, 1664, and 1680.[42–44] All six sites of tyrosine sulfation appear to modulate factor VIII cofactor function. Sulfation at tyrosines 346 and 1664 increases factor VIII activity by increasing the rate of thrombin cleavage.[44] Sulfation at tyrosines 718, 719, and 723 increases the intrinsic activity of factor VIIIa.[44] Sulfation at Tyr 1680 increases the affinity of factor VIII for VWF, as discussed below.[42–44]

The structure and topography of factor VIII have been studied by ultracentrifugation, fluorescence energy transfer, and electron microscopy. Factor VIII is an asymmetrical particle with M_r of 250,000 or 285,000.[45, 46] The A2 domain

of the heavy chain and the A3 domain of the light chain are closely approximated[47] and form a compact globular core of 10 to 14 nm in diameter.[48] The connecting region or B domain appears to form an elongated 5 to 14 nm extension from the core that is lost on activation of factor VIII by thrombin.[48] This general model is consistent with the model proposed for the factor VIII A domains based on the crystallographic structure of ceruloplasmin.[32]

Association of Factor VIII With von Willebrand Factor

Factor VIII binds to VWF with a K_d of approximately 0.4 nmol[49] and circulates in the blood as a non-covalent complex with VWF. The interaction is disrupted by high ionic strength[13, 14] or by phospholipids,[50, 51] suggesting that it involves both electrostatic and hydrophobic components. The binding site on factor VIII requires two regions of the light chain. One necessary structure is within an acidic amino acid segment at the amino terminus of the light chain, particularly amino acid residues between Ser 1669 and Arg 1689,[42] and optimal binding requires sulfation of Tyr 1680.[42–44] The C2 domain is also required for VWF binding,[49] and synthetic peptide 2303–2332, corresponding to a previously identified phospholipid binding site on factor VIII, inhibits this interaction.[52]

▼ BIOSYNTHESIS AND METABOLISM OF FACTOR VIII

The liver is the major site of factor VIII synthesis, and liver transplantation completely corrects factor VIII deficiency due to hemophilia A.[53, 54] Factor VIII mRNA has also been detected in human liver, spleen, lymph node, pancreas, muscle, fetal heart, placenta, and kidney.[20, 55, 56] Allotransplantation of whole spleen in humans with severe hemophilia A was reported to increase factor VIII levels to 30 to 36 per cent of normal,[57] although spleen transplantation did not increase factor VIII levels in hemophilic dogs. The physiological significance of other potential extrahepatic sites of factor VIII synthesis is not known.

Within the liver, it continues to be controversial which cell types synthesize factor VIII. Factor VIII antigen and mRNA have been found variably in either hepatocytes or sinusoidal endothelium.[56, 58, 59] Recent quantitative PCR assays on highly purified cells from mouse liver suggest that hepatocytes contain 80 to 85 per cent and sinusoidal endothelial cells contain 15 to 20 per cent of the total factor VIII mRNA, and that Kupffer cells contain no factor VIII mRNA.[60] Murine sinusoidal endothelial cells[60] and human hepatocytes[58] have been shown to synthesize active factor VIII in culture.

Studies of recombinant factor VIII synthesis indicate that the protein is expressed at relatively low levels because it is not transported efficiently from the endoplasmic reticulum to the Golgi apparatus. The factor VIII primary translation product is translocated into the endoplasmic reticulum, where N-linked glycosylation and disulfide bond formation is initiated. A substantial fraction of the molecules form a complex with protein chaperones including immunoglobulin heavy chain–binding protein (BiP/GRP78), calnexin, and calreticulin, and they are retained at least transiently in the endoplasmic reticulum.[61, 62] Some of the retained material is degraded, and the remainder is transported to the Golgi apparatus where glycosylation is completed and selected tyrosine residues are sulfated. In the Golgi or a later compartment, the single-chain factor VIII precursor is cleaved after Arg 1648 to generate the amino terminus of the light chain. Inclusion of VWF in the extracellular medium promotes the secretion of the factor VIII light chain and its metal ion–dependent association with the heavy chain. In the absence of VWF, the secreted free light and heavy chains do not readily form a stable complex and are degraded. Thus, extracellular VWF may be required for optimal assembly of the factor VIII heavy and light chains into a stable complex.[27]

The normal metabolism of factor VIII depends on complex formation with VWF, which not only may promote the assembly of the factor VIII heavy and light chains but also stabilizes factor VIII in the circulation. Injected factor VIII/ VWF complex is cleared from circulation with a half-disappearance time of about 12 hours.[63, 64] The kinetic patterns are biphasic and are identical to the clearance of the coadministered VWF.[63] In contrast, if factor VIII (essentially free of VWF) is administered to patients with severe VWF deficiency, the factor VIII is rapidly eliminated with a half-time of approximately 2.4 hours,[64] confirming the role of VWF in stabilizing factor VIII. Factor VIII and factor VIII/ VWF complex show similar clearance patterns in patients with hemophilia A, demonstrating that exogenous factor VIII can associate with and be stabilized by endogenous VWF.[64] At steady state, the mean normalized plasma clearance rate for factor VIII/VWF complex is 5 ml/kg/h, suggesting a daily synthesis of about 120 units per kilogram body weight.[65]

▼ BIOLOGICAL FUNCTION OF FACTOR VIII

The role of factor VIII in blood coagulation has been defined during several decades of study.[66, 67] Factor VIII is a component of the intrinsic pathway of blood coagulation, so called because all of the components required for blood clotting by this pathway are found in blood plasma, that is, they are "intrinsic" to the blood. Factor VIII does not have any known catalytic activity but participates as a cofactor in the proteolysis of factor X by factor IXa (Fig. 21–2). The reaction requires calcium ions and a phospholipid membrane surface. The phospholipid requirement is presumably met in vivo by platelet membranes or other cellular membranes. For in vitro clotting of plasma, phospholipid vesicles will suffice, and most of our knowledge of factor VIII biochemis-

try is derived from studies of clotting in systems containing phospholipid.

Regulation of Factor VIIIa Activity

An enormous number of molecular reactions may directly or indirectly affect the procoagulant function of factor VIII. Factor VIII requires activation to participate optimally in the activation of factor X, and this is accomplished by limited proteolysis. Once generated, activated factor VIII (factor VIIIa) is inactivated by proteolytic and non-proteolytic mechanisms that may be influenced by many positive and negative effectors.

Proteolytic Activation of Factor VIII. Human factor VIII is activated up to approximately 40-fold by digestion with thrombin, so that the production of small amounts of thrombin results in the explosive feedback amplification of further thrombin generation.[25, 68] Two-chain factor VIII is rapidly cleaved by thrombin after Arg 740 to liberate carbohydrate-rich connecting peptide fragments of variable size (see Fig. 21–1). The product is a heterodimer consisting of fragments of M_r 90,000 (heavy chain) and approximately 80,000 (light chain), and it probably corresponds to the smallest form of unactivated factor VIII found in plasma. The connecting region or B domain may, therefore, be unnecessary for factor VIII function. In fact, deletion of the B domain is compatible with the biosynthesis of factor VIII species with apparently normal binding to VWF and normal procoagulant activity in vivo.[69]

On further digestion, thrombin cleaves after Arg 372 of the 90,000-dalton heavy chain, between the A1 and A2 domains, to generate 50,000-dalton and 43,000-dalton fragments.[25] Thrombin also cleaves after Arg 1689, just before the A3 domain in the 80,000-dalton light chain, to give a 73,000-dalton fragment and an amino-terminal light chain fragment that probably dissociates from the complex.[25] This cleavage destroys or releases the binding site for VWF.[49, 70, 71] The final product, factor VIIIa, is a heterotrimer that consists of a 50,000-dalton A1 chain, a 43,000-dalton A2 chain, and a 73,000-dalton A3-C1-C2 chain[71-73] (see Fig. 21–1). Similar changes in structure accompany the activation of the homologous factor V by thrombin, except that factor V lacks a cleavage site between domains A1 and A2 so that factor Va is a heterodimer.[30]

The role of specific cleavages in the activation of factor VIII has been determined by use of site-directed mutagenesis to make individual cleavage sites resistant to thrombin. Substitution of Arg 740 and Arg 1648 by isoleucine prevents cleavage at these sites by thrombin but does not prevent activation. Thus, proteolytic excision of the B domain apparently is unnecessary for activation of factor VIII. In contrast, mutation of either Arg 372 or Arg 1689 yields molecules with low intrinsic factor VIIIa activity that are, however, resistant to activation by thrombin.[72]

Thrombin cleaves several bonds in factor VIII to generate factor VIIIa, and this product is not stable. Therefore, the kinetics of factor VIII activation by thrombin is complex. As the factor VIII concentration is increased, the rate of activation by low concentrations of thrombin shows saturation, with a half-maximal rate at approximately 0.08 U factor VIII per milliliter (≈60 pmol).[73] Because this value is approximately 10-fold lower than the average plasma

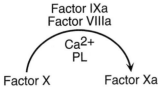

Figure 21–2. The activation of factor X by factor IXa in the presence of factor VIIIa, calcium ions, and phospholipid (PL).

concentration of factor VIII (1 U/ml, ≈0.7 nmol), the concentration of factor VIII is probably not limiting under most conditions that initiate clotting in vivo.

Factor Xa also activates factor VIII[17, 68] (see Fig. 21–1). Factor Xa acts at all of the sites that are cleaved by thrombin. Factor Xa probably also cleaves human factor VIII at the same site as activated protein C (APC) as well as at another site in the factor VIII light chain, after Arg 1721, that is not cleaved by either thrombin or APC.[25] The binding of factor VIII to VWF appears to inhibit activation of factor VIII by factor Xa but to have no effect on activation by thrombin.[74]

Proteolytic and Non-Proteolytic Inactivation of Factor VIIIa. Under most conditions, thrombin-activated factor VIIIa is intrinsically unstable, and factor VIIIa activity decays in what appears to be a first-order process without further proteolytic cleavage.[8, 45, 68] This loss of activity is apparently accompanied by spontaneous dissociation of the 43 kDa A2 domain heavy chain fragment from the factor VIIIa A1/A2/A3-C1-C2 heterotrimer,[75] and active factor VIIIa can be reconstituted from purified inactive A1/A3-C1-C2 heterodimer and A2 domains. Dissociation of the A2 chain is inhibited at high concentrations of factor VIIIa, low ionic strength, and low pH.[76, 77] Under approximately physiological conditions, however, human factor VIIIa activity decays with a half-life of several minutes. Factor VIIIa is stabilized by association with factor IXa and phospholipid.[78] However, factor IXa can proteolytically inactivate factor VIIIa by cleaving it after Arg 336, and the relative rates of A2 dissociation and factor IXa cleavage depend on the local concentration of factor IXa.[79] The importance in vivo of the non-proteolytic loss of factor VIIIa activity, relative to proteolytic destruction, remains unknown.

Factor VIIIa is also degraded and inactivated by APC, as discussed in Chapter 18. Protein C is activated by thrombin in a reaction that is markedly accelerated by the endothelial cell surface cofactor thrombomodulin.[80] Protein C deficiency is associated with severe thrombotic disease,[81] demonstrating that this feedback mechanism for the inactivation of factor VIIIa and factor Va is physiologically important. This anticoagulant mechanism is discussed in Chapter 19.

APC can degrade factors V and VIII as well as their activated forms in a reaction that is stimulated about 50-fold by phospholipid and calcium.[17, 82, 83] However, thrombin-activated factors Va and VIIIa are much better substrates for APC than the native factors are.[82, 84, 85] APC cleaves either the heavy chain of factor VIII or the heavy chain–derived fragments of factor VIIIa after Arg 336 at the carboxyl end

of domain A1 and Arg 562 within domain A2 (see Fig. 21–1).[85] Factor Xa can also cleave factor VIII after Arg 336, and this concordance may explain the ability of factor Xa to inactivate factor VIIIa.[25] APC also appears to cleave the heavy chain of factor VIII after Arg 740, which is the junction of domains A2 and B.[85] APC does not cleave the light chain of factor VIII or factor VIIIa.[25, 85]

Efficient cleavage of factor VIII or VIIIa by APC requires binding to a site light chain, possibly to a segment including amino acids 2009 to 2018 within domain A3 (see Fig. 21–1).[32, 86, 87] Association of the heavy chain with the light chain is necessary for recognition and cleavage of the heavy chain; free heavy chain is not a substrate for APC.[86]

The sensitivity to proteolysis of factor VIII and factor VIIIa may be regulated by interactions with other components of the factor X–activating complex and by other proteases in the blood. For example, VWF inhibits the cleavage of factor VIII by APC,[88] and factor IXa protects factor VIII or VIIIa from degradation by APC.[89, 90] Granulocyte proteases destroy factor VIII or factor VIIIa in a reaction that is inhibited by the presence of factor IXa.[91] Plasmin destroys factor VIII,[92] provided that inhibition by α_2-antiplasmin is overcome, as may occur systemically in disseminated intravascular coagulation or locally in the clot environment. However, such an interaction between plasmin and factor VIII has not been demonstrated to affect clotting in vivo.

Coagulation on Artificial Surfaces

Interactions Within the Intrinsic Factor X–Activating Complex. The four known parts of the optimal factor Xa–generating complex are calcium ions, a phospholipid surface, factor IXa, and factor VIIIa. The role of each of these components can be illustrated by reconstructing the complete system in stages.

During clotting through the intrinsic pathway in vitro, factor IXa activates factor X by cleavage of a single specific peptide bond. The mechanism of factor IXa action is discussed in a later section (Biological Function of Factor IX). Factor VIIIa, phospholipid, and calcium ions act as cofactors that accelerate the rate of factor X cleavage. In the absence of cofactors, bovine factor IXa has a low but measurable activity toward factor X (Table 21–1). The addition of phospholipid alone has no effect on this reaction, and the addition of calcium ions alone results in a modest eightfold increase in the catalytic efficiency. If both calcium ions and phospholipid are added together, the K_m decreases dramatically by 3000-fold to 5000-fold into the range of plasma factor X

Table 21–1. Activation of Bovine Factor X by Bovine Factor IXa

Composition of Reaction*	$K_m$app (µmol)	V_{max} (mol Xa/mol IXa·min)	Catalytic Efficiency (Relative)
IXa	299	0.0022	(1)
IXa, Ca^{2+}	181	0.0105	8
IXa, Ca^{2+}, PL	0.058	0.0247	58,000
IXa, Ca^{2+}, PL, VIIIa	0.063	500	1 × 10^9

* Where indicated, reactions contained Ca^{2+}, ≅10 mmol/l; phospholipid (PL), 10 µmol/l; factor VIIIa, 11 U/ml. Relative catalytic efficiency is V_{max}/K_m, normalized to the value for factor IXa alone.

Adapted from van Dieijen, G., Tans, G., Rosing, J., and Hemker, H. C.: The role of phospholipid and factor VIIIa in the activation of bovine factor X. J. Biol. Chem. 256:3433, 1981. With permission from the American Society for Biochemistry and Molecular Biology.

concentrations (approximately 0.2 μmol), but the maximal rate of reaction increases only an additional twofold. However, if factor VIIIa is then added, the K_m for factor X stays roughly constant, whereas the V_{max} of the reaction increases more than 20,000-fold.[93] Qualitatively similar results have been reported for the human system.[94, 95] Presumably, the stoichiometric interaction between factors VIIIa and IXa[96] enhances the V_{max} of factor IXa, whereas the calcium-dependent binding of factors IXa and X to the phospholipid surface lowers the apparent K_m for factor X in the complete reaction system by increasing the local concentration of reactants.

Factor IXa binds to factor VIII or VIIIa with high affinity ($K_d \approx 11$ to 15 nmol in the absence of phospholipid)[97] through at least two sites (see Plate 21–1). The serine protease domain of factor IXa binds to a site in domain A2 that appears to include the segment Ser 558–Gln 565.[98, 99] The first epidermal growth factor (EGF) domain of factor IXa binds to a site in the factor VIII A3 domain that appears to include the segment Glu 1811–Lys 1818.[100] Binding of factor IXa to factor VIII is inhibited by VWF, but cleavage of the factor VIII light chain after Arg 1689 abolishes this effect. Thus, exposure of the factor IXa binding site requires dissociation of the factor VIII/VWF complex.[97] Binding of factor IXa to both the A/A3-C1-C2 dimer and the A2 chain of factor VIIIa may also explain how factor IXa slows the dissociation of the A2 subunit and thereby stabilizes factor VIIIa activity.

Phospholipid Requirement. Factor VIII and factor VIIIa bind tightly to phospholipid vesicles that contain sufficient phosphatidylserine with a K_d of approximately 2 nmol.[101] Specific, high-affinity binding depends on structural features of the phosphatidylserine head group rather than simply its negative charge.[102] This interaction is mediated by the factor VIII light chain and appears to require a segment of domain C2.[103]

Coagulation on Biological Surfaces

During clotting in vivo, reactions that are moderately well understood in reconstituted solutions occur in the presence of cellular components that may profoundly alter them. In particular, platelets are normally inert until activated by thrombin. After thrombin activation, platelets demonstrate considerable procoagulant activity, perhaps serving the role in vivo that phospholipid vesicles fill for in vitro assays. In addition, the endothelial cell lining of the vascular system has both procoagulant and anticoagulant properties that can be modulated by the adjacent blood.

Hemostatic Reactions at the Platelet Surface. Platelets not only provide procoagulant phospholipid on demand but also have specific receptors for some clotting factors and secrete additional factors during the platelet release reaction. Hemostatic interactions of platelets are also discussed in Chapter 24.

The distribution of phospholipid types across the platelet plasma membrane is asymmetrical, with essentially all of the negatively charged phosphatidylserine confined to the cytoplasmic leaflet.[104] In the resting platelet, the phospholipid exposed to the blood is devoid of procoagulant activity, whereas that exposed to the cytoplasm is extremely active.

Activation of platelets causes the redistribution of coagulantly active phosphatidylserine to the outer leaflet.[105]

Binding of factor VIII to platelets is stimulated approximately 20-fold on thrombin activation, and there are about 450 sites per platelet with a K_d of approximately 3 nmol.[106] This binding affinity is similar to that of factor VIII binding to phospholipids, and phospholipids compete for binding of factor VIII to platelet-derived microparticles.[107] Factor V and factor VIII appear to bind with comparable affinity to different sites on activated platelets or platelet microparticles, although high concentrations of factor Va can inhibit factor VIII binding.[106, 107] VWF inhibits the binding of factor VIII to activated platelets, with an apparent dissociation constant of 0.44 nmol for the factor VIII/VWF interaction.[108]

Hemostatic Reactions at the Endothelial Cell Surface. Endothelial cells can affect blood clotting on their surface through many mechanisms. They contain proteoglycans that accelerate the inactivation of thrombin by antithrombin.[109, 110] Endothelial cells secrete prostacyclin, a potent inhibitor of platelet aggregation,[111] and tissue plasminogen activator, an initiator of fibrinolysis.[112] They also express thrombomodulin, a plasma membrane protein that binds thrombin, promoting the activation of protein C and inhibiting the procoagulant activities of thrombin. The protein C anticoagulant system is discussed in Chapter 19. Thus, the anticoagulant properties of endothelium are maintained by several independent pathways.

Several mechanisms have been described by which endothelial cells might enhance rather than inhibit thrombosis. Intact resting endothelial cells lack tissue factor activity but can express tissue factor in response to stimulation with thrombin[113] or endotoxin[114] and therefore could mediate the activation of factor X by the extrinsic pathway under some conditions. In addition, several components of the intrinsic factor X–activating complex can bind to endothelial cells, which contain specific high-affinity surface receptors for factor IX/IXa and factor X.[115–117] As a consequence, most of the factor X–activating complex could be preassembled on the cell surface. If these clot-promoting activities of endothelium prove to occur in vivo, it will be interesting to learn how the opposing anticoagulant and thrombotic functions of the endothelium are regulated.

▼ MOLECULAR BIOLOGY OF FACTOR VIII

The factor VIII gene is near the tip of the long arm of the X chromosome at Xq28, only about 1 Mb proximal to the telomere and about 7.5 Mb distal to the fragile site at Xq27.3, and approximately 200 kb distal to the glucose-6-phosphate dehydrogenase locus[118, 119] (Fig. 21–3). The factor VIII gene spans about 186 kb of DNA and contains 25 introns and 26 exons[20, 22] (see Fig. 21–1). Accordingly, it constitutes about 0.1 per cent of the X chromosome. The large B domain of factor VIII is encoded by exon 14, which is 3106 nucleotides long.

The factor VIII gene has an additional unusual structural feature that contributes to the pathogenesis of hemophilia. The largest intron, intron 22, is 32.4 kb in length and contains another gene of unknown function termed *F8A* that produces a 1.8 kb transcript.[120] A transcribed sequence homologous to *F8A* is present in the mouse.[120] A second

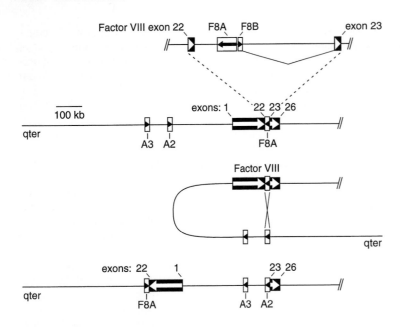

Figure 21–3. Recombination as a cause of severe hemophilia A. This diagram represents the mechanism of factor VIII gene inversion caused by intrachromosomal crossing over between homologous A gene sequences. The arrowheads indicate the direction of gene transcription. The *F8B* transcript includes a short first exon that is spliced as indicated to exon 23 of factor VIII. The orientation of *F8A* is opposite to that of A2 and A3, so that alignment and recombination of *F8A* with either homologue inverts the intervening segment.[134] The rearrangement depicted between *F8A* and the distal A3 sequence is referred to as type 1. The analogous rearrangement involving the proximal A2 sequence is referred to as type 2.

transcript in the opposite direction originates from the same promoter region and includes the downstream exons 23 to 26 of the factor VIII gene.[121] Two other homologues of *F8A* and several kilobases of flanking DNA sequence are present approximately 400 kb telomeric to the factor VIII gene[119, 120] (see Fig. 21–3). As discussed in a later section, recombination among the *F8A* homologues is the most common cause of severe hemophilia A.

▼ FACTOR VIII DEFICIENCY (HEMOPHILIA A)

Clinical Features of Hemophilia

So-called classical hemophilia, or hemophilia A, is an X-linked inherited disease characterized by deficient factor VIII activity. The prevalence of hemophilia A is approximately 100 per million males (e.g., see references 122 and 123). The residual factor VIII activity found in hemophilic plasma is variable. For clinical purposes, the factor VIII deficiency is classified as severe (<1 per cent), moderate (1 to 5 per cent), and mild (5 to 30 per cent) according to the percentage of factor VIII activity assayed relative to normal plasma.

Manifestations of hemophilia A include spontaneous bleeding into joints, muscles, and brain; delayed but prolonged bleeding from minor cuts; and severe bleeding from lacerations. Spontaneous bleeding is generally limited to patients with less than 5 per cent of normal factor VIII activity. Symptoms begin soon after birth and are lifelong but can be ameliorated by aggressive treatment of spontaneous or traumatic bleeding with various forms of factor VIII. The continuing evolution of home therapy for hemophilia has markedly decreased the dependence of hemophiliacs on hospital facilities.[124, 125] Most patients with hemophilia can now lead relatively normal lives, handling routine bleeding by self-administration of factor VIII preparations. Before effective factor VIII concentrates were widely used, patients with frequent hemarthroses developed crippling joint deformities by their second decade. Although skeletal problems have been largely eliminated in patients participating in

modern home-care programs, spontaneous intracranial bleeding and other internal bleeding still cause mortality.

Classification and Molecular Defects in Hemophilia A

Patients with hemophilia A have different degrees of factor VIII deficiency, but the severity of the deficiency varies little among those affected in any given hemophilia pedigree.[126] The qualitative heterogeneity of hemophilia was first directly demonstrated by the discovery of two classes of patients with severe factor VIII deficiency. About three fourths have no detectable factor VIII by both activity and antigen assays and are termed cross-reacting material negative (CRM−). The remainder have decreased or absent factor VIII activity with detectable factor VIII antigen. Patients with equal decrements of factor VIII antigen and activity are sometimes classified as CRM reduced (CRMred). Patients with disproportionately decreased factor VIII activity compared with antigen, consistent with the production of an immunologically recognizable but dysfunctional protein, are classified as CRM+.[9, 10, 127, 128]

The molecular basis for hemophilia A has been elucidated at the level of gene structure in many cases. An astonishing number of patients, at least 2500, have been studied since 1984. An extensive data base of factor VIII mutations has been published and should be consulted for references on individual mutations.[129, 130] This continuously updated resource is available online at the URL http://europium.mrc.rpms.ac.uk. The following summary of specific mutations reflects the state of this data base as of September 1999.

Chromosome Rearrangements. Until recently, the characterization of mutations in hemophilia A posed a conundrum: DNA sequencing disclosed causative mutations in essentially all patients with mild or moderate hemophilia A, but no abnormality could be found in about half of patients with severe disease.[131] This anomaly was explained by the discovery of a single, novel gene rearrangement in about 40 per cent of patients with severe hemophilia A. The mutation is an inversion near the tip of the X chromosome caused by intrachromosomal homologous recombination between *F8A* in intron 22 and one of its two homologues that are telomeric to the factor VIII gene[132, 133] (see Fig. 21–3). The distal homologue A3 is the recombination partner in about 84 per cent of cases, and the proximal homologue A2 accounts for most of the remainder.[134] Rare persons have three *F8A* homologues upstream of the factor VIII gene rather than two, and recombination in this more complex background has occurred in about 1 per cent of patients with severe hemophilia.[134] These events reverse the orientation of exons 1 to 22 and separate them from exons 23 to 26 by about 200 to 500 kb. Because these inversions occur almost exclusively during male meiosis, almost all mothers of patients with factor VIII inversions are carriers.[134, 135]

Deletions and Insertions. At least 92 large deletions (0.2 to more than 210 kb) have been reported. No identical large gene deletions have been found in unrelated patients, and no segment of the factor VIII gene appears to be strikingly susceptible to deletion or insertion events. Such deletions account for about 5 per cent of cases of severe hemophilia A and appear to represent examples of nonhomologous recombination. Three patients with moderate hemophilia have deletions involving exon 22[136] or exons 23 to 24.[137, 138] The moderate phenotype may be explained by inframe splicing around the deleted exons and secretion of a partially active factor VIII protein. Approximately 38 per cent of patients with large deletions have had factor VIII inhibitors (28 of 74 tested). At least 64 distinct small deletions (1 to 86 bp) have been reported, most of which cause a frameshift that should lead to premature termination of translation; only 7 among 49 tested patients have had an inhibitor.

Twenty short insertions (1 to 13 bp) have been described, all in patients with severe hemophilia but no inhibitors (with one exception). Two additional families with severe hemophilia A were described in which the factor VIII gene was mutated by the insertion of a long interspersed element (LINE-1).[139] One of these patients had a significant factor VIII inhibitor. Approximately 50,000 to 100,000 LINE-1 repeats are distributed throughout the genome, and they apparently move to new sites by a process similar to the retrotransposition of retroviruses.[140] In both families, the LINE-1 insertions occurred de novo in the affected males, suggesting that they were derived from an actively transposing LINE-1 element. The probable functional progenitor LINE-1 element was subsequently identified on chromosome 22, cloned, and shown to encode a functional reverse transcriptase. Such functional LINE-1 elements were proposed to provide the reverse transcriptase necessary for the dispersal of various interspersed sequences with properties that suggest derivation from reverse transcripts, including LINE elements, *Alu* repeats, and processed pseudogenes.[141, 142]

Nucleotide Substitutions. At least 324 single nucleotide substitutions from 727 unrelated patients have been collected in the factor VIII mutation data base, including 13 splice site, 46 nonsense, and 267 missense mutations.[129, 130] Six of the potential splice site mutations have been proposed to create alternative splice sites; an effect of one such mutation on splicing has been demonstrated directly.[143] All but two of the patients with nonsense mutations had severe hemophilia. Although nonsense mutations generally cause premature termination of translation, they may rarely affect splicing instead so that the exon containing the nonsense codon is skipped.[144] Of the 33 nonsense mutations for which information was available, 14 (42 per cent) were associated with inhibitor formation. In contrast, inhibitors developed in no patients with splice site mutations and in only approximately 2 per cent of patients with missense mutations.[130]

Missense mutations are often compatible with the synthesis of significant, possibly normal, quantities of factor VIII proteins with variable functional defects, and about half of patients with missense mutations have mild or moderate hemophilia. The resultant CRM+ or CRMred hemophilia phenotype sometimes can be understood in terms of the known structure-function relationships of normal factor VIII. For example, mutations have been identified that substitute either His or Cys for Arg 372[145, 146] or Arg 1689[147, 148] and so prevent proteolytic activation by thrombin; these mutations cause mild to severe CRM+ hemophilia A. As discussed under Association of Factor VIII With von Willebrand Factor, studies of recombinant mutant factor VIII with the substitution Tyr 1680 → Phe indicate that sulfation of Tyr 1680 is required for optimal binding to VWF.[42, 43] The identical mutation is found in patients with mild[149] or moderate[150] hemophilia A. The low factor VIII level of 2 to 10 per cent in these patients appears to be explained by reduced binding to VWF, causing reduced stability of the mutant factor VIII in the circulation.

The distribution of single nucleotide mutations suggests a mechanism by which they probably occur. There are 69 CG dinucleotides in the coding region of the factor VIII cDNA sequence, and to date at least 326 apparently independent C to T transitions have been reported in 35 of them. For comparison, 401 additional point mutations have been reported at 272 other positions.[130] Thus, approximately 45 per cent of reported factor VIII point mutations are C to T transitions occurring in CG dinucleotides, and identical mutations in some sites have occurred independently in many patients. In the factor VIII gene, the likelihood of mutation at CG dinucleotides is estimated to be increased 10-fold to 20-fold relative to other dinucleotides.[151] The cytidine residues in CG dinucleotides are frequently methylated in human genomic DNA, and the resultant 5'-methylcytidine may undergo spontaneous deamination to yield thymidine. This mechanism appears to explain why CG dinucleotides are hot spots for mutation in many genes, including the factor VIII gene.[152]

The origin of hemophilia A mutations shows an interesting dependence on the type of mutation. As discussed above, the common recombination/inversion events occur almost exclusively during male meiosis.[135] Point mutations also occur 5-fold to 10-fold more often in male gametes, whereas deletions are at least 5-fold more common in female gametes. On average, the male to female ratio of mutation frequencies appears to be approximately 3.6.[153]

Prenatal Diagnosis and Carrier Detection in Hemophilia A

At present, the best methods for the genetic analysis of hemophilia A are based on the detection of DNA sequence variations within or near the factor VIII gene. These typically employ DNA probes to identify the causative mutation itself,

DNA sequence polymorphisms within the factor VIII gene, or restriction fragment length polymorphisms (RFLPs) at loci closely linked to the factor VIII gene. Informative DNA markers cannot be identified for all families, and a combination of DNA-based methods and assays of plasma factor VIII may be required for optimal carrier detection and prenatal diagnosis. Fetal samples for DNA extraction can be obtained by chorionic villus sampling at 10 to 14 weeks of gestation or by amniocentesis between 10 and 20 weeks of gestation.[154] Factor VIII does not cross the placenta, and fetal blood suitable for factor VIII levels can be obtained by fetoscopy after about 18 weeks of gestation.[154]

In the most favorable cases, the mutation in the factor VIII gene can be identified directly. Identification of the genetic lesion itself makes both carrier detection and prenatal diagnosis unambiguous. Because inversions due to recombination between *F8A* sequences cause approximately 40 per cent of severe hemophilia A, analysis for these mutations will often be informative.[134]

If the causative mutation is unknown, intragenic DNA sequence polymorphisms are the best alternative markers for genetic studies. At least 11 polymorphisms have been reported within intronic regions of the factor VIII gene.[130, 155, 156] An additional 14 sequence polymorphisms are known within factor VIII exons, among which 4 change the encoded amino acid sequence and the remainder are silent.[130] For these markers to be useful, a given pedigree must contain at least one affected male with a heterozygous mother. The likelihood of demonstrating heterozygosity increases with the number of available polymorphic markers. There is some variation among races in the allelic frequencies of polymorphisms, so that no single combination of markers is necessarily optimal for all families. The utility of certain marker combinations is also limited by linkage disequilibrium. Nevertheless, analysis with the available intragenic polymorphisms has provided useful diagnostic information in at least 95 per cent of women tested.[154, 155]

If intragenic DNA markers are not informative, extragenic RFLPs can be employed. There are several highly polymorphic, extragenic RFLP marker systems that are closely linked to the factor VIII locus, among which two or three have been used extensively for genetic analysis of hemophilia A.[154, 155] For example, about 95 per cent of women are heterozygous at the St14(DXS52) locus, and this marker system is informative in almost all pedigrees.[157, 158] The utility of extragenic markers is limited by a significant probability ($\approx$5 per cent) of recombination between the polymorphic locus and the mutation in the factor VIII gene. To maximize the likelihood of identifying rare individuals in whom such recombination has occurred, diagnoses based on extragenic RFLPs should be checked by assays of plasma factor VIII.

For families with a single sporadic case of hemophilia A, the use of linked DNA polymorphic markers cannot identify with certainty relatives who carry the mutant allele. Approximately one sixth of patients with hemophilia A are found in families with no known prior history of the disease.[159] This is consistent with the calculation of Haldane[160] that about one third of cases of X-linked recessive disorders are due to spontaneous mutations, provided that the population is at equilibrium and affected persons have low fertility. Because factor VIII gene mutations are about 3.6-fold more

common in male gametes, most but not all mothers of isolated patients with hemophilia are carriers.[153] Therefore, in the first subsequent generation, DNA marker studies can exclude carrier status or hemophilia A but generally cannot prove that a female is a carrier or that a male fetus will have hemophilia. In practice, the probability is approximately 0.85 that the mother of a sporadic case will be a carrier of hemophilia.[154]

Because of this uncertainty, genetic counseling for these families may depend on the analysis of plasma factor VIII levels. Heterozygous carriers of hemophilia A often have plasma factor VIII levels intermediate between those of hemophiliacs and unaffected persons in their family, but several factors conspire to make factor VIII levels alone an unreliable index for distinguishing carriers from normal females. Factor VIII levels in carrier women may vary owing to differences in selective X-chromosome inactivation (lyonization) during development. A number of physiological mechanisms may cause transient or sustained elevations of factor VIII, and assays of factor VIII activity are also subject to significant uncertainty. Even in normal males, the level of factor VIII varies widely, and genetic analysis suggests that there are several normal alleles at the factor VIII locus, or linked to it, that cause inheritable differences in normal factor VIII activity.[161] Non-linked modifiers of factor VIII activity also exist, such as ABO blood type.[162, 163] Consequently, even with the best available methods to measure and to analyze plasma factor VIII levels, between 6 and 20 per cent of women will still be misclassified either as normal or as carriers.[163, 164]

Differential Diagnosis of Inherited Factor VIII Deficiency

Severe von Willebrand Disease. Patients with VWD type 1 ordinarily have a decrease in factor VIII levels that parallels their modest deficiency of VWF. Patients who have severe VWD type 3 occasionally have levels of factor VIII that are low enough to be classified as severe deficiency (<1 per cent). In contrast to hemophilia A, however, patients with VWD type 3 have extremely low levels of VWF antigen and ristocetin cofactor activity and markedly prolonged skin bleeding times. VWD type 3 can also be distinguished from hemophilia A by its autosomal recessive mode of inheritance, but this is not possible in many families.

von Willebrand Disease Type 2N. A recessive but autosomally inherited mimic of hemophilia A occurs if the factor VIII binding site on VWF is altered without affecting other VWF functions. This disorder, VWD type 2N, is discussed in more detail under Classification and Molecular Defects in von Willebrand Disease.

Combined Factor V and Factor VIII Deficiency. Factor V and factor VIII deficiency has rarely occurred in the same individual through chance inheritance of both parahemophilia and hemophilia A. However, in most cases, combined factor V and factor VIII deficiency is apparently due to a homozygous or compound heterozygous abnormality at a single autosomal locus. At least 60 apparently unrelated families have been described with this combined deficiency.[165] About 40 per cent appear to have originated around the Mediterranean basin, and consanguinity is present in two thirds. The populations with the highest disease frequency are Asians and Sephardic Jews in Israel. This is the fourth autosomal recessive bleeding disorder known to be relatively frequent in Jewish communities. The other diseases include factor XI deficiency in Ashkenazi Jews (frequency, 1 in 190); Glanzmann thrombasthenia in Iraqi Jews (frequency, 1 in 6400); and factor VII deficiency with the Dubin-Johnson syndrome in Iranian, Moroccan, and Iraqi Jews.[166]

Heterozygous carriers of factor V/factor VIII deficiency are almost always asymptomatic and have normal levels of factor V and factor VIII. Affected homozygotes have roughly equal decreases of factors V and VIII, usually 5 to 25 per cent of normal, and the residual factor V and factor VIII molecules appear to be normal.[165, 166]

Combined deficiency of factors V and VIII is caused by inactivating mutations in ERGIC-53, a component of the endoplasmic reticulum–Golgi intermediate compartment that is homologous to certain lectins.[167, 168] The biological function of ERGIC-53 is not known, although it is proposed to function as a molecular chaperone for the transport from the endoplasmic reticulum to the Golgi compartment of a specific subset of secreted proteins, including coagulation factors V and VIII.

Treatment of Hemophilia A

Treatment of bleeding with factor VIII preparations carries many well-recognized risks. The major ones are the transmission of infectious agents and the development of alloantibody inhibitors of factor VIII activity.

Viral Infections in Hemophilia A. Before the application of viral inactivation methods to factor concentrates in 1985, nearly all transfused hemophiliacs had abnormal liver function test results or serological evidence of viral hepatitis[169] and a substantial fraction had cirrhosis or chronic active hepatitis,[170] mostly due to hepatitis C (non-A, non-B hepatitis).[171] The delta agent (a defective virus that can replicate only in the presence of hepatitis B virus) also causes hepatitis in hemophiliacs.[172] Infection with the human immunodeficiency virus (HIV) has been a major transfusion-associated risk. In one study of 908 U.S. patients with hemophilia A who were transfused between 1978 and 1985, almost two thirds had serological evidence of HIV infection.[173] The risk of transfusion-associated infection has been reduced greatly by changes in the manufacturing of plasma-derived clotting factor concentrates, and the risk is reduced further by the use of recombinant clotting factors.

Several methods have been employed to inactivate hepatitis viruses and HIV-1 in blood products. These include various forms of heating or pasteurization and treatment with detergents and organic solvents. In the United States, all plasma clotting factor preparations that are derived from large numbers of donors have been subjected to at least one virucidal treatment. This includes factor VIII concentrates, highly purified factor VIII, prothrombin complex concentrates, and activated prothrombin complex concentrates, all of which may be manufactured from the pooled plasma of 10,000 or more donors. In contrast, virtually none of the products derived from single donors or from relatively small numbers of donors, such as cryoprecipitate, is so treated. Current methods for the treatment of factor VIII concentrates apparently prevent transmission of HIV, hepatitis B, and hepatitis C.[174, 175]

Following the widespread use of virucidally treated concentrates, some previously unrecognized transfusion-associated infections have emerged. In particular, hepatitis A virus and parvovirus B19 are relatively resistant to inactivation because they lack lipid envelopes, and both apparently have been transmitted by factor VIII concentrates.[176–178]

Factor VIII Preparations for Treatment of Hemophilia A. Low-purity factor VIII concentrates may occasionally have other side effects, including skin test anergy[179] and decreased CD4 lymphocyte levels,[180] that have been attributed to the large variety and amount of contaminating proteins in such concentrates. Rarely, factor VIII concentrates have also been associated with allergic reactions or the development of pulmonary hypertension.[181]

Plasma-derived factor VIII preparations that are essentially free of extraneous proteins have been in use since the late 1980s. These products are prepared by immunoaffinity chromatography, with use of monoclonal antibodies to either factor VIII or VWF. The resultant "monoclonal" factor VIII has a specific activity of more than approximately 2000 units/mg, exclusive of added albumin. Recombinant human factor VIII of similar purity has been commercially available since the early 1990s. Plasma-derived and recombinant products have similar pharmacokinetics, efficacy, and safety.[182–184] Recombinant factor VIII is thought to have a lower risk of viral transmission because the only plasma-derived constituent is albumin. No cases of HIV or hepatitis transmission are known for recombinant factor VIII, although possible instances of parvovirus B19 seroconversion have been reported.[184]

Alternatives to Blood Product Therapy. Factor VIII levels in normal individuals and those with mild to moderate hemophilia A are elevated by a variety of stimuli, including estrogens, catecholamines, neurological stress, chronic inflammation, liver disease, and hyperthyroidism (reviewed in Bloom[185]). Consequently, pharmacological agents have been sought that mimic these effects. The most useful adjunct to factor replacement at present is 1-deamino-(8-D-arginine)-vasopressin (DDAVP), a synthetic analogue of antidiuretic hormone that lacks vasoconstrictor activity. DDAVP stimulates the release of preformed factor VIII and VWF from storage sites into the circulation, elevating plasma levels threefold to sixfold.[186] There are also transient increases in tissue plasminogen activator activity.[187, 188]

The reservoir of VWF is most likely endothelial cells located throughout the vasculature, but the source that accounts for the immediate rise in factor VIII is unknown. Coexpression of factor VIII and VWF in cultured endothelial cells leads to colocalization and storage of both proteins in secretory granules (Weibel-Palade bodies).[189] Although factor VIII and VWF colocalization has not yet been reported in vivo, both proteins may be stored as a complex in a subset of endothelial cells from which they could be released together in response to DDAVP or other stimuli.

The elevations in VWF and factor VIII are maximal at 30 to 90 minutes after a dose of DDAVP and decrease with kinetic properties similar to those of transfused factor VIII/VWF complex. Often, but not uniformly, repeated administration of DDAVP elicits diminishing responses, which seems likely to reflect progressive depletion of stored factors rather than the desensitization of receptors.[187, 190] In patients with severe VWD who have undetectable plasma VWF antigen, DDAVP does not cause an increase in factor VIII levels. Therefore, the factor VIII response obtained for patients with mild deficiency of either factor VIII or VWF is probably secondary to the induction of VWF release. In suitable patients with either hemophilia A or VWD, DDAVP given intravenously, subcutaneously, or intranasally has been used successfully to treat hemarthroses and other spontaneous bleeding and as coverage for minor surgical procedures without the use of factor VIII concentrates.[187, 191, 192]

Antibody Inhibitors of Factor VIII. In approximately 15 to 25 per cent of patients with hemophilia A, therapy is associated with the development of alloantibodies that inhibit factor VIII activity and interfere with subsequent factor replacement therapy.[193, 194] Rarely, autoantibodies to factor VIII may occur in a non-hemophilic person, causing acquired factor VIII deficiency.

Alloantibody inhibitors of factor VIII occur mostly among patients with severe CRM− hemophilia A who have deletions or nonsense mutations in the factor VIII gene.[129, 130] Although inhibitors do occur rarely in patients with CRMred or CRM+ hemophilia A, they are more often transient or of low titer in such patients. The development of inhibitors clearly depends on more than the nature of the factor VIII mutation alone. The extent and location of a factor VIII gene deletion do not correlate with the occurrence of factor VIII inhibitors; patients with and without inhibitors have been found to have similar deletions. Similarly, patients with and without inhibitors have been found with identical nonsense mutations.

In patients who develop inhibitors, the nature of the antibody response is at least partly under genetic control, and several studies have suggested an association between histocompatibility antigen patterns and the development of inhibitors.[195–198] A substantial fraction (15 to 30 per cent) of previously untransfused patients develop transient low-titer inhibitory antibodies that disappear despite continued factor replacement therapy and are of no apparent clinical significance.[182, 195, 199] Other patients with inhibitors appear to fall into two major groups. Inhibitors developing in adults after lifelong exposure to factor VIII are most often of low titer (<6 Bethesda U/ml), and marked increases in the inhibitor titer generally do not occur after treatment with factor VIII; these patients are classified as low responders. More commonly, inhibitors develop after relatively brief exposure to factor VIII (e.g., less than 50 "exposure days") and occasionally after a single treatment with factor VIII. Most such inhibitors develop before the age of 30 years with the greatest risk before the age of 5 years, are of high titer, and show dramatic increases in titer after additional treatment with factor VIII; such patients are classified as high responders.[193, 195]

Alloantibody inhibitors are most often of restricted polyclonal origin and are usually immunoglobulin G (IgG). The majority of inhibitors contain an excess of subclass IgG4 antibodies and usually have at least one component of another IgG subclass.[200] Despite the large size of the factor VIII polypeptide, which offers many potential epitopes for the induction of antibody responses, a small subset of epitopes appear to be recognized by most of the clinically significant inhibitors. For example, one major epitope is within the amino-terminal half of domain A2, and another is within domain C2 of the light chain.[201–203]

There are no fully satisfactory methods to eliminate factor VIII antibodies (reviewed in Hoyer[204] and Aledort[170]). Inhibitors have been suppressed in some patients by treatment with various combinations of corticosteroids, immunosuppressive drugs, and intravenous immune globulin. Prolonged therapy with factor VIII, with or without accompanying immunosuppressive therapy, has induced immune tolerance to factor VIII in some patients. Extracorporeal absorption of inhibitor antibodies on protein A–agarose has been helpful in a few reported cases. The limited number of immunodominant factor VIII epitopes suggests a potential therapeutic use of recombinant factor VIII fragments either for the neutralization of inhibitor antibodies or for the induction of immune tolerance.

Circumvention of Factor VIII Inhibitors. Low-titer inhibitors can be overcome by increased doses of factor VIII. If the antibodies are of sufficiently high titer, effective treatment of bleeding episodes with factor VIII concentrates becomes impossible.

Current methods for circumventing inhibitors fall into two categories: administration of animal factor VIII that does not react with human inhibitors, and "bypassing" inhibitors by generating fibrin through pathways that are independent of factor VIII.

Porcine Factor VIII. Alloantibody inhibitors of human factor VIII are often less potent inhibitors of heterologous factor VIII. For this reason, bovine or porcine preparations have been used sporadically for more than 35 years in the treatment of hemophilia A to circumvent these inhibitors.[205] Heterologous blood products have the additional potential advantage that they are not known to transmit viral diseases to humans. However, the VWF in most bovine or porcine factor VIII preparations aggregates human platelets in vivo, sometimes causing severe thrombocytopenia[205] or allergic reactions.[206]

These problems are reduced by the use of a highly purified concentrate of porcine factor VIII that is relatively free of VWF.[207, 208] Allergic transfusion reactions occur in less than 3 per cent of treated patients.[208] A transient decrease in platelet count occurs in some patients, occasionally with a nadir below 100,000/ml; this appears to be due to residual contamination with porcine VWF. The major factors limiting the utility of porcine factor VIII are cross-reactivity with anti–human factor VIII inhibitors and the induction of significant anti-porcine inhibitors in a majority of patients.

Prothrombin Complex Concentrates. Examination of the intrinsic and extrinsic clotting cascades suggests that factor VIII deficiency might be bypassed by delivering factor VIIa to activate factor X by the extrinsic mechanism, factor Xa itself, or thrombin. So-called prothrombin complex concentrates (PCCs) contain all of these components as well as many unactivated zymogens (prothrombin, factor VII, factor IX, factor X, and protein C) and variable amounts of factor VIII.[209, 210] These concentrates have been used for decades as a source of factor IX for the treatment of hemophilia B, and they had been used sporadically by the late 1960s to treat bleeding in patients with hemophilia A and factor VIII inhibitors. "Activated" prothrombin complex concentrates (APCCs) that contain relatively more of the activated factors and less of their zymogens were prepared specifically for the treatment of patients with factor VIII inhibitors and reported to be effective.[211]

By 1981, the efficacy of both PCCs[212] and APCCs[213] was demonstrated in blinded clinical trials; APCCs may be somewhat more efficacious.[213] Since then, these agents have been used widely. Immediate complications are uncommon but have included thromboembolism, myocardial infarction, and disseminated intravascular coagulation.[212] Anamnestic rises of the factor VIII inhibitor titer occur in many patients.[214, 215]

Factor VIIa. Factor VIIa is one candidate for the effective component in PCCs. A large fraction of the factor VII in PCCs has been proteolytically activated, and this fraction is even higher in APCCs.[216] The procoagulant activity of factor VIIa is dependent on tissue factor, and factor VIIa does not combine with antithrombin in the absence of heparin.[217] Therefore, injected factor VIIa might be able to reach a site of injury in an active form and combine there with liberated tissue factor. This could lead to the local activation of factor X by the extrinsic pathway, without causing significant systemic effects, and potentially could bypass the normal hemostatic requirement for factor VIII activity.

Limited clinical experience suggests that recombinant factor VIIa is effective for the treatment of bleeding in the majority of patients with hemophilia A and high-titer inhibitors. Conditions treated successfully include hemarthroses and muscle hematomas,[218] retropharyngeal hemorrhage,[219] and intracranial hemorrhage.[220, 221] Factor VIIa has also been used as coverage for minor and major surgery.[222, 223]

Gene Therapy for Hemophilia A

Preclinical development of gene therapy for hemophilia A has employed mouse and dog models. The approximately 9 kb factor VIII cDNA is too large to insert into many viral vectors, and gene therapy efforts have used human factor VIII variants from which the B domain has been deleted. A retroviral vector pseudotyped with the vesicular stomatitis virus G glycoprotein was injected intravenously into newborn factor VIII–deficient mice. Normal or supranormal levels of human factor VIII were achieved in some mice, their hemostatic defect was corrected, and factor VIII expression was sustained for at least 14 months.[224] Adenoviral vectors containing a similar B domain–deleted factor VIII were administered to hemophilic dogs, and therapeutic levels of human factor VIII were achieved; levels declined after 1 or 2 weeks, apparently because of a human factor VIII–specific inhibitor antibody response.[225] Similar adenoviral vectors were also administered to mice with targeted inactivation of the factor VIII gene,[226] and factor VIII levels of approximately 2 U/ml were attained for 7 weeks; levels declined thereafter but still were approximately 0.1 U/ml at 40 weeks.[227] Human clinical trials are in progress using retroviral vectors or genetically modified autologous fibroblasts.

Factor IX and Hemophilia B

Like factor VIII, factor IX participates in the middle phase of the intrinsic pathway of blood coagulation (see Fig. 21–2). It circulates in plasma as an inactive zymogen that is activated through proteolytic cleavage by factor XIa or by a complex of factor VIIa and tissue factor. Activated factor IXa then forms a complex with factor VIIIa, a phospholipid surface, and calcium to activate factor X. The clinical similarity of severe hemophilia A (factor VIII deficiency) and hemophilia B (factor IX deficiency) can therefore be rationalized as the result of deficient function of the intrinsic factor X–activating complex, arising by mutations affecting independent components of that complex.

▼ PURIFICATION AND STRUCTURAL CHARACTERIZATION OF FACTOR IX

Assays for Factor IX

Factor IX was first assayed as a component, present both in normal plasma and in plasma from patients with hemophilia A, that corrected the clotting in vitro of plasma from patients with hemophilia B.[4, 5] Unlike factor VIII, factor IX activity is not destroyed during clotting, and normal serum will also correct hemophilia B plasma. Synthetic peptide substrates with adequate specificity for factor IXa are not widely available. Consequently, assays for factor IX still generally involve a determination of the time required for a clot to form in factor IX–deficient plasma. This assay is relatively insensitive and not totally specific for factor IX. One unit of factor IX activity is defined as the amount found in 1 ml of pooled normal plasma.

Factor IXa can be assayed by modification of the factor VIII assays employing purified components. The factor IXa–mediated generation of factor Xa that is dependent on calcium, phospholipid, and factor VIII is determined as described in Assays for Factor VIII.

Heterologous polyclonal and monoclonal antibodies as well as alloantibodies to human factor IX have been reported. With use of such reagents, assays of factor IX antigen by Laurell rocket, radiometric, and enzyme-linked immunosorbent methods have been described.[228]

Purification of Factor IX

Factor IX is difficult to purify for several reasons. The concentration of factor IX in plasma is low, approximately 2 to 3 μg/ml, or approximately 40 to 60 nmol/l. The zymogen form of factor IX is susceptible to cleavage by several blood proteases that may be activated during the collection of blood or during purification procedures. In addition, factor IX belongs to a large family of proteins related to trypsin, many of which occur in blood plasma and tend to copurify. Among these, seven are known that have not only homologous protease-like domains but also another homologous amino-terminal domain that contains 10 to 20 γ-carboxyglutamic acid (Gla) residues. These are discussed in Chapter 18 and include prothrombin, factor VII, factor X, protein C, protein S, and protein Z.

Purification of bovine[229] and human[230] factor IX to homogeneity with efficient resolution from factor VII, factor X, and prothrombin was first achieved by salt gradient elution from heparin-agarose, for which factor IX has the highest affinity. Pure factor IX has a specific activity of approximately 325 to 500 U/mg.[231]

Structure of Factor IX

Human factor IX is composed of a single polypeptide chain of 415 amino acid residues and has a molecular weight of approximately 55,000. Comparison of the factor IX amino acid sequence with other vitamin K–dependent clotting factors, and with more distantly related serine proteases, reveals striking similarities of sequence that reflect the evolution of this protein family from a common ancestor (see Chapter 18). On the basis of these homologies, factor IX can be considered to have four distinct domains. Starting at the amino-terminal tyrosine, these include (1) the Gla domain, (2) the growth factor domain, (3) the activation peptide domain, and (4) the catalytic domain (Fig. 21–4). In addition, the factor IX precursor contains a signal peptide (prepeptide) as well as a short propeptide that is required for efficient post-translational carboxylation of glutamic acid residues. The crystallographic structure of porcine factor IXa has been determined (see Plate 21–2) and provides a useful framework for discussing the structure and function of this protease.

Approximately 20 per cent of the mass of factor IX is carbohydrate. There are two N-glycosylation sites at asparagine residues 157 and 167, within the activation peptide.[232] In 35 per cent of factor IX molecules, the activation peptide is also incompletely modified by O-linked oligosaccharides attached to Thr 159, Thr 169, and Thr 172.[233, 234] The first EGF-like domain has two unusual O-linked oligosaccharides: (xylosyl)$_{1-2}$-glucose is attached to Ser 53,[235] and a tetrasaccharide is linked to Ser 61 through a fucose residue.[236, 237] Similar oligosaccharides are found in certain EGF-like domains of other hemostatic proteases; the function of these O-glycans in the first EGF-like domain is unknown,[238] and they are not conserved in porcine factor IX (see Plate 21–2).

The Gla domain corresponds to amino acid residues 1 through 47 (see Fig. 21–4 and Plate 21–2). In this region, all 12 of the glutamic acid residues are carboxylated to yield γ-carboxyglutamic acid.[239] The structure of the factor IX Gla domain has been determined by nuclear magnetic resonance spectroscopy.[240] The Gla residues are required for the calcium-dependent binding of factors IX and IXa to phospholipid membranes, and amino acid residues 1 to 11 are particularly important for binding.[241] In addition, both factor IX and factor IXa bind to cell-associated collagen IV on endothelial cells,[242, 243] and this binding also depends on specific structural features within residues 3 to 11 of the Gla domain.[244]

The number of calcium ions bound by the Gla domain has not been determined precisely but is estimated to be 9.[245] The homologous Gla domains of other vitamin K–dependent proteins show considerable sequence conservation, which is consistent with the conserved calcium-binding function of this region in all of these proteins.

The growth factor domain of factor IX corresponds approximately to residues 48 through 127 (see Fig. 21–4 and Plate 21–2). This section consists of two tandemly arranged segments that are homologous to EGF. Among serine proteases, similar EGF-like domains are found in factor X, tissue plasminogen activator, urokinase, protein C, and factor XII.[246] However, prothrombin, which does have a homologous Gla domain and catalytic domain, has an unrelated domain in the position corresponding to the growth factor domain of factor IX. This segment of prothrombin is instead homologous to the "kringles" of plasminogen.[247] Interestingly, factor XII, tissue plasminogen activator, and urokinase have both kringle and EGF-like domains.[247] EGF-like domains are found in many other proteins that have no known role in hemostasis.[248] The corresponding gene segments have been shuffled and rearranged in several ways to yield the domain patterns observed in these diverse proteins.

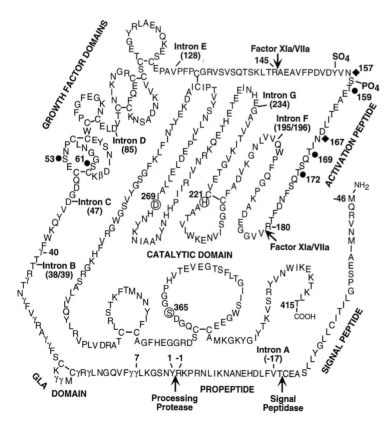

Figure 21–4. Structure of human profactor IX showing the location of the seven introns (A to G) of the factor IX gene. The factor IX precursor contains a 46 amino acid signal peptide and an 18 amino acid propeptide. The sites of cleavage by signal peptidase and a processing protease are indicated. The formation of factor IXa is due to the removal of an activation peptide following cleavage after Arg 145 and Arg 180. The amino acid residues of the catalytic triad His 221, Asp 269, and Ser 365 are circled. The single-letter code for amino acids is used, plus γ for γ-carboxyglutamic acid and β for β-hydroxyaspartic acid. Also indicated are sites of N-linked glycosylation (♦), O-linked glycosylation (●), sulfation of Tyr 155 (SO$_4$), and phosphorylation of Ser 158 (PO$_4$). (Adapted and redrawn from Yoshitake, S., Schach, B.G., Foster, D.C., Davie, E.W., and Kurachi, K.: Nucleotide sequence of the gene for human factor IX [antihemophilic factor B]. Biochemistry 24:3736, 1985.)

In addition to γ-carboxyglutamic acid, factor IX contains another unusual residue, β-hydroxyaspartic acid, present at position 64 in the first EGF-like domain.[249] This amino acid is produced by the post-translational hydroxylation of aspartic acid. About 25 per cent of human factor IX contains β-hydroxyaspartic acid at this position; the remainder contains aspartic acid. In bovine factor IX, however, there is one equivalent of β-hydroxyaspartic acid in the first growth factor domain. β-Hydroxyaspartic acid or the similarly modified β-hydroxyasparagine has been found at the same location within the first EGF-like domains of many vitamin K–dependent proteins, and also in EGF-like domains of many otherwise unrelated proteins, as discussed in Chapter 18. The function of β-hydroxyaspartic acid and β-hydroxyasparagine in these proteins is not known. In the case of factor IX, the first EGF-like domain binds calcium ions and Asp 64 is necessary for high-affinity binding; however, modification of Asp 64 to β-hydroxyaspartic acid is not required.[250]

The activation peptide domain of factor IX contains 35 residues and is the least conserved domain among serine proteases. Variations in this region presumably contribute to the selective activation of these enzymes by proteases that recognize a specific amino acid sequence. In addition to O-linked glycosylation, the activation peptide is post-translationally modified by sulfation of Tyr 155 and phosphorylation of Ser 158.[234] Factor XIa cleaves factor IX at two sites in this region, after Arg 145 and Arg 180 (see Fig. 12–4). Only the cleavage at the second site, however, results in expression of factor IXa catalytic activity. The sequence surrounding this arginine residue is the only highly conserved sequence in this domain among serine protease zymogens.

The catalytic domain of factor IX is a typical serine protease, and like trypsin, the active site of factor IXa contains a catalytic triad composed of His 221, Asp 269, and Ser 365 (see Fig. 21–4 and Plate 21–2). The amino acid sequence surrounding these active site residues is highly conserved among this family of enzymes. As in trypsin, an acidic residue, Asp 359, is located in the bottom of the substrate-binding pocket and results in specificity for cleavage at basic amino acid residues. Many of the serine protease zymogens share a common mechanism of proteolytic activation. Cleavage of the Arg-Val bond after Arg 180 in the activation peptide of factor IX allows the new amino-terminal Val residue to interact with Asp 364, which is adjacent to the active site Ser. This interaction causes a conformational change in the protein, increasing its catalytic activity.[251] Within the serine protease family, the similarities in protein structure and function are mirrored by features of gene organization, as is discussed in Molecular Biology of Factor IX.

▼ BIOSYNTHESIS AND METABOLISM OF FACTOR IX

Factor IX is synthesized primarily in the liver.[232] In common with other secreted proteins, the initial factor IX translation product contains an amino-terminal extension that is present as a preproleader sequence containing 46 (or 41 or 39) amino acids. The prepeptide or signal peptide is cleaved during translation between amino acid residues −18 and −19 by a specific signal peptidase in the rough endoplasmic reticulum. Further proteolytic processing to remove the 18 amino acid propeptide generates the mature polypeptide found in plasma with amino-terminal tyrosine.

The factor IX propeptide functions as a recognition element for propeptide cleavage and for the vitamin K–dependent carboxylase that catalyzes the conversion of glutamic acid residues to γ-carboxyglutamic acid. Certain features of the factor IX propeptide sequence are highly conserved among the vitamin K–dependent clotting factors and appear to be required for efficient carboxylation. These include amino acid residues Val −16, Ala −10, and (less dramatically) Leu −6.[252, 253] Additional conserved residues are required for efficient cleavage of the propeptide, and these include Arg −1, Arg −2, Arg −4, and Leu −6.[253, 254] The propeptide, therefore, contains two independent although possibly overlapping recognition motifs: a region near the amino terminus for the carboxylase, and a region near the carboxyl terminus for the propeptide-processing protease.

The post-translational synthesis of β-hydroxyaspartic acid is catalyzed by a specific α-ketoglutarate–dependent dioxygenase.[255] On the basis of alignment of EGF-like repeats that contain hydroxylated aspartic acid or asparagine residues, a consensus sequence has been proposed for the recognition of potential substrates by this enzyme.[256] Factor IX synthesized in the presence of suitable dioxygenase inhibitors does not contain β-hydroxyaspartic acid but nevertheless appears to have normal γ-carboxyglutamic acid content, blood clotting activity, and cell binding activity.[257] The function of β-hydroxyaspartic acid at position 64 remains, therefore, unknown.

Infusion of ^{125}I-labeled factor IX into patients with hemophilia B is followed by a rapid initial clearance of factor IX with a t½ of approximately 50 minutes, consistent with distribution of the infused protein into a space approximately three times larger than the plasma volume.[258] The rapid clearance phase is followed by slower disappearance, with a t½ of approximately 23 hours for factor IX activity. Unlabeled factor IX clearance in patients with hemophilia B shows a similar pattern.[259] The mean normalized plasma clearance rate of factor IX was estimated to be about 3.4 ml/kg/h, suggesting a daily turnover of approximately 82 units per kilogram of body weight[65] or approximately 164 μg of factor IX per kilogram of body weight assuming a specific activity of 500 U/mg.

▼ BIOLOGICAL FUNCTION OF FACTOR IX

The interactions of factor IX in the intrinsic factor X–activating complex, in solution, and on cell surfaces are discussed in the preceding corresponding section for factor VIII. The following section emphasizes features of factor IX structure that are important for these reactions.

Proteolytic Activation of Factor IX

During activation of factor IX by limited proteolysis, two peptide bonds are cleaved, as shown in Figure 21–5. There are two possible routes to the final factor IXa product, but

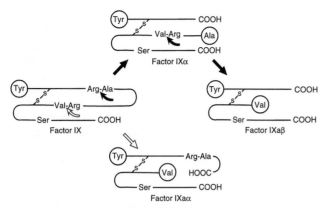

Figure 21–5. Proteolytic activation of factor IX. Amino-terminal residues of the heavy and light chains are shown in circles. The locations of bonds cleaved by activating proteases and the active site serine residue are indicated. The two polypeptide chains of factor IXa, factor IXaα, and factor IXaβ are joined by at least one disulfide bond. The reactions of the upper pathway are catalyzed by either factor XIa or by the factor VIIa/tissue factor complex in the presence of calcium ions. The reaction of the lower pathway is catalyzed by the RVV-X protease of Russell's viper venom, which cleaves the peptide bond indicated by the open curved arrow. (Adapted from Lindquist, P.A., Fujikawa, K., and Davie, E.W.: Activation of bovine factor IX [Christmas factor] by factor XIa [activated plasma thromboplastin antecedent] and a protease from Russell's viper venom. J. Biol. Chem. 253:1902, 1978.)

only one path appears to have a significant rate. When factor IX is activated by factor XIa or factor VIIa/tissue factor, the Arg 145–Ala bond is cleaved rapidly, generating a two-chain form of factor IX that is catalytically inactive and called factor IXα. The rate-limiting step in factor IX activation by either protease is the conversion of factor IXα to factor IXaβ by cleavage after Arg 180 in the activation peptide.[260, 261] The RVV-X protease from Russell's viper venom produces factor IXaα by cleaving only the Arg 180–Val bond. Activation of factor IX by either factor XIa or RVV-X requires the presence of divalent cations, such as calcium, that apparently interact in a complex manner with several metal binding sites on factor IX.[262] High concentrations of factor Xa apparently can cleave factor IX at both sites, although so slowly that feedback activation of factor IX by factor Xa is not likely to be important in vivo.[263]

The two activated enzymes, factor IXaα and factor IXaβ, do not have equivalent coagulant properties. Whereas both have similar activity toward small synthetic substrates, factor IXaα seems to interact with phospholipid less effectively than factor IXaβ does. As a result, factor IXaα is far less active than factor IXaβ for the activation of factor X in a reaction containing factor VIIIa, calcium ions, and phospholipid.[264]

Both factor VIIa and factor XIa are important activators of factor IX in vivo. The concentration of circulating factor IX activation peptide is markedly reduced in congenital factor VII deficiency but not in factor XI deficiency, indicating that factor VIIa/tissue factor accounts for most factor IX cleavage under basal conditions.[265] During the initial phase of blood clotting, the factor VIIa/tissue factor complex generates a burst of factor IXa and factor Xa but then is inhibited rapidly by tissue factor pathway inhibitor, a Kunitz-type protease inhibitor. The subsequent factor IXa generation that sustains blood clotting appears to depend on factor XIa.[266]

The Role of Factor IXa in the Intrinsic Factor X–Activating Complex

Activated factor IXa specifically cleaves the heavy chain of factor X, generating factor Xa (see Fig. 21–2). The same site is cleaved during activation of factor X by the factor VIIa/tissue factor complex or by a Russell's viper venom protease, RVV-X. Factor Xa appears to be able to cleave this site autocatalytically as well, although this reaction is extremely slow and probably insignificant in vivo. In the absence of the cofactors factor VIII and tissue factor, the rate of autoactivation of factor X may be comparable to that of cleavage by factor IXa or factor VIIa.[264]

The K_m of factor IXa for its substrate, factor X, is lowered at least 5000-fold in the presence of both calcium ions and a suitable phospholipid surface (see Table 21–1). The addition of factor VIIIa causes little change in the K_m of the reaction but accelerates the catalytic rate (V_{max}) by a factor of more than 200,000. Thus, the complete factor X–activating complex, composed of factor IXa, factor VIIIa, phospholipid, and calcium, can activate factor X at a rate above 10^9 times that of factor IXa alone, as shown with bovine reagents.[93] Under most conditions, therefore, the activation of factor X by this mechanism appears to be absolutely dependent on both factor VIIIa and factor IXa. Thus, it is not surprising that hemophilia A and B are clinically indistinguishable.

Inactivation of Factor IXa

The rate of clearance of factor IXa in humans in vivo has not been reported. In mice, human factor IXa disappears from the circulation in a biphasic manner. Initially, there is rapid clearance of about 60 per cent of the injected dose in less than 5 minutes, perhaps reflecting rapid binding of factor IXa to endothelial cell receptors. The remaining factor IXa is cleared with a half-life similar to that of factor IX, which is about 24 hours in humans. However, within 2 minutes after injection, more than half of the circulating factor IXa is complexed to antithrombin. These data indicate that the half-life of free factor IXa is extremely short. Antithrombin/factor IXa complexes are cleared primarily by the liver, through a receptor that apparently also binds to α_1-antitrypsin/protease complexes.[267] In human plasma in vitro, factor IXa is rapidly inactivated by antithrombin, and this reaction is markedly accelerated by heparin.[268] Among other plasma protease inhibitors, α_1-antitrypsin and α_2-macroglobulin do not react with factor IXa.[267]

▼ MOLECULAR BIOLOGY OF FACTOR IX

The factor IX locus is near the terminus of the long arm of the human X chromosome, just proximal to the locus for the fragile X mental retardation syndrome locus at q27.3.[269] The factor IX gene (Fig. 21–6) is approximately 33.5 kb in length and consists of eight exons (I to VIII) separated by seven introns (A to G). The presumed region does not have a classical TATA sequence in the usual position relative to the transcription initiation site.[270, 271] The exons range in length from a short 25 nt (exon III) to a long 1935 nt (exon VIII). The introns range from 188 nt (intron B) to 9473 nt (intron

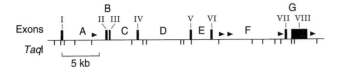

Figure 21–6. Map of the human factor IX gene. The region of the X chromosome containing the gene is represented. The scale is in kilobases of DNA. Exons are numbered (I to VIII), and introns are designated by letter (A to G). The location and orientation of *Alu* repeats are shown by arrowheads. The locations of *Taq*I restriction sites are shown.

F). Five *Alu* sequences are within or adjacent to the gene. The positions of all seven introns within the coding sequence of the factor IX gene are similar to those of the genes for human protein C,[272] factor VII,[273] and factor X.[274] The location of the first three introns of factor IX is also conserved in the prothrombin gene.[275]

The introns divide the factor IX gene into regions that roughly correspond to structural or functional domains of the protein (see Fig. 21–4). A similar pattern is observed for the gene structure of many other proteins that share homologous domains with factor IX.[247]

▼ FACTOR IX DEFICIENCY (HEMOPHILIA B)

Clinical Features of Hemophilia B

X chromosome–linked factor IX deficiency, or hemophilia B, is approximately 20 per cent as common as hemophilia A, with a prevalence of 15 per million males.[122, 123] As in hemophilia A, the residual activity of factor IX in hemophilia B varies among affected kindreds, and the disease is classified as severe (<1 per cent), moderate (1 to 5 per cent), or mild (6 to 30 per cent) on the basis of the amount of factor IX activity assayed in the patient's plasma. About one third to one half of affected kindreds have severe disease. As previously mentioned, the symptoms and clinical course of hemophilia B and hemophilia A are indistinguishable.

Replacement therapy for hemophilia B is similar in principle to that for hemophilia A. For unknown reasons, the incidence of such inhibitors is much lower in hemophilia B than in hemophilia A. Antibodies to factor IX develop in 1 to 2 per cent of treated patients with hemophilia B and 2.5 to 4 per cent of those with severe disease.[276, 277]

Classification and Molecular Defects in Hemophilia B

As in hemophilia A, patients with hemophilia B can be divided into several immunologically defined groups. More than 50 per cent have no detectable factor IX antigen and are termed cross-reacting material negative (CRM − or hemophilia B −). The remaining patients possess some protein that can be recognized by one or more antibodies to normal factor IX and are therefore CRM + or hemophilia B +. Both CRM + and CRM − groups can be further subdivided, indicating that a wide variety of genetic lesions can produce factor IX deficiency. More than 694 different mutations causing hemophilia B have been characterized at the level of DNA sequence, and these provide insight into the mechanisms underlying spontaneous mutation as well as the pathophysiology of hemophilia B. These mutations have been collected in a data base that is continuously updated and is accessible online at URL http://www.umds.ac.uk/molgen/haemBdatabase.htm.[278] Mutations have been identified in every class of gene structural element except for the poly(A) addition site.

Mutations that result in severe, CRM − hemophilia B tend to be due to large gene deletions, frameshift mutations, and nonsense mutations (causing premature termination of translation). The inability to synthesize part or all of the factor IX polypeptide appears to be associated with an increased risk for the development of factor IX inhibitors, probably because the appropriate epitopes are not expressed to establish tolerance. Large deletions or more complex rearrangements account for 2 to 5 per cent of patients with hemophilia B.[278] At least 42 patients with large partial or total gene deletions have been described.[279–281] Among 39 patients with deletions for whom appropriate data were reported, 15 had developed inhibitors.[279] Among 330 patients with characterized frameshift and nonsense mutations, inhibitors were reported in 17 (5 per cent).[278] In contrast, among at least 1160 patients with missense mutations, only 2 patients were found to have inhibitors[279, 282]; only 1 of these was CRM +.[282] Only 1 of 103 patients with splice site mutations reportedly had an inhibitor.[278]

A small minority of patients with CRM + hemophilia B (≈5 per cent) shows an equal decrement of factor IX activity and antigen, and these variants are sometimes referred to as CRMred. This phenotype may be due to mutations that decrease the synthesis of an otherwise normal factor IX; decreased factor IX secretion and increased catabolism are alternative mechanisms. Hemophilia B Leyden is an unusual CRMred variant in which the plasma level of factor IX is not stable. Affected males begin life with low factor IX levels (usually <1 per cent) and suffer from typical spontaneous bleeding. Around the onset of puberty, factor IX levels begin to rise, with subsequent cessation of bleeding. By adulthood, the factor IX level may be 20 to 60 per cent of normal.[283] The mutations associated with the hemophilia B Leyden phenotype cluster within nucleotides −20 to +13, around a major transcription initiation site.[278] These mutations appear to cause abnormal developmental regulation of factor IX expression, although the mechanism of this effect is not known. Some of these mutations disrupt a binding site for CCAAT/enhancer binding protein (C/EBP) between nucleotides +1 and +18[284] or for hepatic nuclear factor-4 (HNF-4) between nucleotides −34 and −10.[285] Recovery from hemophilia B Leyden during puberty appears to depend on an androgen response element that overlaps the HNF-4 site.[286]

Most CRM + patients have excess factor IX antigen, indicating that they produce a functionally defective factor IX. The characterization of these mutations has provided substantial information regarding the structure-function relationships of factor IX.

Propeptide cleavage is prevented by mutations at Arg −4 or Arg −1. These mutations result in moderate to severe hemophilia B, with mildly decreased to normal factor IX antigen levels. The presence of the uncleaved propeptide appears to interfere with the γ-carboxylation[287, 288] or function[289] of the adjacent Gla domain.

Several mutations within the Gla domain have been described that interfere with calcium binding or function of this domain.[278] Factor IX Zutphen contains an interesting mutation in this region, Cys 18 → Arg, that prevents the formation of the normal disulfide bond between Cys 18 and Cys 23. The mutant protein circulates in the blood at normal antigen levels, with α_1-microglobulin disulfide bonded probably to Cys 23.[290, 291]

Mutations within the growth factor domains of factor IX often cause hemophilia B+ of varying severity; a few such mutations appear to cause equal decreases in factor IX antigen and activity (CRMred). In general, the mechanism by which mutations in these domains cause hemophilia B is not known, although several mutations in domain EGF-1 are suggested to alter either the binding of calcium ions or an important calcium-dependent protein conformation. Mutagenesis studies demonstrate that conserved residues Asp 47, Asp 49, Gln 50, Asp 64, and Tyr 69 contribute to high-affinity calcium ion binding by domain EGF-1[292]; and substitutions have been identified at each of these residues in patients with hemophilia B.[278] The effect of mutations on calcium ion binding is not always predictable, however. The mutation Asp 47 → Glu causes severe hemophilia B[293] and moderately reduces the affinity of domain EGF-1 for calcium ions.[292] In contrast, the mutation Asp 47 → Gly causes mild hemophilia B but does not alter the affinity of calcium ion binding, and it is proposed to indirectly affect the interaction of factor IXa with factor VIIIa or factor X.[294]

Mutations within the activation peptide region confirm the importance for factor IX function of proteolytic cleavage after both Arg 145 and Arg 180. The substitution Arg 145 → His, first described in factor IX Chapel Hill,[295, 296] yields a protein that is activated slowly by factor XIa to a species resembling factor IXaα. Factor IX Chapel Hill has about 8 per cent of normal coagulant activity, and after activation to factor IXaα, it has 20 to 33 per cent specific clotting activity compared with normal factor IXaβ.

Several mutations have been described that inhibit or prevent cleavage of the Arg 180–Val bond. These include Arg 180 → Gln, Arg 180 → Trp, Val 181 → Phe, Val 182 → Phe, and Val 182 → Leu.[278] Patients with these mutations have a surprising laboratory phenotype, referred to as hemophilia B$_M$. This variant was reported in 1967 by Hougie and Twomey,[297] who described two brothers with hemophilia B who had normal prothrombin times with use of human (or rabbit) brain thromboplastin as the source of tissue factor but markedly prolonged prothrombin times with use of ox brain thromboplastin. Normal factor IX at similar concentrations does not prolong the ox brain prothrombin time. The variant was called hemophilia B$_M$, after the family name of the index cases—Murphy. This case provided the first evidence for heterogeneity in CRM+ hemophilia B, approximately 10 per cent of which may be classified as hemophilia B$_M$.[298, 299]

Several mutations in the catalytic domain of factor IX that destroy catalytic activity also prolong the ox brain prothrombin time and cause hemophilia B$_M$. A common mechanism may explain the similar effects of these disparate mutations: the catalytically inactive abnormal factor appears to competitively inhibit the activation of factor X by the (human) factor VIIa/(ox brain) tissue factor complex.[300, 301]

Prenatal Diagnosis and Carrier Detection in Hemophilia B

The detection of female carriers of hemophilia B has many problems in common with the detection of carriers of hemo-

philia A, previously discussed. On the basis of assays of plasma factor IX alone, even the best statistical methods will misclassify a fraction of prospective mothers. Prenatal diagnosis by fetoscopy has been successful but is complicated by the relatively low levels of factor IX even in normal fetal blood.[302]

Reliable genotype assignment for potential carriers and for prenatal diagnosis is generally accomplished by methods based on detection of DNA sequence variations. The available marker systems include both intragenic and linked extragenic DNA sequence polymorphisms.[154] Strong linkage disequilibrium limits the utility of some of these polymorphisms. Certain polymorphisms show striking variations in frequency among ethnic groups, and the optimal choices among marker systems must take this into account. Because the complete sequence of the factor IX gene is known,[271] the causative mutation can be identified in almost all cases by polymerase chain reaction analysis and DNA sequencing. For an increasing number of patients, therefore, the molecular defect can be detected directly from samples obtained by amniocentesis or biopsy of chorionic villi[154]; this approach permits unambiguous prenatal diagnosis and identification of carriers without the need to identify informative matings in the pedigree.

Treatment of Hemophilia B

PCCs are widely used for the treatment of bleeding in hemophilia B. As discussed under Treatment of Hemophilia A, these preparations contain a mixture of partially purified vitamin K–dependent blood clotting factors. PCCs are prepared with one or more virucidal treatments and do not appear to transmit HIV or viral hepatitis B and C.[175] Treatment of hemophilia with PCCs has been associated with thrombotic complications, however, including myocardial infarction,[303] venous thrombosis,[304] and disseminated intravascular coagulation.[305] The pathophysiological mechanism of these complications is not known with certainty but may depend on the presence of large amounts of activated clotting factors or phospholipids. Highly purified factor IX concentrates containing low concentrations of contaminating clotting factors are now available. Clinical studies indicate that these purified preparations have markedly decreased thrombogenicity compared with PCCs.[306, 307]

As for hemophilia A, recombinant DNA technology has provided a product for the treatment of hemophilia B that should be free of many potential risks associated with human plasma derivatives. Recombinant human factor IX expressed in CHO cells is commercially available, and clinical experience to date suggests that it is safe and effective. Recombinant and plasma-derived factor IX have a similar elimination half-life of approximately 18 hours, but the initial recovery of recombinant factor IX in vivo is decreased modestly by about 28 per cent compared with plasma-derived factor IX.

The development of a factor IX inhibitor is rare in hemophilia B but can be an extremely serious problem. Agents used for the treatment of bleeding in patients with hemophilia A and factor VIII inhibitors have also been used in patients with hemophilia B and factor IX inhibitors. These include APCCs[308] and recombinant factor VIIa.[218, 221-223]

Gene Therapy for Hemophilia B

Definitive correction of hemophilia B could be achieved, in principle, by the introduction of an active normal factor IX gene into some tissue of the patient. Hemophilia B is an attractive model disease for the development of such somatic cell gene therapy because relatively modest levels of factor IX expression would significantly ameliorate bleeding symptoms, and organ-specific targeting of gene expression may not be required. Preliminary steps toward this goal have been achieved. Mouse models of factor IX deficiency have been produced that show utility for the development of gene therapy.[309–311] Vectors based on adenovirus have been used to achieve sustained expression of normal levels of factor IX in mice by transduction of liver cells in vivo[309]; a similar strategy produced complete but transient correction of factor IX deficiency in hemophilia B dogs.[312] An adeno-associated virus vector injected intramuscularly in mice has yielded stable expression of normal levels of human factor IX,[313] and human clinical trials are in progress using a similar strategy.

von Willebrand Factor and von Willebrand Disease

In 1926, Eric von Willebrand described a bleeding disorder that differed from hemophilia by having an autosomal dominant mode of inheritance, a prolonged skin bleeding time, a normal platelet count, and severe mucocutaneous bleeding rather than spontaneous deep tissue bleeding.[314, 315] Von Willebrand and subsequent workers considered this to be a platelet or vessel wall disorder until 1953, when patients with VWD were discovered to have reduced factor VIII activity, suggesting a plasma abnormality.[316–318] Subsequent transfusion studies confirmed that a factor in either normal or hemophilic plasma could correct the bleeding time in VWD.[319, 320] Thus, as in the hemophilias, VWF was first recognized through its absence in an inherited bleeding disease.

▼ PURIFICATION AND STRUCTURAL CHARACTERIZATION OF VON WILLEBRAND FACTOR

Assays for von Willebrand Factor

The first in vitro assay for VWF activity, described in 1963, was based on the retention of platelets by glass beads.[321, 322] In blood of normal individuals, most of the platelets will adhere to glass, whereas in blood of patients with severe VWD, only a small fraction will adhere. This defect can be corrected by the addition of normal plasma. The glass bead retention assay is technically cumbersome, sensitive to variations in technique, and not specific for VWF. Nevertheless, it was useful in the diagnosis of VWD and was the basis for the first documented purification of VWF in 1972.[323]

A more practical assay was developed in 1971 when Howard and Firkin[324] discovered that the antibiotic ristocetin caused platelet aggregation in normal platelet-rich plasma but not in that from patients with VWD. Normal VWF is now routinely assayed by measuring the ristocetin-induced aggregation of platelets. Ristocetin cofactor activity (VWF:RCo) is assayed by mixing a suitably diluted plasma sample, washed platelets (usually formalin fixed), and a standard concentration of ristocetin. Platelet agglutination is followed by measuring the increase in light transmission through the platelet suspension as a function of time, and

the slopes obtained are compared with those for dilutions of a reference plasma standard. One unit of ristocetin cofactor activity is the amount of 1 ml of normal plasma, and the sensitivity of this assay is approximately 0.03 U/ml.[325] In a variation of this principle, the ristocetin-induced platelet aggregation (RIPA) assay employs the patient's platelet-rich plasma; the rate and extent of platelet aggregation are determined at different concentrations of added ristocetin and compared with those obtained with normal platelet-rich plasma.

A component with similar platelet aggregating activity has been identified in the venom of snakes belonging to the *Bothrops* genus, particularly *B. jararaca*.[326] This factor, termed botrocetin, acts by a mechanism different from that of ristocetin but can be employed in similar assays of botrocetin cofactor activity (VWF:BCo).[327] In certain variants of VWD, the RIPA, VWF:RCo, or VWF:BCo activity may be paradoxically increased (see von Willebrand Disease).

Several immunoassay methods are commonly employed to quantitate VWF antigen (VWF:Ag). The Laurell rocket method can detect 0.01 to 0.03 U/ml of VWF, and a modification with ^{125}I-labeled antibody is 100-fold more sensitive.[328] Immunoassays employing radiometric[329, 330] or enzymatic detection have been described with sensitivities of 0.002 to approximately 0.0002 U/ml.

Information about VWF multimer distribution in either plasma or platelets can be obtained by electrophoresis through agarose or agarose/acrylamide copolymer gels in the presence of the detergent sodium dodecyl sulfate. The separated VWF multimers are visualized by reaction with either ^{125}I-labeled antibody to VWF followed by autoradiography[331–333] or by immunoenzymatic methods. The patterns observed for normal plasma and for several variants of VWD are shown in Figure 21–7.

Assays have been described of VWF binding to collagen[334] and to heparin,[335] but they are not widely used in clinical laboratories. Assays of factor VIII/VWF binding

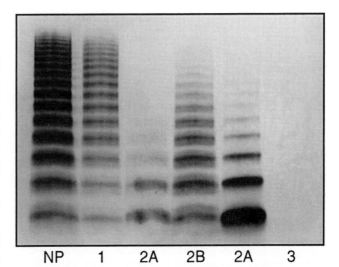

Figure 21–7. VWF multimer patterns in von Willebrand disease. Samples of plasma from a normal individual (N) and from patients with VWD types 1, 2A, and 3 were electrophoresed through a 1.3 per cent agarose/sodium dodecyl sulfate gel, and VWF was detected by Western blotting. (From Sadler, J.E.: von Willebrand disease. *In* Bloom, A.L., Forbes, C.D., Thomas, D.P., and Tuddenham, E.G.D. [eds.]: Haemostasis and Thrombosis. 3rd Ed. Edinburgh, Churchill Livingstone, 1994, pp. 843–857.)

have identified several patients with defects in this interaction. Such patients can have symptomatic factor VIII deficiency, as discussed in von Willebrand Disease Type 2N.

Purification of von Willebrand Factor

Factor VIII and VWF copurify through many different manipulations. Consequently, purification methods for these two proteins are similar. In most procedures, factor VIII and VWF are concentrated by cryoprecipitation and are copurified further by gel filtration chromatography on a 2 to 6 per cent agarose matrix. Both proteins co-elute in the void volume. If desired, factor VIII can be removed by rechromatography in 0.5M CaCl$_2$.[336] Additional chromatography steps are required to remove contaminating fibrinogen and fibronectin. In this fashion, VWF can be purified from plasma about 10,000-fold to near homogeneity with a specific VWF:Ag activity of 150 to 200 U/mg and VWF:RCo activity of approximately 110 U/mg.[336]

Structure of von Willebrand Factor

VWF consists predominantly of a single type of subunit with an apparent molecular weight (M$_r$) of about 250,000. Minor components with lower molecular weight (mainly M$_r$ 189,000, 176,000, 140,000, and 120,000) are present that are proteolytic fragments of the M$_r$ 250,000 subunit.[336, 337]

Multimers of VWF differ in size by a constant number of subunits. This basic repeating unit is a dimer of M$_r$ 250,000 subunits.[337–339] High-resolution electrophoresis methods show that each multimer of plasma VWF consists of a major band associated with several discrete but faint "satellite" bands; this heterogeneity appears to be due mostly to proteolytic degradation during circulation of VWF in the blood.[336, 337]

The VWF primary translation product is a precursor protein of 2813 amino acid residues (M$_r$ ≈ 360,000) that consists of a 22 amino acid signal peptide, a 741 amino acid (M$_r$ ≈ 95,000) propeptide, and the 2050 amino acid (M$_r$ ≈ 260,000) mature subunit (reviewed in Sadler[340]). The propeptide is also known as von Willebrand antigen II,[341] and it circulates in blood independently of VWF, possibly as a non-covalently associated homodimer.[342, 343] The amino acid residues of the prepropeptide region and the mature subunit are often numbered separately. The VWF precursor contains several types of repeated domains or motifs that are shared with other proteins and together account for more than 95 per cent of the sequence.[340] These domains are arranged in the order D1-D2-D'-D3-A1-A2-A3-D4-B1-B2-B3-C1-C2-CK (Fig. 21–8).

The amino acid composition of VWF is remarkable for the high content of half-cystine residues. These are clustered predominantly in two regions near the amino terminus and carboxyl terminus of the subunit. The pairing of 53 half-cystine residues has been reported.[344, 345]

VWF contains about 15 to 19 per cent carbohydrate, and 10 Thr/Ser and 12 Asn glycosylation sites have been identified in the mature VWF subunit[346] (see Fig. 21–8). The N-linked oligosaccharides are heterogeneous and include both complex-type and high-mannose structures. In addition, some of the N-linked oligosaccharides carry ABO blood group determinants.[347] Additional N-linked oligosaccharides

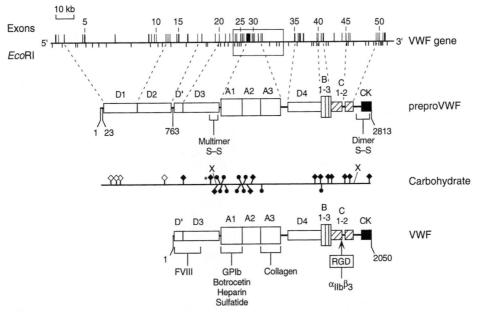

Figure 21–8. VWF gene and protein structure. *VWF gene:* The 52 exons of the VWF gene are indicated by bars above the line, and every fifth exon is numbered. *Eco*RI sites are indicated by tics below the line. The box encloses a region of the gene that is represented by an imperfect copy in a pseudogene located on chromosome 22. *preproVWF:* The dashed lines indicate the correspondence between the gene structure and the encoded primary translation product. The repeated domains are labeled D1, D2, D', D3, A1, A2, A3, D4, B1–3, C1–2, and CK. Amino acid residues in preproVWF are numbered consecutively 1 to 763; residues 1 to 22 are the signal peptide, residues 23 to 763 are the propeptide, and residues 764 to 2813 are the mature subunit. The locations of intersubunit disulfide bonds (S—S) are indicated. *Carbohydrate:* Sites of N-glycosylation shown to be used are indicated by filled diamonds, and potential sites of N-glycosylation in the propeptide are indicated by open diamonds. Two potential sites that are not used are indicated by ×. One site of N-glycosylation labeled with an asterisk occurs in the sequence Asn-Ser-Cys. Sites of O-glycosylation are indicated by filled circles. *VWF:* Amino acid residues in the mature subunit are separately numbered 1 to 2050. The sites of interaction with selected ligands are shown. Activated platelet integrin α$_{IIb}$β$_3$ binds VWF through a segment that includes the tripeptide sequence Arg-Gly-Asp (RGD) in domain C1.

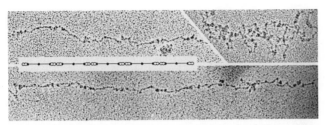

Figure 21–9. Electron micrograph of rotary shadowed human von Willebrand factor. The long, straight molecules are shown approximately on register with a repeat of about 120 nm, as illustrated in the schematic representation of VWF multimer structure *(inset)*. Tangled molecules *(upper right)* were observed most frequently and probably reflect the conformation in solution. (Adapted from Fowler, W.E., Fretto, L.J., Hamilton, K.K., Erickson, H.P., and McKee, P.A.: Substructure of human von Willebrand factor. J. Clin. Invest. 76:1491, 1985; courtesy of Harold Erickson, Duke University.)

are attached to some of the four potential glycosylation sites in the propeptide. The O-linked oligosaccharides appear to consist mainly of typical disialylated tetrasaccharides with the structure NeuAc(α2,3)Gal(β1,3)[NeuAc(α2,6)]Gal-NAc.[348]

One or both of the N-linked oligosaccharides at Asn 384 and Asn 468 are sulfated. Additional sulfate is found on N-linked oligosaccharides of the propeptide.[349]

VWF in solution is extremely asymmetrical.[46] Electron micrographs show that VWF consists of long, flexible filaments of approximately 2 nm containing small, regularly spaced nodules. The filaments range in length from 50 to more than 1800 nm[350] (Fig. 21–9).

▼ BIOSYNTHESIS AND METABOLISM OF VON WILLEBRAND FACTOR

VWF is synthesized by endothelial cells[351] and also by mega-karyocytes.[352] By immunochemical staining, it is localized to endothelial cells, subendothelial connective tissue,[353, 354] syncytiotrophoblast of placenta,[355] and platelet α granules.[356] In severe VWD, VWF is absent from both platelets and endothelial cells.[357, 358] Transfusion studies[358, 359] and bone marrow transplantation[360] in severe VWD suggest that there is no significant movement of plasma VWF into the subendothelium of intact blood vessels or into platelets. Thus, the observed tissue localization probably reflects local synthesis rather than absorption from plasma. Histochemical methods for the localization of VWF have been useful in the identification of endothelial cells and platelet precursors in normal and malignant tissues.

The biosynthesis of VWF is a complex process.[340, 361] In the endoplasmic reticulum, the signal peptide is cleaved from the primary translation product, N-linked glycosylation is initiated, and monomeric pro-VWF species rapidly form dimers through interchain disulfide bonds between carboxyl-terminal CK or cystine-knot domains. The superfamily of proteins containing CK domains includes several growth factors related to transforming growth factor-β (TGF-β) that share a tendency to dimerize through a specific disulfide bond.[340, 362] Alignment of VWF with TGF-β and mutagenesis studies indicate that the intersubunit disulfide probably involves Cys 2010.[363]

Pro-VWF dimers have free sulfhydryl groups that disap-

pear when additional disulfide bonds are formed between dimers after transit to the Golgi apparatus.[364] The resultant multimers contain intersubunit disulfide bonds that appear to involve at least one of the three cysteines at positions 459, 462, and 464.[365] An additional intersubunit disulfide links Cys 379 to Cys 379 on adjacent subunits.[345]

Multimerization depends on the presence of the VWF propeptide. The mechanism underlying this requirement has not been determined but may involve catalysis of protein disulfide exchange.[366] Assembly into multimers coincides approximately with cleavage of the propeptide, probably by the processing protease furin or a related subtilisin-like serine protease.[339, 364, 367] All VWF species except the intracellular dimer and monomer consist primarily of subunits of M_r of about 250,000 with only a small percentage of pro-VWF polypeptides. The final processing of complex-type N-linked oligosaccharides (including sulfation of some structures) and additional O-linked glycosylation also occur in the Golgi apparatus.[368]

Mature intracellular VWF is stored in subcellular organelles that are unique to endothelium, Weibel-Palade bodies (Fig. 21–10). These vesicles are 0.1 to 0.2 μm wide and up to 4 μm long, and they have longitudinal striations that appear to be closely packed multimers of VWF. In cross-section, the striations are seen to correspond to closely packed 150 to 200 ÅÅ tubules. Weibel-Palade bodies appear to be derived from the Golgi apparatus.[369, 370] Targeting to this organelle depends on features of both the propeptide and the mature subunit because neither is directed to storage granules when expressed individually.[371–373] The cleaved propeptide is packaged into Weibel-Palade bodies together with VWF multimers, with a stoichiometry of one propeptide per mature subunit.[342]

Two pathways have been identified for VWF release from cultured endothelial cells. For convenience, these can be called the constitutive and the regulated pathways.[361] Constitutive secretion requires continuing protein synthesis and is not dependent on extracellular calcium ions or intracellular cyclic adenosine monophosphate levels.[374] In cultured endothelial cells, the majority of VWF is secreted constitutively and consists mainly of dimers and small multimers.[375]

Regulated secretion of VWF is stimulated by treatment of endothelial cells with thrombin,[376] epinephrine,[377] histamine,[378] fibrin,[379] complement proteins C5b–9,[380] the calcium ionophore A23187, or the tumor promoter phorbol myristate acetate.[374] VWF secreted by the regulated pathway consists of large multimers and is associated with depletion of the Weibel-Palade bodies.[375] In contrast to constitutive secretion, regulated secretion of VWF does not require protein synthesis and does depend on extracellular calcium influx.[374, 375]

The plasma level of VWF antigen is about 10 μg/ml,[343] but this level may range from 40 to 240 per cent of the mean in normal individuals.[381] Approximately 15 per cent of the total circulating protein is within platelets.[382] Plasma levels of VWF are about 25 per cent lower in persons of blood type O compared with all other ABO blood types, and this variation should be considered in the establishment and interpretation of normal ranges for the diagnosis of VWD. There are additional smaller increases correlated with age,[381] and variations may be associated with Lewis blood type (secretor status).[383]

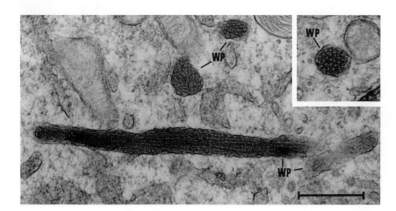

Figure 21–10. Electron micrograph of Weibel-Palade bodies in cultured human endothelial cells. Longitudinal striations are clearly seen in several membrane-delimited Wei-bel-Palade bodies (WP). A cross-section *(inset)* shows that the striations represent closely packed tubules. These are composed principally of VWF. The scale bar indicates 0.5 μm. (From Sadler, J.E.: Biochemistry and genetics of von Willebrand factor. Annu. Rev. Biochem. 67:395, 1998; courtesy of Elisabeth Cramer, Hôpital Henri Mondor, Creteil, France.)

A variety of physiological stresses are associated with transient changes in VWF and factor VIII levels. Most of these, such as exercise, trauma, and surgery, probably result from adrenergic stimulation. The vasopressin analogue DDAVP or growth hormone also causes an acute increase in plasma VWF, and the endogenous hormones may exert a similar influence in some diseases of the nervous system. The mechanism of DDAVP action in vivo appears to be indirect because cultured endothelial cells do not respond to it.[384, 385] Sustained elevation of VWF or factor VIII has been noted in several chronic conditions, including pregnancy, oral estrogen therapy, hyperthyroidism, inflammatory states, renal disease, diabetes, cancer, liver disease, and atherosclerosis (reviewed by Bloom[185]).

VWF is removed from the circulation in a biphasic fashion. An initial rapid disappearance phase with an apparent half-time of about 3 hours is followed by slower clearance with a half-time of about 12 to 20 hours.[63, 343] These kinetic patterns are observed in normal individuals as well as in patients with hemophilia A. In the latter group, the clearance of ^{125}I-labeled VWF parallels the clearance of factor VIII given as cryoprecipitate.[63] This is consistent with the observation that VWF binds to factor VIII in vivo and protects it from catabolism.[64] The clearance of VWF depends to some extent on its multimeric state. Larger multimers (found in cryoprecipitate) disappear faster than do the dimer and small multimers (found in cryosupernatant).[63]

▼ BIOLOGICAL FUNCTION OF VON WILLEBRAND FACTOR

VWF has two well-characterized functions. It is a carrier in plasma for factor VIII, as discussed in Factor VIII and Hemophilia A, and it promotes platelet adhesion to damaged blood vessels.

Platelet adhesion can be observed and quantitated in vitro by perfusing a platelet suspension over a segment of blood vessel from which the endothelium has been removed.[386, 387] In this model system, platelet adhesion depends on VWF in the perfusate. This requirement is demonstrated most easily at high wall shear rates. At the lower shear rates characteristic of large veins and arteries, platelet adhesion is less dependent on VWF (reviewed in Ruggeri[388]). VWF already present in the subendothelium and that circulating in the perfusate both seem to be required for optimal platelet adhesion.[389, 390]

VWF acts as a bridge to connect two surfaces that otherwise may not interact, namely, the platelet membrane and subendothelial connective tissue. Thus, the process of platelet adhesion to the blood vessel wall can be analyzed as two distinct binding interactions that imply separate protein functional domains and corresponding "receptors." The interactions of VWF with platelet membrane proteins are described in Chapter 24.

Interaction of von Willebrand Factor With the Vessel Wall

The primary physiological target for VWF in the subendothelium has not been identified with certainty and there may be more than one. VWF, fibronectin, and collagens types III, IV, and V all seem to colocalize in the extracellular matrix.[391, 392] VWF binds to polymers of various purified collagens of type I, II, III, IV, V, and VI but not to denatured collagen (gelatin) or to elastin.[393–395] However, VWF appears to bind normally to extracellular matrix that is made deficient in fibrillar collagens either by digestion with collagenase or by treatment of cells with α,α'-dipyridyl, a collagen synthesis inhibitor.[391, 392] In addition, monoclonal antibodies to VWF have been identified that inhibit binding to collagens type I and III but not to subendothelial matrix. Conversely, monoclonal antibodies to VWF have been identified that inhibit binding to subendothelial matrix but not to fibrillar collagens.[396] Thus, some type of subendothelial collagen may be a receptor in vivo, but it may not be a fibrillar collagen. Collagen type VI is a logical candidate because it contains large noncollagenous domains and is relatively resistant both to collagenase[397] and to α,α'-dipyridyl.[398]

Interaction of von Willebrand Factor With Platelet Glycoprotein Ib

VWF immobilized in subendothelial connective tissue is the initial target with which circulating platelets interact at the site of vascular injury. The platelet glycoprotein Ib/IX/V complex is the only membrane protein on resting platelets with significant affinity for VWF. The binding site on gpIb has been localized to a 42 kDa amino-terminal fragment of the gpIbα chain. The interaction of gpIbα with VWF is distinguished by rapid binding kinetics that is favorable for decelerating and snaring platelets from the flowing blood.[388] The platelets can then be firmly immobilized by interactions mediated by other adhesive receptors that have higher affinity but also much slower reaction kinetics. These later interactions may include integrin-dependent binding to collagen (mediated by $\alpha_2\beta_1$) or to fibrinogen or fibrin, or possibly to an integrin binding site on VWF itself (mediated by $\alpha_{IIb}\beta_3$).[399]

Influence of Multimer Size on von Willebrand Factor Function

Among the species present in plasma or concentrates, the VWF multimers that are the most active in ristocetin-induced platelet aggregation[400] and are preferentially adsorbed onto collagen[401] are composed of more than four or five dimers.[336] Furthermore, adhesion of platelets to subendothelium in perfusion chambers is promoted by the larger multimers in cryoprecipitate but not by the small multimers in commercial factor VIII concentrates.[402] Thus, for naturally occurring multimers, larger size correlates with higher binding activity, perhaps because of increased valency or steric constraints. The smaller multimers contain a higher proportion of proteolytic fragments of subunits than do larger multimers,[336] and this damage may contribute to their decreased function.

Functional Domains of the von Willebrand Factor Subunit

Binding sites on VWF for several macromolecules have been localized to discrete segments of the mature subunit polypeptide. In many cases, these binding sites appear to correlate with specific repeated domains (see Fig. 21–8).

Factor VIII Binding. The factor VIII binding site is located within the amino-terminal 272 amino acid residues of the VWF subunit,[403] which includes domain D' and part of domain D3. Proper construction of this binding site appears to depend on the propeptide-mediated formation of amino-terminal intersubunit disulfide bonds and also requires proteolytic removal of the propeptide.[404] With the possible exception of the terminal subunits in VWF multimers,[404] all subunits of solution-phase VWF multimers appear capable of binding factor VIII with a stoichiometry of one factor VIII per VWF subunit, and with a similar K_d of 200 to 400 pmol that is independent of multimer size.[405, 406] Binding of VWF to surfaces markedly decreases the stoichiometry of factor VIII binding.[405] The association rate constant for factor VIII/VWF binding is approximately 6×10^6 M^{-1} s^{-1}, indicating that exogenous factor VIII should bind endogenous VWF in vivo with a half-life for complex formation of only about 2 seconds.[406]

The mapping of epitopes for monoclonal antibodies that inhibit factor VIII binding[407–409] and the locations of mutations found in patients with defective factor VIII binding (discussed below) suggest that the binding site involves several discontinuous segments within the first 100 residues of VWF. The amino-terminal 272 amino acid residues of VWF also contain a heparin binding site, but this site appears not to be accessible in the intact protein.[410]

Domain A1. The crystallographic structure of the VWF A1 domain (see Plate 21–3) indicates that it consists of a five-stranded parallel β sheet with a short sixth antiparallel strand on one edge, enclosed by three amphipathic α helices on each side in an open $\alpha\beta$ sheet or dinucleotide-binding fold.[411, 412] This basic architecture is shared by homologous A-like domains from the α chains of certain integrins for which three-dimensional structures have been determined, including $\alpha_2\beta_1$,[413] $\alpha_M\beta_3$,[414] and $\alpha_L\beta_3$.[415] The integrin A domains contain a metal ion binding site at the "top" of the structure (see Plate 21–3), whereas the VWF A1 domain does not because the coordinating amino acid residues are not conserved. The site on VWF that interacts with platelet gpIb is located with VWF domain A1.[365] Alanine-scanning mutagenesis of charged residues[416] suggests that this binding site is located near the top and includes Lys 599 in the third α helix. The snake venom protein botrocetin binds to domain A1 and thereby promotes VWF binding to platelet gpIb.[417] Residues implicated by mutagenesis in botrocetin binding[416, 418] include Arg 636 and Lys 667, suggesting that botrocetin interacts with helices 4 and 5 adjacent to the gpIb binding site. Mutations at residues Arg 629 and Arg 632 affect both botrocetin binding and ristocetin-induced gpIb binding and may be involved in interaction with either ligand. The A1 domain also contains binding sites for heparin[419] and sulfatides[420] and a minor binding site for fibrillar collagens.[421, 422] Although both heparin and sulfatides contain sulfated carbohydrate moieties, they do not appear to bind competitively to the same site.[420] The functional relationships among these clustered binding sites are not understood in detail.

Domain A3. Mutagenesis and peptide inhibition studies indicate that the major collagen binding site is located in domain A3.[421–424] The crystallographic structure of the A3 domain has been determined, and it is similar in structure to the VWF A1 domain.[425, 426] The collagen binding surface has not yet been localized.

Integrin Binding. The VWF binding site for integrin $\alpha_{IIb}\beta_3$ (gpIIb/IIIa complex) of activated platelets is located near the carboxyl end of domain C1 and includes the tetrapeptide sequence Arg–Gly–Asp 1746.[427] Arg-Gly-Asp sequences also occur in fibronectin, fibrinogen, and vitronectin, and these proteins compete with VWF for binding to $\alpha_{IIb}\beta_3$. Several integrin receptors besides $\alpha_{IIb}\beta_3$ also recognize ligands that contain Arg-Gly-Asp sequences but often exhibit striking specificity that depends on other structural features of the ligand. Arg-Gly-Asp–dependent interactions are required for the cell attachment activity of many integrins.[428]

Pathophysiology of von Willebrand Factor

Atherosclerosis. Factor VIII and VWF levels correlate with the risk of atherosclerosis in humans but do not appear to be independent of other cardiovascular risk factors.[429] Therefore, the relationship of these hemostatic variables to the pathogenesis of atherosclerosis is uncertain. Both normal and von Willebrand pigs developed similar coronary artery lesions in response to increased dietary cholesterol, catheter-induced injury, or increased arterial shear stress.[430, 431] Despite having similar atherosclerotic lesions, however, von Willebrand pigs were markedly less susceptible to occlusive coronary or carotid artery thrombosis in a Goldblatt clamp model.[360, 432] Thus, in this pig model, VWF may participate in thrombotic events at atherosclerotic lesions but not in their development. Whether the same is true in humans is unknown.

Hemolytic-Uremic Syndrome and Thrombotic Thrombocytopenic Purpura. Thrombotic thrombocytopenic purpura (TTP) is a disease of unknown cause characterized by microangiopathic hemolytic anemia, thrombocytopenia, and widespread small vessel thrombosis with ischemia. The hemolytic-uremic syndrome (HUS) resembles TTP, but it tends to affect children rather than adults and the vascular lesions tend to be more severe in the kidneys, causing renal failure. Complex abnormalities of VWF multimer structure have been reported in TTP[433, 434] and HUS.[435] Congenital or acquired deficiency of a VWF cleaving plasma protease was reported in patients with TTP, suggesting that some of the changes in VWF multimer structure may be caused by altered proteolysis.[436, 437] Whether the abnormal VWF multimers participate in the pathogenesis of TTP and HUS or are markers for endothelial cell damage remains unknown.

▼ MOLECULAR BIOLOGY OF VON WILLEBRAND FACTOR

The gene for VWF is located near the tip of the short arm of chromosome 12 at 12p13.2.[438, 439] For most genes, the frequency of meiotic recombination is higher in females than in males, but the VWF gene lies within a short chromosomal interval for which recombination is higher in males.[440]

The VWF gene is approximately 180 kb in length and consists of 52 exons separated by 51 introns[441] (see Fig. 21–8). The gene contains at least 18 *Alu* repeats and one LINE-1 repeat. The 5′ flanking region contains an AT-rich sequence resembling a TATA element. The exons range in length from 40 nt (exon 50) to 1379 nt (exon 28), and the introns range in length from 97 nt (intron 29) to approximately 19.9 kb (intron 6). Except for the A domains, segments of the VWF gene that encode homologous repeated domains tend to have similar intron-exon organization, and this is consistent with the evolution of this gene in part by repeated gene segment duplications. Some functional elements of the VWF promoter have been defined by transfection of cells in culture[442–444] and in transgenic animals.[445]

A partial unprocessed VWF pseudogene is located on chromosome 22q11.2.[446] The pseudogene is 21 to 29 kb in length and corresponds to 12 exons (exons 23 to 34) and associated introns of the gene. The presence of splice site and nonsense mutations indicates that the VWF pseudogene cannot give rise to a functional transcript. The pseudogene has diverged from the gene approximately 3.1 per cent in nucleotide sequence, suggesting a recent evolutionary origin near the time of divergence of humans and great apes from other primates.[447]

Homologues of VWF repeated domains occur in many otherwise unrelated proteins, indicating that they have been dispersed throughout the genome by duplication and exon shuffling (reviewed in Sadler[340]). At least 46 VWF A domains have been found among 22 active genes belonging to several protein superfamilies. Selected examples are the complement serine protease zymogens factor B and complement component C2; several collagens, including all three chains (α_1, α_2, α_3) of heterotrimeric collagen type VI and the α_1 chains of homotrimeric collagens type VII, XII, and XIV; and a subset of integrin α subunits, including those of five leukocyte adhesion receptors ($\alpha_M\beta_3$, $\alpha_L\beta_3$, $\alpha_x\beta_2$, $\alpha_d\beta_2$, and $\alpha_E\beta_7$), the platelet collagen receptor ($\alpha_2\beta_1$, also known as gpIa/IIa), and another integrin collagen receptor ($\alpha_1\beta_1$). Many of these proteins contain several A domains; an extreme case is collagen VI(α_3) with up to 12 A domains. Additional representatives of VWF A domains are found in certain invertebrate and protozoan proteins.[340]

VWF C and CK domains occur in several epithelial mucins, frequently in combination with one or more VWF B or D domains (reviewed in Sadler[340]). These proteins tend to form disulfide-linked homodimers or oligomers. For VWF and porcine submaxillary mucin,[448] dimerization has been shown to be mediated by the carboxyl-terminal CK domains. The VWF CK domains are also homologous to the large neurotrophin family of growth factors that includes TGF-β.[449] Most neurotrophin family members are dimeric,[362] suggesting that CK domains function as dimerization motifs in several contexts.

▼ VON WILLEBRAND DISEASE

Clinical Features of von Willebrand Disease

VWD appears to be the most common inherited bleeding disorder, although its prevalence is not known precisely. Inherited abnormalities of VWF can be detected by laboratory testing in approximately 8000 per million population, most of whom are asymptomatic.[450] Clinically significant VWD appears to affect approximately 100 persons per million population.[451] The recognition that VWD is relatively common has followed the discovery of many mildly affected persons, and the true prevalence is probably still higher because such cases may escape diagnosis.

The typical bleeding episodes in VWD are consistent with platelet dysfunction. The most common symptoms are bruising, epistaxis, menorrhagia, oral bleeding, and severe bleeding after trauma or surgery. Gastrointestinal bleeding is less common but may be recurrent and intractable. Unlike in hemophilia A, deep tissue bleeding and hemarthrosis are uncommon.

Classification and Molecular Defects in von Willebrand Disease

VWD is classified into three major categories according to whether the residual VWF is qualitatively normal (type 1) or abnormal (type 2); if the protein is essentially undetectable, the disease is designated type 3. Qualitative type 2 VWD is further subdivided into four variants (2A, 2B, 2M, and 2N), which are based on details of the phenotype. These six categories correspond to distinct pathophysiological mechanisms, and they are intended to correlate with distinct clinical features and therapeutic requirements.[452]

Many distinct mutations causing VWD have been characterized at the level of DNA sequence.[453] Amino acid sequence polymorphisms are common within VWF, and many occur close to mutations that cause VWD.[454] The high prevalence of polymorphisms must be considered when sequence changes identified in patients are proposed to be mutations that cause VWD. An online data base of mutations and polymorphisms in the VWF gene is maintained at the University of Michigan Division of Molecular Medicine and Genetics. The data base is updated continuously and can be accessed at URL http://mmg2.im.med.umich.edu/vWF.

VWD Type 1. In VWD type 1, all sizes of multimer are present (see Fig. 21–7); the VWF antigen is decreased (usually 5 to 30 per cent), and it appears to be structurally and functionally normal. This is the most common form of VWD, accounting for approximately three fourths of cases, and it is inherited as an autosomal dominant disorder. Most patients with VWD type 1 have only mild or moderate bleeding symptoms.

Diagnosis of VWD type 1 can be difficult because the bleeding symptoms are nonspecific and moderately low VWF levels are common. In part, this difficulty is due to the strong influence of ABO blood type on VWF concentration and the broad range of normal values independent of blood group. The high extreme is illustrated by persons of blood type AB who have VWF plasma levels of 1.23 U/ml with a range (± 2 SD) of 0.64 to 2.38 U/ml; the corresponding values in blood type O are a mean of 0.75 U/ml and a range (± 2 SD) of 0.36 to 1.57 U/ml.[381] Evidence that low VWF levels and bleeding are coinherited within a family is reassuring, but the diagnosis is often uncertain in practice.

VWD type 1 is often caused by heterozygous deletion, frameshift, or nonsense mutations that are also observed in patients with severe VWD type 3, as discussed below. In such families, VWD often appears to have low penetrance and chance coinheritance of another mutation for a distinct VWD phenotype can tip the hemostatic balance in favor of symptoms. For example, compound heterozygosity for VWD type 1 and VWD type 2N was found to be associated with bleeding in several patients whose relatives with either single mutant allele were asymptomatic.[455]

In a few relatively rare families, VWD type 1 is inherited as a dominant trait with high penetrance and unusually low VWF levels. Because VWF is multimeric, a strongly dominant phenotype could be explained if a product of the abnormal gene interfered with the biosynthesis or secretion of the normal subunits. One such mechanism was proposed on the basis of studies of a patient with the mutation Cys 386 → Arg.[456] The mutant pro-VWF subunits were retained in the endoplasmic reticulum and reduced the secretion of coexpressed normal VWF subunits. If dimerization of pro-VWF subunits were random, retention of mutant homodimers and heterodimers in the endoplasmic reticulum would reduce the amount of normal pro-VWF dimers arriving in the Golgi to approximately 25 per cent of the total. Any tendency to favor heterodimerization would exacerbate the phenotype. This dominant negative mechanism may explain some unexpectedly severe VWD type 1 phenotypes.[456]

VWD Type 2. Qualitative abnormalities of VWF may be identified from a discrepancy between measures of VWF:Ag and selected VWF binding functions in vitro. VWD type 2 is further divided into subtypes on the basis of the nature of the structural or functional defect.

VWD Type 2A. The largest VWF multimers are required for effective hemostasis, and any mechanism that depletes plasma of them can cause bleeding. VWD type 2A refers to variants in which the largest VWF multimers are absent, and VWF-dependent platelet functions are decreased. This subtype accounts for approximately three fourths of all VWD type 2.

VWD type 2A is usually inherited as a dominant trait caused by single amino acid substitutions within VWF domain A2 (Fig. 21–11). Depending on the mutation, the

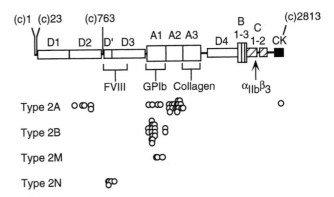

Figure 21–11. Mutations in VWD type 2. Amino acid residues are numbered by codon number (c)1 to (c)2813. References to the individual mutations can be found in the data base of VWD mutations[453] maintained by David Ginsburg (University of Michigan) and accessible at http://mmg2.im.med.umich.edu/vWF. (From Sadler, J.E.: Biochemistry and genetics of von Willebrand factor. Annu. Rev. Biochem. 67:395, 1998; with permission.)

absence of large VWF multimers in plasma (see Fig. 21–7) is due to either impaired multimer assembly within the Golgi apparatus or increased proteolytic destruction of large multimers in the circulation.[457, 458] At present, there is no explanation for the association of specific mutations with either mechanism. In either case, plasma VWF contains increased quantities of proteolytically degraded subunits that are cleaved between Tyr 842 and Met 843 in domain A2.[459, 460] The mutation Cys 2010 → Arg was identified in a patient with dominant VWD type 2A (originally designated type IID) and impairs multimer assembly by preventing the formation of pro-VWF dimers within the endoplasmic reticulum. The mutant pro-VWF monomers are transported to the Golgi, where they form nonfunctional "head-to-head" dimers.[363] Certain mutations within the VWF propeptide are associated with recessive inheritance of VWD type 2A (originally designated type IIC). These mutations impair multimer assembly in the Golgi apparatus, possibly by interfering with the normal function of the VWF propeptide in promoting intersubunit disulfide bond formation.[461] All of these type 2A variants are united by a common pathophysiological mechanism in which the lack of large VWF multimers prevents effective VWF-dependent platelet adhesion.

VWD Type 2B. VWD type 2B is characterized by increased affinity of the mutant VWF for platelets.[462] This variant is relatively uncommon, accounting for less than about 20 per cent of VWD type 2, or less than 5 per cent of all VWD. VWF levels may be normal or low, and VWF:RCo may be normal or low. The characteristic laboratory abnormality occurs in the RIPA test. Platelet-rich plasma of patients with VWD type 2B shows exaggerated platelet aggregation at low concentrations of ristocetin, whereas in VWD type 2A, there is markedly decreased sensitivity to all concentrations of ristocetin.

VWD type 2B is a dominant disorder. Plasma VWF is usually deficient in large multimers (see Fig. 21–7), but the platelet multimer pattern is normal.[331] An important clinical feature of this variant is thrombocytopenia that occasionally may be chronic[463] and often is exacerbated by the stress of pregnancy or surgery. The deficiency of large plasma multimers and the thrombocytopenia appear to be secondary effects of a gain of function mutation. The large plasma VWF multimers bind spontaneously to platelets[462] and are cleared[464]; the residual small multimers are not hemostatically effective. The administration of DDAVP causes the secretion of a full range of multimers that can be detected transiently in plasma.[464, 465] DDAVP can also induce transient severe thrombocytopenia.[466]

At least 14 different mutations have been identified in patients with VWD type 2B.[453, 467, 468] Five of these mutations are C → T transitions within CG dinucleotides, and four of them account for more than 90 per cent of the patients studied so far. All of these mutations cluster within a small region on one side of domain A1 (see Plate 21–3). This cluster appears to mark the location of a regulatory site that normally inhibits the binding of domain A1 to platelet gpIb. Mutations in this site may relieve the inhibition and cause constitutive binding to gpIb, thereby causing the observed dominant gain of function phenotype.

VWD Type 2M. VWD type 2M (M for multimer) includes variants in which platelet adhesion is impaired but the VWF multimer distribution is normal. Such a phenotype might be produced by mutations that inactivate binding sites for ligands either on platelets or in connective tissue. So far, the known type 2M mutations are confined to domain A1 and impair binding to platelet gpIb. Laboratory test results for these patients were similar to those in VWD type 2A with disproportionately low values of VWF:RCo, but the size distribution of plasma VWF multimers was essentially normal.[469–472]

VWD Type 2N. Factor VIII/VWF binding is required for normal factor VIII survival in the circulation, and a decrease in affinity between factor VIII and VWF results in accelerated clearance of factor VIII. As discussed under Classification and Molecular Defects in Hemophilia A, the Tyr 1680 → Phe mutation, within the VWF binding site of the factor VIII light chain, causes X chromosome–linked recessive hemophilia A by this mechanism. Mutations in the factor VIII binding site on VWF cause a similar phenotype that is inherited as an autosomal recessive condition. Platelet-dependent functions of VWF are preserved and the multimer pattern is normal, but factor VIII levels are low, usually less than 10 per cent, and the binding of factor VIII to plasma VWF is markedly decreased or absent.[473, 474] This variant is named VWD type 2N after Normandy, the birth province of one index case (reviewed in Mazurier[475]).

The prevalence of VWD type 2N is not known precisely, but screening of clinic patients suggests that a small percentage of patients with apparent mild hemophilia A actually have VWD type 2N.[476] Between 1990 and 1997 in France, 51 unrelated patients with VWD type 2N were identified.[477] Several of these patients had been misdiagnosed with mild hemophilia A or as hemophilia A carriers with extreme lyonization.

Correct diagnosis has significant implications for genetic counseling and therapy. For example, treatment with highly purified factor VIII is appropriate in hemophilia A but is associated with low recovery and rapid clearance in VWD type 2N.[475] The diagnosis of VWD type 2N should be considered in any patient with congenital factor VIII deficiency in whom the condition is not obviously X chromo-some linked or in whom initial therapy with pure factor VIII or DDAVP gives unexpectedly poor results.

VWD Type 3. VWD type 3 is an autosomal recessive disorder with a low prevalence of 0.5 to 3 per million; the rate is higher in Scandinavian countries and lower in western Europe.[478] The prevalence in the United States and in Israel may be intermediate, approximately 1.4 to 1.6 per million.[478, 479] Bleeding symptoms are generally severe and lifelong. Plasma VWF antigen is usually undetectable (see Fig. 21–7) but may be present at low concentrations (1 to 5 per cent of normal). The factor VIII level is usually less than 10 per cent and is sometimes less than 1 per cent of normal, which is low enough to be associated with hemarthrosis and spontaneous soft tissue bleeding. The heterozygous relatives of patients with VWD type 3 may have normal or mildly reduced levels of VWF; they are usually asymptomatic but some have VWD type 1, as illustrated in the first case reports by von Willebrand.[314]

Most patients with VWD type 3 appear to be compound heterozygous for mutant VWF alleles with large deletions, frameshifts, or nonsense mutations that cannot express significant quantities of the protein; homozygosity has been demonstrated in a few consanguineous families.[453, 480–482] The mutation in the original family of von Willebrand is a single nucleotide insertion in exon 18 that leads to a frameshift and premature termination within the propeptide.[483]

Prenatal Diagnosis and Genetic Counseling in von Willebrand Disease

A prevalence of approximately 1.5 per million for VWD type 3 implies a prevalence of heterozygous "carriers" of approximately 2500 per million. However, the prevalence of symptomatic VWD type 1 is less than 10 per cent of this value. Thus, the inheritance of a single null VWF allele does not reliably cause disease. The factors that distinguish symptomatic from asymptomatic carriers of a given VWF mutation are largely unknown. Consequently, genetic counseling of patients with the milder variants of VWD is difficult and imprecise. Because of the relatively mild phenotype, most families affected with VWD type 1 do not choose to alter their reproductive plans, and prenatal diagnosis is not necessary.

In families affected with more severe VWD variants that exhibit clear inheritance patterns, genetic counseling is facilitated by the accurate identification of mutant VWF alleles. If the causative mutation is not known, intragenic DNA sequence polymorphisms can be used to follow the inheritance of mutant VWF alleles. A large number of useful marker systems have been identified throughout the VWF gene,[454] and these have been used for linkage analysis and prenatal diagnosis. The most useful marker known is a highly polymorphic variable number of tandem repeats within intron 40. At least 98 alleles were identified, and the heterozygosity was calculated to be about 98 per cent in a European population.[484]

Differential Diagnosis of von Willebrand Disease

Inheritable symptomatic abnormalities of the structure, function, or concentration of VWF are grouped together as

VWD. This diagnosis applies to patients with bleeding tendencies that range from trivial to life-threatening, whose symptoms may be characteristic of platelet dysfunction or of hemophilia. Consequently, many conditions of different pathogenesis may resemble some form of VWD. These include a variety of congenital and acquired platelet disorders that may present with similar patterns of bleeding.

Hemophilia A. Appropriate laboratory testing and family studies can usually exclude hemophilia A. However, mild hemophilia associated with aspirin ingestion may be easily confused with VWD. The similarities between hemophilia A and VWD type 2N have been discussed in previous sections (Differential Diagnosis of Inherited Factor VIII Deficiency and VWD Type 2N).

Acquired von Willebrand Syndrome. Many cases have been reported of spontaneous bleeding associated with decreased VWF occurring in adults without a prior personal or family history of abnormal bleeding.[485, 486] Most have occurred in the setting of a recognized autoimmune, myeloproliferative, or lymphoproliferative disease, suggesting an immunological basis for the syndrome. However, some patients do not have an underlying disease that is known to be associated with immune dysfunction, and antibodies to VWF have been demonstrated in less than half. The multimer pattern in plasma may be normal or may show absence of large multimers. Aside from the patient's history, there may be no way to distinguish this syndrome from congenital VWD by assays of plasma factor VIII or VWF. However, platelet-associated VWF is characteristically normal in quantity, ristocetin cofactor activity, and multimer distribution. Furthermore, both the endogenous VWF released by infusion of DDAVP and the exogenous VWF administered in cryoprecipitate have a shortened half-life in the acquired von Willebrand syndrome. The syndrome frequently resolves if the underlying illness is controlled.

Platelet-Type VWD or Pseudo-VWD. Platelet-type VWD or pseudo-VWD is nearly an exact mimic of VWD type 2B, but the defect is in the platelet rather than in the VWF.[487–489] It is autosomally inherited, and heterozygotes are clinically affected. The bleeding time is prolonged, and platelet adhesion to damaged endothelium is reduced. The VWF multimer pattern shows a decrease in large multimers, and RIPA is increased in platelet-rich plasma. In addition, the platelet-associated VWF appears to be normal in quantity and multimer distribution. DDAVP induces an increase in large plasma multimers, but they are cleared rapidly, and thrombocytopenia may occur transiently.[490] However, the patient's plasma does not show disproportionately high ristocetin cofactor activity with normal platelets, whereas the patient's platelets spontaneously aggregate when they are added to normal or hemophilic plasma, and they adsorb normal VWF in the absence of ristocetin.[488, 489, 491] Mutations causing platelet-type VWD or pseudo-VWD have been characterized within the VWF binding domain of platelet gpIbα.[492–495]

Other Disorders. Patients with VWD type 2B may have chronic or intermittent thrombocytopenia associated with large platelets, and platelet survival is decreased with increased clearance by the spleen. This has led to the erroneous diagnosis of chronic autoimmune thrombocytopenia; two such patients were described who were treated inappropriately with splenectomy.[463, 496] Thrombocytopenia associated with pregnancy has been reported in at least eight patients with VWD type 2B; in four, this was misdiagnosed as autoimmune thrombocytopenia and treated with corticosteroids[497, 498] or intravenous immune globulin.[499, 500] VWD type 2B is also associated with postoperative thrombocytopenia[501] and has presented as thrombocytopenia in infancy.[502, 503]

Treatment of von Willebrand Disease

The therapeutic response of bleeding in severe VWD type 3 emphasizes the different roles of factor VIII and VWF in hemostasis. Hemarthrosis, soft tissue hemorrhage, and postoperative bleeding respond to elevations of factor VIII; mucocutaneous bleeding responds to increases in VWF. The bleeding patient with VWD usually needs increases in both factors, and how they are provided depends on the severity of bleeding and the subtype of VWD.

DDAVP. DDAVP is the agent of choice for responsive patients with VWD who require support for only a few days. The use of DDAVP in hemophilia A is discussed in Treatment of Hemophilia A.

The efficacy of DDAVP correlates with the subtype of VWD. It is generally effective in VWD type 1 but not in severe VWD type 3. Therapeutic efficacy in VWD type 2 variants is variable, but patients who respond consistently can be identified by test infusions of DDAVP.[504] Occasional patients with type 2A disease respond, although most do not.[504–506] As expected, administration of DDAVP to patients with VWD type 2N increases the level of VWF but often does not significantly change the factor VIII level.[507, 508] Experience is limited in patients with VWD type 2M, but the nature of the functional defect makes a useful response unlikely.

In VWD type 2B, DDAVP causes transient thrombocytopenia that may be severe, with the appearance of circulating platelet aggregates,[466] and several reports indicated that the bleeding usually was not shortened.[464–466] These findings led to the recommendation that DDAVP not be used in VWD type 2B.[466, 505] Although thrombosis has occurred in a few patients with atherosclerosis who were treated with DDAVP, no such episodes have been reported in VWD type 2B, and the relative risk of thrombosis is not known. Nevertheless, DDAVP has been reported to control bleeding in some VWD type 2B patients without causing clinically significant decrements in platelet count.[503, 509–512] Thus, the use of DDAVP may be appropriate in selected patients with this variant.

Factor VIII/VWF Complex. Patients with VWD who require support for more than a few days, or who undergo major surgery, can be treated with products that contain factor VIII/VWF complex. At present, the most suitable preparations are plasma-derived concentrates of intermediate or high purity that contain both VWF and factor VIII.[513–515] These products are virucidally treated and have a low or absent risk of transmitting viral hepatitis or HIV.[174, 175] Cryoprecipitate is also effective but carries an unacceptable risk of transmitting viral illnesses.

As factor VIII preparations for hemophilia A have become ever more highly purified, they have also become less suitable for the treatment of VWD because they do not treat the deficiency of functional VWF that characterizes many subtypes of VWD. In particular, "monoclonal" or recombinant factor VIII is inappropriate therapy in VWD type 3 and type 2N, because the transfused factor VIII cannot be stabilized by endogenous VWF.[516]

Purified or Recombinant VWF. A highly purified VWF preparation that is essentially free of factor VIII has been used in a few patients with VWD.[517-519] The product exhibits good recovery and a normal half-life in vivo. The increment in factor VIII depends on endogenous synthesis, so that factor VIII levels rise in a delayed fashion and peak approximately 20 hours after the first dose of VWF. For this reason, pure VWF may be useful in preparation for elective surgical procedures that can be scheduled to coincide with the factor VIII response. However, treatment of acute bleeding would require supplementation of pure VWF with additional factor VIII.

Recombinant VWF is under development as a therapeutic product and has undergone preliminary testing in animal models including VWF-deficient dogs.[520]

Antibody Inhibitors of von Willebrand Factor. Antibodies to VWF develop rarely in patients with VWD. All of the reported examples have occurred in VWD type 3. In this subgroup, the prevalence of alloantibodies is about 7.5 per cent,[485] which is similar to the prevalence of alloantibodies in hemophilia A. Deletions within the VWF gene appear to predispose patients to the development of alloantibody inhibitors.[453, 521-523] In contrast to hemophilia A and hemophilia B, the inhibitors that develop in VWD tend to be polyclonal precipitating antibodies. The affected patients often suffer severe side effects from replacement therapy, such as back pain, abdominal pain, and hypotension, consistent with acute serum sickness[485] or anaphylaxis.[524]

Mucosal bleeding in such patients is often difficult to control because infused VWF is rapidly neutralized.[485, 525] Elevation of factor VIII levels is easier to achieve, so that soft tissue and joint hemorrhages usually respond to therapy. A sustained elevation of factor VIII is not obtained, however, unless plasma VWF levels can be increased despite the presence of antibody.[526]

Animal Models of von Willebrand Disease

Pigs with VWD have been used extensively to study VWD and VWF biology, but their utility is limited by their expense, genetic heterogeneity, and slow breeding cycle. A small animal model of VWD type 3 was produced by gene targeting in the mouse.[527]

REFERENCES

1. Rosner, F.: Hemophilia in the Talmud and rabbinic writings. Ann. Intern. Med. 70:833, 1969.
2. Otto, J.E.: An account of an hemorrhagic disposition existing in certain families. Med. Repository 6:1, 1803.
3. Patek, A.J., Jr., and Taylor, F.H.L.: Hemophilia. II. Some properties of a substance obtained from normal human plasma effective in accelerating the coagulation of hemophilic blood. J. Clin. Invest. 16:113, 1937.
4. Aggeler, P.M., White, S.G., Glendenning, M.B., Page, E.W., Leake, T.B., and Bates, G.: Plasma thromboplastin component (PTC) deficiency: a new disease resembling hemophilia. Proc. Soc. Exp. Biol. Med. 79:692, 1952.
5. Biggs, R., Douglas, A.S., Macfarlane, R.G., Dacie, J.V., Pitney, W.R.,

Merskey, C., and O'Brien, J.R.: Christmas disease. Br. Med. J. 2:1378, 1952.
6. Barrowcliffe, T.W.: Methodology of the two-stage assay of factor VIII (VIII:C). Scand. J. Haematol. Suppl. 41:25, 1984.
7. Suomela, H., Blömback, M., and Blömback, B.: The activation of factor X evaluated by using synthetic substrates. Thromb. Res. 10:267, 1977.
8. Hultin, M.B., and Nemerson, Y.: Activation of factor X by factors IXa and VIII: a specific assay for factor IXa in the presence of thrombin-activated factor VIII. Blood 52:928, 1978.
9. Lazarchick, J., and Hoyer, L.W.: Immunoradiometric measurement of the factor VIII procoagulant antigen. J. Clin. Invest. 62:1048, 1978.
10. Peake, I.R., Bloom, A.L., Giddings, J.C., and Ludlam, C.A.: An immunoradiometric assay for procoagulant factor VIII antigen: results in haemophilia, von Willebrand's disease and fetal plasma and serum. Br. J. Haematol. 42:269, 1979.
11. Legaz, M.E., Schmer, G., Counts, R.B., and Davie, E.W.: Isolation and characterization of human factor VIII (antihemophilic factor). J. Biol. Chem. 248:3946, 1973.
12. Hershgold, E.J., Davison, A.M., and Janzen, M.E.: Isolation and some chemical properties of human factor VIII (antihemophilic factor). J. Lab. Clin. Med. 77:185, 1971.
13. Weiss, H.J., and Hoyer, L.W.: Von Willebrand factor: dissociation from antihemophilic factor procoagulant activity. Science 182:1149, 1973.
14. Griggs, T.R., Cooper, H.A., Webster, W.P., Wagner, R.H., and Brinkhous, K.M.: Plasma aggregating factor (bovine) for human platelets: a marker for study of antihemophilic and von Willebrand factors. Proc. Natl. Acad. Sci. USA 70:2814, 1973.
15. Fulcher, C.A., and Zimmerman, T.S.: Characterization of the human factor VIII procoagulant protein with a heterologous precipitating antibody. Proc. Natl. Acad. Sci. USA 79:1648, 1982.
16. Fulcher, C.A., Roberts, J.R., and Zimmerman, T.S.: Thrombin proteolysis of purified factor VIII procoagulant protein: correlation of activation with generation of a specific polypeptide. Blood 61:807, 1983.
17. Vehar, G.A., and Davie, E.W.: Preparation and properties of bovine factor VIII (antihemophilic factor). Biochemistry 19:401, 1980.
18. Fass, D.N., Knutson, G.J., and Katzmann, J.A.: Monoclonal antibodies to porcine factor VIII coagulant and their use in the isolation of active coagulant protein. Blood 59:594, 1982.
19. Knutson, G.J., and Fass, D.N.: Porcine factor VIII:C prepared by affinity interaction with von Willebrand factor and heterologous antibodies: sodium dodecyl sulfate polyacrylamide gel analysis. Blood 59:615, 1982.
20. Toole, J.J., Knopf, J.L., Wozney, J.M., Sultzman, L.A., Buecker, J.L., Pittman, D.D., Kaufman, R.J., Brown, E., Showemaker, C., Orr, E.C., Amphlett, G.W., Foster, W.B., Coe, M.L., Knutson, G.J., Fass, D.N., and Hewick, R.M.: Molecular cloning of a cDNA encoding human antihaemophilic factor. Nature 312:342, 1984.
21. Vehar, G.A., Keyt, B., Eaton, D., Rodriguez, H., O'Brien, D.P., Rotblat, F., Oppermann, H., Keck, R., Wood, W.I., Harkins, R.N., Tuddenham, E.G.D., Lawn, R.M., and Capon, D.J.: Structure of human factor VIII. Nature 312:337, 1984.
22. Gitschier, J., Wood, W.I., Goralka, T.M., Wion, K.L., Chen, E.Y., Eaton, D.H., Vehar, G.A., Capon, D.J., and Lawn, R.M.: Characterization of the human factor VIII gene. Nature 312:326, 1984.
23. Wood, W.I., Capon, D.J., Simonsen, C.C., Eaton, D.L., Gitschier, J., Keyt, B., Seeburg, P.H., Smith, D.H., Hollingshead, P., Wion, K.L., Delwart, E., Tuddenham, E.G.D., Vehar, G.A., and Lawn, R.M.: Expression of active human factor VIII from recombinant DNA clones. Nature 312:330, 1984.
24. Fulcher, C.A., Roberts, J.R., Holland, L.Z., and Zimmerman, T.S.: Human factor VIII procoagulant protein. Monoclonal antibodies define precursor-product relationships and functional epitopes. J. Clin. Invest. 76:117, 1985.
25. Eaton, D., Rodriguez, H., and Vehar, G.A.: Proteolytic processing of human factor VIII. Correlation of specific cleavages by thrombin, factor Xa, and activated protein C with activation and inactivation of factor VIII coagulant activity. Biochemistry 25:505, 1986.
26. Tuddenham, E.G., Trabold, N.C., Collins, J.A., and Hoyer, L.W.: The properties of factor VIII coagulant activity prepared by immunoadsorbent chromatography. J. Lab. Clin. Med. 93:40, 1979.
27. Kaufman, R.J., Wasley, L.C., and Dorner, A.J.: Synthesis, processing, and secretion of recombinant human factor VIII expressed in mammalian cells. J. Biol. Chem. 263:6352, 1988.

28. Church, W.R., Jernigan, R.L., Toole, J., Hewick, R.M., Knopf, J., Knutson, G.J., Nesheim, M.E., Mann, K.G., and Fass, D.N.: Coagulation factors V and VIII and ceruloplasmin constitute a family of structurally related proteins. Proc. Natl. Acad. Sci. USA 81:6934, 1984.

29. Fass, D.N., Hewick, R.M., Knutson, G.J., Nesheim, M.E., and Mann, K.G.: Internal duplication and sequence homology in factors V and VIII. Proc. Natl. Acad. Sci. USA 82:1688, 1985.

30. Kane, W.H., and Davie, E.W.: Blood coagulation factors V and VIII: structural and functional similarities and their relationship to hemorrhagic and thrombotic disorders. Blood 71:539, 1988.

31. Pan, Y., DeFay, T., Gitschier, J., and Cohen, F.E.: Proposed structure of the A domains of factor VIII by homology modelling. Nat. Struct. Biol. 2:740, 1995.

32. Pemberton, S., Lindley, P., Zaitsev, V., Card, G., Tuddenham, E.G., and Kemball-Cook, G.: A molecular model for the triplicated A domains of human factor VIII based on the crystal structure of human ceruloplasmin. Blood 89:2413, 1997.

33. Poole, S., Firtel, R.A., Lamar, E., and Rowekamp, W.: Sequence and expression of the discoidin I gene family in *Dictyostelium discoideum*. J. Mol. Biol. 153:273, 1981.

34. Stubbs, J.D., Lekutis, C., Singer, K.L., Bui, A., Yuzuki, D., Srinivasan, U., and Parry, G.: cDNA cloning of a mouse mammary epithelial cell surface protein reveals the existence of epidermal growth factor–like domains linked to factor VIII–like sequences. Proc. Natl. Acad. Sci. USA 87:8417, 1990.

35. Takahashi, N., Ortel, T.L., and Putnam, F.W.: Single-chain structure of human ceruloplasmin: the complete amino acid sequence of the whole molecule. Proc. Natl. Acad. Sci. USA 81:390, 1984.

36. Xue, J., Kalafatis, M., and Mann, K.G.: Determination of the disulfide bridges in factor Va light chain. Biochemistry 32:5917, 1993.

37. Xue, J., Kalafatis, M., Silveira, J.R., Kung, C., and Mann, K.G.: Determination of the disulfide bridges in factor Va heavy chain. Biochemistry 33:13109, 1994.

38. McMullen, B.A., Fujikawa, K., Davie, E.W., Hedner, U., and Ezban, M.: Locations of disulfide bonds and free cysteines in the heavy and light chains of recombinant human factor VIII (antihemophilic factor A). Protein Sci. 4:740, 1995.

39. Esmon, C.T.: The subunit structure of thrombin-activated factor V. Isolation of activated factor V, separation of subunits, and reconstitution of biological activity. J. Biol. Chem. 254:964, 1979.

40. Tagliavacca, L., Moon, N., Dunham, W.R., and Kaufman, R.J.: Identification and functional requirement of Cu(I) and its ligands within coagulation factor VIII. J. Biol. Chem. 272:27428, 1997.

41. Sudhakar, K., and Fay, P.J.: Effects of copper on the structure and function of factor VIII subunits—evidence for an auxiliary role for copper ions in cofactor activity. Biochemistry 37:6874, 1998.

42. Leyte, A., van Schijndel, H.B., Niehrs, C., Huttner, W.B., Verbeet, M.P., Mertens, K., and van Mourik, J.A.: Sulfation of Tyr1680 of human blood coagulation factor VIII is essential for the interaction of factor VIII with von Willebrand factor. J. Biol. Chem. 266:740, 1991.

43. Pittman, D.D., Wang, J.H., and Kaufman, R.J.: Identification and functional importance of tyrosine sulfate residues within recombinant factor VIII. Biochemistry 31:3315, 1992.

44. Michnick, D.A., Pittman, D.D., Wise, R.J., and Kaufman, R.J.: Identification of individual tyrosine sulfation sites within factor VIII required for optimal activity and efficient thrombin cleavage. J. Biol. Chem. 269:20095, 1994.

45. Hoyer, L.W., and Trabold, N.C.: The effect of thrombin on human factor VIII. Cleavage of the factor VIII procoagulant protein during activation. J. Lab. Clin. Med. 97:50, 1981.

46. Barlow, G.H., Martin, S.E., and Marder, V.J.: Sedimentation analysis of von Willebrand and factor VIIIC protein using partition cells in the analytical ultracentrifuge. Blood 63:940, 1984.

47. Fay, P.J., and Smudzin, T.M.: Intersubunit fluorescence energy transfer in human factor VIII. J. Biol. Chem. 264:14005, 1989.

48. Mosesson, M.W., Fass, D.N., Lollar, P., DiOrio, J.P., Parker, C.G., Knutson, G.J., Hainfeld, J.F., and Wall, J.S.: Structural model of porcine factor VIII and factor VIIIa molecules based on scanning transmission electron microscope (STEM) images and STEM mass analysis. J. Clin. Invest. 85:1983, 1990.

49. Saenko, E.L., and Scandella, D.: The acidic region of the factor VIII light chain and the C2 domain together form the high affinity binding site for von Willebrand factor. J. Biol. Chem. 272:18007, 1997.

50. Andersson, L.-O., and Brown, J.E.: Interaction of factor VIII–von Willebrand factor with phospholipid vesicles. Biochem. J. 200:161, 1981.

51. Lajmanovich, A., Hudry-Clergeon, G., Freyssinet, J.M., and Marguerie, G.: Human factor VIII procoagulant activity and phospholipid interaction. Biochim. Biophys. Acta 678:132, 1981.

52. Saenko, E.L., and Scandella, D.: A mechanism for inhibition of factor VIII binding to phospholipid by von Willebrand factor. J. Biol. Chem. 270:13826, 1995.

53. Marchioro, T.L., Hougie, C., Ragde, H., Epstein, R.B., and Thomas, E.D.: Hemophilia: role of organ homografts. Science 163:188, 1969.

54. Bontempo, F.A., Lewis, J.H., Gorenc, T.J., Spero, J.A., Ragni, M.V., Scott, J.P., and Starzl, T.E.: Liver transplantation in hemophilia A. Blood 69:1721, 1987.

55. Rall, L.B., Bell, G.I., Caput, D., Truett, M.A., Masiarz, F.R., Najarian, R.C., Valenzuela, P., Anderson, H.D., Din, N., and Hansen, B.: Factor VIII:C synthesis in the kidney. Lancet 1:44, 1985.

56. Wion, K.L., Kelly, D., Summerfield, J.A., Tuddenham, E.G., and Lawn, R.M.: Distribution of factor VIII mRNA and antigen in human liver and other tissues. Nature 317:726, 1985.

57. Liu, D.L., Xia, S., Tang, J., Qin, X., and Liu, H.: Allotransplantation of whole spleen in patients with hepatic malignant tumors or hemophilia A. Operative technique and preliminary results [see comments]. Arch. Surg. 130:33, 1995.

58. Ingerslev, J., Christiansen, B.S., Heickendorff, L., and Petersen, C.M.: Synthesis of factor VIII in human hepatocytes in culture. Thromb. Haemost. 60:387, 1988.

59. Stel, H.V., van der Kwast, T.H., and Veerman, E.C.I.: Detection of factor VIII/coagulant antigen in human liver tissue. Nature 303:530, 1983.

60. Do, H., Healey, J.F., Waller, E.K., and Lollar, P.: Expression of factor VIII by murine liver sinusoidal endothelial cells. J Biol. Chem. 274:19587, 1999.

61. Pittman, D.D., Tomkinson, K.N., and Kaufman, R.J.: Post-translational requirements for functional factor V and factor VIII secretion in mammalian cells. J. Biol. Chem. 269:17329, 1994.

62. Pipe, S.W., Morris, J.A., Shah, J., and Kaufman, R.J.: Differential interaction of coagulation factor VIII and factor V with protein chaperones calnexin and calreticulin. J. Biol. Chem. 273:8537, 1998.

63. Over, J., Sixma, J.J., Bouma, B.N., Bolhuis, P.A., Vlooswijk, R.A., and Beeser-Visser, N.H.: Survival of [125]iodine-labeled factor VIII in patients with von Willebrand's disease. J. Lab. Clin. Med. 97:332, 1981.

64. Tuddenham, E.G., Lane, R.S., Rotblat, F., Johnson, A.J., Snape, T.J., Middleton, S., and Kernoff, P.B.: Response to infusions of polyelectrolyte fractionated human factor VIII concentrate in human haemophilia A and von Willebrand's disease. Br. J. Haematol. 52:259, 1982.

65. Noe, D.A., Bell, W.R., Ness, P.M., and Levin, J.: Plasma clearance rates of coagulation factors VIII and IX in factor-deficient individuals. Blood 67:969, 1986.

66. Kaufman, R.J.: Biological regulation of factor VIII activity. Annu. Rev. Med. 43:325, 1992.

67. Lollar, P.: Structure and function of factor VIII. Adv. Exp. Med. Biol. 386:3, 1995.

68. Rapaport, S.I., Schiffman, S., Patch, M.J., and Ames, S.B.: The importance of activation of antihemophilic globulin and proaccelerin by traces of thrombin in the generation of intrinsic prothrombinase activity. Blood 21:221, 1963.

69. Pittman, D.D., Alderman, E.M., Tomkinson, K.N., Wang, J.H., Giles, A.R., and Kaufman, R.J.: Biochemical, immunological, and in vivo functional characterization of B-domain–deleted factor VIII. Blood 81:2925, 1993.

70. Cooper, H.A., Reisner, F.F., Hall, M., and Wagner, R.H.: Effects of thrombin treatment of preparations of factor VIII and the Ca²⁺-dissociated small active fragment. J. Clin. Invest. 56:751, 1975.

71. Hill-Eubanks, D.C., Parker, C.G., and Lollar, P.: Differential proteolytic activation of factor VIII–von Willebrand factor complex by thrombin. Proc. Natl. Acad. Sci. USA 86:6508, 1989.

72. Pittman, D.D., and Kaufman, R.J.: Proteolytic requirements for thrombin activation of anti-hemophilic factor (factor VIII). Proc. Natl. Acad. Sci. USA 85:2429, 1988.

73. Broden, K., Andersson, L.-O., and Sandberg, H.: Kinetics of activation of human factor VIII by thrombin. Thromb. Res. 19:299, 1980.

74. Koedam, J.A., Hamer, R.J., Beeser-Visser, N.H., Bouma, B.N., and Sixma, J.J.: The effect of von Willebrand factor on activation of factor VIII by factor Xa. Eur. J. Biochem. 189:229, 1990.

75. Lollar, P., and Parker, E.T.: Structural basis for the decreased procoagulant activity of human factor VIII compared to the porcine homolog. J. Biol. Chem. 266:12481, 1991.

76. Lollar, P., and Parker, C.G.: pH-dependent denaturation of thrombin-activated porcine factor VIII. J. Biol. Chem. 265:1688, 1990.

77. Fay, P.J., Haidaris, P.J., and Smudzin, T.M.: Human factor VIIIa subunit structure. Reconstruction of factor VIIIa from the isolated A1/A3-C1-C2 dimer and A2 subunit. J. Biol. Chem. 266:8957, 1991.

78. Lollar, P., Knutson, G.J., and Fass, D.N.: Stabilization of thrombin-activated porcine factor VIII:C by factor IXa phospholipid. Blood 63:1303, 1984.

79. Fay, P.J., Beattie, T.L., Regan, L.M., O'Brien, L.M., and Kaufman, R.J.: Model for the factor VIIIa–dependent decay of the intrinsic factor Xase. Role of subunit dissociation and factor IXa–catalyzed proteolysis. J. Biol. Chem. 271:6027, 1996.

80. Esmon, C.T., and Owen, W.G.: Identification of an endothelial cell cofactor for thrombin-catalyzed activation of protein C. Proc. Natl. Acad. Sci. USA 78:2249, 1981.

81. Griffin, J.H., Evatt, B., Zimmerman, T.S., Kleiss, A.J., and Wideman, C.: Deficiency of protein C in congenital thrombotic disease. J. Clin. Invest. 68:1370, 1981.

82. Marlar, R.A., Kleiss, A.J., and Griffin, J.H.: Mechanism of action of human activated protein C, a thrombin-dependent anticoagulant enzyme. Blood 59:1067, 1982.

83. Kisiel, W., Canfield, W.M., Ericsson, L.H., and Davie, E.W.: Anticoagulant properties of bovine plasma protein C following activation by thrombin. Biochemistry 16:5824, 1977.

84. Kisiel, W.: Human plasma protein C: isolation, characterization, and mechanism of activation by α-thrombin. J. Clin. Invest. 64:761, 1979.

85. Fay, P.J., Smudzin, T.M., and Walker, F.J.: Activated protein C–catalyzed inactivation of human factor VIII and factor VIIIa. Identification of cleavage sites and correlation of proteolysis with cofactor activity. J. Biol. Chem. 266:20139, 1991.

86. Fay, P.J., and Walker, F.J.: Inactivation of human factor VIII by activated protein C: evidence that the factor VIII light chain contains the activated protein C binding site. Biochim. Biophys. Acta 994:142, 1989.

87. Walker, F.J., Scandella, D., and Fay, P.J.: Identification of the binding site for activated protein C on the light chain of factors V and VIII. J. Biol. Chem. 265:1484, 1990.

88. Koedam, J.A., Meijers, J.C., Sixma, J.J., and Bouma, B.N.: Inactivation of human factor VIII by activated protein C. Cofactor activity of protein S and protective effect of von Willebrand factor. J. Clin. Invest. 82:1236, 1988.

89. Bertina, R.M., Cupers, R., and van Wijngaarden, A.: Factor IXa protects activated factor VIII against inactivation by activated protein C. Biochem. Biophys. Res. Commun. 125:177, 1984.

90. Walker, F.J., Chavin, S.I., and Fay, P.J.: Inactivation of factor VIII by activated protein C and protein S. Arch. Biochem. Biophys. 252:322, 1987.

91. Varadi, K., and Elodi, S.: Increased resistance of factor IXa–factor VIII complex against inactivation by granulocyte proteases. Thromb. Res. 19:571, 1980.

92. Holmberg, L., Ljung, R., and Nilsson, I.M.: The effects of plasmin and protein Ca on factor VIII:C and VIII:CAg. Thromb. Res. 31:41, 1983.

93. van Dieijen, G., Tans, G., Rosing, J., and Hemker, H.C.: The role of phospholipid and factor VIIIa in the activation of bovine factor X. J. Biol. Chem. 256:3433, 1981.

94. Griffith, M.J., Reisner, H.M., Lundblad, R.L., and Roberts, H.R.: Measurement of human factor IXa activity in an isolated factor X activation system. Thromb. Res. 27:289, 1982.

95. Hultin, M.B.: Role of human factor VIII in factor X activation. J. Clin. Invest. 69:950, 1982.

96. van Dieijen, G., van Rijn, J.L., Govers-Riemslag, J.W., Hemker, H.C., and Rosing, J.: Assembly of the intrinsic factor X activating complex—interactions between factor IXa, factor VIIIa and phospholipid. Thromb. Haemost. 53:396, 1985.

97. Lenting, P.J., Donath, M.J.S.H., van Mourik, J.A., and Mertens, K.: Identification of a binding site for blood coagulation factor IXa on the light chain of human factor VIII. J. Biol. Chem. 269:7150, 1994.

98. Fay, P.J., Beattie, T., Huggins, C.F., and Regan, L.M.: Factor VIIIa A2 subunit residues 558–565 represent a factor IXa interactive site. J. Biol. Chem. 269:20522, 1994.

99. O'Brien, L.M., Medved, L.V., and Fay, P.J.: Localization of factor IXa and factor VIIIa interactive sites. J. Biol. Chem. 270:27087, 1995.

100. Lenting, P.J., van de Loo, J.-W.H.P., Donath, M.J.S.H., van Mourik, J.A., and Mertens, K.: The sequence Glu1811–Lys1818 of human blood coagulation factor VIII comprises a binding site for activated factor IX. J. Biol. Chem. 271:1935, 1996.

101. Gilbert, G.E., Furie, B.C., and Furie, B.: Binding of human factor VIII to phospholipid vesicles. J. Biol. Chem. 265:815, 1990.

102. Gilbert, G.E., and Drinkwater, D.: Specific membrane binding of factor VIII is mediated by O-phospho-L-serine, a moiety of phosphatidylserine. Biochemistry 32:9577, 1993.

103. Foster, P.A., Fulcher, C.A., Houghten, R.A., and Zimmerman, T.S.: Synthetic factor VIII peptides with amino acid sequences contained within the C2 domain of factor VIII inhibit factor VIII binding to phosphatidylserine. Blood 75:1999, 1990.

104. Zwaal, R.F.: Membrane and lipid involvement in blood coagulation. Biochim. Biophys. Acta 515:163, 1978.

105. Bevers, E.M., Comfurius, P., van Rijn, J.L., Hemker, H.C., and Zwaal, R.F.: Generation of prothrombin-converting activity and the exposure of phosphatidylserine at the outer surface of platelets. Eur. J. Biochem. 122:429, 1982.

106. Nesheim, M.E., Pittman, D.D., Wang, J.H., Slonosky, D., Giles, A.R., and Kaufman, R.J.: The binding of ^{35}S-labeled recombinant factor VIII to activated and unactivated human platelets. J. Biol. Chem. 263:16467, 1988.

107. Gilbert, G.E., Sims, P.J., Wiedmer, T., Furie, B., Furie, B.C., and Shattil, S.J.: Platelet-derived microparticles express high affinity receptors for factor VIII. J. Biol. Chem. 266:17261, 1991.

108. Nesheim, M., Pittman, D.D., Giles, A.R., Fass, D.N., Wang, J.H., Slonosky, D., and Kaufman, R.J.: The effect of plasma von Willebrand factor on the binding of human factor VIII to thrombin-activated human platelets. J. Biol. Chem. 266:17815, 1991.

109. Teien, A.N., Abildgaard, U., and Hook, M.: The anticoagulant effect of heparan sulfate and dermatan sulfate. Thromb. Res. 8:859, 1976.

110. Hatton, M.W., Berry, L.R., and Regoeczi, E.: Inhibition of thrombin by antithrombin III in the presence of certain glycosaminoglycans found in the mammalian aorta. Thromb. Res. 13:655, 1978.

111. Weksler, B.B., Ley, C.W., and Jaffe, E.A.: Stimulation of endothelial cell prostacyclin production by thrombin, trypsin, and the ionophore A 23187. J. Clin. Invest. 62:923, 1978.

112. Loskutoff, D.J., and Edgington, T.S.: Synthesis of a fibrinolytic activator and inhibitor by endothelial cells. Proc. Natl. Acad. Sci. USA 74:3903, 1977.

113. Brox, J.H., Osterud, B., Bjorklid, E., and Fenton, J.W., II: Production and availability of thromboplastin in endothelial cells: the effects of thrombin, endotoxin and platelets. Br. J. Haematol. 57:239, 1984.

114. Lyberg, T., Galdal, K.S., Evensen, S.A., and Prydz, H.: Cellular cooperation in endothelial cell thromboplastin synthesis. Br. J. Haematol. 53:85, 1983.

115. Stern, D.M., Drillings, M., Nossel, H.L., Hurlet-Jensen, A., LaGamma, K.S., and Owen, J.: Binding of factors IX and IXa to cultured vascular endothelial cells. Proc. Natl. Acad. Sci. USA 80:4119, 1983.

116. Stern, D.M., Drillings, M., Kisiel, W., Nawroth, P., Nossel, H.L., and LaGamma, K.S.: Activation of factor IX bound to cultured bovine aortic endothelial cells. Proc. Natl. Acad. Sci. USA 81:913, 1984.

117. Heimark, R.L., and Schwartz, S.M.: Binding of coagulation factors IX and X to the endothelial cell surface. Biochem. Biophys. Res. Commun. 111:723, 1983.

118. Poustka, A., Dietrich, A., Langenstein, G., Toniolo, D., Warren, S.T., and Lehrach, H.: Physical map of human Xq27–qter: localizing the region of the fragile X mutation. Proc. Natl. Acad. Sci. USA 88:8302, 1991.

119. Freije, D., and Schlessinger, D.: A 1.6-Mb contig of yeast artificial chromosomes around the human factor VIII gene reveals three regions homologous to probes for the DXS115 locus and two for the DXYS64 locus. Am. J. Hum. Genet. 51:66, 1992.

120. Levinson, B., Kenwrick, S., Lakich, D., Hammonds, G., Jr., and Gitschier, J.: A transcribed gene in an intron of the human factor VIII gene. Genomics 7:1, 1990.

121. Levinson, B., Kenwrick, S., Gamel, P., Fisher, K., and Gitschier, J.: Evidence for a third transcript from the human factor VIII gene. Genomics 14:585, 1992.

122. Ghirardini, A., Schinaia, N., Chiarotti, F., De Biasi, R., Rodeghiero, F., and Binkin, N.: Epidemiology of hemophilia and of HIV infection in Italy. GICC. Gruppo Italiano Coagulopatie Congenite. J. Clin. Epidemiol. 47:1297, 1994.

123. Larsson, S.A., Nilsson, I.M., and Blomback, M.: Current status of

Swedish hemophiliacs. I. A demographic survey. Acta Med. Scand. 212:195, 1982.

124. Jones, P.K., and Ratnoff, O.D.: The changing prognosis of classic hemophilia (factor VIII "deficiency"). Ann. Intern. Med. 114:641, 1991.

125. Smith, P.S., Keyes, N.C., and Forman, E.N.: Socioeconomic evaluation of a state-funded comprehensive hemophilia-care program. N. Engl. J. Med. 306:575, 1982.

126. Graham, J.B., McLendon, W.W., and Brinkhous, K.M.: Mild hemophilia: an allelic form of the disease. Am. J. Med. 225:46, 1953.

127. Denson, K.W., Biggs, R., Haddon, M.E., Borrett, R., and Cobb, K.: Two types of haemophilia (A+ and A−): a study of 48 cases. Br. J. Haematol. 17:163, 1969.

128. Hoyer, L.W., and Breckenridge, R.T.: Immunologic studies of antihemophilic factor (AHF, factor VIII): cross-reacting material in a genetic variant of hemophilia A. Blood 32:962, 1968.

129. Tuddenham, E.G., Schwaab, R., Seehafer, J., Millar, D.S., Gitschier, J., Higuchi, M., Bidichandani, S., Connor, J.M., Hoyer, L.W., Yoshioka, A., Peake, I.R., Olek, K., Kazazian, H.H., Lavergne, J.-M., Giannelli, F., Antonarakis, S.E., and Cooper, D.N.: Haemophilia A: database of nucleotide substitutions, deletions, insertions and rearrangements of the factor VIII gene, second edition. Nucleic Acids Res. 22:4851, 1994.

130. Kemball-Cook, G., Tuddenham, E.G.D., and Wacey, A.I.: The factor VIII Structure and Mutation Resource Site: HAMSTeRS version 4. Nucleic Acids Res. 26:216, 1998.

131. Higuchi, M., Kazazian, H.H., Jr., Kasch, L., Warren, T.C., McGinniss, M.J., Phillips, J.A.D., Kasper, C., Janco, R., and Antonarakis, S.E.: Molecular characterization of severe hemophilia A suggests that about half the mutations are not within the coding regions and splice junctions of the factor VIII gene. Proc. Natl. Acad. Sci. USA 88:7405, 1991.

132. Lakich, D., Kazazian, H.H., Jr., Antonarakis, S.E., and Gitschier, J.: Inversions disrupting the factor VIII gene are a common cause of severe haemophilia A. Nat. Genet. 5:236, 1993.

133. Naylor, J., Brinke, A., Hassock, S., Green, P.M., and Giannelli, F.: Characteristic mRNA abnormality found in half the patients with severe haemophilia A is due to large DNA inversions. Hum. Mol. Genet. 2:1773, 1993.

134. Antonarakis, S.E., Rossiter, J.P., Young, M., Horst, J., de Moerloose, P., Sommer, S.S., Ketterling, R.P., Kazazian, H.H., Jr., Negrier, C., Vinciguerra, C., Gitschier, J., Goossens, M., Girodon, E., Ghanem, N., Plassa, F., Lavergne, J.M., Vidaud, M., Costa, J.M., Laurian, Y., Lin, S.-W., Lin, S.-R., Shen, M.-C., Lillicrap, D., Taylor, S.A.M., Windsor, S., Valleix, S.V., Nafa, K., Sultan, Y., Delpech, M., Vnencak-Jones, C.L., Phillips, J.A., III, Ljung, R.C.R., Koumbarelis, E., Gialeraki, A., Mandalaki, T., Jenkins, P.V., Collins, P.W., Pasi, K.J., Goodeve, A., Peake, I., Preston, F.E., Schwartz, M., Scheibel, E., Ingerslev, J., Cooper, D.N., Millar, D.S., Kakkar, V.V., Giannelli, F., Naylor, J.A., Tizzano, E.F., Baiget, M., Domenech, M., Altisent, C., Tusell, J., Beneyto, M., Lorenzo, J.I., Gaucher, C., Mazurier, C., Peerlinck, K., Matthijs, G., Cassiman, J.J., Vermylen, J., Mori, P.G., Acquila, M., Caprino, D., and Inaba, H.: Factor VIII gene inversions in severe hemophilia A: results of an international consortium study. Blood 86:2206, 1995.

135. Rossiter, J.P., Young, M., Kimberland, M.L., Hutter, P., Ketterling, R.P., Gitschier, J., Horst, J., Morris, M.A., Schaid, D.J., de Moerloose, P., Sommer, S.S., Kazazian, H.H., Jr., and Antonarakis, S.E.: Factor VIII gene inversions causing severe hemophilia A originate almost exclusively in male germ cells. Hum. Mol. Genet. 3:1035, 1994.

136. Youssoufian, H., Antonarakis, S.E., Aronis, S., Tsiftis, G., Phillips, D.G., and Kazazian, H.H., Jr.: Characterization of five partial deletions of the factor VIII gene. Proc. Natl. Acad. Sci. USA 84:3772, 1987.

137. Wehnert, M., Herrmann, F.H., and Wulff, K.: Partial deletions of factor VIII gene as molecular diagnostic markers in haemophilia A. Dis. Markers 7:113, 1989.

138. Lavergne, J.M., Bahnak, B.R., Vidaud, M., Laurian, Y., and Meyer, D.: A directed search for mutations in hemophilia A using restriction enzyme analysis and denaturing gradient gel electrophoresis. A study of seven exons in the factor VIII gene of 170 cases. Nouv. Rev. Fr. Hematol. 34:85, 1992.

139. Kazazian, H.H., Jr., Wong, C., Youssoufian, H., Scott, A.F., Phillips, D.G., and Antonarakis, S.E.: Haemophilia A resulting from de novo insertion of L1 sequences represents a novel mechanism for mutation in man. Nature 332:164, 1988.

140. Singer, M.F., Krek, V., McMillan, J.P., Swergold, G.D., and Thayer, R.E.: LINE-1: a human transposable element. Gene 135:183, 1993.

141. Dombroski, B.A., Mathias, S.L., Nanthakumar, E., Scott, A.F., and Kazazian, H.H., Jr.: Isolation of an active human transposable element. Science 254:1805, 1991.

142. Mathias, S.L., Scott, A.F., Kazazian, H.H., Jr., Boeke, J.D., and Gabriel, A.: Reverse transcriptase encoded by a human transposable element. Science 254:1808, 1991.

143. Tavassoli, K., Eigel, A., Pollmann, H., and Horst, J.: Mutational analysis of ectopic factor VIII transcripts from hemophilia A patients: identification of cryptic splice site, exon skipping and novel point mutations. Hum. Genet. 100:508, 1997.

144. Dietz, H.C., Valle, D., Francomano, C.A., Kendzior, R.J., Jr., Pyeritz, R.E., and Cutting, G.R.: The skipping of constitutive exons in vivo induced by nonsense mutations. Science 259:680, 1993.

145. Arai, M., Inaba, H., Higuchi, M., Antonarakis, S.E., Kazazian, H.H., Jr., Fujimaki, M., and Hoyer, L.W.: Direct characterization of factor VIII in plasma: detection of a mutation altering a thrombin cleavage site (arginine-372→histidine). Proc. Natl. Acad. Sci. USA 86:4277, 1989.

146. Shima, M., Ware, J., Yoshioka, A., Fukui, H., and Fulcher, C.A.: An arginine to cysteine amino acid substitution at a critical thrombin cleavage site in a dysfunctional factor VIII molecule. Blood 74:1612, 1989.

147. Gitschier, J., Kogan, S., Levinson, B., and Tuddenham, E.G.: Mutations of factor VIII cleavage sites in hemophilia A. Blood 72:1022, 1988.

148. Schwaab, R., Ludwig, M., Kochhan, L., Oldenburg, J., McVey, J.H., Egli, H., Brackmann, H.H., and Olek, K.: Detection and characterisation of two missense mutations at a cleavage site in the factor VIII light chain. Thromb. Res. 61:225, 1991.

149. Higuchi, M., Wong, C., Kochhan, L., Olek, K., Aronis, S., Kasper, C.K., Kazazian, H.H., Jr., and Antonarakis, S.E.: Characterization of mutations in the factor VIII gene by direct sequencing of amplified genomic DNA. Genomics 6:65, 1990.

150. Schwaab, R., Oldenburg, J., Schwaab, U., Johnson, D.J.D., Schmidt, W., Olek, K., Brackman, H.H., and Tuddenham, E.G.D.: Characterization of mutations within the factor VIII gene of 73 unrelated mild and moderate haemophiliacs. Br. J. Haematol. 91:458, 1995.

151. Youssoufian, H., Antonarakis, S.E., Bell, W., Griffin, A.M., and Kazazian, H.H., Jr.: Nonsense and missense mutations in hemophilia A: estimate of the relative mutation rate at CG dinucleotides. Am. J. Hum. Genet. 42:718, 1988.

152. Cooper, D.N., and Krawczak, M.: The mutational spectrum of single base-pair substitutions causing human genetic disease: patterns and predictions. Hum. Genet. 85:55, 1990.

153. Becker, J., Schwaab, R., Moller-Taube, A., Schwaab, U., Schmidt, W., Brackmann, H.H., Grimm, T., Olek, K., and Oldenburg, J.: Characterization of the factor VIII defect in 147 patients with sporadic hemophilia A: family studies indicate a mutation type–dependent sex ratio of mutation frequencies. Am. J. Hum. Genet. 58:657, 1996.

154. Peake, I.R., Lillicrap, D.P., Boulyjenkov, V., Briet, E., Chan, V., Ginter, E.K., Kraus, E.M., Ljung, R., Mannucci, P.M., Nicolaides, K., and Tuddenham, E.G.D.: Report of a joint WHO/WFH meeting on the control of haemophilia: carrier detection and prenatal diagnosis. Blood Coagul. Fibrinolysis 4:313, 1993.

155. Lalloz, M.R., McVey, J.H., Pattinson, J.K., and Tuddenham, E.G.: Haemophilia A diagnosis by analysis of a hypervariable dinucleotide repeat within the factor VIII gene. Lancet 338:207, 1991.

156. Kogan, S., and Gitschier, J.: Mutations and a polymorphism in the factor VIII gene discovered by denaturing gradient gel electrophoresis. Proc. Natl. Acad. Sci. USA 87:2092, 1990.

157. Oberle, I., Camerino, G., Heilig, R., Grunebaum, L., Cazenave, J.P., Crapanzano, C., Mannucci, P.M., and Mandel, J.L.: Genetic screening for hemophilia A (classic hemophilia) with a polymorphic DNA probe. N. Engl. J. Med. 312:682, 1985.

158. Richards, B., Heilig, R., Oberle, I., Storjohann, L., and Horn, G.T.: Rapid PCR analysis of the St14 (DXS52) VNTR. Nucleic Acids Res. 19:1944, 1991.

159. Barrai, I., Cann, H.M., Cavalli-Sforza, L.L., Barbujani, G., and De Nicola, P.: Segregation analysis of hemophilia A and B. Am. J. Hum. Genet. 37:680, 1985.

160. Haldane, J.B.S.: The rate of spontaneous mutation of a human gene. J. Genet. 31:317, 1935.

161. Filippi, G., Mannucci, P.M., Coppola, R., Farris, A., Rinaldi, A., and

Siniscalco, M.: Studies on hemophilia A in Sardinia bearing on the problems of multiple allelism, carrier detection, and differential mutation rate in the two sexes. Am. J. Hum. Genet. 36:44, 1984.

162. Kerr, C.B., Preston, A.E., Barr, A., and Biggs, R.: Further studies on the inheritance of factor VIII. Br. J. Haematol. 12:212, 1966.

163. Graham, J.B., Rizza, C.R., Chediak, J., Mannucci, P.M., Briet, E., Ljung, R., Kasper, C.K., Essien, E.M., and Green, P.P.: Carrier detection in hemophilia A: a cooperative international study. I. The carrier phenotype. Blood 67:1554, 1986.

164. Green, P.P., Mannucci, P.M., Briet, E., Ljung, R., Kasper, C.K., Essien, E.M., Chediak, J., Rizza, C.R., and Graham, J.B.: Carrier detection in hemophilia A: a cooperative international study. II. The efficacy of a universal discriminant. Blood 67:1560, 1986.

165. Seligsohn, U.: Combined factor V and VIII deficiency. *In* Seghatchian, M.J., and Savidge, G.F. (eds.): Factor VIII—von Willebrand Factor. Vol. II. Boca Raton, FL, CRC Press, 1989, pp. 89–100.

166. Seligsohn, U., Zivelin, A., and Zwang, E.: Combined factor V and factor VIII deficiency among non-Ashkenazi Jews. N. Engl. J. Med. 307:1191, 1982.

167. Nichols, W.C., Seligsohn, U., Zivelin, A., Terry, V.H., Arnold, N.D., Siemieniak, D.R., Kaufman, R.J., and Ginsburg, D.: Linkage of combined factors V and VIII deficiency to chromosome 18q by homozygosity mapping. J. Clin. Invest. 99:596, 1997.

168. Nichols, W.C., Seligsohn, U., Zivelin, A., Terry, V.H., Hertel, C.E., Wheatley, M.A., Moussalli, M.J., Hauri, H.P., Ciavarella, N., Kaufman, R.J., and Ginsburg, D.: Mutations in the ER-Golgi intermediate compartment protein ERGIC-53 cause combined deficiency of coagulation factors V and VIII. Cell 93:61, 1998.

169. Schulman, S., and Wiechel, B.: Hepatitis, epidemiology and liver function in hemophiliacs in Sweden. Acta Med. Scand. 215:249, 1984.

170. Aledort, L.M., Levine, P.H., Hilgartner, M., Blatt, P., Spero, J.A., Goldberg, J.D., Bianchi, L., Desmet, V., Scheuer, P., Popper, H., and Berk, P.D.: A study of liver biopsies and liver disease among hemophiliacs. Blood 66:367, 1985.

171. Makris, M., Preston, F.E., Triger, D.R., Underwood, J.C., Choo, Q.L., Kuo, G., and Houghton, M.: Hepatitis C antibody and chronic liver disease in haemophilia. Lancet 335:1117, 1990.

172. Rizzetto, M., Morello, C., Mannucci, P.M., Gocke, D.J., Spero, J.A., Lewis, J.H., Van Thiel, D.H., Scaroni, C., and Peyretti, F.: Delta infection and liver disease in hemophilic carriers of hepatitis B surface antigen. J. Infect. Dis. 145:18, 1982.

173. Goedert, J.J., Kessler, C.M., Aledort, L.M., Biggar, R.J., Andes, W.A., White, G.C.D., Drummond, J.E., Vaidya, K., Mann, D.L., Eyster, M.E., Ragni, M.V., Lederman, M.M., Cohen, A.R., Bray, G.L., Rosenberg, P.S., Friedman, R.M., Hilgartner, M.W., Blattner, W.A., Kroner, B., and Gail, M.H.: A prospective study of human immunodeficiency virus type 1 infection and the development of AIDS in subjects with hemophilia. N. Engl. J. Med. 321:1141, 1989.

174. Schimpf, K., Brackmann, H.H., Kreuz, W., Kraus, B., Haschke, F., Schramm, W., Moesseler, J., Auerswald, G., Sutor, A.H., Koehler, K., Hellstern, P., Muntean, W., and Scharrer, I.: Absence of anti-human immunodeficiency virus types 1 and 2 seroconversion after the treatment of hemophilia A or von Willebrand's disease with pasteurized factor VIII concentrate. N. Engl. J. Med. 321:1148, 1989.

175. Mannucci, P.M.: Clinical evaluation of viral safety of coagulation factor VIII and IX concentrates. Vox Sang. 64:197, 1993.

176. Hepatitis A among persons with hemophilia who received clotting factor concentrate—United States, September–December 1995. MMWR Morb. Mortal. Wkly. Rep. 45:29, 1996.

177. Mannucci, P.M., Gdovin, S., Gringeri, A., Colombo, M., Mele, A., Schinaia, N., Ciavarella, N., Emerson, S.U., and Purcell, R.H.: Transmission of hepatitis A to patients with hemophilia by factor VIII concentrates treated with organic solvent and detergent to inactivate viruses. The Italian Collaborative Group. Ann. Intern. Med. 120:1, 1994.

178. Santagostino, E., Mannucci, P.M., Gringeri, A., Azzi, A., Morfini, M., Musso, R., Santoro, R., and Schiavoni, M.: Transmission of parvovirus B19 by coagulation factor concentrates exposed to 100 degrees C heat after lyophilization. Transfusion 37:517, 1997.

179. Brettler, D.B., Forsberg, A.D., Brewster, F., Sullivan, J.L., and Levine, P.H.: Delayed cutaneous hypersensitivity reactions in hemophiliac subjects treated with factor concentrate. Am. J. Med. 81:607, 1986.

180. Carr, R., Veitch, S.E., Edmond, E., Peutherer, J.F., Prescott, R.J., Steel, C.M., and Ludlam, C.A.: Abnormalities of circulating lymphocyte subsets in haemophiliacs in an AIDS-free population. Lancet 1:1431, 1984.

181. Goldsmith, G.H., Jr., Baily, R.G., Brettler, D.B., Davidson, W.R., Jr., Ballard, J.O., Driscol, T.E., Greenberg, J.M., Kasper, C.K., Levine, P.H., and Ratnoff, O.D.: Primary pulmonary hypertension in patients with classic hemophilia. Ann. Intern. Med. 108:797, 1988.

182. Bray, G.L., Gomperts, E.D., Courter, S., Gruppo, R., Gordon, E.M., Manco-Johnson, M., Shapiro, A., Scheibel, E., White, G., 3rd, and Lee, M.: A multicenter study of recombinant factor VIII (recombinate): safety, efficacy, and inhibitor risk in previously untreated patients with hemophilia A. The Recombinate Study Group. Blood 83:2428, 1994.

183. Mannucci, P.M., Brettler, D.B., Aledort, L.M., Lusher, J.M., Abildgaard, C.F., Schwartz, R.S., and Hurst, D.: Immune status of human immunodeficiency virus seropositive and seronegative hemophiliacs infused for 3.5 years with recombinant factor VIII. The Kogenate Study Group. Blood 83:1958, 1994.

184. Aygoren-Pursun, E., and Scharrer, I.: A multicenter pharmacosurveillance study for the evaluation of the efficacy and safety of recombinant factor VIII in the treatment of patients with hemophilia A. German Kogenate Study Group. Thromb. Haemost. 78:1352, 1997.

185. Bloom, A.L.: The biosynthesis of factor VIII. Clin. Haematol. 8:53, 1979.

186. Mannucci, P.M., Ruggeri, Z.M., Pareti, F.I., and Capitanio, A.: 1-Deamino-8-D-arginine vasopressin: a new pharmacological approach to the management of haemophilia and von Willebrand's diseases. Lancet 1:869, 1977.

187. Mannucci, P.M., Bettega, D., and Cattaneo, M.: Patterns of development of tachyphylaxis in patients with haemophilia and von Willebrand disease after repeated doses of desmopressin (DDAVP). Br. J. Haematol. 82:87, 1992.

188. Wall, U., Jern, S., Tengborn, L., and Jern, C.: Evidence of a local mechanism for desmopressin-induced tissue-type plasminogen activator release in human forearm. Blood 91:529, 1998.

189. Rosenberg, J.B., Foster, P.A., Kaufman, R.J., Vokac, E.A., Moussalli, M., Kroner, P.A., and Montgomery, R.R.: Intracellular trafficking of factor VIII to von Willebrand factor storage granules. J. Clin. Invest. 101:613, 1998.

190. Rodeghiero, F., Castaman, G., Di Bona, E., and Ruggeri, M.: Consistency of responses to repeated DDAVP infusions in patients with von Willebrand's disease and hemophilia A. Blood 74:1997, 1989.

191. Mannucci, P.M.: Desmopressin (DDAVP) in the treatment of bleeding disorders: the first 20 years. Blood 90:2515, 1997.

192. Rose, E.H., and Aledort, L.M.: Nasal spray desmopressin (DDAVP) for mild hemophilia A and von Willebrand disease. Ann. Intern. Med. 114:563, 1991.

193. Scharrer, I., and Neutzling, O.: Incidence of inhibitors in haemophiliacs. A review of the literature. Blood Coagul. Fibrinolysis 4:753, 1993.

194. Aledort, L.: Inhibitors in hemophilia patients: current status and management. Am. J. Hematol. 47:208, 1994.

195. McMillan, C.W., Shapiro, S.S., Whitehurst, D., Hoyer, L.W., Rao, A.V., and Lazerson, J.: The natural history of factor VIII:C inhibitors in patients with hemophilia A: a national cooperative study. II. Observations on the initial development of factor VIII:C inhibitors. Blood 71:344, 1988.

196. Lippert, L.E., Fisher, L.M., and Schook, L.B.: Relationship of major histocompatibility complex class II genes to inhibitor antibody formation in hemophilia A. Thromb. Haemost. 64:564, 1990.

197. Aly, A.M., Aledort, L.M., Lee, T.D., and Hoyer, L.W.: Histocompatibility antigen patterns in haemophilic patients with factor VIII antibodies. Br. J. Haematol. 76:238, 1990.

198. Hay, C.R., Ollier, W., Pepper, L., Cumming, A., Keeney, S., Goodeve, A.C., Colvin, B.T., Hill, F.G., Preston, F.E., and Peake, I.R.: HLA class II profile: a weak determinant of factor VIII inhibitor development in severe haemophilia A. UKHCDO Inhibitor Working Party. Thromb. Haemost. 77:234, 1997.

199. Lusher, J.M., Arkin, S., Abildgaard, C.F., and Schwartz, R.S.: Recombinant factor VIII for the treatment of previously untreated patients with hemophilia A. Safety, efficacy, and development of inhibitors. Kogenate Previously Untreated Patient Study Group. N. Engl. J. Med. 328:453, 1993.

200. Fulcher, C.A., Mahoney, S.D.G., and Zimmerman, T.S.: FVIII inhibitor IgG subclass and FVIII polypeptide specificity determined by immunoblotting. Blood 69:1475, 1987.

201. Healey, J.F., Lubin, I.M., Nakai, H., Saenko, E.L., Hoyer, L.W., Scandella, D., and Lollar, P.: Residues 484–508 contain a major

determinant of the inhibitory epitope in the A2 domain of human factor VIII. J. Biol. Chem. 270:14505, 1995.

202. Scandella, D., Gilbert, G.E., Shima, M., Nakai, H., Eagleson, C., Felch, M., Prescott, R., Rajalakshmi, K.J., Hoyer, L.W., and Saenko, E.: Some factor VIII inhibitor antibodies recognize a common epitope corresponding to C2 domain amino acids 2248 through 2312, which overlap a phospholipid-binding site. Blood 86:1811, 1995.

203. Prescott, R., Nakai, H., Saenko, E.L., Scharrer, I., Nilsson, I.M., Humphries, J.E., Hurst, D., Bray, G., and Scandella, D.: The inhibitor antibody response is more complex in hemophilia A patients than in most nonhemophiliacs with factor VIII autoantibodies. Recombinate and Kogenate Study Groups. Blood 89:3663, 1997.

204. Hoyer, L.W.: Factor VIII inhibitors. Curr. Opin. Hematol. 2:365, 1995.

205. Macfarlane, R.G., Mallam, P.C., Witts, L.J., Bidwell, E., Honey, G.E., and Taylor, K.B.: Surgery in haemophilia, the use of animal antihaemophilic globulin in thirteen cases. Lancet 2:251, 1957.

206. Erskine, J.G., and Davidson, J.F.: Anaphylactic reaction to low-molecular-weight porcine factor VIII concentrates. Br. Med. J. 282:2011, 1981.

207. Brettler, D.B., Forsberg, A.D., Levine, P.H., Aledort, L.M., Hilgartner, M.W., Kasper, C.K., Lusher, J.M., McMillan, C., and Roberts, H.: The use of porcine factor VIII concentrate (Hyate:C) in the treatment of patients with inhibitor antibodies to factor VIII. A multicenter US experience. Arch. Intern. Med. 149:1381, 1989.

208. Hay, C.R., Lozier, J.N., Lee, C.A., Laffan, M., Tradati, F., Santagostino, E., Ciavarella, N., Schiavoni, M., Fukui, H., Yoshioka, A., Teitel, J., Mannucci, P.M., and Kasper, C.K.: Safety profile of porcine factor VIII and its use as hospital and home-therapy for patients with haemophilia-A and inhibitors: the results of an international survey. Thromb. Haemost. 75:25, 1996.

209. Hultin, M.B.: Studies of factor IX concentrate therapy in hemophilia. Blood 62:677, 1983.

210. Mannucci, P.M., and Vigano, S.: Protein C concentrates for therapeutic use. Lancet 1:875, 1983.

211. Kurczynski, E.M., and Penner, J.A.: Activated prothrombin concentrate for patients with factor VIII inhibitors. N. Engl. J. Med. 291:164, 1974.

212. Lusher, J.M., Shapiro, S.S., Palascak, J.E., Rao, A.V., Levine, P.H., and Blatt, P.M.: Efficacy of prothrombin-complex concentrates in hemophiliacs with antibodies to factor VIII: a multicenter therapeutic trial. N. Engl. J. Med. 303:421, 1980.

213. Sjamsoedin, L.J., Heijnen, L., Mauser-Bunschoten, E.P., van Geijlswijk, J.L., van Houwelingen, H., van Asten, P., and Sixma, J.J.: The effect of activated prothrombin-complex concentrate (FEIBA) on joint and muscle bleeding in patients with hemophilia A and antibodies to factor VIII. A double-blind clinical trial. N. Engl. J. Med. 305:717, 1981.

214. Hilgartner, M., Aledort, L., Andes, A., and Gill, J.: Efficacy and safety of vapor-heated anti-inhibitor coagulant complex in hemophilia patients. FEIBA Study Group. Transfusion 30:626, 1990.

215. Negrier, C., Goudemand, J., Sultan, Y., Bertrand, M., Rothschild, C., and Lauroua, P.: Multicenter retrospective study on the utilization of FEIBA in France in patients with factor VIII and factor IX inhibitors. French FEIBA Study Group. Factor Eight Bypassing Activity. Thromb. Haemost. 77:1113, 1997.

216. Seligsohn, U., Kasper, C.K., Osterud, B., and Rapaport, S.I.: Activated factor VII: presence in factor IX concentrates and persistence in the circulation after infusion. Blood 53:828, 1979.

217. Broze, G.J., Jr., and Majerus, P.W.: Purification and properties of human coagulation factor VII. J. Biol. Chem. 255:1242, 1980.

218. Bech, R.M.: Recombinant factor VIIa in joint and muscle bleeding episodes. Haemostasis 26(suppl. 1):135, 1996.

219. Macik, B.G., Hohneker, J., Roberts, H.R., and Griffin, A.M.: Use of recombinant activated factor VII for treatment of a retropharyngeal hemorrhage in a hemophilic patient with a high titer inhibitor. Am. J. Hematol. 32:232, 1989.

220. Schmidt, M.L., Gamerman, S., Smith, H.E., Scott, J.P., and DiMichele, D.M.: Recombinant activated factor VII (rFVIIa) therapy for intracranial hemorrhage in hemophilia A patients with inhibitors. Am. J. Hematol. 47:36, 1994.

221. Rice, K.M., and Savidge, G.F.: NovoSeven (recombinant factor VIIa) in central nervous systems bleeds. Haemostasis 26(suppl. 1):131, 1996.

222. Ingerslev, J., Freidman, D., Gastineau, D., Gilchrist, G., Johnsson, H., Lucas, G., McPherson, J., Preston, E., Scheibel, E., and Shuman, M.: Major surgery in haemophilic patients with inhibitors using recombinant factor VIIa. Haemostasis 26(suppl. 1):118, 1996.

223. Smith, O.P., and Hann, I.M.: rVIIa therapy to secure haemostasis during central line insertion in children with high-responding FVIII inhibitors. Br. J. Haematol. 92:1002, 1996.

224. VandenDriessche, T., Vanslembrouch, V., Goovaerts, I., Zwinnen, H., Vanderhaeghen, M.-L., Collen, D., and Chuah, M.K.L.: Long-term expression of human coagulation factor VIII and correction of hemophilia A after in vivo retroviral gene transfer in factor VIII-deficient mice. Proc. Natl. Acad. Sci. USA 96:10379, 1999.

225. Connelly, S., Mount, J., Mauser, A., Gardner, J.M., Kaleko, M., McClelland, A., and Lothrop, C.D., Jr.: Complete short-term correction of canine hemophilia A by in vivo gene therapy. Blood 88:3846, 1996.

226. Bi, L., Lawler, A.M., Antonarakis, S.E., High, K.A., Gearhart, J.D., and Kazazian, H.H., Jr.: Targeted disruption of the mouse factor VIII gene produces a model of haemophilia A. Nat. Genet. 10:119, 1995.

227. Connelly, S., Andrews, J.L., Gallo, A.M., Kayda, D.B., Qian, J., Hoyer, L., Kadan, M.J., Gorziglia, M.I., Trapnell, B.C., McClelland, A., and Kaleko, M.: Sustained phenotypic correction of murine hemophilia A by in vivo gene therapy. Blood 91:3273, 1998.

228. Thompson, A.R.: Radioimmunoassay of factor IX. In Bloom, A.L. (ed.): The Hemophilias. Vol. 5. Edinburgh, Churchill Livingstone, 1982, pp. 122–136.

229. Fujikawa, K., Thompson, A.R., Legaz, M.E., Meyer, R.G., and Davie, E.W.: Isolation and characterization of bovine factor IX (Christmas factor). Biochemistry 12:4938, 1973.

230. Andersson, L.-O., Borg, H., and Miller-Andersson, M.: Purification and characterization of human factor IX. Thromb. Res. 7:451, 1975.

231. DiScipio, R.G., Hermodson, M.A., Yates, S.G., and Davie, E.W.: A comparison of human prothrombin, factor IX (Christmas factor), factor X (Stuart factor), and protein S. Biochemistry 16:698, 1977.

232. Kurachi, K., and Davie, E.W.: Isolation and characterization of a cDNA coding for human factor IX. Proc. Natl. Acad. Sci. USA 79:6461, 1982.

233. Agarwala, K.L., Kawabata, S., Takao, T., Murata, H., Shimonishi, Y., Nishimura, H., and Iwanaga, S.: Activation peptide of human factor IX has oligosaccharides O-glycosidically linked to threonine residues at 159 and 169. Biochemistry 33:5167, 1994.

234. Bond, M., Jankowski, M., Patel, H., Karnik, S., Strang, A., Xu, B., Rouse, J., Koza, S., Letwin, B., Steckert, J., Amphlett, G., and Scoble, H.: Biochemical characterization of recombinant factor IX. Semin. Hematol. 35(suppl. 2):11, 1998.

235. Nishimura, H., Kawabata, S., Kisiel, W., Hase, S., Ikenaka, T., Takao, T., Shimonishi, Y., and Iwanaga, S.: Identification of a disaccharide (Xyl-Glc) and a trisaccharide (Xyl2-Glc) O-glycosidically linked to a serine residue in the first epidermal growth factor–like domain of human factors VII and IX and protein Z and bovine protein Z. J. Biol. Chem. 264:20320, 1989.

236. Nishimura, H., Takao, T., Hase, S., Shimonishi, Y., and Iwanaga, S.: Human factor IX has a tetrasaccharide O-glycosidically linked to serine 61 through the fucose residue. J. Biol. Chem. 267:17520, 1992.

237. Harris, R.J., van Halbeek, H., Glushka, J., Basa, L.J., Ling, V.T., Smith, K.J., and Spellman, M.W.: Identification and structural analysis of the tetrasaccharide NeuAc alpha(2→6)Gal beta(1→4)GlcNAc beta(1→3)Fuc alpha 1→O-linked to serine 61 of human factor IX. Biochemistry 32:6539, 1993.

238. Harris, R.J., and Spellman, M.W.: O-linked fucose and other post-translational modifications unique to EGF modules. Glycobiology 3:219, 1993.

239. DiScipio, R.G., and Davie, E.W.: Characterization of protein S, a gamma-carboxyglutamic acid containing protein from bovine and human plasma. Biochemistry 18:899, 1979.

240. Freedman, S.J., Furie, B.C., Furie, B., and Baleja, J.D.: Structure of the calcium ion-bound γ-carboxyglutamic acid–rich domain of factor IX. Biochemistry 34:12126, 1995.

241. Freedman, S.J., Blostein, M.D., Baleja, J.D., Jacobs, M., Furie, B.C., and Furie, B.: Identification of the phospholipid binding site in the vitamin K–dependent blood coagulation protein factor IX. J. Biol. Chem. 271:16227, 1996.

242. Cheung, W.F., van den Born, J., Kuhn, K., Kjellen, L., Hudson, B.G., and Stafford, D.W.: Identification of the endothelial cell binding site for factor IX. Proc. Natl. Acad. Sci. USA 93:11068, 1996.

243. Wolberg, A.S., Stafford, D.W., and Erie, D.A.: Human factor IX binds to specific sites on the collagenous domain of collagen IV. J. Biol. Chem. 272:16717, 1997.

244. Cheung, W.F., Hamaguchi, N., Smith, K.J., and Stafford, D.W.: The binding of human factor IX to endothelial cells is mediated by residues 3–11. J. Biol. Chem. 267:20529, 1992.
245. Li, L., Darden, T.A., Freedman, S.J., Furie, B.C., Furie, B., Baleja, J.D., Smith, H., Hiskey, R.G., and Pedersen, L.G.: Refinement of the NMR solution structure of the γ-carboxyglutamic acid domain of coagulation factor IX using molecular dynamics simulation with initial Ca²⁺ positions determined by a genetic algorithm. Biochemistry 36:2132, 1997.
246. Stenflo, J.: Structure-function relationships of epidermal growth factor modules in vitamin K–dependent clotting factors. Blood 78:1637, 1991.
247. Patthy, L.: Modular design of proteases of coagulation, fibrinolysis, and complement activation: implications for protein engineering and structure-function studies. Methods Enzymol. 222:10, 1993.
248. Davis, C.G.: The many faces of epidermal growth factor repeats. New Biol. 2:410, 1990.
249. McMullen, B.A., Fujikawa, K., and Kisiel, W.: The occurrence of β-hydroxyaspartic acid in the vitamin K–dependent blood coagulation zymogens. Biochem. Biophys. Res. Commun. 115:8, 1983.
250. Sunnerhagen, M.S., Persson, E., Dahlqvist, I., Drakenberg, T., Stenflo, J., Mayhew, M., Robin, M., Handford, P., Tilley, J.W., Campbell, I.D., and Brownlee, G.G.: The effect of aspartate hydroxylation on calcium binding to epidermal growth factor–like modules in coagulation factors IX and X. J. Biol. Chem. 268:23339, 1993.
251. Sigler, P.B., Blow, D.M., Matthews, B.W., and Henderson, R.: Structure of crystalline α-chymotrypsin. II. A preliminary report including a hypothesis for the activation mechanism. J. Mol. Biol. 35:143, 1968.
252. Jorgensen, M.J., Cantor, A.B., Furie, B.C., Brown, C.L., Shoemaker, C.B., and Furie, B.: Recognition site directing vitamin K–dependent γ-carboxylation resides on the propeptide of factor IX. Cell 48:185, 1987.
253. Handford, P.A., Winship, P.R., and Brownlee, G.G.: Protein engineering of the propeptide of human factor IX. Protein Eng. 4:319, 1991.
254. Bristol, J.A., Furie, B.C., and Furie, B.: Propeptide processing during factor IX biosynthesis. Effect of point mutations adjacent to the propeptide cleavage site. J. Biol. Chem. 268:7577, 1993.
255. Jia, S., VanDusen, W.J., Diehl, R.E., Kohl, N.E., Dixon, R.A., Elliston, K.O., Stern, A.M., and Friedman, P.A.: cDNA cloning and expression of bovine aspartyl (asparaginyl) β-hydroxylase. J. Biol. Chem. 267:14322, 1992.
256. Stenflo, J., Lundwall, A., and Dahlbäck, B.: β-Hydroxyasparagine in domains homologous to the epidermal growth factor precursor in vitamin K–dependent protein S. Proc. Natl. Acad. Sci. USA 84:368, 1987.
257. Derian, C.K., VanDusen, W., Przysiecki, C.T., Walsh, P.N., Berkner, K.L., Kaufman, R.J., and Friedman, P.A.: Inhibitors of 2-ketoglutarate–dependent dioxygenases block aspartyl β-hydroxylation of recombinant human factor IX in several mammalian expression systems. J. Biol. Chem. 264:6615, 1989.
258. Smith, K.J., and Thompson, A.R.: Labeled factor IX kinetics in patients with hemophilia-B. Blood 58:625, 1981.
259. Zauber, N.P., and Levin, J.: Factor IX levels in patients with hemophilia B (Christmas disease) following transfusion with concentrates of factor IX or fresh frozen plasma (FFP). Medicine (Baltimore) 56:213, 1977.
260. Lindquist, P.A., Fujikawa, K., and Davie, E.W.: Activation of bovine factor IX (Christmas factor) by factor XIa (activated plasma thromboplastin antecedent) and a protease from Russell's viper venom. J. Biol. Chem. 253:1902, 1978.
261. Bajaj, S.P., Rapaport, S.I., and Russell, W.A.: Redetermination of the rate-limiting step in the activation of factor IX by factor XIa and by factor VIIa/tissue factor. Explanation for different electrophoretic radioactivity profiles obtained on activation of ³H- and ¹²⁵I-labeled factor IX. Biochemistry 22:4047, 1983.
262. Byrne, R., Amphlett, G.W., and Castellino, F.J.: Metal ion specificity of the conversion of bovine factors IX, IXα, and IXaα to bovine factor IXaβ. J. Biol. Chem. 255:1430, 1980.
263. Kalousek, F., Konigsberg, W., and Nemerson, Y.: Activation of factor IX by activated factor X: a link between the extrinsic and intrinsic coagulation systems. FEBS Lett. 50:382, 1975.
264. Link, R.P., and Castellino, F.J.: Kinetic comparison of bovine blood coagulation factors IXaα and IXaβ toward bovine factor X. Biochemistry 22:4033, 1983.
265. Bauer, K.A., Kass, B.L., ten Cate, H., Hawiger, J.J., and Rosenberg, R.D.: Factor IX is activated in vivo by the tissue factor mechanism. Blood 76:731, 1990.
266. Broze, G.J., Jr.: Tissue factor pathway inhibitor and the revised theory of coagulation. Annu. Rev. Med. 46:103, 1995.
267. Fuchs, H.E., Trapp, H.G., Griffith, M.J., Roberts, H.R., and Pizzo, S.V.: Regulation of factor IXa in vitro in human and mouse plasma and in vivo in the mouse. Role of the endothelium and the plasma proteinase inhibitors. J. Clin. Invest. 73:1696, 1984.
268. Rosenberg, J.S., McKenna, P.W., and Rosenberg, R.D.: Inhibition of human factor IXa by human antithrombin. J. Biol. Chem. 250:8883, 1975.
269. Purrello, M., Alhadeff, B., Esposito, D., Szabo, P., Rocchi, M., Truett, M., Masiarz, F., and Siniscalco, M.: The human genes for hemophilia A and hemophilia B flank the X chromosome fragile site at Xq27.3. EMBO J. 4:725, 1985.
270. Anson, D.S., Choo, K.H., Rees, D.J., Giannelli, F., Gould, K., Huddleston, J.A., and Brownlee, G.G.: The gene structure of human anti-haemophilic factor IX. EMBO J. 3:1053, 1984.
271. Yoshitake, S., Schach, B.G., Foster, D.C., Davie, E.W., and Kurachi, K.: Nucleotide sequence of the gene for human factor IX (antihemophilic factor B). Biochemistry 24:3736, 1985.
272. Foster, D.C., Yoshitake, S., and Davie, E.W.: The nucleotide sequence of the gene for human protein C. Proc. Natl. Acad. Sci. USA 82:4673, 1985.
273. O'Hara, P.J., Grant, F.J., Haldeman, B.A., Gray, C.L., Insley, M.Y., Hagen, F.S., and Murray, M.J.: Nucleotide sequence of the gene coding for human factor VII, a vitamin K–dependent protein participating in blood coagulation. Proc. Natl. Acad. Sci. USA 84:5158, 1987.
274. Leytus, S.P., Foster, D.C., Kurachi, K., and Davie, E.W.: Gene for human factor X: a blood coagulation factor whose gene organization is essentially identical with that of factor IX and protein C. Biochemistry 25:5098, 1986.
275. Degen, S.J., and Davie, E.W.: Nucleotide sequence of the gene for human prothrombin. Biochemistry 26:6165, 1987.
276. Rizza, C.R., and Spooner, R.J.: Treatment of haemophilia and related disorders in Britain and Northern Ireland during 1976–80: report on behalf of the directors of haemophilia centres in the United Kingdom. Br. Med. J. 286:929, 1983.
277. Sultan, Y.: Prevalence of inhibitors in a population of 3435 hemophilia patients in France. French Hemophilia Study Group. Thromb. Haemost. 67:600, 1992.
278. Giannelli, F., Green, P.M., Sommer, S.S., Poon, M.-C., Ludwig, M., Schwaab, R., Reitsma, P.H., Goossens, M., Yoshioka, A., Figueiredo, M.S., and Brownlee, G.G.: Haemophilia B: database of point mutations and short additions and deletions—eighth edition. Nucleic Acids Res. 26:265, 1998.
279. Thompson, A.R.: Molecular biology of the hemophilias. Prog. Hemost. Thromb. 10:175, 1991.
280. Ketterling, R.P., Vielhaber, E.L., Lind, T.J., Thorland, E.C., and Sommer, S.S.: The rates and patterns of deletions in the human factor IX gene. Am. J. Hum. Genet. 54:201, 1994.
281. Saad, S., Rowley, G., Tagliavacca, L., Green, P.M., Giannelli, F., and Centres, U.H.: First report on UK database of haemophilia B mutations and pedigrees. UK Haemophilia Centres. Thromb. Haemost. 71:563, 1994.
282. Ludwig, M., Sabharwal, A.K., Brackmann, H.H., Olek, K., Smith, K.J., Birktoft, J.J., and Bajaj, S.P.: Hemophilia B caused by five different nondeletion mutations in the protease domain of factor IX. Blood 79:1225, 1992.
283. Briet, E., Bertina, R.M., van Tilburg, N.H., and Veltkamp, J.J.: Hemophilia B Leyden: a sex-linked hereditary disorder that improves after puberty. N. Engl. J. Med. 306:788, 1982.
284. Crossley, M., and Brownlee, G.G.: Disruption of a C/EBP binding site in the factor IX promoter is associated with haemophilia B. Nature 345:444, 1990.
285. Reijnen, M.J., Sladek, F.M., Bertina, R.M., and Reitsma, P.H.: Disruption of a binding site for hepatocyte nuclear factor 4 results in hemophilia B Leyden. Proc. Natl. Acad. Sci. USA 89:6300, 1992.
286. Crossley, M., Ludwig, M., Stowell, K.M., De Vos, P., Olek, K., and Brownlee, G.G.: Recovery from hemophilia B Leyden: an androgen-responsive element in the factor IX promoter. Science 257:377, 1992.
287. Diuguid, D.L., Rabiet, M.J., Furie, B.C., Liebman, H.A., and Furie, B.: Molecular basis of hemophilia B: a defective enzyme due to an

unprocessed propeptide is caused by a point mutation in the factor IX precursor. Proc. Natl. Acad. Sci. USA 83:5803, 1986.

288. Ware, J., Diuguid, D.L., Liebman, H.A., Rabiet, M.J., Kasper, C.K., Furie, B.C., Furie, B., and Stafford, D.W.: Factor IX San Dimas. Substitution of glutamine for Arg-4 in the propeptide leads to incomplete γ-carboxylation and altered phospholipid binding properties. J. Biol. Chem. 264:11401, 1989.

289. Bentley, A.K., Rees, D.J., Rizza, C., and Brownlee, G.G.: Defective propeptide processing of blood clotting factor IX caused by mutation of arginine to glutamine at position −4. Cell 45:343, 1986.

290. Bertina, R.M., and van der Linden, I.K.: Factor IX Zutphen. A genetic variant of blood coagulation factor IX with an abnormally high molecular weight. J. Lab. Clin. Med. 100:695, 1982.

291. Wojcik, E.G., van den Berg, M., van der Linden, I.K., Poort, S.R., Cupers, R., and Bertina, R.M.: Factor IX Zutphen: a Cys18→Arg mutation results in formation of a heterodimer with α₁-microglobulin and the inability to form a calcium-induced conformation. Biochem. J. 311:753, 1995.

292. Handford, P.A., Mayhew, M., Baron, M., Winship, P.R., Campbell, I.D., and Brownlee, G.G.: Key residues involved in calcium-binding motifs in EGF-like domains. Nature 351:164, 1991.

293. Bottema, C.D.K., Ketterling, R.P., Yoon, H.-S., and Sommer, S.S.: The pattern of factor IX germ-line mutation in Asians is similar to that of Caucasians. Am. J. Hum. Genet. 47:835, 1990.

294. McCord, D.M., Monroe, D.M., Smith, K.J., and Roberts, H.R.: Characterization of the functional defect in factor IX Alabama. Evidence for a conformational change due to high affinity calcium binding in the first epidermal growth factor domain. J. Biol. Chem. 265:10250, 1990.

295. Noyes, C.M., Griffith, M.J., Roberts, H.R., and Lundblad, R.L.: Identification of the molecular defect in factor IX Chapel Hill: substitution of histidine for arginine at position 145. Proc. Natl. Acad. Sci. USA 80:4200, 1983.

296. Braunstein, K.M., Noyes, C.M., Griffith, M.J., Lundblad, R.L., and Roberts, H.R.: Characterization of the defect in activation of factor IX Chapel Hill by human factor XIa. J. Clin. Invest. 68:1420, 1981.

297. Hougie, C., and Twomey, J.J.: Haemophilia B_M: a new type of factor-IX deficiency. Lancet 1:698, 1967.

298. Parekh, V.R., Mannucci, P.M., and Ruggeri, Z.M.: Immunological heterogeneity of haemophilia B: a multicentre study of 98 kindreds. Br. J. Haematol. 40:643, 1978.

299. Girolami, A., Dal Bo Zanon, R., Saltarin, P., Quaino, V., Altinier, G., Ripa, T., Marchetti, A., and Stocco, D.: Incidence, significance, and subtypes of hemophilia BM in a large population of hemophilia B patients. Blut 44:41, 1982.

300. Østerud, B., Kasper, C.K., Lavine, K.K., Prodanos, C., and Rapaport, S.I.: Purification and properties of an abnormal blood coagulation factor IX (factor IXB_m)/kinetics of its inhibition of factor X activation by factor VII and bovine tissue factor. Thromb. Haemost. 45:55, 1981.

301. Bertina, R.M., van der Linden, I.K., Mannucci, P.M., Reinalda-Poot, H.H., Cupers, R., Poort, S.R., and Reitsma, P.H.: Mutations in hemophilia B_m occur at the Arg¹⁸⁰-Val activation site or in the catalytic domain of factor IX. J. Biol. Chem. 265:10876, 1990.

302. Terwiel, J.P., Veltkamp, J.J., Bertina, R.M., and Muller, H.P.: Coagulation factors in the human fetus of about 20 weeks of gestational age. Br. J. Haematol. 45:641, 1980.

303. Agrawal, B.L., Zelkowitz, L., and Hletko, P.: Acute myocardial infarction in a young hemophiliac patient during therapy with Factor IX concentrate and epsilon aminocaproic acid. J. Pediatr. 98:931, 1981.

304. Abildgaard, C.F.: Hazards of prothrombin-complex concentrates in treatment of hemophilia. N. Engl. J. Med. 304:670, 1981.

305. Ohga, S., Saito, M., Matsukazi, A., Kai, T., and Ueda, K.: Disseminated intravascular coagulation in a patient with haemophilia B during factor IX replacement therapy. Br. J. Haematol. 84:343, 1993.

306. Shapiro, A.D., Ragni, M.V., Lusher, J.M., Culbert, S., Koerper, M.A., Bergman, G.E., and Hannan, M.M.: Safety and efficacy of monoclonal antibody purified factor IX concentrate in previously untreated patients with hemophilia B. Thromb. Haemost. 75:30, 1996.

307. Thomas, D.P., Hampton, K.K., Dasani, H., Lee, C.A., Giangrande, P.L., Harman, C., Lee, M.L., and Preston, F.E.: A cross-over pharmacokinetic and thrombogenicity study of a prothrombin complex concentrate and a purified factor IX concentrate. Br. J. Haematol. 87:782, 1994.

308. Hilgartner, M.W., Knatterud, G.L.: The use of factor eight inhibitor by-passing activity (FEIBA Immuno) product for treatment of bleeding episodes in hemophiliacs with inhibitors. Blood 61:36, 1983.

309. Kung, S.H., Hagstrom, J.N., Cass, D., Tai, S.J., Lin, H.F., Stafford, D.W., and High, K.A.: Human factor IX corrects the bleeding diathesis of mice with hemophilia B. Blood 91:784, 1998.

310. Wang, L., Zoppe, M., Hackeng, T.M., Griffin, J.H., Lee, K.F., and Verma, I.M.: A factor IX–deficient mouse model for hemophilia B gene therapy. Proc. Natl. Acad. Sci. USA 94:11563, 1997.

311. Lin, H.F., Maeda, N., Smithies, O., Straight, D.L., and Stafford, D.W.: A coagulation factor IX–deficient mouse model for human hemophilia B. Blood 90:3962, 1997.

312. Kay, M.A., Landen, C.N., Rothenberg, S.R., Taylor, L.A., Leland, F., Wiehle, S., Fang, B., Bellinger, D., Finegold, M., Thompson, A.R., Read, M., Brinkhous, K.M., and Woo, S.L.C.: In vivo hepatic gene therapy: complete albeit transient correction of factor IX deficiency in hemophilia B dogs. Proc. Natl. Acad. Sci. USA 91:2353, 1994.

313. Herzog, R.W., Hagstrom, J.N., Kung, S.-H., Tai, S.J., Wilson, J.M., Fisher, K.J., and High, K.A.: Stable gene transfer and expression of human blood coagulation factor IX after intramuscular injection of recombinant adeno-associated virus. Proc. Natl. Acad. Sci. USA 94:5804, 1997.

314. von Willebrand, E.A.: Hereditär pseudohemofili. Fin. Laekaresaellsk. Hand. 68:87, 1926.

315. von Willebrand, E.A.: Über hereditäre Pseudohæmophilie. Acta Med. Scand. 76:521, 1931.

316. Alexander, B., and Goldstein, B.: Dual hemostatic defect in pseudohemophilia. J. Clin. Invest. 32:551, 1953.

317. Larrieu, M.J., and Soulier, J.P.: Déficit en facteur antihémophilique A chez une fille associé à un trouble saignement. Rev. Hematol. 8:361, 1953.

318. Quick, A.J., and Hussey, C.V.: Hemophilic condition in the female. J. Lab. Clin. Med. 42:929, 1953.

319. Nilsson, I.M., Blombäck, M., Jorpes, E., Blombäck, B., and Johansson, S.-A.: v. Willebrand's disease and its correction with human plasma fraction 1-0. Acta Med. Scand. 159:179, 1957.

320. Cornu, P., Larrieu, M.J., Caen, J., and Bernard, J.: Transfusion studies in von Willebrand's disease: effect on bleeding time and factor VIII. Br. J. Haematol. 9:189, 1963.

321. Salzman, E.W.: Measurement of platelet adhesiveness: a simple in vitro technique demonstrating an abnormality in von Willebrand's disease. J. Lab. Clin. Med. 62:724, 1963.

322. Zucker, M.B.: In vitro abnormality of the blood in von Willebrand's disease correctable by normal plasma. Nature 197:601, 1963.

323. Bouma, B.N., Wiegerinck, Y., Sixma, J.J., van Mourik, J.A., and Mochtar, I.A.: Immunological characterization of purified anti-haemophilic factor A (factor VIII) which corrects abnormal platelet retention in von Willebrand's disease. Nat. New Biol. 236:104, 1972.

324. Howard, M.A., and Firkin, B.G.: Ristocetin—a new tool in the investigation of platelet aggregation. Thromb. Diath. Haemorrh. 26:362, 1971.

325. Macfarlane, D.E., Stibbe, J., Kirby, E.P., Zucker, M.B., Grant, R.A., and McPherson, J.: A method for assaying von Willebrand factor (ristocetin cofactor). Thromb. Diath. Haemorrh. 34:306, 1975.

326. Read, M.S., Shermer, R.W., and Brinkhous, K.M.: Venom coagglutinin: an activator of platelet aggregation dependent on von Willebrand factor. Proc. Natl. Acad. Sci. USA 75:4514, 1978.

327. Brinkhous, K.M., and Read, M.S.: Use of venom coagglutinin and lyophilized platelets in testing for platelet-aggregating von Willebrand factor. Blood 55:517, 1980.

328. Koutts, J., Walsh, P.N., Plow, E.F., Fenton, J.W.D., Bouma, B.N., and Zimmerman, T.S.: Active release of human platelet factor VIII–related antigen by adenosine diphosphate, collagen, and thrombin. J. Clin. Invest. 62:1255, 1978.

329. Hoyer, L.W.: Immunologic studies of antihemophilic factor (AHF, factor VIII). IV. Radioimmunoassay of AHF antigen. J. Lab. Clin. Med. 80:822, 1972.

330. Ruggeri, Z.M., Mannucci, P.M., Jeffcoate, S.L., and Ingram, G.I.: Immunoradiometric assay of factor VIII related antigen, with observations in 32 patients with von Willebrand's disease. Br. J. Haematol. 33:221, 1976.

331. Ruggeri, Z.M., and Zimmerman, T.S.: Variant von Willebrand's disease. Characterization of two subtypes by analysis of multimeric composition of factor VIII/von Willebrand factor in plasma and platelets. J. Clin. Invest. 65:1318, 1980.

332. Hoyer, L.W., and Shainoff, J.R.: Factor VIII–related protein circulates in normal human plasma as high molecular weight multimers. Blood 55:1056, 1980.

333. Ruggeri, Z.M., and Zimmerman, T.S.: The complex multimeric composition of factor VIII/von Willebrand factor. Blood 57:1140, 1981.

334. Favaloro, E.J., Facey, D., and Grispo, L.: Laboratory assessment of von Willebrand factor. Use of different assays can influence the diagnosis of von Willebrand's disease, dependent on differing sensitivity to sample preparation and differential recognition of high molecular weight VWF forms. Am. J. Clin. Pathol. 104:264, 1995.

335. de Romeuf, C., and Mazurier, C.: Heparin binding assay of von Willebrand factor (vWF) in plasma milieu—evidence of the importance of the multimerization degree of vWF. Thromb. Haemost. 69:436, 1993.

336. Chopek, M.W., Girma, J.P., Fujikawa, K., Davie, E.W., and Titani, K.: Human von Willebrand factor: a multivalent protein composed of identical subunits. Biochemistry 25:3146, 1986.

337. Dent, J.A., Galbusera, M., and Ruggeri, Z.M.: Heterogeneity of plasma von Willebrand factor multimers resulting from proteolysis of the constituent subunit. J. Clin. Invest. 88:774, 1991.

338. Counts, R.B., Paskell, S.L., and Elgee, S.K.: Disulfide bonds and the quaternary structure of factor VIII/von Willebrand factor. J. Clin. Invest. 62:702, 1978.

339. Lynch, D.C., Zimmerman, T.S., Kirby, E.P., and Livingston, D.M.: Subunit composition of oligomeric human von Willebrand factor. J. Biol. Chem. 258:12757, 1983.

340. Sadler, J.E.: Biochemistry and genetics of von Willebrand factor. Annu. Rev. Biochem. 67:395, 1998.

341. Fay, P.J., Kawai, Y., Wagner, D.D., Ginsburg, D., Bonthron, D., Ohlsson-Wilhelm, B.M., Chavin, S.I., Abraham, G.N., Handin, R.I., Orkin, S.H., Montgomery, R.R., and Marder, V.J.: Propolypeptide of von Willebrand factor circulates in blood and is identical to von Willebrand antigen II. Science 232:995, 1986.

342. Wagner, D.D., Fay, P.J., Sporn, L.A., Sinha, S., Lawrence, S.O., and Marder, V.J.: Divergent fates of von Willebrand factor and its propolypeptide (von Willebrand antigen II) after secretion from endothelial cells. Proc. Natl. Acad. Sci. USA 84:1955, 1987.

343. Borchiellini, A., Fijnvandraat, K., ten Cate, J.W., Pajkrt, D., van Deventer, S.J., Pasterkamp, G., Meijer-Huizinga, F., Zwart-Huinink, L., Voorberg, J., and van Mourik, J.A.: Quantitative analysis of von Willebrand factor propeptide release in vivo: effect of experimental endotoxemia and administration of 1-deamino-8-D-arginine vasopressin in humans. Blood 88:2951, 1996.

344. Marti, T., Rösselet, S.J., Titani, K., and Walsh, K.A.: Identification of disulfide-bridged substructures within human von Willebrand factor. Biochemistry 26:8099, 1987.

345. Dong, Z., Thoma, R.S., Crimmins, D.L., McCourt, D.W., Tuley, E.A., and Sadler, J.E.: Disulfide bonds required to assemble functional von Willebrand factor multimers. J. Biol. Chem. 269:6753, 1994.

346. Titani, K., Kumar, S., Takio, K., Ericsson, L.H., Wade, R.D., Ashida, K., Walsh, K.A., Chopek, M.W., Sadler, J.E., and Fujikawa, K.: Amino acid sequence of human von Willebrand factor. Biochemistry 25:3171, 1986.

347. Matsui, T., Titani, K., and Mizuochi, T.: Structures of the asparagine-linked oligosaccharide chains of human von Willebrand factor. Occurrence of blood group A, B, and H(O) structures. J. Biol. Chem. 267:8723, 1992.

348. Samor, B., Michalski, J.C., Mazurier, C., Goudemand, M., De Waard, P., Vliegenthart, J.F., Strecker, G., and Montreuil, J.: Primary structure of the major O-glycosidically linked carbohydrate unit of human von Willebrand factor. Glycoconj. J. 6:263, 1989.

349. Carew, J.A., Browning, P.J., and Lynch, D.C.: Sulfation of von Willebrand factor. Blood 76:2530, 1990.

350. Fowler, W.E., Fretto, L.J., Hamilton, K.K., Erickson, H.P., and McKee, P.A.: Substructure of human von Willebrand factor. J. Clin. Invest. 76:1491, 1985.

351. Jaffe, E.A., Hoyer, L.W., and Nachman, R.L.: Synthesis of von Willebrand factor by cultured human endothelial cells. Proc. Natl. Acad. Sci. USA 71:1906, 1974.

352. Nachman, R., Levine, R., and Jaffe, E.A.: Synthesis of factor VIII antigen by cultured guinea pig megakaryocytes. J. Clin. Invest. 60:914, 1977.

353. Bloom, A.L., Giddings, J.C., and Wilks, C.J.: Factor VIII on the vascular intima: possible importance in haemostasis and thrombosis. Nat. New Biol. 241:217, 1973.

354. Hoyer, L.W., De los Santos, R.P., and Hoyer, J.R.: Antihemophilic factor antigen. Localization in endothelial cells by immunofluorescent microscopy. J. Clin. Invest. 52:2737, 1973.

355. Maruyama, I., Bell, C.E., and Majerus, P.W.: Thrombomodulin is found on endothelium of arteries, veins, capillaries, and lymphatics, and on syncytiotrophoblast of human placenta. J. Cell Biol. 101:363, 1985.

356. Cramer, E.M., Meyer, D., le Menn, R., and Breton-Gorius, J.: Eccentric localization of von Willebrand factor in an internal structure of platelet α-granule resembling that of Weibel-Palade bodies. Blood 66:710, 1985.

357. Holmberg, L., Mannucci, P.M., Turesson, I., Ruggeri, Z.M., and Nilsson, I.M.: Factor VIII antigen in the vessel walls in von Willebrand's disease and haemophilia A. Scand. J. Haematol. 13:33, 1974.

358. Howard, M.A., Montgomery, D.C., and Hardisty, R.M.: Factor-VIII–related antigen in platelets. Thromb. Res. 4:617, 1974.

359. Mannucci, P.M., Pareti, F.I., Holmberg, L., Nilsson, I.M., and Ruggeri, Z.M.: Studies on the prolonged bleeding time in von Willebrand's disease. J. Lab. Clin. Med. 88:662, 1976.

360. Nichols, T.C., Samama, C.M., Bellinger, D.A., Roussi, J., Reddick, R.L., Bonneau, M., Read, M.S., Bailliart, O., Koch, G.G., Vaiman, M., et al.: Function of von Willebrand factor after crossed bone marrow transplantation between normal and von Willebrand disease pigs: effect on arterial thrombosis in chimeras. Proc. Natl. Acad. Sci. USA 92:2455, 1995.

361. Wagner, D.D.: Cell biology of von Willebrand factor. Annu. Rev. Cell Biol. 6:217, 1990.

362. McDonald, N.Q., and Hendrickson, W.A.: A structural superfamily of growth factors containing a cystine knot motif. Cell 73:421, 1993.

363. Schneppenheim, R., Brassard, J., Krey, S., Budde, U., Kunicki, T.J., Holmberg, L., Ware, J., and Ruggeri, Z.M.: Defective dimerization of von Willebrand factor subunits due to a Cys → Arg mutation in type IID von Willebrand disease. Proc. Natl. Acad. Sci. USA 93:3581, 1996.

364. Wagner, D.D., and Marder, V.J.: Biosynthesis of von Willebrand protein by human endothelial cells: processing steps and their intracellular localization. J. Cell Biol. 99:2123, 1984.

365. Fujimura, Y., Titani, K., Holland, L.Z., Russell, S.R., Roberts, J.R., Elder, J.H., Ruggeri, Z.M., and Zimmerman, T.S.: von Willebrand factor. A reduced and alkylated 52/48-kDa fragment beginning at amino acid residue 449 contains the domain interacting with platelet glycoprotein Ib. J. Biol. Chem. 261:381, 1986.

366. Mayadas, T.N., and Wagner, D.D.: Vicinal cysteines in the prosequence play a role in von Willebrand factor multimer assembly. Proc. Natl. Acad. Sci. USA 89:3531, 1992.

367. Rehemtulla, A., and Kaufman, R.J.: Preferred sequence requirements for cleavage of pro–von Willebrand factor by propeptide-processing enzymes. Blood 79:2349, 1992.

368. Vischer, U.M., and Wagner, D.D.: von Willebrand factor proteolytic processing and multimerization precede the formation of Weibel-Palade bodies. Blood 83:3536, 1994.

369. Weibel, E.R., and Palade, G.E.: New cytoplasmic components in arterial endothelia. J. Cell Biol. 23:101, 1964.

370. Wagner, D.D., Olmsted, J.B., and Marder, V.J.: Immunolocalization of von Willebrand protein in Weibel-Palade bodies of human endothelial cells. J. Cell Biol. 95:355, 1982.

371. Wagner, D.D., Saffaripour, S., Bonfanti, R., Sadler, J.E., Cramer, E.M., Chapman, B., and Mayadas, T.N.: Induction of specific storage organelles by von Willebrand factor propolypeptide. Cell 64:403, 1991.

372. Voorberg, J., Fontijn, R., Calafat, J., Janssen, H., van Mourik, J.A., and Pannekoek, H.: Biogenesis of von Willebrand factor–containing organelles in heterologous transfected CV-1 cells. EMBO J. 12:749, 1993.

373. Hop, C., Fontijn, R., van Mourik, J.A., and Pannekoek, H.: Polarity of constitutive and regulated von Willebrand factor secretion by transfected MDCK-II cells. Exp. Cell Res. 230:352, 1997.

374. Loesberg, C., Gonsalves, M.D., Zandbergen, J., Willems, C., van Aken, W.G., Stel, H.V., Van Mourik, J.A., and de Groot, P.G.: The effect of calcium on the secretion of factor VIII–related antigen by cultured human endothelial cells. Biochim. Biophys. Acta 763:160, 1983.

375. Sporn, L.A., Marder, V.J., and Wagner, D.D.: Inducible secretion of large, biologically potent von Willebrand factor multimers. Cell 46:185, 1986.

376. Levine, J.D., Harlan, J.M., Harker, L.A., Joseph, M.L., and Counts, R.B.: Thrombin-mediated release of factor VIII antigen from human umbilical vein endothelial cells in culture. Blood 60:531, 1982.

377. Vischer, U.M., and Wollheim, C.B.: Epinephrine induces von Willebrand factor release from cultured endothelial cells: involvement of cyclic AMP–dependent signalling in exocytosis. Thromb. Haemost. 77:1182, 1997.

378. Hamilton, K.K., and Sims, P.J.: Changes in cytosolic Ca^{2+} associated with von Willebrand factor release in human endothelial cells exposed to histamine. Study of microcarrier cell monolayers using the fluorescent probe indo-1. J. Clin. Invest. 79:600, 1987.

379. Ribes, J.A., Ni, F., Wagner, D.D., and Francis, C.W.: Mediation of fibrin-induced release of von Willebrand factor from cultured endothelial cells by the fibrin β-chain. J. Clin. Invest. 84:435, 1989.

380. Hattori, R., Hamilton, K.K., McEver, R.P., and Sims, P.J.: Complement proteins C5b-9 induce secretion of high molecular weight multimers of endothelial von Willebrand factor and translocation of granule membrane protein GMP-140 to the cell surface. J. Biol. Chem. 264:9053, 1989.

381. Gill, J.C., Endres-Brooks, J., Bauer, P.J., Marks, W.J., and Montgomery, R.R.: The effect of ABO blood group on the diagnosis of von Willebrand disease. Blood 69:1691, 1987.

382. Nachman, R.L., and Jaffe, E.A.: Subcellular platelet factor VIII antigen and von Willebrand factor. J. Exp. Med. 141:1101, 1975.

383. Ørstavik, K.H., Kornstad, L., Reisner, H., and Berg, K.: Possible effect of Secretor locus on plasma concentration of factor VIII and von Willebrand factor. Blood 73:990, 1989.

384. Moffat, E.H., Giddings, J.C., and Bloom, A.L.: The effect of desamino-D-arginine vasopressin (DDAVP) and naloxone infusions on factor VIII and possible endothelial cell (EC) related activities. Br. J. Haematol. 57:651, 1984.

385. Booth, F., Allington, M.J., and Cederholm-Williams, S.A.: An in vitro model for the study of acute release of von Willebrand factor from human endothelial cells. Br. J. Haematol. 67:71, 1987.

386. Weiss, H.J., Turitto, V.T., and Baumgartner, H.R.: Effect of shear rate on platelet interaction with subendothelium in citrated and native blood. I. Shear rate–dependent decrease of adhesion in von Willebrand's disease and the Bernard-Soulier syndrome. J. Lab. Clin. Med. 92:750, 1978.

387. Sakariassen, K.S., Bolhuis, P.A., and Sixma, J.J.: Human blood platelet adhesion to artery subendothelium is mediated by factor VIII–von Willebrand factor bound to the subendothelium. Nature 279:636, 1979.

388. Ruggeri, Z.M.: von Willebrand factor. J. Clin. Invest. 99:559, 1997.

389. Turitto, V.T., Weiss, H.J., Zimmerman, T.S., and Sussman, I.I.: Factor VIII/von Willebrand factor in subendothelium mediates platelet adhesion. Blood 65:823, 1985.

390. Stel, H.V., Sakariassen, K.S., de Groot, P.G., van Mourik, J.A., and Sixma, J.J.: Von Willebrand factor in the vessel wall mediates platelet adherence. Blood 65:85, 1985.

391. Hormia, M., Lehto, V.P., and Virtanen, I.: Factor VIII–related antigen. A pericellular matrix component of cultured human endothelial cells. Exp. Cell Res. 149:483, 1983.

392. Wagner, D.D., Urban-Pickering, M., and Marder, V.J.: Von Willebrand protein binds to extracellular matrices independently of collagen. Proc. Natl. Acad. Sci. USA 81:471, 1984.

393. Santoro, S.A.: Adsorption of von Willebrand factor/factor VIII by the genetically distinct interstitial collagens. Thromb. Res. 21:689, 1981.

394. Morton, L.F., Griffin, B., Pepper, D.S., and Barnes, M.J.: The interaction between collagens and factor VIII/von Willebrand factor: investigation of the structural requirements for interaction. Thromb. Res. 32:545, 1983.

395. Rand, J.H., Patel, N.D., Schwartz, E., Zhou, S.L., and Potter, B.J.: 150-kD von Willebrand factor binding protein extracted from human vascular subendothelium is type VI collagen. J. Clin. Invest. 88:253, 1991.

396. de Groot, P.G., Ottenhof-Rovers, M., van Mourik, J.A., and Sixma, J.J.: Evidence that the primary binding site of von Willebrand factor that mediates platelet adhesion on subendothelium is not collagen. J. Clin. Invest. 82:65, 1988.

397. von der Mark, H., Aumailley, M., Wick, G., Fleischmajer, R., and Timpl, R.: Immunochemistry, genuine size and tissue localization of collagen VI. Eur. J. Biochem. 142:493, 1984.

398. Colombatti, A., and Bonaldo, P.: Biosynthesis of chick type VI collagen. II. Processing and secretion in fibroblasts and smooth muscle cells. J. Biol. Chem. 262:14461, 1987.

399. Savage, B., Saldivar, E., and Ruggeri, Z.M.: Initiation of platelet adhesion by arrest onto fibrinogen or translocation on von Willebrand factor. Cell 84:289, 1996.

400. Martin, S.E., Marder, V.J., Francis, C.W., and Barlow, G.H.: Structural studies of the functional heterogeneity of von Willebrand protein polymers. Blood 57:313, 1981.

401. Aihara, M., Kimura, A., Chiba, Y., and Yoshida, Y.: Plasma collagen cofactor correlates with von Willebrand factor antigen and ristocetin cofactor but not with bleeding time. Thromb. Haemost. 59:485, 1988.

402. Sixma, J.J., Sakariassen, K.S., Beeser-Visser, N.H., Ottenhof-Rovers, M., and Bolhuis, P.A.: Adhesion of platelets to human artery subendothelium: effect of factor VIII–von Willebrand factor of various multimeric composition. Blood 63:128, 1984.

403. Foster, P.A., Fulcher, C.A., Marti, T., Titani, K., and Zimmerman, T.S.: A major factor VIII binding domain resides within the amino-terminal 272 amino acid residues of von Willebrand factor. J. Biol. Chem. 262:8443, 1987.

404. Bendetowicz, A.V., Morris, J.A., Wise, R.J., Gilbert, G.E., and Kaufman, R.J.: Binding of factor VIII to von Willebrand factor is enabled by cleavage of the von Willebrand factor propeptide and enhanced by formation of disulfide-linked multimers. Blood 92:529, 1998.

405. Vlot, A.J., Koppelman, S.J., van den Berg, M.H., Bouma, B.N., and Sixma, J.J.: The affinity and stoichiometry of binding of human factor VIII to von Willebrand factor. Blood 85:3150, 1995.

406. Vlot, A.J., Koppelman, S.J., Meijers, J.C., Dama, C., van den Berg, H.M., Bouma, B.N., Sixma, J.J., and Willems, G.M.: Kinetics of factor VIII–von Willebrand factor association. Blood 87:1809, 1996.

407. Bahou, W.F., Ginsburg, D., Sikkink, R., Litwiller, R., and Fass, D.N.: A monoclonal antibody to von Willebrand factor (vWF) inhibits factor VIII binding. Localization of its antigenic determinant to a nonadecapeptide at the amino terminus of the mature vWF polypeptide. J. Clin. Invest. 84:56, 1989.

408. Jorieux, S., Gaucher, C., Pietu, G., Cherel, G., Meyer, D., and Mazurier, C.: Fine epitope mapping of monoclonal antibodies to the NH$_2$-terminal part of von Willebrand factor (vWF) by using recombinant and synthetic peptides: interest for the localization of the factor VIII binding domain. Br. J. Haematol. 87:113, 1994.

409. Pietu, G., Ribba, A.S., Cherel, G., Siguret, V., Obert, B., Rouault, C., Ginsburg, D., and Meyer, D.: Epitope mapping of inhibitory monoclonal antibodies to human von Willebrand factor by using recombinant cDNA libraries. Thromb. Haemost. 71:788, 1994.

410. Fretto, L.J., Fowler, W.E., McCaslin, D.R., Erickson, H.P., and McKee, P.A.: Substructure of human von Willebrand factor. Proteolysis by V8 and characterization of two functional domains. J. Biol. Chem. 261:15679, 1986.

411. Celikel, R., Varughese, K.I., Madhusudan, Yoshioka, A., Ware, J., and Ruggeri, Z.M.: Crystal structure of the von Willebrand factor A1 domain in complex with the function blocking NMC-4 Fab. Nat. Struct. Biol. 5:189, 1998.

412. Emsley, J., Cruz, M., Handin, R., and Liddington, R.: Crystal structure of the von Willebrand Factor A1 domain and implications for the binding of platelet glycoprotein Ib. J. Biol. Chem. 273:10396, 1998.

413. Emsley, J., King, S.L., Bergelson, J.M., and Liddington, R.C.: Crystal structure of the I domain from integrin α$_2$β$_1$. J. Biol. Chem. 272:28512, 1997.

414. Lee, J.O., Rieu, P., Arnaout, M.A., and Liddington, R.: Crystal structure of the A domain from the α-subunit of integrin CR3 (CD11b/CD18). Cell 80:631, 1995.

415. Qu, A.D., and Leahy, D.J.: Crystal structure of the I-domain from the Cd11a/Cd18 (LFA-1, α(L)β$_2$) integrin. Proc. Natl. Acad. Sci. USA 92:10277, 1995.

416. Matsushita, T., and Sadler, J.E.: Identification of amino acid residues essential for von Willebrand factor binding to platelet glycoprotein Ib. Charged-to-alanine scanning mutagenesis of the A1 domain of human von Willebrand factor. J. Biol. Chem. 270:13406, 1995.

417. Andrews, R.K., Gorman, J.J., Booth, W.J., Corino, G.L., Castaldi, P.A., and Berndt, M.C.: Cross-linking of a monomeric 39/34-kDa dispase fragment of von Willebrand factor (Leu-480/Val-481–Gly-718) to the N-terminal region of the alpha-chain of membrane glycoprotein Ib on intact platelets with bis(sulfosuccinimidyl) suberate. Biochemistry 28:8326, 1989.

418. Kroner, P.A., and Frey, A.B.: Analysis of the structure and function of the von Willebrand factor A1 domain using targeted deletions and alanine-scanning mutagenesis. Biochemistry 35:13460, 1996.

419. Fujimura, Y., Titani, K., Holland, L.Z., Roberts, J.R., Kostel, P., Ruggeri, Z.M., and Zimmerman, T.S.: A heparin-binding domain of human von Willebrand factor. Characterization and localization to a tryptic fragment extending from amino acid residue Val-449 to Lys-728. J. Biol. Chem. 262:1734, 1987.

420. Christophe, O., Obert, B., Meyer, D., and Girma, J.P.: The binding domain of von Willebrand factor to sulfatides is distinct from those interacting with glycoprotein Ib, heparin, and collagen and resides between amino acid residues Leu 512 and Lys 673. Blood 78:2310, 1991.

421. Roth, G.J., Titani, K., Hoyer, L.W., and Hickey, M.J.: Localization of binding sites within human von Willebrand factor for monomeric type III collagen. Biochemistry 25:8357, 1986.

422. Pareti, F.I., Niiya, K., McPherson, J.M., and Ruggeri, Z.M.: Isolation and characterization of two domains of human von Willebrand factor that interact with fibrillar collagen types I and III. J. Biol. Chem. 262:13835, 1987.

423. Kalafatis, M., Takahashi, Y., Girma, J.P., and Meyer, D.: Localization of a collagen-interactive domain of human von Willebrand factor between amino acid residues Gly 911 and Glu 1,365. Blood 70:1577, 1987.

424. Lankhof, H., van Hoeij, M., Schiphorst, M.E., Bracke, M., Wu, Y.P., Ijsseldijk, M.J., Vink, T., de Groot, P.G., and Sixma, J.J.: A3 domain is essential for interaction of von Willebrand factor with collagen type III. Thromb. Haemost. 75:950, 1996.

425. Bienkowska, J., Cruz, M., Atiemo, A., Handin, R., and Liddington, R.: The von Willebrand factor A3 domain does not contain a metal ion–dependent adhesion site motif. J. Biol. Chem. 272:25162, 1997.

426. Huizinga, E.G., van der Plas, R.M., Kroon, J., Sixma, J.J., and Gros, P.: Crystal structure of the A3 domain of human von Willebrand factor: implications for collagen binding. Structure 5:1147, 1997.

427. Berliner, S., Niiya, K., Roberts, J.R., Houghten, R.A., and Ruggeri, Z.M.: Generation and characterization of peptide-specific antibodies that inhibit von Willebrand factor binding to glycoprotein IIb-IIIa without interacting with other adhesive molecules. Selectivity is conferred by Pro1743 and other amino acid residues adjacent to the sequence Arg1744-Gly1745-Asp1746. J. Biol. Chem. 263:7500, 1988.

428. Ruoslahti, E.: RGD and other recognition sequences for integrins. Annu. Rev. Cell Dev. Biol. 12:697, 1996.

429. Folsom, A.R., Wu, K.K., Rosamond, W.D., Sharrett, A.R., and Chambless, L.E.: Prospective study of hemostatic factors and incidence of coronary heart disease: the Atherosclerosis Risk in Communities (ARIC) Study. Circulation 96:1102, 1997.

430. Griggs, T.R., Bauman, R.W., Reddick, R.L., Read, M.S., Koch, G.G., and Lamb, M.A.: Development of coronary atherosclerosis in swine with severe hypercholesterolemia. Lack of influence of von Willebrand factor or acute intimal injury. Arteriosclerosis 6:155, 1986.

431. Nichols, T.C., Bellinger, D.A., Reddick, R.L., Koch, G.G., Sigman, J.L., Erickson, G., du Laney, T., Johnson, T., Read, M.S., and Griggs, T.R.: von Willebrand factor does not influence atherogenesis in arteries subjected to altered shear stress. Arterioscler. Thromb. Vasc. Biol. 18:323, 1998.

432. Nichols, T.C., Bellinger, D.A., Tate, D.A., Reddick, R.L., Read, M.S., Koch, G.G., Brinkhous, K.M., and Griggs, T.R.: von Willebrand factor and occlusive arterial thrombosis. A study in normal and von Willebrand's disease pigs with diet-induced hypercholesterolemia and atherosclerosis. Arteriosclerosis 10:449, 1990.

433. Moake, J.L., Rudy, C.K., Troll, J.H., Weinstein, M.J., Colannino, N.M., Azocar, J., Seder, R.H., Hong, S.L., and Deykin, D.: Unusually large plasma factor VIII:von Willebrand factor multimers in chronic relapsing thrombotic thrombocytopenic purpura. N. Engl. J. Med. 307:1432, 1982.

434. Kelton, J.G., Moore, J., Santos, A., and Sheridan, D.: The detection of a platelet-agglutinating factor in thrombotic thrombocytopenic purpura. Ann. Intern. Med. 101:589, 1984.

435. Moake, J.L., Byrnes, J.J., Troll, J.H., Rudy, C.K., Weinstein, M.J., Colannino, N.M., and Hong, S.L.: Abnormal VIII:von Willebrand factor patterns in the plasma of patients with the hemolytic-uremic syndrome. Blood 64:592, 1984.

436. Furlan, M., Robles, R., Solenthaler, M., Wassmer, M., Sandoz, P., and Lammle, B.: Deficient activity of von Willebrand factor–cleaving protease in chronic relapsing thrombotic thrombocytopenic purpura. Blood 89:3097, 1997.

437. Furlan, M., Robles, R., Solenthaler, M., and Lammle, B.: Acquired deficiency of von Willebrand factor–cleaving protease in a patient with thrombotic thrombocytopenic purpura. Blood 91:2839, 1998.

438. Ginsburg, D., Handin, R.I., Bonthron, D.T., Donlon, T.A., Bruns, G.A.P., Latt, S.A., and Orkin, S.H.: Human von Willebrand factor (vWF): isolation of complementary DNA (cDNA) clones and chromosomal localization. Science 228:1401, 1985.

439. Kuwano, A., Morimoto, Y., Nagai, T., Fukushima, Y., Ohashi, H., Hasegawa, T., and Kondo, I.: Precise chromosomal locations of the genes for dentatorubral-pallidoluysian atrophy (DRPLA), von Willebrand factor (F8vWF) and parathyroid hormone–like hormone (PTHLH) in human chromosome 12p by deletion mapping. Hum. Genet. 97:95, 1996.

440. O'Connell, P., Lathrop, G.M., Law, M., Leppert, M., Nakamura, Y., Hoff, M., Kumlin, E., Thomas, W., Elsner, T., Ballard, L., Goodman, P., Azen, E., Sadler, J.E., Cai, G.Y., Lalouel, J.-M., and White, R.: A primary genetic linkage map for human chromosome 12. Genomics 1:93, 1987.

441. Mancuso, D.J., Tuley, E.A., Westfield, L.A., Worrall, N.K., Shelton-Inloes, B.B., Sorace, J.M., Alevy, Y.G., and Sadler, J.E.: Structure of the gene for human von Willebrand factor. J. Biol. Chem. 264:19514, 1989.

442. Jahroudi, N., Ardekani, A.M., and Greenberger, J.S.: An NF1-like protein functions as a repressor of the von Willebrand factor promoter. J. Biol. Chem. 271:21413, 1996.

443. Schwachtgen, J.-L., Janel, N., Barek, L., Duterque-Coquillaud, M., Ghysdael, J., Meyer, D., and Kerbiriou-Nabias, D.: Ets transcription factors bind and transactivate the core promoter of the von Willebrand factor gene. Oncogene 15:3091, 1997.

444. Schwachtgen, J.-L., Remacle, J.E., Janel, N., Brys, R., Huylebroeck, D., Meyer, D., and Kerbiriou-Nabias, D.: Oct-1 is involved in the transcriptional repression of the von Willebrand factor gene promoter. Blood 92:1247, 1998.

445. Aird, W.C., Jahroudi, N., Weiler-Guettler, H., Rayburn, H.B., and Rosenberg, R.D.: Human von Willebrand factor gene sequences target expression to a subpopulation of endothelial cells in transgenic mice. Proc. Natl. Acad. Sci. USA 92:4567, 1995.

446. Patracchini, P., Calzolari, E., Aiello, V., Palazzi, P., Banin, P., Marchetti, G., and Bernardi, F.: Sublocalization of von Willebrand factor pseudogene to 22q11.22–q11.23 by in situ hybridization in a 46,X,t(X;22)(pter;q11.21) translocation. Hum. Genet. 83:264, 1989.

447. Mancuso, D.J., Tuley, E.A., Westfield, L.A., Lester-Mancuso, T.L., Le Beau, M.M., Sorace, J.M., and Sadler, J.E.: Human von Willebrand factor gene and pseudogene: structural analysis and differentiation by polymerase chain reaction. Biochemistry 30:253, 1991.

448. Perez-Vilar, J., and Hill, R.L.: The carboxyl-terminal 90 residues of porcine submaxillary mucin are sufficient for forming disulfide-bonded dimers. J. Biol. Chem. 273:6982, 1998.

449. Meitinger, T., Meindl, A., Bork, P., Rost, B., Sander, C., Haasemann, M., and Murken, J.: Molecular modelling of the Norrie disease protein predicts a cystine knot growth factor tertiary structure. Nat. Genet. 5:376, 1993.

450. Rodeghiero, F., Castaman, G., and Dini, E.: Epidemiological investigation of the prevalence of von Willebrand's disease. Blood 69:454, 1987.

451. Holmberg, L., and Nilsson, I.M.: von Willebrand's disease. Eur. J. Haematol. 48:127, 1992.

452. Sadler, J.E.: A revised classification of von Willebrand disease. Thromb. Haemost. 71:520, 1994.

453. Ginsburg, D., and Sadler, J.E.: von Willebrand disease: a database of point mutations, insertions, and deletions. Thromb. Haemost. 69:177, 1993.

454. Sadler, J.E., and Ginsburg, D.: A database of polymorphisms in the von Willebrand factor gene and pseudogene. Thromb. Haemost. 69:185, 1993.

455. Eikenboom, J.C., Reitsma, P.H., Peerlinck, K.M.J., and Briët, E.: Recessive inheritance of von Willebrand's disease type I. Lancet 341:982, 1993.

456. Eikenboom, J.C.J., Matsushita, T., Reitsma, P.H., Tuley, E.A., Castaman, G., Br iët, E., and Sadler, J.E.: Dominant type 1 von Willebrand disease caused by mutated cysteine residues in the D3 domain of von Willebrand factor. Blood 88:2433, 1996.

457. Lyons, S.E., Bruck, M.E., Bowie, E.J.W., and Ginsburg, D.: Impaired intracellular transport produced by a subset of type IIA von Willebrand disease mutations. J. Biol. Chem. 267:4424, 1992.

458. Lyons, S.E., Cooney, K.A., Bockenstedt, P., and Ginsburg, D.: Characterization of Leu777Pro and Ile865Thr type IIA von Willebrand disease mutations. Blood 83:1551, 1994.

459. Zimmerman, T.S., Dent, J.A., Ruggeri, Z.M., and Nannini, L.H.: Subunit composition of plasma von Willebrand factor. Cleavage is present in normal individuals, increased in IIA and IIB von Willebrand disease, but minimal in variants with aberrant structure of individual oligomers (types IIC, IID, and IIE). J. Clin. Invest. 77:947, 1986.

460. Dent, J.A., Berkowitz, S.D., Ware, J., Kasper, C.K., and Ruggeri, Z.M.: Identification of a cleavage site directing the immunochemical detection of molecular abnormalities in type IIA von Willebrand factor. Proc. Natl. Acad. Sci. USA 87:6306, 1990.

461. Gaucher, C., D iéval, J., and Mazurier, C.: Characterization of von Willebrand factor gene defects in two unrelated patients with type IIC von Willebrand disease. Blood 84:1024, 1994.

462. Ruggeri, Z.M., Pareti, F.I., Mannucci, P.M., Ciavarella, N., and Zimmerman, T.S.: Heightened interaction between platelets and factor VIII/von Willebrand factor in a new subtype of von Willebrand's disease. N. Engl. J. Med. 302:1047, 1980.

463. Saba, H.I., Saba, S.R., Dent, J., Ruggeri, Z.M., and Zimmerman, T.S.: Type IIB Tampa: a variant of von Willebrand disease with chronic thrombocytopenia, circulating platelet aggregates, and spontaneous platelet aggregation. Blood 66:282, 1985.

464. Ruggeri, Z.M., Lombardi, R., Gatti, L., Bader, R., Valsecchi, C., and Zimmerman, T.S.: Type IIB von Willebrand's disease: differential clearance of endogenous versus transfused large multimer von Willebrand factor. Blood 60:1453, 1982.

465. Ruggeri, Z.M., Mannucci, P.M., Lombardi, R., Federici, A.B., and Zimmerman, T.S.: Multimeric composition of factor VIII/von Willebrand factor following administration of DDAVP: implications for pathophysiology and therapy of von Willebrand's disease subtypes. Blood 59:1272, 1982.

466. Holmberg, L., Nilsson, I.M., Borge, L., Gunnarsson, M., and Sjorin, E.: Platelet aggregation induced by 1-desamino-8-D-arginine vasopressin (DDAVP) in type IIB von Willebrand's disease. N. Engl. J. Med. 309:816, 1983.

467. Holmberg, L., Dent, J.A., Schneppenheim, R., Budde, U., Ware, J., and Ruggeri, Z.M.: von Willebrand factor mutation enhancing interaction with platelets in patients with normal multimeric structure. J. Clin. Invest. 91:2169, 1993.

468. Ribba, A.S., Christophe, O., Derlon, A., Cherel, G., Siguret, V., Lavergne, J.M., Girma, J.P., Meyer, D., and Pietu, G.: Discrepancy between IIA phenotype and IIB genotype in a patient with a variant of von Willebrand disease. Blood 83:833, 1994.

469. Howard, M.A., Salem, H.H., Thomas, K.B., Hau, L., Perkin, J., Coghlan, M., and Firkin, B.G.: Variant von Willebrand's disease type B—revisited. Blood 60:1420, 1982.

470. Rabinowitz, I., Tuley, E.A., Mancuso, D.J., Randi, A.M., Firkin, B.G., Howard, M.A., and Sadler, J.E.: von Willebrand disease type B: a missense mutation selectively abolishes ristocetin-induced von Willebrand factor binding to platelet glycoprotein Ib. Proc. Natl. Acad. Sci. USA 89:9846, 1992.

471. Mancuso, D.J., Kroner, P.A., Christopherson, P.A., Vokac, E.A., Gill, J.C., and Montgomery, R.R.: Type 2M:Milwaukee-1 von Willebrand disease: an in-frame deletion in the Cys509-Cys695 loop of the von Willebrand factor A1 domain causes deficient binding of von Willebrand factor to platelets. Blood 88:2559, 1996.

472. Hillery, C.A., Mancuso, D.J., Sadler, J.E., Ponder, J.W., Jozwiak, M.A., Christopherson, P.A., Gill, J.C., Scott, J.P., and Montgomery, R.R.: Type 2M von Willebrand disease: F606I and I662F mutations in the glycoprotein IB binding domain selectively impair ristocetin- but not botrocetin-mediated binding of von Willebrand factor to platelets. Blood 91:1572, 1998.

473. Nishino, M., Girma, J.-P., Rothschild, C., Fressinaud, E., and Meyer, D.: New variant of von Willebrand disease with defective binding to factor VIII. Blood 74:1591, 1989.

474. Mazurier, C., Dieval, J., Jorieux, S., Delobel, J., and Goudemand, M.: A new von Willebrand factor (vWF) defect in a patient with factor VIII (FVIII) deficiency but with normal levels and multimeric patterns of both plasma and platelet vWF. Characterization of abnormal vWF/FVIII interaction. Blood 75:20, 1990.

475. Mazurier, C.: von Willebrand disease masquerading as haemophilia A. Thromb. Haemost. 67:391, 1992.

476. Schneppenheim, R., Budde, U., Krey, S., Drewke, E., Bergmann, F., Lechler, E., Oldenburg, J., and Schwaab, R.: Results of a screening for von Willebrand disease type 2N in patients with suspected haemophilia A or von Willebrand disease type 1. Thromb. Haemost. 76:598, 1996.

477. Meyer, D., Fressinaud, E., Gaucher, C., Lavergne, J.M., Hilbert, L., Ribba, A.S., Jorieux, S., and Mazurier, C.: Gene defects in 150 unrelated French cases with type 2 von Willebrand disease: from the patient to the gene. INSERM Network on Molecular Abnormalities in von Willebrand Disease. Thromb. Haemost. 78:451, 1997.

478. Mannucci, P.M., Bloom, A.L., Larrieu, M.J., Nilsson, I.M., and West, R.R.: Atherosclerosis and von Willebrand factor. I. Prevalence of severe von Willebrand's disease in western Europe and Israel. Br. J. Haematol. 57:163, 1984.

479. Weiss, H.J., Ball, A.P., and Mannucci, P.M.: Incidence of severe von Willebrand's disease. N. Engl. J. Med. 307:127, 1982.

480. Zhang, Z.P., Lindstedt, M., Falk, G., Blombäck, M., Egberg, N., and Anvret, M.: Nonsense mutations of the von Willebrand factor gene in patients with von Willebrand disease type III and type I. Am. J. Hum. Genet. 51:850, 1992.

481. Zhang, Z.P., Blombäck, M., Egberg, N., Falk, G., and Anvret, M.: Characterization of the von Willebrand factor gene (VWF) in von Willebrand disease type III patients from 24 families of Swedish and Finnish origin. Genomics 21:188, 1994.

482. Schneppenheim, R., Krey, S., Bergmann, F., Bock, D., Budde, U., Lange, M., Linde, R., Mittler, U., Meili, E., Mertes, G., Olek, K., Plendl, H., and Simeoni, E.: Genetic heterogeneity of severe von Willebrand disease type III in the German population. Hum. Genet. 94:640, 1994.

483. Zhang, Z.P., Blömback, M., Nyman, D., and Anvret, M.: Mutations of von Willebrand factor gene in families with von Willebrand disease in the Aland Islands. Proc. Natl. Acad. Sci. USA 90:7937, 1993.

484. Gaucher, C., Mercier, B., and Mazurier, C.: von Willebrand disease family studies: comparison of three methods of analysis of the von Willebrand factor gene polymorphism related to a variable number tandem repeat sequence in intron 40. Br. J. Haematol. 82:73, 1992.

485. Mannucci, P.M., and Mari, D.: Antibodies to factor VIII–von Willebrand factor in congenital and acquired von Willebrand's disease. In Hoyer, L.W. (ed.): Factor VIII Inhibitors. New York, Alan R. Liss, 1984, pp. 109–122.

486. Mohri, H., Motomura, S., Kanamori, H., Matsuzaki, M., Watanabe, S., Maruta, A., Kodama, F., and Okubo, T.: Clinical significance of inhibitors in acquired von Willebrand syndrome. Blood 91:3623, 1998.

487. Takahashi, H.: Studies on the pathophysiology and treatment of von Willebrand's disease. IV. Mechanism of increased ristocetin-induced platelet aggregation in von Willebrand's disease. Thromb. Res. 19:857, 1980.

488. Weiss, H.J., Meyer, D., Rabinowitz, R., Pietu, G., Girma, J.P., Vicic, W.J., and Rogers, J.: Pseudo–von Willebrand's disease. An intrinsic platelet defect with aggregation by unmodified human factor VIII/von Willebrand factor and enhanced adsorption of its high-molecular-weight multimers. N. Engl. J. Med. 306:326, 1982.

489. Miller, J.L., and Castella, A.: Platelet-type von Willebrand's disease: characterization of a new bleeding disorder. Blood 60:790, 1982.

490. Takahashi, H., Nagayama, R., Hattori, A., and Shibata, A.: Platelet aggregation induced by DDAVP in platelet-type von Willebrand's disease. N. Engl. J. Med. 310:722, 1984.

491. Miller, J.L., Boselli, B.D., and Kupinski, J.M.: In vivo interaction of von Willebrand factor with platelets following cryoprecipitate transfusion in platelet-type von Willebrand's disease. Blood 63:226, 1984.

492. Miller, J.L., Cunningham, D., Lyle, V.A., and Finch, C.N.: Mutation in the gene encoding the α chain of platelet glycoprotein Ib in platelet-type von Willebrand disease. Proc. Natl. Acad. Sci. USA 88:4761, 1991.

493. Russell, S.D., and Roth, G.J.: Pseudo–von Willebrand disease: a mutation in the platelet glycoprotein Ib alpha gene associated with a hyperactive surface receptor. Blood 81:1787, 1993.

494. Murata, M., Russell, S.R., Ruggeri, Z.M., and Ware, J.: Expression of the phenotypic abnormality of platelet-type von Willebrand disease in a recombinant glycoprotein Ibα fragment. J. Clin. Invest. 91:2133, 1993.

495. Moriki, T., Murata, M., Kitaguchi, T., Anbo, H., Handa, M., Watanabe, K., Takahashi, H., and Ikeda, Y.: Expression and functional characterization of an abnormal platelet membrane glycoprotein Ib alpha (Met239→Val) reported in patients with platelet-type von Willebrand disease. Blood 90:698, 1997.

496. Sakariassen, K.S., Nieuwenhuis, H.K., and Sixma, J.J.: Differentiation of patients with subtype IIb-like von Willebrand's disease by means of perfusion experiments with reconstituted blood. Br. J. Haematol. 59:459, 1985.

497. Rick, M.E., Williams, S.B., Sacher, R.A., and McKeown, L.P.: Thrombocytopenia associated with pregnancy in a patient with type IIB von Willebrand's disease. Blood 69:786, 1987.

498. Giles, A.R., Hoogendoorn, H., and Benford, K.: Type IIB von Willebrand's disease presenting as thrombocytopenia during pregnancy. Br. J. Haematol. 67:349, 1987.

499. Valster, F.A.A., Feijen, H.L., and Hutten, J.W.: Severe thrombocytopenia in a pregnant patient with platelet-associated IgM, and known von Willebrand's disease; a case report. Eur. J. Obstet. Gynecol. Reprod. Biol. 36:197, 1990.

500. Ieko, M., Sakurama, S., Sagawa, A., Yoshikawa, M., Satoh, M., Yasukouchi, T., and Nakagawa, S.: Effect of a factor VIII concentrate on type IIB von Willebrand's disease–associated thrombocytopenia presenting during pregnancy in identical twin mothers. Am. J. Hematol. 35:26, 1990.

501. Hultin, M.B., and Sussman, I.I.: Postoperative thrombocytopenia in type IIB von Willebrand disease. Am. J. Hematol. 33:64, 1990.

502. Donnér, M., Holmberg, L., and Nilsson, I.M.: Type IIB von Willebrand's disease with probable autosomal recessive inheritance and presenting as thrombocytopenia in infancy. Br. J. Haematol. 66:349, 1987.

503. Mauz-Korholz, C., Budde, U., Kruck, H., Korholz, D., and Gobel, U.: Management of severe chronic thrombocytopenia in von Willebrand's disease type 2B. Arch. Dis. Child. 78:257, 1998.

504. Rodeghiero, F., Castaman, G., and Mannucci, P.M.: Clinical indications for desmopressin (DDAVP) in congenital and acquired von Willebrand disease. Blood Rev. 5:155, 1991.

505. de la Fuente, B., Kasper, C.K., Rickles, F.R., and Hoyer, L.W.: Response of patients with mild and moderate hemophilia A and von Willebrand's disease to treatment with desmopressin. Ann. Intern. Med. 103:6, 1985.

506. Gralnick, H.R., Williams, S.B., McKeown, L.P., Rick, M.E., Maisonneuve, P., Jenneau, C., and Sultan, Y.: DDAVP in type IIA von Willebrand's disease. Blood 67:465, 1986.

507. Lopez-Fernandez, M.F., Blanco-Lopez, M.J., Castiñeira, M.P., and Batlle, J.: Further evidence for recessive inheritance of von Willebrand disease with abnormal binding of von Willebrand factor to factor VIII. Am. J. Hematol. 40:20, 1992.

508. Mazurier, C., Gaucher, C., Jorieux, S., Goudemand, M., and the Collaborative Group: Biological effect of desmopressin in eight patients with type 2N ('Normandy') von Willebrand disease. Br. J. Haematol. 88:849, 1994.

509. Kyrle, P.A., Niessner, H., Dent, J., Panzer, S., Brenner, B., Zimmerman, T.S., and Lechner, K.: IIB von Willebrand's disease: pathogenetic and therapeutic studies. Br. J. Haematol. 69:55, 1988.

510. Fowler, W.E., Berkowitz, L.R., and Roberts, H.R.: DDAVP for type IIB von Willebrand disease. Blood 74:1859, 1989.

511. Casonato, A., Pontara, E., Dannhaeuser, D., Bertomoro, A., Sartori, M.T., Zerbinati, P., and Girolami, A.: Re-evaluation of the therapeutic efficacy of DDAVP in type IIB von Willebrand's disease. Blood Coagul. Fibrinolysis 5:959, 1994.

512. McKeown, L.P., Connaghan, G., Wilson, O., Hansmann, K., Merryman, P., and Gralnick, H.R.: 1-Desamino-8-arginine-vasopressin corrects the hemostatic defects in type 2B von Willebrand's disease. Am. J. Hematol. 51:158, 1996.

513. Rodeghiero, F., Castaman, G., Meyer, D., and Mannucci, P.M.: Replacement therapy with virus-inactivated plasma concentrates in von Willebrand disease. Vox Sang. 62:193, 1992.

514. Berntorp, E.: Plasma product treatment in various types of von Willebrand's disease. Haemostasis 24:289, 1994.

515. Scharrer, I., Vigh, T., and Aygoren-Pursun, E.: Experience with Haemate P in von Willebrand's disease in adults. Haemostasis 24:298, 1994.

516. Morfini, M., Mannucci, P.M., Tenconi, P.M., Longo, G., Mazzucconi, M.G., Rodeghiero, F., Ciavarella, N., De Rosa, V., and Arter, A.: Pharmacokinetics of monoclonally-purified and recombinant factor VIII in patients with severe von Willebrand disease. Thromb. Haemost. 70:270, 1993.

517. Goudemand, J., Mazurier, C., Marey, A., Caron, C., Coupez, B., Mizon, P., and Goudemand, M.: Clinical and biological evaluation in von Willebrand's disease of a von Willebrand factor concentrate with low factor VIII activity. Br. J. Haematol. 80:214, 1992.

518. Meriane, F., Zerhouni, L., Djeha, N., Goudemand, M., and Mazurier, C.: Biological effects of a S/D-treated, very high purity, von Willebrand factor concentrate in five patients with severe von Willebrand disease. Blood Coagul. Fibrinolysis 4:1023, 1993.

519. Smith, M.P., Rice, K.M., Bromidge, E.S., Lawn, M., Beresford-Webb, R., Spence, K., Khair, K., Hann, I., and Savidge, G.F.: Continuous infusion therapy with very high purity von Willebrand factor concentrate in patients with severe von Willebrand disease. Blood Coagul. Fibrinolysis 8:6, 1997.

520. Turecek, P.L., Gritsch, H., Pichler, L., Auer, W., Fischer, B., Mitterer, A., Mundt, W., Schlokat, U., Dorner, F., Brinkman, H.J.M., van Mourik, J.A., and Schwarz, H.P.: In vivo characterization of recombinant von Willebrand factor in dogs with von Willebrand disease. Blood 90:3555, 1997.

521. Shelton-Inloes, B.B., Chehab, F.F., Mannucci, P.M., Federici, A.B., and Sadler, J.E.: Gene deletions correlate with the development of alloantibodies in von Willebrand disease. J. Clin. Invest. 79:1459, 1987.

522. Ngo, K.-Y., Glotz, V.T., Koziol, J.A., Lynch, D.C., Gitschier, J., Ranieri, R.P., Ciavarella, N., Ruggeri, Z.M., and Zimmerman, T.S.: Homozygous and heterozygous deletions of the von Willebrand factor gene in patients and carriers of severe von Willebrand's disease. Proc. Natl. Acad. Sci. USA 85:2753, 1988.

523. Peake, I.R., Liddell, M.B., Moodie, P., Standen, G., Mancuso, D.J., Tuley, E.A., Westfield, L.A., Sorace, J.M., Sadler, J.E., Verweij, C.L., and Bloom, A.L.: Severe type III von Willebrand's disease caused by deletion of exon 42 of the von Willebrand factor gene: family studies that identify carriers of the condition and a compound heterozygous individual. Blood 75:654, 1990.

524. Bergamaschini, L., Mannucci, P.M., Federici, A.B., Coppola, R., Guzzoni, S., and Agostoni, A.: Posttransfusion anaphylactic reactions in a patient with severe von Willebrand disease: role of complement and alloantibodies to von Willebrand factor. J. Lab. Clin. Med. 125:348, 1995.

525. Mannucci, P.M., Ruggeri, Z.M., Ciavarella, N., Kazatchkine, M.D., and Mowbray, J.F.: Precipitating antibodies to factor VIII/von Willebrand factor in von Willebrand's disease: effects on replacement therapy. Blood 57:25, 1981.

526. Bloom, A.L., Peake, I.R., Furlong, R.A., and Davies, B.L.: High potency factor VIII concentrate: more effective than cryoprecipitate in a patient with von Willebrand's disease and inhibitor. Thromb. Res. 16:847, 1979.

527. Denis, C., Methia, N., Frenette, P.S., Rayburn, H., Ullman-Culleré, M., Hynes, R.O., and Wagner, D.D.: A mouse model of severe von Willebrand disease: defects in hemostasis and thrombosis. Proc. Natl. Acad. Sci. USA 95:9524, 1998.

528. Kraulis, P.J.: MOLSCRIPT: a program to produce both detailed and schematic plots of protein structures. J. Appl. Crystallogr. 24:946, 1991.

529. Brandstetter, H., Bauer, M., Huber, R., Lollar, P., and Bode, W.: X-ray structure of clotting factor IXa: active site and module structure related to Xase activity and hemophilia B. Proc. Natl. Acad. Sci. USA 92:9796, 1995.

22 The Molecular Basis of Fibrin
Russell F. Doolittle

▼ ▼

Fibrin is the primary material of blood clots. Its deposition is essential for preserving the integrity of the hemovascular system, but its inopportune occurrence can lead to stoppages that cause heart attacks, strokes, and other circulatory malfunctions. Clearly, its formation and destruction are matters of life and death. Its molecular countenance includes the soluble precursor called fibrinogen, the insoluble polymer itself, and the debris resulting from lysis referred to as fibrin split products. These different states can be viewed in terms of a naturally regulated life cycle: the biosynthesis of the precursor, a dormant period before activation by thrombin, the conversion to an insoluble polymer, the dissolution of the polymeric fibrin gel by plasmin during the fibrinolytic stage, and the stimulation of further biosynthesis by cytokines.

Although we could begin our discussion at any stage of this cycle and continue around, it seems logical to start with a consideration of the structure of the fibrinogen molecule. This provides a molecular frame of reference for all subsequent interactions. From there, we can move forward to the details of fibrin formation, then to fibrinolysis, and finally return to biosynthesis and regulation. Throughout, we must remain aware of how these central components interact with the many other participants in the clotting process. Fibrinogen binds many coagulation proteins in advance of any need for clotting, for example. Fibrin, on the other hand, exhibits different binding sites that attract other interactants, and fibrin degradation products uniquely recognize receptors that are apparently ignored by fibrinogen and fibrin. Not every aspect of these many interactions is understood at present; our knowledge is still incomplete. Nonetheless, a reasonable scenario of events can be drawn. The reader must constantly keep in mind the overall aspect, even amid the morass of atomic detail.

The chapter also includes a brief review of variant human fibrinogens and a consideration of how these defective molecules helped to elucidate many of the structure-function relationships discussed in the other sections. Some comments are also offered on the expression of fibrinogen in recombinant systems and the potential for site-directed mutagenesis as a tool for addressing questions of structure and function.

Fibrinogen: The Precursor of Fibrin

Fibrinogen is a large, complex glycoprotein that occurs in blood plasma at levels of 3 to 4 mg/ml (10^{-5} mol/l). The molecular mass of the molecule found in humans is 340,000 daltons.* As will become clear, clotting depends on fibrinogen molecules colliding effectively after activation by thrombin. The data in Table 22–1 can be used to estimate that a volume increment of plasma measuring 100 nm on a side (one trillionth of a cubic millimeter) contains, on the average, eight or nine fibrinogen molecules. The nearest neighboring fibrinogens are only 50 to 100 nm apart, or as little as one or two molecular lengths. If no other macromolecules

*It must be understood that fibrinogen and fibrin, like all proteins, differ to a degree from organism to organism. The focus in this chapter is on the proteins found in humans. However, much can be learned from comparisons with the equivalent proteins from other species. As a general rule, features found universally are likely to be more important than idiosyncratic differences. Accordingly, occasional comparisons are made to emphasize certain key structure-function relationships.

Table 22–1. Some Properties of Human Fibrinogen

Molecular mass	340,000
Percentage α helix	33
Molecular dimensions (approx.)	60 × 450 Å
Diffusion constant ($D_{20,w}$)	2.09×10^{-7} cm²/sec
Frictional coefficient (f/f_o)	2.34
Sedimentation coefficient ($S_{20,w}$)	7.9
Extinction coefficient	15.1
Partial specific volume	0.715
Isoelectric point	5.5
Calculated net charge at pH 7.3	−20
Percentage carbohydrate	3
Subunit formula	$\alpha_2\ \beta_2\ \gamma_2$

Adapted from Doolittle, R.F.: Structural aspects of the fibrinogen-fibrin conversion. Adv. Protein Chem. 27:1, 1973.

Table 22–2. Relative Concentrations of Some Proteins in Blood Plasma*

Protein	Molecular Weight	μg/ml	Molarity	Per 1,000 Molecules of Fibrinogen
Albumin	70,000	40,000	6×10^{-4}	60,000
α_1-Antitrypsin	54,000	2,900	5×10^{-5}	5,000
Fibrinogen	340,000	3,500	1×10^{-5}	1,000
Antithrombin III	65,000	250	4×10^{-6}	400
α_2-Macroglobulin	730,000	2,600	4×10^{-6}	350
Plasminogen	90,000	150	1.7×10^{-6}	170
Prothrombin	72,000	100	1.4×10^{-6}	140
α_2-Antiplasmin	70,000	70	1×10^{-6}	100
Fibronectin	440,000	350	8×10^{-7}	80
Factor X	56,000	10	2×10^{-7}	20
Factor XIII†	320,000	30	1×10^{-7}	10
Factor IX	56,000	5	9×10^{-8}	10
Factor V†	330,000	10	3×10^{-8}	3
Thrombospondin†	450,000	8	2×10^{-8}	2
Factor VII	50,000	0.5	1×10^{-8}	1
Factor VIII	330,000	0.1	3×10^{-10}	(0.03)

* Taken from data presented in references 281 and 282.
† Found in much higher concentrations in platelets.

were in the way, each fibrinogen molecule would bump into another approximately every 5 msec. The volume increment described, however, contains about 500 albumin molecules and about 100 molecules of assorted other proteins, including—again on the average—one each of prothrombin and plasminogen (Table 22–2). The timely activation of these dictates the events of interest.

▼ SIZE AND SHAPE OF FIBRINOGEN

The unraveling of the structure of fibrinogen during the course of the last half-century is a fascinating story, the early phases of which have been recounted elsewhere.[1-3] Here, I offer only a brief outline of how a working model of fibrinogen was developed.

One of the earliest insights into the structure was accomplished by X-ray fiber diffraction. Concentrated solutions of fibrinogen are viscous enough that they can be drawn out to form fibers, and it was of interest to compare their diffraction patterns with those of fibrin. Indeed, the diffraction patterns of fibrinogen and fibrin were indistinguishable, suggesting that fibrin was nothing more than polymerized fibrinogen units.[4] Most surprising, however, the patterns were also the same as those observed for fibrous proteins like keratin and myosin. These diffraction patterns were subsequently found to be characteristic of α helices wound into "coiled coils."[5] When hydrodynamic studies were performed on fibrinogen, however, its character was found to be more globular than fibrous. When these data were taken together with some early electron microscope studies,[6] it was suggested that the data best fit a molecule with an extended nodular structure.[7]

The electron micrographs published by Hall and Slayter[8] in 1959 provided the first true representation of fibrinogen (Fig. 22–1). Those shadow-cast specimens revealed an extended triglobular structure 475 ± 25 Å in length, the central globule of which was slightly smaller than the terminal ones. The regions connecting the globules could not be resolved, but it was conjectured that they might consist of the coiled

α helices detected by the fiber diffraction study mentioned above.[9]

An important development in discovering the structure of fibrinogen was the purification of a set of stable core fragments generated by the action of plasmin.[10] When preparations of fibrinogen digested with plasmin were applied directly to a diethylaminoethyl (DEAE) cellulose column, a series of peaks emerged that were labeled A to E. Of these, D and E were found to account for the bulk of the mass; the mass ratio of D to E was approximately 4:1. It was subsequently shown that short-term digestions with plasmin yielded transient intermediates, the principal ones of which were denoted X and Y.[11] This study led to the proposal that the stable core fragment E must correspond to the central module observed in the electron microscope and that the fragments D were the terminal ones (Fig. 22–2). Thus, fragment X is a degradation product in which two fragments D remain connected to an E, whereas fragment Y represents a further digested product in which a single fragment D is connected to the fragment E.[12] In retrospect, the minor peaks A to C from the DEAE chromatography represented a variety of peptides chipped away from the native molecule. As much as two thirds of each α chain is lost during the

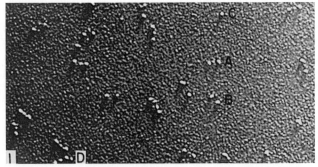

Figure 22–1. Metal-shadowed fibrinogen molecules. (From Hall, C.E., and Slayter, H.S.: The fibrinogen molecule: its size, shape and mode of polymerization. J. Biophys. Biochem. Cytol. 5:11, 1959; with permission.)

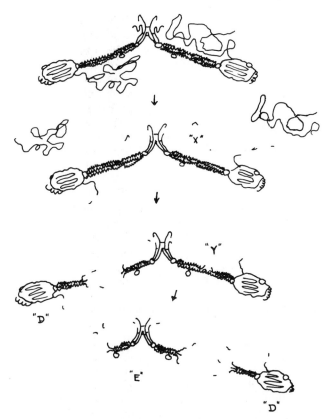

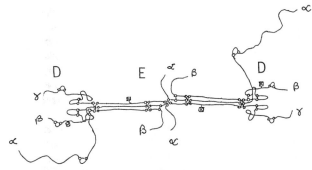

Figure 22–3. Diagrammatic arrangement of six chains in fibrinogen, showing elaborate interconnection by interchain and intrachain disulfide bonds. The approximate locations of cysteines are signified by circles. Squares indicate attached carbohydrate clusters. Regions corresponding to fragments D and E are denoted by capital letters. (Modified from Hoeprich, P.D., and Doolittle, R.F.: Dimeric half-molecules of human fibrinogen are joined through disulfide bonds in an antiparallel orientation. Biochemistry 22:2049, 1983; with permission.)

Figure 22–2. Plasmin degradation of fibrinogen. Plasmin degradation of fibrinogen yields the intermediate fragments denoted X and Y and the terminal fragments D and E. Numerous species of each occur, depending on the exact conditions of the digestion.

noted before, the protein has several well-defined regions* that can be visualized in the electron microscope (Fig. 22–4) and isolated by treating the native protein with appropriate proteases.

▼ AMINO ACID SEQUENCE STUDIES

The proposal that fragments D and E correspond to the major globules of a trimodular molecule was completely

---

conversion to fragment X,[13] an observation that gave rise to the notion of a pair of extended and easily removed polar protuberances.[2]

▼ SUBUNIT ARRANGEMENT

Each fibrinogen molecule is composed of three pairs of nonidentical but homologous polypeptide chains, $\alpha_2\beta_2\gamma_2$,* the molecular masses of which are 67,000, 55,000, and 48,000 daltons, respectively.[14] The six chains are arranged in a manner such that all six amino termini are gathered in the central part of the molecule (Fig. 22–3). All together, there are 29 disulfide bonds,[15] which fall into three classes: three symmetrical connections between the two dimeric halves of the protein, two sets of seven interchain bonds (one of which, as discussed later, may cross from one half of the dimer to the other), and two other sets of six intrachain bonds. Although crystal structure determinations were begun in the early 1970s,[16] progress during the next 20 years was agonizingly slow.[17] In the interim, models of fibrinogen were fashioned on the basis of electron microscopy, physical chemistry, and a host of indirect biochemical studies.[18] As

---

*These fragments are sometimes referred to as domains. Formally, a domain is defined as that part of a protein that can fold independently of neighboring sequences. In this chapter, I will be less exacting and use the term casually for any definable region. I also invoke the terms macrodomain for large regions that are doubtless composed of more than one classic domain and subdomain for smaller regions associated with particular functions.

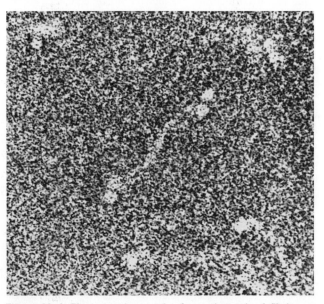

Figure 22–4. Electron micrograph of negative-stained fibrinogen molecule. Note the presence of two distinct domains in the terminal globule region. (From Williams, R.C.: Band patterns seen by electron microscopy in ordered arrays of bovine and human fibrinogen and fibrin after negative staining. Proc. Natl. Acad. Sci. USA 80:1570, 1983; with permission.)

---

*The combinations Aα and Bβ are used by some to describe fibrinogen α and β chains with their fibrinopeptides still attached.

borne out by biochemical and amino acid sequence studies. In particular, a fragment was obtained from fibrinogen treated with cyanogen bromide (which cleaves exclusively at methionine residues) that contained all six amino terminals[19] and cross-reacted immunologically with fragment E.[20, 21] Subsequent amino acid sequence studies on the individual polypeptide chains revealed that each chain contains a skein of amino acids with a rhythmic polarity characteristic of α helices, in each case bounded by braces of cysteines. It was proposed that these stretches, which amounted to about 110 amino acids in each chain, were the coiled coil connectors.[22] Because an α helix translates 1.5 Å per residue, the lengths of the proposed connectors would be about 150 Å, in good agreement with the estimates made from electron microscopy. Models were built that showed how the three chains in each half of the molecule could be mutually bound by disulfide rings at each end of the coiled coils.[23]

The sequence of human fibrinogen was completed in 1979,[24–27] and the information was illuminating well beyond the delineation of the regions corresponding to the coiled coils and the general boundaries of the major fragments. Most interesting was that it confirmed that the three nonidentical chains were descended from a common ancestor. In this regard, although the homology of the β and γ chains persists through their entire lengths, the α chains are radically different in their carboxyl-terminal two thirds (Fig. 22–5). Evidently some kind of crossing over event or "exon shuffle" occurred during the evolution of the α chain since the original gene duplications.

▼ DNA SEQUENCE STUDIES

The advent of recombinant DNA technology in the late 1970s set the stage for a surge of data that both confirmed the protein sequence determined for human fibrinogen, with some minor corrections,[28–31] and provided sequences for fi-

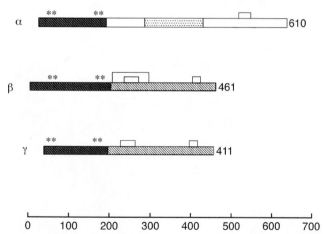

Figure 22–5. Schematic comparison of α (610 residues), β (461 residues), and γ (411 residues) chains from human fibrinogen. All three chains are homologous in the amino-terminal regions that contain the coiled coils *(dark striped shading).* The β and γ chains also have homologous globular carboxyl domains *(light striped shading).* The α chain has a completely different carboxyl-terminal region, including a sector composed of ten 13-residue imperfect repeats *(dotted shading).* Asterisks denote interchain disulfides that make up disulfide rings. Intrachain disulfides are shown with simple lines.

brinogens from a number of other species, including rat,[32] bovine,[33] chicken,[34, 35] frog,[36] and lamprey.[37–39] Moreover, the recombinant studies on human fibrinogen provided an explanation for a minor form of the γ chain and also uncovered a wholly unexpected α chain extension,[28, 31] topics that are taken up in our discussion of fibrinogen biosynthesis.

The comparative data proved useful in assessing those features of fibrinogen most critical to its function. For example, in all known cases save one, the bond cleaved by thrombin during the release of fibrinopeptides is an arginylglycine linkage. The exception is found in the case of the cleavage of fibrinopeptide B from chicken fibrinogen, in which case the bond is arginyl-alanine.[34] More important, the site exposed by the release of the fibrinopeptide A is universally Gly-Pro-Arg. Accordingly, the complementary sites for polymerization must also be highly conserved.

▼ CARBOHYDRATE MOIETIES

Most mammalian fibrinogens contain about 3 per cent carbohydrate. In the case of human fibrinogen, two asparagine-linked carbohydrate clusters occur in each half-molecule, one on the β chain at residue Asn 364, and another on the γ chain at residue Asn 52. In both instances, the carbohydrate is a biantennary-type cluster composed of N-acetyl glucosamines, mannoses, galactoses, and terminal sialic acids.[40] Fibrinogens from some other species have carbohydrate in other positions, including a cluster on the α chain of chicken fibrinogen[41] and clusters elsewhere on the β and γ chains of lamprey fibrinogen,[37, 38] and even its fibrinopeptide B.[42]

▼ THE WORKING MODEL

For the most part, the results of peptide chemistry studies were in good accord with the structures observed by electron microscopists. One matter that is not entirely resolved has to do with the precise localization of the carboxyl-terminal regions of the α chains. The triglobular structure observed in electron micrographs corresponds well to what might be expected from a fragment X molecule, but where would the exposed carboxyl-terminal regions of the α chains be? It was initially suggested that these regions, which account for a quarter of the mass of the native protein, were "free-swimming appendages," and they were often drawn in schematic depictions as randomly dispersed out and away from the terminal globules (see Figs. 22–2 and 22–3). In support of this depiction, it can be noted that these regions are readily cleaved from fibrinogen by a variety of proteases,[13] they have little or no defined secondary structure,[43] and they vary greatly from species to species, both in sequence and in overall length.[2, 44] Also, at least one published electron micrograph shows chains extending from the terminal globules,[45] and in another, immunostaining was used to show the α chain middle region lying out and away from the main body of the molecule.[46] Nevertheless, there have been persistent reports that these regions fold back on the triglobular molecule and either contribute to the central globule[47, 48] or form a fourth, less readily resolved module.[49] Support for this position has been provided by experiments dealing with fibrin formation itself, and an attractive model has been described whereby the carboxyl-terminal domains of α chains dissociate from an intramolecular mode in fibrinogen to form intermolecular attachments in fibrin.[50]

Meanwhile, numerous other studies have been conducted on the terminal macrodomain corresponding to fragment D, and in this case, all sides seem in general agreement. As shown clearly in some electron micrographs (see Fig. 22–4), the terminal globule contains two well-defined modules.[51] Of course, it had been presumed long before these pictures that the terminal globule must contain two discrete domains because of the homology of the β and γ carboxyl-terminal regions.[26, 52] Subsequent degradation studies coupled with microcalorimetry have subdivided each of these into two even smaller domains.[53, 54]

▼ CALCIUM BINDING

Fibrinogen has three "high-affinity" binding sites for calcium.[55, 56] High affinity for an extracellular protein means dissociation constants (K_d) of the order of 10^{-5} mol/l. The extracellular concentration of calcium ions in vertebrate animals is of the order of 2.5×10^{-3} mol/l, about one third of which is bound to assorted proteins at "low-affinity" sites that are only fractionally occupied. Under these conditions, the high-affinity sites ought to be fully occupied. Fibrinogen has low-affinity sites also, which may bear on the process of fibrin formation.

Two of the high-affinity binding sites are situated on the fragment D portions of the molecule. The third site has not been determined with any certainty, but circumstantial evidence suggests that it may involve the carboxyl-terminal regions of α chains.[57] The basis for this conjecture is that fragment X apparently has only two high-affinity binding sites, although there is some dispute about this observation.[58]

In contrast, the evidence linking calcium binding to large molecular weight fragment D took several lines. First, when fibrinogen is digested by plasmin in the absence of calcium ions, the γ chain is degraded to a significantly greater extent than when calcium is present.[59] The portion removed in its absence amounts to the carboxyl-terminal 109 residues. In addition, calcium ions tend to protect the intrachain disulfide involving γ chain residues 326 and 329 from reduction.[60] Finally, it was reported that the cyanogen bromide fragment spanning residues 311 to 336 can bind terbium.[61] Terbium (element number 65) can bind to calcium binding sites and has the advantage that it is fluorescent and easily detected under appropriate conditions. All these results were borne out by an X-ray structure determination of the γ chain domain that showed calcium coordinated to the side chains of residues Asp γ318 and Asp γ320 and backbone atoms for residues Phe γ322 and Gly γ324.[62] These results were confirmed by X-ray structures of fragments D and double-D, which also revealed loosely bound calcium in a homologous setting in the β chain.[63, 64]

▼ X-RAY CRYSTALLOGRAPHY

High-resolution X-ray structure determinations have done much more than reveal calcium binding sites, of course.

Indeed, virtually every aspect of fibrinogen structure is now being re-examined in the light of these structures. The first of the high-resolution structures to be reported was the 30 kDa carboxyl domain of the γ chain[62]; it was followed shortly thereafter by the 86 kDa fragment D.[63] Although much of the pre–X-ray work was confirmed by these structures—and many critical details added—there were some unexpected findings. Among the most interesting was the revelation that the coiled coil portion of fragment D has a fourth α helix running in the opposite direction.[63] Thus, the α chain abruptly reverses its course right in the middle of one of the disulfide ring interconnections and heads back toward the central part of the native molecule (see Plate 22–1). This could be interpreted as support for the view that the carboxyl-terminal domains of α chains are nestled together in the central region.[47, 48]

Beyond that, the X-ray structure unequivocally identified which of the two domains in the terminal globule is β and which is γ. The β chain is oriented such that a portion is folded back next to the coiled coils; as expected, the γ chain domains constitute the ends of the molecule. Both domains have obvious "holes" corresponding to anticipated polymerization sites. The relative arrangement of the two domains is such that the γ chain hole is near the very end of the molecule, but the β chain equivalent is oriented in the opposite direction back near the middle of the coiled coil (see Plate 22–1). As it happens, the important segment corresponding to the last 15 residues of the γ chain is highly mobile and was not discernible in the X-ray structures.[62–64]

A reconstruction of the equivalent of fragment X (which lacks the carboxyl-terminal regions of the α chains) is presented in Plate 22–2; it is based on the X-ray structure of fragment D and structural inferences about fragment E as well as overall dimensions drawn from electron microscopy[8] and a low-resolution X-ray structure.[17] In keeping with my goal to relate structure and function at the atomic level, I refer to this model throughout the remainder of the chapter, bearing in mind that at the moment only the fragment D portions are known at atomic resolution.

Fibrin Formation

Fibrin formation is marked by the transition from a collection of soluble molecules (fibrinogen) to the extended polymeric network that forms the gel. The gel state results from the network's trapping bulk water and all the solutes and particles suspended therein (Fig. 22–6). Electron micrographs of fibrin show the constituent fibrous strands to be thick or thin and more or less branched, depending on the solution conditions during polymerization. If the strands are sufficiently thick, staining reveals a uniformly banded pattern with a repeat distance of 225 Å, which is equivalent to half the length of a fibrinogen molecule (Fig. 22–7). Such observations, taken together with other considerations, long ago led to the reasonable conclusion that the fundamental polymerization events occur by a half-staggered molecule overlap.[65] It is noteworthy that fibrinogen itself can be packed into the same arrangement, even without the removal of the fibrinopeptides, merely by sedimentation into a glassy pellet in the ultracentrifuge.[66] Clearly, the shape of the mole-

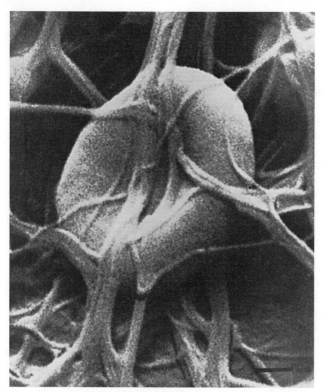

Figure 22–6. Scanning electron micrograph of fibrin strands entangling an erythrocyte. (From Bernstein, E., and Kairenin, E.: Science 173:cover photo, 1971. Copyright 1971 by the AAAS; with permission.)

cules is conducive to a half-staggered overlap even when the molecules are merely crowded together.

▼ THROMBIN ACTION

Fibrinogen is converted into fibrin as a result of thrombin cleaving peptides from the amino-terminal ends of the α and β chains[67]; the released peptides are referred to as the fibrinopeptides A and B, respectively. In human fibrinogen, the cleavages occur at arginyl-glycine bonds. Thrombin is a member of the trypsin serine protease family; it has a narrow specificity, almost always being restricted to particular arginyl linkages. In addition to fibrinogen, it cleaves other proteins involved in blood clotting, including factors V, VIII, and XIII, a receptor on the surface of platelets, and, when complexed with thrombomodulin, protein C.

The rates of release of the fibrinopeptides A and B can be markedly different; in humans, the fibrinopeptide A is released significantly faster than the fibrinopeptide B under typical physiological conditions.[68] Because the exposure of the glycyl-prolyl-argininyl segment corresponding to α chain residues 17 to 19 is the initiating feature of polymerization,

only the release of the fibrinopeptide A is required for clot formation. As a result, certain snake venom enzymes (reptilase, for example) can clot fibrinogen even though they release only the fibrinopeptides A.[69] Thus, these three newly exposed residues, referred to from here on as Gly-Pro-Arg, constitute a conceptual "knob" that binds to a resident hole elsewhere in neighboring fibrin(ogen) molecules.[70, 71] The detailed nature of these knob/hole interactions has now been revealed by several X-ray structures.[63, 64, 72]

Several different interactions actually occur during the propagation of the fibers that form the gel network. The first of these involves the knob/hole interactions between individual molecules that have lost at least one of their fibrinopeptides A. As the resulting dimers add more units, a second kind of interaction necessarily occurs between fibrin units in an end-to-end fashion (see Plates 22–3 and 22–4). The end-to-end forces are relatively weak, and fibrinogen molecules do not ordinarily associate in advance of thrombin provocation. The key feature of fibrin formation is each double-knobbed central domain pinning together two other fibrinogen molecules.[63]

Unitary additions continue until the oligomers contain 15 to 20 units, a stage at which they are referred to as protofibrils.[73] A model of a protofibril based on the X-ray structures of fragments is depicted in Plate 22–5. Protofibrils are still in the solution phase; it is their aggregation with each other that effects gelation. Moreover, they may aggregate in both a lengthwise and a widthwise manner, depending on the solution conditions[74] and whether the fibrinopeptides B have been released. With regard to the latter, circumstantial evidence has largely borne out the early suggestion that release of fibrinopeptide A gives rise to a linear mode of polymerization, whereas removal of the fibrinopeptide B facilitates lateral associations.[75] It has been shown that the rate of release of fibrinopeptide B greatly depends on oligomerization.[76] Fibrin has different properties, depending on the relative rates of the two kinds of association; faster lengthwise propagation leads to finer fibers and transparent clots, and more lateral growth leads to coarser fibers and opaque clots.[77]

▼ INITIAL INTERACTION OF FIBRIN MONOMERS

The removal of the fibrinopeptides A from the amino termini of the fibrinogen α chains gives rise to an entity denoted fibrin monomer, the spontaneous polymerization of which leads to fibrin.[78] Remarkably, small peptides beginning with the sequence Gly-Pro-Arg are able to prevent the polymerization of fibrin monomers.[70] They do this by binding to complementary sites (holes) that are themselves always available and do not need to be uncovered by the action of thrombin. Equilibrium dialysis showed that each molecule of fibrinogen has two such sites for Gly-Pro-Arg knobs, one

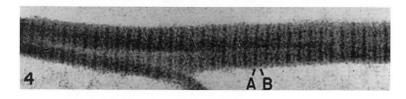

Figure 22–7. Negatively stained fibrin strands. The 225 Å repeated striations are shown. (From Hall, C.E., and Slayter, H.S.: The fibrinogen molecule: its size, shape and mode of polymerization. J. Biophys. Biochem. Cytol. 5:11, 1959; with permission.)

per fragment D, which is to say one on each of the terminal domains.[71] Moreover, only full-size fragments D bound these peptides. Smaller fragments D generated in the absence of calcium ions and lacking the carboxyl-terminal 109 residues of the γ chain (i.e., residues 303 to 411) do not bind Gly-Pro-Arg peptides, and the inference was drawn that the hole must be at least partly constructed from this region. Indeed, affinity labeling studies subsequently showed that tyrosine γ363 is the only side chain labeled by bound Gly-Pro-Arg–derivatized peptides.[79, 80]

Interestingly, peptides beginning with Gly-His-Arg, the sequence exposed by the release of the fibrinopeptide B, also bind to fibrinogen, but they are not nearly as effective in preventing polymerization. The initial observation[70] was that Gly-His-Arg-Pro does not inhibit the association of fibrin monomers at all, but subsequent reports have shown that this peptide can have an effect under certain conditions.[81] For example, it was found that the Gly-His-Arg peptides are effective in delaying clotting brought about by snake venom enzymes that release only the fibrinopeptide B.[82] There is also general agreement that Gly-His-Arg peptides can potentiate the action of Gly-Pro-Arg peptides.[83] The B-type peptides also bind to fragments D of all sizes and independent of the size of the γ chain. Furthermore, binding is greatly enhanced by the presence of calcium ions.[84] This observation was initially at odds with the evidence that the high-affinity calcium binding site resides in the γ chain portion of fragment D, and it was brought into proper perspective only when X-ray structures showed that calcium can also bind to a site on the β chain portion of fragment D.[64]

Remarkably, peptides beginning with the sequence Gly-Pro-Arg are also able to dissociate fibrin clots, so long as the clots have not been stabilized by factor XIII.[85] Further, the physical properties of clots exposed to these peptides change radically as the peptides diffuse into them.[86, 87] In spite of this impressive clot-preventing and gel-reversing power, Gly-Pro-Arg–based peptides have not been used in clinical settings, presumably because they are rapidly cleared from the circulation. Attempts to synthesize derivatives that bind to albumin and that, as a result, might have longer half-lives in vivo have been only modestly successful.[88] Nonetheless, Gly-Pro-Arg peptides have proved useful in in vitro settings, where they can prevent clot formation during studies of other aspects of the coagulation scheme[89, 90] as well as in studies of fibrin formation itself.[91]

▼ ASSOCIATION OF PROTOFIBRILS

The details of protofibril association have been difficult to unravel. Much circumstantial evidence has accumulated that implicates the removal of fibrinopeptides B, for example, but it is evident, also, that protofibrils associate when fibrinogen is clotted by snake venom enzymes that release only the fibrinopeptide A. Numerous factors may enter in, including both general electrostatic effects and specific interatomic interactions. The presence of sialic acid residues, for example, can slow associations by way of electrostatic repulsion, and removal with a sialidase accelerates fibrin formation.[92] On another front, there is a long history of calcium ions being involved in fibrin formation.[93] Although fibrin can be formed in the absence of calcium ions, the gel structure is significantly weaker than that formed in its presence.[94]

Considerable evidence has been reported for the involvement of the carboxyl domains of α chains in the association of protofibrils. The findings take three directions. First, fibrinogen lacking its αC domains polymerizes significantly more slowly than normal.[95, 96] Second, monoclonal antibodies to sites on the αC domain interfere with the later stages of polymerization.[97] Finally, purified fragments corresponding to regions in the αC domain can inhibit polymerization.[98, 99] These findings are somewhat surprising given the wide variability of this domain from species to species. Nonetheless, the following scenario has been proposed. In fibrinogen, the αC domains are associated intramolecularly, but after the removal of the fibrinopeptides B, they are somehow less restrained and can interact on an intermolecular basis. The details of these interactions remain vague.

Fibrin formation can be arrested at the protofibril stage by keeping the concentration of thrombin as the rate-limiting component and then adding an inhibitor of thrombin just before the onset of gelation.[100] The solution of rod-like oligomers can be passed over an appropriate gel filtration column to remove the inhibitor and most of the thrombin. If additional thrombin is then added, gelation occurs in the usual way. Conditions can also be prescribed such that gelation occurs merely by the addition of physiological amounts of calcium ion or tiny amounts of zinc.[101]

▼ FIBRIN STABILIZATION

Although the forces involved in the polymerization process are non-covalent, fibrin clots formed under physiological conditions are reinforced by the addition of covalent cross-links catalyzed by the calcium-dependent transglutaminase commonly known as factor XIII.[102] The enzyme, which occurs in both a plasma and a platelet form, circulates as a precursor and is itself activated by a thrombin-catalyzed cleavage. The activated form is referred to as factor XIIIa. Early evidence that the bulk of the circulating zymogen is bound to fibrinogen[103] was refined by the discovery that the zymogen binds exclusively to a minor form of fibrinogen with anomalously extended γ chains.[104] The association ensures the availability of this relatively infrequent protein (see Table 22–2) when polymerization occurs. The active enzyme ordinarily begins its action on the propagating protofibrils, introducing cross-links between specific lysine side chains and glutamine acceptors in neighboring units. The result of such a union is referred to as an ε-amino(γ-glutamyl)lysine isopeptide.

These isopeptide linkages actually occur in two different settings. In the first, the carboxyl-terminal segments of γ chains in neighboring molecules are reciprocally linked.[105, 106] Virtually all units of the fibrin clot are joined in this fashion. In the second situation, α chains are linked into multimeric arrays[107]; only a small fraction of molecules are ordinarily involved in this process, and it has been supposed that they link protofibrils laterally. Cross-linked fibrin is considerably more stable than non–cross-linked, as reflected in its mechanical and elastic properties.[108–110] It is also considerably more resistant to fibrinolysis.[111]

X-ray structures have not been as informative about the cross-linking situation as hoped. First, as noted above, the structure of the γ chain carboxyl domain was ambiguous about the whereabouts of the carboxyl terminus.[62] The structures of cross-linked double-D were equally vague, the cross-links themselves being absent from electron density maps.[63, 64] Apparently, the carboxyl-terminal segments are exposed and highly mobile, even after the incorporation of the cross-links. The X-ray structures have shown, nonetheless, that the units are linked end-to-end on the opposite faces of the fibrin units from where they are pinned together by the Gly-Pro-Arg knobs from the central domain of other units (see Plates 22–3 to 22–5). This is consistent with the factor XIII needing to have access to position itself during the cross-linking process (see Plate 22–6).

With regard to the cross-linking of α chains, a long and frustrating effort has been under way to pin down the exact locations of the links.[112] The difficulty stems from there being a relatively large number of potential lysine donors in the carboxyl region of the chain,[113] more than half of which have been shown to combine with surrogate glutamine acceptors under the influence of factor XIII.[114] On the other hand, there is a virtual absence of glutamine acceptors in the same region. There is, however, a scant number of glutamines in the central region of the α chain, almost all of which have been shown to be capable of incorporating small molecule surrogate donors,[113] and it appears that the excess of potential donors over acceptors gives rise to a mixed system of cross-links.[114]

In spite of this apparent confusion, significant progress has been made. Several studies have used antibodies to block specific regions of the α chain and shown an inhibition of cross-linking.[115] Other studies have taken advantage of human variant fibrinogens that lack portions of the α chain to show diminished cross-linking.[116] Also, studies on recombinant α chains spanning specific regions have pinpointed several residues that either are or are not involved.[117] Those residues now known to be involved in cross-links include α chain glutamines at positions 221, 237, and 328 and lysines at 539, 556, 580, and 601.[117]

Cross-linking plays an important role in wound healing, and although persons with genetically defective factor XIII do not always experience clotting problems, their healing wounds tend to ooze.[118] In this regard, fibronectin can be cross-linked to fibrin, in which capacity it may serve as a bridge for invading fibroblasts destined to deposit collagen fibers.[119-121] This union is known to involve lysine donors from the fibrin α chain carboxyl regions and glutamine acceptor sites situated near the fibronectin amino termini.[122] Electron micrographs of fibronectin that has been cross-linked to fibrinogen by factor XIIIa show fully extended molecules bridged at their extremities,[123] an observation that argues against the notion of fibrinogen α chains being firmly folded back on the central domain.

▼ CONFORMATIONAL CHANGES

In the simplest instance, one could imagine that fibrin might be indistinguishable from fibrinogen except for the absence of the fibrinopeptides and those surface groups hidden by the units being packed together. This being the case, fibrin might be expected to lack some immunological features present in fibrinogen merely because they were shielded by the packing arrangement. Conceivably, also, the newly exposed knobs in fibrin might occasionally protrude from the polymer and be detectable by suitable antibodies. Indeed, antibodies to both the Gly-Pro-Arg and Gly-His-Arg knobs have been obtained that react uniquely with fibrin.[124-126] Antibodies have also been obtained that can recognize fragments D that have been cross-linked by factor XIIIa.[127]

In addition to these covalent differences between fibrinogen and fibrin, more subtle distinctions are possible as a result of conformational adjustments made during packing, and even though most of the molecule remains accessible to solvent, certain structural features may be covered or uncovered. Numerous immunochemical and labeling experiments have been conducted during the years in attempts to identify such shifting features and to measure the magnitude of the effect. Studies of this kind are of interest on two counts. First, they contribute to our understanding of what happens when fibrinogen is transformed into fibrin. Second, it is of obvious utility in clinical settings to have tests that distinguish circulating fibrin from fibrinogen.

The changes often remain elusive. For example, γ chain residues 312 to 324 were reported to be a fibrin-specific epitope.[128] This is a region involved in the tight binding of a calcium ion and not far from where the Gly-Pro-Arg knob itself binds, and its inaccessibility to antibodies in fibrinogen might conceivably have reflected adjustments made during polymerization. Comparison of these regions in the X-ray structures of fragments D and double-D have not revealed any significant differences, however.[63] Indeed, if anything, the region is less accessible in the double-D fragment from fibrin than in fragment D from fibrinogen.

Fibrinolysis

Fibrin clots are not meant to be permanent structures. Rather, they are temporary sealants that are ordinarily displaced as a part of the normal wound healing process. The dismantling of the clot, whether it is the scaffolding at a wound site or a circulating thrombus, is primarily the role of plasmin; the conversion of plasminogen to plasmin sets the pace of dissolution. Plasminogen occurs in the plasma in two different forms easily distinguished by their amino termini: native Glu-plasminogen and a clipped form lacking 76 residues, Lys-plasminogen. Only the Lys- form binds to fibrinogen, and that weakly.[129] Both forms bind fibrin, but the Lys- form does so much more tightly, even though both have the five characteristic kringle domains[130] that confer unique binding properties. In either case, it appears to be kringle 4 that has a high-affinity binding site for lysine.[131] Note that this binding site is not in the protease portion of the protein, although—perhaps not coincidentally—the enzyme also has a substrate-binding pocket that leads to preferential cleavage after lysine side chains.[132] It is the non-catalytic lysine binding site that is used when plasminogen is purified by affinity chromatography,[133] however, and it is also the principal binding site for ε-aminocaproic acid, a well-known competitive inhibitor of fibrinolysis.

Although a number of early studies had targeted lysines in fibrin as essential for lysis,[134, 135] it was Christenson[136] who pointed out that carboxyl-terminal lysines in proteolyzed fibrin must be most attractive to plasminogen, because only such lysines have the features inherent in ε-aminocaproic acid. The happy result is that as plasmin degrades the fibrin clot, it provides more carboxyl-terminal lysines that can attract additional plasminogen molecules.[137] An interesting countermeasure to this process has evolved among primates. There is an entity known as lipoprotein(a), the apoprotein of which is composed of 37 copies of kringle 4, a single copy of kringle 5, and an inactive serine protease domain,[138] clearly an aberrant descendant of plasminogen. As plasmin chews its way into fibrin (or fibrinogen), it also facilitates the binding of the lipoprotein(a) to these same sites.[139] Elevated concentrations of lipoprotein(a) have been associated with increased risk for thrombosis.[140]

▼ PLASMINOGEN ACTIVATION

Plasminogen can be converted to plasmin either by limited proteolysis or by the binding action of specific bacterial activator proteins like streptokinase; physiologically, the most important process is limited proteolysis by tissue plasminogen activator (t-PA) released from damaged endothelial cells.[141] Should plasminogen be converted to plasmin in the open circulation, the plasmin is promptly inactivated by α_2-antiplasmin.[142] Only when the activation takes place within the relatively safe confines of a clot does plasmin have free rein. To ensure that this happens, t-PA itself contains kringle domains, one of which has been found to have a high-affinity binding site for lysine[143, 144] and is likely to be responsible for the preferential binding of t-PA to lysines in fibrin.[145] It has been shown that t-PA on its own is not effective in activating plasminogen, but fibrin and various fibrin breakdown products are able to increase the activation process by 50-fold.[146] Fibrinogen is wholly inactive in this capacity, so the activity must be attributed to some feature that is exposed during fibrin formation. The activating region has been localized to α chain residues 154 to 159,[147] another region found to be immunologically detectable in fibrin but not in fibrinogen.[148] It was initially presumed that the key residue was lysine 157, but in a puzzling and somewhat anticlimactic result, it was found that the lysine can be acetylated with impunity and that a number of other residues, including glutamate, can serve equally well in synthetic peptide analogues.[149] X-ray studies on fragment D have shown that this region of the α chain, which is located in the coiled coil, is wholly inaccessible, its outside side chains being shielded by the reverse course taken by the chain as it forms a helix proceeding in the opposite direction.[63] The initial conjecture was that the fourth helix must pull away during fibrin formation, thereby exposing the putative activation site. Unhappily, the site was also shown to be inaccessible in the crystal structure of double-D isolated from fibrin.[63] The possibility remains that the fourth helix really does move away during polymerization but then snaps back into its shielding groove after fibrinolysis. More work is needed on this problem.

▼ PHYSICAL CONSIDERATIONS

Whatever the exact mechanism of activation, the major problem to be confronted for dissolution is access to the inside of the clot. Although fibrin gels are relatively open meshworks that allow diffusion in and out, the fibrils themselves may be as much as several hundred molecules in diameter (see Fig. 22–6). There is a good deal of open space within the fibrils also, a consequence of the nodular structure of the individual units.[150] Even with an overlapping half-molecule stagger in which the terminal globules of one unit fit into the interglobular space of another, enough open space should remain for ensuring that the coiled coils are mostly exposed to solvent. Nonetheless, plasmin may be large enough to be excluded and may have to digest its way in from the outside.

In any event, the coarser the fibers, the more porous and accessible they are and the faster they are destroyed by plasmin.[151] Almost anything that leads to coarse clots facilitates lysis. For example, synthetic polymers used as plasma expanders induce coarser clots that are lysed much more rapidly than normal.[152, 153] Whether such clots are as effective in hemostasis is another matter.

Differences in accessibility dictated by the nature of molecular packing in the clot may explain another apparent paradox about fibrinolysis. Aspirin has been reported to be directly involved in accelerating fibrinolysis, an effect attributable to the acetylation of lysines on fibrinogen.[154] Everything said heretofore might lead one to expect that any modification of lysines would slow the action of plasmin. If lysine modifications lead to coarser clots, however, the paradox might be resolved.

With regard to the actual dissolution of the fibrin clot, the mode of attack for plasmin is similar to the assault on fibrinogen described earlier. The critical breakpoints are situated in the central regions of the coiled coils (Fig. 22–8), and in a kind of reverse rendering of the polymerization process, solution occurs at the level of oligomers, long before the last of the individual units is cleaved.[155] The final core fragments are similar to those found when fibrinogen is digested with plasmin, except that cross-linked fibrin does not contain monomeric fragment D units but instead contains D-dimers, the result of the γγ cross-links. Furthermore, under physiological conditions, these dimeric units can remain bound to fragment E with its knobs still positioned in their complementary holes, the overall entity being called D_2E.[156, 157] The fact that such an entity is not found when non–cross-linked fibrin is lysed is a reflection of the modest strength of interaction between the holes and knobs.

▼ BREAKDOWN PRODUCTS AS INHIBITORS OF CLOTTING

It has long been appreciated that fibrinogen and fibrin breakdown products can inhibit the spontaneous polymerization of fibrin monomers.[158] Indeed, fibrinogen itself can terminate growing fibrin oligomers once thrombin is cleared from the system, the lack of an exposed knob bringing the polymerization to a halt. Among the breakdown products, fragment D ought to be the most effective terminator, because it has the necessary hole to participate in oligomer formation but lacks a knob to let the process continue. As might be expected, D-dimer is only about half as effective as fragment D (on a weight basis) in the inhibition of clotting.[159] In this regard, the moiety D_2E should not be an effective inhibitor because all its sites are occupied, but an equilibrium between

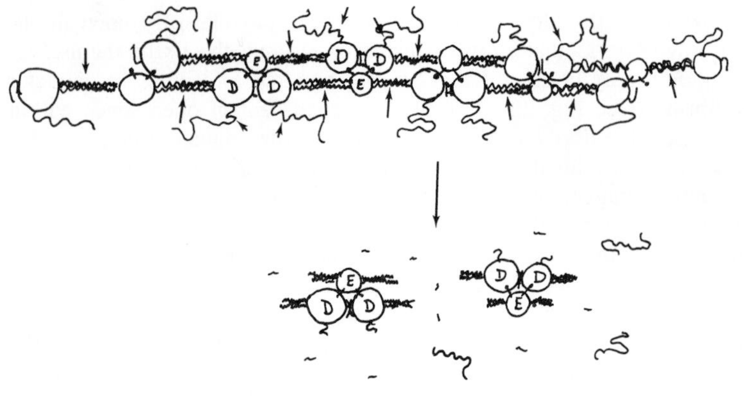

Figure 22–8. Destruction and solubilization of fibrin resulting from plasmin attack on central regions of coiled coil connectors. (Adapted from Doolittle, R.F.: Fibrinogen and fibrin. In Bloom, A.L., and Thomas, D.P. : Haemostasis and Thrombosis. 2nd ed. London, Churchill Livingstone, 1987, pp. 192–215; with permission.)

the D$_2$E form, on the one hand, and D$_2$ and free E, on the other, is likely. As a result, the transient D$_2$ can bind to growing fibrin units and be inhibitory under physiological conditions.

Although there may be some question about just how important fibrin split products are in self-limiting clots formed under ordinary circumstances, fibrinogen split products are certainly of great importance in some clinical settings. Thus, in the case of disseminated intravascular coagulation, plasmin is generated in disproportional amounts, and a massive destruction of fibrinogen ensues with a concomitant release of fragment D and resulting hemorrhage.[160] Certain snake venoms can produce a similar result by attacking fibrinogen directly.[161]

Fibrinogen Biosynthesis

The principal site of fibrinogen biosynthesis in mammals is the liver. At one point, it was thought that fibrinogen might also be made in the precursors of platelets, megakaryocytes,[162] but subsequent attempts to demonstrate mRNAs in megakaryocyte cultures have not upheld the original reports.[163, 164] All of the substantial amount of fibrinogen found in platelets is apparently the result of sequestration.

The half-life of fibrinogen in the general circulation is less than 4 days, doubtless a reflection of its continuous conversion to fibrin and damage by other forms of limited proteolysis that leads to its removal from the circulation. At one point, it was thought that fibrin and fibrinogen degradation products played a role in the subsequent stimulation of fibrinogen biosynthesis, and numerous studies were conducted to test that premise.[165–169] Current thinking, however, postulates that lysis products do not have any significant impact on fibrinogen biosynthesis.[170]

As is well known, fibrinogen is one of the "acute phase proteins," the biosynthesis of which is markedly increased in times of trauma and insult. The provocative stresses range from inflammation to pregnancy and the responding proteins from α_1-antitrypsin to α_2-macroglobulin. Time-honored strategies for provoking the synthesis of acute phase proteins experimentally include the subdural administration of turpentine to laboratory rodents to effect localized inflammation and the administration of snake venom enzymes to bring about massive degradation of fibrinogen. The first method was used by Bouma and colleagues[171] to increase mRNA levels sufficiently to show that the three chains of fibrinogen

are made on separate messages. The other method was used by Crabtree and Kant[172] in the first successful cloning of fibrinogen messages. The known extracellular agents that stimulate synthesis of acute phase proteins include interleukin-6 (originally called hepatocyte-stimulating factor) and other cytokines,[173] which in turn bind to gp130 receptors on hepatocytes[174] and stimulate the manufacture of fibrinogen and other proteins. The intracellular signaling process includes the involvement of the Jak (protein tyrosine kinase)[175] and STAT (signal transduction and activator of transcription)[176] pathways, the endgame involving factors that bind to appropriate DNA promoters.[177] It has long been realized, also, that glucocorticoids play a synergistic role in this process.[178–180]

▼ GENE ARRANGEMENT

In mammals, the three chains of fibrinogen are encoded by single-copy genes lying relatively near each other. In humans, the three genes encompass a 50 kb region on chromosome 4.[181] The α chain gene is situated between the γ chain and β chain genes. Interestingly, the β chain gene lies in the opposite orientation with its coding sequence on the other strand relative to the other two genes. The inversion may have occurred at the time of the duplication that gave rise to the initial β chain. In spite of the inverted arrangement, all three genes are coordinately regulated and made under control of the same signals.[172]

All together, there are 20 introns in the three human fibrinogen genes: four in the α chain gene and eight each in the β chain and γ chain genes. Two of these are common to all three genes, a reflection of their common ancestry. The β and γ chain genes have an additional intron in common also. One of the consequences of intron distribution involves the potential for alternative splicing that can lead to minor or genetically defective forms of human fibrinogen.

▼ ALTERNATIVE PROCESSING

Even though there is only a single gene for each of the three non-identical chains in human fibrinogen, at least three different versions of the protein are made. One of the alternative forms accounts for 5 to 10 per cent of the total fibrinogen and is distinguished by having a slightly longer version of the γ chain, denoted γ'.[182, 183] The mechanism accounting for this form was first predicted on the basis of studies of a patient with a hereditary dysfibrinogenemia. Thus, fibrinogen Paris I was found to have an abnormality near the carboxyl terminus of the γ chain; it was present in both the major and minor forms, indicating that both were the result of the same gene.[184]

The γ′ chain is the result of alternative splicing during the maturation of the message.[185–187] In a predictable fraction of messages, a splice of the last exon does not occur; a "readthrough" into the last intron occurs instead. The result is a γ chain in which the last four amino acids are replaced with a 24-residue alternative version. Subsequently, the chain is subjected to limited proteolysis that removes the last four residues at the carboxyl terminus.[188] The γ′ fibrinogen forms fibrin in a normal way and is even cross-linked by factor XIII to produce γγ dimers.[183] It is not found in platelets, however, suggesting that the carboxyl terminus itself is involved in the sequestration process. As noted above, the minor form turns out to bind factor XIII,[104] ensuring that cross-linking can get under way immediately when fibrin formation is begun.

Another form of fibrinogen results from alternative splicing in the α chain. The α chain gene contains an open reading frame near its 3′ end that was overlooked during the initial gene characterization. In fact, it was incidentally found during the characterization of a chicken α chain cDNA.[35] Remarkably, the second open reading frame encoded a sequence that was homologous to the carboxyl-terminal regions of β and γ chains.[35] It was subsequently discovered that a splice site exists near the end of the α chain and that a small fraction of chains is generated that express the extra domain.[189–191] These extended chains are referred to as αE chains and the fibrinogens in which they occur as fibrinogen-420,[191] a reflection of the larger molecular weight resulting from the extra αEC domains. The function of fibrinogen-420 is unknown, but an X-ray structure of the αEC domain has revealed a well-defined binding cleft, and sequence comparison has suggested that the domain may be involved in binding some form of carbohydrate.[192] In lampreys (primitive fish), this alternative form of α chain is the result of a separate gene rather than alternative splicing.[193]

▼ BIOASSEMBLY OF FIBRINOGEN

A number of logistical problems are associated with the assembly of a heterohexameric protein. The number of chains being made at any moment must be kept about the same, and they must find each other, form the appropriate disulfide bonds, and be processed properly before release into the circulation. Molecular chaperones are needed to facilitate the process.[194, 195] In addition, although transcription of all three genes is coordinated, α chains are half again as long as γ chains, and their translation ought to take proportionately longer. The balance seems to be met at least partly by degradation of excess chains.[196]

The chains must initially associate as dimers and then go on to form trimers, which are in effect half-molecules. The driving force for this preassembly is the stability derived from the formation of coiled coils.[18, 197] The next step involves the joining of the half-molecules across the central dyad.[198] Site mutagenesis studies have shown that there is

likely to be an additional disulfide connection between the two dimeric halves of the molecule, compared with what had been worked out by protein chemists, in that the central αβ connections cross from one half-molecule to the other.[199] The fully formed hexamers are then transported to the endoplasmic reticulum where they are glycosylated, phosphorylated, and sulfated.

▼ POST-TRANSLATIONAL MODIFICATIONS

All three chains of fibrinogen are made in precursor forms with signal peptides that are cleaved during secretion into the endoplasmic reticulum.[200] Time course studies indicate that carbohydrate is added at somewhat different stages, the γ chain cluster being added before the β chain cluster.[201] Disulfide bonds are formed at an early stage, before the addition of phosphate or sulfates, which occurs after translocation to the endoplasmic reticulum but before secretion from the cell.[202]

As implied before, fibrinogen contains both sulfate and phosphate groups that are added post-translationally. In many vertebrate species, but not primates, the fibrinopeptides B contain a sulfated tyrosine, a relatively uncommon residue in proteins. Interestingly, the minor form of human fibrinogen resulting from alternative splicing of the γ chain has a sulfated tyrosine in the carboxyl-terminal extension.[203]

Human fibrinogen contains partially phosphorylated serines at two different locations in the α chain: one at position 3 in the fibrinopeptide A, the other in the central region at position 345.[204] The phosphate at position α3 has been shown to enhance the binding of fibrinogen to thrombin.[205]

Fetal fibrinogen contains more phosphoserine than the adult form, perhaps the result of less extracellular dephosphorylation rather than an increase in incorporation.[204] Although phosphorylation is usually thought of as an intracellular process, the intimate association of fibrinogen and platelets may lead to specific extracellular phosphorylation. Platelets have an ectokinase, and they release adenosine triphosphate (ATP) during their activation, thereby providing the necessary wherewithal.[206] It has been shown that fibrinogen incubated with blood, radioactive ATP, and magnesium ions is indeed phosphorylated.[207] Moreover, the fibers in fibrin gels formed from such phosphorylated fibrinogen are altered, and subsequent fibrinolysis may be affected as well.

Finally, studies of cDNA (prepared from mRNA) revealed that the α chain contains a 15-residue carboxyl-terminal extension that is not present in circulating fibrinogen.[31] The peptide is cleaved before or during secretion from the hepatocyte.[208] I have already noted that a minor form of the γ chain is proteolytically trimmed before or during excretion.[188]

Genetically Defective Fibrinogens

Variant human fibrinogens have contributed much to our understanding of fibrinogen-fibrin biochemistry, in many instances providing important insights into structure-function relationships. Hundreds of such variants have already been identified, some because of their clinical consequences; many others in which the clinical manifestation is mild or absent have been found during routine screening, mostly revealed by long in vitro thrombin times. It is noteworthy that total afibrinogenemia is not automatically fatal; persons so afflicted often live into adulthood before some chance trauma overwhelms secondary hemostatic provisions.[209]

Technical problems are often involved in pinning down the molecular basis of a dysfibrinogenemia. In many cases, the abnormal protein is made in diminished amounts. Moreover, most persons found to have variant fibrinogens are heterozygotes.[210] The autosomal dominant nature of many dysfibrinogenemias, whereby there is a clinical manifestation in the heterozygote, is readily explained by the fact that even a small amount of a fibrinogen lacking either a knob or a hole (but not both, of course) can cap a growing fibrin polymer and inhibit clotting. Curiously, defects associated with knobs are much more likely to exhibit bleeding than are those associated with holes.

In principle, there ought to be as many kinds of genetically defective fibrinogen molecules as there are definable structural dependencies in the native molecule. Some may be strictly architectural, preventing proper folding and assembly, for example. Many are known in which the release of one or the other fibrinopeptide is inhibited, and many others in which some stage of the polymerization event is prevented. Still others may involve interactions with other clotting and lysis components or cells. Variants are systematically catalogued,[211] and the subject is regularly reviewed.[211–214] Here, I highlight only a few of the more graphic and interesting cases (Table 22–3).

Table 22–3. Some Genetically Defective Fibrinogens

Type	Designation*	Changed Residues	Reference
Variant fibrinopeptides A	Lille	α7 D → N	217
	Rouen	α12 G → V	210
Thrombin cleavage points	Petoskey*	α16 R → H	216
	Metz*	α16 R → C	231
	Seattle*	β14 R → C	234
	Ise	β15 G → C	235
A knob	Kanazawa	α18 P → L	210
	Detroit	α19 R → S	215
	Munchen	α19 R → N	210
	Canterbury	α20 V → D	243
γ Chain hole	Matsumoto I	γ364 D → H	224
	Nagoya	γ329 Q → R	221
	Milano I	γ330 D → V	230
	Kyoto III	γ330 D → Y	222
D:D interface	Tokyo II	γ275 R → C	227, 228
	Bergamo II*	γ275 R → H	210
Deletion	Vlissingen	γ319–320 (del)	238
	New York	β9–72 (del)	230
Insertion	Paris	Insert 15 residues after γ350	236, 237
Carbohydrate obstruction	Asahi	γ310 M → T	218
	Caracas II	α434 S → N	219
	Pontoise	β335 A → T	220
Albumin obstruction	Nijmegen	β44 R → C	232

* The designates marked with an asterisk have been found in numerous other cities also.

The first variant fibrinogen to have its molecular basis identified was fibrinogen Detroit,* a case in which severely restricted fibrin formation was found to be correlated with the replacement of the arginine residue at α19 by serine.[215] This is a classic case of a defective knob. In the interval since that initial report, several other replacements have been found at that same position (see Table 22–3).

Other vulnerable locations are the peptide bonds attacked by thrombin. Interestingly, the arginine at α16 is often replaced by histidine and the glycine at α17 by cysteine (see Table 22–3). Unexpectedly, thrombin cleaves the bond in the former case, albeit at a much slower rate.[216] Some instances are also known in which the arginyl-glycine bond is unaffected, but substitution within the fibrinopeptide itself influences the binding of thrombin and can lead to slow release.[217]

▼ THREE-DIMENSIONAL CONSIDERATIONS

Before the availability of X-ray structures, considerable attention was focused on those variant fibrinogens exhibiting defective fibrin formation and especially those with changes in their γ chain carboxyl-terminal domains. Thus, although the knob of the initial knob/hole interaction was well defined, the hole had not been identified with any precision. Amino acid replacements at assorted positions in the section spanning γ chain residues 268 to 375 were all reported to interfere with polymerization. In theory, these variants could have fallen into two general classes: those that disrupted the binding pocket, on the one hand, and those that interfered with abutment of fibrin units at the D:D interface, on the other (see Table 22–3). Other kinds of obstruction could also occur, including substitutions leading to unpaired cysteine side chains or the introduction of anomalous carbohydrate attachment sites.[218–220]

All of these mutations were brought into sharper focus with the advent of X-ray structures of the γC domain[62] and fragments D and double-D from fibrinogen and fibrin,[63] respectively (see Plate 22–7). As it happened, the residues at γ329 (fibrinogen Nagoya[221]), γ330 (fibrinogens Kyoto III[222] and Milano I[223]), and γ364 (fibrinogens Matsumoto I[224] and Melun[225]) were found to be structurally part of the binding cleft,[214] whereas the arginine at γ275 (as in fibrinogens Tokyo II,[226, 227] Osaka II,[228] and eight others) is a principal site of interaction at the D:D interface, as had been predicted on the basis of biochemical experiments.[227, 229]

Although there have been many variants of human fibrinogen reported in which the interaction of the α chain knob (Gly-Pro-Arg) and its γ chain hole has been compromised, there is a dearth of such variants for the corresponding interaction involving the β chain knob (Gly-His-Arg) and the β chain hole. Two things can be cautiously concluded from these findings: first, the clinical consequence of not having the β chain knob/hole interaction is slight; and second, routine thrombin times are not much affected by that interaction.

*As in the case of variant human hemoglobins, variant fibrinogens are named after the city in which they were first found. When more than one variant is found in the same city, an appropriate number is appended.

▼ A DIDACTIC CASE: CYSTEINE CHANGES

A good example of how genetic variants can be informative about a protein's structure is afforded by those fibrinogens with replacements involving cysteine. As noted in an earlier section, all the cysteine residues in fibrinogen are involved in disulfide bonds. This is true of most plasma proteins, of course, only a few of which have odd numbers of cysteines and a free sulfhydryl group as a result. Albumin is one of these exceptions, having 17 disulfide bonds and a single free cysteine.

If any of the cysteines in fibrinogen were to be replaced, its partner would be unpaired and, depending on its location, might react with a molecule of free cysteine, with some other protein containing a free sulfhydryl, or with another molecule like itself, or it could conceivably maintain the free sulfhydryl. A similar situation would exist if any other amino acid in fibrinogen were replaced by a cysteine. In fact, both kinds of variant are known (see Table 22–3). In the case of fibrinogen New York, an entire exon amounting to 64 amino acids is absent from the β chain.[230] Amazingly, these fibrinogen molecules are still able to assemble into six-chained structures, even though the 64-residue β chain skein contains a cysteine residue that is ordinarily bound to one in an α chain. Apparently the unpaired cysteines at α32 are able to find each other and form an additional bond between the two halves of the molecule.

There are some other changes involving a cysteine in which a new disulfide bond occurs. In fibrinogen Metz, the arginine at position α16 is changed to cysteine, and again, the two α chains in every fibrinogen molecule become linked by an additional disulfide.[231] In contrast, in fibrinogen Nijmegen, the arginine at β44 is changed to cysteine, and the result is the formation of an external disulfide bond to the free sulfhydryl in plasma albumin.[232] This observation is consistent with this portion of the β chain being highly exposed, it being common knowledge that one of the first bonds cleaved by plasmin is β42–43.[233]

Albumin has also been found disulfide-bonded to fibrinogen IJmuiden, a case in which the arginine at β14 is replaced with cysteine.[233] The same replacement was reported previously in fibrinogens Seattle and Christchurch II.[234] In contrast, replacement of the adjacent glycine by cysteine at β15 (fibrinogen Ise[235]) does not lead to an attachment to albumin, and the new sulfhydryl in this case is capped with free cysteine. This is also known to be the case in fibrinogens Tokyo II and Osaka II, in which cases the arginine at γ275 is replaced with cysteine and, as noted above, an impairment of the D:D interaction is experienced.

▼ INSERTIONS, DELETIONS, AND FRAMESHIFTS

Not all variant fibrinogens involve simple amino acid replacements, of course. Indeed, one of the first variants ever discovered, fibrinogen Paris,[236] turns out to be the result of a point mutation in an intron that brings about the insertion of 15 amino acids in the γ chain.[237] Correspondingly, there are variants in which residues are deleted. In fibrinogen Vlissingen,[238] for example, six bases are missing, and as a consequence, two γ chain amino acids involved in calcium binding are deleted. In the case of fibrinogen Marburg,[239] a

single base change leading to a stop codon terminates the α chain prematurely. The resulting absence of residues 461 to 610 leads to significantly weakened clot structures.

Aberrations can also result from frameshifts. A case has been reported[240] in which a single base deletion in the α chain results in a frameshift at residue 524 whereby the remaining 97 amino acids are replaced by a new set of 23 with a distinctly hydrophobic character. The unexpected clinical consequence is severe renal amyloidosis. Amyloidosis, a situation in which an abnormal protein accumulates as a result of a lessened solubility that leads to amyloid-like fibers, can also occur in some variant fibrinogens in which certain polar amino acids in the carboxyl region of the fibrinogen α chain are replaced with nonpolar ones.[241, 242]

Anomalies can occur in fibrinogen variants in remarkably subtle ways, as the following example should make clear. In fibrinogen Canterbury,[243] the valine at position α20 is changed to an aspartic acid. This is a relatively exposed part of the molecule, located only four residues past the junction initially cleaved by thrombin at the onset of fibrin formation. The change results in an arginyl-aspartate peptide bond that can be cleaved by the intracellular liver enzyme furin, and as a consequence, a defective fibrinogen molecule is secreted that lacks both the fibrinopeptide A and the A knob.

▼ SITE-DIRECTED MUTAGENESIS

As valuable as naturally occurring variants have been, they may soon be overshadowed by site-directed mutagenesis experiments with recombinant fibrinogens expressed in recombinant systems. The first experiments in this area were limited to making individual chains in bacterial expression systems,[244] but it was not long before a number of laboratories succeeded in generating clottable fibrinogen in eukaryotic expression systems in which all three non-identical chains were assembled appropriately.[245, 246] At this point, expression of fibrinogen or pieces thereof is routine, and designated amino acids can be replaced at will.[247] The power of this approach in exploring the nature of disulfide attachments between individual chains as well as between the dimeric halves of the protein has already been noted.[199]

▼ STUDIES ON KNOCKOUT MICE

Although naturally occurring variant fibrinogens have been extremely useful in relating structure and function, they are limited in their occurrence, and most are heterozygous. Site-directed mutagenesis can be aimed at any change the experimenter chooses, but observations are limited to the in vitro situation. Gene knockouts in mice, on the other hand, allow changes to be imposed and observed in vivo. In these experiments, recombinant constructs are usually injected into blastocysts to generate chimeric animals that can be bred to produce, first, heterozygotes and then, in subsequent generations, homozygotes.

Mouse strains have been developed in which the fibrinogen α chain was disrupted, and as a result, they have no circulating fibrinogen at all.[248] Indeed, there is no trace of any of the three chains in the plasma, and the blood is completely incoagulable. So far as can be told, most of such animals survive their prenatal development, and indeed, depending on their genetic background, most have a not greatly reduced life span. In this regard, they resemble humans who are afibrinogenemic.[209] Significant numbers do experience serious bleeding problems, however, especially abdominal hemorrhages. Moreover, female mice in which the fibrinogen genes are knocked out cannot carry fetal offspring to term.[248]

Knockout mice have shed light on other aspects of the clotting and lysis problem as well. For example, mice deprived of their plasminogen gene are seriously compromised and have greatly reduced life spans.[249] Not only do they have a vast range of thrombotic events, but their wound healing is greatly delayed. When such mice are crossed with fibrinogen-deficient mice, however, these morbid events are wholly reversed, and the progeny are indistinguishable from mice lacking only fibrinogen.[250] That wound healing should be poor in plasminogen-deficient mice but normal in mice lacking both plasminogen and fibrinogen points up the complexity of the process. Moreover, the lack of thrombotic events in the mice lacking both proteins demonstrates that the primary role of plasminogen is definitely fibrinolysis.[250]

Molecular Ecology of Fibrinogen and Fibrin

Fibrinogen and fibrin interact with a wide variety of proteins and cells. I have already touched on involvements with thrombin,[230] factor XIII,[103] plasminogen,[129] apolipoprotein(a),[139] t-PA,[149] and fibronectin.[121] Some other proteins that might warrant mention include thrombospondin and certain protease inhibitors. Let us review the list briefly.

Naturally, thrombin has a great affinity for fibrinogen. Less appreciated is that thrombin also has a marked affinity for fibrin, a property that helps keep its action localized to the region of the clot.[251, 252] I have already called attention to the fact that fibrin, but not fibrinogen, activates t-PA and binds plasminogen and apolipoprotein(a). Also, in this game of point and counterpoint, inhibitors of plasmin and plasminogen activators associate with fibrinogen. For example, the serine protease inhibitor known as α_1-antitrypsin (a misnomer in that its physiological target is obviously not trypsin) is occasionally linked to fibrinogen by a disulfide bond[253]; even more important, another inhibitor, α_2-antiplasmin, can be cross-linked by factor XIIIa into an acceptor site in the same general region of the fibrinogen molecule.[254]

Thrombospondin is a large thrombin-sensitive glycoprotein that occurs in minute quantities in the circulating blood plasma but is released from activated platelets in significant amounts.[255, 256] It interacts with a number of proteins besides thrombin and has been found to be an inhibitor of plasmin as well.[257] It also binds to fibrinogen and influences the nature of fibrin clots, perhaps by regulating the extent of fiber branching.[258, 259] The regions of fibrin(ogen) that are involved in this interaction have been reported to include α chain residues 113 to 126 and β chain residues 243 to 252.[260] The first of these is situated in the middle region of the coiled coils, whereas the second is a part of the terminal macrodomain. The X-ray structure of fragment D[63] reveals that β chain residues 243 to 252 are a part of a loop about

80 Å away from the site implicated on the α chain (see Plate 22–1).

▼ THE INTERACTION OF FIBRINOGEN WITH PLATELETS

Fibrinogen is an essential cofactor in the adhesion of platelets to each other and to the endothelial lining of the circulatory system. A number of agents, including adenosine diphosphate, epinephrine, thrombin, and collagen, stimulate the exposure of fibrinogen receptors on the platelet surface. The primary receptor is the glycoprotein IIb/IIIa, an adhesion protein involved in the binding of other plasma proteins as well.[261] The cell adhesion machinery appears to involve a combinatorial binding system that achieves its remarkable specificity by requiring two recognition components on every protein bound. One of these is the common tripeptidyl sequence Arg-Gly-Asp (RGD); the other, which imposes the bulk of the specificity, is peculiar to the bound protein.

Fibrinogen and fibrin both bind to platelets, but their plasmin degradation products do not.[262] This implies that the two components of a two-site recognition system become separated during the digestion. Consistent with this is the observation that α chains and γ chains have both been implicated in the binding.[263] The specificity binding site has been localized to the carboxyl-terminal 15 residues of the γ chain.[263] It will be recalled that this is the region of the molecule that first becomes cross-linked by factor XIII and that is situated at the tip of the fibrinogen molecule. As such, it is ideally located for bridge formation between platelets. The location of the alleged RGD site is more problematic.

Human α chains contain two widely separated RGD sequences, one at residues 95 to 97 and the other at 572 to 574. Given that the two γ chain sites are indeed located 450 Å apart at the extremes of the molecule, it might be anticipated that the α chain site would be situated terminally also, and not in the coiled coil region, which encompasses residues 50 to 160 (see Plate 22–2). As it happens, the site near the α chain carboxyl terminus (α chain residues 572 to 574) is not conserved from species to species, being absent in the rat, for example. This is not what one expects for an essential interaction site. Rat fibrinogen does have an RGD at α chain positions 280 to 282, however, as well as one in the coiled coil region. At one point, some investigators thought that both RGD sites in human α chains contributed to the interaction,[264] whereas others favored the notion that only the site near the carboxyl terminus was needed.[265] That at least one RGD site was essential to the interaction seemed to be borne out by the observation that trigamin, an RGD-containing peptide found in certain snake venoms, is a powerful inhibitor of the fibrinogen binding to platelets.[266]

Site-directed mutagenesis experiments did not support either view, however, in that recombinant fibrinogen in which one or the other RGD sequence was removed had no effect on fibrinogen binding to platelets.[267] The conclusion was that fibrinogen binding to platelets is primarily through the γ chain carboxyl-terminal segment. Interestingly, inbred mice in which the terminal five residues of the γ chain were deleted suffer serious bleeding episodes, and their fibrinogen does not bind effectively to platelets.[268]

▼ INTERACTIONS WITH OTHER CELLS

When provoked or damaged, the endothelial cells that line the vascular system also bind fibrinogen and fibrin.[269] Originally it was thought that the principal binding sites on fibrinogen were the same as those involved in the binding to platelets.[265] In this case, however, site-directed mutagenesis studies have shown that the α chain RGD at residues 572 to 574 is the principal adhesion site and that the γ chain apparently does not play a role.[270]

Fibrin also binds to other cells of the circulatory system, including macrophages.[271] Fibronectin has been implicated in the process.[271] The central domain of fibrinogen has been reported to be the principal site of interaction, specifically the Gly-Pro-Arg knob exposed by thrombin.[272]

▼ INTERACTION OF FIBRINOGEN WITH BACTERIA

Fibrinogen is unique among the plasma proteins in being able to "clump" certain strains of *Staphylococcus aureus*.[273] The interactive site on fibrinogen has been localized to the carboxyl-terminal segment of γ chains, precisely the region involved in fibrin cross-linking and, more relevant, the site required for binding to platelets.[274, 275] That no other parts of fibrinogen are needed for clumping was dramatically demonstrated by construction of an artificial "clumper."[275] Thus, synthetic peptides corresponding to the terminal 15 residues of the γ chain can be coupled to carriers like albumin, and these constructs clump the bacteria in the complete absence of fibrinogen.

The question arises as to whether the phenomenon of "staph-clumping" is to the advantage of the bacterium or the host. On the one hand, it might be supposed that coating bacteria with fibrin, as opposed to fibrinogen, might lead to increased phagocytosis. On the other hand, fibrinogen coating might be part of an evasive strategy on the part of the bacterium. There is good reason to favor the latter. First, not all mammalian species have fibrinogens capable of clumping these bacteria; the carboxyl-terminal sequences differ to the extent that no interactions occur, at least not with the strains tested. It seems more likely that the bacterium has been able to mimic the action of the platelet receptor than that the host has learned to bind the bacterium. If this were the case, the host could not change its site without compromising its ability to bind platelets. Staphylococcal bacteria are also able to bind to fibrin thrombi, but in this case, the interaction appears to be mediated by fibronectin, another protein with a binding site for these bacteria.[276] The fact that fibrinogen can clump these bacteria in vitro may be misleading. Experiments conducted under more physiological conditions reveal that fibrinogen actually serves as a bridging molecule in the adherence of staphylococci to endothelial cells.[277]

Fibrinogen also binds to other bacteria, including many *Streptococcus* strains. The evidence in this realm strongly favors a protective action whereby phagocytosis of the coated bacterium is inhibited[278]; apparently these bacteria bind fibrinogen to avoid phagocytosis by host cells.[279] Preliminary experiments suggest that the β chain of fibrinogen contains the primary binding site.[279]

Finally, some pathogenic strains of *Bacteroides* have been found to bind fibrinogen specifically. Surprisingly, different strains appear to bind to different parts of the molecule, the fragment D region in one case and the coiled coil region in another.[280]

Concluding Remark

Fibrinogen is a highly differentiated protein. Although its primary functions are clot formation and platelet aggregation, it interacts with a wide variety of other proteins and cells. Its complex structure reflects these diverse actions. As much as possible, this chapter has tried to correlate structure and function by identifying those parts of the protein that are involved in polymerization, cross-linking, lysis, and binding to other proteins and cells. The availability of high-resolution X-ray structures for some core fragments, but not yet the whole molecule, means that some of these phenomena are better understood than others.

In the end, we see fibrinogen as a protein shaped by natural selection to polymerize in various forms, depending on circumstances, and more or less vulnerable to lytic attack, depending on the assembled force of plasminogen and plasminogen activators arrayed against a counterforce of protease inhibitors. It is a molecule that can seal off wounds and prevent the invasion of some bacteria while in other instances providing a safe haven for others. Virtually every aspect of its character reflects the delicate balance between sickness and health, or even life and death.

REFERENCES

1. Scheraga, H.A., and Laskowski, M., Jr.: The fibrinogen-fibrin conversion. Adv. Protein Chem. 12:1, 1957.
2. Doolittle, R.F.: Structural aspects of the fibrinogen-fibrin conversion. Adv. Protein Chem. 27:1, 1973.
3. Doolittle, R.F.: Fibrinogen and fibrin. *In* Bloom, A.L., and Thomas, D.P. (eds.): Haemostasis and Thrombosis. 2nd ed. London, Churchill Livingstone, 1987, pp. 192–215.
4. Bailey, K., Astbury, W.T., and Rudall, K.M.: Fibrinogen and fibrin as members of the keratin-myosin group. Nature 151:716, 1943.
5. Crick, F.H.C.: The packing of α-helices: simple coiled coils. Acta Crystallogr. 6:689, 1953.
6. Siegel, B.M., Mernan, J.P., and Scheraga, H.A.: The configuration of native and partially polymerized fibrinogen. Biochim. Biophys. Acta 11:329, 1953.
7. Shulman, S.: The size and shape of bovine fibrinogen studies of sedimentation, diffusion and viscosity. J. Am. Chem. Soc. 75:5846, 1953.
8. Hall, C.E., and Slayter, H.S.: The fibrinogen molecule: its size, shape and mode of polymerization. J. Biophys. Biochem. Cytol. 5:11, 1959.
9. Cohen, C.: Invited discussion at 1960 Symposium on Protein Structure. J. Polymer Sci. 49:144, 1961.
10. Nussenzweig, V., Seligmann, M., Pelimont, J., and Grabar, P.: Les produits de degradation du fibrinogene humain par la plasmine. Ann. Inst. Pasteur 100:377, 1961.
11. Marder, V.J., Shulman, N.R., and Carroll, W.R.: High molecular weight derivatives of human fibrinogen produced by plasmin. I. Physicochemical and immunological characterization. J. Biol. Chem. 244:2111, 1969.
12. Marder, V.J.: Physicochemical studies of intermediate and final products of plasmin digestion of human fibrinogen. Thromb. Diath. Haemorrh. Suppl. 39:187, 1970.
13. Mills, D., and Karpatkin, S.: Heterogeneity of human fibrinogen: possible relation to proteolysis by thrombin and plasmin as studied by SDS-polyacrylamide gel electrophoresis. Biochem. Biophys. Res. Commun. 40:206, 1970.

14. McKee, P.A., Rogers, L.A., Marler, E., and Hill, R.B.: The subunit polypeptides of human fibrinogen. Arch. Biochem. Biophys. 116:271, 1966.

15. Henschen, A.: Number and reactivity of disulfide bonds in fibrinogen and fibrin. Arkiv Kemi 22:355, 1964.

16. Tooney, N.M., and Cohen, C.: Microcrystals of a modified fibrinogen. Nature 237:23, 1972.

17. Rao, S.P.S., Poojary, M.D., Elliott, B.W., Jr., Melanson, L.A., Oriel, B., and Cohen, C.: Fibrinogen structure in projection at 18 Å resolution electron density by co-ordinated cryo-electron microscopy and X-ray crystallography. J. Mol. Biol. 222:89, 1991.

18. Doolittle, R.F.: Fibrinogen and fibrin. Annu. Rev. Biochem. 53:195, 1984.

19. Blombäck, B., Blombäck, M., Henschen, A., Hessel, B., Iwanaga, S., and Woods, K.R.: N-terminal disulfide knot of human fibrinogen. Nature 218:130, 1968.

20. Marder, V.J.: Identification and purification of fibrinogen degradation products produced by plasmin: considerations on the structure of fibrinogen. Scand. J. Haematol. Suppl. 13:21, 1971.

21. Kowalska-Loth, B., Gardlund, B., Egberg, N., and Blombäck, B.: Plasmic degradation products of human fibrinogen. II. Chemical and immunologic relation between fragment E and N-DSK. Thromb. Res. 2:423, 1973.

22. Doolittle, R.F., Cassman, K.G., Cottrell, B.A., Friezner, S.J., and Takagi, T.: Amino acid sequence studies on the α-chain of human fibrinogen. The covalent structure of the α-chain portion of fragment D. Biochemistry 16:1710, 1977.

23. Doolittle, R.F., Goldbaum, D.M., and Doolittle, L.R.: Designation of sequences involved in the "coiled coil" interdomainal connector in fibrinogen: construction of an atomic scale model. J. Mol. Biol. 120:311, 1978.

24. Henschen, A., and Lottspeich, F.: Amino acid sequence of human fibrin. Preliminary note on the γ-chain sequence. Hoppe Seylers Z. Physiol. Chem. 358:935, 1977.

25. Henschen, A., and Lottspeich, F.: Amino acid sequence of human fibrin. Preliminary note on the completion of the β-chain sequence. Hoppe Seylers Z. Physiol. Chem. 358:1643, 1977.

26. Watt, K.W.K., Takagi, T., and Doolittle, R.F.: Amino acid sequence of the β-chain of human fibrinogen: homology with the γ-chain. Proc. Natl. Acad. Sci. USA 75:1731, 1978.

27. Doolittle, R.F., Watt, K.W.K., Cottrell, B.A., Strong, D.D., and Riley, M.: The amino acid sequence of the α-chain of human fibrinogen. Nature 280:464, 1979.

28. Kant, J.A., Lord, S.T., and Crabtree, G.R.: Partial mRNA sequences for human A α, B β, and γ-fibrinogen chains: evolutionary and functional implications. Proc. Natl. Acad. Sci. USA 80:3953, 1983.

29. Chung, D.W., Chan, W.-Y., and Davie, E.W.: Characterization of a complementary deoxyribonucleic acid coding for the γ chain of human fibrinogen. Biochemistry 22:3250, 1983.

30. Chung, D.W., Que, B.G., Rixon, M.W., Mace, M., Jr., and Davie, E.W.: Characterization of complementary deoxyribonucleic acid and genomic deoxyribonucleic acid for the β chain of human fibrinogen. Biochemistry 22:3244, 1983.

31. Rixon, M.W., Chan, W.-Y., Davie, E.W., and Chung, D.W.: Characterization of a complementary deoxyribonucleic acid coding for the α chain of human fibrinogen. Biochemistry 22:3237, 1983.

32. Crabtree, G.R., and Kant, J.A.: Molecular cloning of cDNA for the α, β and γ chains of rat fibrinogen. J. Biol. Chem. 257:7277, 1981.

33. Chung, D.W., Rixon, M.W., MacGillivray, R.T.A., and Davie, E.W.: Characterization of a cDNA clone coding for the β chain of bovine fibrinogen. Proc. Natl. Acad. Sci. USA 78:1466, 1981.

34. Weissbach, L., Oddoux, C., Procyk, R., and Grieninger, G.: The β chain of chicken fibrinogen contains an atypical thrombin cleavage site. Biochemistry 30:3290, 1991.

35. Weissbach, L., and Grieninger, G.: Bipartite mRNA for chicken α-fibrinogen potential encodes an amino acid sequence homologous to β- and γ-fibrinogens. Proc. Natl. Acad. Sci. USA 87:5198, 1990.

36. Pastori, R.L., Moskaitis, J.E., Smith, L.H., Jr., and Schoenberg, D.R.: Estrogen regulation of Xenopus laevis γ-fibrinogen gene expression. Biochemistry 29:2599, 1990.

37. Strong, D.D., Moore, M., Cottrell, B.A., Bohonus, V.L., Pontes, M., Evans, B., Riley, M., and Doolittle, R.F.: Lamprey fibrinogen γ chain: cloning, cDNA sequencing and general characterization. Biochemistry 24:92, 1985.

38. Bohonus, V., Doolittle, R.F., Pontes, M., and Strong, D.D.: Comple-

mentary DNA sequence of lamprey fibrinogen β chain. Biochemistry 25:6512, 1986.

39. Wang, Y.Z., Patterson, J., Gray, J.E., Yu, C., Cottrell, B.A., Shimizu, A., Graham, D., Riley, M., and Doolittle, R.F.: Complete sequence of the lamprey fibrinogen α chain. Biochemistry 28:9801, 1989.

40. Townsend, R.R., Hilliker, E., Li, Y.-T., Laine, R.A., Bell, W.R., and Lee, Y.C.: Carbohydrate structure of human fibrinogen. J. Biol. Chem. 257:9704, 1982.

41. Grieninger, G., Plant, P.W., and Kossoff, H.S.: Glycosylated A α chains in chicken fibrinogen. Biochemistry 23:5888, 1984.

42. Doolittle, R.F., and Cottrell, B.A.: Lamprey fibrinopeptide B is a glycopeptide. Biochem. Biophys. Res. Commun. 60:1090, 1974.

43. Huseby, R.M., Mosesson, M.W., and Murray, M.: Studies of the amino acid composition and conformation of human fibrinogen: comparison of fractions I-4 and I-8. Physiol. Chem. Phys. 2:374, 1970.

44. Murakawa, M., Okamura, T., Kamura, T., Shibuya, T., Harada, M., and Niho, Y.: Diversity of primary structure of the carboxy-terminal regions of mammalian fibrinogen A α-chains. Thromb. Haemost. 69:351, 1993.

45. Rudee, M.L., and Price, T.M.: Observation of the α-chain extensions of fibrinogen through a new electron microscope specimen preparation technique. Ultramicroscopy 7:193, 1981.

46. Price, T.M., Strong, D.D., Rudee, M.L., and Doolittle, R.F.: Shadow-cast electron microscopy of fibrinogen with antibody fragments bound to specific regions. Proc. Natl. Acad. Sci. USA 78:200, 1981.

47. Mosesson, M.W., Hainfeld, J., Wall, J., and Haschemeyer, R.H.: Identification and mass analysis of human fibrinogen molecules and their domains by scanning transmission electron microscopy. J. Mol. Biol. 153:695, 1981.

48. Erickson, H.P., and Fowler, W.E.: Electron microscopy of fibrinogen, its plasmic fragments and small polymers. Ann. N. Y. Acad. Sci. 408:146, 1983.

49. Weisel, J.W., Stauffacher, C.V., Bullitt, E., and Cohen, C.: A model for fibrinogen: domains and sequence. Science 230:1388, 1985.

50. Veklich, Y.I., Gorkun, O.V., Medved, L.V., Nieuwenhuizen, W., and Weisel, J.W.: Carboxyl-terminal portions of the α chains of fibrinogen and fibrin. Localization by electron microscopy and the effects of isolated αC fragments on polymerization. J. Biol. Chem. 268:13577, 1993.

51. Williams, R.C.: Band patterns seen by electron microscopy in ordered arrays of bovine and human fibrinogen and fibrin after negative staining. Proc. Natl. Acad. Sci. USA 80:1570, 1983.

52. Doolittle, R.F., and Laudano, A.P.: Synthetic peptide probes and the location of fibrin polymerization sites. Protides Biol. Fluids 28:311, 1980.

53. Privalov, P.L., and Medved, L.V.: Domains in the fibrinogen molecule. J. Mol. Biol. 159:665, 1982.

54. Medved, L.V., Litinovich, S.V., and Privalov, P.L.: Domain organization of the terminal parts in the fibrinogen molecule. FEBS Lett. 202:298, 1986.

55. Marguerie, G., Chagniel, G., and Suscillon, M.: The binding of calcium to bovine fibrinogen. Biochim. Biophys. Acta 490:94, 1977.

56. Purves, L.R., Lindsey, G.G., and Franks, J.J.: Role of calcium in the structure and interactions of fibrinogen. S. Afr. J. Sci. 74:202, 1978.

57. Marguerie, G., and Ardaillou, N.: Potential role of the A α chain in the binding of calcium to human fibrinogen. Biochim. Biophys. Acta 701:410, 1982.

58. Nieuwenhuizen, W., and Gravesen, M.: Anticoagulant and calcium-binding properties of high molecular weight derivatives of human fibrinogen, produced by plasmin (fragments X). Biochim. Biophys. Acta 668:81, 1981.

59. Haverkate, F., and Timan, G.: Protective effect of calcium in the plasmin degradation of fibrinogen and fibrin products D. Thromb. Res. 10:803, 1977.

60. Lawrie, J.S., and Kemp, G.: The presence of a Ca^{2+} bridge within the γ chain of human fibrinogen. Biochim. Biophys. Acta 577:415, 1979.

61. Dang, C.V., Ebert, R.F., and Bell, W.R.: Localization of a fibrinogen calcium binding site between γ-subunit positions 311 and 336 by terbium fluorescence. J. Biol. Chem. 260:9713, 1985.

62. Yee, V.C., Pratt, K.P., Cote, H.C., LeTrong, I., Chung, D.W., Davie, E.W., Stenkamp, R.E., and Teller, D.C.: Crystal structure of a 30 kDa C-terminal fragment from the γ chain of human fibrinogen. Structure 5:125, 1997.

63. Spraggon, G., Everse, S., and Doolittle, R.F.: Crystal structures of fragment D from human fibrinogen and its crosslinked counterpart from fibrin. Nature 359:455, 1997.

64. Everse, S.J., Spraggon, G., Veerapandian, L., Riley, M., and Doolittle, R.F.: Crystal structure of fragment double-D from human fibrin with two different bound ligands. Biochemistry 37:8637, 1998.
65. Ferry, J.D.: The mechanism of polymerization of fibrin. Proc. Natl. Acad. Sci. USA 38:566, 1952.
66. Stryer, L., Cohen, C., and Langridge, R.: Axial period of fibrinogen and fibrin. Nature 197:793, 1963.
67. Bailey, K., Bettelheim, F.R., Lorand, L., and Middlebrook, W.R.: Action of thrombin in the clotting of fibrinogen. Nature 167:233, 1951.
68. Blombäck, B., Hessel, B., Hogg, D., and Therkildsen, L.: A two-step fibrinogen-fibrin transition in blood coagulation. Nature 275:501, 1978.
69. Blombäck, B., Blombäck, M., and Nilsson, I.M.: Coagulation studies on reptilase, an extract of the venom from Bothrops jararaca. Thromb. Diath. Haemorrh. 1:1, 1957.
70. Laudano, A.P., and Doolittle, R.F.: Synthetic peptide derivatives which bind to fibrinogen and prevent the polymerization of fibrin monomers. Proc. Natl. Acad. Sci. USA 75:3085, 1978.
71. Laudano, A.P., and Doolittle, R.F.: Studies on synthetic peptides that bind to fibrinogen and prevent fibrin polymerization. Structural requirements, numbers of binding sites and species differences. Biochemistry 19:1013, 1980.
72. Pratt, K.P., Cote, H.C.F., Chung, D.W., Stenkamp, R.E., and Davie, E.W.: The fibrin polymerization pocket: three-dimensional structure of a 30-kDA C-terminal γ chain fragment complexed with the peptide Gly-Pro-Arg-Pro. Proc. Natl. Acad. Sci USA 94:7176, 1997.
73. Hantgan, R.R., and Hermans, J.: Assembly of fibrin. A light scattering study. J. Biol. Chem. 254:11272, 1979.
74. Weisel, J.W.: Fibrin assembly. Lateral aggregation and the role of the two pairs of fibrinopeptides. Biophys. J. 50:1079, 1986.
75. Laurent, T.C., and Blömback, B.: On the significance of the release of two different peptides from fibrinogen during clotting. Acta Chem. Scand. 12:1875, 1958.
76. Hurlet-Jensen, A., Cummins, H.Z., Nossel, H.L., and Liu, C.Y.: Fibrin polymerization and release of fibrinopeptide B by thrombin. Thromb. Res. 27:419, 1982.
77. Ferry, J.D., and Morrison, P.R.: The conversion of human fibrinogen to fibrin under various conditions. J. Am. Chem. Soc. 69:380, 1947.
78. Donnelly, T.H., Laskowski, M., Jr., Notley, N., and Scheraga, H.A.: Equilibria in the fibrinogen-fibrin conversion. II. Reversibility of the polymerization steps. Arch. Biochem. Biophys. 56:369, 1955.
79. Shimizu, A., Nagel, G., and Doolittle, R.F.: Photoaffinity labeling of the primary fibrin polymerization site. I. Isolation and characterization of a labeled cyanogen bromide fragment corresponding to γ337–γ379. Proc. Natl. Acad. Sci. USA 89:2888, 1992.
80. Yamazumi, K., and Doolittle, R.F.: Photoaffinity labeling of the primary fibrin polymerization site. II. Localization of the label to tyrosine γ363. Proc. Natl. Acad. Sci. USA 89:2893, 1992.
81. Pandya, B.V., Gabriel, J.L., O'Brien, J., and Budzynski, A.Z.: Polymerization site in the β chain of fibrin: mapping of the Bβ 1–55 sequence. Biochemistry 30:162, 1991.
82. Furlan, M., Rupp, C., and Beck, E.A.: Inhibition of fibrin polymerization by fragment D is affected by calcium, Gly-Pro-Arg and Gly-His-Arg. Biochim. Biophys. Acta 742:25, 1982.
83. Laudano, A.P., Cottrell, B.A., and Doolittle, R.F.: Synthetic peptides modeled on fibrin polymerization sites. Ann. N. Y. Acad. Sci. 408:315, 1983.
84. Laudano, A.P., and Doolittle, R.F.: Influence of calcium ion on the binding of fibrin amino-terminal peptides to fibrinogen. Science 212:457, 1981.
85. Bale, M.D., Muller, M.F., and Ferry, J.D.: Effects of fibrinogen-binding tetrapeptides on mechanical properties of fine fibrin clots. Proc. Natl. Acad. Sci. USA 82:1410, 1985.
86. Schindlauer, G., Bale, M.D., and Ferry, J.D.: Interaction of fibrinogen-binding tetrapeptides with fibrin oligomers and fine fibrin clots. Biopolymers 25:1315, 1986.
87. Shimizu, A., Schindlauer, G., and Ferry, J.D.: Interaction of the fibrinogen-binding tetrapeptide Gly-Pro-Arg-Pro with fine clots and oligomers of α-fibrin; comparisons with a β-fibrin. Biopolymers 27:775, 1988.
88. Kuyas, C., and Doolittle, R.F.: Gly-Pro-Arg-Pro derivatives that bind to human plasma albumin and prevent fibrin formation. Thromb. Res. 43:4851, 1986.
89. Harfenist, E.J., Guccione, M.A., Packham, M.A., and Mustard, J.F.: The use of the synthetic peptide, Gly-Pro-Arg-Pro, in the preparation of thrombin-degranulated rabbit platelets. Blood 59:952, 1982.
90. Almus, F.E., Rao, L.V.M., and Rapaport, S.I.: Functional properties of factor VIIA/tissue factor formed with purified tissue factor and with tissue factor expressed on cultured endothelial cells. Thromb. Haemost. 62:1067, 1989.
91. Mihalyi, E.: Clotting of fibrinogen. Calcium binding to fibrin during clotting and its dependence on release of fibrinopeptide B. Biochemistry 27:967, 1988.
92. Martinez, J., Palascak, J., and Peters, C.: Functional and metabolic properties of human asialofibrinogen. J. Lab. Clin. Med. 89:367, 1977.
93. Boyer, M.H., Shainoff, J.R., and Ratnoff, O.D.: Acceleration of fibrin polymerization by calcium ions. Blood 39:382, 1972.
94. Donovan, J.W., and Mihalyi, E.: Clotting of fibrinogen. I. Scanning calorimetric study of the effect of calcium. Biochemistry 24:3434, 1985.
95. Medved, L.V., Gorkun, O.V., Manyakov, V.F., and Belitser, V.A.: The role of fibrinogen αC-domains in the fibrin assembly process. FEBS Lett. 181:109, 1985.
96. Holm, B., Brosstad, F., Kierulf, P., and Godal, H.C.: Polymerization properties of two normally circulating fibrinogens, HMW and LMW. Evidence that the COOH-terminal end of the α-chain is of importance for fibrin polymerization. Thromb. Res. 39:595, 1985.
97. Cierniewski, C.S., and Budzynski, A.: Involvement of the α chain in fibrin clot formation. Effect of monoclonal antibodies. Biochemistry 31:4284, 1992.
98. Lau, H.K.F.: Anticoagulant function of a 24-Kd fragment isolated from human fibrinogen Aα chains. Blood 81:3277, 1993.
99. Gorkun, O.V., Veklich, Y.I., Medved, L.V., Henschen, A.H., and Weisel, J.W.: Role of the αC domains of fibrin in clot formation. Biochemistry 33:6986, 1994.
100. Janmey, P.A., and Ferry, J.D.: Gel formation by fibrin oligomers without addition of monomers. Biopolymers 25:1337, 1986.
101. Marx, G.: Protofibrin clots induced by calcium and zinc. Biopolymers 26:911, 1987.
102. Ichinose, A.: The physiology and biochemistry of factor XIII. In Bloom, A.L., Forbes, C.D., Thomas, D.P., and Tuddenham, E.G.D. (eds.): Haemostasis and Thrombosis. 3rd ed. London, Churchill Livingstone, 1994, pp. 531–546.
103. Greenberg, C.S., and Shuman, M.A.: The zymogen forms of blood coagulation factor XIII bind specifically to fibrinogen. J. Biol. Chem. 257:6096, 1982.
104. Siebenlist, K.R., Meh, D.A., and Mosesson, M.W.: Plasma factor XIII binds specifically to fibrinogen molecules containing γ' chains. Biochemistry 35:10448, 1996.
105. Chen, R., and Doolittle, R.F.: Isolation, characterization and location of a donor-acceptor unit from crosslinked fibrin. Proc. Natl. Acad. Sci. USA 66:472, 1970.
106. Chen, R., and Doolittle, R.F.: γ γ Cross-linking sites in human and bovine fibrin. Biochemistry 10:4486, 1971.
107. McKee, P.A., Mattock, P., and Hill, R.L.: Subunit structure of human fibrinogen, soluble fibrin, and cross-linked insoluble fibrin. Proc. Natl. Acad. Sci. USA 66:738, 1970.
108. Gerth, C., Roberts, W.W., and Ferry, J.D.: Rheology of fibrin clots. II. Linear viscoelastic behavior in shear creep. Biophys. Chem. 2:208, 1974.
109. Nelb, G.W., Kamykowski, G.W., and Ferry, J.D.: Kinetics of ligation of fibrin oligomers. J. Biol. Chem. 255:6398, 1980.
110. Bale, M.D., Janmey, P.A., and Ferry, J.D.: Kinetics of formation of fibrin oligomers. II. Size distributions of ligated oligomers. Biopolymers 21:2265, 1982.
111. Gaffney, P.J., and Whitaker, A.N.: Fibrin crosslinks and lysis rates. Thromb. Res. 14:85, 1979.
112. Doolittle, R.F., Cassman, K.G., Cottrell, B.A., and Friezner, S.J.: Amino acid sequence studies on the α chain of human fibrinogen. Isolation and characterization of two linked α-chain cyanogen bromide fragments from fully cross-linked fibrin. Biochemistry 16:1715, 1977.
113. Cottrell, B.A., Strong, D.D., Watt, K.W.K., and Doolittle, R.F.: Amino acid sequence studies on the α chain of human fibrinogen. Exact location of cross-linking acceptor sites. Biochemistry 18:5405, 1979.
114. Sobel, J.H., and Gawinowicz, M.A.: Identification of the α chain lysine donor sites involved in factor XIIIa fibrin cross-linking. J. Biol. Chem. 271:19288, 1996.
115. Mitkevich, O.V., Sobel, J.H., Shainoff, J.R., Vlasik, T.N., Kalantarov, G.F., Trakht, I.N., Streltsova, Z.A., and Samokhin, G.P.: Monoclonal antibody directed to a fibrinogen Aα #529–539 epitope inhibits α-chain crosslinking by transglutaminases. Blood Coagul. Fibrinolysis 7:85, 1996.

116. Sobel, J.H., Trakht, I., Wu, H.Q., Rudchenko, S., and Egbring, R.: α-Chain cross-linking in fibrin(ogen) Marburg. Blood 86:989, 1995.

117. Matsuka, Y.V., Medved, L.V., Migliorini, M.M., and Ingham, K.C.: Factor XIIIa–catalyzed cross-linking of recombinant αC fragments of human fibrinogen. Biochemistry 35:5810, 1996.

118. Duckert, F.: Documentation of the plasma factor XIII deficiency in man. Ann. N. Y. Acad. Sci. 202:190, 1972.

119. Mosher, D.F.: Cross-linking of cold-insoluble globulin by fibrin-stabilizing factor. J. Biol. Chem. 250:6614, 1975.

120. Ruoslahti, E., and Vaheri, A.: Interaction of soluble fibroblast surface antigen with fibrinogen and fibrin. J. Exp. Med. 141:497, 1975.

121. Mosher, D.F., Schad, P.E., and Kleinman, H.K.: Cross-linking of fibronectin to collagen by blood coagulation factor XIIIₐ. J. Clin. Invest. 64:781, 1979.

122. Mosher, D.F., and Johnson, R.B.: Specificity of fibronectin-fibrin cross-linking. Ann. N. Y. Acad. Sci. 408:583, 1983.

123. Erickson, H.P., Carrell, N., and McDonagh, J.: Fibronectin molecule visualized in electron microscopy: a long, thin, flexible strand. J. Cell Biol. 91:673, 1981.

124. Pacella, B.L., Jr., Hui, K.Y., Haber, E., and Matsueda, G.R.: Induction of fibrin-specific antibodies by immunization with synthetic peptides that correspond to amino termini of thrombin cleavage sites. Mol. Immunol. 20:521, 1983.

125. Hui, K.Y., Haber, E., and Matsueda, G.R.: Monoclonal antibodies to a synthetic fibrin-like peptide bind to human fibrin but not fibrinogen. Science 222:1129, 1983.

126. Scheefers-Borchel, U., Muller-Berghaus, G., Fuhge, P., Eberle, R., and Heimburger, N.: Discrimination between fibrin and fibrinogen by a monoclonal antibody against a synthetic peptide. Proc. Natl. Acad. Sci. USA 82:7091, 1985.

127. Wilner, G.D., Mudd, M.S., Hsieh, K.-H., and Thomas, D.W.: Monoclonal antibodies to fibrinogen: modulation of determinants expressed in fibrinogen by γ-chain cross-linking. Biochemistry 21:2687, 1982.

128. Schielen, W.J.G., Adams, H.P.H.M., van Leuven, K., Moskuilen, M., Tesser, G.I., and Nieuwenhuizen, W.: The sequence γ-(312–324) is a fibrin-specific epitope. Blood 77:2169, 1991.

129. Lucas, M.A., Fretto, L.J., and McKee, P.A.: The binding of human plasminogen to fibrin and fibrinogen. J. Biol. Chem. 258:4249, 1983.

130. Söttrup-Jensen, L., Claeys, H., Zajdel, M., Petersen, T.E., and Magnusson, S.: The primary structure of human plasminogen: isolation of two lysine-binding fragments and one 'mini'-plasminogen (MW38000) by elastase-catalyzed-specific limited proteolysis. In Davidson, J.F., Rowan, R.M., Samama, M.M., and Desnoyers, P.C. (eds.): Progress in Chemical Fibrinolysis and Thrombolysis. Vol. 3. New York, Raven Press, 1978, pp. 191–209.

131. Rejante, M., Elliott, B.W., Jr., and Llinas, M.: A ¹H-NMR study of plasminogen kringle 4 interactions with intact and partially digested fibrinogen. Fibrinolysis 5:87, 1991.

132. Weinstein, M.J., and Doolittle, R.F.: Differential specificities of thrombin, plasmin and trypsin with regard to synthetic and natural substrates and inhibitors. Biochim. Biophys. Acta 258:577, 1972.

133. Deutsch, D.G., and Mertz, E.T.: Plasminogen: purification from human plasma by affinity chromatography. Science 170:1095, 1970.

134. Radcliffe, R.: A critical role of lysine residues in the stimulation of tissue plasminogen activator by denatured proteins and fibrin clots. Biochim. Biophys. Acta 743:422, 1983.

135. Varadi, A., and Patthy, L.: β(Leu₁₂₁-Lys₁₂₂) segment of fibrinogen is in a region essential for plasminogen binding by fibrin fragment E. Biochemistry 23:2108, 1983.

136. Christensen, U.: C-terminal lysine residues of fibrinogen fragments essential for binding to plasminogen. FEBS Lett. 182:43, 1985.

137. Fleury, V., and Angles-Cano, E.: Characterization of the binding of plasminogen to fibrin surfaces: the role of carboxy-terminal lysines. Biochemistry 30:7630, 1991.

138. McClean, J.W., Tomlinson, J.E., Kuang, W.J., Eaton, D.L., Chen, E.Y., Fless, G.M., Scanu, A.M., and Lawn, R.M.: cDNA sequence of human apolipoprotein(a) is homologous to plasminogen. Nature 330:132, 1987.

139. Harpel, P.C., Gordon, B.R., and Parker, T.S.: Plasmin catalyzes binding of lipoprotein(a) to immobilized fibrinogen and fibrin. Proc. Natl. Acad. Sci. USA 86:3847, 1989.

140. Scanu, A.M.: Lipoprotein(a). A potential bridge between the fields of atherosclerosis and thrombosis. Arch. Pathol. Lab. Med. 112:1045, 1988.

141. Rijken, D.C., Hoylaerts, M., and Collen, D.: Fibrinolytic properties of one-chain and two-chain human extrinsic (tissue-type) plasminogen activator. J. Biol. Chem. 257:2920, 1982.

142. Wiman, B., and Collen, D.: On the mechanism of reaction between human α₂-antiplasmin and plasmin. J. Biol. Chem. 254:9291, 1979.

143. Ichinose, A., Takio, K., and Fujikawa, K.: Localization of the binding site of tissue-type plasminogen activator to fibrin. J. Clin. Invest. 78:163, 1986.

144. Verheijen, J.H., Caspers, M.P.M., Chang, G.T.G., de Munk, G.A.W., Pouwels, P.H., and Enger-Valk, B.E.: Involvement of finger domain and kringle 2 domain of tissue-type plasminogen activator in fibrin binding and stimulation of activity by fibrin. EMBO J. 5:3525, 1986.

145. de Vos, A.M., Ultsch, M.H., Kelly, R.F., Padmanabhan, K., Tulinsky, A., Westbrook, M.L., and Kossiakoff, A.A.: Crystal structure of the kringle 2 domain of tissue plasminogen activator at 2.4-Å resolution. Biochemistry 31:270, 1992.

146. Nieuwenhuizen, W., Vermond, A., Voskuilen, M., Traas, D.W., and Verheijen, J.H.: Identification of a site in fibrin(ogen) which is involved in the acceleration of plasminogen activation by tissue-type plasminogen activator. Biochim. Biophys. Acta 748:86, 1983.

147. Voskuilen, M., Vermond, A., Veeneman, G.H., van Boom, J.H., Klasen, E.A., Zegers, N.D., and Nieuwenhuizen, W.: Fibrinogen lysine residue Aα 157 plays a crucial role in the fibrin-induced acceleration of plasminogen activation, catalyzed by tissue-type plasminogen activator. J. Biol. Chem. 262:5944, 1987.

148. Schielen, W.J.G., Voskuilen, M., Tesser, G.I., and Nieuwenhuizen, W.: The sequence A α-(148–160) in fibrin, but not in fibrinogen, is accessible to monoclonal antibodies. Proc. Natl. Acad. Sci. USA 86:8951, 1989.

149. Schielen, W.J.G., Adams, H.P.H.M., Voskuilen, M., Tesser, G.J., and Nieuwenhuizen, W.: Structural requirements of position A α-157 in fibrinogen for the fibrin-induced rate enhancement of the activation of plasminogen by tissue-type plasminogen activator. Biochem. J. 276:655, 1991.

150. Carr, M.E., Jr., and Hermans, J.: Size and density of fibrin fibers from turbidity. Macromolecules 11:46, 1978.

151. Carr, M.E., Jr., and Hardin, C.L.: Large fibrin fibers enhance urokinase-induced plasmin digestion of plasma clots. Blood 70(suppl. 1):400a, 1987.

152. Hunter, R.L., Bennett, B., and Check, I.J.: The effect of poloxamer 188 on the rate of in vitro thrombolysis mediated by t-PA and streptokinase. Fibrinolysis 4:117, 1990.

153. Carr, M.E., Jr., Powers, P.L., and Jones, M.R.: Effects of poloxamer 188 on the assembly, structure and dissolution of fibrin clots. Thromb. Haemost. 66:565, 1991.

154. Bjornsson, T.D., Schneider, D.E., and Berger, H., Jr.: Aspirin acetylates fibrinogen and enhances fibrinolysis. Fibrinolytic effect is independent of changes in plasminogen activator levels. J. Pharmacol. Exp. Ther. 250:154, 1989.

155. Francis, C.W., Marder, V.J., and Barlow, G.H.: Plasmic degradation of crosslinked fibrin. J. Clin. Invest. 66:1033, 1980.

156. Hudry-Clergeon, G., Paturel, L., and Suscillon, M.: Identification d'un complexe (D-D) . . . e dans les produits de dégradation de la fibrine bovine stabilisée par le facteur XIII. Pathol. Biol. (Paris) 22(suppl.):47, 1974.

157. Gaffney, P.J., and Joe, F.: The lysis of crosslinked human fibrin by plasmin yields initially a single molecular complex, D dimer-E. Thromb. Res. 15:673, 1979.

158. Latallo, Z.S., Fletcher, A.P., Alkjaersig, N., and Sherry, S.: Inhibition of fibrin polymerization by fibrinogen proteolysis products. Am. J. Physiol. 202:681, 1962.

159. Haverkate, F., Timan, G., and Nieuwenhuizen, W.: Anticlotting properties of fragments D from human fibrinogen and fibrin. Eur. J. Clin. Invest. 9:253, 1979.

160. Brozowic, M.: Disseminated intravascular coagulation. In Bloom, A.L., and Thomas, D.P. (eds.): Haemostasis and Thrombosis. 2nd ed. London, Churchill Livingstone, 1987, pp. 535–541.

161. Lakier, J.B., and Fritz, V.V.: Consumptive coagulopathy caused by a boomslang bite. S. Afr. Med. J. 43:1052, 1969.

162. Leven, R., Schick, P.K., and Budzynski, A.: Fibrinogen biosynthesis in isolated guinea pig megakaryocytes. Blood 65:501, 1982.

163. Louache, F., Debili, N., Cramer, E., Breton-Gorius, J., and Vainchenker, W.: Fibrinogen is not synthesized by human megakaryocytes. Blood 77:311, 1991.

164. Lange, W., Luig, A., Dölken, G., Mertelsmann, R., and Kanz, L.: Fibrinogen γ-chain mRNA is not detected in human megakaryocytes. Blood 78:20, 1991.

165. Ritchie, D.G., Levy, B.A., Adams, M.A., and Fuller, G.M.: Regulation of fibrinogen synthesis by plasmin-derived fragments of fibrinogen and fibrin: an indirect feedback pathway. Proc. Natl. Acad. Sci. USA 79:1530, 1982.

166. Hatzfeld, J.A., Hatzfeld, A., and Maigne, J.: Fibrinogen and its fragment D stimulate proliferation of human hemopoietic cells in vitro. Proc. Natl. Acad. Sci. USA 79:6280, 1982.

167. Bell, W.R., Kessler, C.M., and Townsend, R.F.: Stimulation of fibrinogen biosynthesis by fibrinogen fragments D and E. Br. J. Haematol. 53:599, 1983.

168. Qureshi, G.D., Guzelian, P.S., Vennart, R.M., and Evans, H.J.: Stimulation of fibrinogen synthesis in cultured rat hepatocytes by fibrinogen fragment E. Biochim. Biophys. Acta 844:288, 1985.

169. LaDuca, F.M., Tinsley, L.A., Dang, C.V., and Bell, W.R.: Stimulation of fibrinogen synthesis in cultured rat hepatocytes by fibrinogen degradation product fragment D. Proc. Natl. Acad. Sci. USA 86:8788, 1989.

170. Wang, Y., and Fuller, G.M.: The putative role of fibrin fragments in the biosynthesis of fibrinogen by hepatoma cells. Biochem. Biophys. Res. Commun. 175:562, 1991.

171. Bouma, H., III, Kwan, S.-W., and Fuller, G.M.: Radioimmunological identification of polysomes synthesizing fibrinogen polypeptide chains. Biochemistry 14:4787, 1975.

172. Crabtree, G.R., and Kant, J.A.: Coordinate accumulation of the mRNA for the α, β, and γ chains of fibrinogen after defibrination with Malayan pit viper venom. J. Biol. Chem. 257:7277, 1982.

173. Evans, E., Courtois, G.M., Kilian, P.L., Fuller, G.M., and Crabtree, G.R.: Induction of fibrinogen and a subset of acute phase response genes involves a novel monokine which is mimicked by phorbol esters. J. Biol. Chem. 262:10850, 1987.

174. Wang, Y., and Fuller, G.M.: Biosynthetic and glycosylation events of the IL-6 receptor β-subunit. J. Cell. Biochem. 57:610, 1995.

175. Wang, Y., and Fuller, G.M.: Interleukin-6 and ciliary neurotrophic factor trigger janus kinase activation and early gene response in rat hepatocytes. Gene 162:280, 1995.

176. Tian, S.S., Taplet, P., Sincich, C., Stein, R.B., Rosen, J., and Lamb, P.: Multiple signaling pathways induced by granulocyte colony-stimulating factor involving activation of JAKs, STAT5 and/or STAT3 are required for regulation of three distinct classes of immediate early genes. Blood 88:4435, 1996.

177. Courtois, G., Baumhueter, S., and Crabtree, G.R.: Purified hepatocyte nuclear factor I interacts with a family of hepatocyte-specific promoters. Proc. Natl. Acad. Sci. USA 85:7937, 1988.

178. Plant, P.W., and Grieninger, G.: Noncoordinate synthesis of the fibrinogen subunits in hepatocytes cultured under hormone-deficient conditions. J. Biol. Chem. 261:2331, 1986.

179. Otto, J.M., Grenett, H.E., and Fuller, G.M.: The coordinated regulation of fibrinogen gene transcription by hepatocyte-stimulating factor and dexamethasone. J. Cell Biol. 105:1067, 1987.

180. Zhang, Z., Jones, S., Hagood, J.S., Fuentes, N.L., and Fuller, G.M.: STAT3 acts as a co-activator of glucocorticoid receptor signaling. J. Biol. Chem. 272:30607, 1997.

181. Kant, J., Fornace, A.J., Saxe, D., McBride, O.W., and Crabtree, G.R.: Organization and evolution of the human fibrinogen locus on chromosome four. Proc. Natl. Acad. Sci. USA 82:2344, 1985.

182. Francis, C.W., Marder, V.J., and Martin, S.E.: Demonstration of a large molecular weight variant of the gamma chain of normal human plasma fibrinogen. J. Biol. Chem. 255:5599, 1980.

183. Wolfenstein-Todel, C., and Mosesson, M.W.: Human plasma fibrinogen heterogeneity: evidence for an extended carboxyl-terminal sequence in a normal gamma chain variant (gamma'). Proc. Natl. Acad. Sci. USA 77:5069, 1980.

184. Wolfenstein-Todel, C., and Mosesson, M.W.: Carboxy-terminal amino acid sequence of a human fibrinogen γ-chain variant (γ'). Biochemistry 20:6146, 1981.

185. Crabtree, G.R., and Kant, J.A.: Organization of the rat gamma-fibrinogen gene: alternative mRNA splice patterns produce the gamma A and gamma B (gamma') chains of fibrinogen. Cell 31:159, 1982.

186. Chung, D.W., and Davie, E.W.: γ and γ' chains of human fibrinogen are produced by alternative mRNA processing. Biochemistry 23:4232, 1984.

187. Fornace, A.J., Cummings, D.E., Comeau, C.M., Kant, J.A., and Crabtree, G.R.: Structure of the human γ-fibrinogen gene. Alternate mRNA splicing near the 3' end of the gene products γA and γB forms of γ-fibrinogen. J. Biol. Chem. 259:12826, 1984.

188. Francis, C.W., Muller, E., Henschen, A., Simpson, P.J., and Marder, V.J.: Carboxyl-terminal amino acid sequences of the two variant forms of the γ chain of human plasma fibrinogen. Proc. Natl. Acad. Sci. USA 85:3358, 1988.

189. Fu, Y., Weissbach, L., Plant, P.W., Oddoux, C., Cao, Y., Liang, T.J., Roy, S.N., Redman, C.M., and Grieninger, G.: Carboxy-terminal-extended variant of the human fibrinogen α subunit: a novel exon conferring marked homology to β and γ subunits. Biochemistry 31:11968, 1992.

190. Fu, Y., and Grieninger, G.: Fib420: a normal human variant of fibrinogen with two extended α chains. Proc. Natl. Acad. Sci. USA 91:2625, 1994.

191. Fu, Y., Cao, Y., Hertzberg, K.M., and Grieninger, G.: Fibrinogen α genes: conservation of bipartite transcripts and carboxy-terminal-extended α subunits in vertebrates. Genomics 30:71, 1995.

192. Spraggon, G., Applegate, D., Everse, S.J., Zhang, J.-Z., Veerapandian, L., Redman, C., Doolittle, R.F., and Grieninger, G.: Crystal structure of a recombinant αEC domain from human fibrinogen-420. Proc. Natl. Acad. Sci. USA 95:9099, 1998.

193. Pan, Y., and Doolittle, R.F.: cDNA sequence of a second fibrinogen α chain in lamprey: an archetypal version alignable with full-length β and γ chains. Proc. Natl. Acad. Sci. USA 89:2066, 1992.

194. Yu, S., Sher, B., Kudryk, B., and Redman, C.M.: Fibrinogen precursors. Order of assembly of fibrinogen chains. J. Biol. Chem. 259:10574, 1984.

195. Roy, S.N., Procyk, R., Kudryk, B.J., and Redman, C.M.: Assembly and secretion of recombinant human fibrinogen. J. Biol. Chem. 266:4758, 1991.

196. Roy, S., Yu, S., Banerjee, D., Overton, O., Mukhopadhyay, G., Oddoux, C., Grieninger, G., and Redman, C.: Assembly and secretion of fibrinogen. Degradation of individual chains. J. Biol. Chem. 267:23151, 1992.

197. Huang, S., Cao, Z., Chung, D.W., and Davie, E.W.: The role of βγ and αγ complexes in the assembly of human fibrinogen. J. Biol. Chem. 271:27942, 1996.

198. Xu, W.-F., Chung, D.W., and Davie, E.W.: The assembly of human fibrinogen. J. Biol. Chem. 271:27948, 1996.

199. Huang, S., Cao, Z., and Davie, E.W.: The role of amino-terminal disulfide bonds in the structure and assembly of human fibrinogen. Biochem. Biophys. Res. Commun. 190:488, 1993.

200. Nickerson, J.M., and Fuller, G.M.: In vitro synthesis of rat fibrinogen: identification of preAα, preBβ, and preγ polypeptides. Proc. Natl. Acad. Sci. USA 78:303, 1981.

201. Nickerson, J.M., and Fuller, G.M.: Modification of fibrinogen chains during synthesis: glycosylation of Bβ and γ chains. Biochemistry 20:2818, 1981.

202. Kudryk, B., Okada, M., Redman, C.M., and Blombäck, B.: Biosynthesis of dog fibrinogen. Characterization of nascent fibrinogen in the rough endoplasmic reticulum. Eur. J. Biochem. 125:673, 1982.

203. Hirose, S., Oda, K., and Ikehara, Y.: Tyrosine O-sulfation of the fibrinogen γB chain in primary culture of rat hepatocytes. J. Biol. Chem. 263:7426, 1988.

204. Seydewitz, H.H., Kaiser, C., Rothweiler, H., and Witt, I.: The location of a second in vivo phosphorylation site in the A α-chain of human fibrinogen. Thromb. Res. 33:487, 1984.

205. Maurer, M.C., Peng, J.L., An, S.S., Trosset, Y., Henschen-Edman, A., and Scheraga, H.A.: Structural examination of the influence of phosphorylation on the binding of fibrinopeptide A to thrombin. Biochemistry 37:5888, 1998.

206. Nauk, V.P., Kornecki, E., and Ehrlich, Y.H.: Phosphorylation and dephosphorylation of human platelet surface proteins by an ecto-protein kinase/phosphatase system. Biochim. Biophys. Acta 1092:256, 1991.

207. Martin, S.C., Forsberg, P.-O., and Eriksson, S.D.: The effects of in vitro phosphorylation and dephosphorylation on the thrombin-induced gelation and plasmin degradation of fibrinogen. Thromb. Res. 61:243, 1991.

208. Farrell, D.H., Huang, S., and Davie, E.W.: Processing of the carboxyl 15-amino acid extension in the α-chain of fibrinogen. J. Biol. Chem. 268:10351, 1993.

209. Crabtree, G.R.: The molecular biology of fibrinogen. In Stamatoyannopoulos, G., Nienhuis, A.W., Leder, P., and Majerus, P.W. (eds.): Molecular Basis of Blood Diseases. Philadelphia, W.B. Saunders Co., 1985, pp. 631–655.

210. Ebert, R.F.: Index of Variant Human Fibrinogens. Boca Raton, FL, CRC Press, 1994.

211. Galanakis, D.K.: Inherited dysfibrinogenemia: emerging abnormal structure associations with pathologic and nonpathologic dysfunctions. Semin. Thromb. Haemost. 19:386, 1993.

212. Haverkate, F., and Samama, M.: Familial dysfibrinogenemia and thrombophilia. Report on a study of the SSC subcommittee on fibrinogen. Thromb. Haemost. 73:151, 1995.

213. Matsuda, M.: The structure-function relationship of hereditary dysfibrinogens. Int. J. Haematol. 64:167, 1996.

214. Everse, S.J., Spraggon, G., and Doolittle, R.F.: A three-dimensional consideration of variant human fibrinogens. Thromb. Haemost. 80:1, 1998.

215. Blombäck, M., Blombäck, B., Mammen, E.F., and Prasad, A.S.: Fibrinogen Detroit—a molecular defect in the N-terminal disulphide knot of human fibrinogen? Nature 218:134, 1968.

216. Higgins, D.L., and Shafer, J.A.: Fibrinogen Petoskey, a dysfibrinogenemia characterized by replacement of Arg-A α 16 by a histidyl residue. Evidence for thrombin-catalyzed hydrolysis at a histidyl residue. J. Biol. Chem. 256:12013, 1981.

217. Denninger, M.H., Finlayson, J.S., Raemer, L.A., Porquet-Gernez, A., Goudeman, M., and Menache, D.: Congenital dysfibrinogenaemia: fibrinogen Lille. Thromb. Res. 13:453, 1978.

218. Yamazumi, K., Shimura, K., Terukina, S., Takahashi, N., and Matsuda, M.: A γ methionine-310 to threonine substitution and consequent N-glycosylation at γ asparagine-308 identified in a congenital dysfibrinogenemia associated with posttraumatic bleeding, fibrinogen Asahi. J. Clin. Invest. 83:1590, 1989.

219. Maekawa, H., Yamazumi, K., Muramatsu, S., Kaneko, M., Hirata, H., Takahashi, N., de Bosch, N.B., Carvajal, Z., Ojeda, A., Arocha-Pinango, C.L., and Matsuda, M.: An A α Ser-434 to N-glycosylated Asn substitution in a dysfibrinogen, fibrinogen Caracas II, characterized by impaired fibrin gel formation. J. Biol. Chem. 266:11575, 1991.

220. Kaudewitz, H., Henschen, A., Soria, J., and Soria, C.: Fibrinogen Pontoise—a genetically abnormal fibrinogen with defective fibrin polymerisation but normal fibrinopeptide release. In Lane, D.A., Henschen, A., and Jasani, M.K. (eds.): Fibrinogen-Fibrin Formation and Fibrinolysis. Vol. 4. Berlin, Walter de Gruyter, 1986, pp. 91–96.

221. Miyata, T., Furukawa, K., Iwanaga, S., Takamatsu, J., and Saito, H.: Fibrinogen Nagoya, a replacement of glutamine-329 by arginine in the γ-chain that impairs the polymerization of fibrin monomer. J. Biochem. 105:10, 1989.

222. Terukina, S., Yamazumi, K., Okamoto, K., Yamashita, H., Ito, Y., and Matsuda, M.: Fibrinogen Kyoto III: a congenital dysfibrinogen with a γ-aspartic acid-330 to tyrosine substitution. Blood 74:2681, 1989.

223. Reber, P., Furlan, M., Rupp, C., Kehl, M., Henschen, A., Mannucci, P., and Beck, E.: Characterization of fibrinogen Milano I: amino acid exchange γ330 Asp→Val impairs fibrin polymerization. Blood 67:1751, 1986.

224. Okumura, N., Furihata, K., Terasawa, F., Nakagoshi, R., Ueno, I., and Katsuyama, T.: Fibrinogen Matsumoto I; a γ364 Asp→His (GAT-CAT) substitution associated with defective fibrin polymerization. Thromb. Haemost. 75:887, 1996.

225. Bentolila, S., Samama, M.M., Conard, J., Horellou, M.H., and Ffrench, P.: Association of dysfibrinogenemia and thrombosis. Apropos of a family (fibrinogen Melun) and review of the literature [in French]. Ann. Med. Interne (Paris) 146:575, 1995.

226. Matsuda, M., Baba, M., Morimoto, K., and Nakamikawa, C.: An abnormal fibrinogen with an impaired polymerization site on the aligned DD domain of fibrin molecules. J. Clin. Invest. 72:1034, 1983.

227. Matsuda, M., Nakamikawa, C., Baba, M., and Morimoto, K.: Fibrinogen Tokyo II: an abnormal fibrinogen with an impaired polymerization site on the aligned DD domain of fibrin molecules. In Henschen, A., Hessel, B., McDonagh, J., and Saldeen, T. (eds.): Fibrinogen—Structural Variants and Interactions. Berlin, Walter de Gruyter, 1985, pp. 213–222.

228. Terukina, S., Matsuda, M., Hirata, H., Takeda, Y., Miyata, T., Takao, T., and Shimonishi, Y.: Substitution of γArg-275 by Cys in an abnormal fibrinogen, "fibrinogen Osaka II"; evidence for a unique solitary cystine structure at the mutation site. J. Biol. Chem. 263:13579, 1988.

229. Mosesson, M., Siebenlist, K., DiOrio, J., Matsuda, M., Hainfeld, J.F., and Wall, J.S.: The role of fibrinogen D domain intermolecular association sites in the polymerization of fibrin and fibrinogen Tokyo II (γ275 Arg→Cys). J. Clin. Invest. 96:1053, 1995.

230. Liu, C.Y., Koehne, J.A., and Morgan, F.J.: Characterization of fibrinogen New York I. J. Biol. Chem. 260:4390. 1985.

231. Mosesson, M.W., Siebenblist, K.R., Diorio, J.P., Hainfeld, J., Wall,

J.S., Soria, J., Soria, C., and Samama, M.: Evidence that proximal NH₂-terminal portions of fibrinogen Metz (A α 16 Arg → Cys) A α chains are oriented in the same direction. In Müller-Berghaus, G. (ed.): Fibrinogen and Its Derivatives. Amsterdam, Elsevier Science, 1986, pp. 3–15.

232. Koopman, J., Haverkate, F., Grimbergen, J., Engesser, L., Nováková, I., Kerst, A., and Lord, S.T.: Formation of fibrinogen-albumin and fibrinogen-fibrinogen complexes in abnormal fibrinogens by disulfide bridges. Fibrinogen IJmuiden (B β Arg 14 → Cys) and Nijmegen (B β Arg 44 → Cys). Proc. Natl. Acad. Sci. USA 89:3478, 1992.

233. Takagi, T., and Doolittle, R.F.: Amino acid sequence studies on plasmin-derived fragments of human fibrinogen: amino-terminal sequences of intermediate and terminal fragments. Biochemistry 14:940, 1975.

234. Kaudewitz, H., Henschen, A., Pirkle, H., Heaton, D., Soria, J., and Soria, C.: Structure function relationships in abnormal fibrinogen with Bβ 14 Arg → Cys substitution; fibrinogens Seattle I and Christchurch II [abstract 1901]. Thromb. Haemost. 58:515, 1987.

235. Yoshida, N., Wada, H., Morita, K., Hirata, H., Matsuda, M., Yamazumi, K., Asakura, S., and Shirakawa, S.: A new congenital abnormal fibrinogen Ise characterized by the replacement of B β glycine-15 by cysteine. Blood 77:1958, 1991.

236. Menache, D.: Constitutional and abnormal fibrinogen. Thromb. Diath. Haemorrh. Suppl. 13:173, 1964.

237. Rosenberg, J.B., Newman, P.J., Mosesson, M.W., Guillen, M.-C., and Amrani, D.L.: Paris I dysfibrinogenemia: a point mutation in intron results in insertion of a 15 amino acid sequence in the fibrinogen γ chain. Thromb. Haemost. 69:217, 1993.

238. Koopman, J., Haverkate, F., Briet, E., and Lord, S.T.: A congenitally abnormal fibrinogen (Vlissingen) with a 6-base deletion in the γ-chain gene, causing defective calcium binding and impaired fibrin polymerization. J. Biol. Chem. 266:13456, 1991.

239. Koopman, J., Haverkate, F., Grimbergen, J., Egbring, R., and Lord, S.T.: Fibrinogen Marburg: a homozygous case of dysfibrinogenemia, lacking amino acids Aα 461–610 (Lys 461 AAA → Stop TAA). Blood 80:1972, 1992.

240. Uemichi, T., Liepnieks, J.J., Yamada, T., Gertz, M.A., Bang, N., and Benson, M.D.: A frame shift mutation in the fibrinogen Aα chain gene in a kindred with renal amyloidosis. Blood 87:4197, 1996.

241. Benson, M.D., Liepnieks, J., Uemichi, T., Wheeler, G., and Correa, R.: Hereditary renal amyloidosis associated with a mutant fibrinogen α-chain. Nat. Genet. 3:252, 1993.

242. Uemichi, T.M., Liepnieks, J.J., and Benson, M.D.: Hereditary renal amyloidosis with a novel variant fibrinogen. J. Clin. Invest. 93:731, 1994.

243. Brennan, S.O., Hammonds, B., and George, P.M.: Aberrant hepatic processing causes removal of activation peptide and primary polymerisation site from fibrinogen Canterbury (A α 20 Val → Asp). J. Clin. Invest. 96:2854, 1995.

244. Lord, S.T.: Expression of a cloned human fibrinogen cDNA in Escherichia coli: synthesis of an A alpha polypeptide. DNA 4:33, 1985.

245. Farrell, D.H., Mulvihill, E.R., Huang, S., Chung, D.W., and Davie, E.W.: Recombinant human fibrinogen and sulfation of the γ' chain. Biochemistry 30:9414, 1991.

246. Roy, S.N., Procyk, R., Kudryk, B.J., and Redman, C.M.: Assembly and secretion of recombinant human fibrinogen. J. Biol. Chem. 266:4758, 1991.

247. Lord, S.T., Strickland, E., and Jaycock, E.: Strategy for recombinant multichain protein synthesis: fibrinogen B β chain variants and thrombin substrates. Biochemistry 35:2342, 1996.

248. Suh, T.T., Holmback, K., Jensen, N.J., Daugherty, C.C., Small, K., Simon, D.I., Potter, S.S., and Degen, J.L.: Resolution of spontaneous bleeding but failure of pregnancy in fibrinogen-deficient mice. Genes Dev. 9:2020, 1995.

249. Bugge, T.H., Flick, M.J., Daugherty, C.C., and Degen, J.L.: Plasminogen deficiency causes severe thrombosis but is compatible with development and reproduction. Genes Dev. 9:794, 1995.

250. Bugge, T.H., Kombrinck, K.W., Flick, M.J., Daugherty, C.C., Danton, J.J.S., and Degen, J.L.: Loss of fibrinogen rescues mice from the pleiotropic effects of plasminogen deficiency. Cell 87:709, 1996.

251. Al-Mondhiry, H.A.B., Bilezikian, S.B., and Nossel H.L.: Fibrinogen "New York"—an abnormal fibrinogen associated with thromboembolism: functional evaluation. Blood 45:607, 1975.

252. Liu, C.Y., Nossel, H.L., and Kaplan, K.L.: The binding of thrombin by fibrin. J. Biol. Chem. 254:10421, 1979.

253. Laurell, C.-B., and Thulin, E.: Complexes in human plasma between α_1-antitrypsin and IgA, and α_1-antitrypsin and fibrinogen. Scand. J. Immunol. 4(suppl. 2):7, 1975.

254. Kimura, S., and Aoki, N.: Cross-linking site in fibrinogen for α_2-plasmin inhibitor. J. Biol. Chem. 261:15591, 1986.

255. Baenziger, N.L., Brodie, G.N., and Majerus, P.W.: A thrombin sensitive protein of human platelet membranes. Proc. Natl. Acad. Sci. USA 68:240, 1971.

256. Lawler, J.W., Slayter, H.S.L., and Coligan, J.E.: Isolation and characterization of high molecular weight glycoprotein from human platelets. J. Biol. Chem. 253:8609, 1978.

257. Hogg, P.J., Stenflo, J., and Mosher, D.F.: Thrombospondin is a slow tight-binding inhibitor of plasmin. Biochemistry 31:265, 1992.

258. Tuszynski, G.P., Srivastava, S., Switalska, I., Holt, J.C., Cierniewski, C.S., and Niewiarowski, S.: The interaction of human platelet thrombospondin with fibrinogen. J. Biol. Chem. 260:12240, 1985.

259. Bale, M.D., and Mosher, D.F.: Effects of thrombospondin on fibrin polymerization and structure. J. Biol. Chem. 261:862, 1986.

260. Bacon-Baguley, T., Ogilvie, M.L., Gartner, T.K., and Walz, D.A.: Thrombospondin binding to specific sequences within the Aα- and Bβ-chains of fibrinogen. J. Biol. Chem. 265:2317, 1990.

261. Plow, E.F., Srouji, A.H., Meyer, D., Marguerie, G., and Ginsberg, M.H.: Evidence that three adhesive proteins interact with a common recognition site on activated platelets. J. Biol. Chem. 259:5388, 1984.

262. Holt, J.C., Mahmoud, M., and Gaffney, P.J.: The ability of fibrinogen fragments to support ADP-induced platelet aggregation. Thromb. Res. 16:427, 1979.

263. Hawiger, J., Timmons, S., Kloczewiak, M., Strong, D.D., and Doolittle, R.F.: γ and α chains of human fibrinogen possess sites reactive with human platelet receptors. Proc. Natl. Acad. Sci. USA 79:2068, 1982.

264. Hawiger, J., Kloczewiak, M., Bednarek, M.A., and Timmons, S.: Platelet receptor recognition domains on the α chain of human fibrinogen: structure-function analysis. Biochemistry 28:2909, 1989.

265. Cheresh, D.A., Berliner, S.A., Vicente, V., and Ruggeri, Z.M.: Recognition of distinct adhesive sites on fibrinogen by related integrins on platelets and endothelial cells. Cell 58:945, 1989.

266. Huang, T.-F., Holt, J.C., Lukasiewicz, H., and Niewiarowski, S.: Trigramin. A low molecular weight peptide inhibiting fibrinogen interaction with platelet receptors expressed on glycoprotein IIb-IIIa complex. J. Biol. Chem. 262:16157, 1987.

267. Farrell, D.H., and Thiagarajan, P.: Binding of recombinant fibrinogen mutants to platelets. J. Biol. Chem. 269:226, 1994.

268. Holmbäck, K., Danton, M.J.S., Suh, T.T., Daugherty, C.C., and Degen, J.L.: Impaired platelet aggregation and sustained bleeding in mice lacking the fibrinogen motif bound by integrin $\alpha_{IIb}\beta_3$. EMBO J. 15:5760, 1996.

269. Cheresh, D.A.: Human endothelial cells synthesize and express an Arg-Gly-Asp–directed adhesion receptor involved in attachment to fibrinogen and von Willebrand factor. Proc. Natl. Acad. Sci. USA 84:6471, 1987.

270. Thiagarajan, P., Rippon, A.J., and Farrell, D.H.: Alternative adhesion sites in human fibrinogen for vascular endothelial cells. Biochemistry 35:4169, 1996.

271. Blystone, S.D., Weston, L.K., and Kaplan, J.E.: Fibronectin dependent macrophage fibrin binding. Blood 78:2900, 1991.

272. Gonda, S.R., and Shainoff, J.R.: Adsorptive endocytosis of fibrin monomer by macrophages: evidence of a receptor for the amino terminus of the fibrin α chain. Proc. Natl. Acad. Sci. USA 79:4565, 1982.

273. Duthie, E.S.: The action of fibrinogen on certain pathogenic cocci. J. Gen. Microbiol. 13:383, 1955.

274. Hawiger, J., Timmons, S., Strong, D.D., Cottrell, B.A., Riley, M., and Doolittle, R.F.: Identification of a region of human fibrinogen interacting with staphylococcal clumping factor. Biochemistry 21:1407, 1982.

275. Strong, D.D., Laudano, A.P., Hawiger, J., and Doolittle, R.F.: Isolation, characterization, and synthesis of peptides from human fibrinogen that block the staphylococcal clumping reaction and construction of a synthetic clumping particle. Biochemistry 21:1414, 1982.

276. Toy, P.T.C.Y., Lai, L.-W., Drake, T.A., and Sande, M.A.: Effect of fibronectin on adherence of *Staphylococcus aureus* to fibrin thrombi in vitro. Infect. Immun. 48:83, 1985.

277. Cheung, A.L., Krishnan, M., Jaffe, E.A., and Fischetti, V.A.: Fibrinogen acts as a bridging molecule in the adherence of *Staphylococcus aureus* to cultured human endothelial cells. J. Clin. Invest. 87:2236, 1991.

278. Poirier, T.P., Kehoe, M.A., Whitnack, E., Dockter, M.E., and Beachey, E.H.: Fibrinogen binding and resistance to phagocytosis of *Streptococcus sanguis* expressing cloned M protein of *Streptococcus pyogenes*. Infect. Immun. 57:29, 1989.

279. Traore, M.Y., Valentin-Weigand, P., Chhatwal, G.S., and Blobel, H.: Inhibitory effects of fibrinogen on phagocytic killing of streptococcal isolates from humans, cattle and horses. Vet. Microbiol. 28:295, 1991.

280. Lantz, M.S., Allen, R.D., Bounelis, P., Switalski, L.M., and Hook, M.: *Bacteroides gingivalis* and *Bacteroides intermedius* recognize different sites on human fibrinogen. J. Bacteriol. 172:716, 1990.

281. Putnam, F.W.: Perspectives—past, present, and future. *In* Putnam, F.W. (ed.): The Plasma Proteins. 2nd ed. Vol. 1. New York, Academic Press, 1975, pp. 1–55.

282. Putnam, F.W.: Alpha, beta, gamma, omega—the structure of the plasma proteins. *In* Putnam, F.W. (ed.): The Plasma Proteins. 2nd ed. Vol. 4. New York, Academic Press, 1984, pp. 45–166.

23 Fibrinolysis and the Control of Hemostasis

▼▼▼▼ H. R. Lijnen and D. Collen

▼ ▼

Introduction

Mammalian blood contains an enzymatic system capable of dissolving blood clots. This system, called the fibrinolytic or plasminogen/plasmin system, plays a role not only in the removal of fibrin from the vascular bed but also in other biological phenomena such as reproduction, embryogenesis, cell invasion, angiogenesis, and brain function. In addition, the fibrinolytic system may participate in thrombosis, restenosis, atherosclerosis, neoplasia, metastasis, and chronic lung or kidney inflammatory disorders.[1-4]

The fibrinolytic system (Fig. 23–1) contains a proenzyme, plasminogen, that by the action of plasminogen activators is converted to the active enzyme plasmin, which in turn digests fibrin to soluble degradation products. Two immunologically distinct physiological plasminogen activators (PAs) have been identified: the tissue-type PA (t-PA) and the urokinase-type PA (u-PA). t-PA-Mediated plasminogen activation is mainly involved in the dissolution of fibrin in the circulation.[1] u-PA Binds to a specific cellular receptor (u-PAR), resulting in enhanced activation of cell-bound plas-

minogen. The main role of u-PA appears to be in the induction of pericellular proteolysis via the degradation of matrix components or via activation of latent proteases or growth factors during events such as tissue remodeling and repair, macrophage function, ovulation, embryo implantation, and tumor invasion.[2, 3, 5] A u-PAR-independent function of u-PA has also been demonstrated in fibrin clearance[6] and in arterial neointima formation.[3] Inhibition of the fibrinolytic system may occur either at the level of the PA, by specific plasminogen activator inhibitors (PAIs), or at the level of plasmin, mainly by α₂ antiplasmin. Physiological fibrinolysis is regulated by specific molecular interactions between its main components as well as by controlled synthesis and release, presumably primarily from endothelial cells, of PAs and PAIs.

The physiological plasminogen activators, t-PA and single-chain u-PA (scu-PA), activate plasminogen preferentially at the fibrin surface. Plasmin, associated with the fibrin surface, is protected from rapid inhibition by α₂ antiplasmin and may thus efficiently degrade the fibrin of a thrombus.[1, 7] Some of the properties of the main components of the

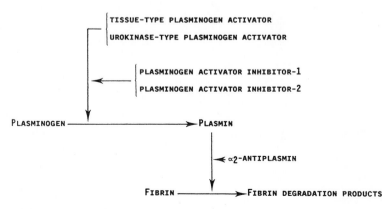

Figure 23–1. Schematic Representation of the Fibrinolytic System. The proenzyme plasminogen is activated to the active enzyme plasmin by tissue-type or urokinase-type plasminogen activator. Plasmin degrades fibrin into soluble fibrin degradation products. Inhibition of the fibrinolytic system may occur at the level of the plasminogen activators, by plasminogen activator inhibitors, or at the level of plasmin, mainly by α₂ antiplasmin.

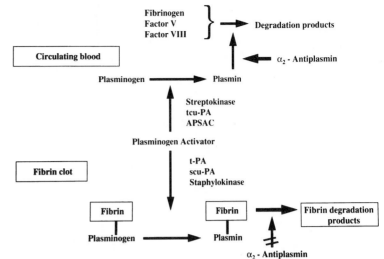

Figure 23–2. Molecular Interactions Determining the Fibrin Specificity of Plasminogen Activators. Non-fibrin-specific plasminogen activators (streptokinase, tcu-PA, APSAC) activate both plasminogen in the fluid phase and fibrin-associated plasminogen. Fibrin-specific plasminogen activators (t-PA, scu-PA, staphylokinase, and to a lesser extent reteplase) preferentially activate fibrin-associated plasminogen.

fibrinolytic system are summarized in Table 23–1, and the molecular interactions determining the fibrin specificity are illustrated in Figure 23–2.

Components of the Fibrinolytic System

▼ PLASMINOGEN

Physicochemical Properties. Human plasminogen (Fig. 23–3) is a single-chain glycoprotein with M_r of 92,000, present in plasma at a concentration of 1.5 to 2 μM. It is synthesized by the liver and cleared from the circulation (via the liver) with a half-life of about 2.2 days. It consists of 791 amino acids and contains five homologous triple-loop structures or "kringles."[8]

Native plasminogen, with NH_2-terminal glutamic acid ("Glu-plasminogen"), is readily converted by limited plasmic digestion to modified forms commonly designated "Lys-plasminogen." This conversion occurs by hydrolysis of the Arg^{68}-Met^{69}, Lys^{77}-Lys^{78}, or Lys^{78}-Val^{79} peptide bonds. Plasminogen is converted to plasmin by cleavage of the Arg^{561}-Val^{562} peptide bond. The plasmin molecule is a two chain trypsin-like serine proteinase with an active site composed

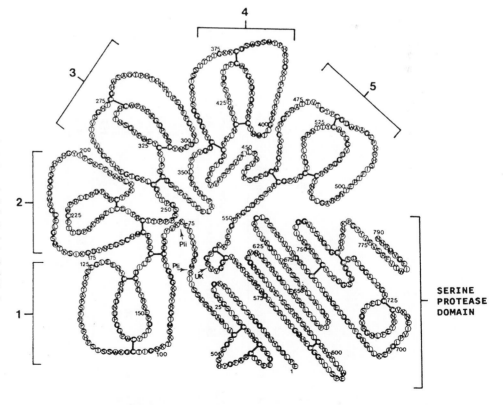

Figure 23–3. Schematic Representation of the Primary Structure of Plasminogen. *Pli,* indicates plasmic cleavage sites for conversion of Glu-plasminogen to Lys-plasminogen; *UK,* cleavage site for plasminogen activators, yielding plasmin. The amino acids are represented by their single-letter symbols and black bars indicate disulfide bonds. The cDNA sequence has revealed that the protein contains 791 amino acids, as a result of the presence of an extra isoleucine at position 65. (Modified from Forsgren, M., et al.: FEBS Lett. 213:254, 1987.)

1-5 : KRINGLE DOMAINS

Table 23–1. Some Properties of the Main Components of the Fibrinolytic System

	M_r (kDa)	Carbohydrate Content (%)	Number of Amino Acids	Catalytic Triad	Reactive Site	Plasma Concentration (mg/l)	Gene Length (kb)	mRNA (kb)	Exons (Number)	Chromosomal Location
Plasminogen	92	2	791	—	—	200	52.5	2.7	19	6
Plasmin	85	2	±715	His[603], Asp[646], Ser[741]	—	—	—	—	—	—
t-PA	68	7	530 (527)*	His[322], Asp[371], Ser[478]	—	0.005	36.6	2.7	14	8
u-PA	54	7	411	His[204], Asp[255], Ser[356]	—	0.008	6.4	2.4	11	10
u-PAR	55–60	± 35	313	—	—	—	23	1.4	7	19
α_2 Antiplasmin	70	13	464	—	Arg[376]-Met[377]	70	16	2.2	10	18
PAI-1	52	ND	379	—	Arg[346]-Met[347]	0.05	12.2	2.4;3.2	9	7
PAI-2	47; 60	ND	393	—	Arg[358]-Thr[359]	<0.005	16.5	1.9	8	18

*The numbering of amino acid residues is usually based on the initially determined incorrect value.
t-PA, tissue-type plasminogen activator; u-PA, urokinase-type plasminogen activator; u-PAR, u-PA receptor; PAI-1, plasminogen activator inhibitor 1; PAI-2, plasminogen activator inhibitor 2; ND, not determined.

of His[603], Asp[646], and Ser[741].[8] Activation of Glu-plasminogen in human plasma appears to occur primarily by direct cleavage of the Arg[561]-Val[562] peptide bond, without generation of Lys-plasminogen intermediates.[9]

The kringles of plasminogen contain lysine binding sites, which interact specifically with amino acids such as lysine and 6-aminohexanoic acid. The lysine binding sites located in the kringle 1–3 region mediate the specific binding of plasminogen to fibrin and the interaction of plasmin with α_2 antiplasmin and play a crucial role in the regulation of fibrinolysis.[7, 10] A plasminogen fragment containing kringle 1–4 (angiostatin) has been reported to have antiangiogenic properties.[11]

Gene Structure. The coding region of the human plasminogen complementary DNA (cDNA) contains an amino-terminal sequence of 19 amino acids with the characteristics of a signal sequence and a mature protein sequence of 791 amino acids.[8] The plasminogen gene spans 52.5 kb, containing 19 exons, and is located on the long arm of chromosome 6 at band q26 or q27.[12, 13] Each of the five kringles is encoded by two separate exons with a single intron in the middle of each structure. The gene organization for the light chain of plasminogen is similar to that of other serine proteinases, such as t-PA, urokinase, and factor XII.[13] The gene coding for plasminogen is also closely related to that of apolipoprotein (a): The 5'-untranslated and flanking sequences contain extensive regions of near identify.[14]

Polymorphism. The heterogeneity of plasminogen in human plasma appears to be genetically controlled. Plasminogen is coded by an autosomal gene with 2 common (Plg*A and Plg*B) and about 11 rare alleles.[15] The allele frequencies differ substantially in various racial groups but are fairly

constant within one race.[16] In the European populations the distribution is roughly the following: common *PLG** A = 0.70, common *PLG** B = 0.28, and rare *PLG** = 0.020. The *PLG* B variant found in Japanese (allele frequency 0.022) was shown to have a normal antigen level but reduced activity to approximately 40 per cent of normal.[17]

▼ PLASMINOGEN ACTIVATORS

Tissue-Type Plasminogen Activator

Physicochemical Properties. Tissue-type plasminogen activator (t-PA) is a serine proteinase with M_r about 70,000, originally isolated as a single polypeptide chain of 527 amino acids (Fig. 23–4).[18] It was subsequently shown that native t-PA contains an NH$_2$-terminal extension of three amino acids (Gly-Ala-Arg-). t-PA Is converted by plasmin to a two chain form by hydrolysis of the Arg[275]-Ile[276] peptide bond. The NH$_2$-terminal region is composed of several domains with homologies to other proteins: a finger domain comprising residues 4–50, a growth factor domain comprising residues 50–87, and two kringles comprising residues 87–176 and 176–262. The region constituted by residues 276–527 represents the serine proteinase part with the catalytic site, composed of His[322], Asp[371], and Ser[478].[18] These distinct domains in t-PA are involved in several functions of the enzyme, including its binding to fibrin, fibrin-specific plasminogen activation, rapid clearance in vivo, and binding to endothelial cell receptors. Binding of t-PA to fibrin is mediated via the finger and second kringle domains.[19] The t-PA molecule comprises three potential N-glycosylation sites, at Asn[117], Asn[184], and Asn[448]. t-PA Preparations usually

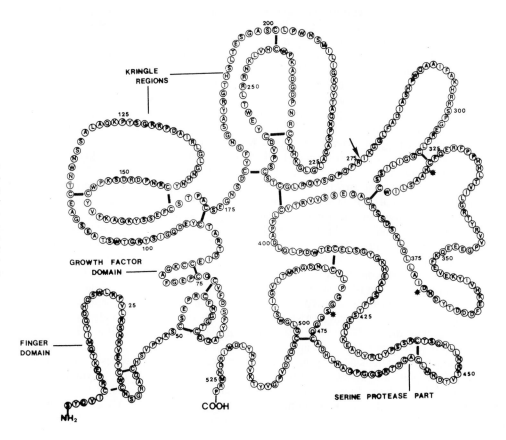

Figure 23–4. Schematic Representation of the Primary Structure of t-PA. The amino acids are represented by their single-letter symbols and black bars indicate disulfide bonds. The active site residues His[322], Asp[371], and Ser[478] are indicated with an asterisk. The arrow indicates the plasmin cleavage site for conversion of single-chain t-PA to two-chain t-PA.

contain a mixture of variant I (with all three glycosylation sites) and variant II (lacking carbohydrate at Asn[184]).[18] In contrast to the single-chain precursor form of most serine proteinases, single-chain t-PA is enzymatically active. Amino acid Lys[156] was shown to contribute directly to the enzymatic activity of the single-chain molecule, by forming a salt bridge with Asp[194] that selectively stabilizes the active conformation.[20]

Gene Structure. The human t-PA gene is localized on chromosome 8 (bands 8.p.12 → q.11.2),[21] and more than 36 kb of its sequence has been determined. It consists of 14 exons, and the intron-exon organization suggests that the assembly occurred according to the "exon shuffling" principle, whereby the distinct structural domains are encoded by a single exon or by adjacent exons.[22] The proximal promoter sequences contain typical TATA and CAAT boxes and potential recognition sequences for transcription factors (e.g., AP1, NF1, Sp1, AP2); consensus sequences of a cyclic adenosine monophosphate–(cAMP)-responsive element and of a AP2 binding site, which may have a cooperative effect on constitutive t-PA gene expression, have been identified.[23]

The complete 2530-base pair cDNA sequence of mature t-PA contains a single reading frame, beginning with the ATG codon at nucleotides 85 to 87.[18] This ATG probably serves as the site of translation initiation and is followed, 562 codons later, by a TGA termination triplet at nucleotides 1771 to 1773. The NH₂-terminal amino acid is preceded by 20 to 23 amino acids (residues -35 to -13), which probably constitute a hydrophobic signal peptide involved in the secretion of t-PA. The remaining hydrophobic amino acids immediately preceding the start of mature t-PA (residues -14 to -1) may constitute a "pro" sequence similar to that found for serum albumin.

Synthesis and Secretion. Vascular endothelial cells synthesize and secrete t-PA into the circulating blood. The plasma concentration of t-PA antigen is about 5 ng/ml. Stimulation of vascular endothelium by venous occlusion, infusion of desmopressin acetate (DDAVP) or epinephrine, and physical exercise result in rapid release (within minutes) of t-PA. This response probably reflects release from cellular storage pools, although such a storage pool has not been conclusively identified.

A variety of agents have been shown to increase the synthesis of t-PA by cultured endothelial cells, including thrombin, histamine, butyrate, phorbol myristate acetate (PMA), basic fibroblast growth factor, activated protein C, butanol and alcohol derivatives, and retinoids. However, only histamine, butyrate, or a combination of cAMP with protein kinase C agonists exclusively stimulates t-PA synthesis without affecting plasminogen activator inhibitor 1 (PAI-1) synthesis.[24, 25]

The mechanisms involved in the stimulatory effect of these various agents on t-PA synthesis appear to be different and are now gradually elucidated. Recently, a functional retinoic acid response element (RARE), which consists of a direct repeat of the GGTCA motif spaced by 5 nucleotides (DR5), has been localized 7.3 kb upstream of the transcription start site of the human t-PA gene. This element mediates the direct regulation by retinoic acid in human fibrosarcoma, endothelial, and neuroblastoma cells.[26] Vasoactive substances, such as histamine and thrombin, bind to specific receptors and activate phospholipase C, which acts on phosphatidylinositol biphosphate to produce diacylglycerol. Diacylglycerol activates membrane-bound protein kinase C, which plays an important role in the regulation of t-PA synthesis. This is suggested by the findings that direct activation of protein kinase C by phorbol esters induces t-PA synthesis, whereas suppression of protein kinase C impairs the increase in t-PA synthesis by histamine and by PMA.[27] The increase of t-PA induced by histamine, thrombin, and PMA in endothelial cells is paralleled by increased levels of messenger RNA (mRNA), as a result of enhanced transcription of the t-PA gene.[28] Overexpression of t-PA in endothelial cells using viral expression vectors could increase local fibrinolysis and may become useful for in vivo therapeutic interventions.

Pharmacokinetic Properties. Rapid clearance of t-PA in man (initial half-life of 6 min) is the result of interaction with several receptor systems. Liver endothelial cells have a mannose receptor that recognizes the high mannose-type carbohydrate side chain at Asn[117] in the kringle 1 domain, whereas liver parenchymal cells contain a calcium-dependent receptor that interacts mainly with the growth factor domain of t-PA.[29] In addition, the low density lipoprotein receptor-related protein (LRP), expressed in high copy number on hepatocytes, binds free t-PA and complexes with PAI-1.[30]

Urokinase-Type Plasminogen Activator

Physicochemical Properties. Urokinase-type plasminogen activator (u-PA) is secreted as a single-chain molecule (scu-PA, prourokinase) that can be converted to a two chain form (tcu-PA). scu-PA Is a serine proteinase of 411 amino acids, with active site triad His[204], Asp[255], and Ser[356].[31] The molecule contains an NH₂-terminal growth factor domain and one kringle structure homologous to the five kringles found in plasminogen and the two kringles in t-PA (Fig. 23–5).[32] u-PA Contains only one N-glycosylation site (at Asn[302]) and contains a fucosylated threonine residue at position 18. Conversion of scu-PA to tcu-PA occurs after proteolytic cleavage at position Lys[158]-Ile[159] by plasmin, but also by kallikrein, trypsin, cathepsin B, human T-cell associated serine proteinase 1, and thermolysin. A fully active tcu-PA derivative is obtained after additional proteolysis by plasmin at position Lys[135]-Lys[136]. A low molecular weight form of scu-PA (32 kDa) can be obtained by selective cleavage at position Glu[143]-Leu[144];[33] this cleavage can be obtained with matrix metalloproteinase 7. In contrast, scu-PA is converted to an inactive two chain molecule by thrombin after proteolytic cleavage at position Arg[156]-Phe[157]. This inactivation is strongly enhanced in the presence of thrombomodulin and is dependent on the 0-linked glucosaminoglycan of thrombomodulin.[34]

Gene Structure. The cDNA of u-PA has been isolated and the nucleotide sequence determined.[32] The cDNA sequence contains an open reading frame that starts with ATG at nucleotide positions 77 to 79 and extends for 1293 nucleotides until a TGA stop codon is reached at positions 1370 to 1372. The open reading frame is preceded by at least 76 nucleotides of 5′-untranslated mRNA, very rich in G/C nucleotides. Beyond the termination codon, the cDNA extends for another 932 nucleotides. The sequence includes two AATAAAA polyadenylation signals (positions 2271–2276 and 2284–2289), preceding the polyadenylation site at posi-

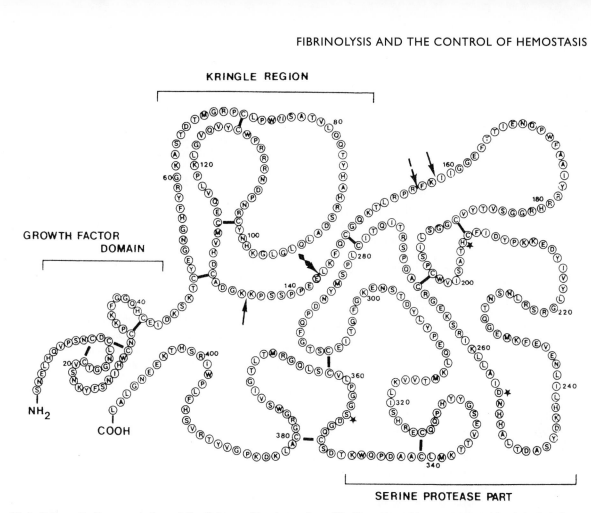

Figure 23–5. Schematic Representation of the Primary Structure of scu-PA. The amino acids are represented by their single letter symbols and black bars indicate disulfide bonds. The active site residues His[204], Asp[255], and Ser[356] are indicated with an asterisk. The arrows indicate the plasmin cleavage sites for conversion of M_r 54,000 scu-PA to M_r 54,000 tcu-PA (Lys[158]-Ile[159]) and of M_r 54,000 tcu-PA to M_r 33,000 tcu-PA (Lys[135]-Lys[136]), for conversion to inactive M_r 54,000 tcu-PA by thrombin (Arg[156]-Phe[157]) and for conversion to M_r 32,000 scu-PA (Glu[143]-Leu[144]).

tion 2304. The human u-PA gene is 6.4 kb long and located on chromosome 10.[21] It contains 11 exons, and the intron-exon organization of the gene closely resembles that of the t-PA gene.[35] However, exons III, VIII, and IX of t-PA are totally, and exon IV partially, missing in the u-PA gene; this accounts for the absence of a finger domain and a second kringle in u-PA. Exon II of the u-PA gene codes for a signal peptide consisting of 20 amino acids; exons III and IV code for the growth factor domain and exons V and VI for the kringle region. The 5′ region of exon VII, which codes for the peptide connecting the light and the heavy chain, is 39 bp longer than the corresponding exon X of the t-PA gene. The 3′-region of exon VII and exons VIII to XI code for the heavy chain.

Pharmacokinetic Properties. Whereas the synthesis of t-PA occurs mainly in endothelial cells, immunocytochemical staining of tissues indicates that many cells of different origin (i.e., fibroblasts, epithelial cells, pneumocytes) produce u-PA.[36] The scu-PA concentration in human plasma ranges between 2 and 20 ng/ml.

The main mechanism of removal of u-PA from the blood (initial half-life in man of 4 to 5 min) appears to be hepatic clearance. scu-PA Is taken up in the liver via a recognition site on parenchymal cells and is subsequently degraded in the lysosomes.[37]

Streptokinase and Anisoylated Plasminogen-Streptokinase Activator Complex

Physicochemical Properties. Streptokinase is a non-enzyme protein produced by several strains of hemolytic streptococci. It consists of a single polypeptide chain of 47 to 50 kDa containing 414 amino acids.[38] Streptokinase activates plasminogen indirectly after a three step mechanism.[39] In the first step, streptokinase forms an equimolar complex with plasminogen, which undergoes a conformational change, resulting in the exposure of an active site in the plasminogen moiety. In the second step, this active site catalyzes the activation of plasminogen to plasmin. In a third step, plasminogen-streptokinase molecules are converted to plasmin-streptokinase complexes.

The equimolar plasminogen-streptokinase complex converts rapidly to the plasmin-streptokinase complex by proteolytic cleavage of both the plasminogen and the streptokinase moieties. In human plasminogen, the Arg[561]-Val[562] and the Lys[77]-Lys[78] peptide bonds are cleaved, and a major proteolytic derivative of 36 kDa is generated from streptokinase.[40] The active site residues in the plasmin-streptokinase complex are the same as those in the plasmin molecule. The main differences between the enzymatic properties of plasmin and those of the plasmin-streptokinase complex are found in their interaction with plasminogen and with α_2 antiplasmin. Plasmin, in contrast to its complex with streptokinase, is unable to activate plasminogen, and it is rapidly neutralized by α_2 antiplasmin, which does not inhibit the plasmin(ogen)-streptokinase complex.

The elimination half-life of streptokinase in man is approximately 20 min (initial half-life of 4 min and terminal half-life of 30 min).[41] The level of antistreptokinase antibodies from previous infections with β hemolytic streptococci varies greatly among individuals. A few days after streptokinase administration, the antistreptokinase titer rises rapidly to 50 to 100 times the preinfusion value and remains high for at least 4 to 6 months, during which period renewed thrombolytic treatment with streptokinase or compounds containing streptokinase is impractical.

Anisoylated plasminogen-streptokinase activator complex (APSAC) was constructed with the intention to control the enzymatic activity of the plasmin(ogen)-streptokinase complex by a specific reversible chemical protection of its catalytic center. This approach should prevent premature neutralization of the agent in the blood stream and enable its activation to proceed in a controlled and sustained manner.[42] Anistreplase (APSAC, Eminase) is an equimolar non-covalent complex between human Lys-plasminogen and streptokinase. The acylated catalytic center is located in the COOH-terminal region of plasminogen, whereas the lysine binding sites are contained within the NH$_2$-terminal region of the molecule. Reversible blocking of the catalytic site by acylation delays the formation of plasmin but has no influence on the lysine binding sites involved in binding of the complex to fibrin, although the affinity of plasminogen for fibrin is very weak. Deacylation starts immediately after dissolution of the lyophilized material and proceeds gradually after intravenous injection. Deacylation uncovers the catalytic center, which converts plasminogen to plasmin. This deacylation of the complex occurs both in the circulation and at the fibrin surface, and the fibrin specificity of thrombolysis by anistreplase is only marginal. In patients with acute myocardial infarction treated with anistreplase, half-lives of 90 to 112 minutes were reported for the plasma clearance of fibrinolytic activity.[43]

Staphylokinase

Staphylokinase, a plasminogen activator produced by certain strains of *Staphylococcus aureus,* was shown to have profibrinolytic properties more than four decades ago. Natural staphylokinase has been purified from *Staphylococcus aureus* strains that were transformed with bacteriophages containing the *staphylokinase* gene or that had undergone lysogenic conversion to staphylokinase production. In addition, the *staphylokinase* gene has been cloned from the bacteriophages *sakϕC* and *sak42D* as well as from the genomic DNA (*sak*STAR) of a lysogenic *S. aureus* strain.[44]

The *staphylokinase* gene encodes a protein of 163 amino acids with amino acid 28 corresponding to the NH$_2$-terminal residue of the mature protein, which consists of 136 amino acids in a single polypeptide chain without disulfide bridges. The mature proteins SakSTAR, SakϕC, and Sak42D differ in only three amino acids: Amino acid 34 is Ser in SakSTAR but Gly in SakϕC and Sak42D; amino acid 36 is Gly in SakSTAR and in SakϕC, but Arg in Sak42D; and amino

acid 43 is His in SakSTAR and in SakϕC, but Arg in Sak42D.[44]

In patients with acute myocardial infarction treated with an intravenous infusion of 10 mg staphylokinase (SakSTAR) over 30 minutes, the postinfusion disappearance of staphylokinase-related antigen from plasma occurred in a biphasic manner with a $t\frac{1}{2}\alpha$ of 6.3 minutes and a $t\frac{1}{2}\beta$ of 37 minutes, corresponding to a plasma clearance of 270 ml/min.[45]

▼ INHIBITORS OF THE FIBRINOLYTIC SYSTEM

Inhibition of the fibrinolytic system may occur at the level of plasmin or at the level of the plasminogen activators. α_2 Antiplasmin is the main physiological plasmin inhibitor in human plasma, whereas inhibition of the physiological plasminogen activators t-PA and u-PA occurs mainly by plasminogen activator inhibitor 1 (PAI-1) and plasminogen activator inhibitor 2 (PAI-2). Inhibition of fibrinolysis may also result from interference with the binding of plasminogen to fibrin by interaction with other plasma proteins (cf. below).

α_2 Antiplasmin

α_2 Antiplasmin is the main physiological plasmin inhibitor in human plasma, whereas plasmin formed in excess of α_2 antiplasmin may be neutralized by α_2 macroglobulin. α_2 Antiplasmin, a M_r 67,000 single-chain glycoprotein containing 464 amino acids and 13 per cent carbohydrate, is present in plasma at a concentration of about 1 μM. It is synthesized by the liver and cleared from the circulation (via the liver) with a half-life of 2.6 days. The reactive site of the inhibitor is the Arg^{376}-Met^{377} peptide bond. α_2 Antiplasmin is unique among serpins (serine proteinase inhibitors) in having a COOH-terminal extension of 51 amino acid residues.[46] This extension contains a secondary binding site that reacts with the lysine binding sites of plasminogen and plasmin. The plasminogen-binding form of α_2-antiplasmin becomes partly converted in the circulating blood to a non-plasminogen-binding, less reactive form (about 30 per cent of the total), which lacks the 26 COOH-terminal residues. Two forms of α_2 antiplasmin were detected in about equal amounts in purified preparations of the inhibitor[47]: a native 464 residue long inhibitor with NH$_2$-terminal methionine (Met^1-α_2 antiplasmin) and a 12 amino acids shorter form with NH$_2$-terminal asparagine (Asn^{13}-α_2 antiplasmin). It is not known whether Asn^{13}-α_2 antiplasmin is present in the circulating blood or whether it is generated in vitro. The NH$_2$-terminal Gln^{14} residue of α_2 antiplasmin can cross-link to Aα-chains of fibrin, in a process that requires Ca^{2+} and is catalyzed by activated coagulation factor XIII.[48]

α_2-Antiplasmin forms an inactive 1:1 stoichiometric complex with plasmin (Fig. 23–6). The inhibition of plasmin (P) by α_2 antiplasmin (A) can be represented by two consecutive reactions: a fast, second-order reaction producing a reversible inactive complex (PA), which is followed by a slower first-order transition resulting in an irreversible inactive complex (PA').

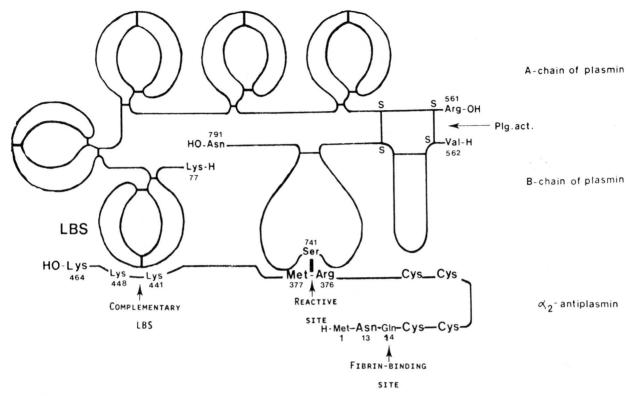

Figure 23–6. Schematic Representation of the Plasmin-α_2-Antiplasmin Complex. LSBI, high-affinity lysine binding site; Plg.act, site of cleavage by plasminogen activators.

This model can be represented by

$$ P + A \underset{k_{-1}}{\overset{k_1}{\rightleftharpoons}} \quad PA \overset{k_2}{\longrightarrow} PA' $$

The second-order rate constant of the inhibition is very high ($k_1 = 2\text{--}4 \times 10^7 \text{ M}^{-1} \text{ s}^{-1}$), but this high inhibition rate depends on the presence of free lysine binding sites and a free active site in the plasmin molecule and on the availability of a plasminogen binding site and of the reactive site peptide bond in the inhibitor. The half-life of plasmin molecules generated at the fibrin surface, which have both their lysine binding sites and active site occupied, is two to three orders of magnitude longer than that of free plasmin.[49]

The gene for human α_2 antiplasmin, located on chromosome 17p13, is approximately 16 kb and contains 10 exons.[50, 51] The NH$_2$-terminal region of the protein, comprising the fibrin cross-linking site, is encoded by exon IV, whereas both the reactive site and the plasminogen-binding site in the COOH-terminal region are encoded by exon X. A restriction fragment length polymorphism (RFLP), associated with the presence of two alleles, A and B, has been identified in the α_2-antiplasmin gene; allele B is the result of a 720 bp deletion in intron VIII.[52]

Plasminogen Activator Inhibitors

Plasminogen Activator Inhibitor I

Physicochemical Properties. Plasminogen activator 1 (PAI-1) was first identified in conditioned media of cultured human endothelial cells and subsequently in plasma, platelets, placenta, and conditioned media of fibrosarcoma cells and hepatocytes.[53] In healthy individuals, highly variable plasma levels of both PAI activity and PAI-1 antigen have been observed. PAI activity ranges from 0.5 to 47 U/ml (t-PA neutralizing units, 1 mg active PAI-1 corresponds to 700,000 units) with 80 per cent of the values below 6 U/ml. PAI-1 antigen ranges between 6 and 85 ng/ml (geometric mean 24 ng/ml). PAI-1 levels are strongly elevated in several thromboembolic disease states. (See Pathophysiology of Fibrinolysis.) PAI-1 is a single-chain glycoprotein with M_r about 52,000 consisting of 379 amino acids. The complementary DNA (cDNA) sequence reveals that PAI-1 is a member of the serpin family with reactive site peptide bond Arg^{346}-Met^{347}.[54] The PAI-1 gene, located on chromosome 7, bands q21.3-q22, is approximately 12.2 kb, and consists of nine exons.[55] As a result of alternative polyadenylation that yields an additional 3' untranslated region, a messenger RNA (mRNA) species of 3.2 kb occurs in addition to one of 2.4 kb.

PAI-1 is stabilized by binding to a plasminogen activator inhibitor binding protein identified as protein S or vitronectin.[56] The PAI-1 binding site on vitronectin was mapped to the region comprising residues Lys^{348} to Arg^{370}.[57]

PAI-1 reacts very rapidly with single-chain and two-chain t-PA and with two-chain u-PA, with second-order inhibition rate constants of the order of 10^7 M^{-1} s^{-1}, but it does not react with scu-PA.[53, 58] Like other serpins, PAI-1 inhibits its target proteinases by formation of a 1:1 stoichiometric reversible complex, followed by covalent binding between the hydroxyl group of the active site serine residue of the proteinase and the carboxyl group of the P1 residue at the reactive center ("bait region") of the serpin. The rapid inhibition of both t-PA and u-PA by PAI-1 involves a reversible high affinity second site interaction that does not depend on a functional active site.[59] The sequence 350–355 of PAI-1, which contains three negatively charged amino acids, interacts with highly positively charged regions in t-PA (residues 296–304)[60] or in u-PA (residues 179–184).[61] In the presence of fibrin, single-chain t-PA is protected from rapid inhibition by PAI-1.[59] It has, however, also been reported that PAI-1 binds to fibrin and that fibrin-bound PAI-1 may inhibit t-PA mediated clot lysis.[62]

PAI-1 occurs as an active inhibitory form that spontaneously converts to a latent form that can be partially reactivated by denaturing agents. The structural basis of the latency in PAI-1 has been resolved by determination of the structure by single-crystal X-ray diffraction. Part of the reactive center loop is inserted in the major β sheet of PAI-1 and is therefore not accessible to the target enzyme (locked conformation). Reactivation of latent PAI-1 by denaturants results in partial elimination of this insertion.[63] A molecular form of intact PAI-1 that has been isolated does not form stable complexes with t-PA but is cleaved at the P1-P1′ peptide bond (substrate PAI-1).[64] The X-ray structure of the cleaved substrate variant shows that it has a new β strand (s4A) formed by insertion of the NH$_2$-terminal portion of the reactive site loop into β sheet A subsequent to cleavage.[65] Thus, inhibitory PAI-1 may convert not only to latent PAI-1, which can be reactivated, but also to substrate PAI-1, which is irreversibly degraded by its target proteinases. This observation may thus have implications for the regulation of the fibrinolytic system.

Synthesis and Secretion. PAI-1 mRNA has been demonstrated in a large variety of tissues, suggesting that common cells in these tissues, such as endothelial or smooth muscle cells, may be the site of production. PAI-1 is found in plasma, platelets, placenta, and the extracellular matrix. Except for platelets, which contain essentially inactive PAI-1, PAI-1 is not stored within cells but is rapidly and constitutively secreted after synthesis. PAI-1 exhibits a circadian variation; its plasma concentration is highest in the morning and lowest in the late afternoon and evening, whereas t-PA exhibits an opposite diurnal variation.

Synthesis and secretion of PAI-1 can be modulated by various agonists such as hormones, growth factors, endotoxin, cytokines, and phorbol esters. Although post-transcriptional regulation of PAI-1 mRNA levels has been suggested, most studies on the regulation of PAI-1 expression demonstrated an effect at the transcriptional level. Alterations in mRNA stability may also contribute to increased PAI-1 levels in some cells. In endothelial cells PAI-1 gene expression is stimulated by lipopolysaccharide, interleukin-1 (IL-1), tumor necrosis factor α, transforming growth factor β, basic fibroblast growth factor, phorbol esters, thrombin, very low density lipoprotein, Lp(a), insulin, or proinsulin. Only a few studies have reported a downregulation of PAI-1 synthesis in endothelial cells, either by forskolin or by endothelial cell growth factor combined with heparin.[24, 25] Studies on the mechanism of the induction by phorbol esters suggested that it is mediated by two regulatory DNA sequences in the proximal promotor of the PAI-1 gene, which were called Box A and Box B.[66] Recently, the DNA encoding a novel transcription factor that selectively interacts with Box B and that is also involved in basal expression of PAI-1 was characterized. This factor has conserved helicase and RING finger domains and was called helicase-like transcription factor (HLTF).[67]

Plasminogen Activator Inhibitor 2

Plasminogen activator inhibitor 2 (PAI-2) levels in plasma are very low but are drastically elevated during pregnancy. PAI-2 exists in two different forms with comparable inhibitory properties that are derived from a single mRNA: an intracellular non-glycosylated form with M_r 47,000 and pI 5.0 and a secreted glycosylated form with M_r 60,000 and pI 4.4. The function of intracellular PAI-2 is unclear because its main target enzyme (u-PA) occurs extracellularly. It may constitute a storage pool from which PAI-2 can be secreted upon cell injury. The precise (patho)physiological role of PAI-2 remains to be determined.

PAI-2 is a serpin of 393 amino acids with reactive site peptide bond Arg[358]-Thr[359]. The PAI-2 gene, located on chromosome 18 bands q21–23, spans 16.5 kb and contains eight exons. The structure of the gene is different from that of the PAI-1 gene but is similar to that of the chicken ovalbumin gene.[68]

PAI-2 inhibits two-chain u-PA about 10-fold more slowly than PAI-1; it also efficiently inhibits two-chain t-PA and less efficiently single-chain t-PA, but it does not inhibit single-chain u-PA.[53] Secretion of PAI-2 is regulated by endotoxin and by phorbol esters that stimulate the gene transcription of PAI-2 more than 50-fold.[53]

Thrombin Activatable Fibrinolysis Inhibitor

The thrombin activatable fibrinolysis inhibitor (TAFI) is a M_r 60,000 single-chain protein, identical to plasma procarboxypeptidase B, occurring at a concentration of 75 nM.[69, 70] Thrombin, trypsin, or plasmin converts the protein to an active carboxypeptidase B. Activated TAFI suppresses fibrinolysis, most likely by removing COOH-terminal lysine residues from (partially degraded) fibrin, thereby preventing additional binding of plasminogen and/or t-PA to fibrin.[71]

▼ UROKINASE-TYPE PLASMINOGEN ACTIVATOR RECEPTOR

The specific cell surface receptor for u-PA is a heterogeneously glycosylated protein of M_r 50,000 to 60,000, synthesized as a 313 amino acid polypeptide, anchored to the plasma membrane by a glycosyl phosphatidylinositol (GPI) moiety that is attached at amino acid 282, 283, or 284. The u-PA receptor (u-PAR) molecule is composed of three distantly related structural domains, of which the NH$_2$-terminal domain is involved in binding u-PA; it binds all forms of u-PA containing an intact growth factor domain.[24]

Mechanisms of Fibrin-Specific Fibrinolysis

The fibrin specificity of the physiological plasminogen activators t-PA and scu-PA has triggered great interest in their use as thrombolytic agents. Fibrin-specific fibrinolysis has also been observed with the bacterial protein staphylokinase. The mechanism underlying the fibrin specificity of these agents is, however, different and is discussed below (see Fig. 23–2).

▼ TISSUE-TYPE PLASMINOGEN ACTIVATOR

In the Presence of Fibrin

Tissue-type plasminogen activator (t-PA) is a poor enzyme in the absence of fibrin, but the presence of fibrin strikingly enhances the activation rate of plasminogen.[72] During fibrinolysis, fibrinogen and fibrin itself are continuously modified by cleavage with thrombin or plasmin. Thrombin-catalyzed formation of desA-fibrin monomer, and desA-fibrin polymerization are essential for stimulation of plasminogen activation by t-PA. Optimal stimulation is only obtained after early plasmin cleavage in the COOH-terminal Aα-chain and the NH_2-terminal Bβ chain of fibrin, yielding fragment X polymer.[73] Kinetic data support a mechanism in which fibrin provides a surface to which t-PA and plasminogen adsorb in a sequential and ordered way, yielding a cyclic ternary complex (Fig. 23–7).[72] Formation of this complex results in an enhanced affinity of t-PA for plasminogen, yielding an up to three orders of magnitude higher catalytic efficiency for plasminogen activation. In agreement with this mechanism, the increase in fibrin stimulation after formation of fibrin X polymers is associated with an enhanced binding of t-PA and plasminogen, which is mediated in part by COOH-terminal lysine residues generated by plasmin cleavage. Interaction of these COOH-terminal lysines with lysine binding sites on t-PA and plasminogen may allow an improved alignment as well as allosteric changes of the t-PA and plasminogen moieties, thus enhancing the rate of plasminogen activation.

Proteins that compete with plasminogen for binding to

lysine residues on fibrin, such as lipoprotein (a) (Lp[a]),[74] or that remove these lysine residues, such as activated TAFI, may thereby have an antifibrinolytic action.[71]

At the Cell Surface

A striking analogy exists between the role of fibrin and that of cell surfaces in plasminogen activation. Many cell types bind plasminogen activators and plasminogen, resulting in enhanced plasminogen activation and protection of bound plasmin from inhibition by α_2 antiplasmin. Gangliosides,[75] as well as a class of membrane proteins with COOH-terminal lysine residues such as α-enolase,[76] play a role in binding of plasminogen to cells. The catalytic efficiency of t-PA for activation of cell bound plasminogen is about 10-fold higher than in solution, possibly as a result of conversion of the plasminogen conformation to the more readily activatable Lys-plasminogen-like structure. Alternatively, it was shown that vascular cells have the capacity to regulate pericellular fibrinolysis by modulating the expression of plasminogen receptors; increased receptor occupancy results in enhanced plasminogen activation by t-PA.[77]

A M_r 40,000 membrane protein (related to annexin II) was proposed as the functional t-PA receptor on human umbilical vein endothelial cells.[78] Cell surface bound t-PA retains its enzymatic activity and is protected from inhibition by PAI-1. Assembly of plasminogen and plasminogen activators at the endothelial cell surface thus provides a focal point for plasmin generation.

▼ UROKINASE-TYPE PLASMINOGEN ACTIVATOR

In the Presence of Fibrin

In contrast to two-chain u-PA (tcu-PA), the single-chain molecule (scu-PA) displays very low activity toward low molecular weight chromogenic substrates, but it appears to

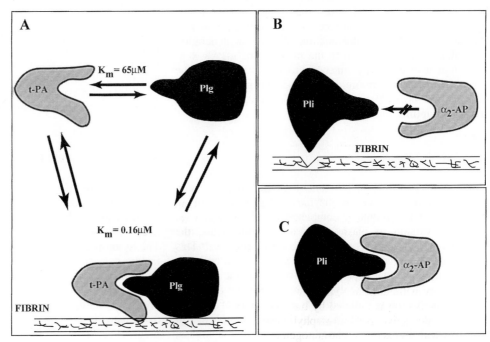

Figure 23–7. Schematic Representation of the Molecular Interactions That Regulate t-PA Mediated Plasminogen Activation at the Fibrin Surface. *A*, t-PA in circulating plasma has a low affinity for plasminogen *(Plg)* (K_m = 65 μM) and no efficient activation occurs. Both t-PA and plasminogen bind to fibrin and in this ternary complex t-PA has a high affinity for plasinogen (K_m = 0.16 μM). *B*, plasmin formed at the fibrin surface is protected from rapid inhibition by α_2 antiplasmin (α_2-AP) and efficiently degrades fibrin. *C*, in plasma, in the absence of fibrin plasmin is very rapidly inhibited by α_2 antiplasmin.

have some intrinsic plasminogen activating potential, which represents ≤ 0.5 per cent of the catalytic efficiency of tcu-PA.[79, 80] Other investigators, however, have claimed that scu-PA has no measurable intrinsic amidolytic or plasminogen activator activities.[81] The occurrence of a transitional state of scu-PA with a higher catalytic efficiency for native plasminogen than tcu-PA has also been postulated.[82] In plasma, in the absence of fibrin, scu-PA is stable and does not activate plasminogen; in the presence of a fibrin clot, scu-PA, but not tcu-PA, induces fibrin-specific clot lysis.[79] scu-PA Does not bind to a significant extent to fibrin, but its intrinsic activity toward fibrin-bound plasminogen may contribute to its fibrin specificity. In addition, plasma α_2 antiplasmin prevents conversion of scu-PA to tcu-PA outside the clot and thus preserves fibrin specificity.[83] Fibrin fragment E-2 selectively promotes the activation of plasminogen by scu-PA, mainly by enhancing the catalytic rate constant of the activation.[84] Scu-PA is an inefficient activator of plasminogen bound to internal lysine residues on intact fibrin but has a higher activity toward plasminogen bound to newly generated COOH-terminal lysine residues on partially degraded fibrin.[85] Thus, the fibrin specificity of scu-PA does not require its conversion to tcu-PA but is mediated by enhanced binding of plasminogen to partially digested fibrin.[86]

At the Cell Surface

The binding of scu-PA to urokinase-type plasminogen activator receptor (u-PAR) at the cell surface is believed to be crucial for its activity under physiological conditions. Binding results in strongly enhanced plasmin generation, which is due to effects on both the activation of plasminogen[87] and the feedback activation of scu-PA to tcu-PA by generated plasmin.[88] Both of these effects are also critically dependent on the cellular binding of plasminogen. Cell associated plasmin is protected from rapid inhibition by α_2 antiplasmin, which further favors the activation of receptor-bound scu-PA.[87] This system can, however, be efficiently inhibited by both PAI-1 and PAI-2.[89] The observation that direct anchorage of u-PA to the cell surface (using a GPI-anchored u-PA mutant) leads to a potentiation of plasmin generation equivalent to that observed in the presence of u-PAR suggests that u-PAR mainly functions to localize u-PA at the cell surface.[90] Furthermore, a u-PAR-independent function of u-PA has been demonstrated in fibrin clearance and in arterial neointima formation in mice.[3, 6]

▼ STAPHYLOKINASE

Staphylokinase forms a 1:1 stoichiometric complex with plasmin(ogen). It is not an enzyme, and generation of an active site in its equimolar complex with plasminogen requires conversion of plasminogen to plasmin. Thus, the plasmin-staphylokinase complex is the active enzyme.[44] This is in contrast with streptokinase, which produces a complex with plasminogen that exposes the active site in the plasminogen moiety without proteolytic cleavage. Kinetic data suggest that activation is initiated by trace amounts of plasmin that generate active plasmin-staphylokinase complex.[91] In mixtures with an excess of plasminogen over staphylokinase,

the generated complex converts excess plasminogen to plasmin.

In a buffer milieu, α_2 antiplasmin rapidly inhibits the plasmin-staphylokinase complex if the lysine binding sites in the plasmin moiety of the complex are available. Fibrin, but not fibrinogen, reduces the inhibition rate of the complex by α_2 antiplasmin by competing for interaction with the lysine binding site(s).[92] However, staphylokinase dissociates from the complex after neutralization by α_2 antiplasmin and is recycled to other plasmin(ogen) molecules.[93] Thus, extensive systemic plasminogen activation with staphylokinase would be expected in plasma, which is inconsistent with its observed fibrin specificity. This may be explained by the finding that in the absence of fibrin, no significant amounts of plasmin-staphylokinase complex are generated because traces of plasmin are inhibited by α_2 antiplasmin. In the presence of fibrin, generation of the complex is facilitated because traces of fibrin-bound plasmin are protected from α_2 antiplasmin and, furthermore, inhibition of the complex by α_2 antiplasmin at the clot surface is delayed more than 100-fold.[92] Recycling of staphylokinase to fibrin-bound plasmin, after slow neutralization of the complex, results in even more efficient generation of the complex. In addition, staphylokinase does not bind to a significant extent to plasminogen in circulating plasma but binds with high affinity to plasmin and to plasminogen, which is bound to partially degraded fibrin.[94] The molecular interactions involved in regulation of the fibrin specificity of staphylokinase are schematically illustrated in Figure 23–8.[44]

Pathophysiology of Fibrinolysis

The physiological importance of the fibrinolytic system is demonstrated by the association between abnormal fibrinolysis and a tendency toward bleeding or thrombosis. Impairment of fibrinolysis may be associated with thrombosis. It may be due to a defective synthesis and/or release of t-PA from the vessel wall, to a deficiency or functional defect in the plasminogen molecule, or to increased levels of inhibitors of t-PA or of plasmin. On the other hand, excessive fibrinolysis due to increased levels of t-PA or to α_2 antiplasmin deficiency may result in bleeding tendency. Recently, the generation of mice that over- or underexpress components of the fibrinolytic system has allowed establishment of its role in several biological processes.[3, 95]

▼ α_2 ANTIPLASMIN DEFICIENCY AND BLEEDING

The first case of congenital homozygous α_2 antiplasmin deficiency was described in a patient who presented with a hemorrhagic diathesis. Several cases of heterozygosity have been described with no or only mild bleeding symptoms.[96] The α_2 antiplasmin levels in all heterozygotes described thus far are consistently between 40 and 60 per cent of normal. Antigen and activity levels usually correspond well, suggesting that the deficiency is due to decreased synthesis of a normal α_2 antiplasmin molecule. The bleeding tendency in these patients may be due to premature lysis of hemostatic plugs, because in the absence of α_2 antiplasmin, the half-life

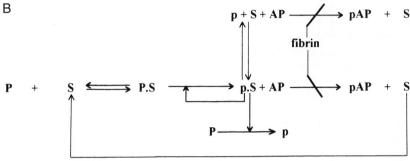

Figure 23–8. Schematic Representation of the Molecular Interactions That Regulate the Fibrin-Specificity of Staphylokinase. *A*, plasminogen *(P)* and staphylokinase *(S)* produce an inactive stoichiometric complex *(P.S)*. In the absence of α_2 antiplasmin *(AP)* the activation reaction is initiated by traces of plasmin *(p)*, which generate active plasmin-staphylokinase complex *(p.S)*. In a plasma milieu in the absence of fibrin, AP inhibits formation of p.S by formation of inactive plasmin-α_2-antiplasmin complex (pAP). *B*, in a plasma milieu in the presence of fibrin, inhibition of traces of p by AP is markedly delayed, thus allowing generation of active p.S complex. Inhibition of generated p.S at the fibrin surface by AP is strongly delayed and thus conversion of P.S to p.S and activation of excess P to p can occur. Slow inhibition of p.S by AP in the presence of fibrin results in generation of pAP, whereby S dissociates from p.S and can be recycled to other P molecules.

of plasmin molecules generated on the fibrin surface may be considerably prolonged.

The molecular defect in α_2 antiplasmin Okinawa was identified as a trinucleotide deletion in exon VII leading to deletion of Glu[137] in the protein.[97] In α_2 antiplasmin Nara insertion of a cytidine nucleotide in exon X leads to a shift in the reading frame of the mRNA resulting in deletion of the COOH-terminal 12 amino acids of native α_2 antiplasmin and replacement with 178 unrelated amino acids.[98] These mutations may lead to the deficiency by affecting the folding of the protein into the native configuration and thereby blocking its intracellular transport from the endoplasmatic reticulum to the Golgi complex.

A dysfunctional α_2 antiplasmin molecule (α_2 antiplasmin Enschede) associated with a serious bleeding tendency has been found in two siblings in a Dutch family. The ability of the protein to bind reversibly to plasminogen was not affected, but it was converted from an inhibitor of plasmin into a substrate. The molecular defect of α_2 antiplasmin Enschede consists of the insertion of an extra alanine residue (GCG insertion) somewhere between amino acid residues 365 and 359 (four Ala residues), 7 to 10 positions on the NH_2-terminal side of the P1 residue (Arg[376]) in the reactive site of α_2-antiplasmin.[99]

Acquired α_2 antiplasmin deficiency associated with enhanced fibrinolysis has been reported in some conditions, including liver disease,[100] disseminated intravascular coagulation, and/or fibrinolysis and acute promyelocytic leukemia.[101] α_2 Antiplasmin levels may be significantly reduced in patients undergoing thrombolytic therapy, as a result of systemic activation of the fibrinolytic system.[102]

▼ PLASMINOGEN ACTIVATOR INHIBITOR I AND THROMBOSIS

Several lines of evidence suggest that increased PAI-1 levels may promote fibrin deposition in vivo. In an experimental rabbit model of jugular vein thrombosis, inhibition of PAI-1 with the use of a monoclonal antibody resulted in promotion of endogenous thrombolysis and inhibition of thrombus ex-

tension.[103] Mice transgenic for the human PAI-1 gene develop venous thrombosis at the tip of the tail within 3 days after birth, but no arterial thrombosis.[104] Furthermore, transgenic mice that totally lack functional PAI-1 lyse experimental pulmonary emboli at a faster rate than controls.[105] In man, increased levels of PAI activity resulting in a decreased fibrinolytic capacity have been reported in several thrombotic disease states, including venous thromboembolism, obesity, sepsis, coronary artery disease, and acute myocardial infarction.[106–110]

Genetic variation at a polymorphic locus of the PAI-1 gene is associated with differences in plasma PAI-1 levels,[111] and a single base pair insertion/deletion polymorphism in the PAI-1 promoter region has been suggested to play an important role in the regulation of the expression of the PAI-1 gene.[112] A 4G allele of this common 4G/5G polymorphism may be a risk factor for myocardial infarction,[113] although this relationship was not definitely confirmed in a large multicenter study.[114] Thus, the homozygous form of the 4G allele is associated with increased PAI-1 antigen levels, but the relation to thrombotic disease remains to be more clearly established.

Defective fibrinolysis in patients with spontaneous or recurrent venous thrombosis may be due to a low concentration of t-PA or to an increased level of PAI-1.[108, 109] Increased PAI-1 levels were reported in patients with a history of idiopathic deep vein thrombosis and/or pulmonary embolism as compared with healthy controls, but this difference was no longer evident after adjustment for body mass index.[115] In the Physician's Health Study,[116] PAI-1 levels in patients who developed venous thrombosis during a 5 year follow-up period were not different from those of controls. The association between enhanced PAI-1 levels and symptomatic venous thrombosis thus requires further study.

High plasma PAI-1 levels in patients with acute myocardial infarction or unstable angina were found to be predictive for recurrent (within 3 years) myocardial infarction in some studies[117, 118] but not in others.[119, 120] In a prospective study in patients with angina pectoris, high basal levels of t-PA antigen but not PAI activity were associated with an increased risk of myocardial infarction.[121, 122] In the Physician's Health

Study, increased t-PA antigen levels were predictive for myocardial infarction within the 5 year follow-up period, but this association disappeared after adjustment for body mass index, high density lipoprotein (HDL) cholesterol, and blood pressure.[123] Local high concentrations of PAI-1 have been observed in coronary arteries with atherogenic lesions and may contribute to the development of vessel wall damage.[124–127]

In the prospective European Concerted Action on Thrombosis (ECAT) study, 10 fibrinolytic variables were measured in 3043 patients with angina pectoris recruited from 18 European centers.[128, 129] A first analysis after adjustment for other non-fibrinolytic coronary risk factors suggested that an increased risk of coronary events within 2 years was associated with higher baseline concentrations of t-PA antigen but not of PAI-1 activity and antigen levels. The prognostic value of the fibrinolytic variables determined in the ECAT study was recently re-examined after separate adjustment for clusters of markers of insulin resistance, inflammation, or endothelial cell damage.[130] These adjustments affected the prognostic value of PAI-1 and t-PA levels differently. Factors involved in the insulin resistance syndrome strongly affected PAI-1 and to a lesser extent t-PA antigen; the latter was primarily influenced by inflammation and endothelial cell damage.

Thus, t-PA antigen levels may constitute a biological marker of coronary heart disease, influenced by a variety of pathophysiological pathways including inflammation. In contrast, PAI levels that determine fibrinolytic activity and that are mainly dependent on the metabolic status emerge as a risk factor predictive for the future development of atherothrombosis.

▼ PLASMINOGEN DEFICIENCY AND THROMBOSIS

Two major types of plasminogen deficiency have been described. In type I deficiency, both plasminogen antigen and functional activity are reduced in parallel, suggesting reduced synthesis of a normally functioning plasminogen molecule (hypoplasminogenemia). In type II deficiency, plasminogen antigen levels are normal or only slightly reduced, whereas the activity is greatly reduced, suggesting an abnormally functioning plasminogen molecule (dysplasminogenemia).

Hypoplasminogenemia

Congenital plasminogen deficiency as a cause of thrombosis, characterized by a parallel decrease of functional and immunoreactive plasminogen, has been reported in only a few cases. In these patients, other investigated hemostatic parameters were normal; thus they apparently represent true isolated plasminogen deficiencies associated with severe thromboembolic complications.[96]

Acquired plasminogen deficiency has been observed in several clinical conditions, including liver disease and sepsis (25 to 45 per cent of normal activity). Possible mechanisms for acquired plasminogen deficiency in severe liver disease are depressed hepatic synthesis of the protein or increased consumption.[96]

Homozygous type I plasminogen deficiency has recently been described in patients with ligneous conjunctivitis, a rare and unusual form of chronic pseudomembranous conjunctivitis caused by massive fibrin deposition within the extravascular space of mucous membranes.[131] In several patients a homozygous point mutation was identified as a probable cause of the deficiency.[132, 133] Replacement therapy with Lys-plasminogen was shown to be successful.[133] The finding that plasminogen deficient mice also develop ligneous conjunctivitis supports a causal role of plasminogen in the disease.[134]

Dysplasminogenemia

Abnormalities in the plasminogen molecule may result in defective conversion to plasmin. Those are classified as type 1 dysplasminogenemia, with normal antigen level, and type 2 dysplasminogenemia-hypoplasminogenemia, with antigen level decreased to 60 to 70 per cent of normal. The molecular defect in the plasminogen molecule may be an active site defect, which may be combined with charge mutation(s) or kinetic defects.

The absence of proteolytic activity in plasmin(ogen) Tochigi is due to a single amino acid substitution, Ala[600] to Thr, near the His residue of the active site.[135] Characterization of the abnormal gene revealed that GCT (coding for Ala[600]) was replaced by ACT (coding for Thr).[136] This Ala to Thr substitution in the plasmin light chain disturbs the active site charge relay system, leading to loss of enzymatic activity. Two additional abnormal plasminogens with the same molecular defect, plasminogen Tochigi II and plasminogen Nagoya, have been identified in other members of the same family.[137] Similar cases (normal plasminogen antigen level but 50 per cent reduced activity) with thrombotic complications have been reported. In all these cases the propositus was identified after suffering from thrombotic complications, whereas other family members with the same plasminogen abnormality have, in general, not had clinical symptoms of thrombosis.[96]

Three types of human plasminogen variants (Chicago I, II, and III) were identified in young males with a history of recurrent deep vein thrombosis. Plasminogen Chicago I and II both have an activation defect characterized by a higher Michaelis constant and impaired plasminogen activator binding although cleavage of the Arg[560]-Val[561] peptide bond is normal. Plasminogen Chicago III has both an impaired affinity for plasminogen activators and an impaired cleavage of the Arg[560]-Val[561] peptide bond.[138, 139] All these dysplasminogenemias thus are characterized by a lowered ratio of functional to immunoreactive plasminogen.

Two independent studies have shown that disruption of the *plasminogen* gene in mice causes a severe thrombotic phenotype but is compatible with development and reproduction.[140, 141] Plasminogen deficiency indeed did not appear to compromise embryonic development and viability of the mice and did not drastically affect male fertility. Homozygous plasminogen-deficient mice display a greatly reduced spontaneous lysis of pulmonary plasma clots, and young animals develop multiple spontaneous thrombotic lesions in liver, stomach, colon, rectum, lung, pancreas, and other tissues. Restoration of normal plasminogen levels in these mice by bolus administration of plasminogen resulted in normalization of the thrombolytic potential toward experimentally induced pulmonary emboli and in removal of endogenous fibrin deposits in the liver, thus establishing conclusively that in vivo fibrin dissolution is critically dependent on the plasminogen/plasmin system.[142]

▼ PLASMINOGEN ACTIVATOR DEFICIENCY AND THROMBOSIS

Impairment of fibrinolysis due to deficient synthesis and/or release of t-PA from the vessel wall may be associated with a tendency to thrombosis. A deficient fibrinolytic response may be caused by a deficient release of t-PA from the vessel wall, but also by an increased rate of neutralization. Defective release of t-PA from the vessel wall during venous occlusion and/or decreased t-PA content in walls of superficial veins is found in about 70 per cent of patients with idiopathic recurrent venous thrombosis.[143]

To date, genetic deficiencies of t-PA or u-PA have not been reported in man. Mice with single or double deficiency of t-PA or u-PA are normal at birth, suggesting that neither t-PA nor u-PA, individually or in combination, is required for normal embryonic development. Double-deficient mice are able to reproduce but are significantly less fertile than wild-type mice or mice with a single deficiency of t-PA or u-PA; this may be due to the poor general health of these animals or to the presence of large fibrin deposits in their gonads.[144] The direct role of plasminogen activators in clearing fibrin deposits is supported by the observation that t-PA-deficient and t-PA–:u-PA-deficient mice have virtually no endogenous spontaneous thrombolytic potential, and that u-PA-deficient and t-PA–:u-PA-deficient mice suffer occasional or extensive spontaneous fibrin deposition, respectively.[144]

▼ ENHANCED PLASMINOGEN ACTIVATOR ACTIVITY AND BLEEDING

Excessive fibrinolysis due to increased t-PA activity levels may be associated with a bleeding tendency. A life-long hemorrhagic disorder associated with enhanced fibrinolysis, due to increased levels of circulating plasminogen activator, has been described in only a few patients.[145, 146]

Alternatively, excessive fibrinolysis due to decreased PAI-1 levels has been reported in a few cases and was apparently associated with bleeding complications.[147, 148] A complete deficiency of PAI-1 has been reported in a young girl who had several episodes of major hemorrhage, all in response to trauma or surgery. The protein lacks the 169 COOH-terminal amino acid region of mature PAI-1, which includes the Arg^{346}-Met^{347} reactive site peptide bond.[149]

Recently, the effect of *PAI*-1 gene disruption on organ development and reproduction and on hemostasis, thrombosis, and thrombolysis has been investigated in mice. Surprisingly, PAI-1-deficient mice are viable and fertile and have no significant organ abnormalities, demonstrating that reproduction and development can proceed normally in the absence of PAI-1.[105] Lysis of a pulmonary plasma clot was significantly faster in homozygous PAI-1-deficient mice as compared with wild-type mice, consistent with an inhibitory role of PAI-1 on plasminogen activation in vivo. Homozygous PAI-1-deficient mice developed venous thrombi sig-

nificantly less frequently than wild-type mice after local injection of endotoxin in the footpad, although a similar extent of inflammation was observed. Thus, these findings suggest a significant role for PAI-1 in the development of venous thrombosis. As discussed above, studies in man did not allow conclusive determination of whether the acute phase reactant PAI-1 was the cause or consequence of thrombotic phenomena.

Clinical Aspects of Thrombolysis

▼ OVERVIEW

Cardiovascular diseases, comprising acute myocardial infarction, stroke, and venous thromboembolism, have, as their immediate underlying cause, thrombosis of critically situated blood vessels with loss of blood flow to vital organs. One approach to the treatment of thrombosis consists of infusing thrombolytic agents (plasminogen activators) to dissolve the blood clot and to restore tissue perfusion and oxygenation. Currently, six thrombolytic agents are available for clinical use: streptokinase, anisoylated plasminogen streptokinase activator complex (APSAC), two-chain urokinase-type plasminogen activator (tcu-PA), recombinant single-chain u-PA (rscu-PA, prourokinase, saruplase), recombinant tissue-type plasminogen activator (rt-PA, alteplase) and a domain deletion mutant of rt-PA (r-PA, reteplase). Streptokinase, APSAC, tcu-PA, and to a large extent reteplase induce extensive systemic plasmin generation; α_2 antiplasmin inhibits circulating plasmin but may become exhausted during thrombolytic therapy, since its plasma concentration is only about half that of plasminogen. As a result plasmin, which has a broad substrate specificity, degrades several plasma proteins, such as fibrinogen; coagulation factors V, VIII, and XII; and von Willebrand factor. These thrombolytic agents are, therefore, considered to be non-fibrin-specific. In contrast, the physiological plasminogen activators, t-PA and to a lesser extent scu-PA, are fibrin-specific, as discussed above: That is, they dissolve the fibrin component of a thrombus without an associated systemic lytic state.

In patients with acute myocardial infarction, reduction of infarct size, preservation of ventricular function, and reduction in mortality rate have been demonstrated with streptokinase, recombinant t-PA (rt-PA) and APSAC. The Global Utilization of Streptokinase and t-PA for Occluded Coronary Arteries (GUSTO) trial has established a correlation between early coronary patency and reduction in mortality rate.[150] Nevertheless, all available thrombolytic agents still suffer significant shortcomings, including large therapeutic doses, short plasma half-lives, limited efficacy and fibrin specificity, reocclusion, and bleeding complications.[1, 151, 152] Other problems are the still limited impact of aspirin and heparin on the speed of thrombolysis or on the resistance to lysis and the fact that they do not consistently prevent reocclusion. Nevertheless, early administration of aspirin was reported to produce a surprising 23 per cent reduction in mortality rate in patients with acute myocardial infarction (AMI), and it is now routinely administered with the thrombolytic agent. The optimal dose of aspirin in patients with AMI is uncertain; it has been recommended to give 325 mg as soon as the diagnosis is established and 75 to 325 mg per day thereafter.

For thrombolytic therapy with rt-PA, it is recommended that intravenous (IV) heparin should be administered concurrently as a bolus of 5000 U followed by an infusion rate of 1000 U/hour (1200 U/hour if the body weight is above 80 kg), to be adjusted to maintain the aPTT at 1.5 to 2 times the control value.[153] It is not clearly established whether patients receiving streptokinase and aspirin benefit from heparin.

Fibrinolytic drugs can also exert procoagulant effects through generation of plasmin, which may activate the coagulation system, resulting in a delay of apparent thrombolysis, failure of initial recanalization, and rapid reocclusion. Thus, vigorous concomitant anticoagulation is needed, at least with fibrin-specific thrombolytic agents. Specific reduction of platelet aggregation is presently being explored with monoclonal antibodies or synthetic peptides against the platelet receptor GPIIb/IIIa. Another approach is the use of selective inhibitors of thrombin, of factor Xa, or of factor VIIa (an overview of the use of concomitant antithrombotic therapy has been published.[153]). Furthermore, in some trials it has been suggested that direct percutaneous transluminal coronary angioplasty (PTCA) and coronary artery bypass graft (CABG) surgery, when feasible, may be comparable or even superior to thrombolytic therapy.[154–156] (An overview on the use of PTCA and CABG has been published.[153])

At present the search for better thrombolytic agents or regimens continues. Recent approaches to improve the thrombolytic properties of plasminogen activators include the production of mutant plasminogen activators, of chimeric molecules comprising portions of different plasminogen activators, of antibody-targeted plasminogen activators using fibrin-specific or platelet-specific monoclonal antibodies, and of plasminogen activators from animal or bacterial sources.[19, 157, 158]

▼ THROMBOLYTIC THERAPY

Thrombolytically treated non-cardiac disorders include deep vein thrombosis, pulmonary embolism, peripheral arterial occlusion, and acute ischemic stroke. In patients with a recent proximal deep vein thrombosis of the leg or pelvis, prevention of the postphlebitic syndrome may be an advantage of thrombolysis over heparin therapy. For treatment of occlusive thrombi, the optimal dose regimens of streptokinase, urokinase, and alteplase are not definitively established. Acute massive pulmonary embolism with hypotension or shock has been treated with thrombolytic agents, followed, depending on the early outcome, by pulmonary embolectomy. It has not been proved unequivocally that thrombolysis is superior to heparin treatment of subacute intermediate pulmonary embolism, whereas major acute pulmonary embolism with hemodynamic instability generally responds well to thrombolysis. Peripheral arterial occlusion is generally treated with catheter-directed and intraoperative intraarterial bolus or short-term infusions of thrombolytic agents. The efficacy and safety of intravenous thrombolysis for the treatment of major ischemic stroke is being tested in clinical trials. Despite an increased incidence of symptomatic intracerebral hemorrhage, alteplase improved clinical outcome at 3 months if administered within 3 hours of the onset of ischemic stroke[159] and before extended infarct signs were

detectable on cerebral computed tomography (CT).[160] Trials with streptokinase were terminated early because of excess rate of mortality, mainly after hemorrhagic conversion of the cerebral infarct.[161–163]

The recognition that thrombosis within the infarct related coronary artery plays a major role in the pathogenesis of acute myocardial infarction and the observation that early administration of thrombolytic agents results in recanalization of occluded coronary arteries have provided the basis for the development of thrombolytic therapy in acute myocardial infarction.[164, 165] Clinical trials have shown that the size of infarction and the resultant mortality rate are decreased and that myocardial function is preserved if reperfusion is achieved within a time window that was initially thought to be only up to 6 hours, whereas subsequent studies have shown a benefit if reperfusion is achieved in up to 12 hours.[166] In the larger clinical trials, an approximate 25 per cent reduction in mortality rate from acute myocardial infarction has been demonstrated with streptokinase, alteplase, or APSAC.[153]

Current indications for thrombolytic therapy, according to the Task Force on Myocardial Reperfusion of the International Society and Federation of Cardiology and World Health Organization, are chest pain consistent with the diagnosis of acute myocardial infarction and at least 0.1 mm of ST-segment elevation in at least two contiguous electrocardiographic (ECG) leads when treatment can be initiated within 12 hours of pain onset. Contraindications include history of a serious bleeding tendency; recent acute internal hemorrhages; major surgery, trauma, or delivery within 10 days; traumatic cardiopulmonary resuscitation; vascular puncture in a non-compressible site; and uncontrolled hypertension. Furthermore, previous use of streptokinase or APSAC is a contraindication for their repeated administration, because of their immunogenicity.[153]

Comparative clinical trials of streptokinase and rt-PA have shown a difference in efficacy for early coronary artery recanalization.[167] Early patency (Thrombolysis in Myocardial Infarction [TIMI] flow grade 2 or 3), confirmed by coronary angiography at 90 minutes after the start of therapy, is approximately 22 per cent with placebo, 53 per cent with streptokinase, and 75 per cent with alteplase (up to 85 per cent with the accelerated regimen; see below).[168] The efficacy of the other thrombolytic agents for early recanalization is probably intermediate between that of streptokinase and that of rt-PA.[153] With streptokinase, a catch-up phenomenon occurs within 3 hours, bringing infarct-related coronary artery patency up to 75 to 80 per cent at 3 hours with both streptokinae and rt-PA.[169]

Presently available thrombolytic agents and some new agents that have shown promise in animal models of venous or arterial thrombosis and in pilot studies in patients with AMI are discussed below.

Tissue-Type Plasminogen Activator and Variants

The recommended dose of recombinant t-PA (alteplase [Activase, Actilyse]) for the treatment of acute myocardial infarction was 100 mg administered IV as 60 mg in the first hour (of which 10 mg was administered as a bolus over the first 1 to 2 minutes), 20 mg over the second hour, and 20 mg over the third hour. Later it was proposed to give the same total dose of 100 mg but "front loaded," starting with a bolus of 15 mg followed by 50 mg in the next 30 minutes and the remaining 35 mg in the following hour.[170] In the GUSTO trial, a dose of 15 mg intravenous bolus of alteplase followed by 0.75 mg/kg over 30 minutes (not to exceed 50 mg) and then 0.50 mg/kg over 60 minutes (not to exceed 35 mg) was utilized.[150] Immediate aspirin (160 to 325 mg) and IV heparin (5000 U bolus and 1000 U/hour, monitored by aPTT) are given. The accelerated regimen in the GUSTO trial was associated with a significantly lower mortality rate than that of streptokinase (6.3 versus 7.3 per cent, $p = 0.001$), but with a slightly higher incidence (0.1 per cent) of survival with disabling stroke. Overall, fewer complications were seen with alteplase, including allergic reactions, clinical indicators of left ventricular dysfunction, and arrhythmias. The survival benefit was largest in patients <75 years, with anterior infarction and <4 hours from onset of symptoms. In the COBALT trial, double-bolus administration of rt-PA (50 mg given 30 minutes apart) was evaluated in patients with myocardial infarction.[171] For catheter-directed local thrombolysis with alteplase in patients with recent peripheral arterial occlusion, a dose of 0.05 to 0.10 mg/kg per hour over an 8 hour period is usually recommended.[158]

By deletion or substitution of functional domains, by site-specific point mutations, and/or by alteration of the carbohydrate composition, mutants of rt-PA have been produced with higher fibrin specificity, more zymogenicity, slower clearance from the circulation, and resistance to plasma proteinase inhibitors. During thrombolytic therapy there is a vast excess of t-PA over PAI-1 in the circulation, but critical lysis occurs at the surface of an arterial thrombus, where the local PAI-1 concentration can be very high.[172] Therefore, mutants with resistance to PAI-1 may be useful to reduce reocclusion. In addition, mutants with prolonged half-life may allow thrombolysis by bolus administration at a reduced dose. Several mutants and variants of t-PA have been evaluated at the preclinical level in animal models of venous and arterial thrombosis and in pilot studies, mainly in patients with acute myocardial infarction. A systematic comparison of domain deletion and substitution variants in experimental animal models, however, led us to conclude that these would not constitute superior thrombolytic agents.[173]

Reteplase (BM 06.022) is a single-chain non-glycosylated deletion variant consisting only of the kringle 2 and the proteinase domain of human t-PA; it contains amino acids 1–3 and 176–527 of rt-PA (deletion of Val[4]-Glu[175]; cf. Fig. 23–4). The Arg[275]-Ile[276] plasmin cleavage site is maintained.[174] The plasminogen activating potential of reteplase is similar to that of rt-PA in the absence of fibrin, but fourfold lower in the presence of a fibrin-like stimulator.[174] Reteplase and t-PA are inhibited by PAI-1 to a similar degree. Pharmacokinetic analysis of plasma activity in the rabbit revealed a half-life of 19 minutes for reteplase and 2 minutes for alteplase, with a 4.3-fold slower plasma clearance for reteplase than for alteplase.[175] In healthy human volunteers[176] and in patients with acute myocardial infarction[177] an initial half-life of 14 to 18 minutes was observed for reteplase, as compared with 5 to 6 minutes for alteplase. Different doses of reteplase in patients with acute myocardial infarction were evaluated in two open non-ran-

domized pilot trials.[178, 179] The randomized angiographic RAPID I trial showed that reteplase, when given as a double bolus of 10 plus 10 MU 30 minutes apart, achieves more rapid, complete, and sustained thrombolysis (TIMI grade 3 flow) than standard dose alteplase (100 mg over 3 hours).[180] In the RAPID II trial, the same reteplase dose regimen appeared to achieve higher rates of early reperfusion than front-loaded alteplase.[181] In the INJECT study, a double-blind randomized trial in patients with acute myocardial infarction, administration of two boluses of 10 MU reteplase given 30 minutes apart only showed a small and not statistically significant benefit over administration of streptokinase (1.5 MU IV over 60 min).[182] In the definitive GUSTO-III trial, no clinical benefit of reteplase over alteplase could be demonstrated, leading to the conclusion that both agents are equivalent.[183]

In TNK-rt-PA, replacement of Asn[117] with Gln (N117Q) deletes the glycosylation site in kringle 1, whereas substitution of Thr[103] by Asn (T103N) reintroduces a glycosylation site at a different site; these modifications substantially decrease the plasma clearance rate. In addition, the amino acids Lys[296]-His[297]-Arg[298]-Arg[299] were each replaced with Ala (cf. Fig. 23–4).[184] TNK-rt-PA has a similar ability to wild-type rt-PA to bind to fibrin and to lyse fibrin clots in a plasma milieu.[184] It has an enhanced fibrin specificity, resistance to inhibition by PAI-1, and slower plasma clearance.[185] It has increased thrombolytic potency on platelet-rich clots in rabbits, preserves fibrinogen, and is effective upon bolus administration at half the dose of rt-PA.[184, 186] Similar results were obtained in a combined arterial and venous thrombosis model in the dog[187] and in a rabbit carotid artery thrombosis model.[188] In patients with acute myocardial infarction, TNK-rt-PA has a plasma clearance of about 150 ml/min and a half-life of 17 minutes, as compared to 570 ml/min and 3 minutes for wild-type rt-PA.[189] In the Thrombolysis in Myocardial Infarction (TIMI) 10A trial, a phase 1 dose-ranging pilot study in patients with acute myocardial infarction, single bolus TNK-rt-PA was administered over 5 to 10 seconds with doses ranging from 5 to 50 mg.[189] The agent was fibrin-specific and had an initial patency and safety profile at the 30 to 50 mg doses that appeared encouraging. In the TIMI-10B trial, a larger phase 2 efficacy trial, a single bolus of 40 mg TNK-t-PA yielded similar TIMI-3 flow rates at 90 minutes to accelerated rt-PA, with faster and more complete reperfusion.[190] In the ASSENT-1 phase 2 safety trial an intracranial hemorrhage rate of 0.76 per cent was observed with the 40 mg dose, an acceptable rate considering the fact that nearly 15 per cent of the patients were above 75 years.[191]

Lanoteplase is a deletion mutant of t-PA (without the finger and growth factor domains) in which glycosylation at Asn[117] is lacking.[192] When it was given as a single bolus of 120 U/kg in the Intravenous n-PA for Treating Infarcting Myocardium Early (InTIME-1) trial, higher infarct-related vessel patency rates were obtained than with alteplase.[193]

Different molecular forms of the *Desmodus* salivary plasminogen activator (DSPA) have been characterized. Two high molecular weight forms, DSPAα1 (43 kDa) and DSPAα2 (39 kDa), exhibit about 85 per cent homology to human t-PA but contain neither a kringle 2 domain nor a plasmin-sensitive cleavage site. DSPAβ lacks the finger domain and DSPAγ lacks the finger and epidermal growth factor domains.[194–196] DSPAα1 and DSPAα2 have a specific activity in vitro that is equal to or higher than that of rt-PA, relative PAI-1 resistance, and greatly enhanced fibrin specificity with a strict requirement for polymeric fibrin as a cofactor.[194–196] In several animal models of thrombolysis, DSPAα1 has a 2.5 times higher potency and four- to eightfold slower clearance rate than t-PA.[197–201] Recombinant DSPAα1 produced in mammalian cell culture may be suitable for bolus administration, whereby its long half-life and high specific activity may allow a reduction of the therapeutic dose.

Streptokinase and Anisoylated Plasminogen-Streptokinase Activator Complex

The initial dose of streptokinase must be adequate to neutralize the plasma levels of antistreptococcal antibodies: The streptokinase-antibody complex thus formed is rapidly cleared from the circulation. The initial dose for an individual patient can be determined by the streptokinase resistance test, but, more practically in patients with AMI, a standard intravenous dose of 1.5 million units is given over 30 to 60 minutes combined with aspirin (160 to 325 mg daily). The safety and efficacy of this regimen in terms of mortality rate reduction were demonstrated in International Study of Infarct Survival (ISIS)-2,[202] Gruppo Italiano per lo Studio della Sopravvivenza nell'Infarto Miocardico (GISSI-2),[203] and ISIS-3.[204] It is associated with moderate efficacy for early coronary artery recanalization: about 55 per cent patency (TIMI flow grade 2 or 3) at 90 minutes with a catch-up to about 80 per cent at 3 hours. It is less efficient for mortality rate reduction in patients treated within the first 6 hours than accelerated alteplase with IV heparin; no significant difference was observed in patients > 75 years old, in patients with small inferior infarcts, and in patients presenting more than 4 hours after the onset of symptoms.[150] Patients in the Global Utilization of Streptokinase and t-PA for Occluded Coronary Arteries (GUSTO-I) trial who survived the first 30 days after treatment with alteplase had significantly fewer major complications during the hospital course than those treated with streptokinase.[205]

The recommended dose of anistreplase (APSAC) in acute myocardial infarction is 30 units (1 mg = 1 unit and 30 mg contains approximately 1,100,000 units of streptokinase) to be given IV as a bolus injection over 3 to 5 minutes, in combination with 160 mg per day of aspirin. In aggregate, comparative studies indicate that the efficacy for coronary thrombolysis (angiographic patency) of anistreplase is comparable to or somewhat higher than that of intravenous streptokinase but lower than that of intracoronary streptokinase.[206] In trials comparing anistreplase (30 units) with IV streptokinase (1.5×10^6 U over 60 minutes), the same decrease in fibrinogen levels and incidence of adverse events were observed.[207] Since anistreplase contains streptokinase, it causes immunization; the antibody titer may increase up to 60-fold within 2 to 3 weeks and remain high for 3 months.[207, 208]

Urokinase-Type Plasminogen Activator

In patients with acute myocardial infarction (two-chain) urokinase is administered either as a 2×10^6 units bolus or as a 3×10^6 units infusion over 90 minutes.[209] Since the 1980s, an initial intravenous dose of 4000 units/kg body weight over 10 minutes followed by the same maintenance dose per kilogram hourly has been recommended for the treatment of acute major pulmonary embolism. At present, a bolus dose in the right atrium of 15,000 units/kg of body weight has been recommended in this indication; an intravenous infusion of 3×10^6 units of urokinase (1×10^6 units over 10 minutes and 2×10^6 units over the next 110 minutes) has also been tested.

With a preparation containing 160,000 IU/mg of saruplase (full-length unglycosylated human recombinant scu-PA obtained from *Escherichia coli*), the dose used successfully in patients with acute myocardial infarction (PRIMI Study) was 20 mg given as a bolus and 60 mg over the next 60 minutes, immediately followed by an intravenous heparin infusion (20 U/kg per hour) for 72 hours. This was associated with earlier reperfusion, higher patency rates, and moderately less fibrinogen breakdown than administration of streptokinase.[210] In the LIMITS Study in patients with acute myocardial infarction, the same dose regimen of saruplase was used, but with a prethrombolytic heparin bolus of 5000 IU and an IV heparin infusion for 5 days starting 30 minutes after completion of thrombolysis.[211] A recombinant glycosylated form of scu-PA (A-74187) has been evaluated in patients with acute myocardial infarction using 60 or 80 mg monotherapy or 60 mg primed with a preceding bolus of 250,000 IU of recombinant tcu-PA, always combined with aspirin and IV heparin.[212] Further studies with saruplase revealed similar TIMI grade 2 and 3 flows to those of a 3 hour infusion of rt-PA (SESAM),[213] whereas in the COMPASS[214] study 30 day mortality rates were lower with saruplase (80 mg/60 minutes) than with streptokinase (5.7 per cent versus 6.7 per cent), with, however, an increased rate of intracranial hemorrhage (0.7 versus 0.3 per cent).

Staphylokinase

In the first pilot recanalization studies, patients with acute myocardial infarction were given 10 mg IV SakSTAR as a 1 mg bolus followed by infusion of 9 mg over 30 minutes.[45] In an open randomized multicenter trial (STAR trial) SakSTAR was compared with accelerated weight-adjusted rt-PA in 100 patients with acute myocardial infarction.[215] Twenty-five patients received 10 mg SakSTAR intravenously over 30 min, and, after a prospectively planned interim analysis, 23 patients were given 20 mg over 30 minutes, with an initial 10 per cent bolus in all patients. rt-PA was given to 52 patients, as a 15 mg intravenous bolus, followed by 0.75 mg/kg body weight over 30 minutes (not to exceed 50 mg), and by 0.5 mg/kg up to 35 mg over the next 60 minutes (total maximum dose of 100 mg over 90 minutes). TIMI grade 3 at 90 minutes was obtained in 58 per cent of patients treated with rt-PA and in 62 per cent of patients treated with SakSTAR (in 50 per cent of patients receiving 10 mg and in 74 per cent receiving 20 mg). The differences in 90 minute patency among the three groups were not statistically significant, probably because of the small numbers of patients. SakSTAR was highly fibrin-specific, as revealed by virtually unaltered levels of plasma fibrinogen, plasminogen, and α2-antiplasmin, whereas rt-PA caused a 30 per cent drop of fibrinogen and a 60 per cent decrease of plasminogen and

α_2 antiplasmin levels at 90 minutes. No strokes, allergic reactions, or other side effects were recorded.

A pilot study of bolus staphylokinase (Sak42D) infusion (20 mg over 5 minutes) for coronary thrombolysis was performed in 12 patients with evolving transmural myocardial infarction. TIMI grade 3 flow at 60 minutes was obtained in 7 patients (58 per cent). Administration of a second bolus (10 mg over 5 minutes), as prospectively determined, to the remaining 5 patients, resulted in TIMI grade 3 flow in 3 of those at 90 minutes, yielding an overall TIMI grade 3 flow rate of 83 per cent at 90 minutes.[216] The encouraging experience obtained in this pilot study inspired a multicenter randomized trial in patients with evolving myocardial infarction, comparing accelerated rt-PA with a double bolus of 15 mg Sak42D given 30 minutes apart.[217] TIMI perfusion grade 3 at 90 minutes was achieved in 68 per cent of patients treated with staphylokinase versus 57 per cent of patients treated with rt-PA (p = not significant). Double bolus Sak42D was, however, significantly more fibrin-specific, whereas the distribution of in-hospital events did not significantly differ in the groups.[217]

In a pilot study in 30 patients with peripheral arterial occlusion, intra-arterial catheter-directed SakSTAR was given as a bolus of 1 mg, followed by a continuous infusion of 0.5 mg per hour, or as a 2 mg bolus followed by an infusion of 1 mg per hour, together with heparin. Complete recanalization was obtained in 83 per cent of the patients after about 7.0 mg SakSTAR infused over 9 hours.[218]

The rather low-grade antigenicity of staphylokinase, as suggested by early dog and baboon experiments, unfortunately is not extended to patients. The vast majority of patients with either myocardial infarction or peripheral arterial occlusion developed neutralizing antibodies to Sak-STAR, albeit after a long lag phase of 7 to 12 days, that remained elevated well above pretreatment levels for several months after administration.[219] Therefore, the restriction to single use probably applies both to streptokinase and to staphylokinase. The absence of cross-reactivity to streptokinase of antibodies elicited by SakSTAR, and vice versa, suggest that the consecutive use of both plasminogen activators may be feasible.[220] Furthermore, variants of recombinant staphylokinase with reduced immunogenicity have been obtained by site-directed mutagenesis.[221–225] Thus, substitution mutagenesis in SakSTAR of clusters of two or three charged amino acids with alanine identified two variants (with approximately 50 per cent reduced specific activity), SakSTAR.M38 (with K35, E38, K74, E75, and R77 substituted with A) and SakSTAR.M89 (with K74, E75, R77, E80, and D82 substituted with A) that did not recognize approximately one third of the antibodies elicited in patients by treatment with wild-type SakSTAR. In patients with peripheral arterial occlusion given doses of 6.5 to 12 mg of compound, SakSTAR.M38 and SakSTAR.M89 induced significantly fewer neutralizing antibodies and staphylokinase-specific immunoglobulin G (IgG) than wild-type SakSTAR.[222]

Further studies revealed that SakSTAR (K74) (with a single substitution of Lys[74] with Ala) had an intact specific activity but did not absorb 40 per cent of the antibodies induced in patients by treatment with wild-type SakSTAR. Intra-arterial administration in patients with peripheral arterial occlusion of SakSTAR (K74) or SakSTAR (K74ER) (with Lys[74], Glu[75], and Arg[77] replaced by Ala) induced signif-

icantly fewer circulating neutralizing antibodies than administration of SakSTAR, while maintaining intact thrombolytic potency.[224, 225]

These variants provide proof of the concept that reduction of the immunogenicity and immunoreactivity of recombinant staphylokinase by protein engineering may be feasible.

REFERENCES

1. Collen, D., and Lijnen, H. R.: Basic and clinical aspects of fibrinolysis and thrombolysis. Blood 78:3114, 1991.
2. Blasi, F.: Urokinase and urokinase receptor: A paracrine/autocrine system regulating cell migration and invasiveness. BioEssays 15:105, 1993.
3. Carmeliet, P., and Collen, D.: Gene manipulation and transfer of the plasminogen and coagulation system in mice. Semin. Thromb. Hemost. 22:525, 1996.
4. Vassalli, J. D., Sappino, A. P., and Belin, D.: The plasminogen activator/plasmin system. J. Clin. Invest. 88:1067, 1991.
5. Bachmann, F.: The plasminogen-plasmin enzyme system. In Colman, R. W., Hirsch, J., Marder, V. J., and Salzman, E. W. (eds.): Hemostasis and Thrombosis. Philadelphia, J. B. Lippincott, 1993.
6. Bugge, T. H., Flick, M. J., Danton, M. J., Daugherty, C. C., Romer, J., Dano, K., Carmeliet, P., Collen, D., and Degen, J. L.: Urokinase-type plasminogen activator is effective in fibrin clearance in the absence of its receptor or tissue-type plasminogen activator. Proc. Natl. Acad. Sci. USA 93:5899, 1996.
7. Collen, D.: On the regulation and control of fibrinolysis. Thromb. Haemost. 43:77, 1980.
8. Forsgren, M., Raden, B., Israelsson, M., Larsson, K., and Heden, L. O.: Molecular cloning and characterization of a full-length cDNA clone for human plasminogen. FEBS Lett. 213:254, 1987.
9. Holvoet, P., Lijnen, H. R., and Collen, D.: A monoclonal antibody specific for Lys-plasminogen: Application to the study of the activation pathways of plasminogen in vivo. J. Biol. Chem. 260:12106, 1985.
10. Wiman, B., and Collen, D.: Molecular mechanism of physiological fibrinolysis. Nature 272:549, 1978.
11. O'Reilly, M. S., Holmgren, L., Shing, Y., Chen, C., Rosenthal, R. A., Moses, M., Lane, W. S., Cao, Y., Sage, E. H., and Folkman, J.: Angiostatin: A novel angiogenesis inhibitor that mediates the suppression of metastases by a Lewis lung carcinoma. Cell 79:315, 1994.
12. Murray, J. C., Buetow, K. H., Donovan, M., Hornung, S., Motulsky, A. G., Disteche, C., Dyer, K., Swisshelm, K., Anderson, J., Giblett, E., Sadler, E., Eddy, R., and Shows, T. B.: Linkage disequilibrium of plasminogen polymorphisms and assignment of the gene to human chromosome 6q26–6q27. Am. J. Hum. Genet. 40:338, 1987.
13. Petersen, T. E., Martzen, M. R., Ichinose, A., and Davie, E. W.: Characterization of the gene for human plasminogen, a key proenzyme in the fibrinolytic system. J. Biol. Chem. 265:6104, 1990.
14. Wade, D. P., Clarke, J. G., Lindahl, G. E., Liu, A. C., Zysow, B. R., Meer, K., Schwartz, K., and Lawn, R. M.: 5' Control regions of the apolipoprotein(a) gene and members of the related plasminogen gene family. Proc. Natl. Acad. Sci. USA 90:1369, 1993.
15. Raum, D., Marcus, D., and Alper, C. A.: Genetic polymorphism of human plasminogen. Am. J. Hum. Genet. 32:681, 1980.
16. Dimo-Simonin, N., Brandt-Casadevall, C., and Gujer, H. R.: Gene frequencies of plasminogen in Switzerland. Hum. Hered. 35:343, 1985.
17. Kera, Y., Nishimukai, H., Yamasawa, K., and Komura, S.: Comparative study of phenotypes on activity and plasma concentration in the genetic system of plasminogen. Hum. Hered. 33:52, 1983.
18. Pennica, D., Holmes, W. E., Kohr, W. J., Harkins, R. N., Vehar, G. A., Ward, C. A., Bennett, W. F., Yelverton, E., Seeburg, P. H., Heyneker, H. L., Goeddel, D. V., and Collen, D.: Cloning and expression of human tissue-type plasminogen activator cDNA in E. coli. Nature 301:214, 1983.
19. Lijnen, H. R., and Collen, D.: Strategies for the improvement of thrombolytic agents. Thromb. Haemost. 66:88, 1991.
20. Tachias, K., and Madison, E. L.: Converting tissue type plasminogen

activator into a zymogen: Important role of Lys 156. J. Biol. Chem. 272:28, 1997.

21. Rajput, B., Degen, S. F., Reich, E., Waller, E. K., Axelrod, J., Eddy, R. L., and Shows, T. B.: Chromosomal locations of human tissue plasminogen activator and urokinase genes. Science 230:672, 1985.

22. Patthy, L.: Evolution of the proteases of blood coagulation and fibrinolysis by assembly from modules. Cell 41:657, 1985.

23. Medcalf, R. L., Ruegg, M., and Schleuning, W. D.: A DNA motif related to the cAMP-responsive element and an exon-located activator protein-2 binding site in the human tissue-type plasminogen activator gene promoter cooperate in basal expression and convey activation by phorbol ester and cAMP. J. Biol. Chem. 265:14618, 1990.

24. Lijnen, H. R., Bachmann, F., Collen, D., Ellis, V., Pannekoek, H., Rijken, D. C., and Thorsen, S.: Mechanisms of plasminogen activation. J. Intern. Med. 236:415, 1994.

25. Lijnen, H. R., and Collen, D.: Mechanisms of physiological fibrinolysis. Bailliere's Clin. Haematol. 8:277, 1995.

26. Bulens, F., Ibanez Tallon, I., Van Acker, P., De Vriese, A., Nelles, L., Belayew, A., and Collen, D.: Retinoic acid induction of human tissue-type plasminogen activator gene expression via a direct repeat element (DR5) located at -7 kilobases. J. Biol. Chem. 270:7167, 1995.

27. Levin, E. G., and Santell, L.: Stimulation and desensitization of tissue plasminogen activator release from human endothelial cells. J. Biol. Chem. 263:9360, 1988.

28. Levin, E. G., Marotti, K. R., and Santell, L.: Protein kinase C and the stimulation of tissue plasminogen activator release from human endothelial cells: Dependence on the elevation of messenger RNA. J. Biol. Chem. 264:16030, 1989.

29. Kuiper, J., Van't Hof, A., Otter, M., Biessen, E. A., Rijken, D. C., and van Berkel, T. J.: Interaction of mutants of tissue-type plasminogen activator with liver cells: Effect of domain deletions. Biochem. J. 313:775, 1996.

30. Orth, K., Madison, E. L., Gething, M. J., Sambrook, J. F., and Herz, J.: Complexes of tissue-type plasminogen activator and its serpin inhibitor plasminogen-activator inhibitor type 1 are internalized by means of the low density lipoprotein receptor-related protein/alpha 2-macroglobulin receptor. Proc. Natl. Acad. Sci. USA 89:7422, 1992.

31. Günzler, W. A., Steffens, G. J., Otting, F., Kim, S. M. A., Frankus, E., and Flohé, L.: The primary structure of high molecular mass urokinase from human urine: The complete amino acid sequence of the A chain. Hoppe-Seyler Z. Physiol. Chem. 363:1155, 1982.

32. Holmes, W. E., Pennica, D., Blaber, M., Rey, M. W., Günzler, W. A., Steffens, G. J., and Heyneker, H. L.: Cloning and expression of the gene for pro-urokinase in Escherichia coli. Biotechnology 3:923, 1985.

33. Stump, D. C., Lijnen, H. R., and Collen, D.: Purification and characterization of a novel low molecular weight form of single-chain urokinase-type plasminogen activator. J. Biol. Chem. 261:17120, 1986.

34. de Munk, G. A., Parkinson, J. F., Groeneveld, E., Bang, N. U., and Rijken, D. C.: Role of the glycosaminoglycan component of thrombomodulin in its acceleration of the inactivation of single-chain urokinase-type plasminogen activator by thrombin. Biochem. J. 290:655, 1993.

35. Riccio, A., Grimaldi, G., Verde, P., Sebastio, G., Boast, S., and Blasi, F.: The human urokinase-plasminogen activator gene and its promoter. Nucleic Acids Res. 13:2759, 1985.

36. Larsson, L. I., Skriver, L., Nielsen, L. S., Grondahl Hansen, J., Kristensen, P., and Dano, K.: Distribution of urokinase-type plasminogen activator immunoreactivity in the mouse. J. Cell Biol. 98:894, 1984.

37. Kuiper, J., Rijken, D. C., de Munk, G. A. W., and van Berkel, T. J.: In vivo and in vitro interaction of high and low molecular weight single-chain urokinase-type plasminogen activator with rat liver cells. J. Biol. Chem. 267:1589, 1992.

38. Jackson, K. W., and Tang, J.: Complete amino acid sequence of streptokinase and its homology with serine proteases. Biochemistry 21:6620, 1982.

39. Reddy, K. N. N.: Mechanism of activation of human plasminogen by streptokinase. In Kline, D. L., and Reddy, K. N. N. (eds.): Fibrinolysis. Boca Raton, Fla., CRC Press, 1980.

40. Siefring, G. E., Jr., and Castellino, F. J.: Interaction of streptokinase with plasminogen: Isolation and characterization of a streptokinase degradation product. J. Biol. Chem. 251:3913, 1976.

41. Staniforth, D. H., Smith, R. A. G., and Hibbs, M.: Streptokinase

and anisoylated streptokinase plasminogen complex: Their action on haemostasis in human volunteers. Eur. J. Clin. Pharmacol. 24:751, 1983.

42. Smith, R. A., Dupe, R. J., English, P. D., and Green, J.: Fibrinolysis with acyl-enzymes: A new approach to thrombolytic therapy. Nature 290:505, 1981.

43. Nunn, B., Esmail, A., Fears, R., Ferres, H., and Standring, R.: Pharmacokinetic properties of anisoylated plasminogen streptokinase activator complex and other thrombolytic agents in animals and in humans. Drugs 33 (Suppl. 3):88, 1987.

44. Lijnen, H. R., and Collen, D.: Staphylokinase, a fibrin-specific bacterial plasminogen activator. Fibrinolysis 10:119, 1996.

45. Collen, D., and Van de Werf, F.: Coronary thrombolysis with recombinant staphylokinase in patients with evolving myocardial infarction. Circulation 87:1850, 1993.

46. Holmes, W. E., Nelles, L., Lijnen, H. R., and Collen, D.: Primary structure of human alpha 2-antiplasmin, a serine protease inhibitor (serpin). J. Biol. Chem. 262:1659, 1987.

47. Bangert, K., Johnsen, A. H., Christensen, U., and Thorsen, S.: Different N-terminal forms of alpha 2-plasmin inhibitor in human plasma. Biochem. J. 291:623, 1993.

48. Kimura, S., and Aoki, N.: Cross-linking site in fibrinogen for alpha 2-plasmin inhibitor. J. Biol. Chem. 261:15591, 1986.

49. Wiman, B., and Collen, D.: On the kinetics of the reaction between human antiplasmin and plasmin. Eur. J. Biochem. 84:573, 1978.

50. Kato, A., Hirosawa, S., Toyota, S., Nakamura, Y., Nishi, H., Kimura, A., Sasazuki, T., and Aoki, N.: Localization of the human alpha 2-plasmin inhibitor gene (PLI) to 17p13. Cytogenet. Cell Genet. 62:190, 1993.

51. Hirosawa, S., Nakamura, Y., Miura, O., Sumi, Y., and Aoki, N.: Organization of the human alpha 2-plasmin inhibitor gene. Proc. Natl. Acad. Sci. USA 85:6836, 1988.

52. Miura, O., Sugahara, Y., Nakamura, Y., Hirosawa, S., and Aoki, N.: Restriction fragment length polymorphism caused by a deletion involving Alu sequences within the human alpha 2-plasmin inhibitor gene. Biochemistry 28:4934, 1989.

53. Kruithof, E. K. O.: Plasminogen activator inhibitors—a review. Enzyme 40:113, 1988.

54. Pannekoek, H., Veerman, H., Lambers, H., Diergaarde, P., Verweij, C. L., van Zonneveld, A. J., and van Mourik, J. A.: Endothelial plasminogen activator inhibitor (PAI): A new member of the Serpin gene family. EMBO J. 5:2539, 1986.

55. Klinger, K. W., Winqvist, R., Riccio, A., Andreasen, P. A., Sartorio, R., Nielsen, L. S., Stuart, N., Stanislovitis, P., Watkins, P., Douglas, R., Grzeschik, H. K., Alitalo, K., Blasi, F., and Danø, K.: Plasminogen activator inhibitor type 1 gene is located at region q21.3-q22 of chromosome 7 and genetically linked with cystic fibrosis. Proc. Natl. Acad. Sci. USA 84:8548, 1987.

56. Declerck, P. J., De Mol, M., Alessi, M. C., Baudner, S., Paques, E. P., Preissner, K. T., Muller-Berghaus, G., and Collen, D.: Purification and characterization of a plasminogen activator inhibitor 1 binding protein from human plasma: Identification as a multimeric form of S protein (vitronectin). J. Biol. Chem. 263:15454, 1988.

57. Gechtman, Z., Sharma, R., Kreizman, T., Fridkin, M., and Shaltiel, S.: Synthetic peptides derived from the sequence around the plasmin cleavage site in vitronectin: Use in mapping the PAI-1 binding site. FEBS Lett. 315:293, 1993.

58. Thorsen, S., Philips, M., Selmer, J., Lecander, I., and Astedt, B.: Kinetics of inhibition of tissue-type and urokinase-type plasminogen activator by plasminogen-activator inhibitor type 1 and type 2. Eur. J. Biochem. 175:33, 1988.

59. Chmielewska, J., Ranby, M., and Wiman, B.: Kinetics of the inhibition of plasminogen activators by the plasminogen-activator inhibitor: Evidence for "second-site" interactions. Biochem. J. 251:327, 1988.

60. Madison, E. L., Goldsmith, E. J., Gerard, R. D., Gething, M. J., and Sambrook, J. F.: Serpin-resistant mutants of human tissue-type plasminogen activator. Nature 339:721, 1989.

61. Adams, D. S., Griffin, L. A., Nachajko, W. R., Reddy, V. B., and Wei, C. M.: A synthetic DNA encoding a modified human urokinase resistant to inhibition by serum plasminogen activator inhibitor. J. Biol. Chem. 266:8476, 1991.

62. Wagner, O. F., de Vries, C., Hohmann, C., Veerman, H., and Pannekoek, H.: Interaction between plasminogen activator inhibitor type 1 (PAI-1) bound to fibrin and either tissue-type plasminogen activator (t-PA) or urokinase-type plasminogen activator (u-PA): Bind-

ing of t-PA/PAI-1 complexes to fibrin mediated by both the finger and the kringle-2 domain of t-PA. J. Clin. Invest. 84:647, 1989.

63. Mottonen, J., Strand, A., Symersky, J., Sweet, R. M., Danley, D. E., Geoghegan, K. F., Gerard, R. D., and Goldsmith, E. J.: Structural basis of latency in plasminogen activator inhibitor-1. Nature 355:270, 1992.

64. Declerck, P. J., De Mol, M., Vaughan, D. E., and Collen, D.: Identification of a conformationally distinct form of plasminogen activator inhibitor-1, acting as a noninhibitory substrate for tissue-type plasminogen activator. J. Biol. Chem. 267:11693, 1992.

65. Aertgeerts, K., De Bondt, H. L., De Ranter, C. J., and Declerck, P. J.: Mechanisms contributing to the conformational and functional flexibility of plasminogen activator inhibitor-1. Nat. Struct. Biol. 2:891, 1995.

66. Descheemaeker, K. A., Wyns, S., Nelles, L., Auwerx, J., Ny, T., and Collen, D.: Interaction of AP-1-, AP-2-, and Sp1-like proteins with two distinct sites in the upstream regulatory region of the plasminogen activator inhibitor-1 gene mediates the phorbol 12-myristate 13-acetate response. J. Biol. Chem. 267:15086, 1992.

67. Ding, H., Descheemaeker, K., Marynen, P., Nelles, L., Carvalho, T., Carmo Fonseca, M., Collen, D., and Belayew, A.: Characterization of a helicase-like transcription factor involved in the expression of the human plasminogen activator inhibitor-1 gene. DNA Cell Biol. 15:429, 1996.

68. Ye, R. D., Ahern, S. M., Le Beau, M. M., Lebo, R. V., and Sadler, J. E.: Structure of the gene for human plasminogen activator inhibitor-2: The nearest mammalian homologue of chicken ovalbumin. J. Biol. Chem. 264:5495, 1989.

69. Bajzar, L., Manuel, R., and Nesheim, M. E.: Purification and characterization of TAFI, a thrombin-activable fibrinolysis inhibitor. J. Biol. Chem. 270:14477, 1995.

70. Eaton, D. L., Malloy, B. E., Tsai, S. P., Henzel, W., and Drayna, D.: Isolation, molecular cloning, and partial characterization of a novel carboxypeptidase B from human plasma. J. Biol. Chem. 266:21833, 1991.

71. Nesheim, M., Wang, W., Boffa, M., Nagashima, M., Morser, J., and Bajzar, L.: Thrombin, thrombomodulin and TAFI in the molecular link between coagulation and fibrinolysis. Thromb. Haemost. 78:386, 1997.

72. Hoylaerts, M., Rijken, D. C., Lijnen, H. R., and Collen, D.: Kinetics of the activation of plasminogen by human tissue plasminogen activator: Role of fibrin. J. Biol. Chem. 257:2912, 1982.

73. Thorsen, S.: The mechanism of plasminogen activation and the variability of the fibrin effector during tissue-type plasminogen activator-mediated fibrinolysis. Ann. NY Acad. Sci. 667:52, 1992.

74. Harpel, P. C., Gordon, B. R., and Parker, T. S.: Plasmin catalyzes binding of lipoprotein (a) to immobilized fibrinogen and fibrin. Proc. Natl. Acad. Sci. USA 86:3847, 1989.

75. Miles, L. A., Dahlberg, C. M., Levin, E. G., and Plow, E. F.: Gangliosides interact directly with plasminogen and urokinase and may mediate binding of these fibrinolytic components to cells. Biochemistry 28:9337, 1989.

76. Miles, L. A., Dahlberg, C. M., Plescia, J., Félez, J., Kato, K., and Plow, E. F.: Role of cell-surface lysines in plasminogen binding to cells: Identification of alpha-enolase as a candidate plasminogen receptor. Biochemistry 30:1682, 1991.

77. Félez, J., Miles, L. A., Fàbregas, P., Jardi, M., Plow, E. F., and Lijnen, H. R.: Characterization of cellular binding sites and interactive regions within reactants required for enhancement of plasminogen activation by t-PA on the surface of leukocytic cells. Thromb. Haemost. 76:577, 1996.

78. Hajjar, K. A., Jacovina, A. T., and Chacko, J.: An endothelial cell receptor for plasminogen/tissue plasminogen activator. I. Identity with annexin II. J. Biol. Chem. 269:21191, 1994.

79. Gurewich, V., Pannell, R., Louie, S., Kelley, P., Suddith, R. L., and Greenlee, R.: Effective and fibrin-specific clot lysis by a zymogen precursor form of urokinase (pro-urokinase): A study in vitro and in two animal species. J. Clin. Invest. 73:1731, 1984.

80. Lijnen, H. R., Van Hoef, B., Nelles, L., and Collen, D.: Plasminogen activation with single-chain urokinase-type plasminogen activator (scu-PA): Studies with active site mutagenized plasminogen (Ser740→Ala) and plasmin-resistant scu-PA (Lys158→Glu). J. Biol. Chem. 265:5232, 1990.

81. Husain, S. S.: Single-chain urokinase-type plasminogen activator does not possess measurable intrinsic amidolytic or plasminogen activator activities. Biochemistry 30:5797, 1991.

82. Liu, J. N., Pannell, R., and Gurewich, V.: A transitional state of pro-

urokinase that has a higher catalytic efficiency against glu-plasminogen than urokinase. J. Biol. Chem. 267:15289, 1992.

83. Declerck, P. J., Lijnen, H. R., Verstreken, M., and Collen, D.: Role of alpha 2-antiplasmin in fibrin-specific clot lysis with single-chain urokinase-type plasminogen activator in human plasma. Thromb. Haemost. 65:394, 1991.

84. Liu, J. N., and Gurewich, V.: Fragment E-2 from fibrin substantially enhances pro-urokinase-induced Glu-plasminogen activation: A kinetic study using the plasmin-resistant mutant pro-urokinase Ala-158-rpro-UK. Biochemistry 31:6311, 1992.

85. Fleury, V., Gurewich, V., and Anglés-Cano, E.: A study of the activation of fibrin-bound plasminogen by tissue-type plasminogen activator, single chain urokinase and sequential combinations of the activators. Fibrinolysis 7:87, 1993.

86. Fleury, V., Lijnen, H. R., and Angles Cano, E.: Mechanism of the enhanced intrinsic activity of single-chain urokinase-type plasminogen activator during ongoing fibrinolysis. J. Biol. Chem. 268:18554, 1993.

87. Ellis, V., Behrendt, N., and Dano, K.: Plasminogen activation by receptor-bound urokinase: A kinetic study with both cell-associated and isolated receptor. J. Biol. Chem. 266:12752, 1991.

88. Ellis, V., Scully, M. F., and Kakkar, V. V.: Plasminogen activation initiated by single-chain urokinase-type plasminogen activator: Potentiation by U937 monocytes. J. Biol. Chem. 264:2185, 1989.

89. Ellis, V., Wun, T. C., Behrendt, N., Ronne, E., and Dano, K.: Inhibition of receptor-bound urokinase by plasminogen-activator inhibitors. J. Biol. Chem. 265:9904, 1990.

90. Lee, S. W., Ellis, V., and Dichek, D. A.: Characterization of plasminogen activation by glycosylphosphatidylinositol-anchored urokinase. J. Biol. Chem. 269:2411, 1994.

91. Collen, D., Schlott, B., Engelborghs, Y., Van Hoef, B., Hartmann, M., Lijnen, H. R., and Behnke, D.: On the mechanism of the activation of human plasminogen by recombinant staphylokinase. J. Biol. Chem. 268:8284, 1993.

92. Silence, K., Collen, D., and Lijnen, H. R.: Regulation by alpha 2-antiplasmin and fibrin of the activation of plasminogen with recombinant staphylokinase in plasma. Blood 82:1175, 1993.

93. Silence, K., Collen, D., and Lijnen, H. R.: Interaction between staphylokinase, plasmin(ogen), and alpha 2-antiplasmin: Recycling of staphylokinase after neutralization of the plasmin-staphylokinase complex by alpha 2-antiplasmin. J. Biol. Chem. 268:9811, 1993.

94. Sakharov, D. V., Lijnen, H. R., and Rijken, D. C.: Interactions between staphylokinase, plasmin(ogen), and fibrin: Staphylokinase discriminates between free plasminogen and plasminogen bound to partially degraded fibrin. J. Biol. Chem. 271:27912, 1996.

95. Carmeliet, P., and Collen, D.: Role of the plasminogen/plasmin system in thrombosis, hemostasis, restenosis and atherosclerosis: Evaluation in transgenic animals. Trends Cardiovasc. Med. 5:117, 1995.

96. Lijnen, H. R., and Collen, D.: Congenital and acquired deficiencies of components of the fibrinolytic system and their relation to bleeding or thrombosis. Fibrinolysis 3:67, 1989.

97. Miura, O., Sugahara, Y., and Aoki, N.: Hereditary alpha 2-plasmin inhibitor deficiency caused by a transport-deficient mutation (alpha 2-PI-Okinawa). Deletion of Glu137 by a trinucleotide deletion blocks intracellular transport. J. Biol. Chem. 264:18213, 1989.

98. Miura, O., Hirosawa, S., Kato, A., and Aoki, N.: Molecular basis for congenital deficiency of alpha 2-plasmin inhibitor: A frameshift mutation leading to elongation of the deduced amino acid sequence. J. Clin. Invest. 83:1598, 1989.

99. Holmes, W. E., Lijnen, H. R., Nelles, L., Kluft, C., Nieuwenhuis, H. K., Rijken, D. C., and Collen, D.: An alanine insertion in alpha 2-antiplasmin "Enschede" abolishes its plasmin inhibitory activity. Science 238:209, 1987.

100. Aoki, N., and Yamanaka, T.: The alpha2-plasmin inhibitor levels in liver diseases. Clin. Chim. Acta 84:99, 1978.

101. Avvisati, G., ten Cate, J. W., Sturk, A., Lamping, R., Petti, M. G., and Mandelli, F.: Acquired alpha-2-antiplasmin deficiency in acute promyelocytic leukaemia. Br. J. Haematol. 70:43, 1988.

102. Collen, D., Bounameaux, H., De Cock, F., Lijnen, H. R., and Verstraete, M.: Analysis of coagulation and fibrinolysis during intravenous infusion of recombinant human tissue-type plasminogen activator in patients with acute myocardial infarction. Circulation 73:511, 1986.

103. Levi, M., Biemond, B. J., van Zonneveld, A. J., ten Cate, J. W., and Pannekoek, H.: Inhibition of plasminogen activator inhibitor-1 activity results in promotion of endogenous thrombolysis and inhibition of thrombus extension in models of experimental thrombosis. Circulation 85:305, 1992.

104. Erickson, L. A., Fici, G. J., Lund, J. E., Boyle, T. P., Polites, H. G., and Marotti, K. R.: Development of venous occlusions in mice transgenic for the plasminogen activator inhibitor-1 gene. Nature 346:74, 1990.

105. Carmeliet, P., Stassen, J. M., Schoonjans, L., Ream, B., van den Oord, J. J., De Mol, M., Mulligan, R. C., and Collen, D.: Plasminogen activator inhibitor-1 gene-deficient mice. II. Effects on hemostasis, thrombosis, and thrombolysis. J. Clin. Invest. 92:2756, 1993.

106. Juhan Vague, I., Moerman, B., De Cock, F., Aillaud, M. F., and Collen, D.: Plasma levels of a specific inhibitor of tissue-type plasminogen activator (and urokinase) in normal and pathological conditions. Thromb. Res. 33:523, 1984.

107. Mellbring, G., Dahlgren, S., Wiman, B., and Sunnegardh, O.: Relationship between preoperative status of the fibrinolytic system and occurrence of deep vein thrombosis after major abdominal surgery. Thromb. Res. 39:157, 1985.

108. Nilsson, I. M., Ljungner, H., and Tengborn, L.: Two different mechanisms in patients with venous thrombosis and defective fibrinolysis: Low concentration of plasminogen activator or increased concentration of plasminogen activator inhibitor. Br. Med. J. 290:1453, 1985.

109. Juhan Vague, I., Valadier, J., Alessi, M. C., Aillaud, M. F., Ansaldi, J., Philip Joet, C., Holvoet, P., Serradimigni, A., and Collen, D.: Deficient t-PA release and elevated PA inhibitor levels in patients with spontaneous or recurrent deep venous thrombosis. Thromb. Haemost. 57:67, 1987.

110. Landin, K., Stigendal, L., Eriksson, E., Krotkiewski, M., Risberg, B., Tengborn, L., and Smith, U.: Abdominal obesity is associated with an impaired fibrinolytic activity and elevated plasminogen activator inhibitor-1. Metabolism 39:1044, 1990.

111. Dawson, S., Hamsten, A., Wiman, B., Henney, A., and Humphries, S.: Genetic variation at the plasminogen activator inhibitor-1 locus is associated with altered levels of plasma plasminogen activator inhibitor-1 activity. Arterioscler. Thromb. 11:183, 1991.

112. Dawson, S. J., Wiman, B., Hamsten, A., Green, F., Humphries, S., and Henney, A. M.: The two allele sequences of a common polymorphism in the promoter of the plasminogen activator inhibitor-1 (PAI-1) gene respond differently to interleukin-1 in HepG2 cells. J. Biol. Chem. 268:10739, 1993.

113. Eriksson, P., Kallin, B., van 't Hooft, F. M., Bavenholm, P., and Hamsten, A.: Allele-specific increase in basal transcription of the plasminogen-activator inhibitor 1 gene is associated with myocardial infarction. Proc. Natl. Acad. Sci. USA 92:1851, 1995.

114. Ye, S., Green, F. R., Scarabin, P. Y., Nicaud, V., Bara, L., Dawson, S. J., Humphries, S. E., Evans, A., Luc, G., and Cambou, J. P.: The 4G/5G genetic polymorphism in the promoter of the plasminogen activator inhibitor-1 (PAI-1) gene is associated with differences in plasma PAI-1 activity but not with risk of myocardial infarction in the ECTIM study. Thromb. Haemost. 74:837, 1995.

115. Grimaudo, V., Bachmann, F., Hauert, J., Christe, M. A., and Kruithof, E. K.: Hypofibrinolysis in patients with a history of idiopathic deep vein thrombosis and/or pulmonary embolism. Thromb. Haemost. 67:397, 1992.

116. Ridker, P. M., Vaughan, D. E., Stampfer, M. J., Manson, J. E., Shen, C., Newcomer, L. M., Goldhaber, S. Z., and Hennekens, C. H.: Baseline fibrinolytic state and the risk of future venous thrombosis: A prospective study of endogenous tissue-type plasminogen activator and plasminogen activator inhibitor. Circulation 85:1822, 1992.

117. Hamsten, A., de Faire, U., Walldius, G., Dahlen, G., Szamosi, A., Landou, C., Blomback, M., and Wiman, B.: Plasminogen activator inhibitor in plasma: Risk factor for recurrent myocardial infarction. Lancet 2:3, 1987.

118. Gram, J., and Jespersen, J.: A selective depression of tissue plasminogen activator (t-PA) activity in euglobulins characterises a risk group among survivors of acute myocardial infarction. Thromb. Haemost. 57:137, 1987.

119. Cimminiello, C.: Tissue-type plasminogen activator and risk of myocardial infarction. Lancet 342:48, 1993.

120. Jansson, J. H., Nilsson, T. K., and Johnson, O.: von Willebrand factor in plasma: A novel risk factor for recurrent myocardial infarction and death. Br. Heart J. 66:351, 1991.

121. Jansson, J. H., Nilsson, T. K., and Olofsson, B. O.: Tissue plasminogen activator and other risk factors as predictors of cardiovascular events in patients with severe angina pectoris. Eur. Heart J. 12:157, 1991.

122. Jansson, J. H., Olofsson, B. O., and Nilsson, T. K.: Predictive value of tissue plasminogen activator mass concentration on long-term mortality in patients with coronary artery disease: A 7-year follow-up. Circulation 88:2030, 1993.

123. Ridker, P. M., Vaughan, D. E., Stampfer, M. J., Manson, J. E., and Hennekens, C. H.: Endogenous tissue-type plasminogen activator and risk of myocardial infarction. Lancet 341:1165, 1993.

124. Salomaa, V., Stinson, V., Kark, J. D., Folsom, A. R., Davis, C. E., and Wu, K. K.: Association of fibrinolytic parameters with early atherosclerosis: The ARIC Study: Atherosclerosis Risk in Communities Study. Circulation 91:284, 1995.

125. Schneiderman, J., Sawdey, M. S., Keeton, M. R., Bordin, G. M., Bernstein, E. F., Dilley, R. B., and Loskutoff, D. J.: Increased type 1 plasminogen activator inhibitor gene expression in atherosclerotic human arteries. Proc. Natl. Acad. Sci. USA 89:6998, 1992.

126. Lupu, F., Bergonzelli, G. E., Heim, D. A., Cousin, E., Genton, C. Y., Bachmann, F., and Kruithof, E. K.: Localization and production of plasminogen activator inhibitor-1 in human healthy and atherosclerotic arteries. Arterioscler. Thromb. 13:1090, 1993.

127. Chomiki, N., Henry, M., Alessi, M. C., Anfosso, F., and Juhan Vague, I.: Plasminogen activator inhibitor-1 expression in human liver and healthy or atherosclerotic vessel walls. Thromb. Haemost. 72:44, 1994.

128. Van de Loo, J. C. W., Haverkate, F., and Thompson, S. G.: Hemostatic factors and the risk of myocardial infarction. N. Engl. J. Med. 332:389, 1995.

129. Thompson, S. G., Kienast, J., Pyke, S. D., Haverkate, F., and van de Loo, J. C.: Hemostatic factors and the risk of myocardial infarction or sudden death in patients with angina pectoris: European Concerted Action on Thrombosis and Disabilities Angina Pectoris Study Group. N. Engl. J. Med. 332:635, 1995.

130. Juhan-Vague, I., Pyke, S. D. M., Alessi, M.-C., Jespersen, J., Haverkate, F., Thompson, S. G., on behalf of the ECAT Study Group: Fibrinolytic factors and the risk of myocardial infarction or sudden death in patients with angina pectoris. Circulation 94:2057, 1996.

131. Mingers, A. M., Heimburger, N., Zeitler, P., Kreth, H. W., and Schuster, V.: Homozygous type I plasminogen deficiency. Semin. Thromb. Hemost. 23:259, 1997.

132. Schuster, V., Mingers, A. M., Seidenspinner, S., Nussgens, Z., Pukrop, T., and Kreth, H. W.: Homozygous mutations in the plasminogen gene of two unrelated girls with ligneous conjunctivitis. Blood 90:958, 1997.

133. Schott, D., Dempfle, C. E., Beck, P., Liermann, A., Mohr-Pennert, A., Azuma, H., Schuster, V., Kramer, M. D., Schwarz, H. P., Liesenhoff, H., and Niessen, K. H.: Successful therapy with Lys-plasminogen in homozygous type 1 plasminogen deficiency (Abstract 70). Fibrinolysis Proteolysis 11 (Suppl. 3):20, 1997.

134. Drew, A. F., Kaufman, A. H., Kombrinck, K. W., Daugherty, C. C., Degen, J. L., and Bugge, T. H.: Ligneous conjunctivitis in plasminogen-deficient mice (Abstract 72). Fibrinolysis Proteolysis 11 (Suppl. 3):21, 1997.

135. Miyata, T., Iwanaga, S., Sakata, Y., and Aoki, N.: Plasminogen Tochigi: Inactive plasmin resulting from replacement of alanine-600 by threonine in the active site. Proc. Natl. Acad. Sci. USA 79:6132, 1982.

136. Ichinose, A., Espling, E. S., Takamatsu, J., Saito, H., Shinmyozu, K., Maruyama, I., Petersen, T. E., and Davie, E. W.: Two types of abnormal genes for plasminogen in families with a predisposition for thrombosis. Proc. Natl. Acad. Sci. USA 88:115, 1991.

137. Miyata, T., Iwanaga, S., Sakata, Y., Aoki, N., Takamatsu, J., and Kamiya, T.: Plasminogens Tochigi II and Nagoya: Two additional molecular defects with Ala-600→Thr replacement found in plasmin light chain variants. J. Biochem. (Tokyo) 96:277, 1984.

138. Wohl, R. C., Summaria, L., and Robbins, K. C.: Physiological activation of the human fibrinolytic system: Isolation and characterization of human plasminogen variants, Chicago I and Chicago II. J. Biol. Chem. 254:9063, 1979.

139. Wohl, R. C., Summaria, L., Chediak, J., Rosenfeld, S., and Robbins, K. C.: Human plasminogen variant Chicago III. Thromb. Haemost. 48:146, 1982.

140. Ploplis, V. A., Carmeliet, P., Vazirzadeh, S., Van Vlaenderen, I., Moons, L., Plow, E. F., and Collen, D.: Effects of disruption of the plasminogen gene on thrombosis, growth, and health in mice. Circulation 92:2585, 1995.

141. Bugge, T. H., Flick, M. J., Daugherty, C. C., and Degen, J. L.: Plasminogen deficiency causes severe thrombosis but is compatible with development and reproduction. Genes Dev. 9:794, 1995.

142. Lijnen, H. R., Carmeliet, P., Bouché, A., Moons, L., Ploplis, V. A., Plow, E. F., and Collen, D.: Restoration of thrombolytic potential in plasminogen-deficient mice by bolus administration of plasminogen. Blood 88:870, 1996.

143. Isacson, S., and Nilsson, I. M.: Defective fibrinolysis in blood and vein walls in recurrent "idiopathic" venous thrombosis. Acta Chir. Scand. 138:313, 1972.

144. Carmeliet, P., Schoonjans, L., Kieckens, L., Ream, B., Degen, J., Bronson, R., De Vos, R., van den Oord, J. J., Collen, D., and Mulligan, R. C.: Physiological consequences of loss of plasminogen activator gene function in mice. Nature 368:419, 1994.

145. Booth, N. A., Bennett, B., Wijngaards, G., and Grieve, J. H.: A new life-long hemorrhagic disorder due to excess plasminogen activator. Blood 61:267, 1983.

146. Aznar, J., Estelles, A., Vila, V., Reganon, E., Espana, F., and Villa, P.: Inherited fibrinolytic disorder due to an enhanced plasminogen activator level. Thromb. Haemost. 52:196, 1984.

147. Schleef, R. R., Higgins, D. L., Pillemer, E., and Levitt, L. J.: Bleeding diathesis due to decreased functional activity of type 1 plasminogen activator inhibitor. J. Clin. Invest. 83:1747, 1989.

148. Diéval, J., Nguyen, G., Gross, S., Delobel, J., and Kruithof, E. K.: A lifelong bleeding disorder associated with a deficiency of plasminogen activator inhibitor type 1. Blood 77:528, 1991.

149. Fay, W. P., Shapiro, A. D., Shih, J. L., Schleef, R. R., and Ginsburg, D.: Brief report: Complete deficiency of plasminogen-activator inhibitor type 1 due to a frame-shift mutation. N. Engl. J. Med. 327:1729, 1992.

150. The GUSTO investigators: An international randomized trial comparing four thrombolytic strategies for acute myocardial infarction. N. Engl. J. Med. 329:673, 1993.

151. Collen, D., and Lijnen, H. R.: Molecular basis of fibrinolysis, as relevant for thrombolytic therapy. Thromb. Haemost. 74:167, 1995.

152. Collen, D.: Towards improved thrombolytic therapy. Lancet 342:34, 1993.

153. Schlant, R. C.: Reperfusion in acute myocardial infarction. Circulation 90:2091, 1994.

154. Grines, C. L., Browne, K. F., Marco, J., Rothbaum, D., Stone, G. W., O'Keefe, J., Overlie, P., Donohue, B., Chelliah, N., Timmis, G. C., Vlietstra, R. E., Strzelecki, M., Puchrowicz-Uchocki, S., and O'Neill, W. W.: A comparison of immediate angioplasty with thrombolytic therapy for acute myocardial infarction: The Primary Angioplasty in Myocardial Infarction Study Group. N. Engl. J. Med. 328:673, 1993.

155. Zijlstra, F., de Boer, M. J., Hoorntje, J. C., Reiffers, S., Reiber, J. H., and Suryapranata, H.: A comparison of immediate coronary angioplasty with intravenous streptokinase in acute myocardial infarction. N. Engl. J. Med. 328:680, 1993.

156. Gibbons, R. J., Holmes, D. R., Reeder, G. S., Bailey, K. R., Hopfenspirger, M. R., and Gersh, B. J.: Immediate angioplasty compared with the administration of a thrombolytic agent followed by conservative treatment for myocardial infarction: The Mayo Coronary Care Unit and Catheterization Laboratory Groups. N. Engl. J. Med. 328:685, 1993.

157. Madison, E. L.: Probing structure-function relationships of tissue-type plasminogen activator by site-specific mutagenesis. Fibrinolysis 8 (Suppl. 1):221, 1994.

158. Verstraete, M., Lijnen, H. R., and Collen, D.: Thrombolytic agents in development. Drugs 50:29, 1995.

159. The National Institute of Neurological Disorders and Stroke rt-PA Stroke Study Group: Tissue plasminogen activator for acute ischemic stroke. N. Engl. J. Med. 333:1581, 1995.

160. Hacke, W., Kaste, M., Fieschi, C., Toni, D., Lesaffre, E., von Kummer, R., Boysen, G., Bluhmki, E., Hàxter, G., Mahagne, M. H., for the ECASS Study Group: Intravenous thrombolysis with recombinant tissue plasminogen activator for acute hemispheric stroke: The European Cooperative Acute Stroke Study (ECASS). JAMA 274:1017, 1995.

161. Multicentre Acute Stroke Trial—Italy (MAST-I) Group: Randomised controlled trial of streptokinase, aspirin, and combination of both in treatment of acute ischaemic stroke. Lancet 346:1509, 1995.

162. The Multicenter Acute Stroke Trial—Europe Study Group: Thrombolytic therapy with streptokinase in acute ischemic stroke. N. Engl. J. Med. 335:145, 1996.

163. Donnan, G. A., Davis, S. M., Chambers, B. R., Gates, P. C., Hankey, G. J., McNeil, J. J., Rosen, D., Stewart-Wynne, E. G., and Tuck, R. R.: Trials of streptokinase in severe acute ischaemic stroke. Lancet 345:578, 1995.

164. De Wood, M. A., Spores, J., Notske, R., Mouser, L. T., Burroughs, R., Golden, M. S., and Lang, H. T.: Prevalence of total coronary occlusion during the early hours of transmural myocardial infarction. N. Engl. J. Med. 303:897, 1980.

165. Rentrop, K. P.: Thrombolytic therapy in patients with acute myocardial infarction. Circulation 71:627, 1985.

166. Braunwald, E.: Myocardial reperfusion, limitation of infarct size, reduction of left ventricular dysfunction, and improved survival: Should the paradigm be expanded? Circulation 79:441, 1989.

167. Chesebro, J. H., Knatterud, G., and Braunwald, E.: Thrombolytic therapy. Correspondence. N. Engl. J. Med. 319:1544, 1988.

168. Collen, D.: Coronary thrombolysis: Streptokinase or recombinant tissue-type plasminogen activator? Ann. Intern. Med. 112:529, 1990.

169. The GUSTO Angiographic Investigators: The effects of tissue plasminogen activator, streptokinase, or both on coronary-artery patency, ventricular function, and survival after acute myocardial infarction. N. Engl. J. Med. 329:1615, 1993.

170. Neuhaus, K. L., Feuerer, W., Jeep-Tebbe, S., Niederer, W., Vogt, A., and Tebbe, U.: Improved thrombolysis with a modified dose regimen of recombinant tissue-type plasminogen activator. J. Am. Coll. Cardiol. 14:1566, 1989.

171. Van de Werf, F., on behalf of the COBALT Investigators: Randomized study of continuous infusion vs double bolus administration of alteplase (rt-PA): The COBALT trial (Abstract 511). Circulation 94 (Suppl.):I89, 1996.

172. Fay, W. P., Eitzman, D. T., Shapiro, A. D., Madison, E. L., and Ginsburg, D.: Platelets inhibit fibrinolysis in vitro by both plasminogen activator inhibitor-1-dependent and -independent mechanisms. Blood 83:351, 1994.

173. Collen, D., Lijnen, H. R., Vanlinthout, I., Kieckens, L., Nelles, L., and Stassen, J. M.: Thrombolytic and pharmacokinetic properties of human tissue-type plasminogen activator variants, obtained by deletion and/or duplication of structural/functional domains, in a hamster pulmonary embolism model. Thromb. Haemost. 65:174, 1991.

174. Kohnert, U., Rudolph, R., Verheijen, J. H., Weening Verhoeff, E. J., Stern, A., Opitz, U., Martin, U., Lill, H., Prinz, H., and Lechner, M.: Biochemical properties of the kringle 2 and protease domains are maintained in the refolded t-PA deletion variant BM 06.022. Protein Eng. 5:93, 1992.

175. Martin, U., Fischer, S., Kohnert, U., Opitz, U., Rudolph, R., Sponer, G., Stern, A., and Strein, K.: Thrombolysis with an *Escherichia coli*–produced recombinant plasminogen activator (BM 06.022) in the rabbit model of jugular vein thrombosis. Thromb. Haemost. 65:560, 1991.

176. Martin, U., von Mollendorff, E., Akpan, W., Kientsch Engel, R., Kaufmann, B., and Neugebauer, G.: Dose-ranging study of the novel recombinant plasminogen activator BM 06.022 in healthy volunteers. Clin. Pharmacol. Ther. 50:429, 1991.

177. Müller, M., Haerer, W., Ellbrück, D., and for the GRECO Study Group: Pharmacokinetics and effects on the hemostatic system of bolus application of a novel recombinant plasminogen activator in AMI patients (Abstract 63). Fibrinolysis 6 (Suppl. 2): 26, 1992.

178. Neuhaus, K. L., von Essen, R., Vogt, A., Tebbe, U., Rustige, J., Wagner, H. J., Appel, K. F., Stienen, U., Konig, R., and Meyer Sabellek, W.: Dose finding with a novel recombinant plasminogen activator (BM 06.022) in patients with acute myocardial infarction: Results of the German Recombinant Plasminogen Activator Study. J. Am. Coll. Cardiol. 24:55, 1994.

179. Tebbe, U., von Essen, R., Smolarz, A., Limbourg, P., Rox, J., Rustige, J., Vogt, A., Wagner, J., Meyer Sabellek, W., and Neuhaus, K. L.: Open, noncontrolled dose-finding study with a novel recombinant plasminogen activator (BM 06.022) given as a double bolus in patients with acute myocardial infarction. Am. J. Cardiol. 72:518, 1993.

180. Smalling, R. W., Bode, C., Kalbfleisch, J., Sen, S., Limbourg, P., Forycki, F., Habib, G., Feldman, R., Hohnloser, S., and Seals, A.: More rapid, complete, and stable coronary thrombolysis with bolus administration of reteplase compared with alteplase infusion in acute myocardial infarction: RAPID Investigators. Circulation 91:2725, 1995.

181. Bode, C., Smalling, R. W., Berg, G., Burnett, C., Lorch, G., Kalbfleisch, J. M., Chernoff, R., Christie, L. G., Feldman, R. L., Seals, A. A., and Weaver, W. D.: Randomized comparison of coronary thrombolysis achieved with double-bolus reteplase (recombinant plasminogen activator) and front-loaded, accelerated alteplase (recombinant tissue plasminogen activator) in patients with acute myocardial infarction: The RAPID II Investigators. Circulation 94:891, 1996.

182. International Joint Efficacy Comparison of Thrombolytics: Randomised, double-blind comparison to reteplase double-bolus administration with streptokinase in acute myocardial infarction (INJECT): Trial to investigate equivalence. Lancet 346:329, 1995.

183. The GUSTO-III investigators: A comparison of reteplase with alteplase for acute myocardial infarction. N. Engl. J. Med. 337:1118, 1997.

184. Keyt, B. A., Paoni, N. F., Refino, C. J., Berleau, L., Nguyen, H., Chow, A., Lai, J., Pena, L., Pater, C., Ogez, J., Etcheverry, T., Botstein, D., and Bennett, W. F.: A faster-acting and more potent form of tissue plasminogen activator. Proc. Natl. Acad. Sci. USA 91:3670, 1994.

185. Paoni, N. F., Keyt, B. A., Refino, C. J., Chow, A. M., Nguyen, H. V., Berleau, L. T., Badillo, J., Pena, L. C., Brady, K., Wurm, F. M., Ogez, J., and Bennett, W. F.: A slow clearing, fibrin-specific, PAI-1 resistant variant of t-PA (T103N, KHRR 296–299 AAAA). Thromb. Haemost. 70:307, 1993.

186. Refino, C. J., Paoni, N. F., Keyt, B. A., Pater, C. S., Badillo, J. M., Wurm, F. M., Ogez, J., and Bennett, W. F.: A variant of t-PA (T103N, KHRR 296–299 AAAA) that, by bolus, has increased potency and decreased systemic activation of plasminogen. Thromb. Haemost. 70:313, 1993.

187. Collen, D., Stassen, J. M., Yasuda, T., Refino, C., Paoni, N., Keyt, B., Roskams, T., Guerrero, J. L., Lijnen, H. R., Gold, H. K., and Bennett, W. F.: Comparative thrombolytic properties of tissue-type plasminogen activator and of a plasminogen activator inhibitor-1-resistant glycosylation variant, in a combined arterial and venous thrombosis model in the dog. Thromb. Haemost. 72:98, 1994.

188. Benedict, C. R., Refino, C. J., Keyt, B. A., Pakala, R., Paoni, N. F., Thomas, G. R., and Bennett, W. F.: New variant of human tissue plasminogen activator (t-PA) with enhanced efficacy and lower incidence of bleeding compared with recombinant human TPA. Circulation 92:3032, 1995.

189. Cannon, C. P., McCabe, C. H., Gibson, C. M., Ghali, M., Sequeira, R. F., McKendall, G. R., Breed, J., Modi, N. B., Fox, N. L., Tracy, R. P., Love, T. W., and Braunwald, E.: TNK-tissue plasminogen activator in acute myocardial infarction: Results of the Thrombolysis in Myocardial Infarction (TIMI) 10A dose-ranging trial. Circulation 95:351, 1997.

190. Cannon, C. P., McCabe, C. H., Gibson, M. C., Adgey, J. A., Sweiger, M. J., Sequeira, R. F., Muller, H. S., McCluskey, E. R., Fox, N. L., Van de Werf, F., and Braunwald, E.: TNK-tissue plasminogen activator compared with front-loaded tissue plasminogen activator in acute myocardial infarction: Primary results of the TIMI-10B trial. Circulation 96 (Suppl. I):206, 1997.

191. Van de Werf, F., and for the ASSENT-1 Investigators: The preliminary results of the ASSENT-1 trial. Presented at the XIXth Congress of the European Society of Cardiology, Stockholm, August 24–28, 1997.

192. Larsen, G. R., Timony, G. A., Horgan, P. G., Barone, K. M., Henson, K. S., Argus, L. B., and Stoudemire, J. B.: Protein engineering of novel plasminogen activators with increased thrombolytic potency in rabbits relative to activase. J. Biol. Chem. 266:8156, 1991.

193. Thadani, U.: INTIME trial. Presented at the Tenth Annual Myocardial Reperfusion Symposium, American College of Cardiology, Anaheim, CA, March 15, 1997.

194. Gardell, S. J., Hare, T. R., Bergum, P. W., Cuca, G. C., O'Neill Palladino, L., and Zavodny, S. M.: Vampire bat salivary plasminogen activator is quiescent in human plasma in the absence of fibrin unlike human tissue plasminogen activator. Blood 76:2560, 1990.

195. Kratzschmar, J., Haendler, B., Langer, G., Boidol, W., Bringmann, P., Alagon, A., Donner, P., and Schleuning, W. D.: The plasminogen activator family from the salivary gland of the vampire bat Desmodus rotundus: Cloning and expression. Gene 105:229, 1991.

196. Bergum, P. W., and Gardell, S. J.: Vampire bat salivary plasminogen activator exhibits a strict and fastidious requirement for polymeric fibrin as its cofactor, unlike human tissue-type plasminogen activator: A kinetic analysis. J. Biol. Chem. 267:17726, 1992.

197. Gardell, S. J., Ramjit, D. R., Stabilito, II, Fujita, T., Lynch, J. J., Cuca, G. C., Jain, D., Wang, S. P., Tung, J. S., Mark, G. E., and Shebuski, R. J.: Effective thrombolysis without marked plasminemia after bolus intravenous administration of vampire bat salivary plasminogen activator in rabbits. Circulation 84:244, 1991.

198. Mellot, M. J., Stabilito, I. I., Holahan, M. A., Cuca, G. C., Wang, S., Li, P., Barrett, J. S., Lynch, J. J., and Gardell, S. J.: Vampire bat salivary plasminogen activator promotes rapid and sustained reperfusion without concomitant systemic plasminogen activation in a canine model of arterial thrombosis. Arterioscler. Thromb. 12:212, 1992.

199. Mellot, M. J., Ramjit, D. R., Stabilito, I. I., Hare, T. R., Senderak, E. T., Lynch, J. J., and Gardell, S. J.: Vampire bat salivary plasminogen activator evokes minimal bleeding relative to tissue-type plasminogen activator as assessed by a rabbit criticle bleeding time model. Thromb. Haemost. 73:478, 1995.

200. Witt, W., Baldus, B., Bringmann, P., Cashion, L., Donner, P., and Schleuning, W. D.: Thrombolytic properties of Desmodus rotundus (vampire bat) salivary plasminogen activator in experimental pulmonary embolism in rats. Blood 79:1213, 1992.

201. Witt, W., Maass, B., Baldus, B., Hildebrand, M., Donner, P., and Schleuning, W. D.: Coronary thrombolysis with Desmodus salivary plasminogen activator in dogs: Fast and persistent recanalization by intravenous bolus administration. Circulation 90:421, 1994.

202. The I.S.A.M. Study Group: A prospective trial of intravenous streptokinase in acute myocardial infarction (I.S.A.M.): Mortality, morbidity, and infarct size at 21 days. N. Engl. J. Med. 314:1465, 1986.

203. Gruppo Italiano per lo Studio della Sopravvivenza nell'Infarto Miocardico: GISSI-2: A factorial randomised trial of alteplase versus streptokinase and heparin versus no heparin among 12,490 patients with acute myocardial infarction. Lancet 336:65, 1990.

204. Third International Study of Infarct Survival Collaborative Group: ISIS-3: A randomised comparison of streptokinase vs. tissue plasminogen activator vs. anistreplase and of aspirin plus heparin vs. aspirin alone among 41,299 cases of suspected acute myocardial infarction: ISIS-3. Lancet 339:753, 1992.

205. Califf, R. M., White, H. D., Van de Werf, F., Sadowski, Z., Armstrong, P. W., Vahanian, A., Simoons, M. L., Simes, R. J., Lee, K. L., Topol, E. J., for the GUSTO-I Investigators: One-year results from the Global Utilization of Streptokinase and t-PA for Occluded Coronary Arteries (GUSTO-I) trial. Circulation 94:1233, 1996.

206. Verstraete, M.: Thrombolytic treatment in acute myocardial infarction. Circulation 82:II96, 1990.

207. Hoffmann, J.J.M.L., Bonnier, J.J.R.M., de Swart, J.B.R.M., Cutsers, P., and Vijgen, P.: Systemic effects of anisoylated plasminogen streptokinase activator complex and streptokinase therapy in acute myocardial infarction. Drugs 33 (Suppl 3):242, 1987.

208. Jalihal, S., and Morris, G. K.: Antistreptokinase titres after intravenous streptokinase. Lancet 335:184, 1990.

209. Mathey, D. G., Schofer, J., Sheehan, F. H., Becher, H., Tilsner, V., and Dodge, H. T.: Intravenous urokinase in acute myocardial infarction. Am. J. Cardiol. 55:878, 1985.

210. PRIMI Trial Study Group: Randomised double-blind trial of recombinant prourokinase against streptokinase in acute myocardial infarction. Lancet 1:863, 1989.

211. Tebbe, U., Windeler, J., Boesl, I., Hoffmann, H., Wojcik, J., Ashmawy, M., Rudiger Schwarz, E., von Loewis, P., Rosemeyer, P., and Hopkins, G.: Thrombolysis with recombinant unglycosylated single-chain urokinase-type plasminogen activator (saruplase) in acute myocardial infarction: Influence of heparin on early patency rate (LIMITS study). J. Am. Coll. Cardiol. 26:365, 1995.

212. Weaver, W. D., Hartmann, J. R., Anderson, J. L., Reddy, P. S., Sobolski, J. C., and Sasahara, A. A.: New recombinant glycosylated prourokinase for treatment of patients with acute myocardial infarction: Prourokinase Study Group. J. Am. Coll. Cardiol. 24:1242, 1994.

213. Bär, F. W., Meyer, J., Vermeer, F., Michels, R., Charbonnier, B., Haerten, K., Spiecker, M., Macaya, C., Hanssen, M., Heras, M., Boland, J. P., Morice, M. C., Dunn, F. G., Uebis, R., Hamm, C., Ayzenberg, O., Strupp, G., Withagen, A. J., Klein, W., Windeler, J., Hopkins, G., Barth, H., and von Fisenne, M. J.: Comparison of saruplase and alteplase in acute myocardial infarction: SESAM Study Group. Am. J. Cardiol. 79:727, 1997.

214. Tebbe, U., Michels, R., Adgey, J., Boland, J., Caspi, A., Charbonnier, B., Windelez, J., Barth, H., Groves, R., Hopkins, G., Fennell, W., Betriu, A., Ruda, M., and Miczoch, J.: Randomized, double-blind study comparing saruplase with streptokinase therapy in acute myocardial infarction: the COMPASS equivalence trial J. Am. Coll. Cardiol. 31:487, 1998.

215. Vanderschueren, S., Barrios, L., Kerdsinchai, P., Van den Heuvel, P., Hermans, L., Vrolix, M., De Man, F., Benit, E., Muyldermans, L., Collen, D., and Van de Werf, F.: A randomized trial of recombinant staphylokinase versus alteplase for coronary artery patency in acute myocardial infarction. Circulation 92:2044, 1995.

216. Vanderschueren, S., Collen, D., and Van de Werf, F.: A pilot study on bolus administration of recombinant staphylokinase for coronary artery thrombolysis. Tromb. Haemost. 76:541, 1996.

217. Vanderschueren, S., Dens, J., Kerdsinchai, P., Desmet, W., Vrolix, M., De Man, F., Van den Heuvel, P., Hermans, L., Collen, D., and Van de Werf, F.: Randomized coronary patency trial of double-bolus recombinant staphylokinase versus front-loaded alteplase in acute myocardial infarction. Am. Heart J. 134:213, 1997.

218. Vanderschueren, S., Stockx, L., Wilms, G., Lacroix, H., Verhaeghe, R., Vermylen, J., and Collen, D.: Thrombolytic therapy of peripheral arterial occlusion with recombinant staphylokinase. Circulation 92:2050, 1995.

219. Vanderschueren, S.M.F., Stassen, J. M., and Collen, D.: On the immunogenicity of recombinant staphylokinase in patients and in animal models. Thromb. Haemost. 72:297, 1994.

220. Declerck, P. J., Vanderschueren, S., Billiet, J., Moreau, H., and Collen, D.: Prevalence and induction of circulating antibodies against recombinant staphylokinase. Thromb. Haemost. 71:129, 1994.

221. Collen, D., Bernaerts, R., Declerck, P., De Cock, F., Demarsin, E., Jenne, S., Laroche, Y., Lijnen, H. R., Silence, K., and Verstreken, M.: Recombinant staphylokinase variants with altered immunoreactivity. I: Construction and characterization. Circulation 94:197, 1996.

222. Collen, D., Moreau, H., Stockx, L., and Vanderschueren, S.: Recombinant staphylokinase variants with altered immunoreactivity. II: Thrombolytic properties and antibody induction. Circulation 94:207, 1996.

223. Vanderschueren, S., Stassen, J. M., and Collen, D.: Comparative antigenicity of recombinant wild-type staphylokinase (SakSTAR) and a selected mutant (SakSTAR.M38) in a baboon thrombolysis model. J. Cardiovasc. Pharmacol. 27:809, 1996.

224. Collen, D., De Cock, F., Demarsin, E., Jenné, S., Lasters, I., Laroche, Y., Warmerdam, P., and Jespers, L.: Recombinant staphylokinase variants with altered immunoreactivity. III. Species variability of antibody binding patterns. Circulation 95:455, 1997.

225. Collen, D., Stockx, L., Lacroix, H., Suy, R., and Vanderschueren, S.: Recombinant staphylokinase variants with altered immunoreactivity. IV. Identification of variants with reduced antibody induction but intact potency. Circulation 95:463, 1997.

24 Platelets

▼▼▼▼ Philip W. Majerus

▼ ▼

Platelets are small discoid anucleate cells 2 to 3 μm in diameter with a cell volume of approximately 10 fl. In man they circulate at a concentration of 250,000 ± 100,000 cells/μl of blood. The primary function of platelets is to prevent hemorrhage resulting from defects in blood vessel walls by forming an aggregate at the site of injury. In addition to primary hemostasis, they participate in reactions of blood coagulation, inflammation, and wound healing. In this chapter, I discuss the physiological and biochemical characteristics of platelets, pointing out disease mechanisms as they apply to this discussion. Much has been learned recently, since platelets have become popular tools for cell biology research. They contain receptors, have a secretion mechanism, are motile, and provide readily accessible human tissue for study.

Much of what is known about platelet function relates to participation of platelets in hemostasis, and therefore, the pathophysiological processes of bleeding disorders due to platelet dysfunction are reasonably well understood. However, the greatest importance of platelets in human disease is in their role in the pathogenesis of atherosclerosis and thrombosis. For example, in England in 1973, 33 patients died of bleeding disorders whereas 100,000 died of thrombosis.[1] Unfortunately, there is currently no definition of the abnormalities in platelet function that predispose to or cause these common disorders. Discovery of such abnormalities is the challenge of the future in platelet research.

Biology of Platelet Production

▼ MEGAKARYOCYTE DIFFERENTIATION

Platelets are formed from large bone marrow cells called megakaryocytes by a remarkable and relatively poorly understood process. The stem cell that is the progenitor of megakaryocytes is morphologically unidentified and has been defined in experiments in which it has been cloned and differentiated in vitro, both in soft agar[2, 3] and by a plasma clot assay.[4, 5] As megakaryocytes proliferate they enlarge and undergo extensive DNA replication without mitosis.[6] The polyploid cells subsequently undergo endomitosis to form multilobed nuclei with 4 to 64 times the haploid amount of DNA[7] (Fig. 24–1), most commonly 16 or 32N. Why these cells are polyploid is completely obscure. Only after DNA replication has ceased do the cells begin to show cytoplasmic differentiation with production of the components that constitute the mature platelet. During this time, a number of

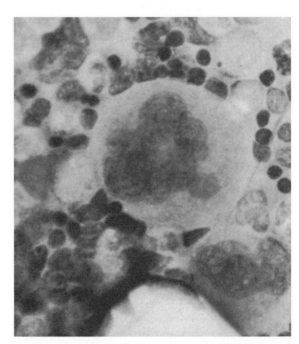

Figure 24–1. Human Megakaryocyte Stained with Wright's Stain with Two Polyploid Cells Shown. (Original magnification 700 ×.)

platelet proteins appear, including fibrinogen,[8] coagulation factor V,[9] platelet factor IV,[10] platelet-derived growth factor,[11] von Willebrand factor (vWF),[12] and some platelet glycoproteins[13] (including glycoproteins Ib, IIb, and IIIa, which are discussed later).

With continued maturation the megakaryocyte cytoplasm develops an extensive membrane system termed demarcation membranes,[14, 15] formed by invagination of the plasma membrane. They communicate with the cell exterior as shown by staining with extracellular tracers such as horseradish peroxidase. The mature megakaryocyte is located directly adjacent to bone marrow sinusoidal endothelial cells. As the extensive demarcation membrane system forms, megakaryocytes develop long filopodia (2.5 $\times$ 120 μm) that directly penetrate the endothelial cytoplasm and extend into the marrow capillaries.[16] These projections then fragment to produce mature platelets. Several thousand platelets are ultimately produced from the cytoplasm of a single mature megakaryocyte. Whether the ploidy of the parent cell has any influence on the number and/or quality of platelets produced is not clear. In rare instances, large fragments appear to break off, and even entire megakaryocytes can enter the circulation and lodge in pulmonary capillaries. In this way, a small percentage of platelet production occurs outside the marrow. In some disorders of bone marrow structure or function, increased numbers of megakaryocyte fragments circulate.

▼ THROMBOCYTOPOIESIS

The production of platelets depends on a variety of hematopoietic cytokines, the most important of which is thrombopoietin. The proliferation and maturation of megakaryocytes are stimulated by early acting cytokines that are not linage specific, including interleukin-3 (IL-3), granulocyte-macrophage colony stimulating factor (GM-CSF), and stem cell factor.[17] However, the development of megakaryocytes is dependent on thrombopoietin.[17] Thrombopoietin is a 332 amino acid glycoprotein that is homologous (23 per cent identity) to its erythroid counterpart erythropoietin. It is encoded by a gene in chromosome 3q27 and has been cloned by several laboratories.[18–22] The thrombopoietin receptor is also homologous to the erythropoietin receptor and is expressed on platelets, megakaryocytes, and endothelial cells.[23] There are only about 200 sites/platelet with a kD of 0.5 nM.[24, 25] Thrombopoietin stimulates platelet production in animals and man and its plasma levels are inversely related to platelet count, as expected.[26] It appears that platelet production is regulated by the thrombopoietin receptor in a novel way. Thus thrombopoietin binds to platelet receptors and is internalized and degraded, decreasing the plasma concentration available to stimulate megakaryocyte proliferation and differentiation.[27, 28] Therefore, when platelet counts are high, thrombopoietin binds to its receptor and is degraded, lowering plasma levels. When thrombocytopenia occurs, binding and degradation decrease and plasma levels rise, thus stimulating platelet production. In fact, it may be that patients with thrombocytopenia respond to lower doses of thrombopoietin for this reason. In thrombopoietin receptor knock out mice thrombopoietin levels are elevated, thrombo-

poietin has a prolonged life span, and the mice are thrombocytopenic.[29]

Thrombopoietin is effective in raising platelet counts in animals and in a few early clinical trials in man also seems to be effective in raising platelet counts or decreasing the time of thrombocytopenia after chemotherapy for cancer.[30, 31] The clinical utility of this cytokine remains to be shown. Several laboratory studies suggest that thrombopoietin increases platelet reactivity to agonists, raising the possibility that it might predispose to thrombosis.[32] Patients with clinically significant thrombocytopenia requiring transfusion of platelets (i.e., <10,000–20,000/ml) have not yet been treated with thrombopoietin.

Recently another hematopoietic cytokine, interleukin-11 (IL-11), has been approved for use in treating thrombocytopenia induced by chemotherapy. IL-11 stimulates megakaryocytopoiesis independently of thrombopoietin and its receptor[33] and has been shown to increase platelet counts and shorten the period of thrombocytopenia after chemotherapy in randomized trials.[34, 35]

▼ PLATELET HOMEOSTASIS

In normal man platelet numbers are maintained at a constant level. The total body platelet mass determines platelet production rather than the circulating platelet number. Normally, approximately one third of platelets are not circulating but remain in the splenic circulation. Thus, asplenic individuals have elevated circulating platelet counts. In disorders that result in splenomegaly a larger fraction of platelets reside in the spleen, resulting in lower numbers of circulating platelets. However, the splenic platelets are available for mobilization, and, therefore, patients with splenomegaly often have decreased numbers of circulating platelets without altered hemostasis. Platelets are produced at a rate of approximately 40,000/μl of blood/day with a life span of 7 to 10 days.[7] Platelet consumption is by a combination of "senescence" and utilization in hemostatic reactions. Autologous platelet survival can be measured by radiolabeling cells in vitro with either ^{51}Cr or ^{111}In and reinfusing them.[36] Increased platelet consumption, as evidenced by decreased survival rate, has been reported in some patients with atherosclerosis or thrombosis; however, this parameter is not regularly associated with vascular disease and its measurement in patients suspected to have vascular disease is of no practical value. In man the time required for differentiation of megakaryocyte precursors to circulating platelets is 4 to 5 days. The best calculations estimate that the marrow can increase platelet production 5- to 10-fold in disease states, thereby maintaining normal platelet numbers despite increased consumption. Diseases associated with decreased platelet numbers result from either decreased production or increased destruction. These include decreased production due to marrow aplasia or infiltration and increased destruction due to autoimmune disorders in which antibody mediated platelet destruction occurs. In general, spontaneous bleeding does not occur until platelet numbers are reduced to at least one tenth of normal.

A variety of disorders are associated with increased platelet numbers; these include so-called reactive thrombocytosis seen in patients with trauma, infections, iron deficiency, and cancer. Mechanisms for increased platelets in these cases are unknown. In myeloproliferative diseases with abnormal marrow function such as myelofibrosis, polycythemia vera, chronic granulocytic leukemia, and primary thrombocytosis, elevated platelet numbers also occur and platelet function is often abnormal despite the increased numbers. Soft agar assays of progenitors of megakaryocytes indicate that these patients produce many more megakaryocyte colonies than normal.[37]

▼ PLATELET STRUCTURE AND METABOLISM

The structure of human platelets is illustrated in Figure 24–2. These cells are free floating and discoid. They contain an intricate system of channels continuous with the plasma membrane that is similar to the demarcation system of the megakaryocyte. This is termed the open canalicular system.[38] The anatomical features of the platelet are similar to those of a sponge, giving these cells an enormous surface area compared with a sphere of comparable size (i.e., ~20 μ³ for a sphere versus 150 μ³ for a platelet, as estimated from the density of cell surface lectin binding sites).[39] Platelets have a dense tubular membrane system thought to be analogous to the sarcoplasmic reticulum of smooth muscle,[38] which serves to pump and release Ca²⁺. They also contain at least

three distinct types of secretory granules: dense, α, and lysosomes.[40] The α granules contain coagulation factors, such as fibrinogen, factor V,[41] high molecular weight kininogen, and von Willebrand factor (vWF). They also contain a number of other proteins and peptides, whose functions are discussed later, including platelet-derived growth factor (PDGF), platelet factor IV, β thromboglobulin, thrombin-sensitive protein (thrombospondin [TSP]), and P selectin. α Granules also contain low concentrations of all plasma proteins, suggesting import by fluid phase endocytosis.[42]

Many of the proteins found in platelet α granules are packaged after synthesis in the precursor megakaryocyte. A number of α granule proteins have been shown to be synthesized de novo by megakaryocytes, including coagulation factor V,[9] platelet factor IV,[10] and vWF.[12] Other proteins contained in α granules, including immunoglobulin G (IgG), albumin, and fibrinogen, are taken up from plasma by a novel endocytotic mechanism.[43–47] Fibronectin, factor V, and high molecular weight kininogen may also be taken up by this mechanism as their concentration in α granules exceeds that of plasma.[42] α Granule proteins are secreted in response to agonists except P selectin, which is an integral membrane protein that becomes a cell surface protein as α granule membranes fuse with plasma membranes during secretion. P selectin binds a receptor on neutrophils called P selectin glycoprotein ligand¹ (PSGL-1), a disulfide-linked homodi-

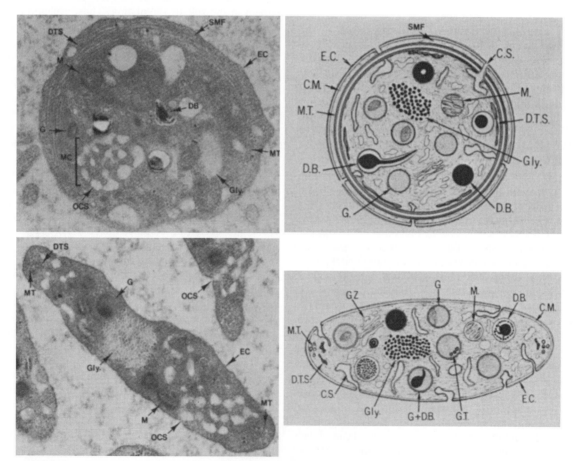

Figure 24–2. Platelet Structure. Diagrams and electron micrographs of thin sections (original magnification 60,000 ×) represent platelets cut in cross section and in the equatorial plane. *CM*, plasma membrane; *CS, OCS*, open canalicular membranes; *DTS*, dense tubular system; *DB*, dense body; *EC*, surface glycoproteins; *Gly*, glycogen granules; *G*, granules; *MT*, microtubules; *M*, mitochondria; *SMF*, microfilaments.

meric mucin-like glycoprotein, and promotes their adhesion to platelets.[47] The physiological role of this phenomenon is uncertain.[48]

Although some α granule proteins are unique to platelets (i.e., PDGF and platelet factor IV), others are major plasma proteins (i.e., fibrinogen, coagulation factor V, and lipoprotein associated coagulation inhibitor). It is a mystery why these latter proteins are packaged in platelets when platelets circulate in a fluid that contains 5 to 10 times as much of these proteins. It has been suggested that agonist-induced secretion from α granules may serve to elevate the local concentration of critical proteins in wounds.[49] A number of the plasma proteins contained in α granules, including histidine-rich glycoprotein,[50] fibronectin,[51] high molecular weight kininogen,[52] and α_1 protease inhibitor,[53] have been proposed to be important in platelet physiological processes. Agonist-induced platelet secretion results in liberation of these molecules, although the meager quantities render any physiological importance problematic.

Another type of secretory granule in platelets is termed the dense body. This organelle contains Ca^{2+} and Mg^{2+} ions, adenosine triphosphate (ATP), adenosine diphosphate (ADP), and smaller amounts of other nucleotides plus several vasoactive amines, particularly 5-hydroxytryptamine (serotonin). The third secretory granule is a lysosome-containing lysosomal enzyme similar to those found in other cells.

Platelets are anucleate and do not contain genomic DNA, although they contain mitochondria and small amounts of messenger RNA (mRNA) that have been amplified by polymerase chain reaction.[54] Platelets do not synthesize protein except after activation by thrombin in a novel activation of translation by an unknown mechanism.[55] Platelets do carry out most reactions of carbohydrate[56] and lipid metabolism[57, 58] that occur in other cells.

Physiology of Platelet Plug Formation

▼ PLATELET ADHESION TO FOREIGN SURFACES

In the circulation, platelets are free-floating cells that do not adhere to each other or to vascular endothelium. When platelets are exposed to a non-endothelial surface, they adhere, flatten, and spread on the surface. In this process platelet shape changes dramatically from a disc to a spiny sphere with long, fine filopodia that may be several times the length of a platelet. Presumably the excess surface membrane required to form the filopodia is obtained from the canalicular membrane system. Under pathological conditions of endothelial injury or wounds, the major non-endothelial surface to which platelets adhere is collagen fibrils. Experimental study of the adherence of platelets to collagen in vitro indicates that fibrillar collagen is required.[59] Collagen monomers or fragments of collagen chains do not support platelet adhesion. The platelet collagen receptor is a dimeric 110/150 kDa glycoprotein that was previously designated glycoprotein Ia/IIa but is now called VLA-2 as it is one of the integrins present on many cells.[60] No inherited abnormalities of this putative receptor have been found. VLA-2 alone does not induce platelet aggregation and secretion, and this process requires a "coreceptor," most likely glycoprotein

VI.[61] Under conditions of shear, in vivo, collagen may not bind directly to platelets because a plasma protein, vWF, is required to support platelet adhesion to subendothelial surfaces. Among current hypotheses, the best is that vWF, under conditions of high flow and shear, first adheres to subendothelial collagen fibers, a process that leads to an alteration in the conformation of the vWF (or its receptor), allowing it to bind to a specific receptor site on platelets. Congenital lack of either vWF (von Willebrand's disease; see Chapter 21) or the platelet receptor (Bernard-Soulier syndrome; see von Willebrand Factor Receptor, page 774) leads to a hemorrhagic diathesis characterized by abnormal platelet adherence.[62] Since the extracellular matrix contains collagen fibers in most loci, platelets readily adhere to wound surfaces. Intact endothelium presumably has no such luminal collagen fibers. Whether other features of endothelial surface proteins are also important in the non-thrombogenicity of this tissue is unknown. Endothelial cells also produce an icosanoid mediator, prostacyclin, that further inhibits platelet adhesion.

▼ PLATELET AGGREGATION

Most of the platelets that accumulate at sites of injury do not adhere directly to subendothelial structures but rather to each other. The process of platelet-platelet adherence is termed aggregation and has properties distinct from those of adhesion. Platelet aggregation has been studied in vitro by measuring the aggregation of stirred suspensions of platelets by monitoring changes in optical density (Fig. 24–3). Platelet aggregation can be triggered experimentally by several potential physiological agonists, the most important of which are adenosine diphosphate (ADP) and thrombin. Other potential agonists include epinephrine, thromboxane A_2, and platelet-activating factor (PAF).[63–65] In all systems studied, platelet aggregation requires both fibrinogen and ADP.[64] In the case of agonists such as thrombin and PAF that stimulate the secretion of platelet granule contents, ADP and fibrinogen are provided by their secretion. In vitro addition of ADP alone to a stirred platelet suspension causes aggregation only in the presence of added fibrinogen. Full aggregation and modest secretion (equivalent to one fourth of the α granules and dense bodies) occurs in response to ADP only when thromboxane A_2 is formed. Thus, when platelets are taken from subjects who have ingested aspirin (thereby blocking cyclooxygenase and subsequent thromboxane production; see Production of Icosanoids, page 770), no secretion and only partial, reversible aggregation are observed with ADP (this has been termed "first-phase" aggregation).

There are two general types of agonists for platelet aggregation:[64]

1. *Weak agonists*, such as ADP and epinephrine, cause aggregation only when thromboxane production occurs in the platelet. With these agonists, secretion follows and depends on platelet aggregation (i.e., if platelets are not stirred during the experiment to promote cell-cell contact, secretion does not occur). Furthermore, secretion is incomplete in response to these agonists.

2. *Strong agonists*, such as thrombin, collagen, and

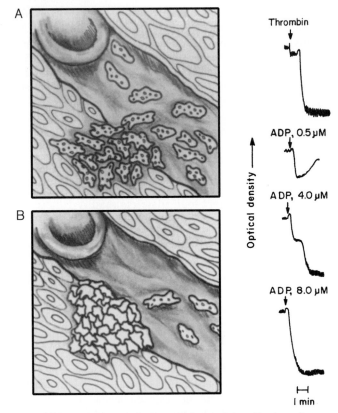

Figure 24–3. Platelet Adhesion and Aggregation. Platelets adhere to subendothelial structures at sites of vascular injury *(A)*. Other platelets then aggregate to each other at the site to form a physical plug *(B)*. The in vitro aggregation of platelets is determined by stirring platelet suspensions in a spectrophotometer and measuring aggregation as changes in optical density. As cells aggregate, optical density decreases. Strong agonists such as thrombin produce rapid, irreversible aggregation, as shown in the upper tracing on the right. ADP, 0.5 μM, produces transient, reversible aggregation; ADP, 4 μM, produces aggregation in two phases, the second of which follows secretion; ADP, 8 μM, produces rapid, irreversible aggregation.

be secreted. Full ADP aggregation is dependent on thromboxane A_2 production.[68] There is a thromboxane A_2 receptor on platelets, but how this moiety, or thromboxane itself, enhances fibrinogen binding in the presence of ADP is unknown.

Other proteins have also been postulated to link fibrinogen or fibrin monomers to each other, including thrombospondin and fibronectin. Thrombospondin is an α granule protein that is secreted when platelets are activated.[69, 70] It is a 440 kDa trimeric protein that is disulfide linked[71] and that binds to the platelet surface after secretion.[71] This protein interacts with fibrinogen, and there is evidence that thrombospondin may serve a bridging function between fibrinogen molecules on adjacent platelets.[72–74] However, the importance of thrombospondin in platelet aggregation is uncertain, since patients with congenital deficiency of α granules with less than 10 per cent of normal thrombospondin (gray platelet syndrome) do not have severely deranged platelet aggregation[75] and thrombospondin "knockout" mice have normal bleeding times and platelet aggregation in response to thrombin.[76] Another proposed function for thrombospondin is that it binds to platelets and then to a plasma protein named histidine-rich glycoprotein to anchor this protein (a known heparin antagonist) to activated platelets. In this way local coagulation reactions may be protected from inhibition by heparin.[77]

Although the measurement of platelet aggregation in vitro has been useful experimentally both in defining the requirements for aggregation and in classifying various hemorrhagic disorders, it is not a very useful test in medical practice. Abnormal platelet aggregation in vitro does not necessarily predict a clinically significant bleeding diathesis. The most direct demonstration of this point is that normal subjects who have taken aspirin have abnormal aggregation for several days thereafter without any significant bleeding disorder. Similarly, attempts to utilize "hyperaggregability" or hypersensitivity of platelets to in vitro stimuli as a predictor of future or current in vivo thrombotic events have been unsuccessful.

Physiological Generation of a Hemostatic Plug

After platelets adhere to collagen, these adherent platelets are activated to secrete ADP, generate thromboxane A_2, and activate coagulation reactions leading to the production of thrombin. These agonists in turn recruit other platelets to aggregate, ultimately forming a physical plug that obstructs the wound surface. Upon this surface a fibrin clot forms and contracts to seal the vessel wall or wound.

▼ PLATELET SECRETION

Platelet secretion of α granules and dense body contents follows platelet aggregation by the agonists previously listed. There is also partial secretion of lysosomal enzymes. Strong agonists result in secretion of 70 to 90 per cent of α granule and dense body contents. Secretion appears to be triggered by contraction of a circumferential band of microtubules that condenses the platelet granules into the center of the cell. Here the granule membranes fuse with membranes of the

platelet-activating factor, cause secretion equally well with or without aggregation (i.e., reaction is the same with or without stirring) and do not depend on thromboxane A_2 production. Thus, thrombin-induced aggregation and secretion occur even in aspirin-treated platelets. At low concentrations of strong agonists, secretion is both aggregation- and thromboxane A_2–dependent. The molecular basis for these two apparently distinct mechanisms for platelet secretion is unknown.

Fibrinogen is required for platelet aggregation; it binds to receptors on activated platelets and appears to provide part of the mechanism linking platelets to each other.[65] Whereas vWF appears to link platelets to the subendothelial surface, fibrinogen links platelets to each other. It has been proposed that polymerization of fibrinogen (fibrin monomers) links one platelet to another. Fibrinogen alone does not support platelet aggregation, implying that fibrinogen receptors are not available on unstimulated cells.[66, 67] Addition of ADP makes fibrinogen binding sites appear by a mechanism that has not been elucidated. Upon addition of ADP to platelets, aggregation appears to precede secretion so that ADP does not act by causing α granule proteins to surface-connected open canalicular membrane.[78] The secretion is analogous to squeezing of water out of a sponge. The physiological characteristics of platelet motility required for shape change and secretion are discussed in the following section in the analysis of clot reaction.

▼ PLATELET CONTRACTION

After the platelet-fibrin hemostatic plug is formed, it decreases in volume by a process that depends on the contractile apparatus of the platelet. Platelet reactions that depend on the contractile system include filopodium formation, lamellipodium formation, secretion, and clot retraction. The cytoskeleton of the platelet consists of actin filaments, microtubules (which are made up of tubulin), and a variety of associated proteins.[79] Platelets contain a smooth muscle–type contractile system. Actin, a 42 kDa protein, comprises approximately 15 per cent of soluble platelet protein.[80, 81] There are six separate genes for actin,[82, 83] producing different proteins in skeletal, cardiac, and various smooth muscle–containing cells, of which β and γ types are expressed in platelets.[81] Actin exists in two forms: as monomers, referred to as G actin, and as a double-helical polymeric form, termed F actin.[84] In unstimulated platelets, approximately 50 per cent of actin is F actin.[85] Platelet myosin has a molecular weight of 460 kDa and consists of dimers of myosin heavy chains (200 kDa) and two types of light chains (20 kDa and 16 kDa).[84] The head of the myosin heavy chain contains the adenosine triphosphatase (ATPase) and actin-binding sites. The ATPase is active only when the 20 kDa light chain is phosphorylated.[86, 87] The phosphorylation of the light chain controls the contractile process and is catalyzed by myosin light chain kinase, a calcium ion and calmodulin-dependent enzyme.[88, 89] In unstimulated platelets, the myosin light chains are unphosphorylated. Upon activation by thrombin, they are phosphorylated within a few seconds, thereby initiating the contractile process. Most of the forces generated by contracting platelets are transmitted through the actin filaments, since actin, present at 100 times the concentration of myosin, composes the majority of the mass of the cytoskeleton.[79]

Study of the polymerization of actin has been facilitated by the recognition that actin filaments have a polarity that is demonstrated by adding heavy meromyosin to preparations of actin filaments. The myosin "decorates" the actin filaments in a characteristic way, producing an arrowhead-like structure with a pointed and a barbed end of the filament.[90] Actin filaments can grow by addition of monomers to either end of the filament, although growth is approximately fivefold faster at the barbed end, which is also the end that abuts the plasma membrane.[91, 92] In vitro, in physiological salts, the critical concentration of G actin that leads to spontaneous polymerization is ~30 μM. The concentration of actin within platelets is ~10 times this concentration, suggesting that actin should be fully polymerized in unstimulated platelets. However, such is not the case, indicating that platelets have a mechanism for preventing actin polymerization. Several regulating mechanisms have been proposed.[84] G actin binds to profilin, a basic protein of 16 kDa, in a 1:1 complex of relatively low affinity. Platelets contain sufficient profilin to bind approximately one half of the total actin in the cell,

which is the proportion of G actin in the unstimulated cells.[93] This complex may serve as an actin buffer such that when conditions favor rapid polymerization of actin, the complex dissociates and actin filaments can grow.[94, 95] Phosphatidylinositol 4,5-bisphosphate (PtdIns [4, 5] P_2) binds profilin with high affinity ($K_d < 0.1$ μM) with a stoichiometry of 5 moles of PtdIns (4, 5) P_2/mole of profilin and thereby frees actin to polymerize.[96] It is possible that this function is served by the polyphosphorylated 3-phosphate-containing phosphatidylinositols in vivo. A second mechanism to inhibit polymerization is mediated by proteins that bind to the ends of actin filaments, thereby capping them and preventing further growth. Several proteins have been proposed as possible barbed-end capping proteins, including vinculin and α actinin, and capping protein.[80] Gelsolin, a 90 kDa protein found in platelets and leukocytes, is a barbed-end capping protein. However, gelsolin may act to regulate actin polymerization in stimulated rather than in resting cells, since this molecule requires μM calcium ions for activity.[97] In unstimulated platelets, the calcium ion concentration is ~0.1 μM, rising to several micromolar concentration upon activation. Targeted deletion of gelsolin in mice results in abnormal shape change in response to thrombin, but actin polymerization is nearly normal.[98]

The state of actin polymerization in platelets has been measured experimentally in two ways. G actin forms a 1:1 complex with deoxyribonuclease (DNase) I, blocking its action on DNA. The proportion of G actin in platelets can be measured as the DNAse inhibitory activity in platelet lysates, and total actin is measured after actin filament depolymerization in guanidine.[85] A second method involves Triton detergent extraction of platelets, whereby the actin filaments remain as an insoluble residue that can be measured by subsequent sodium dodecyl sulfate (SDS) and polyacrylamide gel electrophoresis.[99] These methods have been used to demonstrate that actin filaments grow rapidly upon platelet activation to contain ~75 per cent of the total actin. It appears that the filaments grow mainly from the barbed end, thereby pushing the membrane out into filapodia, with the pointed end pressing against the central circumferential band of microtubles, compressing the granules to the center of the cell. SDS gel electrophoresis of platelet Triton residues after thrombin activation indicates that a number of other proteins become rapidly associated with the actin network after platelet activation, including myosin, actin-binding protein, and a platelet membrane glycoprotein designated IIb/IIIa. (See Fibrinogen Receptor [Glycoprotein IIb/IIIa], page 772.) Whether actin is anchored directly to this membrane glycoprotein or via other putative actin-membrane-anchoring proteins such as ankyrin, vinculin, or α actinin remains to be elucidated. The function of actin-binding protein (a 270 kDa dimeric protein) in the control of actin polymerization is also unclear. Actin-binding protein tends to promote actin bundle formation and may also serve to cross-link actin filaments. The function of this protein may be modulated by proteolysis by a calcium ion–activated protease calpain that occurs in platelets.[95, 97–100] These reactions leading to clot retraction are all dependent on the activation of small guanosine triphosphate (GTP) binding proteins, as indicated in Figure 24–4.

Once platelets are activated, they aggregate and secrete their granule contents. Coagulation reactions then occur on

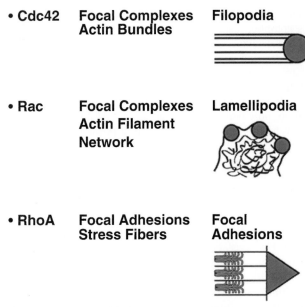

- **Cdc42** Focal Complexes Filopodia
  Actin Bundles

- **Rac** Focal Complexes Lamellipodia
  Actin Filament
  Network

- **RhoA** Focal Adhesions Focal
  Stress Fibers Adhesions

Figure 24–4. Small Guanine Nucleotide Binding Proteins That Mediate Platelet Motility and Clot Retraction. G proteins mediate specific reactions in platelet motility. Cdc42, Rac, and Rho[100] must be activated by binding GTP for each of the processes depicted. (Figure courtesy of J. E. Fox, Cleveland Clinic Foundation, Cleveland, Ohio.)

the platelet surface and finally clot reaction occurs by action of myosin ATPase acting through actin filaments. The actin filaments are anchored to the membrane glycoprotein IIb/IIIa at focal adhesions, which are, in turn, linked to fibrin strands outside the cell. In this way platelet contraction can effectively diminish the volume of the much larger fibrin clot. A congenital disorder with defective clot retraction is Glanzmann's thrombasthenia. (See Fibrinogen Receptor [Glycoprotein IIb/IIIa], page 772.)

▼ ROLE OF PLATELETS IN COAGULATION REACTIONS

The sequence of coagulation reactions that is most widely accepted is called the waterfall, or cascade, hypothesis.[101] However, the current scheme is quite different (Chapter 20), in that the extrinsic system of factor VII and tissue factor is the initial stimulus that sets off the coagulation system.

Platelets potentially participate in a number of coagulation reactions. A major reaction that occurs on the platelet surface is the process of prothrombin activation. In this reaction, factor X_a catalyzes the conversion of prothrombin to thrombin in the presence of a cofactor, factor Va.[102] This reaction occurs on a platelet surface receptor for factors X_a and V_a, which is described on page 776.

A number of experiments have indicated that phospholipids and coagulation factor V_a can replace platelets in prothrombin activation in vitro. Additionally, phospholipid can substitute for platelets in various assays that measure the time required to clot activated plasma after addition of Ca^{2+}. For example, addition of Russell's viper venom to plasma activates factor X (all of the factor X in plasma), and the clotting time of such activated plasma can be shortened by addition of either platelets or phospholipids. Thus,

it has been proposed that the entity in the platelet that promotes the conversion of prothrombin to thrombin is a phospholipoprotein on the platelet surface, which previously had been called platelet factor 3.[103] A variety of empirical tests have been devised to measure this substance, but none utilizes physiological amounts of the various components. In vivo, <1 per cent of factor X is activated to factor X_a. At such low factor X_a concentrations, platelet surface prothrombin activation occurs 15- to 20-fold faster than that which occurs on an optimal phospholipid surface.[104–108] Once a prothrombinase complex is organized on its platelet receptor, it is protected from inactivation by plasma protease inhibitors.[104, 109] The anticoagulant heparin that acts by activating antithrombin III is unable to inhibit factor X_a once it is bound to the platelet surface. Thus, coagulation reactions once started in the area of a hemostatic plug are not blocked by heparin anticoagulation. This may explain the relative ineffectiveness of heparin in preventing arterial thromboses.

Platelets have other mechanisms that also protect ongoing surface coagulation reactions. Platelets secrete platelet factor IV, a 31 kDa tetrameric polypeptide that serves to bind heparin and thereby prevent its anticoagulant action.[110, 111] Similarly, thrombospondin, which is also secreted by platelets, binds to the platelet surface and then binds histidine-rich glycoprotein, which binds heparin and blocks its anticoagulant effect.[77] Therefore, in the immediate platelet milieu, coagulation factors are protected from inhibition.

Prothrombin activation is readily studied in vitro, since all the prothrombin (1 μM) in plasma is activated during this process. Since a large amount of thrombin is formed, it is easily measured. Attempts to define a role for platelets in the activation of factor X itself have been difficult, since a small amount (<1 per cent) is activated during coagulation reactions in vitro. Thus, attempts to add factors IX_a, VIII_a, and X to platelets to demonstrate a specific platelet catalyzed activation reaction have been thus far largely unsuccessful.[112] Platelets do accelerate factor XI activation. Thrombin activates factor XI very poorly and platelets participate in a 50-fold acceleration of the activation.[113] There are 1000 binding sites for factor XI on platelets.[113] Deficiency of factor XII does not result in a bleeding disorder, suggesting that it is not required for factor XI activation. Patients who are factor XI–deficient do bleed, and therefore it is clear that factor XI_a is important for hemostasis. Platelets also contain factor XIII, the enzyme that cross-links fibrin clots. This moiety, however, is contained in the platelet cytoplasm and is not secreted when platelets are activated. Thus, it is difficult to envision a role of platelet factor XIII in hemostasis.

▼ PRODUCTION OF ICOSANOIDS

Platelets produce icosanoid mediators (oxygenated derivatives of arachidonic acid) in response to activation[114] (Fig. 24–5). Arachidonic acid (5,8,11,14-eicosatetraenoic acid) is the major polyunsaturated fatty acid in man. This fatty acid is essential, since we are unable to desaturate fatty acids to form the 14 position double bond found in arachidonate. Dietary linoleate (9,12-octadecadienoic acid) is the major arachidonate precursor in man. Linoleate is converted to arachidonate in liver by desaturases. Many cells that produce icosanoids, including platelets, lack desaturase enzymes and

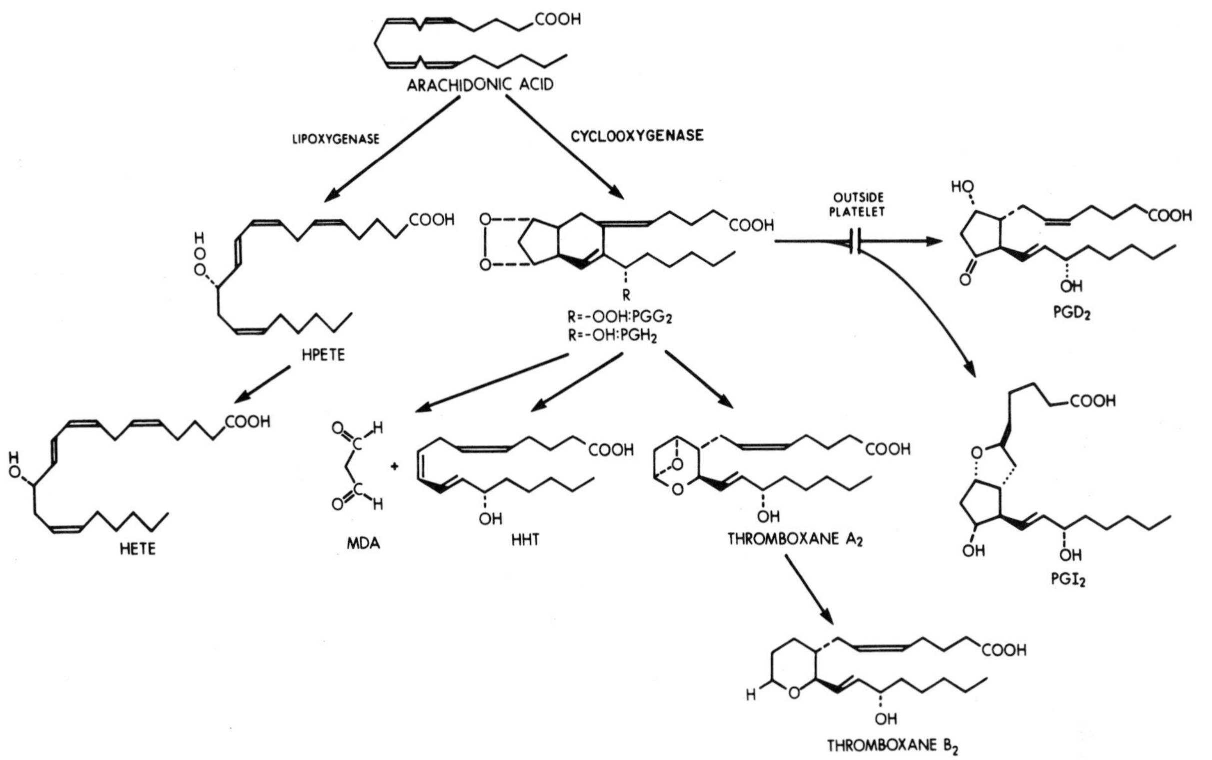

Figure 24–5. Arachidonate Metabolism in Platelets. Note that conversion of PGH$_2$ to PGI$_2$ and PGD$_2$ does not occur within platelets. The icosanoids listed can be divided into those that stimulate platelet aggregation (thromboxane A$_2$, PGH$_2$) and those that inhibit it (PGI$_2$, PGD$_2$).

therefore depend on uptake from plasma for icosanoid precursor fatty acids.[115, 116] In unstimulated platelets, free arachidonate is present in only trace quantities compared with those of other long chain fatty acids. Low free arachidonate levels prevent its metabolism by the unstimulated cell. These levels are maintained when arachidonate bound to albumin is added to platelets; arachidonate is esterified into phospholipids without the production of oxygenated metabolites. Other icosanoid precursor fatty acids are also readily incorporated into cellular phospholipids. In contrast, dietary fatty acids that are not icosanoid precursors such as palmitic, stearic, oleic, and linoleic acids are esterified into platelet phospholipids at a relatively low rate.[117] As a result significant pools of these fatty acids exist within the cell. These findings are explained by the fact that platelets contain a unique long chain acyl–coenzyme A (CoA) synthetase that is specific for icosanoid precursor fatty acids.[118–120] This enzyme has a very high affinity for these fatty acids and prevents accumulation of free acids in unstimulated cells, ensuring sufficient substrate for icosanoid production. Human plasma contains <1 per cent of total free fatty acid as polyunsaturated fatty acids. Therefore, cells require a high affinity uptake system. Most human cells contain the icosanoid precursor-specific acyl-CoA synthetase.[121, 122]

Icosanoid synthesis requires free non-esterified arachidonate, since the oxygenating enzymes do not act on phospholipid-bound fatty acid. The quantity of icosanoid produced upon stimulation of the platelet depends on the nature of the stimulus as well as on the content of arachidonate in the platelets. Activation by agonists, such as ADP and epinephrine, results in liberation of only small amounts of arachidonate, whereas high concentrations of thrombin pro-

duce much larger amounts. The control of icosanoid production depends on phospholipase activity that liberates the fatty acid from phospholipids. Receptor mediated activation of a cytosolic phospholipase A$_2$ triggers arachidonate release in platelets and most other cells. In macrophages this enzyme accounts for almost all release as cells from mice with deletion of this gene fail to synthesize icosanoids in response to agonists.[123–126]

Arachidonate, once liberated from the stimulated platelet, is either converted directly to icosanoids, as outlined in Figure 24–5, or liberated from the cell as free arachidonate, providing a potential substrate for adjacent cells to produce alternative icosanoid mediators.

Lipoxygenase Pathway

Platelets contain a cytosolic 12-lipoxygenase.[127] The enzyme eliminates a proton at carbon 10 of arachidonate, leading to insertion of molecular oxygen at carbon 12 to form 12-hydroperoxyarachidonate (12-HPETE).[128] Subsequently, 12-HPETE is converted to 12-HETE by a peroxidase enzyme. The role of these compounds (which are released from platelets) in platelet physiological processes remains unclear, although recent studies of platelets from mice with targeted deletion of 12-lipoxygenase indicate that the platelets are hyperaggregated by ADP, a response that is abated by addition of 12-HETE to platelet-rich plasma prior to addition of ADP.[129] These mice are also sensitive to ADP injections that cause thrombosis and death. This study suggests that 12-HETE functions to inhibit ADP aggregation without effect on secretion or responses to other agonists.

Cyclooxygenase Pathway

Cyclooxygenase (COX-1), a 72 kDa glycoprotein, is a membrane-bound enzyme that has been localized to the endoplasmic reticulum in fibroblasts[130] and to the dense tubular system in platelets.[131] cDNA's encoding cyclooxygenase has been isolated from a variety of tissues including human platelets and a megakaryocyte precursor cell line.[132, 133] Cyclooxygenase is the first enzyme in a pathway leading to production of a variety of active mediators, including thromboxane A_2,[134] which is the most potent vasoconstrictor known (100 times the potency of angiotensin II), and an agonist that stimulates platelet aggregation and secretion.[135] Cyclooxygenase catalyzes the abstraction of a proton at carbon 13 of arachidonate and related polyunsaturated fatty acids; catalysis is followed by the insertion of two molecules of oxygen. In the case of arachidonate, the product is a cyclic endoperoxide, prostaglandin G_2 (PGG_2). The enzyme also catalyzes a second reaction, in which PGG_2 is peroxidized to PGH_2.[136] In platelets these products are not secreted from cells under physiological conditions but are directly metabolized to other compounds. PGH_2 is converted to thromboxane A_2 by thromboxane synthase.[137] This compound is labile ($t_{1/2}$ = 30 seconds in water) and degrades spontaneously to the inactive metabolite, thromboxane B_2. The latter compound is measured experimentally as evidence of platelet activation, either by radioimmunoassay or by radiochromatography. Thromboxane synthase also forms two other compounds from arachidonic acid in amounts approximately equal to that of thromboxane A_2. These are 12-L-hydroxy-5,8,10-heptadecatrienoic acid (HHT) and malonaldehyde. No function has been elucidated for these latter compounds, although malonaldehyde could act as a physiological cross-linking agent.

In other cells the cyclic endoperoxide, PGH_2, is the precursor of different icosanoids, including PGI_2, which is discussed later, and the stable icosanoids PGE_2, PGD_2, and $PGF_{2\alpha}$. Formation of PGE_2 and PGD_2 is catalyzed by isomerase enzymes not present in platelets.[138, 139] Small amounts of these compounds can be formed by non-enzymatic breakdown of the labile endoperoxide, PGH_2. Thus, in platelets the major products (>90 per cent) of endoperoxide metabolism are thromboxane A_2, HHT, and malonaldehyde. However, PGD_2 is of interest since it is a potent inhibitor of platelet function. Albumin catalyzes production of PGD_2 from PGH_2.[140] This may be of physiological significance in preventing unwanted actions of PGH_2, as outlined in the following. Platelets contain an enzyme that converts PGD_2 to 15-keto-PGD_2, an inactive metabolite.[141]

Aspirin in Platelet Function

Aspirin induces a mild hemostatic defect in man, as evidenced by prolongation of skin bleeding time and impaired platelet aggregation measured in vitro. The aspirin defect results from decreased thromboxane A_2 production. Aspirin inhibits icosanoid production by a unique mechanism; it acetylates cyclooxygenase covalently on a single serine residue (S/536).[142, 143] Aspirin inhibition of the enzyme is prevented by arachidonate in a competitive manner, suggesting that aspirin blocks the substrate binding site.[144] The inhibition is due to steric inhibition by the bulky acetyl group and not to inhibition of catalysis. Thus mutant cyclooxygenase

with S to A mutation at position 536 remains active, and substitution of bulky amino acids at this position inhibits activity.[145, 146] The covalent modification of the enzyme is permanent; therefore, the cell must synthesize new enzyme in order to recover the capacity of producing products. Since unstimulated platelets are incapable of protein synthesis, the defect is permanent, lasting for the life of the platelet (7 to 10 days).[147] This results in a unique pharmacological mechanism of aspirin in platelets whereby the action of repeated doses of the drug is cumulative as residual active enzyme is repeatedly exposed to aspirin. In the steady state (i.e., after several weeks of aspirin therapy), complete inactivation of platelet cyclooxygenase is achieved by extremely low doses of aspirin, much less than those required for other actions of the drug (<80 mg/day yields complete inactivation).[148-150] This has led to clinical trials of low-dose aspirin as an antithrombotic agent. (See Icosanoids, page 780.) Using this strategy, it is possible selectively to block platelet cyclooxygenase and not the same enzyme in other tissues. A second cyclooxygenase gene encoding a putative "inflammatory cyclooxygenase" has been discovered by molecular cloning (COX-2). COX-2 is 60 per cent identical to COX-1 (especially around the S modified by aspirin). Its expression is induced by cytokines and inhibited by corticosteroids.[151-153]

Cyclooxygenase Deficiency

"Aspirin-like" functional defects in subjects with mild bleeding are among the most common problems seen in clinical practice. It is extremely difficult to distinguish congenital cyclooxygenase deficiency from prior aspirin ingestion, since the effects of aspirin persist for several days after the drug is ingested. Approximately 15 patients have been reported to have congenital cyclooxygenase deficiency.[154-158] This defect leads to a mild aspirin-like bleeding disorder characterized by a long skin bleeding time, easy bruising, and abnormal platelet aggregation in vitro. Serious hemorrhage has rarely been a problem in these patients. In none of the cases described to date is a pattern of inheritance demonstrated with multiple family members affected. In a few cases, radioimmunoassay of cyclooxygenase antigen indicates that true deficiency does exist.[158, 159] Measurement of cyclooxygenase antigen is currently the only certain way to diagnose cyclooxygenase deficiency.

It is not known whether cyclooxygenase deficiency affects only platelets or all tissues. In one case cyclooxygenase in an excised vein was also found to be deficient, implying that prostacyclin production by blood vessels was also ablated. Despite deficiency of the antithrombotic icosanoid prostacyclin, this patient had no obvious thrombotic tendency. If cyclooxygenase deficiency is present in all tissues, this would imply that essential fatty acid deficiency,[160] which leads to multiple organ dysfunctions, including sterility and a renal concentration defect, must be due to inability to generate products of pathways other than cyclooxygenase.

Platelet Membrane Receptors and Their Disorders

▼ FIBRINOGEN RECEPTOR (GLYCOPROTEIN IIb/IIIa)

On the basis of measurement of fibrinogen binding, there are approximately 45,000 fibrinogen receptors per platelet.

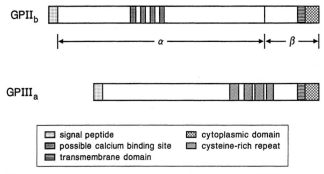

Figure 24–6. Model of Structure of Glycoprotein IIb/IIIa. Amino terminus on the left. α and β chains of GPIIb are indicated.

This receptor has been isolated by immunoaffinity chromatography of a detergent-solubilized platelet membrane extract using monoclonal antibodies.[161, 162] It is a heterodimeric membrane glycoprotein and a member of the gene family of adhesive proteins called integrins[163, 164] (Fig. 24–6). The subunits are homologous but separate gene products designated glycoproteins IIb and IIIa. Glycoprotein IIb is synthesized as a single polypeptide that is post-translationally cleaved into a heavy chain of 871 amino acids and a disulfide linked light chain of 137 amino acids.[165, 166] The heavy chain contains four repeated motifs homologous to calcium binding domains of calmodulin.[166] Glycoprotein IIIa consists of 762 amino acids with a single transmembrane domain near the carboxy-terminus. It contains four cysteine-rich repeats similar to the ligand binding domains of other receptors such as the low density lipoprotein (LDL) receptor.[167, 168] The two chains form a calcium dependent dimer in the membrane. They contain 15 per cent carbohydrate with a high content of mannose residues, suggesting the presence of both N-linked and high mannose oligosaccharide units.[162] The genes encoding these proteins are located together on chromosome 17q21-23.[167] The fibrinogen receptor, glycoprotein IIb/IIIa, also links the extracellular fibrin matrix to the platelet contractile apparatus.[99] Hence, glycoprotein IIb/IIIa links fibrinogen on the cell exterior with the contractile proteins of the cell interior. The former allows platelet aggregation[169] and the latter clot retraction (Fig. 24–7). It also has been demonstrated that fibrinogen binds to isolated glycoprotein IIb/IIIa,[170] and a photoactivatable derivative of fibrinogen becomes linked to this glycoprotein in ADP-activated platelets.[171] These data suggest that glycoprotein IIb/IIIa is

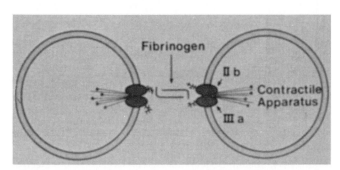

Figure 24–7. Model for the Function of Platelet Membrane Glycoprotein IIb/IIIa. When platelets are activated, IIb/IIIa binds contractile proteins on the cell interior and fibrinogen on the cell exterior.

the fibrinogen receptor and is required for normal platelet aggregation. There are at least two sites in fibrinogen that bind to the receptor. One is located at the carboxy-terminal end of the γ chain of fibrinogen[172] in the so-called fragment D domain. This was shown by demonstrating that the binding of fibrinogen to platelets was blocked by low concentrations of a synthetic pentadecapeptide comprising residues 397 to 411 of the γ chain and by showing direct binding of fragment D of fibrinogen to solubilized glycoprotein IIb-IIIa in vitro.[173] Further cross-linking studies indicate that the fibrinogen peptide binds to a site on glycoprotein IIb (GPIIb) at amino acids 294–314.[174] Peptides from this region inhibit both platelet aggregation and binding of fibrinogen to platelets.[175, 176] The other site on fibrinogen is a pair of RGD sequences. The binding site for RGD is in GPIIIa, and peptides containing RGD sequences inhibit fibrinogen binding to its receptor and thereby inhibit platelet aggregation. A new class of antithrombotic agents based on inhibition of the fibrinogen receptor have been developed. A monoclonal antibody against glycoprotein IIb-IIIa has been approved for use in coronary angioplasty.[177] Several non-peptide inhibitors that mimic the RGD sequence appear promising as antithrombotic drugs.[178]

Binding of fibrinogen to its receptor requires prior exposure of platelets to an agonist, and maximal binding occurs with the same concentrations of fibrinogen and calcium ions required for optimal platelet aggregation. It is unclear how agonists such as ADP lead to development of fibrinogen binding sites.

Glanzmann's Thrombasthenia

One of the most common inherited disorders of platelet function is Glanzmann's thrombasthenia, a disorder due to the absence of the platelet fibrinogen receptor. The initial clue to the pathogenesis of this disorder was derived from study of an antibody obtained from the serum of a multiply transfused thrombasthenic patient.[179] This patient's antibody reacted with normal but not thrombasthenic platelets. The antibody arose from the fact that the patient was not tolerant to the normal fibrinogen receptor glycoprotein IIb/IIIa.[180] It was later shown that the antibody precipitated glycoprotein IIb/IIIa and, most importantly, when added to normal platelets, induced a thrombasthenia-like functional defect in vitro. Direct binding studies of monoclonal antibodies to the fibrinogen receptor indicate absence of the receptor in patients with thrombasthenia with 50 per cent levels in obligate heterozygotes[161] (Fig. 24–8). Other monoclonal antibodies that block platelet aggregation and fibrinogen binding to normal platelets have been isolated.[181–184] Mutations that cause thrombasthenia have been found in both subunits. In the common Iraqi-Jewish disease all six families studied had a common 11 base deletion in exon 12 of GPIIIa.[185] This resulted in a frameshift and protein termination just outside the membrane spanning domain. In three of five Arab families studied, a 13 base deletion encompassing the splice acceptor site of exon 4 of GPIIb causes a 6 amino acid deletion that includes a cysteine residue. The deletion must be critical to protein folding as these patients have no detectable protein.[185] Definition of the mutations in patients has found about 50 mutations almost equally distributed between the two subunits.[186] Thus both subunits are required for

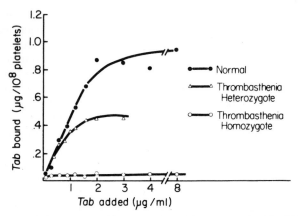

Figure 24–8. Binding of Monoclonal Antiglycoprotein IIb/IIIa (Tab) to Normal and Thrombasthenic Platelets.

fibrinogen binding and the binding site on glycoprotein IIb resides in the amino terminal third of the molecule.[187]

The diagnosis of Glanzmann's thrombasthenia depends on the following criteria: (1) mucocutaneous bleeding, which is usually present from birth; (2) history of bleeding in siblings compatible with autosomal recessive inheritance; (3) normal platelet count and morphological features with prolonged bleeding time*; absent clot retraction, and absent platelet aggregation by ADP, epinephrine, collagen, and thrombin but normal aggregation by ristocetin in the presence of von Willebrand factor (vWF).[188] The functional abnormalities in platelet aggregation and clot retraction are explained by the functions of the fibrinogen receptor protein.

Other proteins, including fibronectin,[189] vWF,[190–193] and thrombospondin,[194] bind to glycoprotein IIb/IIIa. Binding of these molecules has been demonstrated by using pure proteins and washed human platelets. The evidence that they bind to the same receptor site is that they compete with fibrinogen for binding, and binding is diminished or absent when platelets from thrombasthenic patients are used. These findings are of uncertain physiological significance. This is particularly true in the case of vWF, since patients with the disease thrombasthenia do not have defective platelet adhesion, implying that adhesion mediated by vWF occurs through binding to a different receptor from glycoprotein IIb/IIIa. In the presence of plasma, where high concentrations of fibrinogen are found, vWF does not bind to human platelets in the absence of ristocetin.[195]

The P1^A1 antigen is a platelet-specific alloantigen present in 98 per cent of the population.[196] It is absent or reduced in patients with thrombasthenia, since the antigen resides on the IIIa subunit of glycoprotein IIb/IIIa.[197] Individuals who lack P1^A1 antigen but are otherwise normal have normal levels of glycoprotein IIb/IIIa.[197] The P1^A1 antigen is not required for normal function of the protein, and family studies of individuals carrying both thrombasthenia and P1^A1 gene mutations simultaneously indicate that the genes are inherited and that they segregate independently.[198]

Von Willebrand Factor Receptor

A role for von Willebrand factor (vWF) in platelet function was elucidated fortuitously through studies of a toxic antibi-

---

*Bleeding time is measured clinically by determining the time of bleeding after a standardized skin incision 5 mm long by 1 mm deep.

otic, ristocetin, that caused thrombocytopenia.[199] Ristocetin was found to aggregate platelets in vitro in a reaction that required plasma vWF. Ristocetin does not aggregate platelets in plasma of patients with von Willebrand's disease, nor does it aggregate platelets from patients lacking the receptor for vWF. As with thrombasthenia, the elucidation of the vWF receptor has been greatly facilitated by studies of patients congenitally lacking this moiety who suffer from Bernard-Soulier syndrome. Binding studies using purified radiolabeled vWF have confirmed the presence of receptors for human vWF on platelets of normal individuals but not on platelets of Bernard-Soulier patients.[200–202] The vWF receptor is unique in that it does not bind its ligand unless the platelets are subjected to shear stress mediated by flow of blood. This is presumed to be due to a shear-induced conformation change in either vWF or the receptor.[203]

Nurden and Caen fractionated Bernard-Soulier platelet membrane proteins by electrophoresis in SDS and demonstrated a decrease in a major glycoprotein of M_r 155,000[204] (Fig. 24–9). This glycoprotein has been designated glycoprotein I or Ib; there are 25,000 molecules per normal platelet.[205] Studies using crossed immunoelectrophoresis of solubilized platelets clearly demonstrate that glycoprotein Ib is absent in most Bernard-Soulier platelets.[206] Intermediate levels of the glycoprotein have been reported in obligate heterozygotes.[207, 208]

The vWF receptor is a complex structure that contains four polypeptides, which are designated glycoprotein Ib_α (GPIb$_\alpha$), glycoprotein IB_β (GPIb$_\beta$), glycoprotein IX (GPIX), and glycoprotein V (GPV) (Fig. 24–10). All four components of the receptor contain closely related leucine-rich repeat motifs that are highly conserved but of unknown function.[203] GPIB$_\alpha$ and GPIb$_\beta$ form a dimeric disulfide-linked heterodimer of 610 and 181 amino acids, respectively.[166, 203] GPIX and GPV form non-covalent complexes with the proteins that is based on coimmunoprecipitation of all of the proteins by antisera against any one of them.[209] Glycoprotein IX contains 160 amino acids[210] with a single transmembrane domain near the carboxy-terminus and is encoded by a gene

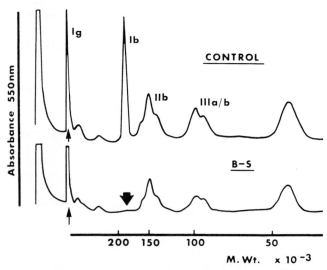

Figure 24–9. Sodium Dodecyl Sulfate Polyacrylamide Gel Electrophoresis of Normal (Top) and Bernard-Soulier Platelets. The gel was stained with periodic acid–Schiff reagent and was scanned by densitometry. Note the absence of glycoprotein Ib indicated by the heavy arrow.

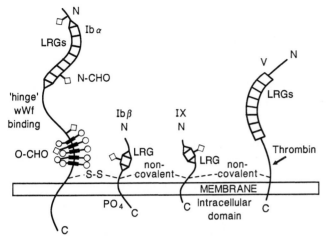

Figure 24–10. Model of von Willebrand Factor Receptor Inserted into Cell Membrane (see text for details). *LRG,* leucine-rich repeats; *Ibₐ,* glycoprotein Ib_{gₐ}; *Ib_B,* glycoprotein Ib_{B}; *IX,* glycoprotein IX; *V,* glycoprotein V.

on chromosome 3 that is apparently not linked to the genes for the other subunits of the receptor.[211] Glycoprotein V (M_r 82,000) contains 544 amino acids, 15 leucine-rich motifs, and a single membrane spanning domain.[212–214]

Bernard-Soulier Syndrome

In 1948 Bernard and Soulier reported a 5 month old infant with a history of spontaneous mucocutaneous bleeding beginning shortly after birth.[215] The patient had a prolonged bleeding time, and his platelets appeared abnormally large on peripheral blood smear. The patient had a sister who died of hemorrhage at the age of 3 years. Over 100 patients with this syndrome have been reported, all with an autosomal recessive inheritance pattern. In most of these cases, the platelet aggregation defect or membrane glycoprotein deficiency has been demonstrated. The diagnosis is established by the finding of mucocutaneous bleeding, a family history compatible with autosomal recessive inheritance, and the following laboratory findings: decreased platelet count with giant platelets on blood smear (Fig. 24–11), normal clot retraction, absent platelet aggregation with vWF plus ristocetin, and normal platelet aggregation with physiological agonists. The degree of bleeding varies among patients even within a family, but most experience episodes severe enough to require transfusion. Unlike patients with coagulation factor abnormalities, these patients do not suffer from hemarthroses. The mechanism for formation of large platelets in the disease is unknown. Perhaps the lack of the vWF receptor affects the demarcation of platelets in the megakaryocyte.

Whether all four proteins are required for vWF receptor function awaits further definition of the mutations in Bernard-Soulier syndrome. Most patients have mutations of GPIbₐ, although several mutations in GPIX have been reported.[216] A single promoter mutation in a GATA motif of GPIB_B has been reported, but no mutations in glycoprotein V have been found.[217] In fact, GPV is not required for cell surface expression of the other three components.[218]

The antibiotic ristocetin is required for in vitro vWF binding and vWF-induced aggregation. Reports that platelet activation would allow binding of vWF without ristocetin do not measure the physiologically significant binding of vWF, as this binding is to glycoprotein IIb/IIIa. (See Fibrinogen Receptor [Glycoprotein IIb/IIIa], page 772.) The requirement for ristocetin to demonstrate binding presumably reflects some conformational change induced in either vWF or the receptor that allows binding. Absence of either the vWF receptor in Bernard-Soulier syndrome or plasma vWF in von Willebrand's disease results in failure of platelet aggregation in platelet-rich plasma in the presence of ristocetin. Although ristocetin-induced aggregation is an in vitro phenomenon, it is the manifestation of a more physiological interaction of platelets with exposed subendothelial surfaces. Platelets adhere to surfaces coated with von Willebrand factor under shear conditions without added ristocetin. Other cells transfected with the von Willebrand factor receptor also adhere provided that they express GPIb_{2α}, GPIb_B, and GPIX.[219]

▼ THROMBIN RECEPTOR

Platelets contain high-affinity binding sites for thrombin, and the binding of thrombin to these sites correlates with the

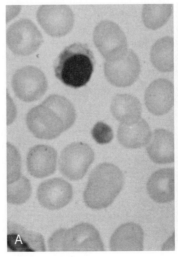
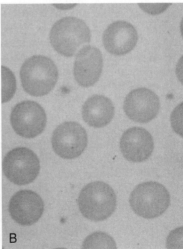

Figure 24–11. Peripheral Blood Smear from a Patient with Bernard-Soulier Syndrome (A) Compared with That from a Normal Subject (B). Note giant platelet compared with a lymphocyte; normal film shows several normal platelets.

activation of platelets by thrombin.[101] Thrombin receptors are specific for thrombin; they do not bind prothrombin or prethrombin II.[220] The latter has the same amino acid sequence as thrombin and lacks only a single internal cleavage that converts this single-chain precursor to the active enzyme. Thrombin inactivated with diisopropylfluorophosphate (DFP) also binds to the receptor but does not cause platelet activation. Thus, it was clear that platelet activation requires proteolysis of some membrane component. The pattern of activation of platelets by thrombin does not suggest an enzymatic reaction but rather a ligand-receptor interaction, since small concentrations of thrombin result in rapid partial activation of platelets rather than slow complete activation, as might be predicted by turnover of a small amount of enzyme. The isolation of cDNA encoding three distinct thrombin receptors explains the properties described above. They are designated for protease activated receptors 1, 3, and 4 (PAR1, PAR3, and PAR4). The receptors are 27 per cent similar in amino acid sequence with seven membrane spanning domains similar to other receptors coupled to trimeric G proteins such as adrenergic receptors.[221–225] The receptors are activated by a novel mechanism wherein thrombin cleaves a single bond between R41/S42 (PAR1) and K38/T39 (PAR3) R47/G48 (PAR4) to liberate a new amino-terminal sequence that serves as a tethered ligand to activate the receptor. Synthetic peptides with the PAR1 or PAR4 sequence but not those of PAR3 sequence are thrombin agonists for human platelets. The receptors are coupled to Gq trimeric G proteins in activating platelets.[224] No congenital abnormality of these receptors has yet been identified, and their relative importance is uncertain.

▼ FACTOR X_a–FACTOR V_a RECEPTOR

Prothrombin activation occurs on the platelet surface. Platelets bind factor X_a with high affinity (K_d = 30 to 70 pM),[104–108, 226] and bound factor X_a catalyzes the activation of prothrombin 300,000 times faster than factor X_a in solution. Factor X_a binds to 200 to 300 sites on the platelet surface. The binding is specific for factor X_a, since neither the zymogen factor X nor other coagulation factors displace bound factor X_a. Factor X_a binding requires either exogenous factor V_a or stimulation of the release reaction to release platelet factor V, which is then converted to factor V_a.[105, 220] Human platelets contain ~0.3 μg factor V/10^8 platelets,[227, 228] which when converted to factor V_a is about 10 times the amount required to saturate the factor X_a–factor V_a receptor sites.[226] Although factor X_a can bind to unstimulated platelets, no binding occurs in the absence of factor V_a. Since factor V_a is formed by thrombin, which also activates platelets, it seems likely that physiological factor X_a binding occurs only when platelets are activated. Although platelets contain cytoplasmic proteases that can activate factor V, there is no evidence that they do so during platelet activation.[229] The fact that prothrombin activation normally occurs on the platelet surface is suggested by studies of patients with congenital factor V deficiency, since clinical severity correlates with platelet, rather than plasma, levels of factor V.[230]

The factor X_a receptor has not been isolated, and, therefore, its protein nature can only be inferred. Factors X_a and V_a appear to interact in binding to platelets, as each stimulates the binding of the other.[231–233] The stoichiometry of binding is one factor X_a/factor V_a.[232]

It has been assumed that the platelet component to which factors X_a and V_a bind are negatively charged phospholipids, analogous to phospholipids used in in vitro coagulation assays. However, although they are required to accelerate prothrombin activation, there is no evidence that acidic phospholipids are exposed in the outer leaflet of the plasma membrane of platelets. Furthermore, phospholipids can substitute for platelets in prothrombin activation only when factor X_a is present in relatively high concentrations, and the affinity of phospholipid for factor X_a, even in the presence of factor V_a, is much less than that of the platelet receptor. When platelets are damaged by vigorous stirring or by addition of calcium ionophore A23187, accelerated prothrombin activation can be demonstrated.[112] The factor X_a concentration dependence of this reaction suggests that it reflects phospholipids rather than the physiological platelet receptor. Further evidence that the platelet receptor is not merely phospholipid is that a monoclonal antibody to factor V_a blocks platelet-, but not phospholipid-stimulated, prothrombin activation.[230] A single patient with an abnormal platelet factor X_a receptor, who has 25 per cent of the normal number of factor X_a receptor sites and suffers from a moderately severe lifelong bleeding disorder, has been described.[226] In contrast, a patient who developed an autoantibody directed against acidic phospholipids has been described; this antibody blocks prothrombin activation in the presence of acidic phospholipids and has no effect on platelet surface prothrombin activation in vitro, and the patient has no bleeding diathesis.[234] Further characterization of the platelet factor X_a receptor has been hindered by the fact that few of these moieties exist on the platelet. If, for example, the factor X_a receptor has a molecular weight of 100,000, it would represent only 0.003 per cent of platelet membrane protein.

▼ ICOSANOID RECEPTORS

Platelets appear to have three distinct icosanoid receptors—two inhibitory and one stimulatory. All are seven membrane spanning G protein coupled receptors that are about 30–40 per cent identical in amino acid sequence.[235]

The inhibitory icosanoids act at a PGI_2/PGE_1 receptor and at a PGD_2 receptor.[236–238] These inhibitors block platelet function by stimulating adenylate cyclase, thereby elevating platelet cAMP levels. That platelets contain two distinct inhibitory receptors is indicated by direct ligand binding studies. PGI_2 and PGE_1 both bind to platelets; they compete with each other but not with PGD_2, which also binds to platelets. PGD_2 binding is not inhibited by either PGI_2 or PGE_1. Experiments showing specific agonist desensitization also support the concept of separate PGI_2/PGE_1 and PGD_2 receptors; exposure of platelets to PGD_2 inhibits subsequent responses to PGD_2 but not to PGI_2 or PGE_1.[239, 240] Although distinct receptors are present, they appear to be coupled to the same adenylate cyclase molecules, since the increases in cAMP stimulated by these substances are not additive. PGI_2 is the most potent inhibitory icosanoid, with 50 per cent of maximal inhibition of platelet function at about 1 nM. PGD_2 and PGE_1 are 50- and 25-fold less potent, respectively. Most patients with myeloproliferative disorders have relative refractoriness to PGD$_2$ and have reduced numbers of PGD$_2$ receptors.[241] Whether this defect contributes to the increased thromboses in these patients is uncertain. Responses to PGI$_2$ in these patients are normal.

The agonists for the stimulatory icosanoid receptor, cyclic endoperoxide PGH$_2$ and thromboxane A$_2$, are both labile, thereby precluding direct binding studies. However, there are selective PGH$_2$/thromboxane A$_2$ receptor antagonists, such as 13-azaprostanoic acid, which have allowed demonstration of high-affinity binding sites on platelet membranes.[242] The platelet thromboxane A$_2$ receptor has been isolated by affinity chromatography,[243] and a cDNA encoding the receptor has been isolated from megakaryocyte cell line and placental cDNA libraries.[244] The receptor comprises 343 amino acids and is a member of the seven membrane spanning receptor family with distant homology to the rhodopsin and adrenergic receptors. Three unrelated patients with a mild congenital "aspirin-like" bleeding disorder have been reported.[245–247] Platelets of affected individuals do not undergo secretion or second-wave aggregation in response to ADP and epinephrine. These platelets also fail to aggregate or undergo the release reaction in response to arachidonic acid, PGH$_2$, or cyclic endoperoxide analogues. Thromboxane A$_2$ formation from added arachidonate is normal as determined by levels of thromboxane B$_2$. Rapid addition of arachidonate-stimulated platelet-rich plasma from normal subjects (which contains thromboxane A$_2$) fails to aggregate the platelets from affected patients, whereas arachidonate-stimulated platelets from patients aggregate aspirin-treated normal platelets. Thromboxane receptor antagonists could prove to be useful as antithrombotic agents.[248]

▼ ADENOSINE DIPHOSPHATE RECEPTOR

Purinergic receptors respond to extracellular nucleotides as agonists. There are two general classes of such receptors: P2X receptors, which are ligand-gated ion channels, and P2Y receptors, which are classical seven membrane spanning G protein coupled receptors. Many examples of both classes

have been cloned from various tissues. Platelets contain three distinct ADP receptors, of which cDNA has been cloned for two. Platelets contain a P2X1 receptor subtype that allows for transmembrane calcium uptake in response to ADP.[249] Selective inhibitors of this receptor do not inhibit platelet aggregation in response to ADP, and thus the role of this receptor in platelet physiological processes is unclear. Platelets also contain P2Y1[250–252] receptors that are coupled to G$_q$ trimeric G protein. ADP activation of this receptor evokes platelet shape change, phosphatidylinositol turnover with inositol trisphosphate production, and calcium mobilization. There is another P2Y-type receptor in platelets, not yet identified by molecular cloning, that is coupled to G$_i$ and that leads to inhibition of adenyl cyclase in response to ADP.[253, 254] The thienopyridine antithrombotic agent ticlopidine acts by blocking this receptor.[253] On the basis of pharmacological studies using selective antagonists it seems clear that activation of both receptors is required to cause ADP induced platelet aggregation[255] (Fig. 24–12). Thus inhibitors of the P2Y1 receptor block platelet shape change, calcium mobilization, phosphatidylinositol turnover, and platelet aggregation with no effect on adenyl cyclase. Conversely inhibitors of the G$_i$ coupled receptor have no effect on the above responses but inhibit the ability of ADP to block adenyl cyclase, and they also inhibit platelet aggregation. Thus it appears that two distinct systems must be activated to evoke platelet aggregation in response to ADP. Consistent with these results are studies of mice with targeted deletion of the Gαq.[256] In homozygous knockout mice there is failure of shape change, aggregation, and the other responses evoked by the P2Y1 receptor in response to ADP. Interestingly, responses to other agonists such as thrombin and collagen also fail to evoke responses in these platelets, suggesting that all signal through a Gαq coupled receptor. In this regard it is interesting that platelets have at least two thrombin receptors that may be coupled to discrete G proteins. Patients with failure of ADP induced platelet aggregation have been reported. One had decreased platelet Gαq,[257] and in another platelet function suggested defective P2Y1 receptor signaling.[258]

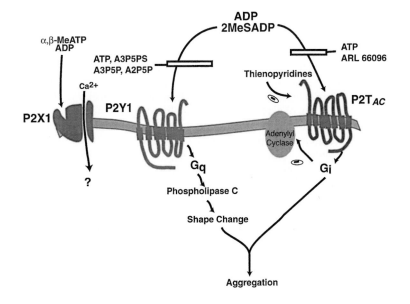

Figure 24–12. Platelet ADP Receptors. Three types of platelet ADP receptors are depicted. A3P5PS, A3P5P, and A2p5p are ADP analogue inhibitors of the P2Y1 receptor. ARP 66096 and thienopyridines are inhibitors of the P2Tac receptor that leads to inhibition of adenylate cyclase.

Stimulus-Secretion Coupling in Platelet Activation

The mechanism by which cells are activated when cell surface receptors are occupied by a ligand is a fundamental, unsolved problem. Platelets have been used extensively for studies of stimulus-response coupling, and much of what is currently known has been elucidated in these cells.

▼ ROLE OF Ca²⁺ IN PLATELET ACTIVATION

The current view of platelet activation by agonists involves several interrelated systems. Ca^{2+} fluxes are thought to mediate several reactions. In unstimulated platelets, the cytosolic Ca^{2+} concentration is estimated to be ~0.1 μM. When cells are maximally stimulated by thrombin or collagen, levels rise to 1 to 5 μM, as measured with the fluorescent indicator Quin-2.[259] Lesser rises in calcium follow stimulation by ADP (~3 μM).[253] Extracellular Ca^{2+} is not required for activation of human platelets. The source of Ca^{2+} is thought to be the platelet-dense tubular system, which is analogous to the sarcoplasmic reticulum in muscle. Upon platelet activation inositol 1,4,5-triphosphate levels rise in response to phospholipase C activation. This binds to IP_3 receptors, which render these membranes permeable to Ca^{2+}, releasing it to the cytoplasm.[260] Ca^{2+} is then reaccumulated by a Ca^{2+}-transporting ATPase.[261] Platelet dense granules also contain Ca^{2+}, which is secreted when platelets are activated. This Ca^{2+} is not thought to participate in platelet activation per se.[262]

The Ca^{2+} signal serves to trigger phosphatidylinositol breakdown (see Phosphoinositide-Derived Messengers in Platelet Activation, page 779), to initiate protein phosphorylation by a Ca^{2+}-dependent protein kinase (protein kinase C), and to activate myosin light chain kinase. The latter enzyme phosphorylates the myosin light chain, which is required for platelet contraction. Other reactions that are stimulated by Ca^{2+} include proteolysis by a Ca^{2+}-dependent protease, calpain, which is found in the platelet cytosol, and the glycogenolysis that occurs within seconds of platelet activation.[262]

▼ PROTEIN PHOSPHORYLATION

A second system of platelet activation involves protein phosphorylation reactions. When platelets are activated by thrombin two major proteins are rapidly phosphorylated.[263] These are the myosin light chain and a 40 kDa protein, pleckstrin.[264] The latter phosphorylation is catalyzed by a ubiquitous protein kinase designated protein kinase C, which is the major protein kinase in platelets.[265] The enzyme is activated by acidic phospholipids, diglyceride, and Ca^{2+}. The lipids serve to increase the enzyme's affinity for Ca^{2+}, allowing activity to occur at lower Ca^{2+} concentrations. Protein kinase C also phosphorylates the myosin light chain, although at a different site and with a much slower time course than that catalyzed by myosin light chain kinase.[266, 267] Platelets also contain cAMP-dependent protein kinase, which presumably catalyzes a number of inhibitory platelet protein phosphorylations since elevation of cAMP level inhibits platelet activation.

Platelets also contain large amounts of protein tyrosine phosphate.[268, 269] Thrombin, collagen, and other strong platelet agonists stimulate rapid tyrosine phosphorylation of a variety of platelet proteins.[270–273] Addition of vanadate, a protein tyrosine phosphatase inhibitor, to permeabilized platelets induces secretion and increased tyrosine phosphorylation.[274] The specific targets of tyrosine phosphorylation in platelets include many cytoskeletal proteins including the cytoplasmic tail of GPIIIa. This phosphorylation is essential for the attachment of the fibrinogen receptor to the cytoskeleton, thereby allowing clot retraction to occur.[275] Platelets have been found to contain multiple different protein tyrosine phosphatases through molecular cloning from a megakaryocyte cDNA library.[276, 277] Activation of receptors that are protein tyrosine kinases stimulates the formation of novel metabolites of phosphatidylinositol (as described below) and is associated with formation of complexes between receptors and phosphatidylinositol 3-kinase. Thrombin stimulation of platelets is associated with formation of complexes containing phosphatidylinositol 3-kinase even though this receptor is not a tyrosine kinase.[278] The role of these complexes in platelet activation is unknown.

▼ CYCLIC ADENOSINE MONOPHOSPHATE

Agents that elevate cAMP levels inhibit platelet activation. cAMP blocks platelet function at a very early stage, since most platelet responses are inhibited, including aggregation, secretion, appearance of fibrinogen receptors, and phosphoinositide turnover.[262] High cAMP levels stimulate calcium uptake by the platelet dense tubular system, thereby diminishing any stimulatory Ca^{2+} signal.[279] cAMP may also inhibit the stimulatory phosphorylation reactions catalyzed by protein kinase C and myosin light chain kinase.[280] It may be that the rate of change and direction of change in Ca^{2+} concentration, rather than the actual level of Ca^{2+}, determine platelet activation. Degradation of polyphosphoinositides is partially resistant to inhibition by cAMP.[281, 282]

As in other cells, cAMP levels are controlled by a complex system. Adenylate cyclase that forms cAMP from ATP is essentially inactive in the absence of the stimulatory guanine-nucleotide binding regulatory protein designated G_s.[283] There is also an inhibitory guanine-nucleotide binding protein designated G_i. Each of these proteins has α, β, and γ subunits, and they are activated by communication with receptors occupied by appropriate agonists. The β and γ subunits of G_s and G_i are the same. Guanosine triphosphate (GTP) binding to the stimulatory G protein leads to dissociation of the α from βγ subunits, resolving free $G_{s\alpha}$, which activates adenylate cyclase. Conversely, dissociation of G_i releases free βγ, which, when present in excess, can bind $G_{s\alpha}$ and thereby lead to inhibition of adenylate cyclase. Some agents activate inhibitory receptors and others stimulatory receptors. GTP hydrolysis to guanosine diphosphate (GDP) results in reversal of activation of these proteins. Another enzyme that controls cAMP levels is cyclic nucleotide phosphodiesterase. Inhibition of this enzyme elevates cAMP and inhibits platelet function. Many inhibitors of platelet function act by raising cAMP levels, such as the adenylate cyclase stimulators PGE_1, PGI_2, and PGD_2 and phosphodiesterase inhibitors such as the antithrombotic agent dipyridamole. It

H
|
H — C — O ①⁻·R
|
H — C — O ②⁻·ARACHIDONATE
| O
| ‖
H — C — O ③⁻·P — O   H
| ‖   HO OH   OH(P)
H   H
                 OH   H
              H   H
                 H   OH(P)

Figure 24–13. Phosphatidylinositol. This phospholipid and its phosphorylated forms serve as storehouses for messenger molecules. P, 4 and 5 positions, which contain phosphate groups in some molecules. When the molecule is broken down by phospholipase C (reaction 1), inositol phosphates and diglyceride are the two products. Lipase reactions (reactions 2 and 3) subsequently liberate arachidonate from diglyceride.

▼ PHOSPHOINOSITIDE-DERIVED MESSENGERS IN PLATELET ACTIVATION

The phosphoinositides are minor phospholipids contained in all cells (Fig. 24–13). They serve as storage forms for messenger molecules and as messenger molecules themselves. The responses of cells to external stimuli are mediated by a variety of messenger molecules. Three such molecules produced as a result of phosphoinositide metabolism are diglyceride, inositol trisphosphate, and arachidonic acid.[290] These substances have properties common to second messengers such as cAMP. Their production is initiated by specific agonists, they are potent activators of other cellular reactions, and they are rapidly degraded to inactive compounds.

Phosphoinositide Metabolism

Phosphoinositides are ubiquitous components of eukaryotic membranes. In platelets phosphatidylinositol comprises about 5 to 7 per cent of phospholipids, phosphatidylinositol-4 phosphate 1 per cent, and phosphatidylinositol-4,5-diphosphate 0.4 per cent. The phosphoinositides are in equilibrium with each other through a "futile cycle" of kinases and phosphatases, as shown in Figure 24–14. Phosphoinositides undergo rapid breakdown in response to receptor-mediated cell activation.[290] All three phosphoinositides are degraded by a phospholipase C to form diglyceride and one of the inositol phosphates.[291] The inositol phosphates are produced in both cyclic and non-cyclic forms, as shown in Figure 24–14. There are multiple phospholipase C enzymes in mammalian tissues, as deduced from direct protein isolation and molecular cloning studies.[292–294] Seven of the 10 known phospholipase C isoenzymes are expressed in human platelets.[295] The different phospholipase C enzymes are coupled to receptors by different G proteins. Gq couples β forms of enzyme,[295–298] and γ forms are activated by tyrosine kinase receptors.[293] The inositol phosphates are subsequently con-

has been difficult to prove that platelet agonists actually lower basal cAMP levels, although most can decrease pharmacologically elevated cAMP levels. Since cAMP turns over in platelets with a t1/2 of less than 1 second,[284] it is apparent that perturbations in adenylate cyclase or phosphodiesterase can have rapid effects that may determine the threshold of platelets to activation, if not actually trigger the activation reaction. Most platelet agonists inhibit adenylate cyclase in cell-free preparations. These include ADP,[285] epinephrine,[286] and platelet-activating factor.[287] Thrombin inhibits adenylate cyclase, as assayed in platelet membranes isolated after treatment of intact cells with thrombin.[288] All of these inhibitions are mediated through receptors coupled to G_i.[289] Epinephrine presumably acts bound to an α_2 receptor that is coupled to a guanine-nucleotide inhibitory protein, as has been reported in other systems.

Figure 24–14. Pathway for Inositol Phosphate Metabolism. Top: *PI*, phosphatidylinositol; *PI₄P*, phosphatidylinositol 4-phosphate; *PI₃P*, phosphatidylinositol 3-phosphate; *PI₃,₄P₂*, phosphatidylinositol 3, 4-bisphosphate; *PI₃,₄,₅P₃*, phosphatidylinositol 3, 4, 5-trisphosphate; *PI₄,₅P₂*, phosphatidylinositol 4, 5-bisphosphate. Bottom: *I*, inositol; *P*, phosphate. The numbers preceding P refer to positions of phosphates on the inositol ring, and those following P, the number of phosphate groups. *PA*, phosphatidic acid; *CDP-DG*, cytidine diphosphate diacylglycerol; *PKC*, protein kinase C; *MG*, 2 monoacylglycerol.

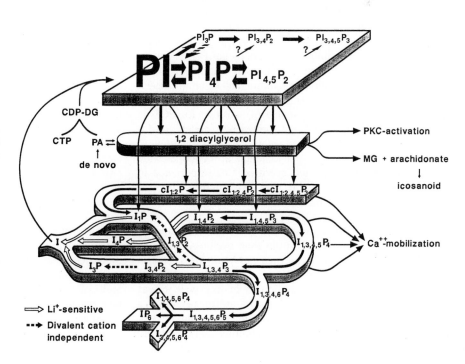

verted to a host of inositol phosphates and subsequently degraded to inositol, which is utilized for resynthesis of phosphoinositides. The diglyceride is either hydrolyzed by lipases[299] to monoglyceride, which is further hydrolyzed to free arachidonate and glycerol, or phosphorylated by diglyceride kinase to form phosphatidic acid. Phosphatidic acid is then converted to phosphatidylinositol, completing the so-called phosphatidylinositol cycle.

Phosphatidylinositols containing phosphate esters in the 3 position of inositol include phosphatidylinositol 3-phosphate, phosphatidylinositol 3,4-bisphosphate, and phosphatidylinositol 3,4,5-trisphosphate (see Figure 24–14).[300] Phosphatidylinositol 3-phosphate is present in cells under all conditions, whereas the polyphosphorylated 3-phosphate containing phosphatidylinositols are formed transiently in response to agonists, such as thrombin in the case of platelets. The functions of these compounds in signaling reactions include activation of protein kinases such as PKC and AKT and stimulation of actin polymerization.[301-303] Production of phosphatidylinositol 3,4-bisphosphate and phosphatidylinositol 3,4,5-trisphosphate occurs by several pathways including action of kinases and phosphatases.[300, 304, 305]

Platelet–Vessel Wall Interactions in the Control of Hemostasis

▼ ICOSANOIDS

Icosanoid mediators transmit signals between platelets and cells of the vessel wall. When stimulated, platelets produce thromboxane A_2, which causes vasoconstriction of blood vessels, thereby promoting hemostasis. Conversely, endothelial cells produce PGI_2 or prostacyclin, which elevates platelet cAMP levels, thereby inhibiting platelet function; furthermore, it causes vasodilatation. Thus, PGI_2 and thromboxane have opposite actions. On this basis it has been proposed that vascular homeostasis is determined by a balance of thromboxane A_2 and PGI_2, and that the occurrence of thrombotic diseases might be influenced by factors that alter this balance. This concept implies that aspirin might have paradoxical effects, since inhibition of endothelial PGI_2 by aspirin might actually promote thrombosis. Endothelial cells have receptors for thrombin, bradykinin, and histamine. Each of these agonists stimulates arachidonate release and conversion to PGI_2. An alternative source of substrate for PGI_2 is cyclic endoperoxides, which are formed by platelets. Endoperoxides may escape from platelets and be converted to PGI_2 by endothelium. The phenomenon of "endoperoxide steal" has been demonstrated in vitro;[114] its importance in vivo is uncertain, although it may explain the action of thromboxane synthetase inhibitors, as outlined in the following.

Early in vitro studies suggested that platelet cyclooxygenase is more sensitive to aspirin than cyclooxygenase in vascular tissue and that because of new enzyme synthesis by endothelium, vascular PGI_2 production was restored quickly after aspirin administration.[114] In this way it was proposed that there might be doses of aspirin at which a selective effect on platelet cyclooxygenase could be obtained. A large number of studies exploring this possibility indicate that although platelet cyclooxygenase is more sensi-

tive to aspirin than that in the endothelium, even low doses of aspirin inhibit PGI_2 synthesis in part. High doses of aspirin, however, do not completely block PGI_2 production.

The concept of a balance between PGI_2 and thromboxane implies that PGI_2 is produced by normal endothelium. Several studies suggest that this is not the case. FitzGerald et al.[306, 307] estimate that circulating PGI_2 levels are ~3 pg/ml, which is 10-fold lower than the minimal amount that inhibits platelet function. It is of course possible that local concentrations of PGI_2 at sites of endothelial injury may reach higher physiologically important concentrations. Follow-up evaluation of patients with rheumatoid arthritis treated with large doses of aspirin does not uncover an increase in thrombosis or atherosclerosis. Furthermore, patients with congenital cyclooxygenase deficiency, who may lack PGI_2, do not suffer from thrombotic episodes. Patients with atherosclerosis are not PGI_2-deficient but have higher than normal levels of urinary PGI_2 metabolites. Thus, there is not evidence that inhibition of PGI_2 production is an undesirable side effect of pharmacological inhibition of thromboxane A_2 (TxA_2) production. In fact, a number of clinical trials indicate that aspirin has a clinically useful antithrombotic effect. Meta-analysis has been used to evaluate the results of 25 trials of aspirin for prevention of death in myocardial infarction. This analysis showed that aspirin had no effect on non-vascular mortality rate but reduced vascular mortality rate by 15 per cent and non-fatal vascular events (stroke, myocardial infarction) by 30 per cent. Low doses of 150–300 mg/day were effective.[308] An alternative antithrombotic therapy, utilizing selective inhibitors of thromboxane synthetase, is also under investigation. Unfortunately, these drugs allow accumulation of cyclic endoperoxides (Fig. 24–15) in platelets, and the endoperoxides are themselves potent platelet-aggregating agents. In fact, these drugs may act primarily by stimulating the production of PGI_2 by endoperoxide steal and also by stimulating the conversion of PGH_2 to PGD_2 by albumin in plasma.

▼ CONTROL OF THROMBOSIS BY VASCULAR CELLS

Endothelial cells inhibit thrombosis by influencing both coagulation and fibrinolysis. Protein C is a vitamin K–dependent plasma protein, described in Chapter 18. In vitro it is activated to protease that exhibits potent anticoagulant activity through the selected proteolysis of factors V_a and VIII_a. The activation of protein C by thrombin, the only known physiological activator, is slow. Endothelial cells contain a cell surface protein designated thrombomodulin that acts as a cofactor for the activation of protein C, increasing the catalytic activity of thrombin more than 1000-fold[309-313] (Fig. 24–16). This endothelial protein has the unique quality of converting thrombin from a coagulation factor to a major anticoagulant moiety. Thrombomodulin is localized to endothelial cells (and the syncytiotrophoblast of placenta, which is also exposed to blood).[314] When thrombin is generated in areas of vascular damage outside the vessel wall, procoagulant reactions occur, whereas inside the adjacent damaged vascular wall, thrombin is converted to an anticoagulant moiety maintaining the fluidity of blood within the vascular channel. Thrombomodulin-stimulated protein C activation is

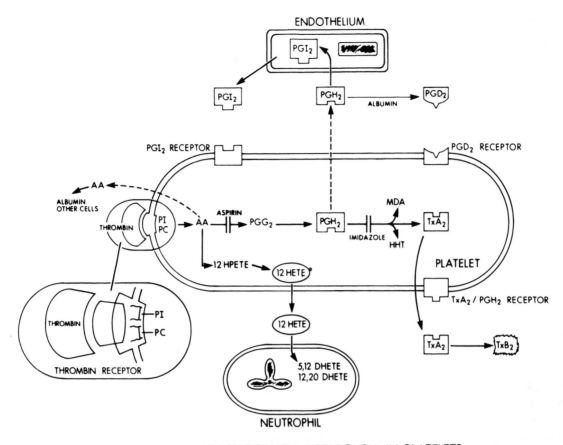

ARACHIDONATE METABOLISM IN PLATELETS

Figure 24–15. The Pathways for Liberation of Arachidonate and Its Conversion to PGH₂ Are Shared by Endothelial Cells and Platelets. PGH₂ is metabolized differently in the two cells to produce the aggregating agent thromboxane A₂ and the antiaggregating agent prostacyclin. Inhibition of cyclooxygenase by drugs can affect the production of both mediators.

modulated by coagulation factor V_a, which is itself a substrate for activated protein C (APC).[315, 316] In the presence of factor V_a, thrombomodulin activity is stimulated approximately threefold.[317] Once APC is formed, the heavy chain of factor V_a is degraded, and the remaining light chain serves to inhibit thrombomodulin activity. This is a feedback mechanism whereby factor V_a promotes its own destruction, and once the anticoagulant function is destroyed, the residual light chain blocks further activation of protein C.

Vascular endothelium also contains heparin molecules,[318, 319] which greatly accelerate the inactivation of coagulation factors by antithrombin III, as discussed further in

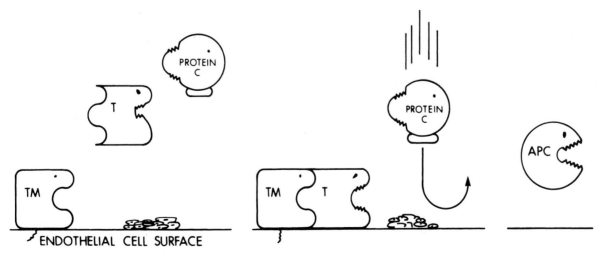

Figure 24–16. Mechanism of Endothelial Thrombomodulin-Stimulated Protein C Activation. Thrombomodulin binding of thrombin is postulated to result in a conformational change in thrombin that renders protein C a good substrate.

Chapter 20. Another reaction important in inhibiting pathological thrombotic reactions is the production of tissue plasminogen activator by endothelial cells, as described in Chapter 23.

▼ PLATELET-DERIVED GROWTH FACTOR

Platelet-derived growth factor is a glycoprotein that has been isolated in two forms, one of 31 kDa, and the other of 28 kDa, which is smaller either because of differences in glycosylation.[320] The two forms of PDGF have equivalent activity, and both are dimeric polypeptide chains linked by multiple interchain disulfide bridges. Human serum contains ~50 ng/ml of PDGF, whereas none is contained in plasma.[321] This growth factor appears to be the major growth-promoting component in serum. PDGF is contained in platelet α granules and is secreted at sites of platelet activation. In this way PDGF promotes wound healing, since it is a potent mitogen for cells of mesenchymal origin, including fibroblasts, glial cells, and smooth muscle cells.[322] When PDGF is added to plasma, it rapidly binds to α_2 macroglobulin.[323] This may serve as a clearance mechanism to prevent biologically active PDGF from entering the systemic circulation at sites of injury.

In addition to stimulating cell proliferation, PDGF acts as a potent chemotactic protein for inflammatory cells, including neutrophils and monocytes, and certain other cells, such as smooth muscle cells and fibroblasts. PDGF attracts these cells to sites of injury, thereby furthering the repair process. The action of PDGF in wound healing may be its primary physiological function in vertebrates[324]; however, this molecule is also involved in atherogenesis.[325] In a number of models of atherosclerosis it is clear that platelets are required for lesion development. This has led to the hypothesis that PDGF, when released intravascularly or into the vessel wall, leads to aberrant proliferation of smooth muscle cells, with formation of atherosclerotic lesions. For this reason, inhibitors of PDGF function are currently being sought.

PDGF stimulates target cells by binding to specific cell surface receptors.[326] Many responses follow rapidly, including enhancement of glycolysis, stimulation of amino acid transport, increased protein synthesis, increased turnover of phosphoinositides, and production of icosanoids.[320] Increased DNA synthesis and cell proliferation then occur. The plasma membrane receptor for PDGF has been identified as a 180 kDa glycoprotein.[327] This molecule has intrinsic and PDGF-stimulated protein tyrosine kinase activity. The PDGF receptor kinase can also serve as a substrate for its own kinase activity and stimulates phosphorylation of other intracellular substrates. The mechanism by which tyrosine phosphorylation leads to cell proliferation has not been elucidated. The tyrosine-specific protein kinase activity of the PDGF receptor protein suggests a parallel to the biological activities observed in various retrovirus-transformed cells. Several retroviral transforming factors are tyrosine-specific protein kinases. The discovery that the α chain of PDGF is highly homologous to the retroviral transforming protein of the simian sarcoma virus[328, 329] has led to the development of the concept that normal growth factors may act as oncogenes, as described in Chapter 26.

▼ PLATELET-ACTIVATING FACTOR

Platelet-activating factor (PAF) is a potent lipid mediator produced by vascular endothelium[330, 331] and several other cell types, including stimulated neutrophils and macrophages.[332, 333] It was discovered as a product of IgE-sensitized rabbit basophils.[334] PAF administered parenterally to animals causes bronchoconstriction, vasodilatation, and hypotension, and neutrophil and platelet aggregation and secretion.[335] Obviously, the physiological function of this mediator does not include its access to the systemic circulation. Platelets have high-affinity receptors (K_d ~ 1 nM) for PAF,[336] and binding of PAF to these receptors correlates with the action of PAF on platelets. The PAF receptor contains 342 amino acids, has seven membrane spanning domains, and shows homology to other such receptors.[337, 338] PAF is a strong platelet agonist, stimulating aggregation and secretion as thrombin does.[339, 340]

Endothelial cells produce PAF in response to thrombin[330, 331] and to leukotrienes,[341] implying receptor-mediated production. The PAF thus formed remains associated with the cells. At sites of vascular injury where thrombin is generated, PAF synthesized by endothelial cells may serve to activate platelets and leukocytes locally, causing them to adhere to sites of injury. Platelets themselves produce very small amounts of PAF in response to the Ca^{2+} ionophore A23187.[342, 343] Whether this is of physiological significance is uncertain, since thrombin-induced platelet activation does not result in PAF formation.[340]

PAF is 1-0-alkyl-2-acetyl-sn-glycerol-3-phosphoryl choline[344] (Fig. 24–17). The PAF produced by polymorphonuclear leukocytes contains primarily a 16 carbon saturated alkyl moiety[328] in the 1 position, although 18 carbon PAF is very active and may be produced in other cells. The acetyl moiety is most important; fatty acids in the 2 position of four carbons or greater are inactive.[344] The synthesis of PAF is initiated by the activation of cytosolic phospholipase A_2, the same enzyme that initiates arachidonate release.[125] The lysophospholipid product of this reaction is then esterified by PAF acetyl transferase to form active PAF. PAF is degraded by plasma and cellular forms of PAF acetylhydrolases.[345] Antagonists of these enzymes may prove to be useful as antiplatelet or anti-inflammatory agents. The duration of PAF action is short, implying mechanisms for rapid inactivation of the mediator. Degradation of PAF to lyso PAF is catalyzed by acetyl hydrolase enzymes that are contained both in plasma[347] and in cells.[348] cDNA encoding both cellular and plasma PAF has been isolated,[345] and the X-ray crystal structure of the former has been solved.[349] This metal ion independent lipases have an active site motif of GXSXG

PAF

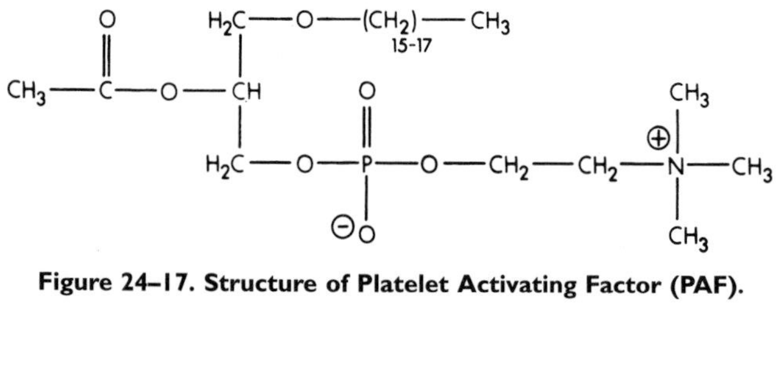

Figure 24–17. Structure of Platelet Activating Factor (PAF).

common to many lipases. They have a trypsin-like catalytic trend of Ser-His-Asp.

REFERENCES

1. Editorial. Lancet 2:133, 1973.
2. Metcalf, D., MacDonald, H. R., Odartchenko, N., and Sordat, B.: Growth of mouse megakaryocyte colonies in vitro. Proc. Natl. Acad. Sci., USA 72:1744, 1975.
3. Nakeff, A., and Daniels-McQueen, S.: In vitro colony assay for a new class megakaryocyte precursor: Colony forming unit megakaryocyte. Proc. Soc. Exp. Biol. Med. 151:587, 1976.
4. McLeod, D. L., Shreeve, M. M., and Axelrad, A. A.: Induction of megakaryocyte colonies with platelet formation in vitro. Nature 261:492, 1976.
5. Vainchenker, W., Bouquet, J., Guichard, J., and Breton-Gorius, J.: Megakaryocyte colony formation from human bone marrow precursors. Blood 54:940, 1979.
6. Ebbe, S., and Stohlman, F.: Megakaryocytopoiesis in the rat. Blood 26:20, 1965.
7. Penington, D. G.: Formation of platelets. In Dingle, J. T., and Gordon, J. L. (eds.): Platelets in Pathology and Biology—2. Amsterdam, Elsevier North Holland Biomedical Press, 1982.
8. Mosesson, M. W., Homandberg, G. A., and Amrani, D. L.: Human platelet fibrinogen gamma chain structure. Blood 63:990, 1984.
9. Chiu, C. P., Schick, P., and Colman, R. W.: Biosynthesis of coagulation factor V in isolated guinea pig megakaryocytes. J. Clin. Invest. 75:339, 1985.
10. Ryo, R., Nakeff, A., Huang, S. S., Ginsberg, M., and Deuel, T. F.: Platelet factor IV synthesis in a megakaryocyte enriched rabbit bone marrow culture. J. Cell Biol. 96:515, 1983.
11. Chernoff, A. R., Levine, R. F., and Goodman, D. S.: Origin of platelet derived growth factor in megakaryocytes in guinea pigs. J. Clin. Invest. 65:926, 1980.
12. Nachman, R. L., Levine, R. F., and Jaffe, E. A.: Synthesis of vWF in cultured guinea pig megakaryocytes. J. Clin. Invest. 60:914, 1977.
13. Rabellino, E. M., Levene, R. B., Leung, L. L. K., and Nachman, R. L.: Human megakaryocytes. II. Expression of platelet proteins in early marrow megakaryocytes. J. Exp. Med. 154:88, 1981.
14. Shaklai, M., and Tavassoli, M.: Demarcation membrane system in rat megakaryocyte and the mechanism of platelet formation: A membrane reorganization process. J. Ultrastruct. Res. 62:270, 1978.
15. Tavassoli, M.: Megacaryocyte-platelet axis and the process of platelet formation and release. Blood 55:537, 1980.
16. Radley, J. M., and Scurfield, G.: The mechanism of platelet release. Blood Cells 56:996, 1980.
17. Kaushansky, K.: Thrombopoietin: Understanding and manipulating platelet production. Annu. Rev. Med. 48:1, 1997.
18. deSauvage, F. J., Hass, P. E., Spencer, S. E., et al: Stimulation of megakaryocytopoiesis and thrombopoiesis by the c-Mpl ligand. Nature 369:533, 1994.
19. Lok, S., Kaushansky, K., Holly, R., et al.: Cloning and expressing of murine thrombopoietin cDNA and stimulation of platelet production in vivo. Nature 369:565, 1994.
20. Bartley, T. D., Bogenberger, J., Hunt, P., et al.: Identification and cloning of a megakaryocyte growth and development factor that is a ligand for the cytokine receptor Mpl. Cell 77:1117, 1994.
21. Sohma, Y., Akahori, H., Seki, N., et al.: Molecular cloning and chromosomal localization of the human thrombopoietin gene. FEBS Lett. 353:57, 1994.
22. Kuter, D. J., Beeler, D. L., and Rosenberg, R. D.: The purification of megapoietin: A physiological regulator of megakaryocyte growth and platelet production. Proc. Natl. Acad. Sci. USA 91:11104, 1994.
23. Vigon, I., Mornon, J-P., Cocault, L., et al.: Molecular cloning and characterization of MPL, the human homolog of the v-impl oncogene: Identification of a member of the hematopoietic growth factor receptor superfamily. Proc. Natl. Acad. Sci. USA 89:5640, 1992.
24. Fielder, P. J., Gurney, A. L., Stefanich, E., Marian, M., Moore, M. W., Carver-Moore, K., and de Sauvage, F. J.: Regulation of thrombopoietin levels by c-mpl–mediated binding to platelets. Blood 87:2154, 1996.
25. Broundy, V. C., Lin, N. L., Sabath, D. F., Papayannopoulou, T., and Kaushansky, K.: Human platelets display high-affinity receptors for thrombopoietin. Blood 89:1896, 1997.
26. Nochol, J., Hokom, M., Hornkohl, S., et al.: Megakaryocyte growth and development factor: Analysis of the in vitro effects on human megakaryopoiesis and endogenous serum levels during chemotherapy induced thrombocytopenia. J. Clin. Invest. 95:2973, 1995.
27. Stefanich, E., Senn, T., Widmer, R., Fratino, C., Keller, G.-A., and Fielder, P. J.: Metabolism of thrombopoietin (TPO) in vivo: Determination of the binding dynamics for TPO in mice. Blood, 89:4063, 1997.
28. Fielder, P. J., Hass, P., Magel, M., Stefanich, E., Widmer, R., Bennett, G. L., Keller, G-A., de Sauvage, F. J., and Eaton, D.: Human platelets as a model for the binding and degradation of thrombopoietin. Blood 89:2782, 1997.
29. Gurney, A. L., Carver-Moore, K., de Sauvage, F. J., and Moore, M. W.: Thrombocytopenia in c-mpl-deficient mice. Science 265:1445, 1994.
30. Vadham-Raj, S., Murray, L. J., Bueso-Ramos, C., Patel, S., Reddy, S. P., Hoots, W. K., Johnston, T., Papadopolouys, N. E., Hittelman, W. N., Johnston, D. A., Yang, T. A., Paton, V. E., Cohen, R. L., Hellmann, S. D., Benjamin, R. S., and Broxmeyer, H. E.: Stimulation of megakaryocyte and platelet production by a single dose of recombinant human thrombopoietin in patients with cancer. Ann. Intern. Med. 126:673, 1997.
31. Fanucchi, M., Glaspy, J., Crawford, J., Garst, J., Figlin, R., Sheridan, W., Menchaca, D., Tomita, D., Ozer, H., and Harker, L.: Effects of polyethylene glycol-conjugated recombinant human megakaryocyte growth and development factor on platelet counts after chemotherapy for lung cancer. N. Engl. J. Med. 336:405, 1997.
32. Oda, A., Miyakawa, Y., Druker, B. J., Ozaki, K., Yabusaki, K., Shirawawa, Y., Handa, M., Kato, T., Miyazaki, H., Shimosaka, A., and Ikeda, Y.: Thrombopoietin primes human platelet aggregation induced by shear stress and by multiple agonists. Blood 87:4664, 1996.
33. Weich, N. S., Wang, A., Fitzgerald, M., Neben, T. Y., Donaldson, D., Giannotti, J., Yetz-Aldape, J., Leven, R. M., and Turner, K. J.: Recombinant human interleukin-11 directly promotes megakaryocytopoiesis in vitro. Blood 90:3893, 1997.
34. Isaacs, C., Robert, N. J., Bailey, F. A., Schuster, M. W., Overmoyer, B., Graham, M., Cai, B., Beach, K. J., Loewy, J. W., and Kaye, J. A.: Randomized placebo-controlled study of recombinant human interleukin-11 to prevent chemotherapy-induced thrombocytopenia in patients with breast cancer receiving dose-intensive cyclophosphamide and doxorubicin. J. Clin. Oncol. 15:3368, 1997.
35. Tepler, E., Elias, L., Smith, J. W. II, Hussein, M., Rosen, G., Chang, A.Y.C., Moore, J. O., Gordon, M. S., Kuca, B., Beach, K. J., Loewy, J. W., Garnick, M. B., and Kaye, J. A. A randomized placebo-controlled trial of recombinant human interleukin-11 in cancer patients with severe thrombocytopenia due to chemotherapy. Blood 87:3067, 1996.
36. Heaton, W. A., Davis, H. H., Welsh, M. J., Mathias, C. J., Joist, H. J., Sherman, L. A., and Siegel, B. A.: Indium 111: A new radionuclide label for studying human platelet kinetics. Br. J. Haematol. 42:613, 1979.
37. Gerwitz, A. M., Bruno, E., Elwell, J., and Hoffman, R.: In vitro studies of megakaryocytopoiesis in thrombocytopenic disorders of man. Blood 61:384, 1983.
38. White, J. G., and Gerrard, J. M.: Anatomy and structural organization of the platelet. In Colman, R. W., Hirsh, J., Marder, V. J., and Salzman, E. W. (eds.): Hemostasis and Thrombosis. Philadelphia, J. B. Lippincott Co., 1982.
39. Feagler, J. R., Tillack, T. W., Chaplin, D. D., and Majerus, P. W.: The effects of thrombin of phytohemagglutinin receptor sites in human platelets. J. Cell Biol. 60:541, 1974.
40. Kaplan, K. L.: Platelet granule proteins: Localization and secretion. In Dingle, J. T., and Gordon, J. L. (eds.): Platelets in Pathology and Biology. Amsterdam, Elsevier/North Holland, 1981.
41. Chesney, C. M., Pifer, D., and Colman, R. W.: Subcellular localization and secretion of factor V from human platelets. Proc. Natl. Acad. Sci. USA 78:5180, 1981.
42. George, J. N.: Platelet IgG: Its significance for the evaluation of thrombocytopenia and for understanding the origin of alpha granule proteins. Blood 76:859, 1990.
43. Handagama, P. J., Shuman, M. A., and Bainton, D. F.: Incorporation of intravenously injected albumin, IgG, and fibrinogen into guinea pig megakaryocyte. J. Clin. Invest. 84:73, 1989.
44. Handgamma, P. J., Rappolee, D. A., Werb, Z., Levin, J., Bainton, D.

F.: Platelet α-granule fibrinogen, albumin, and immunoglobulin G are not synthesized by rat and mouse megadaryocytes. J. Clin. Invest. 86:1364, 1990.

45. Handagama, P., Scarborough, R. M., Shuman, M. A., Bainton, D. F.: Endocytosis of fibrinogen into megakaryocytes and platelet α-granules is mediated by $\alpha_{IIb}\beta_3$ (Glycoprotein IIb-IIa). Blood 82:135, 1993.

46. Handagama, P., Bainton, D. F., Jacques, Y., Conn, M. T., Lazarus, R. A., Shuman, M. A.: Kistrin, an integrin antagonist, blocks endocytosis of fibrinogen into guinea pig megakaryocyte and platelets α-granules. J. Clin. Invest. 91:193, 1993.

47. Moore, K. L.: Structure and function of P-selectin glycoprotein ligand-1. Leuk. Lymphoma 29:1, 1998.

48. McEver, R. P.: Leukocyte interactions mediated by selectins. Thromb. Hemost. 66:80, 1991.

49. Novotny, W. F., Girard, T. J., Miletich, J. P., Broze, G. J.: Platelets secrete a coagulation inhibitor functionally and antigenically similar to the lipoprotein associated coagulation inhibitor. Blood 72:2020, 1988.

50. Leung, L.L.K., Harpel, P. C., Nachman, R. L., and Rabellino, E. M.: Histidine rich glycoprotein is present in human platelets and is released following thrombin stimulation. Blood 62:1016, 1983.

51. Ginsberg, M. H., Painter, R. G., Forsyth, J., Birdwell, C., and Plow, E. F.: Thrombin-increased expression of fibronectin antigen on the platelet surface. Proc. Natl. Acad. Sci. USA 77:1049, 1980.

52. Schmaier, A. H., Zuckerberg, A., Silverman, C., Kuchibhotla, J., Tuszynski, G. P., and Colman, R. W.: High-molecular weight kininogen: A secreted platelet protein. J. Clin. Invest. 71:1477, 1983.

53. Nachman, R. L., and Harpel, P. C.: Platelet α_2 macroglobulin and α1 antitrypsin. J. Biol. Chem. 251:4514, 1976.

54. Newman, P. J., Gorski, J., White, G. C., Gidwitz, S., Cretney, C. J., Aster, R. H.: Enzymatic amplification of platelet-specific RNA using the polermase chain reaction. J. Clin. Invest. 82:739, 1998.

55. Weyrich, A. S., Dixon, D. A., Pabla, R., Elstad, M. R., McIntyre, T. M., Prescott, S. M., Zimmerman, G. A.: Signal-dependent translation of a regulatory protein, Bcl-3, in activated human platelets. Proc. Natl. Acad. Sci. USA 95:5556, 1998.

56. Akkerman, J.W.N.: Regulation of carbohydrate metabolism in platelets: A review. Thromb. Haemost. 39:712, 1979.

57. Majerus, P. W., Smith, M. B., and Clamon, G. H.: Lipid metabolism in human platelets. I. Evidence for a complete fatty acid synthesizing system. J. Clin. Invest. 48:156, 1969.

58. Lewis, N., and Majerus, P. W.: Lipid metabolism in human platelets. II. De novo phospholipid synthesis and the effect of thrombin on the pattern of synthesis. J: Clin. Invest. 48:2114, 1969.

59. Puett, D., Wasserman, B. K., Ford, J. D., and Cunningham, L. W.: Collagen mediated platelet aggregation: Effects of collagen modification involving the protein and carbohydrate moieties. J. Clin. Invest. 52:2495, 1973.

60. Hemler, M. E.: VLA proteins in the integrin family. Annu. Rev. Immunol. 8:365, 1990.

61. Kehrel, B., Wierwille, S., Clemetson, K. J., Anders, O., Steiner, M., Knight, C. G., Farndale, R. W., Okuma, M., Barnes, M. J.: Glycoprotein VI is a major collagen receptor for platelet activation: It recognizes the platelet-activating quaternary structure of collagen, whereas CD36, glycoprotein IIb/IIIa, and von Willebrand factor do not. Blood 15:491, 1998.

62. Baumgartner, H. R., Tshopp, T. B., and Weiss, H. J.: Platelet interaction with collagen fibrils in flowing blood. II. Impaired adhesion-aggregation in bleeding disorder. Thromb. Haemost. 37:17, 1977.

63. Gaarder, A., Jonsen, J., Laland, S., Hellem, A., and Owren, P. A.: ADP in red cells as a factor in the adhesiveness of human blood platelets. Nature 192:531, 1961.

64. Charo, I. F., Feinman, R. D., and Detwiler, T. C.: Interactions of platelet aggregation and secretion. J. Clin. Invest. 60:866, 1977.

65. Shattil, S. J., and Bennett, J. S.: Platelets and their membranes in hemostasis: Physiology and pathophysiology. Ann. Intern. Med. 94:108, 1980.

66. Bennett, J. S. and Vilaire, G.: Exposure of platelet fibrinogen receptors by ADP and epinephrine. J. Clin. Invest. 64:1393, 1979.

67. Marguerie, G. A., Plow, E. F., and Edgington, T. S.: Human platelets possess an inducible and saturable receptor for fibrinogen. J. Biol. Chem. 254:5357, 1979.

68. Bennett, J. S., Vilaire, G., and Burch, J. W.: A role for prostaglandins and thromboxanes in the exposure of platelet fibrinogen receptors. J. Clin. Invest. 68:981, 1981.

69. Baenziger, N. L., Brodie, G. N., and Majerus, P. W.: Isolation and

properties of a thrombin-sensitive protein of human platelets. J. Biol. Chem. 247:2723, 1972.

70. Margossian, S. S., Lawler, J. W., and Slayter, H. S.: Physical characterization of platelet thrombospondin. J. Biol. Chem. 256:7495, 1981.

71. Phillips, D. R., Jennings, L. K., and Prasanna, H. R.: Ca^{++} mediated associated of glycoprotein-G (thrombin sensitive protein, thrombospondin) with human platelets. J. Biol. Chem. 255:11629, 1980.

72. Gartner, T. K., Gerrard, J. M., White, J. G., and Williams, D. C.: Fibrinogen is the receptor for the endogenous lectin of human platelets. Nature 289:688, 1981.

73. Jaffe, E. A., Leung, L.L.K., Nachman, R. L., Levin, R. I., and Mosher, D. F.: Thrombospondin is the endogenous lectin of human platelets. Nature 295:246, 1982.

74. Leung, L.L.K., and Nachman, R. L.: Complex formation of platelet thrombospondin with fibrinogen. J. Clin. Invest. 70:542, 1982.

75. Gerrard, J. M., Phillips, D. R., Rai, G.H.R., Plow, E. F., Walz, D. A., Ross, R., Harker, L. A., and White, J. G.: Biochemical studies of two patients with gray platelet syndrome. J. Clin. Invest. 66:102, 1980.

76. Lawler, J., Sunday, M., Thibert, B., Duquette, M., George, E. L., Rayburn, H., Hynes, R. O.: Thrombospondin-1 is required for normal murine pulmonary hemeostasis and its absence causes pneumonia. J. Clin. Invest. 101:982, 1998.

77. Leung, L.L.K., Nachman, R. L., and Harpel, P. C.: Complex formation of platelet thrombospondin with histidine-rich glycoprotein. J. Clin. Invest. 73:5, 1984.

78. Stenberg, P. A., Shuman, M. A., Levine, S. P., and Bainton, D. F.: Redistribution of alpha-granules and their contents in thrombin-stimulated platelets. J. Cell Biol. 98:748, 1984.

79. Lin, S. E., and Stossel, T. P.: The microfilament network of the platelet. In Spaet, T. H. (ed.): Progress in Hemostasis and Thrombosis. Vol. 6. New York, Grune & Stratton, 1982.

80. Barlalow, K., Witke, W., Kwiatkowski, D. J., and Hartwig, J. H.: Coordinated regulation of platelet actin filament barbed ends by gelsolin and capping protein. J. Cell Biol. 134:389, 1996.

81. Gordon, D. J., Boyer, J. L., and Korn, E. D.: Comparative biochemistry of non-muscle actins. J. Biol. Chem. 252:8300, 1977.

82. Vanderkerchkove, J., and Weber, K.: Comparisons of actins from calf thymus, bovine brain, and SV40-transformed mouse 3T3 cells with rabbit skeletal muscle actin. Eur. J. Biochem. 90:451, 1978.

83. Hanukoglu, I., Tanese, N., and Fuchs, E.: cDNA Sequence of a human cytoplasmic actin. J. Mol. Biol. 163:673, 1983.

84. Korn, E. D.: Biochemistry of actomyosin-dependent cell motility (a review). Proc. Natl. Acad. Sci. USA 75:588, 1978.

85. Carlsson, L., Markey, F., Blikstad, I., Persson, T., and Lindberg, U.: Reorganization of actin in platelets stimulated by thrombin as measured by the DNAse I inhibition assay. Proc. Natl. Acad. Sci. USA 76:6376, 1979.

86. Adelstein, R. S., and Conti, M. A.: Phosphorylation of platelet myosin increases actin-activated ATPase activity. Nature 256:597, 1975.

87. Daniel, J. L., Molish, I. R., and Holmson, H.: Myosin phosphorylation in intact platelets. J. Biol. Chem. 256:7510, 1981.

88. Adelstein, R. S., and Eisenberg, E.: Regulation and kinetics of the actin-myosin-ATP interaction. Annu. Rev. Biochem. 49:921, 1980.

89. Adelstein, R. S., and Klee, C. B.: Purification and characterization of smooth muscle myosin light chain kinase. J. Biol. Chem. 256:7501, 1981.

90. Ishikawa, H., Bischoff, R., and Holtzer, H.: Formation of arrowhead complexes with heavy meromyosin in a variety of cell types. J. Cell Biol. 43:312, 1969.

91. Pollard, T. D., and Mooseker, M. S.: Direct measurement of actin polymerization rate constants by electron microscopy of actin filaments nucelated by isolated microvillous cores. J. Cell Biol. 88:654, 1981.

92. Tilney, L. G., Bonder, E. M., and DeRosier, D. J.: Actin filaments elongate from their membrane-associated ends. J. Cell Biol. 90:485, 1981.

93. Carlsson, L., Nystrom, L. E., Sundkvist, I., et al.: Actin polymerizability is influenced by profilin, a low MW protein in nonmuscle cells. J. Mol. Biol. 115:465, 1977.

94. Markey, F., Persson, T., and Lindberg, U.: Characterization of platelet extracts before and after stimulation with respect to the possible role of profilactin as microfilament precursor. Cell 23:145, 1981.

95. Fox, J.E.B., and Phillips, D. R.: Polymerization and organization of actin filaments within platelets. Semin. Hematol. 20:243, 1983.

96. Hartwig, J. H., Barkalow, K.: Polyphosphoinositide synthesis and platelet shape change. Curr. Opin. Hematol. 4:351, 1997.

97. Lind, S. E., Yin, H. L., and Stossel, T. P.: Human platelets contain gelsolin, a regulator of actin filament length. J. Clin. Invest. 69:1384, 1982.

98. Witke, W., Sharpe, A. H., Hartwig, J. H., Azuma, T., Stossel, T. P., Kwiatkowski, D. J.: Hemostatic, inflammatory, and fibroblast responses are blunted in mice lacking gelsolin. Cell 81:41, 1995.

99. Fox, J.E.B., Reynolds, C. C., and Phillips, D. R.: Calcium-dependent proteolysis occurs during platelet aggregation. J. Biol. Chem. 258:9973, 1983.

100. Nobes, C. D., and Hall, A.: Rho, rac, and cdc42 GTPases regulate the assembly of multimolecular focal complexes associated with actin stress fibers, lamellipodia, and filopodia. Cell 81:53, 1995.

101. Majerus, P. W., and Miletich, J. P.: Relationships between platelets and coagulation factors in hemostasis. Annu. Rev. Med. 29:41, 1978.

102. Milstone, J. H.: Thrombokinase as prime activator of prothrombin: Historical perspectives and present status. Fed. Proc. 63:742, 1964.

103. Marcus, A. J.: Recent advances in platelet lipid metabolism research. Ann. NY Acad. Sci. 201:102, 1972.

104. Miletich, J. P., Jackson, C. M., and Majerus, P. W.: Properties of the factor X_a binding site on human platelets. J. Biol. Chem. 253:6908, 1978.

105. Miletich, J. P., Jackson, C. M., and Majerus, P. W.: Interaction of coagulation factor X_a with human platelets. Proc. Natl. Acad. Sci. USA 74:4033, 1977.

106. Dahlback, B., and Stenflo, J.: Binding of bovine coagulation factor X_a to platelets. Biochemistry 17:4938, 1978.

107. Kane, W. H., Lindhout, M.L.J., Jackson, C. M., and Majerus, P. W.: Factor V_a–dependent binding of factor X_a to human platelets. J. Biol. Chem. 255:1170, 1980.

108. Tracy, P. B., Peterson, J. M., Neshiem, M. E., McDuffie, F. C., and Mann, K. G.: Interaction of coagulation factor V and factor V_a with platelets. J. Biol. Chem. 254:10354, 1979.

109. Teitel, J. M., and Rosenberg, R. D.: Protection of factor X_a from neutralization by the heparin-antithrombin complex. J. Clin. Invest. 71:1383, 1983.

110. Deuel, T. F., Keim, P. S., Farmer, M., and Heinrikson, R. L.: Amino acid sequence of human platelet factor IV. Proc. Natl. Acad. Sci. USA 74:2256, 1977.

111. Hermodson, M., Schmer, G., and Kurachi, K.: Isolation, crystallization and primary amino acid sequence of platelet factor IV. J. Biol. Chem. 252:6276, 1977.

112. Hemker, H. C., Van Rijn, J.L.M.L., Rosing, J., Van Dieijen, G., Bevers, E. W., and Zwaal, R.F.S.: Platelet membrane involvement in blood coagulation. Blood Cells 9:303, 1983.

113. Baglia, F. A., and Walsh, P. N.: Prothrombin is a cofactor for the binding of factor XI to the platelet surface and for platelet-mediated factor XI activation by thrombin. Biochemistry 37:2271, 1998.

114. Majerus, P. W.: Arachidonate metabolism in vascular disorders. J. Clin. Invest. 72:1521, 1983.

115. Needleman, S. W., Spector, A. A., and Hoak, J. C.: Enrichment of human platelet phospholipids with linoleic acid diminishes thromboxane release. Prostaglandins 124:607, 1982.

116. Kaduce, T. L., Hoak, J. C., and Fry, G. L.: Utilization of arachidonic and linoleic acids by cultured human endothelial cells. J. Clin. Invest. 68:1003, 1981.

117. Neufeld, E. J., Wilson, D. B., Sprecher, H., and Majerus, P. W.: High affinity esterification of eicosanoid precursor fatty acids by platelets. J. Clin. Invest. 72:214, 1983.

118. Wilson, D. B., Prescott, S. M., and Majerus, P. W.: Discovery of an arachidonoyl Coenzyme A synthetase in human platelets. J. Biol. Chem. 257:3510, 1982.

119. Neufeld, E. J., Bross, T. E., and Majerus, P. W.: A mutant $HSDM_1C_1$ fibrosarcoma line selected for defective eicosanoid precursor uptake lacks arachidonate-specific acyl-CoA synthetase. J. Biol. Chem. 259:1986, 1984.

120. Neufeld, E. J., Sprecher, H., Evans, R. W., and Majerus, P. W.: Fatty acid structural requirements for activity of arachidonoyl-CoA synthetase. J. Lipid Res. 25:288, 1984.

121. Kang, M. J., Fujino, T., Sasano, H., Minekura, H., Yabuki, N., Nagura, H., Iijima, H., and Yamamoto, T. T.: A novel arachidonate-preferring acyl-CoA synthetase is present in steroidogenic cells of the rat adrenal, ovary, and testis. Proc. Natl. Acad. Sci. USA 94:2880, 1997.

122. Cao, Y., Traer, E., Zimmerman, G. A., McIntyre, T. M., and Prescott, S. M.: Cloning, expression, and chromosomal localization of human long-chain fatty acid-CoA ligase 4 (FACL4). Genomics 49:327, 1998.

123. Bonventre, J. V., Huang, Z., Taheri, M. R., O'Leary, E., Li, E., Moskowitz, M. A., and Sapirstein, A.: Reduced fertility and post-ischaemic brain injury in mice deficient in cytosolic phospholipase A2. Nature 390:622, 1997.

124. Uozumi, N., Kume, K., Nagase, T., Nakatani, N., Ishii, S., Tashiro, F., Komagata, Y., Maki, K., Ikuta, K., Ouchi, Y., Miyazaki, J., and Shimizu, T.: Role of cytosolic phospholipase A_2 in allergic response and parturition. Nature 390:618, 1997.

125. Leslie, C. C.: Properties and regulation of cytosolic phospholipase A_2. J. Biol. Chem. 272:16709, 1997.

126. Borsch-Haubold, A. G., Bartoli, F., Asselin, J., Dudler, T., Kramer, R. M., Apitz-Castro, R., Watson, S. P., and Gelb, M. H.: Identification of the phosphorylation sites of cytosolic phospholipase A_2 in agonist-stimulated human platelets and HeLa cells. J. Biol. Chem. 273:4449, 1998.

127. Nugteren, D. H.: Arachidonate lipoxygenase in blood platelets. Biochem. Biophys. Acta 380:299, 1975.

128. Hamberg, M., and Hamberg, G.: On the mechanism of the oxygenation of arachidonic acid by human platelet lipoxygenase. Biochem. Biophys. Res. Commun. 95:1090, 1980.

129. Johnson, E. N., Brass, L. F., Funk, C. D.: Increased platelet sensitivity to ADP in mice lacking platelet-type 12-lipoxygenase. Proc. Natl. Acad. Sci., USA, 95:3100, 1998.

130. Rollins, T. E., and Smith, W. L.: Subcellular localization of prostaglandin-forming cyclooxygenase in Swiss mouse 3T3 fibroblasts by electron microscopic immunocytochemistry. J. Biol. Chem. 255:4872, 1980.

131. Gerrard, J. M., White, J. G., Rao, G.H.R., and Townsend, D.: Localization of platelet prostaglandin production in the platelet dense tubular system. Am. J. Pathol. 83:283, 1976.

132. Funk, C. D., Funk, L. B., Kennedy, M. E., Pong, A. S., and Fitzgerald, G. A.: Human platelet/erythroleukemia cell prostaglandin G/H synthase: cDNA Cloning, expression, and gene chromosomal assignment. FASEB J. 5:2304, 1991.

133. Takahashi, Y., Ueda, N., Yoshimoto, T., Yamamoto, S., Yokoyama, C., Miyata, A., Tanabe, T., Fuse, I., Hattori, A., and Shibata, A.: Immunoaffinity purification and cDNA cloning of human platelet prostaglandin endoperoxide synthase. Biochem. Biophys. Res. Commun. 182:433, 1992.

134. Hamberg, M., Svensson, J., and Samuelsson, B.: Thromboxanes: A new group of biologically active compounds derived from prostaglandin peroxides. Proc. Natl. Acad. Sci. USA 72:2994, 1975.

135. Samuelsson, B.: Prostaglandins, thromboxanes, and leukotrienes: Formation and biological rules. Harvey Lect. 75:1, 1981.

136. Roth, G. J., Machuga, E. T., and Strittmatter, P.: The heme-binding properties of prostaglandin synthetase from sheep vesicular gland. J. Biol. Chem. 256:10018, 1981.

137. Hammarstrom, S., and Falardeau, P.: Resolution of prostaglandin endoperoxide synthase and thromboxane synthase of human platelets. Proc. Natl. Acad. Sci. USA 74:3691, 1977.

138. Monen, P., Buytenhek, M., and Nugteren, D. H.: Purification of PGH-PGE isomerase from sheep vesicular glands. Methods Enzymol. 86:84, 1982.

139. Shiemizu, T., Yamamoto, S., and Hayaishi, O.: Purification of PGH-PGD isomerase from rat brain. Methods Enzymol. 86:73, 1982.

140. Watanabe, T., Narumiya, S., Shimizu, T., and Hayaishi, O.: Characterization of the biosynthetic pathway of prostaglandin D_2 in human platelet-rich plasma. J. Biol. Chem. 257:14847, 1982.

141. Watanabe, T., Shimizu, T., Narumiya, S., and Hayaishi, O.: NADP-linked 15-hydroxyprostaglandin dehydrogenase for prostaglandin D_2 in human blood platelets. Arch. Biochem. Biophys. 216:372, 1982.

142. Roth, G. J., Stanford, N., and Majerus, P. W.: The acetylation of prostaglandin synthetase by aspirin. Proc. Natl. Acad. Sci. USA 72:3073, 1975.

143. Roth, G. J., Machuga, E. T., and Ozols, J.: Isolation and covalent structure of the aspirin-modified, active-site region of prostaglandin synthetase. Biochemistry 22:4672, 1983.

144. Smith, W. L., and Dewitt, D. L.: Prostaglandin endoperoxide H synthases-1 and -2. Adv. Immunol. 62:167, 1996.

145. DeWitt, D. L., El-Harith, E. A., Draimer, S. A., Andrews, M. J., Yao, E. F., Armstrong, R. L., and Smith, W. L.: The aspirin and heme-binding sites of ovine and murine prostaglandin endoperoxide synthases. J. Biol. Chem. 265:5192, 1990.

146. Shimokawa, T., and Smith, W. L.: Prostaglandin endoperoxide synthase: The aspirin acetylation region. J. Biol. Chem. 267:12387, 1992.

147. Burch, J. W., Stanford, N., and Majerus, P. W.: Inhibition of platelet prostaglandin cyclooxygenase by oral aspirin. J. Clin. Invest. 61:314, 1978.

148. Harter, H. R., Burch, J. W., Majerus, P. W., Stanford, N., Delmez, J. A., Anderson, C. G., and Weerts, C. A.: The prevention of thrombosis by low-dose aspirin. N. Engl. J. Med. 301:577, 1979.

149. Patrignani, P., Filabozzi, P., and Patrono, C.: Selective cumulative inhibition of platelet thromboxane production by low-dose aspirin in healthy subjects. J. Clin. Invest. 69:1366, 1982.

150. FitzGerald, G. A., Oates, J. A., Hawiger, J., Maas, R. L., Roberts, L. J. II, Lawson, S. A., and Brash, A. R.: Endogenous biosynthesis of prostacyclin and thromboxane and platelet function during chronic administration of aspirin in man. J. Clin. Invest. 71:676, 1983.

151. Xie, W., Chipman, J. G., Robertson, D. L., Erikson, R. L., and Simmons, D. L.: Expression of a mitogen-responsive gene encoding prostaglandin synthase is regulated by mRNA splicing. Proc. Natl. Acad. Sci. USA 88:2692, 1991.

152. Kujubu, D. A., Fletcher, B. S., Varnum, B. C., Lim, R. W., and Herschmann, H. R.: TIS10, a phorbol ester tumor promoter–inducible mRNA from Swiss 3T3 cells, encodes a novel prostaglandin synthase/cyclooxygenase homologue. J. Biol. Chem. 266:12866, 1991.

153. Obanion, M. K., Winn, V. D., and Young, D. A.: cDNA cloning and functional activity of a glucocorticoid-regulated inflammatory cyclooxygenase. Proc. Natl. Acad. Sci. USA 89:4888, 1992.

154. Malmsten, C., Hamber, M., Svensson, J., and Samuelsson, B.: Physiological role of an endoperoxide in human platelets: Haemostatic defect due to platelet cyclooxygenase deficiency. Proc. Natl. Acad. Sci. USA 72:1466, 1975.

155. Weiss, H. J., and Lages, B. A.: Possible congenital defect in thromboxane synthetase. Lancet 1:760, 1977.

156. LaGarde, M., Byron, P. A., Vargaftig, B. B., and Dechavenue, M.: Impairment of platelet thromboxane A_2 generation and of the platelet release reaction in two patients with congenital deficiency of platelet cyclooxygenase. Br. J. Haematol. 38:251, 1978.

157. Pareti, F. I., Mannucci, P. M., and D'Angelo, A.: Congenital deficiency of thromboxane and prostacyclin. Lancet 1:898, 1980.

158. Matijevic-Aleksic, N., McPhedran, P., Wu, K. K.: Bleeding disorder due to platelet prostaglandin H synthase-1 (PGHS-1) deficiency. Br. J. Haematol. 92:212, 1996.

159. Roth, G. J., and Machuga, E. T.: Radioimmune assay of human platelet prostaglandin synthetase. J. Lab. Clin. Med. 99:187, 1982.

160. Laposata, M., Prescott, S. M., Bross, T. E., and Majerus, P. W.: Development and characterization of a tissue culture cell line with essential fatty acid deficiency. Proc. Natl. Acad. Sci. USA 79:7654, 1982.

161. McEver, R. P., Baenziger, N. L., and Majerus, P. W.: Isolation and quantitation of the platelet membrane glycoprotein defect in thrombasthenia using a monoclonal hybridoma antibody. J. Clin. Invest. 66:1311, 1980.

162. McEver, R. P., Baenziger, J. U., and Majerus, P. W.: Isolation and structural characterization of the polypeptide subunits of membrane glycoprotein IIb-IIIa from human platelets. Blood 59:80, 1982.

163. Hynes, R. O.: Integrins: Versatility, modulation, and signaling in cell adhesion. Cell 69:11, 1992.

164. Ruoslahti, E.: Integrins. J. Clin. Invest. 87:1, 1991.

165. Poncz, M., Eisman, R., Heidenreich, R., Silver, S. M., Vilaire, G., Surrey, S., Schwartz, E. and Bennett, J. S.: Structure of the platelet membrane glycoprotein IIb. J. Biol. Chem. 262:8476, 1987.

166. Kieffer, N. and Phillips, D. R.: Platelet membrane glycoproteins: Functions in cellular interactions. Annu. Rev. Cell Biol. 6:329, 1990.

167. Rosa, J-P., Bray, P. F., Gayet, O., Johnston, G. I., Cook, R. G., Jackson, K. W., Shuman, M. A. and McEver, R. P.: Cloning of glycoprotein IIIa cDNA from human erythroleukemia cells and localization of the gene to chromosome 17. Blood 72:593, 1988.

168. Fitzgerald, L. A., Steiner, B., Rall, S. C., Lo, S. S., and Phillips, D. R.: Protein sequence of endothelial cell glycoprotein IIIa derived from a cDNA clone: Identify with platelet glycoprotein IIIa and similarity with "integrin." J. Biol. Chem. 262:3936, 1987.

169. Tollefsen, D. T., and Majerus, P. W.: Inhibition of human platelet aggregation by monovalent antifibrinogen antibody fragments. J. Clin. Invest. 55:1259, 1975.

170. Nachman, R. L., and Leung, L.L.K.: Complex formation of platelet membrane glycoproteins IIb-IIIa with fibrinogen. J. Clin. Invest. 69:263, 1982.

171. Bennett, J. S., Vilaire, G., and Cines, D. B.: Identification of the fibrinogen receptor on human platelets by photoaffinity labeling. J. Biol. Chem. 257:8049, 1982.

172. Kloczewiak, M., Timmons, S., Lukas, J., and Hawiger, J.: Platelet receptor recognition site on human fibrinogen. Biochemistry 23:1767, 1984.

173. Nachman, R. L., Leung, L.L.K., Kloczewiak, M., and Hawiger, J.: Complex formation to platelet membrane glycoprotein IIb-IIIa with fibrinogen D domain. J. Biol. Chem. 259:8584, 1984.

174. D'Souze, S. E., Ginsberg, M. H., Burke, T. A., and Plow, E. F.: The ligand binding site of the platelet integrin receptor GPIIb-IIIa is proximal to the second calcium binding domain of its α subunit. J. Biol. Chem. 265:3440, 1990.

175. D'Souze, S. E., Ginsberg, M. H., Matsueda, G. R., and Plow, E. F.: A discrete sequence in a platelet integrin is involved in ligand recognition. Nature 350:66, 1991.

176. Taylor, D. B. and Gartner, T. K.: A peptide corresponding to GPIIb 300–312, a presumptive fibrinogen γ chain binding site on the platelet integrin GP IIb/IIIa, inhibits the adhesion of platelets to at least four adhesive ligands. J. Biol. Chem. 167:11729, 1992.

177. EPIC Investigators: Use of a monoclonal antibody directed against the platelet glycoprotein IIb/IIIa receptor in high-risk coronary angioplasty. N. Engl. J. Med. 330:956, 1994.

178. Coller, B. S.: Monitoring platelet GP IIb/IIIa antagonist therapy. Circulation 97:5, 1998.

179. Degos, L., Dautigny, A., Brouet, J. C., Colombani, M., Ardaillou, N., Caen, J. P., and Colombani, J.: A molecular defect in thrombasthenic platelets. J. Clin. Invest. 56:326, 1975.

180. Hagen, I., Nurden, A., Bjerrum, O. J., Solum, N. O., and Caen, J. P.: Immunochemical evidence for protein abnormalities in platelet from patients with Glanzmann's thrombasthenia and Bernard-Soulier syndrome. J. Clin. Invest. 65:722, 1980.

181. McEver, R. P., Bennett, E. B., and Martin, M. N.: Identification of two structurally and functionally distinct sites on human platelet membrane glyco protein IIb-IIIa using monoclonal antibodies. J. Biol. Chem. 258:5269, 1983.

182. Pidard, D., Montgomery, R. R., Bennett, J. S., and Kunicki, T. J.: Interaction of AP-2, a monoclonal antibody specific for the human glycoprotein IIb-IIIa complex, with intact platelets. J. Biol. Chem. 258:12582, 1983.

183. DiMinno, G., Thiagarajan, P., Perussia, B., Martinez, J., Shapiro, S., Trinchieri, G., and Murphy, S.: Exposure of platelet fibrinogen binding sites by collagen, arachidonate, and ADP: Inhibition by a monoclonal antibody to the glycoprotein IIb-IIIa complex. Blood 61:140, 1983.

184. Coller, B. S., Peershke, E. I., Scudder, L. E., and Sullivan, C. A.: A murine monoclonal antibody that completely blocks the binding of fibrinogen to platelets produces a thrombasthenic-like state in normal platelets and binds to glycoprotein IIb-IIIa. J. Clin. Invest. 72:325, 1983.

185. Newman, P. J., Seligsohn, U., Lyman, S. and Coller, B. S.: The molecular genetic basis of Glanzmann thrombasthenia in the Iraqi-Jewish and Arab populations in Israel. Proc. Natl. Acad. Sci. USA 88:3160, 1991.

186. Grimaldi, C. M., Chen, F., Wu, C., Weiss, H. J., Coller, B. S., French, D. L.: Glycoprotein IIb Leu214Pro mutation produces Glanzmann thrombasthenia with both quantitative and qualitative abnormalities in GPIIb/IIIa. Blood, 91:1562, 1998.

187. Loftus, J. C., Halloran, C. E., Ginsberg, M. H., Feigen, L. P., Zablocki, J. A., Smith, J. W.: The amino-terminal one-third of $\alpha_{IIb}\beta_3$. J. Biol. Chem. 271:2033, 1996.

188. George, J. N., Nurden, A. T., and Phillips, D. R.: Molecular defects that cause abnormalities of platelet vessel wall interactions. N. Engl. J. Med. 311:1084, 1984.

189. Ginsberg, M. H., Forsyth, J., Lightsey, A., Chediak, J., and Plow, E. F.: Reduced surface expression and binding of fibronectin by thrombin-stimulated thrombasthenic platelets. J. Clin. Invest. 71:619, 1983.

190. Ruggeri, Z. M., Bader, R., and de Marco, L.: Glanzmann's thrombasthenia: Deficient binding of vWF to thrombin-stimulated platelets. Proc. Natl. Acad. Sci. USA 79:6038, 1982.

191. Ruggeri, Z. M., de Marco, L., Gatti, L., Bader, R., and Montgomery, R. F.: Platelets have more than one binding site for vWF. J. Clin. Invest. 72:1, 1983.

192. Fujimoto, T., and Hawiger, J.: ADP induces binding of vWF to human platelets. Nature 297:154, 1982.

193. Fujimoto, T., Ohara, S., and Hawiger, J.: Thrombin-induced exposure and PGI2 inhibition of the receptor for factor VIII/vWF on human platelets. J. Clin. Invest. 69:1212, 1982.

194. Bajt, M. L., Ginsberg, M. H., Frelinger, A. L., Berndt, M. C., Loftus, J. C.: A spontaneous mutation of integrin $\alpha_{IIb}\beta_3$ (GPIIb/IIIa) helps define a ligand binding site. J. Biol. Chem. 76:3789, 1992.

195. Schullek, J., Jordan, J., and Mongomery, R. R.: Interaction of vWF with human platelets in plasma milieu. J. Clin. Invest. 73:421, 1984.

196. Van Loghem, J. J., Jr., Dorfmeijer, H., and Van der Hart, M.: Serological and genetic studies on a platelet antigen (ZW). Vox Sang. 4:161, 1959.

197. Kunicki, T. J., and Aster, R. H.: Deletion of the platelet-specific alloantigen Pl^{A1} from platelets in Glanzmann's thrombasthenia. J. Clin. Invest. 61:1225, 1978.

198. Kunicki, T. J., Picard, D., Cazenave, J. P., Nurden, A. J., and Caen, J. P.: Inheritance on the human platelet alloantigen Pl^{A1} in type one thrombasthenia. J. Clin. Invest. 67:717, 1981.

199. Howard, M. A., and Firkin, B. G.: Ristocetin: A new tool in the investigation of platelet aggregation. Thromb. Diath. Haemorrh. 26:362, 1971.

200. Kao, K. J., Pizzo, S. V., and McKee, P. A.: Demonstration and characterization of specific binding sites for factor VIII/vWF on human platelets. J. Clin. Invest. 63:656, 1979.

201. Moake, J. L., Olson, J. D., Tang, S. S., Funicella, T., and Peterson, D. M.: Binding of radioiodinated human vWF to Bernard-Soulier, thrombasthenic, and von Willebrand's disease platelets. Thromb. Res. 19:21, 1980.

202. Ruan, C., Tobelem, G., McMichael, A. J., Drouet, L., Legrand, Y., Degos, L., Kieffer, L., Lee, H., and Caen, J. P.: Monoclonal antibody to human platelet glycoprotein. Br. J. Haematol. 49:511, 1981.

203. Roth, G. J.: Developing relationships: Arterial platelet adhesion, GPIb, and leucine-rich glycoproteins. Blood, 77:5, 1991.

204. Nurden, A. T., and Caen, J. P.: Specific roles for platelet surface glycoproteins in platelet function. Nature 255:720, 1975.

205. Coller, B. S., Peerschke, E. I., Scudder, L. E., and Sullivan, C. A.: Studies with murine monoclonal antibody that abolishes ristocetin-induced binding of von Willebrand factor to platelets: Additional evidence in support of GP Ib as a platelet receptor for von Willebrand factor. Blood 61:99, 1983.

206. Nurden, A. T., Dupuis, D., Kunicki, T. J., and Caen, J. P.: Analysis of the glycoprotein and protein composition of Bernard-Soulier platelets by single and two-dimensional SDS-polyacrylamide gel electrophoresis. J. Clin. Invest. 67:1431, 1981.

207. Berndt, M. C., Gregory, C., Chong, B. H., Zola, H., and Castaldi, P. A.: Additional glycoprotein defects in Bernard-Soulier syndrome: Confirmation of genetic basis by parental analysis. Blood 62:800, 1983.

208. George, J. N., Reimann, T. A., Moake, J. L., Morgan, R. K., Cimo, P. A., and Sears, D. A.: Bernard-Soulier disease: A study of four patients and their parents. Br. J. Haematol. 48:459, 1981.

209. Modderman, P. W., Admiraal, L. G., Sonnenberg, A., and von dem Borne, A.E.G.K.: Glycoproteins V and Ib-IX form a noncovalent complex in the platelet membrane. J. Biol. Chem. 267:364, 1992.

210. Hickey, M. J., Williams, S. A., and Roth, G. J.: Human platelet glycoprotein IX: An adhesive prototype of leucine-rich glycoproteins with flank-center-flank structures. Proc. Natl. Acad. Sci. USA 86:6773, 1989.

211. Hickey, M. J., Deaven, L. L., and Roth, G. J.: Human platelet glycoprotein IX: Characterization of cDNA and localization of the gene to chromosome 3. FEBS Lett. 274:89, 1990.

212. Roth, G. J., Church, T. A., McMullen, B. A., and Williams, S. A.: Human platelet glycoprotein V: A surface leucine-rich glycoprotein related to adhesion. Biochem. Biophys. Res. Commun. 170:153, 1990.

213. Shimomura, T., Fujimura, K., Maehama, S., Takemoto, M., Oda, K., Fujikimoto, T., Oyama, R., Suzuki, M., Ichihara-Tanake, K., Titani, K., and Kuramoto, A.: Rapid purification and characterization of human platelet glycoprotein V: The amino acid sequence contains leucine-rich repetitive modules as in glycoprotein Ib. Blood 75:2349, 1990.

214. Lanza, F., Morales, M., de La Salle, C., Cazenave, J. P., Clemetson, K. J., Shimomura, T., and Phillips, D. R.: Cloning and characterization of the gene encoding the human platelet glycoprotein V: A member of the leucine-rich glycoprotein family cleaved during thrombin-induced platelet activation. J. Biol. Chem., 268:20801, 1993.

215. Bernard, J.: History of congenital hemorrhagic thrombocytopathic dystrophy. Blood Cells 9:179, 1983.

216. Kenny, D., Jonsson, O. G., Morateck, P. A., and Montgomery, R. R.: Naturally occurring mutations in glycoprotein Ibα that result in defective ligand binding and synthesis of a truncated protein. Blood, 92:175, 1998.

217. Ludlow, L. B., Schick, B. P., Budarf, M. L., Driscoll, D. A., Zackai, E. H., Cohen, A., and Konkle, B. A.: Identification of a mutation in a GATA binding site of the platelet glycoprotein Ibβ promoter resulting in the Bernard-Soulier syndrome. J. Biol. Chem. 271:22076, 1996.

218. Li, C. Q., Dong, J., Lanza, F., Sanan, D. A., Sae-Tung, G., Lopez, J. A.: Expression of platelet glycoprotein (GP) V in heterologous cells and evidence for its association with GP Ibα in forming a GP Ib-IX-V complex on the cell surface. J. Biol. Chem. 270P:16302, 1995.

219. Roth, G. J.: Molecular defects in the Bernard-Soulier syndrome: Assessment of receptor genes, transcripts and proteins. C. R. Acad. Sci. III 319:819, 1996.

220. Tollefsen, D., Jackson, C. M., and Majerus, P. W.: Binding of the products of prothrombin activation to human platelets. J. Clin. Invest. 56:241, 1975.

221. Vu, T-K H., Hung, D. T., Wheaton, V. I., and Coughlin, S. R.: Molecular cloning of a functional thrombin receptor reveals a novel proteolytic mechanism of receptor activation. Cell 64:1057, 1991.

222. Coughlin, S. R., Vu, T-K H., Hung, D. T., and Wheaton, V. I.: Characterization of a functional thrombin receptor. J. Clin. Invest., 89:351, 1992.

223. Ishihara, H., Connolly, A. J., Zeng, D., Kahn, M. L., Zheng, Y. W., Timmons, C., Tram, T., and Coughlin, S. R.: Protease-activated receptor 3 is a second thrombin receptor in humans. Nature 386:502, 1997.

224. Verrall, S., Ishii, M., Chen, M., Wang, L., Tram, T., and Coughlin, S. R.: The thrombin receptor second cytoplasmic loop confers coupling to Gq-like G proteins in chimeric receptors. J. Biol. Chem. 272:6898, 1997.

225. Xu, W. F., Andersen, H., Whitmore, T. E., Presnell, S. R., Yee, D. P., Ching, A., Gilbert, T., Davie, E. W., and Foster, D. C.: Cloning and characterization of human protease–activated receptor 4. Proc. Natl. Acad. Sci. USA 95:6642, 1998.

226. Miletich, J. P., Kane, W. H., Hofmann, S. L., and Majerus, P. W.: Deficiency of factor X_a–factor V_a binding sites on the platelets of a patient with a bleeding disorder. Blood 54:1015, 1979.

227. Kane, W. H., Lindhout, M. J., Jackson, C. M., and Majerus, P. W.: Factor V_a–dependent binding of Factor Xa to human platelets. J. Biol. Chem. 255:1170, 1980.

228. Tracy, P. B., Eide, L. L., Bowie, J. W., and Mann, K. G.: Radioimmunoassay of factor V in human plasma and platelets. Blood 60:59, 1982.

229. Kane, W. H., Mruk, J. S., and Majerus, P. W.: Activation of coagulation factor V by a platelet protease. J. Clin. Invest. 70:1092, 1982.

230. Miletich, J. P., Majerus, D. W., and Majerus, P. W.: Patients with congenital factor V deficiency have decreased factor X_a binding sites on their platelets. J. Clin. Invest. 62:824, 1978.

231. Kane, W. H., and Majerus, P. W.: The interaction of human coagulation factor V_a with platelets. J. Biol. Chem. 257:3963, 1982.

232. Tracy, P. B., Nesheim, M. E., and Mann, K. G.: Factor V_a–dependent factor X_a binding to unstimulated platelets. J. Biol. Chem. 256:743, 1981.

233. Higgins, D. L., and Mann, K. G.: The interaction of bovine factor V and factor V–derived peptides with phospholipid vesicles. J. Biol. Chem. 258:6503, 1983.

234. Thiagarajan, P., Shapiro, S. S., and De Marco, L.: Monoclonal immunoglobulin Mλ coagulation inhibitor with phospholipid specificity: Mechanism of a lupus anticoagulant. J. Clin. Invest. 66:397, 1980.

235. Armstrong, R. A.: Platelet prostanoid receptors. Pharmacol. Ther. 72:171, 1996.

236. Siegl, A. M., Smith, J. B., and Silver, M. J.: Specific binding sites for prostaglandin D_2 on human platelets. Biochem. Biophys. Res. Commun. 90:291, 1979.

237. Siegl, A. M., Smith, J. B., Silver, M. J., Nicolaou, K. C., and Ahren, D.: Selective binding site for [^{3}H] prostacylin on platelets. J. Clin. Invest. 63:215, 1979.

238. Schafer, A. I., Cooper, B., O'Hara, D., and Handin, R. I.: Identification of platelet receptors for prostaglandin I_2 and D_2. J. Biol. Chem. 254:2914, 1979.

239. Cooper, B., Schafer, A. I., Puchalsky, D., and Handin, R. I.: Desensitization of prostaglandin-activated platelet adenylate cyclase. Prostaglandins 17:561, 1979.

240. Miller, O. V., and Gorman, R. R.: Evidence for distinct prostaglandin I_2 and D_2 receptors in human platelets. J. Pharmacol. Exp. Ther. 210:134, 1979.

241. Cerpes, B., and Ahern, D.: Characterization of the platelet PGD$_2$ receptor. J. Clin. Invest. 64:586, 1979.

242. Hung, S. G., Ghali, N. I., Venton, D. L., and Le Breton, G. C.: Specific binding of the thromboxane A$_2$ antagonist 13-azaprostanoic acid to human platelet membranes. Biochim. Biophys. Acta 728:171, 1983.

243. Ushikubi, F., Nakajima, M., Hirata, M., Okuma, M., Fujiwara, M. and Narumiya, S.: Purification of the thromboxane A$_2$/prostaglandin H$_2$ receptor from human blood platelets. J. Biol. Chem. 264:16496, 1989.

244. Hirata, M., Yasunori, H., Ushikubi, F., Yokota, Y., Kageyama, R., Nakanishi, S., and Narumiya, S.: Cloning and expression of a cDNA for a human thromboxane A$_2$ receptor. Nature 349:617, 1991.

245. Wu, K. K., Le Breton, G. C., Tai, H. -H., and Chen, Y.-C.: Abnormal platelet response to thromboxane A$_2$. J. Clin. Invest. 67:1801, 1981.

246. Lages, B., Malmsten, C., Weiss, H. J., and Samuelsson, B.: Impaired platelet response to thromboxane-A$_2$ and defective calcium mobilization in a patient with a bleeding disorder. Blood 57:545, 1981.

247. Samama, M., Lecrubier, C., Conard, J., Hotchen, M., Breton-Gorius, M., Vargaftig, B., Chignard, M., Legarde, M., and Dechavanne, M.: Constitutional thrombocytopathy with subnormal response to thromboxane A$_2$. Br. J. Haematol. 48:293, 1981.

248. Gresele, P., Arnout, J., Janssens, W., Deckmyn, H., Lemmens, J., and Vermylen, J.: BM13.177, a selective blocker of platelet and vessel wall thromboxane receptors is active in man. Lancet 1:991, 1984.

249. Sun, B., Li, J. Okahara, K., and Kambayashi, J.: P2X1 purinoceptor in human platelets: Molecular cloning and functional characterization after heterologous expression. J. Biol. Chem. 273:11544, 1998.

250. Leon, C., Hechler, B., Vial, C., Leray, C., Cazenave, J. P., and Gachet, C.: The P2Y1 receptor is an ADP receptor antagonized by ATP and expressed in platelets and megakaryoblastic cells. FEBS Lett. 403:26, 1997.

251. Jin, J., Daniel, J. L., and Kunapuli, S. P.: Molecular basis for ADP-induced platelet activation. II. The P2Y1 receptor mediates ADP-induced intracellular calcium mobilization and shape change in platelets. J. Biol. Chem. 273:2030, 1998.

252. Savi, P., Beauverger, P., Labouret, C., Delfaud, M., Salel, V., Kaghad, M., and Herbert, J. M.: Role of P2Y1 purinoceptor in ADP-induced platelet activation. FEBS Lett. 422:291, 1998.

253. Daniel, J. L., Dangelmaier, C., Jin, J., Ashby, B., Smith, J. B., and Kunapuli, S. P.: Molecular basis for ADP-induced platelet activation. I. Evidence for three distinct ADP receptors on human platelets. J. Biol. Chem. 273:2024, 1998.

254. Hechler, B., Leon, C., Vial, C., Vigne, P., Frelin, C., Cazenave, J. P., and Gachet, C.: The P2Y1 receptor is necessary for adenosine 5'-diphosphate-induced platelet aggregation. Blood 92:152, 1998.

255. Jin, J., and Kunapuli, S. P.: Coactivation of two different G protein–coupled receptors is essential for ADP-induced platelet aggregation. Proc. Natl. Acad. Sci., USA 95:8070, 1998.

256. Offermanns, S., Toombs, C. F., Hu, Y-H., and Siomon, M. I.: Defective platelet activation in Gα$_q$-deficient mice. Nature 389:183, 1997.

257. Gabbeta, J., Yang, X., Kowalska, M. A., Sun, L., Dhanasekaran, N., and Rao, A. K.: Platelet signal transduction defect with Gα subunit dysfunction and diminished Galphaq in a patient with abnormal platelet responses. Proc. Natl. Acad. Sci. USA 94:8750, 1997.

258. Nurden, P., Savi, P., Heilmann, E., Bihour, C., Herbert, J. M., Maffrand, J. P., and Nurden, A.: An inherited bleeding disorder linked to a defective interaction between ADP and its receptor on platelets: Its influence in glycoprotein IIb–IIIa complex function. J. Clin. Invest. 95:1612, 1995.

259. Rink, T. J., Smith, S. W., and Tsien, R. Y.: Cytoplasmic free Ca^{2+} in human platelets: Ca^{2+} thresholds and Ca-independent activation for shape-change and secretion. FEBS Let. 148:21, 1982.

260. Berridge, M. J.: Inositol trisphosphate and calcium signalling. Nature 361:315, 1993.

261. Cutler, L., Rodan, G., and Feinstein, M. B.: Cytochemical localization of adenylate cyclase and of calcium ion, magnesium ion–activated ATPases in the dense tubular system of human blood platelets. Biochim. Biophys. Acta 542:357, 1978.

262. Huang, E. M., and Detwiler, T. C.: Stimulus-response coupling mechanisms. In Phillips, D. R., and Shuman, J. A. (eds.): The Biochemistry of Platelets. New York, Academic Press, 1986.

263. Lyons, R. M., Stanford, N. L., and Majerus, P. W.: Thrombin-induced protein phosphorylation in human platelets. J. Clin. Invest. 56:924, 1975.

264. Tyers, M., Rachubinski, R. A., Steward, M. I., Varrichio, A. M., Shorr,

R. G., Haslam, R. J., and Harley, C. B.: Molecular cloning and expression of the major protein kinase C substrate of platelets. Nature 333:470, 1998.

265. Takai, Y., Kishimoto, A., Iwasa, Y., Kawahara, Y., Mori, T., and Nishizuka, Y.: Calcium-dependent activation of multifunctional protein kinase by membrane phospholipids. J. Biol. Chem. 254:3692, 1979.

266. Naka, M., Nishikawa, M., Adelstein, R. S., and Hidaka, H.: Phorbol ester–induced activation of human platelets is associated with protein kinase C phosphorylation of myosin light chains. Nature 306:490, 1983.

267. Nishikawa, M., Sellers, J. R., Adelstein, R. S., and Hidaka, H.: Protein kinase C modulates in vitro phosphorylation of the smooth muscle heavy meromyosin by myosin light chain kinase. J. Biol. Chem. 259:8808, 1984.

268. Brugge, J., Cotton, P., Lustig, A., Yonemoto, W., Lipsich, L., Cousens, P., Barrett, J. N., Nonner, D., and Keane, R. W.: Characterization of the altered form of the c-src gene product in neuronal cells. Genes Dev. 1:287, 1987.

269. Golden, A., Nemeth, S. P., and Brugge, J. S.: Blood platelets express high levels of the pp66$^{c\text{-}src}$-specific tyrosine kinase activity. Proc. Natl. Acad. Sci. USA 83:852, 1986.

270. Ferrell, J. E., Jr., and Martin, S.: Platelet tyrosine-specific protein phosphorylation is regulated by thrombin. Mol. Cell. Biol. 8:3603, 1988.

271. Golden, A., and Brugge, J. S.: Thrombin treatment induces rapid changes in tyrosine phosphorylation in platelets. Proc. Natl. Acad. Sci. USA 86:901, 1989.

272. Nakamura, S., and Yamamura, H.: Thrombin and collagen induce rapid phosphorylation of a common set of cellular proteins on tyrosine in human platelets. J. Biol. Chem. 263:7089, 1989.

273. Law, D. B., Nannizzi-Alaimo, L., and Phillips, D. R.: Outside-in integrin signal transduction: Alpha IIb β 3-(GP IIb IIIa) tyrosine phosphorylation induced by platelet aggregation. J. Biol. Chem. 271:10811, 1996.

274. Lerea, K. M., Tonks, N. K., Krebs, E. G., Fischer, E. H., and Glomset, J. A.: Vanadate and molybdate increase tyrosine phosphorylation in a 50-kilodalton protein and stimulate secretion in electropermeabilized platelets. Biochemistry 28:9286, 1989.

275. Jenkins, A. L., Nannizzi-Alaimo, L., Silver, D., Sellers, J. R., Ginsberg, M. H., Law, D. A., and Phillips, D. R.: Tyrosine phosphorylation of the beta3 cytoplasmic domain mediates integrin-cytoskeletal interactions. J. Biol. Chem. 273:13878, 1998.

276. Gu, M., York, J. D., Warshawsky, I., and Majerus, P. W.: Identification, cloning, and expression of a cytosolic megakaryocyte protein-tyrosine-phosphatase with sequence homology to cytoskeletal protein 4.1. Proc. Natl. Acad. Sci. USA 88:5867, 1991.

277. Gu, M., Warshawsky, I., and Majerus, P. W.: Cloning and expression of a cytosolic megakaryocyte protein-tyrosine-phosphatase with sequence homology to retinaldehyde-binding protein and yeast SEC14p. Proc. Natl. Acad. Sci. USA 89:2980, 1992.

278. Mitchell, C. A., Jefferson, A. B., Bejeck, B. E., Brugge, J. S., Deuel, T. F., and Majerus, P. W.: Thrombin-stimulated immunoprecipitation of phosphatidylinositol 3-kinase from human platelets. Proc. Natl. Acad. Sci. USA 87:9396, 1990.

279. Feinstein, M. B., Egan, J. J., Shaafi, R. I., and White, J.: The cytoplasmic concentration of free calcium in platelets is controlled by stimulators of cyclic AMP production (PGD$_2$, PGE$_1$, forskolin). Biochem. Biophys. Res. Commun. 113:598, 1983.

280. Feinstein, M. B., Egan, J. J., and Opas, E. E.: Reversal of thrombin induced myosin phosphorylation and the assembly of cytoskeletal structure in platelets by the adenylate cyclase stimulants prostaglandin D$_2$ and forskolin. J. Biol. Chem. 258:1260, 1983.

281. Billah, M. M., and Lapetina, E. G.: Degradation of phosphatidylinositol 4, 5-bisphosphate is insensitive to Ca^{++} mobilization in stimulated platelets. Biochem. Biophys. Res. Commun. 109:1217, 1982.

282. Billah, M. M., and Lapetina, E. G.: Platelet-activating factor stimulates metabolism of phosphoinositides in horse platelets: Possible relationship to Ca^{++} mobilization during stimulation. Proc. Natl. Acad. Sci. USA 80:965, 1983.

283. Gilman, A. G.: G proteins and dual control of adenylate cyclase. Cell 36:577, 1984.

284. Walseth, T. F., Gander, J. E., Eide, S. J., Krick, T. P., and Goldberg, N. D.: ^{18}O labeling of adenine nucleotide α-phosphoryls in platelets: Contribution of phosphodiesterase-catalyzed hydrolysis of cAMP. J. Biol. Chem. 258:1544, 1983.

285. Cooper, D. M. F., and Rodbell, M.: ADP is a potent inhibitor of human platelet membrane adenulate cyclase. Nature 282:517, 1979.

286. Steer, M. L., and Wood, A.: Regulation of human platelet adenylate cyclase by epinephrine, prostaglandin E_1, and guanine nucleotides: Evidence for separate guanine nucleotide sites mediating stimulation and inhibition. J. Biol. Chem. 254:10791, 1979.

287. Haslam, R. J., and Vanderwal, M.: Inhibition of platelet adeynlate cyclase by 1-0-alkyl-2-0-acetyl-sn-glyceryl-3-phosphocholine (platelet activating factor). J. Biol. Chem. 257:6879, 1982.

288. Brodie, G. N., Baenziger, N. L., Chase, L. P., and Majerus, P. W.: The effects of thrombin on adenyl cyclase activity and a membrane protein from human platelets. J. Clin. Invest. 51:81, 1972.

289. Brass, L. F., and Woolkalis, M. J.: Dual regulation of cyclic AMP formation by thrombin in HEL cells, a leukaemic cell line with megakaryocytic properties. Biochem. J. 281:73, 1992.

290. Majerus, P. W., Neufeld, D. J., and Wilson, D. B.: Production of phosphoinositide-derived messengers. Cell 37:701, 1984.

291. Wilson, D. B., Bross, T. E., Hofmann, S. L., and Majerus, P. W.: Hydrolysis of polyphosphoinosidites by purified sheep seminal vesicle phospholipase C enzymes. J. Biol. Chem. 259:11718, 1984.

292. Bansal, V. S., and Majerus, P. W.: Phosphatidylinositol-derived precursors and signals. Annu. Rev. Cell Biol. 6:41, 1990.

293. Majerus, P. W., Ross, T. S., Cunningham, T. W., Caldwell, K. K., Jefferson, A. B., and Bansal, V. S.: Recent insights into phosphatidylinositol signaling. Cell 63:459, 1990.

294. Majerus, P. W.: Inositol phosphate biochemistry. Annu. Rev. Biochem. 61:225, 1992.

295. Lee, S. B., Rao, A. K., Lee, K. H., Yang, X., Bae, Y. S., Rhee, S. G.: Decreased expression of phospholipase C-β 2 isozyme in human platelets with impaired function. Blood 88:1684, 1996.

296. Pang, I. H., and Sternweis, P. C.: Purification of unique α subunits of GTP-binding regulatory proteins (G proteins) by affinity chromatography with immobilized $\beta\gamma$ subunits. J. Biol. Chem. 265:18707, 1990.

297. Strathmann, M., and Simon, M. I.: G protein diversity: A distinct class of α subunits is present in vertebrates and invertebrates. Proc. Natl. Acad. Sci. USA 87:9113, 1990.

298. Taylor, S. J., Smith, J. A., and Exton, J. H.: Purification from bovine liver membranes of a guanine nucleotide–dependent activator of phosphoinositide-specific phospholipase C. J. Biol. Chem. 265:17150, 1990.

299. Prescott, S. M., and Majerus, P. W.: Characterization of 1, 2-diacylglycerol hydrolysis in human platelets: Demonstration of an arachidonoyl-monoacylglycerol intermediate. J. Biol. Chem. 258:764, 1983.

300. Carpenter, C. L., and Cantley, L. C.: Phosphoinositide kinases. Biochemistry 29:11147, 1990.

301. Banfic, H., Downes, C. P., and Rittenhouse, S. E.: Biphasic activation of α/Akt in platelets: Evidence for stimulation both by phosphatidylinositol 3,4-bisphosphate, produced via a novel pathway, and by phosphatidylinositol 3,4,5-trisphosphate. J. Biol. Chem. 273:11630, 1998.

302. Toker, A., Bachelot, C., Chen, C. S., Falck, J. R., Hartwig, J. H., Cantley, L. C., and Kovacsovics, T. J.: Phosphorylation of the platelet p47 phosphoprotein is mediated by the lipid products of phosphoinositide 3-kinase. J. Biol. Chem. 270:29525, 1995.

303. Hartwig, J. H., Kung, S., Kovacsovics, T., Janmey, P. A., Cantley, L. C., Stossel, T. P., and Toker, A.: D3 phosphoinositides and outside-in integrin signaling by glycoprotein IIb–IIIa mediate platelet actin assembly and filopodial extension induced by phorbol 12-myristate 13-acetate. J. Biol. Chem. 271:32986, 1996.

304. Zhang, X., Loijens, J. C., Boronenkov, I. V., Parker, G. J., Norris, F. A., Majerus, P. W., and Anderson, R. A.: Phosphatidylinositol-4-phosphate 5-kinase isoenzymes catalyze the synthesis of 3-phosphate-containing phosphatidylinositol signaling molecules. J. Biol. Chem. 272:17756, 1997.

305. Norris, F. A., Atkins, R. C., and Majerus, P. W.: Inositol polyphosphate 4-phosphatase is inactivated by calpain-mediated proteolysis in stimulated human platelets. J. Biol. Chem. 272:10987, 1997.

306. FitzGerald, G. A., Brash, A. R., Falardeau, P., and Oates, J. A.: Estimated rate of prostacyclin secretion into the circulation of normal man. J. Clin. Invest. 68:1271, 1981.

307. FitzGerald, G. A., Brash, A. R., Oates, J. A., and Pedersen, A. K.: Endogenous prostacyclin biosynthesis and platelet function during selective inhibition of thromboxane synthase in man. J. Clin. Invest. 71:1336, 1983.

308. Antiplatelet Trialists Collaboration: Secondary prevention of vascular disease by prolonged antiplatelet treatment. Br. Med. J. 296:320, 1988.

309. Esmon, C. T., and Owen, W. G.: Identification of an endothelial cell cofactor for thrombin-catalyzed activation of protein C. Proc. Natl. Acad. Sci. USA 78:2249, 1981.

310. Esmon, N. L., Owen, W. G., and Esmon, C. T.: Isolation of a membrane-bound cofactor for thrombin-catalyzed activation of protein C. J. Biol. Chem. 257:859, 1981.

311. Owen, W. G., and Esmon, C. T.: Functional properties of an endothelial cell cofactor for thrombin-catalyzed activation of protein C. J. Biol. Chem. 256:5532, 1981.

312. Salem, H. H., Maruyama, I., Ishii, H., and Majerus, P. W.: Isolation and characterization of thrombomodulin from human placenta. J. Biol. Chem. 259:12246, 1984.

313. Dittman, W. A., and Majerus, P. W.: Structure and function of thrombomodulin: A natural anticoagulant. Blood 74:1, 1990.

314. Maruyama, I., Bell, C. E., and Majerus, P. W.: Thrombomodulin is found on endothelium of arteries, veins, capillaries, lymphatics, and on syncytiotrophoblast of human placenta. J. Cell. Biol. 101:363, 1985.

315. Salem, H. H., Broze, G. J., Miletich, J. P., and Majerus, P. W.: Human coagulation factor V_a is a cofactor for the activation of protein C. Proc. Natl. Acad. Sci. USA 80:1584, 1983.

316. Salem, H. H., Esmon, N. L., Esmon, C. T., and Majerus, P. W.: The effects of thrombomodulin and coagulation factor V_a-light chain on protein C activation in vitro. J. Clin. Invest. 73:968, 1984.

317. Maruyama, I., Salem, H. H., and Majerus, P. W.: Coagulation factor V_a binds to human umbilical vein endothelial cells and accelerates protein C activation. J. Clin. Invest. 74:224, 1984.

318. Marcum, J. A., and Rosenberg, R. D.: Anticoagulantly active heparin molecules from vascular tissue. Biochemistry 33:1730, 1984.

319. Marcum, J. A., McKenney, J. B., and Rosenberg, R. D.: Acceleration of thrombin-antithrombin complex formation via heparin molecules bound to the endothelium. J. Clin. Invest. 74:341, 1984.

320. Deuel, T. F., and Huang, J. S.: Platelet derived growth factor structure, function and roles in normal transformed cells. J. Clin. Invest. 74:669, 1984.

321. Huang, J. S., Huang, S. S., and Deuel, T. F.: Human platelet–derived growth factor: Radioimmunoassay and discovery of a specific plasma-binding protein. J. Cell. Biol. 97:383, 1983.

322. Deuel, T. F., Kawahara, R. S., Mustoe, T. A., and Pierce, G. F.: Growth factors and wound healing: Platelet-derived growth factor as a model cytokine. Annu. Rev. Med. 42:567, 1991.

323. Huang, J. S., Huang, S. S., and Deuel, T. F.: Specific covalent binding of platelet-derived growth factor to human plasma α_2-macroglobulin. Proc. Natl. Acad. Sci. USA 81:342, 1984.

324. Deuel, T. F., Kawahara, R. S., Mustoe, T. A., Pierce, A. F.: Growth factors and wound healing: PDGF as a model cytokine, Annu. Rev. Med. 42:567, 1991.

325. Ross, R., and Glomset, J.: The pathogenesis of atherosclerosis. N. Engl. J. Med. 296:369, 1976.

326. Huang, J. S., Huang, S. S., Kennedy, B., and Deuel, T. F.: Platelet-derived growth factor: Specific binding to target cells. J. Biol. Chem. 257:8130, 1982.

327. Williams, L. T.: Signal transduction by the PDGF receptor. Science 243:1564, 1989.

328. Waterfield, M. D., Scrace, G. T., Whittle, N., Stroobant, P., Johnsson, A., Wasteson, A., Westermark, B., Heldin, C-H., Huang, J. S., and Deuel, T. F.: Platelet-derived growth factor is structurally related to the putative transforming protein p28[sis] of simian sarcoma virus. Nature 304:35, 1983.

329. Doolittle, R. F., Hunkapiller, M. W., Hood, L. E., Devare, Robbins, K. C., Aaronson, S. A., and Antoniades, H. N.: Simian sarcoma virus onc gene, v-sis, is derived from the gene encoding a platelet-derived growth factor. Science 221:275, 1983.

330. Prescott, S. M., Zimmerman, G. A., and McIntyre, T. M.: Human endothelial cells in culture produce platelet-activating factor (1-alkyl-2-acetyl-sn-glycero-3-phosphocholine) when stimulated with thrombin. Proc. Natl. Acad. Sci. USA 81:3534, 1984.

331. Camussi, G., Aglietta, M., Malavasi, F., Tetta, C., Piscibello, W., Sanavio, W., and Bussolino, F.: The release of PAF from human endothelial cells in culture. J. Immunol. 131:2397, 1983.

332. Lynch, J. M., Lotner, G. Z., Betz, S. J., and Henson, P. M.: The release of a platelet-activating factor by stimulated rabbit neutrophils. J. Immunol. 123:1219, 1979.

333. Mencia-Huerta, J. M., and Benveniste, J.: Platelet-activating factor (PAF-acether) and macrophages. Cell. Immunol. 57:281, 1981.

334. Benveniste, J., Henson, P. M., and Cochrane, C. G.: Leukocyte-

dependent histamine release from rabbit platelets: The role of IgE, basophils and a platelet-activating factor. J. Exp. Med. 136:1356, 1972.

335. Pinchard, R. N., McManus, L. M., Hanahan, D. J., and Halowen, M.: Immunopharmacology of PAF. *In* Newball H. H. (ed.): Immunopharmacology of the Lung. New York, Marcel Dekker, 1983.

336. Hwang, S-B., Lee, C-S. C., Cheah, M. J., and Shen, T. Y.: Specific receptor sites for 1-0-alkyl-2-0-acetyl-sn-glycero-3-phosphocholine (platelet activating factor) on rabbit platelet and guinea pig smooth muscle membranes. Biochemistry 22:4756, 1983.

337. Hondo, Z. I., Nakamura, M., Mike, I., Minami, M., Watanabe, T., Seyama, Y., Okado, H., Toh, H., Ito, K., Miyamoto, T., and Shimizu, T.: Cloning by functional expression of platelet-activating factor receptor from guinea pit lung. Nature 49:342, 1991.

338. Ye, R. D., Prossnitz, E. R., Zou, A., and Cochrane, C. G.: Characterization of a human cDNA that encodes a functional receptor for platelet activating factor. Biochem. Biophys. Res. Commun. 180:105, 1991.

339. McManus, L. M., Hanahan, D. J., and Pinckard, R. N.: Human platelet stimulation of acetyl glyceryl ether phosphorylcholine. J. Clin. Invest. 67:903, 1981.

340. Marcus, A. J., Safier, L. B., Ullman, H. L., Wong, T. H., Broekman, J., Weksler, B. B., and Kaplan, K. L.: Effects of acetyl glyceryl ether phosphorylcholine in human platelet function in vitro. Blood 58:1027, 1981.

341. McIntyre, T. M., Zimmerman, G. A., and Prescott, S. M.: Leukotrienes C_4 and D_4 stimulate human endothelial cells to synthesize PAF and bind neutrophils. Proc. Natl. Acad. Sci. USA 83:2204, 1986.

342. Chignard, M., LeCouedic, J. P., Vargaftig, B. B., and Benveniste, J.: PAF secretion from platelets. Br. J. Haematol. 46:455, 1980.

343. Alam, I., Smith, J. B., and Silver, J. J.: Human and rabbit platelets form PAF in response to calcium ionophore. Thomb. Res. 30:71, 1983.

344. Demopoulos, C. A., Pinchard, R. N., and Hanahan, D. J.: Platelet-activating factor. Evidence of 1-0-alkyl-2-acetyl-sn-glyceryl-3-phosphorylcholine as the active component (a new class of lipid chemical mediators). J. Biol. Chem. 254:9355, 1979.

345. Stafforini, D. M., McIntyre, T. M., Zimmerman, G. A., and Prescott, S. M.: Platelet-activating factor acetylhydrolases. J. Biol. Chem. 272:17895, 1997.

346. Clay, K. L., Murphy, R. C., Andres, J. L., Lynch, J., and Henson, P. M.: Structure elucidation of PAF derived from human neutrophils. Biochem. Biophys. Res. Commun. 121:815, 1984.

347. Blank, M. L., Hall, M. N. Cress, E. A., and Snyder, F.: Inactivation of PAF by a plasma hydrolase. Biochem. Biophys. Res. Commun. 113:666, 1983.

348. Blank, M. L., Lee, T., Fitzgerald, V., and Snyder, F.: A specific acetyl-hydrolase for PAF. J. Biol. Chem. 256:175, 1981.

349. Ho, Y. S., Swenson, L., Derewenda, U., Serre, L., Wei, Y., Dauter, Z., Hattori, M., Adachi, T., Aoki, J., Arai, H., Inoue, K., and Derewenda, Z. S.: Brain acetylhydrolase that inactivates platelet-activating factor is a G-protein-like trimer. Nature 385:89, 1997.

Part VI
MOLECULAR ONCOLOGY

25 Molecular Aspects of Oncogenesis
Douglas R. Lowy and Linda Wolff

▼ ▼

Introduction

The period since the early 1970s has witnessed a veritable revolution in our understanding of cancer at the molecular level. Although many important questions remain, it is now possible to describe, at least in broad terms, the molecular mechanisms that regulate normal cell growth and how their breakdown ultimately leads to cancer.[1-4]

As more has been learned about the pathogenesis of cancer, it has become clear that specific molecular events underlie malignant progression. One important generalization is that the progression from normal cells to malignancy represents a multistep process, rather than arising directly as the result of a single change in a normal cell. This experimental finding correlates with the observation that many tumors develop after a series of distinguishable stages, that malignant tumors are usually clonal, and that molecular analysis of tumors often reveals multiple genetic abnormalities. Another important paradigm is that in those instances in which it has been possible to analyze tumor progression in detail, many of the steps have turned out to represent genetic changes. The vast majority of these genetic alter-

ations have been found to involve one of two broad classes of genes: tumor suppressor genes and proto-oncogenes. As their name implies, tumor suppressor genes function to inhibit inappropriate growth of the target cell, and inactivation of these inhibitory genes can promote cancer. Proto-oncogenes, by contrast, stimulate growth of the target cell, prevent growth arrest, or prevent programmed cell death. Activated proto-oncogenes with increased capacity to cause continued inappropriate growth are often called transforming genes or oncogenes. Malignant cells are therefore usually found to have lost the function of one or more tumor suppressor genes and/or to possess increased activity of one or more proto-oncogenes.[2, 5, 6] Point mutations, gene deletions, and chromosomal translocations often underlie these functional changes.

This chapter deals with three major themes: normal and abnormal cell growth, proto-oncogenes and their activation to oncogenes, and tumor suppressor genes and their inactivation. Growth control and the basic functions of these genes are critical to understanding the molecular pathways that lead to malignancy. The chapter does not deal directly with genes that may contribute to tumorigenesis by increasing the susceptibility of cells to mutation without having a direct effect on growth regulation, such as those mutated in nucleotide excision repair syndromes, although alteration of such genes can also have pathogenic significance.[7] This presentation seeks to include some historical background and general principles and emphasizes experimental systems. Although many examples are from hematopoietic systems, the discussion is not restricted to the hematopoietic organ system.

Background: Tumor Viruses, Familial Cancers, and Cell Cycle Control

Much of our current picture of the molecular mechanisms that control growth and oncogenesis stems from work carried out in seemingly unrelated areas, such as tumor viruses, familial cancer, and the growth of cultured somatic cells and of yeast. Tumor viruses have been intensively studied because their capacity to induce neoplastic disease in animals can often be correlated with their ability to alter the growth properties of cultured cells. Most tumor viruses contain genes known as viral oncogenes, which are growth stimulatory. There are two major classes of tumor viruses: oncogenic retroviruses, which contain RNA as their genetic material, and DNA tumor viruses, whose genomes are DNA.[8-10] Studies on both classes of tumor viruses have made significant contributions to our current understanding of molecular oncogenesis. The recognition that viral oncogenes could induce tumors provided an experimental basis for the hypothesis that a limited number of specific genes might be responsible for cancer. Tumor viruses also provided an experimental approach for analyzing the pathogenesis of neoplasia induced by the introduction of a limited number of well defined genes.

Inquiry into the origin of retroviral oncogenes led to the discovery that normal cells contain proto-oncogenes, from which the oncogenes of retroviruses are derived.[3, 11] This critically important observation helped to unify the thinking of investigators in various fields of cancer research. The relationship between viral oncogenes and their normal cellular counterparts formed the conceptual basis for studies in which tumor-derived transforming genes were identified by extracting DNA from tumor cells and introducing the DNA into recipient cells. As with retroviral oncogenes, the transforming genes identified in human tumors were modified versions of proto-oncogenes.[3, 12-15]

The analysis of certain familial cancers helped draw attention to the significance of tumor suppressor genes in neoplasia.[4, 16-18] The genes responsible for several syndromes with a heritable predisposition to neoplasia have been found to encode proteins that ordinarily exert a negative effect on cell growth. In contrast to the genetically dominant oncogenes, which promote growth of the tumors in which they are found, it is through their loss of function that the tumor suppressor genes contribute to uncontrolled proliferation of the target cells.

DNA tumor virus oncogenes, which, unlike retroviral oncogenes, are virus-specific genes, provided further insights into the biological functions of tumor suppressor genes.[19] The oncoproteins encoded by these viruses have been found in many instances to target cellular tumor suppressor genes and to inactivate them. Thus they have historically provided

novel approaches to probe the function and inactivation of such genes.

Studies begun on the cell division cycle (CDC) in yeast have provided a picture of the normal cell cycle and led to the identification of numerous genes involved in regulating cell growth.[20, 21] One of the most intriguing aspects of these studies has been the recognition that many of these growth control genes have been conserved through evolution and exist in mammalian cells as well. The evolutionary conservation of factors regulating cell growth underscores the principle that this type of control is a fundamental requirement for all life forms and cell types. Since cancer results from the failure to maintain normal growth control, this conservation of function means that elucidating the molecular basis of growth and its regulation in any organism may have relevance to human neoplasia.

Cancer Is a Disease of Abnormal Growth

Although molecular oncologists seek to define events and pathways that are of general importance in the development of cancer, it is clear that cancer is a collection of literally hundreds of distinct disease processes that can affect virtually any cell type. The unifying feature is that all types of cancer result from excessive, improperly regulated cell growth, ultimately at the expense of the organism. To place abnormal growth in perspective, aspects of normal growth are briefly reviewed.

▼ NORMAL CELL GROWTH

The Cell Cycle

When cells grow and divide, they must ensure that each progeny cell receives a full complement of DNA and a sufficient amount of other essential components (e.g., mitochondria, ribosomes) to be viable after separation. To accomplish this process, all growing eukaryotic cells cycle through a highly ordered series of events that are commonly divided into four phases: G_1, S, G_2, and M (Fig. 25–1). DNA replica-

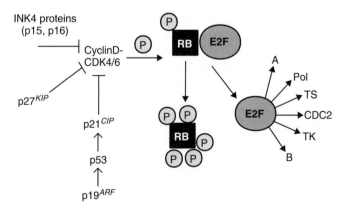

Figure 25–1. The Cell Cycle and Its Positive Regulatory Components. Resting cells in G_0 are triggered by growth factors and their receptors to enter the G_1 phase of the cell cycle. Cyclins D, E, and A accumulate and activate their associated kinases (CDKs), which positively regulate progression (see also Fig. 25–2). A restriction point is shown and depicted in more detail in Figure 25–2. Cyclins A and B are involved in the G_2 to M transition.

tion and histone protein synthesis are carried out during the synthetic (S) phase of the cell cycle, and the physical process of cell division occurs in the mitotic (M) phase. These two phases are separated by two gap (G) phases, with G_1 preceding S and G_2 preceding M. Higher eukaryotic cells that are growth arrested in response to nutrient deprivation or differentiation are said to have entered the G_0 state, a period in which cells are no longer preparing for cell division or increasing their mass.

The entry into and exit from each phase of the cell cycle are tightly regulated. Elucidation of the mechanisms that underlie this regulation came initially from studies in lower eukaryotes, including genetic analysis of CDC mutants of yeasts.[22, 23] Compared with higher eukaryotes, yeast has several important advantages as an experimental organism, including its short generation time, the ease with which mutant strains with stable phenotypes can be isolated, and the efficiency with which specific genes can be targeted for disruption and replacement. Mammalian cells regulate their cell cycle by similar mechanisms, although the complexity of this regulation is even greater than in yeast.[24, 25]

The mechanisms underlying cell cycle control have turned out to be highly relevant to understanding how oncogenes and tumor suppressors can influence cell growth. Regulation of the cell cycle is based on two evolutionarily conserved families of proteins, cyclin-dependent protein kinases (Cdk's) and cyclins. As first shown in fission yeast *Schizosaccharomyces pombe*, the Cdk's such as p34[cdc2] (Cdk1 in mammals) induce downstream events in the cell cycle by phosphorylating proteins on serine or threonine. Their activity is controlled by a series of cyclins that undergo a cycle of synthesis and degradation in each cell division. Most of the cyclins, which were originally identified in developing invertebrates, are either G_1 or G_2 specific, trigger activation of specific Cdk's, and help to regulate the transition from G_1 to S and from G_2 to M (Fig. 25–2).

Cancer cells often have dysregulated cell cycle progression due to alterations of genes involved in what is called restriction point control (see Fig. 25–2), although deregulation of other checkpoints of the cell cycle also occurs in tumors.[26] Until the restriction point is reached, late in the G_1 phase, normal cells are responsive to stimulation by extracellular mitogenic growth factors as well as to inhibition by antiproliferative cytokines. Once cells pass through this important control point, they become refractory to the external growth regulatory signals, as a self-perpetuating program drives the cells through to division.[25] Passage through the restriction point is controlled principally by Cdk4 and Cdk6, which phosphorylate critical substrates required for entry into S phase. The regulation of these Cdk's is complex, as their activity relies on cyclin D as well as on activating phosphorylations and dephosphorylations.[27]

Well studied targets of the Cdk's include the retinoblastoma tumor suppressor protein (pRB) and its family members p130 and p107.[25, 28, 29] As a group, the RB family controls gene expression mediated by the E2F family of transcription factors (see Fig. 25–2), which in turn regulate the expression of several genes that are important to S phase entry, including cyclin E, DNA polymerase-α, and thymidine synthetase. In the absence of Cdk phosphorylation, hypophosphorylated pRB is bound to E2F, and these proteins together repress transcription of E2F target genes; it may

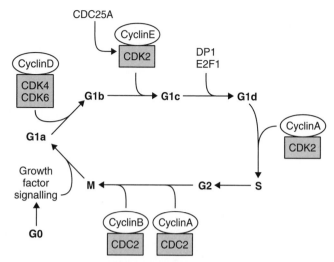

Figure 25–2. RB and Restriction Point Control of Cell Cycle Progression. Hypophosphorylated RB binds to the transcription factor E2F, resulting in transcriptional repression of E2F-regulated genes. When RB is hyperphosphorylated by cyclin D-CDK4/6, E2F is released and triggers expression of genes such as DNA polymerase-α (pol), thymidine kinase (TK), thymidylate synthase (TS), CDC2, cyclin (E), and cyclin A (A). This is an irreversible process because of feedback loops, not shown here. The kinase activity of cyclin D-CDK4/6 is negatively regulated by INK4 proteins such as p15 and p16 as well as p21 and p27. In addition, a protein p19[ARF], encoded by the same locus as p16, stabilizes p53 transcription factor, which in turn positively regulates transcription of the gene encoding p21.

also inhibit transcription of other growth stimulatory genes.[30] Upon cytokine stimulation, the Cdk's phosphorylate pRB, causing it to dissociate from E2F, which can then activate transcription of its target genes.

pRB is not required for cell division but functions in tissue homeostasis so that the proper number of cells is maintained. Other tumor suppressors also act as negative regulators of the restriction point pathway. The Ink4 family of proteins can directly inhibit cyclin D–dependent kinase activity and induce G_1 phase arrest, and their loss is associated with a variety of malignancies. The CIP/KIP proteins, such as p21 and p27, are also potent Cdk inhibitors.

Extracellular Growth Signals: Positive and Negative

Multicellular organisms are faced with the problem of maintaining a vast array of different cell types with the proper balance of growing and differentiated cells. The best studied mechanism for accomplishing this task is through the production of soluble factors that act on a specific subset of cells by modulating their growth state.[31] These growth factors, cytokines, and hormones can have positive or negative effects on cell proliferation and may also induce differentiation of the target cells.[32] In some instances, removal of growth factors may place cells in a resting phase; in others, withdrawal from growth factor stimulation may lead to initiation of programmed cell death, termed apoptosis, which occurs in embryonic development[33] and hematopoiesis.[34]

Nerve growth factor (NGF) and epidermal growth factor (EGF) were the first polypeptide factors to be identified.[35, 36] Subsequent work has led to the discovery of a large number of factors that, taken together, can regulate the growth of virtually all known cell types. By helping to maintain the delicate balance between differentiation and regeneration, these diffusible factors play a key role in normal growth control.

Mitogenic growth factors are required for cells in G_0 to re-enter the cell cycle and for cells in G_1 to commit to S phase.[25, 31] The expression of many genes is altered by growth factor stimulation. These include the G_1 cyclins, a group of so-called immediate early and early response genes, which include at least three proto-oncogenes, c-*fos*, c-*jun*, and c-*myc*.[37–39] The induction of immediate early and early gene transcription occurs, respectively, within about 20 seconds and 2 minutes of growth factor treatment. Their induction does not require new protein synthesis, therefore serving to emphasize the efficiency with which the responding cell can transmit signals from the cell surface to the nucleus. Alterations in the regulated production of mitogenic factors or in the target cell that responds to them have been shown to contribute to a wide variety of neoplasms, as discussed in later sections of this chapter.

In mouse fibroblasts such as BALB 3T3, it was demonstrated that application of a single growth factor is not sufficient to induce mitogenic stimulation of quiescent (G_0) cells. Mitogenesis in these cells requires two classes of factors, termed competence and progression factors.[40] Competence factors, such as platelet derived growth factor (PDGF) or fibroblast growth factor (FGF), are required to initiate re-entry into the cell cycle. EGF and insulin-like growth factor type 1 (IGF-1) are called progression factors because they facilitate commitment to mitosis by driving the cell from G_1 to S via activation of the cell cycle machinery. Although the requirement for more than one growth factor to initiate mitogenesis does not apply to all cells, it may be relevant to at least some hematopoietic cells, including B cells and T cells.[41]

Humoral factors that regulate hematopoietic cell growth are often referred to as cytokines, which are secreted molecules that contribute to intercellular signaling.[42] Several cytokines, such as granulocyte-macrophage colony-stimulating factor (GM-CSF) and granulocyte (G)-CSF, are extracellular mitogens for myeloid cells. Several of the interleukins (ILs), including IL-2, IL-4, IL-7, and IL-10, stimulate proliferation of specific types of lymphocytes. A limited number of cytokines, such as IL-3, can induce growth of cells from multiple lineages. In addition to stimulating proliferation, cytokines often activate specific differentiation-related features or functions in hematopoietic cells.

Some cytokines can oppose proliferation by inducing differentiation and/or growth arrest in cells, and loss of response to this type of humoral regulator could be potentially oncogenic. Cytokines of this type include IL-6 and leukemia inhibitory factor (LIF), which can induce growth arrest of certain myeloid leukemic cells lines, as well as interferons (IFNs) and transforming growth factor beta (TGFβ), both of which are potent negative regulators of growth in multiple lineages.[42]

Receptors Transduce Extracellular Signals

The ability of target cells to respond to extracellular factors requires the expression of receptor proteins that can specifically bind to a given factor or group of factors. The extracellular factors are often referred to as ligands because their activities require that they bind to their cognate, cell associated receptors. The receptors are the key to triggering a cell's response to a growth modulator, since they serve as both a binding target for the ligand and a signaling switch for the cell.

In most cases, receptors are found at the cell surface; many contain an extracellular ligand-binding domain, a membrane-spanning region, and a cytoplasmic tail that allow for signal transduction from the exterior to the interior of the cell (Fig. 25–3). Polypeptide factors such as EGF, GM-CSF, and ILs activate their cognate cell surface receptors by binding to their extracellular moiety. By contrast, the receptors for steroid hormones are found inside cells, as these ligands can readily diffuse into cells.[43]

Many of the cell surface associated receptors, such as the EGF receptor (EGFR) or the receptor for colony-stimulating factor 1 (CSF-1R), possess an intrinsic protein kinase activity that is triggered by receptor dimerization after ligand binding to the receptor.[44–47] Alternatively, receptors including the majority of hematopoietic cytokine receptors are noncovalently associated with a cytoplasmic kinase that is activated by ligand-receptor interaction.[42] Other receptors may alter protein phosphorylation in the opposite direction, by regulating protein phosphatases.[48, 49] The diversity of receptor

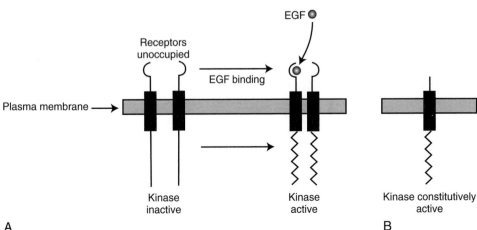

A

B

Figure 25–3. Regulated and Constitutive Activation of the EGF Receptor. *A*, Binding of EGF to the extracellular region of the receptor produces a conformational change (and dimerization) that results in the activation of the intracellular kinase domain. *B*, Truncation of the *EGFR* gene (as is found in the case of v-*erbB*) results in loss of the ligand-binding domain, triggering a constitutive activation of the kinase.

types and the signals that they generate underscore the complex nature of growth regulation in a multicellular organism.

Signal Transduction Pathways

In addition to their effects on cell growth, hormones, growth factors, and cytokines must modulate a wide variety of other processes in the target cell, including cellular metabolism and cytoskeletal changes. Many changes occur as a consequence of signal-induced alterations in gene expression. A further constraint is that these responses must occur within a short period. To carry out these diverse functions, cells have developed signal transduction pathways through a variety of cellular intermediates that link cell-surface receptors to the cytoplasm and ultimately to the nucleus. The components of these pathways provide the amplification of the response to the ligand required to elicit the rapid, yet profound, changes in the state of the target cell. The fundamental nature of these signal transduction pathways is underscored by the finding that many of them are highly conserved in evolution. Furthermore, most of the identified oncogenes represent gain of function mutants of components of these pathways.[50]

The role of tyrosine phosphorylation in signaling was first studied in growth factor receptors such as PDGFR and EGFR.[45–47] After ligand binding, many growth factor receptors, including PDGF, EGF, CSF-1, and stem cell factor (SCF) receptors, form dimers and undergo conformational changes that activate the receptor-associated protein kinase activity, which is required for receptor function. In almost all cases, the receptor kinase activity is specific for the phosphorylation of tyrosine residues; this tyrosine kinase activity is in contrast to that of most protein kinases, which phosphorylate serine and threonine residues. The activated receptors often phosphorylate themselves (at tyrosine residues) and then begin to associate with and phosphorylate cellular substrate proteins. Phosphorylated tyrosine residues on receptors or other proteins can serve as critical docking sites for a network of proteins implicated in signal transduction, from those that induce cytoskeletal changes to those that alter gene transcription. For example, the translocation of signaling proteins from their cytosolic location in unstimulated cells to a membrane associated location may serve as the critical trigger for their activation.[45, 46, 51]

As noted above, most members of the hematopoietic cytokine receptor family do not have intrinsic tyrosine kinase activity. Instead, stimulation of their receptors induces the activation of specific cytoplasmic kinases that are bound to the receptors, leading to phosphorylation of downstream target proteins. Examples of tyrosine kinases that are implicated in hematopoietic signaling are the Jak kinases and Src-related kinases such as Lck, Fyn, Lyn, Hck, and Syk.[52]

The Jak-Stat pathway represents a rapid and direct mechanism of signaling to the nucleus.[53, 54] When Jak kinases are activated after ligand binding to the receptor, the Jak kinases phosphorylate members of a family of proteins called signal transducers and activators of transcription (Stat's). The Stat proteins are able to dimerize upon activation, enter the nucleus, and activate transcription by binding to specific sites in the DNA. Each cytokine receptor activates a specific set of Jak's and Stat's that can function in the stimulation of growth and/or differentiation.

The ligand-stimulated production of "second messengers" represents a distinct set of responses to growth-modulating agents. The second messengers are small, often diffusible molecules, such as cyclic nucleotides, sugar phosphates, ions, or lipid metabolites, which have diverse effects on cell metabolism. They are released in a regulated manner, after the activation of receptor-associated or receptor-stimulated enzymes. After their production, the second messengers bind to and activate specific intracellular target molecules, which constitute the next step in this type of signal transduction pathway. The EGF-induced activation of the enzyme phospholipase C-γ(PLC-γ) is an example of this process.[55] The tyrosine kinase activity of the EGF receptor phosphorylates PLC-γ on tyrosine, increasing the enzymatic activity of PLC-γ, which in turn cleaves membrane phosphatidylinositols to yield two classes of intracellular second messengers, diacylglycerol and inositol phosphates. Diacylglycerol is an activator of the serine/threonine-specific protein kinase C (PK-C), which is also activated by phorbol esters that are tumor promoters.[56] Release of inositol phosphate results in the elevation of intracellular calcium levels, which induces changes in a wide variety of metabolic pathways and cellular processes.[57]

An alternative paradigm for the ligand-induced production of second messengers is provided by the G-protein-coupled receptor family.[58] These hormone-binding receptors, typified by their seven membrane-spanning segments, do not themselves possess an enzymatic activity. Instead, these receptors exist at the cell surface as a complex with a heterotrimeric G protein (which is composed of three subunits, α, β, and γ).[59] The activity of the G protein is regulated by guanine nucleotide binding. Activation of the receptor induces the α subunit of the G protein to exchange guanosine diphosphate (GDP) for guanosine triphosphate (GTP), thereby leading to the α subunit's dissociating from the other two subunits and activating an effector enzyme. Effector enzymes whose activities are regulated in these systems include adenylate cyclase and certain phospholipases.

Both the protein phosphorylation cascades and the production of second messengers described above contribute to changes in the growth state of the target cell, with each receptor activating its particular constellation of molecules. The activation of cytoplasmic protein kinases such as PK-C, the c-*raf* proto-oncogene product, and cyclic adenosine monophosphate– (AMP)–dependent protein kinase (PK-A) is associated with the induction of specific changes in gene expression due at least in part to altered phosphorylation of nuclear transcriptional factors such as the *jun* proto-oncogene product. Thus the changes triggered by binding of an extracellular ligand are relayed to the interior of the cell and ultimately affect gene expression.[60, 61]

▼ ABNORMAL CELL GROWTH

Abrogation of Normal Growth Restraints and Resistance to Differentiation

Cancer results from the ability of neoplastic cells to grow in inappropriate settings, as manifested by invasion and metastasis. Cell culture methods have made it possible to compare the in vitro growth properties of tumor-derived cells with those of non-cancerous cells. These comparisons have revealed that many "cancer-like" properties of the tumor cells are reflected in their in vitro growth characteristics. Furthermore, as methods became available to induce the in vitro transformation of cultured cells with tumor viruses, chemical carcinogens, and oncogenes, it became clear that in vitro transformed cells and cells derived from tumors shared many properties that were distinct from those of normal cells. These observations implied that experimental studies of cultured cells could provide insight into mechanisms that underlie tumorigenesis.

Elucidation of the differences between normal and transformed cells came initially from experiments in fibroblasts. Many oncogenes shown to cause leukemia or to transform other cells can visibly alter the properties of fibroblasts. Fibroblasts normally adhere on a substratum and form a monolayer of flat, non-refractile cells (anchorage dependence)[62] whose growth ceases when the monolayer becomes confluent, a process referred to as contact inhibition or density dependent inhibition.[63] The normal cells are also non-invasive, in that they are unable to pass through a thick membranous structure such as a basement membrane.

These growth restraints are often lacking in tumor-derived cells or cells transformed by certain oncogenes (e.g., activated versions of the proto-oncogenes c-*abl*, c-*ras*, c-*fms*, c-*src*). In contrast to normal cells, many transformed fibroblasts are capable of growth when suspended in agar.[64] When allowed to grow on a substratum, the transformed cells may continue to divide and reach a much higher density than normal cells. The ability of transformed cell fibroblasts to overgrow a monolayer formed the basis for "focus" assays with tumor viruses, and later with transfected oncogenes (Fig. 25–4); a focus of transformed cells arises when a cell in monolayer culture becomes transformed and overgrows the surrounding contact-inhibited cells.[65] In addition, most transformed cells can invade and penetrate membranes, in contrast to normal cells. Normal and transformed cells tend to progress through S, G_2, and M phases at similar rates, but the length of G_1 may be significantly shorter for transformed cells. Furthermore, transformed cells are often resistant to extracellular signals that would render normal cells quiescent or inhibit their growth.

Differentiation represents another normal requirement of cells; complex, multicellular organisms demand a variety of differentiated cell types performing highly specialized functions. In many instances, fully differentiated cells are unable to proliferate. Such "terminal differentiation," which in erythroid cells and keratinocytes even includes loss of the nucleus, is obviously incompatible with tumor growth. Many tumors therefore arise from populations of stem cells or progenitors that are intermediate in maturation and blocked in their drive toward differentiation. Leukemias often conform to this pattern, with the acute forms being much less able to express differentiated functions than the chronic forms.[66]

A further manifestation of the transformed phenotype is a distinctive change in the shape and appearance of fibroblasts and certain epithelial cell lines, often referred to as morphological transformation. The transformed morphological features are characterized by decreased adherence to the substratum and a rounded appearance of the cells, both of which make the cell appear more refractile in the light microscope. Several biochemical alterations contribute to the rounded morphological characteristics and the decreased adhesiveness of transformed cells, including reduced expression of extracellular matrix proteins, such as fibronectin, that normally promote adhesion of cells to the substratum.[67, 68] There are also disruption of the cytoskeleton and a reduction in focal adhesion plaques, which are areas of close apposition between the cellular cytoskeleton and the substratum. The microfilament system, which is composed of actin filament bundles, many of which terminate at the sites of focal adhesions, is notably affected.[69]

Transformed hematopoietic cells possess some of the same characteristics, particularly loss or changes in adhesiveness. For example, partially transformed hematopoietic progenitor cells in patients with chronic myelogenous leukemia (CML) are prematurely released from the bone marrow into the circulation.[70] In vitro, the progenitors are deficient in the ability to adhere to bone marrow stroma or to be regulated by it. The changes in adhesive properties probably result from expression of the Bcr-Abl oncoprotein, which is a product of the Philadelphia chromosome that is characteristic of CML.

The biological differences between normal and transformed (or tumor-derived) cells can be assayed in vivo as well as in vitro. In contrast to normal cells, transformed cells are often capable of forming tumors in susceptible hosts. One widely used system tests the ability of inoculated cells to form tumors in nude *(nu/nu)* mice, whose genetic defect in thymic development impairs their cell-mediated immunity so that they do not reject cells from heterologous species, including human cells. Nude mice therefore provide a rapid

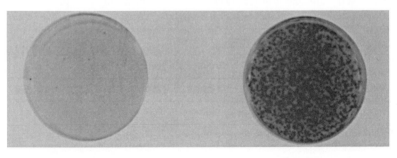

Control
Dish

Focal
Transformation

Figure 25–4. Assay for Focal Transformation in vitro. Established mouse fibroblasts grown in a monolayer culture in Petri dishes were either left untreated (control dish) or subjected to transformation by the introduction of a viral transforming gene (focal transformation). Cells in the control dish are contact inhibited, whereas the transformed cells in the other dish continue to grow and form foci, visualized here by staining the cells.

assay system for the in vivo growth of non-syngeneic tumor cells, without the risk of rejection that would occur in normal animals. Additional in vivo assays that can often distinguish transformed or tumor-derived cells from normal cells are based on the ability of the former to induce angiogenesis or to metastasize in the experimental animal. These in vivo assays, in conjunction with in vitro transformation systems and molecular biological techniques, have permitted investigation of the role of specific molecules in many aspects of neoplasia.

The use of transgenic animals, especially mice, has also permitted experimental assessment of the in vivo relevance of specific genetic changes to tumorigenesis. These studies involve either creating a transgene containing a potential oncogene under control of a promoter whose tissue-specific expression can usually be predicted or disrupting a potential tumor suppressor gene via gene targeting methods.[71, 72] In either case, animals can be observed for their incidence and type of tumors, which can be compared with those arising in control animals. The multistep process of tumor formation can be studied in transgenic animals by performing molecular analysis of the resulting tumors, by treating the mice with carcinogens, or by creating animals with lesions affecting more than one gene.

Acquisition of Growth Factor Independence

Another hallmark of normal cells is their strict dependence on growth factors for continued proliferation. Many of these factors have now been identified, although it is still common for cells to be grown in animal serum, which contains a wide variety of incompletely defined polypeptide, steroid, and other growth-modulating agents. Compared with that of normal cells, the growth of transformed or tumor-derived cells usually displays greatly reduced requirements for serum or growth factors. Often a tumor cell line of a given cell type survives and continues to divide in the absence of growth factors that are required for the growth of normal cells of the corresponding cell type.[31]

At least four mechanisms can account for the reduced dependence on serum or growth factors. In some instances, the tumor cell synthesizes one or more of the required growth factors. This "autocrine" production of ligand by the tumor cells continually activates the appropriate receptors, thus abrogating the requirement for exogenous ligand.[73] In other cases, the number of receptors expressed in the tumor cells may be abnormally high, thereby endowing greater activity to lower concentrations of ligand. In still other instances, there may be specific gain-of-function mutations involving oncogene products that are receptors or a part of the normal cellular signal transduction machinery. These mutations result in the constitutive activation of signaling pathways that would normally require activation by a ligand. The functional inactivation of tumor suppressor gene products represents a fourth mechanism for reduced dependence on serum and growth factors. Since these genes normally restrain cell growth, loss of their inhibitory activity can make certain signals sufficient to stimulate the growth of cells lacking these restraints, although these same signals would be insufficient to stimulate growth of normal cells.

Resistance to Apoptosis

Research carried out over the past decade has indicated that the regulation of programmed cell death (known descriptively as apoptosis) represents a significant feature of tumorigenesis.[74–76] Through this work, it has become apparent that the acquisition of genetic changes that are antiapoptotic is crucial to the development of many leukemias and other malignancies. In addition, antiapoptotic mechanisms in tumors can contribute to resistance to chemotherapy, as many antineoplastic agents mediate their effects by inducing apoptosis.[74, 77, 78]

Apoptosis is an intrinsic suicide program of cells that can be triggered when cells are exposed to certain physiological or pathological stimuli, internal or external. Programmed cell death is utilized by multicellular organisms in conjunction with proliferation to control cell numbers in tissues. In mammals, this process is most obvious in the hematopoietic system, where the size of each lineage and its subpopulations of more or less differentiated cells is continually regulated. It appears that apoptosis is the default program of many hematopoietic cell populations and that several cytokines can prevent apoptosis for maintenance of functional populations. Amazingly, in the normal control of T-cell populations, 95 per cent of T cells die in the thymus during maturation. Programmed cell death functions both to control cell numbers as well as to rid the organism of harmful autoreactive clones.

Cells programmed to die undergo specific characteristic morphological changes, which include condensation of chromatin, blebbing of membranes, and loss of the nuclear envelope.[76] Since chromosomal DNA is cleaved between nucleosomes, as a result of activation of a specific endonuclease, populations of cells undergoing apoptosis can be detected by an analysis of DNA that reveals a characteristic "DNA ladder."[79]

Programmed cell death occurs through a pathway that is highly conserved in evolution. Studies in the nematode *Caenorhabditis elegans* led to the isolation of the first genes involved in apoptosis.[80] For example, in *C. elegans* the *ced*-3 and *ced*-4 genes promote apoptosis, whereas the *ced*-9 gene is antiapoptotic. Each of these genes has counterparts in mammalian cells, namely, the interleukin-1 beta (IL-1β) converting enzyme (ICE) family, *Apaf*-1, and the *Bcl*-2 gene family, respectively. ICE is a member of a family of highly regulated cysteine proteases that work in a cascade and are the main effectors of the death program.[81, 82]

Many extracellular and intracellular factors can contribute to apoptosis (proapoptotic factors), whereas others can inhibit programmed cell death (antiapoptotic factors) (Fig. 25–5), with cell fate being determined by the predominance of pro- or antiapoptotic signals. The physiological context may also determine whether a given signal is pro- or antiapoptotic. Extracellular proapoptotic signals include Fas ligand (FasL), which can induce peripheral T cells to apoptose, as well as tumor necrosis factor α (TNF-α). Both ligands stimulate receptors that in turn activate the caspase cascade.[82] Apoptotic events can be triggered from the inside of the cell after expression of gene products such as the p53 tumor suppressor gene product, the Myc proto-oncoprotein, or inhibited by members of the Bcl-2 family, such as Bax, Bclx$_s$, or Bad.[75]

	Extracellular	Intracellular
Pro-apoptotic factors	Fas ligand TNF	p53 Myc Bax Bad
Anti-apoptotic factors	Growth factors Cytokines	Bcl-2 Bcl-x

Figure 25–5. Examples of Extracellular and Intracellular Factors That Negatively or Positively Regulate the Apoptotic Process.

Since apoptosis can protect the organism from potentially oncogenic events, such as the expression of a single oncogene whose protein functions intracellularly, the acquisition of antiapoptotic mechanisms plays an important role in neoplastic development. Cell survival not only allows the cells to accumulate, but also increases the time during which somatic mutations or other genetic abnormalities can occur, therefore also potentially contributing to oncogenesis.

Instructive results have been obtained from studies of the c-Myc oncoprotein, whose forced expression in fibroblasts can trigger the induction of apoptosis, thus potentially preventing the development of a transformed cell. The coexpression of the antiapoptotic Bcl-2 protein, or of serum growth factors, can protect the cells from apoptosis. This phenomenon has in vivo relevance, as the combined overexpression of c-Myc and Bcl-2 in the lymphocytes of transgenic mice leads to rapid tumor development, compared with that of mice that express only one of the two transgenes.[83] In the context of multistep tumorigenesis, Bcl-2 prevents the apoptosis that would be induced by Myc alone. Through this process, Bcl-2 greatly increases the efficiency with which Myc can drive the abnormal proliferation in the lymphocytes. The ability of the p53 tumor suppressor protein to induce apoptosis provides at least a partial explanation for the high frequency with which the normal function of this protein is abrogated in tumors. In CML, Bcr-Abl may have antiapoptotic properties, as this oncoprotein can protect cells from apoptosis after cytokine removal.[84]

Resistance of tumor cells to senescence may represent another phenomenon of importance to tumorigenesis.[85] Even when all the requirements for their growth are provided, normal cells cultured in vitro are capable of only a limited number of doublings before they undergo a "crisis" period and begin to die, by a mechanism that is distinct from apoptosis.[85] A small proportion of rodent cells survive the crisis period and give rise to established (or "immortalized") cell lines (e.g., the murine NIH 3T3 line). In rodent cells, such immortalization is usually associated with mutation of the p53 tumor suppressor protein (or of genes activated by p53) or the Ink4a genes.[86] In non-established cells, introduction of an activated oncogene such as one encoding an activated Ras oncoprotein leads to the rapid induction of senescence; inactivation of p53 or Ink4a permits the oncoprotein to be highly transforming. Established cells retain many properties of normal cells, but they can proliferate indefinitely without further crisis. Although it is very difficult to establish a human cell line in this way, many cell lines derived from human and animal tumors are found to be immortalized.

One limitation to the indefinite proliferation of normal somatic cells results from the progressive loss of telomers at the ends of chromosomes. This phenomenon, whose genetic properties were first elucidated in yeast, is abrogated in cancer cells, which have been adapted to express constitutively the genes required to maintain their telomer length.[87]

Tumor Progression: Mutations and Epigenetic Phenomena

Evidence from experimental and human cancer suggests that malignancy usually results only after a cell has undergone a series of genetic and perhaps some epigenetic changes.[1, 5, 15] In principle, each change should provide a selective growth advantage to the cell, compared with the progenitor cells lacking that change. This process results in the continual "progression" of the tumor, in which subsets of cells arise that have increasingly autonomous growth characteristics. Many of these changes involve alterations in cell cycle progression, loss of differentiation, and resistance to apoptosis or senescence, and others may allow for escape from an immune response directed against the incipient tumor cells. During the progression of the tumor, there may be several mutational events, such as those that allow for growth factor independence, reduced positional dependence of growth, and increased invasiveness. These altered growth properties may result from gain-of-function changes in proto-oncogenes, amplification (increased copy number) of these loci, or loss of function changes in tumor suppressor genes.

Some tumor types may be associated with a consistent constellation of mutated genes, suggesting that each of these mutant genes serves an important and specific role in the tumor that cannot be easily duplicated by alterations in other genes.[6] Certain in vitro cell transformation assays that depend upon cooperation between more than one transforming gene appear to reflect analogous requirements, since only some combinations of genes induce transformation in these assay systems.[88] In those oncogenic viruses that contain more than one viral oncogene, the combination of oncogenes in the virus can be shown to cooperate with each other by in vitro cell transformation assays or in vivo tumorigenesis assays.

In addition to genetic alterations, a separate type of change may occur that involves the altered expression of certain growth-regulating gene products. For example, there may be increased expression of cell-surface receptors for a growth factor, which, as noted earlier, may enhance the sensitivity of the tumor cells to this factor. Such alterations are referred to as epigenetic, since they do not involve a change in the genetic information in the cell but merely in the way in which the information is expressed. Changes in methylation in the regions associated with gene promoter could account for such changes in expression.[89, 90] Tumor suppressors such as Ink4a have repeatedly been shown to be hypermethylated in tumors and can be correlated with an absence of expression.[91]

Genomic instability also occurs commonly during malignant progression. The instability can often be attributed to inactivation of the p53 tumor suppressor and/or loss of cell cycle checkpoint control, resulting in gross karyotypic abnormalities as well as subtle genetic alterations.[25, 92, 93] The chromosomal changes may augment the genetic or epigenetic changes described above. For example, portions of chromosomes may be deleted, resulting in a loss of tumor suppressor genes, and other portions may be duplicated, resulting in amplification of proto-oncogenes. Gene conversion events are also common; this process often represents another mode of gene amplification, since it may result in a cell's being converted from being heterozygous for a mutant allele to becoming homozygous for the allele. The net result of these processes' occurring together within the tumor cell population is the continual progression of the tumor to a more oncogenic state.

Oncogenes and Proto-Oncogenes

▼ RETROVIRUSES AND THE DISCOVERY AND DEFINITION OF ONCOGENES

The term *oncogene* originally referred to the ability of retroviruses to induce stable, tumorigenic changes in infected cells.[94] In the 1970s, the term came to refer more precisely to retroviral genes that could dramatically alter the growth properties of cells in which they were expressed. The essential feature of these genes was that they could stimulate inappropriate growth of their target cells.[3, 95] Oncogenes induced cellular transformation in vitro, particularly in fibroblasts or epithelial cells, as described in the previous section, or in vivo by causing neoplastic disease in target cells that expressed it. The term was also applied to the transforming genes of DNA tumor viruses, which are discussed later.

Since retroviruses are endogenous to chickens, mice, and many other species, it was initially unclear whether viral oncogenes represented altered versions of viral replication genes or were composed of cell-derived genetic information. The recognition that retroviral oncogenes (collectively abbreviated as v-*onc*) were derived from cellular genes (abbreviated c-*onc*) led to reference to the normal cellular homologues of viral oncogenes as proto-oncogenes.[3, 95] When altered versions of c-*onc* were identified in cancers, the term *oncogene* was expanded to include these genes as well. In this chapter and elsewhere, *oncogene* is now used even more broadly, to include any gene that has the ability to stimulate cell growth or allow expansion of a cell population in a tumor system. Sometimes the demonstration of a gene's transforming nature requires coexpression of a cooperating oncogene. A normal growth factor receptor whose activation stimulates cell growth would be considered a proto-oncogene, whereas a constitutively active version of this receptor would be termed an *oncogene*. Genes that inhibit apoptosis can also be considered proto-oncogenes.

▼ DNA TUMOR VIRUSES

Several groups of DNA-containing viruses have oncogenic potential (Table 25–1).[96, 97] Genes that alter cell growth have been identified for Epstein-Barr virus.[98] In a few cases hepatitis B DNA has been found to integrate near host genes,

Table 25–1. DNA Viruses Associated with Naturally Occurring Malignant Tumors

Virus Group	Virus	Tumor (Host Species)
Hepadenavirus	Hepatitis B	Hepatocellular carcinoma (humans, woodchuck)
Herpesvirus	Epstein-Barr virus	African Burkitt's lymphoma, nasopharyngeal carcinoma (humans)
	Marek's disease virus	T-cell lymphoma (chickens)
Papovaviruses Papillomavirus	Several HPV types (especially 5, 8, 16, 18, 31, 33)	Squamous cell carcinoma, cervical carcinoma, and others (humans, rabbits, cows)
Polyoma/SV40	Polyoma	Various (mice)

such as c-*myc*, which are implicated in cell growth or differentiation, sometimes leading to expression of a fusion protein composed of a viral and a cellular gene.[99, 100] As discussed below, analogous alterations have been studied much more extensively with retroviruses.

Some of the most revealing molecular genetic and biochemical analyses of the DNA tumor virus oncogenes and their encoded protein products have been made for adenoviruses and papovaviruses, especially polyomavirus, SV40, and papillomaviruses.[8, 97, 101, 102] The contribution of these studies includes demonstrating that cooperation between oncogenes is important, that viral oncoproteins can contribute to transformation by modulating the activity of cellular proteins, and that certain oncoproteins encoded by these viruses function primarily by inactivating the proteins encoded by tumor suppressor genes.

Papillomaviruses are classified as large papovaviruses (see Table 25–1), but there are major structural and biological differences between the papillomaviruses and the small papovaviruses, such as SV40 and polyoma. These DNA viruses normally replicate through a lytic life cycle, in which death of the host cell is associated with complete viral replication and the release of progeny virus. Cell transformation by these viruses therefore represents a form of incomplete (abortive) infection.

Some DNA tumor viruses, such as the papillomaviruses, induce tumors in their natural host, whereas others, such as SV40 and adenoviruses, only induce tumors in heterologous hosts. Tumorigenesis by these latter viruses results from abortive infection in a heterologous host. Integration of viral DNA into the host genome is often required for transformation by DNA tumor viruses, although papillomaviruses and Epstein-Barr virus are exceptions to this generalization. However, viral DNA integration into the genome of the host cell is not a normal part of the virus life cycle of DNA tumor viruses, in contrast to that of retroviruses.

Cooperative Roles of Viral Transforming Genes

Molecular dissection of the genomes of the adeno- and papovaviruses has been combined with transformation assays to identify the genes responsible for their transforming function. This analysis has indicated that each virus contains at least two transforming genes. In every case, the genes are located within the viral genome's "early" region, so named because these genes, which encode non-structural viral proteins, are expressed soon after infection of the cell. These transforming genes have coevolved with the virus and participate in virus replication, in contrast to retroviral oncogenes. Analysis of conditional mutants has shown that maintenance of the transformed phenotype depends on the continued activity of these genes.[8, 101–103]

The adeno- and papovaviruses can be infectious for resting cells, since they contain genes that, as part of the viral life cycle, induce DNA synthesis of resting cells. The normal roles for many of the transforming gene products include the induction of cellular DNA synthesis, initiation of viral DNA synthesis, and regulation of viral and cellular gene expression. Given that entry into S phase and control of gene expression represent major ways in which cell growth is controlled, it is perhaps not surprising that viral gene products that alter these functions can induce transformation.

The two major transforming genes of adenoviruses are *E1A* and *E1B*, which encode nuclear proteins. The SV40 early region encodes two gene products, designated small t and large T, of 17 kDa and 94 kDa, respectively. Large T, which is located in the nucleus, is the major transforming gene for cultured cells, although small t may enhance the transformed phenotype.[104] Polyoma virus is similar to SV40 in the size and structural organization of its genome. As with SV40, the early region of polyoma virus encodes two proteins from alternately spliced messenger RNAs (mRNAs); they are called small t and large T proteins, respectively, although they are structurally distinct from the SV40 proteins. An additional protein, designated middle T, is also encoded by this region of polyoma. Transformation of primary cells by polyoma requires the expression of both large T and middle T. Middle T can transform certain established cells; large T can extend the life span of primary cells (immortalization) without morphologically transforming them.[105]

The genital human papillomavirus (HPV) types and the bovine papillomavirus type 1 (BPV) are the papillomaviruses that have been studied most intensively.[106] BPV, which induces large benign fibropapillomas, has two major transforming genes, *E5* and *E6*. *E5* encodes a 44 amino acid non-nuclear membrane-associated protein. The *E6* product is a 16 kDa protein that is found, at least partially, in the nucleus.

Although the tumors induced by HPV are generally benign (warts), certain HPVs (especially types 16 and 18) have also been implicated in malignancy, especially cervical cancer. Other genital HPV types, such as 6 and 11, that infect the cervix and other genital tissues are not associated with cervical malignancy.[103] This difference has led to designation of viruses such as HPV-6 and HPV-11 as low risk, and those such as HPV-16 and -18 as "high risk." The genital HPVs contain two principal transforming genes, *E6* and *E7*, both of which encode nuclear proteins. DNA from high risk HPVs can immortalize primary human epithelial cells, whereas DNA from low-risk HPV types yields negative findings in such assays. Genetic analysis has shown that the *E6* and *E7* genes from a high-risk HPV type cooperate to induce immortalization.[107] The keratinocyte immortalization assay appears to be measuring a function related to the

pathogenesis of HPV associated cervical cancer, since non-mutated forms of *E6* and *E7* are preferentially retained and expressed in cervical carcinomas and in cell lines derived from them.[96]

As noted above, cooperation between the oncogenes of these viruses is a hallmark of their transforming capacity.[71, 88] If non-established human cells are transfected adenovirus E1A, in the absence of E1B, or with a high-risk HPV-E7, in the absence of a high-risk E6, the cells undergo a brief period of increased cell growth, followed by apoptosis. By contrast, if they receive E1B alone or E6 alone, they remain viable and are protected from senescence, but they do not become morphologically transformed. These findings have led to the notion that certain oncogenes can induce immortalization, that is, they can protect cells from undergoing senescence or apoptosis, whereas other oncogenes are categorized as transforming, since they can stimulate cell proliferation. Expression of a transforming oncogene, in the absence of an immortalization oncogene, triggers signals for the cell to undergo apoptosis. Since efficient transformation therefore requires at least one gene of each type, these systems represent important examples of the multistep nature of tumor pathogenesis.

Analysis of the viral oncoproteins provided important insights about the mechanism underlying cooperation (Fig. 25–6).[19, 103, 108] It was found that adenovirus E1A and HPV

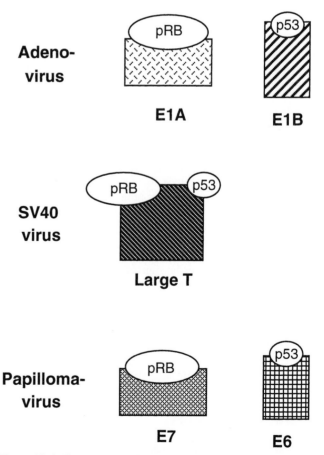

Figure 25–6. Formation of Complexes Between the Products of DNA Tumor Virus Oncogenes and Cellular Proteins. The large T antigen of SV40 binds the products of the *RB* and *p53* tumor suppressors. In the case of the adenoviruses and the papillomaviruses, pRB and p53 binding functions are encoded in different transforming proteins.

E7 were each capable of binding the retinoblastoma tumor suppressor protein, pRB, and adenovirus E1B and HPV E6 formed a complex with another tumor suppressor protein, p53. Further analysis showed that the biological activities of the viral oncoproteins depended on their ability to bind the tumor suppressor proteins and that the binding inactivated the inhibitory functions of the suppressors. The ability of E1A and E7 to stimulate growth arose because inactivation of pRB led to activation of E2F and progression through the cell cycle, as discussed earlier in the section on cell cycle. Furthermore, apoptosis induced by E1A could be shown to have arisen because E1A had induced the expression of p53, which, as noted in the section on apoptosis, is proapoptotic. These results have provided a mechanistic framework for understanding cooperation between these viral oncogenes and have established the paradigm that many oncogenes of DNA tumor viruses act largely by inactivating the function of specific tumor suppressor genes. This analysis of the viral oncoproteins has also explained an apparent paradox of SV40 large T. In contrast to the adenovirus and papillomavirus oncogene system, large T alone is able to immortalize and transform non-established cells. This dual property of large T has arisen because it is able to bind both pRB and p53. Therefore, although papovaviruses, papillomaviruses, and adenoviruses are evolutionarily distinct, a striking convergence is that oncoproteins encoded by all of them bind pRB and p53 (see Fig. 25–6).

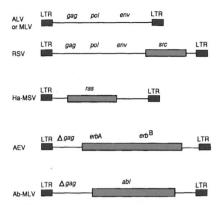

Figure 25–7. Genome Structure of Slowly and Acutely Transforming Retroviruses, as They Appear in the Provirus Form. The 5′ end of the genome is shown on the left, and the 3′ end is shown at the right. Avian leukemia virus (ALV) and murine leukemia virus (MLV) represent weakly oncogenic leukosis viruses that have a full complement of replicative genes, but no v-*onc*. Rous sarcoma virus (RSV) also is replication competent but in addition encodes the v-*src* gene at the 3′ end of the genome. Harvey murine sarcoma virus (Ha-MSV), avian erythroblastosis virus (AEV), and Abelson murine leukemia virus (Ab-MLV) represent replication-defective acutely transforming viruses in which most or all of the replicative genes have been replaced by v-*onc* sequences.

▼ CLASSIFICATION OF RETROVIRUSES

The study of retroviruses has contributed in a major way to understanding of the molecular basis of tumor formation.[3, 9, 95] Since this chapter emphasizes experimental tumor systems, it is relevant to review the classification of retroviruses briefly. This viral family comprises a group of RNA viruses, some members of which can induce cellular transformation or neoplasia. The oncogenic retroviruses can be divided into two broad classes. Some, such as Moloney murine leukemia virus (Mo-MLV) and the avian leukosis virus (ALV), do not possess a cell-derived viral oncogene (Fig. 25–7). These viruses tend to induce neoplastic disease only after a relatively long latency and do not usually induce focal transformation of cultured cells. The second class is known as the acutely transforming retroviruses (see Fig. 25–7; Table 25–2). In susceptible hosts, these viruses typically can induce neoplasia in a matter of days or weeks and often efficiently induce focal transformation of cultured cells. The critical difference between the two classes of viruses is that the acutely transforming retroviruses contain cell-derived oncogenes in addition to (or more often, in the place of) the replicative *gag, pol,* and *env* genes (see Fig. 25–7). Examples of this type of virus include Rous sarcoma virus (RSV), avian erythroblastosis virus (AEV), Harvey murine sarcoma virus (Ha-MSV), and Abelson murine leukemia virus (Ab-MLV).

▼ RETROVIRAL ONCOGENES

Many oncogene-containing retroviruses cause sarcomas or carcinomas; others are capable of inducing lymphomas or leukemias when introduced into animals (e.g., Ab-MLV,

AEV, avian myelocytomatosis virus, avian myeloblastosis virus). Although many v-*onc* genes have not been directly demonstrated to induce disease of the hematopoietic system, they are in general critical components of common proliferation pathways used in cells and therefore can be important elements involved in leukemia cell growth. Most retroviral oncogenes represent gain-of-function mutants of their normal cellular homologues; that means that the v-*onc* and c-*onc* protein products tend to have many similarities. As gain-of-function mutants, the v-*onc* genes are excellent tools for elucidating many biological and biochemical aspects of their normal cellular counterparts. They also continue to be paradigms for how specific changes in the protein products of these genes may subvert their normal function and contribute to oncogenesis.

Many important advances in understanding oncogenes have come from the analysis of RSV (see Fig. 25–7), which was described in 1911.[109] The viral gene (called v-*src*) that accounted for the rapid induction of sarcomas by this virus was the first retroviral oncogene to be identified, although this did not happen for several decades. Identification of v-*src* was made possible largely through unique aspects of the composition of the RSV genome and by the development of cell and virus culture techniques that permitted investigators to examine pure virus strains and their interaction with relatively homogeneous populations of permissive host cells. Identification of retroviral oncogenes and certain cellular oncogenes also depended heavily upon specific aspects of the retrovirus life cycle. Thus to appreciate how these genes were identified, we shall briefly review the genetic organization and life cycle of retroviruses.

▼ RETROVIRUSES: GENOME STRUCTURE AND REPLICATION

The retrovirus genome forms a stable association with the cell by replicating through a DNA intermediate termed a

Table 25–2. Some Acutely Oncogenic Retroviruses, Oncogenes, and Oncoproteins*

Oncogene	Representative Virus	Species	Protein	Function
sis	Simian sarcoma virus	Monkey	p28$^{env\text{-}sis}$	Growth factor
src	Rous sarcoma virus	Chicken	p60^{src}	Tyrosine kinase
abl	Abelson leukemia virus	Mouse	p120$^{gag\text{-}abl}$	Tyrosine kinase
fps†	Fujinami sarcoma virus	Chicken	p140$^{gag\text{-}fps}$	Tyrosine kinase
fes†	Gardner-Arnstein feline sarcoma virus	Cat	p110$^{gag\text{-}fes}$	
fms	McDonough feline sarcoma virus	Cat	p180$^{gag\text{-}fms}$	Tyrosine kinase
fgr	Gardner-Rasheed feline sarcoma virus	Cat	p70$^{gag\text{-}fgr}$	Tyrosine kinase
kit	Hardy-Zuckerman-4 feline sarcoma virus	Cat	p80$^{gag\text{-}kit}$	Tyrosine kinase
yes	Y73 sarcoma virus	Chicken	p90$^{gag\text{-}yes}$	Tyrosine kinase
ros	UR2 sarcoma virus	Chicken	p68$^{gag\text{-}ros}$	Tyrosine kinase
crk	Avian sarcoma virus CT10	Chicken	p47$^{gag\text{-}crk}$	SH2-SH3 adapter
raf	3611 Murine sarcoma virus	Mouse	p75$^{gag\text{-}raf}$	Serine/threonine kinase
	Avian carcinoma virus MH2	Chicken	p100$^{gag\text{-}raf}$	
mos	Moloney sarcoma virus	Mouse	p37$^{env\text{-}mos}$	Serine/threonine kinase
Ha-*ras*	Harvey sarcoma virus	Rat	p21^{ras}H	GTP binding
	Rasheed sarcoma virus	Rat	p29$^{gag\text{-}ras}$H	
Ki-*ras*	Kirsten sarcoma virus	Rat	p21^{ras}K	GTP binding
erbA	Avian erythroblastosis virus	Chicken	p75$^{gag\text{-}erb}$A	Thyroid hormone receptor
erbB	Avian erythroblastosis virus	Chicken	p72^{erb}B	Tyrosine kinase
rel	Reticuloendotheliosis virus	Turkey	p56$^{env\text{-}rel}$	Nuclear
fos	FBJ murine osteogenic sarcoma virus	Mouse	p55^{fos}	Nuclear
ski	Avian SK virus	Chicken	p110$^{gag\text{-}ski\text{-}gag}$	Nuclear
myc	Avian myelocytomatosis virus 29	Chicken	p110$^{gag\text{-}myc}$	Nuclear
jun	Avian sarcoma virus 17	Chicken	p55$^{gag\text{-}jun}$	Nuclear
myb	Avian myeloblastosis virus	Chicken	p45$^{gag\text{-}myb\text{-}env}$	Nuclear
ets	Avian erythroblastosis virus	Chicken	p135$^{gag\text{-}myb\text{-}ets}$	Nuclear

*In several cases, the same oncogene has been transduced by different viruses; only one example for most genes is given.
†*Fps* and *fes* are homologous genes of chicken and cat origin, respectively.

provirus (Fig. 25–8).[9, 10, 110, 111] As an integral part of retrovirus replication, the provirus is integrated into the cellular DNA and thus (irreversibly) forms part of the host cell genome. Proviral integration can occur throughout the host genome. Most retroviruses are not cytotoxic; human immunodeficiency virus (HIV) is an important exception to this rule.

To undergo the complete replicative cycle, the retrovirus requires the products of three viral genes, designated *gag, pol*, and *env* (see Fig. 25–7). *gag* encodes the core proteins of the virion, *pol* the reverse transcriptase[112, 113] and associated activities that catalyze transcription of the viral RNA to the proviral DNA and mediate proviral integration, and *env* the virion envelope glycoprotein. These viral genes are not oncogenes. Their 5′ to 3′ order is *gag-pol-env* both in the viral RNA genome and in the integrated provirus.

Certain sequences are duplicated at the 5′ and 3′ end of the provirus; the duplicated part of the provirus is called the long terminal repeat (LTR) (see Fig. 25–8).[114] Many of the viral elements that are required in *cis-* are located within the LTR, including the major promoter/enhancer region of the provirus and the polyadenylation signal. Another important viral element that is required in *cis-* is the *psi* sequence, which is found just 3′ of the 5′ LTR; *psi* specifies the efficient incorporation (or "packaging") of the viral RNA into virions during the late stages of the replicative cycle.

▼ ACUTELY TRANSFORMING RETROVIRUSES CONTAIN TRANSFORMING GENES

RSV is unique among the acutely transforming retroviruses in that most strains of this virus contain the three replicative genes (and therefore are replication competent), in addition to the transforming *src* gene at the 3′ end of the genome (see Fig. 25–7). The non-defectiveness of RSV facilitated gaining the initial evidence that the highly oncogenic and transforming activities of RSV resided in sequences that were distinct from those required for viral replication.[115–117]

In contrast to RSV, AEV, Ha-MSV, and Ab-MLV bear large deletions in their replicative genes, portions of which are replaced by their respective oncogenes (*erbA* and *erbB*, *ras* or *abl*) (see Fig. 25–7). These latter viruses are therefore replication defective; that is, they are incapable of undergoing a full replicative cycle by themselves. However, they can be propagated through mixed infection with a replication-competent virus of the ALV or MLV type,[118] which can provide the replicative protein products in *trans-*, allowing

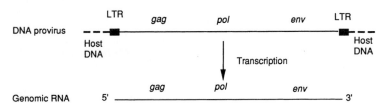

Figure 25–8. Expression of Viral Replicative Genes from the Integrated Provirus of a Weakly Oncogenic Retrovirus. The genomic RNA serves as mRNA for *gag* and *pol* protein synthesis and is packaged into virions. A second spliced mRNA (not shown) is used for translation of the *env* product.

the viral RNA of the acutely oncogenic virus to be incorporated into virions and spread to new cells. Although the replication defectiveness of the acutely oncogenic viruses makes it unlikely for them to persist in the wild, they can be readily propagated in the laboratory.

▼ RELATIONSHIP OF RETROVIRAL ONCOGENES TO PROTO-ONCOGENES

Discovery of Proto-Oncogenes

The first clear evidence that v-*onc* genes were derived from cellular genes came from studies involving v-*src* of RSV. Molecular hybridization studies showed that an RSV "*src*-specific" probe that lacked ALV sequences could hybridize to uninfected cellular DNA from chickens and from other species as well.[11, 119] Other evidence strongly suggested that the *src*-related sequences in cells had functional significance. When poorly oncogenic mutants of RSV that had deletions within v-*src* were injected into chickens, the viruses often reacquired the highly tumorigenic phenotype. This oncogenic change correlated with a recombinational event in the RSV genome; the v-*src* deletion had been repaired by the acquisition of cell-derived sequences that were almost identical to those in wild-type v-*src*.[120]

These experimental results meant that v-*src* and, by implication, other v-*onc* were derived from cellular genes that are conserved in evolution. Indeed when similar analyses were performed, using probes derived from the v-*onc* of other acutely transforming retroviruses, it was found that these genes, like *src*, had cellular homologues.[121] The evolutionary conservation of c-*src* and the other c-*onc* genes made it likely that this class of cellular genes carried out important normal functions in the cell but that these genes could be altered to give rise to dominant transforming genes. Since these cell-derived genes had oncogenic potential as retroviral oncogenes, the cellular homologues of retroviral oncogenes represented prime candidate genes to be involved in the pathogenesis of spontaneous tumors. Many, although not all, of the cellular genes that gave rise to viral oncogenes have subsequently been implicated in human tumors.

The Protein Products of Viral Oncogenes

Identification and analysis of v-*onc* encoded proteins have not only provided enormous insight into how v-*onc*'s transform cells and but also elucidated pathways of cell growth by identifying the functions of their normal cellular homologues.

The v-*src* protein was the first retroviral oncoprotein to be identified, using sera from rabbits in which tumors had been induced with an RSV strain that was infectious for mammalian cells. The v-*src* gene product is a 60 kDa phosphoprotein designated pp60^{v-src}.[122] The sera also recognize the closely related 60 kDa c-*src* product pp60^{c-src}, which is found in normal cells. As antisera that recognized other v-*onc* proteins were developed, proteins related to these products were also identified in normal cells.

Biochemical analysis indicated that there are various classes of viral oncoproteins (see Table 25–2). The first insight into biochemical function was provided by pp60^{v-src},

which was shown to be a protein kinase,[123, 124] suggesting it might transform cells via phosphorylation of critical substrates. The excitement generated by this observation was further enhanced by the subsequent finding that tyrosine was the amino acid phosphorylated on proteins by pp60^{v-src},[125] in contrast to previously described protein kinases, which phosphorylate proteins on serine and threonine residues. Normal cells contain very low levels of phosphotyrosine in their proteins (significantly less than 1 per cent of the total phosphoamino acids), and RSV transformation was associated with a 5- to 10-fold increase in cellular phosphotyrosine. These results therefore implied that cell transformation by v-*src* was mediated by altering the function of cellular substrate proteins that were phosphorylated on tyrosine by pp60^{v-src}.

A protein tyrosine kinase activity was also identified for the v-*abl* oncogene product of Abelson-MLV, the v-*erbB* product of AEV, and several other v-*onc* products. Not all v-*onc* products with kinase activity are tyrosine kinases; the products of the v-*mos* and v-*raf* oncogenes are serine-threonine kinases (see Table 25–2). The protein kinase activities of these oncoproteins and of the v-*onc* proteins with tyrosine kinase activity are essential for their biological activity, since kinase-deficient mutants of these proteins are transformation defective.

Some v-*onc* products, although they are highly transforming, lack a detectable kinase activity and therefore transform cells via other mechanisms. Some, such as the Ras proteins, function through their ability to bind the guanine nucleotide GTP. The v-*sis* product is a growth factor (platelet-derived growth factor [PDGF]). Others, such as those encoded by v-*myc*, v-*fos*, v-*jun*, and v-*myb*, are nuclear proteins that are directly involved in the transcription of mRNA.

From c-*onc* to v-*onc*: Mutation and Overexpression

The demonstration that proto-oncogenes and their products may reside in normal cells raised two related issues: how normal cells are prevented from being transformed, and the nature of the differences between c-*onc* and v-*onc*. Comparisons of c-*onc* and v-*onc* have shown that almost all v-*onc* genes are highly transforming because they function as constitutively active versions of c-*onc*; both mutation and overexpression contribute to the conversion of normal cellular genes to the potent transforming genes found in retroviruses. These findings underlie the dominant paradigms of the field: that proto-oncogenes are normally involved in the regulation of cell growth and that viral oncogenes disrupt the normal balance of growth control because they represent less regulated versions of these proto-oncogenes.[95, 121] Most proto-oncogenes, when overexpressed, are capable of inducing at least immortalization or partial transformation.

Most v-*onc* genes that are mutated are much more potent transforming genes than their normal cellular homologues.[126] A wide variety of structural changes have been found to account for the mutational activation of v-*onc*. These include point mutation that changes single amino acids (exemplified by the v-*ras* genes); deletion of the 5′ end of the gene (v-*raf*); deletion of the 3′ end of the gene (v-*src*); deletion of both 5′ and 3′ sequences (v-*erbB*, which is an activated version of the EGF receptor); and fusion of c-*onc* sequences to portions of viral replicative genes, such as *gag* (v-*abl*). Often more than one of these changes has occurred in a given v-*onc*.

One common consequence of the changes is that mutated protein products, in contrast to their normal counterparts, are more or less constitutively active. In the case of the protein kinases, the structural alterations in the viral oncoprotein remove negative regulatory regions that limit the activity of the normal proteins. In the case of Ras proteins, which ordinarily shuttle between an active, GTP-bound conformation and an inactive, GDP-bound conformation, the mutations serve to maintain them in the active conformation. As these examples illustrate, the structural alterations found in most v-*onc* encoded proteins enhance the function of the normal c-*onc* encoded proteins, rather than investing the v-*onc* products with entirely new biochemical functions.

As noted earlier, the retroviral LTR acts as a strong promoter that contains multiple enhancer elements that result in a high level of expression for genes under their control. Thus when a proto-oncogene is transduced and expressed from the viral LTR, its expression may greatly exceed the normal level of proto-oncogene expression, thereby overwhelming the delicate balance that controls cell proliferation.

Since expression from the viral LTR is constitutive, proto-oncogenes whose level of transcription is normally tightly regulated (e.g., *fos* and *myc*) by the cell cycle or other mechanisms are aberrantly expressed both temporally and quantitatively. Viral transduction of a proto-oncogene may be associated with loss of other steps at which gene expression may normally be regulated, such as mRNA stability and efficiency of translation. When retroviruses are inoculated into an organism, they may infect cell types in which the proto-oncogene that gave rise to their v-*onc* may not be expressed. Although many proto-oncogenes are expressed in virtually all cell types (e.g., c-*ras*), the expression of others is more restricted, so that their expression in inappropriate cells may be related to their activation. For example, transformation may result from expression of a transduced growth factor gene (e.g., v-*sis*) after viral infection of a cell that expresses the cognate receptor, thus forming an aberrant autocrine loop.

Some viral oncoproteins exhibit several differences from their normal cellular counterparts, and experimental analysis can determine the relative contribution of each difference to the overall activity of the oncoprotein. Molecular cloning techniques have been employed to isolate and determine the nucleotide sequence of the v-*onc* genes and their normal cellular homologues.[9] In addition to the obligatory loss of introns in the v-*onc*, these comparisons have revealed a high frequency of deletions and point mutations in v-*onc*. The contribution of these structural changes has then been determined by repairing the mutations, singly or in combination, and determining the activity of these genes. Also, the effects of overexpression have been tested by placing proto-oncogenes under the control of strong promoters, such as LTRs.[127] The development of transgenic mice has enabled investigators to assess the effect of v-*onc* expression in vivo, in a wide variety of different cell types, depending on the promoter used.[71]

Activation of Cellular Oncogenes by Insertional Mutagenesis

As noted earlier, viruses of the ALV or Mo-MLV class, which lack cell-derived oncogenes, are still oncogenic, although they induce neoplasia more slowly than the acute transforming viruses. The long latency between inoculation of these viruses into susceptible animals and the development of malignancy implied that several events, in addition to viral infection, might be required for tumor development. These tumors or leukemias are characteristically monoclonal, in contrast to the polyclonal neoplasias induced by retroviruses that carry oncogenes. The monoclonality can be attributed to the progressive nature of the several events required for malignancy to develop as well as to the infrequency with which the full constellation of changes arise. At each step of this process, there is a clonal expansion of cells resulting from the growth advantage provided by the genetic or epigenetic alteration.

It was initially unclear how retroviruses without oncogenes might induce tumors. The first mechanistic clues were provided by studies of ALV induced bursal lymphomas in chickens. When the integration sites of the ALV sequences were analyzed by Southern blotting experiments, it was found that primary and metastatic tumors in a given animal all contained the same ALV integration site. By itself, this finding was not surprising, since it merely confirmed the clonal origin of the tumors. However, the ALV integration sites in bursal tumors from different animals indicated that the ALV sequences were integrated within the same region of cell DNA in most of the different tumors. Given the almost limitless number of potential integration sites in the host cell genome, finding a common integration site implied that the cells that contained this viral integration site had a selective growth advantage.

Analysis of the viral DNA integration site in the tumor cells showed it contained only a portion of the viral genome, with a large region deleted (Fig. 25–9). The sequences remaining in the tumor cells usually included an LTR but often contained little of the viral replicative genes. This result indicated that although inoculation of the virus was

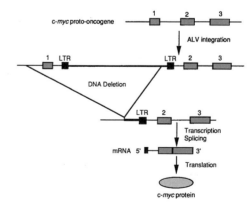

Figure 25–9. Activation of c-*myc* by Proviral Insertion in Avian Bursal Lymphomas. Integration of the ALV provirus is usually followed by a deletion of the non-coding exon 1 of c-*myc* and most of the provirus. The 3' LTR then directs the production of an mRNA species encoding the normal c-*myc* protein. Since the expression of this mRNA lacks the normal control mechanisms that act on c-*myc*, an increase in the level of c-*myc* encoded protein results.

required to induce the lymphomas, neither the expression of viral genes nor viral replication was required for maintenance of the lymphomas.[128] It therefore seemed likely that the retrovirus integration itself might be acting as a mutagenic event, altering the expression of nearby gene(s) that might be involved in the regulation of cell growth. This prediction was fulfilled when it was determined that the common viral integration site was located within the c-*myc* proto-oncogene, the gene that had given rise to the v-*myc* oncogene of an acutely transforming retrovirus.[129] The tumor cells were found to express an mRNA species that began at the viral LTR and encoded the normal protein-coding exons of c-*myc*, resulting in an increased level of the c-*myc* protein product, which in combination with other changes eventually led to the formation of the tumor.

This type of proto-oncogene activation, termed insertional mutagenesis, is not limited to the ALV-induced bursal lymphomas, nor has c-*myc* been the only cellular target identified in this mechanism. In fact, many proto-oncogenes that gave rise to retroviral oncogenes have been found to be targets for insertional mutagenesis by retroviruses that lack their own v-*onc*.

Furthermore, analysis of the cellular sequences surrounding retroviral DNA integration sites has proved to be a rich source for the identification of new genes implicated in tumorigenesis (Table 25–3).[130] The first such example was the *wnt-1* gene (formerly known as *int-1*), which is located at a common integration site identified with mouse mammary tumor virus (MMTV), a mammary tumor inducing virus that lacked an oncogene.[131] Additional studies verified that *wnt-1* was conserved in evolution, had the biological properties of an oncogene in cell transformation experiments, could induce mammary carcinomas when expressed as a transgene in mice, and was the prototype of a multigene family whose members carry out important functions in normal development.[132–134]

Most of the genes affected by retroviral insertional mutagenesis have turned out to be dominant-acting oncogenes, as occurred for ALV and c-*myc*. A partial list of proto-oncogenes activated by this mechanism in carcinomas and in leukemias and lymphomas is given in Table 25–3. Less commonly, the integration event has disrupted the allele of a tumor suppressor gene and led to pathogenic consequences.[135] This latter event occurs much less commonly in retrovirus-induced tumorigenesis, as phenotypic changes usually result only after inactivation of the second allele of the tumor suppressor gene, via a second viral integration event or another mechanism of mutational inactivation. Ad-

Table 25–3. Oncogenes Activated by Retroviral Integration in Hematopoietic and Other Tumors

Oncogene	Gene Product	Retrovirus	Neoplasm
Bmi1	Polycomb group member	M-MuLV and FeLV	Mouse pre-B lymphoma and cat T lymphoma
Ccnd2 (CyclinD)	Cell cycle protein	MuLV	T lymphoma
Csfgm	Growth factor	MuLV, IAP	Myeloid leukemia and cell line
Csfm	Growth factor	MuLV	Mouse monocyte tumor
Csfmr	Growth factor receptor tyr kinase	MuLV	Mouse myeloid leukemia
Egfr/erbB	EGF receptor tyr kinase	ALV	Avian erythroleukemias
Epor	Growth factor receptor	MuLV	Mouse erythroleukemia
ets1	Transcription factor	MuLV	Rat T lymphoma line
Evi1	Transcription factor	MuLV	Mouse myeloid leukemias
Fli1	Transcription factor	MuLV	Mouse erythroleukemia
Gfi1	Transcription factor	MuLV	Rat T and B lymphoma
Hoxb8	Transcription factor	IAP	Myeloid leukemia line
Hoxa7, Hoxa9	Transcription factor	MuLV	Myeloid leukemia
IL3	Growth factor	IAP	Myelomonocytic leukemia
IL5	Growth factor	IAP	Hematopoietic progenitor
IL6	Growth factor	IAP	Plasmacytoma line
IL2rB	Growth factor receptor	IAP	T lymphoma
IL6r	Growth factor receptor	IAP	Plasmacytoma line
IL9r	Growth factor receptor	MuLV	Rat T lymphoma line
Int-2/FGF-3	Growth factor	MMTV	Mouse mammary carcinoma
Int-3	Notch family receptor	MMTV	Mouse mammary carcinoma
Lck	src-Related tyr kinase	MuLV	T lymphoma
Meis1	Transcription factor	MuLV	Myeloid leukemia
mos	Cytoplasmic ser/thr kinase	IAP	Mouse plasmacytomas
Myb	Transcription factor	MuLV	Mouse myeloid leukemias and avian bursal lymphomas
Myc	Transcription factor	ALV	Avian bursal lymphomas
		MuLV and FeLV	Mouse and cat T-cell lymphomas
Nmyc	Transcription factor	MuLV	T lymphoma
Nfe2	Transcription factor	MuLV	Mouse erythroleukemia line
p53	Transcription factor	MuLV	Erythroleukemia and non-T, non-B leukemia
Pim1	Cytoplasmic ser/thr kinase	MuLV	Mouse T and B lymphoma and erythroleukemia
Pim2	Cytoplasmic ser/thr kinase	MuLV	Mouse T and B lymphoma
Prlr	Prolactin receptor	MuLV	Rat T lymphoma
HRas and *Kras*	GTPase	MuLV	Mouse T-cell leukemia and myeloid cell line
Sfpi1	Transcription factor	MuLV	Erythroleukemia
Tiam1	Stimulator of GDP dissociation	MuLV	T lymphoma
Tpl2	Protein kinase	MuLV	Rat T lymphoma line
Wnt-1	Cell-cell communication in development	MMTV	Mouse mammary carcinoma
Wnt-2	Cell-cell communication in development	MMTV	Mouse mammary carcinoma

ditional loci have been identified to be integration sites common to more than one tumor, but the genes that are affected by these integrations remain to be identified.

Retroviruses when integrated immediately 3' or 5' to a cellular gene have been shown to cause increased transcription by providing LTR promoter and enhancer functions or enhancer functions alone. Although the majority of proviruses are integrated either within or proximal to the gene, there are examples of proviruses' activating expression of genes from a distance. A striking example is the activation of c-myc by viral DNA integration in the *Pvt-1/Mlvi-1/Mis-1* locus, which maps 270 kb away from the c-myc locus.[130] Integration within the 3' untranslated region of some genes has resulted in stabilization of mRNA, which represents another form of overexpression.

Although most activations involve overexpression of genes at the transcription level, other examples involve integration within the coding region of the gene, which can cause a structural alteration of the cellular protein. This type of change occurred in ALV induced erythroblastosis, in which proviral insertion in the avian *erbB/EGFR* gene resulted in truncation of the amino-terminal extracellular domain and constitutive activation of the tyrosine kinase activity within its intracellular domain.[2, 136] Another example is activation of the c-myb gene during retroviral integration in a murine model of monocytic leukemia. In that situation, removal of the C-Myb carboxy-terminus, which contains signals for degradation of the protein, resulted in a higher steady-state level of the protein by increasing its half-life.[137]

Activated Oncogenes in Tumors

Many cellular oncogenes have also been identified through analysis of human and animal tumors. One approach has used gene transfer techniques to test the ability of DNA from tumor cells to induce transformation similar to that of viral oncogenes.[2, 15] The other has involved the molecular analysis of specific cytogenetic abnormalities that are characteristic of certain human neoplasms, usually by identifying genes lying at or near chromosomal breakpoints.[92] The latter approach has been most useful in uncovering proto-oncogenes involved in neoplasias of the blood system. As with insertional mutagenesis by retroviruses lacking oncogenes, both of these methods have implicated proto-oncogenes that had originally been identified as the cellular homologues of retroviral oncogenes and have also uncovered previously unidentified proto-oncogenes.

Initially, DNA extracted from chemically transformed murine cell lines was shown to induce morphologically transformed cells, implying the tumor DNA contained dominant-acting transforming sequences.[138] Although DNA from non-transformed cells also gave rise to transformed foci, the frequency was much lower.[139] DNA from certain cell lines derived from human tumors was also able to induce cell transformation.[140] The oncogenes discovered in these early cases turned out to be members of the *ras* gene family (Table 25–4): Ha-*ras* from a bladder tumor cell line[13, 141] and Ki-*ras* from a lung tumor line.[14] When the DNA sequence of the transforming human *ras* genes was compared with that of the normal proto-oncogene, it was found that point mutations had occurred in the tumor-derived genes. These mutations, which affect only a limited number of amino

Table 25–4. Oncogenes Identified by Gene Transfer Techniques

Tumor-Derived Oncogenes Detected by Gene Transfer

Oncogene	Tumor	Type of Alteration
Ha-*ras*, Ki-*ras*, and N-*ras*	Human and rodent carcinomas, sarcomas, neuroblastomas, leukemias, and lymphomas	Point mutation
neu	Rat neuroblastomas and glioblastomas	Point mutation
met	Chemically transformed human osteosarcoma cell line	Recombinant fusion protein
trk	Human colon carcinoma	Recombinant fusion protein

Proto-Oncogenes Activated During the Gene Transfer Process

Oncogene	Activation Mechanism
ret	Recombinant fusion proteins
ros	Recombinant fusion proteins
raf	Recombinant fusion proteins
B-raf	Recombinant fusion proteins
dbl	Recombinant fusion proteins
vav	Recombinant fusion proteins
hst	Aberrant gene expression
fgf-5	Aberrant gene expression
mas	Aberrant gene expression

acids, rendered the mutant *ras* genes much more active biologically. Furthermore, the mutations in the transforming human *ras* genes were similar to those that activated the retroviral *ras* oncogenes. These studies served to establish a closer relationship between c-*onc* and v-*onc* and the biological mechanisms of human cancer.

Many tumor-derived oncogenes have subsequently been isolated from a wide variety of human and animal tumors; several of these genes had not been previously identified as viral oncogenes (see Table 25–4). Some of these transforming genes carried activating mutations that were present in the tumors from which the oncogenes were isolated. For example, the *neu* oncogene (also called *erbB-2*), which is a member of the EGF receptor family, contained an activating point mutation in its transmembrane coding region, leading to constitutive dimerization and activation of the Erb-2 protein.[142]

Molecular analysis of the cytogenic abnormalities in tumors has identified even more cellular oncogenes.[143] Specific karyotypic abnormalities have been noted in a high proportion of some tumor types. Examination of translocation or deletion breakpoints has revealed that many of the genes near these lesions are those present as the v-*onc* of acute transforming retroviruses (e.g., c-myc and bcr-abl). In addition, it has led to the identification of transforming genes that had not been found previously in retroviruses, such as the antiapoptotic gene bcl-2 through analysis of follicular lymphomas.[144] Translocations can cause increased expression of genes near the breakpoint, as exemplified by translocations involving c-myc (see below). However, in leukemias of both the myeloid and lymphoid lineages, the most common activating events have been shown to result in chimeric proteins with portions of the protein originating from two different chromosomes. These chimeric proteins are usually involved in transcription, although an important exception is the Bcr-Abl product described below.

Two striking examples of oncogenes activated by translocation occur in chronic myelogenous leukemia (CML), in which the Philadelphia chromosome represents a translocation between chromosomes 9 and 22, and in Burkitt's lymphoma, associated with a translocation involving chromosome 8 and either chromosome 2, 14, or 22, which are sites of the immunoglobulin genes. Molecular mapping of the sequences near the breakpoints that gave rise to the cytogenetic abnormalities in Burkitt's lymphomas indicated that the proto-oncogene c-*myc* mapped to the region of chromosome 8 that is translocated in the lymphomas. This form of lymphoma is therefore analogous to bursal lymphoma in chickens, in which c-*myc* is activated by ALV proviral insertion. In Burkitt's lymphoma, an increased level of c-*myc* expression was found in the tumor cells, as a result of the *myc* coding sequences' being placed under control of an immunoglobulin regulatory region (Fig. 25–10). Mutation within the first exon of the translocated c-*myc* gene contributed to the efficient transcription of c-*myc* coding sequences,[145, 146] and mutations in its transactivation encoding domain probably also contribute to its oncogenic activity in this disease.[147] An analogous translocation involving c-*myc*, with accompanying mutations, was also found in murine plasmacytomas.[148]

The hypothesis that translocation involving proto-oncogenes contributes to tumor formation gained further support from the discovery that in the Philadelphia chromosome a distinct *abl* protein product with constitutive kinase activity was produced in the CML cells through the fusion of *abl* coding sequences, located near the breakpoint on chromosome 9, to another gene (called *bcr*), located at the breakpoint of chromosome 22.[149, 150] As discussed in greater detail in Chapter 26, the *bcr-abl* fusion protein is remarkably

similar to the v-*abl* protein of A-MLV, in which the constitutive kinase activity is associated with fusion of c-*abl* to viral *gag* sequences.

Amplification of Proto-Oncogenes in Tumors

Gene amplification is an additional way in which proto-oncogenes have been implicated in human cancer. This phenomenon, an increase in the number of copies of a gene per cell, results in increased expression of the oncoprotein. Although gene amplification is not normally found in mammalian development or in somatic cells, situations in which selective pressure is exerted on cells (such as the development of drug resistance) can lead to amplification. As noted earlier, karyotypic abnormalities occur commonly during the progression of tumors. This tendency, coupled with selection for aggressively growing cells, may result in the amplification of genes that confer a growth advantage on cells. Amplified sequences can be found in chromosomes, often as homogeneous staining regions, or in small chromosomes lacking centromeres, termed "double minutes."

The c-*myc* gene was the first proto-oncogene found to be amplified in human tumors, originally in the promyelocytic leukemia line HL-60.[151] A roughly 10-fold increase in the number of c-*myc* copies was shown to correlate with increased transcription of this gene. Subsequent work has identified amplifications of c-*myc* in breast, lung, and stomach cancers, among others.[152] The closely related N-*myc* gene was originally identified as a gene that underwent amplification in neuroblastomas, with N-*myc* amplification in these tumors correlating strongly with a poor clinical prognosis.[153] Similarly, the L-*myc* gene was first identified by virtue of its amplification in lung carcinomas.

Other genes that are frequently found to be amplified in human cancers include *erbB/EGFR* gene, which encodes the EGF receptor, and the related *neu/erbB-2* gene.[154, 155] Overexpression of EGFR or ErbB-2 can result in cell transformation in vitro, in a ligand-dependent manner for *EGFR*[156] and in a ligand-independent mechanism for *Erb-2*.[157] Amplification of the cell cycle regulatory cyclin *D1* gene occurs in several forms of cancer; amplification of the *Cdk4* gene, which is the catalytic partner of *D1*, has been observed in sarcomas and gliomas.[158]

▼ FUNCTIONS OF THE PRODUCTS OF PROTO-ONCOGENES AND ONCOGENES

The proto-oncogene products can be grouped into several major classes, depending on their structure and function (Table 25–5). In this section, the normal functions and biochemical properties of the proto-oncogene products as well as the ways in which their oncogenic properties are unleashed are considered. Only selected examples are discussed. Some recently identified oncogenes, and their mechanism of activation, have been discussed elsewhere.[159]

Growth Factors

Since growth factors and their receptors normally regulate cell growth, it is perhaps not surprising that they each repre-

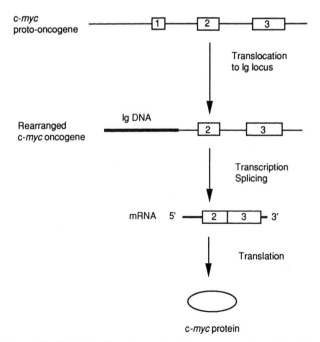

Figure 25–10. Activation of c-*myc* by Rearrangement as a Result of Chromosomal Translocation in Burkitt's Lymphoma. Most tumors display a rearrangement as depicted in the second line: The promoter and first exon of c-*myc* (which is non-coding) are replaced by a portion of the immunoglobulin locus. The strong enhancer present in the immunoglobulin DNA results in the increased expression of normal c-*myc* mRNA and protein.

sent a group of proteins encoded by proto-oncogenes (see Table 25–5). The first direct link between a growth factor and an oncogene was made in 1983, when analysis of the partial amino acid sequence of PDGF showed it shared homology with the product encoded by the v-*sis* transforming gene of simian sarcoma virus (SSV).[160, 161] Further studies of PDGF have revealed that this growth factor is composed of two related polypeptides, A and B, which are encoded by different genes. Biologically active PDGF is a dimer that can consist of A-A, A-B, or B-B type molecules. The gene encoding the PDGF B chain represents the cellular progenitor, c-*sis*, of v-*sis*. In fact, c-*sis* is transforming for those cells that are susceptible to transformation by v-*sis*, and there are no differences at the amino acid level between the mature PDGF-BB product and the v-*sis* product. A PDGF dimer can bind two PDGF receptors, thus directly fostering receptor dimerization and activation.[47]

These findings implied that v-*sis* transforms cells by inducing the overproduction of a growth factor.[162] A further implication of this mechanism was that the target cells for transformation by v-*sis* must express PDGF receptors, since v-*sis* would transform cells by forming a constitutive autocrine loop in cells that expressed the appropriate receptors. This prediction has been borne out experimentally. Fibroblasts, which contain PDGF receptors, are efficiently transformed by SSV, whereas epithelial cells, which lack PDGF receptors, are resistant to transformation by SSV. Furthermore, when cells lacking endogenous PDGF receptors were induced to express these receptors (by gene transfer techniques that introduced a cloned PDGF receptor gene under control of a strong promoter), they became susceptible to transformation by v-*sis*, which activated the tyrosine kinase activity of the PDGF receptors. These results also provided a clear mechanism for the restricted range of potential target cells for v-*sis*.

Autocrine production of other growth factor genes, in the absence of activating mutations, can also induce transformation of cells that express their cognate receptors. These include transforming growth factor α (TGF-α) and members of the fibroblast growth factor (FGF) and *wnt* families.[132, 163, 164] At least some of these factors can induce transformation when applied exogenously to cells, but the factors tend to be more active biologically when produced in an autocrine manner; that implies that they activate their receptors more efficiently by the autocrine than the paracrine route.

Although some cells are normally programmed to express a ligand and its cognate receptor in a controlled manner, the intercellular signaling function of polypeptide growth factors means that the ligand and its receptor are usually produced in different cells. This paracrine relationship between ligand and receptor may be altered in tumors to one of autocrine stimulation, leading to constitutive activation of the receptor. Autocrine production of the growth factor may occur as a primary event involving mutational activation of gene expression after insertional mutagenesis, gene amplification, or chromosomal translocation. It may also occur secondary to epigenetic changes in the regulation of growth factor expression, after activation of another oncogene, as follows *ras* gene activation.[165] Autocrine loops have been documented in human tumors; these include expression of PDGF and its receptor in sarcomas and gliomas, TGF-α and the EGF receptor (the physiological receptor for TGF-

Table 25–5. Functions of Oncogene Products

Growth Factors	
sis	PDGF B-chain growth factor
int-2	FGF-related growth factor
hst (KS3)	FGF-related growth factor
FGF-5	FGF-related growth factor
wnt-1	Growth and differentiation
Growth Factor Receptors	
Tyrosine Kinases	
ros	Membrane associated receptor-like tyrosine kinase
erbB	Truncated EGF receptor tyrosine kinase
neu/erbB-2	Receptor-like tyrosine kinase
fms	Mutant CSF-1 receptor tyrosine kinase
met	Soluble truncated receptor-like tyrosine kinase
trk	Soluble truncated NGF receptor tyrosine kinase
kit (W locus)	Truncaed stem cell receptor tyrosine kinase
sea	Membrane-associated truncated receptor-like tyrosine kinase
ret	Truncated receptor-like protein-tyrosine kinase
Other	
mas	Angiotensin receptor
Cytoplasmic Tyrosine Kinases	
src	Membrane-associated non-receptor tyrosine kinase
yes	Membrane-associated non-receptor tyrosine kinase
fgr	Membrane-associated non-receptor tyrosine kinase
lck	Membrane-associated non-receptor tyrosine kinase
fps/fes	Non-receptor tyrosine kinase
abl/bcr-abl	Non-receptor tyrosine kinase
GTPases	
Ha-ras	Membrane-associated GTP-binding/GTPase
Ki-ras	Membrane-associated GTP-binding/GTPase
N-ras	Membrane-associated GTP-binding/GTPase
gsp	G_s α subunit of heterotrimeric G protein
gip	G_i α subunit of heterotrimeric G protein
Guanine Nucleotide Exchange Factors	
Dbl	GNEF for Cdc42 and Rho
Tiam-1	GNEF for Cdc42 and Rac
Ost	GNEF for Cdc42 and Rho
Adapters	
crk	SH2/SH3 adapter
Cytoplasmic Serine/Threonine Kinases	
raf/mil	Cytoplasmic protein-serine kinase
mos	Cytoplasmic protein-serine kinase (cytostatic factor)
pim-1	Cytoplasmic protein-serine kinase
Other Cytoplasmic Kinase	
PI3K	Regulates phosphoinositols
Nuclear Transcription Factors	
myc	Sequence-specific DNA binding protein
N-myc	Sequence-specific DNA binding protein
L-myc	Sequence-specific DNA binding protein
myb	Sequence-specific DNA binding protein
fos	Combines with c-*jun* product to form AP-1 transcription factor
jun	Sequence-specific DNA binding protein; part of AP-1
rel	Related to NF-κB
ets	Sequence-specific DNA binding protein
ski	Transcription factor?
Antiapoptotic Factors	
bcl-2	

α) in carcinomas, basic FGF and its receptor in melanomas, IL-3, which is activated in a t(5,14) translocation in some pre–B-cell acute lymphoblastic leukemias.[166–168] Tumor cells also produce secretory factors that contribute to invasion and metastasis.[169, 170]

Growth Factor Receptors and Other Receptors

The possible connection between retroviral oncogenes and growth factor receptor signaling systems was first suggested by biochemical studies carried out prior to recognition of the connection between PDGF and v-*sis*. After identification of protein tyrosine kinase activity of the v-*src* and v-*abl* encoded proteins, EGF receptors were found to possess a protein tyrosine kinase activity that was induced when cells carrying these receptors were treated with EGF.[45, 171, 172] Furthermore, when EGF receptors or PDGF receptors were activated by their ligand, the pattern of cellular proteins phosphorylated on tyrosine was similar to that of those phosphorylated in v-*src* transformed cells.[173]

These results implied that a common mechanism might underlie stimulation of cell growth by diffusible polypeptide growth factors and transformation by certain v-*onc* genes. This possibility was confirmed by purification of human EGF receptors, which made it possible to determine the amino acid sequence for peptides from the receptor and to clone the *EGFR* gene molecularly.[174] Comparison of human *EGFR* coding sequence with those of viral oncogenes indicated that v-*erbB* of AEV was probably derived from the avian *EGFR* (leading to *EGFR*'s also being referred to as c-*erbB*). However, the v-*erbB* product differed structurally from the human EGF receptor. The EGF receptor contained a large extracellular ligand-binding domain at its N-terminus, a transmembrane domain, a cytoplasmic kinase domain, and a stretch of amino acids C-terminal to the kinase domain. The v-*erbB* product lacked most of the extracellular domain and some of the C-terminal amino acids; it retained the transmembrane and kinase domains of the EGF receptor (see Fig. 25–3).

Since the extracellular domain of the EGF receptor serves as a ligand-dependent switch that activates the intracellular kinase domain, its absence from the v-*erbB* product suggested that the viral protein might possess a constitutive tyrosine protein kinase activity. Consistent with this hypothesis, v-*erbB* can transform cells in a ligand-independent manner, and the phosphotyrosine containing proteins are similar in v-*erbB* transformed cells and normal cells treated with EGF.[175] Furthermore, in a strain of chickens in which ALV induces erythroblastosis, rather than bursal lymphomas, the common ALV proviral integration site was determined to lie within the *EGFR* gene. In most of the birds with erythroblastosis, the proviral insertion results in constitutive expression of an *EGFR* product that lacks the extracellular domain and has unregulated kinase.[136]

Several other v-*onc* genes also encode modified versions of growth factor receptors (see Tables 25–3 and 25–6). These v-*onc* genes share a similar structural organization in that they encode membrane-spanning regions and intracellular kinase domains that possess the ability to phosphorylate substrate proteins at tyrosine residues. As is true of v-*erbB*, transformation by other receptor-like oncogenes is thought to

involve the constitutive phosphorylation of cellular proteins, resulting in the activation of mitogenic signaling pathways within the cell, although various molecular mechanisms can lead to deregulation.[50] The proto-oncogene c-*fms*, which gave rise to the viral oncogene v-*fms* of the McDonough strain of feline sarcoma virus, was shown to encode the receptor for the hematopoietic growth factor colony-stimulating factor 1 (CSF-1), which is structurally related to PDGFR.[176, 177] Unlike the v-*erbB* product, the v-*fms* product retains its ligand-binding domain and is capable of binding CSF-1. Nevertheless, the tyrosine kinase of the v-*fms* product is constitutively active in the absence of ligand, although this activity can be further increased by exogenous ligand. A point mutation in the extracellular domain was found to be the most important genetic alteration in the conversion of c-*fms* to v-*fms*.[178] Overexpression of normal c-*fms* induces ligand-dependent transformation, but introduction of this point mutation in c-*fms* constitutively activates its encoded kinase activity and renders the protein able to transform cells in the absence of ligand.

The normal versions of several v-*onc* genes that encode receptor protein tyrosine kinases have been implicated in development and are discussed in greater detail in the section Proto-Oncogenes in Development. These include v-*kit*, which is the v-*onc* of another feline sarcoma virus. v-*kit* is derived from the feline *W* gene;[179, 180] in mice, loss of function mutations of *W* are associated with anemia, coat color alteration, and defective gonadal development. Stem cell factor (SCF), which is the ligand for the c-*kit* product, has also been identified.[181–183] The c-*ros* proto-oncogene, which was transduced as the v-*ros* oncogene of an avian sarcoma virus UR2, has been shown to be closely related to the drosophila *sev* gene, which is required for photoreceptor development in drosophila.[184]

Other receptor-like oncogenes, which had been activated by various mechanisms, were initially recognized by gene transfer experiments (Table 25–4).[185] These include *met*, which encodes the receptor for hepatic growth factor,[186] and *trk*, which encodes the high affinity receptor for nerve growth factor[187] as well as *neu/ErbB-2*, whose product is related to EGFR.[142] As with normal receptors, their activity mimics that of growth factor stimulation and depends upon dimerization, protein tyrosine kinase activity, intermolecular phosphorylation of specific tyrosine residues on the receptor, and binding of a constellation of signaling molecules to the activated receptors.[45, 46, 51]

Another mechanism of receptor activation has been identified for the BPV E5 oncoprotein, which can stimulate EGF receptors and PDGF receptors in the absence of ligand.[188, 189] E5, which is only 44 amino acids in length, forms homodimers that can induce dimerization of PDGF receptors via complex formation with the transmembrane region of the receptors.[190]

Some growth factor receptors have been implicated in human cancers, usually as the consequence of an autocrine loop. As discussed in the section on growth factors, production of both ligand and receptor occurs in several types of tumors, allowing autocrine activation. Expression of the ligand is often associated with overexpression of its cognate receptor, as for TGF-α and EGF receptors, since the high level expression of both components is usually more potent than that of only one of them. It is therefore likely that the spontaneous tumors have coordinately selected for overexpression of both ligand and receptor. Coexpression of *SCF* and *c-kit* has been identified in small cell lung cancers.[191] Overexpression of *neu/erbB-2* has also been described in breast cancers, in which it appears to be associated with a poor prognosis in some studies.[154] An interesting feature of ErB-2 is that although it has been difficult to identify an ErbB-2 specific activating ligand, ErbB-2 can form heterodimers with EGFR in response to its ligands, and the tyrosine kinase activity of these heterodimers, as well as their associated biological potency, is greater than that of EGFR homodimers.[192] Truncation of 5′ coding sequences from *TAN-1*, a homologue of the drosophila *notch* gene, which encodes a receptor-like protein, has been identified in some patients with T-cell lymphoblastic lymphoma.[193]

The multiple endocrine neoplasia type 2 (MEN 2) syndrome, which is a dominantly inherited predisposition to the development of medullary thyroid carcinoma and several benign endocrine tumors, represents a germline mutation of the *ret* proto-oncogene, which encodes a receptor protein tyrosine kinase.[194] It is an exception to the general rule that familial cancer syndromes in people usually involve mutated tumor suppressor genes or mutated genes that are implicated in prevention of DNA damage. A variety of mutations in *ret* have been identified in different MEN 2 kindreds; some involve the extracellular portion, and others involve the kinase region of the cytoplasmic domain. The various mutants have increased tyrosine kinase activity, although they range in the degree of activation. A reasonably good correlation has been found between the kinase activity and the severity of the disease in a kindred.

In contrast to the above receptors, some membrane receptors that have been implicated in tumors do not encode tyrosine kinases. As discussed in greater detail in Chapter 26, the erythropoietin (Epo) receptor is a member of this class. It can be mutated to induce Epo-independent transformation of appropriate hematopoietic target cells.[195] The Friend spleen focus forming virus (SFFV) is a replication-defective retrovirus that lacks a cell-derived oncogene but rapidly induces polyclonal splenic enlargement and can convert cell lines from Epo dependence to Epo independence. Further analysis has shown that the SFFV *env* protein, which is a truncated version of a full-length *env* protein, mimics the effects of Epo by binding to and activating the Epo receptor.[196] The non-receptor tyrosine kinases, as described in the next section, may participate in this process.[52, 197]

The *mas* oncogene, which was identified as an artifactually created oncogene in gene transfer experiments (Tables 25–4 and 25–5), encodes a receptor of the seven-transmembrane region family.[198] Subsequent study has revealed that the *mas* product represents a mutated version of the receptor for serotonin 5-HT 1c;[199] stimulation of this receptor by serotonin normally activates PLC.

Cytoplasmic Protein Tyrosine Kinases and Adapter Proteins

A large group of transforming oncogenes encode protein tyrosine kinases that lack membrane-spanning segments and thus are significantly different from the receptor-type kinases described above (see Table 25–5). Many of these transforming genes and the corresponding proto-oncogenes en-

code protein products that are associated with the inner surface of the cell plasma membrane, whereas others are predominantly cytoplasmic. Such non-receptor protein tyrosine kinases are encoded by several retroviral transforming genes including v-*src*, v-*abl*, v-*fps/fes*, v-*fgr*, and v-*yes*. A relatively large number of cellular genes that were not transduced as viral oncogenes also encode non-receptor protein tyrosine kinases. Although many cellular substrates for these enzymes have been identified,[1, 200] it is still unclear which of these targets are responsible for the wide variety of changes induced by expression of the transforming proteins. It is likely, however, that a number of substrates are involved, since these proteins induce wide-ranging effects on cells.

Within the large gene family encoding protein tyrosine kinases, c-*src* is a member of a subfamily that includes c-*yes* and c-*fgr, lck, fyn, lyn, hck,* and *blk.*[201–203] All members of the *Src* subfamily share several structural features (Fig. 25–11), including an amino-terminal membrane-binding domain; a heterogeneous region of about 70 amino acids; two non-catalytic, conserved, Src-homology domains (termed SH2 and SH3); the highly conserved kinase domain (which is considered SH1, comprises about 250 amino acids, and is present in the receptor tyrosine kinases as well); and a C-terminal regulatory region. Each of these regions plays a role in controlling the function of the proteins, as discussed below.[200, 203, 204]

As with the oncogenic versions of receptor kinases, the transforming cytoplasmic protein tyrosine kinases, such as pp60[v-src], are constitutively active enzymes, in contrast to their normal cellular counterparts, which are activated by upstream signals, such as those from receptors or focal adhesions.[205] Although many mutations contribute to the high constitutive activity of v-*src*, one consistent difference between the c-*onc* and v-*onc* proteins encoded by members of the Src subfamily is found downstream from the kinase region itself, at the extreme C-terminus of the protein. In the v-*onc* encoded proteins, these C-terminal amino acids are replaced by other amino acids. Further analysis has shown

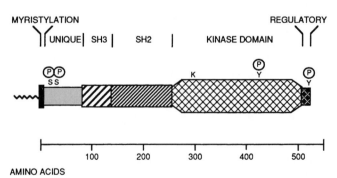

Figure 25–11. Structural Organization of the pp60[c-src] Protein (533 Amino Acids). The N-terminal 7–10 amino acids encode a myristylation domain. The unique region (which includes two sites of serine phosphorylation) varies considerably among the different members of the *Src* subfamily. The SH2 and SH3 domains direct associations of the protein with other cellular proteins and modulate the kinase activity. The kinase domain includes a lysine residue (K) at position 295 that is involved in the binding of ATP and an autophosphorylation site at tyrosine 416 that positively regulates the kinase activity. The C-terminal 19 amino acids of the protein include a tyrosine at position 527 that is phosphorylated and negatively regulates the kinase in vivo (these 19 amino acids are replaced by 12 unrelated amino acids in the v-*src* protein).

that the last dozen C-terminal amino acids encode a region that negatively regulates the kinase activity.

The most important feature of the C-terminus is a tyrosine residue conserved among many non-receptor tyrosine kinases (amino acid 527 of the c-*src* encoded protein). In the c-*onc* proteins, this tyrosine is normally phosphorylated in vivo by an Src-specific kinase, and its phosphorylation correlates with an inactive kinase. Dephosphorylation of tyrosine 527 in vitro stimulates the kinase activity of the c-*src* encoded protein,[206] and mutants of c-*src* in which this codon is changed or deleted (as in v-*src*) display greatly increased transforming function.[207]

It is relevant to note that the middle T antigen of polyomavirus apparently transforms cells via its association with c-Src and other Src subfamily members.[50, 208] This association, which activates the kinase activity of pp60[c-src], occurs through an interaction with the negative regulatory site at the C-terminus of pp60[c-src], probably via dephosphorylation of tyrosine 527. Indeed, the observations on the effects of middle T on pp60[c-src] provided the critical clue to the negative regulatory role of the C-terminal tyrosine 527 of pp60[c-src].

Another tyrosine that is subject to phosphorylation is located in the middle of the kinase domain (residue 416 of the *src* encoded protein). This tyrosine, which is found in all members of the protein tyrosine kinases, is phosphorylated, as a result of autophosphorylation, when the kinase is active.[209] In contrast to that of the C-terminal tyrosine, phosphorylation of this tyrosine increases the kinase activity of the protein.[207]

The N-terminal membrane-association domain, which specifies the covalent addition of myristic acid and palmitic acid to this region of the protein, is required for the protein to bind to the plasma membrane and for the full transforming activity of v-*src*, implying that critical substrates for pp60[v-src] may be located at the plasma membrane. The heterogeneous regions of the different proteins may be involved in the particular intracellular functions that the different members of the *Src* subfamily presumably carry out.

The SH2 and SH3 regions were originally recognized as regions of homology between v-*src* and v-*fps/fes* encoded proteins.[45] Mutation in the SH2 coding region of the v-*fps/fes* gene could drastically alter its transforming function in a way that suggested that this region of the protein might specify interactions of the v-*fps/fes* encoded kinase with substrates or regulatory molecules.[210] In addition, the SH2 regions were evolutionarily conserved in many of the non-receptor tyrosine kinases, again suggesting a functional role for this domain.[211]

A large group of cellular proteins that are not tyrosine kinases have been found to contain SH2 and/or SH3 domains, including several enzymes that play a role in signal transduction.[51, 212, 213] These include PLC-γ, a subunit of phosphatidyl inositol-3 (PI-3) kinase, and the guanosine triphosphatase (GTPase) activating protein (GAP) that interacts with the proteins encoded by the *ras* gene family (see below). A large body of work has demonstrated that the SH2 regions are involved in protein-protein associations. In particular, these regions bind to phosphotyrosine residues in other proteins.

The importance of SH2 regions in regulating protein-protein interactions became clear through the analysis of

membrane-spanning receptor tyrosine kinases.[214] Thus, when a receptor tyrosine kinase is activated by ligand binding and becomes autophosphorylated on tyrosine, SH2-containing proteins, such as PLC-γ, PI-3 kinase, and GAP, associate with the receptor by binding to the area containing the phosphotyrosine.[213, 215] These proteins in turn become phosphorylated by the receptor and may dissociate and form complexes with other SH2-containing proteins.

The signal transduction enzymes mentioned above and the cytoplasmic kinases encoded by c-*src*, c-*yes*, and *fyn* are among the proteins that associate with receptors via this mechanism.[216] In this way, a network of protein-protein associations is built up, thus helping to define the cellular response to the input signal. These findings explain why many of the SH2-containing proteins are tyrosine phosphorylated after growth factor stimulation of cells, or following transformation by tyrosine kinases such as pp60[v-src]. SH3 regions are also implicated in protein-protein interactions, via binding to certain protein rich domains.[51, 213]

The v-*crk* gene of avian sarcoma virus CT10 is relevant to the oncogenic potential of interactions mediated by SH2 and SH3 domains. The v-*crk* encoded protein requires only its SH2 and SH3 regions to function as a transforming gene.[51, 213, 217, 218] Although the v-*crk* product does not encode a kinase, v-*crk*–transformed cells contain elevated levels of phosphotyrosine, and the v-*crk* protein isolated from transformed cells is associated with protein tyrosine kinase activity.[219] Related genes, such as *nck* and *shc*, have also been identified. As with *crk*, they appear to encode SH2-SH3 domains that are not linked to any obvious catalytic activity, suggesting they may function as "adapter" proteins that interact with protein tyrosine kinases.[51, 212, 213] The presence of such adapters suggests that transformation by v-*crk* may result from disruption of a normal network of protein-protein associations regulated by SH2 and SH3 domains. Transformation by v-*crk* might also reflect alterations in the function of protein tyrosine phosphatase(s).

The functional consequence of SH2 interactions may be complex, as shown by analysis of the SH2 region of the c-*src* and v-*src* proteins. Experimental evidence suggests that the low enzymatic activity of pp60[c-src] is associated with the physical interaction between the SH2 region of pp60[c-src] and its C-terminal tail, through the phosphorylation of tyrosine 527 in pp60[c-src].[203, 204, 220] Mutations within the SH2 region tend to activate the biological and enzymatic activity of pp60[c-src], presumably by preventing the interaction between the SH2 region and the C-terminus of the protein.[221] However, if tyrosine 527 is mutated, as occurs in pp60[v-src], mutations within the SH2 region reduce its biological activity, presumably because they reduce the efficiency with which pp60[v-src] interacts with other proteins via its SH2 region. Furthermore, mutations in the SH2 region have been shown to produce a host-cell dependent transformation phenotype. Deletion of a single amino acid within a highly conserved motif in the v-*src* SH2 resulted in a protein that was highly transforming in chicken cells but was defective for rat cell transformation.[222] A similar phenotype resulted from a dipeptide insertion within the SH2 of the v-*fps* oncoprotein.[223]

Taken together, these results suggest a complicated role for the SH2 regions of the cytoplasmic protein tyrosine kinases, involving both modulation of the kinase activity and interaction with host cell substrate proteins. The latter of these functions is likely to be important for all SH2-containing proteins, as the highly conserved FLVRES amino acid motif found in all SH2-containing proteins has been shown to coordinate binding to phosphorylated tyrosine residues. Mutation of these residues in the case of the *abl* oncogene has demonstrated a correlation between binding to tyrosine phosphorylated proteins and transforming function.[224]

Non-receptor protein tyrosine kinases are believed to function in the physiological propagation of signals within the cell. Analysis of Src subfamily members has provided insights into how these molecules may function.[225] The product of the *lck* gene, p56[lck], which is expressed almost exclusively in T cells, has been shown to associate physically with the intracellular portions of the transmembrane cell surface glycoproteins CD4 (of T helper cells) and CD8 (of cytotoxic T cells). As with the Epo receptors, these receptors lack their own kinase domain. The CD4 and CD8 proteins serve as accessory molecules for the T-cell receptor and recognize elements of the major histocompatibility class (MHC) locus that are associated with antigens being presented to the T cells. These findings suggest that the binding of CD4 or CD8 to the MHC transmits a signal via alterations in the activity of the associated p56[lck]. This model for the function of p56[lck] also applies to the IL-2 receptor. Activation of this receptor by ligand results in the activation of p56[lck], which is physically associated with the receptor.[226, 227]

Tyrosine phosphorylation can be reversed by a specific class of phosphatases.[228] As with the protein tyrosine kinases, some of these phosphatases are transmembrane proteins that have a receptor-like structure, whereas others are cytoplasmic. One of the cytoplasmic phosphatases possesses two SH2 domains.[229] The tyrosine phosphatases are highly conserved in evolution, but their precise roles in the control of normal cellular processes and in oncogenesis remain to be clarified. It seems likely that they contribute to both stimulation and inhibition of cell growth. Although their activity should attenuate the growth promoting activity of tyrosine kinases, dephosphorylation of those tyrosines involved in negative regulation, such as tyrosine 527 of pp60[c-src], should have the opposite effect. One of the transmembrane phosphatases, CD45, participates in the activation of T cells by antigen. This activity of CD45 may be mediated by dephosphorylation of the C-terminal tyrosine of the *lck* protein, since this tyrosine is functionally analogous to tyrosine 527 of the c-*src* encoded protein.[228] However, it may be noted that these phosphatases have not yet been directly implicated in tumorigenesis.

Membrane-Associated G Proteins and Their Exchange Factors

Another major class of proto-oncogenes consists of membrane-associated guanine nucleotide binding proteins (see Table 25–5). All of these proteins have in common the ability to bind and hydrolyze GTP. Because they are endowed with these properties, all members of this superfamily contain certain sequence motifs required for these functions.[230, 231] The proteins of this superfamily cycle between an active GTP-bound form and an inactive GDP-bound form. They respond to stimulatory input signals by binding GTP and then hydrolyze the GTP to GDP to attenuate the signal (Fig. 25–12). Rather than encoding their own enzymatic effector function, these proteins regulate the enzymatic activities of other proteins. They participate in a wide variety of cellular processes, including ribosomal translation function, signal transduction by a number of stimuli, trafficking of vesicles, and control of growth and differentiation.

It is common to divide the G protein superfamily into three subfamilies: the prokaryotic and eukaryotic factors for translational initiation and elongation, the Ras-related (low molecular weight) GTP-binding proteins,[232, 233] and the classical or "heterotrimeric" G proteins. Only members of the latter two subfamilies, particularly the Ras proteins, have been directly implicated in oncogenesis.

The *ras* genes were first discovered as the v-Ki-*ras* and v-Ki-*ras* oncogenes of Ha-MSV and Ki-MSV, respectively. A third mammalian *ras* gene (N-*ras*) was identified through gene transfer experiments. Activated *ras* genes have been detected in a large number of gene transfer experiments from human and animal tumors.[234, 235]

The relatively small number of *ras* genes contrasts with the much greater number of growth factors and protein tyrosine kinases. Whereas the latter molecules tend to be expressed in a tissue-specific manner, the *ras* genes are widely expressed; that suggests that they serve to transduce many different extracellular signals. As discussed below, Ras can couple to a variety of signaling systems. Finding mutational activation of *ras* genes in many different forms of cancer, including a variety of hematopoietic tumors,[236] is also consistent with the hypothesis that *ras* is involved in regulating the growth of many cell types.

The normal and oncogenic *ras* genes encode 21 kDa, membrane-associated proteins (p21[ras]), which bind GTP and GDP with high affinity.[232, 233, 237] The Ras proteins can hydrolyze the bound GTP to bound GDP: The GTP-bound protein is biologically active,[238] whereas the GDP-bound form is inactive. As with other oncogenes, oncogenic *ras* genes represent gain-of-function mutants. The proportion of

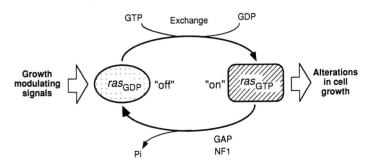

Figure 25–12. The Activation/Inactivation Cycle of p21[ras] and Its Regulation by Cellular Factors. Input signals are transmitted through activated growth factor receptors, resulting in the activation of p21 by stimulating the release of GDP by exchange factors such as Sos, inhibiting GTPase stimulators (GAP, NF1), or both. The binding of GTP to p21 allows the molecule to present its effector domain in a conformation that can be recognized by both GTPase stimulating proteins (GAP, NF1) and target (effector) molecules. The hydrolysis of GTP to GDP returns p21 to the inactive ("off") state.

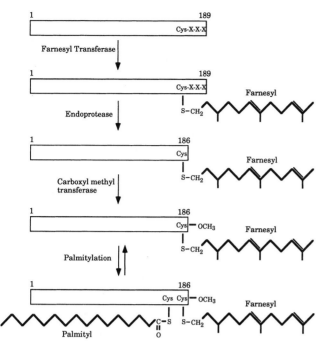

Figure 25–13. Post-Translational Processing of the Mammalian Ras Proteins. The primary translation product is a polypeptide of 189 amino acids *(top)*. Processing begins with the addition of a 15-carbon farnesyl group to the cysteine residue of the C-X-X-X motif. This step can be inhibited by antagonists of the sterol biosynthetic pathway (e.g., lovastatin). Farnesylation is followed by proteolysis of the last three amino acids and carboxymethylation of the C-terminal residue. Some, but not all, Ras proteins can undergo a reversible palmitylation at cysteine residue(s) located just N-terminal to the farnesylated cysteine *(bottom)*. Each of these steps increases the hydrophobicity of the Ras protein and enhances binding to the membrane by Ras.

normal p21^{ras} in the active, GTP-bound state is tightly regulated, representing less than 5 per cent of p21^{ras} in unstimulated cells. By contrast, the activity of oncogenic *ras* mutants, which arise via point mutations involving particular codons, is constitutive because even in unstimulated cells the majority of their mutant proteins are found in the GTP-bound form.

The three mammalian *ras* genes encode closely related proteins, with alternate splicing of c-Ki-*ras* RNA giving rise to two products that differ at the C-terminus.[233] As was the case for pp60$^{v\text{-}src}$, membrane association is critical for *ras* function: Non–membrane localized p21^{ras} is defective in transformation. Whereas membrane association in the *src* encoded proteins is achieved via addition of lipids at the N-terminus, this function is carried out by the C-terminus in p21^{ras},[239] which undergoes a series of enzymatically controlled specific post-translational modifications (Fig. 25–13). These changes include the obligatory addition of a farnesyl residue (an intermediate of sterol metabolism) to p21^{ras} via a conserved cysteine located four amino acids from its C-terminus, followed by proteolytic cleavage of the three amino acids C-terminal to the farnesylated cysteine and carboxy methylation of the cysteine.[240–244] Except for one of the two c-Ki-*ras* encoded products, one or two cysteines of the p21^{ras} proteins, upstream from the farnesylated cysteine, are covalently linked to a palmitate residue. Each modification appears to be required for full biological activity of the protein. In a mouse tumor model based on carrying an

activated *ras* transgene, regression of small tumors has been achieved by a drug that inhibits farnesyl transferase activity, with the goal of inactivating Ras by preventing its membrane association.[245]

As demonstrated from genetic analysis and X-ray crystallography, the majority of the Ras protein represents the catalytic region, which is responsible for the GTP-binding/hydrolysis activities and contains the amino acids implicated in p21^{ras} target function.[233, 246] Oncogenic mutations are located within the catalytic region of the protein. The mutations most commonly found in tumors involve codons 12, 13, and 61. Mutations at these residues impair the intrinsic GTPase activity and render the mutant Ras proteins resistant to regulation by negative regulators of Ras, Ras-GAP (for GTPase activating protein), and neurofibromin, the protein encoded by *NF1*, the tumor suppressor gene responsible for type I neurofibromatosis. Both proteins negatively regulate Ras activity by accelerating the intrinsic GTPase activity of Ras.[233, 246, 247] Ras can also be activated by mutations of residues 116 or 119, which increase the rate of guanine nucleotide dissociation from p21^{ras}.[248, 249]

The proportion of GTP-bound protein rises in response to various extracellular signals, such as PDGF or serum treatment of fibroblasts or activation of the T-cell receptor in T cells (Figs. 25–12 and 25–14).[250–252] The biological importance of these changes in p21^{ras} activity is strongly supported by evidence, obtained with genes or antibodies that specifically interfere with p21^{ras} activity, that *ras* is essential for entry into S phase and for changes in gene expression induced by a variety of growth factors and protein tyrosine kinases.[253, 254] Even viral oncogenes that encode protein tyrosine kinases usually depend upon endogenous Ras for mediating their oncogenic signals, since inhibition of Ras activity can inhibit transformation by v-*src* and related oncogenes.[232, 233, 255] In *Drosophila* photoreceptor development, the *sev* gene, which encodes a receptor tyrosine kinase, activates Ras,[256] as does the let-23 gene, which encodes a receptor tyrosine kinase in the nematode *Caenorhabditis elegans*.[257, 258] Taken together, these findings place Ras in signal transduction pathways downstream from growth factors and protein tyrosine kinases (see Fig. 25–14).

Ras activation by protein tyrosine kinases occurs primar-

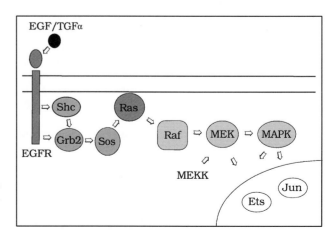

Figure 25–14. Signaling from Growth Factors to the Nucleus via the Ras/Raf/MEK/MAP Kinase Pathway. Similar pathways have also been identified in invertebrates.

ily by stimulation of a Ras-specific exchange factor, Sos, which catalyzes the exchange of GDP for GTP on Ras (Figs. 25–12 and 25–14).[233, 259] Sos is usually activated by localizing to the plasma membrane, via its forming a complex with an activated tyrosine kinase. Rather than this binding being direct between the kinase and Sos, the binding involves at least one adapter protein, Grb-2, which binds directly to Sos, and either to the tyrosine kinase, or to a second adapter protein, Shc, which in turn binds to the tyrosine kinase (see Fig. 25–14).[46, 51] These characteristics probably account for the ability of Ras to couple to so many signaling molecules, since many proteins can bind to Shc or to Grb-2.

Another important feature of Ras is that it has multiple downstream targets that activate functionally distinct pathways. Three of these are discussed here, but other potential downstream targets have also been identified.[260] The best studied immediate downstream targets are the members of the Raf family of serine-threonine kinases, which activate the MAP kinase signaling pathway (see Fig. 25–14). As discussed in greater detail in the next section, the *raf* gene was first identified as the v-*onc* of an acute transforming virus. Ras also binds and activates phosphatidyl inositol 3′ (PI3) kinase, which regulates phospholipids and signals through a different pathway.[261] An acute transforming retrovirus has recently been identified whose v-*onc* represents a constitutively active version of PI3 kinase.[262] Ras also activates the Rho family of GTPases, in part via its activation of PI3′ kinase.[261, 263] This latter family of small G proteins have been implicated in cytoskeletal rearrangement, anchorage-independent growth, and invasion.[263] Full Ras activity seems to require each of these pathways, and perhaps others as well.[260]

The *ras* genes are even more highly conserved in evolution than many other proto-oncogenes, with homologues found in *Saccharomyces cerevisiae* and *S. pombe*.[264, 265] *RAS* is required for *S. cerevisiae* to enter S phase, and *S. cerevisiae* lacking both of their *RAS* genes are non-viable. Mammalian *ras* can restore viability to yeast lacking their yeast *RAS* genes, and a mutant yeast *RAS* can induce transformation of mammalian cells, indicating that conservation of these genes is functional as well as structural. These findings suggested that determining the main target of *RAS* in *S. cerevisiae*, using the power of yeast genetics, would be directly relevant to *ras* in higher eukaryotes. However, although the modulation of adenylate cyclase represents a primary function of *RAS* in *S. cerevisiae*,[266] this function is not directly coupled to *ras* in vertebrate systems. Nevertheless, this system has represented a highly useful model for understanding many aspects of *ras* function, including the positive and negative regulation of its activity, which has many similarities with Ras in mammal cells.[267, 268]

The oncogenic potential of certain guanine nucleotide exchange factors (GNEFs) has also been established.[269, 270] Although attachment of a membrane targeting signal to Sos is sufficient to result in the focal transformation of established rodent cell lines, Sos has not been implicated in tumors, except by virtue of its normal coupling to and activation by tyrosine kinases. However, exchange factors for the Rho family of GTPases have been associated with cell transformation and rarely with tumor formation (see Tables 25–4 and 25–5).[260, 270] Depending on the GNEF in

question, it can activate one or a combination of the Rho family members, whose three prototypic members are Cdc42, Rac, and Rho. Thiam-1, which is a GNEF for Cdc42 and Rac, was identified via retroviral insertional mutagenesis in an aggressive form of T-cell lymphoma. Others, such as the *dbl* and *vav* oncogenes, have been created artifactually (see Table 25–4), and its possible role in tumors remains to be clarified.[271] Overexpression of the *dbl* proto-oncogene can transform established mouse fibroblasts, but the *dbl* oncogene, whose protein product represents an N-terminally truncated version of the normal protein, has much greater transforming activity. The *dbl* proto-oncogene represents the mammalian homologue of the *S. cerevisiae CDC24* gene, which encodes a guanine-nucleotide release factor for the yeast *CDC42* product. Mammalian Dbl has GNEF activity for Rho, as well as for Cdc42.[269, 270] The transforming activity of Dbl requires both its exchange activity, present in its catalytic domain, and it Pleckstrin homology (PH) domain, which is located immediately downstream and probably regulates the membrane association of Dbl.

Genes encoding certain heterotrimeric G proteins have also been implicated in some tumors, although the evidence is less extensive than for *ras* (see Table 25–5). As noted earlier, the heterotrimeric G proteins consist of three subunits, only one of which (the α subunit) actually binds and hydrolyzes GTP.[58, 230, 231, 272] The α subunits are approximately 40 kDa, and their activity is regulated, like that of Ras proteins, by a guanine nucleotide activation cycle. The α subunits are further regulated by their association with the other subunits, termed β and γ, and by their appropriate receptor, which is invariably a member of the seven-transmembrane class. When the receptor becomes activated, the α subunit releases its bound GDP and binds GTP, dissociates from the β-γ complex, and binds to and activates a target effector molecule. Attenuation of the signal is achieved by hydrolysis of the GTP bound to the α subunit, dissociation from the effector, and rebinding to the β-γ receptor complex. An additional layer of complexity exists in this system, for in addition to the α subunits that activate the effector enzyme (G-α_S), there are inhibitory α subunits (G-α_i) that can inhibit the same effector in a GTP-dependent manner.

The effector enzymes that respond to activated G-α subunits include adenylate cyclase, which catalyzes the formation of the second messenger cyclic AMP (cAMP); cGMP phosphodiesterase, which functions in the retina to cleave cGMP in response to light stimulation; and PLC, which hydrolyzes phosphatidyl inositol to release inositol phosphates and diacylglycerol. These enzymes all catalyze the formation of second messengers that in turn alter the activity of protein kinases and other molecules in the interior of the cell. The central position of the α subunits in pathways regulating the formation of second messengers implicated them as potential proto-oncogenes and it has been shown that this may be the case.

The first indication of an altered G-α_S function in a human tumor was the finding that a group of human growth hormone–secreting pituitary adenomas had increased adenylate cyclase activity, and that in purified membrane preparations from these cells, the cyclase activity was unresponsive to normal agonizers.[273] Molecular cloning of the G-α subunits from these tumors revealed the presence of mutations that reduced GTP hydrolysis by G-α_S, resulting in a constitutive, that is, ligand-independent, stimulation of adenylate cyclase in the tumor cells.[274] Another survey of adrenal cortex and ovarian tumors led to the discovery of mutations in a G-α_i subunit in these tumors.[275] Strikingly, some of the mutations mapped to an analogous residue to that found to be mutated in G-α_s in the pituitary tumors, implying that the mutant G-α_i subunits might also have defective GTPase function.

Serine and Threonine Kinases

Although the vast majority of protein phosphorylation in the cell occurs at serine and threonine residues, relatively few genes encoding serine and threonine kinases have been unequivocally implicated as proto-oncogenes, in contrast to the large number of proto-oncogenes that encode receptor and cytoplasmic tyrosine kinases (see Table 25–5). Among these, *raf* and *mos* have been studied in greatest detail.

Many serine and threonine kinases are involved primarily in the regulation of metabolic pathways and processes whose relationship to cell growth may be indirect. Others, such as protein kinase C, are associated with mitogen-associated signal transduction, but their role in oncogenesis remains unclear.[276] These kinases and c-*raf* are part of a group of signal transducers, which also include PI3 kinase, PLC-γ, and GAP, that are often phosphorylated and activated after activation of tyrosine protein kinases.[277]

The c-*raf* gene, which is widely expressed, is the progenitor of retroviral oncogenes present in avian and mammalian retroviruses (see Table 25–2). Two closely related cellular genes, designated A-*raf* and B-*raf*, have also been identified.[278] Their expression is more restricted than that of c-*raf*. The kinase of the c-*raf* product is inducible, whereas that of v-*raf* product is constitutively active. The v-*raf* encoded protein lacks the N-terminus of the c-*raf* product (Fig. 25–15). Systematic deletion of the 5′ end of c-*raf* has demonstrated that the N-terminus of the c-*raf* protein encodes a negative regulatory domain, the removal of which activates its transforming activity and its kinase.[279]

As noted in the previous section, c-*raf* protein functions in the transduction of mitogenic signals in normal cells,[278, 280, 281] as indicated by the finding that treatment of fibroblasts with a number of different growth factors, including EGF and PDGF, induces an increased phosphorylation of c-*raf* protein, as well as an increase in Raf kinase activity.[277, 282] Studies in lymphoid cells yielded similar results when the cells were treated with hematopoietic growth factors such as IL-2, IL-3, GM-CSF, and CSF-1.

The importance of the Raf protein in mitogenic signaling was confirmed in established mouse fibroblasts through the use of a dominant inhibitory mutant of Raf, as well as by antisense *raf* RNA.[283] Expression of the mutant prevents activation of the Raf kinase, and cells expressing the mutant are unable to transduce the mitogenic signals of serum or *O*-tetradecanoylphorbol 13-acetate (TPA) or the transforming signals from an activated Ras protein. The latter result shows that Raf is required for transmission of the Ras signal, which is known to be required for the mitogenic activity of serum. Experiments with neutralizing Ras antibodies have shown that the transforming activity of v-*raf* does not require Ras, in contrast to the dependence of tyrosine protein kinases on Ras.[255] Taken together, these observations placed Raf in the mitogenic signaling pathway, downstream from Ras (see Fig. 25–15).

Activation of the Raf kinase is extremely complex, probably because it can be partially activated by various signals.[281, 284] A main function of Ras is that its binding to Ras recruits Raf from the cytosol, where it is inactive, to the plasma membrane.[285] This membrane localization partially activates Raf, but an active tyrosine kinase, such as v-Src, can further activate Raf, apparently via phosphorylation of tyrosine 340 and/or 341 on Raf.[281] Protein kinase C (PK-C) can also contribute to Raf activation,[278] as stimulation of the Raf kinase by the T-cell receptor depends upon PK-C, as does TPA-dependent activation of Raf. The MAP kinases, also known as MEKs, are important downstream targets of Raf (see Fig. 25–14).

The structure of the PK-C serine and threonine kinases is similar to that of the Raf family (see Fig. 25–15).[56] The classical PK-Cs can be activated physiologically by calcium and diacylglycerol and pharmacologically by phorbol esters such as TPA. Although PK-Cα has been implicated in mitogenic signaling, activation of PK-C is mitogenic for some cells, and Ras activity depends upon PK-C in some cell types. However, PK-Cα has not been identified as an oncogene. Although overexpression of PK-Cα has been reported to render mouse fibroblasts more susceptible to transformation by *ras*,[286] neither wild-type nor mutant PK-Cα appears to be capable of inducing bona fide cell transformation.[287] However, other forms of PK-C have been implicated more directly in Raf activation.[288]

The *mos* oncogene, originally identified as the transforming protein of Mo-MSV, is similar to *raf* in that it encodes a cytoplasmic serine and threonine kinase.[289] However, major differences exist between c-*mos* and c-*raf*, with regard to their expression and to their protein products. Whereas the c-*raf* product is 672 amino acids in length, the c-*mos* gene encodes a much smaller protein of only 343 amino acids that lacks sequences analogous to the N-terminal regulatory domain of the c-*raf* protein. Furthermore, the v-*mos* protein product is structurally similar to the normal c-*mos* encoded protein, and their kinase and biological activities are also similar. The mechanism of activation of *mos*

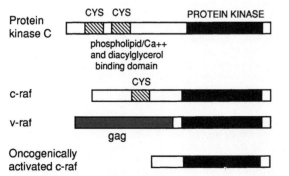

Figure 25–15. Structure of Protein Kinase C and the *raf* Encoded Protein Kinases. The amino-terminus of protein kinase C contains a calcium-binding domain with two cysteine-rich regions (CYS); binding of phospholipids to this region greatly reduces the calcium requirement for activation of the kinase. A similar structure is present in the c-*raf* encoded protein. Oncogenic forms of *raf* found in acutely transforming retroviruses (v-*raf*) or through transfection experiments *(bottom)* contain deletions of the amino-terminus.

therefore involves an increased expression of the normal kinase sequences, rather than truncation.

Expression of c-*mos* is highly restricted, limited mainly to the germ cells.[290] Elegant studies performed in *Xenopus* frog oocytes have shown that *mos* is required for the meiotic maturation of these cells, and that *mos* is a key component of "cytostatic factor," which keeps the mature oocyte arrested at the second meiotic prophase, awaiting fertilization.[291] These observations suggest that the *mos* kinase is involved in cell cycle regulation of the germ cells. Inappropriate expression of *mos* in oncogenesis therefore probably results in abrogation of fundamental cell cycle control mechanisms.

The *pim*-1 gene was detected as a target for insertional mutagenesis in murine lymphomas. It resembles *mos* in that it is also a small gene (encoding a product of 313 amino acids) that is activated by altered expression, rather than by structural mutation.[292]

Nuclear Proto-Oncogenes: Regulators of Transcription

The nucleus represents the control center for many processes that take place within the cell. The regulation of cell growth by the nucleus occurs in two fundamental ways. Most importantly, the pattern of proteins expressed in the cell is determined by nuclear events that control gene transcription, RNA processing, and transport of mature mRNA to the cytoplasm for translation.[60] In addition, DNA synthesis (S phase) as well as the events leading up to mitosis (M) are initiated in the nucleus, in response to diverse signals emanating from the cytoplasm.

Extracellular signals that induce changes in gene expression exert most of these effects through altering gene transcription, although post-transcriptional changes may also play a role. The pattern of gene transcription is controlled principally by the action of transcription factors, which act in concert with each other and with cofactors. Most transcription factors regulate expression of their target genes by interacting directly with specific DNA sequences located within the regulatory region of the gene. A typical transcription factor may be thought of as being composed of four functional regions (Fig. 25–16). One is a regulatory region, which permits the activity of the factor to be positively and negatively controlled. Another is the DNA binding region, which permits the factor to interact preferentially with the specific DNA sequences in its target gene. Most transcription factors bind DNA as oligomers (usually as dimers), which typically form prior to DNA binding. This means that a transcription factor usually has a region that permits it to oligomerize with its appropriate partners. It is common for this region to enable a monomer to form heterodimers by binding to a range of related monomers encoded by other transcription factors, although some factors may only form homodimers. In some factors this region is called a leucine zipper because of the arrangement of leucines within it.[293] The factor also has a signaling region, which contributes the activity of the factor to the transcription complex. The range of factors with which a monomer binds and the other factors present in the transcription complex offer variety and complexity in the effect a given factor may have on transcription of a particular target gene.

A subset of v-*onc* encoded proteins are located in the nucleus. These include the proteins encoded by *myc*, *myb*, *jun*, *fos*, *erbA*, *ski*, *rel*, and *ets* (see Table 25–5).[294–296] Several of these genes, as well as others, are treated in greater detail in Chapter 26 because of their involvement in hematopoietic neoplasms of man. Tables 25–2 and 25–3 also list a number of transcription factors that have been activated by retroviral insertional mutagenesis in experimental models. Although the nuclear localization of these proteins suggests a diversity of potential functions, it is becoming clear that virtually all of these oncogene products act as transcriptional regulators. This conclusion reflects the fundamental nature of transcriptional control in the regulation of cell growth. In many instances, however, most of the relevant genes whose transcription is regulated by these oncogenes remain to be identified.

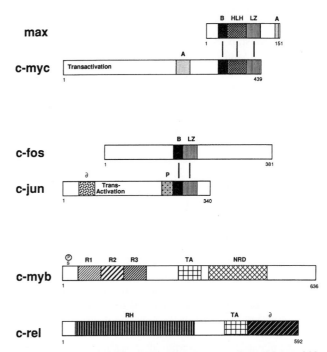

Figure 25–16. Domain Structure and Organization of Several Nuclear Proto-Oncogenes. *Top,* structure of the c-*myc* encoded protein and the associated Max protein. Vertical lines denote the presumed regions of association and DNA binding by Myc-Max heterodimers. B, basic DNA binding region; HLH, helix-loop-helix domain; LZ, leucine-zipper domain; A, acidic region. Both the HLH and LZ domains may be involved in dimer formation by these proteins. *Second from top,* structure of the c-*fos* and c-*jun* encoded proteins. These proteins also contain basic (B) and leucine-zipper (LZ) domains, which are thought to promote dimer formation and DNA binding in this case as well. The c-*jun* product contains two transactivation domains, a more N-terminal domain, and a proline-rich (P) domain near the B/HLH region. Removal of a negative regulatory region (d) of c-*jun* increases transformation by c-*jun* (d is absent in v-*jun*). *Third from top,* structure of the c-*myb* protein. A serine phosphorylation site for CKII is followed by three 52 amino acid repeat regions (R1, R2, R3) that specify DNA binding, a transactivation domain (TA), and a negative regulatory domain (NRD) toward the C-terminus. *Bottom,* structure of the c-*rel* encoded protein. A large N-terminal region of the protein comprises the *rel*-homology (RH) domain, which is conserved among c-*rel*, NF-kB, and *dorsal* proteins. This domain includes regions specifying DNA binding, dimerization, nuclear localization, and binding to inhibitory regulator proteins. The transactivation domain (TA) is found near the C-terminus, followed by a region (δ) that is deleted in v-*rel*. Removal of the δ domain, which encodes a cytoplasmic retention signal (and partially overlaps with the TA domain), activates the transforming function of c-*rel*.

The three well characterized members of the *myc* family are c-*myc*, N-*myc*, and L-*myc*.[297] The c-*myc* gene is a widely expressed early response gene whose transcription is induced within 1–2 minutes after growth arrested cells are stimulated by serum or certain growth factors. It is likely that *myc* regulates the expression of genes in early G_1 that are required for entry into S phase.[298, 299] In this regard, the mitogenic activity of the CSF-1 receptor, when expressed in quiescent fibroblasts, has been shown to depend upon c-*myc* expression.[300]

The *myc* genes are aberrantly expressed in a wide range of malignant tumors, as noted earlier.[152] Although some activated *myc* genes contain mutations in their protein coding sequences, increased (or inappropriate) expression accounts for most of their oncogenic properties. All *myc* genes encode similar phosphoproteins of approximately 60 kDa (see Fig. 25–16).[301] The N-terminal domain of Myc contains a transcriptional transactivation domain. Farther toward the C-terminus is a nuclear localization signal, followed by a series of domains that include a basic region, a helix-loop-helix (HLH) region, and a leucine zipper motif. The basic domain is involved with Myc binding to specific DNA sequences; the HLH and zipper domains direct protein-protein interactions that are required for Myc to dimerize and function as a transcriptional transactivator. Another 21–22 kDa protein, Max, can associate with the Myc, via the HLH and zipper domains, to form heterodimers.[302–304] In contrast to Myc homodimers, which have little DNA-binding activity, the heterodimers bind DNA with greater affinity and function as potent transcriptional activators. Homodimers of Max are inactive in transcriptional activation because these proteins lack the activation domain found in the N-terminus of Myc.

Whereas the Myc proteins have a relatively short half-life and can be induced by the treatment of cells with certain mitogens, the Max proteins are much more stable. Thus the cell can regulate the amount of transcriptionally active Myc-Max heterodimers in response to extracellular signals, with the concentration of c-*myc* (or L-*myc* or N-*myc*) encoded protein in the cell determining its ability to function as transcriptionally active heterodimers.[305] Despite their central role in normal proliferation and in many tumors, Myc target genes are only now being identified.[299] One potentially important target appears to be the *cdc25A* gene, which positively regulates the cell cycle by activating Cdk2.[306]

A dramatic example of convergence in the fields of molecular biology and molecular oncology was provided by studies on AP-1, Fos, and Jun.[295, 296] AP-1 was originally identified as a TPA-inducible DNA binding activity that stimulated transcription of the simian virus 40 (SV40) enhancer. Upon further investigation, both of the major proteins present in purified AP-1 were found to be encoded by proto-oncogenes: c-*jun*, the progenitor of the v-*jun* transforming gene of avian sarcoma virus 17, and c-*fos*, the progenitor of the v-*fos* gene of the FBJ murine osteosarcoma virus.[307] Mutations in the v-*fos* encoded protein leave it constitutively in the nucleus, whereas the nuclear localization of c-*fos* may depend on extracellular signals.[308] However, both c-*fos* and c-*jun* can be activated as transforming genes by overexpression of the non-mutated genes.

In a large number of different cell types c-*fos* and c-*jun* can be rapidly induced by a variety of stimuli, including growth factors, and are thus immediate early response genes.[38, 309] Ras and Raf also induce c-*fos* expression,[310, 311] and suppression of Jun or Fos activity inhibits transformation by Ras; that suggests that Fos and Jun are required for full transformation by oncogenes encoding non-nuclear proteins.[312, 313]

As with the other nuclear oncogenes, cells contain multiple *jun*- and *fos*-related genes. Each *fos* and *jun* gene encodes a protein capable of dimerization and specific binding to the DNA sequence originally identified as the AP-1 binding site.[314] Structural analysis of the c-*jun* encoded protein, which is 340 amino acids, revealed that its C-terminus contains a leucine zipper (for dimerization), a basic region (for specific DNA binding), and a proline-rich transactivation domain (see Fig. 25–16). The N-terminus of the protein contains a regulatory domain that is absent in the v-*jun* product. Phosphorylation of the N-terminal region, which is associated with increased DNA binding and transcriptional activity, can be induced by Ras and MAP kinase, suggesting that this phosphorylation by upstream signals activates the Jun protein.[315, 316]

The c-*jun* proteins can form homodimers that are transcriptional activators or can associate with c-*fos* proteins to form heterodimers that transactivate at least as efficiently as the homodimers. The structure of the c-*fos* protein (381 amino acids) is similar, but not identical, to that of the c-*jun* product in that the protein contains the basic and zipper domains, but these domains are found in the middle of the *fos* protein (see Fig. 25–16). A major difference between the *fos* and *jun* encoded proteins is that the *fos* products are unable to form stable homodimers. Thus, transformation by the v-*fos* encoded protein is dependent on the formation of heterodimers (via the zipper domains) with c-*jun* products to activate transcription. The Fos and Jun proteins also form heterodimers with the more distantly related transcription factors of the cyclic AMP responsive element binding (CREB) factors family, whose DNA binding sequence is similar, but not identical, to that of AP-1.[317, 318] This diversity of interactions presumably serves to fine tune the transcriptional activity of the target genes regulated by these factors.

The v-*myb* gene was first characterized as the transforming gene of avian myeloblastosis virus as described in the literature.[319] The c-*myb* gene has also been activated by ALV and MLV proviral mediated insertional mutagenesis.[320] The c-*myb* gene is a member of a multigene family encoding nuclear phosphoproteins with sequence-specific DNA binding activity.[321] In hematopoietic systems, including lymphoid, myeloid, and erythroid, c-*myb* expression is restricted to immature cells and is downregulated during differentiation. In contrast to many other oncogenes, v-*myb* is not transforming for fibroblasts. Myb functions in proliferation, antiapoptosis, and differentiation. Although its ability to drive proliferation is likely the most important capacity of Myb in tumorigenesis, its ability to prevent apoptosis and perhaps to block differentiation may also contribute to its induction of neoplastic disease.

The c-*myb* encoded protein (see Fig. 25–16), 636 amino acids in length, is highly conserved, with a structural homologue present in yeast.[322] Transcriptional transactivation can be demonstrated for the c-*myb* product in yeast or mammalian cells.[323, 324] An N-terminal DNA binding domain is followed by a centrally located transactivation domain, as shown in Fig. 25–16. A transcriptional modulatory region lies within the C-terminus. It contains phosphorylation sites and a potential protein interaction domain involved in negatively affecting ability of c-Myb to regulate promoters containing Myb binding sites. Removal of the C-terminus, which occurs in some tumors, also results in increased protein stability.[137] However, in the majority of cases, activation of c-*myb* by retroviral insertional mutagenesis involves promoter insertion.[320] This causes the transcription factor to be constitutively expressed even when the cells are differentiating and c-*myb* is normally downregulated.

The *rel* gene represents yet another multigene family of transcriptional regulators with a member that was transduced as a retroviral oncogene. The v-*rel* gene encodes the oncogene product of the Rev-T virus, which causes reticuloendotheliosis in turkeys and B-cell lymphomas in chickens.[325] The c-*rel* gene has a close homologue (for half of the coding region) in the drosophila gene *dorsal*, which controls the establishment of dorsal-ventral axis in the developing embryo. The vertebrate c-*rel* gene is a member of the NF-κB gene family of transcription factors. The transcriptional activity of the proteins encoded by this gene family is regulated by their subcellular localization. Inactive *rel* proteins are sequestered in the cytoplasm by complexing with an inhibitory protein.[326] Their translocation to the nucleus is a prerequisite for their action as transcriptional regulatory factors. Once in the nucleus Rel proteins can both activate and repress transcription under appropriate circumstances. Compared with c-*rel*, the v-*rel* product lacks a large portion of the C-terminal, cytoplasmic-anchoring domain (see Fig. 25–16). On the basis of these findings, v-*rel* has been proposed to transform cells by altering either the regulation of c-*rel* or gene activation by c-*rel*/NF-κB complexes.[327]

Homeobox genes, originally discovered in developmental regulation in *Drosophila*, are strong candidate genes for the regulation of hematopoiesis.[328] Therefore, it is not surprising that activations of transcription factors encoded by these genes have been discovered in models of leukemogenesis.[329] The retrovirus-induced overexpression probably perturbs competency to execute specific differentiation programs. Retrovirally mediated overexpression has been observed for Hoxa7, Hoxa9, or Hoxb8 in murine myeloid tumors (see Table 25–3). There is also frequent activation of a *pbx*-like homeobox gene *(Meis1)* in leukemias with integration in the *Hoxa7* and *Hoxa9* loci, indicating that there can be cooperation between the genes that regulate differentiation.

Cell Cycle and Antiapoptotic Genes

In addition to transcription factors, inappropriate expression of certain cyclins and Cdks, whose role in cell cycle control has been described earlier, has been implicated in some tumors. Their overexpression may help override normal checkpoints of the cell cycle. The *D1* cyclin has been identified as being the most proximate gene on chromosome 11 in the *bcl-1* t(11,14) translocation in patients with CLL.[330] This gene is also amplified and overexpressed in patients with breast cancer and squamous cell cancers of the head and neck.[331] It is overexpressed in parathyroid adenomas, in which analysis of the breakpoints of chromosome 11 inversions in the adenomas has shown that the *D1* coding sequence is juxtaposed to the regulatory region of the parathyroid hormone promoter.[332] In transgenic mice, *D1* has been shown to cooperate with c-*myc* in the induction of lymphomas.[333] A common proviral integration site, *vin-1*, in murine retrovirus induced T-cell leukemias of mice and rats leads to the constitutive expression of *D2* cyclin.[334] Also, the cyclin A gene has been identified as the target for hepatitis B DNA integration in a hepatocellular carcinoma.[100]

Genes that inhibit apoptosis may also be considered potential oncogenes. Indeed, as noted earlier in the chapter, the antiapoptotic gene *Bcl*-2 was originally identified because it was activated via a translocation commonly found in follicular lymphomas.[144] As with cyclin *D1*, a *Bcl*-2 transgene can cooperate with a c-*myc* transgene in the development of murine lymphomas.[71]

Proto-Oncogenes in Development

The evolutionary conservation of proto-oncogenes and their crucial role in normal cell growth suggested that they would participate in embryonic and postembryonic development. Many of these genes have been found to occupy roles in the processes that control development and cell differentiation.[335–338] An in-depth treatment of this topic is far beyond the scope of this chapter, but some approaches and a few specific examples are briefly described.

The molecular identification of genes responsible for naturally occurring mutants represents one approach.[339] As discussed earlier, analysis of the v-*kit* oncogene led to identification of the genes at the white-spotting *(W)* and steel *(Sl)* loci of the mouse.[179–181] Mutations at either the *W* or *Sl* locus are associated with impaired development of hematopoietic, gonadal, and pigment cell lineages, and many naturally occurring mutant alleles at these genetic loci have been identified. Transplantation and coculture experiments involving hematopoietic stem cells and marrow stromal cells from *W* and *Sl* mutants indicated that the defect in *W* mutants is intrinsic to the hematopoietic stem cells, and the defect in *Sl* mutants lies in the stromal cells. These experiments therefore suggested that the *Sl* locus made a factor that stimulated growth of hematopoietic stem cells (and presumably of gonadal and pigment cell precursors as well). The phenotypic similarity between *W* and *Sl* mutants suggested that the *W* locus might be required for the stem cells to respond to the putative *Sl* factor.

The recognition that the c-*kit* encoded protein had the structure of a receptor protein tyrosine kinase, combined with its tissue-specific expression, suggested that c-*kit* might represent the *W* gene. Analysis of different *W* mutants confirmed that the c-*kit* gene was mutated in each instance.[179, 180] The functional consequences of these mutations for the c-*kit* protein include impaired tyrosine kinase activity and failure to synthesize stable protein; these abnormalities have begun to provide insight into the molecular basis for the phenotypic differences associated with various *W* alleles.[340] The recognition that c-*kit* represented the gene at the *W* locus suggested that the putative factor made by the *Sl* locus might be the ligand for the c-*kit* encoded protein. This hypothesis was confirmed by purification of the ligand (SCF) from cells whose culture fluid specifically stimulated cells expressing c-*kit* and by molecular cloning of the gene encoding SCF.[181] As the result of alternate RNA splicing, SCF is expressed as secreted and cell-associated forms; impairment of the cell-associated form is required for the *Sl⁻* mutant phenotype.[341]

The deliberate functional inactivation of proto-oncogenes by gene targeting represents a more direct approach for the assessment of their roles in development.[337, 342] Targeted disruption has now been carried out in the mouse for many proto-oncogenes.

As discussed in earlier sections of the chapter, additional approaches involve the identification of close homologues of proto-oncogenes, or new genes, in simple species such as yeast, *Drosophila*, and the nematode *C. elegans*.[338, 343] The genes can be rapidly analyzed and manipulated in these models.[344] Because the signaling pathways and growth regulation are highly conserved between mammals and lower eukaryotes, the pathways in these model organisms may be directly relevant to mammalian cells. Examples of such conserved pathways are found in development of the R7 photoreceptor cell of the fly and vulval development in the nematode.[257, 345] Pathways that are remarkably similar to the receptor-MAP kinase pathway shown in Figure 25–14 have been identified in both systems. Some of the genes in the pathway were first identified in the model system, leading directly to their subsequent identification in mammals.[256, 257, 345, 346]

Tumor Suppressor Genes

▼ IDENTIFICATION OF TUMOR SUPPRESSOR GENES

Tumor suppressors represent a class of genes that contribute to tumorigenesis through their inactivation (loss of function), in contrast to oncogenes (Table 25–6).[16, 17] This feature suggests that tumor suppressor genes normally serve as negative regulators of cell growth.[347] The tumor suppressor genes, their functions, and the tumors in which they have been implicated have recently been considered in detail.[4] The number of identified tumor suppressor genes continues to expand rapidly, and this section highlights only some of them.

Prior to the molecular identification of tumor suppressor genes, evidence for the existence of such genes came from the analysis of somatic cell hybrids.[348] When tumorigenic cells were fused with normal cells, the hybrids were found to be non-tumorigenic; that finding implied that the tumor cells were lacking a function that could be replaced by the normal cells. Further analysis revealed that the tumor suppressing activity could be localized to specific chromosomes. In some instances, hybrids made between two differ-

ent tumor cell lines were non-tumorigenic, suggesting the existence of multiple recessive tumor suppressor genes. By using microcell fusion, a refined technique by which single chromosomes can be transferred to recipient cells, it has been possible to identify specific regions of chromosomes that harbor tumor suppressor genes. These techniques provided an experimental basis for the belief that cells contained tumor suppressors, but they did not lead directly to the identification of specific genes.[349]

Studies on the inheritance of familial cancers represented another approach that supported the notion that cells contained tumor suppressor genes. Defects in tumor suppressor genes have turned out to be responsible for many of the familial cancer syndromes that are dominantly inherited.

Retinoblastoma was the first of these conditions to be analyzed in detail, and it has turned out to be a paradigm for the identification of tumor suppressor genes. The analysis of familial and sporadic cases of retinoblastoma led Knudsen to propose his "two-hit" hypothesis, which postulated that this form of cancer only developed after two independent loss-of-function mutations.[350] In familial cases, approximately one half of the children in a family have the disease, consistent with inheritance of a single, genetically dominant susceptibility allele, and many afflicted children have independent primary tumors in each eye at an early age. In sporadic cases of retinoblastoma, only a single tumor develops and the average age of onset is older than in familial cases. These characteristics suggested that the genetic basis for the familial form of the disease might be accounted for by inheritance of a defective allele in a critical gene, with retinoblastomas developing after mutational inactivation of a second normal allele (Fig. 25–17). In sporadic cases, the two critical alleles would be normal at birth, so two independent somatic mutations would be required to inactivate both alleles before a retinoblastoma would develop. Since two independent events are much less likely than a single one, this would account for the later onset and unilateral nature of the disease in sporadic cases.

Although this hypothesis was in fact correct, it could not predict the nature of the molecular defects involved in the development of retinoblastoma. For example, the mutations could have involved the activation of two different proto-oncogenes. Instead, subsequent studies have firmly established that both of the genetic lesions involved in retinoblastoma are mutations that inactivate alleles of the same cellular gene, designated *RB* (see Fig. 25–17).

The molecular identification of *RB* was accomplished by positional cloning.[351] This approach involves mapping the phenotype (such as retinoblastoma) to a particular chromosomal location through analysis of affected and unaffected

Table 25–6. Examples of Tumor Suppressor Genes

Gene	Cancer Syndrome	Principal Tumors	Mode of Action
RB1	Retinoblastoma	Retinoblastoma osteosarcoma	Transcriptional regulator/factor
p53	Li-Fraumeni syndrome	Sarcomas, breast and brain tumors	Transcription factor
NF-1	Neurofibromatosis	Neurofibromas, sarcomas, gliomas, myeloid leukemia	Regulates Ras
APC	Familial adenomatous polyposis	Adenomatous polyps, colon cancer	Regulates β catenin function
p16	Familial melanoma and pancreatic cancer	Melanoma, pancreatic cancer	Cyclin-dependent kinase inhibitor
VHL	von Hippel-Lindau syndrome	Renal cell carcinoma	Inhibits transcription elongation
hMSH2	Hereditary non-polyposis colorectal cancer	Colon cancer	Nucleotide mismatch repair

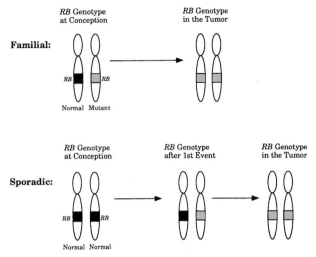

Figure 25–17. Development of Retinoblastoma Through the Mutational Inactivation of RB Function. In the familial form of the disease, the patient inherits one mutant allele and one wild-type (normal) allele. Tumor formation arises after the remaining normal allele is inactivated by a gene conversion event resulting in a homozygous mutant genotype or by a second independent somatic mutation. The sporadic form of the disease occurs when a somatic mutation of one of the normal RB alleles is followed by an inactivation of the second allele, again resulting in a tumor.

family members, cloning the sequences in that region of the chromosome, and identifying a gene within the region in which mutations consistently correlate with the phenotype. The chromosomal localization of *RB* began with the observation that even normal cells from patients with familial retinoblastoma bore deletions in the q14 band of chromosome 13. A similar analysis of sporadic retinoblastoma patients revealed that the same region of chromosome 13 was frequently deleted in the tumor cells, but not the normal cells of these individuals.[352] The next step was identification of a gene in the 13q14 region (the gene encoding esterase D), which served as a linked genetic marker for susceptibility to retinoblastoma,[353] allowing an estimate of its distance from the retinoblastoma susceptibility gene.

The actual identification of the *RB* gene was accomplished by molecular cloning sequences from the 13q14 region that were absent in retinoblastoma patients. Then, DNA segments from adjacent regions of the chromosome and complementary DNAs (cDNAs) were screened for evolutionary conservation and differential expression between normal retinal tissue and tumors.[354–356] These analyses led to the identification of *RB*, which encodes a 928 amino acid protein designated pRB. Retinoblastomas contain internal deletions within this gene, and retinoblastoma lines fail to express pRB.[357]

One of the novel findings arising from the search for the *RB* gene was the nature of the "second hit" at the *RB* locus. Rather than identifying a completely independent second mutation, investigators found that the normal allele was often replaced by a duplicated copy of the mutant allele, as a result of chromosomal non-disjunction, gene conversion, or mitotic recombination. This phenomenon is usually manifested as a loss of heterozygosity when adjacent chromosomal loci (e.g., esterase D) are assayed.[358] Evidence of loss of heterozygosity, usually by Southern blot analysis of restriction fragment length polymorphism (RFLP) in affected

individuals, is now widely used in the mapping of other tumor suppressor loci in a variety of tumor types.

As with many proto-oncogenes, *RB* appears to be expressed in all tissues. However, patients with familial retinoblastoma seem to be at increased risk of development of osteosarcomas, but not other tumors. In the general population, mutations in *RB* have been identified in most cases of small cell carcinoma and some carcinomas of the bladder and breast, in addition to retinoblastomas and osteosarcomas.[17] It remains to be determined what accounts for the association of only certain tumors with alterations in *RB*. Presumably loss of *RB* function in these cell types has greater oncogenic potential than its loss in other cell types.

Gene isolation techniques similar to those just described for the isolation of *RB* are now widespread and have been successfully applied to isolate other tumor suppressor genes (see Table 25–6). Their function is described below.

In contrast to the elegant genetic analyses used to identify *RB* and many other tumor suppressor genes discussed above, identification of *p53* as a tumor suppressor gene occurred via a circuitous route.[359] Study of the *p53* gene began with the observation that a nuclear phosphoprotein of 53 kDa associates with the large T antigen of SV40 in cells transformed by this virus.[360] This association suggested that the p53 protein might play a role in transformation by large T and led to purifying of p53 and cloning of the gene. When the resulting molecular clones encoding p53, which has been isolated from transformed cells, were tested for their biological activity, the *p53* gene was found to immortalize primary cells and functionally substitute for *myc* in *myc* + *ras* cotransformation assays of primary rodent fibroblasts.

Although these results therefore suggested that *p53* was a proto-oncogene, subsequent work showed that molecular clones of *p53* from normal tissues did not function in the transformation assay and that the earlier clones that had been used contained missense mutations in conserved regions of the gene. The non-mutated *p53* clones were actually found to suppress transformation of primary cells by the cooperation of *ras* and either *myc*, adenovirus *E1A*, or mutant *p53*.[361] These findings implied that normal *p53* was an inhibitor of cell growth and that the point mutations identified in *p53* isolated from tumors had functionally inactivated the gene. The designation of *p53* as a tumor suppressor gene was firmly established by finding tumors in which *p53* alleles were absent or clearly inactive.[362]

The *p53* gene is located on the short arm of chromosome 17, where loss of heterozygosity of markers has been associated with many different tumor types. In most instances, this loss of heterozygosity has been mapped to the *p53* gene, with point mutation of evolutionarily conserved codons the most frequent genetic alteration. Of genes known to be involved in human cancer, *p53* is the most commonly altered; abnormalities have been identified in tumors of the bladder, colon, liver, lung, brain, breast, and some leukemias, among others.[16, 363] In addition, the Li-Fraumeni syndrome, a dominantly inherited condition that predisposes affected individuals to several forms of malignancy, has been associated with inactivating germline point mutation of one *p53* allele.[364–366] The normal *p53* allele is inactivated in the tumors that develop in these patients, as with *RB* in familial retinoblastoma.[367] Although patients with Li-Fraumeni syndrome have a higher than expected incidence of several types of malignancy, including breast and brain tumors, it remains to be explained why the range of tumors in Li-Fraumeni syndrome is much narrower than the many different tumor types in which *p53* mutations have been reported.

▼ FUNCTIONS OF TUMOR SUPPRESSOR GENES

RB

RB encodes a 105 kDa nuclear phosphoprotein pRB.[368] The degree of phosphorylation of pRB fluctuates with the cell cycle: high in S and reaching its lowest level during the interval between the end of M and the beginning of G_1. As noted in the section on DNA tumor viruses, an important breakthrough in understanding pRB function came from the recognition that pRB binds to the oncoproteins of several DNA tumor viruses, including adenovirus E1A, SV40 large T, and E7 of certain HPVs (see Fig. 25–6).[19, 108, 369] The observation that SV40 large T complexes preferentially with the hypophosphorylated form of pRB[370] provided the first evidence that the growth inhibitory function of pRB was limited to its hypophosphorylated forms; and implied that hyperphosphorylation of pRB in G_1 led to its inactivation. As discussed in the section devoted to the cell cycle, pRB restrains cells from progressing through G_1 by inhibiting transcription of E2F-dependent target genes and is inactivated by Cdks via hyperphosphorylation during cell cycle progression (see Fig. 25–2).[28] Also pRB binds to several other proteins, which may also represent targets for its activity.[30] The other members of the pRB family, p107 and p130, seem to function similarly to pRB, so it is unclear why their inactivation has not been implicated in human tumors.[29]

p53

The ubiquitous expression of *p53*, its potent growth inhibitory activities, and its inactivation in a variety of tumors all suggested that this gene would serve an essential developmental function. Surprisingly, however, mice carrying disrupted null alleles of *p53* develop normally, but *p53* negative mice develop various tumors at an early age.[371] These experimental observations suggest that a major function of *p53* may be to prevent the development of certain tumors.

Beyond its involvement in the Li-Fraumeni syndrome, *p53* is the most commonly mutated gene in tumors, affected in at least one half of all malignancies, including leukemias.[363, 372] In some tumors, *p53* mutation correlates with a poorer prognosis and resistance to chemotherapy. One striking feature of *p53* is that a point mutation at one of

many different codons can inactivate the protective activities of the wild-type gene. The variety of point mutations that lead to this phenotype, combined with its pleotropic role in protecting cells from potentially tumorigenic changes, as discussed below, probably account for the high frequency with which *p53* is targeted for mutation in cancers.

The p53 protein is a transcriptional regulator that functions as a tetramer (Fig. 25–18) and has many target genes whose transcription it regulates. These include *Bax*, a proapoptotic gene; *WAF1/Cip1*, whose product is a potent inhibitor of Cdk4; and *Mdm2*, a proto-oncogene whose product forms an autoregulatory loop with *p53* by mediating its degradation.[373, 374]

One mechanism by which it interferes with tumor formation is to help maintain the integrity of the cellular genome.[93, 373, 375, 376] *p53* is frequently activated, biochemically and by increased de novo expression, in response to various forms of cellular insults, such as exposure to chemicals or radiation, leading to cell cycle arrest at G_1 and/or G_2 checkpoints.[373, 375, 376] The growth arrest allows the cell to recover from DNA damage through repair mechanisms, thereby reducing the frequency of somatic mutations that could be passed to subsequent cell generations. In addition to serving a critical role in mediating the growth arrest described above, *p53* expression can, in other abnormal contexts, interfere with potentially oncogenic changes by contributing to the induction of apoptosis or senescence. Cells whose *p53* gene function has been inactivated are deficient in all these activities, thus promoting mutations, genomic instability, and resistance to apoptosis.

Depending on the codons involved, three distinct classes of mutant *p53* proteins have been identified. Some function as biologically null, others as dominant inhibitory mutants that interfere with normal *p53* function by complexing with and inactivating the product of the normal *p53* allele (see Fig. 25–18), and a third class behaving as dominant inhibitory mutants that in addition have their own oncogenic activity beyond their ability to inhibit normal *p53*, since they have a transforming phenotype in cells that lack normal *p53*.[377] Since most *p53* mutants have a much longer half-life than the wild type protein, probably because the mutant proteins are resistant to Mdm2-dependent degradation, they can efficiently inhibit the normal *p53*.

NF-I

NF-1 disease is another dominantly inherited disorder, affecting about 1 in 3500 individuals. Approximately 50 per cent of cases appear to represent new mutations, indicating that

Figure 25–18. Mutant p53 Disrupts the Function of Wild-Type p53. *A,* Normal p53 proteins form oligomers that bind to the cellular DNA and alter transcription. *B,* The protein encoded by a mutant *p53* gene has a much longer half-life, so that the level of mutant protein greatly exceeds the level of wild-type protein in the cell. This protein can still form oligomers but no longer binds DNA. Thus it acts as a dominant negatively blocking the function of the wild-type encoded protein. *C,* The presence of two mutant *p53* genes leaves the cell without normally functioning oligomeric complexes.

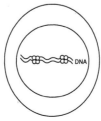
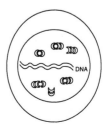
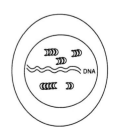

A. Two wild-type p53 genes   B. One mutant and one wild-type gene   C. Two mutant p53 genes

O = wild-type p53   ⊃ = mutant p53

the locus has a high rate of spontaneous mutation. Patients with NF-1 disease are at increased risk of development of pheochromocytomas and a narrow group of malignant tumors that are classified as schwannomas or neurofibrosarcomas; these tumors are associated with mutation of the normal *NF-1* allele. *NF-1* is very large, spanning more than 200 kb; its size may contribute to its high spontaneous mutation rate.[378, 379] Its encoded protein, neurofibromin, is 2818 amino acids in length.

As noted in the section on the *ras* proto-oncogene, the *NF-1* gene is a negative regulator of Ras (see Fig. 25–12). In cell lines derived from malignant schwannomas, an abnormally high proportion of Ras was found to be in the active, GTP-bound form, although the Ras protein in the cell lines was not mutated.[380, 381] The portion of neurofibromin that is responsible for the negative regulation of Ras represents only about 10 per cent of this large protein. The functions of the remainder of the protein have not been clearly identified. One possible clue is that neurofibromin has been found to associate with cytoplasmic microtubules, although the biological significance of this association has not yet been clarified.[382]

APC

The *APC* gene, which is located at chromosome 5q21, encodes a very large 2843 amino acid product whose sequence is related to structural proteins such as intermediate filaments. The gene is interrupted by mutations in patients with familial adenomatous polyposis coli, as well as in some sporadic cases of colorectal carcinoma.[383, 384] The majority of these mutations result in premature termination of the polypeptide chain. As with most tumor suppressor genes, inactivation of the normal *APC* allele is required to manifest pathological consequences. As with many other tumor suppressor genes, a mouse model of this disease has been identified. The dominantly inherited susceptibility of the mice to multiple intestinal neoplasia has been genetically localized to a germ line mutation in one allele of the murine *APC* gene.[385]

Insight into the function of APC has been obtained through identification of β catenin as a binding partner for APC and the finding that this binding can be regulated.[386] Although β catenin is implicated in cell adhesion, it can also stimulate cell growth when it translocates to the nucleus and forms a complex with the transcription factor LEF-1, when it can act as an oncogene.[387] Detailed examination of APC mutants has indicated that their binding to β catenin is impaired. Furthermore, many spontaneous colorectal cancers in which the *APC* gene is normal have mutations in β catenin, which impair its binding to APC.[388] Thus, negative regulation of β catenin represents an important function for APC, and loss of this binding leads to activation of the growth stimulatory properties of β catenin.

Ink4a

Some patients with familial melanoma have been found to have mutations at chromosome 9p21 that involve the *Ink4a* locus discussed in the section dealing with the cell cycle. This complex locus encodes two products, p16 as well as p19ARF.[389] It is believed that the lesions in melanomas are mainly restricted to p16. The *Ink4a* locus, or the related *Ink4b* locus, is mutated in a variety of sporadic tumors, including some hematopoietic malignancies.[390] The p16 protein is a Cdk inhibitor that acts during G_1. The p19ARF protein is also implicated in cell cycle control, but via its influencing the interaction between p53 and Mdm-2. p19ARF increases the activity of p53 by preventing Mdm-2 from inducing p53 degradation. Inactivation of this locus can therefore have profound effects on abrogation of cell growth.

VHL

The von Hippel-Lindau (VHL) syndrome is a dominantly inherited susceptibility to renal carcinoma and less commonly to cancers at other sites. The *VHL* gene, which encodes a 213 amino acid protein, is located at chromosome 3p25.[391] It is also mutated in sporadic kidney tumors. In both sporadic and familial tumors, a large percentage of the VHL mutations encode missense mutants. As with APC, insight into the function of the VHL protein has come from identification of proteins with which it interacts. The normal VHL protein was found to bind two proteins, elongin B and elongin C, both of which are involved in regulating transcriptional elongation, and missense mutants were deficient in binding.[392, 393] The active complex that stimulates transcription is composed of elongins A, B, and C. Since the binding of VHL to elongins B and C, which are regulatory subunits, prevents their forming a complex with the active subunit elongin A, these results support a model in which VHL acts to inhibit transcription elongation. It remains unclear precisely how release of this inhibition by *VHL* mutation leads to transformation, but potential target genes, such as vascular endothelial growth factor, whose expression is increased by VHL mutations, have been identified.[394] The normal VHL protein appears to shuttle between the cytoplasm and nucleus, having the cytoplasmic location when cells are at low density in growth phase, and the latter when they are at high density and have ceased growing.[395] From these findings, it is tempting to speculate that the cytosolic VHL protein is inactive, thus permitting cells to grow, whereas the nuclear VHL is active, inhibiting transcription elongation.

hMSH2 and Related Genes

Hereditary non-polyposis colorectal cancer (HNPCC) is an autosomal dominant disorder.[396, 397] Its manifestations include a high incidence of colorectal cancers, as well as other epithelial tumors. The genes responsible for some kindreds with HNPCC have been identified. Germline mutation at any of four different loci can give rise to the condition. In each case, the gene has turned out to be involved in DNA mismatch repair. The affected genes are *hMSH2, hMLH1, hPMS2,* and *hPMS1.* Inactivation of both alleles of any of the genes leads to a very high rate of spontaneous mutation in cells. The reason that mutation of each gene gives rise to a similar phenotype is that all of four encoded proteins function together in DNA mismatch repair, and each is essential to this process. Although HNPCC is inherited as autosomal dominant, as are the other familial syndromes with lesions in tumor suppressor genes, the DNA mismatch repair genes differ fundamentally from the tumor suppressor genes that have been described above, in that the DNA mismatch repair genes are not directly involved in regulating cell growth. Instead, their high mutator phenotype greatly increases the likelihood that the cells in which their function has been inactivated will develop mutations in growth regulatory genes.

Cancer: Collaboration Among Genes That Regulate Growth

Most of the previous sections have focused on identifying genes that regulate cell growth and viability, with emphasis on the diverse mechanisms by which alterations in a single gene may uncouple the cell from its normal growth controls and drive proliferation. As noted earlier, however, a wealth of evidence indicates that cancer in most instances represents a multistep process that results largely from a series of genetic changes, rather than from a single genetic abnormality. It is theoretically possible that tumors might arise after alterations in a random mixture of genes that regulate cell growth. However, analysis of experimentally induced tumors and of certain human tumors suggests that a pattern and order underlie the constellation of genetic changes that give rise to a particular tumor. This theme is also discussed in Chapter 26.

The observation that efficient transformation of primary rodent fibroblasts requires more than one oncogene, or the combination of an oncogene and inactivation of a tumor suppressor gene, has been noted earlier. Cotransfection of different mixtures of oncogenes in primary rodent cells has led to the general conclusion that efficient transformation by two oncogenes can usually be accomplished if one oncogene efficiently immortalizes cells and the other efficiently transforms established rodent cells.[88] Primary cells transfected with a single "transforming" gene are more likely to have a transformed phenotype if they are grown in the absence of surrounding normal cells. This finding is in agreement with the observation that normal cells, when mixed with transformed cells, can suppress the transformed phenotype in vitro and in vivo.[398, 399] The immortalizing oncogene may help override the inhibitory effect of the normal cells, which could be mediated by the release of growth inhibitory cytokines from the normal cells. Support for this model has been provided by the finding that constitutive expression of c-*myc* can render keratinocytes resistant to the growth inhibitory activity of TGF-β.[400]

We have also noted that many DNA tumor viruses contain more than one oncogene, that the tumorigenic capacity of these viruses usually requires all of their oncogenes to act in concert, and that the encoded oncoproteins, such as adenovirus E1A, may be multifunctional. Retroviruses that carry two oncogenes also represent models for examining cooperation between oncogenes.[401] For example, mutational analysis of AEV (see Fig. 25–7) has shown that v-*erb*B, which encodes a constitutively active transmembrane receptor with protein tyrosine kinase activity, is necessary and sufficient for inducing erythroblastosis.[402] In contrast to tumors caused by wild-type AEV, those resulting from a mutant that lacks v-*erb*A are much less aggressive and include more differentiated cells that express hemoglobin.[403] Although v-*erb*A by itself is not oncogenic, these results dem-

onstrate that it cooperates with v-*erb*B. In appropriate viral constructs, v-*src* and other v-*onc*'s that encode non-receptor protein tyrosine kinases can induce erythroblastosis; v-*erb*A can cooperate with these v-*onc*'s to increase the malignant potential of the tumors and to block the ability of the tumor cells to differentiate.[404]

The use of transgenic animals represents an extremely fruitful approach for studying experimental tumorigenesis in the intact organism. Analysis of the tumorigenic activity of the SV40 large T antigen in transgenic mice has demonstrated the critical role played by the promoter.[71] This oncogene can induce pancreatic, melanocytic, or lymphoid tumors, if the promoter of the transgene is derived, respectively, from the pancreatic elastase gene, the tyrosinase gene, or the immunoglobulin heavy chain gene.[71] Collaboration between oncogenes or combinations of oncogenes and tumor suppressor genes has been shown in transgenic animals.[389]

The relative susceptibility of different strains of mice to tumorigenesis by specific oncogenes can also be probed by the analysis of transgenic mice. For example, mouse strains appear to vary markedly in the efficiency with which an activated *neu* oncogene can induce mammary tumors.[405, 406] The genetic basis for such differences in susceptibility can be explored by examining the differences between transgenic animals derived from different strains.

Although it is possible to induce tumors with a single oncogene, the introduction of two different oncogenes as transgenes usually results in the formation of tumors with much greater efficiency than either transgene alone.[71] Furthermore, the latent period for tumor formation is shorter when two genes are used, and the tumors are often more malignant. As with in vitro transformation studies of primary rodent fibroblastic cells, *myc* and *ras* transgenes in mice have been shown to cooperate in the development of pre–B-cell lymphomas, mammary carcinomas, and hepatic malignancies, with the tumor type determined largely by the promoter used.

Transgenes can also test the oncogenic potential of rearranged genes identified in tumors. As noted earlier, Burkitt's lymphomas often have a translocation that places the c-*myc* gene under the control of the enhancer from the immunoglobulin heavy chain gene. The oncogenic potential of such a chimeric gene has been documented by showing that when introduced as a transgene in mice, it results in B-cell or pre–B-cell tumors.[407] The tumors only develop after a long latency, implying that other genetic changes are required. Mutational activation of endogenous *ras* genes has been detected frequently in these tumors, as might be expected from the cooperation demonstrated between *myc* and *ras* in the development of B-cell tumors.

Molecular evidence from human cancers also supports the hypothesis that several genetic changes are required for malignancy. Alterations of several tumor suppressor genes (*APC, DCC,* and *p53*) and at least one proto-oncogene (K-*ras*) have been implicated in the pathogenesis of colorectal tumors.[6] Inactivation of *APC* is usually the first event, followed by activation of K-*ras* and inactivation of *DCC* and *p53*. Although these events do not occur in all colorectal tumors and probably do not happen in this precise order in every case, analysis of a large number of patients does suggest a general sequence of genetic alterations leading to malignancy. Pathologists have defined a discrete series of stages in the development of metastatic colorectal carcinoma, ranging from hyperproliferation of the epithelium, to benign adenoma, to carcinoma, to the appearance of metastatic variants. Interestingly, the genetic changes detailed above appear to occur at defined stages of the tumor progression.[408]

The examples described in this section, derived from a variety of systems, all point to the involvement of multiple genetic changes during the development of cancer. The epidemiology of cancer, in which the overall incidence shows a dramatic increase with the age of the individual, is in agreement with these findings.

Future Directions

The work described here represents the outcome of efforts aimed at understanding the molecular basis of normal and abnormal cell growth. It reflects the contributions of many fields of inquiry. Taken together, these studies have described a network of intracellular molecules that act in both a positive and a negative manner to control the growth of cells. Since all but the most terminally differentiated cells must respond to a variety of signals, many different players are needed to participate in the growth control network. The result of this requirement is that more than 100 genes have been implicated as proto-oncogenes, and there is a growing list of potential tumor suppressors as well.

One of the major problems of current research is to determine how multiple alterations in these different classes of genes result in different human neoplasms.[4] A more precise delineation of the cellular pathways through which these genes function, the interaction between pathways, and the identity of the components with which their products interact is also needed. It is also important to clarify the molecular mechanisms underlying progression to more aggressive phenotypes. The most fundamental challenge continues to be to translate this enormous, continually expanding body of knowledge of normal and abnormal growth into more effective approaches to prevent and treat various forms of cancer. It seems reasonable to believe that elucidating the fundamental processes that lead to neoplastic disease represents a necessary step toward its eventual control.

REFERENCES

1. Bishop, J. M.: Molecular themes in oncogenesis. Cell 64:235, 1991.
2. Cooper, G. M.: Oncogenes. Boston, Jones & Bartlett Publishers, 1995.
3. Varmus, H., and Weinberg, R. A.: Genes and the Biology of Cancer. New York, Scientific American Library, 1993.
4. Vogelstein, B., and Kinzler, K. W. (eds.): The Genetic Basis of Human Cancer. New York: McGraw-Hill, 1998.
5. Hunter, T.: Cooperation between oncogenes. Cell 64:249, 1991.
6. Vogelstein, B., and Kinzler, K. W.: The multistep nature of cancer. Trends Genet. 9:138, 1993.
7. Bootsma, D., Kraemer, K. H., Cleaver, J. E., and Hoeijmakers, J. H. J.: Nucleotide excision repair syndromes: Xeroderma pigmentosum, Cockayne syndrome, and trichothiodystrophy. *In* Vogelstein, B., Kinzler, K. W. (eds): The Genetic Basis of Human Cancer. New York, McGraw-Hill, 1998.
8. Tooze, J.: Molecular Biology of Tumor Viruses: DNA Tumor Viruses. Cold Spring Harbor, N. Y., Cold Spring Harbor Laboratory, 1981.
9. Weiss, R. A.: RNA Tumor Viruses. 2nd ed. Cold Spring Harbor, N. Y., Cold Spring Harbor Laboratory, 1985.
10. Coffin, J. M., Hughes, S. H., and Varmus, H.: Retroviruses. Plainview, N. Y.: Cold Spring Harbor Laboratory Press, 1997.
11. Stehelin, D., Varmus, H. E., and Bishop, J. M.: DNA related to the transforming gene(s) of avian sarcoma viruses is present in normal avian DNA. Nature 260:170, 1976.
12. Tabin, C. J., Bradley, S. M., Bargman, C. I., et al.: Mechanism of activation of a human oncogene. Nature 300:143, 1982.
13. Santos, E., Tronick, S. R., Aaronson, S. A., Pulciani, S., and Barbacid, M.: T24 human bladder carcinoma oncogene is an activated form of the normal human homologue of BALB- and Harvey-MSV transforming genes. Nature 298:343, 1982.
14. Der, C. J., Krontiris, T. G., and Cooper, G. M.: Transforming genes of human bladder and lung carcinoma cell lines are homologous to the *ras* genes of Harvey and Kirsten sarcoma viruses. Proc. Natl. Acad. Sci. USA 79:3637, 1982.
15. Weinberg, R. A.: Oncogenes and the Molecular Origins of Cancer. Cold Spring Harbor, N. Y., Cold Spring Harbor Laboratory Press, 1989.
16. Marshall, C. J.: Tumor suppressor genes. Cell 64:313, 1991.
17. Weinberg, R. A.: Tumor suppressor genes. Science 254:1138, 1991.
18. Bishop, J. M., and Weinberg, R. A. (eds.): Molecular Oncology. New York, Scientific American, 1996.
19. Whyte, P., Buchkovich, K. J., Horowitz, J. M. et al.: Association between an oncogene and an anti-oncogene: The adenovirus E1A proteins bind to the retinoblastoma gene product. Nature 334:124, 1988.
20. Hartwell, L. H., and Weinert, T. A.: Checkpoints: Controls that ensure the order of cell cycle events. Science 246:629, 1989.
21. Nurse, P.: Ordering S phase and M phase in the cell cycle. Cell 79:547, 1994.
22. Hartwell, L. H.: *Saccharomyces cerevisiae* cell cycle. Bacteriol. Rev. 38:164, 1974.
23. Enoch, T., and Nurse, P.: Coupling M phase and S phase: Controls maintaining the dependence of mitosis on chromosome replication. Cell 65:921, 1991.
24. Pines, J.: Cyclins and cyclin-dependent kinases: A biochemical view. Biochem. J. 308:697, 1995.
25. Sherr, C. J.: Cancer cell cycles. Science 274:1672, 1996.
26. Cahill, D. P., Lengauer, C., Yu, J., et al.: Mutations of mitotic checkpoint genes in human cancers. Nature 392:300, 1998.
27. Nigg, E. A.: Cyclin-dependent protein kinases: Key regulators of the eukaryotic cell cycle. Bioessays 17:471, 1995.
28. Weinberg, R. A.: The retinoblastoma protein and cell cycle control. Cell 81:323, 1995.
29. Mulligan, G., and Jacks, T.: The retinoblastoma gene family: Cousins with overlapping interests. Trends Genet. 15:223, 1998.
30. Taya, Y.: RB kinase and RB-binding proteins: New points of view. Trends Biochem. Sci. 22:14, 1997.
31. Aaronson, S. A.: Growth factors and cancer. Science 254:1146, 1991.
32. Cross, M., and Dexter, T. M.: Growth factors in development, transformation, and tumorigenesis. Cell 64:271, 1991.
33. Yuan, J., and Horvitz, H. R.: The *Caenorhabditis elegans* genes ced-3 and ced-4 act cell autonomously to cause programmed cell death. Dev. Biol. 138:33, 1990.
34. Williams, G. T., Smith, C. A., Spooncer, E., Dexter, T. M., and Taylor, D. R.: Haemopoietic colony stimulating factors promote cell survival by suppressing apoptosis. Nature 343:76, 1990.
35. Levi-Montalcini, R.: The nerve growth factor 35 years later. Science 237:1154, 1987.
36. Carpenter, G., and Cohen, S.: Epidermal growth factor. Annu. Rev. Biochem. 48:193, 1979.
37. Kelly, K., Cochran, B. H., Stiles, C. D., and Leder, P.: Cell-specific regulation of the c-*myc* gene by lymphocytes mitogens and platelet-derived growth factor. Cell 35:603, 1983.
38. Greenberg, M. E., and Ziff, E. B.: Stimulation of 3T3 cells induces transcription of the c-*fos* proto-oncogene. Nature 311:433, 1984.
39. Matsushima, H., Roussel, M. F., Ashmun, R. A., and Sherr, C. J.: Colony stimulating factor 1 regulates novel cyclins during the G_1 phase of the cell cycle. Cell 65:701, 1991.
40. Pardee, A. B.: G_1 events and regulation of cell proliferation. Science 246:603, 1989.
41. Crabtree, G. R.: Contingent genetic regulatory revents in T lymphocyte activation. Science 243:355, 1989.
42. Silvennoinen, O., and Ihle, J. N.: Signaling by the hematopoietic cytokine receptors. Molecular Biology Intelligence Unit, Austin, Tex., R. G. Landes Co., 1996.

43. Green, S., and Chambon, P.: Nuclear receptors enhance our understanding of transcription regulation. Trends Genet. 4:309, 1988.
44. Ullrich, A., and Schlessinger, J.: Signal transduction by receptors with tyrosine kinase activity. Cell 61:203, 1990.
45. van der Greer, P., and Hunter, T.: Receptor protein-tyrosine kinases and their signal transduction pathways. Annu. Rev. Cell Biol. 10:1994, 1994.
46. Lemmon, M. A., and Schlessinger, J.: Regulation of signal transduction and signal diversity by receptor oligomerization. Trends Biochem. Sci. 19:459, 1994.
47. Heldin, C. H.: Dimerization of cell surface receptors in signal transduction. Cell 80:213, 1995.
48. Hunter, T.: Protein-tyrosine phosphatases: The other side of the coin. Cell 58:1013, 1989.
49. Alexander, D. R.: The role of phosphatases in signal transduction. New Biologist 2:1049, 1990.
50. Cantley, L. C., Auger, K. R., Carpenter, C., et al.: Oncogenes and signal transduction. Cell 64:281, 1991.
51. Pawson, T.: Protein modules and signaling networks. Nature 373:573, 1995.
52. Neet, K., and Hunter, T.: Vertebrate non-receptor protein-tyrosine kinase families. Genes Cells 1:147, 1996.
53. Schindler, C., and Darnell, J. E., Jr.: Transcriptional responses to polypeptide ligands: The JAK-STAT pathway. Annu. Rev. Biochem. 64:621, 1995.
54. Ihle, J. N., Nosaka, T., Thierfelder, W., Quelle, F. W., and Shimoda, K.: Jaks and stats in cytokine signaling. Stem Cells 15(Suppl. 1):105, 1997.
55. Nishibe, S., Wahl, M. I., Wedegaertner, P. B., et al.: Selectivity of phospholipase-C phosphorylation by the epidermal growth factor receptor, the insulin receptor, and their cytoplasmic domains. Proc. Natl. Acad. Sci. USA 87:424, 1990.
56. Nishizuka, Y.: Studies and perspectives of protein kinase C. Science 233:305, 1986.
57. Berridge, M. J., and Irvine, R. F.: Inositol phosphates and cell signalling. Nature 341:197, 1989.
58. Collins, S., Caron, M. G., and Lefkowitz, R. J.: From ligand binding to gene expression: New insights into the regulation of G-protein-coupled receptors. Trends Biochem. Sci. 17:37, 1992.
59. Palczewski, K., and Benovic, J. L.: G-protein-coupled receptor kinases. Trends Biochem. Sci. 16:387, 1991.
60. Mitchell, P. J., and Tjian, R.: Transcriptional regulation in mammalian cells by sequence-specific DNA binding proteins. Science 245:371, 1989.
61. Schüle, R., and Evans, R. M.: Cross-coupling of signal transduction pathways: Zinc finger meets leucine zipper. Trends Genet. 7:377, 1991.
62. Abercrombie, M., and Heaysman, J. E. M.: Observations on the social behaviour of cells in tissue culture. II. "Monolayering" of fibroblasts. Exp. Cell Res. 6:293, 1954.
63. Holley, R. W., and Kiernan, J. A.: "Contact inhibition" of cell division in 3T3 Cells. Proc. Natl. Acad. Sci. USA 60:300, 1968.
64. Macpherson, I., and Montagnier, L.: Agar suspension culture for the selective assay of cells transformed by polyoma virus. Virology 23:291, 1964.
65. Temin, H. M., and Rubin, H.: Characteristics of an assay for Rous sarcoma virus and Rous sarcoma cells in tissue culture. Virology 6:669, 1958.
66. Sawyers, C. L., Denny, C. T., and Witte, O. N.: Leukemia and the disruption of normal hematopoiesis. Cell 64:337, 1991.
67. Hynes, R. O.: Cell surface proteins and malignant transformation. Biochim. Biophys. Acta 458:73, 1976.
68. Ruoslahti, E., and Obrink, B.: Review: Common principles in cell adhesion. Exp. Cell Res. 227:1, 1996.
69. Pollack, R., Osborn, M., and Weber, K.: Patterns of organization of actin and myosin in normal and transformed cultured cells. Proc. Natl. Acad. Sci. USA 72:994, 1975.
70. Verfaillie, C. M., Hurley, R., Lundell, B. I., Zhao, C., and Bhatia, R.: Integrin-mediated regulation of hematopoiesis: Do BCR/ABL-induced defects in integrin function underlie the abnormal circulation and proliferation of CML progenitors? Acta Haematol. 97:40, 1997.
71. Adams, J. M., and Cory, S.: Transgenic models of tumor development. Science 254:1161, 1991.
72. Harris, A. W., Strasser, A., Bath, M. L., Elefanty, A. G., and Cory, S.: Lymphomas and plasmacytomas in transgenic mice involving bcl2, myc and v-abl. Curr. Top. Microbiol. Immunol. 224:221, 1997.
73. Sporn, M. B., and Roberts, A. B.: Autocrine growth factors and cancer. Nature 313:745, 1985.
74. Thompson, C. B.: Apoptosis in the pathogenesis and treatment of disease. Science 267:1456, 1995.
75. McKenna, S. L., and Cotter, T. G.: Functional aspects of apoptosis in hematopoiesis and consequences of failure. Adv. Cancer Res. 71:121, 1997.
76. Pan, H., Yin, C., and Van Dyke, T.: Apoptosis and cancer mechanisms. Cancer Surv. 29:305, 1997.
77. Lowe, S. W., Ruley, H. E., Jacks, T., and Housman, D. E.: p53-Dependent apoptosis modulates the cytotoxicity of anticancer agents. Cell 74:957, 1993.
78. Lotem, J., and Sachs, L.: Regulation by bcl-2, c-Myc, and p53 of susceptibility to induction of apoptosis by heat shock and cancer chemotherapy compounds in differentiation-competent and -defective myeloid leukemic cells. Cell Growth Differ. 4:41, 1993.
79. Wyllie, A. H.: Glucocorticoid-induced thymocyte apoptosis is associated with endogenous endonuclease activation. Nature 284:555, 1980.
80. Metzstein, M. M., Stanfield, G. M., and Horvitz, H. R.: Genetics of programmed cell death in C. elegans: Past, present and future. Trends Genet. 14:410, 1998.
81. Fraser, A., and Evan, G.: A license to kill. Cell 85:781, 1996.
82. Villa, P., Kaufmann, S. H., and Earnshaw, W. C.: Caspases and caspase inhibitors. Trends Biochem. Sci. 22:388, 1997.
83. Vaux, D., Cory, S., and Adams, J.: BCL2 gene promotes haematopoietic cell survival and cooperates with c-myc to immortalize pre-B cells. Nature 335:440, 1988.
84. Raitano, A. B., Whang, Y. E., and Sawyers, C. L.: Signal transduction by wild-type and leukemogenic Abl proteins. Biochim. Biophys. Acta 1333:F201, 1997.
85. Campisi, J.: The biology of replicative senescence. Eur. J. Cancer 33:703, 1996.
86. Serrano, M., Lin, A. W., Beach, D., and Lowe, S. W.: Oncogenic ras provokes premature cell senescence associated with accumulation of p53 and p16INK4a. Cell 88:593, 1997.
87. Kim, N. W., Platyszek, M. A., Prowse, K. R., et al.: Specific association of human telomerase activity with immortalization and cancer. Science 266:2011, 1994.
88. Ruley, H. E.: Transforming collaborations between ras and nuclear oncogenes. Cancer Cells 2:258, 1990.
89. Counts, J. L., and Goodman, J. I.: Alterations in DNA methylation may play a variety of roles in carcinogenesis. Cell 83:13, 1995.
90. Jones, P. A.: DNA methylation errors and cancer. Cancer Res 56:2463, 1996.
91. Baylin, S. B., Herman, J. G., Graff, J. R., Vertino, P. M., and Issa, J. P.: Alterations in DNA methylation: A fundamental aspect of neoplasia. Adv. Cancer Res. 72:141, 1998.
92. Solomon, E., Borrow, J., and Goddard, A. D.: Chromosome aberrations and cancer. Science 254:1153, 1991.
93. Gottlieb, T. M., and Oren, M.: p53 In growth control and neoplasia. Biochim. Biophys. Acta 1287:77, 1996.
94. Todaro, G. J., and Huebner, R. J.: The viral oncogene hypothesis: New evidence. Proc. Natl. Acad. Sci. USA 69:1009, 1972.
95. Bishop, J. M.: Viral oncogenes. Cell 42:23, 1985.
96. zur Hausen, H.: Viruses in human cancers. Science 254:1167, 1991.
97. Nevins, J. R., and Vogt, P. K.: Cell transformation by viruses. In Fields, B. N., Knipe, D. M., and Howley, P. M. (eds): Fields Virology. Philadelphia, Lippincott-Raven, 1996.
98. Kieff, E., and Liebowitz, D.: Epstein-Barr virus and its replication, In Fields, B. N., and Knipe, D. M. (eds.): Virology. New York, Raven Press, 1990.
99. Hsu, T.-Y., Möröy, T., Etiemble, J., et al.: Activation of c-myc by woodchuck hepatitis virus insertion in hepatocellular carcinoma. Cell 55:627, 1988.
100. Wang, J., Chenivesse, X., Henglein, B., and Brechot, C.: Hepatitis B virus integration into a cyclin A gene in a hepatocellular carcinoma. Nature 343:555, 1990.
101. Salzman, N. P. (ed.): The Papovaviridae: The polyomaviruses. New York, Plenum Publishing, 1986.
102. Salzman, N. P., and Howley, P. M. (ed.): The Papovaviridae: The papillomaviruses. New York, Plenum Publishing, 1987.
103. Werness, B. A., Münger, K., and Howley, P. M.: Role of the human papillomavirus oncoproteins in transformation and carcinogenic progression. In DeVita, V. T. (ed.): Important Advances in Oncology. Philadelphia, J. B. Lippincott, 1991.

104. Livingston, D. M.: Review: The simian virus 40 large T antigen—a lot packed into a little. Mol. Biol. Med. 4:63, 1987.

105. Rassoulzadegan, M., Cowie, A., Carr, A., et al.: The role of individual polyoma virus early proteins in oncogenic transformation. Nature 300:713, 1982.

106. DiMaio, D.: Transforming activity of bovine and human papillomaviruses. Adv. Cancer Res. 56:133, 1991.

107. Barbosa, M. S., Vass, W. C., Lowy, D. R., and Schiller, J. T.: In vitro activity of the E6 and E7 genes vary among human papillomaviruses of different oncogenic potential. J. Virol. 65:292, 1991.

108. DeCaprio, J. A., Ludlow, J. W., Figge, J., et al.: SV40 Large tumor antigen forms a specific complex with the product of the retinoblastoma susceptibility gene. Cell 54:275, 1988.

109. Rous, P.: Transmission of a malignant new growth by means of a cell-free filtrate. JAMA 56:198, 1911.

110. Varmus, H. E.: Form and function of retroviral proviruses. Science 216:812, 1982.

111. Varmus, H.: Retroviruses. Science 240:1427, 1988.

112. Baltimore, D.: Viral RNA-dependent DNA polymerase. Nature 226:1209, 1970.

113. Temin, H. M., and Mizutani, S.: RNA-dependent DNA polymerase in virions of Rous sarcoma virus. Nature 226:1211, 1970.

114. Temin, H. M.: Function of the retrovirus long terminal repeat. Cell 28:3, 1982.

115. Martin, G. S.: Rous sarcoma virus: A function required for the maintenance of the transformed state. Nature 227:1021, 1970.

116. Duesberg, P. H., and Vogt, P. K.: Differences between the ribonucleic acids of transforming and nontransforming avian tumor viruses. Proc. Natl. Acad. Sci. USA 67:1673, 1970.

117. Vogt, P. K.: Spontaneous segregation of nontransforming viruses from cloned sarcoma viruses. Virology 46:939, 1971.

118. Aaronson, S. A., Jainchill, J. L., and Todaro, G. J.: Murine sarcoma virus transformation of BALB/3T3 cells: Lack of dependence on murine leukemia virus. Proc. Natl. Acad. Sci. USA 66:1236, 1970.

119. Spector, D. H., Smith, K., Padgett, T., et al.: Uninfected avian cells contain RNA related to the transforming gene of avian sarcoma viruses. Cell 13:371, 1978.

120. Wang, L.-H., Halpern, C. C., Nadel, M., and Hanafusa, H.: Recombination between viral and cellular sequences generated transforming sarcoma virus. Proc. Natl. Acad. Sci. USA 75:5812, 1978.

121. Bishop, J. M., and Varmus, H. E.: Functions and origins of retroviral transforming genes. In Weiss, R., et al. (eds.): RNA Tumor Viruses. Cold Spring Harbor, N. Y., Cold Spring Harbor Laboratory, 1982.

122. Brugge, J. S., and Erikson, R. L.: Identification of a transformation-specific antigen induced by an avian sarcoma virus. Nature 269:346, 1977.

123. Collett, M. S., and Erikson, R. L.: Protein kinase activity associated with the avian sarcoma virus src gene product. Proc. Natl. Acad. Sci. USA 75:2021, 1978.

124. Levinson, A. D., Opperman, H., Levintow, L., Varmus, H. E., and Bishop, J. M.: Evidence that the transforming gene of avian sarcoma virus encodes a protein kinase associated with a phosphoprotein. Cell 15:561, 1978.

125. Hunter, T., and Sefton, B. M.: Transforming gene product of Rous sarcoma virus phosphorylates tyrosine. Proc. Natl. Acad. Sci. USA 77:1311, 1980.

126. Parker, R. C., Varmus, H. E., and Bishop, J. M.: Expression of v-src and chicken c-src in rat cells demonstrates qualitative differences between pp60v-src and pp60c-src. Cell 37:131, 1984.

127. Velu, T. J., Vass, V. C., Lowy, D. R., and Tambourin, P. E.: Harvey murine sarcoma virus: Influence of coding and non-coding sequences on cell transformation in vitro and oncogenicity in vivo. J. Virol. 63:1384, 1989.

128. Payne, G. S., Courtneidge, S. A., Crittenden, L. B., et al.: Analysis of avian leukosis virus DNA and RNA in bursal tumors: Viral gene expression is not required for maintenance of the tumor state. Cell 23:311, 1981.

129. Hayward, W. S., Neel, B. G., and Astrin, S. M.: Activation of a cellular onc gene by promoter insertion in ALV-induced lymphoid leukosis. Nature 290:475, 1981.

130. Jonkers, J., and Berns, A.: Retroviral insertional mutagenesis as a strategy to identify cancer genes. Biochim. Biophys. Acta 1287:29, 1996.

131. Nusse, R., and Varmus, H. E.: Many tumors induced by the mouse mammary tumor virus contain a provirus integrated in the same region of the host genome. Cell 31:99, 1982.

132. Brown, A. M. C., Wildin, R. S., Prendergast, T. J., and Varmus, H. E.: A retrovirus vector expressing the putative mammary oncogene int-1 causes partial transformation of a mammary epithelial cell line. Cell 46:1001, 1986.

133. Tsukamoto, A. S., Grosschedl, R., Guzman, R. C., Parslow, T., and Varmus, H. E.: Expression of the int-1 gene in transgenic mice is associated with mammary gland hyperplasia and adenocarcinomas of male and female mice. Cell 55:619, 1988.

134. Nusse, R., and Varmus, H. E.: Wnt genes. Cell 69:1073, 1992.

135. Largaespada, D. A., Shaughnessy, J. D., Jr., Jenkins, N. A., and Copeland, N. G.: Retroviral integration at the Evi-2 locus in BXH-2 myeloid leukemia cell lines disrupts Nf1 expression without changes in steady-state Ras-GTP levels. J. Virol. 69:5095, 1995.

136. Nilsen, T. W., Maroney, P. A., Goodwin, R. G., et al.: c-erbB Activation in ALV-induced erythroblastosis: Novel RNA processing and promoter insertion result in expression of an amino-truncated EGF receptor. Cell 41:719, 1985.

137. Bies, J., and Wolff, L.: Oncogenic activation of c-Myb by carboxyl-terminal truncation leads to decreased proteolysis by the ubiquitin-26S proteasome pathway. Oncogene 14:203, 1997.

138. Shih, C., Shilo, B.-Z., Goldfarb, M. P., Dannenberg, A., and Weinberg, R. A.: Passage of phenotypes of chemically transformed cells via transfection of DNA and chromatin. Proc. Natl. Acad. Sci. USA 76:5714, 1979.

139. Cooper, G. M., Okenquist, S., and Silverman, L.: Transforming activity of DNA of chemically transformed and normal cells. Nature 284:418, 1980.

140. Krontiris, T. G., and Cooper, G. M.: Transforming activity of human tumor DNAs. Proc. Natl. Acad. Sci. USA 78:1181, 1981.

141. Parada, L. F., Tabin, C. J., Shih, C., and Weinberg, R. A.: Human EJ bladder carcinoma oncogene is homologue of Harvey sarcoma virus ras gene. Nature 297:474, 1982.

142. Bargmann, C. I., Hung, M.-C., and Weinberg, R. A.: Multiple independent activations of the neu oncogene by a point mutation altering the transmembrane domain of p185. Cell 45:649, 1986.

143. Rabbits, T. H.: Chromosomal translocations in human cancer. Nature 372, 1994.

144. Finger, L. R., Harvey, R. C., Moore, R. C. A., Showe, L. C., and Croce, C. M.: A common mechanism of chromosomal translocation in T- and B-cell neoplasia. Science 234:982, 1986.

145. Dalla-Favera, R., Bregni, M., Erikson, J., et al.: Human c-myc oncogene is located on the region of chromosome 8 that is translocated in Burkitt lymphoma cells. Proc. Natl. Acad. Sci. USA 79:7824, 1982.

146. Taub, R., Kirsch, I., Morton, C., et al: Translocation of the c-myc gene into the immunoglobin heavy chain locus in human Burkitt lymphoma and murine plasmacytoma cells. Proc. Natl. Acad. Sci. USA 79:7837, 1982.

147. Bhatia, K. K., Huppi, C., Spangler, C., et al.: Point mutations in the c-myc transactivation domain are common in Burkitt's lymphoma and mouse plasmacytoma. Nat. Genet. 5:56, 1993.

148. Shen-Ong, G. L. C., Keath, E. J., Piccoli, S. P., and Cole, M. D.: Novel myc oncogene RNA from abortive immunoglobulin-gene recombination in mouse plasmacytomas. Cell 31:443, 1982.

149. Shtivelman, E., Lifshitz, B., Gale, R. P., and Canaani, E.: Fused transcript of abl and bcr genes in chronic myelogenous leukaemia. Nature 315:550, 1985.

150. Davis, R. L., Konopka, J. B., and Witte, O. N.: Activation of the c-abl oncogene by viral transduction or chromosomal translocation generates c-abl proteins with similar in vitro kinase properties. Mol. Cell. Biol. 5:204, 1985.

151. Collins, S., and Groudine, M.: Amplification of endogenous myc-related DNA sequences in a human myeloid leukemia cell line. Nature 298:679, 1982.

152. DePinho, R. A., Schreiber-Agus, N., and Alt, F. W.: myc Family oncogenes in the development of normal and neoplastic cells. Adv. Cancer Res. 57:1, 1991.

153. Brodeur, G. M., Seeger, R. C., Schwab, M., Varmus, H. E., and Bishop, J. M.: Amplification of N-myc in untreated human neuroblastomas correlates with advanced disease stage. Science 224:1121, 1984.

154. Slamon, D. J., Godolphin, W., Jones, L. A., et al.: Studies of the HER-2/neu proto-oncogene in human breast and ovarian cancer. Science 244:707, 1989.

155. Hendler, F. J., Shum-Slu, A., Oechsli, M., et al., Increased EGF-R1 binding predicts a poor survival in squamous tumors. In Furth, M.,

and Greaves, M. (eds.): Cancer Cells. Vol. 7. Molecular Diagnostics of Human Cancer. Cold Spring Harbor, N. Y., Cold Spring Harbor Laboratory, 1989.

156. Velu, T. J., Beguinot, L., Vass, W. C., et al.: Epidermal growth factor–dependent transformation by a human EGF receptor proto-oncogene. Science 238:1408, 1987.

157. Di Fiore, P. P., Pierce, J. H., Kraus, M. H., et al.: erbB-2 is a potent oncogene when overexpressed in NIH/3T3 cells. Science 237:178, 1987.

158. Hall, M., and Peters, G.: Genetic alterations of cyclins, cyclin-dependent kinases, and Cdk inhibitors in human cancer. Adv. Cancer Res. 68:67, 1996.

159. Hunter, T.: Oncoprotein networks. Cell 88:333, 1997.

160. Doolittle, R. F., Hunkapiller, M. W., Hood, L. E., et al.: Simian sarcoma virus onc gene, v-sis, is derived from the gene (or genes) encoding a platelet-derived growth factor. Science 221:275, 1983.

161. Waterfield, M. D., Scrace, G. T., Whittle, N., et al.: Platelet-derived growth factor is structurally related to the putative transforming protein p28^{sis} of simian sarcoma virus. Nature 304:35, 1983.

162. Beckmann, M. P., Betsholtz, D., Heldin, C.-H., et al.: Comparison of biological properties and transforming potential of human PDGF-A and PDGF-B chains. Science 241:1346, 1988.

163. Rosenthal, A., Lindquist, P. B., Bringman, T. S., Goeddel, D. V., and Derynck, R.: Expression in rat fibroblasts of a human transforming growth factor-α cDNA results in transformation. Cell 46:301, 1986.

164. Derynck, R.: Transforming growth factor α. Cell 54:593, 1988.

165. Shih, T. Y., Weeks, M. O., Young, H. A., and Scolnick, E. M.: p21 of Kirsten murine sarcoma virus is thermolabile in a viral mutant temperature sensitive for maintenance of transformation. J. Virol. 31:546, 1970.

166. Derynck, R., Goeddel, D. V., Ullrich, A., et al.: Synthesis of messenger RNAs for transforming growth factors α and β and the epidermal growth factor receptor by human tumors. Cancer Res. 47:707, 1987.

167. Halaban, R., Kwon, B. S., Ghosh, S., Delli-Bovi, P., and Baird, A.: bFGF is an autocrine growth factor for human melanomas. Oncogene Res. 3:177, 1988.

168. Meeker, T. C., Hardy, D., Willman, C., Hogan, T., and Abrams, J.: Activation of the interleukin-3 gene by chromosome translocation in acute lymphocytic leukemia with eosinophilia. Blood 76:285, 1990.

169. Liotta, L. A., Steeg, P. S., and Stetler-Stevenson, W. G.: Cancer metastasis and angiogenesis: An imbalance of positive and negative regulation. Cell 64:327, 1991.

170. Folkman, J.: Tumor angiogenesis. In Mendelson, J. (ed.): The Molecular Basis of Cancer. Philadelphia, W. B. Saunders Co., 1995.

171. Ushiro, H., and Cohen, S.: Identification of phosphotyrosine as a product of epidermal growth factor–activated protein kinase in A431 cell membranes. J. Biol. Chem. 255:8363, 1980.

172. Hunter, T., and Cooper, J. A.: Epidermal growth factor induces rapid tyrosine phosphorylation of proteins in A431 human tumor cells. Cell 24:741, 1981.

173. Cooper, J. A., Bowen-Pope, D. F., Raines, F., Ross, R., and Hunter, T.: Similar effects of platelet-derived growth factor and epidermal growth factor on the phosphorylation of tyrosine in cellular proteins. Cell 31:263, 1982.

174. Downward, J., Yarden, Y., Mayees, E., et al.: Close similarity of epidermal growth factor receptor and v-erb-B oncogene protein sequences. Nature 307:521, 1984.

175. Gilmore, T., DeClue, J. E., and Martin, G. S.: Protein phosphorylation at tyrosine is induced by the v-erbB gene product in vivo and in vitro. Cell 40:609, 1985.

176. Sherr, C. J., Rettenmeier, C. W., Sacca, R., et al.: The c-fms proto-oncogene product is related to the receptor for the mononuclear phagocyte growth factor, CSF-1. Cell 41:665, 1985.

177. Sherr, C. J.: Mitogenic response to colony-stimulating factor 1. Trends Genet. 7:398, 1991.

178. Roussel, M. F., Downing, J. R., Rettenmier, C. W., and Sherr, C. J.: A point mutation in the extracellular domain of the human CSF-1 receptor (c-fms proto-oncogene product) activates its transforming potential. Cell 55:979, 1988.

179. Chabot, B., Stephenson, D. A., Chapman, V. M., Besmer, P., and Bernstein, A.: The proto-oncogene c-kit encoding a transmembrane tyrosine kinase receptor maps to the mouse W locus. Nature 335:88, 1988.

180. Geissler, E. N., Ryan, M. A., and Housman, D. E.: The dominant-white spotting (W) locus of the mouse encodes the c-kit proto-oncogene. Cell 55:185, 1988.

181. Witte, O. N.: Steel locus defines new multipotent growth factor. Cell 63:5, 1990.

182. Broudy, V. C.: Stem cell factor in hematopoiesis. Blood 90:1345, 1997.

183. Vliagoftis, H., Worobec, A. S., and Metcalfe, D. D.: The protooncogene c-kit and c-kit ligand in human disease. J. Allergy Clin. Immunol. 100:435, 1997.

184. Birchmeier, C., O'Neill, K., Riggs, M., and Wigler, M.: Characterization of the ROS1 cDNA from a human glioblastoma cell line. Proc. Natl. Acad. Sci. USA 87:4799, 1990.

185. Rodrigues, G. A., and Park, M. A.: Oncogenic activation of tyrosine kinases. Curr. Opin. Genet. Dev. 4:14, 1994.

186. Bottaro, D. P., Rubin, J. S., Faletto, D. L., et al.: Identification of the hepatocyte growth factor receptor as the c-met proto-oncogene product. Science 251:802, 1991.

187. Kaplan, D. R., Hempstead, B. L., Martinzanca, D., Chao, M. V., and Parada, L. F.: The trk proto-oncogene product—a signal transducing receptor for nerve growth factor. Science 252:554, 1991.

188. Martin, P., Vass, W. C., Schiller, J. T., Lowy, D. R., and Velu, T. J.: The bovine papillomavirus E5 transforming protein can stimulate the transforming activity of EGF and CSF-1 receptors. Cell 59:21, 1989.

189. Petti, L., Nilson, L. A., and Dimaio, D.: Activation of the platelet-derived growth factor receptor by the bovine papillomavirus-E5 transforming protein. EMBO J 10:845, 1991.

190. Petti, L. M., Reddy, V., Smith, S. O., and DiMaio, D.: Identification of amino acids in the transmembrane and juxtamembrane domains of the platelet-derived growth factor receptor required for productive interaction with the bovine papillomavirus E5 protein. J. Virol. 71:7318, 1997.

191. Hibi, K., Takahashi, T., Sekido, Y., et al.: Coexpression of the stem cell factor and the c-kit genes in small-cell lung cancer. Oncogene 6:2291, 1991.

192. Lenferink, R. E., Pinkas-Kramarski, R., van de Poll, M. L. M., et al.: Differential endocytic routing of homo- and hetero-dimeric ErbB tyrosine kinases confers signaling superiority to receptor heterodimers. EMBO J. 17:3385, 1998.

193. Ellisen, L. W., Bird, J., West, D. C., et al.: TAN-1, the human homolog of the Drosophila notch gene, is broken by chromosomal translocations in T lymphobastic neoplasms. Cell 66:649, 1991.

194. Ponder, B. A. J.: Multiple endocrine neoplasia type 2. In Vogelstein, B., and Kinzler, K. W. (eds.): The Genetic Basis of Human Cancer. New York, McGraw-Hill Book Co., 1998.

195. Yoshimura, A., Longmore, G., and Lodish, H. F.: Point mutation in the exoplasmic domain of the erythropoietin receptor resulting in hormone-independent activation and tumorigenicity. Nature 348:647, 1990.

196. Zon, L. I., Moreau, J.-F., Koo, J.-W., Mathey-Prevot, B., and D'Andrea, A. D.: The erythropoietin receptor transmembrane region is necessary for activation by the Friend spleen focus-forming virus gp55 glycoprotein. Mol. Cell. Biol. 12:2949, 1992.

197. Linnekin, D., Evans, G. A., D'Andrea, A., and Farrar, W. L.: Association of the erythropoietin receptor with protein tyrosine kinase activity. Proc. Natl. Acad. Sci. USA 89:6237, 1992.

198. Young, D., Waitches, G., Birchmeier, C., Fasano, O., and Wigler, M.: Isolation and characterization of a new cellular oncogene encoding a protein with multiple potential transmembrane domains. Cell 45:711, 1986.

199. Jackson, T. R., Blair, L. A. C., Marshall, J., Goedert, M., and Hanley, M. R.: The Mas oncogene encodes an angiotensin receptor. Nature 335:437, 1988.

200. Parsons, J. T., and Weber, M. J.: Genetics of src: Structure and functional organization of a protein tyrosine kinase. Curr. Top. Microbiol. Immunol. 147:80, 1989.

201. Hanks, S. K., Quinn, A. M., and Hunter, T.: The protein kinase family: Conserved features and deduced phylogeny of the catalytic domains. Science 241:42, 1988.

202. Dymecki, S. M., Niederhuber, J. E., and Desiderio, S. V.: Specific expression of a tyrosine kinase gene, blk, in B lymphoid cells. Science 247:332, 1990.

203. Brown, M. T., and Cooper, J. A.: Regulation, substrates and functions of src. Biochim. Biophys. Acta 1287:121, 1996.

204. Williams, J. C., Wierenga, R. K., and Saraste, M.: Insights into Src kinase functions: Structural comparisons. Trends Biochem. Sci. 23:179, 1998.

205. Parsons, J. T., and Parsons, S. J.: Src family protein tyrosine kinases:

Cooperating with growth factor and adhesion signaling pathways. Curr. Opin. Cell Biol. 9:187, 1997.

206. Cooper, J. A., and King, C. S.: Dephosphorylation or antibody binding to the carboxy terminus stimulates pp60$^{c\text{-}src}$. Mol. Cell. Biol. 6:4467, 1986.

207. Kmiecik, T. E., and Shalloway, D.: Activation and suppression of pp60$^{c\text{-}src}$ transforming ability by mutation of its primary sites of tyrosine phosphorylation. Cell 49:65, 1987.

208. Courtneidge, S. A., and Smith, A. E.: Polyoma virus transforming protein associates with the product of the c-src cellular gene. Nature 303:435, 1983.

209. Hanks, S. K., Quinn, A. M., and Hunter, T.: The protein kinase family: Conserved features and deduced phylogeny of the catalytic domains. Science 241:42, 1988.

210. Sadowski, I., Stone, J. C., and Pawson, T.: A non-catalytic domain conserved among cytoplasmic protein-tyrosine kinases modifies the kinase function and transforming activity of Fujinami sarcoma virus p30$^{gag\text{-}fps}$. Mol. Cell. Biol. 6:4396, 1986.

211. Pawson, T.: Non-catalytic domains of cytoplasmic protein-tyrosine kinases: Regulatory elements in signal transduction. Oncogene 3:491, 1988.

212. Koch, C. A., Anderson, D., Moran, M. F., Ellis, C., and Pawson, T.: SH2 and SH3 domains: Elements that control interactions of cytoplasmic signaling proteins. Science 252:668, 1991.

213. Pawson, T., and Schlessinger, J.: SH2 and SH3 domains. Curr. Biol. 3:434, 1993.

214. Heldin, C. H.: SH2 Domains: Elements that control protein interactions during signal transduction. Trends Biochem. Sci. 16:450, 1991.

215. Moran, M. F., Koch, C. A., Anderson, D., et al.: Src Homology region 2 domains direct protein-protein interactions in signal transduction. Proc. Natl. Acad. Sci. USA 87:8622, 1990.

216. Kypta, R. M., Goldberg, Y., Ulug, E. T., and Courtneidge, S. A.: Association between the PDGF receptor and members of the src family of tyrosine kinases. Cell 62:481, 1990.

217. Mayer, B. J., Hamaguchi, M., and Hanafusa, H.: A novel viral oncogene with structural similarity to phospholipase C. Nature 332:272, 1988.

218. Matsuda, M., Mayer, B. J., and Hanafusa, H.: Identification of domains of the v-crk oncogene product sufficient for association with phosphotyrosine-containing proteins. Mol. Cell. Biol. 11:1607, 1991.

219. Mayer, B. J., and Hanafusa, H.: Association of the v-crk oncogene product with phosphotyrosine-containing proteins and protein kinase activity. Proc. Natl. Acad. Sci. USA 87:2638, 1990.

220. Roussel, R. R., Brodeur, S. R., Shalloway, D., and Laudano, A. P.: Selective binding of activated pp60$^{c\text{-}src}$ by an immobilized synthetic phosphopeptide modeled on the carboxyl terminus of pp60$^{c\text{-}src}$. Proc. Natl. Acad. Sci. USA 88:10696, 1991.

221. Hirai, H., and Varmus, H. E.: Site-directed mutagenesis of the Sh2-coding and Sh3-coding domains of C-src produces varied phenotypes, including oncogenic activation of P60C-src. Mol. Cell. Biol. 10:1307, 1990.

222. Verderame, M. F., Kaplan, J. M., and Varmus, H. E.: A mutation in v-src that removes a single conserved residue in the SH-2 domain of pp60$^{v\text{-}src}$ restricts transformation in a host-dependent manner. J. Virol. 63:338, 1989.

223. DeClue, J. E., Sadowski, I., Martin, G. S., and Pawson, T.: A conserved domain regulates interactions of the v-fps protein-tyrosine kinase with the host cell. Proc. Natl. Acad. Sci. USA 84:9064, 1987.

224. Mayer, B., Jackson, P. K., Van Etten, R. A., and Baltimore, D.: Point mutations in the abl SH2 domain coordinately impair phosphotyrosine binding in vitro and transforming activity in vivo. Mol. Cell. Biol. 12:609, 1992.

225. Sefton, B. M.: The lck tyrosine protein kinase. Oncogene 6:683, 1991.

226. Horak, I. D., Gress, R. E., Lucas, P. J., et al.: T-lymphocyte interleukin 2–dependent tyrosine protein kinase signal transduction involves the activation of p56lck. Proc. Natl. Acad. Sci. USA 88:1996, 1991.

227. Hatakeyama, M., Kono, T., Kobayashi, N., and et al.: Interaction of the IL-2 receptor with the src-family kinase p56lck: Identification of novel intermolecular association. Science 252:1523, 1991.

228. Fischer, G. H., Charbonneau, H., and Tonks, N. K.: Protein tyrosine phosphatases: A diverse family of intracellular and transmembrane enzymes. Science 253:401, 1991.

229. Shen, S. H., Bastien, L., Posner, B. I., and Chretien, P.: A protein-tyrosine phosphatase with sequence similarity to the SH2 domain of the protein-tyrosine kinases. Nature 352:736, 1991.

230. Bourne, H. R., Sanders, D. A., and McCormick, F.: The GTPase superfamily: A conserved switch for diverse cell functions. Nature 348:125, 1990.

231. Bourne, H. R., Sanders, D. A., and McCormick, F.: The GTPase superfamily: Conserved structure and molecular mechanism. Nature 349:117, 1991.

232. Boguski, M. S., and McCormick, F.: Proteins regulating Ras and its relatives. Nature 366:643, 1993.

233. Lowy, D. R., and Willumsen, B. M.: Function and regulation of Ras. Annu. Rev. Biochem. 62:851, 1993.

234. Barbacid, M.: ras Genes. Annu. Rev. Biochem. 56:779, 1987.

235. Bos, J. L.: Ras oncogenes in human cancer: A review. Cancer Res. 49:4682, 1989.

236. Rodenhuis, S.: Ras and human tumors. Semin. Cancer Biol. 3:1992.

237. Scolnick, E. M., Papageorge, A. G., and Shih, T. Y.: Guanine nucleotide-binding activity as an assay for src protein of rat-derived murine sarcoma viruses. Proc. Natl. Acad. Sci. USA 76:5355, 1979.

238. Trahey, M., and McCormick, F.: A cytoplasmic protein stimulates normal N-ras p21 GTPase, but does not affect oncogenic mutants. Science 238:542, 1987.

239. Willumsen, B. M., Christensen, A., Hubbert, N. L., Papageorge, A. G., and Lowy, D. R.: The p21 ras C-terminus is required for transformation and membrane association. Nature 310:583, 1984.

240. Hancock, J. F., Magee, A. I., Childs, J. E., and Marshall, C. C.: All ras proteins are polyisoprenylated but only some are palmitoylated. Cell 57:1167, 1989.

241. Hancock, J. F., Paterson, H., and Marshall, C. J.: A polybasic domain or palmitoylation is required in addition to the Caax motif to localize p21 Ras to the plasma membrane. Cell 63:133, 1990.

242. Hancock, J. F., Cadwallader, K., and Marshall, C. J.: Methylation and proteolysis are essential for efficient membrane binding of prenylated p21K-ras(B). EMBO J. 10:641, 1991.

243. Gibbs, J. B.: Ras C-terminal processing enzymes—new drug targets. Cell 65:1, 1991.

244. Kato, K., Der, C. J., and Buss, J. E.: Prenoids and palmitate: Lipids that control the biological activity of Ras proteins. Semin. Cancer Biol. 3:179, 1992.

245. Kohl, N. E., Omer, C. A., Conner, M. W., et al.: Inhibition of farnesyl transferase induces regression of mammary and salivary carcinomas in Ras transgenic mice. Nat. Genet. 1:792, 1995.

246. Wittinghofer, A., Pai, E. F.: The structure of Ras protein: A model for a universal molecular switch. Trends Biochem. Sci. 16:382, 1991.

247. Bollag, G., and McCormick, F.: Regulators and effectors of ras proteins. Annu. Rev. Cell Biol. 7:601, 1991.

248. Sigal, I. S., Gibbs, J. B., D'Alonzo, J. S., et al.: Mutant ras-encoded proteins with altered nucleotide binding exert dominant biological effects. Proc. Natl. Acad. Sci. USA 83:952, 1986.

249. Walter, M., Clark, S. G., and Levinson, A. D.: The oncogenic activation of human p21-ras by a novel mechanism. Science 233:649, 1986.

250. Satoh, T., Endo, M., Nakafuku, M., Nakamura, S., and Kaziro, Y.: Platelet-derived growth factor stimulates formation of active p21Ras. GTP complex in Swiss mouse 3T3-cells. Proc. Natl. Acad. Sci. USA 87:5993, 1990.

251. Gibbs, J. B., Marshall, M. S., Scolnick, E. M., Dixon, R. A. F., and Vogel, U. S.: Modulation of guanine nucleotides bound to ras in NIH3T3 cells by oncogenes, growth factors, and the GTPase activating protein (GAP). J. Biol. Chem. 265:20437, 1990.

252. Downward, J., Graves, J. D., Warne, P. H., Rayter, S., and Cantrell, D. A.: Stimulation of p21ras upon T-cell activation. Nature 346:719, 1990.

253. Mulcahy, L. S., Smith, M. R., and Stacey, D. W.: Requirements for ras proto-oncogene function during serum stimulated growth of NIH 3T3 cells. Nature 313:241, 1985.

254. Medema, R. H., Wubbolts, R., and Bos, J. L.: Two dominant inhibitory mutants of p21(ras) interfere with insulin-induced gene expression. Mol. Cell. Biol. 11:5963, 1991.

255. Smith, M. R., DeGudicibus, S. J., and Stacey, D. W.: Requirement for c-ras proteins during viral oncogene transformation. Nature 320:540, 1986.

256. Simon, M. A., Bowtell, D. D. L., Dodson, G. S., Laverty, T. R., and Rubin, G. M.: Ras1 and a putative guanine nucleotide exchange factor perform crucial steps in signaling by the sevenless protein tyrosine kinase. Cell 67:701, 1991.

257. Kornfield, K.: Vulval development in Caenorhabditis elegans. Trends Genet. 13:55, 1997.

258. Sternberg, P. W., and Han, M.: Genetics of RAS signaling in *C. elegans*. Trends Genet. 14:466, 1998.
259. Feig, L. A.: Guanine-nucleotide exchange factors: A family of positive regulators of Ras and related GTPases. Curr. Opin. Cell Biol. 6:204, 1994.
260. Vojtek, A. B., and Der, C. J.: Increasing complexity of the Ras signaling pathway. J. Biol. Chem. 273:19925, 1998.
261. Rodriguez-Viciana, P., Warne, P. H., Dhand, R., et al.: Phosphatidyl-inositol-3-OH kinase as a direct target of Ras. Nature 370:527, 1994.
262. Chang, H. W., Aoki, M., Fruman, D., et al.: Transformation of chicken cells by the gene encoding the catalytic subunit of PI 3-kinase. Science 276:1848, 1997.
263. Van Aelst, L., and D'Souza-Schorey, C.: Rho GTPases and signaling networks. Genes Dev. 11:2295, 1997.
264. Broach, J. R.: RAS Genes in *Saccharomyces cerevisiae*—signal transduction in search of a pathway. Trends Genet. 7:28, 1991.
265. Powers, S.: Genetic analysis of *ras* homologs in yeasts. Semin. Cancer Biol. 3:1992.
266. Toda, T., Uno, I., Ishikawa, T., et al.: In yeast, *RAS* proteins are controlling elements of adenylate cyclase. Cell 40:27, 1985.
267. Jones, S., Vignais, M. L., and Broach, J. R.: The CDC25 protein of *Saccharomyces cerevisiae* promotes exchange of guanine nucleotides bound to Ras. Mol. Cell. Biol. 11:2641, 1991.
268. Tanaka, K., Lin, B. K., Wood, D. R., and Tamanoi, F.: IRA2, an upstream negative regulator of RAS in yeast, is a RAS GTPase-activating protein. Proc. Natl. Acad. Sci. USA 88:468, 1991.
269. Hart, M. J., Eva, A., Zangrilli, D., et al.: Cellular transformation and guanine nucleotide exchange activity are catalyzed by a common domain on the *dbl* oncogene product. J. Biol. Chem. 269:62, 1994.
270. Cerione, R., and Zheng, Y.: The Dbl family of oncogenes. Curr. Opin. Cell Biol. 6:204, 1996.
271. Eva, A., Vecchio, G., Rao, C. D., Tronick, S. R., and Aaronson, S. A.: The predicted *DBL* oncogene product defines a distinct class of transforming proteins. Proc. Natl. Acad. Sci. USA 85:2061, 1988.
272. Kaziro, Y., Itoh, H., Kozasa, T., Nakafuku, M., and Satoh, T.: Structure and function of signal-transducing GTP-binding proteins. Annu. Rev. Biochem. 60:359, 1991.
273. Vallar, L., Spada, A., and Giannattasio, G.: Altered G_S and adenylate cyclase activity in human GH–secreting pituitary adenomas. Nature 330:566, 1987.
274. Landis, C. A., Masters, S. B., Spada, A., et al.: GTPase inhibiting mutations activate the α chain of G_S and stimulate adenyl cyclase in human pituitary tumours. Nature 340:692, 1989.
275. Lyons, J., Landis, C. A., Harsh, G., et al.: Two G protein oncogenes in human endocrine tumors. Science 249:655, 1990.
276. Thomas, S. M., DeMarco, M., D'Arcangelo, G., Halegoua, S., and Brugge, J. S.: Ras is essential for nerve growth factor–induced and phorbol ester–induced tyrosine phosphorylation of MAP kinases. Cell 68:1031, 1992.
277. Morrison, D. K., Kaplan, D. R., Escobedo, J. A., et al.: Direct activation of the serine/threonine kinase activity of *raf*-1 through tyrosine phosphorylation by the PDGF receptor. Cell 58:649, 1989.
278. Rapp, U. R.: Role of Raf-1 serine/threonine protein kinase in growth factor signal transduction. Oncogene 6:495, 1991.
279. Stanton, V. P., Jr., Nichols, D. W., Laudano, A. P., and Cooper, G. M.: Definition of the human *raf* amino-terminal regulatory region by deletion mutagenesis. Mol. Cell. Biol. 9:639, 1989.
280. Li, P., Wood, K., Mamon, H., Haser, W., and Roberts, T.: Raf-1: A kinase currently without a cause but not lacking in effects. Cell 64:479, 1991.
281. Morrison, D. K., and Cutler, J. R. E.: The complexity of Raf-1 regulation. Curr. Opin. Cell Biol. 9:174, 1997.
282. App, H., Hazan, R., Zilberstein, A., et al.: Epidermal growth factor (EGF) stimulates association and kinase activity of Raf-1 with the EGF receptor. Mol. Cell. Biol. 11:913, 1991.
283. Koch, W., Heidecker, G., Lloyd, P., and Rapp, U. R.: Raf-1 protein kinase is required for growth of induced NIH/3T3 cells. Nature 349:426, 1991.
284. Marais, R., Light, Y., Paterson, H. F., and Marshall, C. J.: Ras recruits Raf-1 to the plasma membrane for activation by tyrosine phosphorylation. EMBO J. 14:313, 1995.
285. Leevers, S. J., Paterson, H. F., and Marshall, C. J.: Requirement for Ras in Raf activation is overcome by targeting Raf to the plasma membrane. Nature 369:411, 1994.
286. Hsiao, W.-L. W., Housey, G. M., Johnson, M. D., and Weinstein, B.
287. Borner, C., Filipuzzi, I., Weinstein, I. B., and Imber, R.: Failure of wild-type or a mutant form of protein kinase C-α to transform fibroblasts. Nature 353:78, 1991.
288. Cai, H., Smmola, U., Wixler, V., et al.: Role of diacylglycerol-regulated protein kinase C isotypes in growth factor activation of the Raf-1 protein kinase. Mol. Cell. Biol. 17:732, 1997.
289. Maxwell, S. A., Arlinghause, R. B.: Serine kinase activity associated with Moloney murine sarcoma virus-124-encoded p37^{mos}. Virology 143:321, 1985.
290. Goldman, D. S., Kiessling, A. A., Millette, C. F., and Cooper, G. M.: Expression of c-*mos* RNA in germ cells of male and female mice. Proc. Natl. Acad. Sci. USA 84:4509, 1987.
291. Sagata, N., Watanabe, N., Vande Woude, G. F., and Ikawa, Y.: The c-*mos* proto-oncogene product is a cytostatic factor responsible for meiotic arrest in vertebrate eggs. Nature 342:512, 1989.
292. Selten, G., Cuypers, H. T., Boelens, W., et al.: The primary structure of the putative oncogene *pim-1* shows extensive homology with protein kinases. Cell 46:603, 1986.
293. Landschulz, W. H., Johnson, P. F., and McKnight, S. L.: The leucine zipper: A hypothetical structure common to a new class of DNA binding proteins. Science 240:1759, 1988.
294. Gutman, A., and Wasylyk, B.: Nuclear targets for transcription regulation by oncogenes. Trends Genet. 7:49, 1991.
295. Lewin, B.: Oncogenic conversion by regulatory changes in transcription factors. Cell 64:303, 1991.
296. Forrest, D., and Curran, T.: Cross signals: Oncogenic transcription factors. Curr. Opin. Genet. Dev. 2:19, 1992.
297. Henriksson, M., and Luscher, B.: Proteins of the Myc network: Essential regulators of cell growth and differentiation. Adv. Cancer Res. 68:109, 1996.
298. Penn, L. J. Z., Laufer, E. M., and Land, H.: C -*M Y C*: Evidence for multiple regulatory functions. Cancer Biol. 1:69, 1990.
299. Grandori, C., and Eisenman, R. N.: Myc target genes. Trends. Biochem. Sci. 22:177, 1997.
300. Roussel, M. F., Cleveland, J. L., Shurtleff, S. A., and Sherr, C. J.: Myc rescue of a mutant CSF-1 receptor impaired in mitogenic signalling. Nature 353:361, 1991.
301. Blackwood, E. M., Kretzner, L., and Eisenman, R. N.: Myc and Max function as a nucleoprotein complex. Curr. Opin. Genet. Dev. 2:227, 1992.
302. Blackwood, E. M., and Eisenman, R. N.: Max: A helix-loop-helix zipper protein that forms a sequence-specific DNA-binding complex with Myc. Science 251:1211, 1991.
303. Prendergast, G. C., Lawe, D., and Ziff, E. B.: Association of Myn, the murine homology of Max, with c-Myc stimulates methylatin-sensitive DNA binding and Ras cotransformation. Cell 65:395, 1991.
304. Kato, G. J., Lee, W. M. F., Chen, L., and Dang, C. V.: Max: Functional domains and interaction with C-myc. Genes Dev. 6:81, 1992.
305. Cole, M. D.: Myc meets its Max. Cell 65:715, 1991.
306. Galaktionov, K., Chen, X., and Beach, D.: Cdc25 cell-cycle phosphatase as a target of c-*myc*. Nature 382:511, 1996.
307. Chiu, R., Boyle, W. J., Meek, J., et al.: The c-*fos* protein interacts with c-*jun*/AP-1 to stimulate transcription of AP-1 responsive genes. Cell 54:541, 1988.
308. Roux, P., Blanchard, J.-M., Fernandez, A., et al.: Nuclear localization of c-*fos* but not v-*fos* protein is controlled by extracellular signals. Cell 63:341, 1990.
309. Müller, R., Bravo, R., Burckhardt, J., and Curran, T.: Induction of c-*fos* gene and protein by growth factors precedes activation of c-*myc*. Nature 312:716, 1984.
310. Stacey, D. W., Watson, T., Kung, H.-F., and Curran, T.: Microinjection of transforming *ras* protein induces c-*fos* expression. Mol. Cell. Biol. 7:523, 1987.
311. Jamal, S., and Ziff, E.: Transactivation of C-fos and beta-actin genes by Raf as a step in early response to transmembrane signals. Nature 344:463, 1990.
312. Ledwith, B. J., Manam, S., Kraynak, A. R., Nichols, W. W., and Bradley, M. O.: Antisense-Fos RNA causes partial reversion of the transformed phenotypes induced by the C-Ha-RAS oncogene. Mol. Cell. Biol. 10:1545, 1990.
313. Smeal, T., Binetruy, B., Mercola, D. A., Birrer, M., and Karin, M.: Oncogenic and transcriptional cooperation with Ha-Ras requires phos-

phorylation of C-Jun on serine-63 and serine-73. Nature 354:494, 1991.

314. Bohmann, D., Bos, T. J., Admon, A., et al.: Human proto-oncogene c-*jun* encodes a DNA binding protein with structural and functional properties of transcription factor AP-1. Science 238:1386, 1987.

315. Binetruy, B., Smeal, T., and Karin, M.: Ha-*ras* augments c-*jun* activity and stimulates phosphorylation of its activation domain. Nature 351:122, 1991.

316. Pulverer, J., Kyriakis, J. M., Avruch, J., Nikolokaki, E., and Woodgett, J. R.: Phosphorylation of c-*jun* mediated by MAP kinases. Nature 353:670, 1991.

317. Hai, T., and Curran, T.: Cross-family dimerization of transcription factors Fos/Jun and ATF/CREB alters DNA-binding specificity. Proc. Natl. Acad. Sci. USA 88:3720, 1991.

318. Kovary, K., and Bravo, R.: Expression of different Jun and Fos proteins during the G0 to G1 transition in mouse fibroblasts: *In vitro* and *in vivo* associations. Mol. Cell. Biol. 11:2451, 1991.

319. Graf, T.: Leukemogenesis: Small diffrences in Myb have large effects. Curr. Biol. 8:R353, 1998.

320. Wolff, L.: Myb-induced transformation. Crit. Rev. Oncog. 7:245, 1996.

321. Weston, K.: Myb proteins in life, death and differentiation. Curr. Opin. Genet. Dev. 8:76, 1998.

322. Lipsick, J. S.: One billion years of Myb. Oncogene 13:223, 1996.

323. Weston, K., and Bishop, J. M.: Transcriptional activation by the v-*myb* oncogene and its cellular progenitor, c-*myb*. Cell 58:85, 1989.

324. Klempnauer, K.-H., Arnold, H., and Biedenkapp, H.: Activation of transcription by v-*myb*: Evidence for two different mechanisms. Genes Dev. 3:1582, 1989.

325. Gilmore, T. D.: Malignant transformation by mutant Rel proteins. Trends Genet. 7:318, 1991.

326. Davis, N., Ghosh, S., Simmons, D. L., et al.: Rel-associated pp40: An inhibitor of the Rel family of transcription factors. Science 253:1991.

327. Ballard, D. W., Walker, W. H., Doerre, S., et al.: The v-*rel* oncogene encodes a kB enhancer binding protein that inhibits NF-kB function. Cell 63:803, 1990.

328. Magli, M. C., Largman, C., and Lawrence, H. J.: Effects of HOX homeobox genes in blood cell differentiation. J. Cell. Physiol. 173:168, 1997.

329. Wolff, L.: Contribution of oncogenes and tumor suppressor genes to myeloid leukemia. Biochim. Biophys. Acta 1332:F67, 1997.

330. Withers, D. A., Harvey, R. C., Faust, J. B., et al.: Characterization of a candidate *bcl*-1 gene. Mol. Cell. Biol. 11:4846, 1991.

331. Lammie, G. A., Vantl, V., Smith, R., et al.: D11S287, a putative oncogene on chromosome 11q13, is amplified and expressed in squamous cell and mammary carcinomas and linked to BCL-1. Oncogene 6:439, 1991.

332. Motokura, T., Bloom, T., Kim, H. G., et al.: A novel cyclin encoded by a bcl1-linked candidate oncogene. Nature 350:512, 1991.

333. Bodrug, S. B. W., Bath, M., et al.: Cyclin D1 transgene impedes lymphocyte maturation and collaborates in lymphomagenesis with the myc gene. EMBO J. 13:2124, 1994.

334. Hanna, Z., Jankowski, M., Tremblay, P., et al.: The *Vin*-1 gene, identified by provirus insertional mutagenesis, corresponds to the G1-phase cyclin D2. Oncogene 8:1661, 1993.

335. Adamson, E. D.: Oncogenes in development. Development 99:449, 1987.

336. Pawson, T., and Bernstein, A.: Receptor tyrosine kinases: Genetic evidence for their role in *Drosophila* and mouse development. Trends Genet. 6:350, 1990.

337. Forrester, L. M., Brunkow, M., and Bernstein, A.: Proto-oncogenes in mammalian development. Curr. Opin. Genet. Dev. 2:38, 1992.

338. Hoffman, F. M., Sternberg, P. W., and Herskowitz, I.: Learning about cancer genes through invertebrate genetics. Curr. Opin. Genet. Dev. 2:45, 1992.

339. Reith, A. D., and Bernstein, A.: Molecular basis of mouse developmental mutants. Genes Dev. 5:1115, 1991.

340. Nocka, K., Tan, J. C., Chiu, E., et al.: Molecular bases of dominant negative and loss of function mutations at the murine c-*kit*/white spotting locus: W[37], W[v], W[41] and W. EMBO J. 9:1805, 1990.

341. Flanagan, J. G., Chan, D. C., and Leder, P.: Transmembrane form of the *Kit* ligand growth factor is determined by alternative splicing and is missing in the SI(d) mutant. Cell 64:1025, 1991.

342. Capecchi, M. R.: Altering the genome by homologous recombination. Science 244:1288, 1989.

343. Hoffmann, F. M.: *Drosophila abl* and genetic redundancy in signal transduction. Trends Genet. 7:351, 1991.

344. Bowen-Pope, D. F., Van Koppen, A., and Schatteman, G.: Is PDGF really important? Testing the hypotheses. Trends Genet. 7:413, 1991.

345. Rubin, G. M.: Signal transduction and the fate of the R7 photoreceptor in *Drosophila*. Trends Genet. 7:372, 1991.

346. Clark, S. G., Stern, M. J., and Horvitz, H. R.: *C. elegans* cell-signalling gene *sem-5* encodes a protein with SH2 and SH3 domains. Nature 356:340, 1992.

347. Boyd, J. A., Barrett, J. C.: Tumor suppressor genes: Possible functions in the negative regulation of cell proliferation. Mol. Carcinogenesis 3:325, 1990.

348. Stanbridge, E. J.: Genetic regulation of tumorigenic expression in somatic cell hybrids. Adv. Viral Oncol. 6:83, 1987.

349. Harris, H.: The analysis of malignancy by cell fusion: The position in 1988. Cancer Res. 48:3302, 1988.

350. Knudson, A. G., Jr.: Mutation and cancer: Statistical study of retinoblastoma. Proc. Natl. Acad. Sci. USA 68:820, 1971.

351. Collins, F. S.: Positional cloning: Let's not call it reverse anymore. Nat. Genet. 1:3, 1992.

352. Francke, U., and Kung, F.: Sporadic bilateral retinoblastoma and 13q chromosomal deletion. Med. Pediatr. Oncol. 2:379, 1976.

353. Sparkes, R. S., Murphree, A. L., Lingua, R. W., et al.: Gene for hereditary retinoblastoma assigned to human chromosome 13 by linkage to esterase D. Science 219:971, 1983.

354. Friend, S. H., Bernards, R., Rogelj, S., et al.: A human DNA segment with properties of the gene that predisposes to retinoblastoma and osteosarcoma. Nature 323:643, 1986.

355. Fung, Y.-K. T., Murphree, A. L., T'Ang, A., et al.: Structural evidence for the authenticity of the human retinoblastoma gene. Science 236:1657, 1987.

356. Lee, W.-H., Bookstein, R., Hong, F., et al.: Human retinoblastoma susceptibility gene: Cloning, identification, and sequence. Science 235:1394, 1987.

357. Horowitz, J. M., Park, S.-H., Bogenmann, E., et al.: Frequent inactivation of the retinoblastoma anti-oncogene is restricted to a subset of human tumor cells. Proc. Natl. Acad. Sci. USA 87:2775, 1990.

358. Cavenee, W. K., Hansen, M. F., Nordenskjold, M., et al.: Genetic origins of mutations predisposing to retinoblastoma. Science 228:501, 1985.

359. Levine, A. J., Momand, J., and Finlay, C. A.: The p53 tumour suppressor gene. Nature 351:453, 1991.

360. Lane, D. P., and Crawford, L. V.: T antigen is bound to a host protein in SV40-transformed cells. Nature 278:261, 1979.

361. Finlay, C. A., Hinds, P. W., and Levine, A. J.: The p53 proto-oncogene can act as a suppressor of transformation. Cell 57:1083, 1989.

362. Mulligan, L. M., Matlashewski, G. J., Scrable, H. J., and Cavenee, W. K.: Mechanisms of p53 loss in human sarcomas. Proc. Natl. Acad. Sci. USA 87:5863, 1990.

363. Hollstein, M., Sidransky, D., Vogelstein, B., and Harris, C. C.: p53 Mutations in human cancers. Science 253:49, 1991.

364. Malkin, D., Li, F. P., Strong, L. C., et al.: Germ line p53 mutations in a familial syndrome of breast cancer, sarcomas, and other neoplasms. Science 250:1233, 1990.

365. Srivastava, S. K., Zou, Z. Q., Pirollow, K., Blattner, W., and Chang, E. H.: Germ-line transmission of a mutated p53 gene in a cancer-prone family with Li-Fraumeni syndrome. Nature 348:747, 1990.

366. Frebourg, T., Kassel, J., Lam, K. T., et al.: Germ-line mutations of the p53 tumor suppressor gene in patients with high risk for cancer inactivate the p53 protein. Proc. Natl. Acad. Sci. USA 89:6413, 1992.

367. Srivastava, S., A., T. Y., Devadas, K., et al.: Detection of both mutant and wild-type p53 protein in normal skin fibroblasts and demonstration of a shared "second hit" on p53 in diverse tumors from a cancer-prone family with Li-Fraumeni syndrome. Oncogene 7:987, 1992.

368. Lee, W.-H., Shew, J.-Y., Hong, F. D., et al.: The retinoblastoma susceptibility gene encodes a nuclear phosphoprotein associated with DNA binding activity. Nature 319:642, 1987.

369. Dyson, N., Howley, P. M., Munger, K., and Harlow, E.: The human papilloma virus-16 E7 oncoprotein is able to bind to the retinoblastoma gene product. Science 243:934, 1989.

370. Ludlow, J. W., DeCaprio, J. A., Huang, C.-M., et al.: SV40 Large T antigen binds preferentially to an underphosphorylated member of the retinoblastoma susceptibility gene product family. Cell 56:57, 1989.

371. Donehower, L. A., Harvey, M., Slagle, B. L., et al.: Mice deficient for p53 are developmentally normal but susceptible to spontaneous tumours. Nature 356:215, 1992.

372. Harris, C. C.: p53: At the crossroads of molecular carcinogenesis risk assessment. Science 262:1980, 1993.

373. Levine, A. J.: p53, The cellular gatekeeper for growth and division. Cell 88:323, 1997.

374. Lane, D. P., and Hall, P. A.: MDM2—arbiter of p53's destruction. Trends Biochem. Sci. 22:372, 1997.

375. Kastan, M. B.: Checkpoint Controls and Cancer. Cold Spring Harbor, N. Y.: Cold Spring Harbor Laboratory Press, 1997.

376. Nurse, P.: Checkpoint pathways come of age. Cell 91:865, 1997.

377. Dittner, D., Pati, S., Zambetti, G., et al.: p53 Gain of function mutations. Nat. Genet. 4:42, 1993.

378. Wallace, M. R., Marchuk, D. A., Andersen, L. B., et al.: Type 1 neurofibromatosis gene: Identification of a large transcript disrupted in three NF1 patients. Science 249:181, 1990.

379. Xu, G. F., O'Connell, P., Viskochil, D., et al.: The neurofibromatosis type-1 gene encodes a protein related to GAP. Cell 62:599, 1990.

380. Basu, T. N., Gutmann, D. H., Fletcher, J. A., et al.: Aberrant regulation of ras proteins in malignant tumour cells from type-1 neurofibromatosis patients. Nature 356:713, 1992.

381. DeClue, J. E., Papageorge, A. G., Fletcher, J. A., et al.: Abnormal regulation of mammalian p21^{ras} contributes to malignant tumor growth in Von Recklinghausen (type-1) neurofibromatosis. Cell 69:265, 1992.

382. Gregory, P. E., Gutmann, D. H., Boguski, M., et al.: The neurofibromatosis type I gene product, neurofibromin, associated with microtubules. Somat. Cell Mol. Genet. 19:265, 1993.

383. Groden, J., Thliveris, A., Samowitz, W., et al.: Identification and characterization of the familial adenomatous polyposis coli gene. Cell 66:589, 1991.

384. Kinzler, K. W., Nilbert, M. C., Su, L.-K., et al.: Identification of FAP locus genes from chromosome 5q21. Science 253:661, 1991.

385. Su, L.-K., Kinzler, K. W., Vogelstein, B., et al.: Multiple intestinal neoplasia caused by a mutation in the murine homolog of the APC gene. Science 256:668, 1992.

386. Rubinfeld, B., Albert, I., Porfiri, E., et al.: Binding of GSK3-beta to the APC-beta-catenin complex and regulation of complex assembly. Science 272:1023, 1996.

387. Behrens, J., von Kries, J. P., Kuhl, M., et al.: Functional interaction of beta-catenin with the transcription factor LEF-1. Nature 382:638, 1996.

388. Morin, P. J., Sparks, A. B., Korinek, V. et al.: Activation of beta-catenin-Tcf signaling in colon cancer by mutations in beta-catenin or APC. Science 275:787, 1997.

389. Chin, L., Pomerantz, J., and DePinho, R. A.: The INK4a/ARF tumor suppressor: One gene—two products—two pathways. Trends Biochem. Sci. 23:291, 1998.

390. Thandla, S., and Aplan, P. D.: Molecular biology of acute lymphocytic leukemia. Semin. Oncol. 24:45, 1997.

391. Duan, D. R., Humphrey, J. S., Chen, D. Y., et al.: Characterization of the VHL tumor suppressor gene product: Localization, complex formation and the effect of natural inactivating mutations. Proc. Natl. Acad. Sci. USA 92:6459, 1995.

392. Duan, D. R., Conaway, J. W., Linehan, W. M., and Klausner, R. D.: Inhibition of transcription elongation by the VHL tumor suppressor protein. Science 269:1402, 1995.

393. Kibel, A., Iliopoulos, O., DeCaprio, J. A., and Kaelin, W. G., Jr.: Binding of the von Hippel-Lindau tumor suppressor protein to elongin B and C. Science 269:1444, 1995.

394. Gnarra, J., Zhou, S., Merrill, M. J., et al.: Post-transcriptional regulation of vascular endothelial growth factor mRNA by the VHL tumor suppressor gene product. Proc. Natl. Acad. Sci. USA 93:10589, 1996.

395. Lee, S., Chen, D. Y. T., Humphrey, J. S., et al.: Nuclear/cytoplasmic localization of the VHL tumor suppressor gene product is determined by cell density. Proc. Natl. Acad. Sci. USA 93:1770, 1996.

396. Kolodner, R. D.: Mismatch repair: Mechanisms and relationship to cancer susceptibility. Trends Biochem. Sci. 20:397, 1995.

397. Boland, C. R.: Hereditary nonpolypopsis colorectal cancer. *In* Vogelstein, B., and Kinzler, K. W. (eds.): The Genetic Basis of Human Cancer. 1998, New York, McGraw-Hill Book Co., 1998.

398. Dotto, G. P., Weinberg, R. A., and Ariza, A.: Malignant transformation of mouse primary keratinocytes by HaSV and its modulation by surrounding normal cells. Proc. Natl. Acad. Sci. USA 85:6389, 1988.

399. Stoker, A. W., Hatier, C., and Bissell, M. J.: The embryonic environment strongly attenuates v-*src* oncogenesis in mesenchymal and epithelial tissues but not in endothelia. Curr. Opin. Cell Biol. 2:864, 1990.

400. Pietenpol, J. A., Stein, R. A., Moran, E., et al.: Transforming growth factor beta 1 suppression of c-*myc* gene transcription: Role in inhibition of keratinocyte proliferation. Proc. Natl. Acad. Sci. USA 87:3758, 1990.

401. Palmieri, S.: Oncogene requirements for tumorigenicity: Cooperative effects between retroviral oncogenes. Curr. Top. Microbiol. Immunol. 148:43, 1989.

402. Graf, T., Ade, N., and Beug, H.: Temperature-sensitive mutant of avian erythroblastosis virus suggests a block of differentiation as mechanism of leukaemogenesis. Nature 257:496, 1978.

403. Graf, T., and Beug, H.: Role of the v-*erbA* and v-*erb-B* oncogenes of avian erythroblastosis virus in erythroid cell transformation. Cell 34:7, 1983.

404. Kahn, P., Frykberg, L., Brady, C., et al.: v-*erbA* Cooperates with sarcoma oncogenes in leukemic cell transformation. Cell 45:349, 1986.

405. Muller, W. J., Sinn, E., Pattengale, P. K., Wallace, R., and Leder, P.: Single-step induction of mammary adenocarcinoma in transgenic mice bearing the activated c-*neu* oncogene. Cell 54:105, 1988.

406. Bouchard, L., Lamarre, L., Tremblay, P. J., and Jolicoeur, P.: Stochastic appearance of mammary tumors in transgenic mice carrying the MMTV/c-*neu* oncogene. Cell 57:931, 1989.

407. Adams, J. M., Harris, A. W., Pinkert, C. A., et al.: The c-*myc* oncogene driven by immunoglobulin enhancers induces lymphoid malignancy in transgenic mice. Nature 318:533, 1985.

408. Fearon, E. R., and Vogelstein, B.: A genetic model for colorectal tumorigenesis. Cell 61:759, 1990.

26 ▼▼▼▼ Mechanisms of Leukemogenesis

Charles L. Sawyers and Owen N. Witte

HEMATOPOIETIC GROWTH FACTORS AS DEFINITIVE PARTICIPANTS IN LEUKEMOGENESIS

RECEPTOR ALTERATIONS IN LEUKEMOGENESIS

INTRACELLULAR SIGNALING MECHANISMS

RAS-CONTROLLED PATHWAYS ARE KEY INTRACELLULAR MEDIATORS OF LEUKEMOGENESIS

TRANSCRIPTION FACTOR TRANSLOCATIONS

TRANSLOCATIONS IN GENES ESSENTIAL FOR HEMATOPOIETIC DEVELOPMENT

TRANSLOCATIONS IN GENES THAT AFFECT HEMATOPOIETIC DIFFERENTIATION

TRANSLOCATIONS THAT TARGET GENES INVOLVED IN HOMEOTIC FUNCTION

TRANSLOCATIONS THAT TARGET GENES AFFECTING APOPTOSIS

ABNORMALITIES IN GENES INVOLVED IN CELL CYCLE PROGRESSION

▼ ▼

In the several years since the last edition of the *Molecular Basis of Blood Diseases* was published, there has been an exponential increase in our knowledge of the molecular events associated with the pathogenesis of human and experimental leukemias and lymphomas. Not surprisingly, the basic principles of molecular oncology apply to leukemias. Genetic damage resulting in positive proliferative signals, loss of tumor suppressor gene function, inhibition of developmental programs, blocks in cell death pathways, resistance to genotoxic agents, and avoidance of host defense mechanisms can all be documented to play a part in the pathogenesis of some type of leukemia. The most obvious genetic changes are defined by the compilation of specific translocations that activate abnormal gene expression and frequently create chimeric structures in a broad range of leukemias and lymphomas. Such translocations provide a molecular definition for a specific type of leukemia and a focus for defining a portion of the potential growth control alterations. A detailed description of each cytogenetic event occurring in human leukemias is not the goal of this chapter. Rather, we hope to use selected examples that unite a specific molecular event to a mechanism or pathway that one can relate to the causation, response to therapy, or progression of disease. We emphasize examples that most directly connect to human disease and restrict examples from the literature on leukemogenesis in experimental animals to those that bridge new concepts or contrast with observations in people.

A substantive understanding of the genesis and progression of any leukemia must depend on a thorough knowledge of the normal growth and differentiation signals used by the pluripotential stem cell, multipotential progenitors, and the lineage-committed intermediates and mature cells that leukemias and lymphomas can mimic. Precise cell surface markers are available to differentiate normal blood cell lineages and precursors from the pluripotential and multipotential elements. Molecularly cloned growth factors and cytokines that expand or restrict subpopulations of hematopoietic cells are readily available and widely used in experimental and clinical settings. Although we have a much better definition of the cellular composition of hematopoietic populations and their comparison to different leukemias, we still lack a fundamental understanding of how the primary decisions of the stem and multi-lineage progenitor cells to restrict their potential are made. The spirited discussion over the role of a random or stochastic process in contrast to an instructional model continues.[1, 2] Our desire to understand the generation of leukemias partly as a perturbation of differentiation is limited by gaps in our understanding of how normal blood elements make these decisions.

The clinical presentation and course of the family of diseases we call leukemia is remarkably diverse. The rapid growth rate and hypercellularity of a childhood acute lymphocytic leukemia starkly contrasts with the more indolent chronic lymphocytic leukemias of older patients. Although their time course of progression without therapy would certainly be different, they both change with time to evolve more aggressive subpopulations with new characteristics of invasion and pathogenesis. A hallmark of all cancers shared by the leukemias is their constant evolution and intercellular competition, limited only by the life span of the host and probably accelerated by our commonly used therapies. As more therapies targeted at specific molecular changes become available, it will be crucial to discriminate the type of leukemia by a specific cytogenetic or molecular event and to define the secondary genetic changes that could limit the effectiveness of a particular therapy.

Hematopoietic Growth Factors as Definitive Participants in Leukemogenesis

During the last two decades, the combined forces of academia and the biotechnology industry have defined and molecularly cloned dozens of hematopoietic growth factors and cytokines that regulate growth and development of blood cells. These factors and their complex range of specificities and mechanisms of action are covered elsewhere in this book, but several trends that relate to the generation of leukemia need discussion.

In various experimental systems, including retroviral transduction into murine bone marrow stem cells and chronic expression from transgenic technology, a hyperproliferative state that can evolve into a leukemic phenotype has been documented when cytokine genes are constitutively expressed.[3, 4] Although the details can vary from factor to factor or with the specific strategy used, the impression gathered is that high doses of any individual factor are needed to see the phenotype and that the pathology is related to cellular excess of specific cell types derived from multiple clones of progenitor cells. These hyperproliferative states are likely produced from hematopoietic elements, which themselves produce the factor in an autocrine loop, and bystander cells responding in the local environment. These same clinical and pathological features can be seen for the autonomous growth of a leukemia, but the time course after genomic insult and evolution from a clone of cells has a very different character.

Much has been published correlating growth factor levels as a participant in the causation and evolution of human leukemia, but few definitive mechanisms linking excessive production of a growth factor to the generation of a leukemia exist. One excellent example is provided by the group of patients with pre-B-cell leukemia associated with the t(5:14) translocation.[5] In these cases, the rearrangement brings the immunoglobulin heavy-chain promoter and enhancer into continuity with the interleukin-3 (IL-3) gene and results in excess production of the factor and presumably a potent autocrine loop to stimulate this immature B-lineage population. IL-3 can function on other cell types, including immature multilineage progenitors and cells in the myeloid lineage, but the pathological outgrowth is largely restricted to the immature B-lineage cells because of the restricted expression pattern of the immunoglobulin gene control elements and the greater effect of an autocrine compared to a paracrine loop. An analogous type of event is seen in a murine myelomonocytic leukemic line called WEHI-3, in which a retroviral-like mobile genetic element called an intracisternal A particle has relocated near the murine IL-3 gene and enhanced its expression resulting in an autocrine loop as a part of the leukemic process.[6]

Such dramatic examples of high-level continuous production of a factor and autocrine stimulation of a specific cell type lead to the simplistic notion that increasing the level of any growth factor is sufficient to drive a leukemic process. However, specific mechanisms have evolved to kinetically regulate the action of growth factors and their receptors. For every phosphorylation event occurring at the receptor level or downstream in a signaling pathway, there are balances with dephosphorylation mechanisms that limit the strength and duration of the signal. Most factor-receptor interactions are intended to induce a change in differentiation or growth status that is not permanent, and downregulation or desensitization by receptor degradation and other mechanisms is used to limit the signal. A particularly good example of this type of mechanism is demonstrated by the family of suppressors of cytokine stimulation (SOCS) genes that are transcriptionally induced by cytokine action but function to bind and inactivate critical components in the signal cascade and limit the persistence of the signal.[7] Studies suggest that SOCS proteins regulate the degradations of JAK family kinases by a ubiquitin-mediated proteolysis mechanism.[8] Each SOCS protein has an SH2 domain that targets interaction with certain phosphotyrosine modified JAKs. In addition, each SOCS protein has a conserved C-terminal motif called the SOCS BOX, which can interact with elongin B or elongin C. The elongin molecules can bind to and activate the ubiquitin-mediated proteolysis process to degrade the targeted JAK kinase and limit the cytokine signal strength and duration. If chronic stimulation by a growth factor is to play a critical role in a leukemogenic process, it must circumvent these countercontrols, which are quantitatively balanced to the strength of the inducing signal.

Another difficulty with the simple model of "add more growth factor and make a leukemia" is the realization that the same receptors that signal for positive proliferation can lead to induction of cell death pathways if the signal strength is not at an optimal level. This is dramatically seen for the immunoglobulin receptor on B lymphocytes, for which high- or low-dose stimulation with antigen or crosslinking reagents can result in cell stasis, proliferation, or death, depending on the co-stimulation of other receptors on the cell surface.[9]

In the mouse and human IL-3 examples cited, the genetic damage alters the expression level of a normal growth factor, which presumably binds to cognate receptors to stimulate the cell. A unique but instructive example comes from the pseudoligand strategy used by the replication defective spleen focus forming virus (SFFV) component of the polycythemia strain of the Friend murine leukemia retrovirus complex.[10] The SFFV component RNA encodes a single glycoprotein with a molecular mass of 55,000 that represents a truncated and mutated version of the class of envelope glycoproteins used by retroviruses in assembly of virions. The SFFV-derived glycoprotein can bind avidly to the erythropoietin (Epo) receptor and stimulate an autocrine loop and cellular hyperplasia. Further genetic damage is necessary to progress to frank leukemia, but the initial phase of the virally induced disease requires this pseudoligand stimulation.[11] Earlier models for activation of the erythropoietin receptor were based on the concept that ligand-induced dimerization was an essential first step in activating the receptor and coupling its output to the JAK/STAT system. However, the binding site for the SFFV glycoprotein is distinct from the hormone-binding cleft. Direct crystallographic evidence and functional analysis have demonstrated that the Epo receptor exists in a preformed dimer conformation, with JAK2 tethered to its cytoplasmic domain.[12, 13] Activation by Epo is related to an allosteric effect rather than the dimerization step. Binding of the SFFV glycoprotein presumably can induce a similar allosteric effect through a different site of interaction and trigger the receptor. It is possible that derivatives of molecules associated with other physiological processes and not previously defined as ligands for hematopoietic growth factor receptors could play a role as pseudoligands. The class of peptide inhibitors of angiogenesis[14-16] derived by fragmentation of a common connective tissue protein normally involved in clotting and adhesion could be viewed as another type of pseudoligand.

It is interesting that the binding site and mechanism of receptor activation must be different for the native erythropoietin molecule and the viral pseudoligand, suggesting that alternative pathways to activate receptors are possible. Small peptides have been defined that can activate the thrombopoietin receptor by binding to sites distinct from the pockets used by the natural ligands but still capable of activating the critical changes in the receptor needed to initiate signaling.[17] Small molecules should eventually replace many of the peptide growth factors now used in clinical practice.

Receptor Alterations in Leukemogenesis

Hematopoietic cells use hundreds of different molecules on their cell surface to receive information from the surrounding environment in the form of soluble molecules, as well as those covalently or noncovalently presented on an adjoining cell surface. In the broadest context, a receptor can be considered as any molecule capable of receiving a signal and participating in transmitting it into the cell. This is relatively easy to visualize for molecules such as transmembrane tyrosine kinase receptors like c-kit, CSF-1 receptor, or the insulin receptor, which bind a specific protein ligand in a cell-surface-bound or soluble form to activate growth and differentiation programs in immature hematopoietic precursors and other cell lineages. The intrinsic tyrosine kinase activity is activated by ligand engagement of the receptor molecules, which causes an allosteric change in shape and multimerization that is transmitted through the transmembrane portion to the intracellular domain, which leads to a program of tyrosine phosphorylation of the receptor, recruitment of other signaling molecules, and further signal transduction.[18]

Receptors for the large family of cytokines that regulate hematopoiesis can have more complicated subunit structures but lack an intrinsic enzyme activity.[19] The intracellular domain of one or more subunit is coupled to kinases such as the JAK family, which can sense the binding of extracellular ligand, become activated, and pass on the signal to molecules such as the STATs to carry the signal into the cell.[20] This pattern of ligand-induced molecular shape change and subunit rearrangement is seen for all classes of receptors for which it has been carefully studied, regardless of the nature of the ligand, which can be a small molecule such as a peptide or a large macromolecular structure such as the surface of a virus particle.

Equally important are the molecular interactions that modify and regulate the efficiency of ligand presentation and hence signal strength to the primary receptor. In the transmembrane multisubunit serine kinase family of receptors used by members of the transforming growth factor-β (TGFβ) family of ligands, a low-affinity but high-capacity interaction helps bind the factor and present it to the portion of the receptor complex with intrinsic enzyme activity.[21] The signals that emanate from this family of receptors can include strong negative effects on cell cycle proliferation and can serve as antagonists of factors that are generally positive influences on the expansion of blood-formed elements.

Because the overall outcome of a cellular decision to divide, differentiate, or die must integrate all these different receptor activities, alterations in receptor function may be expected to feature prominently in human leukemogenesis. Mutations that vary the dosage of a receptor, its ability to multimerize and activate in low or zero ligand concentration, or resist the downregulatory mechanisms that normally limit the duration of signaling for positive acting receptors should set the stage for secondary damage and progression to leukemia. Conversely, inactivation of negative regulatory receptors may change the balance of cell growth analogously to inactivation of a tumor suppressor gene such as *p53* and promote leukemic change. With all this opportunity, why has relatively little direct evidence for the role of receptor activity mutations been accumulated for human leukemias? There is no simple answer, but the complexity of signals emanating from any single receptor that regulate growth and differentiation signals must achieve the right balance to give a net proliferative signal to a clone of cells.

Several excellent examples from the literature on retroviral pathology show how expression of chronic high levels of a specific receptor can produce proliferative changes

and eventually produce leukemias. The myeloproliferative leukemia virus is a rapidly transforming, replication-defective murine retrovirus that expresses the *mpl* oncogene. The normal cellular homologue of mpl is the receptor for the megakaryocyte progenitor growth and differentiation factor thrombopoietin (TPO), which has growth and differentiation effects on red blood cell and platelet precursors.[22] Transfer of this retrovirus into susceptible mouse strains causes a mixed myeloid outgrowth that has all the characteristics expected of a transmissible leukemia. Other examples of naturally occurring retroviral transduction of hematopoietic growth factor receptors include the CSF-1 receptor (*fms* oncogene), the stem cell factor receptor (*kit* oncogene), and the epidermal growth factor (EGF) receptor family member erb-B.[23] In some of these cases, the pathology of the original viral isolate is restricted to nonhematopoietic cell types such as mesenchyme-derived fibroblasts and muscle cells in the causation of sarcomas. The association of these oncogenes with hematopoietic receptors was made from patterns of restricted gene expression and alternative systems of biological analysis. Many engineered examples of retroviral constructs of wild-type or specifically mutated receptors are available in the literature and reinforce the concept that dosage increase or molecular changes that favor ligand-independent allosteric and multimerization changes needed to activate receptors can be sufficient to convert a receptor to oncogenic behavior.

The amplification and hyperexpression of growth factor receptors such as that encoded by the *HER-2/NEU* oncogene in a subgroup of breast cancer patients are well documented and strongly correlate with chance of progression.[24] Amplified expression of other classes of oncogenes such as c-*myc* in human and murine lymphomas and n-*myc* in human neuroblastomas by means of chromosome translocations or amplification of chromosome regions as homogeneous staining regions or double minute chromosomes presage the types of mechanisms expected for growth factor receptors in leukemias.

For human multiple myeloma, there are case reports with chromosomal translocations occurring between the immunoglobulin heavy-chain locus on chromosome 14 and the fibroblast growth factor receptor (type 3), a member of the tyrosine kinase family of receptors, on chromosome 4.[25, 26] Structural analysis of the DNA rearrangements suggest that deregulated expression of the intact receptor would occur and presumably increase its level to that required for ligand independent stimulation. No clear data define the signal transduction pathways affected by the tyrosine kinase activity, but presumably, this receptor can link to pathways functional in late-stage B cells.

Variation in Epo receptor dosage in human erythroleukemias has been reported but not with the consistency or elucidation of the mechanism to give it high value in the causation of the disease. Complementary studies in the murine system using an activating point mutation that leads to ligand-independent signal transduction and leukemias of erythroid precursors after retroviral transduction[27] suggest that this pathway can initiate leukemogenesis in this cell type with optimal stimulation. Several groups have reported autosomal dominant mutations in the Epo receptor associated with familial polycythemia.[28-30] The mutations often result in truncations of the receptor cytoplasmic domain needed for negative regulation of signal transduction. The balance of proliferative versus differentiative effects of the Epo receptor probably plays a role in the outcome of the murine and human mutations, but the nature of these specific signals has not been defined. It would be interesting to compare the results of retroviral transduction of the human polycythemia mutations into murine bone marrow to assess the potential species variation in response from a fundamental difference in the signal complexity emanating from each type of mutant receptor.

The balance between proliferation and terminal maturation to nondividing cells can influence the development of leukemia in the myeloid lineage. Several kindreds presenting with congenital neutropenia with mutations of the granulocyte colony-stimulating factor (G-CSF) receptor that prevent production of neutrophils have been identified. A relatively high proportion of cases progress to myelodysplastic syndromes and myeloid leukemias.[31] The implication is that failure to mature creates a more favorable situation for accumulation of additional genetic damage and hyperproliferation of immature progenitors. Transgenic expression of human G-CSF receptors with mutations found in human patients with congenital neutropenia and acute myelogenous leukemia (AML) has been analyzed.[32, 33] Animals have normal numbers of granulocytes and dramatically heightened responses to G-CSF but no leukemias. Clearly, these types of receptor mutations are not sufficient for oncogenesis.

Specialized receptor systems described in model systems such as *Drosophila* and conserved in mammals function to keep stem cells for specific cell fates in the undifferentiated and highly replicative state.[34] Members of the Notch family of receptors bind to a class of ligands variously called Delta, Jagged, or Serrate, the action of which is modified by

molecules of the Fringe family. Notch receptors are large transmembrane proteins with multiple repeats of EGF-related sequences and another specialized sequence motif called a lin-12 domain in their extracellular domain. The cytoplasmic domain has no obvious enzymatic activity but has about six ankyrin-like repeats, a glutamine-rich segment, and a PEST sequence rich in serine and threonine. The intracellular processing of the Notch receptor is complex and probably involves proteolysis and assembly of a heterodimeric complex on the cell surface.[35–37] Evidence favors a signaling mechanism initiated by cell-cell contact that results in activation of gene sets involved in preventing differentiation (Fig. 26–1).

In a subtype of human T-cell leukemias with a specific translocation between chromosomes 7 and 9, the T-cell-antigen receptor β chain gene rearranges within the human *Notch-1* gene, leading to its truncation within the extracellular EGF repeats.[38] This was originally considered to be an inactivating event, which would have required loss of the other Notch allele or loss of a pathway sensitive to a haploid reduction in gene dosage. Later data have indicated that the truncated allele itself can send a positive growth signal in rodent fibroblast transformation and bone marrow transfer models.[39, 40] The retroviral construct used to transduce the activated Notch alleles into murine bone marrow elements could be expected to be expressed in many cell types, but only T-lineage leukemias were observed in these studies. There is probably a restriction of the action of different Notch alleles in different cell types. Supporting evidence for this comes from the restricted patterns of expression for different Notch alleles, the selective developmental changes of activated Notch alleles,[41] and the isolation of a truncated form of the *Notch-2* allele in a feline retrovirus associated

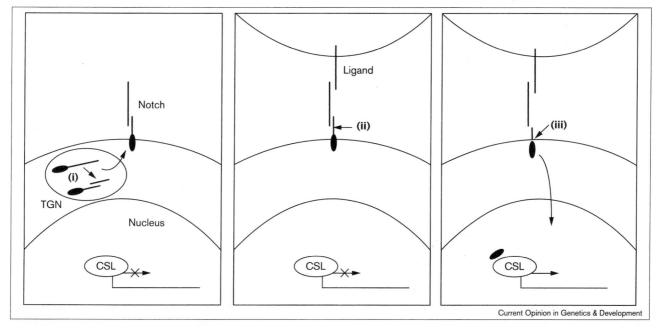

Current Opinion in Genetics & Development

Figure 26–1. Model for Notch signal transduction. A proposed model for Notch signal transduction that involves three independent proteolytic cleavage events. The first cleavage (i) is ligand independent and may occur in the *trans*-Golgi to produce a functional cell surface Notch receptor. After ligand binding, Notch undergoes a second proteolytic event (ii), possibly mediated by a metalloproteinase. After or with the second cleavage, a third cleavage event (iii) generates a soluble cytoplasmic form of Notch that could move to the nucleus to directly interact with and activate CSL protein (a DNA-binding protein that interacts with the cytoplasmic domain of Notch to drive the transcription of responsive genes). (From Weinmaster, G.: Notch signaling: direct or what? Curr. Opin. Genet. Dev. 8:436–442, 1998; with permission.)

with thymic lymphomas,[42] and the rescue of thymoma lines from steroid induced apoptosis by exogenous Notch fragments.[43]

Although the precise nature of the signal sent from the activated *Notch* allele is unknown, evidence favors a model in which ligand-activated or ligand-independent forms are bound with a member of the CSL group of transcription factors, which includes core binding factor and suppressor of hairless. A proteolytic event triggered by specific ligand or occurring spontaneously for the activated receptor form cleaves off an intracellular fragment of the Notch molecule, and it relocates to the nucleus and binds an associated transcription factor to activate gene transcription favoring stem cell renewal and resisting differentiation.[44-46] Other possible pathways could be influenced by the intracellular segment of Notch receptors, which contain multiple-ankyrin repeats, including the NF-κB pathway, which uses inhibitors such as I-κB with a similar overall structure.[47] A more thorough understanding of the nature of such signals for leukemic stem cells would provide important information for planning points of attack for novel therapies.

Certain families of receptors, such as members of the TGFβ superfamily, are known to slow or block hematopoietic cell proliferation for specific lineages. Although the combinatorial possibilities for this large family of ligands and receptors and their effects on different blood cell types is immense, reduction or loss of function of the TGFβ system on certain blood cells such as lymphocytes generally would be predicted to augment cell growth and participate in leukemogenesis. Several correlative examples have been described, including biallelic loss of function of type I TGFβ receptors associated with a subset of chronic lymphocytic leukemias[48] and dominant inhibitory mutants of type II TGFβ receptors in a patient with progression of a cutaneous T-cell lymphoma.[49] The mechanism of dominant inhibition by the mutated allele, which carries a point mutation within the serine kinase domain, appears to be a transdominant blockade of receptor intracellular processing and presentation on the cell surface.

Many receptors are capable of positive and negative growth control for a specific cell type. B lymphocytes use the immunoglobulin antigen–specific receptor to mediate proliferative expansion when the dose of antigen and co-stimuli fall within a critical zone, or it can transmit an apoptotic signal if the balance of signals is not correct.[9] One intriguing mechanism used by the Epstein-Barr virus in its proliferative expansion of B cells is to specifically inactivate the B-cell-antigen receptor by use of a dominant-negative cell surface multimembrane-spanning receptor such as LMP-2 (latent membrane protein type 2).[50, 51] The function of this receptor-like molecule is not to receive a ligand signal from outside the cell, but instead to decoy and bind the various members of the src family of cytoplasmic tyrosine kinases such as lyn, fyn, hck, and blk, which the B-cell-antigen receptor uses to transmit the positive and negative growth signals to downstream pathways. LMP-2 can also send positive signals for growth and development.[52] One might expect to find similar inactivation of the B-cell receptor in human lymphoid malignancies. Mutations and expression variation in the B-cell-antigen receptor–associated molecule called B29 or Igβ, which is essential for signal transduction and B-cell development, have been described in a high percentage of chronic lymphocytic leukemias (CLL).[53] Further work is needed to see what roles these changes in expression and function play in the genesis or progression of CLL but the resemblance to the role of LMP-2 to prevent apoptosis needs further evaluation.

Intracellular Signaling Mechanisms

When a blood cell at any stage of maturation encounters a signal through a cell surface receptor or combination of receptors, it must transmit that information into the cell for a decision process. Many such decisions involve transfer of information to the nucleus to drive gene transcription events associated with cell cycle progression or definitive differentiative changes. However, even in terminally differentiated granulocytes, receptor-mediated interactions regulate cell shape, activation of specific degranulation reactions, and extravasation reactions needed to participate in an inflammatory response. Intracytoplasmic and cytoskeletal changes must be considered along with the transcriptional events associated with oncogenic signal transduction.

The complexity of intracellular signaling pathways, like the combinations of growth factors and their receptors, is almost beyond description. Similar to receptor systems, intracytoplasmic signal transduction can be divided into components that are fixed in concentration (i.e., "hard wired") and those whose expression is regulated in a developmental sequence or in response to specific signals. Some signal transduction molecules are generally expressed in all cell types, and others are tightly restricted in their expression patterns.

When viewed in a global manner, the myriad and interconnected pathways of signal transduction, as seen in the various wall charts provided by companies selling associated reagents, can give the false impression that all the paths defined have equal importance in the cellular outcome for a specific inducing signal. The weight of any particular pathway can only be judged in a genetic test of function. The best understood cases are those in which more genetically tractable organisms, such as yeast, *Drosophila,* or *Caenorhabditis elegans,* have conserved signaling pathways, such as the tyrosine kinase-RAS-MAP kinase cascades.[54] The biochemical definition of a specific component's activation during signal transduction cannot be used as an unambiguous monitor of its relative importance in the final cellular decision.

The specific genetic damage associated with naturally occurring leukemias and other cancers provides a unique opportunity to unite a molecular change with a specific pathway and a biological outcome. A significant limitation is that each event defined, such as a chromosome translocation or point mutation, is part of an evolving process in which the other changes needed to establish the patient's phenotype and help fix a specific mutation into the leukemic clone are unknown. Attempts to create animal models using specific human leukemia–derived oncogenes have improved considerably over the past several years and provide the opportunity to test combinatorial aspects of oncogenesis and the evolution of these complex phenotypes.

As leukemia progresses, the continual process of mutation, selection, and clonal evolution largely determine tumor burden and clinical outcome. What level of change is sufficient to initiate this progression? Because signal transduction cascades are designed to operate with positive signals counterbalanced by downregulatory mechanisms at multiple points along each pathway, it was of interest to determine if elevation of the dosage of a single nonmutated signaling component was sufficient to produce leukemogenesis.

The src family of cytoplasmic tyrosine kinases are key regulators of hematopoietic development and signal response. They help transduce signals from antigen receptors in T and B cells, various cytokine receptors, and other cell surface molecules, including GPI-anchored proteins. More than eight members are expressed in various hematopoietic cell types in a complex pattern.[55] Although many are expressed in a redundant manner within different hematopoietic lineages, specific loss of function mutations created in knockout mice show that certain receptors primarily use one or a limited set of src family kinases as their predominant signal transducer. For example, although the lyn, fyn, and blk kinases are all expressed in B lymphocytes and can be activated by antigen stimulation of the immunoglobulin receptor, only the knockout of lyn has a particularly penetrant phenotype in B-lymphocyte signaling and pathology.[56–58]

The lck member of this family has been extensively studied for its role in T-cell development and signal response. The CD4 and CD8 accessory molecules of the T-cell receptor interact with lck in different types of T cells and serve as a substrate for tyrosine phosphorylation by lck and subsequent signal complex formation with recruitment of other components.[59] Lck can be artificially activated as an oncogene by engineering the deletion or point mutations that alter the highly conserved negative regulatory tyrosine residue located near the carboxy-terminus of the protein, similar to the conversion of cellular src to its viral oncogenic form. Some human T-cell leukemias have a specific joining of the T-cell receptor B-chain control element near the lck locus, which activates transcription and increases expression of the kinase[60, 61] (Fig. 26–2).

To test the role of dosage increase of a nonmutated form of lck, a series of transgenic mice were created that expressed lck from a construct driven by one of the alternative T-cell–specific lck homologous promoters and enhancers.[62] Mice were selected that varied in copy number and were shown to vary in quantitative expression of lck in the thymus in a generally linear manner related to the transgene copy number. At increasing dosage of lck, there was a loss of expression of the CD3 receptor complex on the surface of developing T cells characteristic of less mature cells. At higher dose ranges, thymic leukemias occurred as the animals matured. These studies strongly support the concept that chronic elevation of even a single signal transducer can predispose to malignant progression but must await additional genetic damage to fix a specific clone of cells into a pathway culminating with a frank leukemia.

The processes of chromosome translocation and mRNA splicing can create genetic fusions in which the coding sequences of two proteins are joined and change the control of expression, stability, localization, and function. The chimeric nature of such proteins opens a Pandora's box of signaling possibilities. Each component of the chimera can be viewed as a mutated version of the original protein,

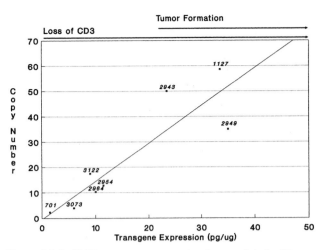

Figure 26–2. *PLGF transgene expression is correlated with copy number and thymic phenotype.* Transgene mRNA levels were determined by solution hybridization assays or by quantitative densitometry. The number of transgene copies integrated into tail DNA was similarly assessed by quantitative densitometry using isolated transgene sequences as standards. Lines above the figure indicate the characteristic phenotypes observed over each dose interval. The level of endogenous *lck* mRNA is indicated at the bottom of the figure. (From Abraham, K.M., et al.: Delayed thymocyte development induced by augmented expression of p56[lck]. J. Exp. Med. 173:1421–1432, 1991; with permission.)

and the overall fusion protein may produce effects neither component alone could accomplish. As discussed in later sections, many examples of chimeric transcription factors created by leukemia-specific translocations have been described. An increasing number of such chimeric structures have been defined in subtypes of leukemias in which one component is derived from a member of the tyrosine kinase family and the second from quite disparate gene families (Table 26–1). Understanding the alternative modes of activation for the tyrosine kinases involved and the common and distinct modes of signal transduction from such chimeras should provide insights for defining the critical pathways used in leukemogenesis (Fig. 26–3).

The landmark description of the Philadelphia chromosome with its highly uniform association with CML and its definition by banding techniques as a balanced translocation between chromosomes 9 and 22 heralded the connection between a unique cytogenetic change and a specific leukemia.[63] The demonstration of the cellular homologue of the abl tyrosine kinase on that part of chromosome 9 retained on the Ph chromosome led to the definition of the DNA structural rearrangement, the large 8.5-kb chimeric mRNA, and chimeric protein structure referred to as P210 Bcr-Abl.[64–66] The rearrangement almost always occurs upstream of the second exon of the *Abl* gene on chromosome 9 and includes all the sequences encoding the Abl SH3 domain through the carboxy terminus. On chromosome 22, the major breakpoint cluster region (M-bcr) in CML occurs within a 5- to 6-kb segment harboring several small exons of the *BCR* gene and can produce some variability in the Bcr-Abl structure that does not seem to have any major consequence on the overall function of the chimera. In the subset of patients with Ph-positive ALL, AML, or occasionally CML, presentation of an alternative breakpoint region (m-bcr) that extends over 100 kb within the first intron of the *BCR* gene

Table 26–1. Tyrosine Kinases Translocations

Disease	Chromosomal Abnormality	Activated Gene	Mechanism of Activation	Predominant Structural Feature*	Invertebrate Homologue	References
CMLL	t(5;12)(q33;p13)	TEL-PDGFRβ	Gene fusion	Tyrosine kinase		76
AML	t(9;12;14)(q34;p13;q22)	TEL-ABL	Gene fusion	Tyrosine kinase		77, 257
Anaplastic large-cell lymphoma	t(2;5)(p23;q35)	NPM-ALK	Gene fusion			258
CML	t(9;22)(q34;q11)	BCR-ABL	Gene fusion	Tyrosine kinase	abl (D)	259–262
ALL	t(9;22)(q34;q11)	BCR-ABL	Gene fusion	Tyrosine kinase	abl (D)	68, 263, 264
T-cell ALL	t(1;7)(p34;q34)	LCK	Relocation to TCRβ locus	Tyrosine kinase		61, 265, 266
T-cell ALL	t(9;12)(p24;p13)	JAK2	Gene fusion	Tyrosine kinase		78, 79
CMML	t(5;7)(q33;q11.2)	HIP1-PDGFβR	Gene fusion	Tyrosine kinase		81
AML	t(5;14)(q33;q32)	CEV14-PDGFβR	Gene fusion	Tyrosine kinase		82

AML, acute myeloid leukemia; ALL, acute lymphoblastic leukemia; APML, acute promyelocytic leukemia; CML, chronic myeloid leukemia; bHLHzip, basic region/helix-loop-helix/leucine; zipper domain, BZIP, basic region/leucine zipper domain.

*Based on analysis of DNA-binding/protein interaction domain. For gene fusions, the partner contributing this structural feature is given in parenthesis.

Adapted from Look, A.T.: Genes altered by chromosomal translocations in leukemias and lymphomas. *In* Vogelstein B, Kinzler K, eds.: The Genetic Basis of Human Cancer. McGraw-Hill Book Co., 1998; with permission.

is used that generates a shorter chimeric mRNA and a P185 (or alternatively named P190) Bcr-Abl protein associated with more aggressive biology.[67, 68]

When these different forms of Bcr-Abl were compared in biological tests of function, they were both able to induce transformation responses in rodent fibroblasts and pre-B-cells, relieve growth factor requirements for a variety of hematopoietic cell lines, and create in vivo leukemias with characteristics of CML or various acute leukemias.[69–75] CML models used enriched populations of hematopoietic stem cells and retroviral delivery of Bcr-Abl to initiate the disease. Mice developed a chronic-like phase with multilineage involvement that could evolve into a blast crisis phase with lymphoid or myeloid dominance after transplantation into syngeneic hosts. There was a clear increase in potency of the P185 form when directly compared with the P210 form in several systems that could be directly related to the increase in specific activity of the tyrosine kinase.

These chimeric structures of the *Bcr-Abl* oncogenes were strikingly similar to the previously described Gag-Abl fusion protein structure expressed from the Abelson murine leukemia virus.[63] In this case, viral transduction had recombined a murine retroviral group antigen gene sequence with a portion of the cellular Abl tyrosine kinase. In the Gag-Abl fusion, the recombination occurs within the Abl SH3 domain, and further mutations within the kinase domain have been selected which augment kinase activation. Although the precise definition of the alternative structural changes for the *Gag-Abl* and *Bcr-Abl* genes are beyond the scope of this chapter, the common thread of deletion and substitution of amino-terminal sequences that mediate changes in cellular localization and kinase activity are evident.

Over the past several years, additional examples of chromosome translocations associated with specific forms of leukemia and lymphoma bear a striking similarity to the general form of *Bcr-Abl* (see Table 26–1). In chronic myelo-

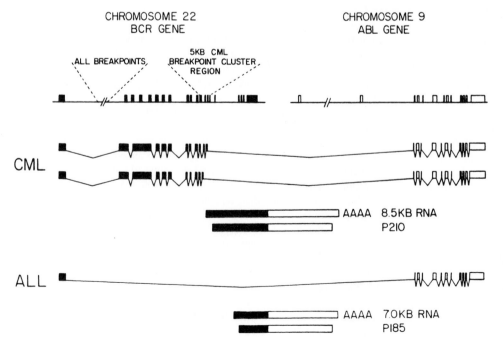

Figure 26–3. Production of the P210 and P185 proteins. The approximate genomic structures of the *BCR* and *ABL* genes are shown, with exonic sequences depicted by the open or blackened boxes. The two breakpoint cluster regions and the resulting chimeric RNA and protein products are identified. Translocation of the *ABL* oncogene to the CML breakpoint cluster region (bcr) in the middle of the *BCR* gene results in the expression of 8.5-kb BCR-ABL RNA and the P210 protein. *ABL* translocation to the ALL bcr in the 5′ portion of the *BCR* gene results in the expression of the 7.0-kb BCR-ABL message and the P185 protein. (From Clark, S.S., et al.: Molecular Pathogenesis, 1989; with permission.)

monocytic leukemias, the t(5;12) translocation generates a fusion between a portion of the *Tel* gene (a member of the Ets family of transcription factors) and a portion of the intracytoplasmic domain of the platelet-derived growth factor type B (PDGFB) chain receptor tyrosine kinase.[76] The *Tel* gene can also recombine by the t(12;19) found in some in acute myeloid leukemias with the *Abl* gene,[77] and the *Jak2* kinase in a series of alternative exon fusion chimeras seen in different myeloid and lymphoid leukemias with the t(9;12) cytogenetic marker.[78, 79] The *Npm* (nucleophosmin) gene can fuse to *Alk*, a member of the receptor family of tyrosine kinases in the t(2;5) rearrangement found in large cell anaplastic lymphomas.[80] Additional rearrangements creating fusion proteins between the Huntintin disease gene protein and the PDGF receptor in the t(5;7) translocation of myelomonocytic leukemia and the *Cev* gene in acute myeloid leukemias with the t(5;14) translocation have been published.[81, 82] Although no specific genomic sequence relationships that would mediate such recombinations have been clearly defined, it is noteworthy that the *Tel* gene appears quite promiscuous in its rearrangements. Additional chromosome juggling involving *Tel* is seen in its rearrangements with another transcription factor AML1 (discussed in a later section).

A common feature of all these tyrosine kinase rearrangement partners is their ability to mediate an oligomerization of the chimeric structure. This is reminiscent of the key role that ligand-induced oligomerization plays in the activation of native receptor tyrosine kinases. Such oligomerizations frequently initiate a chain of events, including autophosphorylations and transphosphorylations, which amplify the activation by directly altering the kinase activity and

leading to the assembly of other signaling components on the decorated receptor. In the case of Bcr, a coiled-coiled type of protein oligomerization domain located near the amino terminus is essential for the activation of the Abl kinase activity and all biological activities of the chimera.[83, 84] Tel uses a helix-loop-helix type dimerization domain, but the resulting effects on the PDGF receptor or Abl kinase segments are similar[85] (Fig. 26–4).

It is interesting to consider in more detail our understanding of the normal functions of the *Bcr* and *Abl* genes and how they relate to the roles they play in the oncogenic fusion. The *Bcr* gene is generally expressed in all tissues and has one known relative detectable by cross-hybridization but with limited structural homology. In addition to the Bcr amino-terminal oligomerization domain, it has a region rich in phosphoserine residues that can serve as a unique interaction site for SH2 domains,[86] a novel form of serine kinase activity,[87] a segment with homology to the *Db1* protooncogene, a pleckstrin homology domain, and GTPase-activating domain function with specificity for the small G proteins Rac and Rho.[88] With this abundance of signaling machinery, it is surprising to see the limited phenotype of Bcr null mice. The only definitive problem in such animals is the excessive oxidative burst from granulocytes and related cells causing tissue injury after endotoxin shock.[89] This is probably mediated by the loss of GAP activity to downregulate pathways controlled by the small G protein Rac in this cell type. In the alternative Philadelphia chromosome translocations seen in CML and ALL, the reciprocal translocation events would largely be composed of the first exon of *Abl* and portions of the *Bcr* gene. Several groups have demonstrated that the Abl-Bcr chimeric products are expressed in Ph chromosome

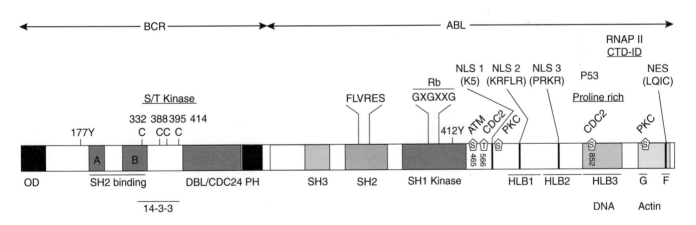

Figure 26–4. Complex signal transduction events associated with BCR-ABL. The *Bcr-Abl* oncogene uses direct physical interaction and substrate phosphorylations to influence a broad range of signal transduction pathways that mediate proliferative, anti-apoptotic, and cytoskeletal changes which combine to produce its leukemogenic effects.

leukemias and are probably enzymatically active for GAP function.[90] However, no specific oncogenic biology related to expression of these reciprocal products is known, and in vitro transformation assays and animal models of CML driven by the Bcr-Abl product do not appear to require their expression.

The cellular form of Abl can be produced with alternative first exon choices and is generally expressed in all tissues. The Abl tyrosine kinase domain is regulated in a complex manner by an amino-terminal SH3/SH2 domain unit and a more carboxy-terminal segment that includes general DNA binding activity, signals for nuclear import and export, a proline-rich region that can bind many SH3 domain–containing proteins, and regions for cytoskeletal interaction.[91–94] Myriad potential regulators have been defined by physical binding, including co-immunoprecipitation and yeast two-hybrid strategies. The precise function of the Abl protein has been hard to define, but evidence for involvement in processes as disparate as cell cycle regulation, pol II transcription, apoptosis, and response to genotoxic shock has been reported.[95–97] The phenotype of Abl-null mice is complex, with some cell-autonomous defects in lymphoid cell development and a host of generalized problems, including neonatal wasting, poor fecundity, and early death, that cannot be easily reconciled with the lengthy list of potential mediators.[98, 99]

What features of the individual components found in the chimera of Bcr-Abl make the new structure signal in an oncogenic manner? Much effort has defined the structural features of Bcr-Abl most critical for transformation and connected them to activation of several signaling pathways. Foremost is the enzymatic activity of the tyrosine kinase and its regulatory domains. Mutation of a major autophosphorylation site within the catalytic domain's activation loop sequence blocks much of the biological activity.[100] Loss of function of the SH2 domain by deletion or mutation of the FLVRES motif prevents efficient downstream tyrosine kinase signaling, whereas mutations in SH3 are generally positive activators of kinase activity and biological function.[101, 102]

It is more difficult to define the role of the multiple motifs found in the large last exon of Abl on the chimera. The nuclear localization and export signals, general DNA binding, and actin-interaction motifs probably play a role in the efficiency of transformation in in vitro systems. In addition to its oncogenic properties, Abl tyrosine kinases can promote cell cycle stasis,[103] and deletion of the carboxy-terminal domain can lessen its cellular toxicity and enhance transformation in some experimental settings.

The very large number of Abl-interacting proteins that can putatively connect to an array of downstream pathways allows almost any cellular signal to be potentially influenced by Bcr-Abl.[104–108] Evidence for interaction or activation with Ras pathway regulators such as PI3 kinase and others is available. Some binding proteins, such as Rin 1,[109] can affect the potency of kinase signaling and biological response in experimental transformation models.

Most of Bcr, except the oligomerization domain and the two serine-rich domains of the first exon, can be deleted with some retention of activity. An interesting site at residue Y177 can serve as a phosphorylation site for the Abl kinase, mediate binding of the Grb-2 signal transducer, and provide one of several connections for the kinase to the Ras pathways.[100, 110]

An alternative approach has been to link the effects of Bcr-Abl in experimental tests of transformation function to specific signaling pathways by correlating downstream activation of a pathway component or transcriptional response and showing that dominant negative inhibition of one pathway component limited the response of the cell.[111] Such approaches have implicated the Ras/MAP kinase cascades, activation of Jnk, Myc, Cyclin D1, NF-κB, PI3 kinase, PLC-γ, certain STAT proteins, anti-apoptotic effects involving Bcl-2, mitochondrial cytochrome *c* release and caspase function, cytoskeletal changes, and other mechanisms as being important for Bcr-Abl–mediated transformation.[112–124] The high level of tyrosine kinase activity can activate many pathways that appear to work in a coordinated manner to create the final leukemic phenotype, but it is not possible to quantitatively value each of the proposed downstream pathways, because a wide variety of experimental settings have been used.

Although the Tel-Abl, Tel-PDGF, and Npm-Alk fusions have not been studied as extensively, there are some interesting similarities in their patterns of signal transduction compared with Bcr-Abl. Alternative activation of the Abl tyrosine kinase by Tel or Bcr seems to result in very similar patterns of downstream activation. A single, small-molecule tyrosine kinase inhibitor can negatively influence signaling by Bcr-Abl, Tel-Abl, and Tel-PDGF receptor chimeras, even though the Abl and PDGF receptor structures are distinct.[125] Work has demonstrated common activation of STAT-1 and -5 by Bcr-Abl, Tel-Abl, Tel-PDGFB, and Tel-Jak2.[115, 126, 127] It is likely that all four of these kinases can directly phosphorylate the STAT proteins and send signals to the nucleus for new gene transcription.

Because many different signaling pathways are activated by the Bcr-Abl oncogene, the job of deciphering which are the quantitatively important signals critical for the creation of CML phenotype is a difficult task. One hint that a specific set of signals is most dominant in creation of the phenotype comes from the remarkable observation that genetic knockout of a single gene for interferon consensus sequence binding protein (ICSBP) can produce mice with a remarkable phenotype of the CML syndrome, including progression to blast crisis of alternative lineages.[128] Production of this factor in various myeloid leukemias, including CML, is low or absent compared with normal progenitors.[129] ICSBP can regulate immune interferon production and responses to intracellular pathogens. Even in the heterozygous state, a reduction in this nuclear factor can result in abnormal hematopoiesis and an eventual leukemic picture. The clinical observation that the chronic phase of CML patients can be effectively suppressed by treatment with interferon-α provides an interesting echo to these murine studies—something in the growth regulation of immature hematopoietic precursors is responding to the level of interferon pathway function, although the mechanistic details are not yet clear.[130]

Ras-Controlled Pathways Are Key Intracellular Mediators of Leukemogenesis

The small G protein Ras and its relatives are highly conserved signal transduction components for connecting various classes of receptors to cytoplasmic pathways. They regulate almost every aspect of cellular life, including proliferation in response to growth factors, cytoskeletal changes, differentiation programs, and cell death, depending on the specific experimental context. Direct binding and activation downstream of various tyrosine kinase receptors and other families of receptors can be mediated by cellular connector proteins such as Shc and Grb-2, whose assembly is regulated by tyrosine phosphorylation. Ras proteins are activated and inactivated for their role in signal transduction by the differential conformation they assume by exchanging GTP for GDP in their nucleotide binding pocket and its subsequent hydrolysis. The activated form can interact with a broad range of effector molecules, including those important in activating several kinase cascades such as Raf and MEKK1, production of PI and other lipid mediators such as PI3 kinase and some isoforms of PKC, and other members of the small G protein family.[131] This cycle is regulated by a multitude of cellular factors that can accelerate the activation of Ras by facilitating the exchange of nucleotides, as well as those that accelerate its inactivation by enhancing the hydrolysis of GTP. Mutations of any of the regulatory components that result in a prolongation of the GTP bound state, sensitize the system to Ras-dependent signals, or bypass the Ras control point could in theory give a sustained proliferative signal and participate in a leukemogenic process.[54]

Mutations of Ras at specific positions that are critical for GTP hydrolysis or its regulation are often found mutated in human cancer. In myelodysplastic syndrome and acute myelogenous leukemia, a specific allele called N-*Ras* is found mutated at a frequency of 40 per cent or more of the cases in some studies when analyzed by polymerase chain reaction (PCR) amplification and direct sequence analysis. As many as 50 per cent of patients with atypical CML lacking the Ph chromosome can show such activating *Ras* mutations.[132] It is not known whether Ras mutations are the initiating event in these processes or complement the progression of disease. The association of disordered hematopoiesis and Ph-negative CML with *Ras* mutations suggests that this genetic lesion alone would not be sufficient to explain the acute myeloid leukemias with which it is also associated.

A remarkable conservation of signal transduction pathways from yeast to man is seen in the connection between cell surface receptors, Ras and other small G proteins, and sets of protein kinases known as the MAP kinases, cascades of which are organized into scaffolded assemblies in the cytoplasm that connect to specific nuclear transcription events.[133] Particularly important for hematopoietic cells is the role that Ras pathways play in the response to extracellular growth and differentiation factors. A well-documented connection between these pathways and the genesis of human leukemias is provided by the role of mutations of the *NF1* gene in juvenile myelomonocytic leukemias (previously referred to as juvenile or childhood CML).

The *NF1* gene was first described in association with the pathology of neurofibromatosis, and its genetics suggested a tumor suppressor mode of action for cells in the peripheral nervous system. Children with NF1 mutations had a several hundred-fold higher risk of developing myeloid leukemias.[134] Homozygous inactivation of *NF1* was observed in leukemic cells from these patients. Subsequently, patients without clinical neurofibromatosis but suffering from juvenile myelomonocytic leukemias were shown to have a high frequency of *NF1* inactivation as well.[135] Analysis of the sequence of the *NF1* gene and direct functional studies of its protein product neurofibromin showed that it could act as a Gap (GTPase activating protein) or antagonist of Ras signal transduction. Loss of *NF1* presumably leads to prolonged Ras signaling and potentiates the effects of added extracellular growth factors, leading to proliferative effects and an increased chance of secondary genetic damage.[136]

Leukemic cells from these patients and hematopoietic cells from *NF1* knockout mice show greater responses to multiple growth factors, including GM-CSF, IL-3, and stem cell factor.[137] Strikingly, the myeloproliferative syndrome of NF1 knockout mouse fetal liver stem cells can be corrected by transplantation into mice deficient for production of GM-CSF.[138] This demonstrates that NF1-mediated pathogenesis is modified by the dosage of GM-CSF signaling and points directly to a target for therapeutic intervention in this subtype of leukemia.

A powerful experimental model to define new pathways and regulators of the leukemic phenotype comes from the use of retroviruses as insertional mutagens. The ability to activate gene transcription dependent on the chance insertion of a retroviral genome has been used to identify numerous proto-oncogenes that can contribute to the pathogenesis of T-cell–derived lymphomas in the mouse. This mutagenesis approach and an in vitro protocol that selected for variants with enhanced invasiveness into fibroblast monolayers defined a gene called *TIAM-1* which connects to the Ras family of small G proteins. TIAM-1 has the sequence characteristics of a group of regulators called GDP/GTP exchange factors, which includes the proto-oncogene *Dbl*, used to help Ras family members become activated.[130] TIAM-1 belongs to the subfamily that regulates the Rho-type small G proteins, which are positive effectors for cytoskeletal rearrangements needed for cell motility, an important component of metastatic and invasive phenotypes. Rho can also participate in sending signals for nuclear transcriptional events associated with proliferation. Increased dosage of the TIAM-1 exchanger would increase the rate of Rho activation and hence its effectiveness of signaling.

Transcription Factor Translocations

During the 4 years since the previous edition of this chapter, the number of transcription factors identified at the sight chromosome translocations has continued to grow (Tables 26–2 to 26–4). Lymphoid and myeloid leukemias can be grouped according to the frequency of specific translocations (Fig. 26–6). In each group, a random (or perhaps better stated as yet to be defined) fraction of 25 to 35 per cent cases occurs. Future efforts will define new molecular partners involved in human leukemia-associated translocations. A comprehensive review of this list is not possible here, but other reviews can be consulted.[140, 141] Whereas earlier versions of this list resembled a collection of seemingly unrelated genes, progress in the biological characterization of specific examples and the discovery of related genes targeted by novel translocations has allowed the emergence of several common themes. We divide these examples into genes that primarily play a role in hematopoietic development, hematopoietic differentiation, homeotic patterning, or apoptosis (Fig. 26–5).

Table 26–2. Transcription Factor Translocations in Lymphoid Leukemias and Lymphomas

Disease	Chromosomal Abnormality	Activated Gene	Mechanism of Activation	Predominant Structural Feature*	Invertebrate Homologue	References
B-cell ALL/Burkitt's lymphoma	t(8;14)(q24;q32)	MYC	Relocation to IgH locus	bHLHzip		142, 143, 267
	t(2;8)(p12;q24)	MYC	Relocation to IgL locus	bHLHzip		268–271
	t(8;22)(q24;q11)	MYC	Relocation to IgL locus	bHLHzip		272, 273
Pre-B-cell ALL	t(1;19)(q23;p13)	E2A-PBX1	Gene fusion	Homeodomain (PBX1)	exd (D), ceh-20 (C)	198, 199
Pro-B-cell ALL	t(17;19)(q22;p13)	E2A-HLF	Gene fusion	BZIP (HLF)	giant (D), ces-2 (C)	216, 217
Pro-B-cell ALL	t(12;21)(p13;q22)	TEL-AML1	Gene fusion	Runt homology (AML1)	runt (D)	162, 163, 274–276
T-cell ALL	t(8;14)(q24;q11)	MYC	Relocation to TCRα/δ locus	bHLHzip		277–279
	t(7;19)(q35;p13)	LYL1	Relocation to TCRβ locus	bHLH		280
	t(1;14)(p32;q11)	TAL1	Relocation to TCRα/δ locus	bHLH		281–283
	t(7;9)(q35;q34)	TAL2	Relocation to TCRβ locus	bHLH		283
	t(11;14)(p15;q11)	LMO1 (RBTN1)	Relocation to TCRα/δ locus	Cysteine-rich		284, 285
	t(11;14)(p13;q11)	LMO2 (RBTN2)	Relocation to TCRα/δ locus	Cysteine-rich		286, 287
	t(7;11)(q35;p13)	LMO2 (RBTN2)	Relocation to TCRβ locus	Cysteine-rich		
	t(10;14)(q24;q11)	HOX11	Relocation to TCRα/δ locus	Homeodomain		144, 288–290
	t(7;10)(q35;q24)	HOX11	Relocation to TCRβ locus	Homeodomain		
Diffuse B-cell lymphoma (large cell)	t(3;14)(q27;q32)	BCL6	Relocation to IgH locus	Zinc finger (BCL6)	tramtrack (D)	291–294
	t(3;4)(q27;p11)	BCL6	Relocation to TTF locus	Zinc finger (BCL6)	tramtrack (D)	292, 295
B-CLL	t(14;19)(q23;q13)	BCL3	Relocation to IgH locus	IκB		224–226
B-cell lymphoma	t(10;14)(q24;q32)	LYT10	Relection to IgH locus	Rel homology	dorsal (D)	223
Lymphoplasmacytoid B-cell lymphoma	t(9;14)(p13;q32)	PAX5	Relocation to IgH locus	Paired Homeobox	paired (D)	296

AML, acute myeloid leukemia; ALL, acute lymphoblastic leukemia; APML, acute promyelocytic leukemia; CML, chronic myeloid leukemia; bHLHzip, basic region/helix-loop-helix/leucine zipper domain, BZIP, basic region/leucine zipper domain.
*Based on analysis of DNA-binding/protein interaction domain. For gene fusions, the partner contributing this structural feature is given in parenthesis.

Table 26–3. Transcription Factor Translocations in Myeloid Leukemias

Disease	Chromosomal Abnormality	Activated Gene	Mechanism of Activation	Predominant Structural Feature*	Invertebrate Homologue	References
AML (granulocytic)	t(8;21)(q22;q22)	AML1-ETO	Gene fusion	Runt homology (AML1)	runt (D)	145, 146, 297, 298
Myelodysplasia	t(3;21)(q26;q22)	AML1-EAP	Gene fusion	Runt homology (AML1)	runt (D)	147
CML (blast crisis)	t(3;21)(q26;q22)	AML1-EVI1	Gene fusion	Runt homology (AML1)	runt (D)	148
AML (undifferentiated)	inv(3)(121,q26)	EVI1	Aberrant expression	Zinc finger	evil (D)	299, 300
AML (myelomonocytic)	inv(16)(p13;q22)	CBFβ-MYH11	Gene fusion	Complex with AML1 (CBFβ)		158
AML (promyelocytic)	t(15;17)(q21;q21)	PML-RARα	Gene fusion	Zinc finger (RARα)		164–166, 301, 302
AML (promyelocytic)	t(11;17)(q23;q21)	PLZF-RARα	Gene fusion	Zinc finger (RARα)		303
AML (promyelocytic)	t(5;17)(q32;q12)	NPM-RARα	Gene fusion	Zinc finger (RARα)		304
AML	t(16;21)(p11;q22)	FUS-ERG (TLS-ERG)	Gene fusion	Ets-like (ERG)		305
AML	t(12;22)(p13;q11)	TEL-MN1	Gene fusion	Ets-like (TEL)		306
AML	t(16;21)(q24;q22)	AML1-MTG16	Gene fusion	Runt homology		307
AML	inv(8)(p11;q13)	MoZ-TIF2	Gene fusion	Nuclear receptor co-activator		308, 309
AML	t(8;16)(p11;p13)	MOZ-CBP	Gene fusion	Nuclear receptor co-activator		310
AML	t(11;16)(q23;p13)	MLL-CBP	Gene fusion	Nuclear receptor co-activator		311, 312
AML	t(2;11)(q31;p15)	NUP98-HOXD13	Gene fusion	Homeotic gene		313
AML	t(7;11)(p15;p15)	NUP98-HOXA9	Gene fusion	Homeotic gene		314, 315
AML	unv(11)(p15;q31)	NUP98-DDX10	Gene fusion	RNA helicase		316

AML, acute myeloid leukemia; ALL, acute lymphoblastic leukemia; APML, acute promyelocytic leukemia; CML, chronic myeloid leukemia; bHLHzip, basic region/helix-loop-helix/leucine zipper domain; BZIP, basic region/leucine zipper domain.
*Based on analysis of DNA-binding/protein interaction domain. For gene fusions, the partner contributing this structural feature is given in parenthesis.

Table 26–4. Transcription Factor Translocations in Mixed-Lineage Leukemias

Disease	Chromosomal Abnormality	Activated Gene	Mechanism of Activation	Predominant Structural Feature*	Invertebrate Homologue	References
Pro-B-cell ALL	t(4;11)(q21;q23)	MLL-AF4	Gene fusion	A-T hook (MLL)	trithorax (D)	183, 186, 317
AML (monocytic)	t(9;11)(q21;q23)	MLL-AF9	Gene fusion	A-T hook (MLL)	trithorax (D)	318
ALL/AML	t(11;19)(q23;q13.3)	MLL-ENL	Gene fusion	A-T hook (MLL)	trithorax (D)	184, 318, 319
AML	t(11;19)(q23;13.1)	MLL-ELL	Gene fusion	A-T hook (MLL)	trithorax (D)	319, 320
AML	t(1;11)(q21;q23)	MLL-AF1Q	Gene fusion	A-T hook (MLL)	trithorax (D)	321
AML	t(1;11)(1p32;q23)	MLL-AFIP	Gene fusion	A-T hook (MLL)	trithorax (D)	322
AML	t(6;11)(q27;q23)	MLL-AF6	Gene fusion	A-T hook (MLL)	trithorax (D)	323
AML	t(10;11)(p12;q23)	MLL-AF10	Gene fusion	A-T hook (MLL)	trithorax (D)	324
AML	t(11;17)(q23;q21)	MLL-AF17	Gene fusion	A-T hook (MLL)	trithorax (D)	325
AML	t(X;11)(q13;q23)	MLL-AFX1	Gene fusion	A-T hook (MLL)	trithorax (D)	326, 327
AML	t(10;11)(p11;q23)	MLL-ABl-1	Gene fusion	A-T hook (MLL)	trithorax (D)	328
AML	t(11;22)(q23;q11.2)	MLL-hCDCrel	Gene fusion	Abl substrate (Abil) AT hook (MLL) GTP binding protein of DiGeorge syndrome		329

AML, acute myeloid leukemia; ALL, acute lymphoblastic leukemia; APML, acute promyelocytic leukemia; CML, chronic myeloid leukemia; bHLHzip, basic region/helix-loop-helix/leucine zipper domain; BZIP, basic region/leucine zipper domain.
*Based on analysis of DNA-binding/protein interaction domain. For gene fusions, the partner contributing this structural feature is given in parenthesis.

Mechanistically, translocations can alter the transcription factor target gene in two ways. In numerous lymphoid leukemias, one partner in the translocation is the immunoglobulin or T-cell receptor locus, which creates a strong transcriptional signal adjacent to the target gene without directly affecting its structure. The resulting leukemias develop as a consequence of increased dosage of the transcription factor target because of high-level overexpression of the normal gene product. Among the best examples are the well-characterized translocation of the c-*Myc* gene in Burkitt's lymphoma to any of the three immunoglobulin loci (heavy chain, lambda light chain, kappa light chain) and the *Hox11* homeobox gene, which is constitutively expressed in T-cell leukemias/lymphomas as a consequence of fusion to the T-cell receptor locus[142–144] (see Table 26–2). Similar to the previous examples involving the cytoplasmic tyrosine kinase Lck, transgenic expression of *Myc* or *Hox11* in the appropriate tissue compartment predisposes the animal to develop leukemia.

A more frequent mechanism for transcription factor deregulation by chromosome translocations in leukemia is through the creation of fusion genes, analogous to the tyrosine kinase fusions involving Abl, PDGFR, and Jak. The transcription factor gene fusions can function as oncogenes by distinct mechanisms. Many of these genes play essential roles in hematopoietic development or differentiation, and the fusion proteins interfere with this function. Because most of the genes targeted by these translocations were previously undefined, detailed characterization of the mechanism of leukemogenesis has shed new light on the molecular basis of normal hematopoietic development. These mechanistic insights have allowed novel therapeutic paradigms to be considered, some of which are in clinical testing.

Translocations in Genes Essential for Hematopoietic Development

When the breakpoints of the two most common translocations found in acute myeloid leukemias [t(8;21) and inv (16)] were cloned, an unexpected finding was the discovery that these two translocations target distinct subunits of the same transcription factor complex. Core binding factor (CBF) consists of α and β subunits, which bind DNA and regulate transcription from a number of genes involved in hematopoietic differentiation. The t(8;21) translocation targets the α subunit of CBF, also known as AML1, and creates a fusion protein with a second gene on chromosome 8 called *ETO* (eight twenty-one).[145, 146] The translocation product retains the DNA binding domain of AML1, which is highly related to the *Drosophila* homeotic gene *runt*, but the transactivation domain is lost as a consequence of fusion to the *ETO* gene (Fig. 26–6).

Structurally, analogous translocations involving AML1 have been reported in blast crisis of CML and in myelodysplastic syndromes associated with t(3;21) translocations, as well as in therapy-related AML associated with t(16;21) translocations.[147, 148] In each case, the *AML1* transactivation domain is removed and replaced with sequences from *EVI1*, *EAP*, or *MDS1* on chromosome 3 or *MTG16*, an *ETO* homologue, on chromosome 16. Because the common theme in each of these distinct translocations is fusion of the AML1 DNA binding domain to apparently unrelated proteins, it has been proposed that their oncogenicity is a consequence of loss of function in association with dominant negative inhibition of the remaining wild-type allele.

However, the experimental evidence supports the concept that gain-of-function effects of the fusion gene also play a role. In transfection experiments, wild-type AML1 activates transcription from the promoters of a number of CBF-responsive genes such as those for IL-3, GM-CSF, and the colony-stimulating factor-1 receptor. *AML1/ETO, AML1/EVI1,* and *AML/MDS1* function as dominant negative mutations, because all suppress the stimulatory effect of wild-type *AML1* in this assay.[149–151] Similar conclusions can be made from knockout and knockin experiments in which the *AML1* genomic locus is altered in the germline of mice. Homozygous deletion of *AML1* causes embryonic lethality because of severe defects in hematopoiesis, demonstrating that *AML1* is essential for hematopoiesis.[152] A similar pheno-

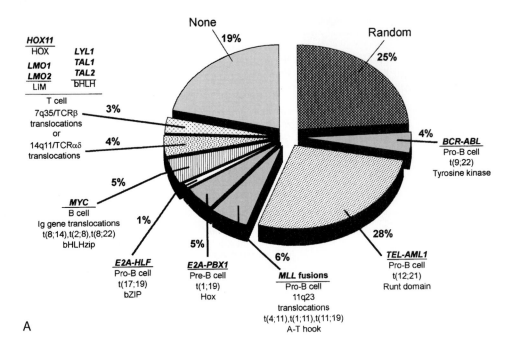

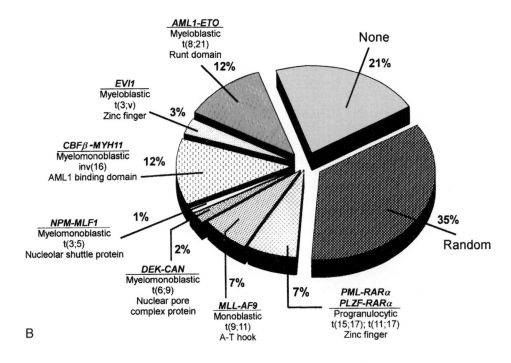

Figure 26–5. A, Distribution of translocation-generated fusion genes among the commonly recognized immunologic subtypes of ALL in children and young adults. Key domains for DNA binding and protein-protein interaction of transcription factors are shown; an exception is the tyrosine kinase domain indicated for BCR-ABL. The section labeled "random" refers to sporadic rearrangements that have so far been observed only in leukemic cells from single cases. **B,** Distribution of translocation-generated fusion genes among the various morphological subtypes of AML in children and young adults. The section labeled "random" refers to sporadic rearrangements that so far have been observed only in the leukemic cells from single cases. Key domains for DNA binding and protein-protein interaction are given for transcription factors, or the type of gene affected for nontranscription factors. (From Look, A.T.: *In* Vogelstein, B., Kinzler K., eds. The Genetic Basis of Human Cancer. Genes altered by chromosomal translocations in leukemias and lymphomas. McGraw-Hill Book Co., 1998; with permission.)

type is obtained when the *AML1/ETO* fusion is introduced by homologous recombination as a single-copy gene into the mouse germline,[153] providing compelling evidence for transdominant activity. The story may not be so simple, because analysis indicates that AML1/ETO may do more than recapitulate the AML1 knockout phenotype. Hematopoietic progenitors from some knockin mice have dysplastic morphology and altered self-renewal capacity,[154] consistent with leukemogenic potential for AML1/ETO.

The collective data support the following model. *AML1/ETO* impairs normal hematopoieses through inhibition of wild-type *AML1* and generates novel signals that alter growth. Precisely how *AML1/ETO* generates these new signals remains to be determined. One hypothesis comes from the observation that *ETO* may encode a transcriptional repressor through recruitment of a complex of proteins with histone deacetylase activity to the promoter.[155] Because most of the *ETO* coding region is retained in the fusion protein, it is likely that *AML1/ETO* may also function to repress transcription. AML1/ETO can block transcription from a range of promoters, including those dependent on C/EBP-α or Ets-1 in a manner that requires the ETO domain.[156, 157] The gain-of-function model also provides a potential explanation for the distinct clinical phenotypes associated with

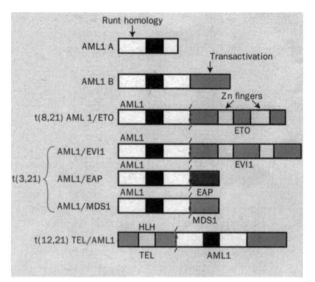

Figure 26–6. Structural features of fusion proteins involving AML1. Fusion proteins created by t(8;21) and t(3;21) translocations (AML1/ETO, AML1/EVI1, AML1/EAP, AML1/MDS1) have lost the AML1 transactivation domain. In the fusion protein (TEL/AML1) created by the t(12;21) translocation, the TEL gene is fused to the NH2-terminal end of the entire AML1 gene. AML1A, truncated isoform; AML1B, full-length AML1 protein. (From Sawyers, C.L.S.: Lancet 349:196–200, 1997; with permission.)

the different AML1 fusion proteins found in AML and myelodysplastic syndromes.

The critical importance of the CBF complex in hematopoietic development and its subversion in leukemogenesis is illustrated further by studies of the inv(16) translocation. Whereas the t(8;21) translocation targets the CBF-α subunit, the inv(16) translocation targets the CBF-β subunit[158] (Fig. 26–7).

CBF-β which does not bind DNA and does not encode a transcriptional activation domain, physically associates

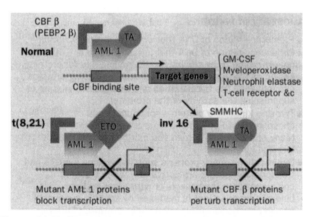

Figure 26–7. Proposed mechanism for disruption of transcriptional activity of AML1 by AML1 or CBPβ fusion proteins. Top, Transcriptional activation of target genes by AML1/CBFβ transcription-factor complex. TA, transactivation domain. **Bottom left,** Postulated mechanism for the suppressive effect of AML1 fusion proteins on activity of AML1 target genes. AML1/ETO competes with native AML1 for binding on activity of AML1 target genes. AML1/ETO competes with native AML1 for binding to CBFβ and crates inactive transcription complexes. **Bottom right,** CBFβ/SMMHC fusion protein formed by the inversion 16 translocation competes with native CBFβ for binding to AML1. (From Sawyers, C.L.S.:. Lancet 349: 196–200, 1997; with permission.)

with the DNA binding α subunit (AML1) and promotes high-affinity interaction of AML1 with consensus DNA binding sites. Analogous to AML1 homozygous disruption of the CBF-β gene in mice causes embryonic lethality by a block in fetal liver hematopoiesis, indicating that both genes are essential partners for proper hematopoietic development.[159] The inv(16) translocation fuses the smooth muscle myosin heavy-chain gene (SMHHC) to the C terminus of CBF-β, creating a chimeric protein which retains the ability to bind AML1 and can form high-molecular-weight multimers through coiled-coiled domain interactions of the myosin tail. Evidence suggests that CBF-β/SMMHC can sequester AML1 in the cytoplasm and block CBF-dependent transcription.[160] As with *AML1/ETO*, knockin experiments demonstrate that introduction of a single copy of CBF-β/ SMMHC into the mouse germline produces an embryonic lethal phenotype that resembles the CBF-α and CBF-β knockouts, providing compelling genetic evidence for a dominant negative effect.[161] However, CBF-β/SMMHC knockin embryos also had elevated levels of circulating erythroblasts derived from the yolk sac, a phenotype not observed in the AML1 or CBF-β knockouts. Together with the observations from the *AML1/ETO* knockin studies, these observations argue for a leukemogenic mechanism beyond simple loss of CBF function. This hypothesis is further supported by the clinically distinct phenotypes of t(8;21)– and inv(16)–associated AML.

In addition to the AML-associated t(8;21) translocation, AML1 is targeted by the t(12;21) translocation in childhood acute lymphocytic leukemia.[162] The consequence is fusion of the N-terminal portion of the *TEL* gene (discussed previously in the context of tyrosine kinase translocations) to the DNA binding and transactivation domains of *AML1* (see Fig. 26–8). The TEL/AML1 fusion protein differs substantially from AML1/ETO in that the transactivation domain is not replaced by foreign sequences. Despite this major structural distinction, early studies suggest that TEL/AML1 may also function to inhibit CBF-dependent transcription, but the mechanistic details are unclear. Curiously, the t(12;21) translocation is extremely difficult to visualize using standard cytogenetic techniques; therefore, fluorescent in situ hybridization (FISH) studies are required to ensure its detection. An accurate molecular diagnosis is of major importance, because children whose leukemias contain the t(12;21) translocation have a more favorable prognosis and may require less extensive therapy than is typically prescribed for childhood ALL.[163]

Translocations in Genes That Affect Hematopoietic Differentiation

One of the great success stories in modern hematology is the discovery of a link between the molecular phenotype of the t(15;17) translocation found in acute promyelocytic leukemia (APL) and the dramatic clinical response of these patients to all-*trans* retinoic acid (ATRA) therapy. This translocation fuses the PML gene on chromosome 15 to the RARα gene on chromosome 17.[164–166] RARα is a well-characterized member of the nuclear hormone receptor family and contains distinct transactivation, DNA-binding, and ligand-binding domains. Retinoids induce differentiation signals in a wide range of tissues, including hematopoietic cells, through activation of RARα in complex with an auxiliary protein RXR, which heterodimerizes with a number of nuclear hormone receptors. PML encodes a novel protein localized to a unique nuclear structure of unknown function known as the PML oncogenic domain (POD) that is disrupted in APL cell.[167–169] Evidence suggests that PML functions as a tumor suppressor gene, because homozygous disruption of the gene in mice predisposes these animals to tumor formation in response to chemical carcinogens.[155] Wild-type PML appears to function in the retinoid acid signaling pathway, because cells from the PML knockout mice are resistant to retinoid-mediated differentiation effects.

As a consequence of the t(15;17) translocation, the PML, gene is fused to the DNA and ligand-binding domains of RAR, creating a chimeric PML/RAR protein (Fig. 26–8). Although a reciprocal fusion mRNA (RAR/PML) can be detected, it is clear from transgenic mouse studies that PML/RAR is sufficient to induce leukemias.[170, 171] When transgene expression is directed to the appropriate myeloid/monocytic cellular compartment, the mice develop a close phenocopy of human promyelocytic leukemia. A number of attempts to create PML/RAR transgenic models using promoters that function earlier in hematopoietic development met with failure, presumably because of transgenic toxicity. In addition to pointing out the practical need to test multiple promoters when establishing transgene models, this experience suggests that leukemic transformation by certain oncogenes is subject to defined lineage and differentiation stage requirements.

One biologic consequence of PML/RAR expression is to block the differentiation response of hematopoietic cells to ligands such as vitamin D or retinoic acid.[172] Since PML/RAR retains the structural motifs in RAR required for complex formation with the auxiliary nuclear receptor RXR, one straightforward model to explain the leukemogenic activity

of PML/RAR is through competition with wild-type RAR for binding to RXR. This model is also consistent with the discovery of the other RAR translocations such as PLZF/RAR and NPM/RAR in patients with APL who lack the typical t(15;17) translocation. PLZF/RAR also forms heterodimers with RXR and blocks RXR-dependent transcription analogous to PML/RAR.[173, 174] The fact that all fusion proteins retain the same region of RAR and produce comparable clinical phenotypes argues that disruption of wild-type RAR function plays a major role in the genesis of APL.

Progress defining the role of co-activators and co-repressors in the regulation of nuclear receptor function has provided exciting insights into how RAR fusion proteins impair RAR function. Co-activators bind directly to hormone receptors in response to ligand binding and allow the assembly of multiprotein complexes with histone acetyltransferase domains that activate transcription through acetylation of histones in chromatin. Conversely, negative regulation of nuclear receptors is mediated by co-repressors, which also bind directly to the hormone receptor and inhibit transcription by recruitment of proteins with histone deacetylase activity. PML/RAR and PLZF/RAR are constitutively bound to the nuclear co-repressor NCoR, raising the possibility that both fusion proteins inhibit RAR-dependent transcription by active repression.[175–178] Exposure to pharmacologic doses of retinoid acid induces a conformational change that favors binding between PML/RAR and co-activators over co-repressors. The role of transcriptional repression in the oncogenicity of RAR fusion proteins is further supported by experiments showing that tricostatin A, an inhibitor of histone deacetylase, restores RAR-dependent transcription in PML/RAR expressing cells (Fig. 26–9).

These insights are important because they raise the possibility that therapeutic strategies targeting the transcriptional repression machinery may be effective in APL patients, including those resistant to ATRA. Clinical studies suggest that phenyl butyrate, another inhibitor of histone deacetylase, has some activity in APL patients who relapse after ATRA treatment (R. Warrel, Memorial Sloan-Kettering, personal communication).

Despite progress in understanding the molecular basis for PML/RAR-induced leukemias, the mechanism for the success of retinoic acid therapy in APL is less clear. Because all of the RAR fusion proteins associated with APL retain the ligand-binding domain of RAR, they are presumably capable of responding to retinoic acid. However, APL patients expressing alternative fusions such as PLZF/RAR are resistant to retinoic acid therapy. One potential explanation comes from the fact that PLZF encodes a POZ (pox virus and zinc finger) domain that can mediate binding to a co-repressor complex.[175, 176] Although retinoic acid can bind PML/RAR and PLZF/RAR and displace RAR-associated co-repressors, a second co-repressor complex bound to the PLZF part of the PLZF/RAR fusion remains intact and continues to inhibit transcription. The failure of PLZF/RAR-expressing patients to respond to ATRA may be caused by persistent transcriptional repression mediated by PLZF. This hypothesis is consistent with the experimental observation that tricostatin A, but not ATRA, can reverse PLZF/RAR-mediated repression of retinoic acid target genes.

More insight into the clinical efficacy of ATRA has come from the analysis of APL patients with PML/RAR-

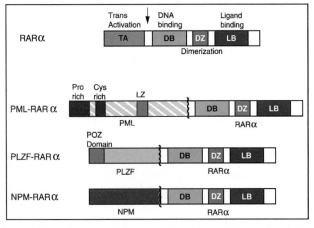

Figure 26–8. Structural features of retinoic acid receptor fusion proteins. Three different chromosome translocations fuse the C-terminal portion of the RAR protein (*top*) to N-terminal sequences of PML, PLZF, or NPM. The DNA binding domain, dimerization domain, and ligand binding domain of the RAR protein are retained in each fusion protein. TA, transactivation; DB, DNA binding; DZ, dimerization; LB, ligand binding; LZ, leucine zipper; RAR, retinoic acid receptor; PML, promyelocytic leukemia; PLZF, promyelocytic leukemia zinc finger; NPM, nucleophosmin. (From Sawyers, C.L.: Molecular genetics of acute leukemias. *In* Lee, et al., Wintrobe's Clinical Hematology. 10th ed. Baltimore, Williams & Wilkins, 1999, pp. 1998–2008; with permission.)

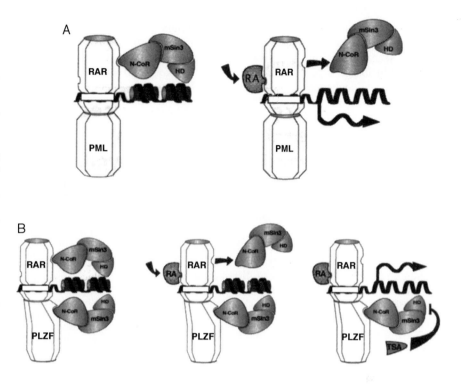

Figure 26–9. A model for the interactions of AP fusion proteins with the N-CoR-mSin3-histodeacetylase (HD) complex. **A,** DNA-bound PM RAR-α interacts with N-CoR (or SMRT) and recruits the mSin3-HD complex, decreasing histone acetylation and producing repressive chromatin organization and transcriptional repression. RA induces dissociation of the N-CoR-mSin3-HD complex, recruitment of coactivators with histone acetyltransferase activity (not shown), increased levels of acetylation, chromatin remodeling, and transcriptional activation. **B,** PLZF RAR-α has two N-CoR binding sites that, even the presence of RA, recruit the N-CoR-mSin3-HD complex and maintain transcription repression. TSA inhibits HD activity within the N-CoR complex, increasing histone acetylation, possibly through RA-recruited coactivators, and leading to transcription activation. (From Grighani, F.: Nature 391:815–818, 1998; with permission.)

expressing leukemias that relapse after initial responses to ATRA. A subset of these patients develop mutations in the hormone-binding domain of the PML/RAR fusion protein that are predicted to impair binding to ATRA.[179] Although these observations strongly support the idea that ATRA functions as a ligand for the PML/RAR fusion protein, it remains unclear why only the all-*trans* isomer of retinoic acid produces clinical responses and why pharmacologic doses are required. Advances in understanding the molecular profile of nuclear receptor function should clarify these issues and lead to additional RAR-directed treatment strategies.

Translocations That Target Genes Involved in Homeotic Function

Normal hematopoiesis is characterized by the sequential activation and suppression of different sets of homeotic genes at distinct stages of differentiation. Constitutive expression of a single *Hox* gene in mouse models perturbs this ordered pattern of differentiation and creates a phenotype that closely resembles human myelodysplasia or leukemia.[180, 181] Several examples of *Hox* gene translocations have been described in human leukemias that led to constitutive expression of the wild-type protein or production of a Hox fusion protein. Although the mechanistic details of the human translocations are yet to be defined, the WEHI-3 murine leukemia example discussed earlier in the context of overproduction of the growth factor IL-3 is particularly instructive. In addition to IL-3, WEHI-3 cells constitutively express Hox2.4 as a consequence of a second intracisternal particle integration.[182] In a reconstitution experiment in mice, it was found that both genes, *IL-3* and *Hox2.4,* must be overexpressed to recapitulate the leukemia, indicating a critical role for the *Hox* genes.[6]

In addition to these examples directly affecting the level of *Hox* gene expression, fusion genes have been described in human leukemias that indirectly affect *Hox* gene function. One example comes from the cloning of the myeloid lymphoid leukemia gene (MLL, also called HRX or ALL1) on chromosome 11q24. The most common MLL translocations are t(4;11) and t(11;19) in ALL and t(9;11) in AML (see Table 26–1), but more than 30 other translocation partners have been described. MLL encodes a 430-kd protein whose C terminus is homologous to the *Drosophila* homeotic protein trithorax, encoded by a master gene that positively regulates *Hox* gene expression in flies.[183–187] The N terminus of MLL contains three A-T hook regions, which function as DNA-binding domains, and a region with homology to the noncatalytic domain of methyltransferase. Knockout studies confirm that MLL functions as a homeotic gene in mice, because homozygous deletion produces an embryonic lethal phenotype associated with branchial arch dysplasia, aberrant somite development, and absent *Hox* gene expression.[188–191] Heterozygous mice are viable but have hematopoietic abnormalities, including anemia and thrombocytopenia.

Similar to the CBF system, the mechanism by which 11q24 translocations induce leukemia appears to be loss of wild-type MLL function and gain of additional signals from sequences provided by the partner chromosome (see Table 26–4). Structural analysis of the translocation breakpoints indicates a consistent pattern of MLL truncation proximal to the trithorax homology domain, thereby creating presumably nonfunctional alleles. The fact that such a large number of apparently unrelated translocation partners exist, some of which add very little additional amino acid sequence to the truncated MLL, led to the hypothesis that loss of trithorax function may be a primary mode of leukemogenesis. However, a growing body of evidence suggest this is not the case. First, distinct translocations are associated with a specific leukemia subtype, suggesting that the translocation partner defines the clinical leukemia phenotype or that certain translocations only occur in progenitors committed to a specific lineage. Second, knockin experiments demonstrate that the *MLL/AF9* fusion gene generated by the t(9;11) translocation induces myeloid leukemias in mice, whereas an MLL protein truncated at the AF9 junction but without fusion of AF9 sequences does not, indicating that the AF9 sequences play a critical role.[192] This conclusion is also consistent with the fact that heterozygous MLL knockout mice do not develop leukemias. Third, retroviral transfer experiments into murine bone marrow using the MLL-ENL fusion protein created by the t(11;19) translocation show that both the MLL and ENL domains are required for the immortalization phenotype observed in myelomonocytic progenitor cells.[193]

With experimental evidence supporting a critical role for the translocation partner in the leukemia phenotypes observed with MLL fusion genes, it remains problematic to explain how such a large number of different fusion proteins can give related phenotypes. One emerging theme is that many of the MLL translocation partners encode proteins involved in modulating gene expression. For example, the AF4, AF9, and ENL proteins targeted by the t(4;11), t(9;11), and t(11;19) translocations, respectively, appear to function directly as transcription factors.[194, 195] In the t(11;16) translocation MLL is fused to a well-characterized transcriptional co-activator CBP, which integrates signaling through a number of transcription factors. Another t(11;19) translocation targets ELL, an RNA polymerase II elongation factor that could modulate gene expression at a posttranscriptional level.[196] Because all of the fusion proteins retain the DNA-binding motif of MLL, it is possible to envision a transformation model whereby transcriptional regulation of MLL target genes is perturbed as a consequence of replacement of the trithorax domain with other transcriptional regulatory proteins. Much work remains to be done, but structure and function analysis of MLL-ENL supports this model, because mutations in the DNA-binding motif of MLL or the transcriptional activation domain of ENL impaired transforming activity.[197] Another area that needs further exploration is whether haplo insufficiency of the MLL partner gene contributes to the leukemia phenotype.

A second example is the t(1;19) translocation that creates a chimeric transcription factor that contains the transactivation domain of the *E2A* gene fused to the DNA-binding domain of the homeotic gene *PBX1*[198, 199] (Fig. 26–10). *E2A* encodes three differentially spliced genes that are members of the basic helix-loop-helix (bHLH) family of transcription factors. E2A proteins play a critical regulatory role during B-cell development, because *E2A* knockout mice show arrested B-cell development.[200, 201] *PBX1* encodes the mammalian homologue of the *Drosophila* homeotic gene *extradenticle*.[202] PBX1 can bind DNA directly, but it prefers to form heterodimers with other homeobox containing Hox proteins and bind DNA.[203, 204] The *E2A-PBX1* fusion gene has enhanced transcriptional activity on artificial promoters that contain PBX1 DNA-binding sites compared with PBX1.[205] These observations argue that the oncogenic activity of E2A/PBX1 is a consequence of dysregulated PBX1 activity driven by the E2A transactivation domain. This model is supported by mutational analysis. E2A-PBX1 transforms fibroblasts[206] and hematopoietic cells[207, 208] in a manner that requires E2A and the Hox interaction domain of PBX1.[209] Further support

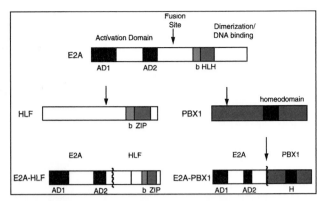

Figure 26–10. Structural features of E2A fusion proteins. The N terminus of the *E2A* gene encodes a transcriptional activation domain that is translocated to HLF or PBX1 by chromosome translocations in ALL. In the case of E2A-HLF, the DNA binding and dimerization domains of E2A are replaced by similar domains in HLF. For E2A-PBX1, the same DNA binding and dimerization domains of E2A are replaced with the DNA binding homeodomain of PBX1. AD, activation domain; HLH, basic helix-loop-helix domain (DNA binding and dimerization); ZIP, basic leucine zipper domain (DNA binding and dimerization); H, homeodomain. (From Sawyers, C.L.: Molecular genetics of acute leukemias. *In* Lee, et al., eds: Wintrobe's Clinical Hematology, 10th ed. Baltimore, Williams & Wilkins, 1999, pp. 1998–2008; with permission.)

comes from the identification of target genes transcriptionally regulated by E2A/PBX1, which are associated with developmentally regulated, lineage-specific expression.[210]

The phenotype of E2A/PBX1 expression in murine hematopoietic cells suggests that a primary effect of the fusion gene is to block cellular differentiation. Retroviral introduction of E2A/PBX1 into mouse bone marrow blocked myeloblast differentiation and produced acute myeloid leukemias.[207] Transgenic expression of E2A/PBX1 in lymphoid cells induced T-cell lymphomas with phenotypes consistent with developmental arrest at the CD4/CD8 double-positive stage of thymocyte development.[208] Curiously, E2A/PBX1 is associated exclusively with B-cell leukemias in humans, underscoring the importance of timed expression of the fusion gene in the appropriate target cell to achieve a precise phenocopy of the human disease in mouse models.

Translocations That Target Genes Affecting Apoptosis

Since the initial discovery of the *Bcl-2* gene as the target of the t(14;18) translocation in follicular lymphoma,[211, 212] it has become clear that perturbation of the normal process of programmed cell death can lead to transformation. The primary consequence of the *Bcl-2* translocation is constitutive expression of the wild-type protein by the immunoglobulin heavy-chain enhancer. Because the initial description that Bcl-2 can protect hematopoietic cells from apotosis after cytokine withdrawal,[213] it is clear that Bcl-2 functions to protect against cell death in response to many stimuli. Its etiologic role in cancer is well established through clinical studies of a range of human cancers showing alterations in Bcl-2 protein levels and through the use of transgenic models showing B-lymphocyte hyperplasia and rapid progression to lymphoma when combined with other oncogenic insults.

Bcl-2 is one of a growing family of structurally related

proteins that function as regulators of apoptosis, and evidence is mounting that abnormalities in other members can also occur in hematopoietic maligancies. Overexpression of the homologue Bcl-X_L occurs in the erythroid precursors of patients with polycythemia vera, a myeloproliferative disorder leading to expansion of the red cell compartment.[214] Whereas Bcl-2 and Bcl-X_L function as inhibitors of apoptosis, other Bcl-2 family members such as Bax and Bad are pro-apoptotic proteins that induce cell death by binding to Bcl-2 and Bcl-X_L and blocking their function. Cell survival in multiple tissue types is determined primarily by the relative levels of pro- and anti-apoptotic Bcl-2 family members. Just as overexpression of the anti-apoptotic Bcl-2 and Bcl-X_L proteins is associated with many human cancers, loss-of-function abnormalities in pro-apoptotic proteins are beginning to be appreciated as an alternative mechanism of oncogenesis. Mutations in Bax have been reported for a subset of human ALL cell lines.[215]

In addition to alterations in the levels or activity of Bcl-2 family members, a number of translocations in human leukemia and lymphoma target genes also affect the apoptotic pathway. One example is the t(17;19) translocation in pediatric ALL, which fuses the transcriptional activation domain of E2A to the DNA-binding and dimerization domain of another transcription factor called hepatic leukemia factor (HLF).[216, 217] E2A/HLF is structurally and functionally analogous to E2A-PBX1 in that the oncogenicity of E2A-HLF requires the transactivation function of E2A and the dimerization and DNA-binding properties of HLF.[218] HLF is not normally expressed in hematopoietic cells; therefore, the oncogenic activity of E2A-HLF is likely to result from the inappropriate expression of HLF target genes. Studies indicate that the primary effect of E2A/HLF in hematopoietic cells is to block apoptosis in response to growth factor withdrawal[219] or p53 activation.[220] Mechanistic studies link E2A-HLF directly to the Bcl-2 pathway. HLF is homologous to the nematode apoptosis pathway gene *Ces-2*, which encodes a transcriptional repressor that induces a cell death program by suppressing expression of survival genes upstream of Bcl-2.[221] Because E2A-HLF protects cells from apoptosis, it is postulated that fusion to E2A most likely converts HLF from a repressor to an activator of cell survival genes. This model is supported by the observation that a dominant-negative mutant of E2A-HLF induces programmed cell death selectively in cells with a t(17;19) translocation.[219]

Translocations involving the NF-κB proteins and NF-κB regulators also appear to function as leukemia oncogenes by affecting apoptosis. NF-κB, originally identified as an activity responsible for transcriptional activation of the Ig-κ light-chain gene, is a component of a signal transduction pathway that is activated by a number of diverse stimuli. The DNA-binding activity is mediated by a two-subunit complex known as the p65/p50 heterodimer. NF-κB activity is regulated in part by a family of cytoplasmic anchor proteins known as inhibitors of NF-κB (I-κB). NF-κB proteins have been implicated in carcinogenesis by multiple mechanisms. The p65 subunit is homologous to the Rel protein, which was originally identified as an avian oncogene that induces bursal lymphomas.[222] The p50 subunit is targeted by the t(10;14) translocation in non-Hodgkin lymphoma.[223] These retroviral transduction and chromosome translocation events generate gain-of-function p65/p50 alleles, which are

postulated to contribute to the genesis of leukemia or lymphoma by enhanced NF-κB activity. Studies of knockout mice lacking the p50 or p65 subunits of NF-κB have provided insights into the mechanism of NF-κB-induced oncogenicity. Cells lacking p50 or p65 are exquisitely sensitive to apoptosis in response to external stimuli such as tumor necrosis factor, indicating that a major function of NF-κB is to protect cells from apoptosis. Analogous to Bcl-2 overexpression, excess NF-κB activity is presumed to permit cell survival at inappropriate times, predisposing these cells to secondary oncogenic events.

A confusing wrinkle in this model has come from the cloning of the t(14;19) translocation found in some patients with CLL. These leukemic cells constitutively express the Bcl-3 gene as a consequence of fusion to the promoter and enhancer regions of the IgH locus. Bcl-3 is a member of the family of proteins that inhibit p50/p65 NF-κB, known as I-κB.[224–226] Because Bcl-3 presumably inhibits the anti-apoptotic function of NF-κB, it is difficult to envision how it may function as an oncogene. This apparent paradox is partly resolved through studies showing that Bcl-3 does not function as a classic cytoplasmic anchor for NF-κB. Rather, it seems that Bcl-3 can activate transcription from certain NF-κB sites by relieving transcriptional repression mediated by specific NF-κB isoforms that lack transactivation domains.[227–229] Transgenic models support the oncogenic potential of Bcl-3 overexpression as these mice develop lymphadenopathy and splenomegaly.[230] Bcl-3 also appears to play a critical role in B-cell function, because knockout mice have defects in germinal center formation and in the production of specific antibodies.[231, 232] Further work is required to understand how perturbations in this family of proteins lead to hematopoietic malignancy.

Abnormalities in Genes Involved in Cell Cycle Progression

Tremendous advances in the cell cycle field have led to the identification of several evolutionarily conserved pathways that serve as checkpoints to regulate cell cycle entry and progression at appropriate times. One such pathway regulates the G_1/S-phase checkpoint and involves cyclin-dependent kinases (Cdks), D cyclins, Cdk inhibitors such as p16, and the retinoblastoma (Rb) gene product.[233] In normal proliferating cells, the level of cyclin D1 protein is tightly regulated and rises during late G_1, where it serves as a co-factor to activate cyclin-dependent kinase 4 (Cdk4). A critical substrate of the Cdk4/cyclin D complex is the tumor suppressor protein Rb, which blocks G_1 progression by sequestration of the E2F family of transcription factors. When active E2F induces transcription from S-phase genes. Phosphorylation of Rb by Cdk4/cyclin D releases E2F and allows cell cycle progression (Fig. 26–11).

Numerous examples of mutations or expression changes in the positive and negative regulators of this pathway have been described in human cancers. In the case of hematologic malignancies, among the best examples is the Bcl-1 gene, which is constitutively expressed in a subset of B-cell lymphomas as a consequence of translocation to an immunoglobulin-enhancer locus[234–236] (Table 26–5). Bcl-1 encodes cyclin D1,[237, 238] one of three D-type cyclins that function in

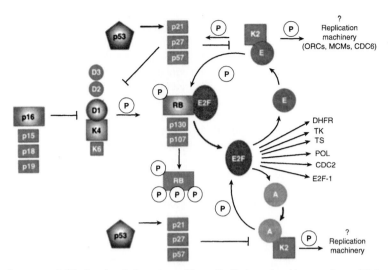

Figure 26–11. Restriction point control. RB phosphorylation triggered by cyclin D–dependent kinases releases RB-bound E2F. Rather than illustrating the many E2F-DP heterodimers that are differentially regulated by various RB family members, E2F "activity" is shown for simplicity. E2F triggers the expression of dihydrofolate reductase (DHFR), thymidine kinase (TK), thymidylate synthase (TS), DNA polymerase-α (POL), CDC2, cyclin E and possibly cyclin A, and E2F-1 itself. This establishes a positive feedback loop, promoting RB phosphorylation by cyclin E-CDK2, contributing to the irreversibility of the restriction point transition and ultimately making it mitogen independent. In parallel, cyclin E-CDK2 may oppose the inhibitory action of p27[KIP1] by phosphorylating it. This allows cyclin A-CDK2 and possibly cyclin E-CDK2 to start the S phase. Possible CDK substrates include those of the origin-recognition complex (ORC), minichromosome maintenance proteins (MCMs), and CDC6, all of which assemble into preinitiation complexes. After cells enter the S phase, cyclin A-CDK2 phosphorylates DP-1 and inhibits E2F binding to DNA. Like p27, p53-inducible p21[CIP1] can induce G arrest by inhibiting the cyclin D-, E-, and A-dependent kinases. In contrast, INK4 proteins antagonize only the cyclin D–dependent kinases. The proteins most frequently targeted in human cancers are highlighted. Arrows depicting inhibitory phosphorylations (P) or inactivating steps are shown in red, and those depicting activating steps are shown in black. (From Sherr, C.J.: Science 274:1672–1677, 1996; with permission.)

cell cycle progression from G_1 to S phase. Constitutive expression of cyclin D accelerates entry into S phase and predisposes to tumor formation in transgenic mice.[239] Abnormalities of other members of this G_1/S pathway have been identified in human leukemias and lymphomas. Deletions or loss of function mutations in the Cdk inhibitor p16 occur with high frequency in T-cell leukemias,[240, 241] and Rb mutations have been reported in megakaryocytic blast crisis of CML.[242]

The *Myc* gene, described previously for its role in Burkitt's lymphoma due to targeting by translocations involving one of three distinct immunoglobulin loci, also plays a critical role in the G_1/S transition.[243] Constitutive expression of *Myc* leads to enhanced S-phase entry and, ultimately, oncogenesis in a range of model systems. *Myc* encodes a transcription factor that binds DNA and activates gene expression through heterodimer formation with the Myc-related protein Max. Recent work has defined a larger family

Table 26–5. Transcription Factor Translocations Involving Other Genes

Disease	Chromosomal Abnormality	Activated Gene	Mechanism of Activation	Predominant Structural Feature*	Invertebrate Homologue	References
Centrocytic B-cell lymphoma	t(11;14)(q13;q32)	Cyclin D1	Relocation to IgH locus	GI Cyclin		234, 235, 238, 330–333
Follicular B-cell lymphoma	t(14;18)(q32;q21)	BCL2	Relocation to IgH locus	Anti-apoptotic domain	ced-9 (C)	212, 333–335
AML	t(6;9)(p23;q34)	DEK-CAN	Gene fusion	Nucleoporin (CAN)		336
AML	t(9;9)(q43;q34)	SET-CAN	Gene fusion	Nucleoporin (CAN)		258
AML	t(7;11)(p15;p15)	NUP98-HOXA9	Gene fusion	Nucleoporin (NUP98)		314, 315
AML	t(3;5)(q35;q35)	NPM-MLF1	Gene fusion	Nucleoporin shuttle protein (NPM)		337
AML	t(10;11)(p13;q14)	CALM-AFIO	Gene fusion	Clathrin assembly (CALM)	cezf (C)	338
T-Pro-ALL	t(x;14)(q28;q11)	C6.1B	Relocation to TCRα/δ locus	Unknown		339
T-cell ALL	t(7;9)(q34;q34)	TANI	Relocation to TCRβ locus	ECF cysteine repeats	notch (D), lin-12 (C)	38
Pre-B ALL	t(5;14)(q31;q32)	IL-3	Relocation to IgH locus	Growth factor		5, 340
T-cell lymphoma	t(4;16)(q26;p13)	IL2-BCM	Gene fusion	Growth factor		341

AML, acute myeloid leukemia; ALL, acute lymphoblastic leukemia; APML, acute promyelocytic leukemia; CML, chronic myeloid leukemia; bHLHzip, basic region/helix-loop-helix/leucine zipper domain; BZIP, basic region/leucine zipper domain.
*Based on analysis of DNA-binding/protein interaction domain. For gene fusions, the partner contributing this structural feature is given in parenthesis.

of Myc-related proteins such as Mad and Mxi1, which regulate Myc target genes in a positive or negative fashion through the formation of heterodimers with Max. Similar to the Bcl-2 family proteins that regulate apoptosis, the relative levels of activating (Myc) and repressive (Mad) family members plays a critical role in determining the transcriptional outcome. The negative regulation of Myc target genes appears to be a consequence of active repression of transcription by Mad/Max complexes through histone deacetylation rather than the lack of a positive transactivation signal. Mad binds Myc target sequences in conjunction with Max and recruits histone deacetylase activity to the promoter through complex formation with Sin3 (see Fig. 26–10).[244, 245] Evidence is beginning to accumulate that loss of function mutations in these negative regulators of Myc may play a role in human cancer. Mxi1 is located on chromosome 10q23, a region which is lost in multiple tumor types, and mice lacking Mxi1 as a consequence of targeted deletion develop cancers.[246, 247]

Another important regulator of the G_1/S transition, p53, also plays a role in hematopoietic malignancies. Patients with Li-Fraumini syndrome inherit germline mutations in *p53*[248] and develop leukemias and lymphomas with high frequency.[249] Somatic *p53* mutations occur in acute leukemia or lymphoma, as well as the blast crisis of CML.[250] Mutations in other genes that regulate *p53* also occur in human hematopoietic tumors. Patients with ataxia telangiectasia inherit germline mutations in *ATM*, a gene that functions upstream of *p53* as a sensor of DNA damage. As with Li-Fraumini syndrome these patients also have an increased risk for developing leukemias.[251] Another recently identified regulator of *p53*, p19 ARF, is also likely to play a role in hematologic malignancies. ARF functions as an upstream activator of *p53* by directly blocking the inhibitory effects of Mdm2 on p53.[252–254] Because ARF is encoded by the same gene as p16 but translated in an alternate reading frame,[225] it can be assumed that loss of function mutations in ARF occur with a frequency comparable to mutations in p16. ARF mutations have already been found with high frequency in other tumor types, and ARF-deficient mice develop cancers.[256]

Summary

With the identification of a multitude of genes targeted by chromosomal breakpoints in human leukemia and lymphoma, an initially complex list of seemingly unrelated proteins indicates that a small number of common pathways become abnormally regulated during leukemogenesis. The fact that many leukemias express tyrosine kinase fusions, *NF1* deletions, or *Ras* mutations suggests that deregulation of the Ras pathway is a common oncogenic event. Insights from the *RAR, AML1,* and *MLL* translocations, showing aberrant assembly of transcriptional co-activator or co-repressor complexes, indicate that perturbations in histone acetylation and deacetylation at the promoter of genes critical for proper hematopoiesis also affect the oncogenic process. As we refine our understanding of the mechanistic details required for leukemogenesis by each translocation target, a future challenge is the translation of these findings to therapy in the clinical arena. One near-term step is the application of molecular diagnostics using FISH or PCR to the clinical evaluation of newly diagnosed leukemia and lymphoma patients. Knowing the molecular phenotype can provide important prognostic information and ultimately, as is the case for PML-RAR, dictates therapy. In the longer term, it is expected that new therapeutic strategies will be developed that specifically target the pathways deregulated by leukemia translocations. The first such attempts using tyrosine kinase inhibitors against the Abl fusion proteins in Ph chromosome–positive leukemias are in phase I clinical testing.

ACKNOWLEDGMENTS

We thank Stephane Wong and Janusz Kabarowski for their assistance in the preparation of figures, Shirley Quan for computer support, and J.C. White and Lisa Dove for their clerical assistance in the preparation of this manuscript. The citations selected for this chapter represent a small fraction of the vast literature on human and experimental leukemia. In many cases, recent reviews or articles were chosen over initial references to provide the interested reader with an overview of the subject. We hope those authors whose work was not directly cited will understand. CLS is supported by the National Cancer Institute and is a Scholar of the Leukemia Society of America. ONW gratefully acknowledges the support of the Howard Hughes Medical Institute and the National Cancer Institute for the work in his laboratory.

REFERENCES

1. Metcalf, D.: Lineage commitment and maturation in hematopoietic cells: the case for extrinsic regulation. Blood 92:345B, 1998.
2. Enver, T., Heyworth, C.M., and Dexter, T.M.: Do stem cells play dice? Blood 92:348, 1998.
3. Hawley, T.S., Fong, A.Z.C., Griesser, H., Lyman, S.D., and Hawley, R.G.: Leukemic predisposition of mice transplanted with gene-modified hematopoietic precursors expressing flt3 ligand. Blood 92:2003, 1998.
4. Rich, B.E., Campos-Torres, J., Tepper, R.I., Moreadith, R.W., and Leder, P.: Cutaneous lymphoproliferation and lymphomas in interleukin 7 transgenic mice. J. Exp. Med. 177:305, 1993.
5. Meeker, T.C., Hardy, D., Willman, C., Hogan, T., and Abrams, J.: Activation of the interleukin-3 gene by chromosome translocation in acute lymphocytic leukemia with eosinophilia. Blood 76:285, 1990.
6. Perkins, A., Kongsuwan, K., Visvader, J., Adams, J.M., and Cory, S.: Homeobox gene expression plus autocrine growth factor production elicits myeloid leukaemia. Proc. Natl. Acad. Sci. USA 87:8398, 1990.
7. Nicholson, S.E., and Hilton, D.J.: The SOCS proteins: a new family of negative regulators of signal transduction. J. Leukoc. Biol. 63:665, 1998.
8. Zhang, J.G., Farley, A., Nicholson, S.E., Willson, T.A., Zugaro, L.M., Simpson, R.J., Moritz, R.L., Cary, D., Richardson, R., Hausmann, G., Kile, B.J., Kent, S.B., Alexander, W.S., Metcalf, D., Hilton, D.J., Nicola, N.A., and Baca, M.: The conserved SOCS box motif in suppressors of cytokine signaling binds to elongins B and C and may couple bound proteins to proteasomal degradation. Proc. Natl. Acad. Sci. USA 96:2071, 1999.
9. Goodnow, C.C.: Balancing immunity and tolerance: deleting and tuning lymphocyte repertoires. Proc. Natl. Acad. Sci. USA 93:2264, 1996.
10. Li, J-P., D'Andrea, A.D., Lodish, H.F., and Baltimore, D.: Activation of cell growth by binding of Friend spleen focus-forming virus gp55 glycoprotein to the erythropoietin receptor. Nature 343:762, 1990.
11. Ben-David, Y., and Bernstein, A.: Friend virus–induced erythroleukemia and the multistage nature of cancer. Cell 66:831, 1991.
12. Livnah, O., Stura, E.A., Middleton, S.A., Johnson, D.L., Jolliffe, L.K., and Wilson, I.A.: Crystallographic evidence for preformed dimers of erythropoietin receptor before ligand activation. Science 283:987, 1999.

13. Remy, I., Wilson, I.A., and Michnick, S.W.: Erythropoietin receptor activation by a ligand-induced conformation change. Science 283:990, 1999.

14. Ding, Y.H., Javaherian, K., Lo, K.M., Chopra, R., Boehm, T., Lanciotti, J., Harris, B.A., Li, Y., Shapiro, R., Hohenester, E., Timpl, R., Folkman, J., and Wiley, D.C.: Zinc-dependent dimers observed in crystals of human endostatin. Proc. Natl. Acad. Sci. USA 95:10443, 1998.

15. O'Reilly, M.S., Boehm, T., Shing, Y., Fukai, N., Vasios, G., Lane, W.S., Flynn, E., Birkhead, J.R., Olsen, B.R., and Folkman, J.: Endostatin: an endogenous inhibitor of angiogenesis and tumor growth. Cell 88:277, 1997.

16. O'Reilly, M.S., Holmgren, L., Shing, Y., Chen, C., Rosenthal, R.A., Moses, M., Lane, W.S., Cao, Y., Sage, E.H., and Folkman, J.: Angiostatin: a novel angiogenesis inhibitor that mediates the suppression of metastases in a Lewis lung carcinoma. Cell 79:315, 1994.

17. Cwirla, S.E., Balasubramanian, P., Duffin, D.J., Wagstrom, C.R., Gates, C.M., Singer, S.C., Davis, A.M., Tansik, R.L., Mattheakis, L.C., Boytos, C.M., Schatz, P.J., Baccanari, D.P., Wrighton, N.C., Barrett, R.W., and Dower, W.J.: Peptide agonist of the thrombopoietin receptor as potent as the natural cytokine. Science 276:1696, 1997.

18. Weiss, A., and Schlessinger, J.: Switching signals on or off by receptor dimerization. Cell 94:277, 1998.

19. Baird, P.N., D'Andrea, R.J., and Goodall, G.J.: Cytokine receptor genes: structure, chromosomal location, and involvement in human disease. Leuk. Lymphoma 18:373, 1995.

20. Schindler, C., and Darnell, J.E.J.: Transcriptional responses to polypeptide ligands. The JAK-STAT pathway. Annu. Rev. Biochem. 64:621, 1995.

21. Massague, J., and Weis-Garcia, F.: Serine/threonine kinase receptors: mediators of transforming growth factor beta family signals. Cancer Surv 27:41, 1996.

22. Kaushansky, K.: Thrombopoietin. N. Engl. J. Med. 339:746, 1998.

23. Rosenberg, N., and Jolicoeur, P.: Retroviral pathogenesis. In Coffin, J.M., Hughes, S.H., and Varmus, H.E., eds: Retroviruses. Plainview, Cold Spring Harbor Laboratory Press, 1997, p. 475.

24. Slamon, D.J., Clark, G.M., Wong, S.G., Levin, W.J., Ullrich, A., and McGuire, W.L.: Human breast cancer: correlation of relapse and survival with amplification of the HER-2/neu oncogene. Science 235:177, 1987.

25. Richelda, R., Ronchetti, D., Baldini, L., Cro, L., Viggiano, L., Marzella, R., Rocchi, M., Otsuki, T., Lombardi, L., Maiolo, A.T., and Neri, A.: A novel chromosomal translocation t(4;14)(p16.3;q32) in multiple myeloma involves the fibroblast growth-factor receptor 3 gene. Blood 90:4062, 1997.

26. Chesi, M., Nardini, E., Brents, L.A., Schrock, E., Ried, T., Kuehl, W.M., and Bergsagel, P.L.: Frequent translocation t(4;14)(p16.3;q32.3) in multiple myeloma is associated with increased expression and activating mutations of fibroblast growth factor receptor 3. Nat. Genet. 16:260, 1997.

27. Longmore, G.D., and Lodish, H.F.: An activating mutation in the murine erythropoietin receptor induces erythroleukemia in mice: a cytokine receptor superfamily oncogene. Cell 67:1089, 1991.

28. Le Couedic, J.P., Mitjavila, M.T., Villeval, J.L., Feger, F., Gobert, S., Mayeux, P., Casadevall, N., and Vainchenker, W.: Missense mutation of the erythropoietin receptor is a rare event in human erythroid malignancies. Blood 87:1502, 1996.

29. Furukawa, T., Narita, M., Sakaue, M., Otsuka, T., Kuroha, T., Masuko, M., Azegami, T., Kishi, K., Takahashi, M., Utsumi, J., Koike, T., and Aizawa, Y.: Primary familial polycythaemia associated with a novel point mutation in the erythropoietin receptor. Br. J. Haematol. 99:222, 1997.

30. Kralovics, R., Indrak, K., Stopka, T., Berman, B.W., Prchal, J.F., and Prchal, J.T.: Two new EPO receptor mutations: truncated EPO receptors are most frequently associated with primary familial and congenital polycythemias. Blood 90:2057, 1997.

31. Dong, F., Brynes, R.K., Tidow, N., Welte, K., Lowenberg, B., and Touw, I.P.: Mutations in the gene for the granulocyte colony-stimulating-factor receptor in patients with acute myeloid leukemia preceded by severe congenital neutropenia. N. Engl. J. Med. 333:487, 1995.

32. McLemore, M.L., Poursine-Laurent, J., and Link, D.C.: Increased granulocyte colony-stimulating factor responsiveness but normal resting granulopoiesis in mice carrying a targeted granulocyte colony-simulating factor receptor mutation derived from a patient with severe congenital neutropenia. J. Clin. Invest. 102:483, 1998.

33. Hermans, M.H., Antonissen, C., Ward, A.C., Mayen, A.E., Ploemacher, R.E., and Touw, I.P.: Sustained receptor activation and hyperproliferation in response to granulocyte colony-stimulating factor (G-CSF) in mice with a severe congenital neutropenia/acute myeloid leukemia-derived mutation in the G-CSF receptor gene. J. Exp. Med. 189:683, 1999.

34. Artavanis-Tsakonas, S., Matsuno, K., and Fortini, M.E.: Notch signaling. Science 268:225, 1995.

35. Logeat, F., Bessia, C., Brou, C., LeBail, O., Jarriault, S., Seidah, N.G., and Israel, A.: The Notch1 receptor is cleaved constitutively by a furin-like convertase. Proc. Natl. Acad. Sci. USA 95:8108, 1998.

36. Weinmaster, G.: The ins and outs of notch signaling. Mol. Cell. Neurosci. 9:91, 1997.

37. Weinmaster, G.: Notch signaling: direct or what? Curr. Opin. Genet. Dev. 8:436, 1998.

38. Ellisen, L.W., Bird, J., West, D.C., Soreng, A.L., Reynolds. T.C., Smith, S.D., and Sklar, J.: TAN-1, the human homolog of the drosophila Notch gene, is broken by chromosomal translocations in T lymphoblastic neoplasms. Cell 66:649, 1991.

39. Capobianco, A.J., Zagouras, P., Blaumueller, C.M., Artavanis-Tsakonas, S., and Bishop, J.M.: Neoplastic transformation by truncated alleles of human NOTCH1/TAN1 and NOTCH2. Mol. Cell. Biol. 17:6265, 1997.

40. Pear, W.S., Aster, J.C., Scott, M.L., Hasserjian, R.P., Soffer, B., Sklar, J., and Baltimore, D.: Exclusive development of T cell neoplasms in mice transplanted with bone marrow expressing activated Notch alleles. J. Exp. Med. 183:2283, 1996.

41. Robey, E., Chang, D., Itano, A., Cado, D., Alexander, H., Lans, D., Weinmaster, G., and Salmon, P.: An activated form of Notch influences the choice between CD4 and CD8 T cell lineages. Cell 87:483, 1996.

42. Rohn, J.L., Lauring, A.S., Linenberger, M.L., and Overbaugh, J.: Transduction of Notch2 in feline leukemia virus-induced thymic lymphoma. J. Virol. 70:8071, 1998.

43. Deftos, M.L., He, Y.W., Ojala, E.W., and Bevan, M.J.: Correlating notch signaling with thymocyte maturation. Immunity 9:777, 1998.

44. Lu, F.M., and Lux, S.E.: Constitutively active human Notch1 binds to the transcription factor CBF1 and stimulates transcription through a promoter containing a CBF1-responsive element. Proc. Natl. Acad. Sci. USA 93:5663, 1996.

45. Struhl, G., and Adachi, A.: Nuclear access and action of notch in vivo. Cell 93:649, 1998.

46. Schroeter, E.H., Kisslinger, J.A., and Kopan, R.: Notch-1 signalling requires ligand-induced proteolytic release of intracellular domain. Nature 393:382, 1998.

47. Guan, E., Wang, J., Laborda, J., Norcross, M., Baeuerle, P.A., and Hoffman, T.: T cell leukemia-associated human notch/translocation-associated Notch homologue has IkappaB-like activity and physically interacts with nuclear factor kappaB proteins in T cells. J. Exp. Med. 183:2025, 1996.

48. DeCoteau, J.F., Knaus, P.I., Yankelev, H., Reis, M.D., Lowsky, R., Lodish, H.F., and Kadin, M.E.: Loss of functional cell surface transforming growth factor beta (TGF-beta) type 1 receptor correlates with insensitivity to TGF-beta in chronic lymphocytic leukemia. Proc. Natl. Acad. Sci. USA 94:5877, 1997.

49. Knaus, P.I., Lindemann, D., DeCoteau, J.F., Perlman, R., Yankelev, H., Hille, M., Kadin, M.E., and Lodish, H.F.: A dominant inhibitory mutant of the type II transforming growth factor beta receptor in the malignant progression of a cutaneous T-cell lymphoma. Mol. Cell. Biol. 16:3480, 1996.

50. Longnecker, R., Miller, C.L., Tomkinson, B., Miao, X-Q., and Kieff, E.: Deletion of DNA encoding the first five transmembrane domains of Epstein-Barr virus latent membrane proteins 2A and 2B. J. Virol 67:5068, 1993.

51. Miller, C.L., Burkhardt, A.L., Lee, J.H., Stealey, B., Longnecker, R., Bolen, J.B., and Kieff, E.: Integral membrane protein 2 of epstein-barr virus regulates reactivation from latency through dominant negative effects on protein-tyrosine kinases. Immunity 2:155, 1995.

52. Caldwell, R.G., Wilson, J.B., Anderson, S.J., Longnecker, R.: Epstein-Barr virus LMP2A drives B cell development and survival in the absence of normal B cell receptor signals. Immunity 9:405, 1998.

53. Thompson, A.A., Talley, J.A., Do, H.N., Kagan, H.L., Kunkel, L., Berenson, J., Cooper, M.D., Saxon, A., and Wall, R.: Aberrations of the B-cell receptor B29 (CD79b) gene in chronic lymphocytic leukemia. Blood 90:1387, 1997.

54. Sternberg, P.W., and Alberola-Ila, J.: Conspiracy theory: RAS and RAF do not act alone. Cell 95:447, 1998.

55. Neet, K., and Hunter, T.: Vertebrate non-receptor protein-tyrosine kinase families. Genes Cells 1:147, 1996.

56. Hibbs, M.L., Tarlinton, D.M., Armes, J., Grail, D., Hodgson, G., Maglito, R., Stacker, S.A., and Dunn, A.R.: Multiple defects in the immune system of Lyn-deficient mice, culminating in autoimmune disease. Cell 83:301, 1995.

57. Nishizumi, H., Taniuchi, I., Yamanashi, Y., Kitamura, D., Llic, D., Mori, S., Watanabe, T., and Yamamoto, T.: Impaired proliferation of peripheral B cells and indication of autoimmune disease in (Ilyn)-deficient mice. Immunity 3:549, 1995.

58. Chan, V.W.F., Meng, F., Soriano, P., DeFranco, A.L., and Lowell, C.A.: Characterization of the B lymphocyte populations in lyn-deficient mice and the role of lyn in signal initiation and down-regulation. Immunity 7:69, 1997.

59. Alberola-Ila, J., Takaki, S., Kerner, J.D., and Perlmutter, R.M.: Differential signaling by lymphocyte antigen receptors. In Paul W.E., Fathman C.G., Metzger H, eds.: Annual Review of Immunology, vol. 15. Palo Alto, Annual Reviews, 1997, p. 125.

60. Marth, J.D., Disteche, C., Pravtcheva, D., Ruddle, F., Krebs, E.G., and Perlmutter, R.M.: Localization of a lymphocyte-specific protein tyrosine kinase gene (lck) at a site of frequent chromosomal abnormalities in human lymphoma. Proc. Natl. Acad. Sci. USA. 83:7400, 1986.

61. Tycko, B., Smith, S.D., and Sklar, J.: Chromosomal translocations joining LCK and TCRB loci in human T cell leukemia. Exp. Med. 174:867, 1991.

62. Abraham, K.M., Levin, S.D., Marth, J.D., Forbush, K.A., and Perlmutter, R.M.: Thymic tumorigenesis induced by overexpression of p56^{lck}. Proc. Natl. Acad. Sci. USA 88:3977, 1991.

63. Rosenberg, N., and Witte, O.N.: The viral and cellular forms of the Abelson (abl) oncogene. Adv. Virus Res. 39:39, 1988.

64. Groffen, J., Stephenson, J.R., Heisterkamp, N., de Klein, A., Bartram, C.R., and Grosveld, G.: Philadelphia chromosomal breakpoints are clustered within a limited region, bcr, on chromosome 22. Cell 36:93, 1984.

65. Shtivelman, E., Lifshitz, B., Gale, R.P., Roe, B.A., and Canaani, E.: Fused transcript of abl and bcr genes in chronic myelogenous leukaemia. Nature 315:550, 1985.

66. Konopka, J.B., Watanabe, S.M., and Witte, O.N.: An alteration of the human c-abl protein in K562 leukemia cells unmasks associated tyrosine kinase activity. Cell 37:1035, 1984.

67. Hermans, A., Heisterkamp, N., von Lindern, M., van Baal, S., Meijer, D., van der Plas, D., Wiedemann, L.M., Groffen, J., Bootsma, D., and Grosveld, G.: Unique fusion of bcr and c-abl genes in Philadelphia chromosome positive acute lymphoblastic leukemia. Cell 51:33, 1987.

68. Clark, S.S., McLaughlin, J., Crist, W.M., Champlin, R., and Witte, O.N.: Unique forms of the abl tyrosine kinase distinguish Ph1-positive CML from Pb1-positive. ALL. Science 235:85, 1987.

69. McLaughlin, J., Chianese, E., and Witte, O.N.: Alternative forms of the BCR-AB1 oncogene have quantitatively different potencies for stimulation of immature lymphoid cells. Mol. Cell. Biol. 9:1866, 1989.

70. Lugo, T.G., Pendergast, A., Muller, A.J., and Witte, O.N.: Tyrosine kinase activity and transformation potency of bcr-abl oncogene products. Science. 247:1079, 1990.

71. Daley, G.Q., Van Etten, R.A., and Baltimore, D.: Induction of chronic myelogenous leukemia in mice by the P210$^{bcr/abl}$ gene of the Philadelphia chromosome. Science 247:824, 1990.

72. Kelliher, M.A., McLaughlin, J., Witte, O.N., and Rosenberg, N.: Induction of a chronic myelogenous leukemia-like syndrome in mice with v-abl and BCR/ABL. Proc. Natl. Acad. Sci. USA 87:6649, 1990.

73. Daley, G.Q., Van Etten, R.A., and Baltimore, D.: Blast crisis in a murine model of chronic myelogenous leukemia. Proc. Natl. Acad. Sci. USA 88:11335, 1991.

74. Gishizky, M.L., Johnson-White, J., and Witte, O.N.: Efficient transplantation of BCR/ABL induced chronic myelogenous leukemia-like syndrome in mice. Proc. Natl. Acad. Sci. USA 90:3755, 1993.

75. Pear, W.S., Miller, J.P., Xu, L., Pui, J.C., Soffer, B., Quackenbush, R.C., Pendergast, A.M., Bronson, R., Aster, J.C., Scott, M.L., and Baltimore, D.: Efficient and rapid induction of a chronic myelogenous leukemia-like myeloproliferative disease in mice receiving P210 bcr/abl-transduced bone marrow. Blood 92:3780, 1998.

76. Golub, T.R., Barker, G.F., Lovett, M., Gilliland, D.G.: Fusion of PDGF receptor beta to a novel ets-like gene, tel, in chronic myelomonocytic leukemia with t(5;12) chromosomal translocation. Cell 77:307, 1994.

77. Golub, T.R., Goga, A., Barker, G.F., Afar, D.E., McLaughlin, J., Bohlander, S.K., Rowley, J.D., Witte, O.N., and Gilliland, D.G.: Oligomerization of the ABL tyrosine kinase by the ETS protein TEL in human leukemia. Mol. Cell. Biol. 16:4107, 1996.

78. Lacronique, V., Boureux, A., Valle, V.D., Poirel, H., Quang, C.T., Mauchauffé, M., Berthou, C., Lessard, M., Berger, R., Ghysdael, J., and Bernard, O.A.: A TEL-JAK2 fusion protein with constitutive kinase activity in human leukemia. Science 278:1309, 1997.

79. Peeters, P., Raynaud, S.D., Cools, J., Wlodarska, I., Grosgeorge, J., Philip, P., Monpoux, F., Van Rompaey, L., Baens, M., Van den Berghe, H., and Marynen, P.: Fusion of TEL, the ETS-variant gene 6 (ETV6), to the receptor-associated kinase JAK2 as a result of t(9;12) in a lymphoid and t(9;15;12) in a myeloid leukemia. Blood 90:2535, 1997.

80. Morris, S.W., Kirstein, M.N., Valentine, M.B., Dittmer, K.G., Shapiro, D.N., Saltman, D.L., and Look, A.T.: Fusion of a kinase gene, ALK, to a nucleolar protein gene, NPM, in non-Hodgkin's Lymphoma. Science 263:1281, 1994.

81. Ross, T.S., Bernard, O.A., Berger, R., and Gilliland, D.G.: Fusion of Huntingtin interacting protein 1 to platelet-derived growth factor beta receptor (PDGFbetaR) in chronic myelomonocytic leukemia with t(5;7)(q33;q11.2). Blood 91:4419, 1998.

82. Abe, A., Emi, N., Tanimoto, M., Terasaki, H., Marunouchi, T., and Saito, H.: Fusion of the platelet-derived growth factor receptor beta to a novel gene CEV14 in acute myelogenous leukemia after clonal evolution. Blood 90:4271, 1997.

83. McWhirter, J.R., Galasso, D.L., and Wang, J.Y.J.: A coiled-coil oligomerization domain of Bcr is essential for the transforming function of Bcr-Abl oncoproteins. Mol. Cell. Biol. 13:7587, 1993.

84. Muller, A.J., Young, J.C., Pendergast, A-M., Pondel, M., Landau, N.R., Littman, D.R., and Witte, O.N.: BCR first exon sequences specifically activate Bcr/Abl tyrosine kinase oncogene of Philadelphia chromosome positive human leukemias. Mol. Cell. Biol. 11:1785, 1991.

85. Jousset, C., Carron, C., Boureux, A., Quang, C.T., Qury, C., Dusanter-Fourt, I., Charon, M., Levin, J., Bernard, O., and Ghysdael, J.: A domain of TEL conserved in a subset of ETS proteins defines a specific oligomerization interface essential to the mitogenic properties of the TEL-PDGFR beta oncoprotein. EMBO J. 16:69, 1997.

86. Pendergast, A.M., Muller, A.J., Havlik, M.H., Maru, Y., and Witte, O.N.: BCR sequences essential for transformation by the BCR/ABL oncogene bind to the ABL SH2 regulatory domain in a non-phosphotyrosine-dependent manner. Cell 66:161, 1991.

87. Maru, Y.M., and Witte, O.N.: The BCR gene encodes a novel serine/threonine kinase activity within a single exon. Cell 67:459, 1991.

88. Diekmann, D., Brill, S., Garrett, M.D., Totty, N., Hsuan, J., Monfries, C., Hall, C., Lim, L., and Hall, A.: Bcr encodes a GTPase activating protein for p21^{rac}. Nature 351:400, 1991.

89. Voncken, J.W., Van Schaick, H., Kaartinen, V., Deemer, K., Coates, T., Landing, B., Pattengale, P., Dorseuil, O., Bokoch, G.M., Groffen, J., and Heisterkamp, N.: Increased neutrophil respiratory burst in bcr-null mutants. Cell 80:719, 1995.

90. Diamond, J., Goldman, J.M., and Melo, J.V.: BCR-ABL, ABL-BCR, BCR, and ABL genes are all expressed in individual granulocyte-macrophage colony-forming unit colonies derived from blood of patients with chronic myeloid leukemia. Blood 85:2171, 1995.

91. McWhirter, J.R., and Wang, J.Y.J.: An actin-binding function contributes to transformation by the bcr-abl oncoprotein of Philadelphia chromosome-positive human leukemias. EMBO J.12:1533, 1993.

92. Taagepera, S., McDonald, D., Loeb, J.E., Whitaker, L.L., McElroy, A.K., Wang, J.Y.J., and Hope, T.J.: Nuclear-cytoplasmic shuttling of C-ABL tyrosine kinase. Proc. Natl. Acad. Sci. USA 95:7457, 1998.

93. Van Etten, R.A., Jackson, P.K., Baltimore, D., Sanders, M.C., Matsudaira, P.T., and Janmey, P.A.: The COOH terminus of the c-Abl tyrosine kinase contains distinct F- and G-actin binding domains with bundling activity. J. Cell Biol. 124:325, 1994.

94. Wen, S.T., Jackson, P.K., and Van Etten, R.A.: The cytostatic function of c-Abl is controlled by multiple nuclear localization signals and requires the p53 and Rb tumor suppressor gene products. EMBO J. 15:1583, 1996.

95. Baskaran, R., Wood, L.D., Whitaker, L.L., Canman, C.E., Morgan, S.E., Xu, Y., Barlow, C., Baltimore, D., Wynshaw-Boris, A., Kastan, M.B., and Wang, J.Y.J.: Ataxia telangiectasia mutant protein activates c-Abl tyrosine kinase in response to ionizing radiation. Nature 387:516, 1997.

96. Nishii, K., Kabarowski, J.H., Gibbons, D.L., Griffiths, S.D., Titley, I.,

Wiedemann, L.M., and Greaves, M.F.: ts BCR-ABL kinase activation confers increased resistance to genotoxic damage via cell cyle block. Oncogene 13:2225, 1996.

97. Welch, P.J., and Wang, J.Y.J.: A C-terminal protein-binding domain in the retinoblastoma protein regulates nuclear c-Abl tyrosine kinase in the cell cyle. Cell 75:779, 1993.

98. Schwartzberg, P.L., Stall, A.M., Hardin, J.D., Bowdish, K.S., Humaran, T., Boast, S., Harbison, M.L., Robertson, E.J., and Goff, S.P.: Mice homozygous for the ablm1 mutation show poor viability and depletion of selected B and T cell populations. Cell 65:1165, 1991.

99. Tybulewicz, V.L.J., Crawford, C.E., Jackson, P.K., Bronson, R.T., and Mulligan, R.C.: Neonatal lethality and lymphopenia in mice with a homozygous disruption of the c-abl proto-oncogene. Cell 65:1153, 1991.

100. Pendergast, A.M., Gishizky, M.L., Havlik, M.H., and Witte, O.N.: SH1 domain autophosphorylation of P210 BCR/ABL is required for transformation but not growth factor independence. Mol. Cell. Biol. 13:1728, 1993.

101. Goga, A., Lui, X., Hambuch, T.M., Senechal, K., Berk, A.J., Witte, O.N., and Sawyers, C.L.: P53 dependent growth suppression by the c-Abl nuclear tyrosine kinase. Oncogene 11:791, 1995.

102. Mayer, B.J., and Baltimore, D.: Mutagenic analysis of the roles of SH2 and SH3 domains in regulation of the Abl tyrosine kinase. Mol. Cell. Biol. 14:2883, 1994.

103. Sawyers, C.L., McLaughlin, J., Goga, A., Havlik, M., and Witte, O.: The nuclear tyrosine kinase c-Abl negatively regulates cell growth. Cell 77:121, 1994.

104. Carpino, N., Wisniewski, D., Strife, A., Marshak, D., Kobayashi, R., Stillman, B., and Clarckson, B.: P62^{+doc}: a constitutively tyrosine-phosphorylated GAP-associated protein in chronic myelogenous leukemia progenitor cells. Cell 88:197, 1997.

105. Senechal, K., Halperm, J., and Sawyers, C.L.: The CRKL adaptor protein transforms fibroblasts and functions in transformation by the BCR-ABL oncogene. J. Biol. Chem. 271:23255, 1996.

106. Wen, S.T., and Van Etten, R.A.: The PAG gene product, a stress-induced protein with antioxidant properties, is an Abl SH3-binding protein and a physiological inhibitor of c-Abl tyrosine kinase activity. Genes Dev. 11:2456, 1997.

107. Yamanashi, Y., and Baltimore, D.: Identification of the Abl- and rasGAP-associated 62 kDa protein as a docking protein, Dok. Cell 88:205, 1997.

108. Zhu, J., and Shore, S.K.: c-ABL tyrosine kinase activity is regulated by association with a novel SH3-domain-binding protein. Mol. Cell. Biol. 16:7054, 1996.

109. Afar, D.E.H., Han, L., McLaughlin, J., Wong, S., Dhaka, A., Parmar, K., Rosenberg, N., Witte, O.N., and Colicelli, J.: Regulation of the oncogenic activity of BCR-ABL by a tightly bound substrate protein RIN1. Immunity 6:773, 1997.

110. Puil, L., Liu, J., Gish, G., Mbamalu, G., Bowtell, D., Pelicci, P.G., Arlinghaus, R., and Pawson, T.: Bcr-Abl oncoproteins bind directly to activators of the Ras signalling pathway. EMBO J. 13:764, 1994.

111. Sattler, M., and Salgia, R.: Activation of hematopoietic growth factor signal transduction pathways by the human oncogene BCR/ABL. Nature 8:63, 1997.

112. Afar, D.E.H., McLaughlin, J., Sherr, C.J., Witte, O.N., and Roussel, M.F.: Signaling by ABL oncogenes through cyclin D1. Proc. Natl. Acad. Sci. USA 92:9540, 1995.

113. Amarante-Mendes, G.P., Kim, C.N., Linda Liu, Y.H., Perkins, C.L., Green, D.R., and Bhalla, K.: Bcr-Abl exerts its antiapoptotic effect against diverse apoptotic stimuli through blockage of mitochondrial release of cytochrome C and activation of caspase-3. Blood 91:1700, 1998.

114. Andoniou, C.E., Thien, C.B., and Langdon, W.Y.: Tumour induction by activated abl involves tyrosine phosphorylation of the product of the cbl oncogene. EMBO J. 13:4515, 1994.

115. Carlesso, N., Frank, D.A., and Griffin, J.D.: Tyrosyl phosphorylation and DNA binding activity of signal transducers and activators of transcription (STAT) proteins in hematopoietic cell lines transformed by Bcr/Abl. J. Exp. Med. 183:811, 1996.

116. Dubrez, L., Eymin, B., Sordet, O., Droin, N., Turhan, A.G., and Solary, E.: BCR-ABL delays apoptosis upstream of procaspase-3 activation. Blood 91:2415, 1998.

117. Goga, A., McLaughlin, J., Afar, D.E.H., Saffran, D.C., and Witte, O.N.: Alternative signals to RAS for hematopoietic transformation by the BCR-ABL oncogene. Cell 82:981, 1995.

118. Kabarowski, J.H., Allen, P.B., and Wiedemann, L.: A temperature sensitive p210 BCR-ABL mutant defines the primary consequences of BCR-ABL tyrosine kinase expression in growth factor dependent cells. EMBO J. 13:5887, 1994.

119. Odai, H., Sasaki, K., Iwamatsu, A., Nakamoto, T., Ueno, H., Yamagata, T., Mitani, K. Yazaki, Y., and Hirai, H.: Purification and molecular cloning of SH2- and SH3-containing inositol polyphosphate-5-phophatase, which is involved in the signaling pathway of granulocyte-macrophage colony-stimulating factor, erythropoietin, and Bcr-Abl. Blood 89:2745, 1997.

120. Raitano, A.B., Halpern, J.R., Hambuch, T.M., and Sawyers, C.L.: The Bcr-Abl leukemia oncogene activates Jun kinase and requires Jun for transformation. Proc. Natl. Acad. Sci. USA 92:11746, 1995.

121. Sanchez-Garcia, I., and Grutz, G.: Tumorigenic activity of the BCR-ABL oncogenes is mediated by BCL2. Proc. Natl. Acad. Sci. USA 92:5287, 1995.

122. Sattler, M., Salgia, R., Shrikhande, G., Verma, S., Choi, J.L., Rohrschneider, L.R., and Griffin, J.D.: The phosphatidylinositol polyphosphate 5-phosphatase SHIP and the protein tyrosine phosphatase SHP-2 form a complex in hematopoietic cells which can be regulated by BCR/ABL and growth factors. Oncogene 15:2379, 1997.

123. Sawyers, C.L., McLaughlin, J., and Witte, O.N.: Genetic requirement for ras in the transformation of fibroblasts and hematopoietic cells by the (IBcr-Abl) oncogene. J. Exp. Med. 181:307, 1995.

124. Skorski, T., Bellacosa, A., Nieborowska-Skorska, M., Majewski, M., Martinez, R., Choi, J.K., Trotta, R., Wlodarski, P., Perrotti, D., Chan, T.O., Wasik, M.A., Tsichlis, P.N., and Calabretta B.: Transformation of hematopoietic cells by BCR/ABL requires activation of a PI-3k/Akt-dependent pathway. EMBO J. 16:6151, 1997.

125. Carroll, M., Ohno-Jones, S., Tamura, S., Buchdunger, E., Zimmermann, J., Lyndon, N.B., Gilliland, D.G., and Druker, B.J.: CPG 57148, a tyrosine kinase inhibitor, inhibits the growth of cells expressing BCR-ABL, TEL-ABL, and TEL-PDGFR fusion proteins. Blood 90:4947, 1997.

126. Carroll, M., Ohno-Jones, S., Tamura, S., Buchdunger, E., Zimmermann, J., Lydon, N.B., Gilliland, D.G., and Druker, B.J.: CGP 57148, a tyrosine kinase inhibitor, inhibits the growth of cells expressing BCR-ABL, TEL-ABL, and TEL-PDGFR fusion proteins. Blood 90:4947, 1997.

127. Shuai, K., Halpern, J., ten Hoeve, J., Rao, X., and Sawyers, C.L.: Constitutive activation of STAT5 by the BCR-ABL oncogene in chronic myelogenous leukemia. Oncogene 13:247, 1996.

128. Holtschke, T., Lohler, J., Kanno, Y., Fehr, T., Giese, N., Rosenbauer, F., Lou, J., Knobeloch, K.P., Gabriele, L., Waring, J.F., Bachmann, M.F., Zinkernagel, R.M., Morse, H.C.I., Ozato, K. and Horak, I.: Immunodeficiency and chronic myelogenous leukemia-like syndrome in mice with a targeted mutation of the ICSBP gene. Cell 87:307, 1998.

129. Schmidt, M., Nagel, S., Proba, J., Thiede, C., Ritter, M., Waring, J.F., Rosenbauer, F. Huhn, D., Wittig, B., Horak, I., and Neubauer, A.: Lack of interferon consensus sequence binding protein (ICSBP) transcripts in human myeloid leukemias. Blood 91:22, 1998.

130. The Italian Cooperative Study Group: CML: Long-term follow-up of the Italian trial of interferon-alpha versus conventional chemotherapy in chronic myeloid leukemia. Blood 92:1541, 1998.

131. Hunter, T.: Oncoprotein Networks. Cell 88:333, 1997.

132. Cogswell, P.C., Morgan, R., Dunn, M., Neubauer, A., Nelson, P., Poland-Johnston, N.K., Sandberg, A.A., and Liu, E.: Mutations of the Ras protooncogenes in chronic myelogenous leukemia: a high frequency of Ras mutations in bcr/abl rearrangement-negative chronic myelogenous leukemia. Blood 74:2629, 1989.

133. Elion, E.A.: Routing MAP kinases cascades. Science 281:1625, 1998.

134. Side, L., Taylor, B., Cayouette, M., Conner, E., Thompson, P., Luce, M., and Shannon, K.: Homozygous inactivation of the NF1 gene in bone marrow cells from children with neurofibromatosis type 1 and malignant myeloid disorders. N. Engl. J. Med. 336:1713, 1997.

135. Side, L.E., Emanuel, P.D., Taylor, B., Franklin, J., Thompson, P., Castleberry, R.P., and Shannon, K.M.: Mutations of the NF1 gene in children with juvenile myelomonocytic leukemia without clinical evidence of neurofibromatosis, type 1. Blood 92:267, 1998.

136. Bollag, G., Clapp, D.W., Shih, S., Adler, F., Zhang, Y.Y., Thompson, P., Lange, B.J., Freedman, M.H., McCormick, F., Jacks, T., and Shannon, K.: Loss of NF1 results in activation of the Ras signaling pathway and leads to aberrant growth in haematopoietic cells. Nat. Genet. 12:144, 1996.

137. Zhang, Y.Y., Vik, T.A., Ryder, J.W., Srour, E.F., Jacks, T., Shannon, K., and Clapp, D.W.: NF1: regulates hematopoietic progenitor cell growth and ras signaling in response to multiple cytokines. Blood 187:1893, 1998.

138. Birnbaum, R., O'Marcaigh, A., Wardak, Z., Zhang, Y., Dranoff, G., Jacks, T., Clapp, D.W., and Shannon, K.M.: Interaction between NF1 and GMCSF in leukemogenesis and hematopoietic engraftment. Blood 90:411a, 1997.

139. Habets, G.G.M., Scholtes, E.H.M., Zuydgeest, D., Kammen, R.A.V.D., Stam, J.C., Berns, A., and Collard, J.G.: Identification of an invasion-inducing gene. *Tiam-1*, that encodes a protein with homology to GDP-GTP exchangers for Rho-like proteins. Cell 77:537, 1994.

140. Look, A.T.: Oncogenic transcription factors in the human acute leukemias. Science 278:1059, 1997.

141. Tenen, D.G., Hromas, R., Licht, J.D., and Zhang, D.E.: Transcription factors, normal myeloid development, and leukemia. Blood 90:489, 1998.

142. Taub, R., Kirsch, I., Morton, C., Lenoir, G., Swan, D., Tronick, S., Aaronson, S., and Leder, P.: Translocation of the c-myc gene into the immunoglobulin heavy chain locus in human Burkitt lymphoma and murine plasmacytoma cells. Proc. Natl. Acad. Sci. USA 79:7837, 1982.

143. Dalla-Favera, R., Bregni, M., Erikson, J., Patterson, D., Gallo, R.C., and Croce, C.M.: Human c-myc onc gene is located on the region of chromosome 8 that is translocated in Burkitt lymphoma cells. Proc. Natl. Acad. Sci. USA 79:7824, 1982.

144. Hatano, M., Roberts, C.W.M., Minden, M., Crist, W.M., and Korsmeyer, S.J.: Deregulation of a homeobox gene, HOX11, by the t(10;14) in T cell leukemia. Science 253:79, 1991.

145. Erickson, P., Gao, J., Chang, K-S., Look, T., Whisenant, E., Raimondi, S., Lasher, R., Trujillo, J., Rowley, J., and Drabkin, H.: Identification of breakpoints in t(8;21) acute myelogenous leukemia and isolation of a fusion transcript, AML1/ETO, with similarity to drosophila segmentation gene, runt. Blood 80:1825, 1992.

146. Miyoshi, H., Shimizu, K., Kozu, T., Maseki, N., Kaneko, Y., and Ohki, M.: t(8;21) Breakpoints on chromosome 21 in acute myeloid leukemia are clustered within a limited region of a single gene, AML1. Proc. Natl. Acad. Sci. USA 88:10431, 1991.

147. Nucifora, G., Begy, C.R., Erickson, P., Drabkin, H.A., and Rowley, J.D.: The 3;21 translocation in myelodysplasia results in a fusion transcript between the AML1 gene and the gene for EAP, a highly conserved protein associated with the Epstein-Barr virus small RNA EBER 1. Proc. Natl. Acad. Sci. USA 90:7784, 1993.

148. Mitani, K., Ogawa, S., Tanaka, T., Miyoshi, H., Kurokawa, M., Mano, H., Yazaki, Y., Ohki, M., and Hirai, H.: Generation of the *AML1-EVI-1* fusion gene in the t(3;21)(q26;q22) causes blastic crisis in chronic myelocytic leukemia. EMBO J. 13:504, 1994.

149. Meyers, S., Lenny, N., and Hiebert, S.W.: The t(8;21) fusion protein interferes with AML-1B-dependent transcriptional activation. Mol. Cell. Biol. 15:1974, 1995.

150. Zent, C.S., Mathieu, C., Claxton, D.F., Zhang, D.E., Tenen, D.G., Rowley, J.D., and Nucifora, G.: The chimeric genes AML1/MDS1 and AML1/EAP inhibit AML1B activation at the CSF1R promoter, but only AML1/MDS1 has tumor-promoter properties. Proc. Natl. Acad. Sci. USA 93:1044, 1996.

151. Frank, R., Zhang, J., Uchida, H., Meyers, S., Hiebert, S.W., and Nimer, S.D.: The AM1/ETO fusion protein blocks transactivation of the GM-CSF promoter by AML1B. Oncogene 11:2667, 1995.

152. Okuda, T., Deursen, J.V., Hiebert, S.W., Grosveld, G., and Downing, J.R.: AML1, the target of multiple chromosomal translocations in human leukemia, is essential for normal fetal liver hematopoiesis. Cell 84:321, 1996.

153. Yergeau, D.A., Hetherington, C.J., Wang, Q., Zhang, P., Sharpe, A.H., Binder, M., Marin-Padilla, M., Tenen, D.G., Speck, N.A., and Zhang, D.E.: Embryonic lethality and impairment of haematopoiesis in mice heterozygous for an AML1-ETO fusion gene. Nat. Genet. 15:303, 1997.

154. Okuda, T., Cai, Z., Yang, S., Lenny, N., Lyu, C.J., van Deursen, J.M., Harada, H., and Downing, J.R.: Expression of a knocked-in AML1-ETO leukemia gene inhibits the establishment of normal definitive hematopoiesis and directly generates dysplastic hematopoietic progenitors. Blood 91:3134, 1998.

155. Wang, Z.G., Delva, L., Gaboli, M., Rivi, R., Giorgio, M., Cordon-Cardo, C., Grosveld, F., and Pandolfi, P.P.: Role of PML in cell growth and the retinoic acid pathway. Nature 279:1547, 1998.

156. Westendorf, J.J., Yamamoto, C.M., Lenny, N., Downing, J.R., Selsted, M.E., and Hiebert, S.W.: The t(8;21) fusion product, AML-1-ETO, associates with C/EBP-alpha, inhibits C/EBP-alpha-dependent transcription, and blocks granulocytic differentiation. Mol. Cell. Biol. 18:322, 1998.

157. Lutterbach, B., Sun, D., Schuetz, J., and Hiebert, S.W.: The MYND motif is required for repression of basal transcription from the multidrug resistance 1 promoter by the t(8;21) fusion protein. Mol. Cell. Biol. 18:3604, 1998.

158. Liu, P., Tarl, S.A., Hajra, A., Claxton, D.F., Marlton, P., Freedman, M., Siciliano, M.J., and Collins, F.S.: Fusion between transcription factor CBFalpha/PEBP2alpha and a myosin heavy chain in acute myeloid leukemia. Science 261:1041, 1993.

159. Wang, Q., Stacy, T., Miller, J.D., Lewis, A.F., Gu, T-L., Huang, X., Bushweller, J.H., Bories, J-C., Alt, F.W., Ryan, G., Liu, P.P., Wynshaw-Boris, A., Binder, M., Marin-Padilla, M., Sharpe, A.H., and Speck, N.A.: The CBFβ subunit is essential for CBFα2 (AML 1) function in vivo. Cell 87:697, 1996.

160. Kanno, Y., Kanno, T., Sakakura, C., Bae, S.C., and Ito, Y.: Cytoplasmic sequestration of the polyomavirus enhancer binding protein 2 (PEBP2)/Core binding factor alpha (CBFalpha) subunit by the leukemia-related PEBP2/CBFbeta-SMMHC fusion protein inhibits PEBP2/CBF-mediated transactivation. Mol. Cell. Biol. 18:4252, 1998.

161. Castilla, L.H., Wijmenga, C., Wang, Q., Stacy, T., Speck, N.A., Eckhaus, M., Marin-Padilla, M., Collins, F.S., Wynshaw-Boris, A., and Liu, P.P.: Failure of embryonic hematopoiesis and lethal hemorrhages in mouse embryos heterozygous for a knocked-in leukemia gene CBFB-MYH11. Cell 87:687, 1996.

162. Golub, T.R., Barker, G.F., Bohlander, S.K., Hiebert, S.W., Ward, D.C., Bray-Ward, P., Morgan, E., Raimondi, S.C., Rowley, J.D., and Gilliland, D.G.: Fusion of the TEL gene on 12p13 to the AML1 gene on 21q22 in acute lymphoblastic leukemia. Proc. Natl. Acad. Sci. USA 92:4917, 1995.

163. Shurtleff, S.A., Buijs, A., Behm, F.G., Rubnitz, J.E., Raimondi, S.C., Hancock, M.L., Chan, G.C., Pui, C.H., Grosveld, G., and Downing, J.R.: TEL/AML1 fusion resulting from a cryptic t(12;21) is the most common genetic lesion in pediatric ALL and defines a subgroup of patients with an excellent prognosis. Leukemia 9:1985, 1995.

164. Borrow, J., Goddard, A.D., Sheer, D., and Solomon, E.: Molecular analysis of acute promyelocytic leukemia breakpoint cluster region on chromosome 17. Science 249:1577, 1990.

165. de The, H., Chomienne, C., Lanotte, M., Degos, L., and Dejean, A.: The t(15;17) translocation of acute promyelocytic leukemia fuses the retinoic acid receptor gene to a novel transcribed locus. Nature 347:558, 1990.

166. Longo, L., Pandolfi, P.P., Biondi, A., Rambaldi, A., Mencarelli, A., Lo Coco, F., Diverio, D., Pegoraro, L., Avanzi, G., Tabilio, A., Zangrilli, D., Alcalay, M., Donti, E., Grignani, F., and Pelicci, P.G.: Rearrangements and aberrant expression of the retinoic acid receptor alpha gene in acute promyelocytic leukemias. J. Exp. Med. 172:1571, 1990.

167. Dyck, J.A., Maul, G.G., Miller, W.H.J., Chen, J.D., Kakizuka, A., and Evans, R.M.: A novel macromolecular structure is a target of the promyelocyte-retinoic acid receptor oncoprotein. Cell 76:333, 1994.

168. Koken, M.H., Puvion-Dutilleul, F., Guillemin, M.C., Viron, A., Linares-Cruz, G., Stuurman, N., de Jong, L., Szostecki, C., Calvo, F., Chomienne, C., Degos, L., Puvion, E., and de The, H.: The t(15;17) translocation alters a nuclear body in a retinoic acid-reversible fashion. EMBO J. 13:1073, 1994.

169. Weis, K., Rambaud, S., Lavau, C., Jansen, J., Carvalho, T., Carmo-Fonseca, M., Lamond, A., and Dejean, A.: Retinoic acid regulates aberrant nuclear localization of PML-RAR alpha in acute promyelocytic leukemia cells. Cell 76:345, 1994.

170. Brown, D., Kogan, S., Lagasse, E., Weissman, I., Alcalay, M., Pelicci, P.G., Atwater, S., and Bishop, J.M.: A *PMLRARalpha* transgene initiates murine acute promyelocytic leukemia. Proc. Natl. Acad. Sci. USA 94:2551, 1997.

171. He, L-Z., Tribioli, C., Rivi, R., Peruzzi, D., Pelicci, P.G., Soares, V., Cattoretti, G., and Pandolfi, P.P.: Acute leukemia with promyelocytic features in PML/RARalpha transgenic mice. Proc. Natl. Acad. Sci. USA 94:5302, 1997.

172. Grignani, F., Ferrucci, P.F., Testa, U., Talamo, G., Fagioli, M., Alcalay, M., Mencarelli, A., Grignani, F., Peschle, C., Nicoletti, I., and Pelicci, P.: The acute promyelocytic leukemia-specific PML-RAR alpha fusion protein inhibits differentiation and promotes survival of myeloid precursor cells. Cell 74:423, 1993.

173. Licht, J.D., Shaknovich, R., English, M.A., Melnick, A., Li, J.Y., Reddy, J.C., Dong, S., Chen, S.J., Zelent, A., and Waxman, S.: Reduced and altered DNA-binding and transcriptional properties of the PLZF-retinoic acid receptor-alpha chimera generated in t(11;17)-associated acute promyelocytic leukemia. Oncogene 12:323, 1998.

174. Dong, S., Zhu, J., Reid, A., Strutt, P., Guidez, F., Zhong, H.J., Wang, Z.Y., Licht, J., Waxman, S., Chomienne, C., Chen, Z., Zelent, A., and Chen, S.J.: Amino-terminal protein-protein interaction motif (POZ-domain) is responsible for activities of the promyelocytic leukemia zinc finger-retinoic acid receptor-alpha fusion protein. Proc. Natl. Acad. Sci. USA 93:3624, 1996.

175. Lin, R.J., Nagy, L., Inoue, S., Shao, W., Miller, W.H., J., and Evans, R.M.: Role of the histone deacetylase complex in acute promyelocytic leukaemia. Nature 391:811, 1998.

176. Grignani, F., De Matteis, S., Nervi, C., Temassoni, L., Gelmetti, V., Cioce, M., Fanelli, M., Ruthardt, M., Ferrara, F.F., Zamir, I., Seiser, C., Grignani, F., Lazar, M.A., Minucci, S., and Pelicci, P.G.: Fusion proteins of the retinoic acid receptor-alpha recruit histone deacetylase in promyelocytic leukaemia. Nature 391:815, 1998.

177. Hong, S-H., David, G., Wong, C-W., Dejean, A., and Privalsky, M.L.: SMRT corepressor interacts with PLZF and with the PML-retinoic acid receptor alpha (RARalpha) and PLZF-RARalpha oncoproteins associated with acute promyelocytic leukemia. Proc. Natl. Acad. Sci. USA 94:9028, 1997.

178. Guidez, F., Ivins, S., Zhu, J., Söderström, M., Waxman, S., and Zelent, A.: Reduced retinoic acid-sensitivities of nuclear receptor corepressor binding to PML- and PLZF-RARalpha underlie molecular pathogenesis and treatment of acute promyelocytic leukemia. Blood 91:2634, 1998.

179. Ding, W., Li, Y-P., Nobile, L.M., Grills, G., Carrera, I., Paietta, E., Tallman, M.S., Wiernik, P.H., and Gallagher, R.E.: Leukemic cellular retinoic acid resistance and missense mutations in the PML-RAR fusion gene after relapse of acute promyelocytic leukemia from treatment with all-trans retinoic acid and intensive chemotherapy. Blood 92:1172, 1998.

180. Thorsteinsdottir, U., Sauvageau, G., Hough, M.R., Dragowska, W., Lansdorp, P.M., Lawrence, H.J., Largman, C., and Humphries, R.K.: Overexpression of HOXA10 in murine hematopoietic cells perturbs both myeloid and lymphoid differentiation and leads to acute myeloid leukemia. Mol. Cell. Biol. 17:495, 1997.

181. Kroon, E., Krosl, J., Thorsteinsdottir, U., Baban, S., Buchberg, A.M., and Sauvageau, G.: Hoxa9 transforms primary bone marrow cells through specific collaboration with Meis 1a but not Pbx1b. EMBO J. 17:3714, 1998.

182. Blatt, C., Aberdam, D., Schwartz, R., and Sachs, L.: DNA rearrangement of a homeobox gene in myeloid leukaemic cells. EMBO J. 7:4283, 1988.

183. Domer, P.H., Fakharzadeh, S.S., Chen, C-S., Jockel, J., Johansen, L., Silverman, G.A., Kersey, J.H., and Korsmeyer, S.J.: Acute mixed-lineage leukemia t(4;11)(q21;q23) generates an MLL-AF4 fusion product B. Proc. Natl. Acad. Sci. 90:7884, 1993.

184. Tkachuk, D.C., Kohler, S., and Cleary, M.L.: Involvement of a homolog of Drosophila trithorax by 11q23 chromosomal translocations in acute leukemias. Cell 71:691, 1992.

185. Ziemin-van der Poel, S., McCabe, N.R., Gill, H.J., Espinosa, R., III, Patel, Y., Harden, A., Rubinelli, P., Smith, S.D., LeBeau, M.M., Rowley, J.D., and Diaz, M.O.: Identification of a gene. *MLL,* that spans the breakpoint in 11q23 translocations associated with human leukemias. Proc. Natl. Acad. Sci. USA 88:10735, 1991.

186. Gu, Y., Nakamura, T., Alder, H., Prasad, R., Canaani, O., Cimino, G., Croce, C.M., and Canaani, E.: The t(4;11) chromosome translocation of human acute leukemias fuses the ALL-1 gene, related to *Drosophila trithorax,* tot he AF-4 gene. Cell 71:701, 1992.

187. Djabali, M., Selleri, L., Parry, P., Bower, M., Young, B.D., and Evans, G.A.: A trithorax-like gene is interrupted by chromosome 11q23 translocations in acute leukaemias. Nat. Genet. 2:113, 1992.

188. Yu, B.D., Hess, J.L., Horning, S.E., Brown, G.A., and Korsmeyer, S.J.: Altered Hox expression and segmental identity in Mll-mutant mice. Nature 378:505, 1995.

189. Yu, B.D., Hanson, R.D., Hess, J.L., Horning, S.E., and Korsmeyer, S.J.: MLL, a mammalian trithorax-group gene, functions as a transcriptional maintenance factor in morphogenesis. Proc. Natl. Acad. Sci. USA 95:10632, 1998.

190. Hess, J.L., Yu, B.D., Li, B., Hanson, R., and Korsmeyer, S.J.: Defects in yolk sac hematopoiesis in Mll-Null embryos. Blood 90:1799, 1997.

191. Yagi, H., Deguchi, K., Aono, A., Tani, Y., Kishimoto, T., and Komori, T.: Growth disturbance in fetal liver hematopoiesis of Mll-mutant mice. Blood 92:108, 1998.

192. Corral, J., Lavenir, I., Impey, H., Warren, A.J., Forster, A., Larson, T.A., Bell, S., McKenzie, A.N.J., King, G., and Rabbitts, T.H.: An MLL-AF9 fusion gene made by homologous recombination causes acute leukemia in chimeric mice: a method to create fusion oncogenes. Cell 85:853, 1996.

193. Lavau, C., Szilvassy, S.J., Slany, R., and Cleary, M.L.: Immortalization and leukemic transformation of a myelomonocytic precursor by retrovirally transduced HRX-ENL. EMBO J. 16:4226, 1997.

194. Rubnitz, J.E., Morrissey, J., Savage, P.A., and Cleary, M.L.: ENL, the gene fused with HRX in t(11;19) leukemias, encodes a nuclear protein with transcriptional activation potential in lymphoid and myeloid cells. Blood 84:1747, 1994.

195. Prasad, R., Yano, Y., Sorio, C., Nakamura, T., Rallapalli, R., Gu, Y., Leshkowitz, D., Croce, C.M., and Canaani, E.: Domains with transcriptional regulatory protein activity within in the ALL1 and AF 4 proteins involved in acute leukemia. Proc. Natl. Acad. Sci. USA 92:12160, 1995.

196. Shilatifard, A., Lane, W.S., Jackson, K.W., Conaway, R.C., and Conaway, J.W.: An RNA polymerase II elongation factor encoded by the human ELL gene. Science 271:1873, 1996.

197. Slany, R.K., Lavau, C., and Cleary, M.L.: The oncogenic capacity of hrx-enl requires the transcriptional transactivation activity of enl and the dna binding motifs of hrx. Mol. Cell. Biol. 18:122, 1998.

198. Nourse, J., Mellentin, J.D., Galili, N., Wilkinson, J., Stanbridge, E., Smith, S.D., and Cleary, M.L.: Chromosomal translocation t(1;19) results in synthesis of a homeobox fusion mRNA that codes for a potential chimeric transcription factor. Cell 60:535, 1990.

199. Kamps, M.P., Murre, C., Sun, X-H., and Baltimore, D.: A new homeobox gene contributes the DNA binding domain of the t(1;19) translocation protein in pre-B ALL. Cell 60:547, 1990.

200. Bain, G., Maandag, E.C.R., Izon, D.J., Amsen, D., Kruisbeek, A.M., Weintraub, B.C., Krop, I., Schlissel, M.S., Feeney, A.J., Roon, M.V., Valk, M.V.D., Riele, H.P.J.T., Berns, A., and Murre, C.: E2A protein are required for proper B cell development and initiation of immunoglobulin gene rearrangements. Cell 79:885, 1994.

201. Zhuang, Y., Soriano, P., and Weintraub, H.: The helix-loop-helix gene E2A is required for B cell formation. Cell 79:875, 1994.

202. Rauskolb, C., Peifer, M., and Wieschaus, E.: Extradenticle, a regulator of homeotic gene activity, is a homology of the homeobox-containing human proto-oncogene pbx1. Cell 74:1101, 1993.

203. Chang, C.P., Shen, W.F., Rozenfeld, S., Lawrence, H.J., Largman, C., and Cleary, M.L.: Pbx proteins display hexapeptide-dependent cooperative DNA binding with a subset of Hox proteins. Genes Dev 9:663, 1995.

204. Lu, O., and Kamps, M.P.: Structural determinants within Pbx1 that mediate cooperative DNA binding with pentapeptide-containing Hox proteins: proposal for a model of a Pbx1-Hox-DNA complex. Mol. Cell. Biol. 16:1632, 1996.

205. Van Dijk, M.A., Voorhoeve, P.M., and Murre, C.: Pbx1 is converted into a transcriptional activator upon acquiring the N-terminal region of E2A in pre-B-cell acute lymphoblastoid leukemia. Proc. Natl. Acad. Sci. USA 90:6061, 1993.

206. Kamps, M.P., Look, A.T., and Baltimore, D.: The human t(1;19) translocation in pre-B ALL produces multiple nuclear E2A-Pbx1 fusion proteins with differing transforming potentials. Genes Dev. 5:358, 1991.

207. Kamps, M.P., and Baltimore, D.: E2A-Pbx1, the t(1;19) translocation protein of human pre-B-cell acute lymphocytic leukemia, causes acute myeloid leukemia in mice. Mol. Cell. Biol. 13:351, 1993.

208. Dedera, D.A., Waller, E.K., LeBrun, D.P., Sen-Majumdar, A., Stevens, M.E., Barsh, G.S., and Cleary, M.L.: Chimeric homeobox gene *E2A-PBX1* induces proliferation, apoptosis, and malignant lymphomas in transgenic mice. Cell 74:833, 1993.

209. Monica, K., LeBrun, D.P., Dedera, D.A., Brown, R., and Cleary, M.L.: Transformation properties of the E2a-Pbx1 chimeric oncoprotein: fusion with E2a is essential, but the Pbx1 homeodomain is dispensable. Mol. Cell. Biol. 14:8304, 1994.

210. Fu, X., and Kamps, M.P.: E2a-Pbx1 induces aberrant expression of tissue-specific and developmentally regulated genes when expressed in NTH 3T3 fibroblasts. Mol. Cell. Biol. 7:1503, 1997.

211. Tsujimoto, Y., Cossman, J., Jaffe, E., and Croce, C.M.: Involvement of the bcl-2 gene in human follicular lymphoma. Science 228:1440, 1985.

212. Cleary, M.L., Smith, S.D., and Sklar, J.: Cloning and structural analysis of cDNAs for bcl-2 and a hybrid bcl-2/immunoglobulin transcript resulting from the t(14;18) translocation. Cell 47:19, 1986.

213. Vaux, D.L., Cory, S., and Adams, J.M.: Bcl-2 gene promotes haemopoietic cell survival and cooperates with c-myc to immortalize pre-B cells. Nature 335:440, 1988.

214. Silva, M., Richard, C., Benito, A., Sanz, C., Olalla, I., and Fernandez-Luna, J.L.: Expression of Bcl-x in erythroid precursors from patients with polycythemia vera. N. Engl. J. Med. 338:564, 1998.

215. Meijerink, J.P.P., Mensink, E.J.B.M., Wang, K., Sedlak, T.W., Slöetjes, A.W., Witte, T.D., Waksman, G., and Korsmeyer, S.J.: Hematopoietic malignancies demonstrate loss-of-function mutations of BAX. Blood 91:2991, 1998.

216. Hunger, S.P., Ohyashiki, K., Yoyama, K., and Cleary, M.L.: Hlf, a novel hepatic bZIP protein, shows altered DNA-binding properties following fusion to E2A in t(17;19)-acute lymphoblastic leukemia. Genes Dev. 6:1608, 1992.

217. Inaba, T., Roberts, W.M., Shapiro, L.H., Jolly, K.W., Raimondi, S.C., Smith, S.D., and Look, A.T.: Fusion of the leucine zipper gene HLF to the E2A gene in human acute B-lineage leukemia. Science 257:531, 1992.

218. Yoshihara, T., Inaba, T., Shapiro, L.H., Kato, J.Y., and Look, A.T.: E2A-HLF-mediated cell transformation requires both the trans-activation domains of E2A and the leucine zipper dimerization domain of HLF. Mol. Cell. Biol. 15:3247, 1995.

219. Inaba, T., Inukai, T., Yoshihara, T., Seyschab, H., Ashmun, R.A., Canman, C.E., Laken, S.J., Kastan, M.B., and Look, A.T.: Reversal of apoptosis by the leukaemia-associated E2A-HLF chimaeric transcription factor. Nature 382:541, 1996.

220. Altura, R.A., Inukai, T., Ashmun, R.A., Zambetti, G.P., Roussel, M.F., and Look, A.T.: The chimeric E2A-HLF transcription factor abrogates p53-induced apoptosis in myeloid leukemia cells. Blood 92:1397, 1998.

221. Metzstein, M.M., Hengartner, M.O., Tsung, N., Ellis, R.E., and Horvitz, H.R.: Transcriptional regulator of programmed cell death encoded by Caenorhabditis elegans gene ces-2. Nature 382:545, 1996.

222. Gilmore, T.D.: Role of rel family genes in normal and malignant lymphoid cell growth. Cancer Surv. 15:69, 1992.

223. Neri, A., Chang, C-C., Lombardi, L., Salina, M., Corradini, P., Maiolo, A.T., Chaganti, R.S.K., and Dalla-Favera, R.: B cell lymphoma-associated chromosomal translocation involves candidate oncogene lyt-10, homologous to NF-kappaB p50. Cell 67:1075, 1991.

224. Ohio, H., Takimoto, G., and McKeithan, T.W.: The candidate proto-oncogene bcl-3 is related to genes implicated in cell lineage determination and cell cycle control. Cell 60:991, 1990.

225. Wulczyn, F.G., Naumann, M., and Scheiderelt, C.: Candidate proto-oncogene bcl-3 encodes a subunit-specific inhibitor of transcription factor NF-kappa B. Nature 358:597, 1992.

226. Kerr, L.D., Duckett, C.S., Wamsley, P., Zhang, Q., Chiao, P., Nabel, G., McKeithan, T.W., Baeuerle, P.A., and Verma, I.M.: The proto-oncogene bcl-3 encodes an I kappa B protein. Genes Dev. 6:2352, 1992.

227. Zhang, Q.D.J., Karin, M., and McKeithan, T.W.: BCL3 encodes a nuclear protein which can alter the subcellular location of NF-kappa B proteins. Mol. Cell. Biol. 14:3915, 1994.

228. Bours, V., Franzoso, G., Azarenko, V., Park, S., Kanno, T., Brown, K., and Siebenlist, U.: The oncoprotein Bcl-3 directly transactivates through kappa B motifs via association with DNA-binding p50B homodimers. Cell 72:729, 1993.

229. Fujita, T., Nolan, G.P., Liou, H.C., Scott, M.L., and Baltimore, D.: The candidate protooncogene bcl-3 encodes a transcriptional coactivator that activates through NF-kappa B p50 homodimers. Genes Dev. 7:1354, 1993.

230. Ong, S.T., Hackbarth, M.L., Degenstein, L.C., Baunoch, D.A., Anastasi, J., and McKeithan, T.W.: Lymphadenopathy, splenomegaly, and altered immunoglobulin production in BCL3 transgenic mice. Oncogene 16:2333, 1998.

231. Franzoso, G., Carlson, L., Scharton-Kersten, T., Shores, E.W., Epstein, S., Grinberg, A., Tran, T., Shacter, E., Leonardi, A., Anver, M., Love, P., Sher, A., and Siebenlist, U.: Critical roles for the Bcl-3 oncoprotein in T cell–mediated immunity, splenic microarchitecture, and germinal center reactions. Immunity 6:479, 1998.

232. Schwarz, E.M., Krimpenfort, P., Berns, A., and Verma, I.M.: Immunological defects in mice with a targeted disruption in Bcl-3. Genes Dev. 11:187, 1997.

233. Sherr, C.J.: Cancer cell cycles. Science 274:1672, 1996.

234. Tsujimoto, Y., Yunis, J., Onorato-Showe, L., Erikson, J., Nowell, P.C., and Croce, C.M.: Molecular cloning of the chromosomal breakpoint of B-cell lymphomas and leukemias with the t(11;14) chromosome translocation. Science 224:1403, 1984.

235. Erikson, J., Finan, J., Tsujimoto, Y., Nowell, P.C., and Croce, C.M.: The chromosome 14 breakpoint in neoplastic B cells with the t(11;14) translocation involves the immunoglobulin heavy chain locus. Proc. Natl. Acad. Sci. USA 81:4144, 1984.

236. Tsujimoto, Y., Jaffe, E., Cossman, J., Gorham, J., Nowell, P.C., and Croce, C.M.: Clustering of breakpoints on chromosome 11 in human B-cell neoplasms with the t(11;14) chromosome translocation. Nature 315:340, 1985.

237. Motokura, T., Bloom, T., Kim, H.G., Juppner, H., Ruderman, J.V., Kronenberg, H.M., and Arnold, A.: A novel cyclin encoded by a bcl-linked candidate oncogene. Nature 350:512, 1991.

238. Rosenberg, C.L., Wong, E., Petty, E.M., Bale, A.E., Tsujimoto, Y., Harris, N.L., and Arnold, A.: PRAD1, a candidate BCL1 oncogene: mapping and expression in centrocytic lymphoma. Proc. Natl. Acad. Sci. USA 88:9638, 1991.

239. Wang, T.C., Cardiff, R.D., Zukerberg, L., Lees, E., Arnold, A., and Schmidt, E.V.: Mammary hyperplasia and carcinoma in MMTV-cyclin D1 transgenic mice. Nature 369:669, 1994.

240. Okuda, T., Shurtleff, S.A., Valentine, M.B., Raimondi, S.C., Head, D.R., Behm, F., Curcio-Brint, A.M., Liu, Q., Pui, C.-H., Sherr, C.J., Beach, D.L., Thomas, A., and Downing, J.R.: Frequent deletion of p16^{INK4a}/MTS1 and p15^{INK4b}/MTS2 in pediatric acute lymphoblastic leukemia. Blood 85:2321, 1995.

241. Ogawa, S., Hangaishi, A., Miyawaki, S., Hirosawa, S., Miura, Y., Takeyama, K., Kamada, N., Ohtake, S., Uike, N., Shimazaki, C., Toyama, K., Hirano, M., Mizoguchi, H., Kobayashi, Y., Furusawa, S., Saito, M., Emi, N., Yazaki, Y., Ueda, R., and Hirai, H.: Loss of the cyclin-dependent kinase 4-inhibitor (p16; MTS1) gene is frequent in and highly specific to lymphoid tumors in primary human hematopoietic malignancies. Blood 86:1548, 1995.

242. Towatari, M., Adachi, K., Kato, H., and Saito, H.: Absence of the human retinoblastoma gene product in the megakaryoblastic crisis of chronic myelogenous leukemia. Blood 78:2178, 1991.

243. Eisenman, R.N., and Cooper, J.A.: Beating a path to MYC. Nature 378:438, 1995.

244. Laherty, C.D., Yang, W.M., Sun, J.M., Davie, J.R., Seto, E., and Eisenman, R.N.: Histone deacetylases associated with the mSin3 corepressor mediate mad transcriptional repression. Cell 89:349, 1997.

245. Ayer, D.E., Laherty, C.D., Lawrence, Q.A., Armstrong, A.P., and Eisenman, R.N.: Mad proteins contain a dominant transcription repression domain. Mol. Cell. Biol. 16:5772, 1996.

246. Eagle, L.R., Yin, X., Brothman, A.R., Williams, B.J., Atkin, N.B., and Prochownik, E.V.: Mutation of the MXI1 gene in prostate cancer. Nat. Genet. 9:249, 1995.

247. Schreiber-Agus, N., Meng, Y., Hoang, T., Hou, J., Chen, K., Greenberg, R., Cordon-Cardo, C., Lee, H.W., and DePinho, R.A.: Role of Mxi1 in ageing organ systems and the regulation of normal and neoplastic growth. Nature 393:483, 1998.

248. Srivastava, S., Zou, Z.Q., Pirollo, K., Blattner, W., and Chang, E.H.: Germ-line transmission of a mutated p53 gene in a cancer-prone family with Li-Fraumeni syndrome. Nature 348:747, 1990.

249. Li, F.P.: Cancer families: human models of susceptibility to neoplasia—the Richard and Hinda Rosenthal Foundation Award lecture. Cancer Res. 48:5381, 1988.

250. Ahuja, H., Bar-Eli, M., Arlin, Z., Advani, S., Allen, S.L., Goldman, J., Snyder, D., Foti, A., and Cline, M.: The spectrum of molecular alterations in the evolution of chronic myelocytic leukemia. J. Clin. Invest. 87:2042, 1991.

251. Saxon, A., Stevens, R.H., and Golde, D.W.: T-cell leukemia in ataxia telangiectasia. N. Engl. J. Med. 301:945, 1979.

252. Kamijo, T., Weber, J.D., Zambetti, G., Zindy, F., Roussel, M.F., and Sherr, C.J.: Functional and physical interactions of the ARF tumor suppressor with p53 and Mdm2. Proc. Natl. Acad. Sci. USA 95:8292, 1998.

253. Zhang, Y., Xiong, Y., and Yarbrough, W.G.: ARF promotes MDM2 degradation and stabilizes p53: ARF-INK4a locus deletion impairs both the Rb and p53 tumor suppression pathways. Cell 92:725, 1998.

254. Pomerantz, J., Schreiber-Agus, N., Liegeois, N.J., Silverman, A., Alland, L., Chin, L., Potes, J., Chen, K., Orlow, I., Lee, H.W., Cordon-Cardo, C., and DePinho, R.A.: The Ink4a tumor suppressor gene

product, p19Arf, interacts with MDM2 and neutralizes MDM2's inhibition of p53. Cell 92:713, 1998.

255. Quelle, D.E., Zindy, F., Ashmun, R.A., and Sherr, C.A.: Alternative reading frames of the INK4a tumor suppressor gene encode two unrelated proteins capable of inducing cell cycle arrest. Cell 83:993, 1995.

256. Kamijo, T., Zindy, F., Roussel, M.F., Quelle, D.E., Downing, J.R., Ashmun, R.A., Grosveld, G., and Sherr, C.J.: Tumor suppression at the mouse INK4a locus mediated by the alternative reading frame product p19ARF. Cell 91:649, 1997.

257. Papadopoulos, P., Ridge, S.A., Boucher, C.A., and Stocking, C.: The novel activation of *ABL* by fusion to an *ets*-related gene, *TEL*[1]. Cancer Res. 55:34, 1995.

258. von Lindern, M., Breems, D., van Baal, S., Adriaansen, H., and Grosveld, G.: Characterization of the translocation breakpoint sequences of two DEK-CAN fusion genes present in t(6;9) acute myeloid leukemia and a SET-CAN fusion gene found in a case of acute undifferentiated leukemia. Genes Chromosomes Cancer 5:227, 1992.

259. Bartram, C.R., de Klein, A., Hagemeijer, A., van Agthoven, T., van Kessel, A.G., Bootsma, D., Grosveld, G., Ferguson-Smith, M.A., Davies, T., Stone, M., Heisterkamp, N., Stephenson, J.R., and Groffen, J.: Translocation of c-abl oncogene correlates with the presence of a Philadelphia chromosome in chronic myelocytic leukaemia. Nature 306:277, 1983.

260. Heisterkamp, N., Stephenson, J.R., Groffen, J., Hansen, P.F., de Klein, A., Bartram, C.R., and Grosveld, G.: Localization of the c-abl oncogene adjacent to a translocation break point in chronic myelocytic leukaemia. Nature 306:239, 1983.

261. Groffen, J., Stephenson, J.R., Heisterkamp, N., de Klein, A., Bartram, C.R., and Grosveld, G.: Philadelphia chromosomal breakpoints are clustered within a limited region, bcr, on chromosome 22. Cell 36:93, 1984.

262. Heisterkamp, N., Stam, K., Groffen, J., de Klein, A., and Grosveld, G.: Structural organization of the bcr gene and its role in the Ph[1] translocation. Nature 315:758, 1985.

263. Chan, L.C., Karhi, K.K., Rayter, S.I., Heisterkamp, N., Eridani, S., Powles, R., Lawler, S.D., Groffen, J., Foulkes, J.G., Greaves, M.F., and Wiedemann, L.M.: A novel abl protein expressed in Philadelphia chromosome positive acute lymphoblastic leukaemia. Nature 325:635, 1987.

264. Kurzrock, R., Shtalrid, M., Romero, P., Kloetzer, W.S., Talpas, M., Trujillo, J.M., Blick, M., Beran, M., and Gutterman, J.U.: A novel c-abl protein product in Philadelphia-positive acute lymphoblastic leukaemia. Nature 325:631, 1987.

265. Burnett, R.C., David, J.C., Harden, A.M., Le Beau, M.M., Rowley, J.D., and Diaz, M.O.: The LCK gene is involved in the t(1;7)(p34;q34) in the T-cell acute lymphoblastic leukemia derived cell line, HSB-2. Genes Chromosomes Cancer 3:461, 1991.

266. Wright, D.D., Sefton, B.M., and Kamps, M.P.: Oncogenic activation of the Lck protein accompanies translocation of the LCK gene in the human HSB2 T-cell leukemia. Mol. Cell. Biol. 14:2429, 1994.

267. Adams, J.M., Gerondakis, S., Webb, E., Corcoran, L.M., and Cory, S.: Cellular myc oncogene is altered by chromosomal translocation to an immunoglobulin locus in murine plasmacytomas and is rearranged similarly in human Burkitt lymphomas. Proc. Natl. Acad. Sci. USA 80:1982, 1983.

268. Emanuel, B.S., Selden, J.R., Chaganti, R.S., Jhanwar, S., Nowell, P.C., and Croce, C.M.: The 2p breakpoint of a 2;8 translocation in Burkitt lymphoma interrupts the V kappa locus. Proc. Natl. Acad. Sci. USA 81:2444, 1984.

269. Erikson, J., Nishikura, K., ar-Rushdi, A., Finan, J., Emanuel, B., Lenoir, G., Nowell, P.C., and Croce, C.M.: Translocation of an immunoglobulin kappa locus to a region 3' of an unrearranged c-myc oncogene enhances c-myc transcription. Proc. Natl. Acad. Sci. USA 80:7581, 1984.

270. Rappold, G.A., Hameister, H., Cremer, T., Adolph, S., Henglein, B., Freese, U.K., Lenoire, G.M., and Bornkamm, G.W.: C-myc and immunoglobulin kappa light chain constant genes are on the 8q+ chromosome of three Burkitt lymphoma lines with t(2;8) translocations. EMBO J. 3:2951, 1984.

271. Taub, R., Kelly, K., Battey, J., Latt, S., Lenoir, G.M., Tantravahi, U., Tu, Z., and Leder, P.: A novel alteration in the structure of an activated c-myc gene in a variant t(2;8) Burkitt lymphoma. Cell 37:511, 1984.

272. Hollis, G.F., Mitchell, K.F., Battey, J., Potter, H., Taub, R., Lenoir, G.M., and Leder, P.: A variant translocation places the lambda immu-

noglobulin genes 3' to the c-myc oncogene in Burkitt's lymphoma. Nature 307:752, 1984.

273. Croce, C.M., Thierfelder, W., Erikson, J., Nishikura, K., Finan, J., Lenoir, G.M., and Nowell, P.C.: Transcriptional activation of an unrearranged and untranslocated c-myc oncogene by translocation of a C lambda locus in Burkitt. Proc. Natl. Acad. Sci. USA 80:6922, 1983.

274. Romana, S.P., Mauchauffe, M., Le Coniat, M., Chumakov, I., Le Paslier, D., Berger, R., and Bernard, Q.A.: The t(12;21) of acute lymphoblastic leukemia results in a tel-AML1 gene fusion. Blood 85:3662, 1995.

275. Romana, S.P., Poirel, H., Leconiat, M., Flexor, M.A., Mauchauffe, M., Jonveaux, P., Macintyre, E.A., Berger, R., and Bernard, O.A.: High frequency of t(12;21) in childhood B-lineage acute lymphoblastic leukemia. Blood 86:4263, 1995.

276. Liang, D.C., Chou, T.B., Chen, J.S., Shurtleff, S.A., Rubnitz, J.E., Downing, J.R., Pui, C.H., and Shih L.Y.: High incidence of TEL/AML1 fusion resulting from a cryptic t(12;21) in childhood B-lineage acute lymphoblastic leukemia in Taiwan. Leukemia 10:991, 1996.

277. Finger, L.R., Harvey, R.C., Moore, R.C., Showe, L.C., and Croce, C.M.: A common mechanism of chromosomal translocation in T- and B-cell neoplasia. Science 234:982, 1986.

278. McKeithan, T.W., Shima, E.A., Le Beau, M.M., Minowada, J., Rowley, J.D., and Diaz, M.O.: Molecular cloning of the breakpoint junction of a human chromosomal 8;14 translocation involving the T-cell receptor alpha-chain gene and sequences on the 3' side of MYC. Proc. Natl. Acad. Sci. USA 83:6636, 1986.

279. Shima, E.A., Le Beau, M.M., McKeithan, T.W., Minowada, J., Showe, L.C., Mak, T.W., Minden, M.D., Rowley, J.D., and Diaz, M.O.: Gene encoding the alpha chain of the T-cell receptor is moved immediately downstream of c-myc in a chromosomal 8;14 translocation in a cell line from a human T-cell leukemia. Proc. Natl. Acad. Sci. USA 83:3439, 1986.

280. Mellentin, J.D., Smith, S.D., and Cleary, M.L.: Lyl-l, a novel gene altered by chromosomal translocation in T cell leukemia, codes for a protein with a helix-loop-helix DNA binding motif. Cell 58:77, 1989.

281. Begley, C.G., Aplan, P.D., Davey, M.P., Nakahara, K., Tchorz, K., Kurtzberg, J., Hershfield, M.S., Haynes, B.F., Cohen, D.I., Waldmann, T.A., and Kirsch, I.R.: Chromosomal translocation in a human leukemic stem-cell line disrupts the T-cell antigen receptor delta-chain diversity region and results in a previously unreported fusion transcript. Proc. Natl. Acad. Sci. USA 86:2031, 1989.

282. Chen, Q., Cheng, J.-T., Tsai, L.-H., Schneider, N., Buchanan, G., Carroll, A., Crist, W., Ozanne, B., Siciliano, M.J., and Baer, R.: The tal gene undergoes chromosome translocation in T cell leukemia and potentially encodes a helix-loop-helix protein. EMBO J. 9:415, 1990.

283. Xia, Y., Brown, L., Tsan, J., Siciliano, M.J., Espinosa, R., III, Le Beau, M.M., and Baer, R.J.: TAL2, a helix-loop-helix gene activated by the (7;9)(q34;32) translocation in human T-cell leukemia. Proc. Natl. Acad. Sci. USA 88:11416, 1991.

284. McGuire, E.A., Hockett, R.D., Pollock, K.M., Bartholdi, M.F., O'Brien, S.J., and Korsmeyer, S.J.: The t(11;14)(p15;q11) in a T-cell acute lymphoblastic leukemia cell line activates multiple transcripts, including Ttg-1, a gene encoding a potential zinc finger protein. Mol. Cell. Biol. 9:2124, 1989.

285. Greenberg, J.M., Boehm, T., Sofroniew, M.V., Keynes, R.J., Barton, S.C., Norris, M.L., Surani, M.A., Spillantini, M.-G., and Rabbitts, T.H.: Segmental and developmental regulation of a presumptive T-cell oncogene in the central nervous system. Nature 344:158, 1990.

286. Boehm, T., Foroni, L., Kaneko, Y., Perutz, M.F., and Rabbitts, T.H.: The rhombotin family of cysteine-rich *LIM*-domain oncogenes: distinct members are involved in T-cell translocations to human chromosomes 11p15 and 11p13. Proc. Natl. Acad. Sci. USA 88:4367, 1991.

287. Royer-Pokora, B., Loos, U., and Ludwig, W.D.: TTG-2, a new gene encoding a cysteine-rich protein with the *LIM* motif, is overexpressed in acute T-cell leukaemia with the t(11;14)(p13;q11). Oncogene 6:1887, 1991.

288. Kennedy, M.A., Gonzalez-Sarmiento, R., Kees, U.R., Lampert, F, Dear, N., Boehm T., and Rabbitts, T.H.: *HOX11*, a homeobox-containing T-cell oncogne on human chromosome 10q24. Proc. Natl. Acad. Sci. USA 88:8900, 1991.

289. Lu, M., Gong, Z., Shen, W., and Ho, A.D.: The tcl-3 proto-oncogene altered by chromosomal translocation in T-cell leukemia codes for a homeobox protein, EMBO J. 10:2905, 1991.

290. Dube, I.D., Kamel-Reid, S., Yuan, C.C., Lu, M., Wu, X., Corpus, G., Raimondi, S.C., Crist, W.M., Carroll, A.J., Minowada, J., and Baker,

J.B.: A novel human homeobox gene lies at the chromosome 10 breakpoint in lymphoid neoplasias with chromosomal translocation t(10;14). Blood 78:2996, 1991.

291. Ye, B.H., Rao, P.H., Chaganti, R.S., and Dalla-Favera, R.: Cloning of bcl-6, the locus involved in chromosome translocations affecting band 3q27 in B-cell lymphoma. Cancer Res. 53:2732, 1993.

292. Kerckaert, J.P., Deweindt, C., Tilly, H., Quief, S., Lecocq, G., and Bastard, C.: LAZ3, a novel zinc-finger encoding gene, is disrupted by recurring chromosome 3q27 translocations in human lymphomas. Nat. Genet. 5:66, 1993.

293. Miki, T., Kawamata, N., Hirosawa, S., and Aoki, N.: Gene involved in the 3q27 translocation associated with B-cell lymphoma, BCL5, encodes a Kruppel-like zinc-finger protein. Blood 83:26, 1994.

294. Ye, B.H., Lista, F., Coco, F.L., Knowles, D.M., Offit, K., Chaganti, R.S. K., and Dalla-Favera, R.: Alternations of a zinc finger-encoding gene, BCL-6, in diffuse large-cell lymphoma. Science 262:747, 1993.

295. Dallery, E., Galiegue-Zouitina, S., Collyn-d'Hooghe, M., Quief, S., Denis, C., Hildebrand, M.P., Lantoine, D., Deweindt, C., Tilly, H., Bastard, C., and Kerckaert, J.-P.: TTF, a gene encoding a novel small G protein, fuses to the lymphoma-associated LAZ3 gene by t(3;4) chromosomal translocation. Oncogene 10:2171, 1995.

296. Iida, S., Rao, P.H., Nallasivam, P., Hibshoosh, H., Butler, M., Louie, D.C., Dyomin, V., Ohno, H., Chaganti, R.S., and Dalla-Favera, R.: The t(9;14)(p13;q32) chromosomal translocation association with lymphoplasmacytoid lymphoma involves the PAX-5 gene. Blood 88:4110, 1996.

297. Gao, J., Erickson, P., Gardiner, K., Le Beau, M.M., Diaz, M.O., Patterson, D., Rowley, J.D., and Drabkin, H.A.: Isolation of a yeast artificial chromosome spanning the 8;21 translocation breakpoint t(8;21)(q22;q22.3) in acute myelogeneous leukemia. Proc. Natl. Acad. Sci. USA 88:4882, 1991.

298. Shimizu, K., Miyoshi, H., Kozu, T., Nagata, J., Enomoto, K., Maseki, N., Kaneko, Y., and Ohki, M.: Consistent disruption of the AML1 gene occurs within a single intron in the t(8;21) chromosomal translocation. Cancer Res. 52:6945, 1992.

299. Morishita, K., Parganas, E., Bartholomew, C., Sacchi, N., Valentine, M.B., Raimondi, S.C., Le Beau, M.M., and Ihle, J.N.: The human Evi-1 gene is located on chromosome 3q24-q28 but is not rearranged in three cases of acute nonlymphocytic leukemias containing t(3;5)(q25;q34) translocations. Oncol. Res. 5:221, 1990.

300. Morishita, K., Parganas, E., Willman, C.L., Whittaker, M.H., Drabkin, H., Oval, J., Taetle R., Valentine, M.B., and Ihle, J.N.: Activation of *EVI1* gene expression in human acute myelogenous leukemias by translocations spanning 300-400 kilobases on chromosome band 3q26. Proc. Natl. Acad. Sci. USA 89:3937, 1992.

301. de The, H., Lavau, C., Marchio, A., Chomienne, C., Degos, L., and Dejean, A.: The PML-RARα fusion mRNA generated by the t(15;17) translocation in acute promyelocytic leukemia encodes a functionally altered RAR. Cell 66:675, 1991.

302. Kakizuka, A., Miller, W.H.J., Umesono, K., Warrell, R.P.J., Frankel, S.R., Murty, V.V.V.S., Dmitrovsky, E., and Evans, R.M.: Chromosomal translocation t(15;17) in human acute promyelocytic leukemia fuses RARα with a novel putative transcription factor, PML. Cell 66:663, 1991.

303. Chen, Z., Brand, N.J., Chen, A., Chen, S.-J., Tong, J.-H., Wang, Z.-Y., Waxman, S., and Zelent, A.: Fusion between a novel Kruppel-like zinc finger gene and the retinoic acid receptor-α locus due to a variant t(11;17) translocation associated with acute promyelocytic leukaemia. EMBO J. 12:1161, 1993.

304. Redner, R.L., Rush, E.A., Faas, S., Rudert, W.A., and Corey, S.J.: The t(5;17) variant of acute promyelocytic leukemia expresses a nucleophosmin-retinoic acid receptor fusion. Blood 87:882, 1996.

305. Ichikawa, H., Shimizu, K., Hayashi, Y., and Ohki, M.: An RNA-binding protein gene, TLS/FUS, is fused to ERG in human myeloid leukemia with t(16;21) chromosomal translocation. Cancer Res. 54:2865, 1994.

306. Buijs, A., Sherr, S., van Baal, S., van Bezouw, S., van der Plas, D., Geurts van Kessel, A., Riegman, P., Lekanne, D.R., Zwarthoff, E., Hagemeijer, A., and Grosveld, G.: Translocation (12;22)(p13;q11) in myeloproliferative disorders results in fusion of the ETS-like TEL gene on 12p13 to the MN1 gene on 22q11. Oncogene 11:809, 1995.

307. Gamou, T., Kitamura, E., Hosoda, F., Shimizu, K., Shinohara, K., Hayashi, Y., Nagase, T., Yokoyama, Y., and Ohki, M.: The partner gene of AML1 in t(16;21) myeloid malignancies is a novel member of the MTG8(ETO) family. Blood 91:4028, 1998.

308. Carapeti, M., Aguiar, R.C.T., Goldman, J.M., and Cross, N.C.P.: A novel fusion between MOZ and the nuclear receptor coactivator TIF2 in acute myeloid leukemia. Blood 91:3127, 1998.

309. Liang, J., Prouty, L., Williams, B.J., Dayton, M.A., and Blanchard, K.L.: Acute mixed lineage leukemia with an inv(8)(p11q13) resulting in fusion of the genes for MOZ and TIF2. Blood 92:2118, 1998.

310. Borrow, J., Stanton, V.P.J., Andresen, J.M., Becher, R., Behm, F.G., Chaganti, R.S. K., Civin, C.I., Disteche, C., Dube, I., Frischauf, A.M., Horsman, D., Mitelman, F., Volinia, S., Watmore, A.E., and Housman, D.E.: The translocation t(8;16)(p11;p13) of acute myeloid leukaemia fuses a putative acetyltransferase to the CREB-binding protein. Nat. Genet. 14:33, 1996.

311. Taki, T., Sako, M., Tsuchida, M., and Hayashi, Y.: The t(11;16)(q23;p13) translocation in myelodysplastic syndrome fuses the MLL gene to the CBP gene. Blood 89:3945, 1997.

312. Sobulo, O.M., Borrow, J., Tomek, R., Reshmi, S., Harden, A., Schleg-elberger, B., Housman, D., Doggett, N.A., Rowley, J.D., and Zeleznik-Le, N.J.: MLL is fused to CBP, a histone acetyltransferase, in therapy-related acute myeloid leukemia with a t(11;16)(q23;p13.3). Proc. Natl. Acad. Sci. USA 94:8732, 1997.

313. Raza-Egilmez, S.Z., Jani-Sait, S.N., Grossi, M., Higgins, M.J., Shows, T.B., and Aplan, P.D.: NUP98-HOXD13 gene fusion in therapy-related acute myelogenous leukemia. Cancer Res. 58:4269, 1998.

314. Nakamura, T., Largaespada, D.A., Lee, M.P., Johnson, L.A., Ohya-shiki, K., Toyama, K., Chen, S.J., Willman, C.L., Chen, I.M., Fein-berg, A.P., Jenkins, N.A., Copeland, N.G., and Shaughnessy, J.D., Jr.: Fusion of the nucleoporin gene NUP98 to HOXA9 by the chromosome translocation t(7;11)(p15;p15) in human myeloid leukaemia. Nat. Genet. 12:154, 1996.

315. Borrow, J., Shearman, A.M., Stanton, V.P.J., Becher, R., Collins, T., Williams, A.J., Dube, I., Katz, F., Kwong, Y.L., Morris, C., Ohyashiki, K., Toyama, K., Rowley, J., and Housman, D.E.: The t(7;11)(p15;p15) translocation in acute myeloid leukaemia fuses the genes for nucleo-porin NUP98 and class I homeoprotein HOXA9. Nat. Genet. 12:159, 1996.

316. Arai, Y., Hosoda, F., Kobayashi, H., Arai, K., Hayashi, Y., Kamada, N., Kaneko, Y., and Ohki, M.: The inv(11)(p15q22) translocation of de novo and therapy related myeloid malignancies results in fusion of the nucleoporin gene, *NUP98*, with the putative RNA helicase gene, *DDX10*. Blood 89:3936, 1997.

317. Morrissey, J., Tkachuk, D.C., Milatovich, A., Francke, U., Link, M., and Cleary, M.L.: A serine/proline-rich protein is fused to HRX in t(4;11) acute leukemias. Blood 81:1124, 1993.

318. Nakamura, T., Alder, H., Gu, Y., Prasad, R., Canaani, O., Kamada, N., Gale, R.P., Lange, B., Crist, W.M., Nowell, P.C., Croce, C.M., and Canaani, E.: Genes on chromosomes 4, 9, and 19 involved in 11q23 abnormalities in acute leukemia share sequence homology and/or common motifs. Proc. Natl. Acad. Sci. USA 90:4631, 1993.

319. Thirman, M.J., Levitan, D.A., Kobayashi, H., Simon, M.C., and Row-ley, J.D.: Cloning of ELL, a gene that fuses to MLL in a t(11;19)(q23;p13.1) in acute myeloid leukemia. Proc. Natl. Acad. Sci. USA 91:12110, 1994.

320. Mitani, K., Kanda, Y., Ogawa, S., Tanaka, T., Inazawa, J., Yazaki, Y., and Hirai, H.: Cloning of several species of MLL/MEN chimeric cDNAs in myeloid leukemia with t(11;19)(q23;p13.1) translocation. Blood 85:2017, 1995.

321. Tse, W., Zhu, W., Chen, H.S., and Cohen, A.: A novel gene, A F1q, fused to MLL in t(1;11) (q21;q23), is specifically expressed in leuke-mic and immature hematopoietic cells. Blood 85:650, 1995.

322. Bernard, O.A., Mauchauffe, M., Mecucci, C., Van den Berghe, H., and Berger, R.: A novel gene, AF-1p, fused to HRX in t(1;11)(p32;q23), is not related to AF-4, AF-9 nor ENL. Oncogene 9:1039, 1994.

323. Prasad, R., Gu, Y., Alder, H., Nakamura, T., Canaani, O., Saito, H., Huebner, K., Gale, R.P., Nowell, P.C., Kuriyama, K., Miyazaki, Y., and Croce, C.M.: Cloning of the ALL-1 fusion partner, the AF-6 gene, involved in acute myeloid leukemias with the t(6;11) chromosome translocation. Cancer Res. 53:5624, 1993.

324. Chaplin, T., Ayton, P., Bernard, O.A., Saha, V., Della Valle, V., Hillion, J., Gregorini, A., Lillington, D., Berger, R., and Young, B.D.: A novel class of zinc finger/leucine zipper genes identified from the molecular cloning of the t(10;11) translocation in acute leukemia. Blood 85:1435, 1995.

325. Prasad, R., Leshkowitz, D., Gu, Y., Alder, H., Nakamura, T., Saito, H., Huebner, K., Berger, R., Croce, C.M., and Canaani, E.: Leucine-zipper dimerization motif encoded by the AF17 gene fused to ALL-1 (MLL) in acute leukemia. Proc. Natl. Acad. Sci. USA 91:8107, 1994.

326. Parry, P., Wei, Y., and Evans, G.: Cloning and characterization of the t(X;11) breakpoint from a leukemic cell line identify a new member of the forkhead gene family. Genes Chromosomes Cancer 11:79, 1994.

327. Borkhardt, A., Repp, R., Haas, O.A., Leis, T., Harbott, J., Kreuder, J., Hammermann, J., Henn, T., and Lampert, F.: Cloning and characterization of AFX, the gene that fuses to MLL in acute leukemias with a t(X;11)(q13;q23). Oncogene 14:195, 1997.

328. Taki, T., Shibuya, N., Taniwaki, M., Hanada, R., Morishita, K., Bessho, F., Yanagisawa, M., and Hayashi, Y.: Abi-1, a human homolog to mouse abl-interactor 1, fuses the MLL gene in acute myeloid leukemia with t(10;11)(p11.2;q23). Blood 92:1125, 1998.

329. Megonigal, M.D., Rappaport, E.F., Jones, D.H., Williams, T.M., Lovett, B.D., Kelly, K.M., Lerou, P.H., Moulton, T., Budarf, M.L., and Felix, C.A.: t(11;22)(q23;q11.2) In acute myeloid leukemia of infant twins fuses MLL with hCDCrel, a cell division cycle gene in the genomic region of deletion in DiGeorge and velocardiofacial syndromes. Proc. Natl. Acad. Sci. USA 95:6413, 1998.

330. Lammie, G.A., Fantl, V., Smith, R., Schuuring, E., Brookes, S., Michalides, R., Dickson, C., Arnold, A., and Peters, G.: D11S287, a putative oncogene on chromosome 11q13, is amplified and expressed in squamous cell and mammary carcinomas and linked to BCL-1. Oncogene 6:439, 1991.

331. Withers, D.A., Harvey, R.C., Faust, J.B., Melnyk, O., Carey, K., and Meeker, T.C.: Characterization of a candidate bcl-1 gene. Mol. Cell. Biol. 11:4846, 1991.

332. Brookes, S., Lammie, G.A., Schuuring, E., Dickson, C., and Peters, G.: Linkage map of a region of human chromosome band 11q13 amplified in breast and squamous cell tumors. Genes Chromosomes Cancer 4:290, 1992.

333. Tsujimoto, Y., Gorham, J., Cossman, J., Jaffe, E., and Croce, C.M.: The t(14;18) chromosome translocations involved in B-cell neoplasms result from mistakes in VDJ joining. Science 229:1390, 1985.

334. Bakhshi, A., Jensen, J.P., Goldman, P., Wright, J.J., McBride, O.W., Epstein, A.L., and Korsmeyer, S.J.: Cloning the chromosomal breakpoint to t(14;18) human lymphomas: clustering around JH on chromosome 14 and near a transcriptional unit on 18. Cell 41:899, 1985.

335. Cleary, M.L., and Sklar J.: Nucleotide sequence of a t(14;18) chromosomal breakpoint in follicular lymphoma and demonstration of a breakpoint cluster region near a transcriptionally active locus on chromosome 18. Proc. Natl. Acad. Sci. USA 82:7439, 1985.

336. von Lindern, M., Fornerod, M., van Baal, S., Jaegle, M., de Wit, T., Buijs, A., and Gresveld, G.: The translocation (6;9), associated with a specific subtype of acute myeloid leukemia, results in the fusion of two genes, dek and can, and the expression of a chimeric, leukemia-specific dek can mRNA. Mol. Cell. Biol. 12:1687, 1992.

337. Yoneda-Kato, N., Look, A.T., Kirstein, M.N., Valentine, M.B., Raimondi, S.C., Cohen, K.J., Carroll, A.J., and Morris, S.W.: The t(3;5)(q25.1;q34) of myelodysplastic syndrome and acute myeloid leukemia produces a novel fusion gene, NPM-MLF1. Oncogene 12:265, 1996.

338. Dreyline, M.H., Martinez-Climent, J.A., Zheng, M., Mao, J., Rowley, J.D., and Bohlander, S.K.: The t(10;11)(p13;q14) in the U937 cell line results in the fusion of the AF10 gene and CALM, encoding a new member of the AP-3 clathrin assembly protein family. Proc. Natl. Acad. Sci. USA 93:4804, 1996.

339. Fisch, P., Forster, A., Sherrington, P.D., Dyer, M.J., and Rabbitts, T.H.: The chromosomal translocation t(X;14)(q28;q11) in T-cell prolymphocytic leukaemia breaks within one gene and activates another. Oncogene 8:3271, 1993.

340. Grimaldi, J.C., and Meeker, T.C.: The t(5;14) chromosomal translocation in a case of acute lymphocytic leukemia joins the interleukin-3 gene to the immunoglobulin heavy chain gene. Blood 73:2081, 1989.

341. Laabi, Y., Gras, M.P., Carbonnel, F., Brouet, J.C., Berger, R., Larsen, C.J., and Tsapis, A.: A new gene, BCM, on chromosome 16 is fused to the interleukin 2 gene by a t(4;16)(q26;p13) translocation in a malignant T cell lymphoma. EMBO J. 11:3897, 1992.

Part VII
VIRUSES

27 The Molecular and Biological Properties of the Human Immunodeficiency Virus

Eric O. Freed and Malcolm A. Martin

Introduction

During the late 1970s and early 1980s, physicians in several large American cities began to encounter previously healthy male patients who presented with symptoms of immunological dysfunction. This new and unusual syndrome was characterized by generalized lymphadenopathy, opportunistic infections (most typically *Pneumocystis carinii* pneumonia, mucosal candidiasis, and disseminated cytomegalovirus infections), and Kaposi's sarcoma. In June 1981, the disease was first brought to the attention of the general medical community when the Centers for Disease Control described five Los Angeles area men with severely impaired immune systems in the *Morbidity and Mortality Weekly Report*.[1] This notification was followed by several reports[2-4] of immunocompromised homosexual men or intravenous drug users with T lymphocytes that responded poorly to antigen and mitogen stimulation in functional assays. Within several months it became clear that an immunodeficiency disease was also affecting other groups, including hemophiliacs, transfusion recipients, recent Haitian immigrants, and sexual partners and/or children of members of the various risk groups.

The epidemiological pattern that emerged suggested that the new disease was acquired from contaminated blood or after sexual intercourse with an affected individual. Between late 1981 and early 1983, numerous microorganisms were proposed as the etiological agent responsible for the acquired immunodeficiency syndrome (AIDS), as the disease was soon called. A strong case was made for members of the herpesvirus family, particularly cytomegaloviruses (CMVs), which were known to replicate efficiently in human lymphocytes and were frequently present in clinical specimens collected from AIDS patients.[4, 5] Others favored a retroviral cause because of the presence of antibodies thought to be specific for human T-cell leukemia virus type 1 (HTLV-1) in some AIDS patients.[6-10] In 1983, scientists at the Pasteur Institute isolated an agent from the lymph nodes of an asymptomatic individual who had generalized lymphadenopathy of unknown origin.[11] During its growth in vitro, the lymphadenopathy-associated virus (LAV) generated progeny virions that were shown to contain reverse transcriptase activity and exhibited electron microscopic features typical of retroviruses. Unlike previously described and intensively studied retroviruses of diverse vertebrate origin, LAV was highly cytopathic during its replication in human peripheral blood lymphocytes, specifically killing the CD4-positive lymphocytes in the culture.[12] Other groups isolated similar T-cell cytopathic viruses from peripheral blood lymphocytes of AIDS patients in 1984[13-15] and obtained convincing serological evidence that linked exposure to LAV-like retroviruses and immunodeficient individuals from the various groups at risk.[16-18] The new retrovirus, associated with AIDS in the United States, Europe, and Central Africa, was named human immunodeficiency virus (HIV)[19] (and subsequently HIV-1). In 1986, a related, but immunologically distinct human retrovirus (now called HIV-2), recovered from individuals residing in West Africa, was also shown to cause AIDS.[20, 21]

The Classification, Genomic Organization, and Proteins Encoded by Human Immunodeficiency Virus

Progress in unraveling the structure and function of the numerous HIV genes has been nothing less than phenomenal. It was facilitated by the early identification of (1) human

T leukemia cell lines that would produce high titers of progeny virus while undergoing a highly cytopathic infection frequently associated with the formation of "ballooning" syncytia (Fig. 27–1A) or (2) infectable continuous CD4-positive human cell lines that chronically released virus without exhibiting evidence of cell killing.[15, 22–24] In these early studies, electron microscopic analyses of the released HIV-1 revealed the presence of 100 to 120 nm particles containing a bullet-shaped cylindrical core, a virion morphologic characteristic reminiscent of that previously described for visna virus (Fig. 27–1B).[12, 25–28] The efficient production of virus particles permitted the isolation of HIV genomic RNA, which was used to generate the complementary DNA (cDNA) probes needed for the cloning of viral DNA from productively infected cells. Molecular clones of proviral DNA were quickly obtained, and subsequent analyses indicated that HIV-1 possessed a genomic organization that not only was related to that of other replication-competent retroviruses but placed it, taxonomically, in the lentivirus genus.[29–36] However, in contrast to previously sequenced prototypical retroviruses such as avian leukosis and Moloney murine leukemia viruses, which contained only three genes encoding their structural proteins (group-specific antigen [*gag*], polymerase [*pol*], and envelope [*env*],[37, 38] the HIV genome included several additional and overlapping open reading frames of unknown function (Fig. 27–2).[33, 34, 36, 39]

Retroviruses are members of a larger group of related eukaryotic retrotransposable elements[40–43] that have the capacity to generate DNA copies of their RNA genomes by using the viral encoded enzyme reverse transcriptase. When portions of their *pol* and *gag* genes are analyzed, five major retroviral genera become evident: (1) "foamy" viruses or spumaviruses; (2) mammalian C-type oncoviruses; (3) bovine leukemia virus (BLV)/HTLV leukemia viruses; (4) a heterogeneous group including Rous sarcoma/avian leukosis and the A-, B-, and D-type viruses; and (5) lentiviruses, including HIV-1 and HIV-2 and closely related simian viruses[30] (Fig. 27–3A). As their name suggests, lentiviruses were known to cause slow, unremitting disease in sheep, horses, and cattle, affecting various lineages of hematopoietic cells, particularly lymphocytes and differentiated macrophages. Sequence information from geographically diverse HIV-1 isolates permitted a more precise assessment of their evolution and phylogenetic relationship to other lentiviruses (Fig. 27–3B).

The structures of retroviral genomes are known to differ from one another with respect to whether translational access to the *pol* gene occurs through ribosomal frameshifting[44] or suppression of a termination codon (e.g., murine leukemia virus [MuLV])[45] and whether the virus-encoded protease occupies a reading frame separate from *gag* and *pol* (e.g., see HTLV-1 in Fig. 27–2).[46–48] Although an extra open reading frame, now known to encode a superantigen, was identified within the 3' long terminal repeat (LTR) of mouse mammary tumor virus proviral DNA,[49–51] the existence of additional, functionally important retroviral genes was generally unappreciated until the discovery and genomic analysis of HTLV-1.[47] The sequencing of HTLV-I proviral DNA revealed the presence of three short overlapping open reading frames, located between the *env* gene and the 3' LTR, one of which encoded a transactivator of transcription, the Tax protein[52–54] (see Fig. 27–2). Despite the similarity of their

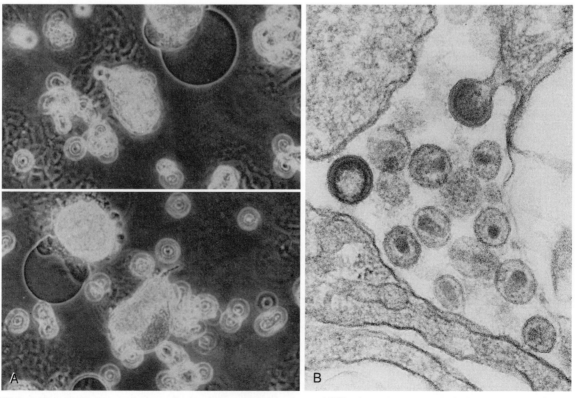

Figure 27–1. *A,* Typical ballooning syncytia visualized in CEM cells, 8 days after an HIV-1 infection at an input multiplicity of approximately 1 × 10⁻³. (The photomicrograph was kindly provided by Dr. Thomas Folks.) *B,* Electron micrograph depicting particles in the process of budding, with an uncondensed core, and several with bullet-shaped nucleoid cores (108,000×). (This photomicrograph was kindly provided by Dr. Jan Orenstein.)

RETROVIRAL GENOMIC ORGANIZATION

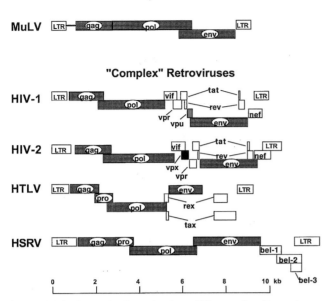

Figure 27–2. Genomic Organization of Mammalian Retroviruses. The genes of Moloney murine leukemia virus (MuLV), human T-cell leukemia virus (HTLV), human spumavirus (HSRV), and human immunodeficiency virus type I (HIV-1) and type 2 (HIV-2), derived from nucleotide sequences of molecular clones,[36, 37, 47, 59, 790, 791] are depicted as they are arranged in their respective proviral DNAs. The position of the protease *(pro)* open reading frame is shown when it differs from that of the *pol* gene. The sizes of the different proviral DNAs are shown in proportion to the 9.7 kb HIV provirus.

genomic organizations, the two human immunodeficiency viruses can be readily distinguished from one another on the basis of a single unique open reading frame: HIV-1 contains the *vpu* gene[55, 56] and HIV-2 encodes the *vpx* gene product (see Fig. 27–2).[57–59] Analyses of human and simian immunodeficiency virus (SIV) genomes have also indicated that HIV-2 is more closely related to the SIVs than to HIV-1 (see Fig. 27–3B).[60–63]

Three of the primary HIV-1 translation products, all encoding structural proteins, are initially synthesized as polyprotein precursors that are subsequently processed by viral or cellular proteases into mature particle-associated proteins (Fig. 27–4A). The 55/41 kDa Gag precursors are cleaved into the matrix (MA), capsid (CA), nucleocapsid (NC), and p6 proteins. The 180 kDa Gag/Pol polyprotein gives rise to the protease (PR), heterodimeric reverse transcriptase (RT), and integrase (IN) proteins, whereas proteolytic digestion by a cellular enzyme(s) converts the glycosylated 160 kDa Env precursor to the gp120 surface (SU) and gp41 transmembrane (TM) cleavage products. The remaining six HIV-1 encoded proteins (Vif, Vpr, Tat, Rev, Vpu, and Nef) are the primary translation products of spliced messenger RNAs (mRNAs).

The relationships between HIV-1 precursor polyproteins and their final protein products have been deduced from pulse-chase/immunoprecipitation experiments of the type shown in Figure 27–4B. Thus, the declining levels of the intracellular 55 kDa Gag precursor are temporally associated with increasing amounts of the 24 kDa CA released into the

medium. A similar inverse relationship is observed between the intracellular gp160 and released gp120 envelope proteins. Note that little if any of the gp160 precursor appears in the medium.

During its evolution, HIV has incorporated multiple sequence elements into its RNA genome that do not encode viral proteins but nonetheless are required for the balanced and coordinated production of progeny virions. Many of these so-called *cis*-acting elements (Fig. 27–5) are present in other replication competent retroviral genomes and a few are unique to the primate lentiviruses. The transfer RNA (tRNA^{Lys}) primer binding site (pbs), required to initiate the reverse transcription reaction, and the major splice donor are situated near the 5′ end of the viral RNA, whereas the polypurine tract (PPT), used for the synthesis of plus-strand viral DNA, and the polyadenylation (PA) signal are located near the 3′ terminus. The canonical encapsidation signal (ψ), consisting of four stem loops, maps between nucleotides 242 and 351 (2001) and contains a GCGCGC motif (DIS) (Fig. 27–5B), which initiates the dimerization of HIV genomes that are incorporated into progeny particles. In addition to an element (FS) that mediates a translational shift from the *gag* into the *pol* reading frame and is present in most other retroviral genomes, the HIV RNA folds into two additional complex structures (TAR and RRE) involved in RNA synthesis and transport. It has also been reported that the TAR element is required for the efficient initiation of reverse transcription.[64] Multiple RNA elements (IR), associated with the nuclear retention/instability of HIV transcripts, are also scattered throughout genes encoding structural proteins.

The Virus Life Cycle: Overview

Because in vivo HIV infections are limited to man and chimpanzee,[65–67] most current knowledge about virus replication derives from infections carried out in tissue culture systems. As is the case for all other retroviruses, the ultimate objectives of the HIV replicative cycle are (1) to generate two copies of its RNA genome; (2) to synthesize an internal nucleocapsid structure, consisting of Gag proteins, which encases viral genomic RNA; (3) to produce a series of particle-associated enzymes (protease, reverse transcriptase, and integrase) encoded by the *pol* gene; and (4) to incorporate viral RNA and an outer lipoprotein membrane, containing viral envelope glycoproteins, into progeny virions.

The principal cellular targets for HIV are CD4+ T lymphocytes and CD4+ cells of macrophage lineage. In vivo, most T lymphocytes circulating in the blood or residing in lymphoid tissues are resting in the G₀ phase of the cell cycle; potential macrophage targets exist as non-dividing cells in G₁.[68] In the laboratory, the cell types commonly used to study HIV infections include activated human peripheral blood mononuclear cells (PBMCs); non-dividing, adherent primary human monocyte derived macrophage (MDM); and continuous human CD4+ T-cell leukemia lines noted earlier. Resting human PBMCs generally do not support productive HIV infections unless they are stimulated with mitogens and propagated in the presence of interleukin-2 (IL-2).[69–71] Although it is still unclear whether the reverse transcription or the integration step of the HIV-1 replication cycle is impaired in unstimulated T lymphocytes, there is general

PHYLOGENETIC RELATIONSHIPS (RT)
OF REPRESENTATIVE RETROVIRUSES

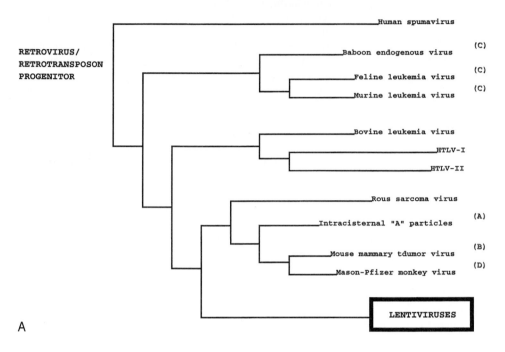

A

LENTIVIRUS PHYLOGENY

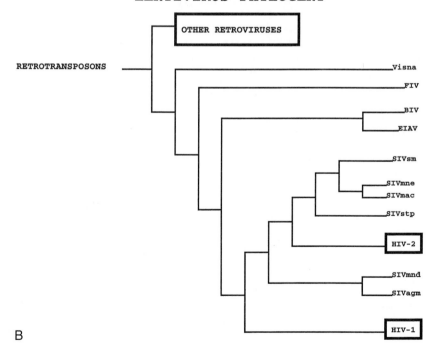

B

Figure 27–3. Phylogenetic Relationships of Representative Retroviruses. *A,* Different retrovirus subfamilies were related to one another on the basis of sequences encoding reverse transcriptase.[30] The letters in parentheses refer to different retrovirus morphological types. *B,* The relationship of the non-primate lentiviruses to themselves and to the primate lentivirus group is based on reverse transcriptase[30]; the relationships between the primate lentiviruses are based on gag sequences.[792] FIV, feline immunodeficiency virus; BIV, bovine immunodeficiency virus; EIAV, equine infectious anemia virus; SIV$_{sm}$, simian immunodeficiency virus, sooty mangabey; SIV$_{mne}$, simian immunodeficiency virus, pig-tailed macaque; SIV$_{mac}$, simian immunodeficiency virus, rhesus macaque; SIV$_{stp}$, simian immunodeficiency virus, stump-tailed macaque; SIV$_{mnd}$, simian immunodeficiency virus, mandrill; SIV$_{agm}$, simian immunodeficiency virus, African green monkey. (Adapted from Doolittle, R. F., Feng, D. F., McClure, M. A., and Johnson, M. S.: Retrovirus phylogeny and evolution. Curr. Top. Microbiol. Immunol. 157:1, 1990; and Khan, A. S., et al.: A highly divergent simian immunodeficiency virus recovered from stored stump-tailed macaque tissues. J. Virol. 65:7061, 1991; with permission.)

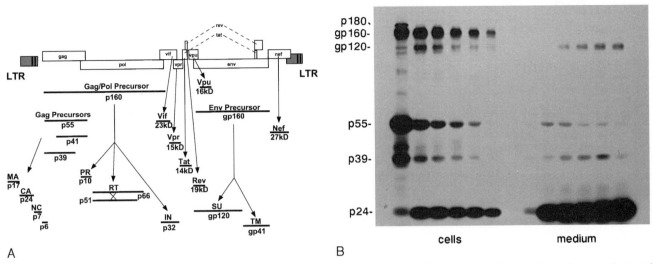

A   B

Figure 27–4. HIV-Encoded Proteins. *A,* The location of the HIV genes, the sizes of primary (in some cases polyproteins) translation products, and the processed mature viral proteins are indicated. *B,* A pulse-chase labeling experiment illustrating precursor-product relationships of the viral-encoded structural proteins. HeLa cells were pulse labeled for 30 minutes with ^{35}S-methionine, 2 days after transfection with an infectious molecular clone of HIV, and then maintained in complete medium for the indicated times (hours). Samples of the cell lysates and supernatant medium (containing released virions) were immunoprecipitated with the serum from an AIDS patient, and the resultant proteins were resolved by polyacrylamide gel electrophoresis. Note that increasing amounts of gp120 and p24 appear in the medium as the amounts of intracellular gp160 and p55 Gag precursor proteins diminish. No gp160 is detected in the medium. p180, Gag/Pol precursor polyprotein; gp160, envelope precursor polyprotein; gp120, the mature glycosylated surface (SU) envelope protein; p55, the Gag precursor polyprotein; p39, Gag precursor polyprotein; p24, processed Gag capsid (CA) protein. The first lane in the two panels depicts the radioactivity incorporated during the 30 minute pulse (P) period, and the other five show the distribution of the label at the indicated times (hours) after the pulse.

agreement that no viral proteins or progeny virions are produced.[72, 73] Activation of resting PBMCs up to 14 days after an initial abortive infection is still able to resurrect a productive infection.[74] In contrast, the non-dividing MDMs are susceptible to infection by so-called macrophage-tropic HIV isolates and release viral progeny capable of infecting both activated human T lymphocytes and cells of non-dividing macrophage lineages. The capacity to infect non-proliferating macrophage distinguishes members of the lentivirus subfamily from other retroviruses.

The primate lentivirus replicative cycle (Fig. 27–6) begins with adsorption of virus particles to CD4 molecules on the surface of susceptible cells.[75–77] Although binding of virions to CD4 is essential for HIV infectivity, their subsequent interaction with a coreceptor belonging to the family of seven membrane spanning CC or CXC of chemokine receptors is required for membrane fusion and entry.[78–82] The two most important of these coreceptors are CXCR4 (previously called fusin or LESTR) and CCR5. The direct fusion of input virions with the plasma membrane of infected cells has in fact been documented by electron microscopy.[83] Adsorbed subviral particles enter the cytoplasm of the infected cell and, after partial uncoating, initiate the reverse transcription of the viral RNA genome. Unfortunately, investigations of these early events in the virus life cycle have been greatly hampered by the very high retrovirus particle/infectivity ratios (>100:1). Thus, simply monitoring the fate of tagged viral proteins during the entry and uncoating steps is unlikely to provide useful information about biologically active particles.

As is the case for other retroelements,[84–87] the partially double-stranded DNA reverse transcript is transported

through the cytoplasm and into the nucleus as a component of a nucleoprotein/preintegration complex (PIC) containing Gag and Pol proteins. This poorly understood process is not the result of simple diffusion and very likely depends on host factors to transport the PICs actively from the plasma membrane to the nuclear pore. These "early" steps in the retrovirus replication cycle undoubtedly require the participation of multiple cellular factors for their successful completion. After the import of the PIC into the nucleus, full length copies of the reverse transcript are integrated into the chromosomal DNA of the infected cell, a step required for efficient viral RNA synthesis and infectious particle production.[88–91] HIV and other lentiviral PICs are able to enter the interphase nucleus of non-dividing macrophage arrested in the G_1 phase of the cell cycle. This is not the case for members of other retroviral genera, which require the nuclear membrane disassembly associated with mitosis to transport the PIC from the cytoplasm to the nucleus.

In activated T lymphocytes, integrated copies of HIV DNA serve as a template for RNA polymerase II (Pol II)–directed viral RNA synthesis. The coordinate interaction of the HIV encoded Tat protein with the cellular transcriptional transactivator proteins NF-κB and Sp1 ensures the production of high levels of viral RNA. Unspliced or partially spliced HIV transcripts are exported from the nucleus to the cytoplasm by a unique transport mechanism mediated by the shuttling Rev protein. The subsequent translation of Gag and Gag-Pol polyproteins occurs on free cytoplasmic ribosomes whereas the gp160 Env precursor is synthesized in the endoplasmic reticulum. Each is transported via independent pathways to the plasma membrane. HIV, like all other retroviruses except type B and type D viruses and the

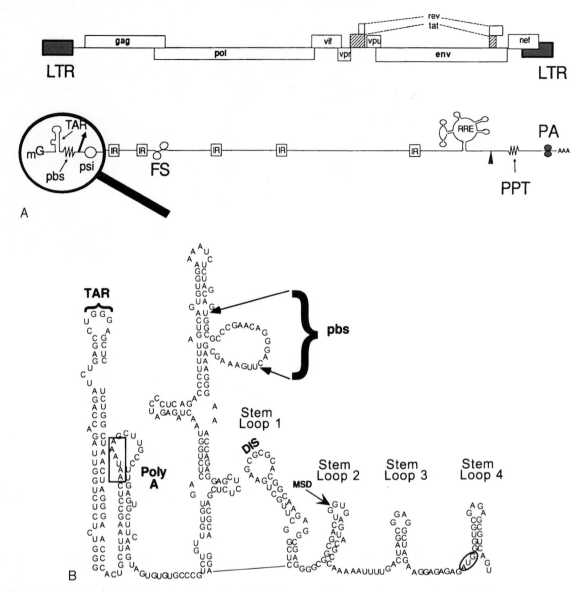

Figure 27–5. Cis-Acting Elements Incorporated into the HIV-1 Genome. A, The cis elements present in HIV-1 genomic RNA have been aligned with a map (top) depicting the genomic organization of HIV-1. ₘG, Methyl capped terminal G residue at 5′ terminus of viral RNA; TAR, Tat-responsive stem-bulge-loop structure; pbs, binding site for the tRNA^Lys primer; psi, major packaging site; IR, RNA instability/nuclear retention elements; FS, frameshift motif; RRE, Rev-responsive element; PPT, polypurine tract, the initiation sequence for second-strand DNA synthesis; PA, polyadenylation signal; large arrow, major splice donor. B, Possible secondary structure at the 5′ terminus of HIV-1 mRNAs. The polyadenylation addition signal is boxed, the pbs is situated between the arrowheads. DIS, dimer initiation site; MSD, major splice donor. (Modified from Clever, J., Sassetti, C., and Parslow, T. G.: RNA secondary structure and binding sites for gag gene products in the 5′ packaging signal of human immunodeficiency virus type 1. J. Virol. 69:2101, 1995; with permission.)

spumaviruses, does not assemble progeny particles intracellularly. Instead, the Gag and Gag-Pol polyproteins, in association with dimers of genomic RNA, condense at the plasma membrane to form an electron-dense "bud" that gives rise to a spherical immature particle containing the mature TM and SU envelope glycoproteins. Proteolytic processing of the Gag and Pol proteins by the HIV protease during or immediately after particle release generates the cone-shaped nucleoid characteristic of mature HIV virions.

As noted in the description of its infectious cycle, HIV uses the same replicative strategy employed by simple retroviruses, which contain genomes consisting of only three genes encoding structural proteins. During its evolution, HIV has acquired six additional genes to carry out functions that

are either mediated by analogous cellular factors present in cells infected by simple retroviruses or uniquely required for replication, transmission, and survival in hematopoietic cells. Several of the HIV accessory proteins (Vif, Vpr, Vpu, and Nef) are not required for replication in cultured human T cells, although virus infectivity may be affected up to several thousand–fold, depending on the accessory gene mutated and the infected cell studied. In view of their conservation, however, these gene products must be required for HIV replication in vivo; their precise function(s) remains to be elucidated.

For many retroviruses, the determinants of tropism reside in the external envelope glycoprotein and the LTR.[92–95] Although changes in the LTR may modulate the efficiency

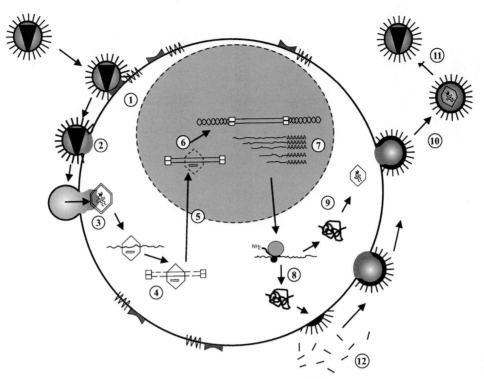

Figure 27–6. The Retrovirus Replicative Cycle. A typical retrovirus infection begins with the adsorption of cell-free virions to cells and their interactions with both the CD4 and chemokine receptors (step 1). In the case of HIV, virus entry (step 2) is a pH-independent process that follows the fusion of virus and cellular membranes and results in the partial uncoating (step 3) of incoming virions. Reverse transcription occurs within subviral particles in the cytoplasm of infected cells (step 4), and the double-stranded DNA product is transported to the nucleus (step 5), where integration into chromosomal DNA (step 6) is mediated by the virus-encoded integrase *(white bar),* a component of a subviral nucleoprotein complex. The integrated viral DNA serves as a template for DNA-dependent RNA polymerase and leads to the production of mRNAs (step 7) that are translated into viral proteins in the cytoplasm of infected cells (step 8). Envelope (step 8) and Gag plus Gag/Pol (step 9) polyproteins are transported via independent pathways to the plasma membrane, where progeny virus particles begin "budding" from cells and are released as immature particles (step 10). Subsequent proteolysis by the virion-encoded protease generates mature particles (step 11) containing a characteristic condensed core *(upper right).* Non-virion-associated gp 120 envelope protein is also released from cells (step 12).

of replication in a variety of T-cell types, the principal determinant of HIV host range resides in the envelope glycoproteins.

The Molecular Biology of Human Immunodeficiency Virus Replication

Most of what is currently known about the function of HIV proteins and their contribution to virus replication in infected individuals has been learned through a variety of in vitro tissue culture systems in which cells are transfected with molecularly cloned viral genes or infected with preparations of virus. In some studies, lymphocytes or epithelial cells have been transfected with plasmids expressing individual HIV proteins to monitor their (1) intracellular location and transport, (2) interaction with other viral or cellular proteins, and (3) binding to *cis*-acting elements associated with the viral genome or proviral DNA. In related experiments, CD4 positive or negative cells have been transfected with plasmids expressing multiple viral gene products or full-length molecular clones of HIV DNA to study virion assembly or to prepare wild-type or mutant virus stocks.

These experimental approaches are to be contrasted with infections of CD4 positive cells in which the spread of HIV progeny through the culture, in successive cycles of

replication, is measured. In such infectivity studies, both primary human cells (PBMCs and MDMs) and continuous CD4⁺ T leukemia cell lines are used. Assays have also been developed to monitor single cycles of infection in those special instances (e.g., pseudotyped HIV inocula) in which newly produced virus particles would be incapable of sustaining a spreading infection. Two general classes of virus inocula are commonly used for infectivity assays: (1) primary virus strains, isolated from HIV infected persons and not extensively propagated in tissue culture, which are able to infect human PBMC and, to a lesser degree, human MDM; (2) T-cell line (TCL) adapted virus strains that are able to enter and replicate in PBMC and CD4⁺ T leukemia cell lines (but not human MDM), utilize the CXCR4 chemokine coreceptor, and frequently induce syncytium formation during productive infections.

▼ THE HUMAN IMMUNODEFICIENCY VIRUS LONG TERMINAL REPEAT

The retroviral LTR is a useful starting point for understanding the complex interplay between HIV and its principal target, the human CD4 positive mononuclear cell. LTRs are generated during the process of reverse transcription and therefore only exist as "repeats" in viral DNA.[96–98] During the replicative cycle, LTR sequences perform a multitude of functions in the context of both viral DNA and genomic RNA (see Fig. 25–7). DNA and RNA sequences, mapping to the R region of the LTR, participate directly in one of the earliest steps of reverse transcription by forming intermolecular DNA-RNA hybrid "bridges" that link the short newly synthesized minus DNA strand with the 3′ end of the genomic RNA template.[99–101] This short (~200 nucleotides [nt]) single-stranded LTR product, called "strong-stop" DNA, allows reverse transcription to extend into U3 sequences after a "jump" to a second RNA template and reverse transcribe the remainder of the retroviral genome. The LTR also plays a critical role at the integration step of the virus life cycle. LTR sequences (known as *att* sequences), located at the termini of the full-length linear viral DNA products of the reverse transcription reaction, mediate precise integration into the chromosomal DNA of host cells.[102, 103] Other HIV LTR sequences, located in the U5 region, contribute to the packaging of progeny RNA genomes during virus assembly.[104]

The major function of the retroviral LTR, in the context of integrated viral DNA, is the regulation of viral RNA synthesis.[105–108] The core promoter and adjacent regulatory elements, both of which recruit the cellular transcriptional machinery to the start site of viral RNA synthesis, are located within the U3 region and function in the context of the 5′ LTR (Fig. 27–7). The polyadenylation signal (AATAAA) and polyadenylation addition site are also positioned in the R region but are active only as components of the 3′ LTR. In contrast to bacteria, in which the complete transcriptional apparatus consists of a single RNA polymerase complex containing four essential subunits, eukaryotic cells contain three different polymerizing enzymes; the RNA Pol II holoenzyme, responsible for transcribing cellular genes,

utilizes more than 30 additional proteins to select the DNA site at which RNA synthesis is initiated. Furthermore, during the assembly of a functional eukaryotic transcription complex, components other than Pol II must be recruited to the promoter.

Like other eukaryotic promoters, the integrated HIV LTR contains several elements that facilitate the loading of Pol II on the DNA. The initial recognition of the HIV promoter requires the participation of several general transcription factors (GTFs), including transcription factor II D (TFIID), which bind to the TATA element and adjacent viral DNA sequences. In the HIV LTR, the TATA element is located −29 to −24 nt upstream of the transcriptional start site. The multicomponent TFIID complex includes the TATA binding protein (TBP), which structurally resembles a horse saddle and markedly bends DNA after attachment.[109, 110] This generates a nucleation site upon which a transcriptional complex can be assembled. The bound TFIID is then recognized by a single GTF, TFIIB, which recruits Pol II to the promoter, a critical interaction that definitively establishes the transcription start site.[111, 112] Nonetheless, the nascent complex is functionally unable to initiate RNA synthesis. Two other GTFs (TFIIE and TFIIH), which modify Pol II allosterically and allow the transcription complex to initiate RNA polymerization and "escape" from the promoter, must be incorporated.[113–115] TFIIH possesses a kinase activity that phosphorylates a unique region within the largest Pol II subunit, the C-terminal domain (CTD). The CTD of human Pol II contains 52 tandem heptapeptide repeats (YSPTSPS) and can be phosphorylated on serine, threonine, and/or tyrosine residues. Taken together, these results suggest that hyperphosphorylation of the CTD induces a conformational change in Pol II that permits the transcription complex to clear the promoter and generate elongated RNA molecules.

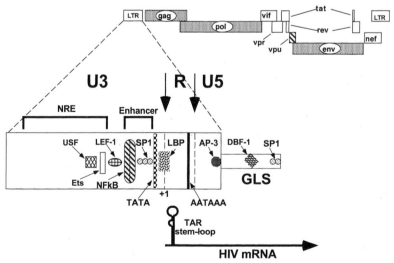

Figure 27–7. Structure of the HIV-1 Long Terminal Repeat (LTR). The HIV-1 LTR, a duplicated 630⁺ bp component of integrated proviral DNA, is subdivided into regions associated with termini of the viral RNA genome. The R (repeat) region is defined as a 96 bp nt repeat present at the 3′ and 5′ termini of HIV-1 genomic RNA; U5 is an 84 nt segment located adjacent to the R region at the 5′ end of the viral genome; U3 is a 454 nt segment situated adjacent to the R region at the 3′ end of the viral RNA. The 5′ LTR and adjacent *gagi* leader sequence (GLS) are expanded to show functionally important binding sites for transcriptional regulatory proteins. The "enhancer" domain contains three Sp 1 binding elements and two NF-κB binding motifs. The transcription start site is located at map position " + 1," which is defined as the border between U3 and R. The negative regulatory element (NRE) is situated between positions −410 and −157 and contains binding sites for USF and the Ets proteins. The TATA site is positioned 22 bp upstream of the transcription initiation site. LBP, leader binding protein; TAR, Tat transactivation response region; AATAAA, polyadenylation signal. An HIV RNA transcript, which is initiated at the first nucleotide within the R region (designated " + 1") and contains the TAR element near its 5′ terminus, is shown at the bottom.

Basal levels of RNA synthesis are thought to reflect the sporadic assembly of functionally competent transcription complexes at the promoter. In eukaryotic cells, regulatory transcriptional factors, which bind to DNA elements near the promoter, can modulate the basal rate of RNA synthesis in response to physiological cues. These regulatory factors function in a combinatorial fashion via protein-protein interactions to recruit GTFs such as TBP and TFIIB, as well as the Pol II enzyme itself, to the promoter. This results in the more frequent assembly of stable transcription complexes that can readily escape the promoter and generate full-length primary transcripts.

As is the case for other eukaryotic cellular promoters, the HIV LTR contains its own ensemble of DNA elements to which transcriptional regulatory factors bind (see Fig. 27–7). Some of these were identified from mutagenesis studies of LTR-driven reporter gene constructs, some were found as a result of gel-retardation or DNA footprinting experiments, and others were discovered from searches of nucleotide sequence databases. Although early studies of HIV LTR–directed expression of reporter genes suggested that a large domain (−410 to −157) within U3, designated the negative regulatory element (NRE), might "silence" viral gene activity,[116, 117] there is little convincing evidence that the NRE plays a significant role during virus replication. Binding sites for upstream factor (USF), erythroblast transformation sequence (Ets), and lymphocyte enhancer-binding factor (LEF-1) are located within this region and represent potentially important regulatory elements for HIV-1 replication in PBMCs.[118] It is also worth noting that the U5 portion of the HIV LTR and the Gag leader, both of which are situated *downstream* of the transcription start site, also contains cognate binding sites for cellular factors that potentially regulate RNA synthesis during productive infection.

The LTRs of HIV and other primate lentiviruses contain three tandemly arranged binding sites for the constitutively expressed Sp1 transcription factor[119, 120] that are situated upstream of a canonical Pol II TATA box (see Fig. 27–7). The Sp1 and TATA elements constitute the HIV-1 core promoter and must be present for basal levels of LTR-directed RNA synthesis. Sp1 was originally isolated from HeLa cells and shown to bind to the multiple GGGCGG motifs (GC box) associated with the 21 base pair (bp) repeats

in simian virus 40 (SV40) DNA, activating both early and late SV40 transcription in vitro.[121, 122] Functional analyses of HIV LTR driven reporter constructs have shown that mutations of individual or pairs of Sp1 sites had little, if any, effect on the basal or Tat-transactivated levels of expression.[120] Mutation of all three HIV Sp1 sites, however, markedly reduced the response to Tat.[120, 123] The role of the Sp1 elements in the context of infectious virus is quite variable, depending on the cell type used for infection.[124–126] Mutations that functionally inactivate all three Sp1 motifs eliminated detectable replication in Jurkat cells, delayed progeny virus production in CEM and H9 cells, and had little effect on infectivity in activated PBMCs.

Adjacent to the Sp1 binding sites, tandem recognition sites for the NF-κB/Rel family of transcription factors constitute an activatable enhancer in the HIV-1 LTR (see Fig. 27–7).[127] The LTRs of HIV-2 and SIV, retaining the triplicated Sp1 motifs, contain only a single NF-κB binding site. NF-κB was originally described as a nuclear factor, induced by lipopolysaccharide or phorbol esters in mature B cells, which bound to the enhancer for the κ light chain gene and activated its transcription.[128] Subsequent work has shown that a variety of immunologically relevant cellular genes, including interleukin-2 (IL-2), β interferon, granulocyte-macrophage colony-stimulating factor (GM-CSF), tumor necrosis factor α (TNF-α), IL-2 receptor α chain, T-cell receptor β chain, and class I major histocompatibility complex (MHC), can be activated by NF-κB.[129] All of these genes contain an upstream canonical NF-κB-binding site (GGGRNNYYCC). It is therefore not surprising that primate lentiviruses, which may reside for many years and replicate in the T cells and/or macrophages of their infected hosts, have incorporated the NF-κB-binding motif upstream of their respective transcriptional start sites.

NF-κB is a member of a large family of cellular transcription factors, which include the c-Rel protein of chickens and the dorsal gene product of *Drosophila*, a regulator of pattern development in embryos.[130, 131] Selected members of this NF-κB/Rel gene family are shown diagrammatically in Figure 27–8. Several contain a highly conserved N-terminal Rel homology domain (RHD), approximately 300 residues in size, that includes DNA binding and dimerization regions and a nuclear localization signal (NLS). A conserved protein

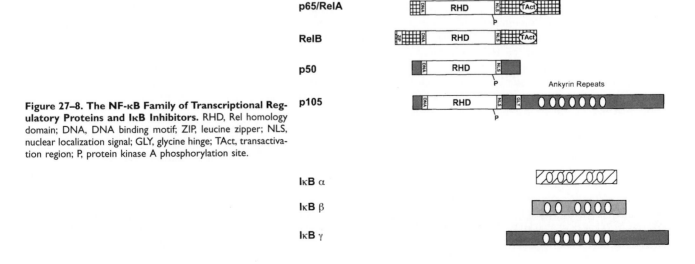

Figure 27–8. The NF-κB Family of Transcriptional Regulatory Proteins and IκB Inhibitors. RHD, Rel homology domain; DNA, DNA binding motif; ZIP, leucine zipper; NLS, nuclear localization signal; GLY, glycine hinge; TAct, transactivation region; P, protein kinase A phosphorylation site.

kinase A site is present in several but not all RHDs. The p65/Rel A protein contains a potent transcription activation domain located downstream from its RHD. Rel B has two activation domains: one associated with a leucine zipper–like region and a second located at the C-terminus.[132, 133] Both domains are required for full Rel B transactivation activity. The p50 protein is derived from the p105 precursor, which contains a glycine-rich hinge linked to an ankyrin repeat domain; the p65/Rel A protein, in contrast, is a primary translation product. The inhibitory IκB proteins all contain multiple 30 to 34 amino acid ankyrin motifs, which provide the interface for binding to various species of NF-κB.

NF-κB "binding activity" was originally attributed to the p50-p65/Rel A heterodimer, the most abundant and functionally active form of NF-κB in human T cells.[134] Because the various members of the c-Rel family are capable of forming dimeric NF-κB molecules, a heterogeneous population of homo- and heterodimers, with different functional specificities, could potentially bind two NF-κB sites present in the HIV-1 LTR. NF-κB functional activity is controlled by its intracellular location. In the cytoplasm, NF-κB dimers are complexed to IκB proteins or other Rel family members containing ankyrin repeats, such as the unprocessed p105 protein, and cannot be imported into the nucleus.[135–137] The binding of IκBα to the RHD of the p65 subunit of heterodimeric NF-κB results in its sequestration in the cytoplasm, perhaps because of a masking of the p65 NLS.[138, 139] Nearly all of the T cells encountered by HIV in vivo are in a resting state and lack NF-κB binding activity. A variety of inducers including cytokines and growth factors (TNF-α, IL-1, platelet derived growth factor [PDGF]), T-cell mitogens (phorbol esters, lectins, calcium ionophores), bacterial lipopolysaccharides, cyclohexamide, DNA damage inducing agents, viral encoded transactivating proteins (HTLV-1 Tax, adenovirus E1A), and oxidative stress can activate Rel/NF-κB.[129] Activation or induction of mammalian T cells results in the phosphorylation of the bound IκB, the rapid degradation of IκB via the ubiquitin pathway, and the translocation of NF-κB into the nucleus, where it can function to activate eukaryotic genes.[137, 140, 141] Convergent signal transducing pathways associated with T-cell activation including those initiated at the IL-1 and TNF receptors have been experimentally studied for their contributions to NF-κB activation.[142–144]

The nuclei of activated human T lymphocytes and T-cell lines contain NF-κB capable of binding to cognate sites in the HIV-1 LTR and stimulating both basal and Tat-induced levels of expression, as monitored with reporter genes in transient transfection assays.[117, 127] When the NF-κB motifs are altered in the context of HIV, infectivity is altered, depending on the type of mutant constructed and the endogenous cellular levels of NF-κB. Deletion of both HIV-1 NF-κB binding motifs resulted in no[124] or modest[126] delays in peak virus production in activated human PBMC, whereas point mutations affecting specific nucleotides involved in NF-κB recognition but not the spatial organization of the HIV promoter/enhancer reduced progeny virus production more than 10-fold.[145] The replication of HIV-1 NF-κB mutants in human T-cell lines was found to be inversely proportional to basal levels of cellular NF-κB. It is likely that the binding of other transcription factors can compensate for the absence of NF-κB at the HIV promoter in these virus mutants. The simultaneous mutation of the two NF-κB motifs

and the three Sp1 sites completely abolishes HIV-1 replication,[124, 126] a result consistent with a report demonstrating that the cooperative interaction of NF-κB and Sp1 promotes the binding of both factors to the HIV-1 LTR and induces transcriptional activation.[146] A synthesis of all of these results is that NF-κB mediates a more rapid and robust production of HIV-1 progeny in activated human T lymphocytes.

The integration of retroviral DNAs during productive viral infections results in the packaging of the provirus and its associated LTR into chromatin. This deposition of nucleosomes on the viral DNA template imposes yet another level of complexity on our present understanding of regulated HIV gene expression as deduced from experiments in which naked DNA is transfected into mammalian cells. DNA footprinting studies have shown that chromatin in the vicinity of the HIV promoter is organized into two large nucleosome-free regions that encompass promoter/enhancer sequences (-250 to $+11$) and a downstream segment that includes the 3′ portions of U5 and the Gag leader ($+150$ to $+250$), respectively.[147, 148] These two deoxyribonuclease (DNase) I hypersensitive regions are separated by a nucleosome that becomes disrupted after transcription activation of the HIV-1 LTR. The downstream nucleosome-free region contains binding sites for three different transcription factors: Ap-3, downstream binding factor–1 (DBF-1), and Sp1 (see Fig. 27–7). Mutagenesis of these binding motifs effectively eliminates the downstream nucleosome-free region and markedly inhibits the transcriptional activity of the integrated HIV-1 promoter in the context of both stably integrated LTR constructs and mutagenized virus.[149, 150] These results suggest that factors binding downstream of the transcription start site contribute to the native chromatin structure of the integrated HIV-1 promoter. Studies of in vitro assembled chromatin have verified the presence of only the upstream nucleosome-free region, which encompasses the NF-κB, Sp1, and TATA binding sites.[151]

Proteins encoded by several heterologous animal viruses are also capable of transactivating the HIV LTR.[117, 152–155] Although this effect has been touted by some as indicating a role of these viruses in disease progression, the coinfection of human T cells by HIV and other viruses has been difficult to document in cells isolated from seropositive individuals. On the basis of tropism for CD4-positive human mononuclear cells, agents capable of directly or indirectly transactivating the HIV LTR would include human T-cell leukemia virus type 1 (HTLV-1), human cytomegalovirus (HCMV), human herpesvirus type 6 (HHV-6), and possibly human adenoviruses.[156] In the case of HTLV-1, it has been proposed that the elevated levels of NF-κB induced by the viral-encoded Tax protein[157, 158] activate HIV replication by binding to the two NF-κB motifs in its LTR.

▼ HUMAN IMMUNODEFICIENCY VIRUS–ENCODED REGULATORY PROTEINS

Tat

Although the mechanism underlying Tat transactivation of HIV LTR–directed expression has been hotly debated for several years, it is now generally agreed that Tat is an extremely potent transactivator that increases the steady-state levels of viral RNA several hundred–fold by directing the formation of a more processive Pol II transcription complex in infected cells. Tat is an indispensable viral protein; when the *tat* gene of an infectious molecular proviral clone of HIV is mutagenized, no detectable progeny virions are produced.[159, 160] HIV-1 Tat is a nuclear protein[161, 162] containing 101 amino acid residues encoded by two exons (Fig. 27–9). A shorter 72 amino acid "single-exon" HIV-1 Tat protein possesses all of the transcriptional activating properties of full-length Tat, as measured in tissue culture infections or in LTR-driven reporter gene experiments.[159, 163–165] The termination codon after the first Tat exon is highly conserved among different HIV-1 isolates,[166] suggesting that the "one exon" and "two exon" Tat proteins mediate different functions during productive viral infections in vivo.

As previously noted, RNA synthesis in eukaryotic cells is usually modulated by transcription activator proteins that bind to DNA motifs located *upstream* of their respective promoters and recruit GTFs and the Pol II holoenzyme to the transcription initiation complex. Visna virus, another member of the lentivirus genus, in fact encodes a DNA-binding Tat protein, which interacts with Ap-1 sites located in its LTR.[167] HTLV-1/HTLV-2 and the human spumaviruses encode their own transactivating proteins, designated Tax and Bel-1, respectively (see Fig. 27–2), which interact (indirectly, in the case of Tax) with LTR elements, also situated

upstream of the transcriptional start site[168–170] (see Chapter 28). In contrast, the immediate target of all primate lentiviral Tat transactivating proteins maps to sequences *downstream* of the start site for viral RNA synthesis.[116] This unusually located transactivation response region, or TAR element, also differs from typical binding sites for Pol II transactivators because it is inactive when present (1) in an inverted orientation, (2) 5' to the promoter, or (3) downstream of the transcription termination site (i.e., in the U5 region of the 3' LTR).[116, 164, 171–175] These unusual properties were subsequently reconciled when it was demonstrated that TAR functioned not as a component of DNA, but as an RNA element (see Fig. 27–7).[176]

The HIV-1 TAR encompasses the 5'-terminal 59 nt of all viral RNAs and folds into a stable stem-loop structure (see Fig. 27–9). Subsequent work has shown that the minimal TAR element (mapping between bases +19 and +42) contains two critical components: a U-rich trinucleotide bulge and a G-rich loop.[171–174, 177–179] Interestingly, the HIV-2 TAR forms a double stem-loop structure, each arm of which also possesses the U-rich bulge and G-rich loop (see Fig. 27–9).[180] Sequences located in both the hexanucleotide loop and the bulge of the HIV-1 TAR are required for Tat function.[161, 174, 177–179, 181, 182] In vitro, purified preparations of Tat bind to TAR RNA (at a ratio of 1:1) with high affinity (12 mM) and moderate specificity.[183] Tat binds to both wild-type

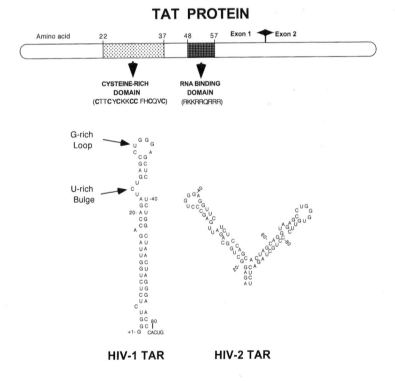

TAT PROTEIN

Figure 27–9. Tat and Its Response Element TAR. Schematic representation of the HIV-1 Tat protein *(top)* with the cysteine-rich activation and RNA-binding domains indicated. The stem-bulge-loop configurations of HIV-1 and HIV-2 TAR elements are shown in the middle; the release of prematurely terminated HIV-1 transcriptional complexes from the DNA template in the absence of Tat is depicted at the bottom.

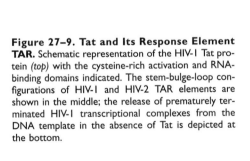

HIV-1 TAR   **HIV-2 TAR**

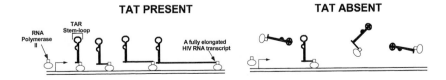

TAT PRESENT   **TAT ABSENT**

or "loop" mutants of TAR but not to TAR elements containing alterations affecting the bulge region.[171, 172, 178, 181, 184–186] Modification of the invariant "bulge" U_{+23} nucleotide and elimination of the base pairs immediately above and below the bulge (see Fig. 27–9) significantly reduce the binding of Tat to TAR.[186] Nuclear magnetic resonance (NMR) studies have shown that the binding of a large Tat peptide to TAR causes the major groove in the RNA duplex structure to widen, thereby generating multiple points of contact involving critical nucleotides (viz., U_{23}) and several groups in the phosphate backbone.[187] This distortion of the TAR structure also brings the loop and bulge regions into close proximity, an effect that may facilitate the interactions of proteins binding to these TAR domains.

The functional organization of the HIV-1 Tat protein has been deduced from TAR binding and transcriptional activation experiments using both wild-type and mutagenized derivatives of the Tat protein. The Tat activation (or effector) domain encompasses the amino-terminal 48 residues, which include (1) a string of highly acidic amino acids (residues 1 to 21), (2) a cysteine-rich region (7 invariant, 6 of which are required for function, between positions 22 and 37), and (3) a hydrophobic core segment (amino acids 41 to 47), which is highly conserved among different HIV isolates (see Fig. 27–9). Mutations in these portions of Tat drastically reduce transactivation activity.[181, 182] The RNA binding domain of the Tat protein has been mapped to a lysine/arginine-rich region between residues 48 and 57 (see Fig. 27–9); peptides containing this segment bind to the TAR bulge region with somewhat less affinity and specificity than do purified preparations of Tat.[188] A nuclear/nucleolar localization signal (GRKKR) also overlaps the RNA-binding region of Tat.[162, 182]

At first glance, the functional organization of HIV-1 Tat is highly reminiscent of that of many other transcriptional regulatory proteins, which contain modular nucleic acid binding and activation domains. However, a growing body of work has revealed that Tat/TAR interactions are more complex in vivo and involve the participation of cellular cofactors. This became apparent in experiments showing that the arginine-rich domain of the Tat protein did not function as an independent RNA-binding module in vivo. These experiments indicated that (1) the targeting of a heterologous protein to TAR in transfected cells required both the RNA binding and activation regions of Tat[189]; (2) the Tat RNA binding domain did not function as a transdominant negative inhibitor of wild-type Tat, as did the analogous domain of other RNA binding proteins such as HIV Rev (see below), and this finding implied that the Tat RNA binding region was neither autonomous nor able to form functional Tat/TAR interactions in vivo[190]; (3) wild-type TAR decoys, but not TAR mutants with changes limited to the G-rich loop, rendered CEM cells resistant to HIV infection.[191] The failure of excess Tat protein to relieve this blockade suggested that a loop-binding cellular cofactor(s), present in limiting amounts, was required for stable Tat/TAR interaction in vivo.

Other studies demonstrated that Tat chimeric proteins, which could be targeted to the promoter via heterologous (non-TAR) RNA binding sites, also exhibited high levels of transactivation.[192–194] This implied that, if necessary, Tat could function in the absence of TAR and recruit cellular factor(s) to the transcription complex. It was also reported

that the inefficient Tat transactivation observed in rodent cells could be overcome if Tat were delivered to the promoter using a surrogate RNA binding site.[195–197] This latter result indicated that a cellular cofactor for Tat transactivation is indeed present in rodent cells but cannot be recruited to or bind TAR. Collectively, these findings are consistent with a model in which Tat uses its transactivation domain to recruit a cellular cofactor(s) to TAR; in such a scenario, Tat would bind to the TAR bulge and the cofactor(s) to the TAR loop.

The hallmark of HIV LTR–directed RNA synthesis in the absence of Tat is the accumulation of prematurely terminated transcripts, 100 to 200 nt in size, which are converted to longer RNA species when Tat is expressed (see Fig. 27–9, bottom).[173, 198–201] This Tat-deficient phenotype has been observed in in vitro transcription experiments, after transient transfection of LTR-driven reporter gene constructs, and in cells harboring integrated HIV proviruses with mutated Tat genes. Because the expression of Tat in many of these experimental systems markedly stimulated transcriptional elongation, attention shifted to the possible involvement of the CTD of Pol II, which, as noted earlier, is converted to a hyperphosphorylated form in highly processive transcription complexes. This line of reasoning was also consistent with the reported inhibition of Tat-stimulated transcription by the purine nucleoside analogue 5,6-dichloro-1-β-D ribofuranosylbenzimidazole (DRB), which blocks RNA chain elongation by inactivating protein kinases.[202] Reports showing that the Pol II CTD was required for Tat-mediated transactivation of viral RNA synthesis also supported such a model.[203–206]

An important observation linking all of these findings was the reported coimmunoprecipitation of a cellular kinase activity with both the full-length HIV-1 and HIV-2 Tat proteins and, most interestingly, the activation domain (residues 1 to 48) of HIV-1 Tat.[207, 208] This enzymatic activity, named Tat associated kinase (TAK), also phosphorylated a 42 kDa protein present in the immunoprecipitate from HeLa cells. Other experiments, which examined Tat-stimulated Pol II processivity in cell-free systems, suggested that Tat interacted with components of the TFIIH complex to enhance transcriptional elongation.[205, 209] Subsequent studies, however, revealed that the Tat-directed TAK could hyperphosphorylate the CTD of Pol II, independently of TFIIH (and its associated CDK8). This activity was also inhibited by DRB.[206, 208, 210] It was later shown that Tat binds with high affinity to a Pol II CTD kinase complex[211] related to the *Drosophila* multicomponent transcriptional elongation factor P-TEFb.[212, 213] P-TEFb shares no subunits in common with the TFIIH elongation factor complex and regulates the transition from abortive to fully processive transcriptional elongation.[214] The active kinase present in the homologous human complex (TAK) was identified as a CDCα-related human protein kinase containing a Pro-Ile-Thr-Ala-Leu-Arg-Glu motif (PITARLE), a 42–43 kDa cyclin-dependent kinase. After depletion of the TAK complex with antibodies directed against PITARLE (renamed CDK9), the residual activity for Tat-simulated RNA chain elongation was, in fact, reduced nearly 100-fold.[211, 215] The identification of novel Tat inhibitors, which specifically abolished CDK9 activity in vivo and in vitro, and the demonstrated dominant negative effects of a CDK9 mutant on Tat transactivation[215] provided strong additional evidence that Tat functioned to regulate transcription elongation.

Although, as noted above, earlier results had shown that the TAK complex interacted with the activation domain of HIV-1 Tat, the CDK9 catalytic subunit itself failed to bind to Tat in in vitro assays. Equally perplexing was the identification of TAK activity in nuclear extracts migrating not as the 42kDa CDK9, but as a 110 kDa complex.[206] This suggested the existence of a possible cyclin-related partner for CDK9 that could provide substrate specificity. These unresolved issues were clarified with the isolation of the "missing link"—an 87 kDa protein from nuclear extracts that bound to wild-type HIV-1 Tat but not to a Tat mutant protein containing a non-functional activation domain.[216] Sequencing of a complementary DNA (cDNA) clone encoding the 87 kDa protein revealed the presence of an amino-terminal cyclin box that was nearly 40 per cent identical to human cyclin C. The new protein, now named cyclin T, is encoded by a single gene mapping to human chromosome 12. Biochemical and functional studies demonstrated that (1) cyclin T is bound to CDK9 in nuclear extracts, (2) cyclin T promotes Pol II mediated transcription directed by the HIV-1 LTR, (3) recombinant cyclin T interacts directly with wild type but not the mutated transcriptional activation domain of the HIV-1 Tat protein, (4) cyclin T itself does *not* bind to TAR RNA, (5) the binding of Tat to TAR RNA is markedly enhanced in the presence of cyclin T, and (6) the Tat/cyclin T complex only binds to TAR RNA in which both the loop and the bulge are intact, whereas Tat alone requires only the trinucleotide bulge for stable TAR interaction. Augmentation of the notoriously poor Tat transactivation of HIV-1 LTR directed gene activity in rodent cells after overexpression of human cyclin T lends added credence to its role as a Tat cofactor.[216]

A model of HIV Tat transactivation is shown in Figure 27–10. Tat interacts, via its activation domain, with the cyclin T subunit of cyclin T/CDK9, a component of the TAK transcription elongation complex present in the nuclei of virus-infected cells. The binding of cyclin T/CDK9 to Tat most likely induces a conformational change in Tat structure, which alters its affinity and specificity for binding to TAR RNA. Thus, the function of Tat is to recruit a critical elonga-

tion factor (the TAK complex) to a promoter-proximal location where it can hyperphosphorylate the Pol II CTD, thereby stimulating transcriptional processivity. The functional contributions of other factors, reported to interact with the HIV Tat protein or TAR RNA, are presently unknown.[198, 209, 217–221]

Possible extracellular roles for Tat have been suggested from studies showing that Tat is taken up by cultured cells, enters the nucleus, and transactivates genes linked to the HIV LTR.[222] Tat purified from *Escherichia coli* has also been reported to inhibit antigen-induced, but not mitogen-induced, proliferation of peripheral blood mononuclear cells.[223] In a similar vein, low concentrations of Tat exhibit a modest stimulatory effect on a tissue culture model of AIDS-Kaposi sarcoma cells.[224] The significance of these extracellular Tat activities in HIV-infected individuals is currently unclear.

Rev

Like other primary RNA transcripts synthesized in eukaryotic cells, HIV pre-mRNAs undergo a series of modifications (capping, 3′-end cleavage, polyadenylation, and splicing) prior to their export to the cytoplasm. Retroviruses utilize cellular machinery to carry out these functions. With few exceptions, the introns present in primary cellular RNA transcripts must be removed prior to transport from the nucleus to the cytoplasm to prevent their translation into non-functional proteins; interference with the splicing of introns has been reported to cause nuclear sequestration of eukaryotic pre-mRNAs and their subsequent degradation.[225, 226] This requirement poses an obvious problem for replication-competent retroviruses like HIV, which must export a variety of intron-containing mRNAs into the cytoplasm, including the unspliced 9.2 kb primary transcript (for encapsidation into progeny virions and production of Gag and Pol proteins) and several other partially spliced mRNAs.

To generate *env* mRNAs, all retroviruses must splice their primary RNA transcripts to remove upstream *gag* and *pol* sequences. For simple retroviruses such as the avian leukosis viruses and MuLVs, this is the only splicing reaction that the viral pre-mRNA undergoes (Fig. 27–11, top). In contrast, the splicing of HIV RNA is an extremely complex

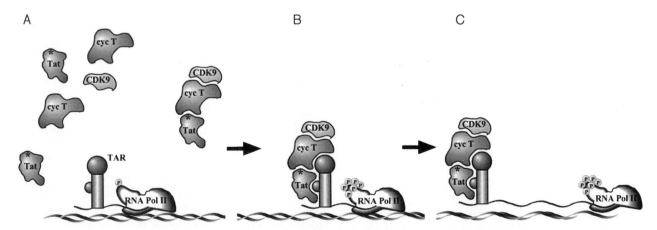

Figure 27–10. Tat Promotes the Phosphorylation of the Carboxy-Terminal Domain (CTD) of RNA Pol II. *A,* In the absence of Tat binding to TAR, the processivity of the RNA Pol II complex is inefficient. *B,* When the activation domain (*) of Tat interacts with the cyclin T (cyc T)/CDK9 complex, the conformation of Tat may change, greatly increasing its affinity and specificity for TAR RNA. *C,* By recruiting the TAK complex (containing cyc T and CDK9), Tat mediates phosphorylation of the CTD and promoter clearance (elongation) of transcriptional complex.

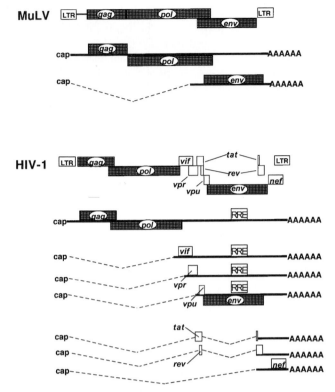

Figure 27–11. Retrovirus Splicing Patterns. In contrast to murine retroviruses (top), which generate only two mRNA species (the unspliced *gag/pol* and the singly spliced *env*), HIV-1 produces several alternatively spliced mRNAs ranging from the unspliced *gag/pol* to the multiply spliced *tat, rev,* and *nef* RNA transcripts. The genomic organization of the proviral DNA, the location of coding sequences, and the position of the Rev-responsive element (RRE), in mRNAs encoding viral structural proteins, are indicated. The dashed lines connect splice donors and acceptors; alternative forms of Tat, Rev, and Nev mRNAs, some of which contain short upstream non-coding exons, are not shown.

27–12). The functional significance of multiply spliced mRNAs encoding the same viral protein, as well as the hierarchy of HIV splice site usage, are not presently understood.

In part, retroviruses solve the eukaryotic cellular requirement for the removal of all intronic sequences from pre-mRNAs prior to nuclear export by incorporating suboptimal splice sites into their genomes. Interestingly, the substitution of "strong" splice sites for weak ones in the genomic RNAs of simple retroviruses results in the overproduction of the proteins encoded by spliced mRNAs and the generation of replication-incompetent particles.[232–234] More recent work, however, suggests that *cis*-acting viral RNA elements interact with cellular proteins to promote the transport of even the simple retroviral genomic RNAs out of the nucleus.[235, 236]

Complex retroviruses, such as HIV, have dealt with the restriction to the nuclear export of unspliced and incompletely spliced transcripts by expressing a novel reading frame encoding the Rev protein. The existence of Rev was discovered by accident when it was noted that *tat* cDNAs, supplied in trans-, did not completely correct a previously constructed HIV *tat* mutant.[237] Thus, although high levels of the completely spliced viral mRNAs were restored in both the nucleus and the cytoplasm after transfection of wild-type *tat,* unspliced and partially spliced transcripts (as well as their encoded proteins) were markedly reduced or undetectable in the cytoplasm. The observed defect was later shown to reflect the absence of the HIV Rev protein, which is encoded by a reading frame that overlaps that of *tat* (see Fig. 27–2 or 27–4) and which had been simultaneously inactivated by the mutation initially thought to affect only *tat.*[237] Subsequent studies revealed that in the absence of Rev, the unspliced *gag/pol* and the partially spliced *vif, vpr,* and *vpu/env* mRNAs fail to accumulate in the cytoplasm, thereby rendering the Rev mutant viruses replication incompetent.[237–241]

HIV Rev is a 19 kDa, predominantly nucleolar phospho-

process because of the presence of both constitutive and alternatively used splice donor and splice acceptor motifs (Fig. 27–11, bottom). Three general classes of HIV mRNAs have been identified during productive virus infections: (1) unspliced genomic RNA, which serves as the mRNA for synthesis of Gag and Pol proteins; (2) partially spliced RNAs, approximately 4.3 to 5.5 kb in size, which are translated into Vif, Vpr, Vpu, and Env proteins; and (3) multiply spliced viral mRNAs ranging from 1.7 to 2.0 kb in size, which encode the Tat, Rev, and Nef proteins. The first two classes of viral mRNA contain spliceable introns yet are efficiently exported from the nucleus into the cytoplasm.

Analyses of viral mRNAs by polymerase chain reaction (PCR) have demonstrated the existence of more than 30 different HIV transcripts in virus producing cells.[227–231] These mRNAs are generated as a consequence of alternative selection of the 5 splice donors and the more than 10 splice acceptors embedded in the HIV genomic RNA. Varied use of these diverse splicing signals gives rise to several sets of different RNAs that serve as alternative templates for the translation of the same protein. For example, 12 different *rev,* 5 different *nef,* 8 different *tat,* and 16 different *env* mRNAs have been identified.[231] This HIV mRNA diversity is due, in part, to the variable inclusion of two upstream 50 and 74 nt non-coding exons in these spliced RNAs (Fig.

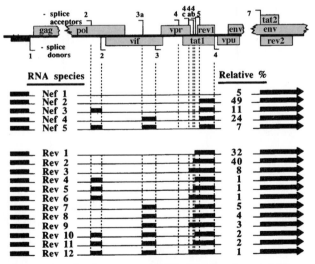

Figure 27–12. The Structure and Relative Abundance of Alternatively Spliced HIV-1 *rev* and *nef* mRNAs. Semiquantitative RT PCR of the *rev* and *nef* transcripts present in HIV-1 producing cells was carried out by using random primers.[231] The black rectangles represent regions of the HIV-1 genome retained in the alternatively spliced *rev* and *nef* RNAs; the relative proportion of each mRNA is indicated at the right.

protein containing 116 amino acid residues. Like Tat, Rev is encoded by two exons and contains two functional regions: (1) an arginine-rich domain that mediates RNA binding, Rev multimerization, and nuclear localization; and (2) a hydrophobic segment, located between residues 73 and 84, that contains several leucine residues, now known to promote nuclear export (Fig. 27–13).[242, 243] Unlike *tat,* both coding exons of *rev* are required for function.[229, 244]

The HIV Rev protein regulates the expression and utilization of viral gene products by binding to a *cis*-acting target, the rev response element (RRE), present in all of the unspliced and partially spliced viral mRNAs (see Fig. 27–11). The RRE, located in a 250 nt segment of the *env* gene, is a complex RNA structure containing multiple stem loops branching from a large central bubble[239, 241, 245] (see Fig. 27–13). The RRE must be present *within* a Rev-responsive transcript and in the *sense* orientation for Rev responsiveness.[245, 246] Nuclease protection, chemical modification, and mutagenesis studies indicate that Rev specifically interacts with a 60[+] nt portion of the RRE, designated stem loop 2 (see Fig. 27–13).[242, 247–251] This region of the RRE binds to Rev even when isolated from the complete RRE structure and mediates Rev responsiveness in functional assays.[252] The determinants for high-affinity binding of Rev

to RRE reside in the central purine-rich "bubble" in stem loop 2, which contains unusual G:G and G:A base pairs that distort the duplex RNA structure and widen the major groove to accommodate the Rev protein.[242, 247, 253–256] NMR analyses have shown that the α-helical, arginine-rich 17 residue peptide from the RNA binding domain of Rev burrows deep into the major groove of a stem loop 2 oligonucleotide, stabilizing the non–Watson-Crick base pairs through specific interactions involving the arginine side chains.[257] It has been proposed that Rev initially binds with high affinity to nucleotides in the RRE loop 2 bubble as a monomer, thereby generating a nucleation point for the multimerization of additional Rev molecules through both protein-protein and protein-RNA interactions.[253, 258–260] HTLV-1, an evolutionarily and biologically distinct retrovirus from HIV, encodes a transactivating protein, Rex, which can functionally substitute for HIV Rev (see Chapter 28). In contrast to Rev, however, HTLV-1 Rex binds to stem loops 4 and 5 of the HIV-1 RRE (see Fig. 27–13) rather than to stem loop 2.[261, 262] Although not yet developed into usable antiviral agents, some aminoglycosides have been shown both to block the binding of HIV Rev to its RRE target and to inhibit the production of progeny virions.[263]

Mutations affecting either the RNA binding or the leucine-rich domains of the Rev protein result in loss of function. Thus, mutants mapping to the leucine-rich region are able to bind to the RRE but are functionally inactive. They interfere with the transactivation mediated by wild-type Rev, exerting a *trans*-dominant effect in assays for Rev function.[243, 264, 265]

Rev-deficient HIV mutants are unable to synthesize the Gag, Pol, and Env viral proteins. Although the total viral RNA levels are normal in cells infected with Rev mutants, the *gag/pol, env, vif,* and *vpr* mRNAs are either absent or markedly underrepresented in the cytoplasm, whereas the completely spliced *tat, rev,* and *nef* mRNAs are usually the only species detected in that cellular compartment.[237, 239, 241, 266] This pattern of RNA expression initially led to proposals that the function of the Rev protein might be to regulate the splicing, facilitate the transport, counter the intrinsic instability, or augment the translation of RRE-containing HIV RNAs. For example, it was known that regions within the *gag, pol,* and *env* HIV RNAs contain sequences (designated IR in Fig. 27–5) that severely inhibit the expression of covalently linked reporter genes by altering RNA transport to the cytoplasm or decreasing RNA stability.[245, 267, 268] Rev is able to reverse these effects, provided that the RRE is present in such transcripts.

It should be noted that a constitutive transport element (CTE) from the genomes of type D retroviruses such as Mason-Pfizer monkey virus (M-PMU), and simian retrovirus 1, can functionally substitute for the Rev protein and facilitate the nuclear export of unspliced or partially spliced HIV RNAs.[269, 270] Mutational and biochemical analyses have shown that the CTE is an extended 165 nt stem loop containing two internal bubble structures that are rotated 180° relative to one another.[271, 272] CTEs presumably bind to cellular factors that mediate nucleocytoplasmic transport.

Subsequent evaluations of the HIV RNA expression pattern showed that the ratios of unspliced (or partially spliced) to completely spliced viral transcripts in the nucleus did not change in the presence or absence of Rev.[239, 241]

REV PROTEIN

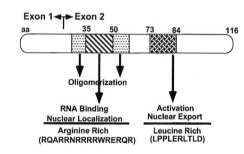

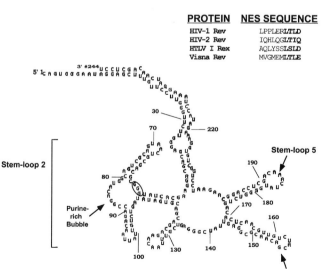

Figure 27–13. Rev and Its Response Element, RRE. A schematic representation of the HIV-I Rev protein with RNA-binding, activation, and oligomerization domains is shown at the top. The structure of the RRE is presented at the bottom with the targets of HIV-I Rev (stem loop 2) and HTLV I Rex (stem loops 4 and 5) indicated. The "bulged" G residues are circled. The sequence of the leucine-rich nuclear export signal (NES) present in other retroviral Rev/Rex proteins is also shown.

Rather, the hallmark of insufficient Rev expression was a superabundance of the 1.7 to 2.0 kb completely spliced RNAs and greatly reduced or no detectable RRE-containing mRNAs only in the cytoplasmic compartment.

Because the splicing of viral RNA in the nucleus was not affected by Rev, attention shifted to the role of Rev in HIV RNA transport. The first unambiguous demonstration that Rev could promote the nuclear export of viral RNA was in experiments in which purified Rev protein and RRE-containing RNA molecules were microinjected into cell nuclei.[273, 274] These studies showed that the RRE-containing unspliced RNA substrates were transported to the cytoplasm only in the presence of Rev. Interestingly, the excised exon (containing the RRE element), derived from other transcripts that did undergo splicing, was also detected in the cytoplasm, indicating that Rev was able to mediate nuclear export without inhibiting RNA splicing.[275] Subsequent microinjection studies revealed that the leucine-rich Rev domain was indeed a nuclear export signal (NES) because when it was fused to bovine serum albumin (BSA), it promoted the transport of the NES/BSA complex into the cytoplasm.[273, 274] NES/BSA fusion proteins, containing a mutated, non-functional leucine-rich Rev domain, remained in the nucleus after microinjection. The nuclear export mediated by the Rev NES in these studies was also shown to be energy dependent and blocked by high concentrations of NES/BSA, implying that the amounts of nucleocytoplasmic transporting proteins were limiting. Surprisingly, the nuclear to cytoplasmic transport of 5S ribosomal RNA (rRNA) and spliceosomal U small nuclear RNAs (snRNAs), but not Pol II–derived cellular mRNAs, was also inhibited by high concentrations of NES/BSA conjugates. Taken together, these results are consistent with the Rev effector domain's functioning as a nuclear export signal that directs RRE-containing viral RNAs to the cytoplasm via a pathway not used by cellular mRNAs.

The bidirectional passage of proteins between the nucleus and cytoplasm occurs through the nuclear pore complex and depends on the presence of NLS and NES transport signals. The energy-dependent and saturable properties of this process implied the participation of transport "receptor" factors. For nuclear import, the interaction of proteins bearing an NLS with members of the β importin family mediated their transport to, and translocation through, the nuclear pore.[276] Studies of HIV Rev and related viral and cellular proteins bearing leucine-rich NES motifs (see Fig. 27–13, middle) have been at the forefront in elucidating the analogous receptor proteins involved in nuclear export. The latter have again turned out to be β importin family members, the best studied of which is called chromosome region maintenance 1 (CRM1) or exportin 1.[277, 278] The energy required for transport in and out of the nucleus is provided by the small guanosine triphosphatase (GTPase) Ran and associated proteins.[279]

One of the earliest reports linking the Rev NES mechanistically to the nuclear export machinery showed that the antibiotic leptomycin B blocked the nuclear export of Rev-dependent RNAs in HeLa cells and human PBMCs.[280] A follow-up study, carried out in *Xenopus* oocytes, showed that leptomycin B inhibited the transport of both the Rev protein and several U snRNAs out of the nucleus.[277] Additional reports demonstrating that leptomycin B binds directly to CRM1 and that overexpression of CRM1 eliminates the

leptomycin B blockade of Rev NES nuclear export, implicated Crm 1 as the long-sought "export receptor" for proteins containing the leucine-rich NES. This conclusion was supported by studies showing that CRM1/exportin (1) shuttled between the nucleus and cytoplasm, (2) possessed a Ran(GTP) binding domain, and (3) interacted with the phenylalanine-glycine (FG) repeats present in nucleoporin proteins.[277, 278, 281] All of this work was consistent with exportin forming a trimeric complex (Rev NES/CRM1/Ran[GTP]) that interacted with nucleoporins during egress from the nucleus. Although other Rev-interacting factors[282–284] have been reported, their role(s) in Rev function remains to be elucidated.

The role of Rev in nuclear to cytoplasmic transport of unspliced or partially spliced HIV RNAs is shown diagrammatically in Figure 27–14. During the early, postintegration phase of the virus life cycle, the HIV pre-mRNA transported to the cytoplasm consists almost entirely of intronless transcripts encoding the Tat, Rev, and Nef proteins. When sufficient quantities of newly synthesized Rev accumulate in the nucleus, Rev multimers, assembled on RRE-containing viral RNAs, cooperatively interact with exportin and the GTP-bound form of Ran. This complex is then translocated through the nuclear pore to the cytoplasm, where it is dissociated by Ran(GTP)-associated proteins (Ran Gap and RanBP1[279, 285]). The unspliced and partially spliced HIV-1 RNA "cargo" released in the cytoplasm is incorporated into progeny virions or translated into viral proteins. The HIV Rev protein utilizes its NLS, which binds to importin β, to shuttle back into the nucleus, where Rev is released from the complex after the interaction of importin β with Ran(GTP). In this transport scheme, the higher concentrations of Ran(GTP) in the nucleus facilitates the formation of the Rev NES/exportin export complex and dissociates the Rev NLS/importin β complex.

▼ HUMAN IMMUNODEFICIENCY VIRUS–ENCODED STRUCTURAL AND OTHER NON-REGULATORY PROTEINS

Gag

Most enveloped virus particles consist of a nucleocapsid core surrounded by an outer lipoprotein shell or envelope. The retrovirus core is encoded by the group specific antigen (*gag*) gene, which, in the case of HIV, directs the synthesis of a 55 kDa Gag precursor. This polyprotein (also known as p55) is released from cells as a component of the immature virus particle and is ultimately cleaved by the viral protease (PR) into the mature 17 kDa matrix (MA), 24 kDa capsid (CA), 7 kDa nucleocapsid (NC) protein and the Pro-rich C-terminal p6 protein (see Fig. 27–4*A*).[286, 287] As noted previously, the mRNA for p55 is the unspliced 9.2 kb transcript (see Fig. 27–11), which requires Rev for its expression in the cytoplasm. Retroviral Gag proteins have three principal functions during virus assembly: (1) forming the structural inner framework of the virion, (2) encapsidating the viral genome, and (3) acquiring a lipid bilayer and associated glycoproteins during particle release. These processes require that Gag proteins participate in protein/protein, protein/RNA, and protein/lipid interactions. As is the case for other replication competent retroviruses, the HIV-1 Gag proteins

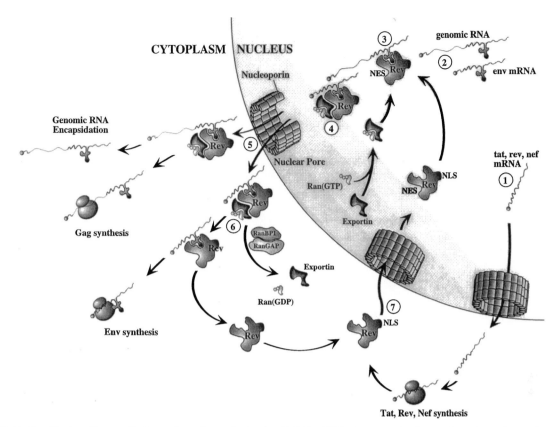

Figure 27–14. Rev Nuclear Export Pathway. Intronless multiply spliced HIV-1 mRNAs (*tat, rev,* and *nef*) use a Rev-independent pathway to exit the nucleus *(1)*. When sufficient amounts of Rev accumulate in the nucleus, Rev multimers bind to RRE-containing unspliced or partially spliced viral mRNAs *(2* and *3)*. Rev/RRE RNAs then bind to a complex consisting of exportin associated with the GTP-bound form of RAN *(4)* and are transported to and translocated through the nuclear pore *(5)*. In the cytoplasm *(6)*, RanBP1/Ran GAP mediate the dissociation of exportin/Ran(GDP) from Rev/RRE RNA. After the removal of Rev from intron containing HIV-1 transcripts, the full-length viral RNA may be encapsidated into progeny virions and other mRNAs may be translated into viral proteins. Using its nuclear localization signal (NLS), Rev recycles back into the nucleus *(7)* in association with importin β.

are critical for virus assembly and release, virion stability, and many of the early steps in the subsequent replication cycle, including uncoating, reverse transcription, and integration.[288]

The HIV p55 Gag precursor oligomerizes after its translation and is targeted to the plasma membrane, where particle assembly is initiated. In most cell types, lentiviruses and the C-type oncoretroviruses assemble progeny virions at the plasma membrane. In contrast, B- and D-type retrovirus particles are formed in the cytoplasm and are subsequently transported to the plasma membrane, where they are released from the cell. Particle formation by all types of retrotransposable elements is a self-assembly process[289, 290]; in the case of HIV-1, particles have been generated in vaccinia, baculovirus, and SV40 expression systems.[291–295] Only the Gag precursor polypeptide is needed for particle formation[296]; there is no requirement for genomic RNA or the envelope, reverse transcriptase, or protease proteins. However, the production of *infectious* virions requires the copackaging with Gag of the Env glycoproteins, the viral RNA genome, and the Gag-Pol polyprotein precursor Pr160. Proteolytic processing by PR subsequent to budding results in the condensation of the immature nucleoid into the cone-shaped core characteristic of mature HIV particles (see Fig. 27–1*B*).

Matrix

The matrix (MA) domain of p55 (Fig. 27–15*A*) serves several important functions in the viral life cycle. After Gag

synthesis, MA directs p55 to the plasma membrane via a multipartite membrane binding signal. The affinity of the MA domain for membrane is provided in part by a myristic acid moiety covalently attached to the N-terminal Gly of MA (see Fig. 27–15*A*). Mutation of this residue significantly impairs binding of Gag to membrane and abolishes virus assembly in most systems.[297–300] Sequences in MA downstream of the myristate group also contribute to membrane binding. Structural studies of HIV-1 MA (as well as MA of BLV, HTLV-2, and M-PMV) suggest that a highly basic patch of residues clusters on the face of MA that is predicted to juxtapose the lipid bilayer.[301–306] It has been proposed that these basic residues interact with the negatively charged acidic phospholipids on the inner leaflet of the lipid bilayer, thereby stabilizing membrane interaction.[302, 307] Mutations affecting these basic residues can be detrimental to virus assembly.[307–309] The mechanism by which Gag traffics and binds specifically to the plasma membrane rather than intracellular membranes is still unclear. Deletion of a large portion of MA,[310] as well as single amino acid changes near the center of the protein,[300] cause virus assembly to be redirected to cytoplasmic compartments.

After Gag binds the plasma membrane, it assembles into particles that bud from the cell. During the process of budding, the viral Env glycoproteins are incorporated into the nascent virions. MA seems to play a crucial role in this process as well; small deletions,[311] insertions,[312] and specific point mutations[313, 314] in MA block Env incorporation without

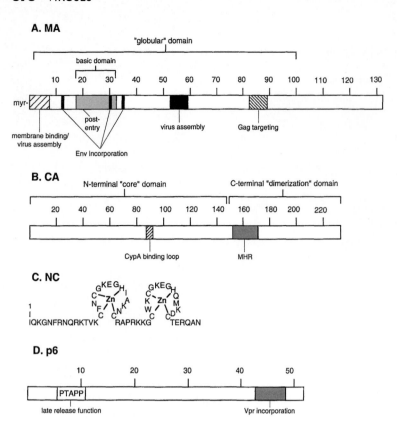

A. MA

Figure 27–15. Linear Representation of the HIV-1 Gag Proteins, with Domains Indicated. Amino acid positions are shown over each diagram. *A*, MA: domains in which point mutations affect virus assembly, membrane binding, Gag targeting, postentry steps, and Env incorporation are shown. The region of MA that forms the main globular domain is indicated; the C-terminus of MA projects away from the plane of the membrane. *B*, CA: The N-terminal "core" and C-terminal "dimerization" domains, visualized by structural analyses, are indicated. The CypA binding region and MHR are shown. *C*, NC: The amino acid sequence is indicated and the two zinc finger domains are shown. *D*, p6: The N-terminal region involved in virus release, and the C-terminal Vpr-interacting sequence are indicated. (From Freed, E. O.: HIV-1 Gag proteins: Diverse functions in the virus life cycle. Virology 251:1, 1998; with permission.)

perturbing assembly and release. Interestingly, the block to Env incorporation imposed by MA mutations can be reversed by pseudotyping virions with heterologous Env glycoproteins containing short cytoplasmic tails, or by removing sequences within the long cytoplasmic tail of the HIV-1 TM glycoprotein gp41.[313–315] These results suggest that a specific interaction takes place between MA and gp41. Although a direct interaction has been difficult to demonstrate in virus-infected cells, in vitro data supporting a direct MA/gp41 interaction have been reported.[316] X-ray crystallographic analysis of MA structure suggests that MA may form trimers that assemble into a higher-order lattice containing holes into which the long cytoplasmic tail of gp41 could insert.[302]

In addition to its function in virus assembly and Env incorporation, MA has also been proposed to play a role early in the virus life cycle, after Env-induced membrane fusion between the lipid bilayers of the viral envelope and the host cell plasma membrane. These early postfusion steps, which are collectively referred to as uncoating, are poorly understood, and it is not clear mechanistically what role MA might play in this process. However, it has been observed that mutations in MA impair the synthesis of viral DNA early post infection, suggesting an early postentry block.[317–319] It has also been observed that MA mutants with this "early" defect display impaired endogenous RT activity and increased Gag membrane binding.[319]

Lentiviruses, including HIV-1, are unique among retroviruses in their ability to infect non-dividing cells. It has been proposed that the basic domain of MA, discussed above in the context of membrane binding, plays a role in translocating the viral preintegration complex to the nucleus.[320–322] It was also reported that phosphorylation of a Tyr residue at the C-terminus of MA is required for infectivity in

fully differentiated (non-dividing) macrophages.[323] However, many aspects of this work have not been widely reproduced,[309, 324–328] leaving in question the role of MA in nuclear localization of the viral preintegration complex.

Capsid

Like MA, capsid (CA) has been implicated both in late (assembly and release) and early steps in virus replication. Mutations within CA produce a range of phenotypes: Those in the C-terminal third of the protein elicit assembly defects,[329–331] whereas more N-terminal changes generally do not affect the efficiency of virus production, but rather inhibit proper virion maturation after release and severely impair infectivity.[330–333] These results have led to the proposal that the C-terminus of CA promotes Gag multimerization, whereas the N-terminus plays a role in core condensation and morphogenesis. The major homology region (MHR), which is highly conserved among retroviral CA proteins, is located near the middle of CA (see Fig. 27–15*B*). Mutations in this domain disrupt virus assembly, maturation, and infectivity.[334]

Using a yeast two-hybrid system, it was demonstrated that HIV-1 Gag binds members of the cyclophilin family of proteins, which function in the cell as peptidyl-prolyl *cis-trans*-isomerases.[335] Further investigation indicated that one of these proteins, cyclophilin A, is specifically incorporated into HIV-1 virions[336, 337]; this incorporation is mediated by an interaction between cyclophilin A and a proline-rich region near amino acid 90 of CA.[337] Treatment of infected cells with cyclosporin A or its analogues or mutation of CA residues that participate in the interaction blocks the incorporation of cyclophilin A into virions and reduces virus infectivity. Mutant or drug-treated virions, which are impaired for cyclophilin A incorporation, are blocked at an early step in the virus life cycle, apparently after membrane fusion but before the initiation of reverse transcription.[338] Unfortunately, although cyclosporin A and its analogues impair virus infectivity, variants that are resistant to, or even dependent upon, the drugs quickly emerge.[339] Although currently available data suggest that cyclophilin A complexed with CA enhances virion infectivity, the mechanism by which this occurs is unclear.

At this time, structural data for the entire CA protein have not been obtained. However, solution NMR and X-ray crystallographic information is available for two domains of CA: the N-terminal "core" domain (residues 1–145)[340–342] and the C-terminal "dimerization" domain (residues 151–231)[343] (see Fig. 27–15B). Both domains are globular, with a high helical content. Residues 146–151 appear to assist in forming a high-affinity capsid interface, which, in conjunction with a more N-terminal β-hairpin interface, is postulated to drive the formation of higher-order CA interactions during assembly. In the crystal, the CA assembles into continuous planar strips.[340] Cyclophilin A binds an exposed loop formed by CA residues 85–93.[340] The MHR forms a complex hydrogen bonding network that may stabilize the overall structure of the C-terminal domain.[343]

Several studies have reported that HIV-1 CA, when expressed in vitro, is capable of assembling into tubular or spherical particles.[344, 345] CA-NC fusion proteins form tubular structures in vitro at protein concentrations lower than those required to form similar particles with CA alone; in the case of CA-NC, tube formation appears to be dependent upon the presence of RNA.[346] Interestingly, adding as few as four residues of MA to the N-terminus of CA converts in vitro particle formation from cylinders to spheres. This observation led to the suggestion that PR-mediated processing at the MA-CA junction causes a major refolding of the N-terminal portion of CA and that this refolding is critical in promoting the morphological changes that occur during core condensation.[345]

Nucleocapsid

The third major domain synthesized as part of the Gag precursor is the nucleocapsid (NC) (see Fig. 27–15C). The principal function of NC involves the specific encapsidation of full-length, unspliced (genomic) RNA into virions, although, as is the case with the other Gag proteins, NC appears to serve multiple functions during the virus life cycle. With the exception of the spumaretroviruses, all retroviral NC proteins contain one or two zinc finger motifs. Unlike most cellular zinc finger domains, those of retroviruses are of the CCHC type (Cys-X_2-Cys-X_4-His-X_4-Cys, where X is any amino acid). HIV-1 NC contains two zinc finger motifs, which bind zinc tightly both in vitro and in virions.[347] Mutations that abrogate zinc binding abolish genome encapsidation and virus infectivity.[348] Other mutations within the zinc finger domains increase the level of spliced versus unspliced viral RNA encapsidated into virions.[349] NC also contains two clusters of basic residues flanking the first zinc finger; mutations in these basic sequences impair the binding of NC to RNA in vitro[350] and RNA encapsidation into virions.[351] The specificity of genome encapsidation results from an interaction between NC and an approximately 120 nucleotide sequence located between the 5′ LTR and the Gag initiation codon (see Fig. 27–5). This sequence, known as the packaging signal or ψ site, folds into a series of four stem loops. It appears that this secondary structure, rather than the primary nucleotide sequence itself, confers RNA encapsidation specificity.[352] Recently, the structure of the HIV-1 NC protein complexed with a portion of the ψ site was determined by NMR spectroscopy.[353]

Many HIV-1 NC mutations cause defects in virus assembly and release,[354, 355] and a heterologous sequence known to mediate protein-protein interactions has been reported to replace NC functionally in virus assembly.[356] These results suggest a role for NC in Gag multimerization, a function mapping largely to the N-terminal basic domain, rather than the zinc fingers.[293, 332, 357] Furthermore, NC appears to play a role in the tight packing of Gag in virions, leading to the production of particles with a density characteristic of retroviral particles.[358] It is suspected that NC-RNA interactions are critical for promoting Gag multimerization; according to this model, RNA provides a template along which molecules of p55 can align and pack.[346] The apparent role of both NC and CA (discussed above) in Gag multimerization implies that assembly of HIV-1 particles involves cooperative interactions between multiple domains within the Gag precursor.

In addition to its roles in RNA encapsidation and Gag assembly, other functions for HIV-1 NC have been observed. For example, retroviral NC proteins have long been known to possess nucleic acid annealing properties.[359] This aspect of NC function contributes to RNA dimerization, binding of the tRNA^{Lys} primer to the primer binding site, initiation of reverse transcription from the tRNA^{Lys} primer, and strand transfers during reverse transcription.[359–361] Mutations in NC also reportedly affect virion structure[362] and impair early steps in the virus life cycle, apparently by destabilizing newly reverse transcribed viral DNA.[363] Interestingly, studies conducted with the Moloney murine leukemia virus demonstrated that changing the single CCHC zinc finger motif to CCCC or CCHH had no effect on zinc binding or RNA encapsidation but profoundly impaired virus infectivity. Again, the block appeared to impair an early step post infection.[364]

Because NC participates in multiple steps in the virus life cycle, and because the retroviral CCHC-type zinc finger motif is relatively rare among cellular proteins, NC presents an attractive target for antivirals. Promising anti-NC compounds include the disulfide benzamides that cause zinc to be "ejected" from retroviral zinc fingers at low micromolar concentrations.[365–367] These compounds effectively inhibit virus replication in culture without significant cytotoxicity. Recently 14 compounds that demonstrated anti-NC activity in vitro were tested for their effect on MuLV replication in vivo. One of these compounds, aldrithiol 2, delayed the onset of MuLV-induced disease and reduced virus loads in infected mice.[368]

p6

In addition to the MA, CA, and NC domains described above, retroviral *gag* genes encode a variety of open reading frames that are generally unique to a particular genus of retroviruses.[296] HIV-1 encodes a Pro-rich 6 kDa protein, known as p6, at the C-terminus of Pr55^{Gag} (see Figs. 27–4A and 27–15D). Mutation of p6, specifically within a highly conserved Pro-Thr-Ala-Pro-Pro (PTAPP) motif, has been reported to block a late step in virus assembly such that virions accumulate at the plasma membrane but fail to release efficiently.[369, 370] Interestingly, mutation of PR largely reverses this defect,[370] suggesting a functional interplay between p6 and PR function, and perhaps explaining why some groups, using Gag-only expression systems, failed to detect a requirement for p6 in virus assembly. p6 also functions to direct the incorporation of Vpr into virions.[371, 372]

In addition to HIV-1 p6, domains encoded by other retroviral Gag proteins serve analogous "late" functions in virus release. These include p2b of Rous sarcoma virus[373] and p9 of equine infectious anemia virus (EIAV).[374] Interestingly, these "late" domains appear to function independently of their position in Gag and can be exchanged from one retrovirus to another.[375] It has been proposed that these proteins interact with host cell plasma membrane proteins, thereby facilitating the final release step during virus budding.[376]

Pol

Downstream of *gag* lies the most highly conserved region of the HIV genome, the *pol* gene, which encodes three enzymes: protease (PR), reverse transcriptase (RT)/RNaseH, and integrase (IN) (see Fig. 27–4A). The functions of RT and IN are required for several events during the early steps of virus infection; PR plays a critical role late in the life cycle by mediating the production of mature, infectious virions. In most retroviruses, the *pol* gene products are derived by enzymatic cleavage of a Gag-Pol fusion protein (160 kDa in size for HIV). This fusion protein (also referred to as Gag-Pro-Pol) is produced either by ribosomal frameshifting (the most common mechanism) or termination suppression (the mechanism used by the mammalian type C retroviruses). In some retroviruses (e.g., M-PMV and HTLV) the gene encoding PR lies in a reading frame distinct from both *gag* and *pol*; in such cases two frameshifting events are required to enter *pol*. The frameshifting or suppression of termination mechanism for Gag-Pol expression ensures that the *pol*-derived proteins are expressed at a low level, approximately 5–10 per cent that of Gag.[377, 378] If the requirement for frameshifting in the HIV genome is eliminated by the insertion of a single nucleotide, the Gag-Pol precursor is overexpressed. This results in the proteolytic processing of the Gag and Gag-Pol polyproteins intracellularly, the release of free CA and RT from cells, and a block in the production of progeny virions.[379] Like p55 Gag, the N-terminus of the Gag-Pol fusion protein is myristylated and targeted to the plasma membrane.

Protease

The sequence encoding the retroviral protease (PR) is always located between the *gag* and *pol* genes; in the HIV genome, it is encoded by the *pol* open reading frame (see Fig. 27–4A). In the avian type C oncoretroviruses, PR is expressed as part of the Gag precursor.[296] The proteolytic digestion of the Gag and Pol precursors is required to generate infectious virions, a process that occurs during or immediately after particle

release. PR-mutant HIV-1 virions are non-infectious and appear doughnut-shaped in the electron microscope (EM), lacking the bullet shaped core characteristic of mature virions (see Fig. 27–1B).[380, 381] Retroviral PRs are related to cellular "aspartic" proteases such as renin, using two apposed Asp residues to coordinate a water molecule that catalyzes the hydrolysis of a peptide bond in the target protein.[382, 383] Because of their small size relative to that of cellular aspartic proteases, retroviral proteases function as dimers, with each monomer forming half of the active site.[384, 385] Crystallography of HIV-1 PR indicates that the substrate binding site is located within a cleft formed between the two monomers.[386, 387] Like their cellular homologues, the HIV PR dimer contains "flaps" that overhang the binding site and may stabilize the substrate within the cleft; the active site Asp residues lie in the center of the dimer.

The PR cleavage sites in retroviral Gag and Gag-Pol precursors are not identical. The proteolytic processing of model proteins and substrate analogues by the HIV PR indicates that the binding cleft can accommodate a peptide approximately seven residues in length; synthetic peptides of this size are cleaved in vitro.[388–390] The cleavage of different scissile bonds within the p55 polyprotein by HIV PR is highly ordered; processing at the amino terminus of NC is the most rapid in vitro, whereas the cleavage converting p25 to p24 CA is the slowest.[391, 392] Mutations in Gag that disrupt the ordered nature of PR-mediated processing severely disrupt virus assembly.[393–395] Furthermore, HIV-1 mutants engineered to synthesize a linked PR dimer (i.e., a duplicated PR-coding region) exhibit rapid, premature processing of Gag and Gag-Pol polyproteins and a block in virus production.[396]

Compounds that inhibit HIV-1 PR function have proved to be the most effective antiviral drugs developed to date. The PR inhibitor saquinavir (also known as Ro 31–8959) mimics a sequence frequently found at Gag and Gag-Pol cleavage sites. The interaction of this peptidomimetic compound with PR locks it in a transition state configuration that renders PR inactive at low drug concentrations.[397, 398] When PR inhibitors are used to treat HIV-infected patients, virus loads decline precipitously, but drug-resistant variants soon emerge. Longer-lasting benefits are achieved with so-called triple therapy, in which a PR inhibitor (e.g., indinavir or saquinavir) is combined with two RT inhibitors (e.g., zidovudine [AZT] and lamivudine [3TC]) (see below).

Reverse Transcriptase

By definition, retroviruses possess the ability to convert their single-stranded RNA genomes into double-stranded DNA after infection.[399, 400] The enzyme that catalyzes this reaction is reverse transcriptase (RT), in conjunction with its associated RNAse H activity. The mature HIV-1 RT holoenzyme is a heterodimer of 66 and 51 kDa subunits; the 51 kDa subunit is derived from the N-terminus of the 66 kDa subunit (see Figs. 27–4A and Fig. 27–16A). Retroviral RTs have three enzymatic activities: (1) RNA-directed DNA polymerase (for "negative" strand DNA synthesis), (2) RNase H (for degradation of the genomic RNA present in DNA/RNA hybrid intermediates), and (3) DNA-directed DNA polymerase (for second or "positive" strand DNA synthesis

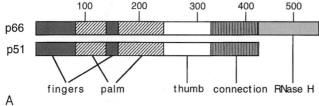

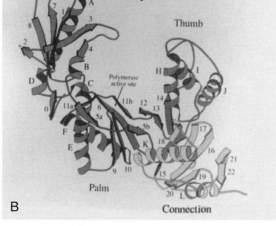

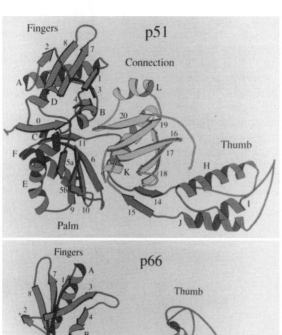

Figure 27–16. Structure of HIV-1 RT. *A*, Linear representation of the major domains within p66 and p51. *B*, Ribbon diagram of p66 and p51, with functional domains indicated. β sheets are numbered, and α helices are indicated by letter. Reprinted with permission. (From Jacobo-Molina, A., Ding, J., Nanni, R. G., Clark, A. D., Jr., Lu, X., Tantillo, C., Williams, R. L., Kamer, G., Ferris, A. L., Clark, P., Hizi, A., Hughes, S. H., and Arnold, E.: Crystal structure of human immunodeficiency virus type 1 reverse transcriptase complexed with double-stranded DNA at 3.0 Å resolution shows bent DNA. Proc. Natl. Acad. Sci. USA 90:6320, 1993; with permission.)

to generate a double-stranded DNA substrate for integration). As is true for other DNA polymerase reactions, reverse transcription is primer dependent; retroviruses employ specific tRNAs for this function. HIV and the other lentivirus RTs utilize tRNA^{Lys}, which binds to the primer binding site (*pbs* in Fig. 27–5) to initiate negative strand DNA synthesis.

The 560 residue p66 subunit of HIV-1 RT contains all the sequence information needed for enzymatic activity: an N-terminal 166 amino acid polymerase domain and a C-terminal ~120 amino acid RNase H domain.[401–405] The pro-

teolytic cleavage (by the HIV PR) of the RNase H domain from one subunit of the p66 homodimer generates a functional RT heterodimer. Even though each subunit possesses an intact active site for the DNA polymerization reaction, both monomeric forms of the HIV RT are enzymatically inert.[406] The processed p66/p51 heterodimer has 10 times greater polymerizing activity than the p66 homodimer, reflecting the possible steric hindrance of an extra 15 kDa RNase H domain. The p51 homodimer has virtually no measurable RT activity.[401, 407–411] The elucidation of the crystal structure of HIV-1 RT indicates that the p66/p51 heterodimer is an asymmetrical structure containing single active DNA polymerizing, RNase H, and tRNA binding sites.[412] The 66 kDa domain can be visualized as a right hand, with the polymerase active site within the palm and the template-binding cleft formed by the palm, fingers, and thumb[413, 414] (see Fig. 27–16B). The p51 subunit does not form a polymerizing cleft, and the two aspartic acid residues constituting its active site are buried within the molecule.

The high rate of variation among HIV populations poses one of the fundamental challenges to effective control of this pathogen.[415, 416] Retroviruses are highly variable because of (1) the error-prone nature of the enzymatic activity of RT, which lacks exonucleolytic proofreading activity, and (2) high rates of recombination. Retroviral mutation rates have been measured both in vitro[417, 418] and in vivo.[419–422] The in vitro mutation rate for HIV-1 RT is approximately 40-fold higher than the in vivo rate, suggesting that the in vitro reaction lacks factor(s) that increase fidelity.[419] The total HIV-1 in vivo mutation rate (a composite of substitutions, frameshifts, simple deletions, and deletions with insertions) was measured at 3×10^{-5} per cycle of replication. Since the HIV-1 genome is approximately 10 kbp in length, this corresponds to 0.3 errors per genome per cycle of replication.[419] Using similar methods, in vivo mutation rates for other retroviruses (e.g., spleen necrosis virus, murine leukemia virus, and bovine leukosis virus) were observed to be between 2-fold and 10-fold lower than that of HIV-1.[416]

As discussed above, retroviral virions contain two copies of single-stranded RNA. Template switching, which is an essential element of reverse transcription, appears to have selected for a low affinity between RT and template.[423] As a result, *intermolecular* template switches (from one RNA to the other) occur frequently during reverse transcription.[415] Template switching can occur when RT encounters a break in the template ("forced copy choice")[424] or can occur in the absence of strand breaks.[425] These intermolecular template jumps, which do not require homology between the two RNAs, lead to high levels of recombination and significantly contribute to high genomic variability.

RT has long been a target in the search for antiviral compounds. Several have been developed, including the nucleoside analogues (e.g., 3′-azido-3′-deoxythymidine [AZT or zidovudine], dideoxyinosine [ddI], and dideoxycytidine [ddC]) and the nonnucleoside inhibitors (e.g., nevirapine). Unfortunately, resistance to these compounds develops rapidly in patients. Mutations affecting two regions of RT were associated with isolates that exhibited reduced sensitivity to AZT.[426–428] On the basis of the crystallographic data, these revertant changes would be predicted to affect the interaction of RT with the RNA template.[412] In vitro, the degree of AZT resistance can be correlated with amino acid substitutions in the RT; partially resistant isolates have subsets of the four mutations. The picture is not as clear-cut in vivo because of the presence of genotypic mixtures of HIV with variable sensitivities to AZT.

Integrase

A hallmark of retrovirus replication is the insertion of a DNA copy of the viral genome (the product of reverse transcription) into the host cell chromosome. The integrated viral DNA (the "provirus") serves as the template for the synthesis of viral RNAs and is maintained as part of the host cell genome for the lifetime of the infected cell. Integration is required for the establishment of a productive infection; retroviral mutants deficient in the ability to integrate into the host cell chromosome are non-infectious in all target cell types, including primary monocyte-derived macrophages.[91, 429]

The integration of viral DNA is mediated by integrase (IN), a 32 kDa protein generated by proteolytic cleavage of the C-terminal portion of the HIV-1 Gag-Pol polyprotein (see Fig. 27–4A). Unintegrated, flush-ended linear viral DNA is the immediate precursor to integrated proviral DNA.[85, 430] In all retroviral systems, integration proceeds in four steps (Fig. 27–17): (1) in a reaction known as 3'-end processing, IN removes two nucleotides from the 3' termini of both strands of full-length viral DNA, generating a preintegration substrate with 3'-recessed ends; (2) IN catalyzes a staggered cleavage of the cellular target; (3) in a strand transfer reaction, the 3' recessed ends of viral DNA are joined to the 5' "overhanging" termini of the cleaved cellular DNA; and (4) cellular repair machinery fills the gap, thereby completing the integration reaction.[431–435] The integrated HIV provirus is flanked by a 5 bp direct repeat and terminates with the dinucleotides 5'-TG and CA-3'.

Retroviral IN proteins are composed of three distinct domains: an N-terminal zinc-finger-containing domain, a core domain, and a relatively non-conserved C-terminal domain (Fig. 27–18). The N-terminal domain has been shown to bind zinc[436]; binding to this ion appears to stabilize IN

INTEGRATION OF HIV DNA

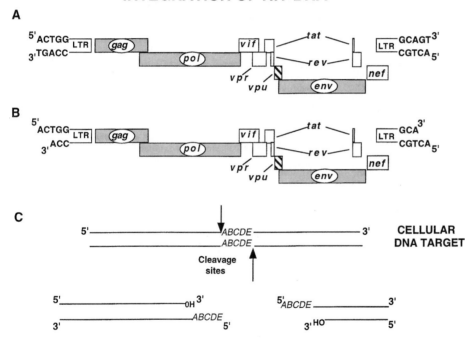

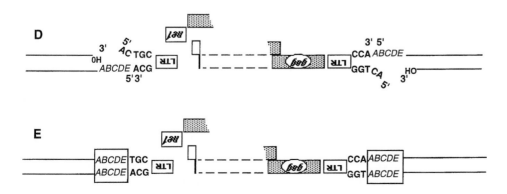

Figure 27–17. Integration of HIV-1 DNA. Two nucleotides are removed from the 3' ends of each strand of the full-length viral DNA by HIV IN (A and B), and 5 bp staggered cuts are made in the cellular DNA target (C). The recessed ends of the viral DNA are then joined to the protruding termini of the digested cellular DNA (D), and the remaining "gap" is filled in by cellular repair enzymes (E). The 5 bp "target site duplication" in cellular DNA is boxed.

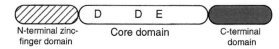

Figure 27–18. Linear Representation of HIV-1 IN. The N-terminal zinc finger domain, core domain, and C-terminal domain are shown, as are the highly conserved Asp and Glu residues that form the D-D-35-E motif.

structure, promote IN multimerization, and enhance catalytic activity.[437] Because of solubility problems, it has not yet been possible to crystallize the entire 288 amino acid HIV-1 IN protein. However, the crystal structure of the catalytically active core (amino acid residues 50–212) of HIV-1 IN has been determined.[438] The crystal structure of the core domain of Rous sarcoma virus (RSV) IN has also been solved.[439] Each monomer of HIV-1 IN is composed of a five-stranded β sheet flanked by helices; this structure bears striking resemblance to other polynucleotidyl transferases including RNase H and the bacteriophage MuA transposase.[438, 440] Three highly conserved residues are found in analogous positions in other polynucleotidyl transferases; in HIV-1 IN these are Asp[64,] Asp[116,] and Glu[152,] the so-called D,D-35-E motif (see Fig. 27–18). Mutations at these positions block integration both in vivo and in vitro.[441, 442] It is currently not clear what role the C-terminal region of IN plays; it exhibits DNA-binding activity and reportedly contains a bipartite nuclear localization sequence involved in the transport of viral DNA to the nucleus.[443]

During reverse transcription and transport of viral DNA to the nucleus, the viral nucleic acid remains associated with a high molecular weight complex composed of both viral and, presumably, cellular proteins.[84, 85] The complex that carries the viral DNA to the nucleus is referred to as the preintegration complex (PIC). Lentiviruses are unique among retroviruses in that the host cell does not have to pass through mitosis for productive infection to occur; the lentiviral PIC must therefore contain determinants that facilitate its transport to, and across, the nuclear membrane. Much effort has been directed at determining the composition of the HIV-1 PIC. Although controversy remains concerning the determinants of nuclear localization (see sections on MA and Vpr), some agreement has been reached on which viral proteins are found in the HIV-1 PIC.

In addition to RT and IN, MA, Vpr, and NC have been reported to be present in HIV-1 PICs, whereas CA is absent.[323, 444, 445] The non-histone chromosomal protein high-mobility groups (HMG) I(Y) can also be isolated from HIV-1 PICs,[446] and the human homologue of the yeast protein SNF5 stimulates HIV-1 IN activity in vitro.[447] The latter protein, which functions as a transcriptional activator, was postulated to promote integration by targeting viral DNA to transcriptionally active regions of the host chromosome.[447]

In in vitro assays, purified IN is capable of performing the 3'-end processing and strand transfer reactions and also catalyzes a reaction, known as disintegration, that in essence is the strand transfer reaction in reverse.[448] The disintegration reaction can also be carried out by the catalytic core of IN.[436] The development of in vitro assays to monitor IN activity makes it possible to screen for agents that block this critical step in the HIV life cycle.[85, 449–452] Several classes of agents inhibit IN activity in vitro; these include polyanions, nucleotide analogues, and DNA binding compounds.[452] PICs, iso-

lated from newly infected cells, are able to direct integration that more closely mimics the reaction occurring in infected cells (i.e., PICs direct the joining of both viral DNA termini to cellular DNA rather than only one end, as observed with purified IN). An evaluation of the effect of inhibitors on integration in vitro revealed that many compounds that blocked activity of purified IN were not inhibitory in assays using purified PICs.[453] Since PICs perform reactions that more faithfully reproduce authentic integration, and since they contain additional viral and cellular proteins, they should prove more useful than purified IN in identifying compounds that will exhibit anti-integration activity in vivo and in understanding the fundamentals of integration itself.

Env

The HIV envelope (Env) glycoproteins play a major role in the virus life cycle. They contain the determinants that (1) interact with the CD4 receptor and coreceptor, (2) mediate a fusion reaction between the lipid bilayer of the viral envelope and the host cell plasma membrane, and (3) specify the tropism for cells of the lymphocytic or monocyte/macrophage lineages. In addition, the HIV Env proteins contain epitopes that elicit immune responses that are important from both diagnostic and vaccine development perspectives.

The synthesis of the HIV Env is directed by the singly spliced 4.3 kb Vpu/Env bicistronic mRNA (see Fig. 27–11); translation occurs on polyribosomes associated with the rough endoplasmic reticulum (ER). The 160 kDa polyprotein precursor (gp160) is an integral membrane protein that is anchored to cell membranes by a hydrophobic stop-transfer signal in the domain destined to be the mature transmembrane (TM) envelope glycoprotein, gp41 (see Fig. 27–19). gp160 is cotranslationally glycosylated and rapidly undergoes oligomerization in the ER. Subsequently, gp160 is transported to the Golgi apparatus, where, like other retroviral envelope precursor proteins, it is proteolytically cleaved by cellular enzymes to the mature surface (SU) glycoprotein gp120 and TM glycoprotein gp41[454–457] (Fig. 27–19). The cellular enzyme responsible for cleavage of retroviral Env precursors after a highly conserved Lys/Arg-X-Lys/Arg-Arg motif is furin or a furin-like protease.[458] Cleavage of gp160 is required for Env-induced fusion activity and virus infectivity.[455, 457, 459] Subsequent to gp160 cleavage, gp120 and gp41 form a weak, non-covalent association that is critical for the transport of the Env complex from the Golgi apparatus to the cell surface.[459]

The HIV Env glycoprotein complex, in particular the SU (gp120) domain, is very heavily glycosylated. Approximately half the molecular mass of gp160 is composed of oligosaccharide side chains. Most of this glycosylation is N-linked (i.e., attached to Asn in Asn-X-Ser/Thr sequences), but O-linked glycosylation has also been reported.[460] As shown in Figure 27–19, gp120 contains interspersed conserved (C1 to C5) and variable (V1 to V5) domains.[461, 462] HIV-1 isolates of diverse geographic origin may exhibit >85% amino acid identity within conserved domains of gp120, whereas only 20% to 30% of the residues may be conserved within hypervariable regions.[462, 463] In contrast, the cysteines present in the gp120 of different isolates are highly conserved and form disulfide bonds that link the first four variable regions in large loops.[464] None of the disulfide

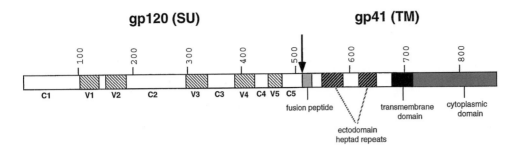

Figure 27–19. Linear Representation of HIV-1 Env Structure. The five variable (V1–V5) and conserved (C1–C5) domains of gp120 are indicated. In gp41, the fusion peptide, ectodomain heptad repeats, membrane-spanning (transmembrane) sequence, and cytoplasmic tail are shown. The arrow represents the site of gp160 cleavage to gp120 and gp41. Amino acid positions are indicated above the bar.

bonds joins gp120 to gp41. The gp120s of different HIV-1 isolates also contain more than 20 N-linked glycosylation sites, which are linked to complex or hybrid/high mannose-type oligosaccharides.[464]

The major cell-surface receptor for SIV/HIV is CD4, the first retroviral receptor protein identified.[24, 69, 465, 466] On T lymphocytes, the normal function of CD4 is to interact with class II major histocompatibility complex (MHC) molecules in class II MHC–restricted T-cell responses. CD4 is a 55 kDa member of the immunoglobulin (Ig) superfamily, consisting of a highly charged cytoplasmic domain, a single hydrophobic membrane-spanning domain, and four extracellular Ig-like domains.[467] The high-affinity CD4 binding site for gp120 has been localized to a small segment of the N-terminal extracellular domain, analogous to the second complementarity determining region (CDR-2) loop of an Ig kappa chain variable domain.[468–470] In vitro mutagenesis and antibody blocking studies have localized the CD4 binding determinant of Env to the C3 and C4 domains of gp120,[471–473] although a more discontinuous, conformation-dependent domain is clearly required for high-affinity gp120/CD4 binding.[473, 474] The recent crystallization of a gp120 "core" domain (from which variable loops had been removed) complexed with fragments of CD4 or a neutralizing antibody[475, 476] has further refined our understanding of the gp120/CD4 interaction. Of particular significance is the observation that the CD4 binding site in gp120 is deeply recessed and flanked by heavily glycosylated variable regions.[476]

The HIV-1 Env glycoprotein binds CD4 not only during the early phase of infection, but also during transport of Env to the surface of CD4-positive cells.[22] This intracellular association of gp160 and CD4 results in a downmodulation of CD4 from the cell surface; as a result, Env-expressing cells are partially resistant to further infection.[477] This process, known as superinfection interference, was described many years ago for other retroviruses.[478]

The identification of CD4 as the primary receptor for HIV raised the hope that soluble forms of CD4 (sCD4) might display antiviral effects in vivo. In fact, sCD4 can effectively inhibit syncytium formation and HIV infectivity in tissue culture systems, primarily by inducing gp120 shedding.[479] Unfortunately, this strong inhibitory effect is generally limited to laboratory-adapted isolates. Primary strains are neutralized poorly by sCD4, and sCD4 therapy of HIV infected individuals has little if any effect on the levels of p24 antigenemia or viremia.[480–482]

A primary function of viral Env glycoproteins, in addition to receptor binding, is to promote a membrane fusion reaction between the lipid bilayers of the viral envelope and

host cell membranes (Fig. 27–20). This membrane fusion event enables the viral nucleocapsid to gain entry into the host cell cytoplasm. A number of regions in both gp120 and gp41 have been implicated, directly or indirectly, in Env-mediated membrane fusion. Studies on the HA$_2$ hemagglutinin protein of the orthomyxoviruses and the F protein of the paramyxoviruses indicated that a highly hydrophobic domain at the N-terminus of these proteins, referred to as the "fusion peptide," played a critical role in membrane fusion.[483] Mutational analyses demonstrated that an analogous domain was located at the N-terminus of the HIV-1,[484] HIV-2,[485] and SIV[486] TM glycoproteins (see Fig. 27–19); non-hydrophobic substitutions within this region of gp41 greatly reduced or blocked syncytium formation and resulted in the production of non-infectious progeny virions. C-terminal to the fusion peptide are two leucine zipper–like heptad repeat domains[487, 488] (see Fig. 27–19). Mutations in the N-terminal leucine zipper–like motif impair infectivity,[489] and peptides derived from these sequences exhibit potent antiviral activity in culture.[490, 491] It has been proposed that these heptad repeat domains interact with each other in an antiparallel fashion to generate a homotrimeric coiled-coil that bears striking resemblance in overall structure to the fusion-competent (low-pH-induced) form of influenza HA$_2$. These results highlight the existence of fundamental similarities in the mechanism by which enveloped viruses induce membrane fusion (see Fig. 27–20) and suggest that peptides derived from the gp41 ectodomain leucine zipper–like sequences may display antiviral activity in vivo.

The fusion function of HIV is not limited to gp41. The V3 loop of gp120 (see Fig. 27–19), which elicits isolate-specific neutralizing antibodies, has also been shown to be an essential player in the membrane fusion reaction. Mutations throughout the V3 loop of HIV-1 block syncytium formation and virus infectivity without perturbing the processing, transport, and CD4 binding properties of gp120.[492–494] The analogous domain of the HIV-2 Env glycoprotein is also required for fusion and infectivity.[485] In addition to V3, the V1/V2 region appears to participate in some manner in the fusion reaction, as illustrated by the observations that mutations in these variable loops impair fusion[495] and antibodies that bind this region can neutralize virus infectivity.[496, 497]

The mechanism by which retroviral Env glycoproteins are incorporated into budding virions remains incompletely characterized. Several lines of evidence suggest that Env glycoproteins are incorporated into virions by active recruitment via a direct interaction between Env and MA: (1) data were presented in 1984 that the Env and Gag proteins of the Rous sarcoma virus could be chemically cross-linked[498]; (2) mutations in the HIV-1 and M-PMV MA could block HIV-

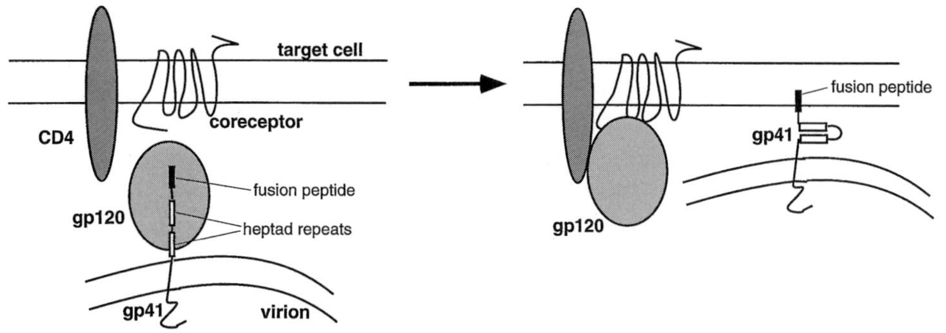

Figure 27–20. Highly Schematic Representation of the Transition from "Resting" (Left Side) to "Fusogenic" (Right Side) Env Conformation. In the resting conformation, the gp41 fusion peptide is buried and the ectodomain heptad repeats assume an extended conformation. After interaction of gp120 with CD4 and coreceptor, the fusion peptide is exposed and inserts into the lipid bilayer of the target cell while the heptad repeats interact in an antiparallel fashion to form a coiled coil. Note: Only monomeric gp120 and gp41 are shown; in reality, both gp120 and gp41 are associated in a higher-order (probably trimeric) complex.

1 Env incorporation,[311–314, 499] and this incorporation defect could be reversed by pseudotyping virions with heterologous Env glycoproteins or by removing the gp41 cytoplasmic tail[313, 314]; (3) HIV-1 MA directed the incorporation of HIV-1 Env into particles containing HIV-1/visna chimeric Gag[312]; (4) HIV-1 Env could direct basolateral budding of Gag in polarized epithelial cells[500, 501]; and (5) direct binding between HIV-1 MA and peptides derived from the gp41 cytoplasmic tail was reportedly detected in vitro.[316] Some evidence, however, supports a more passive mode of Env incorporation. Heterologous Env proteins (e.g., those of MuLV, HTLV, and vesicular stomatitis virus) can be incorporated into HIV-1 virions and can confer infectivity,[502–504] and the entire cytoplasmic tails of RSV and HIV-1 can be removed without blocking Env incorporation.[313, 314, 505, 506] A model that is consistent with currently available data would propose that Env incorporation (and incorporation of cellular membrane proteins) can occur in the absence of an interaction with Gag; however, the incorporation of *full-length* HIV-1 Env requires a specific interaction between the gp41 cytoplasmic tail and MA. The function of the unusually long lentiviral cytoplasmic tail is presently unknown. However, it is clear that the long tail plays a role in infectivity that is distinct from its putative function in Env incorporation.[314, 507]

Distinct HIV/SIV isolates display a striking pattern of selective tropism for subsets of CD4+ cells. Many laboratory-adapted isolates (e.g., HIV-1$_{IIIB}$, HIV-1$_{Lai}$, or HIV-1$_{SF-2}$) readily infect activated human peripheral blood lymphocytes (PBLs) and T-cell lines but cannot replicate efficiently in primary human monocyte-derived macrophages, which are major in vivo HIV/SIV targets in the brain, spinal cord, lung, and lymph nodes. In contrast, the host range of macrophage-tropic (M-tropic) strains of HIV, isolated from asymptomatic individuals, is usually limited to PBLs and cells of the monocyte/macrophage lineage; continuous T-cell lines are usually refractory to infection by these isolates.[508–511] Over time, the virus present in an infected individual gradually changes and cytopathic isolates capable of inducing syncytia and infecting PBLs and T-cell lines (but not macrophages) become more prevalent. In fact, the evolution of isolates from primarily M-tropic to T-cell line (T-) tropic variants appears to play a major role in disease progres-

sion.[512] The determinants of M- versus T-tropism reside primarily in the V3 loop of gp120[513–515]; however, amino acids located in the V1/V2 domain may be required for full infectivity of recombinant viruses.[515]

In most cell systems CD4 expression is a prerequisite for infection. However, soon after the identification of CD4 as the major HIV/SIV receptor, it was recognized that CD4 is not sufficient for HIV-induced membrane fusion and virus entry. Mouse cells expressing human CD4 were not infectable,[466] whereas CD4+ mouse/human cell hybrids could be induced to fuse upon expression of HIV-1 Env.[516, 517] Furthermore, as mentioned above, different HIV-1 isolates displayed cell-type tropism such that they preferentially infected only a subset of CD4+ cells (i.e., T-cell lines versus macrophages). These observations suggested that secondary receptor(s), or coreceptor(s), expressed on human cells functioned in concert with CD4 in the membrane fusion process. However, more than a decade of research failed to identify convincingly such a coreceptor. Recently, though, a number of studies, outlined below, have demonstrated that members of the chemokine receptor family of seven-transmembrane domain proteins provided the long-sought coreceptor function. One impetus for this discovery was the observation that several β chemokines produced by CD8+ T cells (i.e., regulated on activation, normal T expressed and selected [RANTES], macrophage inflammatory protein [MIP-1α], and MIP-1β) could suppress infection by certain strains of HIV-1, HIV-2, and SIV.[518] This finding simultaneously led a number of investigators to test whether the cell-surface proteins that bound these molecules, the β chemokine receptors, could function as HIV-1 coreceptors (Fig. 27–21). The results indicated that the β chemokine receptor CCR-5 could in fact render CD4+ non-human cells permissive for infection by M-tropic isolates of HIV-1.[79, 80, 519] In an independent approach, the α chemokine receptor CXCR4 (originally designated fusin) was identified as the primary coreceptor for T-tropic isolates of HIV-1.[78] The strategy used to make this finding was based on the screening of a human library for cDNAs that could confer upon non-human cells the ability to fuse with HIV-1 Env-expressing cells.

Since the initial discovery of CCR5 and CXCR4 as major coreceptors for M-tropic and T-tropic HIV-1 isolates,

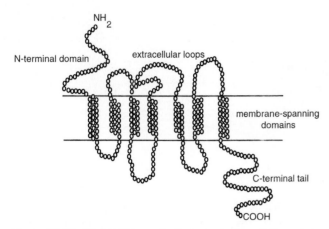

Figure 27–21. Highly Schematic Representation of Coreceptor Structure. The N-terminal and C-terminal domains, the extracellular loops, and the seven membrane-spanning domains are shown.

respectively, these and other coreceptors have been the focus of one of the most active areas of HIV/SIV research. A number of additional findings have refined our understanding of which molecules serve as coreceptors for a range of HIV-1, HIV-2, and SIV isolates; how these proteins interact with gp120; which domains are critical to coreceptor function; and what are the implications of coreceptor gene mutations for susceptibility to HIV infection and disease progression. Although a detailed discussion of these topics is beyond the scope of this chapter, a summary of some of the more important findings follows.[520] (1) In addition to CCR5 and CXCR4, certain strains of HIV-1 also use CCR2b and CCR3 as coreceptors.[79, 81, 521] (2) Signaling through the β chemokine receptors is not required for coreceptor function.[522–524] (3) SIV and HIV-2 generally use CCR5 as a coreceptor, although CXCR4 can also be utilized.[525, 526] Interestingly, certain isolates of HIV-2 use coreceptors in a CD4-independent manner, that is, as primary receptors.[527, 528] In fact, the designation of the chemokine receptors as "coreceptors" may be a misnomer; the observation of CD4-independent SIV/HIV-2 infection, together with the finding that feline immunodeficiency viruses utilize the chemokine receptors but not CD4,[529] suggest that the use of the chemokine receptors in lentiviral infection may have predated the involvement of CD4. (4) Dual-tropic HIV-1 isolates, which in culture can infect both T-cell lines and macrophages, can use multiple coreceptors, suggesting that they may represent evolutionary intermediates between M-tropic and T-tropic strains.[81, 530] (5) Direct interactions between coreceptor and gp120 have been detected; this interaction is greatly stimulated by, or is dependent upon, the presence of CD4.[531–534] (6) It is clear that, in an isolate-dependent fashion, multiple domains in the N-terminal domain and extracellular loops of CCR5 and CXCR4 can play a role in coreceptor function and that the gp120-coreceptor interaction is complex.[521, 535–541] (7) Although it is currently not known which domain(s) of gp120 is responsible for coreceptor interaction, the V3 loop appears to play a major role, consistent with its function in influencing HIV-1 tropism.[542] In fact, single amino acid changes in the V3 loop have been reported to shift coreceptor usage.[543] (8) A variety of findings, including the observations that some HIV-1 strains utilize CCR5 yet cannot infect

macrophages[544, 545] and that some isolates infect macrophages in a CCR5-independent manner,[546] indicate that coreceptors other than those mentioned above may play a vital role in HIV/SIV infection both in culture and in vivo. Indeed, a number of additional coreceptors, named Bonzo (STRL33), BOB, ChemR1 (CCR8), V28, gpr1, and gpr15, have been demonstrated to serve as coreceptors for HIV/SIV fusion and infection in culture.[547–551]

It has been recognized for several years that certain individuals, despite persistent high-risk behavior, remain uninfected.[552] The discovery of CCR5, CXCR4, and related molecules as HIV coreceptors prompted investigators to test whether these individuals might have inherited mutant coreceptor alleles. In some instances, this turned out to be the case. One mutant CCR5 allele, which is relatively common in white populations, contains a 32 base pair deletion and encodes a truncated protein that is not efficiently expressed at the cell surface and cannot function as an HIV-1 coreceptor.[546, 553–556] Homozygotes for this mutation are extremely rare among HIV-1 infected individuals, highlighting the protective benefits of inheriting a mutant form of CCR5. Some evidence suggests that heterozygosity at this allele may confer some protective benefits, particularly in slowing disease progression.[553–555] It was also recently reported that an inherited CCR2 mutation causes a delay in disease progression, perhaps as a result of its linkage with the CCR5 gene regulatory region.[557, 558] It should be emphasized, however, that mutations in genes for currently recognized coreceptors appear to be present in only a minority of multiply exposed, uninfected individuals, suggesting the existence of other mechanisms of protection from HIV infection. Indeed, the analysis of a large number of hemophiliacs exposed to HIV-1-contaminated factor VIII revealed that protection correlated not with CCR5 mutations but rather with high levels of β chemokine production.[559] Additionally, mutations in the gene encoding the ligand for CXCR4 stromal-derived factor (SDF-1) were demonstrated to confer some protection from disease progression.[560]

The identification of HIV coreceptors presents novel opportunities for antiviral therapy. A derivative of RANTES was synthesized by modifying its N-terminus with aminooxypentane. This molecule, known as (AOP)-RANTES, does not induce chemotaxis but potently inhibits infection by a variety of HIV-1 isolates.[561] The bicyclam AMD3100 was found to inhibit entry of HIV-1 isolates using CXCR4 as a coreceptor, and a chemokine agonist encoded by human herpesvirus 8 (Kaposi's sarcoma associated virus) was reported to inhibit virus entry through CCR3, CCR5, and CXCR4.[562] Undoubtedly, much effort in the near future will be focused on further elucidating the mechanism of coreceptor function, identifying and characterizing novel coreceptors, and using knowledge gained in these studies to develop coreceptor-based antiviral therapies.

Vif

The virus infectivity factor (*vif*) gene, present in all lentiviruses except equine infectious anemia virus,[563] overlaps with the *pol* and *vpr* genes of HIV-1 (see Fig. 27–4A). Early reports indicated that Vif was not required for efficient virus production but was necessary for the generation of fully infectious virions.[237, 564, 565] In subsequent studies it became apparent that the phenotype of *vif*-defective mutants was strikingly cell-type dependent, and that this phenotype was imposed by the cell type in which virus was produced.[566, 567] This led to the suggestion that cell types "permissive" for Vif-defective viruses (e.g., HeLa, COS, SupT1, and Jurkat) express a factor that substitutes for Vif function. To date, however, no such factor has been identified.

The Vif⁻ defect, although imposed in the producer cell, becomes apparent at an early postentry step in the virus life cycle. Vif-defective virions, produced from "non-permissive" cell types, fail to reverse transcribe their genomes efficiently after infection,[568–570] perhaps as a result of instability of the complex in which reverse transcription takes place.[571] Vif-defective virions have also been reported to display morphological abnormalities evident by EM[572] and defects in endogenous RT reactions.[573] Some investigators reported that Vif mutation causes a defect in Gag processing, such that Vif⁻ virions contain increased levels of the Gag precursor p55.[574, 575] An effect of Vif on Gag processing has also been observed in vitro.[576] However, a detailed analysis of Vif⁻ virions obtained from non-permissive cells failed to reveal any effect of Vif mutation on viral protein composition.[577] Although a small amount of Vif has been detected in virions,[577–580] the biological implications of this observation remain unclear.

Vpu

The signature of the HIV-1 family of primate lentiviruses is the presence of the *vpu* gene; it is absent from HIV-2 and all SIVs examined to date with the exception of the highly HIV-1-related SIV$_{cpz}$ (see Fig. 27–2). Vpu is a small integral membrane phosphoprotein (81 amino acid residues) that is produced at intracellular levels comparable to those of Gag proteins in virus-infected cells.[56, 581–583] Vpu has not been detected in virus particles. Vpu mutants are defective in the release of viral proteins and progeny virions; the intracellular synthesis and processing of HIV-1 proteins are unaffected. The demonstration that Vpu and the Env precursor polyprotein are expressed from the same bicistronic mRNA (see Fig. 27–11) has focused attention on the possible functional interaction of Vpu and gp160.[584] As discussed above, HIV infection leads to the downregulation of CD4 expression from the cell surface, in part because of the formation of intracellular gp160/CD4 complexes that are retained in the ER.[22, 585, 586] It has been demonstrated that Vpu interferes with gp160/CD4 complex formation by inducing the degradation of CD4 in the ER.[587, 588] The mechanism by which Vpu induces CD4 degradation appears to involve proteosome function[589]; recently, a host cell factor, named βTrCP, was shown to interact with Vpu and connect CD4 to the proteosomal degradative machinery.[590]

The two major functions of Vpu (enhancement of virus release and CD4 downregulation) are apparently separable. Mutation of Vpu phosphoacceptor sites or deletion of the Vpu cytoplasmic domain eliminated its ability to downregulate CD4 but only partially inhibited its role in virus release.[591, 592] Interestingly, although *vpu* is expressed only by HIV-1 genomes, it has the ability to enhance the release of widely divergent retroviruses.[593]

Vpr

The *vpr* gene, which overlaps with *vif* at its 5′ end, encodes a 14 kDa protein that is incorporated at high levels in virus particles[594–596] (see Fig. 27–4A) and is reportedly present in the viral preintegration complex.[323] Initially, it was observed that Vpr transactivated expression from the HIV-1 LTR.[595, 596] Subsequently, several additional functions for Vpr were proposed. A number of groups have reported that Vpr arrests cells in the G$_2$ phase of the cell cycle,[597–600] apparently by inhibiting the activity of the cyclin-dependent Ser/Thr kinase p34^{cdc2}.[601, 602] Vpr also was observed to induce differentiation of rhabdomyosarcoma cells[603] and arrest growth in yeast.[604, 605] Although the biological implications of these functions are unclear, it has been suggested that increased HIV LTR-driven transcription in the G$_2$ phase of the cell cycle could provide a rationale for the evolution of a Vpr cell cycle arrest function.[606, 607] This Vpr-induced enhancement of LTR-driven transcription is apparently mediated by the p300 transcriptional coactivator.[607]

Vpr has also been reported to play a role in targeting the viral preintegration complex to the nucleus in non-dividing cells.[321, 322, 328, 608] However, Vpr is clearly not the sole determinant of nuclear localization, since *vpr*-defective mutants can still grow, albeit at lower levels, in cultures of non-dividing primary human monocyte–derived macrophages.[309, 609, 610] Interestingly, in HIV-2, SIV$_{sm}$, and SIV$_{mac}$, the putative functions of HIV-1 Vpr (cell-cycle arrest and infection of non-dividing cells) seem to be performed by two proteins: Vpr and the related Vpx. In these closely related primate lentiviruses, Vpx is required for efficient infection of non-dividing cells, whereas Vpr induces cell cycle arrest but has no role in nuclear targeting.[611] In the SIVagm system, in which Vpr but no Vpx is expressed, Vpr appears to mediate both functions.[612] Although Vpr may enhance virus replication in culture, it has been demonstrated that a *vpr*-deleted clone of SIV$_{mac}$ is infectious, and pathogenic, in rhesus macaques.[613]

Nef

The Nef gene, present only in primate lentiviruses, overlaps approximately one half of the 3′ LTR and encodes a 27 kDa membrane-associated, myristylated phosphoprotein (see Fig. 27–4A). The *nef* mRNA is the first transcript detected in HIV-infected human T-cell lines[227] but is dispensable for virus replication in tissue culture systems. It was originally reported that Nef downregulated virus replication by affecting a target in the negative regulatory element (NRE) that restricted transcription directed by the HIV LTR.[614] Subsequent studies, however, failed to confirm these results.[615] It was also suggested that Nef is related to G proteins such as *ras,* possessing guanosine triphosphate (GTP) binding and guanosine triphosphatase (GTPase) activities, and therefore might function as a modulator of intracellular second messenger signaling pathways.[616] Subsequent work has not corroborated these biochemical properties.[617–619] Structural studies indicate that Nef is composed of two major domains: a relatively disordered N-terminal region and a compact C-terminal core.[620, 621]

Although the functions of the Nef protein remain to be completely elucidated, it is clear that deletion of the *nef* gene has a profound effect in the SIV/rhesus macaque animal model system. Nef has been shown to be required for (1) the maintenance of a large number of circulating mononuclear cells containing SIV proviral DNA and (2) the development of immunodeficiency.[622] In monkeys inoculated with *nef*-deleted virus, high-level antibody responses developed but produced no detectable circulating virus. These results imply that Nef plays a critical role in initiating and sustaining SIV infection in vivo. In its absence, virus replication and spread are severely compromised. Although very low levels of progeny virus production were adequate to elicit antibody production in animals inoculated with *nef*-deleted SIV, they were insufficient to induce disease.

Although it is currently not clear why *nef*-deleted SIV mutants display markedly reduced pathogenicity in vivo, several lines of evidence suggest that Nef is involved in signal transduction. Both HIV and SIV Nef contain a highly conserved consensus binding site for the SH3 domain of Src kinases (Pro-*X*-*X*-Pro [PXXP, where *X* is any amino acid]), and Nef has been reported either to activate or to inhibit T-cell signaling.[623, 624] The identification of a naturally occurring mutant *nef* allele has provided some important clues about Nef function. A strain of SIV$_{mac}$ known as SIV$_{pbj14}$ induces a rapidly fatal disease in infected macaques characterized by marked T lymphocyte proliferation, retrafficking of T cells to the gastrointestinal tract, and severe diarrhea. In culture, SIV$_{pbj14}$ causes extensive T lymphocyte activation and displays the unusual ability to replicate efficiently in resting PBMCs.[625] These features are the result of an Arg to Tyr mutation that creates a sequence reminiscent of an immunoreceptor tyrosine-based activation motif (ITAM). ITAMs, present in the cytoplasmic domains of T-cell and B-cell receptors, are essential for lymphocyte activation,[626] and the putative ITAM of SIV$_{pbj14}$ reportedly activates T-cell signaling.[627] SIV$_{pbj14}$ Nef may thus have a greatly enhanced property possessed by wild-type Nef, namely, the ability to activate T-cell proliferation. In fact, a role for wild-type HIV-1 and SIV Nef in lymphocyte activation has been reported.[628] Nef has also been shown to be required for HIV-1 replication and pathogenicity in severe combined immunodeficient (SCID) mice that have had human fetal thymus and liver implants.[629]

Together with the HIV-1 Env and Vpu proteins, Nef possesses the capacity to downregulate cell-surface expression of CD4,[616, 630] apparently by inducing rapid CD4 endocytosis.[631, 632] Despite its name (nef, for "negative factor"), Nef stimulates virus infectivity, a phenomenon that is distinct from its ability to downregulate CD4.[633, 634] This enhancement of virus infectivity appears to be manifested at an early step in the virus life cycle, since *nef*-deleted mutants fail to reverse transcribe their genomes efficiently after infection.[633, 635–637] Interestingly, this defect can be partially suppressed by pseudotyping with the vesicular stomatitis G glycoprotein (VSV-G).[638] VSV-G directs entry via fusion in a low pH endosome after endocytosis,[639] whereas HIV-1 Env generally mediates entry via direct fusion at the plasma membrane. These observations suggest that the role Nef plays in an early postentry step is dependent upon the mode of HIV-1 entry. In addition to reducing cell-surface CD4 expression, Nef has been reported to downregulate major histocompatibility complex (MHC) class I molecule expression from the cell surface.[640] Intriguingly, MHC class I downregulation may prevent cytotoxic T lymphocytes

(CTLs) from recognizing and eliminating virus-infected cells, thus providing HIV and SIV with a mechanism for evading at least one aspect of the host immune response.[641]

It was reported by several groups that Nef is incorporated into virions.[642–644] However, as is the case for Vif, it is not clear what, if any, function is served by virion incorporation, particularly since HIV-1 Nef is incorporated with equivalent efficiency into HIV-1 and MuLV virions.[644] However, one might imagine that for a protein whose functions include T-cell activation, virion incorporation would be a most useful property.

A summary of the major proposed functions of the HIV-1 accessory proteins is presented in Table 27–1.

Human Immunodeficiency Virus Life Cycle: Clinical Perspectives

Because HIV-1 infections in vivo are limited to humans and chimpanzees, our understanding of how the virus replicates, spreads to various tissues, and ultimately induces disease has been limited, for the most part, to retrospective analyses of clinical specimens collected from seropositive individuals. Thus, although valuable information about the structure and function of the numerous HIV proteins had accrued from elegant biochemical analyses and transfection studies, and important insights had emerged about the interplay between viral and cellular proteins during productive infections of cultured human lymphocytes and macrophages, knowledge about virus replication in vivo was largely incomplete. Questions pertaining to the biological characteristics of HIV-1 in its natural microenvironments such as lymph nodes, spleen, microglia in the central nervous system, Langerhans cells in the skin, and tissue macrophages were difficult if not impossible to answer with available in vitro systems. Studies of contemporaneous HIV replication in vivo were initially hindered by the lack of assays sensitive enough to detect extremely low levels of infectious virus, viral nucleic acids, and viral proteins. This impediment has gradually been surmounted with the development of sensitive molecular diagnostic tools. The extent of virus replication and tissue location of virion production during all phases of the HIV-1 life cycle in vivo is now amenable to rigorous investigation. Consequently, the mechanisms responsible for sustaining virus production for a decade or more and the cellular factors that become dysfunctional during the irrevocable clinical progression to AIDS can now be exhaustively examined.

HIV-1 is transmitted hetero- or homosexually in vaginal secretions and semen, after transfusions of contaminated blood and blood products, and from infected mothers to their infants. There is no evidence that HIV has ever been transmitted by direct contact through intact skin, by insects, or through the administration of processed biological products such as gamma globulin.[645, 646] Although there are several published reports that HIV-1 directly infects cultured gastrointestinal or genitourinary tract epithelial cells,[647–649] it is more likely that the virus gains entry as a result of mucosal injury during receptive anal intercourse or microtrauma attending heterosexual vaginal intercourse[650]; genital ulceration, secondary to sexually transmitted disease, has been clearly linked to HIV-1 transmission.[651] Partner studies indicate that virus-infected individuals exhibiting severe im-

Table 27–1. HIV-1 Accessory Proteins

Protein	Major Proposed Functions	Comments
Vif	Enhancement of virus infectivity	Phenotype markedly cell-type specific Incorporated at low levels in virions
Vpu	Increased particle release CD4 degradation	Not detected in virions
Vpr	Cell cycle arrest Nuclear import of preintegration complex	Incorporated at high levels in virions
Nef	CD4 downregulation MHC class I downregulation Enhancement of virus infectivity Increased virus load in vivo Lymphocyte activation	Incorporated at low levels in virions

mune dysfunction and high levels of circulating virus are more likely to transmit HIV than are asymptomatic persons.[652, 653] The probability of transmission for different types of interpersonal contacts has been reported to be 1 per 3 to 4 for untreated mother to infant (pre- and postpartum); 1 per 100 to 500 for a single anal receptive sexual contact; 1 per 500 to 1000 for a single male-to-female vaginal sexual contact; 1 per 1000 to 1500 for a single female-to-male vaginal sexual contact; 3 to 4 per 1000 for a single percutaneous exposure to HIV-infected blood; and 1 per 40,000 to 250,000 for exposure to blood obtained from undetected, yet HIV-1 infected seronegative donors (Fig. 27–22).[654–659] The use of condoms unquestionably decreases sexual transmission and the administration of AZT reduces the perinatal spread of HIV by nearly 70 per cent.[660–662]

Primary HIV infections present as an acute, self-limited mononucleosis-like syndrome several weeks after exposure to the virus and may be accompanied by fever, malaise, pharyngitis, rash, lymphadenopathy, and gastrointestinal and occasionally neurological symptoms.[663–665] Virus has been isolated from PBMC, plasma, and the cerebrospinal fluid of individuals recently infected with HIV.[664, 666, 667] Relatively high titers (10^1 to 10^4 tissue culture infectious units per milliliter of plasma) of cell-free, circulating infectious virus have been measured at times that coincide with symptoms of the febrile illness.[480, 668] This viremia is frequently associated with a marked, but transient, CD4+ T lymphocyte loss and inversion of the CD4/CD8 ratio.[669] The immunological response to the acute HIV-1 syndrome involves both arms of the immune system and results in a rapid decline of the viremia. Although antibodies to HIV-1 Gag and Env proteins can be detected 2 to 4 weeks after the onset of symptoms,[670, 671] a cytotyoxic T lymphocyte (CTL) response, which occurs prior to the appearance of neutralizing antibodies, has been temporally linked with falling virus loads.[672–674] In some individuals this immunological response effectively reduces the virus load to a level at which cell-free HIV is not recoverable from the plasma until much later in the clinical course. Nonetheless, specific anti-HIV-1 antibodies can be detected by enzyme-linked immunosorbent assay

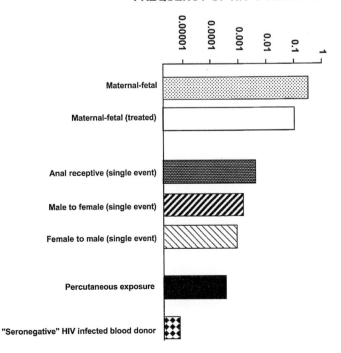

FREQUENCY OF HIV-1 TRANSMISSION

Figure 27–22. HIV-1 Transmission Frequencies by Various Routes.

(ELISA) within 3 months of exposure and continue to be synthesized throughout the entire infection.

The relatively asymptomatic clinical course after initial exposure to HIV is characterized by extremely low numbers of HIV-infected PBMCs (e.g., 1 per 10^4 to 10^6 cells) in the peripheral blood, the absence of detectable plasma viremia, and levels of CD4-positive cells greater than 500/mm.[653, 675-677] A robust CTL response has been correlated with these low virus loads and the absence of clinical symptoms.[678, 679] The lack of significant virus production during this period has led some to propose that HIV-1 is not the cause of AIDS[680] and others to suggest an HIV latency model based on the herpes simplex virus (HSV) paradigm, in which dormant HSV genomes reside in dorsal root ganglia until they are activated to initiate new rounds of replication. During this period, clinical symptoms are mild (fatigue, lymphadenopathy) to non-existent even though CD4+ T cell levels gradually decline.[681] Prior to the introduction of effective antiretroviral drugs, the average duration of the symptomatic phase of HIV-1 infection was estimated to be 8 to 10 years (Fig. 27–23).[682-684] More recently, the length of this clinically latent state has increased, in part, as a result of the availability of potent combinations of antiviral agents and better treatments for opportunistic infections.[685, 686]

The emergence of the symptomatic stage of HIV infection is associated with increasing viral burdens and a significant decline of CD4+ cell numbers to below 500/mm³. AIDS defining neoplasms and opportunistic viral (cytomegalovirus [CMV], HSV, HHV-8 [associated with Kaposi's sarcoma]); bacterial (*Mycobacterium avium*), protozoal (*Pneumocystis carinii, Toxoplasma gondii, Cryptosporidia*); and fungal (*Candida albicans*) infections generally appear when CD4+ T lymphocyte levels fall to below 200 cells/mm³. Although slowly replicating, macrophage-tropic, CCR5-utilizing HIV-1 variants can be recovered during all phases of in vivo infection, the virus isolated in approximately 50 per cent of AIDS patients exhibits a syncytium inducing (SI) phenotype and readily replicates to high titers in continuous human T leukemia cell lines (T-cell line tropic).[512, 687] During

the very late stage of HIV infection, CD8+ CTLs, which had previously been maintained at normal or even elevated levels, also decline markedly.[688]

A small percentage (1 to 5 per cent) of virus-infected individuals are clinically healthy 10 to 15 years after their initial exposure to HIV-1. These so-called long-term non-progressors have virus loads that are significantly lower than those of asymptomatic seropositive persons who progress to AIDS and have stable CD4+ T lymphocyte levels in the 600 to 1200 cells/mm³ range.[689, 690] Broadly reactive neutralizing antibodies and potent CTL activity can be demonstrated in a majority of these individuals, and their lymph node architecture remains largely intact.[690-692] Although a defective *nef* gene has been reported to be present in the virus recovered from a cohort of healthy blood donor/transfusion recipients 11 to 15 years after infection,[693] no single common HIV-1 genetic determinant has been linked to the well-being of a majority of long-term non-progressors. The roles of the immune system in successfully controlling the HIV-1 infection as well as the genetic characteristics (e.g., mutations affecting chemokine receptors[556-558, 560]) of long-term non-progressors require additional study.

The second human immunodeficiency virus, HIV-2, was initially isolated from individuals residing in West Africa.[21] HIV-2 infections are prevalent in areas with socioeconomic ties to West Africa: Fewer than 100 cases have been identified in the United States since 1992.[694, 695] Although the genomic organization of HIV-2 is similar to that of HIV-1 (see Fig. 27–2), it is genetically more closely related to the SIVs, lacking the *vpu* gene, present only in HIV-1. Compared with that caused by HIV-1, clinical disease induced by HIV-2 is slow to develop. Natural history studies have indicated that the decline of CD4+ T lymphocytes (below 400 cells/mm³) may be 10-fold slower[696] and the rate of heterosexual and perinatal transmission of HIV-2 is considerably lower than that of HIV-1.[697-699] The HIV-2 associated disease-free interval in a cohort of Senegalese commercial sex workers cannot be calculated because it is so long.[696, 700] In this cohort, HIV-2 had no effect on survival.[701]

During the early years of the epidemic, the detection and quantitation of cell-free and cell-associated HIV-1 in infected individuals were fraught with many difficulties. At that time, HIV-1 levels in vivo were determined solely by the isolation of virus using the highly labor-intensive, limiting dilution cocultivation procedure. Viral DNA, present in the PBMCs collected from asymptomatic infected individuals, was undetectable by standard Southern blot analyses. The introduction of in situ hybridization techniques, though tedious to perform, revealed that only extraordinarily low numbers (1 per 10^5 to 10^6) of circulating cells were infected with virus.[676, 702] A major breakthrough in molecular diagnostics occurred with the application of DNA polymerase chain reaction (PCR) to quantitate HIV-1 DNA in infected individuals at various stages of virus infection.[676, 677] The subsequent use of reverse transcriptase (RT) PCR to measure virion RNA provided a rapid and sensitive procedure to monitor HIV-1 circulating in the blood and obviated the need for quantitative virus isolation in patient management. Quantitative-competitive (QC) RNA PCR was used to demonstrate the high virus burdens in individuals with advanced clinical disease.[653, 703] During the acute HIV-1 infection, viral RNA levels of 10^6 copies/ml of blood or greater were commonly

CLINICAL COURSE OF AN HIV INFECTION

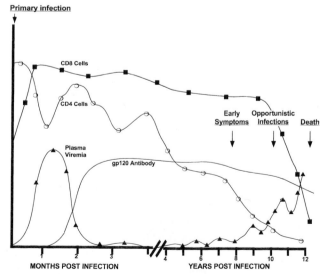

Figure 27–23. HIV-I Clinical Course.

measured.[704] In asymptomatic seropositive individuals, virus loads fell to the 10^3 to 10^6 copies/ml range, values that were 100- to 1000-fold higher than the titers of infectious virus, recovered by cocultivation. HIV-1 RNA levels, measured after the resolution of the primary infection (the "set point"), were shown to be predictive of the subsequent clinical course (Fig. 27–24).[705] Collectively, the multitude of studies measuring viral RNA levels during all phases of in vivo HIV-1 infections laid to rest models of microbiological latency and, in retrospect, were consistent with reports describing the emergence of resistant HIV-1 variants that appeared after the institution of antiretroviral therapy.

Most virus isolated at the time of seroconversion and during the extended asymptomatic phase of in vivo infection replicates slowly in vitro and is macrophage tropic.[706–708] Nucleotide sequence analyses have revealed that the virus transmitted to a new recipient is quite homogeneous and represents a minor variant of the genetically heterogeneous HIV-1 swarm present in the donor.[707–709] Virus isolates exhibiting increased cytopathicity, tropism for T-cell lines, and a syncytium-inducing phenotype are typically recovered from individuals with high levels of circulating viral RNA, CD4+ T lymphocyte depletion, and clinical progression.[512, 687, 710] Several studies monitoring the longitudinal evolution of HIV-1 in individuals with different clinical outcomes have reported that *env* sequences evolve more slowly in persons experiencing rapid CD4+ T-cell loss.[711–713] Whether this inverse relationship merely reflects the selective pressure imposed by a relatively intact and still functional immune system or some other unrecognized facet of virus-host interaction is not presently known.

The advent of potent anti-HIV-1 drugs (viz., protease inhibitors), capable of significantly reducing the steady-state levels of virus production in vivo, coupled with the availability of sensitive techniques to measure HIV-1 RNA in the blood, provided the means to quantitate virus production and clearance in infected persons rigorously. Thus, the administration of a protease plus an RT inhibitor,[714] or simply a protease inhibitor alone,[715] to AIDS patients resulted in a 100-fold reduction of viral RNA levels over a 2-week interval. Since both antiretroviral agents prevent subsequent rounds of infection, the decline of viral RNA was a measure of the intrinsic decay rate of HIV-1 in the blood. The exponential loss of circulating virus and associated rise in the number of CD4+ cells were consistent with the continuous production of progeny virions and what were interpreted to be very substantial daily losses ($1–2 \times 10^9$ cells) of infected CD4+ T lymphocytes. A follow-up study, using a similar approach to carefully examine viral dynamics immediately after the start of antiviral therapy, concluded that the half-life for HIV-1 in the blood was less than 6 hours and that of productively infected cells was 1 to 2 days (Fig. 27–25, right).[716] Taken together, these values suggested that 10^8 to 10^{10} virus particles are released each day from 10^8 infected cells. Thus, the HIV-1 detected in circulating blood is recently produced, has a short half-life, and is generated in cells that are rapidly turning over.

In a subsequent study, the clearance of virus and infected cells was analyzed in HIV-1 infected individuals treated with a combination of two RT inhibitors and a single protease inhibitor, which reduced the virus load to undetectable levels (20 to 500 RNA copies/ml of blood).[717] Careful analysis indicated that HIV RNA decay in the blood was biphasic: the initial, previously reported rapid phase, with a half-life of approximately 0.6 day, followed by a slower second phase with a half-life of 6 to 25 days. The second phase of HIV-1 clearance, thought to represent the decay of a chronically virus-producing reservoir in vivo, such as tissue macrophage or follicular dendritic cells, contributes only a fraction of the progeny virions generated each day.

T lymphocyte subset analysis of cells collected before and after highly active antiretroviral therapy (HAART) has raised questions about whether the rapid and substantial elevation of CD4+ T-cell number observed subsequent to antiviral therapy is actually reflective of sustained and vigorous pretreatment proliferation of CD4+ T lymphocytes. Rigorous immunophenotyping, combined with mathematical modeling, has revealed that the marked increases of T lymphocytes during the first 3 to 4 weeks of HAART are restricted to activated CD4+ and CD8+ memory cells; levels of naive T cells slowly rise over a 6 month period.[718, 719] Because activated memory cells reside in peripheral lymphoid tissue such as lymph nodes, these results are more compatible with a redistribution than a proliferation model of T-cell reconstitution. It has been proposed that reduced virus loads effected by HAART dampen the immune response and ultimately result in the release of both B and T cells, previously trapped in lymphoid organs, into the circulating blood.[719, 720]

The elegant analyses of HIV-1 production and clearance in vivo emphasize a major accomplishment of the HIV-1 research effort: the development of effective and clinically useful antiretroviral agents directed against the viral encoded enzymes, reverse transcriptase, and protease. When used as monotherapy, several of these drugs have provided clinical benefit, if only for the short term. As is the case for other antimicrobials used to treat chronic infectious diseases, the

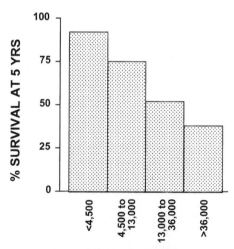

VIRAL LOAD AFTER SEROCONVERSION
(RNA copies/ml plasma)

Figure 27–24. The Relationship Between HIV Load and Survival. Viral RNA levels in the plasma were determined by RT PCR at the setpoint after acute infection and correlated with survival without AIDS. (Data from Mellors, J. W., Rinaldo, C. R., Jr., Gupta, P., White, R. M., Todd, J. A., and Kingsley, L. A.: Prognosis in HIV-1 infection predicted by the quantity of virus in plasma. Science 272:1167, 1996; with permission.)

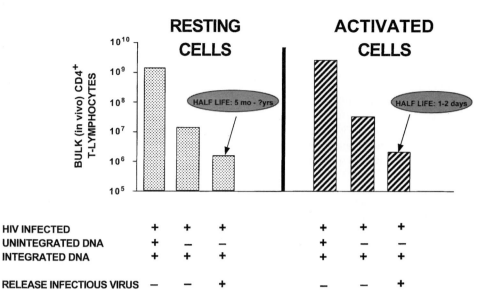

Figure 27–25. Frequencies and Properties of Resting (Memory) and Activated CD4⁺ T Lymphocytes in HIV-1 Infected Individuals.

effectiveness of these agents has been limited by the appearance of drug resistant HIV-1 variants. For the nucleoside analogue AZT, which is metabolically activated by phosphorylation within cells, the stepwise accumulation of four or five specific mutations (affecting residues 41, 67, 70, 215, and 219) invariably occurs within 6 to 12 months of therapy in patients with severe clinical disease.[428, 721] This is to be contrasted with the extremely rapid appearance of highly resistant virus in patients treated with the nucleoside 3TC. The substitution of the single methionine residue to valine at codon 184 of the HIV-1 RT results in a >500-fold increase in resistance to 3TC.[722, 723] Interestingly, the Val[184] mutation results in only a slight growth disadvantage compared with wild-type HIV-1, but more importantly it suppresses AZT resistance in different combinations of the five established AZT mutational backgrounds.[724] When administered to HIV-1 infected individuals, AZT plus 3TC induces a substantially greater reduction of circulating virus and sustained CD4⁺ T lymphocyte increases, compared with treatment with AZT alone, even though the Val[184] mutation emerges during therapy.[724, 725]

HIV-1 protease inhibitors, introduced into clinical use in 1995, are more potent antiviral agents than the RT inhibitors. After administration, they frequently induce marked declines of plasma viral RNA levels to approximately 1 per cent of baseline values, which are associated with a concomitant increase in CD4⁺ cell numbers.[715, 726] When used in monotherapy regimens, HIV-1 variants with reduced sensitivity, containing an ordered accumulation of multiple mutations affecting not only the protease gene but Gag substrate cleavage sites as well,[727–729] invariably appear. In general, the rate of resistance to protease inhibitors is inversely related to the plasma levels of the drug, and the HIV-1 variants that emerge may be less fit than the pretherapy virus.[728, 730]

The realization that the 3TC-induced Val[184] change in the HIV-1 RT resensitized AZT-resistant virus to AZT, coupled with the availability of potent new protease inhibitors, led to the simultaneous administration of AZT, 3TC, and a protease inhibitor, a three-drug combination now referred to as highly active antiretroviral therapy (HAART). Triple

combination therapy commonly results in sustained reductions of plasma viral RNA to undetectable levels,[731, 732] although HIV-1 resistance has been observed in a substantial number of HAART recipients. As had been shown previously for antiretroviral agents used in monotherapy regimens, resistant HIV-1 variants, preexisting at low frequencies as integrated proviral DNA copies, emerge; these variants are insensitive to triple combination therapy.[733–736] Nonetheless, the CD4⁺ T lymphocyte counts continue to rise in a large fraction of HAART recipients in the face of little if any reduction of the HIV-1 viremia.

Triple drug therapy has already had a major impact on HIV-1 morbidity and mortality rates. Between 1995 and 1997, the mortality rate in eight U.S. cities declined from 29.4 to 8.8 per 100 person-years.[737] In infected individuals with a history of experiencing a CD4⁺ T-cell count of less than 100 cells/ml on at least one occasion, the incidence of three major opportunistic infections (*Pneumocystis carinii* pneumonia, cytomegalovirus retinitis, and *Mycobacterium avium* disease complex) fell nearly sixfold.

The successful clinical response to intensive antiretroviral therapies led some to predict that HIV-1 could be completely eradicated. For example, on the basis of the 1 to 4 week "second phase" decay of virus in the blood, it was suggested that total suppression of HIV-1 would be obtained after 2 to 3 years of HAART.[716] Unfortunately, such an optimistic outcome does not appear to be forthcoming. Several reports have shown that despite the absence of detectable plasma viral RNA after long-term (2.5 years) triple drug therapy, HIV-1 was still recoverable from patients on HAART using enhanced cocultivation techniques.[738–740]

As noted earlier, non-dividing CD4⁺ T cells, which constitute the bulk of this T lymphocyte subset in lymph nodes and blood, are arrested in G_0 and refractory to HIV-1 infection. It is now appreciated that a small fraction, yet a formidable total number of resting lymphocytes in seropositive individuals harbor integrated, replication-competent copies of proviral DNA that can be activated to release infectious virus.[741] Standard and inverse DNA PCR analyses of the HIV DNA present in highly purified samples of resting CD4⁺ T lymphocytes from infected donors revealed that (1)

0.5 per cent of the cells contained viral DNA (both integrated and non-integrated forms), (2) 0.005 per cent of the cells carried only integrated viral DNA, and (3) about 10 per cent of the cells harboring integrated viral DNA could be induced to produce infectious virus.[742] The frequencies of non-dividing CD4+ cells containing integrated copies of HIV-1 proviruses were similar in the circulating blood and lymph nodes. Further analyses indicated that the integrated viral DNA resided in CD45RO+ CD4+ T cells, a lymphocyte phenotype characteristic of non-dividing memory cells. No correlation was observed between the number of these resting virus-infected cells and the levels of HIV-1 RNA in the blood or the numbers of circulating CD4+ T cells.[742] It was estimated that a total of up to 1×10^6 infected resting CD4+ memory cells, capable of releasing replication competent HIV for many months to years, are present in seropositive individuals (see Fig. 27–25).[742]

Even though it is not presently known how the resting CD4+ memory cells become infected, this reservoir of latent, non-expressing proviral DNA represents a formidable challenge for virus eradication. One study has suggested that CD45RO+ CD4+ T cells are long-lived (5.5 months),[743] but the actual turnover rate of this T lymphocyte subset may be considerably greater. The observation that the number of HIV-1 infected memory cells remains unchanged during triple drug therapy implies that this virus reservoir is extremely stable and/or may be continuously replenished with newly infected cells.[738]

Prospects for a Human Immunodeficiency Virus–I Vaccine

In contrast to the successful development and clinical use of potent antiretroviral agents for treating HIV-1 infections, progress in obtaining effective prophylactic vaccines has been frustratingly slow. The correlates of protective immunity against the primate lentivirus infection remain to be elucidated. There have been only a few examples of consistent vaccine-induced protection against a virus challenge; for the most part these have not been associated with a specific immunological mechanism.

Much of our current understanding about immunity to these agents derives from human and subhuman primate responses to ongoing primate lentiviral infections. HIV Env glycoproteins are quite immunogenic, eliciting the antibodies detected in a variety of assays used for serological screening.[454, 744] The most immunodominant region of the envelope has been mapped to a seven amino acid peptide located in the extracellular domain of gp41 that reacts with 100 per cent of sera from HIV-infected individuals.[745, 746] Antibodies directed to this gp41 epitope are of diagnostic importance only because they exhibit no demonstrable virus-neutralizing activity. In contrast, gp120 elicits two types of neutralizing antibodies that may be relevant for vaccine development. Isolate-specific antibodies appear after the initial exposure to HIV in recently infected persons or may be synthesized in mice, rabbits, goats, and chimpanzees after immunization with virus, intact gp120, or its peptide subunits.[747–750] HIV type-specific antibodies (1) bind with high affinity to linear epitopes situated in the V3 loop, (2) do *not* block the interaction of gp120 with CD4, and (3) may inhibit

syncytium formation and virus entry.[751–754] Type-specific antibodies characteristically neutralize only a single HIV isolate; amino acid changes introduced into the V3 loop and/or certain other regions of gp120 allow such variants to escape neutralization. The second category of neutralizing antibody elicited by gp120 appears months to years after a primary HIV infection and may neutralize different virus isolates.[755–757] This broadly neutralizing activity is directed to discontinuous conformational epitopes in gp120, rather than only the V3 loop, and may also interfere with binding to CD4. In general, primary viral isolates are more difficult to neutralize than tissue culture adapted HIV-1 strains, and the levels of circulating neutralizing antibodies in seropositive individuals are quite low.[758, 759]

As noted earlier, the resolution of the primary lentivirus infection is temporally related to the emergence of virus-specific CTLs, which appear prior to neutralizing antibodies. The humoral response observed, readily measured by ELISA and immunoblotting, is of obvious diagnostic importance. However, the direct binding of antibody to HIV-1 particles or to native viral envelope glycoproteins, expressed on the surface of productively infected cells, has been difficult to demonstrate.[760] Another confounding, yet consistent, finding has been the inevitable progression to disease despite the presence of robust humoral and cellular immune responses.

Because HIV-1 can only infect humans and the endangered great apes (and only rarely induces disease in chimpanzees[761]), the SIV/macaque monkey system has been the principal model employed in vaccine experiments involving the primate lentiviruses. African monkeys, such as the African green monkey, are endemically infected with SIV and do not develop immunodeficiency. In contrast, their close Asian macaque relatives (viz., rhesus monkeys, pig-tailed macaques, and cynomolgus monkeys) develop disease after inoculation with SIV characterized by CD4+ T-cell depletion, opportunistic infections, wasting, and a variety of malignancies. Asian macaques also exhibit hierarchical susceptibilities to SIV; pig-tailed macaques are the most readily infectable and cynomolgus monkeys the least. Typically, in rhesus monkeys AIDS develops after inoculation with a pathogenic SIV within a 1 to 2 year period,[762] a time frame considerably more rapid than that reported for HIV-1 infections of man.[683, 684] Although SIV and HIV-1 share a similar genomic organization and possess Gag proteins that are structurally and immunologically related, their envelope glycoproteins are quite divergent and do not cross-react in serological assays (Fig. 27–26). Thus, commonly used vaccine strategies, based on the immunogenicity of HIV-1 gp120 or gp160, cannot be directly tested in the SIV/macaque system.

Because a plethora of SIV isolates, exhibiting a continuum of replicative and pathogenic potentials, have been used as challenge viruses for different species of Asian macaques in vaccine experiments conducted since the 1980s, the results obtained have been quite variable and difficult to interpret. In most experiments, animals have been inoculated intravenously with sufficient amounts of a cell-free SIV to induce disease in all of the animals under study. Whether such a regimen appropriately models the potential routes of exposure and inoculum size for HIV-1 infections of humans remains unresolved.

Chimeric viruses that include the *tat, rev, vpu,* and *env*

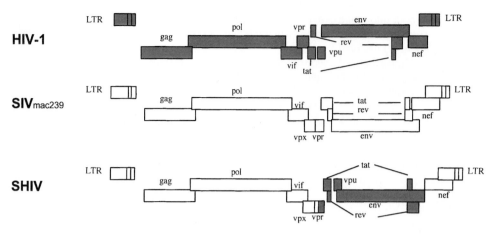

Figure 27–26. Genomic Organization of HIV, SIV, and SHIV Lentiviruses.

genes of HIV-1, engrafted into a genetic background of SIV, have been developed to evaluate the protective effects of HIV-1 envelope-induced immune responses directly (see Fig. 27–26). Although the initially developed SIV/HIV-1 (SHIV) chimeric viruses only replicated to low titers and failed to induce disease in inoculated animals,[763] more recent SHIV derivatives readily replicate to high titers in vivo and cause severe, irreversible CD4+ T lymphocyte depletion in a matter of weeks.[764–766]

A variety of vaccine strategies, shown to elicit protective immunity against other microorganisms in man, have been evaluated in both the HIV-1/chimpanzee and SIV-SHIV/macaque model systems. These include live attenuated virus, recombinant vector, subunit, and the more recently developed DNA vaccines. The generation of neutralizing antibody, the parameter shown to be associated with protective immunity conferred by virtually all known effective viral vaccines, has been difficult to achieve after immunization by any of these approaches. Furthermore, the modest levels of neutralizing antibodies in some HIV-1 infected individuals are frequently unable to block autologous virus infections or inhibit the replication of other primary virus isolates in ex vivo assays.

Vaccination with live attenuated virus vaccines (or an equivalent low-level, non-pathogenic chronic infection) has been the one approach that has consistently elicited protection against a subsequent challenge with primate lentiviruses.[767–770] Historically, adult macaque monkeys, inoculated with SIV containing a disrupted *nef* gene, produced low levels of circulating virus and failed to develop immunodeficiency.[622] Most interestingly, animals persistently infected with such a *nef*-defective virus resisted infection and did not develop clinical disease after intravenous challenge with the pathogenic wild-type parental SIV.[768] Several studies have suggested that the protection induced by live attenuated primate lentiviral vaccines is directly related to the replicative capacity of the weakened virus.[767, 771] Recent work has also demonstrated that rhesus macaques previously vaccinated with a live attenuated SIV resist a subsequent challenge with SHIV, a lentivirus bearing a non-cross-reactive Env protein (see Fig. 27–26), suggesting that envelope-induced immune responses may not be required for the protection observed.[772, 773] In addition, no neutralizing antibodies directed against the SHIV challenge virus were detected in these protected monkeys. Although virus-specific

cellular immune responses have been measured in some macaques immunized with live attenuated SIV vaccines, the mechanism(s) responsible for the protection observed has not yet been elucidated.

The requirement for persistent low level replication of live attenuated lentiviruses for protective immunity has raised concern about their possible reversion to virulence and/or natural or induced fluctuations in immune function during the lifetime of vaccinees that might permit uncontrolled viral replication. Unlike live attenuated polioviruses, which are not efficiently transported from the gastrointestinal tract to the spinal cord and central nervous system and, therefore, rarely cause neurological disease, attenuation of lentiviruses, thus far, solely involves impaired replicative capacity. Reports of immunodeficiency induced in newborn monkeys after vaccination with SIVs harboring multiple deleted genes[774] emphasize how difficult it may be to sustain low virus loads in otherwise healthy immunized individuals.

Replication-competent viral and bacterial vectors, expressing individual or multiple lentiviral proteins, have also been used as experimental vaccines in primate lentiviral systems. This has primarily involved vaccinia virus recombinants, which induce both cellular and humoral immune responses.[775, 776] In the frequently studied "prime and boost" regimen, the inoculation of recombinant vaccinia virus expressing lentiviral Env and/or Gag proteins is followed by immunization with purified viral proteins.[777] This vaccine approach has resulted in protection[778] or delay of disease development[779, 780] after challenge with some strains of SIV. A more recent embellishment has been use of avian poxviruses, which cannot complete their replicative cycle in human cells, to deliver potentially immunogenic lentiviral proteins to vaccinees.[781]

Subunit vaccines, used prophylactically in humans to protect against hepatitis B and influenza virus induced disease, have proved disappointing when applied to lentiviral infections. They have failed to elicit CTL responses or neutralizing antibodies consistently.[782–784] When administered to human volunteers, preparations of HIV-1 gp120 or gp160 envelope proteins did not protect against subsequent viral infections or disease development.[785]

The subcutaneous or intradermal inoculation of purified DNA encoding the influenza virus nucleoprotein has been reported to protect mice and ferrets from a subsequent influenza virus challenge.[786, 787] Although some resistance to infection has been reported after DNA vaccination of subhuman primates with plasmid constructs expressing the HIV-1 Env protein, the levels of immunogen expressed in vivo were generally low and the replicative properties of the challenge virus strains used in such studies were not robust.[788, 789]

An emerging consensus is that an effective lentiviral vaccine may require combinations of multiple vaccine strategies to elicit both cellular and humoral immunity. Because other protective human vaccines block disease development and not the initial virus infection, it has been proposed that by blunting the primary infection, an effective HIV-1 vaccine would greatly impair virus dissemination throughout the body and allow the immune system sufficient time to mount an effective and durable response. This could result in low virus loads, prolongation of the asymptomatic phase, increased survival rate, and reduced transmission of HIV-1 to uninfected individuals.

ACKNOWLEDGMENTS

The authors are deeply indebted to Ms. Carol Ball for invaluable editorial assistance in collating, researching, compiling, proofreading, editing, and updating the entire manuscript and bibliography. We also appreciate Dr. Michael Cho's help in creating Figures 27–10 and 27–14.

REFERENCES

1. CDC: Pneumocystis pneumonia–Los Angeles. MMWR 30:250, 1981.
2. Masur, H., Michelis, M. A., Greene, J. B., Onorato, I., Vande Stouwe, R. A., Holzman, R. S., Wormser, G., Brettman, L., Lange, M., Murray, H. W., and Cunningham-Rundles, S.: An outbreak of community-acquired *Pneumocystis carinii* pneumonia: Initial manifestation of cellular immune dysfunction. N. Engl. J. Med. 305:1431, 1981.
3. Gottlieb, M. S., Schroff, R., Schanker, H. M., Weisman, J. D., Fan, P. T., Wolf, R. A., and Saxon, A.: *Pneumocystis carinii* pneumonia and mucosal candidiasis in previously healthy homosexual men: Evidence of a new acquired cellular immunodeficiency. N. Engl. J. Med. 305:1425, 1981.
4. Siegal, F. P., Lopez, C., Hammer, G. S., Brown, A. E., Kornfeld, S. J., Gold, J., Hassett, J., Hirschman, S. Z., Cunningham-Rundles, C., Adelsberg, B. R., Parham, D. M., Siegal, M., Cunningham-Rundles, S., and Armstrong, D.: Severe acquired immunodeficiency in male homosexuals, manifested by chronic perianal ulcerative herpes simplex lesions. N. Engl. J. Med. 305:1439, 1981.
5. Quinnan, G. V., Jr., Masur, H., Rook, A. H., Armstrong, G., Frederick, W. R., Epstein, J., Manischewitz, J. F., Macher, A. M., Jackson, L., Ames, J., Smith, H. A., Parker, M., Pearson, G. R., Parrillo, J., Mitchell, C., and Straus, S. E.: Herpesvirus infections in the acquired immune deficiency syndrome. JAMA 252:72, 1984.
6. Gelmann, E. P., Popovic, M., Blayney, D., Masur, H., Sidhu, G., Stahl, R. E., and Gallo, R. C.: Proviral DNA of a retrovirus, human T-cell leukemia virus, in two patients with AIDS. Science 220:862, 1983.
7. Essex, M., McLane, M. F., Lee, T. H., Falk, L., Howe, C. W. S., Mullins, J. I., Cabradilla, C., and Francis, D. P.: Antibodies to cell membrane antigens associated with human T-cell leukemia virus in patients with AIDS. Science 220:859, 1983.
8. Gallo, R. C., Sarin, P. S., Gelmann, E. P., Robert-Guroff, M., Richardson, E., Kalyanaraman, V. S., Mann, D., Sidhu, G. D., Stahl, R. E., Zolla-Pazner, S., Leibowitch, J., and Popovic, M.: Isolation of human T-cell leukemia virus in acquired immune deficiency syndrome (AIDS). Science 220:865, 1983.
9. Jaffe, H. W., Francis, D. P., McLane, M. F., Cabradilla, C., Curran, J. W., Kilbourne, B. W., Lawrence, D. N., Haverkos, H. W., Spira, T. J., Dodd, R. Y., Gold, J., Armstrong, D., Ley, A., Groopman, J., Mullins, J., Lee, T. H., and Essex, M.: Transfusion-associated AIDS: Serologic evidence of human T-cell leukemia virus infection of donors. Science 223:1309, 1984.
10. Schüpbach, J., Sarngadharan, M. G., and Gallo, R. C.: Antigens on HTLV-infected cells recognized by leukemia and AIDS sera are related to HTLV viral glycoprotein. Science 224:607, 1984.
11. Barré-Sinoussi, F., Chermann, J. C., Rey, F., Nugeyre, M. T., Chamaret, S., Gruest, J., Dauguet, C., Axler-Blin, C., Vézinet-Brun, F., Rouzioux, C., Rozenbaum, W., and Montagnier, L.: Isolation of a T-lymphotropic retrovirus from a patient at risk for acquired immune deficiency syndrome (AIDS). Science 220:868, 1983.
12. Montagnier, L., Chermann, J. C., Barré-Sinoussi, F., Chamaret, S., Gruest, J., Nugeyre, M. T., Rey, F., Dauguet, C., Axler-Blin, C., Vézinet-Brun, F., Rouzioux, C., Saimot, G.-A., Rozenbaum, W., Gluckman, J. C., Klatzmann, D., Vilmer, E., Griscelli, C., Foyer-Gazengel, C., and Brunet, J. B.: A new human T-lymphotropic retrovirus: Characterization and possible role in lymphadenopathy and acquired immune deficiency syndromes. *In* Gallo, R. C., Essex, M. E., and Gross, L. (eds.): Human T-Cell Leukemia/Lymphoma Virus: The Family of Human T-Lymphotropic Retroviruses: Their Role in Malignancies and Association with AIDS. Cold Spring Harbor, N.Y., Cold Spring Harbor Laboratory, 1984.
13. Levy, J. A., Hoffman, A. D., Kramer, S. M., Landis, J. A., Shimabukuro, J. M., and Oshiro, L. S.: Isolation of lymphocytopathic retroviruses from San Francisco patients with AIDS. Science 225:840, 1984.
14. Gallo, R. C., Salahuddin, S. Z., Popovic, M., Shearer, G. M., Kaplan, M., Haynes, B. F., Palker, T. J., Redfield, R., Oleske, J., Safai, B., White, G., Foster, P., and Markham, P. D.: Frequent detection and isolation of cytopathic retroviruses (HTLV-III) from patients with AIDS and at risk for AIDS. Science 224:500, 1984.
15. Popovic, M., Sarngadharan, M. G., Read, E., and Gallo, R. C.: Detection, isolation, and continuous production of cytopathic retroviruses (HTLV-III) from patients with AIDS and pre-AIDS. Science 224:497, 1984.
16. Sarngadharan, M. G., Popovic, M., Bruch, L., Schüpbach, J., and Gallo, R. C.: Antibodies reactive with human T-lymphotropic retroviruses (HTLV-III) in the serum of patients with AIDS. Science 224:506, 1984.
17. Schüpbach, J., Popovic, M., Gilden, R. V., Gonda, M. A., Sarngadharan, M. G., and Gallo, R. C.: Serological analysis of a subgroup of human T-lymphotropic retroviruses (HTLV-III) associated with AIDS. Science 224:503, 1984.
18. Vilmer, E., Barre-Sinoussi, F., Rouzioux, C., Gazengel, C., Brun, F. V., Dauguet, C., Fischer, A., Manigne, P., Chermann, J. C., Griscelli, C., and Montagnier, L.: Isolation of new lymphotropic retrovirus from two siblings with haemophilia B, one with AIDS. Lancet 1:753, 1984.
19. Coffin, J., Haase, A., Levy, J. A., Montagnier, L., Oroszlan, S., Teich, N., Temin, H., Toyoshima, K., Varmus, H., Vogt, P., and Weiss, R.: Human immunodeficiency viruses (letter). Science 232:697, 1986.
20. Clavel, F., Mansinho, K., Chamaret, S., Guetard, D., Favier, V., Nina, J., Santos-Ferreira, M.-O., Champalimaud, J.-L., and Montagnier, L.: Human immunodeficiency virus type 2 infection associated with AIDS in West Africa. N. Engl. J. Med. 316:1180, 1987.
21. Clavel, F., Guetard, D., Brun-Vezinet, F., Chamaret, S., Rey, M.-A., Santos-Ferreira, M. O., Laurent, A. G., Dauguet, C., Katlama, C., Rouzioux, C., Klatzmann, D., Champalimaud, J. L., and Montagnier, L.: Isolation of a new human retrovirus from West African patients with AIDS. Science 233:343, 1986.
22. Hoxie, J. A., Alpers, J. D., Rackowski, J. L., Huebner, K., Haggarty, B. S., Cedarbaum, A. J., and Reed, J. C.: Alterations in T4 (CD4) protein and mRNA synthesis in cells infected with HIV. Science 234:1123, 1986.
23. Folks, T., Benn, S., Rabson, A., Theodore, T., Hoggan, M. D., Martin, M., Lightfoote, M., and Sell, K.: Characterization of a continuous T-cell line susceptible to the cytopathic effects of the acquired immunodeficiency syndrome (AIDS)–associated retrovirus. Proc. Natl. Acad. Sci. USA 82:4539, 1985.
24. Dalgleish, A. G., Beverley, P. C. L., Clapham, P. R., Crawford, D. H., Greaves, M. F., and Weiss, R. A.: The CD4 (T4) antigen is an essential component of the receptor for the AIDS retrovirus. Nature 312:763, 1984.
25. Gonda, M. A., Wong-Staal, F., Gallo, R. C., Clements, J. E., Narayan, O., and Gilden, R. V.: Sequence homology and morphologic similarity of HTLV-III and visna virus, a pathogenic lentivirus. Science 227:173, 1985.
26. Gelderblom, H. R.: Assembly and morphology of HIV: Potential effect of structure on viral function (editorial). AIDS 5:617, 1991.

27. Gelderblom, H. R., Özel, M., Gheysen, D., Reupke, H., Winkel, T., Herz, U., Grund, C., and Pauli, G.: Morphogenesis and fine structure of lentivirses. *In* Schellekens, H., and Horzinek, M. C. (eds.): Animal Models in AIDS. Amsterdam, Elsevier, 1990.

28. Gelderblom, H. R., Hausmann, E. H. S., Özel, M., Pauli, G., and Koch, M. A.: Fine structure of human immunodeficiency virus (HIV) and immunolocalization of structural proteins. Virology 156:171, 1987.

29. Alizon, M., Sonigo, P., Barré-Sinoussi, F., Chermann, J.-C., Tiollais, P., Montagnier, L., and Wain-Hobson, S.: Molecular cloning of lymphadenopathy-associated virus. Nature 312:757, 1984.

30. Doolittle, R. F., Feng, D. F., McClure, M. A., and Johnson, M. S.: Retrovirus phylogeny and evolution. Curr. Top. Microbiol. Immunol. 157:1, 1990.

31. Hahn, B. H., Shaw, G. M., Arya, S. K., Popovic, M., Gallo, R. C., and Wong-Staal, F.: Molecular cloning and characterization of the HTLV-III virus associated with AIDS. Nature 312:166, 1984.

32. Luciw, P. A., Potter, S. J., Steimer, K., Dina, D., and Levy, J. A.: Molecular cloning of AIDS-associated retrovirus. Nature 312:760, 1984.

33. Ratner, L., Haseltine, W., Patarca, R., Livak, K. J., Starcich, B., Josephs, S. F., Doran, E. R., Rafalski, J. A., Whitehorn, E. A., Baumeister, K., Ivanoff, L., Petteway, S. R., Jr., Pearson, M. L., Lautenberger, J. A., Papas, T. S., Ghrayeb, J., Chang, N. T., Gallo, R. C., and Wong-Staal, F.: Complete nucleotide sequence of the AIDS virus, HTLV-III. Nature 313:277, 1985.

34. Sanchez-Pescador, R., Power, M. D., Barr, P. J., Steimer, K. S., Stempien, M. M., Brown-Shimer, S. L., Gee, W. W., Renard, A., Randolph, A., Levy, J. A., Dina, D., and Luciw, P. A.: Nucleotide sequence and expression of an AIDS-associated retrovirus (ARV-2). Science 227:484, 1985.

35. Shaw, G. M., Hahn, B. H., Arya, S. K., Groopman, J. E., Gallo, R. C., and Wong-Staal, F.: Molecular characterization of human T-cell leukemia (lymphotropic) virus type III in the acquired immune deficiency syndrome. Science 226:1165, 1984.

36. Wain-Hobson, S., Sonigo, P., Danos, O., Cole, S., and Alizon, M.: Nucleotide sequence of the AIDS virus, LAV. Cell 40:9, 1985.

37. Shinnick, T. M., Lerner, R. A., and Sutcliffe, J. G.: Nucleotide sequence of Moloney murine leukaemia virus. Nature 293:543, 1981.

38. Schwartz, D. E., Tizard, R., and Gilbert, W.: Nucleotide sequence of Rous sarcoma virus. Cell 32:853, 1983.

39. Muesing, M. A., Smith, D. H., Cabradilla, C. D., Benton, C. V., Lasky, L. A., and Capon, D. J.: Nucleic acid structure and expression of the human AIDS/lymphadenopathy retrovirus. Nature 313:450, 1985.

40. Rogers, J. H.: The origin and evolution of retroposons. Int. Rev. Cytol. 93:188, 1985.

41. Doolittle, R. F., Feng, D.-F., Johnson, M. S., and McClure, M. A.: Origins and evolutionary relationships of retroviruses. Q. Rev. Biol. 64:1, 1989.

42. Weiner, A. M., Deininger, P. L., and Efstratiadis, A.: Nonviral retroposons: Genes, pseudogenes, and transposable elements generated by the reverse flow of genetic information. Annu. Rev. Biochem. 55:631, 1986.

43. Xiong, Y., and Eickbush, T. H.: Origin and evolution of retroelements based upon their reverse transcriptase sequences. EMBO J. 9:3353, 1990.

44. Jacks, T., and Varmus, H. E.: Expression of the Rous sarcoma virus *pol* gene by ribosomal frameshifting. Science 230:1237, 1985.

45. Yoshinaka, Y., Katoh, I., Copeland, T. D., and Oroszlan, S.: Murine leukemia virus protease is encoded by the *gag-pol* gene and is synthesized through suppression of an amber termination codon. Proc. Natl. Acad. Sci. USA 82:1618, 1985.

46. Power, M. D., Marx, P. A., Bryant, M. L., Gardner, M. B., Barr, P. J., and Luciw, P. A.: Nucleotide sequence of SRV-1, a type D simian acquired immune deficiency syndrome retrovirus. Science 231:1567, 1986.

47. Seiki, M., Hattori, S., Hirayama, Y., and Yoshida, M.: Human adult T-cell leukemia virus: Complete nucleotide sequence of the provirus genome integrated in leukemia cell DNA. Proc. Natl. Acad. Sci. USA 80:3618, 1983.

48. Moore, R., Dixon, M., Smith, R., Peters, G., and Dickson, C.: Complete nucleotide sequence of a milk-transmitted mouse mammary tumor virus: Two frameshift suppression events are required for translation of *gag* and *pol*. J. Virol. 61:480, 1987.

49. Dickson, C., and Peters, G.: Protein-coding potential of mouse mammary tumor virus genome RNA as examined by in vitro translation. J. Virol. 37:36, 1981.

50. Marrack, P., Kushnir, E., and Kappler, J.: A maternally inherited superantigen encoded by a mammary tumour virus. Nature 349:524, 1991.

51. Frankel, W. N., Rudy, C., Coffin, J. M., and Huber, B. T.: Linkage of *Mls* genes to endogenous mammary tumour viruses of inbred mice. Nature 349:526, 1991.

52. Haseltine, W. A., Sodroski, J., Patarca, R., Briggs, D., Perkins, D., and Wong-Staal, F.: Structure of 3' terminal region of type II human T lymphotropic virus: Evidence for new coding region. Science 225:419, 1984.

53. Nagashima, K., Yoshida, M., and Seiki, M.: A single species of pX mRNA of human T-cell leukemia virus type I encodes *trans*-activator p40^x and two other phosphoproteins. J. Virol. 60:394, 1986.

54. Chen, I. S. Y., Slamon, D. J., Rosenblatt, J. D., Shah, N. P., Quan, S. G., and Wachsman, W.: The *x* gene is essential for HTLV replication. Science 229:54, 1985.

55. Cohen, E. A., Terwilliger, E. F., Sodroski, J. G., and Haseltine, W. A.: Identification of a protein encoded by the *vpu* gene of HIV-1. Nature 334:532, 1988.

56. Strebel, K., Klimkait, T., and Martin, M. A.: A novel gene of HIV-1, *vpu*, and its 16-kilodalton product. Science 241:1221, 1988.

57. Kappes, J. C., Morrow, C. D., Lee, S.-W., Jameson, B. A., Kent, S. B. H., Hood, L. E., Shaw, G. M., and Hahn, B. H.: Identification of a novel retroviral gene unique to human immunodeficiency virus type 2 and simian immunodeficiency virus SIV$_{MAC}$. J. Virol. 62:3501, 1988.

58. Henderson, L. E., Sowder, R. C., Copeland, T. D., Benveniste, R. E., and Oroszlan, S.: Isolation and characterization of a novel protein (X-ORF product) from SIV and HIV-2. Science 241:199, 1988.

59. Guyader, M., Emerman, M., Sonigo, P., Clavel, F., Montagnier, L., and Alizon, M.: Genome organization and transactivation of the human immunodeficiency virus type 2. Nature 326:662, 1987.

60. Hirsch, V. M., Olmsted, R. A., Murphey-Corb, M., Purcell, R. H., and Johnson, P. R.: An African primate lentivirus (SIV$_{sm}$) closely related to HIV-2. Nature 339:389, 1989.

61. Gojobori, T., Moriyama, E. N., Ina, Y., Ikeo, K., Miura, T., Tsujimoto, H., Hayami, M., and Yokoyama, S.: Evolutionary origin of human and simian immunodeficiency viruses. Proc. Natl. Acad. Sci. USA 87:4108, 1990.

62. Smith, T. F., Srinivasan, A., Schochetman, G., Marcus, M., and Myers, G.: The phylogenetic history of immunodeficiency viruses. Nature 333:573, 1988.

63. Miura, T., Sakuragi, J.-i., Kawamura, M., Fukasawa, M., Moriyama, E. N., Gojobori, T., Ishikawa, K.-i., Mingle, J. A. A., Nettey, V. B. A., Akari, H., Enami, M., Tsujimoto, H., and Hayami, M.: Establishment of a phylogenetic survey system for AIDS-related lentiviruses and demonstration of a new HIV-2 subgroup. AIDS 4:1257, 1990.

64. Harrich, D., Ulich, C., and Gaynor, R. B.: A critical role for the TAR element in promoting efficient human immunodeficiency virus type 1 reverse transcription. J. Virol. 70:4017, 1996.

65. Alter, H. J., Eichberg, J. W., Masur, H., Saxinger, W. C., Gallo, R., Macher, A. M., Lane, H. C., and Fauci, A. S.: Transmission of HTLV-III infection from human plasma to chimpanzees: An animal model for AIDS. Science 226:549, 1984.

66. Fultz, P. N., McClure, H. M., Swenson, R. B., McGrath, C. R., Brodie, A., Getchell, J. P., Jensen, F. C., Anderson, D. C., Broderson, J. R., and Francis, D. P.: Persistent infection of chimpanzees with human T-lymphotropic virus type III/lymphadenopathy-associated virus: a potential model for acquired immunodeficiency syndrome. J. Virol. 58:116, 1986.

67. Gajdusek, D. C., Amyx, H. L., Gibbs, C. J., Jr., Asher, D. M., Rodgers-Johnson, P., Epstein, L. G., Sarin, P. S., Gallo, R. C., Maluish, A., Arthur, L. O., Montagnier, L., and Mildvan, D.: Infection of chimpanzees by human T-lymphotropic retroviruses in brain and other tissues from AIDS patients (letter). Lancet 1:55, 1985.

68. Hamilton, J. A., Vairo, G., and Cocks, B. G.: Inhibition of S-phase progression in macrophages is linked to G1/S-phase suppression of DNA synthesis genes. J. Immunol. 148:4028, 1992.

69. McDougal, J. S., Mawle, A., Cort, S. P., Nicholson, J. K. A., Cross, G. D., Scheppler-Campbell, J. A., Hicks, D., and Sligh, J.: Cellular tropism of the human retrovirus HTLV-III/LAV. I. Role of T cell activation and expression of the T4 antigen. J. Immunol. 135:3151, 1985.

70. Zagury, D., Bernard, J., Leonard, R., Cheynier, R., Feldman, M., Sarin, P. S., and Gallo, R. C.: Long-term cultures of HTLV-III–infected T cells: A model of cytopathology of T-cell depletion in AIDS. Science 231:850, 1986.

71. Gowda, S. D., Stein, B. S., Mohagheghpour, N., Benike, C. J., and Engleman, E. G.: Evidence that T cell activation is required for HIV-1 entry in CD4+ lymphocytes. J. Immunol. 142:773, 1989.

72. Stevenson, M., Stanwick, T. L., Dempsey, M. P., and Lamonica, C. A.: HIV-1 replication is controlled at the level of T cell activation and proviral integration. EMBO J. 9:1551, 1990.

73. Zack, J. A., Cann, A. J., Lugo, J. P., and Chen, I. S. Y.: HIV-1 production from infected peripheral blood T cells after HTLV-I induced mitogenic stimulation. Science 240:1026, 1988.

74. Zack, J. A., Arrigo, S. J., Weitsman, S. R., Go, A. S., Haislip, A., and Chen, I. S. Y.: HIV-1 entry into quiescent primary lymphocytes: Molecular analysis reveals a labile, latent viral structure. Cell 61:213, 1990.

75. Engleman, E. G., Benike, C. J., Glickman, E., and Evans, R. L.: Antibodies to membrane structures that distinguish suppressor/cytotoxic and helper T lymphocyte subpopulations block the mixed leukocyte reaction in man. J. Exp. Med. 153:193, 1981.

76. Reinherz, E. L., Kung, P. C., Goldstein, G., and Schlossman, S. F.: Separation of functional subsets of human T cells by a monoclonal antibody. Proc. Natl. Acad. Sci. USA 76:4061, 1979.

77. Reinherz, E. L., and Schlossman, S. F.: The differentiation and function of human T lymphocytes. Cell 19:821, 1980.

78. Feng, Y., Broder, C. C., Kennedy, P. E., and Berger, E. A.: HIV-1 entry cofactor: Functional cDNA cloning of a seven-transmembrane, G protein–coupled receptor. Science 272:872, 1996.

79. Choe, H., Farzan, M., Sun, Y., Sullivan, N., Rollins, B., Ponath, P. D., Wu, L., Mackay, C. R., LaRosa, G., Newman, W., Gerard, N., Gerard, C., and Sodroski, J.: The β-chemokine receptors CCR3 and CCR5 facilitate infection by primary HIV-1 isolates. Cell 85:1135, 1996.

80. Deng, H., Liu, R., Ellmeier, W., Choe, S., Unutmaz, D., Burkhart, M., Di Marzio, P., Marmon, S., Sutton, R. E., Hill, C. M., Davis, C. B., Peiper, S. C., Schall, T. J., Littman, D. R., and Landau, N. R.: Identification of a major co-receptor for primary isolates of HIV-1. Nature 381:661, 1996.

81. Doranz, B. J., Rucker, J., Yi, Y., Smyth, R. J., Samson, M., Peiper, S. C., Parmentier, M., Collman, R. G., and Doms, R. W.: A dual-tropic primary HIV-1 isolate that uses fusin and the β-chemokine receptors CKR-5, CKR-3, and CKR-2b as fusion cofactors. Cell 85:1149, 1996.

82. Moore, J. P., Trkola, A., and Dragic, T.: Co-receptors for HIV-1 entry. Curr. Opin. Immunol. 9:551, 1997.

83. Stein, B. S., Gowda, S. D., Lifson, J. D., Penhallow, R. C., Bensch, K. G., and Engleman, E. G.: pH-independent HIV entry into CD4-positive T cells via virus envelope fusion to the plasma membrane. Cell 49:659, 1987.

84. Bowerman, B., Brown, P. O., Bishop, J. M., and Varmus, H. E.: A nucleoprotein complex mediates the integration of retroviral DNA. Genes Dev. 3:469, 1989.

85. Brown, P. O., Bowerman, B., Varmus, H. E., and Bishop, J. M.: Correct integration of retroviral DNA in vitro. Cell 49:347, 1987.

86. Fuetterer, J., and Hohn, T.: Involvement of nucleocapsids in reverse transcription: A general phenomenon? Trends Biochem. Sci. 12:92, 1987.

87. Fujiwara, T., and Mizuuchi, K.: Retroviral DNA integration: Structure of an integration intermediate. Cell 54:497, 1988.

88. Hippenmeyer, P. J., and Grandgenett, D. P.: Requirement of the avian retrovirus p32 DNA binding protein domain for replication. Virology 137:358, 1984.

89. Donehower, L. A., and Varmus, H. E.: A mutant murine leukemia virus with a single missense codon in pol is defective in a function affecting integration. Proc. Natl. Acad. Sci. USA 81:6461, 1984.

90. Panganiban, A. T., and Temin, H. M.: The retrovirus pol gene encodes a product required for DNA integration: Identification of a retrovirus int locus. Proc. Natl. Acad. Sci. USA 81:7885, 1984.

91. Schwartzberg, P., Colicelli, J., and Goff, S. P.: Construction and analysis of deletion mutations in the pol gene of Moloney murine leukemia virus: A new viral function required for productive infection. Cell 37:1043, 1984.

92. Holland, C. A., Hartley, J. W., Rowe, W. P., and Hopkins, N.: At least four viral genes contribute to the leukemogenicity of murine retrovirus MCF 247 in AKR mice. J. Virol. 53:158, 1985.

93. Oliff, A., Signorelli, K., and Collins, L.: The envelope gene and long terminal repeat sequences contribute to the pathogenic phenotype of helper-independent Friend viruses. J. Virol. 51:788, 1984.

94. Rosen, C. A., Haseltine, W. A., Lenz, J., Ruprecht, R., and Cloyd, M. W.: Tissue selectivity of murine leukemia virus infection is determined by long terminal repeat sequences. J. Virol. 55:862, 1985.

95. Li, Y., Golemis, E., Hartley, J. W., and Hopkins, N.: Disease specificity of nondefective Friend and Moloney murine leukemia viruses is controlled by a small number of nucleotides. J. Virol. 61:693, 1987.

96. Varmus, H. E., Heasley, S., Kung, H.-J., Oppermann, H., Smith, V. C., Bishop, J. M., and Shank, P. R.: Kinetics of synthesis, structure and purification of avian sarcoma virus–specific DNA made in the cytoplasm of acutely infected cells. J. Mol. Biol. 120:55, 1978.

97. Shank, P. R., Hughes, S. H., Kung, H.-J., Majors, J. E., Quintrell, N., Guntaka, R. V., Bishop, J. M., and Varmus, H. E.: Mapping unintegrated avian sarcoma virus DNA: Termini of linear DNA bear 300 nucleotides present once or twice in two species of circular DNA. Cell 15:1383, 1978.

98. Hsu, T. W., Sabran, J. L., Mark, G. E., Guntaka, R. V., and Taylor, J. M.: Analysis of unintegrated avian RNA tumor virus double-stranded DNA intermediates. J. Virol. 28:810, 1978.

99. Stoll, E., Billeter, M. A., Palmenberg, A., and Weissmann, C.: Avian myeloblastosis virus RNA is terminally redundant: Implications for the mechanism of retrovirus replication. Cell 12:57, 1977.

100. Coffin, J. M., and Haseltine, W. A.: Terminal redundancy and the origin of replication of Rous sarcoma virus RNA. Proc. Natl. Acad. Sci. USA 74:1908, 1977.

101. Collett, M. S., and Faras, A. J.: Avian retrovirus RNA-directed DNA synthesis: Transcription at the 5′ terminus of the viral genome and the functional role for the viral terminal redundancy. Virology 86:297, 1978.

102. Colicelli, J., and Goff, S. P.: Mutants and pseudorevertants of Moloney murine leukemia virus with alterations at the integration site. Cell 42:573, 1985.

103. Panganiban, A. T., and Temin, H. M.: The terminal nucleotides of retrovirus DNA are required for integration but not virus production. Nature 306:155, 1983.

104. Murphy, J. E., and Goff, S. P.: Construction and analysis of deletion mutations in the U5 region of Moloney murine leukemia virus: Effects on RNA packaging and reverse transcription. J. Virol. 63:319, 1989.

105. Sealey, L., and Chalkley, R.: At least two nuclear proteins bind specifically to the Rous sarcoma virus long terminal repeat enhancer. Mol. Cell. Biol. 7:787, 1987.

106. Speck, N. A., and Baltimore, D.: Six distinct nuclear factors interact with the 75-base-pair repeat of the Moloney murine leukemia virus enhancer. Mol. Cell. Biol. 7:1101, 1987.

107. Cordingley, M. G., Riegel, A. T., and Hager, G. L.: Steroid-dependent interaction of transcription factors with the inducible promoter of mouse mammary tumor virus in vivo. Cell 48:261, 1987.

108. Fujisawa, J., Seiki, M., Sato, M., and Yoshida, M.: A transcriptional enhancer sequence of HTLV-I is responsible for trans-activation mediated by p40c of HTLV-I. EMBO J. 5:713, 1986.

109. Nikolov, D. B., Hu, S. H., Lin, J., Gasch, A., Hoffmann, A., Horikoshi, M., Chua, N. H., Roeder, R. G., and Burley, S. K.: Crystal structure of TFIID TATA-box binding protein. Nature 360:40, 1992.

110. Kim, J. L., Nikolov, D. B., and Burley, S. K.: Co-crystal structure of TBP recognizing the minor groove of a TATA element. Nature 365:520, 1993.

111. Ha, I., Roberts, S., Maldonado, E., Sun, X., Kim, L. U., Green, M., and Reinberg, D.: Multiple functional domains of human transcription factor IIB: Distinct interactions with two general transcription factors and RNA polymerase II. Genes Dev. 7:1021, 1993.

112. Li, Y., Flanagan, P. M., Tschochner, H., and Kornberg, R. D.: RNA polymerase II initiation factor interactions and transcription start site selection. Science 263:805, 1994.

113. Lu, H., Zawel, L., Fisher, L., Egly, J. M., and Reinberg, D.: Human general transcription factor IIH phosphorylates the C-terminal domain of RNA polymerase II. Nature 358:641, 1992.

114. Ohkuma, Y., and Roeder, R. G.: Regulation of TFIIH ATPase and kinase activities by TFIIE during active initiation complex formation. Nature 368:160, 1994.

115. Serizawa, H., Conaway, J. W., and Conaway, R. C.: An oligomeric form of the large subunit of transcription factor (TF) IIE activates phosphorylation of the RNA polymerase II carboxyl-terminal domain by TFIIH. J. Biol. Chem. 269:20750, 1994.

116. Rosen, C. A., Sodroski, J. G., and Haseltine, W. A.: The location of *cis*-acting regulatory sequences in the human T cell lymphotropic virus type III (HTLV-III/LAV) long terminal repeat. Cell 41:813, 1985.

117. Siekevitz, M., Josephs, S. F., Dukovich, M., Peffer, N., Wong-Staal, F., and Greene, W. C.: Activation of the HIV-1 LTR by T cell mitogens and the trans-activator protein of HTLV-I. Science 238:1575, 1987.

118. Kim, J. Y., Gonzalez-Scarano, F., Zeichner, S. L., and Alwine, J. C.: Replication of type 1 human immunodeficiency viruses containing linker substitution mutations in the −201 to −130 region of the long terminal repeat. J. Virol. 67:1658, 1993.

119. Garcia, J. A., Wu, F. K., Mitsuyasu, R., and Gaynor, R. B.: Interactions of cellular proteins involved in the transcriptional regulation of the human immunodeficiency virus. EMBO J. 6:3761, 1987.

120. Harrich, D., Garcia, J., Wu, F., Mitsuyasu, R., Gonzalez, J., and Gaynor, R.: Role of SP1-binding domains in in vivo transcriptional regulation of the human immunodeficiency virus type 1 long terminal repeat. J. Virol. 63:2585, 1989.

121. Dynan, W. S., and Tjian, R.: The promoter-specific transcription factor Sp1 binds to upstream sequences in the SV40 early promoter. Cell 35:79, 1983.

122. Gidoni, D., Kadonaga, J. T., Barrera-Saldana, H., Takahashi, K., Chambon, P., and Tjian, R.: Bidirectional SV40 transcription mediated by tandem Sp1 binding interactions. Science 230:511, 1985.

123. Berkhout, B., and Jeang, K.-T.: Functional roles for the TATA promoter and enhancers in basal and Tat-induced expression of the human immunodeficiency virus type 1 long terminal repeat. J. Virol. 66:139, 1992.

124. Leonard, J., Parrott, C., Buckler-White, A. J., Turner, W., Ross, E. K., Martin, M. A., and Rabson, A. B.: The NF-κB binding sites in the human immunodeficiency virus type 1 long terminal repeat are not required for virus infectivity. J. Virol. 63:4919, 1989.

125. Parrott, C., Seidner, T., Duh, E., Leonard, J., Theodore, T. S., Buckler-White, A., Martin, M. A., and Rabson, A. B.: Variable role of the long terminal repeat Sp1-binding sites in human immunodeficiency virus replication in T lymphocytes. J. Virol. 65:1414, 1991.

126. Ross, E. K., Buckler-White, A. J., Rabson, A. B., Englund, G., and Martin, M. A.: Contribution of NF-κB and Sp1 binding motifs to the replicative capacity of human immunodeficiency virus type 1: Distinct patterns of viral growth are determined by T-cell types. J. Virol. 65:4350, 1991.

127. Nabel, G., and Baltimore, D.: An inducible transcription factor activates expression of human immunodeficiency virus in T cells. Nature 326:711, 1987.

128. Queen, C., and Baltimore, D.: Immunoglobulin gene transcription is activated by downstream sequence elements. Cell 33:741, 1983.

129. Miyamoto, S., and Verma, I. M.: Rel/NF-κB/IκB story. Adv. Cancer. Res. 66:255, 1995.

130. Bours, V., Villalobos, J., Burd, P. R., Kelly, K., and Siebenlist, U.: Cloning of a mitogen-inducible gene encoding a κB DNA-binding protein with homology to the *rel* oncogene and to cell-cycle motifs. Nature 348:76, 1990.

131. Ghosh, S., Gifford, A. M., Riviere, L. R., Tempst, P., Nolan, G. P., and Baltimore, D.: Cloning of the p50 DNA binding subunit of NF-κB: Homology to *rel* and *dorsal*. Cell 62:1019, 1990.

132. Dobrzanski, P., Ryseck, R. P., and Bravo, R.: Both N- and C-terminal domains of RelB are required for full transactivation: Role of the N-terminal leucine zipper-like motif. Mol. Cell. Biol. 13:1572, 1993.

133. Ryseck, R.-P., Bull, P., Takamiya, M., Bours, V., Siebenlist, U., Dobrzanski, P., and Bravo, R.: RelB, a new Rel family transcription activator that can interact with p50-NF-κB. Mol. Cell. Biol. 12:674, 1992.

134. Baeuerle, P. A., and Baltimore, D.: A 65-kD subunit of active NF-κB is required for inhibition of NF-κB by IκB. Genes Dev. 3:1689, 1989.

135. Baeuerle, P. A., and Baltimore, D.: Activation of DNA-binding activity in an apparently cytoplasmic precursor of the NF-κB transcription factor. Cell 53:211, 1988.

136. Inoue, J.-i., Kerr, L. D., Kakizuka, A., and Verma, I. M.: IκBγ, a 70 kd protein identical to the C-terminal half of p110 NF-κB: A new member of the IκB family. Cell 68:1109, 1992.

137. Kerr, L. D., Inoue, J.-i., Davis, N., Link, E., Baeuerle, P. A., Bose, H. R., Jr., and Verma, I. M.: The rel-associated pp40 protein prevents DNA binding of Rel and NF-κB: Relationship with IκBβ and regulation by phosphorylation. Genes Dev. 5:1464, 1991.

138. Beg, A. A., Ruben, S. M., Scheinman, R. I., Haskill, S., Rosen, C. A., and Baldwin, A. S., Jr.: IκB interacts with the nuclear localization sequences of the subunits of NF-κB: A mechanism for cytoplasmic retention. Genes Dev. 6:1899, 1992.

139. Ganchi, P. A., Sun, S. C., Greene, W. C., and Ballard, D. W.: IκB/MAD-3 masks the nuclear localization signal of NF-κ Bp65 and requires the transactivation domain to inhibit NF-κB p65 DNA binding. Mol. Biol. Cell. 3:1339, 1992.

140. Brown, K., Park, S., Kanno, T., Franzoso, G., and Siebenlist, U.: Mutual regulation of the transcriptional activator NF-κB and its inhibitor, IκB-α. Proc. Natl. Acad. Sci. USA 90:2532, 1993.

141. Palombella, V. J., Rando, O. J., Goldberg, A. L., and Maniatis, T.: The ubiquitin-proteasome pathway is required for processing the NF-κB1 precursor protein and the activation of NF-κB. Cell 78:773, 1994.

142. Rothe, M., Sarma, V., Dixit, V. M., and Goeddel, D. V.: TRAF2-mediated activation of NF-κB by TNF receptor 2 and CD40. Science 269:1424, 1995.

143. Cheng, G., and Baltimore, D.: TANK, a co-inducer with TRAF2 of TNF- and CD40L-mediated NF-κB activation. Genes Dev. 10:963, 1996.

144. Cao, Z., Henzel, W. J., and Gao, X.: IRAK: A kinase associated with the interleukin-1 receptor. Science 271:1128, 1996.

145. Chen, B. K., Feinberg, M. B., and Baltimore, D.: The κB sites in the human immunodeficiency virus type 1 long terminal repeat enhance virus replication yet are not absolutely required for viral growth. J. Virol. 71:5495, 1997.

146. Perkins, N. D., Edwards, N. L., Duckett, C. S., Agranoff, A. B., Schmid, R. M., and Nabel, G. J.: A cooperative interaction between NF-κB and Sp1 is required for HIV-1 enhancer activation. EMBO J. 12:3551, 1993.

147. Verdin, E.: DNase I-hypersensitive sites are associated with both long terminal repeats and with the intragenic enhancer of integrated human immunodeficiency virus type 1. J. Virol. 65:6790, 1991.

148. Verdin, E., Paras, P., Jr., and Van Lint, C.: Chromatin disruption in the promoter of human immunodeficiency virus type 1 during transcriptional activation. EMBO J. 12:3249, 1993.

149. El Kharroubi, A., and Martin, M. A.: *cis*-acting sequences located downstream of the human immunodeficiency virus type 1 promoter affect its chromatin structure and transcriptional activity. Mol. Cell. Biol. 16:2958, 1996.

150. Van Lint, C., Amella, C. A., Emiliani, S., John, M., Jie, T., and Verdin, E.: Transcription factor binding sites downstream of the human immunodeficiency virus type 1 transcription start site are important for virus infectivity. J. Virol. 71:6113, 1997.

151. Pazin, M. J., Sheridan, P. L., Cannon, K., Cao, Z., Keck, J. G., Kadonaga, J. T., and Jones, K. A.: NF-κB-mediated chromatin reconfiguration and transcriptional activation of the HIV-1 enhancer in vitro. Genes Dev. 10:37, 1996.

152. Nelson, J. A., Reynolds-Kohler, C., Oldstone, M. B. A., and Wiley, C. A.: HIV and HCMV coinfect brain cells in patients with AIDS. Virology 165:286, 1988.

153. Gendelman, H. E., Phelps, W., Feigenbaum, L., Ostrove, J. M., Adachi, A., Howley, P. M., Khoury, G., Ginsberg, H. S., and Martin, M. A.: Trans-activation of the human immunodeficiency virus long terminal repeat sequence by DNA viruses. Proc. Natl. Acad. Sci. USA 83:9759, 1986.

154. Davis, M. G., Kenney, S. C., Kamine, J., Pagano, J. S., and Huang, E.-S.: Immediate-early gene region of human cytomegalovirus transactivates the promoter of human immunodeficiency virus. Proc. Natl. Acad. Sci. USA 84:8642, 1987.

155. Lusso, P., Ensoli, B., Markham, P. D., Ablashi, D. V., Salahuddin, S. Z., Tschachler, E., Wong-Staal, F., and Gallo, R. C.: Productive dual infection of human CD4⁺ T lymphocytes by HIV-1 and HHV-6. Nature 337:370, 1989.

156. Nelson, J. A., Ghazal, P., and Wiley, C. A.: Role of opportunistic viral infections in AIDS. AIDS 4:1, 1990.

157. Leung, K., and Nabel, G. J.: HTLV-1 transactivator induces interleukin-2 receptor expression through an NF-κB-like factor. Nature 333:776, 1988.

158. Ballard, D. W., Böhnlein, E., Lowenthal, J. W., Wano, Y., Franza, B. R., and Greene, W. C.: HTLV-I tax induces cellular proteins that activate the κB element in the IL-2 receptor α gene. Science 241:1652, 1988.

159. Dayton, A. I., Sodroski, J. G., Rosen, C. A., Goh, W. C., and Haseltine, W. A.: The *trans*-activator gene of the human T cell lymphotropic virus type III is required for replication. Cell 44:941, 1986.

160. Fisher, A. G., Feinberg, M. B., Josephs, S. F., Harper, M. E., Marselle,

L. M., Reyes, G., Gonda, M. A., Aldovini, A., Debouk, C., Gallo, R. C., and Wong-Staal, F.: The *trans*-activator gene of HTLV-III is essential for virus replication. Nature 320:367, 1986.

161. Wright, C. M., Felber, B. K., Paskalis, H., and Pavlakis, G. N.: Expression and characterization of the *trans*-activator of HTLV-III/ LAV virus. Science 234:988, 1986.

162. Hauber, J., Perkins, A., Heimer, E. P., and Cullen, B. R.: Trans-activation of human immunodeficiency virus gene expression is mediated by nuclear events. Proc. Natl. Acad. Sci. USA 84:6364, 1987.

163. Sodroski, J., Patarca, R., Rosen, C., Wong-Staal, F., and Haseltine, W.: Location of the *trans*-activating region on the genome of human T-cell lymphotropic virus type III. Science 229:74, 1985.

164. Muesing, M. A., Smith, D. H., and Capon, D. J.: Regulation of mRNA accumulation by a human immunodeficiency virus *trans*-activator protein. Cell 48:691, 1987.

165. Cullen, B. R.: *Trans*-activation of human immunodeficiency virus occurs via a bimodal mechanism. Cell 46:973, 1986.

166. Korber, B., Foley, B., Leitner, T., McCutchan, F., Hahn, B., Mellors, J. W., Myers, G., and Kuiken, C. (eds.): Human Retroviruses and AIDS 1997. Los Alamos, N. Mex., Los Alamos National Laboratory, 1997.

167. Hess, J. L., Small, J. A., and Clements, J. E.: Sequences in the visna virus long terminal repeat that control transcriptional activity and respond to viral *trans*-activation: Involvement of AP-1 sites in basal activity and *trans*-activation. J. Virol. 63:3001, 1989.

168. Keller, A., Partin, K. M., Löchelt, M., Bannert, H., Flügel, R. M., and Cullen, B. R.: Characterization of the transcriptional *trans* activator of human foamy retrovirus. J. Virol. 65:2589, 1991.

169. Brady, J., Jeang, K.-T., Duvall, J., and Khoury, G.: Identification of p40x-responsive regulatory sequences within the human T-cell leukemia virus type I long terminal repeat. J. Virol. 61:2175, 1987.

170. Paskalis, H., Felber, B. K., and Pavlakis, G. N.: Cis-acting sequences responsible for the transcriptional activation of human T-cell leukemia virus type I constitute a conditional enhancer. Proc. Natl. Acad. Sci. USA 83:6558, 1986.

171. Hauber, J., and Cullen, B. R.: Mutational analysis of the *trans*-activation-responsive region of the human immunodeficiency virus type I long terminal repeat. J. Virol. 62:673, 1988.

172. Jakobovits, A., Smith, D. H., Jakobovits, E. B., and Capon, D. J.: A discrete element 3' of human immunodeficiency virus 1 (HIV-1) and HIV-2 mRNA initiation sites mediates transcriptional activation by an HIV *trans* activator. Mol. Cell. Biol. 8:2555, 1988.

173. Kao, S.-Y., Calman, A. F., Luciw, P. A., and Peterlin, B. M.: Anti-termination of transcription within the long terminal repeat of HIV-1 by *tat* gene product. Nature 330:489, 1987.

174. Selby, M. J., Bain, E. S., Luciw, P. A., and Peterlin, B. M.: Structure, sequence, and position of the stem-loop in *tar* determine transcriptional elongation by *tat* through the HIV-1 long terminal repeat. Genes Dev. 3:547, 1989.

175. Peterlin, B. M., Luciw, P. A., Barr, P. J., and Walker, M. D.: Elevated levels of mRNA can account for the trans-activation of human immunodeficiency virus. Proc. Natl. Acad. Sci. USA 83:9734, 1986.

176. Berkhout, B., Silverman, R. H., and Jeang, K.-T.: Tat *trans*-activates the human immunodeficiency virus through a nascent RNA target. Cell 59:273, 1989.

177. Berkhout, B., and Jeang, K.-T.: *trans* Activation of human immunodeficiency virus type 1 is sequence specific for both the single-stranded bulge and loop of the *trans*-acting-responsive hairpin: A quantitative analysis. J. Virol. 63:5501, 1989.

178. Feng, S., and Holland, E. C.: HIV-1 *tat trans*-activation requires the loop sequence within *tar.* Nature 334:165, 1988.

179. Roy, S., Parkin, N. T., Rosen, C., Itovitch, J., and Sonenberg, N.: Structural requirements for *trans* activation of human immunodeficiency virus type 1 long terminal repeat-directed gene expression by *tat:* Importance of base pairing, loop sequence, and bulges in the *tat*-responsive sequence. J. Virol. 64:1402, 1990.

180. Emerman, M., Guyader, M., Montagnier, L., Baltimore, D., and Muesing, M. A.: The specificity of the human immunodeficiency virus type 2 transactivator is different from that of human immunodeficiency virus type 1. EMBO J. 6:3755, 1987.

181. Garcia, J. A., Harrich, D., Soultanakis, E., Wu, F., Mitsuyasu, R., and Gaynor, R. B.: Human immunodeficiency virus type 1 LTR TATA and TAR region sequences required for transcriptional regulation. EMBO J. 8:765, 1989.

182. Ruben, S., Perkins, A., Purcell, R., Joung, K., Sia, R., Burghoff, R., Haseltine, W. A., and Rosen, C. A.: Structural and functional characterization of human immunodeficiency virus *tat* protein. J. Virol. 63:1, 1989.

183. Dingwall, C., Ernberg, I., Gait, M. J., Green, S. M., Heaphy, S., Karn, J., Lowe, A. D., Singh, M., and Skinner, M. A.: HIV-1 *tat* protein stimulates transcription by binding to a U-rich bulge in the stem of the TAR RNA structure. EMBO J. 9:4145, 1990.

184. Dingwall, C., Ernberg, I., Gait, M. J., Green, S. M., Heaphy, S., Karn, J., Lowe, A. D., Singh, M., Skinner, M. A., and Valerio, R.: Human immunodeficiency virus 1 tat protein binds trans-activation-responsive region (TAR) RNA in vitro. Proc. Natl. Acad. Sci. USA 86:6925, 1989.

185. Roy, S., Delling, U., Chen, C.-H., Rosen, C. A., and Sonenberg, N.: A bulge structure in HIV-1 TAR RNA is required for Tat binding and Tat-mediated *trans*-activation. Genes Dev. 4:1365, 1990.

186. Weeks, K. M., Ampe, C., Schultz, S. C., Steitz, T. A., and Crothers, D. M.: Fragments of the HIV-1 Tat protein specifically bind TAR RNA. Science 249:1281, 1990.

187. Aboul-ela, F., Karn, J., and Varani, G.: The structure of the human immunodeficiency virus type-1 TAR RNA reveals principles of RNA recognition by Tat protein. J. Mol. Biol. 253:313, 1995.

188. Cordingley, M. G., LaFemina, R. L., Callahan, P. L., Condra, J. H., Sardana, V. V., Graham, D. J., Nguyen, T. M., LeGrow, K., Gotlib, L., Schlabach, A. J., and Colonno, R. J.: Sequence-specific interaction of Tat protein and Tat peptides with the transactivation-responsive sequence element of human immunodeficiency virus type 1 *in vitro*. Proc. Natl. Acad. Sci. USA 87:8985, 1990.

189. Luo, Y., Madore, S. J., Parslow, T. G., Cullen, B. R., and Peterlin, B. M.: Functional analysis of interactions between Tat and the trans-activation response element of human immunodeficiency virus type 1 in cells. J. Virol. 67:5617, 1993.

190. Madore, S. J., and Cullen, B. R.: Genetic analysis of the cofactor requirement for human immunodeficiency virus type 1 Tat function. J. Virol. 67:3703, 1993.

191. Sullenger, B. A., Gallardo, H. F., Ungers, G. E., and Gilboa, E.: Analysis of trans-acting response decoy RNA-mediated inhibition of human immunodeficiency virus type 1 transactivation. J. Virol. 65:6811, 1991.

192. Tiley, L. S., Madore, S. J., Malim, M. H., and Cullen, B. R.: The VP16 transcription activation domain is functional when targeted to a promoter-proximal RNA sequence. Genes Dev. 6:2077, 1992.

193. Selby, M. J., and Peterlin, B. M.: *Trans*-activation by HIV-1 Tat via a heterologous RNA binding protein. Cell 62:769, 1990.

194. Southgate, C., Zapp, M. L., and Green, M. R.: Activation of transcription by HIV-1 Tat protein tethered to nascent RNA through another protein. Nature 345:640, 1990.

195. Hart, C. E., Ou, C.-Y., Galphin, J. C., Moore, J., Bacheler, L. T., Wasmuth, J. J., Petteway, S. R., Jr., and Schochetman, G.: Human chromosome 12 is required for elevated HIV-1 expression in human-hamster hybrid cells. Science 246:488, 1989.

196. Newstein, M., Stanbridge, E. J., Casey, G., and Shank, P. R.: Human chromosome 12 encodes a species-specific factor which increases human immunodeficiency virus type 1 *tat*-mediated *trans*activation in rodent cells. J. Virol. 64:4565, 1990.

197. Alonso, A., Cujec, T. P., and Peterlin, B. M.: Effects of human chromosome 12 on interactions between Tat and TAR of human immunodeficiency virus type 1. J. Virol. 68:6505, 1994.

198. Marciniak, R. A., Garcia-Blanco, M. A., and Sharp, P. A.: Identification and characterization of a HeLa nuclear protein that specifically binds to the trans-activation-response (TAR) element of human immunodeficiency virus. Proc. Natl. Acad. Sci. USA 87:3624, 1990.

199. Feinberg, M. B., Baltimore, D., and Frankel, A. D.: The role of Tat in the human immunodeficiency virus life cycle indicates a primary effect on transcriptional elongation. Proc. Natl. Acad. Sci. USA 88:4045, 1991.

200. Laspia, M. F., Rice, A. P., and Mathews, M. B.: HIV-1 Tat protein increases transcriptional initiation and stabilizes elongation. Cell 59:283, 1989.

201. Toohey, M. G., and Jones, K. A.: In vitro formation of short RNA polymerase II transcripts that terminate within the HIV-1 and HIV-2 promoter-proximal downstream regions. Genes Dev. 3:265, 1989.

202. Marciniak, R. A., and Sharp, P. A.: HIV-1 Tat protein promotes formation of more-processive elongation complexes. EMBO J. 10:4189, 1991.

203. Chun, R. F., and Jeang, K.-T.: Requirements for RNA polymerase II

carboxyl-terminal domain for activated transcription of human retroviruses human T-cell lymphotropic virus I and HIV-1. J. Biol. Chem. 271:27888, 1996.

204. Okamoto, H., Sheline, C. T., Corden, J. L., Jones, K. A., and Peterlin, B. M.: Trans-activation by human immunodeficiency virus Tat protein requires the C-terminal domain of RNA polymerase II. Proc. Natl. Acad. Sci. USA 93:11575, 1996.

205. Parada, C. A., and Roeder, R. G.: Enhanced processivity of RNA polymerase II triggered by Tat-induced phosphorylation of its carboxy-terminal domain. Nature 384:375, 1996.

206. Yang, X., Herrmann, C. H., and Rice, A. P.: The human immunodeficiency virus Tat proteins specifically associate with TAK in vivo and require the carboxyl-terminal domain of RNA polymerase II for function. J. Virol. 70:4576, 1996.

207. Herrmann, C. H., and Rice, A. P.: Specific interaction of the human immunodeficiency virus Tat proteins with a cellular protein kinase. Virology 197:601, 1993.

208. Herrmann, C. H., and Rice, A. P.: Lentivirus Tat proteins specifically associate with a cellular protein kinase, TAK, that hyperphosphorylates the carboxyl-terminal domain of the large subunit of RNA polymerase II: Candidate for a Tat cofactor. J. Virol. 69:1612, 1995.

209. Garcia-Martinez, L. F., Mavankal, G., Neveu, J. M., Lane, W. S., Ivanov, D., and Gaynor, R. B.: Purification of a Tat-associated kinase reveals a TFIIH complex that modulates HIV-1 transcription. EMBO J. 16:2836, 1997.

210. Herrmann, C. H., Gold, M. O., and Rice, A. P.: Viral transactivators specifically target distinct cellular protein kinases that phosphorylate the RNA polymerase II C-terminal domain. Nucleic Acids Res. 24:501, 1996.

211. Zhu, Y., Pe'ery, T., Peng, J., Ramanathan, Y., Marshall, N., Marshall, T., Amendt, B., Mathews, M. B., and Price, D. H.: Transcription elongation factor P-TEFb is required for HIV-1 tat transactivation in vitro. Genes Dev. 11:2622, 1997.

212. Marshall, N. F., and Price, D. H.: Control of formation of two distinct classes of RNA polymerase II elongation complexes. Mol. Cell Biol. 12:2078, 1992.

213. Marshall, N. F., and Price, D. H.: Purification of P-TEFb, a transcription factor required for the transition into productive elongation. J. Biol. Chem. 270:12335, 1995.

214. Marshall, N. F., Peng, J., Xie, Z., and Price, D. H.: Control of RNA polymerase II elongation potential by a novel carboxyl-terminal domain kinase. J. Biol. Chem. 271:27176, 1996.

215. Mancebo, H. S., Lee, G., Flygare, J., Tomassini, J., Luu, P., Zhu, Y., Peng, J., Blau, C., Hazuda, D., Price, D., and Flores, O.: P-TEFb kinase is required for HIV Tat transcriptional activation in vivo and in vitro. Genes Dev. 11:2633, 1997.

216. Wei, P., Garber, M. E., Fang, S. M., Fischer, W. H., and Jones, K. A.: A novel CDK9-associated C-type cyclin interacts directly with HIV-1 Tat and mediates its high-affinity, loop-specific binding to TAR RNA. Cell 92:451, 1998.

217. Marciniak, R. A., Calnan, B. J., Frankel, A. D., and Sharp, P. A.: HIV-1 Tat protein trans-activates transcription in vitro. Cell 63:791, 1990.

218. Gaynor, R., Soultanakis, E., Kuwabara, M., Garcia, J., and Sigman, D. S.: Specific binding of a HeLa cell nuclear protein to RNA sequences in the human immunodeficiency virus transactivating region. Proc. Natl. Acad. Sci. USA 86:4858, 1989.

219. Gatignol, A., Buckler-White, A., Berkhout, B., and Jeang, K.-T.: Characterization of a human TAR RNA-binding protein that activates the HIV-1 LTR. Science 251:1597, 1991.

220. Sune, C., Hayashi, T., Liu, Y., Lane, W. S., Young, R. A., and Garcia-Blanco, M. A.: CA150, a nuclear protein associated with the RNA polymerase II holoenzyme, is involved in Tat-activated human immunodeficiency virus type 1 transcription. Mol. Cell. Biol. 17:6029, 1997.

221. Zhou, Q., and Sharp, P. A.: Tat-SF1: Cofactor for stimulation of transcriptional elongation by HIV-1 Tat. Science 274:605, 1996.

222. Frankel, A. D., and Pabo, C. O.: Cellular uptake of the Tat protein from human immunodeficiency virus. Cell 55:1189, 1988.

223. Viscidi, R. P., Mayur, K., Lederman, H. M., and Frankel, A. D.: Inhibition of antigen-induced lymphocyte proliferation by Tat protein from HIV-1. Science 246:1606, 1989.

224. Ensoli, B., Barillari, G., Salahuddin, S. Z., Gallo, R. C., and Wong-Staal, F.: Tat protein of HIV-1 stimulates growth of cells derived from Kaposi's sarcoma lesions of AIDS patients. Nature 345:84, 1990.

225. Gruss, P., Lai, C. J., Dhar, R., and Khoury, G.: Splicing as a requirement for biogenesis of functional 16S mRNA of simian virus 40. Proc. Natl. Acad. Sci. USA 76:4317, 1979.

226. Chung, S., and Perry, R. P.: Importance of introns for expression of mouse ribosomal protein gene rpL32. Mol. Cell. Biol. 9:2075, 1989.

227. Guatelli, J. C., Gingeras, T. R., and Richman, D. D.: Alternative splice acceptor utilization during human immunodeficiency virus type 1 infection of cultured cells. J. Virol. 64:4093, 1990.

228. Robert-Guroff, M., Popovic, M., Gartner, S., Markham, P., Gallo, R. C., and Reitz, M. S.: Structure and expression of tat-, rev-, and nef-specific transcripts of human immunodeficiency virus type 1 in infected lymphocytes and macrophages. J. Virol. 64:3391, 1990.

229. Schwartz, S., Felber, B. K., Benko, D. M., Fenyö, E.-M., and Pavlakis, G. N.: Cloning and functional analysis of multiply spliced mRNA species of human immunodeficiency virus type 1. J. Virol. 64:2519, 1990.

230. Furtado, M. R., Balachandran, R., Gupta, P., and Wolinsky, S. M.: Analysis of alternatively spliced human immunodeficiency virus type-1 mRNA species, one of which encodes a novel TAT-ENV fusion protein. Virology 185:258, 1991.

231. Purcell, D. F., and Martin, M. A.: Alternative splicing of human immunodeficiency virus type 1 mRNA modulates viral protein expression, replication, and infectivity. J. Virol. 67:6365, 1993.

232. Arrigo, S., and Beemon, K.: Regulation of Rous sarcoma virus RNA splicing and stability. Mol. Cell. Biol. 8:4858, 1988.

233. Katz, R. A., Kotler, M., and Skalka, A. M.: cis-Acting intron mutations that affect the efficiency of avian retroviral RNA splicing: Implication for mechanisms of control. J. Virol. 62:2686, 1988.

234. Miller, C. K., Embretson, J. E., and Temin, H. M.: Transforming viruses spontaneously arise from nontransforming reticuloendotheliosis virus strain T-derived viruses as a result of increased accumulation of spliced viral RNA. J. Virol. 62:1219, 1988.

235. McNally, L. M., and McNally, M. T.: SR protein splicing factors interact with the Rous sarcoma virus negative regulator of splicing element. J. Virol. 70:1163, 1996.

236. Ogert, R. A., Lee, L. H., and Beemon, K. L.: Avian retroviral RNA element promotes unspliced RNA accumulation in the cytoplasm. J. Virol. 70:3834, 1996.

237. Sodroski, J., Goh, W. C., Rosen, C., Dayton, A., Terwilliger, E., and Haseltine, W.: A second post-transcriptional trans-activator gene required for HTLV-III replication. Nature 321:412, 1986.

238. Emerman, M., Vazeux, R., and Peden, K.: The rev gene product of the human immunodeficiency virus affects envelope-specific RNA localization. Cell 57:1155, 1989.

239. Felber, B. K., Hadzopoulou-Cladaras, M., Cladaras, C., Copeland, T., and Pavlakis, G. N.: rev Protein of human immunodeficiency virus type 1 affects the stability and transport of the viral mRNA. Proc. Natl. Acad. Sci. USA 86:1495, 1989.

240. Hammarskjöld, M.-L., Heimer, J., Hammarskjöld, B., Sangwan, I., Albert, L., and Rekosh, D.: Regulation of human immunodeficiency virus env expression by the rev gene product. J. Virol. 63:1959, 1989.

241. Malim, M. H., Hauber, J., Le, S.-Y., Maizel, J. V., and Cullen, B. R.: The HIV-1 rev trans-activator acts through a structured target sequence to activate nuclear export of unspliced viral mRNA. Nature 338:254, 1989.

242. Malim, M. H., Tiley, L. S., McCarn, D. F., Rusche, J. R., Hauber, J., and Cullen, B. R.: HIV-1 structural gene expression requires binding of the Rev trans-activator to its RNA target sequence. Cell 60:675, 1990.

243. Mermer, B., Felber, B. K., Campbell, M., and Pavlakis, G. N.: Identification of trans-dominant HIV-1 rev protein mutants by direct transfer of bacterially produced proteins into human cells. Nucleic Acids Res. 18:2037, 1990.

244. Sadaie, M. R., Rappaport, J., Benter, T., Josephs, S. F., Willis, R., and Wong-Staal, F.: Missense mutations in an infectious human immunodeficiency viral genome: Functional mapping of tat and identification of the rev splice acceptor. Proc. Natl. Acad. Sci. USA 85:9224, 1988.

245. Rosen, C. A., Terwilliger, E., Dayton, A., Sodroski, J. G., and Haseltine, W. A.: Intragenic cis-acting art gene-responsive sequences of the human immunodeficiency virus. Proc. Natl. Acad. Sci. USA 85:2071, 1988.

246. Hadzopoulou-Cladaras, M., Felber, B. K., Cladaras, C., Athanassopoulos, A., Tse, A., and Pavlakis, G. N.: The rev (trs/art) protein of human immunodeficiency virus type 1 affects viral mRNA and protein expression via a cis-acting sequence in the env region. J. Virol. 63:1265, 1989.

247. Dayton, E. T., Powell, D. M., and Dayton, A. I.: Functional analysis of CAR, the target sequence for the Rev protein of HIV-1. Science 246:1625, 1989.

248. Heaphy, S., Dingwall, C., Ernberg, I., Gait, M. J., Green, S. M., Karn, J., Lowe, A. D., Singh, M., and Skinner, M. A.: HIV-1 regulator of virion expression (Rev) protein binds to an RNA stem-loop structure located within the Rev response element region. Cell 60:685, 1990.

249. Holland, S. M., Ahmad, N., Maitra, R. K., Wingfield, P., and Venkatesan, S.: Human immunodeficiency virus Rev protein recognizes a target sequence in Rev-responsive element RNA within the context of RNA secondary structure. J. Virol. 64:5966, 1990.

250. Kjems, J., Brown, M., Chang, D. D., and Sharp, P. A.: Structural analysis of the interaction between the human immunodeficiency virus Rev protein and the Rev response element. Proc. Natl. Acad. Sci. USA 88:683, 1991.

251. Olsen, H. S., Nelbock, P., Cochrane, A. W., and Rosen, C. A.: Secondary structure is the major determinant for interaction of HIV *rev* protein with RNA. Science 247:845, 1990.

252. Huang, X., Hope, T. J., Bond, B. L., McDonald, D., Grahl, K., and Parslow, T. G.: Minimal Rev-response element for type 1 human immunodeficiency virus. J. Virol. 65:2131, 1991.

253. Heaphy, S., Finch, J. T., Gait, M. J., Karn, J., and Singh, M.: Human immunodeficiency virus type 1 regulator of virion expression, rev, forms nucleoprotein filaments after binding to a purine-rich "bubble" located within the rev-responsive region of viral mRNAs. Proc. Natl. Acad. Sci. USA 88:7366, 1991.

254. Holland, S. M., Chavez, M., Gerstberger, S., and Venkatesan, S.: A specific sequence with a bulged guanosine residue(s) in a stem-bulge-stem structure of Rev-responsive element RNA is required for *trans* activation by human immunodeficiency virus type 1 Rev. J. Virol. 66:3699, 1992.

255. Bartel, D. P., Zapp, M. L., Green, M. R., and Szostak, J. W.: HIV-1 Rev regulation involves recognition of non–Watson-Crick base pairs in viral RNA. Cell 67:529, 1991.

256. Kjems, J., Frankel, A. D., and Sharp, P. A.: Specific regulation of mRNA splicing in vitro by a peptide from HIV-1 Rev. Cell 67:169, 1991.

257. Battiste, J. L., Mao, H., Rao, N. S., Tan, R., Muhandiram, D. R., Kay, L. E., Frankel, A. D., and Williamson, J. R.: α Helix-RNA major groove recognition in an HIV-1 rev peptide-RRE RNA complex. Science 273:1547, 1996.

258. Wingfield, P. T., Stahl, S. J., Payton, M. A., Venkatesan, S., Misra, M., and Steven, A. C.: HIV-1 Rev expressed in recombinant *Escherichia coli:* Purification, polymerization, and conformational properties. Biochemistry 30:7527, 1991.

259. Zapp, M. L., Hope, T. J., Parslow, T. G., and Green, M. R.: Oligomerization and RNA binding domains of the type 1 human immunodeficiency virus Rev protein: A dual function for an arginine-rich binding motif. Proc. Natl. Acad. Sci. USA 88:7734, 1991.

260. Zemmel, R. W., Kelley, A. C., Karn, J., and Butler, P. J.: Flexible regions of RNA structure facilitate co-operative Rev assembly on the Rev-response element. J. Mol. Biol. 258:763, 1996.

261. Hanly, S. M., Rimsky, L. T., Malim, M. H., Kim, J. H., Hauber, J., Duc Dodon, M., Le, S.-Y., Maizel, J. V., Cullen, B. R., and Greene, W. C.: Comparative analysis of the HTLV-I Rex and HIV-1 Rev *trans*-regulatory proteins and their RNA response elements. Genes Dev. 3:1534, 1989.

262. Solomin, L., Felber, B. K., and Pavlakis, G. N.: Different sites of interaction for Rev, Tev, and Rex proteins within the Rev-responsive element of human immunodeficiency virus type 1. J. Virol. 64:6010, 1990.

263. Zapp, M. L., Stern, S., and Green, M. R.: Small molecules that selectively block RNA binding of HIV-1 Rev protein inhibit Rev function and viral production. Cell 74:969, 1993.

264. Malim, M. H., Böhnlein, S., Hauber, J., and Cullen, B. R.: Functional dissection of the HIV-1 Rev *trans*-activator—derivation of a *trans*-dominant repressor of Rev function. Cell 58:205, 1989.

265. Venkatesh, L. K., and Chinnadurai, G.: Mutants in a conserved region near the carboxy-terminus of HIV-1 Rev identify functionally important residues and exhibit a dominant negative phenotype. Virology 178:327, 1990.

266. Feinberg, M. B., Jarrett, R. F., Aldovini, A., Gallo, R. C., and Wong-Staal, F.: HTLV-III expression and production involve complex regulation at the levels of splicing and translation of viral RNA. Cell 46:807, 1986.

267. Schwartz, S., Felber, B. K., and Pavlakis, G. N.: Distinct RNA sequences in the *gag* region of human immunodeficiency virus type 1 decrease RNA stability and inhibit expression in the absence of Rev protein. J. Virol. 66:150, 1992.

268. Maldarelli, F., Martin, M. A., and Strebel, K.: Identification of post-transcriptionally active inhibitory sequences in human immunodeficiency virus type 1 RNA: Novel level of gene regulation. J. Virol. 65:5732, 1991.

269. Bray, M., Prasad, S., Dubay, J. W., Hunter, E., Jeang, K.-T., Rekosh, D., and Hammarskjöld, M.-L.: A small element from the Mason-Pfizer monkey virus genome makes human immunodeficiency virus type 1 expression and replication Rev-independent. Proc. Natl. Acad. Sci. USA 91:1256, 1994.

270. Zolotukhin, A. S., Valentin, A., Pavlakis, G. N., and Felber, B. K.: Continuous propagation of RRE(-) and Rev(-)RRE(-) human immunodeficiency virus type 1 molecular clones containing a cis-acting element of simian retrovirus type 1 in human peripheral blood lymphocytes. J. Virol. 68:7944, 1994.

271. Ernst, R. K., Bray, M., Rekosh, D., and Hammarskjöld, M.-L.: Secondary structure and mutational analysis of the Mason-Pfizer monkey virus RNA constitutive transport element. RNA 3:210, 1997.

272. Tabernero, C., Zolotukhin, A. S., Valentin, A., Pavlakis, G. N., and Felber, B. K.: The posttranscriptional control element of the simian retrovirus type 1 forms an extensive RNA secondary structure necessary for its function. J. Virol. 70:5998, 1996.

273. Fischer, U., Huber, J., Boelens, W. C., Mattaj, I. W., and Luhrmann, R.: The HIV-1 Rev activation domain is a nuclear export signal that accesses an export pathway used by specific cellular RNAs. Cell 82:475, 1995.

274. Wen, W., Meinkoth, J. L., Tsien, R. Y., and Taylor, S. S.: Identification of a signal for rapid export of proteins from the nucleus. Cell 82:463, 1995.

275. Fischer, U., Meyer, S., Teufel, M., Heckel, C., Luhrmann, R., and Rautmann, G.: Evidence that HIV-1 Rev directly promotes the nuclear export of unspliced RNA. EMBO J. 13:4105, 1994.

276. Powers, M. A., and Forbes, D. J.: Cytosolic factors in nuclear transport: What's importin? Cell 79:931, 1994.

277. Fornerod, M., Ohno, M., Yoshida, M., and Mattaj, I. W.: CRM1 is an export receptor for leucine-rich nuclear export signals. Cell 90:1051, 1997.

278. Stade, K., Ford, C. S., Guthrie, C., and Weis, K.: Exportin 1 (Crm1p) is an essential nuclear export factor. Cell 90:1041, 1997.

279. Gorlich, D., and Mattaj, I. W.: Nucleocytoplasmic transport. Science 271:1513, 1996.

280. Wolff, B., Sanglier, J. J., and Wang, Y.: Leptomycin B is an inhibitor of nuclear export: Inhibition of nucleo-cytoplasmic translocation of the human immunodeficiency virus type 1 (HIV-1) Rev protein and Rev-dependent mRNA. Chem. Biol. 4:139, 1997.

281. Neville, M., Stutz, F., Lee, L., Davis, L. I., and Rosbash, M.: The importin-β family member Crm1p bridges the interaction between Rev and the nuclear pore complex during nuclear export. Curr. Biol. 7:767, 1997.

282. Bogerd, H. P., Fridell, R. A., Madore, S., and Cullen, B. R.: Identification of a novel cellular cofactor for the Rev/Rex class of retroviral regulatory proteins. Cell 82:485, 1995.

283. Fritz, C. C., Zapp, M. L., and Green, M. R.: A human nucleoporin–like protein that specifically interacts with HIV Rev. Nature 376:530, 1995.

284. Bevec, D., Jaksche, H., Oft, M., Wohl, T., Himmelspach, M., Pacher, A., Schebesta, M., Koettnitz, K., Dobrovnik, M., Csonga, R., Lottspeich, F., and Hauber, J.: Inhibition of HIV-1 replication in lymphocytes by mutants of the Rev cofactor eIF-5A. Science 271:1858, 1996.

285. Nigg, E. A.: Nucleocytoplasmic transport: Signals, mechanisms and regulation. Nature 386:779, 1997.

286. di Marzo Veronese, F., Copeland, T. D., Oroszlan, S., Gallo, R. C., and Sarngadharan, M. G.: Biochemical and immunological analysis of human immunodeficiency virus *gag* gene products p17 and p24. J. Virol. 62:795, 1988.

287. Mervis, R. J., Ahmad, N., Lillehoj, E. P., Raum, M. G., Salazar, F. H. R., Chan, H. W., and Venkatesan, S.: The *gag* gene products of human immunodeficiency virus type 1: Alignment within the *gag* open reading frame, identification of posttranslational modifications, and evidence for alternative gag precursors. J. Virol. 62:3993, 1988.

288. Freed, E. O.: HIV-1 Gag proteins: Diverse functions in the virus life cycle. Virology 251:1, 1998.

289. Garfinkel, D. J., Boeke, J. D., and Fink, G. R.: Ty element transposition: Reverse transcriptase and virus-like particles. Cell 42:507, 1985.

290. Kawai, S., and Hanafusa, H.: Isolation of defective mutant of avian sarcoma virus. Proc. Natl. Acad. Sci. USA 70:3493, 1973.

291. Ross, E. K., Fuerst, T. R., Orenstein, J. M., O'Neill, T., Martin, M. A., and Venkatesan, S.: Maturation of human immunodeficiency virus particles assembled from the *gag* precursor protein requires in situ processing by *gag-pol* protease. AIDS Res. Hum. Retroviruses 7:475, 1991.

292. Smith, A. J., Cho, M.-I., Hammarskjöld, M.-L., and Rekosh, D.: Human immunodeficiency virus type 1 Pr55^gag and Pr160^gag-pol expressed from a simian virus 40 late replacement vector are efficiently processed and assembled into viruslike particles. J. Virol. 64:2743, 1990.

293. Gheysen, D., Jacobs, E., de Foresta, F., Thiriart, C., Francotte, M., Thines, D., and De Wilde, M.: Assembly and release of HIV-1 precursor Pr55^gag virus-like particles from recombinant baculovirus-infected insect cells. Cell 59:103, 1989.

294. Karacostas, V., Nagashima, K., Gonda, M. A., and Moss, B.: Human immunodeficiency virus-like particles produced by a vaccinia virus expression vector. Proc. Natl. Acad. Sci. USA 86:8964, 1989.

295. Shioda, T., and Shibuta, H.: Production of human immunodeficiency virus (HIV)–like particles from cells infected with recombinant vaccinia viruses carrying the *gag* gene of HIV. Virology 175:139, 1990.

296. Wills, J. W., and Craven, R. C.: Form, function, and use of retroviral gag proteins (editorial). AIDS 5:639, 1991.

297. Göttlinger, H. G., Sodroski, J. G., and Haseltine, W. A.: Role of capsid precursor processing and myristoylation in morphogenesis and infectivity of human immunodeficiency virus type 1. Proc. Natl. Acad. Sci. USA 86:5781, 1989.

298. Bryant, M., and Ratner, L.: Myristoylation-dependent replication and assembly of human immunodeficiency virus 1. Proc. Natl. Acad. Sci. USA 87:523, 1990.

299. Pal, R., Reitz, M. S., Jr., Tschachler, E., Gallo, R. C., Sarngadharan, M. G., and di Marzo Veronese, F.: Myristoylation of gag proteins of HIV-1 plays an important role in virus assembly. AIDS Res. Hum. Retroviruses 6:721, 1990.

300. Freed, E. O., Orenstein, J. M., Buckler-White, A. J., and Martin, M. A.: Single amino acid changes in the human immunodeficiency virus type 1 matrix protein block virus particle production. J. Virol. 68:5311, 1994.

301. Massiah, M. A., Starich, M. R., Paschall, C., Summers, M. F., Christensen, A. M., and Sundquist, W. I.: Three-dimensional structure of the human immunodeficiency virus type 1 matrix protein. J. Mol. Biol. 244:198, 1994.

302. Hill, C. P., Worthylake, D., Bancroft, D. P., Christensen, A. M., and Sundquist, W. I.: Crystal structures of the trimeric human immunodeficiency virus type 1 matrix protein: Implications for membrane association and assembly. Proc. Natl. Acad. Sci. USA 93:3099, 1996.

303. Christensen, A. M., Massiah, M. A., Turner, B. G., Sundquist, W. I., and Summers, M. F.: Three-dimensional structure of the HTLV-II matrix protein and comparative analysis of matrix proteins from the different classes of pathogenic human retroviruses. J. Mol. Biol. 264:1117, 1996.

304. Conte, M. R., Klikova, M., Hunter, E., Ruml, T., and Matthews, S.: The three-dimensional solution structure of the matrix protein from the type D retrovirus, the Mason-Pfizer monkey virus, and implications for the morphology of retroviral assembly. EMBO J. 16:5819, 1997.

305. Matthews, S., Mikhailov, M., Burny, A., and Roy, P.: The solution structure of the bovine leukaemia virus matrix protein and similarity with lentiviral matrix proteins. EMBO J. 15:3267, 1996.

306. McDonnell, J. M., Fushman, D., Cahill, S. M., Zhou, W., Wolven, A., Wilson, C. B., Nelle, T. D., Resh, M. D., Wills, J., and Cowburn, D.: Solution structure and dynamics of the bioactive retroviral M domain from Rous sarcoma virus. J. Mol. Biol. 279:921, 1998.

307. Zhou, W., Parent, L. J., Wills, J. W., and Resh, M. D.: Identification of a membrane-binding domain within the amino-terminal region of human immunodeficiency virus type 1 Gag protein which interacts with acidic phospholipids. J. Virol. 68:2556, 1994.

308. Yuan, X., Yu, X., Lee, T. H., and Essex, M.: Mutations in the N-terminal region of human immunodeficiency virus type 1 matrix protein block intracellular transport of the Gag precursor. J. Virol. 67:6387, 1993.

309. Freed, E. O., Englund, G., and Martin, M. A.: Role of the basic domain of human immunodeficiency virus type 1 matrix in macrophage infection. J. Virol. 69:3949, 1995.

310. Facke, M., Janetzko, A., Shoeman, R. L., and Krausslich, H. G.: A large deletion in the matrix domain of the human immunodeficiency virus *gag* gene redirects virus particle assembly from the plasma membrane to the endoplasmic reticulum. J. Virol. 67:4972, 1993.

311. Yu, X., Yuan, X., Matsuda, Z., Lee, T. H., and Essex, M.: The matrix protein of human immunodeficiency virus type 1 is required for incorporation of viral envelope protein into mature virions. J. Virol. 66:4966, 1992.

312. Dorfman, T., Mammano, F., Haseltine, W. A., and Gottlinger, H. G.: Role of the matrix protein in the virion association of the human immunodeficiency virus type 1 envelope glycoprotein. J. Virol. 68:1689, 1994.

313. Freed, E. O., and Martin, M. A.: Virion incorporation of envelope glycoproteins with long but not short cytoplasmic tails is blocked by specific, single amino acid substitutions in the human immunodeficiency virus type 1 matrix. J. Virol. 69:1984, 1995.

314. Freed, E. O., and Martin, M. A.: Domains of the human immunodeficiency virus type 1 matrix and gp41 cytoplasmic tail required for envelope incorporation into virions. J. Virol. 70:341, 1996.

315. Mammano, F., Kondo, E., Sodroski, J., Bukovsky, A., and Gottlinger, H. G.: Rescue of human immunodeficiency virus type 1 matrix protein mutants by envelope glycoproteins with short cytoplasmic domains. J. Virol. 69:3824, 1995.

316. Cosson, P.: Direct interaction between the envelope and matrix proteins of HIV-1. EMBO J. 15:5783, 1996.

317. Yu, X., Yu, Q. C., Lee, T. H., and Essex, M.: The C terminus of human immunodeficiency virus type 1 matrix protein is involved in early steps of the virus life cycle. J. Virol. 66:5667, 1992.

318. Casella, C. R., Raffini, L. J., and Panganiban, A. T.: Pleiotropic mutations in the HIV-1 matrix protein that affect diverse steps in replication. Virology 228:294, 1997.

319. Kiernan, R. E., Ono, A., Englund, G., and Freed, E. O.: Role of matrix in an early postentry step in the human immunodeficiency virus type 1 life cycle. J. Virol. 72:4116, 1998.

320. Bukrinsky, M. I., Haggerty, S., Dempsey, M. P., Sharova, N., Adzhubel, A., Spitz, L., Lewis, P., Goldfarb, D., Emerman, M., and Stevenson, M.: A nuclear localization signal within HIV-1 matrix protein that governs infection of non-dividing cells. Nature 365:666, 1993.

321. Heinzinger, N. K., Bukinsky, M. I., Haggerty, S. A., Ragland, A. M., Kewalramani, V., Lee, M. A., Gendelman, H. E., Ratner, L., Stevenson, M., and Emerman, M.: The Vpr protein of human immunodeficiency virus type 1 influences nuclear localization of viral nucleic acids in nondividing host cells. Proc. Natl. Acad. Sci. USA 91:7311, 1994.

322. von Schwedler, U., Kornbluth, R. S., and Trono, D.: The nuclear localization signal of the matrix protein of human immunodeficiency virus type 1 allows the establishment of infection in macrophages and quiescent T lymphocytes. Proc. Natl. Acad. Sci. USA 91:6992, 1994.

323. Gallay, P., Swingler, S., Song, J., Bushman, F., and Trono, D.: HIV nuclear import is governed by the phosphotyrosine-mediated binding of matrix to the core domain of integrase. Cell 83:569, 1995.

324. Freed, E. O., and Martin, M. A.: HIV-1 infection of non-dividing cells (letter). Nature 369:107, 1994.

325. Freed, E. O., Englund, G., Maldarelli, F., and Martin, M. A.: Phosphorylation of residue 131 of HIV-1 matrix is not required for macrophage infection. Cell 88:171, 1997.

326. Bukrinskaya, A. G., Ghorpade, A., Heinzinger, N. K., Smithgall, T. E., Lewis, R. E., and Stevenson, M.: Phosphorylation-dependent human immunodeficiency virus type 1 infection and nuclear targeting of viral DNA. Proc. Natl. Acad. Sci. USA 93:367, 1996.

327. Fouchier, R. A., Meyer, B. E., Simon, J. H., Fischer, U., and Malim, M. H.: HIV-1 infection of non-dividing cells: Evidence that the amino-terminal basic region of the viral matrix protein is important for Gag processing but not for post-entry nuclear import. EMBO J. 16:4531, 1997.

328. Nie, Z., Bergeron, D., Subbramanian, R. A., Yao, X.-J., Checroune, F., Rougeau, N., and Cohen, E. A.: The putative alpha helix 2 of human immunodeficiency virus type 1 Vpr contains a determinant which is responsible for the nuclear translocation of proviral DNA in growth-arrested cells. J. Virol. 72:4104, 1998.

329. Chazal, N., Carriere, C., Gay, B., and Boulanger, P.: Phenotypic characterization of insertion mutants of the human immunodeficiency virus type 1 Gag precursor expressed in recombinant baculovirus-infected cells. J. Virol. 68:111, 1994.

330. Dorfman, T., Bukovsky, A., Ohagen, A., Hoglund, S., and Gottlinger, H. G.: Functional domains of the capsid protein of human immunodeficiency virus type 1. J. Virol. 68:8180, 1994.

331. Reicin, A. S., Paik, S., Berkowitz, R. D., Luban, J., Lowy, I., and Goff, S. P.: Linker insertion mutations in the human immunodeficiency virus type 1 *gag* gene: Effects on virion particle assembly, release, and infectivity. J. Virol. 69:642, 1995.

332. Jowett, J. B., Hockley, D. J., Nermut, M. V., and Jones, I. M.: Distinct signals in human immunodeficiency virus type 1 Pr55 necessary for RNA binding and particle formation. J Gen. Virol. 73:3079, 1992.

333. Wang, C. T., and Barklis, E.: Assembly, processing, and infectivity of human immunodeficiency virus type 1 gag mutants. J. Virol. 67:4264, 1993.

334. Mammano, F., Ohagen, A., Hoglund, S., and Gottlinger, H. G.: Role of the major homology region of human immunodeficiency virus type 1 in virion morphogenesis. J. Virol. 68:4927, 1994.

335. Luban, J., Bossolt, K. L., Franke, E. K., Kalpana, G. V., and Goff, S. P.: Human immunodeficiency virus type 1 Gag protein binds to cyclophilins A and B. Cell 73:1067, 1993.

336. Thali, M., Bukovsky, A., Kondo, E., Rosenwirth, B., Walsh, C. T., Sodroski, J., and Gottlinger, H. G.: Functional association of cyclophilin A with HIV-1 virions. Nature 372:363, 1994.

337. Franke, E. K., Yuan, H. E., and Luban, J.: Specific incorporation of cyclophilin A into HIV-1 virions. Nature 372:359, 1994.

338. Braaten, D., Franke, E. K., and Luban, J.: Cyclophilin A is required for an early step in the life cycle of human immunodeficiency virus type 1 before the initiation of reverse transcription. J. Virol. 70:3551, 1996.

339. Aberham, C., Weber, S., and Phares, W.: Spontaneous mutations in the human immunodeficiency virus type 1 *gag* gene that affect viral replication in the presence of cyclosporins. J. Virol. 70:3536, 1996.

340. Gamble, T. R., Vajdos, F. F., Yoo, S., Worthylake, D. K., Houseweart, M., Sundquist, W. I., and Hill, C. P.: Crystal structure of human cyclophilin A bound to the amino-terminal domain of HIV-1 capsid. Cell 87:1285, 1996.

341. Gitti, R. K., Lee, B. M., Walker, J., Summers, M. F., Yoo, S., and Sundquist, W. I.: Structure of the amino-terminal core domain of the HIV-1 capsid protein. Science 273:231, 1996.

342. Momany, C., Kovari, L. C., Prongay, A. J., Keller, W., Gitti, R. K., Lee, B. M., Gorbalenya, A. E., Tong, L., McClure, J., Ehrlich, L. S., Summers, M. F., Carter, C., and Rossmann, M. G.: Crystal structure of dimeric HIV-1 capsid protein. Nat. Struct. Biol. 3:763, 1996.

343. Gamble, T. R., Yoo, S., Vajdos, F. F., von Schwedler, U. K., Worthylake, D. K., Wang, H., McCutcheon, J. P., Sundquist, W. I., and Hill, C. P.: Structure of the carboxyl-terminal dimerization domain of the HIV-1 capsid protein. Science 278:849, 1997.

344. Ehrlich, L. S., Agresta, B. E., and Carter, C. A.: Assembly of recombinant human immunodeficiency virus type 1 capsid protein in vitro. J. Virol. 66:4874, 1992.

345. von Schwedler, U. K., Stemmler, T. L., Klishko, V. Y., Li, S., Albertine, K. H., Davis, D. R., and Sundquist, W. I.: Proteolytic refolding of the HIV-1 capsid protein amino-terminus facilitates viral core assembly. EMBO J. 17:1555, 1998.

346. Campbell, S., and Vogt, V. M.: Self-assembly in vitro of purified CA-NC proteins from Rous sarcoma virus and human immunodeficiency virus type 1. J. Virol. 69:6487, 1995.

347. Bess, J. W., Jr., Powell, P. J., Issaq, H. J., Schumack, L. J., Grimes, M. K., Henderson, L. E., and Arthur, L. O.: Tightly bound zinc in human immunodeficiency virus type 1, human T-cell leukemia virus type I, and other retroviruses. J. Virol. 66:840, 1992.

348. Gorelick, R. J., Henderson, L. E., Hanser, J. P., and Rein, A.: Point mutants of Moloney murine leukemia virus that fail to package viral RNA: Evidence for specific RNA recognition by a "zinc finger–like" protein sequence. Proc. Natl. Acad. Sci. USA 85:8420, 1988.

349. Zhang, Y., and Barklis, E.: Nucleocapsid protein effects on the specificity of retrovirus RNA encapsidation. J. Virol. 69:5716, 1995.

350. Schmalzbauer, E., Strack, B., Dannull, J., Guehmann, S., and Moelling, K.: Mutations of basic amino acids of NCp7 of human immunodeficiency virus type 1 affect RNA binding in vitro. J. Virol. 70:771, 1996.

351. Poon, D. T., Wu, J., and Aldovini, A.: Charged amino acid residues of human immunodeficiency virus type 1 nucleocapsid p7 protein involved in RNA packaging and infectivity. J. Virol. 70:6607, 1996.

352. McBride, M. S., and Panganiban, A. T.: Position dependence of functional hairpins important for human immunodeficiency virus type 1 RNA encapsidation in vivo. J. Virol. 71:2050, 1997.

353. De Guzman, R. N., Wu, Z. R., Stalling, C. C., Pappalardo, L., Borer, P. N., and Summers, M. F.: Structure of the HIV-1 nucleocapsid protein bound to the SL3 psi-RNA recognition element. Science 279:384, 1998.

354. Dorfman, T., Luban, J., Goff, S. P., Haseltine, W. A., and Gottlinger, H. G.: Mapping of functionally important residues of a cysteine-histidine box in the human immunodeficiency virus type 1 nucleocapsid protein. J. Virol. 67:6159, 1993.

355. Hong, S. S., and Boulanger, P.: Assembly-defective point mutants of the human immunodeficiency virus type 1 Gag precursor phenotypically expressed in recombinant baculovirus-infected cells. J. Virol. 67:2787, 1993.

356. Zhang, Y., Qian, H., Love, Z., and Barklis, E.: Analysis of the assembly function of the human immunodeficiency virus type 1 gag protein nucleocapsid domain. J. Virol. 72:1782, 1998.

357. Hoshikawa, N., Kojima, A., Yasuda, A., Takayashiki, E., Masuko, S., Chiba, J., Sata, T., and Kurata, T.: Role of the *gag* and *pol* genes of human immunodeficiency virus in the morphogenesis and maturation of retrovirus-like particles expressed by recombinant vaccinia virus: An ultrastructural study. J. Gen. Virol. 72:2509, 1991.

358. Bennett, R. P., Nelle, T. D., and Wills, J. W.: Functional chimeras of the Rous sarcoma virus and human immunodeficiency virus gag proteins. J. Virol. 67:6487, 1993.

359. Darlix, J.-L., Lapadat-Tapolsky, M., de Rocquigny, H., and Roques, B. P.: First glimpses at structure-function relationships of the nucleocapsid protein of retroviruses. J. Mol. Biol. 254:523, 1995.

360. Li, X., Quan, Y., Arts, E. J., Li, Z., Preston, B. D., de Rocquigny, H., Roques, B. P., Darlix, J. L., Kleiman, L., Parniak, M. A., and Wainberg, M. A.: Human immunodeficiency virus type 1 nucleocapsid protein (NCp7) directs specific initiation of minus-strand DNA synthesis primed by human tRNA(Lys3) in vitro: Studies of viral RNA molecules mutated in regions that flank the primer binding site. J. Virol. 70:4996, 1996.

361. Guo, J., Henderson, L. E., Bess, J., Kane, B., and Levin, J. G.: Human immunodeficiency virus type 1 nucleocapsid protein promotes efficient strand transfer and specific viral DNA synthesis by inhibiting TAR-dependent self-priming from minus-strand strong-stop DNA. J. Virol. 71:5178, 1997.

362. Ottmann, M., Gabus, C., and Darlix, J. L.: The central globular domain of the nucleocapsid protein of human immunodeficiency virus type 1 is critical for virion structure and infectivity. J. Virol. 69:1778, 1995.

363. Berthoux, L., Pechoux, C., Ottmann, M., Morel, G., and Darlix, J. L.: Mutations in the N-terminal domain of human immunodeficiency virus type 1 nucleocapsid protein affect virion core structure and proviral DNA synthesis. J. Virol. 71:6973, 1997.

364. Gorelick, R. J., Chabot, D. J., Ott, D. E., Gagliardi, T. D., Rein, A., Henderson, L. E., and Arthur, L. O.: Genetic analysis of the zinc finger in the Moloney murine leukemia virus nucleocapsid domain: Replacement of zinc-coordinating residues with other zinc-coordinating residues yields noninfectious particles containing genomic RNA. J. Virol. 70:2593, 1996.

365. Rice, W. G., Supko, J. G., Malspeis, L., Buckheit, R. W., Jr., Clanton, D., Bu, M., Graham, L., Schaeffer, C. A., Turpin, J. A., Domagala, J., Gogliotti, R., Bader, J. P., Halliday, S. M., Coren, L., Sowder, R. C., Arthur, L. O., and Henderson, L. E.: Inhibitors of HIV nucleocapsid protein zinc fingers as candidates for the treatment of AIDS. Science 270:1194, 1995.

366. Tummino, P. J., Scholten, J. D., Harvey, P. J., Holler, T. P., Maloney, L., Gogliotti, R., Domagala, J., and Hupe, D.: The in vitro ejection of zinc from human immunodeficiency virus (HIV) type 1 nucleocapsid protein by disulfide benzamides with cellular anti-HIV activity. Proc. Natl. Acad. Sci. USA 93:969, 1996.

367. Turpin, J. A., Terpening, S. J., Schaeffer, C. A., Yu, G., Glover, C. J., Felsted, R. L., Sausville, E. A., and Rice, W. G.: Inhibitors of human immunodeficiency virus type 1 zinc fingers prevent normal processing of gag precursors and result in the release of noninfectious virus particles. J. Virol. 70:6180, 1996.

368. Ott, D. E., Hewes, S. M., Alvord, W. G., Henderson, L. E., and Arthur, L. O.: Inhibition of Friend virus replication by a compound that reacts with the nucleocapsid zinc finger: Antiretroviral effect demonstrated in vivo. Virology 243:242, 1998.

369. Gottlinger, H. G., Dorfman, T., Sodroski, J. G., and Haseltine, W. A.: Effect of mutations affecting the p6 Gag protein on human immunodeficiency virus particle release. Proc. Natl. Acad. Sci. USA 88:3195, 1991.

370. Huang, M., Orenstein, J. M., Martin, M. A., and Freed, E. O.: p6[Gag]

is required for particle production from full-length human immunodeficiency virus type 1 molecular clones expressing protease. J. Virol. 69:6810, 1995.

371. Paxton, W., Connor, R. I., and Landau, N. R.: Incorporation of Vpr into human immunodeficiency virus type 1 virions: Requirement for the p6 region of gag and mutational analysis. J. Virol. 67:7229, 1993.

372. Kondo, E., Mammano, F., Cohen, E. A., and Gottlinger, H. G.: The p6^{gag} domain of human immunodeficiency virus type 1 is sufficient for the incorporation of Vpr into heterologous viral particles. J. Virol. 69:2759, 1995.

373. Wills, J. W., Cameron, C. E., Wilson, C. B., Xiang, Y., Bennett, R. P., and Leis, J.: An assembly domain of the Rous sarcoma virus Gag protein required late in budding. J. Virol. 68:6605, 1994.

374. Puffer, B. A., Parent, L. J., Wills, J. W., and Montelaro, R. C.: Equine infectious anemia virus utilizes a YXXL motif within the late assembly domain of the Gag p9 protein. J. Virol. 71:6541, 1997.

375. Parent, L. J., Bennett, R. P., Craven, R. C., Nelle, T. D., Krishna, N. K., Bowzard, J. B., Wilson, C. B., Puffer, B. A., Montelaro, R. C., and Wills, J. W.: Positionally independent and exchangeable late budding functions of the Rous sarcoma virus and human immunodeficiency virus Gag proteins. J. Virol. 69:5455, 1995.

376. Garnier, L., Wills, J. W., Verderame, M. F., and Sudol, M.: WW domains and retrovirus budding (letter). Nature 381:744, 1996.

377. Oppermann, H., Bishop, J. M., Varmus, H. E., and Levintow, L.: A joint produce of the genes gag and pol of avian sarcoma virus: A possible precursor of reverse transcriptase. Cell 12:993, 1977.

378. Hayman, M. J.: Viral polyproteins in chick embryo fibroblasts infected with avian sarcoma leukosis viruses. Virology 85:241, 1978.

379. Park, J., and Morrow, C. D.: Overexpression of the gag-pol precursor from human immunodeficiency virus type 1 proviral genomes results in efficient proteolytic processing in the absence of virion production. J. Virol. 65:5111, 1991.

380. Peng, C., Ho, B. K., Chang, T. W., and Chang, N. T.: Role of human immunodeficiency virus type 1–specific protease in core protein maturation and viral infectivity. J. Virol. 63:2550, 1989.

381. Kohl, N. E., Emini, E. A., Schleif, W. A., Davis, L. J., Heimbach, J. C., Dixon, R. A. F., Scolnick, E. M., and Sigal, I. S.: Active human immunodeficiency virus protease is required for viral infectivity. Proc. Natl. Acad. Sci. USA 85:4686, 1988.

382. Toh, H., Kikuno, R., Hayashida, H., Miyata, T., Kugimiya, W., Inouye, S., Yuki, S., and Saigo, K.: Close structural resemblance between putative polymerase of a *Drosophila* transposable genetic element 17.6 and pol gene product of Moloney murine leukaemia virus. EMBO J. 4:1267, 1985.

383. Skalka, A. M.: Retroviral proteases: First glimpses at the anatomy of a processing machine. Cell 56:911, 1989.

384. Hansen, J., Billich, S., Schulze, T., Sukrow, S., and Moelling, K.: Partial purification and substrate analysis of bacterially expressed HIV protease by means of monoclonal antibody. EMBO J. 7:1785, 1988.

385. Kotler, M., Danho, W., Katz, R. A., Leis, J., and Skalka, A. M.: Avian retroviral protease and cellular aspartic proteases are distinguished by activities on peptide substrates. J. Biol. Chem. 264:3428, 1989.

386. Lapatto, R., Blundell, T., Hemmings, A., Overington, J., Wilderspin, A., Wood, S., Merson, J. R., Whittle, P. J., Danley, D. E., Geoghegan, K. F., Hawrylik, S. J., Lee, S. E., Scheld, K. G., and Hobart, P. M.: X-ray analysis of HIV-1 proteinase at 2.7 Å resolution confirms structural homology among retroviral enzymes. Nature 342:299, 1989.

387. Wlodawer, A., Miller, M., Jaskólski, M., Sathyanarayana, B. K., Baldwin, E., Weber, I. T., Selk, L. M., Clawson, L., Schneider, J., and Kent, S. B. H.: Conserved folding in retroviral proteases: Crystal structure of a synthetic HIV-1 protease. Science 245:616, 1989.

388. Miller, M., Schneider, J., Sathyanarayana, B. K., Toth, M. V., Marshall, G. R., Clawson, L., Selk, L., Kent, S. B. H., and Wlodawer, A.: Structure of complex of synthetic HIV-1 protease with a substrate-based inhibitor at 2.3 Å resolution. Science 246:1149, 1989.

389. Erickson, J., Neidhart, D. J., VanDrie, J., Kempf, D. J., Wang, X. C., Norbeck, D. W., Plattner, J. J., Rittenhouse, J. W., Turon, M., Wideburg, N., Kohlbrenner, W. E., Simmer, R., Helfrich, R., Paul, D. A., and Knigge, M.: Design, activity, and 2.8 Å crystal structure of a C_2 symmetric inhibitor complexed to HIV-1 protease. Science 249:527, 1990.

390. Billich, S., Knoop, M.-T., Hansen, J., Strop, P., Sedlacek, J., Mertz, R., and Moelling, K.: Synthetic peptides as substrates and inhibitors of human immune deficiency virus-1 protease. J. Biol. Chem. 263:17905, 1988.

391. Tritch, R. J., Cheng, Y.-S. E., Yin, F. H., and Erickson-Viitanen, S.: Mutagenesis of protease cleavage sites in the human immunodeficiency virus type 1 gag polyprotein. J. Virol. 65:922, 1991.

392. Erickson-Viitanen, S., Manfredi, J., Viitanen, P., Tribe, D. E., Tritch, R., Hutchison, C. A., III, Loeb, D. D., and Swanstrom, R.: Cleavage of HIV-1 gag polyprotein synthesized in vitro: Sequential cleavage by the viral protease. AIDS Res. Hum. Retroviruses 5:577, 1989.

393. Krausslich, H. G., Facke, M., Heuser, A. M., Konvalinka, J., and Zentgraf, H.: The spacer peptide between human immunodeficiency virus capsid and nucleocapsid proteins is essential for ordered assembly and viral infectivity. J. Virol. 69:3407, 1995.

394. Pettit, S. C., Moody, M. D., Wehbie, R. S., Kaplan, A. H., Nantermet, P. V., Klein, C. A., and Swanstrom, R.: The p2 domain of human immunodeficiency virus type 1 Gag regulates sequential proteolytic processing and is required to produce fully infectious virions. J. Virol. 68:8017, 1994.

395. Wiegers, K., Rutter, G., Kottler, H., Tessmer, U., Hohenberg, H., and Kräusslich, H.-G.: Sequential steps in human immunodeficiency virus particle maturation revealed by alterations of individual Gag polyprotein cleavage sites. J. Virol. 72:2846, 1998.

396. Kräusslich, H.-G.: Human immunodeficiency virus proteinase dimer as component of the viral polyprotein prevents particle assembly and viral infectivity. Proc. Natl. Acad. Sci. USA 88:3213, 1991.

397. Craig, J. C., Duncan, I. B., Hockley, D., Grief, C., Roberts, N. A., and Mills, J. S.: Antiviral properties of Ro 31–8959, an inhibitor of human immunodeficiency virus (HIV) proteinase. Antiviral Res. 16:295, 1991.

398. Roberts, N. A., Martin, J. A., Kinchington, D., Broadhurst, A. V., Craig, J. C., Duncan, I. B., Galpin, S. A., Handa, B. K., Kay, J., Kröhn, A., Lambert, R. W., Merrett, J. H., Mills, J. S., Parkes, K. E. B., Redshaw, S., Ritchie, A. J., Taylor, D. L., Thomas, G. J., and Machin, P. J.: Rational design of peptide-based HIV proteinase inhibitors. Science 248:358, 1990.

399. Temin, H. M., and Mizutani, S.: RNA-dependent DNA polymerase in virions of Rous sarcoma virus. Nature 226:1211, 1970.

400. Baltimore, D.: RNA-dependent DNA polymerase in virions of RNA tumour viruses. Nature 226:1209, 1970.

401. Hansen, J., Schulze, T., Mellert, W., and Moelling, K.: Identification and characterization of HIV-specific RNase H by monoclonal antibody. EMBO J. 7:239, 1988.

402. Prasad, V. R., and Goff, S. P.: Linker insertion mutagenesis of the human immunodeficiency virus reverse transcriptase expressed in bacteria: Definition of the minimal polymerase domain. Proc. Natl. Acad. Sci. USA 86:3104, 1989.

403. Johnson, M. S., McClure, M. A., Feng, D.-F., Gray, J., and Doolittle, R. F.: Computer analysis of retroviral pol genes: Assignment of enzymatic functions to specific sequences and homologies with nonviral enzymes. Proc. Natl. Acad. Sci. USA 83:7648, 1986.

404. Hizi, A., Barber, A., and Hughes, S. H.: Effects of small insertions on the RNA-dependent DNA polymerase activity of HIV-1 reverse transcriptase. Virology 170:326, 1989.

405. Larder, B., Purifoy, D., Powell, K., and Darby, G.: AIDS virus reverse transcriptase defined by high level expression in *Escherichia coli*. EMBO J. 6:3133, 1987.

406. Restle, T., Muller, B., and Goody, R. S.: Dimerization of human immunodeficiency virus type 1 reverse transcriptase: A target for chemotherapeutic intervention. J. Biol. Chem. 265:8986, 1990.

407. Becerra, S. P., Kumar, A., Lewis, M. S., Widen, S. G., Abbotts, J., Karawya, E. M., Hughes, S. H., Shiloach, J., and Wilson, S. H.: Protein-protein interactions of HIV-1 reverse transcriptase: Implication of central and C-terminal regions in subunit binding. Biochemistry 30:11707, 1991.

408. Lowe, D. M., Aitken, A., Bradley, C., Darby, G. K., Larder, B. A., Powell, K. L., Purifoy, D. J. M., Tisdale, M., and Stammers, D. K.: HIV-1 reverse transcriptase: Crystallization and analysis of domain structure by limited proteolysis. Biochemistry 27:8884, 1988.

409. Tisdale, M., Ertl, P., Larder, B. A., Purifoy, D. J., Darby, G., and Powell, K. L.: Characterization of human immunodeficiency virus type 1 reverse transcriptase by using monoclonal antibodies: Role of the C terminus in antibody reactivity and enzyme function. J. Virol. 62:3662, 1988.

410. Hizi, A., McGill, C., and Hughes, S. H.: Expression of soluble, enzymatically active, human immunodeficiency virus reverse transcriptase in *Escherichia coli* and analysis of mutants. Proc. Natl. Acad. Sci. USA 85:1218, 1988.

411. Le Grice, S. F. J., Naas, T., Wohlgensinger, B., and Schatz, O.: Subunit-selective mutagenesis indicates minimal polymerase activity in heterodimer-associated p51 HIV-1 reverse transcriptase. EMBO J. 10:3905, 1991.

412. Kohlstaedt, L. A., Wang, J., Friedman, J. M., Rice, P. A., and Steitz, T. A.: Crystal structure at 3.5 Å resolution of HIV-1 reverse transcriptase complexed with an inhibitor. Science 256:1783, 1992.

413. Arnold, E., Jacobo-Molina, A., Nanni, R. G., Williams, R. L., Lu, X., Ding, J., Clark, A. D., Jr., Zhang, A., Ferris, A. L., Clark, P., Hizi, A., and Hughes, S. H.: Structure of HIV-1 reverse transcriptase/DNA complex at 7 Å resolution showing active site locations. Nature 357:85, 1992.

414. Jacobo-Molina, A., Ding, J., Nanni, R. G., Clark, A. D., Jr., Lu, X., Tantillo, C., Williams, R. L., Kamer, G., Ferris, A. L., Clark, P., Hizi, A., Hughes, S. H., and Arnold, E.: Crystal structure of human immunodeficiency virus type 1 reverse transcriptase complexed with double-stranded DNA at 3.0 Å resolution shows bent DNA. Proc. Natl. Acad. Sci. USA 90:6320, 1993.

415. Pathak, V. K., and Hu, W.-S.: "Might as well jump!" Template switching by retroviral reverse transcriptase, defective genome formation, and recombination. Semin. Virol. 8:141, 1997.

416. Mansky, L. M.: Retrovirus mutation rates and their role in genetic variation. J. Gen. Virol. 79:1337, 1998.

417. Bebenek, K., Abbotts, J., Roberts, J. D., Wilson, S. H., and Kunkel, T. A.: Specificity and mechanism of error-prone replication by human immunodeficiency virus-1 reverse transcriptase. J. Biol. Chem. 264:16948, 1989.

418. Roberts, J. D., Bebenek, K., and Kunkel, T. A.: The accuracy of reverse transcriptase from HIV-1. Science 242:1171, 1988.

419. Mansky, L. M., and Temin, H. M.: Lower in vivo mutation rate of human immunodeficiency virus type 1 than that predicted from the fidelity of purified reverse transcriptase. J. Virol. 69:5087, 1995.

420. Mansky, L. M., and Temin, H. M.: Lower mutation rate of bovine leukemia virus relative to that of spleen necrosis virus. J. Virol. 68:494, 1994.

421. Parthasarathi, S., Varela-Echavarria, A., Ron, Y., Preston, B. D., and Dougherty, J. P.: Genetic rearrangements occurring during a single cycle of murine leukemia virus vector replication: Characterization and implications. J. Virol. 69:7991, 1995.

422. Pathak, V. K., and Temin, H. M.: Broad spectrum of in vivo forward mutations, hypermutations, and mutational hotspots in a retroviral shuttle vector after a single replication cycle: Deletions and deletions with insertions. Proc. Natl. Acad. Sci. USA 87:6024, 1990.

423. Temin, H. M.: Retrovirus variation and reverse transcription: Abnormal strand transfers result in retrovirus genetic variation. Proc. Natl. Acad. Sci. USA 90:6900, 1993.

424. Coffin, J. M.: Structure, replication, and recombination of retrovirus genomes: Some unifying hypotheses. J. Gen. Virol. 42:1, 1979.

425. Julias, J. G., Hash, D., and Pathak, V. K.: E-vectors: Development of novel self-inactivating and self-activating retroviral vectors for safer gene therapy. J. Virol. 69:6839, 1995.

426. Richman, D. D., Guatelli, J. C., Grimes, J., Tsiatis, A., and Gingeras, T.: Detection of mutations associated with zidovudine resistance in human immunodeficiency virus by use of the polymerase chain reaction. J. Infect. Dis. 164:1075, 1991.

427. Larder, B. A., and Kemp, S. D.: Multiple mutations in HIV-1 reverse transcriptase confer high-level resistance to zidovudine (AZT). Science 246:1155, 1989.

428. Larder, B. A., Darby, G., and Richman, D. D.: HIV with reduced sensitivity to zidovudine (AZT) isolated during prolonged therapy. Science 243:1731, 1989.

429. Englund, G., Theodore, T. S., Freed, E. O., Engleman, A., and Martin, M. A.: Integration is required for productive infection of monocyte-derived macrophages by human immunodeficiency virus type 1. J. Virol. 69:3216, 1995.

430. Colicelli, J., and Goff, S. P.: Sequence and spacing requirements of a retrovirus integration site. J. Mol. Biol. 199:47, 1988.

431. Brown, P. O., Bowerman, B., Varmus, H. E., and Bishop, J. M.: Retroviral integration: Structure of the initial covalent product and its precursor, and a role for the viral IN protein. Proc. Natl. Acad. Sci. USA 86:2525, 1989.

432. Farnet, C. M., and Haseltine, W. A.: Integration of human immunodeficiency virus type 1 DNA in vitro. Proc. Natl. Acad. Sci. USA 87:4164, 1990.

433. Grandgenett, D. P., and Vora, A. C.: Site-specific nicking at the avian retrovirus LTR circle junction by the viral pp32 DNA endonuclease. Nucleic Acids Res. 13:6205, 1985.

434. Roth, M. J., Schwartzberg, P. L., and Goff, S. P.: Structure of the termini of DNA intermediates in the integration of retroviral DNA: Dependence on IN function and terminal DNA sequence. Cell 58:47, 1989.

435. Leavitt, A. D., Rose, R. B., and Varmus, H. E.: Both substrate and target oligonucleotide sequences affect in vitro integration mediated by human immunodeficiency virus type 1 integrase protein produced in Saccharomyces cerevisiae. J. Virol. 66:2359, 1992.

436. Bushman, F. D., Engelman, A., Palmer, I., Wingfield, P., and Craigie, R.: Domains of the integrase protein of human immunodeficiency virus type 1 responsible for polynucleotidyl transfer and zinc binding. Proc. Natl. Acad. Sci. USA 90:3428, 1993.

437. Zheng, R., Jenkins, T. M., and Craigie, R.: Zinc folds the N-terminal domain of HIV-1 integrase, promotes multimerization, and enhances catalytic activity. Proc. Natl. Acad. Sci. USA 93:13659, 1996.

438. Dyda, F., Hickman, A. B., Jenkins, T. M., Engelman, A., Craigie, R., and Davies, D. R.: Crystal structure of the catalytic domain of HIV-1 integrase: Similarity to other polynucleotidyl transferases. Science 266:1981, 1994.

439. Bujacz, G., Jaskolski, M., Alexandratos, J., Wlodawer, A., Merkel, G., Katz, R. A., and Skalka, A. M.: High-resolution structure of the catalytic domain of avian sarcoma virus integrase. J. Mol. Biol. 253:333, 1995.

440. Rice, P., and Mizuuchi, K.: Structure of the bacteriophage Mu transposase core: A common structural motif for DNA transposition and retroviral integration. Cell 82:209, 1995.

441. LaFemina, R. L., Schneider, C. L., Robbins, H. L., Callahan, P. L., LeGrow, K., Roth, E., Schleif, W. A., and Emini, E. A.: Requirement of active human immunodeficiency virus type 1 integrase enzyme for productive infection of human T-lymphoid cells. J. Virol. 66:7414, 1992.

442. Engelman, A., and Craigie, R.: Identification of conserved amino acid residues critical for human immunodeficiency virus type 1 integrase function in vitro. J. Virol. 66:6361, 1992.

443. Gallay, P., Hope, T., Chin, D., and Trono, D.: HIV-1 infection of nondividing cells through the recognition of integrase by the importin/karyopherin pathway. Proc. Natl. Acad. Sci. USA 94:9825, 1997.

444. Bukrinsky, M. I., Sharova, N., McDonald, T. L., Pushkarskaya, T., Tarpley, W. G., and Stevenson, M.: Association of integrase, matrix, and reverse transcriptase antigens of human immunodeficiency virus type 1 with viral nucleic acids following acute infection. Proc. Natl. Acad. Sci. USA 90:6125, 1993.

445. Karageorgos, L., Li, P., and Burrell, C.: Characterization of HIV replication complexes early after cell-to-cell infection. AIDS Res. Hum. Retroviruses 9:817, 1993.

446. Farnet, C. M., and Bushman, F. D.: HIV-1 cDNA integration: Requirement of HMG I(Y) protein for function of preintegration complexes in vitro. Cell 88:483, 1997.

447. Kalpana, G. V., Marmon, S., Wang, W., Crabtree, G. R., and Goff, S. P.: Binding and stimulation of HIV-1 integrase by a human homolog of yeast transcription factor SNF5. Science 266:2002, 1994.

448. Chow, S. A., Vincent, K. A., Ellison, V., and Brown, P. O.: Reversal of integration and DNA splicing mediated by integrase of human immunodeficiency virus. Science 255:723, 1992.

449. Bushman, F. D., and Craigie, R.: Activities of human immunodeficiency virus (HIV) integration protein in vitro: Specific cleavage and integration of HIV DNA. Proc. Natl. Acad. Sci. USA 88:1339, 1991.

450. Fujiwara, T., and Craigie, R.: Integration of mini-retroviral DNA: A cell-free reaction for biochemical analysis of retroviral integration. Proc. Natl. Acad. Sci. USA 86:3065, 1989.

451. Katz, R. A., Merkel, G., Kulkosky, J., Leis, J., and Skalka, A. M.: The avian retroviral IN protein is both necessary and sufficient for integrative recombination in vitro. Cell 63:87, 1990.

452. Farnet, C. M., and Bushman, F. D.: HIV cDNA integration: Molecular biology and inhibitor development. AIDS 10:S3, 1996.

453. Farnet, C. M., Wang, B., Lipford, J. R., and Bushman, F. D.: Differential inhibition of HIV-1 preintegration complexes and purified integrase protein by small molecules. Proc. Natl. Acad. Sci. USA 93:9742, 1996.

454. Allan, J. S., Coligan, J. E., Barin, F., McLane, M. F., Sodroski, J. G., Rosen, C. A., Haseltine, W. A., Lee, T. H., and Essex, M.: Major glycoprotein antigens that induce antibodies in AIDS patients are encoded by HTLV-III. Science 228:1091, 1985.

455. McCune, J. M., Rabin, L. B., Feinberg, M. B., Lieberman, M., Kosek, J. C., Reyes, G. R., and Weissman, I. L.: Endoproteolytic cleavage of gp160 is required for the activation of human immunodeficiency virus. Cell 53:55, 1988.

456. Dewar, R. L., Vasudevachari, M. B., Natarajan, V., and Salzman, N. P.: Biosynthesis and processing of human immunodeficiency virus type 1 envelope glycoproteins: Effects of monensin on glycosylation and transport. J. Virol. 63:2452, 1989.

457. Freed, E. O., Myers, D. J., and Risser, R.: Mutational analysis of the cleavage sequence of the human immunodeficiency virus type 1 envelope glycoprotein precursor gp160. J. Virol. 63:4670, 1989.

458. Hallenberger, S., Bosch, V., Angliker, H., Shaw, E., Klenk, H. D., and Garten, W.: Inhibition of furin-mediated cleavage activation of HIV-1 glycoprotein gp160. Nature 360:358, 1992.

459. Willey, R. L., Klimkait, T., Frucht, D. M., Bonifacino, J. S., and Martin, M. A.: Mutations within the human immunodeficiency virus type 1 gp160 envelope glycoprotein alter its intracellular transport and processing. Virology, 184:319, 1991.

460. Bernstein, H. B., Tucker, S. P., Hunter, E., Schutzbach, J. S., and Compans, R. W.: Human immunodeficiency virus type 1 envelope glycoprotein is modified by O-linked oligosaccharides. J. Virol. 68:463, 1994.

461. Modrow, S., Hahn, B. H., Shaw, G. M., Gallo, R. C., Wong-Staal, F., and Wolf, H.: Computer-assisted analysis of envelope protein sequences of seven human immunodeficiency virus isolates: Prediction of antigenic epitopes in conserved and variable regions. J. Virol. 61:570, 1987.

462. Willey, R. L., Rutledge, R. A., Dias, S., Folks, T., Theodore, T., Buckler, C. E., and Martin, M. A.: Identification of conserved and divergent domains within the envelope gene of the acquired immunodeficiency syndrome retrovirus. Proc. Natl. Acad. Sci. USA 83:5038, 1986.

463. Myers, G., Foley, B., Mellors, J. W., Korber, B., Jeang, K.-T., and Wain-Hobson, S. (eds.). Human Retroviruses and AIDS 1996: Part I. Nucleic Acid Alignment and Sequences—Nucleotide HMMER Alignments of HIV-1 *tat*—Alignment of HIV-1 *tat* Consensus Sequences. Los Alamos, N. Mex., Los Alamos National Laboratory, 1996.

464. Leonard, C. K., Spellman, M. W., Riddle, L., Harris, R. J., Thomas, J. N., and Gregory, T. J.: Assignment of intrachain disulfide bonds and characterization of potential glycosylation sites of the type 1 recombinant human immunodeficiency virus envelope glycoprotein (gp120) expressed in Chinese hamster ovary cells. J. Biol. Chem. 265:10373, 1990.

465. Klatzmann, D., Champagne, E., Chamaret, S., Gruest, J., Guetard, D., Hercend, T., Gluckman, J.-C., and Montagnier, L.: T-lymphocyte T4 molecule behaves as the receptor for human retrovirus LAV. Nature 312:767, 1984.

466. Maddon, P. J., Dalgleish, A. G., McDougal, J. S., Clapham, P. R., Weiss, R. A., and Axel, R.: The T4 gene encodes the AIDS virus receptor and is expressed in the immune system and the brain. Cell 47:333, 1986.

467. Maddon, P. J., Molineaux, S. M., Maddon, D. E., Zimmerman, K. A., Godfrey, M., Alt, F. W., Chess, L., and Axel, R.: Structure and expression of the human and mouse T4 genes. Proc. Natl. Acad. Sci. USA 84:9155, 1987.

468. Clayton, L. K., Hussey, R. E., Steinbrich, R., Ramachandran, H., Husain, Y., and Reinherz, E. L.: Substitution of murine for human CD4 residues identifies amino acids critical for HIV-gp120 binding. Nature 335:363, 1988.

469. Arthos, J., Deen, K. C., Chaikin, M. A., Fornwald, J. A., Sathe, G., Sattentau, Q. J., Clapham, P. R., Weiss, R. A., McDougal, J. S., Pietropaolo, C., Axel, R., Truneh, A., Maddon, P. J., and Sweet, R. W.: Identification of the residues in human CD4 critical for the binding of HIV. Cell 57:469, 1989.

470. Ryu, S.-E., Kwong, P. D., Truneh, A., Porter, T. G., Arthos, J., Rosenberg, M., Dai, X., Xuong, N.-h., Axel, R., Sweet, R. W., and Hendrickson, W. A.: Crystal structure of an HIV-binding recombinant fragment of human CD4. Nature 348:419, 1990.

471. Kowalski, M., Potz, J., Basiripour, L., Dorfman, T., Goh, W. C., Terwilliger, E., Dayton, A., Rosen, C., Haseltine, W., and Sodroski, J.: Functional regions of the envelope glycoprotein of human immunodeficiency virus type 1. Science 237:1351, 1987.

472. Lasky, L. A., Nakamura, G., Smith, D. H., Fennie, C., Shimasaki, C., Patzer, E., Berman, P., Gregory, T., and Capon, D. J.: Delineation of a region of the human immunodeficiency virus type 1 gp120 glycoprotein critical for interaction with the CD4 receptor. Cell 50:975, 1987.

473. Olshevsky, U., Helseth, E., Furman, C., Li, J., Haseltine, W., and Sodroski, J.: Identification of individual human immunodeficiency virus type 1 gp120 amino acids important for CD4 receptor binding. J. Virol. 64:5701, 1990.

474. Cordonnier, A., Riviere, Y., Montagnier, L., and Emerman, M.: Effects of mutations in hyperconserved regions of the extracellular glycoprotein of human immunodeficiency virus type 1 on receptor binding. J. Virol. 63:4464, 1989.

475. Wyatt, R., Kwong, P. D., Desjardins, E., Sweet, R. W., Robinson, J., Hendrickson, W. A., and Sodroski, J. G.: The antigenic structure of the HIV gp120 envelope glycoprotein. Nature 393:705, 1998.

476. Kwong, P. D., Wyatt, R., Robinson, J., Sweet, R. W., Sodroski, J., and Hendrickson, W. A.: Structure of an HIV gp120 envelope glycoprotein in complex with the CD4 receptor and a neutralizing human antibody. Nature 393:648, 1998.

477. Stevenson, M., Meier, C., Mann, A. M., Chapman, N., and Wasiak, A.: Envelope glycoprotein of HIV induces interference and cytolysis resistance in CD4+ cells: Mechanism for persistence in AIDS. Cell 53:483, 1988.

478. Rubin, H.: A virus in chick embryos which induces resistance in vitro to infection with Rous sarcoma virus. Proc. Natl. Acad. Sci. USA 46:1105, 1960.

479. Moore, J. P., McKeating, J. A., Weiss, R. A., and Sattentau, Q. J.: Dissociation of gp120 from HIV-1 virions induced by soluble CD4. Science 250:1139, 1990.

480. Daar, E. S., Li, X. L., Moudgil, T., and Ho, D. D.: High concentrations of recombinant soluble CD4 are required to neutralize primary human immunodeficiency virus type 1 isolates. Proc. Natl. Acad. Sci. USA 87:6574, 1990.

481. Kahn, J. O., Allan, J. D., Hodges, T. L., Kaplan, L. D., Arri, C. J., Fitch, H. F., Izu, A. E., Mordenti, J., Sherwin, S. A., Groopman, J. E., and Volberding, P. A.: The safety and pharmacokinetics of recombinant soluble CD4 (rCD4) in subjects with the acquired immunodeficiency syndrome (AIDS) and AIDS-related complex: A phase 1 study. Ann. Intern. Med. 112:254, 1990.

482. Schooley, R. T., Merigan, T. C., Gaut, P., Hirsch, M. S., Holodniy, M., Flynn, T., Liu, S., Byington, R. E., Henochowicz, S., Gubish, E., Spriggs, D., Kufe, D., Schindler, J., Dawson, A., Thomas, D., Hanson, D. G., Letwin, B., Liu, T., Gulinello, J., Kennedy, S., Fisher, R., and Ho, D. D.: Recombinant soluble CD4 therapy in patients with the acquired immunodeficiency syndrome (AIDS) and AIDS-related complex: A phase I–II escalating dosage trial. Ann. Intern. Med. 112:247, 1990.

483. White, J. M.: Membrane fusion. Science 258:917, 1992.

484. Freed, E. O., Myers, D. J., and Risser, R.: Characterization of the fusion domain of the human immunodeficiency virus type 1 envelope glycoprotein gp41. Proc. Natl. Acad. Sci. USA 87:4650, 1990.

485. Freed, E. O., and Myers, D. J.: Identification and characterization of fusion and processing domains of the human immunodeficiency virus type 2 envelope glycoprotein. J. Virol. 66:5472, 1992.

486. Bosch, M. L., Earl, P. L., Fargnoli, K., Picciafuoco, S., Giombini, F., Wong-Staal, F., and Franchini, G.: Identification of the fusion peptide of primate immunodeficiency viruses. Science 244:694, 1989.

487. Gallaher, W. R., Ball, J. M., Garry, R. F., Griffin, M. C., and Montelaro, R. C.: A general model for the transmembrane proteins of HIV and other retroviruses. AIDS Res. Hum. Retroviruses 5:431, 1989.

488. Delwart, E. L., Mosialos, G., and Gilmore, T.: Retroviral envelope glycoproteins contain a "leucine zipper"–like repeat. AIDS Res. Hum. Retroviruses 6:703, 1990.

489. Chen, S. S., Lee, C. N., Lee, W. R., McIntosh, K., and Lee, T. H.: Mutational analysis of the leucine zipper–like motif of the human immunodeficiency virus type 1 envelope transmembrane glycoprotein. J. Virol. 67:3615, 1993.

490. Wild, C., Oas, T., McDanal, C., Bolognesi, D., and Matthews, T.: A synthetic peptide inhibitor of human immunodeficiency virus replication: Correlation between solution structure and viral inhibition. Proc. Natl. Acad. Sci. USA 89:10537, 1992.

491. Wild, C. T., Shugars, D. C., Greenwell, T. K., McDanal, C. B., and Matthews, T. J.: Peptides corresponding to a predictive α-helical domain of human immunodeficiency virus type 1 gp41 are potent inhibitors of virus infection. Proc. Natl. Acad. Sci. USA 91:9770, 1994.

492. Freed, E. O., and Risser, R.: Identification of conserved residues in the human immunodeficiency virus type 1 principal neutralizing determinant that are involved in fusion. AIDS Res. Hum. Retroviruses 7:807, 1991.

493. Freed, E. O., Myers, D. J., and Risser, R.: Identification of the principal neutralizing determinant of human immunodeficiency virus type 1 as a fusion domain. J. Virol. 65:190, 1991.

494. Page, K. A., Stearns, S. M., and Littman, D. R.: Analysis of mutations in the V3 domain of gp160 that affect fusion and infectivity. J. Virol. 66:524, 1992.

495. Sullivan, N., Thali, M., Furman, C., Ho, D. D., and Sodroski, J.: Effect of amino acid changes in the V1/V2 region of the human immunodeficiency virus type 1 gp120 glycoprotein on subunit association, syncytium formation, and recognition by a neutralizing antibody. J. Virol. 67:3674, 1993.

496. Fung, M. S., Sun, C. R., Gordon, W. L., Liou, R. S., Chang, T. W., Sun, W. N., Daar, E. S., and Ho, D. D.: Identification and characterization of a neutralization site within the second variable region of human immunodeficiency virus type 1 gp120. J. Virol. 66:848, 1992.

497. McKeating, J. A., Shotton, C., Cordell, J., Graham, S., Balfe, P., Sullivan, N., Charles, M., Page, M., Bolmstedt, A., Olofsson, S., Kayman, S. C., Wu, Z., Pinter, A., Dean, C., Sodroski, J., and Weiss, R. A.: Characterization of neutralizing monoclonal antibodies to linear and conformation-dependent epitopes within the first and second variable domains of human immunodeficiency virus type 1 gp120. J. Virol. 67:4932, 1993.

498. Gebhardt, A., Bosch, J. V., Ziemiecki, A., and Friis, R. R.: Rous sarcoma virus p19 and gp35 can be chemically crosslinked to high molecular weight complexes: An insight into virus assembly. J. Mol. Biol. 174:297, 1984.

499. Rhee, S. S., and Hunter, E.: A single amino acid substitution within the matrix protein of a type D retrovirus converts its morphogenesis to that of a type C retrovirus. Cell 63:77, 1990.

500. Owens, R. J., Dubay, J. W., Hunter, E., and Compans, R. W.: Human immunodeficiency virus envelope protein determines the site of virus release in polarized epithelial cells. Proc. Natl. Acad. Sci. USA 88:3987, 1991.

501. Lodge, R., Gottlinger, H., Gabuzda, D., Cohen, E. A., and Lemay, G.: The intracytoplasmic domain of gp41 mediates polarized budding of human immunodeficiency virus type 1 in MDCK cells. J. Virol. 68:4857, 1994.

502. Lusso, P., di Marzo Veronese, F., Ensoli, B., Franchini, G., Jemma, C., DeRocco, S. E., Kalyanaraman, V. S., and Gallo, R. C.: Expanded HIV-1 cellular tropism by phenotypic mixing with murine endogenous retroviruses. Science 247:848, 1990.

503. Lusso, P., Lori, F., and Gallo, R. C.: CD4-independent infection by human immunodeficiency virus type 1 after phenotypic mixing with human T-cell leukemia viruses. J. Virol. 64:6341, 1990.

504. Landau, N. R., Page, K. A., and Littman, D. R.: Pseudotyping with human T-cell leukemia virus type I broadens the human immunodeficiency virus host range. J. Virol. 65:162, 1991.

505. Perez, L. G., Davis, G. L., and Hunter, E.: Mutants of the Rous sarcoma virus envelope glycoprotein that lack the transmembrane anchor and cytoplasmic domains: Analysis of intracellular transport and assembly into virions. J. Virol. 61:2981, 1987.

506. Wilk, T., Pfeiffer, T., and Bosch, V.: Retained in vitro infectivity and cytopathogenicity of HIV-1 despite truncation of the C-terminal tail of the *env* gene product. Virology 189:167, 1992.

507. Gabuzda, D. H., Lever, A., Terwilliger, E., and Sodroski, J.: Effects of deletions in the cytoplasmic domain on biological functions of human immunodeficiency virus type 1 envelope glycoproteins. J. Virol. 66:3306, 1992.

508. Gartner, S., Markovits, P., Markovitz, D. M., Kaplan, M. H., Gallo, R. C., and Popovic, M.: The role of mononuclear phagocytes in HTLV-III/LAV infection. Science 233:215, 1986.

509. Collman, R., Hassan, N. F., Walker, R., Godfrey, B., Cutilli, J., Hastings, J. C., Friedman, H., Douglas, S. D., and Nathanson, N.: Infection of monocyte-derived macrophages with human immunodeficiency virus type 1 (HIV-1): Monocyte-tropic and lymphocyte-tropic strains of HIV-1 show distinctive patterns of replication in a panel of cell types. J. Exp. Med. 170:1149, 1989.

510. Cheng-Mayer, C., Weiss, C., Seto, D., and Levy, J. A.: Isolates of human immunodeficiency virus type 1 from the brain may constitute a special group of the AIDS virus. Proc. Natl. Acad. Sci. USA 86:8575, 1989.

511. Schuitemaker, H., Kootstra, N. A., de Goede, R. E. Y., de Wolf, F., Miedema, F., and Tersmette, M.: Monocytotropic human immunodeficiency virus type 1 (HIV-1) variants detectable in all stages of HIV-1 infection lack T-cell line tropism and syncytium-inducing ability in primary T-cell culture. J. Virol. 65:356, 1991.

512. Tersmette, M., Gruters, R. A., de Wolf, F., de Goede, R. E. Y., Lange, J. M. A., Schellekens, P. T. A., Goudsmit, J., Huisman, H. G., and Miedema, F.: Evidence for a role of virulent human immunodeficiency virus (HIV) variants in the pathogenesis of acquired immunodeficiency syndrome: Studies on sequential HIV isolates. J. Virol. 63:2118, 1989.

513. O'Brien, W. A., Koyanagi, Y., Namazie, A., Zhao, J.-Q., Diagne, A., Idler, K., Zack, J. A., and Chen, I. S. Y.: HIV-1 tropism for mononuclear phagocytes can be determined by regions of gp120 outside the CD4-binding domain. Nature 348:69, 1990.

514. Shioda, T., Levy, J. A., and Cheng-Mayer, C.: Macrophage and T cell-line tropisms of HIV-1 are determined by specific regions of the envelope gp120 gene. Nature 349:167, 1991.

515. Westervelt, P., Gendelman, H. E., and Ratner, L.: Identification of a determinant within the human immunodeficiency virus 1 surface envelope glycoprotein critical for productive infection of primary monocytes. Proc. Natl. Acad. Sci. USA 88:3097, 1991.

516. Dragic, T., Charneau, P., Clavel, F., and Alizon, M.: Complementation of murine cells for human immunodeficiency virus envelope/CD4-mediated fusion in human/murine heterokaryons. J. Virol. 66:4794, 1992.

517. Broder, C. C., Dimitrov, D. S., Blumenthal, R., and Berger, E. A.: The block to HIV-1 envelope glycoprotein-mediated membrane fusion in animal cells expressing human CD4 can be overcome by a human cell component(s). Virology 193:483, 1993.

518. Cocchi, F., DeVico, A. L., Garzino-Demo, A., Arya, S. K., Gallo, R. C., and Lusso, P.: Identification of RANTES, MIP-1α, and MIP-1β as the major HIV-suppressive factors produced by CD8+ T cells. Science 270:1811, 1995.

519. Alkhatib, G., Combadiere, C., Broder, C. C., Feng, Y., Kennedy, P. E., Murphy, P. M., and Berger, E. A.: CC CKR5: A RANTES, MIP-1α, MIP-1β receptor as a fusion cofactor for macrophage-tropic HIV-1. Science 272:1955, 1996.

520. Doms, R. W., and Peiper, S. C.: Unwelcomed guests with master keys: How HIV uses chemokine receptors for cellular entry. Virology 235:179, 1997.

521. Rucker, J., Samson, M., Doranz, B. J., Libert, F., Berson, J. F., Yi, Y., Smyth, R. J., Collman, R. G., Broder, C. C., Vassart, G., Doms, R. W., and Parmentier, M.: Regions in β-chemokine receptors CCR5 and CCR2b that determine HIV-1 cofactor specificity. Cell 87:437, 1996.

522. Atchison, R. E., Gosling, J., Monteclaro, F. S., Franci, C., Digilio, L., Charo, I. F., and Goldsmith, M. A.: Multiple extracellular elements of CCR5 and HIV-1 entry: Dissociation from response to chemokines. Science 274:1924, 1996.

523. Alkhatib, G., Locati, M., Kennedy, P. E., Murphy, P. M., and Berger, E. A.: HIV-1 coreceptor activity of CCR5 and its inhibition by chemokines: Independence from G protein signaling and importance of coreceptor downmodulation. Virology 234:340, 1997.

524. Farzan, M., Choe, H., Martin, K. A., Sun, Y., Sidelko, M., Mackay, C. R., Gerard, N. P., Sodroski, J., and Gerard, C.: HIV-1 entry and macrophage inflammatory protein-1βeta-mediated signaling are independent functions of the chemokine receptor CCR5. J. Biol. Chem. 272:6854, 1997.

525. Chen, Z., Zhou, P., Ho, D. D., Landau, N. R., and Marx, P. A.: Genetically divergent strains of simian immunodeficiency virus use CCR5 as a coreceptor for entry. J. Virol. 71:2705, 1997.

526. Kirchhoff, F., Pohlmann, S., Hamacher, M., Means, R. E., Kraus, T., Uberla, K., and Di Marzio, P.: Simian immunodeficiency virus variants with differential T-cell and macrophage tropism use CCR5 and an unidentified cofactor expressed in CEMx174 cells for efficient entry. J. Virol. 71:6509, 1997.

527. Endres, M. J., Clapham, P. R., Marsh, M., Ahuja, M., Turner, J. D., McKnight, A., Thomas, J. F., Stoebenau-Haggarty, B., Choe, S., Vance, P. J., Wells, T. N., Power, C. A., Sutterwala, S. S., Doms, R. W., Landau, N. R., and Hoxie, J. A.: CD4-independent infection by HIV-2 is mediated by fusin/CXCR4. Cell 87:745, 1996.

528. Reeves, J. D., McKnight, A., Potempa, S., Simmons, G., Gray, P. W., Power, C. A., Wells, T., Weiss, R. A., and Talbot, S. J.: CD4-independent infection by HIV-2 (ROD/B): Use of the 7-transmembrane receptors CXCR-4, CCR-3, and V28 for entry. Virology 231:130, 1997.

529. Willett, B. J., Picard, L., Hosie, M. J., Turner, J. D., Adema, K., and Clapham, P. R.: Shared usage of the chemokine receptor CXCR4 by the feline and human immunodeficiency viruses. J. Virol. 71:6407, 1997.

530. Simmons, G., Wilkinson, D., Reeves, J. D., Dittmar, M. T., Beddows,

S., Weber, J., Carnegie, G., Desselberger, U., Gray, P. W., Weiss, R. A., and Clapham, P. R.: Primary, syncytium-inducing human immunodeficiency virus type 1 isolates are dual-tropic and most can use either Lestr or CCR5 as coreceptors for virus entry. J. Virol. 70:8355, 1996.

531. Lapham, C. K., Ouyang, J., Chandrasekhar, B., Nguyen, N. Y., Dimitrov, D. S., and Golding, H.: Evidence for cell-surface association between fusin and the CD4-gp120 complex in human cell lines. Science 274:602, 1996.

532. Trkola, A., Dragic, T., Arthos, J., Binley, J. M., Olson, W. C., Allaway, G. P., Cheng-Mayer, C., Robinson, J., Maddon, P. J., and Moore, J. P.: CD4-dependent, antibody-sensitive interactions between HIV-1 and its co-receptor CCR-5. Nature 384:184, 1996.

533. Wu, L., Gerard, N. P., Wyatt, R., Choe, H., Parolin, C., Ruffing, N., Borsetti, A., Cardoso, A. A., Desjardin, E., Newman, W., Gerard, C., and Sodroski, J.: CD4-induced interaction of primary HIV-1 gp120 glycoproteins with the chemokine receptor CCR-5. Nature 384:179, 1996.

534. Hill, C. M., Deng, H., Unutmaz, D., Kewalramani, V. N., Bastiani, L., Gorny, M. K., Zolla-Pazner, S., and Littman, D. R.: Envelope glycoproteins from human immunodeficiency virus types 1 and 2 and simian immunodeficiency virus can use human CCR5 as a coreceptor for viral entry and make direct CD4-dependent interactions with this chemokine receptor. J. Virol. 71:6296, 1997.

535. Picard, L., Simmons, G., Power, C. A., Meyer, A., Weiss, R. A., and Clapham, P. R.: Multiple extracellular domains of CCR-5 contribute to human immunodeficiency virus type 1 entry and fusion. J. Virol. 71:5003, 1997.

536. Edinger, A. L., Amedee, A., Miller, K., Doranz, B. J., Endres, M., Sharron, M., Samson, M., Lu, Z. H., Clements, J. E., Murphey-Corb, M., Peiper, S. C., Parmentier, M., Broder, C. C., and Doms, R. W.: Differential utilization of CCR5 by macrophage and T cell tropic simian immunodeficiency virus strains. Proc. Natl. Acad. Sci. USA 94:4005, 1997.

537. Potempa, S., Picard, L., Reeves, J. D., Wilkinson, D., Weiss, R. A., and Talbot, S. J.: CD4-independent infection by human immunodeficiency virus type 2 strain ROD/B: The role of the N-terminal domain of CXCR-4 in fusion and and entry. J. Virol. 71:4419, 1997.

538. Brelot, A., Heveker, N., Pleskoff, O., Sol, N., and Alizon, M.: Role of the first and third extracellular domains of CXCR-4 in human immunodeficiency virus coreceptor activity. J. Virol. 71:4744, 1997.

539. Lu, Z., Berson, J. F., Chen, Y., Turner, J. D., Zhang, T., Sharron, M., Jenks, M. H., Wang, Z., Kim, J., Rucker, J., Hoxie, J. A., Peiper, S. C., and Doms, R. W.: Evolution of HIV-1 coreceptor usage through interactions with distinct CCR5 and CXCR4 domains. Proc. Natl. Acad. Sci. USA 94:6426, 1997.

540. Bieniasz, P. D., Fridell, R. A., Aramori, I., Ferguson, S. S., Caron, M. G., and Cullen, B. R.: HIV-1-induced cell fusion is mediated by multiple regions within both the viral envelope and the CCR-5 coreceptor. EMBO J. 16:2599, 1997.

541. Farzan, M., Choe, H., Vaca, L., Martin, K., Sun, Y., Desjardins, E., Ruffing, N., Wu, L., Wyatt, R., Gerard, N., Gerard, C., and Sodroski, J.: A tyrosine-rich region in the N terminus of CCR5 is important for human immunodeficiency virus type 1 entry and mediates an association between gp120 and CCR5. J. Virol. 72:1160, 1998.

542. Cocchi, F., DeVico, A. L., Garzino-Demo, A., Cara, A., Gallo, R. C., and Lusso, P.: The V3 domain of the HIV-1 gp120 envelope glycoprotein is critical for chemokine-mediated blockade of infection. Nat. Med. 2:1244, 1996.

543. Speck, R. F., Wehrly, K., Platt, E. J., Atchison, R. E., Charo, I. F., Kabat, D., Chesebro, B., and Goldsmith, M. A.: Selective employment of chemokine receptors as human immunodeficiency virus type 1 coreceptors determined by individual amino acids within the envelope V3 loop. J. Virol. 71:7136, 1997.

544. Cheng-Mayer, C., Liu, R., Landau, N. R., and Stamatatos, L.: Macrophage tropism of human immunodeficiency virus type 1 and utilization of the CC-CKR5 coreceptor. J. Virol. 71:1657, 1997.

545. Dittmar, M. T., McKnight, A., Simmons, G., Clapham, P. R., Weiss, R. A., and Simmonds, P.: HIV-1 tropism and co-receptor use (letter). Nature 385:495, 1997.

546. Rana, S., Besson, G., Cook, D. G., Rucker, J., Smyth, R. J., Yi, Y., Turner, J. D., Guo, H.-H., Du, J.-G., Peiper, S. C., Lavi, E., Samson, M., Libert, F., Liesnard, C., Vassart, G., Doms, R. W., Parmentier, M., and Collman, R. G.: Role of CCR5 in infection of primary macrophages and lymphocytes by macrophage-tropic strains of human immunodeficiency virus: Resistance to patient-derived and prototype isolates resulting from the Δccr5 mutation. J. Virol. 71:3219, 1997.

547. Deng, H. K., Unutmaz, D., Kewal Ramani, V. N., and Littman, D. R.: Expression cloning of new receptors used by simian and human immunodeficiency viruses. Nature 388:296, 1997.

548. Alkhatib, G., Liao, F., Berger, E. A., Farber, J. M., and Peden, K. W.: A new SIV co-receptor, STRL33 (letter). Nature 388:238, 1997.

549. Liao, F., Alkhatib, G., Peden, K. W., Sharma, G., Berger, E. A., and Farber, J. M.: STRL33, a novel chemokine receptor-like protein, functions as a fusion cofactor for both macrophage-tropic and T cell line–tropic HIV-1. J. Exp. Med. 185:2015, 1997.

550. Farzan, M., Choe, H., Martin, K., Marcon, L., Hofmann, W., Karlsson, G., Sun, Y., Barrett, P., Marchand, N., Sullivan, N., Gerard, N., Gerard, C., and Sodroski, J.: Two orphan seven-transmembrane segment receptors which are expressed in CD4-positive cells support simian immunodeficiency virus infection. J. Exp. Med. 186:405, 1997.

551. Rucker, J., Edinger, A. L., Sharron, M., Samson, M., Lee, B., Berson, J. F., Yi, Y., Margulies, B., Collman, R. G., Doranz, B. J., Parmentier, M., and Doms, R. W.: Utilization of chemokine receptors, orphan receptors, and herpesvirus-encoded receptors by diverse human and simian immunodeficiency viruses. J. Virol. 71:8999, 1997.

552. Paxton, W. A., Martin, S. R., Tse, D., O'Brien, T. R., Skurnick, J., VanDevanter, N. L., Padian, N., Braun, J. F., Kotler, D. P., Wolinsky, S. M., and Koup, R. A.: Relative resistance to HIV-1 infection of CD4 lymphocytes from persons who remain uninfected despite multiple high-risk sexual exposures. Nat. Med. 2:412, 1996.

553. Liu, R., Paxton, W. A., Choe, S., Ceradini, D., Martin, S. R., Horuk, R., MacDonald, M. E., Stuhlmann, H., Koup, R. A., and Landau, N. R.: Homozygous defect in HIV-1 coreceptor accounts for resistance of some multiply-exposed individuals to HIV-1 infection. Cell 86:367, 1996.

554. Samson, M., Libert, F., Doranz, B. J., Rucker, J., Liesnard, C., Farber, C.-M., Saragosti, S., Lapoumeroulie, C., Cognaux, J., Forceille, C., Muyldermans, G., Verhofstede, C., Burtonboy, G., Georges, M., Imai, T., Rana, S., Yi, Y., Smyth, R. J., Collman, R. G., Doms, R. W., Vassart, G., and Parmentier, M.: Resistance to HIV-1 infection in caucasian individuals bearing mutant alleles of the CCR-5 chemokine receptor gene. Nature 382:722, 1996.

555. Dean, M., Carrington, M., Winkler, C., Huttley, G. A., Smith, M. W., Allikmets, R., Goedert, J. J., Buchbinder, S. P., Vittinghoff, E., Gomperts, E., Donfield, S., Vlahov, D., Kaslow, R., Saah, A., Rinaldo, C., Detels, R., Hemophilia Growth and Development Study, Multicenter AIDS Cohort Study, Multicenter Hemophilia Cohort Study, San Francisco City Cohort, ALIVE Study, and O'Brien, S. J.: Genetic restriction of HIV-1 infection and progression to AIDS by a deletion allele of the CKR5 structural gene. Science 273:1856, 1996.

556. Huang, Y., Paxton, W. A., Wolinsky, S. M., Neumann, A. U., Zhang, L., He, T., Kang, S., Ceradini, D., Jin, Z., Yazdanbakhsh, K., Kunstman, K., Erickson, D., Dragon, E., Landau, N. R., Phair, J., Ho, D. D., and Koup, R. A.: The role of a mutant CCR5 allele in HIV-1 transmission and disease progression. Nat. Med. 2:1240, 1996.

557. Smith, M. W., Dean, M., Carrington, M., Winkler, C., Huttley, G. A., Lomb, D. A., Goedert, J. J., O'Brien, T. R., Jacobson, L. P., Kaslow, R., Buchbinder, S., Vittinghoff, E., Vlahov, D., Hoots, K., Hilgartner, M. W., Hemophilia Growth and Development Study (HGDS), Multicenter AIDS Cohort Study (MACS), Multicenter Hemophilia Cohort Study (MHCS), San Francisco City Cohort (SFCC), ALIVE Study, and O'Brien, S. J.: Contrasting genetic influence of CCR2 and CCR5 variants on HIV-1 infection and disease progression. Science 277:959, 1997.

558. Kostrikis, L. G., Huang, Y., Moore, J. P., Wolinsky, S. M., Zhang, L., Guo, Y., Deutsch, L., Phair, J., Neumann, A. U., and Ho, D. D.: A chemokine receptor CCR2 allele delays HIV-1 disease progression and is associated with a CCR5 promoter mutation. Nat. Med. 4:350, 1998.

559. Zagury, D., Lachgar, A., Chams, V., Fall, L. S., Bernard, J., Zagury, J. F., Bizzini, B., Gringeri, A., Santagostino, E., Rappaport, J., Feldman, M., O'Brien, S. J., Burny, A., and Gallo, R. C.: C-C chemokines, pivotal in protection against HIV type 1 infection. Proc. Natl. Acad. Sci. USA 95:3857, 1998.

560. Winkler, C., Modi, W., Smith, M. W., Nelson, G. W., Wu, X., Carrington, M., Dean, M., Honjo, T., Tashiro, K., Yabe, D., Buchbinder, S., Vittinghoff, E., Goedert, J. J., O'Brien, T. R., Jacobson, L. P., Detels, R., Donfield, S., Willoughby, A., Gomperts, E., Vlahov, D., Phair, J., ALIVE Study, Hemophilia Growth and Development Study (HGDS), Multicenter AIDS Cohort Study (MACS), Multicenter Hemophilia Cohort Study (MHCS), San Francisco City Cohort (SFCC), and O'Brien, S. J.: Genetic restriction of AIDS pathogenesis by an SDF-1 chemokine gene variant. Science 279:389, 1998.

561. Simmons, G., Clapham, P. R., Picard, L., Offord, R. E., Rosenkilde, M. M., Schwartz, T. W., Buser, R., Wells, T. N. C., and Proudfoot, A. E.: Potent inhibition of HIV-1 infectivity in macrophages and lymphocytes by a novel CCR5 antagonist. Science 276:276, 1997.

562. Kledal, T. N., Rosenkilde, M. M., Coulin, F., Simmons, G., Johnsen, A. H., Alouani, S., Power, C. A., Luttichau, H. R., Gerstoft, J., Clapham, P. R., Clark-Lewis, I., Wells, T. N. C., and Schwartz, T. W.: A broad-spectrum chemokine antagonist encoded by Kaposi's sarcoma–associated herpesvirus. Science 277:1656, 1997.

563. Kawakami, T., Sherman, L., Dahlberg, J., Gazit, A., Yaniv, A., Tronick, S. R., and Aaronson, S. A.: Nucleotide sequence analysis of equine infectious anemia virus proviral DNA. Virology 158:300, 1987.

564. Strebel, K., Daugherty, D., Clouse, K., Cohen, D., Folks, T., and Martin, M. A.: The HIV 'A' (sor) gene product is essential for virus infectivity. Nature 328:728, 1987.

565. Fisher, A. G., Ensoli, B., Ivanoff, L., Chamberlain, M., Petteway, S., Ratner, L., Gallo, R. C., and Wong-Staal, F.: The sor gene of HIV-1 is required for efficient virus transmission in vitro. Science 237:888, 1987.

566. Gabuzda, D. H., Lawrence, K., Langhoff, E., Terwilliger, E., Dorfman, T., Haseltine, W. A., and Sodroski, J.: Role of vif in replication of human immunodeficiency virus type 1 in CD4+ T lymphocytes. J. Virol. 66:6489, 1992.

567. Sakai, H., Shibata, R., Sakuragi, J.-I., Sakuragi, S., Kawamura, M., and Adachi, A.: Cell-dependent requirement of human immunodeficiency virus type 1 Vif protein for maturation of virus particles. J. Virol. 67:1663, 1993.

568. Sova, P., and Volsky, D. J.: Efficiency of viral DNA synthesis during infection of permissive and nonpermissive cells with vif-negative human immunodeficiency virus type 1. J. Virol. 67:6322, 1993.

569. von Schwedler, U., Song, J., Aiken, C., and Trono, D.: Vif is crucial for human immunodeficiency virus type 1 proviral DNA synthesis in infected cells. J. Virol. 67:4945, 1993.

570. Courcoul, M., Patience, C., Rey, F., Blanc, D., Harmache, A., Sire, J., Vigne, R., and Spire, B.: Peripheral blood mononuclear cells produce normal amounts of defective Vif-human immunodeficiency virus type 1 particles which are restricted for the preretrotranscription steps. J. Virol. 69:2068, 1995.

571. Simon, J. H., and Malim, M. H.: The human immunodeficiency virus type 1 Vif protein modulates the postpenetration stability of viral nucleoprotein complexes. J. Virol. 70:5297, 1996.

572. Hoglund, S., Ohagen, A., Lawrence, K., and Gabuzda, D.: Role of Vif during packing of the core of HIV-1. Virology 201:349, 1994.

573. Goncalves, J., Korin, Y., Zack, J., and Gabuzda, D.: Role of Vif in human immunodeficiency virus type 1 reverse transcription. J. Virol. 70:8701, 1996.

574. Borman, A. M., Quillent, C., Charneau, P., Dauguet, C., and Clavel, F.: Human immunodeficiency virus type 1 Vif-mutant particles from restrictive cells: Role of Vif in correct particle assembly and infectivity. J. Virol. 69:2058, 1995.

575. Simm, M., Shahabuddin, M., Chao, W., Allan, J. S., and Volsky, D. J.: Aberrant Gag protein composition of a human immunodeficiency virus type 1 Vif mutant produced in primary lymphocytes. J. Virol. 69:4582, 1995.

576. Kotler, M., Simm, M., Zhao, Y. S., Sova, P., Chao, W., Ohnona, S. F., Roller, R., Krachmarov, C., Potash, M. J., and Volsky, D. J.: Human immunodeficiency virus type 1 (HIV-1) protein Vif inhibits the activity of HIV-1 protease in bacteria and in vitro. J. Virol. 71:5774, 1997.

577. Fouchier, R. A., Simon, J. H., Jaffe, A. B., and Malim, M. H.: Human immunodeficiency virus type 1 Vif does not influence expression or virion incorporation of gag-, pol-, and env-encoded proteins. J. Virol. 70:8263, 1996.

578. Liu, H., Wu, X., Newman, M., Shaw, G. M., Hahn, B. H., and Kappes, J. C.: The Vif protein of human and simian immunodeficiency viruses is packaged into virions and associates with viral core structures. J. Virol. 69:7630, 1995.

579. Karczewski, M. K., and Strebel, K.: Cytoskeleton association and virion incorporation of the human immunodeficiency virus type 1 Vif protein. J. Virol. 70:494, 1996.

580. Camaur, D., and Trono, D.: Characterization of human immunodeficiency virus type 1 Vif particle incorporation. J. Virol. 70:6106, 1996.

581. Terwilliger, E. F., Cohen, E. A., Lu, Y., Sodroski, J. G., and Haseltine, W. A.: Functional role of human immunodeficiency virus type 1 vpu. Proc. Natl. Acad. Sci. USA 86:5163, 1989.

582. Klimkait, T., Strebel, K., Hoggan, M. D., Martin, M. A., and Orenstein, J. M.: The human immunodeficiency virus type 1–specific protein vpu is required for efficient virus maturation and release. J. Virol. 64:621, 1990.

583. Strebel, K., Klimkait, T., Maldarelli, F., and Martin, M. A.: Molecular and biochemical analyses of human immunodeficiency virus type 1 vpu protein. J. Virol. 63:3784, 1989.

584. Schwartz, S., Felber, B. K., Fenyö, E.-M., and Pavlakis, G. N.: Env and Vpu proteins of human immunodeficiency virus type 1 are produced from multiple bicistronic mRNAs. J. Virol. 64:5448, 1990.

585. Stevenson, M., Zhang, X., and Volsky, D. J.: Downregulation of cell surface molecules during noncytopathic infection of T cells with human immunodeficiency virus. J. Virol. 61:3741, 1987.

586. Crise, B., Buonocore, L., and Rose, J. K.: CD4 is retained in the endoplasmic reticulum by the human immunodeficiency virus type 1 glycoprotein precursor. J. Virol. 64:5585, 1990.

587. Willey, R. L., Maldarelli, F., Martin, M. A., and Strebel, K.: Human immunodeficiency virus type 1 Vpu protein regulates the formation of intracellular gp160-CD4 complexes. J. Virol. 66:226, 1992.

588. Willey, R. L., Maldarelli, F., Martin, M. A., and Strebel, K.: Human immunodeficiency virus type 1 Vpu protein induces rapid degradation of CD4. J. Virol. 66:7193, 1992.

589. Schubert, U., Anton, L. C., Bacik, I., Cox, J. H., Bour, S., Bennink, J. R., Orlowski, M., Strebel, K., and Yewdell, J. W.: CD4 glycoprotein degradation induced by human immunodeficiency virus type 1 Vpu protein requires the function of proteasomes and the ubiquitin-conjugating pathway. J. Virol. 72:2280, 1998.

590. Margottin, F., Bour, S. P., Durand, H., Selig, L., Benichou, S., Richard, V., Thomas, D., Strebel, K., and Benarous, R.: A novel human WD protein, h-βTrCp, that interacts with HIV-1 Vpu connects CD4 to the ER degradation pathway through an F-box motif. Mol. Cell. 1:565, 1998.

591. Schubert, U., and Strebel, K.: Differential activities of the human immunodeficiency virus type 1–encoded Vpu protein are regulated by phosphorylation and occur in different cellular compartments. J. Virol. 68:2260, 1994.

592. Schubert, U., Bour, S., Ferrer-Montiel, A. V., Montal, M., Maldarelli, F., and Strebel, K.: The two biological activities of human immunodeficiency virus type 1 Vpu protein involve two separable structural domains. J. Virol. 70:809, 1996.

593. Gottlinger, H. G., Dorfman, T., Cohen, E. A., and Haseltine, W. A.: Vpu protein of human immunodeficiency virus type 1 enhances the release of capsids produced by gag gene constructs of widely divergent retroviruses. Proc. Natl. Acad. Sci. USA 90:7381, 1993.

594. Yuan, X., Matsuda, Z., Matsuda, M., Essex, M., and Lee, T. H.: Human immunodeficiency virus vpr gene encodes a virion-associated protein. AIDS Res. Hum. Retroviruses 6:1265, 1990.

595. Cohen, E. A., Dehni, G., Sodroski, J. G., and Haseltine, W. A.: Human immunodeficiency virus vpr product is a virion-associated regulatory protein. J. Virol. 64:3097, 1990.

596. Cohen, E. A., Terwilliger, E. F., Jalinoos, Y., Proulx, J., Sodroski, J. G., and Haseltine, W. A.: Identification of HIV-1 vpr product and function. J. Acquir. Immune. Defic. Syndr. 3:11, 1990.

597. Jowett, J. B., Planelles, V., Poon, B., Shah, N. P., Chen, M. L., and Chen, I. S.: The human immunodeficiency virus type 1 vpr gene arrests infected T cells in the G2 + M phase of the cell cycle. J. Virol. 69:6304, 1995.

598. Rogel, M. E., Wu, L. I., and Emerman, M.: The human immunodeficiency virus type 1 vpr gene prevents cell proliferation during chronic infection. J. Virol. 69:882, 1995.

599. Planelles, V., Jowett, J. B., Li, Q. X., Xie, Y., Hahn, B., and Chen, I. S.: Vpr-induced cell cycle arrest is conserved among primate lentiviruses. J. Virol. 70:2516, 1996.

600. Bartz, S. R., Rogel, M. E., and Emerman, M.: Human immunodeficiency virus type 1 cell cycle control: Vpr is cytostatic and mediates G2 accumulation by a mechanism which differs from DNA damage checkpoint control. J. Virol. 70:2324, 1996.

601. He, J., Choe, S., Walker, R., Di Marzio, P., Morgan, D. O., and Landau, N. R.: Human immunodeficiency virus type 1 viral protein R (Vpr) arrests cells in the G2 phase of the cell cycle by inhibiting p34cdc2 activity. J. Virol. 69:6705, 1995.

602. Re, F., Braaten, D., Franke, E. K., and Luban, J.: Human immunodeficiency virus type 1 Vpr arrests the cell cycle in G2 by inhibiting the activation of p34cdc2-cyclin B. J. Virol. 69:6859, 1995.

603. Levy, D. N., Fernandes, L. S., Williams, W. V., and Weiner, D. B.:

Induction of cell differentiation by human immunodeficiency virus 1 vpr. Cell 72:541, 1993.

604. Macreadie, I. G., Castelli, L. A., Hewish, D. R., Kirkpatrick, A., Ward, A. C., and Azad, A. A.: A domain of human immunodeficiency virus type 1 Vpr containing repeated H(S/F)RIG amino acid motifs causes cell growth arrest and structural defects. Proc. Natl. Acad. Sci. USA 92:2770, 1995.

605. Zhao, Y., Cao, J., O'Gorman, M. R., Yu, M., and Yogev, R.: Effect of human immunodeficiency virus type 1 protein R (*vpr*) gene expression on basic cellular function of fission yeast *Schizosaccharomyces pombe*. J. Virol. 70:5821, 1996.

606. Goh, W. C., Rogel, M. E., Kinsey, C. M., Michael, S. F., Fultz, P. N., Nowak, M. A., Hahn, B. H., and Emerman, M.: HIV-1 Vpr increases viral expression by manipulation of the cell cycle: A mechanism for selection of Vpr in vivo. Nat. Med. 4:65, 1998.

607. Felzien, L. K., Woffendin, C., Hottiger, M. O., Subramanian, R. A., Cohen, E. A., and Nabel, G. J.: HIV transcriptional activation by the accessory protein, VPR, is mediated by the p300 co-activator. Proc. Natl. Acad. Sci. USA 95:5281, 1998.

608. Popov, S., Rexach, M., Zybarth, G., Reiling, N., Lee, M. A., Ratner, L., Lane, C. M., Moore, M. S., Blobel, G., and Bukrinsky, M.: Viral protein R regulates nuclear import of the HIV-1 pre-integration complex. EMBO J. 17:909, 1998.

609. Kawamura, M., Ishizaki, T., Ishimoto, A., Shioda, T., Kitamura, T., and Adachi, A.: Growth ability of human immunodeficiency virus type 1 auxiliary gene mutants in primary blood macrophage cultures. J. Gen. Virol. 75:2427, 1994.

610. Theodore, T. S., Englund, G., Buckler-White, A., Buckler, C. E., Martin, M. A., and Peden, K. W.: Construction and characterization of a stable full-length macrophage-tropic HIV type 1 molecular clone that directs the production of high titers of progeny virions. AIDS Res. Hum. Retroviruses 12:191, 1996.

611. Fletcher, T. M. III, Brichacek, B., Sharova, N., Newman, M. A., Stivahtis, G., Sharp, P. M., Emerman, M., Hahn, B. H., and Stevenson, M.: Nuclear import and cell cycle arrest functions of the HIV-1 Vpr protein are encoded by two separate genes in HIV-2/SIV(SM). EMBO J. 15:6155, 1996.

612. Campbell, B. J., and Hirsch, V. M.: Vpr of simian immunodeficiency virus of African green monkeys is required for replication in macaque macrophages and lymphocytes. J. Virol. 71:5593, 1997.

613. Hoch, J., Lang, S. M., Weeger, M., Stahl-Hennig, C., Coulibaly, C., Dittmer, U., Hunsmann, G., Fuchs, D., Müller, J., Sopper, S., Fleckenstein, B., and Überla, K. T.: *vpr* Deletion mutant of simian immunodeficiency virus induces AIDS in rhesus monkeys. J. Virol. 69:4807, 1995.

614. Ahmad, N., and Venkatesan, S.: *Nef* protein of HIV-1 is a transcriptional repressor of HIV-1 LTR. Science 241:1481, 1988.

615. Kim, S., Ikeuchi, K., Byrn, R., Groopman, J., and Baltimore, D.: Lack of a negative influence on viral growth by the *nef* gene of human immunodeficiency virus type 1. Proc. Natl. Acad. Sci. USA 86:9544, 1989.

616. Guy, B., Kieny, M. P., Riviere, Y., Le Peuch, C., Dott, K., Girard, M., Montagnier, L., and Lecocq, J.-P.: HIV F/3′ *orf* encodes a phosphorylated GTP-binding protein resembling an oncogene product. Nature 330:266, 1987.

617. Nebreda, A. R., Bryan, T., Segade, F., Wingfield, P., Venkatesan, S., and Santos, E.: Biochemical and biological comparison of HIV-1 NEF and *ras* gene products. Virology 183:151, 1991.

618. Matsuura, Y., Maekawa, M., Hatori, S., Ikegami, N., Hayashi, A., Yamazaki, S., Morita, C., and Takebe, Y.: Purification and characterization of human immunodeficiency virus type 1 *nef* gene product expressed by a recombinant baculovirus. Virology 184:580, 1991.

619. Kaminchik, J., Bashan, N., Pinchasi, D., Amit, B., Sarver, N., Johnston, M. I., Fischer, M., Yavin, Z., Gorecki, M., and Panet, A.: Expression and biochemical characterization of human immunodeficiency virus type 1 *nef* gene product. J. Virol. 64:3447, 1990.

620. Grzesiek, S., Bax, A., Clore, G. M., Gronenborn, A. M., Hu, J. S., Kaufman, J., Palmer, I., Stahl, S. J., and Wingfield, P. T.: The solution structure of HIV-1 Nef reveals an unexpected fold and permits delineation of the binding surface for the SH3 domain of Hck tyrosine protein kinase. Nat. Struct. Biol. 3:340, 1996.

621. Lee, C. H., Saksela, K., Mirza, U. A., Chait, B. T., and Kuriyan, J.: Crystal structure of the conserved core of HIV-1 Nef complexed with a Src family SH3 domain. Cell 85:931, 1996.

622. Kestler, H. W. III, Ringler, D. J., Mori, K., Panicali, D. L., Sehgal, P.

K., Daniel, M. D., and Desrosiers, R. C.: Importance of the *nef* gene for maintenance of high virus loads and for development of AIDS. Cell 65:651, 1991.

623. Harris, M.: From negative factor to a critical role in virus pathogenesis: The changing fortunes of Nef. J. Gen. Virol. 77:2379, 1996.

624. Ratner, L., and Niederman, T. M.: Nef. Curr. Top. Microbiol. Immunol. 193:169, 1995.

625. Du, Z., Lang, S. M., Sasseville, V. G., Lackner, A. A., Ilyinskii, P. O., Daniel, M. D., Jung, J. U., and Desrosiers, R. C.: Identification of a nef allele that causes lymphocyte activation and acute disease in macaque monkeys. Cell 82:665, 1995.

626. Howe, L. R., and Weiss, A.: Multiple kinases mediate T-cell-receptor signaling. Trends Biochem. Sci. 20:59, 1995.

627. Luo, W., and Peterlin, B. M.: Activation of the T-cell receptor signaling pathway by Nef from an aggressive strain of simian immunodeficiency virus. J. Virol. 71:9531, 1997.

628. Alexander, L., Du, Z., Rosenzweig, M., Jung, J. U., and Desrosiers, R. C.: A role for natural simian immunodeficiency virus and human immunodeficiency virus type 1 nef alleles in lymphocyte activation. J. Virol. 71:6094, 1997.

629. Jamieson, B. D., Aldrovandi, G. M., Planelles, V., Jowett, J. B., Gao, L., Bloch, L. M., Chen, I. S., and Zack, J. A.: Requirement of human immunodeficiency virus type 1 nef for in vivo replication and pathogenicity. J. Virol. 68:3478, 1994.

630. Garcia, J. V., and Miller, A. D.: Serine phosphorylation–independent downregulation of cell-surface CD4 by *nef*. Nature 350:508, 1991.

631. Aiken, C., Konner, J., Landau, N. R., Lenburg, M. E., and Trono, D.: Nef induces CD4 endocytosis: Requirement for a critical dileucine motif in the membrane-proximal CD4 cytoplasmic domain. Cell 76:853, 1994.

632. Rhee, S. S., and Marsh, J. W.: Human immunodeficiency virus type 1 Nef-induced down-modulation of CD4 is due to rapid internalization and degradation of surface CD4. J. Virol. 68:5156, 1994.

633. Chowers, M. Y., Pandori, M. W., Spina, C. A., Richman, D. D., and Guatelli, J. C.: The growth advantage conferred by HIV-1 *nef* is determined at the level of viral DNA formation and is independent of CD4 downregulation. Virology 212:451, 1995.

634. Goldsmith, M. A., Warmerdam, M. T., Atchison, R. E., Miller, M. D., and Greene, W. C.: Dissociation of the CD4 downregulation and viral infectivity enhancement functions of human immunodeficiency virus type 1 Nef. J. Virol. 69:4112, 1995.

635. Miller, M. D., Warmerdam, M. T., Gaston, I., Greene, W. C., and Feinberg, M. B.: The human immunodeficiency virus-1 *nef* gene product: A positive factor for viral infection and replication in primary lymphocytes and macrophages. J. Exp. Med. 179:101, 1994.

636. Aiken, C., and Trono, D.: Nef stimulates human immunodeficiency virus type 1 proviral DNA synthesis. J. Virol. 69:5048, 1995.

637. Schwartz, O., Marechal, V., Danos, O., and Heard, J. M.: Human immunodeficiency virus type 1 Nef increases the efficiency of reverse transcription in the infected cell. J. Virol. 69:4053, 1995.

638. Aiken, C.: Pseudotyping human immunodeficiency virus type 1 (HIV-1) by the glycoprotein of vesicular stomatitis virus targets HIV-1 entry to an endocytic pathway and suppresses both the requirement for Nef and the sensitivity to cyclosporin A. J. Virol. 71:5871, 1997.

639. Matlin, K. S., Reggio, H., Helenius, A., and Simons, K.: Pathway of vesicular stomatitis virus entry leading to infection. J. Mol. Biol. 156:609, 1982.

640. Schwartz, O., Marechal, V., Le Gall, S., Lemonnier, F., and Heard, J. M.: Endocytosis of major histocompatibility complex class I molecules is induced by the HIV-1 Nef protein. Nat. Med. 2:338, 1996.

641. Collins, K. L., Chen, B. K., Kalams, S. A., Walker, B. D., and Baltimore, D.: HIV-1 Nef protein protects infected primary cells against killing by cytotoxic T lymphocytes. Nature 391:397, 1998.

642. Pandori, M. W., Fitch, N. J., Craig, H. M., Richman, D. D., Spina, C. A., and Guatelli, J. C.: Producer-cell modification of human immunodeficiency virus type 1: Nef is a virion protein. J. Virol. 70:4283, 1996.

643. Welker, R., Kottler, H., Kalbitzer, H. R., and Krausslich, H. G.: Human immunodeficiency virus type 1 Nef protein is incorporated into virus particles and specifically cleaved by the viral proteinase. Virology 219:228, 1996.

644. Bukovsky, A. A., Dorfman, T., Weimann, A., and Gottlinger, H. G.: Nef association with human immunodeficiency virus type 1 virions and cleavage by the viral protease. J. Virol. 71:1013, 1997.

645. Goedert, J. J., and Blattner, W. A.: The epidemiology and natural history of human immunodeficiency virus. *In* DeVita, V. T., Jr., Hell-

man, S. and Rosenberg, S. A. (eds.): AIDS: Etiology, Diagnosis, Treatment, and Prevention. Philadelphia, J. B. Lippincott Co., 1988.

646. Blanche, S., Rouzioux, C., Moscato, M.-L. G., Veber, F., Mayaux, M.-J., Jacomet, C., Tricoire, J., Deville, A., Vial, M., Firtion, G., de Crepy, A., Douard, D., Robin, M., Courpotin, C., Ciraru-Vigneron, N., le Deist, F., Griscelli, C., and the HIV Infection in Newborns French Collaborative Study Group: A prospective study of infants born to women seropositive for human immunodeficiency virus type 1. N. Engl. J. Med. 320:1643, 1989.

647. Adachi, A., Koenig, S., Gendelman, H. E., Daugherty, D., Gattoni-Celli, S., Fauci, A. S., and Martin, M. A.: Productive, persistent infection of human colorectal cell lines with human immunodeficiency virus. J. Virol. 61:209, 1987.

648. Moyer, M. P., Huot, R. I., Ramirez, A., Jr., Joe, S., Meltzer, M. S., and Gendelman, H. E.: Infection of human gastrointestinal cells by HIV-1. AIDS Res. Hum. Retroviruses 6:1409, 1415, 1990.

649. Furuta, Y., Eriksson, K., Svennerholm, B., Fredman, P., Horal, P., Jeansson, S., Vahlne, A., Holmgren, J., and Czerkinsky, C.: Infection of vaginal and colonic epithelial cells by the human immunodeficiency virus type 1 is neutralized by antibodies raised against conserved epitopes in the envelope glycoprotein gp120. Proc. Natl. Acad. Sci. USA 91:12559, 1994.

650. de Vincenzi, I.: A longitudinal study of human immunodeficiency virus transmission by heterosexual partners: European Study Group on Heterosexual Transmission of HIV. N. Engl. J. Med. 331:341, 1994.

651. Mayer, K. H., and Anderson, D. J.: Heterosexual HIV transmission. Infect. Agents Dis. 4:273, 1995.

652. Goedert, J. J., Eyster, M. E., Biggar, R. J., and Blattner, W. A.: Heterosexual transmission of human immunodeficiency virus: Association with severe depletion of T-helper lymphocytes in men with hemophilia. AIDS Res. Hum. Retroviruses 3:355, 1987.

653. Ho, D. D., Moudgil, T., and Alam, M.: Quantitation of human immunodeficiency virus type 1 in the blood of infected persons. N. Engl. J. Med. 321:1621, 1989.

654. Goedert, J. J., Mendez, H., Drummond, J. E., Robert-Guroff, M., Minkoff, H. L., Holman, S., Stevens, R., Rubinstein, A., Blattner, W. A., Willoughby, A., and Landesman, S. H.: Mother-to-infant transmission of human immunodeficiency virus type 1: Association with prematurity or low anti-gp120. Lancet 2:1351, 1989.

655. Padian, N., Marquis, L., Francis, D. P., Anderson, R. E., Rutherford, G. W., O'Malley, P. M., and Winkelstein, W., Jr.: Male-to-female transmission of human immunodeficiency virus. JAMA 258:788, 1987.

656. CDC: Update: Human immunodeficiency virus infections in health-care workers exposed to blood of infected patients. MMWR 36:285, 1987.

657. Blattner, W. A.: HIV epidemiology: Past, present, and future. FASEB J. 5:2340, 1991.

658. Tokars, J. I., Marcus, R., Culver, D. H., Schable, C. A., McKibben, P. S., Bandea, C. I., and Bell, D. M. (for the CDC Cooperative Needlestick Surveillance Group): Surveillance of HIV infection and zidovudine use among health care workers after occupational exposure to HIV-infected blood. Ann. Intern. Med. 118:913, 1993.

659. Holmberg, S. D.: Risk factors for sexual transmission of human immunodeficiency virus. In DeVita, V. T., Jr., Hellman, S. and Rosenberg, S. A. (eds.): AIDS: Etiology, Diagnosis, Treatment, and Prevention. Philadelphia, Lippincott-Raven Publishers, 1997.

660. Weller, S. C.: A meta-analysis of condom effectiveness in reducing sexually transmitted HIV. Soc. Sci. Med. 36:1635, 1993.

661. Dunn, D. T., Newell, M. L., Ades, A. E., and Peckham, C. S.: Risk of human immunodeficiency virus type 1 transmission through breastfeeding. Lancet 340:585, 1992.

662. St. Louis, M. E., Kamenga, M., Brown, C., Nelson, A. M., Manzila, T., Batter, V., Behets, F., Kabagabo, U., Ryder, R. W., and Oxtoby, M.: Risk for perinatal HIV-1 transmission according to maternal immunologic, virologic, and placental factors. JAMA 269:2853, 1993.

663. Cooper, D. A., Gold, J., Maclean, P., Donovan, B., Finlayson, R., Barnes, T. G., Michelmore, H. M., Brooke, P., and Penny, R. (for the Sydney AIDS Study Group): Acute AIDS retrovirus infection: Definition of a clinical illness associated with seroconversion. Lancet 1:537, 1985.

664. Ho, D. D., Sarngadharan, M. G., Resnick, L., di Marzo Veronese, F., Rota, T. R., and Hirsch, M. S.: Primary human T-lymphotropic virus type III infection. Ann. Intern. Med. 103:880, 1985.

665. Tindall, B., and Cooper, D. A.: Primary HIV infection: Host responses and intervention strategies (editorial). AIDS 5:1, 1991.

666. Gaines, H., Albert, J., von Sydow, M., Sönnerborg, A., Chiodi, F., Ehrnst, A., Strannegård, Ö., and Åsjö, B.: HIV antigenaemia and virus isolation from plasma during primary HIV infection (letter). Lancet 1:1317, 1987.

667. Goudsmit, J., de Wolf, F., Paul, D. A., Epstein, L. G., Lange, J. M. A., Krone, W. J. A., Speelman, H., Wolters, E. C., Van Der Noordaa, J., Oleske, J. M., Van Der Helm, H. J., and Coutinho, R. A.: Expression of human immunodeficiency virus antigen (HIV-Ag) in serum and cerebrospinal fluid during acute and chronic infection. Lancet 2:177, 1986.

668. Clark, S. J., Saag, M. S., Decker, W. D., Campbell-Hill, S., Roberson, J. L., Veldkamp, P. J., Kappes, J. C., Hahn, B. H., and Shaw, G. M.: High titers of cytopathic virus in plasma of patients with symptomatic primary HIV-1 infection. N. Engl. J. Med. 324:954, 1991.

669. Gaines, H., von Sydow, M. A., von Stedingk, L. V., Biberfeld, G., Bottiger, B., Hansson, L. O., Lundbergh, P., Sonnerborg, A. B., Wasserman, J., and Strannegaard, O. O.: Immunological changes in primary HIV-1 infection. AIDS 4:995, 1990.

670. Gaines, H., von Sydow, M., Sönnerborg, A., Albert, J., Czajkowski, J., Pehrson, P. O., Chiodi, F., Moberg, L., Fenyö, E. M., Åsjö, B., and Forsgren, M.: Antibody response in primary human immunodeficiency virus infection. Lancet 1:1249, 1987.

671. Cooper, D. A., Imrie, A. A., and Penny, R.: Antibody response to human immunodeficiency virus after primary infection. J. Infect. Dis. 155:1113, 1987.

672. Borrow, P., Lewicki, H., Hahn, B. H., Shaw, G. M., and Oldstone, M. B.: Virus-specific CD8+ cytotoxic T-lymphocyte activity associated with control of viremia in primary human immunodeficiency virus type 1 infection. J. Virol. 68:6103, 1994.

673. Koup, R. A., Safrit, J. T., Cao, Y., Andrews, C. A., McLeod, G., Borkowsky, W., Farthing, C., and Ho, D. D.: Temporal association of cellular immune responses with the initial control of viremia in primary human immunodeficiency virus type 1 syndrome. J. Virol. 68:4650, 1994.

674. Safrit, J. T., Andrews, C. A., Zhu, T., Ho, D. D., and Koup, R. A.: Characterization of human immunodeficiency virus type 1–specific cytotoxic T lymphocyte clones isolated during acute seroconversion: Recognition of autologous virus sequences within a conserved immunodominant epitope. J. Exp. Med. 179:463, 1994.

675. CDC: Classification system for human T-lymphotropic virus type III/lymphadenopathy–associated virus infections. Ann. Intern. Med. 105:234, 1986.

676. Schnittman, S. M., Psallidopoulos, M. C., Lane, H. C., Thompson, L., Baseler, M., Massari, F., Fox, C. H., Salzman, N. P., and Fauci, A. S.: The reservoir for HIV-1 in human peripheral blood is a T cell that maintains expression of CD4. Science 245:305, 1989.

677. Schnittman, S. M., Greenhouse, J. J., Psallidopoulos, M. C., Baseler, M., Salzman, N. P., Fauci, A. S., and Lane, H. C.: Increasing viral burden in CD4+ T cells from patients with human immunodeficiency virus (HIV) infection reflects rapidly progressive immunosuppression and clinical disease. Ann. Intern. Med. 113:438, 1990.

678. Musey, L., Hughes, J., Schacker, T., Shea, T., Corey, L., and McElrath, M. J.: Cytotoxic-T-cell responses, viral load, and disease progression in early human immunodeficiency virus type 1 infection. N. Engl. J. Med. 337:1267, 1997.

679. Ogg, G. S., Jin, X., Bonhoeffer, S., Dunbar, P. R., Nowak, M. A., Monard, S., Segal, J. P., Cao, Y., Rowland-Jones, S. L., Cerundolo, V., Hurley, A., Markowitz, M., Ho, D. D., Nixon, D. F., and McMichael, A. J.: Quantitation of HIV-1-specific cytotoxic T lymphocytes and plasma load of viral RNA. Science 279:2103, 1998.

680. Duesberg, P.: HIV is not the cause of AIDS. Science 241:514, 1988.

681. Lang, W., Perkins, H., Anderson, R. E., Royce, R., Jewell, N., and Winkelstein, W., Jr.: Patterns of T lymphocyte changes with human immunodeficiency virus infection: From seroconversion to the development of AIDS. J. Acquir. Immune Defic. Syndr. 2:63, 1989.

682. Curran, J. W., Jaffe, H. W., Hardy, A. M., Morgan, W. M., Selik, R. M., and Dondero, T. J.: Epidemiology of HIV infection and AIDS in the United States. Science 239:610, 1988.

683. Moss, A. R., and Bacchetti, P.: Natural history of HIV infection. AIDS 3:55, 1989.

684. Rutherford, G. W., Lifson, A. R., Hessol, N. A., Darrow, W. W., O'Malley, P. M., Buchbinder, S. P., Barnhart, J. L., Bodecker, T. W., Cannon, L., Doll, L. S., Holmberg, S. D., Harrison, J. S., Rogers, M. F., Werdegar, D., and Jaffe, H. W.: Course of HIV-1 infection in a cohort of homosexual and bisexual men: An 11 year follow up study. Br. Med. J. 301:1183, 1990.

685. Lemp, G. F., Hirozawa, A. M., Cohen, J. B., Derish, P. A., McKinney, K. C., and Hernandez, S. R.: Survival for women and men with AIDS. J. Infect. Dis. 166:74, 1992.

686. Seage, G. R., III, Oddleifson, S., Carr, E., Shea, B., Makarewicz-Robert, L., van Beuzekom, M., and De Maria, A.: Survival with AIDS in Massachusetts, 1979 to 1989. Am. J. Public Health 83:72, 1993.

687. Cheng-Mayer, C., Seto, D., Tateno, M., and Levy, J. A.: Biologic features of HIV-1 that correlate with virulence in the host. Science 240:80, 1988.

688. Klein, M. R., van Baalen, C. A., Holwerda, A. M., Kerkhof Garde, S. R., Bende, R. J., Keet, I. P., Eeftinck-Schattenkerk, J. K., Osterhaus, A. D., Schuitemaker, H., and Miedema, F.: Kinetics of Gag-specific cytotoxic T lymphocyte responses during the clinical course of HIV-1 infection: A longitudinal analysis of rapid progressors and long-term asymptomatics. J. Exp. Med. 181:1365, 1995.

689. Cao, Y., Qin, L., Zhang, L., Safrit, J., and Ho, D. D.: Virologic and immunologic characterization of long-term survivors of human immunodeficiency virus type 1 infection. N. Engl. J. Med. 332:201, 1995.

690. Pantaleo, G., Menzo, S., Vaccarezza, M., Graziosi, C., Cohen, O. J., Demarest, J. F., Montefiori, D., Orenstein, J. M., Fox, C., Schrager, L. K., Margolick, J. B., Buchbinder, S., Giorgi, J. V., and Fauci, A. S.: Studies in subjects with long-term nonprogressive human immunodeficiency virus infection. N. Engl. J. Med. 332:209, 1995.

691. Lifson, A. R., Buchbinder, S. P., Sheppard, H. W., Mawle, A. C., Wilber, J. C., Stanley, M., Hart, C. E., Hessol, N. A., and Holmberg, S. D.: Long-term human immunodeficiency virus infection in asymptomatic homosexual and bisexual men with normal CD4+ lymphocyte counts: Immunologic and virologic characteristics. J. Infect. Dis. 163:959, 1991.

692. Rinaldo, C., Huang, X.-L., Fan, Z., Ding, M., Beltz, L., Logar, A., Panicali, D., Mazzara, G., Liebmann, J., Cottrill, M., and Gupta, P.: High levels of anti-human immunodeficiency virus type 1 (HIV-1) memory cytotoxic T-lymphocyte activity and low viral load are associated with lack of disease in HIV-1-infected long-term nonprogressors. J. Virol. 69:5838, 1995.

693. Deacon, N. J., Tsykin, A., Solomon, A., Smith, K., Ludford-Menting, M., Hooker, D. J., McPhee, D. A., Greenway, A. L., Ellett, A., Chatfield, C., Lawson, V. A., Crowe, S., Maerz, A., Sonza, S., Learmont, J., Sullivan, J. S., Cunningham, A., Dwyer, D., Dowton, D., and Mills, J.: Genomic structure of an attenuated quasi species of HIV-1 from a blood transfusion donor and recipients. Science 270:988, 1995.

694. O'Brien, T. R., George, J. R., and Holmberg, S. D.: Human immunodeficiency virus type 2 infection in the United States: Epidemiology, diagnosis, and public health implications. JAMA 267:2775, 1992.

695. Onorato, I. M., O'Brien, T. R., Schable, C. A., Spruill, C., and Holmberg, S. D.: Sentinel surveillance for HIV-2 infection in high-risk U.S. populations. Am. J. Public Health 83:515, 1993.

696. Marlink, R., Kanki, P., Thior, I., Travers, K., Eisen, G., Siby, T., Traore, I., Hsieh, C.-C., Dia, M. C., Gueye, E.-H., Hellinger, J., Gueye-Ndiaye, A., Sankale, J.-L., Ndoye, I., Mboup, S., and Essex, M.: Reduced rate of disease development after HIV-2 infection as compared to HIV-1. Science 265:1587, 1994.

697. Kanki, P. J., Travers, K. U., MBoup, S., Hsieh, C.-C., Marlink, R. G., Gueye-NDiaye, A., Siby, T., Thior, I., Hernandez-Avila, M., Sankale, J.-L., NDoye, I., and Essex, M. E.: Slower heterosexual spread of HIV-2 than HIV-1. Lancet 343:943, 1994.

698. Gayle, H. D., Gnaore, E., Adjorlolo, G., Ekpini, E., Coulibaly, R., Porter, A., Braun, M. M., Zabban, M.-L. K., Andou, J., Timite, A., Assi-Adou, J., and DeCock, K. M.: HIV-1 and HIV-2 infection in children in Abidjan, Côte d'Ivoire. J. Acquir. Immune. Defic. Syndr. 5:513, 1992.

699. Andreasson, P. A., Dias, F., Naucler, A., Andersson, S., and Biberfeld, G.: A prospective study of vertical transmission of HIV-2 in Bissau, Guinea-Bissau. AIDS 7:989, 1993.

700. Dufoort, G., Courouce, A. M., Ancelle-Park, R., and Bletry, O.: No clinical signs 14 years after HIV-2 transmission via blood transfusion (letter). Lancet 2:510, 1988.

701. Poulsen, A. G., Aaby, P., Larsen, O., Jensen, H., Naucler, A., Lisse, I. M., Christiansen, C. B., Dias, F., and Melbye, M.: 9-Year HIV-2-associated mortality in an urban community in Bissau, west Africa. Lancet 349:911, 1997.

702. Koenig, S., Gendelman, H. E., Orenstein, J. M., Dal Canto, M. C., Pezeshkpour, G. H., Yungbluth, M., Janotta, F., Aksamit, A., Martin, M. A., and Fauci, A. S.: Detection of AIDS virus in macrophages in brain tissue from AIDS patients with encephalopathy. Science 233:1089, 1986.

703. Piatak, M., Jr., Saag, M. S., Yang, L. C., Clark, S. J., Kappes, J. C., Luk, K. C., Hahn, B. H., Shaw, G. M., and Lifson, J. D.: High levels of HIV-1 in plasma during all stages of infection determined by competitive PCR. Science 259:1749, 1993.

704. Daar, E. S., Moudgil, T., Meyer, R. D., and Ho, D. D.: Transient high levels of viremia in patients with primary human immunodeficiency virus type 1 infection. N. Engl. J. Med. 324:961, 1991.

705. Mellors, J. W., Rinaldo, C. R., Jr., Gupta, P., White, R. M., Todd, J. A., and Kingsley, L. A.: Prognosis in HIV-1 infection predicted by the quantity of virus in plasma. Science 272:1167, 1996.

706. Schuitemaker, H., Koot, M., Kootstra, N. A., Dercksen, M. W., de Goede, R. E., van Steenwijk, R. P., Lange, J. M., Schattenkerk, J. K., Miedema, F., and Tersmette, M.: Biological phenotype of human immunodeficiency virus type 1 clones at different stages of infection: Progression of disease is associated with a shift from monocytotropic to T-cell-tropic virus population. J. Virol. 66:1354, 1992.

707. Zhang, L. Q., MacKenzie, P., Cleland, A., Holmes, E. C., Brown, A. J., and Simmonds, P.: Selection for specific sequences in the external envelope protein of human immunodeficiency virus type 1 upon primary infection. J. Virol. 67:3345, 1993.

708. Zhu, T., Mo, H., Wang, N., Nam, D. S., Cao, Y., Koup, R. A., and Ho, D. D.: Genotypic and phenotypic characterization of HIV-1 patients with primary infection. Science 261:1179, 1993.

709. Clark, S. J., and Shaw, G. M.: The acute retroviral syndrome and the pathogenesis of HIV-1 infection. Semin. Immunol. 5:149, 1993.

710. Connor, R. I., Mohri, H., Cao, Y., and Ho, D. D.: Increased viral burden and cytopathicity correlate temporally with CD4+ T-lymphocyte decline and clinical progression in human immunodeficiency virus type 1–infected individuals. J. Virol. 67:1772, 1993.

711. Wolinsky, S. M., Korber, B. T., Neumann, A. U., Daniels, M., Kunstman, K. J., Whetsell, A. J., Furtado, M. R., Cao, Y., Ho, D. D., and Safrit, J. T.: Adaptive evolution of human immunodeficiency virus-type 1 during the natural course of infection. Science 272:537, 1996.

712. Ganeshan, S., Dickover, R. E., Korber, B. T., Bryson, Y. J., and Wolinsky, S. M.: Human immunodeficiency virus type 1 genetic evolution in children with different rates of development of disease. J. Virol. 71:663, 1997.

713. Delwart, E. L., Pan, H., Sheppard, H. W., Wolpert, D., Neumann, A. U., Korber, B., and Mullins, J. I.: Slower evolution of human immunodeficiency virus type 1 quasispecies during progression to AIDS. J. Virol. 71:7498, 1997.

714. Wei, X., Ghosh, S. K., Taylor, M. E., Johnson, V. A., Emini, E. A., Deutsch, P., Lifson, J. D., Bonhoeffer, S., Nowak, M. A., Hahn, B. H., Saag, M. S., and Shaw, G. M.: Viral dynamics in human immunodeficiency virus type 1 infection. Nature 373:117, 1995.

715. Ho, D. D., Neumann, A. U., Perelson, A. S., Chen, W., Leonard, J. M., and Markowitz, M.: Rapid turnover of plasma virions and CD4 lymphocytes in HIV-1 infection. Nature 373:123, 1995.

716. Perelson, A. S., Neumann, A. U., Markowitz, M., Leonard, J. M., and Ho, D. D.: HIV-1 dynamics in vivo: Virion clearance rate, infected cell life-span, and viral generation time. Science 271:1582, 1996.

717. Perelson, A. S., Essunger, P., Cao, Y., Vesanen, M., Hurley, A., Saksela, K., Markowitz, M., and Ho, D. D.: Decay characteristics of HIV-1–infected compartments during combination therapy. Nature 387:188, 1997.

718. Autran, B., Carcelain, G., Li, T. S., Blanc, C., Mathez, D., Tubiana, R., Katlama, C., Debre, P., and Leibowitch, J.: Positive effects of combined antiretroviral therapy on CD4+ T cell homeostasis and function in advanced HIV disease. Science 277:112, 1997.

719. Pakker, N. G., Notermans, D. W., de Boer, R. J., Roos, M. T., de Wolf, F., Hill, A., Leonard, J. M., Danner, S. A., Miedema, F., and Schellekens, P. T.: Biphasic kinetics of peripheral blood T cells after triple combination therapy in HIV-1 infection: A composite of redistribution and proliferation. Nat. Med. 4:208, 1998.

720. Roederer, M.: Getting to the HAART of T cell dynamics. Nat. Med. 4:145, 1998.

721. Kellam, P., Boucher, C. A., and Larder, B. A.: Fifth mutation in human immunodeficiency virus type 1 reverse transcriptase contributes to the development of high-level resistance to zidovudine. Proc. Natl. Acad. Sci. USA 89:1934, 1992.

722. Boucher, C. A., Cammack, N., Schipper, P., Schuurman, R., Rouse, P., Wainberg, M. A., and Cameron, J. M.: High-level resistance to

(−) enantiomeric 2′-deoxy-3′-thiacytidine in vitro is due to one amino acid substitution in the catalytic site of human immunodeficiency virus type 1 reverse transcriptase. Antimicrob. Agents Chemother. 37:2231, 1993.

723. Tisdale, M., Kemp, S. D., Parry, N. R., and Larder, B. A.: Rapid in vitro selection of human immunodeficiency virus type 1 resistant to 3′-thiacytidine inhibitors due to a mutation in the YMDD region of reverse transcriptase. Proc. Natl. Acad. Sci. USA 90:5653, 1993.

724. Larder, B. A., Kemp, S. D., and Harrigan, P. R.: Potential mechanism for sustained antiretroviral efficacy of AZT-3TC combination therapy. Science 269:696, 1995.

725. Eron, J. J., Benoit, S. L., Jemsek, J., MacArthur, R. D., Santana, J., Quinn, J. B., Kuritzkes, D. R., Fallon, M. A., and Rubin, M. for the North American HIV Working Party: Treatment with lamivudine, zidovudine, or both in HIV-positive patients with 200 to 500 CD4+ cells per cubic millimeter. N. Engl. J. Med. 333:1662, 1995.

726. Markowitz, M., Mo, H., Kempf, D. J., Norbeck, D. W., Bhat, T. N., Erickson, J. W., and Ho, D. D.: Selection and analysis of human immunodeficiency virus type 1 variants with increased resistance to ABT-538, a novel protease inhibitor. J. Virol. 69:701, 1995.

727. Doyon, L., Croteau, G., Thibeault, D., Poulin, F., Pilote, L., and Lamarre, D.: Second locus involved in human immunodeficiency virus type 1 resistance to protease inhibitors. J. Virol. 70:3763, 1996.

728. Molla, A., Korneyeva, M., Gao, Q., Vasavanonda, S., Schipper, P. J., Mo, H. M., Markowitz, M., Chernyavskiy, T., Niu, P., Lyons, N., Hsu, A., Granneman, G. R., Ho, D. D., Boucher, C. A., Leonard, J. M., Norbeck, D. W., and Kempf, D. J.: Ordered accumulation of mutations in HIV protease confers resistance to ritonavir. Nat. Med. 2:760, 1996.

729. Zhang, Y. M., Imamichi, H., Imamichi, T., Lane, H. C., Falloon, J., Vasudevachari, M. B., and Salzman, N. P.: Drug resistance during indinavir therapy is caused by mutations in the protease gene and in its Gag substrate cleavage sites. J. Virol. 71:6662, 1997.

730. Zennou, V., Mammano, F., Paulous, S., Mathez, D., and Clavel, F.: Loss of viral fitness associated with multiple Gag and Gag-Pol processing defects in human immunodeficiency virus type 1 variants selected for resistance to protease inhibitors in vivo. J. Virol. 72:3300, 1998.

731. Gulick, R. M., Mellors, J. W., Havlir, D., Eron, J. J., Gonzalez, C., McMahon, D., Richman, D. D., Valentine, F. T., Jonas, L., Meibohm, A., Emini, E. A., and Chodakewitz, J. A.: Treatment with indinavir, zidovudine, and lamivudine in adults with human immunodeficiency virus infection and prior antiretroviral therapy. N. Engl. J. Med. 337:734, 1997.

732. Hammer, S. M., Squires, K. E., Hughes, M. D., Grimes, J. M., Demeter, L. M., Currier, J. S., Eron, J. J., Jr., Feinberg, J. E., Balfour, H. H., Jr., Deyton, L. R., Chodakewitz, J. A., and Fischl, M. A., for the AIDS Clinical Trials Group 320 Study Team: A controlled trial of two nucleoside analogues plus indinavir in persons with human immunodeficiency virus infection and CD4 cell counts of 200 per cubic millimeter or less. N. Engl. J. Med. 337:725, 1997.

733. Havlir, D. V., Eastman, S., Gamst, A., and Richman, D. D.: Nevirapine-resistant human immunodeficiency virus: Kinetics of replication and estimated prevalence in untreated patients. J. Virol. 70:7894, 1996.

734. Lech, W. J., Wang, G., Yang, Y. L., Chee, Y., Dorman, K., McCrae, D., Lazzeroni, L. C., Erickson, J. W., Sinsheimer, J. S., and Kaplan, A. H.: In vivo sequence diversity of the protease of human immunodeficiency virus type 1: Presence of protease inhibitor–resistant variants in untreated subjects. J. Virol. 70:2038, 1996.

735. Roberts, N. A., Craig, J. C., and Sheldon, J.: Resistance and cross-resistance with saquinavir and other HIV protease inhibitors: theory and practice (editorial). AIDS 12:453, 1998.

736. Mohri, H., Singh, M. K., Ching, W. T., and Ho, D. D.: Quantitation of zidovudine-resistant human immunodeficiency virus type 1 in the blood of treated and untreated patients. Proc. Natl. Acad. Sci. USA 90:25, 1993.

737. Palella, F. J., Jr., Delaney, K. M., Moorman, A. C., Loveless, M. O., Fuhrer, J., Satten, G. A., Aschman, D. J., and Holmberg, S. D.: Declining morbidity and mortality among patients with advanced human immunodeficiency virus infection: HIV Outpatient Study Investigators. N. Engl. J. Med. 338:853, 1998.

738. Finzi, D., Hermankova, M., Pierson, T., Carruth, L. M., Buck, C., Chaisson, R. E., Quinn, T. C., Chadwick, K., Margolick, J., Brookmeyer, R., Gallant, J., Markowitz, M., Ho, D. D., Richman, D. D., and Siliciano, R. F.: Identification of a reservoir for HIV-1 in patients on highly active antiretroviral therapy. Science 278:1295, 1997.

739. Wong, J. K., Hezareh, M., Gunthard, H. F., Havlir, D. V., Ignacio, C. C., Spina, C. A., and Richman, D. D.: Recovery of replication-competent HIV despite prolonged suppression of plasma viremia. Science 278:1291, 1997.

740. Chun, T. W., Stuyver, L., Mizell, S. B., Ehler, L. A., Mican, J. A., Baseler, M., Lloyd, A. L., Nowak, M. A., and Fauci, A. S.: Presence of an inducible HIV-1 latent reservoir during highly active antiretroviral therapy. Proc. Natl. Acad. Sci. USA 94:13193, 1997.

741. Chun, T. W., Finzi, D., Margolick, J., Chadwick, K., Schwartz, D., and Siliciano, R. F.: In vivo fate of HIV-1–infected T cells: Quantitative analysis of the transition to stable latency. Nat. Med. 1:1284, 1995.

742. Chun, T. W., Carruth, L., Finzi, D., Shen, X., DiGiuseppe, J. A., Taylor, H., Hermankova, M., Chadwick, K., Margolick, J., Quinn, T. C., Kuo, Y. H., Brookmeyer, R., Zeiger, M. A., Barditch-Crovo, P., and Siliciano, R. F.: Quantification of latent tissue reservoirs and total body viral load in HIV-1 infection. Nature 387:183, 1997.

743. McLean, A. R., and Michie, C. A.: In vivo estimates of division and death rates of human T lymphocytes. Proc. Natl. Acad. Sci. USA 92:3707, 1995.

744. Barin, F., McLane, M. F., Allan, J. S., Lee, T. H., Groopman, J. E., and Essex, M.: Virus envelope protein of HTLV-III represents major target antigen for antibodies in AIDS patients. Science 228:1094, 1985.

745. Gnann, J. W., Jr., Nelson, J. A., and Oldstone, M. B. A.: Fine mapping of an immunodominant domain in the transmembrane glycoprotein of human immunodeficiency virus. J. Virol. 61:2639, 1987.

746. Kennedy, R. C., Henkel, R. D., Pauletti, D., Allan, J. S., Lee, T. H., Essex, M., and Dreesman, G. R.: Antiserum to a synthetic peptide recognizes the HTLV-III envelope glycoprotein. Science 231:1556, 1986.

747. Weiss, R. A., Clapham, P. R., Weber, J. N., Dalgleish, A. G., Lasky, L. A., and Berman, P. W.: Variable and conserved neutralization antigens of human immunodeficiency virus. Nature 324:572, 1986.

748. Arthur, L. O., Pyle, S. W., Nara, P. L., Bess, J. W., Jr., Gonda, M. A., Kelliher, J. C., Gilden, R. V., Robey, W. G., Bolognesi, D. P., Gallo, R. C., and Fischinger, P. J.: Serological responses in chimpanzees inoculated with human immunodeficiency virus glycoprotein (gp120) subunit vaccine. Proc. Natl. Acad. Sci. USA 84:8583, 1987.

749. Matthews, T. J., Langlois, A. J., Robey, W. G., Chang, N. T., Gallo, R. C., Fischinger, P. J., and Bolognesi, D. P.: Restricted neutralization of divergent human T-lymphotropic virus type III isolates by antibodies to the major envelope glycoprotein. Proc. Natl. Acad. Sci. USA 83:9709, 1986.

750. Putney, S. D., Matthews, T. J., Robey, W. G., Lynn, D. L., Robert-Guroff, M., Mueller, W. T., Langlois, A. J., Ghrayeb, J., Petteway, S. R., Jr., Weinhold, K. J., Fischinger, P. J., Wong-Staal, F., Gallo, R. C., and Bolognesi, D. P.: HTLV-III/LAV–neutralizing antibodies to an *E. coli*–produced fragment of the virus envelope. Science 234:1392, 1986.

751. Rusche, J. R., Javaherian, K., McDanal, C., Petro, J., Lynn, D. L., Grimaila, R., Langlois, A., Gallo, R. C., Arthur, L. O., Fischinger, P. J., Bolognesi, D. P., Putney, S. D., and Matthews, T. J.: Antibodies that inhibit fusion of human immunodeficiency virus–infected cells bind a 24-amino acid sequence of the viral envelope, gp120. Proc. Natl. Acad. Sci. USA 85:3198, 1988.

752. Linsley, P. S., Ledbetter, J. A., Kinney-Thomas, E., and Hu, S. L.: Effects of anti-gp120 monoclonal antibodies on CD4 receptor binding by the *env* protein of human immunodeficiency virus type 1. J. Virol. 62:3695, 1988.

753. Nara, P. L., Robey, W. G., Arthur, L. O., Asher, D. M., Wolff, A. V., Gibbs, C. J., Jr., Gajdusek, D. C., and Fischinger, P. J.: Persistent infection of chimpanzees with human immunodeficiency virus: Serological responses and properties of reisolated viruses. J. Virol. 61:3173, 1987.

754. Skinner, M. A., Langlois, A. J., McDanal, C. B., McDougal, J. S., Bolognesi, D. P., and Matthews, T. J.: Neutralizing antibodies to an immunodominant envelope sequence do not prevent gp120 binding to CD4. J. Virol. 62:4195, 1988.

755. Profy, A. T., Salinas, P. A., Eckler, L. I., Dunlop, N. M., Nara, P. L., and Putney, S. D.: Epitopes recognized by the neutralizing antibodies of an HIV-1-infected individual. J. Immunol. 144:4641, 1990.

756. Steimer, K. S., Scandella, C. J., Skiles, P. V., and Haigwood, N. L.: Neutralization of divergent HIV-1 isolates by conformation-dependent human antibodies to gp120. Science 254:105, 1991.

757. Thali, M., Olshevsky, U., Furman, C., Gabuzda, D., Posner, M., and Sodroski, J.: Characterization of a discontinuous human immunodeficiency virus type 1 gp120 epitope recognized by a broadly reactive neutralizing human monoclonal antibody. J. Virol. 65:6188, 1991.

758. Weiss, R. A., Clapham, P. R., Cheingsong-Popov, R., Dalgleish, A. G., Carne, C. A., Weller, I. V. D., and Tedder, R. S.: Neutralization of human T-lymphotropic virus type III by sera of AIDS and AIDS-risk patients. Nature 316:69, 1985.

759. Trkola, A., Ketas, T., Kewalramani, V. N., Endorf, F., Binley, J. M., Katinger, H., Robinson, J., Littman, D. R., and Moore, J. P.: Neutralization sensitivity of human immunodeficiency virus type 1 primary isolates to antibodies and CD4-based reagents is independent of coreceptor usage. J. Virol. 72:1876, 1998.

760. Parren, P. W., Mondor, I., Naniche, D., Ditzel, H. J., Klasse, P. J., Burton, D. R., and Sattentau, Q. J.: Neutralization of human immunodeficiency virus type 1 by antibody to gp120 is determined primarily by occupancy of sites on the virion irrespective of epitope specificity. J. Virol. 72:3512, 1998.

761. Novembre, F. J., Saucier, M., Anderson, D. C., Klumpp, S. A., O'Neil, S. P., Brown, C. R., II, Hart, C. E., Guenthner, P. C., Swenson, R. B., and McClure, H. M.: Development of AIDS in a chimpanzee infected with human immunodeficiency virus type 1. J. Virol. 71:4086, 1997.

762. Kestler, H., Kodama, T., Ringler, D., Marthas, M., Pedersen, N., Lackner, A., Regier, D., Sehgal, P., Daniel, M., King, N., and Desrosiers, R.: Induction of AIDS in rhesus monkeys by molecularly cloned simian immunodeficiency virus. Science 248:1109, 1990.

763. Shibata, R., Kawamura, M., Sakai, H., Hayami, M., Ishimoto, A., and Adachi, A.: Generation of a chimeric human and simian immunodeficiency virus infectious to monkey peripheral blood mononuclear cells. J. Virol. 65:3514, 1991.

764. Reimann, K. A., Li, J. T., Veazey, R., Halloran, M., Park, I.-W., Karlsson, G. B., Sodroski, J., and Letvin, N. L.: A chimeric simian/human immunodeficiency virus expressing a primary patient human immunodeficiency virus type 1 isolate env causes an AIDS-like disease after in vivo passage in rhesus monkeys. J. Virol. 70:6922, 1996.

765. Joag, S. V., Li, Z., Foresman, L., Stephens, E. B., Zhao, L. J., Adany, I., Pinson, D. M., McClure, H. M., and Narayan, O.: Chimeric simian/human immunodeficiency virus that causes progressive loss of CD4+ T cells and AIDS in pig-tailed macaques. J. Virol. 70:3189, 1996.

766. Shibata, R., Maldarelli, F., Siemon, C., Matano, T., Parta, M., Miller, G., Fredrickson, T., and Martin, M. A.: Infection and pathogenicity of chimeric simian-human immunodeficiency viruses in macaques: Determinants of high virus loads and CD4 cell killing. J. Infect. Dis. 176:362, 1997.

767. Marthas, M. L., Sutjipto, S., Higgins, J., Lohman, B., Torten, J., Luciw, P. A., Marx, P. A., and Pedersen, N. C.: Immunization with a live, attenuated simian immunodeficiency virus (SIV) prevents early disease but not infection in rhesus macaques challenged with pathogenic SIV. J. Virol. 64:3694, 1990.

768. Daniel, M. D., Kirchhoff, F., Czajak, S. C., Sehgal, P. K., and Desrosiers, R. C.: Protective effects of a live attenuated SIV vaccine with a deletion in the nef gene. Science 258:1938, 1992.

769. Almond, N., Kent, K., Cranage, M., Rud, E., Clarke, B., and Stott, E. J.: Protection by attenuated simian immunodeficiency virus in macaques against challenge with virus-infected cells. Lancet 345:1342, 1995.

770. Shibata, R., Siemon, C., Cho, M. W., Arthur, L. O., Nigida, S. M., Jr., Matthews, T., Sawyer, L. A., Schultz, A., Murthy, K. K., Israel, Z., Javadian, A., Frost, P., Kennedy, R. C., Lane, H. C., and Martin, M. A.: Resistance of previously infected chimpanzees to successive challenges with a heterologous intraclade B strain of human immunodeficiency virus type 1. J. Virol. 70:4361, 1996.

771. Desrosiers, R. C., Lifson, J. D., Gibbs, J. S., Czajak, S. C., Howe, A. Y., Arthur, L. O., and Johnson, R. P.: Identification of highly attenuated mutants of simian immunodeficiency virus. J. Virol. 72:1431, 1998.

772. Cranage, M. P., Whatmore, A. M., Sharpe, S. A., Cook, N., Polyanskaya, N., Leech, S., Smith, J. D., Rud, E. W., Dennis, M. J., and Hall, G. A.: Macaques infected with live attenuated SIVmac are protected against superinfection via the rectal mucosa. Virology 229:143, 1997.

773. Shibata, R., Siemon, C., Czajak, S. C., Desrosiers, R. C., and Martin, M. A.: Live, attenuated simian immunodeficiency virus vaccines elicit potent resistance against a challenge with a human immunodeficiency virus type 1 chimeric virus. J. Virol. 71:8141, 1997.

774. Baba, T. W., Jeong, Y. S., Pennick, D., Bronson, R., Greene, M. F.,

and Ruprecht, R. M.: Pathogenicity of live, attenuated SIV after mucosal infection of neonatal macaques. Science 267:1820, 1995.

775. Hu, S.-L., Fultz, P. N., McClure, H. M., Eichberg, J. W., Thomas, E. K., Zarling, J., Singhal, M. C., Kosowski, S. G., Swenson, R. B., Anderson, D. C., and Todaro, G.: Effect of immunization with a vaccinia-HIV env recombinant on HIV infection of chimpanzees. Nature 328:721, 1987.

776. Shen, L., Chen, Z. W., Miller, M. D., Stallard, V., Mazzara, G. P., Panicali, D. L., and Letvin, N. L.: Recombinant virus vaccine-induced SIV-specific CD8+ cytotoxic T lymphocytes. Science 252:440, 1991.

777. Hu, S. L., Klaniecki, J., Dykers, T., Sridhar, P., and Travis, B. M.: Neutralizing antibodies against HIV-1 BRU and SF2 isolates generated in mice immunized with recombinant vaccinia virus expressing HIV-1 (BRU) envelope glycoproteins and boosted with homologous gp160. AIDS Res. Hum. Retroviruses 7:615, 1991.

778. Hu, S. L., Abrams, K., Barber, G. N., Moran, P., Zarling, J. M., Langlois, A. J., Kuller, L., Morton, W. R., and Benveniste, R. E.: Protection of macaques against SIV infection by subunit vaccines of SIV envelope glycoprotein gp160. Science 255:456, 1992.

779. Israel, Z. R., Edmonson, P. F., Maul, D. H., O'Neil, S. P., Mossman, S. P., Thiriart, C., Fabry, L., Van Opstal, O., Bruck, C., Bex, F., Burny, A., Fultz, P. N., Mullins, J. I., and Hoover, E. A.: Incomplete protection, but suppression of virus burden, elicited by subunit simian immunodeficiency virus vaccines. J. Virol. 68:1843, 1994.

780. Hirsch, V. M., Fuerst, T. R., Sutter, G., Carroll, M. W., Yang, L. C., Goldstein, S., Piatak, M., Jr., Elkins, W. R., Alvord, W. G., Montefiori, D. C., Moss, B., and Lifson, J. D.: Patterns of viral replication correlate with outcome in simian immunodeficiency virus (SIV)–infected macaques: Effect of prior immunization with a trivalent SIV vaccine in modified vaccinia virus Ankara. J. Virol. 70:3741, 1996.

781. Paoletti, E.: Applications of pox virus vectors to vaccination: An update. Proc. Natl. Acad. Sci. USA 93:11349, 1996.

782. Giavedoni, L. D., Planelles, V., Haigwood, N. L., Ahmad, S., Kluge, J. D., Marthas, M. L., Gardner, M. B., Luciw, P. A., and Yilma, T. D.: Immune response of rhesus macaques to recombinant simian immunodeficiency virus gp130 does not protect from challenge infection. J. Virol. 67:577, 1993.

783. Daniel, M. D., Mazzara, G. P., Simon, M. A., Sehgal, P. K., Kodama, T., Panicali, D. L., and Desrosiers, R. C.: High-titer immune responses elicited by recombinant vaccinia virus priming and particle boosting are ineffective in preventing virulent SIV infection. AIDS Res. Hum. Retroviruses 10:839, 1994.

784. Mascola, J. R., Snyder, S. W., Weislow, O. S., Belay, S. M., Belshe, R. B., Schwartz, D. H., Clements, M. L., Dolin, R., Graham, B. S., Gorse, G. J., Keefer, M. C., McElrath, M. J., Walker, M. C., Wagner, K. F., McNeil, J. G., McCutchan, F. E., and Burke, D. S. for the National Institute of Allergy and Infectious Diseases AIDS Vaccine Evaluation Group: Immunization with envelope subunit vaccine products elicits neutralizing antibodies against laboratory-adapted but not primary isolates of human immunodeficiency virus type 1. J. Infect. Dis. 173:340, 1996.

785. Connor, R. I., Korber, B. T., Graham, B. S., Hahn, B. H., Ho, D. D., Walker, B. D., Neumann, A. U., Vermund, S. H., Mestecky, J., Jackson, S., Fenamore, E., Cao, Y., Gao, F., Kalams, S., Kunstman, K. J., McDonald, D., McWilliams, N., Trkola, A., Moore, J. P., and Wolinsky, S. M.: Immunological and virological analyses of persons infected by human immunodeficiency virus type 1 while participating in trials of recombinant gp120 subunit vaccines. J. Virol. 72:1552, 1998.

786. Ulmer, J. B., Donnelly, J. J., Parker, S. E., Rhodes, G. H., Felgner, P. L., Dwarki, V. J., Gromkowski, S. H., Deck, R. R., DeWitt, C. M., Friedman, A., Hawe, L. A., Leander, K. R., Martinez, D., Perry, H. C., Shiver, J. W., Montgomery, D. L., and Liu, M. A.: Heterologous protection against influenza by injection of DNA encoding a viral protein. Science 259:1745, 1993.

787. Donnelly, J. J., Friedman, A., Martinez, D., Montgomery, D. L., Shiver, J. W., Motzel, S. L., Ulmer, J. B., and Liu, M. A.: Preclinical efficacy of a prototype DNA vaccine: Enhanced protection against antigenic drift in influenza. Nat. Med. 1:583, 1995.

788. Letvin, N. L., Montefiori, D. C., Yasutomi, Y., Perry, H. C., Davies, M. E., Lekutis, C., Alroy, M., Freed, D. C., Lord, C. I., Handt, L. K., Liu, M. A., and Shiver, J. W.: Potent, protective anti-HIV immune responses generated by bimodal HIV envelope DNA plus protein vaccination. Proc. Natl. Acad. Sci. USA 94:9378, 1997.

789. Boyer, J. D., Ugen, K. E., Wang, B., Agadjanyan, M., Gilbert, L.,

Bagarazzi, M. L., Chattergoon, M., Frost, P., Javadian, A., Williams, W. V., Refaeli, Y., Ciccarelli, R. B., McCallus, D., Coney, L., and Weiner, D. B.: Protection of chimpanzees from high-dose heterologous HIV-1 challenge by DNA vaccination. Nat. Med. 3:526, 1997.

790. Maurer, B., Bannert, H., Darai, G., and Flügel, R. M.: Analysis of the primary structure of the long terminal repeat and the gag and pol genes of the human spumaretrovirus. J. Virol. 62:1590, 1988.

791. Flügel, R. M., Rethwilm, A., Maurer, B., and Darai, G.: Nucleotide sequence analysis of the *env* gene and its flanking regions of the human spumaretrovirus reveals two novel genes. EMBO J. 6:2077, 1987.

792. Khan, A. S., Galvin, T. A., Lowenstine, L. J., Jennings, M. B., Gardner, M. B., and Buckler, C. E.: A highly divergent simian immunodeficiency virus (SIV$_{stm}$) recovered from stored stump-tailed macaque tissues. J. Virol. 65:7061, 1991.

793. Clever, J., Sassetti, C., and Parslow, T. G.: RNA secondary structure and binding sites for *gag* gene products in the 5′ packaging signal of human immunodeficiency virus type 1. J. Virol. 69:2101, 1995.

28 ▼▼▼▼ Viral Pathogenesis of Hematological Disorders

B19 Parvoviruses
Neal Young

▼ ▼

B19 parvovirus is the only member of the important family of Parvoviridae that is known to cause disease in humans. Illnesses due to parvovirus infection range from a relatively innocuous rash illness of childhood to fatal fetal infection. Despite its relatively recent discovery, many aspects of B19 parvovirus are well understood; this chapter emphasizes virus structure, replication strategy, gene expression, antigenicity, tissue tropism, pathogenesis, and host immune response.

Yvonne Cossart, a virologist working in London in the mid-1970s, discovered B19 parvovirus while investigating laboratory assays for hepatitis B.[1] She used an immunoelectrophoretic technique in which sera from blood bank donors, serving as a source of antigen, were reacted with samples from patients with hepatitis, used as a source of antibody. In comparison with more specific assays, she noted a number of apparently false-positive reactions. When she excised the precipitin lines from the agarose and examined them by electron microscopy, she noted particles typical in appearance of parvoviruses (Fig. 28–1). (One of the viremic blood bank donor's serum had been encoded "B19"—there is no parvovirus A or B1–18!) Using the same assay system, British colleagues found antibodies in a high proportion of normal adults.[2] Subsequently, evidence of acute infection, immunoglobulin (Ig) M or viral antigen, was seroepidemiologically linked to transient aplastic crisis of sickle cell anemia[3] and fifth disease in normal children.[4] The genetic material of the particles present in acute phase sera could be characterized as single-stranded DNA, allowing classification of the agent as a proper member of the Parvoviridae family.[5, 6] In the mid-1980s, the virus was cloned by Cotmore and Tattersall at Yale[7] and sequenced by Astell's laboratory in Vancouver.[8] About the same time, B19 parvovirus was first cultivated in vitro with use of human bone marrow cells by Ozawa and colleagues[9] at the National Institutes of Health; human erythroid progenitors remain the most convenient productive tissue culture system, and inoculation of these cells has allowed a description of the molecular biology of B19. A few cell lines that support viral replication have proved useful for assay of neutralizing antibodies.[10] Expression of B19 parvovirus capsid proteins by use of recombinant technology has been useful for development of clinical assays for specific parvovirus antibodies, and engineered capsids should be suitable for a human vaccine.[11, 12]

Whereas the rash illness due to acute parvovirus infection in children is fortunately innocuous, B19 is not always so benign; aplastic crisis and persistent infection can terminate fatally, and the arthropathy that follows infection in adult women may have substantial morbidity. The full spectrum of B19 parvovirus illness is probably still unknown. Assay of some tissues, like the heart in myocarditis, for parvovirus infection may be difficult; on the other hand, overinterpretation of modestly elevated IgM values and especially of positive polymerase chain reaction test results has led to false assignment of diseases to this agent. In addition to their clinical relevance, parvoviruses are intrinsically worthy of examination. The laboratory study of this virus has increased our understanding of the interactions among pathogenic virus, target cell, and host immune system, especially in the hematopoietic system. Fuller discussions of the Parvoviridae and B19 parvovirus are found in textbook chapters and monographs.[13–18]

The Parvoviruses

The Parvoviridae, small, single-stranded DNA viruses, are common animal pathogens. Feline panleukopenia virus was one of the first viruses experimentally demonstrated to cause disease in animals; this virus infects cat hematopoietic and lymphocytic cells and causes often fatal neutropenia.[19–21] The canine, mink, and feline parvoviruses are similar enough to one another at the nucleotide and amino acid level to be grouped as host range variants.[22, 23] These parvoviruses are striking for the recent development of tropism for some species, like mink and dogs, and their host-dependent behavior. Canine parvovirus suddenly appeared among dogs

---

All material in this chapter is in the public domain, with the exception of any borrowed figures or tables.

worldwide in the pandemic of 1978,[22] and more recently the virus spread to isolated wolf populations in Michigan's Upper Peninsula.

There are interesting examples of the variety of clinical syndromes resulting from infection of animal parvoviruses in different hosts. Feline panleukopenia virus causes congenital ataxia in kittens that is due to a remarkably specific attack on cells of the developing fetal cerebellum.[24] Canine parvovirus is notorious for myocarditis in puppies, which is rare in kittens. Feline panleukopenia virus often kills cats because of marrow myeloid hypoplasia and neutropenia, which does not usually occur in dogs.[22, 25] Tropism for bone marrow hematopoietic progenitors may be a common feature of parvovirus biology: minute virus of mice suppresses murine progenitor and stem cell proliferation[26, 27]; feline panleukopenia virus infects cat myeloid progenitor cells[28]; and Aleutian disease virus replicates in mink lymphocytes.[29]

▼ PHYSICAL FEATURES

Parvoviruses are defined by their size, symmetry, and genetic material. *Parvum* is Latin for small, and the parvoviruses are among the smallest viruses, usually 15 to 28 nm in diameter. In the electron microscope, they show icosahedral symmetry; the specific arrangement of viral proteins in the capsid has been determined by X-ray crystallography, described below. The absence of a lipid envelope contributes to the high heat stability of parvoviruses, a major factor in their extremely contagious behavior. Each parvovirus capsid contains a single copy of the viral genome, composed of about 5000 bases of single-stranded DNA (Fig. 28–2). (For convenient reference, the entire genome is equated to 100 map units.) Parvoviruses have molecular weights ranging from 1.55 to 1.97 × 10[6], about half of which represents DNA; their buoyant density in cesium chloride density gradients ranges from 1.36 to 1.43 g/ml, the less dense particles representing empty capsids.

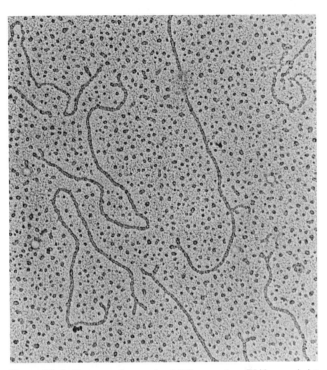

Figure 28–2. Electron micrograph of B19 parvovirus DNA annealed in vitro showing terminal hairpin structures. (Courtesy of B.J. Cohen.)

▼ TAXONOMY

The classification of Parvoviridae family is based on morphology and functional characteristics.[30] The family has recently been subdivided into two subfamilies, separating the insect viruses in subfamily Densovirinae from the animal parvoviruses in Parvovirinae. Parvovirinae contains three genuses. Most vertebrate disease-causing parvoviruses are autonomous parvoviruses (genus Parvovirus), meaning that they replicate in the absence of helper virus. Adeno-associated viruses occupy the genus Dependovirus and require coinfection of target cells with adenovirus or herpesviruses for replication. The adeno-associated viruses infect human tissue culture cells and also human beings. Adeno-associated viral DNA has been detected in cervical tissue and abortuses,[31] but in general, the viruses are regarded as nonpathogenic.[32] Adeno-associated viruses remain latent in the absence of helper virus, and they have the remarkable property of site-specific integration into chromosome 19 in some cell lines.[33] The autonomous viruses have been hypothesized to have evolved from a defective parvovirus, originally a cellular transposon that functioned by interfering with viral infections[34]; consistent with this hypothesis is the striking genetic homology between goose and duck parvoviruses and human adeno-associated virus.[35, 36]

Because of its distinctive biological properties, genomic organization, and capsid structure, B19 parvovirus has been placed in a new, fourth genus, Erythrovirus. Sequence homology suggests that B19 parvovirus, minute virus of mice, and adeno-associated virus are equally different from each other and presumably separated at about the same evolutionary point in time.[8] B19 parvovirus behaves like an autonomous virus, but its genomic organization and extremely limited tissue host range suggest a close relationship also to

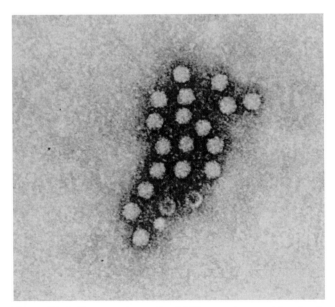

Figure 28–1. Electron micrograph of B19 parvovirus particles showing icosahedral symmetry and empty capsids, both characteristic of members of the Parvoviridae family. (Courtesy of Y. Cossart.)

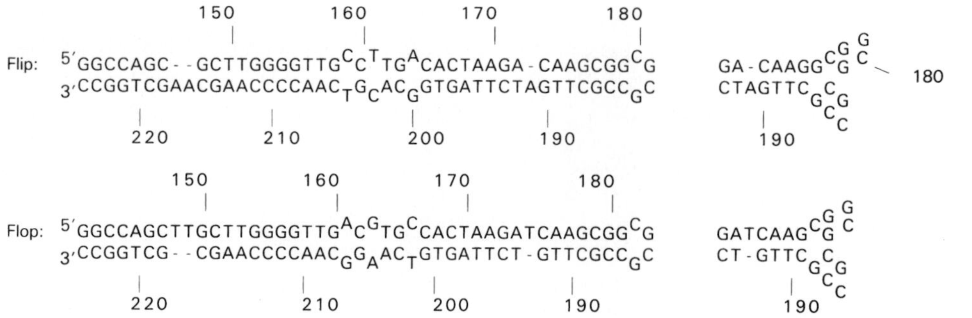

```
            150         160         170         180
             |           |           |           |
Flip:  5'GGCCAGC- -GCTTGGGGTTGᶜCᵀTGᴬCACTAAGA-CAAGCGGᶜG          GA-CAAGGᶜᴳᴳ
       3'CCGGTCGAACGAACCCCAACᵀGᶜACᴳGTGATTCTAGTTCGCCᴳC              Gᶜ~ 180
                                                               CTAGTTCᴳ Gᶜᴳ
             |           |           |           |                    ᶜᶜ
            220         210         200         190                   |
                                                                     190

            150         160         170         180
             |           |           |           |
Flop:  5'GGCCAGCTTGCTTGGGGTTGᴬCᴳTGᶜCACTAAGATCAAGCGGᶜG          GATCAAGᶜᴳᴳ
       3'CCGGTCG- -CGAACCCCAACᴳᴳᴬACᵀGTGATTCT-GTTCGCCᴳC                 Gᶜ
                                                               CT-GTTCᴳ Gᶜᴳ
             |           |           |           |                    ᶜᶜ
            220         210         200         190                   |
                                                                     190
```

Figure 28–3. Schematic of the palindromic nucleotide sequences that form the terminal hairpin structures of B19 parvovirus; alternative conformations are shown.

the adeno-associated viruses. Genus Erythrovirus ultimately will also include several simian parvoviruses that are most closely related genetically to B19, infect erythroid progenitor cells in vitro, and cause anemia in their respective monkey hosts.[37–39]

B19 Parvovirus

▼ GENOMIC ORGANIZATION

Most vertebrate parvoviruses, including B19, have a similar genomic organization; the capsid proteins are encoded by genes on the right side of the genome, the non-structural proteins by genes on the left side. At both ends of the genome are terminal repeat sequences, palindromes of variable length and symmetry according to the species of virus (Fig. 28–3). These inverted repeat elements serve as the double-stranded matrix needed to initiate DNA synthesis, and they are therefore required for virus propagation.[13, 40] Somewhat surprisingly, the terminal repeats also appear to be necessary and sufficient for other virus functions, including not only replication but also packaging of DNA. B19 has the longest terminal repeats among the parvoviruses, 365 nucleotides, rivaled only by human adeno-associated virus and bovine parvovirus.[41] In both B19 parvovirus and adeno-associated virus, the 5' and 3' ends have identical sequences.[40] The length, the presence of several long direct repeat sequences, the high content of guanosine-cytosine pairs, and the resulting strong secondary structure of the

B19 parvovirus terminal repeat sequences have made them resistant to molecular cloning in bacteria with only a single report of full-length cloning of a presumably infectious virus.[42]

▼ DNA STRUCTURE AND REPLICATION

Replication of parvovirus single-stranded DNA is initiated from the short double-stranded regions contained in the self-annealing, terminal hairpin structures. For B19 parvovirus, DNA synthesis proceeds from the long palindromes to produce high molecular weight intermediates through a rolling hairpin model.[41, 43] Parvovirus DNA replicative intermediates correspond to duplexes equivalent to twofold or fourfold the original single-stranded template.[9] High molecular weight replicative intermediates can be detected directly by Southern analysis (of DNA extracted under low salt conditions) or after restriction enzyme digestion (of DNA extracted with normal salt concentration); asymmetrical fragments are obtained after *Bam*HI digestion, resulting in characteristic doublets on electrophoresis and hybridization (Fig. 28–4). DNA analysis thus allows determination of both presence and propagation of parvovirus in tissue culture and clinical samples.

Late events in parvovirus DNA replication include exonuclease cleavage of the large DNAs, resolution of the hairpin structures, and packaging of the newly synthesized DNA single strands into capsids.[41] Binding of cellular pro-

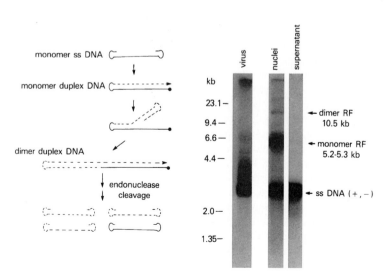

Figure 28–4. Restriction enzyme analysis of DNA from erythroid cells infected with B19 parvovirus. On this Southern analysis, high molecular weight replicating monomers and dimers are present in the nuclei but not in the cytosol or cytoplasm or in the supernatant of cultures, which contain only virions.

teins and parvovirus non-structural proteins to DNA is involved in these processes for animal parvoviruses and in adeno-associated virus, but the mechanics of these events have not been determined for B19 parvoviruses in their target cells.

▼ RNA TRANSCRIPTION

Whereas the scheme of DNA replication of B19 parvovirus is broadly similar to that of other autonomous parvoviruses, the pattern of RNA transcription for B19 parvovirus sets it apart from most of the other Parvoviridae[41] (Figs. 28–5 and 28–6). B19 parvovirus transcription is unusual in several important features: (1) the large number of transcripts, (2) the extent of splicing and the large size of the introns removed, (3) the failure to coterminate all transcripts at the far right side of the genome, (4) the use of unusual polyadenylation signals for termination of transcripts in the middle of the genome, (5) the use of a single strong promoter at the far left side (at map unit 6, thus termed P_6) with an accompanying leader sequence to initiate transcription of all RNA species, and (6) the abundant production of two short RNA species with coding potential but uncertain importance in viral replication[44] (see Fig. 28–5). Because the TATA box in the middle of the genome does not represent a functional promoter either in bone marrow targets or in transfected cells,[45, 46] B19 parvovirus is denied the use of multiple promoters and enhancer elements to regulate transcript abundance. The control of the relative quantities of the minor and major capsid proteins, which are derived from overlapping sequences on the right side of the genome, is in part modulated by multiple upstream AUG codons that are present before the authentic transcription initiation codon; these spurious triplets reduce the efficiency of translation. The upstream AUG codons are removed by splicing of the VP2 RNA, greatly improving translation of the major capsid protein.[47]

▼ NON-STRUCTURAL PROTEIN

The gene for non-structural protein is fairly homologous among the parvoviruses, consistent with its required role in virus propagation.[8, 14, 41] Non-structural protein is generally restricted to the nucleus and binds to DNA. Nickase, helicase, and endonuclease activities have been assigned to non-structural protein of adeno-associated virus, but the non-structural protein genes do not share homology with known cellular toxins or pore-forming proteins. Parvovirus non-structural proteins are pleiotropic: they are required for parvovirus replication, including resolution of the terminal hairpin structures; they are needed for RNA transcription; they function as enhancer elements for the parvovirus structural gene promoter and for their own promoter; they are required for excision of the parvoviral genome from transfecting plasmid; and they may "lead" the DNA strand into the preformed capsid. The non-structural proteins also cause host cell death[48, 49]; they can suppress heterologous promoter function, and they are the mediators of parvovirus "oncosuppressive" effects in a variety of cell culture systems.[50]

Mutation and deletion analyses of the non-structural protein gene have not allowed separation or assignment of the protein's functions to specific regions, and multiple activities can be abolished with an appropriate single amino acid substitution.[51] For B19's promoter, functional importance has been assigned to binding sites for regulatory factors including YY1,[52] nucleotide triphosphates,[53] and GATA-1 and the glucocorticoid receptor.[54] Non-structural protein gene expression precedes capsid protein gene expression and DNA synthesis for B19 parvovirus[55] (as for minute virus of mice[56]), corresponding to the early and late events of virus replication observed for many other viruses.

▼ STRUCTURAL PROTEINS

The two or three capsid proteins are derived from overlapping reading frames and thus share substantial amino acid

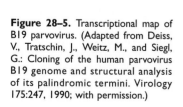

Figure 28–5. Transcriptional map of B19 parvovirus. (Adapted from Deiss, V., Tratschin, J., Weitz, M., and Siegl, G.: Cloning of the human parvovirus B19 genome and structural analysis of its palindromic termini. Virology 175:247, 1990; with permission.)

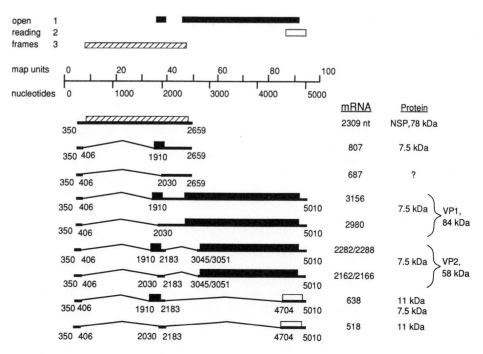

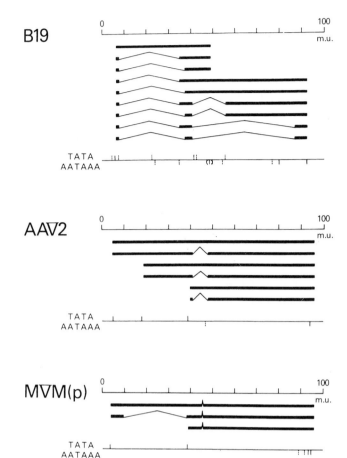

B19

AAV2

MVM(p)

TATA
AATAAA

Figure 28–6. Comparison of the transcriptional maps of representative parvovirus species. There is no middle promoter in the B19 parvovirus genome.

identity; for example, in B19 parvovirus, the minor capsid protein differs from the major capsid protein by an additional 226 amino acid extension at the amino terminus. By convention, the longest and least abundant minor capsid species is denoted VP1, and the shorter major capsid proteins are denoted VP2 and VP3. The B19 virion is composed of 60 capsid proteins, 5 to 10 per cent of which are VP1 and the remainder VP2. For animal parvoviruses, tissue tropism[57] and host range specificity[23] have been mapped to a few nucleotides within the capsid genes. The canine/feline differences are located on the virus surface in exposed loop regions and may affect binding. For murine parvovirus, tissue tropism (for fibroblast or lymphocyte) is determined in the nucleus, after viral entry and before replication,[58] suggesting multiple functional effects for the structural as well as non-structural proteins.

▼ CAPSID STRUCTURE

With the solution at the atomic level of the structure of canine parvovirus, the three-dimensional organization of capsid proteins has been determined in detail[59, 60] (Fig. 28–7). The central structural motif of an eight-stranded, antiparallel β barrel is similar to that of many other DNA and RNA viruses of the same size and symmetry; the β barrels form

the capsid, and insertions form the viral surface. For canine and feline parvoviruses, the insertions between the β sheets are extensive and form large loops on the capsid surface. An unusual feature is the large protrusion on the threefold axes, which forms a spike on the surface made up of VP2 loop regions that are important as antigen recognition sites for neutralizing antibodies. There are deep canyons about the fivefold axes that, by analogy with other viruses, were predicted to be binding sites for receptors (but see below).

The structure of the human virus has been inferred from studies of empty B19 parvovirus capsids, synthesized in a baculovirus system, with molecular replacement using the defined canine structure.[60] For uncertain reasons, the crystallographic structure has been solved only to relatively low resolution.[61] Surprisingly, even at 8 Å resolution and also by cryoelectron microscopic examination,[62] major differences have been observed between B19 and canine parvoviruses, most important the absence of the major threefold axis spike and the open cylindrical structures at the fivefold axes (Fig. 28–8). The unique region of VP1, an amino-terminal extension of VP2, is too infrequently represented in an individual capsid to be visualized by either method but has been shown by other techniques to be external to the capsid surface (see below). The presence of VP1 is not required for capsid formation, and full-length VP1 proteins alone form a capsid structure inefficiently.[63]

▼ B19 IN CELL CULTURE

B19 parvovirus is extraordinarily tropic for human erythroid cells. Viral replication occurs at high levels only in erythroid progenitor cells,[9] and replicative double-stranded DNA forms can be detected in the bone marrow of infected patients.[64] In tissue culture, B19 parvovirus has been propagated in the erythroid cells of human bone marrow[65] and fetal liver,[66, 67] in cultured cells from a patient with erythroleukemia,[68] and in a few human megakaryocytoblastoid cell lines derived from patients with leukemia.[10, 69] Erythroid colony formation by the late erythroid progenitor cell (the CFU-E) and the more primitive erythroid progenitor (the burst-forming unit or BFU-E) is strongly inhibited by virus, whereas myelopoiesis (granulocyte-macrophage colony formation by the CFU-GM progenitor) is unaffected even by high concentrations of virus.[70–72] Susceptibility of marrow cells increases with erythroid differentiation,[73] and virus propagation in all culture systems is dependent on the presence of erythropoietin. For the UT-7 cell line, adaptation to growth during months in erythropoietin is required before virus can be propagated,[10] suggesting that cell susceptibility to virus is related to the hormone's sustained effects on erythroid differentiation and not to more transient alterations in cell metabolism. In these chronically infected cells, virus is latent although not integrated into the genome; cell synchronization induces virus replication, transcription, and protein production.[74]

B19 parvovirus is directly cytotoxic to the host cell and induces characteristic light[65] and electron[75] microscopic morphological changes in erythroid precursors. The virus' cytopathic effect is manifest as giant pronormoblasts, first recognized by Owren[76] in 1948 in the bone marrow of patients with transient aplastic crisis and reproduced in tissue

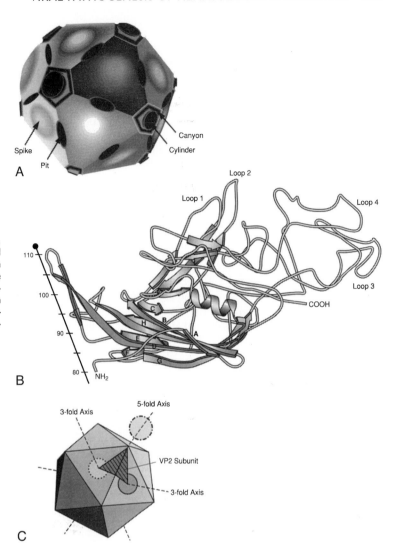

Figure 28–7. The structure of canine parvovirus. *A,* Schematic of the surface structure. *B,* Arrangement of β barrel sheets (A to H) and α helices (loops 1 to 3). *C,* Diagram showing placement of one of the 60 capsid proteins and the axes of symmetry of the capsid. (Adapted from Agbandje-McKenna, M., and Rossmann, M.G.: The structure of human parvovirus B19. *In* Anderson, L.J., and Young, N.S. [eds.]: Human Parvovirus B19. Basel, Karger, 1997, p. 3; with permission.)

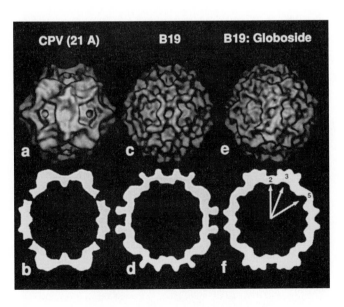

Figure 28–8. Cryoelectron microscopic imaging of canine parvovirus (*a* and *b*) compared with B19 viral capsids alone (*c* and *d*) and complexed with the cellular receptor globoside (*e* and *f*). Surface views are shown above, cross-sections below. B19 lacks the prominent channels and spikes apparent for canine parvovirus, and globoside creates extra densities on the threefold depression. (From Chapman, P.R., Agbandje-McKenna, M., Kajigaya, S., Brown, K.E., Young, N.S., Baker, T.S., and Rossmann, M.G.: Cryo-electron microscopy studies of empty capsids of human parvovirus B19 complexed with its cellular receptor. Proc. Natl. Acad. Sci. USA 93:7502, 1996; with permission.)

culture infection.[65] Giant pronormoblasts are early erythroid cells with a diameter of about 25 to 32 μm, nuclear inclusions or multiple nucleoli, and cytoplasmic vacuolization; these cells are scattered throughout the aspirate smear of infected bone marrow and striking for their disproportionate size (Fig. 28–9). Late erythroid cells are absent from infected tissue culture or clinical specimens. There may be subtle dysplastic alterations in myeloid and megakaryocytic cells. Infected late erythroid progenitors from tissue culture inoculations show cytopathic ultrastructural changes on electron microscopy, including characteristic margination of chromatin, pseudopod formation, vacuolization, and viral particles in lacunae within the chromatin (Fig. 28–10).

Virus toxicity is the result of expression of the single non-structural protein of the virus.[48] (On the other hand, cell lines can express the parvovirus capsid proteins without any effect on cell proliferation.[77]) In permissive erythroid progenitor cells, the major RNA species that accumulate encode the capsid proteins.[45] In contrast, when the viral genome is transfected into non-permissive cells, the pattern of RNA transcription is altered so that the non-structural protein transcript is overrepresented.[78] A functional "block" in virus transcription in these non-permissive cells has been localized to the middle of the parvovirus genome by RNAase protection experiments.[78] Predominant transcription of the non-structural protein gene in non-permissive cells, corresponding to abortive infection, may explain reduction of megakaryocytic progenitor number in vitro, and of platelet and white cell levels in infected persons, in the absence of the ability of the virus to productively infect these cells[79] (Fig. 28–11).

▼ CELLULAR RECEPTOR

The cellular receptor for B19 parvovirus is erythrocyte P antigen. The receptor's discovery was based on the observation of clumping of erythrocytes by B19, a familiar property of viruses. Red cell membranes were tested with use of inhibition of hemagglutination as an assay; activity resided in the lipid rather than protein fraction and was further purified to neutral glycosphingolipid and ultimately to a tetrahexose ceramide, globoside or erythrocyte P antigen.[80] Virus binds with high affinity to the abundant globoside on the red cell surface, and either a monoclonal antibody to P antigen or an excess of free globoside protects erythroid progenitor cells from parvovirus infection in vitro. By cryo-electron microscopy, the binding sites for globoside have been visualized in depressions along the threefold axis of

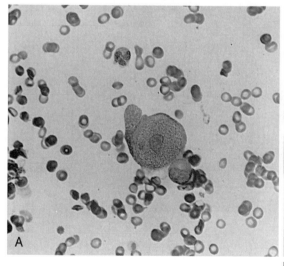

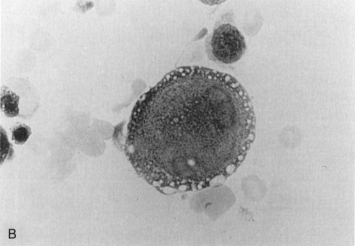

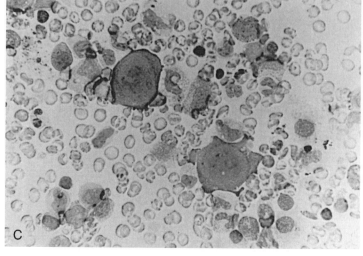

Figure 28–9. Giant pronormoblasts in B19 parvovirus–infected bone marrow erythroid progenitors from a patient (A) and after in vitro inoculation of bone marrow culture (B and C).

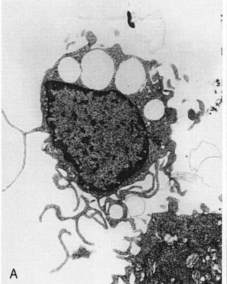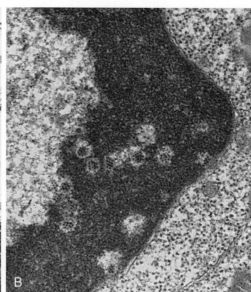

Figure 28–10. Electron micrographs of an early erythroid precursor infected with B19 parvovirus. *A,* Margination of nuclear chromatin, vacuolization, and pseudopod formation in the cytoplasm. *B,* Virus particles are present in lacunae within the marginated chromatin.

symmetry (and not, as predicted, in the canyon regions of the fivefold axis)[81] (see Fig. 28–8).

The P blood group antigen system, which was discovered by Landsteiner and Levine in 1927, contains two common antigens (P and P_1) and the less common antigen P^k; some rare individuals, denoted as p phenotype, lack all three antigens. Erythrocytes from donors who lack P antigen do not hemagglutinate B19 parvovirus.[80] When sera from p phenotype individuals, concentrated in Amish communities, were tested for antibody to B19 parvovirus, none contained IgG, indicating an absence of past infection.[82] Bone marrow from p individuals could not be infected by the virus, and erythroid progenitor cells grew normally at viral concentra-

tions that completely inhibited normal donors' colony formation. Thus, the genetic absence of the cellular receptor for the virus confers resistance to parvovirus infection.

Identification of the receptor explains the tissue tropism of B19 parvovirus. Although globoside is ubiquitous as a cytoplasmic component, it is present on the surface of only a few cell types, including not only erythrocytes but also erythroid progenitor cells, some megakaryocytes, endothelial cells, fetal liver and cardiac tissue, and some cells of the placenta. Involvement of these tissues in parvovirus infection has been observed (see below). For example, expression of P antigen and viral capsid proteins have been colocalized by immunohistochemistry of bone marrow from infected patients.[83] One as yet inadequately tested prediction from the discovery of the receptor is that paroxysmal cold hemoglobinuria, a severe hemolytic anemia of childhood that commonly follows a viral infection, is a post–parvovirus B19 disease.

Epidemiology

B19 parvovirus is a common infection in humans. Virus-specific IgG antibody appears in the first 2 weeks after inoculation, persists for life, and is the most convenient marker of past exposure.[84] About 50 per cent of adults have IgG antibody to B19 parvovirus; the proportion increases to more than 90 per cent in the elderly. An annual seroconversion rate of 1.5 per cent was estimated from studies of serial samples from women of childbearing age.[85] Thus, most individuals acquire immunity during childhood, but susceptibility continues in others throughout adult life. Seroprevalence of IgG antibody is similarly high worldwide, except among some isolated Brazilian[86] and African[87] tribal populations.

Fifth disease is seasonal, with peak occurrence in spring and summer. Both fifth disease and transient aplastic crisis appear to cycle in approximately 3- to 4-year periods. Epidemics of fifth disease in normal children and clusters of transient aplastic crisis in patients with underlying hemolysis

Figure 28–11. Transcription is related to permissivity of B19 parvovirus. Permissive cells allow full-length transcription of both the nonstructural and the capsid gene RNAs. Capsid RNAs are the predominant RNA species in erythroid cells. Non-permissive cells have a functional transcriptional block in the middle of the genome that results in relative overexpression of non-structural protein RNA and cell death without viral propagation.

occur concurrently, but they are frequently recognized and treated by different physician specialists.[88] Whereas IgG antibody to B19 parvovirus is common, viral antigen is found rarely in normal persons; only 1 of 24,000 blood donors contained a high titer of virus in one purposeful screen.[89] However, viral DNA is more easily detected by the polymerase chain reaction and has been present in 0.03 to 0.6 per cent of blood donors in other blood bank screens.[90, 91] (Virus was found in 7 of 53 patients tested years after an acute infection by use of this method[92]—persistence of viral sequences at low levels in blood and tissues in normal individuals is important in interpreting the role of the virus in disease; see below.)

B19 parvovirus is excreted from the nasopharynx, and the major route of transmission is probably through the upper airway; there is little evidence of virus excretion in feces or urine.[93] In epidemics, the attack rate is high; between 10 and 60 per cent of susceptible schoolchildren develop fifth disease in school outbreaks,[85, 94] and for school and daycare personnel, parvovirus infections occurred in 20 to 30 per cent.[95] Sibling to sibling transfer is probably a major path of transmission.[85]

Although viremia is rare in the general population, B19 parvovirus can be transmitted in transfused blood products,[96] and almost all coagulation factor concentrates contain detectable B19 parvovirus sequences.[90] Parvoviruses, including B19, are heat resistant and can withstand the usual thermal treatment to destroy viral infectivity. Parvovirus has been transmitted by dry- and steam-heated,[97] heated lyophilized,[98] chromatographically purified,[99] and solvent detergent–inactivated[97] blood products, but hemophiliacs who received factor VIII concentrate that had been heated to 80°C for 72 hours had a lower rate of seroconversion than did those who had received unheated concentrate.[100] Screening of blood donors to avoid transmission in pooled products is impractical.[96] Nosocomial transmission from infected patients to medical staff can occur,[101] but outbreaks on a hospital ward may be indistinguishable from coincident community epidemics; infection of susceptible staff by patients is not inevitable,[102] and the risk of transmission may be decreased by handwashing.[103]

Clinical Syndromes

▼ FIFTH DISEASE

Acute infection with B19 parvovirus causes the childhood exanthem fifth disease (erythema infectiosum).[88, 104] Children with fifth disease are usually not very ill. The characteristic rash—the "slapped cheek" facial erythema and a lacy, reticular, evanescent maculopapular eruption over the trunk and proximal extremities (Fig. 28–12)—combined with its contagious character allows recognition of parvovirus infection in the individual patient and of the epidemic in the community. Parvovirus proteins were detected by immunofluorescence of epidermal cells in one affected child.[105]

Adults with fifth disease suffer joint pains or frank arthritis, alone or in combination with a rash, more often than do affected children, and symptoms that mimic rheumatoid arthritis[106, 107] or fibromyalgia[108] can occasionally persist for months and even years. However, B19 parvovirus does

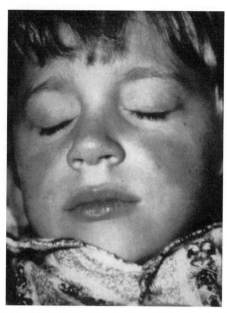

Figure 28–12. "Slapped cheek" rash in a child with typical erythema infectiosum. (From Anderson, M.J., Higgins, P.G., Davis, L.R., et al.: Experimental parvoviral infection in humans. J. Infect. Dis. 152:257, 1985; with permission.)

not cause rheumatoid arthritis.[109, 110] Acute parvovirus infection in adults most often is asymptomatic or produces only a non-specific influenza-like illness.[111]

▼ TRANSIENT APLASTIC CRISIS

This was the first human parvovirus illness identified, and the clear clinical relationship between acute virus infection and a specific form of marrow failure led to hematologists' interest in this pathogen. In persons with underlying hemolysis, acute B19 infection causes transient aplastic crisis, an abrupt cessation of erythropoiesis characterized by reticulocytopenia, absent erythroid precursors in the bone marrow, and precipitous worsening of anemia. The aregenerative quality of anemic crisis was recognized early from observations on hereditary spherocytosis in large Scandinavian kindreds, later appreciated also for other persons with underlying hemolysis. Owren[76] introduced the term "aplastic crisis" and stressed the relationship of anemic crisis to preceding infection and the temporary quality of red cell failure. Transient aplastic crisis occurs as a unique event in the life of patients with a variety of forms of underlying hemolysis, not only sickle cell disease but also erythrocyte membrane defects, enzymopathies, and thalassemias. Transient aplastic crisis can also occur under conditions of erythroid stress, such as hemorrhage and iron deficiency, and after bone marrow transplantation.[112, 113] In retrospect, parvovirus infection was almost certainly responsible for cases of transient erythropoietic failure that were blamed on kwashiorkor, folic acid deficiency, some drugs (especially immunosuppressive agents), and bacterial infections.[112] It is not accidental that many of the reported cases of aplastic crisis occurred in hospitalized patients, because the virus can be transmitted nosocomially (see above). Parvovirus infection was probably responsible for cases of aplastic anemia (five of six cases of which occurred in sickle cell patients and were restricted to anemia only) that once were imputed to glue sniffing.[114]

Although suffering from an ultimately self-limited illness, the patient with an aplastic crisis may be acutely and profoundly ill. Symptoms can include not only the dyspnea and fatigue of worsened anemia but extreme lassitude, confusion, and congestive heart failure; death can occur. Aplastic crisis may be the first evidence of hereditary spherocytosis in a patient with compensated hemolysis.[115] Transient aplastic crisis,[116–118] as well as experimental parvovirus infection in humans,[119] is often associated with variable degrees of neutropenia and thrombocytopenia, which may dominate the clinical picture.[120–122] In one patient with transient aplastic crisis, the marrow was strikingly myelodysplastic.[123] Rarely, transient aplastic crisis may be complicated by bone marrow necrosis.[124, 125] Typical transient aplastic crisis is readily treated by blood transfusion. Atypically, transient pancytopenia[121, 126, 127] and a case of typical severe aplastic anemia[128] have been reported to follow acute parvovirus infection. Pancytopenia due to acute marrow failure with hemophagocytosis, which can occur after many different viral infections, has also been noted after parvovirus infection.[129–132] More tenuously linked are cases of idiopathic thrombocytopenic purpura,[133] because both this syndrome and IgM antibody to parvovirus are not uncommon in pediatric populations.

Community-acquired aplastic crisis is almost always due to parvovirus infection.[134, 135] B19 parvovirus infection should be the presumptive diagnosis in transient aplastic crisis and sought in any patient with anemia due to an abrupt cessation of erythropoiesis. (Transient erythroblastopenia of childhood, temporary red cell failure production in very young, hematologically normal children, is not associated with B19 parvovirus seroconversion.[136, 137]) Patients with transient aplastic crisis are often viremic at presentation, with concentrations of viral genomes as high as 10^{14} per milliliter as determined by DNA dot blot hybridization of serum[138, 139]; IgM antibody appears during the first week of convalescence and is a specific indicator of recent infection.[140] Testing for IgG antibody is not helpful; IgG to parvovirus is present in about 50 per cent of the adult population, and IgG may not be found in early serum specimens in transient aplastic crisis. Both IgG and IgM antibody to parvovirus can be measured in capture immunoassays.[2, 84]

▼ HYDROPS FETALIS DUE TO B19 PARVOVIRUS

In utero infection is a cause of non-immune hydrops fetalis, in which death occurs as a result of severe anemia[141, 142] (Fig. 28–13). Hydropic infants born of mothers infected with parvovirus show leukoerythroblastosis, iron deposition in the liver, and viral cytopathic alterations of erythroblasts in the liver; virus has been demonstrated by DNA hybridization and protein immunoblot, mainly in the liver.[143, 144] The risk of a fatal outcome for the fetus is highest if infection occurs during the first two trimesters; although the probability of stillbirth has not been quantitated, it almost certainly is low. In a prospective British study of 190 seropositive women, there was significant excess fetal loss during the second trimester, and the risk of fetal death due to B19 parvovirus was estimated at 9 per cent with a transplacental transmission rate of 33 per cent.[145] Similar findings came from a

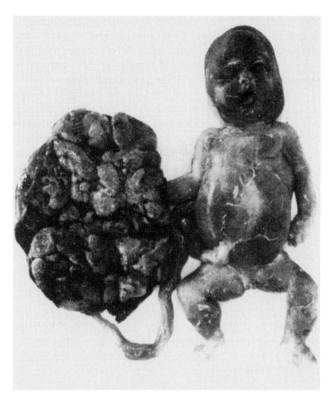

Figure 28–13. Hydropic fetus and placenta after intrauterine B19 parvovirus infection. (From Caul, O.E., Usher, J.M., and Burton, A.P.: Intrauterine infection with human parvovirus B19: a light and electron microscopy study. J. Med. Virol. 24:55, 1988; with permission.)

retrospective American study.[146] These and other[147, 148] series show that normal infants were born even when the umbilical cord blood tested positive for specific IgM antibody. An increased risk of spontaneous abortion during the first trimester is being investigated in several large epidemiological surveys; a preliminary estimate is that about 5 per cent of infected women suffered spontaneous fetal abortions.[149]

Whereas the overall risk of a poor outcome to pregnancy is low, the concern of the potentially exposed pregnant mother is not. Parvovirus infection is contagious. Pregnant women are commonly exposed to fifth disease through other children in the household, at schools and daycare centers, and as nursing and medical personnel. About half of the pregnant population has acquired protective immunity, as determined by assay for IgG antibody to parvovirus, although the protective value of pre-existing antibody has been questioned.[150] Evidence of seroconversion should be sought in exposed women who entered pregnancy lacking antiparvovirus antibodies. Hydrops can be detected by ultrasound examination, and suspected hydrops can be treated with intrauterine red blood cell transfusion,[151] although not always with a successful outcome.[152] The utility of this type of intervention, or of the administration of commercial immunoglobulins containing antiparvovirus antibodies, will need to be determined.

▼ CONGENITAL INFECTION

Parvovirus infection of the fetus need not be fatal but may persist after birth.[148, 153–155] Brown and colleagues described three infants who were infected with parvovirus during the second trimester; despite treatment, in utero blood transfusion or exchange transfusion at birth, all were born with chronic anemia that resembled congenital pure red cell or dyserythropoietic anemia.[156] Congenital infection is distinctive among parvovirus syndromes in the low level of viral infection; virus was detected in the bone marrow by gene amplification but did not circulate. Presumably, infection early in ontogeny allows efficient suppression of red cell production. In one case that terminated fatally, virus was present in other tissues obtained at autopsy, including thymus, brain, heart, liver, and spleen, suggesting the possibility of parvovirus effects on other organ systems after in utero infection. Exposure of the fetal immune system to virus early in pregnancy would be predicted to result in tolerance to the capsid proteins and absence of an antibody response despite continued virus production.

No congenital physical malformations have been consistently associated with intrauterine parvovirus infection, either prospectively or in retrospective analysis of banked fetal tissue, although viral infection of myocardial cells was shown by in situ hybridization at autopsy of one hydropic infant[157] and immune thrombocytopenia observed in another viremic newborn[153]; liver disease[158] and eye abnormalities[159] have also been reported.

▼ PERSISTENT INFECTION

Patients with persistent B19 parvovirus infection have pure red cell aplasia. Persistently infected patients have failed to mount a neutralizing antibody response to the virus, and they lack the immune complex–mediated symptoms of fifth disease, fever, rash, and polyarthralgia/polyarthritis. Persistent parvovirus infection and pure red cell aplasia have been documented in four populations of patients: patients with congenital immunodeficiency (Nezelof syndrome),[64, 160, 161] children with lymphoblastic leukemia and other cancers in remission on chemotherapy,[162–164] patients with the acquired immunodeficiency syndrome (AIDS),[165] and recipients of bone marrow and solid organ transplants.[166–173] Defective antibody production also occurs in other diseases associated with pure red cell aplasia, like chronic lymphocytic leukemia, and some of these cases may also represent occult viral infection (because parvovirus infection was unrecognized previously in AIDS[174–177] and leukemia[178]). In a retrospective, systematic assay of marrow and blood samples from patients who had presented with a diagnosis of chronic pure red cell aplasia, 14 per cent were considered likely to have been chronically infected with B19 parvovirus.[179] In another study, however, 30 per cent of patients who suffered chronic anemia of diverse causes had evidence of viral infection by IgM antibody or gene amplification for DNA, without distinguishing clinical features such as reticulocytopenia,[180] suggesting irrelevance of the laboratory tests to the pathophysiological process. Even within populations infected by human immunodeficiency virus type 1 (HIV-1), the prevalence and role of B19 parvovirus have been debated. In assays by direct DNA hybridization of blood, B19 parvovirus infection is unusual among homosexual men (1 to 2 per cent positive).[181] However, among anemic HIV-1–infected men, 5 of 30 showed evidence of parvovirus infection with concor-

dance among DNA hybridization and serological studies and bone marrow morphology.[181] A Swedish study showed B19 virus by gene amplification in 5 of 69 retrovirus-infected patients.[182] Virus may be more prevalent in bone marrow; B19 was detected by gene amplification in 13 of 61 patients in an Irish study[183] and by immunohistochemistry in 7 of 81 New York patients, all of whom were either anemic or pancytopenic.[184]

The anemia of persistent parvovirus infection is severe, and the patients are dependent on erythrocyte transfusions. The bone marrow should contain some giant pronormoblasts, the cytopathic sign of parvovirus infection, although these are infrequent. The anemia may be intermittent, with periods of relapse associated with viremia and remission with spontaneous disappearance of virus from the circulation, possibly due to depletion of the erythroid target cell population. On occasion, as in transient aplastic crisis, neutropenia, thrombocytopenia, or pancytopenia dominates the clinical presentation.[164, 185, 186] The diagnosis is established by detection of B19 parvovirus genome in the serum, blood, or bone marrow cells by dot blot hybridization; polymerase chain reaction amplification of viral DNA may be necessary in rare cases.[187] Antibody testing is not useful in the diagnosis of persistent infection (see below). Persistent parvovirus infection may be the dominant manifestation of some inherited immunodeficient states, although multiple immune system defects usually are apparent once directed testing of T- and B-cell function is performed.

Effective therapy consists of infusion of commercial immunoglobulin preparations, which are a good source of neutralizing antibodies because most of the adult population has been exposed to the virus. One patient with congenital immunodeficiency was cured by a 10-day course followed by intermittent injections until virus had disappeared from his serum.[165] Patients with AIDS respond to a 5- to 10-day course but may relapse some months later; they respond to a second course.[165] In an occasional patient, virus may disappear from the circulation yet anemia persist.[188] In general, circulating viral concentrations are sufficiently high in chronic infection to be detected by direct DNA hybridization tests. Indeed, patients with AIDS have had high virus titers, orders of magnitude above those measured in other patients with chronic parvovirus infection.[165] Measurement of serum virus is helpful in predicting relapse in these patients and may assist in determining optimal maintenance regimens.

▼ OTHER SYNDROMES

Parvovirus has been less confidently linked to a variety of other diseases. Only recently has it become appreciated that circulating parvovirus DNA can persist and be detected by gene amplification methods, especially with sensitive nested versions of the polymerase chain reaction, in normal individuals who have apparently normal immune system function, for years after an acute infection, usually without evidence of clinical disease or with atypical symptoms.[92, 189, 190] Fewer studies of visceral tissue have been performed, but virus may be harbored in reticuloendothelial and other organs as well (see below).

Thus, in many instances, initial positive reports of disease association, which were based solely on results from gene amplification methodology, have been refuted by more complete studies with appropriate controls, including Kawasaki disease,[191] Henoch-Schönlein purpura,[192] chronic neutropenia in children,[193, 194] and juvenile rheumatoid arthritis.[195] Other suggestive associations, based mainly on case reports and polymerase chain reaction assays, that require rigorous examination include B19 parvovirus with myocarditis[196–198]; systemic vasculitis, in syndromes resembling Wegener's granulomatosis and polyarteritis nodosa[199]; fulminant hepatitis and subsequent aplastic anemia[200]; chronic fatigue syndrome[201]; and even diabetes mellitus![202]

Immune Response

▼ NORMAL RESPONSE

Both virus-specific IgM and IgG antibodies are made after experimental[119] and natural[140] B19 parvovirus infection.[203] After intranasal inoculation of volunteers, virus can first be detected at days 5 to 6 and levels peak at days 8 to 9 (Fig. 28–14). Virus is rarely detected in patients with clinical fifth disease because the manifestations are secondary to immune complex formation, and patients therefore present to medical attention after the period of viremia has passed. IgM antibody to virus appears about 10 to 12 days after experimental inoculation; IgM antibody may be present in patients with transient aplastic crisis at the time of reticulocyte nadir and during the subsequent 10 days. IgG antibody appears in normal volunteers about 2 weeks after inoculation; in patients with transient aplastic crisis, IgG is not present at the time of reticulocyte depression but appears rapidly with recovery. IgM antibody may be found in serum samples for several months after exposure.[204] IgG presumably persists for life and protects against second infection. Antibody-producing cells apparently of recipient origin persist for years after allogeneic marrow transplantation.[205] IgA antibodies to B19 parvovirus can also be detected and presumably play a role in protection against infection by the natural nasopharyngeal route.[206]

▼ CELLULAR IMMUNE RESPONSE

Attempts to measure lymphocyte proliferation in response to intact parvovirus virions have been unsuccessful.[207] However, one group succeeded in measuring a cellular immune response to the viral proteins if not to intact virions. Peripheral blood mononuclear cells from seropositive donors proliferated in response to recombinant capsid proteins, and the immune response was class II restricted, implicating a role for helper lymphocytes in the response to B19 parvovirus infection.[208]

The possible importance of the cellular immune response in B19 infection is suggested by analogy with other parvoviruses. T-cell responses limit rat parvovirus infection.[209] Delayed hypersensitivity to canine virus can be passively transferred by lymphocytes exposed to virus in vitro; T cells proliferate and secrete interleukin-2 in response to soluble viral antigen, and T-cell epitopes map to the major capsid protein.[210] For Aleutian disease virus, lymphocyte responses probably represent pathological phenomena.[211]

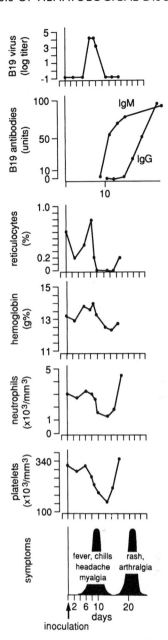

Figure 28–14. Virological, immunological, and clinical course after B19 infection in a normal host.

Many animal parvoviruses infect lymphocytes in vivo and replicate in lymphocytes and macrophages in vitro, including minute virus of mice,[212] porcine parvovirus,[213] feline panleukopenia virus,[214] and Aleutian disease virus.[215]

▼ B-CELL NEUTRALIZING EPITOPES

Several regions containing neutralizing epitopes have been localized to linear sequences of B19 parvovirus[203]: one region at the amino terminus of VP2 at amino acids 38 to 87[216] and six others distributed within the carboxyl-terminal half of VP2 (amino acids 253–272, 309–330, 328–344, 359–382, 449–468, 491–515[217, 218]); neutralizing epitopes are also found in the unique region of VP1.[219] Some of the neutralizing epitopes of VP2, by analogy with the three-dimensional structure of canine parvovirus,[59] correspond to external loops of the protein present on the virus surface as major protrusions or spikes.[219] Anti-VP2 antibodies directed against sequences in the β barrel central core structure are produced in animals immunized with VP2-only–containing empty capsids, but these antibodies fail to neutralize virus activity.[220] Similarly, peptides derived from VP2 sequence, although effective in eliciting binding antibodies, do not induce production of neutralizing antibodies; in contrast, even short sequences derived from the VP1 unique region elicit marked neutralizing antibody responses.[221, 222] Nevertheless, both anti-VP2 and anti-VP1 specificities are present in normal human convalescent antisera, and sera that predominate in either one or the other specificity effectively neutralize virus; however, VP1 is the major antigen recognized on immunoblot by late convalescent phase antiserum or in commercial immunoglobulin preparations.[207]

Antisera raised to the unique region of VP1 as a single large 226 amino acid polypeptide or to shorter fragments can precipitate empty capsids and also neutralize virus activity, indicating that most of the unique region is external to the virus surface.[223] (The entire unique region can be substituted with heterologous protein, which retains its native conformation, functional activity, and external topography on the capsid.[224]) The unique region of VP1 thus appears to contain the most readily detectable linear neutralizing epitopes of B19 parvovirus. The majority of monoclonal antibodies that neutralize B19 parvovirus do not recognize peptide sequences within the capsid proteins and presumably bind to conformationally determined epitopes.[216] Whereas VP2 contains neutralizing epitopes, these are not presented to the immune system in VP2-only empty capsids,[11] suggesting that the conformation of some VP2 determinants is altered by insertion of one or two VP1 molecules per 60 protein subunit capsid.[220] A further alteration probably occurs with insertion of DNA into empty capsids containing both proteins, because many monoclonal antibodies raised to virions and screened by enzyme-linked immunosorbent assay (ELISA) fail to recognize VP1 plus VP2 empty capsids in the same test.[216]

▼ IMMUNITY AND DISEASE

The pattern of disease that follows parvovirus infection is the result of balance between virus, marrow target cell, and the immune response (Fig. 28–15). Bone marrow depression in parvovirus infection occurs during the early viremic phase and under normal conditions is terminated by a neutralizing antibody response. In acute infection, the period of viremia is abbreviated, usually 1 to 3 days, and virus titers can be extremely high (10^{11} to 10^{14} genome copies per milliliter).[138, 139] By contrast, in persistent infection, virus can be demonstrated in serum samples obtained months apart; the viral titer is often lower (10^6 genome copies per milliliter), although AIDS patients may have serum concentrations as high as in an acute infection. The immune response terminates viremia, but antiparvovirus antibodies also produce the clinical manifestations of rash and joint pains, which are secondary to immune complex formation (fifth disease symptoms can be precipitated by treatment of persistent infection with immunoglobulin). On occasion, the immune response is aberrant and includes rheumatoid factor and antibodies to lymphocytes and nuclear antigen.[225–227] In patients with hyperactive erythropoiesis, larger amounts of virus may be produced and the immune response may be weak, perhaps resulting in relatively greater quantities of antigen to antibody and little immune complex formation (rash and joint pains are rare in patients with transient aplastic crisis[116]). In both persistent infection in children and adults and in utero infection, failure to mount a neutralizing antibody response allows parvovirus to persist and causes chronic anemia.[187] The humoral response appears to be dominant in controlling human parvovirus infection; not only does normal recovery from infection correlate with the appearance of circulating specific antivirus antibody, but administration of commercial immunoglobulins can cure or ameliorate persistent parvovirus infection in immunodeficient patients.

Persistent B19 parvovirus infection is the result of failure to produce effective neutralizing antibodies by the immunosuppressed host or in the normally immunodeficient fetus.

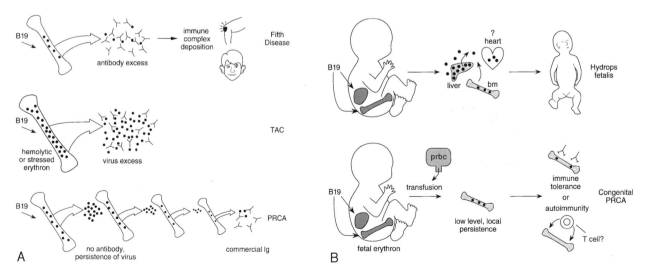

Figure 28–15. Pathogenesis of human diseases caused by B19 parvovirus in children and adults (A) and in the fetus (B). TAC, transient aplastic crisis; PRCA, pure red cell aplasia; bm, bone marrow; prbc, packed red blood cells.

Antibodies to parvovirus, as determined in immunoassays or ELISA, are not present in most patients, but a pattern of antibody response suggestive of early infection (IgM antibody and IgG antibody directed to the major capsid protein) may be found in congenital immunodeficiency.[207] A poor reaction on immunoblot testing is a consistent finding and correlates with low neutralizing activity for the virus in erythroid colony assays.[207] These results suggest that the linear epitopes detected by immunoblotting are functionally important, and the clinical findings in persistent infection are analogous to animal data showing dependence of a neutralizing antibody response on presentation of specific epitopes, particularly the amino-terminal region of the minor capsid protein. Perhaps because of the limited epitopes presented to the immune system by B19 parvovirus, the congenital immunodeficiency states associated with persistent infection may be clinically subtle, with susceptibility largely restricted to parvovirus.

▼ PASSIVE IMMUNITY AND VACCINE DEVELOPMENT

Antibodies play a dominant role in the normal immune response to parvovirus, and antibodies are protective in both passive and active immunizations. Convalescent antiserum can protect puppies against canine parvovirus infection,[228] and commercial immunoglobulin from normal donors can cure or ameliorate persistent B19 parvovirus infection in immunosuppressed human patients.[160, 165] Human convalescent phase antisera[207] and commercial immunoglobulin preparations[229] contain neutralizing antibodies to parvovirus, as assessed in vitro by use of erythroid colony systems.

Parvovirus infection can be prevented in animals by vaccination. A human vaccine would be useful, at a minimum, to prevent transient aplastic crisis in persons with hemolysis and to protect the fetus in seronegative pregnant women; universal vaccination might be more efficient and would eliminate the risk of chronic red cell aplasia with acquired immunosuppression as well as the wide range of parvovirus-related illnesses, the full spectrum of which is unknown. Effective vaccines have been produced for animals with use of attenuated or fixed virus preparations, including feline,[230] canine,[22] and porcine[231] parvoviruses. Antisera raised against peptide fragments of canine parvovirus, determined to contain neutralizing epitopes, have also been protective in a dog model.[232, 233]

Prospects for a B19 parvovirus vaccine are good. The immunogen will be recombinant capsid rather than attenuated or killed virus, owing to the difficulty of propagating B19 parvovirus in tissue culture and the potential danger of inadvertently modifying its tissue range for the worse by in vitro selection. Recombinant B19 parvovirus capsids produced in baculovirus are suitable to induce neutralizing antibodies in inoculated animals[11, 234]; in primates, the choice of adjuvant appears important.[12] The presence of VP1 protein in the capsid immunogen is critical for the production of antibodies that neutralize virus activity in vitro. Capsids with supernormal VP1 content are more efficient in inducing neutralizing activity in immunized animals, and neutralization correlates with anti-VP1 reactivity on immunoblot.[234]

Conclusion

The basic biology of B19 parvovirus is well understood and directly relevant to human diseases caused by this agent. B19 parvovirus is cytotoxic to human erythroid target cells, but serious disease results only if the host's erythroid marrow is stressed or immunity is inadequate. The antibody response limits virus propagation in the human host, and a restricted number of viral epitopes presented to the immune system may allow the virus to elude some genetically deficient immune systems. Development of recombinant empty capsids should provide a basis for vaccination and prevention of parvovirus disease.

Outstanding and interesting questions remain. What is the exact molecular basis of altered transcription in erythroid cells and its relation to tissue tropism? How is virus uncoated? Does virus persist in non-erythroid cells? Does the virus kill cells outside of the bone marrow? The history of virology suggests that the answers to these questions will have implications not only for B19 parvovirus but for normal cell function too.

REFERENCES

1. Cossart, Y.E., Field, A.M., Cant, B., et al: Parvovirus-like particles in human sera. Lancet 1:72, 1975.
2. Cohen, B.J., Mortimer, P.P., and Pereira M.S.: Diagnostic assays with monoclonal antibodies for the human serum parvovirus-like virus (SPLV). J. Hyg. 91:113, 1983.
3. Pattison, J.R., Jones, S.E., Hodgson, J., et al: Parvovirus infections and hypoplastic crisis in sickle cell anemia. Lancet 1:664, 1981.
4. Anderson, M.J., Jones, S.E., Fisher-Hoch, S.P., Lewis, E., Hall, S.M., Bartlett, C.L., Cohen, B.J., Mortimer, P.P., and Pereira M.S.: Human parvovirus, the cause of erythema infectiosum (fifth disease)? Lancet 1:1378, 1983.
5. Summers, J., Jones, S.E., and Anderson, M.J.: Characterization of the genome of the agent of erythrocyte aplasia permits its classification as a human parvovirus. J. Gen. Virol. 64:2527, 1983.
6. Clewley, J.P.: Biochemical characterization of a human parvovirus. J. Gen. Virol. 65:241, 1984.
7. Cotmore, S.F., and Tattersall, P.: Characterization and molecular cloning of a human parvovirus genome. Science 226:1161, 1984.
8. Shade, R.O., Blundell, M.C., Cotmore, S.F., Tattersall, P., and Astell, C.R.: Nucleotide sequence and genome organization of human parvovirus B19 isolated from the serum of a child during aplastic crisis. J. Virol. 58:921, 1986.
9. Ozawa, K., Kurtzman, G., and Young, N.S.: Replication of the B19 parvovirus in human bone marrow cultures. Science 233:883, 1986.
10. Shimomura, S., Komatsu, N., Frickhofen, N., Anderson, S., Kajigaya, S., and Young, N.S.: First continuous propagation of B19 parvovirus in a cell line. Blood 79:18, 1992.
11. Kajigaya, S., Fujii, H., Field, A.M., Rosenfeld, S., Anderson, L.J., Shimada, T., and Young, N.S.: Self-assembled B19 parvovirus capsids, produced in a baculovirus system, are antigenically and immunogenically similar to native virions. Proc. Natl. Acad. Sci. USA 88:4646, 1991.
12. Bostic, J.R., Brown, K.E., Donahue, R.E., Young, N.S., and Koenig, S.: Marked enhancement of anti-parvoviral B19 functional antibody responses in rodents and primates with different virus-like particle (VLP)/adjuvant formulations [abstract]. Blood 90(suppl. 1):10b, 1997.
13. Berns, K.I.: Parvovirus replication. Microbiol. Rev. 54:316, 1990.
14. Berns, K.I.: Parvoviruses: the viruses and their replication. In Fields, B.N., Knipe, D.M., Howley, P.M., Chanock, R.M., Melnick, J.L., Monath, T.P., Roizman, B., and Straus, S.E. (eds.): Fields Virology. Philadelphia, Lippincott-Raven, 1996, p. 2173.
15. Berns, K.I. (ed.): The Parvoviruses. New York, Plenum, 1984.
16. Brown, K.E., Young, N.S., and Liu, J.M.: Molecular, cellular and clinical aspects of parvovirus B19 infection. Crit. Rev. Oncol. Hematol. 16:1, 1994.

17. Anderson, L.J., and Young, N.S. (eds.): Human Parvovirus B19. Basel, Karger, 1997.
18. Young, N.S.: Parvoviruses. *In* Fields, B.N., Knipe, D.M., Howley, P.M., Chanock, R.M., Melnick, J.L., Monath, T.P., Roizman, B., and Straus, S.E. (eds.): Fields Virology. Philadelphia, Lippincott-Raven, 1996, p. 2199.
19. Hammon, W.D., and Enders, J.F.: A virus disease of cats, principally characterized by aleucocytosis, enteric lesions and the presence of intranuclear inclusion bodies. J. Exp. Med. 69:327, 1939.
20. Lawrence, J.S., Syverton, J.T., Shaw, J.S., and Smith, F.P.: Infectious feline agranulocytosis. Am. J. Pathol. 16:333, 1940.
21. Kurtzman, G.J., Platanias, L., Lustig, L., Frickhofen, N., and Young, N.S.: Feline parvovirus propagates in cat bone marrow cultures and inhibits hematopoietic colony formation in vitro. Blood 74:71, 1989.
22. Parrish, C.R.: Emergence, natural history, and variation of canine, mink, and feline parvoviruses. Adv. Virus Res. 38:403, 1990.
23. Truyen, U., Gruenberg, A., Chang, S.-F., Obermaier, B., Veijalainen, P., and Parrish, C.R.: Evolution of the feline-subgroup parvoviruses and the control of canine host range in vivo. J. Virol. 69:4702, 1995.
24. Ramirez, J.C., Fairen, A., and Almendral, J.M.: Parvovirus minute virus of mice strain i multiplication and pathogenesis in the newborn mouse brain are restricted to proliferative areas and to migratory cerebellar young neurons. J. Virol. 70:8109, 1996.
25. Macartney, L., McCandlish, I.A.P., Thompson, H., and Cornwell, H.J.C.: Canine parvovirus enteritis 1: clinical, haematological and pathological features of experimental infection. Vet. Rec. 115:201, 1984.
26. Segovia, J.C., Real, A., Bueren, J.A., and Almendral, J.M.: In vitro myelosuppressive effects of the parvovirus minute virus of mice (MVMi) on hematopoietic stem and committed progenitor cells. Blood 77:980, 1991.
27. Segovia, J.C., Bueren, J.A., and Almendral, J.M.: Myeloid depression follows infection of susceptible newborn mice with the parvovirus minute virus of mice (strain i). J. Virol. 69:3229, 1995.
28. Kurtzman, G.: Feline panleucopenia virus. *In* Young, N.S. (ed.): Viruses and Bone Marrow. New York, Marcel Dekker, 1993, p. 119.
29. Mori, S., Wolfinbarger, J.B., Miyazawa, M., and Bloom, M.E.: Replication of Aleutian mink disease parvovirus in lymphoid tissues of adult mink: involvement of follicular dendritic cells and macrophages. J. Virol. 65:952, 1991.
30. Murphy, F.A., Fauquet, C.M., Bishop, D.H.L., Ghabrial, S.A., Jarvis, A.W., Martelli, G.P., Mayo, M.A., and Summers, M.D. (eds.): Virus Taxonomy. Classification and Nomenclature of Viruses. New York, Springer-Verlag, 1995.
31. Tobiasch, E., Rabreau, M., Geletneky, K., Larüe-Charlus, S., Severin, F., Becker, N., and Schlehofer, J.R.: Detection of adeno-associated virus DNA in human genital tissue and in material from spontaneous abortion. J. Med. Virol. 44:215, 1994.
32. Berns, K.I., and Giraud, C.: Adenovirus and adeno-associated virus vectors for gene therapy. Ann. N. Y. Acad. Sci. 772:95, 1996.
33. Linden, R.M., Winocour, E., and Berns, K.I.: The recombination signals for adeno-associated virus site-specific integration. Proc. Natl. Acad. Sci. USA 93:7966, 1996.
34. Fisher, R.E., and Mayor, H.D.: The evolution of defective and autonomous parvoviruses. J. Theor. Biol. 149:429, 1991.
35. Brown, K.E., Green, S.W., and Young, N.S.: Goose parvovirus (GPV)—an autonomous member of the dependovirus genus? Virology 210:283, 1995.
36. Zádori, Z., Stefancsik, R., Rauch, T., and Kisary, J.: Analysis of the complete nucleotide sequences of goose and muscovy duck parvoviruses indicates common ancestral origin with adeno-associated virus 2. Virology 212:562, 1995.
37. Brown, K.E., O'Sullivan, M.G., and Young, N.S.: Simian parvovirus. Semin. Virol. 6:339, 1995.
38. O'Sullivan, M.G., Anderson, D.K., Goodrich, J.A., Tulli, H., Green, S.W., Young, N.S., and Brown, K.E.: Experimental infection of cynomolgus monkeys with simian parvovirus. J. Virol. 71:4517, 1997.
39. O'Sullivan, M.G., Anderson, D.K., Lund, J.E., and Brown, W.P.: Clinical and epidemiological features of simian parvovirus infection in cynomolgus macaques with severe anemia. Lab. Anim. Sci. 46:291, 1996.
40. Tattersall, P., and Cotmore, S.F.: Reproduction of autonomous parvovirus DNA. *In* Tijssen, P. (ed.): Handbook of Parvoviruses. Vol. 1. Boca Raton, FL, CRC Press, 1990, p. 123.
41. Astell, C.R., Luo, W., Brunstein, J., and Amand, J.: B19 parvovirus:

42. Deiss, V., Tratschin, J., Weitz, M., and Siegl, G.: Cloning of the human parvovirus B19 genome and structural analysis of its palindromic termini. Virology 175:247, 1990.
43. Astell, C.R.: Terminal hairpins of parvovirus genomes and their role in DNA replication. *In* Tijssen, P. (ed.): Handbook of Parvoviruses. Vol. 1. Boca Raton, FL, CRC Press, 1990, p. 59.
44. St. Amand, J., Beard, C., Humphries, K., and Astell, C.R.: Analysis of splice junctions and in vitro and in vivo translation potential of the small, abundant B19 parvovirus RNAs. Virology 183:133, 1991.
45. Ozawa, K., Ayub, J., Yu-Shu, H., Kurtzman, G., Shimada, T., and Young, N.: Novel transcription map for the B19 (human) pathogenic parvovirus. J. Virol. 61:2395, 1987.
46. Liu, J.M., Fujii, H., Green, S.W., Komatsu, N., Young, N.S., and Shimada, T.: Indiscriminate activity from the B19 parvovirus P6 promoter in nonpermissive cells. Virology 182:361, 1991.
47. Ozawa, K., Ayub, J., and Young, N.S.: Translational regulation of B19 parvovirus capsid protein production by multiple upstream AUG triplets. J. Biol. Chem. 263:10922, 1988.
48. Ozawa, K., Ayub, J., Kajigaya, S., Shimada, T., and Young, N.S.: The gene encoding the nonstructural protein of B19 (human) parvovirus may be lethal in transfected cells. J. Virol. 62:2884, 1988.
49. Caillet-Fauquet, P., Perros, M., Branderburger, A., Spegelaere, P., and Rommelaere, J.: Programmed killing of human cells by means of an inducible clone of parvoviral genes encoding non-structural proteins. EMBO J. 9:2989, 1990.
50. Rommelaere, J., and Tattersall, P.: Oncosuppression by parvoviruses. *In* Tijssen, P. (ed.): Handbook of Parvoviruses. Vol. 2. Boca Raton, FL, CRC Press, 1990, p. 41.
51. Li, X., and Rhode, S.L., III: Mutation of lysine 405 to serine in the parvovirus H-1 NS1 abolishes its functions for viral DNA replication, late promoter trans activation, and cytotoxicity. J. Virol. 64:4654, 1990.
52. Momoeda, M., Kawase, M., Janes, S.W., Miyamura, K., Young, N.S., and Kajigaya, S.: The transcriptional regulator YY1 binds to the 5′ terminal region of B19 parvovirus and regulates P6 promoter activity. J. Virol. 68:7159, 1994.
53. Momoeda, M., Wong, S., Kawase, M., Young, N.S., and Kajigaya, S.: A putative NTP-binding domain in the nonstructural protein of B19 parvovirus is required for cytotoxicity. J. Virol. 68:8443, 1994.
54. Chang, T.J., Scher, B., Waxman, S., and Scher, W.: GATA-1 and the glucocorticoid receptor can influence transcriptional regulation of erythrotropic viral sequences: Friend leukemia virus and B19 parvovirus. Mol. Cell. Diff. 2.:289, 1994.
55. Shimomura, S., Wong, S., Komatsu, N., Kajigaya, S., and Young, N.S.: Early and late gene expression in UT-7 cells infected with B19 parvovirus. Virology 194:149, 1993.
56. Clemens, K.E., and Pintel, D.J.: The two transcriptional units of the autonomous parvovirus minute virus of mice are transcribed in a temporal order. J. Virol. 62:1448, 1988.
57. Ball-Goodrich, L.J., Moir, R.D., and Tattersall, P.: Parvoviral target cell specificity: acquisition of fibrotropism by a mutant of the lymphotropic strain of minute virus of mice involves multiple amino acid substitutions within the capsid. Virology 184:175, 1991.
58. Previsani, N., Fontana, S., Hirt, B., and Beard, P.: Growth of the parvovirus of mice MVMp3 in EL4 lymphocytes is restricted after cell entry and before viral DNA amplification: cell-specific differences in virus uncoating in vitro. J. Virol. 71:7769, 1997.
59. Tsao, J., Chapman, M.S., Agbandje, M., Keller, W., Smith, K., Wu, H., Luo, M., Smith, T.J., Rossmann, M.G., Compans, R.W., and Parrish, C.R.: The three-dimensional structure of canine parvovirus and its functional implications. Science 251:1456, 1991.
60. Agbandje-McKenna, M., and Rossmann, M.G.: The structure of human parvovirus B19. *In* Anderson, L.J., and Young, N.S. (eds.): Human Parvovirus B19. Basel, Karger, 1997, p. 3.
61. Agbandje, M., Kajigaya, S., McKenna, R., Rossmann, M.G., and Young, N.S.: The structure of human parvovirus B19 at 8 Å resolution. Virology 203:106, 1994.
62. Chapman, M.S., and Rossmann, M.G.: Structure, sequence, and function correlations among parvoviruses. Virology 194:491, 1993.
63. Wong, S., Momoeda, M., Field, A., Kajigaya, S., and Young, N.S.: Formation of empty B19 parvovirus capsids by the truncated minor capsid protein. J. Virol. 68:4690, 1994.
64. Kurtzman, G., Ozawa, K., Hanson, G.R., Cohen, B., Oseas, R., and

biochemical and molecular features. *In* Anderson, L.J., and Young, N.S. (eds.): Human Parvovirus B19. Basel, Karger, 1997, p. 16.

Young, N.: Chronic bone marrow failure due to persistent B19 parvovirus infection. N. Engl. J. Med. 317:287, 1987.

65. Ozawa, K., Kurtzman, G., and Young, N.: Productive infection by B19 parvovirus of human erythroid bone marrow cells in vitro. Blood 70:384, 1987.

66. Yaegashi, N., Shiraishi, H., Takeshita, T., Nakamura, M., Yajima, A., and Sugamura, K.: Propagation of human parvovirus B19 in primary culture of erythroid lineage cells derived from fetal liver. J. Virol. 63:2422, 1989.

67. Brown, K.E., Mori, J., Cohen, B.J., and Field, A.M.: In vitro propagation of parvovirus B19 in primary foetal liver cultures. J. Gen. Virol. 72(pt. 3):741, 1991.

68. Takahashi, T., Ozawa, K., Mitani, K., Miyazono, K., Asano, S., and Takaku, F.: B19 parvovirus replicates in erythroid leukemic cells in vitro [letter]. J. Infect. Dis. 160:548, 1989.

69. Munshi, N.C., Zhou, S., Woody, M.J., Morgan, D.A., and Srivastava, A.: Successful replication of parvovirus B19 in the human megakaryocytic cell line MB-02. J. Virol. 67:562, 1993.

70. Mortimer, P.P., Humphries, R.K., Moore, J.G., Purcell, R.H., and Young, N.S.: A human parvovirus-like virus inhibits hematopoietic colony formation in vitro. Nature 302:426, 1983.

71. Takahashi, M., Koike, T., and Moriyama, Y.: Inhibition of erythropoiesis by human parvovirus-containing serum from a patient with hereditary spherocytosis in aplastic crisis. Scand. J. Haematol. 37:118, 1986.

72. Srivastava, A., and Lu, L.: Replication of B19 parvovirus in highly enriched hematopoietic progenitor cells from normal human bone marrow. J. Virol. 62:3059, 1988.

73. Takahashi, T., Ozawa, K., Takahashi, K., Asano, S., and Takaku, F.: Susceptibility of human erythropoietic cells to B19 parvovirus in vitro increases with differentiation. Blood 75:603, 1990.

74. Shimomura, S., Wong, S., Brown, K.E., Komatsu, N., Kajigaya, S., and Young, N.S.: Early and late gene expression in UT-7 cells is infected with B19 parvovirus. Virology 194:149, 1993.

75. Young, N.S., Harrison, M., Moore, J.G., Mortimer, P.P., and Humphries, R.K.: Direct demonstration of the human parvovirus in erythroid progenitor cells infected in vitro. J. Clin. Invest. 74:2024, 1984.

76. Owren, P.A.: Congenital hemolytic jaundice: the pathogenesis of the "hemolytic crisis." Blood 3:231, 1948.

77. Kajigaya, S., Shimada, T., Fujita, S., and Young, N.S.: A genetically engineered cell line that produces empty capsids of B19 (human) parvovirus. Proc. Natl. Acad. Sci. USA 86:7601, 1989.

78. Liu, J., Green, S., Shimada, T., and Young, N.S.: A block in full-length transcript maturation in cells nonpermissive for B19 parvovirus. J. Virol. 66:4686, 1992.

79. Srivastava, A., Bruno, E., Briddell, R., Cooper, R., Srivastava, C., van Besien, K., and Hoffman, R.: Parvovirus B19–induced perturbation of human megakaryocytopoiesis in vitro. Blood 76:1997, 1990.

80. Brown, K.E., Anderson, S.M., and Young, N.S.: Erythrocyte P antigen: cellular receptor for B19 parvovirus. Science 262:114, 1993.

81. Chapman, P.R., Agbandje-McKenna, M., Kajigaya, S., Brown, K.E., Young, N.S., Baker, T.S., and Rossmann, M.G.: Cryo-electron microscopy studies of empty capsids of human parvovirus B19 complexed with its cellular receptor. Proc. Natl. Acad. Sci. USA 93:7502, 1996.

82. Brown, K.E., Hibbs, J.R., Gallinella, G., Anderson, S.M., Lehman, E.H., McCarthy, M., and Young, N.S.: Resistance to parvovirus B19 due to lack of virus receptor (erythrocyte P antigen). N. Engl. J. Med. 330:1192, 1994.

83. Kerr, J.R., Mcquaid, S., and Coyle, P.V.: Expression of P antigen in parvovirus B-19 infected bone marrow. N. Engl. J. Med. 332:128, 1995.

84. Erdman, D.D.: Human parvovirus B19: laboratory diagnosis. In Anderson, L.J., and Young, N.S. (eds.): Human Parvovirus B19. Basel, Karger, 1997, p. 93.

85. Koch, W.C., and Adler, S.P.: Human parvovirus B19 infections in women of childbearing age and within families. Pediatr. Infect. Dis. J. 8:83, 1989.

86. de Freitas, R.B., Wong, D., Boswell, F., de Miranda, M.F., Linhares, A.C., Shirley, J., and Desselberger, U.: Prevalence of human parvovirus (B19) and rubellavirus infections in urban and remote rural areas in northern Brazil. J. Med. Virol. 32:203, 1990.

87. Schwarz, L., Gurtler, L.G., Zoulek, G., Deinhardt, F., and Roggendorf, M.: Seroprevalence of human parvovirus B19 infection. Int. J. Med. Microbiol. 271:231, 1989.

88. Chorba, T.L., Coccia, P., Holman, R.C., Tattersall, P., Anderson, L.J., Sudman, J., Young, N.S., Kurczynski, E., Saarinen, U.M., Moir, R.,

Lawrence, D.N., Jason, J.M., and Evatt, B.: Role of parvovirus B19 in aplastic crisis and erythema infectiosum (fifth disease). J. Infect. Dis. 154:383, 1986.

89. Cohen, B.J., Field, A.M., Gudnadottir, S., Beard, S., and Barbara, J.A.J.: Blood donor screening for parvovirus B19. J. Virol. Methods 30:233, 1990.

90. McOmish, F., Yap, P.L., Jordan, A., Hart, H., Cohen, B.J., and Simmonds, P.: Detection of parvovirus B19 in donated blood: a model system for screening by polymerase chain reaction. J. Clin. Microbiol. 31:323, 1993.

91. Yoto, Y., Kudoh, T., Haseyama, K., Suzuki, N., Oda, T., Katoh, T., Takahashi, T., Sekiguchi, S., and Chiba, S.: Incidence of human parvovirus B19 DNA detection in blood donors. Br. J. Haematol. 91:1017, 1995.

92. Kerr, J.R., Curran, M.D., Moore, J.E., Coyle, P.V., and Ferguson, W.P.: Persistent parvovirus B19 infection [letter]. Lancet 345:1118, 1995.

93. Anderson, M.J., Higgins, P.G., Davis, L.R., et al.: Experimental parvoviral infection in humans. J. Infect. Dis. 152:257, 1985.

94. Plummer, A.F., Hammond, W.G., and Forward, K.: An erythema infectiosum–like illness caused by human parvovirus infection. N. Engl. J. Med. 313:74, 1985.

95. Gillespie, S.M., Cartter, M.L., Asch, S., Rokos, J.B., Gary, G.W., Tsou, C.J., Hall, D.B., Anderson, L.J., and Hurwitz, E.S.: Occupational risk of human parvovirus B19 infection for school and day-care personnel during an outbreak of erythema infectiosum. JAMA 263:2061, 1990.

96. Luban, N.L.: Human parvoviruses: implications for transfusion medicine. Transfusion 34:821, 1994.

97. Yee, T.T., Cohen, B.J., Pasi, K.J., and Lee, C.A.: Transmission of symptomatic parvovirus B19 infection by clotting factor concentrate. Br. J. Haematol. 93:457, 1996.

98. Santagostino, E., Mannucci, P.M., Gringeri, A., Azzi, A., Morfini, M., Musso, R., Santoro, R., and Schiavoni, M.: Transmission of parvovirus B19 by coagulation factor concentrates exposed to 100°C heat after lyophilization. Transfusion 37:517, 1997.

99. Azzi, A., Ciappi, S., Zakvrzewska, K., Morfini, M., Mariani, G., and Mannucci, P.M.: Human parvovirus B19 infection in hemophiliacs first infused with two high-purity, virally attenuated factor VIII concentrates. Am. J. Hematol. 39:228, 1992.

100. Williams, M.D., Beddall, A.C., Pasi, K.J., Mortimer, P.P., and Hill, F.G.H.: Transmission of human parvovirus B19 by coagulation factor concentrates. Vox Sang. 58:177, 1990.

101. Bell, L.M., Naides, S.J., Stoffman, P., Hodinka, R.L., and Plotkin, S.A.: Human parvovirus B19 infection among hospital staff members after contact with infected patients. N. Engl. J. Med. 321:485, 1989.

102. Dowell, S.F., Török, T.J., Thorp, J.A., Hedrick, J., Erdman, D.D., Zaki, S.R., Hinkle, C.J., Bayer, W.L., and Anderson, L.J.: Parvovirus B19 infection in hospital workers: community or hospital acquisition. J. Infect. Dis. 172:1076, 1995.

103. Seng, C., Watkins, P., Morse, D., Barret, S.P., Zambon, M., Andrews, N., Atkins, M., Hall, S., Lau, Y.K., and Cohen, B.J.: Parvovirus B19 outbreak on an adult ward. Epidemiol. Infect. 113:345, 1994.

104. Balfour, H.H., Jr.: Erythema infectiosum (fifth disease): clinical review and description of 91 cases seen in an epidemic. Clin. Pediatr. 8.:721, 1969.

105. Schwartz, T., Wiersbitzky, S., and Pambor, M.: Detection of parvovirus B19 in a skin biopsy of a patient with erythema infectiosum. J. Med. Virol. 43:171, 1994.

106. Reid, D.M., Reid, T.M.S., Rennie, J.A.N., Brown, T., and Eastmond, C.J.: Human parvovirus-associated arthritis: a clinical and laboratory description. Lancet 1:422, 1985.

107. White, D.G., Woolf, A.D., Mortimer, P.P., Cohen, B.J., Blake, D.R., and Bacon, P.A.: Human parvovirus arthropathy. Lancet 1:419, 1985.

108. Leventhal, L.J., Naides, S.J., and Freundlich, B.: Fibromyalgia and parvovirus infection. Arthritis Rheum. 34:1319, 1991.

109. Nikkari, S., Luukkainen, R., Möttönen, T., Meurman, O., Hannonen, P., Skurnik, M., and Toivanen, P.: Does parvovirus B19 have a role in rheumatoid arthritis? Ann. Rheum. Dis. 53:106, 1994.

110. Hajeer, A.H., MacGregor, A.J., Rigby, A.S., Ollier, W.E.R., Carthy, D., and Silman, A.J.: Influence of previous exposure to human parvovirus B19 infection in explaining susceptibility to rheumatoid arthritis: an analysis of disease discordant twin pairs. Ann. Rheum. Dis. 53:137, 1994.

111. Woolf, A.D., Campion, G.V., Chishick, A., Wise, S., Cohen, B.J., Klouda, P.T., Caul, O., and Dieppe, P.A.: Clinical manifestation of human parvovirus B19 in adults. Arch. Intern. Med. 149:1153, 1989.

112. Young, N.: Hematologic and hematopoietic consequences of B19 parvovirus infection. Semin. Hematol. 25:159, 1988.

113. Weiland, H.T., Salimans, M.M.M., Fibbe, W.E., Kluin, P.M., and Cohen, B.J.: Prolonged parvovirus B19 infection with severe anaemia in a bone marrow transplant recipient [letter]. Br. J. Haematol. 710:300, 1989.

114. Powars, D.: Aplastic anemia secondary to glue sniffing. N. Engl. J. Med. 273:700, 1965.

115. Lefrère, J.J., Courouce, A.-M., Bertrand, Y., Girot, R., and Soulier, J.-P.: Human parvovirus and aplastic crisis in chronic hemolytic anemias: a study of 24 observations. Am. J. Hematol. 23:271, 1986.

116. Nunoue, T., Koike, T., Koike, R., Sanada, M., Tsukada, T., Mortimer, P.P., and Cohen, B.J.: Infection with human parvovirus (B19), aplasia of the bone marrow and a rash in hereditary spherocytosis. J. Infect. 14:67, 1987.

117. Kurtzman, G., Gascon, P., Caras, M., Cohen, B., and Young, N.: B19 parvovirus replicates in circulating cells of acutely infected patients. Blood 71:1448, 1988.

118. Doran, H.M., and Teall, A.J.: Neutropenia accompanying erythroid aplasia in human parvovirus infection [letter]. Br. J. Haematol. 69:287, 1988.

119. Anderson, M.J., Higgins, P.G., Davis, L.R., Willman, J.S., Jones, S.E., Kidd, I.M., Pattison, J.R., and Tyrrell, D.A.J.: Experimental parvoviral infection in humans. J. Infect. Dis. 152:257, 1985.

120. Pont, J., Puchhammer-Stöckl, E., Chott, A., Popow-Kraupp, T., Keinzer, H., Postner, G., and Honetz, N.: Recurrent granulocytic aplasia as clinical presentation of a persistent parvovirus B19 infection. Br. J. Haematol. 80:160, 1992.

121. Saunders, P.W.G., Reid, M.M., and Cohen, B.J.: Human parvovirus induced cytopenias: a report of five cases [letter]. Br. J. Haematol. 63:407, 1986.

122. Gautier, E., Bourhis, J.H., Bayle, C., Cartron, J., Pico, J.L., and Tchernia, G.: Parvovirus B19 associated neutropenia. Treatment with Rh G-CSF. Hematol. Cell. Ther. 39:85, 1997.

123. Baurmann, H., Schwarz, T.F., Oertel, J., Serke, S., Roggendorf, M., and Huhn, D.: Acute parvovirus B19 infection mimicking myelodysplastic syndrome of the bone marrow. Ann. Hematol. 43:45, 1992.

124. Conrad, M.E., Studdard, H., and Anderson, L.J.: Case report: aplastic crisis in sickle cell disorders: bone marrow necrosis and human parvovirus infection. Am. J. Med. Sci. 295:212, 1988.

125. Pardoll, D.M., Rodeheffer, R.J., Smith, R.R.L., and Charache, S.: Aplastic crisis due to extensive bone marrow necrosis in sickle cell disease. Arch. Intern. Med. 142:2223, 1982.

126. Frickhofen, N., Raghavachar, A., Heit, W., Heimpel, H., and Cohen, B.J.: Human parvovirus infection [letter]. N. Engl. J. Med. 314:646, 1986.

127. Hanada, T., Koike, K., Takeya, T., Nagasawa, T., Matsunaga, Y., and Takita, H.: Human parvovirus B19–induced transient pancytopenia in a child with hereditary spherocytosis. Br. J. Haematol. 70:113, 1988.

128. Hamon, M.D., Newland, A.C., and Anderson, M.J.: Severe aplastic anaemia after parvovirus infection in the absence of underlying haemolytic anaemia [letter]. J. Clin. Pathol. 41:1242, 1988.

129. Caul, O.E., Usher, J.M., and Burton, A.P.: Intrauterine infection with human parvovirus B19: a light and electron microscopy study. J. Med. Virol. 24:55, 1988.

130. Boruchoff, E.S., Woda, A.B., Pihan, A.G., Durbin, A.W., Burstein, D., and Blacklow, R.N.: Parvovirus B19–associated hemophagocytic syndrome. Arch. Intern. Med. 150:897, 1990.

131. Shirono, K., and Tsuda, H.: Parvovirus B19–associated haemophagocytic syndrome in healthy adults. Br. J. Haematol. 89:923, 1995.

132. Yufu, Y., Matsumoto, M., Miyamura, T., Nishimura, J., Nawata, H., and Ohshima, K.: Parvovirus B19–associated haemophagocytic syndrome with lymphadenopathy resembling histiocytic necrotizing lymphadenitis (Kikuchi's disease). Br. J. Haematol. 96:868, 1997.

133. Lefrère, J.J., Courouce, A.M., and Kaplan, C.: Parvovirus and idiopathic thrombocytopenic purpura [letter]. Lancet 1:279, 1989.

134. Serjeant, G.R., Topley, J.M., Mason, K., Serjeant, B.E., Pattison, J.R., Jones, S.E., and Mohamed, R.: Outbreak of aplastic crises in sickle cell anaemia associated with parvovirus-like agent. Lancet 2:595, 1981.

135. Rao, K.R.P., Patel, A.R., Anderson, M.J., Hodgson, J., Jones, S.E., and Pattison, J.R.: Infection with parvovirus-like virus and aplastic crisis in chronic hemolytic anemia. Ann. Intern. Med. 98:930, 1983.

136. Young, N.S., Mortimer, P.P., Moore, J.G., and Humphries, R.K.: Characterization of a virus that causes transient aplastic crisis. J. Clin. Invest. 73:224, 1984.

137. Wodzinski, M.A., and Lilleyman, J.S.: Transient erythroblastopenia of childhood due to human parvovirus B19 infection. Br. J. Haematol. 73:127, 1989.

138. Anderson, M.J., Jones, S.E., and Minson, A.C.: Diagnosis of human parvovirus infection by dot-blot hybridization using cloned viral DNA. J. Med. Virol. 15:163, 1985.

139. Clewley, J.P.: Detection of human parvovirus using a molecularly cloned probe. J. Med. Virol. 15:173, 1985.

140. Saarinen, U.M., Chorba, T.L., Tattersall, P., Young, N.S., Anderson, L.J., Palmer, E., and Coccia, P.F.: Human parvovirus B19–induced epidemic acute red cell aplasia in patients with hereditary hemolytic anemia. Blood 67:1411, 1986.

141. Hall, C.J.: Parvovirus B19 infection in pregnancy. Arch. Dis. Child. Fetal Neonatal Ed. 71:F4, 1994.

142. Levy, R., Weissman, A., Blomberg, G., and Hagay, Z.J.: Infection by parvovirus B19 during pregnancy: a review. Obstet. Gynecol. Surv. 52:254, 1997.

143. Anand, A., Gray, E.S., Brown, T., Clewley, J.P., and Cohen, B.J.: Human parvovirus infection in pregnancy and hydrops fetalis. N. Engl. J. Med. 316:183, 1987.

144. Cotmore, S.F., McKie, V.C., Anderson, L.J., Astell, C.R., and Tattersall, P.: Identification of the major structural and nonstructural proteins encoded by human parvovirus B19 and mapping of their genes by procaryotic expression of isolated genomic fragments. J. Virol. 60:548, 1986.

145. Public Health Laboratory Service Working Party on Fifth Disease: Prospective study of human parvovirus (B19) infection in pregnancy. Br. Med. J. 300:1166, 1990.

146. Anderson, L.J., and Hurwitz, E.S.: Human parvovirus B19 and pregnancy. Clin. Perinatol. 15:273, 1988.

147. Guidozzi, F., Ballot, D., and Rothberg, A.D.: Human B19 parvovirus infection in an obstetric population. A prospective study determining fetal outcome. J. Reprod. Med. 39:36, 1994.

148. Koch, W.C., Adler, S.P., and Harger, J.: Intrauterine parvovirus B19 infection may cause an asymptomatic or recurrent postnatal infection. Pediatr. Infect. Dis. J. 12:747, 1993.

149. Rodis, J.F., Quinn, D.L., Gary, G.W., Jr., and Anderson, L.J.: Management and outcomes of pregnancies complicated by human B19 parvovirus infection: a prospective study. Am. J. Obstet. Gynecol. 163(pt. 1):1168, 1990.

150. Cassinotti, P., Schultze, D., Wieczorek, K., Schonenberger, R., and Siegl, G.: Parvovirus B19 infection during pregnancy and development of hydrops fetalis despite the evidence for pre-existing anti-B19 antibody: how reliable are serological results? Clin. Diagn. Virol. 2.:87, 1994.

151. Schwarz, T.F., Roggendorf, M., Hottentrager, B., Deinhardt, F., Enders, G., Gloning, K.P., Schramm, T., and Hansmann, M.: Human parvovirus B19 infection in pregnancy [letter]. Lancet 2:566, 1988.

152. Panero, C., Azzi, A., Carbone, C., Pezzati, M., Mainardi, G., and di Lollo, S.: Fetoneonatal hydrops from human parvovirus B19. Case report. J. Perinat. Med. 22:257, 1994.

153. Wright, I.M., Williams, M.L., and Cohen, B.J.: Congenital parvovirus infection. Arch. Dis. Child. 66:253, 1991.

154. Belloy, M., Morinet, F., Blondin, G., Courouce, A.M., Peyrol, Y., and Vilmer, E.: Erythroid hypoplasia due to chronic infection with parvovirus B19. N. Engl. J. Med. 322:633, 1990.

155. Donders, G.G.G., Van Lierde, S., van Elsacker-Niele, A.M.W., Moerman, P., Goubau, P., and Vandenberghe, K.: Survival after intrauterine parvovirus B19 infection with persistence in early infancy: a two-year follow-up. Pediatr. Infect. Dis. J. 13:234, 1994.

156. Brown, K.E., Green, S.W., Antunez-de-Mayolo, J., Bellanti, J.A., Smith, S.D., Smith, T.J., and Young, N.S.: Congenital anemia following transplacental B19 parvovirus infection. Lancet 343:895, 1994.

157. Porter, H.J., Quantrill, A.M., and Fleming, K.A.: B19 parvovirus infection of myocardial cells [letter]. Lancet 1:535, 1988.

158. White, F.V., Jordan, J., Dickman, P.S., and Knisely, A.S.: Fetal parvovirus B19 infection and liver disease of antenatal onset in an infant with Ebstein's anomaly. Pediatr. Pathol. Lab. Med. 15:121, 1995.

159. Hartwig, N.G., Vermeij-Keers, C., Van Elsacker-Niele, A.M., and Fleuren, G.J.: Embryonic malformations in a case of intrauterine parvovirus B19 infection. Teratology 39:295, 1989.

160. Kurtzman, G., Frickhofen, N., Kimball, J., Jenkins, D.W., Nienhuis, A.W., and Young, N.S.: Pure red-cell aplasia of 10 years' duration due to persistent parvovirus B19 infection and its cure with immunoglobulin therapy. N. Engl. J. Med. 321:519, 1989.

161. Gahr, M., Pekrun, A., and Eiffert, H.: Persistence of parvovirus B19-DNA in blood of a child with severe combined immunodeficiency associated with chronic pure red cell aplasia. Eur. J. Pediatr. 150:470, 1991.

162. Kurtzman, G., Cohen, B., Myers, P., Amanullah, A., and Young, N.: Persistent B19 parvovirus infection as a cause of severe anemia in children with acute lymphocytic leukemia in remission. Lancet 2:1159, 1988.

163. Rao, S.P., Miller, S.T., and Cohen, B.J.: B19 parvovirus infection in children with malignant solid tumors receiving chemotherapy. Med. Pediatr. Oncol. 22:255, 1994.

164. Mihal, V., Dusek, J., Hajduch, M., and Cohen, B.J.: Transient aplastic crisis in a leukemic child caused by parvovirus B19 infection. Pediatr. Hematol. Oncol. 13:173, 1996.

165. Frickhofen, N., Abkowitz, J., Safford, M., Berry, J.M., Antunez-de-Mayolo, J., Astrow, A., Cohen, R., Halperin, I., King, L., Mintzer, D., Cohen, B., and Young, N.S.: Persistent parvovirus infection in patients infected with human immunodeficiency virus type 1 (HIV-1): a treatable cause of anemia in AIDS. Ann. Intern. Med. 113:926, 1990.

166. Corbett, T.J., Saw, H., Popat, U., MacMahon, E., Cohen, B.J., Knowles, W.A., Beard, S., and Prentice, H.G.: Successful treatment of parvovirus B19 infection and red cell aplasia occurring after an allogeneic bone marrow transplant. Bone Marrow Transplant. 16:711, 1995.

167. Nield, G., Anderson, M., Hawes, S., and Colvin, B.T.: Parvovirus infection after renal transplant [letter]. Lancet 2:1226, 1986.

168. Nour, B., Green, M., Michaels, M., Reyes, J., Tzakis, A., Gartner, J.C., McLoughlin, L., and Starzl, T.E.: Parvovirus B19 infection in pediatric transplant patients. Transplantation 56:835, 1993.

169. Thio, K., and Janner, D.: Aplastic anemia in a cardiac transplant recipient. Pediatr. Infect. Dis. J. 15:1139, 1996.

170. Ndimbie, O.K., Frezza, E., Jordan, J.A., Koch, W., and Van Thiel, D.H.: Parvovirus B19 in anemic liver transplant recipients. Clin. Diagn. Lab. Immunol. 3:756, 1996.

171. Itala, M., Kotilainen, P., Nikkari, S., Remes, K., and Nikoskelainen, J.: Pure red cell aplasia caused by B19 parvovirus infection after autologous blood stem cell transplantation in a patient with chronic lymphocytic leukemia [letter]. Leukemia 11:171, 1997.

172. Bertoni, E., Rosati, A., Zanazzi, M., Azzi, A., Zakrzewska, K., Guidi, S., Fanci, R., and Salvadori, M.: Aplastic anemia due to B19 parvovirus infection in cadaveric renal transplant recipients: an underestimated infectious disease in the immunocompromised host. J. Nephrol. 10:152, 1997.

173. Mathias, R.S.: Chronic anemia as a complication of parvovirus B19 infection in pediatric kidney transplant patient. Pediatr. Nephrol. 11:355, 1997.

174. Berner, Y.N., Green, L., and Handzel, Z.T.: Erythroblastopenia in acquired immunodeficiency syndrome (AIDS) [letter]. Acta Haematol. 70:273, 1983.

175. Mintzer, D., and Reilly, R.: Pure red cell aplasia associated with human immunodeficiency virus infection: response to intravenous systemic gammaglobulin [abstract]. Blood 70:124a, 1987.

176. Gottlieb, F., and Deutsch, J.: Red cell aplasia responsive to immunoglobulin therapy as initial manifestation of human immunodeficiency virus infection. Am. J. Med. 92:331, 1992.

177. Zuckerman, M.A., Williams, I., Bremner, J., Cohen, B., and Miller, R.F.: Persistent anaemia in HIV-infected individuals due to parvovirus B19 infection. AIDS 8:1191, 1994.

178. Sallan, S.E., and Buchanan, G.R.: Selective erythroid aplasia during therapy for acute lymphoblastic leukemia. Pediatrics 59:895, 1977.

179. Frickhofen, N., Chen, Z.J., Young, N.S., Cohen, B.J., Heimpel, H., and Abkowitz, J.L.: Parvovirus B19 as a cause of acquired chronic pure red cell aplasia. Br. J. Haematol. 87:818, 1994.

180. Heegaard, E.D., Myhre, J., Hornsleth, A., Gundestrup, M., and Boye, H.: Parvovirus B19 infections in patients with chronic anemia. Haematologica 82:402, 1997.

181. Abkowitz, J.L., Brown, K.E., Wood, R.W., Kovach, N.L., Green, S.W., and Young, N.S.: Clinical relevance of parvovirus B19 as a cause of anemia in patients with human immunodeficiency virus infection. J. Infect. Dis. 176:269, 1997.

182. Gyllensten, K., Sönnerborg, A., Jorup-Rönström, C., Halvarsson, M., and Yun, Z.: Parvovirus B19 infection in HIV-1 infected patients with anemia. Infection 22:356, 1994.

183. Kerr, J.R., Kane, D., Crowley, B., Leonard, N., O'Briain, S., Coyle, P.V., and Mulcahy, F.: Parvovirus B19 infection in AIDS patients. Int. J. STD AIDS 8:184, 1997.

184. Liu, W., Ittmann, M., Liu, J., Schoentag, R., Tierno, P., Greco, M.A., Sidhu, G., Nierodzik, M., and Wieczorek, R.: Human parvovirus B19 in bone marrows from adults with aquired aplastic immunodeficiency syndrome: a comparative study using in situ hybridization and immunohistochemistry. Hum. Pathol. 28:760, 1997.

185. De Renzo, A., Azzi, A., Zakrewska, K., Cicoira, L., Notaro, R., and Rotoli, B.: Cytopenia caused by parvovirus in an adult ALL patient. Haematologica 79:259, 1994.

186. Nigro, G., Gattinara, G.C., Mattia, S., Caniglia, M., and Fridell, E.: Parvovirus-B19–related pancytopenia in children with HIV infection [letter]. Lancet 340:115, 1992.

187. Frickhofen, N., and Young, N.S.: Persistent parvovirus B19 infections in humans. Microb. Pathog. 7:319, 1989.

188. Bowman, C.A., Cohen, B.J., Norfolk, D.R., and Lacey, C.J.N.: Red cell aplasia associated with human parvovirus B19 and HIV infection: failure to respond clinically to intravenous immunoglobulin [letter]. AIDS 4:1038, 1990.

189. Faden, H., Gary, G.W.J., and Anderson, L.J.: Chronic parvovirus infection in a presumably immunologically healthy woman. Clin. Infect. Dis. 15:595, 1992.

190. Sasaki, T., Murai, C., Muryoi, T., Takahashi, Y., Munakata, Y., Sugamura, K., and Abe, K.: Persistent infection of human parvovirus B19 in a normal subject. Lancet 346:851, 1995.

191. Nigro, G., Eufemia, D., Zerbini, M., Krzysztofiak, A., Finocchiaro, R., and Giardini, O.: Parvovirus B19 infection in a hypogammaglobulinemic infant with neurologic disorders and anemia: successful immunoglobulin therapy. Pediatr. Infect. Dis. J. 13:1019, 1994.

192. Ferguson, P.J., Saulsbury, F.T., Dowell, S.F., Török, T.J., Erdman, D.D., and Anderson, L.J.: Prevalence of human parvovirus B19 infection in children with Henoch-Schönlein purpura. Arthritis Rheum. 39:880, 1996.

193. McClain, K., and Mahoney, D.H., Jr.: Lack of evidence for parvovirus B19 viraemia in children with chronic neutropenia [letter]. Br. J. Haematol. 88:895, 1994.

194. Hartman, K.R., Brown, K.E., Green, S.W., and Anderson, S.: Lack of evidence for parvovirus B19 viraemia in children with chronic neutropenia [letter]. Br. J. Haematol. 84:895, 1994.

195. Soderlund, M., von Essen, R., Haapasaari, J., Kiistala, U., Kiviluoto, O., and Hedman, K.: Persistence of parvovirus B19 DNA in synovial membranes of young patients with and without chronic arthopathy. Lancet 349:1063, 1997.

196. Saint-Martin, J., Choulot, J.J., Bonnaud, E., Morinet, F.: Myocarditis caused by parvovirus [letter]. J. Pediatr. 116:1007, 1990.

197. Knisely, A.S., O'Shea, P.A., Anderson, L.J., Jr., and Gary, G.W.: Parvovirus B19 infection myocarditis and death in a 3-year-old boy. Pediatr. Pathol. 8:665, 1996.

198. Malm, C., Fridell, E., and Jansson, K.: Heart failure after parvovirus B19 infection. Lancet 341:1408, 1993.

199. Finkel, T.H., Török, T.J., Ferguson, P.J., Durigon, E.L., Zaki, S.R., Leung, D.Y.M., Harbeck, R.J., Gelfand, E.W., Saulsbury, F.T., Hollister, J.R., and Anderson, L.J.: Chronic parvovirus B19 infection and systemic necrotising vasculitis: opportunistic infection or aetiological agent? Lancet 343:1255, 1994.

200. Langnas, A.N., Markin, R.S., Cattral, M.S., and Naides, S.J.: Parvovirus B19 as a possible causative agent of fulminant liver failure and associated aplastic anemia. Hepatology 22:1661, 1995.

201. Jacobson, S.K., Daly, J.S., Thorne, G.M., and McIntosh, K.: Clinical parvovirus B19 infection resulting in chronic fatigue syndrome: case history and review. Clin. Infect. Dis. 24:1048, 1997.

202. Kasuga, A., Harada, R., and Saruta, T.: Insulin-dependent diabetes mellitus associated with parvovirus B19 infection. Ann. Intern. Med. 125:700, 1996.

203. Kajigaya, S., and Momoeda, M.: Immune response to B19 infection. In Anderson, L.J., and Young, N.S. (eds.): Human Parvovirus B19. Basel, Karger, 1997, p. 120.

204. Anderson, L.J., Tsou, C., Parker, R.A., Chorba, T.L., Wulff, H., Tattersall, P., and Mortimer, P.P.: Detection of antibodies and antigens of human parvovirus B19 by enzyme-linked immunosorbent assay. J. Clin. Microbiol. 24:522, 1986.

205. Ang, H.A., Apperley, J.F., and Ward, K.N.: Persistence of antibody to human parvovirus B19 after allogeneic bone marrow transplantation: role of prior recipient immunity. Blood 89:4646, 1997.

206. Erdman, D.D., Usher, M.J., Tsou, C., Caul, E.O., Gary, G.W., Kajigaya, S., Young, N.S., and Anderson, L.J.: Human parvovirus B19 specific IgG, IgA, and IgM antibodies and DNA in serum specimens from persons with erythema infectiosum. J. Med. Virol. 35:110, 1991.

207. Kurtzman, G., Cohen, R., Field, A.M., Oseas, R., Blaese, R.M., and Young, N.: The immune response to B19 parvovirus infection and an antibody defect in persistent viral infection. J. Clin. Invest. 84:1114, 1989.

208. von Poblotzki, A., Gerdes, C., Reiscl, U., Wolf, H., and Modrow, S.: Lymphoproliferative responses after infection with human parvovirus B19. J. Virol. 70:7327, 1996.

209. Jacoby, R.O., Johnson, E.A., Paturzo, F.X., Gaertner, D.J., Brandsma, J.L., and Smith, A.L.: Persistent rat parvovirus infection in individually housed rats. Arch. Virol. 117:193, 1991.

210. Rimmelzwaan, G.F., Van der Heijden, R.W.J., Tijhaar, E., Poelen, M.C.M., Carlson, J., Osterhaus, A.D.M.E., and UytdeHaag, F.G.C.M.: Establishment and characterization of canine parvovirus-specific murine CD4+ T cell clones and their use for the delineation of T cell epitopes. J. Gen. Virol. 71:1095, 1990.

211. Alexandersen, S., Bloom, M.E., and Perryman, S.: Nucleotide sequence and genomic organization of Aleutian mink disease parvovirus (ADV): sequence comparisons between a nonpathogenic and a pathogenic strain. J. Virol. 62:2903, 1988.

212. Tattersall, P., and Bratton, J.: Reciprocal productive and restrictive virus-cell interactions of immunosuppressive and prototype strains of minute virus of mice. J. Virol. 46:944, 1983.

213. Harding, M.J., and Molitor, T.: Porcine parvovirus: replication in and inhibition of selected cellular functions of swine alveolar macrophages and peripheral blood lymphocytes. Arch. Virol. 101:105, 1988.

214. Carlson, J.H., Scott, F.W., and Duncan, J.R.: Feline panleukopenia III. Development of lesions in the lymphoid tissue. Vet. Pathol. 15:383, 1978.

215. Porter, D.D., and Larsen, A.E.: Mink parvovirus infections. In Tijssen, P. (ed.): Handbook of Parvoviruses. Vol. 2. Boca Raton, FL, CRC Press, 1990, p. 87.

216. Yoshimoto, K., Rosenfeld, S., Frickhofen, N., Kennedy, D., Kajigaya, S., and Young, N.S.: A second neutralizing epitope of B19 parvovirus implicates the spike region in the immune response. J. Virol. 65:7056, 1991.

217. Sato, H., Hirata, J., Kuroda, N., Shiraki, H., Maeda, Y., and Okochi, K.: Identification and mapping of neutralizing epitopes of human parvovirus B19 by using human antibodies. J. Virol. 65:5845, 1991.

218. Sato, H., Hirata, J., Furukawa, M., Kuroda, N., Shiraki, H., Maeda, Y., and Okochi, K.: Identification of the region including the epitope for a monoclonal antibody which can neutralize human parvovirus B19. J. Virol. 65:1667, 1991.

219. Rosenfeld, S.R., Yoshimoto, K., Anderson, S., Kajigaya, S., Young, N.S., Warrener, P., Bonsal, G., and Collett, M.: The unique region of the minor capsid protein of human parvovirus B19 is exposed on the virion surface. J. Clin. Invest. 89:2023, 1992.

220. Rosenfeld, S.J., Kajigaya, S., Young, N.S., Ayub, J., and Saxinger, C.: Subunit interaction in B19 parvovirus empty capsids. Arch. Virol. 136:9, 1994.

221. Saikawa, T., Momoeda, M., Anderson, S., Kajigaya, S., and Young, N.S.: Neutralizing linear epitopes of B19 parvovirus cluster in the VP1 unique and VP1-VP2 junction region. J. Virol. 67:3004, 1993.

222. Anderson, S., Momoeda, M., Kawase, M., Kajigaya, S., and Young, N.S.: Peptides derived from the unique region of B19 parvovirus minor capsid protein elicit neutralizing antibodies in rabbits. Virology 206:626, 1995.

223. Kawase, M., Momoeda, M., Young, N.S., and Kajigaya, S.: Most of the VP1 unique region of B19 parvovirus is located on the capsid surface. Virology 211:359, 1995.

224. Miyamura, K., Kajigaya, S., Momoeda, M., Young, N.S., and Smith-Gill, S.J.: Parvovirus particles as platform for protein presentation. Proc. Natl. Acad. Sci. USA 91:8507, 1994.

225. Cohen, B.J., Buckley, M.M., and Clewley, P.J.: Human parvovirus infection in early rheumatoid and inflammatory arthritis. Ann. Rheum. Dis. 45:832, 1986.

226. Vigeant, P., Ménard, H.-A., and Boire, G.: Chronic modulation of the autoimmune response following parvovirus B19 infection. J. Rheumatol. 21:1165, 1995.

227. Soloninka, C.A., Anderson, M.J., and Laskin, C.A.: Anti-DNA and antilymphocyte antibodies during acute infection with human parvovirus B19. J. Rheumatol. 16:777, 1989.

228. Meunier, P.C., Cooper, B.J., Appel, M.J.G., Lanieu, M.E., and Slauson, D.O.: Pathogenesis of canine parvovirus enteritis: sequential virus distribution and passive immunization studies. Vet. Pathol. 22:617, 1985.

229. Takahashi, M., Koike, T., Moriyama, Y., and Shibata, A.: Neutralizing activity of immunoglobulin preparation against erythropoietic suppression of human parvovirus [letter]. Am. J. Hematol. 37:68, 1991.

230. Davis, E.V., Gregory, G.G., and Beckenhauer, W.H.: Infectious feline panleukopenia. Developmental report of a tissue culture origin formalin-inactivated vaccine. Vet. Med. Small Anim. Clin. 65:237, 1970.

231. Pye, D., Bates, J., Edwards, S.J., and Hollingworth, J.: Development of a vaccine preventing parvovirus-induced reproductive failure in pigs. Aust. Vet. J. 67:179, 1979.

232. Rimmelzwaan, G.F., Carlson, J., UytdeHaag, F.G., and Osterhaus, A.D.: A synthetic peptide derived from the amino acid sequence of canine parvovirus structural proteins which defines a B cell epitope and elicits antiviral antibody in BALB c mice. J. Gen. Virol. 71:2741, 1990.

233. Langeveld, J.P.M., Casal, J.I., Cortés, E., van de Wetering, G., Boshuizen, R.S., Schaaper, W.M.M., Dalsgaard, K., and Meloen, R.H.: Effective induction of neutralizing antibodies with the amino terminus of VP2 of canine parvovirus as a synthetic peptide. Vaccines 12:1473, 1994.

234. Bansal, G.P., Hatfield, J., Dunn, F.E., Warrener, P., Young, J.F., Top, F.H., Collett, M.C., Anderson, S., Rosenfeld, S., Kajigaya, S., and Young, N.S.: Immunogenicity studies of recombinant human parvovirus B19 proteins. Vaccines 167:1034, 1992.

Retroviruses (HTLVs)

Mitsuaki Yoshida

▼ ▼

Introduction to Retroviruses

▼ GENERAL DESCRIPTION

Retroviruses constitute a unique family of RNA viruses that contain reverse transcriptase, which on infection transcribes genomic RNA into DNA. The cores of the viral particles contain, in addition to genomic RNA, Gag protein and reverse transcriptase. Enveloping the core is a membrane, similar to the plasma membrane of host cells, on which viral Env (envelope) glycoprotein is exposed. The interaction of Env protein with a receptor on a target cell is required for infection. On infection, the RNA genome is reverse-transcribed into DNA, which is then integrated into host cell DNA by covalent linkage to form proviral DNA. The proviral genomes can be maintained in infected cells as cellular DNA sequences whether or not viral replication occurs.

Rous sarcoma virus was found in transmissible sarcomas of chickens in 1910. Since then, retroviruses have been isolated from many species of animals, and those from mice and chickens have been investigated extensively. The viruses may be transmitted in two ways: horizontally from host to host by replication and infection (exogenous viruses) and vertically to successive generations of hosts by transmission of proviral genomes through germ cells (endogenous viruses). Studies of retroviruses, of wide interest because of their tumorigenic properties, have led to the discovery of oncogenes. Retroviruses have also been of interest in connection with autoimmune and various neurological diseases.

▼ VIRAL REPLICATION

The viral particle contains two copies of a single-stranded, positive RNA, which is dimerized in the 5′ region. After incorporation of a viral particle by a cell, the reverse transcriptase in the viral core reverse-transcribes the genomic RNA to complementary DNA (cDNA) (Fig. 28–16). The cDNA is then converted to double-stranded DNA and integrated into the host's chromosomal DNA. The integrated DNA, or "provirus," has a repeating sequence (long terminal repeat [LTR]) at both ends, which contains many elements essential to viral gene expression and replication. Details of the mechanism of replication have been presented elsewhere.[1]

Integrated proviruses are transcribed by the cellular machinery, the integration itself being necessary for retroviral gene expression and replication. A subpopulation of the viral transcripts is spliced into subgenomic mRNA, and both spliced and unspliced RNAs are translated into viral proteins. The genomic RNA (unspliced RNA) and viral proteins are assembled at specific sites under the plasma membrane, and the particles are released from cells by budding. In general, retroviral replication is not especially harmful to cells, and infected cells can commonly be used to establish virus-producing cell lines. The integrated proviruses are stable and are transmitted to daughter cells whether or not the proviral genome is expressed.

Retroviruses can infect a wide range of cellular types in vitro. The receptors for a few retroviruses have been identified as membrane proteins,[2, 3] and their expression in many types of cells is consistent with the array of cells at risk of retroviral infection. The receptors for most viruses have not been identified, however. In contrast to the broad specificity

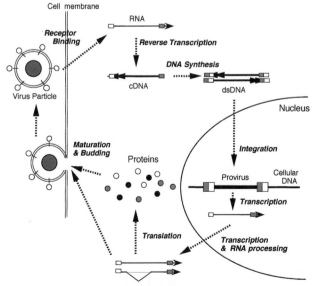

Figure 28–16. Replication cycle of retroviruses. Open and closed boxes at the termini of the RNA and proviral genomes stand for the U5 and U3 sequences, respectively, and the fused sequences at both termini of the proviral genome are the long terminal repeats.

of retroviral infection, the viruses are able to induce tumors in relatively few tissues.

▼ GENOMIC STRUCTURES

All retroviruses can be placed in one of two groups, dependent on whether they carry host-derived oncogenes (Fig. 28–17; see reference 1). Retroviruses not containing oncogenes are generally competent in replication and have *gag*, *pol*, and *env* genes in their genomes. Because they can induce leukemia or lymphoma after a long period of latency, these viruses are called chronic leukemia viruses. For a long time, the question of how retroviruses without oncogenes could induce tumors was perplexing, but it is now established that LTRs at the proviral termini activate expression of adjacent cellular genes. When by chance a provirus is integrated in the vicinity of a proto-oncogene, tumorigenesis follows. This "promoter-insertion mechanism of viral carcinogenesis" operates in a variety of tumor systems, as exemplified by *myc* activation by avian leukemia virus (ALV) in B-cell lymphoma,[4] *erb* B activation by ALV in chicken erythroblastosis,[5] and *int*1 and *int*2 activation by mouse mammary tumor virus in mouse mammary tumors.[6] The enhancer/promoter in the LTR is responsible for gene activation, and thus integration of the provirus into certain regions is sufficient for activation of a cellular proto-oncogene.[7] Because proviral integration is not site specific, repeated integration through viral replication is usually required before the provirus appears in a tumorigenic site. This explains the long period of latency between infection and tumorigenesis.

The second group of retroviruses carry an oncogene acquired from a cellular proto-oncogene.[1] In the acquisition of this oncogene, a portion of the RNA composing the *gag*,

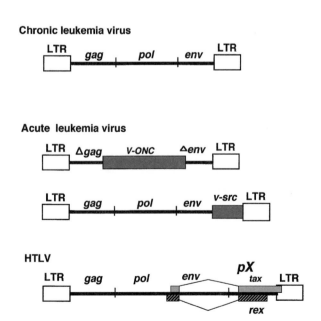

Figure 28–17. Genomic structure of retroviruses. The constitutions of the genomes are illustrated in the provirus DNA forms. The open boxes are the long terminal repeats, and the closed boxes are the viral oncogenes that were acquired from the cellular genes. Those of the HTLV genome, however, are specific to the viruses.

pol, and *env* genes is deleted. Consequently, acute sarcoma/leukemia viruses are generally replication defective, and they must infect cells in company with a chronic leukemia virus, which acts as a "helper" in replication. One exception is Rous sarcoma virus, which has the oncogene *src* between *env* and the 3′ LTR. The acute leukemia viruses transform cells using the protein encoded by the viral oncogene. Thus, cellular transformation requires viral gene expression but not viral replication or site-specific integration, and tumor development is rapidly induced. The tissue specificity of retroviral tumorigenesis is restricted by either the class of oncogene in the viral genome or the promoter activity of the integrated LTR, as well as by the nature of the viral receptors of the host cells.

Human Retroviruses

Retroviruses have been recognized in a variety of animals, but only recently have they been isolated from humans. The human T-cell leukemia virus (HTLV), human immunodeficiency virus (HIV), human endogenous viruses, and human foamy viruses are distributed among four groups of retroviruses. I review here the replication and pathology of HTLV and related viruses, with particular attention devoted to HTLV-1. With some exception, observations on HTLV-1 are applicable to other members of the HTLV group.

▼ HTLVs AND DISEASES

Human T-cell leukemia virus type 1 (HTLV-1) is the etiological agent in adult T-cell leukemia (ATL).[8, 9] ATL was first described in 1977 in Japan[10] as a unique T-cell malignant neoplasm (see Pathogenesis). The clustering of patients with this disease in Kyushu and Shikoku in southwestern Japan strongly suggested an infectious agent. The human retrovirus HTLV was reported in the United States in 1980 after characterization of reverse transcriptase in cultured T cells established from a T-cell lymphoma.[11] Establishment of a T-cell line with use of cells from an ATL patient was achieved independently in Japan by cocultivation of cord blood lymphocytes and peripheral lymphocytes from an ATL patient.[12, 13] In these cultures, retrovirus-like particles were detected at the outer cell membrane of T cells. Furthermore, the sera of ATL patients were found to contain antibodies that reacted specifically with the cell line established from the ATL patient.[14] These early observations, soon confirmed by extensive epidemiological studies,[15, 16] suggested that a *human retrovirus* existed in association with ATL. Direct proof of the presence of a retrovirus in ATL patients and its relationship to the patients' antibodies was obtained through characterization of the viral genome[17–19] and seroepidemiological surveys.[14, 20] Because the viral genome has an extra sequence, pX, in addition to the *gag*, *pol*, and *env* genes, HTLV was classified as a distinct type of retrovirus[19] (see Fig. 28–17).

After characterization of HTLV, another virus, HTLV-2, immunologically similar to the known HTLV (HTLV-1) retrovirus, was isolated from a patient with hairy T-cell leukemia.[21, 22] Identical over about 60 per cent of their genomic sequences,[23] HTLV-1 and HTLV-2 are clearly distinct.

HTLV-2 has been isolated from only three patients with hairy T-cell leukemia, and its association with this disease may be fortuitous.

An animal virus similar to HTLV-1, simian T-cell leukemia virus (STLV), was isolated from various species of non-human primates,[24, 25] including the Japanese macaque, African green monkey, pig-tailed macaque, gorilla, and chimpanzee. The STLVs share a 90 to 95 per cent identity of genomic sequence with HTLV-1 and are also similar to each other.[26] In some colonies of Japanese macaques, 60 to 70 per cent of all individuals are STLV positive, whereas in other, sometimes neighboring colonies, virtually all animals are STLV negative. Although STLV is widely distributed in monkeys, no typically leukemic animals have been observed. A few cases of a leukemia-like disease have been noted in STLV-infected monkeys,[27] but an etiological connection between STLV and disease remains to be established.

Another member of the HTLV group is bovine leukemia virus (BLV).[28] This virus infects and replicates in B cells of cows and induces B-cell lymphoma. BLV also infects lymphocytes of sheep and induces leukemia in these animals after a short latent period.

▼ EPIDEMIOLOGY

The sera of nearly all ATL patients contain circulating antibodies to HTLV-1 proteins.[14] These antibodies are easily detected by indirect immunostaining of cells infected with HTLV-1, by enzyme-linked immunosorbent assay (ELISA), by a particle agglutination assay, or by Western blotting. HTLV-1 antibodies are also detectable in some healthy adults[15, 16]; such asymptomatic, seropositive individuals are defined as carriers of the virus. In fact, HTLV-1 can be isolated from them by the establishment of infected cell lines.[29] With use of the polymerase chain reaction (PCR), HTLV-1 DNA sequences in circulating lymphocytes can be detected in nearly all seropositive people. Thus, antibodies to HTLV-1 proteins are reliable indicators of HTLV-1 infection and replication.

Geographical Clustering. HTLV-1 antibodies are present in 5 to 15 per cent of adults clustered in southwestern Japan,[15] the Caribbean islands and South America,[16] Central Africa,[30] and Papua New Guinea and the Solomon Islands in Melanesia[31] (Fig. 28–18). However, the prevalence of healthy, seropositive adults varies significantly by version and even from village to village within endemic areas. For example, in a given isolated island in Kyushu, Japan, 30 to 40 per cent of people older than 40 years might be infected, whereas the prevalence may be far lower on a neighboring island.[32] Significantly, the diseases ATL and HAM/TSP (see HAM/TSP and Other Diseases) are also clustered and overlap HTLV-1 in distribution. ATL patients and healthy carriers are found sporadically all over the world, but most live in or have moved from areas of endemicity. These epidemiological findings indicate a close association of HTLV-1 with ATL and HAM/TSP. In the case of ATL, it has been proposed that infection by HTLV-1 early in life is of significance to the later development of leukemia.

HTLV-2 is frequently isolated in the United States from intravenous drug abusers and persons infected with HIV,[33] but its pathogenic relation is not clear. HTLV-2 was recently

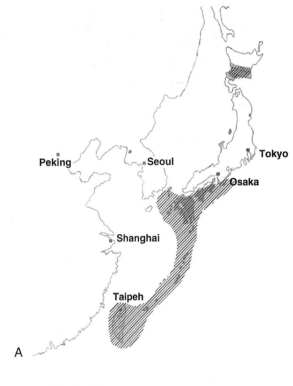

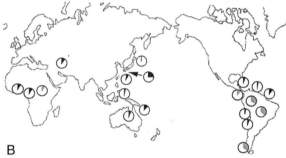

Figure 28–18. Geographical distribution of HTLV-1 in Japan *(A)* and the distribution of seroprevalence rate of antibodies to HTLV-1 (black) and HTLV-2 (gray) in the world scale *(B)*. (*B* reconstructed from the original by Tajima, K.: Worldwide distribution of HTLV. Jpn. J. Cancer Res. 89:cover page, 1998; with permission.)

found to be endemic in South America,[34-36] particularly clustering in the highlands, and also among the Pygmy in Africa.[37] HTLV-2 might have been maintained in these areas until today's spreading into the United States and European countries. Infections with HTLV types 1 and 2 are mutually exclusive in these endemic areas.

Age-Dependent Prevalence. The prevalence of virus carriers increases between 20 and 40 to 50 years of age, reaching a maximum between 50 and 60 years. The prevalence is 1.6 times higher in women than in men (Fig. 28–19). The increased prevalence in adulthood in women is attributed to sexual transmission of HTLV-1 from husbands to wives, but transmission from wives to husbands is infrequent.

The age-dependent increase of antibody prevalence was somewhat mysterious. Cohort studies in islands in Japan during 10 years revealed that seroconversion of adults from antibody-negative to positives is rare except among wives

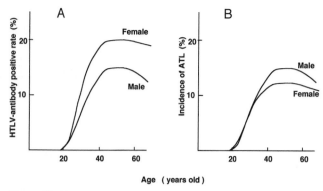

Figure 28–19. Schematic illustration of seropositive rates (A) and incidence of ATL (B) as a function of age. Increases of antibodies to HTLV-1 and the incidence of ATL are in parallel, but their relative ratios are different between men and women. The seropositive rate before 20 years of age is not zero.

of positive husbands and does not explain the drastic increase of seroprevalence in the population around 40 to 50 years old.[38] It is now accepted that the age-dependent increase is due to the reduction of infection risk at an early stage of lives.[38] Artificial milk started to be popular around 40 years ago in these areas in Japan and thus reduced the incidence of breast milk–borne infection of HTLV-1.

Familial Aggregation. HTLV-1 infection was frequently observed in family members: spouse and sisters and brothers. Although the familial aggregation was originally believed to indicate a genetic predisposition to HTLV-1 infection, viral transmission from husband to wife through semen and mother to child through breast milk is the more likely explanation.

Genomic Stability. Molecular analyses demonstrated that the viral genome is well conserved in Japan and the Caribbean area.[39] Viral isolates from Africa and Papua New Guinea show only limited variation.[31] Retroviral genomes are thought to be unstable relative to those of other viruses owing to reverse transcription. The stability of HTLV-1 is in sharp contrast to the highly labile genome of HIV. Genomic conservation may be selected to the low replicative competency of HTLV-1 in vivo.[40]

Nevertheless, the HTLV-1 genome is highly variable within infected individuals.[41–43] The viral sequences of the pX and LTR isolated from individuals show various base substitutions and multiple clones within a single individual. In most carriers and HAM/TSP patients, more than half of the independent clones are variants, and mutations are almost random in type and position.[42] On the other hand, clones isolated from ATL patients do not show such sequence variation, probably reflecting the clonal expansion of leukemic cells in ATL patients. The genome of HTLV-1, therefore, mutates frequently during viral replication in vivo, but these variants appear not to be efficiently transmitted to recipients. Neither the mechanism responsible for high mutation rates nor preferential transmission of the prototype is well understood.

▼ HTLV-1 INFECTION AND EXPRESSION

In Vitro Infection and Transformation

Cell-free viral particles of HTLV-1 have extremely low infectivity in vitro. However, cocultivation with virus-produc-

ing cells can result in transmission of HTLV-1 to a variety of human cells (Fig. 28–20; see references 12 and 13), including T and B lymphocytes, fibroblasts, and epithelial cells, as well as cells from monkeys, rats,[44] rabbits,[45] and hamsters. In infected cells, the provirus is integrated into random sites in the chromosomal DNA, and most of the viral genes are expressed. However, in non–T cell lines, the integrated provirus is latent and viral genes are silent. HTLV-1 infection in culture usually induces the fusion of many infected cells to form syncytia.

Only T cells with the CD4+ marker are immortalized on infection of peripheral blood cells with HTLV-1.[12, 13, 46] Immortalized cells express high levels of the α chain of the interleukin-2 (IL-2) receptor (IL-2Rα)[47] and proliferate in an IL-2–dependent fashion. Furthermore, established cell lines tend to acquire IL-2–independent growth. Phenotypes of the cells immortalized in vitro mimic those of leukemic cells in vivo to some extent[48] (see Adult T-Cell Leukemia). Immortalization by HTLV-1 appears unique to this virus[49]; animal retroviruses that do not carry an oncogene neither immortalize nor transform cells in vitro. Because immortalization of T cells by HTLV-2 and STLV has been reported, this profound effect on proliferation may be a general property conferred on T cells by HTLVs. A contribution of pX to immortalization has been proposed.

In Vivo Transmission

Despite the broad range of cell types that can be infected in vitro by HTLV-1, cells of both ATL patients and asymptomatic viral carriers infected in vivo are almost exclusively T cells with the CD4+ phenotype (see Fig. 28–20). These infected cells, irrespective of whether they are leukemic, do

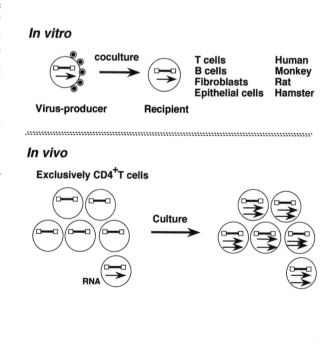

Figure 28–20. Comparison of HTLV-1 infection and expression in vivo and in vitro. In vitro transmission requires cocultivation with virus-producing cells. Infected cells in vivo are mostly CD4+ T cells, but not expressing the viral genome.

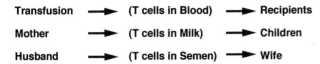

Figure 28–21. Transmission of HTLV-1 in three major pathways. In these pathways, transfer of infected living cells into recipients is essential for efficient viral transmission.

not express viral information—even as RNA—at significant levels.[40] They can express their viral genes after several hours' culture in vitro,[50] demonstrating that the latency in vivo is not a function of a defect in the integrated provirus. By reverse-PCR for mRNA, more than 99 per cent of infected cells fail to express viral genes in vivo.[42] It was previously suspected that viral gene suppression is linked to the lack of replication of infected T cells in peripheral blood. However, no significant viral expression is demonstrable in either enlarged lymph nodes or skin lesions in which some populations of malignant cells are dividing.[51]

Viral transmission can occur through blood transfusion, the sharing of contaminated needles by intravenous drug abusers, nursing of infants by infected mothers, and sexual relations (Fig. 28–21).

Blood Transfusion. HTLV-1 is readily transmitted by blood cell products. Retrospective studies of blood transfusions showed that 60 to 70 per cent of recipients of fresh, seropositive blood were infected with HTLV-1.[52] No recipients of fresh, seropositive plasma were infected, indicating that the transfer of infected cells from donor to recipient is required for viral transmission, analogous to in vitro infectivity. Surprisingly, HTLV-1 infection acquired through transfusion seems not to induce ATL (see Sexual Transmission, below) but can cause HAM/TSP.[53] Therefore, exclusion of HTLV-1–positive blood in the blood bank can protect against both HTLV-1 infection and development of HAM/TSP.

Intravenous Drug Abuse. In some areas of the United States and Jamaica,[54] HTLV-1 antibodies have been found in up to 20 per cent of intravenous drug abusers as the result of the sharing of unsterilized needles. Surprisingly, PCR studies of DNA indicate that a large proportion of the infecting viruses were HTLV-2.

Mother to Child. Viral transmission from mother to child was originally suggested by epidemiological evidence; most mothers of seropositive children were carriers of the virus, and about 30 per cent of the children of infected mothers were themselves seropositive.[55–57] Neonatal infection was initially suspected, but surveys of lymphocytes in cord blood samples from a large number of children born to seropositive mothers have excluded this possibility. Instead, breast milk is the likely source of transmissible virus.[56, 57] Milk taken from seropositive mothers and given to adult marmosets leads to the appearance of antibodies in these monkeys,[58] and cessation of breast-feeding by seropositive mothers has drastically reduced the seroconversion rates of their children (see Prevention of HTLV-1 Infection).

Sexual Transmission. Wives with seropositive husbands are usually seropositive. However, the husbands of seropositive wives show the same antibody frequency as do other men of the region. From these data, it is likely that virus is transmitted from husband to wife but not from wife

to husband.[32] Infected T cells found in semen from men infected with HTLV-1 probably transmit virus. Epidemiological studies show that the rate of seropositivity is higher in women than in men, but the sex-specific incidence of ATL does not mirror this difference; HTLV-1 infections sexually transmitted to women are thought not to lead to development of ATL (see Fig. 28–19).

▼ MOLECULAR BIOLOGY OF HTLV-1 GENE EXPRESSION

HTLV-1 Genome

The HTLV-1 proviral genome was cloned from leukemic cell DNA acquired from an ATL patient,[18, 19] and the complete nucleotide sequence was determined.[19] The proviral genome is 9032 bp long and contains, in common with other retroviruses, *gag*, *pol*, and *env* genes and 3′ and 5′ LTRs. The presence of a so-called pX region on the 3′ side of the *env* gene distinguishes the HTLV-1 genome from those of other retroviruses (see Fig. 28–17). In recognition of this distinction, HTLV-1 is placed into a distinct group of pX-bearing retroviruses that includes HTLV-2, STLV, and BLV. The pX sequence is not, like retroviral oncogenes, of cellular origin but a virus-specific sequence essential to replication.

Retroviral LTRs regulate viral gene expression and replication. The pX region of HTLV contains additional, overlapping, regulatory genes (Fig. 28–22): *tax*, *rex*, and a gene whose function remains unknown. The products of the genes are p40[tax],[59–62] p27[rex],[63, 64] and p21[x].[51, 63, 64] The Tax protein, or p40[tax], is a *trans*-activator of proviral transcriptional initiation[65–68] and is essential to viral gene expression and replication. The Tax protein also *trans*-activates transcription of some cellular genes associated with T-cell proliferation[69] (see below). The second protein, p27[rex], is a *trans*-acting modulator of RNA processing, which induces unspliced *gag* and *env* mRNAs.[70, 71] Without *rex* gene function, all HTLV-1 transcripts are doubly spliced into an mRNA encoding Tax and Rex proteins,[72] effectively preventing production of viral structural proteins. Thus, Rex is also essential for HTLV-1 gene expression and replication. A protein of unknown function, p21[x],[64] is composed of the same sequence as the C-terminal portion of p27[rex]. The regulatory system in HTLVs is unique, operating at the levels of transcription and RNA

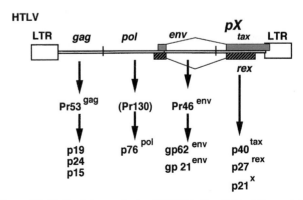

Figure 28–22. Protein products of HTLV-1. Gag, Pol, and Env proteins are processed from the precursors, and the pX proteins are encoded by independent genes overlapping in the pX sequence.

processing and exerting control of both qualitative and quantitative aspects of gene expression.[72] They have similarities to the Tat and Rev systems of HIV, which are also essential for viral replication.[73, 74]

The pX sequence also possibly encodes various proteins when the sequence is alternatively spliced.[75, 76] Some of these products were characterized by use of expression vectors.[77] However, these protein products have yet to be identified in infected cells or cell lines, and therefore their physiological significance is unknown.

Transcription

Retroviral LTR sequences lie at both termini of the integrated proviral genome and contain elements needed for efficient transcriptional initiation and termination: a TATA box, a transcriptional enhancer, and a poly(A) signal, all of which consist of short nucleotide sequences. Because these elements are recognized by cellular transcriptional factors for RNA polymerase II, expression of the retrovirus depends on the cellular machinery of the host.

In addition to LTR-associated regulators, HTLV-1 contains the *tax* gene, which acts in *trans* to stimulate viral transcription.[65–68] *Trans*-activation of the LTR by the Tax protein increases viral gene expression more than 200-fold. *Trans*-activation requires a transcriptional enhancer in the LTR, which is composed of three direct repeats of a 21 bp sequence[78–81] containing an imperfect cyclic adenosine monophosphate (cAMP) response element (CRE) (Fig. 28–23). Tax is a protein containing a zinc finger motif,[82] but it does not bind directly to the 21 bp sequence. Perhaps Tax interacts with a cellular protein that then binds to enhancer DNA to mediate *trans*-activation of viral transcription. The viral Tax is essential for an efficient viral replication.

Tax activates cellular as well as viral genes[69, 83] (see Fig. 28–23), including the genes for IL-2,[69] IL-2Rα,[69] granulocyte-macrophage colony-stimulating factor (GM-CSF),[84] the proto-oncogenes c-*fos*[85] and c-*jun*,[86] and the genes for parathyroid hormone–related protein (PTHrP)[87] and major histocompatibility complex class I antigen.[88] These mechanisms of the *trans*-activation and their implication are discussed later (see Molecular Biology of Pathogenesis).

RNA Processing

Although *trans*-activation by Tax might lead one to expect an efficient replication, HTLV-1 replication is highly restricted in vivo. This restriction is, in part, a function of the *rex* gene, the second pX gene.[71, 72] For replication of HTLV-1, three species of HTLV-1 mRNA are required: genomic (unspliced) RNA as *gag* and *pol* mRNA; a 4.2 kb, singly spliced, subgenomic RNA as *env* mRNA; and a 2.1 kb, doubly spliced mRNA for the expression of Tax and Rex proteins. A certain balance of expression of these three unspliced and spliced mRNAs is essential to efficient HTLV replication.[89] The process for expression differs from host cell mRNA, in which splicing is not generally a means of regulation of the expression levels but is of qualitative alteration. In the quantitative regulation of viral mRNA, expression is controlled post-transcriptionally by p27[rex] (Fig. 28–24).

A defect in the proviral *rex* gene leads to production of completely spliced *tax/rex* mRNA,[72] whereas expression of additional *rex* genes complements the defect, instituting production of *gag* and *env* mRNAs. Clearly, Rex protein is required for the expression of unspliced mRNA and production of viral structural proteins, and therefore Rex is essential to viral replication. In return, the activity of Rex reduces the level of spliced mRNA that encodes regulatory proteins, a reduction resulting in a lower level of Tax protein and, eventually, viral transcription. Thus, Rex produces a *trans*-acting positive signal for the expression of viral structural proteins but a negative signal for total viral gene expression. In short, Rex exerts feedback control of viral gene expression. Because Tax and Rex are encoded by a single species of spliced mRNA, activation by Tax is always followed by the negative effect of Rex.

The mechanism by which Rex functions is not clearly understood. Rex requires a *cis*-acting element (RxRE) consisting of 205 nucleotides located in the 3′ region of the viral RNA[90] (see Fig. 28–23). The unique secondary structure of this element allows Rex protein to bind to it. A nuclear export signal in Rex protein[91] suggests transport of Rex/RNA complex into the cytoplasm irrespective of RNA processing. However, Rex seems to exert its influence not only through simple activation of nuclear transport. First, Rex can induce unspliced RNA of some constructs even in the nucleus.[92] Second, the action of Rex is affected by mutations in the splicing signals that do not contribute to nuclear transport of RNA.[92] These observations suggest that some process

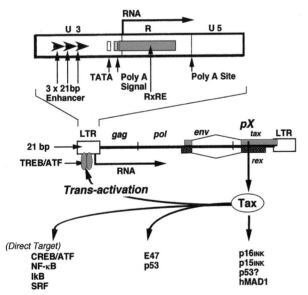

Figure 28–23. Summary of pleiotropic function of Tax protein. Elements for *trans*-activation and *trans*-repression of the viral genome are summarized above the viral genome, and effects on cellular targets are listed under the arrows from Tax.

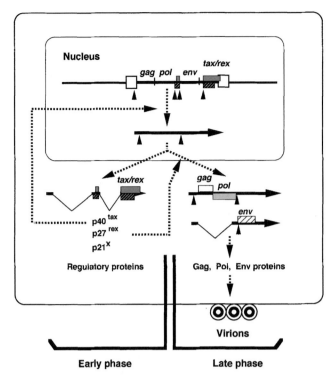

Figure 28–24. RNA processing of HTLV-1 transcripts and the effects of Tax and Rex on expression. Tax activates transcription of the genome into RNA, and Rex induces *gag* and *env* mRNA, reducing *tax/rex* mRNA.

operating in the nucleus before transport may also be a target for Rex regulation. Confusing the issue is the fact that the effect of Rex may vary, depending on the RNA construct used in the analysis.[92]

HIV has a gene, *rev*, strikingly similar in function to *rex* in HTLV-1.[73] In the HIV system, Rev binds to RvRE, which has a unique secondary structure[93] and is found in the *env* coding sequence.[94] Binding of Rev is thought to activate transport of unspliced RNA to the cytoplasm.[95] Surprisingly, Rex can also interact with HIV RvRE to regulate HIV gene expression,[96] thus indicating that similar mechanisms are involved in the regulation of RNA processing by Rex and Rev.

Trans-Regulation of Viral Replication

The combination of the two regulatory genes *tax* and *rex* produces time-dependent positive and negative effects: Tax regulates viral transcription, then Rex modulates expression of subgenomic mRNA species at the level of RNA processing and, finally, represses the expression of Tax. This unique regulatory system in the HTLV group is required for the replication and survival of this type of virus.

The initial genetic expression of HTLV produces Tax, which *trans*-activates transcription, causing proviral DNA in the cell to further enhance its own expression. The accumulated Rex protein induces expression of unspliced mRNA, leading to an abundance of mRNA molecules and maximal production of viral antigens, which are targets of the host's immune response, before the negative regulation by Rex becomes effective (see Fig. 28–24). Sequential regulation by

tax and *rev* leads to transient viral replication, and infected cells can escape the host's immunological defenses. The cellular factors involved in long periods of latency have not been identified.

Some cell lines infected in vitro with HTLV-1 do express viral genes efficiently.[11, 12, 17] These established cell lines usually contain multiple copies (generally 10 or so) of defective proviruses,[39] in some of which expression of Tax is insensitive to suppression by Rex. Thus, disrupted Tax/Rex regulation accounts for continuous expression of viral proteins, one of which, Tax, is probably essential for in vitro immortalization of infected T cells. Accordingly, the presence of many defective proviruses and efficient viral expression in established T-cell lines are explained. Other retroviruses do not have the equivalent of the *tax/rex* gene, and regulation of their genetic expression is effected by unknown mechanisms.

▼ PATHOGENESIS

Adult T-Cell Leukemia

Clinical Features

The onset of ATL is observed in individuals between 20 and 70 years of age, with the peak rate in middle age (40 to 60 years)[97] (see Fig. 28–19). The male to female incidence ratio is 1.4:1. Symptoms vary from patient to patient. Frequent are skin lesions, lymphadenopathy, hepatomegaly and splenomegaly, and infiltration of leukemic cells into the lungs and other organs.[97] Antibodies to HTLV-1 proteins are commonly present in serum, as are increased levels of serum lactate dehydrogenase and hypercalcemia.

In addition to the typical, acute form of ATL, smoldering, chronic, and acute (lymphoma-associated) types have been recognized.[97] In smoldering ATL, patients commonly have one to several percentages of morphologically abnormal T cells in their peripheral blood but do not show other signs of severe illness and are thus thought to be in an early stage of ATL development. The abnormal cells are not aggressively malignant but are HTLV-1 infected and expanded clonally. Some patients with chronic ATL have high levels of HTLV-1–infected leukemic cells but can remain asymptomatic for some time. Their leukemic cells also carry clonally integrated HTLV-1 proviruses. The acute form or phase of ATL is aggressive and resistant to treatment; consequently, most patients with acute ATL die within 6 months of onset.

ATL Cells

Leukemic cells are CD4+ T cells.[48] In morphological appearance, they usually demonstrate a highly lobulated nucleus (Fig. 28–25). These cells unfailingly carry integrated HTLV-1 proviruses, and the site of integration is monoclonal in a given ATL patient.[8] In 70 to 80 per cent of cases of ATL, one copy of complete provirus on average is integrated into each leukemic cell; on occasion, one or two copies of defective provirus are integrated into the DNA of a single cell. Conservation of the pX region, even in defective proviruses,[98] is thought to reflect the important role of pX in tumorigenesis. Alternatively, because the viral sequences at the 5' region are deleted more frequently than those at

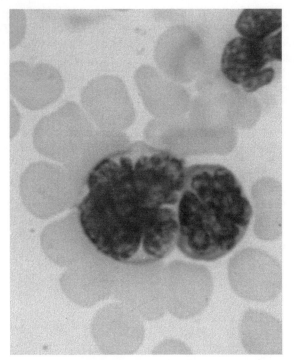

Figure 28–25. Typical morphological appearance of leukemic T cells *(center)* **from a patient with ATL.** Peripheral blood cells were stained with Giemsa solution, and a highly lobulated nucleus is characteristic.

the 3′ region during one cycle replication of HTLV-1,[99] conservation of the pX region at the 3′ region may simply reflect the spontaneous deletion, but not selection by gene function.

Leukemic cells express a high level of IL-2Rα on their surfaces. Production of PTHrP, IL-1β, or GM-CSF by tumor cells has also been reported. In almost all cases, leukemic cells carry aberrant chromosomes; there are frequently multiple abnormalities, such as trisomy of chromosome 7,[100] and 14q11,[101] 14q32,[102] and 6q15 translocations, in a single cell. No abnormality common to all cells was identified in systematic studies in Japan.[103] Most frequent was the abnormality involving 14q32 found in 25 per cent of ATL patients.[101]

Viral Involvement in Leukemogenesis

The etiological role of HTLV-1 in the development of ATL has been demonstrated by seroepidemiological, molecular biological, and in vitro studies: (1) ATL and HTLV-1 are identical in geographical distribution, and most ATL patients are infected with HTLV-1. (2) Leukemic cells from ATL patients are infected with HTLV-1 and show monoclonal integration of proviral DNA, indicating that leukemic cells originate from a single HTLV-1–infected cell.[8] (3) Infection by HTLV-1 can immortalize T cells in vitro. The immunological phenotypes and morphology of immortalized T cells are similar to those of leukemic cells,[12, 17] indicating that the transforming capacity of HTLV-1 plays a critical role in leukemogenesis.

It is estimated that there are approximately 1 million carriers of HTLV-1 in Japan, and about 500 cases of ATL arise each year. About 2 to 5 per cent of all carriers of

HTLV-1 are thought to develop ATL during their life span,[104] an estimated incidence higher than initially predicted. No significant difference in incidence of ATL was found in two endemic areas of Japan, Kyushu (south) and Hokkaido (north), suggesting that no other exogenous factor is involved in development of ATL.

Whereas most cases of ATL are associated with HTLV-1 infection, ATL "unrelated to HTLV-1 infection" has been described.[105] Patients with this disease are indistinguishable either clinically or hematologically from patients with typical ATL, but they lack HTLV-1 antibodies and their leukemic cells carry no HTLV-1 proviral DNA. The etiology of this disease has not been determined.

HAM/TSP and Other Diseases

During epidemiological screening for HTLV-1 antibodies, some populations of patients with neurological disease were found to be strongly antibody positive. These patients had a slowly progressive myelopathy known in tropical zones as tropical spastic paraparesis (TSP)[106, 107] and, in endemic areas of Japan, as HTLV-1–associated myelopathy (HAM).[108, 109]

The unique clinical appearance of HAM/TSP stems from chronic, symmetrical, bilateral involvement of the pyramidal tracts, mainly at the thoracic level of the spinal cord, and symptoms include progressive spastic paresis with bladder dysfunction but minimal sensory deficits. HTLV-1–infected T cells infiltrate the cerebrospinal fluid and spinal cord.[109]

Patients with HAM/TSP frequently have titers of HTLV-1 antibodies 10 times higher than those of asymptomatic carriers or ATL patients.[110] Because Japanese patients have certain common HLA types, an association of HAM/TSP with particular histocompatibility antigens has been proposed.[110] Asymptomatic members of families of HAM/TSP patients who have the same HLA haplotypes will also have high titers of HTLV-1 antibodies. Thus, certain HLA types appear to be associated with a vigorous immune response to HTLV-1 infection. Despite this response, most HAM/TSP patients harbor much larger populations of infected cells than do HTLV-1 carriers at large,[111] an observation attributed to infection of activated T cells.

In the spinal cord of HAM/TSP patients, infiltration of many T cells can be demonstrated by in situ hybridization. Possible mechanisms of tissue damage include secretion of lymphokines such as tumor necrosis factor by infected T cells that would damage the central nervous system[112, 113] and cross-reactivity of T-cell clones for epitopes of nervous system tissues.[114] However, the details of pathogenesis of HAM/TSP are still unclear.

Transfusion of seropositive blood can lead to HAM/TSP after an average interval of 2 years.[53] However, recently developed procedures for screening for seropositive blood have greatly reduced the risk of acquiring HAM/TSP by this route.

Through induction of immunodeficiency, HTLV-1 infection is associated with many diseases other than ATL and HAM/TSP: chronic lung diseases, monoclonal gammopathy, chronic renal failure, strongyloidiasis, non-specific dermatomycosis, and HTLV-1–associated lymphadenitis and uveitis. Further systematic studies are required to elucidate the exact relationships of these diseases with HTLV-1 infection.

Molecular Biology of Pathogenesis

ATL cells are infected with HTLV-1, and the site for the provirus integration is monoclonal. However, no common site of integration has been observed among ATL patients.[115] In this characteristic, HTLV-1 differs from chronic retroviruses in tumor cells of other animals, in which integration is usually adjacent to a proto-oncogene (see above). Thus, *cis*-activation of a human cellular gene by an LTR of an integrated HTLV-1 provirus is not involved in the development of ATL. Consequently, a *trans*-acting function of HTLV-1 is postulated in leukemogenesis.[115]

Tax, a *trans*-regulator of HTLV-1, is the leading candidate for this activity in ATL.[83] Tax can immortalize T cells in an IL-2–dependent fashion,[116] transform rat embryonic cells in cooperation with c-*ras*,[117–119] and induce mesenchymal tumors in *tax*-transgenic mice.[120, 121] Through identification of the cellular targets of Tax, pleiotropic functions of Tax have been shown to include transcriptional *trans*-activation and functional enhancement of growth-promoting genes and *trans*-repression and functional suppression of growth-inhibitory genes.

Trans-Activation of Transcription

Tax responds to specific enhancers to activate transcription of viral and cellular genes, including the 21 bp enhancer in the LTR of HTLV-1,[78, 79, 81] the NF-κB binding site in the gene for IL-2Rα,[122, 123] and the serum response element in c-*fos* and c-*egr* genes.[124] More enhancers will be identified, because some of the activated genes have no response element or binding sequences related to the known enhancers. *Trans*-activation is mediated by either activation of the enhancer binding protein or inactivation of inhibitors of transcription factors.

Enhancer Binding Proteins. Tax protein has a single copy of the zinc finger motif but itself does not bind directly to DNA. Instead, Tax was found to bind to other enhancer binding proteins. Target molecules include three categories of DNA-binding proteins (Fig. 28–26). In the first group are CREB (cAMP response element [CRE] binding protein[125, 126]), CREM (CRE modulator protein[126]), ATF-1,[125] and ATF-2,[127] which bind to the 21 bp enhancer in the HTLV-1 LTR. The second target is the NF-κB family of proteins, such as p50, p65, c-Rel, and p52, which bind to the NF-κB binding site[128–132] in the IL-2Rα gene. The third protein is serum response factor, which binds to the serum response element[124] in the c-*fos* or c-*egr* gene. These transcription factors are regulated by phosphorylation; thus, transcription is signal dependent. However, Tax binding enables activation of these factors without specific phosphorylation and thus without any extracellular signals.

It is not well understood how Tax binding to these various transcription factors manages to bypass the normal regulation exercised by phosphorylation. Several possible explanations are acceleration of dimerization of the DNA-binding proteins,[133] stabilization of the complex between DNA and enhancer binding proteins,[134] and recruitment of other transcription factors into the transcriptional complexes.[135] One attractive model is the recruitment of CBP (CREB binding protein) onto the enhancer/CREB complexes.[135] In the absence of Tax, CBP, a histone-acetylating enzyme,[136] binds to CREB only when it is phosphorylated by protein kinase A,[137, 138] and CREB/P-CBP complex on the enhancer would acetylate histones bound to nearby DNA, breaking up nucleosome structure of DNA. However, Tax can bind to both CREB and CBP, forming a ternary complex of CREB/Tax/CBP without phosphorylation of CREB and thus activate transcription even in the absence of an external signal.[136] This simple binding hypothesis needs further careful characterization, however, because the prototype CRE and some mutants of the 21 bp enhancer to which CREB can still bind are not *trans*-activated by Tax.[139] Some additional signal from the enhancer DNA sequence seems to be required for activation.

Transcriptional Inhibitors. NF-κB proteins are activated by Tax binding in the nucleus.[128–132] However, in resting cells, NF-κB proteins are complexed with IκB and remain an inactive complex in the cytoplasm[140, 141] (see Fig. 28–18). On stimulation, IκB proteins are phosphorylated and rapidly degraded, and the released NF-κB then migrates into the nucleus by virtue of its nuclear translocation signal and binds to a specific DNA sequence.[142] NF-κB precursors such as p100 and p105 also function as inhibitors of NF-κB.[143]

Tax is able to bind to IκBα[144] and IκBγ,[145] and also to p100[146, 147] and p105,[148] and the binding results in destabilization of IκB/NF-κB complexes (see Fig. 28–26). Tax can bypass the effect of phosphorylation of IκB. It has been reported that Tax induces phosphorylation of IκB followed by its degradation. Activation of a protein kinase activity by Tax[149] suggests the former, but the binding of Tax to a component of the proteasomes is more consistent with the latter mechanism.[150] Whatever the molecular pathway, Tax downregulates the transcriptional inhibitor IκB in the cytoplasm. In activation of the NF-κB system, Tax exerts its effects through two independent processes targeting activators, NF-κB, and their inhibitors, IκB.

Basic Transcription Factors. Besides activation of specific enhancer binding proteins, Tax also binds to and enhances the activity of some basic transcription factors, such as transcription factor TFIIA[151] and the TATA-binding protein (TBP).[152] Tax binding to TBP increases recruitment of TBP onto the TATA sequence located close to the enhancer. Tax binding to these general transcription factors may contribute to the enhancement of transcription.

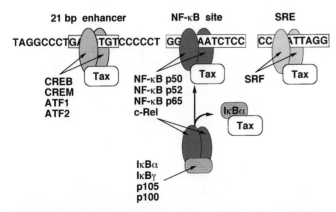

Figure 28–26. Binding of Tax protein to cellular enhancer binding proteins and to regulators of the enhancer binding proteins. Tax binding can activate the transcriptional activities without responsive phosphorylation.

Trans-Repression of Transcription

The proliferation of cells is controlled by a combination of activating and suppressing regulators. Tax is able to *trans*-repress transcription of specific genes as well as to *trans*-activate some other specific genes. Initially, *trans*-repression by Tax was described for DNA polymerase β,[153] a repair enzyme required for damaged DNA. Downregulation of this enzyme would result in accumulation of mutations in HTLV-1–infected cells. Consistent with this prediction, a higher mutation rate was directly demonstrated in cells expressing Tax protein.[186]

Tax was demonstrated to *trans*-repress transcription of the p18[INK],[187] *NF1*,[154] *lck*,[155] and *bax* genes.[156] Tax also *trans*-represses many p53-target genes.[188, 189] p18[INK] is a member of inhibitors of cyclin-dependent kinase (CDK) 4, thus *trans*-repression of this gene expression would result in activation of CDK4. The *trans*-repression is mediated through a transcription factor, E47, which binds to E-box element of the p18[INK] promoter.[190] A transcription factor p53 is also involved in *trans*-repression of its target genes in a similar fashion to E47.[189] This effect is equivalent to a functional suppression of the tumor suppressor protein, p53.

NF1 is a tumor suppressor gene in neurofibromatosis[157] and a negative regulator of Ras function.[158] Downregulation of *NF1* would thus result in a constitutive activation of Ras similar to activated *ras* oncogene. Such an effect would explain the high prevalence of neurofibromatosis in Tax transgenic mice.[121] Remarkably, a single protein, Tax, is able to *trans*-repress tumor suppressor gene *NF1* on the one hand and also to *trans*-activate proto-oncogenes and cytokine genes on the other hand.

Lck is an Src-related tyrosine kinase that is closely linked to CD4/8 molecules under the cell membrane of T cells.[159] Therefore, downregulation of *lck* might impair some T cell–specific signals for differentiation and immune responses.[155] Tax also *trans*-represses expression of *bax* gene,[156] the protein product of which accelerates apoptosis. Repression of this gene, therefore, may be responsible for phenotypes of HTLV-1–infected cells resistant to apoptosis; resistance to apoptosis would also contribute to survival of leukemogenic progenitor cells.

Inhibition of Tumor Suppressor Proteins

Cells are stimulated to proliferate or are otherwise arrested at G_0 or G_1 phase. Some tumor suppressor genes are able to arrest cells at a specific phase of the cell cycle, and spontaneous mutations or deletions in these genes are frequently observed in tumor cells. Tax was shown to bind directly to some tumor suppressor proteins, p16[INK] and p15[INK],[160, 161] and to inhibit their suppressor activities[162] (Fig. 28–27). Tax binding to p16[INK] or p15[INK] blocks their inhibitory actions on cyclin-dependent kinases 4 and 6,[163, 164] thus in turn activating the kinases.[162] On activation of cyclin-dependent kinases 4 and 6, Rb is phosphorylated and no longer binds E2F, thus releasing active E2F,[165–167] which then binds to target DNA sequences to initiate expression of various genes for DNA synthesis. In fact, cells arrested at G_1 by the expression of p16[INK] were efficiently triggered to enter S phase by expression of Tax.[162] p16[INK] is also proposed to play roles in cell senescence.[168] Binding of Tax to p16[INK] might be a possible mechanism for immortalization of in-

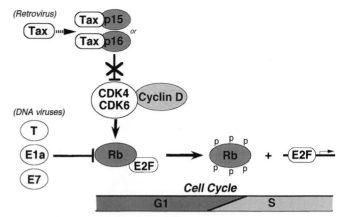

Figure 28–27. Inactivation of tumor suppressor proteins p16 and p15 by Tax-activating cyclin-dependent kinases. Targeting of Rb protein by DNA tumor viruses is also compared.

fected cells. p16[INK] is frequently deleted in many human tumor cells, particularly melanoma and hematopoietic tumors.[165] Tax-induced functional inactivation of p16[INK] would be analogous to structural deletion in contributing to the development of ATL. The p16[INK] gene is deleted in many T-cell lines but not in HTLV-1–infected T-cell lines, supporting significance in immortalization in vitro. Observations in vivo are somewhat different from those in cell lines. Some cases of ATL had deletion of p16[INK] in their tumor cells,[169] thus arguing against the importance of p16[INK] inactivation in vivo. Preliminary analysis, however, suggests less frequent deletion of p16[INK] in the chronic phase of ATL than in the acute phase (unpublished data). Tax-mediated inactivation of p16[INK] might play a role in vivo in cell immortalization and malignant transformation. Other members of the INK family, p18 and p19,[170] were neither bound nor inhibited by Tax, although these members also contain similar domains of ankyrin motifs.

The effect of Tax on another tumor suppressor protein, p53, has also been described; p53 expressed in HTLV-1–infected T-cell lines is stabilized and less active.[171, 172] p53 is a cell cycle checkpoint gene, whose expression is induced by chromosomal DNA damage. Its functional impairment suggests abnormal cell cycle progression through the checkpoint. The function of p53 is suppressed by Tax through *trans*-repression of p53-directed transcription, although Tax does not bind directly to p53 itself.[190] Tax of HTLV-1 binds to the human homologue (HsMAD1) of the yeast mitotic checkpoint protein MAD1.[173] HsMAD1 is a component of the mitotic checkpoint system that prevents anaphase and commitment to cellular division until chromosomal alignment is properly completed. Therefore, abrogation of the mitotic checkpoint function of HsMAD1 may be linked to abnormal cell division and accumulation of chromosome abnormalities.

Perspectives in Pathogenesis

Common Transforming Strategy With DNA Tumor Viruses. Tax appears to be pleiotropic in affecting cellular proliferation and other functions, properties of Tax unique to the HTLV family among retroviruses. HTLV-1 uses a common strategy with DNA tumor viruses to induce abnormal cell growth: interaction with p16^{INK} and p15^{INK}, which are upstream regulators of Rb, and interaction with CBP/ p300. Transforming proteins of DNA tumor viruses also bind to Rb and CPB/p300.[167, 174, 175] Tax targets p16^{INK} and p15^{INK}, the upstream regulators of Rb, and abrogates the Rb signaling pathway, which suppresses cell cycle. Rb is well characterized as a target of transforming proteins of DNA tumor viruses.[167] T antigens of SV40[176] and polyomavirus,[177] E1A of adenoviruses,[178] and E7 of human papillomaviruses[179] all bind to Rb protein and inactivate it, releasing an active transcription factor, E2F.[77] Therefore, HTLV-1 Tax and various transforming proteins of DNA tumor viruses inactivate the same signaling pathway targeting different molecules. It is surprising that regulatory proteins required for the replication of totally unrelated RNA and DNA viruses use the same signaling pathway to modulate cellular proliferation. Rb is a negative regulator for the transcription factor E2F, which is responsible for DNA synthesis in S phase. Targeting Rb would be an advantage for DNA viruses, because it would enhance replication of their own genomic DNA. Retroviruses reproduce their genome by transcription. However, they also increase their proviral copy numbers along with the expansion of infected cells. Because replication of HTLV-1 is highly restricted in vivo, HTLV-1 probably developed a method for induction of DNA synthesis for cell proliferation and to counter the negative regulation of cell cycle through Rb.

Extending this argument, p16^{INK} and Rb genes are frequently deleted in spontaneous human tumors, but their deletions are mutually exclusive.[169, 180, 181] As an analogy of these spontaneous deletions, the virally induced functional inactivation of either p16^{INK} or Rb protein would be primarily responsible for the induction of tumors.

Low Expression of Tax In Vivo. The pleiotropic functions of Tax thus far identified in vitro are all consistent with its role as an etiological factor for ATL. However, an unexplained phenomenon is the extremely low expression of Tax in vivo. Infected T cells in peripheral blood do not produce significant amounts of Tax protein, irrespective of their transformation status. The persistent prevalence of antibodies to viral proteins implies continuous expression of the viral proteins in infected individuals. Viral expression at mRNA is detected only by the sensitive reverse PCR method,[40] not by any other technique, and more than 95 per cent of infected cells are absolutely negative for expression

of viral message. Yet, most leukemic cells do express IL-2Rα[47] and other Tax-responsive genes and proliferate abnormally in vivo.

There may be several explanations for these seemingly contradictory or inconsistent observations. First, Tax plays essential roles in early stages of transformation but is no longer required for maintenance of the transformed state. Second, low levels of Tax may be sufficient for the maintenance of abnormal phenotypes in infected cells, although against this possibility is the finding that the majority of infected cells are absolutely negative for Tax expression. Third, a certain level of Tax might be transiently expressed in a small population of infected cells at one time and in another cell population at another (Fig. 28–28).

When primary cells from infected individuals are cultured, the expression of viral genes is induced quickly, within a few hours in many cases. Therefore, the latent state is not intrinsic to the provirus, nor are the suppressive factors for viral expression in vivo antibodies to viral antigens.[182] However, the suppression was not reproducible in reconstituted systems, and the mechanisms for the in vivo latency are not further elucidated.

The extremely low expression of Tax in cells in vivo is in contrast to transforming genes of DNA tumor viruses, which are actively expressed and responsible for maintenance of the transformed phenotypes. For example, human papillomavirus E6/E7 gene products are present in HeLa cell lines maintained for long periods, and their repression inhibits cell growth.[183]

Clonal Expansion of Infected T Cells. Another point in question is the clonal burst of infected T cells. Growth stimulation through the pleiotropic functions of Tax would result in a random population of proliferating cells, because Tax stimulates growth of most infected T cells. As leukemic cells are always monoclonal, an additional genetic event is postulated to trigger the clonal selection of infected T cells. Although nothing is known about precise second events or whether clonal selection is even associated with the viral function, that a further alteration is necessary for leukemia is consistent with the long delay in ATL development after HTLV-1 infection.

▼ PREVENTION OF HTLV-1 INFECTION

Infection by HTLV-1 induces production of antibodies to viral proteins, and infection can be diagnosed by the pres-

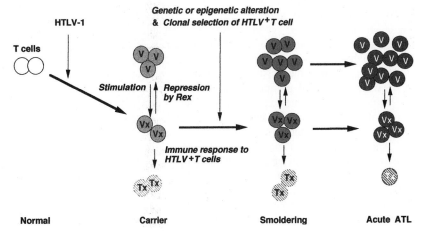

Figure 28–28. Proposed phase transition of HTLV-1–infected T cells from the carrier state to malignant ATL. Polyclonally proliferated cells can undergo rejection by host immune response, repression of viral expression by Rex function, or clonal expansion leading to leukemogenesis by an unknown mechanism.

ence of these antibodies. Assay kits for ELISA, Western blotting, and particle agglutination have been produced. Extracts of HTLV-1–infected cells are used in commercially available kits, and assays employing recombinant proteins have also been developed. Each system has its advantages and disadvantages, but results can be checked by Western blotting or indirect immunostaining of infected cells, although both of these methods require optimization.

Transfusion of seropositive blood results in transmission of HTLV-1 to most recipients,[52] but with the introduction of HTLV-1 screening systems in blood banks, seropositive blood is now excluded in Japan, viral transmission through transfusion has been greatly reduced, and transfusion-related HAM/TSP has been effectively prevented. Application of these preventives to populations in all endemic areas is important to eliminate HTLV-1 infection.

The major natural route of viral transmission is from mother to child by infected T cells in breast milk.[56, 57] Curiously, mothers with high levels of antibodies to Tax protein transmit the virus to their offspring at a higher rate than do those with low titers of Tax antibodies.[184] Efficient replication of HTLV-1 possibly stimulates antibody production, but antibodies do not, in fact, significantly inhibit viral replication.

Because breast milk is the major source of infection, avoidance of breast-feeding should prevent infection of children. This possibility is being tested with seropositive mothers in Nagasaki City, Japan. By consent, pregnant women are surveyed for HTLV-1 antibodies; those who are seropositive are asked not to breast feed. Preliminary results indicate a drastic reduction in the incidence of seropositive children, from about 30 per cent to just a small percentage. The early success of this trial provides direct evidence for viral transmission through milk and raises the possibility of eliminating ATL in the next few generations.

Unfortunately, not all children of seropositive mothers who were not breast fed remained seronegative. Perhaps these few cases reflect the protocol deviations. However, studies using animal models suggest other pathways of viral transmission. For example, when female rats were infected with HTLV-1 by injection of rat cells infected in vitro, they transmitted the virus to their pups; even some pups that were transferred to uninfected foster mothers immediately after birth were infected.

Studies of children of seropositive mothers indicate that some carry HTLV-1 proviral DNA, but they have no circulating antibodies to HTLV-1 after 6 months of age (and no longer carry passively acquired maternal antibodies).[185] These studies are based on PCR, which is capable of detecting even one molecule of HTLV-1 DNA per cell, and further analyses are required for confirmation. Nonetheless, these findings imply the existence of unknown mechanisms of viral infection and unique immunological properties of the host, a level of gene expression too low to result in an immunological response, or insufficient numbers of proviral copies to foster production of antibodies.

Another aspect for prevention of HTLV-1–associated diseases is an inhibition of viral replication in carriers. Malignant transformation does not require the viral replication, but reduced numbers of infected T cells would imply the reduction of progenitor cells for ATL. HTLV-1 is able to replicate even in the presence of antibodies against the viral proteins; therefore, the development of immunological strategies is needed. Furthermore, the integrated proviruses with long latency would be a barrier for targeting of any type of treatment. Further investigations are essential for comprehension of HTLV-1 viral infection, replication, and pathogenesis to achieve prevention of HTLV-1 infection in humans.

REFERENCES

1. Weiss, R., Teich, N., Varmus, H., and Coffin, J. (eds.): RNA Tumor Viruses. Cold Spring Harbor, NY, Cold Spring Harbor Laboratory, 1985.
2. Johann, S.V., Gibbons, J.J., and O'Hara, B.: GLVR1, a receptor for Gibbon ape leukemia virus, is homologous to a phosphate permease of *Neurospora crassa* and is expressed at high levels in the brain and thymus. J. Virol. 66:1635, 1992.
3. Dalgleish, A.G., Beverly, C.L., Calpman, P.R., Crawford, D.H., Greaves, M.F., and Weiss, R.A.: The CD4 antigen is an essential component of the receptor for the AIDS retrovirus. Nature 312:763, 1985.
4. Hayward, W.S., Neel, B.G., and Astrin, S.: Activation of a cellular onc gene by promoter insertion in ALV-induced lymphoid leukosis. Nature 290:475, 1981.
5. Fung, Y.K., Lewis, W.G., Crittenden, L.B., and Kung, H.J.: Activation of the cellular oncogene c-*erb* B by LTR insertion: molecular basis for induction of erythroblastosis by avian leukosis virus. Cell 33:375, 1983.
6. Nusse, R., and Varmus, H.E.: Many tumors induced by the mouse mammary tumor virus contain a provirus integrated in the same region of the host genome. Cell 31:99, 1982.
7. Chatis, P.A., Holland, C.A., Hartley, J.W., Rowe, W.P., and Hopkins, N.: Role for the 3′ end of the genome in determining disease specificities of Friend and Moloney leukemia viruses. Proc. Natl. Acad. Sci. USA 80:4408, 1983.
8. Yoshida, M., Seiki, M., Yamaguchi, K., and Takatsuki, K.: Monoclonal integration of HTLV in all primary tumors of adult T-cell leukemia suggests causative role of HTLV in the disease. Proc. Natl. Acad. Sci. USA 81:2534, 1984.
9. Yoshida, M.: Multiple targets of HTLV-1 for dysregulation of host cells. Semin. Virol. 7:394, 1996.
10. Uchiyama, T., Yodoi, J., Sagawa, K., Takatsuki, K., and Uchino, H.: Adult T cell leukemia: clinical and hematological features of 16 cases. Blood 50:481, 1977.
11. Poiesz, B.J., Ruscetti, F.W., Gazdar, A.F., Bunn, P.A., Minna, J.D., and Gallo, R.C.: Detection and isolation of type C retrovirus particles from fresh and cultured lymphocytes of a patient with cutaneous T-cell lymphoma. Proc. Natl. Acad. Sci. USA 77:7415, 1980.
12. Miyoshi, I., Kubonishi, I., Yoshimoto, S., Akagi, T., Ohtsuki, Y., Shiraishi, Y., Nagata, K., and Hinuma, Y.: Type C virus particles in a cord T cell line derived by cocultivating normal human cord leukocytes and human leukemic T cells. Nature 294:770, 1981.
13. Miyoshi, I., Kubonishi, I., Sumida, M., Hiraki, S., Kimura, I., Miyamoto, K., and Sato, J.: A novel T cell line derived from adult T cell leukemia. Jpn. J. Cancer Res. (Gann) 71:155, 1980.
14. Hinuma, Y., Nagata, K., Misaka, M., Nakai, M., Matsumoto, T., Kinoshita, K., Shirakawa, S., and Miyoshi, I.: Adult T cell leukemia: antigen in an ATL cell line and detection of antibodies to the antigen in human sera. Proc. Natl. Acad. Sci. USA 78:6476, 1981.
15. Hinuma, Y., Komoda, H., Chosa, T., Kondo, T., Kohara, M., Takenaka, T., Kikuchi, M., Ichimaru, M., Yunoki, K., Sato, I., Matsuo, R., Takiuchi, Y., Uchino, H., and Hamaoka, M.: Antibodies to adult T-cell leukemia-virus-associated antigen (ATLA) in sera from patients with ATL and controls in Japan: a nation-wide sero-epidemiologic study. Int. J. Cancer 29:631, 1982.
16. Blattner, W., Kalyanaraman, V.S., Robert-Guroff, M., Lister, T.A., Galton, D.A., Sarin, P.S., Crawford, M.H., Catovsky, D., Greaves, M., and Gallo, R.C.: The human type C retrovirus, HTLV in Blacks from the Caribbean region, and relationship to adult T-cell leukemia/lymphoma. Int. J. Cancer 30:257, 1982.
17. Yoshida, M., Miyoshi, I., and Hinuma, Y.: Isolation and characteriza-

tion of retrovirus from cell lines of human adult T cell leukemia and its implication in the diseases. Proc. Natl. Acad. Sci. USA 79:2031, 1982.

18. Seiki, M., Hattori, S., and Yoshida, M.: Human adult T-cell leukemia virus: molecular cloning of the provirus DNA and the unique terminal structure. Proc. Natl. Acad. Sci. USA 79:6899, 1982.

19. Seiki, M., Hattori, S., Hirayama, Y., and Yoshida, M.: Human adult T cell leukemia virus: complete nucleotide sequence of the provirus genome integrated in leukemia cell DNA. Proc. Natl. Acad. Sci. USA 80:3618, 1983.

20. Kalyanaraman, V.S., Sarngadharan, M.G., Nakao, Y., Ito, Y., Aoki, T., and Gallo, R.C.: Natural antibodies to the structural protein (p24) of the human T cell leukemia (lymphoma) retrovirus found in sera of leukemia patients in Japan. Proc. Natl. Acad. Sci. USA 79:1653, 1982.

21. Kalyanaraman, V.S., Sarngadharan, M.G., Robert-Guroff, M., Miyoshi, I., Blayney, D., Golde, D., and Gallo, R.C.: A new subtype of human T cell leukemia virus (HTLV-II) associated with a T cell variant of hairy T cell leukemia. Science 218:571, 1982.

22. Chen, I.S.Y., McLaghlin, J., Gasson, J.C., Clark, S.C., and Golde, D.W.: Molecular characterization of genome of a novel human T cell leukemia virus. Nature 305:502, 1983.

23. Shimotohno, K., Golde, D.W., Miwa, M., Sugimura, T., and Chen, I.S.Y.: Nucleotide sequence analysis of the long terminal repeat of human T-cell leukemia virus type II. Proc. Natl. Acad. Sci. USA 81:1079, 1984.

24. Miyoshi, I., Yoshimoto, S., Fujishita, M., Ohtsuki, Y., Taguchi, H., Shiraishi, Y., Akagi, T., and Minezawa, M.: Isolation in culture of a type C virus from Japanese monkey seropositive to adult T cell leukemia-associated antigens. Jpn. J. Cancer Res. (Gann) 74:323, 1983.

25. Ishikawa, K., Fukusawa, M., Tsujimoto, H., Else, J.G., Ishakia, M., Ubhi, N.K., Ishida, T., Takenaka, O., Kawamoto, Y., and Shotake, T.: Serological survey and virus isolation of simian T cell leukemia/T-lymphotropic virus type I (STLV-I) in nonhuman primates in their native countries. Int. J. Cancer 40:233, 1987.

26. Komuro, A., Watanabe, T., Miyoshi, I., Hayami, M., Tsujimoto, H., Seiki, M., and Yoshida, M.: Detection and characterization of simian retroviruses homologous to human T-cell leukemia virus type I. Virology 138:373, 1984.

27. Tsujimoto, H., Seiki, M., Nakamura, H., Watanabe, T., Sakakibara, I., Sasagawa, A., Honjo, S., Hayami, M., and Yoshida, M.: Adult T-cell leukemia-like disease in monkey naturally infected with simian retrovirus related to human T-cell leukemia virus type I. Jpn. J. Cancer Res. (Gann) 76:911, 1985.

28. Sagata, N., Yasunaga, T., Tsuzuku-Kawamura, J., Ohishi, K., Ogawa, Y., and Ikawa, Y.: Complete nucleotide sequence of the genome of bovine leukemia virus. Its evolutionary relationship. Proc. Natl. Acad. Sci. USA 82:677, 1985.

29. Gotoh, Y., Sugimura, K., and Hinuma, Y.: Healthy carriers of a human retrovirus, adult T cell leukemia virus (ATLV): demonstration by clonal culture of ATLV carrying T cells from peripheral blood. Proc. Natl. Acad. Sci. USA 79:4780, 1982.

30. Ratner, L., Josephs, S.F., Starcich, B., Hahn, B., Shaw, G.M., Gallo, R.C., and Wong-Staal, F.: Nucleotide sequence analysis of a variant of human T cell leukemia virus (HTLV-Ib) provirus with a deletion in pX-I. J. Virol. 54:781, 1985.

31. Yanagihara, R., Nerurkar, V.R., and Ajdukiewicz, A.B.: Comparison between strains of human T lymphotropic virus type I isolated from inhabitants of the Solomon Islands and Papua New Guinea. J. Infect. Dis. 164:443, 1991.

32. Tajima, K., Tominaga, S., Suchi, T., Kawagoe, T., Komoda, H., Hinuma, Y., Oda, T., and Fujita, K.: Epidemiological analysis of the distribution of antibody to adult T cell leukemia virus associated antigen: possible horizontal transmission of adult T cell leukemia virus. Jpn. J. Cancer Res. (Gann) 73:893, 1982.

33. Lee, H., Swanson, P., Shorty, V.S., Zackk, J.A., Rosenblatt, J.D., and Chen, I.S.Y.: High rate of HTLV-II infection in seropositive IV drug abusers in New Orleans. Science 244:471, 1989.

34. Switzer, W.M., Black, F.L., Pieniazek, D., Biggar, R.J., Lal, R.B., and Heneine, W.: Endemicity and phylogeny of the human T cell lymphotropic virus type II subtype A from the Kayapo Indians of Brazil: evidence for limited regional dissemination. AIDS Res. Hum. Retroviruses 12:635, 1996.

35. Hjelle, B., Zhu, S.W., Takahashi, H., Ijichi, S., and Hall, W.W.: Endemic human T cell leukemia virus type II infection in southwestern US Indians involves two prototype variants of virus. J. Infect. Dis. 168:737, 1993.

36. Zaninovic, V., Sanzon, F., Lopez, F., Velandia, G., Blank, A., Blank, M., Fujiyama, C., Yashiki, S., Matsumoto, D., Katahira, Y., et al.: Geographic independence of HTLV-I and HTLV-II foci in the Andes Highland, the Atlantic coast, and the Orinoco of Colombia. AIDS Res. Hum. Retroviruses 10:97, 1994.

37. Gessain, A., Mauclere, P., Froment, A., Biglione, M., Le Hesran, J.Y., Tekaia, F., Millan, J., and de The, G.: Isolation and molecular characterization of a human T-cell lymphotropic virus type II (HTLV-II), subtype B, from a healthy Pygmy living in a remote area of Cameroon: an ancient origin for HTLV-II in Africa. Proc. Natl. Acad. Sci. USA 92:4041, 1995.

38. Takezaki, T., Tajima, K., Komoda, H., and Imai, J.: Incidence of human T lymphotropic virus type I seroconversion after age 40 among Japanese residents in an area where the virus is endemic. J. Infect. Dis. 171:559, 1995.

39. Watanabe, T.: HTLV type I (U.S. isolate) and ATLV (Japanese isolate) are the same species of human retrovirus. Virology 133:238, 1984.

40. Kinoshita, T., Shimoyama, M., Tobinai, K., Ito, M., Ito, S., Ikeda, S., Tajima, K., Shimotohno, K., and Sugimura, T.: Detection of mRNA for the tax_1/rex_1 gene of human T cell leukemia virus type I in fresh peripheral blood mononuclear cells of adult T-cell leukemia patients and viral carriers by using the polymerase chain reaction. Proc. Natl. Acad. Sci. USA 86:5620, 1989.

41. Niewiesk, S., Daenke, S., Parker, C.E., Taylor, G., Weber, J., Nightingale, S., and Bangham, C.R.: The transactivator gene of human T-cell leukemia virus type I is more variable within and between healthy carriers than patients with tropical spastic paraparesis. J. Virol. 68:6778, 1994.

42. Saito, M., Furukawa, Y., Kubota, R., Usuku, K., Izumo, S., Osame, M., and Yoshida, M.: Mutation rates in LTR of HTLV-1 in HAM/TSP patients and the carriers are similarly high to Tax/Rex-coding sequence. J. Neurovirol. 2:330, 1996.

43. Saito, M., Furukawa, Y., Kubota, R., Usuku, K., Sonoda, S., Izumo, S., Osame, M., and Yoshida, M.: Frequent mutation in pX region of HTLV-1 is observed in HAM/TSP patients, but is not specifically associated with the central nervous system lesions. J. Neurovirol. 1:286, 1995.

44. Tateno, M., Kondo, N., Itoh, T., Chubachi, T., Togashi, T., and Yoshiki, T.: Rat lymphoid cell lines with human T cell leukemia virus production. I. Biological and serological characterization. J. Exp. Med. 159:1105, 1984.

45. Miyoshi, I., Yoshimoto, S., Taguchi, H., Kubonishi, I., Fujishita, M., Ohtsuki, Y., Shiraishi, Y., and Akagi, T.: Transformation of rabbit lymphocytes with adult T cell leukemia virus. Jpn. J. Cancer Res. (Gann) 74:1, 1983.

46. Popovic, M., Lange-Wantzin, G., Sarin, P.S., Mann, D., and Gallo, R.C.: Transformation of human umbilical cord blood T cells by human T cell leukemia/lymphoma virus. Proc. Natl. Acad. Sci. USA 80:5402, 1983.

47. Wano, Y., Uchiyama, T., Fukui, K., Maeda, M., Uchino, H., and Yodoi, J.: Characterization of human interleukin 2 receptor (Tac antigen) in normal and leukemic T cells. Co-expression of normal and aberrant receptors on HUT 102 cells. J. Immunol. 132:3005, 1984.

48. Hattori, T., Uchiyama, T., Tobinai, K., Takatsuki, K., and Uchino, H.: Surface phenotype of Japanese adult T-cell leukemia cells characterized by monoclonal antibodies. Blood 58:645, 1981.

49. Chen, I.S., Quan, S.G., and Golde, D.W.: Human T-cell leukemia virus type II transforms normal human lymphocytes. Proc. Natl. Acad. Sci. USA 80:7006, 1983.

50. Hinuma, Y., Gotoh, Y., Sugamura, K., Nagata, K., Goto, T., Nakai, M., Kamada, N., Matsumoto, T., and Kinoshita, K.: A retrovirus associated with human adult T cell leukemia: in vitro activation. Jpn. J. Cancer Res. (Gann) 73:341, 1982.

51. Yoshida, M.: Expression of the HTLV-1 genome and its association with a unique T-cell malignancy. Biochim. Biophys. Acta 970:145, 1987.

52. Okochi, K., Sato, H., and Hinuma, Y.: A retrospective study on transmission of adult T cell leukemia virus by blood transfusion: seroconversion in recipients. Vox Sang. 46:245, 1983.

53. Osame, M., Izumo, S., Tagata, A., Matsumoto, M., Matsumoto, T., Sonoda, S., Tara, M., and Shibata, Y.: Blood transfusion and HTLV-1 associated myelopathy. Lancet 2:104, 1986.

54. Robert-Guroff, M., Weiss, S.H., Giron, J.A., Jennings, A.M., Ginzgurg, H.M., Margolis, I.B., Blattner, W.A., and Gallo, R.C.: Prevalence of antibodies to HTLV-I, -II and -III in intravenous drug abusers from an AIDS endemic region. JAMA 255:3133, 1986.

55. Kusuhara, K., Sonoda, S., Takahashi, K., Tokunaga, K., Fukushige, J., and Ueda, K.: Mother to child transmission of human T cell leukemia virus type I (HTLV-I): a fifteen year follow up in Okinawa. Int. J. Cancer 40:755, 1987.

56. Hino, S., Yamaguchi, K., Katamine, S., Sugiyama, H., Amagasaki, T., Kinoshita, K., Yoshida, Y., Doi, H., Tsuji, Y., and Miyamoto, T.: Mother to child transmission of human T cell leukemia virus type I. Jpn. J. Cancer Res. (Gann) 76:474, 1985.

57. Kinoshita, K., Amagasaki, T., Hino, S., Dio, H., Yamanouchi, K., Ban, N., Momita, S., Ikeda, S., Kamihira, S., Ichimaru, M., Katamine, S., Miyamoto, T., Tsuji, Y., Ishimaru, T., Yamabe, T., Ito, M., Kamura, S., and Tsuda, T.: Milk-borne transmission of HTLV-1 from carrier mothers to their children. Jpn. J. Cancer Res. (Gann) 78:674, 1987.

58. Yamanouchi, K., Kinoshita, K., Moriuchi, R., Katamine, S., Amagasaki, T., Ikeda, S., Ichimaru, M., Miyamoto, T., and Hino, S.: Oral transmission of human T-cell leukemia virus type-I into a common marmoset (Callithrix jacchus) as an experimental model for milk-borne transmission. Jpn. J. Cancer Res. (Gann) 76:481, 1985.

59. Kiyokawa, T., Seiki, M., Imagawa, K., Shimizu, F., and Yoshida, M.: Identification of a protein (p40x) encoded by a unique sequence pX of human T-cell leukemia virus type I. Jpn. J. Cancer Res. (Gann) 75:747, 1984.

60. Haseltine, W.A., Sodroski, J., Patarca, R., Briggs, D., Perkins, D., and Wong-Staal, F.: Structure of 3' terminal region of type II human T lymphotropic virus: evidence for new coding region. Science 225:419, 1984.

61. Lee, T.H., Coligan, J.E., Sodroski, J., Haseltine, W.A., Salahuddin, S.Z., Wong-Staal, F., Gallo, R.C., and Essex, M.: Antigens encoded by the 3' terminal region of human T cell leukemia virus: evidence for a functional gene flanked by the env gene and 3'LTR. Science 226:57, 1984.

62. Slamon, D.J., Press, M.F., Souza, L.M., Cline, M.J., Golde, D.W., Gasson, J.C., and Chen, I.S.Y.: Studies of the putative transforming protein of the type I human T cell leukemia virus. Science 228:1427, 1985.

63. Kiyokawa, T., Seiki, M., Iwashita, S., Imagawa, K., Shimizu, F., and Yoshida, M.: P27x-III and p21x-III, proteins encoded by the pX sequence of human T-cell leukemia virus type I. Proc. Natl. Acad. Sci. USA 82:8359, 1985.

64. Nagashima, K., Yoshida, M., and Seiki, M.: A single species of pX mRNA of HTLV-1 encodes trans-activator p40x and two other phosphoproteins. J. Virol. 60:394, 1986.

65. Sodroski, J.G., Rosen, C.A., and Haseltine, W.A.: Trans-acting transcriptional activation of the long terminal repeat of human T lymphotropic viruses in infected cells. Science 225:381, 1984.

66. Fujisawa, J., Seiki, M., Kiyokawa, T., and Yoshida, M.: Functional activation of long terminal repeat of human T-cell leukemia virus type I by trans-activator. Proc. Natl. Acad. Sci. USA 82:2277, 1985.

67. Felber, B.K., Paskalis, H., Kleinman-Ewing, C., Wong-Staal, F., and Pavlakis, G.N.: The pX protein of HTLV-1 is a transcriptional activator of its long terminal repeats. Science 229:675, 1985.

68. Chen, I.S.Y., Slamon, D.J., Rosenblatt, J.D., Shah, N.P., Quan, S.G., and Wachsman, W.: The x gene is essential for HTLV replication. Science 229:54, 1985.

69. Inoue, J., Seiki, M., Taniguchi, T., Tsuru, S., and Yoshida, M.: Induction of interleukin 2 receptor gene expression by p40x encoded by human T-cell leukemia virus type I. EMBO J. 5:2883, 1986.

70. Inoue, J., Seiki, M., and Yoshida, M.: The second pX product p27x-III of HTLV-1 is required for gag gene expression. FEBS Lett. 209:187, 1986.

71. Inoue, J., Yoshida, M., and Seiki, M.: Transcriptional (p40x) and post-transcriptional (p27x-III) regulators are required for the expression and replication of human T cell leukemia virus type I genes. Proc. Natl. Acad. Sci. USA 84:3635, 1987.

72. Hidaka, M., Inoue, M., Yoshida, M., and Seiki, M.: Post-transcriptional regulator (rex) of HTLV-1 initiates expression of viral structural proteins but suppresses expression of regulatory proteins. EMBO J. 7:519, 1988.

73. Feinberg, M.B., Jarrett, R.F., Aldovini, A., Gallo, R.C., and Wong-Staal, F.: HTLV-III expression and production involve complex regulation at the levels of splicing and translation of viral RNA. Cell 46:807, 1986.

74. Knight, D.M., Flomerfelt, F.A., and Gyrayab, J.: Expression of art/trs protein of HIV and study of its role in viral envelope synthesis. Science 236:837, 1987.

75. Berneman, Z.N., Gartenhaus, R.B., Reitz, M.S., Jr., Blattner, W.A., Manns, A., Hanchard, B., Ikehara, O., Gallo, R.C., and Klotman, M.E.: Expression of alternatively spliced human T-lymphotropic virus type I pX mRNA in infected cell lines and in primary uncultured cells from patients with adult T-cell leukemia/lymphoma and healthy carriers. Proc. Natl. Acad. Sci. USA 89:3005, 1992.

76. Ciminale, V., Pavlakis, G.N., Derse, D., Cunningham, C.P., and Felber, B.K.: Complex splicing in the human T-cell leukemia virus (HTLV) family of retroviruses: novel mRNAs and proteins produced by HTLV type I. J. Virol. 66:1737, 1992.

77. Franchini, G., Mulloy, J.C., Koralnik, I.J., Lo Monico, A., Sparkowski, J.J., Andresson, T., Goldstein, D.J., and Schlegel, R.: The human T-cell leukemia/lymphotropic virus type I p12I protein cooperates with the E5 oncoprotein of bovine papillomavirus in cell transformation and binds the 16-kilodalton subunit of the vacuolar H^+ ATPase. J. Virol. 67:7701, 1993.

78. Fujisawa, J., Seiki, M., Sato, M., and Yoshida, M.: A transcriptional enhancer of HTLV-1 is responsible for trans-activation mediated by p40x of HTLV-1. EMBO J. 5:713, 1986.

79. Shimotohno, K., Takano, M., Teruuchi, T., and Miwa, M.: Requirement of multiple copies of a 21-nucleotide sequence in the U3 regions of human T-cell leukemia virus type I and type II long terminal repeats for trans-acting activation of transcription. Proc. Natl. Acad. Sci. USA 83:8112, 1986.

80. Fujisawa, J., Toita, M., and Yoshida, M.: A unique enhancer element for the trans-activator (p40tax) of human T cell leukemia virus type 1 from cAMP and TPA-responsive elements. J. Virol. 63:3234, 1989.

81. Paskalis, H., Felber, B.K., and Pavlakis, G.N.: Cis-acting sequences responsible for the transcriptional activation of a human T-cell leukemia virus type I constitute a conditional enhancer. Proc. Natl. Acad. Sci. USA 83:6558, 1986.

82. Seiki, M., Hikikoshi, A., Taniguchi, T., and Yoshida, M.: Expression of the pX gene of HTLV-1: general splicing mechanism in the HTLV family. Science 228:1532, 1985.

83. Yoshida, M., and Seiki, M.: Recent advances in the molecular biology of HTLV-1: trans-activation of viral and cellular genes. Annu. Rev. Immunol. 5:541, 1987.

84. Miyatake, S., Seiki, M., Malefijt, R.D., Heike, T., Fujisawa, J., Takebe, Y., Nishida, J., Shlomai, J., Yokota, T., Yoshida, M., Arai, K., and Arai, N.: Activation of T cell–derived lymphokine genes in T cells and fibroblasts: effects of human T cell leukemia virus type I p40^{tax} protein and bovine papilloma virus encoded E2 protein. Nucleic Acids Res. 16:6547, 1988.

85. Fujii, M., Sassone-Corsi, P., and Verma, I.M.: C-fos promoter trans-activation by the tax$_1$ protein of human T-cell leukemia virus type I. Proc. Natl. Acad. Sci. USA 85:8526, 1988.

86. Fujii, M., Niki, T., Mori, T., Matsuda, T., Matsui, M., Nomura, N., and Seiki, M.: HTLV-1 Tax induces expression of various immediate early serum responsive genes. Oncogene 6:1023, 1991.

87. Watanabe, T., Yamaguchi, K., Takatsuki, K., Osame, M., and Yoshida, M.: Constitutive expression of parathyroid hormone–related protein (PTHrP) gene in HTLV-1 carriers and adult T cell leukemia patients which can be trans-activated by HTLV-1 tax gene. J. Exp. Med. 172:759, 1990.

88. Sawada, M., Suzumura, A., Yoshida, M., and Marunouchi, T.: Human T-cell leukemia virus type I trans activator induces class I major histocompatibility complex antigen expression in glial cells. J. Virol. 64:4002, 1990.

89. Yoshida, M., and Seiki, M.: Molecular biology of HTLV-1: biological significance of viral genes in its replication and leukemogenesis. In Gallo, R.C., and Wong-Shaal, F. (eds.): Retrovirus Biology and Human Disease. New York, Marcel Dekker, 1989, p. 161.

90. Toyoshima, H., Itoh, M., Inoue, J., Seiki, M., Takaku, F., and Yoshida, M.: Secondary structure of the HTLV-1 rex responsive element is essential for rex regulation of RNA processing and transport of unspliced RNAs. J. Virol. 64:2825, 1990.

91. Palmeri, D., and Malim, M.H.: The human T-cell leukemia virus type 1 posttranscriptional trans-activator Rex contains a nuclear export signal. J. Virol. 70:6442, 1996.

92. Inoue, J., Itoh, M., Akizawa, T., Toyoshima, H., and Yoshida, M.: HTLV-1 Rex protein accumulates unspliced RNA in the nucleus as well as in cytoplasm. Oncogene 6:1753, 1991.

93. Malim, M.H., Hauber, J., Fenrick, R., and Cullen, B.R.: Immunodeficiency virus rev trans-activator modulates the expression of the viral regulatory genes. Nature 335:181, 1988.

94. Zapp, M.L., and Green, M.R.: Sequence-specific RNA binding by the HIV-1 Rev protein. Nature 342:714, 1989.
95. Malim, M.H., Hauber, J., Le, S.-Y., Maizel, J.V., and Cullen, B.R.: The HIV-1 rev *trans*-activator acts through a structured target sequence to activate nuclear export of unspliced viral mRNA. Nature 338:254, 1989.
96. Rimsky, L., Hauber, J., Dukovich, M., Malim, M.H., Langlois, A., Cullen, B.K., and Greene, W.C.: Functional replacement of the HIV-1 rev protein by the HTLV-1 rex protein. Nature 335:738, 1988.
97. Takatsuki, K., Yamaguchi, K., Kawano, F., Hattori, T., Nishimura, H., Tsuda, H., Sanada, I., Nakada, K., and Itai, Y.: Clinical diversity in adult T-cell leukemia/lymphoma. Cancer Res. 45(suppl.):4644, 1985.
98. Yoshida, M., Seiki, M., Hattori, S., and Watanabe, T.: Genome structure of human T cell leukemia virus and its involvement in the development of adult T-cell leukemia. *In* Human T-cell Leukemia/Lymphoma Virus. Cold Spring Harbor, NY, Cold Spring Harbor Laboratory, 1984, p. 141.
99. Hiramatsu, K., and Yoshikura, H.: Frequent partial deletion of human adult T-cell leukemia virus type I proviruses in experimental transmission: pattern and possible implication. J. Virol. 58:508, 1986.
100. Ueshima, T., Fukuhara, S., Hattori, T., Uchiyama, T., Takatsuku, K., and Uchino, H.: Chromosome studies in adult T cell leukemia in Japan: significance of trisomy 7. Blood 58:420, 1981.
101. Sadamori, N., Nishino, K., Kusano, M., Tomonaga, Y., Tagawa, M., Yao, E., Sasagawa, I., Nakamura, H., and Ichimaru, M.: Significance of chromosome 14 anomaly at band 14q11 in Japanese patients with adult T cell leukemia. Cancer 58:2244, 1986.
102. Miyamoto, K., Tomita, N., Ishii, A., Nonaka, H., Kondo, T., Tanaka, T., and Katasjima, K.: Chromosome abnormalities of leukemia cells in adult patients with T cell leukemia. J. Natl. Cancer Inst. 73:353, 1984.
103. Correlation of chromosome abnormalities with histologic and immunologic characteristics in non-Hodgkin's lymphoma and adult T cell leukemia-lymphoma. Fifth International Workshop on Chromosomes in Leukemia-Lymphoma. Blood 70:1554, 1987.
104. Tajima, K.: The 4th nation-wide study of adult T-cell leukemia/lymphoma (ATL) in Japan: estimates of risk of ATL and its geographical and clinical features. The T- and B-cell Malignancy Study Group. Int. J. Cancer 45:237, 1990.
105. Shimoyama, M., Kagami, Y., Shimotohno, K., Miwa, M., Minato, K., Tobinai, K., Suemasu, K., and Sugimura, T.: Adult T-cell leukemia/lymphoma not associated with human T-cell leukemia virus type I. Proc. Natl. Acad. Sci. USA 83:4524, 1986.
106. Gessain, A., Barin, F., Vernant, J.C., Gout, O., Maurs, L., Calender, A., and de The, G.: Antibodies to human T lymphotropic virus type 1 in patients with tropical spastic paraparesis. Lancet 2:407, 1985.
107. Rodgers-Johnson, P., Gajdusek, D.C., Morgan, O., Zaninovic, V., Sarin, P., and Graham, D.S.: HTLV-I and HTLV-III antibodies and tropical spastic paraparesis. Lancet 2:1247, 1985.
108. Osame, M., Matsumoto, M., Usuku, K., Izumo, S., Ijichi, N., Amitani, H., Tara, M., and Igata, A.: Chronic progressive myelopathy associated with elevated antibodies to human T-lymphotropic virus type 1 and adult T-cell leukemia-like cells. Ann. Neurol. 21:117, 1987.
109. Osame, M., Usuku, K., Izumo, S., Ijichi, N., Amitani, H., Igata, A., Matsumoto, M., and Tara, M.: HTLV-1 associated myelopathy, a new clinical entity. Lancet 1:1031, 1986.
110. Usuku, K., Sonoda, S., Osame, M., Yashiki, S., Takahashi, K., Matsumoto, M., Sawada, T., Tsuji, K., Tara, M., and Igata, A.: HLA haplotype-linked high immune responsiveness against HTLV-1 in HTLV-1–associated myelopathy: comparison with adult T-cell leukemia/lymphoma. Ann. Neurol. 23:143, 1988.
111. Yoshida, M., Osame, M., Kawai, H., Toita, M., Kuwasaki, N., Nishida, Y., Hiraki, Y., Takahashi, K., Nomura, K., Sonoda, S., Eiraku, N., Ijichi, S., and Usuku, K.: Increased replication of HTLV-1 in HTLV-1–associated myelopathy. Ann. Neurol. 26:331, 1989.
112. Matsuda, M., Tsukada, N., Miyagi, K., and Yanagisawa, N.: Increased levels of soluble tumor necrosis factor receptor in patients with multiple sclerosis and HTLV-1–associated myelopathy. J. Neuroimmunol. 52:33, 1994.
113. Mendez, E., Kawanishi, T., Clemens, K., Siomi, H., Soldan, S.S., Calabresi, P., Brady, J., and Jacobson, S.: Astrocyte-specific expression of human T-cell lymphotropic virus type 1 (HTLV-1) Tax: induction of tumor necrosis factor alpha and susceptibility to lysis by CD8+ HTLV-1–specific cytotoxic T cells. J. Virol. 71:9143, 1997.
114. Tsuchida, T., Parker, K.C., Turner, R.V., McFarland, H.F., Coligan, J.E., and Biddison, W.E.: Autoreactive CD8+ T-cell responses to

human myelin protein-derived peptides. Proc. Natl. Acad. Sci. USA 91:10859, 1994.
115. Seiki, M., Eddy, R., Shows, T.B., and Yoshida, M.: Nonspecific integration of the HTLV provirus genome into adult T-cell leukemia cells. Nature 309:640, 1984.
116. Grassman, R., Dengler, C., Muller-Fleckenstein, I., Fleckenstein, B., McGuire, K., Dokhelar, M., Sodroski, J., and Haseltine, W.: Transformation to continuous growth of primary human T lymphocytes by human T cell leukemia virus type I X-region genes transduced by a herpesvirus saimiri vector. Proc. Natl. Acad. Sci. USA 86:3351, 1989.
117. Tanaka, A., Takahashi, C., Yamaoka, S., Nosaka, T., Maki, M., and Hatanaka, M.: Oncogenic transformation by the *tax* gene of human T cell leukemia virus type I in vitro. Proc. Natl. Acad. Sci. USA 87:1071, 1990.
118. Willems, L., Heremans, H., Chen, G., Portetelle, D., Billiau, A., Burny, A., and Kettmenn, R.: Cooperation between bovine leukemia virus transactivator and Ha-*ras* oncogene product in cellular transformation. EMBO J. 9:1577, 1990.
119. Pozzatti, R., Vogel, J., and Jay, G.: The human T-lymphotropic virus type I *tax* gene can cooperate with the *ras* oncogene to induce neoplastic transformation of cells. Mol. Cell. Biol. 10:413, 1990.
120. Nerenberg, M., Hinrichs, S.H., Reynolds, R.K., Khoury, G., and Jay, G.: The *tat* gene of human T lymphotropic virus type I induces mesenchymal tumors in transgenic mice. Science 237:1324, 1987.
121. Hinrichs, S., Nerenberg, M., Reynolds, R.K., Khoury, G., and Jay, G.: A transgenic mouse model for human neurofibromatosis. Science 237:1324, 1987.
122. Leung, K., and Nabel, G.J.: HTLV-1 transactivator induces interleukin-2 receptor expression through an NF-κB–like factor. Nature 333:776, 1988.
123. Lowenthal, J.W., Böhnlein, E., Ballard, D.W., and Greene, W.: Regulation of interleukin 2 receptor alpha subunit (Tac or CD25 antigen) gene expression: binding of inducible nuclear proteins to discrete promoter sequences correlates with transcriptional activation. Proc. Natl. Acad. Sci. USA 85:4468, 1988.
124. Fujii, M., Tsuchiya, H., Chuhjo, T., Akizawa, T., and Seiki, M.: Interaction of HTLV-1 Tax1 with p67SRF causes the aberrant induction of cellular immediate early genes through CArG boxes. Genes Dev. 6:2066, 1992.
125. Zhao, L.J., and Giam, C.Z.: Human T-cell lymphotropic virus type I (HTLV-I) transcriptional activator, Tax, enhances CREB binding to HTLV-I 21-base-pair repeats by protein-protein interaction. Proc. Natl. Acad. Sci. USA 89:7070, 1992.
126. Suzuki, T., Fujisawa, J.I., Toita, M., and Yoshida, M.: The *trans*-activator tax of human T-cell leukemia virus type 1 (HTLV-1) interacts with cAMP-responsive element (CRE) binding and CRE modulator proteins that bind to the 21-base-pair enhancer of HTLV-1. Proc. Natl. Acad. Sci. USA 90:610, 1993.
127. Franklin, A.A., Kubik, M.F., Uittenbogaard, M.N., Brauweiler, A., Utaisincharoen, P., Matthews, M.A., Dynan, W.S., Hoeffler, J.P., and Nyborg, J.K.: Transactivation by the human T-cell leukemia virus Tax protein is mediated through enhanced binding of activating transcription factor-2 (ATF-2), ATF-2 response and cAMP element-binding protein (CREB). J. Biol. Chem. 268:21225, 1993.
128. Suzuki, T., Hirai, H., Fujisawa, J., Fujita, T., and Yoshida, M.: A *trans*-activation Tax of human T-cell leukemia virus type 1 binds to NF-κB p50 and serum response factor (SRF) and associates with enhancer DNAs of the NF-κB site and CArG box. Oncogene 8:2391, 1993.
129. Suzuki, T., Hirai, H., and Yoshida, M.: Tax protein of HTLV-1 interacts with the Rel homology domain of NF-κB p65 and c-Rel proteins bound to the NF-κB binding site and activates transcription. Oncogene 9:3099, 1994.
130. Kanno, T., Brown, K., and Siebenlist, U.: Evidence in support of a role for human T-cell leukemia virus type I Tax in activating NF-κB via stimulation of signaling pathways. J. Biol. Chem. 270:11745, 1995.
131. Munoz, E., and Israel, A.: Activation of NF-κB by the Tax protein of HTLV-1. Immunobiology 193:128, 1995.
132. Beraud, C., Sun, S.C., Ganchi, P., Ballard, D.W., and Greene, W.C.: Human T-cell leukemia virus type I Tax associates with and is negatively regulated by the NF-κB2 p100 gene product: implications for viral latency. Mol. Cell. Biol. 14:1374, 1994.
133. Petropoulos, L., Lin, R., and Hiscott, J.: Human T cell leukemia virus type 1 tax protein increases NF-κB dimer formation and antagonizes the inhibitory activity of the IκB alpha regulatory protein. Virology 225:52, 1996.

134. Adya, N., Zhao, L.J., Huang, W., Boros, I., and Giam, C.Z.: Expansion of CREB's DNA recognition specificity by Tax results from interaction with Ala-Ala-Arg at positions 282–284 near the conserved DNA-binding domain of CREB. Proc. Natl. Acad. Sci. USA 91:5642, 1994.

135. Kwok, R.P., Laurance, M.E., Lundblad, J.R., Goldman, P.S., Shih, H., Connor, L.M., Marriott, S.J., and Goodman, R.H.: Control of cAMP-regulated enhancers by the viral transactivator Tax through CREB and the co-activator CBP. Nature 380:642, 1996.

136. Ogryzko, V.V., Schiltz, R.L., Russanova, V., Howard, B.H., and Nakatani, Y.: The transcriptional coactivators p300 and CBP are histone acetyltransferases. Cell 87:953, 1996.

137. Gonzalez, G.A., and Montminy, M.: Cyclic AMP stimulates somatostatin gene transcription by phosphorylation of CREB at serine 133. Cell 59:675, 1989.

138. Chrivia, J.C., Kwok, R.P., Lamb, N., Hagiwara, M., Montminy, M.R., and Goodman, R.H.: Phosphorylated CREB binds specifically to the nuclear protein CBP. Nature 365:855, 1993.

139. Fujisawa, J., Toita, M., and Yoshida, M.: A unique enhancer element for the *trans* activator (p40tax) of human T-cell leukemia virus type I that is distinct from cyclic AMP- and 12-*O*-tetradecanoylphorbol-13-acetate-responsive elements. J. Virol. 63:3234, 1989.

140. Baeuerle, P.A., and Baltimore, D.: IκB: a specific inhibition of the NF-κB transcription factor. Science 242:540, 1988.

141. Baeuerle, P.A., and Baltimore, D.: Activation of DNA-binding activity in an apparently cytoplasmic precursor of the NF-κB transcription factor. Cell 53:211, 1988.

142. Beg, A.A., Ruben, S.M., Scheinman, R.I., Haskill, S., Rosen, C.A., and Baldwin, A.S., Jr.: IκB interacts with the nuclear localization sequences of the subunits of NF-κB: a mechanism for cytoplasmic retention. Genes Dev. 6:1899, 1992.

143. Fan, C.-M., and Maniatis, T.: Generation of p50 subunit of NF-κB by processing of p105 through an ATP-dependent pathway. Nature 354:395, 1991.

144. Suzuki, T., Hirai, H., Murakami, T., and Yoshida, M.: Tax protein of HTLV-1 destabilizes the complexes of NF-κB and IκB-α and induces nuclear translocation of NF-κB for transcriptional activation. Oncogene 10:1199, 1995.

145. Hirai, H., Suzuki, T., Fujisawa, J., Inoue, J., and Yoshida, M.: Tax protein of human T-cell leukemia virus type I binds to the ankyrin motifs of inhibitory factor κB and induces nuclear translocation of transcription factor NF-κB proteins for transcriptional activation. Proc. Natl. Acad. Sci. USA 91:3584, 1994.

146. Beraud, C., Sun, S.-C., Ganchi, P., Ballard, D.W., and Greene, W.C.: Human T-cell leukemia virus type I Tax associates with and is negatively regulated by the NF-κB2 p100 gene product: implications for viral latency. Mol. Cell. Biol. 14:1374, 1994.

147. Murakami, T., Hirai, H., Suzuki, T., Fujisawa, J., and Yoshida, M.: HTLV-1 Tax enhances NF-κB2 expression and binds to the products p52 and p100, but does not suppress the inhibitory function of p100. Virology 206:1066, 1995.

148. Hirai, H., Fujisawa, J., Suzuki, T., Ueda, K., Muramatsu, M., Tsuboi, A., Arai, N., and Yoshida, M.: Transcriptional activator Tax of HTLV-1 binds to the NF-κB precursor p105. Oncogene 7:1737, 1992.

149. Lindholm, P.F., Tamami, M., Makowski, J., and Brady, J.N.: Human T-cell lymphotropic virus type 1 Tax1 activation of NF-κB: involvement of the protein kinase C pathway. J. Virol. 70:2525, 1996.

150. Beraud, C., and Greene, W.C.: Interaction of HTLV-I Tax with the human proteasome: implications for NF-κB induction. J. Acquir. Immune Defic. Syndr. Hum. Retrovirol. 13:S76, 1996.

151. Clemens, K.E., Piras, G., Radonovich, M.F., Choi, K.S., Duvall, J.F., DeJong, J., Roeder, R., and Brady, J.N.: Interaction of the human T-cell lymphotropic virus type 1 tax transactivator with transcription factor IIA. Mol. Cell. Biol. 16:4656, 1996.

152. Caron, C., Rousset, R., Beraud, C., Moncollin, V., Egly, J.M., and Jalinot, P.: Functional and biochemical interaction of the HTLV-I Tax1 transactivator with TBP. EMBO J. 12:4269, 1993.

153. Jeang, K.T., Widen, S.G., Semmes, O.J., 4th, and Wilson, S.H.: HTLV-I *trans*-activator protein, tax, is a *trans*-repressor of the human beta-polymerase gene. Science 247:1082, 1990.

154. Feigenbaum, L., Fujita, K., Collins, F.S., and Jay, G.: Repression of the NF1 gene by Tax may explain the development of neurofibromas in human T-lymphotropic virus type 1 transgenic mice. J. Virol. 70:3280, 1996.

155. Lemasson, I., Robert-Hebmann, V., Hamaia, S., Duc Dodon, M., Gazzolo, L., and Devaux, C.: Transrepression of *lck* gene expression by human T-cell leukemia virus type 1–encoded p40tax. J. Virol. 71:1975, 1997.

156. Brauweiler, A., Garrus, J.E., Reed, J.C., and Nyborg, J.K.: Repression of *bax* gene expression by the HTLV-1 Tax protein: implications for suppression of apoptosis in virally infected cells. Virology 231:135, 1997.

157. Goldberg, N.S., and Collins, F.S.: The hunt for the neurofibromatosis gene. Arch. Dermatol. 127:1705, 1991.

158. Martin, G.A., Viskochil, D., Bollag, G., McCabe, P.C., Crosier, W.J., Haubruck, H., Conroy, L., Clark, R., O'Connell, P., Cawthon, R.M., Innis, M.A., and McCormick, F.: The GAP-related domain of the neurofibromatosis type 1 gene product interacts with ras p21. Cell 63:843, 1990.

159. Zamoyska, R., Derham, P., Gorman, S.D., von Hoegen, P., Bolen, J.B., Veillette, A., and Parnes, J.R.: Inability of CD8 alpha' polypeptides to associate with p56lck correlates with impaired function in vitro and lack of expression in vivo. Nature 342:278, 1989.

160. Serrano, M, Hannon, G.J., and Beach, D.: A new regulatory motif in cell-cycle control causing specific inhibition of cyclin D/CDK4. Nature 366:704, 1993.

161. Guan, K.L., Jenkins, C.W., Li, Y., Nichols, M.A., Wu, X., O'Keefe, C.L., Matera, A.G., and Xiong, Y.: Growth suppression by p18, a p16INK4/MTS1- and p14INK4B/MTS2-related CDK6 inhibitor, correlates with wild-type pRb function. Genes Dev. 8:2939, 1994.

162. Suzuki, T., Kitao, S., Matsushime, H., and Yoshida, M.: HTLV-1 Tax protein interacts with cyclin-dependent kinase inhibitor p16INK4A and counteracts its inhibitory activity towards CDK4. EMBO J. 15:1607, 1996.

163. Grana, X., and Reddy, E.P.: Cell cycle control in mammalian cells: role of cyclins, cyclin dependent kinases (CDKs), growth suppressor genes and cyclin-dependent kinase inhibitors (CKIs). Oncogene 11:211, 1995.

164. Sherr, C.J., and Roberts, J.M.: Inhibitors of mammalian G1 cyclin-dependent kinases. Genes Dev. 9:1149, 1995.

165. Dowdy, S.F., Hinds, P.W., Louis, K., Reed, S.I., Arnord, A., and Weinberg, R.A.: Physical interactions of the retinoblastoma protein with human cyclins. Cell 73:499, 1993.

166. Ewen, M.E., Sluss, H.K., Sherr, C.J., Matsushime, H., Kato, J., and Livingston, D.M.: Functional interaction of the retinoblastoma protein with mammalian D-type cyclins. Cell 73:487, 1993.

167. Nevins, J.R.: E2F: a link between the Rb tumor suppressor protein and viral oncoproteins. Science 258:424, 1992.

168. Serrano, M., Lee, H.W., Chin, L., Cordon-Cardo, C., Beach, D., and DePinho, R.A.: Role of the INK4a locus in tumor suppression and cell mortality. Cell 85:27, 1996.

169. Hangaishi, A., Ogawa, S., Imamura, N., Miyawaki, S., Miura, Y., Uike, N., Shimazaki, C., Emi, N., Takeyama, K., Hirosawa, S., Kamada, N., Kobayashi, Y., Takemoto, Y., Kitani, T., Toyama, K., Ohtake, S., Yazaki, Y., Ueda, R., and Hirai, H.: Inactivation of multiple tumor-suppressor genes involved in negative regulation of the cell cycle, MTS1/p16INK4A/CDKN2, MTS2/p15INK4B, p53, and Rb genes in primary lymphoid malignancies. Blood 87:4949, 1996.

170. Chan, F.K., Zhang, J., Cheng, L., Shapiro, D.N., and Winoto, A.: Identification of human and mouse p19, a novel CDK4 and CDK6 inhibitor with homology to p16ink4. Mol. Cell. Biol. 15:2682, 1995.

171. Akagi, T., Ono, H., Tsuchida, N., and Shimotohno, K.: Aberrant expression and function of p53 in T-cells immortalized by HTLV-I Tax1. FEBS Lett. 406:263, 1997.

172. Cereseto, A., Diella, F., Mulloy, J.C., Cara, A., Michieli, P., Grassmann, R., Franchini, G., and Klotman, M.E.: p53 functional impairment and high p21waf/cip1 expression in human T-cell lymphotropic/leukemia virus type I–transformed T cells. Blood 88:1551, 1996.

173. Jin, D.Y., Spencer, F., and Jeang, K.T.: Human T cell leukemia virus type 1 oncoprotein Tax targets the human mitotic checkpoint protein MAD1. Cell 93:81, 1998.

174. Eckner, R., Ludlow, J.W., Lill, N.L., Oldread, E., Arany, Z., Modjtahedi, N., DeCaprio, J.A., Livingston, D.M., and Morgan, J.A.: Association of p300 and CBP with simian virus 40 large T antigen. Mol. Cell. Biol. 16:3454, 1996.

175. Arany, Z., Newsome, D., Oldread, E., Livingston, D.M., and Eckner, R.: A family of transcriptional adaptor proteins targeted by the E1A oncoprotein. Nature 374:81, 1995.

176. Ludlow, J.W., DeCaprio, J.A., Huang, C.M., Lee, W.H., Paucha, E., and Livingston, D.M.: SV40 large T antigen binds preferentially to

an underphosphorylated member of the retinoblastoma susceptibility gene product family. Cell 56:57, 1989.

177. Dyson, N., Buchkovich, K., Whyte, P., and Harlow, E.: The cellular 107K protein that binds to adenovirus E1A also associates with the large T antigens of SV40 and JC virus. Cell 58:249, 1989.

178. Whyte, P., Buchkovich, K.J., Horowitz, J.M., Friend, S.H., Raybuck, M., Weinberg, R.A., and Harlow, E.: Association between an oncogene and an anti-oncogene: the adenovirus E1A proteins bind to the retinoblastoma gene product. Nature 334:124, 1988.

179. Dyson, N., Howley, P.M., Munger, K., and Harlow, E.: The human papilloma virus-16 E7 oncoprotein is able to bind to the retinoblastoma gene product. Science 243:934, 1989.

180. Cayuela, J.M., Madani, A., Sanhes, L., Stern, M.H., and Sigaux, F.: Multiple tumor-suppressor gene 1 inactivation is the most frequent genetic alteration in T-cell acute lymphoblastic leukemia. Blood 87:2180, 1996.

181. Nobori, T., Miura, K., Wu, D.J., Lois, A., Takabayashi, K., and Carson, D.A.: Deletions of the cyclin-dependent kinase-4 inhibitor gene in multiple human cancers. Nature 368:753, 1994.

182. Tochikura, T., Iwahashi, M., Matsumoto, T., Koyanagi, Y., Hinuma, Y., and Yamamoto, N.: Effect of human serum anti-HTLV antibodies on viral antigen induction in vitro cultured peripheral lymphocytes from adult T-cell leukemia patients and healthy virus carriers. Int. J. Cancer 36:1, 1985.

183. von Knebel Doeberitz, M., Rittmuller, C., zur Hausen, H., and Durst, M.: Inhibition of tumorigenicity of cervical cancer cells in nude mice by HPV E6-E7 anti-sense RNA. Int. J. Cancer 51:831, 1992.

184. Hino, S., Doi, H., Yoshikumi, H., Sugiyama, H., Ishimaru, T., Yamabe, T., Tsuji, Y., and Miyamoto, T.: HTLV-1 carrier mothers with high titer antibody are at high risk as a source of infection. Jpn. J. Cancer Res. (Gann) 78:1156, 1986.

185. Saito, S., Ando, Y., Furuki, K., Kakimoto, K., Tanigawa, T., Moriyama, I., Ichijo, M., Nakamura, M., Ohtani, K., and Sugamua, K.: Detection of HTLV-I genome in sero-negative infants born to HTLV-I seropositive mothers by polymerase chain reaction. Jpn. J. Cancer Res. (Gann) 80:808, 1989.

186. Miyake, H., Suzuki, T., Hirai, H., and Yoshida, M.: Trans-activator Tax of human T-cell leukemia virus type 1 enhances mutation frequency of the cellular genome. Virology 253:155, 1999.

187. Suzuki, T., Narita, T., Uchida-Toita, M., and Yoshida, M.: Downregulation of INK4 family of cyclin-dependent kinase inhibitors by Tax protein of HTLV-1 through two distinct mechanisms. Virology 259:384, 1999.

188. Mulloy, J.C., Kislyakova, T., Cereseto, A., Casareto, L., LoMonico, A., Fullen, J., Lorenzi, M.V., Cara, A., Nicot, C., Giam, C., and Franchini, G.: Human T-cell lymphotropic/leukemia virus type 1 Tax abrogates p53-induced cell cycle arrest and apoptosis through its CREB/ATF functional domain. J. Virol. 72:8852, 1998.

189. Pise-Masison, C.A., Choi, K.S., Radonovich, M., Dittmer, J., Kim, S.J., and Brady, J.N.: Inhibition of p53 transactivation function by the human T-cell lymphotropic virus type 1 Tax protein. J. Virol. 72:1165, 1998.

190. Suzuki, T., Kitao, S., Matsushime, H., and Yoshida, M.: Tax protein of HTLV-1 inhibits CBP/p300-mediated transcription by interfering with recruitment of CBP/p300 onto DNA element of E-box or p53 binding site. Oncogene 18:4137, 1999.

Herpesviruses

Eric Bruening and Bill Sugden

STRUCTURAL PROPERTIES OF HERPESVIRUSES

LATENT AND LYTIC INFECTIONS BY HERPESVIRUSES

INFECTION BY HUMAN CYTOMEGALOVIRUS IN CELL CULTURE

INFECTION BY EPSTEIN-BARR VIRUS IN CELL CULTURE

INFECTIONS IN THE HUMAN HOST
  ▼ Human Cytomegalovirus as a Pathogen
    Early History

Clinical Manifestations of HCMV Infections
Pathophysiology of HCMV-Associated Mononucleosis
Treatment of HCMV-Associated Diseases
  ▼ Epstein-Barr Virus as a Pathogen
    Early History
    Clinical Manifestations of EBV Infections
    Molecular and Cellular Analyses of EBV-Associated B-Lymphoid Diseases
    Treatment of EBV-Associated Lymphoid Diseases

▼ ▼

Herpesviruses cause a variety of diseases in many animals, including humans. Chickenpox and infectious mononucleosis usually appear soon after infection, whereas herpetic cold sores, retinitis in immunocompromised patients, and Burkitt's lymphoma can arise years after first infection with a specific herpesvirus. Varied disease manifestations reflect disparate virus/host relationships. The outcome of an infection with any herpesvirus depends on the cell tropism of the virus, the molecular details of its life cycle, and the host's immune response. The ability to prevent herpesviral diseases or to intervene in ongoing infections requires an appreciation of the viral life cycle and the host's reaction to that infection. Understanding of the pathophysiological process has led to vaccines that prevent herpesvirus-induced lymphoma in chickens and chickenpox in children and to antiviral drugs that are effective in the treatment of human herpesviral diseases. Additional, successful therapies will follow only from an increased understanding of the modus operandi of these viruses as cellular parasites and the host's responses to them.

Herpesviruses take their insalubrious name (meaning "creeping, slimy liquid") from lesions that some of them induce. They compose a large family of viruses with members capable of infecting species from channel catfish to people. Members share similarities in virion structure; the virus particles are enveloped and contain glycoproteins within their lipid coat. The envelope covers an amorphous layer termed the tegument or matrix, which itself covers an icosahedral structure of 162 protein capsomers. This structure houses a DNA genome as the kernel of these viruses. The virion DNA genomes are all duplex, linear molecules that range in length from 134,000 bp for channel catfish virus (CCV)[1] to between 230,000 and 235,000 bp for human cytomegalovirus (HCMV).[2] Therefore, HCMV is currently distinguished as having the largest genome of any known virus. Clinical isolates of HCMV can have clusters of genes not present in the sequenced laboratory strain, thus providing further complexity to genomic analyses.[3]

The family Herpesviridae has been divided into three subfamilies on the basis of differing biological properties.[4] The alphaherpesviruses can have a broad host range and are usually neurotropic; they include human herpes simplex viruses type 1 and type 2 (HSV-1 and HSV-2) and human varicella-zoster virus (VZV). The betaherpesviruses have a restricted host range and a protracted replicative cycle. For example, the betaherpesvirus HCMV can be clinically identified by its efficient propagation only in human fibroblast strains, and its plaques require 7 to 14 days to form in these cells. By way of contrast, HSV-1 yields plaques in a variety of cells in 2 to 3 days. The gammaherpesviruses are characterized both by their having a limited host range and by their infecting lymphoid cells in vivo and in cell culture. Epstein-Barr virus (EBV) is a member of this subfamily in the human. HCMV and EBV are herpesviruses that are described in detail* because they both are human pathogens and infect hematopoietic cells in vivo and in vitro.

Structural Properties of Herpesviruses

The large size of the viral DNA indicates that herpesviruses encode much information. Many of their genes are devoted to the regulation of and coding for structural proteins of the viral particle. This amount of viral genetic information is consistent with the complexity of the large structure of the viral particles. Viral particles range in size from 150 to 300 nm, just below the limit of resolution of a light microscope. They are pleomorphic, and stocks of HCMV, for example, contain an array of particles, some of which lack envelopes and others DNA.[5] Infectious particles are presumed to be fully enveloped and must contain viral DNA; DNA alone can also be infectious in vitro.[6] The size and density of herpesviral particles make them difficult to purify because intact and fragmented cellular membrane-bound organelles copurify with them; a "purified" sample of virus can never be assumed to be free of cellular contaminants, and this lack of purity makes analyses of viral components difficult. In studies of HSV-1, the high rate of viral replication (10^9 infectious units or 10^{11} particles per milliliter of cell culture fluid) in cell culture means that on purification, viral particles predominate over cellular debris. The well-studied structure derived for the HSV-1 particle has served as a paradigm for that of other herpesviruses.

Particles of herpesviruses are surrounded by lipid envelopes derived from the cells in which the viruses assemble. Herpesviruses encode an array of glycoproteins that are embedded in these lipid bilayers. These glycoproteins are of particular interest both as targets for the humoral immune response and as the required viral ligands for the cellular receptors that mediate viral binding and entry into cells. The glycoproteins in viral envelopes can be detected by labeling

their sugar moieties in partially purified viral preparations.[7] These proteins elicit neutralizing antibodies in immunized animals[8] and in infected human beings.[9] One glycoprotein encoded by EBV, gp340, serves not only to elicit neutralizing antibodies[10] and a cellular immune response,[11] but also to bind a cellular glycoprotein, CD21. CD21 is a receptor for the C3d component of complement and for EBV.[12, 13] gp340 of EBV has been tested as a vaccine against EBV in marmosets as a purified glycoprotein[14] or expressed in a vaccinia viral vector[15] and found to afford some protection.

Beneath the herpesviral envelope is an amorphous layer of material termed the tegument or matrix. Nevertheless, this portion of the viral particle contains specific proteins. For example, a polypeptide of 33 kDa is present in the tegument of HCMV and can bind either the Fc moiety of human immunoglobulin or β_2-microglobulin[16] (Fig. 28–29). The tegument in turn covers the core or nucleocapsid, which is icosahedral and composed of 162 subunits or capsomers. Although several proteins form these subunits, a single major polypeptide within the HCMV nucleocapsid accounts for 90 per cent of its mass.[3, 17]

The nucleocapsids house the polyamine-coated DNA genome of herpesviruses.[18] These linear, double-stranded molecules encode between 100 and 200 genes. As the structures of viral particles of herpesviruses are related, so too are their DNAs. Homologues for 30 open reading frames in HCMV are found in EBV[3]; other related tracts of open reading frames have been identified in these two viral genomes, although they display different relative orientations.[19] This clustering of related genes is consistent with the evolution of HCMV and EBV from a common ancestor.[3]

The structures of virion DNA molecules from indepen-

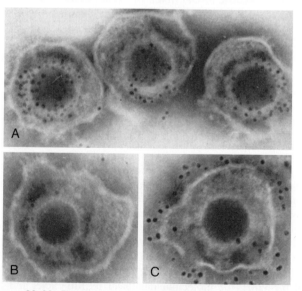

Figure 28–29. Electron microscopic detection of specific viral antigens localizes them to specific regions of HCMV particles. The virion envelope, the amorphous tegument within it, and the nucleocapsid that houses the viral DNA are clearly visible. The antigens are detected by coupling antibodies to them with colloidal gold, which is electron dense. A viral antigen that binds the Fc portion of immunoglobulin proteins is localized to the tegument in A. This viral antigen does not efficiently bind the Fab portion of immunoglobulin in B. A viral glycoprotein is localized to the virion envelope in C. This study was performed by L. M. Stannard and D. R. Hardie (J. Virol. 65:3411–3415, 1991).

---

*Two excellent reviews have served as general sources for this description: *Cytomegalovirus Biology and Infection*, second edition, by M. Ho (Plenum Medical Book Company, New York), 1991; and *Virology*, by B. N. Fields, D. M. Knipe, and P. M. Howley (Raven Press, New York), 1996.

dent isolates of EBV are highly conserved, and variations are usually detected only in the length of repeated sequences.[20] In contrast, the structures of HCMV genomes exhibit a striking, defined heterogeneity (Fig. 28–30). HCMV DNA from a cloned viral stock is composed of four variants or isomers that arise in the infected host cell. The HCMV genome contains two pairs of inverted repeats, with one member of each pair at the ends of the linear molecules and the other member of each pair juxtaposed internally. Recombination between the pairs of the inverted repeats yields the isomers found not only in HCMV stocks but also among other herpesviruses (e.g., HSV-1, HSV-2, and VZV). Not all herpesviruses generate different isomers of their DNAs (e.g., EBV), and the role of isomerization in the viral life cycle is uncertain; for example, mutants of HSV-1 that do not isomerize their DNAs replicate well in cell culture.[21]

Latent and Lytic Infections by Herpesviruses

Herpesviruses can latently infect their human hosts. This form of infection, in fact, is pathognomonic for this family of viruses. Latent infections are defined operationally as an inability to detect the virus easily in an infectious form in the host much of the time. With increasingly sensitive molecular analyses, this operational definition has had to be qualified but is retained as an approximate description of the non-productive phase of herpesviruses' life cycles in their human hosts. Latent infections occur after primary infections in which the introduced virus is amplified by infecting cells of the host lytically; that is, the virus infects some cells, progeny virus is produced, the cells die and lyse, and progeny virus is released. This initial lytic or productive infection is eventually limited by the host's immune response. Latent infections may ensue.

Latent and lytic types of infection have in vitro counterparts. HCMV infects human fibroblast strains lytically. EBV infects human B lymphocytes latently and induces them to

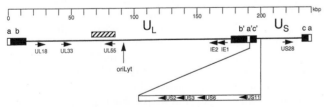

Figure 28–30. The viral genome of HCMV is depicted along with some of its genetic elements discussed in the text. The long and short unique regions (U_L and U_S) are flanked by repeated and inverted regions (a, b, c, and a', b', c') through which the genome rearranges to yield four possible isomers. Replication is initiated from the lytic origin (*oriLyt*) and thought to proceed by a rolling circle mechanism. Concatemers are resolved into unit length genomes within the "a" sequence and packaged into maturing particles. HCMV and EBV share blocks of sequence homology. The hatched box indicates such a region, which is contiguous in HCMV but separated into two distinct regions in the EBV genome. Horizontal arrows indicate open reading frames of some of the genes discussed in the text. The most well studied of these are the immediate early complex of IE1 and IE2, which serve transcriptional regulatory functions. A cluster of genes including US3 and US11 affects the immune response of the host. The viral homologue of MHC class I, UL18, lies within the long unique region. Two well-characterized G-coupled receptor homologues are also indicated (UL33 and US28).

proliferate, and only rarely do these latently infected B lymphoblasts convert spontaneously to support a productive infection. It may seem odd that a latent infection takes place in cell culture in the absence of an immune response. For EBV in people, however, the initial productive infection may occur in non-lymphoid cells.[22] Infection of B lymphocytes in vitro would, therefore, reflect a virus/host cell relationship that is primarily latent in the host, too.

Infection by Human Cytomegalovirus in Cell Culture

HCMV infects early passage human fibroblast strains efficiently in culture. The virus initially associates with cells through an interaction with cell surface heparan sulfate[23]; however, additional events involving viral glycoproteins are surely required for its entry. For example, the gB glycoprotein (UL55) of HCMV, which is the major neutralizing determinant recognized by antibodies in human sera,[24] when expressed in cells induces their fusion,[25] indicating that this viral protein contributes to the association of enveloped HCMV with the plasma membrane of the host cell. After binding and fusion of the virus particle to the plasma membrane of the cell, the released nucleocapsid makes its way to the nucleus, where it can be detected within minutes of exposure to virus.[26]

The viral genetic information is now at the site in which it can be expressed, but as with most animal DNA viruses, the expression of HCMV genes is well regulated. Some regulation is achieved by components of the virus particle that influence expression of specific viral genes.[27, 28] Among the three viral proteins that compose the tegument is the phosphorylated product of the UL82 gene that activates transcription of immediate early viral genes and enhances the infectivity of HCMV DNA.[29] Cellular transcription factors also participate in the regulation of the first set of HCMV genes to be expressed in infected cells. These α or immediate early (IE) genes are transcribed from distinct regions of HCMV DNA.[30, 31] Much work has been done on the *cis*-acting sequences, which affect the transcription of one cluster of HCMV immediate early genes[32–34] (see Fig. 28–30), showing that several cellular transcription factors bind to and regulate the promoter of these genes. HCMV immediate early promoter functions in a wide variety of cell types and presumably contributes to HCMV's capacity to infect fibroblasts, epithelial cells, and hematopoietic cells in vivo. Products of the immediate early genes of HCMV themselves perform regulatory functions. They can increase or decrease expression from viral promoters.[35–38] The IE1 72 kDa protein positively regulates some promoters by associating with cellular E2F1[39]; the IE2 gene product inhibits its own transcription, perhaps by preventing binding of a positively acting cellular protein.[40] The immediate early genes contribute to the viral life cycle not only by downregulating their own expression but also by inducing expression of the next two temporal sets of viral genes, termed β or early and γ or late genes.[41, 42] Products of the early genes contribute to the machinery required to synthesize viral DNA, and products of the late genes include virion structural proteins.[2] One viral protein, pp65, encoded by the UL83 gene, made late during infection accumulates to become the most abundant

HCMV protein in productively infected cells and forms part of the matrix of the virus particle. Detection of pp65 has served as a convenient diagnostic marker for productively infected cells in seropositive transplant recipients because its abundance allows more sensitive detection than do assays for infectious HCMV.[43]

Nevertheless, the protracted life cycle of HCMV in fibroblasts is not readily explained by transcriptional controls of the sets of viral genes expressed sequentially. Similar controls are found in alphaherpesviruses, which rapidly traverse their life cycles. A post-transcriptional control for processing viral RNAs late in infection may retard the life cycle of HCMV.[44] In addition, a mechanism for regulating translation of some HCMV mRNAs has been posited to affect the life cycle of this betaherpesvirus.[45, 46] The UL4 gene of HCMV, for example, is regulated by a small upstream open reading frame whose translation inhibits that of UL4 in *cis* by its polypeptide's failing to be released from the ribosome.[47]

Once the early RNAs of HCMV are transcribed and translated, viral DNA synthesis begins. A stretch of viral DNA has been identified in the HCMV genome that supports replication when it is inserted into plasmid vectors that are introduced into HCMV-infected cells.[48] Eleven viral genes are required to support the function of this putative origin of viral DNA synthesis[49]; a small, non-polyadenylated RNA transcribed within this putative origin may contribute to its function, too.[50]

With the onset of viral DNA synthesis, the final stages of the productive cycle of HCMV take place. Virions are assembled in the nucleus and encapsidate newly synthesized DNA. They derive their envelope from the nuclear membrane, as has been suggested for HSV-1 (HSV-1 is often observed to be fully enveloped while still in the cytoplasm of the infected cell).[51] Endosomes may also contribute to the formation of the viral envelope.[52] The productively infected cells die and release virus, but it is not clear whether cell lysis is the general means by which herpesviruses exit from the cell; secretory pathways may allow escape before cellular lysis.[53]

The study of a productive infection of human fibroblasts by HCMV in cell culture forms one basis for our understanding of this virus/host cell relationship at a molecular level, but it can provide only a limited appreciation of the complexity of infection in human hosts by HCMV. A variety of viral genes exist that have no obvious role in infections in cell culture but are likely to provide a selective advantage to HCMV in its human host. For example, analysis of the DNA of HCMV indicates that it encodes 54 open reading frames or exons for glycoproteins among its 200 genes.[2] One of these glycoproteins, encoded by the US9, has been shown to promote the lateral spread of infection in polarized retinal pigmented epithelium.[54] HCMV also encodes three genes (see Fig. 28–30) whose products are related to the rhodopsin family of receptors, all of which transduce signals by coupling to G proteins.[55, 56] The putative G-coupled receptors of HCMV are thought to function much as their cellular counterparts do in transducing extracellular signals. One of these putative G-coupled receptors, US28, is a β-chemokine receptor that has the potential to modulate the inflammatory response to HCMV infection.[57] Another HCMV-encoded G protein-coupled receptor, UL33, has been partially character-

ized; although it is dispensable for replication in tissue culture, UL33 has been demonstrated to be present in the virion particle,[58] and its homologues in mouse or rat CMVs are required by rodent CMVs for their replication in animal hosts.[59, 60]

A second class of viral genes (see Fig. 28–30) also not required for infection of fibroblasts in cell culture inhibit the host's immune response to HCMV. This class includes viral gene products that inhibit the function of major histocompatibility complex (MHC) class I molecules by distinct means at different times of the viral life cycle as well as one that may inhibit recognition of infected cells by natural killer (NK) cells. Immediately after infection, the US3 gene of HCMV is expressed. Its protein binds newly synthesized MHC class I heavy chains in the endoplasmic reticulum and, by retaining them, prevents their movement to the Golgi apparatus and ultimately to the cell surface.[61] Expression of the US11 gene leads to the degradation of newly synthesized class I heavy chains at an early stage of infection.[62, 63] By 72 hours after infection, the US6 gene product is synthesized maximally and inhibits the transporter associated with antigen processing (TAP), so that processed antigenic peptides cannot be loaded onto newly synthesized, remaining class I heavy chains in the lumen of the endoplasmic reticulum.[64–66] The failure of infected cells to present MHC class I antigens means that peptides derived from the HCMV-encoded proteins cannot be displayed on the cell surface, either to generate a new cytotoxic T-lymphocyte response or to elicit killing by previously primed cells. Further, the UL18 gene of HCMV encodes a homologue of MHC class I antigens that associates with β₂-microglobulin[67] and can bind peptides[68]; when expressed in HLA-A, B, and C minus mutant cells in culture, UL18 inhibits NK-mediated cell killing.[69, 70] The downregulation of MHC class I antigens at the infected cell surface by at least three viral genes would elicit a cytotoxic NK response that is inhibited by the action of a fourth viral gene. Clearly, HCMV has evolved multiple strategies to evade immune response, thereby facilitating its persistence in most of us for most of our lives!

Previous studies of infection of fibroblasts by HCMV in vitro also provide a limited perspective because HCMV infects cells other than fibroblasts in vivo. Studies in cell culture are therefore now being extended to characterize infections of additional cell types by HCMV in vitro. Multiple observations, for example, indicate that HCMV is maintained in blood cells latently. Monocytes freshly isolated from the blood of seropositive donors may contain viral DNA but do not express viral RNAs characteristic of productive infection.[71] On differentiation into macrophages after treatment with a phorbol ester and hydrocortisone, the cells do support expression of lytic viral RNAs as detected by reverse transcription and polymerase chain reaction (PCR) analysis.[71] When peripheral blood mononuclear cells from two seropositive donors are mixed to yield monocyte-derived macrophages that have been stimulated allogeneically in vitro, the cells support production and release of infectious HCMV.[72] Reactivation from a latent infection by allogeneic stimulation may contribute to the many HCMV infections that arise after transfusions and allogeneic tissue transplantations. HCMV can productively infect macrophages after treatment of adherent monocytes with concanavalin A,[73] consistent with HCMV's latency being dependent on the

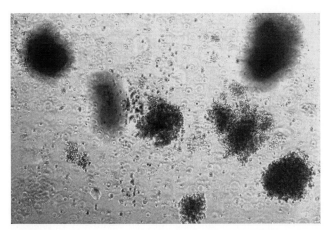

Figure 28–31. A colony of cells that express β-galactosidase encoded by a recombinant HCMV and that arose from a single stem cell is shown. The stem cell termed a colony-forming unit was isolated from bone marrow and infected in vitro. The infected bone marrow cells were dispersed as single cells in methylcellulose in an optimal cytokine environment for colony outgrowth. After 14 days, the X-gal substrate was added to identify cells expressing the viral transgene. Colonies like those shown here, which stained blue, were almost exclusively of myelomonocytic lineage. Staining of each cell within a positive colony indicates that HCMV was transmitted latently to daughter cells. Coculture of these colonies with fibroblast cultures, which support a lytic infection, recovered HCMV genetically marked like the input virus.

differentiated state of the host monocyte. This dependency is further illustrated by studies in vitro with bone marrow progenitor cells identified as being CD34+. Isolated and purified CD34+ cells can be infected with HCMV such that 50 per cent of the CD34+ cells express a β-galactosidase marker encoded by the virus 48 hours after infection[74] (Fig. 28–31). These cells do not appear to support productive infection in vitro because they can be induced to differentiate and survive to express their β-galactosidase marker.[74] CD34+ cells freshly isolated from HCMV-seropositive donors contain HCMV DNA but do not express an immediate early RNA characteristic of lytic infection.[75] Bone marrow progenitor cells therefore can be infected by HCMV in vitro, and presumably in vivo, to yield latently infected stem cells, which on differentiation to macrophages support productive infection if appropriately activated. Many studies also indicate that HCMV infects in vivo a wide variety of human cell types in addition to hematopoietic cells and that the outcome of these infections depends dramatically on the specific cell infected.[76]

Infection by Epstein-Barr Virus in Cell Culture

Whereas infection of fibroblast strains by HCMV yields a productive outcome for the virus, infection of B lymphocytes by EBV in general is non-productive. This difference is only heightened on consideration of the fates of the two infected host cells. Human fibroblast strains have a limited life span in culture of 50 to 100 cell divisions. HCMV replicates best in those fibroblasts that have been in culture for only a few generations and that proliferate efficiently, and these cells are killed by HCMV. EBV, on the other hand, infects non-proliferating, primary B lymphocytes that exhibit no proliferative capacity in culture. On infection with EBV, these cells

are induced to proliferate and yield progeny capable of proliferating indefinitely in cell culture. Although EBV "immortalizes" infected B lymphocytes efficiently, these immortalized cells only rarely yield progeny virus.[77, 78]

As the outcome of infection by EBV differs so strikingly from that of HCMV, so do many (but not all) stages of the viral life cycle. EBV binds to its cellular receptor CD21 through the viral gp340.[12, 79] EBV binds also to the HLA-DR β chain[80] on B lymphocytes by a complex of viral glycoproteins, gH, gL, and gp42, which are all essential for infection of this cell type.[81] The virus is internalized into cell vacuoles, where nucleocapsids are released from their envelopes.[82] The nucleocapsids migrate to the nucleus, where the viral DNA is circularized and transcribed. Whether EBV brings into the cells proteins that affect transcription of its DNA is unknown. During the first 72 hours after infection, viral RNA synthesis from one strand occurs from a single promoter termed Wp and then switches to a second promoter, Cp[83] (Fig. 28–32). By 72 to 96 hours after infection, products from a third promoter on the opposite strand can

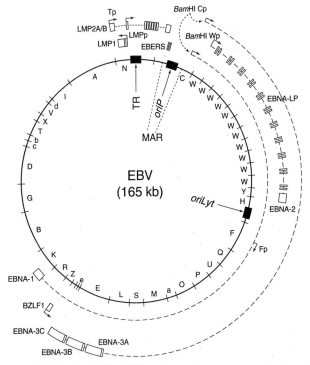

Figure 28–32. The DNA of EBV is depicted as a circular molecule as it would be found in cells immortalized by infection in vitro or in lymphoma cells isolated from patients. The letters inside the circle denote viral DNA fragments generated by its digestion with BamHI endonuclease. The black boxes represent critical cis-acting elements; the open boxes represent translated exons found in mature mRNAs. The origin of plasmid DNA replication, oriP, lies between the terminal repeats (TR), which are fused from the linear virion DNA, and two promoters, Cp and Wp, which direct clockwise transcription. Early after infection, these transcripts originate from Wp and later from Cp. Primary clockwise transcripts from these promoters are often long and are differentially spliced to yield multiple, distinct mRNAs encoding Epstein-Barr nuclear antigens or EBNAs. The origin of DNA replication used during the lytic phase (oriLyt) of EBV's life cycle maps approximately 40,000 bp away from oriP. LMP-1 is translated from a short, spliced, counterclockwise transcript that maps between promoters for clockwise transcription of LMP-2A and LMP-2B. These viral proteins are found in the plasma membrane of infected cells. BZLF-1 is a critical, positive regulator of EBV's escape from latency and an ensuing productive infection.

be detected. The primary transcripts range from 3 to 100 kb, and some are multiply spliced.[84-86] The transcripts are translated into 10 or 11 proteins,[87] but the remaining 90 or so open reading frames of EBV are not expressed. As those viral genes characteristic of the latent phase of the viral life cycle are expressed, dramatic changes in the host cell occur, induced by the actions of some or all of the latent viral genes. The small resting B lymphocyte swells to a lymphoblast, expresses new cellular antigens,[88, 89] and traverses the cell cycle. The circularized EBV DNA now replicates in synchrony with cell DNA.[90] The virus uses a plasmid origin of replication, *oriP*; one viral protein, Epstein-Barr nuclear antigen 1 (EBNA-1) (see Fig. 28–32); and additional cellular enzymes needed for DNA synthesis.[91-93] The B lymphoblast now proliferates efficiently, maintains EBV DNA as a plasmid that expresses a small subset of its genes, and efficiently yields cellular progeny that over time are found to be immortalized. These immortalized, proliferating B cells are both the hosts for and the result of the latent phase of EBV's life cycle in cell culture.

The multiple viral genes that contribute to the latent phase of EBV cells (see Fig. 28–32) are both essential for viral pathogenicity, because of effects on the infected B cell, and useful as markers for this stage of infection. The EBNA-2 gene of EBV, a major viral transcriptional regulator of viral and cellular genes during latent infection, is expressed early after infection. EBNA-2 is required for immortalization of infected cells.[94, 95] The gene product acts not by direct interaction with DNA but by binding to a cellular protein variously termed CBF-1, RBPJκ, or Su(H), which itself binds site-specifically to DNA sequences in a few known viral and cellular promoters.[96] EBNA-2 on binding to Su(H) provides its own transactivation domain, which associates with cellular TFIIB and TAF40 to promote transcription.[97] A second important viral gene, EBNA-1, is expressed after and positively regulated by EBNA-2. EBNA-1 is both a transcriptional activator and essential for replication of EBV plasmid DNA; EBNA-1 binds to the EBV plasmid origin of DNA synthesis[98] to mediate maintenance of the viral genome in proliferating cells.[99] As might be expected, EBNA-1 is expressed in infected cells of all EBV-associated diseases.[100, 101] EBNA-1 positively regulates promoters for its own synthesis and that of EBNA-2[102] and latent membrane protein LMP-1.[103] A third viral gene central to latency, LMP-1, encodes a protein that is located at the plasma membrane,[104] is also required for immortalization of cells by EBV,[105] and affects signaling from the membrane.[106-108] LMP-1 is often expressed in EBV-positive Hodgkin's disease[109] along with EBNA-1 and small viral RNAs termed EBERs.[110] The EBERs are not required for immortalization of infected B cells,[111] and although their role in EBV's life cycle is not clear, they are expressed abundantly[112] and therefore serve as readily detected diagnostic markers for EBV in this lymphoma.[113] Another diagnostic viral gene, LMP-2A, is also not essential for immortalization of B-lymphoid cells[114] but contributes to maintaining the latent phase of the viral life cycle.[115] LMP-2A encodes the only viral gene clearly expressed in the non-proliferating cells in which EBV resides in the blood of seropositive healthy donors.[116] The characterization of the viral genes expressed during the latent phase of EBV's life cycle has helped both to elucidate the mechanism by which EBV immortalizes B

lymphocytes and to identify viral markers diagnostic of tumor cells.

Were EBV only to immortalize infected B lymphocytes, the result of the infection, although of importance for a human host, would be a dead end for the virus. EBV also undergoes productive infection in these immortalized cells, albeit inefficiently. Between 0.1 and 0.001 per cent of cells in different clones of EBV-immortalized B lymphoblasts spontaneously convert to support a productive infection in each cell generation.[78] The immediate cause of this conversion is not known, but an early event is the induction of a viral gene, BZLF-1 (see Fig. 28–32), a transcriptional activator that induces several viral genes that collectively regulate expression of the remaining 90 or so open reading frames of EBV.[117-119] From this stage on, the ensuing lytic phase of EBV's life cycle is similar to the latter stages of productive infection of fibroblasts by HCMV. The early genes of EBV are expressed, some of which encode enzymes necessary for viral DNA synthesis.[120] Late genes are subsequently activated; some encode virion structural proteins.[120] Concurrent with the expression of late genes, EBV DNA is synthesized. In contrast to DNA synthesis that occurs during the latent phase of the viral life cycle, an origin different from *oriP* is used for lytic DNA synthesis, termed *oriLyt* (see Fig. 28–32), which yields large concatemeric structures, presumably by a rolling circle mechanism.[121] Binding of *oriLyt* to the product of BZLF-1 in multiple positions is essential for *oriLyt* function.[122] In addition to BZLF-1, six other viral genes are required for *oriLyt*-mediated DNA synthesis[123]; these EBV genes are homologues of HCMV genes that support DNA synthesis. The DNA products of EBV's lytic mode of DNA synthesis are cleaved and packaged into viral nucleocapsids in the nucleus. Cleavage depends both on specific sites at the termini of virion DNA[94] and on the capacity of the nucleocapsid to accommodate the DNA.[124] The assembly of complete virions and their exit from their host cells are presumed to mimic those processes of HCMV in fibroblasts.

Infections in the Human Host

Diseases associated with herpesviruses can result from either the latent or lytic phases of their life cycles. Symptoms can result from cell lysis and the immune response to infection; alternatively, pathological processes can result from changes in the latently infected cell. We shall use our understanding of the lytic and latent phases of viral life cycles gleaned from studies in cell culture to analyze the molecular bases of blood diseases associated with HCMV and EBV.

▼ HUMAN CYTOMEGALOVIRUS AS A PATHOGEN

Early History

As with most animal viruses, the history of HCMV is short. Scattered observations of human tissues that may have been infected by HCMV and that displayed characteristic structures now interpreted to be cytomegalic inclusions have been reported since the beginning of the 20th century.[125] The advent of cell culture in the 1940s allowed the isolation of HCMV in the middle 1950s.[126] Much work has gone into mapping the prevalence of the virus and serological studies to associate it with specific human diseases. Most infections with HCMV are benign. Ferreting out the conditions that lead to disease has been difficult and continues today.

Clinical Manifestations of HCMV Infections

Most people in the world are eventually infected by HCMV, as determined by their antibodies to HCMV-associated antigens. Infection occurs in affluent countries later in life than in Third World countries, but more than half of all screened populations are infected by age 50 years.[125] Historically, the first syndrome associated with HCMV infections was cytomegalic inclusion disease. Cytomegalic inclusion disease occurs in certain fatal infections in which affected tissues show large cells with polymorphic inclusions in their nuclei (Fig. 28–33). A search for the causative agent of cytomegalic inclusion disease led to the isolation of HCMV.[126] Intranuclear inclusions caused by HCMV result from synthesis and compartmentalization of late viral gene products and are indicative of productive infection. Although most infections by HCMV are clinically silent, some result in disease.

Primary infections during pregnancy with HCMV are associated with several sequelae, including mental retardation of the child. The magnitude of this problem has been addressed in Great Britain by a 7-year prospective study of more than 10,000 women[127]: 58 per cent of the women were seropositive when first tested; 0.75 per cent of those studied had primary infections during their pregnancies, and 20 per cent of their children had congenital infections. Twelve per cent of the congenitally infected children by 4 years of age became severely retarded, although they displayed no gross problems at birth. Extrapolating from these data, approximately 1 or 2 per 10,000 live births can be expected to develop mental retardation as a result of primary infection with HCMV.[127] Primary infection at any time during pregnancy increases the risk of inducing mental retardation.[127]

Both primary infection and reactivation with HCMV can cause interstitial pneumonitis. In most cases, this pneumonitis arises in immunocompromised patients as the result of immunosuppressive therapy or the acquired immune deficiency syndrome (AIDS). HCMV-associated pneumonitis may be difficult to diagnose because it can mimic gram-negative bacterial pneumonia or contribute to a bacterial lung infection.[125] For treatment of pneumonitis, HCMV must be rapidly and accurately detected,[128] using semiquantitative applications of PCR as the most sensitive assay.[129] This method potentially allows HCMV-associated pneumonia to be predicted in immunocompromised hosts.[130]

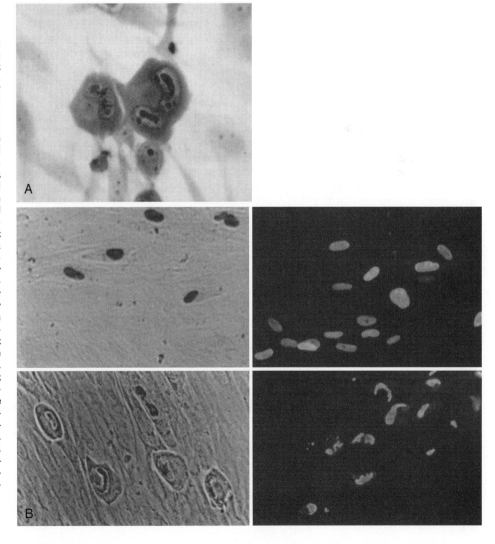

Figure 28–33. HCMV infects human fibroblasts in cell culture and produces inclusion bodies late in infection that are pathognomonic for cytomegalic inclusion disease in vivo. Simian CMV infects established monkey epithelial cells and produces similar inclusion bodies in them. *A*, Monkey epithelial cells infected with simian CMV are fixed and stained with hematoxylin and eosin to reveal the cytomegalic inclusion bodies within their nuclei. *B*, A strain of human fibroblasts is infected with HCMV. The upper two panels show infected cells fixed and stained with monoclonal antibodies to an immediate early protein of HCMV; that on the upper left is visualized with a horseradish peroxidase (HRP)-mediated reaction, and that on the upper right by immunofluorescence. The nuclei of the infected cells are uniformly stained. The lower two panels show infected cells fixed and stained with monoclonal antibodies to a late protein of HCMV; that on the lower left is visualized with HRP, and that on the lower right with immunofluorescence. The nuclei are not uniformly stained; rather, the staining is compartmentalized to the inclusion bodies within the nuclei, indicating that cytomegalic inclusions contain viral proteins expressed late in the viral life cycle. These analyses were performed by Dr. A. Lakeman of the University of Alabama with monoclonal antibodies developed by Dr. W. Britt from the University of Alabama.

HCMV-associated pneumonitis is often fatal. In one study of bone marrow recipients, 84 per cent of those who developed pneumonitis died.[131] This extraordinarily high rate may reflect the association between graft-versus-host disease (GvHD) and HCMV infection,[132] in which GvHD itself would be a major contributor to mortality.

Primary infection with HCMV in the normal population can cause a mononucleosis-like syndrome[133] characterized by high fever, mild lymphocytosis, some atypical lymphocytes, and mild hepatitis.[125] HCMV is usually distinguished from the more common EBV-associated mononucleosis by negative testing for heterophil antibodies (antibodies to foreign antigens such as horse red blood cells). In all other respects, the courses of HCMV- and EBV-associated mononucleosis are similar.[134] HCMV-associated mononucleosis also results from transfusions.[135] When seronegative recipients are transfused with blood from seropositive donors, the risk of seroconverting is on the order of 1 per cent per unit of blood transfused.[136, 137] Only 20 per cent of graft recipients who are seronegative, are immunosuppressed, and receive both transfusions and a kidney from seropositive donors have been found to develop HCMV-associated mononucleosis.[138]

Pathophysiology of HCMV-Associated Mononucleosis

Mononucleosis is the predominant blood disease associated with HCMV. The major evidence that HCMV is etiological is correlative, because the disease follows immediately on infection, determined by seroconversion. What is not clear is what virus/host cell relationships take place in the patient to cause the syndrome. Specifically, what cells are infected? What is the outcome of these infections? What is the immune response to these infections?

Multiple types of blood cells can be infected by HCMV in vitro including proliferating T cells,[139] bone marrow progenitor CD34$^+$ cells,[74] and monocyte-derived macrophages.[73] Different blood cells that were freshly isolated from donors have been found to contain viral DNA and to express viral RNA. In six of six seropositive donors, HCMV DNA was detected by use of sensitive nested PCR in mature monocytes (CD14$^+$ cells) and in CD3$^+$ T cells in one of these donors.[140] Blood cells from immunocompromised donors have also been analyzed by nested PCR to detect HCMV DNA and with a combination of reverse transcription and PCR to detect both early and late viral RNA. In one study, B cells (CD19$^+$), T cells (CD4$^+$ or CD8$^+$), monocytes (CD14$^+$), and granulocytes (CD16$^+$) were separated by flow cytometry and found to contain HCMV DNA at different frequencies and at different levels.[141] Granulocytes (CD16$^+$) were most often positive and harbored the highest levels of viral DNA. Both early and late viral RNAs were detected in some HCMV DNA-positive lymphocytes, monocytes, and granulocytes.[141] Interpretations of these findings must be tempered with the recognition that some positive assays may result from contamination of impure cell populations. However, many distinct hematopoietic cells are likely to be infected with HCMV under different conditions in vivo. Whereas studies do not allow identification of a single cell type as being a specific host for infection by HCMV, the major atypical lymphocyte in HCMV-associated mononucleosis is

a CD8$^+$ T cell[142]; these cells are probably cytotoxic effector cells targeted to some HCMV-infected blood cells.

Two hypotheses must be tested: that HCMV-associated mononucleosis results from productive infections of hematopoietic cells and that CD8$^+$ cells are the predominant atypical lymphocytes in this disease because they are amplified to kill the HCMV-infected cells. An attractive idea is that monocyte-derived macrophages, which support infection in vitro[72, 73] and are the predominant HCMV-positive cell type in immunocompetent hosts,[140] contribute to HCMV-associated mononucleosis.

Treatment of HCMV-Associated Diseases

High fever in HCMV-associated mononucleosis in adults often requires treatment. However, HCMV-associated diseases in immunocompromised patients usually require immediate intervention. HCMV pneumonitis is often fatal, and HCMV-associated retinitis in AIDS patients is usually progressive. In both syndromes, HCMV infection is productive. The most effective treatment to date is to limit the productive infection by inhibiting viral DNA replication. One of the four genes of HCMV that are homologues of HSV-1 genes involved in DNA replication encodes a DNA polymerase[2] that is inhibited by the nucleoside analogue ganciclovir (9-[1,3-dihydroxy-2-propoxymethyl]guanine) once it is phosphorylated by cellular kinases.[143] Treatment of HCMV-associated retinitis with ganciclovir is remarkably effective,[144] therapy of established HCMV pneumonitis less so.[145] Ganciclovir has been combined with immune globulin for prophylaxis and for the early treatment of HCMV infection in bone marrow recipients.[146, 147]

The use of ganciclovir has attendant problems. First, cellular DNA polymerases are also inhibited by phosphorylated forms of ganciclovir,[143] and at higher doses of inhibitor, more uninfected cells are affected deleteriously. Second, prolonged use of ganciclovir selects for mutants of HCMV that are resistant to it.[148] Third, intravenously administered ganciclovir has an associated toxicity; however, a recently available oral formulation is effective at reducing HCMV-associated disease in solid organ transplant recipients without significant toxicity.[149]

HCMV-associated diseases are most severe in immunosuppressed patients and particularly so in seronegative transplant recipients.[150] The treatment of transplant recipients has focused on providing them some form of protective immunity. Passive immunization through administration of hyperimmune globulin in combination with ganciclovir has proved effective in reducing the severity of post-transplantation sequelae. When given prophylactically, this combination reduced HCMV-associated disease to a level similar to that found in seropositive patients.[151, 152]

Immune protection against HCMV has also been provided at a cellular level. Bone marrow recipients can acquire an HCMV-associated pneumonia with a mortality rate as high as 50 to 80 per cent. Recipients with a slow reconstitution of their cytotoxic T cells (CD8$^+$) are most likely to develop this pneumonia.[153, 154] One experimental, effective approach to minimize these pneumonias is to amplify donor cytotoxic T cells that are specific to HCMV-infected cells in vitro and to infuse the T cells into the recipient after the initial transplant.[155] The use of specific, cytotoxic T cells expanded in vitro appears to avoid GvHD that develops when unselected T cells are infused into recipients.

▼ EPSTEIN-BARR VIRUS AS A PATHOGEN

Early History

Not only is EBV's history brief, but so too is the medical community's recognition of some of the diseases with which it is associated. Its discovery, however, is a marvelous tale.[156] Dennis Burkitt identified a formerly unrecognized childhood tumor prevalent in East Africa in the mid-1950s[157] and from his clever investigations postulated that it was caused by a vector-borne virus.[158] Epstein and his colleagues developed the means to propagate cells from these childhood tumors (now known as Burkitt's lymphomas), which had to be flown from East Africa to England for study, and they identified in rare cells in these cultures a new virus—Epstein-Barr virus.[159] Soon after the identification of EBV, acute observation and serendipity were coupled by the Henles, who noted that a laboratory colleague seroconverted to express antibodies to EBV on developing infectious mononucleosis.[160] This finding paved the way for retrospective and prospective epidemiological surveys that have established EBV as the causative agent of the heterophil-positive form of infectious mononucleosis.[161, 162]

Clinical Manifestations of EBV Infections

Most infections with EBV are clinically silent. In developing countries and among the poor, children are usually infected asymptomatically in early life after the protection from maternally acquired antibodies has waned. In industrialized societies, many are first infected as adolescents, in whom primary infection can result in heterophil-positive infectious mononucleosis. The usual presentation is sore throat, fever, and malaise for 2 to 3 weeks. During the acute phase of infectious mononucleosis, EBV-infected B lymphocytes can be detected in the peripheral blood; in extreme cases, up to 20 per cent have been found to be infected.[163] Some infected cells are proliferating[164] and constitute a portion of the atypical lymphocytes characteristic of infectious mononucleosis.[165, 166] EBV-infected, proliferating B lymphocytes secrete immunoglobulins[167] that are presumably the source of the heterophil antibodies. T lymphocytes proliferate in response to EBV-infected cells and also contribute to the atypical lymphocytes. The large number of proliferating lymphocytes may contribute to the generalized lymphadenopathy and the splenomegaly frequently associated with infectious mononucleosis. In most cases, the acute phase of the disease passes within 3 weeks. During convalescence, the number of atypical cells declines to undetectable levels in the blood, and the infection in a few of these cells is latent. However, people often shed EBV in their saliva for weeks to months after recovering from infectious mononucleosis.[168, 169]

Young children in some regions of the world, including East Africa and New Guinea, in which malaria is endemic, can develop Burkitt's lymphoma 7 to 48 months after infection by EBV.[170, 171] The tumor is often recognized clinically as a mass of the jaw and usually has colonized several additional sites when diagnosed. These additional sites may include the orbit and the abdomen, but not often the bone marrow.[172] Sporadic Burkitt's lymphoma, not usually associated with EBV or malaria, occurs throughout the world at about 1 per 1,000,000 children per year or 1 per cent of the frequency of Burkitt's lymphoma in East Africa and New Guinea. In contrast to endemic Burkitt's lymphoma, sporadic cases usually do not present as a mass of the jaw and often involve the bone marrow.[172]

In EBV-positive Burkitt's lymphoma, the tumor mass grows rapidly and contains proliferating cells with mitotic figures. Tumor cells express at least one viral protein, EBNA-1,[173, 174] and a set of viral RNAs whose function is unknown,[175] and they usually contain multiple copies of the viral genome in plasmid form.[176] Tumor cells express monoclonal surface immunoglobulin and express a single X-linked glucose-6-phosphate dehydrogenase isozyme in heterozygous females.[177, 178] These findings indicate that endemic Burkitt's lymphoma is clonal in origin with EBV infecting a precursor to the tumor cell. These tumor cells can be propagated readily in cell culture, and over time they can express all the viral genes characteristic of the latent phase of EBV's life cycle, in addition to EBNA-1.[100] In general, Burkitt's lymphoma tumor cells, of all origins, usually display a striking, characteristic karyotype, a chromosomal translocation that juxtaposes one of the three immunoglobulin loci with the c-*myc* locus.[179, 180] This rearrangement leads to the expression only of the translocated c-*myc* allele at a level similar to that of non-rearranged c-*myc* in B lymphoblasts immortalized by EBV in vitro.[181]

EBV is also causally associated with B-cell lymphomas in immunocompromised hosts. Patients can be congenitally immunodeficient, such as males who have an X-linked lymphoproliferative syndrome[182]; iatrogenically immunosuppressed, such as graft recipients[183, 184]; or immunocompromised, as in AIDS.[185] In all cases, the EBV-associated lymphoma cells express EBV antigens, are polyclonal, and lack the characteristic chromosomal translocations between immunoglobulin loci and that of c-*myc*.

As the association of EBV with B-cell lymphomas has become better appreciated, additional hematopoietic tumors have been found to contain EBV DNA and viral gene products, especially some T-cell lymphomas and Hodgkin's lymphomas. Eight of 21 post-transplantation T-cell lymphomas surveyed were found to be EBV positive.[186] In one study of tumors of the salivary gland, one site found to support productive infection by EBV in vivo, all three identified T-cell lymphomas were found to contain EBV DNA and to express its small nuclear RNAs (EBERs).[187] Two T-cell lymphomas that developed in patients with chronic, active EBV infection were found to express three viral gene products, EBNA-1, LMP-1, and LMP-2.[188] These findings indicate that EBV can be found in some T cells and probably contributes to the evolution of T-cell lymphomas that harbor it. The frequency of these tumors and the role of EBV in their etiology remain to be established. Evidence for EBV in Hodgkin's disease is more extensive than that for T-cell lymphomas. A survey of 14 studies encompassing more than 1500 patients with Hodgkin's disease has found EBV in 40 per cent of the cases, as determined by expression of EBERs, LMP-1, or both.[189] EBV is particularly common in Hodgkin's lymphomas classified as being of mixed cellularity[189] and in those that arise in immunocompromised hosts. In 13 of 13 patients with Hodgkin's disease infected with HIV, the Reed-Sternberg cells contained EBV-encoded EBERs.[190] When EBERs are detected by in situ hybridization in some Reed-Sternberg cells of a tumor, they are usually detected in all,[110] indicating that infection with EBV is likely to be an early event in the evolution of the tumor. EBNA-1 is also expressed in EBV-positive Hodgkin's disease,[101] consistent with the viral DNA being maintained as a plasmid in the cells. The frequent association of EBV with Hodgkin's disease, its presence in the majority of mixed cellularity cases, and its ubiquity in all tumor cells when it is present in any combine to make it likely that EBV contributes causally to a significant subset of Hodgkin's lymphomas. However, the prospective epidemiological surveys that might support a causal role for EBV in this tumor have not been undertaken and may be impractical given the widespread distribution of EBV in adults.

There are also non-lymphoid diseases associated with EBV. Some AIDS patients develop oral hairy leukoplakia, a productive infection of mucosal epithelial cells by EBV.[191] The affected tissue consists of stratified squamous epithelium. EBV is not detected in the basal layer of this tissue, but in the upper layers the BZLF-1 gene of EBV is expressed, and productively amplified viral DNA can be detected.[192] Some carcinomas have been found to be latently infected with EBV. In a large survey of 1000 gastric carcinomas in Japan, 70 primary tumors were EBV positive and expressed only EBNA-1 in the tumor cells.[193]

In East Asia as well as in areas in which Burkitt's lymphoma is endemic, infection of epithelial cells in the post-nasal space with EBV is associated with a common form of nasopharyngeal carcinoma[194]; between 50,000 and 100,000 new cases develop each year. EBNA-1 is expressed in the tumor cells,[195, 196] which contain multiple copies of viral plasmid DNAs.[197] That the tumor cells proliferate in vivo to kill the host while maintaining multiple viral genomes indicates that this disease represents predominantly a latent infection. A prospective seroepidemiological study indicates that antibodies of the immunoglobulin A class to EBV-associated early antigens constitute a major risk factor for the development of nasopharyngeal carcinoma.[198] This finding, therefore, causally associates EBV with nasopharyngeal carcinoma. EBV stands out among human tumor viruses for the diversity of neoplasms, of both lymphoid and epithelial origin, with which it is associated.

Molecular and Cellular Analyses of EBV-Associated B-Lymphoid Diseases

How does infection of human B lymphocytes by one virus lead to such different results—a self-limiting proliferation, infectious mononucleosis, or a rapidly dividing Burkitt's lymphoma? Even a partial answer is instructive, because it illustrates the various contexts in which EBV contributes to diseases of the blood.

First, although different strains of EBV exist, it is clear that no one strain has been specifically associated with a disease manifestation.[199] The A and B strains of EBV differ at multiple loci and yield infected cells with different growth properties, but each is associated with all the diseases caused by EBV. Second, in infectious mononucleosis, although many infected B lymphocytes are induced to proliferate in vivo[164] and continue to proliferate on explantation into cell culture,[200] an effective cytotoxic response to these infected cells has been documented.[201–203] Viral targets for this response include many genes of EBV, other than EBNA-1, that are characteristic of latent infection. The dramatic immune response in vivo leads to a diminution of infected B lymphocytes in the peripheral blood of convalescing patients, although once infected, most people with EBV retain some small number of infected cells in their blood. These persisting EBV-positive cells can be detected long after convalescence by tissue culture of lymphoid cells, in the presence of cyclosporine to inhibit a cytotoxic response to the proliferating, infected cells[204] or by introducing them into SCID mice (mice inbred to display a particular severe combined immunodeficiency), in which they grow as lethal polyclonal tumors.[205] The EBV-positive lymphoid cells isolated from the peripheral blood of normal donors are small resting CD19$^+$, CD23$^-$ cells present at levels of 1 per million B cells[206]; these cells express primarily LMP-2A.[116]

The importance of an effective, cell-mediated response to EBV-infected cells in limiting infectious mononucleosis can also be inferred from the course of primary infections in immunocompromised hosts. EBV seronegative bone marrow recipients, for example, can develop polyclonal EBV-associated lymphomas 2 to 3 months after receiving grafts from EBV seropositive donors[207]; the malignant neoplasm is of donor origin. The persistence of EBV-infected cells in the healthy host is probably important as a stimulus to the immune response and constitutively limits reinfections throughout life. Many people shed EBV in their saliva, and thus reinoculation is probably common.[168]

What differs in the infection of children destined to develop Burkitt's lymphoma? A prospective seroepidemiological survey has found that children with abnormally high titers of antibodies to EBV late proteins have an increased risk for development of Burkitt's lymphoma compared with matched control subjects,[170, 171] indicating that a robust infection with EBV is a major risk determinant. Chronic malaria is endemic among children where Burkitt's lymphoma is found[208, 209]; and malaria induces T-cell immunosuppression such that the host cannot efficiently kill EBV-infected B lymphocytes.[210, 211] For example, children in the Gambia have five times more EBV-positive cells in their peripheral blood as measured by limiting dilution assays during the acute phase of malaria than during convalescence from this parasite.[212] Thus, it appears that those destined to develop Burkitt's lymphoma have both a robust infection with EBV and an impaired immune response that only inefficiently limits the proliferation of infected cells.

Several known molecular alterations occur in the clone of EBV-infected cells that develops into a tumor. They most likely occur after infection in a rare cell among the large population of cells induced to proliferate by EBV. One of three immunoglobulin loci is juxtaposed to the c-myc locus[180] in greater than 90 per cent of cases, and mutations occur in the tumor suppressor gene termed p53 in 40 to 75 per cent of the cases studied.[213, 214] These mutations are usually followed by subsequent events that inactivate the expression of the wild-type p53 allele.[213, 214] Because of their ubiquity, these mutations can be assumed to provide the mutant cell a selective advantage in vivo; one such hypothetical advantage might be to allow the EBV-infected cell to continue to proliferate in the absence of expression of some of the EBV genes required for immortalization, such as EBNA-2 and LMP-1. Cells in which the growth-promoting functions of these viral genes were substituted by those of cellular genes would escape the T cell-mediated cytotoxicity directed against these viral gene products. For example, conditional mutants have been used to demonstrate that EBNA-2 is required for EBV-infected cells to proliferate,[215] and EBNA-2 is a target for cytotoxic T cells.[216] Consistent with this model, EBNA-1, which is required to maintain the viral DNA as a plasmid in proliferating cells,[92, 99, 217] is not a target for the immune system and is expressed in Burkitt's lymphomas.[100] EBNA-1 contains a repeat element that inhibits its processing for display as an antigen by HLA class I molecules.[218, 219] Probably the translocated c-*myc* functionally substitutes for EBNA-2, LMP-1, and other required viral genes; efficient expression of c-*myc* has been shown to support proliferation of an EBV-positive cell in which EBNA-2 has been rendered conditionally non-functional.[220] Whether or not this hypothesis proves correct, several rare events must occur in one clone of cells for its evolution into Burkitt's lymphoma. Only in those regions of the world in which chronic malaria and early infection with EBV overlap is the frequency of these rare events high enough to yield the 1 case of Burkitt's lymphoma per 10,000 children characteristic of these regions.

Treatment of EBV-Associated Lymphoid Diseases

The symptoms of EBV-associated infectious mononucleosis are usually mild and readily treated with bed rest. Those infrequent cases that are complicated by respiratory obstruction or hemolytic anemia respond to administration of corticosteroids. Rare cases that progress to splenic rupture are treated surgically. In other instances of EBV infections, antiviral therapy may be used. For example, one treatment is directed against the lytic phase of the EBV life cycle. Acyclovir (9-[(2-hydroxyethoxy)methyl]guanine), once phosphorylated in the cell, is recognized by EBV DNA polymerase, is incorporated into a growing DNA chain, and terminates that chain.[221] In immunosuppressed patients who develop a syndrome similar to infectious mononucleosis, in which the proliferating B lymphocytes are karyotypically normal, treatment with acyclovir is successful in resolving the disease.[222] Acyclovir will be useful for treating only those EBV-associated lymphoid diseases in which the lytic cycle is required to maintain the disease.

Lymphomas associated with EBV in general and Burkitt's lymphoma in particular are not responsive to antiviral therapies. The one viral protein consistently expressed in tumor cells is EBNA-1, but no therapies designed to inhibit its function have been developed. Burkitt's lymphomas are treated with combination chemotherapy and, for large tumor masses, radiation.[172] Response rates to these therapies in African cases are high,[172] with 60 per cent to 90 per cent 2-year tumor-free rates, depending on the extent of the tumor at the time of treatment. One hope for treating EBV-associated lymphomas grows out of identification of epitopes in latently expressed viral proteins that are recognized by cyto-

toxic T lymphocytes.[223, 224] These epitopes, if they can be used to stimulate appropriately responding cytotoxic T lymphocytes, might serve as a vaccine to engender the desired immune responses to tumor cells expressing particular viral proteins. The epitopes must be delivered such that they can be recognized[225]; they must be extensive enough so that the HLA repertoire of the patient includes alleles that recognize the presented epitopes; and the cellular transporter proteins that carry the antigenic peptides into the lumen of the endoplasmic reticulum must function. At least in Burkitt's lymphoma cells, the two components of this transporter, TAP-1 and TAP-2, appear to be downregulated,[226] perhaps by EBV-encoded or cellular interleukin-10.[227]

EBV lymphomas arise in transplant recipients who are immunosuppressed to minimize rejection of their grafts,[228, 229] often with cyclosporin A, a drug that limits proliferation of cytotoxic T lymphocytes directed against EBV-infected cells.[230] A monitored reduction of immunosuppressive drugs in patients developing EBV-positive, post-transplantation lymphomas may allow an increase in their cytotoxic T-lymphocyte response sufficient to eliminate the tumors. An experimental approach that has proved successful is to treat bone marrow transplant recipients with adoptive cellular immunotherapy.[231] Cytotoxic T lymphocytes from donor cells are expanded in vitro with EBV-infected autologous B cells as stimulators. These cells are administered after the transplant and do not contribute to GvHD.[231] In 36 patients tested, none developed lymphomas after transplantation, whereas five were expected to develop EBV-associated lymphoproliferations on the basis of historical experience.[231] Adoptive cellular immunotherapy is obviously not currently practical as routine therapy, but its success underscores the role of cytotoxic T lymphocytes in limiting EBV-associated lymphoproliferative diseases.

Our appreciation for the molecular mechanisms by which EBV immortalizes B lymphocytes is growing rapidly. On the basis of the identification and functional characterization of many viral proteins, new families of antiviral drugs will be developed to limit non-malignant EBV-induced lymphoproliferations. As these drugs are developed, concomitant directed research may also contribute to antiviral therapies applicable to EBV-associated malignant neoplasms.

REFERENCES

1. Davison, A.J.: Channel catfish virus: a new type of herpesvirus. Virology 186:9, 1992.
2. Chee, M.S., Bankier, A.T., Beck, S., Bohni, R., Brown, C.M., Cerny, R., Horsnell, T., Hutchison, C.A., III, Kouzarides, T., Martignetti, J.A., Preddie, E., Satchwell, S.C., Tomlinson, P., Weston, K.M., and Barrell, B.G.: Analysis of the protein-coding content of the sequence of human cytomegalovirus strain AD169. Curr. Top. Microbiol. Immunol. 154:125, 1990.
3. Cha, T.A., Tom, E., Kemble, G.W., Duke, G.M., Mocarski, E.S., and Spaete, R.R.: Human cytomegalovirus clinical isolates carry at least 19 genes not found in laboratory strains. J. Virol. 70:78, 1996.
4. Roizman, B., Carmichael, L.E., Deinhardt, F., de-The, G., Nahmias, A.J., Plowright, W., Rapp, F., Sheldrick, P., Takahashi, M., and Wolf, K.: Herpesviridae: definition, provisional nomenclature and taxonomy. Intervirology 16:201, 1981.
5. Stinski, M.F.: Human cytomegalovirus: glycoproteins associated with virions and dense bodies. J. Virol. 19:594, 1976.
6. Lakeman, A.D., and Osborn, J.E.: Size of infectious DNA from human and murine cytomegalovirus. J. Virol. 30:414, 1979.

7. Farrar, G.H., and Oram, J.D.: Characterization of the human cytomegalovirus envelope glycoproteins. J. Gen. Virol. 65:1991, 1984.

8. Rasmussen, L., Nelson, M., Neff, M., and Merigan, T.C., Jr.: Characterization of two different human cytomegalovirus glycoproteins which are targets for virus neutralizing antibody. Virology 163:308, 1988.

9. Matsumoto, Y., Sugano, T., Miyamoto, C., and Masuho, Y.: Generation of hybridomas producing human monoclonal antibodies against human cytomegalovirus. Biochem. Biophys. Res. Commun. 137:273, 1986.

10. Yao, Q.Y., Rowe, M., Morgan, A.J., Sam, C.K., Prasad, U., Dang, H., Zeng, Y., and Rickinson, A.B.: Salivary and serum IgA antibodies to the Epstein-Barr virus glycoprotein gp340: incidence and potential for virus neutralization. Int. J. Cancer 48:45, 1991.

11. Wallace, L.E., Wright, J., Ulaeto, D.O., Morgan, A.J., and Rickinson, A.B.: Identification of two T-cell epitopes on the candidate Epstein-Barr virus vaccine glycoprotein gp340 recognized by CD4+ T-cell clones. J. Virol. 65:3821, 1991.

12. Fingeroth, J.D., Weis, J.J., Tedder, T.F., Strominger, J.L., Biro, P.A., and Fearon, D.T.: Epstein-Barr virus receptor of human b lymphocytes is the C3d receptor CR2. Proc. Natl. Acad. Sci. USA 81:4510, 1984.

13. Nemerow, G.R., Mold, C., Schwend, V.K., Tollefson, V., and Cooper, N.R.: Identification of gp350 as the viral glycoprotein mediating attachment of Epstein-Barr virus (EBV) to the EBV/C3d receptor of B cells: sequence homology of gp350 and C3 complement fragment C3d. J. Virol. 61:1416, 1987.

14. Morgan, A.J., Allison, A.C., Finerty, S., Scullion, F.T., Byars, N.E., and Epstein, M.A.: Validation of a first-generation Epstein-Barr virus vaccine preparation suitable for human use. J. Med. Virol. 29:74, 1989.

15. Mackett, M., Cox, C., Pepper, S.D., Lees, J.F., Naylor, B.A., Wedderburn, N., and Arrand, J.R.: Immunisation of common marmosets with vaccinia virus expressing Epstein-Barr virus (EBV) gp340 and challenge with EBV. J. Med. Virol. 50:263, 1996.

16. Stannard, L.M., and Hardie, D.R.: An Fc receptor for human immunoglobulin G is located within the tegument of human cytomegalovirus. J. Virol. 65:3411, 1991.

17. Gibson, W.: Protein counterparts of human and simian cytomegaloviruses. Virology 128:391, 1983.

18. Gibson, W., and Roizman B.: Compartmentalization of spermine and spermidine in the herpes simplex virion. Proc. Natl. Acad. Sci. USA 68:2818, 1971.

19. Kouzarides, T., Bankier, A.T., Satchwell, S.C., Weston, K., Tomlinson, P., and Barrell, B.G.: Large-scale rearrangement of homologous regions in the genomes of HCMV and EBV. Virology 157:397, 1987.

20. Kintner, C., and Sugden, B.: Conservation and progressive methylation of Epstein-Barr viral DNA sequences in transformed cells. J. Virol. 38:305, 1981.

21. Jenkins, F.J., and Roizman, B.: Herpes simplex virus 1 recombinants with noninverting genomes frozen in different isomeric arrangements are capable of independent replication. J. Virol. 59:494, 1986.

22. Sixbey, J.W.: Epstein-Barr virus and epithelial cells. In Klein, G. (ed.): Advances in Viral Oncology. Vol. 8. New York, Raven Press, 1989, pp. 187–202.

23. Compton, T., Nowlin, D.M., and Cooper, N.R.: Initiation of human cytomegalovirus infection requires initial interaction with cell surface heparan sulfate. Virology 193:834, 1993.

24. Britt, W.J., Vugler, L., Butfiloski, E.J., and Stephens, E.B.: Cell surface expression of human cytomegalovirus (HCMV) gp55–116 (gB): use of HCMV-recombinant vaccinia virus–infected cells in analysis of the human neutralizing antibody response. J. Virol. 64:1079, 1990.

25. Tugizov, S., Navarro, D., Paz, P., Wang, Y., Qadri, I., and Pereira, L.: Function of human cytomegalovirus glycoprotein b: syncytium formation in cells constitutively expressing gB is blocked by virus-neutralizing antibodies. Virology 201:263, 1994.

26. Smith, J.D., and De Harven, E.: Herpes simplex virus and human cytomegalovirus replication in WI-38 cells. II. An ultrastructural study of viral penetration. J. Virol. 14:945, 1974.

27. Batterson, W., Furlong, D., and Roizman, B.: Molecular genetics of herpes simplex virus VIII. Further characterization of a temperature-sensitive mutant defective in release of viral DNA and in other stages of the viral reproductive cycle. J. Virol. 45:397, 1983.

28. Preston, C.M., Frame, M.C., and Campbell, M.E.M.: A complex formed between cell components and an HSV structural polypeptide binds to a viral immediate early gene regulatory DNA sequence. Cell 52:425, 1988.

29. Baldick, C.J., Jr., Marchini, A., Patterson, C.E., and Shenk, T.: Human cytomegalovirus tegument protein pp71 (ppUL82) enhances the infectivity of viral DNA and accelerates the infectious cycle. J. Virol. 71:4400, 1997.

30. Wathen, M.W., and Stinski, M.F.: Temporal patterns of human cytomegalovirus transcription: mapping the viral RNAs synthesized at immediate early, early, and late times after infection. J. Virol. 41:462, 1982.

31. Weston, K.: An enhancer element in the short unique region of human cytomegalovirus regulates the production of a group of abundant immediate early transcripts. Virology 162:406, 1988.

32. Thomson, D.R., Stenberg, R.M., Goins, W.F., and Stinski, M.F.: Promoter-regulatory region of the major immediate early gene of human cytomegalovirus. Proc. Natl. Acad. Sci. USA 81:659, 1984.

33. Hennighausen, L., and Fleckenstein, B.: Nuclear factor 1 interacts with five DNA elements in the promoter region of the human cytomegalovirus major immediate early gene. EMBO J. 5:1367, 1986.

34. Ghazal, P., and Nelson, J.A.: Enhancement of RNA polymerase II initiation complexes by a novel DNA control domain downstream from the cap site of the cytomegalovirus major immediate-early promoter. J. Virol. 65:2299, 1991.

35. Cherrington, J.M., and Mocarski, E.S.: Human cytomegalovirus ie1 transactivates the α promoter-enhancer via an 18-base-pair repeat element. J. Virol. 63:1435, 1989.

36. Malone, C.L., Vesole, D.H., and Stinski, M.F.: Transactivation of a human cytomegalovirus early promoter by gene products from immediate-early gene IE2 and augmentation by IE1: mutational analysis of the viral proteins. J. Virol. 64:1498, 1990.

37. Pizzorno, M., O'Hare, P., Sha, L., La Femina, R.L., and Hayward, G.S.: Trans-activation and autoregulation of gene expression by the immediate-early region 2 gene products of human cytomegalovirus. J. Virol. 62:1167, 1988.

38. Pizzorno, M.C., and Hayward, G.S.: The IE2 gene products of human cytomegalovirus specifically down-regulate expression from the major immediate-early promoter through a target sequence located near the cap site. J. Virol. 64:6154, 1990.

39. Margolis, M.J., Pajovic, S., Wong, E.L., Wade, M., Jupp, R., Nelson, J.A., and Azizkhan, J.C.: Interaction of the 72-kilodalton human cytomegalovirus IE1 gene product with E2F1 coincides with E2F-dependent activation of dihydrofolate reductase transcription. J. Virol. 69:7759, 1995.

40. Macias, M.P., Huang L., Lashmit, P.E., and Stinski, M.F.: Cellular or viral protein binding to a cytomegalovirus promoter transcription initiation site: effects on transcription. J. Virol. 70:3628, 1996.

41. Staprans, S.I., Rabert, D.K., and Spector, D.H.: Identification of sequence requirements and trans-acting functions necessary for regulated expression of a human cytomegalovirus early gene. J. Virol. 62:3463, 1988.

42. Depto, A.S., and Stenberg, R.M.: Regulated expression of the human cytomegalovirus pp65 gene: octamer sequence in the promoter is required for activation by viral gene products. J. Virol. 63:1232, 1989.

43. Boeckh, M., Gooley, T.A., Myerson, D., Cunningham, T., Schoch, G., and Bowden, R.A.: Cytomegalovirus pp65 antigenemia-guided early treatment with ganciclovir versus ganciclovir at engraftment after allogeneic marrow transplantation: a randomized double-blind study. Blood 88:4063, 1996.

44. Goins, W.F., and Stinski, M.F.: Expression of a human cytomegalovirus late gene is posttranscriptionally regulated by a 3′-end-processing event occurring exclusively late after infection. Mol. Cell. Biol. 6:4202, 1986.

45. Geballe, A.P., Spaete, R.R., and Mocarski, E.S.: A cis-acting element within the 5′ leader of a cytomegalovirus (beta) transcript determines kinetic class. Cell 46:865, 1986.

46. Geballe, A.P., and Mocarski, E.S.: Translational control of cytomegalovirus gene expression is mediated by upstream AUG codons. J. Virol. 62:3334, 1988.

47. Cao, J., and Geballe, A.P.: Inhibition of nascent-peptide release at translation termination. Mol. Cell. Biol. 16:7109, 1996.

48. Anders, D.G., and Punturieri, S.M.: Multicomponent origin of cytomegalovirus lytic-phase DNA replication. J. Virol. 65:931, 1991.

49. Pari, G.S., and Anders, D.G.: Eleven loci encoding trans-acting factors are required for transient complementation of human cytomegalovirus oriLyt-dependent DNA replication. J. Virol. 67:6979, 1993.

50. Huang, L., Zhu, Y., and Anders, D.G.: The variable 3′ ends of a human cytomegalovirus oriLyt transcript (SRT) overlap an essential, conserved replicator element. J. Virol. 70:5272, 1996.

51. Schwartz, J., and Roizman, B.: Concerning the egress of herpes simplex virus from infected cells: electron and light microscope observations. Virology 38:42, 1969.

52. Tooze, J., Hollinshead, M., Reis, B., Radsak, K., and Kern, H.: Progeny vaccinia and human cytomegalovirus particles utilize early endosomal cisternae for their envelopes. Eur. J. Cell Biol. 60:163, 1993.

53. Johnson, D.C., and Spear, P.G.: Monensin inhibits the processing of herpes simplex virus glycoproteins, their transport to the cell surface, and the egress of virions from infected cells. J. Virol. 43:1102, 1982.

54. Maidji, E., Tugizov, S., Jones, T., Zheng, Z., and Pereira, L.: Accessory human cytomegalovirus glycoprotein US9 in the unique short component of the viral genome promotes cell-to-cell transmission of virus in polarized epithelial cells. J. Virol. 70:8402, 1996.

55. Chee, M.S., Satchwell, S.C., Preddie, E., Weston, K.M., and Barrell, B.G.: Human cytomegalovirus encodes three G protein–coupled receptor homologues. Nature 344:774, 1990.

56. Welch, A.R., McGregor, L.M., and Gibson, W.: Cytomegalovirus homologs of cellular G protein–coupled receptor genes are transcribed. J. Virol. 65:3915, 1991.

57. Gao, J.L., and Murphy, P.M.: Human cytomegalovirus open reading frame US28 encodes a functional beta chemokine receptor. J. Biol. Chem. 269:28539, 1994.

58. Margulies, B.J., Browne, H., and Gibson, W.: Identification of the human cytomegalovirus G protein–coupled receptor homologue encoded by UL33 in infected cells and enveloped virus particles. Virology 225:111, 1996.

59. Davis-Poynter, N.J., Lynch, D.M., Vally, H., Shellam, G.R., Rawlinson, W.D., Barrell, B.G., and Farrell, H.E.: Identification and characterization of a G protein–coupled receptor homolog encoded by murine cytomegalovirus. J. Virol. 71:1521, 1997.

60. Beisser, P.S., Vink, C., Van Dam, J.G., Grauls, G., Vanherle, S.J., and Bruggeman, C.A.: The R33 G protein–coupled receptor gene of rat cytomegalovirus plays an essential role in the pathogenesis of viral infection. J. Virol. 72:2352, 1998.

61. Ahn, K., Angulo, A., Ghazal, P., Peterson, P.A., Yang, Y., and Fruh, K.: Human cytomegalovirus inhibits antigen presentation by a sequential multistep process. Proc. Natl. Acad. Sci. USA 93:10990, 1996.

62. Jones, T.R., Hanson, L.K., Sun, L., Slater, J.S., Stenberg, R.M., and Campbell, A.E.: Multiple independent loci within the human cytomegalovirus unique short region down-regulate expression of major histocompatibility complex class I heavy chains. J.Virol. 69:4830, 1995.

63. Wiertz, E.J., Jones, T.R., Sun, L., Bogyo, M., Geuze, H.J., and Ploegh, H.L.: The human cytomegalovirus US11 gene product dislocates MHC class I heavy chains from the endoplasmic reticulum to the cytosol. Cell 84:769, 1996.

64. Ahn, K., Gruhler, A., Galocha, B., Jones, T.R., Wiertz, E.J., Ploegh, H.L., Peterson, P.A., Yang, Y., and Fruh, K.: The ER-luminal domain of the HCMV glycoprotein US6 inhibits peptide translocation by TAP. Immunity 6:613, 1997.

65. Hengel, H., Koopmann, J.O., Flohr, T., Muranyi, W., Goulmy, E., Hammerling, G.J., Koszinowski, U.H., and Momburg, F.: A viral ER-resident glycoprotein inactivates the MHC-encoded peptide transporter. Immunity 6:623, 1997.

66. Lehner, P.J., Karttunen, J.T., Wilkinson, G.W., and Cresswell, P.: The human cytomegalovirus US6 glycoprotein inhibits transporter associated with antigen processing–dependent peptide translocation. Proc. Natl. Acad. Sci. USA 94:6904, 1997.

67. Browne, H., Smith, G., Beck, S., and Minson, T.: A complex between the MHC class I homologue encoded by human cytomegalovirus and β_2 microglobulin. Nature 347:770, 1990.

68. Fahnestock, M.L., Johnson, J.L., Feldman, R.M., Neveu, J.M., Lane, W.S., and Bjorkman, P.J.: The MHC class I homolog encoded by human cytomegalovirus binds endogenous peptides. Immunity 3:583, 1995.

69. Reyburn, H.T., Mandelboim, O., Vales-Gomez, M., Davis, D.M., Pazmany, L., and Strominger, J.L.: The class I MHC homologue of human cytomegalovirus inhibits attack by natural killer cells. Nature 386:514, 1997.

70. Farrell, H.E., Vally, H., Lynch, D.M., Fleming, P., Shellam, G.R., Scalzo, A.A., and Davis-Poynter, N.J.: Inhibition of natural killer cells by a cytomegalovirus MHC class I homologue in vivo. Nature 386:510, 1997.

71. Taylor-Wiedeman, J., Sissons, P., and Sinclair, J.: Induction of endogenous human cytomegalovirus gene expression after differentiation of monocytes from healthy carriers. J. Virol. 68:1597, 1994.

72. Soderberg-Naucler, C., Fish, K.N., and Nelson, J.A.: Reactivation of latent human cytomegalovirus by allogeneic stimulation of blood cells from healthy donors. Cell 91:119, 1997.

73. Ibanez, C.E., Schrier, R., Ghazal, P., Wiley, C., and Nelson, J.A.: Human cytomegalovirus productively infects primary differentiated macrophages. J. Virol. 65:6581, 1991.

74. Maciejewski, J.P., Bruening, E.E., Donahue, R.E., Mocarski, E.S., Young, N.S., and St. Jeor, S.C.: Infection of hematopoietic progenitor cells by human cytomegalovirus. Blood 80:170, 1992.

75. Mendelson, M., Monard, S., Sissons, P., and Sinclair, J.: Detection of endogenous human cytomegalovirus in CD34$^+$ bone marrow progenitors. J. Gen. Virol. 77:3099, 1996.

76. Sinzger, C., Grefte, A., Plachter, B., Gouw, A.S., The, T.H., and Jahn, G.: Fibroblasts, epithelial cells, endothelial cells and smooth muscle cells are major targets of human cytomegalovirus infection in lung and gastrointestinal tissues. J. Gen. Virol. 76:741, 1995.

77. Wilson, G., and Miller, G.: Recovery of Epstein-Barr virus from nonproducer neonatal human lymphoid cell transformants. Virology 95:351, 1979.

78. Sugden, B.: Expression of virus-associated functions in cells transformed in vitro by Epstein-Barr virus: Epstein-Barr virus cell surface antigen and virus-release from transformed cells. *In* Purtillo, D.T. (ed.): Immune Deficiency and Cancer. New York, Plenum, 1984, pp. 165–177.

79. Nemerow, G.R., Wolfert, R., McNaughton, M.E., and Cooper, N.R.: Identification and characterization of the Epstein-Barr virus receptor on human b lymphocytes and its relationship to the C3d complement receptor (CR2). J. Virol. 55:347, 1985.

80. Spriggs, M.K., Armitage, R.J., Comeau, M.R., Strockbine, L., Farrah, T., Macduff, B., Ulrich, D., Alderson, M.R., Mullberg, J., and Cohen, J.I.: The extracellular domain of the Epstein-Barr virus BZLF2 protein binds the HLA-DR beta chain and inhibits antigen presentation. J. Virol. 70:5557, 1996.

81. Li, Q., Spriggs, M.K., Kovats, S., Turk, S.M., Comeau, M.R., Nepom, B., and Hutt-Fletcher, L.M.: Epstein-Barr virus uses HLA class II as a cofactor for infection of B lymphocytes. J. Virol. 71:4657, 1997.

82. Nemerow, G.R., and Cooper, N.R.: Early events in the infection of human B lymphocytes by Epstein-Barr virus: the internalization process. Virology 132:186, 1984.

83. Woisetschlaeger, M., Yandava, C.N., Furmanski, L.A., Strominger, J.L., and Speck, S.H.: Promoter switching in Epstein-Barr virus during the initial stages of infection of B-lymphocytes. Proc. Natl. Acad. Sci. USA 87:1725, 1990.

84. Bodescot, M., and Perricaudet, M.: Epstein-Barr virus mRNAs produced by alternative splicing. Nucleic Acids Res. 14:7103, 1986.

85. Laux, G., Perricaudet, M., and Farrell, P.: A spliced Epstein-Barr virus gene expressed in immortalized lymphocytes is created by circularization of the linear viral genome. EMBO J. 7:769, 1988.

86. Speck, S.H., and Strominger, J.L.: Transcription of Epstein-Barr virus in latently infected, growth-transformed lymphocytes. *In* Klein G. (ed.): Advances in Viral Oncology. Vol. 8. New York, Raven Press, 1989, pp. 133–150.

87. Kieff, E.: Epstein-Barr virus and its replication. *In* Fields, B.N., Knipe, D.M., and Howley, P.M. (eds.): Virology. 3rd ed. New York, Raven Press, 1996, pp. 2343–2396.

88. Kintner, C., and Sugden, B.: Identification of antigenic determinants unique to the surfaces of cells transformed by Epstein-Barr virus. Nature 294:458, 1981.

89. Gregory, G.D., Kirchgens, C., Edwards, C.F., Young, L.S., Rowe, M., Forster, A., Rabbitts, T.H., and Rickinson, A.B.: Epstein-Barr virus–transformed human precursor B Cell lines: altered growth phenotype of lines with germline or rearranged but non-expressed heavy chain genes. Eur. J. Immunol. 17:1199, 1987.

90. Adams, A., Pozos, T.C., and Purvey, H.V.: Replication of latent Epstein-Barr virus genomes in normal and malignant lymphoid cells. Int. J. Cancer 44:560, 1989.

91. Yates, J., Warren, N., Reisman, D., and Sugden, B.: A cis-Acting element from the Epstein-Barr viral genome that permits stable replication of recombinant plasmids in latently infected cells. Proc. Natl. Acad. Sci. USA 81:3806, 1984.

92. Lupton, S., and Levine, A.J.: Mapping genetic elements of Epstein-Barr virus that facilitate extrachromosomal persistence of Epstein-Barr virus–derived plasmids in human cells. Mol. Cell. Biol. 5:2533, 1985.

93. Gahn, T.A., and Schildkraut, C.L.: The Epstein-Barr virus origin of plasmid replication, *oriP*, contains both the initiation and termination sites of DNA replication. Cell 58:527, 1989.

94. Hammerschmidt, W., and Sugden, B.: Genetic analysis of immortalizing functions of Epstein-Barr virus in human B-lymphocytes. Nature 340:393, 1989.

95. Cohen, J.I., Wang, F., Mannick, J., and Kieff, E.: Epstein-Barr virus nuclear protein 2 is a key determinant of lymphocyte transformation. Proc. Natl. Acad. Sci. USA 86:9558, 1989.

96. Henkel, T., Ling, P.D., Hayward, S.D., and Peterson, M.G.: Mediation of Epstein-Barr virus EBNA2 transactivation by recombination signal-binding protein J kappa. Science 265:92, 1994.

97. Tong, X., Wang, F., Thut, C.J., and Kieff, E.: The Epstein-Barr virus nuclear protein 2 acidic domain can interact with TFIIB, TAF40, and RPA70 but not with TATA-binding protein. J. Virol. 69:585, 1995.

98. Rawlins, D.R., Milman, G., Hayward, S.D., and Hayward, G.S.: Sequence-specific DNA binding of the Epstein-Barr virus nuclear antigen (EBNA-1) to clustered sites in the plasmid maintenance region. Cell 42:859, 1985.

99. Aiyar, A., Tyree, C., and Sugden, B.: Submitted for publication.

100. Rowe, M., Rowe, D.T., Gregory, C.D., Young, L.S., Farrell, P.J., Rupani, H., and Rickinson, A.B.: Differences in B cell growth phenotype reflect novel patterns of Epstein-Barr virus latent gene expression in Burkitt's lymphoma cells. EMBO J. 6:2743, 1987.

101. Grasser, F.A., Murray, P.G., Kremmer, E., Klein, K., Remberger, K., Feiden, W., Reynolds, G., Niedobitek, G., Young, L.S., and Mueller-Lantzsch, N.: Monoclonal antibodies directed against the Epstein-Barr virus–encoded nuclear antigen 1 (EBNA1): immunohistologic detection of EBNA1 in the malignant cells of Hodgkin's disease. Blood 84:3792, 1994.

102. Sugden, B., and Warren, N.: A promoter of Epstein-Barr virus that can function during latent infection can be transactivated by EBNA-1, a viral protein required for viral DNA replication during latent infection. J. Virol. 63:2644, 1989.

103. Gahn, T.A., and Sugden, B.: An EBNA-1-dependent enhancer acts from a distance of 10 kilobase pairs to increase expression of the Epstein-Barr virus LMP gene. J. Virol. 69:2633, 1995.

104. Liebowitz, D., Wang, D., and Kieff, E.: Orientation and patching of the latent infection membrane protein encoded by Epstein-Barr virus. J. Virol. 58:233, 1986.

105. Kaye, K.M., Izumi, K.M., and Kieff, E.: Epstein-Barr virus latent membrane protein 1 is essential for B-lymphocyte growth transformation. Proc. Natl. Acad. Sci. USA 90:9150, 1993.

106. Mosialos, G., Birkenbach, M., Yalamanchili, R., VanArsdale, T., Ware, C., and Kieff, E.: The Epstein-Barr virus transforming protein LMP1 engages signaling proteins for the tumor necrosis factor receptor family. Cell 80:389, 1995.

107. Mitchell, T., and Sugden, B.: Stimulation of NF-κB–mediated transcription by mutant derivatives of the latent membrane protein of Epstein-Barr virus. J. Virol. 69:2968, 1995.

108. Kieser, A., Kilger, E., Gires, O., Ueffing, M., Kolch, W., and Hammerschmidt, W.: Epstein-Barr virus latent membrane protein-1 triggers AP-1 activity via the c-Jun N-terminal kinase cascade. EMBO J. 16:6478, 1997.

109. Herbst, H., Dallenbach, F., Hummel, M., Niedobitek, G., Pileri, S., Muller-Lantzsch, N., and Stein, H.: Epstein-Barr virus latent membrane protein expression in Hodgkin and Reed-Sternberg cells. Proc. Natl. Acad. Sci. USA 88:4766, 1991.

110. Wu, T.C., Mann, R.B., Charache, P., Hayward, S.D., Staal, S., Lambe, B.C., and Ambinder, R.F.: Detection of EBV gene expression in Reed-Sternberg cells of Hodgkin's disease. Int. J. Cancer 46:801, 1990.

111. Swaminathan, S., Tomkinson, B., and Kieff, E.: Recombinant Epstein-Barr virus with small RNA (EBER) genes deleted transforms lymphocytes and replicates in vitro. Proc. Natl. Acad. Sci. USA 88:1546, 1991.

112. Arrand, J.R., and Rymo, L.: Characterization of the major Epstein-Barr virus–specific RNA in Burkitt lymphoma-derived cells. J. Virol. 41:376, 1982.

113. Brousset, P., Meggetto, F., Chittal, S., Bibeau, F., Arnaud, J., Rubin, B., and Delsol, G.: Assessment of the methods for the detection of Epstein-Barr virus nucleic acids and related gene products in Hodgkin's disease. Lab. Invest. 69:483, 1993.

114. Longnecker, R., Miller, C.L., Miao, X.Q., Tomkinson, B., and Kieff, E.: The last seven transmembrane and carboxy-terminal cytoplasmic domains of Epstein-Barr virus latent membrane protein 2 (LMP2) are dispensable for lymphocyte infection and growth transformation in vitro. J. Virol. 67:2006, 1993.

115. Miller, C.L., Lee, J.H., Kieff, E., and Longnecker, R.: An integral membrane protein (LMP2) blocks reactivation of Epstein-Barr virus from latency following surface immunoglobulin crosslinking. Proc. Natl. Acad. Sci. USA 91:772, 1994.

116. Qu, L., and Rowe, D.T.: Epstein-Barr virus latent gene expression in uncultured peripheral blood lymphocytes. J. Virol. 66:3715, 1992.

117. Countryman, J., and Miller, G.: Activation of expression of latent Epstein-Barr herpesvirus after gene transfer with a small cloned subfragment of heterogeneous viral DNA. Proc. Natl. Acad. Sci. USA 82:4085, 1985.

118. Grogan, E., Jenson, H., Countryman, J., Heston, L., Gradoville, L., and Miller, G.: Transfection of a rearranged viral DNA fragment, WZ het, stably converts latent Epstein-Barr viral infection to productive infection in lymphoid cells. Proc. Natl. Acad. Sci. USA 84:1332, 1987.

119. Takada, K., Shimizu, N., Sakuma, S., and Ono, Y.: Transactivation of the latent Epstein-Barr virus (EBV) genome after transfection of the EBV DNA fragment. J. Virol. 57:1016, 1986.

120. Baer, R., Bankier, A.T., Biggin, M.D., Deininger, P.L., Farrell, P.J., Gibson, T.J., Hatfull, G., Hudson, G.S., Satchwell, S.C., Seguin, C., Tuffnell, P.S., and Barrell, B.G.: DNA sequence and expression of the B95-8 Epstein-Barr virus genome. Nature 310:207, 1984.

121. Hammerschmidt, W., and Sugden, B.: Identification and characterization of oriLyt, a lytic origin of DNA replication of Epstein-Barr virus. Cell 55:427, 1988.

122. Schepers, A., Pich, D., and Hammerschmidt, W.: A transcription factor with homology to the AP-1 family links RNA transcription and DNA replication in the lytic cycle of Epstein-Barr virus. EMBO J. 12:3921, 1993.

123. Fixman, E.D., Hayward, G.S., and Hayward, S.D.: Trans-acting requirements for replication of Epstein-Barr virus ori-Lyt. J. Virol. 66:5030, 1992.

124. Bloss, T.A., and Sugden, B.: Optimal lengths for DNAs encapsidated by Epstein-Barr virus. J. Virol. 68:8217, 1994.

125. Ho, M.: Cytomegalovirus. 2nd ed. New York, Plenum, 1991.

126. Weller, T.H.: Cytomegalovirus: the difficult years. J. Infect. Dis. 122:532, 1970.

127. Griffiths, P.D., and Baboonian, C.: A prospective study of primary cytomegalovirus infection during pregnancy: final report. Br. J. Obstet. Gynecol. 91:307, 1984.

128. Paradis, I.L., Grgurich, W.F., Dummer, J.S., Dekker, A., and Dauber, J.H.: Rapid Detection of cytomegalovirus pneumonia from lung lavage cells. Am. Rev. Respir. Dis. 138:697, 1988.

129. Kulski, J.K.: Quantitation of human cytomegalovirus DNA in leukocytes by end-point titration and duplex polymerase chain reaction. J. Virol. Methods 49:195, 1994.

130. Rasmussen, L., Morris, S., Zipeto, D., Fessel, J., Wolitz, R., Dowling, A., and Merigan, T.C.: Quantitation of human cytomegalovirus DNA from peripheral blood cells of human immunodeficiency virus-infected patients could predict cytomegalovirus retinitis. J. Infect. Dis. 171:177, 1995.

131. Meyers, J.D., Flournoy, N., and Thomas, E.D.: Risk factors for cytomegalovirus infection after human marrow transplantation. J. Infect. Dis. 153:478, 1986.

132. Neiman, P.E., Reeves, W., Ray, G., Flournoy, N., Lerner, K.G., Sale, G.E., and Thomas, E.D.: A prospective analysis of interstitial pneumonia and opportunistic viral infection among recipients of allogeneic bone marrow grafts. J. Infect. Dis. 136:754, 1977.

133. Klemola, E., von Essen, R., Henle, G., and Henle, W.: Infectious-mononucleosis–like disease with negative heterophil agglutination test. Clinical features in relation to Epstein-Barr virus and cytomegalovirus antibodies. J. Infect. Dis. 121:608, 1970.

134. Lajo, A., Borque, C., Del Castillo, F., and Martin-Ancel, A.: Mononucleosis caused by Epstein-Barr virus and cytomegalovirus in children: a comparative study of 124 cases. Pediatr. Infect. Dis. J. 13:56, 1994.

135. Lang, D.J., and Hanshaw, J.B.: Cytomegalovirus infection and the postperfusion syndrome (recognition of primary infections in four patients). N. Engl. J. Med. 280:1145, 1969.

136. Wilhelm, J.A., Matter, L., and Schopfer, K.: The risk of transmitting cytomegalovirus to patients receiving blood transfusions. J. Infect. Dis. 154:169, 1986.

137. Preiksaitis, J.K., Brown, L., and McKenzie, M.: The risk of cytomegalovirus infection in seronegative transfusion recipients not receiving exogenous immunosuppression. J. Infect. Dis. 157:523, 1988.

138. Weir, M.R., Henry, M.L., Blackmore, M., Smith, J., First, M.R., Irwin, B., Shen, S., Genemans, G., Alexander, J.W., Corry, R.J., Nghiem, D.D., Ferguson, R.M., Kittur, D., Shield, C.F., Sommer, B.G., and

Williams, G.M.: Incidence and morbidity of cytomegalovirus disease associated with a seronegative recipient receiving seropositive donor-specific transfusion and living-related donor transplantation. A multicenter evaluation. Transplantation 45:111, 1988.

139. Braun, R.W., and Reiser, H.C.: Replication of human cytomegalovirus in human peripheral blood T cells. J. Virol. 60:29, 1986.

140. Taylor-Wiedeman, J., Sissons, J.G., Borysiewicz, L.K., and Sinclair, J.H.: Monocytes are a major site of persistence of human cytomegalovirus in peripheral blood mononuclear cells. J. Gen. Virol. 72:2059, 1991.

141. Meyer-Konig, U., Hufert, F.T., and von Laer, D.M.: Infection of blood and bone marrow cells with the human cytomegalovirus in vivo. Leuk. Lymphoma 25:445, 1997.

142. Felsenstein, D., Carney, W.P., Iacoviello, V.R., and Hirsch, M.S.: Phenotypic properties of atypical lymphocytes in cytomegalovirus-induced mononucleosis. J. Infect. Dis. 152:198, 1985.

143. Mar, E.C., Chiou, J.F., Cheng, Y.C., and Huang, E.S.: Inhibition of cellular DNA polymerase alpha and human cytomegalovirus-induced DNA polymerase by the triphosphates of 9-(2-hydroxyethoxymethyl)-guanine and 9-(1,3-dihydroxy-2-propoxymethyl)guanine. J. Virol. 53:776, 1985.

144. Mills, J., Jacobson, M.A., O'Donnell, J.J., Cederberg, D., and Holland, G.N.: Treatment of cytomegalovirus retinitis in patients with AIDS. Rev. Infect. Dis. 10(suppl. 3):S522, 1988.

145. Erice, A., Jordan, M.C., Chace, B.A., Fletcher, C., Chinnock, B.J., and Balfour, H.H., Jr.: Ganciclovir treatment of cytomegalovirus disease in transplant recipients and other immunocompromised hosts. J.A.M.A. 257:3082, 1987.

146. Reed, E.C., Bowden, R.A., Dandliker, P.S., Lilleby, K.E., and Meyers, J.D.: Treatment of cytomegalovirus pneumonia with ganciclovir and intravenous cytomegalovirus immunoglobulin in patients with bone barrow transplants. Ann. Intern. Med. 109:783, 1988.

147. Emanuel, D., Cunningham, I., Jules-Elysee, K., Brockstein, J.A., Kernan, N.A., Laver, J., Stover, D., White, D.A., Fels, A., Polsky, B., Castro-Malaspina, H., Peppard, J.R., Bartus, P., Hammerling, U., and O'Reilly, R.J.: Cytomegalovirus pneumonia after bone marrow transplantation successfully treated with the combination of ganciclovir and high-dose intravenous immune globulin. Ann. Intern. Med. 109:777, 1988.

148. Erice, A., Chou, S., Biron, K.K., Stanat, S.C., Balfour, H.H., Jr., and Jordan, M.C.: Progressive disease due to ganciclovir-resistant cytomegalovirus in immunocompromised patients. N. Engl. J. Med. 320:289, 1989.

149. Gane, E., Saliba, F., Valdecasas, G.J., O'Grady, J., Pescovitz, M.D., Lyman, S., and Robinson, C.A.: Randomised trial of efficacy and safety of oral ganciclovir in the prevention of cytomegalovirus disease in liver-transplant recipients. Lancet 350:1729, 1997.

150. Snydman, D.R., Werner, B.G., Heinze-Lacey, B., Berardi, V.P., Tilney, N.L., Kirkman, R.L., Milford, E.L., Cho, S.I., Bush, H.L., Jr., Levey, A.S., Strom, T.B., Carpenter, C.B., Levey, R.H., Harmon, W.E., Zimmerman, C.E., Shapiro, M.E., Steinman, T., LoGerfo, F., Idelson, B., Schröter, G.P.J., Levin, M.J., McIver, J., Leszczynski, J., and Grady, G.F.: Use of cytomegalovirus immune globulin to prevent cytomegalovirus disease in renal-transplant recipients. N. Engl. J. Med. 317:1049, 1987.

151. Steinmuller, D.R., Novick, A.C., Streem, S.B., Graneto, D., and Swift, C.: Intravenous immunoglobulin infusions for the prophylaxis of secondary cytomegalovirus infection. Transplantation 49:68, 1990.

152. Metselaar, H.J., Rothbarth, P.H., Brouwer, R.M., Wenting, G.J., Jeekel, J., and Weimar, W.: Prevention of cytomegalovirus-related death by passive immunization. A double-blind placebo-controlled study in kidney transplant recipients treated for rejection. Transplantation 48:264, 1989.

153. Quinnan, G.V., Jr., Kirmani, N., Rook, A.H., Manischewitz, J.F., Jackson, L., Moreschi, G., Santos, G.W., Saral, R., and Burns, W.H.: Cytotoxic T cells in cytomegalovirus infection: HLA-restricted T-lymphocyte and non–T-lymphocyte cytotoxic responses correlate with recovery from cytomegalovirus infection in bone-marrow-transplant recipients. N. Engl. J. Med. 307:7, 1982.

154. Reusser, P., Riddell, S.R., Meyers, J.D., and Greenberg, P.D.: Cytotoxic T-lymphocyte response to cytomegalovirus after human allogeneic bone marrow transplantation: pattern of recovery and correlation with cytomegalovirus infection and disease. Blood 78:1373, 1991.

155. Walter, E.A., Greenberg, P.D., Gilbert, M.J., Finch, R.J., Watanabe, K.S., Thomas, E.D., and Riddell, S.R.: Reconstitution of cellular immunity against cytomegalovirus in recipients of allogeneic bone marrow by transfer of T-cell clones from the donor. N. Engl. J. Med. 333:1038, 1995.

156. Epstein, M.A.: Historical Background; Burkitt's Lymphoma and Epstein-Barr Virus. Lyon, IARC Press, 1985, pp. 17–27. IARC scientific publication 60.

157. Burkitt, D.: A sarcoma involving the jaws in African children. Br. J. Surg. 46:218, 1958.

158. Burkitt, D.: Determining the climatic limitations of a children's cancer common in Africa. Br. Med. J. 2:1019, 1962.

159. Epstein, M.A., Achong, B.G., and Barr, Y.M.: Virus particles in cultured lymphoblasts from Burkitt's lymphoma. Lancet 1:702, 1964.

160. Henle, G., Henle, W., and Diehl, V.: Relation of Burkitt's tumor-associated herpes-type virus to infectious mononucleosis. Proc. Natl. Acad. Sci. USA 59:94, 1968.

161. Niederman, J.C., McCollum, R.W., Henle, G., and Henle, W.: Infectious mononucleosis. J.A.M.A. 203:205, 1968.

162. Evans, A.S.: The transmission of EB viral infections. In Hooks, J.J., and Jordan, G.W. (eds.): Viral Infections in Oral Medicine. New York, Elsevier North Holland, 1982, pp. 211–225.

163. Robinson, J.E., Smith, D., and Niederman, J.: Plasmacytic differentiation of circulating Epstein-Barr virus–infected B lymphocytes during acute infectious mononucleosis. J. Exp. Med. 153:235, 1981.

164. Robinson, J., Smith, D., and Niederman, J.: Mitotic EBNA-positive lymphocytes in peripheral blood during infectious mononucleosis. Nature 287:334, 1980.

165. Giuliano, V.J., Jasin, H.E., and Ziff, M.: The nature of the atypical lymphocyte in infectious mononucleosis. Clin. Immunol. Immunopathol. 3:90, 1974.

166. Klein, G., Svedmyr, E., Jondal, M., and Persson, P.O.: EBV-determined nuclear antigen (EBNA)–positive cells in the peripheral blood of infectious mononucleosis patients. Int. J. Cancer 17:21, 1976.

167. Bird, A.G., and Britton S.: A new approach to the study of human B lymphocyte function using an indirect plaque assay and a direct B cell activator. Immunol. Rev. 45:41, 1979.

168. Miller, G., Niederman, J.C., and Andrews, L.-L.: Prolonged oropharyngeal excretion of Epstein-Barr virus after infectious mononucleosis. N. Engl. J. Med. 288:229, 1973.

169. Niederman, J.C., Miller, G., Pearson, H.A., Pagano, J.S., and Dowaliby, J.M.: Infectious mononucleosis. Epstein-Barr virus shedding in saliva and the oropharynx. N. Engl. J. Med. 294:1355, 1976.

170. de-Thé, G., Geser, A., Day, N.E., Tukei, P.M., Williams, E.H., Beri, D.P., Smith, P.G., Dean, A.G., Bornkamm, G.W., Feorino, P., and Henle, W.: Epidemiological evidence for causal relationship between Epstein-Barr virus and Burkitt's lymphoma from Ugandan prospective study. Nature 274:756, 1978.

171. Geser, A., de Thé, G., Lenoir, G., Day, N.E., and Williams, E.H.: Final case reporting from the Ugandan prospective study of the relationship between EBV and Burkitt's lymphoma. Int. J. Cancer 29:397, 1982.

172. Magrath, I.T.: Malignant non-Hodgkin's lymphomas. In Pizzo, P.A., and Poplach, D.G. (eds.): Principles and Practice of Pediatric Oncology. Philadelphia, J.B. Lippincott, 1989, pp. 415–456.

173. Lindahl, T., Klein, G., Reedman, B.M., Johansson, B., and Singh, S.: Relationship between Epstein-Barr virus (EBV) DNA and the EBV-determined nuclear antigen (EBNA) in Burkitt lymphoma biopsies and other lymphoproliferative malignancies. Int. J. Cancer 13:764, 1974.

174. Gregory, C.D., Rowe, M., and Rickinson, A.B.: Different Epstein-Barr virus–B Cell interactions in phenotypically distinct clones of a Burkitt's lymphoma cell line. J. Gen. Virol. 71:1481, 1990.

175. Tao, Q., Robertson, K.D., Manns, A., Hildesheim, A., and Ambinder, R.F.: Epstein-Barr virus (EBV) in endemic Burkitt's lymphoma: molecular analysis of primary tumor tissue. Blood 91:1373, 1998.

176. Lindahl, T., Adams, A., Bjursell, G., Bornkamm, G.W., Kaschka-Dierich, C., and Jehn, U.: Covalently closed circular duplex DNA of Epstein-Barr virus in a human lymphoid cell line. J. Mol. Biol. 102:511, 1976.

177. Fialkow, P.J., Klein, G., Gartler, S.M., and Clifford, P.: Clonal origin for individual Burkitt tumors. Lancet 1:384, 1970.

178. Gunven, P., Klein, G., Klein, E., Norin, T., and Singh, S.: Surface immunoglobulins on Burkitt's lymphoma biopsy cells from 91 patients. Int. J. Cancer 25:711, 1980.

179. Zech, L., Haglund, U., Nilsson, K., and Klein, G.: Characteristic chromosomal abnormalities in biopsies and lymphoid-cell lines from patients with Burkitt and non-Burkitt lymphomas. Int. J. Cancer 17:47, 1976.

180. Klein, G.: Specific chromosomal translocations and the genesis of B-cell–derived tumors in mice and men. Cell 32:311, 1983.

181. Spencer, C.A., and Groudine, M.: Control of c-*myc* Regulation in normal and neoplastic cells. Adv. Cancer Res. 56:1, 1991.

182. Purtilo, D.T., Sakamoto, K., Saemundsen, A.K., Sullivan, J.L., Synnerholm, A.C., Anvret, M., Pritchard, J., Sloper, C., Sieff, C., Pincott, J., Pachman, L., Rich, K., Cruzi, F., Cornet, J.A., Collins, R., Barnes, N., Knight, J., Sandstedt, B., and Klein, G.: Documentation of Epstein-Barr Virus infection in immunodeficient patients with life-threatening lymphoproliferative diseases by clinical, virological, and immunopathological studies. Cancer Res. 41:4226, 1981.

183. Crawford, D.H., Thomas, J., Janossy, G., Sweny, P., Fernando, O.N., Moorhead, J.F., and Thompson, J.H.: Epstein Barr virus nuclear antigen positive lymphoma after cyclosporin a treatment in patients with renal allograft. Lancet 1:1355, 1980.

184. Hanto, D.W., Frizzera, G., Purtilo, D.T., Sakamoto, K., Sullivan, J.L., Saemundsen, A.K., Klein, G., Simmons, R.L., and Najarian, J.S.: Clinical spectrum of lymphoproliferative disorders in renal transplant recipients and evidence for the role of the Epstein-Barr virus. Cancer Res. 41:4253, 1981.

185. Ernberg, I.: Epstein-Barr virus and acquired immunodeficiency syndrome. *In* Klein G. (ed.): Advances in Viral Oncology. Vol. 8. New York, Raven Press, 1989, pp. 203–217.

186. Dockrell, D.H., Strickler, J.G., and Paya, C.V.: Epstein-Barr virus–induced T cell lymphoma in solid organ transplant recipients. Clin. Infect. Dis. 26:180, 1998.

187. Wen, S., Mizugaki, Y., Shinozaki, F., and Takada, K.: Epstein-Barr virus (EBV) infection in salivary gland tumors: lytic EBV infection in nonmalignant epithelial cells surrounded by EBV-positive T-lymphoma cells. Virology 227:484, 1997.

188. Kanegane, H., Bhatia, K., Gutierrez, M., Kaneda, H., Wada, T., Yachie, A., Seki, H., Arai, T., Kagimoto, S.I., Okazaki, M., Oh-ishi, T., Moghaddam, A., Wang, F., and Tosato, G.: A syndrome of peripheral blood T-cell infection with Epstein-Barr virus (EBV) followed by EBV-positive T-cell lymphoma. Blood 91:2085, 1998.

189. Glaser, S.L., Lin, R.J., Stewart, S.L., Ambinder, R.F., Jarrett, R.F., Brousset, P., Pallesen, G., Gulley, M.L., Khan, G., O'Grady, J., Hummel, M., Preciado, M.V., Knecht, H., Chan, J.K., and Claviez, A.: Epstein-Barr virus–associated Hodgkin's disease: epidemiologic characteristics in international data. Int. J. Cancer 70:375, 1997.

190. Siebert, J.D., Ambinder, R.F., Napoli, V.M., Quintanilla-Martinez, L., Banks, P.M., and Gulley, M.L.: Human immunodeficiency virus–associated Hodgkin's disease contains latent, not replicative, Epstein-Barr virus. Hum. Pathol. 26:1191, 1995.

191. Greenspan, J.S., Greenspan, D., Lennette, E.T., Abrams, D.I., Conant, M.A., Peterson, V., and Freese, U.K.: Replication of Epstein-Barr virus within the epithelial cells of oral "hairy" leukoplakia, an AIDS-associated lesion. N. Engl. J. Med. 313:1564, 1985.

192. Young, L.S., Lau, R., Rowe, M., Niedobitek, G., Packham, G., Shanahan, F., Rowe, D.T., Greenspan, D., Greenspan, J.S., Rickinson, A.B., and Farrell, P.J.: Differentiation-associated expression of the Epstein-Barr virus BZLF1 transactivator protein in oral hairy leukoplakia. J. Virol. 65:2868, 1991.

193. Imai, S., Koizumi, S., Sugiura, M., Tokunaga, M., Uemura, Y., Yamamoto, N., Tanaka, S., Sato, E. and Osato, T.: Gastric carcinoma: monoclonal epithelial malignant cells expressing Epstein-Barr virus latent infection protein. Proc. Natl. Acad. Sci. USA 91:9131, 1994.

194. Klein, G., Giovanella, B.C., Lindahl, T., Fialkow, P.J., Singh, S., and Stehlin, J.S.: Direct evidence for the presence of Epstein-Barr virus DNA and nuclear antigen in malignant epithelial cells from patients with poorly differentiated carcinoma of the nasopharynx. Proc. Natl. Acad. Sci. USA 71:4737, 1974.

195. Tugwood, J.D., Lau, W.-H., Sai-Ki, O., Tsao, S.-Y., Martin, W.M.C., Shiu, W., Desgranges, C., Jones, P.H., and Arrand, J.R.: Epstein-Barr virus–specific transcription in normal and malignant nasopharyngeal biopsies and in lymphocytes from healthy donors and infectious mononucleosis patients. J. Gen. Virol. 68:1081, 1987.

196. Young, L.S., Dawson, C.W., Clark, D., Rupani, H., Busson, P., Tursz, T., Johnson, A., and Rickinson, A.B.: Epstein-Barr virus gene expression in nasopharyngeal carcinoma. J. Gen. Virol. 69:1051, 1988.

197. Kaschka-Dierich, C., Adams, A., Lindahl, T., Bornkamm, G.W., Bjursell, G., and Klein, G.: Intracellular forms of Epstein-Barr virus DNA in human tumour cells in vivo. Nature 260:302, 1976.

198. Zeng, Y., Zhang, L.G., Wu, Y.C., Huang, Y.S., Huang, N.Q., Li, J.Y., Wang, Y.B., Jiang, M.K., Fang, Z., and Meng, N.N.: Prospective studies on nasopharyngeal carcinoma in Epstein-Barr virus IgA/VCA antibody-positive persons in Wuzhou City, China. Int. J. Cancer 36:545, 1985.

199. Sugden, B.: Comparison of Epstein-Barr viral DNAs in Burkitt lymphoma biopsy cells and in cells clonally transformed in vitro. Proc. Natl. Acad. Sci. USA 74:4651, 1977.

200. Hinuma, Y., and Katsuki, T.: Colonies of EBNA-positive cells in soft agar from peripheral leukocytes of infectious mononucleosis patients. Int. J. Cancer 21:426, 1978.

201. Svedmyr, E., and Jondal, M.: Cytotoxic effector cells specific for B cell lines transformed by Epstein-Barr virus are present in patients with infectious mononucleosis. Proc. Natl. Acad. Sci. USA 72:1622, 1975.

202. Murray, R.J., Kurilla, M.G., Griffin, H.M., Brooks, J.M., Mackett, M., Arrand, J.R., Rowe, M., Burrows, S.R., Moss, D.J., Kieff, E., and Rickinson, A.B.: Human cytotoxic T-cell responses against Epstein-Barr virus nuclear antigens demonstrated by using recombinant vaccinia viruses. Proc. Natl. Acad. Sci. USA 87:2906, 1990.

203. Burrows, S.R., Sculley, T.B., Misko, I.S., Schmidt, C., and Moss, D.J.: An Epstein-Barr virus–specific cytotoxic T cell epitope in EBV nuclear antigen 3 (EBNA 3). J. Exp. Med. 171:345, 1990.

204. Yao, Q.Y., Rickinson, A.B., and Epstein, M.A.: A re-examination of the Epstein-Barr virus carrier state in healthy seropositive individuals. Int. J. Cancer 35:35, 1985.

205. Mosier, D.E., Baird, S.M., Kirven, M.B., Gulizia, R.J., Wilson, D.B., Kubayashi, R., Picchio, G., Garnier, J.L., Sullivan, J.L., and Kipps, T.J.: EBV-associated B-cell lymphomas following transfer of human peripheral blood lymphocytes to mice with severe combined immune deficiency. Curr. Top. Microbiol. Immunol. 166:317, 1990.

206. Miyashita, E.M., Yang, B., Lam, K.M., Crawford, D.H., and Thorley-Lawson, D.A.: A novel form of Epstein-Barr virus latency in normal B cells in vivo. Cell 80:593, 1995.

207. Schubach, W.H., Hackman, R., Neiman, P.E., Miller, G., and Thomas, E.D.: A monoclonal immunoblastic sarcoma in donor cells bearing Epstein-Barr virus genomes following allogeneic marrow grafting for acute lymphoblastic leukemia. Blood 60:180, 1982.

208. Morrow, R.H., Kisuule, A., Pike, M.C., and Smith, P.G.: Burkitt's lymphoma in the Mengo Districts of Uganda: epidemiologic features and their relationship to malaria. J. Natl. Cancer Inst. 56:479, 1976.

209. Facer, C.A., and Playfair, J.H.L.: Malaria, Epstein-Barr virus, and the genesis of lymphomas. Adv. Cancer Res. 53:33, 1989.

210. Moss, D.J., Burrows, S.R., Castelino, D.J., Kiane, R.G., Pope, J.H., Rickinson, A.B., Alpers, M.P., and Heywood, P.F.: A comparison of Epstein-Barr virus–specific T-cell immunity in malaria-endemic and -nonendemic regions of Papua New Guinea. Int. J. Cancer 31:727, 1983.

211. Whittle, H.C., Brown, J., Marsh, K., Greenwood, B.M., Seidelin, P., Tighe, H., and Wedderburn, L.: T-cell control of Epstein-Barr virus–infected B cells is lost during *P. falciparum* malaria. Nature 312:449, 1984.

212. Lam, K.M., Syed, N., Whittle, H., and Crawford, D.H.: Circulating Epstein-Barr virus–carrying B cells in acute malaria. Lancet 337:876, 1991.

213. Gaidano, G., Ballerini, P., Gong, J.Z., Inghirami, G., Neri, A., Newcomb, E.W., Magrath, I.T., Knowles, D.M., and Dalla-Favera, R.: p53 mutations in human lymphoid malignancies: association with Burkitt lymphoma and chronic lymphocytic leukemia. Proc. Natl. Acad. Sci. USA 88:5413, 1991.

214. Farrell, P.J., Allan, G.J., Shanahan, F., Vousden, K.H., and Crook, T.: p53 is frequently mutated in Burkitt's lymphoma cell lines. EMBO J. 10:2879, 1991.

215. Kempkes, B., Spitkovsky, D., Jansen-Durr, P., Ellwart, J.W., Kremmer, E., Delecluse, H.J., Rottenberger, C., Bornkamm, G.W., and Hammerschmidt, W.: B-cell proliferation and induction of early G1-regulating proteins by Epstein-Barr virus mutants conditional for EBNA2. EMBO J. 14:88, 1995.

216. Schmidt, C., Burrows, S.R., Sculley, T.B., Moss, D.J., and Misko, I.S.: Nonresponsiveness to an immunodominant Epstein-Barr virus–encoded cytotoxic T-lymphocyte epitope in nuclear antigen 3A: implications for vaccine strategies. Proc. Natl. Acad. Sci. USA 88:9478, 1991.

217. Yates, J.L., Warren, N., and Sugden, B.: Stable replication of plasmids derived from Epstein-Barr virus in various mammalian cells. Nature 313:812, 1985.

218. Levitskaya, J., Coram, M., Levitsky, V., Imreh, S., Steigerwald-Mul-

len, P.M., Klein, G., Kurilla, M.G., and Masucci, M.G.: Inhibition of antigen processing by the internal repeat region of the Epstein-Barr virus nuclear antigen-1. Nature 375:685, 1995.

219. Levitskaya, J., Sharipo, A., Leonchiks, A., Ciechanover, A., and Masucci, M.G.: Inhibition of ubiquitin/proteasome-dependent protein degradation by the Gly-Ala Repeat domain of the Epstein-Barr virus nuclear antigen 1. Proc. Natl. Acad. Sci. USA 94:12616, 1997.

220. Polack, A., Hortnagel, K., Pajic, A., Christoph, B., Baier, B., Falk, M., Mautner, J., Geltinger, C., Bornkamm, G.W., and Kempkes, B.: c-myc Activation renders proliferation of Epstein-Barr virus (EBV)–transformed cells independent of EBV nuclear antigen 2 and latent membrane protein 1. Proc. Natl. Acad. Sci. USA 93:10411, 1996.

221. Colby, B.M., Shaw, J.E., Elion, G.B., and Pagano, J.S.: Effect of acyclovir [9-(2-hydroxyethoxymethyl)guanine] on Epstein-Barr virus DNA replication. J. Virol. 34:560, 1980.

222. Hanto, D.W., Frizzera, G., Gajl-Peczalska, K.J., Balfour, H.H., Jr., Simmons, R.L., and Najarian, J.S.: Acyclovir therapy of Epstein-Barr virus–induced posttransplant lymphoproliferative diseases. Transplant. Proc. 17:89, 1985.

223. Moss, D.J., Schmidt, C., Elliott, S., Suhrbier, A., Burrows, S., and Khanna, R.: Strategies involved in developing an effective vaccine for EBV-associated diseases. Adv. Cancer Res. 69:213, 1996.

224. Rickinson, A.B., and Moss, D.J.: Human cytotoxic T lymphocyte responses to Epstein-Barr virus infection. Annu. Rev. Immunol. 15:405, 1997.

225. Thomson, S.A., Burrows, S.R., Misko, I.S., Moss, D.J., Coupar, B.E., and Khanna, R.: Targeting a polyepitope protein incorporating multiple class II–restricted viral epitopes to the secretory/endocytic pathway facilitates immune recognition by CD4$^+$ cytotoxic T lymphocytes: a novel approach to vaccine design. J. Virol. 72:2246, 1998.

226. Rowe, M., Khanna, R., Jacob, C.A., Argaet, V., Kelly, A., Powis, S., Belich, M., Croom-Carter, D., Lee, S., Burrows, S.R., et al.: Restoration of endogenous antigen processing in Burkitt's lymphoma cells by Epstein-Barr virus latent membrane protein-1: coordinate up-regulation of peptide transporters and HLA-class I antigen expression. Eur. J. Immunol. 25:1374, 1995.

227. Zeidler, R., Eissner, G., Meissner, P., Uebel, S., Tampe, R., Lazis, S., and Hammerschmidt, W.: Downregulation of TAP1 in B lymphocytes by cellular and Epstein-Barr virus–encoded interleukin-10. Blood 90:2390, 1997.

228. Boubenider, S., Hiesse, C., Goupy, C., Kriaa, F., Marchand, S., and Charpentier, B.: Incidence and consequences of post-transplantation lymphoproliferative disorders. J. Nephrol. 10:136, 1997.

229. Haque, T., Thomas, J.A., Parratt, R., Hunt, B.J., Yacoub, M.H., and Crawford, D.H.: A prospective study in heart and lung transplant recipients correlating persistent Epstein-Barr virus infection with clinical events. Transplantation 64:1028, 1997.

230. York, L.J., and Qualtiere, L.F.: Cyclosporin abrogates virus-specific T-cell control of EBV-induced B-cell lymphoproliferation. Viral Immunol. 3:127, 1990.

231. Heslop, H.E., and Rooney, C.M.: Adoptive cellular immunotherapy for EBV lymphoproliferative disease. Immunol. Rev. 157:217, 1997.

Part VIII

GENE THERAPY

29 Gene Therapy for Hematopoietic Diseases

▼▼▼▼ Brian P. Sorrentino and Arthur W. Nienhuis

▼ ▼

Gene therapy has been considered for blood disorders since the first discovery of a molecular lesion leading to hematological disease, the amino acid substitution in β globin causing sickle cell anemia. At that time, the tools for gene cloning and gene transfer did not exist, but the concept that disease-causing molecular lesions could be treated by gene replacement was formed. As described in the other chapters of this book, knowledge of the molecular basis for blood disorders has exploded during the past decade. Investigators are continuing to develop strategies as to how this new information can be used for treatment, and the field of experimental hematopoietic gene therapy has grown enormously as a result. A wide range of disorders is now being considered for therapeutic intervention (Table 29–1). Whereas it is true that no unequivocal cures have yet been demonstrated, the concept that genetic modification may be used for treatment is well established. Gene therapy has proved to be effective, and in some cases curative, in animal models of blood disorders such as Jak3 deficiency, hemophilia A and hemophilia B, cancer, and metabolic storage diseases. Promising results have been obtained in clinical gene therapy trials for chronic granulomatous disease, adenosine deaminase deficiency, and modulation of graft-versus-host disease. Clinical proof of principle for gene therapy is likely to come in the near future.

Significant obstacles remain to the general implementation of gene therapy and are the focus of ongoing studies. Current vector systems have flaws that impede efficient gene transfer and expression in many cases, and new vector systems are being developed to address these limitations. Efficient and stable modification of hematopoietic stem cells remains a difficult goal, prompting efforts to understand more about their biology and their complex interactions with gene therapy vectors. The increasing availability of animal models for human blood disorders has facilitated progress in these areas and has allowed stringent preclinical testing of specific gene therapy strategies. Hematologists have played a major role in the development of human gene therapy to date and are likely to remain important contributors to this promising area of medical research.

The Science of Gene Therapy for Hematopoietic Disorders

▼ CRITICAL RELATIONSHIPS BETWEEN THE BIOLOGY OF STEM CELLS AND TRANSDUCTION WITH RETROVIRAL VECTORS

A major area of current research in gene therapy for hematopoietic disorders is focused on developing conditions that allow efficient transduction of repopulating human hematopoietic stem cells. Stem cells are a highly desired target for gene therapy applications for several reasons. By definition, stem cells can replace the entire hematopoietic system in patients undergoing ablation of hematopoiesis with irradiation or cytotoxic drugs. Therefore, the ability to stably insert exogenous genes into stem cells ex vivo would allow transplantation of these transduced cells and genetic modification of all hematopoietic lineages. The inserted gene will be stable for the lifetime of the patient because of the high capacity of stem cells to undergo self-renewing divisions in vivo. Mature T lymphocytes are an alternative target in certain instances in which modification of myeloid cells is unnecessary,[1] such as the immunodeficiency syndromes[2–4] and the modulation of antihost immune responses.[5] Unlike myeloid progenitors, targeted lymphoid progenitors persist in vivo for extended periods.[4, 6] However, considering the increasing number of hematological diseases being ascribed to single-gene defects at the level of stem cells and the wide range of disorders that could potentially be amenable to stem

Supported in part by the ASSISI Foundation Grant 94-000; National Heart, Lung, and Blood Institute Program Project Grant PO1 HL 53749; Cancer Center Support CORE Grant P30 CA 21765; and the American Lebanese Syrian Associated Charities (ALSAC).

Table 29–1. Hematological and Immune Disorders Potentially Amenable to Hematopoietic Cell–Directed Gene Therapy

Disorders	Therapeutic Genes	Target Cells
Inherited immunodeficiency		Stem cells or T lymphocytes
Severe combined immunodeficiency (SCID)	Common gamma chain, Janus kinase 3, adenosine deaminase	
Combined immunodeficiency	Purine nucleoside phosphorylase	
X-linked agammaglobulinemia	Bruton tyrosine kinase	
Wiskott-Aldrich	WAS	
Chronic granulomatous disease	Components of phagocytic oxidase system (phox 91, 47, 67, 22)	Stem cells
Acquired Immunodeficiency		Stem cells or T lymphocytes
AIDS	Transdominant mutants, antisense RNA, or ribozymes directed against HIV gene products	
Lysosomal storage disease		Stem cells
Gaucher	Glucocerebrosidase	Neural cells
GM$_1$ gangliosidosis	β-Galactosidase	
Galactosialidosis	Protective protein	
Hurler	α-Iduronidase	
MPS-VI	Arylsulfase B	
Fabry	α-Galactosidase A	
Hemoglobinopathies		Stem cells
Sickle cell anemia	β-like globins, erythroid transcription factors	
Thalassemia	α or β globins	
Fanconi anemia	FAA, FAC	Stem cells
Relapsed chronic myelogenous leukemia	Thymidine kinase from herpes simplex virus	Allogeneic T lymphocytes
Chemotherapy-induced hematopoietic suppression	Drug resistance genes, such as MDR1, DHFR, or MGMT	Stem cells
Hemophilia	Factor VIII, factor IX	Liver, muscle

cell targeting, the hematopoietic stem cell will remain a highly desirable target for gene therapy vectors.

Retroviral vectors are the most widely used system for introducing exogenous genes into stem cells. Despite the fact that these vectors are efficient at transducing murine hematopoietic stem cells, it became clear in the early 1990s that conditions resulting in efficient transduction in mice could not be directly extrapolated for the transduction of human stem cells. Strategies proven to be effective in the mouse transplant system were incorporated into the initial clinical marking protocols, such as the use of replication-defective murine retroviruses as gene transfer vectors[7–10] and the use of early-acting hematopoietic cytokines to support the culture of stem cells.[11, 12] In general, these trials resulted in less than 1 per cent vector-marked cells in the peripheral blood after the transplant procedure.[13–15] An important exception was the 10 to 15 per cent marked cells observed in pediatric cancer patients who received autologous hematopoietic cells that had been transduced with short periods of culture with vector supernatants in the absence of cytokines.[16] Although the lack of efficient stem cell marking in these trials was disappointing, it did focus the field on the nature of the biological differences between human and murine stem cells that were underlying the relative differences in transduction frequency. Significant progress has been made in understanding these differences and has suggested alternative approaches for achieving efficient stable transduction of human repopulating stem cells. It has become clear that there is a critical relationship between interactions of retroviral vectors with the hematopoietic stem cell target and the ex vivo conditions used to enhance this transduction process. The following section of this chapter focuses on these relationships, with emphasis on current approaches to overcome the biological barriers of stem cell transduction.

Limitations to Retrovirus-Mediated Transduction of Stem Cells

Standard laboratory techniques for transfection of mammalian cells use physical methods of gene transfer, such as electroporation and calcium phosphate–mediated DNA uptake. These methods cannot be employed for transduction of stem cells because of their relative inefficient DNA transfer rate; but perhaps more important, the integration efficiency of the DNA construct is low. In contrast, murine retroviruses are efficient vectors for gene transfer, and at least in dividing cells, the integration efficiency mediated by the viral integrase protein is high. Therefore, most transduced stem cells will have the vector genome stably integrated into the host cell DNA, thereby resulting in the stable persistence of vector sequences in the progeny of stem cells. For these reasons, much attention has been focused on the use of murine retroviral vectors for hematopoietic stem cell transduction.

Retroviruses contain a single-stranded RNA genome that is converted into a double-stranded DNA molecule through the action of the viral enzyme reverse transcriptase. The observation that RNA tumor viruses could incorporate a cellular proto-oncogene, and stably integrate these sequences into an infected target cell, led to the discovery that these viruses could be used as gene transfer vehicles for eukaryotic cells.[17] Breakthroughs in this area were the construction of replication-defective retroviral vectors that could be used to transmit and express a cloned gene of interest and the development of cellular systems to package the vector genome into infectious particles.[18, 19] These packaging cell lines stably express the viral *gag*, *pol*, and *env* proteins required for encapsidation of the vector genome but cannot package the defective helper genome itself (Fig. 29–1). These systems have evolved to allow efficient production

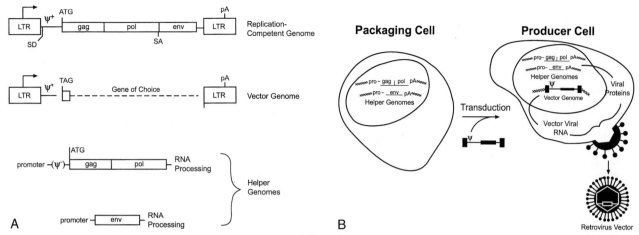

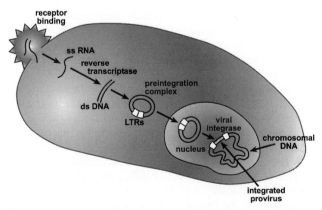

Figure 29–1. Packaging of murine retroviral vectors. *A*, Retroviral vector and packaging genomes. Shown at the top is the structure of the wild-type replication-competent genome from a murine retrovirus. The 5′ LTR directs transcriptional initiation *(arrow)*, and the 3′ LTR contains the polyadenylation (pA) sequence. The ψ packaging sequence is required for incorporation of the genome into viral particles. The relative locations of the viral *gag, pol,* and *env* genes are shown, with the translational start site for *gag* indicated by the ATG initiation codon. Also shown are splice donor (SD) and acceptor (SA) sites that result in a spliced subgenomic transcript. Vector genomes are made by deleting the viral genes and inserting an exogenous gene in their place. The ψ packaging sequence and the upstream portion of *gag* are retained to enable efficient encapsidation of the vector genome. The initiation codon has been mutated to reduce the probability of generating replication-competent retrovirus as a result of recombination between the vector and packaging genomes. Helper genomes are generated by expressing the *gag, pol,* and *env* genes from two separate plasmids under control of exogenous promoters and RNA processing elements. The ψ packaging sequence has been deleted in these helper genomes so that their transcripts are not encapsidated. *B*, Packaging and producer cells. Packaging cells are made by stably inserting the helper genomes into mammalian cells. The vector genome is then stably inserted, typically by transduction with the vector genome, to derive vector-producing cells. In these cells, transcomplementation of the genomic vector RNA by viral proteins results in infectious but replication-incompetent vector particles that are released into the medium. (Adapted from Sorrentino, B.P., and Nienhuis, A.W.: The hematopoietic system as a target for gene therapy. *In* Friedmann, T. [ed.]: The Development of Gene Therapy. Cold Spring Harbor, NY, Cold Spring Harbor Laboratory Press, 1999; with permission.)

of recombinant vector particles with a minimal chance of inadvertent production of wild-type virus through recombination events.[20–22]

In considering the barriers to hematopoietic stem cell transduction, it is important to understand the events leading to transduction of target cells and the stable incorporation of the proviral genome (Fig. 29–2). The retroviral particle first binds to the cell through a specific interaction of the retrovi-

Figure 29–2. The retroviral life cycle. Binding of the virus to the cell is mediated by specific interactions with the viral envelope and cellular receptors. The diploid RNA genome is released into the cytoplasm, where a double-stranded complementary DNA is formed through the action of viral reverse transcriptase. A circular double-stranded DNA intermediate is incorporated as part of the preintegration complex, which gains access to the nuclear contents either during mitosis or by direct nuclear transmigration in the case of lentiviruses. The proviral genome is subsequently integrated into the chromosomal DNA, a reaction mediated by the viral integrase protein. After integration, the provirus will be stably passed to subsequent daughter cells following host cell division.

ral envelope protein with a corresponding cellular receptor expressed on the surface of the target cell. Various types of retroviruses use different envelope proteins that will in part determine their cellular tropism. For instance, ecotropic retroviruses are defined by an envelope protein that specifically interacts with an amino acid transport molecule expressed exclusively on the surface of rodent cells.[23, 24] In contrast, amphotropic retroviruses are coated with an envelope protein that recognizes a phosphate transporter expressed on a wide variety of mammalian cells,[25, 26] including most human cells. This is particularly relevant given that gene therapy vectors can be packaged with a variety of envelope proteins, and as discussed later, these pseudotypes have an important impact on the stem cell transduction efficiency. After binding to the cell, the viral envelope fuses with the cell membrane, resulting in release of a viral preintegration complex into the cytoplasm. Reverse transcription is completed in the cytoplasm, and a double-stranded DNA genome, called the provirus, is generated. In the case of murine retroviruses, the preintegration complex comes into contact with the nuclear DNA during mitoses, when the nuclear membrane breaks down before cell division. In the case of lentiviruses such as the human immunodeficiency virus (HIV), the preintegration complex contains karyophilic signals that allow the preintegration complex to traverse the nuclear pores, resulting in nuclear access in non-dividing cells.[27] In either case, once contact with the cellular chromatin has been obtained, the provirus is integrated into the chromosomal DNA through the actions of the viral integrase protein, which facilitates the nicking of cellular DNA and the processing of the proviral termini.

A number of steps in this process present proven or potential barriers to the stable transduction of human hematopoietic stem cells. One important obstacle is the low level of expression of certain retroviral receptors on the surface of human stem cells. As a result, commonly used vectors cannot gain access to the stem cell cytoplasm. A second recognized barrier is that most repopulating stem cells are deeply quiescent[28, 29] and do not divide during the transduction period. Therefore, even stem cells that were initially transduced may not undergo integration of the proviral genome. This problem is compounded by the relatively short half-life of the murine retroviral preintegration complex in non-dividing cells.[30] Quiescent stem cells also appear to be limited in their ability to synthesize the proviral cDNA through cytoplasmic reverse transcription,[31] perhaps because of limiting amounts of nucleotide precursors that are available for cDNA synthesis. The unique biological properties of stem cells present significant barriers for retrovirus-mediated gene transfer (Fig. 29–3). Development of successful vector systems and transduction protocols must address these limitations.

Expression of Retroviral Receptors on Hematopoietic Stem Cells

One important explanation for the difference in transduction efficiencies between murine and human stem cells is that the ecotropic vectors, which efficiently target murine stem cells, cannot be used to transduce human cells. The human homologue of the amino acid transporter is not capable of binding the ecotropic envelope of the virus and facilitating transduction.[32, 33] The phosphate transport molecule that serves as a receptor of amphotropic virus is expressed in a wide variety of species, including mice and humans.[34] Amphotropic vectors effectively transduce human myeloid progenitor cells.[35–37] Despite this finding, recent work has shown that the level of amphotropic receptor expression in both mouse and human stem cells is low and correlates with the relative inefficiency of stem cell transduction with amphotropic vectors.[38] These results support that ampho-

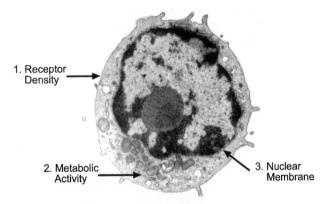

1. Receptor Density
2. Metabolic Activity
3. Nuclear Membrane

Figure 29–3. Biological barriers to stem cell transduction. Shown is an electron micrograph of a CD34$^+$, CD38$^-$ human hematopoietic cell. The first barrier to stem cell transduction occurs at the level of the cell membrane and is due to limiting degrees of expression of retroviral receptor molecules. The second potential barrier occurs in the cytoplasm, where limiting amounts of nucleotide precursors associated with the G$_0$ state of the cell cycle may limit formation of the cDNA provirus. The third barrier occurs at the level of nuclear entry for the preintegration complex. Because mitosis is required for transduction with murine retroviral vectors, nuclear access is limited in most repopulating cells owing to cell cycle quiescence. (Photomicrograph courtesy of G. Murti.)

tropic receptor expression is a major limitation for transduction of human stem cells.

A number of approaches are being explored to circumvent the limitation imposed by the level of amphotropic receptor expression. Culture of hematopoietic cells in the presence of cytokines increases binding of amphotropic virus, presumably by upregulating expression of the amphotropic receptor.[39] Another technique for increasing amphotropic receptor expression is culture in phosphate-free media, which appears to upregulate expression through feedback regulation of phosphate transporter expression.[40] This strategy has been associated with an increased transduction frequency of lymphocytes with use of amphotropic vectors.[41] In vivo administration of cytokines results in increased receptor expression in bone marrow–derived stem cells, suggesting that cytokine-mobilized stem cells may be particularly amenable to transduction with amphotropic vectors.[42] Studies in non-human primates suggest that up to 10 per cent of cytokine-mobilized repopulating cells can be transduced with an amphotropic vector.[43] A large increase in receptor expression has also been noted in human umbilical cord blood samples that had been cryopreserved and thawed.[42] Altogether, these results suggest that amphotropic receptor expression is regulated by external cues and that expression levels can be modulated with a number of experimental manipulations.

A second general approach has been the use of pseudotyped retroviral vectors containing alternative envelope proteins that interact with receptors that are more abundant on stem cells. The most extensively studied alternative envelope protein is derived from the gibbon ape leukemia virus (GALV). The GALV envelope binds to a phosphate receptor that is closely related to the amphotropic receptor but has a distinct expression pattern.[44] A packaging line is available for producing high-titer vectors with the GALV pseudotype[45] and has been used to study these vectors for their ability to transduce hematopoietic stem cells from primates. It has been shown that a relatively high proportion of human stem cells can be transduced with GALV-pseudotyped vectors as assayed by repopulation of immunodeficient mice with genetically modified human cells.[46] Furthermore, a direct comparison of amphotropic and GALV vectors in transplanted baboons has suggested a modest advantage for GALV-pseudotyped vectors that was associated with higher levels of GALV receptor expression.[47] It is still unclear whether GALV vectors have a unique advantage for stem cell gene transfer, considering that comparable transduction efficiencies have been achieved in transplanted rhesus macaques with use of standard amphotropic retroviral vectors.[43]

Another envelope protein being studied for pseudotyping is the G protein from the vesicular stomatitis virus (VSV-G). This protein mediates viral binding through a ubiquitous membrane phospholipid thought to be present on all cells, as reflected by the extremely broad host range of wild-type VSV. A second important advantage is that VSV-G–pseudotyped particles are stable and, in contrast to standard murine leukemia virus vectors, can be highly concentrated by ultracentrifugation, allowing transduction to occur at high multiplicity of infections.[48] VSV-G–pseudotyped murine vectors have been used to transduce both CD34$^+$ hematopoietic cells and lymphocytes[31, 49, 50]; however, it is still unclear whether these vectors have the ability to efficiently transduce repopulating stem cells. Addressing this question will be facilitated by the availability of stable packaging lines, which produce high-titer vectors by regulated expression of the toxic VSV-G protein.[51–53] The other important use of VSV-G envelope is for pseudotyping HIV vectors,[54] as discussed below.

Cell Cycle Quiescence as a Block to Stable Transduction of Stem Cells

Another barrier to efficient stem cell transduction is the low proportion of stem cells that are passing through S-phase at any given point in time. The commonly used vectors based on murine oncoretroviruses cannot transduce non-dividing cells owing to the barrier imposed by the intact nuclear membrane.[55] Investigators are currently pursuing several approaches to circumvent this obstacle. One strategy is to induce stem cell self-renewal divisions in vitro, at a time when the cells are exposed to the vector. A challenging aspect of this approach is finding conditions that cause amplification of stem cells rather than divisions associated with commitment and differentiation. A second strategy is to use vectors that are capable of integrating into non-dividing cells. Lentiviruses such as HIV possess this property, so that much current effort is being directed at developing HIV-based vector systems.

Induction of Cycling in Stem Cells to Enhance Transduction

Despite the number of hematopoietic cytokines that have been identified to date, no single cytokine has been shown to direct stem cell amplification during in vitro culture. In the murine system, combinations of early-acting myeloid cytokines allow modest increases in the number of repopulating stem cells during 4- to 6-day periods.[12, 56] For this reason, mouse gene transfer protocols typically employ combinations of interleukin (IL)–3, IL-6, and stem cell factor (SCF) during ex vivo culture to facilitate retroviral stem cell transduction. When this strategy is combined with other maneuvers to increase stem cell cycling, such as treating donor mice with 5-fluorouracil (5-FU),[57] high levels of stem cell transduction can be routinely achieved with use of ecotropic retroviral vectors.[11, 58, 59]

Progress is being made in deriving culture conditions that lead to cycling and expansion of human repopulating cells, and it is anticipated that these conditions will be useful for enhancing transduction of human stem cells. Normally, only a small proportion of primitive human cells enter cycle during long-term culture, with only half of the primitive cells cycling after 30 days in culture.[28] In contrast, more mature myeloid progenitors rapidly proliferate for at least 3 weeks in the presence of early-acting myeloid cytokines.[36, 60] Significant expansion of earlier progenitor cells, defined as long-term culture initiating cells (LTC-ICs), can also be obtained in myeloid suspension cultures.[61, 62] However, expansion of LTC-ICs does not necessarily correlate with changes in the number of repopulating stem cells, as defined by engraftment in non-obese diabetic mice with severe combined immune deficiency (NOD/SCID).[63] Modest expansion of NOD/SCID repopulating cells (SRCs) from human umbilical cord blood can be obtained by culturing CD34+ cells for 4 days in serum-free media containing high concentrations of early-acting cytokines.[64] The lack of serum

in the transduction cultures may be an important factor in avoiding a quantitative loss of stem cells because of serum-induced differentiation.[65]

A novel approach for promoting cell cycle progression of human stem cells in culture is direct molecular modulation of the cell cycle machinery. A complex regulatory network of cyclin-dependent kinases and inhibitors of their function control cell cycle progression in many types of cells.[66, 67] Recent work has shown that it is possible to downregulate the levels of cyclin-dependent kinase inhibitors to drive hematopoietic stem cells into cycle and thereby increase their transducibility with murine retroviral vectors. In cultures of human CD34+ cells, antisense oligonucleotides directed against p27 (Kip-1) mRNA were used together with an antibody against transforming growth factor-β (TGF-β). Neutralization of TGF-β resulted in downregulation of p15 (INK4B), a potent inhibitor of G_1 cell cycle progression, and the antisense block to p27 synthesis has been previously shown to promote cell cycle progression in fibroblasts.[68] This strategy was shown to significantly enhance transduction of primitive human hematopoietic cells, as defined by engraftment of transduced cells in immune deficient mice.[69] Further advances in the understanding of the molecular mechanisms that control stem cell self-renewal divisions should prove useful in deriving new approaches to stem cell transduction.

Another variable related to the kinetics of stem cell cycling is the timing of vector application. Because primitive cells enter cycle relatively late during culture, application of vector at late time points during the transduction protocol is important for achieving a higher transduction frequency of primitive cells.[70] Earlier exposure of quiescent cells to vector particles appears to block transduction at later time points when the cells are in cycle,[71] presumably owing to downmodulation of the retroviral receptor before cells are prepared to divide and allow integration of the vector genome. At least in part because of these factors, "pre-stimulating" stem cells for 2 to 5 days in vector-free culture results in substantial increases in retroviral transduction.[57, 72, 73] Relatively efficient transduction of human umbilical cord blood SRCs has been achieved by pre-stimulating cells for three days in serum-free cultures supplemented with hematopoietic cytokines, before transduction with a murine retroviral vector.[46]

Another approach for increasing the transducibility of stem cells involves treating the host with hematopoietic cytokines before collecting cells for transduction. The basis for this approach was derived from the observation that mice treated with SCF and granulocyte colony-stimulating factor (G-CSF) display a large amplification of stem cells in the bone marrow and the peripheral blood.[74, 75] These cytokine-mobilized peripheral blood stem cells were more efficiently transduced than post–5-FU bone marrow stem cells,[74] perhaps in part because of induction of cycling as a result of the cytokine treatment. We now know that the amphotropic receptor is also induced by cytokine mobilization. Post-cytokine bone marrow stem cells are also excellent targets for gene transfer.[76] When rhesus monkey stem cells were mobilized from the blood and bone marrow with SCF and G-CSF and transduced with an amphotropic retroviral vector, as many as 5 per cent of the peripheral blood cells were marked with the vector 1 year after transplantation.[76] More recent studies in the rhesus model have shown even greater degrees of marking with use of cytokine-mobilized peripheral blood CD34+ cells.[43]

Lentiviral Vectors to Overcome the G_0 Block

In contrast to murine oncoretroviruses, lenti-retroviruses such as HIV possess the ability to infect non-dividing cells with subsequent integration of their genome. On the basis of this property, much current effort is being focused on exploring lentiviral vector systems for the transduction of quiescent hematopoietic stem cells. Despite the natural resistance to use of a human pathogen as a vector system, initial results appear promising, and HIV vectors may offer an important methodology for stem cell gene therapy.

Much that is known about lentiviruses is derived from the study of HIV, the pathological entity responsible for the acquired human immunodeficiency syndrome. It has long been known that HIV can infect non-dividing macrophages in vivo and that this intrinsic property allows infection of other quiescent cell types.[77] This biological property is due to the ability of the HIV preintegration complex to traverse the nuclear pores and gain access to the nuclear chromatin without the requirement for mitotic breakdown of the nuclear envelope.[30] These karyophilic properties are mediated by a nuclear localization signal within the matrix protein of *gag*[27, 78, 79] and by the HIV accessory protein designated Vpr.[80] Attempts to incorporate these elements into Moloney-based murine vectors have failed to yield a chimeric virus with the ability to infect non-dividing cells.[81]

Initial HIV vectors relied on the native envelope protein and could transduce only cells expressing the native HIV receptor, CD4.[82] Subsequent HIV-based vectors were created by replacing a portion of the viral envelope coding sequences with a reporter gene and pseudotyping the vector with the VSV-G envelope protein. Unlike Moloney-based vectors, HIV vectors have been used to efficiently infect a variety of growth-arrested cells in vitro, including primary human macrophages and terminally differentiated neurons.[83, 84] The ability of HIV-based vectors to transduce non-dividing cells has allowed efficient in vivo targeting of both retinal and brain cells in rats, prompting the development of lentiviral vectors for neurological gene therapy applications.[85–87] These studies also showed that reverse transcription was the rate-limiting step for transduction but that the efficiency of transduction can be improved by pretreating the vector with deoxynucleoside triphosphates to promote partial cDNA synthesis within the virion before infection.[85, 87]

As a first step toward achieving human hematopoietic stem cell transduction, several groups have shown that VSV-G–pseudotyped HIV vectors efficiently transduce human hematopoietic cells in vitro, including peripheral blood lymphocytes,[88] primary human macrophages,[89] and CD34+ progenitors.[54, 84] These results have been extended to show that HIV vectors can transduce more primitive and quiescent human hematopoietic cells characterized by the CD34+, CD38− phenotype,[90] a population that is highly refractory to transduction with Moloney-based vectors. A recent report documented the ability of a VSV-G–pseudotyped HIV vector to transduce cells (SRC) capable of establishing hematopoiesis in immunodeficient mice. Human umbilical cord blood cells were transduced with a green fluorescent protein

(GFP)–expressing HIV vector, in a simple 5-hour transduction protocol done in the absence of exogenous cytokines. After injection into NOD/SCID mice, between 2 and 20 per cent of the engrafted human cells expressed the GFP marker gene, at times ranging from 7 to 22 weeks after transplantation.[91] Relatively high levels of transduced myeloid progenitors were also noted in the bone marrow of the transplanted mice. These results demonstrate the capacity of HIV vectors for human stem cell transduction and suggest that transduction can be achieved with minimal ex vivo manipulation of stem cells. Future studies will be needed to determine whether HIV vectors will result in higher transduction efficiencies than those that have been achieved with use of optimal conditions for murine retroviral vectors.[43, 46, 92]

Hematopoietic Stromal Elements to Enhance Transduction With Retroviral Vectors

Hematopoietic stem cells are maintained in vivo in intimate contact with a complex hematopoietic microenvironment consisting of mesenchyme-derived stromal cells, extracellular matrix molecules, and vascular elements. Increasing knowledge of stem cell/microenvironment interactions has led to testing of various stromal elements in stem cell transduction protocols. Mesenchymal stromal cells can be established in culture from bone marrow aspirates by periodically removing non-adherent hematopoietic cells and allowing bone marrow–derived fibroblasts to adhere to the tissue culture plate. Transduction in the presence of adherent stroma has a number of theoretical advantages, such as allowing interactions with membrane-bound molecules that are supportive of stem cell viability and expressed on the surface of the stromal cells.[93] In vitro studies have demonstrated improved transduction efficiency of LTC-ICs when human bone marrow cells were transduced in the presence of stroma.[94] Transduction in the context of long-term stromal cultures resulted in relatively high levels of gene transfer into canine repopulating cells.[95] Stromal cultures have also been shown to increase gene transfer efficiency in primate experiments, but to a much lesser degree. In rhesus monkey experiments, an increase in marking was noted when transduction was done in the presence of autologous marrow stroma and soluble hematopoietic cytokines.[43] A similar beneficial effect of stroma on cytokine-supported transduction has been noted in a clinical marking trial of adult cancer patients.[14] In contrast, when similar patients received cells transduced in the presence of autologous marrow stroma but without added cytokines, no long-term marking was noted.[96] Taken together, these results suggest that stromal cells can augment human stem cell transduction to a limited degree but that additional cytokine support increases transduction frequency.

Extracellular matrix molecules in the bone marrow have also been investigated for potential use in stem cell transduction protocols. One molecule in particular, fibronectin, has clearly emerged as an important mediator of gene transfer. On the basis of the observation that stem cells and primitive progenitors bind to fibronectin,[97] various peptide fragments of fibronectin have been studied as facilitators of retrovirus-mediated transduction. Culture of human hematopoietic cells with retroviral vectors in the presence of the carboxyl-terminal 30/35 kDa fragment of fibronectin significantly enhanced gene transfer into human myeloid progenitors and LTC-ICs.[98] The mechanism for this effect is in part due to colocalization of the retroviral particles and hematopoietic cells to distinct but closely approximate binding motifs on the fibronectin molecule[99, 100] (Fig. 29–4). Fibronectin may also act by inducing proliferation of hematopoietic stem cells through binding to very late antigen (VLA)–4 and VLA-5, integrin molecules expressed on the surface of stem cells.[101, 102] The net results of these effects are a significant increase in stem cell transduction relative to what can be achieved with simple supernatant transduction alone.[103] A recombinant human fibronectin fragment designated CH-296 is available and contains both the stem cell binding motif and the binding site for the vector particles. This fragment has been used to achieve significant levels of stem cell transduction in a baboon transplant model with a GALV-pseudotyped vector.[92] The ease of use afforded by the CH-296 fragment, together with the reproducible increase in transduction efficiency of primitive hematopoietic cells, has led to the widespread use of this fibronectin fragment in stem cell transduction protocols.

▼ METHODS FOR SELECTION AND AMPLIFICATION OF TRANSDUCED STEM CELLS

One broad approach for overcoming low stem cell transduction efficiencies is to selectively amplify the subset of stem cells that contain the vector. If successfully accomplished, this approach can compensate for inefficient stem cell transduction and can theoretically be used with any vector system. This strategy relies on the use of a dominant selectable marker within the vector. This marker can be a gene conferring drug resistance, a phenotypic marker that allows cell sorting of transduced cells, or a construct giving a direct proliferative advantage to the transduced cells. If the selectable marker is not itself a therapeutic gene, a second

therapeutic gene can be incorporated into the selectable vector. The feasibility of this approach has been validated in preclinical murine models using retroviral vectors, and it is now being tested in large animal models and in clinical trials. Selection of transduced stem cells can ultimately be combined with methods for achieving more efficient transduction, and it seems likely that both of these complementary efforts will be required to achieve a high number of corrected cells, especially in populations of patients in which myeloablative conditioning is not clinically appropriate.

Pretransplantation Sorting of Transduced Cells Expressing a Marker Gene

One method for enrichment of transduced hematopoietic cells involves the use of fluorescence-activated cell sorting (FACS) to isolate stem cells that are expressing vector sequences. Hematopoietic cells are first transduced with a vector expressing a marker that can be detected by FACS and are subsequently sorted to isolate vector-expressing cells. This vector-expressing population is then used to reconstitute lethally irradiated animals. Stem cells that remain untransduced are discarded from the graft, so that the reconstituted hematopoietic system should consist mostly, if not entirely, of transduced cells.

This strategy was initially employed in the mouse transplant model using the human cell surface antigen CD24 as the selectable marker. Transplant of these sorted CD24-expressing cells into lethally irradiated mice resulted in high proportions of CD24-expressing myeloid and lymphoid cells for up to 4 months after transplantation.[104] The proportion of CD24-expressing peripheral blood cells was even higher when a murine stem cell virus (MSCV)–based vector was used, approaching 90 per cent CD24+ positive cells in the bone marrow. This increase in expressing cells seen with the MSCV vector reflected less frequent silencing of expression in vivo with the MSCV versus the murine myeloproliferative sarcoma virus (MPSV) vector.[105] More recent work in the murine system has used GFP as a marker.[106] This natural fluorochrome, expressed as an intracellular protein, eliminates the need for antibody staining, providing greater sensitivity.[107] In vitro studies have been done in human CD34+ hematopoietic cells, in which sorting for cells expressing a transferred murine CD24 gene resulted in a large enrichment for myeloid progenitors and LTC-ICs that expressed a linked neo^R gene.[108] As a step toward applying this method, vectors coexpressing both a CD24 and a glucocerebrosidase cDNA have been tested for use in gene therapy for Gaucher disease.[109]

Several potential problems limit the clinical application of this approach. In a clinical setting, the proportion of transduced stem cells may be low, with limiting numbers of cells within the transduced graft. Pretransplantation sorting would therefore yield an insufficient number of stem cells for achieving hematopoietic engraftment. This limitation could be circumvented if an effective method for in vitro stem cell amplification were available and could subsequently be employed. A second limitation is that sorting cannot reduce competition from endogenous stem cells residing in the host, so that this strategy cannot be used in cases in which myeloablation is not justified. In contrast, methods

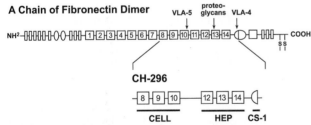

Figure 29–4. Fibronectin molecules for facilitating retrovirus-mediated stem cell transduction. The top diagram shows the structure of the A chain of a fibronectin dimer and the lower diagram the recombinant CH-296 fragment used to enhance stem cell transduction. Fibronectin repeats are indicated as enclosed areas, and the type III repeats are numbered 1 to 14. The VLA-5 binding domain is indicated (CELL) and contains the Arg-Gly-Asp (RGD) recognition sequence that mediates adhesion of hematopoietic stem cells to the fibronectin fragment. The VLA-4 binding sequence is designated CS-1 and may also play an important role in stem cell binding. Retroviral particles adhere to repeats 12 to 14. The colocalization of stem cells and virus particles, along with possible direct effects of CH-296 on stem cell maintenance, results in enhancement of stem cell transduction. (Adapted from Hanenberg, H., Xiao, X.L., Dilloo, D., Hashino, K., Kato, I., and Williams, D.A.: Colocalization of retrovirus and target cells on specific fibronectin fragments increases genetic transduction of mammalian cells. Nat. Med. 2:876, 1996; with permission.)

for the selection of transduced cells in vivo provide for this possibility.

In Vivo Selection With Drug Resistance Genes

In vivo stem cell selection is a strategy whereby selective outgrowth of transduced stem cells is achieved within the host at some time after transplantation (Fig. 29–5). This goal can be achieved by any means that gives transduced stem cells an in vivo proliferative advantage over their untransduced counterparts. The most widely explored technique is to incorporate a drug resistance gene into the vector, so that transduced stem cells have a survival advantage when the host is treated with the relevant cytotoxic drug. An alternative approach, detailed in the next section, is the use of growth-promoting genes, such as engineered cytokine receptors, that can be directly activated with non-toxic compounds. In either case, the advantages are that the host can be safely engrafted with an adequate number of stem cells and the minority of transduced stem cells can be potentially

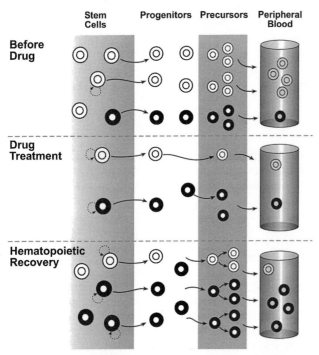

Figure 29–5. In vivo selection of stem cells transduced with a drug resistance gene vector. This schematic depicts how stem cell selection with cytotoxic drugs can result in increased proportions of modified cells in the peripheral blood. Cells that contain a vector expressing a drug resistance gene are indicated with dark fill, whereas unmodified cells are open. Various stages of hematopoietic maturation are indicated, and progression through these compartments is shown with solid arrows. Stem cell self-renewal divisions are shown as broken arrows. Before drug administration, a minority of cells contains the transferred drug resistance gene. When the animal is treated with the appropriate cytotoxic drug, stem cells expressing the resistance vector have a significant survival advantage and therefore are enriched by drug treatment. In the recovery phase, cell expansion results in an increased number and proportion of cells containing the drug resistance vector. If selection has occurred at the stem cell level, increased numbers of genetically modified cells will be seen in all hematopoietic compartments and will be stable over time. (Adapted from Sorrentino, B.P.: Drug resistance gene therapy. *In* Brenner M.K., and Moen, R.C. [eds.]: Gene Therapy in Cancer. New York, Marcel Dekker, 1996; with permission.)

expanded in an incremental fashion in their natural environment. In vivo selection therefore aims to exploit the physiological stem cell expansion that occurs in vivo in response to stem cell depletion.[110]

Significant effort has been focused on drug resistance genes as dominant selectable markers for transduced stem cells. The key requirements for this approach are that (1) the cytotoxic drugs used result in significant depletion of unmodified hematopoietic stem cells, (2) the resistance gene is expressed at significant levels in the primitive stem cells, (3) the drug selection regimen can be tolerated without excessive toxicity, and (4) the resistance gene is suitable for generating bicistronic vectors containing a linked therapeutic gene. The first gene to be studied for in vivo selection was the human multidrug resistance 1 *(MDR1)* gene.[111] The product of *MDR1* is P-glycoprotein, a transmembrane pump that extrudes many types of chemotherapeutic drugs out of the cell, thereby conferring a drug resistance phenotype.[112] In vitro studies with an *MDR1* retrovirus,[112, 113] and work with an *MDR1* transgenic mouse line,[114, 115] confirmed the hypothesis that enforced expression of P-glycoprotein would protect hematopoietic cells from a variety of cytotoxic drugs. In later studies using mice that had been transplanted with bone marrow cells transduced with an *MDR1* retroviral vector, treatment with taxol resulted in increases in the number and proportion of transduced hematopoietic cells in the peripheral blood.[116, 117] These studies provided the first evidence that a drug resistance gene could be used for the in vivo selection of transduced hematopoietic cells and served as the rationale for developing clinical trials testing this approach.

In clinical trials, adult cancer patients received *MDR1*-transduced cells as part of an autologous transplant treatment protocol and were subsequently treated with taxol on the basis of clinical indications. The results have been disappointing regarding selection, with no evidence of enrichment for transduced cells seen after taxol treatment.[14, 15] There are several potential explanations for the lack of selection in these trials, including the absence of engraftment of transduced stem cells, potential rearrangement of the vector,[118] and a lack of selective pressure within the stem cell compartment.[119] Another concern is the demonstration that transduction with an *MDR1* vector during cytokine-mediated expansion was associated with the development of a myeloproliferative syndrome in mice transplanted with the expanded, genetically modified cells.[120] Future efforts at developing *MDR1* as a selectable marker for stem cells will have to address these important concerns.

Another system for stem cell selection uses variants of dihydrofolate reductase (DHFR) for conferring resistance to antifolate drugs such as methotrexate (MTX) and trimetrexate (TMTX). The advantages of this system are that (1) the *DHFR* cDNA is small (690 bp) and stable in retroviral vectors, (2) antifolates are relatively non-toxic and are known to be tolerated in allogeneic transplant patients, and (3) single amino acid substitutions in the enzyme active site result in variant enzymes that confer high levels of cellular resistance to antifolate drugs.[121–123] In particular, a variant of human *DHFR* containing a leucine to tyrosine substitution in codon 22[124] confers a 100-fold increase in resistance to TMTX in transduced hematopoietic cells.[59] Despite these advantages, earlier studies of *DHFR*-mediated selection in transplanted mice have given equivocal and conflicting results.[125, 126] It is now clear that the drug regimen used for selection is a critical component of the selection strategy. Antifolates such as MTX and TMTX do not exert selective pressure in the stem cell compartment because their toxicity is restricted to more mature hematopoietic cells.[127] This limitation can be overcome by giving TMTX together with drugs that inhibit the uptake and salvage of extracellular nucleosides. One such inhibitor, nitrobenzylmercaptopurine-riboside 5′-monophosphate (NBMPR-P), can dramatically sensitize normal murine stem cells to the effects of TMTX.[128] This observation has led to the use of a combination of TMTX and NBMPR-P for selection of *DHFR*-transduced stem cells. Mice transplanted with varying proportions of cells transduced with bicistronic *DHFR* vectors were treated with several courses of TMTX and NBMPR-P.[129] Significant enrichments for vector-expressing peripheral blood cells were noted in all hematopoietic lineages after drug treatment (Fig. 29–6). Secondary transplant experiments confirmed that selection had occurred at the level of primitive stem cells.[129] These studies established the feasibility of the *DHFR* system for stem cell selection and provided strong proof that genetically modified hematopoietic stem cells can be selectively enriched by post-transplantation chemotherapy. Experiments are now in progress to determine whether this *DHFR* system can be used for stem cell selection in non-human primates.

The third system for stem cell selection uses DNA alkyltransferase genes to confer protection against nitrosourea drugs such as BCNU and CCNU. These genes encode DNA repair proteins that are expressed at high levels in drug-resistant tumor cells and provide cellular resistance by removing cytotoxic DNA adducts induced by drug treatment.[130] Several observations have led to pursuit of these genes as selectable markers for stem cells. First, hematopoietic cells generally express low levels of alkyltransferases[131] but can be made to be highly drug resistant by retrovirus-mediated transfer of various alkyltransferase cDNAs.[132–135] A second advantage is that nitrosoureas exert strong selective pressure within the stem cell compartment, as evidenced by the prolonged and cumulative myelosuppression associated with their use in cancer therapy. Retroviral vectors containing various human methylguanine methyltransferase (MGMT) cDNAs have been tested as selectable markers in transplanted mice. In one study, selection of transduced myeloid progenitors in the bone marrow was noted after treatment with BCNU.[136] Similar results have been obtained in mice transduced with a variant of *MGMT* and subsequently treated with BCNU together with O-6-benzylguanine, a pharmacological potentiator of nitrosourea toxicity.[137] In currently open clinical trials, investigators will be determining whether selection can be obtained in cancer patients undergoing transplantation with transduced autologous CD34[+] cells and subsequent treatment with nitrosourea chemotherapy.

Positive Selection Systems

Another approach for amplifying transduced stem cells is based on the enforced expression of growth-promoting genes such as cytokine receptors. These systems are based on the hypothesis that enforced expression of mitogenic receptors will allow the selective outgrowth of transduced stem cells in the presence of the appropriate ligand. To provide a means for controlling the proliferation of transduced cells, a variety of ligand-binding domains have been used to replace the extracellular portion of the cytokine receptor, so that receptor dimerization and activation can be controlled by the pharmacological administration of specific ligands (Fig. 29–7). An intrinsic advantage of this approach is that relatively non-toxic substances may in principle be used for selection, and thereby the host toxicity associated with cytotoxic drugs can be avoided.

A recently characterized system uses the binding domain for the drug FK-506 to allow receptor activation with a dimeric form of the drug, designated FK-1012.[138] Receptors that are responsive to FK-1012 have been engineered with use of hematopoietic receptors for erythropoietin,[139] thrombopoietin,[140] or the c-*kit* ligand.[141] These constructs have been retrovirally transferred to several hematopoietic cell types and have resulted in ligand-specific, cytokine-indepen-

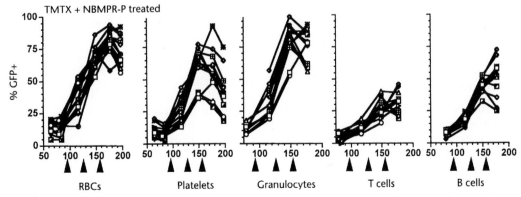

Figure 29–6. Enrichment for vector-expressing peripheral blood cells in mice treated with trimetrexate and a nucleoside transport inhibitor. Mice were transplanted with bone marrow cells that had been transduced with a retroviral vector expressing both a resistance-conferring *DHFR* gene and the enhanced green fluorescent protein (EGFP) marker. The proportions of EGFP-expressing peripheral blood cells were determined for the indicated hematopoietic lineages by flow cytometry. Each line represents serial determinations from an individual animal. The x-axis indicates the post-transplantation day on which the analysis was performed. Drug treatments consisted of a 5-day course with trimetrexate and the nucleoside transport inhibitor NBMPR-P and are indicated on the x-axis as bold arrowheads. The increases seen with drug treatment were statistically significant for all lineages. (Adapted from Allay, J.A., Persons, D.A., Galipeau, J., Riberdy, J.M., Ashmun, R.A., Blakley, R.L., and Sorrentino, B.P.: In vivo selection of retrovirally transduced hematopoietic stem cells. Nat. Med. 4:1136, 1998; with permission.)

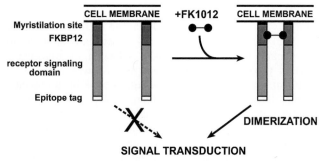

SIGNAL TRANSDUCTION

Figure 29–7. Chimeric cytokine receptors for the selective expansion of transduced hematopoietic cells. Selective amplification of transduced cells may be possible by introducing cytokine receptors that can be specifically activated by synthetic drugs. This schematic shows one such strategy for achieving this goal. The cytoplasmic portion of a hematopoietic cytokine receptor is fused to the binding domain from the FK-506–binding protein FKBP12. This binding domain can also recognize a lipid-soluble dimeric form of the drug designated FK-1012. The myristylation-targeting domain from c-*src* is used to direct localization to the inner surface of the cell membrane. FK-1012 is then used as a pharmacological mediator of dimerization to bring together the two FK-506–binding domains. In the absence of FK-1012, the fusion protein is unable to dimerize and is therefore unable to initiate the signal transduction cascade. Addition of FK-1012 results in dimerization and thereby mediates a proliferative signal in cells that have been transduced with this construct. The receptor fragment can be from the erythropoietin, thrombopoietin, or stem cell factor receptors. (Courtesy of Dr. C. A. Blau.)

dent growth in vitro. In one study, culture of transduced murine bone marrow cells with FK-1012 resulted in a 1 million–fold expansion of clonogenic myeloid cells, showing that sustained activation of the chimeric receptor led to dramatic amplification of primitive multipotent cells.[140] The hormone-binding domain of the estrogen receptor has also been used to generate a variant G-CSF receptor that allowed estrogen-induced growth of murine myeloid cells in vitro.[142] Future studies will determine whether these positive selection systems can be used for amplification of pluripotent stem cells in vivo. This possibility is suggested by earlier experiments showing that transgenic mice expressing an activated form of the erythropoietic receptor displayed a modest increase in primitive myeloid cells when treated with exogenous erythropoietin.[143]

▼ VECTOR SYSTEMS OF GENE THERAPY FOR HEMATOPOIETIC DISORDERS

Gene Expression Using Murine Retroviral Vectors

Although much work with murine retroviral vectors has focused on increasing stem cell transduction efficiencies, another important area of investigation has been the improvement of vector expression. One problem is that cells can methylate sequences within the retroviral promoter, resulting in silencing of transcription over time. In mice transplanted with Moloney leukemia virus vectors, progressive silencing of vector expression was seen in splenic progenitor colonies after serial transplantation.[144] Silencing has been reported to occur in promoters from other types of viral vectors and appears to be mediated, at least in part, at the level of chromatin structure.[145] With use of embryonic carcinoma (EC) cells and embryonic stem (ES) cells as

models for vector silencing, a number of newer vectors have been described that are relatively resistant to transcriptional silencing. Using derivatives of the murine MPSV, several investigators have derived vectors that are stably expressed in EC and ES cells.[146–148] These MPSV-based vectors resist silencing by virtue of mutations in the U3 enhancer region of the long terminal repeat (LTR),[149] by an alteration in the 5′ untranslated region encompassing the tRNA binding site,[147, 148, 150] and in one case by an intentional insertion of a bacterial demethylating sequence in the promoter region.[148] A number of vectors have been generated that incorporate these *cis*-acting elements and in general give high levels of expression in primary hematopoietic cells.[151–153] One particularly useful variant is MSCV.[154] When directly compared with the parental MPSV vector for in vivo silencing, the MSCV promoter led to the most stable long-term expression in murine serial transplant experiments.[105] Furthermore, evidence that MSCV vectors can be used for in vivo stem cell selection[129] provides proof that they can drive expression of exogenous genes in primitive stem cells. Splicing of the retroviral transcript also facilitates exogenous gene expression.[155] The MFG series of vectors use the normal 5′ and 3′ splice sites to generate a subgenomic mRNA, in which the exogenous gene is inserted at the position of the viral *env* initiation codon.[156] By use of MFG vectors expressing the human adenosine deaminase gene, high-level expression has been obtained in the hematopoietic cells of transplanted mice.[157]

It is often desirable to express more than one exogenous gene from a single vector, as in the case of vectors containing a selectable marker gene and a second linked therapeutic gene. A variety of designs have been tested for creating multigene vectors (Fig. 29–8). A second gene can be expressed by using an internal promoter located between the retroviral LTRs; however, drug selection for gene expression can lead to suppression of the second transcriptional unit.[158] One approach to this problem is to place one of the exogenous genes within the 3′ LTR, generating in target cells two copies of the exogenous gene that lie outside the transcriptional unit of the vector.[159] A variant of this idea is to introduce a deletional mutation in the 3′ LTR sequence to create a "self-inactivating vector" that lacks promoter activity in target cells.[160, 161] In certain instances, fusion proteins can be created that retain both functional activities of the parent gene products.[162] A more recently developed method for creating double-gene retroviral vectors is the use of internal ribosomal entry sequences (IRESs). These viral sequences allow ribosomal access to downstream coding sequences[163] and thereby circumvent potential issues of transcriptional interference by directing efficient translation of both genes from a single bicistronic transcript.[164] High-level expression from IRES-containing vectors has been documented in a number of cases,[106, 165–167] including vectors that express three independent coding sequences from two different IRESs.[168]

Lentiviral Vectors

As discussed above, lentiviral vectors may be particularly well suited for hematopoietic stem cell transduction because of their ability to stably transduce non-dividing cells. Analogous to murine retroviral vectors, HIV vector genomes have

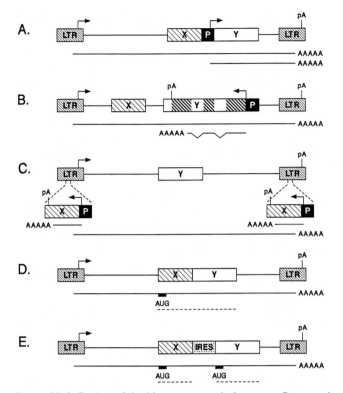

that transcription from the LTR requires *trans*-activation from the Tat protein. Although these vectors resulted in high levels of gene expression in human cells,[88] the anticipated use of tissue-specific promoters and the potential toxic effects of *tat* expression in target cells justified the development of HIV vectors lacking the *tat* coding sequences. In target cells transduced with *tat*-less vectors, the exogenous gene is expressed from a heterologous internal promoter that is not subject to potential transcriptional interference by the inactive LTR promoter[83] (see Fig. 29–9). Further modifications of the vector genome designed to improve safety include promoter deletions resulting in self-inactivating vectors[169] and chimeric promoters that are *tat* independent.[170]

Vector packaging is also accomplished in much the same way as for murine retroviral vectors, by use of packaging constructs that provide the necessary viral proteins in *trans* but which themselves cannot be packaged because of alterations in the genome. Early versions of packaging constructs contained all the viral genes except for the gp160 envelope.[83, 88] It has been shown that the *vif, vpr, vpu,* and *nef* accessory genes are not necessary for packaging or for the capacity to transduce at least some types of non-dividing cells. On the basis of these observations, a minimal packaging construct has been described that contains only the *gag, pol, tat,* and *rev* genes. This packaging system increases the

Figure 29–8. Design of double-gene retroviral vectors. Diagrams *A* to *E* show five different designs for expressing two different coding sequences (X and Y) using retroviral vectors. *A,* Vector containing a downstream internal promoter (P). The transcript initiated in the LTR will lead to efficient translation of gene X but not Y. A second transcript is initiated from the internal promoter that leads to expression of gene Y. With this design, mRNA expression from one transcription unit can negatively affect the other. *B,* Vector containing a second gene inserted antisense to the retroviral promoter. This design permits inclusion of introns in gene Y (open areas). This strategy is used to express globin genes and can be used for other genes in which introns contain transcriptional regulatory elements or where splicing of the second transcript will enhance gene expression. *C,* Double-copy vectors. These vectors are constructed by inserting a copy of gene X into the U3 region of the 3' LTR. The inserted gene is then duplicated in the 5' LTR region before insertion into the target cell genome. Note that gene X requires an internal promoter for expression and is located outside the retroviral transcription unit, thereby providing insulation from potential transcriptional interference. *D,* Fusion of coding sequences. A single chimeric polypeptide can be generated by fusion of the coding sequences from two genes. In this case, a single transcript and translational initiation site are sufficient for expression. This approach is limited to cases in which the two gene products have the same subcellular localization and bifunctional chimeras can be generated. *E,* Bicistronic vector containing an internal ribosomal entry sequence (IRES). This design leads to expression of a single mRNA transcript from which both genes can be efficiently translated. The IRES directs ribosomal entry at the downstream initiation codon. Note that the expression of both gene products is physically linked and therefore codominant. (Adapted from Sorrentino, B.P.: Drug resistance gene therapy. *In* Brenner M.K., and Moen, R.C. [eds.]: Gene Therapy in Cancer. New York, Marcel Dekker, 1996; with permission.)

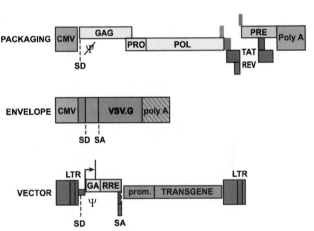

Figure 29–9. Genomes for the generation of pseudotyped HIV vectors. A second-generation packaging genome is shown that expresses the *gag, pol,* and *protease* genes to form the protein core of the vector. The *tat* and *rev* genes are also included and required for generation of vector particles. The *env* gene is deleted together with the accessory genes *env, vif, vpr, vpu,* and *nef.* The packaging construct in expressed from the CMV promoter and includes a heterologous polyadenylation signal, design features that decrease the chance of recombination with the vector. Downstream from the splice donor, the construct has a 39 bp deletion in the ψ packaging sequence so that the packaging transcript cannot be incorporated into vector particles. The outer envelope for the virus is encoded by a separate plasmid that contains the gene for the VSV-G protein. This protein is chosen to provide broad host cell tropism and because the stability of this envelope protein allows concentration of vector particles by ultracentrifugation. The vector genome contains both HIV LTRs, the complete HIV leader sequence with the 5' splice donor site (SD), and approximately 360 bp of the *gag* gene including the ψ packaging sequence. Also included for efficient packaging is a fragment of the *env* gene containing the *rev* response element (RRE) and the splice acceptor (SA) sites from the third exon of the *tat* and *rev* genes. The transgene is inserted downstream of the SA site and is driven by an internal promoter (prom). (Adapted with permission from Naldini, L., and Verma, I.M.: Lentiviral vectors. *In* Friedmann, T. [ed.]: The Development of Gene Therapy. Cold Spring Harbor, NY, Cold Spring Harbor Laboratory Press, 1999; with permission.)

been designed that do not express any viral genes but retain the *cis*-acting sequences necessary for the production of infectious particles. These sequences are the HIV LTRs, the upstream ψ packaging sequence and part of *gag* gene, and a fragment of the HIV envelope gene that contains the *rev* response element and a splice acceptor site (Fig. 29–9). Initial vectors were made that used the retroviral LTR for expression of the exogenous gene of interest. This design required that the *tat* gene be included in the vector, given safety of HIV vectors by deleting accessory genes known to be virulence factors for the wild-type virus.[171, 172] Modifications to prevent the packaging genome from being incorporated into the vector particles include replacement of the viral LTR with a promoter from cytomegalovirus, a deletion in the ψ packaging sequence, and substitution of a mammalian polyadenylation sequence in place of the 3′ LTR. A separate plasmid is required to provide envelope protein and generate pseudotyped vector particles. The most commonly used envelope is the VSV-G protein, which allows vectors to be concentrated by ultracentrifugation in a manner similar to VSV-G–pseudotyped Moloney-based vectors.[54]

Vector preparations have typically been made by transient cotransfection of vector, packaging, and envelope constructs. Titers of about 10^5 to 10^6 particles per milliliter can be obtained for most vectors and increased to between 10^7 and 10^8 plaque-forming units per milliliter with concentration. One problem with producing a stable producer line is the toxicity of some of the packaging proteins, most notably the VSV-G envelope and the viral protease. A report describes a stable packaging line in which this limitation was overcome by controlling expression of the HIV trans-complementing proteins and the VSV-G envelope with a tetracycline-regulated system.[173] In summary, significant progress has been made in developing HIV vector systems, with particular emphasis on design features that enhance safety for potential future clinical trials.

Foamy Virus Vectors

Another retrovirus being considered for gene therapy is human foamy virus (HFV), which is a member of the spumavirus family. Although HFV was originally isolated from a patient's nasopharyngeal carcinoma tissue, seropositivity in humans is thought to be extremely rare.[174] Vectors have been constructed by deleting the viral genes from the genome but retaining the LTRs and the packaging signal, analogous to the design of murine retroviral vectors. These vectors have demonstrated a number of desirable properties for hematopoietic applications, including integration in a wide variety of cell types, resistance to serum inactivation, a relatively large packaging capacity for exogenous genes, and enhanced ability to transduce stationary cells.[175] The transcriptional activation of the HFV LTR requires trans-complementation with viral protein Bel-1.[176] This requirement ensures that the LTR will be transcriptionally silenced in target cells and decreases both the risk of inadvertent replication-competent virus production in vivo and the possibility of transcriptional interference when internal promoters are used. A variety of hematopoietic cell types have been transduced with HFV vectors, including human primary hematopoietic progenitors, and the transduction efficiency appears relatively high as assessed by a variety of in vitro assays.[177] Progress has been made in defining the critical cis-acting sequences required for packaging of the HFV vector genome.[178] Stable vector packaging lines have not yet been developed but represent an important goal for gene therapy applications.

Adeno-Associated Virus Vectors

Adeno-associated virus (AAV) is a replication-defective parvovirus that is non-pathogenic in humans. Vectors derived from AAV are under development for a variety of human disease applications, including hematopoietic disorders. The single-stranded DNA genome of AAV contains coding sequences for the structural *cap* and non-structural *rep* proteins, flanked by two 145 bp inverted terminal repeats. These inverted terminal repeats are the only *cis*-acting sequences necessary for replication and encapsidation of recombinant AAV vector particles, so that vectors can be generated by replacing the *rep* and *cap* genes with exogenous sequences.[179] Because the AAV lytic cycle requires coinfection with wild-type adenovirus, vector production has been accomplished by adenoviral infection of cells transfected with both the vector plasmid and a plasmid expressing the AAV *rep* and *cap* genes. Recombinant particles are then purified from the supernatant of the cells by ultracentrifugation, with titers reaching 10^{10-11} vector units per milliliter. One disadvantage of this production method is contamination with helper adenovirus, which can potentially result in host immune responses directed against transduced target cells.[180] This limitation has been circumvented by construction of helper plasmids that contain the *trans*-complementing genes of adenovirus (Fig. 29–10), thereby eliminating the need for adenoviral infection.[181, 182] One goal for the future is to develop stable packaging lines that express these adenoviral helper proteins together with the other necessary helper functions required for AAV vector production.

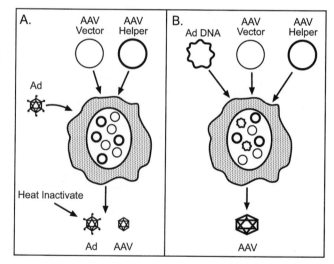

Figure 29–10. Methods for production of AAV vectors. *A*, The classical method for generating AAV vectors. To generate virus, cells are cotransfected with an AAV vector plasmid and an AAV helper plasmid that expresses the *rep* and *cap* genes. Adenoviral infection is required to provide other essential helper functions for recombinant AAV replication. This system results in coproduction of wild-type adenovirus and AAV vector particles. The wild-type adenovirus can be removed by purification over cesium chloride gradients or by heating the AAV preparation at 56°C for 30 minutes. These methods do not completely remove all adenovirus capsid components, and the resulting contamination can lead to unintended immune responses in vivo. *B*, Adenovirus-free AAV production using an adenovirus miniplasmid. This technique uses a third plasmid that provides essential adenovirus helper functions for AAV production, thereby circumventing the need for infection with wild-type adenovirus. The adenovirus miniplasmid contains the E2A, E4, and VA genes from adenovirus, and the human 293 cells provide the required E1A and E1B proteins. Because some of the early and most of the late adenovirus genes are missing from this construct, no wild-type adenovirus is produced. (Adapted from Samulski, R., et al.: Adeno-associated viral vectors. In Friedmann, T. [ed.]: The Development of Gene Therapy. Cold Spring Harbor, NY, Cold Spring Harbor Laboratory Press, 1999; with permission.)

The increasingly well understood interactions between AAV vectors and targeted host cells are important in considering gene therapy applications. Studies have indicated that the cellular uptake of AAV virions is mediated through an interaction with heparan sulfate molecules present on the cell surface.[183] Although the nearly ubiquitous appearance of membrane-associated heparan sulfate is consistent with the broad host range of AAV vectors, there is evidence that other cellular coreceptors are required,[184–186] which may limit AAV tropism. After cellular entry, the single-stranded DNA vector genome is converted to a double-stranded molecule, a step required for expression of the episomal vector and for integration of the vector genome (Fig. 29–11). A number of factors are known to enhance transduction with AAV vectors, presumably by affecting this process of DNA duplex formation. These factors include the expression of the adenoviral E1 and E4 proteins[187, 188] and induction of DNA repair with DNA-damaging agents.[189–191] Conversely, a phosphorylated cellular protein has been identified that inhibits second-strand DNA synthesis, and the levels of this phosphoprotein are a determinant of transduction efficiency in hematopoietic cell types.[192] After the single-stranded genome is converted to a double-stranded form, expression of the vector can commence, independent of integration into the host cell chromosome. Expression from these episomal templates accounts for a significant proportion of the overall gene expression in cases in which unselected populations of cells were analyzed.[193–195]

Because wild-type AAV virus often integrates within a preferred site on human chromosome 19,[196] it was initially hoped that AAV vectors would display site-specific integration and thereby be less likely to result in insertional mutagenesis or attenuated expression because of position effects. It is now clear that AAV vectors often integrate randomly,[197, 198] perhaps in part owing to the absence of *rep* protein expression in the target cell.[199] A more important issue for gene therapy is the absolute frequency of integration in transduced cells. In hematopoietic cells as well as in certain other cell types, integration into the host genome occurs only in a minority of clones in which the vector was initially expressed.[193, 195] In one study, integration in erythroleukemia cells was associated only with a high ratio of vector particles to target cells (multiplicity of infection).[194] Interestingly, the average integrated copy number was increased by inclusion in the vector of a regulatory element from the human β globin gene cluster.[194] Further understanding of the determinants of integration frequency will be especially important for the development of AAV vectors for hematopoietic stem cell transduction, a setting in which episomal vector copies would be rapidly diluted during the proliferation of stem cell progeny.

One advantage provided by AAV vectors is that they can efficiently transmit and express human globin gene constructs and therefore may be useful for the treatment of hemoglobinopathies. Unlike murine retroviral vectors in which the inclusion of critical transcriptional control elements from the β globin locus control region (LCR) often leads to rearrangements, AAV vectors incorporating LCR elements are stable and express exogenous globin genes at high levels in erythroleukemia cell lines.[197, 200–202] With the subsequent demonstration that AAV vectors efficiently transduced human CD34$^+$ myeloid progenitors from a variety of sources,[203–206] investigators have gone on to test AAV-globin vectors in primary human erythroid cells. These studies confirmed that a variety of exogenous globin genes can be efficiently transmitted to primary erythroid progenitors with use of AAV vectors and that these genes are expressed at potentially therapeutic levels.[194, 207] Another example of AAV-mediated transfer of a therapeutic gene to human CD34$^+$ cells involves the treatment of Fanconi anemia. An AAV vector containing the *FACC* gene was used for the in vitro correction of CD34$^+$ myeloid progenitors derived from a Fanconi anemia patient.[208] The clinical implementation of either of these strategies will require transduction of repopulating hematopoietic stem cells, with efficient integration of the vector genome. Although transduction of murine stem cells has been demonstrated with use of an AAV vector,[209] it is still not clear whether the efficiency of stem cell transduction will be adequate for clinical application. A transplant study in rhesus monkeys showed that when CD34$^+$ cells were targeted in vitro with an AAV-globin vector and then reinfused into two irradiated monkeys, approximately 1 in 10^5 circulating blood cells contained the vector.[210] Clearly, increased transduction efficiency will be necessary for using AAV vectors in human stem cell targeting. One important consideration is the high degree of patient to patient variability in the transduction efficiency of bone marrow–derived human CD34$^+$ cells.[211]

A potentially more immediate application of AAV vectors is in the treatment of the hemophilias.[212, 213] One approach has been to directly inject vectors into skeletal muscle

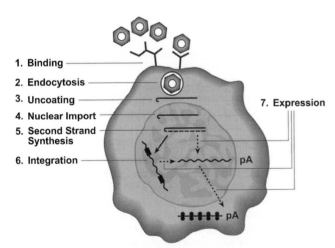

1. Binding
2. Endocytosis
3. Uncoating
4. Nuclear Import
5. Second Strand Synthesis
6. Integration
7. Expression

Figure 29–11. Transduction with AAV vectors and expression in cells. Binding of AAV to the cell surface most likely occurs through a two-step process, first by binding of virus particles to heparan sulfate proteoglycans, followed by interaction with specific cell surface peptides such as the human fibroblast growth factor receptor 1 or $\alpha_v\beta_5$ integrin. After endocytosis and uncoating, the single-stranded DNA genome is transported to the nucleus. In the nucleus, a double-stranded DNA genome is formed through a process known as second-strand synthesis. This rate-limiting step for expression and integration is controlled by a variety of cellular and viral factors. The double-stranded episomal genome serves as a template for gene expression and in some cases may be the only source of vector gene expression. The double-stranded vector genome can also integrate into the host cell chromosome, usually at random positions but sometimes at a specific site on chromosome 19. The efficiency of integration is much less than that associated with retroviral vectors and is dependent on high multiplicities of infection. Expression from the integrated template will be stable in proliferating cell populations, in contrast to expression from episomal templates.

sites to express secreted forms of deficient clotting factors. Because AAV vectors can achieve sustained in vivo expression in muscle tissue,[214 215] they are particularly well suited for this strategy. The liver is another in vivo target for AAV-hemophilia vectors. In vivo transduction of hepatocytes has been achieved in several preclinical animal models by intravenous injections or direct administration into the portal circulation.[216–218] The therapeutic issues specific to hemophilia gene therapy are discussed in detail later in this chapter. In summary, the potential impact of AAV vectors on a wide range of blood diseases, together with the unique advantages of AAV as a vector system, ensures that AAV vectors will continue to be an important area in gene therapy for hematopoietic disorders.

Adenoviral Vectors

Because of the extensive cellular proliferation that accompanies hematopoiesis, effective hematopoietic cell gene therapy requires integration of the vector genome into repopulating stem cells. For this reason, non-integrating vectors such as those based on adenovirus currently play a relatively minor role in stem cell gene therapy. It is conceivable that transient expression of exogenous genes in primitive hematopoietic cells could be of use, either therapeutically or experimentally. In these cases, adenovirus vectors would be a rational choice. Primary human hematopoietic cells have been transduced with adenovirus vectors.[219, 220] In one study, vector expression was noted in a significant proportion of quiescent CD34$^+$, CD38$^-$ cells immediately after transduction,[221] suggesting that adenovirus vectors could be used for the transient expression of foreign genes during ex vivo culture. A more widespread application of adenoviral vectors is their use in gene therapy for hemophilia and cancer immunotherapy. Given the potential impact of these applications, a considerable amount of effort is being expended on developing and testing adenoviral vector systems.

Of the 50 known serotypes of human adenovirus, most vectors have been based on the adenovirus 2 and 5 serotypes. The relatively complex 36 kb double-stranded DNA genome encodes a multitude of viral genes (Fig. 29–12). The genome is flanked by inverted terminal repeats, and a packaging signal necessary for encapsidation is located in the 5′ region of the genome. Four groups of genes designated E1 to E4 are expressed early in the replication cycle. After DNA replication, late genes encompassing the structural proteins are expressed. The first generation of adenoviral vectors was created by inserting exogenous genes in place of the endogenous E1 genes. Because the E1 genes are required for viral transcription and replication, the vector is replication defective in target cells. Packaging is accomplished by introducing vector plasmids into 293 cells, which provide the E1 region gene products in *trans* and are therefore permissive for vector growth. Titers of 10^{11} particles per milliliter can be routinely achieved with this system.

Vector particles initially bind to cells through an interaction with the knob region of the adenovirus fiber protein with a cellular receptor (CAR) that binds both adenovirus and group B coxsackieviruses.[222, 223] Subsequent vector internalization requires binding of the viral penton base with specific $\alpha_v\beta_3$ or $\alpha_v\beta_5$ integrins, a step that leads to receptor-mediated endocytosis of the vector particle.[224] After cell entry, the viral endosome is disrupted and the adenoviral DNA subsequently transported to the nucleus. Significant progress has been made in targeting adenovirus vectors to specific cell types. Targeting has been accomplished by modifying viral capsid proteins to enable binding to specific cellular targets[225–227] or through the use of bispecific antibodies that bind both the adenovirus vector and cell surface epitopes.[228–230] T lymphocytes, which do not express the CAR receptor or α_v integrins, have been targeted with these techniques. Transduction of primary T lymphocytes was achieved by use of an antibody binding the CD3 receptor of T cells and the adenovirus vector.[231]

Hematopoietic cells lack the CAR receptor and are relatively refractory to adenovirus vector transduction.[232] This property can be exploited to enact efficient purging of tumor cells from bone marrow grafts. A 10^6 log depletion of myeloma tumor cells was achieved by first transducing grafts with an adenovirus vector expressing herpes simplex virus thymidine kinase (HSV-TK) from a tumor-specific promoter, followed by ganciclovir treatment. Normal bone marrow–derived progenitors were not transduced with the adenovirus vector and were not reduced in number by ganciclovir treatment.[233] Conversely, it may be possible to increase targeting of hematopoietic cells when it is therapeutically desirable.

For applications requiring persistent in vivo expression of transduced cells, it has become apparent that a major problem with adenovirus vectors is the induction of a potent host immune response.[180, 234–237] Because E1-deleted vectors continue to express low levels of antigenic viral proteins, new vectors have been designed that are deleted of various combinations of E1, E2, E3, and E4.[238–241] Although these vectors resulted in decreased immune responses in some studies, clearance of transduced cells in vivo was still noted, in part because of persistent low levels of viral gene expression. It was also clear that in multiple instances, the immune response was directed against the product of the transgene itself.[241–243] Recent work has shown that the potent immunogenicity of adenovirus vectors, at least when they are administered intramuscularly, can be attributed to the relatively efficient transduction of dendritic cells.[244] A number of strategies are currently being explored for eliminating or overcoming host immune responses, including the generation of "gutless" vectors that contain no viral proteins,[245–248] inclusion of immunosuppressive genes from the E3 region,[249] treatment of the host with immunosuppressive therapies,[242, 250, 251] and use of vectors with alternative adenovirus serotypes.[252] Deletion of all the viral genes also increases the space available for inserting exogenous DNA fragments up to 28 kb,[253] an important advantage in the gene therapy for hemophilia B. This increased capacity for exogenous genes also allows the inclusion of large genomic fragments that include endogenous regulatory regions that allow tissue-specific transcription.[254]

In summary, adenovirus vectors are extremely efficient at transducing a wide variety of non-dividing cells and can be administered directly in vivo into muscle, liver, and lung tissue. These properties support the continued development of adenovirus vectors for hemophilia as well as for other non-hematopoietic diseases such as cystic fibrosis and muscular dystrophy. A critical limitation is the potent immune response mounted by the host, which results in transient gene

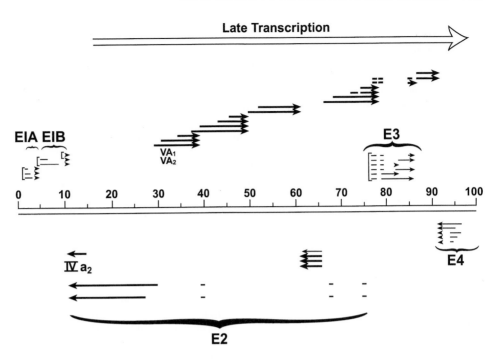

Figure 29–12. Adenovirus transcription map. This schematic diagram depicts the general transcription map of adenovirus. The early region transcription units are E1A, E1B, E2, E3, and E4, and their transcripts are indicated as light arrows. Vectors are made by deleting various combinations of these regions and inserting exogenous genes in their place. The primary major late transcript is indicated by the open arrow, and processed late mRNAs are shown as bold arrows. The locations of the VA RNAs, which are transcribed by RNA polymerase III, are also shown. Also shown is the location of the pIVa2 transcript, which is expressed at an intermediate time. The genome length units correspond to 360 bp, and the entire genome length is about 36 kb.

expression and resistance to multiple treatment applications. Significant advances have been made in vector design and in understanding the biology of the immune responses. Standard adenovirus vectors are inefficient for transduction of hematopoietic cells, but this may be an advantage for purging of hematopoietic grafts, and targeting strategies may be able to overcome inefficient transduction of hematopoietic cells when it is desirable.

Other Non-Integrating Vectors

SV40 pseudovirion vectors are being considered as non-integrating vectors for hematopoietic cell targeting. Infectious particles can be generated by transfecting COS cells with circular plasmid vectors and wild-type SV40 DNA.[255] This system produces recombinant particles in titers ranging between 10^4 and 10^5 particles per milliliter. Primary human bone marrow cells have been efficiently transduced with an *MDR1*-expressing SV40 pseudovirion vector, and 87 to 97 per cent of cells expressed the transferred gene.[256] One limitation of this vector system is the presence of high titers of wild-type SV40 virus in the vector stocks. Although SV40 is thought to be non-pathogenic in humans, testing of these vectors in human trials will require generation of helper-free stocks. The availability of an in vitro packaging system that relies on vector assembly by recombinant capsid proteins may result in the generation of vector particles more appropriate for clinical use.[257]

Another non-integrating system based on the herpes simplex virus has been used for hematopoietic cell transduction. With use of a disabled infectious single-cycle vector (DISC-HSV), normal human hematopoietic cells and leukemic blasts were transduced and shown to express a transferred β-galactosidase marker gene.[258] Given the general difficulty in transducing leukemic blasts, this vector system offers an advantage for inducing immune responses against leukemia. A DISC-HSV vector that expressed a GM-CSF gene was used to induce an antileukemia immune response

in a murine leukemia model.[258] On the basis of these results, DISC-HSV vectors are being considered for human vaccine trials.

Disease-Specific Applications and Clinical Trials

In the late 1980s, the first human gene therapy trial was developed and initiated by investigators at the National Institutes of Health.[259–263] In five patients, tumor-infiltrating lymphocytes were marked with a murine retroviral vector containing a *neoR* gene and subsequently reinfused. Marked lymphocytes were detected in the peripheral circulation for several months, and subsequent tumor biopsy samples confirmed homing of the marked lymphocytes to tumor deposits in vivo.[264] This pioneering work demonstrated several important principles that were instrumental in the conception and design of future studies. First, the regulatory process for human gene therapy trials was established, and precedents were set for establishing the safety of clinical vector preparations. Second, the concept was proved that marking with genetic vectors could serve as a powerful tool for tracking manipulated autologous cells after reinfusion into patients. Some of the most interesting subsequent trials employed this design to address medically relevant biological questions. Third, because no adverse effects were noted with the gene marking procedure, this study started what is now considered an extensive safety record for the clinical use of genetic vectors.

Numerous clinical trials were developed, and by 1995, there were more than 200 approved gene therapy studies under way throughout the world. It is now perceived that this plunge into human trials was in some ways premature owing to limitations in the available vector delivery systems and perhaps also because of lack of scientific rigor in the design of some trials. In the last 3 to 4 years, the field has recognized that although effective gene therapy for several diseases may come in the near future, more work is needed to develop better gene delivery systems, to test gene therapy strategies vigorously in appropriate animal models of human disease, and to further elucidate the basic molecular mechanisms of candidate diseases. Arguably, no single disorder has yet been cured by gene therapy, and gene therapy is not the standard of care for any disorder. Despite these qualifications, the lessons learned from the initial clinical experience have focused investigators on several key obstacles to truly effective therapy. In this light, the following section reviews the results from previous gene therapy trials targeting hematological diseases and reviews the scientific basis for pursuing gene therapy in specific blood disorders.

▼ MARKING STUDIES

Some of the most informative clinical trials have used neo^R-expressing murine retroviral vectors to mark and track hematopoietic cells after therapeutic infusions. One important principle demonstrated by these studies is that pluripotent repopulating cells can be transduced with retroviral vectors in patients, albeit at a low level, and that gene-modified myeloid cells can persist for prolonged periods after transplantation. In pediatric cancer patients undergoing autologous transplantation, a simple 6-hour transduction of bone marrow mononuclear cells was performed using one of two amphotropic Moloney leukemia virus neo^R vectors. After transplantation, marking was detected in both myeloid and lymphoid cells in most patients, and it has been stable for more than 5 years after transplantation.[16] In adult cancer patients, stem cell marking has been more difficult to achieve. In older patients with multiple myeloma or breast cancer, CD34$^+$ cells from both peripheral blood and bone marrow were marked with genetically distinguishable vectors and reinfused after high-dose conditioning therapy. Although some patients showed stable marking for greater than 18 months, the average vector copy number was generally less than 0.001 genomes per cell.[13] The relatively higher level of marking in the pediatric study is not simply related to differences in the transduction protocol, given that 6-hour cytokine-free transductions have resulted in poor marking in adult patients.[96] Although there are a number of potential explanations for the relatively increased marking seen in the pediatric studies, one interesting possibility is that different classes of repopulating cells were marked in adult versus pediatric patients. Immunopurified CD34$^+$ cells were transduced in the adult studies, whereas whole bone marrow mononuclear cells were used for marking in the pediatric trials. The demonstration that a human CD34$^-$ stem cell exists and that CD34$^-$ stem cells are more primitive than CD34$^+$ repopulating cells[65, 265] suggests the possibility that the increased marking seen in the pediatric trials could have been due to transduction of a primitive cell that is excluded by the CD34 selection process.

These and other marking studies have also yielded important information regarding the use of autologous stem cell transplantation for cancer treatment. With certain malignant neoplasms, it is known that the relapse rate after autologous transplantation is higher than that seen after allogeneic transplantation. An important issue is whether this difference is solely due to the graft-versus-tumor effect associated with allogeneic transplants or whether relapse is in part related to contaminating tumor cells in the autologous graft. Marking studies have unequivocally demonstrated that tumor cell contamination of the graft can contribute to relapse in pediatric patients with acute myelogenous leukemia[266] or with metastatic neuroblastoma[267] and in adult patients with chronic myelogenous leukemia.[268] In the neuroblastoma study, analysis of tumor cells for proviral integration sites showed that at least 200 tumor cells from the graft had contributed to relapse.[267]

Retroviral marking has also been used in the allogeneic setting to address other transplant-related questions. A significant problem associated with HLA-mismatched grafts, and with T cell–depleted grafts, has been the development of lymphoproliferative disorders associated with Epstein-Barr virus (EBV) infection. This disorder can now be treated with cytotoxic T lymphocytes (CTLs) derived from the donor, which are specific for EBV-infected cells from the patient. When retrovirally transduced, EBV-specific CTLs were administered to pediatric transplant patients, marked cells were found to accumulate in disease sites and to induce complete and sustained antitumor responses.[269–271] Marked autologous CTLs are also being tested for use in patients with advanced Hodgkin's disease, a disorder also associated with EBV infection.[272] The use of retroviral vectors to stably transduce lymphocytes also provides a means to modulate allogeneic immune responses with "suicide" gene vectors, as discussed later in this chapter.

▼ GENETIC DISEASES

SCID due to Adenosine Deaminase Deficiency

Severe combined immunodeficiency (SCID), a rare and genetically heterogeneous disorder that usually presents in infants shortly after birth, is characterized by profound defects in cellular and humoral immunity. In the 1970s, homozygous deficiency of the enzyme adenosine deaminase (ADA) was identified as a cause of SCID.[273, 274] The fact that this disorder was treatable with allogeneic stem cell transplantation suggested that it could also be treated by gene transfer into autologous stem cells or long-lived lymphocytes. Despite its rarity, ADA deficiency was chosen as an early target disease for gene therapy for several reasons. In patients lacking enzyme activity, there is an accumulation of deoxyadenosine triphosphate, a compound that is toxic to developing lymphocytes. Early clinical studies showed that red blood cell transfusions could partially restore immune function, indicating that the ADA-positive erythrocytes could rescue lymphoid function in *trans* by providing an enzymatic "sink" for the toxic metabolite. A related point is that high levels of regulated expression of the exogenous ADA vector were not thought to be necessary for phenotypic correction. Either T lymphocytes[1, 6] or pluripotent stem cells[275] were considered to be appropriate targets for corrective vectors, and significant degrees of *ADA* gene transfer and expression had been accomplished in large animal models.[276, 277] As a result of these considerations, several human *ADA* gene therapy trials were initiated in the early 1990s.

In a study done at the National Institutes of Health, two children with ADA deficiency were treated with infusions of transduced autologous T lymphocytes. Lymphocytes were collected from patients being treated with pegylated (PEG)–ADA enzyme infusions and then transduced in vitro with an amphotropic Moloney leukemia virus–based retroviral vector. Repeated infusions of transduced T lymphocytes were given during a 2-year period. During the second year of treatment, one patient had up to 30 per cent transduced lymphocytes in circulation; the second patient had significantly lower numbers of genetically modified cells.[4] Both patients showed improved immune function while receiving therapy, with increases in T-lymphocyte numbers and improved humoral immune responses despite decreasing doses of exogenous ADA enzyme. Japanese investigators have similarly treated a patient with transduced T cells and reported lymphocyte marking between 10 and 20 per cent associated with improvement in immune function.[278, 279] However, ADA enzyme therapy was not withdrawn from any of these patients, making it difficult to fully evaluate the clinical impact of the gene therapy procedure.

In another study, Italian investigators treated two patients with simultaneous infusions of transduced lymphocytes and bone marrow cells, each targeted with one of two genetically distinguishable ADA vectors. A double-copy retroviral vector was used to transmit two copies of the *ADA* cDNA under control of an *ADA* promoter fragment. Repetitive infusions were given during a 1- to 2-year treatment period and resulted in between 2 and 5 per cent vector-expressing lymphocytes in vivo.[3] Similar to the results of the National Institutes of Health study, both patients showed significant improvement in immune function despite a reduction in the dose of exogenous PEG-ADA enzyme. After infusion of transduced cells was completed, there was an increase in the proportion of marked T-cell clones that were derived from the transduced bone marrow cells, suggesting that bone marrow stem cells were a better target for achieving long-term, stable correction.

Another study reported treatment of three newborn patients, in whom ADA deficiency was prenatally diagnosed, with retrovirally transduced, CD34[+] autologous cord blood cells given as a single infusion on the fourth day of life. Gene-modified cells were detected in the peripheral blood and bone marrow for more than 4 years after treatment; however, the frequency of such cells was only between 1 in 3000 and 1 in 100,000.[280] Expression of the ADA vector was documented in transduced bone marrow progenitors studied 18 months after infusion. PEG-ADA infusions were stopped in one patient 4 years after the initiation of gene therapy. A significant enrichment for transduced T lymphocytes was seen, indicating that corrected T cells had a survival advantage over their untransduced counterparts that was unmasked by withdrawal of exogenous enzyme.[281] In contrast, no advantage for transduced cells was seen in B lymphocytes or natural killer (NK) cells. Clinical immune function deteriorated in this patient, mandating reinstitution of PEG-ADA therapy.

Although it is disappointing that none of these trials demonstrated unequivocal clinical correction resulting from gene therapy, some benefit appears to have been associated with the gene therapy procedures. Currently available vectors and improved transduction conditions promise better success in future trials.

SCID due to Defects in Cytokine Signaling Pathways

Defects in cytokine signaling pathways account for the majority of SCID cases.[282] Mutations affecting the common gamma chain (γ_c) gene, a common component of the receptors for IL-2, IL-4, IL-7, IL-9, and IL-15, are responsible for X-linked SCID[283, 284] and account for almost 50 per cent of SCID cases. With ligand-induced receptor dimerization, a cytoplasmic protein known as Janus kinase 3 (Jak3) associates with the γ_c and becomes phosphorylated (Fig. 29–13), an event that is required for signaling.[285, 286] Mutations in Jak3 that lead to loss of function have been shown to cause autosomal recessive SCID[287, 288] and account for about 8 per cent of all cases. Patients with genetic defects in γ_c or in Jak3 present with an indistinguishable phenotype characterized by low numbers of T lymphocytes, relatively high numbers of B lymphocytes, and low numbers of NK cells.[282] Unlike in SCID due to ADA deficiency, there is no option for drug treatment in these patients, and the only currently available therapy is allogeneic transplantation. Because of the generally good results obtained when a parent is used as a stem cell donor, transplants are available to practically all patients; however, many patients suffer from delayed reconstitution of T-cell function and persistent humoral immunodeficiency.[289–291] Gene therapy is now being considered as a potential alternative treatment option for both γ_c and Jak3 deficiency.

Preclinical experiments have supported the use of gene

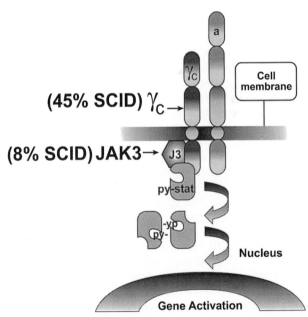

Figure 29–13. Cytokine signaling components involved in the pathogenesis of SCID. A schematic diagram of the IL-7 receptor is shown. The common gamma chain (γ_c) is a shared component of the receptors for IL-2, IL-4, IL-7, IL-9, and IL-15. Mutations in the γ_c gene are the cause of X-linked SCID and account for 45 per cent of all SCID cases. Ligand binding to the receptor leads to phosphorylation and activation of a cytoplasmic tyrosine kinase designated Janus kinase 3 (Jak3). Mutations in Jak3 result in a genetically recessive form of SCID that accounts for about 8 per cent of all cases. Association of Jak3 with the γ_c is required for cytokine signaling and normal lymphoid development. Jak3 activation leads to phosphorylation and dimerization of STAT proteins, with subsequent activation of downstream genes in the nucleus. Both the γ_c and Jak3 are candidates for gene replacement to treat SCID.

transfer to treat these signaling defects. Retroviral vectors containing either a γ_c or a Jak3 cDNA have been used to correct the biochemical defects in B-cell lines from SCID patients.[292–294] Although an important first step, these in vitro experiments did not address several critical issues regarding the plausibility of gene therapy for these disorders. Early development of lymphocytes could require tightly regulated expression of Jak3 or the γ_c, which would not be expected with the use of retroviral vectors in vivo. Second, enforced expression of a cytokine signaling component without normal regulation could result in abnormal development or even neoplasia. Other questions are whether an adequate number of gene-corrected cells can be provided to confer significant restoration of immunity and whether the reconstituted immune system would respond normally to an immune challenge.

To address these questions, our group has used a mouse model of Jak3 deficiency[295] to test the effects of retrovirus-mediated Jak3 gene replacement. Using a retroviral vector that expressed Jak3 under control of the MPSV promoter, Jak3-deficient stem cells were transduced ex vivo and subsequently transplanted into Jak3-deficient mice that had been lethally irradiated. After reconstitution, all transplanted mice showed significant increases in the number of T and B lymphocytes, in serum levels of immunoglobulins G and A, and in the ability to generate an antigen-specific immunoglobulin G response.[296] A second finding was that Jak3-transduced lymphoid progenitors had a survival advantage in vivo over their untransduced counterparts, suggesting that low numbers of Jak3-corrected stem cells may be sufficient for restoring immune function. We have found that significant levels of immune reconstitution can be achieved in unablated newborn mice injected with transduced cells from the newborn liver (Bunting and Sorrentino, unpublished observations), indicating that it may be possible to achieve correction in patients while avoiding the toxic effects of myeloablative conditioning. We have also used the murine model to test whether gene therapy could protect from a viral pathogen, given that viral infections are a common cause of morbidity and mortality in patients with SCID. When mice were challenged with a laboratory strain of influenza virus, a significant survival advantage was seen (Fig. 29–14) in mice that received cells transduced with the Jak3 vector. This protection from lethality was associated with normal antiviral immune responses, including generation of virus-specific cytotoxic T lymphocytes, formation of anti-influenza G immunoglobulins, and long-term persistence of memory cells in lymphoid organs.[297] We have not seen any abnormality specifically associated with enforced Jak3 production, indicating that tight regulation of Jak3 gene expression is not required in vivo to maintain normal hematopoiesis. The availability of animal models for γ_c deficiency[284, 298, 299] should allow analogous studies to be done with γ_c vectors. Toward this goal, normal dogs have been reconstituted with cells expressing high levels of a transferred human γ_c cDNA.[300]

These preclinical studies show that SCID due to Jak3 deficiency and perhaps γ_c deficiency as well may be particularly well suited for gene therapy. The robust levels of immune reconstitution in vivo, the strong selective advantage in vivo for corrected cells, and the availability of vectors

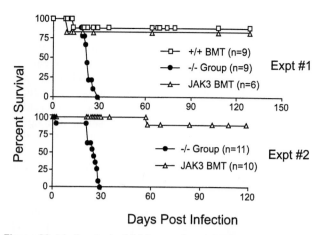

Figure 29–14. Survival of Jak3-transduced SCID mice after challenge with influenza virus. Jak3-deficient bone marrow cells were transduced with a Jak3-expressing retroviral vector and transplanted into irradiated Jak3-deficient recipients (Jak3 BMT). After hematopoietic reconstitution, mice were inoculated intranasally with a laboratory strain of influenza virus. Shown are the survival curves for mice in two independent experiments. As controls, mock-transduced marrow cells from Jak3-deficient mice were used for transplants (−/− group) as well as untransduced marrow cells from normal mice (+/+ BMT). (Adapted from Bunting, K.D., Flynn, K.J., Riberdy, J.M., Doherty, P.C., and Sorrentino, B.P.: Virus-specific immunity after gene therapy in a murine model of severe combined immunodeficiency. Proc. Natl. Acad. Sci. USA 96:232, 1999; with permission.)

that confer long-term expression in vivo all increase the hope of successful clinical implementation.

Chronic Granulomatous Disease

Another inherited immunodeficiency that is being considered for gene therapy is chronic granulomatous disease (CGD), a disorder of granulocyte function that affects about 1 in 200,000 people. Patients with this disorder suffer recurrent life-threatening infections due to a lack of NADPH oxidase (*phox*) function required for killing of opsonized pathogens by phagocytes. Defects in any one of four genes can lead to CGD. Two thirds of the cases are caused by mutations in the X-linked gp91-*phox* gene,[301] and about one third of the cases are due to autosomal recessive mutations in the p47-*phox* gene. Other rarer forms of CGD are due to defects in p22-*phox* and p67-*phox*, additional components of the NADPH oxidase complex. Although CGD can be cured by allogeneic bone marrow transplantation, this approach is not widely used because of the toxicity of transplant conditioning and the lack of matched related donors for most cases. For these reasons, gene therapy is being considered as an alternative approach.

Retroviral vectors expressing various *phox* cDNAs have been constructed and validated by use of in vitro assays.[302–306] The availability of mouse models for the gp91-*phox* and p47-*phox* deficiency[307, 308] have allowed testing of these vectors in an in vivo model system. With use of gp91-*phox*–deficient mice, bone marrow cells were transduced with a corrective vector and transplanted into lethally irradiated recipients. After reconstitution, superoxide production was detected in 50 to 80 per cent of the circulating granulocytes. Furthermore, these transplanted mice were significantly protected from pulmonary fungal infections after inhalation of *Aspergillus fumigatus* spores.[309] In similar studies with p47-*phox*–

deficient mice, bone marrow cells transduced with a retroviral vector were infused into sublethally irradiated recipient mice[310] to determine whether correction could be obtained with a less intensive conditioning regimen. Four weeks after transplantation, about 12 per cent of the granulocytes were corrected, with levels falling to about 3 per cent at 14 weeks. Although these levels of marking were relatively low, they were sufficient for conferring protection against *Burkholderia cepacia*, a bacterial pathogen.[311] On the basis of these animal model studies and data from female carriers of X-linked CGD, it is predicted that gene correction of at least 5 per cent of the circulating granuloctyes will be required for clinical benefit.

The results from two clinical trials of CGD gene therapy have been reported. In the first trial, five adult patients with p47-*phox* deficiency were treated with retrovirally transduced hematopoietic cells. Peripheral blood CD34+ cells were first mobilized with G-CSF and subsequently transduced with a murine retroviral vector that expressed human p47-*phox*. The transduced cells were administered as two infusions during 2 days, with a total of between 0.1 and 4.7 cells per kilogram given to each patient. None of the patients received any form of myeloablative conditioning. Oxidase-positive granulocytes appeared in all five patients and ranged in concentration from 1 in 2000 to 1 in 50,000 of total peripheral blood granulocytes.[312] Corrected cells were detectable for as long as 6 months in some patients. In one patient who developed pneumonia, oxidase-positive cells were detected in the empyema fluid, indicating that gene-corrected cells could localize to a site of infection. In a second study, the same investigators have treated unablated X-linked CGD patients with a protocol that was more efficient in obtaining engraftment of corrected cells. The main differences in this protocol were the use of the CH-296 fibronectin fragment for transduction, the use of a 293 cell–based amphotropic producer clone,[313] and the administration of higher numbers of transduced cells. Three to 4 weeks after each of two gene therapy cycles, between 1 in 500 and 1 in 1700 oxidase normal neutrophils were noted.[314]

There has been substantial progress toward gene therapy for CGD, and it seems likely that effective protocols for this disorder are close at hand. The main focus is now to achieve an adequate number of corrected cells in vivo, presumably greater than 5 per cent of the total granulocytes. This may be accomplished by the use of subablative conditioning regimens that have tolerable toxicity, through the use of vectors that include a selectable marker allowing amplification of genetically modified cells in vivo, and through continued progress in the transduction and expansion of stem cells.

Metabolic Storage Diseases

Metabolic storage diseases are a diverse group of disorders in which mutations in the genes for various metabolic enzymes lead to toxic substrate accumulations in a variety of tissues. Because many of these diseases are treatable with allogeneic bone marrow transplantation, gene therapy is being considered as an alternative approach. Each of these enzyme deficiencies has unique biological properties that influence the potential success of a gene replacement approach. For example, in some of these diseases, transduced cells can "cross-correct" defective cells in *trans*,[315, 316] predicting reversal of the disease phenotype even when a significant proportion of the hematopoietic cells remain untransduced. The emergence of mouse models for metabolic storage disorders[317] will allow preclinical testing of gene therapy strategies, as has been done in a mouse model of Sly syndrome.[318]

One critical issue is whether stem cell–targeted gene therapy will be corrective for the neurological manifestations of these diseases. For example, deficiency of glucocerebrosidase in Gaucher disease leads to a deleterious accumulation of glucocerebroside in macrophages and macrophage-derived cells within various organs. Pathological changes are typically noted in the bone marrow, spleen, liver, and brain. In animal model studies, transfer of glucocerebrosidase vectors into repopulating stem cells has been demonstrated, with significant levels of vector-encoded glucocerebrosidase expression documented in hematopoietic organs after transplantation.[58, 319–321] Rapid appearance of marked macrophages was seen in the bone marrow, spleen, peripheral blood, liver, and lung. In contrast, engraftment of microglial cells in the central nervous system (CNS) occurred relatively late, with approximately 20 per cent of the microglial cells in the brain expressing the glucocerebrosidase vector 6 to 8 months after transplantation.[322] Another important aspect may be the distribution of modified microglial cells within the CNS. In mice transplanted with transgenic marrow expressing a β-galactosidase marker, the modest numbers of donor microglial cells that were found in the brain were predominantly located in perivascular and leptomeningeal sites, but not in the parenchyma of the brain.[323] Another study showed more diffuse infiltration with marrow-derived glial cells, but the absolute numbers of cells engrafting the brain were relatively low.[324] Direct targeting of the CNS with corrective vectors may be necessary.[87, 325]

Two gene therapy clinical trials have been initiated for Gaucher disease. Both trials use retroviral vectors to transduce autologous CD34+ cells obtained from the blood or bone marrow. Patients received infusions of transduced cells without any form of myeloablative conditioning. Early results from these trials have shown that less than 1 per cent of circulating leukocytes contained the glucocerebrosidase vector after infusion of transduced CD34+ cells.[326–328] Higher numbers of transduced cells will presumably be required to achieve clinical benefit. Toward this goal, bicistronic vectors that include a selectable marker have been proposed for the enrichment of glucocerebrosidase-expressing cells before infusion[109, 329] or the in vivo selection of corrected cells after transplantation.[166, 330]

Fanconi Anemia

Fanconi anemia is an autosomal recessive disorder characterized by bone marrow failure, congenital skeletal abnormalities, and an increased incidence of malignant neoplasms. A diversity of genetic lesions can cause this disease, as evidenced by the identification of at least eight complementation groups by use of in vitro cellular assays. The genes for complementation groups A *(FAA)* and C *(FAC)* have been cloned[331, 332] and account for 15 per cent and 65 per cent of cases, respectively. Retroviral vectors expressing either the *FAC* or *FAA* cDNAs have been used to transduce cells derived from patients with Fanconi anemia and to correct the defect in DNA repair.[333, 334] In vitro correction has also been reported with use of an AAV vector expressing the FAC protein.[208] These in vitro studies showed a growth advantage for transduced myeloid progenitors, suggesting that corrected stem cell clones could have a natural selective advantage in vivo. On the basis of these results, three Fanconi anemia group C patients have been treated with multiple infusions of retrovirally transduced peripheral blood CD34+ cells, given without any preceding myeloablation. Preliminary results have shown transient increases in bone marrow cellularity and expansion in the numbers of myeloid progenitors in treated patients.[335] Further follow-up is necessary to determine whether there was a selective advantage for transduced stem cells and whether this approach can be developed into a clinically effective procedure.

Hemoglobinopathies

Sickle cell anemia and severe β thalassemia are among the most common inherited single-gene defects worldwide, so that effective gene therapy for these disorders would have a tremendous medical impact. These diseases were the first hematopoietic disorders to be considered for gene therapy, and they remain important targets for stem cell–directed gene therapy.[336] Several general strategies have been pursued. Addition of functional β globin gene could be curative for β thalassemia, but competition from the sickle β chain for hemoglobin assembly may reduce the effectiveness of this approach for treating sickle cell anemia. High-level expression of a fetal γ globin gene would be preferable, given the preferential assembly of α with γ globin chains, and considering that hemoglobin F or mixed tetramers containing α and β^S chains are not incorporated into sickle hemoglobin polymers. Recombinant β-like globin chains are available that have potent antisickling properties.[337] A third possibility is transfer of genes that reactivate expression of the γ globin genes. Modulation of erythroid transcription factor activity, such as erythroid Kruppel-like factor, may be one potential means for influencing the developmental switch from fetal to adult hemoglobin expression.[338, 339] Another possibility would be supplying an engineered transcription factor that could induce expression of the normally silent δ globin gene.[340]

Derivation of a therapeutic vector for β thalassemia and sickle cell anemia has proved to be challenging. A general problem with retroviral vectors designed to express β-like globin genes has been difficulty in achieving high-level, erythroid-specific expression. Early vectors were constructed by use of the endogenous globin promoter to drive the genomic β globin gene, which was inserted in reverse orientation to the LTR-driven transcript. Although these vectors were able to transduce repopulating mouse stem cells, expression of the transferred globin gene in erythroid cells was only about 1 per cent of that of the endogenous murine β globin genes.[341–343] It became clear with the discovery of the upstream LCR[344] that high-level expression would require incorporation of LCR elements into the vector construct. As the active sequences within the LCR were mapped in transgenic mouse experiments,[345–350] it was possible to include "miniature" LCR constructs into retroviral vectors. Unfortunately, LCR elements generally rendered these glo-

bin vectors unstable, so that frequent rearrangements and low titers made the derivation of useful clones extremely difficult.[351–353]

Modifications of both the LCR constructs and the globin gene itself led to derivation of high-titer globin vectors that expressed potentially therapeutic levels of human globin in murine erythroleukemia cells.[353–357] In most of these experiments, there was significant variation in the degree of globin expression among individual clones, indicating that the degree of vector expression was dependent on the position of integration.[358] These position effects are likely to be responsible, at least in part, for the variable and modest levels of globin expression obtained when these vectors are tested in mouse transplant experiments.[354, 359] Authentic mouse models of sickle cell anemia[360] and severe β thalassemia[361, 362] have been developed and will be valuable for the preclinical testing of future globin vectors.

In contrast to retroviral vectors, AAV vectors provide a more stable system for the transfer of LCR-globin constructs. An AAV vector containing the human γ globin gene linked to the LCR core elements from hypersensitive sites 2, 3, and 4 has been used to transduce primary human erythroid progenitors. In transduced colonies, expression of the marked γ globin mRNA was between 4 and 71 per cent that of the endogenous γ globin genes and was associated with a significant increase in the hemoglobin F content of pooled erythroid colonies.[207] A limitation with these vectors, which was recognized in later experiments, was that integration of the vector genome was infrequent, and expression was mostly from non-integrated vector copies. Inclusion of the 3′ regulatory element downstream of the human ^{A}γ gene was shown to facilitate the integration of the vector genome in head-to-tail tandem arrays.[194] Therefore, it remains an open question whether AAV vectors can be used to achieve stable integration of globin transgenes into reconstituting hematopoietic stem cells. Transduction of primitive hematopoietic cells has been reported[203, 205, 209]; however, the efficiency of stable transduction may be prohibitively low.[210]

▼ CANCER TREATMENT

The majority of clinical gene therapy trials have focused on treatment of a wide variety of cancers. Many of these trials aim to induce antitumor responses by modifying tumor cells with immune-modulatory genes. Because this large area is not specific to hematopoietic applications and has been reviewed elsewhere,[363, 364] it is not discussed here. Instead, we focus on two cancer applications that specifically modify hematopoietic cells to gain an advantage in cancer treatment. The first is the use of suicide gene vectors in allogeneic bone marrow transplantation to modulate the activity of alloreactive donor lymphocytes. Second, we discuss chemoprotection strategies in which drug resistance genes are used to protect hematopoiesis from the toxic effects of anticancer drugs.

Modulation of Allogeneic Immune Responses in Bone Marrow Transplantation

It is now known that a significant component of the antitumor effect seen with allogeneic bone marrow transplantation is due to immune destruction of tumor cells mediated by donor-derived lymphocytes. This graft-versus-malignancy effect has been noted in chronic myelogenous leukemia, acute leukemia, lymphoma, and multiple myeloma. In a similar fashion, infusion of donor lymphocytes can result in second remissions in patients who relapse after transplantation. The ability to use these allogeneic responses is limited by the occurrence of graft-versus-host-disease (GvHD), a donor cell–mediated immune attack on normal host tissues that can lead to significant morbidity and mortality. Investigators have used a gene therapy approach to control GvHD in the setting of donor lymphocyte infusions, with the goal of increasing the efficacy of treatment with alloreactive T lymphocytes.

The basic strategy is to transduce donor lymphocytes in vitro with a selectable retroviral vector that also contains the gene encoding HSV-TK. The HSV-TK gene serves as a suicide gene by conferring sensitivity to the relatively inert antiviral drug ganciclovir.[365] The lymphocytes are then expanded and selected for vector expression, either with G418 for vectors containing the neo[R] gene or by cell sorting for vectors expressing a truncated nerve growth factor (tNGF) gene. These cells are then infused into patients as an antitumor treatment. If GvHD develops, ganciclovir is administered to selectively kill the donor lymphocytes that express the HSV-TK suicide vector. The HSV-TK suicide system has been well characterized for killing transduced tumor cells and provides an effective system for the in vivo elimination of transduced cells with little toxicity to normal tissues.[366] The feasibility of treating GvHD with this system has been established in murine transplantation experiments, in which lymphoid-specific expression of the HSV-TK gene was achieved in transgenic donor mice.[367, 368]

Encouraging results from a clinical trial testing this approach have been reported. In eight patients with a variety of post-transplantation malignant neoplasms, allogeneic lymphocytes were collected from the original donor and transduced with a retroviral vector expressing both the HSV-TK and tNGF cDNAs. The lymphocytes were then selected for tNGF expression and infused at varying doses into the patients. The proportion of marked cells in the peripheral circulation ranged from less than 0.001 per cent to 13.4 per cent, and marked cells were detectable for up to 12 months after the last infusion.[5] Five of the eight patients showed antitumor responses after infusion of the gene-modified donor lymphocytes. Three of these responding patients subsequently developed GvHD and were treated with ganciclovir. In two patients, the proportion of transduced lymphocytes fell below the level of polymerase chain reaction detection within 24 hours of ganciclovir administration. This disappearance of transduced cells was accompanied by a complete regression of all signs of acute GvHD. Furthermore, these patients remained in complete remission from their malignant disease despite the lysis of allogeneic lymphocytes. The other patient displayed clinical improvement from chronic GvHD with ganciclovir treatment and was noted to have a persistent although reduced level of transduced donor lymphocytes after treatment.

These studies show that the allogeneic response can be modulated in a clinically beneficial way. Several questions regarding this approach are now being addressed. Two of these patients have developed an immune response to the

HSV-TK/neo[R] gene product that resulted in the unwanted elimination of transduced cells. Generation of improved vectors that lack the neo[R] gene and that confer higher levels of ganciclovir sensitivity may circumvent this limitation.[369] A second issue is that ex vivo expansion of cells can compromise the alloreactivity of the donor lymphocytes. This effect can be avoided by specific changes in the ex vivo culture and stimulation of lymphocytes during the transduction procedure.[370, 371] Studies are also in progress to determine whether this approach can be used during the initial transplantation procedure by depleting the graft of T cells, transducing the T cells with a suicide vector, and then adding back these modified lymphocytes to the stem cell graft before transplantation.

Transfer of Drug Resistance Genes to Protect From Chemotherapy-Induced Myelosuppression

One of the first applications to be suggested for stem cell gene transfer was the use of drug resistance genes to protect hematopoiesis from the toxic effects of cytotoxic drugs. Protection of mice from the toxic effects of MTX was achieved by transduction of hematopoietic stem cells with a retroviral vector expressing a murine DHFR cDNA.[125, 372] Since these studies, numerous other drug resistance genes have been proposed for use in myeloprotection including human variants of DHFR,[59, 123] the human MDR1 gene,[116, 373] DNA alkyltransferase genes,[132, 133, 374] the gene for class 1 aldehyde dehydrogenase,[375, 376] and genes for other drug-detoxifying enzymes.[377, 378] Clinical trials have now begun to test this approach for intensifying cancer chemotherapy.

MDR1 Gene Transfer

The human MDR1 gene product, P-glycoprotein, is a transmembrane drug efflux pump that confers cellular resistance to many different xenobiotic anticancer drugs.[112] The feasibility of MDR1 gene transfer for chemoprotection was first demonstrated in transgenic mouse experiments, in which expression of the MDR1 transgene was shown to protect against myelosuppression associated with many commonly used antineoplastic drugs.[115, 379] Later studies showed that mice could also be protected by transfer of MDR1-expressing retroviral vectors.[116, 117, 380] With the demonstration that human CD34[+] cells could be transduced with MDR1 vectors and rendered relatively drug resistant,[381, 382] clinical trials to test this approach were begun.

In a trial at M.D. Anderson Cancer Center, 20 patients with either ovarian or breast cancer underwent transplantation with CD34[+] cells that were transduced with an amphotropic MDR1 retroviral vector by one of two different transduction protocols. Three to 4 weeks after transplantation, MDR1-transduced hematopoietic cells were detected in five of the eight patients who received cells that were transduced in the presence of stromal monolayers.[14] The concentration of MDR1-marked cells in these patients was about 1 in 1000. No marked cells were seen in any of the 10 patients who received cells transduced in suspension without stromal cell support. A second study done at Columbia University also examined retrovirus-mediated MDR1 transduction of hematopoietic cells in adult cancer patients. CD34[+] cells were transduced and reinfused together with unmanipulated cells after high-dose chemotherapy. Although between 20 and 50 per cent of granulocyte-macrophage colony-forming units were transduced in the pretransplantation graft, marked cells were detected in only two of five patients after hematopoietic reconstitution.[15] In these two patients, the proportion of transduced cells was less than 1 in 1000 on analysis between 3 and 10 weeks after transplantation.

The small numbers of *MDR1*-transduced cells seen in these initial trials are unlikely to be sufficient for conferring hematopoietic protection. The scaled-up vector preparations used in these studies had relatively low titers, ranging from 2×10^4 to 1×10^5 colony-forming units per milliliter. Higher titer vectors should be useful for increasing the proportion of transduced cells. Second, the low numbers of transduced cells seen in the Columbia study may have been due to competition from the concurrently infused unmanipulated cells, which would be predicted to have an engraftment advantage.[383] A third area that can be optimized is the stability of the vector genome. The *MDR1* cDNA is prone to rearrangements because of cryptic RNA splicing sites within the coding sequence.[118] The availability of alternative *MDR1* cDNAs that are less susceptible to rearrangements should provide an advantage in this regard.[165] Newer vectors have also been characterized that are optimized for *MDR1* expression in hematopoietic cells and should give enhanced chemoprotection when adequate numbers of transduced cells are obtained.[152, 153, 384]

There are several concerns regarding the ultimate safety of *MDR1* gene therapy for cancer. One issue that applies to all forms of drug resistance gene therapy is the potential for the inadvertent transduction of occult tumor cells that may contaminate the hematopoietic graft. Although this has not been observed in the clinical trials to date and is likely to have little effect on the overall outcome if it occurs in the setting of advanced disease, it does represent a potential limitation of this general approach. The use of tumor cell–purging protocols may provide a means to overcome this limitation.[385, 386] A second concern is the possibility that enforced expression of the *MDR1* cDNAs could induce hematopoietic abnormalities such as leukemia. This concern stems from the recent observation that transplanted mice that received ex vivo expanded, *MDR1*-transduced cells developed a myeloproliferative disorder resembling chronic myelogenous leukemia.[120] It is not yet clear whether the observed hematopoietic abnormality was dependent on the ex vivo expansion of cells after *MDR1* transduction or specific to the modified *MDR1* cDNA used in these experiments. More information regarding the safety of *MDR1* gene transfer is necessary for further development of *MDR1*-mediated chemoprotection.

DHFR Genes for Myeloprotection

Antifolate drugs such as MTX are used to treat a wide variety of malignant neoplasms; however, their use is associated with dose-limiting myelosuppression and gastrointestinal toxicity. One commonly employed means to circumvent these toxicities is the use of 5-formyltetrahydrofolate (leucovorin) after antifolate administration. Although leucovorin "rescue" clearly reduces toxicity to normal host tissues, animal model and clinical trials have shown that leucovorin

administration can also protect tumor cells,[387, 388] so that the value of this approach for increasing the therapeutic index of antifolate drugs has been questioned.[389, 390] An alternative approach is the use of drug-resistant *DHFR* variants for protecting bone marrow cells from drug-induced toxicity. Numerous studies in mice have shown that significant protection from myelosuppression can be achieved by retrovirus-mediated transfer of *DHFR* genes to murine stem cells.[59, 125, 126, 372, 391–393] Protection from myelosuppression has also been associated with a secondary sparing from gastrointestinal toxicity,[394] showing that significant increases in dose intensity could be achieved with use of *DHFR* vectors. A study in mice bearing implanted breast tumors demonstrated that *DHFR*-mediated hematopoietic protection allowed increased doses of MTX to be administered and that these increased doses resulted in improved tumor responses.[395] It is encouraging that partial protection can be obtained when as little as 10 per cent of myeloid cells express the vector,[396] suggesting that clinically therapeutic effects may be achieved in conjunction with currently available gene transfer protocols. The availability of newer human *DHFR* variants with high protective capacities[397] should allow increased marrow protection in the face of relatively high drug doses.

Alkyltransferase Genes for Nitrosourea Protection

A third major system being evaluated for hematopoietic protection is the use of alkyltransferase genes for protection against nitrosourea-induced hematopoietic toxicity. Nitrosoureas, such as BCNU and CCNU, are DNA-damaging agents that alkylate guanine residues at the O-6 position, which ultimately leads to cell death by a variety of mechanisms. These drugs are toxic to hematopoietic cells, particularly stem cells, and cause prolonged bone marrow suppression as the major dose-limiting toxicity. Cellular protection can be conferred by expression of DNA alkyltransferase genes, such as the human methylguanine-DNA methyltransferase gene *(MGMT)*. These proteins function as scavengers for alkyl residues and, by removing these DNA adducts, protect cells from cytotoxic downstream events. Overexpression of *MGMT* is an important cause of tumor cell resistance to nitrosourea therapy.[398] Hematopoietic progenitors express low levels of endogenous alkytransferase,[131, 399] suggesting that *MGMT*-expressing vectors could be used to protect hematopoietic cells.

Retroviral vectors expressing a variety of alkyltransferase genes have been tested in mouse transplant experiments. Vectors expressing the wild-type human *MGMT* cDNA were shown to result in engraftment with drug-resistant myeloid progenitors[133] and in protection from the myelosuppressive effects of BCNU.[132] BCNU protection has also been demonstrated in transplanted mice with use of a vector that expressed the bacterial *ada* gene.[134] *MGMT* gene transfer can also ameliorate BCNU-induced immunosuppression[400] and increase overall survival in heavily BCNU-treated mice.[401] In vitro studies show that *MGMT* vectors can also protect human CD34+ hematopoietic cells from drug toxicity.[402]

Studies have focused on the use of mutant *MGMT* genes for conferring resistance to O-6-benzylguanine (BG) and nitrosourea combinations. Administration of BG can potentiate the tumoricidal effects of nitrosoureas by stoichiometrically depleting cells of wild-type *MGMT* activity.[403] However, the use of BG to sensitize tumor cells is limited by the fact that hematopoietic cells are also sensitized,[131] predicting that BG together with BCNU would be limited by severe myelosuppression. There is now evidence that this limitation can be circumvented by transfer of *MGMT* genes that contain amino acid substitutions conferring resistance to BG-induced inactivation.[404] One such mutant, bearing a glycine to alanine substitution at amino acid 156, has been tested for hematopoietic protection. A retroviral vector expressing this variant was used to transduce mouse stem cells, and transplanted mice were protected from the lethal effects of BCNU administered together with BG.[137] This vector has also been used to confer protection to human hematopoietic cells in vitro.[135] Therefore, it may be possible to sensitize tumor cells to nitrosoureas by use of BG, while simultaneously protecting against hematopoietic toxicity with a vector expressing a *MGMT* variant. Clinical trials testing this approach have just begun at the University of Indiana and at Case Western Reserve University.

▼ HEMOPHILIA

Hemophilia, an X-linked recessive disorder that affects about 1 in 5000 males, is characterized by recurrent bleeding into soft tissues and joint spaces. The majority of cases are due to a deficiency in clotting factor VIII, whereas about 20 per cent of cases are due to deficiency in factor IX (hemophilia A and hemophilia B, respectively). Acute bleeding can be effectively treated with intravenous administration of factor concentrates; however, this type of therapy does not prevent bleeding or eliminate the chronic manifestations of the disease. Clinical experience with factor replacement has indicated that continuous maintenance of factor levels at a small percentage of the normal level would greatly reduce spontaneous bleeding and would be of significant clinical benefit. Toward this goal, gene therapy is being actively pursued as a potentially curative modality.

In contrast to many of the other blood disorders being considered for gene therapy, hematopoietic cells are not a target for hemophilia vectors. The liver is the native site of factor VIII and factor IX production and is one important target for hemophilia vectors. Skeletal muscle is the other organ that is being considered for hemophilia gene therapy. Accordingly, because these tissues are composed of predominantly postmitotic cells, adenovirus and AAV are the vectors of choice on the basis of their ability to transduce nondividing cells. Transduction of liver cells has been achieved in a dog model with use of retroviral vectors,[405] but surgery and partial hepatectomy were required for transduction, making this approach unappealing for clinical application.

Adenovirus vectors expressing factor IX have been studied for in vivo transduction of hepatocytes. When a factor IX–expressing adenoviral vector was injected into the portal circulation of hemophilia B dogs, therapeutic levels of factor IX were detected for short periods in the treated animals.[406] A major cause of the decline in factor levels was a host T cell–mediated immune response directed against virally transduced cells, and vector expression could be prolonged by treatment with immunosuppressive drugs.[407] Adenovirus vectors have also been used to correct a mouse model of hemophilia B,[408] with strain-dependent immune responses

also noted.[409] Direct hepatic toxicity has been described as another limitation associated with the systemic administration of adenovirus vectors.[410] This toxicity may be overcome by using the newest generation of adenovirus vectors, in which all the viral genes have been deleted.[254]

AAV vectors appear to be better suited for transducing hepatocytes with factor IX constructs. Immune responses are less of a problem with AAV vectors, in part because AAV vectors do not express any wild-type viral genes. High levels of human factor IX have been achieved in vivo in mice by transducing the liver with recombinant AAV vectors.[217, 218] Analogous experiments in the canine model for hemophilia B have been reported. Two factor IX–deficient dogs were treated by intraportal administration of an AAV vector expressing human factor IX. Both animals showed partial correction of the whole blood clotting time and of the activated partial thromboplastin time.[212] This was associated with factor IX levels of between 0.5 and 1 per cent of normal, and partial correction of the coagulation defect was sustained for at least 8 months. There were no inhibitors detected against factor IX in these treated dogs, although an expected humoral response to the AAV virions was observed.

Direct injection of AAV vectors into skeletal muscle sites is also being tested for hemophilia gene therapy. Initial marking studies done in mice have shown that muscle fiber transduction with AAV vectors resulted in sustained expression of a transferred β-galactosidase gene.[215] Further studies with AAV vectors expressing human factor IX showed that humoral immune responses could result in loss of factor IX expression both in mice[411] and in hemophilia B dogs.[412] However, when AAV vectors containing the canine factor IX cDNA were injected intramuscularly into hemophiliac dogs, more sustained degrees of factor IX expression and partial clotting time correction were noted. Of the five dogs treated, one animal had a sustained level of factor IX that was equivalent to 1.4 per cent of normal human plasma levels.[213] Two of the five dogs showed transient immune responses against canine factor IX that were not thought to be clinically significant.

These results in the canine animal model of hemophilia B are highly encouraging. Future work will likely focus on increasing the levels of factor IX obtained in vivo, on defining the extent and significance of the immune response associated with AAV vectors, and on developing the methodology to scale up vector production for adapting this approach for human patients. Parallel efforts in hemophilia A are under way. Because the factor VIII cDNA is significantly larger than the factor IX cDNA, it may not be possible to develop AAV vectors given the 4.5 kb packaging constraint. A deleted form of the factor VIII cDNA has been described that can be packaged in retroviral vectors[413, 414] but that is still above the packaging limits of AAV vectors. An adenovirus vector containing a human factor VIII cDNA has been constructed and administered intravenously to factor VIII–deficient dogs. High levels of human factor VIII were found in the serum within 48 hours; however, expression was transient owing to development of a factor VIII antibody.[415] More sustained levels of factor VIII production have been achieved by use of adenovirus vectors in a mouse model of hemophilia A. Therapeutic levels of factor VIII expression were noted for more than 9 months after intravenous administration of the adenovirus vector, and treated mice were resistant to the bleeding associated with tail clipping.[416]

Summary

Gene transfer has become an important component of experimental hematology. Work in animal models has unequivocally established that genetic diseases can be effectively treated by gene transfer methodologies. Rapid progress is being made in the development of vector systems suitable for gene insertion into desired targets in humans, such as hematopoietic stem cells, muscle, and liver. Concurrently, the biological barriers to gene transfer into such cells and tissues are coming to be understood. The initial clinical trials that have now been completed have provided information that will be useful in planning future protocols. During the next decade, we anticipate increasing success in use of gene transfer methodologies for the treatment of human hematological diseases.

ACKNOWLEDGMENTS

We would like to thank Drs. Elio Vanin, Victor Garcia, and Christopher Walsh for their helpful discussions and insights. We also want to thank Betty Ciullo and Jean Johnson for their help in organizing and preparing this manuscript.

REFERENCES

1. Culver, K., Cornetta, K., Morgan, R., Morecki, S., Aebersold, P., Kasid, A., Lotze, M., Rosenberg, S.A., Anderson, W.F., and Blaese, R.M.: Lymphocytes as cellular vehicles for gene therapy in mouse and man. Proc. Natl. Acad. Sci. USA 88:3155, 1991.
2. Ferrari, G., Rossini, S., Giavazzi, R., Maggioni, D., Nobili, N., Soldati, M., Ungers, G., Mavilio, F., Gilboa, E., and Bordignon, C.: An in vivo model of somatic cell gene therapy for human severe combined immunodeficiency. Science 251:1363, 1991.
3. Bordignon, C., Notarangelo, L.D., Nobili, N., Ferrari, G., Casorati, G., Panina, P., Mazzolari, E., Maggioni, D., Rossi, C., and Servida, P.: Gene therapy in peripheral blood lymphocytes and bone marrow for ADA-immunodeficient patients. Science 270:470, 1995.
4. Blaese, R.M., Culver, K.W., Miller, A.D., Carter, C.S., Fleisher, T., Clerici, M., Shearer, G., Chang, L., Chiang, Y., and Tolstoshev, P.: T lymphocyte-directed gene therapy for ADA-SCID: initial trial results after 4 years. Science 270:475, 1995.
5. Bonini, C., Ferrari, G., Verzeletti, S., Servida, P., Zappone, E., Ruggieri, L., Ponzoni, M., Rossini, S., Mavilio, F., Traversari, C., and Bordignon, C.: HSV-TK gene transfer into donor lymphocytes for control of allogeneic graft-versus-leukemia. Science 276:1719, 1997.
6. Culver, K.W., Morgan, R.A., Osborne, W.R., Lee, R.T., Lenschow, D., Able, C., Cornetta, K., Anderson, W.F., and Blaese, R.M.: In vivo expression and survival of gene-modified T lymphocytes in rhesus monkeys. Hum. Gene Ther. 1:399, 1990.
7. Williams, D.A., Lemischka, I.R., Nathan, D.G., and Mulligan, R.C.: Introduction of new genetic material into pluripotent haematopoietic stem cells of the mouse. Nature 310:476, 1984.
8. Dick, J.E., Magli, M.C., Huszar, D., Phillips, R.A., and Bernstein, A.: Introduction of a selectable gene into primitive stem cells capable of long-term reconstitution of the hemopoietic system of W/Wv mice. Cell 42:71, 1985.
9. Eglitis, M.A., Kantoff, P., Gilboa, E., and Anderson, W.F.: Gene expression in mice after high efficiency retroviral-mediated gene transfer. Science 230:1395, 1985.
10. Keller, G., Paige, C., Gilboa, E., and Wagner, E.F.: Expression of a foreign gene in myeloid and lymphoid cells derived from multipotent haematopoietic precursors. Nature 318:149, 1985.
11. Luskey, B.D., Rosenblatt, M., Zsebo, K., and Williams, D.A.: Stem cell factor, interleukin-3, and interleukin-6 promote retroviral-mediated gene transfer into murine hematopoietic stem cells. Blood 80:396, 1992.
12. Bodine, D.M., Karlsson, S., and Nienhuis, A.W.: Combination of interleukins 3 and 6 preserves stem cell function in culture and enhances retrovirus-mediated gene transfer into hematopoietic stem cells. Proc. Natl. Acad. Sci. USA 86:8897, 1989.
13. Dunbar, C.E., Cottler-Fox, M., O'Shaughnessy, J.A., Doren, S., Carter, C., Berenson, R., Brown, S., Moen, R.C., Greenblatt, J., and Stewart, F.M.: Retrovirally marked CD34-enriched peripheral blood and bone marrow cells contribute to long-term engraftment after autologous transplantation. Blood 85:3048, 1995.
14. Hanania, E.G., Giles, R.E., Kavanagh, J., Fu, S.Q., Ellerson, D., Zu, Z., Wang, T., Su, Y., Kudelka, A., Rahman, Z., Holmes, F., Hortobagyi, G., Claxton, D., Bachier, C., Thall, P., Cheng, S., Hester, J., Ostrove, J.M., Bird, R.E., Chang, A., Korbling, M., Seong, D., Cote, R., Holzmayer, T., Deisseroth, A., and Mechetner, E.: Results of MDR-1 vector modification trial indicate that granulocyte/macrophage colony-forming unit cells do not contribute to posttransplant hematopoietic recovery following intensive systemic therapy. Proc. Natl. Acad. Sci. USA 93:15346, 1996.
15. Hesdorffer, C., Ayello, J., Ward, M., Kaubisch, A., Vahdat, L., Balmaceda, C., Garrett, T.D., Fetell, M., Reiss, R., Bank, A., and Antman, K.: Phase I trial of retroviral-mediated transfer of the human MDR1 gene as marrow chemoprotection in patients undergoing high-dose chemotherapy and autologous stem-cell transplantation. J. Clin. Oncol. 16:165, 1998.
16. Brenner, M.K., Rill, D.R., Holladay, M.S., Heslop, H.E., Moen, R.C., Buschle, M., Krance, R.A., Santana, V.M., Anderson, W.F., and Ihle, J.N.: Gene marking to determine whether autologous marrow infusion restores long-term haemopoiesis in cancer patients. Lancet 342:1134, 1993.
17. Tabin, C.J., Hoffmann, J.W., Goff, S.P., and Weinberg, R.A.: Adaptation of a retrovirus as a eucaryotic vector transmitting the herpes simplex virus thymidine kinase gene. Mol. Cell. Biol. 2:426, 1982.
18. Watanabe, S., and Temin, H.M.: Construction of a helper cell line for avian reticuloendotheliosis virus cloning vectors. Mol. Cell. Biol. 3:2241, 1983.
19. Mann, R., Mulligan, R.C., and Baltimore, D.: Construction of a retrovirus packaging mutant and its use to produce helper-free defective retrovirus. Cell 33:153, 1983.
20. Miller, A.D., and Rosman, G.J.: Improved retroviral vectors for gene transfer and expression. Biotechniques 7:980, 1989.
21. Markowitz, D., Goff, S., and Bank, A.: Construction and use of a safe and efficient amphotropic packaging cell line. Virology 167:400, 1988.
22. Danos, O., and Mulligan, R.C.: Safe and efficient generation of recombinant retroviruses with amphotropic and ecotropic host ranges. Proc. Natl. Acad. Sci. USA 85:6460, 1988.
23. Kim, J.W., Closs, E.I., Albritton, L.M., and Cunningham, J.M.: Transport of cationic amino acids by the mouse ecotropic retrovirus receptor. Nature 352:725, 1991.
24. Wang, H., Kavanaugh, M.P., North, R.A., and Kabat, D.: Cell-surface receptor for ecotropic murine retroviruses is a basic amino-acid transporter. Nature 352:729, 1991.
25. Miller, D.G., and Miller, A.D.: A family of retroviruses that utilize related phosphate transporters for cell entry. J. Virol. 68:8270, 1994.
26. Miller, D.G., Edwards, R.H., and Miller, A.D.: Cloning of the cellular receptor for amphotropic murine retroviruses reveals homology to that for gibbon ape leukemia virus. Proc. Natl. Acad. Sci. USA 91:78, 1994.
27. Bukrinsky, M.I., Haggerty, S., Dempsey, M.P., Sharova, N., Adzhubel, A., Spitz, L., Lewis, P., Goldfarb, D., Emerman, M., and Stevenson, M.: A nuclear localization signal within HIV-1 matrix protein that governs infection of non-dividing cells. Nature 365:666, 1993.
28. Hao, Q.L., Thiemann, F.T., Petersen, D., Smogorzewska, E.M., and Crooks, G.M.: Extended long-term culture reveals a highly quiescent and primitive human hematopoietic progenitor population. Blood 88:3306, 1996.
29. Goodell, M.A., Brose, K., Paradis, G., Conner, A.S., and Mulligan, R.C.: Isolation and functional properties of murine hematopoietic stem cells that are replicating in vivo. J. Exp. Med. 183:1797, 1996.
30. Lewis, P.F., and Emerman, M.: Passage through mitosis is required for oncoretroviruses but not for the human immunodeficiency virus. J. Virol. 68:510, 1994.

31. Agrawal, Y.P., Agrawal, R.S., Sinclair, A.M., Young, D., Maruyama, M., Levine, F., and Ho, A.D.: Cell-cycle kinetics and VSV-G pseudotyped retrovirus-mediated gene transfer in blood-derived CD34+ cells. Exp. Hematol. 24:738, 1996.

32. Yoshimoto, T., Yoshimoto, E., and Meruelo, D.: Molecular cloning and characterization of a novel human gene homologous to the murine ecotropic retroviral receptor. Virology 185:10, 1991.

33. Yoshimoto, T., Yoshimoto, E., and Meruelo, D.: Identification of amino acid residues critical for infection with ecotropic murine leukemia retrovirus. J. Virol. 67:1310, 1993.

34. Kozak, S.L., Siess, D.C., Kavanaugh, M.P., Miller, A.D., and Kabat, D.: The envelope glycoprotein of an amphotropic murine retrovirus binds specifically to the cellular receptor/phosphate transporter of susceptible species. J. Virol. 69:3433, 1995.

35. Fink, J.K., Correll, P.H., Perry, L.K., Brady, R.O., and Karlsson, S.: Correction of glucocerebrosidase deficiency after retroviral-mediated gene transfer into hematopoietic progenitor cells from patients with Gaucher disease. Proc. Natl. Acad. Sci. USA 87:2334, 1990.

36. Flasshove, M., Banerjee, D., Mineishi, S., Li, M.X., Bertino, J.R., and Moore, M.A.: Ex vivo expansion and selection of human CD34+ peripheral blood progenitor cells after introduction of a mutated dihydrofolate reductase cDNA via retroviral gene transfer. Blood 85:566, 1995.

37. Eglitis, M.A., Kohn, D.B., Moen, R.C., Blaese, R.M., and Anderson, W.F.: Infection of human hematopoietic progenitor cells using a retroviral vector with a xenotropic pseudotype. Biochem. Biophys. Res. Commun. 151:201, 1988.

38. Orlic, D., Girard, L.J., Jordan, C.T., Anderson, S.M., Cline, A.P., and Bodine, D.M.: The level of mRNA encoding the amphotropic retrovirus receptor in mouse and human hematopoietic stem cells is low and correlates with the efficiency of retrovirus transduction. Proc. Natl. Acad. Sci. USA 93:11097, 1996.

39. Crooks, G.M., and Kohn, D.B.: Growth factors increase amphotropic retrovirus binding to human CD34+ bone marrow progenitor cells. Blood 82:3290, 1993.

40. Chien, M.L., Foster, J.L., Douglas, J.L., and Garcia, J.V.: The amphotropic murine leukemia virus receptor gene encodes a 71-kilodalton protein that is induced by phosphate depletion. J. Virol. 71:4564, 1997.

41. Bunnell, B.A., Muul, L.M., Donahue, R.E., Blaese, R.M., and Morgan, R.A.: High-efficiency retroviral-mediated gene transfer into human and nonhuman primate peripheral blood lymphocytes. Proc. Natl. Acad. Sci. USA 92:7739, 1995.

42. Orlic, D., Girard, L.J., Anderson, S.M., Pyle, L.C., Yoder, M.C., Broxmeyer, H.E., and Bodine, D.M.: Identification of human and mouse hematopoietic stem cell populations expressing high levels of mRNA encoding retrovirus receptors. Blood 91:3247, 1998.

43. Tisdale, J.F., Hanazono, Y., Sellers, S.E., Agricola, B.A., Metzger, M.E., Donahue, R.E., and Dunbar, C.E.: Ex vivo expansion of genetically marked rhesus peripheral blood progenitor cells results in diminished long-term repopulating ability. Blood 92:1131, 1998.

44. Miller, A.D.: Cell-surface receptors for retroviruses and implications for gene transfer. Proc. Natl. Acad. Sci. USA 93:11407, 1996.

45. Miller, A.D., Garcia, J.V., von Suhr, N., Lynch, C.M., Wilson, C., and Eiden, M.V.: Construction and properties of retrovirus packaging cells based on gibbon ape leukemia virus. J. Virol. 65:2220, 1991.

46. Schilz, A.J., Brouns, G., Knobeta, H., Ottmann, O.G., Hoelzer, D., Fauser, A.A., Thrasher, A.J., and Grez, M.: High efficiency gene transfer to human hematopoietic SCID-repopulating cells under serum-free conditions. Blood 92:3163, 1998.

47. Kiem, H.P., Heyward, S., Winkler, A., Potter, J., Allen, J.M., Miller, A.D., and Andrews, R.G.: Gene transfer into marrow repopulating cells: comparison between amphotropic and gibbon ape leukemia virus pseudotyped retroviral vectors in a competitive repopulation assay in baboons. Blood 90:4638, 1997.

48. Burns, J.C., Friedmann, T., Driever, W., Burrascano, M., and Yee, J.K.: Vesicular stomatitis virus G glycoprotein pseudotyped retroviral vectors: concentration to very high titer and efficient gene transfer into mammalian and nonmammalian cells. Proc. Natl. Acad. Sci. USA 90:8033, 1993.

49. von Kalle, C., Kiem, H.P., Goehle, S., Darovsky, B., Heimfeld, S., Torok-Storb, B., Storb, R., and Schuening, F.G.: Increased gene transfer into human hematopoietic progenitor cells by extended in vitro exposure to a pseudotyped retroviral vector. Blood 84:2890, 1994.

50. Gallardo, H.F., Tan, C., Ory, D., and Sadelain, M.: Recombinant retroviruses pseudotyped with the vesicular stomatitis virus G glyco-

protein mediate both stable gene transfer and pseudotransduction in human peripheral blood lymphocytes. Blood 90:952, 1997.

51. Yang, Y., Vanin, E.F., Whitt, M.A., Fornerod, M., Zwart, R., Schneiderman, R.D., Grosveld, G., and Nienhuis, A.W.: Inducible, high-level production of infectious murine leukemia retroviral vector particles pseudotyped with vesicular stomatitis virus G envelope protein. Hum. Gene Ther. 6:1203, 1995.

52. Chen, S.T., Iida, A., Guo, L., Friedmann, T., and Yee, J.K.: Generation of packaging cell lines for pseudotyped retroviral vectors of the G protein of vesicular stomatitis virus by using a modified tetracycline inducible system. Proc. Natl. Acad. Sci. USA 93:10057, 1996.

53. Ory, D.S., Neugeboren, B.A., and Mulligan, R.C.: A stable human-derived packaging cell line for production of high titer retrovirus/vesicular stomatitis virus G pseudotypes. Proc. Natl. Acad. Sci. USA 93:11400, 1996.

54. Akkina, R.K., Walton, R.M., Chen, M.L., Li, Q.X., Planelles, V., and Chen, I.S.: High-efficiency gene transfer into CD34+ cells with a human immunodeficiency virus type 1–based retroviral vector pseudotyped with vesicular stomatitis virus envelope glycoprotein G. J. Virol. 70:2581, 1996.

55. Miller, D.G., Adam, M.A., and Miller, A.D.: Gene transfer by retrovirus vectors occurs only in cells that are actively replicating at the time of infection. Mol. Cell. Biol. 10:4239, 1990.

56. Bodine, D.M., Crosier, P.S., and Clark, S.C.: Effects of hematopoietic growth factors on the survival of primitive stem cells in liquid suspension culture. Blood 78:914, 1991.

57. Bodine, D.M., McDonagh, K.T., Seidel, N.E., and Nienhuis, A.W.: Survival and retrovirus infection of murine hematopoietic stem cells in vitro: effects of 5-FU and method of infection. Exp. Hematol. 19:206, 1991.

58. Correll, P.H., Kew, Y., Perry, L.K., Brady, R.O., Fink, J.K., and Karlsson, S.: Expression of human glucocerebrosidase in long-term reconstituted mice following retroviral-mediated gene transfer into hematopoietic stem cells. Hum. Gene Ther. 1:277, 1990.

59. Spencer, H.T., Sleep, S.E., Rehg, J.E., Blakley, R.L., and Sorrentino, B.P.: A gene transfer strategy for making bone marrow cells resistant to trimetrexate. Blood 87:2579, 1996.

60. Shapiro, F., Yao, T.J., Raptis, G., Reich, L., Norton, L., and Moore, M.A.: Optimization of conditions for ex vivo expansion of CD34+ cells from patients with stage IV breast cancer. Blood 84:3567, 1994.

61. Petzer, A.L., Zandstra, P.W., Piret, J.M., and Eaves, C.J.: Differential cytokine effects on primitive (CD34+CD38−) human hematopoietic cells: novel responses to Flt3-ligand and thrombopoietin. J. Exp. Med. 183:2551, 1996.

62. Zandstra, P.W., Conneally, E., Petzer, A.L., Piret, J.M., and Eaves, C.J.: Cytokine manipulation of primitive human hematopoietic cell self-renewal. Proc. Natl. Acad. Sci. USA 94:4698, 1997.

63. Gan, O.I., Murdoch, B., Larochelle, A., and Dick, J.E.: Differential maintenance of primitive human SCID-repopulating cells, clonogenic progenitors, and long-term culture-initiating cells after incubation on human bone marrow stromal cells. Blood 90:641, 1997.

64. Bhatia, M., Bonnet, D., Kapp, U., Wang, J.C., Murdoch, B., and Dick, J.E.: Quantitative analysis reveals expansion of human hematopoietic repopulating cells after short-term ex vivo culture. J. Exp. Med. 186:619, 1997.

65. Bhatia, M., Bonnet, D., Murdoch, B., Gan, O.I., and Dick, J.E.: A newly discovered class of human hematopoietic cells with SCID-repopulating activity. Nat. Med. 4:1038, 1998.

66. Sherr, C.J.: Mammalian G1 cyclins. Cell 73:1059, 1993.

67. Sherr, C.J., and Roberts, J.M.: Inhibitors of mammalian G1 cyclin-dependent kinases. Genes Dev. 9:1149, 1995.

68. Coats, S., Flanagan, W.M., Nourse, J., and Roberts, J.M.: Requirement of p27Kip1 for restriction point control of the fibroblast cell cycle. Science 272:877, 1996.

69. Dao, M.A., Taylor, N., and Nolta, J.A.: Reduction in levels of the cyclin-dependent kinase inhibitor p27(kip-1) coupled with transforming growth factor beta neutralization induces cell-cycle entry and increases retroviral transduction of primitive human hematopoietic cells. Proc. Natl. Acad. Sci. USA 95:13006, 1998.

70. Veena, P., Traycoff, C.M., Williams, D.A., McMahel, J., Rice, S., Cornetta, K., and Srour, E.F.: Delayed targeting of cytokine-nonresponsive human bone marrow CD34+ cells with retrovirus-mediated gene transfer enhances transduction efficiency and long-term expression of transduced genes. Blood 91:3693, 1998.

71. Hanenberg, H., Hashino, K., Konishi, H., Hock, R.A., Kato, I., and

Williams, D.A.: Optimization of fibronectin-assisted retroviral gene transfer into human CD34+ hematopoietic cells. Hum. Gene Ther. 8:2193, 1997.

72. Bertolini, F., de Monte, L., Corsini, C., Lazzari, L., Lauri, E., Soligo, D., Ward, M., Bank, A., and Malavasi, F.: Retrovirus-mediated transfer of the multidrug resistance gene into human haemopoietic progenitor cells. Br. J. Haematol. 88:318, 1994.

73. Breems, D.A., Van Driel, E.M., Hawley, R.G., Siebel, K.E., and Ploemacher, R.E.: Stroma-conditioned medium and sufficient prestimulation improve fibronectin fragment-mediated retroviral gene transfer into human primitive mobilized peripheral blood stem cells through effects on their recovery and transduction efficiency. Leukemia 12:951, 1998.

74. Bodine, D.M., Seidel, N.E., Gale, M.S., Nienhuis, A.W., and Orlic, D.: Efficient retrovirus transduction of mouse pluripotent hematopoietic stem cells mobilized into the peripheral blood by treatment with granulocyte colony-stimulating factor and stem cell factor. Blood 84:1482, 1994.

75. Bodine, D.M., Seidel, N.E., and Orlic, D.: Bone marrow collected 14 days after in vivo administration of granulocyte colony-stimulating factor and stem cell factor to mice has 10-fold more repopulating ability than untreated bone marrow. Blood 88:89, 1996.

76. Dunbar, C.E., Seidel, N.E., Doren, S., Sellers, S., Cline, A.P., Metzger, M.E., Agricola, B.A., Donahue, R.E., and Bodine, D.M.: Improved retroviral gene transfer into murine and rhesus peripheral blood or bone marrow repopulating cells primed in vivo with stem cell factor and granulocyte colony-stimulating factor. Proc. Natl. Acad. Sci. USA 93:11871, 1996.

77. Lewis, P., Hensel, M., and Emerman, M.: Human immunodeficiency virus infection of cells arrested in the cell cycle. EMBO J. 11:3053, 1992.

78. Gallay, P., Swingler, S., Aiken, C., and Trono, D.: HIV-1 infection of nondividing cells: C-terminal tyrosine phosphorylation of the viral matrix protein is a key regulator. Cell 80:379, 1995.

79. Gallay, P., Swingler, S., Song, J., Bushman, F., and Trono, D.: HIV nuclear import is governed by the phosphotyrosine-mediated binding of matrix to the core domain of integrase. Cell 83:569, 1995.

80. Heinzinger, N.K., Bukinsky, M.I., Haggerty, S.A., Ragland, A.M., Kewalramani, V., Lee, M.A., Gendelman, H.E., Ratner, L., Stevenson, M., and Emerman, M.: The Vpr protein of human immunodeficiency virus type 1 influences nuclear localization of viral nucleic acids in nondividing host cells. Proc. Natl. Acad. Sci. USA 91:7311, 1994.

81. Deminie, C.A., and Emerman, M.: Functional exchange of an oncoretrovirus and a lentivirus matrix protein. J. Virol. 68:4442, 1994.

82. Shimada, T., Fujii, H., Mitsuya, H., and Nienhuis, A.W.: Targeted and highly efficient gene transfer into CD4+ cells by a recombinant human immunodeficiency virus retroviral vector. J. Clin. Invest. 88:1043, 1991.

83. Naldini, L., Blomer, U., Gallay, P., Ory, D., Mulligan, R., Gage, F.H., Verma, I.M., and Trono, D.: In vivo gene delivery and stable transduction of nondividing cells by a lentiviral vector. Science 272:263, 1996.

84. Reiser, J., Harmison, G., Kluepfel-Stahl, S., Brady, R.O., Karlsson, S., and Schubert, M.: Transduction of nondividing cells using pseudotyped defective high-titer HIV type 1 particles. Proc. Natl. Acad. Sci. USA 93:15266, 1996.

85. Blomer, U., Naldini, L., Kafri, T., Trono, D., Verma, I.M., and Gage, F.H.: Highly efficient and sustained gene transfer in adult neurons with a lentivirus vector. J. Virol. 71:6641, 1997.

86. Miyoshi, H., Takahashi, M., Gage, F.H., and Verma, I.M.: Stable and efficient gene transfer into the retina using an HIV-based lentiviral vector. Proc. Natl. Acad. Sci. USA 94:10319, 1997.

87. Naldini, L., Blomer, U., Gage, F.H., Trono, D., and Verma, I.M.: Efficient transfer, integration, and sustained long-term expression of the transgene in adult rat brains injected with a lentiviral vector. Proc. Natl. Acad. Sci. USA 93:11382, 1996.

88. Parolin, C., Taddeo, B., Palu, G., and Sodroski, J.: Use of cis- and trans-acting viral regulatory sequences to improve expression of human immunodeficiency virus vectors in human lymphocytes. Virology 222:415, 1996.

89. Poeschla, E., Corbeau, P., and Wong-Staal, F.: Development of HIV vectors for anti-HIV gene therapy. Proc. Natl. Acad. Sci. USA 93:11395, 1996.

90. Uchida, N., Sutton, R.E., Friera, A.M., He, D., Reitsma, M.J., Chang, W.C., Veres, G., Scollay, R., and Weissman, I.L.: HIV, but not murine leukemia virus, vectors mediate high efficiency gene transfer into freshly isolated G₀/G₁ human hematopoietic stem cells. Proc. Natl. Acad. Sci. USA 95:11939, 1998.

91. Miyoshi, H., Smith, K.A., Mosier, D.E., Verma, I.M., and Torbett, B.E.: Efficient transduction of human CD34+ cells that mediate long-term engraftment of NOD/SCID mice by HIV vectors. Science 283:682, 1999.

92. Kiem, H.P., Andrews, R.G., Morris, J.A., Peterson, L., Heyward, S., Allen, J.M., Rasko, J.E., Potter, J., and Miller, A.D.: Improved gene transfer into baboon marrow repopulating cells using recombinant human fibronectin fragment CH-296 in combination with interleukin-6, stem cell factor, FLT-3 ligand, and megakaryocyte growth and development factor. Blood 92:1878, 1998.

93. Toksoz, D., Zsebo, K.M., Smith, K.A., Hu, S., Brankow, D., Suggs, S.V., Martin, F.H., and Williams, D.A.: Support of human hematopoiesis in long-term bone marrow cultures by murine stromal cells selectively expressing the membrane-bound and secreted forms of the human homolog of the steel gene product, stem cell factor. Proc. Natl. Acad. Sci. USA 89:7350, 1992.

94. Moore, K.A., Deisseroth, A.B., Reading, C.L., Williams, D.E., and Belmont, J.W.: Stromal support enhances cell-free retroviral vector transduction of human bone marrow long-term culture-initiating cells. Blood 79:1393, 1992.

95. Bienzle, D., Abrams-Ogg, A.C., Kruth, S.A., Ackland-Snow, J., Carter, R.F., Dick, J.E., Jacobs, R.M., Kamel-Reid, S., and Dube, I.D.: Gene transfer into hematopoietic stem cells: long-term maintenance of in vitro activated progenitors without marrow ablation. Proc. Natl. Acad. Sci. USA 91:350, 1994.

96. Emmons, R.V., Doren, S., Zujewski, J., Cottler-Fox, M., Carter, C.S., Hines, K., O'Shaughnessy, J.A., Leitman, S.F., Greenblatt, J.J., Cowan, K., and Dunbar, C.E.: Retroviral gene transduction of adult peripheral blood or marrow-derived CD34+ cells for six hours without growth factors or on autologous stroma does not improve marking efficiency assessed in vivo. Blood 89:4040, 1997.

97. Williams, D.A., Rios, M., Stephens, C., and Patel, V.P.: Fibronectin and VLA-4 in haematopoietic stem cell–microenvironment interactions. Nature 352:438, 1991.

98. Moritz, T., Patel, V.P., and Williams, D.A.: Bone marrow extracellular matrix molecules improve gene transfer into human hematopoietic cells via retroviral vectors. J. Clin. Invest. 93:1451, 1994.

99. Hanenberg, H., Xiao, X.L., Dilloo, D., Hashino, K., Kato, I., and Williams, D.A.: Colocalization of retrovirus and target cells on specific fibronectin fragments increases genetic transduction of mammalian cells. Nat. Med. 2:876, 1996.

100. van der Loo, J.C., Xiao, X., McMillin, D., Hashino, K., Kato, I., and Williams, D.A.: VLA-5 is expressed by mouse and human long-term repopulating hematopoietic cells and mediates adhesion to extracellular matrix protein fibronectin. J. Clin. Invest. 102:1051, 1998.

101. Schofield, K.P., Humphries, M.J., de Wynter, E., Testa, N., and Gallagher, J.T.: The effect of alpha4 beta1-integrin binding sequences of fibronectin on growth of cells from human hematopoietic progenitors. Blood 91:3230, 1998.

102. Yokota, T., Oritani, K., Mitsui, H., Aoyama, K., Ishikawa, J., Sugahara, H., Matsumura, I., Tsai, S., Tomiyama, Y., Kanakura, Y., and Matsuzawa, Y.: Growth-supporting activities of fibronectin on hematopoietic stem/progenitor cells in vitro and in vivo: structural requirement for fibronectin activities of CS1 and cell-binding domains. Blood 91:3263, 1998.

103. Moritz, T., Dutt, P., Xiao, X., Carstanjen, D., Vik, T., Hanenberg, H., and Williams, D.A.: Fibronectin improves transduction of reconstituting hematopoietic stem cells by retroviral vectors: evidence of direct viral binding to chymotryptic carboxy-terminal fragments. Blood 88:855, 1996.

104. Pawliuk, R., Kay, R., Lansdorp, P., and Humphries, R.K.: Selection of retrovirally transduced hematopoietic cells using CD24 as a marker of gene transfer. Blood 84:2868, 1994.

105. Pawliuk, R., Eaves, C.J., and Humphries, R.K.: Sustained high-level reconstitution of the hematopoietic system by preselected hematopoietic cells expressing a transduced cell-surface antigen. Hum. Gene Ther. 8:1595, 1997.

106. Persons, D.A., Allay, J.A., Allay, E.R., Smeyne, R.J., Ashmun, R.A., Sorrentino, B.P., and Nienhuis, A.W.: Retroviral-mediated transfer of the green fluorescent protein gene into murine hematopoietic cells facilitates scoring and selection of transduced progenitors in vitro and identification of genetically modified cells in vivo. Blood 90:1777, 1997.

107. Persons, D.A., Allay, J.A., Riberdy, J.M., Wersto, R.P., Donahue, R.E., Sorrentino, B.P., and Nienhuis, A.W.: Utilization of the green fluorescent protein gene as a marker to identify and track genetically-modified hematopoietic cells. Nat. Med. 4:1201, 1998.

108. Conneally, E., Bardy, P., Eaves, C.J., Thomas, T., Chappel, S., Shpall, E.J., and Humphries, R.K.: Rapid and efficient selection of human hematopoietic cells expressing murine heat-stable antigen as an indicator of retroviral-mediated gene transfer. Blood 87:456, 1996.

109. Migita, M., Medin, J.A., Pawliuk, R., Jacobson, S., Nagle, J.W., Anderson, S., Amiri, M., Humphries, R.K., and Karlsson, S.: Selection of transduced CD34$^+$ progenitors and enzymatic correction of cells from Gaucher patients, with bicistronic vectors. Proc. Natl. Acad. Sci. USA 92:12075, 1995.

110. Iscove, N.N., and Nawa, K.: Hematopoietic stem cells expand during serial transplantation in vivo without apparent exhaustion. Curr. Biol. 7:805, 1997.

111. Chen, C.J., Chin, J.E., Ueda, K., Clark, D.P., Pastan, I., Gottesman, M.M., and Roninson, I.B.: Internal duplication and homology with bacterial transport proteins in the mdr1 (P-glycoprotein) gene from multidrug-resistant human cells. Cell 47:381, 1986.

112. Pastan, I., and Gottesman, M.M.: Multidrug resistance. Annu. Rev. Med. 42:277, 1991.

113. Pastan, I., Gottesman, M.M., Ueda, K., Lovelace, E., Rutherford, A.V., and Willingham, M.C.: A retrovirus carrying an MDR1 cDNA confers multidrug resistance and polarized expression of P-glycoprotein in MDCK cells. Proc. Natl. Acad. Sci. USA 85:4486, 1988.

114. Galski, H., Sullivan, M., Willingham, M.C., Chin, K.V., Gottesman, M.M., Pastan, I., and Merlino, G.T.: Expression of a human multidrug resistance cDNA (MDR1) in the bone marrow of transgenic mice: resistance to daunomycin-induced leukopenia. Mol. Cell. Biol. 9:4357, 1989.

115. Mickisch, G.H., Licht, T., Merlino, G.T., Gottesman, M.M., and Pastan, I.: Chemotherapy and chemosensitization of transgenic mice which express the human multidrug resistance gene in bone marrow: efficacy, potency, and toxicity. Cancer Res. 51:5417, 1991.

116. Sorrentino, B.P., Brandt, S.J., Bodine, D., Gottesman, M., Pastan, I., Cline, A., and Nienhuis, A.W.: Selection of drug-resistant bone marrow cells in vivo after retroviral transfer of human MDR1. Science 257:99, 1992.

117. Podda, S., Ward, M., Himelstein, A., Richardson, C., de la Flor-Weiss, E., Smith, L., Gottesman, M., Pastan, I., and Bank, A.: Transfer and expression of the human multiple drug resistance gene into live mice. Proc. Natl. Acad. Sci. USA 89:9676, 1992.

118. Sorrentino, B.P., McDonagh, K.T., Woods, D., and Orlic, D.: Expression of retroviral vectors containing the human multidrug resistance 1 cDNA in hematopoietic cells of transplanted mice. Blood 86:491, 1995.

119. Blau, C.A., Neff, T., and Papayannopoulou, T.: Cytokine prestimulation as a gene therapy strategy: implications for using the MDR1 gene as a dominant selectable marker. Blood 89:146, 1997.

120. Bunting, K.D., Galipeau, J., Topham, D., Benaim, E., and Sorrentino, B.P.: Transduction of murine bone marrow cells with an MDR1 vector enables ex vivo stem cell expansion, but these expanded grafts cause a myeloproliferative syndrome in transplanted mice. Blood 92:2269, 1998.

121. McIvor, R.S., and Simonsen, C.C.: Isolation and characterization of a variant dihydrofolate reductase cDNA from methotrexate-resistant murine L5178Y cells. Nucleic Acids Res. 18:7025, 1990.

122. Simonsen, C.C., and Levinson, A.D.: Isolation and expression of an altered mouse dihydrofolate reductase cDNA. Proc. Natl. Acad. Sci. USA 80:2495, 1983.

123. Banerjee, D., Schweitzer, B.I., Volkenandt, M., Li, M.X., Waltham, M., Mineishi, S., Zhao, S.C., and Bertino, J.R.: Transfection with a cDNA encoding a Ser31 or Ser34 mutant human dihydrofolate reductase into Chinese hamster ovary and mouse marrow progenitor cells confers methotrexate resistance. Gene 139:269, 1994.

124. Lewis, W.S., Cody, V., Galitsky, N., Luft, J.R., Pangborn, W., Chunduru, S.K., Spencer, H.T., Appleman, J.R., and Blakley, R.L.: Methotrexate-resistant variants of human dihydrofolate reductase with substitutions of leucine 22. Kinetics, crystallography, and potential as selectable markers. J. Biol. Chem. 270:5057, 1995.

125. Corey, C.A., DeSilva, A.D., Holland, C.A., and Williams, D.A.: Serial transplantation of methotrexate-resistant bone marrow: protection of murine recipients from drug toxicity by progeny of transduced stem cells. Blood 75:337, 1990.

126. Zhao, S.C., Li, M.X., Banerjee, D., Schweitzer, B.I., Mineishi, S., Gilboa, E., and Bertino, J.R.: Long-term protection of recipient mice from lethal doses of methotrexate by marrow infected with a double-copy vector retrovirus containing a mutant dihydrofolate reductase. Cancer Gene Ther. 1:27, 1994.

127. Blau, C.A., Neff, T., and Papayannopoulou, T.: The hematological effects of folate analogs: implications for using the dihydrofolate reductase gene for in vivo selection. Hum. Gene Ther. 7:2069, 1996.

128. Allay, J.A., Spencer, H.T., Wilkinson, S.L., Belt, J.A., Blakley, R.L., and Sorrentino, B.P.: Sensitization of hematopoietic stem and progenitor cells to trimetrexate using nucleoside transport inhibitors. Blood 90:3546, 1997.

129. Allay, J.A., Persons, D.A., Galipeau, J., Riberdy, J.M., Ashmun, R.A., Blakley, R.L., and Sorrentino, B.P.: In vivo selection of retrovirally transduced hematopoietic stem cells. Nat. Med. 4:1136, 1998.

130. Brent, T.P., Houghton, P.J., and Houghton, J.A.: O6-Alkylguanine-DNA alkyltransferase activity correlates with the therapeutic response of human rhabdomyosarcoma xenografts to 1-(2-chloroethyl)-3-(trans-4-methylcyclohexyl)-1-nitrosourea. Proc. Natl. Acad. Sci. USA 82:2985, 1985.

131. Gerson, S.L., Phillips, W., Kastan, M., Dumenco, L.L., and Donovan, C.: Human CD34$^+$ hematopoietic progenitors have low, cytokine-unresponsive O6-alkylguanine-DNA alkyltransferase and are sensitive to O6-benzylguanine plus BCNU. Blood 88:1649, 1996.

132. Moritz, T., Mackay, W., Glassner, B.J., Williams, D.A., and Samson, L.: Retrovirus-mediated expression of a DNA repair protein in bone marrow protects hematopoietic cells from nitrosourea-induced toxicity in vitro and in vivo. Cancer Res. 55:2608, 1995.

133. Allay, J.A., Dumenco, L.L., Koc, O.N., Liu, L., and Gerson, S.L.: Retroviral transduction and expression of the human alkyltransferase cDNA provides nitrosourea resistance to hematopoietic cells. Blood 85:3342, 1995.

134. Harris, L.C., Marathi, U.K., Edwards, C.C., Houghton, P.J., Srivastava, D.K., Vanin, E.F., Sorrentino, B.P., and Brent, T.P.: Retroviral transfer of a bacterial alkyltransferase gene into murine bone marrow protects against chloroethylnitrosourea cytotoxicity. Clin. Cancer Res. 1:1359, 1995.

135. Reese, J.S., Koc, O.N., Lee, K.M., Liu, L., Allay, J.A., Phillips, W.P.J., and Gerson, S.L.: Retroviral transduction of a mutant methylguanine DNA methyltransferase gene into human CD34 cells confers resistance to O6-benzylguanine plus 1,3-bis(2-chloroethyl)-1-nitrosourea. Proc. Natl. Acad. Sci. USA 93:14088, 1996.

136. Allay, J.A., Davis, B.M., and Gerson, S.L.: Human alkyltransferase-transduced murine myeloid progenitors are enriched in vivo by BCNU treatment of transplanted mice. Exp. Hematol. 25:1069, 1997.

137. Davis, B.M., Reese, J.S., Koc, O.N., Lee, K., Schupp, J.E., and Gerson, S.L.: Selection for G156A O^6-methylguanine DNA methyltransferase gene-transduced hematopoietic progenitors and protection from lethality in mice treated with O^6-benzylguanine and 1,3-bis(2-chloroethyl)-1-nitrosourea. Cancer Res. 57:5093, 1997.

138. Spencer, D.M., Wandless, T.J., Schreiber, S.L., and Crabtree, G.R.: Controlling signal transduction with synthetic ligands. Science 262:1019, 1993.

139. Blau, C.A., Peterson, K.R., Drachman, J.G., and Spencer, D.M.: A proliferation switch for genetically modified cells. Proc. Natl. Acad. Sci. USA 94:3076, 1997.

140. Jin, L., Siritanaratkul, N., Emery, D.W., Richard, R.E., Kaushansky, K., Papayannopoulou, T., and Blau, C.A.: Targeted expansion of genetically modified bone marrow cells. Proc. Natl. Acad. Sci. USA 95:8093, 1998.

141. Jin, L., Asano, H., and Blau, C.A.: Stimulating cell proliferation through the pharmacologic activation of c-kit. Blood 91:890, 1998.

142. Ito, K., Ueda, Y., Kokubun, M., Urabe, M., Inaba, T., Mano, H., Hamada, H., Kitamura, T., Mizoguchi, H., Sakata, T., Hasegawa, M., and Ozawa, K.: Development of a novel selective amplifier gene for controllable expansion of transduced hematopoietic cells. Blood 90:3884, 1997.

143. Kirby, S.L., Cook, D.N., Walton, W., and Smithies, O.: Proliferation of multipotent hematopoietic cells controlled by a truncated erythro-poietin receptor transgene. Proc. Natl. Acad. Sci. USA 93:9402, 1996.

144. Challita, P.M., and Kohn, D.B.: Lack of expression from a retroviral vector after transduction of murine hematopoietic stem cells is associated with methylation in vivo. Proc. Natl. Acad. Sci. USA 91:2567, 1994.

145. Chen, W.Y., Bailey, E.C., McCune, S.L., Dong, J.Y., and Townes,

T.M.: Reactivation of silenced, virally transduced genes by inhibitors of histone deacetylase. Proc. Natl. Acad. Sci. USA 94:5798, 1997.

146. Franz, T., Hilberg, F., Seliger, B., Stocking, C., and Ostertag, W.: Retroviral mutants efficiently expressed in embryonal carcinoma cells. Proc. Natl. Acad. Sci. USA 83:3292, 1986.

147. Grez, M., Akgun, E., Hilberg, F., and Ostertag, W.: Embryonic stem cell virus, a recombinant murine retrovirus with expression in embryonic stem cells. Proc. Natl. Acad. Sci. USA 87:9202, 1990.

148. Challita, P.M., Skelton, D., el-Khoueiry, A., Yu, X.J., Weinberg, K., and Kohn, D.B.: Multiple modifications in *cis* elements of the long terminal repeat of retroviral vectors lead to increased expression and decreased DNA methylation in embryonic carcinoma cells. J. Virol. 69:748, 1995.

149. Hilberg, F., Stocking, C., Ostertag, W., and Grez, M.: Functional analysis of a retroviral host-range mutant: altered long terminal repeat sequences allow expression in embryonal carcinoma cells. Proc. Natl. Acad. Sci. USA 84:5232, 1987.

150. Weiher, H., Barklis, E., Ostertag, W., and Jaenisch, R.: Two distinct sequence elements mediate retroviral gene expression in embryonal carcinoma cells. J. Virol. 61:2742, 1987.

151. Baum, C., Eckert, H.G., Stockschlader, M., Just, U., Hegewisch-Becker, S., Hildinger, M., Uhde, A., John, J., and Ostertag, W.: Improved retroviral vectors for hematopoietic stem cell protection and in vivo selection. J. Hematother. 5:323, 1996.

152. Eckert, H.G., Stockschlader, M., Just, U., Hegewisch-Becker, S., Grez, M., Uhde, A., Zander, A., Ostertag, W., and Baum, C.: High-dose multidrug resistance in primary human hematopoietic progenitor cells transduced with optimized retroviral vectors. Blood 88:3407, 1996.

153. Hildinger, M., Fehse, B., Hegewisch-Becker, S., John, J., Rafferty, J.R., Ostertag, W., and Baum, C.: Dominant selection of hematopoietic progenitor cells with retroviral MDR1 co-expression vectors. Hum. Gene Ther. 9:33, 1998.

154. Hawley, R.G., Fong, A.Z., Burns, B.F., and Hawley, T.S.: Transplantable myeloproliferative disease induced in mice by an interleukin 6 retrovirus. J. Exp. Med. 176:1149, 1992.

155. Krall, W.J., Skelton, D.C., Yu, X.J., Riviere, I., Lehn, P., Mulligan, R.C., and Kohn, D.B.: Increased levels of spliced RNA account for augmented expression from the MFG retroviral vector in hematopoietic cells. Gene Ther. 3:37, 1996.

156. Dranoff, G., Jaffee, E., Lazenby, A., Golumbek, P., Levitsky, H., Brose, K., Jackson, V., Hamada, H., Pardoll, D., and Mulligan, R.C.: Vaccination with irradiated tumor cells engineered to secrete murine granulocyte-macrophage colony-stimulating factor stimulates potent, specific, and long-lasting anti-tumor immunity. Proc. Natl. Acad. Sci. USA 90:3539, 1993.

157. Riviere, I., Brose, K., and Mulligan, R.C.: Effects of retroviral vector design on expression of human adenosine deaminase in murine bone marrow transplant recipients engrafted with genetically modified cells. Proc. Natl. Acad. Sci. USA 92:6733, 1995.

158. Emerman, M., and Temin, H.M.: Genes with promoters in retrovirus vectors can be independently suppressed by an epigenetic mechanism. Cell 39:459, 1984.

159. Hantzopoulos, P.A., Sullenger, B.A., Ungers, G., and Gilboa, E.: Improved gene expression upon transfer of the adenosine deaminase minigene outside the transcriptional unit of a retroviral vector. Proc. Natl. Acad. Sci. USA 86:3519, 1989.

160. Yu, S.F., von Ruden, T., Kantoff, P.W., Garber, C., Seiberg, M., Ruther, U., Anderson, W.F., Wagner, E.F., and Gilboa, E.: Self-inactivating retroviral vectors designed for transfer of whole genes into mammalian cells. Proc. Natl. Acad. Sci. USA 83:3194, 1986.

161. Hawley, R.G., Covarrubias, L., Hawley, T., and Mintz, B.: Handicapped retroviral vectors efficiently transduce foreign genes into hematopoietic stem cells. Proc. Natl. Acad. Sci. USA 84:2406, 1987.

162. Germann, U.A., Chin, K.V., Pastan, I., and Gottesman, M.M.: Retroviral transfer of a chimeric multidrug resistance–adenosine deaminase gene. FASEB J. 4:1501, 1990.

163. Jang, S.K., Davies, M.V., Kaufman, R.J., and Wimmer, E.: Initiation of protein synthesis by internal entry of ribosomes into the 5' nontranslated region of encephalomyocarditis virus RNA in vivo. J. Virol. 63:1651, 1989.

164. Morgan, R.A., Couture, L., Elroy-Stein, O., Ragheb, J., Moss, B., and Anderson, W.F.: Retroviral vectors containing putative internal ribosome entry sites: development of a polycistronic gene transfer system and applications to human gene therapy. Nucleic Acids Res. 20:1293, 1992.

165. Galipeau, J., Benaim, E., Spencer, H.T., Blakley, R.L., and Sorrentino, B.P.: A bicistronic retroviral vector for protecting hematopoietic cells against antifolates and P-glycoprotein effluxed drugs. Hum. Gene Ther. 8:1773, 1997.

166. Aran, J.M., Gottesman, M.M., and Pastan, I.: Drug-selected coexpression of human glucocerebrosidase and P-glycoprotein using a bicistronic vector. Proc. Natl. Acad. Sci. USA 91:3176, 1994.

167. Sugimoto, Y., Aksentijevich, I., Murray, G.J., Brady, R.O., Pastan, I., and Gottesman, M.M.: Retroviral coexpression of a multidrug resistance gene (MDR1) and human alpha-galactosidase A for gene therapy of Fabry disease. Hum. Gene Ther. 6:905, 1995.

168. Lieu, F.H., Hawley, T.S., Fong, A.Z., and Hawley, R.G.: Transmissibility of murine stem cell virus-based retroviral vectors carrying both interleukin-12 cDNAs and a third gene: implications for immune gene therapy. Cancer Gene Ther. 4:167, 1997.

169. Zufferey, R., Dull, T., Mandel, R.J., Bukovsky, A., Quiroz, D., Naldini, L., and Trono, D.: Self-inactivating lentivirus vector for safe and efficient in vivo gene delivery. J. Virol. 72:9873, 1998.

170. Dull, T., Zufferey, R., Kelly, M., Mandel, R.J., Nguyen, M., Trono, D., and Naldini, L.: A third-generation lentivirus vector with a conditional packaging system. J. Virol. 72:8463, 1998.

171. Zufferey, R., Nagy, D., Mandel, R.J., Naldini, L., and Trono, D.: Multiply attenuated lentiviral vector achieves efficient gene delivery in vivo. Nat. Biotechnol. 15:871, 1997.

172. Kim, V.N., Mitrophanous, K., Kingsman, S.M., and Kingsman, A.J.: Minimal requirement for a lentivirus vector based on human immunodeficiency virus type 1. J. Virol. 72:811, 1998.

173. Kafri, T., van Praag, H., Ouyang, L., Gage, F.H., and Verma, I.M.: A packaging cell line for lentivirus vectors. J. Virol. 73:576, 1999.

174. Ali, M., Taylor, G.P., Pitman, R.J., Parker, D., Rethwilm, A., Cheing-song-Popov, R., Weber, J.N., Bieniasz, P.D., Bradley, J., and McClure, M.O.: No evidence of antibody to human foamy virus in widespread human populations. AIDS Res. Hum. Retroviruses 12:1473, 1996.

175. Russell, D.W., and Miller, A.D.: Foamy virus vectors. J. Virol. 70:217, 1996.

176. Bieniasz, P.D., Erlwein, O., Aguzzi, A., Rethwilm, A., and McClure, M.O.: Gene transfer using replication-defective human foamy virus vectors. Virology 235:65, 1997.

177. Hirata, R.K., Miller, A.D., Andrews, R.G., and Russell, D.W.: Transduction of hematopoietic cells by foamy virus vectors. Blood 88:3654, 1996.

178. Erlwein, O., Bieniasz, P.D., and McClure, M.O.: Sequences in pol are required for transfer of human foamy virus-based vectors. J. Virol. 72:5510, 1998.

179. Samulski, R.J., Chang, L.S., and Shenk, T.: Helper-free stocks of recombinant adeno-associated viruses: normal integration does not require viral gene expression. J. Virol. 63:3822, 1989.

180. Yang, Y., and Wilson, J.M.: Clearance of adenovirus-infected hepatocytes by MHC class I–restricted CD4+ CTLs in vivo. J. Immunol. 155:2564, 1995.

181. Xiao, X., Li, J., and Samulski, R.J.: Production of high-titer recombinant adeno-associated virus vectors in the absence of helper adenovirus. J. Virol. 72:2224, 1998.

182. Ferrari, F.K., Xiao, X., McCarty, D., and Samulski, R.J.: New developments in the generation of Ad-free, high-titer rAAV gene therapy vectors. Nat. Med. 3:1295, 1997.

183. Summerford, C., and Samulski, R.J.: Membrane-associated heparan sulfate proteoglycan is a receptor for adeno-associated virus type 2 virions. J. Virol. 72:1438, 1998.

184. Mizukami, H., Young, N.S., and Brown, K.E.: Adeno-associated virus type 2 binds to a 150-kilodalton cell membrane glycoprotein. Virology 217:124, 1996.

185. Qing, K., Mah, C., Hansen, J., Zhou, S., Dwarki, V., and Srivastava, A.: Human fibroblast growth factor receptor 1 is a co-receptor for infection by adeno-associated virus 2. Nat. Med. 5:71, 1999.

186. Summerford, C., Bartlett, J.S., and Samulski, R.J.: α-V β-5 integrin: a co-receptor for adeno-associated virus type 2 infection. Nat. Med. 5:78, 1999.

187. Ferrari, F.K., Samulski, T., Shenk, T., and Samulski, R.J.: Second-strand synthesis is a rate-limiting step for efficient transduction by recombinant adeno-associated virus vectors. J. Virol. 70:3227, 1996.

188. Fisher, K.J., Gao, G.P., Weitzman, M.D., DeMatteo, R., Burda, J.F., and Wilson, J.M.: Transduction with recombinant adeno-associated virus for gene therapy is limited by leading-strand synthesis. J. Virol. 70:520, 1996.

189. Russell, D.W., Alexander, I.E., and Miller, A.D.: DNA synthesis and topoisomerase inhibitors increase transduction by adeno-associated virus vectors. Proc. Natl. Acad. Sci. USA 92:5719, 1995.

190. Alexander, I.E., Russell, D.W., Spence, A.M., and Miller, A.D.: Effects of gamma irradiation on the transduction of dividing and nondividing cells in brain and muscle of rats by adeno-associated virus vectors. Hum. Gene Ther. 7:841, 1996.

191. Ni, T.H., McDonald, W.F., Zolotukhin, I., Melendy, T., Waga, S., Stillman, B., and Muzyczka, N.: Cellular proteins required for adeno-associated virus DNA replication in the absence of adenovirus coinfection. J. Virol. 72:2777, 1998.

192. Qing, K., Khuntirat, B., Mah, C., Kube, D.M., Wang, X.S., Ponnazhagan, S., Zhou, S., Dwarki, V.J., Yoder, M.C., and Srivastava, A.: Adeno-associated virus type 2–mediated gene transfer: correlation of tyrosine phosphorylation of the cellular single-stranded D sequence–binding protein with transgene expression in human cells in vitro and murine tissues in vivo. J. Virol. 72:1593, 1998.

193. Bertran, J., Miller, J.L., Yang, Y., Fenimore-Justman, A., Rueda, F., Vanin, E.F., and Nienhuis, A.W.: Recombinant adeno-associated virus-mediated high-efficiency, transient expression of the murine cationic amino acid transporter (ecotropic retroviral receptor) permits stable transduction of human HeLa cells by ecotropic retroviral vectors. J. Virol. 70:6759, 1996.

194. Hargrove, P.W., Vanin, E.F., Kurtzman, G.J., and Nienhuis, A.W.: High-level globin gene expression mediated by a recombinant adeno-associated virus genome that contains the 3′ gamma globin gene regulatory element and integrates as tandem copies in erythroid cells. Blood 89:2167, 1997.

195. Malik, P., McQuiston, S.A., Yu, X.J., Pepper, K.A., Krall, W.J., Podsakoff, G.M., Kurtzman, G.J., and Kohn, D.B.: Recombinant adeno-associated virus mediates a high level of gene transfer but less efficient integration in the K562 human hematopoietic cell line. J. Virol. 71:1776, 1997.

196. Kotin, R.M., Linden, R.M., and Berns, K.I.: Characterization of a preferred site on human chromosome 19q for integration of adeno-associated virus DNA by non-homologous recombination. EMBO J. 11:5071, 1992.

197. Walsh, C.E., Liu, J.M., Xiao, X., Young, N.S., Nienhuis, A.W., and Samulski, R.J.: Regulated high level expression of a human gamma-globin gene introduced into erythroid cells by an adeno-associated virus vector. Proc. Natl. Acad. Sci. USA 89:7257, 1992.

198. Kearns, W.G., Afione, S.A., Fulmer, S.B., Pang, M.C., Erikson, D., Egan, M., Landrum, M.J., Flotte, T.R., and Cutting, G.R.: Recombinant adeno-associated virus (AAV-CFTR) vectors do not integrate in a site-specific fashion in an immortalized epithelial cell line. Gene Ther. 3:748, 1996.

199. Bertran, J., Yang, Y., Hargrove, P., Vanin, E.F., and Nienhuis, A.W.: Targeted integration of a recombinant globin gene adeno-associated viral vector into human chromosome 19. Ann. N. Y. Acad. Sci. 850:163, 1998.

200. Miller, J.L., Walsh, C.E., Ney, P.A., Samulski, R.J., and Nienhuis, A.W.: Single-copy transduction and expression of human gamma-globin in K562 erythroleukemia cells using recombinant adeno-associated virus vectors: the effect of mutations in NF-E2 and GATA-1 binding motifs within the hypersensitivity site 2 enhancer. Blood 82:1900, 1993.

201. Einerhand, M.P., Antoniou, M., Zolotukhin, S., Muzyczka, N., Berns, K.I., Grosveld, F., and Valerio, D.: Regulated high-level human beta-globin gene expression in erythroid cells following recombinant adeno-associated virus-mediated gene transfer. Gene Ther. 2:336, 1995.

202. Zhou, S.Z., Li, Q., Stamatoyannopoulos, G., and Srivastava, A.: Adeno-associated virus 2–mediated transduction and erythroid cell–specific expression of a human beta-globin gene. Gene Ther. 3:223, 1996.

203. Lubovy, M., McCune, S., Dong, J.Y., Prchal, J.F., Townes, T.M., and Prchal, J.T.: Stable transduction of recombinant adeno-associated virus into hematopoietic stem cells from normal and sickle cell patients. Biol. Blood Marrow Transplant. 2:24, 1996.

204. Goodman, S., Xiao, X., Donahue, R.E., Moulton, A., Miller, J., Walsh, C., Young, N.S., Samulski, R.J., and Nienhuis, A.W.: Recombinant adeno-associated virus–mediated gene transfer into hematopoietic progenitor cells. Blood 84:1492, 1994.

205. Fisher-Adams, G., Wong K.K.J., Podsakoff, G., Forman, S.J., and Chatterjee, S.: Integration of adeno-associated virus vectors in CD34⁺ human hematopoietic progenitor cells after transduction. Blood 88:492, 1996.

206. Zhou, S.Z., Cooper, S., Kang, L.Y., Ruggieri, L., Heimfeld, S., Srivastava, A., and Broxmeyer, H.E.: Adeno-associated virus 2–mediated high efficiency gene transfer into immature and mature subsets of hematopoietic progenitor cells in human umbilical cord blood. J. Exp. Med. 179:1867, 1994.

207. Miller, J.L., Donahue, R.E., Sellers, S.E., Samulski, R.J., Young, N.S., and Nienhuis, A.W.: Recombinant adeno-associated virus (rAAV)–mediated expression of a human gamma-globin gene in human progenitor-derived erythroid cells [published erratum appears in Proc. Natl. Acad. Sci. USA 92:646, 1995]. Proc. Natl. Acad. Sci. USA 91:10183, 1994.

208. Walsh, C.E., Nienhuis, A.W., Samulski, R.J., Brown, M.G., Miller, J.L., Young, N.S., and Liu, J.M.: Phenotypic correction of Fanconi anemia in human hematopoietic cells with a recombinant adeno-associated virus vector. J. Clin. Invest. 94:1440, 1994.

209. Ponnazhagan, S., Yoder, M.C., and Srivastava, A.: Adeno-associated virus type 2–mediated transduction of murine hematopoietic cells with long-term repopulating ability and sustained expression of a human globin gene in vivo. J. Virol. 71:3098, 1997.

210. Schimmenti, S., Boesen, J., Claassen, E.A., Valerio, D., and Einerhand, M.P.: Long-term genetic modification of rhesus monkey hematopoietic cells following transplantation of adenoassociated virus vector–transduced CD34⁺ cells. Hum. Gene Ther. 9:2727, 1998.

211. Ponnazhagan, S., Mukherjee, P., Wang, X.S., Qing, K., Kube, D.M., Mah, C., Kurpad, C., Yoder, M.C., Srour, E.F., and Srivastava, A.: Adeno-associated virus type 2–mediated transduction in primary human bone marrow–derived CD34⁺ hematopoietic progenitor cells: donor variation and correlation of transgene expression with cellular differentiation. J. Virol. 71:8262, 1997.

212. Snyder, R.O., Miao, C., Meuse, L., Tubb, J., Donahue, B.A., Lin, H.F., Stafford, D.W., Patel, S., Thompson, A.R., Nichols, T., Read, M.S., Bellinger, D.A., Brinkhous, K.M., and Kay, M.A.: Correction of hemophilia B in canine and murine models using recombinant adeno-associated viral vectors. Nat. Med. 5:64, 1999.

213. Herzog, R.W., Yang, E.Y., Couto, L.B., Hagstrom, J.N., Elwell, D., Fields, P.A., Burton, M., Bellinger, D.A., Read, M.S., Brinkhous, K.M., Podsakoff, G.M., Nichols, T.C., Kurtzman, G.J., and High, K.A.: Long-term correction of canine hemophilia B by gene transfer of blood coagulation factor IX mediated by adeno-associated viral vector. Nat. Med. 5:56, 1999.

214. Kessler, P.D., Podsakoff, G.M., Chen, X., McQuiston, S.A., Colosi, P.C., Matelis, L.A., Kurtzman, G.J., and Byrne, B.J.: Gene delivery to skeletal muscle results in sustained expression and systemic delivery of a therapeutic protein. Proc. Natl. Acad. Sci. USA 93:14082, 1996.

215. Fisher, K.J., Jooss, K., Alston, J., Yang, Y., Haecker, S.E., High, K., Pathak, R., Raper, S.E., and Wilson, J.M.: Recombinant adeno-associated virus for muscle directed gene therapy. Nat. Med. 3:306, 1997.

216. Koeberl, D.D., Alexander, I.E., Halbert, C.L., Russell, D.W., and Miller, A.D.: Persistent expression of human clotting factor IX from mouse liver after intravenous injection of adeno-associated virus vectors. Proc. Natl. Acad. Sci. USA 94:1426, 1997.

217. Nakai, H., Herzog, R.W., Hagstrom, J.N., Walter, J., Kung, S.H., Yang, E.Y., Tai, S.J., Iwaki, Y., Kurtzman, G.J., Fisher, K.J., Colosi, P., Couto, L.B., and High, K.A.: Adeno-associated viral vector–mediated gene transfer of human blood coagulation factor IX into mouse liver. Blood 91:4600, 1998.

218. Snyder, R.O., Miao, C.H., Patijn, G.A., Spratt, S.K., Danos, O., Nagy, D., Gown, A.M., Winther, B., Meuse, L., Cohen, L.K., Thompson, A.R., and Kay, M.A.: Persistent and therapeutic concentrations of human factor IX in mice after hepatic gene transfer of recombinant AAV vectors. Nat. Genet. 16:270, 1997.

219. Watanabe, T., Kuszynski, C., Ino, K., Heimann, D.G., Shepard, H.M., Yasui, Y., Maneval, D.C., and Talmadge, J.E.: Gene transfer into human bone marrow hematopoietic cells mediated by adenovirus vectors. Blood 87:5032, 1996.

220. Frey, B.M., Hackett, N.R., Bergelson, J.M., Finberg, R., Crystal, R.G., Moore, M.A., and Rafii, S.: High-efficiency gene transfer into ex vivo expanded human hematopoietic progenitors and precursor cells by adenovirus vectors. Blood 91:2781, 1998.

221. Neering, S.J., Hardy, S.F., Minamoto, D., Spratt, S.K., and Jordan, C.T.: Transduction of primitive human hematopoietic cells with recombinant adenovirus vectors. Blood 88:1147, 1996.

222. Bergelson, J.M., Cunningham, J.A., Droguett, G., Kurt-Jones, E.A.,

Krithivas, A., Hong, J.S., Horwitz, M.S., Crowell, R.L., and Finberg, R.W.: Isolation of a common receptor for coxsackie B viruses and adenoviruses 2 and 5. Science 275:1320, 1997.

223. Tomko, R.P., Xu, R., and Philipson, L.: HCAR and MCAR: the human and mouse cellular receptors for subgroup C adenoviruses and group B coxsackieviruses. Proc. Natl. Acad. Sci. USA 94:3352, 1997.

224. Wickham, T.J., Mathias, P., Cheresh, D.A., and Nemerow, G.R.: Integrins alpha v beta 3 and alpha v beta 5 promote adenovirus internalization but not virus attachment. Cell 73:309, 1993.

225. Dmitriev, I., Krasnykh, V., Miller, C.R., Wang, M., Kashentseva, E., Mikheeva, G., Belousova, N., and Curiel, D.T.: An adenovirus vector with genetically modified fibers demonstrates expanded tropism via utilization of a coxsackievirus and adenovirus receptor-independent cell entry mechanism. J. Virol. 72:9706, 1998.

226. Krasnykh, V., Dmitriev, I., Mikheeva, G., Miller, C.R., Belousova, N., and Curiel, D.T.: Characterization of an adenovirus vector containing a heterologous peptide epitope in the HI loop of the fiber knob. J. Virol. 72:1844, 1998.

227. Wickham, T.J., Tzeng, E., Shears, L.L., Roelvink, P.W., Li, Y., Lee, G.M., Brough, D.E., Lizonova, A., and Kovesdi, I.: Increased in vitro and in vivo gene transfer by adenovirus vectors containing chimeric fiber proteins. J. Virol. 71:8221, 1997.

228. Wickham, T.J., Segal, D.M., Roelvink, P.W., Carrion, M.E., Lizonova, A., Lee, G.M., and Kovesdi, I.: Targeted adenovirus gene transfer to endothelial and smooth muscle cells by using bispecific antibodies. J. Virol. 70:6831, 1996.

229. Goldman, C.K., Rogers, B.E., Douglas, J.T., Sosnowski, B.A., Ying, W., Siegal, G.P., Baird, A., Campain, J.A., and Curiel, D.T.: Targeted gene delivery to Kaposi's sarcoma cells via the fibroblast growth factor receptor. Cancer Res. 57:1447, 1997.

230. Douglas, J.T., Rogers, B.E., Rosenfeld, M.E., Michael, S.I., Feng, M., and Curiel, D.T.: Targeted gene delivery by tropism-modified adenoviral vectors. Nat. Biotechnol. 14:1574, 1996.

231. Wickham, T.J., Lee, G.M., Titus, J.A., Sconocchia, G., Bakacs, T., Kovesdi, I., and Segal, D.M.: Targeted adenovirus-mediated gene delivery to T cells via CD3. J. Virol. 71:7663, 1997.

232. Huang, S., Kamata, T., Takada, Y., Ruggeri, Z.M., and Nemerow, G.R.: Adenovirus interaction with distinct integrins mediates separate events in cell entry and gene delivery to hematopoietic cells. J. Virol. 70:4502, 1996.

233. Teoh, G., Chen, L., Urashima, M., Tai, Y., Celi, L.A., Chen, D., Chauhan, D., Ogata, A., Finberg, R.W., Webb, I.J., Kufe, D.W., and Anderson, K.C.: Adenovirus vector–based purging of multiple myeloma cells. Blood 92:4591, 1999.

234. Li, Q., Kay, M.A., Finegold, M., Stratford-Perricaudet, L.D., and Woo, S.L.: Assessment of recombinant adenoviral vectors for hepatic gene therapy. Hum. Gene Ther. 4:403, 1993.

235. Yang, Y., Nunes, F.A., Berencsi, K., Furth, E.E., Gonczol, E., and Wilson, J.M.: Cellular immunity to viral antigens limits E1-deleted adenoviruses for gene therapy. Proc. Natl. Acad. Sci. USA 91:4407, 1994.

236. Brody, S.L., Metzger, M., Danel, C., Rosenfeld, M.A., and Crystal, R.G.: Acute responses of non-human primates to airway delivery of an adenovirus vector containing the human cystic fibrosis transmembrane conductance regulator cDNA. Hum. Gene Ther. 5:821, 1994.

237. Simon, R.H., Engelhardt, J.F., Yang, Y., Zepeda, M., Weber-Pendleton, S., Grossman, M., and Wilson, J.M.: Adenovirus-mediated transfer of the CFTR gene to lung of nonhuman primates: toxicity study. Hum. Gene Ther. 4:771, 1993.

238. Engelhardt, J.F., Ye, X., Doranz, B., and Wilson, J.M.: Ablation of E2A in recombinant adenoviruses improves transgene persistence and decreases inflammatory response in mouse liver. Proc. Natl. Acad. Sci. USA 91:6196, 1994.

239. Goldman, M.J., Litzky, L.A., Engelhardt, J.F., and Wilson, J.M.: Transfer of the CFTR gene to the lung of nonhuman primates with E1-deleted, E2a-defective recombinant adenoviruses: a preclinical toxicology study. Hum. Gene Ther. 6:839, 1995.

240. Bett, A.J., Krougliak, V., and Graham, F.L.: DNA sequence of the deletion/insertion in early region 3 of Ad5 dl309. Virus Res. 39:75, 1995.

241. Gao, G.P., Yang, Y., and Wilson, J.M.: Biology of adenovirus vectors with E1 and E4 deletions for liver-directed gene therapy. J. Virol. 70:8934, 1996.

242. Dai, Y., Schwarz, E.M., Gu, D., Zhang, W.W., Sarvetnick, N., and Verma, I.M.: Cellular and humoral immune responses to adenoviral vectors containing factor IX gene: tolerization of factor IX and vector antigens allows for long-term expression. Proc. Natl. Acad. Sci. USA 92:1401, 1995.

243. Morral, N., O'Neal, W., Zhou, H., Langston, C., and Beaudet, A.: Immune responses to reporter proteins and high viral dose limit duration of expression with adenoviral vectors: comparison of E2a wild type and E2a deleted vectors. Hum. Gene Ther. 8:1275, 1997.

244. Jooss, K., Yang, Y., Fisher, K.J., and Wilson, J.M.: Transduction of dendritic cells by DNA viral vectors directs the immune response to transgene products in muscle fibers. J. Virol. 72:4212, 1998.

245. Fisher, K.J., Choi, H., Burda, J., Chen, S.J., and Wilson, J.M.: Recombinant adenovirus deleted of all viral genes for gene therapy of cystic fibrosis. Virology 217:11, 1996.

246. Parks, R.J., and Graham, F.L.: A helper-dependent system for adenovirus vector production helps define a lower limit for efficient DNA packaging. J. Virol. 71:3293, 1997.

247. Chen, H.H., Mack, L.M., Kelly, R., Ontell, M., Kochanek, S., and Clemens, P.R.: Persistence in muscle of an adenoviral vector that lacks all viral genes. Proc. Natl. Acad. Sci. USA 94:1645, 1997.

248. Morsy, M.A., Gu, M., Motzel, S., Zhao, J., Lin, J., Su, Q., Allen, H., Franlin, L., Parks, R.J., Graham, F.L., Kochanek, S., Bett, A.J., and Caskey, C.T.: An adenoviral vector deleted for all viral coding sequences results in enhanced safety and extended expression of a leptin transgene. Proc. Natl. Acad. Sci. USA 95:7866, 1998.

249. Ilan, Y., Droguett, G., Chowdhury, N.R., Li, Y., Sengupta, K., Thummala, N.R., Davidson, A., Chowdhury, J.R., and Horwitz, M.S.: Insertion of the adenoviral E3 region into a recombinant viral vector prevents antiviral humoral and cellular immune responses and permits long-term gene expression. Proc. Natl. Acad. Sci. USA 94:2587, 1997.

250. Jooss, K., Yang, Y., and Wilson, J.M.: Cyclophosphamide diminishes inflammation and prolongs transgene expression following delivery of adenoviral vectors to mouse liver and lung. Hum. Gene Ther. 7:1555, 1996.

251. Ilan, Y., Prakash, R., Davidson, A., Jona, Droguett, G., Horwitz, M.S., Chowdhury, N.R., and Chowdhury, J.R.: Oral tolerization to adenoviral antigens permits long-term gene expression using recombinant adenoviral vectors. J. Clin. Invest. 99:1098, 1997.

252. Mack, C.A., Song, W.R., Carpenter, H., Wickham, T.J., Kovesdi, I., Harvey, B.G., Magovern, C.J., Isom, O.W., Rosengart, T., Falck-Pedersen, E., Hackett, N.R., Crystal, R.G., and Mastrangeli, A.: Circumvention of anti-adenovirus neutralizing immunity by administration of an adenoviral vector of an alternate serotype. Hum. Gene Ther. 8:99, 1997.

253. Kochanek, S., Clemens, P.R., Mitani, K., Chen, H.H., Chan, S., and Caskey, C.T.: A new adenoviral vector: replacement of all viral coding sequences with 28 kb of DNA independently expressing both full-length dystrophin and beta-galactosidase. Proc. Natl. Acad. Sci. USA 93:5731, 1996.

254. Schiedner, G., Morral, N., Parks, R.J., Wu, Y., Koopmans, S.C., Langston, C., Graham, F.L., Beaudet, A.L., and Kochanek, S.: Genomic DNA transfer with a high-capacity adenovirus vector results in improved in vivo gene expression and decreased toxicity. Nat. Genet. 18:180, 1998.

255. Oppenheim, A., Peleg, A., Fibach, E., and Rachmilewitz, E.A.: Efficient introduction of plasmid DNA into human hemopoietic cells by encapsidation in simian virus 40 pseudovirions. Proc. Natl. Acad. Sci. USA 83:6925, 1986.

256. Rund, D., Dagan, M., Dalyot-Herman, N., Kimchi-Sarfaty, C., Schoenlein, P.V., Gottesman, M.M., and Oppenheim, A.: Efficient transduction of human hematopoietic cells with the human multidrug resistance gene 1 via SV40 pseudovirions. Hum. Gene Ther. 9:649, 1998.

257. Sandalon, Z., Dalyot-Herman, N., Oppenheim, A.B., and Oppenheim, A.: In vitro assembly of SV40 virions and pseudovirions: vector development for gene therapy. Hum. Gene Ther. 8:843, 1997.

258. Dilloo, D., Rill, D., Entwistle, C., Boursnell, M., Zhong, W., Holden, W., Holladay, M., Inglis, S., and Brenner, M.: A novel herpes vector for the high-efficiency transduction of normal and malignant human hematopoietic cells. Blood 89:119, 1997.

259. Anderson, W.F.: Musings on the struggle—part I. The "phonebook." Hum. Gene Ther. 3:251, 1992.

260. Anderson, W.F.: Musings on the struggle—part V. Beginning the N2/TIL protocol. Hum. Gene Ther. 5:427, 1994.

261. Anderson, W.F.: Musings on the struggle—part IV. Aftermath of the RAC meeting. Hum. Gene Ther. 4:555, 1993.

262. Anderson, W.F.: Musings on the struggle—part III. The October 3 RAC meeting. Hum. Gene Ther. 4:401, 1993.

263. Anderson, W.F.: Musings on the struggle—part II. The N2-TIL protocol. Hum. Gene Ther. 4:237, 1993.

264. Rosenberg, S.A., Aebersold, P., Cornetta, K., Kasid, A., Morgan, R.A., Moen, R., Karson, E.M., Lotze, M.T., Yang, J.C., and Topalian, S.L.: Gene transfer into humans—immunotherapy of patients with advanced melanoma, using tumor-infiltrating lymphocytes modified by retroviral gene transduction. N. Engl. J. Med. 323:570, 1990.

265. Goodell, M.A., Rosenzweig, M., Kim, H., Marks, D.F., DeMaria, M., Paradis, G., Grupp, S.A., Sieff, C.A., Mulligan, R.C., and Johnson, R.P.: Dye efflux studies suggest that hematopoietic stem cells expressing low or undetectable levels of CD34 antigen exist in multiple species. Nat. Med. 3:1337, 1997.

266. Brenner, M.K., Rill, D.R., Moen, R.C., Krance, R.A., Mirro, J.J., Anderson, W.F., and Ihle, J.N.: Gene-marking to trace origin of relapse after autologous bone-marrow transplantation. Lancet 341:85, 1993.

267. Rill, D.R., Santana, V.M., Roberts, W.M., Nilson, T., Bowman, L.C., Krance, R.A., Heslop, H.E., Moen, R.C., Ihle, J.N., and Brenner, M.K.: Direct demonstration that autologous bone marrow transplantation for solid tumors can return a multiplicity of tumorigenic cells. Blood 84:380, 1994.

268. Deisseroth, A.B., Zu, Z., Claxton, D., Hanania, E.G., Fu, S., Ellerson, D., Goldberg, L., Thomas, M., Janicek, K., and Anderson, W.F.: Genetic marking shows that Ph+ cells present in autologous transplants of chronic myelogenous leukemia (CML) contribute to relapse after autologous bone marrow in CML. Blood 83:3068, 1994.

269. Rooney, C.M., Smith, C.A., Ng, C.Y., Loftin, S., Li, C., Krance, R.A., Brenner, M.K., and Heslop, H.E.: Use of gene-modified virus-specific T lymphocytes to control Epstein-Barr-virus–related lymphoproliferation. Lancet 345:9, 1995.

270. Heslop, H.E., Ng, C.Y., Li, C., Smith, C.A., Loftin, S.K., Krance, R.A., Brenner, M.K., and Rooney, C.M.: Long-term restoration of immunity against Epstein-Barr virus infection by adoptive transfer of gene-modified virus-specific T lymphocytes. Nat. Med. 2:551, 1996.

271. Rooney, C.M., Smith, C.A., Ng, C.Y., Loftin, S.K., Sixbey, J.W., Gan, Y., Srivastava, D.K., Bowman, L.C., Krance, R.A., Brenner, M.K., and Heslop, H.E.: Infusion of cytotoxic T cells for the prevention and treatment of Epstein-Barr virus–induced lymphoma in allogeneic transplant recipients. Blood 92:1549, 1998.

272. Roskrow, M.A., Suzuki, N., Gan, Y., Sixbey, J.W., Ng, C.Y., Kimbrough, S., Hudson, M., Brenner, M.K., Heslop, H.E., and Rooney, C.M.: Epstein-Barr virus (EBV)–specific cytotoxic T lymphocytes for the treatment of patients with EBV-positive relapsed Hodgkin's disease. Blood 91:2925, 1998.

273. Parkman, R., Gelfand, E.W., Rosen, F.S., Sanderson, A., and Hirschhorn, R.: Severe combined immunodeficiency and adenosine deaminase deficiency. N. Engl. J. Med. 292:714, 1975.

274. Hirschhorn, R., Beratis, N., and Rosen, F.S.: Characterization of residual enzyme activity in fibroblasts from patients with adenosine deaminase deficiency and combined immunodeficiency: evidence for a mutant enzyme. Proc. Natl. Acad. Sci. USA 73:213, 1976.

275. Kantoff, P.W., Gillio, A.P., McLachlin, J.R., Bordignon, C., Eglitis, M.A., Kernan, N.A., Moen, R.C., Kohn, D.B., Yu, S.F., and Karson, E.: Expression of human adenosine deaminase in nonhuman primates after retrovirus-mediated gene transfer. J. Exp. Med. 166:219, 1987.

276. van Beusechem, V.W., Kukler, A., Heidt, P.J., and Valerio, D.: Long-term expression of human adenosine deaminase in rhesus monkeys transplanted with retrovirus-infected bone-marrow cells. Proc. Natl. Acad. Sci. USA 89:7640, 1992.

277. Bodine, D.M., Moritz, T., Donahue, R.E., Luskey, B.D., Kessler, S.W., Martin, D.I., Orkin, S.H., Nienhuis, A.W., and Williams, D.A.: Long-term in vivo expression of a murine adenosine deaminase gene in rhesus monkey hematopoietic cells of multiple lineages after retroviral mediated gene transfer into CD34+ bone marrow cells. Blood 82:1975, 1993.

278. Egashira, M., Ariga, T., Kawamura, N., Miyoshi, O., Niikawa, N., and Sakiyama, Y.: Visible integration of the adenosine deaminase (ADA) gene into the recipient genome after gene therapy. Am. J. Med. Genet. 75:314, 1998.

279. Onodera, M., Ariga, T., Kawamura, N., Kobayashi, I., Ohtsu, M., Yamada, M., Tame, A., Furuta, H., Okano, M., Matsumoto, S., Kotani, H., McGarrity, G.J., Blaese, R.M., and Sakiyama, Y.: Successful peripheral T-lymphocyte–directed gene transfer for a patient with severe combined immune deficiency caused by adenosine deaminase deficiency. Blood 91:30, 1998.

280. Kohn, D.B., Weinberg, K.I., Nolta, J.A., Heiss, L.N., Lenarsky, C., Crooks, G.M., Hanley, M.E., Annett, G., Brooks, J.S., and el-Khoureiy, A.: Engraftment of gene-modified umbilical cord blood cells in neonates with adenosine deaminase deficiency. Nat. Med. 1:1017, 1995.

281. Kohn, D.B., Hershfield, M.S., Carbonaro, D., Shigeoka, A., Brooks, J., Smogorzewska, E.M., Barsky, L.W., Chan, R., Burotto, F., Annett, G., Nolta, J.A., Crooks, G.M., Kapoor, N., Elder, M., Ara, D., Owen, T., Madsen, E., Snyder, F.F., Bastian, J., Muul, L., Blaese, R.M., Weinberg, K., and Parkman, R.: T lymphocytes with a normal ADA gene accumulate after transplantation of transduced autologous umbilical cord blood CD34+ cells in ADA-deficient SCID neonates. Nat. Med. 4:775, 1998.

282. Buckley, R.H., Schiff, R.I., Schiff, S.E., Markert, M.L., Williams, L.W., Harville, T.O., Roberts, J.L., and Puck, J.M.: Human severe combined immunodeficiency: genetic, phenotypic, and functional diversity in one hundred eight infants. J. Pediatr. 130:378, 1997.

283. Noguchi, M., Yi, H., Rosenblatt, H.M., Filipovich, A.H., Adelstein, S., Modi, W.S., McBride, O.W., and Leonard, W.J.: Interleukin-2 receptor gamma chain mutation results in X-linked severe combined immunodeficiency in humans. Cell 73:147, 1993.

284. Cao, X., Shores, E.W., Hu-Li, J., Anver, M.R., Kelsall, B.L., Russell, S.M., Drago, J., Noguchi, M., Grinberg, A., Bloom, E.T., et al.: Defective lymphoid development in mice lacking expression of the common cytokine receptor gamma chain. Immunity 2:223, 1995.

285. Miyazaki, T., Kawahara, A., Fujii, H., Nakagawa, Y., Minami, Y., Liu, Z.J., Oishi, I., Silvennoinen, O., Witthuhn, B.A., Ihle, J.N., et al.: Functional activation of Jak1 and Jak3 by selective association with IL-2 receptor subunits. Science 266:1045, 1994.

286. Russell, S.M., Johnston, J.A., Noguchi, M., Kawamura, M., Bacon, C.M., Friedmann, M., Berg, M., McVicar, D.W., Witthuhn, B.A., Silvennoinen, O., et al.: Interaction of IL-2R beta and gamma c chains with Jak1 and Jak3: implications for XSCID and XCID. Science 266:1042, 1994.

287. Russell, S.M., Tayebi, N., Nakajima, H., Riedy, M.C., Roberts, J.L., Aman, M.J., Migone, T.S., Noguchi, M., Markert, M.L., Buckley, R.H., et al.: Mutation of Jak3 in a patient with SCID: essential role of Jak3 in lymphoid development. Science 270:797, 1995.

288. Macchi, P., Villa, A., Gillani, S., Sacco, M.G., Frattini, A., Porta, F., Ugazio, A.G., Johnston, J.A., Candotti, F., and O'Shea, J.J.: Mutations of Jak-3 gene in patients with autosomal severe combined immune deficiency (SCID). Nature 377:65, 1995.

289. Fischer, A., Landais, P., Friedrich, W., Morgan, G., Gerritsen, B., Fasth, A., Porta, F., Griscelli, C., Goldman, S.F., Levinsky, R., et al.: European experience of bone-marrow transplantation for severe combined immunodeficiency. Lancet 336:850, 1990.

290. Buckley, R.H., Schiff, S.E., Schiff, R.I., Roberts, J.L., Markert, M.L., Peters, W., Williams, L.W., and Ward, F.E.: Haploidentical bone marrow stem cell transplantation in human severe combined immunodeficiency. Semin. Hematol. 30:92, 1993.

291. Haddad, E., Landais, P., Friedrich, W., Gerritsen, B., Cavazzana-Calvo, M., Morgan, G., Bertrand, Y., Fasth, A., Porta, F., Cant, A., Espanol, T., Muller, S., Veys, P., Vossen, J., and Fischer, A.: Long-term immune reconstitution and outcome after HLA-nonidentical T-cell–depleted bone marrow transplantation for severe combined immunodeficiency: a European retrospective study of 116 patients. Blood 91:3646, 1998.

292. Candotti, F., Johnston, J.A., Puck, J.M., Sugamura, K., O'Shea, J.J., and Blaese, R.M.: Retroviral-mediated gene correction for X-linked severe combined immunodeficiency. Blood 87:3097, 1996.

293. Candotti, F., Oakes, S.A., Johnston, J.A., Notarangelo, L.D., O'Shea, J.J., and Blaese, R.M.: In vitro correction of JAK3-deficient severe combined immunodeficiency by retroviral-mediated gene transduction. J. Exp. Med. 183:2687, 1996.

294. Taylor, N., Uribe, L., Smith, S., Jahn, T., Kohn, D.B., and Weinberg, K.: Correction of interleukin-2 receptor function in X-SCID lymphoblastoid cells by retrovirally mediated transfer of the gamma-c gene. Blood 87:3103, 1996.

295. Nosaka, T., van Deursen, J.M., Tripp, R.A., Thierfelder, W.E., Witthuhn, B.A., McMickle, A.P., Doherty, P.C., Grosveld, G.C., and Ihle, J.N.: Defective lymphoid development in mice lacking Jak3. Science 270:800, 1995.

296. Bunting, K.D., Sangster, M.Y., Ihle, J.N., and Sorrentino, B.P.: Restoration of lymphocyte function in Janus kinase 3–deficient mice by retroviral-mediated gene transfer. Nat. Med. 4:58, 1998.

297. Bunting, K.D., Flynn, K.J., Riberdy, J.M., Doherty, P.C., and Sorrentino, B.P.: Virus-specific immunity after gene therapy in a murine model of severe combined immunodeficiency. Proc. Natl. Acad. Sci. USA 96:232, 1999.

298. DiSanto, J.P., Muller, W., Guy-Grand, D., Fischer, A., and Rajewsky, K.: Lymphoid development in mice with a targeted deletion of the interleukin 2 receptor gamma chain. Proc. Natl. Acad. Sci. USA 92:377, 1995.

299. Henthorn, P.S., Somberg, R.L., Fimiani, V.M., Puck, J.M., Patterson, D.F., and Felsburg, P.J.: IL-2R gamma gene microdeletion demonstrates that canine X-linked severe combined immunodeficiency is a homologue of the human disease. Genomics 23:69, 1994.

300. Whitwam, T., Haskins, M.E., Henthorn, P.S., Kraszewski, J.N., Kleiman, S.E., Seidel, N.E., Bodine, D.M., and Puck, J.M.: Retroviral marking of canine bone marrow: long-term, high-level expression of human interleukin-2 receptor common gamma chain in canine lymphocytes. Blood 92:1565, 1998.

301. Dinauer, M.C., Orkin, S.H., Brown, R., Jesaitis, A.J., and Parkos, C.A.: The glycoprotein encoded by the X-linked chronic granulomatous disease locus is a component of the neutrophil cytochrome *b* complex. Nature 327:717, 1987.

302. Sekhsaria, S., Gallin, J.I., Linton, G.F., Mallory, R.M., Mulligan, R.C., and Malech, H.L.: Peripheral blood progenitors as a target for genetic correction of p47phox-deficient chronic granulomatous disease. Proc. Natl. Acad. Sci. USA 90:7446, 1993.

303. Li, F., Linton, G.F., Sekhsaria, S., Whiting-Theobald, N., Katkin, J.P., Gallin, J.I., and Malech, H.L.: CD34+ peripheral blood progenitors as a target for genetic correction of the two flavocytochrome b558 defective forms of chronic granulomatous disease. Blood 84:53, 1994.

304. Kume, A., and Dinauer, M.C.: Retrovirus-mediated reconstitution of respiratory burst activity in X-linked chronic granulomatous disease cells. Blood 84:3311, 1994.

305. Cobbs, C.S., Malech, H.L., Leto, T.L., Freeman, S.M., Blaese, R.M., Gallin, J.I., and Lomax, K.J.: Retroviral expression of recombinant p47phox protein by Epstein-Barr virus–transformed B lymphocytes from a patient with autosomal chronic granulomatous disease. Blood 79:1829, 1992.

306. Weil, W.M., Linton, G.F., Whiting-Theobald, N., Vowells, S.J., Rafferty, S.P., Li, F., and Malech, H.L.: Genetic correction of p67phox deficient chronic granulomatous disease using peripheral blood progenitor cells as a target for retrovirus mediated gene transfer. Blood 89:1754, 1997.

307. Pollock, J.D., Williams, D.A., Gifford, M.A., Li, L.L., Du, X., Fisherman, J., Orkin, S.H., Doerschuk, C.M., and Dinauer, M.C.: Mouse model of X-linked chronic granulomatous disease, an inherited defect in phagocyte superoxide production. Nat. Genet. 9:202, 1995.

308. Jackson, S.H., Gallin, J.I., and Holland, S.M.: The p47phox mouse knock-out model of chronic granulomatous disease. J. Exp. Med. 182:751, 1995.

309. Bjorgvinsdottir, H., Ding, C., Pech, N., Gifford, M.A., Li, L.L., and Dinauer, M.C.: Retroviral-mediated gene transfer of gp91phox into bone marrow cells rescues defect in host defense against *Aspergillus fumigatus* in murine X-linked chronic granulomatous disease. Blood 89:41, 1997.

310. Mardiney, M., and Malech, H.L.: Enhanced engraftment of hematopoietic progenitor cells in mice treated with granulocyte colony-stimulating factor before low-dose irradiation: implications for gene therapy. Blood 87:4049, 1996.

311. Mardiney, M., Jackson, S.H., Spratt, S.K., Li, F., Holland, S.M., and Malech, H.L.: Enhanced host defense after gene transfer in the murine p47phox-deficient model of chronic granulomatous disease. Blood 89:2268, 1997.

312. Malech, H.L., Maples, P.B., Whiting-Theobald, N., Linton, G.F., Sekhsaria, S., Vowells, S.J., Li, F., Miller, J.A., DeCarlo, E., Holland, S.M., Leitman, S.F., Carter, C.S., Butz, R.E., Read, E.J., Fleisher, T.A., Schneiderman, R.D., Van Epps, D.E., Spratt, S.K., Maack, C.A., Rokovich, J.A., Cohen, L.K., and Gallin, J.I.: Prolonged production of NADPH oxidase-corrected granulocytes after gene therapy of chronic granulomatous disease. Proc. Natl. Acad. Sci. USA 94:12133, 1997.

313. Davis, J.L., Witt, R.M., Gross, P.R., Hokanson, C.A., Jungles, S., Cohen, L.K., Danos, O., and Spratt, S.K.: Retroviral particles produced from a stable human-derived packaging cell line transduce target cells with very high efficiencies. Hum. Gene Ther. 8:1459, 1997.

314. Malech, H.L., Horwitz, M.E., Linton, G.F., Theobald-Whiting, N., Brown, M.R., Farrell, C.J., Butz, R.E., Carter, C.S., DeCarlo, E.,

Miller, J.A., Van Epps, D.E., Read, E.J., and Fleisher, T.A.: Extended production of oxidase normal neutrophils in X-linked chronic granulomatous disease (CGD) following gene therapy with gp91phox transduced CD34+ cells [abstract]. Blood 92:690a, 1998.

315. Braun, S.E., Pan, D., Aronovich, E.L., Jonsson, J.J., McIvor, R.S., and Whitley, C.B.: Preclinical studies of lymphocyte gene therapy for mild Hunter syndrome (mucopolysaccharidosis type II). Hum. Gene Ther. 7:283, 1996.

316. Braun, S.E., Aronovich, E.L., Anderson, R.A., Crotty, P.L., McIvor, R.S., and Whitley, C.B.: Metabolic correction and cross-correction of mucopolysaccharidosis type II (Hunter syndrome) by retroviral-mediated gene transfer and expression of human iduronate-2-sulfatase. Proc. Natl. Acad. Sci. USA 90:11830, 1993.

317. Hahn, C.N., del Pilar, M., Schroder, M., Vanier, M.T., Hara, Y., Suzuki, K., and d'Azzo, A.: Generalized CNS disease and massive GM1-ganglioside accumulation in mice defective in lysosomal acid beta-galactosidase. Hum. Mol. Genet. 6:205, 1997.

318. Wolfe, J.H., Sands, M.S., Barker, J.E., Gwynn, B., Rowe, L.B., Vogler, C.A., and Birkenmeier, E.H.: Reversal of pathology in murine mucopolysaccharidosis type VII by somatic cell gene transfer. Nature 360:749, 1992.

319. Correll, P.H., Colilla, S., Dave, H.P., and Karlsson, S.: High levels of human glucocerebrosidase activity in macrophages of long-term reconstituted mice after retroviral infection of hematopoietic stem cells. Blood 80:331, 1992.

320. Correll, P.H., Colilla, S., and Karlsson, S.: Retroviral vector design for long-term expression in murine hematopoietic cells in vivo. Blood 84:1812, 1994.

321. Xu, L.C., Karlsson, S., Byrne, E.R., Kluepfel-Stahl, S., Kessler, S.W., Agricola, B.A., Sellers, S., Kirby, M., Dunbar, C.E., and Brady, R.O.: Long-term in vivo expression of the human glucocerebrosidase gene in nonhuman primates after CD34+ hematopoietic cell transduction with cell-free retroviral vector preparations. Proc. Natl. Acad. Sci. USA 92:4372, 1995.

322. Krall, W.J., Challita, P.M., Perlmutter, L.S., Skelton, D.C., and Kohn, D.B.: Cells expressing human glucocerebrosidase from a retroviral vector repopulate macrophages and central nervous system microglia after murine bone marrow transplantation. Blood 83:2737, 1994.

323. Kennedy, D.W., and Abkowitz, J.L.: Kinetics of central nervous system microglial and macrophage engraftment: analysis using a transgenic bone marrow transplantation model. Blood 90:986, 1997.

324. Eglitis, M.A., and Mezey, E.: Hematopoietic cells differentiate into both microglia and macroglia in the brains of adult mice. Proc. Natl. Acad. Sci. USA 94:4080, 1997.

325. Kaplitt, M.G., Leone, P., Samulski, R.J., Xiao, X., Pfaff, D.W., O'Malley, K.L., and During, M.J.: Long-term gene expression and phenotypic correction using adeno-associated virus vectors in the mammalian brain. Nat. Genet. 8:148, 1994.

326. Barranger, J.A., Rice, E.O., Dunigan, J., Sansieri, C., Takiyama, N., Beeler, M., Lancia, J., Lucot, S., Scheirer-Fochler, S., Mohney, T., Swaney, W., Bahnson, A., and Ball, E.: Gaucher's disease: studies of gene transfer to haematopoietic cells. Baillieres Clin. Haematol. 10:765, 1997.

327. Barranger, J.A., Rice, E., Sansieri, C., Bahnson, A., Mohney, T., Swaney, W., Takiyama, N., Dunigan, J., Beeler, M., Lucot, S., Schierer-Fochler, S., and Ball, E.: Transfer of the glucocerebrosidase gene to CD34 cells and their autologous transplantation in patients with Gaucher disease [abstract]. Blood 90:405a, 1997.

328. Dunbar, C.E., Kohn, D.B., Schiffmann, R., Barton, N.W., Nolta, J.A., Wells, S., Esplin, J., Pensiero, M., Emmons, R.V., Leitman, S., Kreps, C.B., Carter, C., Kimball, J., Young, N.S., Brady, R.O., and Karlsson, S.: Retroviral gene transfer of the glucocerebrosidase gene into PB or BM CD34+ cells from patients with Gaucher disease: results from a clinical trial [abstract]. Blood 90:237a, 1997.

329. Medin, J.A., Migita, M., Pawliuk, R., Jacobson, S., Amiri, M., Kluepfel-Stahl, S., Brady, R.O., Humphries, R.K., and Karlsson, S.: A bicistronic therapeutic retroviral vector enables sorting of transduced CD34+ cells and corrects the enzyme deficiency in cells from Gaucher patients. Blood 87:1754, 1996.

330. Aran, J.M., Licht, T., Gottesman, M.M., and Pastan, I.: Complete restoration of glucocerebrosidase deficiency in Gaucher fibroblasts using a bicistronic MDR retrovirus and a new selection strategy. Hum. Gene Ther. 7:2165, 1996.

331. Strathdee, C.A., Gavish, H., Shannon, W.R., and Buchwald, M.: Cloning of cDNAs for Fanconi's anaemia by functional complementation. Nature 356:763, 1992.

332. Lo Ten Foe, J.R., Rooimans, M.A., Bosnoyan-Collins, L., Alon, N., Wijker, M., Parker, L., Lightfoot, J., Carreau, M., Callen, D.F., Savoia, A., Cheng, N.C., van Berkel, C.G., Strunk, M.H., Gille, J.J., Pals, G., Kruyt, F.A., Pronk, J.C., Arwert, F., Buchwald, M., and Joenje, H.: Expression cloning of a cDNA for the major Fanconi anaemia gene, FAA. Nat. Genet. 14:320, 1996.

333. Walsh, C.E., Grompe, M., Vanin, E., Buchwald, M., Young, N.S., Nienhuis, A.W., and Liu, J.M.: A functionally active retrovirus vector for gene therapy in Fanconi anemia group C. Blood 84:453, 1994.

334. Fu, K., Foe, J.R., Joenje, H., Rao, K.W., Liu, J.M., and Walsh, C.E.: Functional correction of Fanconi anemia group A hematopoietic cells by retroviral gene transfer. Blood 90:3296, 1997.

335. Liu, J.M., Kim, S., Read, E.J., Dokal, I., Carter, C.S., Leitman, S.F., Pensiero, M., Young, N.S., and Walsh, C.E.: Experimental trial of gene therapy for group C Fanconi anemia patients: 2 year follow-up [abstract]. Blood 90:239a, 1997.

336. Sadelain, M.: Genetic treatment of the haemoglobinopathies: recombinations and new combinations. Br. J. Haematol. 98:247, 1997.

337. McCune, S.L., Reilly, M.P., Chomo, M.J., Asakura, T., and Townes, T.M.: Recombinant human hemoglobins designed for gene therapy of sickle cell disease. Proc. Natl. Acad. Sci. USA 91:9852, 1994.

338. Wijgerde, M., Gribnau, J., Trimborn, T., Nuez, B., Philipsen, S., Grosveld, F., and Fraser, P.: The role of EKLF in human beta-globin gene competition. Genes Dev. 10:2894, 1996.

339. Perkins, A.C., Gaensler, K.M., and Orkin, S.H.: Silencing of human fetal globin expression is impaired in the absence of the adult beta-globin gene activator protein EKLF. Proc. Natl. Acad. Sci. USA 93:12267, 1996.

340. Donze, D., Jeancake, P.H., and Townes, T.M.: Activation of delta-globin gene expression by erythroid Krupple-like factor: a potential approach for gene therapy of sickle cell disease. Blood 88:4051, 1996.

341. Karlsson, S., Bodine, D.M., Perry, L., Papayannopoulou, T., and Nienhuis, A.W.: Expression of the human beta-globin gene following retroviral-mediated transfer into multipotential hematopoietic progenitors of mice. Proc. Natl. Acad. Sci. USA 85:6062, 1988.

342. Dzierzak, E.A., Papayannopoulou, T., and Mulligan, R.C.: Lineage-specific expression of a human beta-globin gene in murine bone marrow transplant recipients reconstituted with retrovirus-transduced stem cells. Nature 331:35, 1988.

343. Bender, M.A., Gelinas, R.E., and Miller, A.D.: A majority of mice show long-term expression of a human beta-globin gene after retrovirus transfer into hematopoietic stem cells. Mol. Cell. Biol. 9:1426, 1989.

344. Grosveld, F., van Assendelft, G.B., Greaves, D.R., and Kollias, G.: Position-independent, high-level expression of the human beta-globin gene in transgenic mice. Cell 51:975, 1987.

345. Philipsen, S., Talbot, D., Fraser, P., and Grosveld, F.: The beta-globin dominant control region: hypersensitive site 2. EMBO J. 9:2159, 1990.

346. Talbot, D., Philipsen, S., Fraser, P., and Grosveld, F.: Detailed analysis of the site 3 region of the human beta-globin dominant control region. EMBO J. 9:2169, 1990.

347. Pruzina, S., Hanscombe, O., Whyatt, D., Grosveld, F., and Philipsen, S.: Hypersensitive site 4 of the human beta globin locus control region. Nucleic Acids Res. 19:1413, 1991.

348. Philipsen, S., Pruzina, S., and Grosveld, F.: The minimal requirements for activity in transgenic mice of hypersensitive site 3 of the beta globin locus control region. EMBO J. 12:1077, 1993.

349. Liu, D., Chang, J.C., Moi, P., Liu, W., Kan, Y.W., and Curtin, P.T.: Dissection of the enhancer activity of beta-globin 5′ DNase I–hypersensitive site 2 in transgenic mice. Proc. Natl. Acad. Sci. USA 89:3899, 1992.

350. Caterina, J.J., Ryan, T.M., Pawlik, K.M., Palmiter, R.D., Brinster, R.L., Behringer, R.R., and Townes, T.M.: Human beta-globin locus control region: analysis of the 5′ DNase I hypersensitive site HS 2 in transgenic mice. Proc. Natl. Acad. Sci. USA 88:1626, 1991.

351. Novak, U., Harris, E.A., Forrester, W., Groudine, M., and Gelinas, R.: High-level beta-globin expression after retroviral transfer of locus activation region–containing human beta-globin gene derivatives into murine erythroleukemia cells. Proc. Natl. Acad. Sci. USA 87:3386, 1990.

352. Chang, J.C., Liu, D., and Kan, Y.W.: A 36-base-pair core sequence of locus control region enhances retrovirally transferred human beta-globin gene expression. Proc. Natl. Acad. Sci. USA 89:3107, 1992.

353. Leboulch, P., Huang, G.M., Humphries, R.K., Oh, Y.H., Eaves, C.J., Tuan, D.Y., and London, I.M.: Mutagenesis of retroviral vectors trans-

354. Plavec, I., Papayannopoulou, T., Maury, C., and Meyer, F.: A human beta-globin gene fused to the human beta-globin locus control region is expressed at high levels in erythroid cells of mice engrafted with retrovirus-transduced hematopoietic stem cells. Blood 81:1384, 1993.

355. Takekoshi, K.J., Oh, Y.H., Westerman, K.W., London, I.M., and Leboulch, P.: Retroviral transfer of a human beta-globin/delta-globin hybrid gene linked to beta locus control region hypersensitive site 2 aimed at the gene therapy of sickle cell disease. Proc. Natl. Acad. Sci. USA 92:3014, 1995.

356. Sadelain, M., Wang, C.H., Antoniou, M., Grosveld, F., and Mulligan, R.C.: Generation of a high-titer retroviral vector capable of expressing high levels of the human beta-globin gene. Proc. Natl. Acad. Sci. USA 92:6728, 1995.

357. Ren, S., Wong, B.Y., Li, J., Luo, X.N., Wong, P.M., and Atweh, G.F.: Production of genetically stable high-titer retroviral vectors that carry a human gamma-globin gene under the control of the alpha-globin locus control region. Blood 87:2518, 1996.

358. Rivella, S., and Sadelain, M.: Genetic treatment of severe hemoglobinopathies: the combat against transgene variegation and transgene silencing. Semin. Hematol. 35:112, 1998.

359. Raftopoulos, H., Ward, M., Leboulch, P., and Bank, A.: Long-term transfer and expression of the human beta-globin gene in a mouse transplant model. Blood 90:3414, 1997.

360. Ryan, T.M., Ciavatta, D.J., and Townes, T.M.: Knockout-transgenic mouse model of sickle cell disease. Science 278:873, 1997.

361. Yang, B., Kirby, S., Lewis, J., Detloff, P.J., Maeda, N., and Smithies, O.: A mouse model for beta 0-thalassemia. Proc. Natl. Acad. Sci. USA 92:11608, 1995.

362. Ciavatta, D.J., Ryan, T.M., Farmer, S.C., and Townes, T.M.: Mouse model of human beta zero thalassemia: targeted deletion of the mouse beta maj- and beta min-globin genes in embryonic stem cells. Proc. Natl. Acad. Sci. USA 92:9259, 1995.

363. Jaffee, E.M., and Pardoll, D.M.: Considerations for the clinical development of cytokine gene-transduced tumor cell vaccines. Methods 12:143, 1997.

364. Pardoll, D.M.: Cancer vaccines. Nat. Med. 4:525, 1998.

365. Moolten, F.L.: Tumor chemosensitivity conferred by inserted herpes thymidine kinase genes: paradigm for a prospective cancer control strategy. Cancer Res. 46:5276, 1986.

366. Culver, K.W., Ram, Z., Wallbridge, S., Ishii, H., Oldfield, E.H., and Blaese, R.M.: In vivo gene transfer with retroviral vector-producer cells for treatment of experimental brain tumors. Science 256:1550, 1992.

367. Helene, M., Lake-Bullock, V., Bryson, J.S., Jennings, C.D., and Kaplan, A.M.: Inhibition of graft-versus-host disease. Use of a T cell–controlled suicide gene. J. Immunol. 158:5079, 1997.

368. Cohen, J.L., Boyer, O., Salomon, B., Onclercq, R., Charlotte, F., Bruel, S., Boisserie, G., and Klatzmann, D.: Prevention of graft-versus-host disease in mice using a suicide gene expressed in T lymphocytes. Blood 89:4636, 1997.

369. Verzeletti, S., Bonini, C., Marktel, S., Nobili, N., Ciceri, F., Traversari, C., and Bordignon, C.: Herpes simplex virus thymidine kinase gene transfer for controlled graft-versus-host disease and graft-versus-leukemia: clinical follow-up and improved new vectors. Hum. Gene Ther. 9:2243, 1998.

370. Contassot, E., Ferrand, C., Certoux, J.M., Reynolds, C.W., Jacob, W., Chiang, Y., Cahn, J.Y., Herve, P., and Tiberghien, P.: Retrovirus-mediated transfer of the herpes simplex type I thymidine kinase gene in alloreactive T lymphocytes. Hum. Gene Ther. 9:73, 1998.

371. Contassot, E., Murphy, W., Angonin, R., Pavy, J.J., Bittencourt, M.C., Robinet, E., Reynolds, C.W., Cahn, J.Y., Herve, P., and Tiberghien, P.: In vivo alloreactive potential of ex vivo–expanded primary T lymphocytes. Transplantation 65:1365, 1998.

372. Williams, D.A., Hsieh, K., Desilva, A., and Mulligan, R.C.: Protection of bone marrow transplant recipients from lethal doses of methotrexate by the generation of methotrexate-resistant bone marrow. J. Exp. Med. 166:210, 1987.

373. McLachlin, J.R., Eglitis, M.A., Ueda, K., Kantoff, P.W., Pastan, I.H., Anderson, W.F., and Gottesman, M.M.: Expression of a human complementary DNA for the multidrug resistance gene in murine hematopoietic precursor cells with the use of retroviral gene transfer. J. Natl. Cancer Inst. 82:1260, 1990.

374. Dumenco, L.L., Warman, B., Hatzoglou, M., Lim, I.K., Abboud, S.L., and Gerson, S.L.: Increase in nitrosourea resistance in mammalian cells by retrovirally mediated gene transfer of bacterial O6-alkylguanine-DNA alkyltransferase. Cancer Res. 49:6044, 1989.

375. Magni, M., Shammah, S., Schiro, R., Bregni, M., Siena, S., DiNicola, M., Dalla-Favera, R., and Gianni, A.M.: Gene therapy for drug-induced myelotoxicity: induction of cyclophosphamide resistance by aldehyde dehydrogenase-1 gene transfer [abstract]. Blood 84:A1414, 1994.

376. Moreb, J., Schweder, M., Suresh, A., and Zucali, J.R.: Overexpression of the human aldehyde dehydrogenase class I results in increased resistance to 4-hydroperoxycyclophosphamide. Cancer Gene Ther. 3:24, 1996.

377. Letourneau, S., Greenbaum, M., and Cournoyer, D.: Retrovirus-mediated gene transfer of rat glutathione S-transferase Yc confers in vitro resistance to alkylating agents in human leukemia cells and in clonogenic mouse hematopoietic progenitor cells. Hum. Gene Ther. 7:831, 1996.

378. Neff, T., and Blau, C.A.: Forced expression of cytidine deaminase confers resistance to cytosine arabinoside and gemcitabine. Exp. Hematol. 24:1340, 1996.

379. Mickisch, G.H., Aksentijevich, I., Schoenlein, P.V., Goldstein, L.J., Galski, H., Stahle, C., Sachs, D.H., Pastan, I., and Gottesman, M.M.: Transplantation of bone marrow cells from transgenic mice expressing the human MDR1 gene results in long-term protection against the myelosuppressive effect of chemotherapy in mice. Blood 79:1087, 1992.

380. Hanania, E.G., Fu, S., Roninson, I., Zu, Z., Deisseroth, A.B., and Gottesman, M.M.: Resistance to taxol chemotherapy produced in mouse marrow cells by safety-modified retroviruses containing a human MDR-1 transcription unit. Gene Ther. 2:279, 1995.

381. Ward, M., Richardson, C., Pioli, P., Smith, L., Podda, S., Goff, S., Hesdorffer, C., and Bank, A.: Transfer and expression of the human multiple drug resistance gene in human CD34+ cells. Blood 84:1408, 1994.

382. Hanania, E.G., Fu, S., Zu, Z., Hegewisch-Becker, S., Korbling, M., Hester, J., Durett, A., Andreeff, M., Mechetner, E., Holzmayer, T., Roninson, I.B., Giles, R.E., Berenson, R., Heimfeld, S., and Deisseroth, A.B.: Chemotherapy resistance to taxol in clonogenic progenitor cells following transduction of CD34 selected marrow and peripheral blood cells with a retrovirus that contains the MDR-1 chemotherapy resistance gene. Gene Ther. 2:285, 1995.

383. Peters, S.O., Kittler, E.L., Ramshaw, H.S., and Quesenberry, P.J.: Ex vivo expansion of murine marrow cells with interleukin-3 (IL-3), IL-6, IL-11, and stem cell factor leads to impaired engraftment in irradiated hosts. Blood 87:30, 1996.

384. Baum, C., Hegewisch-Becker, S., Eckert, H.G., Stocking, C., and Ostertag, W.: Novel retroviral vectors for efficient expression of the multidrug resistance (mdr-1) gene in early hematopoietic cells. J. Virol. 69:7541, 1995.

385. Shpall, E.J., Jones, R.B., Bast, R.C., Jr., Rosner, G.L., Vandermark, R., Ross, M., Affronti, M.L., Johnston, C., Eggleston, S., Tepperburg, M., et al.: 4-Hydroperoxycyclophosphamide purging of breast cancer from the mononuclear cell fraction of bone marrow in patients receiving high-dose chemotherapy and autologous marrow support: a phase I trial. J. Clin. Oncol. 9:85, 1991.

386. Shpall, E.J., Bast, R.C., Jr., Joines, W.T., Jones, R.B., Anderson, I., Johnston, C., Eggleston, S., Tepperberg, M., Edwards, S., and Peters, W.P.: Immunomagnetic purging of breast cancer from bone marrow for autologous transplantation. Bone Marrow Transplant. 7:145, 1991.

387. Sirotnak, F.M., Moccio, D.M., and Dorick, D.M.: Optimization of high-dose methotrexate with leucovorin rescue therapy in the L1210 leukemia and sarcoma 180 murine tumor models. Cancer Res. 38:345, 1978.

388. Browman, G.P., Goodyear, M.D., Levine, M.N., Russell, R., Archibald, S.D., and Young, J.E.: Modulation of the antitumor effect of methotrexate by low-dose leucovorin in squamous cell head and neck cancer: a randomized placebo-controlled clinical trial. J. Clin. Oncol. 8:203, 1990.

389. Ackland, S.P., and Schilsky, R.L.: High-dose methotrexate: a critical reappraisal. J. Clin. Oncol. 5:2017, 1987.

390. Kamen, B.A., and Weitman, S.D.: High-dose methotrexate: is it warranted? Pediatr. Hematol. Oncol. 11:135, 1994.

391. Li, M.X., Banerjee, D., Zhao, S.C., Schweitzer, B.I., Mineishi, S., Gilboa, E., and Bertino, J.R.: Development of a retroviral construct containing a human mutated dihydrofolate reductase cDNA for hematopoietic stem cell transduction. Blood 83:3403, 1994.

392. Vinh, D.B., and McIvor, R.S.: Selective expression of methotrexate-resistant dihydrofolate reductase (DHFR) activity in mice transduced with DHFR retrovirus and administered methotrexate. J. Pharmacol. Exp. Ther. 267:989, 1993.

393. May, C., James, R.I., Gunther, R., and McIvor, R.S.: Methotrexate dose-escalation studies in transgenic mice and marrow transplant recipients expressing drug-resistant dihydrofolate reductase activity. J. Pharmacol. Exp. Ther. 278:1444, 1996.

394. May, C., Gunther, R., and McIvor, R.S.: Protection of mice from lethal doses of methotrexate by transplantation with transgenic marrow expressing drug-resistant dihydrofolate reductase activity. Blood 86:2439, 1995.

395. Zhao, S.C., Banerjee, D., Mineishi, S., and Bertino, J.R.: Post-transplant methotrexate administration leads to improved curability of mice bearing a mammary tumor transplanted with marrow transduced with a mutant human dihydrofolate reductase cDNA. Hum. Gene Ther. 8:903, 1997.

396. Allay, J.A., Galipeau, J., Blakley, R.L., and Sorrentino, B.P.: Retroviral vectors containing a variant dihydrofolate reductase gene for drug protection and in vivo selection of hematopoietic cells. Stem Cells (Dayt) 16(suppl. 1):223, 1998.

397. Patel, M., Sleep, S.E., Lewis, W.S., Spencer, H.T., Mareya, S.M., Sorrentino, B.P., and Blakley, R.L.: Comparison of the protection of cells from antifolates by transduced human dihydrofolate reductase mutants. Hum. Gene Ther. 8:2069, 1997.

398. Erickson, L.C., Laurent, G., Sharkey, N.A., and Kohn, K.W.: DNA cross-linking and monoadduct repair in nitrosourea-treated human tumour cells. Nature 288:727, 1980.

399. Gerson, S.L., Miller, K., and Berger, N.A.: O6 alkylguanine-DNA alkyltransferase activity in human myeloid cells. J. Clin. Invest. 76:2106, 1985.

400. Maze, R., Kapur, R., Kelley, M.R., Hansen, W.K., Oh, S.Y., and Williams, D.A.: Reversal of 1,3-bis(2-chloroethyl)-1-nitrosourea–induced severe immunodeficiency by transduction of murine long-lived hemopoietic progenitor cells using O6-methylguanine DNA methyltransferase complementary DNA. J. Immunol. 158:1006, 1997.

401. Maze, R., Carney, J.P., Kelley, M.R., Glassner, B.J., Williams, D.A., and Samson, L.: Increasing DNA repair methyltransferase levels via bone marrow stem cell transduction rescues mice from the toxic effects of 1,3-bis(2-chloroethyl)-1-nitrosourea, a chemotherapeutic alkylating agent. Proc. Natl. Acad. Sci. USA 93:206, 1996.

402. Allay, J.A., Koc, O.N., Davis, B.M., and Gerson, S.L.: Retroviral-mediated gene transduction of human alkyltransferase complementary DNA confers nitrosourea resistance to human hematopoietic progenitors. Clin. Cancer Res. 2:1353, 1996.

403. Gerson, S.L., Zborowska, E., Norton, K., Gordon, N.H., and Willson, J.K.: Synergistic efficacy of O6-benzylguanine and 1,3-bis(2-chloroethyl)-1-nitrosourea (BCNU) in a human colon cancer xenograft completely resistant to BCNU alone. Biochem. Pharmacol. 45:483, 1993.

404. Crone, T.M., Goodtzova, K., Edara, S., and Pegg, A.E.: Mutations in human O6-alkylguanine-DNA alkyltransferase imparting resistance to O6-benzylguanine. Cancer Res. 54:6221, 1994.

405. Kay, M.A., Rothenberg, S., Landen, C.N., Bellinger, D.A., Leland, F., Toman, C., Finegold, M., Thompson, A.R., Read, M.S., and Brinkhous, K.M.: In vivo gene therapy of hemophilia B: sustained partial correction in factor IX–deficient dogs. Science 262:117, 1993.

406. Kay, M.A., Landen, C.N., Rothenberg, S.R., Taylor, L.A., Leland, F., Wiehle, S., Fang, B., Bellinger, D., Finegold, M., Thompson, A.R., et al.: In vivo hepatic gene therapy: complete albeit transient correction of factor IX deficiency in hemophilia B dogs. Proc. Natl. Acad. Sci. USA 91:2353, 1994.

407. Fang, B., Eisensmith, R.C., Wang, H., Kay, M.A., Cross, R.E., Landen, C.N., Gordon, G., Bellinger, D.A., Read, M.S., and Hu, P.C.: Gene therapy for hemophilia B: host immunosuppression prolongs the therapeutic effect of adenovirus-mediated factor IX expression. Hum. Gene Ther. 6:1039, 1995.

408. Lin, H.F., Maeda, N., Smithies, O., Straight, D.L., and Stafford, D.W.: A coagulation factor IX–deficient mouse model for human hemophilia B. Blood 90:3962, 1997.

409. Kung, S.H., Hagstrom, J.N., Cass, D., Tai, S.J., Lin, H.F., Stafford, D.W., and High, K.A.: Human factor IX corrects the bleeding diathesis of mice with hemophilia B. Blood 91:784, 1998.

410. Lieber, A., He, C.Y., Meuse, L., Schowalter, D., Kirillova, I., Winther, B., and Kay, M.A.: The role of Kupffer cell activation and viral gene expression in early liver toxicity after infusion of recombinant adenovirus vectors. J. Virol. 71:8798, 1997.

411. Herzog, R.W., Hagstrom, J.N., Kung, S.H., Tai, S.J., Wilson, J.M., Fisher, K.J., and High, K.A.: Stable gene transfer and expression of human blood coagulation factor IX after intramuscular injection of recombinant adeno-associated virus. Proc. Natl. Acad. Sci. USA 94:5804, 1997.

412. Monahan, P.E., Samulski, R.J., Tazelaar, J., Xiao, X., Nichols, T.C., Bellinger, D.A., Read, M.S., and Walsh, C.E.: Direct intramuscular injection with recombinant AAV vectors results in sustained expression in a dog model of hemophilia. Gene Ther. 5:40, 1998.

413. Chuah, M.K., Vandendriessche, T., and Morgan, R.A.: Development and analysis of retroviral vectors expressing human factor VIII as a potential gene therapy for hemophilia A. Hum. Gene Ther. 6:1363, 1995.

414. Dwarki, V.J., Belloni, P., Nijjar, T., Smith, J., Couto, L., Rabier, M., Clift, S., Berns, A., and Cohen, L.K.: Gene therapy for hemophilia A: production of therapeutic levels of human factor VIII in vivo in mice. Proc. Natl. Acad. Sci. USA 92:1023, 1995.

415. Connelly, S., Mount, J., Mauser, A., Gardner, J.M., Kaleko, M., McClelland, A., and Lothrop, C.D.J.: Complete short-term correction of canine hemophilia A by in vivo gene therapy. Blood 88:3846, 1996.

416. Connelly, S., Andrews, J.L., Gallo, A.M., Kayda, D.B., Qian, J., Hoyer, L., Kadan, M.J., Gorziglia, M.I., Trapnell, B.C., McClelland, A., and Kaleko, M.: Sustained phenotypic correction of murine hemophilia A by in vivo gene therapy. Blood 91:3273, 1998.

▼▼▼▼ INDEX

Note: Page numbers in *italics* refer to illustrations; page numbers followed by t refer to tables.

A

Abelson murine leukemia virus, 801, *801, 802t*
Abetalipoproteinemia, acanthocytosis in, 294
abl, 807
v-*abl,* 810
ABO blood group system, 315t, 331–339
  A phenotype of, 336–339, *337,* 338t
  A subgroups of, 335–336
  B(A) phenotype in, 336
  B phenotype of, 336–339, *337,* 338t
  B subgroups of, 335–336
  cis-AB phenotype in, 335–336
  erythrocyte expression of, 334–335
  factor VIII levels and, 339
  functions of, 339
  glycosyltransferases of, 334, *334*
  Helicobacter pylori infection and, 339
  IgM antibodies against, 335
  molecular genetics of, 336–339, *336, 337,* 338t
  O phenotype of, 336, *337,* 338t, 339
  oligosaccharide structure of, 331–334, *332–334*
  von Willebrand factor levels and, 339
Acanthocytosis, 294, 303
Aceruloplasminemia, 379
Acquired immunodeficiency syndrome (AIDS), 888–893, *889–892.* See also *Human immunodeficiency virus 1 (HIV-1).*
  chemokines in, 524–525, *525*
  clinical features of, 889
  gene therapy in, 970t
  hairy leukoplakia in, 960
  treatment of, 891–892
Actin, 282, *282*
  integrin binding of, 488
  of cytoskeleton, 281, *281*
  of platelets, 769
α-Actinin, 286
  integrin binding of, 488
Acyclovir, in Epstein-Barr virus infection, 961
Adaptor proteins, in T-cell activation, 475
Adducin, 282, *282*
  spectrin binding to, 291
Adeno-associated virus vectors, hepatocyte transduction with, 991–992
  stem cell transduction with, 980–982, *980, 981*
Adenocarcinoma, Hb F in, 160
Adenosine deaminase deficiency, gene therapy in, 984–985
Adenosine diphosphate, platelet interaction with, 497, 768
  platelet receptor for, 777, *777*

Adenosine monophosphate, cyclic (cAMP), in platelet activation, 778–779
  in thrombomodulin regulation, 629
Adenoviral vectors, hepatocyte transduction with, 991
  immunogenicity of, 982
  stem cell transduction with, 982–983, *983*
Adenoviruses, transforming genes of, 800, *800*
Adult T-cell leukemia, 941–942
  CD4⁺ T cells in, 941–942, *942*
  clinical features of, 941
  HTLV-1 in, 942
  pathogenesis of, 943–945, *943, 944*
  prevention of, 945–946
  smoldering, 941
  Tax protein in, 943–945, *943–945*
African iron overload, 379
Agammaglobulinemia, X-linked, gene therapy in, 970t
Aiolos proteins, 92
Akt (protein kinase B), 110
Albumin, plasma concentration of, 720t
Alcoholism, hemoglobin in, 234
Aldrithiol 2, antiretroviral activity of, 879
Alkyltransferase, genes for, for in vivo stem cell selection, 976–977
  in gene therapy, 990–991
All-*trans*-retinoic acid therapy, in acute promyelocytic leukemia, 845, 846
Alteplase, 754–755
Alveolar macrophage, granulocyte-macrophage colony-stimulating factor effect on, 29
AMD3100, anti-HIV-1 activity of, 886
Amegakaryocytic thrombocytopenia, 57
AML1-EAP, 842t
AML1-ETO, 842t, 843–844, *844,* 845, *845*
AML1-EVI1, 842t, 843, *845*
AML1-MDS1, 843, *845*
AML1-MTG16, 842t
Amplification refractory mutation system analysis, in thalassemia, 217–218, *218*
Amyloidosis, renal, fibrinogen mutation in, 731
Anaplastic lymphoma kinase, 105
Anemia, aplastic, growth factors in, 51–52
  Hb F in, 159–160
  paroxysmal nocturnal hemoglobinuria and, 564, 573–574
  erythropoietin and, 28, 48–49
  Fanconi, gene therapy in, 970t, 981, 987–988
  genes for, 51
  growth factors in, 51
  Hb F in, 159–160
  hemolytic. See also *Paroxysmal nocturnal hemoglobinuria.*

Anemia *(Continued)*
  Heinz body, 259–261, *260*
  in hereditary elliptocytosis, 297
  in hereditary spherocytosis, 296
  in α thalassemia, 192–193. See also α *Thalassemia.*
  in β thalassemia, 202–203, 210. See also β *Thalassemia.*
  in B19 parvovirus infection, 926
  in Hb Constant Spring, 195
  in Hb H disease, 194
  in hereditary spherocytosis, 296
  of chronic disease, 50–51, *50*
  renal failure–related, 48–49
  sideroblastic, 381
  spur cell, 294
Anergy, 449, 476
Angiogenesis, 3–5
  chemokines in, 527–528
Angiopoietin-I, in hematopoiesis, 4
Anion exchanger-1. See *Band 3 (anion exchanger-1, protein 3).*
Anisoylated plasminogen-streptokinase activator complex, in myocardial infarction, 756
  physicochemical properties of, 746
Anistreplase, in myocardial infarction, 756
Ankyrin (protein 2.1), 282, *282*
  band 3 binding to, 283, *284*
  cytoskeleton interaction with, 281, *281,* 290–291, *290*
  deficiency of, 303
  isoforms of, 290–291
  nonerythroid tissue expression of, 304
  protein 4.2 binding to, 291
  spectrin binding to, 290–291, *290*
  structure of, 290, *290*
Antibodies. See also *Immune receptors; Immunoglobulin(s).*
  anti-A, 335
  anti-B, 335
  anti-B19 parvovirus, 927–929, *927, 928*
  anti-factor VIII, 690
  anti-factor IX, 696
  anti-HTLV-1, 937, 941
  anti-Lewis, 343
  anti-P₁, 349
  anti-Rh, 316–317
  anti-von Willebrand factor, 706
Anticoagulation, 614–636, *615.* See also *C4b-binding protein; Protein C; Protein S; Thrombomodulin.*
Antigen processing, 459–478. See also *Lymphocyte(s), T; T-cell antigen receptors.*
  B-cell in, 408–409, *408,* 446, *447,* 450–451
  class I HLA molecules in, 461–462, *461–464, 464–467, 466*

1/29/2008

ISBN 0-7216-7671-5

90038